CURRENT THERAPY IN ORAL AND MAXILLOFACIAL SURGERY

SHAHROKH C. BAGHERI, DMD, MD, FACS

Chief, Division of Oral and Maxillofacial Surgery
Department of Surgery
Northside Hospital
Georgia Oral and Facial Surgery, and Eastern Surgical Associates and Consultants
Atlanta, Georgia

Clinical Associate Professor
Department of Oral and Maxillofacial Surgery
Georgia Health Sciences University
Augusta, Georgia

Clinical Assistant Professor
Department of Surgery
School of Medicine
Emory University
Atlanta, Georgia

R. BRYAN BELL, DDS, MD, FACS

Medical Director
Oral, Head and Neck Cancer Program
Providence Cancer Center
Robert W. Franz Cancer Research Center
Providence Portland Medical Center

Attending Surgeon and Director of Resident Education
Trauma Service/Oral and Maxillofacial Surgery Service
Legacy Emanuel Medical Center

Affiliate Associate Professor
Oregon Health and Science University

Head and Neck Surgical Associates Partner
Portland, Oregon

HUSAIN ALI KHAN, DMD, MD

Attending Surgeon, Division of Oral and Maxillofacial Surgery
Department of Surgery
Northside Hospital
Georgia Oral and Facial Surgery, and Eastern Surgical Associates and Consultants
Atlanta, Georgia

Clinical Associate Professor
Department of Oral and Maxillofacial Surgery
Georgia Health Sciences University
Augusta, Georgia

ELSEVIER
SAUNDERS

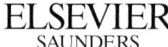

3251 Riverport Lane
St. Louis, Missouri 63043

CURRENT THERAPY IN ORAL AND MAXILLOFACIAL SURGERY   ISBN: 978-1-4160-2527-6

Vice President and Publisher: Linda Duncan
Executive Editor: John Dolan
Senior Developmental Editor: Courtney Sprehe
Publishing Services Manager: Julie Eddy
Project Manager: Richard Barber
Design Direction: Kim Denando

Printed in the United States

Last digit is the print number: 9   8   7   6   5   4   3   2   1

This book is dedicated to ...

My family—Nooshin, Shaheen, Bijan; my parents—Parviz, Ladan; and my brother, Homayoun. It is through their love and support that I derive my energy and passion for life.

All students and surgeons throughout the world, who help improve on the life of others by their skills, dedication, and knowledge of surgery.

My mentors and educators that influenced my career—Drs. Leonard B. Kaban, Robert A. Bays, Sam E. Farish, Thomas B. Dodson, Eric J. Dierks, Bryce E. Potter, and Roger A. Meyer.

My friends and co-editors—Drs. R. Bryan Bell and Husain Ali Khan, who helped realize this most challenging project.

Shahrokh C. Bagheri

I am fortunate to have been surrounded by individuals of much higher quality than myself since boyhood. At home, at school and in my current profession—I am deeply indebted to God, my family, friends, teachers, and colleagues, who have provided me the license, opportunity, and mentorship necessary for a successful surgical career and a fulfilling life.

This book is dedicated to these individuals:

E. Craig Nemec, Bruce Bordeleon, Don A. Hay, Gene R. Huebner, Wayne W. Barkmeier, Lawrence J. Sutton, Sean M. Cerone, Timothy A. Turvey, Raymond P. White, George H. Blakey, John R. Zuniga, Ramon L. Ruiz, Tinerfe J. Tejera, Shawn M. Conrad, Steven A. Bankston, Todd E. Zeigler, Eric J. Dierks, Bryce E. Potter, William B. Long, Leon A. Assael, Robert W. T. Myall, Jason K. Potter, Kevin Arce, Julie Ann Smith, Joshua E. Lubek, Brian L. Schmidt, David L. Hirsch, Shahrokh C. Bagheri and H. Ali Khan for their tutelage, support, and unwavering friendship; as well as the physicians, residents, fellows, nurses, surgical technicians and administrators on the Trauma Service at Legacy Emanuel Medical Center, the Providence Cancer Center, and the Departments of Oral and Maxillofacial Surgery at Oregon Health and Science University and the University of Washington.

My parents—William and Sherry Bell; brother—Adam Bell; sisters—Christine Foreman and Elizabeth Atkins; and in-laws, Franklin and Karen Halvorsen—thank you for your unconditional love.

My family, whom I adore and whose patience, gentleness, and love illuminate my path home at the end of a long day—Heidi, Harrison, and Caroline—thank you for my wonderful life.

R. Bryan Bell

This book is dedicated to ...

My loving wife, Nauzi, for giving me the opportunity to expand beyond myself and raising our beautiful daughter, Layla.

My parents—Zehra and Mazhar; my family—Abbas, Hydar, Qamar, Desh, and my uncle, Abbas, and my aunt, Shahnaz.

My mentors—Mr. Edward Edelstein, Dr. Brian McPherson, Dr. Robert E. Marx, Dr. Mark Stevens, and Dr. Angelo Cuzalina.

My colleague and co-editor, Dr. R. Bryan Bell, for his ongoing hard work and contribution to this text. Special thanks to my friend, colleague, and co-editor, Shahrokh C. Bagheri for his leadership and future vision of this esteemed surgical specialty.

Future surgeons, without which this text has no purpose.

Husain Ali Khan

FOREWORD

In 1956, I became the first oral surgery teaching fellow at MD Anderson Hospital in Houston, Texas. My surgical experience at the country's premier cancer hospital consisted of assisting two world-renowned head and neck cancer surgeons, William McComb and A.J. Ballantyne.

My curiosity and interest were profoundly influenced by observing these two giants of their field perform cancer surgery. Patients were frequently treated by radical neck dissections, concomitant tracheotomy, and radiation and were confined in the hospital for weeks without reconstructive surgery. The patient's quality of life after such a surgery was bleak, and the prognosis was generally dismal.

Fifty-five years after my experiences as an oral surgery resident, I had the privilege of participating in an astounding symposium, *Technological Advances in Head and Neck Oncology and Cranio-Maxillofacial Surgery*, organized and conducted by a very talented and visonary group of surgeons, many of whom are authors or editors (Bryan Bell, for example) in this text. The same type of patients I saw 55 years ago are now diagnosed and treatment-planned with the use of three-dimensional virtual imaging, treated surgically with microvascular reconstruction performed immediately at the time of ablation, and frequently discharged from the hospital within a few days. Oral and maxillofacial surgeons with fellowship training in head and neck oncologic surgery, reconstructive microvascular surgery, and implantology perform the procedures and manage the patients throughout their cancer treatment. Many new and revolutionary techniques have evolved from the science and techniques of maxillofacial surgery described in this book.

The expanded role of oral and maxillofacial surgeons in the treatment of cancer patients is just one example of how research in our field has greatly benefitted patients. The reader of this text will note that it is written by oral and maxillofacial surgeons with advanced training and expertise in a number of subspecialty disciplines: oral surgery, anesthesia, craniomaxillofacial trauma, head and neck surgery, maxillofacial reconstructive surgery, orthognathic surgery, pediatric craniofacial surgery, and facial plastic surgery. All these subspecialty areas certainly overlap the scope of practice of other surgical disciplines. But those who question the role of our specialty in oncologic and reconstructive surgery, cosmetic surgery, or pediatric cleft and craniofacial surgery should be reminded of the paradigm shift in head and neck and craniomaxillofacial (CMF) surgery. Fifty-seven years ago, we were known as oral surgeons. Today, through the evolution of new science, technology, and techniques, we are known as oral and maxillofacial surgeons. Our specialty is poised to move forward to new frontiers. The authors of this book provide answers to clinical questions and stimulate further research and progress in treatment methods founded predominantly on evidence-based interdisciplinary animal and clinical investigations, achieved collaboratively by basic and clinical scientists.

Our specialty continues to derive its standards from selected individuals who emerge to take their place in history. The editors have selected visionaries, creative thinkers, and pioneers who have moved or will move our specialty to new heights. In this dynamic publication, health care practitioners will obtain the scientific knowledge, technical skill, and strategies to manage most simple or complex CMF problems.

I believe that this text defines the current scope of oral and maxillofacial surgery as or more completely than any previous work. When I completed my training, if one wanted a single text to define the specialty's scope of practice, the most frequently referenced was generally Kurt Thoma's text on oral surgery. Drs. Bagheri, Bell, and Khan have today redefined that scope in a way I did not think possible all those years ago at MD Anderson. Through advanced surgical training, laid over a foundation of dentistry and medicine, oral and maxillofacial surgeons have the ideal skill set to optimally manage the entire spectrum of head and neck and CMF problems in a unique manner that is most beneficial to the patient.

PARADIGM SHIFT

Greater new designs have faster, better, and cheaper outcomes. Technological advances have influenced the present and future treatment of virtually all craniomaxillofacial patients. The efficiency, duration, affordability, and convenience of such treatment will be changed forever through technology. A paradigm shift will take place through a global teaching revolution of surgical education by three-dimensional, virtual imaging technology; the power of the Internet; surgical robotics; and computer-assisted and simulated surgery. All who use this text will become a part of the ongoing paradigm shift in oral and maxillofacial surgery and will be forever changed in their approach to treatment of CMF deformity patients.

THE EXPLOSION OF TECHNOLOGY

In this golden era of surgical science and technology is the accelerating and deepening wave of change sweeping through medicine and dentistry. The editors and authors of this book want to stimulate the reader with this wave of new ideas and global information. As the cost of communication goes down each year, the means of communication increase dramatically. From cell phones to computers to iPads, GPS devices, and the Internet, technology has found its way into every corner of the world and crossed the divide between rich and poor.

The pervasiveness of technology is most apparent in the proliferation of cell phones. Thirty years ago the cost of a 3-pound mobile phone with the capacity to make a scant 30 calls was $4000. In sharp contrast, today smart phones provide the customer a 6-ounce, handheld multipurpose instrument for $90. The instrument has more processing power than the North American Defense Command in 1965 or the mainframe computer at the University of Texas Southwestern Medical School used for study of the long face syndrome in 1975 by Dr. Stephen Schendel and colleagues.

The world can be educated about virtually anything with the use of available, powerful, convenient, and affordable technology. Computer-assisted surgical simulation, medical imaging, information-guided therapies, demonstration of workflow at work stations in a digital hospital or office-based setting, digital imaging for virtual CAD/CAM splints, in-office planning for surgical treatment and reconstruction of craniomaxillofacial deformities, electronic imaging, and interdisciplinary electronic communication are precisely described and illustrated. Many of the contributing authors and scientists of this book have already said farewell to standard facebow transfers, plaster model surgery, conventional splints, and traditional bone grafts! They have replaced them with the digital world, tissue engineering, in-office accelerated CMF surgery, and accelerated orthodontics!

Many facial deformities and malocclusions remain untreated, or are managed inefficiently over long periods of time. Sophisticated advancements in CMF surgery, orthognathic and orthodontic techniques, implantology, and microvascular surgery have enabled oral and maxillofacial surgeons to achieve predictable outcomes with convenience, efficiency, and affordability. The paradigm shift in oral and maxillofacial surgery is supported by technological achievements that enable practitioners to enhance the quality of life for their patients.

AFFORDABLE HEALTH CARE FOR EVERYBODY

Americans generally recognize that our nation's health care system has become fragmented, excessively expensive, horridly inefficient, inconvenient, and inequitable. Head and neck surgery, plastic and reconstructive surgery, and oral and maxillofacial surgery specialties will not reach their lofty altruistic goals until innovative science collaborates with health care to solve the dilemma of 50 million citizens in our country without health insurance. Uwe Freihardt, a renowned health care economist, passionately declares that once a nation decides that it has a moral obligation to provide health care for everyone, that it can build a system to meet that obligation. The "impossible dream" of health care for more than half the world's population and some 50 million American citizens can be actualized to eliminate this inequality. An army of talented surgeons and scientists in our specialty will play a pivotal role in attacking this "challenge."

HEALTH NEEDS A HERO

When you provide another with comfort, when you lend a hand, or simply be there for someone who needs help, you transform the health of a country. Big change doesn't require a hero's effort. Just one small act of kindness can make you a hero to someone else. How can you and how will you be involved is the focus of this book.

William H. Bell, DDS

PREFACE

The specialty of oral and maxillofacial surgery (OMFS) has witnessed a rapid expansion of its scope. This has occurred despite the many prevailing academic, financial, and governmental forces that attempt, either actively or through inertia, to hinder expansion of any medical or surgical field of endeavor, whether or not it has demonstrated a need or mission and the where-withal, through research, training, and experience to properly and competently address that need. As in any surgical specialty, expansion of the scope of practice is mostly the result of additional training and adaptation of scientific and clinical research, which eminates from the academic training centers, although innovations and their acceptance into the specialty also result from forward-thinking and skillful surgeons in private practice. The phrase "full scope" is seldom applicable to any single surgeon since the magnitude of surgical procedures under the umbrella of OMFS overwhelms the intellectual and technical skill capacities of any one professional. The name change of the specialty in 1978 was most appropriate at that time. However, when examining the contents of this first edition of *Current Therapy in Oral and Maxillofacial Surgery,* it may be suggested that another name change, or at a minimum some modification to encompass the added anatomy of the cranium and neck, is on the horizon.

This text is a sampling of the most current therapy in oral and maxillofacial surgery by some of the specialty's foremost and distinguished surgeons/authors, writing on their particular areas of interest and expertise, providing recent treatment strategies, and opening a window into the future of the profession. The material is organized into the many subcategories or, in some cases, subspecialties that have evolved from the parent profession of oral surgery. Each section begins with a synopsis of pertinent historic and anatomic factors. The majority of the text is focused on the current approaches to the disease processes, highlighting surgical techniques and potential complications. When possible, an evidence-based approach to writing has been emphasized. However, at the end of each chapter, particular "Pearls and Pitfalls" that are based on the culmination of the authors' experience are listed. Although we have tried to include all the OMFS subcategories, the intent of this book is not to be a comprehensive text of surgery. Subjects were selected to address particular surgical or management problems that are relevant to the advancement of the field and are applicable to modern practice.

It is the authors' fervent hope that the important information presented in this book will improve the care of oral and maxillofacial surgery patients throughout the world. An additional goal is to stimulate the reader to search for and/or develop further innovations in our exciting and challenging surgical specialty.

Shahrokh C. Bagheri
R. Bryan Bell
Husain Ali Khan

ACKNOWLEDGMENTS

The time-consuming work of reviewing manuscripts and contributing our own chapters would not have been possible without the understanding and support of our family and colleagues. We are deeply grateful to numerous individuals in Atlanta and Portland for their patience with missed deadlines and delayed correspondence due to the necessarily intrusive mix of scholarly activity and clinical practice. In particular, we would like to thank the following individuals for their support and confidence:

Kevin Arce, Leon Assael, Gary Boloux, Angelo Cuzalina, Eric Dierks, Sam Farish, Henry Ferguson, Eugene Kelly, William Long, Josh Lubek, Jay Malmquist, Roger Meyer, Rod Nichols, Bob Myall, Vincent Perciaccante, Steven Roser, Julie Ann Smith, Martin Steed, Mark Stevens, Jason Potter, Bryce Potter, and Hank Windell.

We have also each had the privilege of working with a group of very talented resident surgeons from the training programs based at Emory University (Dr. Bagheri), Medical College of Georgia (Drs. Bagheri and Khan), Oregon Health & Science University (Dr. Bell), and the University of Washington (Dr. Bell). They provide the stimulus for this project and we would like to acknowledge them as future leaders of oral and maxillofacial surgery:

OHSU: Brett Ueeck, Eric Holmgren, Craig Kindsfater, Brian Woo, David Verschueren, Tim Osborn, Scott Sklenicka, Michael Wilkinson, Saif Al-Bustani, Samuel Bobek.

University of Washington: Forrest Bale, Pardeep Brar, Antonio Caso, Todd Carter, Chad Collins, Michael DaBell, Abe Estess, Ryan Gibson, Steve Huang, Patricia Kelly, Andrew Kramer, Libby Kutcipal, Jarom Luu, Erich Naumann, Jerald Pruner, Tony Rea, Emmanuel Taylor.

Emory University: Nizar Merheb, Nader Elbokle, Donny Quick, Martin Steed, Piyush Patel, Chris Jo, Hussein Ads, William Kapgan, Mehran Mehrabi, Boris Kalika, Deepak Krishnan, Fernando Jimenez, Abtin Shahriari, Brenda Hall, Bruce Anderson, Cang Huynh, Danielle Cunningham, Jaspal Girn, Henry Blair, Shyam Prasad, Jeffrey Wallace, Amy Kuhmichel, David Liang, Mimi Park, Robert "Cory" Ryan, Kael Rogers, Sung-Hee Cho, Jonathan Threadgill, Michael Demo, Anne Stearns, Thao Le. Brian Tallent, Damian Jimenez, Ajay Ganti, Ashley Gibbs, Lisa Tran, James Parelli, Robert Attia, Ibrahim Haron, Justine Moe.

Georgia Health Sciences University: Kyle Hunt, Daniel Scott, Abtin Etezadi, Patrick Walker, Hany Emam, Jeremy Hickson, William Klein, Matt Kikuchi, Sara Akeel, Carlos Pirela.

Modern textbooks are as much about corralling talent as they are about writing. We are indebted to the numerous authors who have contributed their valuable time and expertise to make this project a reality. Since one of our jobs as editors is to ensure the quality and timeliness of the manuscripts, the fact that virtually all of the authors submitted well-organized and contemporary chapters made this task easier.

Finally, we would also like to acknowledge the publishing team at Elsevier for their hard work and dedication toward the completion of this project. We owe a particular debt of gratitude to Courtney Sprehe, who has managed this project from the beginning with patience, confidence, and attention to detail; to Rich Barber in Book Production and to John Dolan, for his vision and dedication to medical/dental education.

Shahrokh C. Bagheri
R. Bryan Bell
Husain Ali Khan

CONTRIBUTORS

Shelly Ambramowicz, DMD, MPH
Instructor in Surgery
Department of Oral and Maxillofacial Surgery
Harvard School of Dental Medicine
Boston, Massachusetts
Attending Surgeon
Department of Plastic and Oral Surgery
Children's Hospital Boston
Boston, Massachusetts

Tara L. Aghaloo, DDS, MD, PhD
Associate Professor
Department of Oral and Maxillofacial Surgery
University of California, Los Angeles
Los Angeles, California

Saif S. Al-Bustani, MD, DMD
Chief Resident
Department of Oral and Maxillofacial Surgery
Oregon Health and Science University
Legacy Emanuel Medicine Center
Portland, Oregon

Rafael E. Alcalde, DDS, PhD
Affiliate Assistant Professor
University of Washington
Seattle, Washington

Kevin Arce, DMD, MD, MCR
Senior Associate Consultant
Division of Oral and Maxillofacial Surgery
Department of Surgery
Mayo Clinic
Rochester, Minnesota

Meredith August, DMD, MD
Associate Professor
Department of Oral and Maxillofacial Surgery
Massachusetts General Hospital
Boston, Massachusetts

Shahid R. Aziz, MD, DMD, FACS
Associate Professor
Department of Oral and Maxillofacial Surgery
New Jersey Dental School
Division of Plastic Surgery
Department of Surgery
New Jersey Medical School
University of Medicine and Dentistry of
    New Jersey
Newark, New Jersey

Shahrokh C. Bagheri, DMD, MD, FACS
Chief, Division of Oral and Maxillofacial Surgery
Department of Surgery
Northside Hospital
Georgia Oral and Facial Surgery, and Eastern
    Surgical Associates and Consultants
Atlanta, Georgia
Clinical Associate Professor
Department of Oral and Maxillofacial Surgery
Georgia Health Sciences University
Augusta, Georgia
Clinical Assistant Professor
Department of Surgery
School of Medicine
Emory University
Atlanta, Georgia

Jonathan S. Bailey, DMD, MD, FACS
Associate Professor
Division of Oral and Maxillofacial Surgery
Division of Head and Neck Cancer
Carle Clinic Association
Urbana, Illinois

Stephen A. Bankston, DMD
Clinical Assistant Professor
Department of Oral and Maxillofacial Surgery
Medical College of Georgia
Augusta, Georgia
Private Practice
Atlanta, Georgia

Jennifer P. Bassiur, DMD
Director
The Center for Oral, Facial, and Head Pain
Assistant Professor of Clinical Dentistry
Section of Hospital Dentistry
Division of Oral and Maxillofacial Surgery
College of Dental Medicine
Columbia University
New York, New York
Assistant Attending
New York Presbyterian Hospital
New York, New York

Brian Thomas Bast, DMD, MD
Associate Clinical Professor
Residency Program Director
Department of Oral and Maxillofacial Surgery
University of California, San Francisco
San Francisco, California

Dale A. Baur, DDS, MD
Associate Professor and Chair
Department of Oral and Maxillofacial Surgery
Case Western Reserve University
Cleveland, Ohio

Steven W. Beadnell, DMD
Adjunct Associate Professor
Department of Oral and Maxillofacial Surgery
School of Dentistry
Oregon Health and Science University
Portland, Oregon
Private Practice
Sunset Oral and Maxillofacial Surgery
Portland, Oregon

Lou S. Belinfante, BS, DDS
Active Staff
Northside Forsyth Hospital
Cumming, Georgia
Northside Hospital
Atlanta, Georgia
Honorary Staff
Emory Adventist Hospital
Smyrna, Georgia
Private Practice
Dawsonville, Georgia

R. Bryan Bell, DDS, MD, FACS
Medical Director
Oral, Head and Neck Cancer Program
Providence Cancer Center
Robert W. Franz Cancer Research Center
Providence Portland Medical Center
Attending Surgeon and Director of Resident
    Education
Trauma Service/Oral and Maxillofacial Surgery
    Service
Legacy Emanuel Medical Center
Affiliate Associate Professor
Oregon Health and Science University
Head and Neck Surgical Associates Partner
Portland, Oregon

Jeffrey Bennett, DMD
Professor and Chair
Department of Oral Surgery and
    Hospital Dentistry
Indiana University School of Dentistry
Indianapolis, Indiana

Steven P. Best, DMD
Resident
Department of Oral and Maxillofacial Surgery
College of Dental Medicine
Broward Medical Center
Nova Southeastern University
Fort Lauderdale, Florida

George H. Blakely III, DDS
Raymond P. White Distinguished Associate
    Clinical Professor
Residency Program Director
Department of Maxillofacial Surgery
School of Dentistry
University of North Carolina Healthcare
Chapel Hill, North Carolina

Remy H. Blanchaert, Jr., DDS, MD
Private Practice
Oral and Maxillofacial Surgery Associates
Wichita, Kansas

Dale S. Bloomquist, DDS, MS
Emeritus Associate Professor and Acting Chairman
Department of Oral and Maxillofacial Surgery
School of Dentistry
University of Washington
Seattle, Washington

Behnam Bohluli, DMD
School of Dentistry
Buali Medical Center
Azad University
Tehran, Iran

Gary F. Bouloux, MD, DDS, MDSc, FRACD(OMS)
Assistant Professor and Director of Research
Department of Oral and Maxillofacial Surgery
Emory University School of Medicine
Atlanta, Georgia

Jimmy James Brown, DDS, MD, FACS
Professor
Department of Otolaryngology
Georgia Health Sciences University
Medical College of Georgia
Augusta, Georgia

Daniel Buchbinder, DMD, MD
Clinical Professor
Department of Oral Maxillofacial Surgery
Chief
Division of Maxillofacial Surgery
Department of Otolaryngology
Director
Residency Program in Oral and Maxillofacial
    Surgery
Beth Israel Center
New York, New York
Jacobi Medical Center
Albert Einstein College of Medicine
Bronx, New York
Institute for Head and Neck and Thyroid Diseases
Continuum Cancer Centers
New York, New York

Tuan Giang Bui, MD, DMD
Fellow
Head and Neck Surgery/Microvascular
    Reconstruction
Providence Portland Hospital
Legacy Emanuel Hospital
Portland, Oregon

John F. Caccamese, Jr., DMD, MD, FACS
Associate Professor and Program Director
Department of Oral-Maxillofacial Surgery
University of Maryland, Baltimore College of
    Dental Surgery
University of Maryland Medical System
Baltimore, Maryland

Johanny Caceres, DDS
Chief Resident
Division of Oral and Maxillofacial Surgery
Jackson Memorial Hospital
University of Miami
Miami, Florida

Aaron Sterling Card, DMD, MD
Resident of Oral and Maxillofacial Surgery
University of Kentucky
Lexington, Kentucky

Eric R. Carlson, DMD, MD, FACS
Professor and Chairman
Department of Oral and Maxillofacial Surgery
Director
Oral and Maxillofacial Surgery Residency Program
University of Tennessee Medical Center
Director
Oral/Head and Neck Oncologic Surgery
    Fellowship Program
University of Tennessee Cancer Institute
Knoxville, Tennessee

Guillermo E. Chacon, DDS
Affiliate Associate Professor
Department of Oral and Maxillofacial Surgery
University of Washington
Seattle, Washington
Attending Staff
Good Samaritan Hospital
Private Practice
Oral and Facial Surgery Center of Puyallup
Puyallup, Washington
Chief
Department of Pediatric Oral and Maxillofacial
    Surgery
Mary Bridge Children's Hospital
Tacoma, Washington

Radhika Chigurupati, DMD, MS
Associate Clinical Professor
Department of Oral and Maxillofacial Surgery
University of California, San Francisco
UCSF Center for Craniofacial Abnormalities
School of Dentistry
UCSF Benioff Children's Hospital and Moffitt
    Medical Center
San Francisco, California

Tarek Victor Copty
Cosmetic Surgeon (ABS, AACS, ABCS)
Private Practice, Copty Surgical Arts
Amman, Jordan

Bernard J. Costello, DMD, MD, FACS
Professor and Program Director
Department of Oral and Maxillofacial Surgery
University of Pittsburgh
Chief
Department of Pediatric Oral and Maxillofacial
    Surgery
Children's Hospital of Pittsburgh
Pittsburgh, Pennsylvania

Larry L. Cunningham, Jr., DDS, MD, FACS
Associate Professor, Residency Director, and Chief
Division of Oral and Maxillofacial Surgery
College of Dentistry
Chandler Medical Center
University of Kentucky
Lexington, Kentucky

Angelo Cuzalina, MD, DDS
AACS Cosmetic Surgery Fellowship Director
Associate Faculty Oklahoma State Medical School
President of the American Academy of Cosmetic
    Surgery 2011
Private Practice, Tulsa Surgical Arts, PC
Tulsa, Oklahoma

Betsy K. Davis, DMD, MS
Director
Maxillofacial Prosthodontic Clinic
Medical University of South Carolina
Charleston, South Carolina

Nagi Demian, DDS, MD
Assistant Professor and Chief of Service
Department of Oral and Maxillofacial Surgery
University of Texas Health Science Center
    at Houston
Lyndon B. Johnson General Hospital
Houston, Texas

Michael M. Demo, DDS
Resident
Emory University
Atlanta, Georgia

Eric J. Dierks, MD, DMD, FACS
Staff Surgeon
The Head and Neck Surgical Associates
Director of Fellowship
Head and Neck Oncologic Surgery
Affiliate Professor
Department of Oral and Maxillofacial Surgery
Oregon Health and Science University
Portland, Oregon
Affiliate Professor
Department of Oral and Maxillofacial Surgery
University of Washington
Seattle, Washington

Michael P. Ding, DDS, MD
Private Practice, Austin Oral and Maxillofacial
    Surgery
Austin, Texas

Thomas B. Dodson, DMD, MPH
Visiting (Attending) Oral and Maxillofacial
    Surgeon
Massachusetts General Hospital
Director
Center for Applied Clinical Investigation
Associate Professor
Department of Oral and Maxillofacial Surgery
Harvard School of Dental Medicine
Boston, Massachusetts

Franklin M. Dolwick, DDS
Professor
Department of Oral and Maxillofacial Surgery
College of Dentistry
University of Florida
Gainesville, Florida

Amir H. Dorafshar, MBChB
Assistant Professor
Department of Plastic and Reconstructive Surgery
The Johns Hopkins Medical Institute
The R. Adams Cowley Shock Trauma Center
University of Maryland Medical Center
Baltimore, Maryland

Connie L. Drisko, DDS
Dean and Merritt Professor
Department of Periodontics
School of Dentistry
Medical College of Georgia
Georgia Health Sciences University
Augusta, Georgia

Sean P. Edwards, MD, DDS, FRCD(C)
Clinical Assistant Professor
Residency Program Director
Chief of Pediatric Maxillofacial Surgery
C.S. Mott Children's Hospital
University of Michigan Health System
Ann Arbor, Michigan

Hany A. Emam, BDS, MSc
Resident
Department of Oral and Maxillofacial Surgery
Medical College of Georgia
Georgia Health Sciences University
Augusta, Georgia

Mark Engelstad, MD, DDS, MHI
Associate Professor
Department of Oral and Maxillofacial Surgery
Oregon Health and Science University
Portland, Oregon

Stephen L. Engroff, MD, DDS
Private Practice, Tri-County Oral-Facial Surgeons
State College, Pennsylvania

Sam E. Farish, DMD
Associate Professor
Division of Oral and Maxillofacial Surgery
Emory University School of Medicine
Atlanta, Georgia

Brian B. Farrell, DDS, MD
Assistant Clinical Professor
Department of Oral and Maxillofacial Surgery
Louisiana State University Health Science Center
New Orleans, Louisiana
Private Practice
University Oral and Maxillofacial Surgery
Charlotte, North Carolina

Tirbod Fattahi, MD, DDS, FACS
Associate Professor of Surgery and Chief
Division of Oral and Maxillofacial Surgery
University of Florida Health Science Center,
    Jacksonville
Jacksonville, Florida

Stephen E. Feinberg, DDS, MS, PhD
Professor in Dentistry and Surgery
Associate Chair of Research in Oral and
    Maxillofacial Surgery
University of Michigan Health System
University of Michigan Medical and Dental
    Schools
Attending Staff in Oral and Maxillofacial Surgery
University of Michigan Hospitals
Ann Arbor, Michigan
Co-Founder
Tissue Regeneration Systems, A Biotechnology
    Company
Ann Arbor, Michigan

Alan L. Felsenfeld, DDS
Professor of Clinical Dentistry
Section of Oral and Maxillofacial Surgery
School of Dentistry
University of California
Los Angeles, California

Rui Fernandes, DMD, MD, FACS
Assistant Professor
Chief of Head and Neck Surgery
Director of Oral and Maxillofacial Residency
Director of Microvascular Fellowship
Divisions of Oral Maxillofacial Surgery and
    Surgical Oncology
Department of Surgery
College of Medicine—Jacksonville
University of Florida
Jacksonville, Florida

Thomas R. Flynn, DMD
Associate Professor of Oral and Maxillofacial
    Surgery
Harvard School of Dental Medicine
Boston, Massachusetts

Judah S. Garfinkle, DMD, MS
Director of Craniofacial Orthodontics
Assistant Professor of Plastic and Reconstructive
    Surgery
Assistant Professor of Orthodontics
Oregon Health and Science University
Private Practice, Limited to Orthodontics
Portland, Oregon

Jaime Gateno, DDS, MD
Chairman
Department of Oral and Maxillofacial Surgery
The Methodist Hospital
Houston, Texas
Professor of Clinical Surgery (Oral and
    Maxillofacial Surgery)
Weill Medical College
Cornell University
New York, New York

Marianela Gonzalez, DDS, MS
Assistant Professor and Director
Undergraduate Oral and Maxillofacial Surgery
    Curriculum
Director
Undergraduate Emergency Oral and Maxillofacial
    Surgery Clinic
Baylor College of Dentistry
Baylor University Medical Center
Dallas, Texas

Phoebe Good, DMD, MS
Division of Orthodontics
University of California, San Francisco
Private Practice, Good and Sears Orthodontics
San Francisco, California

**Reginald H.B. Goodday, DDS, MSc,
FRCD(C), FICD**
Chair
Department of Oral and Maxillofacial Sciences
Dalhousie University
District Chief
Department of Oral and Maxillofacial Surgery
Queen Elizabeth II Health Sciences Center
Halifax, Nova Scotia, Canada

Barry H. Grayson, DDS
Associate Professor of Surgery (Craniofacial
    Orthodontics)
Department of Plastic Surgery
Langone Medical Center
New York University
New York, New York

Curtis Gregoire, DDS, MD, MSc, FRCDC
Associate Professor
Dalhousie University
Halifax, Nova Scotia, Canada

Andres Guerra, DMD
Fellow, Oncologic Surgery
University of Tennessee
Graduate School of Medicine
University of Tennessee Cancer Institute
Knoxville, Tennessee

Cesar A. Guerrero, DDS
Professor
Central University of Venezuela
Santa Rosa Maxillofacial Surgery Center
Caracas, Venezuela

Christopher John Haggerty, DDS, MD
Private Practice
Kansas City, Missouri

Brent R. Hayek, MD
Assistant Professor of Ophthalmology
Section of Oculoplastic and Reconstructive
    Surgery
Emory Eye Center
Atlanta, Georgia

Barry H. Hendler, DDS, MD
Medical Director/Director OMS, Cosmetic Surgery
    Associates
Department of Oral and Maxillofacial Surgery
University of Pennsylvania Health System
Associate Professor
Department of Oral and Maxillofacial Surgery
    and Pharmacology
University of Pennsylvania School of Dental
    Medicine
Philadelphia, Pennsylvania

Mariana Henriquez, DDS
Oral Surgeon
Central University of Venezuela
Santa Rosa Maxillofacial Surgery Center
Caracas, Venezuela

Alan S. Herford, DDS, MD, FACS
Professor and Chair
Department of Oral and Maxillofacial Surgery
Loma Linda University School of Medicine
Loma Linda University Medical Center
Loma Linda, California

Kenji W. Higuchi, DDS, MS, FACD, FICD
Private Practice
Spokane, Washington

David L. Hirsch, DDS, MD, FACS
Assistant Professor
Department of Surgery
Department of Oral and Maxillofacial Surgery
New York University Langone Medical Center
Head of Surgical Service
Head of Surgical Pathology and Reconstruction
Bellevue Hospital Center
New York, New York

Matthew R. Hlavacek, MD, DDS
Assistant Professor
Department of Oral and Maxillofacial Surgery
Assistant Professor
Department of Surgery
Truman Medical Center
University of Missouri—Kansas City
Kansas City, Missouri

Jon D. Holmes, DMD, MD, FACS
Assistant Clinical Professor
Department of Oral and Maxillofacial Surgery
University of Alabama at Birmingham
Private Practice, ClarkHolmes Oral and Facial
    Surgery
Birmingham, Alabama

Michael P. Horan, MD, DDS, PhD
Resident
Department of Oral and Maxillofacial Surgery
Case Western Reserve University
Cleveland, Ohio

Kenji Izumi, DDS, PhD
Associate Professor
Division of Oral Anatomy
Niigata University Graduate School for Medical
    and Dental Sciences
Niigata City, Niigata

Michael S. Jaskolka, DDS, MD
Cleft and Craniomaxillofacial Surgeon
Charleston Area Medical Center
Facial Surgery Center
First Appalachian Craniofacial Disorders
    Specialists (FACES)
Charleston, West Virginia

Don Joondeph, DDS, MS
Professor Emeritus
Department of Orthodontics
University of Washington
Seattle, Washington
Private Practice of Orthodontics
Bellevue, Washington

David Michael Junck, DDS
Oral and Maxillofacial Surgeon
Kishwaukee Community Hospital
Private Practice, Oral and Maxillofacial Surgeons
    for Northern Illinois
Sycamore, Illinois

Leonard B. Kaban, DMD, MD, FACS
Walter C. Guralnick Professor and Chairman
Department of Oral and Maxillofacial Surgery
Harvard School of Dental Medicine
Massachusetts General Hospital
Boston, Massachusetts

Deepak Kademani, DMD, MD, FACS
Associate Professor
Department of Oral and Maxillofacial Surgery
University of Minnesota Medical Center
Minneapolis, Minnesota

Husain Ali Khan, DMD, MD
Attending Surgeon, Division of Oral and
    Maxillofacial Surgery
Department of Surgery
Northside Hospital
Georgia Oral and Facial Surgery, and Eastern
    Surgical Associates and Consultants
Atlanta, Georgia
Clinical Associate Professor
Department of Oral and Maxillofacial Surgery
Georgia Health Sciences University
Augusta, Georgia

David A. Keith BDS, FDSRCS, DMD
Professor of Oral and Maxillofacial Surgery
Harvard School of Dental Medicine
Visiting Oral and Maxillofacial Surgery
Massachusetts General Hospital
Dental Director
Harvard Vanguard Medical Associates
Boston, Massachusetts

Nathan A. Kemalyan, MD, FACS
Medical Director
Oregon Burn Center
Legacy Health System
Portland, Oregon

D. David Kim, DMD, MD, FACS
Associate Professor
Residency and Fellowship Program Director
Department of Oral and Maxillofacial Surgery
Louisiana State University Health Sciences Center,
    Shreveport
Shreveport, Louisiana

King Kim, DMD
Adjunct Clinical Professor
Department of Oral and Maxillofacial Surgery
School of Dental Medicine
Nova Southeastern University/Broward General
    Medical Center
Fort Lauderdale, Florida
Private Practice, New Image Maxillofacial Surgery
Melbourne, Florida

Christopher T. Kirkup, DDS, MS
Assistant Clinical Professor
Indiana University School of Dentistry
Private Practice, Indiana Oral and Maxillofacial
    Surgery Associates
Indianapolis, Indiana

Antonia Kolokythas, DDS
Assistant Professor
Department of Oral and Maxillofacial Surgery
University of Illinois at Chicago
Chicago, Illinois

James A. Kraus, DMD
Former Chief Resident
Tufts University/Tufts Medical Center
Boston, Massachusetts
Cranio-maxillofacial Surgery Fellow
Royal Children's Hospital
Melbourne, Australia

Edward T. Lahey, III, DMD, MD
Assistant Oral and Maxillofacial Surgeon
Instructor
Department of Oral and Maxillofacial Surgery
Massachusetts General Hospital
Harvard School of Dental Medicine
Boston, Massachusetts

David K. Lam, DDS, PhD
Postdoctoral Scholar
Department of Oral and Maxillofacial Surgery
University of California, San Francisco
San Francisco, California

Ahn D. Le, DDS, PhD
Associate Professor
Departments of Endodontics, Oral and
    Maxillofacial Surgery, and Orthodontics
Herman Ostrow School of Dentistry of USC
Center for Craniofacial Molecular Biology
University of Southern California
LAC+USC Health Care Network
California Hospital Medical Center
Los Angeles, California

Janice S. Lee, DDS, MD, FACS
Associate Professor
Department of Clinical Oral and Maxillofacial
    Surgery
University of California, San Francisco
San Francisco, California

Jessica J. Lee, DDS
Associate Professor
Department of Oral and Maxillofacial Surgery
University of Washington
Seattle, Washington

Joyce T. Lee, DDS, MD
Clinical Associate Professor
Division of Oral and Maxillofacial Surgery
Department of Surgery
Emory University School of Medicine
Active Staff
Grady Memorial Hospital
Emory Midtown Hospital
Piedmont Hospital
Atlanta, Georgia

Stanley Yung-Chuan Liu, DDS, MD
Resident of Oral and Maxillofacial Surgery
University of California, San Francisco
San Francisco, California

Joshua Eli Lubek, MD, DDS
Assistant Professor and Fellowship Director
Maxillofacial Oncology and Microvascular
 Surgery
Department of Oral and Maxillofacial Surgery
University of Maryland
Baltimore, Maryland

Gregory J. Mackay, MD, FACS
Associate Clinical Professor
Department of Oral and Maxillofacial Surgery
Medical College of Georgia
Augusta, Georgia
Vice Chief Pediatric Plastic Surgery
Department of Surgery
Childrens' Heathcare of Atlanta
Atlanta, Georgia

**Stephen P.R. Macleod, BDS, MD ChB, FDS
RCS (ED), FDS RCS (ENG), FRCS (ED)**
Associate Professor of Surgery
University of Colorado School of Medicine
Associate Professor of Oral and Maxillofacial
 Surgery
University of Colorado School of Dental Medicine
Aurora, Colorado
Director of Dentistry and Oral and Maxillofacial
 Surgery
Denver Health
Denver, Colorado

Rafael A. Madero-Visbal, MD
Research Fellow
Department of Head and Neck Surgery
M.D. Anderson Cancer Center Orlando
Orlando, Florida

Matthew J. Madsen, DMD, MD
Resident
Department of Oral and Maxillofacial Surgery
University of Louisville
Louisville, Kentucky

Jose M. Marchena, DMD, MD
Private Practice
Newburyport Oral Surgery
Newburyport, Massachusetts
Clinical Assistant Professor
The University of Texas Health Science Center
 at Houston
Houston, Texas

Glen Maron, DDS
Assistant Clinical Professor
Section of Oral and Maxillofacial Surgery
Department of Surgery
Emory University
Atlanta, Georgia

Robert E. Marx, DDS
Professor of Surgery and Chief
Division of Oral and Maxillofacial Surgery
University of Miami Miller School of Medicine
Miami, Florida

Joseph P. McCain, DMD
Professor of Oral and Maxillofacial Surgery
School of Dental Medicine
Nova Southeastern University
Fort Lauderdale, Florida
Chief of Oral and Maxillofacial Surgery
Baptist Hospital
Private Practice
Miami, Florida

Shawn A. McClure, DMD, MD
Associate Professor and Director of Research
Department of Oral and Maxillofacial Surgery
NOVA/NSU College of Dental Medicine
Fort Lauderdale, Florida

Adam P. McCormick, DDS
Chief Resident
Department of Oral and Maxillofacial Surgery
Virginia Commonwealth University Medical
 Center
Richmond, Virginia

Noshir R. Mehta, DMD, MDS, MS
Director
Craniofacial Pain Headache and Sleep Center
Chairman, General Dentistry
Associate Dean International Relations
Tufts University School of Dental Medicine
Boston, Massachusetts

Louis G. Mercuri, DDS, MS
Clinical Professor of Surgery
Division of Oral and Maxillofacial Surgery
Department of Surgery
Loyola University Medical Center
Maywood, Illinois

Roger Albert Meyer, MD, DDS, MS, FACS
Director
Maxillofacial Consultants, Ltd.
Greensboro, Georgia

Michael Miloro, DMD, MD, FACS
Professor, Department Head, and Program
 Director
University of Illinois
Chicago, Illinois

Elena V. Mujica, DDS
Oral Surgeon Resident
Central University of Venezuela
Santa Rosa Maxillofacial Surgery Center
Caracus, Venezuela

**Robert W. T. Myall, BDS, MD, FRCD(C),
FDSRCS**
Professor of Oral and Maxillofacial Surgery
School of Dentistry
Professor of Surgery
School of Medicine
Oregon Health and Science University
Portland, Oregon

**Dimitrios Nikolarakos, BDSc, MBBS,
FRACDS (OMS), FRCS Eng (OMFS)**
Consultant Maxillofacial Surgeon
Thomas Tatum Head and Neck Unit
St. George's Healthcare NHS Trust
London, United Kingdom

Devin Joseph Okay, DDS
Director
Division of Prosthodontics
Beth Israel Medical Center
Private Practice in Prosthodontics
New York, New York

**Robert Andrew Ord, DDS, MD, FRCS,
FACS, MS**
Professor and Chairman
Department of Oral and Maxillofacial Surgery
University of Maryland, Greenbaum Cancer
 Center
University of Maryland Oral and Maxillofacial
 Surgery Associates
Baltimore, Maryland

Felice O'Ryan, DDS
Director, Maxillofacial Surgery
Kaiser Permanente Oakland Medical Center
Oakland, California

Timothy Marx Osborn, DDS, MD
Private Practice, Oral-Facial Surgery Associates
North Adams, Massachusetts

Harry Papadopoulous, DDS, MD
Clinical Associate Professor
Department of Oral Surgery and Hospital
 Dentistry
Indiana University
Indianapolis, Indiana

Bonnie L. Padwa, DMD, MD
Associate Professor
Department of Oral and Maxillofacial Surgery
Harvard School of Medicine
Oral Surgeon-in-Chief
Children's Hospital Boston
Boston, Massachusetts

Zachary S. Peacock, DMD, MD
Former Chief Resident
University of California, San Francisco
San Francisco, California
Assistant in Oral and Maxillofacial Surgery
Massachusetts General Hospital
Boston, Massachusetts

Vincent James Perciaccante, DDS
Clinical Assistant Professor
Emory University School of Medicine
Atlanta, Georgia
Private Practice
Peachtree City, Georgia

Phillip Pirgousis, DMD, MD
Head Neck/Microvascular Fellow
College of Medicine
University of Florida
Jacksonville, Florida

M.A. Pogrel, DDS, MD, FRCS, FACS
Professor and Chairman
Department of Oral and Maxillofacial Surgery
University of California, San Francisco
San Francisco, California

Jeffrey C. Posnick, DMD, MD, FRCS(C), FACS
Clinical Professor of Surgery and Pediatrics
Georgetown University
Washington, DC
Adjunct Professor of Orthodontics
Baltimore College of Dental Surgery
University of Maryland
Baltimore, Maryland
Adjunct Professor of Oral and Maxillofacial
    Surgery
Howard University College of Dentistry
Washington, DC
Director
Posnick Center for Facial Plastic Surgery
Chery Chase, Maryland

Jason K. Potter, MD, DDS
Clinical Assistant Professor
Department of Plastic Surgery
University of Texas Southwestern Medical Center
Dallas, Texas

**David S. Precious CM, DDS, MSc, FRCDC,
FICD, FACD, FADI, FRCS (Eng)**
Dean Emeritus and Professor
Dalhousie University
Halifax, Nova Scotia, Canada

Jeffrey R. Prinsell, DMD, MD
Private Practice, Oral and Maxillofacial Surgery
Marietta, Georgia

Clement Qaqish, DDS, MD
Chief Resident
Department of Oral and Maxillofacial Surgery
University of Maryland Medical Center
Baltimore, Maryland

Pat Ricalde, MD, DDS, FACS
Director
St. Joseph's Craniofacial Center
Private Practice
Tampa, Florida

Helen Rivera, DDS
Oral and Maxillofacial Surgery and Pathology
    Departments
Central University of Venezuela
Caracas, Venezuela

Eduardo D. Rodriguez, MD, DDS
Associate Professor and Chief
Departments of Plastic, Reconstructive,
    and Maxillofacial Surgery
R. Adams Cowley Shock Trauma Center
Johns Hopkins School of Medicine
University of Maryland
Baltimore, Maryland

Juan C. Rodriguez, DDS
Research Fellow
Department of Oral and Maxillofacial Surgery
Case Western Reserve University
Cleveland, Ohio

Steven M. Roser, DMD, MD, FACS
DeLos Hill Professor and Chief
Division of Oral and Maxillofacial Surgery
Emory University School of Medicine
Atlanta, Georgia

Ramon L. Ruiz, DMD, MD
Associate Professor of Surgery
University of Central Florida College of Medicine
Medical Director
Pediatric Craniomaxillofacial Surgery
Pediatric Oral and Maxillofacial Surgery
Arnold Palmer Hospital for Children
Orlando, Florida

Andrew R. Salama, DDS, MD
Assistant Professor
Department of Oral and Maxillofacial Surgery
University of Maryland Medical Center
Baltimore, Maryland

Martin I. Salgueiro, DDS
Assistant Professor
Department of Oral and Maxillofacial Surgery
Medical College of Georgia
Augusta, Georgia

Yoh Sawatari, DDS
Assistant Professor of Clinical Surgery
Division of Oral and Maxillofacial Surgery
Miller School of Medicine
University of Miami
Miami, Florida

Stephen A. Schendel, MD, DDS
Professor Emeritus
Division of Plastic Surgery
Stanford University
Palo Alto, California

Edward R. Schlissel, DDS, MS
Professor Emeritus
Department of General Dentistry
School of Dental Medicine
Stony Brook University
Stony Brook, New York
Clinical Assistant Professor
Department of Surgery
Emory University School of Medicine
Atlanta, Georgia

Brian L. Schmidt, DDS, MD, PhD
Professor
Department of Oral and Maxillofacial Surgery
Director
Bluestone Center for Clinical Research
New York University College of Dentistry
New York, New York

Steven J. Scrivani, DDS, DMedSc
Professor
The Craniofacial Pain and Headache Center
Tufts University School of Dental Medicine
Boston, Massachusetts
Research Associate
Pain and Analgesia Imaging and Neuroscience
    (PAIN) Group
Brain Imaging Center, McLean Hospital
Belmont, Massachusetts

Rabie M. Shanti, DMD
Resident
Department of Oral and Maxillofacial Surgery
New Jersey Dental School
University of Medicine and Dentistry of
    New Jersey
Newark, New Jersey

Thomas D. Shellenberger, DMD, MD
Chief
Department of Head and Neck Surgery
The University of Texas M.D. Anderson
    Cancer Center at Houston
Houston, Texas

Julie Ann Smith, DDS, MD
Assistant Professor and Pre-doctoral Program
    Director
Oregon Health and Science University
Portland, Oregon

Miller H. Smith, MD, DDS
Clinical Fellow, Graduate
Department of Oral Maxillofacial Surgery
University of Michigan Health System
Ann Arbor, Michigan
Current Fellow
NHS Greater Glasgow and Clyde
Southern General Hospital
Glasgow, United Kingdom

Michael J. Spink, DDS, MD
Assistant Professor of Oral and Maxillofacial
    Surgery
Baystate Medical Center
Springfield, Massachusetts

David C. Stanton, DMD, MD, FACS
Associate Professor and Residency Program
    Director
Department of Oral and Maxillofacial Surgery
University of Pennsylvania
Philadelphia, Pennsylvania

Martin B. Steed, DDS
Assistant Professor and Residency Program
    Director
Division of Oral and Maxillofacial Surgery
Department of Surgery
Emory University
Atlanta, Georgia

Mark R. Stevens, DDS
Professor and Chairman
Department of Oral and Maxillofacial Surgery
College of Dental Medicine
Georgia Health Sciences University
Professor (Joint Appointment)
Department of Oral Biology
Faculty Member
Medical College of Georgia Health, Inc.
Medical College of Georgia Children's
    Medical Center
Veterans Administrative Medical Center
Augusta State Prison
Augusta, Georgia

Robert A. Strauss, DDS, MD
Professor and Director
Residency Training Program
Virginia Commonwealth University
    Medical Center
Richmond, Virginia

John F. Teichgraeber, MD, FACS
Professor and Chief
Division of Pediatric Plastic Surgery
Department of Pediatric Surgery
The University of Texas Health Science Center
    at Houston
Houston, Texas

Brinda Thimmappa, MD
Adjunct Assistant Professor
Department of Plastic Surgery
Loma Linda University
Loma Linda, California
Division of Plastic Surgery
Southwest Washington Medical Center
Vancouver, Washington

Paul S. Tiwana, DDS, MD, MS, FACS
Associate Professor and Graduate Program
    Director
Division of Oral and Maxillofacial Surgery
Department of Surgery
University of Texas Southwestern Medical Center
Dallas, Texas

Antwan L. Treadway, DMD
Assistant Professor
Society of Oral and Maxillofacial Surgeons
Medical College of Georgia
Augusta, Georgia
Wellstar Cobb Hospital
Wellstar Douglas Hospital
Austell, Georgia
Northside Hospital
Private Practice, Atlanta Oral and Facial Surgery
Atlanta, Georgia

Robert Gilbert Triplett, DDS, PhD
Texas State Board of Dental Examiners
Regents Professor and Vice Chairman
Department of Oral and Maxillofacial Surgery
Baylor College of Dentistry
Texas A&M Health Science Center
Chief of Dentistry
Department of Surgery
Baylor University Medical Center
Texas Scottish Rite Hospital for Children
Dallas, Texas

Myron R. Tucker, DDS
Adjunct Professor
Louisiana State University Department of Oral and
    Maxillofacial Surgery
New Orleans, Louisiana
Private Practice (Retired)
Charlotte, North Carolina

Timothy A. Turvey, DDS
Professor and Chairman
Department of Oral and Maxillofacial Surgery
University of North Carolina
School of Dentistry
Chapel Hill, North Carolina

Carlos M. Ugalde, DDS, MS
Private Practice
Northwest Oral Maxillofacial and Implant Surgery
Eugene, Oregon

Aaron Vickers, DDS, MD
Resident
Department of Oral and Maxillofacial Surgery
University of Louisville
School of Dentistry
Louisville, Kentucky

Joseph D. Walrath, MD
Associate in Ophthalmology
Division of Oculoplastics
Department of Ophthalmology
Emory University
Atlanta, Georgia

Brent B. Ward, DDS, MD, FACS
Assistant Professor and Fellowship Program
    Director
Section of Oral and Maxillofacial Surgery
University of Michigan
Ann Arbor, Michigan

Jill M. Weber, DDS
Section Head
Oral and Maxillofacial Surgery Head and Neck
    Institute
Cleveland Clinic Foundation
Associate Clinical Professor
Department of Oral and Maxillofacial Surgery
Case School of Dental Medicine
Cleveland, Ohio

Heather B. Westmoreland, MD
Medical Director
Cardiovascular MRI
Northeast Georgia Medical Center
Cardiologist
Northeast Georgia Heart Center, PC
Gainesville, Georgia

Fayette C. Williams, DDS, MD
Clinical Faculty, John Peter Smith Hospital
Department of Oral and Maxillofacial Surgery
Fort Worth, Texas

Larry M. Wolford, DMD
Clinical Professor
Department of Oral and Maxillofacial Surgery
Baylor College of Dentistry
Baylor University Medical Center
Texas A&M University Health Science Center,
    Dallas
Private Practice, Baylor University Medical Center
Dallas, Texas

Ted Wojno, MD
Director
Oculoplastic and Orbital Surgery
Department of Ophthalmology
Emory University School of Medicine
Atlanta, Georgia

Mark E. Wong, DDS
Professor, Chairman and Program Director
University of Texas Health Science Center
    at Houston
Houston, Texas

Brian M. Woo, DDS, MD
Faculty
Department of Oral and Maxillofacial Surgery
University of California, San Francisco—Fresno
Fresno, California

James J. Xia, MD, PhD, MS
Director of Surgical Planning Laboratory
Department of Oral and Maxillofacial Surgery
The Methodist Hospital Research Institute
Houston, Texas
Associate Professor of Surgery
Department of Oral and Maxillofacial Surgery
Weill Medical College
Cornell University
New York, New York
Associate Professor
Departments of Pediatric Surgery and
    Orthodontics
The University of Texas Houston Health
    Science Center
Houston, Texas

A. Maziar Zafari, MD, PhD, FACC, FAHA
Associate Professor of Medicine
Director
Cardiovascular Training Program
Emory University School of Medicine
Atlanta, Georgia
Atlanta Veterans Affairs Medical Center
Decatur, Georgia

TABLE OF CONTENTS

THE PAST

Although the basic principles of surgery apply to the oral and maxillofacial region, several factors have previously distinguished this profession from other surgical disciplines. In addition to surgery, oral and maxillofacial surgeons (OMSs) have embraced the basic and advanced principles of medicine, dentistry, pathology, infectious diseases, and radiology to provide comprehensive patient care. Unlike many areas of medicine that have a medical and a surgical specialty (e.g., neurology and neurosurgery), the surgical counterpart to oral and maxillofacial surgery was previously lacking. The principles of facial trauma care with a focus on dentoalveolar injuries and the treatment of odontogenic infections have dominated the past.

THE PRESENT

The current principles of oral and maxillofacial surgery continue to be dictated by traditional concepts of surgery that are continuously modified to accommodate emerging knowledge and technology. Enhanced understanding of wound healing, biomaterials, minimally invasive surgical techniques, new operations, and other modern advances continue to follow the traditional principles of surgery in a more effective, efficient, and safer routine. The evolution of the non-surgical disciplines of oral and maxillofacial radiology, oral pathology, and oral medicine and the greater integration of the profession with other medical and surgical specialties is noteworthy.

THE FUTURE

As the future inevitably becomes the present, it will bring improved understanding of the biological concepts that allow the application of new principles of surgery that were previously thought to be impossible. Advances in recombinant molecules will aid in wound healing and tissue regeneration. Development of advanced imaging technology will improve diagnostic modalities that may minimize or eliminate the need for tissue biopsies and simplify differential diagnosis. Advancements in robotic surgery will lead to more accurate and efficient surgical care. Suturing may become a relic of the past. The future will also bring new diseases that challenge all existing principles. The magnitude and continuously expanding scope of the specialty will require additional subspecialty training programs. These new specialty interests will find their place among the other surgical specialties. The core training of the OMS is destined to change in preparation for the future challenges of our surgical specialties.

The History of Oral and Maxillofacial Surgery

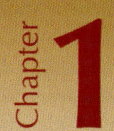
Chapter 1

Lou S. Belinfante

In 1915, while at a national dental meeting, a prominent exodontist from Denver, Colorado, Dr. Menifee Howard, met with a group of other dentists whose main areas of practice were also related to the extraction of teeth, anesthesia, and the ethical aspects of such. They theorized that a new organization would be beneficial to advance their burgeoning areas of expertise. After acquiring the names of other dentists with similar interests from files provided by dental supply houses, a list of interested parties was assembled. Letters were sent out to 125 dentists throughout the country regarding a potential future meeting. On August 6, 1918, in conjunction with the annual meeting in Chicago of the National Dental Association (a circuitous precursor to the modern American Dental Association), a seminal meeting was held, which lasted for 3 days. The deliberations were mostly related to administrative structuring to meet the needs and types of committees desired and the membership of these committees. Also discussed were declarations regarding the advancement of standards, the present status of exodontia and other closely related fields, and imagined future areas of interest. A short time thereafter, a subcommittee met with the trustees of the National Dental Association to petition them for formal recognition of their now conceived specialty. Indeed, recognition was quickly granted, and the nascent group became the American Society of Oral Surgeons and Exodontists.

The pieces of the pie, relative to an officially recognized organization, were starting to fit together. It is important to recognize the enormous scientific and administrative contributions of previous historical giants that led to such a memorable and significant chain of events.

A new specialty was being established that was deeply rooted in dentistry. It initially was associated with the correction of traumatic facial injuries and abnormalities and the treatment of terminally diseased dentitions while using ambulatory anesthetic agents. Like many noteworthy events, a significant number of very dedicated persons along with the timing of certain circumstances, some planned, some serendipitous, turned the concept of the specialty into a reality. Who were some of these prophetic individuals and how did they lay the foundation for such a timely and influential organization?

Simon Hullihen (1810-1857) is considered the first recognized oral surgeon. He designed many instruments and performed a number of operations involving the correction of cleft lips and palates, jaw deformities, and the repair of fractured jaws.

James Garretson (1825-1895) is generally thought of as the father of oral surgery because he named the specialty by writing a book titled *Diseases and Surgery of Mouth, Jaws and Associated Parts,* which later was published as *A System of Oral Surgery.*

Robert Ivey (1881-1974) was instrumental in the development of the multidisciplinary team to treat cleft palates.

Varaztad Kazanjian (1879-1974), who had a dental degree and a prosthetic laboratory background, designed many ingenious devices to aid in the treatment of maxillofacial injuries, especially those sustained during World War I. Later, with an additional medical degree, he made important contributions in the formation of the specialty of plastic surgery.

Truman W. Brophy (1848-1928) was instrumental in determining the educational path for the profession of dentistry. With these rudimentary concepts, the teaching of advanced basic sciences for the study of oral surgery was initiated.

Mathew Cryer (1840-1921), an inventor of many oral surgery instruments, established the first hospital dental service in America at the Philadelphia General Hospital in 1901.

Many other pioneers followed or were contemporaries of the aforementioned individuals. However, there are two other individuals who were noteworthy because of their exceptionally prodigious contributions to the literature—Theodor Blum (1883-1962) and Kurt Thoma (1883-1972).

Blum was very involved with many aspects of oral surgery (107 published articles), but he is most noted for his deep involvement with the New York Institute of Oral Pathology and his discovery that some watchmakers were using their tongues to paint the dials of watches with radium for dial illumination. This exposure to radiation later caused them to develop cancer.

Kurt Thoma, with all due respect to other persons of historical note who helped create the specialty in this era, could probably give new meaning to the words *quintessential* and *Renaissance man* in terms of his immense contributions to the specialty. He was the author of about 300 articles and 8 textbooks. His books encompassed a panoramic range of subjects, including the following titles: *Oral Anesthesia* (1914); *Oral Abscesses* (1916); *Oral Roentgenology* (1917); *Teeth, Diet and Health* (1923); *Clinical Pathology of the Jaws* (1925); *Oral Diagnosis* (1936); *Oral Pathology* (1941); and *Oral Surgery* (1948). The enormity of his involvement with the specialty is illustrated by the broad range of his accomplishments, starting with periodic revisions of his texts. *Oral Surgery,* for example, is a two-volume set, and in 1970, the book was in its fifth edition. In addition to the large number of articles he authored, he edited the oral surgery section of the monthly publication, *Oral Surgery Oral Medicine Oral Pathology.* He attended to his professorial duties at the Massachusetts General Hospital (MGH), Harvard School of Dental Medicine, and later Boston University Graduate School of Dentistry. He still casts a shadow on the field through his students and other colleagues. The author of this paper had the privilege of being one of his students during the years 1966 and 1967.

As a corollary to the process of establishing and defining the specialty, the use of chemical agents to eliminate the pain of surgical procedures was slowly evolving from theory to practice. Four individuals were instrumental in making this happen.

Horace Wells (1815-1848) was a dentist who practiced in Hartford, Connecticut. He practiced, lectured, and demonstrated the use of nitrous oxide during the extraction of teeth. Although he attempted the removal of a tooth under nitrous oxide in the MGH famed domed surgical suite, the procedure failed when the patient muttered during the extraction. Nevertheless, Wells has been credited by the American Dental Association and American Medical Association as the person most closely associated with the discovery of anesthesia.

William Morton (1819-1868), a dentist who later attained a medical degree (although there is a question as to whether he ever obtained dental or medical degrees), worked with Horace Wells in his Hartford office and later in his own in Boston, Massachusetts.

Charles T. Jackson (1805-1880) was a chemist and physician in the Boston area who taught at Harvard. He mentored Wells in the use of ether compounds.

Crawford W. Long (1815-1878) was a physician in Georgia who used ether on a number of his patients while operating.

Morton quickly became frustrated with the use of nitrous oxide because he was unable to achieve the results he hoped for. With the help of Jackson, he started to work with ether compounds, and together they developed the use of sulfuric ether. Later, in front of a medical student group at the MGH in the same room where Wells tried to extract a tooth with the aid of nitrous oxide, Morton gave a patient ether anesthesia while Dr. John C. Warren, a senior surgeon at MGH, painlessly removed a vascular tumor from a patient's neck. After the procedure and with reference to the consistently suitable level of general anesthesia, Dr. Warren uttered his now famous medical phrase, "Gentlemen, this is no humbug." The domed room thereafter became known as the "ether dome." A little over 100 years later in the same city, an anesthesia course was given by Adrian Hubble and Harold Krogh, both oral surgeons, regarding the merits of intravenous barbiturate anesthesia. When the course was over, the chair of the anesthesia department at Tufts University went up to the board and wrote the phrase, "Gentleman, this is no humbug." Today other compounds are used, such as propofol (Diprivan), midazolam (Versed), and ketamine (Ketalar).

Independently, other national and world events gave the nascent specialty a greater scope. Newer methods to treat soft and hard tissue injuries to the face were developed during the American Civil War. Up to that time, maxillofacial wounds, to include the soft and hard tissues, were treated with craniofacial bandages for stabilization. However, Confederate dentists J. B. Bean and C. N. Covey, based upon their knowledge of the occlusion, devised intraoral splints that were successfully used to stabilize maxillomandibular fractured segments. Also, Thomas B. Gunning, a New York City dentist, developed splints that stabilized fractures of the maxillofacial complex. Some of the splints had openings to allow food consumption during the stabilization period. William Seward, Secretary of State in the Lincoln cabinet, fractured his jaw when he fell from his carriage. He was successfully treated by Gunning using one of his splints, after much reluctance on the part of Seward's medical staff, which caused a 1-month delay.

The specialty was maturing with a firm base in anesthesia, trauma, and exodontia. In 1937, for the first time the formation of a certifying board was suggested during the Presidential address at the oral surgery annual meeting. After several years of in-house discussions and committee deliberations, along with strong impetus from major hospital staffs, a formal request was made to the Council on Dental Education of the American Dental Association (ADA) that the specialty be allowed to establish a certifying board. In 1946, with the unanimous approval of the ADA House of Delegates, the Council on Dental Education allowed the formation of a certifying board (ABOS) to proceed with an exam for diplomatic status. Once this action occurred, oral surgery became the first recognized boarded dental specialty. The development of a board, together with the desire for solidification and greater equality of the educational requirements for residency programs, led to changes in 3-year programs that had a separate didactic year. These programs fully integrated the didactic year within the 3-year program, This resulted in greater equality in residency program evaluations. These programs had to meet the suggested standards of the ADA for oral surgery training programs. The standards commission is not just an ADA entity. It is also recognized by the U.S. Department of Education and the Council on Post Secondary Accreditation. The list of standards is the key instrument dictating that the oral surgery resident receive the minimum amount of specialty training needed for proficiency. It speaks for the ADA and requires that all training programs adhere to their suggested requirements for the performance of certain procedures and the amount of time that should be spent with other specialties in the hospital or other settings. If the standards are not met, the program may lose its ADA accreditation.

Another very important aspect that the specialty needed was to secure its proper position in the hospital milieu. However, starting in the 1950s and continuing for approximately the next 30 years, the Joint Commission on Accreditation of Hospitals (JCAH) made it difficult for oral and maxillofacial surgeons to perform procedures that they were well trained for in a hospital setting. The Joint Commission, formerly the Joint Commission on Accreditation of Healthcare Organizations (JCAHO), is a powerful, private sector, U.S.–based, nonprofit organization. It is the accrediting body for most U.S. hospitals. Every fixed number of years, hospitals are inspected by the JCAHO to ensure that they are properly performing their hospital functions.

If The Joint Commission finds that the hospital is not meeting its standards, they have the power to revoke accreditation or reduce the rating of the hospital. This may cause grave economic difficulties for the hospital, because many insurance companies will not allow their policyholders to use the hospital. During the period when the JCAH interfered with the practice of oral surgeons, its corporate members were the American College of Surgeons, American College of Physicians, American Hospital Association, Canadian Medical Association, and American Medical Association.

For years, oral and maxillofacial surgeons had difficulties admitting and discharging their own patients, performing procedures that they were eminently qualified to perform, and attaining committee assignments. They were unable to operate in a hospital operating room without a physician being present and they experienced other irritating roadblocks. The corporate entities took turns denying the ADA membership, "without prejudice." Thousands of letters were sent to the commissioners by oral surgeons asking for membership and the correction of the wrongs inflicted by the organization. At that time, one of the members of the American Association of Oral and Maxillofacial Surgeons (AAOMS) board, Jack Gamble from Louisiana, even drove in a blinding rainstorm for several hours in an effort to convince one of the commissioners to vote for ADA membership. It was not until 1982 that the ADA was offered a corporate seat on the JCAH, after a great many meetings, threatened lawsuits, revision in language that was demeaning to oral surgeons, and just plain wearing down old, misleading, and misunderstood aspects of the specialty. The first ADA commissioner was Charles McCallum, an oral and maxillofacial surgeon from Alabama. With his skills in interpersonal relationships, it was not long before Dr. McCallum became the chairman of the board. He was followed a few years later by another oral and maxillofacial surgeon, Dr. John Helfrick of Texas. Even still, with all the gains that have been made, the Organization only recently cleared up the matter of privileges for oral and maxillofacial surgeons to admit and discharge patients without co-admission with a physician.

It was also during this period that the basic science education of predoctoral candidates in dental schools was strengthened. This occurred in part because of greater outside funding for dental schools, and also because of a renewed interest in research and the greater intellectual sophistication of incoming students.

Other areas that profoundly affected the development of the specialty involved technical innovations. The invention of ultrahigh-speed gas and electric drills and saws by Robert Hall replaced the belt-driven drills. This allowed the surgeon to alter tissues such as teeth and bone more precisely with fingertip pressure. Later, laser energy along with fine-tip, electrically heated points and other configurations greatly assisted the surgeon when modifying and removing soft tissues. The metallurgical development of space-age materials, such as titanium and stronger, harder alloys, gave rise to the use of plates and screws as fixation devices. The newer materials began to replace wire because of their greater strength and the ability to position bony parts with greater ease, accuracy, and stability. Also, the body did not recognize titanium as foreign. For example, if one were performing a procedure to treat vertical maxillary hypoplasia with an interpositional graft to fill the gap, the surgeon could obviate the use of infraorbital suspension wires and multiple additional fixation wires with the use of plates and screws that had greater stability.

In addition, the use of plates and screws made out of lactic acid derivatives that are phagocytized over a longer period than it takes for the bony segments has also gained favor.

Other devices or therapeutic modalities that have improved surgical outcomes are the judicious use of antibiotics, steroids to reduce edema, three-dimensional imaging with and without the production of the anatomic area of interest in the form of a model, hypotensive general anesthesia, advanced bone grafting materials, and blood products to greatly improve graft acceptance. Microneurologic advances and the widespread use of implants to replace teeth and to augment or replace other maxillofacial anatomic entities have also enhanced success rates.

The work of Per-Ingvar Branemark, a Swedish research-oriented orthopedic surgeon, had a profound effect on the specialty and on dentistry as a profession. During the early 1950s, he was working with chemically pure titanium implant chambers to study the blood flow in rabbit bone. When the experiment was completed and it came time to remove the chambers from the bone, he discovered that the bone and titanium had become fully integrated and it was impossible to remove the chamber. He called the discovery "osseointegration," referring to the biological fusion of bone to a foreign substance. Histological analysis revealed that osteoblasts had grown on and into the roughened surface of the titanium implants over time. When this was revealed to his dental colleagues, root form implants were developed. The long-term success was astonishing. The placement of titanium root form implants and other prosthetic devices has greatly affected the specialty and has brought oral and maxillofacial surgery ever closer to the medical profession.

Along with the discovery of osseointegration, newer concepts of bone physiology began to emerge. Many of these newer theories had widespread acceptance that was attributed to Dr. Robert Marx, a Florida oral and maxillofacial surgeon. When root form implants were first used, if there was not enough bone to place the implant exactly where it was needed, the surgeon would make the excuse that he placed the implant in the best possible location considering the paucity of bone available. Dr. Marx helped eliminate the need for this explanation through his basic research in tissue engineering. He was also in the forefront regarding the use of autogenous growth factors for enhanced wound healing, platelet-rich plasma for increasing the success rate of grafts, recombinant bone morphogenetic protein, sinus grafts, intricate major reconstructive procedures, and hyperbaric oxygen therapy. He has also focused on understanding graft physiology, maxillofacial pathology, and lately, bisphosphonate-induced osteonecrosis. In essence, for all the medical and dental disciplines that use this osseous tissue, he has greatly advanced the understanding of bone pathophysiology as well as newer and far-reaching effects for wider applications.

Because of a dearth of orthodontic therapy in the United States during World War II, when surgeons in Europe performed corrective jaw surgery, the resulting occlusions were often not as good as they could have been if orthodontics had been involved. Therefore, in some instances, attempts to refine the occlusion involved two jaw surgeries. The resultant outcomes were better because the surgery treated the maxillofacial defects at their origin. The results improved both the occlusion and facial physiognomy. During the postwar years, the techniques and concepts were refined. Some of the Europeans involved in developing the treatments of these defects were Heinrich Kole, M. Wassmund, Richard Trauner, and Hugo Obwegesser. In 1966, Obwegeser was invited to present his advanced surgical developments in the field of intraoral orthognathics at Walter Reed Army Medical Center by General Robert Shira. His presentation concerning innovative surgeries involving the maxillae and the mandible, along with combinations of techniques, were mind-boggling to the American oral surgeons that were present. He stimulated a tremendous interest in an area of the specialty that at the time involved only one jaw surgery, the mandible. In 1972, Bell and Levy explained through their angiographic studies the blood supply that sustained the osteotomized sections of maxillary surgeries. Their findings revealed why multiple osteotomized sections can survive. After the visit to Walter Reed, and even to this day, orthognathic surgery has become an integral part of OMS residency training.

It was also during this time in the 1970s, with great impetus from AAOMS past presidents Terry Slaughter, Charles McCallum, and Robert Walker, that the name of the specialty changed officially to the American Association of Oral and Maxillofacial Surgeons, and full fellowship required board certification.

Additionally, there is an intellectual stimulant, the *Journal of Maxillofacial Surgery,* that continues to chronicle the magnitude of surgical advancements and presents newer concepts and procedures for the specialty to absorb and improve upon. The journal is a very strong and unifying factor that keeps the membership on the cutting edge.

However, this magnificent publication had trouble getting started. It was first published as a quarterly in 1943. In 1958 it became a bimonthly, and finally in the late 1960s the journal started publishing monthly. During those early years, the editors included such period giants of the specialty as Fred Henny and James Haywood. In 1972, the journal came under the guidance of Dan Laskin, who became the editor-in-chief and held the position for 30 years. His monthly editorials have become legend. Simultaneously, he became the editor of the AAOMS Forum and still maintains that position. One can still feel his presence at the AAOMS Board of Trustees meetings, sitting at the opposite end of the table from the president, correcting manuscripts that were sent to him in the hope of publication in the journal. While editing these papers (which, at times looked like football diagrams in an effort to present the best possible paper for publication), he would simultaneously listen to board discussions, and when asked, he would give an opinion or put some historical situation into perspective. In addition to these aspects of serving the specialty, he is a full-time academician, first at the University of Illinois for over 32 years, and then at the Medical College of Virginia, where he was Professor and Chairman of the Department of Oral and Maxillofacial Surgery for 18 years. He continues to sit on the editorial boards of many noted national and international journals. Even now his energy is boundless, as revealed by his more than 1000 contributions to the literature. He is also author or co-author of 16 books. Dr. Laskin's presence is one of the primary reasons that the specialty has achieved its renowned position in the two worlds of dentistry and medicine. He is a true icon of the specialty.

Another very important step was the establishment of the Oral and Maxillofacial Foundation. The very essence of this sister organization can be found in their mission, which states that they are "dedicated to advancing the long-term development, health and well-being of the oral and maxillofacial surgery specialty and the public it serves through financial support of research and education." Their primary goal is to support the specialty and its cornerstones of education and research. The foundation accomplishes this through funding projects that are the focus of oral surgeons, residents in the specialty, students, and innovative practitioners. Topics include cancer, temporomandibular joint disorders, dental implant technology, and basic biology.

In addition, the foundation funds fellowships that allow young surgeons to develop specialized surgical skills and to broaden their knowledge and judgment in areas of practice. Since the inception of the foundation, 159 grants, research awards, fellowships, and other awards have amounted to over $7 million. The foundation has given out an average of $438,000 per year for new projects and approximately $200,000 per year for ongoing projects.

The Foundation Alliance, composed of spouses, significant others, and friends of oral and maxillofacial surgeons, contributes greatly to the annual meetings and other fund-raising events.

Just a few years ago the president-elect of the AAOMS, Phillip Maloney, a full-time educator with an ancillary hometown private practice, felt that his perceived importance of the foundation could greatly benefit OMS by enlisting a strong campaign of the membership of the AAOMS, captains of industry, and any other interested parties to raise the corpus of foundation monies from approximately $1 million to at least $3 million. It was because of his initiative and foresight that today this amount is in the $9 million range.

During the 1980s, "sky blue sessions" at many AAOMS board meetings raised the questions of who we were and where we were headed relative to our surgical latitudes as well-trained surgeons. Also discussed were such topics as our potential capabilities relative to the current broad scope of practice along with future needs for additional professional degrees. Therefore in 1986, a conference was called by the vice president of the board, to which 50 of the most prominent and influential AAOMS members were invited to discuss advanced and additional degrees and potential increases in the scope of practice. To create a level playing field, some of the individuals who were invited were known to have antagonistic views, either for or against additional degrees.

As a background, it was very common for the oral and maxillofacial surgeon to be called into emergency rooms throughout the country, usually late at night, to address and treat facial fractures and attendant soft tissue lacerations. These might include fractures of the maxilla and mandible, along with orbital, frontal, and nasal fractures. The treatment of these injuries together with the advancement of orthognathic surgery, which routinely surgically altered maxillas, mandibles, and chins and in some cases, augmented midface and other facial deficiencies with alloplastic materials, made the oral and maxillofacial surgeon think about performing similar elective procedures. Why couldn't the well-trained OMS treat, de novo, nasal and eyelid deformities, rhytids of the skin in the form of full face and regional facial areas? At this point, some programs that offered medical degrees in addition to training in oral and maxillofacial surgery were having trouble keeping their M.D. residents in the specialty for the long term. At times, one could find the two-degreed person entering a residency in internal medicine, neurosurgery, plastic surgery, and the like after finishing the OMS residency. The question was how to keep residents in the specialty after they received an M.D. This was addressed at the conference, in part, by altering the sequential timing of the additional degree while finishing the OMS training. A Ph.D. program for those interested in research was also addressed. There were many emotions released at the conference, but in the end, a pathway was found to potentially address the degree issues and alter the scope of the specialty. After the conference, the practice of oral and maxillofacial surgery was permanently altered.

Many double degree programs arose with a true interest in facial cosmetic surgery. The 1988 midwinter meeting, held in Tucson, Arizona, was devoted solely to facial cosmetic surgery. Because of imagined transportation and logistical problems in getting to Tucson, there were real concerns about the potential attendance at the meeting. Also, would the subject matter draw an OMS audience? As it turned out, it was one of the largest turnouts the association ever had for a midwinter event. Afterward, courses and fellowships developed in a number of institutions. To legitimize overall aspects, the AAOMS met with the American Board of Oral and Maxillofacial Surgeons (ABOMS) and the ADA to change the definition of the specialty to recognize the broadened scope. In addition, the ABOMS began to query candidates on their oral and written exams regarding cosmetic topics. The ADA, for its part, incorporated into their standards a requirement that all OMS residents be trained in cosmetic facial surgery procedures.

Despite a dichotomy in training (i.e., medical degree), the scope of practice for U.S. oral and maxillofacial surgeons has been and continues to be essentially the same, regardless of degree. This is changing in some instances, however, because of dedicated fellowship training in head and neck oncologic surgery, microvascular reconstructive surgery, pediatric craniofacial surgery, and cosmetic surgery. One primary reason for this is that faculty at many U.S. training programs have previously lacked experience and training in so-called expanded scope areas, such as head and neck oncology, microvascular surgery, cosmetic surgery, and pediatric cleft and craniofacial surgery. In years past, if an OMS graduate wished to obtain training in any of these areas, then he or she was forced to seek it outside of the specialty, in either otolaryngology or plastic surgery. Recently, however, the development of a number of formally recognized advanced training fellowships has significantly increased the opportunities available to those graduates of U.S. oral and maxillofacial surgery programs who wish to expand their scope of practice. Standing on the shoulders of OMSs trained in the United States in otolaryngology (Eric Dierks and Bryce Potter), plastic surgery (Jeff Posnick), and in Europe (Robert Ord and Joseph Helman), dozens of OMSs trained in North America are now providing comprehensive head and neck, microvascular, and pediatric craniofacial surgery at various training institutions around the country. Just as the development of and training in orthognathic surgery contributed to the evolution of the U.S. specialty from oral surgery to oral and maxillofacial surgery in the late 1960s and 1970s, current fellowship training in head and neck surgery is transforming the specialty today.

When asked to write this chapter on the history and the need for oral and maxillofacial surgery as a specialty, it would seem even to the most casual observer that over these past few years, oral and maxillofacial surgery has achieved its rightful and respected place in the treatment of the entire maxillofacial region. In the history of humankind, no specialty has ever been able to routinely take the entire bony facial skeleton, rearrange and alter it as necessary, and also manipulate the soft tissue facial drape to reduce rhytids, correct redundant facial and periorbital skin defects of the nose and ears, and augment soft tissue defects.

In conclusion, oral and maxillofacial surgery is one of the rarest of all dental or medical specialties. In most instances, the trained OMS takes, reads, and interprets the patient's x-rays; administers local and/or general anesthesia (the safety record of which, for similar surgical procedures, is extraordinary); performs many surgeries in the office, which saves the patient time and money; attracts the best and brightest from the prespecialty pool; receives superior training in maxillofacial trauma (in part because of the amount of time spent studying the occlusion, on which many traumatic reparative procedures are based); treats facial cosmetic defects, treats a variety of head and neck diseases, including oral cancer and reconstruction. ridge preservation and augmentation.

As the contents of this text demonstrate, the unequivocal conclusion is that the future for the specialty is quite exciting, and its practitioners' skills are widely admired by the general public.

BIBLIOGRAPHY

Belinfante LS: Oral and maxillofacial surgery: a new wrinkle, *J Esthet Dent* 9(5):238-245, 1997.

Belinfante LS: Spotlight: oral and maxillofacial surgery, Georgia Dental Association Action September, 1997.

Guralnick WC: A tribute to Kurt H. Thoma, *Oral Surg Oral Med Oral Pathol* 38(4):495-500, 1974.

Guralnick WC: From exodontia to oral and maxillofacial surgery: the evolution of a specialty, *J Mass Dent Soc* 38(3):117-118, 150-151, 1989.

Nelson CL: Oral and maxillofacial surgery develops as a specialty, *J Indiana Dent Assoc* 87(1):73, 2008.

Roberts SL: Oral and maxillofacial surgery. A specialty altered by time and circumstance, *N Y State Dent J* 63(9):46-50, 1997.

Shira RB: Editorial: Dr. Kurt Hermann Thoma, *Oral Surg Oral Med Oral Pathol* 34(3): 373, 1972.

The building of a specialty: oral and maxillofacial surgery in the United States 1918-1998, *J Maxfac Surg* 56(7)(Suppl):3, 1998.

Thoma KH: History of oral surgery: the oldest specialty in dentistry, *Oral Surg Oral Med Oral Pathol* Jan;10(1):1-10, 1957.

Chapter 2

Wound Healing: Repair Biology and Wound and Scar Treatment

Anh D. Le, Jimmy James Brown

BIOLOGY OF WOUND REPAIR

Wound healing is a complex cascade of highly integrated cellular and molecular events that drive the process of tissue restoration, which consists of several distinct but overlapping phases. These stages include hemostasis and inflammation, proliferation, and remodeling (Fig. 2-1).[1,2] Impaired healing in acute and chronic wounds generally occurs when there is a failure to progress through the normal stages of wound repair. Although rates and patterns of healing depend on the local, systemic, and surgical factors of the host, the phases of oral mucosal healing closely approximate those of cutaneous healing.[3] In general, wounds in the oral cavity appear to heal faster than dermal wounds, and they have minimal or no scar formation.

HEMOSTASIS AND INFLAMMATORY PHASE

Severe tissue injury disrupts blood vessels and causes extravasations of blood constituents. Blood coagulation and platelet aggregation generate a fibrin clot within the vessel lumen and provide a provisional matrix for cell migration. Several pro-coagulant factors including fibrinogen, fibronectin, and thrombospondin are secreted by the injured cells and initiate the coagulation cascade. The clot and surrounding wound tissues release pro-inflammatory cytokines and growth factors, including platelet-derived growth factor (PDGF), vascular endothelial growth factor (VEGF), fibroblast growth factor (FGF), epidermal growth factor (EGF), and transforming growth factor-β (TGF-β). Once bleeding is controlled, inflammatory cells migrate into the wound (chemotaxis) and begin to remove apoptotic cells and bacteria from the injured area. Clinical signs include localized edema (swelling), pain (dolor), redness (rubor), and increased warmth (calor) at the wound site. Neutrophils are the predominant inflammatory cells during the early inflammatory phase, but they are rapidly outnumbered by macrophages, derived from mobilized monocytes, and T lymphocytes during the transition to the proliferative phase.

PROLIFERATION PHASE

The proliferation phase is characterized by epithelial proliferation and migration over the provisional matrix. In the reparative dermal tissue, fibroblasts and endothelial cells proliferate and contribute to capillary growth, collagen synthesis, and granulation tissue formation. Fibroblasts are the major cells responsible for the production of collagen, glycoaminoglycans, and proteoglycans, which are major components of the extracellular matrix. Concurrent with these events is the process of angiogenesis, whereby new blood vessels are formed and lymphatics are recanalized in the healing tissues. This essential process reestablishes proper transport of nutrients and oxygen to the local injured sites. Epithelial cells originating from the bulge of hair follicles, sebaceous glands, and the basal layer of the epidermal margins of the wound edges proliferate and resurface the wound. In contrast to skin, the process of reepithelialization progresses more rapidly in an oral mucosal wound. The oral epithelial cells migrate directly onto the moist, exposed surface of the fibrin clot instead of under the dry exudate (scab) of a dermal wound.[2]

MATURATION AND REMODELING PHASE

The remodeling phase is the final stage of tissue repair and is distinguished by a continual turnover of collagen fibers. The tensile strength of the wound is gradually restored as the collagen fibers are realigned and increasingly cross-linked in a well-organized pattern. The maximal tensile strength of a healed wound is reached in 6 to 12 months post-injury, depending on host factors, but it never reaches the initial strength of unwounded tissue. Eventually, active collagen synthesis achieves equilibrium with collagenolysis. The homeostasis can be delayed by disruptive processes such as poor oxygen perfusion,[3] lack of nutrients, and wound infection, which favor collagen breakdown and wound dehiscence.

PRINCIPLES OF WOUND CARE

From a surgical viewpoint the nature of the healing process is determined by several factors, including the nature of the injury, the anatomic site, the type of tissue, the timing of the repair, and orientation of the wound margins. Early primary closure with adequate apposition of the wound margins usually results in healing by primary or first intention, with minimal scar formation. In the presence of wound infection, severe tissue loss, or poor apposition of the wound margins, the healing process is prolonged, with excess granulation and connective tissue formation, also known as healing by second intention. In infected wounds with purulent drainage or in contaminated traumatic wounds, the surgeon may attempt healing by third intention, whereby the wounds are allowed to initially granulate and heal by second intention, followed by delayed primary closure.

WOUND CLOSURE

Wound closure is particularly important in the head and neck region, where the treatment goals are a mechanically sound wound closure and a cosmetically acceptable scar. Most simple wounds, generated by surgical incisions or clean lacerations, heal rapidly by primary intention. Complex wounds, such as burns, avulsions, and infected or contaminated injuries, usually heal more slowly by secondary intention, and may require skin grafts or flaps. Current wound management focuses on eliminating causative factors, providing systemic support to enhance tissue repair, and maintaining a physiologic local wound environment amenable to optimal healing. All wounds should be as clean as possible, and debrided of non-viable tissues or foreign bodies. Ragged wound margins must be revised and undermined to achieve a tension-free closure as appropriate. Depending on the nature of the wound, sutures, suction drains, or pressure dressings may be applied.

Proper suture technique should incorporate three major principles including proper distribution of tension to the deeper layers,

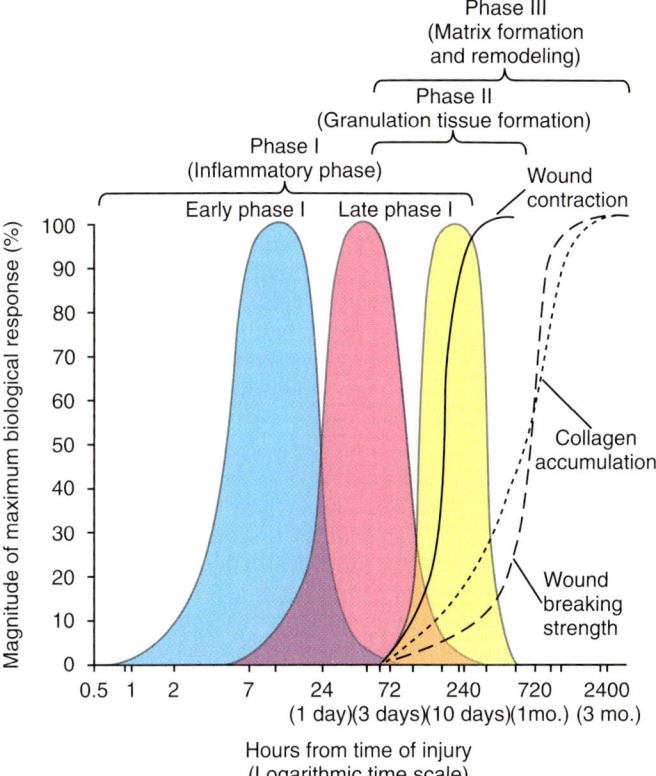

Fig. 2-1 ■ The three overlapping phases of wound healing. (Redrawn from Kloth LC, McCulloch JM: *Wound healing: alternatives in management*, ed 3, Philadelphia, 2002, FA Davis Company, p 4.)

FULL THICKNESS WOUNDS

Full thickness injuries imply a complete loss of the epithelial layer and its appendages leading to the exposure of the subcutaneous (submucosal) tissues. Full thickness wounds can be caused by tumor excision, trauma, burns, infection, radiation, or vascular compromise. These wounds will heal gradually by granulation and epithelialization. The healing process is slow and can be uncomfortable, with high risk of infection until the protective epithelium is fully restored. Healing of the full thickness wounds can be enhanced by grafting the wound bed with an epithelial layer. If the wound bed is clean and well vascularized, a full or partial thickness skin graft can be placed. Depending on the location, a vascularized flap may also be a better choice. Frequent dressing changes and topical antibacterial agents are useful in reducing the risk of infection.

USE OF SKIN SUBSTITUTES

Immediate wound coverage is critical for the acceleration of wound healing and prevention of infection. When the surface area is relatively large, the wound can be covered by synthetic and natural dressings aside from the native skin grafts. The commercially available human skin substitutes are grouped into three major types and serve as excellent alternatives to autografts. The first type consists of grafts of cultured epidermal cells with no dermal components (Epicel, Genzyme Biosurgery, Cambridge, Mass.). The second type has only dermal components (AlloDerm, LifeCell Corp., Woodlands, Texas; Dermagraft, Advanced Biohealing, Inc., La Jolla, Calif.). The third type consists of a bilayer of both dermal and epidermal elements (Apligraf, Organogenesis Inc., Canton, Mass.; Integra; Johnson & Johnson Medical LifeSciences Corp., Plainsboro, NJ). The chief effect of most skin substitutes is to promote wound healing by stimulating the recipient host to produce a variety of wound-healing cytokines and chemokines. The use of cultured skin to cover wounds is particularly attractive, inasmuch as the living cells already can produce the necessary level of growth factors at the appropriate time.

atraumatic handling of tissues, and eversion of wound margins. Where appropriate, closure of the cutaneous wound should be layered. Deep sutures are usually placed in strong, fibrous tissue, such as fascia or dermis, rather than muscle or fat. Wound tensile strength depends on suture integrity in the first few weeks until strong collagen fiber is formed. Hence polyglycolic acid (PGA) sutures are suitable for this purpose. Non-resorbable sutures may be indicated to close wounds under tension. Closure of the dermal (subcutaneous) layer is fundamental for esthetic wound closure. Dermal sutures should be inverted to avoid extrusion of the knots. If the deeper portion of the suture is wider than the portion that crosses the surface, there will be some eversion of the wound margins. Mucosa can be closed with either permanent or resorbable sutures. Skin can be closed with permanent sutures or staples. Depending on the individual wound, simple sutures, horizontal or vertical mattress sutures, half-buried mattress sutures, or running sutures can be used.

PARTIAL THICKNESS WOUNDS

Partial thickness injuries are caused by abrasions or the harvest of skin or mucosal grafts. Such injuries heal primarily by reepithelialization. In the moist environment of the mucosa, similar wounds form a fibrinous pseudomembrane. Dressings may aid in wound epithelialization; increase patient comfort and compliance; and decrease the risk of infection and overall healing time. Gauze dressings impregnated with various antibacterial compounds and occlusive dressing films are often used for this purpose. Wet-to-dry dressings are effective in debriding partial thickness wounds that have become infected. Systemic antibiotics do not work well in this situation and should be used only if there is cellulitis in the surrounding tissues.

PRINCIPLES OF SCAR TREATMENT

Revision of excessive scars resulting from aberrant wound healing is among the most challenging endeavors for the surgeon, particularly in the head and neck region where cosmesis is paramount. There is no single treatment option that stands alone as the best practice model. As a result, a combination of approaches is the best remedy for this challenging problem.[4,5]

SCAR ANALYSIS AND TIMING OF SCAR REVISION

In scar revision, the opportune time for the best outcomes may be lost at the initial wound repair if the assessment and surgical technique are shoddily performed. Therefore attention to the details of primary repair is the key to minimizing unsightly scar formation. Initial management requires a full analysis of location, color, height, thickness, and direction of the scar. In general, the more conspicuous the scar, the greater the challenge the surgeon faces to improve its esthetics. This weighs heavily on the analysis and planning at the beginning of wound management.

The morphology of scars varies among a wide variation of colors, sizes, and shapes. They may be raised, flattened, wide, or narrow, with straight or corrugated borders. Altered sensation such as pruritus, numbness, and even frank pain may accompany scar formation. The location of the scar should be carefully documented with an assessment of the adjoining structures or units of face or neck that may be influenced by its repair. Color matches should be considered

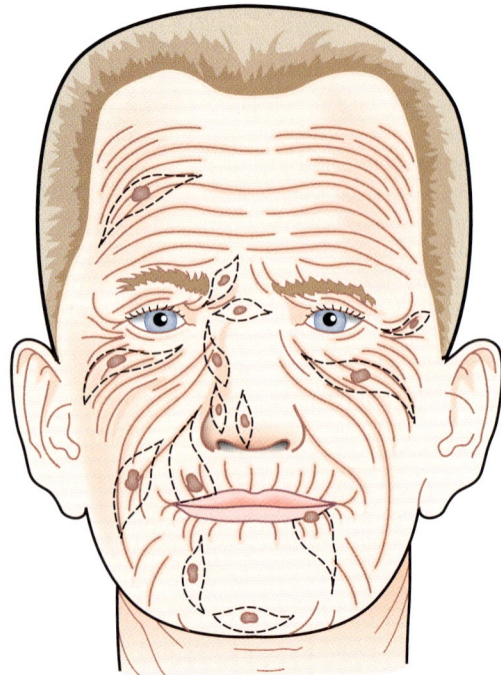

Fig. 2-2 ■ Relaxed skin tension lines with appropriate placement of resection. (Redrawn from Kraissl CJ: The selection of appropriate lines for elective surgical incisions, *Plast Reconstr Surg* 8:1-28, 1951.)

if nearby tissues will be used to facilitate repair. The full three-dimensional configuration of the scar should be documented in units of measure such as millimeters. Also important are the directional tendencies and vector forces influencing the scar, especially with respect to the relaxed skin tension lines of the face and neck[6] (Fig. 2-2).

The timing of scar revision is influenced by a variety of factors. These include the type and location of injury and psychological state of the patient, including his or her realistic expectations of the potential outcomes of revision surgery. Depending on the treatment techniques employed, the timing of revision may vary. In general, scar revision should not be performed until the scar is considered mature. This usually is in the range of 6 to 12 months, though some techniques such as dermabrasion may be performed earlier.

TREATMENT AND RECONSTRUCTIVE GOALS

The reconstructive goal in most situations would be to create a scar that more closely resembles the surrounding tissues, rather than to remove the scar, which may be unrealistic. Other specific reconstructive goals include creating a scar that (1) is flat and level with the surrounding skin, (2) has an appropriate color match, (3) is narrow, (4) is parallel to the favorable skin lines, and (5) avoids straight and unbroken lines. Attention to the details of wound management in its primary repair phase is critical for preventing excessive scarring. The surgeon should remain steadfast to current accepted treatment and reconstructive goals and their realistic expectations of the potential outcomes of revision surgery. An analysis of the scar's psychological impact on the patient and his or her expectation of the outcome of revision is also of utmost importance. Furthermore, the patient should be aware that several secondary procedures may be necessary to achieve optimal results.

SPECIFIC TREATMENT AND TECHNIQUES

A variety of scar modifying techniques may be selected based on the scar analysis, treatment timing, and reconstructive goals. These techniques can be subdivided into three broad categories: excisional,

irregularization, and epithelial abrasion techniques. Multiple techniques combined with appropriate staging usually offer the best outcomes. The patient must be informed that scars cannot be removed, but their unsightly nature can be modified to become more acceptable esthetically and functionally through adroit scar analysis and meticulous techniques.

Excisional Techniques

Fusiform Excision Excisional techniques rely on total removal of the offending scar with subsequent replacement of normal mobilized native skin. This approach conforms to the principle that the simplest procedure is generally the best. The scars to be revised usually fall within the relaxed skin tension lines in favorable areas of the face and neck and may simply be excised in a fusiform fashion. The wound is then closed with dermal approximation and equalization of its margins. Fusiform wounds generally close without redundancy when their opposed angles are 30 degrees or less. Those that have angles greater than 30 degrees should be designed to follow the curvature of a contour line or a relaxed skin tension line that is less noticeable to the casual observer (see Fig. 2-2).

Scar Repositioning In many situations the scar may be oriented contra to normal skin creases or relaxed skin tension lines. This usually creates a more noticeable scar. This scar can be repositioned to fall more favorably along a normal skin crease or behind hair-bearing areas to render it less apparent. An example of a repositioning maneuver is a scar on the exposed region of the cheek that may be shifted to realign in the form of a fusiform excision in the naso-labial fold.

Serial Partial Excision Serial excisions may be used when lack of elasticity of the scar and its surrounding tissues prohibits a one-stage excision and closure without distortion of the proximal anatomic landmarks. This is a staged technique with only partial removal of the scar in the first stage, followed by approximation of remaining scar to adjacent normal tissues. The closure is usually preceded by wide undermining of the wound margins, and the process can be repeated as many times as needed to achieve a more esthetically acceptable scar.

Irregularization Techniques

Z-plasty The Z-plasty is a form of scar irregularization where triangular flaps are transposed on both ends of a linear scar to increase the length and reorient the direction of the scar. It is usually performed on a tightly contracted scar.[7,8] Z-plasties are particularly useful in effacing and elongating webbed scars. Instead of one larger Z-plasty, several small Z-plasties can be performed to obscure and neutralize major forces of contracture that work against satisfactory scar camouflage (Fig. 2-3). The Z-plasty technique should be done with caution when scar lengthening is undesirable. Of note are the angles formed by the three members of the Z-plasty. In general, angles of 30 degrees will theoretically lengthen the scar by 25%, whereas angles of 45 and 60 degrees will lengthen the scar by 50% and 75%, respectively.

W-plasty The W-plasty or so-called zigzag plasty contains uniformly interposed triangular advancement flaps, which create an irregular scar for camouflage. It is particularly useful to reposition scar lines to match directions of relaxed skin tension lines of the face. In areas of facial curvatures such as the mandibular line and forehead, especially when vertical scars are present, the W-plasty technique will interrupt and camouflage the scar by breaking it up

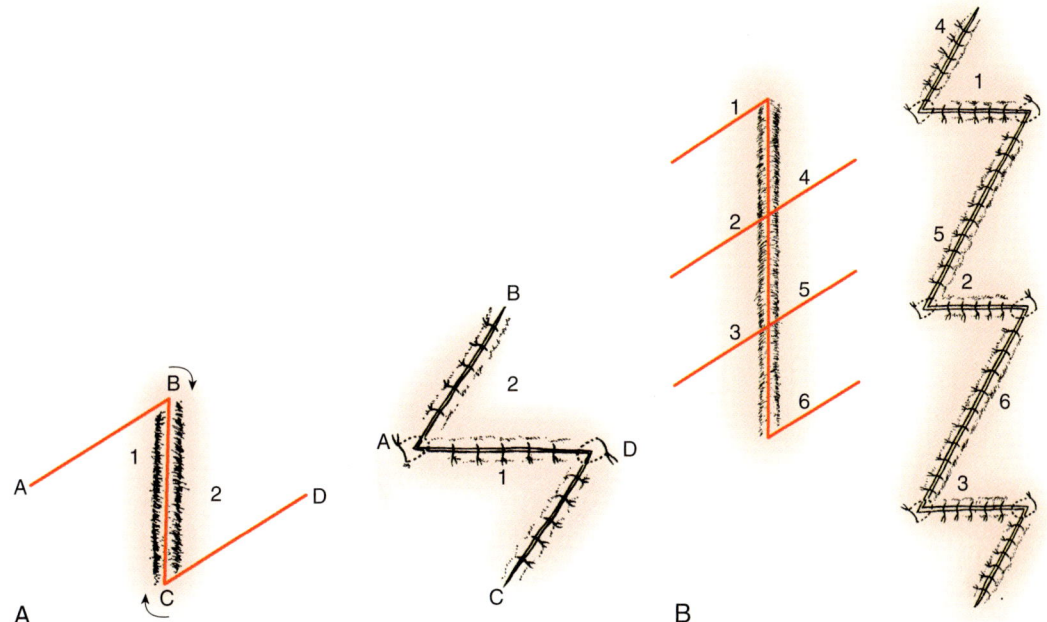

Fig. 2-3 ■ Z-plasty techniques. **A,** Simple Z-plasty. Scar is central limb; direction is changed when flaps are transposed. **B,** Multiple Z-plasties. Tissue length is increased with less distortion. (Adapted from Canale ST, Beaty JH, editors: *Campbell's operative orthopaedics,* ed 11, Philadelphia, 2008, Mosby.)

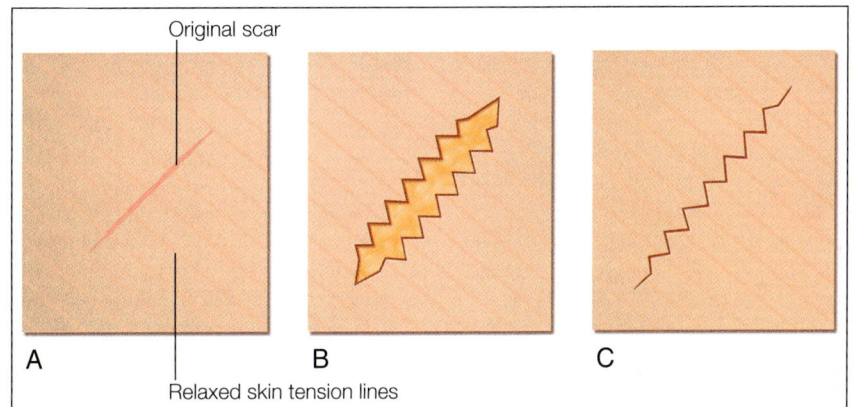

Fig. 2-4 ■ W-plasty shows interruption and irregularization of the scar. (From Arndt KA, editor: *Scar revision—Procedures in cosmetic dermatology,* Philadelphia, 2006, Saunders.)

into smaller components (Fig. 2-4). However, W-plasty usually does not lengthen a constricted scar as much as Z-plasty does, and it requires considerable excision of scar and healthy skin, which can lead to a relatively tight closure and a widened scar.

Geometric Broken-Line Closure Geometric broken-line closure (GBLC) is a scar excision technique that is based on the concept of scar irregularization for camouflage (Fig. 2-5). It is similar to the running W-plasty technique (see Fig. 2-4) except that it incorporates a more random pattern of small flaps of varying sizes and shapes, such as triangles, squares, and half circles. This decreases the predictability of the closure seen in the running W-plasty and thus improves scar camouflage. The W-plasty technique has its greatest shortcoming when it is used on a scar that is too long and thus predictably irregular. The scar will be somewhat more conspicuous. In this situation the GBLC technique will add more unpredictability to the scar line and thus improve camouflage (Fig. 2-6).

Resurfacing Techniques

Epithelial Abrasion Dermabrasion is a form of epithelial abrasion that is useful in the revision of unsightly scars. This technique abrades the superficial epithelial layers of the skin without extending through the dermis and is particularly suited to improve acne scars or pigmented scars. There are many techniques and devices used to improve scar esthetics and camouflage. Devices such as sandpaper disk and the more popular wire brush have been employed since the early 1940s.

Ablative Laser Several laser applications have been utilized to revise the unsightly scar. Among the lasers that have been used for the treatment of scars are carbon dioxide (CO_2), erbium : yttrium-aluminum-garnet (Er : YAG), neodymium : yttrium-aluminum-garnet (Nd : YAG),[9] fractional resurfacing, and pulsed dye laser (PDL).[10] Currently, PDL is considered the laser modality of choice for the revision of raised scars. For atrophic scars, such as those caused by

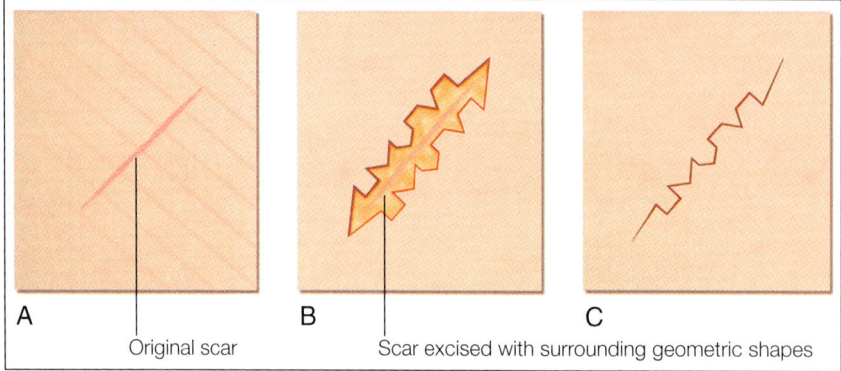

A   B   C
Original scar   Scar excised with surrounding geometric shapes

Fig. 2-5 ■ W-plasty shown with geometric broken-line technique (GBLC). (From Arndt KA, editor: *Scar revision—Procedures in cosmetic dermatology,* Philadelphia, 2006, Saunders.)

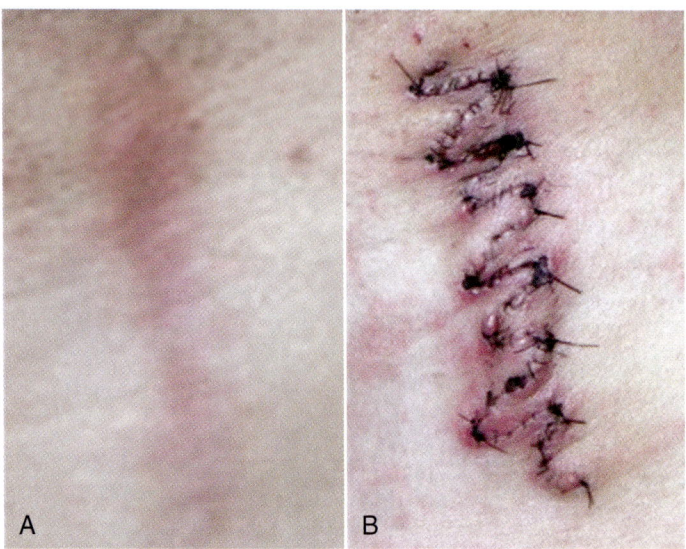

Fig. 2-6 ■ Revision of a neck scar using combination approaches of W-plasties and GBLC techniques. **A,** Preoperative image. **B,** Postoperative image.

acne, the CO_2 and Er:YAG applications appear to be most efficacious for esthetic improvement.

POSTOPERATIVE CARE

The postoperative care for revised scars may call for more stringent adherence to protocol by both physician and surgeon. For example, rest and limitation of function are absolute requirements, so that the postsurgical wound is not subjected to excessive forces or tensions.

After keloid revision, a pressure or elastic dressing may be applied over the area to reduce the chance of recurrence. For other types of scar revision, a lighter dressing may be applied. Sutures are usually removed after 3 to 4 days for facial procedures, and after 5 to 7 days for incisions at some tension-bearing area of the neck. It is usually recommended that the patient avoid activities that would stretch or place tension on the wound, as this may widen the new scar. Avoidance of sun exposure is critical in the first 3 to 6 months, and a sun blocking cream is always recommended when the patient must venture outside.

PEARLS AND PITFALLS

- Wound healing is a strictly regulated cascade of physiologic events that determine the outcome of the healing scars.
- Current wound management focuses on eliminating causative factors, providing systemic support to enhance tissue repair, and maintaining a local wound environment amenable for optimal healing.
- Scar revision and camouflage techniques vary with the type of scar, its location, and its orientation with respect to relaxed skin tension lines.
- A key point is that multiple techniques combined with appropriate staging usually offer the best outcomes.
- Patients must be aware that scars cannot be removed, but their unsightly nature can be modified to become more acceptable through meticulous technique and adroit scar analysis.
- The surgeon should remain steadfast to current accepted treatment and reconstructive goals and have realistic expectations of the potential outcomes of revision surgery.

REFERENCES

1. Singer A, Clark R: Cutaneous wound healing, *N Engl J Med* 341:738-746, 1999.
2. Guo S, DiPietro LA: Factors affecting wound healing, *J Dent Res* 89(3):219-229, 2010.
3. Gustafson GT: Ecology of wound healing in the oral cavity, *Scand J Haematol Suppl* 40:393-409, 1984.
4. Borges AF: Principles of scar camouflage, *Facial Plast Surg* Spring;1(3):181-190, 1984.
5. Thomas JR, Mobley SR: Scar revision and camouflage. In Cummins CW, Flint PW, Haughey BH, et al, editors: *Otolaryngology: head and neck surgery,* ed 4, Philadelphia, 2005, Mosby Elsevier.
6. Borges AF: Relaxed skin tension lines. In Borges AF: *Elective incisions and scar revisions,* Boston, 1973, Little Brown & Co.
7. Borges AF: Z-Plastic scar revision. In Borges AF: *Elective incisions and scar revisions,* Boston, 1973, Little Brown & Co.
8. Skouge JW: Subcutaneous island pedicle flap with Z-plasty: a cosmetic enhancement. *Dermatol Surg* Dec;33(12):1529-1532, 2007.
9. Martins A, Trindade F, Leite L: Facial scars after a road accident—combined treatment with pulsed dye laser and Q-switched Nd:YAG laser, *J Cosmet Dermatol* Sep;7(3):227-229, 2008.
10. Donelan MB, Parrett BM, Sheridan RL: Pulsed dye laser therapy and Z-plasty for facial burn scars: the alternative to excision, *Ann Plast Surg* May;60(5):480-486, 2008.

Flap Classification and Principles of Flap Design for Head and Neck Reconstruction

Andrew R. Salama

Given the myriad of reconstructive options available, it seems easy to theoretically reconstruct even the most complex ablative or traumatic defects, especially since the introduction of microvascular free flaps. The head and neck reconstructive surgeon is faced with the task of conceptualizing a defect, often before it even exists. The challenge arises in choosing the appropriate reconstructive modality for each patient, which begins with the identification of functional goals. Although facial harmony and esthetics are factors in reconstruction of the maxillofacial region, the maintenance of function closely correlates with quality of life outcomes. Considerations in flap design and flap choice are largely based on the characteristics of the anatomic defect. Multiple flap classification systems have been described, and such stratification can be used to direct clinician decision-making. Additionally, flap evolution has closely mirrored the progress of continuing flap reclassification in the literature. This chapter will focus on the classification of flaps and treatment planning with an emphasis on flap choice and free flap design in the reconstruction of oral cavity defects.

ETIOPATHOGENESIS AND CAUSATIVE FACTORS

Reconstruction of the oral cavity is complicated by its anatomic and functional complexity. As the site of entry to the aerodigestive tract, it contains several specialized tissues: the mandible, dentition, tongue, and soft palate. Furthermore it is microbially rich and continuously exposed to saliva.[1] Functional and esthetic reconstruction of major maxillofacial defects requires an in-depth comprehension of the intrinsic anatomy or anatomic subunits to be reconstructed. A guiding principle of reconstruction is to replace absent tissue with qualitatively and quantitatively similar tissue. Ablative defects from both benign and malignant disease are predictable for preoperative planning. Good communication between the ablative and reconstructive surgeons may prevent intraoperative changes to the treatment plan that would potentially affect the outcome. Factors including previous radiotherapy or surgery involving the neck and general medical condition should be incorporated into a reconstructive plan. Elective ablative surgery affords the surgeon ample time to conceptualize and plan a reconstruction, whereas traumatic defects are less predictable and often require temporization to ensure the wound bed is suitable for reconstruction. Historically, reconstruction was typically delayed to permit wound stabilization, facilitate reconstruction, and monitor for disease recurrence. This paradigm has been abandoned by most practitioners and immediate reconstruction is advocated when feasible.

PATHOLOGIC ANATOMY AND FLAP CLASSIFICATION

An ideal classification system aids in communication, treatment planning, and outcome assessment. By definition, a flap is a unit of tissue that is transferred from a donor site to a recipient site while maintaining its blood supply. There are several approaches to the classification of flaps, including donor site or destination, type or types of tissue to be transferred, and blood supply. There is no perfect classification system; however, multiple efforts have been made to standardize terminology in the literature. The evolution of flaps has been mirrored by scientific endeavors to reclassify them.

The most basic means of flap classification is by tissue type. Tolhurst[2] devised the "atomic" system of flap classification, in part based on tissue type. Flaps of any tissue type can be devised, provided there is an underlying reliable vascular supply to maintain physiologic homeostasis in the recipient bed. Single-source tissue flaps typically include skin, fascia, muscle, or bone. Composite tissue flaps include more than one type of tissue, such as osteocutaneous or fasciocutaneous.

Flaps may also be described in terms of their proximity to the recipient site (local, regional, distant). Local flaps involve transfer of tissue from the immediate adjacent anatomic subsite. They are descriptively stratified by the basic geometric movement required to facilitate wound closure: advancement, rotation, or transposition. A tongue flap is considered a local/random flap, whereas a facial artery myomucosal flap is considered a local/axial pattern flap. The majority of local flaps for head and neck reconstruction are used for cutaneous defects (Fig. 3-1).

Regional flaps involve the transposition of tissue from a neighboring anatomic site. They too can be further described by their blood supply; however, the majority have an axial pattern of vascularization. Regional cutaneous flaps including the bipedicled forehead flap with a random pattern of blood supply are not commonly used. Distinction should be drawn between the bipedicled forehead flap and the paramedian forehead. The latter differs from a bipedicle forehead flap in that a vascular pedicle is included in the flap design. The deltopectoral flap, a prototypical regional/cutaneous flap, has an axial pattern blood supply from the second, third, and fourth perforators of the internal mammary artery. The distal one third of the flap, however, has a random pattern. The majority of regional flaps used in contemporary reconstruction of head and neck defects are myocutaneous or muscle-only flaps. The pectoralis major myocutaneous flap (PMMC), introduced by Ariyan in 1979, was quickly adopted as the first-choice reconstructive option, and is still considered a versatile and robust choice.[3] The main advantages of the PMMC are that the surgery is easy, a large amount of soft tissue can

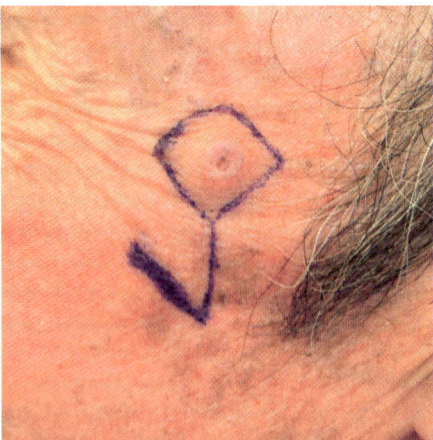

Fig. 3-1 ■ Preoperative image of a rhomboid flap used to reconstruct a cutaneous defect of the cheek before excision of a basal cell carcinoma.

BOX 3-1	Mathes and Nahai[7] Classification of Muscle Blood Supply

Type I: Single vascular pedicle (e.g., vastus lateralis)
Type II: Dominant vascular pedicle(s) and minor vascular pedicle(s) (e.g., trapezius)
Type III: Dominant pedicles (e.g., rectus abdominis)
Type IV: Segmental vascular pedicles (e.g., flexor hallucis longus)
Type V: Dominant vascular pedicle and secondary segmental vascular pedicles (e.g., latissimus dorsi)

BOX 3-2	Cormack and Lamberty[8] Classification of Fasciocutaneous Flaps

Type A: Contains multiple, unnamed fascial perforators
Type B: Contains a single perforator
Type C: Contains multiple small fascial perforators

BOX 3-3	Nakajima[9] Classification of Perforating Vessels to Fasciocutaneous Flaps

Type A: Direct cutaneous
Type B: Direct septocutaneous
Type C: Direct cutaneous branch of a muscular vessel
Type D: Perforating cutaneous branch of a muscular vessel
Type E: Septocutaneous perforator
Type F: Musculocutaneous perforator

---

be obtained, and morbidity at the donor site is low. Although the versatility of free flaps has supplanted the broad use of regional flaps in developed countries, regional flaps are widely used in developed and developing countries alike. Other common and useful regional flaps are derived from the latissimus dorsi muscle, the temporalis muscle, and the temporoparietal fascia; all are reliable for head and neck reconstruction.

Distant flaps may be either free or pedicled. Pedicled distant flaps are infrequently used in head and neck reconstruction, although they do occasionally appear in the contemporary medical literature.[4] Tagliacozzi theorized the use of a distant/pedicled arm flap, the so-called Italian flap, for nasal reconstruction. Free flaps entail transfer of tissue from a remote site with accompanied vascular supply to a recipient bed. Blood flow is reestablished by microvascular anastomosis. Widely adopted after the introduction of the radial forearm free flap (RFFF) in the early 1980s, free flaps have revolutionized head and neck surgery. Innumerable flaps have been described, and their versatility, reliability, and utility for reconstruction are unmatched choices for reconstruction in the head and neck.

Contemporary flap nomenclature and classification is based upon blood supply. Knowledge of the intrinsic blood supply to the skin is recognized as a critical factor in flap success. The recognition that the skin receives its blood supply mainly from vessels that traverse the deep fascia through muscle spawned the evolution of musculocutaneous flaps.[5] Axial pattern flaps are based on a reliable, well-defined vascular pedicle, oriented longitudinally within the flap.[6] The work by Mathes and Nahai[7] helped elucidate the different patterns of blood distribution within muscle flaps; five different patterns were identified based on the principle that muscular blood supply is derived from specific series of arteries and accompanying veins (Box 3-1). The corresponding skin territory of each superficial muscle extends from the insertion to the origin and courses along its borders and may even extend beyond.[6] The skin overlying muscle is perfused by perforating arteries from the muscle. The Mathes and Nahai[7] classification led to a greater understanding of flaps such as the PMMC, in which a reliable skin paddle overlying the muscle is perfused from a specific source vessel. Their work aided surgeons in designing flaps for particular uses based on the pattern of vascularization. Cormack and Lamberty elucidated three vessel subtypes that accounted for many of the cutaneous flaps of the time (Box 3-2). Though the concept was not new, they coined the term *fasciocutaneous* to describe a flap where the skin is supplied by vessels that pass along intermuscular and intercompartmental fascia to reach the skin.

Type A fasciocutaneous flaps contain multiple, unnamed fascial perforators. Type B fasciocutaneous flaps contain a single perforator. Type C fasciocutaneous flaps contain multiple small fascial perforators, but all are fed from a single subfascial vessel that must be transferred with the flap. Nakajima and colleagues[9] expanded on this concept and identified six types of fasciocutaneous perforators, distinguishing between direct and indirect perforators (Box 3-3). The angiosome concept illustrated that arteries closely follow the connective tissue framework of the body. Injection studies by Taylor and Palmer[10] showed that the blood supply to the skin and deep tissues corresponded to a consistent source vessel. The vascular supply to the skin was supplied by direct cutaneous arteries with reinforcement by smaller indirect vessels. Controversy surrounding the use of the term perforator was largely ameliorated following the Fifth International Course on Perforator Flaps in Ghent, Belgium, in 2001. According to Wei and colleagues,[11] a true perforator must pass through a muscle en route to the skin. The nomenclature born from the Ghent conference includes the source artery and the muscle that is traversed by the vessel supplying the skin paddle. The anterior lateral thigh flap would hence be named the lateral circumflex femoral artery perforator flap, with the addition of the vastus lateralis muscle in the notation.

To date, there is no consensus on the classification of flaps. The current trend is to classify free flaps by source vessel. There is little doubt that the classification will continue to evolve with our expanding interest and knowledge of the anatomy and physiology of flaps.

RECONSTRUCTIVE GOALS

Cormack and Lamberty[8] described the components of flap design and suggested the incorporation of the six *C*s: circulation, constituents, conditioning, contiguity, conformation, and construction.[12] A

BOX 3-4	Reconstructive Ladder

Primary closure
Healing by secondary intention
Skin grafting
Local flaps
Regional flaps
Microvascular free flaps

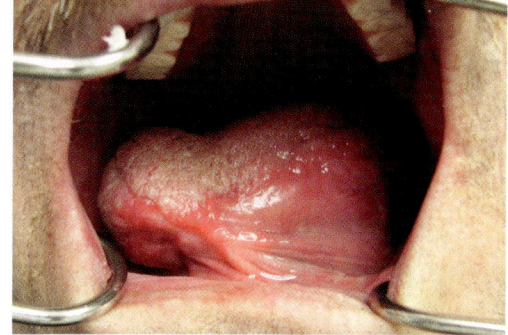

Fig. 3-2 ■ Tethering of the tongue to the floor of the mouth following resection of an early stage squamous cell carcinoma.

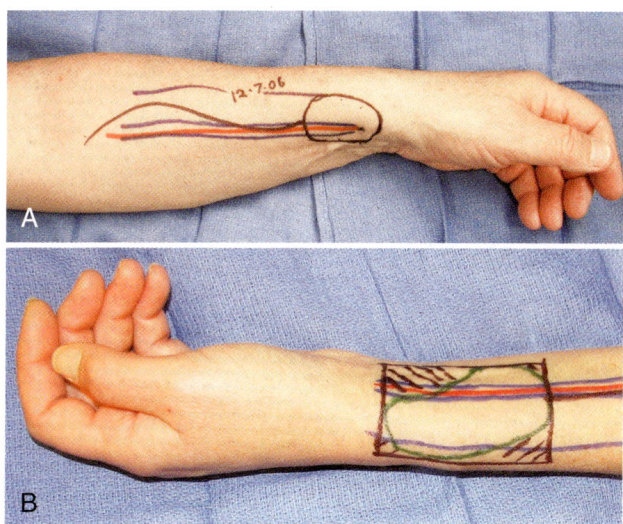

Fig. 3-3 ■ Routine surgical marking for an RFFF. **A,** The skin paddle is centered between the brachioradialis and flexor carpi radialis muscles. **B,** The skin paddle has been extended to include the cephalic vein.

functional reconstructive model identifies the immediate purpose of a reconstructive effort. For instance, reconstruction of a maxillectomy defect should first address isolating the sinus and nasal cavity from the oral cavity, and then address restoring the dentition. Conceptualizing a defect on the basis of its tissue constituents is a logical starting point for the reconstructive surgeon. The reconstructive ladder is a frequently referenced framework that stratifies options by level of complexity (Box 3-4). There are no absolute indications for reconstructing particular defects, and preferences vary by individual surgeon and geographic regions.

The most common defects in the oral maxillofacial region requiring reconstruction involve the lips, tongue, floor of mouth, mandible and maxilla, and buccal mucosa.

SPECIFIC TREATMENT AND TECHNIQUES

The goals of functional tongue reconstruction are to restore the bulk and preserve the mobility of the residual, non-resected tongue. Defects of one third or less are often treated with primary closure, healing by secondary intention, or skin grafting. There is little benefit in objective measures of swallowing efficiency between flaps of any kind and primary closure for smaller glossectomy defects. Articulation and deglutition are affected by preservation of the tip of the tongue and base of the tongue, respectively. Provided that the tip of the tongue can be preserved, speech outcomes with primary closure are often preferable to free flap reconstruction in small (less than one third) glossectomy defects. Suturing the tongue to the floor of the mouth can tether it, which adversely affects speech (Fig. 3-2). Larger defects ranging from one third to one half of the oral tongue are ideally suited for microvascular free flaps or regional flaps. The most commonly used free flaps for this purpose are the RFFF, the lateral arm flap, and the anterior lateral thigh flap (ALT). The submental artery perforator flap has utility as both a free flap and rotational flap, but may have limitations when a neck dissection is performed, because the source vessels are frequently encountered in level I of the neck. Although there is no consensus on which flap has the greatest utility, the workhorse flap for tongue reconstruction remains the RFFF. Based upon the radial artery, its accompanying veins, and occasionally the cephalic vein, the RFFF is a reliable, robust flap that satisfies the needs for intermediately sized defects. Flap design begins with estimation of the defect size that includes both clinical and radiographic examinations. An estimation of the linear dimension of the flap can be gained by direct clinical measurement. Though a 1:1 ratio of resected to reconstructed tissue seems logical, it is safer to harvest a larger flap, accounting for tissue shrinkage of both the tongue and flap. Two-dimensional measurements of the anticipated defect with an additional 20% can be incorporated into the flap design. Tumor depth may be difficult to estimate by CT. MRI is useful for evaluating deeply invasive tumors. It is attractive to design RFFFs in geometric shapes, but there is little evidence to suggest a difference in functional outcomes. Urken and Biller[13] suggested the use of the bilobed flap, which allows for reconstruction of the floor of the mouth and tongue and eliminates a "dog-ear." Alternatively, a wedge of skin in the floor of mouth can be deepithelialized and closed unto itself. The deepithelialized wedge is advantageous because it adds a bulk of fascia in the floor of mouth as an extra layer where oral cutaneous leaks are common. The skin paddle can be rectangular, elliptical, or oval and oriented over the skin of the radial artery, located between the brachioradialis and flexor carpi radialis muscles (Fig. 3-3). Preoperative testing should include a bedside Allen test. This ensures adequacy of the blood supply through the ulnar artery to the hand. The test is considered normal if, after compression of both the ulnar and radial arteries followed by repeated clenching of the fingers to squeeze out the blood, the normal color or a slightly more pronounced red color of the palm of the hands returns in less than 10 seconds after release of only the ulnar artery. A positive Allen test precludes the use of this flap.[14] It is helpful to include the cephalic vein in the flap by extending the skin paddle laterally over the radial surface of the wrist, although the vein can be "captured" and incorporated into the fascial aspect only. The entire flap can be used as a fascia-only flap for either covering a surface or restoring a volume defect (Fig. 3-4). Although the thickness of the RFFF can be variable, it is typically thicker in women. The thickness of the flap in the immediate postoperative period changes, as the flow dynamics in the tissue change from flow-through to end-flow. Additional bulk can be obtained by deepithelializing a portion of the flap and using this portion to create

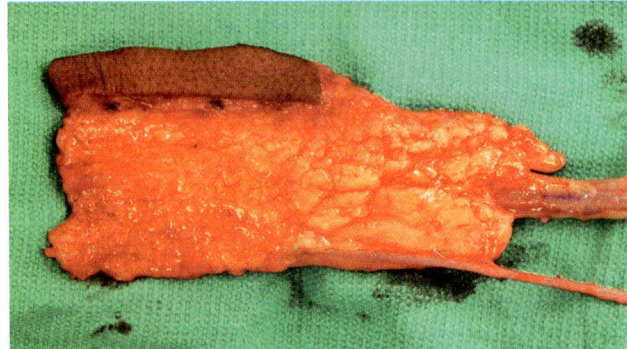

Fig. 3-4 ■ A fasciocutaneous flap that has been largely deepithelialized to restore bulk of a subcutaneous defect. A portion of skin has been left to aid in postoperative monitoring.

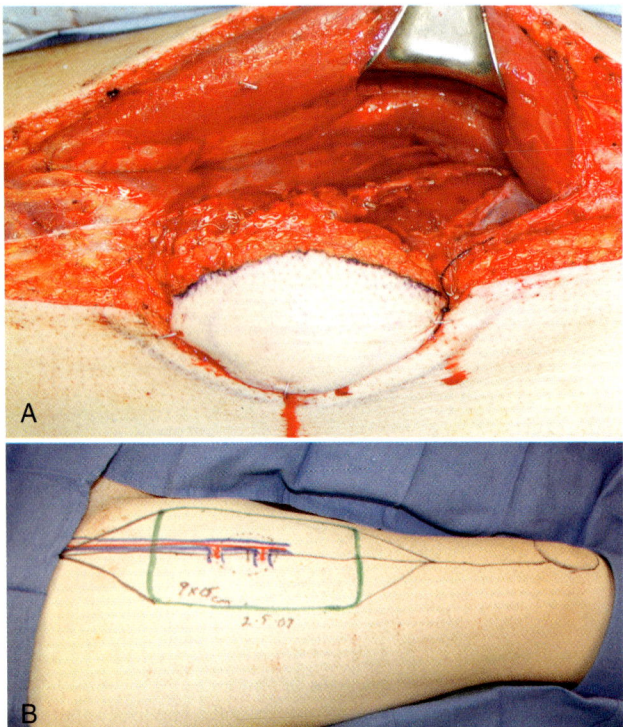

Fig. 3-5 ■ **A,** An elliptical ALT flap raised to facilitate primary closure. **B,** A larger skin paddle designed as an extended hexagon, also to facilitate primary closure of the donor site.

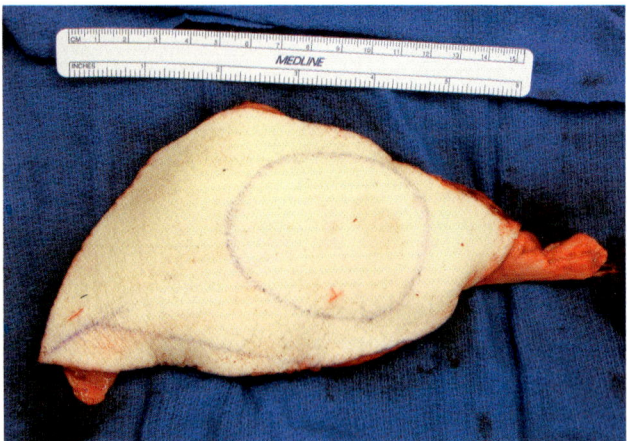

Fig. 3-6 ■ A large ALT flap. The T-shaped marking corresponds to the localization of the perforator, which lies within a 3-cm circle drawn at the midpoint of a line connecting the anterior iliac spine and the lateral border of the patella.

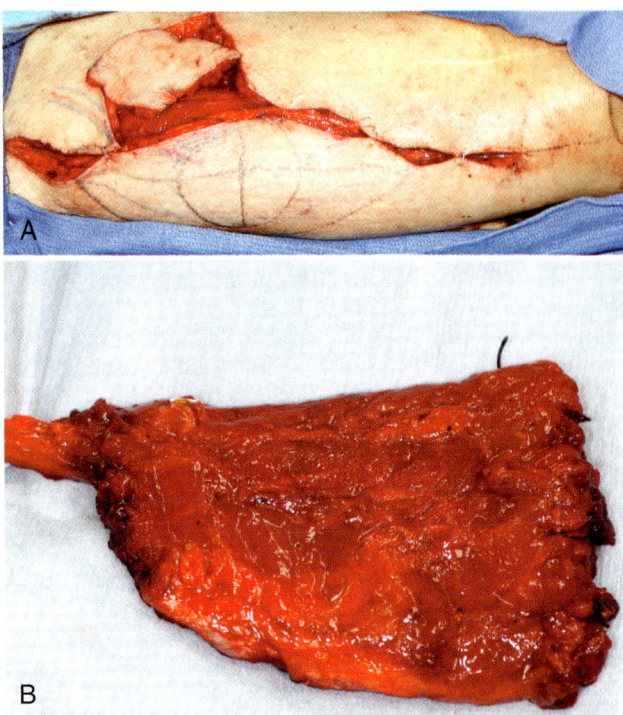

Fig. 3-7 ■ **A,** An anterior medial thigh flap, raised after failure to identify a dominant lateral perforator for a planned ALT flap. **B,** A vastus lateralis flap, used to reconstruct a hemiglossectomy defect in a patient who had neither lateral nor medial perforators.

a laminated flap that is tucked underneath the cutaneous portion. The RFFF can also be designed to include a sensory nerve, the antebrachial cutaneous nerve.

Glossectomy defects greater than one half are best reconstructed with bulkier flaps. The anterior lateral thigh flap, the rectus abdominis flap (RA), and the latissimus dorsi flap (LD) are all suitable candidates. The major disadvantage of the RA and LD is sacrifice of a functional muscular unit and the long-term loss of muscle bulk following denervation. The ALT is well suited for larger tongue resections. It is technically more difficult to raise the ALT because of inconsistency in perforator location and size. Doppler ultrasonography is used to identify a dominant perforator along the lateral intermuscular septum between the vastus lateralis and rectus femoris muscles. The skin paddle is typically an ellipse or extended hexagon because these shapes facilitate primary wound closure (Fig. 3-5). For a larger glossectomy defect, the shape of the flap is less important than the overall volume. The ALT is well suited for chimerism,

provided there are two distinct perforators. Customized, independent skin paddles can be designed after verification of the perforators. Alternatively, a larger flap can be raised and the intervening portion deepithelialized. The perforator need not be geometrically centered, although it is the author's preference to do so (Fig. 3-6). Occasionally, preoperative Doppler testing may be deceptive, and a search for a perforator begins after the medial portion of the flap is elevated. Knowledge of the anatomic variants of the source vessel to the ALT is essential. If a dominant perforator is not found, the anterior medial thigh flap, the tensor fasciae latae flap, and the vastus lateralis flap are viable options within the dissection field (Fig. 3-7). There is often an inverse relationship between size of the lateral and medial perforators to the skin emanating from the lateral circumflex branch of the deep femoral artery. The thickness of the skin over the lateral aspect of the thigh should be evaluated. The ALT can be raised as a suprafascial flap, or can be thinned after flap raising, provided that a 3-cm region of fascia is maintained around the perforator. Attempting to insert a larger, thick flap into a small defect may compromise the venous outflow in the small perforator, resulting in flap demise. It is the author's choice to limit the use of the ALT to hemiglossectomy defects or larger.

There are multiple donor site options for vascularized reconstruction of the mandible and maxilla. The fibula free flap (FFF) has been compared to both the deep circumflex iliac artery flap (DCIA) and the scapula flap in terms of donor site morbidity, pedicle length, and suitability for placement of endosseous implants. The fibula is relatively easy to raise, provides a consistent length of bone up to 25 cm, and can be harvested with either a large skin paddle or multiple skin paddles. There is little doubt that the DCIA provides the greatest degree of bone stock for dental implants. Disadvantages of the DCIA include the relatively short and small caliber vessels and the limitation of the skin paddle. Though the internal oblique muscle can be incorporated as a soft tissue paddle, it is less flexible. The scapula system is a highly diverse source for composite tissue transfer in terms of both bone length and number of distinct skin paddles.

When the fibula is used, flap design should begin with defect analysis, including the anticipated length of the defect, the site of the soft tissue defect (intraoral/extraoral), and the availability of recipient site vessels. The surgeon should also consider whether reconstruction of the condyle will be necessary and how many osteotomies will be needed. Preoperative clinical examination should include evaluation of the extremities for signs of vascular insufficiency. Preoperative magnetic resonance (MR) angiography or CT angiography should be used to evaluate the vascular pattern and distribution to the foot. The use of preoperative testing is controversial, although it seems prudent and cost-effective to evaluate the blood supply to the calf to reduce devascularizing complications.[15,16] An inconclusive MR angiogram or CT angiogram should be confirmed with a conventional angiogram.

There are three major considerations in designing an osteocutaneous free fibula flap: the site of the soft tissue defect, the site of the anastomosis (left or right), and the length of bone required to restore continuity. The amount of bone can be estimated clinically or radiographically. CT and MRI may be helpful in estimating the linear length required (Fig. 3-8). Typically, the maximum amount of bone is harvested, leaving 6 cm of bone proximally and distally, and osteotomies are made following the resection. Osteotomizing bone before the final defect is determined could result in incomplete restoration of continuity, requiring an additional free bone graft. Monocortical fixation is placed on the outward facing surface of the fibula. Irrespective of the side of the planned anastomosis, the vascular pedicle must be oriented on the lingual aspect of the neomandible or neomaxilla.

The choice of the right or left leg can be confusing to the microsurgery neophyte, and algorithms have been devised to assist in this task. The perforators pass within the posterior crural septum situated toward the caudal aspect of the fibula (Fig. 3-9). One must account for the positioning of the flap, the location of the planned anastomosis, and the position and flexibility of the skin paddle. For lateral defects of the mandible, the use of the ipsilateral fibula with the pedicle oriented posteriorly positions the posterior crural septum at the inferior border of the neomandible. This would be ideal for a skin defect but suboptimal for an adjacent mucosal defect, because the skin paddle would have to extend over and above the neomandible. The use of either the contralateral fibula with the pedicle oriented posteriorly or the ipsilateral fibula with the pedicle oriented

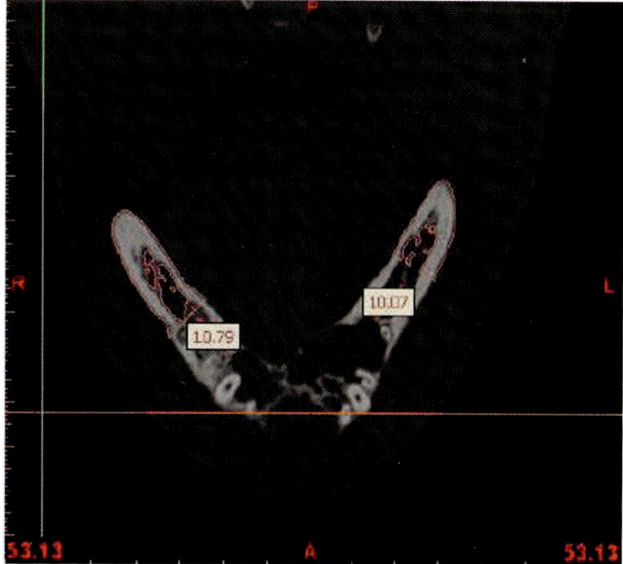

Fig. 3-8 ■ Axial CT image of an ameloblastoma. Linear estimates of the defect were used to construct stereolithographic guides to assist in segmentation of the fibula.

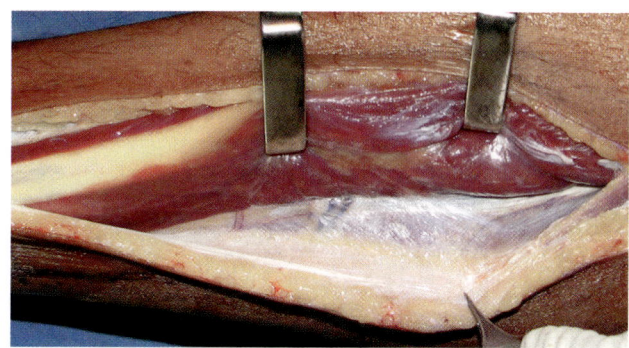

Fig. 3-9 ■ Fibula dissection illustrating a dominant septocutaneous perforator.

anteriorly would place the skin paddle more appropriately for a mucosal defect (Fig. 3-10). This decision-making process can be quite confusing at first, although thoughtful consideration of pedicle location and skin paddle orientation simplifies matters. Through-and-through defects can be reconstructed with two separately designed skin paddles or one large skin paddle that has an intervening segment of deepithelialized tissue (Fig. 3-11). Particular attention should be paid to the linear dimension of the soft tissue component, and a backup plan for obtaining additional soft tissue should be available.

Perforators, either septocutaneous or musculocutaneous, emanating from the peroneal artery should be identified preoperatively by Doppler ultrasonography (Fig. 3-12). On average there are approximately four sizable perforators, although the more proximal perforators are more likely to be fed from the posterior tibial artery. The size of the skin paddle should be estimated from the anticipated defect, again adding 20% for shrinkage of the flap. In spite of the use of Doppler ultrasonography, complete absence of perforators does occur in a minority of patients, which requires the use of an alternative soft tissue skin paddle or use of the contralateral leg. Identification of perforators impacts the design of the skin paddle. The skin paddle should include at least one perforator and can reliably reach sizes as large as 10 cm by 20 cm according to anatomic studies. The perforator does not need to be centered within

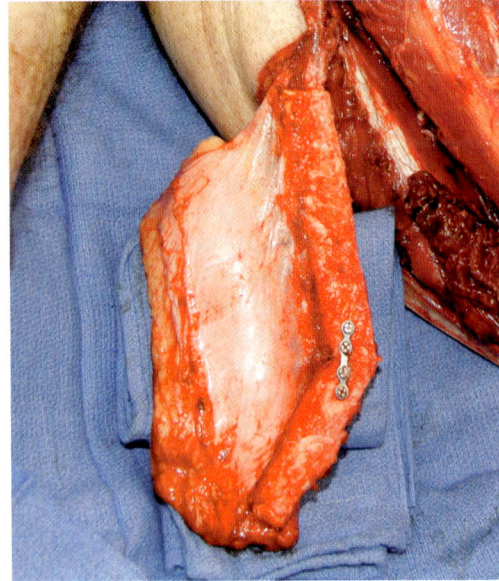

Fig. 3-10 ■ A right osteocutaneous free fibula for reconstruction of a right hemimandible. The skin paddle is oriented medially for obturation of a mucosal defect. The vascular pedicle is oriented anteriorly.

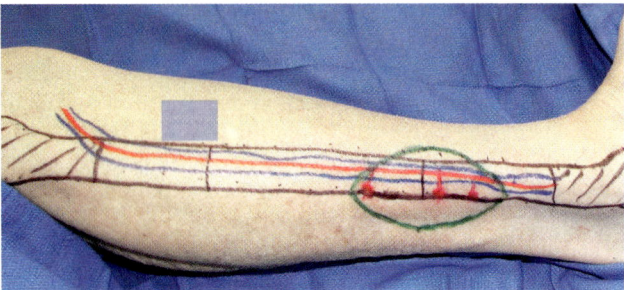

Fig. 3-12 ■ Preoperative surgical markings for an osteocutaneous free fibula flap. Doppler ultrasonography has been used to identify three perforators around which the skin paddle has been designed.

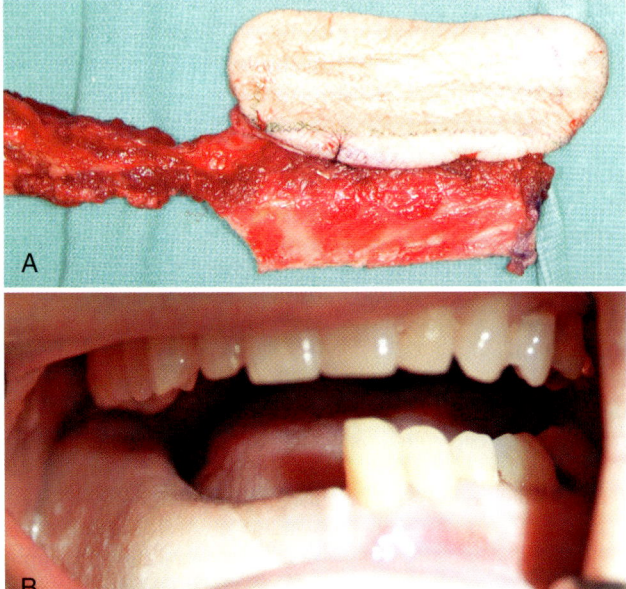

Fig. 3-13 ■ An osteocutaneous free fibula flap (**A**), with a rounded rectangular skin paddle to reconstruct the alveolar mucosa defect (**B**).

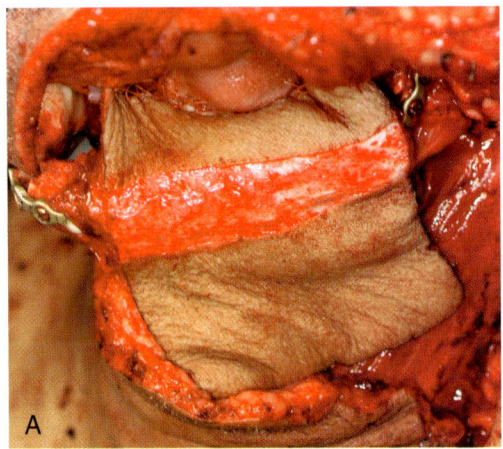

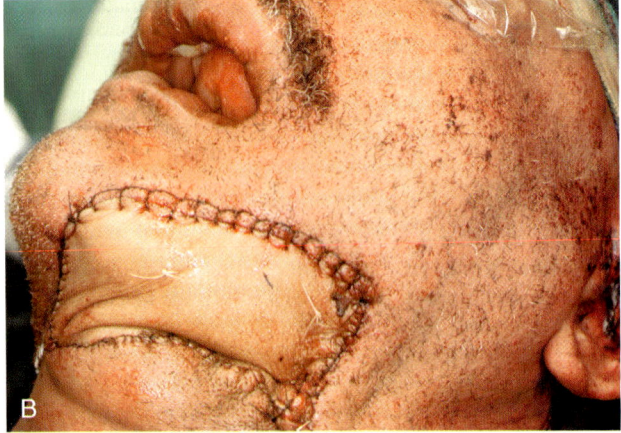

Fig. 3-11 ■ **A,** An osteocutaneous fibula for reconstruction of a composite through-and-through left lateral mandibular defect. An intervening portion of the skin paddle has been deepithelialized. **B,** Tension-free inset of the extraoral portion of the skin paddle.

the skin paddle, and the skin paddle can even be designed in series. Offsetting the bone and skin paddle is helpful in reconstruction of the retromolar fossa, in which a lateral segmental defect is combined with a retromolar fossa and soft palate defect achieving additional reach. The size and shape of the skin paddle is matched to the anticipated defect, although many surgeons use an ellipse as the default shape and either trim or deepithelialize superfluous soft tissue. Composite alveolar resections of the mandible with a limited soft tissue defect can include a narrow rectangular skin paddle to reconstruct the soft tissue formerly occupied by the attached gingiva (Fig. 3-13). The flexor hallucis longus muscle and the soleus muscle can be harvested with the fibula to provide soft tissue augmentation or to be used in place of a skin paddle (Fig. 3-14).

The fibula can be osteotomized into several segments to mimic the native curvature of the mandible. On-the-fly free osteotomies can be performed after the resection is complete. Indexing a titanium reconstruction plate before tumor removal ensures a close approximation of mandibular continuity. Templates can then be fashioned to simulate the segments of the neomandible using surgical rulers, foam sponges, or wooden tongue blades[17] (Fig. 3-15). Particular attention is paid to the angulation of the osteotomies, and bone to bone contact is ideal. Miniplates can be used to secure the neomandible or maxilla before insetting. Computer-assisted modeling can also be used to optimize osteotomy location and angulation.

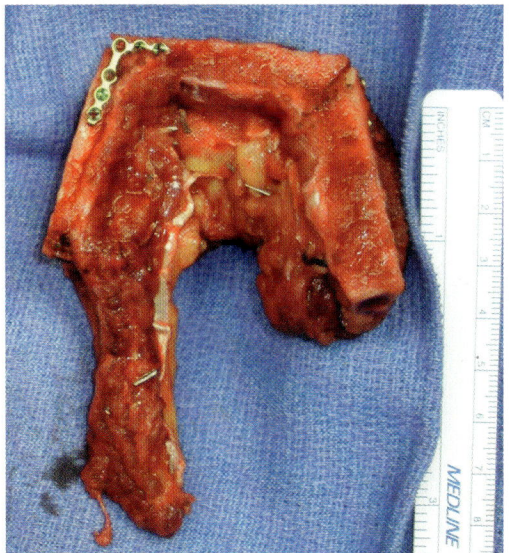

Fig. 3-14 ■ A bone-only fibula used for a total maxillary reconstruction. The flexor hallucis longus muscle is used to reconstruct the hard and soft palate mucosa.

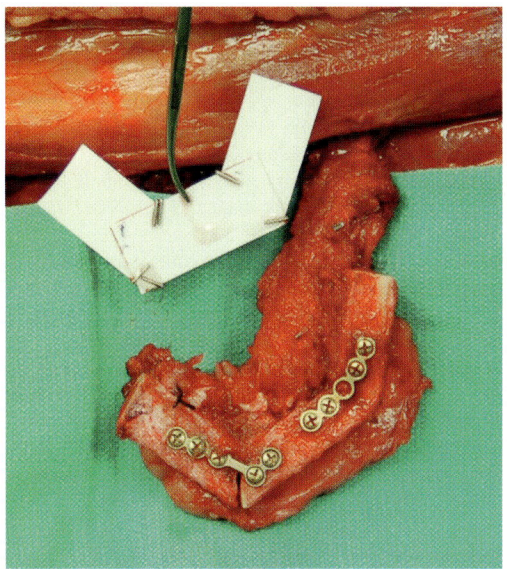

Fig. 3-15 ■ A bone-only fibula flap designed for a symphyseal defect. Surgical rulers have been used to assist in the angles of the osteotomies.

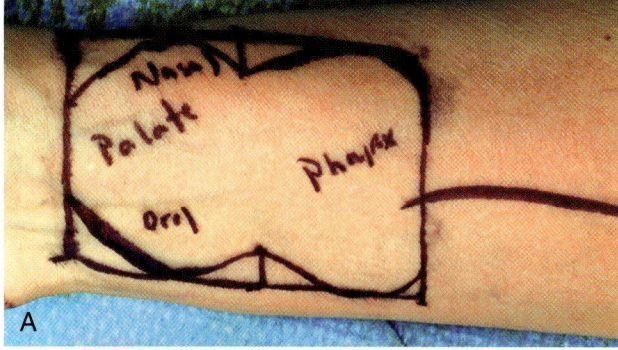

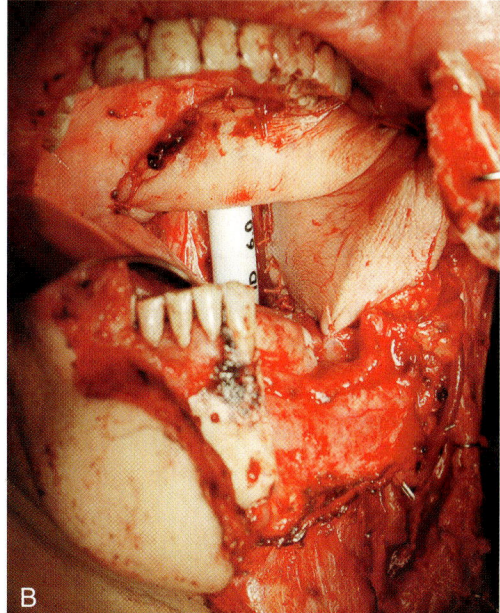

Fig. 3-16 ■ Surgical markings (**A**) for a radial folded forearm flap for reconstruction of the pharynx and soft palate (**B**).

Complex defects requiring multiple osteotomies can be simplified through computer-generated resection templates and cutting guides.

Reconstruction of the ascending ramus and condyle can aptly be reconstructed with the FFF. The condyle should be tapered to more closely approximate the shape of the condyle and to fit into the joint space. Proper positioning of the neocondyle can be difficult to achieve and it is not uncommon for the ramus to be positioned laterally and inferiorly. This can be overcome by drilling a hole through the outer cortex of the neocondyle and securing this to a hole drilled into or over the zygomatic arch.

Composite reconstruction of the maxilla using the fibula is quite similar to reconstruction of the mandible. Positioning and fixation of the maxilla is slightly more difficult. Posterior fixation to the pterygoid plate is extremely difficult to achieve, and cantilevering the maxilla from the piriform rim and zygoma is usually sufficient.

Small, posterolateral defects of the maxilla can be reconstructed with soft tissue only in place of an obturator. This obviates the need for an obturator but does not preclude its use in the future. Soft tissue reconstruction of the anterior maxilla typically does not provide sufficient support of the nose and upper lip. Irreversible collapse of the mid-face commonly occurs and is not often amenable to prosthetic reconstruction.

The anatomy of the soft palate, tonsillar pillar, and glossopharyngeal fold are unique and functionally complex. Some degree of nasal escape can be expected immediately following surgery. The folded RFFF has been suggested as the best choice for replacing both oral and nasal linings and covering the glossopharyngeal fold. The recreation of a functional nasal port is possible, although the mobility of the reconstructed soft palate is limited (Fig. 3-16).

POSTOPERATIVE CARE

Flap choice and flap design are important factors in flap success. Monitoring flaps postoperatively for vascular thrombosis or ischemia has been shown to improve salvage rates.[18] The majority of flap failures are due to venous obstruction caused by hematoma, kinking, flap swelling, and pedicle twisting.[19] Irrespective of monitoring modality, periodic clinical examination for skin color, turgor, and capillary refill coupled with Doppler examination should be performed in the first three days when possible.

PEARLS AND PITFALLS

- Attempts should be made to simplify reconstruction and eliminate elements of potential failure.
  - It is better to harvest more soft tissue than less.
  - Flap design is only one element in flap success.
  - Measure twice, cut once.
- Radial forearm free flap: The RFFF should be designed over the radial artery and cephalic vein when possible, which adds a larger vein for microvascular anastomosis. Geometric designs are of limited value in the reconstruction of the tongue, except when a large portion of the floor of the mouth is resected. A bilobed flap is helpful in these cases to prevent excessive tissue bulk in the floor of the mouth. The ulnar aspect of the flap should be raised first in a suprafascial plane; this creates a safe zone to prevent damage to the ulnar artery. If the ulnar artery is encountered, an ulnar-based flap can be raised.
- Anterior lateral thigh flap: Common errors begin with flap design. Be careful when marking the anterior iliac spine in obese patients, which may shift the anatomic landmark line laterally, causing the surgeon to miss the dominant perforator. Elevate the ALT caudally to cranially, and identify the intermuscular septum between the vastus lateralis and rectus femoris muscles. Do not circumferentially incise the skin paddle until a perforator is found. If a dominant perforator cannot be located, shift toward an anterior medial thigh flap, tensor fascia flap, or vastus lateralis flap.
- Free fibula flap: Radiographic and clinical examination of the extremities are critical in flap choice. Consider previous surgery and radiation exposure and length of bony resection when choosing which vessels will be used for microvascular anastomosis. If skin perforators cannot be located, look proximally and distally. Inform patients that a second flap may be necessary for soft tissue coverage.

REFERENCES

1. Neligan PC, Gullane PJ, Gilbert RW: Functional reconstruction of the oral cavity, *World J Surg* 27(7):856-862, 2003.
2. Tolhurst DE: A comprehensive classification of flaps: the atomic system, *Plast Reconstr Surg* 80(4):608-609, 1987.
3. Ariyan S: The pectoralis major myocutaneous flap. A versatile flap for reconstruction in the head and neck, *Plast Reconstr Surg* 63(1): 73-81, 1979.
4. Wilson DE, Maves MD: Tagliacotian cross-arm flap reconstruction of facial defects, *Otolaryngol Head Neck Surg* 94(2):219-223, 1986.
5. Blondeel P, editor: *Perforator flaps: anatomy, technique and clinical applications*, St Louis, 2006, Quality Medical Publishing.
6. Thorne C, editor: *Grabb and Smith's plastic surgery*, Philadelphia, 2006, Lippincott Williams & Wilkins.
7. Mathes SJ, Nahai F: Classification of the vascular anatomy of muscles: experimental and clinical correlation, *Plast Reconstr Surg* 67(2):177-187, 1981.
8. Cormack GC, Lamberty BG: A classification of fascio-cutaneous flaps according to their patterns of vascularisation, *Br J Plast Surg* 34(2):215-220, 1981.
9. Nakajima H, Fujino T, Adachi S: A new concept of vascular supply to the skin and classification of skin flaps according to their vascularization, *Ann Plast Surg* 16(1):1-19, 1986.
10. Taylor GI, Palmer JH: The vascular territories (angiosomes) of the body: experimental study and clinical applications, *Br J Plast Surg* 40(2):113-141, 1987.
11. Wei FC, Jain V, Suominen S, Chen HC: Confusion among perforator flaps: what is a true perforator flap? *Plast Reconstr Surg* 107(3):874-876, 2001.
12. Cormack GC, editor: *The fasciocutaneous system of vessels*, Edinburgh, 1994, Churchill Livingstone.
13. Urken ML, Biller HF: A new bilobed design for the sensate radial forearm flap to preserve tongue mobility following significant glossectomy, *Arch Otolaryngol Head Neck Surg* 120(1):26-31, 1994.
14. Benit E, Vranckx P, Jaspers L et al: Frequency of a positive Allen's test in 1,000 consecutive patients undergoing cardiac catheterization, *Cathet Cardiovasc Diagn* 38:352-354, 1986.
15. Kelly AM, Cronin P, Hussain HK et al: Preoperative MR angiography in free fibula flap transfer for head and neck cancer: clinical application and influence on surgical decision making, *AJR Am J Roentgenol* 188(1): 268-274, 2007.
16. Rosson GD, Singh NK: Devascularizing complications of free fibula harvest: peronea arteria magna, *J Reconstr Microsurg* 21(8): 533-538, 2005.
17. Fernandes R: An easy method for predictable osteotomies in the vascularized fibula flap for mandibular reconstruction, *J Oral Maxillofac Surg* 65(9):1874-1875, 2007.
18. Devine JC, Potter LA, Magennis P et al: Flap monitoring after head and neck reconstruction: evaluating an observation protocol, *J Wound Care* 10(1):525-529, 2001.
19. Yu P, Chang DW, Miller MJ et al: Analysis of 49 cases of flap compromise in 1310 free flaps for head and neck reconstruction, *Head Neck* 31(1):45-51, 2009.

Principles of Repair and Grafting of Bone and Cartilage

Chapter 4

Tara L. Aghaloo, Alan L. Felsenfeld

Bone grafting in reconstruction of the oral and maxillofacial region is a common procedure, with literature publication starting in the late 1800s and the earliest citations noted in the 1950s.[1-4] Within the oral cavity, bone grafts are subject to wound dehiscence, infection, and graft resorption; donor site morbidity may also occur for autogenous grafts. Although autogenous bone grafts are still the gold standard, clinicians and researchers are constantly investigating other sources for grafting, including allografts, alloplasts, and osteoinductive recombinant proteins to decrease or eliminate the need for a secondary surgical site for hard tissue oral and maxillofacial reconstruction.[5]

In the oral and maxillofacial region, cartilage repair is limited anatomically to the articular disk in the temporomandibular joint (TMJ) and auricular and nasal cartilage. When comparing bone and cartilage repair, it is well accepted that cartilaginous repair and regeneration is much more challenging than bone.[6,7]

ETIOPATHOGENESIS AND CAUSATIVE FACTORS

Congenital and acquired bone defects are common in the oral and maxillofacial region. Cleft palate is the second most common congenital deformity following cardiac anomalies,[8,9] and craniosynostosis occurs in 1 in 3000 live births. Other congenital defects and syndromes such as ectodermal dysplasia, Treacher Collins syndrome, hemifacial microsomia, and many others present with craniofacial bony defects that are challenging to correct or reconstruct. Other defects specific to the jaws, including maxillary and mandibular hypoplasia, are corrected with orthognathic surgery and often require bone grafting. Systemic pathologic conditions that require surgical intervention or bony reconstruction include acromegaly and ankylosing spondylitis. Acquired bone defects from trauma, tumor, infection, surgical procedures, and alveolar bone atrophy are also seen daily in our clinical practices. These bony defects usually require multiple and extensive grafting procedures, which often yield suboptimal anatomic, functional, or esthetic results.

Defects in nasal, auricular, or TMJ articular cartilage are generally caused by traumatic injury, infection, pathology, or degeneration.[6] Difficulties with cartilaginous repair after injury are well known. Cartilage has a limited capacity for self-repair because of its minimal vascular supply and low cellular density.[6,7] In addition, full thickness articular cartilage injuries that affect the underlying bone often heal by the formation of fibrocartilage, which can lead to rapid degradation upon further injury.[7,10] Large defects usually require autologous cartilaginous grafting for nasal and auricular defects, or total joint replacement without an articular disk for the TMJ area, which also often yield suboptimal results.

ANATOMIC CONSIDERATIONS

In performing surgery to repair or reconstruct bone and cartilage in the oral and maxillofacial region, the surgeon must be familiar with normal anatomy of both the injury and the donor sites if autologous tissue grafting will be used. Patients who have been edentulous for many years or have congenitally missing teeth have significant alveolar bone deficiencies. Since the deficiency increases with time, early intervention with bony reconstruction may decrease the continued resorption associated with prolonged edentulism. Another important consideration is the importance of vascularity on wound healing and repair. This is apparent when evaluating the success of bone grafts, where vascularity determines the incorporation of the graft to the recipient bed.[11] When using local flaps, they also must have adequate vascularity for survival. Incisions must be placed in easily manipulated locations and orientations so that the flaps can cover bone grafts without tension to protect the graft from contamination or infection.[12]

For cartilage regeneration, anatomic differences between tissues such as the ear and nose are apparent when compared to load-bearing joints such as the knee and TMJ. Even anatomic differences between load-bearing joints may affect their ability to perform specific functions, especially since the TMJ is composed of fibroelastic cartilage, whereas the knee joint is composed of articular or hyaline cartilage.[13-15] Also, in the treatment of arthritis, significant differences exist between the TMJ and other joints. In some orthopedic situations, possible treatments include fusion, which is never an acceptable option for the TMJ.[6]

DIAGNOSTIC STUDIES

In evaluating bone repair or planning bone reconstruction, adequate radiographs are required. For most of the oral and maxillofacial region, panoramic radiographs and CT scans are a necessity. MRIs are also important in evaluating the anatomy of the articular disk and surrounding soft tissues and detecting potential disk dislocation, with or without reduction upon mouth opening. Bone scans may also be used to rule out continued pathologic activity for certain disease processes. Being able to evaluate the defect and its planned reconstruction in three dimensions is important in restoring esthetics, form, and function to the face or jaws. The advent of three-dimensional (3D) models as tools to aid in complex maxillofacial reconstruction offers more detailed presurgical planning and identification of potential complications.

TREATMENT AND RECONSTRUCTIVE GOALS

The goals of repair and reconstruction are to recapture the normal form, function, and esthetics of the bone and cartilage that existed before injury. Specific for a bone graft, several principles must be followed: (1) remove diseased tissue; (2) establish functional occlusion; (3) restore or maintain adequate vascularity; (4) provide a base for prosthetic reconstruction, with or without dental implants; (5) maintain space; (6) provide soft tissue coverage; (7) maintain stability; and (8) prevent infection.

NORMAL HEALING

NORMAL BONE HEALING (REPAIR)

Bone healing undergoes the same three stages seen with soft tissue healing: inflammatory, fibroplastic, and remodeling. The inflammatory stage begins immediately after injury and lasts up to 5 days. Initially, vasoconstriction allows a blood clot to form, and then cells with inflammatory and phagocytic properties are attracted to the wound site to decrease debris and bacteria accumulation. The fibroplastic stage involves fibroblasts that produce fibrin, which increases wound strength over the next 2 to 3 weeks. Increased vascularity with new budding capillaries is also important in this stage. Increased blood flow brings cells and various factors to induce fibrinolysis as the fibrin network continues to mature. Finally, the remodeling stage involves reorganization and strengthening of the wound, but with significant wound contraction to close the gap.[16]

Extraction sockets heal in a similar manner, but the inflammatory stage takes approximately 2 weeks to form the blood clot, break down debris, and deposit osteoid. The fibroplastic stage occurs during the next 2 weeks, with epithelialization of the socket and formation of woven bone. The remodeling stage lasts 4 to 6 months, during which cortical and trabecular woven bone is resorbed and replaced by lamellar bone.[16] Healing of fractures also follows these three stages, but the process is further classified as healing by primary or secondary intention. Primary intention occurs when the fracture edges are precisely placed without a gap between the segments, which often requires rigid internal fixation and immobilization to promote more rapid healing and decrease scarring and risk of infection.[17] Healing by secondary intention occurs with bone avulsion or imperfect anatomic reduction with a residual space between the two bony edges. In these situations, more collagen deposition is required to bridge the gap, resulting in callus formation with the involvement of periosteal and overlying soft tissue responses.[17] If healing continues with stability, lack of infection, and adequate vascularization, remodeling will occur and the callus will calcify and become bone. The process of creeping substitution occurs here, where the gradual formation of osteoid tissue across the defect slowly matures to normal bone. It is important to understand that healing of a fracture requires specific responses in the bone marrow, cortex, periosteum, and overlying soft tissues.[16] If these do not occur, a fibrous union will result.[16]

NORMAL CARTILAGE HEALING (REPAIR)

The need for cartilage repair usually results from damage caused by trauma, pathologic condition, or arthritis.[18] Although repairing damaged cartilaginous tissue is difficult enough in healthy states, repair in the presence of disease such as arthritis or autoimmune disorders poses a unique challenge. Cartilage healing and repair is significantly more limited than in bone because of its minimal

potential for self-regeneration. Even though cartilage is a metabolically active tissue, it lacks inherent blood and lymphatic vessels. Inflammation does not occur and progenitor cells from the blood or bone marrow cannot access damaged tissue. Therefore cartilage is unable to repair or regenerate itself.[19,20]

Current evidence suggests that additional cartilage on articular surfaces can only form during the first 3 months of postnatal life.[21] Damage to articular cartilage where cartilage and bone are in direct contact extends from the articular surface to the subchondral bone. Damage is accompanied by bleeding into the defect, which activates the normal bone healing process, and inflammation triggers hematoma formation. As the repair process continues with the fibroplastic stage, where fibroblasts begin to increase wound strength, the resultant fibrous tissue is not consistent with the structural and functional properties of articular cartilage.[6] In partial thickness defects where the injury is contained within the articular cartilage, blood and cells cannot access the injury site. In these cartilaginous injuries, the defect remains.[10,22,23] This significant challenge with cartilage healing has clinicians and researchers searching for techniques to successfully regenerate damaged cartilage.

SPECIFIC TREATMENT AND TECHNIQUES

BONE GRAFTING

Bone grafting is a common technique used to treat damaged or missing bone in orthopedic and oral and maxillofacial surgery. Historically, autogenous bone is the gold standard for critical size defects in the craniofacial region.[24,25] Autogenous bone possesses all the important biological processes: osteogenesis, the formation of new bone from transplantation of osteocompetent cells; osteoinduction, formation of new bone from the differentiation and stimulation of undifferentiated mesenchymal stem cells; and osteoconduction, formation of new bone along a scaffold from the host osteocompetent cells at the recipient site.[26] Many donor sites are available for autogenous bone grafts, including extraoral sites such as the iliac crest, tibia, rib, and calvarium, and intraoral sites such as the ramus, chin, and tuberosity. Extraoral sites provide a larger volume of bone than intraoral sites, but they carry greater donor site morbidity.[27-30] Cortical bone, as harvested from the calvarium, has less resorption but a slower revascularization rate than cancellous bone from the iliac crest or tibia.[31] Cancellous bone, also called trabecular bone, provides pluripotent or osteogenic precursor cells and more rapid revascularization of the graft.[32] Alternatively, use of intraoral donor sites decreases the need for hospitalization and lowers cost, but these sites cannot be used to reconstruct large maxillofacial defects.

Since both intraoral and extraoral autogenous bone grafts are limited in quantity and require a second surgical site, the use of bone substitutes continues to increase. Allografts are bone grafts from a donor of the same species. They are usually sterilized by gamma irradiation or ethylene oxide to eliminate disease transmission[33]; however, the risk of interindividual infection is still a concern with the use of allografts.[34,35] Although a large number of studies in the orthopedic and oral and maxillofacial literature document favorable outcomes with the use of allografts, only osteoconductive and potential osteoinductive properties are documented.[36]

Other alternatives to autogenous bone grafts are alloplastic bone substitutes and xenografts. Xenografts are bone grafts from another species, usually bovine, for oral and maxillofacial surgery. Xenografts are deproteinized to remove all organic material, and are often combined with ceramics such as hydroxyapatite. Ceramics also are used as bone substitutes, including various combinations of hydroxyapatite and β-tricalcium phosphate (β-TCP), bioactive glasses, porous hydroxyapatite, calcium sulfate, and calcium carbonate. These materials have no bioactive proteins and possess only osteoconductive properties.[25,37,38] As a result of the lack of inductive properties, alloplast uses are limited to small space-maintaining defects in oral and maxillofacial surgery, based on defect volume, location, and host factors.[39-41]

HARD TISSUE ENGINEERING

In recent years, a new era in reconstructive surgery has begun with the application of tissue engineering, including the use of cells, scaffolds, and growth factors to improve bone healing and regeneration. When engineering a bony construct with this triad of components, it may be possible to create an ideal, easily available, and highly reliable bone graft material with no donor site morbidity and a low risk of infection or antigenicity. Osteogenic or osteoinductive signals could be preserved, the construct could be easily manipulated but remain stable, and vascular supply could be maintained.[42] In evaluating a complex craniofacial defect, a 3D scaffold that can withstand pressures from the overlying soft tissue is necessary to adequately reconstruct the missing hard tissue. These scaffolds must maintain space to allow for tissue regeneration; provide an environment for cell attachment and possibly proliferation, differentiation, or both; and endure functional loading that supports bone growth. The scaffold must be degraded, metabolized, or excreted easily, and be cost-effective when processed to fit complex defects.[43-45] The scaffold also should provide an interface with cell receptors and extracellular matrix to facilitate the functional interaction that allows normal cellular functions to occur.[45] To date, poly-L-lactic acid (PLLA) and poly-L-glycolic acid (PLGA) are commonly used synthetic scaffolds in bone tissue engineering because they are biologically inert and safe to use in humans.[46] In vivo animal studies have shown the ability of these scaffolds to regenerate bone in defects of either critical or non-critical size when incorporated with recombinant growth factors.[47-52] Many other synthetic as well as naturally occurring scaffolds have been successfully used for bone repair and regeneration, including PLGA/polyethylene glycol (PEG), calcium phosphate, collagen, alginate, silk, polycaprolactone, poly(propylene fumarate), and others.[43,44]

In addition to the use of synthetic or naturally occurring scaffolds, their surface properties can be altered, including texture, roughness, hydrophobicity, charge, and chemical composition, to enhance the interaction with cells for improved cell signaling, differentiation, and function.[53-55] Indeed, marrow stromal cells (MSCs) can be induced to convert to an osteogenic phenotype when seated on a porous, dense scaffold.[56] Using the scaffold to create a more favorable microenvironment for interaction with local cells and factors can improve the osteoinductivity of the construct, which is important when scaffolds are used as carriers for temporal and spatial release of growth factors and proteins.

Growth factors and proteins that reside in the extracellular matrix play crucial roles in the bone healing process. Factors such as bone morphogenetic protein-2 (BMP-2), basic fibroblast growth factor (bFGF), platelet-derived growth factor (PDGF), transforming growth factor-β (TGF-β), and vascular endothelial growth factor (VEGF) have shown positive effects in promoting fracture healing.[57-61] BMPs are now well known to induce expression of osteoblast markers and stimulate bone formation in vivo,[62] and are the focus of much of the bone regeneration studies in both translational research and clinical practice. BMPs make up a large portion of the TGF-β superfamily, which regulates key steps in the differentiation, proliferation, and morphogenetic processes of bone and cartilage.[63-65] BMPs are among the most potent regulators of osteoblast differentiation[66] and BMP types 2, 4, 6, and 7 all have osteoinductive properties in vivo.[67,68] BMP-2 released from various carriers has been shown to completely regenerate calvarial defects in the rodent model.[50,52,69,70] In humans, BMP-2 recombinant protein can regenerate mandibular continuity and cleft palate defects, and augment maxillary sinuses, with outcomes that are comparable to those of autogenous particulate bone and marrow.[71-74] These results have led the U.S. Food and Drug Administration (FDA) to approve rhBMP-2 on an absorbable collagen sponge for use in orthopedic surgery for spinal fusion and non-union of tibia fractures, and in oral and maxillofacial surgery for sinus augmentation and localized alveolar ridge defects.

As bone regeneration strategies become more attainable and realistic, the importance of vascularity is apparent. Formation of new vessels and revascularization of a bone graft is crucial to successful regeneration. VEGF is the most potent and widely used regulator of vascularization, with important effects on osteoblasts and osteoclasts during bone repair.[75] Osteoblasts express VEGF receptors, and impaired VEGF-receptor signaling could lead to decreased recruitment and differentiation of osteoblasts.[76,77] Animal studies have shown the ability of VEGF to enhance BMP-2 effects in critical size defects[78] and BMP-2 has been shown to induce osteoblastic differentiation and bone formation that expresses VEGF.[79] To improve bone regeneration, other combinations of growth factors have also been investigated to more closely mimic natural temporal and spatial expression. Chitosan-based scaffolds using VEGF pre-encapsulated in alginate microspheres allowed the delayed release of VEGF, several days after PDGF was released into the defect. Although PDGF increased bone formation over the scaffold alone, the addition of VEGF enhanced both new vessel formation and bone regeneration.[80] Furthermore, sequential release of factors such as VEGF and PDGF are more effective at promoting angiogenesis than simultaneous release.[81]

Soft tissue wound-healing effects of PDGF are well established, especially in diabetics with chronic non-healing ulcers on a lower extremity.[82,83] PDGF has important functions in mitogenesis, angiogenesis, and recruitment of fibroblasts and osteoblasts to assist in wound healing.[84,85] In animal studies, PDGF induced bone regeneration in calvarial defects when implanted on a PLLA scaffold.[86] PDGF has also been shown to improve periodontal defects, which led to FDA approval of PDGF on a tricalcium phosphate carrier for periodontal intrabony defects.[87]

bFGF plays a role in cell proliferation, motility, differentiation, mitogenesis, wound healing, tissue repair, and angiogenesis.[88] Its role in alveolar bone repair and healing mandibular and long bone fractures is well established.[89,90] Recent animal studies have shown preliminary success using bFGF to repair large osteochondral defects, where the regenerated cartilage demonstrated a hyaline-like appearance.[91] Difficulty with cartilage repair and regeneration has been previously mentioned in this chapter, and will be discussed in more detail in a later section.

TGF-β has been studied for decades for its potential role in bone regeneration and repair. It has chemotactic and mitogenic properties important in promoting osteoblast differentiation and inhibiting osteoclastic bone resorption.[85,92] TGF-β also functions in connective tissue repair and formation of vessels, demonstrating bone-specific properties. It is not as potent as BMP-2, a member of the larger TGF-β superfamily. Therefore, much of the research in bone regeneration has focused on BMP-2 as previously discussed.

IGFs are also mitogens for osteoblasts and osteoblast precursors to stimulate differentiation and bone formation.[85] IGF-1 has been shown to improve bone healing in both healthy and diabetic animals[93,94] and to increase bone contact when coated on implants in combination with TGF-β.[95]

In evaluating the ideal growth factor to regenerate bone, the goal of clinicians and researchers is to recapture the normal physiologic process of bone healing and repair. This goal encourages the use of growth factor combinations or more complex scaffolds to release specific factors in a sequential or prolonged fashion. Studies evaluating sustained release of BMP-2 to increase the bioactivity, and lead to improved osteoblastic differentiation in vitro and bone formation in vivo.[69,96-100] Combinations such as VEGF plus BMP-2, BMP-7 plus PDGF, PDGF plus VEGF, PDGF plus IGF-1, and TGF-β plus IGF-1 have all demonstrated enhanced bone healing or regeneration.[80,95,101-103]

In addition to prolonging the release and combining growth factors to improve bone regeneration, the use of cells such as mesenchymal stem cells, alone, transduced with growth factors, or implanted directly with growth factors, is currently under intense investigation.[99] MSCs can be acquired from multiple autologous sources, including iliac crest, tibia, and sternal bone marrow; periosteum; adipose tissue; synovium; skin; pericytes; umbilical cord; peripheral blood; dental pulp; periodontal ligament; deciduous teeth; and apical papillae.[45,104,105] Under appropriate conditions, including osteogenic media (ascorbic acid, β-glycerophosphate, dexamethasone, fetal bovine serum) or treatment with osteoinductive factors such as BMP-2, TGF-β, and IGF-1, MSCs can differentiate into osteoblasts and form bone.[99,104,105] Indeed, animal models of bone marrow stromal cells (BMSCs) with hydroxyapatite/tricalcium phosphate (HA/TCP) or calcium alginate scaffolds significantly induce bone regeneration, better than autologous bone grafts.[106-108]

When recombinant growth factors are delivered, the initial high concentration is not maintained at the site for long periods and therefore limits the amount of bone formation. Gene therapy helps to overcome this limitation, where MSCs can be engineered to express osteoinductive growth factors to regenerate bony defects. This indirect, or ex vivo, gene therapy approach, where the cells are genetically modified outside the body and then reimplanted to deliver factors to a localized defect, has successfully regenerated long bone and craniofacial defects.[109-111] Initial studies used MSCs that were transduced with BMP-2 and then incorporated into a collagen scaffold and implanted into segmental defects in the rat.[110] Since then, other studies used cells from periosteum, fat, and muscle with both viral and non-viral vectors to obtain acceptable bony regeneration.[18] In vivo gene therapy can also be performed, where a gene is directly injected using vectors within a matrix, such as fibrin glue, alginate, or collagen.[23] This technique is simpler and more cost-effective than ex vivo gene therapy because there are no autologous cells or in vitro expansion required.[112] Many in vivo gene therapy studies have successfully regenerated bony defects in small animals when various BMP genes are transferred. However, larger animal models have not yet provided similarly consistent results.[18]

The combination of cells, scaffolds, and differentiation factors holds great promise as an implantable construct for 3D tissue engineering. Most likely, these cocktails will differ in each clinical situation, based on the number of factors required, timing of release, structural support required by the scaffold, cell type and differentiation potential, local environment, and type of pathology or disease. Even though the task seems quite complicated, considerable progress has been made in the field of tissue engineering for craniofacial bone regeneration, including the maxillary sinus, calvarium, and palate.[113-115] Although significantly more research is needed before these techniques can replace current bone grafting procedures, human case reports demonstrate regeneration of large bony defects with combinations of growth factors, scaffolds, and MSCs.[45]

CARTILAGE REGENERATION

Because cartilage healing and repair is extremely limited after injury, reconstruction of ear and nose defects is often performed with cartilaginous transplantation.[116] However, anatomic nasal septal and auricular donor sites are small and long-term results for cartilage grafting are still unknown. So research has focused on cartilage regeneration using gene therapy and engineering principles.[23] Even more challenging are defects in a joint because the roles of a normal anatomic and functional articular surface are more complex. As discussed earlier, tissue engineering and gene therapy have been successful in bone regeneration both in animal models and clinical studies,[24,45] but progress in gene therapy for cartilage regeneration has been slower and more difficult to achieve.[23] In situ regeneration is based on the concept of introducing undifferentiated MSCs to the area of injury via holes drilled through the cartilage and into the subchondral bone. Accessing the bone marrow will attract the MSCs and the blood clot formed in the initial healing stages, providing the appropriate environment for chondrogenic differentiation.[117] Clinically, some studies have shown favorable functional results similar to cell-based therapy with this microfracture technique in humans, even though the regenerated cartilage was not histologically identical to the original.[117-119] Furthermore, factors present in the normal blood clot possess chemotactic properties for MSCs, which have potentially favorable effects for the microfracture technique.[117] However, this process is not usually consistent with articular cartilage formation because it is more similar to normal bone formation.[6]

Autologous chondrocytes can be harvested, grown in vitro, and injected or implanted into cartilaginous defects or areas of damage. Similar to osteogenic differentiation in vitro, chondrogenic differentiation requires a specific set of supplements in culture, including dexamethasone, TGF-β, ascorbic acid, chondroitin sulfate, serum withdrawal, or multilayer culture system.[99,117] In orthopedic surgery, autologous chondrocytes have been used either alone or on a 3D carrier to treat defects in the knee and improve pain from osteoarthritis.[10,120,121] However, the disadvantages of harvesting autologous chondrocytes are similar to those of harvesting autologous bone and bone marrow, including donor site morbidity. Some additional disadvantages of using autologous chondrocytes are dedifferentiation and loss of potential redifferentiation with increased expansion in vitro, and lack of similarities in growth and differentiation with chondrocytes from different anatomic locations.[122]

Similar to bone regeneration methods discussed previously, ex vivo and in vivo gene therapies have been investigated for cartilage regeneration. Mainly chondrocytes or MSCs from multiple autologous sources can be transduced ex vivo with growth factors and implanted or injected into damaged articular or meniscal cartilage.[18,123,124] Animal studies have demonstrated the ability of chondrocytes transduced ex vivo with BMP-7 in a fibrin matrix to repair full thickness articular cartilage defects and MSCs transduced with BMP-7 to repair rabbit osteochondral defects.[125,126] In vivo gene therapy is also under investigation, mostly with viral and non-viral vectors, but fewer data in animal studies are available to evaluate short- and long-term results.[18] Using genes that can be transduced ex vivo into harvested chondrocytes or undifferentiated MSCs, or implanted in vivo, could significantly improve cartilage regeneration. This gene therapy could aid in inducing MSCs down the chondrocyte lineage with TGF-β or Sox-9,[127] improve vascularity with VEGF, promote extracellular matrix deposition with TGF-β or BMP-2,[128] and inhibit osteogenesis, all of which would improve the morphology and function of the damaged or missing cartilaginous tissue.[23]

Despite advancement in the field, acquiring the ability to induce harvested cells to express these specific genes in a temporal fashion in vivo after implantation poses considerable challenges. Specifically for gene therapy, the utility of viral and non-viral vectors must still be assessed. The outcomes of direct in vivo injection of a gene vector have yet to be compared with results from implantation of cells containing genes that were transduced ex vivo. These techniques must all be evaluated to determine the ideal therapy for each defect. The cell type that should be used for cartilage regeneration is also a point for discussion—fully differentiated or immature chondrocytes, undifferentiated MSCs that can be induced to differentiate into chondrocytes, or synovial lining cells in a joint space.[23,122] As mentioned earlier, use of autologous chondrocytes has some disadvantages, which have prompted researchers to investigate other cell sources. MSCs from bone marrow or adipose tissue can be stimulated to differentiate into chondrocytes expressing osterix, Runx2, and type X collagen.[122] Synovial cells have been shown to have superior chondrogenic potential than MSCs from the same patients,[129] but little is known about the role of these cells in the pathogenesis of arthritis.[122]

Great progress has been made in cartilage tissue engineering where an entire ear, trachea, TMJ, and nasal septum have been fabricated and implanted in vivo.[130-133] However, much less work has been done in the oral and maxillofacial region as compared to orthopedic needs elsewhere in the body. Similarly, less favorable cosmetic and functional outcomes are described for cartilage engineering in the head and neck.[116] Interactions between native and regenerated cartilage, as well as between cartilage and subchondral bone, is a challenge, especially in regenerating cartilage in a joint space. Preliminary in vitro studies to differentiate osteochondral cells have been done with MSCs from multiple animal species,[134,135] but much more work is needed to translate these experiments in vivo and to patients. In vivo studies to evaluate chondrocytic differentiation of MSCs adjacent to subchondral bone are also underway, where defect remodeling, histologic bone and cartilage morphology, and functional properties can be studied.[117,136,137] Indeed, chondrocytes respond to external forces by changing their extracellular matrix, and therefore mechanical studies on cells and scaffolds to be used for chondrogenic regeneration are also being conducted.[138-140]

As the progress in understanding cartilage regeneration follows that of bone, it will become more important to understand how to use 3D constructs to provide structural support for larger and more complex defects and to facilitate cell to cell and cell to matrix interactions. Both biologically natural scaffolds, such as blood clots, and artificial scaffolds, such as collagen sponges, fibrin sealants, and hydrogels, have been used to support cartilage regeneration.[117] Moreover, the combination of scaffolds with MSCs and differentiation factors will likely improve cartilage regeneration. Collagen-based or highly porous scaffolds have been shown to favor MSC differentiation into chondrocytes,[116,141] and hydrogels with encapsulated TGF-β have improved chondrocyte differentiation and viability.[142]

PEARLS AND PITFALLS

- Considerable progress has been made in recent years in both bone and cartilage repair and regeneration, as researchers and clinicians are striving to recapture the naturally occurring process of healing.
- Although in vitro, animal, and preliminary human studies have shown good success with these engineering techniques, regenerating multiphasic human tissues or multiple tissues in close proximity involves incredibly complex processes.[143]
- In bone engineering, regenerating cortical and cancellous bone where anatomically and functionally necessary, with new vascularity and 3D support has provided significant challenges that have not yet been overcome.
- Cartilage poses even more difficulty with our current technologies, where the three major zones of cartilage have different structural and functional properties.[144]
- The interaction between cartilage and subchondral bone is a complicating factor, especially when the entire cartilage-bone complex requires regeneration because of trauma or degenerative disease where inflammation or pathology is still present.[145]

REFERENCES

1. Converse JM: Restoration of facial contour by bone grafts introduced through the oral cavity, *Plast Reconstr Surg (1946)* 6(4): 295-300, 1950.
2. Boyne PJ: Use of freeze-dried homogenous bone grafts in the surgical positioning of teeth, *J Oral Surg (Chic)* 15(3):231-237, 1957.
3. Boyne PJ, Losee FL: Use of anorganic heterogenous bone in oral bony defects, *U S Armed Forces Med J* 8(6):789-794, 1957.
4. Losee FL, Boyne PJ: Response of oral tissues to grafts of ethylenediamine-treated heterogeneous bone, *Nature* 179(4564):818, 1957.
5. Bauer TW, Muschler GF: Bone graft materials. An overview of the basic science, *Clin Orthop Relat Res* (371):10-27, 2000.
6. Naujoks C, Meyer U, Wiesmann HP et al: Principles of cartilage tissue engineering in TMJ reconstruction, *Head Face Med* 4:3, 2008.
7. Vinatier C, Gauthier O, Masson M et al: Nasal chondrocytes and fibrin sealant for cartilage tissue engineering, *J Biomed Mater Res A* 89(1):176-185, 2009.
8. Cohen MM Jr: Craniofacial disorders caused by mutations in homeobox genes MSX1 and MSX2, *J Craniofac Genet Dev Biol* 20(1): 19-25, 2000.
9. Bardach J, Morris H: *Multidisciplinary management of cleft lip and palate*, Philadelphia, 1990, WB Saunders.
10. Buckwalter JA: Articular cartilage: injuries and potential for healing, *J Orthop Sports Phys Ther* 28(4):192-202, 1998.
11. Goldberg VM, Stevenson S: The biology of bone grafts, *Semin Arthroplasty* 4(2):58-63, 1993.
12. van Gemert JT, van Es RJ, Van Cann EM, Koole R: Nonvascularized bone grafts for segmental reconstruction of the mandible—A reappraisal, *J Oral Maxillofac Surg* 67(7): 1446-1452, 2009.
13. Bouloux GF: Temporomandibular joint pain and synovial fluid analysis: a review of the literature, *J Oral Maxillofac Surg* 67(11): 2497-2504, 2009.
14. Stratmann U, Schaarschmidt K, Santamaria P: Morphometric investigation of condylar cartilage and disc thickness in the human temporomandibular joint: significance for the definition of ostearthrotic changes, *J Oral Pathol Med* 25(5):200-205, 1996.
15. Mitchell ME, Giza E, Sullivan MR: Cartilage transplantation techniques for talar cartilage lesions, *J Am Acad Orthop Surg* 17(7): 407-414, 2009.
16. Hupp J: Wound repair. In Peterson LE, Hupp JR, Tucker MR, editors: *Contemporary oral and maxillofacial surgery*, St. Louis, 2003, Mosby, pp 49-62.
17. Einhorn TA: The cell and molecular biology of fracture healing, *Clin Orthop Relat Res* 355(Suppl):S7-21, 1998.
18. Evans CH, Ghivizzani SC, Robbins PD: Orthopedic gene therapy in 2008, *Mol Ther* 17(2):231-244, 2009.
19. Chiang H, Jiang CC: Repair of articular cartilage defects: review and perspectives, *J Formos Med Assoc* 108(2):87-101, 2009.

20. Vinatier C, Mrugala D, Jorgensen C et al: Cartilage engineering: a crucial combination of cells, biomaterials and biofactors, *Trends Biotechnol* 27(5):307-314, 2009.

21. Hunziker EB, Kapfinger E, Geiss J: The structural architecture of adult mammalian articular cartilage evolves by a synchronized process of tissue resorption and neoformation during postnatal development, *Osteoarthritis Cartilage* 15(4):403-413, 2007.

22. Hunziker EB: Articular cartilage repair: basic science and clinical progress. A review of the current status and prospects, *Osteoarthritis Cartilage* 10(6):432-463, 2002.

23. Steinert AF, Noth U, Tuan RS: Concepts in gene therapy for cartilage repair, *Injury* 39(Suppl 1):S97-113, 2008.

24. Baltzer AW, Lieberman JR: Regional gene therapy to enhance bone repair, *Gene Ther* 11(4):344-350, 2004.

25. Costantino PD, Hiltzik D, Govindaraj S, Moche J: Bone healing and bone substitutes, *Facial Plast Surg* 18(1):13-26, 2002.

26. Miyazaki M, Tsumura H, Wang JC, Alanay A: An update on bone substitutes for spinal fusion, *Eur Spine J* 18(6):783-799, 2009.

27. Franceschi RT: Biological approaches to bone regeneration by gene therapy, *J Dent Res* 84(12):1093-1103, 2005.

28. Canady JW, Zeitler DP, Thompson SA, Nicholas CD: Suitability of the iliac crest as a site for harvest of autogenous bone grafts, *Cleft Palate Craniofac J* 30(6):579-581, 1993.

29. Frodel JL, Marentette LJ: The coronal approach. Anatomic and technical considerations and morbidity, *Arch Otolaryngol Head Neck Surg* 119(2):201-207; discussion 140, 1993.

30. Frodel JL Jr, Marentette LJ, Quatela VC, Weinstein GS: Calvarial bone graft harvest. Techniques, considerations, and morbidity, *Arch Otolaryngol Head Neck Surg* 119(1): 17-23, 1993.

31. Albrektsson T: Repair of bone grafts. A vital microscopic and histological investigation in the rabbit, *Scand J Plast Reconstr Surg* 14(1):1-12, 1980.

32. Rawashdeh MA, Telfah H: Secondary alveolar bone grafting: the dilemma of donor site selection and morbidity, *Br J Oral Maxillofac Surg* 46(8):665-670, 2008.

33. Bienek C, MacKay L, Scott G et al: Development of a bacteriophage model system to investigate virus inactivation methods used in the treatment of bone allografts, *Cell Tissue Bank* 8(2):115-124, 2007.

34. Buck BE, Malinin TI, Brown MD: Bone transplantation and human immunodeficiency virus. An estimate of risk of acquired immunodeficiency syndrome (AIDS), *Clin Orthop Relat Res* 240:129-136, 1989.

35. Kappe T, Cakir B, Mattes T et al: Infections after bone allograft surgery: a prospective study by a hospital bone bank using frozen femoral heads from living donors, *Cell Tissue Bank* 11(3):253-259, 2010.

36. Boyan BD, Ranly DM, McMillan J et al: Osteoinductive ability of human allograft formulations, *J Periodontol* 77(9):1555-1563, 2006.

37. Hallman M, Thor A: Bone substitutes and growth factors as an alternative/complement to autogenous bone for grafting in implant dentistry, *Periodontol 2000* 47:172-192, 2008.

38. Vaccaro AR, Chiba K, Heller JG et al: Bone grafting alternatives in spinal surgery, *Spine J* 2(3):206-215, 2002.

39. Garofalo GS: Autogenous, allogenetic and xenogenetic grafts for maxillary sinus elevation: literature review, current status and prospects, *Minerva Stomatol* 56(7-8): 373-392, 2007.

40. Enneking WF, Mindell ER: Observations on massive retrieved human allografts, *J Bone Joint Surg Am* 73(8):1123-1142, 1991.

41. Friedlaender GE: Immune responses to osteochondral allografts. Current knowledge and future directions, *Clin Orthop Relat Res* 174:58-68, 1983.

42. Block MS, Kent JN: Sinus augmentation for dental implants: the use of autogenous bone, *J Oral Maxillofac Surg* 55(11):1281-1286, 1997.

43. Kretlow JD, Mikos AG: 2007 AIChE Alpha Chi Sigma Award: From Material to Tissue: Biomaterial Development, Scaffold Fabrication, and Tissue Engineering, *AIChE J* 54(12):3048-3067, 2008.

44. Scheller EL, Krebsbach PH, Kohn DH: Tissue engineering: state of the art in oral rehabilitation, *J Oral Rehabil* 36(5):368-389, 2009.

45. Zaky SH, Cancedda R: Engineering craniofacial structures: facing the challenge, *J Dent Res* 88(12):1077-1091, 2009.

46. Frazza EJ, Schmitt EE: A new absorbable suture, *J Biomed Mater Res* 5(2):43-58, 1971.

47. Bessho K, Carnes DL, Cavin R, Ong JL: Experimental studies on bone induction using low-molecular-weight poly(DL-lactide-co-glycolide) as a carrier for recombinant human bone morphogenetic protein-2, *J Biomed Mater Res* 61(1):61-65, 2002.

48. Boyan BD, Lohmann CH, Somers A et al: Potential of porous poly-D,L-lactide-co-glycolide particles as a carrier for recombinant human bone morphogenetic protein-2 during osteoinduction in vivo, *J Biomed Mater Res* 46(1):51-59, 1999.

49. Hollinger JO, Leong K: Poly(alpha-hydroxy acids): carriers for bone morphogenetic proteins, *Biomaterials* 17(2):187-194, 1996.

50. Aghaloo T, Cowan CM, Chou YF et al: Nell-1-induced bone regeneration in calvarial defects, *Am J Pathol* 169(3):903-915, 2006.

51. Aghaloo TL, Amantea CM, Cowan CM et al: Oxysterols enhance osteoblast differentiation in vitro and bone healing in vivo, *J Orthop Res* 25(11):1488-1497, 2007.

52. Cowan CM, Aghaloo T, Chou YF et al: MicroCT evaluation of three-dimensional mineralization in response to BMP-2 doses in vitro and in critical sized rat cal-

varial defects, *Tissue Eng* 13(3):501-512, 2007.

53. Bottaro DP, Liebmann-Vinson A, Heidaran MA: Molecular signaling in bioengineered tissue microenvironments, *Ann N Y Acad Sci* 961:143-153, 2002.

54. Geckeler K, Wacker R, Martini F et al: Enhanced biocompatibility for SAOS-2 osteosarcoma cells by surface coating with hydrophobic epoxy resins, *Cell Physiol Biochem* 13(3):155-164, 2003.

55. Schneider GB, English A, Abraham M et al: The effect of hydrogel charge density on cell attachment, *Biomaterials* 25(15):3023-3028, 2004.

56. Dadsetan M, Hefferan TE, Szatkowski JP et al: Effect of hydrogel porosity on marrow stromal cell phenotypic expression, *Biomaterials* 29(14):2193-2202, 2008.

57. Fujii H, Kitazawa R, Maeda S et al: Expression of platelet-derived growth factor proteins and their receptor alpha and beta mRNAs during fracture healing in the normal mouse, *Histochem Cell Biol* 112(2): 131-138, 1999.

58. Lee FY, Storer S, Hazan EJ et al: Repair of bone allograft fracture using bone morphogenetic protein-2, *Clin Orthop Relat Res* 397:119-126, 2002.

59. Rundle CH, Miyakoshi N, Ramirez E et al: Expression of the fibroblast growth factor receptor genes in fracture repair, *Clin Orthop Relat Res* 403:253-263, 2002.

60. Schmidmaier G, Wildemann B, Heeger J et al: Improvement of fracture healing by systemic administration of growth hormone and local application of insulin-like growth factor-1 and transforming growth factor-beta1, *Bone* 31(1):165-172, 2002.

61. Street J, Bao M, deGuzman L et al: Vascular endothelial growth factor stimulates bone repair by promoting angiogenesis and bone turnover, *Proc Natl Acad Sci U S A* 99(15):9656-9661, 2002.

62. Spinella-Jaegle S, Roman-Roman S, Faucheu C et al: Opposite effects of bone morphogenetic protein-2 and transforming growth factor-beta1 on osteoblast differentiation, *Bone* 29(4):323-330, 2001.

63. Reddi AH: Morphogenesis and tissue engineering of bone and cartilage: inductive signals, stem cells, and biomimetic biomaterials, *Tissue Eng* 6(4):351-359, 2000.

64. Iwata H, Sakano S, Itoh T, Bauer TW: Demineralized bone matrix and native bone morphogenetic protein in orthopaedic surgery, *Clin Orthop Relat Res* 395:99-109, 2002.

65. Wozney JM: Overview of bone morphogenetic proteins, *Spine (Phila Pa 1976)* 27(16 Suppl 1):S2-8, 2002.

66. Yamaguchi A, Komori T, Suda T: Regulation of osteoblast differentiation mediated by bone morphogenetic proteins, hedgehogs, and Cbfa1, *Endocr Rev* 21(4):393-411, 2000.

67. Gitelman SE, Kobrin MS, Ye JQ et al: Recombinant Vgr-1/BMP-6-expressing tumors induce fibrosis and endochondral bone formation in vivo, *J Cell Biol* 126(6): 1595-1609, 1994.

68. Sampath TK, Maliakal JC, Hauschka PV et al: Recombinant human osteogenic protein-1 (hOP-1) induces new bone formation in vivo with a specific activity comparable with natural bovine osteogenic protein and stimulates osteoblast proliferation and differentiation in vitro, *J Biol Chem* 267(28): 20352-20362, 1992.

69. Chung YI, Ahn KM, Jeon SH et al: Enhanced bone regeneration with BMP-2 loaded functional nanoparticle-hydrogel complex, *J Control Release* 121(1-2):91-99, 2007.

70. Kamakura S, Nakajo S, Suzuki O, Sasano Y: New scaffold for recombinant human bone morphogenetic protein-2, *J Biomed Mater Res A* 71(2):299-307, 2004.

71. Boyne PJ: Application of bone morphogenetic proteins in the treatment of clinical oral and maxillofacial osseous defects, *J Bone Joint Surg Am* 83-A Suppl 1(Pt 2):S146-150, 2001.

72. Herford AS, Boyne PJ: Reconstruction of mandibular continuity defects with bone morphogenetic protein-2 (rhBMP-2), *J Oral Maxillofac Surg* 66(4):616-624, 2008.

73. Dickinson BP, Ashley RK, Wasson KL et al: Reduced morbidity and improved healing with bone morphogenic protein-2 in older patients with alveolar cleft defects, *Plast Reconstr Surg* 121(1):209-217, 2008.

74. Boyne PJ, Lilly LC, Marx RE et al: De novo bone induction by recombinant human bone morphogenetic protein-2 (rhBMP-2) in maxillary sinus floor augmentation, *J Oral Maxillofac Surg* 63(12):1693-1707, 2005.

75. Poh CK, Shi Z, Lim TY et al: The effect of VEGF functionalization of titanium on endothelial cells in vitro. *Biomaterials* 31(7):1578-1585, 2010.

76. Gerber HP, Ferrara N: Angiogenesis and bone growth, *Trends Cardiovasc Med* 10(5):223-228, 2000.

77. Hiratsuka S, Minowa O, Kuno J et al: Flt-1 lacking the tyrosine kinase domain is sufficient for normal development and angiogenesis in mice, *Proc Natl Acad Sci U S A* 95(16):9349-9354, 1998.

78. Kanczler JM, Ginty PJ, White L et al: The effect of the delivery of vascular endothelial growth factor and bone morphogenic protein-2 to osteoprogenitor cell populations on bone formation, *Biomaterials* 31(6):1242-1250, 2010.

79. Kakudo N, Kusumoto K, Wang YB et al: Immunolocalization of vascular endothelial growth factor on intramuscular ectopic osteoinduction by bone morphogenetic protein-2, *Life Sci* 79(19):1847-1855, 2006.

80. De la Riva B, Sanchez E, Hernandez A et al: Local controlled release of VEGF and PDGF from a combined brushite-chitosan system enhances bone regeneration, *J Control Release* 143(1):45-52, 2010.

81. Chen RR, Silva EA, Yuen WW, Mooney DJ: Spatio-temporal VEGF and PDGF delivery patterns blood vessel formation and maturation, *Pharm Res* 24(2):258-264, 2007.

82. Steed DL: Clinical evaluation of recombinant human platelet-derived growth factor for the treatment of lower extremity ulcers, *Plast Reconstr Surg* 117(7 Suppl):143S-149S; discussion 150S-151S, 2006.

83. Mandracchia VJ, Sanders SM, Frerichs JA: The use of becaplermin (rhPDGF-BB) gel for chronic nonhealing ulcers. A retrospective analysis, *Clin Podiatr Med Surg* 18(1):189-209, viii, 2001.

84. Antoniades HN: Human platelet-derived growth factor (PDGF): purification of PDGF-I and PDGF-II and separation of their reduced subunits, *Proc Natl Acad Sci U S A* 78(12):7314-7317, 1981.

85. Marx R: Platelet-rich plasma: a source of multiple autologous growth factors for bone grafts. In Lynch S, Genco R, Marx R, editors: *Tissue engineering: applications in maxillofacial surgery and periodontics*, Chicago, 1999, Quintessence, pp 71-82.

86. Park YJ, Ku Y, Chung CP, Lee SJ: Controlled release of platelet-derived growth factor from porous poly(L-lactide) membranes for guided tissue regeneration, *J Control Release* 51(2-3):201-211, 1998.

87. Howell TH, Fiorellini JP, Paquette DW et al: A phase I/II clinical trial to evaluate a combination of recombinant human platelet-derived growth factor-BB and recombinant human insulin-like growth factor-I in patients with periodontal disease, *J Periodontol* 68(12):1186-1893, 1997.

88. Basilico C, Moscatelli D: The FGF family of growth factors and oncogenes, *Adv Cancer Res* 59:115-165, 1992.

89. Gong Z, Zhou S, Cao J, Gu X: Effects of recombinant human basic fibroblast growth factor on cell proliferation during mandibular fracture healing in rabbits, *Chin J Traumatol* 4(2):110-112, 2001.

90. Kawaguchi H, Kurokawa T, Hanada K et al: Stimulation of fracture repair by recombinant human basic fibroblast growth factor in normal and streptozotocin-diabetic rats, *Endocrinology* 135(2):774-781, 1994.

91. Maehara H, Sotome S, Yoshii T et al: Repair of large osteochondral defects in rabbits using porous hydroxyapatite/collagen (HAp/Col) and fibroblast growth factor-2 (FGF-2), *J Orthop Res* 28(5):677-686, 2010.

92. Mohan S, Baylink DJ: Bone growth factors, *Clin Orthop Relat Res* 263:30-48, 1991.

93. Shen FH, Visger JM, Balian G et al: Systemically administered mesenchymal stromal cells transduced with insulin-like growth factor-I localize to a fracture site and potentiate healing, *J Orthop Trauma* 16(9): 651-659, 2002.

94. Thaller SR, Lee TJ, Armstrong M et al: Effect of insulin-like growth factor type 1 on critical-size defects in diabetic rats, *J Craniofac Surg* 6(3):218-223, 1995.

95. Lamberg A, Bechtold JE, Baas J et al: Effect of local TGF-beta1 and IGF-1 release on implant fixation: comparison with hydroxyapatite coating, *Acta Orthop* 80(4):499-504, 2009.

96. Jung RE, Weber FE, Thoma DS et al: Bone morphogenetic protein-2 enhances bone formation when delivered by a synthetic matrix containing hydroxyapatite/tricalciumphosphate, *Clin Oral Implants Res* 19(2):188-195, 2008.

97. Kempen DH, Lu L, Hefferan TE et al: Retention of in vitro and in vivo BMP-2 bioactivities in sustained delivery vehicles for bone tissue engineering, *Biomaterials* 29(22):3245-3252, 2008.

98. Takahashi Y, Yamamoto M, Yamada K et al: Skull bone regeneration in nonhuman primates by controlled release of bone morphogenetic protein-2 from a biodegradable hydrogel, *Tissue Eng* 13(2):293-300, 2007.

99. Salinas CN, Anseth KS: Mesenchymal stem cells for craniofacial tissue regeneration: designing hydrogel delivery vehicles, *J Dent Res* 88(8):681-692, 2009.

100. Karageorgiou V, Meinel L, Hofmann S et al: Bone morphogenetic protein-2 decorated silk fibroin films induce osteogenic differentiation of human bone marrow stromal cells, *J Biomed Mater Res A* 71(3):528-537, 2004.

101. Zhang Y, Shi B, Li C et al: The synergetic bone-forming effects of combinations of growth factors expressed by adenovirus vectors on chitosan/collagen scaffolds, *J Control Release* 136(3):172-178, 2009.

102. Young S, Patel ZS, Kretlow JD et al: Dose effect of dual delivery of vascular endothelial growth factor and bone morphogenetic protein-2 on bone regeneration in a rat critical-size defect model, *Tissue Eng Part A* 15(9):2347-2362, 2009.

103. Stefani CM, Machado MA, Sallum EA et al: Platelet-derived growth factor/insulin-like growth factor-1 combination and bone regeneration around implants placed into extraction sockets: a histometric study in dogs, *Implant Dent* 9(2):126-131, 2000.

104. Huang GT, Gronthos S, Shi S: Mesenchymal stem cells derived from dental tissues vs. those from other sources: their biology and role in regenerative medicine, *J Dent Res* 88(9):792-806, 2009.

105. Panetta NJ, Gupta DM, Quarto N, Longaker MT: Mesenchymal cells for skeletal tissue engineering. *Panminerva Med* 51(1):25-41, 2009.

106. De Kok IJ, Drapeau SJ, Young R, Cooper LF: Evaluation of mesenchymal stem cells following implantation in alveolar sockets: a canine safety study, *Int J Oral Maxillofac Implants* 20(4):511-518, 2005.

107. Yamada Y, Ueda M, Hibi H, Nagasaka T: Translational research for injectable tissue-engineered bone regeneration using mesenchymal stem cells and platelet-rich plasma: from basic research to clinical case study, *Cell Transplant* 13(4):343-355, 2004.

108. Weng Y, Wang M, Liu W et al: Repair of experimental alveolar bone defects by tissue-engineered bone, *Tissue Eng* 12(6): 1503-1513, 2006.

109. Chang SC, Wei FC, Chuang H et al: Ex vivo gene therapy in autologous critical-size craniofacial bone regeneration, *Plast Reconstr Surg* 112(7):1841-1850, 2003.

110. Lieberman JR, Daluiski A, Stevenson S et al: The effect of regional gene therapy with bone morphogenetic protein-2-producing bone-marrow cells on the repair of

segmental femoral defects in rats, *J Bone Joint Surg Am* 81(7):905-917, 1999.

111. Dai KR, Xu XL, Tang TT et al: Repairing of goat tibial bone defects with BMP-2 gene-modified tissue-engineered bone, *Calcif Tissue Int* 77(1):55-61, 2005.

112. Evans CH, Palmer GD, Pascher A et al: Facilitated endogenous repair: making tissue engineering simple, practical, and economical, *Tissue Eng* 13(8):1987-1993, 2007.

113. Moreau JL, Caccamese JF, Coletti DP et al: Tissue engineering solutions for cleft palates, *J Oral Maxillofac Surg* 65(12):2503-2511, 2007.

114. Shayesteh YS, Khojasteh A, Soleimani M et al: Sinus augmentation using human mesenchymal stem cells loaded into a beta-tricalcium phosphate/hydroxyapatite scaffold, *Oral Surg Oral Med Oral Pathol Oral Radiol Endod* 106(2):203-209, 2008.

115. Tu Q, Valverde P, Li S et al: Osterix overexpression in mesenchymal stem cells stimulates healing of critical-sized defects in murine calvarial bone, *Tissue Eng* 13(10): 2431-2440, 2007.

116. Rotter N, Haisch A, Bucheler M: Cartilage and bone tissue engineering for reconstructive head and neck surgery, *Eur Arch Otorhinolaryngol* 262(7):539-545, 2005.

117. Richter W: Mesenchymal stem cells and cartilage in situ regeneration, *J Intern Med* 266(4):390-405, 2009.

118. Knutsen G, Drogset JO, Engebretsen L et al: A randomized trial comparing autologous chondrocyte implantation with microfracture. Findings at five years, *J Bone Joint Surg Am* 89(10):2105-2112, 2007.

119. Steinwachs MR, Guggi T, Kreuz PC: Marrow stimulation techniques, *Injury* 39(Suppl 1):S26-31, 2008.

120. Brittberg M, Lindahl A, Nilsson A et al: Treatment of deep cartilage defects in the knee with autologous chondrocyte transplantation, *N Engl J Med* 331(14):889-895, 1994.

121. Marlovits S, Zeller P, Singer P et al: Cartilage repair: generations of autologous chondrocyte transplantation, *Eur J Radiol* 57(1):24-31, 2006.

122. van Osch GJ, Brittberg M, Dennis JE et al: Cartilage repair: past and future—Lessons for regenerative medicine, *J Cell Mol Med* 13(5):792-810, 2009.

123. Baragi VM, Renkiewicz RR, Qiu L et al: Transplantation of adenovirally transduced allogeneic chondrocytes into articular cartilage defects in vivo, *Osteoarthritis Cartilage* 5(4):275-282, 1997.

124. Goto H, Shuler FD, Lamsam C et al: Transfer of lacZ marker gene to the meniscus, *J Bone Joint Surg Am* 81(7):918-925, 1999.

125. Mason JM, Breitbart AS, Barcia M et al: Cartilage and bone regeneration using gene-enhanced tissue engineering, *Clin Orthop Relat Res* 379(Suppl):S171-178, 2000.

126. Hidaka C, Goodrich LR, Chen CT et al: Acceleration of cartilage repair by genetically modified chondrocytes over expressing bone morphogenetic protein-7, *J Orthop Res* 21(4):573-583, 2003.

127. Li Y, Tew SR, Russell AM et al: Transduction of passaged human articular chondrocytes with adenoviral, retroviral, and lentiviral vectors and the effects of enhanced expression of SOX9, *Tissue Eng* 10(3-4):575-584, 2004.

128. Shuler FD, Georgescu HI, Niyibizi C et al: Increased matrix synthesis following adenoviral transfer of a transforming growth factor beta1 gene into articular chondrocytes, *J Orthop Res* 18(4):585-592, 2000.

129. Sakaguchi Y, Sekiya I, Yagishita K, Muneta T: Comparison of human stem cells derived from various mesenchymal tissues: superiority of synovium as a cell source, *Arthritis Rheum* 52(8):2521-2529, 2005.

130. Vacanti CA, Paige KT, Kim WS et al: Experimental tracheal replacement using tissue-engineered cartilage, *J Pediatr Surg* 29(2):201-204; discussion 204-205, 1994.

131. Kamil SH, Vacanti MP, Aminuddin BS et al: Tissue engineering of a human sized and shaped auricle using a mold, *Laryngoscope* 114(5):867-870, 2004.

132. Puelacher WC, Mooney D, Langer R et al: Design of nasoseptal cartilage replacements synthesized from biodegradable polymers and chondrocytes, *Biomaterials* 15(10):774-778, 1994.

133. Puelacher WC, Wisser J, Vacanti CA et al: Temporomandibular joint disc replacement made by tissue-engineered growth of cartilage, *J Oral Maxillofac Surg* 52(11):1172-1177; discussion 1177-1178, 1994.

134. Ahmed N, Dreier R, Gopferich A et al: Soluble signalling factors derived from differentiated cartilage tissue affect chondrogenic differentiation of rat adult marrow stromal cells, *Cell Physiol Biochem* 20(5):665-678, 2007.

135. Hwang NS, Varghese S, Puleo C et al: Morphogenetic signals from chondrocytes promote chondrogenic and osteogenic differentiation of mesenchymal stem cells, *J Cell Physiol* 212(2):281-284, 2007.

136. Angele P, Schumann D, Angele M et al: Cyclic, mechanical compression enhances chondrogenesis of mesenchymal progenitor cells in tissue engineering scaffolds, *Biorheology* 41(3-4):335-346, 2004.

137. Steck E, Fischer J, Lorenz H et al: Mesenchymal stem cell differentiation in an experimental cartilage defect: restriction of hypertrophy to bone-close neocartilage, *Stem Cells Dev* 18(7):969-978, 2009.

138. Asanbaeva A, Masuda K, Thonar EJ et al: Mechanisms of cartilage growth: modulation of balance between proteoglycan and collagen in vitro using chondroitinase ABC, *Arthritis Rheum* 56(1):188-198, 2007.

139. McMahon LA, Reid AJ, Campbell VA, Prendergast PJ: Regulatory effects of mechanical strain on the chondrogenic differentiation of MSCs in a collagen-GAG scaffold: experimental and computational analysis, *Ann Biomed Eng* 36(2):185-194, 2008.

140. Terraciano V, Hwang N, Moroni L et al: Differential response of adult and embryonic mesenchymal progenitor cells to mechanical compression in hydrogels, *Stem Cells* 25(11):2730-2738, 2007.

141. Koga H, Muneta T, Ju YJ et al: Synovial stem cells are regionally specified according to local microenvironments after implantation for cartilage regeneration, *Stem Cells* 25(3):689-696, 2007.

142. Park H, Temenoff JS, Tabata Y et al: Injectable biodegradable hydrogel composites for rabbit marrow mesenchymal stem cell and growth factor delivery for cartilage tissue engineering, *Biomaterials* 28(21): 3217-3227, 2007.

143. Sharma B, Elisseeff JH: Engineering structurally organized cartilage and bone tissues, *Ann Biomed Eng* 32(1):148-159, 2004.

144. Cohen NP, Foster RJ, Mow VC: Composition and dynamics of articular cartilage: structure, function, and maintaining healthy state, *J Orthop Sports Phys Ther* 28(4):203-215, 1998.

145. Lumelsky NL: Commentary: engineering of tissue healing and regeneration, *Tissue Eng* 13(7):1393-1398, 2007.

Burns of the Head and Neck

Chapter 5

Nathan A. Kemalyan

Thermal injuries to the skin can be a significant threat to life and health and are the source of considerable long-term disability. The face, head, and neck are among the most highly valued body surface areas in terms of function, appearance, and the person's sense of self. This region conveys the special senses as well as our most important means of communication. It is the portal for nourishment and plays an important role in core body temperature regulation. It contains and protects the central nervous system and conveys the exchange of respiratory gases, and thus deep burns to the head and neck are immediately life-threatening. Burns to the face, in particular, can produce profound acute and chronic disability.

Burns to the face and neck seldom occur in isolation. They are most often part of a larger burn involving adjacent scalp, torso, and upper extremities. A serious burn to the face is among the accepted criteria for transfer of care to a burn center, where multidisciplinary patient-specific care can be delivered.[1]

The skin reacts to thermal injury in prototypical ways, irrespective of the body surface involved. The end common pathway of tissue loss in a deep burn is coagulation necrosis, followed by liquefaction as autolytic and bacterial enzymes separate non-viable tissue from the living margin of the wound. The depth of injury determines the ability of the skin to recover from it. However, skin varies considerably in thickness and density of epidermal appendages. The recovery of sensation and elasticity that is required to maintain full function of underlying motor units also varies according to burn location, so injuries of similar depth can have widely varying effects on the functional outcomes of different surfaces. The face, head, and neck contain several unique regions that confer a very complex set of functional demands on the skin. Skin thickness and elasticity vary widely, and some areas carry a high density of hair follicles. Motion of underlying bones, joints, and muscle units also varies widely. It follows that serious burns on the face, head, and neck exhibit a broad range of functional and cosmetic outcomes.

ETIOPATHOGENESIS AND CAUSATIVE FACTORS

All thermal injuries can be classified in terms of injury mechanism, burn depth (Fig. 5-1), and burn surface area. Hot water scalding mechanisms generally produce partial thickness burns, but may still lead to surgical skin replacement. Scalding with hot oil or other organic compounds often produces deeper burns requiring surgery.

Vapor flash incidents produce burns of varying depth (Fig. 5-2), and many will heal without requiring surgery. Gasoline flash burns (see Fig. 5-2, *B*) are generally deeper than other flash burns and often require skin grafting. Direct contact with flame (see Fig. 5-2, *C*) commonly produces deep burns that will require surgical management. Chemical and electrical burns (Fig. 5-3) vary widely in magnitude, depending on the specific agent and dosage of energy transfer to the tissue.

Appearance of burns varies widely and changes daily, making predictions of burn depth and behavior based on appearance hazardous. The mechanism of injury is more reliable in understanding the dosage of energy delivered. There are no widely accepted diagnostic imaging modalities that will improve on the accuracy of an experienced clinician who can synthesize injury mechanism, appearance, and host factors and then predict burn behavior and appropriate treatment.

The overriding factor that ultimately adversely affects the functional outcome of burn injuries on the head and neck is scar formation. All deeper burns heal with some degree of scarring. Thermal injuries have a unique capacity to produce proliferative, hypertrophic scars. Their formation is quite variable and influenced by inheritable predisposition, age, and burn depth. Additional complicating factors include infection, secondary breakdown of the healing wound, wound closure techniques, and other unknown influences. A hypertrophic scar confers much of the disability associated with burn injury, because it adversely affects durability, pliability, and appearance of the scar, and it prolongs pain and other discomforts.

Our innate inability to regenerate fully functional skin after a deep burn also results in reduced and altered sensation, leaving the host with impaired protective sensation. Loss of hair follicles affects appearance. Loss of sebaceous glands alters epidermal hydration and desquamation. Altered vasomotor control and the loss of sweat glands results in reduced local capacity to dissipate heat and regulate body temperature.

Partial thickness burns healing within 14 days will rarely leave significant functional or cosmetic impairment to the face. Burns healing between 14 and 21 days will often result in changes in texture and pigmentation, but generally do not produce significant scars. The deep partial thickness burn presents the most difficult dilemma to the surgeon. Burns requiring longer than 21 days to heal will always leave some degree of dermal scarring. The range of dysfunction can be very broad, ranging from subtle dermal tightening to horrific hypertrophic scarring resulting in gross functional and cosmetic impairments. Full thickness burns of any size affecting the face, head, and neck will require surgical management.

Burn surgeons generally agree that skin replacement on the face should follow facial cosmetic units (Fig. 5-4). A general rule of thumb favors replacement of a complete cosmetic unit if greater than 50% of that cosmetic unit is involved with deep burn. The exact borders of the burn will be unique to each patient, and there is no substitute for experience in making appropriate decisions that minimize the consequences of both the burn and surgical intervention to close the burn.

The natural history of a shallow flash or scald burn on the face may be complete in as little as 1 week. But if the burn is deep and the scar requires maturation, this period may extend well beyond a year.

27

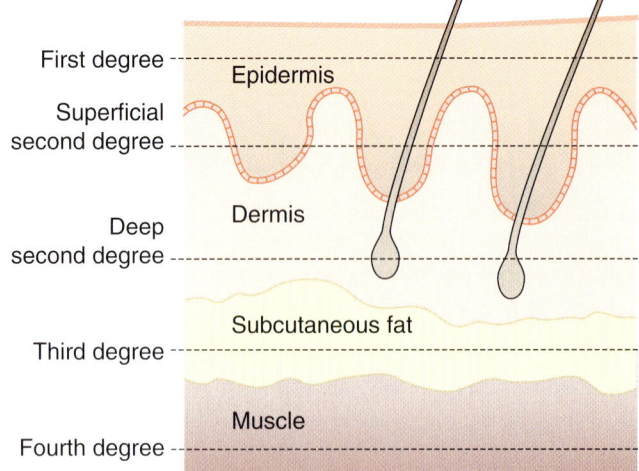

Fig. 5-1 ■ Depths of burn. (From Townsend CM, Beauchamp RD, Evers BM, Mattox K, editors: *Sabiston textbook of surgery*, ed 18, Philadelphia, 2008, Saunders.)

The deeper and larger the burn, the more significant the role of adjunctive measures to manage the consequences of scar. These modalities include active and passive range of motion exercises, manual manipulation of the scar, application of pressure, splinting to combat contracture of the neck, and application of silicone gel. In some cases, early reconstructive surgery in advance of full scar maturation is needed to intervene in severe functional deformities.

EARLY TREATMENT CONSIDERATIONS

The face has greater capacity to dissipate heat, and therefore better tolerance to burn injury, than other body parts. It is endowed with excellent blood flow and a high density of epidermal appendages from which to generate new epidermis. The burned face generates a more potent inflammatory response than similar sized burns elsewhere on the body. Even a shallow facial burn often results in the development of dramatic edema. This may result in temporary loss of eyelid excursion, as well as significant perioral edema affecting speech, eating, and swallowing. Deep burns to the face and neck can result in rapid compromise of the upper airway. Early control of the airway by endotracheal intubation is always a prudent step in the management of a significant burn to the face and neck (Fig. 5-5). Flame burns, vapor flash burns, electrical flash burns, and high-voltage electrical injuries frequently cause pharyngeal and hypopharyngeal edema and thus compromise the upper airway. Edema may result from direct thermal injury to those surfaces or occur secondarily from severe edema of the skin and subcutaneous tissue of the face and neck.

Burns rarely affect vascular circulation to and from the neck and head, except in the rare instance of a circumferential full thickness burn to the neck where escharotomy may be indicated. Burn edema peaks at about 48 hours after injury, after which the rate of resolution will vary according to the depth and breadth of the burn injury. Patients remain intubated until edema has peaked and is resolving, as indicated by air leakage around the endotracheal tube when the cuff is deflated. Patients may require prolonged intubation due to inhalation injury, magnitude of overall burn, or other co-morbidities. Positioning the patient at 30 to 45 degrees with the head up will assist in resolution of edema.

Corneal injury is frequent, but serious corneal injury is rare. Most corneal injuries heal spontaneously in the interval required for skin

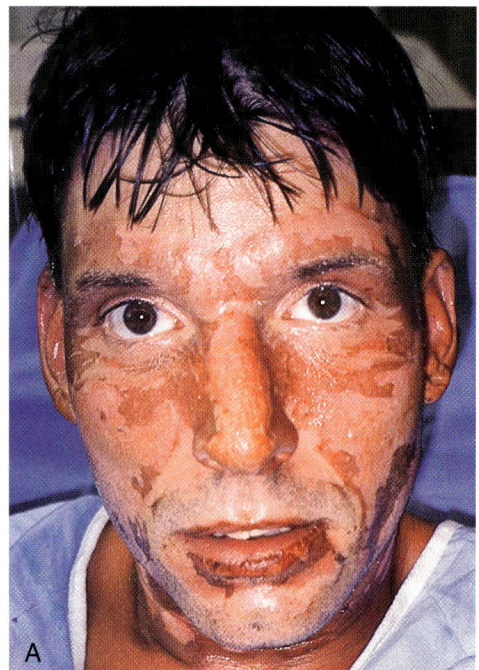

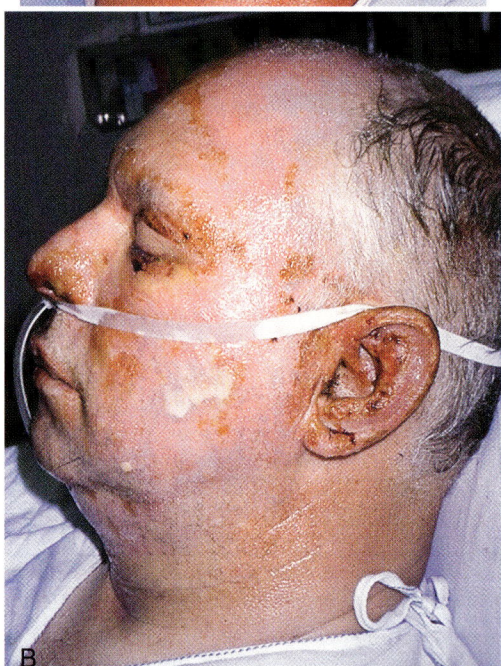

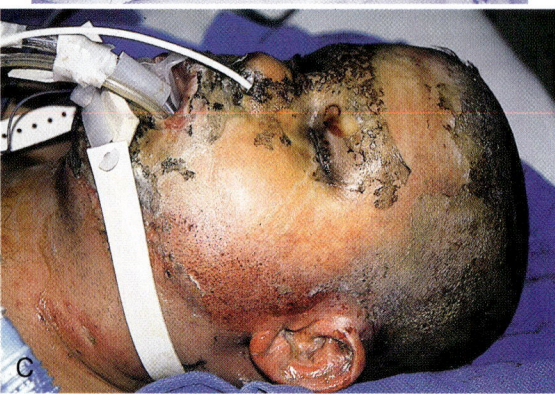

Fig. 5-2 ■ Partial-thickness burns. **A,** Flash burn from gas grill. **B,** Flash burn from throwing gas on a fire. **C,** Deeper partial thickness burn from a house fire. (From Ward Booth P, Eppley BL, Schmelzeisen R: *Maxillofacial trauma and esthetic facial reconstruction,* Edinburgh, 2003, Churchill Livingstone.)

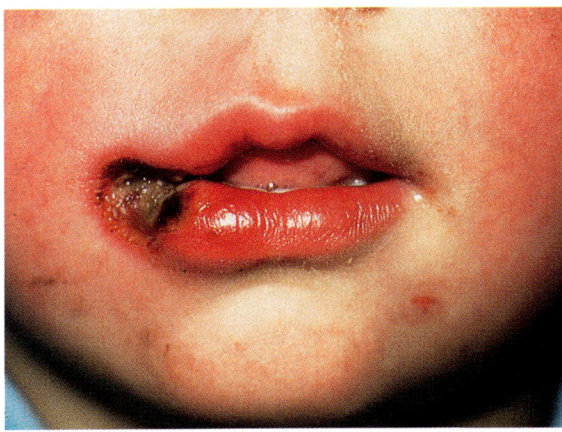

Fig. 5-3 ■ Electric burn. (From Ward Booth P, Eppley BL, Schmelzeisen R: *Maxillofacial trauma and esthetic facial reconstruction*, Edinburgh, 2003, Churchill Livingstone.)

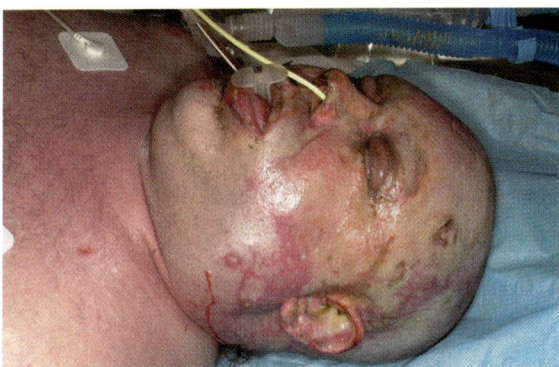

Fig. 5-5 ■ Deep partial thickness face burn, resulting in facial swelling requiring intubation for airway control. (From Monahan FD et al: *Phipps' medical-surgical nursing: health and illness perspectives*, ed 8, St Louis, 2007, Mosby.)

TOPICAL TREATMENT OF BURNS TO THE HEAD, FACE, AND NECK

Daily mechanical cleansing of the burn with a mild soap and tap water solution is a part of the care of every burn. The goal is to remove loose epidermis, dried coagulum, and degenerating eschar. The next task is to maintain a clean, moist, wound-healing environment under a topical antimicrobial agent or dressing. The choice of topical treatment depends on burn depth, location, and practitioner experience.

Shallow burns are adequately treated with petroleum jelly or a petrolatum-based antimicrobial agent, which should be applied with adequate frequency to maintain a glistening surface. These shallow injuries rarely become highly colonized or infected. No gauze dressing is generally required. Petrolatum or Xeroform gauze may be used if frequent application of ointment is not tolerated or is impractical. Deeper burns with attached eschar are better treated with gauze impregnated with topical antimicrobial agents to retain moisture and to mechanically debride the necrotic surface in the process of dressing changes. Silver sulfadiazine remains the most commonly applied topical agent in management of deeper burns. It is compatible with burns around the eyes, ears, and mouth because it is non-toxic to conjunctival and mucosal surfaces. Deep burns to the ear are at some risk of acute bacterial chondritis. They may be treated with topical mafenide acetate cream from the outset. Alternatively, topical mafenide acetate cream can be implemented as a part of the treatment of chondritis when it is recognized. Chondritis is rare and most patients heal adequately when treated with silver sulfadiazine cream, even with focal cartilage exposure. Silver sulfadiazine and mafenide acetate creams are both water based and perform best when held in place with gauze and changed twice daily.

A host of durable silver membranes, biologic skin substitutes, and alloplastic dressings have been developed that can be used to treat facial burns. These are best left to the burn specialist. Essentially all facial burns can be adequately treated with one of the three common topical agents just mentioned.

The scalp and hair-bearing regions of the face deserve special attention. Hair follicles of the male face and scalp are deeply situated, often projecting into the subcutaneous fat. Hair growth resumes well in advance of epidermal regeneration and can interfere significantly with wound hygiene by trapping eschar and coagulum onto the surface of the burn. Orderly healing is facilitated by carefully shaving the hair-bearing surface with generous lubricant and a single-edged razor, taking care to avoid "harvesting" the

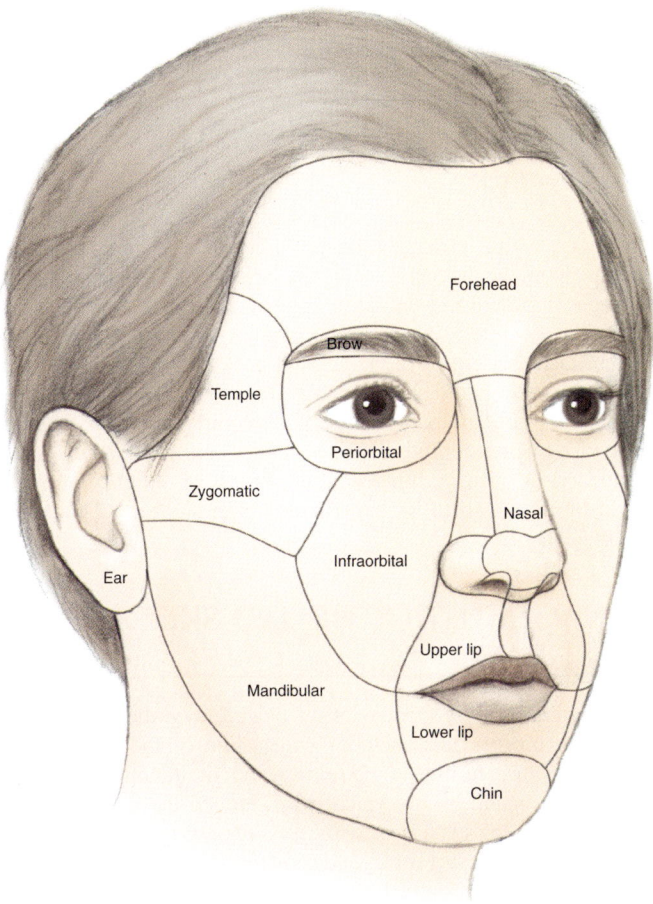

Fig. 5-4 ■ Facial cosmetic units. (From Baker SR: *Local flaps in facial reconstruction*, ed 2, Philadelphia, 2007, Mosby.)

healing. Patients with corneal opacification must have early ophthalmologic consultation and treatment to minimize the chance of permanent impairment in vision.

Early enteral feeding is the preferred method of nourishment in burn victims. This often requires placement of a nasoenteric feeding tube. Nasoenteric and endotracheal tubes are difficult to secure to the burned face, but the use of a nasal bridle and fixation of the orotracheal tube to the dentition can help with this problem.

regenerating epidermis in the process. Attempts at managing deep burns in the presence of intact hair can lead to chronic, painful, and difficult-to-manage wounds. Generally, hair will easily reemerge from the closed surface of a deeper dermal injury once the epidermis becomes stable.

If a deep dermal burn in hair-bearing skin produces hypertrophic scar, chronic and recurrent folliculitis often follows. For this reason, deep dermal burns in hair-bearing areas are sometimes better treated by full thickness excision and skin grafting, particularly when surrounding full thickness burn mandates grafting.

SURGICAL CARE OF THE BURNED FACE, HEAD, AND NECK

Once the decision for skin replacement has been made, excision and split-thickness skin grafting is the primary treatment in the acute setting. Smaller burns may occasionally be excised and primarily closed. The rare burn may be more amenable to composite tissue transfer, such as a free flap as a primary closure technique. Whenever possible, the burn should be grafted with color-matched skin harvested from adjacent areas of the neck or scalp. The scalp is an ideal donor site for many reasons. Hair is rarely transplanted with split thickness skin graft. The scalp donor site heals extraordinarily well, and subsequent hair growth obscures any minor texture of color variation at the donor site. There is considerable debate over details in the conduct of grafting the face and neck. Our practice follows the paradigm described in several publications from the University of Washington burn center. The excision is accompanied by temporary coverage with cryopreserved human allograft. After 5 to 7 days, the allograft is replaced by unmeshed autograft harvested from the color-matched donor site, usually the scalp. Great care is taken to achieve scrupulous hemostasis on the excised burn. The graft is fixed into place with fibrin glue, rapidly absorbing plain gut suture, tape strips, or a combination of these. The use of staples is minimized. Care is taken to place graft-graft junctions along natural lines in the face, or at boundaries of facial cosmetic units. Graft-graft junctions are placed perpendicular to commonly occurring lines of scar contracture if possible. Deep full thickness burns are preferentially covered with a dermal regeneration template such as Integra artificial skin (Integra LifeSciences Corp., Plainsboro, N.J.) (Fig. 5-6), then subsequently autografted to minimize the potential for serious hypertrophic scar and scar contracture. Skin grafts develop their first circulatory connections at 72 hours after placement, and circulation is well established by the fifth postoperative day. Early graft care is aimed at draining hematomas or seromas and avoiding disruption by shearing forces. Most skin grafts are tolerant of soap and water within 1 week.[2]

TRACHEOSTOMY

There are several reasons to consider tracheostomy in the burn victim. Severe burns to the face, head, and neck may be much more easily managed without the prolonged presence of an orotracheal tube. Patients with large body surface area burns, severe inhalation injury, or both will require prolonged ventilatory support. These individuals can undergo a safe, orderly emergence from the sedation and delirium that accompany critical care without concern for an unexpected loss of airway control. The complications of prolonged orotracheal intubation on the glottis can be avoided by early tracheostomy. This must be balanced against tracheostomy-associated complications such as tracheomalacia, tracheal stenosis, tracheal tethering, and other complications that occur with the surgical airway access.

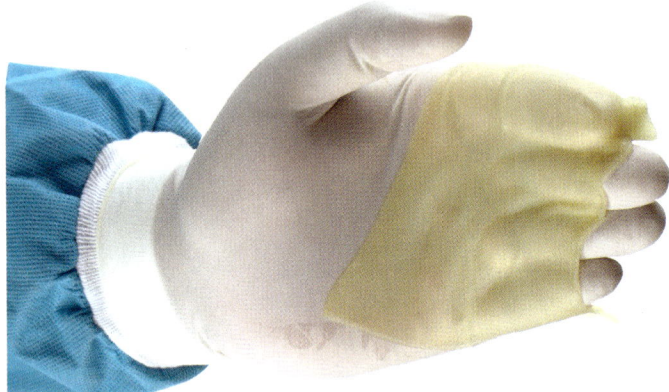

Fig. 5-6 ■ Integra artificial skin. (From Integra LifeSciences Corp., Plainsboro, N.J.)

Placement of a tracheostomy is not mandatory after severe burns to the face and neck but should be considered in patients requiring mechanical ventilation longer than 14 days; those requiring significant skin grafting to the face, head, and neck; and those with severe preexisting cardiopulmonary disease.[3]

Inhalation Injury

Severe burns to the face and neck are often associated with inhalation injury, which increases the mortality of any burn, increases time spent in the intensive care unit and the hospital, results in prolonged mechanical ventilation, and increases the need for tracheostomy. At times, severe inhalation injury interferes with timely surgical management of the facial and neck burn. Almost all burn victims who survive to skin closure will eventually become free of mechanical ventilation, but some will require prolonged maintenance of a tracheostomy because of the chronic sequelae of severe pulmonary or airway injury. Management of inhalation injury should be delegated to an experienced burn surgeon or intensive care specialist.

MANAGEMENT OF HEALED SKIN AND SKIN GRAFT

Deep burns, whether spontaneously healed or grafted, undergo a maturation process that includes contraction of the dermal scar. Scar contracture results in deformity and limitation in range of motion. This manifests in typical ways around the face and neck. Contracture of the eyelids or adjacent skin can result in ectropion and incomplete closure of eyelids, increasing the risk of corneal exposure keratitis. Contracture around the nasal ala can produce alar stenosis or fixed alar flaring. Oral microstomia and limited mandibular excursion occur frequently after grafting the mid and lower face. Confluent burns to the anterior neck require sustained splinting and active range of motion exercises for many months to avoid flexion contracture of the neck. Maintenance of the submental angle requires concerted effort by the patient and burn therapist. Secondary scar release and grafting or more advanced reconstructive adjuncts are often needed. Healed burns, donor sites, and skin grafts should be protected from the ultraviolet rays of the sun until pigmentation has returned to normal. Failure to do so may result in durable hyperpigmentation of injured surfaces. Grafted surfaces require exogenous treatment with emollients because intrinsic lubrication is not possible after loss of sebaceous gland function.

Partial thickness burns with preserved deep dermal sebaceous and sweat glands will grow a crop of microblisters and sebaceous collections until the ducts of these glands reemerge and drain on the skin surface.

It is now possible to construct very close tolerance facial orthoses to exert pressure on facial scars and maintain a position of adequate neck extension. Maturity of facial scars and skin grafts is reached at roughly 1 year after the injury.

RECONSTRUCTIVE CONSIDERATIONS

Cosmetic reconstructive surgery of the burned face is generally withheld until scar maturity has been reached, but functional reconstructive surgery must often precede this stage. Progressive contracture in spite of optimal splinting and therapy may necessitate early intervention. Corneal exposure keratitis, severe microstomia, oral incompetence, and severe progressive neck contracture may all mandate release of immature scar to preserve function even as the scar continues to mature.

Focal hypertrophic scar can often be treated by simple excision and closure. Simple contractures often respond quite favorably to Z-plasty or simple local rotation flaps formed with skin and subcutaneous tissue. Complex burn reconstruction requires all of the skills of a plastic and reconstructive surgeon. Skin expansion, full thickness skin grafting over a large surface area, and composite tissue transfer are often required for the most complex of face and neck reconstructions.

PEARLS AND PITFALLS

- Failure to recognize the potential for airway compromise can lead to patient mortality. When in doubt, one should err on the side of controlling the airway.
- One notable exception is the nasal cannula fire in the oxygen-dependent smoker. These small burns rarely compromise the airway or result in acute deterioration in gas exchange. Intubation may lead to prolonged ventilator dependence, so cautious observation is usually the treatment of choice for this injury.
- Failure to choose skin replacement in a deep partial thickness burn may have profound consequences caused by disfiguring scars. The decision for skin grafting for the face and neck is generally beyond the experience of the practitioner who only occasionally treats burns. For this reason, deep burns to the head, face, and neck are primary indications for referral to a regional burn center.

REFERENCES

1. Carter JE, Neff LP, Holmes JH: Adherence to burn center referral criteria: are patients appropriately being referred? *J Burn Care Res* Jan-Feb;31(1):26-30, 2010.

2. Friedstat JS, Klein MB: Acute management of facial burns, *Clin Plast Surg* Oct;36(4):653-660, 2009.

3. Cochran A: Inhalation injury and endotracheal intubation, *J Burn Care Res* Jan-Feb;30(1):190-191, 2009.

Chapter **6**

Endoscopic Oral and Maxillofacial Surgery

Joseph P. McCain, King Kim

Taking into account the advantages of minimally invasive surgery, such as decreased morbidity, improved visualization and surgical precision, use as adjunctive teaching aid, and accurate documentation, endoscopy techniques have further progressed through scientific advancements. Apparent disadvantages, such as technique sensitivity and need for specialized training, have been improved. Scientific development includes enhancing various types of endoscopes, optics of endoscopic systems, and documentation of procedures.

The types of basic rigid arthroscopic optical systems include the rod-lens system by H.H. Hopkins of Reading, England, and the graded refractory index lens system (GRIN) by Nippon Sheet Glass Company, Osaka, Japan. Optical characteristics are composed of field of view and direction of view. Field of view is the angle drawn from the arthroscope tip to the extreme edge of field or object. Because the arthroscope is in a fluid medium, the field of view angle is approximately 40% less than when measured in air. The direction of view is the angle projected between the normal axis of the arthroscope and a line through the center of the image viewed through the arthroscope.

Optical parameters include the stigmatism of image, which is whether a point in the field is focused as a point in the apparent field. Also, distortion, which is a straight line in the object, is not necessarily reproduced as a straight line in the image. Chronic correction is the displacement of image axially as a function of wavelength or color, and the image may be different sizes as a function of color. Moreover, vignetting is the defect due to optical design, construction, or misalignment, which is caused by bending or displacement of the optical elements. Transmission is when each surface reflects some fraction of the light falling upon it, and each element has some absorption. Veiling glare is the image-forming light reflected by each surface that is in turn re-reflected in part by all surfaces preceding it in the system.

Documentation with photography and video adjuncts have made a major impact in allowing minimally invasive and endoscopic surgical techniques to evolve at an amazing rate. Consequently, oral and maxillofacial surgery has transcended the traditional surgical methods by incorporating endoscopic techniques as a pillar in future considerations and advancement.

SIALOENDOSCOPY

The modern era of diagnosis of conditions involving salivary glands and their treatment starts with Charpy and Poirier in 1904, who performed the first sialographies with mercury, and Arcelin, who used bismuth in 1912 for the same procedure. Herman Kuttner (1870-1932), however, is credited with the most advancements in the development of anatomy, imagery, and surgery of salivary glands.

IMAGERY

The multifactorial scope of imaging in the diagnosis and management of salivary gland obstruction consists of the confirmation of the clinical diagnosis of obstruction, exclusion of salivary gland pathology unrelated to obstruction (inflammatory and autoimmune conditions or tumors), differential diagnosis of obstruction (calculus, mucous plug, or stenosis), suitability for minimally invasive treatment, procedure planning, and monitoring of postoperative progress. Although plain film imaging (Fig. 6-1, *A* and *B*), sialography (Fig. 6-1, *C* and *D*), ultrasound, and scintigraphy contribute to the diagnosis and planning of surgical procedures, from the endoscopist's perspective, computed tomography (CT) (Fig. 6-1, *E*) and magnetic resonance imaging (MRI) are the most relevant.

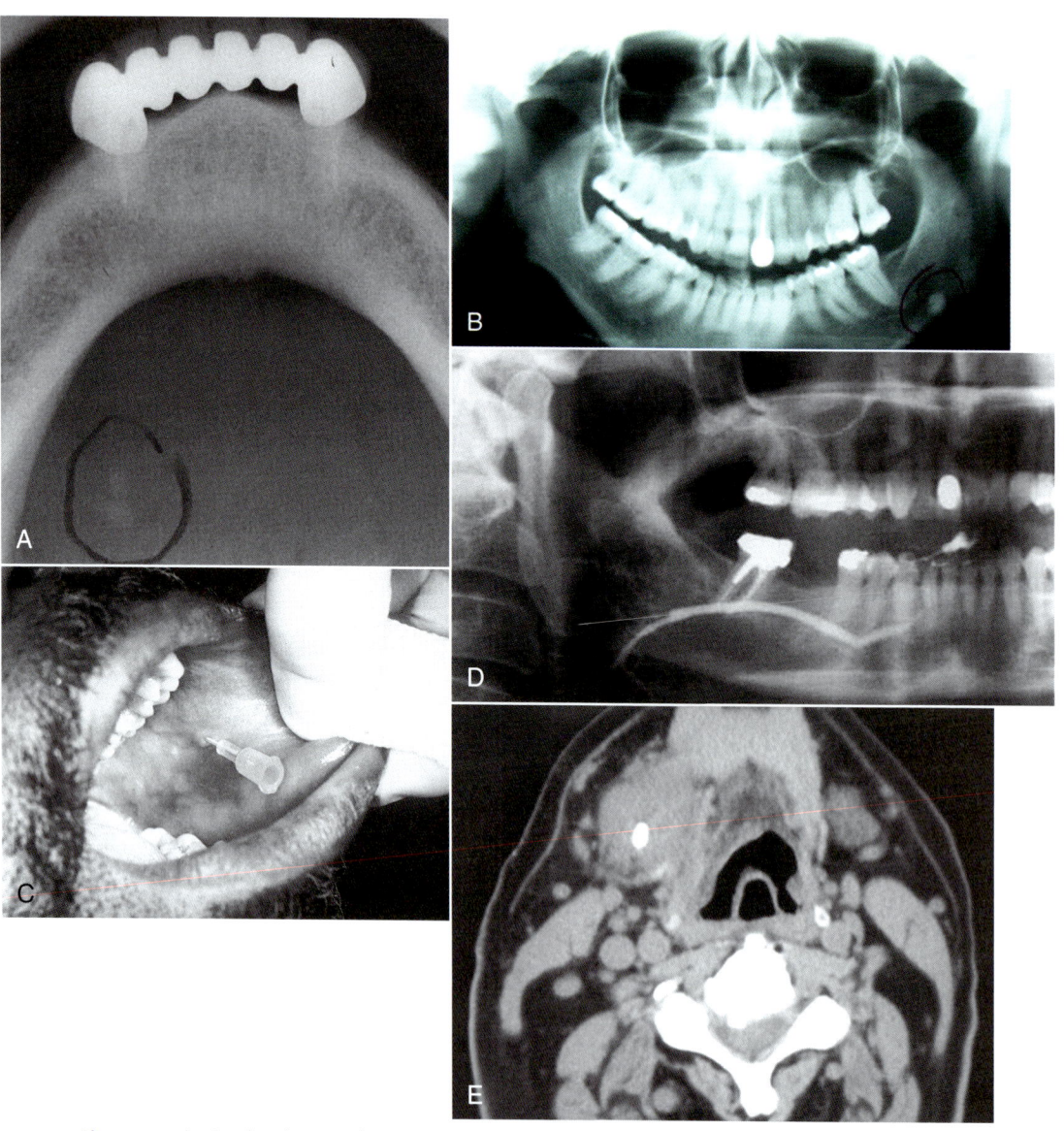

Fig. 6-1 ▪ **A,** Occlusal view of stone on the right floor of the mouth. **B,** Panoramic radiograph of left submandibular sialolith (circumscribed in red marker). **C,** Angiocatheter for administration of contrast substance presialography. **D,** Sialogram of the right submandibular duct. **E,** Axial facial CT of sialolith in the right submandibular duct. (**C,** From Hupp JR, Ellis EE, Tucker MR: *Contemporary oral and maxillofacial surgery,* ed 5, St. Louis, 2008, Mosby.)

SALIVARY CALCULUS (SIALOLITH OR STONE)

LOCATION AND NUMBER

Because most cases of sialadenitis have an obstructive etiology and most obstructions are caused by sialoliths, it is only natural to put more emphasis on the salivary calculus. Statistics show that between 63% and 94% of sialoliths occur in the submandibular gland. Within the submandibular gland, 9% of calculi are found in the gland parenchyma, 90% are in the duct, 60% are located in the hilum, and 30% are in the distal duct. In the parotid gland, 23% of stones are found in the parenchymal system, 13% in the hilum, and 64% in the ductal system. Multiple stones occur in 7% of parotid and 13% in submandibular sialolithiasis. Approximately 5% of patients will present with three or more stones. Parotid sialoliths are smaller, and in most cases, there is more than one. Average stone size in the parotid is between 6 and 8 mm; submandibular stones are slightly larger.

STRUCTURE AND COMPOSITION OF SIALOLITHS

As submandibular glands produce mostly mucous secretions, so the submandibular calculi are 8% inorganic and 94% radiopaque, hence denser and more calcium rich. The parotid gland, on the other hand, has a predominantly serous secretion. Therefore the parotid sialoliths are only 50% inorganic and only 43% radiopaque; they tend to be less dense and less calcium rich. The main minerals present in stones are calcium phosphate and carbonate in the form of hydroxyapatite, with various amounts of whitlockite in submandibular calculi and octacalcium phosphate in parotid calculi. The organic matrix of the sialolith represents 12% of the weight, 5% originating in insoluble proteins and 1% in lipids.

PATHOPHYSIOLOGY

Though the exact cause of sialolithiasis remains somewhat elusive, there are a number of plausible theories, but none have been fully substantiated.

Mechanical Theory

Intermittent stasis secondary to hyposecretion, dehydration, strictures, convolutions, diverticuli, and other possible causes produces a shift in the mucoid element of saliva (hyperviscosity), forming a pseudogel. This gel provides the framework for deposition of salt and organic substances, eventually resulting in a stone.

Metabolic Theory and Phenomenon

Statherin, a calcium-binding protein, prevents primary precipitation of calcium phosphate in solution. Its presence creates a supersaturation of saliva with calcium and phosphate. Increases in the salivary bicarbonate level alter the calcium phosphate solubility and cause the precipitation of calcium and phosphate ions, triggering the calculus formation cascade. Acidic proline-rich proteins reduce secondary precipitation onto hard tissues. Hence a deficit of crystallization inhibitors will also contribute to or accelerate the phenomenon.

Inflammatory Theory

Bacterial ascent into the gland parenchyma causes an acute or chronic inflammatory response. The gland manifests a histologic pattern of chronic inflammation, resulting in hyposecretion or abnormal secretion of saliva and decreased salivary flow. Over time the condition becomes refractory to medical management.

RETURN TO FUNCTION

Secretory function needs to be reestablished as soon as possible to restore viability of the gland. Absence or decreased secretory function will lead to recurrence of inflammation, mucous plug formation, or calculus formation. Human and animal studies have showed that glandular tissue secretory function can be regained even after extensive periods of obstruction and even atrophy. Restitutio ad integrum takes longer for the duct than for the gland. Full functional recovery takes between 6 and 24 months.

HISTORY OF SIALOENDOSCOPY

Sialoendoscopy is a rather recent development of the oral and maxillofacial surgery and otorhinolaryngology specialties. It started in 1990 when Konigsberger and then Gundlach performed the first successful endoscopy-assisted intracorporeal lithotripsy of sialoliths. Immediately afterward in 1991 Katz used a 0.8-mm flexible endoscope for the diagnosis of sialolithiasis as well as mechanical removal of calculi from the major salivary glands. In 1994 Arzoz introduced a 2.1-mm miniurethroscope with a working channel of 1 mm for use as an intracorporeal pneumoballistic lithotripter to fragment the calculus. Nahlieli published his 3-year experience with these techniques in 1997. In 2000 Marchal also reported on sialoendoscopic techniques. In 2001 Zenk reported his initial experiences with a new and highly flexible semirigid sialoendoscope with high quality imaging (6000 pixels). It had an external diameter of 1.1 mm and a working channel of 0.4 mm. In 2004 and 2006 Nahlieli and Nazarian published results of endoscopic treatment of juvenile and chronic recurrent parotitis, and radioactive iodine sialadenitis. Koch, in 2005, presented his experience with the treatment of idiopathic sialadenomegaly. McCain and Troulis published results of the first multicenter comprehensive study of these techniques in the United States in 2007.

INDICATIONS FOR PROCEDURE

Sialoendoscopy fully justifies the coming of age of the endoscopic subspecialties and presents the same tremendous versatility. It is an excellent diagnostic technique for ductal and parenchymal strictures, occlusions, convolutions, and recurrent episodes of idiopathic sialadenomegaly. Interventional sialoendoscopy is an invaluable aid in the sialolithotomy of ductal calculi less than 6 mm in diameter, located as far as the gland hilum. It is also very useful for therapeutic submandibular or parotid lavage. The technique permits endoscopic examination of the ductal system immediately postsialolithotomy from the middle part of the ducts. And lastly, it can be used to successfully manage recurrent pathologic conditions in children.

ARMAMENTARIUM

- **Conic dilators.** The dilators have been specifically designed to gently dilate the papilla without hemorrhage or trauma.
- **Salivary probes.** The probes are available in 12 sizes. The apex design permits atraumatic use of the instrument. The probes have a constant diameter along the working length. Manipulation should be gentle, limiting deep insertion and preventing ductal perforation and movements along false paths (Fig. 6-2, *A*).
- **Hollow rigid bougies.** The bougies allow blind dilation of gross stenosis of the main duct. The guide wire is inserted first under endoscopic control, traversing the stenotic process, and then the sialoendoscope is removed after marking the distance to the

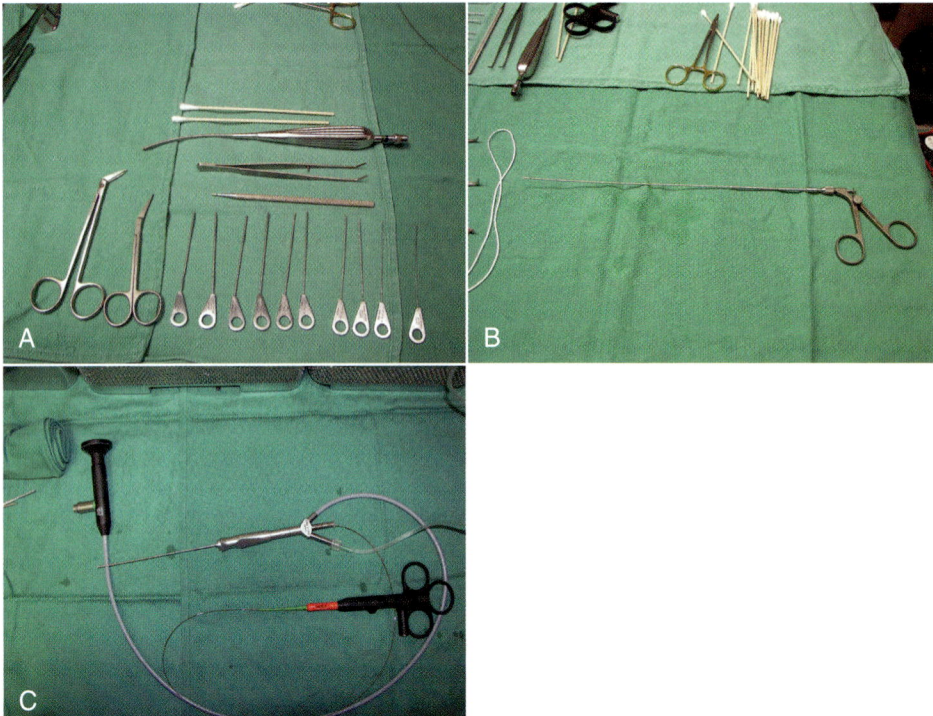

Fig. 6-2 ■ **A,** Part of the sialoendoscopy armamentarium setup: 10 calibrated Marchal salivary probes (#0000-#6), angulated tenotomy scissors, papillotomy scissors, bougie, small Andrews suction-tip, and Q-tips. **B,** Endoscopic forceps. **C,** Holmium laser fiber protruding from the distal end of a Storz-Marchal cannula.

stenosis. The bougies are then inserted sequentially in increasing diameters.

- **Forceps.** This instrument measures 0.8 mm and can be used to retrieve small calculus fragments or to harvest biopsies in the ductal system (Fig. 6-2, *B*).
- **Stone retrieval baskets.** The baskets are available in three sizes, with three, four, or six wires each. Consistent with their denomination, they are used to engage and capture the stone for retrieval or deliver it close to the caruncula, where a papillotomy will facilitate retrieval.
- **Sialoendoscopes.** There are a variety of sialoendoscopes on the market, conveniently classified in two categories: multipurpose and all-in-one. In these authors' experience, the current workhorse of sialoendoscopy is the Storz-Marchal 1.3 mm Universal, because it facilitates the diagnostic and interventional procedures on both Wharton and Stensen ducts. It is a three-channel endoscope with a working channel of 0.6 mm that permits advancement of both baskets and laser fibers (Fig. 6-2, *C*). It prevents insertion of balloon dilators or forceps.

SIALOENDOSCOPE PORTS OF ENTRY

The natural access to the salivary ducts is the *puncta salivaria* (Fig. 6-3), found in most instances at the center of the caruncula or papilla. They will require, in the majority of instances, dilation with lachrymal or ductal probes before insertion of the endoscope. Sometimes dilation of the punctum is impossible by conventional means, and a papillotomy with a CO_2 laser is performed immediately posterior to the orifice. If the papillotomy fails, then surgical dissection and exposure of the anterior portion of the duct via microsurgical technique together with longitudinal incision will facilitate the intraluminal insertion of the scope. Finally, if the stone is somewhat

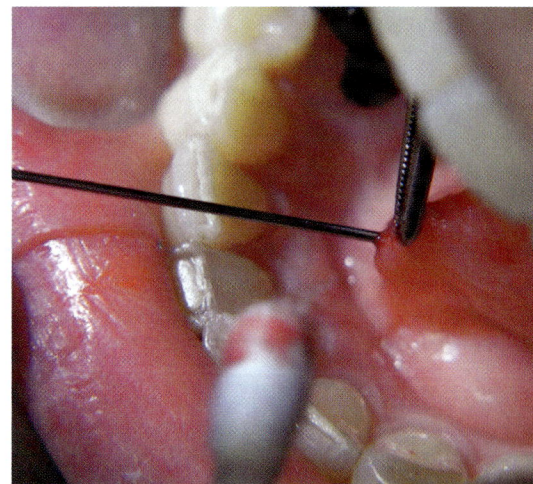

Fig. 6-3 ■ Cannulation of duct through the punctum, at the sublingual caruncula.

visible and palpable, a sialolithotomy incision will permit the intraluminal advancement of the endoscope after calculus retrieval.

This initial step of the procedure is by no means simple. The authors have had numerous opportunities to identify the factors contributing to difficult or unsuccessful duct dilation. Caruncula inflammation, papilla stenosis or calcification, previous gland and/or duct surgery with de novo or pseudoduct opening, preoperative administration of astringents or antisialagogues (parasympathomimetic medications), ductal orifice sphincter spasm, duct stenosis or fibrosis, abnormal duct convolutions, and duct occlusion or obstruction are all factors that can make ductal access and dilation practically impossible.

Ancient Roman wisdom states, "Errare humanum est. Perseverare diabolicum." The free English translation is, "It is human to make mistakes. However, to persevere in the same mistake is diabolical." Duct dilation and catheterization can be extremely frustrating at times. The surgeon has to patiently persevere in his attempts to find the punctum, and then dilate the duct, to the point of becoming diabolical. There is a steep learning curve in acquiring salivary duct stenting skills.

SURGICAL TECHNIQUE

The surgical procedure can be performed with local anesthesia; however, for both patient and surgeon comfort, it should be done with general anesthesia. With the patient in a dorsal supine reflex position, general anesthesia is achieved via nasoendotracheal intubation. The surgeon should inform the anesthesia team that the patient is **NOT** to be given any parasympathomimetic drugs to prevent the antisialagogue effect associated with atropine, glycopyrrolate, and other drugs in this category. In our experience, general anesthetics potentiate hyposalivation even without the administration of such drugs. At this time, we are testing various general anesthesia techniques to rule out the medications with undesired effects toward the procedure, and to identify the ideal general anesthesia.

To expose the caruncula sublingualis, the ventral surface of the tongue must be elevated toward the palate. This can be performed by conventional retraction or by placement of one or two 2-0 silk sutures paramedian through the lingual apex. The papilla is very gently manipulated and instrumented. Our preference is to apprehend with dental pick-ups ("cotton pliers"). No suction should be applied to the papilla, rather saliva should be blotted with Q-tips. After locating the punctum, progressive dilation of the duct is performed with salivary probes of increasing diameter. We favor the calibrated Marchal salivary probes. A duct dilated to a size #3 or #4 probe should accommodate the Storz-Marchal 1.3-mm scope. The scope is then advanced as far proximally into the duct as permitted (to the obstruction or into the gland hilum) (Fig. 6-4, *A*).

Notwithstanding the apparent simplicity and straightforwardness of the technique, extensive elaborative remarks could be made on the subject. The paramount summation is that sialoendoscopy, whether diagnostic or interventional, adheres to the basic principles of endoscopy, where the optical cavity is maintained with closed system irrigation and the navigation is facilitated by duct straightening. The alignment of the duct over the cannula is a "pull-out" maneuver similar to the apprehension of the caruncula with angled pick-ups (see Fig. 6-3) to facilitate dilator insertion.

The versatility of this procedure cannot be overemphasized. Calculi of small diameter can be grasped with forceps, wire baskets (Fig. 6-4, *B*), or graspers, instruments that are manipulated through the working cannula of the endoscope. The obstructive mucous plug or sialolith can be dislodged by gentle retraction and removal of the endoscope. In many situations (calculus of diameter >6 mm) a papillotomy will be necessary for retrieval, because the orifice sphincter will not dilate past 3 to 4 mm in most cases. If the sialolith is too large to be advanced distally toward the duct emergence, it can be morcelized with forceps, then fragments can be removed under irrigation. This particular approach has become quite popular for fixed or impacted calculi. Another approach that we particularly favor is fragmentation of calculi with the holmium laser before removal (Fig. 6-4, *C*). The technique can also be combined with intracorporeal and extracorporeal lithotripsy.

Duct stenting is performed at the end of most sialoendoscopies (invasive or noninvasive) and sialoendoscopically assisted surgeries on salivary glands or ducts. The preferred method is to use 4-0/5-0

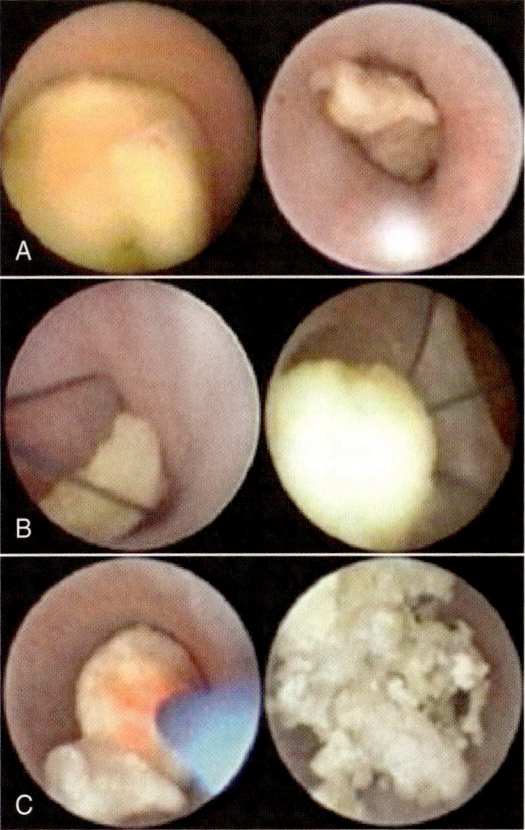

Fig. 6-4 ■ **A,** Endoscopic view of duct with obstructive salivary stones (round and irregular). **B,** Basket retrieval of stone. **C,** Fragmentation of large stone with holmium laser. (From Al-Abri R, Marchal F: Sialendoscopy in the old patients: a new tool or a revolution? *Eur Geriatric Med* 1(2):95-98, 2010.)

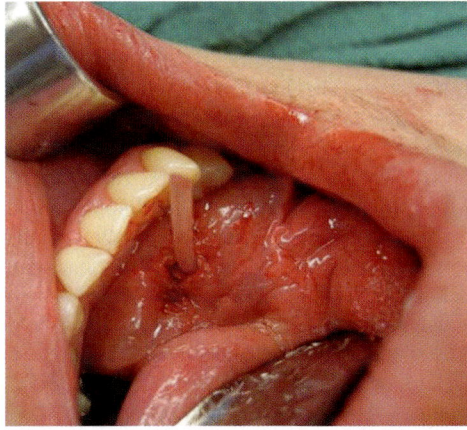

Fig. 6-5 ■ Stenting of duct at the end of surgery.

proline or other nonresorbable suture to secure a polyethylene tube fashioned out of a butterfly catheter at the papilla, de novo orifice, or duct opening (Fig. 6-5). The stent will usually correct most unfavorable angles and convolutions of the Wharton duct around the lingual nerve and the mylohyoid muscle (one of the main causes of obstruction supporting the mechanical theory). It also prevents ductal lumen obstruction by postoperative edema. The stent facilitates physiologic lavage of calculus fragments by saliva. The longer the stent remains in place (the authors remove it at 4 weeks postoperative), the less likely it is that postoperative duct stenosis occurs.

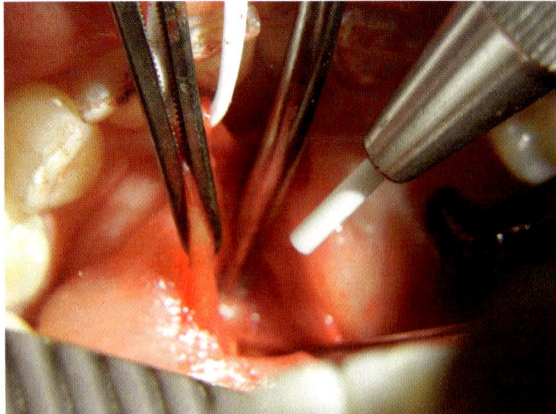

Fig. 6-6 ■ Sialoductoplasty (duct cut-down) with CO_2 laser.

Finally, it prevents the extravasation phenomenon (with subsequent ranula formation) and decreases the possibility of recurrence of sialolithiasis.

SURGICAL TECHNIQUE FOR ENDOSCOPIC INTRAORAL SIALOLITHOTOMY WITH OR WITHOUT SIALODUCTOPLASTY

As previously mentioned in this chapter, frequently the size of the stone will prevent endoscopic retrieval, notwithstanding capture of the sialolith with endoscopic basket or graspers. However, the sialoductoplasty (Fig. 6-6) becomes an easier, faster, and much more precise procedure. In other instances, the obstruction removal is not amenable to or fails pure endoscopic techniques, mostly because of a stenosed duct.

The first steps of the procedure are identical to the standard endoscopic approach. The endoscope is inserted in the duct to locate the obstruction, lavage, and dislodge the calculus from the ductal attachment, if present. The duct is then dissected and isolated from the surrounding tissues to the level of the first mandibular molar for the submandibular gland or the right angle deviation over the masseter for the parotid gland. Next, a longitudinal ductotomy with a CO_2 laser over a salivary probe or endoscope will expose the obstruction. The submandibular gland is impinged cranially, toward the oral cavity, with manual pressure from the submandibular region. With fine hemostats, the duct is extended anteriorly (with very light tension) at the same time. After the obstruction is removed, the proximal duct is explored endoscopically to rule out the presence of additional calculi or fragments, and the ductal system is lavaged as far as the hilum.

DISCUSSION

The authors' data are supported by 7 years' experience with sialo-endoscopy and sialoendoscopically assisted procedures at Miami Baptist Hospital. They feel that presenting a summary of results is extremely relevant for the implementation of these techniques.

Salivary duct dilation and navigation was performed in 100 out of 104 cases (97%). Sialolith retrieval or emulsification was successful in 64 out of 80 attempts (84%). Strictures or mucous plugs were managed in all attempted cases (100%). Ductal stenting was achieved in 77 out of 85 cases attempted (87%). In all, 87 out of 99 cases with chronic sialadenitis achieved symptomatic relief. At the time this chapter was written, 22 out of 104 cases were

deemed failures. Six patients underwent subsequent salivary gland removal (five submandibular and one parotid). Nine patients are asymptomatic and do not desire further intervention. One patient's symptoms resolved with de novo sialoendoscopy and sialolithotomy. Six patients were subsequently treated with transoral sialoductoplasty.

The average sialolith diameter in the cases deemed failures was 1.1 ± 0.4 cm, determined by preoperative CT or radiograph. Twenty-one percent of the ducts could not be explored to the hilum following removal of the obstruction, secondary to strictures and adhesions. In 15% of cases, some extravasation of the irrigating fluid elevated the floor of the mouth. No patients required emergency airway management. In 24% of situations the sialoendoscopy was aborted for the open procedure because the obstruction was not visible or could not be reached with the endoscope. Intraluminal navigation was restricted by convolutions, strictures, mucous plugs, and adhesions. In 27% of the cases, the duct emergence had to be opened via papillotomy with a No. 11 scalpel, both to cannulate the duct and to accommodate passage of large stones.

The authors have had an overall success rate of 28% for pure intraluminal stone retrieval without open intervention. In 62% of patients, open intervention was required and sharp and blunt dissection was used to enter the duct and remove the obstacle under direct vision. The sialolith was visualized near the hilum of the gland, but persistently rolled in and out of the gland, resulting in no stone retrieval by either method (intraluminal or open) in 10% of situations. One patient experienced a transient lingual nerve paresthesia. Another had to remain intubated overnight for observation secondary to extravasation phenomenon.

Although the learning curve is rather steep, endoscopic access to the salivary ductal system for management of sialolithiasis and strictures is feasible. Sialoendoscopy permits a minimally invasive surgical procedure that reduces the unnecessary removal of histologically functional glands and decreases the risk of facial nerve paresis.

CLINICAL ENDOSCOPIC OBSERVATIONS

The authors' clinical endoscopic experience and results concur with those of Nahlieli and Marchal. The following are a few pertinent facts that were apparent during sialoendoscopy that the authors continue to observe and research.

There has been debate over ductal peristalsis, mostly inspired by the spontaneous passage of rather large calculi before any therapeutic maneuvers. Peristalsis could force calculi out of the duct. But increased pressure caused by saliva accumulation proximal to the obstruction, secondary to intraparenchymal hypertension, could also be responsible for dislodging the sialolith from the duct. Possibly a combination of both mechanisms underlie spontaneous passage. However, the presence of smooth muscle fibers within the ductal wall, pseudosphincters beginning at the caruncula for the Wharton duct, respectively adjacent to the ramification inside the Stensen duct, has been documented.

The phenomenon of sialolith impaction was noted to occur distal to the bifurcation in the Wharton duct and masseteric curvature in the Stensen duct. It makes sense to postulate that in cases of long-standing ductal sialolith impaction, a ductal diverticulum will form, which makes calculus fragments or secondary calculi retrieval very difficult. Depending on the amount of muscle fibers in the ductal adventitia, this may not resolve after obstruction removal or disimpaction, or both. In one case of reentry sialoendoscopy, the sialolith was documented by imagery, located via endoscope, but found completely encased in the ductal wall. It was not retrieved because it was very close to the lingual nerve and also because duct stenting had reestablished patency and flow.

Rather infrequently found, with a 2:1 ratio in Stensen and Wharton ducts, ductal polyps obstruct salivary flow. Sialoendoscopy is the only consistent diagnostic method. Polyps may be removed or excised with forceps or baskets. The ratio for ductal strictures in Wharton and Stensen ducts is 2:1, and for convolutions, the ratio is 3.5:1. Other endoscopist-clinicians have mentioned highly infrequent occurrences, such as foreign bodies (hair or plant fragments) and anatomic malformations (hilar pseudopelvic malformation), that we have not yet encountered.

The Bartholin duct or sublingual duct is infrequently found emerging up to 5 mm distal to papilla, in the anterior portion of the Wharton duct. A consistent finding in chronic sialadenitis or long-standing sialolithiasis is the ecchymotic, angiopenic, and matted appearance of the ductal mucosa.

ENDOSCOPICALLY ASSISTED ORBITAL FLOOR FRACTURE REPAIR

ANATOMY ABBREVIATED

The human orbit is a quadrangular pyramid with the peak at the orbital apex, averaging a volume of 30 mL. in the adult, with the globe occupying 7 mL. Maintaining and restoring orbital volume is critical for globe position and visual acuity. The seven osseous components of the orbit are the maxilla, zygomatic, frontal, ethmoid (os planum), lacrimal, palatine, and sphenoid (Fig. 6-7). The maxilla, zygomatic, and palatine form the adult orbital floor. The orbital floor is the shortest of all the walls; 35 to 40 mm does not reach the orbital apex and terminates at the posterior margin of the maxillary sinus. The infraorbital sulcus, canal, and foramen are continuous and tunnel through the maxilla, encasing the terminal maxillary branch of the trigeminal nerve, the infraorbital artery, and infraorbital vein.

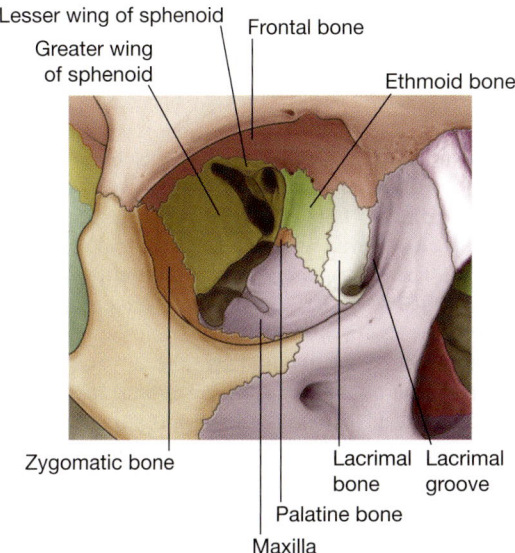

Fig. 6-7 ■ Orbital osseous components: frontal, sphenoid, ethmoid, lacrimal, maxilla, zygoma, and palate (nonlabeled, contained between os planum, maxilla, and sphenomaxillary and sphenoidal fissures). (From Drake R et al: *Gray's anatomy for students*, ed 2, 2010, Churchill Livingstone.)

Labels on Fig. 6-7: Lesser wing of sphenoid; Frontal bone; Greater wing of sphenoid; Ethmoid bone; Zygomatic bone; Lacrimal bone; Lacrimal groove; Palatine bone; Maxilla

MECHANISMS AND CONFIGURATION OF ORBITAL FLOOR FRACTURES

Fractures of the anterior and medial thirds of the orbital floor and medial wall are common because of their thin walls and lack of support. The increased intraorbital pressure is relieved by traumatic expansion of the walls with herniation of orbital contents into the maxillary sinus, the ethmoid air cells, or both.

Linear internal orbital fractures maintain periosteal attachments and rarely herniate orbital contents; however, they result in an increase in orbital volume, hypoglobus, and enophthalmos. Blow-out fractures are the most common. They are 2 cm or less in diameter and most often involve the anterior and medial floor (Fig. 6-8). These as well as the two-wall and complex fractures, or those extending to the posterior orbit, are amenable to pure endoscopic repair. However, the endoscopic-assisted open reduction and internal fixation (ORIF) remains the preferred method for the more complex fractures and those extending to the posterior orbit.

PRESENTATION OF ORBITAL FLOOR FRACTURES

The inherent problems with orbital floor fractures are hypoglobus, enophthalmos, diplopia (secondary to inferior rectus, orbital tissue entrapment, or both), restricted ocular range of motion, orbital emphysema (from communication with the maxillary sinus) (Fig. 6-9), orbital hemorrhage with the risk of compressive optic neuropathy, globe rupture, hyphema, retinal edema, decreased visual acuity, or even amaurosis.

SURGICAL TECHNIQUE

There are four classic approaches to the orbital floor: subciliary, transconjunctival, midtarsal, and transantral. In the traditional periorbital approaches, the posterior margin of the orbital floor defect is often difficult to visualize. The unassisted, conventional techniques require significant manipulation of the orbital tissues, result in inflammation, and increase the risk of ectropion or entropion. The transantral approach can be performed in a transmaxillary or transnasal fashion. These authors favor the transantral/transmaxillary approach.

With the patient under general anesthesia via oral endotracheal intubation, the forced duction test is performed. Access to the lateral antral wall is achieved via a modified Caldwell-Luc incision. The lateral antrostomy is performed next with the positioning of two

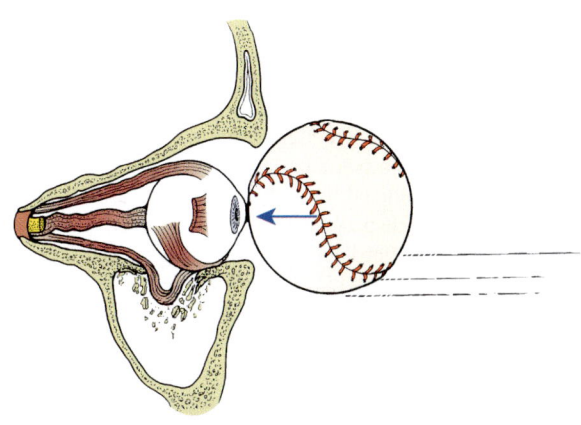

Fig. 6-8 ■ Blunt-force causing orbital blow-out fracture with some of the typical features: bony fragments and orbital contents sagging into the maxillary sinus below. (From Hupp JR, Ellis E, Tucker MR: *Contemporary oral and maxillofacial surgery*, ed 5, St. Louis, 2008, Mosby.)

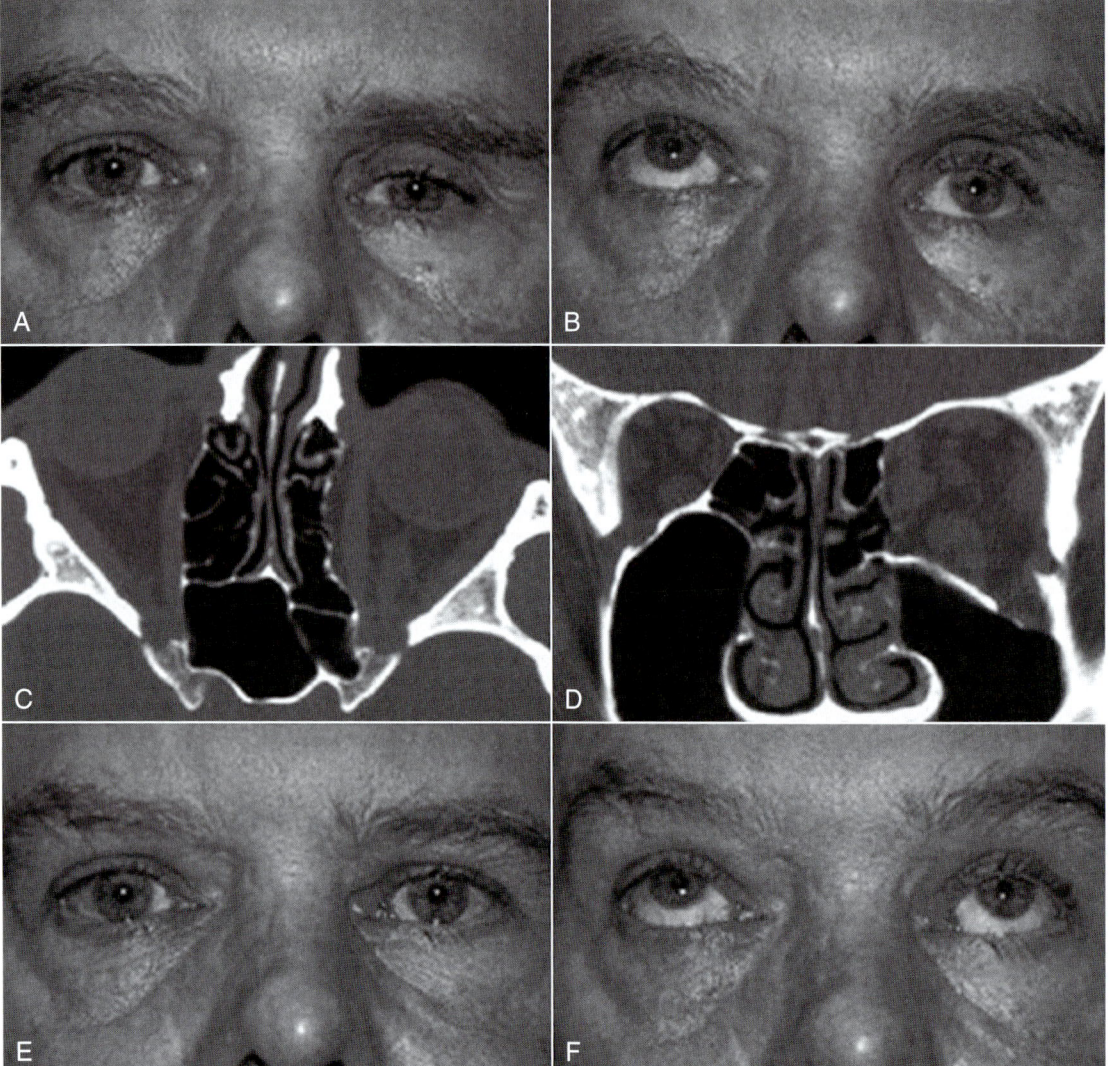

Fig. 6-9 ■ Orbital floor fracture signs. **A** and **B,** OS-hypoglobus/enophthalmos, restricted ocular ROM (upper gaze). **C,** Axial CT confirmation of the sphenoidal fracture and enophthalmos. **D,** Coronal CT confirming hypoglobus and inferior rectus entrapment (note the rounded shape of the muscle as opposed to flattened shape on the contralateral side). **E** and **F,** Postoperative restitutio ad integrum. (From Harris GJ: Orbital blow-out fractures: surgical timing and technique, *Eye* 20:1207-1212, 2006.)

portals, each 6 to 7 mm in diameter, with the posterior osteotomy at the buttress area (Fig. 6-10, *A*). The antrum acts as a natural optical cavity. A 30-degree endoscope, 4 mm in diameter (Karl Storz, Tuttlingen, Germany) with a xenon light source is preferred; however, a 0-, 45-, or 70-degree scope may also be used. The endoscope is inserted through one antrostomy (the vision portal), while instruments are manipulated through the working portal. The fracture site is visualized, inspected, then demucosalized. Each shelf is carefully dissected, and prolapsed orbital fat is repositioned cranially into the orbit. All margins of the fracture are identified (Fig. 6-10, *B* and *C*). All sharp osseous fragments are removed or conformed (Fig. 6-10, *D* and *E*). The fracture is reduced and de novo forced duction testing is performed. Pulse testing is performed under endoscopic vision. Care is taken when manipulating the intraorbital contents from the antrum to avoid impingement of the musculature, periorbita, and optic nerve. The infraorbital nerve and inferior rectus muscle are identified. For the operative situations where orbital contents continue to herniate and the orbital volume requires additional support, a Silastic implant is trimmed, adapted, and stabilized

on the orbital floor (Fig. 6-10, *F* to *I*) so that both orbital volume and ocular globe function are restored. The forced duction and pulse tests are repeated under transantral endoscope inspection. The incision is usually closed with a tight water seal and resorbable interrupted sutures. The postoperative CT will confirm adequate floor position (Fig. 6-10, *J* and *K*). The patient receives sinus precaution instructions.

Based on the intraoperative findings, the surgeon is always prepared to access the orbital floor from a periorbital approach. Possibly one of the greatest advantages of the endoscopic approach is the ease of converting to an endoscopically assisted open approach should the necessity arise.

Some other advantages of endoscopic surgery are direct vision and evaluation of the surgical field, smaller incisions, precise reductions and repairs, and decreased postoperative morbidity, preventing the relatively high complication rate of the transcutaneous and transconjunctival approaches, including poor cosmesis. From the patient perspective, there is no question about the choice, because the advantages by far outweigh the disadvantages. The only

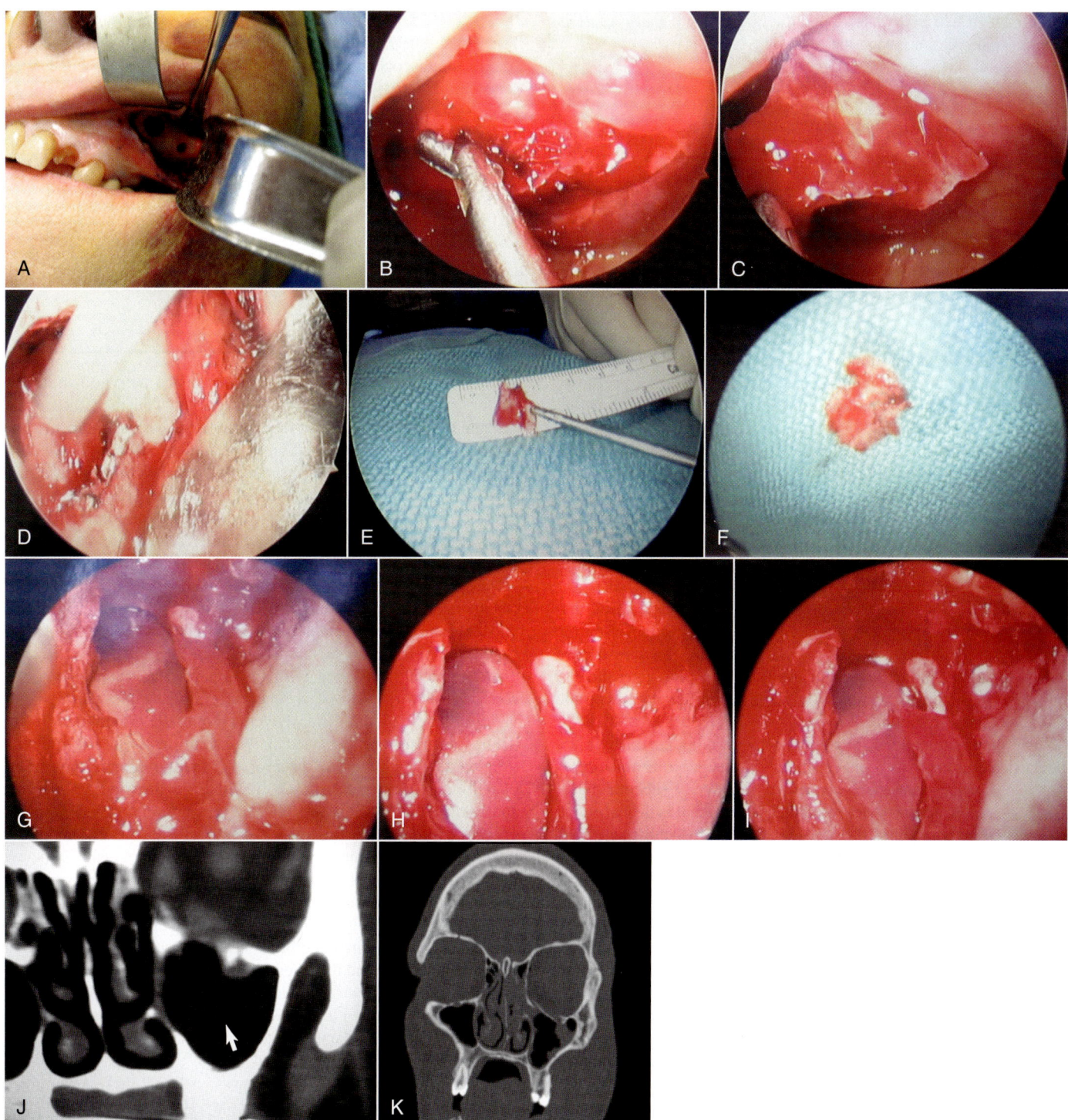

Fig. 6-10 ■ **A,** Exposure of the lateral maxillary sinus wall via modified Caldwell-Luc incision with double antrostomy, posterior portal at the malar buttress. **B** and **C,** Demucosalization and identification of the fracture defect margins. **D** and **E,** Removal of sharp osseous fragments. **F** to **I,** Silastic implant restoring orbital floor defect. **J,** Coronal CT confirming position of implant and orbital floor continuity and level correction. **K,** Postoperative coronal CT of ORIF OS-orbital floor fracture without implant.

disadvantages are increased surgery time, need for advanced surgical skills only achievable through a longer learning curve, and additional costs and manpower. In addition to those just mentioned, there are additional advantages of the endoscopic open reduction with implants for the orbital floor fractures. The displaced orbital floor acts as a scaffold for fracture reduction, maintained by the implant from the antral side. There is no additional intraorbital foreign body, preventing infraorbital interference with the ocular muscles and the infraorbital nerve. The reduction is purely anatomic. This is the only approach, giving the surgeon the ability to ascertain the forced duction test (via endoscope) from an inferosuperior perspective, thus observing the inferior rectus for entrapment or interference during movement. It carries low postoperative morbidity because there is minimal intervention inside the orbit.

ENDOSCOPICALLY ASSISTED OPEN REDUCTION INTERNAL FIXATION OF MANDIBLE CONDYLE FRACTURES

INDICATIONS AND CONTRAINDICATIONS

The topic of closed reduction (CR) versus ORIF of condylar fractures continues to be a subject of dispute between clinicians. The contributions of Zide and Kent to the treatment of this trauma resulted, in the mid 1980s, in development of the gold standard indications and contraindications for the open techniques. According to these authors, the absolute indications for ORIF are dislocation of the condyle into the middle cranial fossa, incorrect occlusion despite closed reduction and intermaxillary fixation (IMF), medial dislocation of condyle, and invasion by foreign body. Subsequently, the same authors have added a few relative indications supportive of ORIF, such as bilateral condylar fractures associated with comminuted fractures of the midface, B/L condyle fractures associated with post-traumatic apertognathia, medical contraindications for IMF (convulsion disorders or psychiatric disorders), B/L condylar fractures in edentulous patients, unilateral fractures without posterior occlusal stop, and loss of vertical dimension.

In a follow-up paper to his benchmark 1983 article, Zide discusses the current experience with condyle fractures, including the Zide/Kent sequence as well as the Haug/Assael "Open vs Closed Treatment of Mandibular Subcondylar Fractures." He states that the only two real indications for ORIF are condylar displacement and ramus height instability.

The contraindications for opening the mandibular condyle are pediatric condylar injury and comminuted intracapsular fractures.

As far as the technique is concerned, in cases of subcondylar or condylar neck fractures where the condyle fragment is displaced but without dislocation, the fractures can be reduced and fixated via intraoral approach assisted with an endoscope. In condylar neck fractures with medial dislocation (Fig. 6-11), endoscopic assisted reduction has proven to be very difficult by intraoral approach alone. A combined intraoral and extraoral approach would be indicated. Though two-plate fixation, adaptation plate fixation, and miniplate fixation have been used for ORIF, most authors agree that the single mini-dynamic compression plate is the most reliable, versatile, and consistent in performance, supported by a biomechanical assessment of performance.

ARMAMENTARIUM

The basic surgical armamentarium includes a 4-mm-diameter straight endoscope with a 30-degree optic lens illuminated by a xenon light source (Karl Storz, Tuttlingen, Germany) (Fig. 6-12), a video system, and a set for condylar fracture fixation system. The endoscope can be incorporated into a specifically designed tissue dissector or a modified posterior border retractor, part of the KLS or Synthes subcondylar fracture instrumentation that also includes the Snowden-Pencer suction tip elevator.

ENDOSCOPICALLY ASSISTED ORIF FOR NONDISLOCATED CONDYLAR FRACTURE

The intraoral mucosal incision is placed at the pterygomandibular raphe, on the anterior border of the ramus. The incision can be extended caudally to the vestibular mucosa corresponding to the mandibular first molar. Creation of an optical cavity follows. The subperiosteal dissection then exposes the lateral part of the mandibular ramus, posterior border, sigmoid notch, and gonial angle. The inferiorly inserting fibers of the temporalis are disconnected from the coronoid process. Next, a sigmoid notch retractor and a modified posterior border retractor are used to provide access for the endoscope and the plate fixation. The endoscope is inserted in the optical chamber, on the lateral aspect of the ramus, to verify the fracture line. Intermaxillary fixation in correct occlusion by means of arch bars is achieved next. The nondislocated or laterally dislocated condylar segment is reduced with instruments that each operator is comfortable with (Snowden-Pencer elevators, angled, straight, or various combinations). After the reduction of the proximal segment, the tip of the elevator is placed on the lateral surface of the fragment to temporarily stabilize its position. A titanium compression miniplate for condylar fixation will be adapted over the condylar segment and ramus (Fig. 6-13, *A* and *B*). The transoral endoscope provides good visibility of the fractured segment and the lower part of the plate. With endoscopic assistance, the condylar segment is fixated with one to three titanium screws via the transbuccal approach. The trocar will be inserted through a 3-mm stab incision in the tragal fold, inferior to the pinna. Precise anatomic reduction of the condylar segment over the mandibular ramus is achieved with a long periosteal elevator and modified condylar distracters. The fixation is then finalized with two to three titanium screws placed in a transbuccal (Fig. 6-13, *C*) or transoral location, using a right-angle screwdriver drill. The maxillary fixation is removed to check for occlusal

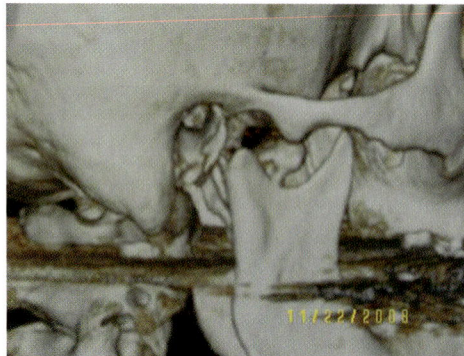

Fig. 6-11 ■ CT-based 3-D reconstruction presenting a right medially displaced subcondylar fracture.

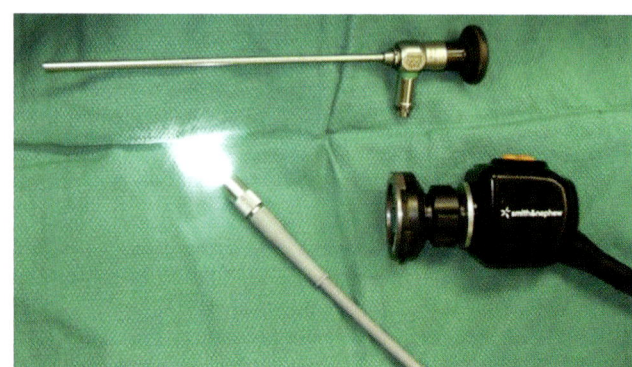

Fig. 6-12 ■ Storz endoscope with 30-degree lens.

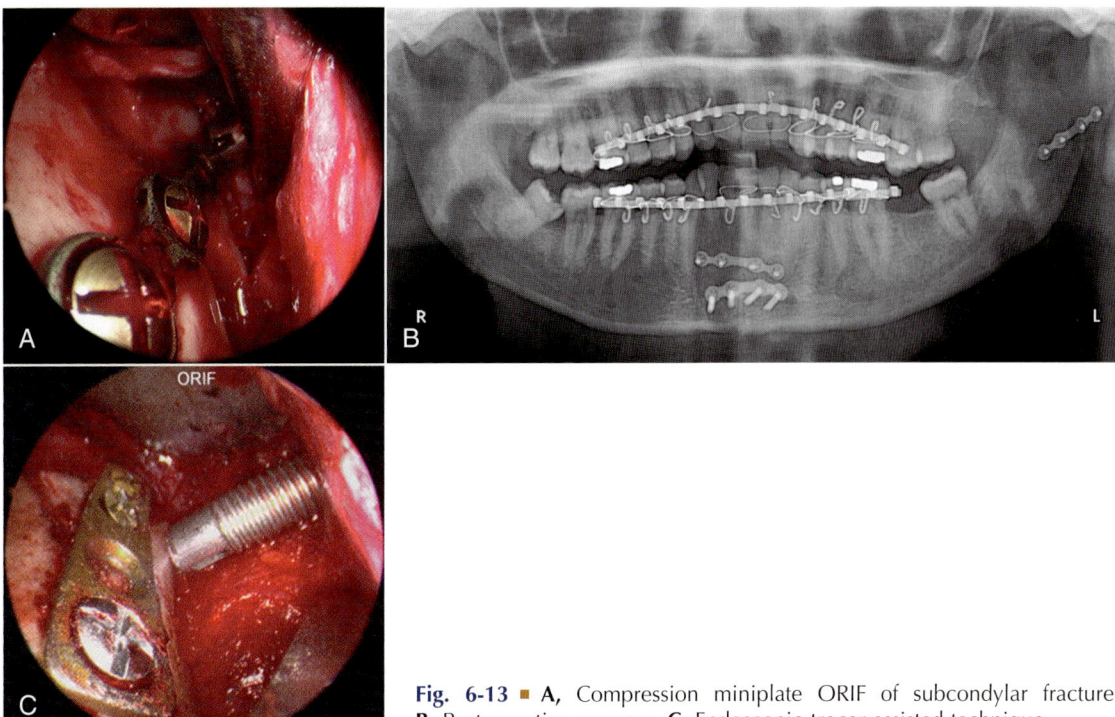

Fig. 6-13 ■ **A,** Compression miniplate ORIF of subcondylar fracture. **B,** Postoperative panorex. **C,** Endoscopic trocar-assisted technique.

shift. The surgical wound is closed primarily when a stable occlusion in retruded contact position is secured.

ENDOSCOPICALLY ASSISTED ORIF FOR DISLOCATED CONDYLAR FRACTURE

The condylar fracture medially dislocated is a contraindication for solely intraoral reduction. There are a variety of facial approaches to the condyle; however, the medially dislocated condylar fracture poses problems for all of them. The ramus fragment typically rises superiorly into the fossa and obscures the view of the dislocated fragment via the submandibular approach. Also, the length of the dissection from the tegument to the fracture site is significant enough to result in poor visibility even with additional light from the endoscope. On the other hand, the retromandibular approach confers good access to the condylar area because it is close to the fracture site. However, the necessary dissection of the marginal mandibular and buccal branches of the facial nerve from the parotid tissues increases the risk of damage to cranial nerve (CN) VII. The conventional preauricular approach leaves obvious facial scars. The next two techniques described are ones that have worked best at the hands of the authors.

The best access to the medially dislocated condyle is via the preauricular approach. Once the zygomatic arch and glenoid fossa are exposed by subperiosteal dissection, the displaced condyle can be mobilized back into the fossa with manipulation forceps. Reduction of the fracture is facilitated by forceful mouth opening to allow the fractured condylar head to be relocated in the fossa. The plate is adapted to the condylar segment and fixated with two to three screws. The endoscope is inserted intraorally and manipulated cranially to visualize the fractured condylar neck and inferior part of the plate. A rather precise anatomic reduction can be achieved by caudal traction on the plate attached to the condylar segment. Further stabilization is facilitated with periosteal elevators, angle elevators,

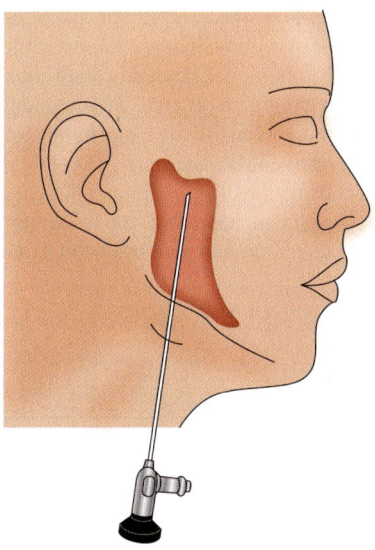

Fig. 6-14 ■ The Troulis technique. (Redrawn from Troulis MJ, Kaban LB: Endoscopic approach to the ramus/condyle unit: clinical applications, *J Oral Maxillofac Surg* 59(5):503-509, 2001.)

modified posterior border retractors, or a combination of these. A 3-mm stab incision in the cutaneous fold inferior to the pinna will accommodate the transbuccal trocar. The final fixation is achieved with two transbuccal screws on the distal segment. The transbuccal trocar route can be avoided by using a right-angle screwdriver drill to apply the screws transorally. The intermaxillary fixation is then removed to evaluate occlusal stability.

In the past few years, the Troulis submandibular approach has gained more favor in the eyes of these authors (Fig. 6-14). It consists of a 1.5-cm subangulomandibular incision approximately 2 cm cervical to the angle. Dissection is carried sharply to the bone and then continued in a subperiosteal plane with suction-assisted endoscopic elevators, such as the Snowden-Pencer elevators, to create an optical space. The 30-degree Karl Storz endoscope can be placed parallel to the posterior border of the ramus, with direct access to the condyle. The anterior and posterior borders of the ramus, the sigmoid notch, the coronoid process, and the posterior body of the mandible are the relevant anatomic landmarks visualized once the scope is in the optic chamber. A curved, long-handled retractor is positioned to maintain the optical cavity. An osseous orifice is trepanned at the angle and a wire is passed to facilitate the distraction of the ramus. The authors prefer a mandibular angle clamp for the same purpose. With the patient in IMF, the distal and proximal fragments are identified through the endoscope. A long-handled, narrow-tipped clamp is used to apprehend the condylar neck and position the condylar head in the fossa. The fracture is reduced and the distracted ramus released, wedging the two segments together. A 2.0-mm (five hole) titanium plate is positioned, then the proximal screws are placed. The plate-holder/introducer is then removed and the plate used to manipulate the proximal segment. Reduction at the posterior border is evaluated and the distal screws are placed with or without the aid of a percutaneous trocar.

ADVANTAGES

The endoscopically assisted technique allows for direct visualization with operating field magnification. It awards such precise anatomic reduction that 85% to 95% of patients regain immediate postoperative function of the mandible with TMJ function restored to unrestricted pretrauma joint movement. All cases of early malocclusion are amenable to two to five days elastic IMF for stabilization of correct occlusion. The technique immediately restores chin point location and jaw line. It prevents lateral deviation with maximal IMO and TMJ luxation of the contralateral side, maintaining condylar head mechanics without remodeling. In the majority of cases, it eliminates the need for postoperative IMF. The small, remotely placed incisions leave minimal, inconspicuous scars. Minimal dissection and manipulation of tissues results in decreased pain, swelling, and overall morbidity; quicker recovery; and shorter hospital stay.

ENDOSCOPICALLY ASSISTED OPEN REDUCTION AND INTERNAL FIXATION OF MANDIBLE ANGLE FRACTURES

The mandible angle fracture (Fig. 6-15) is one of the most common injuries of the maxillofacial complex and may be treated in various ways. The endoscopically assisted technique is indicated, technically, in any angle fracture requiring internal fixation, including but not limited to a Champy plate, superior and inferior border plates, just inferior border plate, or miniplates.

The incision is similar to the one used for the standard intraoral approach for ORIF of the mandibular angle fracture. Next, the subperiosteal dissection will create an optical cavity. The 0-, 30-, or 45-degree, 4-mm diameter scope, xenon light source, and standard mandibular fracture instrumentation are used. Recommended specialized instruments are Minnesota, cheek, and trocar-cheek retractors with an endoscopic sleeve to improve visualization and decrease instrumentation in the cavity. The endoscope visualization of the fracture and inferior border of the mandible are ideal. Superior, tension, and inferior fixation plates are positioned and fixated using a single transbuccal trocar technique (Fig. 6-16, A and B). The optional locking cannula, the authors' preference, also aids in the precise placement of fixation hardware. Once optimal fixation is achieved and reduction confirmed with the endoscope, appropriate documentation is recorded and closure completed (Fig. 6-16, C and D).

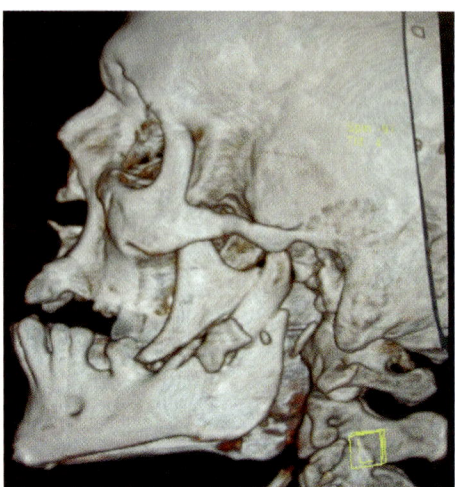

Fig. 6-15 ■ 3-D reconstruction revealing left-condylar-ramus mandibular fracture.

As with all other endoscopically assisted surgical techniques, the advantages by far outweigh the risks. There is no better way of verification for plate placement than the scope view. The angulation for screw placement is ideal (90 degrees). From the soft tissue perspective, there is less stretching and minimal dissection from the mandible. Immediate function of the mandible is less difficult. The reduction is precise enough that the surgeon can confidently remove the arch bars at the end of the procedure. Although initially the surgery will require approximately 2.5 times longer than the conventional technique, duration will decrease with experience. In these authors' hands, the surgical time for an ORIF of an isolated angle fracture averages 45 minutes. As we see it, the only disadvantages of this technique are cost and manpower.

Other endoscopic applications in OMS include the endoscopically assisted ORIF of the isolated zygomatic arch fractures and the endoscopically assisted condylectomy and reconstruction.

ENDOSCOPICALLY ASSISTED ORTHOGNATHIC SURGERY

One of the major advances in oral and maxillofacial surgery in the 1990s was the introduction of the endoscope and lasers, which enables orthognathic surgery to be performed on outpatients. The endoscope facilitates osteotomies and fixation in a poorly accessed maxillofacial region by improving visibility and allowing precise anatomic alignment of the osseous fragments.

INTRAORAL VERTICAL RAMUS OSTEOTOMY/VERTICAL SUBSIGMOID OSTEOTOMY

The intraoral vertical ramus osteotomy/vertical subsigmoid osteotomy (IVRO/VSO) is an osteotomy that is typically performed to correct mandible prognathism. Other indications for this procedure would include malocclusion secondary to malunion of a mandible fracture, condylar hyperplasia with asymmetric prognathism, and mandibular asymmetry secondary to Parry-Romberg syndrome. As in most orthognathic surgical procedures today, IVRO is usually performed transorally. This route has limited visibility and makes application of rigid fixation rather difficult. The role of the endoscope in IVRO/VSO is to facilitate surgical access to the sigmoid

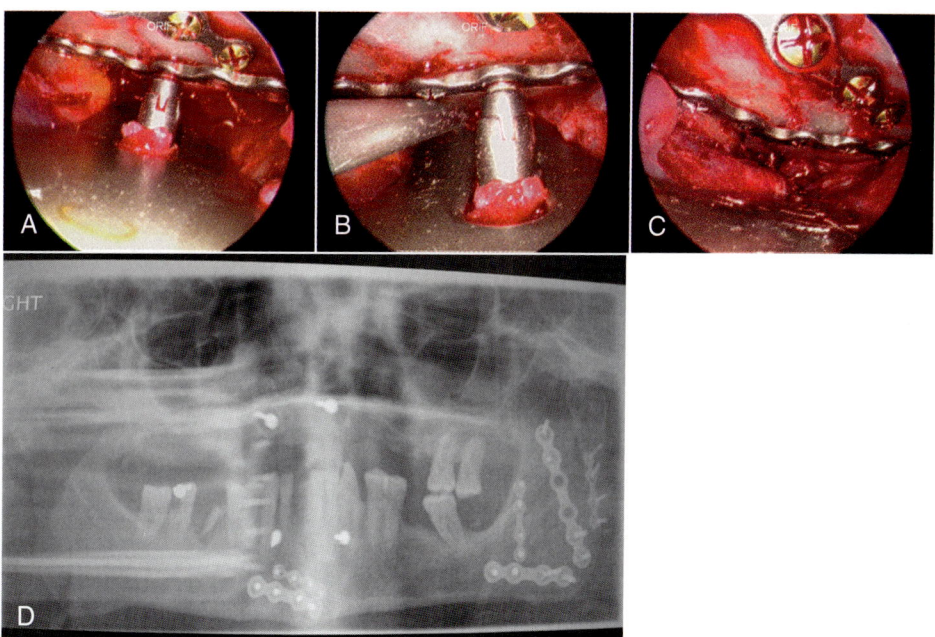

Fig. 6-16 ■ **A** and **B,** Endoscopic placement of tension and fixation plates. **C,** ORIF completed. **D,** Postop panorex.

notch region during osteotomy and segment adaptation and fixation of proximal segments.

SURGICAL TECHNIQUE

The IVRO/VSO technique represents a modified version of the Herbert protocol. The mucosal incision is placed lateral to the external oblique ridge from the ascending ramus to the vestibular mucosa corresponding to the second mandibular molar. The buccinator muscle is then incised closer to its attachment at the external oblique ridge. A mucoperiosteal flap is raised to expose the lateral aspect of the ramus, without any detachment at the medial aspect of the ramus. The adjacent images reveal some of the McCain modifications to standard instruments that facilitate this approach (Fig. 6-17, *A* and *B*). The sigmoid notch and the posterior mandibular border are identified and retracted using a sigmoid notch retractor (Stryker/Leibinger, Irving, Texas) and a posterior border retractor (Stryker/Leibinger), respectively. The anatomic landmarks of the ramus are identified to estimate the position of the mandibular foramen. The osteotomy cut is initiated with an oscillating saw and 70-degree saw blade. The endoscope is then introduced intraoral to assess the completeness of the osteotomy, especially at its superior portion close to the sigmoid notch (Fig. 6-17, *C*). The osteotomy is completed with a curved osteotome. The medial pterygoid muscle is then slightly elevated to facilitate movement of the two segments of the ramus. The proximal (condylar) segment is mobilized lateral to the distal (ramus) segment (Fig. 6-17, *D*). The mandible is then set back according to the prefabricated occlusal splint. The occlusion is temporarily stabilized with IMF.

The endoscope is introduced intraorally to the osteotomy site. The proximal segment is exposed with a posterior border retractor adapted lateral to the distal ramus contour. Any identifiable interferences are adjusted using a large round/oval osteotomy bur to ensure good coaptation of the segments. A titanium miniplate is adapted to bridge over the segments. A 3-mm stab incision in the preauricular fold, inferior to the pinna, allows access for transbuccal trocar. The plate is secured to the proximal segment first through the cannula with 6- to 8-mm titanium screws. A channel retractor is then inserted at the lower border of the proximal segment to allow precise control

of the condyle position in the glenoid fossa. The proximal segment is carefully adapted over the distal segment and fixated in position in the same fashion. At the end of the operation the IMF is released and the occlusion evaluated by manually hinging the condyle at the most retruded contact position.

Postoperative management is identical to that of routine osteotomy patients. The patients were advised to follow a soft diet for the first 6 weeks, and active mandibular opening is advised after 2 weeks. Any minor malocclusion was corrected with guiding orthodontic elastics in the first 6 weeks. The neurosensory status of the inferior alveolar nerve and TMJ status were assessed with a visual analogue scale (VAS) (0 = normal sensation; 10 = anesthesia). Neurosensory assessment of the inferior alveolar nerve (IAN) function at the mental nerve distribution was determined by light touch threshold (with von Frey fibers), two-point discrimination and pain threshold (with a 23-gauge needle attached to the arm of an orthodontic gauge meter). Clinical TMJ changes were evaluated using the McCain VAS and clinical TMJ exam.

DISCUSSION

With setback surgery in the mandible, surgical access to the sigmoid notch region is often limited. Incomplete osteotomy at the sigmoid notch can lead to an unfavorable fracture pattern. After completion of the osteotomy, the proximal segment should normally lie lateral to the distal segment, as opposed to a condylar fracture where a precise interdigitation of the fractured segments is attempted. Meticulous osteoplasty is required to ensure good overlap between the proximal and distal segments before fixation. Clinical experience with the procedure shows that the most likely area of interference is immediately inferior to the sigmoid notch. The endoscope enhances visibility so that an appropriate osteoplasty is performed.

The most technically difficult step of the procedure is the fixation of the plate over the proximal segment, because it is located in the most posterior area of the tunnel/optic cavity, with rather poor intraoral access. Again, the endoscope provides valuable visibility and access. Once fixation of the proximal segment is achieved, control of the condyle position and fixation to the distal segment are relatively easy to perform. For the condyle fracture repair, the use of a

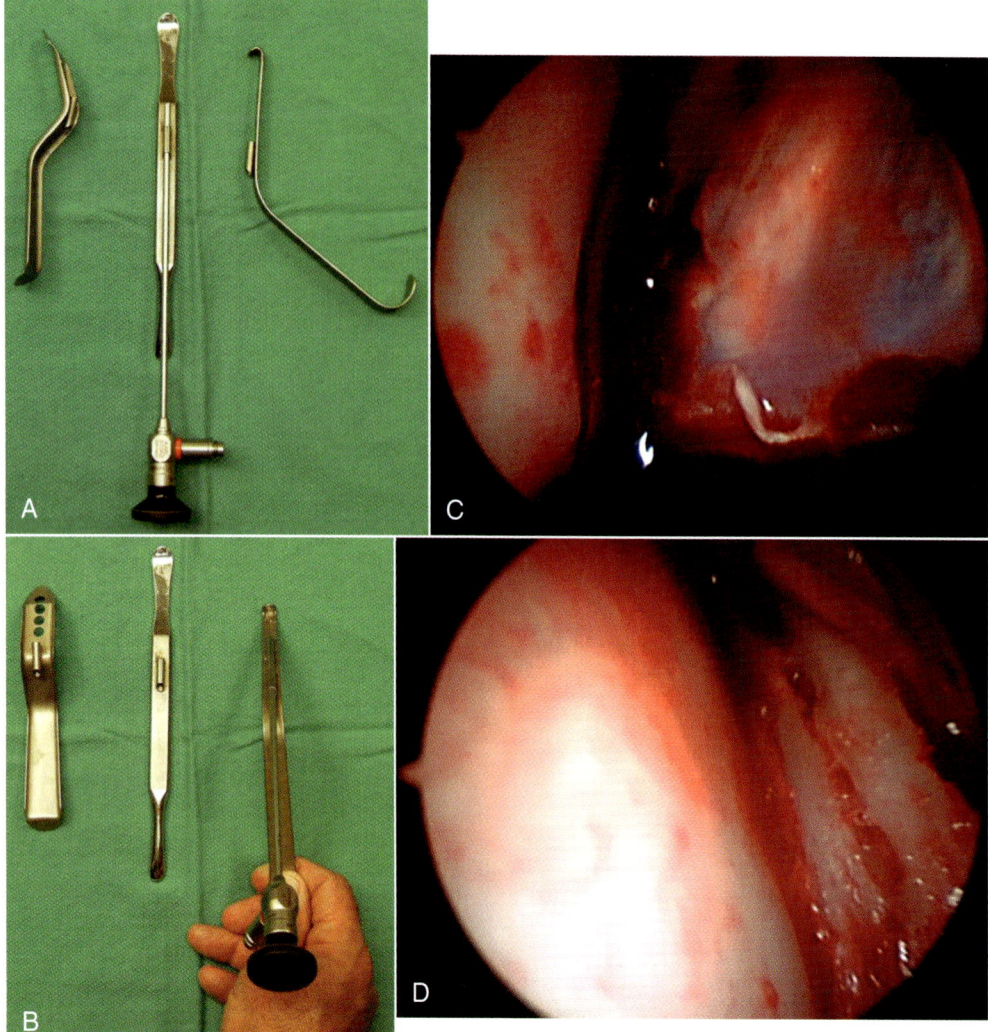

Fig. 6-17 ■ **A** and **B,** Minnesota, Seldin, and channel retractors with McCain's modifications for endoscopic procedures. **C,** Osteotomy at the sigmoid notch. **D,** Lateral positioning of the proximal segment.

right-angle handpiece with self-threading screws is recommended to prevent cutaneous incisions. The analogy does not apply, because longer screws are necessary to stabilize and fixate the two segments of the IVRO/VRO. These segments are much less stable than those caused by a subcondylar fracture. For that reason, a trocar stab incision is used instead. This inconspicuous incision is adequately camouflaged by the pinna.

Notwithstanding claims by other authors that endoscope-assisted rigid fixation of the mandible via intraoral route alone is time-consuming, with potentially increased bleeding and edema, the surgeon who perseveres will quickly improve and achieve a reasonable operation time.

EXTRAORAL VERTICAL RAMUS OSTEOTOMY (EVRO)

The surgeons in favor of the Troulis approach assert that the use of relatively long intraoral incisions and extensive dissections necessary for the introduction of the endoscope in the IVRO/VRO procedure often causes considerable bleeding and significant postoperative swelling. They also suggest that visibility remains difficult and the surgical orientation is parallel to the region of interest.

Experience with the ORIF of subcondylar fractures shows that medially displaced fractures or proximal segments are extremely difficult to reduce or are completely inaccessible via this approach. Lastly, IMF before reduction and fixation of segments limits access, making the procedure very difficult and time-consuming.

SURGICAL TECHNIQUE

A 1.5-cm subangulomandibular incision is placed approximately 2 cm caudal to the angle (Fig. 6-18, *A*). Next, the dissection is carried bluntly to the masseter muscle, which is cut with a needlepoint electrocautery. The inferior border of the mandible is exposed and the dissection is completed in a subperiosteal plane with specially designed, suction-assisted endoscopic elevators (Snowden-Pencer, Tucker, Georgia). A careful dissection in this plane results in a clean and dry optical cavity. The position of the incision and the mobility of the adjacent soft tissues allow the endoscope to be introduced in the wound and oriented parallel to the posterior border of the ramus with direct access to the entire ramus-condyle unit (RCU).

The anatomic landmarks of the RCU are identified: anterior and posterior borders of the ramus, sigmoid notch, coronoid process, and posterior corpus. A long-handled retractor is positioned to maintain the optical cavity, which is irrigated through the appropriate port of the endoscope.

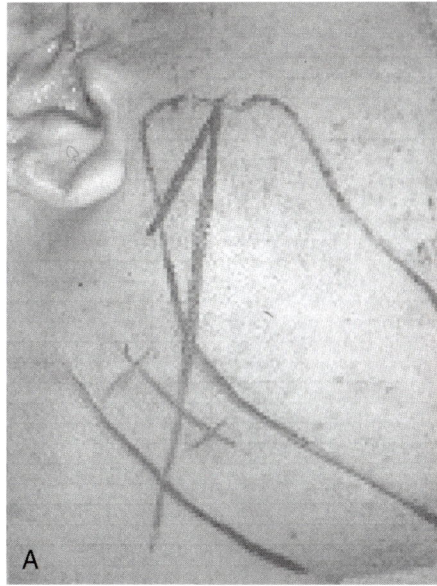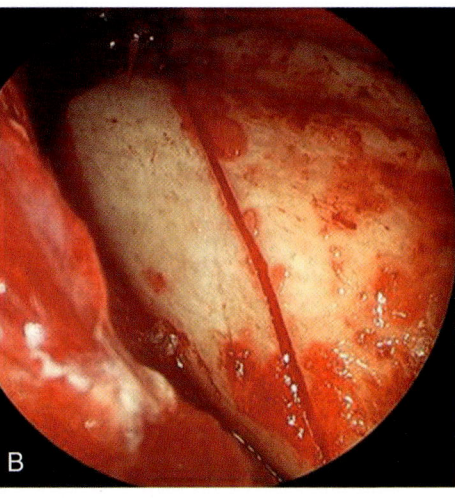

Fig. 6-18 ■ **A,** Patient marked for Troulis technique EVRO. **B,** VRO endoscopically assisted. (**A** from Troulis MJ, Kaban LB: Endoscopic vertical ramus osteotomy: early clinical results, *J Oral Maxillofac Surg* 62(7):824-828, 2004.)

With endoscopic visualization, an osteotomy is executed from the sigmoid notch to the mandibular angle using a long-shaft reciprocating blade (Fig. 6-18, *B*). The medial pterygoid muscle is partially stripped to allow overlap of the proximal and distal segments. When required, a clamp can be used to control the proximal segment. The patient is then wired in maxillomandibular fixation (MMF) in the desired, preplanned occlusion. Three screws, 12- to 14-mm long by 2.0 mm in diameter, are used to secure the segments into position (tetracortical). Screw holes are drilled and screws tapped through the incision or with a percutaneous trocar.

The average operating time for this procedure in experienced hands is approximately 75 minutes per case (B/L). In the majority of cases, trocar access is not required. Typically no patients experience sensory changes related to the IAN; marginal mandibular nerve weakness is unlikely to occur, and if it does, its duration is short (less than a week). TMJ complications are highly infrequent.

DISCUSSION

The Troulis approach significantly reduces the trauma of the dissection and reduces bleeding and swelling because of the well-contained and localized nature of the optical cavity. Both lateral and medial aspects of the ramus are accessible with the technique. Also, MMF can be performed without compromising access. The technique can also be used to place miniature mandible distractors. The EVRO is the appropriate technique for patients with well-developed asymptomatic third molars intimately involved with the IAN. The mandible can be set back and rigid fixation applied, while the third molars can be left in place. Although both IVRO and EVRO are similar low-risk anesthesia/paresthesia procedures involving the IAN, the EVRO offers the advantage of direct visualization as the osteotomy is performed. In the future, this procedure will hopefully be performed in the office under local anesthesia and intravenous sedation.

BILATERAL SAGITTAL SPLIT RAMUS OSTEOTOMY

In 1957 Trauner and Obwegeser started popularizing the intraoral bilateral sagittal split ramus osteotomy (BSSRO). The technique has been modified by Dal Pont (1961), Hansuck (1968), and Epker (1977). Except for the advent of rigid fixation, for over 30 years there have been no improvements to this highly effective procedure.

SURGICAL TECHNIQUE

After making the standard subperiosteal dissection on the ramus superior, medial, and lateral, the next important step is to locate the lingula. This structure can be visualized directly when the soft tissues are adequately retracted medially with a Seldin retractor; however, at times, this is very difficult to achieve. At this time, the 30-degree endoscope is inserted in the subperiosteal pocket, medial to the ramus. Manipulation of the scope will bring the lingula in sight (Fig. 6-19, *A*). If the lingula has already been identified under direct vision, the endoscope confirms its location and the magnified image can be viewed on the monitor. To facilitate medial retraction of the soft tissues while positioning the scope in the area of interest, a Seldin retractor was modified to receive a sleeve attachment that accommodates the endoscope. This allows the endoscope and the Seldin retractor to move as one unit, which makes it easier to retract and view the lingula.

After positive identification of the lingula the operation can proceed on either of two of the following avenues. First, the endoscope can be removed, the lingula protected, and the medial cut can now be performed. Second, the endoscope is left in the field and the surgeon performs the medial osteotomy with direct vision on the monitor (without looking directly into the pocket) (Fig. 6-19, *B* and *C*). After the osteotomy is completed, the osteotomy depth and superior and posterior extent of the cut can all be verified via endoscope. The cut should be through the medial cortex and superior and posterior to the lingula. After the medial osteotomy is checked, a photograph of the osteotomy can be taken with the scope.

The next two steps of the procedure are carried out under direct vision. The lateral osteotomy follows the sagittal osteotomy and the two cuts are connected. A crucial step after the lateral osteotomy consists of verifying the complete osteotomy of the inferior border of the mandible. Per standard technique, the surgeon holds the channel retractor in place while retracting the buccal soft tissues to visualize the inferior border directly. Confirmation of a complete cut may come easy to the experienced surgeon. However, if this cannot be determined or if the inferior border cortex is incompletely removed, the possibility of a "bad split" increases. All the guesswork is eliminated when the 30-degree scope is pistoned in to within

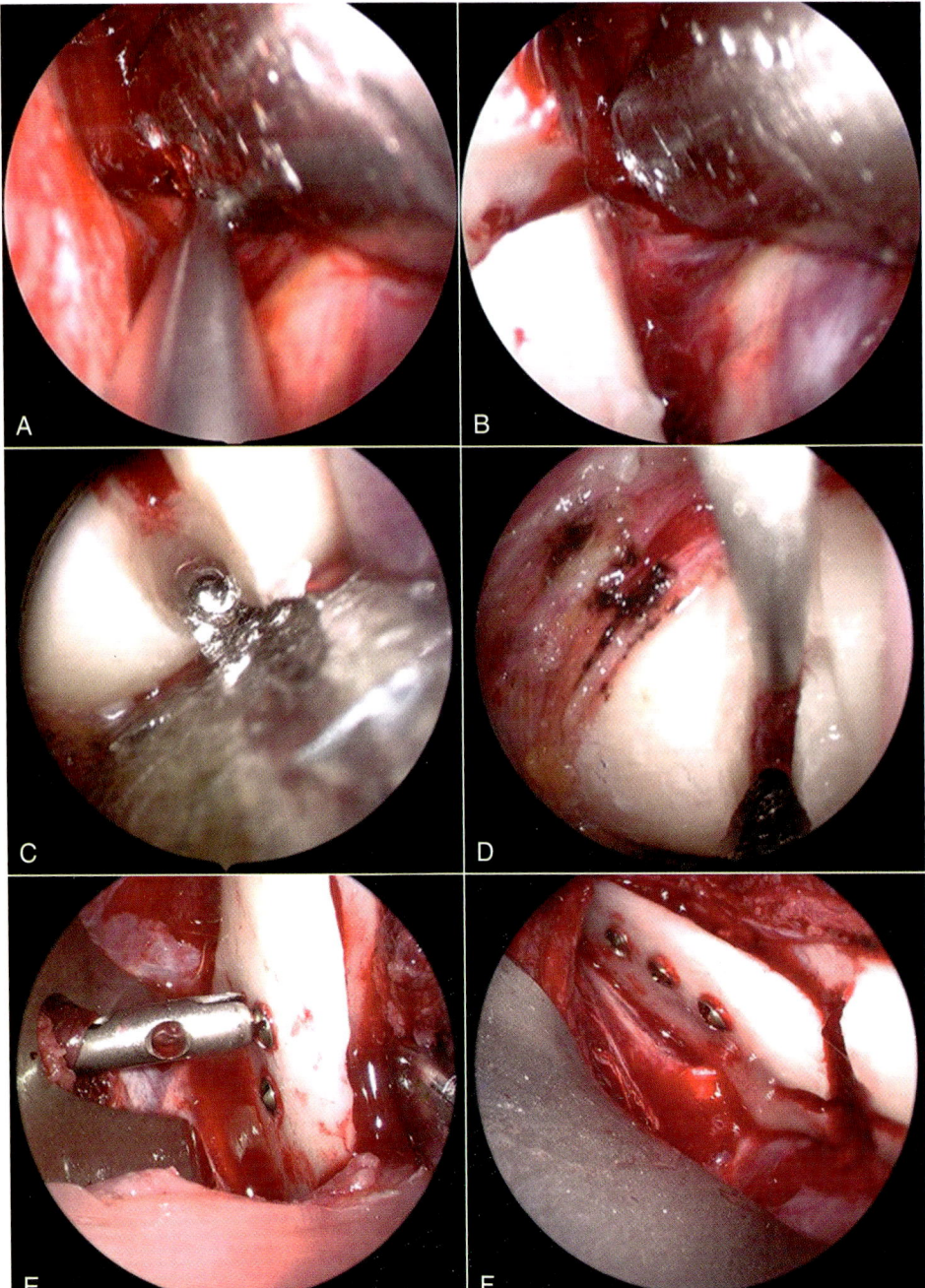

Fig. 6-19 ■ **A,** Endoscopic visualization of lingula. **B,** Medial osteotomy. **C** and **D,** Incomplete versus complete inferior border osteotomy. **E** and **F,** Stabilization and fixation of SSO with bicortical screws.

2 mm of the inferior border osteotomy. The angled scope is more favorable for this position because its shaft is directed in the same path as the lateral osteotomy. Once the end of the scope reaches the inferior border, the angle permits good visualization of the depth of the cut (Fig. 6-19, *D* and *E*). Inevitably, there will be bleeding at the inferior border. The authors' preference is the #3 myringotomy suction tip, because most of the time, it affords a snug fit into the lateral osteotomy. If the inferior border needs fine tuning, the scope can be left in place while the surgeon operates off the monitor and the cut is appropriately completed. If the surgeon is uncomfortable with cutting indirectly, the scope can be removed, the osteotomy completed, and the endoscope can be reinserted for confirmation.

Fixation and stabilization with bicortical screws is performed via endoscope-assisted trocar technique (Fig. 6-19, *F*).

MANAGEMENT OF BSSRO COMPLICATIONS

The complications of BSSRO can be subdivided into such categories as vascular, neural, infectious, occlusal, and dental. They can also manifest as dysfunctional TMJ, undesired fractures (bad split), fixation complications, or any combination of those just listed. The most feared intraoperative complication, the undesired fracture, has been reported in up to 20% of patients. A higher incidence has been reported in cases where the third molars are present. Both proximal and distal segments can fracture.

Most of the BSSRO complications consist of condyle fracture or buccal/lingual plate fracture. The fractures can be individual or comminuted. The most common is the fracture of the buccal cortex. However, the experienced orthognathic surgeon has encountered at least once the horizontal bicortical ramus cut, the distal segment vertical fracture (fracture of the lingual plate), or the fracture of the medial condyle and neck.

Rescue of the unfavorable BSSRO fracture involves completion of the originally planned osteotomy, positioning the mandible into the preplanned occlusion, and fixating the segments with internal fixation devices. Other reconstructive options include aborting the procedure, establishing MMF, assessing the complication pattern with high-resolution CT scans, and allowing the unfavorable fracture to heal before reattempting treatment. Another sequence of options would be completion of the BSSRO in the conventional fashion, followed by MMF or rigid fixation of segments. Lastly, an extraoral approach can be employed via preauricular, retromandibular, or submandibular incisions that will permit visualization, reduction, and fixation with reconstruction plates.

When a comminuted fracture occurs, as, for example, with a large buccal cortical plate fracture plus a separate condylar segment, the limited visualization permits few treatment options. If reoperation after healing is attempted, the delay in treatment may have deleterious consequences. But if immediate repair is attempted through large extraoral facial or cervical incisions, the advantage of direct visualization of the segments requiring reduction has to be weighed against the obvious inherent risks involving facial nerve damage, scarring, or both. This option is unattractive to both the patient and the surgeon.

At this point, enter the endoscope, facilitating visualization of the entire RCU as already presented earlier in this chapter. Comminuted fractures with a subcondylar component are endoscopically treated with ORIF of the condylar segment first. The sagittal split osteotomy (SSO) is then completed along the medial ramus and inferior border. After separation of the proximal and distal segments, the patient is wired in MMF using a prefabricated splint. The segments are then rigidly fixated per standard technique.

LE FORT I OSTEOTOMY

The maxillary sinus is anatomically suited to combine endoscopy with a conservative, small approach. The pneumatized sinus and the thin, translucent osseous walls are an ideal, potential, natural optic cavity for the introduction of the endoscope. Endoscopically assisted, minimally invasive techniques reduce surgical trauma in the maxilla with only minimal osseous denudation. This way the vascular supply of the osteotomized segment(s), so critical for any procedure in the maxillary region, is preserved.

The following endoscopically assisted surgical technique was first attempted on cadavers before its clinical application. The object of the trial was to find an optimal minimally invasive approach to the maxillary sinus and to select the appropriate instrumentation for the Le Fort I osteotomy. Additionally, handling of the endoscope during the procedure was extensively practiced.

SURGICAL TECHNIQUE

The procedure is presently performed under general anesthesia; however, in the near future, local anesthesia in combination with intravenous sedation will replace general anesthesia. The following surgical technique was first performed by J. Wiltfang and P. Kessler from the University of Erlangen-Nuremberg, Germany (Fig. 6-20, A).

A short vertical incision in the vestibular fornix corresponding to the maxillary canine is placed bilaterally (Fig. 6-20, B). The incision is done in full thickness down to the buccal cortical plate of the maxilla. The mucoperiosteum is elevated and the piriform aperture is exposed. The osseous structure of the anterior and laterodorsal maxillary antral wall is exposed via blunt subperiosteal tunneling. A portal is then placed at the union of the anterior and medial maxillary sinus walls, at the exact Le Fort level that facilitates the introduction of the endoscope. Under diaphanoscopy from the endoscope light, first the anterior, then the laterodorsal antral walls are osteotomized with straight and gently curved osteotomes. The position and osteotomy line of the chisels are controlled endoscopically with 30- and 70-degree scopes. After the osteotomy of the medial sinus walls, the pterygoid plates are separated from the maxilla under gentle downward pressure so that a curved osteotome will fit through the antral chamber. The curved osteotome is then directed dorsocaudally to avoid the fracture of the pterygoid process. The technique is versatile and can be modified to accommodate Le Fort I segmental osteotomies (two-, three- or four-piece maxilla).

Although the authors prefer a conventional vestibular incision for the Le Fort I osteotomy, the endoscope remains invaluable in confirming the final pterygoid cuts and the precise location of the palatine vessels after the down fracture. Ultimately, it is very effective in keeping the entire surgical team engaged throughout the procedure, and it is an excellent adjunct in documenting procedure steps and final results (Fig. 6-20, C and D).

TEMPOROMANDIBULAR JOINT ARTHROSCOPY

The TMJ disorders have always been in the focus of attention for the maxillofacial surgeon. The unique characteristics of the TMJ and the pain accompanying TMJ disorders have been treated since the inception of our specialty. The advances in TMJ arthroscopic instrumentation are one of the most important treatment options for TMJ disorders. Much less invasive than open arthrotomy, arthroscopy has been a mainstay in the diagnosis and treatment of TMJ problems in the United States for the past 27 years, with advancements similar or at times superior to those reported in the orthopedic literature.

The authors have been very successful in treating various TMJ conditions. This unique 30-year experience with both conventional and minimally invasive techniques underlies the development of a treatment cascade protocol for the TMJ patient. It is the authors' belief that every patient should benefit from the most conservative treatment possible. The first level of the cascade is medical management, diet modifications, physical therapy, and orthotic treatment. Because the therapeutic approach is analog driven, only the patients who are still symptomatic after the conservative treatment will undergo further treatment. After the initial evaluation (including TMJ-MRI) is complete, the definitive diagnosis will be obtained via the diagnostic arthroscopic lysis and lavage.

The literature supports arthroscopic lysis and lavage as an effective treatment in 70% of patients in Wilkes classification stages II to V. This regimen decreases pain, increases mobility, improves diet, and reduces use of medications. Synovitis and other inflammatory pathologies benefit from laser synovectomy and corticosteroid or hyaluronic acid injection into the retrodiskal tissue, all endoscopically assisted. Additional endoscopic instrumentation can effectively remove adhesions and smooth disk perforation margins. If disk repositioning is needed, a procedure devised by McCain is available. The learning curve for the diskopexy is quite considerable, but its advantages warrant recommendation to patients considering an open procedure. The authors' expertise and results with this

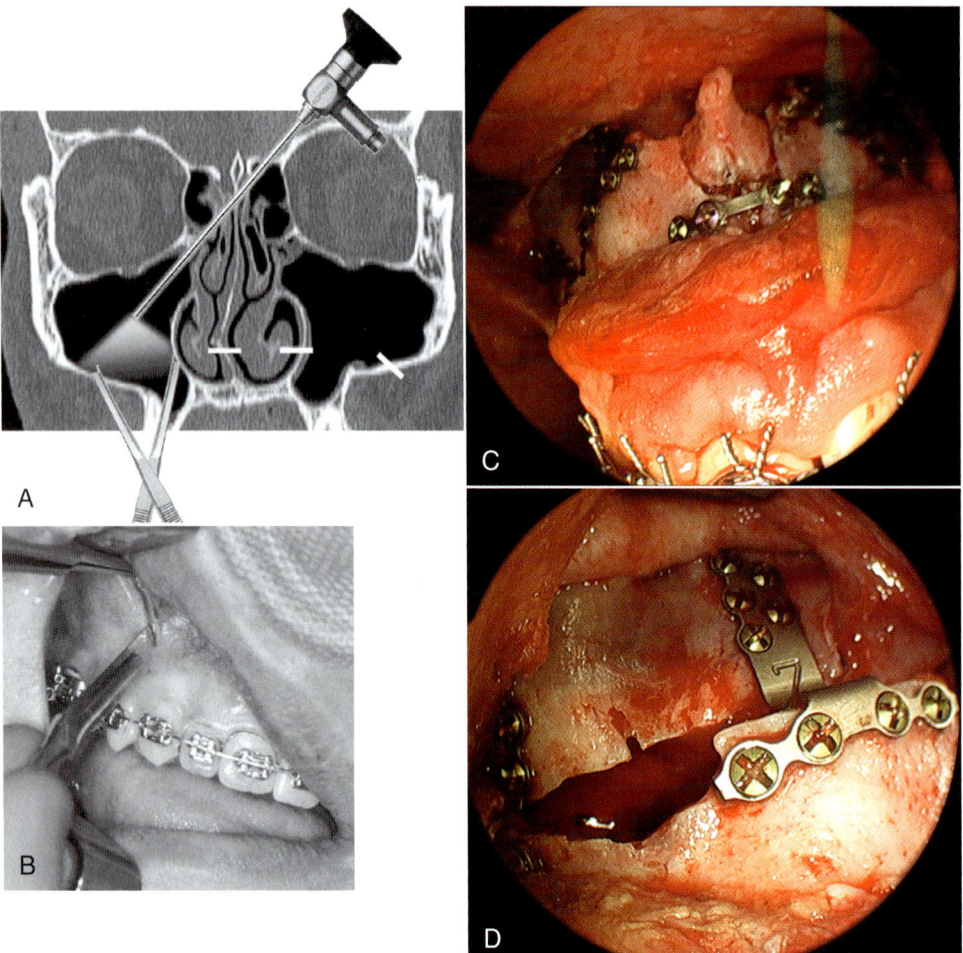

Fig. 6-20 ■ **A,** Wiltfang-Kessler technique. **B,** Vertical canine fornix vestibular incisions. **C** and **D,** Stabilization and fixation of the maxilla after Le Fort I osteotomy. (**A** and **B** from Wiltfang J, Kessler P: Endoscopically assisted Le Fort I osteotomy to correct transverse and sagittal discrepancies of the maxilla, *J Oral Maxillofac Surg* 60:1142-1145, 2002.)

technique make it a highly predictable procedure. At the other end of the spectrum, a hypermobile joint will tend to dislocate or lock open. Except for the block graft or hardware placement, all the other treatments (eminectomy, injection of sclerosing agent or autologous blood, posterior scarification/contracture procedure) can be completed with endoscopic assistance.

OFFICE ARTHROSCOPY

One of the developments in technology is the OnPoint System (Biomet, Jacksonville, Fla.) (Fig. 6-21, *A*). This diagnostic arthroscopy system uses a 1.2-mm, 0-degree scope. The high-quality resolution and portable surgical unit make this operation amenable to the outpatient setting, with significant cost savings for the patient. The armamentarium includes an ergonomic handpiece containing a camera and light source, enabled to record still images and videos. The 1.2-mm disposable scope is the size of an 18-gauge needle. The other instruments included are a single-use cannula, trocar, obturator, and cannula plug. The cannula has an outside diameter of 1.9 mm and a Luer port on the body to connect an irrigation source. The port also permits intra-articular injection.

The patient is prepped and draped in sterile fashion per McCain routine. A small amount of local anesthetic (1 mL) is divided for injection at puncture and insufflation points. Once local anesthesia is achieved, the joint is insufflated with 2 to 3 mL of 0.5%

bupivacaine (Marcaine). With the patient in assisted or unassisted mandibular protrusion, the insufflation needle puncture is placed in the preauricular fold or crease at the level of merger between pinna and tragus. The needle travels craniomedial, oriented toward an imaginary line bisecting the policis nail of surgeon's nondominant hand while palpating the infero-zygomatic concavity resulting from the anterior movement of the condyle (Fig. 6-21, *B*).

FOSSA PORTAL

Immediately afterward, the trocar cannula is introduced into the superior joint space at the fossa portal (Fig. 6-22). This puncture site has to be inside a circle with a 20-mm diameter, centered over the glenoid fossa. The osseous boundaries of this circle are the apex of the articular eminence anteriorly, the middle of the acoustic meatus posteriorly, the posterior portion of the temporal fossa at the anterior segment of the supramastoid crest of the temporal squama, and finally the posterosuperior border of the ramus at condylar neck level inferiorly. The superficial correspondent of the posterior osseous landmark is the middle of the tragus, because it is situated 5 mm anterior to the tragal apex and 5 mm posterior to the anterior wall of the osseous external auditory canal. The authors' observations have placed the peak of the cartilaginous wall of the meatus at the exact level of the posterior aspect of the TMJ capsule. The neurovascular bundle (auriculotemporal nerve, superficial temporal vein and artery) is, in 80% of cases, 5 to 8 mm anterior to the midportion of tragus.

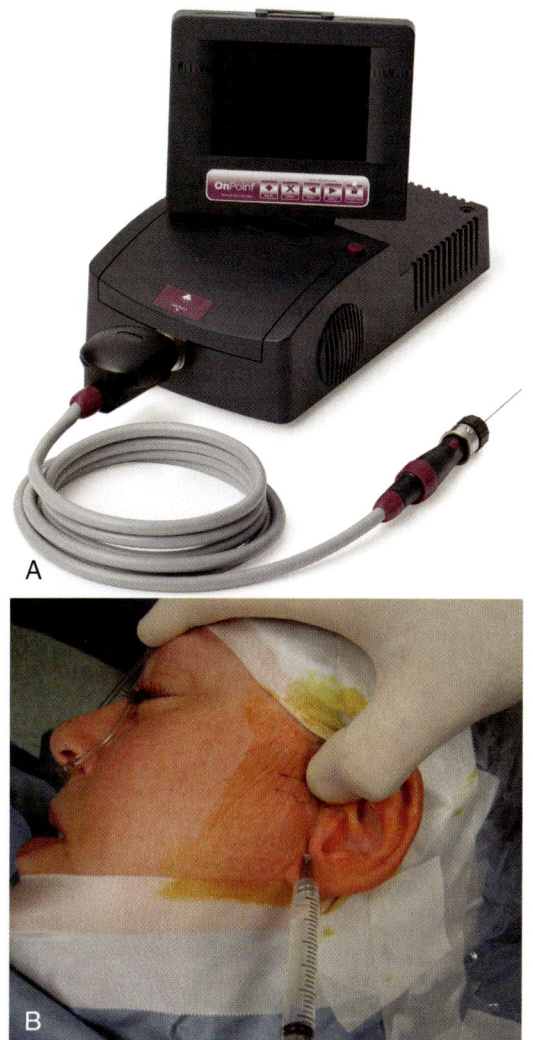

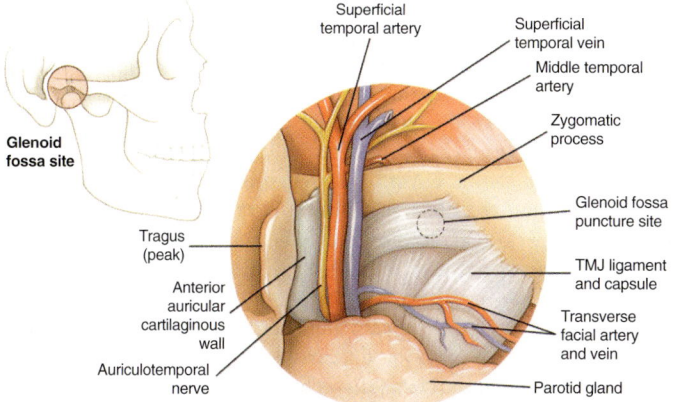

Fig. 6-21 ■ **A,** OnPoint 1.2 mm Scope System. **B,** Joint insufflation. (**A** courtesy Biomet Microfixation, Jacksonville, Fla.)

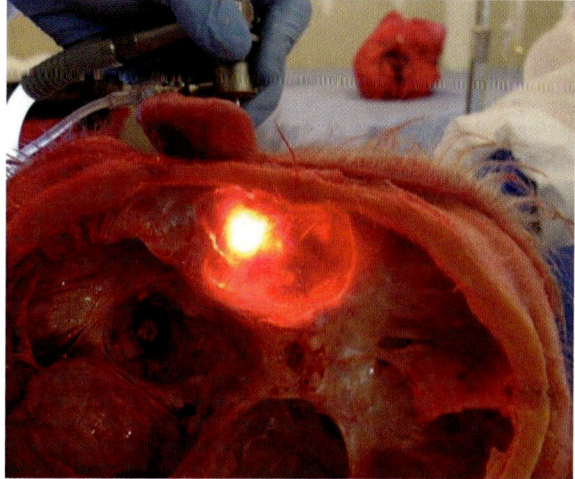

Fig. 6-23 ■ Perforation of the glenoid fossa, dissection.

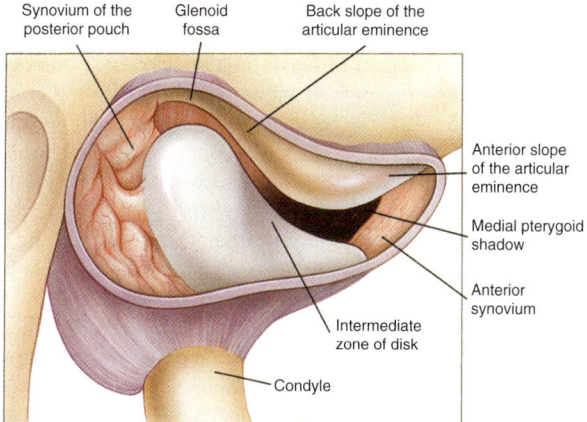

Fig. 6-24 ■ Internal arthroscopic anatomy. (From McCain JP: *Principles and practice of temporomandibular joint arthroscopy,* St. Louis, 1996, Mosby.)

Fig. 6-22 ■ Fossa puncture-related anatomy and landmarks. (From McCain JP: *Principles and practice of temporomandibular joint arthroscopy,* St. Louis, 1996, Mosby.)

DANGER ZONES

Before proceeding with the fossa puncture, then the diagnostic sweep, the surgeon must be cognizant of the "danger zones" and proximity of vital structures associated with this procedure. The three danger zones are the dura mater and temporal lobe situated immediately cranial to the glenoid fossa, with a thickness of 0.5 to 1.5 mm (Fig. 6-23); the tympanum, ossicles, and middle ear; and the entire length of the medial aspect of the capsule represented by the lateral pterygoid. The vital structures that have to be given special consideration are the mandibular division of the trigeminal nerve, especially the lingual and inferior alveolar branches; the auriculotemporal nerve (ATN); and the internal maxillary artery together with all the small branches supplying the capsule.

INTERNAL ARTHROSCOPIC ANATOMY (Fig. 6-24)

POSTERIOR RECESS

The first structure encountered upon entering the joint is the *synovium.* The synovial membrane is mesenchymal in origin and is a continuation of the cambium layer of the periosteum. Similar to other joints, the TMJ synovium covers the capsule and periarticular disk tissues, with the exception of the articular surfaces of the cartilages. The synovial lining is soft and grayish with a translucent background. The normal synovium exhibits mild capillary proliferation, which is diffuse throughout the lining. With the condyle in a forward position, the synovium of the posterior pouch lies flat and tight over the retrodiskal tissue. The *oblique protuberance* is a classic structure of the posterior pouch. With the condyle forward, the oblique protuberance is a fibroelastic band that protrudes into the retrodiskal tissue. It is located $\frac{2}{3}$ medial, from lateral to medial into the joint. With the condyle seated, the synovium buckles and ruffles like an accordion being closed. The synovial tissue attaches from the back portion of the disk. The posterior band of the disk running over the retrodiskal tissue attaches to the posterior aspect of the glenoid fossa at approximately midportion or the superior one third of the posterior wall of the glenoid fossa. The *medial synovial drape* appears normally as a gray, translucent lining. Very distinct striae run superior to inferior, defining the medial synovium. It serves as another classic landmark in the arthroscopic examination. In the background of the medial aspect of the drape, the *pterygoid shadow* reflects with a reddish-purple tinge.

INTERMEDIATE ZONE

In the middle of the joint, the *fibrocartilage* of the glenoid fossa is visible, thin, white, and not very reflective. Anterior to the glenoid fossa and along the back slope of the articular eminence, the fibrocartilage becomes whiter and more reflective of light and also takes on a classic appearance of striae formation that runs anterior to posterior. Changing the angle of view inferiorly, with the condyle forward, part of the *disk* can be seen as milky white, highly reflective, and without striations. With the condyle forward, the disk completely covers the condyle. The clear junction between the synovium and the posterior band of the disk is represented by a red-white line where the capillary proliferation stops and the disk begins. A U-shaped depression or flexure between the synovial junction and the posterior band of the disk can be observed. With the condyle seated, the disk covers the condyle and the flexure deepens significantly to the normal anatomic position of the disk. Toward the most lateral depth of the joint are the *articular eminence* and the trough within the eminence where the disk moves with the condylar translation.

ANTERIOR RECESS

In the anterior pouch, the anterior slope of the articular eminence is evident. The fibrocartilage and anterior band of the disk are both white, reflective, and without striae. The synovium is tightly attached and has a gray, translucent background with mild capillary proliferation widely dispersed throughout. The synovium is also attached tightly to the anterior ascending aspect of the articular eminence. Looking medially, the continuation of the medial synovial drape can be seen. The vertical striae of the drape are nonexistent, whereas the background consistency is deep purple secondary to the reflection of the pterygoid muscle fibers, which are much closer in this area. The lateral synovium is not tightly attached but maintains the same color as the medial synovium. The posteroanterior trough on the medial aspect of the joint is where the synovium descends off the medial synovial drape and then attaches to the disk in the same fashion as the medial trough.

SURGICAL TECHNIQUE

PALPATION OF TMJ ANATOMY

The surgeon palpates the lateral joint anatomy in preparation for the puncture, while the assistant manipulates the jaw. With the condyle seated, the assistant's thumb rolls into the buccal fold away from the occlusal surfaces to allow proper seating of the condyle in maximum occlusal intercuspation. The areas to be palpated are the superficial temporal artery preauricular (puncture must be anterior to artery), the condyle in back-and-forth and side-to-side motion of the mandible, the zygomatic process of the temporal bone, particularly the maximum concavity of the glenoid fossa (the soft tissue depression for the fossa portal puncture is located in this area) and the articular eminence with the condyle seated.

MARKING THE PUNCTURE SITE

The Holmlund-Hellsing line is drawn with deletable marker between the lateral canthus and the apex of tragus. A marking point is made at about the midportion of the external tragus. From this point, approximately 10 mm anterior and 2 mm inferior to the line, the maximum concavity of the fossa is located.

INSUFFLATION

The purpose of joint distention in this particular case is to expand the target area; 3 mL 0.5% bupivacaine in a 3-mL syringe with a 25-gauge, $1\frac{1}{2}$-inch needle are used in the process. A vasoconstrictor should not be used because it could prevent diagnostic evaluation of capillary engorgement or reperfusion hypoxia phenomenon reflecting synovitis. The needle is aimed at the central portion of the back slope of the eminence. Bone is contacted with the tip of the needle. The average joint will take approximately 3 mL. A plunger rebound greater than $\frac{1}{2}$ mL indicates sufficient insufflation. Adequate joint distention is indicated by the amount of pressure on the plunger. Stenosed or fibrotic joints will typically take less fluid and the pressure required to insufflate the joint is increased. Hypermobile joints or those with disk perforations without adhesions may require more fluid.

PUNCTURE

The puncture is placed at the maximum concavity of the glenoid fossa. The cannula is held in the right hand for a right joint puncture or in the left hand for a left joint puncture. The index controls the tip, while the palm of the hand controls the base of the cannula. With the condyle forward, the pollicis nail of the nondominant hand is used to palpate the stable, zygomatic process corresponding to the maximum concavity of the glenoid fossa immediately caudal. The trocar is rotated as it penetrates the skin. This puncture is made deliberately and carefully, so that it penetrates the lateral capsule into the joint space in one pass. If more than one attempt is made, multiple lacerations of the capsule will cause problems with extravasation during the course of the operation. The trocar is then advanced until contact is felt with the osseous structure superior. The instrument should never be passed straight through the capsule without locating the bone. The trocar is used almost in the same fashion as a periosteal elevator after it perforates the temporalis, for the periosteum at the level of the zygomatic bone. The zygomatic arch is felt between the pollicis nail of the nondominant hand and the index finger of the dominant hand. The trocar then steps off the ledge. The distance from the tegument surface to the ledge varies between 5 and 10 mm. If this dissection in not done properly, there is a high probability of invading the posterolateral subsynovial tissue. The trocar is then rotated until a slight pop is felt. It is then inserted approximately 10 to 15 mm. In resting position, the cannula should be angled anterosuperiorly. If it is angled posteriorly or held straight, the cannula could lacerate the cartilaginous anterior wall of the external auditory meatus, possibly perforating the tympanic membrane and violating the middle ear. Upon removal of the trocar from the cannula, the reflux of fluid should confirm capsule perforation. A blunt obturator is inserted and locked into the cannula. The cannula is then angled toward the open joint space. The middle portion of the cannula should, at this point, lever off the lateral aspect of the lateral margin of the glenoid fossa. The cannula should not be inserted more than 20 to 25 mm from tegument to the center of the joint. Before inserting the scope, the joint is backwashed to remove all blood and synovial fluid. The backwashing is continued until the return fluid is clear. The scope can be inserted next. The image on the monitor will confirm correct entry into the joint space. The image may not be very clear because of the absence of outflow.

OUTFLOW NEEDLE PUNCTURE

With the mandible protruded, the scope is stationary and directed to the center of the fossa area of the joint. The assistant insufflates the joint with 2 to 3 mL of fluid to maintain joint distention. The purpose of the outflow needle is to establish patent irrigation and, at the same time, maintain adequate joint distention for intra-articular instrumentation. A 22-gauge, 1½-inch needle is inserted approximately 5 mm anterior and 5 mm inferior to the fossa puncture site, under joint insufflation.

DIAGNOSTIC SWEEP

There are seven anatomic areas examined during the sweep: (1) medial synovial drape; (2) pterygoid shadow; (3) retrodiskal synovium (where the oblique protuberance, the retrodiskal synovial tissue attached to the posterior glenoid process, and the lateral recess of the retrodiskal synovial tissue have to be closely inspected); (4) posterior slope of the articular eminence and glenoid fossa; (5) articular disk; (6) intermediate zone; and (7) anterior recess (with special consideration for the disk-synovium crease, the midportion, the medial anterior corner, and the lateral anterior corner). Losing orientation inside the joint, even for a short time, can be a very frustrating experience for the rookie arthroscopist. Adding to the obstacles of inexperience, intra-articular pathology can deepen the confusion. The easiest method of preventing this confusion is for the operator to be comfortable with the four classic intra-articular anatomic landmarks: medial synovial drape with its distinct superior-to-inferior striae; oblique protuberance of the retrodiskal synovium; posterior slope of the articular eminence with distinct anterior-to-posterior striae; and anterior disk-synovium crease, which is where the anterior synovium and anterior band of the disk meet. This last landmark is where the second or working cannula is placed.

Area 1: Medial Synovial Drape (Fig. 6-25, A)

In many situations the surgeon will run into one of the classic landmarks, typically, the oblique protuberance or the posterior slope of the articular eminence. The drape can be reached by swiveling and pistoning the arthroscope until the drape becomes visible. In acute inflammatory states, capillary proliferation with hyperemia of the medial synovial drape is increased. In addition, erythematous patches (petechiae) may be seen on the drape, or the entire drape may appear erythematous. Occasionally the drape may prolapse or bulge into the joint space. Adhesive phenomena can also be seen. In chronic synovitis, the drape has a fibrotic or whitish appearance.

Area 2: Pterygoid Shadow (Fig. 6-25, B)

The second area to be examined will be reached by swiveling the scope anteriorly and pistoning medially until the shadow comes into view. A medial trough leads from the medial synovial drape anterior to the pterygoid shadow. With pathologic states, the pterygoid shadow looks markedly erythematous and hypervascularized and becomes quite thin. The synovial lining can thin out enough to perforate, allowing herniation of the pterygoid muscle directly into the anteromedial aspect of the superior joint space.

Area 3: Retrodiskal Synovium (Fig. 6-25, C)

The third area to be examined is reached by backtracking along the initial path of the scope. Once the medial synovial drape is visible, the scope is pistoned out (lateral) and swiveled minimally to bring into view both anterior and posterior components of the retrodiskal synovium. In inflammatory pathologic states the synovial tissue shows increased hypervascularity and erythema along with a redundant pattern. *Zone 1: An oblique protuberance* is visualized by pistoning out the scope. It is located about ⅓ of the way lateral from the drape. *Zone 2: Retrodiskal tissue attached to posterior glenoid process* is seen after the scope is swiveled superiorly. *Zone 3: The lateral recess of the retrodiskal synovial tissue* can be accessed by pistoning out from the oblique protuberance.

Area 4: Posterior Slope of the Articular Eminence and Glenoid Fossa (Fig. 6-25, D)

The fourth area of the intra-articular exam is reached in the following manner. From the lateral recess the scope is pistoned out until the periphery of the capsule is visible. From there the scope is advanced so that the capsular fragmentation is no longer visible. To examine the fibrocartilage of the back slope of the eminence, the scope is pistoned in to the most medial aspect of the articular eminence and then slowly pistoned out, backtracking along the previous path. The pathologic change occurring most often in this area is various stages of chondromalacia. To complete the examination of this area, the scope is swiveled superior and posterior. From that position, pistoning out to the joint periphery will permit visualization of the glenoid fossa. When destruction (thinning) of the fibrocartilage is advanced, the underlying bone appears slightly yellow or brownish. In inflammatory states, creeping of the synovial tissue can be observed in the glenoid fossa.

Area 5: Articular Disk (Fig. 6-25, E)

When the examination of the glenoid fossa is complete, the scope should be at the extreme periphery of the joint and in position to examine the fifth area. From this posterolateral position, the posterior band of the disk is located. With the condyle forward, the inspection proceeds in an anterior and inferior direction from this peripheral position. In pathologic states, the synovium creeps onto the surface of the disk. Fragmentation of the disk surface usually indicates that disk perforation is either imminent or present. In cases of disk perforation, the inferior joint space can be examined by introducing the scope through the perforation.

JOINT DYNAMICS AND DISK MOBILITY

The next step of the diagnostic sweep is to examine dynamics and mobility from the posterolateral position. The scope must be at the most peripheral posterolateral position, almost exiting the joint space. If the operator does not ensure the appropriate position of the scope in this instance, damage to the retrodiskal tissues and the disk may occur along with scuffing of the glenoid fossa and the back slope of the eminence. At this time in the operation, the assistant and the surgeon reciprocally manipulate the condyle into a seated position. Disk mobility between the fossa and disk can now be observed, and disk mobility between the condyle and disk can be inferred. In nonpathologic states, the disk should glide smoothly along the articular eminence, without any anteroposterior or mediolateral erratic movements. If an erratic movement is noted in the anteroposterior direction with a simultaneous audible or palpable clicking, then a reducing disk is the most likely situation.

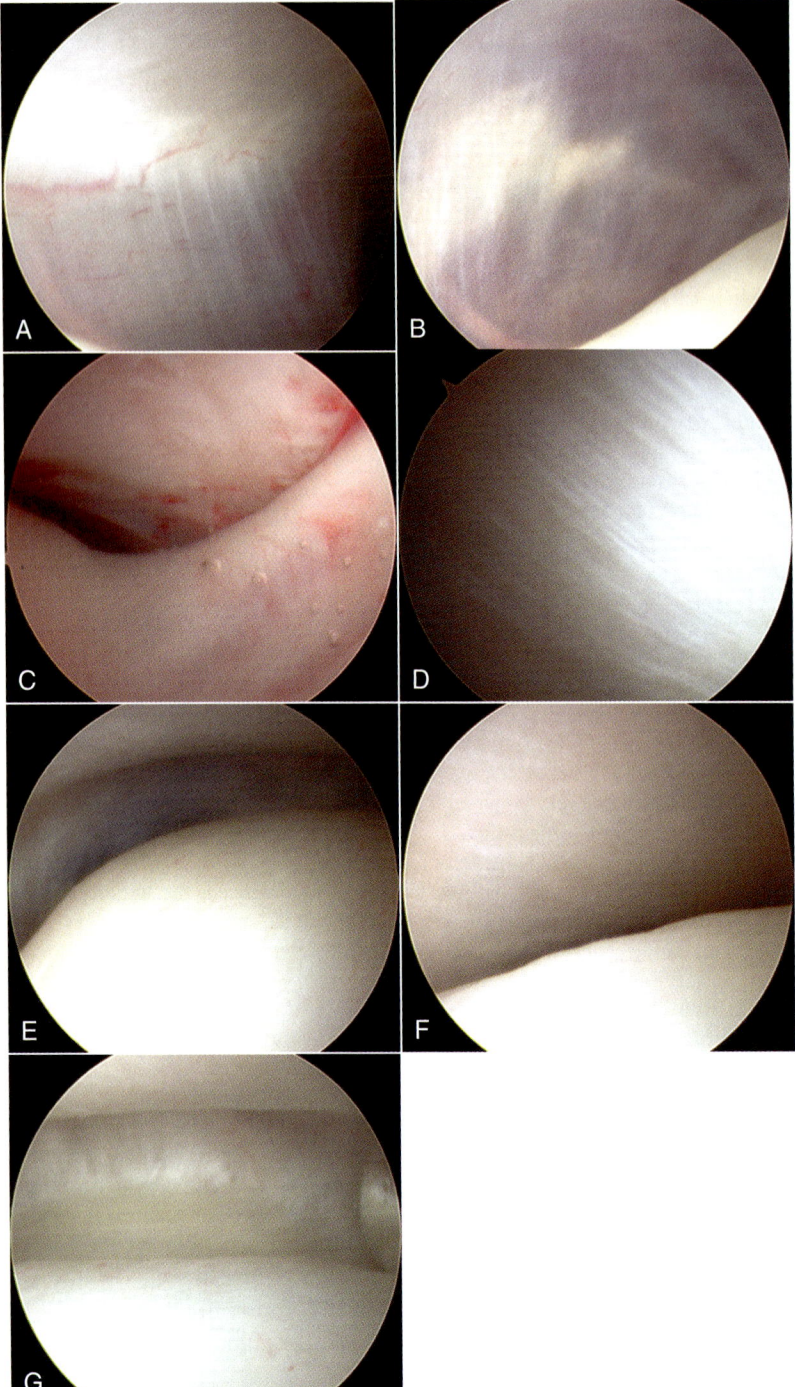

Fig. 6-25 ■ **A,** Medial synovial drape. **B,** Pterygoid shadow. **C,** Retrodiskal synovium with the oblique protuberance. **D,** Posterior slope of the eminence. **E,** Articular disk with 100% roofing. **F,** Intermediate zone. **G,** Anterior recess with puncture bubble.

ARTHROSCOPIC ASSESSMENT OF DISK POSITION

Disk position can be assessed regardless of whether the disk is in a normal position. In normal arthroscopic anatomy, the posterior band of the disk lies adjacent to the back slope of the fibrocartilage of the articular eminence and the glenoid fossa when the condyle is in the forward and seated positions, respectively. To identify the reducing disk, arthroscopic observation is performed first with the condyle forward. In the seated position, the retrodiskal synovium comes into view. The nonreducing disk is determined arthroscopically by observing the roofing of the disk with the condyle forward. In nonroofing situations, the disk is not reducing.

ROOFING

This concept was developed to evaluate the covering of the condyle by the articular disk when the condyle is either forward or seated. An attempt is made to specifically grade the amount of displacement by arthroscopic observation of the disk. The first observation of roofing is made with the condyle forward. When viewed in physiologic disk position, with the condyle 100% roofed by the disk, the posterior band of the disk can be seen lying adjacent to the posterior slope of the articular eminence, thus giving a white-on-white appearance. The disk flexure with its U-shape is prominent; the retrodiskal synovial tissue appears normal, with or without hypervascularity. The second observation of roofing is made with the condyle seated. This assessment reveals the degree of displacement in reducing the disk. Gradations of roofing are ascertained by the arthroscopic view of the posterior band of the disk as it abuts the midportion of the glenoid fossa and the articular eminence. In nonpathologic states, with the condyle 100% roofed, the posterior band of the disk abuts at approximately the midportion of the glenoid fossa or just at the beginning of the back slope of the articular eminence. When evaluating the degree of roofing with the condyle seated, occasionally there are some technical difficulties. In certain instances, the condyle cannot be completely seated into the glenoid fossa because it is obstructed by the tip of the arthroscope, notwithstanding the capsular peripheral position of the scope. In abnormal situations of disk displacement and marked redundant retrodiskal synovium, the arthroscopic view quickly becomes obstructed by the redundant synovium, even though the condyle is seated and the position of the scope maintained. These factors are valuable diagnostic indicators that disk displacement in the seated position is occurring.

Area 6: Intermediate Zone (Fig. 6-25, F)

In order to examine the sixth area, with the condyle forward, the scope is pistoned to facilitate placement at approximately 1 mm away from the interface between the junction of the articular eminence and the articular disk. From this 11 o'clock to 1 o'clock position, the scope follows the path of the articular eminence. Normally this area should have a complete white-on-white appearance, with the fibrocartilage, cranially, white and the disk, caudally, also white. The scope is swiveled, first anterior, moving down the articular eminence, then lateral, positioning it in the lateral synovial trough while observing the intermediate zone. With the condyle forward, the scope is pistoned or swiveled anterior as far as permitted. With disk displacement without reduction, it is paramount to note when disk tissue is first observed. The degree of roofing can be assessed by comparing the white fibrocartilage, cranially, and the red retrodiskal synovium, caudally. The scope is then pistoned as far anterior as permitted to the apex of the articular eminence. When the arthroscope can no longer be moved anteriorly, the condyle is seated. A triangle reflecting an open space and pathway to the anterior recess should be visible. The triangle is limited by the apex of the anterior slope of the articular eminence, the articular disk inferiorly, and the beginning of the anterior synovium anteriorly. Seating the condyle and pistoning the scope into the anterior recess must be precisely coordinated.

Area 7: Anterior Recess (Fig. 6-25, G)

The seventh area is the last one to be examined. Examination can only begin after the condyle is seated and the anterior triangle identified. The arthroscope is pistoned directly into the anterior recess until the midportion of the anterior synovium is visible. At this point, by swiveling and pistoning the scope slightly posterior and inferior, the anterior disk-synovium crease is identified. The crease is examined by following it to the terminal medial point, the most extreme medioanterior corner of the crease and the pterygoid shadow. The scope is then pistoned out along the synovial crease to the periphery of the capsule. At the lateral and anterior limit, the junction between the anterior disk-synovium crease and the lateral synovial capsule can be viewed. In pathosis, the vascularity of the anterior synovial pouch increases and all characteristics of inflammation of synovium are present. Occasionally, synovial redundancy and synovial plicae

are also present. Creeping of synovium onto the articular eminence can also be seen. The disk below in the anterior recess may appear buckled, with the anterior band becoming prominent.

INTRA-ARTICULAR PATHOLOGY

Although the micromolecular aspects of TMJ pathology are beyond the scope of this chapter, a brief review of intra-articular pathology is required.

Synovitis: The acute form consists of inflammation with dilated superficial capillaries but not hyperemia in the early stages, progressively increasing hyperemia, then total obliteration of the superficial vascularity in the most severe stages. For clinical purposes, it is described in stages 1 through 4, with 2 and 3 for the intermediate stages. The chronic form is characterized by synovial hyperplasia with increasing proliferation of tissue folds, particularly in the retrodiskal area.

Fibrosis: Intra-articular hemorrhage results in the formation of a fibrin scaffold for the fibroblasts to migrate upon and produce fibrous adhesions. In addition, pseudodigit villous proliferations are frequently present. The condition can present as fibrous adhesions or total synovial fibrosis.

Pigmented Villonodular Synovitis: This state is characterized by multiple, diffuse, pigmented, nodular villi, which can involve the entire synovium. Typically it occurs following prolonged inflammation stages, most commonly seen with osteoarthritis.

Synovial Chondromatosis: This rare disease of the synovial membrane presents with multiple osteocartilaginous bodies attached to the synovium and others floating freely in the joint space.

Rheumatoid Arthritis: Rheumatoid arthritis is a systemic disease of undetermined etiology. It is considered an autoimmune disease, with a rheumatoid antibody factor, anti-IgG, present in 85% to 90% of patients. From a TMJ perspective, it is characterized by synovial hypervascularity with elongated villous lesions, aggregates of lymphocytes, and dilated capillaries. More than 50% of patients with this disease also have TMJ involvement.

Pseudogout/Chondrocalcinosis: In contrast to gout, where the crystals are deposited in the synovium, synovial villi, and fibrillated and fragmented fibrocartilage (chondromalacia grade III), chondrocalcinosis is characterized by calcium pyrophosphate crystals in the synovium with the articular cartilage unaltered.

Joint Stenosis: In cases of synovitis without any disk or cartilage pathology, some joint stenosis accompanies the condition along with generalized capsulitis. This will restrict the range of motion of the joint. Small intrasynovial adhesions are not likely to restrict joint motion; however, the combination of these adhesions, alteration of synovial fluid mechanics, and generalized capsulitis and stenosis will restrict condylar motion, because of pain and loss of function. In the authors' experience, adhesive synovitis is most commonly diagnosed in the anterior recess, with the posterior recess being the second most common area.

Articular Dysfunction: From an arthroscopic perspective, the discussion will revolve around reducing and nonreducing disks. In the situation of a reducing disk, the posterior band of the disk is visible and accessible for suturing when the condyle is forward. In the nonreducing disk, there is no posterior band seen with the condyle forward. Also, the entire anterior band may be obscured with fibrosis. Obviously, the cases of chronic disk dislocation associated with fibrosis and pseudowall formation will obliterate the disk-synovium crease.

Osteoarthritis (Fig. 6-26): The studies of Boering and Rasmussen seem to support the idea of a natural process of joint aging. Whether this process occurs slowly or rapidly, the operative

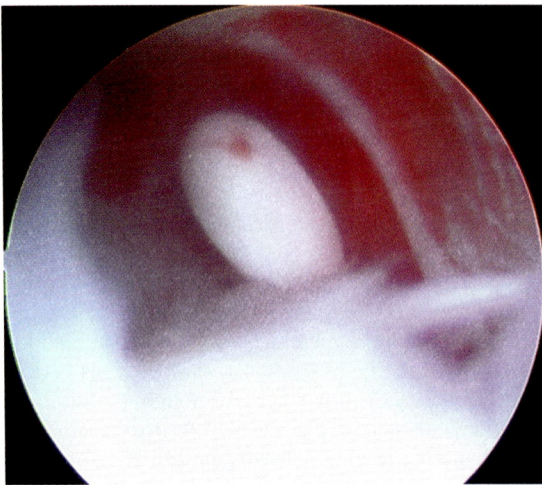

Fig. 6-26 ■ Osteoarthritis and intra-articular loose body.

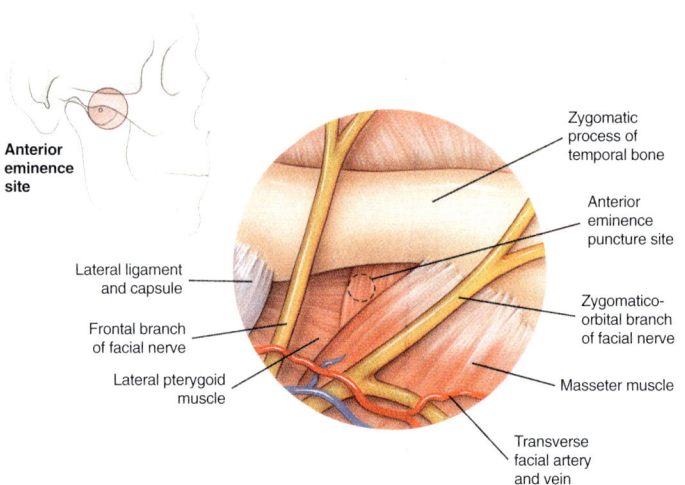

Fig. 6-27 ■ Anterior eminence portal (second puncture). (From McCain JP: *Principles and practice of temporomandibular joint arthroscopy,* St. Louis, 1996, Mosby.)

procedures to treat this condition are limited by joint size, stenosis, pathologic state, and the technical limitations of the surgeon and instrumentation. One of the typical arthroscopic findings when dealing with this entity is articular cartilage degeneration that can be observed along the posterior slope and peak of the articular eminence. A brief discussion of *chondromalacia* along with the classification of this pathognomonic finding will follow next.

Chondromalacia: *Grade I: Softening of cartilage* is caused by digestion of proteoglycan collagenases from injured chondrocytes. Clinically, the cartilage turns opaque white, as opposed to its normal tan appearance. The difference is quite subtle; however, very gentle palpation of the articular cartilage with the scope will reveal its compressibility, friability, and the dimpling or pitting effect of this edematous tissue, evident mostly on the posterior slope of the eminence. *Grade II: Furrowing* is the result of disruption of some of the deep zone collagen fibrils at the calcified and noncalcified cartilage attachment, and hydrated swelling of the proteoglycan-depleted areas along the fibrils in the TMJ. *Grade III: Fibrillation and ulceration* are caused by rupture of the deeper collagen fibrils from their calcified and noncalcified cartilage attachment and then the disruption of the parallel articular surface fibrils. These disruptions result in fibrillar strands of degenerating cartilage that can be observed hanging from the posterior slope and peak of the articular eminence when suspended in the Ringer lactate arthroscopic medium. *Grade IV: Crater formation and subchondral bone exposure* result from progressive breakdown of the deep and superficial fibrils, followed by a breakdown of the intermediate cartilage fibrils.

Arthrofibrosis: We chose to describe this condition separately from the fibrosis described earlier because of the severity of this condition and its association with the severe hypomobility of Wilkes stages IV and V. It also represents one of the most difficult surgical challenges for the TMJ arthroscopist. Correlation with clinical findings compels us to reiterate that severe trismus in the presence of good excursive joint motion should prompt the surgeon in diagnosing an extra-articular condition. Hence the focus should be more on myotomy and fasciotomy procedures, followed by aggressive physical therapy and counseling. The patient with intra-articular degeneration and hypomobility typically presents with minimal opening, minimal excursive motion, and focal joint pain. Documentation of baseline interincisal opening should be done under sedation or anesthesia immediately before the procedure. The entire diagnostic arthroscopy for this condition is very different from what we presented earlier in

the chapter. The surgeon must be particularly careful when puncturing a hypomobile joint. Frequently, the greatest concavity of the glenoid fossa is less evident, and the condyle becomes difficult to palpate, particularly if the lateral pole is degenerated or absent. Also, insufflation of the superior joint compartment is more difficult because the lateral capsular wall distention cannot be palpated and plunger rebound cannot be felt. These are typical signs of joint stenosis and intra-articular fibrosis, or more concisely, arthrofibrosis. The diagnostic sweep is attempted. However, a "white out" of fibrillar tissue makes visualization of structures very difficult. A lysis maneuver is performed blindly to increase the working space. During this initial sweep, it is paramount that the contours of the fossa and eminence are palpated at all times. The joint is again backwashed and the scope reinserted. The glenoid fossa and eminence should be visible at this point, and sometimes the condyle can also be seen. As previously described in this chapter, the next step of the diagnostic sweep is to position the scope medially in the joint, to identify the medial synovial drape. Extreme caution should be exercised so as not to violate this structure and venture too far medially, where the internal maxillary artery and other vital structures can be found. This complication can be prevented by continuous awareness of cannula depth.

ARTHROSCOPIC ARTHROPLASTY

This surgical procedure necessitates the establishment of a second portal to insert the working cannula. Most of the intra-articular instrumentation will be manipulated via this portal.

ANTERIOR EMINENCE PORTAL (Fig. 6-27)

For teaching and visualizing purposes, a circle of 20-mm diameter can be superimposed over the anterior eminence region in the same fashion as for the fossa portal. The boundaries for this circle are the zygomatic process of the temporal arch anteriorly, the apex of the articular eminence of the zygomatic process of the temporal bone posteriorly, the temporal fossa superiorly, and the mandibular sigmoid notch inferiorly. The anatomic structures at this site are as follows, from lateral to medial: the tegument; the superficial parotid fascia; the superior anterior parotid gland lobule; the deep parotid fascia and the most posterior point of intersection of the frontal branch of the facial nerve; the masseter; the masseteric nerve, artery, and vein; the anterolateral aspect of the TMJ capsule; and the lateral pterygoid. Measuring from the midportion of the tragus anterior, the length of the frontal branch of the facial nerve would range from 13 to 40 mm, with a mean of 20 to 25 mm. The zygomatic-orbital branch lies anterior to the frontal branch.

LYSIS AND LAVAGE

In addition to the diagnostic lysis and lavage (L/L), the double puncture arthroscopic L/L emphasizes the lytic aspect more. Using a straight probe, the pouches and recesses of the superior joint space can be directly manipulated. The lysis procedure is designed to distend all pouches and recesses along the capsule to give the physical therapist a head start in postoperative joint manipulation. The sequential lysis of adhesions in the superior joint space proceeds from anterior to posterior, without repeated motion of instruments from the back to the front of the joint, which increases the risk of unnecessary articular surface scuffing. The lysis maneuvers with a probe under direct arthroscopic visualization are performed according to the triangulation techniques. The purpose of the procedure is to restore the volume and architecture of the joint. The probe is first placed in the most medial aspect of the joint, and then swept laterally along the disk-synovium junction with an inferoanterior maneuver. Then, by sweeping medial to lateral along the articular eminence, a superoanterior maneuver is executed to complete the lysis. These maneuvers are repeated until an adequate recess volume is restored. In many instances, the anterior recess lysis is followed by posterior recess lysis. Under direct observation, the probe and the scope are translated back into the posterior pouch. Upon release of lateral adhesions, a marked increase in the range of motion of the condyle occurs immediately. There is one critical observation these authors have made over thousands of procedures performed. Medial wall synovitis is, in many instances, related to the inflammation of the insertion of the superior belly of the lateral pterygoid, causing myalgia, and restricted range of motion of the mandible.

DEBRIDEMENT

There are instances when adhesions cannot be disrupted with the probe, or the fragments of broken adhesions tenaciously remain attached to the walls. A motorized whisker shaver is then used to debride these fragments. Sometimes it is necessary to use an alternating sequence of whisker shaver and bipolar electrocautery to first desiccate and then remove some of the more resilient fragments. In the absence of the debridement, there is a high likelihood of postoperative crepitation in the area.

SYNOVECTOMY

The most effective technique of reduction of redundant synovium is bipolar electrocautery. Redundant synovium most often occurs in the posterior pouch, especially after disk reduction procedures. Occasionally, it may be encountered in the anterior recess. Hypervascularity and redundancy can effectively be reduced with bipolar electrocautery. The McCain-Leibinger bipolar electrocautery easily fits through a 2.0-mm working cannula and is used for synovium reduction purposes. The synovium changes color from bright red to off-white or even a light brown. On occasion, the cauterized and desiccated fragments of synovial tissue fail to vaporize with bipolar electrocautery. For these situations, the holmium laser is used instead.

ANTERIOR RELEASE

Using a blunt probe, a lysis procedure is performed, if necessary, in the anterior recess until the entire disk-synovium crease can be visualized from medial to lateral. Just before commencing the release, the disk-synovium crease is confirmed with a hook probe. If the crease is not properly identified, iatrogenic disk perforation may occur during the anterior release procedure. If the anteroposterior disk dimension appears adequate and the shape of the disk is relatively normal, the release starts in the medial one half of the disk-synovium crease. Using a holmium laser, the synovial capsule is incised just anterior and parallel to the anterior margin of the disk. The surgeon observes the muscle fibers inserting into the disk and capsule. Dissection should be performed to a depth no greater than 5 mm or until the anterior band is freely mobile and is not tethered. Myotomy at the most anteromedial corner should be done cautiously. When the anteromedial synovial drape is incised at the junction with the disk, an artery, approximately 1 to 2 mm in diameter, is usually found directly subjacent to the junction. Arthroscopically, it appears white and tubular. If this vessel is inadvertently incised, copious intra-articular hemorrhaging will occur. This vessel cannot be cauterized or tied off by any current means. To stop the bleeding, all instruments must be removed and constant lateral pressure must be maintained on the joint for 5 minutes, while the condyle is held in a forward and contralateral position. The puncture techniques are then repeated and the joint is lavaged and suctioned free of clots. No further releasing is done in that area and the release is completed laterally. Identification of this artery will prevent this problem, and the myotomy can be carefully completed around the artery. The other potential bleeding points encountered in the lateral pterygoid can be relatively easily controlled with bipolar cautery. The lateral one half to two thirds of the anterior release may be performed more expediently with less risk of hemorrhage. One of the concerns with an excessively deep anterior release is that of avascular necrosis, which can be documented on postoperative MRIs. The most plausible explanation for this complication is that the fibers inserting in the pterygoid fovea (of the condyle) have been transected, causing subsequent venous congestion in the condylar head and, ultimately, changes on the MRI. In light of these observations, the authors surmise that the myotomy should be confined to a depth of 5 mm, so that only the superior head insertion is released. Probing to assess anterior band mobility should be routinely performed during the anterior release. Obviously, the recommendation is to always err on the conservative side.

DISK REDUCTION

Once the anterior release is achieved, the disk is reduced in the anatomic position. To begin the reduction, the blunt probe is introduced and passed posteriorly by following the intermediate zone. Simultaneously, the condyle is distracted anteriorly and contralaterally. Once the probe is positioned in the posterolateral recess, the retrodiskal tissues are depressed posteroinferiorly. Disk reduction should be felt by the surgeon and confirmed arthroscopically. The disk is held in reduced position with the probe and the working cannula while the scope is retracted to a lateral position. Then the probe pressure is released to ascertain passive reduction and positioning of the disk in the anatomic position.

POSTERIOR CAUTERIZATION AND SCARIFICATION (Fig. 6-28)

Once disk reduction is achieved, an increased amount of redundant synovium is noted in the retrodiskal flexure. Even with minor disk repositioning procedures and less evidence of redundancy of posterior synovium, in the absence of diskopexy, this procedure should be performed. Typically, a "reefing" phenomenon occurs, where the retrodiskal tissue is bunched up and needs to be reduced in bulk with bipolar cautery. If not, this fairly large amount of tissue can fibrose

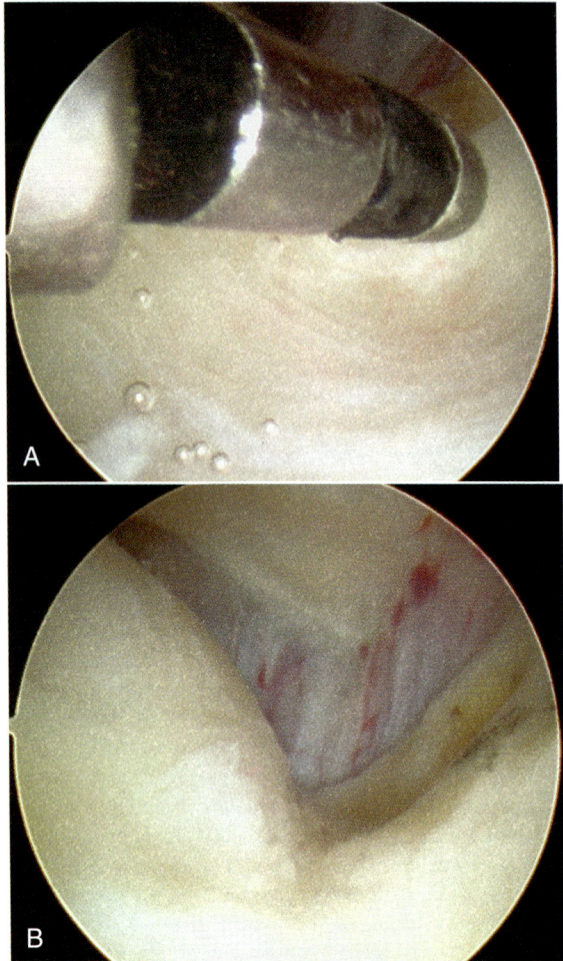

Fig. 6-28 ■ **A** and **B,** Posterior contracture and scarification.

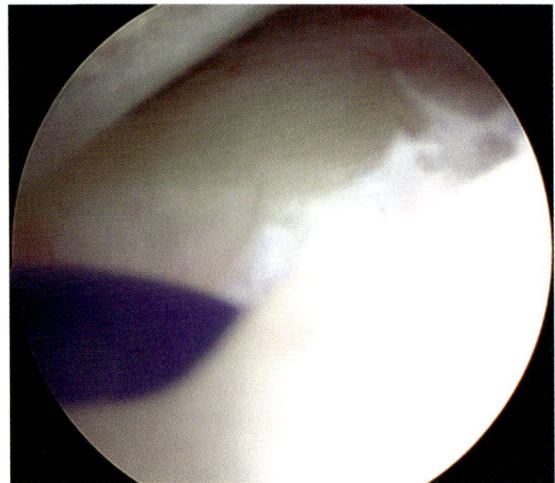

Fig. 6-29 ■ Suture diskopexy.

during healing. During postoperative settling, the disk may then be displaced by this potentially fibrotic mass. Retrodiskal ablation should therefore be performed until a normal-shaped retrodiskal flexure is sculpted. The inflamed synovium is cauterized and the areas of excess tissue bulk ablated with bipolar cautery, laser, or both. Deep electrocautery of the oblique protuberance should then be performed. An examination of the anterior and posterior pouches is then completed.

DISK FUNCTION

Before making the decision to exit the TMJ, joint mechanics have to be reassessed. If disk reduction is inadequate or clicking is noted, the anterior release is revisited with the blunt probe. If tethering is observed, it is most likely in the medial muscle insertion area or in the most lateral extent of the crease. Once the anterior release is extended, disk function is reassessed. If clicking persists or the disk position is not satisfactorily stable, the diskopexy procedure should be considered.

ARTHROSCOPIC DISK SUTURING AND DISKOPEXY

This procedure was developed with the thought that arthroscopic restoration of functional intra-articular anatomy is the best treatment alternative for managing articular dysfunction. The authors believe that symptomatic internal derangements should be restored to a

normal condyle-disk relationship, arresting the natural course of osteoarthritis. The diskopexy is performed to achieve this goal. This technique addresses both the reducing and nonreducing disk.

DISKOPEXY FOR THE REDUCING DISK (Fig. 6-29)

Placement of the Suture Passing Needle

Since it is visible, the surgeon scans the posterior band of the disk to identify the ideal area for suture placement. The best place is at the junction between the middle and medial thirds of the disk. From this point, the arthroscope is swiveled into the lateral recess in preparation for suture passing, while the assistant maintains the condyle in a forward position. The vector technique is applied to determine the exact point of entry of the suture passing needle through the skin. The scope is positioned in the lateral excess directly lateral to the posterior band of the disk. This location will correlate with the lateral pole of the condyle. The depth of the scope is noted, then using an empty cannula, this distance is marked off on the skin. The suture passing needle enters the skin at this point. A 20-gauge, $1\frac{1}{4}$-inch needle threaded with a single #1 polydioxanone suture is passed perpendicular to the skin and advanced until the lateral pole of the condyle is felt with the needle. The needle tip is then walked superiorly until it slides off the head of the condyle. An upward bulging of the posterior band will be noted where the needle is passing through the disk. The suture passing needle is redirected to engage the desired amount of posterior band tissue (a 2- to 3-mm bite of disk fibrocartilage). The needle tip is then advanced and observed in the greatest concavity of the fossa. This area provides the greatest accessibility for suture retrieval.

Placement of the Suture Catching Needle

The suture catching needle is passed percutaneously from the preauricular skin crease at the level of the pinna. This particular instrument is called the Meniscus Mender II (Smith and Nephew) and is provided with an interchangeable obturator and a lasso type of suture retriever. Once it enters the skin, the mender is advanced anteromedially and toward the maximum concavity of the glenoid fossa. As it enters the superior joint space, disk incorporation is carefully avoided as the mender passes. The scope is fixed on the greatest concavity of the glenoid fossa, and once the mender is visualized, it is positioned close to the suture passing needle. At this point, the obturator is removed and the retriever is inserted. The lasso portion is slipped over the 20-gauge needle and the needle is advanced slightly. The suture is advanced through the passing needle and retrieved with the lasso. The suture passing needle and the meniscus mender are removed, leaving the two free ends of the suture exiting the skin. The scope is also removed.

Retrograde Passing of the Anterior Suture End

With a No. 11 blade, two small incisions (~5 mm each) are placed in the preauricular skin crease, away from each other, extending superiorly from the suture exit point. Using a fine straight hemostat, a blunt dissection is performed adjacent to the suture ends and along the tragal cartilage, down to the joint capsule. The anterior suture end must now be passed posterior for final tying. Using a #3 half circle, tapered, French spring eye needle, the anterior suture (lower end) is passed back down its needle tract to the capsule. The suture needle is then redirected posterosuperiorly along the extracapsular fatty tissue. The tip should emerge in the center of the superior blunt dissection wound and is retrieved with an Adson forceps. Passing the needle through the middle of both blunt dissections is a very deliberate move, avoiding any impingement on epidermal or dermal tissue layers. If impingement occurs, a dimple in the skin will form and disk-traction results will not be ideal. This may also lead to impingement of the frontal branch of the facial nerve. The suture is tied down in the extracapsular fatty tissue. A surgeon's knot is used to prevent slippage when cinching the knot down. Once the knot has been cinched down for the first time, the condyle is seated by the assistant and the knot is cinched again. Additional ties are placed in the suture and it is trimmed at the knot. The skin incisions are closed with 6-0 nylon or 5-0 fast gut, one interrupted suture per incision.

DISKOPEXY FOR THE NONREDUCING DISK

In this situation, with the condyle forward, the posterior band is not visible. This is a double puncture technique. After the anterior release, posterior cauterization, and disk reduction are performed as described previously in this chapter, the operator can proceed with the diskopexy. Here are the fine points of this procedure in the nonreducing disk. First, the disk is held in the reduced position with the working cannula and probe, and the scope is pistoned laterally. In preparation for suturing, the surgeon hands the assistant the blunt probe. The assistant now firmly stabilizes the disk in the reduced position. The scope is carefully swiveled laterally from the desired disk suturing point to the lateral recess. In general, this will place the field of view over the lateral pole area, and the working cannula will occupy the lower portion of this field. The suture is passed as previously described. Once the suture passes through the disk, the assistant takes charge of the scope and the reduction probe, and the surgeon retrieves the suture with the meniscus mender. All the other steps of the procedure are performed as described earlier. As for inferior joint space adhesions or anchored disk phenomenon, the arthroscopic surgical techniques for disk repositioning and fixation are predictably repeatable despite some limitations.

ARTHROSCOPIC PROCEDURES FOR MANAGEMENT OF TMJ OSTEOARTHRITIS

Obviously, the purpose of developing these techniques is to provide new therapies for TMJ cartilage destruction and severe synovitis. To achieve treatment goals, a multidisciplinary approach is necessary, including stress management counseling, physical therapy, and orthotic therapy to reduce joint overloading.

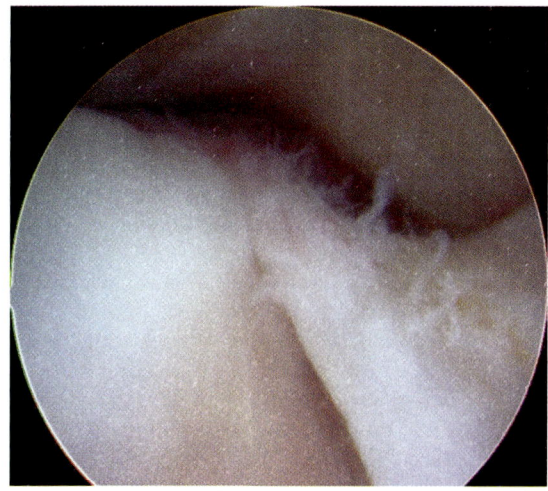

Fig. 6-30 ■ Disk perforation.

RETRODISKAL PERFORATIONS (Fig. 6-30)

Identification and documentation of the retrodiskal perforation should exist from the previous diagnostic arthroscopy. This time the surgeon performs a short diagnostic sweep, and without further delay, using the vector technique previously described, establishes a second portal in the anterior recess. A blunt probe will then be used to ascertain the disk quality and mobility. The anterior disk-synovium junction is identified with a hook probe. The blunt probe and scope are then swiveled into the posterior recess. The perforation is measured, and if visible, the condyle is palpated. A whisker shaver may now be employed to remove any cartilage degeneration that has a "crab meat" appearance on the periphery of the perforation. A better assessment of the size and shape of the perforation can now be done, and the condyle will be easier to see. Now is the time to compare all the MRI and arthroscopic findings and make correlations. If feasible, the anterior release is performed, followed by disk reduction and diskopexy. The suturing technique in this particular situation is modified from the one presented earlier in the incorporation of the perforation into the retrodiskal flexure. Sometimes this cannot be done with just one suture. Additional anterolateral release is indicated, and up to two or three additional sutures can be placed. If despite all attempts, the perforation is not completely closed, the size and position of the residual perforation should be assessed. In the absence of crepitation and osseous contact in the fully seated condyle position, the goal of an interposed soft tissue pad has been met, much like the case of the autogenous dermal graft, temporalis muscle flap graft, conchal graft, or lyophilized or freeze-dried dura graft.

CENTRAL PERFORATIONS

The goals of managing the large central perforation are to not only restore the normal functional anatomy, but also achieve a balance between the loading forces sustained by the condyle, the remainder of the disk, and the glenoid fossa. No diskopexy should be attempted for these cases. Treatment consists of decreasing crepitation, smoothing bone-to-bone contact, and improving joint mobility if indicated. Meniscectomy is reduced only to the diseased portions or the tissue impinging on condylar motion. The first step is debridement of all advanced degenerative fibrocartilage with bipolar or monopolar cautery or a laser instrument. The margins of the disk perforation are trimmed while the degenerative areas of grade III and IV chondromalacia are removed from the eminence. The joint is then lavaged and the joint mechanics are observed arthroscopically. Particular consideration is given to finding bone-to-bone contact areas. Wherever these are noticed, abrasion arthroplasty is performed. Once the area to be reduced is identified, the condyle is translated well past the apex of the articular eminence while the assistant pivots the mandible to the contralateral side. This increases the space between the impinging surfaces to allow instrument access. The area is adjusted and blended into the medial and lateral aspects, and the posterior slope of the eminence is blended into the normal contour of the fossa. The maneuver is repeated until the crepitation is removed or significantly reduced. Osteophytes on the medial aspect of the apex of the eminence are osteoplasticized. Not all medial osseous prominences are removed, because they sometimes provide useful meniscus load-bearing areas. High condylar osteoplasty transperforation may sometimes be necessary. The procedure is terminated once osseous impingement is relieved and crepitation abolished or reduced. Clicking that is intractable or that develops postarthroplasty is usually caused by perforation of the anterior or anteromedial meniscus. The authors manage this problem by trimming the margins of the perforation with a suction punch or laser instrument. In the rare instances where the anterolateral aspects of a perforation need to be adjusted, interchanging the straight- and side-firing laser tips will be necessary.

ARTHROFIBROSIS

With the invaluable information provided by the diagnostic arthroscopy at hand, the surgeon proceeds with a short diagnostic sweep, assessing any changes in the status of joint stenosis or refibrosis of the areas that were previously opened by the lysis and lavage. After assessment of the medial sulcus, the scope is pistoned laterally and swiveled through the intermediate zone into the anterior recess. In most instances this will not be possible for the same reasons mentioned previously (impingement or white out). Using vector triangulation, the second puncture establishes the anterior recess portal. The holmium laser is used to debride the joint. This maneuver is carefully advanced into the anterior recess by contouring along the eminence. As the debridement proceeds anteriorly and more joint space is opened, a third puncture may be necessary to gain adequate access for the procedure. The scope can be switched into the second puncture portal. The limiting factor for the debridement is a normal anterior recess volume. Evidence may reveal that there is no residual disk present. Osteoplasty of the condylar head is performed as described earlier in the chapter. Indiscriminant arthrectomy should be avoided, and surfaces with normal aspect fibrocartilage, synovium, or both should not be violated. The arthrectomy procedure is terminated when a notable improvement in excursive motion is reached. The interincisal opening is reassessed and documented. In bilateral cases, the procedure follows the same pattern in the contralateral joint. The interincisal opening is always documented at the end of the procedure.

COMPLICATIONS OF SURGICAL ARTHROSCOPY

DAMAGE TO CRANIAL NERVE VII AND FACIAL PALSY AND ATONY

When approaching the TMJ for a glenoid fossa portal puncture, the frontotemporal branch of the facial nerve should be anterior, whereas for an eminence or working portal puncture it is located posterior. However, the zygomatic branch of facial nerve may be in jeopardy as well. In the authors' experience, paresis of the frontotemporal branch of the facial nerve occurs in less than 1% of procedures

(reaching a high of 0.73% in early days of arthroscopy). Invariably, these patients had undergone open arthrotomy before the minimally invasive procedure. This suggests scarring of the preauricular tissues, which increases pressure on the nerve branches from joint distention and causes palsy of the frontotemporal and zygomatic facial rami. It manifests as an atony of the orbicularis oculi muscle and the frontal division of the occipitofrontalis muscle, translated in the partial ability to elevate the eyebrow and to completely occlude the superior palpebral sulcus or fold, both in the immediate postoperative period. A definite diagnosis is made 24 hours postoperative. Typically, the duration of signs varies between 1 week and 6 months. An additional mechanism of injury for CN VII with this procedure is extravasation, with or without hematoma formation. Misplacement of the irrigating cannula or joint lavage at excessively high pressure can force solutions beyond the confines of the capsule and into the adjacent tissues. The majority of incidents involving CN VII are compressive (equivalent to neurapraxia described by Seddon and Sutherland), in which injuries include both mechanical deforming forces and ischemic factors. Upon injury, first there is an increased vascular permeability causing subperineural and endoneural edema and leading to connective tissue changes. Perineural and epineural thickening may occur, followed by localized nerve fiber changes, in which some nerves function normally but others exhibit segmental demyelinization. As the magnitude and the duration of compression increases, wallerian degeneration becomes apparent. The peripheral fascicles and nerve fibers are primarily affected, whereas those located more centrally may be spared. Should axonotmesis or neurotmesis occur during puncture, the only factor obstructing nerve regeneration would be cicatricial tissue, which competes with the axonal growth cone to bridge the gap. In the authors' experience, CN VII injuries have a good prognosis for restitutio ad integrum of function.

DAMAGE TO THE CRANIAL NERVE V (AURICULOTEMPORAL, LINGUAL, OR INFERIOR ALVEOLAR) WITH HYPERESTHESIA, DYSESTHESIA, PARESTHESIA, OR ANESTHESIA

The ATN along with the superficial temporal artery and vein are posterior but close to the fossa puncture site. Our present experience has revealed that hemorrhage is uncommon, and if encountered, it is not significant and is stopped with direct pressure. Postoperative anesthesia around the entry sites is a common occurrence that spontaneously resolves within 2 weeks. No hyperesthesia or dysesthesia has been reported. Rotation of the trocar cannula while penetrating the portal sites permits important vital structures to be bypassed and the intracapsular space to be punctured with minimal resistance. This complication stems from a placement too far posterior to the fossa portal as a consequence of operator concern for CN VII damage. When the lingual nerve is concerned, the most immediate proximity to the mandibular condyle report comes from Johansson. On an extensive cadaver study, the mandibular nerve was dissected running vertical from the foramen ovale at approximately 10 mm inferior to the foramen. It then divided into the inferior alveolar and lingual rami, with the latter passing 3.5 mm medial to the condyle. The nerve can be injured if the operator is not cognizant of the intra-articular anatomy and perforates the drape at a distance of more than 35 mm from the tegument. Another possibility is the medial extravasation of irrigation fluid secondary to medial capsular perforation without a proper irrigation system. This perforation may also involve the inferior alveolar nerve. Hyperesthesia of the infraorbital nerve is associated with long operative time, excessive volumes of irrigation fluid, and extravasation of irrigant into the medial tissues. The condition is self-limiting, because the fluid is resorbed into the lymphatic and venous systems. Extravasation is prevented by careful puncture technique, observation of the surgical site, gentle pressure during irrigation, and a patent inflow and outflow system.

DAMAGE TO CRANIAL NERVE VIII AND VESTIBULOCOCHLEAR DYSFUNCTION

Tympanic membrane perforation and ossicle disruption in the middle ear has been reported, including otitis media with subsequent hypoacusis. The middle ear is entered either through the osseous or soft tissue external auditory meatus. If the tympanic membrane is perforated and the ossicles appear in the view field, immediate cessation of procedure and intra-operative ENT/ORL consultation is warranted. The ossicles have a classic melted wax appearance. If no manipulation is performed, the incidence of permanent disruption of ossicles is low and the complication will be limited to the tympanic membrane. Small perforations in the anterior or inferior portions of the tympanum, typically, cause minimal hearing loss and heal uneventfully, without sequelae. Posterior tympanum injuries may dislocate the ossicles and, potentially, result in more significant loss of hearing. All perforations involving more than 30% of the tympanum surface or the posterior portion of it should be managed by an otorhinolaryngologist. Postoperative complaints of severe hearing loss or vertigo are signs of a possible middle ear injury and an ORL/ENT referral should not be delayed. Laceration of the external auditory meatus (EAM) occurs by transfixiation of the canal with the arthroscope at the junction of the tragus and osseous meatus. Minor hemorrhage is controlled with bipolar cautery, whereas the EAM is treated with hydrocortisone suspension drops for up to 2 weeks. If granulation tissue develops at the osseous-cartilaginous junction, bipolar cautery is employed. Baldursson and Blackmer have suggested a correlation between specific sensorineural hearing loss, with a predictable decrease in hearing levels at the 1000 to 2000 Hz range, and TMJ dysfunction or parafunction, or both. In the authors' experience, all patients regained normal hearing levels within 2 months postoperative. This confirms the fact that arthroscopy does not affect hearing levels if no direct trauma to the middle ear has occurred. Ensuring that the scope is not advanced past 20 to 25 mm without accurately checking its position will prevent the occurrence of this complication.

SCUFFING OF FIBROCARTILAGE

The cartilage covering the eminence and fossa is most prone to iatrogenic damage; this is the most common arthroscopic complication. At the time of insufflation, the needle point is directed toward the posterior slope of the eminence, making contact with the fibrocartilage. Also, examination sweeps of the joint cavity, involving translation of the arthroscope along with the cannula, could also release pieces of cartilage into the superior joint space. If scuffing becomes significant, it impairs visibility during arthroscopic procedures to the point of misdiagnosis of chondromalacia by the inexperienced arthroscopist.

DAMAGE TO THE MAXILLARY ARTERY AND ITS COLLATERALS AND ARTERIOVENOUS FISTULA FORMATION

As it courses medial to the condylar neck, the maxillary artery was found immediately lateral to the lateral pterygoid in two thirds of reviewed cases. The authors have encountered this complication, resulting in a left pterygoid AV fistula.

DAMAGE TO THE SUPERFICIAL TEMPORAL VESSELS AND AV FISTULA

Whether profuse or not, all cases of hemorrhage from the superficial temporal artery and vein (STA/STV) intimately related to the posterior aspect of the joint capsule were managed uneventfully by applying controlled pressure. Other authors have reported the formation of an AV fistula. Typically, the patient complains of a constant hissing or whishing sound over the operated TMJ. The fistulectomy and subsequent embolization of the STA were uneventful.

PERFORATION OF THE GLENOID FOSSA

This complication can be consistently prevented by directing the instruments toward the tubercle and away from the fossa. Most violations of the middle cranial fossa will result in CSF leaks that resolve spontaneously. Should the leak persist in the wound or through the incision, a pressure dressing is applied and the patient is hospitalized and the head elevated. Persistence of leak after 48 hours mandates neurosurgical consult and placement of lumbar subarachnoid drain. Head CT with bone windows is obtained to document the site. Surgical dural neuroraphy is very uncommon.

DAMAGE TO THE DISK

Repairs of the meniscus result in a fibrous tissue seal of the surfaces as seen arthroscopically. Core biopsies have shown minimal tissue reaction at the area of repair, consisting of fibrous cell repair with sparse vasculature. There is minimal collagen formation at the repair site and no collagen penetration or angioproliferation into the substance of the repaired meniscus. All needle punctures are filled in and smooth with the meniscus surface 12 weeks postoperative. Exposed nonresorbable sutures are covered with translucent fibrous tissue. The cellular response to meniscal tears has four potential sources: adjacent synovium, capsule vascularity, intra-articular microhemorrhage, and free synovial cells. The adjacent synovium contributes angioblastic and cellular tissue for peripheral meniscal tears. The synovium proliferates in the area and migrates over the disk in a similar way to the pannus noticed on articular cartilage defects. Tears in the lateral one third of the meniscus have abundant vascularity for hemorrhage and angioblastic proliferation. The avascular portion of disk presents fibrous tissue healing response 4 to 6 weeks postoperative.

Hemarthrosis is a consequence of laceration of the STA/STV, severely inflamed synovium and retrodiskal tissue upon entry, and laceration of the pterygoid artery during myotomy for anterior release procedures. Hemorrhage can be significant enough to abort the procedure. When pressure irrigation cannot stop the hemorrhage (despite some clearing of the surgical field) the joint remains congested, prolonging the healing, increasing postoperative discomfort and extending recovery time. While the intra-articular coagulum organizes, it increases the risk of formation of adhesive bands and scarring, reflected clinically in fibrous ankylosis. This limits range of motion of the mandible in all excursions (vertical, protrusive, and lateral). Interincisal opening will be less than 35 mm, and the lateral and protrusive movements will be less than 6 mm. The authors use the following protocol for stopping excessive hemorrhage: (1) The pressure in the irrigation bag is increased. (2) A small amount of Healon (0.5 mL) is injected intra-articularly. (3) Cautery or laser is applied to the bleeding area. (4) Using a 3½-inch spinal needle on a 3-mL syringe, passed through the cannula into the affected area, a small amount of local anesthetic with vasoconstrictor is administered directly into the bleeding site. (5) De novo insufflation of the joint with local anesthetic, transcannula (2% lidocaine with 1/100,000 epinephrine), should stop the hemorrhage. (6) The entire joint is insufflated under pressure, with irrigation fluid while all cannulae are obturated for 5 minutes so that hydrostatic pressure stops blood flow. (7) Should all previous measures be unsuccessful, all instruments are removed from the joint, and direct palmar or digital external pressure is applied for 5 minutes. For added pressure, the condyle is seated in the fossa, particularly if the source of bleeding is in the posterior pouch. If the source is in the anterior pouch, the mandible is manipulated to a protrusive position. The instruments are then reinserted in their original portals and the condition of the joint is reassessed. (8) A #4 catheter balloon is inserted through the working portal and inflated with normal saline. It is left in place for 5 minutes, then deflated and the joint is reassessed. (9) If all measures were unsuccessful, the joint is approached via open technique.

Infection is quasi-infrequent as a consequence of proper sterilization, sterile operating environment, forgiving high vascular tissues, antibiotherapy, and high volume irrigation. The presentation is with erythematous puncture sites and surrounding edematous halos 3 to 5 days postoperative. Administration of a cephalosporin for 7 days resolves the problem. The authors now use a standard protocol for all arthroscopic cases. Preoperative cephalosporin (with the alternative for erythromycin in patients allergic to penicillin) is administered at recommended doses. The antibiotics are administered intravenously while inpatient status is maintained (usually 24 hours). Antibiotics are then given orally for 7 days.

Noninfectious postoperative effusions present with preauricular edema, with a higher level of tenderness to palpation than normally encountered postoperative. The patients are managed with soft diet, joint rest, and application of heat over the affected area. NSAIDs were prescribed as needed. Uneventful, complete resolution of symptoms was evident 4 weeks postoperative. If an effusion persists after 6 weeks, it can be aspirated. If that fails, steroid injection is administered as the last nonsurgical modality. Caution should be exercised to avoid misdiagnosis of this condition, because some effusions develop a few weeks or months after the surgery. Those are an indication of progression of degenerative disease.

INSTRUMENT FAILURE AND LOOSE BODIES

Instrument failure can be attributed to manufacturing defects, misuse, and wear of parts of the instrument itself, all potentially leading to breakage. Backup instruments, including the arthroscope, are mandatory while performing arthroscopy. All instruments with flexible parts should be tested by the surgeon before introduction to the joint (including OnPoint scope, trocar, cannula, scissors, biopsy forceps). Application of excessive force, extreme bending of the scope, especially when negotiating access to the most anterolateral aspect of the superior joint compartment to determine the site for the second puncture, can damage or break the optical system and require replacement or repair. The golden rules include: never force or power-move an instrument; use ferromagnetic instruments; always have a "golden retriever" available; avoid force in removing the instruments; confirm that every movable instrument is closed before removal. If an inadvertent event occurs, Dr. McCain has established a standard protocol (Box 6-1).

BOX 6-1	**Dr. McCain's Protocol for Handling Instrument Failure**

1. Stop the procedure while maintaining the position of the arthroscope and working cannulae.
2. Keep the instrument or foreign body in view.
3. Check the inflow bags to confirm that there is sufficient irrigation fluid to maintain joint distention at all times.
4. Record and measure the depth of the instrument with a scored cannula.
5. Have adequate removal instruments available, including extras.
6. Adjust inflow to ensure optimal visibility.
7. Take a radiograph of the joint if the instrument cannot be inserted arthroscopically.
8. Consider fluoroscopic assistance.
9. Remove the fragment or object.
10. When using a grabber, tips may not fit in the working cannula upon removal. It may be desirable to step up the working cannula to a 3-mm diameter, using a "switch stick," and then perform the retrieval maneuvers. If the foreign body cannot be retrieved, the next arthroscopic attempt should be made in the early postoperative phase (10 days to no longer than 6 weeks postoperative). Should this second attempt fail, the doctor and the patient must review all possible outcomes associated with leaving the foreign body as is. The likelihood of future osteoarthritis or foreign body reaction must be explained to the patient.

PEARLS AND PITFALLS

- Addressing TMJ concerns with surgical procedures should only be initiated after attempts are made in correcting the problem with conservative therapy.
- Be sure to take appropriate preoperative measurements, such as preoperative maximal incisal opening and pain intensity on a visual analog scale. This is crucial in evaluating the efficacy of the procedure performed.
- Be sure to exercise sterile technique for the arthroscopic procedure performed.
- Make sure to draw appropriate landmarks and reference points with an indelible marking pen, before making any punctures. The first puncture should be made 10 mm anterior to and 2 mm inferior to the Holmlund-Helsing line, with the patient's mandible protruded.
- The first puncture should be made through the skin, pointing the sharp trocar in an anterosuperior direction until a pop is heard. The trocar should not be inserted any deeper than 20 to 25 mm from the skin surface.
- Accessing an adequate lavage portal with the second puncture is vital to the procedure. Without it, the patient will experience immense swelling from the irrigating fluid. The lavage portal should be inserted 5 mm anterior to and then 5 mm inferior to the fossa portal.
- The diagnostic sweep should focus on seven anatomic areas: medial synovial drape, pterygoid shadow, retrodiskal synovium, posterior slope of the articular eminence and glenoid fossa, articular disk, intermediate zone, and anterior recess. Examining these areas for pathologic changes will alert the clinician as to the overall condition of the joint and any future treatment that may be necessary.
- Treat the pathology of the TMJ and do not become overzealous. If chondromalacia is visible, use bipolar electrocautery or a disk shaver to remove the pathosis. If the disk is displaced, use diskopexy techniques to reposition and secure the disk into a new position. Central perforations should be managed with meniscectomy of the diseased areas of disk tissue. Smooth bone-to-bone contacts to improve joint mobility, and debride all degenerated tissue. No diskopexy should be attempted for central perforations.

BIBLIOGRAPHY

Anastassov GE, Lee H, Schneider R: Arthroscopic reduction of a high condylar process fracture: a case report, *J Oral Maxillofac Surg* 58(9): 1048-1051, 2000.

Arzoz E, Santiago A, Esnal F, Palomero R: Endoscopic intracorporeal lithotripsy for sialolithiasis, *J Oral Maxillofac Surg* 54(7):847-850, 1996.

Bouloux GF: Temporomandibular joint pain and synovial fluid analysis: a review of the literature, *J Oral Maxillofac Surg* 67(11):2497-2504, 2009.

Chen CT, Chen YR: Endoscopically assisted repair of orbital floor fractures, *Plast Reconstr Surg* 108:2011, 2001.

Cheung LK, Lo J: Endoscope-assisted rigid fixation for intraoral vertical subsigmoid osteotomy: a preliminary clinical study, *J Oral Maxillofac Surg* 68(1):8-14, 2010.

Chossegros C, Cheynet F, Conrath J: Inframtemporal space infection after temporomandibular arthroscopy: an unusual complication, *J Oral Maxillofac Surg* 53(8):949-951, 1995.

de Miranda SL, Abrahão M: Intraoral vertical ramus osteotomy endoscopic surgery, *J Oral Maxillofac Surg* April 65(4):805-808, 2007.

Dimitroulis G: A review of 56 cases of chronic closed lock treated with temporomandibular joint arthroscopy, *J Oral Maxillofac Surg* 60(5):519-524, 2002.

Ducic Y, Verret DJ: Endoscopic transantral repair of orbital floor fractures, *Otolaryngol Head Neck Surg* 140(6):849-854, 2009.

Farwell DG, Strong EB: Endoscopic repair of orbital floor fractures, *Otolaryngol Clin North Am* 40(2):319-328, 2007.

Fernandez R, Fattahi T, Steinberg B, Schare H: Endoscopic repair of isolated orbital floor fracture with implant placement, *J Oral Maxillofac Surg* 65(8):1449-1453, 2007.

Fernandez R, Strong EB: Endoscopic repair of orbital floor fractures, *Oper Tech Otolaryngol Head Neck Surg* 19(3):209-213, 2008.

Goldberg JS, Julian JB, Dachille R: Local subcutaneous atrophy following arthroscopy of the TMJ, *J Oral Maxillofac Surg* 47(9):986-987, 1989.

González Martín-Moro J, Sastre-Pérez J, Fernández IP: Horner syndrome after temporomandibular joint arthroscopy: a new complication. *J Oral Maxillofac Surg* 67(6): 1320-1322, 2009.

González-García R: Arthroscopy surgery for the treatment of chronic closed lock of the temporomandibular joint: a clinical study in 344 arthroscopic procedures, *J Oral Maxillofac Surg* August 66(8):65, 2008.

González-García R: Arthroscopic myotomy of the lateral pterygoid muscle with coablation for the treatment of temporomandibular joint anterior disc displacement without reduction, *J Oral Maxillofac Surg* 67(12):2699-2701, 2009.

González-García R, Rodríguez-Campo FJ, Escorial-Hernández V, et al: Complications of temporomandibular joint arthroscopy: a retrospective analytic study of 670 arthroscopic procedures, *J Oral Maxillofac Surg* 64(11): 1587-1591, 2006.

González-García R, Rodríguez-Campo FJ, Monje F, et al: Influence of the upper joint surface and synovial lining in the outcome of chronic closed lock of the temporomandibular joint treated with arthroscopy, *J Oral Maxillofac Surg* 68(1):35-42, 2010.

González-García R, Sanromán JF, Goizueta-Adame C, et al: Transoral endoscopic-assisted management of subcondylar fractures in 17 patients: an alternative to open reduction with rigid internal fixation and closed reduction with maxillomandibular fixation, *Int J Oral Maxillofac Surg* 38(1):19-25, 2009.

Gundlach P, Scherer H, Hopf J, et al: Endoscopic-controlled laser lithotripsy of salivary calculi: in vitro studies and initial clinical use [in German], *HNO* 38(7):247-250, 1990.

Habu M, Tanaka T, Tomoyose T, et al: Significance of dynamic magnetic resonance sialography in prognostic evaluation of saline solution irrigation of the parotid gland for the treatment of xerostomia, *J Oral Maxillofac Surg*, 768-776, 2009.

Haug RH, Brandt MT: Traditional versus endoscope-assisted open reduction with rigid internal fixation (ORIF) of adult mandibular condyle fractures: a review of the literature regarding current thoughts on management, *J Oral Maxillofac Surg* 62(10):1272-1279, 2004.

Holmlund AB, Axelsson S, Gynther GW: A comparison of discectomy and arthroscopic lysis and lavage for the treatment of chronic closed lock of the temporomandibular joint: a randomized outcome study, *J Oral Maxillofac Surg* September 59(9):972-977, 2001.

Indresano AT: Surgical arthroscopy as the preferred treatment for internal derangements of the temporomandibular joint, *J Oral Maxillofac Surg* 59(3):308-312, 2001.

Israel HA: Technique for placement of a discal traction suture during temporomandibular joint arthroscopy, *J Oral Maxillofac Surg* 47(3):311-313, 1989.

Israel HA, Langevin CJ, Singer MD, Behrman DA: The relationship between temporomandibular joint synovitis and adhesions: pathogenic mechanisms and clinical implications for surgical management, *J Oral Maxillofac Surg* 4(7):1066-1074, 2006.

Katz P: Endoscopy of the salivary glands, *Ann Radiol (Paris)* 34(1-2):110-113, 1991.

Kellman RM: Endoscopically assisted repair of subcondylar fractures of the mandible: an evolving technique, *Arch Facial Plast Surg* 5(3):244-250, 2003.

Kellman RM: Endoscopy in cranio maxillofacial skeletal surgery, *Curr Opin Otolaryngol Head Neck Surg* 9:253-255, 2001.

Kim K, McCain JP: Use of the endoscope in bisagittal split osteotomy, *J Oral Maxillofac Surg* 66(8):1773-1775, 2008.

Kim YK, Im JH, Chung H, Yun PY: Clinical application of ultrathin arthroscopy in the temporomandibular joint for treatment of closed lock patients, *J Oral Maxillofac Surg* 67(5):1039-1045, 2009.

Kincaid BL, Powers DB, Childress RW, Schmitz JP: The use of endoscopy for management of bilateral sagittal split complications, *J Oral Maxillofac Surg* 64(5):846-850, 2006.

Koch M, Zenk J, Bozzato A, et al: Sialoscopy in cases of unclear swelling of the major salivary glands, *Otolaryngol Head Neck Surg* 133(6): 863-868, 2005.

Kondoh T, Westesson PL: Diagnostic accuracy of temporomandibular joint lower-compartment arthroscopy using an ultrathin arthroscope: a postmortem study, *J Oral Maxillofac Surg* 49(6):619-626, 1991.

Konigsberger R, Feyh J, Goetz A, Kastenbauer E: Endoscopically controlled electro hydraulic intracorporeal shock wave lithotripsy (EISL) of salivary stones, *J Otolaryngol* 22(1):12-13, 1993.

Konigsberger R, Feyh J, Goetz A, et al: Endoscopic controlled laser lithotripsy in the treatment of sialolithiasis [in German], *Laryngorhinootologie* 69(6):322-323, 1990.

Kornbrot A, Shaw AS, Toohey MR: Pseudoaneurysm as a complication of arthroscopy: a case report, *J Oral Maxillofac Surg* 49(11): 1226-1228, 1991.

Lauer G, Pradel W, Schneider M, Eckelt U: A new 3-dimensional plate for transoral endoscopic-assisted osteosynthesis of condylar neck fractures, *J Oral Maxillofac Surg* 65(5):964-971, 2007.

Lauer G, Schmelzeisen R: Endoscope-assisted fixation of mandibular condylar process fractures, *J Oral Maxillofac Surg* 57(1): 36-39,1999.

Lee C, Mueller RV, Lee K, Mathes SJ: Endoscopic subcondylar fracture repair: functional, aesthetic, and radiographic outcomes, *Plast Reconstr Surg* 102(5):1434-1443; discussion 1444-1445, 1998.

Lo J, Cheung LK: Endoscopic-assisted rigid fixation of condylar fracture: a technical note, *J Oral Maxillofac Surg* 64(9):1443-1446, 2006.

Maturo SC, Wiseman J, Mair E: Transantral endoscopic repair of orbital floor fractures with the use of flexible endoscope holder: a cadaver study, *Ear Nose Throat J* 87(12):693-695, 2008.

Mazzonetto R, Spagnoli DB: Long-term evaluation of arthroscopic discectomy of the temporomandibular joint using the Holmium YAG laser, *J Oral Maxillofac Surg* 59(9):1018-1023, 2001.

McCain JP: Arthroscopy of the human temporomandibular joint, *J Oral Maxillofac Surg* 46(8):648-655, 1988.

McCain JP: Complications of TMJ arthroscopy, *J Oral Maxillofac Surg* 46(4):256, 1988.

McCain JP: *Principles and practice of temporomandibular joint arthroscopy*, St. Louis, 1996, Mosby.

McCain JP, Balazs EA, de la Rua H: Preliminary studies on the use of a viscoelastic solution in arthroscopic surgery of the temporomandibular joint, *J Oral Maxillofac Surg* 47(11):1161-1168, 1989.

McCain JP, de la Rua H, Le Blanc WG: Correlation of clinical, radiographic, and arthroscopic findings in internal derangements of the TMJ, *J Oral Maxillofac Surg* 47(9):913-921, 1989.

McCain JP, de la Rua H: A modification of the double puncture technique in temporomandibular joint arthroscopy, *J Oral Maxillofac Surg* 48(7):760-761, 1990.

McCain JP, de la Rua H: Foreign body retrieval: a complication of TMJ arthroscopy report of a case, *J Oral Maxillofac Surg* 47(11):1221-1225, 1989.

McCain JP, Goldberg HM, de la Rua H: Preoperative and postoperative audiologic measurements in patients undergoing arthroscopy of the TMJ, *J Oral Maxillofac Surg* 47(10):1026-1027, 1989.

McCain JP, Podrasky AE, Zabiegalski NA: Arthroscopic disc repositioning and suturing: a preliminary report, *J Oral Maxillofac Surg* 50(6):568-579, 1992.

McCain JP, Sanders B, Koslin MG, et al: Temporomandibular joint arthroscopy: a 6-year multicenter retrospective study of 4,831 joints, *J Oral Maxillofac Surg* 50(9):926-930, 1992.

McCain JP: American experience: reconstructive surgery just getting better, *J Oral Maxillofac Surg* 65(9):12-13, 2007.

Miki T, Wada J, Haraoka J, Inaba J: Endoscopic transmaxillary reduction and balloon technique for blowout fractures of the orbital flood, *Minim Invasive Neurosurg* 47(6):359-364, 2004.

Montgomery MT, Van Sickels JE, Harms SE, Thrash WT: Arthroscopic TMJ surgery: effects on signs, symptoms, and disc position, *J Oral Maxillofac Surg* 47(12):1263-1271, 1989.

Moses JJ: TMJ arthroscopic surgery: rationale and technique, *J Oral Maxillofac Surg* 62(Suppl 1):96-97, 2004.

Moses JJ: TMJ Arthroscopic surgery—Current concepts, rationale, and technique, *J Oral Maxillofac Surg* 63(8 Suppl):123-124, 2005.

Murakami KI: Japanese experience: surgical techniques and long-term results, *J Oral Maxillofac Surg* 65(9):11, 2007.

Nahlieli O, Bar T, Shacham R, et al: Management of chronic recurrent parotitis: current therapy, *J Oral Maxillofacial Surg* 62(9):1150-1155, 2004.

Nahlieli O, Bar-Droma E, Zagury A, et al: *J Oral Maxillofac Surg* 65:1751-1757, 2007.

Nahlieli O, Baruchin AM: Endoscopic technique for the diagnosis and treatment of obstructive salivary gland diseases, *J Oral Maxillofac Surg* 57(12):1394-1401, 1999.

Nahlieli O, Baruchin AM: Sialoendoscopy: three years' experience as a diagnostic and treatment modality, *J Oral Maxillofac Surg* 55(9):912-918, 1997.

Nahlieli O, Iro H, McGurk M, Zenk J: *Modern management preserving the salivary glands*, Herzliya, Israel, 2007, Isradon.

Nahlieli O, Nazarian Y: Sialadenitis following radioiodine therapy: a new diagnostic and treatment modality, *Oral Dis* 12(5):476-479, 2006.

Nahlieli O, Neder A, Baruchin AM: Salivary gland endoscopy: a new technique for diagnosis and treatment of sialolithiasis, *J Oral Maxillofac Surg* 52(12):1240-1242, 1994.

Nahlieli O, Shacham R, Shlesinger M, Eliav E: Juvenile recurrent parotitis: a new method of diagnosis and treatment, *Pediatrics* 114(1):9-12, 2004.

Pedroletti F, McCain JP: Endoscopically assisted repair of mandibular angle fractures, *J Oral Maxillofac Surg* 68(4):912-914, 2010.

Perrott DH, Alborzi A, Kaban LB, Helms CA: A prospective evaluation of the effectiveness of temporomandibular joint arthroscopy, *J Oral Maxillofac Surg* 48(10):1029-1032, 1990.

Pham AM, Strong EB: Endoscopic management of facial fractures. *Curr Opin Otolaryngol Head Neck Surg* 14(4):234-241, 2006.

Preisler SA, Koorbusch GF, Olson RA: An acquired arteriovenous fistula secondary to temporomandibular joint arthroscopy: report of a case, *J Oral Maxillofac Surg* 49(2):187-190, 1991.

Rauch S, Gorlin RJ: Diseases of the salivary glands. In Gorlin RJ, Goldman HM, editors: *Oral pathology*, ed 6, St. Louis, 1970, Mosby, pp 997-1003.

Robiony M, Polini F, Costa F, et al: Endoscopically assisted intraoral vertical ramus osteotomy and piezoelectric surgery in mandibular prognathism, *J Oral Maxillofac Surg* 65(10):2119-2124, 2007.

Sandler NA, Andreasen KH, Johns FR: The use of endoscopy in the management of subcondylar fractures of the mandible: a cadaver study, *Oral Surg Oral Med Oral Pathol Oral Radiol Endod* 88(5):529-531, 1999.

Sandler NA: Endoscopic-assisted reduction and fixation of a mandibular subcondylar fracture: report of a case, *J Oral Maxillofac Surg* 59(12):1479-1482, 2001.

Saunders CJ, Whetzel TP, Stokes RB: Transantral endoscopic orbital floor fracture. A cadaver and clinical study, *Plast Reconstr Surg* 100(3):575-581, 1997.

Schmelzeisen R, Cienfuegos-Monroy R, Schön R, et al: Patient benefit from endoscopically assisted fixation of condylar neck fractures—A randomized controlled trial, *J Oral Maxillofac Surg* 67(1):147-158, 2009.

Schoen R, Fakler O, Metzger MC, et al: Preliminary functional results of endoscope-assisted transoral treatment of displaced bilateral condylar mandible fractures, *Int J Oral Maxillofac Surg* 37(2):111-116, 2008.

Schön R, Schramm A, Gellrich NC, Schmelzeisen R: Follow-up of condylar fractures of the mandible in 8 patients at 18 months after transoral endoscopic-assisted open treatment. *J Oral Maxillofac Surg* January 2003 volume 61 issue 1 Pages 49-54.

Segami N, Yamada T, Nishimura M: Thermal injury during temporomandibular joint arthroscopy: a case report, *J Oral Maxillofac Surg* 62(4):508-510, 2004.

Smolka W, Iizuka T: Arthroscopic lysis and lavage in different stages of internal derangement of the temporomandibular joint: correlation of preoperative staging to arthroscopic findings and treatment outcome, *J Oral Maxillofac Surg* 63(4):471-478, 2005.

Strong EB, Kim KK, Diaz RC: Endoscopic approach to orbital blowout fracture repair, *Otolaryngol Head Neck Surg* 131(5):683-695, 2004.

Sugisaki M, Ikai A, Tanabe H: Dangerous angles and depths for middle ear and middle cranial fossa injury during arthroscopy of the temporomandibular joint, *J Oral Maxillofac Surg* 53(7):803-810, 1995.

Tarro AW: Advanced TMJ arthroscopy including use of the holmium: YAG laser, *J Oral Maxillofac Surg* 61(8):130a-131, 2003.

Tarro AW: Minimally invasive TMJ surgery: from arthrocentesis to advanced laser arthroscopy, *J Oral Maxillofac Surg* 63(8):115-116, 2005.

Torres D: Poster 48: Minimally invasive alternative for treatment of recurrent temporomandibular joint dislocation, *J Oral Maxillofac Surg* 67(9):97-98, 2009.

Troulis MJ: Endoscopic management of subcondylar fractures, *J Oral Maxillofac Surg* 61(8): 20-28, 2003.

Troulis MJ: Endoscopic open reduction and internal rigid fixation of subcondylar fractures, *J Oral Maxillofac Surg* 62(10):1269-1271, 2004.

Troulis MJ, Kaban LB: Endoscopic approach to the ramus/condyle unit: clinical applications, *J Oral Maxillofac Surg* 59(5):503-509, 2001.

Troulis MJ, Kaban LB: Endoscopic vertical ramus osteotomy: early clinical results, *J Oral Maxillofac Surg* 62(7):824-828, 2004.

Troulis MJ, Williams WB, Kaban LB: Endoscopic mandibular condylectomy and reconstruction: early clinical results, *J Oral Maxillofac Surg* 62(4):460-465, 2004.

Tsuyama M, Kondoh T, Seto K, Fukuda J: Complications of temporomandibular joint arthroscopy: a retrospective analysis of 301 lysis and lavage procedures performed using the triangulation technique, *J Oral Maxillofac Surg* 58(5):500-505, 2000.

White RD: Arthroscopic lysis and lavage as the preferred treatment for internal derangement of the temporomandibular joint, *J Oral Maxillofac Surg* 59(3):313-316, 2001.

Williams WB, Troulis MJ, Kaban LB: Reduction of subcondylar fractures using endoscopic access, *J Oral Maxillofac Surg* 62:26-27, 2004.

Williams WB: Open reduction and rigid internal fixation of subcondylar fractures using extraoral endoscopic access, *J Oral Maxillofac Surg* 67(9):61, 2009.

Wiltfang J, Kessler P: Endoscopically assisted Le Fort I osteotomy to correct transverse and sagittal discrepancies of the maxilla, *J Oral Maxillofac Surg* 60(10):1142-1145, 2002.

Zenk J, Koch M, Bozzato A, Iro H: Sialoscopy: initial experiences with a new endoscope, *Br J Oral Maxillofac Surg* 42(4):293-298, 2004.

Principles of Microvascular Surgery

Chapter 7

Remy H. Blanchaert Jr.

Microvascular surgery significantly altered the art and science of maxillofacial reconstructive surgery. Microsurgical technique rapidly gained popularity because of the positive impact it has had on the reliability of reconstructive efforts. A significant difference exists between local-regional flaps and microvascular flaps in that the blood supply to the microsurgical flaps is robust. The majority of the microvascular free tissue transfers are oriented directly over a segmental blood supply. The local-regional flaps universally place the most poorly supplied portions of the entire flap at the defect site. In oral cavity reconstruction, that places the most vulnerable tissue in a very challenging environment. Local-regional flaps do not reliably contain the type and volume of bone often required in maxillofacial reconstructions. Additionally, the majority of the volume of tissue transferred in a local-regional flap is nowhere near the recipient site.

The versatility of microvascular flaps allows the reconstructive surgeon to have myriad options to match the specific needs of each circumstance to the techniques and flap chosen. The type (bone, skin, oral-pharyngeal lining), volume, and character of the tissue can be restored by selecting a flap with those desired characteristics. Microvascular flaps will never completely replace traditional local-regional flaps in all instances. The advantages of the technique, specifically reliability, adaptability, and single stage surgery, make microsurgery an extremely useful and necessary technique for the maxillofacial surgeon.

ETIOPATHOGENESIS AND CAUSATIVE FACTORS

Maxillofacial microvascular surgery is used to manage tumors, trauma, and congenital deformities. The majority of these defects or deficiencies contain composite tissues. Mucosa, skin, and bone must all be replaced in these cases if premorbid or normal form and function is to be completely restored. Microsurgery techniques are the only way to completely reconstruct composite tissue defects in one surgical procedure. Restoration of the dentoalveolar complex is critical in all cases of maxillofacial reconstruction, because several studies report that patients' quality of life and self-image are closely tied to the ability to chew and swallow normally. Microvascular flap selection is carried out with the intention of replacing the lost or missing tissue in one surgical setting as much as possible. Experience has demonstrated the suitability of certain flaps in specific situations. It is not possible to use one flap for all purposes.

Tumor resection oftentimes produces similar defects that quickly become familiar to the reconstructive surgeon. For example, all microsurgeons have been faced with the challenge of an anterior mandibular defect after the resection of an advanced cancer on the floor of the mouth. This quickly becomes routine, and the surgeon develops considerable finesse in the manipulation of fibula bone segments to achieve the complex contour of the anterior mandible while simultaneously restoring the volume and mobility of the floor of the mouth with the transferred skin component of the flap. Once the three-dimensional assessment of the defect is mastered, tissue that was lost in the tumor ablation can be more accurately replicated. Oral and oral-pharyngeal tissues are commonly replaced with the free radial forearm flap (FRFF), anterolateral thigh flap (ATF), lateral arm flap, or scapula flap. Composite tissue and bone containing defects are generally restored using the free fibula osteocutaneous flap (FFOF) or the deep circumflex iliac artery (DCIA) flap. Occasionally, the composite tissue defect characteristics require the composite scapula flap.

Trauma reconstruction is quite complex because the defects created by the trauma are widely varied. The majority of the trauma defects that require microvascular technique are avulsive injuries associated with high velocity projectiles or blasts. The maxillofacial microsurgeon draws heavily on the experience gained in tumor reconstruction. The same three-dimensional assessment skills developed in tumor surgery allow the microsurgeon to appropriately plan reconstructions for trauma patients, so that surgical interventions are minimized without sacrificing ideal form. The free fibula and DCIA flaps are commonly used in jaw reconstruction, whereas the free radial forearm flap and scapula composite flap are used to restore other structural elements of the maxillofacial region.

Congenital deformities may on occasion benefit from microsurgical technique as well. Hemifacial microsomia and juvenile rheumatoid arthritis may require restoration of a significant portion of the mandible, in particular the temporomandibular joint. Once again, the experience gained in ablative tumor reconstruction, in which mandibular disarticulation is required, provides the maxillofacial microsurgeon with familiarity in this type of defect.

MICROVASCULAR FLAP ANATOMY

In general, microvascular flap anatomy is based on a named major blood vessel or significant perforating vessel. The vessel anatomy of all the common flaps has been widely studied and reported upon. The diameters of these vessels are in the range of 1.5 to 3 mm. There are two major flaps in which presurgical vessel anatomy assessment is mandatory. The flaps requiring preoperative assessment are the FRFF and the FF. In the cases of the FRFF, the absence of an intact palmar arch could result in ischemia to portions of the hand. This can easily be assessed with the Allen test. The failure to restore normal blood flow to the hand after release of the ulnar artery and exsanguination with both the radial and ulnar arteries occluded signifies an incomplete palmar arch (Fig. 7-1). Another simple and practical test involves occluding the radial artery with a pulse oximeter probe on the thumb of the hand on the planned donor arm. The potential donor leg for the free fibula flap must be assessed for the presence of a peroneal dominant circulation or significant atherosclerotic disease. It is estimated that between 10% and 20% of patients have diminutive anterior tibial or posterior tibial vessels and

TABLE 7-1	Typical Flaps Used in Maxillofacial Surgery Are Described along with Characteristics of the Vascular Pedicle		
FLAP	**VASCULAR PEDICLE**	**VESSEL DIAMETER (mm)**	**PEDICLE LENGTH**
Radial forearm	Radial artery	2.5	Long
	Cephalic vein	—	—
Fibula flap	Peroneal A/V	—	Variable
Rectus abdominis	Deep inferior epigastic A/V	3.4	Long
Gracilis	Branch of adductor A/V	2	Up to 6 cm
DCIA	DCIA/V	2-3	6-8 cm
Scapula	Circumflex scapular A/V	3	Variable
Anterolateral thigh	Profunda femoris A/V	3	Variable
Lateral arm	Posterior radial collateral A/V	2.5	Short

A/V, Artery/vein; *DCIA,* deep circumflex iliac artery.

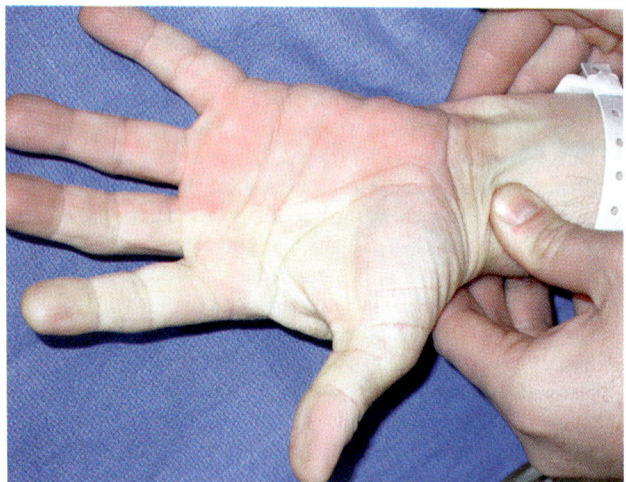

Fig. 7-1 ■ A failed Allen test. Clearly evident is the lack of communication between the radial and ulnar palmar arches.

are reliant on the peroneal artery for perfusion of the distal portions of the lower limb. These conditions could be easily identified by the use of magnetic resonance angiography, which is preferred over arteriography because adequate information can be obtained without the radiation or contrast media exposure. Some maxillofacial microsurgeons have their patients undergo Doppler imaging and mapping of the lateral lower leg to identify the location of septocutaneous perforating vessels to the overlying skin. Studies show the consistent presence of a major perforator with 2 cm of the midpoint of the fibula between the head of the fibula and the lateral malleolus. Additional studies show a predominance of septocutaneous perforators eight tenths of the way along the fibula.

The specific anatomy of the commonly used flaps is discussed in detail in the chapters that follow. For convenience sake, a table summarizing the vascular characteristics of the flaps is included (Table 7-1).

Recipient vessel selection must be considered early in the planning process for maxillofacial microsurgical reconstruction. Previous irradiation, prior surgery, or the presence of fixed adenopathy can greatly alter the availability or suitability of vessels for microsurgical anastomosis. This is quite similar to the need for extremity microsurgeons to select a microvascular technique that ensures that they are outside the "zone of injury" when selecting the location for microsurgical anastomosis.

Commonly used recipient vessels are the internal jugular vein and external carotid artery for end-to-side anastomosis. End-to-end anastomosis is preferred by many maxillofacial microsurgeons. Selection of the most appropriate recipient vessel for end-to-end anastomosis depends on flap pedicle length and size and flap position. Coordination with the ablative surgeon as to the ideal recipient vessel is required to ensure availability and careful handling of the desired recipient vessel. The facial artery and vein are common recipient vessels because their location and size are ideal. On occasion, a common facial-lingual trunk may be too large. Rather than accept the size mismatch or poor location of the vessel, the surgeon may choose another option. The superior thyroid artery is also commonly used; however, the accompanying vein is a difficult vessel to use as a recipient. The external jugular vein is sometimes used if it is available. This vessel has several valves that should be avoided. The transverse cervical artery and vein are also suitable recipient vessels. They are quite reliable and their position and length offer considerable discretion for the anastomosis location. More important is the fact that in previously operated or irradiated sites, these may be the only vessels suitable for end-to-end anastomosis that are outside the area of previous injury. On a similar note the superficial temporal artery and vein are excellent recipient vessels for maxillary reconstruction or face/scalp reconstruction.

DIAGNOSTIC STUDIES

The presurgical evaluation of a maxillofacial patient for microvascular surgery is straightforward. Basically, any patient who can safely undergo an anesthetic for longer than 4 hours is an appropriate surgical candidate. The majority of maxillofacial microsurgery cases are done with ablative tumor surgery. Such patients will have already been evaluated with a prolonged general anesthetic in mind. Trauma patients or those patients undergoing surgery for congenital or developmental anomalies should receive a standard cardiovascular evaluation and anesthesia consultation if indicated.

Any patient suspected to have a hypercoagulable state should be thoroughly evaluated by a hematologist. In extreme situations, such a condition may exclude the patient as a microsurgery candidate.

Site-specific evaluation may be required before flap donor site selection. This subject is addressed in detail in the next section.

TREATMENT AND RECONSTRUCTIVE GOALS

The goals of the maxillofacial microvascular surgeon are to achieve the immediate and complete restoration of premorbid form and function in a challenging array of clinical situations. Accomplishing total reconstruction with a single flap is the norm; however, extremely challenging defects may require more than one flap. The old dogma of a reconstructive ladder should be thrown out for maxillofacial reconstruction other than minor skin defects. The most appropriate flap should be used, whatever the difficulty or complexity.

The immediate restoration of form is an absolute necessity for several reasons. Nowhere is this more evident than mandibular reconstruction. Several studies show that immediate reconstruction of the mandible is more favorable than delayed reconstruction because of dramatic decreases in both costs and complications. Clearly, immediate mandibular reconstruction allows for improved efforts at safe and effective swallowing. Without immediate mandibular reconstruction there is no place for insertion of the suprahyoid muscles which are so important in laryngeal elevation and protected swallowing. In addition, by immediately reconstructing the mandible, the disfiguring impact of scar contraction or subsequent radiation injury on the operated mandible is diminished. Immediate mandibular reconstruction also allows for the early rehabilitation of the masticatory apparatus.

One of the distinct advantages of microsurgical reconstruction of the oral cavity and oral pharynx following ablative tumor resection is the creation of a reliable seal to prevent salivary contamination of the neck, which can lead to wound infection or salivary fistula formation. This advantage is afforded by the almost limitless volume of well-vascularized, flexible soft tissue that can be transferred to the defect. This eliminates the distinct disadvantages of heavy, tethered, immobile pedicled local-regional flaps. Additionally, the arc of rotation of a local-regional flap limits its applicability, whereas a microvascular free flap is much less limited in its placement.

The value of immediate reconstruction with few complications must also be considered in terms of facilitating the prompt completion of adjuvant therapies such as chemotherapy or radiation therapy, or both.

SPECIFIC TREATMENT AND TECHNIQUES

Maxillofacial microsurgical reconstruction requires careful recipient site preparation, accurate three-dimensional flap design, careful flap harvest, flap inset, perfect microsurgical technique, and management of both the donor site and the recipient site. In general, time spent in preparation of the recipient site to facilitate inset and anastomosis is greatly rewarded with comfortable microsurgery and reduced flap ischemia time.

Typically, the microsurgeon must perform some degree of damage control following the ablative surgeon's neck dissection and resection. Experience shows that even the slightest ongoing hemorrhage at the resection site or the neck can lead to wound hematoma and potential flap compromise. The recipient vessels must also be dissected free and evaluated for adequate flow, because they could easily have been damaged by improper handling during the ablative surgery. The defect site must then be scrutinized. On occasion the defect can be simplified with either partial closure in areas of significant tissue redundancy or additional resection to uniform smooth

edges. Once again, the tissue must be carefully evaluated, because rough handling of a wound margin could lead to possible necrosis of the wound edge.

Once the three-dimensional requirements of the flap are determined the design is transferred to the donor site. It is prudent to err only on the side of too large a flap versus too small. A flap that is too small creates tension at the margins and may limit later mobility or range of motion of the native tissues. Where appropriate, the flap may be harvested when blood flow is controlled by tourniquet following exsanguination of the extremity. Tourniquet pressure can typically be set at 75 to 100 mm Hg over the patient's systolic blood pressure. Tourniquet times should, of course, be limited as much as possible. The tourniquet should be released as soon as possible and the flap allowed to reperfuse. Extreme care should be taken to ensure the hemostasis of the flap following harvest because wound hematoma can compromise venous outflow of the flap. It is often possible to modify the bone containing portions of flaps at the donor site if the surgeon so chooses. Some surgeons elect to do so at the defect site because the pedicle geometry can more easily be evaluated. Either way, it is prudent to consider flap modifications, inset, and position of the anastomosis before severing the vascular pedicle.

Flap inset should be completed before anastomosis. Doing so ensures stability of the flap during the microsurgery and defines the vessel geometry and proper pedicle length. Redundancy of the vascular pedicle should be avoided because it can lead to kinked veins. Likewise it is important that the pedicle be in as near its native position as possible. Twisting or rotation should be avoided (Fig. 7-2).

The microvascular anastomosis should then be completed. This is almost always done with the artery first because of its deeper position. A binocular internally lighted microscope is required. Variable field of view and magnification are desirable. A surgical assistant, if used, should be positioned opposite the primary surgeon for the microvascular anastomosis. Appropriate Acland clamps are necessary for end-to-end anastomosis. End-to-side anastomosis will require additional atraumatic vascular clamps. The adventitia of both sides of the anastomosis should be removed and the vessel ends irrigated with heparinized saline solution 1000 units per 100 mL normal saline. Valves within the veins should be widely avoided. Standard suture technique with 9-0 nylon sutures should be completed. Before final sutures are placed, the vessels should be filled

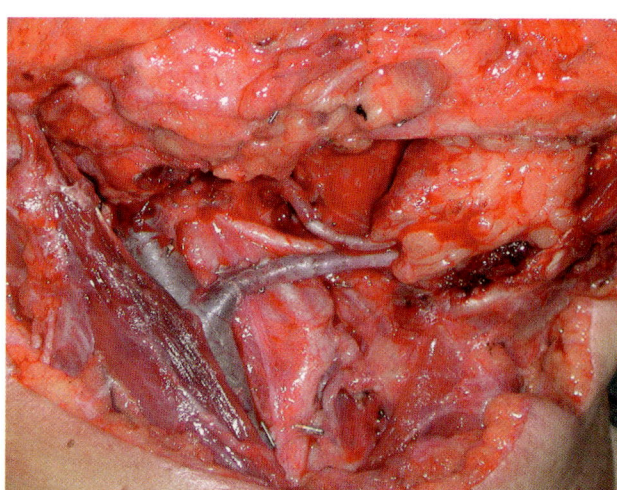

Fig. 7-2 ■ The flap vessels in their native position. The anastomosis is completed at a pedicle length that reduces redundancy yet allows movement of the neck without tension.

with the heparinized saline solution. Interrupted technique is most suitable to vessel size mismatch, whereas continuous technique is more suitable in end-to-side anastomosis. Following release of the vessel clamps the flap and pedicle should be carefully evaluated for perfusion and hemostasis. If the anastomosis and the perfusion of the flap do not look perfect immediately, even if there is the slightest doubt, it is best to redo the anastomosis immediately.

The recipient site should be carefully evaluated for hemostasis before closure over several closed-suction drains. It is important to fix the position of the drains to prevent their movement and potential compression of the flap pedicle. Studies show decreased incidence of infection in head and neck surgery when wound irrigation fluid contains antibiotics. Clindamycin at a concentration of 600 mg per liter of normal saline is recommended. Standard layered closure should be performed.

The donor site is similarly managed with drains and appropriate irrigation. Some donor sites require site-specific management, grafts, or splinting, or a combination of these. The DCIA flap closure should be reinforced with synthetic polypropylene mesh over the muscle closure to prevent hernia formation. Titanium mesh or polypropylene mesh should be used on the medial side of the iliac osteotomy. The FRFF typically requires a split thickness skin graft to cover the donor site. The area should remain splinted with a bolster over the graft for 1 week. The hand should be in the position of maximum function. The free fibula donor site can often be closed primarily; however, undue tension can lead to vascular compromise of the limb. All other flaps are closed primarily with appropriate undermining.

POSTOPERATIVE CARE

It has been shown that the use of anticoagulants after surgery is fraught with risk. The potential for wound hematoma is markedly increased with the use of either low-molecular-weight dextran or heparin. Both of these medications are unnecessary. Antiplatelet therapy can be provided by prescribing a daily aspirin without significant risk of hematoma.

Flap monitoring is viewed by some as unnecessary. Most microsurgeons prefer to have hourly flap perfusion checks. Visual inspection (capillary refill), surface Doppler probes, or implantable Doppler probes can be used. Vessel compression due to hematoma results in the majority of returns to the operating room rather than thrombosis at the anastomosis. An arterial thrombosis will almost always be detectable immediately in the operating room or early postoperatively, whereas a venous thrombosis may be detected much later. A favored flap perfusion assessment technique of the author is to prick the cutaneous elements of the flap with the needle from a tuberculin syringe (Fig. 7-3). The resultant blood should be immediate, bright red, and cease bleeding almost immediately through normal clot formation.

Appropriate postoperative care should maintain stable blood pressures through aggressive therapy if necessary. Sedation may be required. Wound drainage should be maintained until output is negligible. Nutritional support should be instituted as early as possible. Wound evaluation should be conducted serially by the same observer to identify a wound problem as early as possible. Hematoma is the greatest risk in the early postoperative time frame. Wound infection becomes the greatest risk by the third postoperative day. Wound infection must be aggressively managed, because pedicle

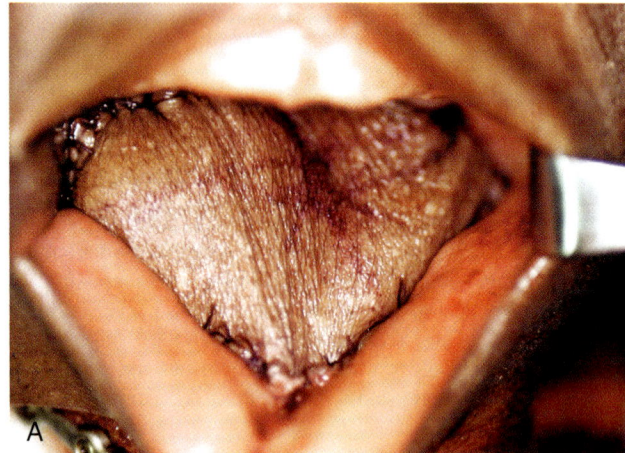

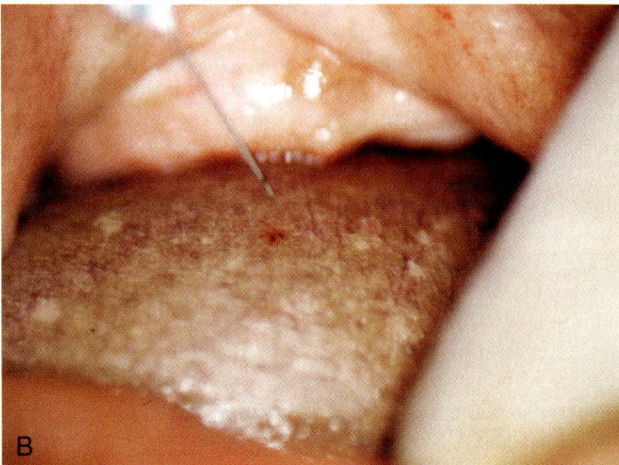

Fig. 7-3 ■ **A,** An inset flap before revascularizaton. **B,** Following reperfusion, the flap is assessed with a needle from a tuberculin syringe. Note the color of the flap, character of the skin, and the color of the blood.

thrombosis is likely to occur if infection remains untreated. Opening the wound and evacuating hematoma or infection should be done in the operating room under sterile conditions. The entire wound should be opened to allow wide visualization and protection of the vascular pedicle.

PEARLS AND PITFALLS

- Prepare the operative field for comfortable microvascular anastomosis using towels or other materials to support the microsurgeon's forearm.
- Always have a "plan B" in mind. The defect may not be what was anticipated, especially in reoperated cases or previously irradiated patients.
- Planning and preparation can save considerable operative time, especially ischemia time.
- Wound hematoma can be devastating to a microvascular flap if it compresses the vascular pedicle. Take great care with hemostasis and drainage of the operative site.
- Wound infection may cause intravascular coagulation of the microvascular flap pedicle. Antibiotic irrigation has been demonstrated to have a positive effect on wound infection.

BIBLIOGRAPHY

Brown MR, McCulloch TM, Funk GF et al: Resource utilization and patient morbidity in head and neck reconstruction, *Laryngoscope* 107:1028-1031, 1997.

Shah JP, Patel SG: *Head & neck surgery & oncology*, ed 3, Edinburgh, 2004, Mosby.

Sullivan MJ, Baker SR, Crompton R, Smith-Wheelock M: Free scapula osteocutaneous flap for mandibular reconstruction, *Arch Otolaryngol Head Neck Surg* 115:1334-1340, 1989.

Urken ML, Cheney ML, Sullivan MJ, Biller HF: *Atlas of regional and free flaps for head and neck reconstruction*, New York, 1995, Raven Press.

Urken ML, Weinberg H, Vickery C, et al: The internal oblique-iliac crest free flap in composite defects of the oral cavity involving bone, skin and mucosa, *Laryngoscope* 101:257-270, 1991.

Vaughan ED: The radial forearm free flap in orofacial reconstruction. Personal experience in 120 consecutive cases, *J Craniomaxillofac Surg* 18:2-7, 1990.

Antibiotic Prophylaxis to Prevent Surgical Site Infections in Oral and Maxillofacial Surgery

Chapter **8**

Julie Ann Smith

The concept of antibiotic prophylaxis to prevent surgical site infections has been well established in orthopedic and general surgery. Antibiotic prophylaxis is defined as the administration of antibiotics before contamination by a surgical incision has occurred, and it is given with the intention of preventing infection.[1,2] In terms of dentistry and oral surgery, there are fairly clearly defined recommendations for antibiotic prophylaxis to prevent infective endocarditis, as well as prosthetic joint infection.[3,4] As far as other disease entities are concerned, such as diabetes, liver disease, lupus, and others, the guidelines for antibiotic prophylaxis in dentistry and oral surgery are less clear.[5,6] The use of antibiotic prophylaxis to prevent surgical site infections in oral and maxillofacial surgical procedures is not entirely clear-cut. In several instances, conflicting information may be found throughout the literature regarding antibiotic prophylaxis in oral and maxillofacial surgery. Peterson set forth these five principles of antibiotic prophylaxis,[7] including the following:

1. The surgical procedure should have a significant risk for infection.
2. The correct antibiotic for the surgical procedure should be selected.
3. The antibiotic level must be high.
4. The timing of antibiotic administration must be correct.
5. The shortest antibiotic exposure must be used.

WOUND CONTAMINATION

Many factors may contribute to the risk for surgical site infection, including the patient's co-morbid conditions and age, quality of tissue at the surgical site, and skill of the surgeon. However, wound contamination is an extremely important factor. Surgical wounds are categorized as clean, clean-contaminated, contaminated, or dirty. Clean wounds (class I) are those that are atraumatic, without inflammation, and without a break in asepsis, and they are closed primarily.

Clean wounds in head and neck surgery have a very low infection rate (<1% to 2% without perioperative antibiotics). Because of this low infection rate, routine antibiotic prophylaxis has not been recommended for clean head and neck surgeries.[8,9,10] In clean-contaminated procedures (class II), a mucosal barrier is crossed or communication with the oral cavity occurs. Infection rates of 10% to 15% have been reported in clean-contaminated oral surgery procedures.[9,10] Examples of class II operations include orthognathic surgery, placement of implants, bone grafting, and non-infected extractions. Prophylactic antibiotics may be of benefit in class II operations. Contaminated wounds (class III) include traumatic injury involving the oral mucosa and can usually be managed with only preoperative antibiotics unless other risk factors for infection are present, in which case postoperative antibiotics may also be necessary.[2] Contaminated wounds may have an infection rate of 20% to 30% without antibiotics.[9,10] Dirty wounds (class IV) are those that are actively infected or the result of trauma in which there has been a delay in treatment and there is communication with the oral cavity and the possible presence of devitalized tissue or foreign bodies. Class IV wounds may have up to a 50% rate of infection and are often managed with preoperative as well as postoperative antibiotics.[2,10]

TIMING OF ADMINISTRATION AND SELECTION OF ANTIBIOTICS

Effective antibiotic prophylaxis must include proper timing of administration, as well as appropriate antibiotic selection and dose. To achieve adequate tissue concentrations, a parenteral prophylactic antibiotic should be administered 30 minutes before incision.[11] It has been demonstrated by Burke[12] and by Miles and colleagues[13] that if antibiotics were not given until 4 or more hours after the injection of bacteria into a surgical site, the site became involved with the same level of inflammation or cellulitis as though no antibiotic had been administered, thus underscoring the importance of pre-procedure antibiotics.

The antibiotic selected should provide coverage against the microbes likely to be encountered in the surgical field and should cover as narrow a spectrum as possible. To cover organisms from the oral cavity, an antibiotic should be effective against streptococci, anaerobic gram-positive cocci, and anaerobic gram-negative rods. When skin structures are involved, *Staphylococcus aureus* and *Staphylococcus epidermidis* should also be covered. Additionally, involvement of sinus and nasal structures would necessitate an antibiotic effective against *Haemophilus influenzae*, diphtheroids, and peptostreptococci.[2] To maintain high levels of antibiotic in tissues, the antibiotic should have a long half-life. In general, the antibiotic that best fulfills these criteria is penicillin. The decision to use antibiotics should be made with careful consideration of the patient's overall physical condition and co-morbid diseases, complexity of the surgical procedure, and the consequences of potential infection. It must be remembered that the use of antibiotics does carry a risk for adverse reactions in up to 7% of patients receiving antibiotics.[14] Potential adverse reactions include allergy, gastrointestinal upset, antibiotic-associated colitis, pseudomembranous colitis, and selection of resistant organisms. This chapter outlines the evidence for and against antibiotic prophylaxis to prevent surgical site infection in the most common oral surgical procedures, including orthognathic surgery, bone grafting, placement of dental implants, extraction of third molars, and management of facial trauma. It is not intended to be a systematic review or a meta-analysis, and in some cases, clear-cut recommendations are difficult to make after reviewing the literature.

ORTHOGNATHIC SURGERY

The use of antibiotic prophylaxis in patients undergoing orthognathic surgery has been a point of controversy for many years (Table 8-1). The overall complication rate associated with orthognathic surgery is low. The reported range of infectious complications has been broad—Alpha and colleagues found a 3.4% to 33.3% infection rate reported in the literature for mandibular osteotomies.[15] Most studies, however, have reported lower infection rates. Alpha and colleagues performed a retrospective evaluation of 1066 mandibular sagittal osteotomies and found a 6.5% incidence of infection requiring plate removal.[15] Similarly, Kim and Park found an infection rate of 1% in their retrospective review of 301 patients who underwent orthognathic surgery.[16] Chow and co-workers found a 9.7% complication rate in a retrospective review of 2910 orthognathic procedures.[17] Of these complications, 7.4% were related to infection. Before their review there was no clear consensus on the necessity for prophylactic antibiotics in orthognathic surgery. In Chow and co-workers' study it was found that patients undergoing surgery on both jaws had a significantly higher risk for infection, with 92.7% of infected patients having surgery on both jaws. However, the duration of the surgery did not correlate with infective risk. In this study 21.6% of infections occurred within the first postoperative week; 51% involved the maxilla (all of which were segmentalized Le Fort I osteotomies) and 49% involved the mandible. It was found that patients who received only one preoperative antibiotic dose had a significantly higher rate of infection than did those who received preoperative and postoperative antibiotics. The duration of postoperative antibiotics ranged from 2 to 14 days and did not significantly affect the infection rate. Furthermore, there was no significant difference between penicillin and non-penicillin antibiotics in preventing postoperative infection. The conclusion of this study was that administration of only a single preoperative dose of antibiotics was not recommended for prophylaxis. In this study patients who had received postoperative antibiotics in addition to a preoperative dose had a lower infection rate than did those who had received only a preoperative dose, although the optimal duration of postoperative antibiotic administration was not as clear, but it was thought that at least 2 postoperative days of antibiotics was useful.[17]

Zijderveld and associates found that a single preoperative dose of antibiotics resulted in a significantly lower risk for infection than in cases in which no antibiotics were given at all.[18] This

TABLE 8-1	Summary of Studies Regarding the Antibiotic Protocol for Orthognathic Surgery			
YEAR	AUTHOR	NUMBER OF PATIENTS	ANTIBIOTIC PROTOCOL	CONCLUSION
2007	Chow et al.	1294	Single preoperative dose vs. preoperative + postoperative doses for varying duration (2-14 days)	Preoperative plus postoperative dosing resulted in fewer infections; ideal duration of postoperative antibiotics unknown, but at least 2 days recommended
1999	Zijderveld et al.	54	Single preoperative dose vs. no antibiotics	Decreased risk for infection when single preoperative dose given. Infection rates: amoxicillin-clavulanate, 11.1%; cefuroxime, 17.6%; no antibiotics, 52.6%
1984	Ruggles and Hann	40	Peri-operative IV antibiotics vs. peri-operative + 2 days postoperative antibiotics	Increased infection when only peri-operative antibiotics used (7.5%)—not a statistically significant difference
1994	Fridrich et al.	30	Peri-operative vs. postoperative antibiotics for 1 week	No significant difference
2003	Lindeboom et al.	70	Single preoperative dose vs. 24-hour dosing	No significant difference between single preoperative dose (5.6%) and 24-hour dosing (2.8%)
1999	Bentley, et al.	30	1 day vs. 5 day	Increased infection when only 1 day of antibiotics administered (60%) vs. 5-day dosing (6.7%)

randomized, double-blind, placebo-controlled study compared single preoperative doses of amoxicillin-clavulanate with cefuroxime and demonstrated an 11.1% infection rate in the amoxicillin-clavulanate group, a 17.6% infection rate in the cefuroxime group, and a 52.6% infection rate in the placebo group. Their conclusion was that antibiotic prophylaxis consisting of a single preoperative dose resulted in a reduced risk for complications and that there was no significant difference between the two antibiotics evaluated, although the power of the study may have been too low to demonstrate a difference between the two antibiotics.[18]

The duration of postoperative prophylactic antibiotics in patients undergoing orthognathic surgery has been examined on numerous occasions. Ruggles and Hann performed a prospective, randomized, double-blind study comparing the use of only peri-operative intravenous antibiotics versus peri-operative plus 2-day postoperative intravenous antibiotics in 40 patients undergoing orthognathic surgery.[19] The study population included 53 osteotomies, with seven patients undergoing simultaneous bone grafting and four patients undergoing simultaneous allograft augmentation. All patients received one preoperative intramuscular dose of penicillin, as well as intravenous penicillin every 3 hours intraoperatively and one dose 3 hours postoperatively. In addition, the study group received 2 additional days of intravenous penicillin every 4 hours, whereas the placebo group received intravenous placebo for 2 days. Patients were monitored for infection, which was defined as meeting any three of the following defined criteria: elevation of body temperature longer than 72 hours or a sudden rise in body temperature postoperatively with return to normal; increasing edema, induration, and erythema of the wound margin and surrounding tissue; unusual surgical site pain; elevated white blood cell count with a leftward shift; or suppurative drainage from surgical site. In three patients, all of whom were in the group receiving only peri-operative antibiotics, an infection with purulent drainage developed 1 to 2 weeks postoperatively. This observed increased number of infections in the group receiving only peri-operative antibiotics versus postoperative antibiotics was not statistically significant. This study was published in 1984, and a limitation of the study may be the fact that intravenous antibiotics were used postoperatively for 2 days. Today, it is unlikely that all orthognathic patients would be hospitalized for 2 days postoperatively to receive intravenous antibiotics.

Fridrich and colleagues performed a prospective study comparing the use of peri-operative antibiotics and postoperative antibiotics for 1 week in 30 orthognathic surgery patients.[20] There was no significant difference in infection rates between the two groups, again indicating that prolonged periods of postoperative antibiotics do not offer an advantage over peri-operative dosing.

The dosing protocol was also examined by Lindeboom and co-workers in a prospective randomized study of prophylactic antibiotic use in patients undergoing bilateral sagittal split osteotomies.[21] Seventy patients undergoing a total of 140 mandibular osteotomies were assigned to either single preoperative dosing or 24-hour dosing with clindamycin. The preoperative dose was administered intravenously 15 minutes before the incision. Postoperatively, patients received either intravenous clindamycin every 6 hours for four doses or intravenous placebo every 6 hours for four doses. Surgical wounds were examined for pain, swelling, erythema, inflammation, or purulence postoperatively. There was a 5.6% infection rate in patients receiving only preoperative antibiotics and a 2.8% infection rate in those receiving antibiotics preoperatively and for 24 hours postoperatively. There was no statistically significant difference in infection rate between these two dosing schedules, and the authors thought that long-term antibiotic prophylaxis was not advantageous in orthognathic surgery.

Bentley and associates performed a prospective, randomized, double-blind trial examining 1-day versus 5-day antibiotic prophylaxis for orthognathic surgery in 30 patients.[22] This study revealed a 60% infection rate in patients receiving antibiotics for 1 day postoperatively versus a 6.7% infection rate in patients receiving 5 days of postoperative antibiotics, which was a significant difference. Of note, however, wire osteosynthesis and maxillo-mandibular fixation (MMF) were used instead of plates and screws, so translation of these results to cases in which plates and screws and no MMF are used is questionable. Additionally, 90% of the infections were found in the mandibular incision, and it was postulated by the authors that perhaps the wound breakdown in these incisions was due to the use of feeding catheters by the patients. Furthermore, as was pointed out in the discussion of this particular article by Abubaker, the definition of infection was rather broad and included purulent drainage, serosanguineous drainage with a positive culture (could be contaminated), spontaneous wound dehiscence, and the surgeon's diagnosis of infection.[23] Although these results seem to be in opposition to those of other studies in which it was suggested that prolonged postoperative antibiotics are not necessary, when taken in consideration with the potential limitations of this study, it does not entirely refute these other studies.

Overall, the evidence is not clear-cut but does seem to support the use of at least peri-operative prophylactic antibiotics to prevent infection in orthognathic surgery. Although the ideal duration of postoperative antibiotics is not definitively known, there is no evidence to support a prolonged duration of postoperative antibiotics.[2]

BONE GRAFTING

Antibiotic prophylaxis of intraoral onlay bone grafting in preparation for dental implant placement has not been studied extensively (Table 8-2). Lindeboom and van den Akker performed a prospective, placebo-controlled, double-blind trial examining antibiotic prophylaxis for onlay bone grafting using a ramal donor site.[24] In their study, 20 patients were randomized to receive either placebo or a single preoperative dose of oral phenethicillin. Patients were observed for 30 days for evidence of infection as demonstrated by either purulence, serosanguineous drainage with a positive culture, spontaneous dehiscence, or pain necessitating wound exploration

TABLE 8-2	Summary of Studies Regarding the Antibiotic Protocol for Bone Grafting			
YEAR	AUTHOR	NUMBER OF PATIENTS	ANTIBIOTIC PROTOCOL	CONCLUSION
2003	Lindeboom and van den Akker	20	Single preoperative dose vs. placebo in ramal onlay bone graft	Higher risk for infection in placebo group, of questionable statistical significance
2006	Lindeboom et al.	150	Preoperative phenethicillin vs. preoperative clindamycin in ramal onlay bone grafts to maxilla	Infection rates: phenethicillin, 5.3%; clindamycin, 2.7%—no statistically significant difference

with a resultant positive wound culture. The trial was ended early when the infection rate was determined to be high and it was found that two patients had recipient site infections, one had a donor site infection, and two had both sites infected. All these patients had been in the placebo group. This study had low power, but the authors concluded that a single preoperative dose of oral antibiotics was efficacious in decreasing the risk for infection in onlay bone grafting. However, the statistical analysis used to evaluate the data from this study was inappropriate, as pointed out in a subsequent letter to the editor written by Brennan and co-authors.[25] The authors of the letter to the editor thought that the results of the study were not statistically significant once the proper statistical analysis was used. In response, Lindeboom and colleagues agreed that their statistical analysis was incorrect, but they thought that at the very least their results were clinically significant.[25]

In a follow-up study, Lindeboom and co-workers performed a randomized prospective, controlled, double-blind trial comparing a single preoperative dose of phenethicillin and a single preoperative dose of clindamycin for prophylaxis of ramal onlay bone grafts involving the maxilla.[26] Antibiotics were administered orally 1 hour before the procedure and the patients were observed for 8 weeks for the development of signs of infection at the recipient site, as defined in the previously mentioned study.[24] This follow-up study[26] did not have a placebo arm, enrolled 150 patients, and had adequate power (80%). The recipient site infection rate in the phenethicillin group was 5.3%, and in the clindamycin group it was 2.7%. This study did not demonstrate a significant difference between the two antibiotics in efficacy in preventing infection in onlay bone grafting.

In light of the limited number of studies of antibiotic prophylaxis in patients undergoing onlay bone grafting, it is difficult to ascertain a conclusion. It seems that based on the findings of Lindeboom and van den Akker,[24] at least a preoperative dose of antibiotics should be considered. Ideally, a prospective, randomized, controlled, double-blind trial with adequate power should be completed to address this question.

Sinus lifting presents another interesting scenario in which systemic antibiotic prophylaxis has not been closely evaluated. It is estimated that infectious complications in sinus lifting could range in frequency from 2% to 7%.[27] Several studies involving local (topical—mostly tetracycline) antibiotic use in bone grafting for oral surgical and periodontal procedures have been performed, but few studies have examined systemic antibiotics in this context. Furthermore, the antibiotics that have been examined are typically those with a broad spectrum of activity rather than antibiotics that target anaerobic bacteria (such as metronidazole), which might be expected to play a role in infection of sinus lift bone grafting. Choukroun and associates performed an interesting study of antibiotic use in sinus lifts.[27] They studied 94 sinus lifts performed with freeze-dried bone graft in 72 patients. Eighty-two sinus lifts were performed with a 0.5% metronidazole solution mixed into the graft material and 12 sinus lifts were performed without metronidazole. All patients received amoxicillin for 6 days postoperatively. The patients were monitored with computed tomography to assess homogeneity of the grafts. Sinus lifts performed with metronidazole were found to be more significantly homogeneous than were those performed without metronidazole. The non-homogeneity within the bone grafts performed without metronidazole was theorized to be potentially associated with bacterial contamination of the graft. Although this study is interesting, more research should be done to examine the use of antibiotic prophylaxis in sinus lift procedures before definitive recommendations on antibiotic prophylaxis can be made.

IMPLANTS

Placement of dental implants poses an interesting scenario because one must consider that bacterial contamination at the time of implant insertion can result in subsequent non-integration and ultimately implant loss. Once a biomaterial, such as titanium, is infected, such infected surfaces are resistant to eradication with antibiotics and are difficult to treat, with removal of the implant often being required.[28] The development of an infection around an implant is potentially influenced by the skill of the surgeon, as well as maintenance of asepsis during the surgery.[29] The most likely bacteria to cause implant infection include streptococci, anaerobic gram-negative rods, anaerobic gram-positive cocci, and anaerobic gram-negative cocci.[10,30] The ideal antibiotic should be bactericidal against the flora expected. Placement of dental implants is considered a class II, or clean-contaminated, surgical procedure. The value of prophylactic antibiotics in implant surgery has been examined in various trials throughout the years (Table 8-3).

Dent and colleagues performed one of the earliest studies examining the use of prophylactic antibiotics in implant surgery as part of the comprehensive Dental Implant Clinical Research Group (DICRG).[10] A total of 2641 implants were studied in this randomized prospective trial. Investigators were permitted to determine whether to provide antibiotics, what type of antibiotic was to be used, and how the antibiotic was to be administered. Preoperative antibiotics were administered to 54.8% of the patients and postoperative antibiotics to 96%. Failure of the implant was recorded either during the healing phase or at phase II surgery. Patients who did not receive preoperative antibiotics exhibited a higher failure rate both during healing and at stage II. Patients who did receive preoperative antibiotics had a 1.4% failure rate as compared with a 4% failure rate observed in patients who did not receive preoperative antibiotics. The risk for failure was two to three times higher if preoperative antibiotics were not used. Although this study supports the use of preoperative antibiotics, it should be noted that it was not a controlled, blinded trial with well-defined parameters.

Laskin and co-workers performed another study as part of the DICRG that monitored patients up to 3 years postoperatively.[31] More than 2900 implants were monitored and implant survival was compared according to whether preoperative antibiotics were administered and also whether sufficient antibiotic doses were used. This was not a blinded study since the investigators were given the discretion to choose whether antibiotics would be used and, if so, what kind and how they would be administered. Fifty-five percent of patients received preoperative antibiotics and 96% received postoperative antibiotics. It was found that the implant failure rate was 4.6% when preoperative antibiotics were used versus 10% when no preoperative antibiotics were used, which was a significant difference. It was also found that the use of chlorhexidine along with preoperative antibiotics increased the survival of implants by 7.8% in comparison to implants in which neither was used. Laskin and co-authors concluded that preoperative antibiotics significantly improved implant survival.[31]

In contrast, Gynther and colleagues thought that preoperative and postoperative antibiotics did not offer any advantage in terms of implant survival.[32] Their study was a retrospective review that covered two separate periods. One hundred forty-seven patients who had 790 implants placed were given preoperative oral antibiotics in addition to postoperative oral antibiotics, and this group was compared with 132 patients who had 664 implants placed but did not receive any antibiotics. The investigators found no significant difference between the two groups with respect to early and late postoperative infections or implant survival. However, this was a

TABLE 8-3	Summary of Studies Regarding the Antibiotic Protocol for Implants			
YEAR	AUTHOR	NUMBER OF IMPLANTS	ANTIBIOTIC PROTOCOL	CONCLUSION
1997	Dent et al.	2641	Practitioner's discretion	Preoperative antibiotics had a 1.4% failure rate, no preoperative antibiotics had a 4% failure rate—significant difference favoring preoperative antibiotics
2000	Laskin et al.	2973	Practitioner's discretion	Preoperative antibiotics had a 4.6% failure rate, no preoperative antibiotics had a 10% failure rate—significant difference favoring preoperative antibiotics
1998	Gynther et al.	790 implants had antibiotics preoperatively + 10 days postoperatively; 664 implants had no antibiotics preoperatively or postoperatively	Preoperative and postoperative antibiotics vs. no antibiotics	No significant difference for early and late infections or implant survival—favored no antibiotic use
2005	Hossein et al.	2236 implants had 1 preoperative dose + 1 week of postoperative antibiotics; 775 implants had 1 preoperative dose + 1 same-day postoperative dose	1-week postoperative dosing vs. 1-day dosing	No significant difference in complications or implant survival, favored 1-day dosing over 1-week postoperative dosing
2005	Binahmed et al.	302 implants had 1 preoperative dose + 1-week postoperative dosing; 445 implants had 1 preoperative dose	Preoperative and postoperative vs. preoperative only	No significant difference in infection or failure rates—favored single dose preoperatively
2007	Mazzoch, et al.	736 implants had no preoperative or postoperative antibiotics	No antibiotics, 3 days of anti-inflammatories	96.2% survival rate with no antibiotic use—similar to success rate in studies using antibiotics
2008	Abu-Ta'a et al.	128 implants had preoperative + 2 days postoperative antibiotics; 119 implants had no antibiotics; strict asepsis protocol for both groups	Preoperative and short-term postoperative antibiotics vs. no antibiotics	No significant difference in infections—antibiotics offer no advantage when aseptic techniques are used
2007	Schwartz and Larson	Review of the literature included 4 studies	Review of various protocols	Studies were of poor quality, with small sample size, and underpowered—conclusion difficult to ascertain
2003	Esposito et al.	Cochrane review of 2 studies	Review of various protocols	Not sufficient evidence to support or discourage use of preoperative antibiotics to prevent complications or failures
2008	Esposito et al.	Cochrane review of 2 studies	Meta-analysis of 2 studies examining antibiotic use vs. no antibiotics	Some evidence to support use of antibiotics 1 hour before surgery to reduce risk for implant failure

retrospective study in which the patients receiving antibiotics were treated between 1980 and 1985 and the patients not receiving antibiotics were treated between 1991 and 1995, which the authors report may have influenced their results somewhat.

Several studies have examined the utility of long-term prophylactic antibiotics versus a single preoperative dose. Hossein and colleagues monitored the implant survival rate in patients receiving a single preoperative dose of antibiotics versus those receiving 1 week of postoperative antibiotics.[33] No significant differences were found between the two groups' rate of complications or implant survival. In conclusion, the investigators thought that single-dose preoperative antibiotics should be used instead of long-term postoperative antibiotics because postoperative antibiotics did not offer an additional advantage. Binahmed and associates found similar results in their prospective study of implant patients given preoperative antibiotics versus those given only postoperative antibiotics.[34] These investigators found that long-term postoperative antibiotics did not result in a lower incidence of infection or implant failure than did a single preoperative antibiotic dose.

Mazzocchi and co-workers retrospectively evaluated 736 implants placed with no preoperative or postoperative antibiotics and found that the survival rate was 96.2%, similar to that in studies in which antibiotics were used.[35] In conclusion, they stated that prophylactic antibiotics may not be beneficial in implant patients.

Abu-Ta'a and colleagues conducted a prospective, randomized, double-blind, controlled clinical trial examining implant patients in which the implants were placed under conditions of strict asepsis.[36] One hundred nineteen implants were placed in patients receiving no antibiotics and 128 implants were placed in patients receiving amoxicillin 1 hour preoperatively and for 2 days postoperatively. An aseptic technique that included a preoperative chlorhexidine rinse and preoperative disinfection of peri-oral skin was followed. Sterile drapes were used, as was a meshed nose guard to prevent contamination from the nasal skin. Additionally, two suctions were used—one for the mouth and a separate one for the wound. Patients were evaluated over a 5-month period and observed for symptoms of infection or inflammation, as well as failure of an implant to integrate. Infection developed in one of those treated with antibiotics and in four patients not given antibiotics. The survival rate of implants placed in patients receiving antibiotics was 100%, whereas it was 96% in those not receiving antibiotics. No significant difference was seen between the two groups with regard to a practitioner's identification of signs and symptoms of inflammation or infection at the time of suture removal. There was a significant difference, however, between the two groups at that time with respect to the patient's perception of pain, swelling, and erythema, but not purulence, thus indicating that the antibiotic regimen used may have reduced postoperative discomfort but did not reduce the incidence of infection. Based on these results, the authors thought that antibiotics did not offer significant additional benefit when placing implants with strict aseptic technique.

Schwartz and Larson conducted a review of the literature concerning antibiotic prophylaxis in implant patients and assessed the quality of existing studies.[37] Of the aforementioned studies, those by Binahmed and colleagues[34] and Laskin and associates[31] were given a quality score of 50% or less in the literature review. The only study that received a quality score greater than 50% was that by Gynther and co-workers,[32] which received a score of 71%. The conclusion of the study by Gynther and co-workers had been that preoperative and postoperative antibiotics do not offer any advantage in implant survival over providing no antibiotics at all.[32] The conclusion of the review of the literature was that the studies evaluating prophylactic antibiotics in implant placement procedures were of poor quality, with small sample sizes and underpowered studies.

Antibiotic prophylaxis for implant placement was reviewed by the Cochrane Collaboration in 2003,[38] and this review was updated in 2008.[29] In the 2003 review it was concluded that there was not sufficient evidence to recommend or discourage the use of preoperative antibiotics to prevent implant failures or complications.[38,39] As part of the 2008 review, a meta-analysis of two trials was conducted. One trial was the previously mentioned study of Abu-Ta'a and colleagues in which the authors concluded that antibiotics do not offer significant additional benefit over placebo when placing implants under strict asepsis.[36] The second study evaluated was a placebo-controlled trial that compared preoperative antibiotics with placebo.[40] A total of 158 patients from each arm in this study were evaluated at 1 week, 2 weeks, and 4 months postoperatively and were assessed for prosthesis and implant failure, adverse events, and complications. Although four times as many patients in the placebo group as in the preoperative antibiotic group experienced implant failure, this finding was not found to be statistically significant. The meta-analysis of these two studies included 410 patients and demonstrated no significant difference in prosthesis failure, postoperative infections, or adverse events when comparing implants placed with antibiotics versus placebo. A statistically significant difference was found with respect to implant losses, with patients receiving antibiotics having fewer implant losses. A 6% implant failure rate in patients not receiving antibiotics was demonstrated in the meta-analysis, and the number needed to treat was 25 to prevent one patient from having an implant failure. In conclusion, the authors of the 2008 update of the Cochrane review thought that there is some evidence to support administering 2 g of amoxicillin 1 hour preoperatively to reduce the likelihood of early implant failure. In consideration of the literature previously mentioned in this section, this recommendation seems to be appropriate.

THIRD MOLARS

The usefulness of antibiotics in preventing infection in the setting of third molar surgery has been a topic of discussion over the years, with multiple trials being performed (Table 8-4). A majority of the literature favors not using antibiotic prophylaxis for third molar extractions. Alveolar osteitis (AO), though not related to bacterial infection, is an inflammatory complication with a reported frequency as high as 25% to 30% in patients undergoing mandibular third molar extraction.[41] The rate of postoperative infection after third molar extraction has been reported to range between 1% and 6%,[42] and other literature reports a range of 2% to 12%.[43] A major principle of antibiotic prophylaxis is that the procedure in question should have a significant risk for infection, and therefore, with such a low infection rate, antibiotic prophylaxis may not be indicated for third molar extraction.

Piecuch and colleagues performed a retrospective review of 2134 patients who had 6713 third molars removed.[44] Patients underwent one of six different types of treatment, including no antibiotics, peri-operative systemic antibiotics, placement of tetracycline powder in the socket, peri-operative systemic antibiotics and tetracycline placement, postoperative antibiotics, and postoperative antibiotics with tetracycline placement. The overall infection rate was low—3.5%. The infection rate associated with maxillary third molar extraction was exceedingly low—0.27%. Infections were stratified according to the level of impaction. Because of the low rate of infection of maxillary third molars, only mandibular impactions were found to demonstrate any significant differences. For erupted mandibular third molars, there was a significant reduction in infection in patients in whom tetracycline was placed in the socket in comparison to patients in whom no antibiotic was used. For soft tissue–impacted third molars, there was no significant difference among any of the treatment groups. For partial bone impactions, systemic perioperative antibiotics and placement of tetracycline in the socket significantly reduced the infection rate. Additionally, tetracycline placed in the socket of partial bone impactions appeared to be more efficacious in preventing infection than did systemic peri-operative antibiotics. Systemic antibiotics, as well as tetracycline placed in the socket, were demonstrated to reduce infection in patients with full bone impactions. Furthermore, tetracycline placed in the socket was more efficacious than systemic perioperative antibiotics in preventing infection when full bone impactions were removed. A limitation of this study was its retrospective and non-randomized design. As can be determined from the data, the degree of impaction seems to have an influence on the infection rate, and different levels of impaction respond to different prophylactic techniques. The authors identified the weakness of their study to be its retrospective and non-randomized nature. They thought that their results supported the idea that antibiotics in some form, administered prophylactically, may be useful in preventing infection after mandibular third molar extraction, as reflected in the aforementioned results.

The use of systemic antibiotics for third molar prophylaxis was examined by Sekhar and associates.[45] In this prospective, randomized, double-blind, controlled study, patients undergoing asymptomatic mandibular third molar removal were included. One hundred twenty-five patients completed the study and had been randomized to either a placebo arm, a single preoperative dose of metronidazole, or 5 postoperative days of metronidazole. Patients were examined 6 days postoperatively and the following parameters were evaluated: pain scores on the second and sixth postoperative days, interincisal opening, and presence or absence of purulence or AO. Their analysis did not reveal any significant differences between the study groups with regard to these parameters, and the authors thought that antibiotic prophylaxis did not reduce morbidity when mandibular third molars were removed.

A somewhat larger study was performed by Poeschl and associates in which 288 patients underwent removal of 528 impacted mandibular third molars.[46] A prospective study was performed in

TABLE 8-4	Summary of Studies Regarding the Antibiotic Protocol for Third Molars			
YEAR	AUTHOR	NUMBER OF THIRD MOLARS OR PATIENTS	ANTIBIOTIC PROTOCOL	CONCLUSION
1995	Piecuch et al.	6713 3rd molars, 2134 patients	No antibiotics vs. several combinations of systemic antibiotics and topical antibiotics	Maxillary 3rd molars: very low infection rate—antibiotics not indicated; mandibular 3rd molars: antibiotics in some form may be useful—degree of impaction is influential in which prophylactic technique is most valuable
2001	Sekar et al.	125 patients, mandibular 3rd molars only	Placebo (n = 34) vs. single preoperative dose (n = 44) vs. 5 days of postoperative antibiotics (n = 47)	Antibiotic prophylaxis does not decrease morbidity after mandibular 3rd molar extraction
2004	Poeschl et al.	528 mandibular 3rd molars, 288 patients	No antibiotics vs. amoxicillin-clavulanate for 5 days postoperatively vs. clindamycin for 5 days postoperatively	No significant difference in healing, pain, MIO, or inflammation—postoperative prophylactic antibiotics not recommended
2005	Arteagoitia et al.	490 mandibular 3rd molars, 490 patients	Postoperative placebo vs. postoperative amoxicillin-clavulanate for 4 days, chlorhexidine rinse for 7 days	Statistically significant decrease in infection/inflammation in antibiotic (1.9%) vs. placebo group (12.9%)—antibiotics useful in reducing infection and inflammation but should not be used in all cases
2008	Ataoglu et al.	150 3rd molars, 150 patients	No antibiotics vs. amoxicillin-clavulanate for 5 days postoperatively vs. amoxicillin-clavulanate for 5 days preoperatively	No significant difference in pain, infection, swelling, AO, or MIO—authors did not recommend routine antibiotic prophylaxis
2007	Halpern and Dodson	118 patients	IV placebo vs. IV antibiotics preoperatively	8.5% infection rate in placebo group and no infections in antibiotic group—prophylactic IV antibiotics decreased frequency of surgical site infection
2007	Kaczmarzyk et al.	86 patients, mandibular 3rd molars requiring bone removal	Placebo (n = 27) vs. single preoperative dose (n = 31) vs. preoperative + 5 days of postoperative antibiotics (n = 28)	No significant difference in postoperative complications, did not support use of prophylactic antibiotics
2007	Ren et al.	2932 patients in 16 trials studying AO; 2396 patients in 12 trials studying surgical site infection	Meta-analysis of RCTs from 1974 to 2007 examining antibiotic prophylaxis to prevent AO and surgical site infections	Preoperative systemic antibiotics reduced incidence of AO and infection in mandibular 3rd molars; authors noted this should not provide rigid guideline
2009	Monaco et al.	59 patients aged 12-19, germectomy of one mandibular 3rd	Preoperative antibiotics vs. no antibiotics; all rinsed with chlorhexidine preoperatively and for 7 days postoperatively	Antibiotics resulted in significant decrease in pain, analgesic use, and wound infection; no significant reduction in swelling or fever; authors concluded antibiotic prophylaxis is beneficial
2005	Caso et al.	7 randomized prospective clinical trials	Meta-analysis of RCTs from 1977 to 2002: 2 studies of preoperative chlorhexidine rinse, 5 studies of rinsing at least on the day of surgery and for several days afterward	No significant reduction in AO from a single preoperative rinse; 3 of 5 studies using multiple postoperative rinses showed significant reduction in AO—minimum number of days of postoperative rinsing is unknown

AO, alveolar osteitis; MIO, maximal incisional opening; RCT, randomized controlled trial.

which patients were randomized to receive either amoxicillin-clavulanate for 5 days postoperatively, clindamycin for 5 days postoperatively, or no antibiotics. All patients rinsed with 0.2% chlorhexidine solution preoperatively. Patients underwent release of any hematoma on postoperative day 2, and any patients who had partial eruption of the third molar had iodoform gauze placed in the site at the time of surgery, which was removed on postoperative day 2. Patients were assessed on postoperative days 2 and 10 and at 4 weeks postoperatively. The following parameters were evaluated: difference in interincisal opening in comparison to preoperatively, infection, dry socket, pain as indicated on a visual analog scale, and side effects. There was no significant difference among these groups with regard to the incidence of infection or dry socket, interincisal opening, or pain. Of note, a large percentage of the dry sockets (69.6%) were associated with partially erupted third molars. The authors concluded that routine oral postoperative antibiotic prophylaxis for asymptomatic third molars is not recommended.

In contrast, Arteagoitia and co-workers found that postoperative administration of amoxicillin-clavulanate after the removal of one mandibular third molar did significantly reduce the incidence of inflammatory and infectious complications in their study of 494 patients.[47] This was a prospective, double-blind, placebo-controlled, randomized clinical trial. Patients were randomized to receive either 4 days of postoperative amoxicillin-clavulanate or no antibiotics. The socket was irrigated with 0.12% chlorhexidine at the conclusion of the procedure. Patients also rinsed with 0.12% chlorhexidine three times per day for 7 days postoperatively. Patients were assessed on postoperative day 7 and whenever necessary during the 8 weeks after surgery. The diagnosis of postoperative infection or inflammation was determined according to specific criteria, including elevated temperature (>37.8° C after 24 hours), intraoral fluctuance/purulence, dry socket, severe pain increasing after 48 hours with inflammation or erythema, or severe pain after postoperative day 7 with inflammation or erythema. Their findings revealed a statistically significant increase in infection and inflammation in the placebo group. The groups had been well matched except for the fact that a greater proportion of teeth in the placebo group required bone removal. Regression analysis showed that only age was a confounding variable—not sex, smoking, depth of impaction, angulation, intervention time, need for sectioning, and need for bone removal. Of note, use of a 0.12% chlorhexidine rinse for 7 days postoperatively may have been a confounder in the overall results. The frequency of infection or inflammation was 1.9% in the group receiving antibiotics and 12.9% in the group not receiving antibiotics. The relative risk ratio for inflammatory complications without the use of postoperative antibiotics was 0.15. The number needed to treat to prevent one infectious or inflammatory complication was 10. Despite these findings, the authors questioned the idea of providing antibiotics to all patients to prevent these complications. In conclusion, they thought that use of clinical judgment was most important, especially with respect to a patient's age inasmuch as older patients had a greater risk for infectious or inflammatory complications.

Ataoglu and associates studied 150 patients undergoing maxillary and mandibular third molar removal.[48] The patients were randomized to receive either 5 days of preoperative amoxicillin-clavulanate, 5 days of postoperative amoxicillin-clavulanate, or no antibiotic. All patients rinsed with 0.12% chlorhexidine preoperatively. Patients were evaluated on postoperative days 2 and 7 and were examined for swelling, infection, AO, interincisal opening, and pain. With regard to these parameters, the authors did not find a significant difference between the three treatment groups. The authors concluded that routine antibiotic prophylaxis is not indicated for third molar surgery.

Intravenous prophylactic antibiotic administration before third molar removal was examined by Halpern and Dodson in a placebo-controlled, double-blind, randomized clinical trial comparing preoperative intravenous administration of penicillin or clindamycin (in penicillin-allergic patients) versus placebo.[49] This study included 118 patients and the outcomes assessed were postoperative inflammation or surgical site infection. The group receiving preoperative antibiotics had no infections or postoperative inflammatory complications. The group receiving placebo had an 8.5% (P = .03) surgical site infection rate and no AO. All infections occurred in patients in whom the removed tooth had been either a partial or complete

bone-impacted mandibular third molar and required bone removal. In conclusion, the authors thought that the use of intravenous prophylactic antibiotics did decrease the incidence of surgical site infections. The number needed to treat was 12. A review of this study by Beirne indicated that it was limited by small sample size but was otherwise a well-designed study.[50]

On the contrary, Kaczmarzyk and co-workers demonstrated that neither preoperative nor postoperative antibiotics were more effective than placebo in preventing inflammatory or infectious complications of mandibular third molar removal.[51] Their study was a prospective, randomized, double-blind, placebo-controlled trial. Eighty-six patients requiring third molar removal were divided into three treatment groups: single-dose preoperative oral clindamycin, multiple-dose clindamycin postoperatively for 5 days in addition to a preoperative dose, and placebo. The following parameters of inflammation were evaluated on postoperative days 1, 2, and 7: trismus, facial swelling, body temperature, lymphadenopathy, AO, and subjective pain assessment. There was no significant difference among the groups with regard to postoperative inflammatory complications, and the authors thought that the results did not support the use of prophylactic antibiotics for the removal of third molars. However, the sample size was small, so perhaps a larger sample size would support different results.

Ren and Malmstrom performed a thorough meta-analysis of randomized controlled clinical trials published between 1974 and 2007 to evaluate antibiotic use for third molar extractions.[43] They evaluated two primary outcomes: AO and surgical site infection. In studies reporting AO as an outcome, there were 2932 patients randomized in 16 trials. AO occurred in 6.2% of patients who received preoperative systemic antibiotics and in 14.4% of those who did not. The number needed to treat to prevent one episode of AO was 13. According to the analysis, there was a statistically significant reduction in the incidence of AO for mandibular third molar extraction when preoperative systemic antibiotics were used. Postoperative antibiotics did not have a statistically significant effect on the incidence of AO. In studies reporting surgical site infection as an outcome, 2396 patients in 12 clinical trials were included. Surgical site infection occurred in 4% of the patients receiving antibiotics and in 6.1% of those not receiving antibiotics. The number needed to treat to prevent one infection was 25. Both penicillin and metronidazole were effective in reducing the frequency of AO, but metronidazole was not as effective as penicillin in prevention of surgical site infection. The meta-analysis suggested that the most effective dosing strategy was to provide preoperative antibiotics 30 to 90 minutes before surgery and to continue them for 3 to 5 days postoperatively. A single preoperative dose was thought to be as effective as multi-day dosing. It was found that antibiotics given after surgery had started was not effective in reducing the incidence of AO or infection. Despite the statistical significance of their findings, the authors ultimately concluded that the decision to provide preoperative antibiotics must be made by carefully weighing the risks versus the benefits of doing so. It was thought that the results should not stand as a rigid guideline for antibiotic prophylaxis and that risk factors should be considered when deciding whether to provide antibiotics. A reasonable approach was believed to be the administration of penicillin 1 hour before the surgical removal of impacted mandibular third molars. The decision to provide postoperative antibiotics should be considered for those with risk factors, including smoking, poor oral hygiene, and advanced age.

A study recently published by Monaco and co-authors examined the use of prophylactic antibiotics in a select population.[52] The study population consisted of 59 healthy patients aged 12 to 19 who underwent removal of mandibular third molars that had not yet exhibited root development (germectomy). Only the right molar of each patient was evaluated. It was thought that by studying such a specific population, the interaction of other co-morbid conditions or variability would be minimized. Patients were randomized to receive either preoperative antibiotics or no antibiotics. Patients were not blinded to the treatment group that they were in. The antibiotic used was amoxicillin, 2 g given orally 1 hour preoperatively. Patients rinsed preoperatively with 0.12% chlorhexidine and rinsed twice daily with 0.20% chlorhexidine for 7 days postoperatively. Patients completed a questionnaire evaluating pain, fever, swelling, trismus, and use of anti-inflammatory medications during the week after surgery. Additionally, the surgeon evaluated the patient for infection at the 1-week follow-up appointment. The authors found a statistically significant reduction in pain, use of analgesics, and wound infection when preoperative antibiotics were used. The authors did not find a statistically significant reduction in swelling or fever. Because of the significant reduction in pain related to the use of prophylactic antibiotics, it was concluded by the authors that antibiotic prophylaxis is of benefit in this younger population.

In view of these and the multitude of other studies that have looked at this question, it is probably best to follow the recommendations of Arteagoitia and co-authors[47] and use clinical judgment when considering whether to administer prophylactic antibiotics to patients undergoing third molar extraction. Prophylactic antibiotics in cases in which infection does not already exist should probably be considered more seriously in older patients, in those with co-morbid conditions that may predispose to a higher risk for infection, and for extractions of partial or full bone-impacted mandibular third molars. Additionally, the use of postoperative antibiotics has not been shown to result in a significant reduction in infections in third molar extractions. Therefore, true antibiotic prophylaxis in which the dose is provided before surgery so that a high tissue concentration can be achieved before surgical contamination offers the best chance for prevention of infection.[2]

Not only has systemic antibiotic prophylaxis been studied extensively in third molar surgery, but the use of chlorhexidine rinses has been studied as well. A meta-analysis by Caso and colleagues examined the use of chlorhexidine to prevent AO.[53] They evaluated seven randomized controlled trials and divided them into two groups: one group of two studies that examined strictly preoperative use of chlorhexidine rinses and a second group of five studies

that examined rinsing at least on the day of surgery and for several days postoperatively. In the group in which only preoperative rinses were used, there did not seem to be a reduction in the frequency of AO. In the group in which postoperative rinses were used, three of the five studies showed a significant reduction in AO in response to rinsing with chlorhexidine both preoperatively once and postoperatively for several days. Some limitations of the meta-analysis included the fact that many of the studies used slightly different rinsing protocols. Additionally, there were differences among studies with regard to the criteria used for diagnosing AO. In this meta-analysis it was not possible to determine the minimum number of days of postoperative rinsing needed to significantly reduce the incidence of AO. In conclusion, postoperative chlorhexidine rinses seem to decrease the risk for AO, but further study is necessary to determine an ideal protocol. An additional consideration should be that, although not as common as antibiotic resistance, chlorhexidine resistance has been reported. For example, there have been reports of resistance to chlorhexidine in strains of *Pseudomonas aeruginosa*, *Proteus mirabilis*, *Escherichia coli*, *Serratia marcescens*, and *Pseudomonas stutzeri*.[54]

FACIAL FRACTURES

Mandibular fractures have a higher rate of infection than maxillary fractures do, and therefore most studies of antibiotic prophylaxis in patients with facial trauma have examined the use of antibiotics for mandibular fractures (Table 8-5). Furthermore, subcondylar fractures rarely become infected, and the highest rate of infection is associated with compound fractures, either open to the mouth or those with teeth in the line of fracture.[55] Chole and Yee performed a randomized controlled trial comparing the use of peri-operative antibiotics with no antibiotics in patients undergoing either open or closed treatment of facial fractures.[55] The study group received one preoperative as well as one postoperative dose of cefazolin, whereas the control group received no antibiotics. When all facial fractures were analyzed, 8.9% of patients in the antibiotic group became infected as opposed to 42.3% of patients in the control group, thus demonstrating a significant reduction in infection related to prophylactic antibiotics. No maxillary or zygoma fractures became infected, and all infections except for one case of meningitis occurred in the mandible at the parasymphysis or the angle. The beneficial effect of prophylactic antibiotics was significant for open

TABLE 8-5	Summary of Studies Regarding Antibiotic Protocol for Facial Fractures			
YEAR	AUTHOR	NUMBER OF PATIENTS	ANTIBIOTIC PROTOCOL	CONCLUSION
1987	Chole and Yee	101 patients: 79 mandible, 18 zygoma, 4 Le Fort fractures	Perioperative vs. no antibiotics for treatment of open or closed fractures	Antibiotic group had an 8.9% infection rate, control group had a 42.2% infection rate; significantly decreased infection rate in open treatment of mandibular angle and parasymphysis fractures when peri-operative antibiotics used
2006	Andreasen et al.	483 patients, 4 randomized studies	Systematic review of studies in 1975-1988 to evaluate the benefit of antibiotics in the treatment of facial trauma	Antibiotics significantly decreased risk for infection in open treatment of compound mandibular fractures; studies supported short-term antibiotic use (<48 h); no indication for antibiotic prophylaxis in treatment of maxillary, zygoma, or condyle fractures
2006	Miles et al.	181 patients, open treatment of mandibular fractures	Preoperative + intraoperative antibiotics vs. preoperative + intraoperative + postoperative antibiotics for 5-7 days	Postoperative antibiotics did not provide additional benefit over peri-operative antibiotics in preventing infection (peri-operative dosing had only a 14% infection rate and postoperative dosing had a 10% infection rate)

reductions only, not for closed reductions. Additionally, there was no significant difference between the infection rate of fractures treated in closed manner (with or without antibiotics) and fractures treated in open manner in which prophylactic antibiotics were given. The authors' conclusion was that prophylactic antibiotics were of benefit in the open treatment of mandibular angle or para-symphysis fractures.

A recent systematic review by Andreasen and co-authors[56] of the use of prophylactic antibiotics in patients with facial fractures, which included the study of Chole and Yee,[55] was also supportive. This review examined whether prophylactic antibiotics prevent infections in jaw fracture treatment; which combination of antibiotic, dose, and length of treatment is ideal; and whether there are situations in which prophylactic antibiotics should not be used. Four randomized studies published between 1975 and 1988 were included in determining the possible benefit of prophylactic antibiotics. However, none of the studies included met the strict criteria for a randomized controlled trial. The authors of the systematic review concluded that in the treatment of compound mandibular fractures, especially those treated in an open manner, prophylactic antibiotics were strongly indicated to reduce the risk for postoperative infection, with risk for infection being reduced approximately three-fold. Additionally, they believed that open treatment of fractures increased the risk for postoperative infection. Again, infections of the maxilla, zygoma, and condylar region were not reported, thus indicating that the infection rate of fractures in these areas is exceedingly low. Two studies (Aderhold, Gerlach and Pape, and Abubaker and Rollert)[56,57] in which short-term treatment (<48 hours) with antibiotics was compared with a longer-term course (>48 hours) were evaluated, and the overall evidence supported the shorter-term use of antibiotics. In Aderhold's 1983 study, open and closed treatment of 120 compound mandibular fractures was evaluated.[56] Forty patients received no antibiotics, 40 received antibiotics for up to 48 hours, and 40 received antibiotics for longer than 48 hours. The highest infection rate was 20% and occurred in patients receiving no antibiotics. Those receiving antibiotics for longer than 48 hours had a 10% infection rate, and those receiving antibiotics for up to 48 hours had the lowest infection rate of 5%. In a separate study, Gerlach and Pape evaluated antibiotic prophylaxis in the open treatment of 200 mandibular fractures.[56] Their study included four groups: a control group receiving no antibiotics, one-shot preoperative antibiotics, 1-day antibiotics with the first dose given preoperatively, and a 3-day course of antibiotics. The control group exhibited a 22% infection rate, whereas the antibiotic groups had infection rates of 6%, 2%, and 8%, respectively. It was concluded that one-shot prophylaxis was appropriate to prevent infections in the open treatment of compound mandibular fractures. In their 2001 study, Abubaker and Rollert examined 1-day versus 5-day prophylaxis of mandibular fractures with penicillin in 30 patients.[57] The 1-day patients received intravenous antibiotics preoperatively and every 4 hours intra-operatively and for 12 hours postoperatively. The 5-day patients received the same regimen plus postoperative antibiotics for 5 days. There was no additional benefit derived from the provision of post-operative antibiotics inasmuch as the patients receiving only 1 day of antibiotics had an infection rate of 12.5% and those receiving 5 days of postoperative antibiotics had an infection rate of 14.3%. A limitation of this study was that the sample size was small, and the authors believed that their study should be considered a pilot study. Additionally, many of the fractures in the study were treated in

closed fashion, and several patients treated in open fashion also underwent MMF. A 1997 study by Heit and colleagues was analyzed in which different antibiotic regimens were compared. They compared penicillin with ceftriaxone and found no difference in prophylactic benefit based on which antibiotic was used.[58] The conclusion of Andreasen and co-authors in their systematic review was that short-term antibiotic prophylaxis (<48 hours and possibly just as a single dose) was beneficial in preventing infection in the open treatment of mandibular fractures and that there is no indication for antibiotic prophylaxis in the treatment of maxillary, zygoma, or condylar fractures because of the low incidence of infections with these types of fractures.[56]

The necessity for postoperative antibiotics in the open treatment of mandibular fractures was recently examined by Miles and co-workers, who studied 181 patients undergoing open treatment of mandible fractures via intraoral incisions, extraoral incisions, or a combined approach.[59] Patients were randomized to receive either only preoperative and intraoperative antibiotics or postoperative antibiotics in addition to preoperative and intraoperative antibiotics. The postoperative regimen included either an intramuscular injection of penicillin G benzathine or 5 or 7 days of oral clindamycin. Patients were monitored for infection for a minimum of 5 weeks. Patients receiving only perioperative antibiotics had a 14% infection rate and those receiving perioperative and postoperative antibiotics had a 10% infection rate—this difference was not statistically significant. Of note, there was a statistically significant increased risk for infection in patients who abused alcohol and tobacco concomitantly. The authors identified their high dropout rate as a potential weakness of the study. A total of 291 patients had been enrolled in the study, but only 181 meet full inclusion criteria, which included adequate follow-up. In conclusion, the authors thought that their results corroborated those of Abubaker and Rollert[57] and that although perioperative antibiotics are of clear benefit in mandibular fractures, there does not seem to be additional benefit derived from providing postoperative antibiotics.

A subsequent study by Lovato and Wagner also corroborated the finding that postoperative antibiotics do not provide additional benefit.[60] Their study consisted of a retrospective chart review of 150 patients who underwent closed or open treatment of either complicated or uncomplicated mandibular fractures and for whom 6 weeks of follow-up data was available. A majority of patients (81.33%) were treated with open reduction. Patients fell into one of two categories: those who received antibiotics only perioperatively for less than 24 hours and those who received antibiotics for more than 24 hours and up to 10 days. There was no standard protocol for antibiotic administration, several different antibiotics were used, and in 18% of the cases reviewed, the antibiotic used was unknown. All patients had received a prescription for postoperative chlorhexidine rinses. The authors found that infection developed in 10.67% of patients receiving antibiotics for the extended period and in 13.33% of patients receiving only perioperative antibiotics. No significant difference was detected between the two groups. Additionally, there was no significant difference in the infection rate in patients treated in open versus closed fashion. Various limitations existed in this study. It was noted by the authors that to detect a difference of 2% between the two groups, it would be necessary to have 1604 subjects in each group and their study had just 75 patients in each group—therefore this study was to be regarded as a pilot study.

PEARLS AND PITFALLS

- In orthognathic surgery, bone grafting, and implant placement, the evidence seems to support at least preoperative antibiotics, although in the case of bone grafting, additional study is warranted.
- In third molar extraction, it is clear that partial or full bone-impacted mandibular third molars are most likely to become infected, but the decision for antibiotic prophylaxis should take into consideration the patient's overall risk factors for infection.
- The most clear-cut evidence seems to be in support of short-term antibiotics in the management of compound mandibular fractures.
- It makes sense that antibiotic prophylaxis is of *potential* benefit in class II operations such as orthognathic surgery, bone grafting, implants, and third molar extraction.

- The more clearly defined benefit of antibiotic prophylaxis in class III operations such as for mandibular fractures is logical.
- There are several challenges in reviewing the literature on this subject. Many studies are retrospective, not blinded or controlled, and of low power.
- Several broad definitions of infection that are not consistent across the board are being evaluated.
- As can be seen, use of antibiotic prophylaxis for oral and maxillofacial surgical procedures is not entirely clear-cut. Ultimately, one's clinical judgment on a case-by-case basis is the most important guide of all.

REFERENCES

1. Stone HH, Haney BB, Kolb LD, et al: Prophylactic and preventive antibiotic therapy: timing, duration, and economics, *Ann Surg* 189:691-698, 1979.
2. Laskin DM: The use of prophylactic antibiotics for the prevention of postoperative infections, *Oral Maxillofac Surg Clin North Am* 15:155-160, 2003.
3. Wilson W, Taubert KA, Gewiz M, et al: Prevention of infective endocarditis, *Circulation* 116:1736-1754, 2007.
4. American Association of Orthopedic Surgeons: Information Statement 1033. Antibiotic prophylaxis for bacteremia in patients with joint replacements. Available at *http://www.aaos.org/about/papers/advistmt/1033.asp*, February 2009.
5. Lockhart PB, Loven B, Brennan MT, et al: The evidence base for the efficacy of antibiotic prophylaxis in dental practice, *J Am Dent Assoc* 138:458-474, 2007.
6. Tong DC, Rothwell BR: Antibiotic prophylaxis in dentistry: a review and practice recommendations, *J Am Dent Assoc* 131:366-374, 2000.
7. Peterson LJ: Antibiotic prophylaxis against wound infections in oral and maxillofacial surgery, *J Oral Maxillofac Surg* 48:617-620, 1990.
8. Johnson JT, Wagner RL: Infection following uncontaminated head and neck surgery, *Arch Otolaryngol Head Neck Surg* 113:368-369, 1987.
9. Resnik RR, Misch C: Prophylactic antibiotic regimens in oral implantology: rationale and protocol, *Implant Dent* 17:142-150, 2008.
10. Dent CD, Olson JW, Farish SE, et al: The influence of preoperative antibiotics on success of endosseous implants up to and including stage II surgery: a study of 2,641 implants, *J Oral Maxillofac Surg* 55(Suppl 5):19-24, 1997.
11. Condon RE, Wittmann DH: The use of antibiotics in general surgery, *Curr Probl Surg* 28:807-949, 1991.
12. Burke JF: The effective period of preventive antibiotic action in experimental incisions and dermal lesions, *Surgery* 50:161-168, 1961.
13. Miles AA, Miles EM, Burke J: The value and duration of defense reaction of the skin to primary lodgment of bacteria, *Br J Exp Pathol* 38:79-86, 1957.
14. Alanis A, Weinstein AJ: Adverse reactions associated with the use of oral penicillins and cephalosporins, *Med Clin North Am* 67:113, 1983.
15. Alpha C, O'Ryan F, Silva A, et al: The incidence of postoperative wound healing problems following sagittal ramus osteotomies stabilized with miniplates and monocortical screws, *J Oral Maxillofac Surg* 64:659-668, 2006.
16. Kim SG, Park SS: Incidence of complications and problems related to orthognathic surgery, *J Oral Maxillofac Surg* 65:2438-2444, 2007.
17. Chow LK, Singh B, Chiu WK, et al: Prevalence of postoperative complications after orthognathic surgery: a 15-year review, *J Oral Maxillofac Surg* 65:984-992, 2007.
18. Zijderveld SA, Smeele LE, Kostense PJ, et al: Preoperative antibiotic prophylaxis in orthognathic surgery: a randomized, double-blind, and placebo-controlled clinical study, *J Oral Maxillofac Surg* 57:1403-1406, 1999.
19. Ruggles JE, Hann JR: Antibiotic prophylaxis in intraoral orthognathic surgery, *J Oral Maxillofac Surg* 42:797-801, 1984.
20. Fridrich KL, Partnoy BE, Zeitler DL: Prospective analysis of antibiotic prophylaxis for orthognathic surgery, *Int J Adult Orthognath Surg* 9:129-131, 1994.
21. Lindeboom JA, Baas EM, Kroon FH: Prophylactic single-dose administration of 600 mg clindamycin versus 4-time administration of 600 mg clindamycin in orthognathic surgery: a prospective randomized study in bilateral mandibular sagittal ramus osteotomies, *Oral Surg Oral Med Oral Pathol Oral Radiol Endod* 95:145-149, 2003.
22. Bentley KG, Head TW, Aiello GA: Antibiotic prophylaxis in orthognathic surgery: a 1-day versus 5-day regimen, *J Oral Maxillofac Surg* 57:226-230, 1999.
23. Abubaker AO: Antibiotic prophylaxis in orthognathic surgery: a 1-day versus 5-day regimen, discussion, *J Oral Maxillofac Surg* 57:230-232, 1999.
24. Lindeboom JA, van den Akker HP: A prospective placebo-controlled double-blind trial of antibiotic prophylaxis in intraoral bone grafting procedures: a pilot study, *Oral Surg Oral Med Oral Pathol Oral Radiol Endod* 96:669-672, 2003.
25. Brennan MT, et al; Lindeboom JA, et al: Letter to the editor and in reply, *Oral Surg Oral Med Oral Pathol Oral Radiol Endod* 97:664-665, 2004.
26. Lindeboom JA, Frenken JW, Tuk JG, et al: A randomized prospective controlled trial of antibiotic prophylaxis in intraoral bone-grafting procedures: preoperative single-dose penicillin versus preoperative single-dose clindamycin, *Int J Oral Maxillofac Surg* 35:433-436, 2006.
27. Choukroun J, Simonpieri A, Del Corso M, et al: Controlling systematic perioperative anaerobic contamination during sinus-lift procedures by using metronidazole: an innovative approach, *Implant Dent* 17:257-263, 2008.
28. Esposito M, Hirsch JM, Lekholm U, et al: Biological factors contributing to failures of osseointegrated oral implants (II): etiopathogenesis, *Eur J Oral Sci* 106:721-764, 1998.
29. Esposito M, Grusovin MG, Talati M, et al: Interventions for replacing missing teeth: antibiotics at dental implant placement to prevent complications (review), *Cochrane Database Syst Rev* 3:CD004152, 2008.
30. Pye AD, Lockhart DEA, Dawson MP, et al: A review of dental implants and infection, *J Hosp Infect* 72:104-110, 2009.
31. Laskin DM, Dent CD, Morris HF, et al: The influence of preoperative antibiotics on success of endosseous implants at 36 months, *Ann Periodontol* 5:166-174, 2000.
32. Gynther GW, Kondell PA, Moberg LE, et al: Dental implant installation without antibiotic prophylaxis, *Oral Surg Oral Med Oral Pathol Oral Radiol Endod* 85:509-511, 1998.
33. Hossein K, Dahlin C, Bengt A: Influence of different prophylactic antibiotic regimens on implant survival rate: a retrospective clinical study, *Clin Implant Dent Relat Res* 7:32-35, 2005.
34. Binahmed A, Stoykewych A, Peterson L: Single preoperative dose versus long-term prophylactic antibiotic regimens in dental implant surgery, *Int J Oral Maxillofac Implants* 20:115-117, 2005.

35. Mazzocchi A, Passi L, Moretti R: Retrospective analysis of 736 implants inserted without antibiotic therapy, *J Oral Maxillofac Surg* 65:2321-2323, 2007.

36. Abu-Ta'a M, Quirynen M, Teughels W, et al: Asepsis during periodontal surgery involving oral implants and the usefulness of perioperative antibiotics: a prospective, randomized, controlled clinical trial, *J Clin Periodontol* 35:58-63, 2008.

37. Schwartz AB, Larson EL: Antibiotic prophylaxis and postoperative complications after tooth extraction and implant placement: a review of the literature, *J Dent* 35:881-888, 2007.

38. Esposito M, Coulthard P, Oliver R, et al: Antibiotics to prevent complications following dental implant treatment, Cochrane Database Syst Rev 3:CD004152, 2003.

39. Reed SG: Inconclusive evidence to recommend prophylactic antibiotics to prevent complications following dental implant treatment, *J Evid Base Dent Pract* 4:210-211, 2004.

40. Esposito M, Cannizzaro G, Bozzoli P, et al: Efficacy of prophylactic antibiotics for dental implants: a multicentre placebo-controlled randomised clinical trial, *Eur J Oral Implant* 1:23-31, 2008.

41. Blum IR: Contemporary views on dry socket (alveolar osteitis): a clinical appraisal of standardization, aetiopathogenesis and management: a critical review, *Int J Oral Maxillofac Surg* 31:309-317, 2002.

42. Zeitler DL: Prophylactic antibiotics for third molar surgery: a dissenting opinion, *J Oral Maxillofac Surg* 53:61-64, 1995.

43. Ren YF, Malmstrom HS: Effectiveness of antibiotic prophylaxis in third molar surgery: a meta-analysis of randomized controlled clinical trials, *J Oral Maxillofac Surg* 65:1909-1921, 2007.

44. Piecuch JF, Arzadon J, Lieblich SE: Prophylactic antibiotics for third molar surgery: a supportive opinion, *J Oral Maxillofac Surg* 53:53-60, 1995.

45. Sekhar CH, Narayanan V, Baig MF: Role of antimicrobials in third molar surgery: prospective, double blind, randomized, placebo-controlled study, *Br J Oral Maxillofac Surg* 39:134-137, 2001.

46. Poeschl PW, Eckel D, Poeschl E: Postoperative prophylactic antibiotic treatment in third molar surgery—a necessity? *J Oral Maxillofac Surg* 62:3-8, 2004.

47. Arteagoitia I, Diez A, Barbier L, et al: Efficacy of amoxicillin/clavulanic acid in preventing infectious and inflammatory complications following impacted mandibular third molar extraction, *Oral Surg Oral Med Oral Pathol Oral Radiol Endod* 100:E11-E18, 2005.

48. Ataoglu H, Oz GY, Candirli C, et al: Routine antibiotic prophylaxis is not necessary during operations to remove third molars, *Br J Oral Maxillofac Surg* 46:133-135, 2008.

49. Halpern LR, Dodson TB: Does prophylactic administration of systemic antibiotics prevent postoperative inflammatory complications after third molar surgery? *J Oral Maxillofac Surg* 65:177-185, 2007.

50. Beirne OR: Article analysis and evaluation: administration of intravenous antibiotics immediately before extraction of wisdom teeth lowers the rate of postsurgical infections, *J Evid Base Dent Pract* 8:26-27, 2008.

51. Kaczmarzyk T, Wichlinski J, Stypulkowska J, et al: Single-dose and multi-dose clindamycin therapy fails to demonstrate efficacy in preventing infectious and inflammatory complications in third molar surgery, *Int J Oral Maxillofac Surg* 36:417-422, 2007.

52. Monaco G, Tavernese L, Agostini R, et al: Evaluation of antibiotic prophylaxis in reducing postoperative infection after mandibular third molar extraction in young patients, *J Oral Maxillofac Surg* 67:1467-1472, 2009.

53. Caso A, Hung LK, Beirne OR: Prevention of alveolar osteitis with chlorhexidine: a meta-analytic review, *Oral Surg Oral Med Oral Pathol Oral Radiol Endod* 99:155-159, 2005.

54. Russell AD: Bacterial resistance to disinfectants: present knowledge and future problems, *J Hosp Infect* 43:S57-S68, 1998.

55. Chole RA, Yee J: Antibiotic prophylaxis for facial fractures, *Arch Otolaryngol Head Neck Surg* 113:1055-1057, 1987.

56. Andreasen JO, Jensen SS, Schwartz O, et al: A systematic review of prophylactic antibiotics in the surgical treatment of maxillofacial fractures, *J Oral Maxillofac Surg* 64:1664-1668, 2006.

57. Abubaker AO, Rollert MK: Postoperative antibiotic prophylaxis in mandibular fractures: a preliminary randomized, double-blind, and placebo-controlled clinical study, *J Oral Maxillofac Surg* 59:1415-1419, 2001.

58. Heit JM, Stevens MR, Jeffords K: Comparison of ceftriaxone with penicillin for antibiotic prophylaxis for compound mandible fractures, *Oral Surg Oral Med Oral Pathol Oral Radiol Endod* 83:423-426, 1997.

59. Miles BA, Potter JK, Ellis E: The efficacy of postoperative antibiotic regimens in the open treatment of mandibular fractures: a prospective randomized trial, *J Oral Maxillofac Surg* 64:576-582, 2006.

60. Lovato C, Wagner JD: Infection rates following perioperative prophylactic antibiotics versus postoperative extended regimen prophylactic antibiotics in surgical management of mandibular fractures, *J Oral Maxillofac Surg* 67:827-832, 2009.

Chapter 9

Tissue Engineering

Miller H. Smith, Kenji Izumi, Stephen E. Feinberg

Oral maxillofacial surgeons have a number of approaches for reconstruction of soft and hard tissue defects. Autogenous, allogeneic, alloplastic, and xenogeneic options have been available for years and are continuing to evolve. The current "gold standards" of autogenous soft and hard tissues have inherent donor site morbidity, which limits their use in certain applications. The field of tissue engineering has exploded not as a means of repair but as a common goal of regeneration whereby tissues are re-established into their pre-injury state with minimal to absent native tissue scar formation while attempting to minimize risk and morbidity. Materials and techniques continue to evolve for effective and unique alternatives of repair and are providing a bridge for the regenerative strategies of the future. Current tissue-engineering goals for any application encourage the re-establishment of three-dimensional form and function while using scaffolds, cells, biologic factors, and both biomechanical and biophysical stimulation to assist in regeneration of tissues through manipulation of the host environment. Knowing the mechanical properties of all hard tissues to be re-established and providing unique microenvironments for each tissue type are essential for recapitulation of the intricate form of the cranio-maxillofacial region. The difficulty in this field, in general, is that specific applications in other regions of the body cannot always be extrapolated to the head and neck.

ETIOPATHOGENESIS/CAUSATIVE FACTORS

A variety of conditions may necessitate either soft or hard tissue reconstruction. There can be a substantial traumatic or ablative defect involving superficial soft tissues and skin. Certain congenital syndromes may also necessitate soft tissue bulk, such as Parry-Romberg syndrome (hemifacial atrophy) and hemifacial microsomia. Hard tissue needs are more wide ranging, depending on the site, and are based on etiology: developmental, traumatic, pathologic, and/or inflammatory. Some wounds prove very difficult to reconstruct because of substantial inflammation, foreign body reaction from previous surgical efforts, scar tissue formation, compromised vascularity, abnormal anatomy, bilateralism, or large composite tissue loss necessitating reconstruction of multiple hard and soft tissue components. An understanding of the specific structural and functional needs of the injured site is imperative before surgery.

RECONSTRUCTIVE GOALS

The ultimate goal of regeneration is to provide esthetics, minimize scarring, and maximize function across all fields. To accomplish this task effectively, several principles must be adhered to, and these may vary between reconstruction of hard and soft tissues.

SOFT TISSUE PRINCIPLES

- Be of appropriate bulk and plasticity
- Reconstruct like tissues (skin, mucosa, muscle, fat, fascia, tendon, ligaments, or a combination thereof)
- Have unrestricted function
- Be reliable with minimal tissue loss during healing
- Possess advantageous scarring characteristics

HARD TISSUE PRINCIPLES

- Replace complex three-dimensional geometries
- Be biocompatible with minimal inflammatory response
- Assume load bearing and unrestricted function
- Be bioabsorbable to allow transition of load to regenerating structures
- Possess mechanical properties similar to those of native tissue
- Allow hard tissue ingrowth
- Be reliable to avoid mechanical failure
- Stimulate site-specific tissue formation to restore function

TREATMENT

The use of scaffolds and constructs is instrumental for regeneration of both soft and hard tissue. Science, to date, has not been able to regenerate complex tissue defects without a framework to build on. These scaffolds can be developed by a variety of means (outlined later) to satisfy site-specific requirements. Although a scaffold itself will also allow minimal promotion of reparative tissues alone, multiple biologic agents (some still yet to be determined) are required to augment the desired tissue response. It is clear that the body possesses complex interdependent interactions during growth, injury, and healing. Manipulation of these interactions could promote the induction of a fetal healing phase that would be ideal to minimize scarring and effectively regenerate the desired tissues.[1]

Modulation of the host environment is desirable to achieve these goals. Inflammation is an innate healing response and is necessary to allow regeneration; however, limiting excessive inflammation is necessary to prevent scar formation, which may be detrimental. It has become clear that a number of inflammatory mediators are important in facilitating a proper healing response, including tumor necrosis factor-α (TNF-α), interleukin-1 (IL-1), and 6 (IL-6). Attempts at decreasing these cytokines with inhibitory agents have been shown to alter the healing response such that the risk for infection is increased and regenerate tissue formation is decreased. More site-specific cytokines continue to be identified, and it is perceivable that their complex modulation (both increase and decrease) may promote appropriate site-specific healing with fewer side effects.[2]

Extensive research has been applied to the evaluation of known biologics, including transplanted cells (undifferentiated stem cells and differentiated progenitor cells), growth factors, and biomechanical and biophysical stimulants (Fig. 9-1). Combining these biologics

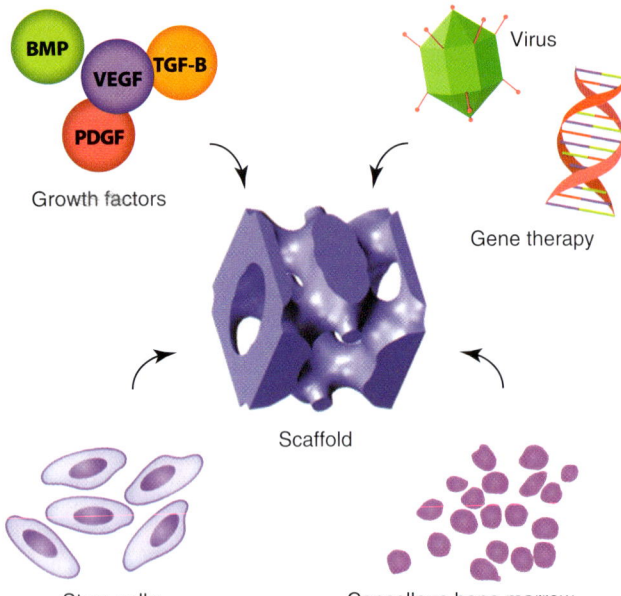

Growth factors

Virus

Gene therapy

Scaffold

Stem cells

Cancellous bone marrow

Fig. 9-1 ■ Various biologics (growth factors and viruses for gene therapy) and progenitor/stem cells can be added and combined with a variety of scaffold materials.

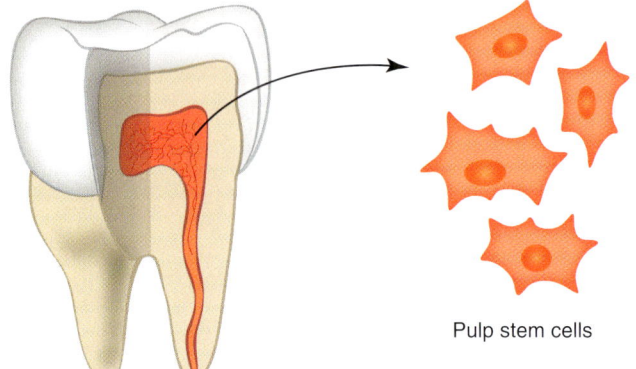

Pulp stem cells

Fig. 9-2 ■ Viable dental pulp from extracted teeth, notably third molars, can be cultured to harvest stem cells.

with basic or complex scaffolds is critical for site-specific soft and hard tissue regeneration. More recently, interest has taken hold in developing an engineered vascular network for blood supply with a composite framework for improved reconstructive options with both hard and soft tissue components.

BIOLOGICS

BIOPHYSICAL AND BIOMECHANICAL STIMULATION

Ultrasound and electrical fields offer a means of biophysical stimulation that enhances bone repair. Ultrasound using low-intensity pulsed signals (30 mW/cm^2) has shown some benefit in accelerating bone healing during fracture repair and distraction procedures.[3] The results of several studies have demonstrated some benefits in improving function, but they are limited in their overall bone-healing response.[4,5] Electromagnetic signals can be provided through direct current, capacitive coupling, inductive coupling, or combinations thereof. Use of direct current is limited because of the creation of an inflammatory-type response. Capacitive coupling (electrical fields exclusively) and inductive coupling (electromagnetic fields) alter cytosolic calcium concentrations through voltage-gated calcium channels and intracellular release, respectively. Pulsed electromagnetic fields have been shown to promote osteoblast formation and the production of osteogenic cytokines such as bone morphogenetic proteins (BMP-2 and BMP-4) and transforming growth factor-β (TGF-β).[6-13] Great interest has been directed toward using this modality with tissue engineering to augment current and future strategies for bone healing.

Promising results have been achieved in nerve repair as well.[8,12] Future investigation is focusing on the use of implantable devices for stimulation during bone repair and reconstruction.[14,15]

DISTRACTION OSTEOGENESIS

Distraction was first described by Ilizarov in 1969 and has given us insight into native bone-healing capacity. By providing steady traction or tension on a stable callus, tissues can be augmented in a variety of ways for condylar, alveolar, and segmental reconstruction.[16-28] Distractor devices have evolved over the years from an external device to more compact internal devices that can be placed intraorally to minimize extraoral scar defects. Further research is being conducted to create smaller bio-expandable devices that possess the appropriate strength and are self-activated by an internal motor mechanism.[29]

CELLULAR DELIVERY

With the use of scaffolds, delivery of biologic agents has been of keen interest to researchers. Stem cells and differentiated progenitor cells have their own indications, depending on location and desired regeneration strategy. A great amount of work is still necessary to idealize treatment outcomes in animals even before trials in humans are conducted. Stem cell therapy continues to be on the forefront given the ability to direct differentiation and enhance tissue regeneration through the provision of specific cell lines. Stem cells located throughout the body can be cultured from various tissue sources to stimulate cell-specific differentiation and expansion.[30,31] Hard tissue regeneration focuses on the pluripotency of bone marrow stromal stem cells (also known as mesenchymal stem cells), hematopoietic stem cells, and adipose stem cells to differentiate into chondrocytes and osteoblasts.[32] Further interest has peaked with harvest and manipulation of dental pulp stem cells, especially those from extracted wisdom and primary teeth (Fig. 9-2). Several for-profit companies have marketed collections of extracted teeth to be made available for future stem cell use:

- National Dental Pulp Laboratory, Inc., Newton, Mass
- BioEden, Inc., Austin, Texas
- StemSave, New York, New York

The non-profit National Stem Cell Bank has been relocated to WiCell (Madison, Wisc.) for cGMP (current good manufacturing practices) research cell lines. These cells can be differentiated and expanded *ex vivo* or relocated and induced within the desired site of reconstruction.[33] Once cells have been delineated, they can be incorporated directly within the fabricated scaffolds by using hydrogels to precisely deliver to the reconstructed area cells that possess characteristics similar to the tissues to be repaired or regenerated.[34-46]

GROWTH FACTORS

More recently, growth factors have been explored for specific applications to manipulate the host environment for promotion of repair and regeneration (Table 9-1). Specific growth factors for head and neck applications include recombinant human bone morphogenetic proteins (rhBMP-2 and rhBMP-7), platelet-derived growth factor

TABLE 9-1	Growth Factors Used in Soft and Hard Tissue Reconstruction	
GROWTH FACTOR	**SOURCE**	**EFFECTS**
BMP	Bone matrix, osteoprogenitor cells (periosteum and ostium), fibroblasts, proliferating chondrocytes	Mesenchymal cells differentiated into osteoblasts, matrix deposition
PDGF	Platelets, keratinocytes, macrophages	Chemotaxis and activation of macrophages and fibroblasts, matrix deposition; migration and proliferation of osteoblasts, cementoblasts, and periodontal ligament
VEGF	Keratinocytes, macrophages	Neovascularization and angiogenesis; indirectly involved with osteoprogenitor cell differentiation
TGF-β	Macrophages, platelets, keratinocytes	Keratinocyte migration, proliferation, remodeling; chondrogenesis
IGF-I	Plasma, platelets	Endothelial cell and fibroblast proliferation
FGF	Macrophages, fibroblasts, endothelial cells	Angiogenesis, fibroblast proliferation

BMP, Bone morphogenetic protein; *FGF*, fibroblast growth factor; *IGF-I*, insulin-like growth factor I; *PDGF*, platelet-derived growth factor; *TGF-β*, transforming growth factor-β; *VEGF*, vascular endothelial growth factor.

(PDGF), vascular endothelial growth factor (VEGF), TGF-β, and insulin-like growth factor type I (IGF-I).[47-63]

Bone Morphogenetic Proteins

rhBMP-7 (OP-1, Stryker, Portage, Mich.) is currently available only for posterolateral and lateral spinal fusions. The Food and Drug Administration (FDA) has authorized the use of rhBMP-2 (Infuse, Medtronic, Minneapolis, Minn.) for sinus lift and alveolar augmentation procedures, although trials are currently being conducted to identify success in other maxillofacial procedures.[52,64-67] BMPs target the undifferentiated mesenchymal stem cell to differentiate into osteoblasts through direct receptor stimulation and signaling.[55]

Platelet-Derived Growth Factor

Ultra-concentrated formulations of PDGF (Gem 21s, Osteohealth, Shirley, NY) have proved beneficial for periodontal defects and small alveolar defects. PDGF has potent chemotactic and mitogenic properties for bone regeneration, with both migration and proliferation of osteoblasts, cementoblasts, and periodontal ligament fibroblasts.[54,68-75] In addition, PDGF has been implicated in promoting soft tissue wound healing through chemotaxis of fibroblasts and subsequent stimulation of proliferation and matrix deposition for wound repair. One such product is marketed for the treatment of non-healing ulcers, especially in diabetics (Regranex, Systagenix Wound Management, Quincy, Mass.).[76-79]

Vascular Endothelial Growth Factor

Neovascularization is up-regulated with VEGF, which is also involved in the differentiation of osteoprogenitor cells through the delivery of nutrients and oxygen to injured areas, as well as secretion of growth factors and cytokines by endothelial cells of the newly developed vessels.[80] The role of VEGF on chondrocytes, osteoclasts, and osteoblasts is well documented, with evolution of endochondral bone formation and improvement of bone mineralization.[81-83]

Other Growth Factors

Other growth factors such as TGF-β, IGF-I, and basic fibroblast growth factor (bFGF) are useful for cartilage and soft tissue promotion.[76,84] Multiple isoforms of TGF-β have been isolated and found to contribute to keratinocyte migration, matrix synthesis, and remodeling, as well as chondrogenesis and bone regeneration with minimal scarring at different stages of the healing cascade. Some may additionally be involved in inflammation and cause fibrosis with scarring. It is therefore critical to further elucidate beneficial formulations for improving wound healing.[76,85] FGF in particular has been shown to be exceptionally useful for soft tissue repair as a result of its promotion of angiogenesis and keratinocyte migration and mitogenesis.[76-79] Combinations of these growth factors are being evaluated and proving to be beneficial for numerous maxillofacial applications.[48,62,86-91] Further large-scale prospective randomized trials are needed to determine the proper concentration and application of these materials. Such materials should be used cautiously; off-label use is not advocated given their substantial systemic effects and risks.

GENE THERAPY

Gene therapy has been investigated by numerous teams for improving delivery and bioavailability of the critical growth factors just listed for both soft tissue and bone regeneration.[56,70,75,83,91-99] Concerns regarding high concentrations of vectors, gene over-expression, or disturbance of native cell signaling have limited mainstream acceptance by the FDA, and gene therapy may therefore not be available for routine human applications for years to come. New technologies have evaluated reactive materials to allow spatial control of the delivery of gene vectors without substantial diffusion to outlying tissues. Such substrate site-specific delivery allows the use of decreased levels of viral vectors for local transduction.[98,99] Any of the aforementioned growth factors can then be delivered directly to the site without worrying about diffusion and can be combined to influence differential tissue regeneration.

SPECIFIC TREATMENT AND TECHNIQUES

SOFT TISSUE RECONSTRUCTION

Oral Mucosa and Skin

A large amount of research is being conducted to identify strategies for minimizing the scarring and donor site morbidity related to skin and mucosal grafting in the head and neck region to treat post-ablative defects and burn injuries, as well as for pre-prosthetic purposes.[76,79,100-102] A variety of approaches have been used in the past, including split- and full-thickness skin grafts, oral mucosa free grafts, and oral connective tissue grafts. Standard, orally harvested

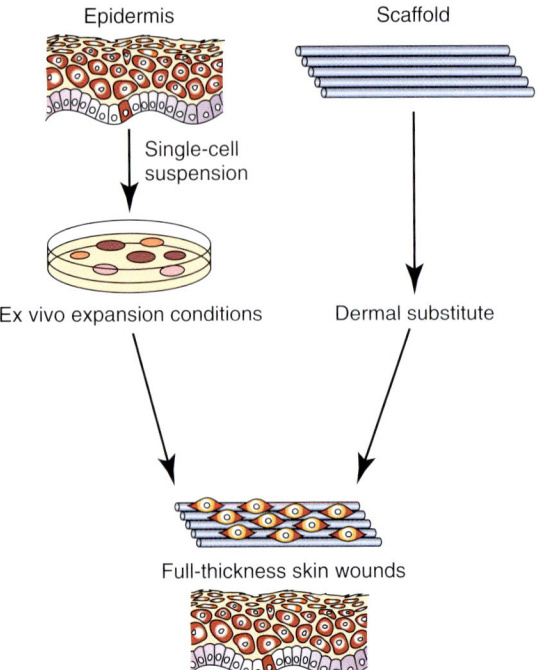

Fig. 9-3 ■ Harvest of a small number of the patient's own keratinocytes from oral mucosa or skin (or both) can be expanded in culture and grown on a dermal scaffold to create a pliable graft material.

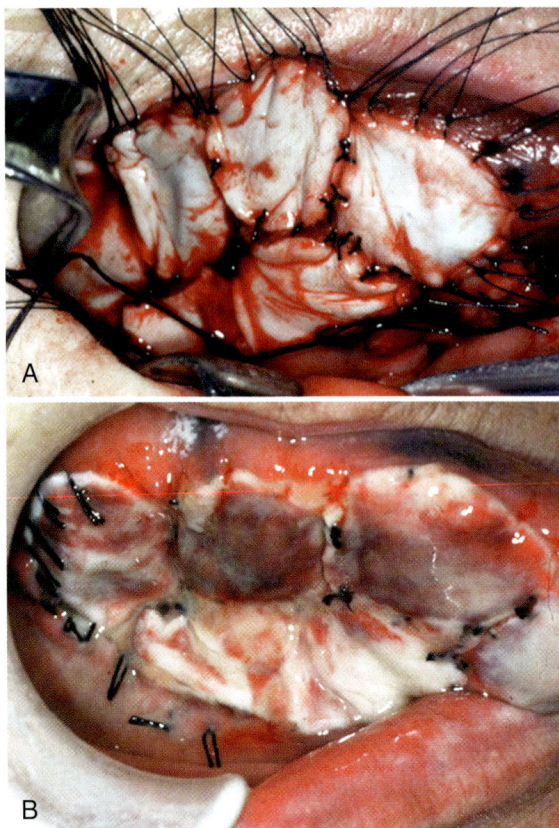

Fig. 9-4 ■ Ex vivo–produced oral mucosa equivalent (EVPOME) grafts can be used to reconstruct various oral defects (**A**); they can obviate the need for other larger donor sites and assist in early repair and healing with minimal scar formation (**B**).

grafts are restricted to the treatment of small defects because of their limited supply and significant discomfort at the donor site. More recently, deepithelialized acellular cadaveric dermal grafts have been used but have demonstrated varied results of healing and scarring in treating lower eyelid,[103] alveolar,[104] and tongue[105] wounds, where they act more as a biologic barrier during the healing process. In addition, because burn victims may have few sites available for graft harvest, cell culture techniques have been investigated for aerosolization and uniform seeding of keratinocytes across the wound bed. Trials are still ongoing to determine effectiveness in humans, but products are currently on the market (CellSpray, Avita Medical Americas, Woburn, Mass.).[106-108]

A newer method of creating a tissue-engineered soft tissue substitute is expansion of a small number of oral keratinocytes onto an underlying dermal scaffold. A soft tissue construct can thereby be prefabricated to provide a variety of options for regeneration of skin and mucosa. Oral keratinocytes are a viable alternative to epidermal (skin) keratinocytes because they have unique characteristics:

1. Heightened growth potential in vitro, thereby necessitating a small donor site
2. Ability of cells to expand for coverage of larger wounds more rapidly
3. Secretion of pro-angiogenic factors, such as VEGF and IL-8, which enhance cell integration at graft sites
4. Secretion of potent antimicrobial peptides (e.g., β-defensins), which may be able to play a role in combating infections

Autogenous oral keratinocytes are harvested through the use of a small tissue punch biopsy and subsequently developed and grown on top of acellular, non-immunogenic, human cadaveric dermis (AlloDerm, LifeCell, Branchburg, NJ), thereby generating an ex vivo–produced oral mucosa equivalent (EVPOME)[105,109-111] (Fig. 9-3). AlloDerm, used as the dermal equivalent for EVPOME, has excellent handling characteristics, provides the grafts with a supple nature, and is an off-the-shelf tissue product well established in the field of oral and maxillofacial surgery. EVPOME is used as a full-thickness mucosa or skin substitute (Fig. 9-4) and has keratinization characteristics identical to those of native oral tissues.

Procedure

A small, 4- to 6-mm tissue punch biopsy specimen is harvested from the oral mucosa 3 to 4 weeks (depending on the size of the grafts needed) before the desired reconstructive surgery. Palatal tissue provides a keratinized mucosa equivalent, whereas the retromolar pad or buccal mucosa provides non-keratinized mucosa equivalent. The harvested tissue is transferred into a culture medium and transported to a cGMP (current Good Manufacturing Practice) facility. The harvested sites can be closed primarily (buccal, retromolar) or have a protective collagen plug sutured into place (palate).

The manufacturing and culturing procedures for EVPOME have been described in detail elsewhere.[105] Briefly, oral keratinocytes are dissociated by soaking the harvested biopsy tissue in 0.04% trypsin solution. The cells are grown in a serum-free culture medium. The lack of xenogeneic cells avoids any cross-contamination of the autogenous oral keratinocytes. Following growth of a sufficient number of keratinocytes over a period of 1 to 2 weeks, cells are seeded onto pieces of type IV collagen–presoaked AlloDerm (cadaveric human dermis) on the roughened side containing an intact basement membrane. For the first 4 days (Fig. 9-5) a composite of keratinocytes and AlloDerm is incubated in a submerged culture. For the next 7 days the composite is raised at an air-liquid interface culture with a higher calcium concentration to promote keratinocyte differentiation (Fig. 9-6). On reaching day 11 after seeding the dermis with keratinocytes, the EVPOME grafts are ready for transplantation (Fig. 9-7).

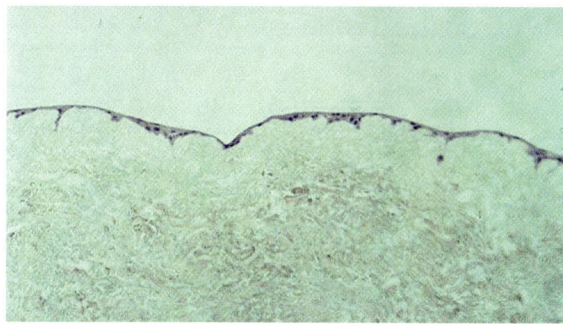

Fig. 9-5 ▪ Early keratinocyte culture with monolayer of epithelial cells grown on the dermal constructs at day 4.

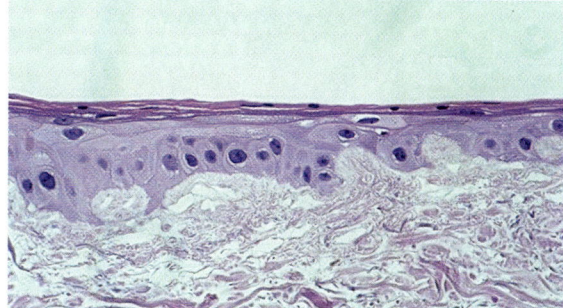

Fig. 9-6 ▪ Expansion and growth, i.e. stratification of the epithelium, of constructs at an air-liquid interface indicative of epithelial maturation/differentiation.

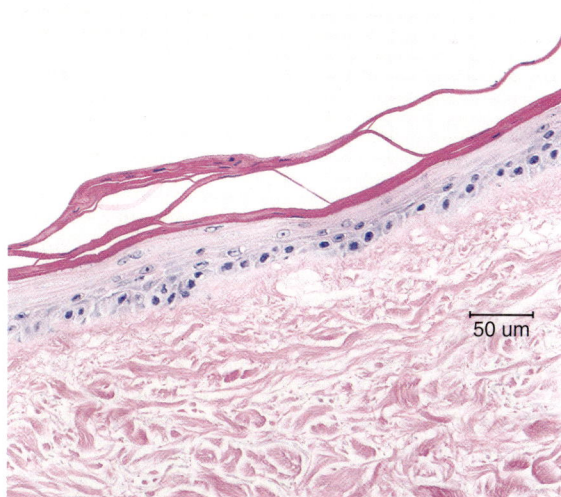

Fig. 9-7 ▪ At culture day 11, the grafts are ready for use with a newly formed stratified epithelial layer with evidence of parakertatinization.

The recipient bed is prepared through conventional surgical procedures such as vestibuloplasty and tumor excision. Hemostasis in the recipient bed is critical for graft success. Additionally, periosteum, if present, must remain intact if at all possible to allow vascular nourishment of the graft (Fig. 9-8). The engineered EVPOME graft is handled with great care and trimmed with a sharp blade to minimize any trauma to the harvested keratinocytes. These grafts are then secured circumferentially and bolstered (pressure dressing)

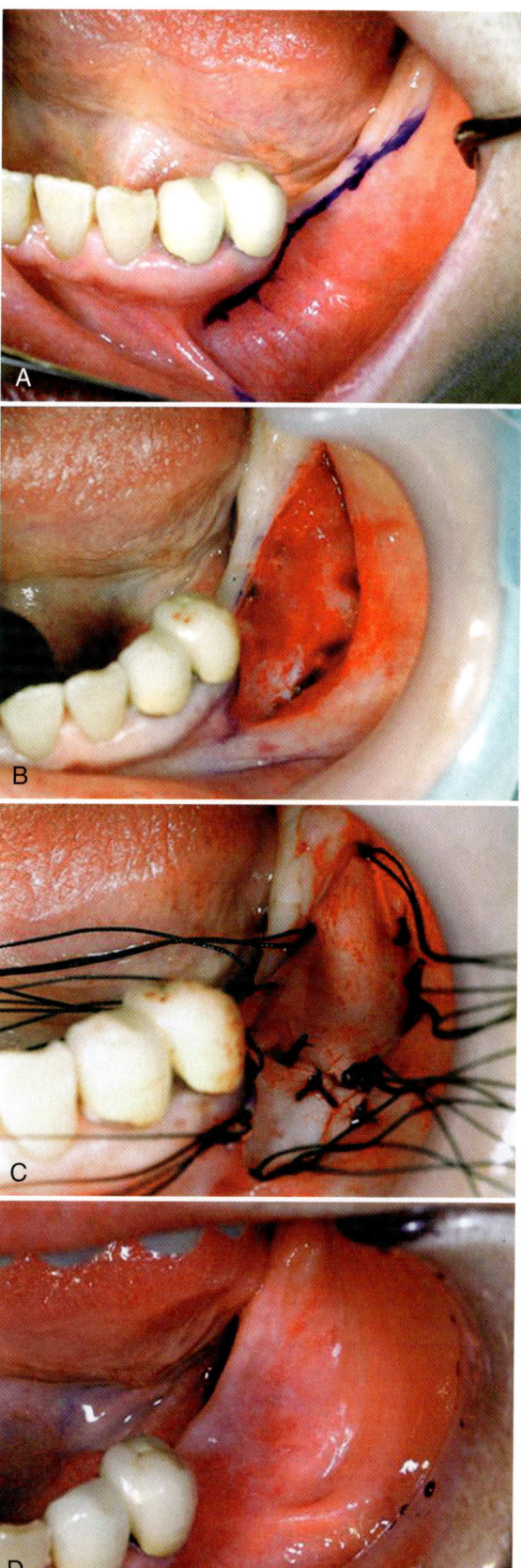

Fig. 9-8 ▪ Maintaining a healthy vascular wound bed (periosteum is maintained when grafting onto bone) is essential for graft success. **A,** Incision through mucosa. **B,** Maintenance of an intact periosteum. **C,** Suturing of the EVPOME in place. **D,** Postgrafting view at 4 weeks.

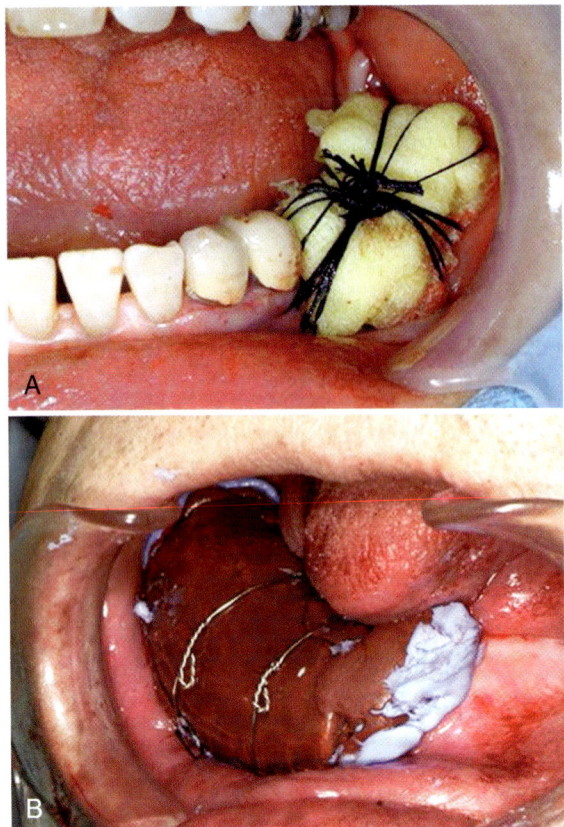

Fig. 9-9 ■ Bolsters (**A**) or stents (**B**) are used to minimize tissue disruption, which would lead to graft failure.

to minimize disruption and hematoma formation underneath the grafts during healing (Fig. 9-9).

Ideally, a number of principles must be adhered to for proper success of a soft tissue EVPOME graft:

- The recipient site must have an intact periosteum or a well-vascularized bed for the graft.
- Vessel inosculation from the underlying capillary network requires stability and immobility of the graft.
- Pressure dressings (bolsters or surgical stents) allow close adaptation to avoid hematoma formation under the graft.

HARD TISSUE RECONSTRUCTION

Osseous and Cartilaginous Tissues

The current gold standards for bone reconstruction include autogenous non-vascularized and vascularized tissues. Selection is dependent on the recipient site and relative size of the defect. Valid options are bone harvested from the calvaria, local regional maxilla and mandible, ribs with or without cartilage (costochondral), iliac crest, radius, fibula, and scapula. Allogeneic (Puros Allograft, Zimmer Dental, Carlsbad, Calif.; Mineross, Biohorizons, Birmingham, Ala.) and xenogeneic (Bio-Oss, Osteohealth, Shirley, New York) bone substitutes are available for smaller defects or as fillers for autogenous tissues. They provide an additional framework for bone regeneration mostly through osteoconduction. The scaffolds themselves work as an osteoconductive framework, but to maximize the potential for cartilage differentiation or osteogenesis, they are combined with a number of osteobiologics. Cells, growth factors, gene vectors, and electromagnetic fields have all been combined with scaffolds to enhance bone and cartilage formation.

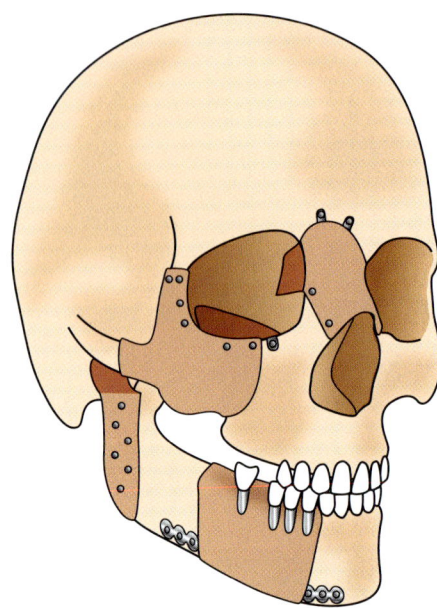

Fig. 9-10 ■ Using rapid prototyped scaffolds, complex three-dimensional shapes can be reconstructed to conform to the intricacies of the facial skeleton.

A number of studies have evaluated membranes (resorbable and non-resorbable, as well as reinforced) for use in guided bone regeneration for isolated tooth defects and larger alveolar defects.[112-114] In essence, a membrane is a type of scaffolding that attempts to allow bone ingrowth and maturation while creating a barrier limiting soft tissue ingrowth. This application is clearly limited to smaller defects but is ever present in the oral surgeon's skill set. More complex scaffolds are being developed with intricate three-dimensional shapes to permit more elaborate esthetic restoration of bone and cartilage. In the past, scaffolds were nonresorbable and used a variety of alloys (including titanium) or polymethylmethacrylate.[115] The current trend is to use a variety of bioabsorbable and biocompatible materials that have been developed for cranio-maxillofacial reconstruction. They focus primarily on regenerating tissues based on the reconstructive goals listed earlier.[116-120] Scaffolds have already been used for the reconstruction of complex three-dimensional geometries to restore form and function and closely mimic the properties of the native tissues (Fig. 9-10). With the use of rapid prototyping technology, scaffolds can be generated that possess reliable strength with a modulus of elasticity favoring either bone or cartilage. Additionally, through a variety of means, biologic agents can be delivered in a consistent manner to offer effective regenerative strategies.[120-123] Some bioresorbable scaffolds are on the market for specific cranial burr hole defects (Osteoplug, Osteopore International, Singapore), and other medical device companies have evolved for scaffold design (Tissue Regeneration Systems, Inc., Ann Arbor, Mich.).

Procedure

Imaging of the region of interest is performed anywhere in the maxillofacial skeleton. Either magnetic resonance imaging or computed tomography (cone beam or conventional multi-slice) can be used to identify the defect preemptively before resection or at the time of reconstruction. The data set is uploaded into a variety of imaging software programs (Analyze, AnalyzeDirect, Inc., Overland Park, Kans; ENVI, ITT Visual Information Solutions, Boulder, Colo.; MIMICS, Materialise, Leuven, Belgium; MATLAB,

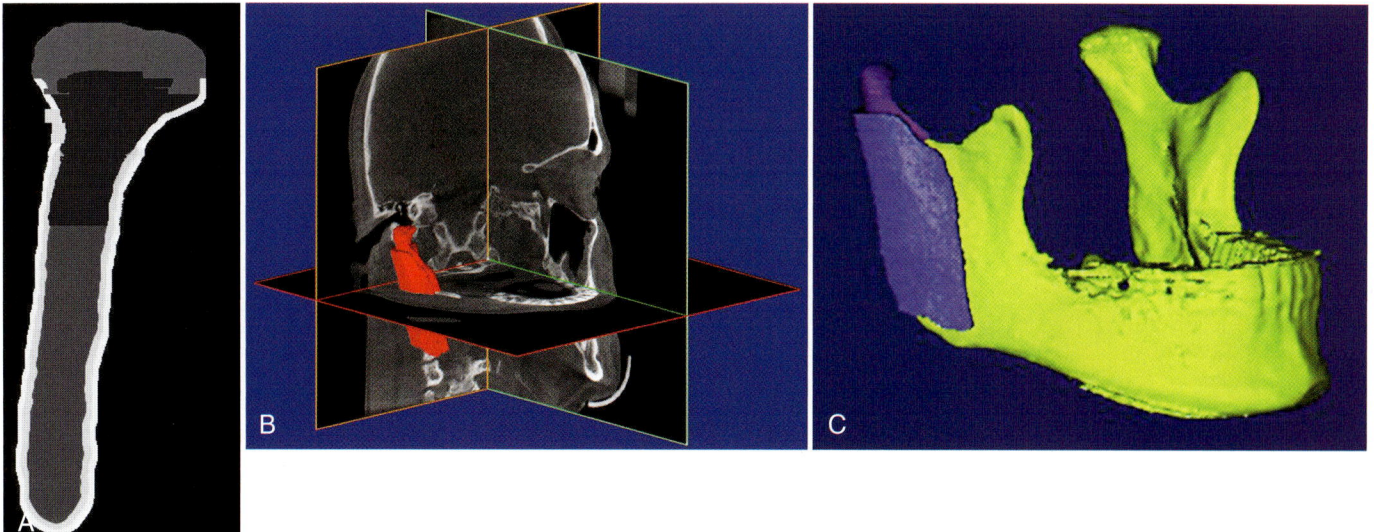

Fig. 9-11 ■ **A,** The area of interest, condylar ramus construct, is mapped and can be constructed by using control objects, mirrored objects, or freehand design. **B** and **C,** Additional areas are identified and the mapping is dilated to allow scaffold fabrication.

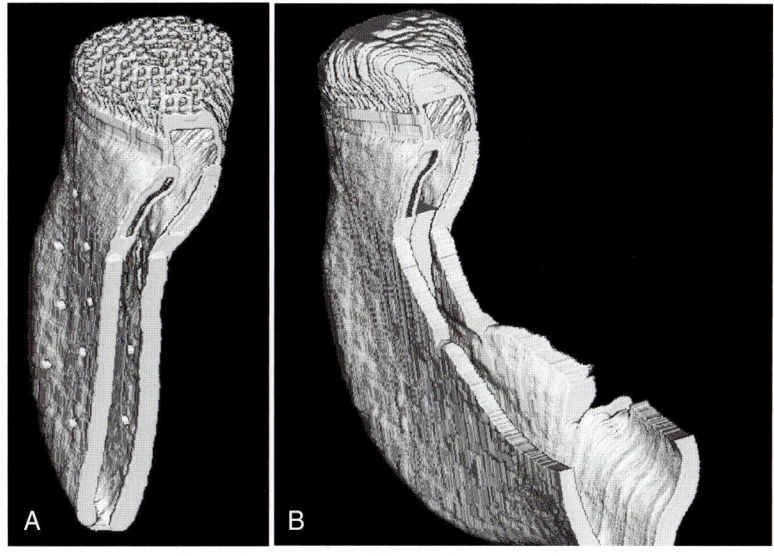

Fig. 9-12 ■ Depending on the area of reconstruction, scaffolds and their sleeves can be customized for reconstruction. **A,** condylar-ramus construct. **B,** Condylar-ramus construct + horizontal ramus of the mandible.

Mathworks, Natick, MA) and is subsequently mapped to develop a macrostructured template (Fig. 9-11). The contralateral normal side can be used for a symmetric mirror image template design, standardized templates can be inserted to reconstruct a defect, or tissues can be computationally designed from scratch. Scaffolds generated from computer-simulated templates can be manufactured and secured to local tissues for stabilization and function[124] (Fig. 9-12). A variety of internal micro-architectures can be applied to the scaffolds to allow variable degrees of porosity and strut structure based on interconnecting spheres or cylinders (Fig. 9-13). One can control the mechanical properties of the scaffold through manipulation of the internal architecture (Fig. 9-14). For example, porosity and tissue ingrowth are inversely proportional to the effective modulus (strength) of the scaffold.[118,120,124-126]

With the scaffold design template, rapid prototyping techniques are used for creation of a layer-by-layer structure.[127] These fabrication methods allow the generation of complex geometric shapes with intricate microstructures and a well-controlled interconnective porous architecture design.[118,125,126] Such techniques include three-dimensional printing, multi-jet modeling, fused deposition modeling, stereolithography, and selective laser sintering.[120,128-130] Other techniques for scaffold fabrication (including salt leaching, solvent casting, membrane lamination, thermal phase separation, and others) have been described but have less reliable external and internal geometries, which can affect the mechanical properties for bone regeneration because of random configuration.[131] However, they can be used for scaffold design in cartilage and soft tissue reconstruction. Selection of the scaffold material is based on the properties desired and the manufacturing methods. Polylactic acid, polyglycolic acid, and polycaprolactone are all FDA-approved materials, and polypropylene fumarate and other polymers are additionally frequently investigated. Each material has a variety of methods for fabrication, with the majority being created via rapid prototyping techniques. The desired tissues to be regenerated will determine the materials needed and the characteristics of the scaffold design. Current research is focusing on temporomandibular joint condylar

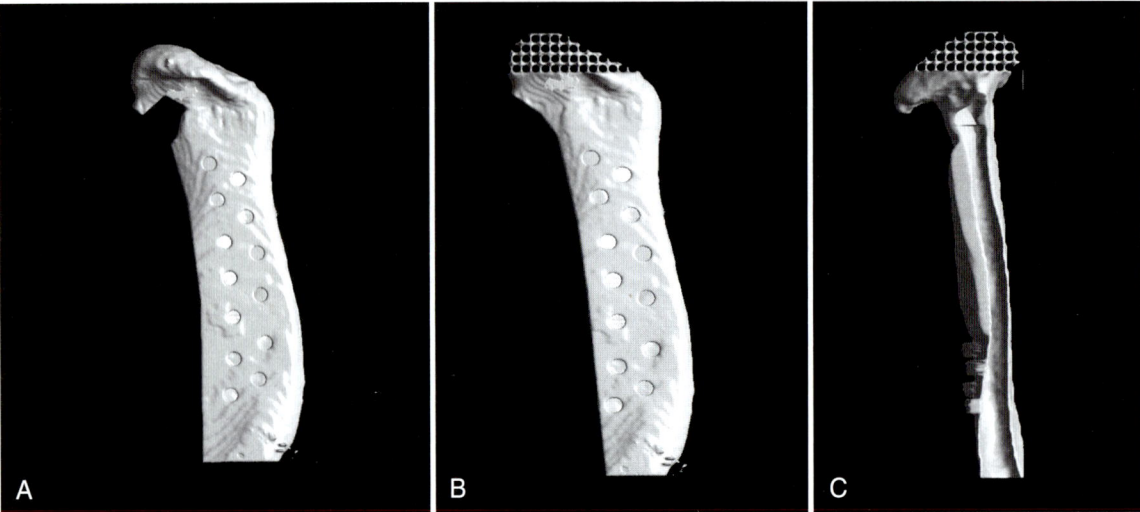

Fig. 9-13 ■ Porous architecture can be applied to the scaffold to meet design requirements to allow decrease in material, ingrowth of cells and vasculature, and to control mechanical strength. Examples of a condylar-ramus construct are shown.

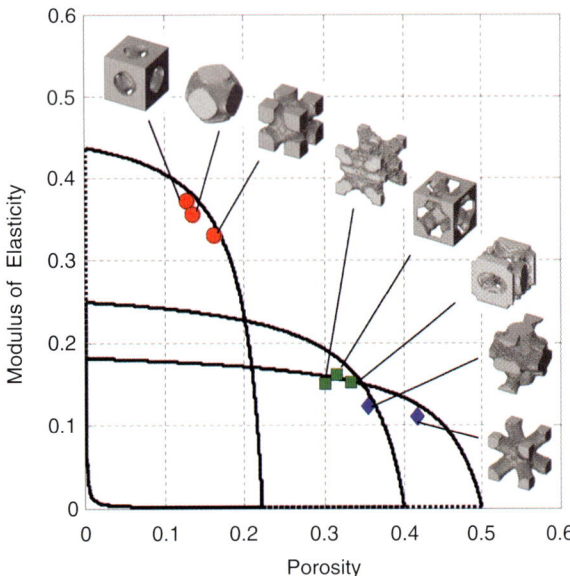

Fig. 9-14 ■ Internal micro-architecture can be manipulated to control porosity and the modulus of elasticity, which are inversely proportional.

reconstruction because the complexity of a functional joint with cartilage and bone requirements can allow similar principles to be manipulated for smaller defects elsewhere in the craniofacial skeleton[123] (Fig. 9-15).

Differentiation of cartilaginous tissues can be achieved by applying dynamic functional loading and strain directly to the scaffolds previously designed. Dynamic compressive forces can increase cartilage formation and improve the properties of the cartilage as a function of the strain applied,[31,132] whereas loss of function can limit cartilage and bone differentiation.[133,134] It is possible to vary the porosity and strut structure at different portions of the scaffold to offer differing moduli of compression along the surface versus internally in the scaffold. This allows cartilaginous tissues to be

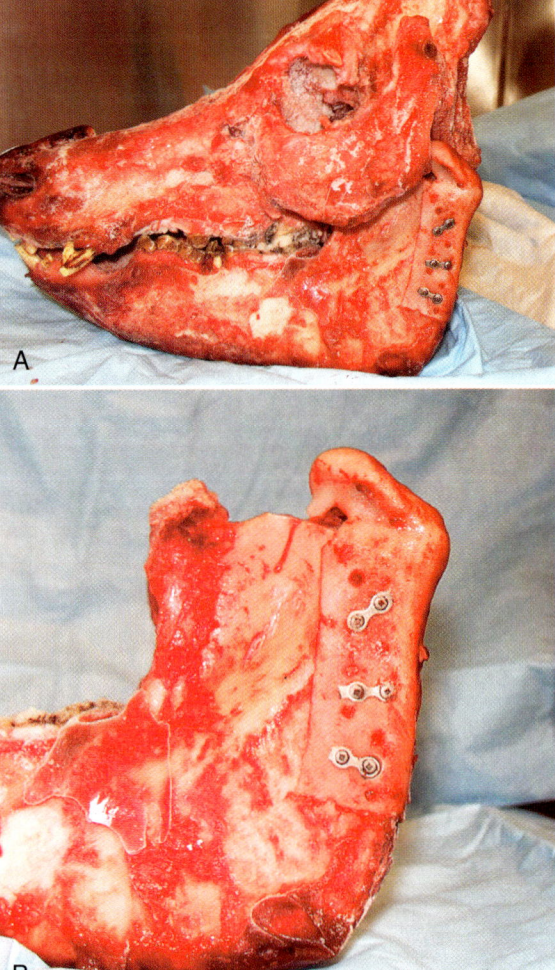

Fig. 9-15 ■ Scaffolds reproduce three-dimensional anatomy and are closely adapted to the native skeleton as is shown with a condylar-ramus construct in a pig mandible. **A,** View of lateral aspect of pig skull. **B,** Close-up of scaffold in place to replace the condylar head.

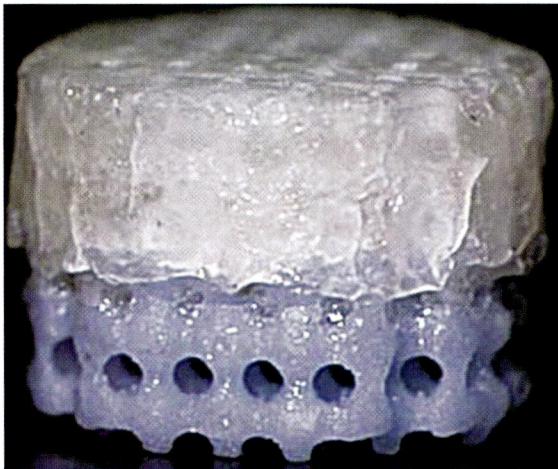

Fig. 9-16 ■ Hydroxyapatite and other osteoconductive materials can be bound to the biodegradable scaffold to confer beneficial properties for bone regeneration and/or cartilage formation.

more favorably produced at the surface while the stiffness internally promotes osseous regeneration.[120,135] Other methods have evaluated combined biphasic scaffolds with prefabricated cartilaginous tissues created for insertion. An interconnective rapid prototyped porous scaffold can be combined with either sponge or hydrogels to offer a more resilient surface coating for cartilage regeneration.[131,136] Temporomandibular joint diskal tissues can additionally be fabricated with these tissue-engineering principles. Further research is necessary to determine the functionality of the implanted disk. Several researchers have applied both scaffold and scaffold-less designs incorporated with cultured chondrocyte cells and growth factors to create a resilient construct with desirable mechanical and biochemical properties.[137-140] The principles of disk regeneration can be transitioned to the creation of ligaments and tendons because of their high collagen and elastin content for composite tissue scaffold design.[141]

Before implantation, a variety of osteoconductive and osteoinductive materials can be used as coatings for the biocompatible, bioresorbable materials. Hydroxyapatite can be coated in a controlled manner onto the underlying polymer. This coating can confer beneficial mechanical properties and increase the stiffness of the scaffold, although porosity must be compromised in this case (Fig. 9-16). Growth factors can then be soaked onto the scaffold framework or covalently bonded to allow more reliable diffusion characteristics. Cells can be seeded into the scaffold as well or may be combined with hydrogels to secure them to the scaffold. The possibilities for scaffold design are endless, and further research will determine a more precise combination of bioabsorbable polymers, growth factors, and autologous cells for site-specific regeneration.

COMPOSITE TISSUE RECONSTRUCTION

Prefabricated Vascularized Flaps

There is a constant need to offer improved reconstructive options with less patient morbidity. Tissue-engineered prefabricated flaps show great promise in offering vascularized composite tissue constructs as alternatives to conventional flaps. Sites can be prepared to provide additional sources of bone and cartilage through the use of cells and growth factors. Patients act as their own bioreactors, and the manufactured tissues can then be harvested for microvascular reconstruction of ablative and traumatic defects.[142-147] Studies are

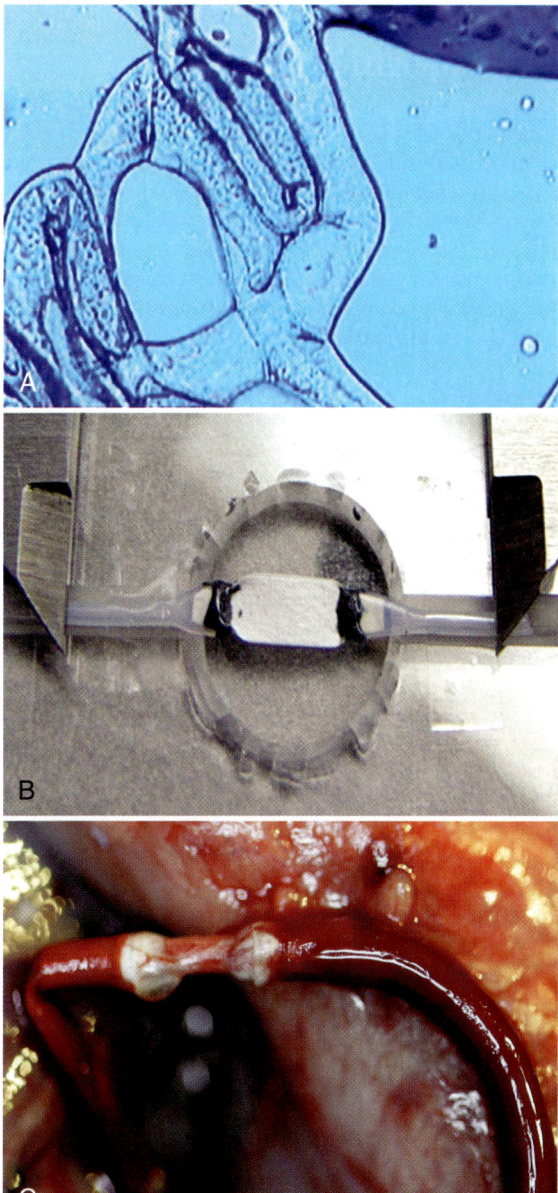

Fig. 9-17 ■ **A,** A microcapillary network manufactured from electrospinning can be constructed in vitro to allow diffusion of nutrients to an underlying composite scaffold. **B,** Microcapillary device prior to placement in vivo. **C,** Attached inflow and outflow vessels can be sutured to native donor vessels; an A-V fistula has been created between the femoral artery and vein in a rat model. One can see perfusion through the fabricated microcapillary network.

presently being conducted at the University of Michigan to develop composite mucocutaneous grafts that would be used for reconstruction of the lips (personal communication, Feinberg, 2010). This involves simultaneous culturing of oral and epidermal skin keratinocytes over the same dermal equivalent. The composite mucocutaneous construct would then be grafted onto a muscular bed in situ so that it can develop its own vascular supply per the technique of Warnke and Terhyeden discussed previously.[143] A major challenge is developing a functional mucocutaneous construct with innervation and function of the muscular core. The current limitations of prefabricated flaps involve donor site morbidity and the need for flap maturation. Primary reconstruction is therefore not an option.

More recently, research is focusing on creating a neocapillary network to use as a framework for creation of an *in vitro* constructed microvascularized flap[148-152] (Fig. 9-17). A soft tissue, hard tissue, or combined scaffold would then be combined with biologics and matured in a laboratory bioreactor. A preshaped composite myo-osseocutaneous microvascular flap could theoretically be custom-manufactured and created beforehand to be used for primary tissue reconstruction and regeneration. Future developments are necessary to evolve the various components and combine them *in vitro* to offer the maxillofacial surgeon unsurpassed alternatives.[153-156]

FUTURE DIRECTIONS

Further research is essential to bring any product to clinical use, and we are only at the beginning of understanding the complex cellular relationships promoting regeneration and modulating scarring. Every individual presents a unique quandary in that host tissues may be affected by a variety of systemic conditions that limit healing capacity. Diabetes, vascular compromise, tobacco use, radiation therapy, and immunologic and infectious conditions all pose difficulties in tissue healing.[77,157-160]

PEARLS AND PITFALLS

- For maxillofacial surgery to advance as a specialty, further research efforts are essential to provide reconstructive options to our patients.
- A primary goal is tissue regeneration to restore a patient to a pre-injury state.
- Adherence to soft tissue and hard tissue goals is important during the design of a regenerative scaffold.
- Innumerable options for combining biologics are available to the reconstructive surgeon; however, the interactions at a cellular level are variable and based on site, concentration, timing of release, and role of inflammatory mediators. Further research and trials are needed to optimize their combined use in therapy.
- Although many options are currently available to the maxillofacial surgeon for specific clinical use, off-label use must be restricted or patients may be at risk for side effects and worsened outcomes.
- Understanding the native tissue requirements is essential for developing both soft and hard tissue constructs.
- Prefabricated microvascular flaps have recently been used for human applications, and future developments can create unparalleled opportunities.
- Modulation of the host environment will allow more reliable outcomes in difficult-to-manage patients.

REFERENCES

1. Dang C, Ting K, Soo C, et al: Fetal wound healing current perspectives, *Clin Plast Surg* 30:13-23, 2003.
2. Mountziaris PM, Mikos AG: Modulation of the inflammatory response for enhanced bone tissue regeneration, *Tissue Eng Part B Rev* 14:179-186, 2008.
3. Ding Y, Li G, Zhang X, et al: Effect of low-intensity pulsed ultrasound on bone formation during mandible distraction osteogenesis in a canine model—a preliminary study, *J Oral Maxillofac Surg* 67:2431-9243, 2009.
4. Busse JW, Bhandari M, Lulkarni AV, et al: The effect of low-intensity pulsed ultrasound therapy on time to fracture healing: a meta-analysis, *CMAJ* 166:437-441, 2002.
5. Busse JW, Kaur J, Mollon B, et al: Low intensity pulsed ultrasonography for fractures: systematic review of randomised controlled trials, *BMJ* 338:b351, 2009.
6. Wilson DH, Jagadeesh P, Newmann PP, et al: The effects of pulsed electromagnetic energy on peripheral nerve regeneration, *Ann N Y Acad Sci* 238:575-585, 1974.
7. Wilson DH, Jagadeesh P: Experimental regeneration in peripheral nerves and the spinal cord in laboratory animals exposed to a pulsed electromagnetic field, *Paraplegia* 14:12-20, 1976.
8. Byers JM, Clark KF, Thompson GC: Effect of pulsed electromagnetic stimulation on facial nerve regeneration, *Arch Otolaryngol Head Neck Surg* 124:383-389, 1998.
9. Aaron RK, Boyan BD, Ciombor DM, et al: Stimulation of growth factor synthesis by electric and electromagnetic fields, *Clin Orthop Relat Res* 419:30-37, 2004.
10. Ciombor DM, Aaron RK: The role of electrical stimulation in bone repair, *Foot Ankle Clin* 10:579-593, vii, 2005.
11. Levin M: Large-scale biophysics: ion flows and regeneration, *Trends Cell Biol* 17:261-270, 2007.
12. Yamada M, Tanemura K, Okada S, et al: Electrical stimulation modulates fate determination of differentiating embryonic stem cells, *Stem Cells* 25:562-570, 2007.
13. Sundelacruz S, Levin M, Kaplan DL: Membrane potential controls adipogenic and osteogenic differentiation of mesenchymal stem cells, *PLoS One* 3:e3737, 2008.
14. Epstein AJ: Electrically conducting polymers: science and technology, *Mater Res Soc Bull* 22:16-23, 1997.
15. Kitzmiller J, Beversdorf D, Hansford D: Fabrication and testing of microelectrodes for small-field cortical surface recordings, *Biomed Microdevices* 8:81-85, 2006.
16. Stucki-McCormick SU: Reconstruction of the mandibular condyle using transport distraction osteogenesis, *J Craniofac Surg* 8:48-52, discussion 53, 1997.
17. Stucki-McCormick SU, Winick R, Winick A: Distraction osteogenesis for the reconstruction of the temporomandibular joint, *N Y State Dent J* 64:36-41, 1998.
18. Drew SJ, Schwartz MH, Sachs SA: Distraction osteogenesis, *N Y State Dent J* 65:26-29, 1999.
19. Stucki-McCormick SU, Fox RM, Mizrahi RD: Reconstruction of a neocondyle using transport distraction osteogenesis, *Semin Orthod* 5:59-63, 1999.
20. Stucki-McCormick SU, Mizrahi RD, Fox RM, et al: Distraction osteogenesis of the mandible using a submerged intraoral device: a report of three cases, *J Oral Maxillofac Surg* 57:192-198, 1999.
21. Hikiji H, Takato T, Matsumoto S, et al: Experimental study of reconstruction of the temporomandibular joint using a bone transport technique, *J Oral Maxillofac Surg* 58:1270-1276; discussion 1277, 2000.
22. Li J, Ying B, Hu J, et al: Reconstruction of mandibular symphyseal defects by trifocal distraction osteogenesis: an experimental study in Rhesus, *Int J Oral Maxillofac Surg* 35:159-164, 2006.
23. Zhu S, Hu J, Li J, et al: Reconstruction of mandibular condyle by transport distraction osteogenesis: experimental study in rhesus monkey, *J Oral Maxillofac Surg* 64:1487-1492, 2006.
24. Cheung LK, Lo J: The long-term effect of transport distraction in the management of temporomandibular joint ankylosis, *Plast Reconstr Surg* 119:1003-1009, 2007.
25. Schwartz HC, Relle RJ: Distraction osteogenesis for temporomandibular joint reconstruction, *J Oral Maxillofac Surg* 66:718-723, 2008.
26. Zhu SS, Hu J, Ying BB, et al: Growth of the mandible after condylar reconstruction using transport distraction osteogenesis: an experimental investigation in goats, *Plast Reconstr Surg* 121:1760-1767, 2008.
27. Cheung LK, Zheng LW, Ma L, et al: Transport distraction versus costochondral graft for reconstruction of temporomandibular joint ankylosis: which is better? *Oral Surg Oral Med Oral Pathol Oral Radiol Endod* 108:32-40, 2009.

28. Schwartz HC: Transport distraction osteogenesis for reconstruction of the ramus-condyle unit of the temporomandibular joint: surgical technique, *J Oral Maxillofac Surg* 67:2197-2200, 2009.

29. Baumgart R, Hinterwimmer S, Krammer M, et al: The bioexpandable prosthesis: a new perspective after resection of malignant bone tumors in children, *J Pediatr Hematol Oncol* 27:452-455, 2005.

30. Mao JJ, Giannobile WV, Helms JA, et al: Craniofacial tissue engineering by stem cells, *J Dent Res* 85:966-979, 2006.

31. Chung C, Burdick JA: Engineering cartilage tissue, *Adv Drug Deliv Rev* 60:243-262, 2008.

32. Ogawa R, Mizuno S: Cartilage regeneration using adipose-derived stem cells, *Curr Stem Cell Res Ther* 5:129-132, 2010.

33. Kanczler JM, Mirmalek-Sani SH, Hanley NA, et al: Biocompatibility and osteogenic potential of human fetal femur–derived cells on surface selective laser sintered scaffolds, *Acta Biomater* 5:2063-2071, 2009.

34. Guo X, Park H, Young S, et al: Repair of osteochondral defects with biodegradable hydrogel composites encapsulating marrow mesenchymal stem cells in a rabbit model, *Acta Biomater* 6:39-47, 2010.

35. Chen F, Mao T, Tao K, et al: Bone graft in the shape of human mandibular condyle reconstruction via seeding marrow-derived osteoblasts into porous coral in a nude mice model, *J Oral Maxillofac Surg* 60:1155-1159, 2002.

36. Abukawa H, Shin M, Williams WB, et al: Reconstruction of mandibular defects with autologous tissue–engineered bone, *J Oral Maxillofac Surg* 62:601-606, 2004.

37. Alhadlaq A, Mao JJ: Mesenchymal stem cells: isolation and therapeutics, *Stem Cells Dev* 13:436-448, 2004.

38. Alhadlaq A, Mao JJ: Tissue-engineered osteochondral constructs in the shape of an articular condyle, *J Bone Joint Surg Am* 87:936-944, 2005.

39. Knippenberg M, Helder MN, Zandieh Doulabi B, et al: Osteogenesis versus chondrogenesis by BMP-2 and BMP-7 in adipose stem cells, *Biochem Biophys Res Commun* 342:902-908, 2006.

40. Shao XX, Hutmacher DW, Ho ST, et al: Evaluation of a hybrid scaffold/cell construct in repair of high-load-bearing osteochondral defects in rabbits, *Biomaterials* 27:1071-1080, 2006.

41. Ando W, Tateishi K, Hart DA, et al: Cartilage repair using an in vitro generated scaffold-free tissue-engineered construct derived from porcine synovial mesenchymal stem cells, *Biomaterials* 28:5462-5470, 2007.

42. Bailey MM, Wang L, Bode CJ, et al: A comparison of human umbilical cord matrix stem cells and temporomandibular joint condylar chondrocytes for tissue engineering temporomandibular joint condylar cartilage, *Tissue Eng* 13:2003-2010, 2007.

43. Nicodemus GD, Villanueva I, Bryant SJ: Mechanical stimulation of TMJ condylar chondrocytes encapsulated in PEG hydrogels, *J Biomed Mater Res A* 83:323-331, 2007.

44. Grayson WL, Chao PH, Marolt D, et al: Engineering custom-designed osteochondral tissue grafts, *Trends Biotechnol* 26:181-189, 2008.

45. Jafarian M, Eslaminejad MB, Khojasteh A, et al: Marrow-derived mesenchymal stem cells–directed bone regeneration in the dog mandible: a comparison between biphasic calcium phosphate and natural bone mineral, *Oral Surg Oral Med Oral Pathol Oral Radiol Endod* 105:e14-e24, 2008.

46. Chum ZZ, Woodruff MA, Cool SM, et al: Porcine bone marrow stromal cell differentiation on heparin-adsorbed poly(ε-caprolactone)–tricalcium phosphate–collagen scaffolds, *Acta Biomater* 5:3305-3315, 2009.

47. Aghaloo T, Cowan CM, Zhang X, et al: The effect of NELL1 and bone morphogenetic protein-2 on calvarial bone regeneration, *J Oral Maxillofac Surg* 68:300-308, 2010.

48. An C, Cheng Y, Yuan Q, et al: IGF-1 and BMP-2 induces differentiation of adipose-derived mesenchymal stem cells into chondrocytes-like cells, *Ann Biomed Eng* 38:1647-1654, 2010.

49. Beck LS, Amento EP, Xu Y, et al: TGF-beta 1 induces bone closure of skull defects: temporal dynamics of bone formation in defects exposed to rhTGF-beta 1, *J Bone Miner Res* 8:753-761, 1993.

50. Bessho K, Carnes DL, Cavin E, et al: BMP stimulation of bone response adjacent to titanium implants in vivo, *Clin Oral Implants Res* 10:212-218, 1999.

51. Vehof JW, Fisher JP, Dean D, et al: Bone formation in transforming growth factor beta-1–coated porous poly(propylene fumarate) scaffolds, *J Biomed Mater Res* 60:241-251, 2002.

52. Peel SA, Hu ZM, Clokie CM: In search of the ideal bone morphogenetic protein delivery system: in vitro studies on demineralized bone matrix, purified, and recombinant bone morphogenetic protein, *J Craniofac Surg* 14:284-291, 2003.

53. Hu ZM, Peel SA, Sandor GK, et al: The osteoinductive activity of bone morphogenetic protein (BMP) purified by repeated extracts of bovine bone, *Growth Factors* 22:29-33, 2004.

54. Nevins M, Giannobile WV, McGuire MK, et al: Platelet-derived growth factor stimulates bone fill and rate of attachment level gain: results of a large multicenter randomized controlled trial, *J Periodontol* 76:2205-2215, 2005.

55. McKay WF, Peckham SM, Badura JM: A comprehensive clinical review of recombinant human bone morphogenetic protein-2 (INFUSE Bone Graft), *Int Orthop* 31:729-734, 2007.

56. Rabie AB, Dai J, Xu R: Recombinant AAV-mediated VEGF gene therapy induces mandibular condylar growth, *Gene Ther* 14:972-980, 2007.

57. Zhou AJ, Peel SA, Clokie CM: An evaluation of hydroxyapatite and biphasic calcium phosphate in combination with Pluronic F127 and BMP on bone repair, *J Craniofac Surg* 18:1264-1275, 2007.

58. Clokie CM, Sandor GK: Reconstruction of 10 major mandibular defects using bioimplants containing BMP-7, *J Can Dent Assoc* 74:67-72, 2008.

59. Elsalanty ME, Por YC, Genecov DG, et al: Recombinant human BMP-2 enhances the effects of materials used for reconstruction of large cranial defects, *J Oral Maxillofac Surg* 66:277-285, 2008.

60. Lin Y, Tang W, Wu L, et al: Bone regeneration by BMP-2 enhanced adipose stem cells loading on alginate gel, *Histochem Cell Biol* 129:203-210, 2008.

61. Schopper C, Moser D, Spassova E, et al: Bone regeneration using a naturally grown HA/TCP carrier loaded with rh BMP-2 is independent of barrier-membrane effects, *J Biomed Mater Res A* 85:954-963, 2008.

62. Springer IN, Niehoff P, Açil Y, et al: BMP-2 and bFGF in an irradiated bone model, *J Craniomaxillofac Surg* 36:210-217, 2008.

63. Hu ZM, Peel SA, Ho SK, et al: Comparison of platelet-rich plasma, bovine BMP, and rhBMP-4 on bone matrix protein expression in vitro, *Growth Factors* 27:280-288, 2009.

64. Boyne PJ, Lilly LC, Marx RE, et al: De novo bone induction by recombinant human bone morphogenetic protein-2 (rhBMP-2) in maxillary sinus floor augmentation, *J Oral Maxillofac Surg* 63:1693-1707, 2005.

65. Springer IN, Açil Y, Kuchenbecker S, et al: Bone graft versus BMP-7 in a critical size defect—cranioplasty in a growing infant model, *Bone* 37:563-569, 2005.

66. Herford AS, Boyne PJ, Rawson E, et al: Bone morphogenetic protein–induced repair of the premaxillary cleft, *J Oral Maxillofac Surg* 65:2136-2141, 2007.

67. Herford AS, Boyne PJ: Reconstruction of mandibular continuity defects with bone morphogenetic protein-2 (rhBMP-2), *J Oral Maxillofac Surg* 66:616-624, 2008.

68. Chang PC, Seol YJ, Cirelli JA, et al: PDGF-B gene therapy accelerates bone engineering and oral implant osseointegration, *Gene Ther* 17:95-104, 2009.

69. Giannobile WV, Lee CS, Tomala MP, et al: Platelet-derived growth factor (PDGF) gene delivery for application in periodontal tissue engineering, *J Periodontol* 72:815-823, 2001.

70. Jin Q, Anusaksathien O, Webb SA, et al: Engineering of tooth-supporting structures by delivery of PDGF gene therapy vectors, *Mol Ther* 9:519-526, 2004.

71. Cooke JW, Sarment DP, Whitesman LA, et al: Effect of rhPDGF-BB delivery on mediators of periodontal wound repair, *Tissue Eng* 12:1441-1450, 2006.

72. Sarment DP, Cooke JW, Miller SE, et al: Effect of rhPDGF-BB on bone turnover during periodontal repair, *J Clin Periodontol* 33:135-140, 2006.

73. Jin Q, Wei G, Lin Z, et al: Nanofibrous scaffolds incorporating PDGF-BB microspheres induce chemokine expression and tissue neogenesis in vivo, *PLoS One* 3:e1729, 2008.

74. Lin Z, Sugai JV, Jin Q, et al: Platelet-derived growth factor-B gene delivery sustains gingival fibroblast signal transduction, *J Periodontal Res* 43:440-449, 2008.

75. Chang PC, Cirelli JA, Jin Q, et al: Adenovirus encoding human platelet-derived growth factor-B delivered to alveolar bone defects exhibits safety and biodistribution profiles favorable for clinical use, *Hum Gene Ther* 20:486-496, 2009.

76. Martin P: Wound healing—aiming for perfect skin regeneration, *Science* 276:75-81, 1997.

77. Adler SC, Kent KJ: Enhancing wound healing with growth factors, *Facial Plast Surg Clin North Am* 10:129-146, 2002.

78. Robson MC: Cytokine manipulation of the wound, *Clin Plast Surg* 30:57-65, 2003.

79. Flock ST, Marchitto KS: Progress towards seamless tissue fusion for wound closure, *Otolaryngol Clin North Am* 38:295-305, 2005.

80. Li QF, Rabie AB: A new approach to control condylar growth by regulating angiogenesis, *Arch Oral Biol* 52:1009-1017, 2007.

81. Rabie AB, Hagg U: Factors regulating mandibular condylar growth, *Am J Orthod Dentofacial Orthop* 122:401-409, 2002.

82. Dai J, Rabie AB: VEGF: an essential mediator of both angiogenesis and endochondral ossification, *J Dent Res* 86:937-950, 2007.

83. Dai J, Rabie AB: Gene therapy to enhance condylar growth using rAAV-VEGF, *Angle Orthod* 78:89-94, 2008.

84. Wang L, Detamore MS: Effects of growth factors and glucosamine on porcine mandibular condylar cartilage cells and hyaline cartilage cells for tissue engineering applications, *Arch Oral Biol* 54:1-5, 2009.

85. Cho TJ, Gerstenfeld LC, Einhorn TA: Differential temporal expression of members of the transforming growth factor beta superfamily during murine fracture healing, *J Bone Miner Res* 17:513-520, 2002.

86. Giannobile WV, Whitson SW, Lynch SE: Non-coordinate control of bone formation displayed by growth factor combinations with IGF-I, *J Dent Res* 76:1569-1578, 1997.

87. Howell TH, Fiorellini JP, Paquette DW, et al: A phase I/II clinical trial to evaluate a combination of recombinant human platelet-derived growth factor-BB and recombinant human insulin-like growth factor-I in patients with periodontal disease, *J Periodontol* 68:1186-1193, 1997.

88. Rasubala L, Yoshikawa H, Nagata K, et al: Platelet-derived growth factor and bone morphogenetic protein in the healing of mandibular fractures in rats, *Br J Oral Maxillofac Surg* 41:173-178, 2003.

89. Alam S, Ueki K, Marukawa K, et al: Expression of bone morphogenetic protein 2 and fibroblast growth factor 2 during bone regeneration using different implant materials as an onlay bone graft in rabbit mandibles, *Oral Surg Oral Med Oral Pathol Oral Radiol Endod* 103:16-26, 2007.

90. Young S, Patel ZS, Kretlow JD, et al: Dose effect of dual delivery of vascular endothelial growth factor and bone morphogenetic protein-2 on bone regeneration in a rat critical-size defect model, *Tissue Eng Part A* 15:2347-2362, 2009.

91. Zhao J, Hu J, Wang S, et al: Combination of beta-TCP and BMP-2 gene–modified bMSCs to heal critical size mandibular defects in rats, *Oral Dis* 16:46-54, 2010.

92. Zhu Z, Lee CS, Tejeda KM, et al: Gene transfer and expression of platelet-derived growth factors modulate periodontal cellular activity, *J Dent Res* 80:892-897, 2001.

93. Chen QP, Giannobile WV: Adenoviral gene transfer of PDGF downregulates gas gene product PDGFalphaR and prolongs ERK and Akt/PKB activation, *Am J Physiol Cell Physiol* 282:C538-C544, 2002.

94. Chang SC, Chuang HL, Chen YR, et al: Ex vivo gene therapy in autologous bone marrow stromal stem cells for tissue-engineered maxillofacial bone regeneration, *Gene Ther* 10:2013-2019, 2003.

95. Anusaksathien O, Jin Q, Zhao M, et al: Effect of sustained gene delivery of platelet-derived growth factor or its antagonist (PDGF-1308) on tissue-engineered cementum, *J Periodontol* 75:429-440, 2004.

96. Schek RM, Hollister SJ, Krebsbach PH: Delivery and protection of adenoviruses using biocompatible hydrogels for localized gene therapy, *Mol Ther* 9:130-138, 2004.

97. Lin CY, Schek RM, Mistry AS, et al: Functional bone engineering using ex vivo gene therapy and topology-optimized, biodegradable polymer composite scaffolds, *Tissue Eng* 11:1589-1598, 2005.

98. Hu WW, Wang Z, Hollister SJ, et al: Localized viral vector delivery to enhance in situ regenerative gene therapy, *Gene Ther* 14:891-901, 2007.

99. Hu WW, Elkasabi Y, Chen HY, et al: The use of reactive polymer coatings to facilitate gene delivery from poly (epsilon-caprolactone) scaffolds, *Biomaterials* 30:5785-5792, 2009.

100. Bannasch H, Fohn M, Unterberg T, et al: Skin tissue engineering, *Clin Plast Surg* 30:573-579, 2003.

101. Bannasch H, Momeni A, Knam F, et al: Tissue engineering of skin substitutes, *Panminerva Med* 47:53-60, 2005.

102. Fohn M, Bannasch H: Artificial skin, *Methods Mol Med* 140:167-182, 2007.

103. Sullivan SA, Dailey RA: Graft contraction: a comparison of acellular dermis versus hard palate mucosa in lower eyelid surgery, *Ophthal Plast Reconstr Surg* 19:14-24, 2003.

104. Bessho K, Murakami K, Iizuka T: The use of a new bilayer artificial dermis for vestibular extension, *Br J Oral Maxillofac Surg* 36:457-459, 1998.

105. Izumi K, Feinberg SE, Iida A, et al: Intraoral grafting of an ex vivo produced oral mucosa equivalent: a preliminary report, *Int J Oral Maxillofac Surg* 32:188-197, 2003.

106. Fraulin FO, Bahoric A, Harrop AR, et al: Autotransplantation of epithelial cells in the pig via an aerosol vehicle, *J Burn Care Rehabil* 19:337-345, 1998.

107. Currie LJ, Martin R, Sharpe JR, et al: A comparison of keratinocyte cell sprays with and without fibrin glue, *Burns* 29:677-685, 2003.

108. Wood FM, Kolybaba ML, Allen P: The use of cultured epithelial autograft in the treatment of major burn wounds: eleven years of clinical experience, *Burns* 32:538-544, 2006.

109. Izumi K, Takacs G, Terashi H, et al: Ex vivo development of a composite human oral mucosal equivalent, *J Oral Maxillofac Surg* 57:571-577, discussion 577-578, 1999.

110. Izumi K, Terashi H, Marcello CL, et al: Development and characterization of a tissue-engineered human oral mucosa equivalent produced in a serum-free culture system, *J Dent Res* 79:798-805, 2000.

111. Izumi K, Song J, Feinberg SE: Development of a tissue-engineered human oral mucosa: from the bench to the bed side, *Cells Tissues Organs* 176:134-152, 2004.

112. Needleman IG, Worthington HV, Giedrys-Leeper E, et al: Guided tissue regeneration for periodontal infra-bony defects, *Cochrane Database Syst Rev* 2:CD001724, 2006.

113. Nickles K, Ratka-Kruger P, Neukranz E, et al: Open flap debridement and guided tissue regeneration after 10 years in infrabony defects, *J Clin Periodontol* 36:976-983, 2009.

114. Parrish LC, Miyamoto T, Fong M, et al: Non-bioabsorbable vs. bioabsorbable membrane: assessment of their clinical efficacy in guided tissue regeneration technique. A systematic review, *J Oral Sci* 51:383-400, 2009.

115. Bonassar LJ, Vacanti CA: Tissue engineering: the first decade and beyond, *J Cell Biochem Suppl* 30-31:297-303, 1998.

116. Hollister SJ, Lin CY, Lin CY, et al: Design and fabrication of scaffolds for anatomic bone reconstruction, *Med J Malaysia* 59(Suppl B):131-132, 2004.

117. Hutmacher DW, Sittinger M, Risbud MV: Scaffold-based tissue engineering: rationale for computer-aided design and solid free-form fabrication systems, *Trends Biotechnol* 22:354-362, 2004.

118. Fang Z, Starly B, Sun W: Computer-aided characterization for effective mechanical properties of porous tissue scaffolds, *Comput Aided Design* 37:65-72, 2005.

119. Hollister SJ: Porous scaffold design for tissue engineering, *Nat Mater* 4:518-524, 2005.

120. Hollister SJ, Lin CY, Saito E, et al: Engineering craniofacial scaffolds, *Orthod Craniofac Res* 8:162-173, 2005.

121. Rohner D, Hutmacher DW, Cheng TK, et al: In vivo efficacy of bone-marrow–coated polycaprolactone scaffolds for the reconstruction of orbital defects in the pig,

J Biomed Mater Res B Appl Biomater 66: 574-580, 2003.

122. Herring SW, Ochareon P: Bone—special problems of the craniofacial region, *Orthod Craniofac Res* 8:174-182, 2005.

123. Smith MH, Flanagan CL, Kempppainen JM, et al: Computed tomography–based tissue-engineered scaffolds in craniomaxillofacial surgery, *Int J Med Robot* 3:207-216, 2007.

124. Hollister SJ, Levy RA, Chu TM, et al: An image-based approach for designing and manufacturing craniofacial scaffolds, *Int J Oral Maxillofac Surg* 29:67-71, 2000.

125. Lin CY, Kikuchi N, Hollister SJ: A novel method for biomaterial scaffold internal architecture design to match bone elastic properties with desired porosity, *J Biomech* 37:623-636, 2004.

126. Wettergreen MA, Bucklen BS, Sun W, et al: Creation of a unit block library of architectures for use in assembled scaffold engineering, *Comput Aided Design* 37:1141-1149, 2005.

127. Christensen AM: Tactile surgical planning using patient-specific anatomic models. In Bell WH, Guerrero CA, editors: *Distraction osteogenesis of the facial skeleton*, Hamilton, Ontario, 2007, BC Decker.

128. Zein I, Hutmacher DW, Tan KC, et al: Fused deposition modeling of novel scaffold architectures for tissue engineering applications, *Biomaterials* 23:1169-1185, 2002.

129. Williams JM, Adewunmi A, Schek RM, et al: Bone tissue engineering using polycaprolactone scaffolds fabricated via selective laser sintering, *Biomaterials* 26:4817-4827, 2005.

130. Partee B, Hollister SJ, Das S: Selective laser sintering process optimization for layered manufacturing of CAPA(R) 6501 polycaprolactone bone tissue engineering scaffolds, *J Manufacturing Sci Eng* 128:531-540, 2006.

131. Taboas JM, Maddox RD, Krebsbach PH, et al: Indirect solid free form fabrication of local and global porous, biomimetic and composite 3D polymer-ceramic scaffolds, *Biomaterials* 24:181-194, 2003.

132. Sundaramurthy S, Mao JJ: Modulation of endochondral development of the distal femoral condyle by mechanical loading, *J Orthop Res* 24:229-241, 2006.

133. Kajikawa A, Hirabayashi S, Harii K: An experimental study on the growth of condylar cartilage, using a new vascularized mandible heterotopic transplant model, *J Oral Maxillofac Surg* 61:239-245, 2003.

134. Kajikawa A, Hirabayashi S, Harii K: A new vascularized mandible heterotopic transplant model for studies on the growth of condylar cartilage, *J Oral Maxillofac Surg* 61:234-238, 2003.

135. Hollister SJ, Maddox RD, Taboas JM: Optimal design and fabrication of scaffolds to mimic tissue properties and satisfy biological constraints, *Biomaterials* 23:4095-4103, 2002.

136. Schek RM, Taboas JM, Hollister SJ, et al: Tissue engineering osteochondral implants for temporomandibular joint repair, *Orthod Craniofac Res* 8:313-319, 2005.

137. Detamore MS, Athanasiou KA: Effects of growth factors on temporomandibular joint disc cells, *Arch Oral Biol* 49:577-583, 2004.

138. Detamore MS, Athanasiou KA: Evaluation of three growth factors for TMJ disc tissue engineering, *Ann Biomed Eng* 33:383-390, 2005.

139. Johns DE, Athanasiou KA: Growth factor effects on costal chondrocytes for tissue engineering fibrocartilage, *Cell Tissue Res* 333:439-447, 2008.

140. Johns DE, Wong ME, Athanasiou KA: Clinically relevant cell sources for TMJ disc engineering, *J Dent Res* 87:548-552, 2008.

141. Johns DE, Athanasiou KA: Design characteristics for temporomandibular joint disc tissue engineering: learning from tendon and articular cartilage, *Proc Inst Mech Eng H* 221:509-526, 2007.

142. Terheyden H, Knak C, Jepsen S, et al: Mandibular reconstruction with a prefabricated vascularized bone graft using recombinant human osteogenic protein-1: an experimental study in miniature pigs. Part I: prefabrication, *Int J Oral Maxillofac Surg* 30:373-379, 2001.

143. Terheyden H, Warnke P, Dunsche A, et al: Mandibular reconstruction with prefabricated vascularized bone grafts using recombinant human osteogenic protein-1: an experimental study in miniature pigs. Part II: transplantation, *Int J Oral Maxillofac Surg* 30:469-478, 2001.

144. Terheyden H, Menzel C, Wang H, et al: Prefabrication of vascularized bone grafts using recombinant human osteogenic protein-1—part 3: dosage of rhOP-1, the use of external and internal scaffolds, *Int J Oral Maxillofac Surg* 33:164-172, 2004.

145. Warnke PH, Springer IN, Wiltfang J, et al: Growth and transplantation of a custom vascularised bone graft in a man, *Lancet* 364:766-770, 2004.

146. Warnke PH, Springer IN, Açil Y, et al: The mechanical integrity of in vivo engineered heterotopic bone, *Biomaterials* 27:1081-1087, 2006.

147. Warnke PH, Wiltfang J, Springer I, et al: Man as living bioreactor: fate of an exogenously prepared customized tissue-engineered mandible, *Biomaterials* 27:3163-3167, 2006.

148. Neumann T, Nicholson BS, Sanders JE: Tissue engineering of perfused microvessels, *Microvasc Res* 66:59-67, 2003.

149. Sun ZC, Zussman E, Yarin AL, et al: Electrospinning of nanofibers from polymer nanofibers by co-electrospinning, *Adv Mater* 15:1929-1936, 2003.

150. Dror Y, Salalha W, Avrahami R, et al: One-step production of polymeric microtubes by co-electrospinning, *Small* 3:1064-1073, 2007.

151. Reneker DH, Yarin AL, Zussman E, et al: Electrospinning of nanofibers from polymer solutions and melts, *Adv Appl Mech* 41:43-195, 2007.

152. Makhoul NM, Zussman E, et al: Development of a microcapillary system for tissue engineering, *J Oral Maxillofac Surg* 66(8 Suppl):45-46, 2008.

153. Frerich B, Lindemann N, Kurtz-Hoffmann J, et al: In vitro model of a vascular stroma for the engineering of vascularized tissues, *Int J Oral Maxillofac Surg* 30:414-420, 2001.

154. Frerich B, Kurtz-Hoffmann J, Lindemann N, et al: Influence of growth hormone on maintenance of capillary-like structures in an in vitro model of stromal vascular tissue—results from morphometric analysis, *Artif Organs* 29:338-341, 2005.

155. Hokugo A, Sawada Y, Sugimoto K, et al: Preparation of prefabricated vascularized bone graft with neoangiogenesis by combination of autologous tissue and biodegradable materials, *Int J Oral Maxillofac Surg* 35:1034-1040, 2006.

156. Fumimoto Y, Matsuyama A, Komoda H, et al: Creation of a rich subcutaneous vascular network with implanted adipose tissue–derived stromal cells and adipose tissue enhances subcutaneous grafting of islets in diabetic mice, *Tissue Eng Part C Methods* 15:437-444, 2009.

157. Greenhalgh DG, Sprugel KH, Murray MJ, et al: PDGF and FGF stimulate wound healing in the genetically diabetic mouse, *Am J Pathol* 136:1235-1246, 1990.

158. Albertson S, Hummel RP 3rd, Breeden M, et al: PDGF and FGF reverse the healing impairment in protein-malnourished diabetic mice, *Surgery* 114:368-372, discussion 372-373, 1993.

159. Greenhalgh DG: Tissue repair in models of diabetes mellitus. A review, *Methods Mol Med* 78:181-189, 2003.

160. Greenhalgh DG: Wound healing and diabetes mellitus, *Clin Plast Surg* 30:37-45, 2003.

Molecular Biology of Head and Neck Cancer: Therapeutic Implications

David K. Lam, Brian L. Schmidt

Head and neck cancer is a major health concern, with more than 540,000 new cases diagnosed and 271,000 disease-related deaths occurring annually worldwide.[1-3] As oral and maxillofacial surgeons providing comprehensive surgical management for head and neck cancer, we are continually challenged with difficulty predicting the capricious clinical behavior of head and neck cancer, recurrence at the primary site following resection, cervical and distant metastasis, and the development of second primary head and neck cancers. Early- to moderate-stage oral squamous cell carcinoma (OSCC) is usually treated surgically along with radiotherapy given with or without chemotherapy postoperatively for high-risk patients.[4] In patients with advanced disease, multidisciplinary non-surgical approaches have increasingly been used to improve disease control, survival, and quality of life.[5-7] However, despite the best combination of surgical and non-surgical approaches, more than 50% of patients with OSCC experience local recurrence or distant metastasis and subsequently have poorer prognoses,[4,8] and therefore more effective therapies are needed for these patients. Our understanding of the molecular biology of head and neck cancer has progressed significantly over the last decade, and the causes and solutions of these clinical challenges have a molecular basis. The development of novel diagnostic and therapeutic approaches to OSCC requires a better understanding of the molecular pathogenesis of OSCC and the molecular events involved in its growth, invasion, and metastasis. Molecular approaches will greatly increase our ability to predict clinical behavior, determine prognosis, guide surgical treatment, and aid cancer surveillance. This chapter focuses on improving our understanding of the molecular mechanisms of head and neck cancer and its therapeutic implications.

MOLECULAR BIOLOGY OF HEAD AND NECK CANCER

Head and neck cancer is a heterogeneous disease that develops through a complex, multi-step process involving genetic alterations, growth regulation, apoptosis, immortalization, angiogenesis, invasion, and metastasis following a series of molecular events influenced by the individual's genetic predisposition and environmental exposure to carcinogens (Fig. 10-1, *A*). Chronic exposure to carcinogens such as alcohol, tobacco, betel quid chewing, and oncogenic viruses may result in genetic alterations that can develop into dysplastic lesions and subsequent invasive OSCC.[9-11] These genetic alterations in oral cancer cells can be divided into two categories. *Dominant changes*, most frequently occurring in proto-oncogenes, result in gain of function. *Recessive changes*, or mutations frequently found in genes in the growth-inhibitory pathway or in tumor suppressor genes, lead to loss of function.[12] As a result of these alterations, cancer cells acquire a cellular growth advantage with autonomous growth, evade growth-inhibitory signals, escape apoptosis, and may replicate infinitely. Cancer cells can also stimulate angiogenesis and thereby allow OSCC to further grow, invade, and metastasize. The timing and accumulation of these genetic alterations resulting in carcinoma are probably critical. Because genetic changes precede phenotypic changes, molecular and genetic analysis might afford the clinician the possibility to intervene earlier and improve the prognosis.

GENETIC ALTERATIONS

Genetic alterations involving the loss of chromosomal material at 3p, 9p, and 17p occurs in a high proportion of dysplastic oral lesions, thus suggesting that these alterations may serve as early markers in oral carcinogenesis, whereas carcinomas more frequently display losses at 8p and 13q and may be associated with later stages of carcinogenesis.[13-15] The chromosome 3p region includes the tumor suppressor genes *FHIT* and *RSSFIA*, which are inactivated by exonic deletion and hypermethylation.[16-19] Loss of chromosomal region 9p21 occurs in 70% to 80% of dysplastic lesions of the oral mucosa.[9,13,16,20,21] The CDKN2A locus region of 9p21 encodes the tumor suppressors p16 and p14^{ARF}, which are often inactivated by promoter hypermethylation.[22] During progression from dysplasia to invasive OSCC, genetic alterations involving the loss of heterozygosity of chromosome region 17p may also occur, as well as *p53* gene mutation.[23,24] Alterations involving *p53* in oral dysplasia are associated with increased genomic instability and generally occur late in the progression from dysplasia to invasive carcinoma.

Oncogenes

Proto-oncogenes are highly regulated genes that encode proteins mediating positive cell growth regulation and cell survival signals. If a proto-oncogene is altered via chromosomal translocation, mutation, gene amplification, or retroviral insertion, it may become an activated "gain-of-function" oncogene that promotes uncontrolled cell proliferation and resultant carcinogenesis.[25-27] Oncogenes may be categorized as (1) growth factors or growth factor receptors, (2) intracellular signal transducers, (3) transcription factors, (4) cell cycle regulators, or (5) those involved in the inhibition of apoptosis.[21] The majority of these oncogenes promote aberrant cell proliferation by overriding various checkpoints of the cell cycle.[28]

Tumor Suppressor Genes

Tumor suppressor genes, or anti-oncogenes, encode proteins that transduce negative cell growth regulation signals such as those involved in cell cycle arrest and apoptosis.[29] In contrast to oncogenes, which are activated by mutation of only one of the two gene copies, tumor suppressor genes are inactivated by point mutations or deletion in both alleles of the gene in a "two-hit" fashion.[30-32] Once tumor suppressor genes are inactivated, the cell escapes stringent cell cycle control and is predisposed to uncontrolled growth and division.[33,34] "Loss of function" of multiple tumor suppressor genes is thought to be the major event leading to the development of malignancy.[32,35]

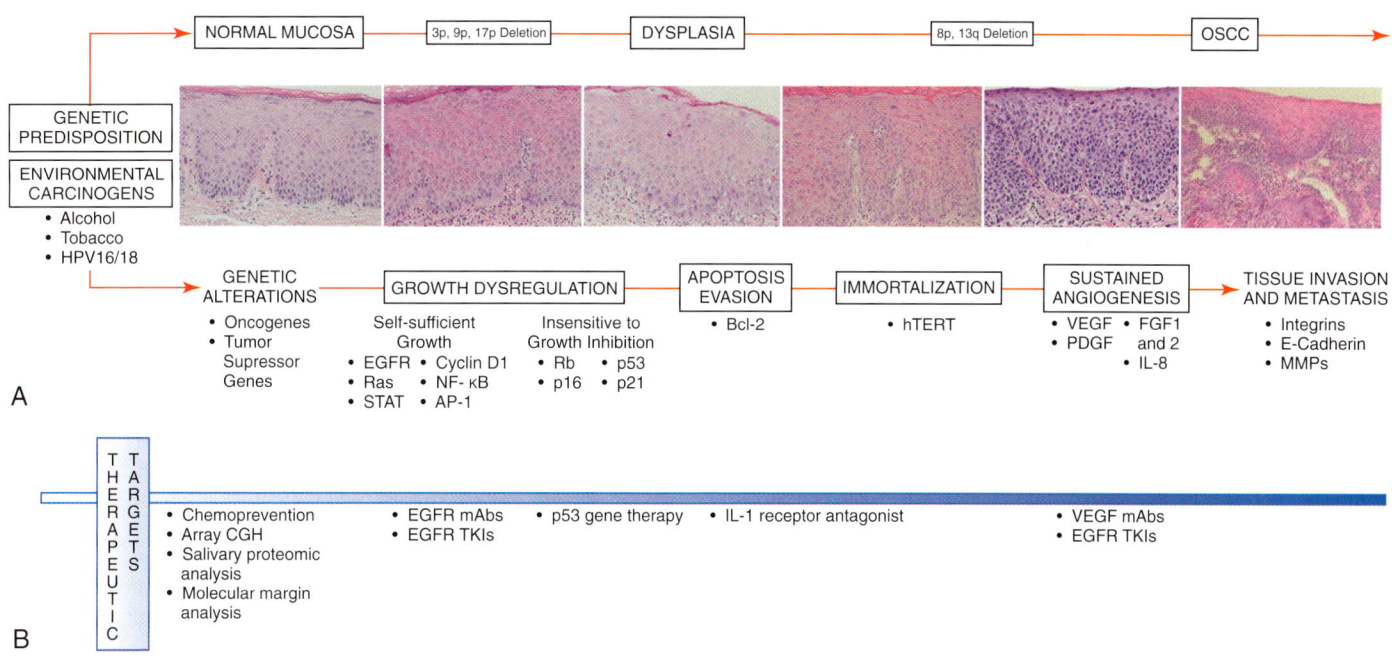

Fig. 10-1 ■ Molecular biology of head and neck cancer and its implications for therapy. **A,** Under the influence of genetic predisposition and environmental carcinogens, head and neck cancer develops through a complex, multi-step process involving genetic alterations, growth regulation, apoptosis, immortalization, angiogenesis, invasion, and metastasis. **B,** With improved understanding of the molecular mediators involved in head and neck carcinogenesis, targeted approaches may provide useful diagnostic, therapeutic, and surveillance strategies. (Photomicrographs courtesy of Dr. Darren Cox.)

Field Cancerization

The entire epithelial layer of the oral cavity may be exposed to various carcinogenic insults and is therefore at increased risk for malignant transformation from the accumulation of genetic alterations of oncogenes and tumor suppressor genes. The theory of "field cancerization" has been developed from the finding of dysplastic epithelium adjacent to invasive oral cancers, which accounts for the high incidence of second primary tumors in patients treated for OSCC.[36] In this model, multifocal oral cancers develop from separate, independent genetic alterations, and many of these second primary tumors have been associated with lower survival rates than occurs with the original tumor.[37,38] In an updated progression model, second or multiple cancers distant from the dysplastic fields have been suggested to be clonally related and derived from the expansion of a common pre-neoplastic progenitor.[39] This occurs when a stem cell located in the basal epithelial layer acquires a genetic alteration and subsequently gives rise to a clonal unit whereby the stem cell and all its daughter cells share the DNA alteration and progress to an expanding field as a result of additional genetic alterations.[40] The resultant mucosal field pushes the normal epithelium aside and may expand to several centimeters in size. These fields may appear as leukoplakia or erythroplakia but often remain clinically undetectable. Clonal selection ultimately results in carcinoma formation within this field of pre-neoplastic cells.

SELF-SUFFICIENCY IN GROWTH SIGNALING

Exogenous growth signals stimulate normal oral keratinocyte proliferation. Growth signals are usually transduced from cell surface receptors that subsequently activate multiple intracellular signaling pathways to result in cell proliferation. This growth signaling may be dysregulated by increases in the level of growth factor receptors or their ligands to promote autocrine stimulation in the absence of exogenous factors during oral carcinogenesis.[41]

Epidermal Growth Factor Receptor

Epidermal growth factor receptor (EGFR) is a member of the membrane-bound receptor tyrosine kinase family. EGF and transforming growth factor-α (TGF-α) are endogenous ligands for EGFR.[42] Following ligand binding, EGFR dimerizes with another EGFR and autophosphorylates, which results in a series of intracellular signaling events that involve activation of the Ras/Raf/mitogen-activated protein kinase (MAPK), signal transducer and activator of transcription (STAT), and protein kinase C (PKC) pathways.[43,44] These signaling events then mediate cell proliferation and survival, invasion, metastasis, and angiogenesis.[45] EGFR overexpression progressively increases from oral premalignant lesions to invasive OSCC. EGFR is overexpressed in 80% to 100% of oral cancers[44,45] and is an independent prognostic marker that correlates with increased tumor size, decreased radiation sensitivity, and increased risk for recurrence.[46-51] However, patients with head and neck cancers overexpressing EGFR may exhibit a higher proportion of complete responses to chemotherapy than those with cancers exhibiting low EGFR expression. This overexpression of EGFR with consequently greater intrinsic proliferative activity is thought to result in greater chemosensitivity in cells undergoing mitogenesis.[52]

Ras Oncogene

Ras (H-*ras*, K-*ras*, N-*ras*) is an important proto-oncogene involved in the regulation of cell growth and transduction of mitogenic cell signaling from the cell surface to the nucleus. The *ras* gene encodes protein p21, which is constitutively activated through mutation.[53] A high incidence of H-*ras* mutations has been found in oral cancer, mostly in Asians and possibly associated with betel nut chewing.[54,55]

STAT Proteins

STAT proteins are latent cytoplasmic transcription factors activated by various extracellular signaling proteins.[56,57] On activation, STAT proteins can up-regulate the transcription of various target genes and result in uncontrolled cellular proliferation, anti-apoptotic responses, and angiogenesis.[58] Activated STAT3 levels may be elevated in oral cancer via up-regulation of the EGFR, TGF-α, Jak, Src, or interleukin-6 (IL-6) signaling pathways.[59,60] Activated STAT3 is highly expressed in poorly differentiated oral cancers and is correlated with metastasis and a poor prognosis.[61]

Cyclin D1

Cyclin D1 is a proto-oncogene that regulates the initiation of DNA synthesis.[62] Overexpression of cyclin D1 occurs in a high percentage of premalignant lesions[63] and oral cancers.[64] Cyclin D1 overexpression is an early event in oral carcinogenesis and is associated with more aggressive tumor behavior, an increased rate of lymph node metastases, and a worse prognosis.[65,66]

Nuclear Factor κB

The nuclear factor κB (NF-κB) is a ubiquitous nuclear transcription factor that regulates many target genes, including immunoregulatory and inflammatory genes, anti-apoptotic genes, and genes that positively regulate cell proliferation.[67] NF-κB1 (p105/p50), NF-κB2 (p100/p52), RelA (p65), c-Rel, and RelB are included in the NF-κB family. NF-κB expression levels increase gradually from premalignant lesions to invasive cancer.[68] Moreover, NF-κB may inhibit apoptosis through the induction of anti-apoptotic proteins and suppress the apoptotic potential of chemotherapeutic agents, thereby leading to chemoresistance.[69]

Activating Protein-1

The activating protein-1 (AP-1) transcription factor family is made up of multiple Jun (cJun, JunB, and JunD) and Fos (cFos, FosB, Fra-1, and Fra-2) members. AP-1 regulates cellular proliferation, differentiation, apoptosis, oncogene-induced transformation, and cancer cell invasion.[70-73] AP-1 activation induces transformation and malignant progression in oral cancer; it is found to be activated in both oral dysplasia and OSCC cell lines and is associated with malignant transformation in squamous epithelial cells.[74,75]

INSENSITIVITY TO GROWTH-INHIBITORY SIGNALS

Growth-inhibitory signals are regulated by interactions of cyclin-dependent kinase (CDK), cyclin, and the retinoblastoma (*Rb*) gene product. The proteins encoded by the tumor suppressor genes *p16*, *p15*, *p21*, and *p53* also act as inhibitors of cell cycle progression, and when their expression is lost, progression through the cell cycle is increased.[76] Loss of growth-inhibitory signals and the development of self-sufficient growth signals via oncogene activation are needed for oral carcinogenesis.

Retinoblastoma Gene

The *Rb* gene product is a crucial regulator of G_1/S cell cycle progression. When normally hypophosphorylated, it complexes with the transcription factor E2F and inhibits E2F-mediated regulation of DNA synthesis.[77] Following mitogen stimulation, Rb is phosphorylated and dissociated from E2F, which allows cell proliferation via E2F activation of c-Myc, cyclin A, and p21WAF-1.[78]

Alterations in Rb expression have been documented in 64% of premalignant lesions and in 66% of OSCC cases,[79] as well as in advanced-stage oral cancers.[80]

p16

The *p16* tumor suppressor gene on chromosome 9p21-22 binds to CDK4 and CDK6 to inhibit cellular proliferation.[81,82] Loss of *p16* occurs in 60% of premalignant lesions and 83% of oral cancers,[22,79,83] thus suggesting that alteration in *p16* is an early event in oral cancer progression.[20,84,85] Reduced *p16* expression in oral cancer has also been correlated with a poorer prognosis.[86]

p53

The *p53* tumor suppressor gene on chromosome 17p13.1 plays a role in cell cycle arrest, cellular differentiation, DNA repair, and apoptosis. It is the most commonly mutated gene and is altered in 25% to 70% of oral cancers.[87-89] *p53* mutations often arise as a result of tobacco or alcohol exposure, and their presence is associated with early recurrence and the development of second primaries.[90] Tumor-associated *p53* mutants may develop the ability to transform cells, increase tumorigenicity, and modulate the sensitivity of cancer cells to chemotherapy and radiation therapy.[91-94] *p53* appears to be mutated at the transition from superficial to invasive carcinoma.[95] In addition to mutation, *p53* can be inactivated by infection with human papillomaviruses such as HPV-16 or HPV-18. Loss of function of *p53* has been associated with both carcinogenesis and a worse overall prognosis in patients with OSCC.[96]

p21

p21 is a cell cycle inhibitor whose expression is transactivated by wild-type, but not by mutant *p53*.[97] *p21* interacts with cyclin/CDK to result in cell cycle arrest and consequently mediates the growth-suppressing and apoptosis-promoting functions of *p53*.[98] Expression of *p21* is increased in premalignant and malignant oral lesions, thus suggesting that alteration of *p21* expression may be an early event in oral carcinogenesis.[99] Altered *p21* expression in oral cancer has also been correlated with a poorer prognosis.[100]

EVASION OF APOPTOSIS

Apoptosis is a form of molecularly programmed cell death in which senescent or altered cells that have become useless or harmful for the multicellular organism are eliminated. A critically important group of apoptosis-regulating proteins is the Bcl-2 family, which is composed of proteins with pro-apoptotic (Bax, Bak) or anti-apoptotic (Bcl-2, Bcl-XL) effects. Alterations in levels of expression of Bcl-2 family members may promote tumor progression and result in resistance to cytotoxic therapies such as chemotherapy and radiation therapy.[101,102] Elevated expression of Bcl-2 or Bcl-XL has been detected in a mouse model of both oral dysplasia and OSCC.[103] Increased levels of Bcl-XL expression with wild-type p53 have been associated with cisplatin resistance in oral cancer cell lines,[104] and Bcl-2/XL inhibitors have been shown to result in growth inhibition and apoptosis.[105] Thus, inhibition of Bcl-XL may be a promising therapeutic strategy for overcoming cisplatin resistance in oral cancer.[104,105]

IMMORTALITY

Normal cells have a limited capacity to replicate themselves. Cancer cells become immortalized and have the capacity to replicate indefinitely by telomere lengthening.[106] Telomeres, or repetitive tandem DNA repeat sequences complexed with telomere-binding proteins, shorten after each round of cell division and thus limit the life span of cells. The enzyme telomerase maintains telomeric repeats by elongating telomeric DNA by reverse transcription, and its activity is determined largely by human telomerase reverse transcriptase (hTERT) levels.[107] Telomerase up-regulation is common in human cancers.[108] Elevated expression of hTERT may serve as an early marker in oral carcinogenesis and is associated with poor treatment outcomes.[109-112]

SUSTAINED ANGIOGENESIS

In the absence of adequate tissue perfusion, tumor growth is limited to 1 to 2 mm³; thus, solid tumors must develop a blood supply for further growth and metastasis.[113] This is accomplished by a shift in balance between pro-angiogenic and anti-angiogenic factors.[113,114] Major pro-angiogenic signals include vascular endothelial growth factor (VEGF), platelet-derived growth factor (PDGF), fibroblast growth factors (FGF-1 and FGF-2), and (interleukin-8) IL-8, whereas anti-angiogenic factors include the interferons, proteolytic fragments such as angiostatin and endostatin, and thrombospondin-1.

Vascular Endothelial Growth Factor

VEGF plays an important role in the regulation of angiogenesis by increasing vessel permeability and endothelial cell growth, proliferation, migration, and differentiation.[115] There are three VEGF receptors: VEGFR-1/Flt-1, VEGFR-2/Flk-1/KDR, and VEGFR-3/Flt-4; these receptors may be activated by six VEGF ligands, including VEGF-A, VEGF-B, VEGF-C, VEGF-D, VEGF-E, and placental growth factor.[115,116] Activation of VEGFR-1 promotes endothelial cell migration without inducing cell proliferation.[116] VEGFR-2 mediates endothelial cell mitogenesis, proliferation, and survival.[117] Expression of VEGF and VEGFR-2 has been correlated with a greater proliferation index and worse survival in head and neck cancer.[118,119] VEGFR-3/Flt-4 is expressed mostly in lymphatic vessels,[120] is activated by VEGF-C and VEGF-D, and regulates lymphangiogenesis.[121-124] Lymphangiogenesis can occur adjacent to or within human cancers and correlates with lymph node metastasis in oral cancer.[125,126] Since oral cancer preferentially metastasizes to regional lymph nodes, the VEGF-C/VEGFR-3 signaling pathway may be an important therapeutic target.

Interleukin-8

IL-8 functions in immune surveillance, inflammation, and angiogenesis and is secreted by leukocytes and tumor cells.[127] IL-8 acts as a potent angiogenic factor in tumors by modulating endothelial cell proliferation and migration.[127,128] Some human OSCC cell lines produce IL-8 constitutively, and IL-8 production by these cell lines is up-regulated in the presence of various cytokines such as epidermal growth factor (EGF) and tumor necrosis factor-α (TNF-α).[129,130] IL-8 has also been found in OSCC cells within tumor specimens, and its expression correlated with increased neovascularity.[131,132]

TISSUE INVASION AND METASTASIS

Head and neck cancer is characterized by local invasion and a propensity for dissemination to locoregional lymph nodes. The first step in cancer cell invasion and metastasis involves increased cell motility, and this process may be associated with an epithelial-mesenchymal transition.[133] Epithelial-mesenchymal transition occurs when epithelial cells change from a polarized epithelium to a fibroblast-like mesenchymal phenotype. This process eventually results in the loss of epithelial integrity, increased migration, local invasion, and metastasis.

Integrins

Integrins are heterodimeric, transmembrane glycoproteins that mediate cell-cell and cell-matrix interactions, and they are critical for the maintenance of tissue integrity and regulation of cell proliferation, growth, differentiation, and migration. Integrin $\alpha_6\beta_4$ has been shown to be associated with early recurrence and metastasis in oral cancer.[134] Expression of $\alpha_V\beta_5$ is lower in OSCC than in normal epithelium,[135,136] whereas $\alpha_V\beta_6$ expression is up-regulated in oral dysplasia, where its expression is correlated with progression to malignant disease.[137] Thus, $\alpha_V\beta_6$ may be useful in predicting malignant transformation.[138]

E-cadherin

E-cadherin aids in the maintenance of tight cell-cell contact in normal oral epithelia and suppresses tumor cell motility, invasion, and metastasis. Decreased E-cadherin expression during epithelial-mesenchymal transition leads to loss of cell-cell adhesion and contributes to cell dissociation with increased motility and invasion of tumor cells.[139,140] Decreased or complete loss of E-cadherin expression has been associated with lymph node metastasis and poor prognosis in oral cancer.[141]

Matrix Metalloproteinases

Matrix metalloproteinases (MMPs), or zinc metalloenzymes involved in extracellular matrix remodeling, consist of the collagenases, gelatinases, stromelysins, stromelysin-like MMPs, membrane-type MMPs, and new MMPs. Malignant cells may use MMPs to dissolve the basement membrane and degrade interstitial stroma to facilitate invasion and metastasis. MMP-2 expression is higher in cell nests of metastatic tumors than in those of non-metastatic tumors in oral cancer, thus suggesting that MMP-2 is a marker predictive of metastasis.[142,143] MMP-3, MMP-10, and MMP-11 have also been implicated in the progression of oral cancer.[144,145]

THERAPEUTIC IMPLICATIONS

With improved understanding of the molecular biology of head and neck cancer, targeted approaches directed against molecular mediators involved in carcinogenesis may provide useful diagnostic, therapeutic, and surveillance strategies (see Fig. 10-1, B).

CHEMOPREVENTION

The field cancerization concept suggests that the multi-focality of oral carcinogenesis may be an important cause of treatment failure. Although primary excision may completely remove an oral carcinoma, the altered field can persist and a second primary tumor may develop in the same field and be clinically indistinguishable from a local recurrence. As the resolution of molecular techniques improves, the clinician might be able to determine whether patients with either extensive or multiple sites of genetically altered mucosa can be managed surgically. In particular, patients with extensive fields may be candidates for chemopreventive approaches in which systemic therapy is administered with the intent of preventing the entire oral epithelium from progressing along the multistep pathway of carcinogenesis.[146]

TARGETING THE EPIDERMAL GROWTH FACTOR RECEPTOR

Various treatment strategies have been developed to disrupt the EGFR signal transduction pathway in OSCC. EGFR monoclonal antibodies (mAbs) have been developed to prevent binding of ligand to EGFR and thus inhibit receptor activation and facilitate receptor degradation.[147] Another monoclonal antibody–targeting strategy uses anti-EGFR monoclonal antibodies conjugated with toxins to stimulate the immune system to selectively attack tumor cells over-expressing EGFR.[148] EGFR tyrosine kinase inhibitors (TKIs) directly interact with the cytoplasmic enzymatic domain of receptor kinases to inhibit their enzymatic activity.

Epidermal Growth Factor Receptor Monoclonal Antibodies

Cetuximab (Erbitux) is one of the first EGFR monoclonal antibodies studied in OSCC. In clinical studies, cetuximab has demonstrated anti-tumor effects both as a single agent and when combined with radiation therapy or chemotherapy.[149] Moreover, in a phase III multi-center trial comparing radiotherapy alone with radiotherapy and cetuximab, the combination therapy resulted in significant improvement in locoregional control and overall survival in patients with locoregionally advanced head and neck cancer.[149] Panitumumab and matuzumab are fully humanized antibodies to EGFR and thus differ from cetuximab, whose murine sequences may elicit hypersensitivity reactions.[150-152] However, further studies of these newer EGFR antibodies are needed to determine their efficacy in treating OSCC.

Tyrosine Kinase Inhibitors

Erlotinib (Tarceva) and gefitinib (Iressa) are small-molecule EGFR TKIs that target the intracellular portion of the receptor. In phase II trials, erlotinib has yielded modest effects in the treatment of recurrent or metastatic head and neck cancer.[153]

TARGETING p53

Gene therapy involves the use of various viral vectors or DNA directly to replace a mutated gene within a tumor with a functionally normal gene. Gene therapy approaches to head and neck premalignant lesions and cancer may involve the following[154]: (1) addition gene therapy, which aims to regulate tumor growth by introducing a wild-type tumor suppressor gene that inactivates the carcinogenic cells; (2) oncolytic viruses, which replicate only in the tumor cells and ultimately kill them; (3) suicide gene therapy, in which the enzyme-encoding gene is introduced into the tumor cell to stimulate the generation of products toxic to the cells; (4) immunotherapy to increase the patient's immune response to the tumor; and (5) introduction of genes to inhibit tumor angiogenesis by using microencapsulated cells for the release of therapeutic proteins to encapsulate recombinant cells.

In a phase I/II clinical trial involving adenoviral vectors, the use of wild-type *p53* gene therapy to treat the cancer cells of patients with recurrent disease has yielded modest antitumor activity in several patients.[155] Another approach has used the ONYX-015 virus, an adenovirus engineered to replicate selectively in p53-deficient cells and leave cells with normal p53 unaffected.[156] In a trial of ONYX-015 used as a mouthwash for chemoprevention in patients with oral dysplasia, reversible responses were evident.[157] Administration of ONYX-015 has also yielded biologic activity in patients with refractory head and neck cancer.[158-160] In particular, intratumoral injection of ONYX-015 with cisplatin and 5-fluorouracil has demonstrated substantial and durable responses.[161,162]

TARGETING VASCULAR ENDOTHELIAL GROWTH FACTOR

Strategies similar to that used in targeting EGFR are also applied to inhibit VEGF. Bevacizumab is a recombinant humanized monoclonal antibody against VEGF that has been used in head and neck cancer. Since EGFR induces angiogenesis via expression of VEGF, it has been demonstrated that inhibition of EGFR results in decreased VEGF secretion and tumor microvessel production in vivo.[163] Thus, combined targeting of VEGF and EGFR is more effective than targeting of either pathway alone.[164,165] The VEGFR TKI AZD2171

(AstraZeneca) has also demonstrated growth inhibition and decreased microvessel density in vivo.[166,167] The VEGF-C/VEGFR-3 signaling system is a key regulator of tumor lymphangiogenesis. Soluble VEGFR-3 protein constructs that neutralize monoclonal antibodies to VEGFR-3 and VEGF-D and small-molecule inhibitors of VEGFR-3 kinase[168,169] are currently under study.

FUTURE DIAGNOSTIC AIDS AND THERAPIES

MICROARRAYS

The findings of the Human Genome Project along with advances in microarray technology have enabled a high-throughput means for investigating the relative roles of specific genes in the pathogenesis of head and neck cancer. Microarray technology may be used in a number of ways, including measuring changes in gene expression, identifying genomic gains and losses, and determining mutations in DNA. The process of determining the level at which a certain gene is expressed is called gene expression analysis.[170] In this technique the immobilized DNA on the chip is cDNA derived from the mRNA of known genes. The control DNA and sample DNA consist of cDNA derived from the mRNA of normal and diseased tissue, respectively. If a particular gene is overexpressed in disease, more sample cDNA than control cDNA will hybridize to the spot representing that expressed gene. As we gain further insight into the gene expression patterns of particular disease states, mRNA may be extracted from diseased tissue from any individual and tested to determine whether the gene expression pattern in that tissue matches the expression pattern of the disease state. Future applications of this technique may not only prove useful for diagnosis but also aid in the development of new therapeutic approaches that are targeted at particular genes expressed in the cancer state.

Microarray technology may also be used to identify cancer-related gains and losses in the chromosomal region across the entire genome via array comparative genomic hybridization (CGH). To date, this technology has been applied primarily to the study of cancer.[171] DNA repair genes play a major role in cancer, and mutations in these genes can produce broken chromosomes that lead to specific chromosomal gains and losses. Changes in chromosomes are related to cancer progression, and the patterns of these changes may be relevant to clinical prognosis. Array CGH allows accurate quantification of variations in DNA copy number over the entire genome and provides reliable detection of single-copy changes from diploid.[171] We performed array CGH on 89 OSCCs and focused on narrow regions of gene amplification to facilitate identification of genetic pathways important in the development of OSCC.[171] Genes involved in integrin signaling, survival, adhesion, and migration, as well as members of the hedgehog and notch pathways, were amplified and overexpressed in OSCC. The development of novel, high-throughput, automated array CGH technology shows great potential utility for the identification of genes and gene products that could provide either therapeutic, prognostic, or diagnostic targets. Arrays will also allow clinicians to monitor the effectiveness of gene-targeted therapy. A comparative array analysis of gene expression in tissues before and after treatment would demonstrate whether the drug is producing the expected changes in gene expression. Resistant cases could be identified early and an alternative approach implemented.

SALIVARY PROTEOMIC ANALYSIS

Proteomics encompasses the identification and quantification of proteins, as well as the modifications, interactions, and activities of these proteins. Cancer is a consequence of genetic and epigenetic alterations that lead to protein dysregulation, which may affect cell division, differentiation, immune recognition, tissue invasion, and metastasis. Proteomic approaches can be used to successfully identify disease markers. Proteomic analysis has been applied to biofluids for the possible diagnosis of cancer and has been used to diagnose various cancers. Using a complex combination of mass spectrometry and bio-informatics, serum analysis was able to diagnose ovarian cancer with a sensitivity of 100%, specificity of 95%, and positive predictive value of 94%[172] and diagnose prostate cancer with a sensitivity of 83% and specificity of 97%.[173] Clearly, for oral cancer, identification of a salivary protein or proteomic pattern would be of considerable assistance in screening patients at risk for oral cancer. We have demonstrated that certain salivary peptides are increased in patients with oral cancer relative to normal controls.[174] Identification and measurement of a salivary biomarker would be particularly beneficial for screening patients at risk for OSCC—such as those with a history of oral cancer, those with alcohol and tobacco use, or those who have a potentially malignant epithelial lesion.

MOLECULAR MARGIN ANALYSIS

Despite the presence of microscopically negative margins, local recurrence develops in 3.9% to 32% of patients with OSCC.[175-177] Currently, there is no rapid and accurate technique available to comprehensively identify and map genetic alterations in specimens for guiding the surgical management of head and neck cancer. Brennan and colleagues demonstrated that histologically normal surgical margins that contain *p53* mutations are associated with a significantly increased incidence of local recurrence.[178] Using an

assay based on highly sensitive polymerase chain reaction, they studied surgical specimens to determine whether occult neoplastic cells could be identified in surgical margins and lymph nodes obtained following resection in 30 patients with head and neck cancer. Local recurrence was found in 5 of 13 (38%) patients with positive margins assessed by this method as compared with no recurrence in patients with negative margins. Moreover, molecular analysis identified neoplastic cells in 6 of 28 (21%) lymph nodes that initially tested negative by traditional histopathologic means. Their study highlights the potential utility of molecular margin analysis whereby after surgical resection, margins could be obtained and analyzed intraoperatively to confirm genetically clear margins.

PEARLS AND PITFALLS

- As our understanding of the molecular biology of head and neck cancer continues to evolve, we may be better able to tailor specific diagnostic and therapeutic applications for individual patients.
- Potential molecular assays may provide assistance to clinicians in (1) screening patients, (2) predicting conversion from premalignancy to malignancy, (3) assessing the status of prognostic tumor indicators, and (4) monitoring patients after therapy.
- Future applications may involve early diagnosis that is simple to make and can easily be implemented by untrained health technicians, immediate evaluation of surgical margins that covers the entire genome, and therapy that is monitored with specific DNA arrays, RNA expression arrays, and proteomics.

REFERENCES

1. Stewart BW, Kleihues P: *World cancer report*, Geneva, 2003, International Agency for Research on Cancer, pp 232-236.
2. Jemal A, Siegel R, Murray T, et al: Cancer statistics, 2006, *CA Cancer J Clin* 56:106-130, 2006.
3. American Cancer Society: *Cancer facts & figures 2008*, Atlanta, 2008, American Cancer Society.
4. Forastiere A, Koch W, Trotti A, et al: Head and neck cancer, *N Engl J Med* 346:1890-1900, 2001.
5. Haraf DJ, Rosen FR, Stenson K, et al: Induction chemotherapy followed by concomitant TFHX chemoradiotherapy with reduced dose radiation in advanced head and neck cancer, *Clin Cancer Res* 9:5936-5943, 2003.
6. Bernier J, Domenge C, Ozsahin M, et al: Postoperative irradiation with or without concomitant chemotherapy for locally advanced head and neck cancer, *N Engl J Med* 350:1945-1952, 2004.
7. Cooper JS, Pajak TF, Forastiere AA, et al: Postoperative concurrent radiotherapy and chemotherapy for high-risk squamous-cell carcinoma of the head and neck, *N Engl J Med* 350:1937-1944, 2004.
8. Khuri FR, Shin DM, Glisson BS, et al: Treatment of patients with recurrent or metastatic squamous cell carcinoma of the head and neck: current status and future directions, *Semin Oncol* 27:25-33, 2000.
9. Perez-Ordonez B, Beauchemin M, Jordan RC: Molecular biology of squamous cell

carcinoma of the head and neck, *J Clin Pathol* 59:445-453, 2006.
10. Choi S, Myers JN: Molecular pathogenesis of oral squamous cell carcinoma: implications for therapy, *J Dent Res* 87:14-32, 2008.
11. Wang F, Arun P, Friedman J, et al: Current and potential inflammation targeted therapies in head and neck cancer, *Curr Opin Pharmacol* 9:389-395, 2009.
12. Bishop JM: Molecular themes in oncogenesis, *Cell* 64:235-248, 1991.
13. Califano J, van der Riet P, Westra W, et al: Genetic progression model for head and neck cancer: implications for field cancerization, *Cancer Res* 56:2488-2492, 1996.
14. Garnis C, Baldwin C, Zhang L, et al: Use of complete coverage array comparative genomic hybridization to define copy number alterations on chromosome 3p in oral squamous cell carcinomas, *Cancer Res* 63:8582-8585, 2003.
15. Masayesva BG, Ha P, Garrett-Mayer E, et al: Gene expression alterations over large chromosomal regions in cancers include multiple genes unrelated to malignant progression, *Proc Natl Acad Sci U S A* 101:8715-8720, 2004.
16. Mao L, Lee JS, Fan YH, et al: Frequent microsatellite alterations at chromosome 9p21 and 3p41 in oral premalignant lesions and their value in cancer risk assessment, *Nat Med* 2:682-685, 1996.
17. Kisielewski AE, Xiao GH, Liu SC, et al: Analysis of the FHIT gene and its product in

squamous cell carcinomas of the head and neck, *Oncogene* 17:83-91, 1998.
18. Hogg RP, Honorio S, Martinez A, et al: Frequent 3p allele loss and epigenetic inactivation of the RASSF1A tumour suppressor gene from region 3p21.3 in head and neck squamous cell carcinoma, *Eur J Cancer* 38:1585-1592, 2002.
19. Dong SM, Sun DI, Benoit NE, et al: Epigenetic inactivation of RASSFIA in head and neck cancer, *Clin Cancer Res* 9:3635-3640, 2003.
20. van der Riet P, Nawroz H, Hruban RH, et al: Frequent loss of chromosome 9p21-22 early in head and neck cancer progression, *Cancer Res* 54:1156-1158, 1994.
21. Sidransky D: Molecular genetics of head and neck cancer, *Curr Opin Oncol* 7:229-233, 1995.
22. Reed AL, Califano J, Cairns P, et al: High frequency of p16(CDKN2/MTS-1/INK4A) inactivation in head and neck squamous cell carcinoma, *Cancer Res* 56:3630-3633, 1996.
23. Nawroz H, van der Riet P, Hruban RH, et al: Allelotype of head and neck squamous cell carcinoma, *Cancer Res* 54:1152-1155, 1994.
24. van Houten VM, Tabor MP, van den Brekel MW, et al: Mutated p53 as a molecular marker for the diagnosis of head and neck cancer, *J Pathol* 198:476-486, 2002.
25. Klein GE, Klein E: Evolution of tumors and impact of molecular oncology, *Nature* 315:190-195, 1985.

26. Alitalo K, Schwab M: Oncogene amplification in tumor cells, *Adv Cancer Res* 47:235-281, 1986.

27. Haluska FG, Tsujimoto Y, Croce CM: Oncogene activation by chromosome translocation in human malignancy, *Annu Rev Genet* 21:321-345, 1987.

28. Field JK: The role of oncogenes and tumour-suppressor genes in the aetiology of oral, head, and neck squamous cell carcinoma, *J R Soc Med* 88:35-39, 1995.

29. Weinberg RA: Tumor suppressor genes, *Science* 254:1138-1146, 1991.

30. Knudson AG Jr: Genetics and the etiology of human cancer, *Adv Hum Genet* 8:1-66, 1977.

31. Vogelstein B, Kinzler KW: The multistep nature of cancer, *Trends Genet* 9:138-141, 1993.

32. Yokota J, Sugimura T: Multiple steps in carcinogenesis involving alteration of multiple tumour suppressor genes, *FASEB J* 7:920-925, 1993.

33. Levine AJ: p53, the cellular gatekeeper for growth and division. *Cell* 88:323-331, 1997.

34. Levine AJ, Momand J, Finlay CA: The p53 tumor suppressor gene, *Nature* 351:453-456, 1991.

35. Lee WH: Tumor suppressor genes—the hope [editorial], *FASEB J* 7:819, 1993.

36. Slaughter DP, Southwick HW, Smejkal W: Field cancerization in oral stratified squamous epithelium: clinical implication of multicentric origin, *Cancer* 6:963-968, 1953.

37. Day GL, Blot WJ, Shore RE, et al: Second cancers following oral and pharyngeal cancers: role of tobacco and alcohol, *J Natl Cancer Inst* 86:131-137, 1994.

38. Cianfriglia F, DiGregorio DA, Manieri A: Multiple primary tumours in patients with oral squamous cell carcinoma, *Oral Oncol* 35:157-163, 1999.

39. Braakhuis BJ, Tabor MP, Kummer JA, et al: A genetic explanation of Slaughter's concept of field cancerization: evidence and clinical implications, *Cancer Res* 63:1727-1730, 2003.

40. Braakhuis BJ, Brakenhoff RH, Leemans CR: A genetic progression model of oral cancer: current evidence and clinical implications, *J Oral Pathol Med* 33:317-322, 2004.

41. Todd R, Chou MY, Matossian K, et al: Cellular source of transforming growth factor-alpha in human oral cancer, *J Dent Res* 70:917-923, 1991.

42. Tzahar E, Waterman H, Chen X, et al: A hierarchical network of inter-receptor interactions determines signal transduction by Neu differentiation factor/neuregulin and epidermal growth factor, *Mol Cell Biol* 16:5276-5285, 1996.

43. Rogers SJ, Harrington KJ, Rhys-Evans P, et al: Biological significance of c-erbB family oncogenes in head and neck cancer, *Cancer Metastasis Rev* 24:47-69, 2005.

44. Kalyankrishna S, Grandis JR: Epidermal growth factor receptor biology in head and neck cancer, *J Clin Oncol* 24:2666-2672, 2006.

45. Reuter CWM, Morgan MA, Eckardt A: Targeting EGF-receptor signaling in squamous cell carcinomas of the head and neck, *Br J Cancer* 96:408-416, 2007.

46. Grandis JR, Melhem MF, Gooding WE, et al: Levels of TGF-alpha and EGFR protein in head and neck squamous cell carcinoma and patient survival, *J Natl Cancer Inst* 90:824-832, 1998.

47. Shin DM, Ro JY, Hong WK, et al: Dysregulation of epidermal growth factor receptor expression in premalignant lesions during head and neck tumorigenesis, *Cancer Res* 54:3153-3159, 1994.

48. Ang KK, Berkey BA, Tu X, et al: Impact of epidermal growth factor receptor expression on survival and pattern of relapse in patients with advanced head and neck carcinoma, *Cancer Res* 62:7350-7356, 2002.

49. Gupta AK, McKenna WG, Weber CN, et al: Local recurrence in head and neck cancer: relationship to radiation resistance and signal transduction, *Clin Cancer Res* 8:885-892, 2002.

50. Chen IH, Chang JT, Liao CT, et al: Prognostic significance of EGFR and Her-2 in oral cavity cancer in betel quid prevalent area cancer prognosis, *Br J Cancer* 89:681-686, 2003.

51. Shiraki M, Odajima T, Ikeda T, et al: Combined expression of p53, cyclin D1 and epidermal growth factor receptor improves estimation of prognosis in curatively resected oral cancer, *Mod Pathol* 18:1482-1489, 2005.

52. Santini J, Formento JL, Francoual M, et al: Characterization, quantification, and potential clinical value of the epidermal growth factor receptor in head and neck squamous cell carcinomas, *Head Neck* 13:132-139, 1991.

53. Todd R, Donoff RB, Wong DTW: The molecular biology of oral cancer: toward a tumour progression model, *J Oral Maxillofac Surg* 55:613-623, 1997.

54. Saranath D, Bhoite LT, Mehta AR, et al: Loss of allelic heterozygosity at the Harvey *ras* locus in human oral carcinomas, *J Cancer Res Clin Oncol* 117:484-488, 1991.

55. Das N, Majumder J, Das Gupta UB: Ras gene mutations in oral cancer in eastern India, *Oral Oncol* 36:76-80, 2000.

56. Darnell JE Jr: STATs and gene regulation, *Science* 277:1630-1635, 1997.

57. Bromberg J, Darnell JE Jr: The role of STATs in transcriptional control and their impact on cellular function, *Oncogene* 19:2468-2473, 2000.

58. Leeman RJ, Lui VW, Grandis JR: STAT3 as a therapeutic target in head and neck cancer, *Expert Opin Biol Ther* 6:231-241, 2006.

59. Bowman T, Garcia R, Turkson J, et al: STATs in oncogenesis, *Oncogene* 19:2474-2488, 2000.

60. Turkson J, Jove R: STAT proteins: novel molecular targets for cancer drug discovery, *Oncogene* 19:6613-6626, 2000.

61. Masuda M, Suzui M, Yasumatu R, et al: Constitutive activation of signal transducers and activators of transcription 3 correlates with cyclin D1 overexpression and may provide a novel prognostic marker in head and neck squamous cell carcinoma, *Cancer Res* 62:3351-3355, 2002.

62. Smith BD, Haffty BG: Molecular markers as prognostic factors for local recurrence and radioresistance in head and neck squamous cell carcinoma, *Radiat Oncol Invest* 7:125-144, 1999.

63. Rousseau A, Lim MS, Lin Z, et al: Frequent cyclin D1 gene amplification and protein overexpression in oral epithelial dysplasias, *Oral Oncol* 37:268-275, 2001.

64. Miyamoto R, Uzawa N, Nagaoka S, et al: Prognostic significance of cyclin D1 amplification and overexpression in oral squamous cell carcinomas, *Oral Oncol* 39:610-618, 2003.

65. Michalides R, van Veelen N, Hart A, et al: Overexpression of cyclin D1 correlates with recurrence in a group of forty-seven operable squamous cell carcinomas of the head and neck, *Cancer Res* 55:975-978, 1995.

66. Mineta H, Miura K, Ogino T, et al: Cyclin D1 overexpression correlates with poor prognosis in patients with tongue squamous cell carcinoma, *Oral Oncol* 36:194-198, 2000.

67. Karin M, Cao Y, Greten FR, et al: NF-κB in cancer: from innocent bystander to major culprit, *Nat Rev Cancer* 2:301-310, 2002.

68. Mishra A, Bharti AC, Varghese P, et al: Differential expression and activation of NF-kappaB family proteins during oral carcinogenesis: role of high-risk human papillomavirus infection, *Int J Cancer* 119:2840-2850, 2006.

69. Nakanishi C, Toi M: Nuclear factor-κB inhibitors as sensitizers to anticancer drugs, *Nat Rev Cancer* 5:297-309, 2005.

70. McDonnell SE, Kerr LD, Matrisian LM: Epidermal growth factor stimulation of stromelysin mRNA in rat fibroblasts requires induction of proto-oncogenes c-fos and c-jun and activation of protein kinase C, *Mol Cell Biol* 10:4284-4293, 1990.

71. Robinson CM, Prime SS, Huntley S, et al: Overexpression of JunB in undifferentiated malignant rat oral keratinocytes enhances the malignant phenotype in vitro without altering cellular differentiation, *Int J Cancer* 91:625-630, 2001.

72. Szabo E, Preis LH, Brown PH, et al: The role of jun and fos gene family members in 12-O-tetradecanoylphorbol-13-acetate–induced hemopoietic differentiation, *Cell Growth Differ* 2:475-482, 1991.

73. Brown PH, Alani R, Preis LH, et al: Suppression of oncogene-induced transformation by a deletion mutant of c-jun, *Oncogene* 8:877-886, 1993.

74. Domann FE Jr, Levy JP, Finch JS, et al: Constitutive AP-1 DNA binding and trans-activating ability of malignant but not benign mouse epidermal cells, *Mol Carcinog* 9:61-66, 1994.

75. Turatti E, da Costa Neves A, de Magalhaes MH, et al: Assessment of c-Jun, c-Fos and cyclin D1 in premalignant and malignant oral lesions, *J Oral Sci* 47:71-76, 2005.

76. Hunter T, Pines J: Cyclin and cancer II: cyclin D and CDK inhibitors come of age, *Cell* 79:573-582, 1994.

77. Lundberg AS, Weinberg RA: Control of the cell cycle and apoptosis, *Eur J Cancer* 35:1886-1894, 1999.

78. Goodger NM, Gannon J, Hunt T, et al: Cell cycle regulatory proteins: an overview with relevance to oral cancer, *Oral Oncol* 33:61-73, 1997.

79. Pande P, Mathur MR, Shukia NK, et al: pRb and p16 protein alterations in human oral tumorigenesis, *Oral Oncol* 34(B):396-403, 1998.

80. Pavelic ZP, Lasmar M, Pavelic L, et al: Absence of retinoblastoma gene product in human primary oral cavity carcinomas, *Eur J Cancer B Oral Oncol* 32(B):347-351, 1996.

81. Serrano M, Hannon GJ, Beach D: A new regulatory motif in cell cycle control causing specific inhibition of cyclin-D/CDK4, *Nature* 366:704-707, 1993.

82. Kamb A, Gruis NA, Weaver-Feldhaus J, et al: A cell cycle regulator potentially involved in genesis of many tumor types, *Science* 264:436-440, 1994.

83. Wu CL, Roz L, McKown S, et al: DNA studies underestimate the major role of CDKN2A inactivation in oral and oropharyngeal squamous cell carcinomas, *Genes Chromosomes Cancer* 25:16-25, 1999.

84. Loughran O, Malliri A, Owens D, et al: Association of CDKN2A/p16INK4A with human head and neck keratinocyte replicative senescence: relationship of dysfunction to immortality and neoplasia, *Oncogene* 13:561-568, 1996.

85. Papadimitrakopoulou V, Izzo J, Lippman SM, et al: Frequent inactivation of p16ink4a in oral premalignant lesions, *Oncogene* 14:1799-1803, 1997.

86. Bova RJ, Quinn DI, Nankervis JS, et al: Cyclin D1 and p16INK4a expression predict reduced survival in carcinoma of the anterior tongue, *Clin Cancer Res* 5:2810-2819, 1999.

87. Boyle JO, Hakim J, Koch W, et al: The incidence of p53 mutations increases with progression of head and neck cancer, *Cancer Res* 53:4477-4480, 1993.

88. Caamano J, Rosvold EA, Bauer B, et al: p53 alterations in human squamous cell carcinomas and carcinoma cell lines, *Am J Pathol* 142:1131-1139, 1993.

89. Baral R, Patnaik S, Das BR: Co-overexpression of p53 and c-myc proteins is linked with advance stages of betel and tobacco related oral squamous cell carcinoma from eastern India, *Eur J Oral Sci* 106:907-913, 1998.

90. Shin DM, Lee JS, Lippman SM, et al: p53 expressions: predicting recurrence and second primary tumors in head and neck squamous cell carcinoma, *J Natl Cancer Inst* 88:519-529, 1996.

91. Sigal A, Rotter V: Oncogenic mutations of the p53 tumor suppressor: the demons of the guardian of the genome, *Cancer Res* 60:6788-6793, 2000.

92. Temam S, Flahault A, Perie S, et al: p53 gene status as a predictor of tumor response to induction chemotherapy of patients with locoregionally advanced squamous cell carcinomas of the head and neck, *J Clin Oncol* 18:385-394, 2000.

93. Warnakulasuriya S, Jia C, Johnson N, et al: p53 and P-glycoprotein expression are significant prognostic markers in advanced head and neck cancer treated with chemo/radiotherapy, *J Pathol* 191:33-38, 2000.

94. Sidransky D, Boyle J, Koch W: Molecular screening: prospects for a new approach, *Arch Otolaryngol Head Neck Surg* 119:1187-1190, 1993.

95. Song H, Xu Y: Gain of function of p53 cancer mutants in disrupting critical DNA damage response pathways, *Cell Cycle* 6:1570-1573, 2007.

96. Cabelguenne A, Blons H, de Waziers I, et al: p53 alterations predict tumor response to neoadjuvant chemotherapy in head and neck squamous cell carcinoma: a prospective series, *J Clin Oncol* 18:1465-1473, 2000.

97. El Deiry WS, Tokino T, Velculescu VE, et al: WAF1, a potential mediator of p53 tumor suppression, *Cell* 75:817-825, 1993.

98. Sherr CJ, Roberts JM: Inhibitors of mammalian G_1 cyclin dependent kinases, *Genes Dev* 9:1149-1163, 1995.

99. Agarwal S, Mathur M, Shukla NK, et al: Expression of cyclin dependent kinase inhibitor p21 waf/cip1 in premalignant and malignant oral lesions: relationship with p53 status, *Oral Oncol* 34:353-360, 1998.

100. Kudo Y, Takata T, Ogawa I, et al: Expression of p53 and p21CIP/WAF1 proteins in oral epithelial dysplasias and squamous cell carcinomas, *Oncol Rep* 6:539-545, 1999.

101. Kroemer G: The proto-oncogene Bcl-2 and its role in regulating apoptosis. *Nat Med* 3:614-620, 1997.

102. Wilson GD, Saunders MI, Dische S, et al: bcl-2 expression in head and neck cancer: an enigmatic prognostic marker, *Int J Radiat Oncol Biol Phys* 49:435-441, 2001.

103. Popovic B, Jekic B, Novakovic I, et al: Bcl-2 expression in oral squamous cell carcinoma, *Ann N Y Acad Sci* 1095:19-25, 2007.

104. Bauer JA, Trask DK, Kumar B, et al: Reversal of cisplatin resistance with a BH3 mimetic, (-)-gossypol, in head and neck cancer cells: role of wild-type p53 and Bcl-XL, *Mol Cancer Ther* 4:1096-1104, 2005.

105. Oliver CL, Bauer JA, Wolter KG, et al: In vitro effects of the BH3 mimetic, (-)-gossypol, on head and neck squamous cell carcinoma cells, *Clin Cancer Res* 10:7757-7763, 2004.

106. Stewart SA, Weinberg RA: Telomerase and human tumorigenesis, *Semin Cancer Biol* 10:399-406, 2000.

107. Shay JW, Wright WE: Telomerase therapeutics for cancer: challenges and new directions, *Nat Rev Drug Discov* 5:577-584, 2006.

108. Hanahan D, Weinberg RA: The hallmarks of cancer, *Cell* 100:57-70, 2000.

109. Mao L, El-Naggar AK, Fan YH, et al: Telomerase activity in head and neck squamous cell carcinoma and adjacent tissues, *Cancer Res* 56:5600-5604, 1996.

110. Kannan S, Tahara H, Yokozaki H, et al: Telomerase activity in premalignant and malignant lesions of human oral mucosa, *Cancer Epidemiol Biomarkers Prev* 6:413-420, 1997.

111. Lee BK, Diebel E, Neukam FW, et al: Diagnostic and prognostic relevance of expression of human telomerase subunits in oral cancer, *Int J Oncol* 19:1063-1068, 2001.

112. Chen HH, Yu CH, Wang JT, et al: Expression of human telomerase reverse transcriptase (hTERT) protein is significantly associated with the progression, recurrence and prognosis of oral squamous cell carcinoma in Taiwan, *Oral Oncol* 43:122-129, 2007.

113. Folkman J: What is the evidence that tumors are angiogenesis dependent? *J Natl Cancer Inst* 82:4-6, 1990.

114. Bouck N, Stellmach V, Hsu H: How tumors become angiogenic, *Adv Cancer Res* 69:135-174, 1996.

115. Ferrara N, Gerber HP, LeCouter J: The biology of VEGF and its receptors, *Nat Med* 9:669-676, 2003.

116. Neufeld G, Cohen T, Gengrinovitch S, et al: Vascular endothelial growth factor (VEGF) and its receptors, *FASEB J* 13:9-22, 1999.

117. Cross MJ, Dixelius J, Matsumoto T, et al: VEGF receptor signal transduction, *Trends Biochem Sci* 28:488-494, 2003.

118. Kyzas PA, Cunta IW, Ioannidis JP: Prognostic significance of vascular endothelial growth factor immunohistochemical expression in head and neck squamous cell carcinoma: a meta-analysis, *Clin Cancer Res* 11:1434-1440, 2005.

119. Kyzas PA, Stefanou D, Batistatou A, et al: Potential autocrine function of vascular endothelial growth factor in head and neck cancer via vascular endothelial growth factor receptor-2, *Mod Pathol* 18:485-494, 2005.

120. Taipale J, Makinen T, Arighi E, et al: Vascular endothelial growth factor receptor-3, *Curr Top Microbiol Immunol* 237:85-96, 1999.

121. Plate K: From angiogenesis to lymphangiogenesis, *Nat Med* 7:151-152, 2001.

122. Skobe M, Hawighorst T, Jackson DG, et al: Induction of tumor lymphangiogenesis by VEGF-C promotes breast cancer metastasis, *Nat Med* 7:192-198, 2001.

123. Alitalo K, Carmeliet P: Molecular mechanisms of lymphangiogenesis in health and disease, *Cancer Cell* 1:219-227, 2002.

124. Shibuya M, Claesson-Welsh L: Signal transduction by VEGF receptors in regulation of angiogenesis and lymphangiogenesis, *Exp Cell Res* 312:549-560, 2006.

125. Beasley NJP, Prevo R, Banerji S, et al: Intratumoral lymphangiogenesis and lymph node metastasis in head and neck cancer. *Cancer Res* 62:1315-1320, 2002.

126. Dadras SS, Paul T, Bertoncini PT, et al: Tumor lymphangiogenesis: a novel prognostic indicator for cutaneous melanoma metastasis and survival, *Am J Pathol* 162:1951-1960, 2003.

127. Koch AE, Polverini PJ, Kunkel SL, et al: Interleukin-8 as a macrophage-derived mediator of angiogenesis, *Science* 258:1798-1801, 1992.

128. Fujimoto J, Sakaguchi H, Aoki I, et al: Clinical implications of expression of interleukin 8 related to angiogenesis in uterine cervical cancers, *Cancer Res* 60:2632-2635, 2000.

129. Cohen RF, Contrino J, Spiro JD, et al: Interleukin-8 expression by head and neck squamous cell carcinoma, *Arch Otolaryngol Head Neck Surg* 121:202-209, 1995.

130. Maruyama K, Zhang JZ, Nihei Y, et al: Regulatory effects of gamma-interferon on IL-6 and IL-8 secretion by cultured human keratinocytes and dermal fibroblasts, *J Dermatol* 22:901-906, 1995.

131. Richards BL, Eisma RJ, Spiro JD, et al: Coexpression of interleukin-8 receptors in head and neck squamous cell carcinoma, *Am J Surg* 174:507-512, 1997.

132. Chen Z, Malhotra PS, Thomas GR, et al: Expression of proinflammatory and proangiogenetic cytokines in patients with head and neck cancer, *Clin Cancer Res* 5:1369-1379, 1999.

133. Thiery JP: Epithelial-mesenchymal transitions in tumor progression, *Nat Rev Cancer* 2:442-454, 2002.

134. Cortesina G, Sacchi M, Bussi M, et al: Integrin expression in head and neck cancers, *Acta Otolaryngol* 115:328-330, 1995.

135. Jones J, Sugiyama M, Watt FM, et al: Integrin expression in normal, hyperplastic, dysplastic, and malignant oral epithelium, *J Pathol* 169:235-243, 1993.

136. Jones JL, Walker RA: Control of matrix metalloproteinase activity in cancer, *J Pathol* 183:377-379, 1997.

137. Hamidi S, Salo T, Kainulainen T, et al: Expression of $\alpha_v\beta_6$ integrin in oral leukoplakia, *Br J Cancer* 82:1433-1440, 2000.

138. Thomas GJ, Nystrom ML, Marshall JF: Alphabeta6 integrin in wound healing and cancer of the oral cavity, *J Oral Pathol Med* 35:1-10, 2006.

139. Takeichi M: Cadherin cell adhesion receptors as a morphogenetic regulator, *Science* 251:1451-1455, 1991.

140. Gumbiner BM: Cell adhesion: the molecular basis of tissue architecture and morphogenesis, *Cell* 84:345-357, 1996.

141. Diniz-Freitas M, Garcia-Caballero T, Antunez-Lopez J, et al: Reduced E-cadherin expression is an indicator of unfavorable prognosis in oral squamous cell carcinoma, *Oral Oncol* 42:190-200, 2006.

142. Kawamata H, Uchida D, Hamano H, et al: Active-MMP2 in cancer cell nests of oral cancer patients: correlation with lymph node metastasis. *Int J Oncol* 13:699-704, 1998.

143. Kurahara S, Shinohara M, Ikebe T, et al: Expression of matrix metalloproteinase-2 relates to lymph node metastasis of squamous cell carcinoma of oral cavity: a clinicopathologic study, *Am J Clin Pathol* 99:18-23, 1999.

144. Muller D, Wolf C, Abecassis J, et al: Increased stromelysin 3 gene expression is associated with increased local invasiveness in head and neck squamous cell carcinomas, *Cancer Res* 53:165-169, 1993.

145. Kusukawa J, Sasaguri Y, Morimatsu M, et al: Expression of matrix metalloproteinase-3 in stage I and II squamous cell carcinoma of the oral cavity, *J Oral Maxillofac Surg* 53:530-534, 1995.

146. Lippman SM, Sudbo J, Hong WK: Oral cancer prevention and the evolution of molecular-targeted drug development, *J Clin Oncol* 23:346-356, 2005.

147. Li S, Schmitz KR, Jeffrey PD, et al: Structural basis for inhibition of the epidermal growth factor receptor by cetuximab, *Cancer Cell* 7:301-311, 2005.

148. Govindan SV, Griffiths GL, Hansen HJ, et al: Cancer therapy with radiolabeled and drug/toxin-conjugated antibodies, *Technol Cancer Res Treat* 4:375-391, 2005.

149. Bonner JA, Harari PM, Giralt J, et al: Radiotherapy plus cetuximab for squamous cell carcinoma of the head and neck, *N Engl J Med* 354:567-578, 2006.

150. Vanhoefer U, Tewes M, Rojo F, et al: Phase I study of the humanized antiepidermal growth factor receptor monoclonal antibody EMD72000 in patients with advanced solid tumors that express the epidermal growth factor receptor, *J Clin Oncol* 22:175-184, 2004.

151. Alekshun T, Garrett C: Targeted therapies in the treatment of colorectal cancers, *Cancer Control* 12:105-110, 2005.

152. Kim GP, Erlichman C: Oxaliplatin in the treatment of colorectal cancer, *Expert Opin Drug Metab Toxicol* 3:281-294, 2007.

153. Soulieres D, Senzer NN, Vokes EE, et al: Multicenter phase II study of erlotinib, an oral epidermal growth factor receptor tyrosine kinase inhibitor, in patients with recurrent or metastatic squamous cell cancer of the head and neck, *J Clin Oncol* 22:77-85, 2004.

154. Ahmed SM, Mubeen, Jigna VR: Molecular biology: an early detector of oral cancers, *Ann Diagn Pathol* 13:140-145, 2009.

155. Clayman GL, el-Naggar AK, Lippman SM, et al: Adenovirus-mediated p53 gene transfer in patients with advanced recurrent head and neck squamous cell carcinoma, *J Clin Oncol* 16:2221-2232, 1998.

156. Bischoff JR, Kirn DH, Williams A, et al: An adenovirus mutant that replicates selectively in p53-deficient human tumor cells, *Science* 274:373-376, 1996.

157. Rudin CM, Cohen EE, Papadimitrakopoulou VA, et al: An attenuated adenovirus, ONYX-015, as mouthwash therapy for premalignant oral dysplasia, *J Clin Oncol* 21:4546-4552, 2003.

158. Ganly I, Kirn D, Eckhardt G, et al: A phase I study of Onyx-015, an E1B attenuated adenovirus, administered intratumorally to patients with recurrent head and neck cancer. *Clin Cancer Res* 6:798-806, 2000.

159. Nemunaitis J, Ganly I, Khuri F, et al: Selective replication and oncolysis in p53 mutant tumors with ONYX-015, an E1B-55kD gene-deleted adenovirus, in patients with advanced head and neck cancer: a phase II trial, *Cancer Res* 60:6359-6366, 2000.

160. Nemunaitis J, Khuri F, Ganly I, et al: Phase II trial of intratumoral administration of ONYX-015, a replication-selective adenovirus, in patients with refractory head and neck cancer, *J Clin Oncol* 19:289-298, 2001.

161. Khuri FR, Nemunaitis J, Ganly I, et al: A controlled trial of intratumoral ONYX-015, a selectively replicating adenovirus, in combination with cisplatin and 5-fluorouracil in patients with recurrent head and neck cancer, *Nat Med* 6:879-885, 2000.

162. Lamont JP, Nemunaitis J, Kuhn JA, et al: A prospective phase II trial of ONYX-015 adenovirus and chemotherapy in recurrent squamous cell carcinoma of the head and neck (the Baylor experience), *Ann Surg Oncol* 7:588-592, 2000.

163. Ciardiello F, Caputo R, Bianco R, et al: Inhibition of growth factor production and angiogenesis in human cancer cells by ZD 1839 (Iressa), a selective epidermal growth factor receptor tyrosine kinase inhibitor, *Clin Cancer Res* 7:1459-1465, 2001.

164. Yigitbasi OG, Younes MN, Doan D, et al: Tumor cell and endothelial cell therapy of oral cancer by dual tyrosine kinase receptor blockade, *Cancer Res* 64:7977-7984, 2004.

165. Prichard CN, Kim S, Yazici YD, et al: Concurrent cetuximab and bevacizumab therapy in a murine orthotopic model of anaplastic thyroid carcinoma, *Laryngoscope* 117:674-679, 2007.

166. Wedge SR, Kendrew J, Hennequin LF, et al: AZD2171: a highly potent, orally bioavailable, vascular endothelial growth factor receptor 2 tyrosine kinase inhibitor for the treatment of cancer, *Cancer Res* 65:4389-4400, 2005.

167. Gomez-Rivera F, Santillan-Gomez AA, Younes MN, et al: The tyrosine kinase inhibitor, AZD2171, inhibits vascular endothelial growth factor receptor signaling and growth of anaplastic thyroid cancer in an orthotopic nude mouse model, *Clin Cancer Res* 13:4519-4527, 2007.

168. Lin J, Lalani AS, Harding TC, et al: Inhibition of lymphogenous metastasis using adeno-associated virus–mediated gene transfer of a soluble VEGFR-3 decoy receptor, *Cancer Res* 65:6901-6909, 2005.

169. Pytowski B, Goldman J, Persaud K, et al: Complete and specific inhibition of adult lymphatic regeneration by a novel VEGFR-3 neutralizing antibody, *J Natl Cancer Inst* 97:14-21, 2005.

170. DeRisi J, Penland L, Brown PO, et al: Use of a cDNA microarray to analyse gene expression patterns in human cancer, *Nat Genet* 14:457-460, 1996.

171. Snijders AM, Schmidt BL, Fridlyand J, et al: Rare amplicons implicate frequent deregulation of cell fate specification pathways in oral squamous cell carcinoma, *Oncogene* 24:4232-4242, 2005.

172. Petricoin EF, Ardekani AM, Hitt BA, et al: Use of proteomic patterns in serum to identify ovarian cancer, *Lancet* 359:572-577, 2002.

173. Adam BL, Qu Y, Davis JW, et al: Serum protein fingerprinting coupled with a pattern-matching algorithm distinguishes prostate cancer from benign prostate hyperplasia and healthy men, *Cancer Res* 62:3609-3614, 2002.

174. Pickering V, Jordan RC, Schmidt BL: Elevated salivary endothelin levels in oral cancer patients—a pilot study, *Oral Oncol* 43:37-41, 2007.

175. Looser KG, Shah JP, Strong EW: The significance of "positive" margins in surgically resected epidermoid carcinomas, *Head Neck Surg* 1:107-111, 1978.

176. Chen TY, Emrich LJ, Driscoll DL: The clinical significance of pathological findings in surgically resected margins of the primary tumor in head and neck carcinoma, *Int J Radiat Oncol Biol Phys* 13:833-837, 1987.

177. Slootweg PJ, Hordijk GJ, Schade Y, et al: Treatment failure and margin status in head and neck cancer. A critical view on the potential value of molecular pathology, *Oral Oncol* 38:500-503, 2002.

178. Brennan JA, Mao L, Hruban RH, et al: Molecular assessment of histopathological staging in squamous-cell carcinoma of the head and neck, *N Engl J Med* 332:429-435, 1995.

Principles of Distraction Osteogenesis

Chapter **11**

Cesar A. Guerrero, Helen Rivera, Elena V. Mujica, Mariana Henriquez, Marianela Gonzalez

Distraction osteogenesis is a relatively new surgical technique based on the principle of "tension stress" that allows lengthening of bone and surrounding soft tissues through progressively controlled fracture separation by means of a distraction device.

The first attempt at lengthening a femoral fracture was performed by Alessandro Codivilla (1905) in Bologna, Italy, but it was not until the 1950s that Gavril Ilizarov from Kurgan, Russia, popularized the method to widen or lengthen limbs. Various publications of animal and clinical trials to increase the size and width of the facial bones can be found in the literature; however, the nineties offered a new stage for the growth and development of distraction osteogenesis in the craniofacial skeleton. After our publications in 1990 and 1992 on mandibular widening, McCarthy in 1992 on craniofacial microsomia, and later Ortiz-Monasterio and Molina on treatment of the mid-face, this new technology has improved and been widely popularized as a result of better instrumentation, miniaturized distraction appliances, multi-vectorial devices, and use of the intraoral, transconjunctival, and coronal approaches to avoid facial scars. Nevertheless, success in surgery and postoperative follow-up is based on sound biologic and biomechanical principles.

BIOLOGIC PRINCIPLES OF DISTRACTION OSTEOGENESIS

PROTOCOL FOR DISTRACTION

Distraction osteogenesis is indicated for patients with deficiencies or bone discontinuity who have adequate blood supply, sufficient quantity and quality of bone, and ideal surrounding tissues; such patients need to be reliable and intelligent to understand and follow the postoperative instructions.

Osteotomy

The incision and reflection of soft tissues to perform the surgery must be as limited as possible so that the blood supply is not diminished, which is mainly responsible for healing and mineralization. The bone cuts are performed under abundant irrigation, ideally with lactated Ringer solution, and every effort is made to avoid overheating of bone and damage to soft tissues. Once the bone is fractured, the soft tissues are carefully and meticulously closed in layers. The presence of the distraction device under the periosteum would limit bone healing, contract the distraction chamber, and permit saliva and contamination into the distraction area. Ideally, the distraction device should be placed away from the osteotomy site.

Latency Period

After the osteotomy is performed and the soft tissues closed carefully, the distraction device must be activated to open the bone gap 1 or 2 mm. This space will fill with blood, which consolidates, and collagen fibers will advance to bridge the gap; between 6 and 7 days is needed for completion of this process. In addition, undifferentiated cells and morphogenetic proteins accumulate on the sides of the fracture. This interval, during which there is no activation of distraction and the patient is maintained on a liquid diet, is called the latency period.

Activation Period

After 7 days of resting while the collagen fibers develop, activation of the appliance is initiated at a rate of 1 mm/day in one treatment or divided into two or three sessions per day or at a rate of 0.5 mm/day for very small bone fragments, such as for alveolar distraction or patients with compromised blood supply. This is called the *rhythm and rate of distraction* (i.e., the amount of activation and how often). The collagen fibers are stretched slowly and progressively until the

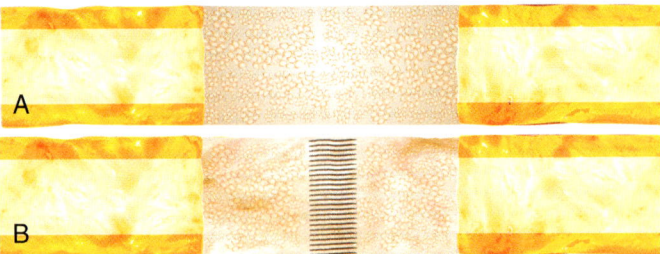

Fig. 11-1 ▪ **A,** Ideal situation in which the bone has been lengthened and all the variables controlled to obtain bone identical to the adjacent bone. The soft tissues must be intact and the protocol followed meticulously. **B,** The fibrous interzone is the last to mineralize.

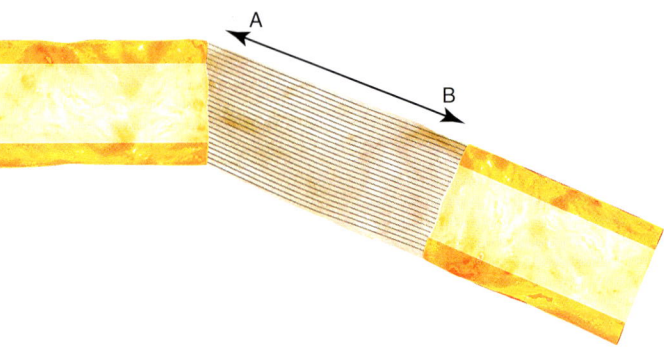

Fig. 11-2 ▪ The collagen fibers will stretch in a straight fashion, from point A to point B.

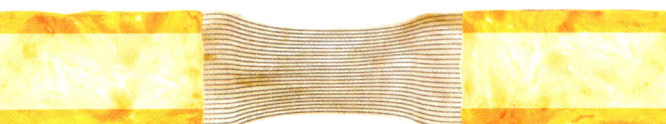

Fig. 11-3 ▪ In longer movements the periosteal layer contracts and creates a defect called an "hourglass" deformity.

desired movement has been accomplished. The space created within the fractured bony parts is called the distraction chamber, and the chamber box has six walls, two limited by bone and four limited by periosteum. The entire chamber is filled with collagen fibers, and nutrients for mineralization are obtained from neighboring tissues. The patient is maintained on a liquid diet until the end of the activation period, at which time acrylic is applied to the distractor to make it rigid, and the diet is advanced to soft foods.

Consolidation

The time between the end of the activation period and complete bone mineralization of the chamber is the consolidation period. Obviously, many variables are involved in this critical period: the quality and quantity of the original bone, the amount of movement, the age of the patient, the rigidity of the appliance, and the surgical site. The new instrumentation and miniaturized distractors allow the surgical devices to be kept in place for much longer periods, which permits mineralization to become advanced before considering removal of the appliance. The basic rule is to remove the distractors once adequate radiopacity is observed on radiographs. Because extraoral appliances were used in the initial period of distraction osteogenesis, there was a tendency to remove the appliances before proper mineralization to avoid the psychological impact and reduce scar formation around the surgical facial pins; major relapse and the need for secondary surgeries were common. Other surgeons suggested that the bone fragments be rigidly fixated once distraction was accomplished, and thus two major surgical interventions were needed.

Intraoral, transconjunctival, and coronal approaches permit surgeons to perform distraction osteogenesis without facial scars and, by using the new miniaturized distraction devices, allow prolongation of the consolidation period without considering removal of the appliances. Once activation is completed, mineralization starts at the two bony walls, with major contributions from the periosteum. Deposition of minerals begin at either end of the chamber (Fig. 11-1, A) and advances into the mid-chamber, with a fibrous island called the fibrous interzone (Fig. 11-1, B) left in the middle. The fibrous interzone reduces slowly and progressively until complete disappearance, after which the consolidation period is completed and the patient is advised to have the distractors removed.

This healing process of mineralization and bone maturation starts after activation is completed, and depending on certain variables, especially the amount of movement and the age of the patient, 2 to 24 months is needed. Creation of a curve or molding of the regenerate bone is not possible because according to the biomechanical concept of lengthening the bone from point A to point B, there is no other bone shape possible but a straight line between the two separated points (Fig. 11-2). In addition, the more extensive the bone movement, the narrower the mid-chamber because the periosteal

layer contracts as the distraction device is activated further; this phenomenon is called the "hourglass deformity" (Fig. 11-3) and is particularly important since this is the weakest point in the bone and the place where post-treatment fractures occur.

Remodeling Period

Once the distractors are removed, patients progress to normal living and daily activities, the healed bone undergoes regular tension from the muscles and normal biting forces, and the soft tissues surrounding the bones exert regular tension over the tissues; this process will transform the bone and allow definitive healing and final reshaping.

The healing process of distraction osteogenesis is variable and depends on the tissues involved in maxillary or mandibular lengthening.

BIOLOGY

BONE LENGTHENING

Once the osteotomy has been performed and the latency and activation periods completed, the distraction chamber, filled with collagen fibers, will undergo cell differentiation. Mesenchymal cells situated in the periphery of the osteotomy gap will invade the chamber and turn into osteoblasts, chondroblasts, or fibroblasts, depending on the magnitude of strain, rigidity of the callus, and movement (Fig. 11-4). Different histologic patterns can be observed in the various stages of bone healing (Figs. 11-5 and 11-6).

The histologic pattern within the distraction chamber is uniform, and bone differentiation and metabolism depend on mechanical loading. Bone healing is achieved by maturation of the collagen template and deposition of osteoid by osteoblast proliferation, and levels of osteocalcin and osteonectin are increased as woven and lamellar bone develops. Even though both the endosteum (both bony walls) and periosteum make contributions to osteoid deposition, the periosteum is more important and justifies a non-invasive surgical technique to keep the periosteal layer intact (Fig. 11-7).

The new tissue forms in a direction parallel to the vector of traction, spindle-shaped fibroblasts appear in the distraction gap, the

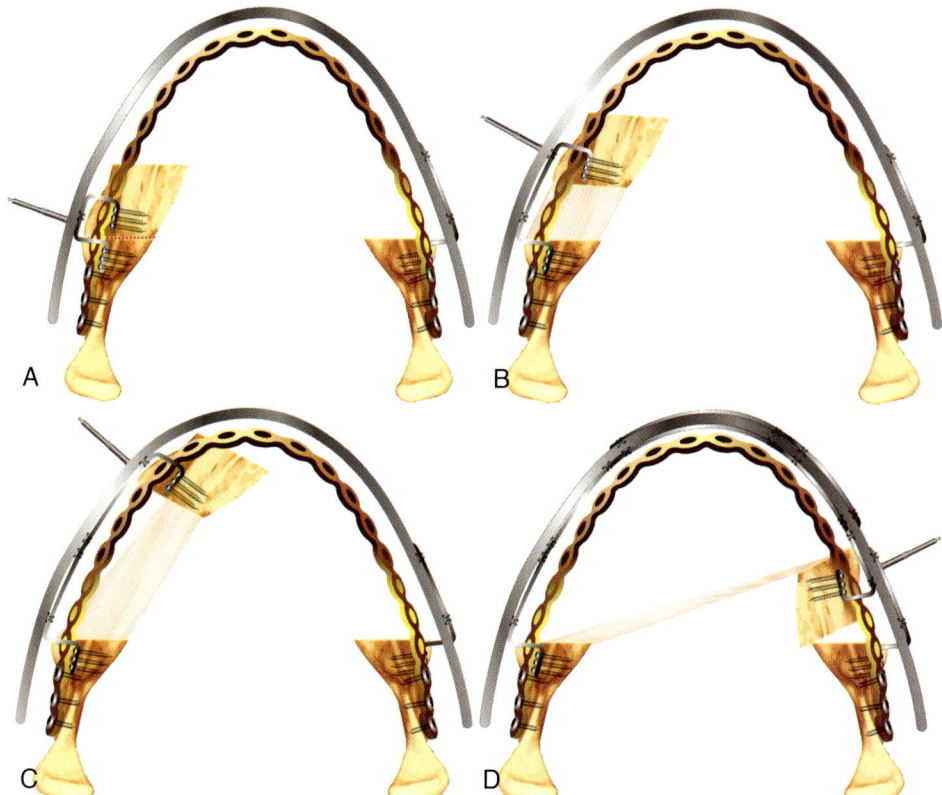

Fig. 11-4 ■ **A,** The distractor device is placed in position and the osteotomy is performed. **B,** After a latency period, activation is performed and collagen fibers begin to stretch in the direction of the distracted segment. **C,** Bone formation depends on the collagen fibers that had been stretched and mineralization, which proceeds from point A to point B. **D,** Understanding the biology is fundamental for predicting the development of new bone. Even though the distraction process proceeded all around the plate, clinically it is a complete failure because of bone across the reconstruction plate, a result contrary to the surgeon's plan.

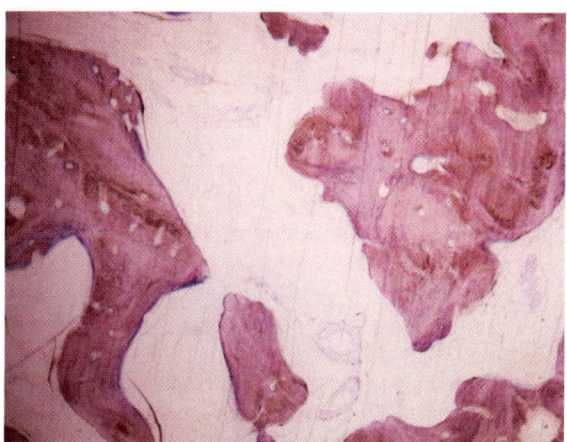

Fig. 11-5 ■ Microscopic examination shows trabecular bone (hematoxylin-eosin stain; ×40) within the distractor chamber.

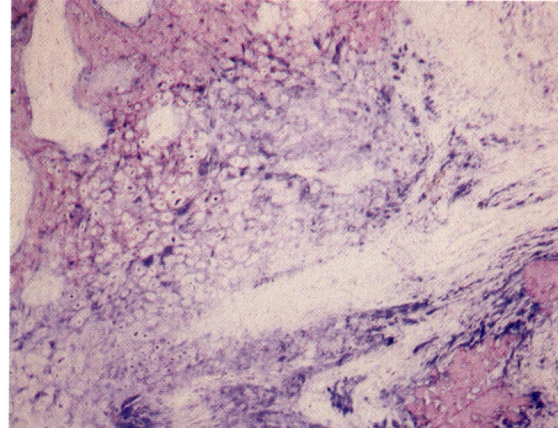

Fig. 11-6 ■ Docking site surgery. During bone transport, the wall facing the defect and traveling through develops fibrous and cartilage tissue that needs to be removed, with activation being continued until bone continuity is reached. The bone edges require perforations to make them bleed, and cancellous bone should be placed for faster consolidation until bone continuity is achieved.

peripheral vascular supply extends into the chamber and starts the process of mineralization, and osteoblasts proliferate within the collagen matrix and initiate osteoid deposition with the creation of bone spicules. In addition, chondroblasts start depositing chondroid, but to a minor degree, depending on the rigidity and stability of the distraction frame; if excess movement is present, more fibrous tissue and cartilage production will be seen. These islands of cartilage will become encased in the bone matrix and are of no clinical significance unless they are abundant. Mineralization occurs from either end

of the bony walls and from the periosteal layer in the periphery and finally bridges the center to eliminate the fibrous interzone, the last area to consolidate. Haversian remodeling is the final stage of cortical healing and results in maturity and mechanical stability (Fig. 11-8).

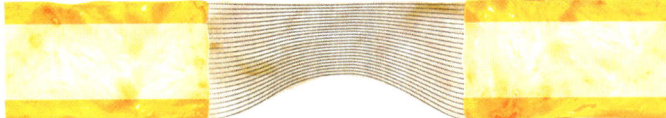

Fig. 11-7 ■ The typical collagen fibers frame after periosteal disruption and diminished blood supply in one wall. When the distractor is applied to the buccal surface and the periosteum is not sewn back, the other remaining three walls will create ideal bone with collapse under the distractor where the layer was interrupted.

MUSCLE LENGTHENING

Most surgeons consider distraction osteogenesis as merely bone lengthening and think that the surrounding tissues should "just" accommodate; however, there are important issues regarding function and relapse that are related to the fact that as muscles lengthen, different healing processes become relevant to the health and position of the bone.

The distraction movement will lengthen striated muscle, and the adaptation is usually well tolerated when the direction is parallel to

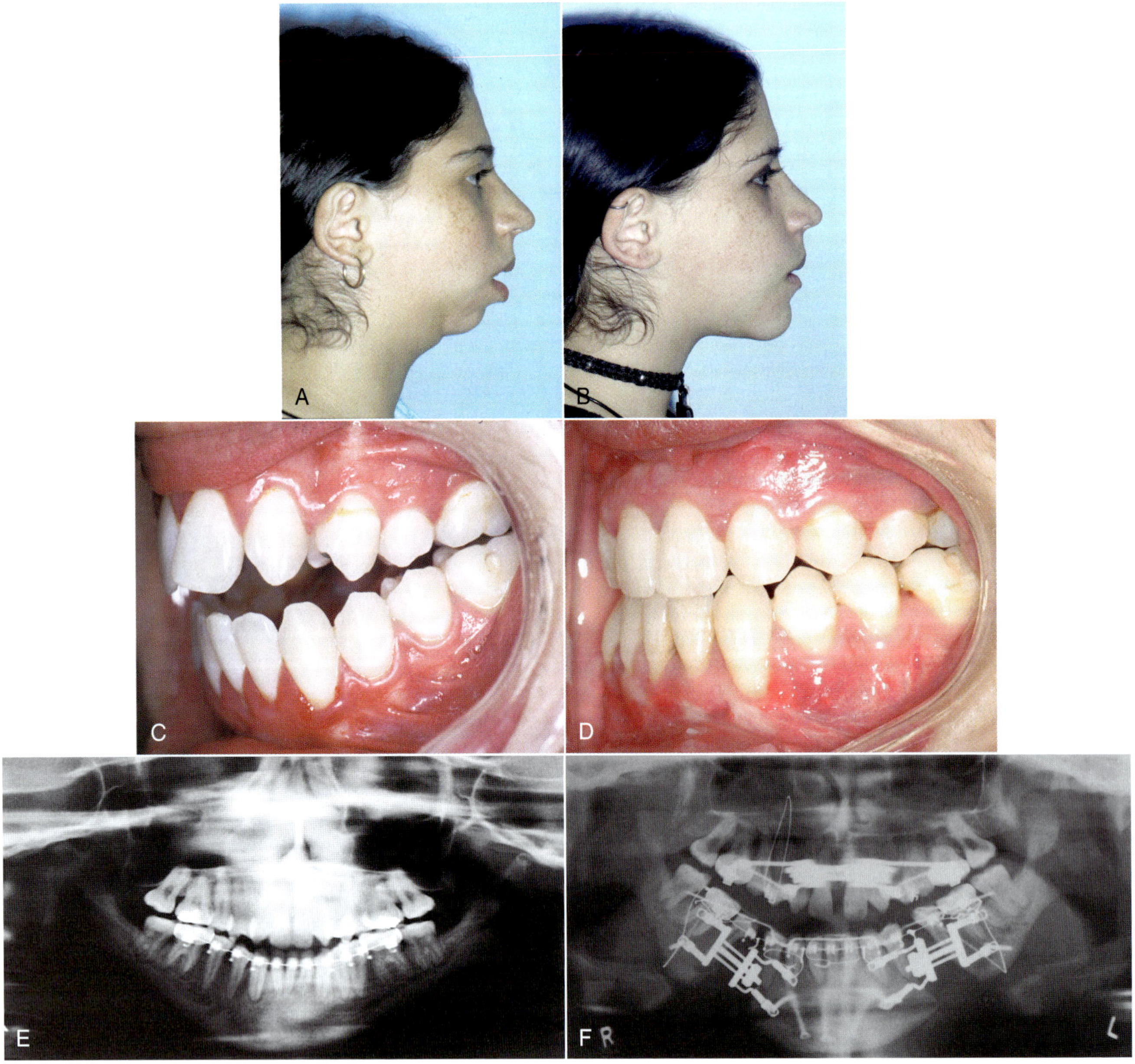

Fig. 11-8 ■ Treacher Collins syndrome and Pierre Robin sequence in an 18-year-old woman. Profile views were obtained preoperatively (**A**) and after mandibular lengthening with combined genioplasty (**B**). Mandibular lengthening of 24 mm at the inferior border of the mandible and 12-mm chin advancement were achieved for a total of 36-mm anterior mandibular movement. Lateral intraoral views were obtained before (**C**) and after (**D**) treatment. **E**, Preoperative panoramic radiograph. **F**, Panoramic radiograph during mandibular and maxillary activation. Observe the radiolucent distraction sites at the premolars and at the maxillary midline.

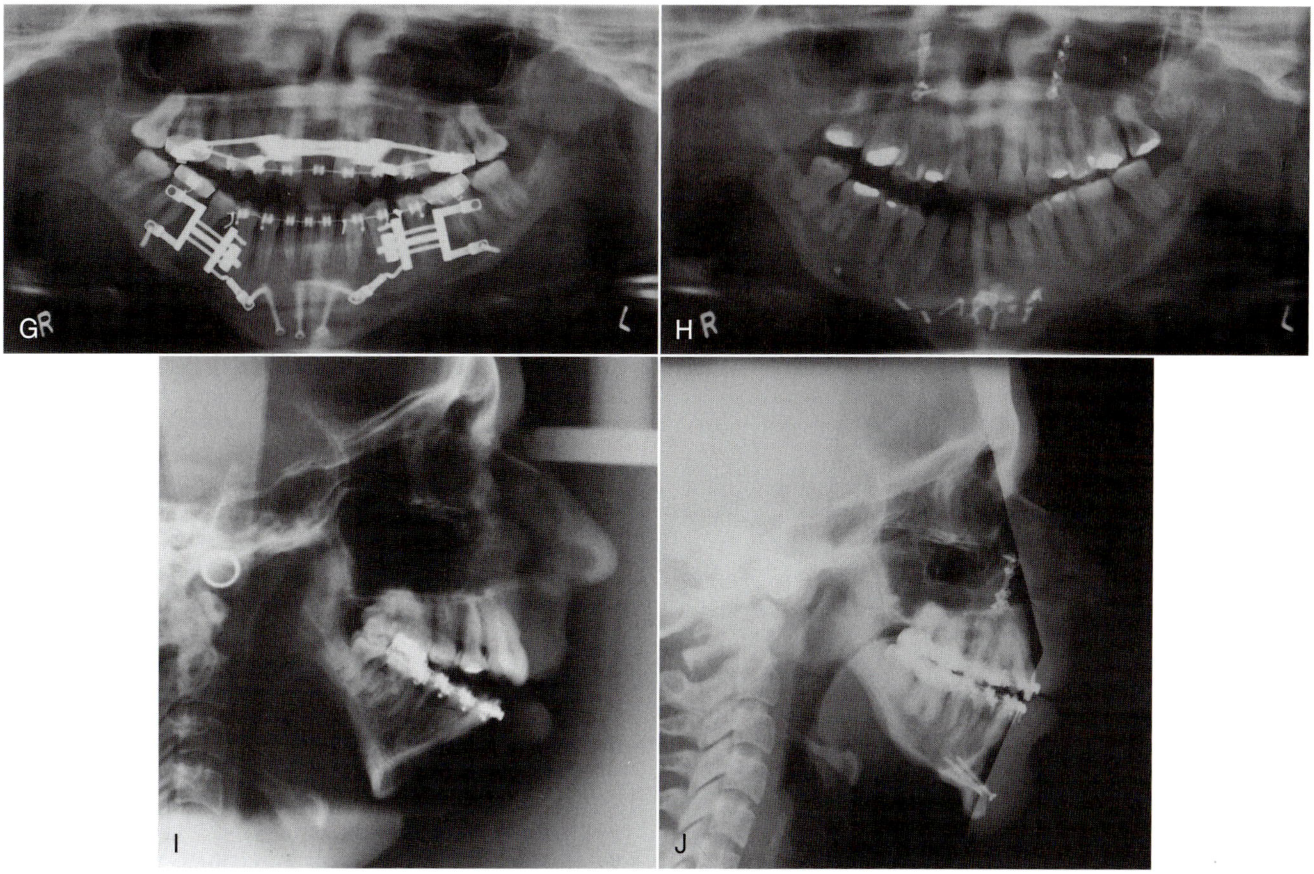

Fig. 11-8, cont'd ■ **G,** Panoramic radiograph after activation for mandibular lengthening and maxillary widening was completed. **H,** Postoperative panoramic radiograph at the 6-year follow-up. Preoperative (**I**) and postoperative (**J**) lateral radiographs show inadequate anatomy for sagittal split osteotomy and reduced bone quantity posterior to the second molar area, which compromises distraction osteogenesis at this level. An anterior open bite is also evident. Mandibular lengthening is performed at the body site, anterior to the mental nerve. This is the ideal surgical technique for a deformed or inadequate mandibular ramus or after previous failures. Differential distraction between the inferior border and alveolar crest permits closure of the open bite and major gnathion-gonion advancements. Double trips were performed to advance the mandible by changing the vector and combining a Le Fort I osteotomy with genioplasty to achieve a true inferior border of the mandible with an increase of 36 mm.

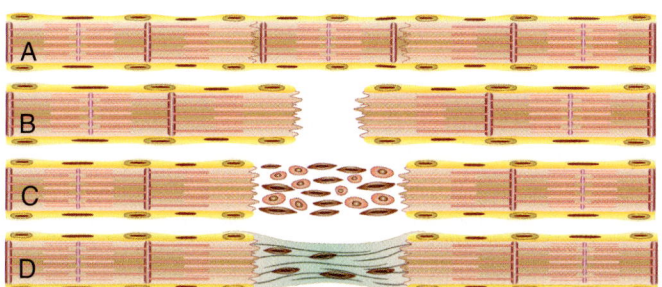

Fig. 11-9 ■ **A,** Ideal muscle regeneration in which sarcomeres increase in number at the origin and insertion. **B,** Rupture of muscle sarcomeres. **C,** Fibroblast migration. **D,** Fibrous tissue invasion and sclerosis formation after muscle rupture caused by exceeding the distraction limits.

the distraction. The areas M and Z (Fig. 11-9, *A*) are stretched initially, and this will create pressure at the origin and insertion of the muscle and stimulate the creation of new sarcomeres at either end of the myotendinous junction, or new ones could be created within the muscle mass, called intercalary new sarcomeres. As distraction

activation continues, the inner pressure of the muscle increases and induces fibers to rupture (Fig. 11-9, *B* and *C*); these fibers may heal by muscle regeneration or by sclerosis and fibrosis (Fig. 11-9, *D*). Staged activations decrease muscle damage since DNA synthesis is higher with multiple small activations, such as four 0.25-mm activations in 24 hours.

After lengthening, mandibular hypomobility develops in some patients secondary to muscle edema and spasm, as well as muscle widening when forces are applied in a plane perpendicular to the insertion of the muscle. Active physiotherapy is mandatory for all patients to achieve the goals of mouth opening and mandibular translation in the early postoperative phase. In any event, there will be situations in which distraction osteogenesis should be performed in different surgical stages to avoid the functional complications and relapse associated with large movements; for any lengthening of more than 25% of the original bone size, several stages should be considered. It is also important to measure the different muscles involved in a predetermined direction. For example, a 20-mm mandibular anteroposterior advancement in the mandibular angle in an 80-mm-long mandible corresponds to bone lengthening of 20%, but the geniohyoid muscle undergoes 35% lengthening and the masseter muscle is widened 40%; both muscles will be very susceptible to contraction, relapse, and diminished functionally postoperatively, and hypomobility usually occurs.

The muscles will increase in length via different mechanisms: increasing numbers of sarcomeres either at the insertion and origin or within the muscle mass. If tolerance is exceeded, fibrous tissue invades the ruptured areas and produces fibrosis and mandibular hypomobility. The ideal rhythm and rate need to be followed and the limit of 25% of the original muscle length not be surpassed.

NERVE LENGTHENING

Nerve lengthening in cranio-maxillofacial surgery is not as important as it would be in orthopedic surgery, where femoral or tibial lengthening of greater than 25% would produce paralysis of the limb, as opposed to paresthesia of the lower lip. However, understanding the physiology and biology associated with distraction may help in reducing this nerve injury problem.

The surgical plan should avoid lengthening the nerve as much as possible; in lengthening of the mandible, performing sagittal split or body osteotomies anterior to the mental nerve would allow major movements without injuring the mandibular nerve. Distraction osteogenesis is usually indicated in clinical situations in which traditional surgery with minor movements would not achieve the desired goal. Avoidance of the mandibular body area where the nerve is in the canal should be the obvious reasoning, and advancing the distal segment anterior to the mental nerve after sagittal split osteotomy should permit the surgeon the desired advancement without needing to deal with the alveolar nerve.

Histologically, there are three possibilities after distraction. First, the nerve may exhibit perineural thickening and decreased surface area of axons, various axonal abnormalities, myelin thickening, and disruption of the lamellar pattern, and there is a direct relationship between the number of millimeters advanced and alterations in the nerve. Second, the nerve can be damaged during surgery and have no axonal connection, with the subsequent development of fibrosis. Third, a distractor screw can be placed within the nerve canal and cause damage to or displace neural structures.

DISTRACTION OSTEOGENESIS AND THE PERIODONTAL LIGAMENT

The periodontal fibers are divided into gingival, transseptal, alveolar crestal, horizontal, oblique, and apical fibers; their main purpose is tooth attachment and support during function. When the osteotomy is planned to be performed between teeth, careful evaluation with orthodontic involvement is necessary. Leaving enough bone between the roots is fundamental, and surgery has to be performed meticulously with the use of thin saws after weakening the bone with a 701 burr and finalizing the cut with a spatula osteotome—all under abundant irrigation to avoid overheating of bone and teeth necrosis. The ideal scenario is a fracture within the bone with two complete bony walls and no perforations in the periodontal ligament (PDL). Even though there is no communication to the PDL, the transseptal fibers will be stretched as the activation proceeds. This interdental tension will incline the teeth into the chamber into immature tissues, with possible complications such as gingival recession, ankylosed teeth, interdental fibrosis, and dental pulp necrosis with changes in color. The orthodontist has to integrate the teeth on either side via brackets secured with a metallic ligature in a figure of eight to ensure the absence of mobility after activation and allow the formation of immature bone that will progress in time to maturity; the soft tissues are lengthened to keep the bone from contacting saliva and to avoid contamination of the developed distraction chamber with food. The

teeth will be moved medially after 10 to 12 weeks of consolidation by controlled, slow progressive movement of about 1 mm/mo per side. Usually, a plastic tooth or pontic (with a bracket) is fixed between the teeth and secured with metallic ligatures to the brackets, and the pontic is reduced on either side every 4 weeks to allow mobilization of the teeth via an elastic chain fixed to the brackets. This movement should not be commenced before 3 months of consolidation so that the teeth can be moved into mature bone. This protocol guarantees excellent bone height, good bone architecture, intact dental roots, and an excess of interdental papillae, the latter being achieved by lengthening of gingival tissue. As the teeth are brought together, there is an excess of interdental gingival tissue, which will mature and contract according to the crestal bone height.

If the osteotomy is performed without enough bone space between the roots, the PDL or the dental root could be exposed to the distraction chamber, the biologic process is different, the collagen fibers will be formed from one side with a much lower level on the tooth side, bone maturation is much stronger on the bone side, and the level on the invaded PDL side is lower. The rhythm of distraction should be slower and the rate decreased to overcome this problem. By distracting the bones in slower fashion, the gingival tissues are maintained at the original good level and the maturation process will also be slower, but the gingival level and tooth movement should be adequate at the end of treatment, with no consequences.

The teeth should be maintained apart by means of metallic ligatures as the distraction process proceeds while avoiding tooth inclination or translation into the distraction chamber; once the bone attains moderate mineralization, the teeth should be moved into the distraction gap slowly and progressively, around 1 mm/mo per side. With inclined teeth that need to be placed upright, moving them into the collagen fiber network before sufficient bone maturation will result in complications, delays in orthodontic treatment, and the aforementioned complications of gingival recession and dental necrosis. In contrast, when orthodontic treatment is not initiated until after 2 months of consolidation because of patient irresponsibility or the orthodontist being afraid of dealing with the patient after surgery, mineralization will continue and convert the regular soft bone into well-calcified and sometimes hypermineralized bone, with subsequent alveolar contraction and decreased bone height; in this situation it is complicated to mobilize the teeth into the newly formed bone, treatment is delayed, and it may even be impossible to completely close the dental diastema.

BONE TRANSPORT

The biology involved in distraction osteogenesis during bone transport is similar to that described at the osteotomy site; however, as the distraction chamber is progressively opened by the activation, the free segment (called a disc or bullet) is traveling across the soft tissues. The planned movement is based on translating the disc to dock into the receiving site and provide bone continuity to the resected or missing bony part.

The bone segment (disc or bullet) travels through soft tissues, and as the bone moves by being pushed with the distractor, cartilage-like tissue develops in the bone wall facing the scar and fibrous tissues secondary to poor blood supply and permanent compression; this round fibrocartilage cannot fuse to the receiving bone to complete the surgical plan. Docking site surgery is necessary to remove the fibrocartilage tissue, make holes in the bone cortex to allow bleeding, and further activate the appliance to unite the two bony segments. Locally obtained cancellous bone is then placed around the area to allow rigid and faster healing (Fig. 11-10). The

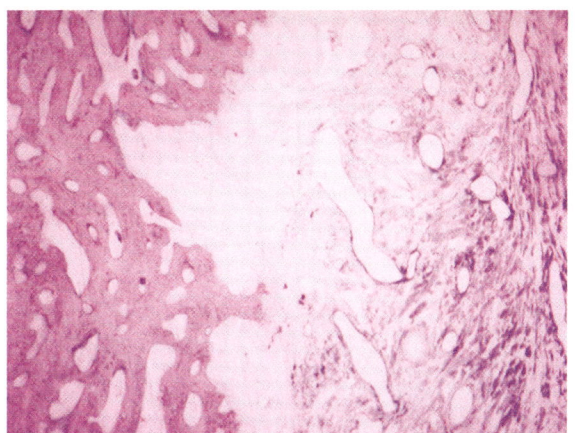

Fig. 11-10 ■ Histologic section of the docking site (hematoxylin-eosin stain; ×40) showing trabecular bone and fibrovascular tissue.

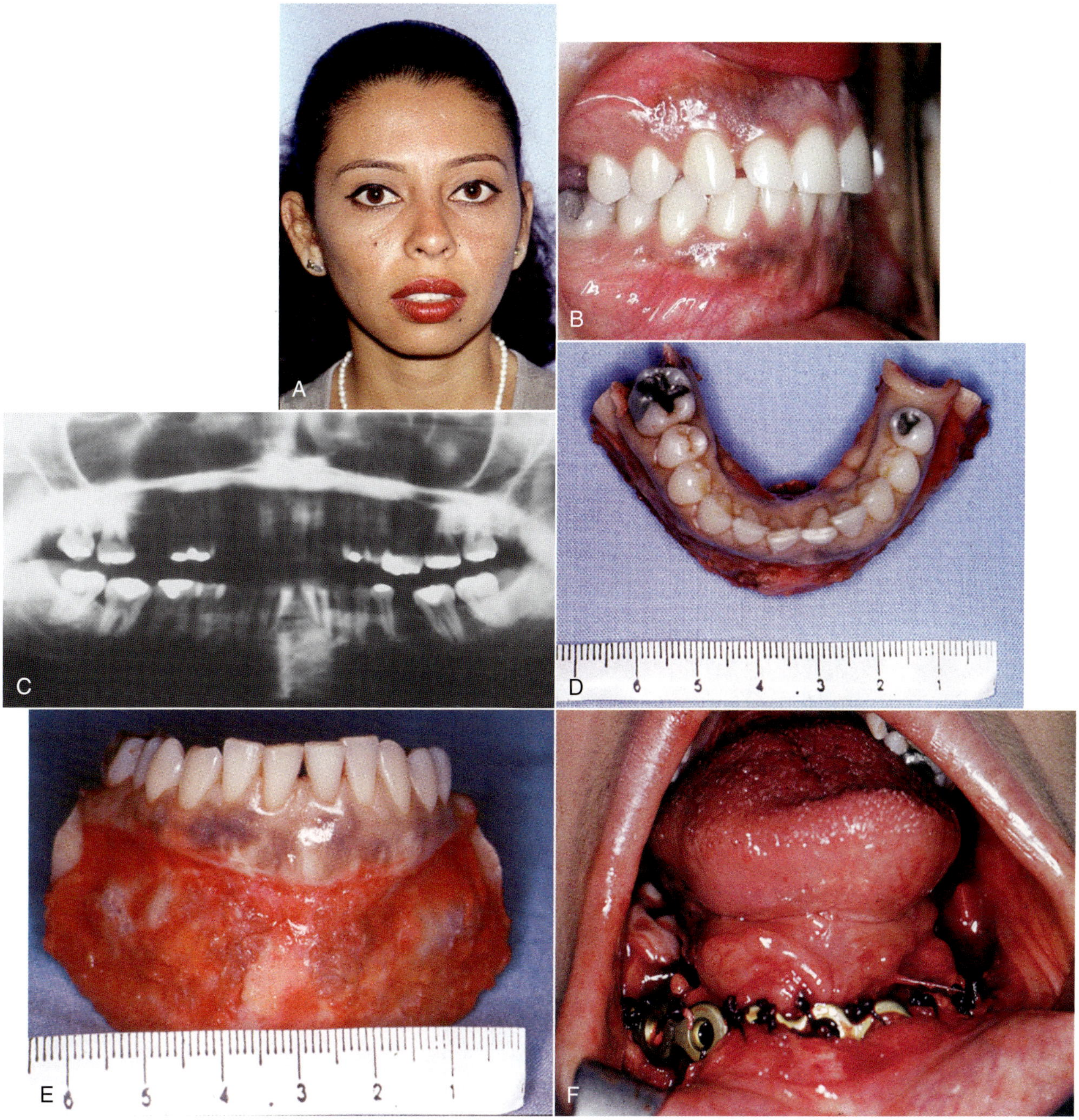

Fig. 11-11 ■ Preoperative frontal (**A**) and dental (**B**) views are shown of a 28-year-old patient with mandibular myxoma. Intraoral removal with immediate reconstruction by bone transport via distraction osteogenesis was performed. **C,** Preoperative panoramic radiograph. **D to F,** Gross mandibular resection specimen. An intraoral view was obtained of the reconstruction plate following the mandibular contour.

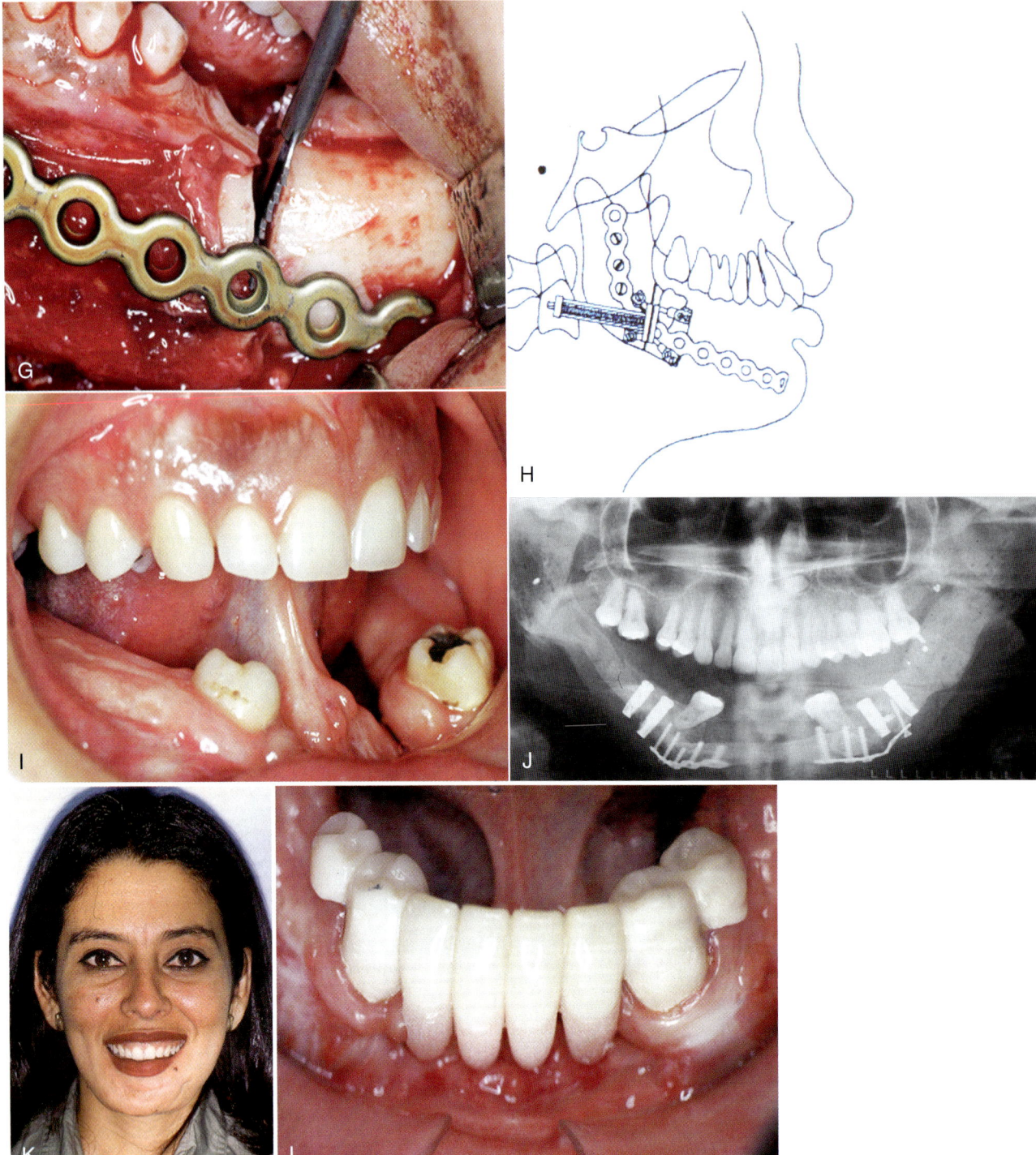

Fig. 11-11, cont'd ■ **G,** Mandibular plate fixed before resection of the lesion to maintain stability and positioning of the segment. **H,** Presurgical planning showing the mandibular reconstruction plate in position, the vertical osteotomy, and an intraoral distractor with the correct vector. **I,** There is no possibility of creating a curve with distraction because the collagen fibers run from point A to point B. **J,** Postoperative panoramic radiograph. Dental implants were inserted a year after surgery and a small bone graft placed in the symphyseal area for bone continuity. At the 10-year follow-up, a postoperative frontal view shows no extraoral scar (**K**), and a dental view (**L**) shows the prosthetic reconstruction placed in the new mandible.

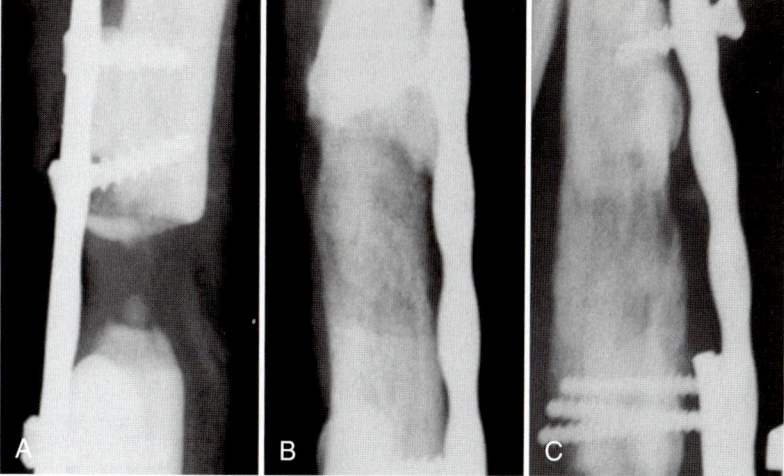

Fig. 11-12 ■ **A,** Group 1: bone discontinuity after partial resection and no surgery. **B,** Group 2: bone healing after bone transport by distraction osteogenesis. **C,** Group 3: bone healing after the application of bone morphogenetic protein-2 in a collagen carrier. Note the better and stronger bone consolidation 80 days after the treatment of a 12-mm bone defect (canine research study). (From Guerrero CA, Rojas A, Figueroa F, et al: Radiographic evaluation of traditional versus rhBMP-2 inducted intraoral bone transport in mandibular reconstruction. In Diner PA, Arnaud E, editors. 4th *International Congress of Maxillofacial and Craniofacial Distraction, Paris, France,* Bologna, Italy, 2003, Monduzzi Editore, pp 391-396.)

reconstruction plate should be left in place until adequate radiopacity is seen on radiographs to ensure mineralization. This process may take months, depending on the age of the patient, amount of movement, and quality and quantity of bone. The distractors should be removed once the activation is finalized and the docking site has been prepared to continue the consolidation period without the presence of the distractors (Fig. 11-11).

NEW MINIATUARIZED INTRAORAL DISTRACTORS

Advances in technology and instrumentation have allowed clinicians to use smaller, more comfortable intraoral devices. These developments have improved surgical outcomes, basically because the appliances may remain in position for longer periods without patient inconvenience and allow a more complete bone consolidation period with no relapse and no complications after removal of the distractors.

The activation devices have also been modified to permit access in remote locations in the facial skeleton and easy removal after finishing by twisting the activation bar in the opposite direction.

Some appliances have internal mechanisms for changing the vector of distraction during the activation phase to ensure adequate occlusion and ideal bone repositioning. In others, the vector can be changed at the end of distraction by removing and replacing certain screws in the anterior plate.

BLOOD MORPHOGENETIC PROTEINS TO SPEED UP MINERALIZATION

Distraction osteogenesis has many advantages over traditional surgery, including the capability of making large movements, avoidance of the multiple failures inherent in traditional surgical treatment, possibility of adjustment after surgery, no metal left in the surgical site at the end of treatment, avoidance of bone grafts, and the ability to perform "minor surgery" in medically compromised patients. However, historically, there have been two major drawbacks. One is the presence of the distractor, which was extraoral at the beginning, with thick, uncomfortable, and difficult-to-handle devices; presently, though, the appliances are small, unnoticeable, multivectoral, easy to manage, and user-friendly. The second problem is the length of the treatment, especially for bone transport. Patients required 12 to 24 months of consolidation before dental implants could be inserted. The need to speed up the healing process is fundamental, and many research projects were initiated to overcome this difficulty, from ultrasound, to automatically activated distraction devices, to application of bone morphogenetic proteins (BMPs).

Recombinant human BMP-2 (rhBMP-2) and rhBMP-7 have been used widely recently to speed up the mineralization process and allow surgeons to reduce the time required for healing and insertion of dental implants in the distraction osteogenesis chambers. The proteins need to be combined with a transporter that progressively and slowly introduces the reconstituted proteins mixed with lyophilized buffer into the chamber to increase mineralization activity and treatment time; thus far, collagen is the most common transporter used, and as it is resorbed, BMP is released into the chamber (Fig. 11-12).

PEARLS AND PITFALLS

- The surgical plan should be executed according to the biologic principles of distraction osteogenesis: maintenance of the blood supply to the maximum extent possible, avoidance of unnecessary stripping, working through tunnels, and avoidance of overheating the bone while performing the osteotomy.
- Corticotomies should not be performed because secondary surgery may be required or the distraction appliance could be dislodged during activation.
- Once the distractors are completely activated, acrylic is placed over the distraction screw to make it more stable and allow the patient to advance to a soft diet.
- The consolidation period varies according to the age of the patient, the amount of movement required, and the quantity and quality of bone.
- As a rule, radiographs must show adequate rigidity before removal of the distractors, which could take months, depending on the patient. Miniaturized devices can be used and be kept in place for months without disturbing the patient's social life, work, or school activities—another reason to not use extraoral appliances. Most maxillo-mandibular deficiencies can be treated with intraoral distraction osteogenesis.
- Use of BMPs may speed up the healing process, especially in cases requiring long movements or bone transport.
- Because mandibular range of motion tends to decrease, physiotherapy is indicated from the beginning.
- Patients must make compromises to undergo treatment: those living far away from the hospital or not able to cooperate properly with the different phases of treatment should not undergo distraction osteogenesis.
- New instrumentation, better technology, and advanced surgical procedures will offer more comfort and superb outcomes in clinical situations in which traditional surgery is limited, is too complicated, or is too expensive, as it is with major bone grafts and unpredictable surgeries.

BIBLIOGRAPHY

Abbott LC: The operative lengthening of the tibia and fibula, *J Bone Joint Surg* 9:128-152, 1927.

Bell WH, Epker BN: Surgical orthodontic expansion of the maxilla, *Am J Orthod* 70:517-528, 1976.

Bell WH, Gonzalez M, Guerrero CA, et al: Intraoral widening of the mandible by distraction osteogenesis: histologic and radiographic assessment, *J Oral Maxillofac Surg* 55:97, 1997.

Bell WH, Gonzalez M, Guerrero C, et al: Distraction histogenesis: effect of intraoral widening on gingival and periodontal ligament. In Arnaud E, Diner PA, editors: *3rd International Congress on Facial Distraction Processes, Paris, France*. Bologna, Italy, 2001, Monduzzi Editore, pp 173-178.

Bell WH, Gonzalez M, Samchukov ML, et al: Intraoral widening and lengthening of the mandible in baboons by distraction osteogenesis, *J Oral Maxillofac Surg* 57:548-562, 1999.

Bell WH, Harper RP, Gonzalez M, et al: Distraction osteogenesis to widen the mandible, *Br J Oral Maxillofac Surg* 35:11-19, 1997.

Block MS, Chang A, Crawford C: Mandibular alveolar ridge augmentation in the dog using distraction osteogenesis, *J Oral Maxillofac Surg* 54:309-314, 1996.

Chin M, Toth BA: Distraction osteogenesis in maxillofacial surgery using internal devices: review of five cases, *J Oral Maxillofac Surg* 54:45-53, 1996.

Codivilla A: On the means of lengthening in the lower limbs, the muscles and tissues which are shortened through deformity, *Am J Orthop Surg* 2:353-363, 1905.

Cohen SR, Holmes RE, Machado L: Midface distraction. In Samchukov ML, Cope JB, Cherkashin AM, editors: *Craniofacial distraction osteogenesis*, St Louis, CV Mosby, 2001, pp 520-530.

Constantino PD, Friedman CD: Bone regeneration within a human segmental mandible defect: a preliminary report, *Am J Otolaryngol* 16:56-65, 1995.

Constantino PD, Shybut G, Fiedeman CD, et al: Segmental mandibular regeneration by distraction osteogenesis. An experimental study. *Arch Otolaryngol Head Neck Surg* 116:535-545, 1990.

DeDeyne PG, Paley D, Herzenberg JE: Muscle and its connective tissue adaptation to distraction osteogenesis [abstract 3]. ASAMI North America, First International Meeting, New Orleans, March 1998.

Fonseca RJ, Walker RV: *Oral and maxillofacial trauma*, Philadelphia, 1991, WB Saunders, p 275.

Gaggl AJ, Schultes GR, Karcher H: Alveolar ridge augmentation with the aid of distraction implants. In Samchucov ML, Cope JB, Cherkashin AM, editors: *Craniofacial distraction osteogenesis*, St Louis, 2001, CV Mosby, pp 401-413.

Gonzalez M, Bell WH, Guerrero CA, et al: Positional changes and stability of bone segments during simultaneous bilateral mandibular lengthening and widening by distraction osteogenesis, *Br J Oral Maxillofac Surg* 39:169-178, 2001.

Gonzalez M, Guerrero CA, Henriquez M, et al: Docking site surgery in bone transport. In Arnaud E, Diner PA, editors: *5th International Congress of Maxillofacial and Craniofacial Distraction, Paris, France*. Bologna, Italy, 2006, Monduzzi Editore, pp 99-104.

Guerrero C: Rapid mandibular expansion, *Rev Venez Ortod* 48:1-2, 1990.

Guerrero CA: Maxillary intraoral distraction osteogenesis. In Arnaud E, Diner PA, editors: *3rd International Congress on Cranial and Facial Bone Distraction Processes, Paris, France*. Bologna, Italy, 2001, Monduzzi Editore, pp 381-387.

Guerrero CA, Bell WH: Intraoral distraction. In McCarthy JG, editor: *Distraction of the craniofacial skeleton*, New York, 1999, Springer-Verlag, pp 219-248.

Guerrero CA, Bell WH, Contasti GI, et al: Mandibular widening by intraoral distraction osteogenesis, *Br J Oral Maxillofac Surg* 35:383-392, 1997.

Guerrero CA, Bell WH, Contasti GI, et al: Intraoral mandibular distraction osteogenesis, *Semin Orthod* 5:35-40, 1999.

Guerrero C, Bell WH, Flores A, et al: Distraccción osteogénica mandibular intraoral. *Odontol Día* 10:116-132, 1995.

Guerrero CA, Bell WH, Gonzalez M, et al: Intraoral distraction osteogenesis. In Fonseca R, editor: *Oral and maxillofacial surgery*, Philadelphia, 2000, WB Saunders, pp 380-402.

Guerrero CA, Bell HW, Gonzalez M: Mandibular remodeling: the fifth stage in distraction osteogenesis healing. In Arnaud E, Diner PA, editors: *3rd International Congress on Cranial and Facial Bone Distraction Processes, Paris, France*. Bologna, Italy, 2001, Monduzzi Editore, pp 267-273.

Guerrero CA, Bell WH, Gonzalez M, et al: Intraoral mandibular bone transport: a case report. In Samchukov ML, Cope JB, Cherkashin AM, editors: *Craniofacial distraction osteogenesis*, St Louis, 2001, CV Mosby, pp 372-375.

Guerrero CA, Bell WH, Gonzalez M, et al: Maxillary advancement combined with posterior palate reposition via distraction osteogenesis: a case report. In Samchukov ML, Cope JB, Cherkashin AM, editors: *Craniofacial distraction osteogenesis*, St Louis, 2001, CV Mosby, pp 531-534.

Guerrero CA, Bell WH, Gonzalez M, et al: Maxillo-mandibular reconstruction by intraoral bone transport. In Arnaud E, Diner PA, editors: *3rd International Congress on Cranial and Facial Bone Distraction Processes, Paris, France*. Bologna, Italy, 2001, Monduzzi Editore, pp 569-574.

Guerrero CA, Bell WH, Meza LS: Intraoral distraction osteogenesis. Maxillary and mandibular lengthening. In Stucki-McCormick SU, guest editor: *Atlas of the oral and maxillofacial Surgery Clinics of North America (distraction osteogenesis)*, 1999, pp 111-151.

Guerrero C, Contasti G: Transverse mandibular deficiency. In Bell WH, editor: *Modern practice in orthognathic and reconstructive surgery*, vol 3, ed 2. Philadelphia, 1992, WB Saunders, pp 2383-2397.

Guerrero CA, Contasti GI, Rodriguez AM, et al: Surgical orthodontics in mandibular widening. In Bell WH, Guerrero CA, editors: *Distraction osteogenesis of the facial skeleton*, Hamilton, Ontario, 2007, BC Decker, pp 153-165.

Guerrero CA, Figueroa F, Bell WH, et al: Surgical orthodontics in mandibular lengthening. In Bell WH, Guerrero CA, editors: *Distraction osteogenesis of the facial skeleton*, Hamilton, Ontario, 2007, BC Decker, pp 373-388.

Guerrero CA, Figueroa F, Gonzalez M: 3-D alveolar distraction osteogenesis. In Diner PA, Arnaud E, editors. *4th International Congress of Maxillofacial and Craniofacial Distraction, Paris, France*, Bologna, Italy, 2003, Monduzzi Editore, pp 37-42.

Guerrero CA, Gonzalez M, Dominguez E: Bone transport by distraction osteogenesis for maxillomandibular reconstruction. In Bell WH, Guerrero CA, editors: *Distraction osteogenesis of the facial skeleton*, Hamilton, Ontario, 2007, BC Decker, pp 501-519.

Guerrero CA, Gonzalez M, Laplana R, et al: Reconstrução do rebordo alveolar mediante distração ostogênica para implantes osseointegrados. In Dinato JC, Polido W, editors: *Implantes osseointegrados: cirugia e prótese*. Brazil, 2001, Artes Mèdicas, pp 423-439.

Guerrero CA, Laplana R, Figueredo N, et al: Surgical implant repositioning: a clinical report, *Int J Oral Maxillofac Implants* 14:48-54, 1999.

Guerrero CA, Lopez P, Figueroa F, et al: Three-dimensional alveolar distraction osteogenesis. In Bell WH, Guerrero CA, editors: *Distraction osteogenesis of the facial skeleton*, Hamilton, Ontario, 2007, BC Decker, pp 475-493.

Guerrero CA, Rojas A, Figueroa F, et al: Radiographic evaluation of traditional versus rhBMP-2 inducted intraoral bone transport in mandibular reconstruction. In Diner PA, Arnaud E, editors. *4th International Congress of Maxillofacial and Craniofacial Distraction, Paris, France*, Bologna, Italy, 2003, Monduzzi Editore, pp 391-396.

Harper RP, Bell WH, Hinton RJ, et al: Reactive changes in the temporomandibular joint after midline osteodistraction, *Br J Oral Maxillofac Surg* 35:20-25, 1997.

Hidding J, Lazar F, Zoeller JE: Vertical distraction of the alveolar process: a new technique for reconstructing the alveolar ridge. In Samchucov ML, Cope JB, Cherkashin AM, editors: *Craniofacial distraction osteogenesis*, St. Louis, 2001, CV Mosby, pp 393-400.

Ilizarov GA: A method of uniting bones in fractures and an apparatus to implement this method. USSR Authorship Certificate 98471, filed 1952.

Ilizarov GA: Basic principles of transosseous compression and distraction osteosynthesis, *Ortop Travmatol Protez* 32(11):7-15, 1971.

Ilizarov GA: The tension-stress effect on the genesis and growth of tissues: Part I. The influence of stability of fixation and soft tissue preservation, *Clin Orthop Relat Res* 230:249-281, 1989.

Ilizarov GA: The tension-stress effect on the genesis and growth of tissues: Part II. The influence of the rate and frequency of distraction, *Clin Orthop Relat Res* 239:263-285, 1989.

Ilizarov GA, Chikorina NK: Electron microscope investigation of the anterior tibial muscle in experimental tibial lengthening. In *Abstracts of First International Symposium on Experimental and Clinical Aspects of Transosseous Osteosynthesis*, Kurgan, USSR, September 1983, pp 20-22.

Ilizarov GA, Kuznetsova B, Peschansky VS, et al: Blood vessels and blood coagulation system in experimental limb lengthening. In *Abstracts of First International Symposium on Experimental and Clinical Aspects of Transosseous Osteosynthesis*, Kurgan, September 1983, USSR, pp 20-22.

Ilizarov GA, Ledioev VI: The course of compact bone reparative regeneration in distraction osteosynthesis under different conditions of bone fragment fixation and experimental study, *Exp Khir Anest* 14:3-12, 1969.

Ilizarov GA, Palienko LA, Schreiner AA: The bone marrow hemopoietic function and its relationship with the activity of osteogenesis upon reparative regeneration under the conditions of crus elongation in dogs, *Ontogonez* 15:146-152, 1984.

Ilizarov GA, Schreiner AA: A new method of close flexion osteoclasis [experimental study], *Orthop Travmatol Protez* 40:9, 1979.

Ilizarov GA, Schreiner AA, Imerlishvili IA, et al: On the problem of improving osteogenesis conditions in limb lengthening. In *Abstracts of First International Symposium on Experimental and Clinical Aspects of Transosseous Osteosynthesis*, Kurgan, USSR, September 1983, pp 20-22.

Jensen OT: Alveolar segmental "sandwich" osteotomies for posterior edentulous mandibular sites for dental implants, *J Oral Maxillofac Surg* 64:471-475, 2006.

Karaharju-Suvanto T, Karaharju EO, Ranta R: Mandibular distraction: an experimental study in sheep, *J Craniomaxillofac Surg* 18:280-282, 1990.

Karp NS, McCarthy JG, Schreiber JS, et al: Membranous bone lengthening: a serial histologic study, *Ann Plast Surg* 29:2-7, 1990.

Karp NS, Thorne CHM, McCarthy JG, et al: Bone lengthening in the craniofacial skeleton, *Ann Plast Surg* 24:231-237, 1990.

Little RM, Riedel RA, Artun J: An evaluation of changes in mandibular anterior alignment from 10 to 20 years post-retention, *Am J Orthod Dentofac Orthop* 93:423-428, 1988.

Makarov MR, Kochutina LN, Birch JG, et al: Muscle histomorphology during distraction osteogenesis. In Stein H, Suk SI, Leung PC, et al, editors: *SIROT 99 International Research Society of Orthopaedic Surgery and Traumatology, Sydney, Australia, April 16-19, 1999*, Tel Aviv, Israel, 1999, Freund Publishing, pp 647-652.

McCarthy JG, Schreiber J, Karp N, et al: Lengthening the human mandible by gradual distraction, *Plast Reconstr Surg* 89:1-8, discussion 9-10, 1992.

McCormick SU, McCarthy JG, Grayson BH, et al: Effect of mandibular distraction on the temporomandibular joint. Part I, *J Craniofac Surg* 6:358-363, 1995.

Michieli S, Miotti B: Lengthening of mandibular body by gradual surgical-orthodontic distraction, *J Oral Surg* 35:187-192, 1977.

Molina F, Ortiz Monasterios F: Mandibular elongation and remodeling by distraction: a farewell to major osteotomies, *Plast Reconst Surg* 96:825-840, discussion 841-842, 1995.

Obwegeser H: Surgical correction of small retro displaced maxillae. "The dish face deformity," *Plast Reconstr Surg* 43:351-365, 1969.

Oda T, Sawaki Y, Ueda M: Experimental alveolar ridge augmentation by distraction osteogenesis using a simple device that permits secondary implant placement, *Int J Oral Maxillofac Implants* 15:95-102, 2000.

Polley JW, Figueroa AA: Management of severe maxillary deficiency in childhood and adolescent through distraction osteogenesis with an external, adjustable, rigid distraction device, *J Craniofac Surg* 8:181-185, discussion 186, 1997.

Razdolsky Y, Dessner S, El-Bialy T: Correction of alveolar ridge deficiency using the ROD-5 distraction device: a case report. In Samchucov ML, Cope JB, Cherkashin AM, editors: *Craniofacial distraction osteogenesis*, St Louis, 2001, CV Mosby, pp 454-4581.

Samchukov ML, Cope JB, Cherkashin AM: *Craniofacial distraction osteogenesis*, St Louis, 2001, CV Mosby.

Samchukov ML, Cope JB, Harper RP, et al: Biomechanical considerations for mandibular lengthening and widening by gradual distraction, *Am J Oral Maxillofac Surg* 56:51-59, 1998.

Schendel SA, Wolford LM, Epker BN: Mandibular deficiency syndrome. III. Surgical advancement of the deficient mandible in growing children: treatment results in twelve patients, *Oral Surg Oral Med Oral Pathol* 45:364-377, 1978.

Snyder CC, Levine GA, Swanson HM, et al: Mandibular lengthening by gradual distraction: preliminary report, *Plast Reconstr Surg* 51:506-508, 1973.

Trauner R, Obwegeser H: The surgical correction of mandibular prognathism and retrognathia with consideration of genioplasty: Part I. Surgical procedures to correct mandibular prognathism and reshaping of the chin, *Oral Surg Oral Med Oral Pathol* 10:677-689, 1957.

Ueda M: Maxillofacial bone distraction processes using osseointegrated implants and an intraoral device. In Diner PA, Vasquez MP, editors. *Proceeding of the International Congress on Cranial and Facial Bone Distraction Processes; 1997 June 19-21; Paris, France*, Bologna, Italy, 1997, Monduzzi Editore, pp 75-84.

12

Principles of Implantology and Osseointegration

Guillermo E. Chacon, Carlos M. Ugalde

Over the course of the past 30 years, oral implantology has constantly evolved to become one of the main focuses of modern dentistry. Today, this treatment modality has been incorporated into the curriculum of most dental schools, which has dramatically improved the availability of professionals trained to treat patients with dental implants. Significant improvements in the success rate and longevity of dental implants have increased awareness and the interest of the public and professional community alike. For most clinical scenarios, implant-retained and implant-supported restorations provide the best alternative for the rehabilitation of partially or completely edentulous patients. When patient satisfaction and oral health–related quality of life are compared in patients treated with dental implants and those treated with conventional prosthetic techniques, satisfaction is always significantly greater in the former group.[1] Additional benefits associated with dental implant therapy include no risk for caries, improved esthetics, maintenance of bone at the edentulous site, and decreased abutment loss (Fig. 12-1).

ETIOPATHOGENESIS/CAUSATIVE FACTORS

There are several major causes of tooth loss; among them are dental caries, periodontal disease, and trauma. The aging process has always been intuitively considered to be an important variable in tooth longevity. However, it was not until the National Institute of Dental and Craniofacial Research ran a study of surveillance of dental health in the United Sates between 1999 and 2002 that this particular point was confirmed. In this study it was found that the mean number of remaining teeth is indeed inversely correlated to the patient's age.[2] Conversely, young age does not necessarily correlate with maintenance of complete dentition. In this same study it was found that the population of young adults between 20 and 39 years of age averages only 27 teeth. If one makes the assumption that all individuals have their third molars removed before the age of 20 (and this is of course a big assumption), this shows that this age group is missing at least one permanent tooth. In the subset of individuals ranging between 40 and 59 years of age, the average number of remaining permanent teeth is 24. Again, not counting the third molars, this is a 15% decline in the number of remaining natural dental units. Finally, in the patient subset 60 years and older, the average number of remaining permanent teeth is just 19. This is a 32% attrition rate of the natural dentition. The same study revealed a similar trend on complete edentulism. In other words, the older the individual, the greater the chance of having natural teeth missing. To this effect, the prevalence was shown to be less than 1% for the young adult group and 25% for the group 60 years or older. If in addition one considers the current life expectancy in the United States, which is 77.9 years,[3] it becomes immediately evident that many senior adults spend almost 25% of their life with significantly

crippled dentition. Interestingly, non-Hispanic black adults have the highest prevalence of edentulism, followed by the non-Hispanic white population, with the Mexican American group having the lowest prevalence.

Education has proved to play a major role in dental health and the resulting number of remaining natural teeth. The population subgroup of individuals without a high school education has an increased prevalence of complete edentulism of 9%, followed by 4% for the group with a high school education and 3.5% for those with an education beyond the high school level. Another important factor to take into account is income level. The population that is more than 200% below the federal poverty level (FPL) has higher additional prevalence (15%) than does the group less than 100% of FPL (5%). Finally, smoking has been associated with poor dental health, with smokers having a higher prevalence of edentulism (14%) than non-smokers (4.5%).

Multiple problems have been associated with edentulism. Even though edentulous patients pursue restorative procedures with complete or partial dentures, this is rarely adequate to compensate for the missing natural structures. The bite force pressure that these individuals are able to generate is approximately 25% less than normal. As a consequence, their food selection is very limited, with significantly less intake of vegetables, carotenes, and fiber and a greater tendency to consume foods high in cholesterol and saturated fat.[4] The combination of poor oral intake, compromised dental function, and malnutrition can lead to debilitation, illness, and potentially decreased life span.[5] In a recent article, David Felton showed that completely edentulous patients have a higher risk for the development of multiple systemic disorders. Edentulism was found to be a global issue, with estimates of an increasing demand for complete denture prostheses in the future. Completely edentulous patients were found to be at higher risk for poor nutrition, for coronary artery plaque formation (odds ratio, 2.32), to be smokers (odds ratio, 2.42), to be asthmatic and edentulous in the maxillary arch (odds ratio, 10.52), to be diabetic (odds ratio, 1.82), to having rheumatoid arthritis (odds ratio, 2.27), and to have certain cancers (odds ratios varying from 1.54 to 2.85, depending on the type of cancer). In addition, chronic residual ridge resorption continues to be the primary intraoral complication of edentulism, and there appear to be few opportunities to reduce bone loss in these patients.[6]

PATHOLOGIC ANATOMY

According to Wolff's law, bone remodels in direct relation to the forces applied to it.[7] Approximately 4% of strain is required to obtain a balance between osseous formation and the resorption process.[8] Following dental extraction, alveolar bone starts to undergo an immediate process of resorption and remodeling.[9] Alveolar bone remodels significantly during the first few months after losing teeth, with a quick reduction of almost 25% of alveolar width and a decrease in alveolar height of 4 mm on average.[10] A marked decrease

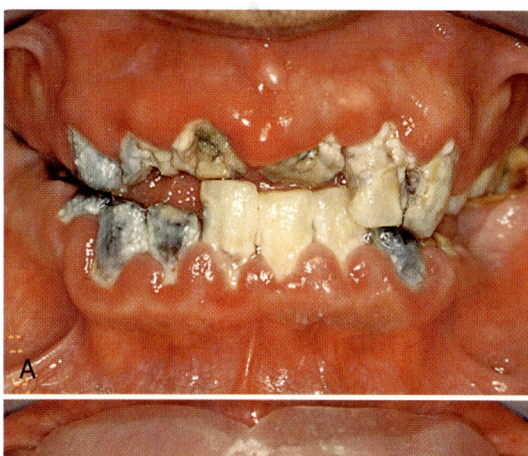

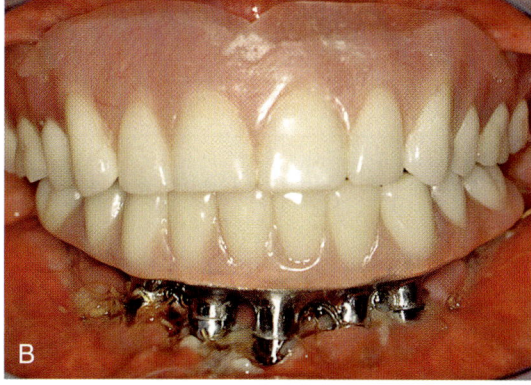

Fig. 12-1 ■ Relatively simple treatment plans can achieve excellent results in implant patients. **A,** Preoperative view showing rampant caries. **B,** The patient underwent full mouth extraction with placement of five mandibular implants and delivery of a conventional maxillary complete denture and an immediately loaded mandibular fixed-detachable (hybrid) bridge.

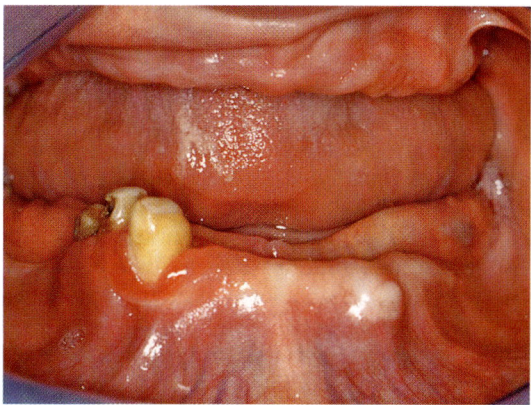

Fig. 12-2 ■ The loss of teeth triggers resorption of the residual alveolar ridges, which can become so distorted that replacement of dentition is prevented unless significant reconstructive procedures are performed.

in blood supply and increased interalveolar distance make the remodeling process appear to be more significant, approximately four-fold for the maxillary ridge in comparison to the mandible.[8] A more recent study suggests that the alveolus may suffer 40% reduction in height and 60% in width within the first 6 months after extraction[11] (Fig. 12-2).

As the intraoral hard structures change, a direct and proportional alteration can be observed in the overlying soft tissues. The soft structures are affected by a progressive decrease in keratinized tissue and attached gingiva. Secondary to the bone loss and apical

migration of the crest of the residual alveolar ridges, muscle insertions become more prominent. In an edentulous patient, the lack of counterpressure provided by the dentition allows the tongue to expand over the residual alveolar ridge and results in tongue hypertrophy as well.

The lack of teeth and bone resorption in edentulous patients cause multiple changes in facial architecture, which ultimately compromises the overall facial esthetics of patients and gives them the classic "old toothless face look." This results mainly from a decrease in facial height as a result of reduced vertical dimension and improper support of the lips and cheeks. Bone resorption and the absence of mandibular teeth decrease the labiomental angle, followed by collapse of the muscular attachment and a counterclockwise rotation of the chin, which gives the patient a pseudo-prognathic appearance. At the same time, a reduction in function of the mandible causes atrophy of the orbicularis oris and buccinator muscles, with the modiolus being displaced posteriorly and medially. Consequently, the patient acquires an aged appearance with hollow cheeks and thin lips. The absence of support of the upper lip increases the columellar-philtrum angle, which increases lip length and gives the impression of a large nose. Finally, a lower attachment of the buccinators and mentalis muscles to the body and symphysis causes tissue sagging and, subsequently, jowls and a "witch's chin" appearance, respectively.

DIAGNOSTIC STUDIES

Traditionally, obtaining dental models of the patient's mouth has been of great value in determining the residual anatomy of the patient. As expected, the information obtained is limited to the structures observed during clinical examination, which may or may not accurately represent what is happening under the surface. Therefore, radiographic imaging can provide the surgeon with valuable information about bone morphology and the position of relevant anatomic structures. Different modalities of radiographic imaging are used for implant dentistry, all of them with specific advantages over the other modalities. The traditional periapical radiograph provides detailed image quality for evaluating bone height and monitoring bone healing around the implant with minimal radiation exposure and operative time, but with very limited information on the surrounding structures. This is usually a good imaging option for individual units in the anterior maxillary and mandibular arches. In situations involving completely edentulous patients, the cephalometric radiograph helps the surgeon determine the anteroposterior implant angulations in the anterior region, as well as the intermaxillary relationships. However, the panoramic radiograph is probably the most common radiographic modality used for surgical dental implant planning because of the overall view of the maxilla and mandible that it provides; however, the image suffers from magnification and positional artifacts (Fig. 12-3).

In 1973 computed tomography (CT) was developed, and advances in this technology led to the introduction of cone beam CT in 1999. This technology produces excellent three-dimensional images of the maxillofacial structures with a fraction of the radiation dose of conventional CT (Fig. 12-4). When CT is used, bone quality can be determined with Hounsfield units, which correspond to the degree of attenuation of a biologic object subjected to a dose of radiation. The Hounsfield unit is also known as the CT number; the value of water corresponds to 0, air to −1000 units, and bone to values approximately higher than 400 units, depending on its density.[12] Another way to measure radiation is by using sieverts (Sv), a unit reflecting the effect of radiation on tissue and named after the Swedish medical physicist Rolf Sievert. It has been established that

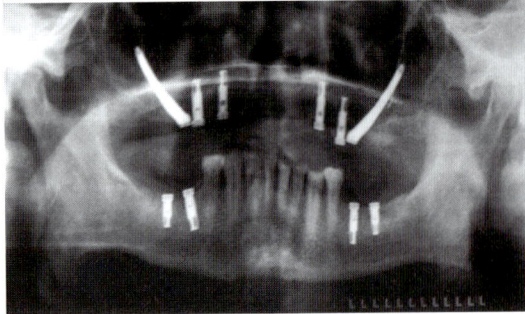

Fig. 12-3 ■ A panoramic radiograph has inherent distortion, which limits its reliability in certain circumstances. The curvature created along the zygomatic implants is a clear example of how much image alteration can occur.

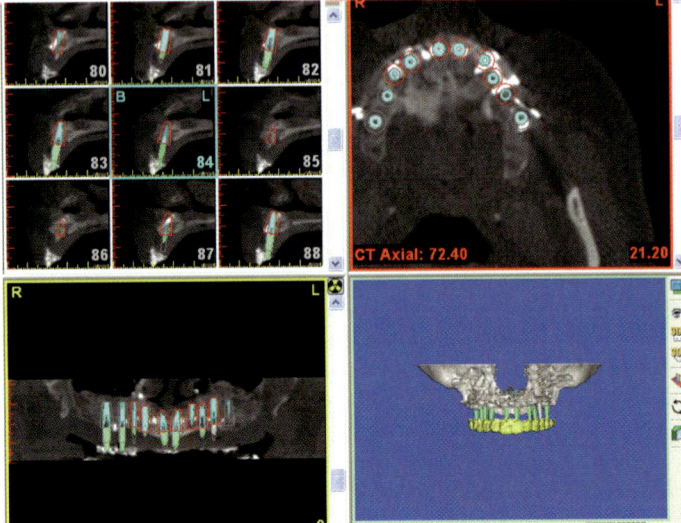

Fig. 12-4 ■ Cone beam computed tomography technology combined with implant treatment planning software allows the clinician to plan the procedure in true three dimensions with zero distortion of the images. Notice the virtual placement of the implants in this particular case.

a full-body equivalent dose of 1 Sv causes nausea and that 2 to 5 Sv causes epilation or hair loss, hemorrhage, and death in many cases. Higher than 3 Sv will lead to a dose that is lethal to 50% of individuals within 30 days ($LD_{50/30}$), and with higher than 6 Sv, survival is unlikely. Table 12-1 summarizes the radiation dose values of different imaging techniques. Notice that the doses are listed in microsieverts (μSv).

The implant surgeon may use any of the imaging modalities just described but must strictly follow the radiation safety principle of "as low as reasonably achievable" (ALARA) to provide the patient with the best possible care.

RECONSTRUCTIVE GOALS

The goal of implant dentistry is to restore normal dental anatomy and function while maintaining residual alveolar bone height and width. In other words, implant-supported restorations should reestablish an adequate esthetic appearance and restore the chewing capacity of the patient. At the same time, once the implant is placed under function, occlusal forces should maintain a balance to favor the alveolar bone remodeling process.

TABLE 12-1	Comparison of Different Commonly Used Imaging Techniques for the Treatment of Dental Implant Patients
RADIATION SOURCE	**RADIATION DOSE**
Daily background radiation	8 μSv
10-second cone beam CT study	34 μSv
20-second cone beam CT study	68 μSv
Panoramic radiograph (average)	10-15 μSv
Digital panoramic radiograph	4.7-14.9 μSv
Highest film panoramic radiograph	26 μSv
Full mouth series	150 μSv
Medical CT study	1200-3300 μSv

From Dr. Sharon Brooks, Department of Radiology, University of Michigan, and Dr. Stuart White, Department of Radiology, University of California, Los Angeles.

SPECIFIC TREATMENTS AND TECHNIQUES

PREOPERATIVE CONSIDERATIONS— PHARMACOLOGY

The use of preoperative antibiotic prophylaxis during dental implant surgery is still controversial. A study comparing preoperative or postoperative antibiotics involving almost 3000 implants demonstrated a higher survival rate in the group receiving preoperative antibiotic prophylaxis.[13] The same results were observed in a similar study involving a similar number of implants.[14] However, other studies have found no statistically significant benefits with the use of prophylactic antibiotics during routine implant placement.[15,16]

DEFINITIONS

Dental implants are restored at different times following initial placement. The literature has multiple names describing the variety of situations involved in dental implant treatment. For this reason, Cochrane and colleagues published a consensus statement of appropriate terms and definitions of these distinctive scenarios.[17]

- Immediate loading: a restoration is placed in occlusion within 48 hours of implant placement.
- Immediate restoration: a restoration that is not in occlusion is inserted within 48 hours of implant placement.
- Conventional loading: the prosthetic component is inserted during a second procedure after a healing period of 3 to 6 months.
- Early loading: a restoration in occlusion is placed after 48 hours of implant placement, but no later than 3 months.
- Delayed loading: the prosthetic component is attached in a second procedure after 3 to 6 months of implant placement.

BASIC TECHNIQUE

Several important considerations must be kept in mind when surgically placing osseointegrated dental implants. As an inert alloplastic device, the fixture has no ability to fight infection, which is why it is of utmost importance to perform the surgical procedures in a way that minimizes the risk for infection, particularly during the critically important immediate postoperative period. A simple but effective way to help in this effort is to carefully prepare and place the surgical fields in accordance with standard aseptic guidelines.[18] A sterile surgical technique must be followed with strong consideration of antibiotic prophylaxis. It has been the common practice of the authors to use the same antibiotic protocol recommended by the American Heart Association for patients at risk for subacute bacterial endocarditis: 2 g of amoxicillin 1 hour before the procedure or 600 mg of clindamycin for penicillin-allergic patients. In addition, a 0.12% chlorhexidine mouth rinse twice daily is started 2 days before the procedure and continued for 5 days after surgery.

Manipulation of soft tissues must be as gentle as possible. This helps reduce the risk for tissue trauma, which translates into easier postoperative recovery. At all times during preparation of the osteotomies, copious irrigation must be used. The implant sites require the use of sharp drills with a progressive increase in size. An intermittent and precise preparation with controlled speed and torque will also assist in minimizing trauma to the bone.[19] These concepts are not new to the field of oral implantology and have been in place since the very early developments of this discipline. All of these concepts have a direct impact on the ability of the clinician to control the temperature at the surgical site. It is of critical importance to maintain the temperature below 47° C and to keep drilling time to less than 1 minute at a time.[20,21]

Finally, avoiding contact of the implant surface aids in the prevention of bacterial seeding. For this reason it is recommended that the implant be retrieved from the sterile vial and carried directly to the osteotomy site without touching the gloves, suction tip, saliva, or other tissues. Once the fixture is inserted to the correct depth, careful repositioning and manipulation of the soft tissues are performed. If sutures are to be used, fine monofilament materials are recommended to avoid entrapment by bacterial plaque as much as possible (Fig. 12-5).

IMMEDIATE PLACEMENT FOLLOWING TOOTH EXTRACTION

In recent years it has become more and more common for patients to want their treatment completed in the shortest possible time. Gone are the days of waiting 9 to 12 months between implantation and second-stage surgery. This is why placing implants during the same surgical encounter in which the extractions are performed has become the preferred approach when clinical conditions allow. It is important to keep in mind that serious controversy still exists regarding the feasibility of this treatment modality, thus making it tremendously important to select each case according to individual conditions.[22] Among the characteristics to be considered are tooth position relative to the free gingival margin, the form of the periodontium, tooth shape, and the position of the osseous crest before the extraction.[23] It is important to point out that a recent review of the literature also found a suggestion that immediate and immediate-delayed implants may be at higher risk than delayed implants for implant failure and complications; conversely, the esthetic outcome might be better when placing implants just after tooth extraction.[24]

There are several practical advantages to immediate postextraction implantation. First and foremost, this approach allows the shortest possible healing time, with a considerable decrease in the time between tooth removal and delivery of the implant crown. Another, but no less important advantage of this treatment modality is the immediate support and stimulation that the fixture gives to the surrounding bone, which significantly reduces bone loss at the alveolar crest level.

It is recommended that any foci of acute infection be eliminated to minimize the possibility of postoperative infection. Chronic conditions such as asymptomatic periapical radiolucency have not been

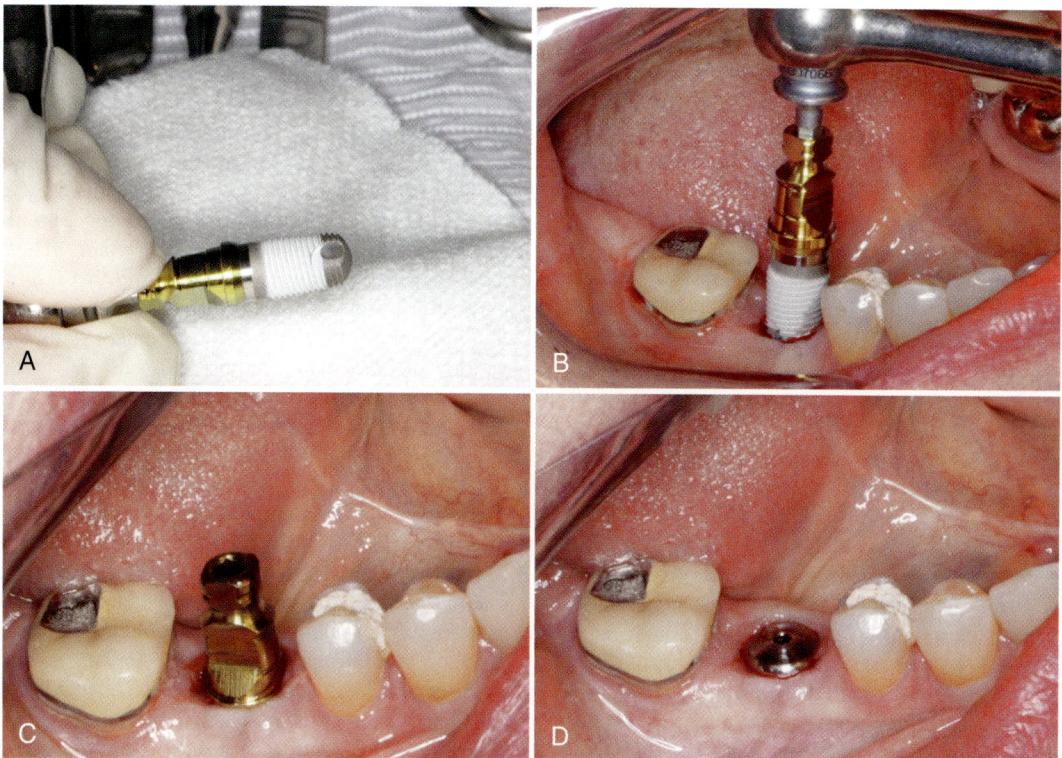

Fig. 12-5 ■ A critical step in prevention of infection is to avoid contamination of the implant body during placement. **A,** Fixture removed from the sterile vial. **B,** Implant inserted into the osteotomy while avoiding contact with instruments, tissues, and saliva. **C,** Implant completely seated with the carrying mount still in place. **D,** Healing abutment placed for a one-stage implant procedure.

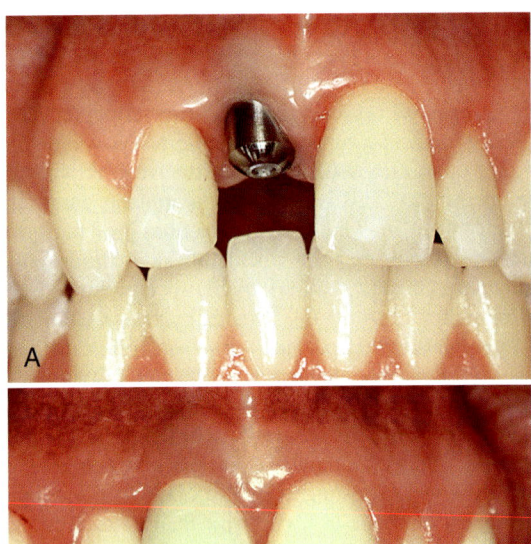

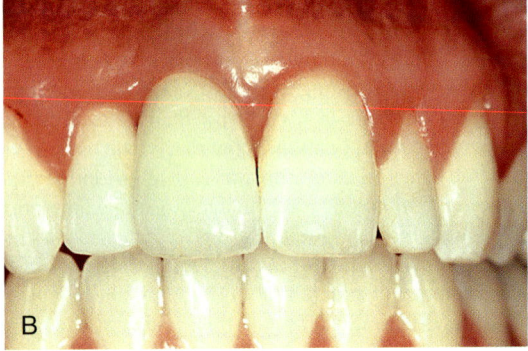

Fig. 12-6 ■ Adequate depth of the implant shoulder allows an adequate emergence profile, which translates into excellent esthetics. **A,** Temporary crown removed. **B,** Final restoration in place 6 months after initial delivery.

shown to be associated with a higher rate of complications and have been shown to provide equally favorable tissue integration of the implants as long as adequate initial implant stability is achieved.[25] This last point is accomplished by anchoring the implant at least 4 mm apical to the anatomic apex of the natural socket. This ensures anchoring of the tip of the fixture in solid bone. However, the clinician has to be mindful of the biomechanical and esthetic effects that such anchoring may have on future restoration. First, the shoulder of the implant should not be placed more than 1 to 2 mm apical to the osseous crest to prevent "die-back" to the level of the implant-crown interface. In addition, the implant platform should be placed no more and no less than 3 mm apical to the cemento-enamel junction of the neighboring teeth, which provides ideal vertical distance for a proper emergence profile and adequate biomechanical occlusal conditions (Fig. 12-6).

IMMEDIATE IMPLANT LOADING

Immediate loading of dental implants has been a hot topic for the past several years. It has been reported as a viable treatment option that increases not only patient comfort and acceptance but also soft tissue esthetics. However, documentation in the literature is insufficient regarding the clinical outcome and the peri-implant bone response of immediately loaded implants versus the conventional loading protocol used for bone of various quality. Romanos and co-workers performed a literature search and analysis in an attempt to demonstrate the survival rate of immediately loaded implants. They included data from histologic and histomorphometric evaluations in which this technique was compared with conventionally loaded implants. The analysis showed high survival rates of immediately loaded implants along with osseointegration, with a high percentage of bone-to-implant contact based on histologic evaluation of human and animal studies of immediately and

conventionally loaded implants.[26] Similarly, many other studies have considered implant survival to be the only measure of success. Bahat and Sullivan suggested that a better analysis should also include the long-term stability of the hard and soft tissues around the implant and other adjacent structures, as well as the long-term stability of all the restorative components.[27]

Although the conventional two-stage protocol has been the standard approach for dental implant therapy and immediate loading is perceived as the new frontier of treatment, in reality, the latter has been in use for more than 20 years. In 1990, a study conducted at the Harvard University School of Dental Medicine by Schnitman, Whörle, and Rubinstein reported on the use of fixed interim prostheses.[28] This has historically been viewed as the first scientifically organized approach for evaluation of the validity of this treatment modality. Unfortunately, a statistically significant number of implants failed, which made the clinicians worry about the practical clinical application of this modality. However, in 1994, Henry and Rosenberg published a preliminary report on a clinical series of immediately loaded implants.[29] They placed six mandibular implants in a series of five patients. The fixtures were immediately loaded with a provisional removable overdenture. The temporary prostheses were kept in place for 7 weeks, at which time they were replaced with the permanent ones. Their results showed a 100% success rate of osseointegration. The main disadvantage of this study was that the patient series was very small, which made it statistically impossible to extrapolate the results and generalize the success of immediate loading. However, it provided a solid base to build on for future researchers.

It was not until 1999 that a clinical trial with a truly large series involving immediately loaded implants was published by the Brånemark group at the University of Gothenburg.[30] In this study, 50 patients received 150 implants using the Brånemark Novum implant system. This system uses a series of surgical jigs to place three implants in the anterior mandible. The implants are then immediately loaded with a fixed-detachable bridge built over two prefabricated titanium bars. Three implants were lost to follow-up and three failed, which resulted in an overall survival rate of 98%. One prosthesis failed, for a prosthetic survival rate of 98%. The average treatment time was approximately 7 hours from the time that the patients arrived for surgery to the time that they left with the final prosthesis in place. At the baseline examination, the marginal bone level was 0.72 mm below the reference point. The average marginal bone loss was 0.2 mm/yr and 0.26 mm between the 3-month and the 1-year visits. The accumulated mean bone loss, including baseline, was −1.25 mm. This was a landmark study that established the validity of immediate loading as a safe and predictable treatment modality in implant dentistry. The main unanswered question that remained at this point was whether this outcome was the result of the precisely manufactured Novum System (Fig. 12-7). Would it be possible to obtain the same level of clinical predictability with a conventional restorative protocol? The answer came in 2001 in two different studies. The first was published by Chow and co-authors.[31] They treated 27 consecutive patients at the Hong Kong Osseointegration Implant Centre between June 1998 and December 2000. This included a total of 123 Brånemark System fixtures that were installed and regularly monitored for 3 to 30 months. Prosthesis stability and marginal bone levels were regularly evaluated clinically and radiographically, respectively, after implant surgery. Fifteen of the 27 patients had been monitored for 1 year or longer. Two patients with eight fixtures withdrew from the study. Two of the 115 remaining fixtures failed, for an overall implant survival rate of 98.3%. Mean marginal bone change was reported for 49 fixtures that had passed the 1-year review. Mean marginal bone loss was

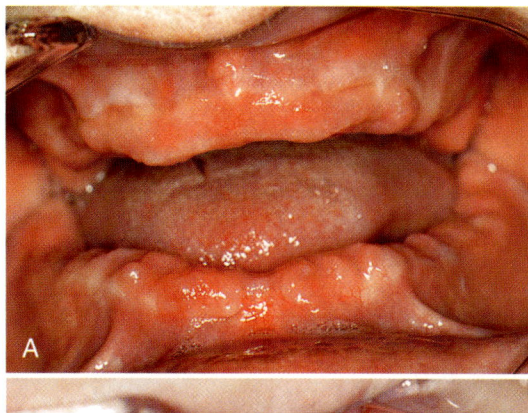
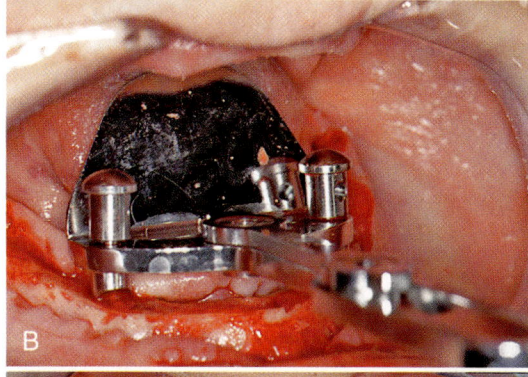
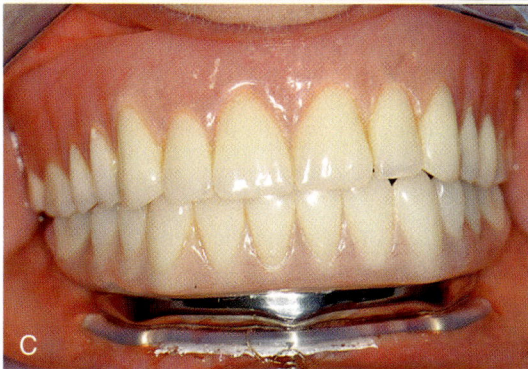

Fig. 12-7 ■ The Brånemark Novum System is designed as an immediate loading solution in which three implants are placed in the anterior mandible for a fixed-detachable bridge. **A,** Preoperative clinical findings. **B,** Use of surgical jigs for precise placement of the three fixtures. **C,** Procedure completed 6 hours after placement of the implants. (Prosthetic photographs courtesy Dr. Edwin McGlumphy.)

0.60 mm ($P < .05$) after 1 year of functional loading. The second landmark study was published by Chiapasco and colleagues.[32] This study compared the results of immediate and delayed loading of implants with implant-retained mandibular overdentures. In their protocol, 10 patients had 40 Brånemark System MKII implants placed in the interforaminal area of the mandible. Standard abutments were immediately screwed to the implants, rigidly connected with a bar, and immediately loaded with an overdenture. An equal group of patients was used as a control. This group received the same type and number of implants in the same area, but the implants were treated via the conventional two-stage protocol. Four to 8 months later, standard abutments were screwed to the implants and the same prosthetic procedure was applied. Each implant was evaluated at the time of prosthetic loading and at 6, 12, and 24 months after the initial loading. Peri-implant bone resorption was evaluated on panoramic radiographs taken 12 and 24 months after the initial prosthetic loading. No significant differences were found between the two groups at 6 and 24 months ($P > .05$). The cumulative success rate of the implants was 97.5% in both groups, which generated a considerable increase in awareness regarding immediate loading in implant dentistry.

At this point there was reasonable scientific evidence of the validity of delivering definitive prosthetic care at the time of implant placement, but such evidence had been accumulated with the Brånemark System only. As a follow-up to the 2001 study, Chiapasco and Gatti compared four different commercially available implant systems: Straumann, Brånemark, Frialoc, and 164 Ha-Ti Mathys.[33] The loading protocol was the same as the one used in the 2001 study. Their treatment group included 82 patients treated with 328 fixtures, 296 of which were monitored from a minimum of 36 months to a maximum of 96 months, with a mean follow-up of 62 months. Seven implants in six different patients were removed because of loss of osseointegration, and 18 implants, though still osseointegrated, did not fulfill the criteria for success because of bone resorption greater than 0.2 mm/yr after the first year of loading. Despite implant losses, all patients maintained their bars supporting overdentures, although in six patients the overdenture was supported by three implants instead of four. The only patient who lost two implants received two new implants, which survived normally. Therefore, the absolute success and survival rates were 91.6% and 97.6%, respectively, whereas the cumulative survival and success rates of implants as determined by life-table analysis were 96.1% and 88.2%, respectively. From this point forward, a wealth of clinical and scientific publications followed and provided additional data to support the validity of the delivery of immediate prosthetic care over freshly placed implants. This has become an accepted treatment modality and, in many cases, the preferred treatment option. In 2004, Castellon and associates categorically stated that delayed loading of implants was once the rule but is now the exception.[34] They went further and stated that there is sufficient evidence to prove that immediate loading is no longer experimental and that it can be recommended as an acceptable treatment alternative. Needless to say, over the past 6 years, the body of evidence has continued to solidify this concept, thus making immediate loading in implant dentistry a key component of everyday practice (Fig. 12-8).

ZYGOMATIC IMPLANTS

The Zygomaticus System, developed as part of the Brånemark System, allows reconstruction of a severely resorbed maxilla without the need for bone grafting. This approach is especially recommended for cases in which the maxillary sinuses extend anteriorly up to the bicuspid area. However, it is of the utmost importance to have sufficient bone in the anterior maxilla to allow the placement of two to four conventional implants in this area. These implants were introduced in 1998 by Professor Per-Ingvar Brånemark and his team at the Institute of Applied Biotechnology from the University of Gothenburg. The track record of this system has paralleled that of its conventional counterpart, including a very high success rate, which has been reported to be between 94% and 100%.[35,36]

Patient selection is extremely important for this particular treatment modality. It is determined by evaluating the available bone volume in three different areas: zone 1 (premaxilla), zone 2 (bicuspid), and zone 3 (molar). Radiographic evaluation must include the width and height of the zygomatic body, the thickness of the schneiderian membrane, and the width of the residual alveolar bone. The maxillary sinus must be free of any disease. Success of the zygomatic implant depends on providing bicortical stabilization at the crestal and cephalad levels. The implant must successfully engage four cortices: lingual cortex, cortical floor of the maxillary sinus, and the inferior and superior portions of the zygoma.[37]

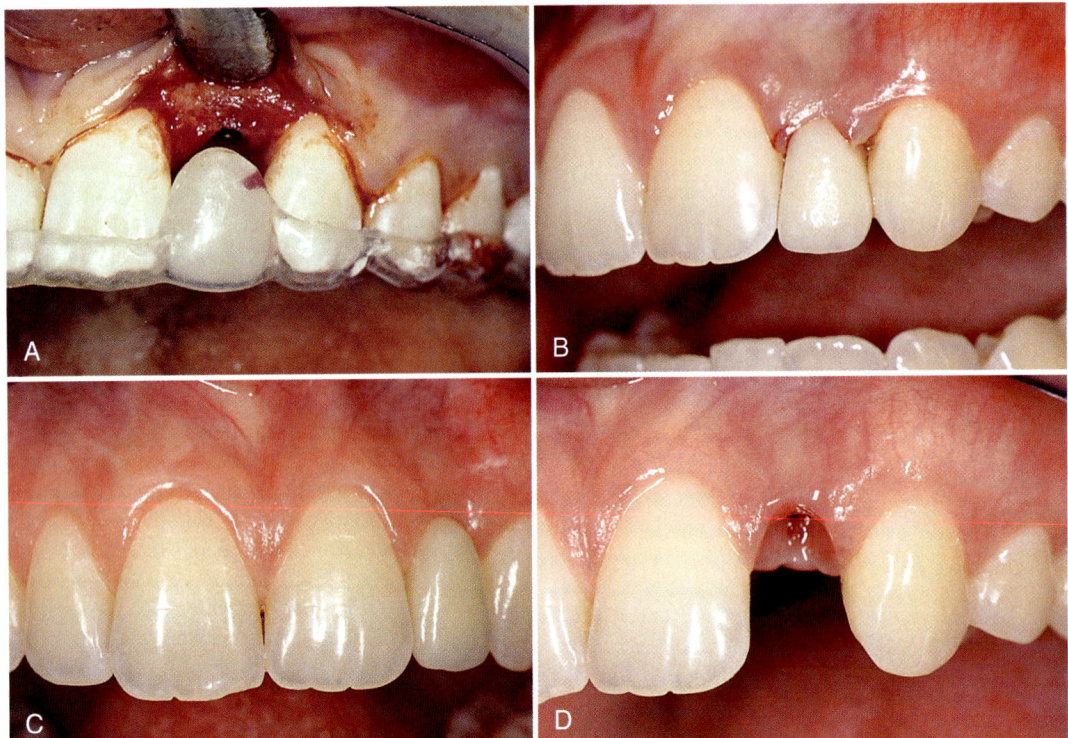

Fig. 12-8 ■ Immediate loading has gained tremendous popularity because of its short treatment time. Case selection is key for the success of this approach. **A,** Implant placement to replace congenitally missing tooth No. 10. Notice the adequate depth of the implant shoulder. **B,** Flap repositioned with delivery of the final restoration. **C,** Four months after placement and crown delivery. **D,** Appearance of the soft tissues after removal of the crown for a hygiene check-up at the 4-month visit. (Prosthetic photographs courtesy Dr. Edwin McGlumphy.)

The surgical procedure requires direct visualization of the base of the zygomatic body. The surgeon must establish a clear view of the pathway of the instruments and determine the length of the zygomatic implants, which ranges between 30 and 52.5 mm. The surgical protocol calls for exposure of the lateral wall of the maxilla in a similar fashion as the degloving exposure performed during maxillary orthognathic surgery. A vertical window is then created on the lateral wall of the maxilla, parallel to the junction with the posterior maxillary wall along the body of the zygomatic buttress. The schneiderian membrane is reflected with maxillary sinus curets; this step is recommended to prevent insertion of the membrane fragments in the zygomatic osteotomy, which may compromise osseointegration. The surgeon must ensure complete visualization of the drill at all times. For this reason, a retractor placed in the incisura zygomatica facilitates the process. The implant site is prepared according to the manufacturer's protocol, which roughly follows the same principles as conventional implant site preparation. The zygomatic implant has a 45-degree platform, which permits it to be made parallel to the anterior implants. However, the head of the fixture consequently normally emerges in a slightly palatal position in the second premolar/first molar area of the maxilla. The insertion tool comes attached to the implant with a single screw, which compensates for the angled platform and permits manipulation along the axis of the fixture. The implant can be inserted either with a handpiece at slow speed and high torque or with a hand wrench. The screw head of the implant is used as a reference, and once adequate position has been confirmed, the screw head is removed along with the insertion tool. After the insertion tool is removed, the prosthetic platform of the implant is identical to the one on the regular Brånemark System implants. Finally, the cover screw is put in place.

Following placement of the zygomatic implants, a total of four and in some cases two implants are placed in the anterior maxilla. The clinician must at all times remember the overriding consideration that these implants must always function within a cross-arch rigid framework (Fig. 12-9).

POSTOPERATIVE CARE

Implant patients are advised to follow routine oral hygiene techniques to maintain ideal conditions around the fixtures and their prosthetic components. In most instances the use of chlorhexidine mouthwash is prescribed. This is of particular importance in cases involving bone grafting. Patients should adhere to a soft diet during the acute recovery period and avoid chewing on the surgically treated sites, especially in cases involving immediate loading, immediate restoration, and early loading. Patients with a removable prosthetic appliance are advised to not wear it until the clinician has had the opportunity to perform the appropriate adjustments (see Fig. 12-9).

With regard to postoperative pain control, the literature is ambiguous on the effect of cyclooxygenase-1 (COX-1)/COX-2 and COX-2–only inhibitors on delayed bone healing.[38-46] The argument revolves around increased levels of prostaglandin E_2 and F_2 during the early phases of bone healing.[47] Nonsteroidal anti-inflammatory drugs or COX-2 inhibitors have been reported to inhibit these two types of prostaglandins. A 2009 study by Alissa and colleagues investigated this particular issue.[48] In this study a total of 61 patients were allocated to the ibuprofen (31 patients) or placebo group (30 patients). Overall, 132 implants were inserted, with 67 being in the ibuprofen group and 65 in the placebo group. The primary outcome

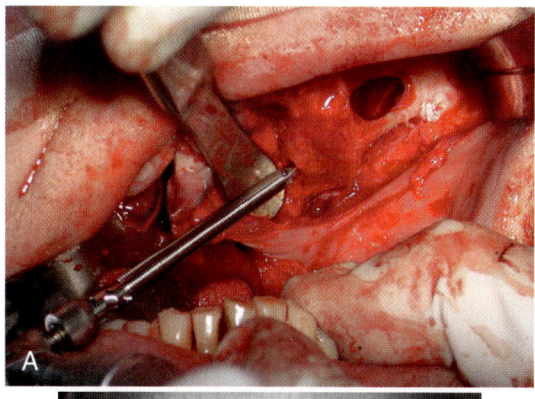

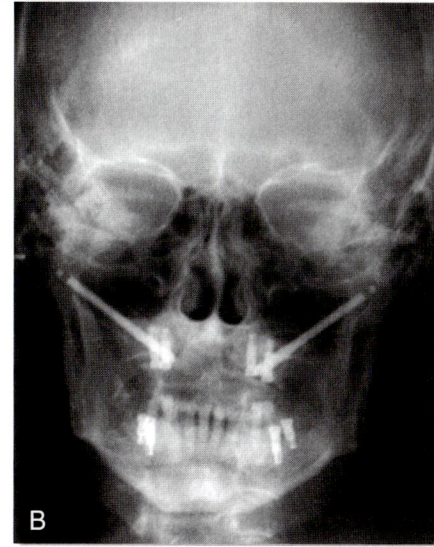

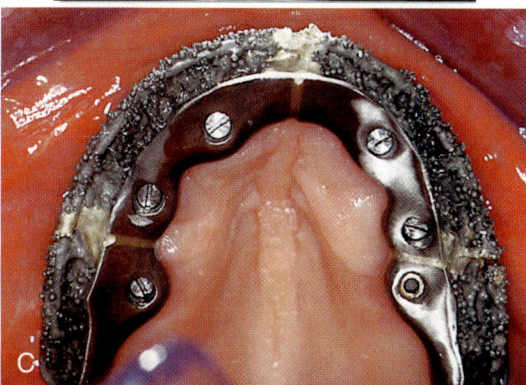

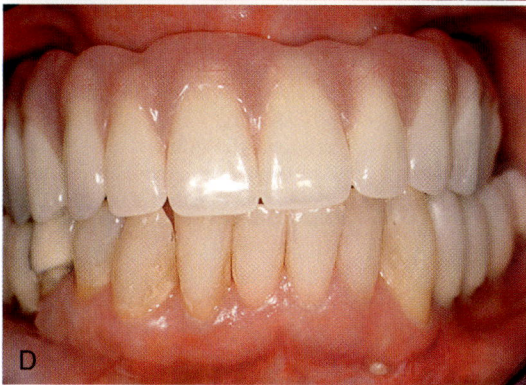

Fig. 12-9 ■ The Zygomaticus implants allow the clinician to place implants in a severely resorbed posterior maxillary without the need for bone grafting. **A,** Zygomaticus implant being delivered to the osteotomy site. This particular one is a 52.5-mm implant. **B,** Radiographic appearance on a posteroanterior skull film. **C,** Metal framework try-in. **D,** Final restoration in place. (Prosthetic photographs courtesy Dr. Edwin McGlumphy.)

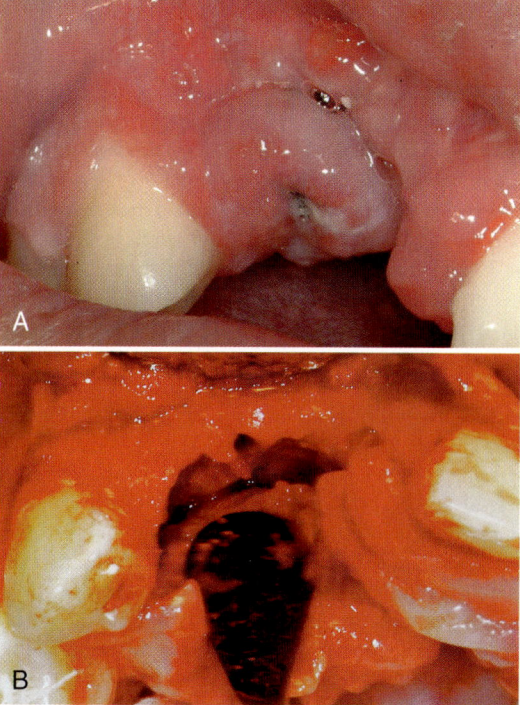

Fig. 12-10 ■ Peri-implantitis is a serious complication that can compromise implant success. **A,** Development of a peri-implant infection during the healing period, 2 months after placement. **B,** The implant had to be removed and the site débrided. Notice the significant amount of bone loss at the site, which will require aggressive reconstruction if a new attempt is to be made to place a new fixture.

measure was change in marginal bone level around the dental implants from baseline (2 weeks after placement) to the 3- and 6-month radiographic examinations. At the end, no statistically significant difference was found between the two groups of patients. For this reason, a short-term course of 5 to 7 days of this medication is recommended. Additional analgesic support through the use of opioid agonists is also advisable in the early postoperative period.

PERI-IMPLANTITIS

Peri-implantitis is an inflammatory process that affects the tissue around an osseointegrated dental implant and results in exaggerated marginal bone loss.[49] Interestingly, the microorganisms associated with this process are different from those typically found in periodontal infectious processes. They include *Porphyromonas gingivalis*, *Porphyromonas intermedia*, and *Actinobacillus actinomycetemcomitans*. Peri-implantitis is considered a multi-factorial condition with susceptibility being closely related to the host's immune response, the presence of systemic disease, and the quality of the local environment around the implant[50] (Fig. 12-10).

The University of Berne in Switzerland described a novel approach for the management of peri-implantitis called cumulative interceptive support therapy.[51] The main goal of this approach is to detect peri-implant infections as early as possible and address the problem with appropriate therapy. The parameters considered are the presence of plaque, bleeding on probing, purulent exudate, peri-implant pockets, and radiographic evidence of bone loss. In normal ideal clinical conditions, implants should not have any of these characteristics. In situations in which these findings are present, supportive therapy is used. It consists of four different protocols: mechanical débridement, antiseptic treatment, antibiotic treatment, and regenerative or resective therapy.

Mechanical débridement is always the first level of therapy and in many instances can be accomplished with rubber cups and polishing paste. In addition, acrylic scalers could also be used for the removal of gross amounts of calculus. The second level of therapy consists of antiseptic treatment. This therapy is added to the cumulative support treatment when bleeding is demonstrated on probing or there are pockets measuring between 4 and 5 mm, with or without the presence of suppuration. The antiseptic recommended is chlorhexidine digluconate at a concentration between 0.1% and 0.2% for 3 to 4 weeks. The next level of treatment consists of antibiotic therapy and is indicated in situations in which probing depth greater than 6 mm is found, with or without the presence of pus, and bleeding is demonstrated on probing. The systemic antibiotics recommended are ornidazole, metronidazole, or metronidazole combined with amoxicillin. Furthermore, topical antibiotics could be used, such as 25% tetracycline fibers. The last level of treatment involves regenerative or resective therapy, which is reserved for patients with severe bone destruction. This treatment requires an environment free of infection, and the surgical goal is to correct the soft tissue, apply guided tissue regeneration, or both. In patients with severe bone loss, implant mobility, or infection that does not respond to the salvage therapy, implant removal is indicated.

SUMMARY

Dental implant therapy has evolved by leaps and bounds over the last 30 years, particularly in the last decade. Groundbreaking research coupled with revolutionary technologic advances has provided the clinician with invaluable tools to deliver never before seen treatment options to replace missing teeth and their surrounding tissues. This chapter has attempted to illustrate some of the most salient points regarding this "implant revolution," but it is not an exhaustive review of all the different treatment options currently available. Such a review would require a complete textbook or a series of them.

There is no question that these are exciting times to be involved in the care of patients in need of dental implants, and of course, the logical question to ask is "what is coming next?"

PEARLS AND PITFALLS

- For the past 30 years, oral implantology has been evolving to become one of the main focuses of modern dentistry.
- Partial and complete edentulism continues to be a growing problem, especially in the patient population 40 years and older.
- The timing of dental implant therapy is essential in attempts to prevent atrophy of the residual alveolar ridges.
- Cone beam CT has become a very useful tool in the diagnosis and management of dental implant patients, particularly for those with severe anatomic and structural compromise. However, image interpretation and translation to the actual clinical scenario continue to rest on the shoulders of the treating clinician.
- Immediate loading of dental implants has proved to be an effective and predictable treatment option. However, case selection continues to be of the utmost importance in preventing undesirable results.
- Postoperative management, including therapy for peri-implantitis, is key to long-term success.
- As surgical professionals, we need to remember that the ultimate goal of implant restoration is that the implant look like and function like a tooth. Proper presurgical planning and sound surgical principles provide us with the opportunity to deliver high-quality care to our patients.

REFERENCES

1. Brennan M, Houston F, O'Sullivan M, et al: Patient satisfaction and oral health–related quality of life outcomes of implant overdentures and fixed complete dentures, *Int J Oral Maxillofac Implants* 25:791-800, 2010.
2. Beltran-Aguilar ED, Barker LK, Canto MT, et al, for the Centers for Disease Control and Prevention (CDC). Surveillance for dental caries, dental sealants, tooth retention, edentulism, and enamel fluorosis—United States, 1988-1994 and 1999-2002, *MMWR Surveill Summ* 54(3):1-43, 2005.
3. Xu J, Kochanek KD, Murphy SL, et al: Deaths—final data 2007, *Natl Vital Stat Rep* 58(19):1-135, 2010.
4. Joshipura KJ, Willett WC, Douglass CW: The impact of edentulousness on food and nutrient intake, *J Am Dent Assoc* 127:459-467, 1996.
5. Hildebrandt GH, Dominguez BL, Schork MA, et al: Functional units, chewing, swallowing, and food avoidance among the elderly, *J Prosthet Dent* 77:588-595, 1997.
6. Felton DA: Edentulism and comorbid factors, *J Prosthodont* 18:88-96, 2009.
7. Wolff J: *Das Gesetz der Transformation der Knochen*, Berlin, 1892, Verlag von August Hirschwald.
8. Roberts WE, Fielder PJ, Rosenoer LM, et al: Nuclear morphometric analysis of osteoblast precursor cells in periodontal ligament, SL-3 rats, *Am J Physiol* 252:R247-R251, 1987.
9. Covani U, Bortolaia C, Barone A, et al: Bucco-lingual crestal bone changes after immediate and delayed implant placement, *J Periodontol* 75:1605-1612, 2004.
10. Tallgren A: The reduction in face height of edentulous and partially edentulous subjects during long-term denture wear. A longitudinal roentgenographic cephalometric study, *Acta Odontol Scand* 24:195-239, 1966.
11. Lekovic V, Camargo PM, Klokkevold PR, et al: Preservation of alveolar bone in extraction sockets using bioabsorbable membranes, *J Periodontol* 69:1044-1049, 1998.
12. Brooks SL: Radiation doses of common dental radiographic examinations: a review, *Acta Stomatolog Croat* 42:202-217, 2008.
13. Laskin DM, Dent CD, Morris HF, et al: The influence of preoperative antibiotics on success of endosseous implants at 36 months, *Ann Periodontol* 5:166-174, 2000.
14. Dent CD, Olson JW, Farish SE, et al: The influence of preoperative antibiotics on success of endosseous implants up to and including stage II surgery: a study of 2,641 implants, *J Oral Maxillofac Surg* 55:19-24, 1997.
15. Morris HF, Ochi S, Plezia R, et al: AICRG, Part III: the influence of antibiotic use on the survival of a new implant design, *J Oral Implantol* 30:144-151, 2004.
16. Mazzocchi A, Passi L, Moretti R: Retrospective analysis of 736 implants inserted without antibiotic therapy, *J Oral Maxillofac Surg* 65:2321-2323, 2007.
17. Cochran DL, Morton D, Weber HP: Consensus statements and recommended clinical procedures regarding loading protocols for endosseous dental implants, *Int J Oral Maxillofac Implants* 19(Suppl):109-113, 2004.
18. Garg AK, Reddi SN, Chacon GE: The importance of asepsis in dental implantology, *Implant Soc J* 5:8-11, 1994.
19. Adell R, Lekholm U, Brånemark P-I: Surgical procedures. In Brånemark P-I, Zarb GA, Albrektsson T, editors: *Tissue-integrated prostheses: osseointegration in clinical dentistry*, Chicago, 1985, Quintessence, pp 211-232.
20. Eriksonn R, Albrektsson T: Temperature thresholds for heat-induced bone tissue injury: a vital-microscopic study in the rabbit, *J Prosthetic Dent* 50:101-107, 1983.
21. Chacon GE, Bower DL, Larsen PE, et al: Heat production by 3 implant drill systems after repeated drilling and sterilization, *J Oral Maxillofac Surg* 64:265-269, 2006.
22. Koh RU, Rudek I, Wang HL: Immediate implant placement: positives and negatives, *Implant Dent* 19:98-108, 2010.
23. Misch CE: Anterior single-tooth replacement: surgical consideration. In Misch CE, editor: *Contemporary implant dentistry*, St Louis, 2008, CV Mosby, pp 739-768.

24. Esposito M, Grusovin MG, Polyzos IP, et al: Timing of implant placement after tooth extraction: immediate, immediate-delayed or delayed implants? A Cochrane systematic review, *Eur J Oral Implantol* 3:189-205, 2010.

25. Siegenthaler DW, Jung RE, Holderegger C, et al: Replacement of teeth exhibiting periapical pathology by immediate implants: a prospective, controlled clinical trial, *Clin Oral Implants Res* 18:727-737, 2007.

26. Romanos G, Fronum S, Hery C, et al: Survival rate of immediately vs delayed loaded implants: analysis of the current literature, *J Oral Implantol* 36:315-324, 2010.

27. Bahat O, Sullivan RM: Parameters for successful implant integration revisited part II: algorithm for immediate loading diagnostic factors, *Clin Implant Dent Relat Res* 12(Suppl 1):e13-e22, 2010.

28. Schnitman PA, Wöhrle PS, Rubenstein JE: Immediate fixed interim prostheses supported by two-stage threaded implants: methodology and results, *J Oral Implant* 15:96-105, 1990.

29. Henry P, Rosenberg I: Single-stage surgery for rehabilitation of the mandible: preliminary results, *Pract Periodont Aesthet Dent* 6:15-22, 1994.

30. Brånemark P-I, Engstrand P, Öhrnell L-O, et al: Brånemark Novum: a new treatment concept for rehabilitation of the edentulous mandible. Preliminary results from a prospective clinical follow-up study, *Clin Implant Dent Relat Res* 1:2-16, 1999.

31. Chow J, Hui E, Liu J, et al: The Hong Kong Bridge Protocol. Immediate loading of mandibular Brånemark fixtures using a fixed provisional prosthesis: preliminary results, *Clin Implant Dent Relat Res* 3:166-174, 2001.

32. Chiapasco M, Abati S, Romeo E, et al: Implant-retained mandibular overdentures with Brånemark System MKII implants: a prospective comparative study between

33. Chiapasco M, Gatti C: Implant-retained mandibular overdentures with immediate loading: a 3- to 8-year prospective study on 328 implants, *Clin Implant Dent Relat Res* 5:29-38, 2003.

34. Castellon P, Block MS, Smith MB, et al: Immediate loading of the edentulous mandible: delivery of the final restoration or a provisional restoration—which method to use? *J Oral Maxillofac Surg* 62(9 Suppl 2):30-40, 2004.

35. Stevenson AR, Austin BW: Zygomatic fixtures—the Sydney experience, *Ann R Australas Coll Dent Surg* 15:337-339, 2000.

36. Higuchi KW: The Zygomaticus fixture: an alternative approach for implant anchorage in the posterior maxilla, *Ann R Australas Coll Dent Surg* 15:28-33, 2000.

37. Nkenke E, Hahn M, Lell M, et al: Anatomic site evaluation of the zygomatic bone for dental implant placement, *Clin Oral Implants Res* 14:72-79, 2003.

38. Dekel S, Lenthall G, Francis MJ: Release of prostaglandins from bone and muscle after tibial fracture. An experimental study in rabbits, *J Bone Joint Surg Br* 63:185-189, 1981.

39. Bo J, Sudmann E, Marton PF: Effect of indomethacin on fracture healing in rats, *Acta Orthop Scand* 47:588-599, 1976.

40. Sudmann E, Hagen T: Indomethacin-induced delayed fracture healing, *Arch Orthop Unfallchir* 85:151-154, 1976.

41. Allen HL, Wase A, Bear WT: Indomethacin and aspirin: effect of nonsteroidal anti-inflammatory agents on the rate of fracture repair in the rat, *Acta Orthop Scand* 51:595-600, 1980.

42. Huo MH, Troiano NW, Pelker RR, et al: The influence of ibuprofen on fracture repair: biomechanical, biochemical, histologic, and

histomorphometric parameters in rats, *J Orthop Res* 9:383-390, 1991.

43. Altman RD, Latta LL, Keer R, et al: Effect of nonsteroidal antiinflammatory drugs on fracture healing: a laboratory study in rats, *J Orthop Trauma* 9:392-400, 1995.

44. Aspenberg P: Postoperative COX inhibitors and late prosthetic loosening—suspicion increases! *Acta Orthop* 76:733-734, 2005.

45. Gregory LS, Forwood MR: Cyclooxygenase-2 inhibition delays the attainment of peak woven bone formation following four-point bending in the rat, *Calcif Tissue Int* 80:176-183, 2007.

46. Tiseo BC, Namur GN, de Paula EJ, et al: Experimental study of the action of COX-2 selective nonsteroidal anti-inflammatory drugs and traditional anti-inflammatory drugs in bone regeneration, *Clinics (Sao Paulo)* 61:223-230, 2006.

47. Funk CD: Prostaglandins and leukotrienes: advances in eicosanoid biology, *Science* 294:1871-1875, 2001.

48. Alissa R, Sakka S, Oliver R, et al: Influence of ibuprofen on bone healing around dental implants: a randomised double-blind placebo-controlled clinical study, *Eur J Oral Implantol* 2:185-199, 2009.

49. Albrektsson T, Isidor E: Consensus report of session W. In Lang NP, Karring T, editors. Proceedings of the First European Workshop on Periodontology, London, 1994, Quintessence, pp 365-369.

50. Alsaadi G, Quirynen M, Komárek A, et al: Impact of local and systemic factors on the incidence of oral implant failures, up to abutment connection, *J Clin Periodontol* 34:610-617, 2007.

51. Lang NP, Wilson TG, Corbet EF: Biological complications with dental implants: their prevention, diagnosis and treatment, *Clin Oral Implants Res* 11(Suppl 1):14, 2000.

THE PAST

Oral surgical procedures dominated the entire specialty upon its birth in 1918. The majority of the procedures were related to exodontia and elimination of odontogenic infections. As a result of increasing experience with dentoalveolar trauma, especially in World War II, the specialty developed a more comprehensive approach to facial trauma care; this was recognized by other specialties. Only in the later part of the 20th century did reconstructive and regenerative oral surgical procedures (implants, bone grafting) flourish.

THE PRESENT

The scope of oral surgical procedures has dramatically expanded to encompass complex dental and bone reconstructive modalities with implants and advanced bone grafting techniques. The influence of other specialties, such as orthodontics, has brought with it the need for elective minor (e.g., exposure of canines) and major (orthognathic) surgical procedures; however, extraction of third molars continues to be a major part of the private oral and maxillofacial surgical practice. Computer-assisted surgery has improved the accuracy and predictability of many procedures. The development of evidence-based medicine challenges the logic behind many routine surgical procedures. With increasing age, the need for geriatric care of patients with complex medical problems has put a greater demand on the profession. In addition, complications of other medical or surgical care, such as osteoradionecrosis, bisphosphonate-related osteonecrosis, and peripheral trigeminal nerve injuries, have been given greater emphasis.

THE FUTURE

The practice of oral surgery will be significantly enhanced by improved tissue regeneration technology using computer-assisted treatment plans and surgery. The ability to selectively and predictably grow tissue, such as bone, mucosa, and nerve tissue, using growth factors and distraction technology, will facilitate reconstruction of currently challenging defects, such as the atrophic mandible. Advances in local anesthetic delivery systems will eliminate the need for needle injections. Soft tissue diagnosis without biopsy can be envisioned using advanced scanning technology as seen in many science fiction movies. The need for basic oral surgical procedures such as exodontia is unlikely to change, especially with increased ease of tooth replacement with computer-assisted implantology. However, exodontia will be facilitated by instrumentation that dissolves or disrupts the periodontal ligaments with minimal intervention. In-office scanners will allow intraoperative visualization of relevant surgical anatomy, such as the lingual or inferior alveolar nerve.

Chapter **13**

Management of Asymptomatic Wisdom Teeth: An Evidence-Based Approach

Thomas B. Dodson

The management of wisdom teeth or third molars (M3s) can be challenging. The purpose of this chapter is to outline an evidence-based approach to the management of asymptomatic, disease-free wisdom teeth.

ANATOMIC AND CLINICAL DEFINITIONS

For the purposes of this chapter, an *impacted tooth* is unlikely to erupt into a useful, functional position due to inadequate space to accommodate the tooth. An impacted tooth may be visible in the mouth. An impacted tooth may not be visible in the mouth but may be palpated with a periodontal probe. In this circumstance, the M3 is unerupted but chronically contaminated due to its communication with the oral cavity. An impacted tooth may not be visible or palpable with a periodontal probe, and it may be evident only on a radiograph.

An *erupted tooth* has reached the occlusal plane and has no evidence of an operculum. An erupted wisdom tooth may or may not be functional. An erupted wisdom tooth may or may not be hygienic, as evidenced by gingival inflammation or plaque accumulation. Please notice, in this chapter, there is no definition of a partially erupted M3. A partially erupted M3 could be considered impacted—that is, a static condition in which the tooth is unlikely to erupt into a useful functional position—or a dynamic condition with the tooth expected to erupt fully.

For the purposes of this chapter, M3s are classified based on the presence (or absence) of patient report of symptoms and the presence (or absence) of disease detected by physical or radiographic examination. Given these two categories, that is, symptom and disease status, M3s can be classified into four groups (Box 13-1). The groups are (1) symptomatic and signs of disease present (Sx+/D+), (2) symptomatic and disease free (Sx+/D−), (3) asymptomatic and disease present (Sx−/D+), and (4) asymptomatic and disease free (Sx−/D−).

The Sx+/D+ (symptomatic, disease present) group is recognized based on history and physical or radiographic examination, for

	DISEASE PRESENT	
SYMPTOMS PRESENT	**YES**	**NO**
Yes	S+/D+	S+/D–
No	S–/D+	S–/D–

S+/D+, Symptoms present/disease present, for instance, symptomatic pericoronitis or caries.

S+/D–, Symptoms present/disease-free, for instance, pain due to eruption ("teething"), but there is adequate room for the tooth to erupt or vague pain without any clinical or radiographic evidence of disease.

S–/D+, Asymptomatic/disease present, for instance, patient has no complaints, but there is clinical evidence of caries, periodontal disease, or radiographic evidence of disease, such as bone loss, resorption, or a space-occupying lesion.

S–/D–, Asymptomatic/disease-free, for instance, patient has no complaints and no disease is evident on clinical or radiographic examination.

instance, symptomatic pericoronitis, caries, or swelling or pain from a secondarily infected cystic lesion. The Sx+/D– (symptomatic, disease-absent) group is more subtle. Clinical examples include pain symptoms from teething in the setting of adequate space for the M3 to erupt into a useful, functional position and vague complaints of pain in the M3 region but no specific disease that explains well the symptoms. The Sx–/D+ (asymptomatic, disease present) group is also recognizable. The patient reports no symptoms, but disease is evident on clinical examination, for instance, soft tissue inflammation, caries, plaque accumulation, and increased probing depths, or on radiographic examination, for instance, cystic lesions, caries, internal resorption, or resorption or caries of adjacent teeth. The Sx–/D– (asymptomatic, disease-absent) group is also readily recognizable. By history, the patient reports no symptoms, and there are no signs of disease evident on physical or radiographic examination. In all of the above settings, the tooth may be erupted or impacted.

GENERAL APPROACHES TO THE MANAGEMENT OF M3s

Sx+/D+

Most patients in this group would benefit from operative intervention, ranging from restorative care to periodontal therapy to extraction, depending on the functional and hygienic status of the tooth and the ease or predictability of delivering care. At one extreme, based on the patient's wishes, an erupted, functional, hygienic, clinically accessible M3 may be treated with the full scope of restorative care, including endodontic, periodontal, and prosthetic treatment. Conversely, many times, extraction may be the preferred option. There may be a role for medical management, for instance, symptomatic relief with antibiotics and analgesics in the setting where extraction may be contraindicated due to risk for nerve injury and the patient refuses coronectomy. Given multiple treatment options, and consistent with the principles of evidence-based care, patient interest, desire, and perception of risks, benefits, and costs need to be incorporated into the clinician's decision-making process.[1,2]

Sx+/D–

While uncommon, there is a cohort of patients who have symptoms and signs of pericoronitis due to tooth eruption, but they appear to have adequate room for the teeth to erupt into a useful, functional position. In this setting, pericoronitis is a side effect of tooth eruption, not disease. Treatment options range from medical management with expectant monitoring to extraction. Discriminating

between teething pain associated with a tooth that will erupt and pericoronitis of an impacted tooth can be challenging.

Predicting which M3s will erupt into a useful, functional position is a challenging and imperfect process.[3,4] As such, both the patient and clinician need to be prepared to admit to an error in prognosis and be prepared to alter the treatment recommendation. For example, despite an initial preference for medical management, after multiple symptomatic episodes, a patient may elect extraction, despite the clinician's assurance that there is a high likelihood that the symptomatic tooth will erupt into a useful, functional position. Alternatively, despite the radiographic assessment of adequate space, the clinician may note an absence of progress in eruption and now recommend extraction over expectant monitoring.

In some cases, pain symptoms may be attributed to the M3s, but there is no demonstrable clinical or radiographic disease. Extraction may be indicated to eliminate M3s from the differential diagnosis.

Sx–/D+

This group of patients will be commonly encountered by oral and maxillofacial surgeons (OMSs). In a cohort of subjects of age 14 to 45 years with asymptomatic M3s, 25% of the study subjects had periodontal disease as evidenced by probing depths of greater than 5 mm.[5] This group may also include patients with asymptomatic carious lesions, pericoronitis, or radiographic evidence of disease, for instance, radiolucent lesions or resorption of the M3 or the adjacent tooth. In this group, treatment is tailored to the patient's needs and desires and ranges from restorative care to extraction.

Sx–/D–

The remainder of this chapter is devoted to one of the more challenging decisions that the practicing OMS faces on a daily basis: how to manage the asymptomatic, disease-free M3. The key clinical question to answer is "Among patients with asymptomatic, disease-free (Sx–/D–) M3s, do those who elect M3 extraction to prevent problems in the future, when compared with those who elect M3 retention, have better outcomes?" Fortunately, there has been a systematic review of the topic summarized in the Cochrane Reviews and the answer is simple: "No evidence was found to support or refute routine prophylactic removal of asymptomatic impacted wisdom teeth in adults."[6]

Given the lack of high-quality evidence to direct care, what is the clinician to do? Evidence-based clinical decision making is not characterized by abandoning clinical responsibility in the absence of high-quality evidence. It is, instead, making clinical decisions with the *best evidence available* while incorporating patient preferences and desires, assessments of risks and benefits, costs and consequences into the decision-making process. In the case of asymptomatic, disease-free M3s, given the lack of evidence supporting M3 retention versus extraction, patient preference is the primary driving force in deciding treatment.[7]

MANAGEMENT OF ASYMPTOMATIC, DISEASE-FREE (Sx–/D–) M3s

When managing Sx–/D– M3s, there are functionally two treatment choices. The first choice is M3 extraction to prevent problems in the future. The second choice is active surveillance and rendering treatment as indicated, for instance, extractions, restorative or periodontal care, or continued surveillance. The elements of active surveillance are undefined, but would include an assessment of patient symptoms and a physical and radiographic examination. Who should be doing the surveillance, for instance, generalist or specialist, and the frequency of visits, for instance, annual or biannual, is undefined.

The risks and costs of M3 removal have been well documented and will not be detailed in this review. Briefly, they include surgical-site infections and other inflammatory complications, bleeding, damage to adjacent teeth or restoration(s), new or persistent periodontal defects on the adjacent teeth, tuberosity or mandibular fractures, retained roots, lingual or mandibular nerve injury, a persistent symptomatic oroantral communication, and need for additional treatment to manage the complication(s). In additiona to the direct costs of care, there are the indirect costs due to loss of productivity at work or school.

The risks and implications of M3 retention are less well detailed. Recent studies involving study cohorts of subjects who have elected to retain their asymptomatic, disease-free teeth have demonstrated that (1) asymptomatic M3s are not necessarily disease free[5]; (2) that retained M3s frequently and unpredictably change position, eruption status, and periodontal status[8,9]; and (3) retained, asymptomatic M3s may be extracted between 30% and 60% of the time.[10-12] As such, patients who elect active surveillance as their preferred treatment are committed to a lifetime of monitoring with its associated costs and no assurance that extraction can be avoided later in life. As a personal observation, the oldest person this author has treated for wisdom tooth problems was 93 years old.

Despite the dearth of data to inform decision making regarding Sx–/D– M3s, two organizations, the American Public Health Association (APHA) and the United Kingdom's National Health Service (NHS), have formally recommended against the removal of M3s when the only treatment goal is to prevent problems in the future.[13,14] As an avid proponent of evidence-based clinical decision making, this author is surprised and disappointed that these two organizations would develop policy recommendations absent compelling data to support or refute treatment alternatives. The APHA policy recommendation is based on a one-sided, biased presentation of research findings, and in this author's opinion, can be generally ignored due to its unscientific summary of the published literature.[15]

The NHS recommendation, however, is based on a thoughtful, considered summary of the available data, requiring a more careful evaluation of its rationale for recommending against the removal of M3s. The fundamental flaw common to both organizations' policy recommendations is that, while carefully assessing the risks of operative intervention, they either ignore completely or fail to account appropriately for the costs and consequences of "prescribing" retention of Sx–/D– M3s.

The NHS's National Institute for Clinical Excellence (NICE) drafted and disseminated guidance for M3 management. Briefly, the guidelines suggest that the practice of prophylactic removal of pathology-free, impacted M3s should be discontinued, and removal of impacted M3s should be limited to patients with evidence of pathology. One episode of pericoronitis is insufficient to warrant removal, unless the episode is particularly severe.[16]

The evidence supporting the NICE recommendation regarding M3 management is low quality. NICE asserts that "there is no reliable research evidence to support a health benefit to patients from prophylactic removal of pathology-free impacted" M3s. There is a fallacy in logic when one uses the absence of data to support one treatment option (prophylactic extraction) as the rationale to support an alternative treatment option (nonoperative treatment). There is a general failure to appreciate the costs and consequences of nonoperative treatment, reflecting an underlying, unproven, and unstated bias that nonoperative treatment is both safer and less expensive than operative treatment.

The sole research document cited by NICE to support its position is a review article that summarizes the effectiveness and cost-effectiveness of prophylactic removal of M3s.[17] The authors reviewed 40 articles. Two articles were randomized controlled trials. One trial concluded that M3 removal to prevent incisor crowding was unwarranted. The other trial, comparing operative versus non-operative M3 management, was ongoing and results were unavailable. There were 34 literature reviews of poor quality. There were four well-executed decision-analysis papers that consistently suggested that a strategy of M3 retention was cheaper and more cost effective than removal of pathology-free M3s.[18-21]

This author's reading of the Song et al paper is that the fundamental basis for the recommendation against prophylactic removal of Sx–/D– M3s was based on the economic analyses. In the setting of evidence-based decision making, a therapeutic clinical decision or policy recommendation based on economic analyses, absent sufficient clinical follow-up or verification studies, is better than expert opinion but is still a very weak level of evidence (2c).[22] Given the significant weight that NICE placed on the economic analyses, a more careful review of these studies is warranted.

The first element to consider when assessing the validity of cost-effectiveness analyses is how "cost" is estimated. As such, the reader must determine if all of the relevant or important costs are included. The paper by Edwards et al concludes that mandibular M3 retention is a less costly and more cost-effective strategy than extraction of pathology-free teeth.[19] Many relevant or important costs are not considered, and the focus of the cost-saving benefits accrue to the NHS (the payor), not the patient (the beneficiary).

One example of a cost oversight is to assume that the cost of managing an asymptomatic, disease-free M3 with retention of the M3 was $0. This assumption seems simplistic at best and disingenuous at worst. It fails to account for the cost of a lifetime of follow-up for patients who retain their M3s. At a minimum, some costs are incurred for serial panoramic imaging required to monitor asymptomatic, disease-free M3s. In a second example, the investigators estimate the cost of an episode of pericoronitis to be £14, the cost of a consultant visit. This cost assumption fails to account for the patient's pain and suffering, the opportunity costs to the patient for missed work or school, and the consultant's opportunity cost for repeat medical management visits, the costs of medical management (antibiotics and analgesics), and any associated imaging costs. In a third example, the analyses assume that the cost of converting from disease-free to diseased M3s is simply the cost of tooth extraction (£458). Globally, this assumption fails to account for patient pain, suffering, and inconvenience of unscheduled time missed from school or work; the opportunity cost of the clinician in re-evaluating a patient; costs of medical management, for instance, antibiotics or analgesics; and management costs of associated complications, for instance, damage to the adjacent second molar and management of an odontogenic cyst or tumor.

Perhaps treatment costs are sufficiently different between the United States and the United Kingdom to make the findings of the analysis not applicable to U.S. surgeons and patients. For example, cost estimates of M3s removed in the United Kingdom included a significant proportion of patients who were treated in a hospital. In the United States, the overwhelming majority of M3 extractions are completed in an office-based ambulatory setting at significantly lower costs than treatment rendered in a hospital.

The second element of cost-effectiveness analyses is the measurement or estimate of "effectiveness." In the analyses of M3 management, effectiveness is measured by patient preference of alternative outcomes, that is, utilities. The assessment of utilities, or patient preferences, can be challenging to implement and difficult to understand by both the research subject and the casual reader of cost-analyses studies. The usual method is to query research subjects regarding a number of health outcomes, for instance, a few days of pain due to pericoronitis or a fractured mandible following the removal of Sx–/D– M3s, and then ask the subjects to rank and weight their preferences.

The abilities of the researcher to develop appropriate health outcome scenarios and of research subjects to rank and weight appropriately the different health care outcomes are critical to estimating treatment effectiveness. If the research subjects cannot appropriately rank or weight their preference for a health outcome, the entire cost-effectiveness analysis is thrown into disarray. For example, in a study measuring patient preferences regarding M3 removal, research subjects reported that having "… fluid-filled sac around your wisdom tooth … was preferable to experiencing … mild discomfort for a few days …" after tooth extraction.[23] In other words, the research subjects preferred having an odontogenic cyst or tumor rather than an elective extraction of a M3. This preference choice makes no sense and leads this author to question the research subjects' abilities to discern among the preferences or even understand their choices and associated consequences.

Good cost-effectiveness analyses include sensitivity analyses to estimate how changes in assumptions change the decision, for instance, a recommendation favoring tooth retention may change to a recommendation favoring extraction. In the Edwards et al study, the sensitivity analyses revealed that this model was only sensitive to the threshold probability estimates for pericoronitis (0.4), periodontal disease (0.17), and unrestorable caries in the adjacent second molar (0.22).[19] For example, if the frequency of periodontal disease is greater than 0.17, the most cost-effective strategy for an asymptomatic mandibular M3 would change from retention to removal. Of note, the current estimate of the prevalence of periodontal disease in a sample of asymptomatic individuals is 0.25.[5]

Overall, the major weakness of all of the studies acknowledged by the Song et al, common to all of the economic analyses was the inability to assess the long-term consequences of nonoperative management. This is not an inconsequential limitation. While most consequences of operative M3 management are short term and easier to measure, for instance, pain, swelling, and loss of work or school, the costs and consequences of a strategy to manage M3s nonoperatively must be assessed over the patient's life span.

The final element in cost-effectiveness analyses is determining how the model behaves in the "real" world. Given the findings of the cost-effectiveness studies, NICE recommends no extraction for asymptomatic, disease-free M3s. An obvious question is "What happens to the M3s over time?" An alternative question is "How often was the recommended or prescribed treatment protocol in error?" Recent studies permit incidence estimates of M3 extractions in samples where the prescribed M3 management strategy was retention. In a 4-year follow-up study of 130 asymptomatic mandibular M3s (*n* = 70, starting at age 20), 34 (26%) were removed due to development of disease (caries, pericoronitis, or pain).[11] Hill and Walker reported on a sample of 228 subjects whose M3s were retained.[10] At the end of five years, 71 (31%) subjects had one or more M3s removed due to developing disease. In a longer follow-up study (12 years, starting at age 20) composed of a sample of 81 students (k = 285 M3s), Venta et al documented that 54 (67%) subjects underwent extraction of one or more M3s due to signs, symptoms, or patient-perceived needs.[12] In all three studies, the authors acknowledged the high incidence of M3 removal in a setting initially prescribing retention of asymptomatic, disease-free M3s, but they claim that these findings were inadequate evidence to support a strategy of prophylactic removal. At a minimum, the relatively high, unanticipated risk for future M3 removal for Sx–/D– teeth warrants

new economic analyses comparing the two treatment strategies: active surveillance or extraction.

Given that it takes a lifetime to determine whether the recommendation to retain M3s is correct begs the question, "What are the consequences of delayed treatment?" Phillips et al demonstrated that age of extraction is associated with an increased risk for prolonged recovery following M3 removal.[24] In the multivariate adjusted model, the odds for a prolonged recovery in a patient greater than age 24 years is 3 to 4 times that of the patient who is less than or equal to 18 years for early or late symptoms, oral function, and pain recovery. The failure of any of the decision analyses papers cited by Song et al to account appropriately for the risk for extraction and the associated increased misery of extraction with increasing age is a major limitation in their usefulness in guiding clinical decision making, let alone making major policy recommendations for an organization (APHA) or a nation (United Kingdom).[13,14,17]

SUMMARY

It was not the purpose of this chapter to refute the NICE recommendation regarding its guidance in the management of asymptomatic, disease-free M3s or to criticize the NHS for adopting this position. This chapter's purpose was to review the evidence regarding the management of asymptomatic, disease-free (S–/D–) M3s. This author concluded that the current evidence regarding the management of Sx–/D– M3s is insufficient to guide treatment recommendations for individual patients, let alone draft local, regional, or national policy. Given the weak scientific basis, alternative explanations driving the motivation to adopt the NICE guidance may be political or a need to ration heath care resources. Both are acceptable rationales for accepting NICE guidance. It should be acknowledged, however, that using politics or economics as a basis for adopting NICE guidance ignores the basic evidence-based medicine principle of explicitly acknowledging and incorporating patient preference into the clinical decision-making process.

In fairness, Song et al acknowledge that the current evidence regarding M3 management is limited and the recommends are (1) implementing a randomized clinical trial "… to compare prophylactic removal with management by deliberate retention, using long-term follow-up" and (2) initiating additional "… decision analysis models that could be used to compare long-term outcomes of prophylactic removal with retention of impacted third molars."[17] Implementing a randomized trial in the United States is probably not feasible for a host of reasons, both ethical and practical, but such a trial could be completed under the auspices of the NHS. However, it is surprising that such a trial is not in place, given the very weak evidence supporting the NICE current guidelines regarding management of asymptomatic, disease-free M3s. It is also concerning the NHS has not funded or supported further economic studies to confirm or refute the previous analyses that only assess the short-term outcomes of retaining asymptomatic, disease-free M3s.

It was not the purpose of this chapter to refute M3 retention as a treatment option for the management of Sx–/D– M3s. The chapter pointed out that the data are currently insufficient to make individual patient recommendations, let alone national policy, regarding the management of Sx–/D– M3s. Among patients with Sx–/D– M3s, this author recommends a careful, unbiased presentation of the risks and benefits of operative and nonoperative management of M3s. Following this discussion, it is incumbent upon the surgeon to seek unambiguously and actively the patient's preference regarding the management choices and to weigh heavily that choice. Regardless of patients' ultimate decisions to retain or extract Sx–/D– M3s, there are substantial data to support their choices.

PEARLS AND PITFALLS

- While the management of asymptomatic, disease-free wisdom teeth is controversial, the best evidence currently available neither supports nor refutes extraction of asymptomatic, disease-free third molars.
- When managing a patient with asymptomatic, disease-free third molars, one must carefully review the risks and benefits of extraction or retention, and heavily weight the patient's treatment preference.
- For patients who elect retention, the frequency of symptoms or disease associated with the retained wisdom teeth is high enough to warrant a regular schedule of follow-up—that is, active surveillance. While details of follow-up protocols are evolving, the current recommendation is a physical and radiographic examination every 12 to 24 months by a health care professional trained to evaluate third molars.
- For patients who elect third molar retention as their preferred treatment choice, no data are available to make a recommendation as to when active surveillance may be discontinued.

REFERENCES

1. Sackett DL, Rosenberg WM, Gray JA, et al: Evidence-based medicine: what it is and what it isn't, *BMJ* 312:71-72, 1996.
2. Montori VM, Guyatt GH: Progress in evidence-based medicine, *JAMA* 300:1814-1816, 2008.
3. Venta I, Murtomaa H, Ylipaavalniemi P: A device to predict lower third molar eruption, *Oral Surg Oral Med Oral Pathol Oral Radiol Endod* 84:598-603, 1997.
4. Venta I, Schou S: Accuracy of the third molar eruption predictor in predicting eruption, *Oral Surg Oral Med Oral Pathol Oral Radiol Endod* 91:638-642, 2001.
5. Blakey GH, Marciani RD, Haug RH, et al: Periodontal pathology associated with asymptomatic third molars, *J Oral Maxillofac Surg* 60:1227-1233, 2002.
6. Mettes TG, Nienhuijs ME, van der Sanden WJ, et al: Interventions for treating asymptomatic impacted wisdom teeth in adolescents and adults, *Cochrane Database Syst Rev* (2):CD003879, 2005.
7. Norwegian Knowledge Centre for the Health Services: *Prophylactic removal of wisdom teeth: SMM-rapprt Nr. 10/2003*, Oslo, 2003, Norwegian Knowledge Centre for the Health Services (NOKC).
8. Phillips C, Norman J, Jaskolka M, et al: Changes over time in position and periodontal status of retained third molars, *J Oral Maxillofac Surg* 65:2011-2017, 2007.
9. Blakey GH, Jacks MT, Offenbacher S, et al: Progression of periodontal disease in the second/third molar region in subjects with asymptomatic third molars, *J Oral Maxillofac Surg* 64:189-193, 2006.
10. Hill CM, Walker RV: Conservative, non-surgical management of patients presenting with impacted lower third molars: a 5-year study, *Br J Oral Maxillofac Surg* 44:347-350, 2006.
11. von Wowern N, Nielsen HO: The fate of impacted lower third molars after the age of 20. A four-year clinical followup, *Int J Oral Maxillofac Surg* 18:277-280, 1989.
12. Venta I, Ylipaavalniemi P, Turtola L: Long-term evaluation of estimates of need for third molar removal, *J Oral Maxillofac Surg* 58:288-291, 2000.
13. Available at Opposition to prophylactic removal of third molars (wisdom teeth). http://www.apha.org/advocacy/policy/policysearch/default.htm?id=1371. Accessed February 28, 2011.
14. Available at Guidance on the extraction of wisdom teeth (TA1). http://egap.evidence.nhs.uk/TA1. Accessed February 28, 2011. Fact-based versus evidenced-based policy positions: confessions of an accidental politician, *J Oral Maxillofac Surg* 67:1153-1154, 2009.
15. Dodson TB: Fact-based versus evidence-based policy positions: Confessions of an accidental politician, *J Oral Maxillofac Surg* 67:1153-1154, 2009.
16. Available at Guidance on the estraction of wisdom teeth http://www.nice.org.uk/nicemedia/live/11385/31993/31993.pdf. Accessed February 28, 2011.
17. Song F, O'Meara S, Wilson P, et al: The effectiveness and cost-effectiveness of prophylactic removal, *Health Technol Assess* 4:1-55, 2000.
18. Brickley M, Kay E, Shepherd JP, Armstrong RA: Decision analysis for lower-third-molar surgery, *Med Decis Making* 15:143-151, 1995.
19. Edwards M, Brickley M, Goodey R, Shepherd J: The cost, effectiveness, and cost-effectiveness of removal and retention of asymptomatic, disease-free third molars, *Br Dent J* 187:380-384, 1999.
20. Tulloch J, Antczak-Bouckoms A: Decision analysis in the evaluation of clinical strategies for the management of mandibular third molars, *J Dent Educ* 51:652-660, 1987.
21. Tulloch J, Antczak-Bouckoms A, Ung N: Evaluation of the costs and relative effectiveness of alternative strategies for the removal of mandibular third molars, *Int J Technol Assess Health Care* 6:505-515, 1990.
22. Available at http://www.cebm.net/index.aspx?o=1025. Accessed July 31, 2009.
23. Liedholm R, Knutsson K, Lyss L, et al: The outcomes of mandibular third molar removal and non-removal: a study of patients' preferences using a multi-attribute method, *Acta Odontol Scand* 58:293-298, 2000.
24. Phillips C, White RP, Shugars DA, Zhou X: Risk factors associated with prolonged recovery and delayed healing after third molar surgery, *J Oral Maxillofac Surg* 61:1436-1448, 2003.

Value of Oral and Maxillofacial Surgeons: Dentistry's Liaisons to Medicine and Hospital Care

Chapter 14

Connie L. Drisko

Of all the oral health providers, oral and maxillofacial surgery (OMFS) is the dental specialty most closely linked to our medical colleagues. However, compared to other head and neck surgeons, oral and maxillofacial surgeons are trained in general dentistry prior to entering the specialty. This training positions them with specific dental knowledge not found in other general surgery or surgical specialties. Experience with the intricacies of the masticatory system, including the anatomy of the dentition and all of the complexities of occlusion and the envelope of motion, allow a more complete approach to treatment planning, and the restoration or replacement of these structures. This in-depth knowledge of the teeth and jaws, as well as the muscles of mastication, the temporomandibular joint, and craniofacial development, makes the oral and maxillofacial surgeon exclusively qualified to treat these conditions among all other health care providers and surgeons. Following trauma—the loss of hard and soft tissues from destructive disease or malformations from craniofacial developmental disorders—oral and maxillofacial surgeons are uniquely qualified to assemble a team of specialists across disciplines to definitively treat and facilitate the restoration and repair of oral and craniofacial structures and to reestablish masticatory, respiratory, and visual function in the case of trauma reconstruction. Enabling patients to return to a healthy state of function, comfort, and esthetics also enhances their quality of life. Teeth or their replacements are an integral predictable part of this reconstruction. Without the leadership and expertise of the oral and maxillofacial surgeon in collaboration with restorative and maxillofacial prosthodontists and other dental specialists, few trauma or cancer patients would be able to achieve optimum esthetics and function.

SCOPE OF TRAINING

The specialty goes far beyond that of general dentistry and most other dental specialties in the scope of training. In addition to having a more lengthy residency than any other specialty, the minimum of 4 years in a residency includes higher levels of "the diagnosis, surgical and adjunctive treatment of diseases, injuries and defects involving both the functional and aesthetic aspects of the hard and soft tissues of the oral and maxillofacial region" (quote from the OMFS website). Part of the intensive hospital-based training includes competency in admission history and physicals, general anesthesia, facial plastic surgery, emergency room training in general trauma, orthognathic surgery, and cancer therapy, including knowledge of postsurgical chemotherapy and radiation therapy. The residency is closely tied to many of the medical and surgical residencies, including training in anesthesia, general surgery, ear-nose-throat (ENT), medicine, hematology, emergency medicine, and many more. The hospital-based residencies provide valuable training ground for the future practice of oral and maxillofacial surgery, but the hospital and the medical system also benefit greatly from the presence of such surgeons, faculty, and residents who bring unique expertise to the

health care team by their in-depth knowledge of the oral and maxillofacial structures and function that no other specialists provide, including plastic surgeons or otolaryngologists. Team approaches to complex cases are often needed, and, when OMFS is included, they provide expertise that will enhance the overall treatment planning and reconstruction of a difficult trauma, developmental defect, or cancer case.

In the past two decades, the field of OMFS has gone through extensive change. One important factor is the development of the dual certification (MD/OMS) that has enhanced the presence of the specialty in the hospital setting and further strengthened the field among the medical specialties. Although not essential, this training path has facilitated research in many areas, including growth and development, dental implants, regenerative medicine, and advancements in maxillofacial reconstruction. The dual certification programs further advanced fellowship training in head and neck oncology, reconstruction, craniofacial syndromes, and facial plastic surgery, among others. This recent expansion of scope is rapidly changing the future of this specialty, which will undoubtedly further strengthen the stance of oral and maxillofacial surgeons in the dental and medical arena.

INTERPROFESSIONAL LIAISONS

Oral and maxillofacial surgeons are an important link in the referral network for primary care providers and are often the first to find life-threatening lesions or conditions during their examinations and routine care. Likewise, physicians often refer patients with jaw pain, oral lesions, and infections to maxillofacial surgeons, because physicians are not always trained to the same extent in the management of oral infections and lesions. Close working relationships with primary care providers allow the best possible approach for managing acute and chronic situations involving the oral and facial structures. Collaboration between dentists and physicians also enhances the capability for the patient to achieve total health. An example is the joint treatment of patients with chronic illness and conditions such as diabetes and cardiovascular, diseases that are negatively affected by oral infections, including abscessed teeth and untreated periodontal disease. Through appropriate interprofessional referrals, patients can access a team of experts in medicine and dentistry that are able to jointly provide education and recommendations for improving overall health through the management of orofacial and systemic diseases and conditions.

TREATING INFECTIONS, TRAUMA, AND CRANIOFACIAL ABNORMALITIES

The ability to manage all ranges of pathologic conditions in and about the oral and maxillofacial region has continued to evolve since the inception of the specialty. This has included an increase in training in many programs from the traditional 4 years to many now offering 7-year residencies. All programs incorporate extensive training in anesthesia administration. This enables the OMF surgeon to provide a more cost-effective and convenient surgery for their patients. Patients who present with complex maxillofacial problems can have these procedures performed in an affordable outpatient setting with the benefit of comfort and safety through pain management techniques provided by the experienced OMF surgeon.

Although many dentists are now able to place implants, those requiring extensive site developments through use of large autogenous grafting from extraoral sites, such as ribs, tibia, and iliac crest, are usually accomplished by OMF surgeons. The recent development of zygomatic implants in the severely atrophied maxilla requires the skills of an OMF surgeon, because knowledge of the zygomatic anatomy is beyond the training of other dental specialists. OMF surgeons are perhaps the best specialists to diagnosis and treat infections in the maxillofacial region, because most of these infections are of an odontogenic origin. Because these infections may also present with life-threatening emergencies, the OMF surgeon is also well suited, having knowledge of securing a compromised airway through tracheotomy in combination with knowledge of the cervical anatomy, to treat, decompress, and drain these infected spaces.

In the maxillofacial trauma arena, OMF surgeons are also well qualified to manage injuries sustained to the craniomaxillofacial region. Most of these facial trauma reconstructions are based on the ability to use the dentition and occlusion for proper anatomic reduction. No other specialist processes this extensive knowledge of the orofacial structures and dentition better than the OMF surgeon. Much of the applied craniofacial knowledge comes from the specialist's ability to correct congenital and acquired oral and maxillofacial deformities due to differences in skeletal growth. The OMF surgeon is adept and understands the importance of the dental reconstruction utilizing root-form implants and dental prostheses to support the oral facial soft tissue, which is essential in restoring the maxillofacial trauma patient to preinjury form. Working closely and communicating with his or her counterpart, the restorative dentist maximizes the reconstruction.

More persons than ever are opting for elective procedures to enhance their esthetics and correct the aging face. Although orthognathic surgery is normally performed to correct significant misalignment of the jaws and teeth and to improve breathing and function, another benefit is the simultaneous improvement of the patient's appearance. Orthodontists are usually needed to interface with the surgeon to achieve the optimum results. Dentists who have esthetics expertise are needed to guide the orientation of the jaws for optimum tooth and gingival display, function, and facial balance. Oral maxillofacial surgeons, especially those who are fellowship–trained, are competent to correct the soft tissue deficits and abnormalities.

In older adults, periodontists and restorative dentists may play a major role in the overall treatment planning process for orthognathic surgery. Working with other dental colleagues gives the oral surgeon a distinct advantage over other surgical specialties, because the OMF surgeon understands the occlusal and functional goals and is better able to contribute to the treatment planning of these complex cases. Their dental knowledge is of even greater importance when trying to correct the jaw alignment of edentulous patients, where there are no teeth to guide the surgeon. Understanding the use of customized, computerized stints and guides for the future placement of implant-supported dentures or a fixed retainer is extremely important to the surgeon doing the anatomical correction and realignment, a procedure best handled by an oral surgeon. Also, orthognathic procedures are sometimes used to correct sleep apnea. It is imperative that the surgeon is knowledgeable in the nonsurgical options available to patients needing treatment for mild forms of sleep apnea so that patients are fully informed regarding their treatment choices.

FACIAL PLASTIC SURGERY AND SKIN TREATMENTS

Because oral and maxillofacial surgeons are trained in facial reconstruction and management of head, neck, and facial trauma, they are also well positioned for performing facial cosmetic procedures on an outpatient basis, including malar augmentation, genioplasty, blepharoplasty, rhytidectomy, facial and neck liposuction, forehead and brow lift, lip enhancement, and rhinoplasty. Skin treatments are also done in oral surgeon's offices, including Botox injections, chemical peels, dermabrasion, laser and injectable fillers, such as Restylane or collagen. However, uncorrected esthetic problems may remain if the surgeon performing these cosmetic procedures is not knowledgeable about the many aspects of improving the patient's overall esthetic appearance by enhancing the smile. Knowledge of the impact of the patient's smile on his or her overall appearance can be extraordinarily helpful in treatment planning and achieving the optimum esthetic result that the patient desires.

ANESTHESIA AND MEDICAL AND DENTAL EMERGENCIES

The ability to provide patients with safe, effective outpatient anesthesia has distinguished the specialty of oral and maxillofacial surgery since its earliest days. Oral surgeons, as the surgical specialists of the dental profession, are trained in all aspects of anesthesia and are frequently asked to be the emergency experts on call in dental practices, dental schools, and other multidisciplinary clinics, including those with other dentists and physicians. They are relied on to be our safety net for treating dental and medical emergencies, because of their extensive training in emergency medicine and airway management as well as their anesthesia experience.

PEARLS AND PITFALLS

- No other specialty in dentistry requires as much expertise in so many areas of medicine and dentistry as oral and maxillofacial surgery.
- Training is not limited to dental management of patients; it also includes the medical management of the patient as well.
- Procedures range from those based in plastic and general surgery, oral and internal medicine, oral and general pathology, cancer therapy, dermatology, and orthopedics.
- OMF surgeons are the interface between medicine and dentistry and perform many of the same functions as a physician, and more.

Removal of Third Molars

Chapter 15

M.A. Pogrel

Third molar removal is the most frequently performed single procedure carried out by many oral and maxillofacial surgeons. Surveys have shown that over 80% of many oral and maxillofacial surgeons' practice is taken up with dentoalveolar surgery, of which about 65% is removal of third molars. Indications for removal of unerupted third molars are identified in the Parameters and Pathways published by the American Association of Oral and Maxillofacial Surgeons and include[1]:

1. Pain
2. Carious tooth
3. Pericoronitis
4. Facilitation of the management of or limitation of progression of periodontal disease
5. Nontreatable pulpal or periapical lesion
6. Acute and/or chronic infection (e.g., cellulitis, abscess)
7. Ectopic position (malposition, supraeruption, traumatic occlusion)
8. Abnormalities of tooth size or shape precluding normal function
9. Facilitation of prosthetic rehabilitation
10. Facilitation of orthodontic tooth movement and promotion of stability of the dental occlusion
11. Tooth in the line of fracture complicating fracture management
12. Tooth involved in surgical treatment of associated cysts and tumors
13. Tooth interfering with orthognathic and/or reconstructive surgery
14. Preventive or prophylactic removal, when indicated, for patients with medical or surgical conditions or treatments (e.g., organ transplants, alloplastic implants, bisphosphonate therapy, chemotherapy, radiation therapy)
15. Clinical findings of pulp exposure by dental caries
16. Clinical findings of fractured tooth or teeth
17. Impacted tooth
18. Internal or external resorption of tooth or adjacent teeth
19. Patient's informed refusal of nonsurgical treatment options
20. Anatomic position causing potential damage to adjacent teeth
21. Use of the third molar as a donor tooth for tooth transplant
22. Tooth impeding the normal eruption of an adjacent tooth
23. Resorption of an adjacent tooth
24. Pathology associated with the tooth follicle
25. Abnormality of size or shape precluding normal function

REMOVAL OF LOWER THIRD MOLARS

Techniques advocated for removal of unerupted or impacted lower third molars usually involve the raising of a buccal flap, which involves an incision down the external oblique ridge to the distobuccal line angle of the second molar, and then down into the buccal sulcus anterolaterally, terminating at the distal aspect of the first molar (Fig. 15-1). If it carries forward any further than this in the buccal sulcus, a small bleeding vessel is often encountered, which can be troublesome. An alternative technique is to take an envelope flap around the gingival margin of the second molar, and even the first molar; sometimes this is augmented with an anterior relaxing incision (Fig. 15-2). In some ways, it is felt to be preferable to utilize the buccal sulcus incision and not to compromise the gingival crevice around the second or first molars. A buccal flap is normally raised, which should not extend further inferior than is necessary, because although further raising this flap may marginally improve access, it does increase postoperative swelling. Techniques today do not advocate raising a lingual flap or placement of a lingual retractor, though advocates of this technique state that raising a lingual flap and placing a lingual retractor give improved access and visibility, and the incidence of permanent lingual nerve problems may decrease. However, it is accepted that placement of a lingual retractor may cause some short-term traction paresthesia to the lingual nerve.[2] Bone removal is normally carried out with a drill, with advocates for either a round bur or a fissure bur. General techniques involve guttering around the lateral aspect of the third molar and also distobuccally. Care must be taken if one proceeds onto the distal aspect of the third molar or distolingually, because the lingual nerve can occasionally be encountered in this area. If the tooth will not now elevate from the socket, most authorities would advocate sectioning the tooth, either horizontally or vertically, depending on its position. Most techniques involve cutting through the tooth approximately two thirds to three quarters of the distance from the buccal to the lingual aspect of the tooth and then placing an instrument in the groove and cracking off the crown of the tooth such that the lingual plate is not penetrated, and therefore not endangering the lingual nerve. By knowing the length of the cutting portion of a fissure bur, one can calculate the correct depth to section the crown of the tooth without risking damage to the lingual nerve. Following removal of the crown, the roots can normally be elevated, although occasionally they may need to be separated and elevated independently. On completion of the tooth removal, the residual follicle should be removed with care, because, on the lingual side, the lingual nerve can occasionally be intimately related to follicular remnants, and in some cases, it is more expedient to leave follicular remnants behind, because the formation of a residual cyst from these remnants is an extremely rare occurrence. Following removal of follicular remnants, the lingual plate should be examined to ensure that it is in continuity and that the lingual nerve is not visible and damaged. The depth of the socket should also be inspected to see if the inferior alveolar nerve can be visualized and if it is intact. If a discontinuity defect of either nerve is seen, immediate repair is advocated. If the nerve is visualized, but not obviously damaged, the patient should still be followed up closely to assess for altered sensation postoperatively.[3] Following debridement of the socket, the current standard of care does not require any material, either autogenous or allogenic,

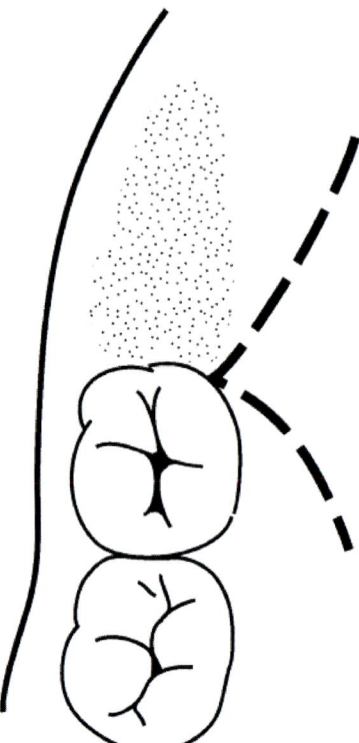

Fig. 15-1 ■ A typical buccal incision with buccal releasing incision for the removal of the lower right third molar. (From Pogrel MA, Goldman KE: Lingual flap retraction for third molar removal. *J Oral Maxillof Surg* 62(9):1125-1130, 2004.)

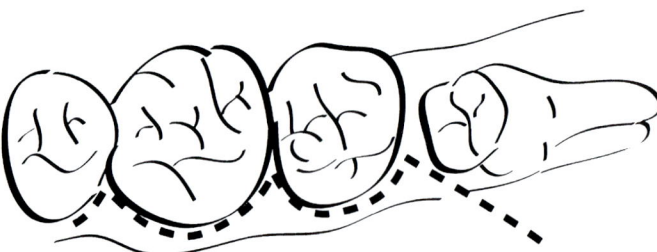

Fig. 15-2 ■ An envelope flap incision for removal of the lower left third molar.

to be placed in the socket, and studies are not yet complete to show whether this is helpful in any way to ensure adequate bone formation in the third molar socket and whether it improves the periodontal condition around the distal aspect of the second molar.[4,5] The residual socket can be sutured, but if sutures are to be placed, they should be superficial only, particularly on the lingual side, to avoid any involvement of a high lingual nerve, which occurs in about 15% of cases.[6-9] A single 3/0 or 4/0 resorbable suture on a reverse cutting needle is preferred. Some authorities prefer not to suture the socket but rather to place a pack with it—for example, Terracortil, an antibiotic/steroid pack. Some substances placed in tooth sockets can be neurotoxic to the inferior alveolar nerve, if it is exposed in the socket. These include tetracycline paste and possibly Surgicel (due to its low pH).[10]

CORONECTOMY

Coronectomy is a technique whereby the crown of the tooth and the coronal portion of the roots are removed, but the apical portion of the roots is retained. It also goes by the names of partial root retention, vital root retention, and partial odontectomy. It may be indicated when the apical portion of the roots of the tooth is in contact with vital structures and their removal might damage these structures. The most frequent example is the roots of the lower third molars and their relationship to the inferior alveolar nerve.

Traditionally, the relationship of the roots of a lower third molar to the inferior alveolar nerve has been judged from a Panorex radiograph, and criteria have been introduced to aid this evaluation.[11-14] More recently, however, the advent of cone beam computed tomography (CBCT) scanning technology has enabled more information to be gathered on the exact relationship in three dimensions.[15-18] It is considered that when the results of the cone beam CT scan might alter the treatment provided that it should be offered to a patient.

Although there are variations in the technique of coronectomy, certain common principles apply.

- The tooth involved should not be mobile.
- There should be no decay or infection involving the roots of the teeth.
- The tooth should be vital or adequately endodontically treated.
- The crown and the coronal portion of the roots should be removed until they are 2 to 3 mm below the surrounding crestal bone. Animal studies have shown that if this rule is followed bone will grow over the retained roots.[19-21]
- No treatment of the exposed pulp is required.[22]
- The retained portion of the root should not be mobilized during the coronectomy procedure.

Patients are normally placed on prophylactic antibiotics so that antibiotics are present in the pulp chamber as the tooth is sectioned. However, there are only a small number of papers describing the results of coronectomy, and not all of them used antibiotics.

In the technique, a buccal incision is made over the external oblique ridge of the mandible as in a conventional third molar approach (shown in Fig. 15-1). Buccal and lingual flaps are then raised and a lingual retractor is placed. The latter is done because the crown of the tooth must be fully sectioned and mobile before removal, and, if a retractor is not used, there is a risk of perforating the lingual plate and possibly damaging the lingual nerve. The lingual retractor should preferably be specifically designed with an appropriate shape and no sharp edges and with an adequate width to fully protect the lingual nerve.[2]

Once the retractor is positioned, a fissure bur is used at an angle of 45 degrees to section the crown. After the crown has been removed, the fissure bur is used to remove a portion of the remaining roots on the buccal side so that they are below the alveolar crest (Fig. 15-3). The exposed pulp is not treated in any way. Primary closure of the socket is felt to be necessary even if a periosteal release has to be performed. A watertight seal is obtained using vertical mattress sutures. A radiograph is normally taken to ensure that tooth and root removal is adequate. The radiograph also serves as a baseline for later radiographs to assess bone formation over the roots.

There are few contraindications to coronectomy, but these do include the following:

- There is acute infection around the tooth to undergo coronectomy.
- There is chronic infection including extensive dental decay and periodontal disease involving the roots of the tooth.
- There is mobility in the tooth.
- In teeth that are horizontally impacted along the course of the inferior alveolar nerve, the risks of damaging the inferior alveolar

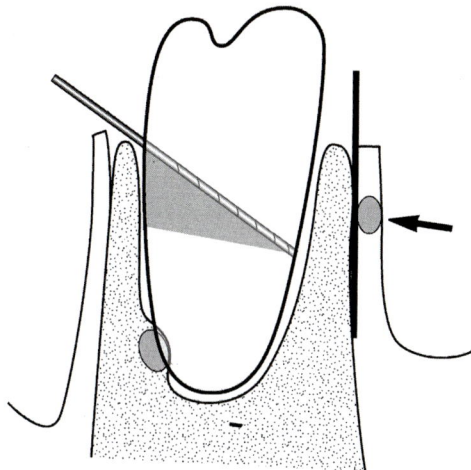

Fig. 15-3 ■ The technique for removal of the lower right third molar. Note the angle of the bur set to approximately 45 degrees and lingual retractor placed protecting the lingual nerve *(arrow)*. The shaded area of root on buccal side is to be removed secondarily. (From Pogrel M, Lee JS, Muff DF: Coronectomy: a technique to protect the inferior alveolar nerve. *J Oral Maxillofac Surg* 62(12):1447-1452, 2004.)

nerve by coronectomy may outweigh the risks of damaging the nerve with tooth removal.

- There are few complications to coronectomy, but among those reported are the following:
  - Postoperative infections. This has only occurred in about 1% of patients and, in some cases, has led to removal of the root fragments.
  - Mobilization of the remaining root fragment during tooth sectioning. If this happens, the root fragment must normally be removed, but if it is mobile, it generally does not affect the nerve.
  - Injury to the inferior alveolar nerve as a result of the coronectomy technique.
  - Subsequent migration of the root fragment. This appears to occur in about 30% of cases, and the migration is always away from the inferior alveolar nerve. Occasionally, these root fragments do appear intraorally, in which case they must be removed, but removal is a fairly simple affair.

There is limited available literature on coronectomy, and if one excludes case reports, only five articles describe the technique in detail.[23-27] All these articles suggest the technique is successful, but all have variations in the technique utilized. Figure 15-4 shows a case where the inferior alveolar nerve appears to groove the third molar on the lingual side on one side and may actually pierce the roots on the other side. Coronectomy was carried out in this case, and there was no involvement of either inferior alveolar or lingual nerves.

REMOVAL OF UPPER THIRD MOLARS

The indications for removal of upper third molars are fewer than those for lower third molars, because they cause few problems and can remain asymptomatic for many years. The two structures of importance around the site of the third molar are the maxillary sinus and the pterygomaxillary space.

Upper third molars are normally approached through an incision along the crest of the maxillary tuberosity back to the distobuccal

aspect of the upper second molar. From there, a releasing incision extends upward and forward into the buccal sulcus. A buccal flap is raised, and there is normally no need to raise a palatal flap. Buccal bone can be removed either with a sharp instrument (e.g., a chisel, periosteal elevator, or dental elevator) if it is very thin, or with a drill if it is more substantial. Once the crown of the tooth has been located, a purchase point should be made at the amelo-cemental junction on the mesial aspect of the tooth, and the tooth can then normally be elevated in an occlusodistal direction. An obstruction should be placed behind the tooth so that when elevated it comes down into the oral cavity rather than being displaced backward into the pterygomaxillary space. A periosteal elevator makes a suitable instrument to place behind the upper third molar, but the surgeon's finger can also be used to guide the tooth into the oral cavity. Sectioning of the tooth is not normally needed. Following removal of the tooth and debridement of the socket, buccal compression is normally used to compress the buccal plate and decrease the size of the socket. One suture is normally all that is required on the distal aspect of the second molar. Healing is usually uneventful.

If the maxillary sinus is encountered during removal of an upper third molar, then a periosteal releasing incision should be made in the buccal flap so that it can be advanced with ease across the socket; vertical mattress sutures should then be employed in order to close the opening, and the patient should be placed on sinus precautions (antibiotics, nasal decongestants, avoid nose blowing) for 10 days. Healing is usually uneventful (Fig. 15-5).

If the tooth is displaced into the pterygomaxillary space, then there is often considerable oozing of blood because the pterygoid venous plexus will often be encountered in this area. If the tooth cannot be recovered directly, then radiographs should be taken, the area packed, and an attempt made to remove the tooth several days later when the initial inflammation has settled and bleeding has ceased. In some cases, unerupted and uninfected teeth can be left indefinitely in the pterygomaxillary space (Fig. 15-6).

IMAGING FOR THIRD MOLARS

Although it is possible to image a third molar utilizing periapical films, it is difficult, because an adequate radiograph must show the whole tooth, its surrounding bone, its relationship to adjacent teeth, its relationship to the inferior alveolar nerve in the case of the lower molars, and its relationship to the sinus in the case of upper third molars. A Panorex-type radiograph more reliably shows these relationships. If there appears to be a close relationship between the inferior alveolar nerve and the lower third molar, then cone beam CT scans may be indicated to assess whether this is a true anatomic relationship or merely superimposition (Fig. 15-7). If it is a true anatomic relationship, then the available alternatives should be discussed with the patient, including electing not to remove the tooth; having facilities available for nerve repair; removing a pathologic lesion only, such as a cyst, and leaving the tooth in place; or carrying out coronectomy.

ANTIBIOTICS AND STEROIDS

The use of antibiotics in conjunction with third molar removal remains controversial, though it is widely practiced. If it is to be of value, the antibiotics should be commenced preoperatively and therefore be truly prophylactic.[28-34] Oral antibiotics can be commenced 1 or more hours prior to extractions, while intravenous antibiotics can be administered immediately preoperatively. The

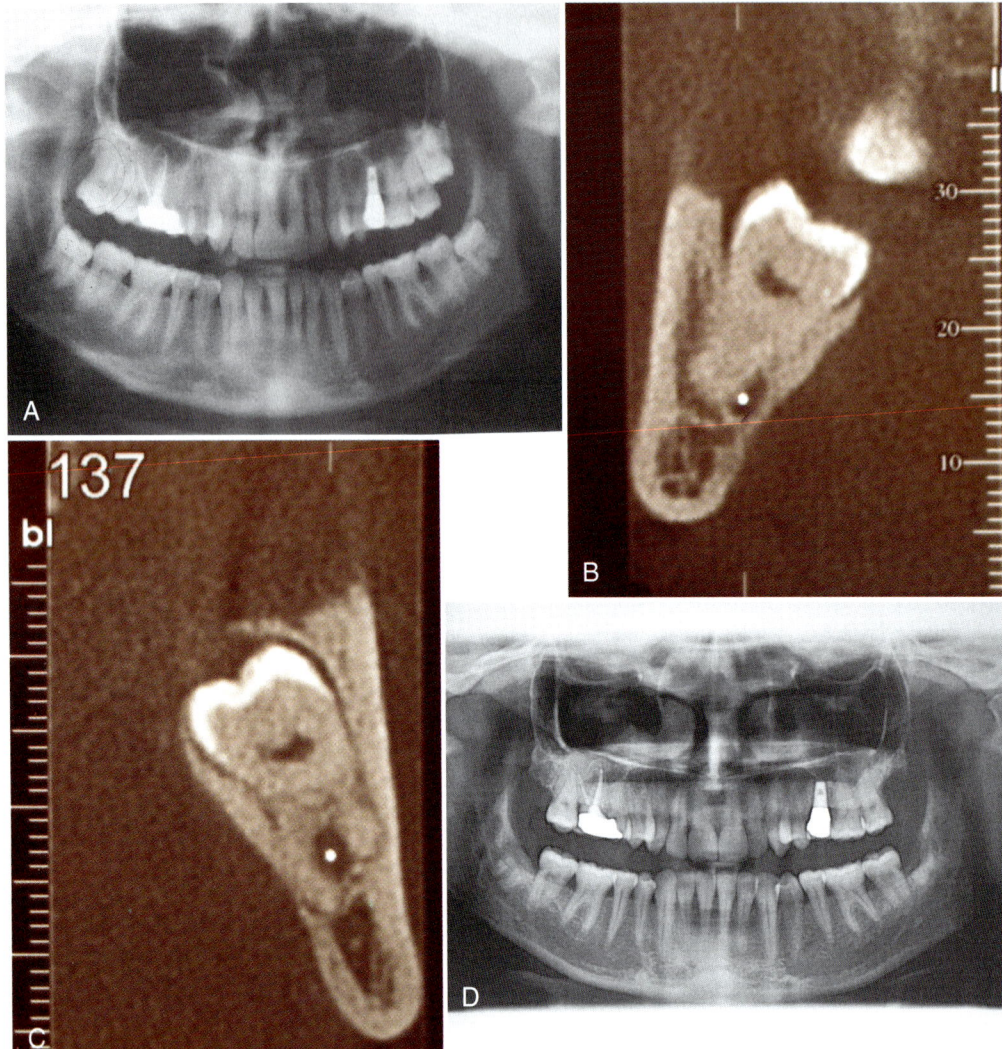

Fig. 15-4 ■ **A,** Panorex radiograph suggesting a close relationship between the inferior alveolar nerve and both lower third molars. **B** and **C,** Coronal cone beam computed tomography (CT) scans indicating a very close relationship between the inferior alveolar nerve and the roots of the lower third molars in three dimensions with the nerve on the lingual side on the right appearing to go through the roots on the left side. **D,** Panorex radiograph showing remaining root fragments following coronectomy. There was no inferior alveolar nerve damage.

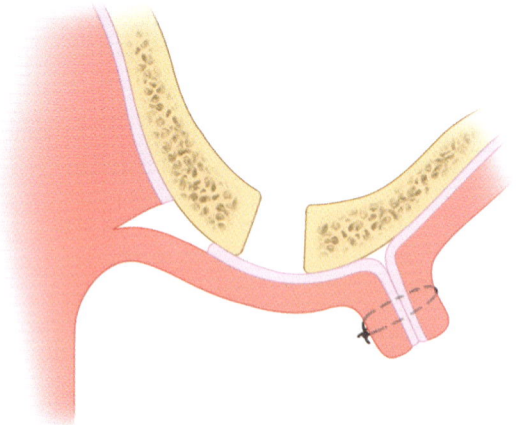

Fig. 15-5 ■ Method of closure of an oroanthral fistula. Incision of the periosteum to allow a tension-free advancement of the buccal flap, with vertical mattress sutures to allow a watertight and substantial repair.

choice of antibiotic remains controversial, but for most patients, penicillin is still the antibiotic of choice, because most oral organisms are still sensitive to it. The duration of prophylactic antibiotics is also controversial, and many authorities would advocate that 24 hours is an adequate period, though others would extend coverage as long as 7 days. There are no set guidelines, though some authorities do advocate prophylactic antibiotics when extensive bone removal occurs, but not for routine extractions or soft tissue impactions.

There is evidence that the use of steroids following third molar removal can decrease swelling and, therefore, decrease discomfort,[35-42] temporary nerve damage,[43] and possibly the amount of time lost from work. The exact steroid to be used and for how long remains controversial. Protocols include dexamethasone or methylprednisolone given intravenously at the time of the procedure and the use of a Decadron or Medrol dose pack, with a decreasing regimen of steroids over a 6-day period. The use of steroids should be weighed against any possible systemic effects, including an increased susceptibility to infections.[44]

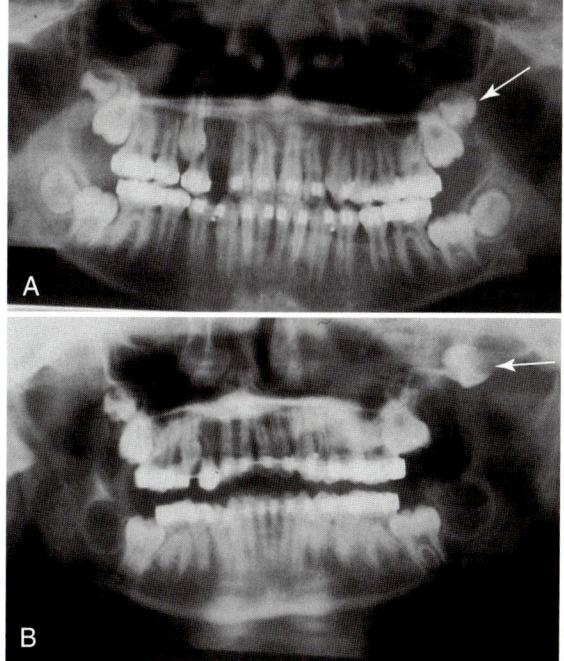

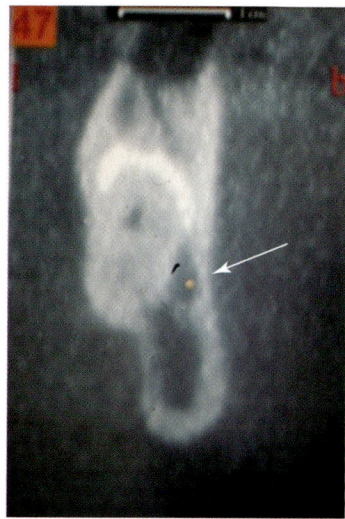

Fig. 15-7 ■ A cone beam computed tomography (CT) scan (coronal slice) showing the relationship of the inferior alveolar nerve to the roots of the lower third molar. Note also the vertical absence of a lingual plate of bone vertical to the lower third molar.

Fig. 15-6 ■ An upper left third molar displaced into the pterygopalatine fossa. **A,** Preoperative. **B,** Postoperative.

PEARLS AND PITFALLS

- The buccal approach is normally favored, but a lingual approach can sometimes be justified, providing an appropriate retractor is employed.
- In selected circumstances, coronectomy is a safe and effective means of avoiding inferior alveolar nerve involvement during lower third molar removal.
- The use of cone beam computed tomography (CBCT) should be employed to determine the relationship of the roots of a lower third molar to the inferior alveolar nerve when its position may determine the proposed treatment plan.
- Immediate closure of a known sinus perforation is recommended following upper third molar removal.
- The use of antibiotics in relationship to third molar removal remains controversial, but if they are to be used, it is preferable that they be commenced preoperatively.

REFERENCES

1. American Association of Oral and Maxillofacial Surgeons. *Parameters of care: clinical practice guidelines for oral and maxillofacial surgery.* Rosemont, Ill, 2007, American Association of Oral and Maxillofacial Surgeons.
2. Pogrel MA, Goldman KE: Lingual flap retraction for third molar removal, *J Oral Maxillofac Surg* 62(9):1125-1130, 2004.
3. Cadra M, Pogrel MA, Robert RC: Nerve evaluation protocol, *California Association of Oral Maxillofacial Surgeons,* Roseville Calif., 2003.
4. Dodson TB: Reconstruction of alveolar bone defects after extraction of mandibular third molars: a pilot study, *Oral Surg Oral Med Oral Pathol Oral Radiol Endod* 82(3):241-247, 1996.
5. Dodson TB: Management of mandibular third molar extraction sites to prevent periodontal defects, *J Oral Maxillofac Surg* 62(10):1213-1224, 2004.
6. Behnia H, Kheradvar A, Shahrokhi M: An anatomic study of the lingual nerve in the third molar region, *J Oral Maxillofac*

Surg 58(6):649-651, 2000; discussion 652-653.
7. Kiesselbach JE, Chamberlain JG: Clinical and anatomic observations on the relationship of the lingual nerve to the mandibular third molar region, *J Oral Maxillofac Surg* 42(9):565-567, 1984.
8. Miloro M, Halkias LE, Slone HW, Chakeres DW: Assessment of the lingual nerve in the third molar region using magnetic resonance imaging, *J Oral Maxillofac Surg* 55(2):134-137, 1997.
9. Pogrel MA, Renaut A, Schmidt B, Ammar A: The relationship of the lingual nerve to the mandibular third molar region: an anatomic study, *J Oral Maxillofac Surg* 53(10):1178-1181, 1995.
10. Zuniga JR, Leist JC. Topical tetracycline-induced neuritis: a case report, *J Oral Maxillofac Surg* 53(2):196-199, 1995.
11. Blaeser BF, August MA, Donoff RB, et al: Panoramic radiographic risk factors for inferior alveolar nerve injury after third molar extraction, *J Oral Maxillofac Surg* 61(4):417-421, 2003.

12. Howe G, Poynton HG: Prevention of damage to the inferior alveolar nerve during the evaluation of mandibular third molars, *Br Dent J* 109:355, 1960.
13. Nakagawa Y, Ishii H, Nomura Y, et al: Third molar position: reliability of panoramic radiography, *J Oral Maxillofac Surg* 65(7):1303-1308, 2007.
14. Rood JP, Shehab BA: The radiological prediction of inferior alveolar nerve injury during third molar surgery, *Br J Oral Maxillofac Surg* 28(1):20-25, 1990.
15. Dodson TB: Role of computerized tomography in management of impacted mandibular third molars, *N Y State Dent J* 71(6):32-35, 2005.
16. Ohman A, Kivijarvi K, Blomback U, Flygare L: Pre-operative radiographic evaluation of lower third molars with computed tomography, *Dentomaxillofac Radiol* 35(1):30-35, 2006.
17. Susarla SM, Dodson TB: Preoperative computed tomography imaging in the management of impacted mandibular third molars, *J Oral Maxillofac Surg* 65(1):83-88, 2007.

18. Tantanapornkul W, Okouchi K, Fujiwara Y, et al: A comparative study of cone-beam computed tomography and conventional panoramic radiography in assessing the topographic relationship between the mandibular canal and impacted third molars, *Oral Surg Oral Med Oral Pathol Oral Radiol Endod* 103(2):253-259, 2007.

19. Cook RT, Hutchens LH, Burkes EJ: Periodontal osseous defects associated with vitally submerged roots, *J Periodontol* 48(5):249-260, 1977.

20. Plata RL, Kelln EE, Linda L: Intentional retention of vital submerged roots in dogs, *Oral Surg Oral Med Oral Pathol* 42(1):100-108, 1976.

21. Whitaker DD, Shankle RJ: A study of the histologic reaction of submerged root segments, *Oral Surg Oral Med Oral Pathol* 37(6):919-935, 1974.

22. Johnson DL, Kelly JF, Flinton RJ, Cornell MT: Histologic evaluation of vital root retention, *J Oral Surg* 32(11):829-833, 1974.

23. Freedman GL: Intentional partial odontectomy: review of cases, *J Oral Maxillofac Surg* 55(5):524-526, 1997.

24. Knutsson K, Lysell L, Rohlin M: Postoperative status after partial removal of the mandibular third molar, *Swed Dent J* 13(1-2):15-22, 1989.

25. O'Riordan BC: Coronectomy (intentional partial odontectomy of lower third molars), *Oral Surg Oral Med Oral Pathol Oral Radiol Endod* 98(3):274-280, 2004.

26. Pogrel MA, Lee JS, Muff DF: Coronectomy: a technique to protect the inferior alveolar nerve, *J Oral Maxillofac Surg* 62(12):1447-1452, 2004.

27. Renton T, Hankins M, Sproate C, McGurk M: A randomised controlled clinical trial to compare the incidence of injury to the inferior alveolar nerve as a result of coronectomy and removal of mandibular third molars, *Br J Oral Maxillofac Surg* 43(1):7-12, 2005.

28. Bulut E, Bulut S, Etikan I, Koseoglu O: The value of routine antibiotic prophylaxis in mandibular third molar surgery: acute-phase protein levels as indicators of infection, *J Oral Sci* 43(2):117-122, 2001.

29. Delilbasi C, Saracoglu U, Keskin A: Effects of 0.2% chlorhexidine gluconate and amoxicillin plus clavulanic acid on the prevention of alveolar osteitis following mandibular third molar extractions, *Oral Surg Oral Med Oral Pathol Oral Radiol Endod* 94(3):301-304, 2002.

30. Foy SP, Shugars DA, Phillips C, et al: The impact of intravenous antibiotics on health-related quality of life outcomes and clinical recovery after third molar surgery, *J Oral Maxillofac Surg* 62(1):15-21, 2004.

31. Monaco G, Staffolani C, Gatto MR, Checchi L: Antibiotic therapy in impacted third molar surgery, *Eur J Oral Sci* 107(6):437-441, 1999.

32. Piecuch JF, Arzadon J, Lieblich SE: Prophylactic antibiotics for third molar surgery: a supportive opinion, *J Oral Maxillofac Surg* 53(1):53-60, 1995.

33. Poeschl PW, Eckel D, Poeschl E: Postoperative prophylactic antibiotic treatment in third molar surgery—a necessity? *J Oral Maxillofac Surg* 62(1):3-8, 2004; discussion 9.

34. Zeitler DL: Prophylactic antibiotics for third molar surgery: a dissenting opinion, *J Oral Maxillofac Surg* 53(1):61-64, 1995.

35. Alexander RE, Throndson RR: A review of perioperative corticosteroid use in dentoalveolar surgery, *Oral Surg Oral Med Oral Pathol Oral Radiol Endod* 90(4):406-415, 2000.

36. Baxendale BR, Vater M, Lavery KM: Dexamethasone reduces pain and swelling following extraction of third molar teeth, *Anaesthesia* 48(11):961-964, 1993.

37. Esen E, Tasar F, Akhan O: Determination of the anti-inflammatory effects of methylprednisolone on the sequelae of third molar surgery, *J Oral Maxillofac Surg* 57(10):1201-1206, 1999; discussion 1206-1208.

38. Hyrkas T, Ylipaavalniemi P, Oikarinen VJ, Paakkari I: A comparison of diclofenac with and without single-dose intravenous steroid to prevent postoperative pain after third molar removal, *J Oral Maxillofac Surg* 51(6):634-636, 1993.

39. Milles M, Desjardins PJ: Reduction of postoperative facial swelling by low-dose methylprednisolone: an experimental study, *J Oral Maxillofac Surg* 51(9):987-991, 1993.

40. Schmelzeisen R, Frolich JC: Prevention of postoperative swelling and pain by dexamethasone after operative removal of impacted third molar teeth, *Eur J Clin Pharmacol* 44(3):275-277, 1993.

41. Schultze-Mosgau S, Schmelzeisen R, Frolich JC, Schmele H: Use of ibuprofen and methylprednisolone for the prevention of pain and swelling after removal of impacted third molars, *J Oral Maxillofac Surg* 53(1):2-7, 1995; discussion 8.

42. Ustün Y, Erdogan O, Esen E, Karsli ED: Comparison of the effects of 2 doses of methylprednisolone on pain, swelling, and trismus after third molar surgery, *Oral Surg Oral Med Oral Pathol Oral Radiol Endod* 96(5):535-939, 2003.

43. Barron RP, Benoliel R, Zeltser R, et al: Effect of dexamethasone and dipyrone on lingual and inferior alveolar nerve hypersensitivity following third molar extractions: preliminary report, *J Orofac Pain* 18(1):62-68, 2004.

44. Tiwana PS, Foy SP, Shugars DA, et al: The impact of intravenous corticosteroids with third molar surgery in patients at high risk for delayed health-related quality of life and clinical recovery, *J Oral Maxillofac Surg* 63(1):55-62, 2005.

Management of the Impacted Canine

Chapter 16

Steven W. Beadnell

The proper eruption and final position of the canine tooth is an essential part of the maturation of the dentition to ensure proper occlusion and optimize the esthetic appearance of the patient's smile. Abnormal eruption or failure of the eruption of the canine can result in malposition and periodontal compromise of adjacent teeth, loss of arch space, internal or external resorption of the canine or adjacent teeth, formation of cysts associated with the impacted tooth, and recurrent infection with a partially erupted canine. Impacted canines complicate orthodontic treatment, potentially compromising the occlusion and esthetic outcome of the case. Early diagnosis, surgical and orthodontic manipulation to prevent impaction and to manage the impacted teeth, is essential in obtaining an optimal outcome for the patient.

ETIOPATHOGENESIS/CAUSATIVE FACTORS

The maxillary canines are the second most frequently impacted teeth after wisdom teeth, with incidence reports in the literature in the range of 1% to 3.5% in the general population. Mandibular canine impaction occurs at a much lower rate, possibly about 0.3%.[1] These rates would be much higher in a cohort of patients undergoing orthodontic treatment. Peck et al, in a review of the literature on palatally impacted canines, reports the incidence of bilateral maxillary canine impaction at 17% to 45%.[2] The rate among female patients is twice as high as among males: 1.17% versus 0.51%.[3]

The anomaly of canine impaction has been attributed to genetic and local factors. Although the actual cause is probably multifactorial, genetic and guidance theories of causation have been proposed. Proponents of the genetic theory—the assumption that the impaction is under genetic influence—identify increased occurrence of other dental anomalies, bilateral occurrence of impaction, familial occurrence, sex differences, and population differences as support for the genetic theory of impaction.[2] The guidance theory is based on more local factors influencing the proper eruption of the canine. Some authors have used the same data proposed by Peck et al to support their guidance theory of impaction.[4] Bishara identified multiple factors that are likely involved in the etiology of the impacted canine: (1) tooth size–arch length discrepancies, (2) prolonged retention or early loss of the deciduous canine, (3) abnormal position of the tooth bud, (4) the presence of an alveolar cleft, (5) ankylosis, (6) cystic or neoplastic formation, (7) dilacerations of the root, (8) iatrogenic, (9) trauma, and (10) idiopathic, including primary failure of eruption.[5] In most cases, it is difficult to identify the precise etiologic factor leading to the impaction of the canine.

Prediction of canine impaction in the maxilla has been evaluated by multiple authors. Warford et al evaluated the prediction of maxillary canine impaction after primary canine extraction in patients less than age 12 years using sector localization and angular measurements based on panographic radiographs.[6] The location of the cusp tip of the canine in question and its relationship to the adjacent lateral incisor was divided into specific sectors: Sector I represents the area distal to a line tangent to the distal heights of contour of lateral incisor crown and root; sector II is mesial to sector I, but distal to the bisector of the lateral incisor's long axis; sector III is mesial to sector II, but distal to the mesial heights of contour of the lateral incisor crown and root; and sector IV includes all areas mesial to sector III (Fig. 16-1).[6] The findings in Warford's study indicate that of the two factors considered for predicting maxillary canine impaction, canine angulation and sector location, the prediction appears to rest almost solely on the sector location of the cusp tip of the erupting canine. As shown by the predictive values for sector location alone—(I) 0.06, (II) 0.38, (III) 0.87, and (IV) 0.99—the more mesial the cusp tip location, the greater the likelihood of impaction. The overall incidence of impaction was 82%, if the canine cusp tip was in sections II, III, or IV.[6] In any patient where the tip of the canine overlaps the root of the lateral incisor in a Panorex film, orthodontic evaluation and possible early intervention would be appropriate.

Ericson also showed that the position of the crown of the canine in relationship to the root of the lateral incisor is a key determinant in the potential for eruption or impaction of the maxillary canine after primary canine extraction. If the crown of the canine was distal to the midline of the lateral incisor root, the canine erupted 92% of the time, whereas if it was mesial to the midline of the root, eruption occurred in 64% of the cases after primary canine extraction (Fig. 16-2).[7]

DIAGNOSTIC STUDIES

Early detection of the potential for canine impaction is important, because early intervention can reduce the treatment time, complexity, and complications. The earliest and most simple method for early detection involves visual inspection and tactile clinical examination by the age of 9 to 10 years. The maxillary and mandibular canine usually erupts around age 10 to 12 years, with a buccal bulge usually palpable at least 1 year before eruption. The diagnosis of an impacted maxillary canine is done using both clinical examination and radiographic assessment (Fig. 16-3). Clinical signs that might indicate canine impaction include over-retained or asymmetry in exfoliation of the primary canine, lack of canine bulge on the buccal aspect of the ridge by age 10 years, asymmetry of the buccal canine bulge, palatal bulge in the canine region, lack of deciduous canine root resorption, and malposition of the adjacent lateral incisor.

Radiographs useful for diagnosis and evaluation of impacted canines include panographic, periapical, occlusal, and lateral cephalometric plain films. Using Clark's rule, plain films can usually assist in the determination of the relative buccal-lingual position of the impacted tooth, that is, if the object moves the same direction as the movement of the beam, then it is on the buccal aspect of the ridge; if movement is in the opposite direction, then it is on the lingual

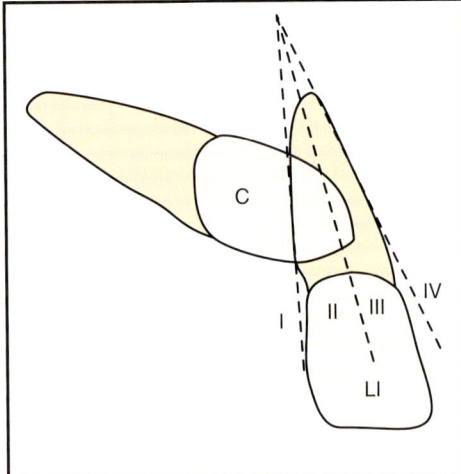

Fig. 16-1 ■ Position of the incisal edge of the impacted canine in relation to the root of the adjacent lateral incisor is divided into sectors I, II, III, IV.

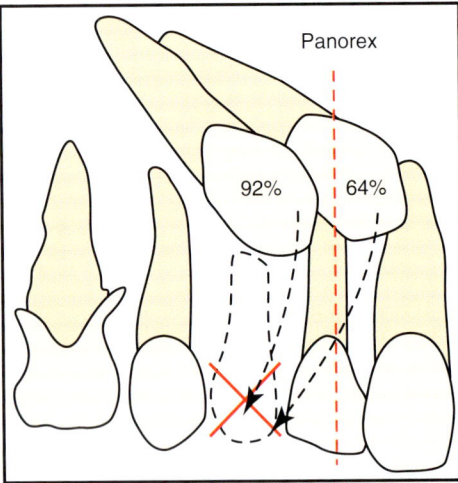

Fig. 16-2 ■ Likehood of canine eruption after primary canine extraction based on canine position in relation to the root of the lateral incisor.

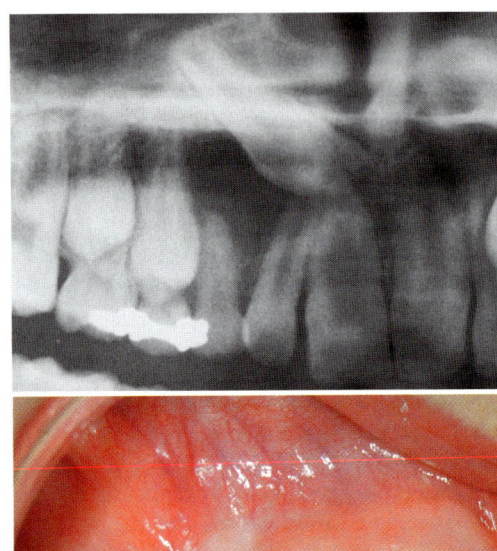

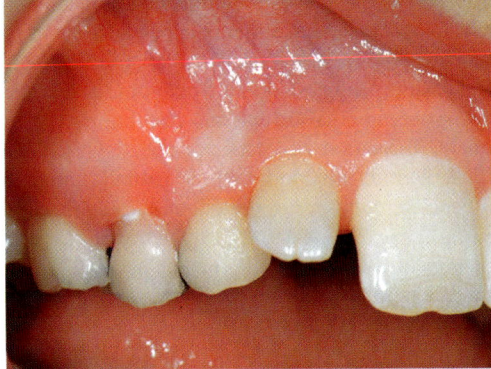

Fig. 16-3 ■ An over-retained primary canine, malposition of the lateral incisor and lack of canine bulge in a 10-year-old patient with impacted tooth #6 with a dentigerous cyst.

aspect of the ridge. Cone beam CT scanning, with or without three-dimensional (3D) reconstruction, provides an opportunity for exact localization of the impacted canine. Walker et al showed the benefits of 3D volumetric imaging of impacted canines, which can demonstrate presence or absence of the canine, size of the follicle, inclination of the long axis of the tooth, relative buccal and palatal positions, amount of the bone covering the tooth, 3D proximity and resorption of roots of adjacent teeth, condition of adjacent teeth, local anatomic considerations, and overall stage of dental development, root form, and the presence of pathology or adverse conditions affecting the impacted tooth.[8] This information assists the orthodontist in planning the mechanics that will be used to guide the eruption of the tooth while minimizing the risks to the adjacent teeth (Fig. 16-4).

Most references note the preponderance of maxillary canine impaction on the palatal (85%) versus buccal (15%) aspect of the ridge. These data have been based on plain film evaluation and primarily on the mode of surgical access to the impacted maxillary canines. Recent evaluation of the canine position by Liu et al, using cone beam CT scanning to definitively determine the position of the impacted maxillary canine results, showed a different distribution: 45.2% impacted buccally, 40.5% impacted palatally, and 14.5%

impacted midalveolus.[9] The majority of maxillary canine impactions are, in fact, most easily approached from the palatal aspect of the ridge, but exact localization to determine the best surgical approach is of paramount importance. The cone beam CT technology allows the precise localization of the impacted tooth.

TREATMENT GOALS/OPTIONS

The treatment goals for management of the impacted canine include:
- Eruption of the impacted canine into the arch with functional occlusion
- Maintenance of an adequate zone of attached tissue on the buccal and lingual aspects of the canine as it is erupted into the mouth
- Esthetic gingival contours once the impacted canine is in position
- Minimizing or avoiding damage to the adjacent teeth, maintaining an intact periodontium

Several factors must be taken into consideration in determining the treatment option chosen for management of the impacted canine, including:
- Patient age
- General dental health and oral hygiene
- Whether space is available within the arch or if it can be established with orthodontic manipulation
- Suitability of the first bicuspid to replace the canine
- Favorability of the position of the impacted canine and the likelihood of being able to get it into position with orthodontic treatment
- Patient motivation for orthodontic treatment
- Medical contraindications for surgery

Pitt et al asked orthodontists to evaluate several factors that will influence the difficulty of treatment in order to develop a "treatment

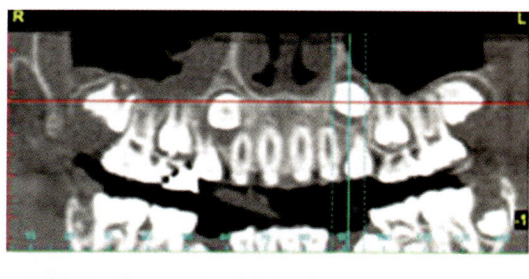
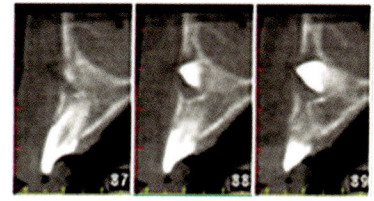
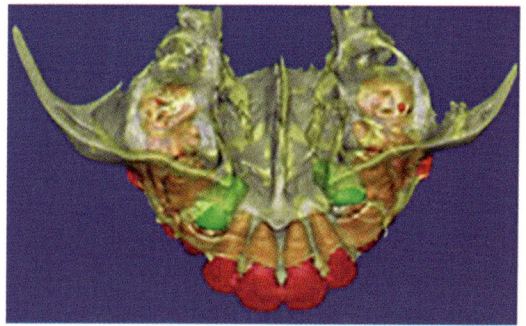
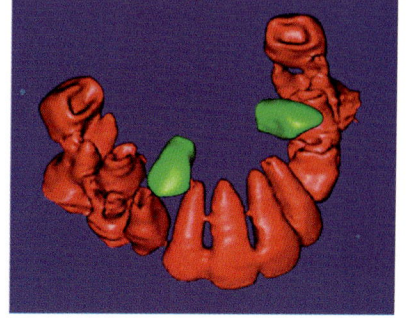

Fig. 16-4 ■ Cone beam CT scan of impacted teeth #6 and #11 (images taken using i-Cat technology, Imaging Sciences International, Hatfield, Pa).

difficulty index" with which to preoperatively evaluate impacted canine cases. Their analysis showed that the horizontal position, as measured by the degree of overlap of the lateral and central incisors by the crown of the impacted canine, is the most important factor in determining the difficulty of aligning the unerupted tooth. Patient age was the next most important factor, followed by vertical height and buccopalatal position.[10] Becker and Chaushu evaluated the effects of age on success of orthodontically erupting impacted canines by looking at 38 matched cases in a series of adults (mean age 29.8 ± 8.6) versus young patients (mean age 13.7 ± 1.3). They found 100% success in the young patients and 69.5% in the adults, with all of the failures being in patients older than age 30 years.[11]

Multiple treatment options are available to manage impacted canines; the treatment is chosen after consultation between the surgical team and treating orthodontist:

- Retention of the impacted canine in place with serial radiographic observation to check for development of asymptomatic pathosis with or without retention of the primary canine
- Extraction of the impacted tooth and retention of the primary canine with restorative procedures to improve its esthetic contours
- Extraction of the impacted tooth and primary canine followed by orthodontic space closure, substituting the first bicuspid for the extracted canine ("bicuspid substitution")
- Extraction of the impacted tooth and primary canine with replacement using an implant-supported crown
- Surgical exposure of the impacted canine with orthodontic alignment of the ectopic tooth after its surgical exposure
- Autotransplantation of the impacted tooth into its anatomic position in the arch after orthodontic pretreatment for space opening

SURGICAL MANAGEMENT OF IMPACTED CANINES

Most of the literature available today is related to the impaction of maxillary canines, reflecting their 20-fold greater occurrence than impacted mandibular canines. The typical management involves orthodontic manipulation to provide adequate space for the tooth in the arch and surgical access to the impacted tooth, with bonding of an orthodontic eruption device consisting of an orthodontic bracket/gold chain combination to the crown of the tooth (Fig. 16-5).

ARMAMENTARIUM FOR EXPOSURE/BONDING PROCEDURE

Instruments and supplies needed for the surgical procedure of exposing and bonding an eruption device to an impacted canine include:

1. Surgical instrumentation to allow incision, flap reflection, and suturing of the soft tissue as required
2. Orthodontic pliers that allow easy grasping, manipulation, and placement of the eruption bracket/chain
3. Eruption devices usually consisting of an orthodontic bracket with attached small gold-link chain
4. Light-cured orthodontic composite/adhesive or cyanoacrylate cement
5. Hemostatic agent, such as Hemodent, and cotton pellets for application/packing around the exposed tooth

Two basic approaches, either a "closed" or "open" technique, are used to provide access to the impacted canine. In the "closed eruption" technique (Fig. 16-6), the crown of the canine is exposed, the orthodontic eruption device is attached to the crown, and the flap is sutured back over the tooth, leaving only the eruption chain exposed for orthodontic manipulation. The eruption chain is usually exited through either the crestal incision or the extraction site of the primary canine and ligated to the archwire or brackets on the adjacent teeth. In the "open eruption" technique (Fig. 16-7), the crown of the impacted tooth is exposed with either an opening cut into the overlying tissue without flap reflection, or a flap is reflected, a window cut in it, and then the flap is repositioned.

After exposure of the impacted tooth, the overlying bone is removed with a bur or curet, and the follicle is minimally debrided to allow access to the tooth. In the closed technique, the eruption bracket/chain is bonded to the tooth at the time of surgery; in the open technique, it can be done at the time of surgery by the surgeon or done at a subsequent appointment with the orthodontist.

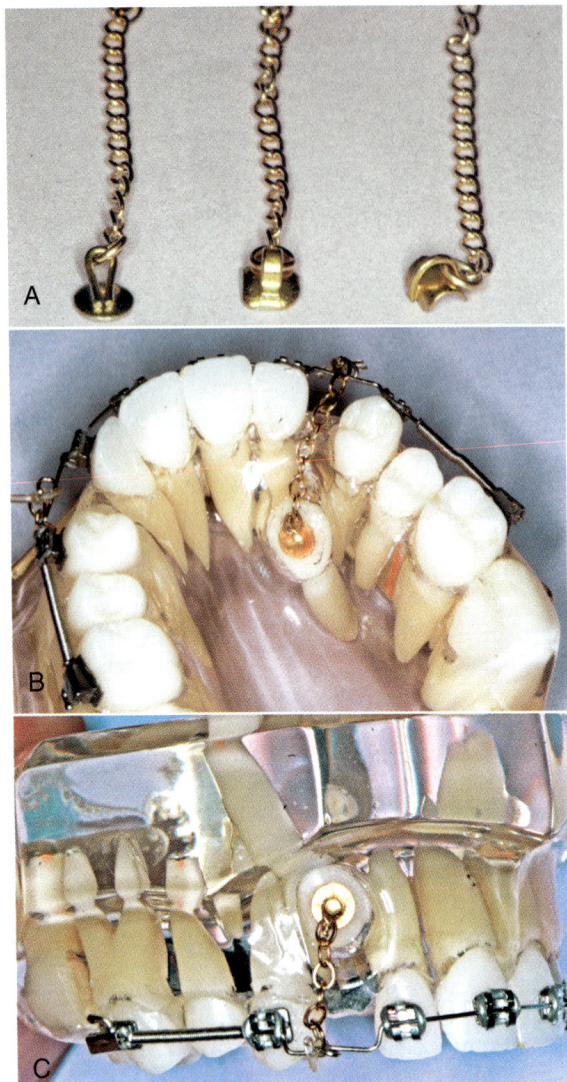

Fig. 16-5 ■ An orthodontic bracket/gold chain combination (**A**) bonded to the crown of the tooth (**B** and **C**).

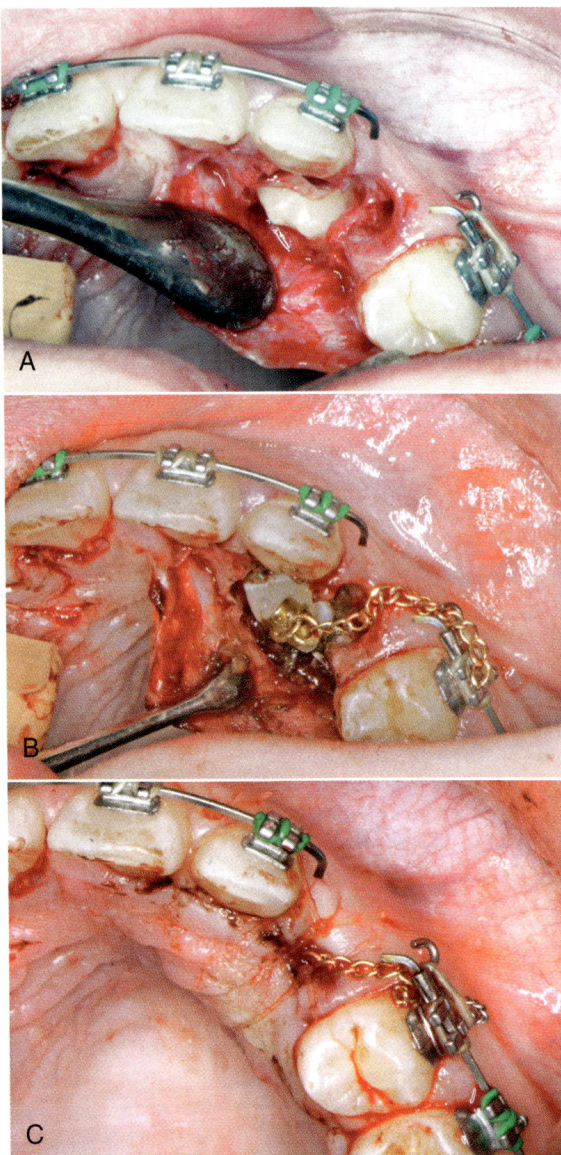

Fig. 16-6 ■ Flap, closed eruption procedure for exposure (**A**) and bonding (**B**) of palatally impacted tooth #11. **C,** Flap sutured back over the tooth, leaving only the eruption chain exposed.

Hemostasis can be achieved using electrosurgery or by packing cotton pellets soaked in hemostatic agents around the exposed tooth. The isolated tooth is then etched for the appropriate period of time (depending on the manufacturer's guidelines), rinsed and dried, and the eruption device bonded to the tooth using a light-cured, acid-etch composite material. Drying the tooth after etching is easily done by drawing air over the surface using the surgical suction tip immediately beside the exposed crown of the tooth. Positioning of the bracket as near to or on the incisal edge of the tooth provides the orthodontist with the best mechanical advantage for positioning of the tooth (Fig. 16-8).

Photographic documentation of the surgical procedure at the time of uncovering is advantageous to the orthodontist, if he or she is not present at the time of the surgery. This allows the orthodontist to fully appreciate the position of the tooth within the alveolus, proximity of the impacted tooth to the adjacent teeth, and the position of the applied orthodontic eruption device on the tooth. Full knowledge of these facets of the surgical procedure are easily documented and provided to the orthodontist through intraoperative photographs. This provides the orthodontist with the appropriate information to plan the proper orthodontic manipulation of the tooth.

Four basic surgical techniques have been described by Kokich and Cooke for managing the impacted canines, each having its clinical situation where it is the appropriate choice.[12,13]

1. Gingivectomy/soft tissue window
2. Apically positioned flap
3. Open eruption—replaced flap with a soft tissue window or tissue excision without flap
4. Closed eruption—replaced flap without a soft tissue window removed

Cooke developed a decision tree to assist in deciding which of these techniques should be applied in specific clinical situations. Factors considered in the selection of surgical techniques include the buccal or palatal/lingual position of the impacted tooth, the adequacy of the zone of keratinized gingival (KG) tissue present, and whether the surgeon/orthodontist prefers the open or closed technique. An expanded version of this decision tree is shown in Figure 16-9.[13]

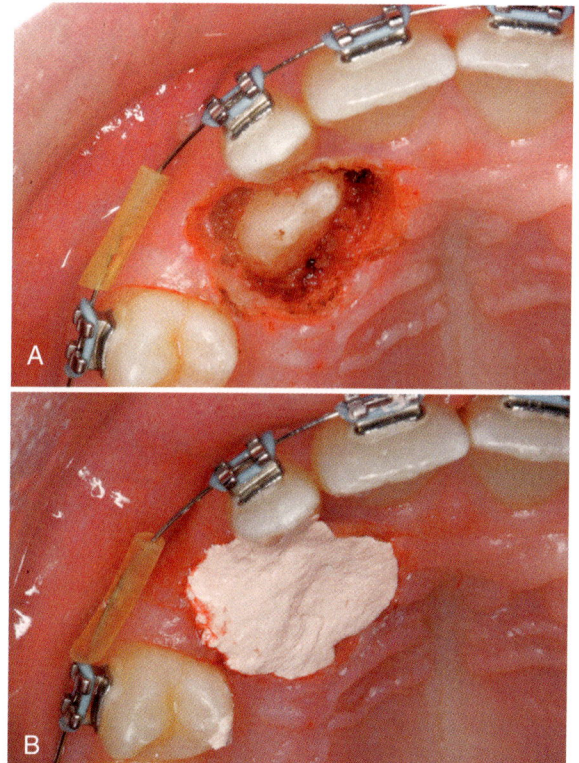

Fig. 16-7 ■ Flapless open procedure (**A**) with periodontal dressing applied (**B**) for palatally impacted tooth #6.

MAXILLARY CANINES

LABIAL/BUCCAL IMPACTIONS

The management of a labially impacted canine is somewhat more challenging, because the appropriate surgical method must be chosen to maintain an adequate zone of attached tissue around the tooth during its eruption. The labially impacted tooth often has a bony dehiscence over the root, resulting in recession of the soft tissue once the tooth is in position. Orthodontic traction must be applied in a manner to avoid buccally directed forces on the tooth.

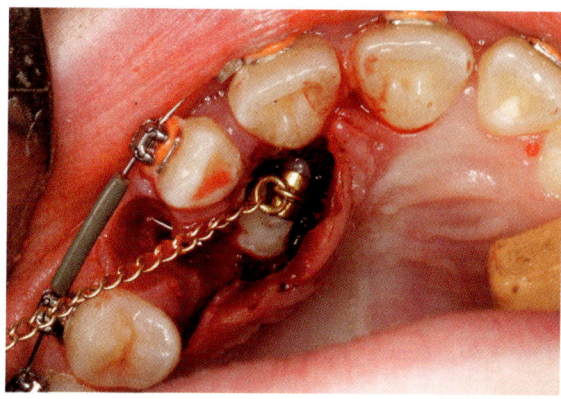

Fig. 16-8 ■ GAC U-Link bracket (DENTSPLY GAC International, Bohemia, NY) bonded to incisal edge of impacted tooth #6.

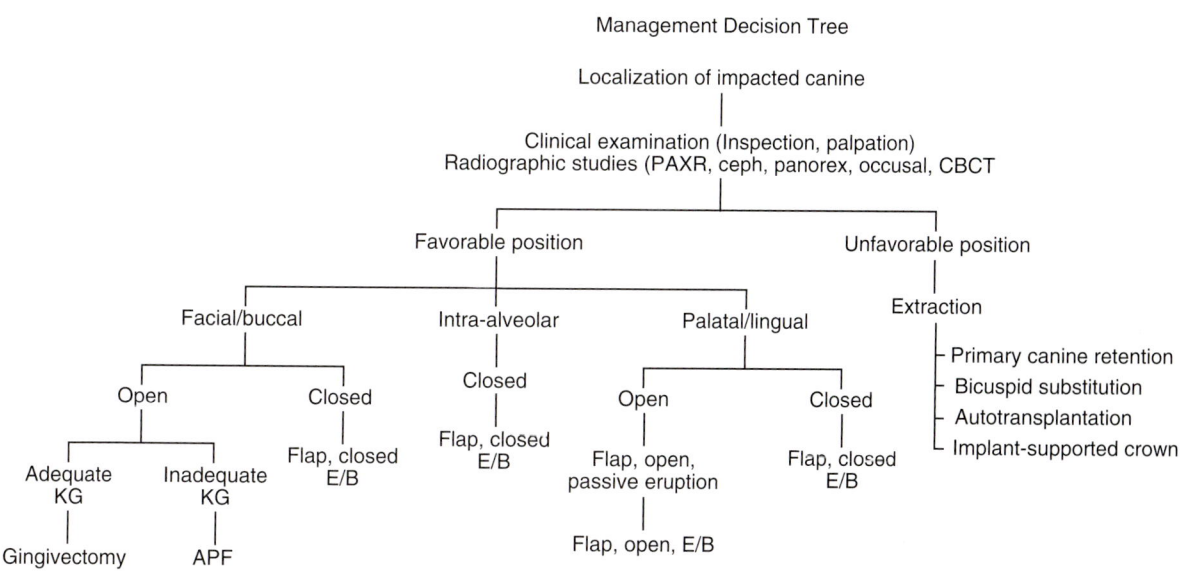

Fig. 16-9 ■ Decision tree to assist in choosing the appropriate surgical technique to correct an impacted canine. (Modified from Cooke J, Wang HL: Canine impactions: incidence and management. *Int J Periodontics Restorative Dent* 26(5):483-491, 2006.)

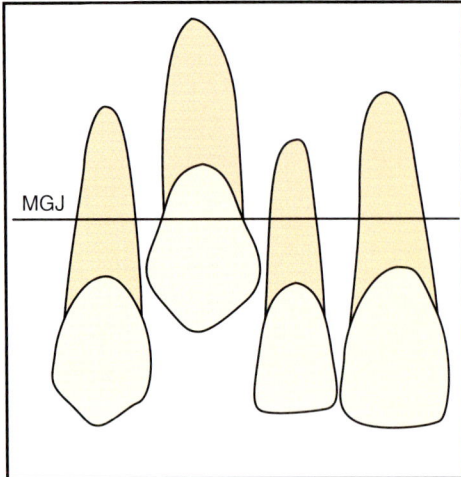

Fig. 16-10 ■ Crown of the impacted tooth in relation to the mucogingival junction should be considered in choosing the method of exposure of the crown.[12]

In these cases, use of a Ballista spring or other orthodontical device—one which pulls the tooth toward the central aspect of the ridge rather than toward the buccal archwire—will result in a more favorable outcome. In managing labially impacted canines, Kokich has identified several factors that influence the decision regarding the best technique for exposure of the tooth: the vertical position of the tooth, the labial or intra-alveolar position, the amount of keratinized gingiva present, and the mesiodistal position of the tooth (Fig. 16-10).[12] The three methods of exposure for a labially impacted canine include gingivectomy, an apically positioned flap, and closed eruption.

If the crown of the impacted tooth is mostly below the mucogingival junction and an adequate zone of attached tissue is present such that a 3-mm wide band of keratinized tissue can be maintained, a gingivectomy exposing one half to two thirds of the crown can be done (Fig. 16-11). It is unusual for this to be the case, because the buccally impacted canine usually has relatively thin, nonkeratinized tissue overlying the crown.

When the labially positioned canine overlaps the lateral/central incisors, an apically positioned flap (APF) allows exposure of the tooth with maintenance of an adequate zone of keratinized gingiva (Fig. 16-12). In canines mesially positioned over the lateral or central incisor, an APF harvesting a 3-mm band of keratinized tissue from the incisor area can be harvested if there is an adequate width of attached tissue overlying the incisors (5 to 6 mm) to allow maintenance of adequate keratinized tissue over the incisors. If there is inadequate keratinized tissue in the incisor region, a pedicled, split-thickness flap from the canine edentulous area can be utilized, but the distance the tissue must be transferred can limit the use of this technique.

With the labially impacted canine in an edentulous area, a conventional APF-harvested keratinized tissue from the crest of the edentulous ridge can be used. Bonding of a bracket onto the buccal surface of the canine at the time of the surgery assists in keeping the flap from migrating coronally over the crown of the tooth. Vermette et al showed that there are some potential esthetic considerations in the selection of apically positioned flaps for buccally impacted canines, sometimes resulting in compromised esthetics and vertical relapse of the repositioned tooth, especially when they are positioned high in the alveolus.[14] Labially impacted canines high in the alveolus can pose a significant challenge, because during the

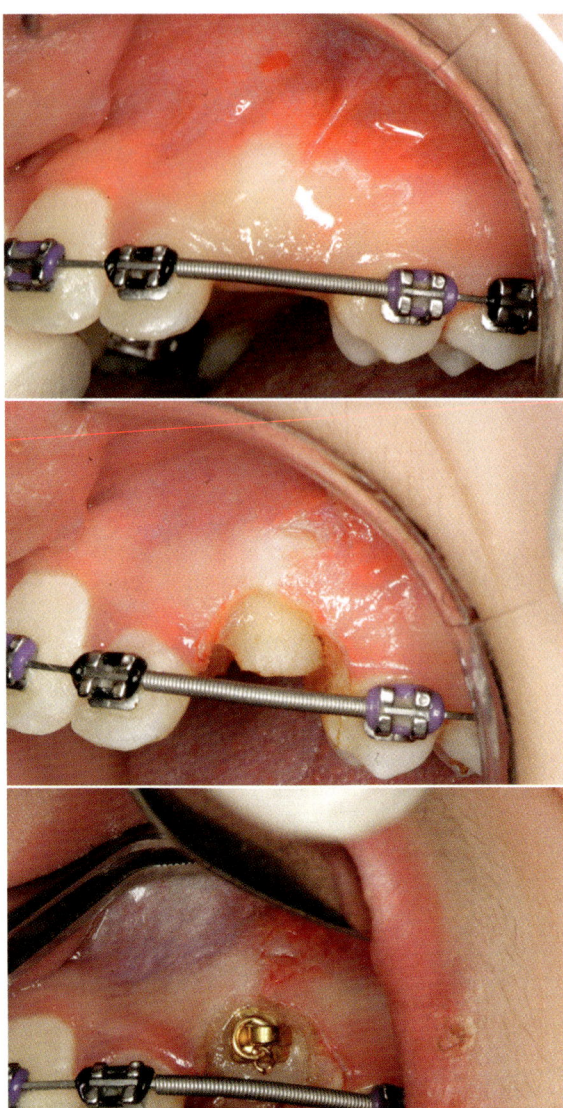

Fig. 16-11 ■ Labially positioned impacted tooth #11 exposed by gingivectomy.

eruption process the dense palatal bone tends to make the tooth move out toward the buccal aspect, possibly creating a dehiscence in the buccal bone and malposition of the tooth. Canines high in the alveolus must be managed by a closed technique with buccal flap reflection, bonding of an eruption device, and repositioning/closure of the flap, because an apically positioned flap is not feasible due to inability to stabilize the flap (Fig. 16-13).

INTRA-ALVEOLAR IMPACTIONS

Intra-alveolar impaction is suspected when the tooth is seen in the edentulous area on a radiograph but the crown is not palpable on the buccal or palatal aspect of the ridge. Intra-alveolar impactions are typically a result of inadequate space in the arch for eruption; pathosis, such as a supernumerary tooth or a dentigerous cyst blocking eruption; or sometimes it is idiopathic. Due to the depth of the crown within the alveolus, gingivectomy and apically positioned flaps are usually not appropriate choices, because the soft tissue will tend to close over the site postsurgically. This tendency can be overcome by application of periodontal dressings over the freshly exposed buccal surface, this being most effective when the tooth is

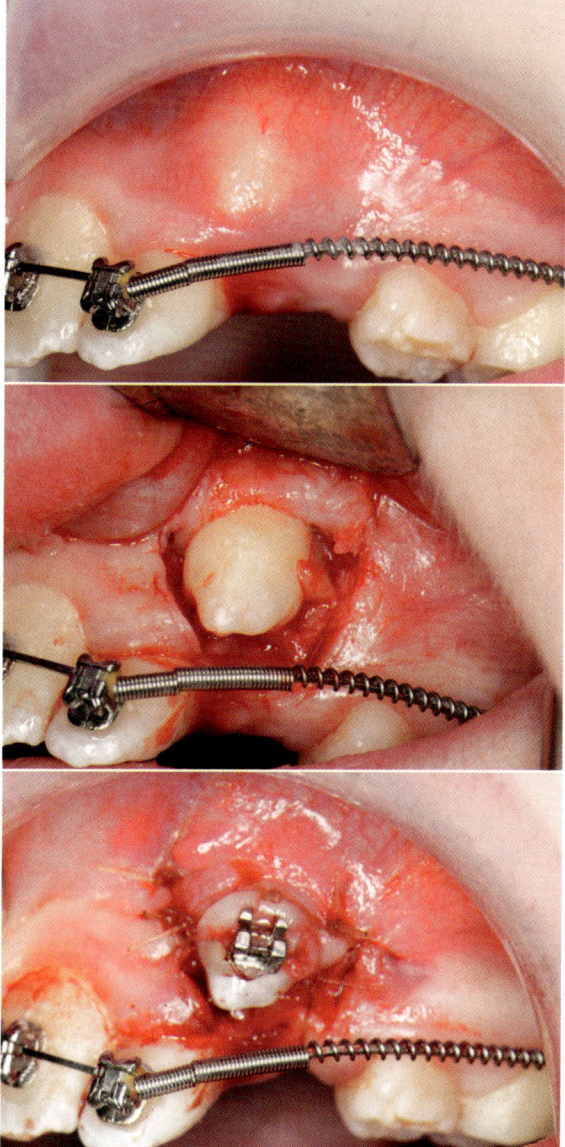

Fig. 16-12 ■ Labially impacted tooth #11 managed with an apically positioned flap.

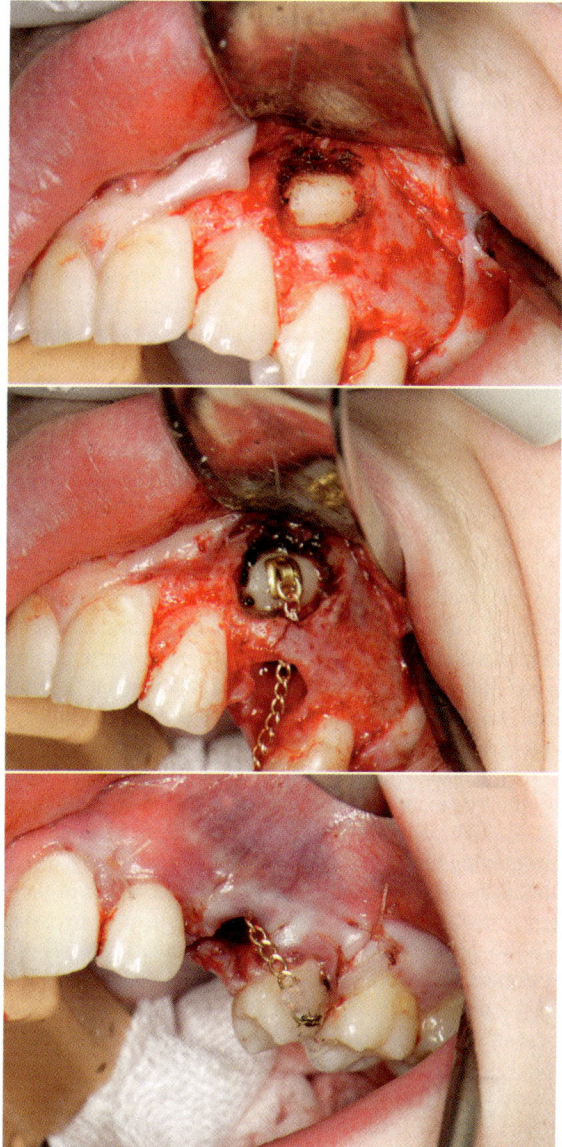

Fig. 16-13 ■ Labially impacted tooth #11 managed with closed, tunnel technique.

toward the buccal aspect of the ridge. In most intra-alveolar cases, a buccal flap procedure with bonding of an eruption bracket/chain device and closure of the flap is the procedure of choice. A tunnel technique, exiting the eruption chain through the extraction socket of the primary canine, as described by Crescini et al, can be used to facilitate eruption of the tooth into the central aspect of the ridge through the keratinized tissue, much like the tooth that erupts naturally.[15]

PALATALLY IMPACTED CANINES

Palatally impacted canines can pose a significant challenge for the orthodontist and surgeon, depending on several factors that determine the prognosis for successful eruption of the tooth into the arch. The decision as to whether to salvage these teeth or consider extraction must be carefully evaluated preoperatively. Motamedi et al evaluated the position of palatally impacted canine teeth in relation to successful eruption, finding that successful eruption seems to be primarily guided by the canine's angulation to the midline, amount of lateral incisor root overlap, and root curvature or anomaly.[16] In a review of 146 cases of palatally impacted canines, the presence of a nondilacerated canine root or lateral incisor root overlap was less than 50%, and a less than 45-degree angulation of the impaction to the midline correlated with a successful outcome. In this series, 70.54% of the canines were successfully orthodontically erupted, the remainder being extracted due to ankylosis or failure to move.[16]

Impacted canines, especially those on the palate, have been shown by several authors to potentially cause resorption of the roots of the adjacent lateral and central incisors. The incidence is variable in studies using plain films, but using cone beam CT scan technology, the assessment of the degree of root resorption should be more accurate. Cone beam CT scans can detect the position of the impacted canine as well as the extent and exact location of the lateral incisor root resorption, which cannot be detected by classic radiographic approaches. Compared with conventional radiographic methods, such as intraoral and panoramic radiographs, the amount of resorption detected by CT scanning was approximately 50% higher, with one study showing a 67% incidence of lateral incisor resorption.[9,17,18]

The treatment options for the palatally impacted canine include open or closed eruption techniques. Access to the canine is typically done by utilizing a sulcular incision along the palatal aspect of the adjacent teeth, usually extending from first bicuspid to the midline, with or without vertical releasing incisions, to access the tooth. In simple palatal impactions that are not deep within the bone, either the open or closed technique can be utilized. In cases of more deeply impacted canines, the open technique is more difficult because it can be challenging to avoid the tissue closing back over the hole, even with periodontal packings used to initially keep the site open. In terms of patient tolerance of the procedure, Chaushu et al compared open versus closed techniques, revealing substantial impairment and recovery time regarding pain and analgesic consumption, oral function (ability to eat and enjoy food, swallowing, and mouth opening), and food accumulation after an open eruption technique.[19] An additional consideration in planning the management is whether the impacted tooth will be allowed to passively erupt once exposed, then brought into the arch using orthodontic manipulation as described by Schmidt and Kokich, or actively erupted by placement of an orthodontic eruption device (bracket/chain) and application of traction on the tooth immediately after the surgical procedure.[12,20] Schmidt and Kokich have advocated for early surgical exposure of palatally impacted maxillary canines with passive eruption onto the palate and subsequent orthodontic manipulation into alignment in the arch. A primary advantage of this technique is it allows early uncovering of the palatally impacted canine and autonomous eruption onto the palate without the orthodontic appliances in place; orthodontic treatment can then be undertaken, shortening the overall time in appliances.[12,20] While there have been several published reports detailing the advantages of the closed versus open technique in terms of the esthetic results and periodontal health of the treated teeth, a review by Parkin et al showed that there is no evidence to support one surgical technique versus the other in terms of dental health, esthetics, economics, and patient factors in palatally impacted maxillary canines.[21]

In cases where the impacted canine is close to the surface, an open or closed technique can be utilized. If the palatal bulge is quite prominent, usually there is no bone overlying the impacted canine, only tissue, and the tooth can simply be exposed by excision of the overlying soft tissue. Either the surgeon can attach the eruption device to the tooth at the time of surgery or the orthodontist can attach it at a later date. The advantage of doing a formal flap procedure to expose the tooth is that it affords the surgeon the opportunity to remove the bone overlying the entire crown of the tooth down to the cementoenamel junction (CEJ), providing access for fenestration of the dense palatal bone between the crown of the impacted tooth and its intended position in the arch, and allowing for better assessment of the proximity of the tooth to the roots of the adjacent lateral and central incisors. After the flap is repositioned, if an open technique is desired, the flap is simply repositioned and a window is cut out of the tissue, leaving the impacted canine exposed. The palatal flap is sutured to the buccal tissue using interdental sutures. If an open technique is used, coverage of the area of exposure using a periodontal dressing or a vacuum-formed palatal stent is done to provide improved patient comfort and to keep the tissue from growing over the site. In more deeply palatally impacted canines, the closed technique is typically used with the chain running subperiosteally, exiting out the crestal incision/primary canine extraction site, or exiting through a small incision in the palatal mucosa made over the bracket. The advantage of the chain exiting through the palatal mucosa overlying the bracket is that the orthodontist can then provide traction in any direction to move the impacted tooth away from the roots of the lateral/central incisors (Fig. 16-14).

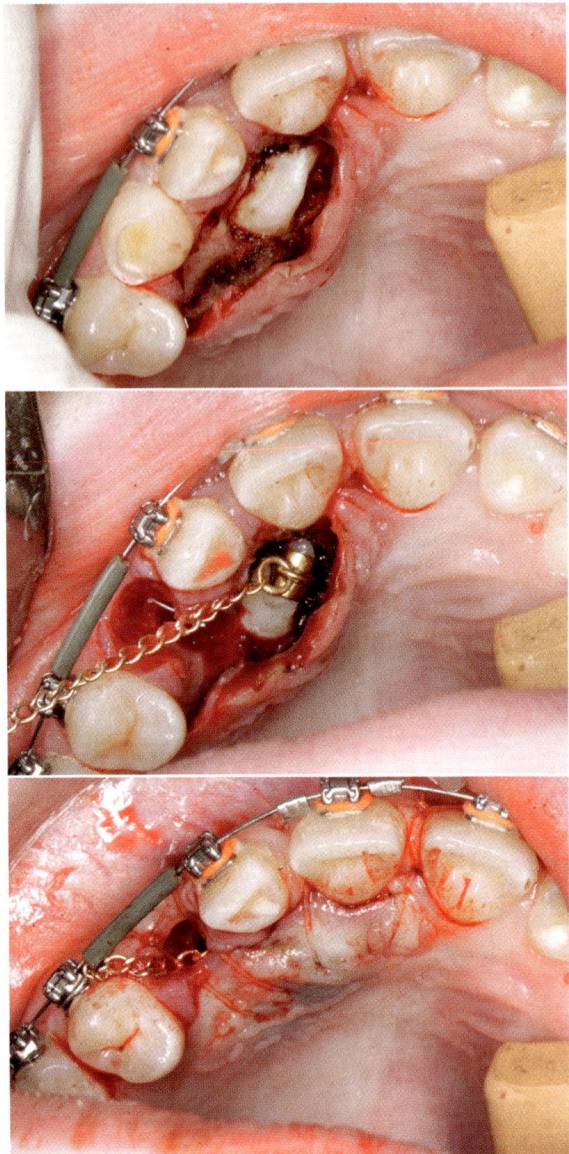

Fig. 16-14 ■ Palatally impacted tooth #6 managed using flap, closed technique.

Palatally impacted teeth immediately adjacent to or against the roots of the lateral and central incisors have the potential complication of resorption of the roots of these teeth during the application of traction for eruption. Care must be taken to avoid dragging the crown of the impacted tooth across the lingual aspect of the incisors as it is brought toward its normal position in the arch. In these cases, initial eruption of the tooth onto the palate is achieved by using lingual buttons placed on the bicuspid or molar region, a transpalatal arch, or a temporary anchorage device. The devices are used as anchorage to first pull the impacted canine palatally and away from the adjacent roots to reduce the likelihood of root resorption. Figure 16-15 shows the preoperative occlusal radiograph, postoperative Panorex views, and clinical photograph in a case of the close proximity of the bilaterally impacted canines to the adjacent roots; palatal temporary anchorage devices were placed and the chains exited through the overlying mucosa to facilitate initial palatal movement of the canines away from the roots of the lateral incisors.

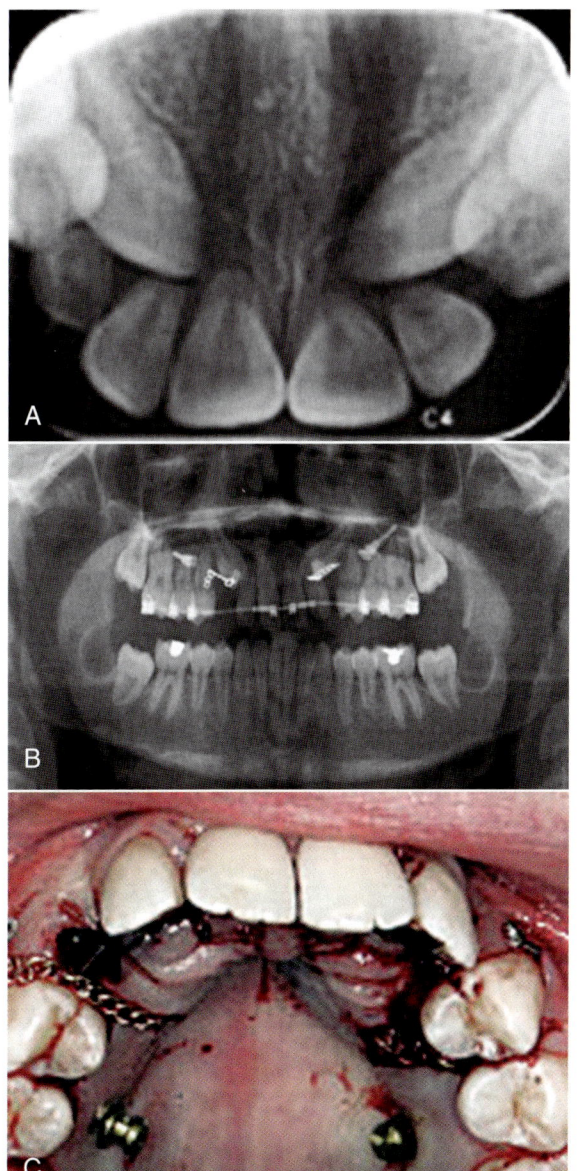

Fig. 16-15 ▪ Palatally impacted teeth #6 and #11 with temporary anchorage devices in place. **A,** Preoperative occlusal radiograph. Postoperative Panorex view (**B**) and clinical photograph (**C**) showing palatal temporary anchorage devices placed with the chains exiting out through the overlying mucosa.

MANDIBULAR CANINES

The incidence of impacted mandibular canines is significantly lower than that of the maxillary canine, and much less documentation of the management of these cases is available in the literature. In a review of 4500 Panorex views from a Turkish cohort, Aydin et al reported the overall incidence of canine impaction to be 3.58% in the maxilla, with an incidence of only 0.44% in the mandible.[22]

The challenge of impacted mandibular canines is the difficulty the orthodontist has in attempting to gain mechanical advantage to move the tooth into the arch, even if the surgeon can apply an orthodontic eruption device on the tooth. Frequently, the impacted mandibular canine is in a horizontal position near the roots of the adjacent teeth; the dense bone in the region, as well as the relative buccal position of these horizontally impacted teeth within the

alveolus, makes it very challenging for the orthodontist to bring the tooth into the arch; therefore, most of the time horizontally positioned teeth should be extracted. Impacted mandibular canines that are in a recoverable position are usually on the buccal aspect of the alveolus or in an intra-alveolar position. Buccally positioned or intra-alveolar impacted mandibular canines can be managed using the techniques described herein for the buccally positioned maxillary canines. The relatively narrow band of keratinized tissue often seen in the anterior mandible makes gingivectomy and apically positioned flaps a less common procedure for the impacted mandibular canine (Fig. 16-16).

COMPLICATIONS OF EXPOSURE/ BONDING PROCEDURES

FAILURE OF ERUPTION

Despite the proper analysis of the case, favorable position of the impacted tooth, application of an eruption device, and proper orthodontic mechanics, some teeth simply cannot be brought into the arch. It is important to counsel patients that exposure/bonding and orthodontic manipulation, while usually highly predictable, cannot be guaranteed in any individual case. If the tooth fails to erupt, treatment options include:

1. Reevaluate the case to assess for supernumerary teeth that may be blocking eruption, expanded follicular space indicating cystic degeneration, and adequacy of space in the arch for eruption.
2. Re-explore the area, check for ankylosis, and make sure there are no impediments to eruption of the tooth. Luxation of the tooth can be undertaken, but the author's experience is that once the tooth becomes ankylosed, the prognosis is very poor even with further surgical manipulation. In cases of ankylosis, corticotomies and distraction of the tooth and bone en bloc sometimes have been reported to be successful.

RESORPTION OF TEETH

The resorption of the adjacent teeth is certainly a possible complication of the orthodontic manipulation of impacted teeth, especially palatally impacted canines lying against the palatal aspect of the lateral or central incisors. During the surgical exposure, care must be taken to preserve the integrity of the bone or soft tissue around these teeth.

Resorption of the impacted tooth, either the crown or the root, has been shown to occur during orthodontic eruption and often results in ankylosis of the tooth. During the exposure of the palatally impacted canines, care must be exercised in bone removal. It has been recommended that bone removal over the crown be undertaken down to the level of the CEJ to facilitate eruption of the tooth, but any exposure or damage to the root will increase the potential for resorption.

BOND/ATTACHMENT FAILURE

The orthodontic eruption device is usually bonded to the impacted tooth using an acid-etch composite or cyanoacrylate type material. Closely following the material manufacturer's instructions and attention to the proper isolation and etching of the tooth will result a good union between the bracket and the tooth. Bond failure is managed by removal of the eruption device and re-exposure and bonding of an additional appliance to the tooth. If great progress in eruption of the tooth has been achieved before bond failure, an open technique may suffice in exposing the tooth for access by the orthodontist.

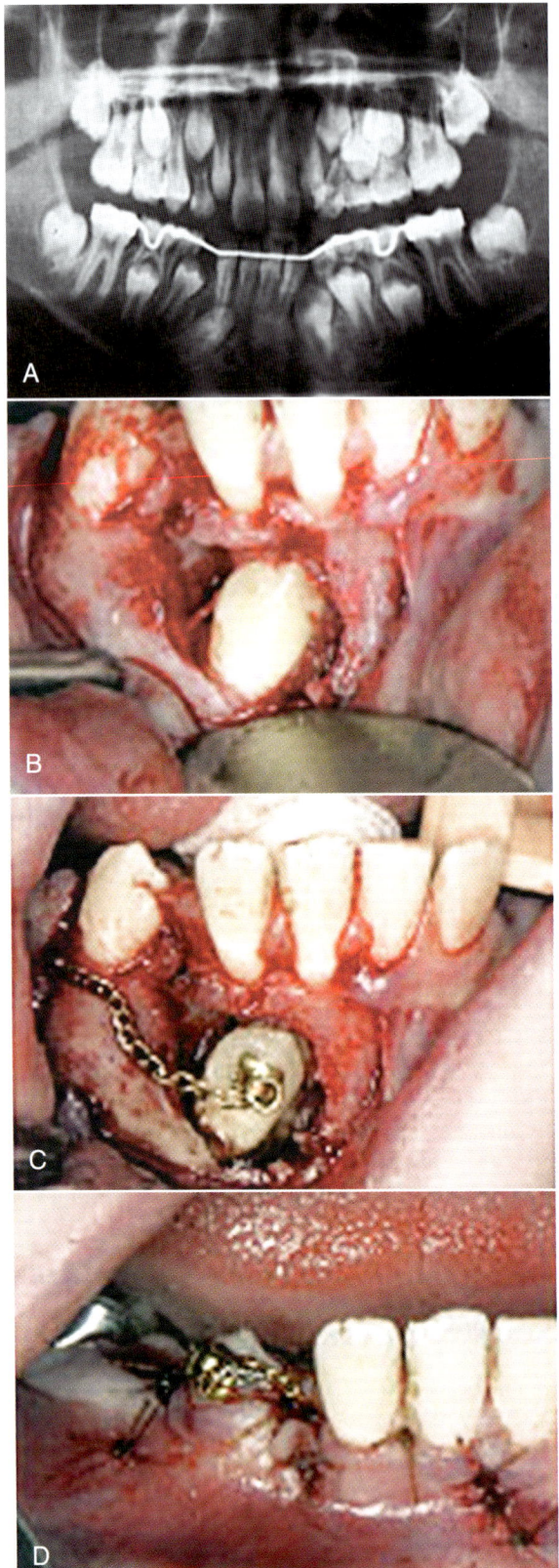

Fig. 16-16 ■ Labially impacted tooth #27 with enlarged follicular space (**A**) managed with flap, closed technique (**B** to **D**).

POSTOPERATIVE CARE

The patient undergoing exposure and bonding of impacted canines usually has a relatively uncomplicated postoperative course. Chaushu et al evaluated the patient's perception of the recovery after both the open and closed eruption technique. The Health-Related Quality of Life questionnaire was given to patients to assess their postoperative course. Severe pain, classified as 8-10/10 scale, and swelling peaked on postoperative day 1 and had mostly resolved by the third postoperative day. Buccolingual tooth location was the most significant predictor variable, with results showing a delayed recovery for patients with buccally impacted teeth. The open eruption technique for palatal impactions significantly delayed the patient's recovery, especially when the need for bone removal was present.[19,23]

Prophylactic antibiotics are usually not necessary for the management of these cases, because postoperative infection has been very unusual in the author's experience. The patient is instructed to perform general oral hygiene measures in a standard fashion and advised to use a 0.12% chlorhexidine mouth rinse twice per day for 7 days postoperatively. The patient is reevaluated at the end of 1 week and then released to the orthodontist to begin the orthodontic manipulation of the impacted tooth.

TREATMENT ALTERNATIVES FOR REPLACEMENT OF NONSALVAGEABLE IMPACTED CANINES

In some cases, it is simply not practical to obtain optimal positioning of the tooth, the risk of the adjacent teeth with orthodontic eruption may be too high, and the patient may not want to undergo extended orthodontic treatment. In these cases, the treatment alternatives include removal of the tooth with bicuspid substitution, retention of the primary canine with contour enhancement using conventional restorative techniques, autotransplantation of the impacted canine, and replacement of the missing canine with an implant-supported crown.

BICUSPID SUBSTITUTION

In cases where the canine is lost, moving the adjacent bicuspid into the position of the canine with orthodontic space closure can be considered. Factors in the decision include the effect on the occlusal scheme, size, and configuration of the adjacent bicuspid and the esthetic demands of the patient. The orthodontist can critically evaluate the situation to determine if an acceptable result can be achieved using this method.

RETENTION OF THE PRIMARY CANINE

The primary canine clinical crown is significantly smaller than the permanent canine. Conventional restorative techniques using adhesive dentistry can be used to reshape/restore the primary canine to a contour that approximates the appearance of the contralateral permanent canine.

AUTOTRANSPLANTATION

Early reports of autotransplantation showed relatively high rates of root resorption that made this an unacceptable alternative treatment. A more recent study by Arikan evaluated the survival rate and periodontal status of 32 transplanted canines during a 5-year period and showed that autotransplantation may be a viable alternative in some cases. Progressive root resorption was observed in only two teeth, and one tooth was extracted during year 4, yielding a 5-year success rate of 93.5%.[24]

IMPLANT-SUPPORTED CROWN

The utilization of osseointegrated implants for the replacement of missing teeth has been shown to have outstanding success overall. Depending on the status of the edentulous ridge after the impacted canine is removed, immediate or delayed implant placement can be undertaken, and the tooth replaced with an implant-supported crown. Garcia has shown that as long as the residual bone in the area is adequate for good initial primary stability of the immediately placed implant, grafting the surgical defect of the adjacent extracted canine results in a favorable outcome.[25]

SUMMARY

The impacted canine can prove to be a challenge for both the surgeon and the orthodontist. Careful preoperative planning of the surgical technique and subsequent orthodontic mechanics utilized to manage the impacted tooth are dictated by clinical and radiographic findings. Alternative treatments that have predictable outcomes can be considered when the impacted canine is determined to be unsalvageable.

PEARLS AND PITFALLS

- Early diagnosis and intervention with impacted canines results in a more favorable outcome.
- Absence of a symmetric canine bulge in the maxillary vestibule by age 9 warrants further radiographic assessment of the position and eruption potential of the unerupted canines.
- During orthodontic eruption of buccally impacted maxillary canines, the tooth tends to ride out toward the buccal, potentially resulting in prominent roots with bony fenestrations and mucogingival defects.
- Maintaining an adequate zone of keratinized gingival on the buccal aspect of the impacted canine as it erupts is essential for achieving optimal esthetics and long-term gingival health.
- Intraoperative photos showing the position of the impacted canine and its relationship to the adjacent teeth assist the orthodontist in the planning of the vectors of traction used to erupt the tooth.

REFERENCES

1. Schubert M, Baumert U: Alignment of impacted maxillary canines: critical analysis of eruption path and treatment time, *J Orofac Orthop* 70:200-212, 2009.
2. Peck S, Peck L, Kataja M: The palatally displaced canine as a dental anomaly of genetic origin, *Angle Orthod* 64(4):249-256, 1994.
3. Bishara SE: Clinical management of impacted maxillary canines, *Semin Orthod* 4(2):87-98, 1998.
4. Becker A: Palatal canine displacement: guidance theory or an anomaly of genetic origin, *Angle Orthod* 65(2):95-102, 1995.
5. Bishara SE: Impacted maxillary canines: a review, *Am J Orthod Dentofacial Orthop* 10:159-171, 1992.
6. Warford JH, Grandhi RK, Tira DE: Prediction of maxillary canine impaction using sectors and angular measurement, *Am J Orthod Dentofacial Orthop* 124(6):651-655, 2003.
7. Ericson S: Early treatment of palatally erupting maxillary canines by extraction of the primary canines, *Eur J Orthod* 1:283-295, 1988.
8. Walker L, Enciso R, Mah J: Three-dimensional localization of maxillary canines with cone-beam computed tomography, *Am J Orthod Dentofacial Orthop* 125(4):418-423, 2005.
9. Liu D, Zhang W, Zhang Z, et al: Localization of impacted maxillary canines and observation of adjacent incisor resorption with cone-beam computed tomography, *Oral Surg Oral Med Oral Pathol Oral Radiol Endod* 105(1):91-98, 2008.
10. Pitt S, Hamdan A, Rock P: A treatment difficulty index for unerupted maxillary canines, *Eur J Orthod* 28:141-144, 2006.

11. Becker A, Chaushu S: Success rate and duration of orthodontic treatment for adult patients with palatally impacted maxillary canines, *Am J Orthod Dentofacial Orthop* 124(5):509-514, 2003.
12. Kokich V: Surgical and orthodontic management of impacted maxillary canines, *Am J Orthod Dentofacial Orthop* 126(3):278-283, 2004.
13. Cooke J, Wang HL: Canine impactions: incidence and management, *Int J Periodontics Restorative Dent* 26(5):483-491, 2006.
14. Vermette ME, Kokich V, Kennedy DB: Uncovering labially impacted teeth: apically positioned flap and closed-eruption technique, *Angle Orthod* 65(1):23-32, 1995.
15. Crescini A, Baccetti T, Rotundo R, et al: Tunnel technique for the treatment of impacted mandibular canines, *Int J Peridontics Restorative Dent* 29(2):213-218, 2009.
16. Motamedi MH, Tabatabaie FA, Navi F, et al: Assessment of radiographic factors affecting surgical exposure and orthodontic alignment of impacted canines of the palate: a 15-year retrospective study, *Oral Surg Oral Med Oral Pathol Oral Radiol Endod* 107:772-775, 2009.
17. Alqerban A, Jacobs R, Lambrechts P, et al: Root resorption of the maxillary lateral incisor caused by impacted canine: a literature review, *Clin Oral Investig* 13(3):247-255, 2009.
18. Walker L, Enciso R, Mah J: Three-dimensional localization of maxillary canines with cone-bean computed tomography, *Am J Orthod Dentofacial Orthop* 128:418-423, 2005.

19. Chaushu S, Becker A, Zeltser R, et al: Patients' perception of recovery after exposure of impacted teeth: a comparison of closed-versus open-eruption techniques, *J Oral Maxillofac Surg* 63:323-329, 2005.
20. Schmidt A, Kokich V: Periodontal response to early uncovering, autonomous eruption, and orthodontic alignment of palatally impacted maxillary canines, *Am J Orthod Dentofacial Orthop* 131:449-455, 2007.
21. Parkin N, Benson PE, Thind B, Shah A: Open versus closed surgical exposure of canine teeth that are displaced in the roof of the mouth, *Cochrane Database Syst Rev* (4):CD006966, 2008.
22. Aydin U, Yilmaz HH, Yildirim D: Incidence of canine impaction and transmigration in a patient population, *Dentomaxillof Radiol* 33:164-169, 2004.
23. Chaushu S, Becker A, Chaushu G: Lingual orthodontic treatment and absolute anchorage to correct an impacted maxillary canine in an adult, *Am J Orthod Dentofacial Orthop* 134:811-819, 2008.
24. Arikan F, Nizam N, Sonmez S: 5-year longitudinal study of survival rate and periodontal parameter changes at sites of maxillary canine autotransplantation, *J Periodontol* 79(4):595-602, 2008.
25. Garcia B, Boronat A, Larrazabal C, Penarrocha M: Immediate implants after the removal of maxillary impacted canines: A clinical series of nine patients, *In J Oral Maxillofac Implants*, 24(2):348-352, 2009.

Implants for Orthodontic Anchorage: Temporary Anchorage Device

Joyce T. Lee

Over the past 3 decades, successful application of dental endosseous implants has been well established in oral and maxillofacial surgery. Since the late 1980s to early 1990s, the use of endosseous implants has expanded to the treatment of orthodontic patients. The principle of placing implants as anchorage devices to facilitate orthodontic movement of teeth, as well as to affect skeletal growth, has broadened the clinical applications of dental implants. Conventional orthodontics for the treatment of dental and facial skeletal discrepancies often involves cumbersome intraoral appliances, such as full arch braces, interarch elastics, and Nance appliances, in addition to extraoral appliances such as headgear. In situations in which patients are partially edentulous or have oligodontia, the lack of teeth can often pose challenges for the orthodontist in devising a treatment plan with the existing dentition to provide sufficient anchorage. Implants placed into the maxillo-mandibular skeleton enable the orthodontist to provide additional anchorage and exert predictable force in all three spatial planes: transverse, vertical, and sagittal. There is a vast amount of literature on the use of implants in orthodontics to treat malaligned teeth by uprighting, extrusion, intrusion, mesialization, and distalization.

Early after their introduction, the literature has been filled with descriptions of different types and designs of anchorage devices for orthodontic purposes that have various shapes and sizes of screws, plates, cylinders, and other components. Some of these implants required a healing period for osseointegration before orthodontic forces could be applied, whereas others were designed to be left and restored with a prosthetic crown on completion of the orthodontic treatment. Several different classifications of osseous anchorage devices have been described by Creekmore and Eklund, Kanomi and Costa, and Cope. Devices with different designs that served the same purpose of assisting in orthodontic treatment lacked uniformity and thus made the nomenclature extremely confusing. In 2005, a meta-analysis conducted by Labanauskaite and colleagues attempted to clarify and further classify these implant devices according to their shape and size (cylindrical, screws, miniplates, and disk shaped), fixation of the implant to the surface of the bone (osseointegrated versus mechanical locking), and clinical applications (orthodontic, orthodontic and restorative/prosthetic, and orthopedic). In a more contemporary approach, the definition of these implants has been narrowed so that it refers specifically to titanium alloy miniscrews or miniplates that are placed as removable temporary anchorage devices (TADs) in the maxilla and mandible to facilitate orthodontic movement. For the purpose of this chapter, we will discuss the type of implants placed solely for the purpose of temporary orthodontic anchorage.

Unlike its predecessor, the conventional endosseous osseointegrated implant, a TAD differs from it in many ways. A TAD is designed to be placed for orthodontic anchorage purposes, and on completion of treatment the implant device is always removed. In addition, the success criteria for TADs are defined differently. The capacity to withstand orthodontic forces throughout treatment, lack of clinically detectable mobility, presence of soft tissue health, and lack of painful symptoms are defined as success. In other words, these anchorage devices do not need to be osseointegrated.

One of the early implant devices on the market for orthodontic anchorage was the palatal implant. In 1995, Block and Hoffman designed a disk-shaped subperiosteal implant with a roughened hydroxyapatite undersurface that could be placed in the hard palate for orthodontic anchorage. This implant required surgical placement through a palatal tunneling technique and a latency period for osseointegration before loading. Although studies documented its success in providing anchorage, this implant did not gain broad application because of multiple disadvantages, including cost, lengthy osseointegration period, and need for a surgical procedure to place and remove the implant. Similarly, Wehrbein and associates devised a cylindrical palatal implant in 1996 for the same purpose. Without doubt, these devices have achieved success and safety in providing anchorage for the placement of implants in the palatal area.

ANATOMIC CONSIDERATIONS

Since 2006, the U.S. Food and Drug Administration has approved the use of TADs in patients who are 12 years and older. Pretreatment planning for these patients includes serial lateral cephalograms or hand-wrist films to assess growth cessation. Placement of anchorage implants in the mid-palatal suture may affect skeletal growth of the maxilla. Recently, cone beam computed tomography (CT) technology has drastically reduced the cost and increased the accessibility and ease of obtaining a three-dimensional volumetric study of areas where bone volume, quality, and proximity to vital structures may be questionable for the placement of palatal implants. CT analysis has revealed that bone density is thickest at the level between the first and second premolars and the first and second molars, thus making these areas ideal for placement. If a situation warrants placement of the anchorage more anteriorly, paramedian placement in the area of the premolars may be more suitable because this will avoid potential injury to the incisive neurovascular bundle. Generally, the incisive canal should be kept at a minimum distance of 1 cm from placement of the implant. Although classified as a temporary orthodontic anchorage device, the early generation of palatal implants required osseointegration and indeed differed from the more recent TAD miniscrews and miniplates.

TAD miniscrews are not osseointegrated. Instead, they rely on mechanical engagement of the screw threads to the cortical alveolar bone. Because of this very crucial difference, loading can be performed immediately at orthodontic forces of less than 2 N. An increase in length and hence surface area of TADs does not add to their stability since they do not engage by the principles of osseointegration. Any screw length greater than 5 to 6 mm and up to 12 mm appears to be sufficient. Unlike screw length, screw diameter is significant in determining the stability of TADs. Miyawaki and co-authors, in an article on the optimal screw dimensions and design of TAD miniscrews, reported that a diameter of no less than 1.2 to 1.4 mm in the maxilla and no greater than 1.4 to 1.8 mm in the mandible provides adequate stability. The recommended difference in screw diameter in the maxilla versus the mandible is due to differences in corticocancellous bone composition. The amount of cortical bone and its density are crucial factors in providing stability to TADs. The thickest portion of the alveolar bone is located between the lateral incisors and canines anteriorly and adjacent to the first molars posteriorly. These sites are ideal for the placement of TADs. Although placement of TADs is possible in areas where there is a high cancellous-to-cortical bone ratio, the hard palate, the infranasal spine, and the maxillary buttress, symphysis, parasymphysis, and retromolar region tend to be more optimal sites given their higher cortical bone content. The TAD miniplate carried over the traditional principles of plating for trauma and osteotomy fixation in oral and maxillofacial surgery. These plates are low profile with one end fixed to bone via screws while the other end emerges transmucosally and has tubes, buttons, notches, and grooves to allow orthodontic attachments (Fig. 17-1).

The ideal site for placement of TADs is in an area where there is thick type D2, three-bone density, sufficient bone volume and clearance from vital structures, thin attached gingival soft tissue, and optimal location for anchorage to support the planned orthodontic forces. Three-dimensional studies indicate that the alveolar bone widens as it approaches the apical portion of the tooth roots.

Clinically, this level is often apical to the mucogingival junction. For optimal placement of TADs, the screw body should engage the thicker portion of the alveolus apically and the screw head should emerge coronally from the mucogingival junction through the attached gingiva (Fig. 17-2).

TAD miniscrews and plates provide both direct and indirect anchorage for orthodontic treatment. Direct anchorage refers to situations in which the implant serves as an anchor for the orthodontic forces applied. Indirect anchorage refers to situations in which the implant stabilizes a tooth or group of teeth, with the entire unit serving as anchorage for the orthodontic forces exerted. TADs are versatile and can readily be used for retraction, protraction, uprighting, and intrusion of teeth. Although Sugawara reported a high relapse rate of 30% in cases in which TADs were used for the intrusion of molars, the amount of forces applied, the treatment period, and the degree of intrusion may have been contributing factors.

TREATMENT AND TECHNIQUES

The surgical protocol for TAD miniplates involves gaining access to bone via a full-thickness mucoperiosteal incision. Two to three monocortical fixation screws are used to secure the plate vertically in between roots of the teeth, and the transmucosal end of the plate is positioned so that it emerges out of the attached gingiva. Placement of TAD miniscrews can be done via a flapless approach. The soft tissue gingiva can be removed with a small punch. The TAD screws can be screwed in place either with a drill or by hand, but a smaller pilot hole may need to be drilled first in dense cortical bone. The TAD miniscrew should be placed at an angle that is ideal in assisting in the planned orthodontic movement. The TAD is placed at a very slight 30- to 45-degree acute angle to the occlusal plane to engage the greatest dimension of bone available and also to allow emergence of the screw head from the attached gingiva. Loading can begin immediately with forces of less than 50 to 250 g, depending on the planned orthodontic movements. Excessive intrusive or torque forces beyond 250 g affect stability and increase the risk for failure. In addition, minimal clearance of 2 mm from any adjacent vital structures and tooth roots is recommended to avoid potential injury. TADs are absolutely contraindicated in patients with a known allergy to titanium alloy. Patients with a history of heavy tobacco use, advanced osteoporosis, uncontrolled immune or metabolic bone disorders (i.e., uncontrolled diabetes), and bisphosphonate use should be evaluated on a case-by-case basis and the underlying problem corrected before TAD placement.

POSTOPERATIVE CARE

Complications of TAD placement include infection, damage to adjacent teeth and neurovascular bundles, perforation of the maxillary sinus, loosening or migration of the implant, and hardware fracture. Perioperative antibiotics are recommended, as well as the use of oral chlorhexidine rinses, similar to the surgical protocol for conventional endosseous implants. Patient compliance in maintaining good oral hygiene is also important to minimize mucosal inflammation. Studies have shown peri-implant mucosal inflammation to be one of the major causes of TAD failure. Care in handling these delicate mini-implants during placement and removal is crucial to avoid shearing the screw head or fracturing the implant.

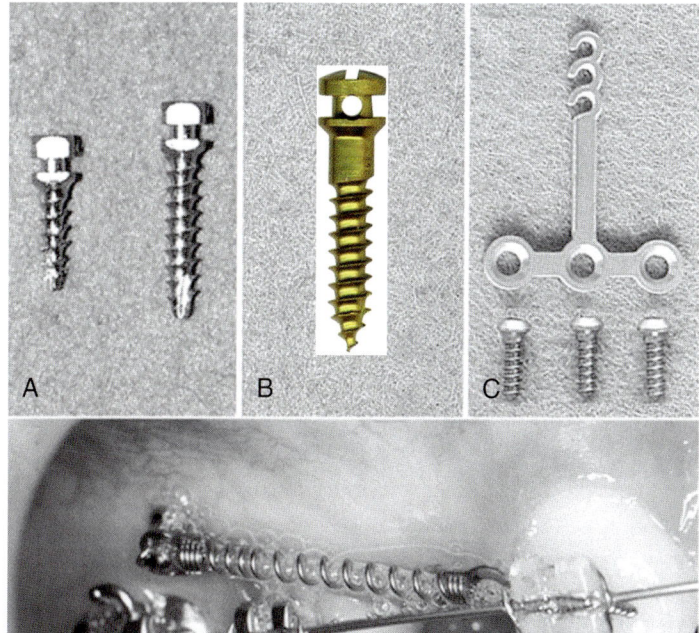

Fig. 17-1 ■ **A** and **B,** Type A titanium screws, 2.0 mm in diameter with variable lengths. **C,** Miniplate with screws, 2 mm in diameter and 5 mm in length. **D,** Clinical use of a type A screw. (**A, C, D** Modified from Kuroda S, Sugawara Y, Deguchi T, et al: Clinical use of miniscrew implants as orthodontic anchorage: success rates and postoperative discomfort, *Am J Orthod Dentofacial Orthop* 131:9-15, 2007; **B,** courtesy KLS Martin L.P., Jacksonville, Fla.)

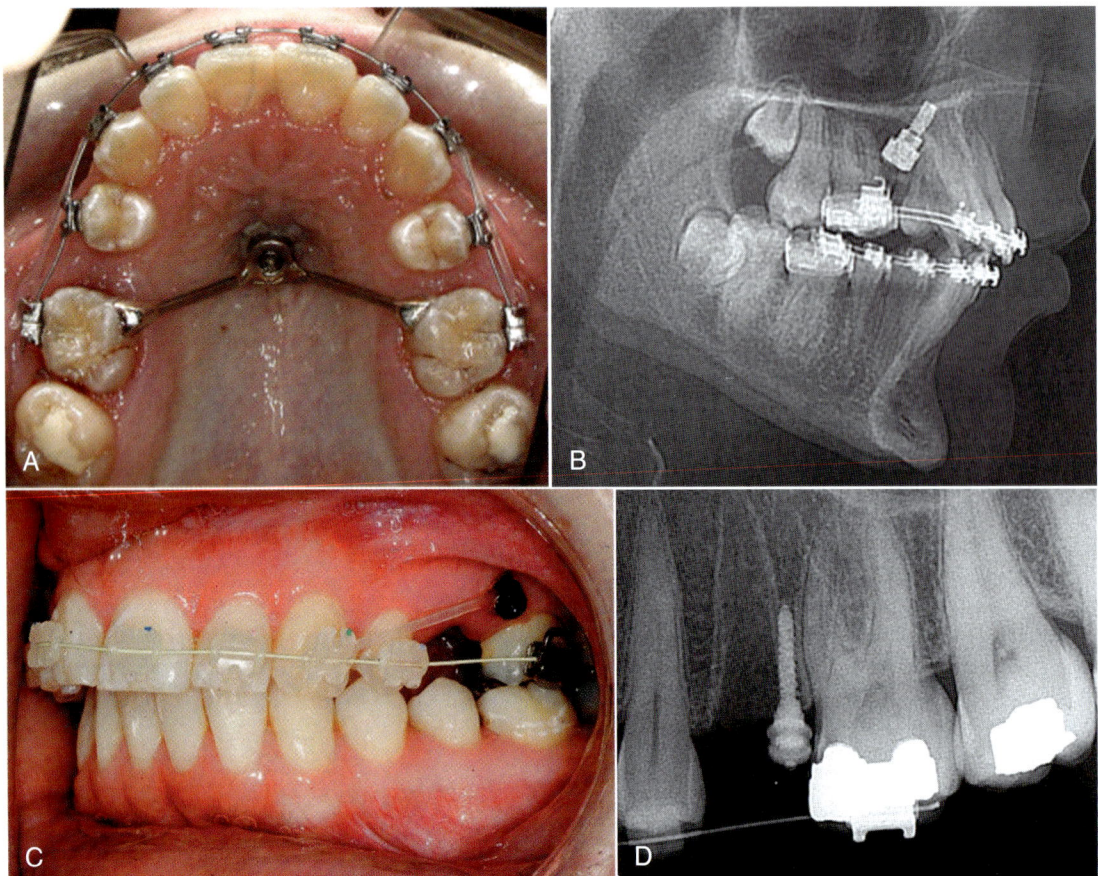

Fig. 17-2 ■ **A,** After the molar distalization phase, the temporary anchorage device is bonded to the first molars to provide anchorage for retraction of the anterior teeth. **B,** Lateral cephalograph of this patient showing the 6-mm intraosseous implant (and healing cap) in the standard anterior palate site and angulated 25 degrees to the vertical plane. **C,** An Aarhus mini-implant inserted in the buccal interproximal region mesial to the first molar and at an angulation of approximately 45 degrees to the vertical axis. This has been loaded immediately with a traction auxiliary to distalize the canine and first premolar. **D,** A postinsertion radiograph confirms the position of the mini-implant in the interproximal bone between the second premolar socket and the first molar roots. (From Prabhu J, Cousley RRJ: Current products and practice: bone anchorage devices in orthodontics, *J Orthod* 33:288-307, 2006.)

PEARLS AND PITFALLS

- The overall success rate of TADs in recent years has risen predictably to 90%.
- The key to success in cases involving the use of TADs is careful planning and a multidisciplinary approach, including a team composed of an orthodontist, a surgeon, and a restorative dentist.
- It is through a team approach that the ideal location (dense cortical bone, emergence from attached gingiva), proper angulation (slight acute angle to the occlusal plane), and appropriate size of the TAD (screw diameter of 1.2 to 1.4 mm in the maxilla and 1.4 to 1.8 mm in the mandible) can be accurately predetermined.
- Orthodontic treatment with TADs increases patients' acceptance of treatment by minimizing the necessity of having to deal with interarch elastics and awkward orthodontic gear.

- TADs offer the possibility of a shorter course of treatment while force is continuously being exerted, whereas conventional orthodontics requires headgear or elastics; the choice may depend heavily on patient compliance.
- Both the placement and removal of TADs are minimally invasive procedures and can often be performed with the patient under local anesthesia.
- Because TADs provide adequate stability, the orthodontist can use these implants immediately after insertion.
- The cost of TADs is far lower than that for conventional osseointegrated implants.

BIBLIOGRAPHY

Bae SM, Park HS, Kyung HM, et al: Clinical application of micro-implant anchorage, *J Clin Orthod* 36:298-302, 2002.

Baumgaertel S: Quantitative investigation of palatal bone depth and cortical bone thickness for mini-implant placement in adults, *Am J Orthod Dentofacial Orthop* 136:104-108, 2009.

Block MS, Hoffman DR: A new device for absolute anchorage for orthodontics, *Am J Orthod Dentofacial Orthop* 107:251-258, 1995.

Celenza F, Hochman MN: Absolute anchorage in orthodontics: direct and indirect implant-assisted modalities, *J Clin Orthod* 34:397-402, 2000.

Chen Y, Kyung HM, Zhao WT, et al: Critical factors for the success of orthodontic mini-implants: a systematic review, *Am J Orthod Dentofacial Orthop* 135:284-291, 2009.

Chen YJ, Chang HH, Lin HY, et al: Stability of miniplates and miniscrews used for orthodontic anchorage: experience with 492 temporary anchorage devices, *Clin Oral Implants Res* 19:1188-1196, 2008.

Cheng SJ, Tseng JY, Lee JJ: A prospective study of the risk factors associated with failure of mini-implant used for orthodontic anchorage, *Int J Oral Maxillofac Implants* 19:100-106, 2004.

Cope JB: Temporary anchorage devices in orthodontics: a paradigm shirt, *Semin Orthod* 11:3-9, 2005.

Cornelis MA, Scheffler NR, Mahy P, et al: Modified miniplates for temporary skeletal anchorage in orthodontics: placement and removal surgeries, *J Oral Maxillofac Surg* 66:1439-1445, 2008.

Costa A, Pasta G, Bergamaschi G: Intraoral hard and soft tissue depths for temporary anchorage devices, *Semin Orthod* 11:10-15, 2005.

Costa A, Raffini M, Melsen B: Miniscrews as orthodontic anchorage: a preliminary report, *Int J Adult Orthod Orthognath Surg* 13:201-209, 1998.

Creekmore TD, Eklund MK: The possibility of skeletal anchorage, *J Clin Orthod* 17:266-269, 1983.

Gapski R, Wang HL, Mascarenhas P, et al: Critical review of immediate implant loading, *Clin Oral Implants Res* 14:515-527, 2003.

Heymann GC, Camilla Tulloch JF: Implantable devices as orthodontic anchorage: a review of current treatment modalities, *J Esthet Restor Dent* 18:68-80, 2006.

Janssen KI, Raghoebar GM, Vissink A, et al: Skeletal anchorage in orthodontics—a review of various systems in animal and human studies, *Int J Oral Maxillofac Implants* 23:75-88, 2008.

Kanomi R: Mini-implant for orthodontic anchorage, *J Clin Orthod* 31:763-767, 1997.

Kravitz ND, Kusnoto B, Tsay TP, et al: The use of temporary anchorage devices for molar intrusion, *J Am Dent Assoc* 138:56-64, 2007.

Kuroda S, Sugawara Y, Deguchi T, et al: Clinical use of miniscrew implants as orthodontic anchorage: success rates and postoperative discomfort, *Am J Orthod Dentofacial Orthop* 131:9-15, 2007.

Labanauskaite B, Jankauskas G, Vasiliauskas A, et al: Implants for orthodontics anchorage. Meta-analysis. *Stomatologica* 7:128-132, 2005.

Leung MT, Lee TC, Rabie AB, et al: Use of mini-screws and miniplates in orthodontics, *J Oral Maxillofac Surg* 66:1461-1466, 2008.

Miyawaki S, Koyama I, Inoue M, et al: Factors associated with the stability of titanium screws placed in the posterior region for orthodontic anchorage, *Am J Orthod Dentofacial Orthop* 124:373-378, 2003.

Ohashi E, Pecho OE, Moron M, et al: Implant vs screw loading protocols in orthodontics: a systematic review. *Angle Orthod* 76:721-727, 2006.

Papadopoulos MA, Tarawneh F: The use of mini-screw implants for temporary skeletal anchorage in orthodontics: a comprehensive review, *Oral Surg Oral Med Oral Pathol Oral Radiol Endod* 103:e6-e15, 2007.

Park HS, Bae SM, Kyung HM, et al: Micro-implant anchorage for treatment of skeletal class I bialveolar protrusion, *J Clin Orthod* 35:417-422, 2001.

Park HS, Jeong SH, Kwon OW: Factors affecting the clinical success of screw implants used as orthodontic anchorage, *Am J Orthod Dentofacial Orthop* 130:18-25, 2006.

Poggio PM, Incorvati C, Velo S, et al: "Safe zones": a guide for miniscrew positioning in the maxillary and mandibular arch, *Angle Orthod* 76:191-197, 2006.

Prabhu J, Cousley RRJ: Current products and practice: bone anchorage devices in orthodontics, *J Orthod* 33:288-307, 2006.

Reynders R, Ronchi L, Bipat S: Mini-implants in orthodontics: a systematic review of the literature, *Am J Orthod Dentofacial Orthop* 135:564.e1-564.e19, discussion 564-565, 2009.

Sándor GK, Daskalogiannakis J, Carmichael RP: Facilitation of orthodontics and orthognathic surgery using dental implants, *Atlas Oral Maxillofac Surg Clin North Am* 16:125-135, 2008.

Straumann USA. 510(k) Summary. Available at: www.fda.gov/cdrh/pdf4/k040469.pdf. Accessed Oct. 24, 2006.

Tseng YC, Hsieh CH, Chen CH, et al: The application of mini-implants for orthodontic anchorage, *Int J Oral Maxillofac Surg* 35:704-707, 2006.

Viwattanatipa N, Thanakitcharu S, Uttraravichien A, et al: Survival analysis of surgical mini-screws as orthodontic anchorage, *Am J Orthod Dentofacial Orthop* 136:29-36, 2009.

Wehrbein H, Glatzmaier J, Mundwiller U, et al: The Orthosystem—a new implant system for orthodontic anchorage in the palate, *J Orofac Orthop* 57:142-153, 1996.

Wu TY, Kuang SH, Wu CH: Factors associated with the stability of mini-implants for orthodontic anchorage: a study of 414 samples in Taiwan, *J Oral Maxillofac Surg* 67:1595-1599, 2009.

Dental Implant Prosthetic Rehabilitation: Autogenous Bone Grafting for Alveolar Defects

Stephen A. Bankston

When Professor Per-Ingvar Brånemark placed the first titanium root-form dental implant in 1965, only patients with adequate bone volume were considered candidates for implant rehabilitation.[1] Patients with atrophy and alveolar deficiencies were restricted to prosthetic reconstruction with conventional prostheses. As dental implants became more popular and their indications for restoration became more diverse, the need to address alveolar deficiencies also grew. Technologic innovations in bone physiology, tissue banking, and surgical techniques have advanced the knowledge and understanding of the reconstruction of alveolar defects.

Since the infancy of dental implants in the late 1960s and 1970s, implant dentistry has grown to greater than a $700 million industry in the United States in 2008.[2] It is estimated that the U.S. dental implant market will exceed $1 billion by the year 2013.[3] The widespread acceptance and increased placement of implants have also led to a significant rise in concomitant reconstructive procedures, including hard and soft tissue grafting. Successful implant osseointegration, stability, and long-term survival require that the implant site have sufficient bone quality and quantity that will withstand loading and occlusal forces. When alveolar ridge deficiencies exist, reconstruction of the defect is required before or concurrent with implant placement. The contemporary oral and maxillofacial surgeon must not only be able to place implants but also possess the knowledge and surgical prowess to address alveolar deficiencies for comprehensive implant reconstruction. Reconstruction of alveolar defects encompasses replacement of hard and soft tissues that have been lost secondary to congenital anomalies, trauma, pathology, atrophy, or other causes. Autogenous grafts are the most widespread and predictable graft materials used for the reconstruction of alveolar defects.

ETIOPATHOGENESIS/CAUSATIVE FACTORS

It was estimated that by the year 2010, 100 million Americans will be missing one or more teeth and that 36 million will be edentulous in one or both arches.[4,5] As teeth are lost, the supporting periodontal structures and bone are also lost, and this creates alveolar defects. Alveolar resorption following tooth loss occurs in a predictable pattern, initially along the labial surface of the alveolar crest. This reduces alveolar width and, later, alveolar height. The majority of the bone loss, estimated to be 40% to 60%, occurs within the first 36 months following the loss of teeth, and the resorption pattern declines to 0.25% to 0.5% annually after the first 3 years.[6] The resulting defects can be manifested as insufficient alveolar bone width, height, or a combination of both deficiencies. Alveolar defects can compromise implant support, function, and esthetics.

A variety of graft materials are available for restoring alveolar defects, including autologous, allogeneic, and xenogeneic grafts and alloplastic materials. When compared with bone substitutes, autogenous bone has more ideal biochemical properties and greater potential for integration with the surrounding tissues. Autogenous grafts are the gold standard by which other graft materials are compared. They are well documented and have been used extensively for reconstructing alveolar defects. Autogenous bone is a connective tissue that has the ability to heal and remodel by cellular regeneration and the production of a mineral matrix, as opposed to collagen deposition and scar formation. Bone cellular regeneration involves osteoprogenitor cells that have the ability to differentiate into bone-forming cell lineages: osteoblasts, osteocytes, and osteoclasts. It is this unique property of cellular regeneration that allows reconstructive surgeons to predictably perform bone grafting.[7]

Autogenous grafts are superior to other graft materials because of their combined osteoconductive, osteoinductive, and osteogenic properties. Osteoconduction is the formation of new bone from adjacent bone or periosteum along a physical matrix. The matrix acts as a scaffold and allows deposition and new bone growth on its surface. With autogenous grafts, the cortical portion of the graft acts as a scaffold and is remodeled and replaced with new bone in a process known as creeping substitution.[8] Osteoinduction describes a process whereby new bone is produced in an area where bone did not exist previously. Osteoinduction is the formation of bone by biochemical stimulation and transformation of undifferentiated pluripotent mesenchymal cells into bone-forming cells. Osteogenesis is the development and formation of new bone from osteoid produced by osteoblasts. Osteogenesis can be induced by osteoprogenitor cells from within the bony defect or by the transfer of live osteoprogenitor cells from the harvest site.[9] The osteogenic property of autogenous grafts is one of the most important characteristics that separate autogenous grafts from all other graft materials. Autogenous grafts also have the advantage of invoking minimal immunologic reactions.

Advancements in gene technology by recombinant techniques have revealed the sequence of many growth factors and other proteins involved in the formation and remodeling of bone. Recombinant human proteins in the form of bone morphogenetic protein (rhBMP-2) have shown the ability to regenerate skeletal tissue and induce new bone formation. Because the growth factors are proteins, a carrier is required for their release at intervals, and the carrier must be degraded with minimal tissue reaction. Although rhBMP-2 has shown considerable promise, additional clinical trials are needed to address the delivery technology, accuracy in dosing, and conditions for stimulation of bone growth.[10]

PATIENT EVALUATION/DIAGNOSTIC STUDIES

Preoperative evaluation consists of a thorough medical and dental examination (Box 18-1). A systems review is performed and all medications noted. The social history is reviewed, including

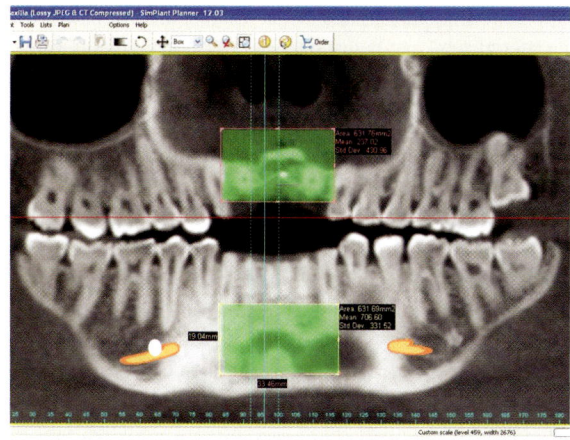

Fig. 18-1 ■ Computed tomographic evaluation of the recipient donor sites using the SimPlant dental software (Materialise Leuven, Belgium).

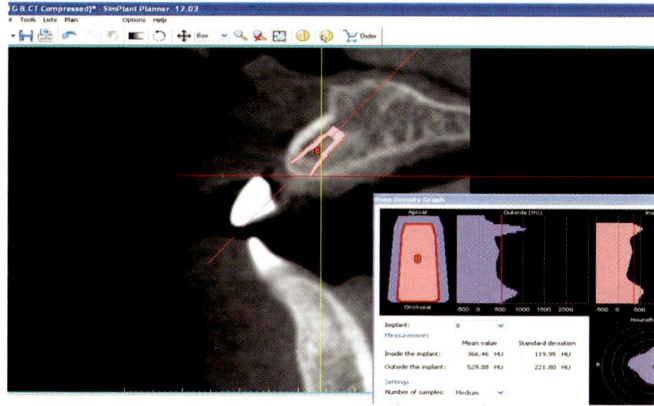

Fig. 18-2 ■ Diagnostic wax-up used for making the computed tomography radiographic template with the SimPlant dental software (Materialise Leuven, Belgium) for planning implant treatment.

BOX 18-1	Preoperative Treatment Planning

- Medical evaluation
- Dental examination
- Radiographic examination: Panorex, periapicals, lateral cephalogram, computed tomography (if available)
- Facial and intraoral photographs
- Mounted models: diagnostic wax-up
- Conference with the restorative dentist or prosthodontist

inquiries about tobacco use. Smoking has been implicated in increased failure rates in bone grafting and implants.[11] The dental examination evaluates occlusion, teeth adjacent to the defect, periodontal status, and gingival architecture. The quantity of keratinized tissue and the thickness of the mucosa are assessed. Thin periodontal biotypes have a higher incidence of recession than do thick biotypes.[12] The endodontic status of teeth adjacent to the recipient site is also evaluated.

The radiographic examination consists of plain films to visualize the alveolar defect and potential donor sites. The films are also used to evaluate the surrounding anatomy, including the tooth roots, maxillary sinus, mental foramen, and inferior alveolar neurovascular bundle. Computed tomography (CT) provides three-dimensional visualization of the alveolar defect and potential donor sites (Fig. 18-1). The images have minimal distortion with superior accuracy of the related anatomy. CT scans provide unsurpassed volumetric analysis of alveolar defects in comparison to plain films. Multiple computer-based software programs are available to analyze the CT scans and aid in planning treatment for implants and bone graft requirements. Stereolithic models can be generated from the CT scan to provide replicas of the craniofacial skeleton. Hounsfield units obtained from the CT scan provide a measure of the bone density at the alveolar defect and donor site.

Facial and intraoral photographs provide valuable information about esthetics, facial contours, and symmetry. The soft tissues can also be evaluated at rest and with animation. Photographs provide a permanent record of the pretreatment conditions that can be compared with the final treatment results. Mounted models provide ridge form and interocclusal relationships between arches. Diagnostic waxing allows visualization of the planned prosthetic outcome. Visualizing the proposed tooth position helps in determining ideal implant placement and graft requirements. The wax-up can also be used as a radiographic template for the CT scan and as a surgical guide for placement of the implant (Fig. 18-2).

After the aforementioned examinations have been performed and the diagnostic data have been compiled and analyzed, a treatment plan can be formulated. Treatment planning incorporates the restorative dentist or prosthodontist and the surgeon. The treatment plan addresses the patient's chief complaint, restorative goals, and any hard or soft tissue deficiencies. The decision to perform bone grafting is driven by the requirements for the prosthesis.

TREATMENT/RECONSTRUCTIVE GOALS

The widespread use of autogenous grafts to reconstruct defects in the maxillofacial region clearly separates oral and maxillofacial surgeons from the other specialties that treat the maxillofacial region. Each alveolar defect is unique and involves specific hard and soft tissue requirements for reconstruction. One of the goals of reconstructing alveolar defects is restoration of alveolar ridge bone height and width to adjacent bone levels. Other reconstruction goals include restoration of osseous bulk to provide strength and soft tissue profile for the implant restoration. Osseous bulk also provides support for facial tissues, including lip support, which can improve facial esthetics. Restoration of the continuity of the maxillary and mandibular arch form is another reconstructive goal because this optimizes the maxillofacial musculature complex. Reconstruction of alveolar defects is imperative to provide support for implants and, ultimately, a functioning prosthesis under loading and occlusal forces.

Selection of the donor site depends on the size, location, and overall geometry of the alveolar defect that is being restored. Harvest site selection should also correlate with the specific hard and soft tissue requirements of the graft. Multiple sites have traditionally been used for reconstruction of alveolar defects, including the iliac crest, tibia, rib, and calvaria. In addition, local intraoral harvest sites such as the mandibular symphysis and ramus buccal shelf have become increasingly popular for reconstructing alveolar defects.

The mandibular symphysis and ramus buccal shelf offer some advantages over distant donor sites, including convenience of surgical access and proximity of the donor and recipient sites. Intraoral donor grafts are often associated with less resorption than that in the iliac crest, tibia, and rib grafts.[13] There are no external cutaneous scars associated with intraoral sites. Morbidity is less with the procedure because of the absence of a distant donor site. There is also a decrease in total operating time with the use of local intraoral donor sites. The procedures require less anesthesia time, and in most cases general anesthesia is not required. With the reduced surgical time and decreased anesthesia requirements, the cost is also correspondingly lower.[14]

The principal disadvantage of intraoral sites is the limited amount of bone that can be harvested for reconstruction. The quality of the bone is typically type I and type II with minimal cancellous marrow available. When larger quantities of bone are required for reconstruction, the iliac crest and tibia are the preferred sites for bone harvest.

SPECIFIC TREATMENT AND TECHNIQUES

PREPARATION OF THE RECIPIENT SITE

The alveolar defect is exposed and the recipient site developed before harvesting the bone graft. This allows the surgeon to thoroughly visualize the defect and determine the size and shape of the graft required for reconstruction of the defect. It also minimizes the amount of time between graft harvest and placement. The incisions for exposure of the alveolar defect are made along the crest of the ridge through the attached gingiva. A broad-based flap design with divergent releasing incisions is created to maximize the vascular supply and allow tension-free closure. A full-thickness mucoperiosteal flap is reflected beyond the margins of the defect. With the alveolar defect exposed, the soft tissue is débrided and uneven bony contours are removed. Preparation of the recipient site is completed by perforation of the cortical plate with multiple holes to increase revascularization of the graft. The perforations also release growth factors such as platelet-derived growth factor and transforming growth factors. Additionally, the cortical perforations facilitate intimate adaptation of the graft to the underlying recipient bed[15] (Fig. 18-3).

DONOR SITES

Mandibular Symphysis

The mandibular symphysis provides the greatest volume of bone of all the intraoral donor sites available. Studies on cadavers have revealed that the site can yield an average block measuring $21 \times 10 \times 7$ mm or greater.[16] A symphysis graft can provide up to 4 to 8 mm of vertical or horizontal augmentation, which can enable reconstruction of up to a three-tooth defect. The symphysis is composed of D-1 and D-2 density bone with varying amounts of trabecular marrow.[17] The bone can be harvested as a block or a particulate graft. Radiographic evaluation of the region is used to help evaluate the donor site. A Panorex, lateral cephalometric radiograph, periapicals, or CT scan (or any combination of these imaging modalities) can be used to identify pertinent anatomic landmarks and help determine the amount of available bone.

One of the principal advantages of the symphysis as a donor site is the ease of surgical access. The vestibular and sulcular incisions are the two classic incisions used for flap design for exposure of the symphysis. The vestibular incision is made in a straight or curvilinear line between the cuspid teeth. The incision is made 0.75 to 1 cm below the mucogingival junction and is confined to the canine area to minimize the risk for injury to the mental nerve. The average distance of the mental foramen is 2.2 cm lateral to the midline of the mandibular skeleton.[18] Disadvantages of this approach include more soft tissue bleeding from the mentalis muscle and possible scar formation. The second popular flap design is made with the sulcular incision. The sulcular incision is reserved for patients with healthy periodontium and a thick periodontal biotype and in those in whom recession would not be an esthetic concern. The incision is made in the sulcus from the second bicuspid to the contralateral second bicuspid. Distal oblique releasing incisions are made in the buccal vestibule proximal to the mental foramina.

A full-thickness mucoperiosteal flap is reflected to expose the mandibular symphysis, bilateral mental foramina, and the inferior border. After the symphysis has been thoroughly exposed and graft dimension requirements verified from the recipient site, the bone can be harvested. The graft should be 2 to 3 mm larger than the recipient site to allow contouring and adaptation of the graft. The osteotomies are confined to 5 mm from the apices of the teeth, 5 mm from the mental foramina, and 5 mm from the inferior border[19] (Fig. 18-4). The osteotomies can be performed with a surgical handpiece and burs or with a saw under copious irrigation. The osteotomies extend through the outer cortex into cancellous bone. In most cases the inferior border of the mandible and the lingual cortex are preserved intact. A single beveled osteotome or chisel is used to complete the osteotomies and remove the bone. A small amount of cancellous marrow can be harvested from the symphysis donor site. The harvested bone is placed in physiologic saline immediately to preserve the osteocompetent cells.

Following harvesting of the graft, hemostatic agents such as Gelfoam (Pfizer Inc., New York), Surgicel (Ethicon Inc., Somerville N.J.), Avitene (Davol Inc., Providence R.I.), or platelet-rich plasma may be placed in the donor site. With larger bone grafts, a bone substitute can be placed in the donor defect to maintain facial contours and allow future secondary harvesting from the site.[20] Layered closure of the donor site with resorbable sutures is performed after the graft has been placed at the recipient site.

The mandibular symphysis is associated with a higher incidence of postoperative complications than seen with other intraoral donor sites. Altered sensation in the anterior teeth, chin, and lip is the most common complaint from patients. The altered sensation is temporary in many instances, and spontaneous recovery occurs in most patients.[21] However, it is crucial to inform the patient of these potential complications preoperatively.

Mandibular Ramus Buccal Shelf

The mandibular ramus buccal shelf is another excellent bone source for reconstructing alveolar defects. Studies of samples from dry skulls have revealed that the ramus buccal shelf can yield a rectangular graft with average dimensions of $37.6 \times 33.2 \times 22.5 \times 9.2$ mm or greater.[22] The graft can provide bone for reconstruction of up to a four-tooth defect. With the possibility of performing bilateral harvest, the reconstructive potential is doubled. The ramus buccal shelf is composed of almost entirely D-1 cortical bone and has minimal cancellous marrow.[23] Such bone morphology is ideal for

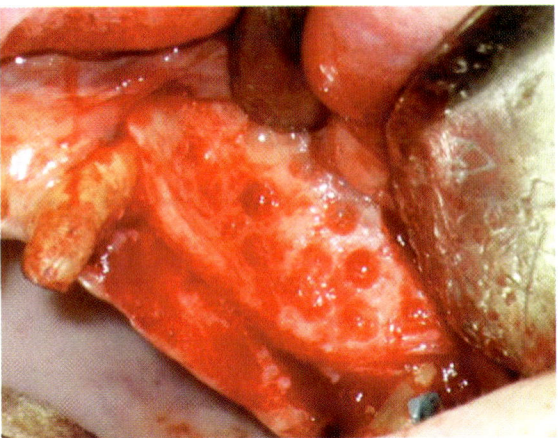

Fig. 18-3 ■ Recipient site preparation with cortical perforations.

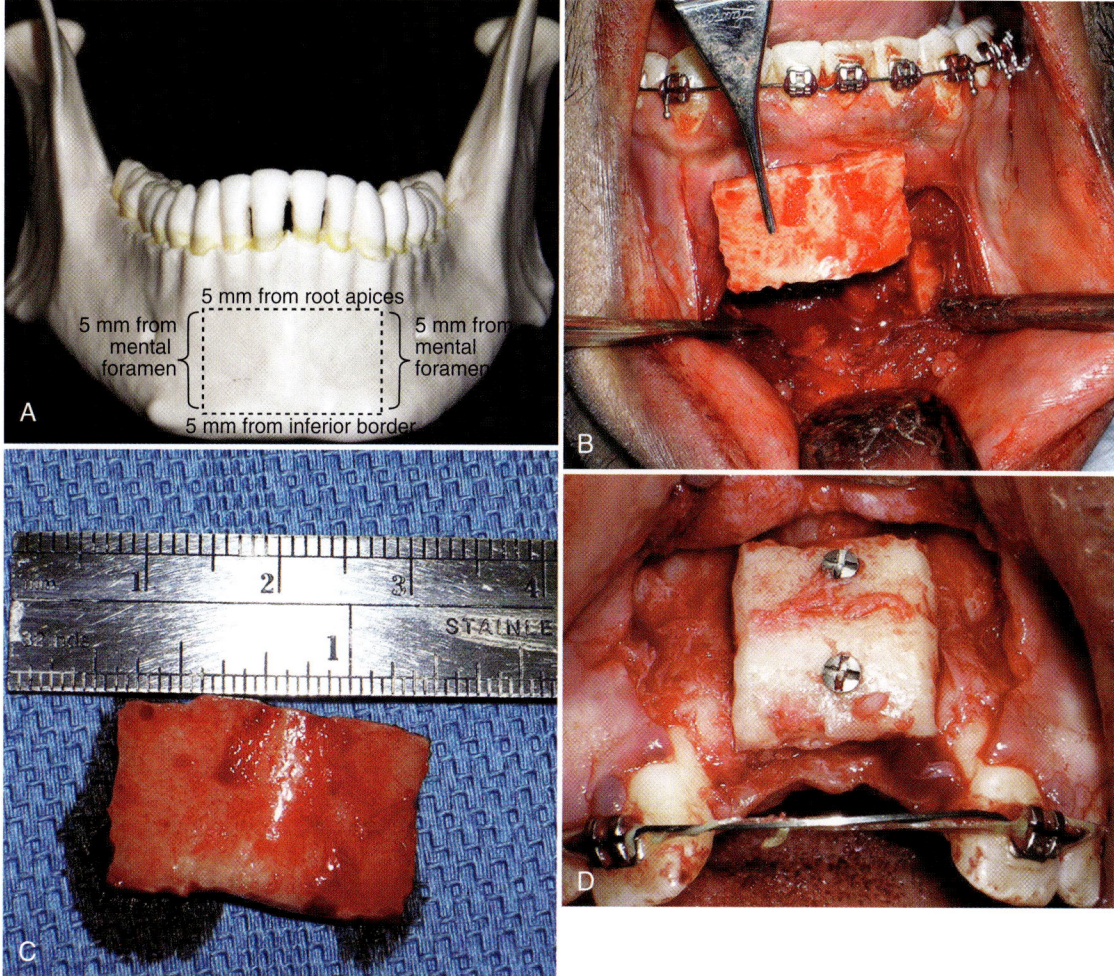

Fig. 18-4 ■ **A,** Borders of the osteotomies for harvest of the mandibular symphysis. **B,** Monocortical bone harvested from the mandibular symphysis. **C,** Cortical bone graft harvested from the mandibular symphysis. **D,** Symphysis graft fixed to the anterior maxilla.

veneer grafts to increase ridge width. A panoramic radiograph or CT is used to evaluate the donor site and identify the course of the inferior alveolar canal. A submentovertex radiograph can also be used to evaluate the thickness of the ramus.

The ramus buccal shelf harvest technique has many features similar to mandibular sagittal ramus osteotomy. The initial incision is analogous to the approach for removing mandibular third molars. A sulcular incision is made around the posterior molar and continued posteriorly and laterally from the retromolar pad. The incision is extended superiorly along the ascending ramus. The incision should not be extended higher than the level of the occlusal plane to minimize possible injury to the buccal nerve and artery or exposure of the buccal fat pad.[24] A full-thickness mucoperiosteal flap is reflected to expose the lateral ramus, external oblique ridge, buccal shelf, and body of the mandible. A notched ramus retractor is used to reflect the flap to the base of the coronoid process.

The anatomic boundaries of the graft are determined by the inferior alveolar canal, the posterior teeth, and coronoid process (Fig. 18-5). The size of the osteotomies is determined by the volumetric graft requirements of the alveolar defect to be reconstructed. Three complete osteotomies and one partial osteotomy are used to harvest the graft. The osteotomies are performed with a surgical handpiece and burs or with a reciprocating saw. The vertical ramus osteotomy is made at the base of the coronoid process, perpendicular to the external oblique ridge through the lateral cortex of the ramus

into the marrow. All osteotomies should just penetrate the cortical bone until bleeding occurs. The osteotomy extends posterior to the level of the antilingula, approximately 10 to 12 mm. The superior external oblique osteotomy is made 5 to 6 mm medial to the external oblique ridge. The osteotomy can be extended superiorly to the base of the coronoid process and anteriorly to the distal aspect of the first molar, depending on the bone volume required to reconstruct the defect. This allows procurement of grafts up to 40 mm in length. The anterior body vertical osteotomy is made in the mandibular body through the buccal cortex just into bleeding marrow. The position of anterior body vertical osteotomy is determined by the length of the superior external oblique osteotomy and the position of the inferior alveolar canal. The inferior osteotomy is used to connect the inferior aspect of the two vertical osteotomies and is created parallel to the external oblique osteotomy. The inferior osteotomy is made with a shallow cut into the buccal cortex to create a line of fracture. An osteotome or chisel is wedged in the superior external oblique osteotomy and used to harvest the graft by fracturing along the inferior osteotomy.[25] The graft is harvested carefully to prevent injury to the underlying inferior alveolar neurovascular bundle. The graft is placed immediately in physiologic saline.

Following harvesting of the graft, all sharp edges around the osteotomy are smoothed. Hemostatic agents can be placed if indicated. The use of bone substitutes is not indicated because they can be irritating to an exposed inferior alveolar nerve and the site will remodel

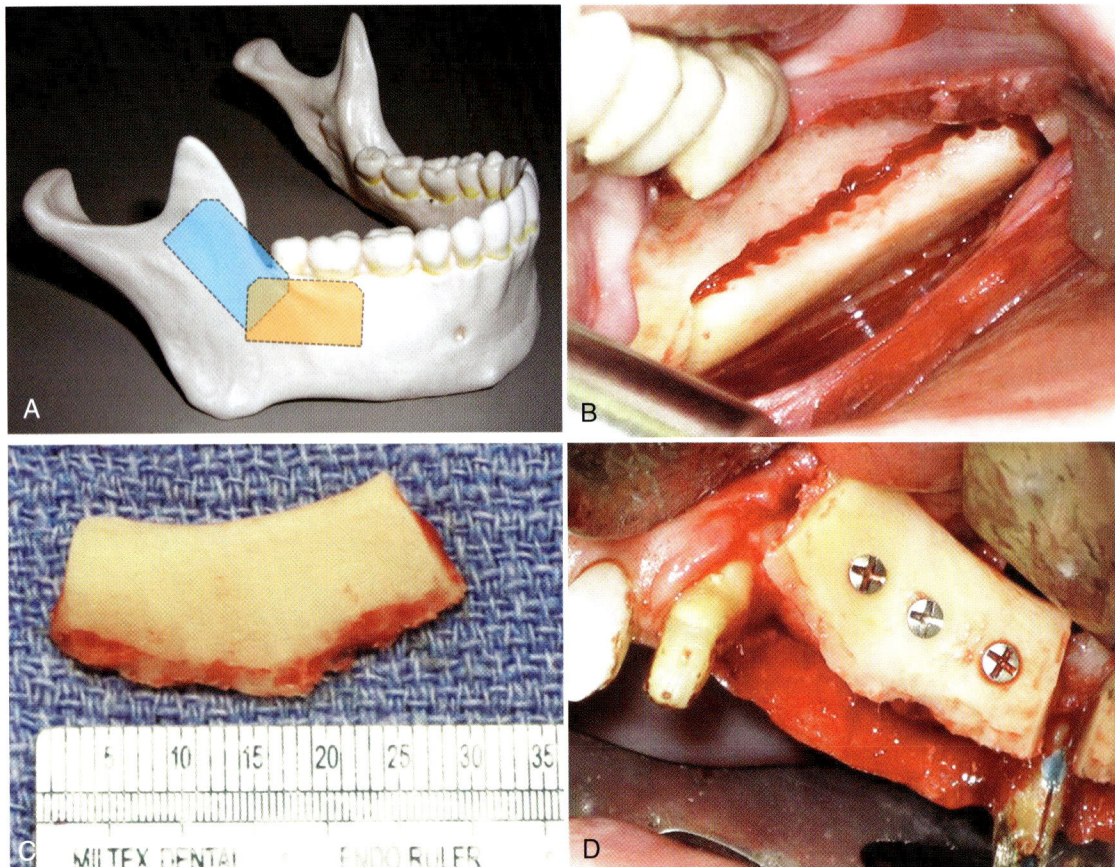

Fig. 18-5 ■ **A,** Borders of the osteotomies for harvest of the mandibular ramus buccal shelf. **B,** Osteotomies prepared for harvest of the mandibular ramus buccal shelf. **C,** Cortical bone graft harvested from the mandibular ramus buccal shelf. **D,** Ramus buccal shelf bone graft fixed to the left maxilla.

without graft material. The donor site is closed with resorbable suture after placement and fixation of the graft at the recipient site.

The incidence of complications is lower with the ramus buccal shelf than with the mandibular symphysis. There are fewer neurosensory complaints despite the greater potential for damage to the inferior alveolar nerve at a more proximal position. There is generally less postoperative edema and pain. Disadvantages of the ramus buccal shelf site are difficulties in surgical access and limitations in size and shape of the graft. There is also an increased incidence of trismus, which usually resolves within weeks.

Anterior Iliac Crest

When larger quantities of bone are required for reconstructing alveolar defects than the intraoral sites can provide, the iliac crest is the preferred donor site. The iliac crest can provide a large amount of cancellous marrow, and the cortical plate can also be harvested, which can provide structural support and contour for the graft. The iliac crest has the greatest cancellous-to-cortical bone ratio, and up to 50 cm³ of cancellous bone can be harvested from a single anterior hip site. When the anterior ilium is used as a donor site, preparation of the recipient site and graft harvest can be performed simultaneously, thereby reducing total operative time.

Radiographic evaluation of the pelvis is performed to help evaluate the donor site. An anteroposterior pelvic radiograph or CT scan can be used to identify pertinent anatomic landmarks and help determine the amount of bone available. Several anatomic landmarks and sensory cutaneous nerves must be identified when harvesting from the anterior iliac crest. The lateral cutaneous branch of the

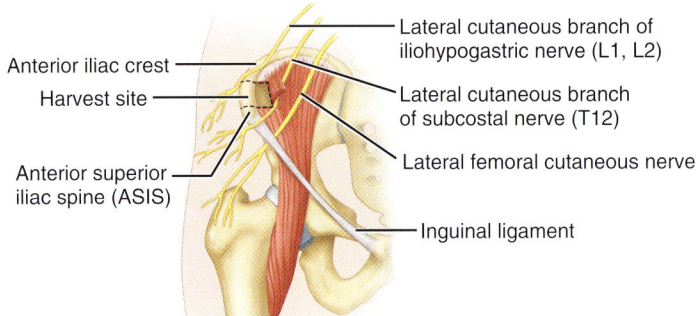

Fig. 18-6 ■ Anatomy for anterior iliac bone harvest. (Adapted from Bagheri SC, Jo C: *Clinical review of oral and maxillofacial surgery,* St. Louis, 2008, Mosby.)

iliohypogastric nerve, which carries sensory fibers for L1 and L2, transverses the area of the iliac tubercle. Because of the course of the nerve and its variability in location, it is the nerve most often injured during harvest of the anterior iliac crest. The lateral cutaneous branch of the subcostal nerve, which carries sensory fibers from T12, courses over the anterior superior spine. The lateral femoral cutaneous nerve is located anteriorly and medially between the psoas major and the iliacus muscles and provides sensation to the skin of the lateral aspect of the thigh[26] (Fig. 18-6).

The surgical approach for harvesting bone from the anterior ilium is designed to avoid the aforementioned sensory cutaneous nerves.

The patient is positioned supine with a roll placed under the buttock to elevate and rotate the iliac crest. A separate surgical setup is used to avoid contamination of the donor and recipient sites. The patient is prepared and draped in standard sterile fashion. The incision is 4 to 6 cm in length and positioned 2 to 3 cm lateral to the iliac crest, depending on the size of the graft needed. The initial incision is made 1.5 to 2 cm posterior to the anterior superior iliac spine and extended posterior to the area of the tubercle. This approach ensures that the incisional scar will be positioned laterally away from the belt line and waistband area. The incision is made parallel to the iliac crest and carried through the skin to subcutaneous tissue. The skin is then retracted and the incision repositioned over the iliac crest. The incision is continued through subcutaneous tissue down to the periosteum of the iliac crest. Subperiosteal dissection with reflection of the iliacus muscle on its medial aspect is preferred over lateral dissection of the tensor fasciae latae muscle, which can result in increased gait disturbances.[27,28] The size and design of the osteotomies are determined by the volumetric graft requirements of the alveolar defect to be reconstructed. In the most common harvest method used, a monocortical cancellous block is harvested and cancellous marrow is removed by curettage from the window that was created (Fig. 18-7). The osteotomies are performed with a surgical saw or osteotomes and a mallet. The marrow is harvested with curets and bone gouges. When the graft has been harvested, it is placed immediately in physiologic saline. The bony edges of the donor site are smoothed and the wound inspected for hemostasis. Hemostatic agents can be placed if indicated. The wound is closed beginning at the periosteum and muscle layers and continued in layered fashion to the skin.

GRAFT RECIPIENT SITE

After harvesting the bone, the graft should be contoured to fit the recipient site. The graft must be stabilized rigidly with two-point fixation to prevent rotation. Low-profile, self-tapping titanium screws 1.0 to 2.0 mm in diameter are ideal for most block grafts. Resorbable screws can also be used for graft fixation and have the advantage of not requiring removal before implant placement. Intimate adaptation of the graft to the host bone is paramount to prevent microrotation and subsequent incomplete bone incorporation. The bony edges of the graft should be smoothed to help prevent wound dehiscence, which is one of the principal complications associated with block grafts. Primary tension-free closure of the wound is crucial for successful incorporation of the graft. The mucosal flap is undermined and the periosteum scored to allow greater advancement of the soft tissue.

A staged approach with delayed implant placement is more predictable and preferred by many clinicians. This allows implants to be placed in increased bone volume in ideal positions with improved initial stability. In the maxilla, at least 4 months is required for graft incorporation, and because of the more cortical nature of the mandible, 5 to 6 months is recommended. Following these guidelines allows implants to be placed into healed grafts that have physiologic and histologic characteristics similar to the recipient bone.

POSTOPERATIVE CARE

Postoperative care of bone graft patients is similar to that for other oral and maxillofacial surgical procedures. Antibiotic prophylaxis is recommended for bone-grafting procedures to help reduce the incidence of postoperative infection. Antibiotics such as amoxicillin, clindamycin, or a cephalosporin can be started preoperatively and continued for at least 1 week postoperatively. Narcotic analgesics

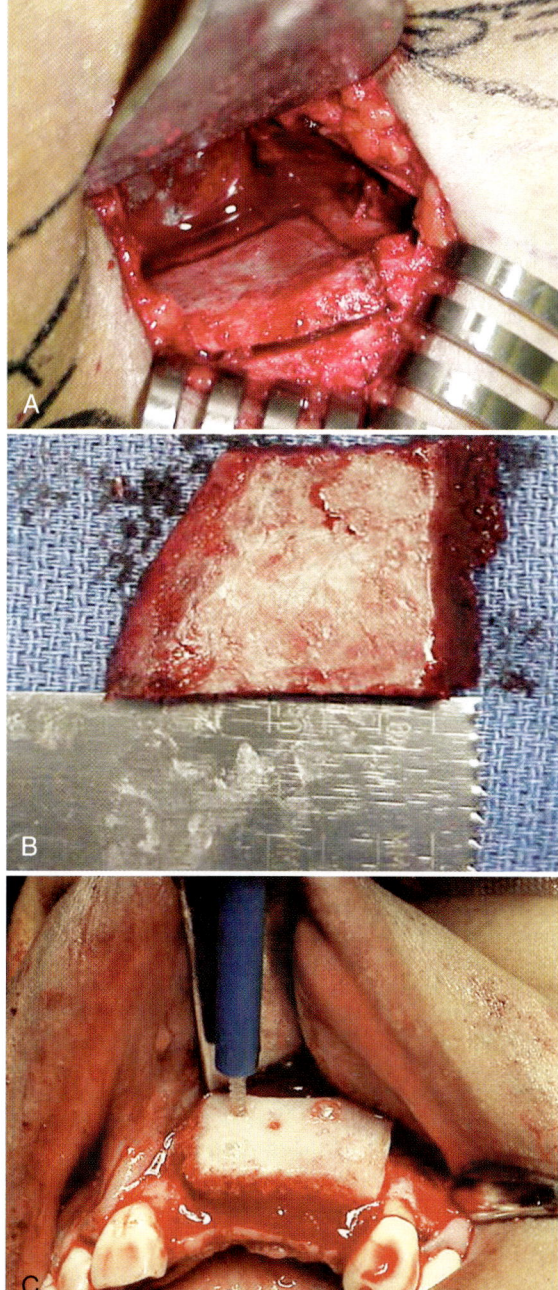

Fig. 18-7 ■ **A,** Medial approach for monocortical harvest of the anterior iliac crest. **B,** Corticocancellous block graft harvested from the anterior iliac crest. **C,** Corticocancellous bone graft fixed with resorbable screws in the anterior maxilla.

and nonsteroidal anti-inflammatory medications are used to control postoperative discomfort. Pressure dressings and the application of ice during the postoperative period are beneficial in reducing postoperative edema and associated soreness. A short course of glucocorticosteroids can also aid in decreasing postoperative edema.

The patient is instructed to maintain meticulous oral hygiene at the surgical sites. Chlorhexidine gluconate germicidal mouth rinse is a useful adjunct to help reduce the bacterial count at the surgical sites. Dentures or other prosthetic appliances should not be worn over the surgical site immediately to decrease the chance of wound dehiscence developing. Close postoperative follow-up is recommended for bone graft patients to monitor healing at the recipient and donor sites.

PEARLS AND PITFALLS

- A comprehensive evaluation and a thorough diagnostic work-up are essential for assessing alveolar defects.
- The decision to perform bone grafting is driven by the requirements for the prosthesis.
- Selection of a donor site is based on the volumetric needs and functional requirements of the graft.
- Extensive understanding of the donor site anatomy and harvesting techniques is required to minimize potential complications.
- Preparation of the recipient site must include cortical perforations, intimate contact of the graft, and two-point fixation for successful graft incorporation.

- Wide releasing incisions, undermining of the flap, and scoring of the periosteum to advance the soft tissue are essential for primary tension-free closure and minimizing postoperative wound dehiscence.
- A staged reconstruction with delayed placement of the implant is more predictable. In the maxilla at least 4 months and in the mandible 5 to 6 months are required for graft incorporation.

REFERENCES

1. Adell R, Lekholm U, Rockler B, et al: A 15-year study of osseointegrated implants in the treatment of the edentulous jaw, *Int J Oral Surg* 10:387-414, 1981.
2. Pechisker A, Zamanian K: *U.S. markets for dental implants & final abutments 2009 report*, Vancouver, BC, Canada, March 2009, iData Research, Inc.
3. Millennium Research Group: *US markets for dental implants 2009 report*. Toronto, Canada.
4. Douglass CW, Watson A: Future needs for fixed and removable partial dentures in the United States, *J Prosthet Dent* 87:9-14, 2002.
5. Kalorama Information: *Implant-based dental reconstruction: the worldwide implant and bone graft market 2005*. Rockville, Md, September 2005, Division of Market Research Group.
6. Ashman A, Rosenlicht J: Ridge preservation: addressing a major problem in dentistry, *Dent Today* 12:80-84, 1993.
7. Marx RE: Bone and bone graft healing, *Oral Maxillofac Surg Clin North Am* 19:455-466, 2007.
8. Schweiberer L, Stutzle H, Mandelkow H: Bone transplantation, historical review, *Arch Orthop Trauma Surg* 109:1-8, 1989.
9. Albrektsson T, Johansson C: Osteoinduction, osteoconduction and osseointegration, *Eur Spine J* 10:96-101, 2001.
10. Wikesjo U, Huang Y, Polimeni G, et al: Bone morphogenetic proteins: a realistic alternative to bone grafting for alveolar reconstruction, *Oral Maxillofac Surg Clin North Am* 19:535-551, 2007.
11. Levin L, Schwartz-Arad D: The effect of cigarette smoking on dental implants and

related surgery, *J Implant Dent* 14:357-363, 2005.
12. Stanford CM: Application of oral implants to the general dental practice, *J Am Dent Assoc* 136:1092-1100, 2005.
13. Jensen J, Sindet-Pedersen S, Oliver AJ: Varying treatment strategies for reconstruction of maxillary atrophy with implants: results in 98 patients, *J Oral Maxillofac Surg* 52:210-216, 1994.
14. Misch CM: Autogenous bone grafting for dental implants. In Fonseca RJ, Turvey TA, Marciani RD, editors: *Oral and maxillofacial surgery*, ed 2, St Louis, 2008, WB Saunders, pp 406-427.
15. Carvalho P, Vasconcellos L, Pi J: Influence of bed preparation on the incorporation of autogenous bone grafts: a study in dogs, *Int J Oral Maxillofac Implants* 15:565-570, 2000.
16. Montazam A, Valauri DV, St-Hilaire H, et al: The mandibular symphysis as a donor site in maxillofacial bone grafting: a quantitative anatomic study, *J Oral Maxillofac Surg* 58:1368-1371, 2000.
17. Pikos MA: Mandibular block autografts for alveolar ridge augmentation, *Atlas Oral Maxillofac Surg Clin North Am* 13:91-107, 2005.
18. Cutright B, Quillopa N, Schubert W: An anthropometric analysis of the key foramina for maxillofacial surgery, *J Oral Maxillofac Surg* 61:354-357, 2003.
19. Misch CM, Misch CE, Resnik RR, et al: Reconstruction of maxillary alveolar defects with mandibular symphysis grafts for dental implants: a preliminary procedural report, *Int J Oral Maxillofac Implants* 7:360-366, 1992.

20. Schwartz-Arad D, Levin L: Symphysis revisited: clinical and histologic evaluation of newly formed bone and reharvesting potential of previously used symphysial donor sites for onlay bone grafting, *J Periodontol* 80:865-869, 2009.
21. Silva FM, Cortez AL, Moreira RW, et al: Complications of intraoral donor sites for bone grafting prior to implant placement, *Implant Dent* 15:420-426, 2006.
22. Gungormus M, Yavuz MS: The ascending ramus of the mandible as a donor site in maxillofacial bone grafting, *J Oral Maxillofac Surg* 60:1316-1318, 2002.
23. Pikos MA: Block autografts for localized ridge augmentation: Part II. The posterior mandible, *Implant Dent* 9:67-75, 2000.
24. Hall HD: Intraoral surgery. In Bell WH, editor. *Modern practice in orthognathic and reconstructive surgery*, Philadelphia, 1992, WB Saunders, pp 2111-2139.
25. Misch CM: Comparison of intraoral donor sites for ridge augmentation prior to implant placement, *Int J Oral Maxillofac Implant* 12:767-776, 1997.
26. Marx RE: Philosophy and particulars of autogenous bone grafting, *Oral Maxillofac Surg Clin North Am* 5:599-612, 1993.
27. Baqain ZH, Anabtawi M, Karaky AA, et al: Morbidity from anterior iliac crest bone harvesting for secondary alveolar bone grafting: an outcome assessment study, *J Oral Maxillofac Surg* 67:570-575, 2009.
28. Marx RE, Morales MJ: Morbidity from bone harvest in major jaw reconstruction: a randomized trial comparing the lateral anterior and posterior approaches to the ilium, *J Oral Maxillofac Surg* 48:196-203, 1988.

Dental Implant Prosthetic Rehabilitation: Allogeneic Grafting/Bone Graft Substitutes in Implant Dentistry

Chapter 19

Mark R. Stevens, Hany A. Emam

Implant dentistry has become an excellent treatment modality since its inception in the modern era of dentistry. It not only allows a fairly conservative and esthetic alternative for treating partial edentulism but also provides a stable functional foundation for treating complete edentulism. Dental implants are a viable treatment option when there is sufficient quantity and quality of bone to achieve the desired functional and esthetic results.

The reduction in bone volume may have occurred as a result of periodontal disease before tooth loss, pneumatization of the maxillary sinus, long-term wearing of ill-fitting dentures, osteoporosis, and the physiologic bone remodeling that occurs after tooth extraction. In the past, the available bone was not modified and dictated the implant position, size, and number. Fewer and short implants were used in areas of deficient bone volume, thereby compromising the long-term treatment outcome. Today, the treatment plan first considers the final prosthesis options, followed by performing the necessary modifications to achieve the ideal environment needed for optimal implant placement.

Several surgical techniques can be used for correction of atrophied alveolar bone to establish the structural base of osseous tissue for supporting dental implants. Such techniques include guided bone regeneration, onlay bone grafting, interpositional bone grafting, distraction osteogenesis, ridge split, and sinus augmentation.[1-3] The three-dimensional pattern of bone loss dictates selection of the optimum technique or techniques necessary to reestablish adequate bone volume and intermaxillary relationships to provide the most favorable biomechanical and esthetic conditions for implant placement.

BONE GRAFT MATERIALS AND MECHANISM OF BONE REGENERATION

Different bone augmentation materials are used for alveolar reconstructive therapy, including autografts, allografts, alloplasts, and xenografts. Bone grafts of any type can regenerate bone through three possible mechanisms: *osteogenesis*, *osteoinduction*, and *osteoconduction*. Grafts may develop bone from one, two, or all three of these mechanisms to varying degrees.

Osteogenesis is new bone formation induced by osteoprogenitor cells that are present in the graft, survive the transplant, proliferate, and differentiate to osteoblasts; this process is called *phase I osteogenesis*. Autogenous bone is the only graft material with osteogenic properties.[4]

Osteoinduction involves new bone formation by stimulation and recruitment of osteoprogenitor cells derived from undifferentiated mesenchymal stem cells at the graft site; this process is called *phase II osteogenesis*. Recruitment and differentiation are accomplished through a cascade of events triggered by graft-derived inducing factors called *bone morphogenic proteins* (BMPs), which are members of the transforming growth factor-β (TGF-β) superfamily.

These BMPs are present in the matrix of the graft and are accessed after the mineral content of the bone graft has been removed by osteoclastic activity. It has been shown that osteoinductive materials can induce bone formation even in ectopic sites (subcutaneous tissue).[5]

Osteoconduction is ingrowth of vascular tissue and mesenchymal stem cells into the scaffold structure presented by the graft material. Bone growth occurs by resorption or apposition from the existing surrounding bone in a process called *creeping substitution*, or *phase III osteogenesis*. Therefore, this process must occur in the presence of bone or undifferentiated mesenchymal cells. Osteoconductive materials do not grow bone when placed in soft tissue. Instead, the material remains relatively unchanged or is resorbed.[6]

TYPES OF BONE GRAFTS

An **autograft**, in which the graft is harvested from the same individual, is considered the gold standard of all bone-grafting materials because it is the only bone graft material that provides the three mechanisms of osteogenesis, osteoinduction, and osteoconduction required for bone regeneration. Autogenous grafts are nonimmunogenic, and their superiority comes from the transfer of osteocompetent cells to provide the osteogenic potential.[7]

Autogenous bone can be harvested from intraoral sites such as the symphysis, maxillary tuberosity, ramus, coronoid process, and debris from osteotomies performed for insertion of the implant. The advantage of harvesting the graft intraorally is the ease of harvesting the bone, which may be present in the same surgical field and thus avoid exposure of another surgical site. Conversely, disadvantages include limitation of the amount of harvested bone. Extraoral bone graft harvesting is used to provide a greater volume of material for patients undergoing major augmentation procedures. Iliac crest, tibia, fibula, and cranial bone are common sites for graft harvesting.[8]

An **allograft** is a graft that is taken from the same species as the host but is genetically dissimilar. The grafts are prepared as fresh, frozen, freeze-dried, mineralized, and demineralized (Table 19-1). Numerous configurations of allograft bone are available, including powder, cortical chips, cancellous cubes, cortical struts, and others. Once the grafts are harvested, they are processed through different methods, including physical débridement, ultrasonic washing, treatment with ethylene oxide, antibiotic washing, gamma irradiation for spore elimination, and freeze-drying. The goal of these steps is to remove the antigenic component and reduce the host's immune response while retaining the biologic characteristics of the graft. However, the mechanical properties of the graft are weakened.[9]

Allogeneic bone is principally osteoconductive, although it may have some osteoinductive capability, depending on how it is processed. In 1965, Marshall Urist described the process of acid demineralization of bone before its implantation by using 0.5 to 0.6 mol/L hydrochloric acid. The organic bone matrix includes BMPs, which

TABLE 19-1	Allografts			
MATERIAL	**COMMERCIAL SOURCE**	**COMPOSITION**	**BONE GROWTH METHOD**	**RESORPTION TIME**
DFDB (demineralized)	Pacific Tissue Bank Grafton MTF DynaGraft	Collagen + growth factors	Mainly osteoinduction, varies according to processing method	±6 mo
FDB (mineralized)	MinerOss Puross	Minerals + collagen	Mainly osteoconduction	1 yr +

DFDB, Demineralized freeze-dried bone; *FDB,* freeze-dried bone.

are factors responsible for the de novo bone formation. BMP is not acid-soluble, but the calcium and phosphate salts of hydroxyapatite (HA) are removed from the bone in the acid-reducing process, and as a result, demineralization of the freeze-dried bone (FDB) more readily exposes the BMPs with their osteopromotive effect. Therefore, FDB is primarily osteoconductive, whereas demineralized freeze-dried bone (DFDB) is believed to be osteoinductive.[10]

The results of studies performed with DFDB are conflicting. Controversy still exists about the osteopromotive effects of DFDB. Some reports raise the question of variability in the concentration of BMPs in the commercially available grafts and conclude that the osteoinductive properties of DFDB are variable from one cadaver to another; in addition, the product fabrication process may have some effect on the osteoinductivity of the allograft if the demineralization process is very sensitive. It has been shown that the osteoinductive properties of the graft are eliminated if the calcium content is less than 2% by weight. Moreover, controversy exists about the use of ethylene oxide for sterilization of the graft because it may be destructive to BMPs.[11]

Demineralized cortical bone was found to have higher concentration of BMPs than trabecular bone does. In addition, membranous cortical bone exhibits greater concentrations of BMPs than endochondral cortical bone does, so the skull represents a better source for inductive proteins than the rest of the skeleton.

Several studies have been conducted to evaluate the safety of allografts. According to the American Association of Tissue Banks, the probability of DFDB containing human immunodeficiency virus is 1 in 2.8 billion, as compared with a risk of 1 in 450,000 with blood transfusions. Rigorous background checks are performed on the donor and family before the donor is accepted into the program. Clinically, biopsy specimens of sites containing allograft from human patients sometimes show chronic inflammatory cells; however, the histologic appearance is nonspecific, and the inflammation cannot be attributed to an immune reaction with certainty.[6]

Xenografts are derived from the inorganic portion of bone of a genetically different species than the host. One of the most popularly used xenografts is bovine bone. It is reported to be good bone bank material, provided that it is completely deproteinated by high temperature processing (1100° C) and all the residual organic material that might provoke an immune response is totally removed.[12]

Concern has been raised over the risk for transmission of disease from cattle to humans through the bone graft material derived from the bovine bone used for dental implants. The recent incidents of bovine spongiform encephalopathy in humans have underscored this likelihood. Results from an analysis conducted by the German Federal Ministry of Health and the Pharmaceutical Research and Manufacturers Association of America showed that the risk for disease transmission was negligible and could be attributed to the stringent protocols followed in sourcing and processing the raw bovine bone used in the commercial products.[13]

TABLE 19-2	Xenografts	
MATERIAL	**BRAND NAME**	**STRUCTURE**
Deproteinized bovine bone mineral	Bio-Oss	Cancellous or cortical
Inorganic ovine HA + cell-binding peptide	PepGen P-15	Peptide + microporous HA
	Osteograft N	Microporous + macroporous
Coral (Ca carbonate)	Biocoral Interpore 200 (Coralline)	Natural coral

HA, Hydroxyapatite.

One of the best-known xenografts is *Bio-Oss* (Osteohealth, Shirley, NY) (Table 19-2). It is processed by having all its organic material removed. This leaves a crystalline structure that practically matches human cancellous bone in structure. In 1992, Klinge and colleagues noted total resorption of Bio-Oss granules at 14 weeks after placement in rabbit skulls.[14] However, Skoglund and co-authors reported that granules were present even after 44 months.[15]

Another popular alternative xenograft is *coralline hydroxyapatite*, which is made from ocean coral. This material was created with the intention of producing a graft material with a more consistent pore size. Coral, which is composed mainly of calcium carbonate, is processed to remove most of the organic content. It is then subjected to high pressure and heat in the presence of an aqueous phosphate solution. When this process is completed, the calcium carbonate skeleton is totally replaced with a calcium phosphate skeleton (hydrothermal exchange). The material is concurrently sterilized in this process.[16]

The generation of biomimetic microenvironments by using scaffolds containing cell recognition sequences in combination with bone cells offers tremendous potential for skeletal tissue regeneration. *PepGen P-15* (DENTSPLY Friadent CeraMed, Lakewood, Colo.) is the first engineered collagen I binding domain for potential osteoblasts and is able to multiply the complete regeneration cascade. It is a combination bone replacement graft material composed of natural inorganic bovine-derived HA matrix coupled with a synthetic cell-binding peptide (P-15) (Figs. 19-1 and 19-2).[17]

Alloplasts are synthetic bone substitutes that possess osteoconductive potential (Box 19-1). The ideal synthetic graft material should be biocompatible and elicit minimal fibrotic changes. The graft should support new bone growth and undergo remodeling. Other features include similar toughness, modulus of elasticity, and compressive strength as the host's cortical or cancellous bone. Many synthetic materials are available, including bioactive glass, glass ionomers, aluminum oxide, calcium sulfate, calcium phosphates as

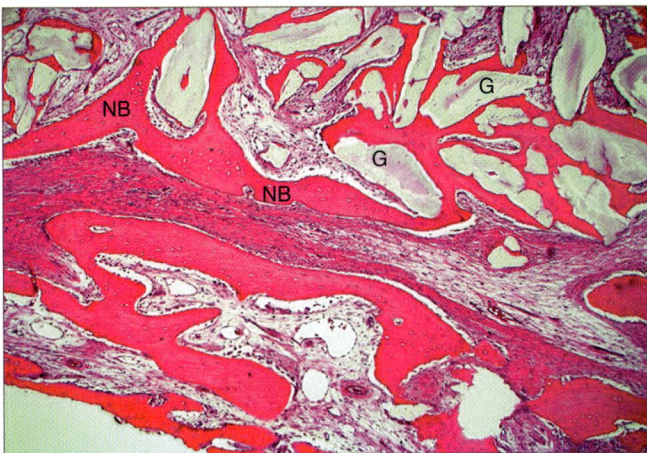

Fig. 19-1 ■ Microphotograph (16 weeks, 5 × 1.25, OP hematoxylin-eosin stain) of newly formed bone (NB) in an interconnecting trabecular pattern (bone bridging) surrounding the remaining graft particles (G, PepGen P-15).

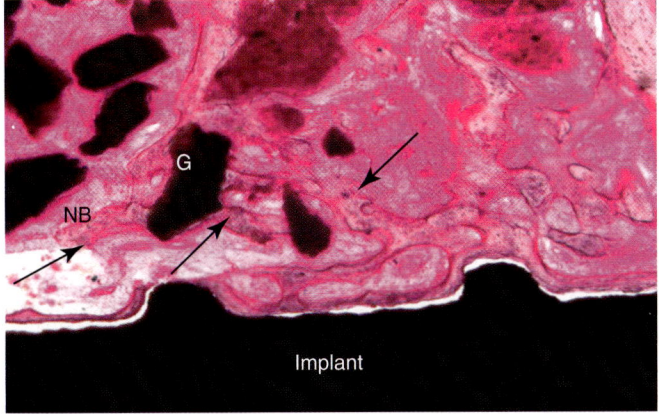

Fig. 19-2 ■ Microphotograph (8 weeks, 5 × 1.6, OP aragon) of newly formed bone (NB) in an interconnecting trabecular pattern (bone bridging—*arrows*) surrounding the remaining graft particles (G, PepGen P-15) supporting a dental implant.

BOX 19-1	Alloplasts

Ceramics
β-Tricalcium phosphate (β-TCP)
Hydroxyapatite (HA) (Bone source, Norian)
Ca_2SO_4 (plaster of paris)
Calcium phosphate cement (Ceredex, α-BSM)
Bioactive glass (PerioGlass, BioGran)

Polymers
Methylmethacrylate (HTR synthetic bone)
Poly-α-hydroxyacids (PLA, PLGA)

α- and β-tricalcium phosphate (TCP), synthetic HA, and synthetic absorbable polymers.[16]

Among the main advantages of synthetic bone substitutes are unlimited supply and avoidance of a secondary surgical procedure for harvesting autogenous bone with its associated morbidity, such as pain, bleeding, paresthesia, infection, dysfunction, and other complications. However, the main disadvantage is lack of the osteoinductive power offered by autogenous grafts, which lead to direct osteogenesis from the implanted viable osteoblasts.

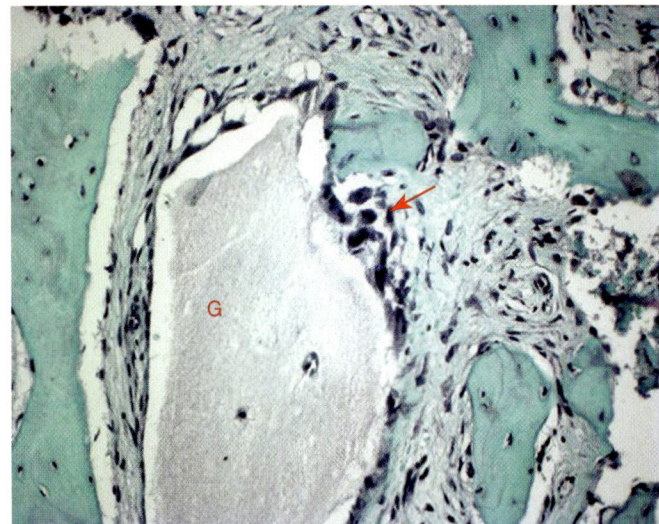

Fig. 19-3 ■ Cell-mediated resorption of multinucleated cells (*arrow*) on the surface of the graft particle (G).

Clinicians may prefer performing grafting procedures with *combination grafts*. This will combine the osteogenic potential of autogenous bone and the unlimited supply offered by bone substitutes, which act as *expanders* or *fillers*. Combination grafts therefore decrease donor site morbidity caused by harvesting a large volume of autogenous bone for extensive reconstructive procedures.

PROPERTIES OF GRAFT MATERIALS

It is important to consider the physical and chemical properties of the graft materials used in augmentation procedures. *Physical properties* include the surface area or form of the product (block, particle), porosity (dense, macroporous, microporous), and crystallinity (crystalline, amorphous). *Chemical properties* are related to the calcium-to-phosphorus ratio, element impurities (such as carbonate), and the pH of the surrounding region. These properties play a role in the rate of resorption and clinical applications of the material.[7]

The larger the particle size, the longer the material will remain at the augmentation site. It has also been reported that the greater the porosity, the more rapidly the graft material is resorbed because committed cells and blood vessels (bone-modeling unit) can invade the spaces between the graft particles and replace the graft with newly formed bone. However, dense HA may lack any microporosity or macroporosity within the particles and take a long time for resorption since the osteoclasts may attack only the surface and cannot penetrate the dense material. With respect to crystallinity, the more highly crystalline the structure is, the harder for the body to break and resorb the graft.[7]

Resorption of bone substitutes may be cell or solution mediated (Fig. 19-3). Cell-mediated resorption requires living cells of the body to resorb the material as osteoclasts. Solution-mediated resorption is a chemical process; impurities such as calcium carbonate permit solution-mediated resorption, which then increases the porosity of the graft. The pH in the region also affects the rate of graft resorption. As pH decreases (because of infection), the HA components are resorbed by solution-mediated resorption. Bone, dense HA, macroporous HA, microporous HA, crystalline HA, or amorphous HA may all be resorbed within a 2-week period.[7]

Close matching of the resorption rate to the bone deposition rate is important. Selection of graft material should be based on the

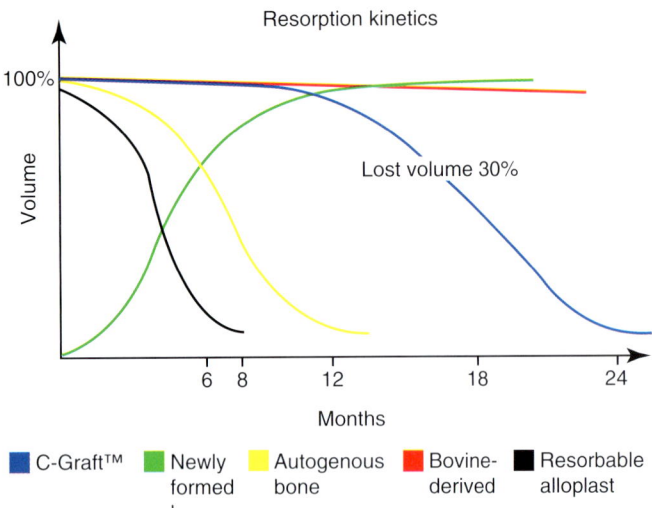

Fig. 19-4 ■ Resorption kinetics of different bone substitutes. (Courtesy Rolf Ewers, MD, DMD, PhD, Chairman, University Hospital for Cranio-Maxillofacial and Oral Surgery, Medical University, Vienna, Austria.)

BOX 19-2	Bone Morphogenetic Proteins Approved for Clinical Use and Indications

rhBMP-2 (Wyeth/Medtronic)
InductOs (CHMP approved)
   Open tibia fracture, 2002
   Interbony spinal fusion, 2005
INFUSE Bone Graft (FDA approved)
   Interbony spinal fusion, 2002
   Open tibial fracture, 2004
   Oral/maxillofacial, 2007
rhOP-1 (Stryker)
OP-1 Implant (FDA, HDE, and CHMP approved)
   Recalcitrant long bone nonunions, 2001/2004
OP-1 Putty (FDA, HDE approved)
   Osteolateral (intertransverse) lumbar spinal fusion revision, 2004
FDA, Food and Drug Administration.

location of the graft site, the soft tissue environment, and its possible role in promoting and supporting future implant osseointegration. A rapidly resorbing scaffold might reestablish a void filled with connective tissue, whereas one that is resorbed too slowly or not at all would impede bone deposition and limit creeping substitution. There are, however, clinical indications in which resorption is not desired but, instead, a permanent implant is preferred, such as craniofacial onlays for cosmetic augmentation (Fig. 19-4).

BONE GROWTH FACTORS

The term *growth factors* encompasses a group of polypeptides of approximately 6 to 45 kD that are involved in cellular proliferation, differentiation, and morphogenesis of tissues and organs during embryogenesis, postnatal growth, and adulthood.[18]

Factors that are involved in the regeneration and induction of bone tissue have attracted attention because they can possibly facilitate skeletal reconstruction. Such factors include platelet-derived growth factor (PDGF), vascular endothelial growth factor (VEGF), insulin-like growth factors (IGFs), TGF-β, BMPs, and platelet-rich plasma (PRP).

Bone morphogenetic proteins, particularly BMP-2, BMP-4, and BMP-7, appear to be the most reliable of all growth factors currently discussed with regard to enhancement of bone regeneration in reconstruction of the facial skeleton (Box 19-2). BMPs stimulate angiogenesis, migration, proliferation, and differentiation of mesenchymal stem cells into bone-forming cells in the area of bone injury. Although a high washout effect of BMPs during the first few hours in most of the carriers used has to be taken into account, this short-term signal appears to be sufficient for initial induction of the cascade of endochondral bone formation to provide bone regeneration in the defects of the various models. Recombinant techniques are now used to provide large amounts of BMPs, which are normally present in very small quantities within the organic matrix of bone (accounting for only approximately 0.1% of the mass of the organic matrix).[19]

The bioactive protein GEM 21S is a combination of bioactive proteins (highly purified recombinant human PDGF [rhPDGF-BB]) and a biocompatible osteoconductive matrix (β-TCP). It is presently being used for periodontal regeneration procedures and offers many times the amount of growth factors normally found in PRP.

The apparent strong desire of clinicians for the use of growth factors to facilitate reconstructive surgical procedures by obviating the need for procurement of autogenous grafts is contrasted by their limited availability for clinical application. This has prompted the application of autogenous growth factors by using PRP derived from the patient's own blood. This preparation has come into wide use recently despite the fact that there is currently controversial scientific evidence about the benefit of using this preparation, especially for reconstructive and preprosthetic bone grafting. According to the characteristics and biologic activity of the growth factors present in PRP, the use of PRP is supposed to increase proliferation of undifferentiated mesenchymal cells and to enhance angiogenesis, which can then support incorporation of the bone graft by increasing the proliferation of osteoprogenitor cells in the graft. In addition, it may improve soft tissue healing by increasing proliferation and matrix synthesis.[20]

Recently, to improve the handling characteristics of graft materials for facilitation of their use in several clinical situations, several commercial suppliers have begun to provide several matrices and delivery systems as *carriers*. Addition of the carrier changes the consistency of the material from a particulate consistency to a more coherent hydrogel form (flow) or clay-like (putty) form that results in ease in handling during surgical application. The carrier must be nontoxic and biocompatible and should not impede any of the steps of the bone-forming cascade. Furthermore, when used with growth factors, it must first bind to the carriers, which permits timed release of the growth factors, facilitates the invasion of blood vessels, enables cellular attachment, and finally, promotes the deposition of new bone.

Sodium hyaluronate, carboxymethylcellulose, poly-α-hydroxy-acids, absorbable collagen sponges, and lecithin are among the carrier materials used. In addition to handling characteristics, it is assumed that the carrier material, when added to a particulate graft form, will provide spaces between these particles (lower packing density), thereby facilitating capillary ingrowth and the creeping substitution process and leading to proper healing with optimal new bone formation in a shorter period (Fig. 19-5).

TREATMENT PLAN AND RECONSTRUCTIVE GOALS

The treatment planning sequence for implant dentistry begins with design of the final prosthesis. After determination of the type of restoration and the number and position of teeth to be restored, patient-associated factors are evaluated. Bone density in the region

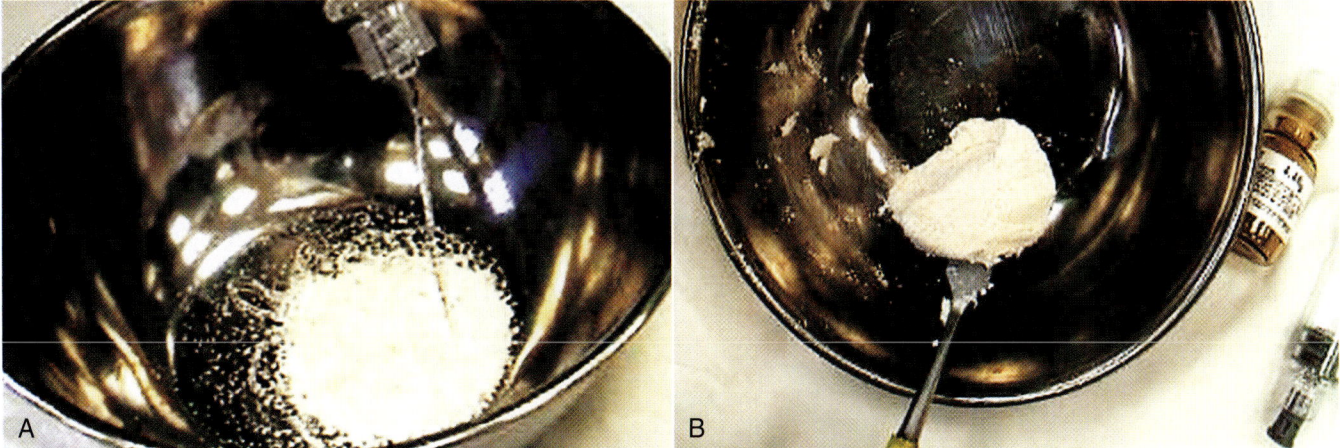

Fig. 19-5 ■ **A** and **B,** Use of a carrier material (sodium hyaluronate) with PepGen P-15 particles to obtain a putty consistency improves the handling characteristics and lowers the packing density between the particles.

of implant placement is also considered. The key implant positions and the number of implants and ideal implant sizes are then selected. Finally, the available bone volume is evaluated for implant placement according to the proposed treatment plan.

Previous studies have shown that the most common cause of implant failure is stress-related failure, especially after loading. Mechanical stress can have both positive and negative consequences for bone tissue and therefore also for maintaining osseointegration of the oral implants. Dental implants function to transfer occlusal loads to the surrounding biologic tissues. If occlusal loads are within the bone's physiologic tolerance zone, osseointegration will be maintained. In contrast, if occlusal loads are excessive and beyond the bone's physiologic tolerance limit, the bone will ultimately be resorbed and failure of osseointegration will result. Thus, as a general rule, the goal of treatment planning should be to minimize and evenly distribute the mechanical stress in the implant system and the surrounding bone.[21]

The magnitude of stress depends on two variables: the *magnitude of force*, which is hard to control by the dentist, and the *functional cross-sectional area*, which participates in load bearing and dissipation of stress. This area should be considered when executing the treatment plan; it should be adequate to allow optimal distribution of stress and prevent concentration of stress around dental implants.

Three types of force may be imposed on dental implants within the oral environment: compression, tension, and shear. Bone is strongest when loaded in compression, 30% weaker when loaded in tension, and 65% weaker when loaded in shear. Considering the *direction* of applied occlusal loads during implant placement is important; implants should be aligned in the oral cavity so that these loads are converted into more favorable compressive loads at the bone-implant interface rather than being converted into tension and shear. Therefore, in the treatment plan, implants should be oriented to receive axial forces parallel to the long axis of the implants as much as possible to avoid the destructive effects of angled forces.[22,23]

From the previous discussion, sufficient amount of bone volume should be available to provide the optimal biomechanical foundation for implant placement. Sufficient bone volume will allow the placement of wide-diameter implants with sufficient length and number as needed by the treatment plan instead of using small, short implants that were used only because of the presence of insufficient bone volume and thus compromising the treatment outcome. Moreover, adequate bone volume allows placing and aligning implants with the optimal axial inclination to receive occlusal forces in a more favorable axial direction.

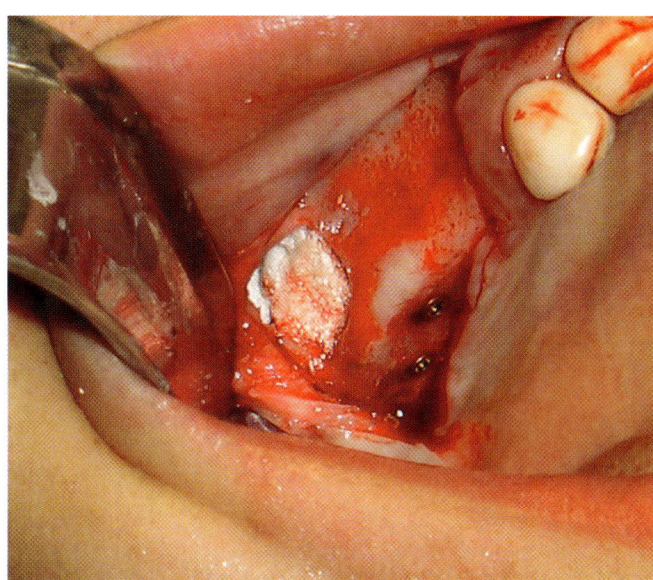

Fig. 19-6 ■ Sinus augmentation procedure using bone substitute material with simultaneous implant placement.

In addition to providing optimal bone volume, bone augmentation procedures offer a means of avoiding injury to vital structures, such as the inferior alveolar canal and the maxillary sinus, which was previously an obstacle when considering implant therapy as a treatment option (Figs. 19-6 to 19-8).

It is worth mentioning that proper selection of the implant design is of paramount importance in achieving long-term success.[24] Some areas in the oral cavity require special consideration, such as the poor-density maxillary posterior edentulous area. Wide-diameter threaded implants with optimal length should be used to increase the bone-implant contact ratio and the surface area for proper distribution of stress at the bone-implant interface. This can be done only with sufficient bone volume to accommodate the selected implants; if not sufficient, bone augmentation procedures will be mandatory.

When considering esthetics, sufficient bone volume is also necessary to achieve the desirable esthetic outcome, especially in the esthetic (anterior) zone. The emergence profile is greatly dependent on the bone surrounding dental implants to allow optimal soft tissue draping around the abutments for ideal esthetic results. Furthermore, the presence of sufficient bone volume allows flexibility in choosing the properly sized implant for a better abutment emergence profile.[25]

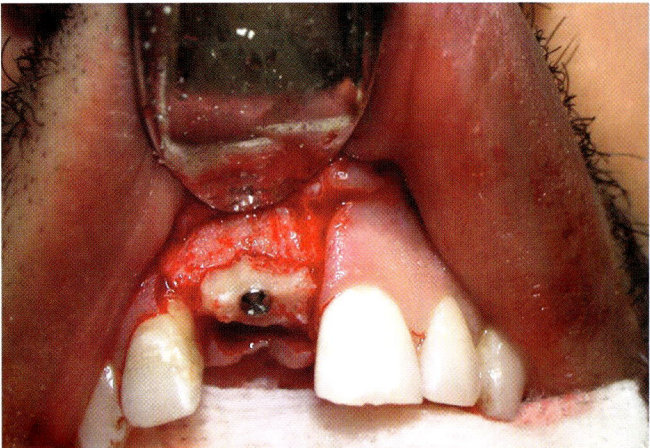

Fig. 19-7 ■ Onlay bone grafting using autogenous bone.

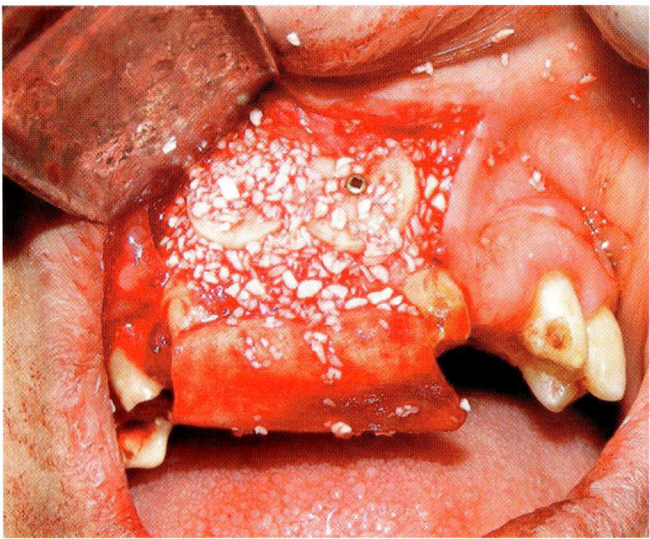

Fig. 19-8 ■ Alveolar bone augmentation using a combination graft and resorbable membrane (autogenous and Bio-Oss).

PEARLS AND PITFALLS

Several factors may improve the success and predictability of bone graft procedures, including the following:

- **Surgical asepsis and absence of infection**—Contamination of bone grafts because of endogenous bacteria, lack of aseptic surgical technique, inadequate soft tissue closure, and salivary exposure may lead to infection with subsequent lowering of pH. Solution-mediated resorption will follow with resultant graft loss. Some clinicians prefer including antibiotics locally within the graft material to guard against bacterial contamination because no blood supply is present early in the graft. Primary soft tissue closure is also mandatory for success of the grafting procedure. It allows healing by primary intention and protects the graft from any surrounding contamination until healing. Dehiscence with graft loss is one of the most common complications in bone-grafting procedures. Therefore, careful surgical flap planning that ensures adequate blood supply to the site with minimal trauma and primary soft tissue closure without tension is required.
- **Maintenance of space**—Creation of a desired contoured space for bone formation is very important in the grafting procedure. If the graft material is resorbed too rapidly in comparison to the time required for bone formation, the site may fill with connective tissue rather than bone. Therefore, the space must be maintained long enough without collapse for bone to fill the desired area. Titanium-reinforced barrier membranes, tent screws elevated above the bone at the desired height and covered with a membrane, and block grafts (covered with a membrane or not) are all used to create and maintain space for bone growth.
- **Graft stability**—For predictable bone augmentation, graft stability is paramount. Bone remodeling and graft healing require a rigid interface for blood clot adhesion with its associated growth factors. If a graft becomes mobile, its vascularity will be compromised, followed by fibrous encapsulation and, frequently, sequestration. If block grafts are used, fixation can be achieved with titanium screws, or the graft can be fixed with the inserted implant itself. If particulate graft is used, it can be covered with a barrier membrane fixed with membrane tacks to avoid dislodgment of the graft particles.
- **Regional acceleratory phenomenon**—The host site during bone augmentation procedures should be decorticated to establish bleeding points in the cortical bone before graft placement. This procedure will provide access to trabecular bone vessels, encourage revascularization, bring growth factors to the graft site, increase the availability of osteogenic cells promoting graft union, and shorten the healing time.

REFERENCES

1. Aghaloo TL, Moy PK: Which hard tissue augmentation techniques are the most successful in furnishing bony support for implant placement? *Int J Oral Maxillofac Implants* 22(Suppl):49-70, 2007.
2. Jensen J, Sindet-Pedersen S, Oliver AJ: Varying treatment strategies for reconstruction of maxillary atrophy with implants: results in 98 patients, *J Oral Maxillofac Surg* 52:210-216, discussion 216-218, 1994.
3. Isaksson S, Alberius P: Maxillary alveolar ridge augmentation with onlay bone-grafts and immediate endosseous implants, *J Craniomaxillofac Surg* 20:2-7, 1992.
4. Giannoudis PV, Dinopoulos H, Tsiridis E: Bone substitutes: an update, *Injury* 36(Suppl 3):S20-S27, 2005.
5. Browaeys H, Bouvry P, De Bruyn H: A literature review on biomaterials in sinus augmentation procedures, *Clin Implant Dent Relat Res* 9:166-177, 2007.
6. Khan SN, Cammisa FP Jr, Sandhu HS, et al: The biology of bone grafting, *J Am Acad Orthop Surg* 13:77-86, 2005.
7. Misch CE, Dietsh F: Bone-grafting materials in implant dentistry, *Implant Dent* 2:158-167, 1993.
8. Clavero J, Lundgren S: Ramus or chin grafts for maxillary sinus inlay and local onlay augmentation: comparison of donor site morbidity and complications, *Clin Implant Dent Relat Res* 5:154-160, 2003.
9. Marx RE: Bone and bone graft healing, *Oral Maxillofac Surg Clin North Am* 19:455-466, v, 2007.
10. Wikesjo UM, Sorensen RG, Kinoshita A, et al: RhBMP-2/alphaBSM induces significant vertical alveolar ridge augmentation and dental implant osseointegration, *Clin Implant Dent Relat Res* 4:174-182, 2002.
11. Zhang M, Powers RM Jr, Wolfinbarger L Jr: Effect(s) of the demineralization process on the osteoinductivity of demineralized bone matrix, *J Periodontol* 68:1085-1092, 1997.
12. Kao ST, Scott DD: A review of bone substitutes, *Oral Maxillofac Surg Clin North Am* 19:513-521, vi, 2007.
13. Sogal A, Tofe AJ: Risk assessment of bovine spongiform encephalopathy transmission through bone graft material derived from bovine bone used for dental applications. *J Periodontol* 70:1053-1063, 1999.
14. Klinge B, Alberius P, Isaksson S, et al: Osseous response to implanted natural bone mineral and synthetic hydroxylapatite ceramic in the repair of experimental skull bone

defects, *J Oral Maxillofac Surg* 50:241-249, 1992.

15. Skoglund A, Hising P, Young C: A clinical and histologic examination in humans of the osseous response to implanted natural bone mineral, *Int J Oral Maxillofac Implants* 12:194-199, 1997.

16. Moore WR, Graves SE, Bain GI: Synthetic bone graft substitutes, *Aust N Z J Surg* 71:354-361, 2001.

17. Nguyen H, Qian JJ, Bhatnagar RS, et al: Enhanced cell attachment and osteoblastic activity by P-15 peptide–coated matrix in hydrogels, *Biochem Biophys Res Commun* 311:179-186, 2003.

18. Schilephake H: Bone growth factors in maxillofacial skeletal reconstruction, *Int J Oral Maxillofac Surg* 31:469-484, 2002.

19. Wikesjo UM, Huang YH, Polimeni G, et al: Bone morphogenetic proteins: a realistic alternative to bone grafting for alveolar reconstruction, *Oral Maxillofac Surg Clin North Am* 19:535-551, vi-vii, 2007.

20. Marx RE, Carlson ER, Eichstaedt RM, et al: Platelet-rich plasma: growth factor enhancement for bone grafts, *Oral Surg Oral Med Oral Pathol Oral Radiol Endod* 85:638-646, 1998.

21. Isidor F: Influence of forces on peri-implant bone, *Clin Oral Implants Res* 7(Suppl 2):8-18, 2006.

22. Misch C: *Contemporary implant dentistry*, ed 3, St Louis, 2008, CV Mosby, pp 200-229.

23. Bidez MW, Misch CE: Issues in bone mechanics related to oral implants, *Implant Dent* 1:289-294, 1992.

24. Rieger MR, Adams WK, Kinzel GL, et al: Finite element analysis of bone-adapted and bone-bonded endosseous implants, *J Prosthet Dent* 62:436-440, 1989.

25. Jivraj S, Chee W: Treatment planning of implants in the aesthetic zone, *Br Dent J* 201:77-89, 2006.

Dental Implant Prosthetic Rehabilitation: Vertical Distraction Osteogenesis

Chapter 20

Glen Maron

A vertical alveolar defect is one of the most challenging conditions faced in oral reconstructive surgery. Over the course of time, several techniques have been introduced in an attempt to solve the esthetic and functional concerns of alveolar bone loss, including guided bone regeneration, onlay grafting, and alveolar distraction. The choice of which technique is the most ideal for future implant placement remains controversial. The ultimate goal of any reconstruction is to achieve a soft tissue profile similar to that of the natural dentition, with absence of fibrous tissue at the site, and the presence of adequate bone for implant placement.

The physiologic challenges in alveolar reconstruction involve soft tissue, bone, and blood supply. As noted by Dr. David Garber, "The tissue is the issue, but the bone sets the tone." This is clearly illustrated in many cases in which the final result of a procedure is compromised because of lack of adequate bone at the site. Frequently, the patient judges the final result on the soft tissue contours and profile and lack of symmetry with respect to the adjacent teeth. Blood supply to the site can be compromised by multiple previous surgeries, scarring, and host factors. When dealing with an alveolar defect, all of these issues must be taken into consideration in choosing which technique will give the best result.

Horizontal defects in both the maxilla and mandible lend themselves well to be treated with traditional grafting techniques, with predictable results. Vertical defects, however, tend to have a higher risk for complications with traditional grafting. Soft tissue defects, infection, inadequate bone volume, and loss of the graft are just some of the issues that frustrate our efforts.

This chapter looks at the uses, techniques, advantages, and disadvantages of alveolar distraction osteogenesis for vertical defects in the maxilla and mandible. It should be remembered, though, that no one technique is perfect and that there will always be alternatives that work better for some clinicians. As Dennis Tarnow is often quoted, "We need to achieve one miracle at a time."

HISTORICAL PERSPECTIVE

As early as 1905, the Italian surgeon Alessandro Codivilla was attempting to distract long bones with various techniques.[1] In 1927, L. C. Abbott reported using distraction to elongate tibial defects.[2] All modern distraction is based on the revolutionary work of the Russian orthopedic surgeon Dr. Gavril Ilizarov.[3] Over a period of 30 years, Ilizarov explored the basic science, defined parameters for clinical application, and improved the instrumentation for the distraction osteogenesis process. Restricted communication between Soviet and Western medical communities limited dissemination of the work outside Russia. Once relations between the former Soviet Union and the West improved, this invaluable work was made widely available. *Distraction osteogenesis* is the biologic process of new bone formation between the surfaces of bone segments that are gradually separated by incremental traction. Specifically, this process is initiated when distraction forces are applied to the callus tissues that connect the divided bone segments, and it continues as long as these tissues are stretched. The traction generates tension that stimulates new bone formation parallel to the vector of distraction. A mechanical apparatus, the distraction device, is used to provide gradual, controlled transport of a mobilized bone segment. When the desired repositioning of the bone segment is achieved, the distraction device is left in a static mode to act as a fixation device.

Displacement of the osseous segment results in positioning of a healthy portion of bone into a previously deficient site. Because the soft tissue is left attached to the transport segment, movement of the bone also results in expansion of the soft tissue adjacent to the bone segment. At the original location of the segment remains a regeneration chamber that has a natural capacity to heal by filling with bone. This propensity of the regeneration chamber to heal by filling with bone instead of fibrous tissue is a function of the surrounding, healthy cancellous bone walls and location within the skeletal functional matrix. As a result of the gradual distraction, the entire housing, including the osseous and soft tissue components, are enlarged in a single, simultaneous process.

ALVEOLAR DISTRACTION

The techniques of distraction apply no matter what bone is being considered for the procedure. Distraction osteogenesis techniques for the craniofacial skeleton have been pioneered by Chin and McCarthy.[4-6] Alveolar distraction devices have now been developed by multiple manufacturers, and all have similar characteristics for application. The advantages of alveolar distraction over other bone-grafting techniques center around several factors, including the movement of vital bone, minimal risk for infection, short treatment times, little or no resorption of bone, and predictable results in which soft tissue is generated along with bone.

MOVEMENT OF VITAL BONE

This technique is the only approach in which the blood supply to the graft is maintained and, therefore, is a vital graft as opposed to a free graft. This greatly reduces the risk for failure or sloughing of the bone. This concept is debated by some since the small segments of bone being moved in alveolar distraction are sometimes stripped of their blood supply when the segment is mobilized. Several authors have reported that these small segments are vulnerable to resorption. However, with careful manipulation of the site, the blood supply can be maintained and the vital segment moved to the desired position.

MINIMAL RISK FOR INFECTION

In a study by Block, Chang, and Crawford, no infections developed in patients undergoing alveolar distraction.[7] However, in 2002, Klesper and colleagues reported two instances of infected devices.[8] Obviously, any time that a foreign body is placed, there is a risk for infection, but this author as well has seen no cases of infection in 12 years of performing the alveolar distraction process and indeed has had several cases in which the titanium plate and segment became partially exposed but were not lost.

SHORTER TREATMENT TIMES

The overall treatment time for alveolar distraction is 3 to 4 months, as opposed to 6 months with traditional grafting techniques. This allows more rapid entry into the implant phase of treatment. Multiple studies have documented that the distracted bone is solid and will accept and undergo successful integration of implants. This shorter treatment time is an advantage in today's era of greater patient expectation and pressure to get to the final result.

PARAMETERS FOR DISTRACTION

When a clinical requirement for significant vertical ridge augmentation exists, distraction osteogenesis can be used successfully with a variety of devices. Thorough assessment and treatment planning are imperative for success. The prerequisites for optimal bone augmentation of defects via distraction osteogenesis are a minimum of 6 to 7 mm of bone height above vital structures, such as neurovascular bundles or air passages/sinus cavities, and a vertical ridge defect of 3 to 8 mm. The height of bone on adjacent teeth acts as a reference point for the extent of vertical gain that can be achieved. Improvement of attachment levels on teeth with distraction has not been successful in the animal model. Therefore, compromised dentition with considerable bone loss may need to be extracted to create a true vertical component of 4 mm within the defect span.

TECHNIQUE

Several good distraction devices are currently available. The author's preference is to use the KLS device as the vector control arm, and external plates aid in stabilizing the segments. For this particular approach, local anesthesia and intravenous sedation are recommended in most cases. A vestibular mucosal incision is also recommended.

The periosteum is released carefully. The vertical distractor is placed in the desired position. The plates are cut carefully and contoured with bending pliers to fit the desired location. The correct vector of distraction is checked and interference with occlusion should be avoided. In this position one hole is drilled on either side of the microplates and one screw (4 or 5 mm) is inserted. The distractor is removed and the osteotomy line is marked with a bur or sterile pencil. The buccal-cortical osteotomy is performed with a Lindemann drill or an oscillating saw.

The segment is completely mobilized lingually or palatally with the use of fine chisels. The distractor is fixed in the same position by using the predrilled holes. Additional screw holes are drilled on the caudal and cranial sides and the screws inserted. The function of the distractor is checked to ensure that it is correct and there is no bony interference with the occlusion, and the soft tissue is closed. X-ray control postoperatively is recommended. After a 5- to 7-day latency period, distraction begins at 0.5 to 1 mm/day. The device selected will determine the amount of turns. Overcorrection of 1 to 2 mm may be considered because of relapse potential (Fig. 20-1).

COMPLICATIONS

VECTOR CONTROL

One major complaint about alveolar distraction is that although early distraction cases showed potential in terms of bone movement and soft tissue benefits, the position of the bone segment was lingual to the desired position and therefore the position of the implants would wind up less than desired. This disadvantage had led many to abandon the use of distraction (Fig. 20-2).

The use of a vector control arm or vector control plate has resolved or at least recognized this issue and allows alteration of the angle and vector of the distraction.

The subtle and not frequently published technique of "torquing" the segment allows one to maintain the correct vector as the segment is being advanced (Fig. 20-3).

OVERDISTRACTION

There can never be enough bone. Usually, the segment will have a knife edge at its most distal point, and this bone is of too poor quality to accept implants. With overdistraction of the segment by 15% to 25%, an ideal bone contour can be achieved, as well as satisfactory tissue to close over the implants at the time of implant surgery.

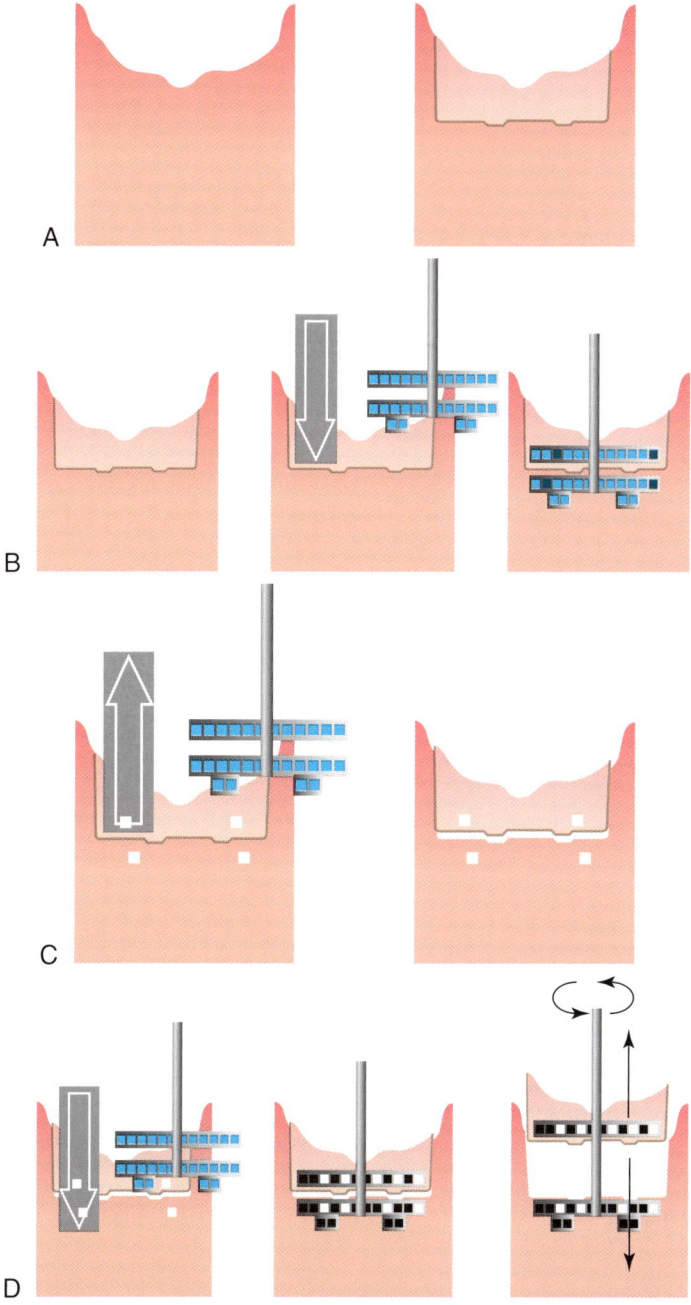

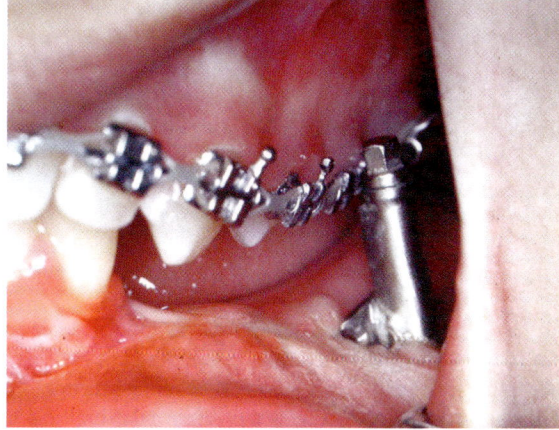

Fig. 20-2 ■ Vector too far towards lingual.

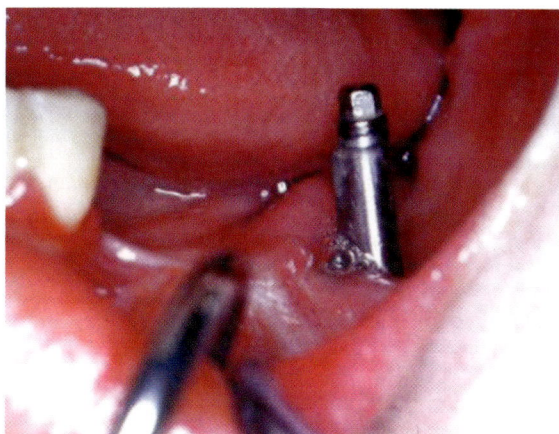

Fig. 20-3 ■ After vector correction.

Fig. 20-1 ■ Surgical step-by-step procedure. **A,** Osteotomy line marked. **B,** Distractor placed. **C,** Distractor removed (*left*) and osteotomy performed (*right*). **D,** Distractor refixed and checked for interference. The fifth step is closure of the wound (not pictured).

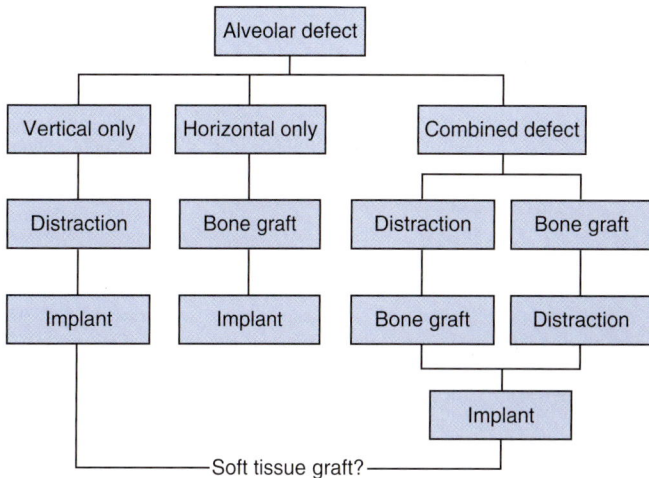

Fig. 20-4 ■ Author's protocol for alveolar reconstruction.

PROTOCOL FOR ALVEOLAR RECONSTRUCTION

Distraction is a tool to be added to the armamentarium of alveolar reconstruction. It is not the only tool, and there are clearly defined indications for using this technique versus traditional grafting. In many cases in which distraction is being used, additional bone grafting, either before or after the procedure, may be required. There may be a need for soft tissue augmentation as well. Figure 20-4 illustrates the author's preferred sequence for dealing with these extremely challenging cases.

For vertical defects, only distraction is an ideal method used by itself. When a horizontal defect is present, any number of traditional grafting techniques will work. However, when there is both a vertical and a horizontal component of the defect, achievement of the ideal result will require combining techniques. The author prefers

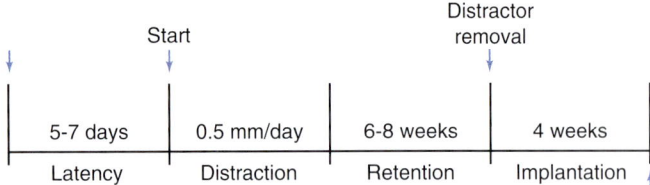

Fig. 20-5 ■ Alveolar distraction time line.

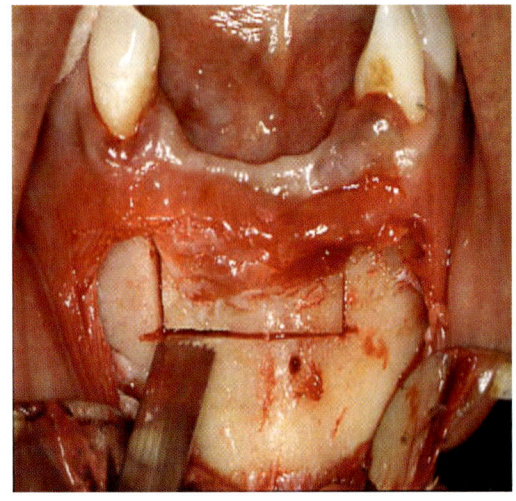

Fig. 20-6 ■ Ensuring divergent cuts.

to perform distraction in these cases first, as long as at least 5 to 7 mm of bone is present. This allows "stretching" of the soft tissue along with the bone, and then horizontal or onlay grafting is easier at the second procedure. Again, it will often take multiple procedures to provide the patient with an acceptable result. The use of distraction is and should remain a viable option in the reconstructive surgeon's armamentarium.

PEARLS AND PITFALLS

- The rate of distraction has traditionally been noted to be 1 mm/day. However, that rate was based on the initial work of Ilizarov and has not been well studied for small segments.
- The recent work of Froum and Rosenberg lends credence to a slower rate of distraction of 0.25 to 0.5 mm/day[9] (Fig. 20-5). The author has found that this slower rate yields less fibrous tissue ingrowth at the site.

- Many colleagues have reported that their patients have difficulty turning the device after only a few days, and this is most likely caused by binding.
- Ensuring that the walls of the osteotomy are parallel or diverge slightly toward the coronal side of the cuts will prevent binding and allow free movement.
- Test-distract the segments at the time of surgery to ensure a smooth and non-binding path (Fig. 20-6).

REFERENCES

1. Codivilla A: On the means of lengthening in the lower limbs, the muscles and tissues which are shortened through deformity, *Am J Orthop Surg* 2:353-369, 1905.
2. Abbott LC: The operative lengthening of the tibia and fibula, *J Bone Joint Surg* 9:128-152, 1927.
3. Ilizarov GA: The principles of the Ilizarov method, *Hosp Jt Dis Orthop Inst* 48:1-11, 1988.
4. Chin M, Ng T, Tom WK: New protocol of alveolar distraction: review of 50 cases. 5th International Congress of Maxillofacial and Craniofacial Distraction, June 2006.
5. Chin M, Toth BA: Distraction osteogenesis in maxillofacial surgery: using internal devices, *J Oral Maxillofac Surg* 54:45-53, 1996.
6. McCarthy JG: Distraction osteogenesis of the craniofacial skeleton, *Plast Reconstr Surg* 107:1812-1827, 2001.
7. Block MS, Chang A, Crawford C: Mandibular alveolar ridge augmentation in the dog using distraction osteogenesis, *J Oral Maxillofac Surg* 54:309-314, 1996.
8. Klesper B, Lazar F, Siessegger M, et al: Vertical distraction osteogenesis of fibula transplants for mandibular reconstruction—a preliminary study, *J Craniomaxillofac Surg* 30:280-285, 2002.
9. Froum SJ, Rosenberg ES, Elian N, et al: Distraction osteogenesis for ridge augmentation: prevention and treatment of complications. Thirty case reports. *Int J Periodontics Restorative Dent* 28:337-345, 2008.

BIBLIOGRAPHY

Buis J, Rousseau P, Soupre V, et al: "Distraction" of grafted alveolar bone in cleft case using endosseous implant, *Cleft Palate Craniofac J* 38:405-409, 2001.

Enislidis G, Fock N, Millesi-Schobel G, et al: Analysis of complications following alveolar distraction osteogenesis and implant placement in the partially edentulous mandible, *Oral Surg Oral Med Oral Pathol Oral Radiol Endod* 100:25-30, 2005.

Jensen OT, Laster Z: Preventing complications arising in alveolar distraction osteogenesis, *J Oral Maxillofac Surg* 60:1217-1218, 2002.

Kanno T, Mitsugi M, Furuki Y, et al: Overcorrection in vertical alveolar distraction osteogenesis for dental implants, *Int J Oral Maxillofac Surg* 36:398-402, 2007.

Saulacic N, Zix J, Iizuka T: Complication rates and associated factors in alveolar distraction osteogenesis: a comprehensive review, *Int J Oral Maxillofac Surg* 38:210-217, 2009.

Dental Implant Prosthetic Rehabilitation: Sinus Grafting

Chapter 21

Antwan L. Treadway, Stephen A. Bankston

If the eyes are "windows to the soul," in an analogous manner the maxillary sinus is a window into the maxilla. The maxillary sinus graft has been the subject of more animal and clinical research trials than any other single bone-grafting site in the maxillofacial region.[1] For their part, the maxillary sinuses assist the other sinuses in decreasing the overall weight of the human skull. Normal and abnormal maxillary sinus anatomy may present challenges to practicing oral and maxillofacial surgeons who intend to place endosseous root-form implants. Root-form implants have revolutionized the potential for not only esthetic restoration but also functional rehabilitation of edentulous maxillary ridges.

Major challenges can face surgeons who intend to place implants if there is inadequate bone in the maxillary antrum to stabilize and integrate the implants. Compartmentalized or septum-divided topography within the sinus may also present challenges in treatment planning and final implementation of designed treatment plans. The advent of computed tomography (CT) specifically designed to assist in avoiding error in estimation of bone height has changed the paradigms of treatment. The surface area available for grafting and even the volume of particulate or block graft required can be scientifically determined before surgery. This presents a major boon for grafting and implant-placing surgeons. In this chapter we will examine the cause of over-pneumatized sinuses and the treatment goals and techniques to deal with this phenomenon.

ETIOPATHOGENIC/CAUSATIVE FACTORS

The maxillary alveolus undergoes progressive, non-reversible bone loss after the removal of a tooth from the alveolar process. Over time this loss results in expansion of the maxillary sinus cavity known as over-pneumatization. This presents a daunting challenge to implant surgeons. There is usually a reduction in the amount of bone available to stabilize a maxillary implant once placed in the maxilla. In Cawood and Howell's treatise on the patterns of maxillary and mandibular resorption in 1988,[2] they devised a classification for edentulous and over-pneumatized maxillas and maxillary sinuses (Fig. 21-1):
- Class 1: Dentate
- Class 2: Immediately after extraction; the alveolus has healed
- Class 3: Well-rounded ridge; width and height are acceptable
- Class 4: Knife edge width; typically acceptable height
Unacceptable width:
- Class 5: Flat ridge; deficient width and height
- Class 6: Depressed ridge with loss of basilar bone and no distinctive pattern

There is increased morbidity in implant therapy if the fixture moves after placement, so one of the linchpin goals for successful implant therapy is primary stability. This tenet is of prime importance in the quest for good osseointegration of the implant fixture. Implants can be placed into over-pneumatized or atrophic maxillas (or both); however, augmentation with either particulate or corticocancellous grafts is usually required.[3] Maxillary sinus cavities that have continued to expand after tooth loss are prevalent in a large section of the populace. The implant surgeon's approach to restoring the area should be discussed with the patient, and all options for treatment (even those nonsurgical) should be broached during the treatment-planning consultation.

An element of paramount importance is maintenance of the integrity of the sinus membrane and its continued function. The lining of the maxillary sinus, known as the schneiderian membrane, is attached to the bordering bone of the maxillary sinus and is characterized by a periosteum overlaid with a thin layer of pseudo-ciliated stratified respiratory epithelium.[4]

The normal thickness of the membrane is 0.3 to 0.8 mm in its natural state.[5] Chronic sinus disease and additional sinus pathology may induce thickening of the mucosa but does not increase its tensile strength. This means that in the presence of disease or with a pristine sinus cavity, the sinus membrane is in danger of perforation unless great care is taken when dissecting and preparing the cavity before grafting. In studies of the histologic changes in the mucosal lining after implant placement, there was no change in the number of glands and goblet cells inside the mucosa.[6]

The aforementioned study was performed without the addition of grafting materials, but extrapolation of the data suggests similar results in situations with grafting materials. A sinus grafted with particulate material may be at increased risk for infection and/or rhinosinusitis, but the membrane amazingly adapts to either challenge. Additional studies have also found that exposure of the implant in the sinus does not always lead to the development of sinus complications.[7] The schneiderian membrane has proved to be an adaptable and amenable ally in restoration of an edentulous posterior maxilla in patients with over-pneumatization and attrition of the residual maxillary alveolus. Implant surgeons can use this adaptability to their advantage, even in patients with membrane tears. In a retrospective study of membrane perforations by Arkedian and colleagues, class II and class III perforations did not statistically change the outcome of implant placement into the grafted sinus.[4] Implants osseointegrated successfully in 94% of patients on average. These numbers suggest adaptability even in the event of perforation when it is properly repaired.[2]

PATHOLOGIC ANATOMY

A properly functioning sinus uses the motility of the ciliated mucosa to move mucus and filter the air that moves across them. The maxillary ostium and mucosal lining contribute to normal function of the maxillary sinus. Maintenance of this anatomic relationship is dependent on careful manipulation of the membrane when it is elevated from the antrum floor. Direct elevation of the sinus in the medial and superior aspect of the sinus must be accomplished carefully to not disturb the ostium and cause blockage or inflammation. As noted in Figure 21-2, the position of the ostium

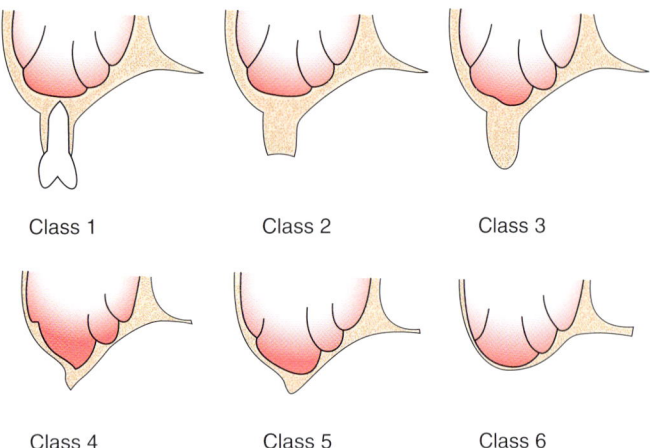

Fig. 21-1 ■ Cawood and Howell's treatise on the patterns of maxillary resorption.[2]

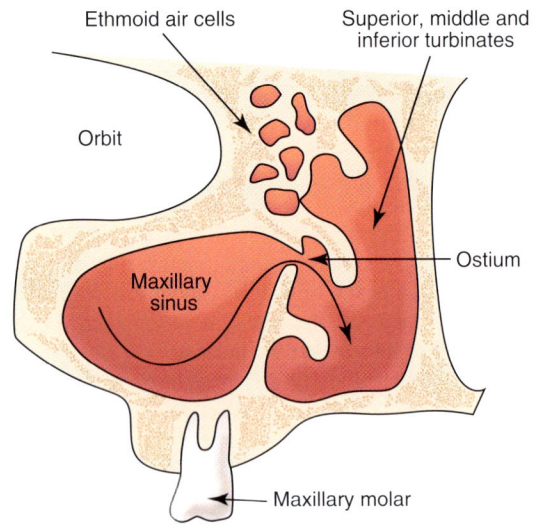

Fig. 21-2 ■ Position of the maxillary ostium.

dictates the limit of dissection in the medial and superior planes of the sinus cavity.

An additional component that must be taken into consideration is the blood supply to the sinus and potential hemorrhage during the surgical procedure. Three arteries supply the maxillary sinus: the infraorbital, posterior superior alveolar, and lateral nasal arteries (posterior). The aforementioned vessels are all a division or branch of the internal maxillary artery. Most bleeding events during sinus surgery can be controlled by direct pressure and subsequent tamponade—however, the anatomy of the region may make it difficult to obtain direct pressure.

The changes in anthropometric measurements of the maxillary sinus are predictable and have been catalogued as mentioned earlier by Cawood and Howell. The pattern of loss of alveolar bone is normal after tooth loss; however, loss of basal bone is described as pathologic.[8]

Common pathology that greatly influences outcomes in the sinus is the presence of sinus polyps, mucoceles, and persistent or refractory sinusitis. Sinus polyps and mucoceles are usually differentiated by their contents. Mucoceles (sometimes known as extravasation

phenomena) are typically filled with fluid or mucin, are generally found along the floor of the sinus cavity, and have a classic smooth, dome-shaped morphology. Polyps are usually more dense in nature and consist of solid cells[9]; they are typically found along the roof and upper portions of the sinus cavity wall. Polyps may also erode bone, which is not a feature of mucoceles.

Refractory sinusitis may have an anatomic origin or be caused by exacerbations of infection and inflammation. Anatomic considerations involve impairment of the sinus lining or, potentially, blockage of the ostium. The different flora that inhabit the sinus may cause prolonged and difficult management challenges for the treating practitioner. *Haemophilus influenzae*, *Streptococcus pneumoniae*, and *Moraxella catarrhalis* are a few of the principal flora that must be addressed in acute and chronic exacerbations of sinusitis. Management of this disease process is discussed further in the section on postoperative care and follow-up in this chapter.

DIAGNOSTIC STUDIES

In the modern age of oral and maxillofacial surgery, the integration of technology into all facets of surgery is an exciting event. Diagnostic modalities have leaped beyond alginate impressions and refractory casts, although the lessons learned with these methods still serve and are part of sound surgical principle. Modern computer simulations and three-dimensional graphics can allow surgeons to visualize all aspects of a surgical area and not be limited by line of sight or unfavorable anatomy. These are exciting times as we forge ahead with more accurate diagnosis to shorten patients' surgical and recovery time.

Proper diagnostic work-up of a patient before grafting is essential for postoperative success and retention of the graft. As with any other surgery or medical treatment, the history and physical examination are the most important tools to gather information regarding any past procedures or trauma to the area in question. Plain films (Panorex and sometimes periapical radiographs) give the grafting surgeon initial insight into the grafting site and indicate potential barriers or hurdles to success. The presence of septa, anatomic limitations, and asymptomatic pathology in and around the sinus cavity may be noted. In some cases, mounted diagnostic casts give weight to the big picture of what the restorative dentist may have to encounter after grafting and implant placement. They can be used to determine whether there is enough interocclusal space and whether orthodontics or additional crowns and bridges may be needed to "open the bite" and provide restored implants.

The advent of CT and digitized radiographs in 1972 has greatly assisted surgeons in proper treatment planning of their surgical case. CT can show up to 200 or more different levels or shades of gray to offer increased information and detail of anatomic structures. In contrast, a panoramic radiograph is limited to about 30 shades of gray in its detail.[10] Refinement of these digitized images by treatment planning software allows the images to be fleshed out into three dimensions and simulated implants to be placed to show their viability in the particular case. Although there are good arguments to support the wider use of CT, there is also the "old-school" line of thought that with mounted models and diagnostic wax-ups, periapical and panoramic radiographs provide good intraoral examination. That money can be saved in the treatment planning of a procedure, if not the time.[11] The density of bone in an area proposed for implant placement may also be determined with CT. The scan will measure the Hounsfield units to determine the density and therefore the ease or difficulty of preparation of the osteotomy site. According to Kraut, approximately 14% of patients seeking mandibular implants and 72% of patients seeking maxillary implants

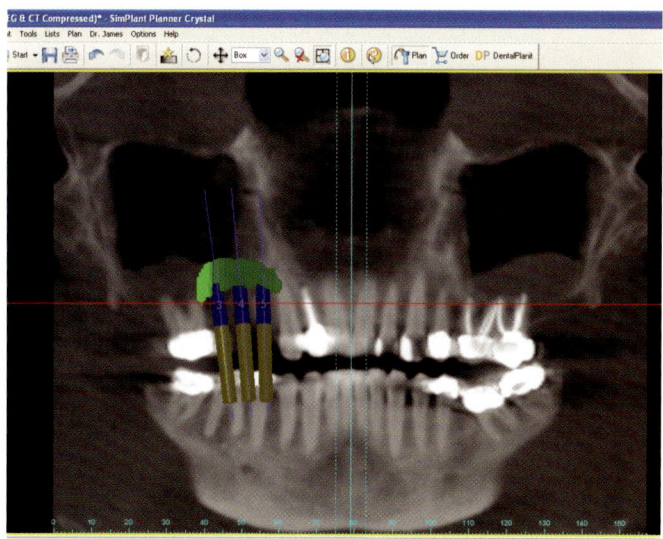

Fig. 21-3 ■ Cone beam computed tomography showing treatment planning software and simulated sinus graft.

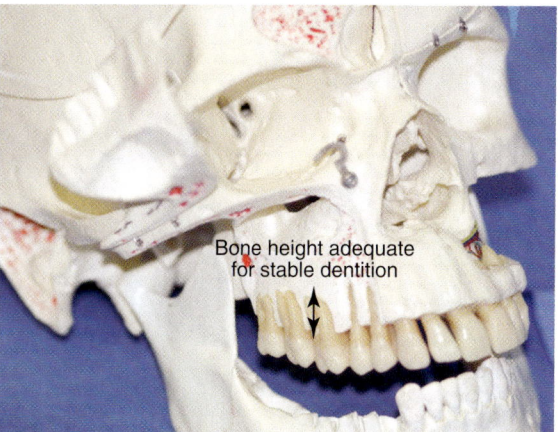

Fig. 21-4 ■ Maxillary sinus showing adequate bone around the roots of the teeth.

benefit from the use of CT in their treatment planning.[10] Although it would be inappropriate and not cost-effective to use CT for all implant planning, it is fast becoming a more commonplace tool in the diagnostic armamentarium (Fig. 21-3).

In the controversy surrounding the use of CT there is always a discussion of the dosimetry of the radiation to which the scanned subject is exposed. The average radiation doses in adults from standard head CT range from 34 to 55 mGy. The bone marrow radiation dose with maxillofacial CT was found to vary between 17 and 21 mGy.[12] Also noted in studies is the interesting fact that even though cumulative dosages for CT may be higher because of its narrower beam, there is less risk for exposure of sensitive organs (i.e., thyroid, gonads).[12] These numbers and studies are correlated with traditional CT and do not take into account the newer cone beam CT. Cone beam CT uses a smaller radiation field than helical (traditional hospital based) scanners do, which results in a 20% decrease in radiation delivered to the patient.[13] Cone beam CT also has the distinct advantage of being free of the magnification and superimposition of structures that occurs with plain film panoramic radiographs.[14] Cone beam technology is associated with less radiation, cheaper cost of analysis, and less wasteful printing of studies.

TREATMENT/RECONSTRUCTIVE GOALS

Facial esthetics demands that as we restore function, we also restore the esthetic units of the face. After the ridge becomes edentulous, there is progressive loss of show of vermilion and a "puckered" appearance of the lower part of the face. This has been described as narrowing of the face, inversion of the lips, and hollowing of the cheeks.[8] This process contributes to a much more elderly appearance and to one of the major esthetic complaints of edentulous patients.

Although a posterior sinus lift does not have a direct effect on esthetics, restoration of the proper vertical dimension of occlusion and the ability to "open up" a closed bite is paramount in successful rehabilitation of edentulous persons.

Placement of single or multiple posterior maxillary implants restores the function of the molar region and its part in deglutition. Maintenance of proper sinus function by adhering to sound surgical principles is also important. The maxillary ostium should be considered and the volume of graft should be preplanned to yield adequate

bone for implant placement (Fig. 21-4). Ironically, a procedure that is now performed to rid patients of dentures had its beginnings after contributions by Boyne[15] and then modernization of the theory by Tatum[16] to enhance the tuberosity for full denture fabrication.

SPECIFIC TREATMENT AND TECHNIQUES

The principal approach to the maxillary antrum is accomplished in one of three common ways:

1. Placement of the traditional antrostomy superiorly as in the traditional Caldwell-Luc position
2. Positioning of the osteotomy on the lateral maxillary wall midway between the alveolar crest and the zygomatic buttress
3. Impacting the floor of the antrum from an inferior approach so that the osseous floor is "infractured" at the inferior level of the antrum[15]

The primary concern with the "infracturing" technique is that dehiscence may lead to fistula formation and significant restorative surgery if not properly executed. For these reasons, some surgeons consider the traditional Caldwell-Luc approach superior to the other approaches—though in many instances not as popular. The design of the window may be ovoid (Fig. 21-5) or rectangular (Fig. 21-6).

A crestal-to-sulcular incision is made around the necks of the teeth or in the dentate maxilla. In an edentulous maxilla, the incision may be made along the crest of the ridge or just slightly to the lingual side when there is an expectation that the soft tissue envelope may be a concern. A full-thickness mucoperiosteal flap is elevated; adequate envelope length is imperative to prevent tears in the flap. These potential tears, if not handled properly, may allow ingress of bacteria and subsequent infection, which can ultimately affect the viability of the graft.

A cortical window is etched out with a rotary instrument while being careful to not go too deep and perforate the schneiderian membrane (Fig. 21-7, A and B). The inferior aspect of the membrane is gently elevated with sinus elevators and the trapdoor is infractured (Fig. 21-7, C and D), along with the membrane superiorly. Particulate or cortical graft may be placed once adequate space is achieved (Fig. 21-7, E). Continued vigilance, even after elevation, is important to prevent membrane perforation and potential graft compromise.

Lateral wall and infracture approaches can be accomplished by several methods and have distinctive advantages and disadvantages. The use of ultrasonic surgery or piezosurgery (or both) may assist the surgeon in maintaining the integrity of the schneiderian membrane during elevation. Ultrasonic surgery has the benefit of an

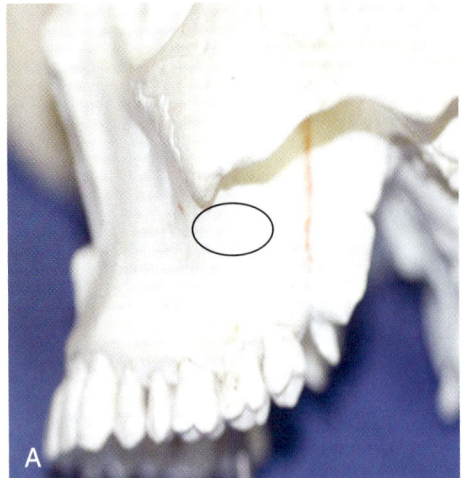

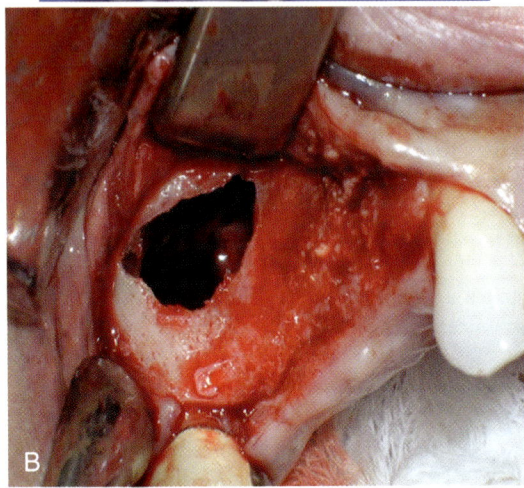

Fig. 21-5 ■ **A,** Ovoid/traditional Caldwell-Luc access to the sinus. **B,** Outline and elevated membrane before grafting.

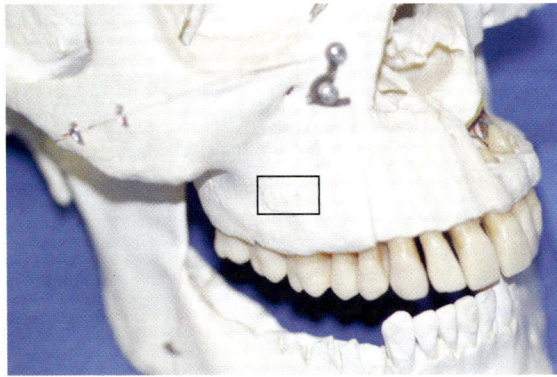

Fig. 21-6 ■ Trapdoor for entry into the maxillary antrum.

instrument that will not tear soft tissue, but it may lack sufficient power to actually osteotomize the bone of the lateral antral wall. Piezosurgery involves the use of several tips for first osteotomizing the wall and then lifting the membrane.[17]

Antral septa may also compromise the surgical outcome and should be assessed whenever noted. The presence of septa in the anterior or posterior aspect of the sinus may be most accurately determined by CT. A bifurcated trapdoor or a "W" may be used to reduce the chance of violating the schneiderian membrane. With the advent of cone beam CT (commonly known as I-CAT—only one of

several brands available), knowledge of the exact location and size of the septa can assist the surgeon planning the osteotomy in recognizing or avoiding this particular stumbling block.[18]

Indirect sinus lift (or the Summers technique) is also a modality that has gained some popularity among experienced surgeons who have developed tactile sensation for the schneiderian membrane. This technique has been adopted and modified since the article discussing it appeared in 1994.[19] Notably, controversy over whether to use or not to use grafting material with the technique still exists. The technique of the authors differs, and one example of our method is presented here.

A tissue punch is used to remove a core of gingival tissue at the ridge. Once the core of tissue is removed, it is placed in saline and preserved in the event that a soft tissue graft will be needed to "plump" up deficient crestal tissue. An osteotomy is prepared just short of the extent of the bone, and then resorbable material (i.e., CollaPlug), which acts as a "shock absorber," is advanced with a sized or calibrated osteotome. The antral floor is infractured right at the osteotomy site, and the compacted bone and resorbable material act to lift the membrane so that the implant can be placed.[17]

The sinus may be grafted with several different types of material. Autogenous grafts are still the "gold standard" and are the only grafts with osteogenic and osteoconductive properties. As noted in Chapter 19, osteogenic, osteoinductive, and osteoconductive properties are elements sought by grafting surgeons.

Even among autogenous sources, the location of the graft site also influences the surgeon's choice. The anterior and posterior ileum, as well as the mandible, are common sites for harvesting autogenous corticocancellous bone (Fig. 21-8). Studies to determine the best type of graft (i.e., cortical versus cancellous), as well as the best sites, have been done. In some recent research, bone obtained from the mandible was found to have higher density at 6 months after grafting than bone obtained from either the anterior or posterior iliac crests.[20] There have also been studies in which it was found that cortical grafts exhibit better implant osseointegration by surface area than particulate grafts do, as alluded to earlier in this chapter.[3]

Another popular and very good site from which to obtain autogenous bone is the tibial plateau. The anterior tibia is rich in cancellous bone and offers a volume of bone that can greatly augment the deficient sinus cavity. One advantage of using the anterior ileum is that the site can be harvested at the same time as oral access to the maxillary antrum is achieved if two surgeons are present. The posterior ileum can be accessed only if the patient is prone, and thus the patient must be turned and redraped during surgery. This site offers a great deal of bone graft volume, more than 50 cm³, with the average amount needed for sinus elevation being 2 to 5 cm³ of bone graft.[2,21]

The tibia offers a readily accessible, more moderate volume of bone to the grafting surgeon (Fig. 21-9). The tubercle of Gerdy is accessed via a small incision, and dissection is carried down to the periosteum. The flap is elevated and the bone is approached with care to ensure that one is not too close to or undermines the plateau.

After making a small access hole in the bone, the cancellous bone can be removed via curettage. This autogenous bone can then be mixed with platelet-rich plasma, augmented with alloplasts, or used in its natural form to pack the surgical cavity created by elevation.

The material consolidates over the next several months, and implants can then be placed into the grafted site when ready (Fig. 21-10, A and B). The finished graft and implant surgery culminate in a stable and healthy periodontium with successfully osseointegrated endosseous implants (Fig. 21-10, C).

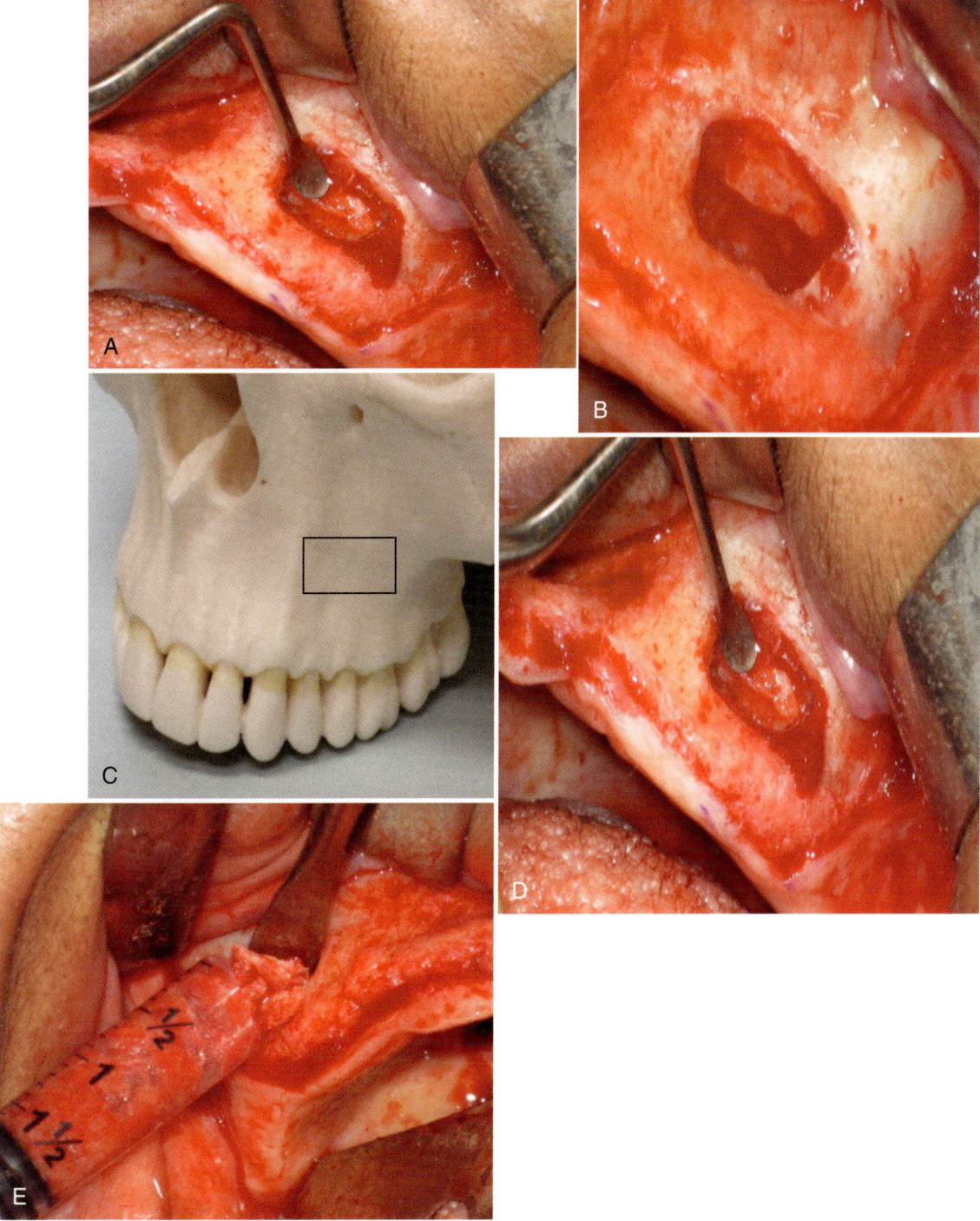

Fig. 21-7 ■ Careful dissection of the schneiderian membrane (**A**) and "infracture" of the trapdoor (**B**) act as a roof for placement of graft material. **C** and **D,** Rectangular trapdoor access before grafting. **E,** Cancellous bone grafted to the right maxillary antrum.

The different graft materials fall into three additional categories after the obvious autograft (from the host): allografts, xenografts, and alloplasts. See Tables 21-1 and 21-2 (adapted from Kao and Scott) for a recent review of these materials and their properties.[22]

The different graft materials have strengths and weaknesses that can be daunting for even the most experienced maxillofacial surgeon. The size and configuration of particulate graft materials and the shape and size of the corticocancellous grafts are of prime importance.

The lack of osteoinductive properties in grafting material has always been an issue that concerns surgeons. The ability to induce bone growth, especially from an exogenous source, is a beneficial attribute. Bone growth is readily induced by bone morphogenetic proteins (BMPs), which can be found in cortical bone. There are 14 BMPs in general, and 3 of them have been the core of research in developing grafting sources. BMP-2, BMP-4, and BMP-7 have garnered the most attention, with BMP-2 being the most commonly favored component. Thanks to recombinant technology and science,

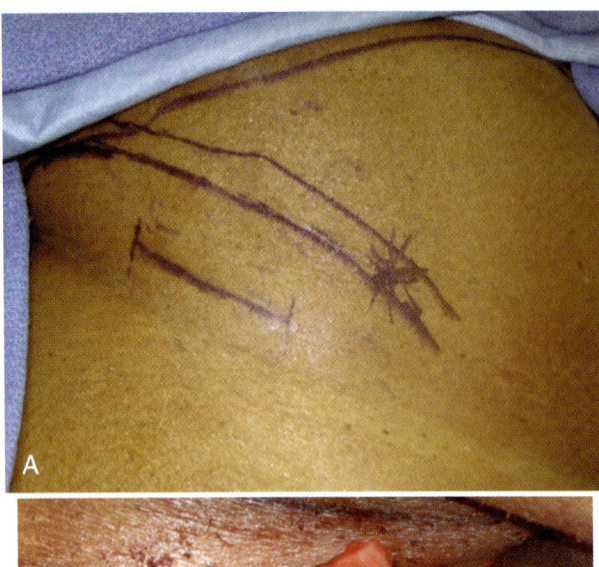

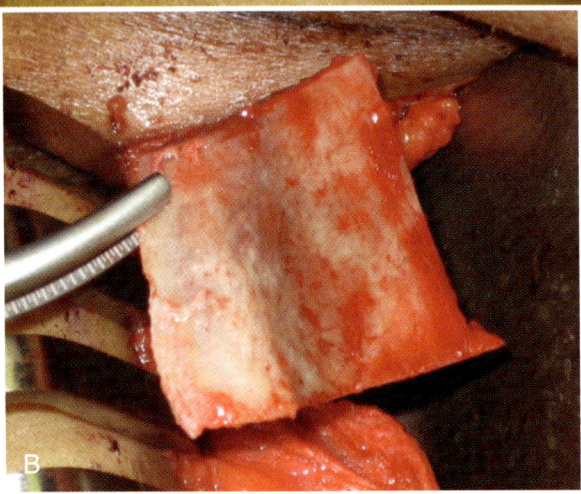

Fig. 21-8 ■ Anterior iliac crest approach (**A**) and corticocancellous block harvest (**B**).

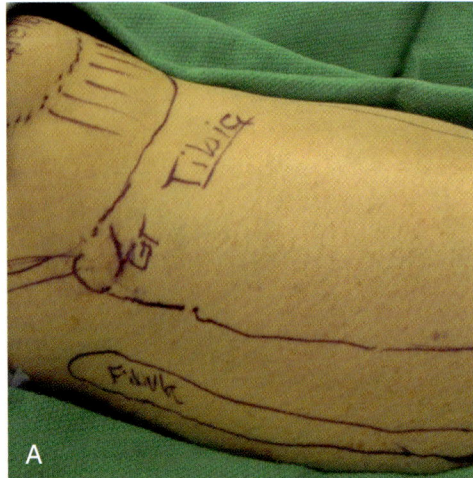

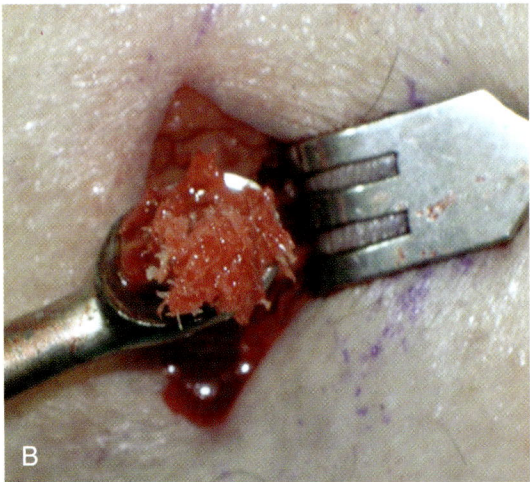

Fig. 21-9 ■ **A** and **B,** Tibial plateau harvest site.

TABLE 21-1	Synopsis of Bone Substitutes	
GRAFT MATERIAL	**CHARACTERISTICS**	**EXAMPLES**
Allograft	A graft taken from a member of the same species as the host but genetically dissimilar	Cadaver cortical/ cancellous bone FDBA DFDBA
Xenograft	Graft derived from a genetically different species from the host	Bio-Oss, coralline HA, red algae
Alloplast (synthetic material)	Fabricated graft material	Calcium sulfate, bioactive glass, HA, NiTi

DFDBA, demineralized freeze-dried bone allograft; FDBA, freeze-dried bone allograft; HA, hydroxyapatite.
From Kao ST, Scott DD: A review of bone substitutes, Oral Maxillofac Surg Clin North Am 19:513-521, 2007.

TABLE 21-2	Characteristics of Bone Graft Materials
CHARACTERISTIC	**GRAFT MATERIAL**
Osteogenesis	Autograft
Osteoinduction	BMP DFDBA DBM Bio-Oss
Osteoconduction	Calcium phosphate Calcium sulfate Collagen FDBA Glass ionomers HA NiTi

BMP, bone morphogenetic protein; DBM, demineralized bone matrix; DFDBA, demineralized freeze-dried bone allograft; FDBA, freeze-dried bone allograft; HA, hydroxyapatite.
From Kao ST, Scott DD: A review of bone substitutes, Oral Maxillofac Surg Clin North Am 19:513-521, 2007.

recombinant human BMP-2 (rhBMP-2) is available for use and study. In a multicenter trial to test the viability of rhBMP-2 versus autogenous particulate grafts, rhBMP-2 on an absorbable collagen sponge was found to result in a comparable amount of bone for implant placement. After a period of 6 months the grafted bone had higher density, but the rhBMP-2–induced bone, which was still maturing at 6 months, gained superior density after loading and additional time (another 6 months).[23]

The soft tissue envelope is rarely a concern when the plan is to use particulate grafts in the inner aspect of the antrum. However,

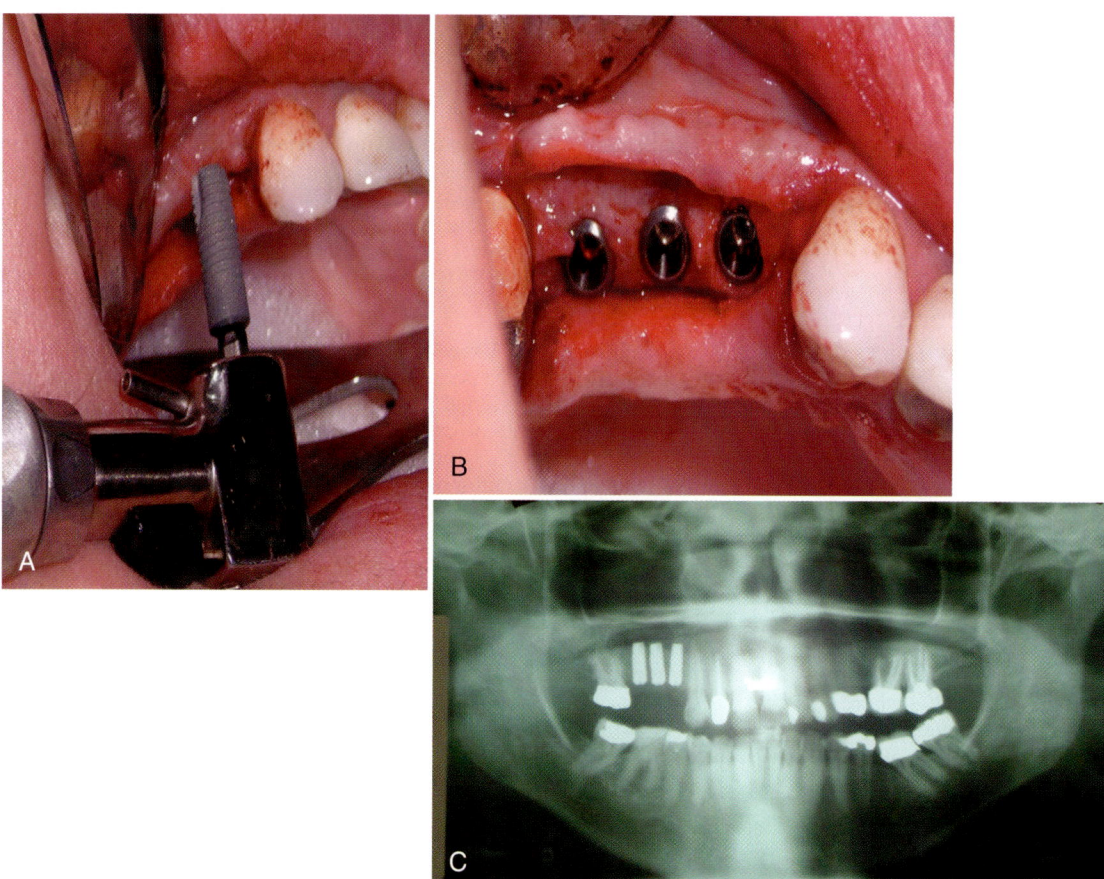

Fig. 21-10 ■ **A** and **B,** Placement of endosseous implants into the grafted site. **C,** Postoperative sinus graft and implant placement at 5 months.

the soft tissue envelope and the ability to undermine tissue and perhaps "steal" tissue from the maxillary vestibule can be used to assist in tension-free closure. The maxillofacial surgeon should be able to close these defects with care and precision.

POSTOPERATIVE CARE

The immediate postoperative care of the maxillary sinus is important for obtaining a successful and beneficial outcome. The patient must be compliant and the surgeon must be vigilant in the postoperative course so that any potential problems do not become disastrous and result in loss of the graft or failure of the endosseous implants.

Experienced surgeons will undoubtedly tell you that there are three main components to successful sinus lifting and subsequent grafting:

1. One must make sure that the patient's nasal passages and sinus pathways are kept pristine and as clear as possible with the administration of an antihistamine or decongestant (or both). Some decongestants may dry the nasal mucosa out to the point of pain, so a short course of decongestant for the initial 4 to 5 days is usually sufficient for the patient to recover from the incipient surgical edema.

2. Instructing patients to avoid blowing their nose is also helpful in the management of a recently grafted sinus. Patients may not be able to comply with refraining from blowing their nose, especially in the presence of significant congestion. The phenomenon of a sneeze can also be devastating to a recently grafted sinus. It is helpful to have patients realize that if they do have to sneeze,

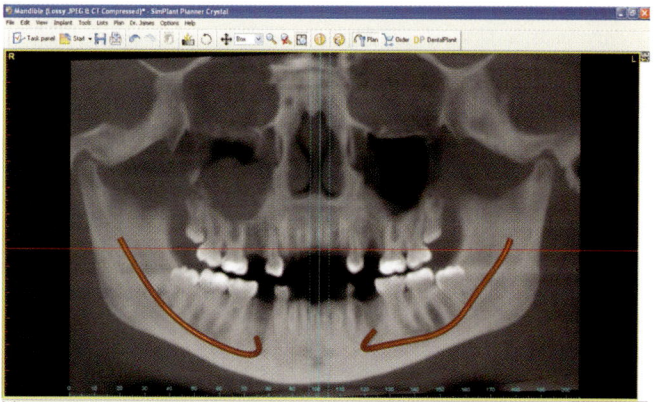

Fig. 21-11 ■ Right maxillary sinusitis.

they should not stifle the sneeze but "let it go" to avoid undue pressure in the sinus cavity from a curtailed sneeze. Continued problems with the sinus and congestion issues should prompt a return visit to the surgeon for immediate firsthand inspection and radiographs to evaluate the surgical site.

3. The bane of any surgery lies in the specter of postoperative infection (Fig. 21-11). The maxillary sinus is colonized by a unique milieu of bacteria. Different species of *Streptococcus, Enterococcus, Peptostreptococcus, Staphylococcus,* and *Actinomyces* inhabit the sinus, along with *Moraxella,* just to name a few, and they are members of the normal and altered flora.

There is even mention in the literature of methicillin-resistant *Staphylococcus aureus* infection after placement of a graft and endosseous implants.[24] Though not commonplace, it is indicative of the serious nature that postoperative infection may pose if not closely monitored. Empiric therapy is not contraindicated; however, culture and sensitivity studies, if they can be performed, set a gold standard for definitive treatment of a draining sinus.

Second-generation cephalosporins, Augmentin, and third- and fourth-generation quinolones (levofloxacin [Levaquin] and moxifloxacin [Avelox]) are also effective in many cases. There is an association with greater postoperative compromise when chronic sinusitis is present. Those with chronic sinusitis need to be evaluated, and it should be eradicated before sinus grafting surgery.[24]

PEARLS AND PITFALLS

- Not only is the design of the trapdoor antrostomy important in maintaining viability of the residual ridge and remaining teeth, but it also plays an important function in achieving proper elevation of the sinus membrane.
- Tears of the sinus membrane larger than 2 mm have a very guarded prognosis. Tears 2 mm or smaller have a good record of healing and survivability.
- Autogenous bone is still the preferred graft material and the gold standard by which others are measured.

- CT can assist the surgeon in determining the size of the implant, the density of the recipient sites, and the quantity of graft material needed during pretreatment planning and thus minimize surgical error.
- CT is the best tool in the armamentarium for identifying the position of the ostium and a variety of other anatomic landmarks.
- Intra-antral septa are prime areas for membrane tears, and "W" or bifurcated trapdoors can eliminate schneiderian membrane tears around these impeding structures.

REFERENCES

1. Jensen OT: *The sinus bone graft,* ed 2. Hanover Park, IL, 2006, Quintessence, p vii.
2. Cawood JI, Howell RA: A classification of the edentulous jaws, *Int J Oral Maxillofac Surg* 17:232-236, 1988.
3. Lee SH, Choi BH, Li J, et al: Comparison of corticocancellous block and particulate bone grafts in maxillary sinus floor augmentation for bone healing around implants, *Oral Surg Oral Med Oral Pathol Oral Radiol Endod* 104:324-328, 2007.
4. Ardekian L, Oved-Peleg E, Mactei E, et al: The clinical significance of sinus membrane perforation during augmentation of the maxillary sinus, *J Oral Maxillofac Surg* 64:277-282, 2006.
5. Morgensen C, Tos M: Quantitative histology of the maxillary sinus, *Rhinology* 15:129-140, 1977.
6. Sul SH, Choi BH, Jeong SM, et al: Histologic changes in the maxillary sinus membrane after sinus membrane elevation and the simultaneous insertion of dental implants without the use of grafting materials, *Oral Surg Oral Med Oral Pathol Oral Radiol Endod* 105(4):e1-e5, 2008.
7. Jung JH, Choi BH, Zhu SJ, et al: The effects of exposing dental implants to the maxillary sinus cavity on sinus complications, *Oral Surg Oral Med Oral Pathol Oral Radiol Endod* 102:602-605, 2006.
8. Sutton DN, Lewis RK, Patel M, et al: Changes in facial form relative to progressive atrophy of the edentulous jaws, *Int J Oral Maxillofac Surg* 33:676-682, 2004.
9. Marx RE, Sterns D: *Oral and maxillofacial pathology; a rationale for diagnosis and treatment,* Hanover Park, 2003, Quintessence, pp 518-519.
10. Kraut R: A case for routine computed tomography imaging of the dental alveolus before implant placement, *J Oral Maxillofac Surg* 59:64-67, 2001.
11. Pieper SP, Lewis SG: A case against routine computed tomography imaging of the dental alveolus before implant placement, *J Oral Maxillofac Surg* 59:68-70, 2001.
12. Tai CE, Sutherland IS, McFadden L: Prospective analysis of secondary alveolar bone grafting using computed tomography, *J Oral Maxillofac Surg* 58:1241-1249, discussion 1250, 2000.
13. Sukovic P: Cone beam computed tomography in craniofacial imaging, *Orthod Craniofac Res* 6(Suppl I):31-36, discussion 179-182, 2003.
14. Angelopoulos C, Thomas S, Hechler S, et al: Comparison between digital panoramic radiography and cone beam computed tomography for the identification of mandibular canal as part of presurgical dental implant assessment, *J Oral Maxillfac Surg* 66:2130-2135, 2008.
15. Boyne PJ: Augmentation of the posterior maxilla by way of sinus grafting procedures: recent research and clinical observations, *Oral Maxillofac Surg Clin North Am* 16:19-31, v-vi, 2004.
16. Tatum H: Maxillary and sinus implant reconstructions, *Dent Clin North Am* 30:207-229, 1986.
17. Raja SV: Management of the posterior maxilla with sinus lift: review of techniques, *J Oral Maxillofac Surg* 67:1730-1734, 2009.
18. Zijderveld SA, van der Bergh JP, Schulten E, et al: Anatomical and surgical findings and complications in 100 consecutive maxillary sinus floor elevation procedures, *J Oral Maxillofac Surg* 66:1426-1438, 2008.
19. Summers RB: A new concept in maxillary implant surgery: the osteotome technique, *Compend Continuous Educ Dent* 15:152, 154-156, 158 passim, quiz 162, 1994.
20. Thowarth M, Srour S, Felszeghy E, et al: Stability of autogenous bone grafts after sinus procedures: a comparative study between anterior and posterior aspects of the iliac crest and an intraoral donor site, *Oral Surg Oral Med Oral Pathol Oral Radiol Endod* 100:278-284, 2005.
21. Doud Galli SK, Lebowitz RA, Giacchi RJ, et al: Chronis sinusitis complicating sinus lift surgery, *Am J Rhinol* 15:181-186, 2001.
22. Kao S, Scott D: A review of bone substitutes, *Oral Maxillofacial Surg Clin North Am* 19:513-521, vi, 2007.
23. Triplett RG, Nevins M, Marx R, et al: Pivotal, randomized, parallel evaluation of recombinant human bone morphogenetic protein-2/absorbable collagen sponge and autogenous bone graft for maxillary sinus floor augmentation, *J Oral Maxillofac Surg* 67:1947-1960, 2009.
24. Ward BB, Terrell JE, Collins JK: Methicillin-resistant *Staphylococcus aureus* sinusitis associated with sinus lift bone grafting and dental implants: a case report, *J Oral Maxillofac Surg* 66:231-234, 2008.

Chapter 22

Reconstruction of the Atrophic Mandible

Michael S. Jaskolka, George H. Blakey III

An atrophic mandible presents a number of reconstructive challenges because of its altered anatomy and physiology. Progressive erosion leads to loss of form and function and predisposes patients to fractures that are difficult to treat. State-of-the-art reconstruction revolves around restoration of mandibular volume in conjunction with placement of endosseous titanium implants to stabilize bone grafts and provide a foundation for prosthetic and functional esthetic rehabilitation. Although the literature is replete with multiple techniques to achieve these goals, the most predictable contemporary protocol involves harvesting of autogenous iliac crest, extraoral bone graft augmentation, and delayed placement of dental implants in conjunction with prosthetic treatment planning.

ETIOPATHOGENESIS/CAUSATIVE FACTORS

Although oral health awareness and prevention of dental disease have reduced rates of tooth loss and complete edentulism in developed countries, growth of the elderly population is likely to be associated with an increase in the overall number of edentulous individuals. The loss of teeth initiates a sequence of physiologic events that leads to the progressive loss of alveolar bone in a predictable pattern that is accelerated by the use of conventional denture prostheses. Over time, this leads to both functional and esthetic changes related to denture stability, chewing, swallowing, speech, and facial soft tissue support. Initially, these alterations may be managed with traditional pre-prosthetic, surgical, and prosthetic techniques, which may allow interim rehabilitation. However, as resorption of the mandible progresses and becomes more severe, these procedures become less successful.

PATHOLOGIC ANATOMY

The progression of alveolar and mandibular atrophy has been well described in the literature. Many different values (including height <10 mm) are used for the definition of an "atrophic" mandible. Because the alveolar bone is resorbed and the vertical dimension of the mandible is reduced to less than 10 mm, it provides poor bone stock for implant restoration, is overly thin and more prone to fracture, provides a limited platform for traditional dentures, and is in a poor relationship to the maxilla (Fig. 22-1).

Mandibular resorption leads to additional anatomic and phenotypic alterations beyond the change in dimension. There is an associated reduction in mucosal surface area, atrophy, and relatively superficial repositioning of the oral and facial musculature, as well as the inferior alveolar neurovascular bundle (Fig. 22-2). Additionally, erosion of the cancellous alveolar bone leaves a dense and primarily cortical basal strut in place. Facial changes include a reduction in vertical dimension and conversion to a class III prognathic relationship secondary to both the pattern of resorption and autorotation of the mandible.

Physiologic changes also occur and may be relevant to the pathology of mandibular resorption, as well as pose important considerations for reconstructive procedures. The aging mandible is associated with decreased osteogenic potential, probably because of reduced peripheral stem cell populations. Moreover, progressive narrowing of the inferior alveolar artery leads to a transition from a centrifugal to a centripetal blood supply of the mandible, thereby resulting in higher relative importance of the periosteum and surrounding tissues for vascular supply.

DIAGNOSTIC STUDIES

A careful extraoral and intraoral examination is paramount for accurate diagnosis and development of an individualized reconstructive treatment plan. However, evaluation is incomplete without the use of radiographic studies. Digital panoramic radiography is the most widely accepted technique. It is readily available, fast, inexpensive, and associated with limited radiation exposure. However, cone beam computed tomography (CBCT) technology is quickly setting the new standard for evaluation of maxillofacial hard tissue and provides three-dimensional data for both diagnosis and treatment planning. Although medical CT provides even more soft tissue information, the cost and radiation dosage should preclude its regular application in this scenario.

TREATMENT/RECONSTRUCTIVE GOALS

The goal of mandibular reconstruction is restoration of form and function. In a severely deficient mandible, it is important to consider the following: (1) bone bulk to strengthen the mandible and protect the neurovascular bundle, (2) a broad convex ridge, (3) ideal ridge relationships, (4) fixed tissue over the denture and implant support areas, and (5) sufficient depth of the facial and lingual vestibules.

Historically, the goals of reconstruction of an atrophic mandible were focused on the provision of a substantial base for conventional denture wear. Attempts began with autogenous solid bone graft augmentation, and a variety of different protocols have been described that use different techniques (e.g., vascularized and nonvascularized), different donor sites (e.g., fibula, rib, ilium, and cranium), different approaches (e.g., intraoral and extraoral), different graft positions (e.g., superior and inferior), and different types of fixation. Several inventive modified osteotomy and bone graft combinations have also been described, including the "sandwich" and "visor" techniques, which are used in combination with autogenous bone grafts.

In an attempt to minimize donor site morbidity, many authors have explored the use of different materials, including a variety of allografts (e.g., cadaveric), xenografts (e.g., bovine), and alloplasts (e.g., hydroxyapatite). Additionally, isolated prosthetic restoration

175

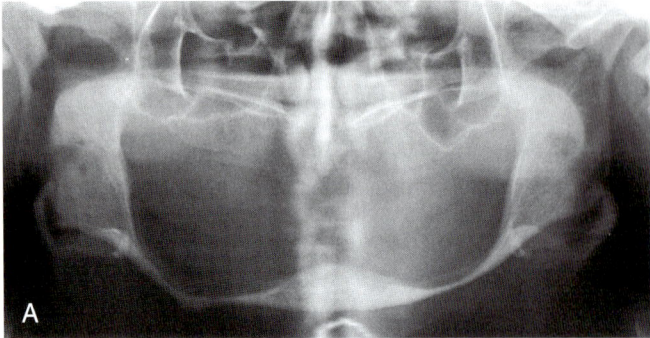

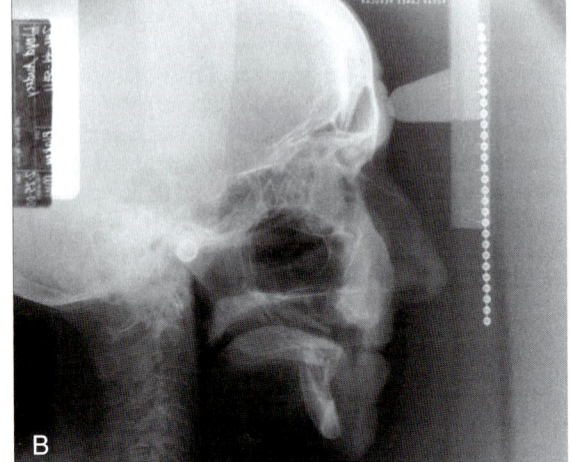

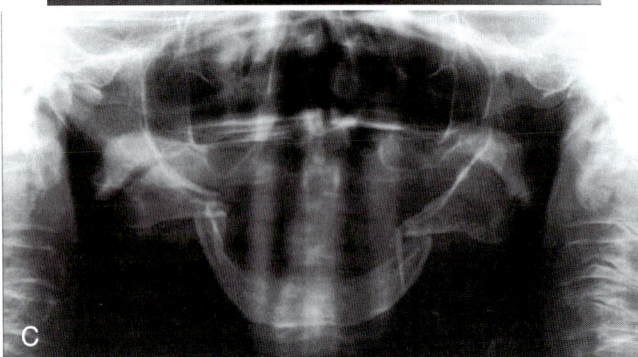

Fig. 22-1 ■ **A,** Panoramic radiograph of a severely atrophic mandible. **B,** Lateral cephalogram depicting a bilateral fracture of the atrophic mandible leading to a typical "bucket handle" deformity. **C,** Panoramic radiograph depicting a bilateral fracture of an atrophic mandible leading to the "bucket handle" deformity.

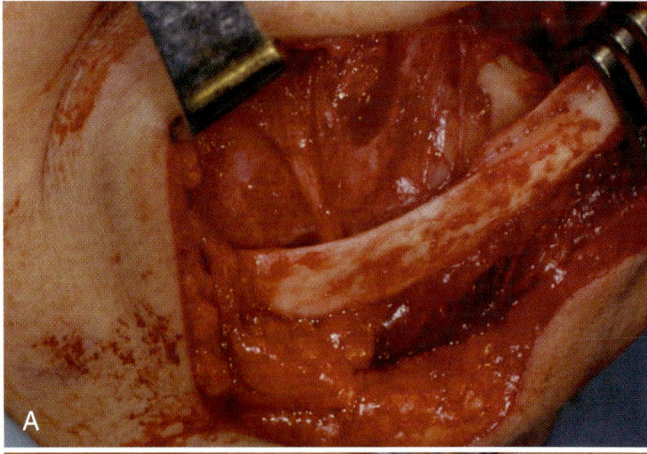

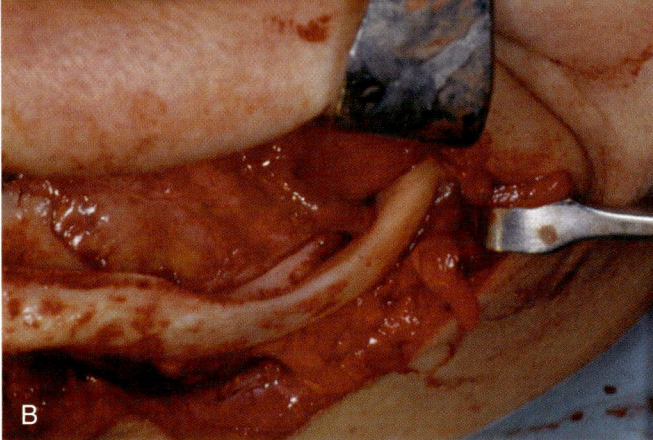

Fig. 22-2 ■ Close-up views of exposure of the right side (**A**) and left side (**B**) of an atrophic mandible and the inferior alveolar neurovascular bundle lying on the superior aspect of the mandible with bone coverage.

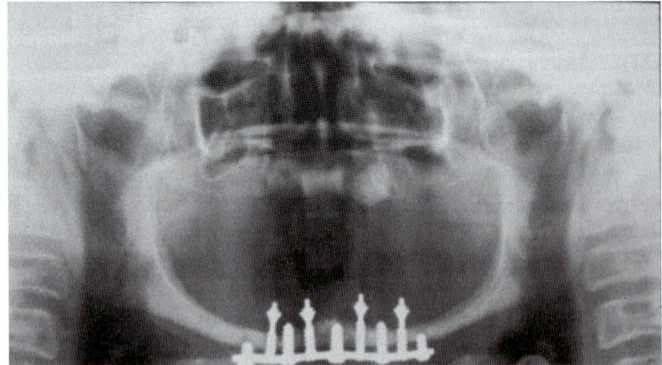

Fig. 22-3 ■ Panoramic radiograph of a failing transmandibular implant.

(e.g., transmandibular implant) has been performed in an attempt to distribute restorative forces and promote bone regeneration (Fig. 22-3). Some failed in the short term because of graft dehiscence and infection, whereas others failed over time secondary to graft resorption, migration, and mandibular fracture. Even in those that were considered "successful," conventional prosthetic rehabilitation was often problematic and short-lived.

The emergence of osseointegrated implants has led to a paradigm shift in the rehabilitation of atrophic mandibles and has served to narrow the goals of mandibular reconstructive surgery. Prosthetic treatment plans that include dental implants provide many options that can be tailored to each individual patient, all of which lead to improved retention, stability, esthetics, and patient satisfaction when compared with conventional dentures. Initial prosthetic treatment planning before surgical intervention is critical to help tailor the surgical treatment plan; for instance, bone augmentation may be

necessary to provide adequate volume for implant placement in ideal orientation and location.

Long-term stabilization of bone grafts and mandibular volume is dictated by successful osseointegration. However, implants are not without pitfalls. Although they have largely banished pre-prosthetic soft tissue surgical procedures to textbooks, implants still require careful soft tissue evaluation and management. The need for adequate depth of the floor of the mouth and labial vestibules is important, and the role of keratinized tissue around the area of emergence is vital for the maintenance of health and longevity. Depending on the prosthetic restorative scheme, the orientation of implants in relation to each other, as well as their location in relation to other stomatognathic components, is critical, and they can be unforgiving to placement error. They also require regular long-term maintenance, which is often cost-prohibitive for many patients.

An atrophic mandible creates specific challenges in implant reconstruction. The limited bone mass increases the possibility of fracture at the time of or following placement. Moreover, the location of the inferior alveolar neurovascular bundle may require additional surgical maneuvers.

SPECIFIC TREATMENT AND TECHNIQUES

Clinical and radiographic evaluation (Fig. 22-4) is followed by preliminary prosthodontic consultation and the development of a final prosthetic treatment plan. This provides useful information to the oral and maxillofacial surgeon regarding the number of implants required for prosthetic restoration and subsequently the volume and location of the required mandibular augmentation. In some cases, supplemental implants should be considered for stabilization of bone grafting and mandibular volume, as well as for providing for possible implant failure or conversion to a more stabilized restoration. Preliminary mounting plus diagnostic wax-up of a restorative treatment plan is also useful for fabrication of a maxillary bone surgical guide for bone graft placement and visualization of ideal contours.

After outlining a prosthetic treatment plan, a finalized surgical treatment plan can be developed. Estimation of the volume of bone graft needed is followed by determination of an appropriate site for bone graft harvest. The ilium is the site of choice for autogenous cancellous bone graft (Fig. 22-5). Up to 50 cm³ of cancellous bone can be harvested from the anterior crest, although this is usually insufficient for substantial bony reconstruction. The posterior iliac crest can provide up to 100 cm³ of cancellous bone, depending on the size of the patient. Although a significant body of literature is dedicated to the positive and negative aspects of anterior and posterior hip graft harvesting, the only significant considerations are the volume of bone required, the additional time needed to position and reposition the patient while under general anaesthesia, and the ability of two surgical teams to work concurrently.

When a significant volume of bone graft is required, general anesthesia is commonly induced on a stretcher and the patient is orally or nasally intubated. The tube is secured and the eyes are taped and well padded. Before incision, 60 to 120 mL of whole blood is drawn for the development of platelet-rich plasma (PRP). A baseline platelet count can assist in the customized preparation of PRP to develop an efficacious aggregate. The patient is positioned and the posterior ilium is harvested as outlined in a step-by-step fashion by Marx. A catheter can be inserted subcutaneously for relief of pain if desired in conjunction with wound closure, but it should be independently covered with an occlusive dressing. The patient is cleaned and antibiotic ointment applied to the wound, which is then covered with a pressure dressing. The patient is next repositioned on the operating room table in the supine position, and a Foley catheter can be inserted at this time if necessary.

If so desired, it can be placed on the maxilla or maxillary prosthesis and used to evaluate the mandibular relationship. The patient is then re-prepared and draped for an extraoral approach, with the lower lip left visible in the operative field. Depending on the extent of the planned reconstruction, an extraoral incision is marked slightly posterior to the submental crease in a curvilinear fashion paralleling the inferior border of the mandible (Fig. 22-6). This in essence is the anterior portion of a high apron flap. Although the majority of the skin incision and dissection of the mandible takes place anterior to the facial artery, care must still be taken to ensure that one remains 2 cm below the inferior border of the mandible to minimize the likelihood of injury to the marginal mandibular branch of the facial nerve.

Frequently, patients will be paralyzed while in the prone position to aid in ventilation, so it is important to confirm return of neuromuscular activity. Local anesthetic with epinephrine can be injected superficially. An incision is made in the skin with a No. 15 blade. A Bovie cautery with a needle tip is used to cut through the subcutaneous tissue to the platysma. Circumferential dissection of the skin flaps helps in achieving a tension-free closure. Anteriorly there are few vital structures; however, a layered approach to the mandible

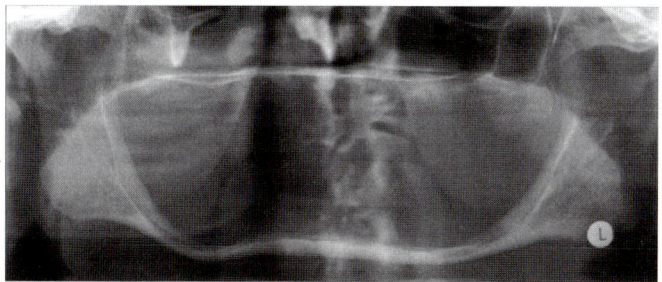

Fig. 22-4 ■ Panoramic radiograph of a severely atrophic mandible.

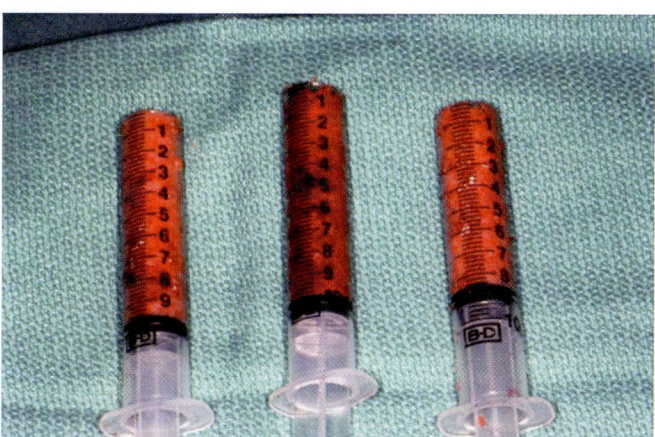

Fig. 22-5 ■ Syringes filled with compressed iliac bone graft.

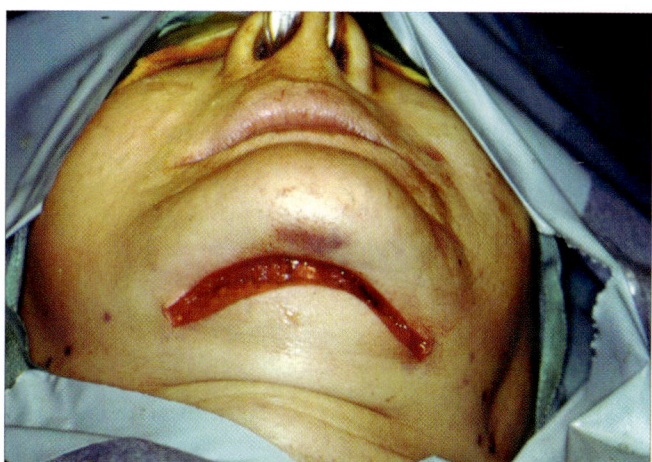

Fig. 22-6 ■ Example of the extent of a typical extraoral incision necessary for augmentation of an atrophic mandible.

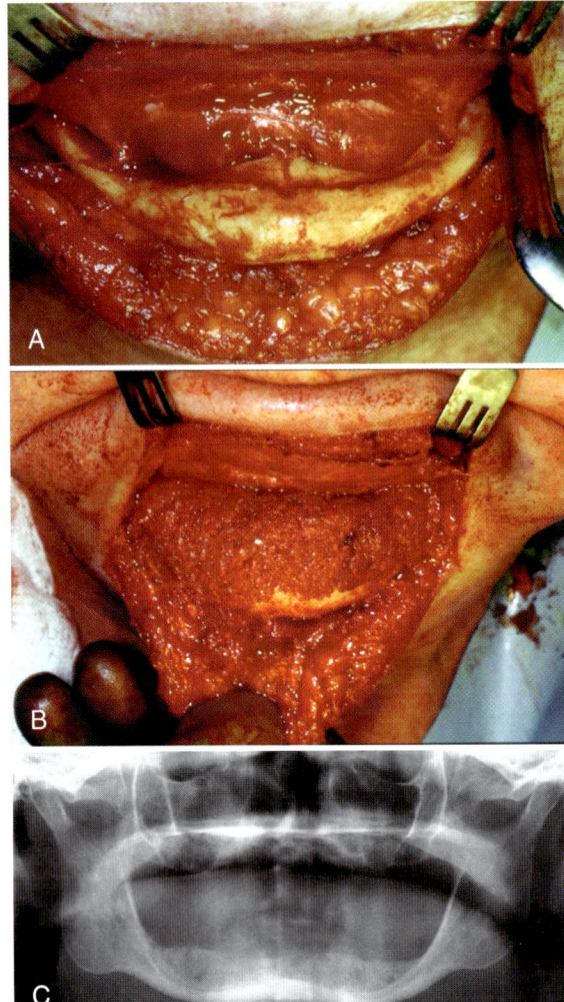

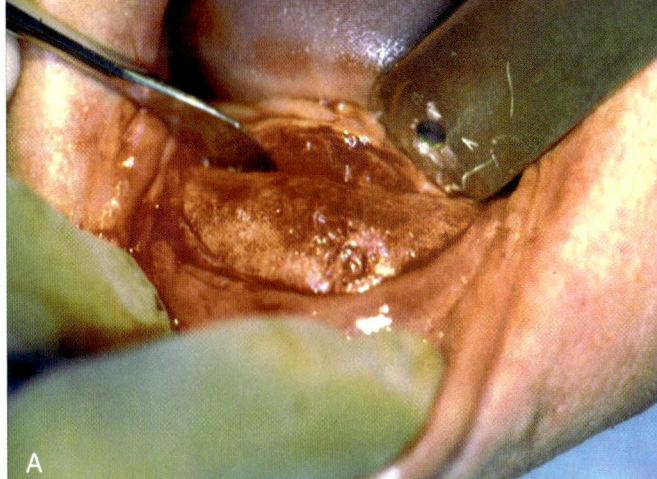

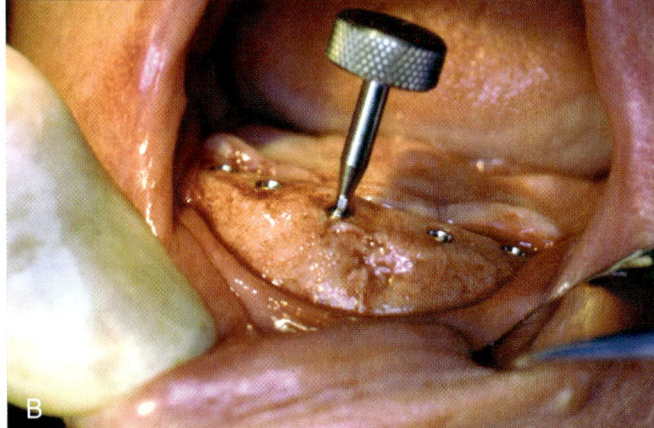

Fig. 22-7 ■ **A,** Typical exposure of an atrophic mandible before bone graft placement. **B,** Placement of an autogenous bone graft with platelet-rich plasma. **C,** Panoramic radiograph following bone graft augmentation of an atrophic mandible with autologous posterior iliac crest and platelet-rich plasma.

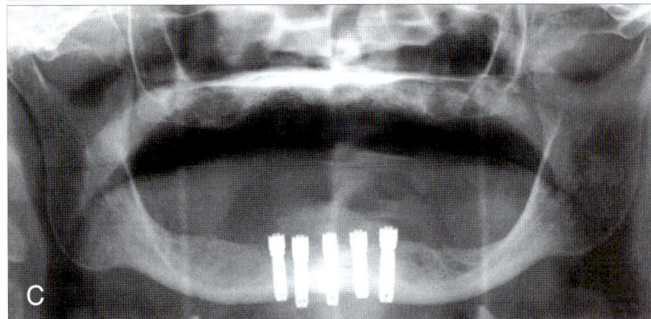

Fig. 22-8 ■ **A,** Transoral exposure of the mandible following bone grafting before placement of endosseous implants. **B,** Transoral placement of five mandibular endosseous implants. **C,** Panoramic radiograph following placement and integration of five endosseous implants in an atrophic mandible previously augmented with autologous posterior iliac crest and platelet-rich plasma.

facilitates hemostasis and a watertight closure. Posteriorly, the platysma is dissected on its deep aspect and divided with a knife after testing with a nerve stimulator. The superficial layer of the deep cervical fascia can then be undermined and divided after testing with a nerve stimulator as well. Anteriorly, dissection is then continued superiorly to the inferior border of the mandible while leaving the digastric and suprahyoid musculature intact. Once identified, a knife or Bovie can be used to cut through the periosteum. Lateral dissection is carried superiorly and posteriorly in a subperiosteal plane, without intraoral perforation. Extension of the dissection may be necessary, depending on the scope of the planned augmentation. Special care must be taken to leave the lingual periosteum and musculature attached to help contain the bone graft. Attention must also be given to the location of the inferior alveolar neurovascular bundle and its point of exit from the native mandible. If it is located on the superior aspect of the mandible, it may be dissected free, positioned laterally, and protected. The PRP is then activated and mixed with the cancellous particulate bone maxraft. This provides excellent working consistency. The bone graft is then packed in the subperiosteal pocket and compressed. If a stent is being used, one

surgical member can change gloves and evaluate the intraoral position of the augmentation before closure. The periosteum may require lateral scoring to allow reapproximation, and the wound can then be closed in layers and covered with antibiotic ointment for dressing. A final intraoral survey is important to ensure that no perforation into the oral cavity has occurred (Fig. 22-7).

An important variation of this technique, as described by Marx, uses primary placement of implants to "tent pole" the tissue for limiting compression of the bone graft by the soft tissue envelope. The biggest drawback of this technique is the potential for placement of an implant in a less than desirable position.

The patient is evaluated postoperatively at regular appointments. Interim prosthesis wear may commence at 2 to 4 weeks, depending on the clinical appearance, with the understanding that wear should be minimized. At approximately 4 months following bone graft augmentation, surgical planning for implant placement can begin. CBCT is performed with a radiographic stent fabricated by the restoring prosthodontist. Depending on graft consolidation, the prosthetic plan and number of implants are finalized. At this time, final evaluation of the depth of the floor of the mouth and labial vestibule, as well as the amount of keratinized tissue, must be made. Any soft tissue surgery should be planned appropriately with the goal of placement of implants under intravenous sedation and local anesthesia at 6 months after bone graft placement (Fig. 22-8).

Following standard implant placement, the patient is again evaluated at regular intervals. Patients are instructed to not wear their prosthesis for 2 weeks and undergo prosthetic relining at this time. After a period of 2 to 4 months of osseointegration, the implants are uncovered and the patient proceeds to final prosthetic restoration.

POSTOPERATIVE CARE

After iliac crest bone grafting, patients are mobilized early and undergo consultation with a physiotherapist on the first postoperative day. The pressure dressing is left in place and changed on the day of discharge unless otherwise saturated. In general, patients remain in the hospital for 1 to 3 postoperative days, often depending on their medical co-morbid conditions. When a subcutaneous catheter is used for pain relief, it is generally empty and removed on the fifth postoperative day at a follow-up appointment.

All patients undergo postoperative panoramic radiographic evaluation. The neck incisions are cleaned with peroxide and water twice a day and kept covered with a thin layer of antibiotic ointment. Patients are prescribed a soft oral diet for the first several weeks.

Analgesics are quickly transitioned from an intravenous to an oral route. Systemic antibiotics are used for a total of 7 days and are also transitioned from an intravenous to an oral route during hospitalization. Systemic steroids are given intravenously for 24 hours in the perioperative period.

PEARLS AND PITFALLS

- Early establishment of a prosthetic treatment plan and ongoing communication with a restorative dentist are key to success.
- The cost of dental implants and prosthetic treatment must be given consideration when developing treatment protocols. Additionally, treatment plans may be staged or designed to allow the future addition of implants and conversion of prostheses.
- Advanced age and multiple co-morbid conditions often go hand in hand with the atrophic mandible patient population. Medical status must be thoroughly evaluated and taken into careful consideration when determining treatment goals, bone graft donor site, anesthetic and medical risks, and the details of perioperative management.
- Successful bone grafting requires careful extraoral anatomic dissection with avoidance of key structures, prevention of intraoral perforation, development of a contained bone graft "pocket," management of the inferior alveolar neurovascular bundle, and evaluation and provision of adequate volume and type of soft tissue.
- Placement of dental implants following bone grafting is a requirement for bone graft maintenance. Distal graft resorption posterior to the region of implant placement must be accounted for and taken into consideration during the initial grafting procedure.
- Techniques continue to rapidly develop. There will probably be a growing role for bone morphogenetic protein and other regenerative technologies in the near future, with the ultimate goal of eliminating morbidity from bone graft harvest.

BIBLIOGRAPHY

Bell RB, Blakey GH, White RP, et al: Staged reconstruction of the severely atrophic mandible with autogenous bone graft and endosteal implants, *J Oral Maxillofac Surg* 60:1135-1141, 2002.

Bradley JC: The clinical significance of age changes in the vascular supply of the mandible, *Int J Oral Surg* 10(Suppl 1):71-76, 1981.

Cawood JI, Howell RA: A classification of the edentulous jaws, *Int J Oral Maxillofac Surg* 17:232-236, 1988.

Cawood JI, Howell RA: Reconstructive preprosthetic surgery. I. Anatomical considerations, *Int J Oral Maxillofac Surg* 20:75-82, 1991.

Ellis E, Zide M: *Surgical approaches to the facial skeleton*, ed 2, Philadelphia, 2006, Lippincott, Williams & Wilkins.

Marx RE: Bone harvest from the posterior ilium, *Atlas Oral Maxillofac Surg Clin North Am* 13:109-118, 2005.

Marx RE, Shellenberger T, Wimsatt J, et al: Severely resorbed mandible: predictable reconstruction with soft tissue matrix expansion (tent pole) grafts, *J Oral Maxillofac Surg* 60:878-888, 2002.

Zygoma Implants in a Compromised Maxilla: Their Use in Both Atrophic and Maxillectomy Patients

Eric J. Dierks, Kenji W. Higuchi

Rehabilitation of major defects in the craniomaxillofacial region is critical in providing improved quality of life for affected patients. Following oncologic resection, traumatic loss, or congenital anomalies of mid-facial and maxillary anatomy, profound difficulties affecting speech, mastication, bolus transportation, and facial esthetics are common.[1] In addition to functional impairment, these conditions are associated with varying degrees of psychosocial problems and compromised social integration.[2] Correction of defects in this region may be accomplished by microvascular free flap transfer as a surgical alternative in selected patients. However, in many instances, autogenous reconstruction may be precluded because of compromised patient tolerance for complex and protracted surgery, absence of a qualified surgical team, or simply patient preference.

Professor Per-Ingvar Brånemark noted a commonality among three groups of patients: those with an atrophic, fully edentulous maxilla, patients with cleft palate deformities, and those who have undergone maxillectomy. He observed that surgeons were invariably confronted with deficient bone volume for anchorage of implants in the region of the defect or the posterior maxilla. In an effort to reduce surgical morbidity and simplify treatment, Brånemark considered the possibility of using the dense compact bone of the zygoma as an anchorage site for an implant-supported prosthesis. After several iterations and based on anatomic measurements[3] and clinical experience, longer machine-surfaced titanium implants with lengths ranging from 35 to 55 mm were developed for clinical trials. Following the initial pilot studies by Brånemark during the years 1989 to 1994 in which use of the zygoma implant was evaluated,[4] retrospective and prospective clinical trials were conducted in multiple centers.[5-7]

In a prospective 16-center evaluation with 3-year follow-up, Kahnberg and co-authors reported a 96.3% survival rate.[7] Malevez and associates retrospectively found a 100% survival rate for 103 zygoma implants in 55 patients after 6 to 48 months of loading.[8] Brånemark and colleagues described their results in 28 consecutive patients with severely resorbed edentulous maxillas; 52 zygoma implants were monitored for 5 to 10 years and had a survival rate of 94% and no significant complications.[5]

Although the zygoma implant penetrates the lateral wall of the maxillary sinus, the health of the maxillary sinus does not appear to be adversely compromised by the presence of the implant. Petrusson performed rhinoscopy and sinuscopy in 14 patients 16 to 64 months after placement of zygoma implants and found no signs of sinus inflammation around the implants.[9] Fifty-two immediately loaded zygoma implants in 26 patients were evaluated via paranasal sinus computed tomography (CT) preoperatively and postoperatively by Davó and co-workers.[10] After an average 21.9 months' follow-up, these authors found that 15% to 20% of patients had asymptomatic mucosal thickening. Two of the maxillary sinuses demonstrated opacity on CT, but following ear, nose, and throat (ENT) evaluation, both merited only follow-up, not surgery. No oral-antral fistulas or other paranasal sinus complications were identified.

The first maxillectomy patient was treated with a zygoma implant by Brånemark and Higuchi in 1999.[11] Since then, multiple centers have effectively used single and multiple zygoma implants in rehabilitating maxillectomy defects.[1,5,12,13]

THE ZYGOMA IMPLANT IN PATIENTS WITH POSTERIOR MAXILLARY ATROPHY

ETIOPATHOGENESIS/CAUSATIVE FACTORS

The exact cause of maxillary atrophy is unclear, but it is related to the premature loss of teeth. The dental root structure introduces functional stress into the alveolar process that stimulates the density and bulk of the adjacent bone. The maxillary sinus enlarges through childhood as the permanent maxillary dentition descends and erupts. The most inferior point of the floor of the maxillary sinus most closely approaches the alveolar crest at the level of the first molar. This pneumatization process of the maxilla generally ends in eruption of the maxillary second molars, but it can restart following extraction of the first or second molars. Pneumatization of an edentulous posterior alveolus produces loss of much of the alveolar bone, which results in a hollow, shell-like alveolar ridge that initially retains its intraoral contour and allows retention of a conventional denture. Long-term denture wearers experience repetitive superimposition of transmucosally applied masticatory forces on the alveolar ridge that results in vertical or horizontal resorption (or both) and resultant loss of the ridge contour. This can progress to flattening of the alveolus or thinning of the ridge to a knife edge shape. The so-called combination syndrome of natural lower anterior teeth opposing an upper full denture can produce severe atrophy and resorption in the anterior maxilla. Maxillary atrophy can occur anteriorly, posteriorly, or both. Patients with atrophy so advanced that the palate is rendered flat pose the greatest challenge to the prosthetic surgical team (Fig. 23-1).

PATHOLOGIC ANATOMY

MAXILLARY ATROPHY

Bedrossian and associates divided the maxilla into three zones of potential atrophy, and their classification aids in understanding the use of zygomatic and other implants in this patient group[14] (Fig. 23-2). Edentulous patients with an eggshell-thin posterior maxillary alveolus (zone 3) who retain 4 mm or less of vertical bone height are not candidates for simultaneous posterior implant placement and sinus lift bone grafting (Fig. 23-3). The 1994 Academy of Osseointegration Sinus Graft Consensus Conference reviewed the results of 2997 implants placed in 1007 grafted sinuses. After a

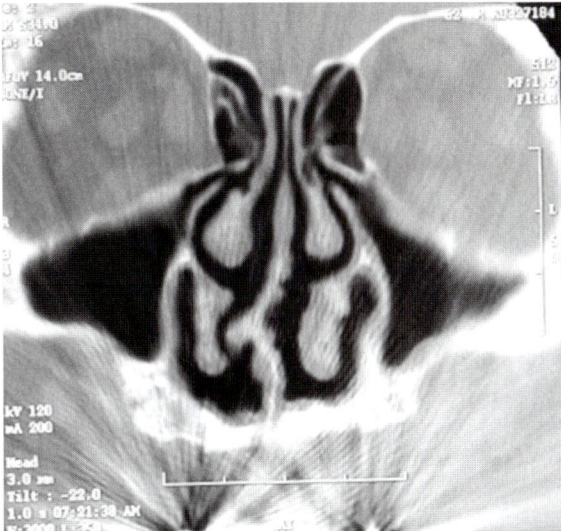

Fig. 23-1 ■ A completely flat palate makes denture construction challenging and denture wear almost impossible.

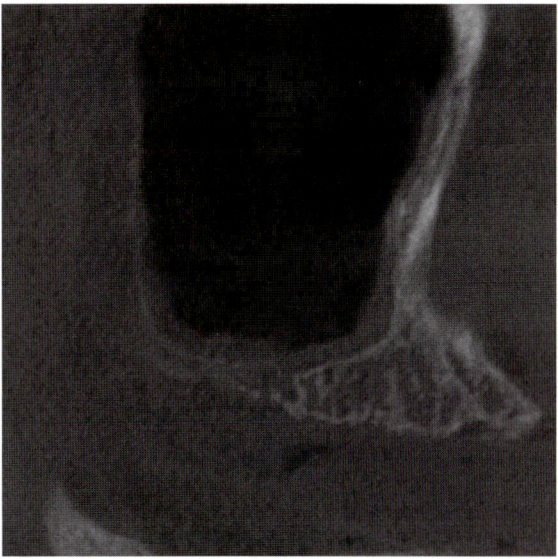

Fig. 23-3 ■ Posterior maxillary atrophy to less than 4 mm as demonstrated on cone beam computed tomography.

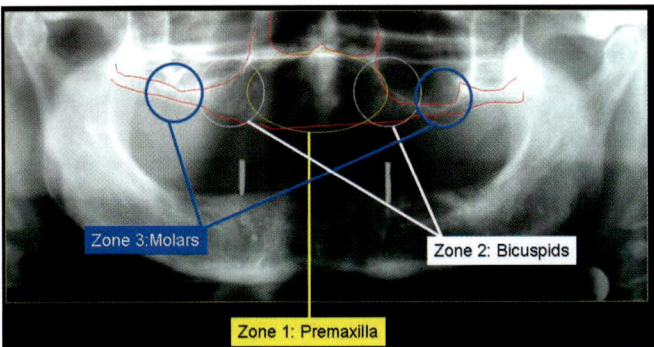

Fig. 23-2 ■ Classification of the three zones of the maxilla.[14]

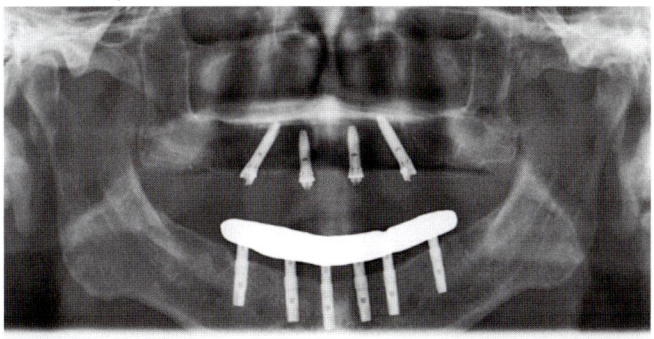

Fig. 23-4 ■ Tilted implants can support a full upper prosthesis on only four implants if there is adequate anterior bone.

minimum 3-year post-restoration follow-up, a 61% failure rate was found when implants were placed simultaneously with sinus lift bone grafts.[15] A recent review of published papers that compared implant survival in the posterior maxilla between grafted sinus floors versus implants placed into native bone showed greater variability in implant survival for implants placed in grafted sinus floors.[16]

The efficacy of tilted implants has been well documented.[17-20] Edentulous patients who are fortunate enough to have adequate bone in the incisor-canine region (zone 1), as well as the premolar region (zone 2), may be candidates for the simpler option of tilting the most distal implants to extend the fixture's location distally to the second premolar–first molar area as described in the "all on 4" technique (Fig. 23-4). Although the "all on 4" technique is generally used with fixed, detachable prostheses, conventional fixed bridgework is also an option with tilted implants combined with mesial conventional implants.[21]

Patients with combined zone 2 and zone 3 atrophy must choose between staged sinus lift bone grafting followed by multiple conventional root-form implants and the graftless, single-stage option of zygoma implants. The zygoma implant may also appeal to patients with zone 2 and 3 atrophy who simply want to expedite their treatment plans. Patients with maxillary atrophy are often elderly and may have medical co-morbid conditions that make them better candidates for a single operation to place all their implants. Such medically fragile patients may be less suitable for a multistep,

multiple-surgery treatment plan involving staged sinus lift grafting followed months later by subsequent conventional root-form implant placement.

THE ZYGOMAS

The paired zygomas occupy the anterolateral corners of the midface. They form most of the floor and the anterolateral walls of the orbit, as well as the roof of each maxillary sinus (Fig. 23-5). Their functional significance is to transmit mandibular masticatory forces generated by the pterygoid-masseteric sling and temporalis musculature vertically from the maxillary molar region to the anterior skull base. The body of the zygoma tends not to change its morphology, even in the presence of severe atrophy of the adjacent maxillary alveolus.

Zygoma Implants

The length of zygoma implants ranges from 30 to 55 mm, and their diameter tapers from 4 mm superiorly to 5 mm at the fixture level (Fig. 23-6, *A*). Implant integration occurs within the thick bone in the body of the zygoma, which produces an integrated length in the range of 15 to 20 mm. Acquisition of an additional zone of integration at the level of the alveolus is welcome, but unnecessary. The path of the zygoma implant lies along the crest of the zygomaticomaxillary buttress (ZMB), and its external hex fixture head emerges in the second premolar–first molar area (Fig. 23-6, *B*). The fixture

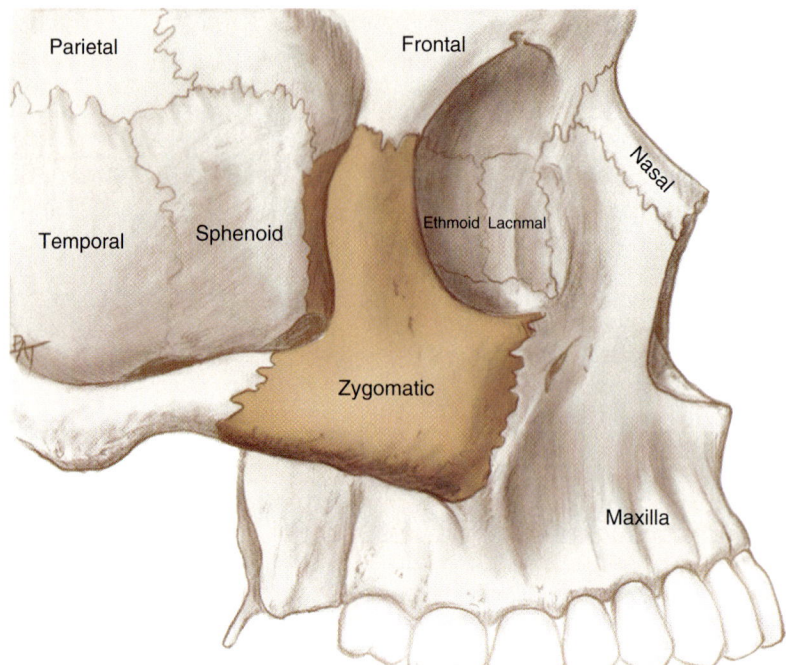

Fig. 23-5 ■ The zygomatic body has adequate bone stock even with coexisting maxillary alveolar atrophy. (From Fehrenbach MJ, Herring SW: *Illustrated anatomy of the head and neck,* ed 3, St. Louis, 2007, Mosby.)

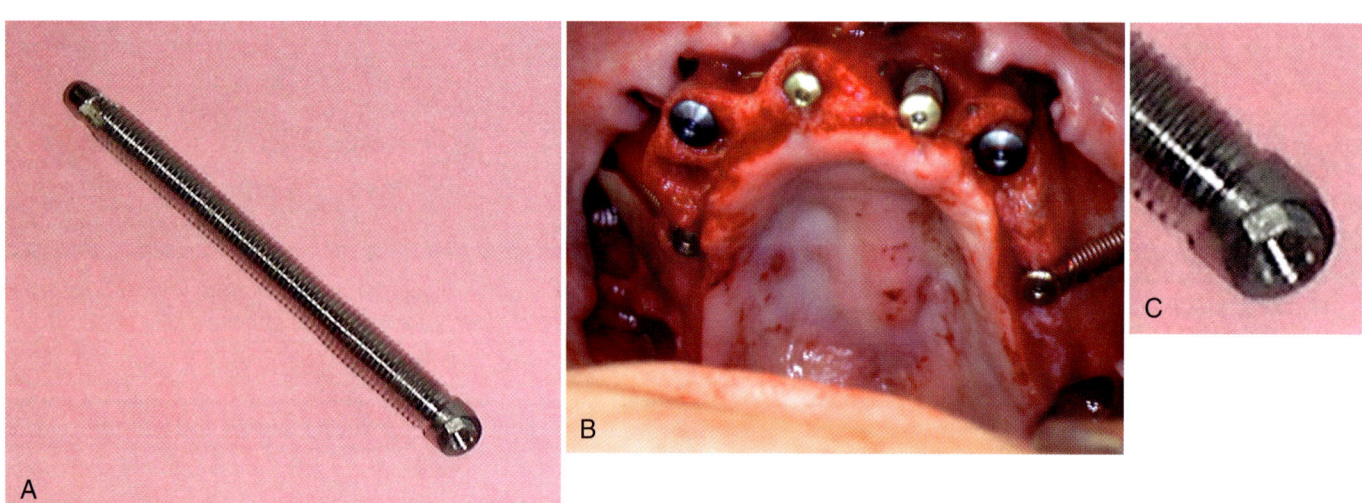

Fig. 23-6 ■ **A,** The Nobel Biocare zygoma implant. **B,** Emergence of the zygoma implant at the second premolar–first molar area. **C,** A 45-degree angulation of the fixture head approximates the occlusal table.

is angulated at 45 degrees (Nobel Biocare, Yorba Linda, Calif.) or 55 degrees (Southern Implants, Irene, South Africa) to orient it roughly parallel to the occlusal plane (Fig. 23-6, *C*). The long moment arm of the zygoma implant makes it inappropriate to use without cross-arch stabilization to other conventional implants (Fig. 23-7) or to anterior conventional implants plus a zygoma implant on the opposite side (Fig. 23-8).

Conventional, edentulous patients are best served by zygoma implants with a fully textured and threaded surface, which allows the potential for optimal integration anywhere along the buried implant shaft. Conversely, maxillectomy patients require daily cleansing of their maxillectomy defects, which are open to the oral cavity. Hygiene considerations of the exposed implant shaft within the maxillectomy defect may be addressed with either a smoothly machined, threaded, but non-textured implant (Nobel Biocare) or an

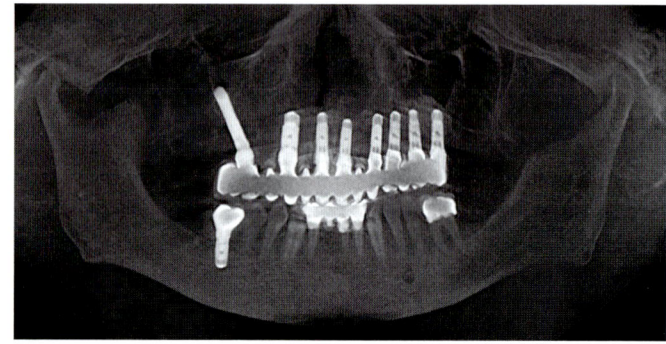

Fig. 23-7 ■ Cross-arch stabilization to the bridge and implants.

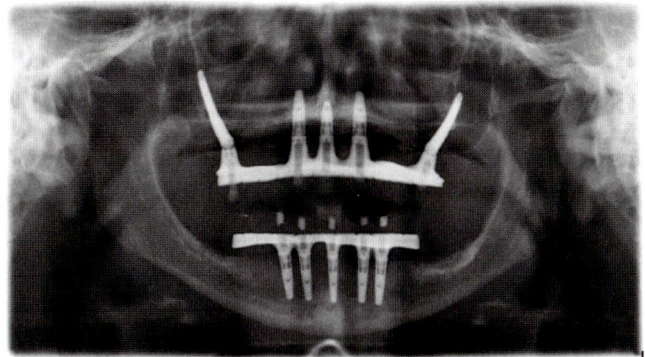

Fig. 23-8 ■ Bilateral zygoma implants connected to three conventional anterior implants.

implant with a smooth, non-threaded shaft extending through the maxillectomy defect with threads only on its apical aspect (Southern Implants).

DIAGNOSTIC STUDIES

HISTORY AND PHYSICAL EXAMINATION

The history and physical examination should focus on the condition of the patient's paranasal sinuses in general and the maxillary sinuses in particular. Acute sinusitis is a contraindication to placement of zygoma implants, but chronic sinusitis is not, provided that the sinusitis is under adequate medical control. Conditions that adversely affect maxillary sinus drainage such as allergic rhinosinusitis, nasal polyps, chronic fungal sinusitis, and severe septal deviation may be reasons for preoperative ENT evaluation. A patient with a previous chronic sinus condition will still probably have that condition following the placement of zygoma implants. Preoperative documentation can be helpful to avoid refocusing the patient's sinus complaints on the zygoma implant.

Physical examination of the oral cavity in contemplation of placement of zygoma implants should include assessment of the patient's ability to open the mouth widely. The presence of mandibular teeth in the canine-premolar area represents a relative contraindication because of their potential for interference with the long path of instrumentation needed to place zygoma implants. Care in retraction and protection of both hard and soft tissues, as well as creative adjustments in the angulation of the drilling and implant placement apparatus, can circumvent the spatial encumbrance of opposing teeth, but such adjustments are much easier under full general endotracheal anesthesia with pharmacologic neuromuscular blockade (Box 23-1).

IMAGING STUDIES

Some form of CT of the maxillofacial structures and paranasal sinuses is helpful in planning surgery, ruling out significant sinus pathology, and optimizing zygoma implant positioning. The low cost and very low levels of radiation associated with cone beam CT make it preferable to medical paranasal sinus CT, but either will suffice. CT measurement from the zygomatic notch to the crest of the maxillary alveolar ridge will help anticipate the length of the zygoma implant but will provide values that tend to be slightly longer than the actual length of the implant required at surgery. CT evaluation of the atrophic anterior maxilla is also of critical importance to the entire treatment plan. In a patient with diffuse maxillary atrophy (zones 1, 2, and 3), it is often the conventional implants

BOX 23-1 Indications and Contraindications for Zygomatic Implants in Patients with Maxillary Atrophy

Indications
Moderate to advanced posterior maxillary alveolar atrophy
Atrophic patient who insists on continuous wear of the denture

Relative Indication
Maxillofacial defects resulting from tumor or trauma

Contraindications
Inability to adequately open the mouth
Acute sinusitis

Relative Contraindications
Unilateral defects
Uncontrolled chronic sinus disease
Presence of mandibular dentition (may interfere with surgical access)

placed in the atrophic anterior maxilla that may be unsuitable for immediate loading. An innovative alternative for such patients can be the use of bilateral, double zygoma implants reported by Schmidt and colleagues[13] for maxillectomy defects and later reported by Maló and co-authors[22] for non-oncologic, diffusely atrophic patients. In patients with non-oncologic, advanced maxillary atrophy, the path of one or both of the double zygoma implants may lie outside the maxillary sinus.

TREATMENT/RECONSTRUCTIVE GOALS

The goal of the zygoma implant is to provide a posterior implant fixture in a patient who is unsuitable for straightforward placement of a conventional root-form implant in this location.

Although the path of a zygoma implant lies partially or totally within the maxillary sinus, its position at the ZMB is remote from the sinus drainage ostium (Fig. 23-9). Treatment with zygoma implants should not predispose to sinus pathology. Endoscopic evaluation of the maxillary sinus after placement of zygoma implants has shown no evidence of infection or inflammation.[9]

Advantages of the zygoma implant in a patient with standard maxillary atrophy include the ability to place the implant along with anterior maxillary implants in one surgical stage, thereby avoiding sinus grafting. Postoperatively, the patient is able to wear a conventional denture over the healing implant if immediate loading is not done. Disadvantages include the more extensive dissection required for placement and the need for the surgeon to be familiar with antral, zygomatic, and orbital anatomy. The need for at least deep intravenous sedation, if not general endotracheal anesthesia, could be viewed as a potential disadvantage.

SPECIFIC TREATMENT AND TECHNIQUES

SURGICAL TECHNIQUES

Brånemark Standard Technique

Zygoma implants are optimally placed in a surgical center or hospital operating room under general nasoendotracheal anesthesia, although the procedure can be done under deep intravenous sedation. Complete mid-facial local anesthesia is especially important if

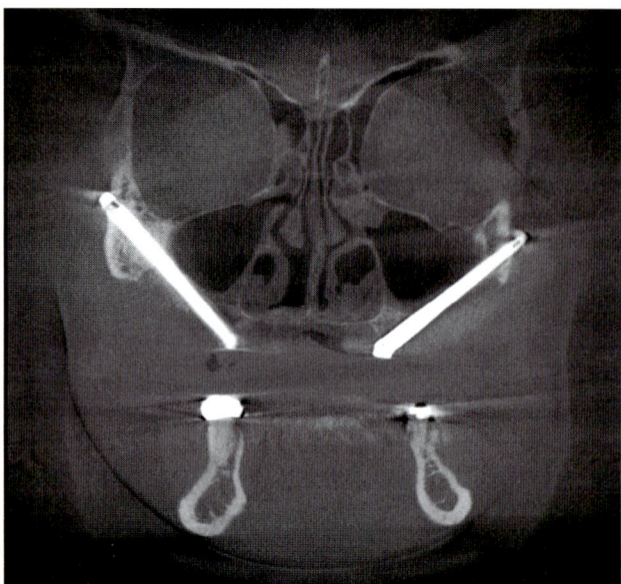

Fig. 23-9 ■ Cone beam computed tomography scan showing the maxillary sinus ostium widely separated from the zygoma implant.

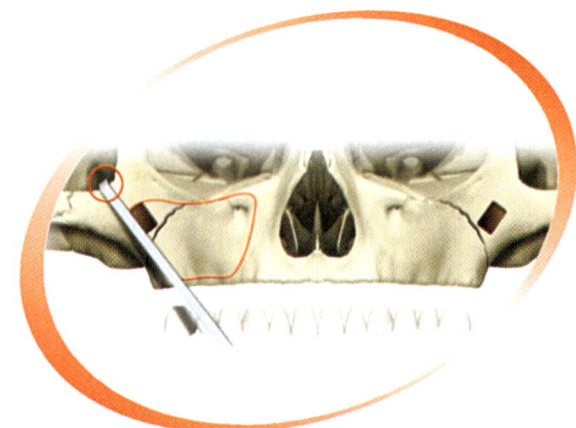

Fig. 23-10 ■ Notch retractor and access hole for the standard Brånemark technique. (Courtesy Nobel Biocare, Yorba Linda, Calif.)

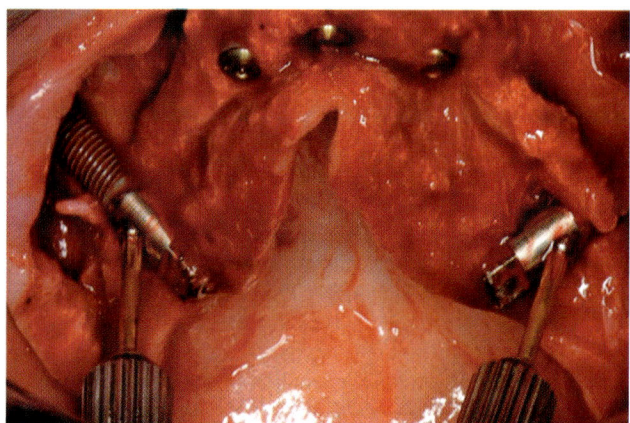

Fig. 23-11 ■ The alignment of the screws retaining the insertion abutment should parallel the anterior conventional implants.

sedation is used.[23] A full crestal incision is made along with anterior midline and bilateral posterolateral relaxing incisions. This allows wide access to the zygomatic body, ZMB, and the anterior maxilla. If condemned maxillary teeth are present, they are removed, followed by appropriate alveolectomy. In a full-arch implant procedure, the anterior implants are placed first. Most such patients will require four conventional anterior implants, although three will suffice. Two are absolutely necessary. Conventional anterior implants should be placed on the palatal aspect of the alveolar ridge, in combination with appropriate alveolectomy and peri-implant grafting as needed.

The standard Brånemark technique for placement of zygoma implants entails full subperiosteal exposure of the lateral aspect of the body of the zygoma. A specialized retractor is placed into the zygomatic notch, at the junction of the zygomatic arch and the lateral orbital rim. The ZMB is traced down to the alveolus, and an emergence hole is created at the base of the ZMB, on the palatal aspect of the ridge. An access hole is then drilled just below the zygomatic body to allow visualization of the drilling process into the zygoma (Fig. 23-10). The mandible is placed in the maximal open position and the lips and other soft tissues are carefully protected. The presence of mandibular dentition makes alignment of the long drills difficult. The standard technique calls for passage of the implant just inside the maxillary sinus wall, within or through the ZMB as it courses into the body of the zygoma. Although elevation of the sinus membrane is recommended, this is rarely feasible or practical. The authors make no attempt to elevate and preserve the sinus membrane, nor to graft for enhancement of the area of integration. The thick bone at the base of the body of the zygoma is drilled to create a flat area into which a round bur is used to create a dimple. The initial 2.9-mm-diameter drill is used first, with the drill hole extended until the tip of the drill exits the zygomatic bone near the zygomatic arch, followed by a transitional pilot drill and, finally, the 3.5-mm drill. The depth gauge is used to determine the length of implant needed. On removal of the implant from its container, the screw retaining the transfer abutment should be loosened and retightened before placement of the implant. The zygoma implant is threaded into position without tapping. The long axis of

the screw that retains the transfer abutment is aligned with the long axis of the anterior implants by placing the driver into its hex fixture and assessing the axis of the driver (Fig. 23-11). The transfer fixture is removed to expose the 45-degree orientation of the implant platform, which now parallels the fixture surfaces of the anterior implants. This standard surgical approach results in the platform lying on the palatal aspect of the alveolar crest, thus necessitating angled or University of California, Los Angeles–type abutments to avoid over-bulking the prosthesis along the palatal aspect of the alveolar ridge. This palatal position of the platform has been a source of criticism of the zygoma implant.

Sinus Slot Technique

A modification termed the sinus slot technique was reported by Stella and Warner[24]; it allows placement of the fixture at or very near the crest of the alveolar ridge. Full lateral soft tissue reflection off the zygomatic body is not necessary, and the zygomatic notch retractor is not used in the technique. The emergence hole is drilled on the crest of the alveolus at the foot of the ZMB. A vertical oblique slot in the ridge of the ZMB is created with a fissure burr and terminates cephalad in the thicker bone of the zygomatic body (Fig. 23-12). Instead of an access hole as in the standard technique, the slot is broadened to taper into a flat surface, which is sculpted into the thicker bone at the base of the zygomatic body. The flat surface

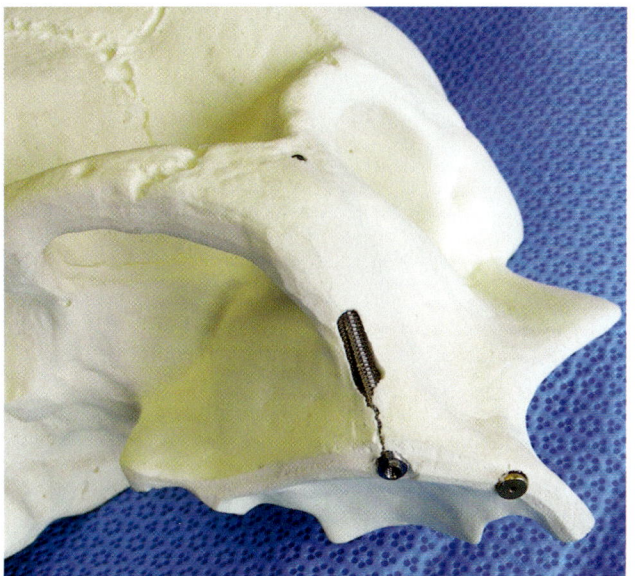

Fig. 23-12 ■ The sinus slot technique.

of the boss will receive a dimple made with the round bur. External finger pressure is used to identify the zygomatic notch by palpation instead of directly viewing it with the notch retractor. The drilling, passage of the implant, and alignment then proceed as with the conventional technique, except that the drill and implant pass through the slot in the ZMB, with the implant often lying partially outside the maxillary sinus. The fixture then lies at or near the alveolar crest.

Another modification of the original technique was described by Boyes-Varley and colleagues.[25] These authors advocate the use of a specific surgical guide and modification of the implant design to increase the platform angulation to 55 degrees rather than the standard 45 degrees. Their technique results in placement of the fixture on the crest of the alveolus with an angulation of the implant that more closely approaches vertical. Computer-aided intraoperative navigation to assist in placement of the zygomatic implant has also been reported.[26]

POSTOPERATIVE CARE

The typical patient with maxillary atrophy can easily undergo placement of zygoma implants on an outpatient basis, whereas an oncologic resection/zygoma implant patient will be hospitalized and receive medically appropriate postoperative care. The typical maxillary atrophy patient should receive perioperative antibiotics beginning with a substantial dose approximately 1 hour before surgery. One gram of cefazolin or 600 mg of clindamycin administered intravenously is a common option. No evidence-based justification exists for beginning antibiotics earlier, and this practice may induce antibiotic resistance. Postoperative antibiotics are optional. Use of decongestants postoperatively is also optional and is unnecessary for patients with healthy sinuses. The role of perioperative chlorhexidine mouth rinses is unclear but they are probably helpful. Facial bruising over the lateral aspect of the malar prominence is not uncommon in patients who have undergone the traditional technique for placing zygoma implants because of the greater degree of dissection in the area. Patients should be advised to refrain from forceful nose blowing and should try to sneeze with the mouth open for approximately 2 weeks following surgery.

ZYGOMA IMPLANTS IN MAXILLECTOMY PATIENTS

ETIOPATHOGENESIS/CAUSATIVE FACTORS

Maxillectomy is necessary for the surgical management of a variety of malignant as well as aggressive, benign neoplastic conditions, including squamous cell carcinoma, minor salivary gland tumors, maxillary ameloblastoma, and many others. Maxillectomy for tumor resection almost always spares the body of the zygoma. Avulsive trauma can also result in significant defects of the maxilla, often with preservation of the zygoma. Simple closure of the maxillectomy defect with a soft tissue free flap does not constitute a maxillary reconstruction. These defects are not completely reconstructed until these patients are rehabilitated with functional oral prostheses.

PATHOLOGIC ANATOMY

The traditional prosthetic management of patients requiring resection of one or both of the paired maxillas has been construction of an obturator prosthesis that would rely on retention provided by a combination of dental clasps and extension of the prosthetic material into undercuts along the periphery of the maxillectomy defect. Before the advent of microvascular osseous free flap reconstruction, maxillectomy prostheses equally tested the prosthodontist's art and the patient's determination. The advent of bone-containing microvascular free flap reconstruction of the maxilla in the 1990s allowed quick restoration of speech, as well as oral intake of soft foods, by sealing off the maxillary sinus from the oral cavity—at the expense of a significantly longer, more complex operation. Complete masticatory rehabilitation took far longer, and these patients routinely suffered without any dental prosthesis for many months or even years as the free flap healed to the adjacent structures and secondary pre-prosthetic surgeries were completed. Two types of free flaps are used for maxillary reconstruction: soft tissue–only flaps, such as the radial forearm flap, which simply seal off the oral-antral communication, and soft tissue plus bone composite flaps, such as the vascularized iliac crest and the fibula flap.

A soft tissue flap such as the radial forearm flap provides no support whatsoever for a prosthesis and serves only to seal off the defect. Terms such as "waterbed" and "trampoline effect" describe the lack of support that a radial forearm flap offers a maxillary prosthesis. Soft tissue plus bone composite flaps such as the iliac crest and fibula carry a soft tissue paddle that seals the defect, as well as bone that heals to the adjacent native maxilla. Postoperatively, most of these patients must do without a functioning temporary prosthesis as the extensive lymphedema of the soft tissue paddle slowly subsides. Soft tissue revision surgery is performed eventually, and conventional dental implants can be placed into the reconstructed bone. As a result, such patients must often wait a year or more before a functioning masticatory system can be restored (Fig. 23-13). Those unfortunate individuals who succumb to their battle with oral cancer may never live to enjoy the social and functional benefits of comprehensive maxillary reconstruction. The zygoma implant can be placed at the time of ablative oncologic surgery, can be loaded immediately, and will greatly expedite oral rehabilitation.

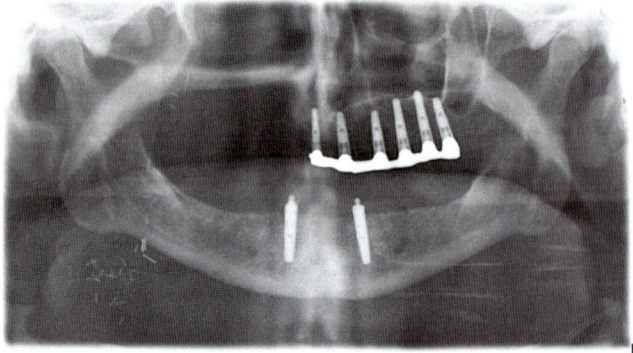

Fig. 23-13 ■ A patient undergoing right maxillectomy required multistep surgery, including a left sinus lift, followed by implant placement. The right zygoma had been resected, thereby precluding the superior result that a zygoma implant could have provided.

DIAGNOSTIC STUDIES

Preoperative imaging of the maxilla and zygoma will usually be part of the oncologic work-up. A maxillectomy patient who is to undergo placement of a zygoma implant or implants following resection will offer the surgeon wide access to the zygomatic body. Maxillectomy patients undergoing secondary placement of zygoma implants often have trismus and scarring of the lips and buccal mucosa, which makes access extremely difficult. Such patients need to be evaluated carefully in regard to their ability to adequately open the mouth and retract the lips and cheeks. Re-opening the Weber-Fergusson incision may be necessary. Zygoma implant surgery for maxillectomy patients is optimally performed in an operating room under general endotracheal anesthesia.

TREATMENT/RECONSTRUCTIVE GOALS

The zygoma implant provides an immediate platform to which a functional dental prosthesis can quickly be attached. This offers maxillectomy patients rapid return to social interaction, as well as a nearly normal diet (Fig. 23-14, *A*). A highly functioning, immediately loaded temporary prosthesis can be fitted on the operating table at the conclusion of the ablative oncologic procedure (Fig. 23-14, *B*). Later, the zygomatic implant can be linked with a Hader bar to anterior or pterygoid implants (or to both) to form the retentive base for a final prosthesis (Fig. 23-14, *C* and *D*). Schmidt and co-authors reported the use of bilateral, dual zygomatic implants to support a total maxillary prosthesis without anterior implants.[13] Soft tissue free flaps and zygomatic implants can be combined. Panagos and Hirsch reported a hybrid immediate reconstruction of a maxillary defect that used a microvascular radial forearm flap with both a zygomatic implant and a pterygoid implant. The implants perforated the flap to support a maxillary prosthesis[27] (Fig. 23-15). The combination of vascularized iliac crest bone with a soft tissue paddle plus zygoma and conventional implants placed at the time of ablative surgery has also been reported.[28] Bilateral zygoma implants combined with a midline frontal implant have likewise been reported for use in supporting a nasal prosthesis.[29] The role of zygoma implants in patients who have previously undergone radiation therapy is unclear; however, a history of previous exposure to radiation is not an absolute contraindication.

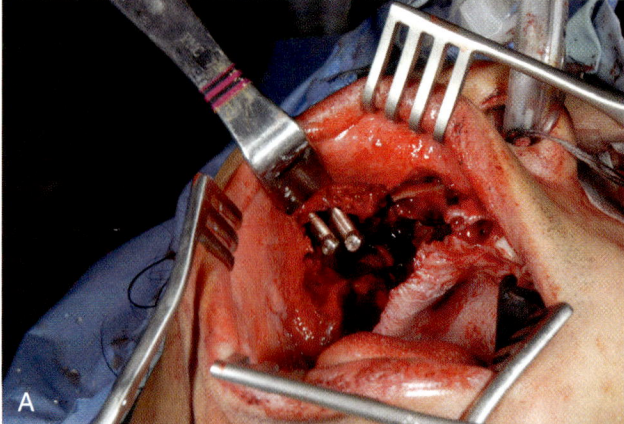

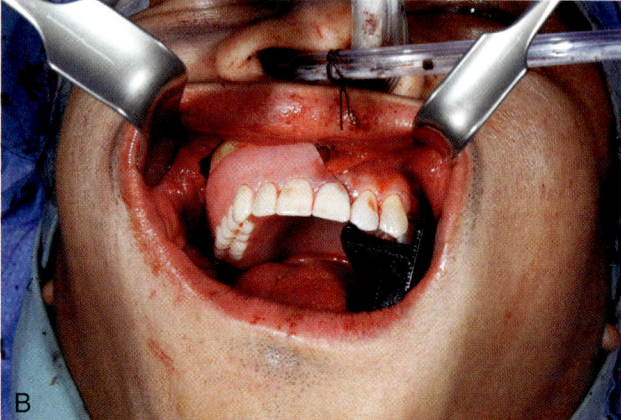

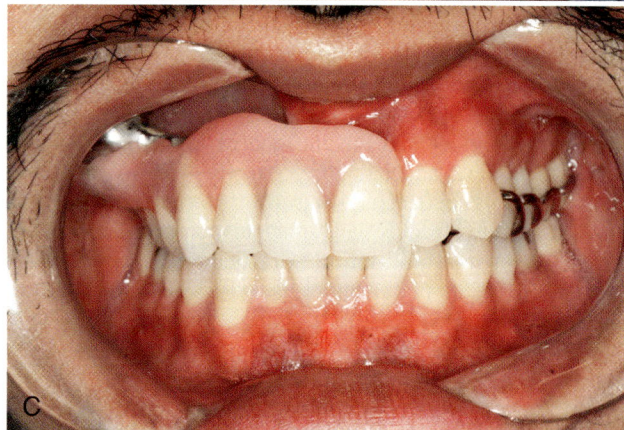

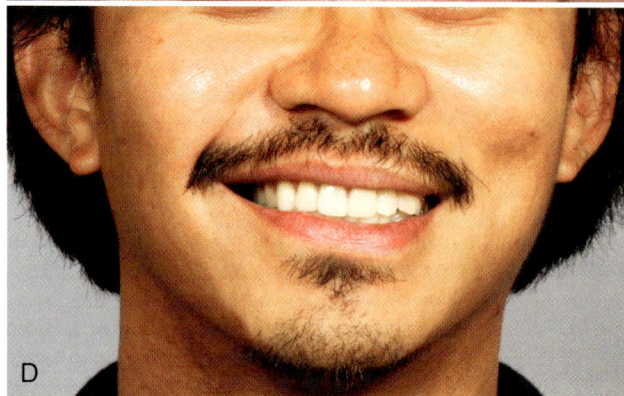

Fig. 23-14 ■ **A,** Placement of paired, unilateral zygoma implants at time of maxillectomy for ameloblastoma. **B,** Immediate provisional prosthesis. **C,** Final prosthesis. **D,** Excellent esthetic and functional result.

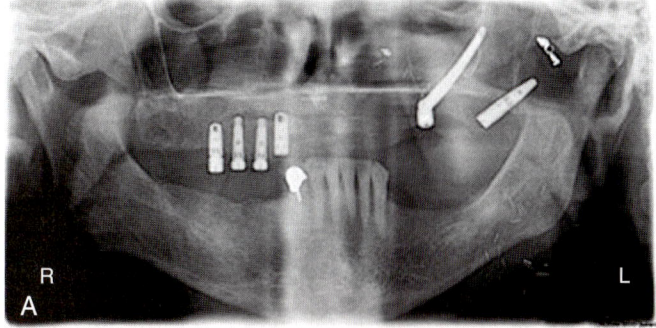

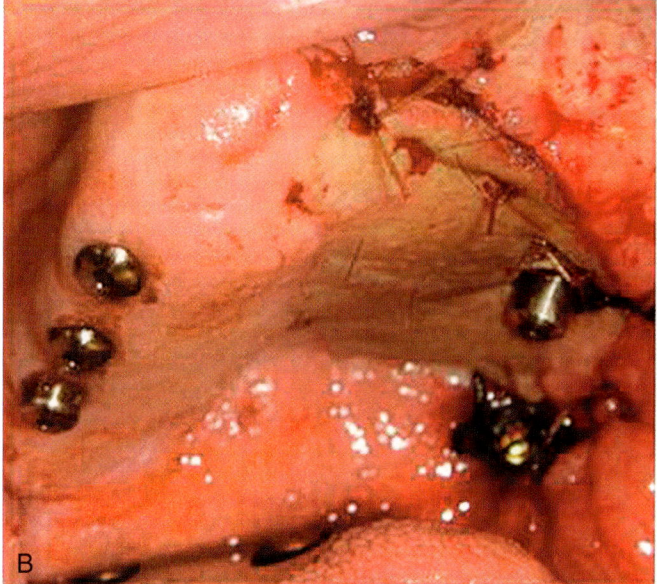

Fig. 23-15 ■ **A,** Zygoma implant plus pterygoid implant with contralateral conventional implants. **B,** Zygoma implant and pterygoid implants penetrating the radial forearm flap for reconstruction after left maxillectomy. (Courtesy David Hirsch, New York.)

SPECIFIC TREATMENT AND TECHNIQUES

SURGICAL TECHNIQUE IN TUMOR PATIENTS

Following maxillectomy, access to the body of the zygoma is rarely a problem, and a Weber-Fergusson approach makes soft tissue retraction easy. A slot is created in the remnant of the ZMB and extended up to the thicker bone of the body of the zygoma, where a flat boss is created, as in the sinus slot technique. The flat boss can be enlarged and angled anteriorly if a second zygoma implant is to be placed. The orientation of double ipsilateral zygoma implants should allow at least 3 mm of bone between each implant. Correct angulation is facilitated by the use of a provisional denture prosthesis or surgical guide, which helps avoid the tendency to place the fixture heads too far to the buccal side. Smooth or nontextured machined-surface zygoma implants offer the advantage of a less sticky surface for secretions to cling to within the open maxillectomy defect.

POSTOPERATIVE CARE

A maxillectomy patient who has undergone placement of zygomatic implants requires no special care for the implants beyond the normal care of the hospitalized patient.

SUMMARY

The zygoma implant is an underused resource that provides a cost-effective, single-stage solution to the problem of inadequate posterior maxillary bone as a result of either atrophy or maxillectomy. A patient with maxillary atrophy can avoid the many months spent waiting for consolidation of a sinus lift bone graft, followed by the time necessary for implant integration before restoration. A maxillectomy patient can experience a greatly expedited and simplified treatment plan that will enable prosthesis construction in as short a time as possible following tumor resection. In both the atrophic and maxillectomy groups of patients, the zygoma implant does not entail any greater prosthetic complexity or cost.

PEARLS AND PITFALLS

The Zygoma Implant in Patients with Posterior Maxillary Atrophy
- Be sure that patients can open their mouth adequately.
- Patients with limited mouth opening or the presence of mandibular dentition may be managed by angling the implant anteriorly so that the fixture emerges at the first premolar area.
- Plan for rigid cross-arch fixation to multiple other implants.
- Before placing the implant, loosen and retighten the screw that retains the transfer abutment. The screw is very tight and can be difficult to remove once the implant is in position.
- Self-retaining plastic photographic cheek retractors are helpful during surgery.
- Design the alveolar crestal incision such that it lies slightly to the palatal side of the crest so that attached tissue will be included in the flap. The attached gingival tissue will ultimately lie lateral to the fixture platform. Mucogingival stress around the platform can potentially allow salivary leakage around the implant into the maxillary sinus.
- Drill the hole for the implant completely through the zygoma so that the bit can be palpated percutaneously.
- Guide the implant into the hole created in the zygoma by viewing through the lateral opening or slot. The implant will tend to be self-directed posterior and medial to the drilled hole. Be sure that the implant has not passed posterior to the zygomatic body into soft tissues.
- The prosthetic design should minimize posterior cantilevering behind the zygomatic implant/

Zygoma Implants in Maxillectomy Patients
- Avoid the tendency to position the fixture head too far to the buccal side. This necessitates extension of the final prosthesis laterally, where it can abrade the buccal mucosa.
- Zygoma implants in maxillectomy patients are often oriented so that the fixture head lies anterior to the usual second premolar–first molar region. This can facilitate placement.
- Previously treated maxillectomy patients often have trismus, which limits the angulation of the instrumentation. Re-opening the Weber-Fergusson facial incision may be helpful.

REFERENCES

1. Weischer T, Schlettler D, Mohr C: Titanium implants in the zygoma as retaining elements after hemimaxillectomy, *Int J Oral Maxillofac Implants* 12:211-214, 1997.

2. Landes CA: Zygoma implant–supported midfacial prosthetic rehabilitation: a 4-year follow-up study including assessment of quality of life, *Clin Oral Implants Res* 16:313-325, 2005.

3. Rigolizzo M, Camilli J, Francischone C, et al: Zygomatic bone: anatomic basis for osseo-integrated implant anchorage, *Int J Oral Maxillofac Implants* 20:441-447, 2005.

4. Higuchi KW: The zygomaticus fixture: an alternative approach for implant anchorage in the posterior maxilla, *Ann R Australas Coll Dent Surg* 15:28-33, 2000.

5. Brånemark P-I, Gröndahl K, Öhrnell L-O, et al: Zygoma fixture in the management of advanced atrophy of the maxilla: technique and long-term results, *Scand J Plast Reconstr Surg Hand Surg* 38:70-85, 2004.

6. Hirsch J-M, Öhrnell L-O, Henry PJ, et al: A clinical evaluation of the zygoma fixture: one year of follow-up at 16 clinics, *J Oral Maxillofac Surg* 62(Suppl 2):22-29, 2004.

7. Kahnberg KE, Henry P, Hirsch J-M, et al: Clinical evaluation of the zygoma implant: 3-year follow-up at 16 clinics, *J Oral Maxillofac Surg* 65:2033-2038, 2007.

8. Malevez C, Abarca M, Durdu F, et al: Clinical outcome of 103 consecutive implants: a 6-48 month follow-up study, *Clin Oral Implants Res* 15:18-22, 2004.

9. Petruson B: Sinuscopy in patients with titanium implants in the nose and sinuses, *Scand J Plast Reconstr Surg Hand Surg* 38:86-93, 2004.

10. Davó R, Malevez C, López-Orellana C, et al: Sinus reactions to immediately loaded zygoma implants, a clinical and radiographic study, *Eur J Oral Implantol* 1:53-60, 2008.

11. Brånemark P-I, Higuchi KW, Oliveira MF: *Rehabilitation of complex cleft palate and craniomaxillofacial defects: the challenge of Bauru*, Carol Stream, Ill., 1999, Quintessence pp 31-37.

12. Boyes-Varley JG, Howes DG, Davidge-Pitts KD, et al: A protocol for maxillary reconstruction following oncology resection using zygomatic implants, *Int J Prosthodont* 20:521-531, 2007.

13. Schmidt BL, Pogrel MA, Young CW, et al: Reconstruction of extensive maxillary defects using zygomaticus implants, *J Oral Maxillofac Surg* 62(Suppl 2):82-89, 2004.

14. Bedrossian E, Sullivan RM, Fortin Y, et al: Fixed-prosthetic implant restoration of the edentulous maxilla: a systematic pretreatment evaluation method, *J Oral Maxillofac Surg* 66:112-122, 2008.

15. Shulman LB, Jensen OT: Academy of Osseointegration, Sinus Graft Consensus Conference. *Int J Oral Maxillofac Implants* 13(Suppl):4, 1998.

16. Graziani F, Donos N, Needleman I, et al: Comparison of implant survival following sinus floor augmentation procedures with implants placed into pristine posterior maxillary bone: a systematic review, *Clin Oral Implants Res* 15:677-682, 2004.

17. Aparicio C, Perales P, Rangert B: Tilted implants as an alternative to maxillary sinus grafting: a clinical, radiologic, and periotest study, *Clin Implant Dent Relat Res* 3:39-49, 2001.

18. Krekmanov L, Kahn M, Rangert B, et al: Tilting of posterior mandibular and maxillary implants for improved prosthesis support, *Int J Oral Maxillofac Implants* 15:405-414, 2000.

19. Malo P, Rangert B, Nobre M: All-on-4 immediate-function concept with Brånemark System implants for completely edentulous maxillae: a 1-year retrospective clinical study. *Clin Implant Dent Relat Res* 7(Suppl 1):S88-S94, 2005.

20. Zampelis A, Rangert B, Heijl L: Tilting of splinted implants for improved prosthodontic support: a two-dimensional finite element analysis, *J Prosthet Dent* 97(6 Suppl):S35-S43, 2007.

21. Calandriello R, Tomatis M: Simplified treatment of the atrophic posterior maxilla via immediate/early function and tilted implants: a prospective 1-year clinical study, *Clin Implant Dent Relat Res* 7(Suppl 1):S1-S12, 2005.

22. Maló P, Nobre Mde A, Petersson U, et al: A pilot study of complete edentulous rehabilitation with immediate function using a new implant design: case series, *Clin Implant Dent Relat Res* 8:223-232, 2006.

23. Zide BM, Swift R: How to block and tackle the face, *Plast Reconstr Surg* 101:840-851, 1998.

24. Stella J, Warner M: Sinus slot technique for simplification and improved orientation of zygomaticus dental implants: a technical note, *Int J Oral Maxillofac Implants* 15:889, 2000.

25. Boyes-Varley JG, Howes DG, Lownie JF, et al: Surgical modifications to the Brånemark zygomaticus protocol in the treatment of the severely resorbed maxilla: a clinical report, *Int J Oral Maxillofac Implants* 18:232-237, 2003.

26. Watziger F, Birkfellner W, Wanschiz F, et al: Placement of endosteal implants in a zygoma after maxillectomy: a cadaver study using surgical navigation, *Plast Reconstr Surg* 107:659-667, 2001.

27. Panagos P, Hirsch DL: Resection of a large, central hemangioma with reconstruction using a radial forearm flap combined with zygomatic and pterygoid implants, *J Oral Maxillofac Surg* 67:630-636, 2009.

28. Hu YJ, Hardiano A, Li SY, et al: Reconstruction of a palatomaxillary defect with vascularized iliac bone combined with a superficial inferior epigastric artery flap and zygomatic implants as anchorage, *Int J Oral Maxillofac Surg* 36:854-857, 2007.

29. Bowden JR, Flood TR, Downie IP: Zygomaticus implants for retention of nasal prosthesis after rhinectomy, *Br J Oral Maxillofac Surg* 44:54-56, 2006.

Efficacy of rhBMP-2 in Association with Dental Implants

Chapter 24

Robert Gilbert Triplett, Mark E. Wong

Endosteal dental implants are highly successful, with numerous reports of success rates in the range of 89% to 99% for both individual and multiple implants. Attempts to improve these excellent results have been realized by altering the surfaces of titanium implants. Surface modifications have not only improved the long-term success of dental implants but have also allowed earlier loading with functional prostheses. These results have been achieved because the properties of biomaterial surfaces play a critical role in modulating the biologic response of the surrounding tissue. Bone morphogenetic proteins (BMPs) are a family of proteins that have been demonstrated experimentally and clinically to exert a positive effect on bone formation. Its commercial form, recombinant human BMP-2 (rhBMP-2), has undergone extensive scientific investigation and has received approval by the Food and Drug Administration (FDA) as a substitute for autogenous bone in maxillofacial and orthopedic applications. It has been demonstrated clinically to form bone in orthopedic sites (the spine and tibia) and the maxillofacial region, such as defects in the maxillary sinus floor and maxillary alveolar bone. Investigators have recently focused on using this bone induction factor in conjunction with dental and orthopedic implants as a means of accelerating bone healing around implants (osseointegration). A number of well-controlled animal studies have investigated the feasibility of using rhBMP-2 in conjunction with dental implants to accelerate the osseous response of the host and to improve healing in less than optimal sites such as type IV bone.[1]

Surgical placement of dental implants initiates a sequence of cellular and molecular events that represents a combined response of wound healing and fracture repair.[2] Proliferation plus differentiation of osteogenic cells (preosteoblasts) into osteoblasts follows activation of periosteal, perivascular, and endosteal lining cells under the influence of local and systemic growth factors. Osteoblastic differentiation initiates the production and mineralization of osteoid, followed by organization of the bone-implant interface.[3] At times, deficiencies in the healing process may result in delayed healing and compromised implant integration. BMPs have undergone extensive study as factors capable of enhancing bone healing and as a substitute for autogenous bone grafts. BMP-2 has been shown to possess chemotactic properties, which results in the attraction of a variety of cellular elements to the site of implantation, and to be a mitogenic agent, whereby it increases the cellular population of important bone-forming cells.[4] BMP-2 can also influence the differentiation and proliferation of mesenchymal progenitor cells into cells of a chondroblastic and osteoblastic lineage.[5] The mode of action, bone-forming capacity, and safety of rhBMP-2 contained on an absorbable collagen sponge (ACS) have been extensively investigated and are well understood (Box 24-1).[1]

SCIENTIFIC INVESTIGATIONS

In animal models, application of rhBMP-2/ACS resulted in induction of normal bone at the site of implantation. The induced bone undergoes remodeling, assumes the appropriate structure for the site with the defect, and displays anisotropic behavior in response to functional loads. Although earlier studies focused on the structure and biologic activity of this protein, over the past 14 years, additional investigations have used rhBMP-2 to accelerate and improve the quality and quantity of osseointegration. Since BMP is highly water-soluble, methods of delivering and retaining the protein have great physiologic significance. Essentially, rhBMP-2 can be combined with a material in one of two ways. Adsorption is a function of surface energy and is the process by which a protein is retained on the surface of a material by virtue of weak van der Waal forces or stronger covalent bonding. The adsorptive ability of a material is characterized by its wettability and can be improved by increasing the contact angle between the two materials. Incorporation is a different method of combining two substances. In this process, a protein is co-precipitated with another material (usually a ceramic) under physiologic conditions to preserve the bioactivity of the protein. Use of this technique to improve a material's integration within biologic tissue is referred to as biomimetic technology. Both adsorption and incorporation can be used to transport and retain rhBMP-2 within the site of a defect. These processes can be used in conjunction with protein carriers or directly with a treated implant surface.

Carrier technology uses an inert material to transport and contain the protein within a defect site and thereby maintain sufficient physiologic concentrations of BMP for promotion of a clinically significant osteogenic response. Characteristics such as the rate of protein release and carrier degradation play important roles in material selection. Studies using different materials with different geometric properties and different methods of attaching the protein to the carrier have met with varying degrees of success. Several studies have investigated these different mechanisms of conveying rhBMP-2 to an implant site, and the results are described in the next section.

THE EFFECT OF CARRIERS

In an effort to investigate the effect of BMP adsorbed onto a collagen sponge on implant osseointegration, Sykaras and colleagues created an edentulous region in the mandible of dogs and placed rhBMP-2/ACS into chambers of hollow basket, press-fit dental implants.[6] One hundred four 3.5×8 mm implants were used, and the animals were divided into two groups to compare the response of bone formation at 2, 4, 8, and 12 weeks. In the treatment group, a concentration of 0.4 mg/mL of rhBMP-2 was placed into the apical hollow chamber of an implant just before insertion. The control group received only

- Water soluble
- Diffuses away unless bound
- Degraded by local proteases
- Binds to collagen, hydrophilic surfaces
- Burst release may upregulate Noggins
- Recruitment of osteoclastic along with osteogenic cells

the implant without either a sponge or rhBMP-2 (Fig. 24-1). The volume of rhBMP-2 delivered by each implant was 20 μg, and the concentration and dose were determined from previous studies on carrier release kinetics by the manufacturer.[7,8] The collagen sponge retained approximately 95% of the rhBMP-2 during the initial impregnation and released the rhBMP-2 in two phases: an initial "burst" phase within hours of implantation and a second prolonged phase governed by the carrier (ACS) and its geometric characteristics.[9]

Uncomplicated healing followed the surgical procedures in all dogs. At the time of sacrifice, 23 implants (22%) were verified to be lost. There were no differences in failure rates between the rhBMP-2–treated implants and the controls (empty hollow baskets) ($P = .05$). Histologic observations confirmed bone regeneration in both treated and control implants. Minimal bone formation was noted at 2 weeks in both groups, and the collagen sponge appeared to occupy most of the hollow chambers in the experimental group (rhBMP-2/ACS) without signs of degradation or infiltration by connective tissue. Branching organized trabeculae of woven bone were seen filling the defect in both groups. At 4 and 8 weeks, fibrous connective tissue was noted to engulf the collagen sponge, with fibroblasts infiltrating the sponge at the periphery. No evidence of local inflammation was found. Collagen sponge fragments were still evident at 12 weeks, thus suggesting slow degradation of the matrix and gradual replacement by bone. Along the side wall of the implant recipient site, increased amounts of host bone were observed in areas apposing the apical perforation (of the implant) in the rhBMP-2–treated sites.

The histomorphometric results of assessment of bone-implant contact (BIC/%) of the hollow chamber surfaces in direct contact with bone are shown in Figure 24-2. At 2 weeks, no statistical difference was found between the two groups. At 4 and 8 weeks, the experimental group showed significantly more bone apposition than did controls. The results of the BIC comparison between the two groups failed to show a statistical difference between the groups at 2 and 4 weeks, but BIC was higher at 8 and 12 weeks. Even though the treated implants exhibited increased bone fill around the hollow cylinders, the area of regenerated bone was statistically lower than the area in the initial host site. This incongruous finding may be due to the walls of the titanium implant preventing the osteoblast progenitor cells from penetrating into the hollow portion of the implant. Another study used histomorphometric and radiographic imaging to evaluate the effect of rhBMP-2 on osseointegration. It was determined that rhBMP-2/ACS confined to the hollow implant chamber does not improve osseointegration along the implant's outer surface, probably because the chamber walls limit diffusion of the signaling protein. Radiographic evaluation resulted in an overestimation of BIC and poor correlation with histomorphometric data.[10]

Since the optimal carrier for rhBMP-2 is still not known, additional investigations have studied carriers other than ACS. One such study examined a synthetic bioabsorbable carrier for rhBMP-2 that was used in supra-ridge osseous defects around dental implants in the dog mandible.[11] After making a standardized circumferential

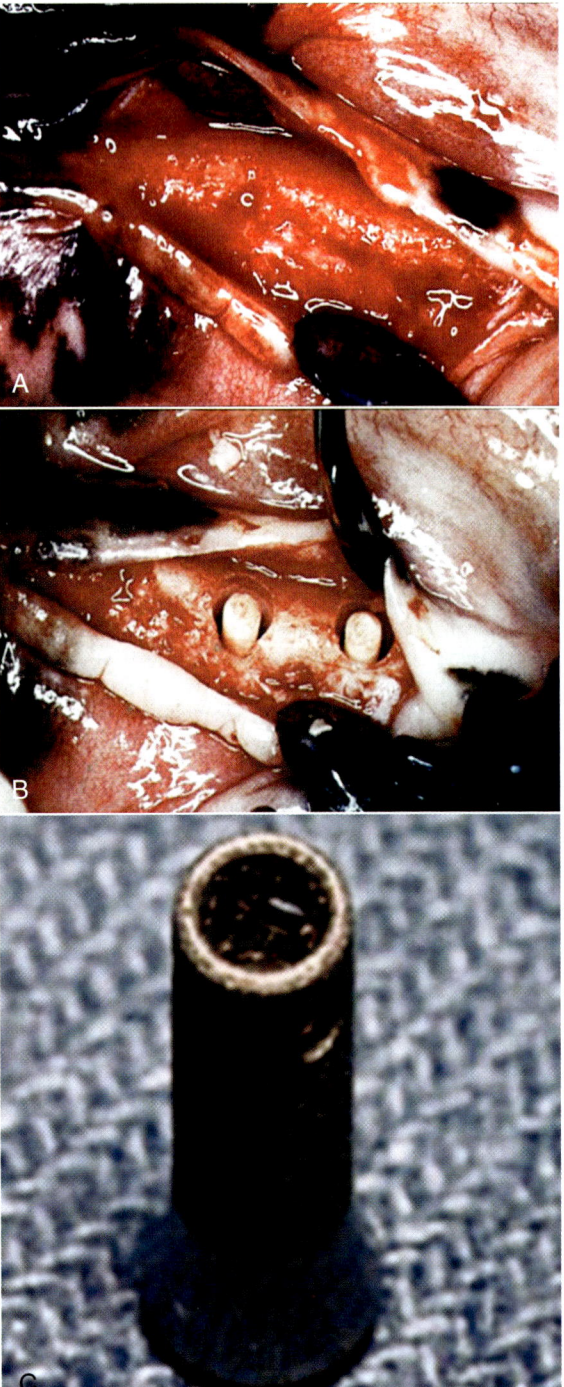

Fig. 24-1 ■ **A,** Dog mandible with alveolar bone exposed in preparation for an implant procedure. **B,** Surgical preparation of the implant site to receive hollow basket implants. **C,** Hollow basket implant that rhBMP-2 could be placed into before insertion onto the mandible.

defect around the coronal 4 mm of each implant, half of the defects received a polylactide/glycolide (PLGA) polymer carrier with or without rhBMP-2, and the other half received a collagen carrier with or without rhBMP-2. In addition, half of the implants were covered with a nonresorbable membrane (expanded polytetrafluoroethylene) to exclude soft tissue, whereas the remaining half were left uncovered. Histomorphometric analysis was performed on the specimens 4 and 12 weeks after implantation to determine the percentage of new bone contact with the implant, the area of new bone, and the percentage of filling of the defect. After 4 weeks, the

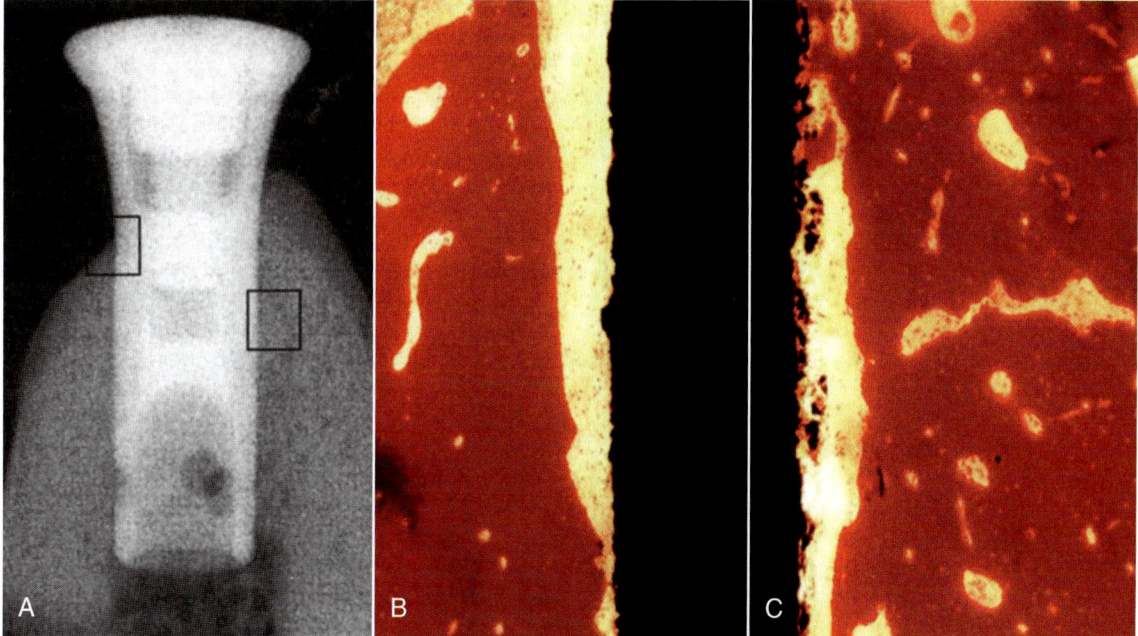

Fig. 24-2 ■ **A,** Radiograph of an implant highlighting two areas of interest. **B,** Photomicrograph showing the relationship of the bone to implant at the coronal portion of the implant. **C,** Photomicrograph showing bone to implant contact mid body of the implant.

rhBMP-2–treated sites with membranes had a significantly higher percentage of BIC, more new bone, and a higher percentage of defect filling than did sites without the rhBMP-2 and without membranes. However, after 12 weeks, there was no statistical difference in membrane-protected sites with or without rhBMP-2 in terms of BIC, new bone formed, or percent defect filling. The PLGA carrier did not perform as well as the ACS carrier when compared between experimental groups.

INCORPORATION OF BONE MORPHOGENETIC PROTEIN WITH COATED IMPLANT SURFACES

Modification of the surface characteristics of titanium implants to improve osteoconductivity has resulted in more rapid dental implant stability. Investigations are under way to combine these surface changes with osteoinductive proteins to further accelerate the bone response. Attempts have recently been made to combine growth factors (rhBMP-2) with the surface of an implant to improve the osseointegrative process. Calcium salts are capable of promoting osteogenic responses through the provision of a calcium-rich local environment. With the development of new technology, calcium phosphate can now be deposited in layers on the implant's surface under physiologic conditions of temperature (37° C) and pH (7.4). This development has allowed the introduction of biomimetic technology into the field of implantology, whereby bioactive agents are incorporated into the three-dimensional crystal latticework following co-precipitation of the protein and mineral salt. This is a reversible chemical reaction that allows the protein (i.e., rhBMP-2) to be gradually released in vivo as the surface layers of the mineral undergo degradation.[12] BMP-2 liberated from biomimetic implant coatings induces and sustains direct ossification in ectopic rat models.[13]

COMPARING METHODS OF BINDING PROTEINS

The efficacy of osteogenic agents such as rhBMP-2 depends on their mode of application. In 2007, Liu and co-workers investigated the osteoinductive efficacy of a BMP-2–bearing calcium phosphate

BOX 24-2	Properties Affecting Protein Absorption (Adhesion of Molecules to a Solid Surface)

- Surface hydrophobicity/surface absorption
- Surface charge—may attack/repel proteins
- Steric concerns
- Surface roughness
- Passive absorption (immersion of material in solution)—early disappearance
- Active absorption (immersion followed by evaporation of solution)
- Burst release

coating as a function of different drug delivery modes.[12,13] In this study, titanium alloy (Ti6Al4V) discs were coated biomimetically with a 22 ± 6.4 (standard deviation) µm layer of calcium phosphate and exposed to three different concentrations of BMP-2 (0.1, 1, and 10 µm/mL). The amount of drug incorporated into the coatings was 0.56 ± 0.03, 0.61 ± 0.05, and 1.70 ± 0.24 µg per implant, respectively.

In group 1, the BMP-2 was adsorbed *onto the surface* of the coating of the implant. In group 2, the BMP-2 was incorporated *into the coating*, and in group 3, the BMP-2 *was both adsorbed onto the coating* and *incorporated into the coating* of the implant. In another group (4), it was adsorbed onto the uncoated metal surface of the implant.

When BMP-2 was adsorbed onto the uncoated metal surface of the titanium alloy implant, it failed to stimulate/induce an osteogenic response. When adsorbed onto a calcium phosphate coating at the same or lower dose, it was osteoinductive. However, the osteoinductivity of the absorbed BMP-2 was significantly lower (5- to 70-fold) than the osteoinductivity of BMP-2 incorporated *into* the calcium phosphate coating (Box 24-2).

When BMP-2 was both adsorbed onto the surface of the implant and incorporated into the calcium phosphate, the osteogenic response was not additive as one might intuitively predict. Instead, the response was markedly compromised by the combination of two methods of protein delivery. At the same dose of BMP, the efficacy was two-fold higher for coatings containing incorporated BMP-2 alone than for those that included BMP-2 adsorbed onto the coating surface. This effect is believed to be linked to burst release of BMP-2 from the adsorbed pool of BMP-2. A burst effect produces a high initial local concentration of BMP-2 that recruits and activates osteoclasts, thereby leading to enhanced bone resorption.[14] The authors also speculated that a rapid supraphysiologic dose of BMP can lead to nonspecific activation and expression of Noggins (homodimers that antagonize BMP activity by blocking the binding epitopes of BMP receptors) that results in inactivation of BMP-2 and depression of bone formation. Studies that measure concentrations of BMP-2 released from adsorbed and incorporated BMP-2 have shown that the concentration liberated into the peri-implant milieu is dramatically different. The entire adsorbed pool of BMP-2 was released by 2 weeks after implantation, whereas the incorporated BMP-2 was more gradually released and much more efficient in stimulating bone formation along the implant surface. Differences in the osteoinductive efficacy of BMP-2 therefore reflect differences in its release kinetics. Most of the adsorbed depot of BMP-2 was liberated in a single, low rapid burst of a few hours' duration, whereas a much smaller remaining portion was released gradually over a period of several days to weeks. BMP-2 is water-soluble and thus susceptible to local protease activity within the interstitial fluid. When it is adsorbed at a low loading dose, most of the released BMP-2 either diffuses away from the implantation site or undergoes nonspecific enzymatic inactivation before it is able to exert an osteoinductive effect. At higher loading doses, however, the peak concentration transiently generated after the initial burst release may be sufficient to promote nonspecific secondary binding to local collagen fibrils.[15] In this case, the osteogenic response is probably elicited by BMP-2 released from a secondary collagen-bound pool or from a small residual from the coating-adsorbed depot, thereby allowing slow release of the protein. When BMP-2 was incorporated into the crystal latticework of a coating at a comparatively lower dose, it was released gradually and at a more constant rate as the coating underwent cell-mediated degradation during the following weeks. The rate of BMP-2 release is believed to be related to the rate of degradation of the coating. Using incorporated BMP, a sustained osteogenic response to a low pharmacologic dose was observed in the implant milieu and proved to be highly efficient in forming bone. The authors concluded that simple manipulation of the mode of drug delivery, such as using a biomimetic calcium phosphate coating, can produce vast improvements in the osteoinductive efficacy of the system.

DISCUSSION

rhBMP-2 has been shown to induce bone regeneration and support dental implant prosthetic reconstruction.[1] Numerous animal and human studies have demonstrated the ability of this signaling protein to induce bone de novo and, in comparative trials with autografts, to stimulate osteogenesis for support of dental implant-borne prostheses as effectively as autografts do.

rhBMP-2 allows surgeons to use an off-the-shelf product to stimulate the regeneration of deficient alveolar bone without the morbidity associated with a host donor site (jaws, hip, or tibia).

In an attempt to improve prosthetic reconstruction of failed and compromised dentition, implants have revolutionized the dentist's ability to restore missing teeth without the progressive loss of alveolar bone associated with conventional removable prostheses. The success rate of dental implants is extremely high and, depending on case selection, ranges from 89% to 99%. Concerted efforts, however, are still being made to further improve implant survival and to accelerate bone formation around dental implants to expedite and improve their mechanical stability and function.

Improvements in surface characteristics have made a significant impact on implant survival, particularly in type III and IV bone. These improvements in the bone-implant interface have also allowed earlier loading (function) of the implant-supported prosthesis.

The ability of rhBMP-2 to stimulate osteogenesis could further enhance the success and early loading of implants and consequently has been a logical area for investigation.

The biologic activity of bone growth factors/signaling proteins such as rhBMP-2 has been summarized as cell attraction/chemotaxis, morphogenesis, proliferation, and osteogenesis. However, there are also other chemical and mechanical factors that affect the ability of growth factors, such as rhBMP-2, to predictably induce bone formation, including (1) binding and release of the protein from a carrier (release kinetics); (2) a microenvironment at the implant site conducive to bone healing; (3) the ability of the cells and growth factors to migrate or diffuse into the microenvironment; (4) space for cells to multiply, differentiate, and form bone; and (5) proper mechanical and biologic factors responsible for bone remodeling.

Currently, rhBMP-2 technology has not developed to the extent that it can be used as a clinically beneficial coating on a dental implant, although early strides have been made in this area. It should be remembered that *unless sufficient physical space is present to allow bone formation, augmentation strategies will not provide any clinical benefit*. The concept of placing rhBMP-2 into an implant site in bone before placement of the implant to overcome poor bone quality has not been substantiated, and experimental efforts using this approach have failed to achieve the desired results.[6]

Currently, Infuse bone graft (rhBMP-2/ACS) is approved by the FDA for clinical use in repairing alveolar defects in the maxilla and augmenting the maxillary sinus floor (bone defect). Off-label use for the reconstruction of other osseous defects is growing rapidly, and Infuse has been used successfully for grafting of alveolar cleft defects, augmentation of alveolar ridges, and reconstruction of segmental mandibular defects (Herford). Carefully controlled trials have demonstrated that Infuse is a good alternative to autogenous bone grafts and performs as well as an autograft in supporting functional prostheses.[1] Whatever the application, it is important that a physically secluded space be available to contain the Infuse (rhBMP-2/ACS) and allow subsequent bone formation.

CONCLUSION

rhBMP-2 is a potent bone signaling molecule for which there is strong scientific evidence of its ability to induce osteogenesis in the maxillofacial skeleton. Its potential for enhancing bone formation in association with dental implants is intriguing. However, to date, the optimal technology for adsorbing or incorporating rhBMP-2 into/onto an implant surface with desirable release kinetics has not been determined. Methods to deliver rhBMP-2 from spaces within dental implants (such as hollow baskets) have not proved beneficial in enhancing osseointegration. Adsorption plus incorporation of the molecule into the implant surface or within a coating has also provided mixed results. Introduction of rhBMP-2 into a secluded space adjacent to a clinically stable, but unloaded dental implant has shown preliminary promise. Clinical trials are in progress and early results suggest that this technique should prove as efficacious as autogenous bone for induction of bone around the implant apex. One of the major challenges in testing the effectiveness of new technology that improves osseointegration is the extremely high success rate of "untreated" implants. Demonstration of a statistically valid, superior outcome with an rhBMP-2–coated implant in a variety of populations, different bone types, and varying bone quantity is a daunting task that requires extremely large sample sizes. The success rate of currently used dental implants will make it more difficult to justify the increased expense of including biomimetic technology to achieve a favorable cost/benefit ratio in the treatment of standard edentulous patients. However, if this technology can allow more rapid loading of implants, improve outcomes in patients with poor-quality bone, and serve as a cost-effective alternative to cases requiring large bone grafts, which are typically performed in a hospital setting, a role for coated implants may be identified.

PEARLS AND PITFALLS

- When rhBMP-2 is implanted into a physiologically active recipient site, it is capable of stimulating bone formation in a manner similar to that of autogenous bone grafts.
- rhBMP-2 stimulates both bone and soft tissue repair. This response can cause significant soft tissue swelling, which can be alarming to patients. Patients should be prepared for this potential postoperative occurrence.
- Space must be available for mesenchymal stem cells to migrate into an osseous defect for differentiation, proliferation, and secretion of osteoid. In the absence of a secluded space, the osteogenic response will be attenuated.
- The suggestion that rhBMP-2/ACS, placed into an implant site at the time of implantation, will improve osseointegration has not been demonstrated in animal studies.

- Implantation of rhBMP-2 into poor-quality bone in the maxillofacial region would (intuitively) seem reasonable. However, no published studies have validated this assumption.
- BMP is water-soluble, and therefore methods of retaining and promoting sustained release of the protein over a period of weeks is essential for a clinically significant osteogenic response.
- Adsorption of rhBMP-2 onto the surface of dental implants may activate both osteoblastic and osteoclastic activity, and evidence of a net beneficial effect is still pending.
- The negative effects of adsorbed rhBMP-2 may be mitigated by using higher doses of BMP or by incorporating BMP into the structure of an implant coating with the use of biomimetic technology.

REFERENCES

1. Triplett RG, Nevins MR, Marx RE, et al: Pivotal, randomized, parallel evaluation of recombinant human bone morphogenetic protein-2/absorbable collagen sponge and autogenous bone graft for maxillary sinus floor augmentation, *J Oral Maxillofac Surg* 67:1947-1960, 2009.
2. Caplan AI, Goldberg VM: Principles of tissue engineered regeneration of skeletal tissues, *Clin Orthop Relat Res* 367(Suppl):512-516, 1999.
3. Chappard D, Aguado E, Hure G, et al: The early remodeling phases around titanium implants: a histomorphometric assessment of bone quality in a 3-and 6-month study in sheep, *Int J Oral Maxillofac Implants* 14:189-196, 1999.
4. Wang EA, Rosen V, D'Allesandro JS, et al: Recombinant human bone morphogenetic protein induces bone formation, *Proc Natl Acad Sci U S A* 87:2220-2224, 1990.
5. Wozney JM: The bone morphogenetic protein family and osteogenesis, *Mol Reprod Dev* 32:160-167, 1992.

6. Sykaras N, Triplett RG, Nunn ME, et al: Effect of recombinant human bone morphogenetic protein-2 on bone regeneration and osseointegration, *Clin Oral Implants Res* 12:339-349, 2001.
7. Wikesjo UM, Guglielmoni P, Promsudthi A, et al: Periodontal repair on dogs: effect of rhBMP-2 concentration on regeneration of alveolar bone and periodontal attachment, *J Clin Periodontol* 16:392-400, 1999.
8. Sigurdsson TJ, Nygaard L, Tatakis DN, et al: Periodontal repair in dogs: evaluation of rhBMP-2 carriers, *Int J Periodontics Restorative Dent* 16:524-537, 1996.
9. Uludag H, D'Augusta D, Palmer R, et al: Characterization of rhBMP-2 pharmacokinetics implanted with biomaterial carriers in the rat ectopic model, *J Biomed Mater Res* 46:193-202, 1999.
10. Sykaras N, Woody RD, Iacopino AM, et al: Osseointegration of dental implants complexed with rhBMP-2: a comparative histomorphometric and radiographic evaluation, *Int J Oral Maxillofac Implants* 19:667-678, 2004.

11. Jones AA, Buser D, Schenk R, et al: The effect of rhBMP-2 around endosseous implants with and without membrane in the canine model, *J Periodontol* 77:1184-1193, 2006.
12. Liu Y, Huse RO, deGroot K, et al: Delivery mode and efficacy of BMP-2 in association with implants, *J Dent Res* 86:84-89, 2007.
13. Liu Y, Enggist L, Kuffer AF, et al: The influence of BMP-2 and its mode of delivery on the osteoconductivity of implant surfaces during the early phase of osseointegration, *Biomaterials* 28:2677-2686, 2007.
14. Ruhe PQ, Boerman DC, Russel FG, et al: Controlled release of rhBMP-2 loaded poly(dl-lactic-co-glycolic acid)/calcium phosphate cement composites in vivo, *J Control Release* 106:162-171, 2005.
15. Hartman EH, Vehof JW, Spauwen PH, et al: Ectopic bone formation in rats: the importance of the carrier, *Biomaterials* 26:1829-1835, 2005.

Chapter 25

Computer-Assisted Implant Surgery

Edward R. Schlissel

The increased availability of computed tomography (CT) and the development of adjunctive software have provided surgeons with new techniques for planning and placement of dental implants. These procedures provide improvements in safety, predictability, and accuracy. Surgeons, restorative dentists, and patients all benefit from the use of reconstructed images, analysis and planning software, and guides for precise osteotomy and placement of implants. Acceleration of prosthetic reconstruction is often possible.

The combination of CT scanning and planning software has also assisted the shift in treatment planning from one that is implant based to one based on the final restoration. By including the biologic principles of implant integration, bone vitality, and soft tissue response, it is possible to develop a plan of treatment that is more likely to result in pleasing functional and esthetic outcomes. The need for hard or soft tissue augmentation of the implant site and for angulated abutments and the possibility of accelerated provisional restoration may be determined before surgery. All these factors are of benefit to the patient, surgeon, and restorative dentist.

ETIOPATHOGENESIS/CAUSATIVE FACTORS

Dental implants must be placed in locations that are biologically suitable and acceptable for restorative needs. Frequently, these sites have questionable bone volume and are in proximity to other teeth or anatomic structures. Undesirable outcomes include damage to the inferior alveolar nerve (IAN), fenestration of buccal or lingual bone, collisions with the roots of teeth, and improper angulation. Planning of implant location before surgery and guidance during osteotomy and implant placement reduce the risk for error.

DIAGNOSTIC STUDIES

For optimal benefit, a sequence of planning appointments is required for collection of data and communication between the surgeon and restorative dentist before and during treatment. It is desirable for all dentists and their office staff involved in the process to understand the benefits of CT-guided planning and placement. They must know the sequence and timing of care and the cost for scans, planning software, and service, as well as surgical and restorative fees. By planning the case to completion before beginning treatment it is much more likely that the proposal to the patient will be accurate and that alternatives can be considered realistically.

The primary focus of implant-based restoration is the final prosthesis. The functional and esthetic requirements must be determined early in the planning process, and the expected results of treatment and alternative plans that may be available must be discussed with the patient.

A comprehensive examination of the oral cavity and a review of systemic conditions and medications must be conducted to determine suitability for implant surgery. The examination should also include an assessment of occlusion. Periapical and panoramic radiographs are helpful, but not definitive. It is not always possible to make accurate three-dimensional evaluations from two-dimensional images. A comparison of conventional radiographs and CT scan data shows the difference (Fig. 25-1).

The customary assessments for implant placement are adequate in some instances, typically when esthetic demands are not high, but to take advantage of planning software and to make a plan based on the desired restoration, additional steps are required. These steps involve making an accurate provisional restoration that can be used as a scanning guide during the CT process.

The foundation of planning for guided implant placement is a set of accurate study models precisely articulated in the correct occlusal relationship. It is important to evaluate the occlusion in maximum intercuspation and in lateral and protrusive excursion. Anticipating occlusal forces can help avoid complications after delivery of the restoration. This procedure is valuable for both single-tooth restorations and full-arch prostheses.

It is the choice of the dentist whether to make the impression with an elastomeric material such as polyvinyl siloxane (PVS) or irreversible hydrocolloid (alginate) and whether to pour the casts with improved stone or die stone. One advantage offered by using PVS is that multiple pours may be made from the same impression, which will be more consistently accurate than reproducing casts made from alginate impressions. This benefit outweighs the increased cost of the material. Dental die stone offers some advantages over improved stone. Die stone is less subject to setting expansion and is more resistant to damage during handling or fitting of the surgical guide.

TREATMENT/RECONSTRUCTIVE GOALS

At the completion of implant integration and placement of the final restoration, the patient must have acceptable function, esthetics, and comfort. The goal of using computer-assisted implant surgery is to make the planning process more predictable and to achieve the desired outcomes more easily and with a reduction in risk.

Current understanding, gained through long clinical experience, provides guidelines for the location and dimensions of implants. The general consensus is that the minimum distance between an implant and an adjacent natural tooth should be 1.5 mm. The distance between implants should be no less than 3 mm. The minimal thickness of bone surrounding the implant on the facial and lingual aspects should be a minimum of 1.0 to 1.5 mm.

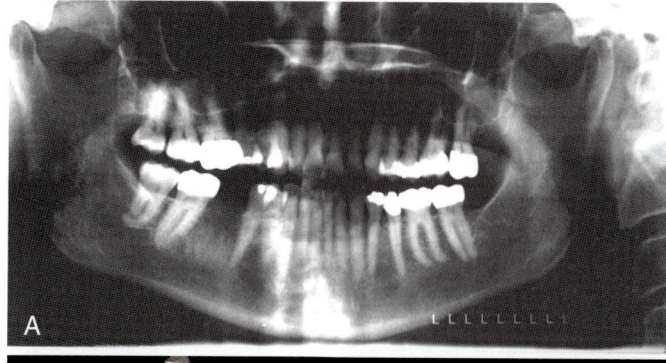

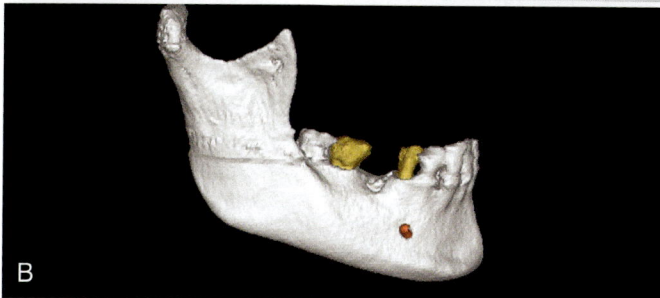

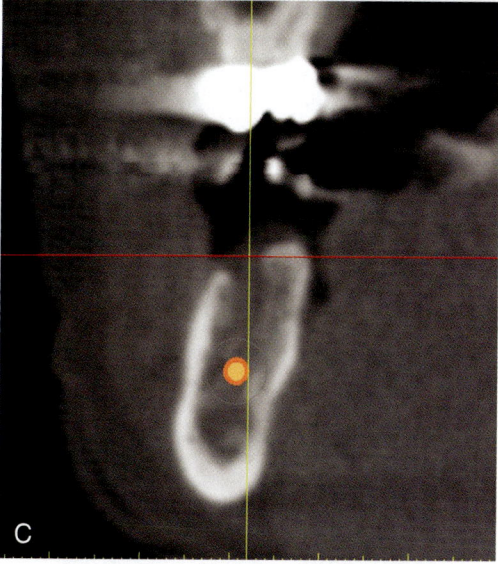

Fig. 25-1 ■ **A,** Panoramic radiograph. **B,** Three-dimensional reconstruction of a cone beam computed tomography (CBCT) scan. **C,** Cross-sectional image from a reconstructed CBCT scan.

SPECIFIC TREATMENT AND TECHNIQUES

The scanning appliance provides the information needed to identify the location of prosthetic teeth and the soft tissue surface. Many popular planning programs use a "double-scan" process. Reference markers are embedded in the appliance or attached to it before the scan is made. The patient is scanned while wearing the appliance, and then the appliance is removed and scanned by itself outside the mouth at a different beam intensity. The software uses the reference markers to correlate the images. With this technique, denture base resin and artificial teeth, which are rendered poorly with scans made at settings to examine bone, can be reconstructed for planning purposes. Soft tissue dimensions may be calculated as the difference between the scan appliance and bone. For this to be accurate, the scan appliance must be well adapted to the soft tissue. One diagnostic model should be used to create an appliance to be worn by the

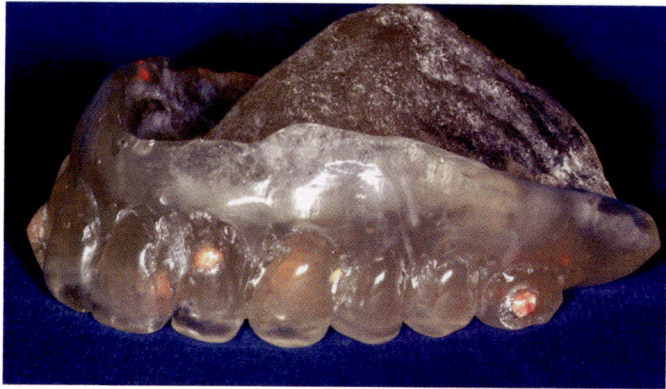

Fig. 25-2 ■ Acrylic resin duplicate denture with gutta percha markers.

patient during the CT scan. Another model should be left unmodified as part of the patient's records. The third model may be used for fabrication of a provisional restoration.

The number and location of markers depend on the software program. The specific nature of the markers should be determined before the scanning appliance is fabricated. Often, the markers are small pieces, approximately 1 mm in diameter, of gutta percha or lead foil (Fig. 25-2).

Some planning software can accommodate a radiopaque guide, which is commonly used in a "single-scan" technique. This process can be accurate but is more labor intensive and may introduce scatter into the CT image if too much barium sulfate is incorporated into the guide. Most radiopaque scan guides are composed of a combination of 10% to 20% barium sulfate by weight in methylmethacrylate. Unless carefully controlled, contraction during polymerization can create gaps at the tissue surface, which would result in poor characterization of the soft tissue surface in the reconstructed image. It is also critical to control the distribution of the barium sulfate in the acrylic resin. Poor mixing before addition of the monomer results in a scan appliance that is not homogeneous and has spots of high radiolucency. This may lead to undesired scatter in the scan data and thus mask critical structures (Fig. 25-3).

The composition and design of the scanning appliance depend on the software that will be used for planning. Consultation with the scan provider and laboratory is essential in the early stages of treatment to avoid problems. Examples of scanning software are Simplant (Materialise, Leuven, Belgium) and NobelGuide (Nobel Biocare, Zurich, Switzerland).

The scan guide prosthesis may be made of conventional denture teeth and resin and may include some wax as long as it is dimensionally stable. If the scan appliance makes contact with soft tissue, careful attention must be directed to adaptation of the intaglio surface. This is of particular concern if an existing denture is used as a scan appliance. If there is any concern about the adaptation, a hard reline should be done before the scan.

It is possible to use a denture record base and final wax-up as a scanning appliance. When planning a full-arch restoration for the maxilla, this is advantageous because it allows assessment of the vertical dimension of occlusion, lip support, need for prosthetic replacement of soft tissue, and the relationship of the upper lip to the alveolar ridge in the high smile position. All these factors are critical in planning the final prosthesis and offering the patient an accurate prediction of the outcome. The arrangement of the teeth for the scan appliance should be approved by the patient and may be incorporated into the final restoration.

It is also possible to use a provisional fixed partial denture as a scanning appliance. Arrangements must be made for the restoration

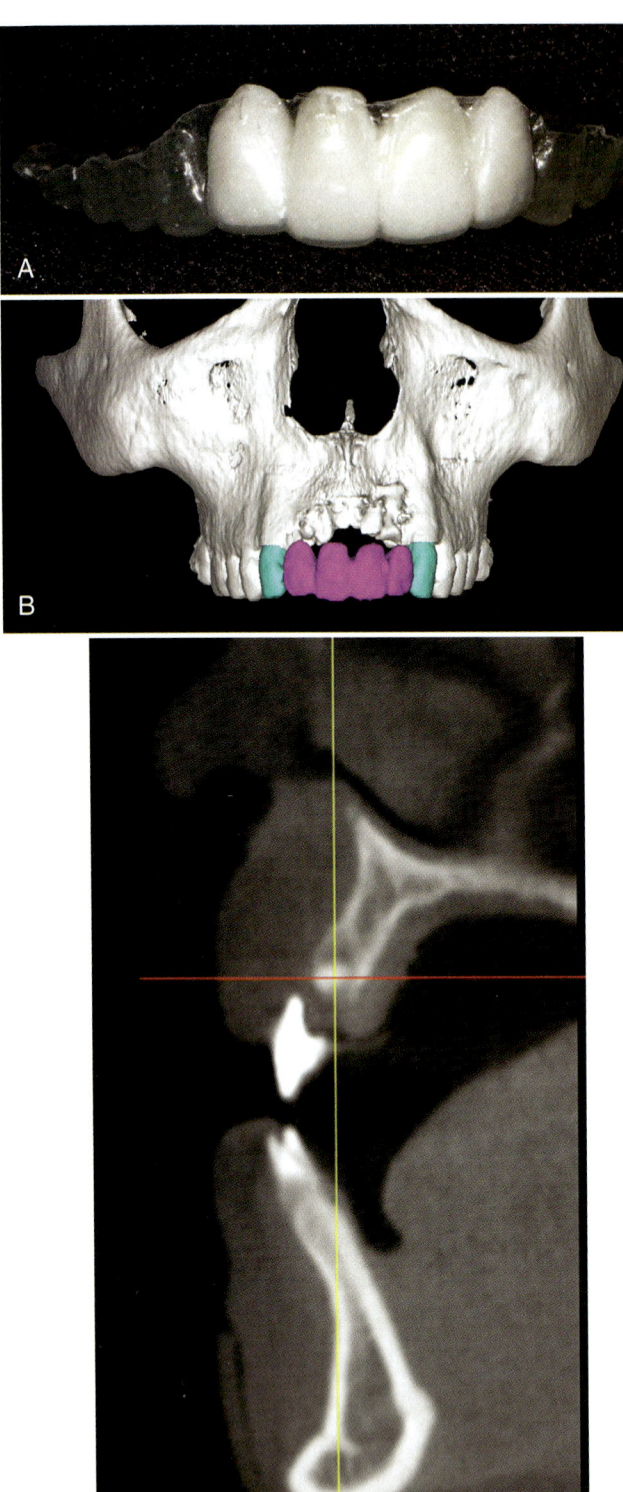

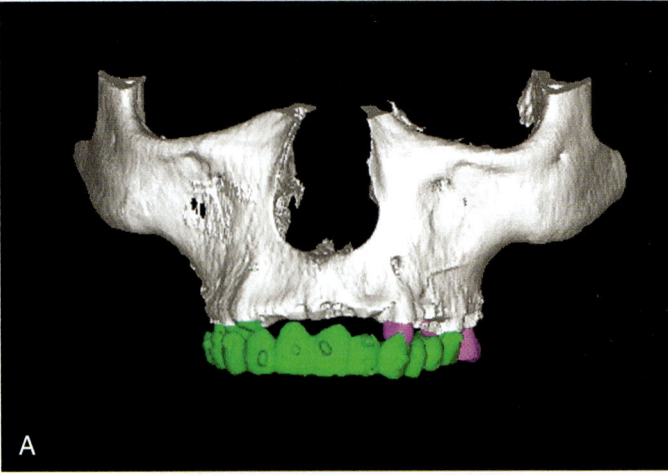

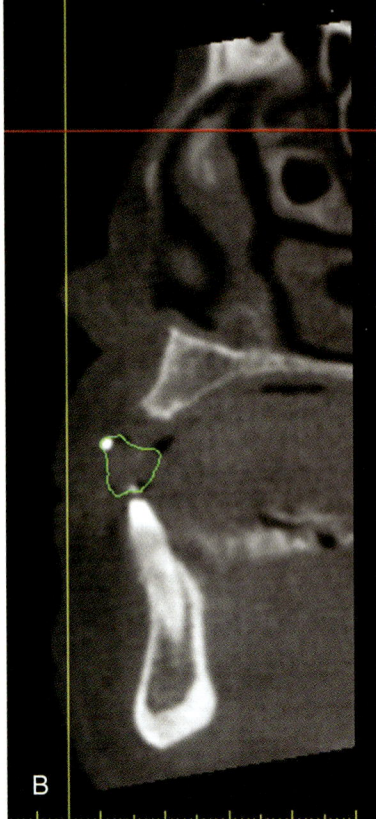

Fig. 25-4 ■ **A,** Three-dimensional reconstruction of a cone beam computed tomography (CBCT) scan with a resin provisional fixed partial denture (note the markers on the surface). **B,** Cross-sectional image from a reconstructed CBCT scan (note the radiopaque marker within the image of the provisional fixed partial denture).

Fig. 25-3 ■ **A,** Radiopaque scan guide. **B,** Three-dimensional reconstruction of a cone beam computed tomography (CBCT) scan with a radiopaque scan guide. **C,** Cross-sectional image from a reconstructed CBCT scan.

to be removed from the patient's mouth during the scan visit so it may be "double-scanned" outside the mouth. A common plan is for the patient to visit the dentist immediately before the scan to have the prosthesis removed and recemented with a product such as paste-consistency denture adhesive. The prosthesis can be removed at the

scan center and be replaced after the scan. The patient would then return to the dentist to have the prosthesis replaced with the appropriate product (Fig. 25-4).

After the scan is completed, the data must be converted into a format that can be used by the planning software. Every product has specific protocols that can be accommodated from the DICOM (digital imaging and communication in medicine) files generated by the scanner. Many dentists, particularly those who have a cone beam computed tomography (CBCT) scanner in their office, prefer to do all image manipulation by themselves. Many other dentists prefer to refer the patient to a scan center, which can also convert the files

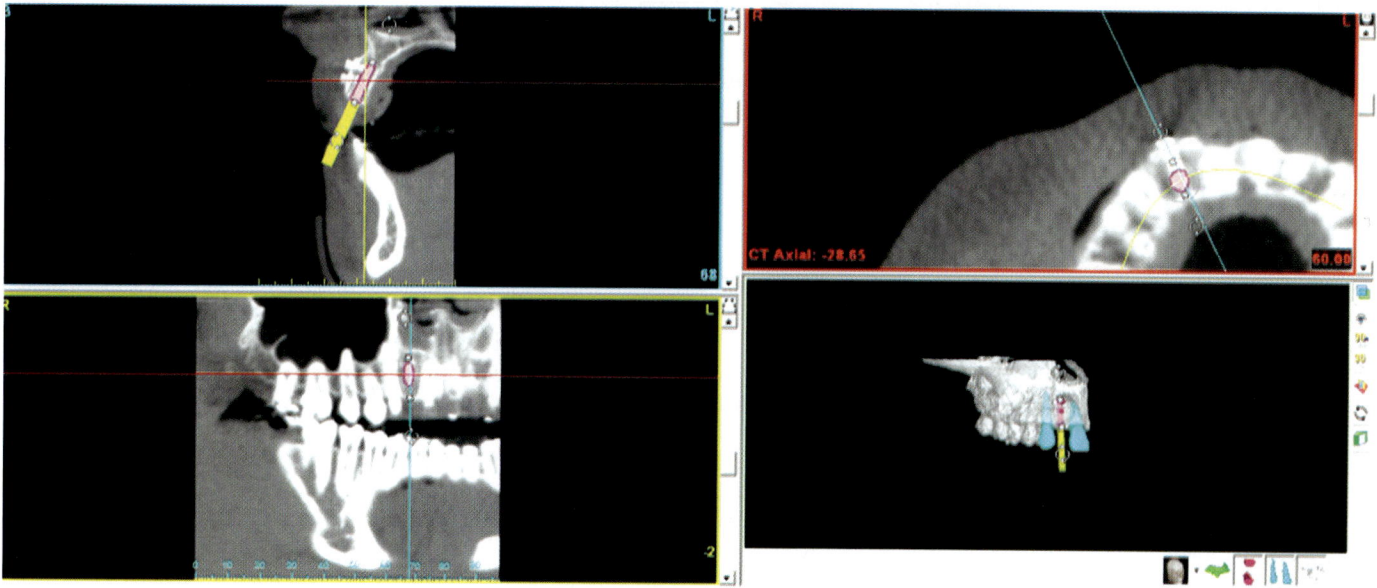

Fig. 25-5 ■ Overview of virtual placement of the implant (note the graft fixation screws, which will be removed before placement of the implant).

for use in scanning software and prepare a preliminary plan of treatment.

After the files have been converted, it is possible to evaluate potential implant sites in the desired prosthetic locations. Virtual implants may be placed, and brand, diameter, shape, and length may be selected. The suitability of each location may be checked for bone volume and density and angulation relative to the planned restoration. With an understanding of the biologic and functional requirements of implants, the plan may be completed (Fig. 25-5).

Planning software also allows the capture of images and videos. These can be very helpful in communication between the surgeon, restorative dentist, laboratory, and patient. Demonstration of the plan to the patient can be a very powerful tool and can be especially useful in helping the patient understand the procedures to follow. Showing a prospective patient a sample video from another case is a very powerful treatment planning aid. This visual demonstration of the process can be much more compelling than a verbal description.

During the planning process it is possible to identify implant sites that need augmentation. The impact on the course of treatment, the cost to the patient, and the need for provisional restorations may be predicted. This may be invaluable in providing the patient with the choices needed to give informed consent.

There are several options for doing the actual planning. Either the surgeon or the restorative dentist may do the plan, or it may be done through a scanning service.

Whoever does the plan, it should be reviewed by the surgeon and restorative dentist before presenting it to the patient or proceeding with the case. Such review may easily be accomplished through an Internet-based conference.

After the plan for treatment has been completed, it is possible to design and fabricate a surgical guide. For patients who are partially edentulous, the guide is supported by teeth. For patients who are completely edentulous in the arch under treatment, the guide may be supported by soft tissue or bone. The surgeon typically makes the choice of technique.

The accuracy of the guide depends on numerous factors, including the precision of the pretreatment model, the dimensional stability of the guide, accuracy in positioning the guide in the mouth, and

the resolution of the scan. Complete understanding of these factors is required to achieve the expected result.

Tooth-supported guides, which are used for partially edentulous patients, must fit the model and the teeth identically. Inaccuracy of the impression or model may result in a guide that does not fit correctly in the mouth. Care must be taken to produce accurate models and to verify seating of the surgical guide in the mouth before surgery begins.

Guides typically include windows to confirm complete seating on the teeth. If the openings provided by the manufacturer are too small or are in locations that are inaccessible for viewing, they may be enlarged or additional openings made. Care should be taken to not reduce the structural integrity of the guide.

It is critical to compare seating of the guide on the model and on the teeth. If any discrepancy exists, the guides must be adjusted until they are identical. There should be no gaps between the guide and supporting teeth on the model or in the mouth. When fully seated, the guide must be stable and not move when manipulated lightly.

Soft tissue–supported guides are more problematic. The base should fit passively and the flanges at all borders should not extend beyond the vestibule or floor of the mouth. Accurate positioning of the guide may be improved by using an occlusal index. This is done before the surgical appointment on a model made with the surgical guide.

Planning a surgical guide for a fully edentulous arch requires the placement of stabilizing pins or screws. They provide improved stability during osteotomy and implant placement. The design must allow these devices to be placed without interference with implant locations and must be accessible for placement during surgery.

The most challenging cases are patients with minimal alveolar ridge height. Maxillary cases, in which the patient has a flat palatal vault, and mandibular cases, in which the floor of the mouth is high, require particular care in guide placement. It is possible to introduce an error in placement that is greater than the margin of safety included in the planning process. This can result in failure. The use of a bite registration can be helpful. Intraoperative radiographs plus visual inspection of the osteotomy sites is advisable.

Bone-supported guides may be used but require considerable manipulation of the soft tissue. Thin spikes of bone must be identified during planning and accommodated before attempting to seat the guide. If not accounted for through bone reduction or relief of the undersurface of the guide, small protuberances may interfere with accurate seating of the guide, which will result in errors in implant placement.

It is often possible to identify the need for adjustments to the ridge during the planning process. In such cases, a bone reduction guide may be made for use before seating of the surgical guide. CT information may be used to contour the implant sites at the time of implant placement.

Based on the plan developed with software, three items may be produced with photopolymerized resin: a duplicate model of the surgical field, a template for guided reduction of undesired bone protuberances, and an osteotomy/implant placement guide (Fig. 25-6).

The surgical procedure begins with reflection of soft tissue and exposure of the bone beyond the dimensions of the two guides. The bone reduction guide is placed and full seating is confirmed. After contouring the ridge to the levels on the guide, that guide is removed, the osteotomy/placement guide is seated and verified, and implant placement proceeds. If desired, bone anchor screws may be added to stabilize the guide during surgery.

It is important to realize that very small bone contours may be below the resolution of the scan. Palpation of the exposed ridge and evaluation of the seating of the guide are critical steps for accurate placement of the guide.

Surgical guides may be made by laser photopolymerization of liquid resin or computer-aided design/computer-aided manufacturing (CAD/CAM) processes. In both cases, dimensional stability and accuracy of fit are critical. The instructions provided by the manufacturer for handling, storage, and disinfection before surgery must be carefully observed. In general, autopolymerizing resins and conventional light-cured composite resins undergo too much contraction during curing to be accurate and fit passively.

Surgical guides must accommodate the sequence of drill diameters necessary for optimal osteotomy. This can be accomplished either by making a series of guides with guide cylinders of different diameter or by making the guide with a large-diameter master cylinder (typically 5.0 mm) and providing sleeves that are inserted and removed during surgery. The accuracy of both systems is improved with precise placement, prevention of movement during use, and accuracy in manufacturing. Use of multiple guides requires careful attention to the placement of each template (Fig. 25-7).

The depth of osteotomy must be controlled during surgery. Traditional techniques require the surgeon to observe markings on the drills during placement. Several manufacturers have developed

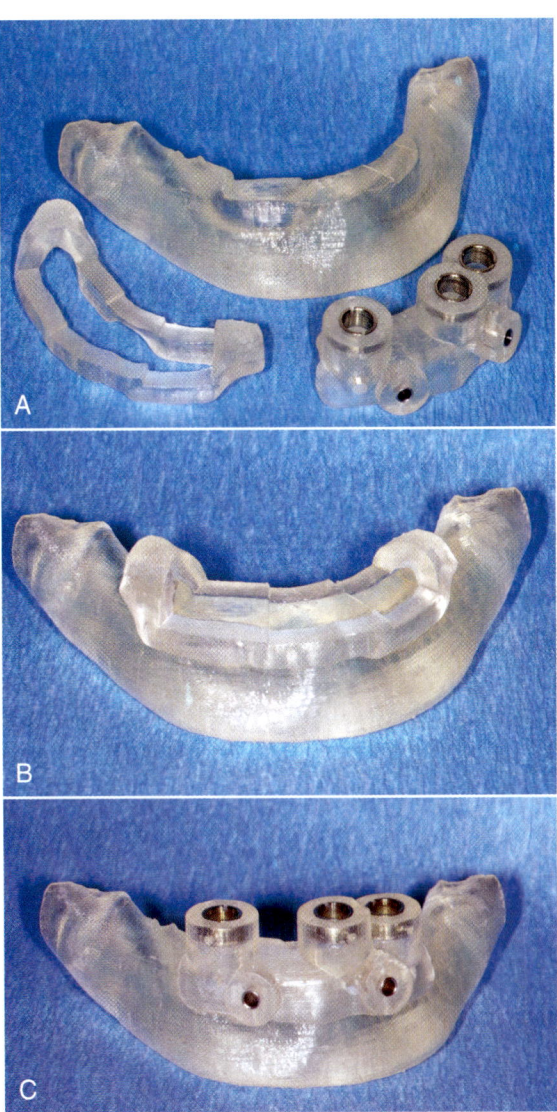

Fig. 25-6 ■ **A,** Replica mandible, bone reduction guide, and osteotomy/placement guide. **B,** Bone reduction guide seated on the model (note the viewing windows to evaluate its placement on the remaining teeth). **C,** Osteotomy/placement guide on the replica mandible (note the sleeves for anchor pins).

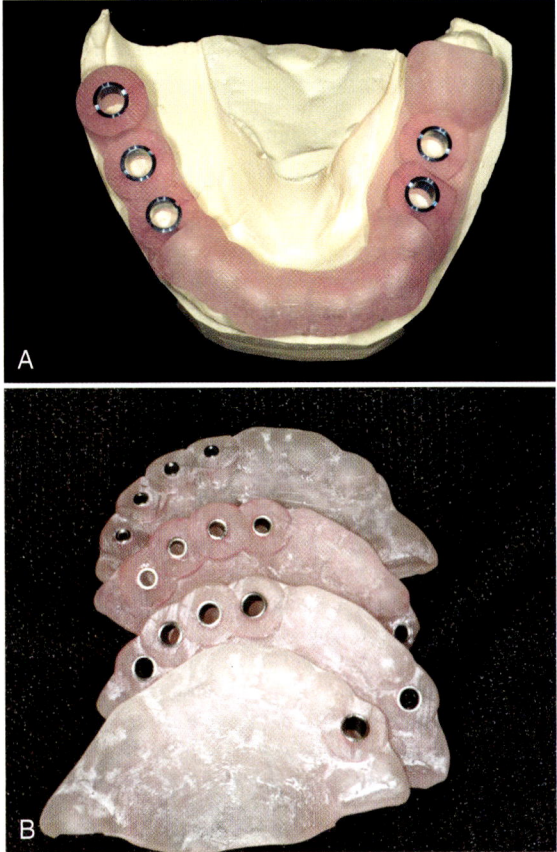

Fig. 25-7 ■ **A,** Osteotomy/placement guide on the model with a single guide for all drills (note the slots in the master cylinders, which may be used to orient implant rotation during placement). **B,** Sequential osteotomy guides, each for a different drill diameter.

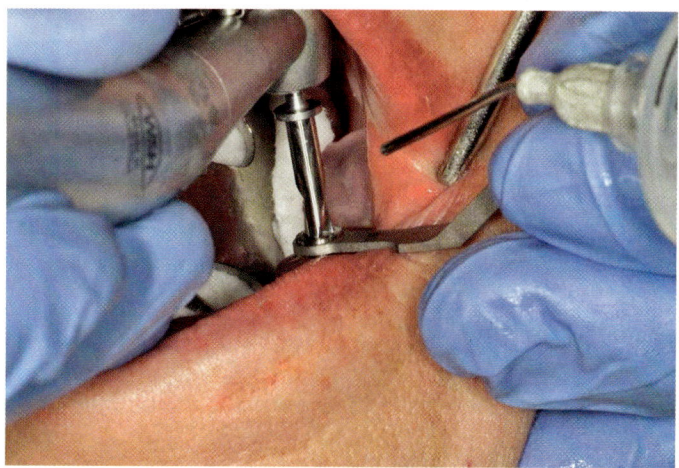

Fig. 25-8 ■ Osteotomy drill being inserted into the placement sleeve, which is within the placement guide (note the depth control collar on the drill).

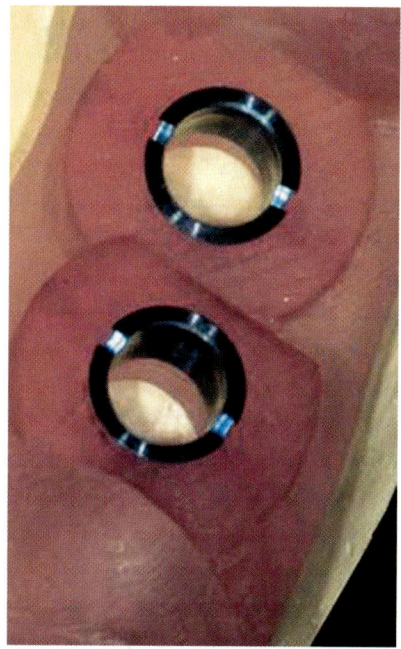

Fig. 25-9 ■ Osteotomy/implant placement guide master cylinders (note the notches, which may be used to align implant rotation during placement).

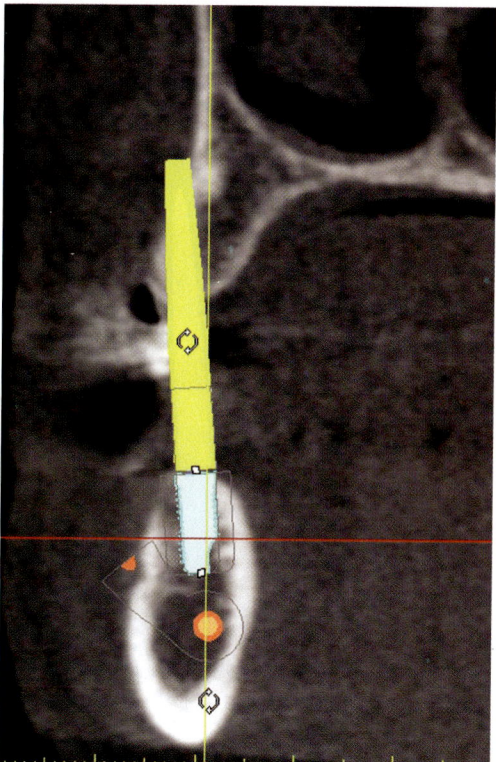

Fig. 25-10 ■ Virtual implant with safety zones around the implant and inferior alveolar nerve.

kits with depth-limiting drills, which makes this step easier to monitor. The planning process results in a drilling sequence that specifies the use of drills of different diameter in the guide until fully seated. This eliminates the need to visually observe the depth of drill penetration and allows more confident use in areas of high concern, such as in the vicinity of the IAN, adjacent teeth, or sites of previous surgery (Fig. 25-8).

It is also possible to deliver implants through a surgical guide. Surgical kits that allow such delivery also provide index marks to locate the position of internal or external retentive features of the implant. This is helpful in cases in which a provisional prosthesis is fabricated before surgery (Fig. 25-9).

The accuracy of the data used for creating a surgical guide is related to the technology and parameters used for the scan and subsequent manipulation during conversion to planning software. Most spiral CT scans achieve a slice thickness of 0.5 mm. Most CBCT scans have a slice thickness of 0.3 mm. These limitations are inherent in the process and must be considered when evaluating implant sites, selecting implant dimensions and location, and determining margins of safety.

Metal objects, including restorations, screws, and plates, can create problems with the scan data. Scatter from metal objects in or close to the area of interest can obscure critical features. The process of filtering the data, which is necessary to decrease the effects of scatter, may reduce the information available for planning. In some cases it may be necessary to remove the metal from the field and repeat the scan.

Planning software allows the identification of critical anatomic structures. The course of the IAN is usually traced. The user of the software may also specify margins of safety around implants. This provides information on collisions between implants, the distance between an implant and adjacent teeth, and proximity to critical structures such as the IAN, incisive canal, and maxillary sinus. Typical settings are 1.5 mm between a tooth and an implant, 3.0 mm between implants, and 2.0 mm between implants and anatomic structures such as the IAN. These dimensions are only a guide and must be adjusted to meet the comfort level of the surgeon, the reliability of the scan data, and the anticipated accuracy in guide positioning. It is prudent to allow additional safety margins for guides that will be placed on soft tissue because the initial position and intraoperative positions may change (Fig. 25-10).

CASE STUDY

Implant manufacturers have developed surgical instrumentation to complement surgical guides constructed with the use of planning software and CT and CBCT data. Some software is used only with one brand of implants; others are adaptable to several brands. All

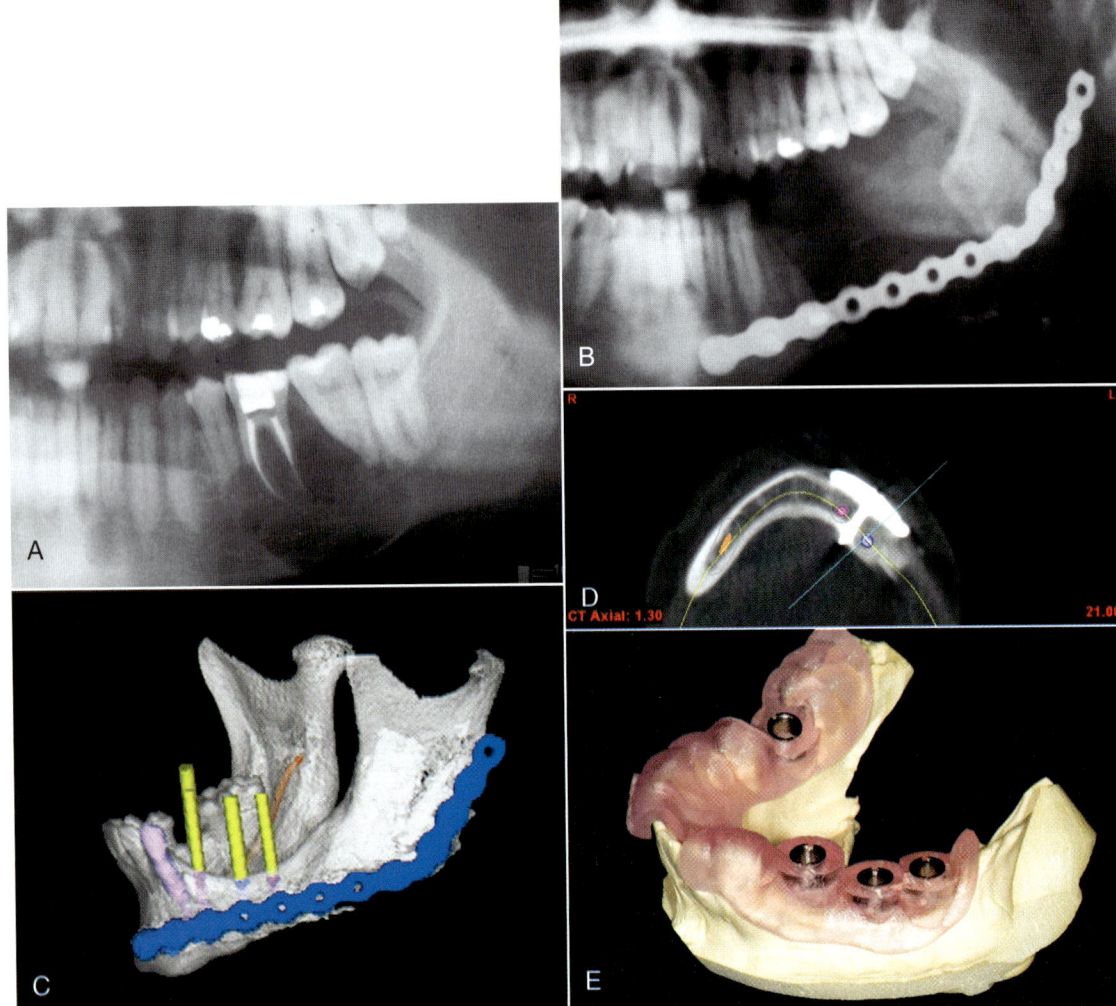

Fig. 25-11 ■ **A,** Panoramic radiograph of a mandibular tumor. **B,** Postsurgical radiograph after tumor resection. **C,** Overview of planned implant locations after healing from mandibular reconstruction. **D,** Axial view of the planned implant locations showing the bar, screw, and safety zones. **E,** Guide for osteotomies and implant placement.

have specific libraries of implants and abutments that can be considered and chosen during the planning process. The clinical protocol for guided placement is specific to the brand of guide and implant, but most steps are common and can be demonstrated by the following case.

A patient was seen by the surgeon with a radiolucency in the left posterior mandible (Fig. 25-11, *A*). The lesion was identified as an ameloblastoma, and surgical resection and placement of a fixation bar followed (Fig. 25-11, *B*). After healing of the wound, an autogenous graft was placed to restore the resected area and provide a base for implants.

After healing, CBCT was performed and a plan for implant placement and restoration was completed (Fig. 25-11, *C* to *E*). It was possible to avoid a fixation screw in the surgical plan and to achieve the desired implant positions and inclinations. The patient requested the placement of an additional implant on the contralateral side, which was unrelated to the original lesion.

Images from the virtual plan were assessed and agreed on by the surgeon and restorative dentist, after which an osteotomy/placement guide was ordered (Fig. 25-11, *F*).

The surgical guide was placed, the position verified, and stability assessed. It was decided that it was not necessary to expose the

surgical sites by elevation of a flap. After excision of soft tissue with a punch, osteotomy proceeded according to the predetermined sequence.

For each diameter drill the specified sleeve was inserted in the master cylinder and the pilot drill advanced to the planned depth. Note the collar on the drill to limit penetration (Fig. 25-11, *G*). After completion of the osteotomy, the first implant was delivered. The surgical handpiece was used until the collar of the implant mount was located just above the master cylinder. Complete seating of the implant was accomplished with a hand driver. The implant mount was left in place to help stabilize the guide (Fig. 25-11, *H*). The next osteotomy was completed and the implants placed in sequence (Fig. 25-11, *I* and *J*) until all implants were placed. Location of the implants was verified with a panoramic radiograph (Fig. 25-11, *K*). The actual locations may be compared with the planned locations.

After osseointegration of the implants, restorations were made (Fig. 25-12). It was the choice of the restorative dentist to make a screw-retained fixed partial denture in the grafted site. Since the patient has no IAN, she has no sensation in that area. It was planned that the prosthesis would be removed periodically for evaluation of the site.

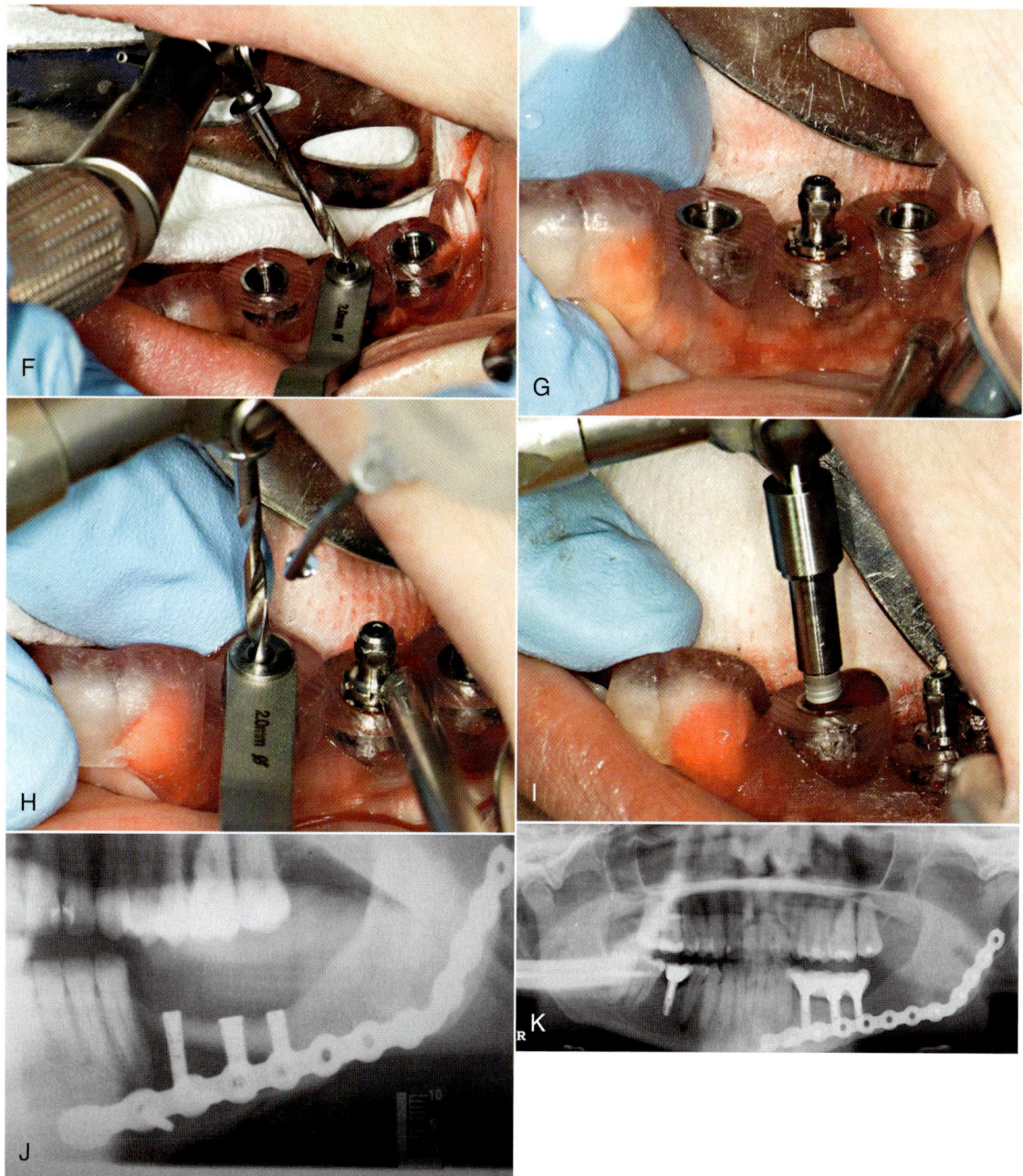

Fig. 25-11, cont'd ▪ **F,** Pilot drill (2.0 mm) and positioning sleeve in the surgical guide (note the depth-limiting collar). **G,** Implant mount seated in the surgical guide. **H,** Second pilot osteotomy. **I,** Second implant being delivered through the guide. **J,** Postsurgical panoramic radiograph showing implants in position and comparison to the virtual plan, part **C. K,** Panoramic radiograph with the restorations in place.

In this case the remaining teeth supported the guide. With soft tissue–supported guides it is possible to compress the underlying soft tissue and tilt the guide during placement of the implants. In patients with a fully edentulous arch, many surgeons prefer to place the most distal implants first and drive them alternately to prevent dislodgment of the guide. The position of the guide should be monitored as each implant is placed.

Guided implant placement is also helpful in areas that are not easily accessible. This illustration shows implants placed in the maxillary tuberosities. The abutments emerge as planned, within the restoration, which is supported by a CAD/CAM-milled titanium bar (see Fig. 25-12).

POSTOPERATIVE CARE

It is often possible to reduce the size of surgical incisions or to complete implant placement with a "flapless" technique. In both cases the postoperative course for the patient is improved over that

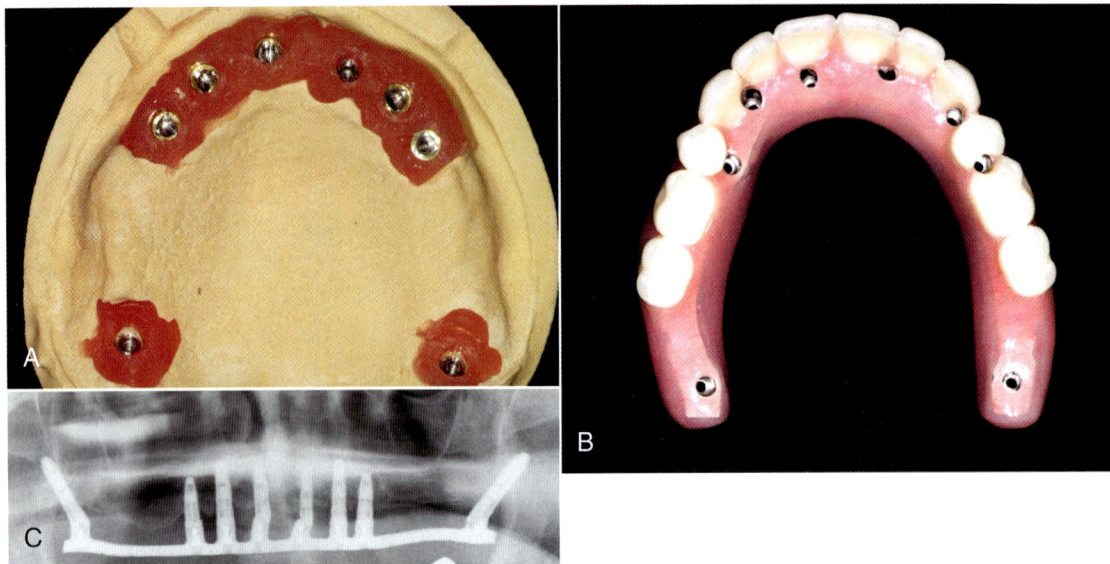

Fig. 25-12 ■ **A,** Gypsum model showing the positions of the implant replicas. **B,** Palatal view of the prosthesis (note the location of the screw access holes). **C,** Panoramic radiograph of the final restoration.

with traditional placement technique. No additional procedures are needed for implants placed with computer-assisted techniques.

If provisional restorations are placed at the time of implant placement, the patient should be evaluated regularly to ensure that occlusal contacts in all positions and excursions are as desired. Adjustment of the provisional restoration should be made as needed.

ACKNOWLEDGMENT

The author thanks his surgical colleagues Dr. S. Bagheri, Dr. R. Wunderle, and Dr. P. J. Schaner III for their guidance and assistance and Mr. Mark Palmer of 360imaging (Atlanta, Georgia) for his support.

PEARLS AND PITFALLS

The implant team, which includes the surgeon, the restorative dentist, the scan center, and the laboratory technical specialist, should all contribute to development of a plan for computer-assisted implant placement. Key points are:
- Accurate pretreatment models
- Development of a plan for final prostheses
- Well-managed scan with an appropriate scan appliance
- Attention to detail when using software to plan implant location
- Accurate placement of the surgical guide
- Care during placement of implants
- Postoperative evaluation and adjustment of provisional restoration as needed

BIBLIOGRAPHY

Almog DM, Benson BW, Wolfgang L, et al: Computerized tomography–based imaging and surgical guidance in oral implantology, *J Oral Implantol* 32:14-18, 2006.

Balshi SF, Wolfinger GJ, Balshi TJ: Surgical planning and prosthesis construction using computer technology and medical imaging for immediate loading of implants in the pterygomaxillary region, *Int J Periodontics Restorative Dent* 26:239-247, 2006.

Di Giacomo GA, Cury PR, de Araujo NS, et al: Clinical application of stereolithographic surgical guides for implant placement, *J Periodontol* 76:503-507, 2005.

Ersoy AE, Turkyilmaz I, Ozan O, et al: Reliability of implant placement with stereolithic surgical guides generated from computed tomography: clinical data from 94 implants, *J Periodontol* 79:1339-1345, 2008.

Hoffman J, Westendorff C, Gomez-Roman G, et al: Accuracy of navigation-guided socket drilling before implant installation compared to the conventional free-hand method in a synthetic edentulous lower jaw model, *Clin Oral Implants Res* 16:609-614, 2005.

Sclar AG: Guidelines for flapless surgery, *J Oral Maxillofac Surg* 65(7 Suppl 1):20-32, 2007.

Tardieu PB, Rosenfeld AL: *Computer-guided implantology*, Chicago, 2009, Quintessence.

Management of the Anticoagulated Patient

Rabie M. Shanti, Shahid R. Aziz

Anticoagulants and antiplatelet agents are increasingly being used for primary and secondary prophylaxis in patients with cardiovascular and cerebrovascular thromboembolic disease and venous thromboembolism. In the United States, it is estimated that 2.3 million patients suffer from atrial fibrillation and that 40% of these patients are receiving anticoagulation therapy.[1] Many clinicians still favor the practice of reducing or temporarily discontinuing use of the anticoagulation agent before any surgical intervention. Management of these patients is a balancing act between maintaining surgical and postsurgical hemostasis and minimizing risk for an embolic event. The most common causes of atrial thromboembolism are valvular heart disease and atrial fibrillation. The risk for arterial thromboembolism in patients with atrial fibrillation is 1% per year for those without any other co-morbid conditions and 17% per year for those older than 75 years.[2,3] Furthermore, nearly 20% of these arterial thromboemboli are fatal in patients with atrial fibrillation.[2] The average rate of such embolic events is reduced by 66% in patients with atrial fibrillation and by 75% in patients with mechanical heart valves with the use of anticoagulation therapy. Thus, there must be an evidence-based rationale for temporarily discontinuing anticoagulation therapy in any patient because of the risk for catastrophic embolic complications.

The most current guidelines all favor continuing anticoagulation therapy during minor surgical procedures. This is based on the belief that the risk for "significant bleeding" in patients taking oral anticoagulants with a stable international normalized ratio (INR) of 1.5 to 4 is very low in comparison to the risk for a thromboembolic event as a result of cessation of the use of the anticoagulant agent. The effects of thrombotic events on systemic health should never be taken lightly; for example, embolic strokes result in a significant neurologic deficit or death in 70% of patients, and thrombosis in a patient with a mechanical heart valve is fatal in 15% of cases.[4,5] Consequently, clinicians should base their decision to discontinue a patient's anticoagulation on solid medical evidence rather than relying on anecdotal evidence or fear of a particular clinical complication (postoperative bleeding).

Warfarin sodium (Coumadin), which was initially marketed as a pesticide against rats and mice, is the most commonly used anticoagulation agent. The mechanism of its action is as follows: warfarin competitively inhibits the enzyme epoxide reductase, which converts the reduced form of vitamin K to the active vitamin K epoxide. By inhibiting epoxide reductase, warfarin diminishes available vitamin K in tissues, which serves as a co-enzyme for glutamyl carboxylase. This is the enzyme that is responsible for the carboxylation of coagulation factors, specifically clotting factors II, VII, IX, and X and endogenous proteins C and S.

Management of an anticoagulated patient is a topic of great significance to the oral and maxillofacial surgeon inasmuch as postoperative hemostasis is a fundamental patient management issue.

Additionally, as the population ages, the practitioner will encounter this particular group of patients at an increasing incidence. Therefore, this chapter will focus on the general principles of management of patients who are receiving anticoagulant and antiplatelet therapy and undergoing oral surgical procedures.

ETIOPATHOGENESIS/CAUSATIVE FACTORS

Several conditions are associated with an increased likelihood for a thromboembolic event, such as the presence of a mechanical heart valve or a history of stroke (Box 26-1). Therefore, the clinician should stratify these patients into high risk, moderate risk, and low risk for experiencing a thromboembolic event by not receiving anticoagulation therapy. Such stratification is based on the type of prosthetic valve, the patient's age, the presence of atrial fibrillation, existing co-morbid conditions, and history of stroke or a thrombotic event. Patients should be stratified according to their risk for thromboembolism rather than being stratified according to the invasiveness of the surgical procedure. Although patients undergoing major reconstructive procedures are obviously at greater risk for postoperative bleeding than those undergoing minor dentoalveolar procedures, regardless of the complexity and invasiveness of the operation being performed, all patients should be properly assessed regarding their risk for thromboembolism. Based on the American College of Chest Physicians (ACCP) guidelines for all the conditions listed in Box 26-1, older-generation aortic valve prostheses, mitral valve prostheses, and a history of transient ischemic attack within the past 6 months pose the greatest risk for thromboembolism (>10%).[6] Patients considered to be within the moderate-risk category have a 4% to 10% per year incidence of thromboembolism, whereas patients in the low-risk category have less than a 4% per year incidence of thromboembolism.[6]

DIAGNOSTIC STUDIES

Before any laboratory study, a thorough review of the patient's medical history should be carried out. The history should focus on the patient's bleeding history and current medications. A quick examination of the upper extremities can be done to rapidly check for ecchymoses, a finding indicative of a potentially anticoagulated state. Likewise, asking simple questions ("when you cut yourself shaving, how long does it take you to stop bleeding") can also easily inform the clinician of potential risk for bleeding. It is important to also ask about the use of herbal supplements; for example, St. John's wort interacts with warfarin and causes a reduction in warfarin's anticoagulation effect.

BOX 26-1 Risk Factors for Thromboembolism

High Risk
- DVT within the past 1 to 3 months
- CVA or TIA within the past 6 months
- Any type of mitral valve prosthesis or older aortic prosthesis

Moderate Risk
- DVT within the past 3 to 12 months
- Active cancer
- Bileaflet aortic valve prosthesis with risk factors (AF, CHF, HTN, DM, >75 years of age)

Low Risk
- Singe DVT event more than 12 months previously with no other risk factors
- Bileaflet aortic valve prosthesis without risk factors (AF, CHF, HTN, DM, >75 years of age)

AF, atrial fibrillation; *CHF*, congestive heart failure; *CVA*, cerebrovascular accident; *DM*, diabetes mellitus; *DVT*, deep venous thrombosis; *HTN*, hypertension; *TIA*, transient ischemic attack.

$$\text{INR} = \left(\frac{\text{plasma prothrombin time (sec)}}{\text{mean normal prothrombin time (sec)}}\right)^{\text{ISI}}$$

Fig. 26-1 ■ Calculation of the international normalized ratio.

Laboratory assessment of an anticoagulated patient should include hemoglobin, hematocrit, partial thromboplastin time, prothrombin time (PT), and the INR. The World Health Organization (WHO) Committee on Biological Standards introduced the INR in 1983 to provide clinicians with a more standardized assessment tool for patients receiving anticoagulation therapy.[7] The INR was developed to standardize the PT. The PT test is based on the sensitivity of various thromboplastins; it is a test of the intrinsic clotting cascade and is the test used to monitor patients taking warfarin. The INR is calculated by comparing the patient's PT with that of a mean of 20 fresh plasma samples from healthy ambulatory patients while using the international sensitivity index to correct for the sensitivity of the various thromboplastins that a laboratory might use[8] (Fig. 26-1). According to the WHO calibration recommendations, laboratory variation is usually within the range of 4%.[8,9] In summary, the INR value should be independent of the laboratory used to measure the INR. With regard to what is an acceptable INR range, there exists a great deal of debate.

TREATMENT GOALS

Management of an anticoagulated patient undergoing oral and maxillofacial surgery has historically been controversial because of early reports of major bleeding after office-based procedures in these patients.[10] There is a plethora of literature on the risk for bleeding in individuals receiving oral anticoagulants while undergoing oral and maxillofacial surgical procedures (i.e., extractions). The rate of postoperative bleeding in the aforementioned patients ranges from 9% to 50%, depending on the study.[11,12] However, as discussed previously, the complications of inappropriately discontinuing anticoagulation therapy, though less frequent, are much greater in severity. Therefore, it is imperative for the clinician to avoid any unnecessary modifications in patients' anticoagulant medications when possible. The goal of management of anticoagulated surgical patients is to assess their risk for suffering a thromboembolic event and appropriately evaluate and manage their bleeding risk. In addition, the oral and maxillofacial surgeon should coordinate management with the patient's physician when adjusting medications.

SPECIFIC TREATMENT AND TECHNIQUES

The first step in the perioperative management of patients taking antithrombotic medications is to assess their risk for a thromboembolic event. As listed previously (see Box 26-1), several conditions increase the likelihood of such an event occurring. The following are strategies for the management of patients requiring anticoagulation or antiplatelet therapy while undergoing office-based/outpatient oral and maxillofacial surgery.

MANAGEMENT OF PATIENTS TAKING WARFARIN

After the use of warfarin is discontinued, the INR will drop in almost all patients to 1.5 within a period of 4 days if the INR was 2.0 to 3.0 before drug discontinuation or within 5 days if the INR was 2.5 to 3.5.[13] Subsequently, when the INR reaches 1.5, the surgical procedure can be carried out without an increased risk for bleeding.[2,13] Patients who have an INR higher than 4.0 should not undergo any nonemergency surgical interventions and should receive an immediate referral to the physician managing their anticoagulation therapy. In the same situation, if the INR is higher than 1.5 after discontinuation of warfarin for 4 to 5 days, a small dose of vitamin K (1 mg IV or vitamin K 2.5 mg) should be administered. However, if the INR is between 1.7 and 2.0, fresh frozen plasma can be given immediately before surgery[7,14] (Fig. 26-2). Even though bleeding is a treatable complication, if the aforementioned recommendations are not implemented, postoperative bleeding can develop and delay the resumption of anticoagulation therapy, thereby resulting in increased risk for a thromboembolic event. Another clinical decision that most clinicians face when managing anticoagulated patients is when the INR should be checked, and the answer is the day before the surgical procedure. Furthermore, after warfarin therapy is resumed, it will take 3 days for the INR to reach 2.0, so warfarin should be started on the night of the procedure, provided that there is no obvious bleeding.[2] Additionally, a variety of U.S. Food and Drug Administration–approved hemostatic agents have been developed for control of local bleeding. These products vary in cost, convenience, and biologic/physical properties; however, very little literature exists on the effectiveness of one over the others. The more commonly used local hemostatic measures in oral and maxillofacial surgery include gelatin sponges (Gelfoam), oxidized cellulose, cyanoacrylate, thrombin, fibrin glue, and collagen fleece. Hemostatic mouthwashes have also been reported to control local bleeding in anticoagulated patients undergoing tooth extraction.[15] The authors favor judicious use of Gelfoam packed into the surgical site (extraction socket) combined with primary closure of the site to maintain hemostasis. If primary closure is not feasible, placement of Gelfoam combined with a "figure-of-eight" suture and cyanoacrylate over the extraction site will also maintain hemostasis. Vicryl sutures are preferred—though resorbable, they will remain intact for days to weeks after surgery, thus allowing healing of the associated soft tissues (Fig. 26-3).

HEPARIN FOR BRIDGING ANTICOAGULATION ("COUMADIN-HEPARIN SWITCHING")

The rationale behind bridging anticoagulation is to minimize the time that the patient spends not receiving anticoagulation therapy during the perioperative period. The decision whether to bridge

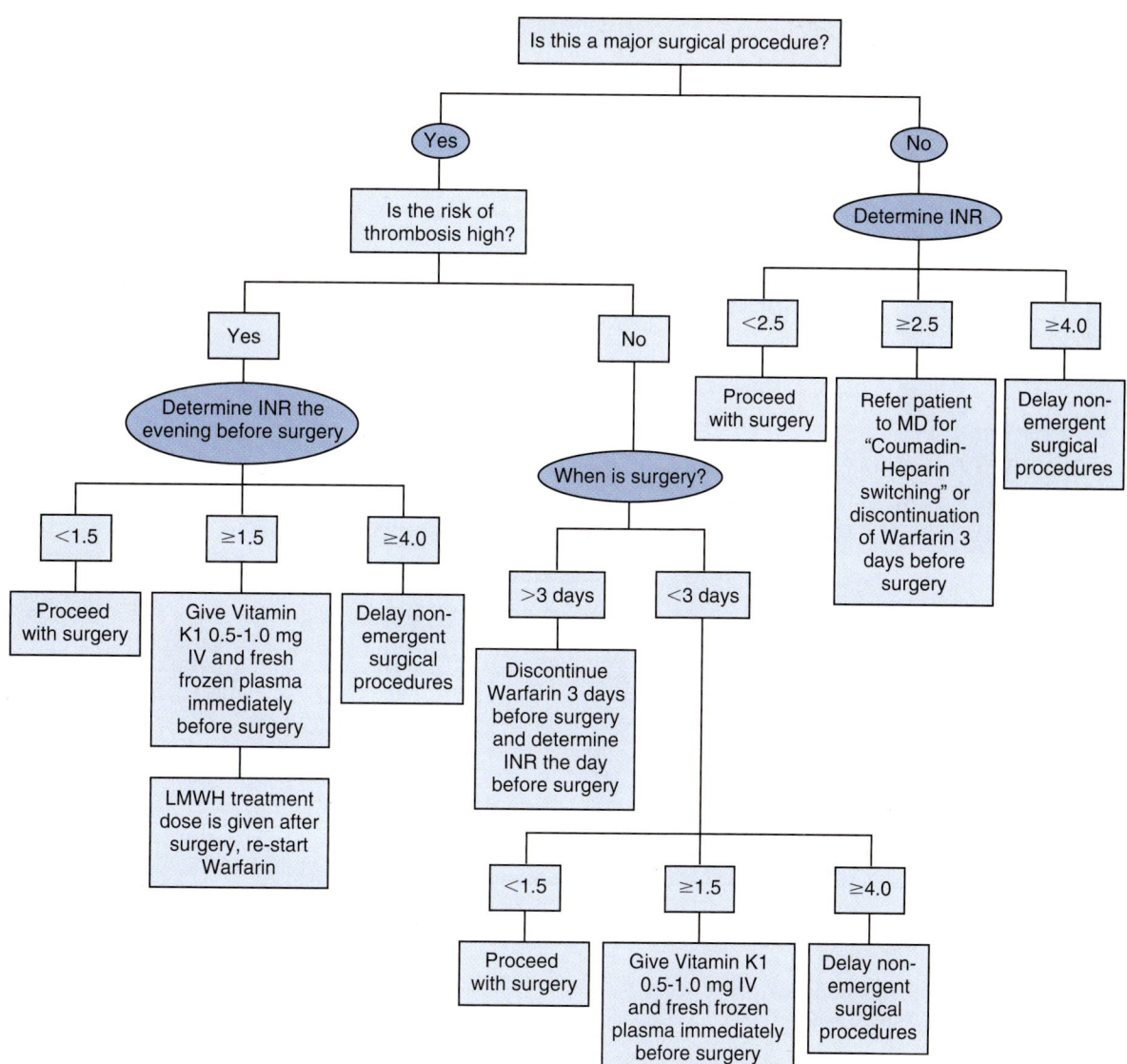

Fig. 26-2 ■ Algorithm for adjusting the international normalized ratio before oral surgery.

should be based on the patient's risk for thromboembolism and associated risk for bleeding.[6] An ideal bridging anticoagulation approach consists of admitting the patient 4 to 5 days before surgery, discontinuing warfarin, and administering unfractionated heparin intravenously while the effects of warfarin recede.[16] Subsequently, the intravenous heparin is discontinued 3 to 4 hours before the surgical procedure to avoid the anticoagulant effects of heparin during the procedure. Postoperatively, warfarin and heparin are restarted, with heparin being administered for 4 to 5 days until a therapeutic range of warfarin is achieved.[16] In clinical practice, however, this approach is impracticable because of several factors, including hospital bed availability and health care cost. Therefore, an alternative approach is carried out in which the patient receives low-molecular-weight heparin (LMWH), which can be administered

subcutaneously in a fixed low dose without laboratory monitoring. When compared with the intravenous unfractionated heparin that is provided in hospitals, LMWH is less costly, and its pharmacologic properties allow it to be used for outpatient treatment. No large cohort study has compared the safety and effectiveness of unfractionated heparin over LMWH in periprocedural anticoagulation in patients undergoing dental or craniomaxillofacial surgical procedures. However, LMWH has been shown to be superior to intravenous unfractionated heparin for other purposes (i.e., venous thromboembolism).[17,18]

Based on the ACCP guidelines, bridging anticoagulation with therapeutic-dose subcutaneous LMWH is recommended for high-risk patients. For moderate-risk patients, the guidelines recommend therapeutic-dose unfractionated heparin, therapeutic-dose LMWH,

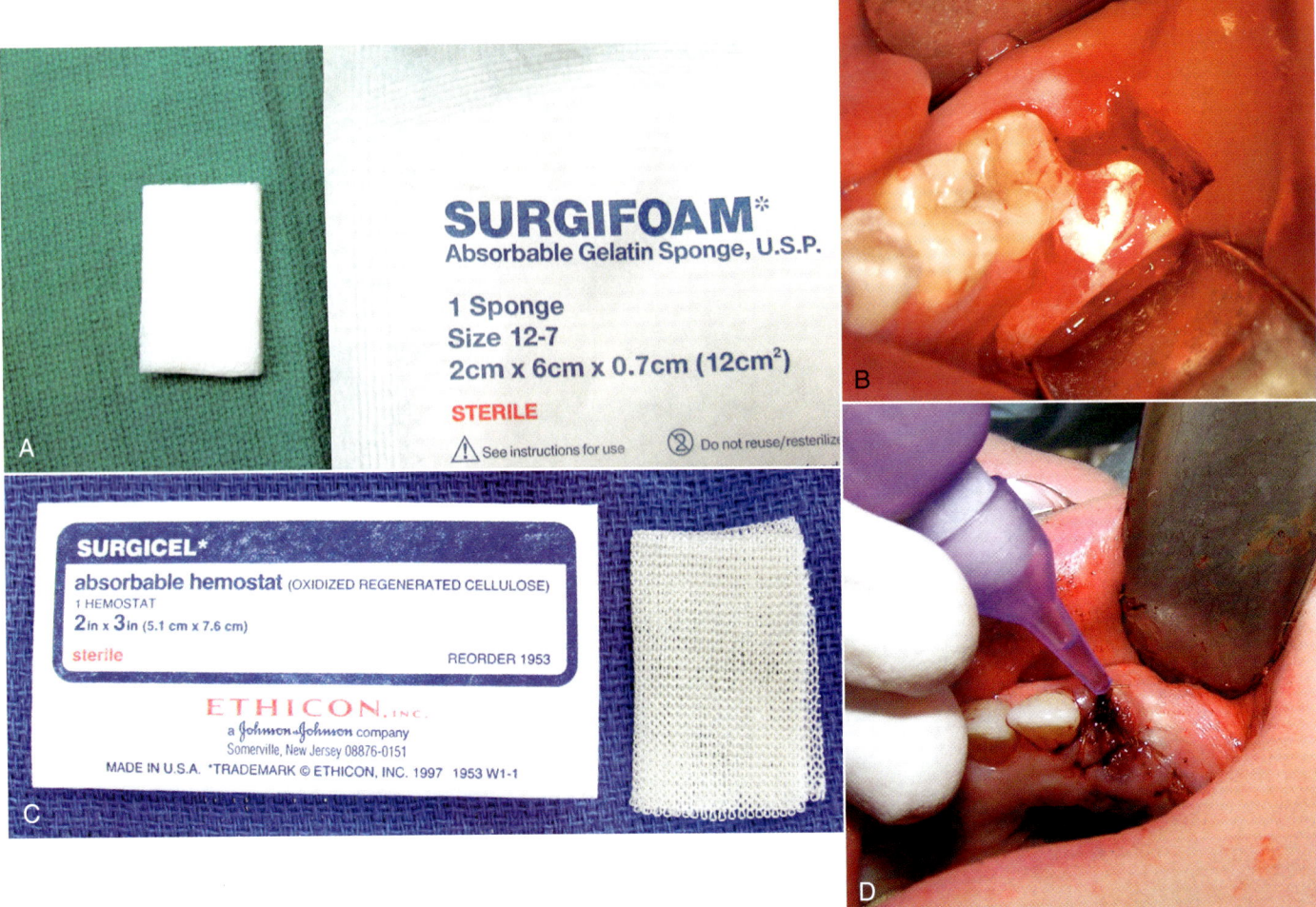

Fig. 26-3 ■ **A,** Absorbable gelatin sponge (Surgifoam/Gelfoam). **B,** Gelfoam placed in the extraction site. **C,** Oxidized regenerated cellulose (Surgicel). **D,** Cyanoacrylate applied over the extraction site.

or low-dose LMWH. Finally, for low-risk patients, the guidelines recommend low-dose LMWH or no bridging anticoagulation. Of importance to note, there is little significant evidence to support the LMWH approach with regard to its safety and efficacy. However, the risk for a thromboembolic event in a high- or moderate-risk patient, especially after the discontinuation of anticoagulant therapy, is justification enough to implement aggressive bridging therapy.

The decision of when to restart warfarin anticoagulation therapy in a patient undergoing bridging anticoagulation is a question commonly faced by clinicians. Regardless of the bridging protocol, the bridging agent should be continued until an INR of 2.0 is achieved so that the patient is not over-anticoagulated. Before restarting any anticoagulation agent the clinician must decide whether the patient is hematologically stable based on the hemostasis achieved intra-operatively and the risk for bleeding that the type of surgery being performed poses. Based on the most current ACCP recommendations, warfarin should be restarted within the first 12 to 24 hours after the procedure if the clinician believes that there is adequate hemostasis.[6] Additionally, restarting warfarin should in no way lead to acute hemorrhage in the patient since at least 48 hours is needed for the anticoagulative effect of warfarin to take place. Additionally, unfractionated heparin and LMWH should also be initiated within

24 hours if the patient has adequate hemostasis. In the case of major surgical procedures, restarting the bridging agent too soon can significantly increase the risk for postoperative bleeding. This is true for minor procedures; however, for major procedure associated with a high risk for postoperative bleeding, the clinician may decide to completely discontinue the unfractionated heparin or therapeutic-dose heparin or delay its use for at least 48 to 72 hours.[6]

MANAGEMENT OF PATIENTS TAKING ANTIPLATELET DRUGS

Antiplatelet drugs have scarce data with regard to their management in surgical patients. The most commonly prescribed antiplatelet agents are clopidogrel (Plavix), dipyridamole (Persantine), and acetylsalicylic acid. Other agents include ticlopidine (Ticlid), abciximab (ReoPro), eptifibatide (Integrilin), and cilostazol (Pletal). Nonsteroidal anti-inflammatory drugs (NSAIDs) or acetylsalicylic acid (aspirin) have not been shown to increase the risk for significant bleeding in patients undergoing certain nonoral and non-maxillofacial surgical procedures (e.g., colonoscopy with biopsy).[2] Although the literature is scant on the management of surgical patients receiving antiplatelet therapy, the majority of the literature and recommendations by scientific advisories (e.g., American Heart Association, American College of Cardiology, American College of Surgeons, and Society for Cardiovascular Angiography and Interventions) do not recommend preoperative cessation of antiplatelet agents. If the decision is made to temporarily discontinue antiplatelet therapy, the standard protocol is to discontinue the antiplatelet agent 7 days before the surgical intervention. This is the amount of time required to restore the total pool of functional platelets.

POSTOPERATIVE CARE

An anticoagulated patient should not be prescribed a non-selective NSAID or cyclooxygenase-2 (COX-2) inhibitor for analgesia following a surgical procedure because of the risk of over-anticoagulation and hemorrhage.[10] Furthermore, there is mounting evidence that COX-2 inhibitors can cause a rise in the INR and increase the risk for gastrointestinal bleeding with concomitant use of warfarin and a nonselective NSAID or COX-2 inhibitor.[10]

The following postoperative instructions should be provided to patients undergoing routine oral surgical procedures and are to be applied in the first 24 hours: (1) avoid spitting or rinsing the mouth; (2) avoid hot foods and liquids; (3) avoid high-pressure sucking since this can transmit high negative pressure to the area of surgery and disturb any formed clot; (4) avoid chewing on the surgical side; (5) avoid manipulating the surgical site with the tongue or foreign objects; and (6) if bleeding occurs, apply digital pressure to the area of bleeding for up to 20 minutes, and if the bleeding persists, the patient should notify the surgeon immediately.

PEARLS AND PITFALLS

- The first step in managing anticoagulated patients is to assess their risk for experiencing a thromboembolic event (see Box 26-1) by stratifying these patients as being at high, moderate, or low risk for such an event. Subsequently, a decision can be made whether to discontinue the anticoagulant preoperatively.
- For patients requiring temporary cessation of anticoagulation therapy, the anticoagulant should be stopped 5 days before surgery and restarted 12 to 24 hours after surgery, unless the patient had a procedure considered to be high risk for postoperative bleeding or the operative site was not hemostatic.
- If the INR is supratherapeutic at 1 to 2 days before surgery and surgery cannot be delayed, for an INR > 2.5 and < 4.0 (vitamin K 1 mg IV or Vitamin K 2.5 mg sc or po) can be given immediately before surgery. Patients who have an INR higher than 4.0 should not undergo any nonemergency surgical interventions and should receive an immediate referral to the physician managing their anticoagulation therapy.
- Because of ease of administration and cost-effectiveness, outpatient subcutaneous LMWH should be administered as a bridging agent instead of the inpatient administration of intravenous unfractionated heparin. LWMH should be discontinued 24 hours before surgery.
- Bleeding is a controllable perioperative complication; therefore, the clinician should use local hemostatic measures liberally and always err on the side of continuing anticoagulation.
- In contrast to anticoagulation agents, antiplatelet agents should be continued only in patients at high risk for cardiac events. In patients who are not at a high risk for such events, the antiplatelet agent should be discontinued at a minimum of 5 days before surgery.
- Management of these patients should be performed in concert with the patient's physician or physicians.

REFERENCES

1. Dunn AS, Turpie AG: Perioperative management of patients receiving oral anticoagulants: a systematic review, *Arch Intern Med* 163:901-908, 2003.
2. Hittelet A, Deviere J: Management of anticoagulants before and after endoscopy, *Can J Gastroenterol* 17:329-332, 2003.
3. Risk factors for stroke and efficacy of antithrombotic therapy in atrial fibrillation. Analysis of pooled data from five randomized controlled trials, *Arch Intern Med* 154:1449-1457, 1994.
4. Tiede DJ, Nishimura RA, Gastineau DA, et al: Modern management of prosthetic valve anticoagulation, *Mayo Clin Proc* 73:665-680, 1998.
5. Longstreth WT Jr, Bernick C, Fitzpatrick A, et al: Frequency and predictors of stroke death in 5,888 participants in the cardiovascular health study, *Neurology* 56:368-375, 2001.
6. Kraai EP, Lopes RD: Perioperative management of anticoagulation: guidelines translated for the clinician, *J Thromb Thrombolysis* 28:16-22, 2009.
7. Hirsh J, Poller L: The international normalized ratio: a guide to understanding and correcting its problems, *Arch Intern Med* 154:282-288, 1994.
8. Beirne OR, Koehler JR: Surgical management of patients on warfarin sodium, *J Oral Maxillofac Surg* 54:1115-1118, 1996.
9. Loeliger EA, van den Besselaar AM, Lewis SM: Reliability and clinical impact of the normalization of the prothrombin times in oral anticoagulant control, *Thromb Haemost* 53:148-154, 1985.
10. Perry DJ, Noakes TJC, Helliwell PS, for the British Dental Society: Guidelines for the management of patients on oral anticoagulants requiring dental surgery, *Br Dent J* 203:389-393, 2007.
11. Al-Mubarak S, Rass MA, Alsuwyed A, et al: Thromboembolic risk and bleeding in patients maintaining or stopping oral anticoagulant therapy during dental extraction, *J Thromb Haemost* 4:689-691, 2006.
12. Randall C: Surgical management of the primary care dental patient on warfarin, *Dent Update* 32:414-416, 2005.
13. White RH, McKittrick T, Hutchinson R, et al: Temporary discontinuation of warfarin therapy: changes in the international normalized ratio, *Ann Intern Med* 122:40-42, 1995.
14. Kearon C, Hirsh J: Management of anticoagulation before and after elective surgery, *N Engl J Med* 336:1506-1511, 1997.
15. Patatanian E, Fugate SE: Hemostatic mouthwashes in anticoagulated patients undergoing dental extraction, *Ann Pharmacother* 40:2205-2210, 2006.
16. Douketis JD, Johnson JA: Low-molecular-weight heparin as bridging anticoagulation during interruption of warfarin, *Arch Intern Med* 164:1319-1326, 2004.
17. van Dongen CJJ, van den Belt AGM: Fixed dose subcutaneous low-molecular-weight heparins versus adjusted dose unfractionated heparin for venous thromboembolism, *Cochrane Database Syst Rev* 4:CD001100, 2004.
18. Mismetti P, Laporte-Simitsides S, Tardy B, et al: Preventions of venous thromboembolism in internal medicine with unfractionated or low-molecular-weight heparins: a meta-analysis of randomized clinical trials, *Thromb Haemost* 83:14-19, 2000.

Chapter 27

The Preoperative Cardiac Evaluation

Heather B. Westmoreland, A. Maziar Zafari

Approximately 27 million patients undergo surgery each year in the United States, and an estimated 8 million have known coronary artery disease (CAD) or risk factors for cardiovascular disease. A substantial number of all deaths in patients undergoing noncardiac surgery are caused by cardiovascular complications. It is estimated that almost 1 million patients will have perioperative cardiovascular complications.[1] Approximately 50,000 of these patients will experience perioperative myocardial infarction (MI), and about 40% will die.[1] The incidence of perioperative MI is increased 10- to 50-fold in patients who have previously experienced coronary events.[2] When considering a patient for non-cardiac surgery, it is important to approximate the risk for postoperative cardiovascular complications. The preoperative evaluation is meant not to "clear" the patient for surgery but to identify obvious or hidden cardiovascular risk and therefore reduce the occurrence of complications.[3]

In the following sections are some very common examples of patients whom a maxillofacial surgeon may see on a daily basis. This chapter is meant to clarify certain cardiovascular scenarios and provide recommendations on how to approach patients with common cardiovascular disorders.

CLINICAL CASES

CASE 1

Mr. H. is a 68-year-old white man with diabetes, hypertension, dyslipidemia, and previous tobacco use. He suffered a small MI two years ago and occasionally has chest discomfort with exertion. Oropharyngeal cancer has recently been diagnosed and he is now scheduled to undergo maxillectomy. *Does he need further evaluation before his elective surgery? What can be done to minimize his risk for perioperative complications?*

CASE 2

Mrs. W. is a 45-year-old African American woman. She has non-ischemic chronic heart failure (HF) with a left ventricular ejection fraction (LVEF) of 25%. She has been maintained on a stable regimen of a beta blocker, angiotensin converting enzyme inhibitor, spironolactone, and a diuretic and had an implantable cardioverter-defibrillator (ICD) placed 3 years ago. She has had no hospitalizations for HF in the past two years. On her way home from work one evening, she was struck head-on in a motor vehicle accident. She was rushed to the local trauma center and found to have extensive maxillofacial trauma. She needs to undergo semi-urgent surgery. *How should her cardiac condition be managed?*

CASE 3

Mr. A. is a 75-year-old Asian-American being seen for preoperative evaluation. He is scheduled for a dental implant in one week. While auscultating his chest, you hear a murmur. When you question Mr. A. about this murmur, he produces an echocardiogram report revealing that he has moderate aortic stenosis. *Should you proceed with surgery next week?*

ETIOLOGY

Perioperative MI is a complex entity that can be precipitated by a number of different pathophysiologic mechanisms. The cardiovascular system of patients who undergo general anesthesia and noncardiac surgical procedures is subject to multiple strains and complications. Patients who were previously stable can decompensate postoperatively, thus leading to significant postoperative morbidity and mortality.[2] Mechanisms by which patients may deteriorate include increases in myocardial oxygen consumption, alterations in coagulation that precipitate thrombosis, and changes in vascular tone and endothelial function.[4] Furthermore, most postoperative MIs are associated with either no chest pain or atypical chest pain. This can be a result of pain medications, residual anesthesia, or other postoperative painful stimuli that may mask angina pectoris.[1]

Most experts agree that the anesthesiologist should choose the type of anesthesia, but there can be risks involved with each type. General anesthesia has been shown to cause changes in arterial and central venous pressure, alter cardiac output, and contribute to the development of arrhythmias. Decreased systemic vascular resistance, a decline in myocardial contractility, a reduction in stroke volume, and an increase in myocardial irritability are all possible mechanisms for these cardiovascular shifts. Induction of general anesthesia lowers systemic arterial pressure by 20% to 30%, endotracheal intubation increases blood pressure by 20 to 30 mmHg, and agents such as nitric oxide lower cardiac output by 15%.[5]

Nongeneral anesthesia can also play a role in cardiovascular compromise. Opioid-based drugs are widely used because of their cardiac safety profile, but increased doses may lead to respiratory depression and the need for mechanical ventilation. Postoperative weaning from mechanical ventilation is associated with myocardial ischemia.[5] Although the use of fentanyl, sufentanil, or alfentanil usually causes less myocardial depression than inhaled anesthetics do, many of these intravenous agents still cause venodilation, which in turn may lead to reduced preload and a further decrease in cardiac output. Other sedatives, including propofol, may compromise cardiac contractility and increase afterload on the right ventricle.[6]

There has been conflicting evidence surrounding the differences or decrease in cardiac risk when using general versus local anesthesia. Both epidural and spinal anesthesia may cause decreases in preload and afterload by sympathetic blockade.[5] Many studies have reported no significant differences in complication rates for regional versus general anesthesia,[7-12] but two studies have demonstrated lower rates of MI in patients who received regional or spinal anesthesia.[13,14]

Thus, it is crucial to identify and optimize medical therapy in patients with chronic HF because such patients are extremely sensitive to these hemodynamic changes. Recognizing this condition before surgery and increasing preoperative volume status helps in applying the Frank-Starling principle, which can offset a potential decrease in cardiac output. Moreover, other inhalational and intravenous anesthetics, when combined with muscle relaxants, frequently sensitize the myocardium to circulating catecholamines, which along with the stress of the surgical procedure, often increases the risk for ventricular arrhythmias.[2]

APPROACH TO THE PATIENT UNDERGOING MAXILLOFACIAL SURGERY

STEPWISE APPROACH

When planning surgery, it is important to approach the patient in a systematic fashion. The American College of Cardiology (ACC) and the American Heart Association (AHA) recommended a stepwise approach to cardiac evaluation in the 2007 Updated Guidelines on Perioperative Cardiovascular Evaluation for Noncardiac Surgery. One should evaluate a patient's current medical conditions and risk-stratify, medically optimize, and monitor the patient perioperatively.[15]

The first decision to consider is whether this is a surgery that can wait. If the answer is no, the surgery must proceed. The preoperative evaluation may need to be limited if the procedure is urgent. Rapid assessment of the 12-lead electrocardiogram (ECG), vital signs, volume status, hematocrit, electrolytes, renal function, and urinalysis should be performed.[15] In this situation, a more complete assessment can be accomplished once the urgent surgery is completed.

If the surgery is elective and non-urgent, a stepwise approach to the patient should be pursued. The first step should be a thorough history. This will help stratify patients into low- or higher-surgical risk categories. The history should inquire about any past episodes of angina pectoris, MI, HF or HF symptoms, and symptomatic arrhythmias as well as whether the patient has a pacemaker or implantable cardiac defibrillator (ICD).[5,15] Related illnesses such as diabetes mellitus, peripheral vascular disease, cerebrovascular disease, renal impairment, and chronic pulmonary disease should also be assessed and documented.[5] If the patient has known CAD, a thorough assessment of any recent change in symptoms is essential. Precise doses of current medications and over-the-counter or herbal drugs are also extremely important.

Risk stratification includes assessment of the risk for complications associated with the individual patient and the patient's co-morbid conditions and the risk for complications associated with the planned surgical procedure. Box 27-1 outlines symptoms or co-morbid conditions that make up the major-, intermediate- and low-risk patient categories.

Major risk is defined as patients with recent MI, unstable angina (defined as Canadian class III or IV), decompensated HF, significant arrhythmias, or severe valvular disease. Patients with major clinical predictors of increased risk may warrant further testing or intervention before surgery or at the least a delay in surgery until these symptoms can be adequately assessed.

Intermediate risk includes patients with previous MI by history or ECG, renal insufficiency, diabetes (especially insulin requiring), compensated HF, or mild angina (defined as Canadian class I or II). Intermediate-risk symptoms demand comprehensive questioning

---

BOX 27-1	Clinical Predictors of Increased Risk for Perioperative Cardiac Complications

Major

Unstable coronary syndromes
- Acute or recent myocardial infarction* with evidence of important ischemic risk by clinical symptoms or noninvasive study
- Unstable or severe† angina (Canadian class III or IV)‡

Decompensated heart failure

Significant arrhythmias
- High-grade atrioventricular block
- Symptomatic ventricular arrhythmias in the presence of underlying heart disease
- Supraventricular arrhythmias with uncontrolled ventricular rate

Severe valvular disease

Intermediate

Mild angina pectoris (Canadian class I or II)

Previous myocardial infarction by history or pathologic Q waves

Compensated or previous heart failure

Diabetes mellitus (particularly insulin dependent)

Renal insufficiency

Minor

Advanced age

Abnormal findings on electrocardiography (left ventricular hypertrophy, left bundle branch block, ST-T abnormalities)

Rhythm other than sinus (e.g., atrial fibrillation)

Low functional capacity (e.g., inability to climb one flight of stairs with a bag of groceries)

History of stroke

Uncontrolled systemic hypertension

---

*The American College of Cardiology National Database Library defines *recent* MI as longer than 7 days but less than or equal to 1 month (30 days); acute MI is MI occurring within 7 days.

†May include "stable" angina in patients who are unusually sedentary.

‡Campeau L: Grading of angina pectoris, *Circulation* 54:522-523, 1976.

From Eagle KA, Berger PB, Calkins H, et al: ACC/AHA guideline update for perioperative cardiovascular evaluation for noncardiac surgery-executive summary: a report of the American College of Cardiology/American Heart Association Task Force on Practice Guidelines (Committee to Update the 1996 Guidelines on Perioperative Cardiovascular Evaluation for Noncardiac Surgery), *J Am Coll Cardiol* 39:542-553, 2002.

---

and careful evaluation regarding the patient's functional status before further testing is needed.[16,17]

Minor risk most often includes patients with advanced age, uncontrolled systemic hypertension, atrial fibrillation, low functional capacity, history of stroke, or findings on the ECG such as left ventricular hypertrophy, ST-T wave abnormalities, or left bundle branch block. These patients also need no further evaluation before surgery unless their functional capacity is very low.[4]

RISK STRATIFICATION

Functional capacity is an extremely useful tool in assessing risk. A patient's functional capacity can be illustrated in metabolic equivalents (METs), which are defined as the oxygen consumption of a 70-kg, 40-year-old man in a resting state.[18] By asking simple, straightforward questions, one can ascertain a patient's ability to perform daily activities, which can correlate with cardiovascular health (Box 27-2). For example, an inability to walk or dress oneself would indicate very low functional capacity at around 1 MET, but scrubbing floors or playing golf may indicate higher functioning

BOX 27-2	Functional Assessment as Defined by METs*

1 MET
Can you take care of yourself?
Eat, dress, or use the toilet?
Walk indoors around the house?
Walk a block or two on level ground at 2 to 3 mph or 3.2 to 4.8 km/h?
Do light work around the house such as dusting or washing dishes?

4 METs
Can you climb a flight of stairs or walk up a hill?
Walk on level ground at 4 mph or 6.4 km/h?
Run a short distance?
Do heavy work around the house such as scrubbing floors or lifting or moving heavy furniture?
Participate in moderate recreational activities such as golf, bowling, dancing, doubles tennis, or throwing a baseball or football?

Greater than 10 METs
Can you participate in strenuous sports such as swimming, singles tennis, football, basketball, or skiing?
METs, metabolic equivalents.

*Data from Hlatky MA, Boineau RE, Higginbotham MB, et al: A brief self-administered questionnaire to determine functional capacity (the Duke Activity Status Index), *Am J Cardiol* 64:651-654, 1989; Fletcher GF, Balady G, Froelicher VF, et al: Exercise standards. A statement for healthcare professionals from the American Heart Association, *Circulation* 91:580-615, 1995; from Eagle KA, Berger PB, Calkins H, et al: ACC/AHA guideline update for perioperative cardiovascular evaluation for noncardiac surgery-executive summary: a report of the American College of Cardiology/American Heart Association Task Force on Practice Guidelines (Committee to Update the 1996 Guidelines on Perioperative Cardiovascular Evaluation for Noncardiac Surgery), *J Am Coll Cardiol* 39:542-553, 2002.

BOX 27-3	Surgical Risk*

High (Reported Cardiac Risk Often Greater than 5%)
Emergency major operations, particularly in the elderly
Aortic and other major vascular surgery
Peripheral vascular surgery
Anticipated prolonged surgical procedures associated with large fluid shifts, blood loss, or both

Intermediate (Reported Cardiac Risk Generally Less than 5%)
Carotid endarterectomy surgery
Head and neck surgery
Intraperitoneal and intrathoracic surgery
Orthopedic surgery
Prostate surgery

Low† (Reported Cardiac Risk Generally Less than 1%)
Endoscopic procedures
Superficial procedure
Cataract surgery
Breast surgery

*Combined incidence of cardiac death and non-fatal myocardial infarction.
†Does not generally require further preoperative cardiac testing.
From Eagle KA, Berger PB, Calkins, et al: ACC/AHA guideline update for perioperative cardiovascular evaluation for noncardiac surgery-executive summary: a report of the American College of Cardiology/American Heart Association Task Force on Practice Guidelines (Committee to Update the 1996 Guidelines on Perioperative Cardiovascular Evaluation for Noncardiac Surgery), *J Am Coll Cardiol* 39:542-553, 2002.

BOX 27-4	Shortcut to Noninvasive Testing in Preoperative Patients If Any Two Factors Are Present

1. Intermediate clinical predictors are present (Canadian class 1 or 2 angina, previous MI based on history or pathologic Q waves, compensated or previous heart failure, diabetes, or renal insufficiency)
2. Poor functional capacity (less than 4 METs)
3. High-risk surgical procedure (emergency major operations,* aortic repair or peripheral vascular surgery, or prolonged surgical procedures with large fluid shifts or blood loss)

*Emergency major operations may require proceeding to surgery immediately without sufficient time for non-invasive testing or preoperative interventions.
METs, metabolic equivalents; MI, myocardial infarction.
Modified with permission from Leppo JA, Dahlberg ST: The question: to test or not to test in preoperative cardiac risk evaluation, *J Nucl Cardiol* 5:332-342, 1998. Copyright © 1998 by the American Society of Nuclear Cardiology. This material may not be reproduced, stored in a retrieval system, or transmitted in any form or by any means without the prior permission of the publisher.
In Eagle KA, Berger PB, Calkins H, et al: ACC/AHA guideline update for perioperative cardiovascular evaluation for noncardiac surgery-executive summary: a report of the American College of Cardiology/American Heart Association Task Force on Practice Guidelines (Committee to Update the 1996 Guidelines on Perioperative Cardiovascular Evaluation for Noncardiac Surgery), *J Am Coll Cardiol* 39:542-543, 2002.

individuals. Patients who fall into the lower MET group may need further testing before surgery. An increased incidence of cardiac complications in non-cardiac surgery is directly related to poor functional capacity.[17]

When assessing a patient before surgery, it is also important to classify the type of surgery that will be performed as high-, intermediate-, or low-risk surgery. Box 27-3 lists several common surgeries and the type of risk with which they are associated. These are stratified in the following manner:

1. High risk involves any type of emergency surgery, aortic or major vascular surgery, peripheral vascular surgery, or a procedure defined as prolonged or associated with large fluid shifts. The cardiac risk reported for these surgeries is usually defined as being greater than 5%.
2. Intermediate risk carries a reported cardiac risk of less than 5% and includes head and neck surgery, carotid endarterectomy, orthopedic surgery, prostate surgery, and intraperitoneal and intrathoracic surgery.
3. Low-risk surgeries typically do not require any further testing before the procedure. Such surgeries include cataract surgery, breast surgery, and superficial and endoscopic procedures.

In an effort to streamline this process, the ACC/AHA guidelines compiled these and other risk factors into a straightforward and easy-to-use algorithm (Fig. 27-1).

In situations in which patients need emergency surgery, have high-risk cardiovascular symptoms, or have previously undergone cardiac revascularization, the preoperative guidelines are reasonably straightforward. However, it seems that the bulk of patients requiring preoperative evaluation fall into the intermediate or minor clinical predictor categories. In an effort to simplify this sometimes difficult decision, Box 27-4 offers a streamlined approach. Essentially, if two of the three factors listed are true, the use of non-invasive cardiac testing is recommended as part of the preoperative evaluation. For example, the presence of either low functional capacity or high surgical risk in a patient with intermediate clinical predictors warrants further non-invasive testing.

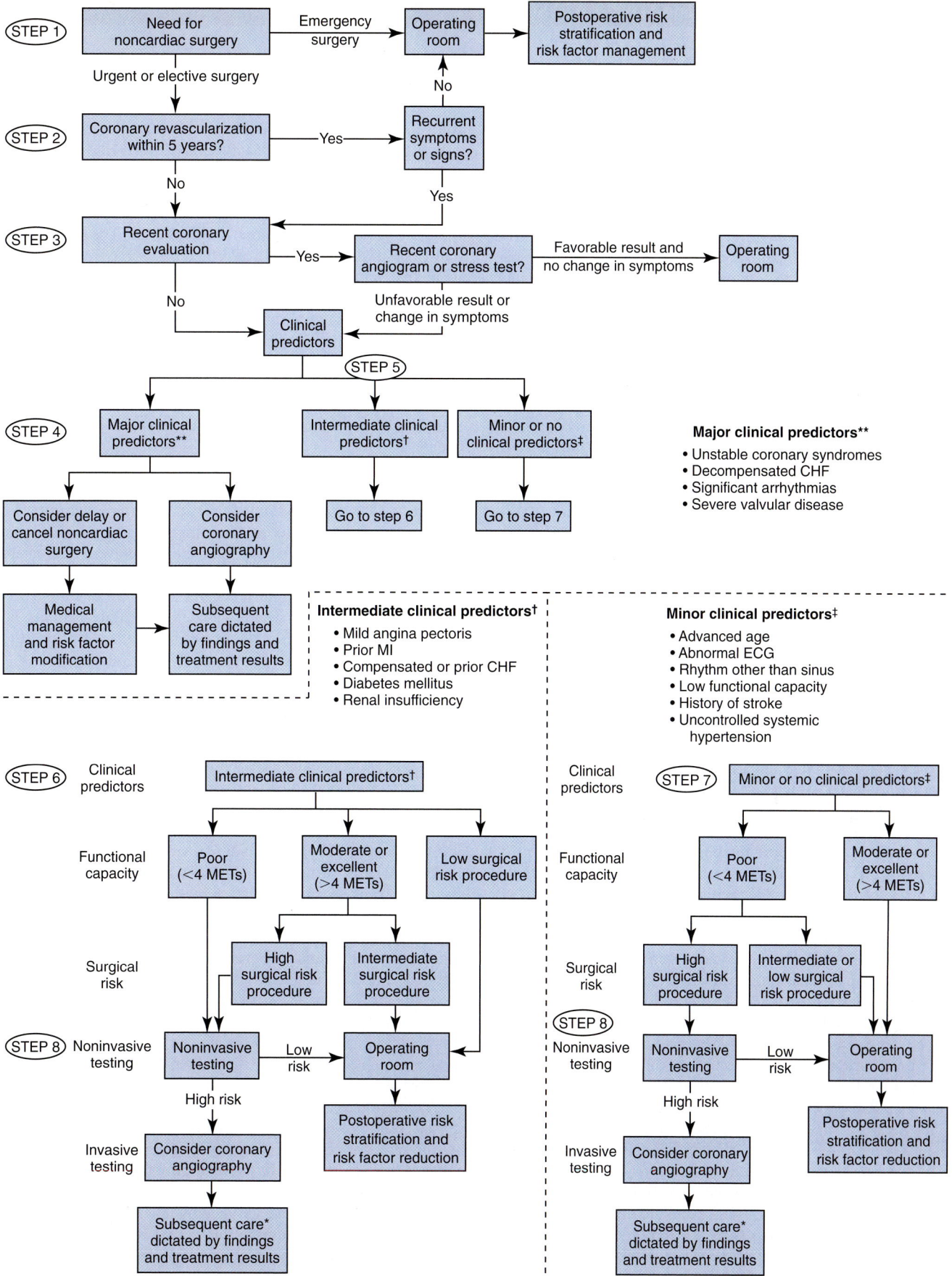

Fig. 27-1 ■ Stepwise approach to preoperative cardiac assessment. The steps are discussed in text. *Subsequent care may include cancellation or delay of surgery, coronary revascularization followed by noncardiac surgery, or intensified care. (From Eagle KA, Berger PB, Calkins H, et al: ACC/AHA guideline update for perioperative cardiovascular evaluation for noncardiac surgery—executive summary: a report of the American College of Cardiology/American Heart Association Task Force on Practice Guidelines [Committee to Update the 1996 Guidelines on Perioperative Cardiovascular Evaluation for Noncardiac Surgery], *J Am Coll Cardiol* 39:542-553, 2002.)

DIAGNOSTIC STUDIES

RESTING LEFT VENTRICULAR FUNCTION

Evaluation of resting LVEF preoperatively can predict risk for complications. This can be accomplished with a myriad of procedures, including echocardiography, contrast-enhanced ventriculography, and radionuclide angiography. The greatest risk for complications has been seen in patients with a resting LVEF of less than 35%. This risk is largely predictive of perioperative or postoperative exacerbation of HF or, in very seriously ill patients, death. These data cannot be extrapolated to predict postoperative ischemic events.[5]

ELECTROCARDIOGRAPHY

In patients with known or documented CAD, the resting ECG can be the single most important test to predict morbidity and mortality before surgery.[19-22] It is important to note that the resting 12-lead ECG cannot recognize increased risk in patients undertaking low-risk surgery.[23] The presence of Q waves is a poor prognostic sign. Their degree and size can offer a rough approximation of LVEF and can estimate long-term mortality.[24,25] ST segments are also helpful in preoperative assessment in that depressions that are horizontal or down-sloping and are greater than 0.5 mm are associated with a decrease in life expectancy. Other findings on the ECG that are linked to diminished longevity are left ventricular hypertrophy with a "strain pattern" and left bundle branch block.[19-22,24-28] If abnormalities are seen on the ECG and noninvasive testing is recommended based on the patient's risk factors, further evaluation may be accomplished through stress testing.

EXERCISE STRESS TESTING

Exercise stress testing can prove to be an objective tool in the quantification of functional capacity. This modality can also detect the presence or inducibility of cardiac arrhythmias and preoperative myocardial ischemia, which can further approximate perioperative cardiac risk and long-term prognosis.[5] In most ambulatory patients, this is the test of choice. However, exercise testing alone is not a very sensitive or specific test for obstructive CAD. Detection of obstructive CAD is dependent on the degree of stenosis and the extent of its distribution. It has been reported that up to half of all patients who have single-vessel disease may undergo exercise ECG stress testing and perform satisfactory levels of exercise without any clinical evidence of disease.[29] The mean sensitivity and specificity of exercise testing for detecting obstructive CAD are 68% and 77%, respectively. The sensitivity and specificity for multivessel disease are 81% and 66% and, for three-vessel or left main coronary disease, 86% and 53%, respectively.[5,30,31] Alternatively, Weiner and colleagues found that a low-risk subset of patients who could tolerate an exercise workload up to or past stage III of the Bruce protocol and have no ECG abnormalities had an annual mortality rate of less than 1% per year.[32] In patients who have significant abnormalities on their resting ECG, the exercise stress ECG will be much less reliable and other studies should be initiated. Examples of such abnormalities include left ventricular hypertrophy with a "strain" pattern, left bundle branch block, and a digitalis effect. In these situations, other diagnostic testing such as exercise echocardiography or exercise myocardial perfusion imaging is preferred.[5]

MYOCARDIAL PERFUSION IMAGING

If a patient cannot exercise, the choice may then be to perform myocardial perfusion imaging with pharmacologic stress. Two modalities that are commonly used are dobutamine stress echocardiography and intravenous dipyridamole/adenosine myocardial perfusion imaging using both thallium 201 and technetium 99m.[5]

The positive predictive value of a myocardial perfusion imaging study has been shown to positively correlate with the pretest cardiac risk of the patient.[33] Several studies have looked at the positive and negative predictive values of stress myocardial perfusion imaging studies before surgery. The majority of these studies involved patients undergoing vascular surgery, which is considered high risk. Ischemia was defined as thallium redistribution. The positive predictive value of these studies is extremely low. However, the negative predictive value is consistently very high at around 99% for MI or death. Patients with fixed defects do have an increase in cardiac risk above that of patients with normal findings on scans, but a test that demonstrates thallium redistribution or ischemia confers more risk.[15] Shaw and colleagues demonstrated in a meta-analysis of dipyridamole thallium imaging for risk stratification before vascular surgery that a reversible myocardial perfusion defect predicts perioperative events, whereas a fixed thallium defect predicts long-term cardiac events.[33]

Dobutamine stress echocardiography is a safe test that can be performed successfully on most patients. The negative and positive predictive values of dobutamine stress echocardiography are similar to the rates established for thallium imaging: low positive but high negative predictive values. The degree to which wall motion abnormality occurs and the extent to which wall motion abnormality occurs at low ischemic thresholds are predictors of long-term and short-term outcomes.[34-36] There is no definitive agreement that hypotension is a predictor of ischemia, but one study did show it to be an independent predictor of perioperative complications.[37]

The ACC/AHA guidelines recommend exercise testing as the first choice in patients who can exercise and have no abnormalities on the resting ECG. If these criteria cannot be met, the next appropriate test is myocardial perfusion imaging or dobutamine stress echocardiography. Avoidance of dipyridamole in patients with bronchospasm or carotid artery disease is recommended. Dobutamine should be avoided in patients with hypertension or hypotension as well as when echocardiographic imaging is limited because of poor visualization (obesity, chronic lung disease).

Occasionally, there are situations in which the patient has many risk factors or symptoms that suggest unstable angina. In these circumstances it may be appropriate to send the patient for coronary angiography rather than to proceed with noninvasive testing. Put simply, referral criteria for coronary angiography before surgery are the same as those for patients not planning to undergo surgery. These criteria include angina that has proved resistant to optimal medical therapy, evidence of significant ischemia on noninvasive testing, and unstable angina or an equivocal result from noninvasive testing in a patient being evaluated for either intermediate- or high-risk noncardiac surgery.[38]

If patients are referred for coronary angiography and a high-risk coronary artery stenosis is identified, it is likely that such a stenosis will be treated by percutaneous coronary intervention. Postoperatively, patients have increased risk for stent thrombosis and bleeding. The risk for coronary stent thrombosis is reduced if the patient completes 4 weeks of dual antiplatelet therapy after bare metal stenting. Bleeding risk is higher during this period, which led to the ACC/AHA recommendation that surgeons should wait at least two weeks, preferably four weeks, after coronary stenting with bare metal stents to perform noncardiac surgery. This time delay allows increased endothelialization of the stent and the completion of the recommended course of dual antiplatelet therapy. Dual platelet therapy is presently regarded as the use of clopidogrel and aspirin for four weeks with a shift to aspirin alone thereafter.[39,40]

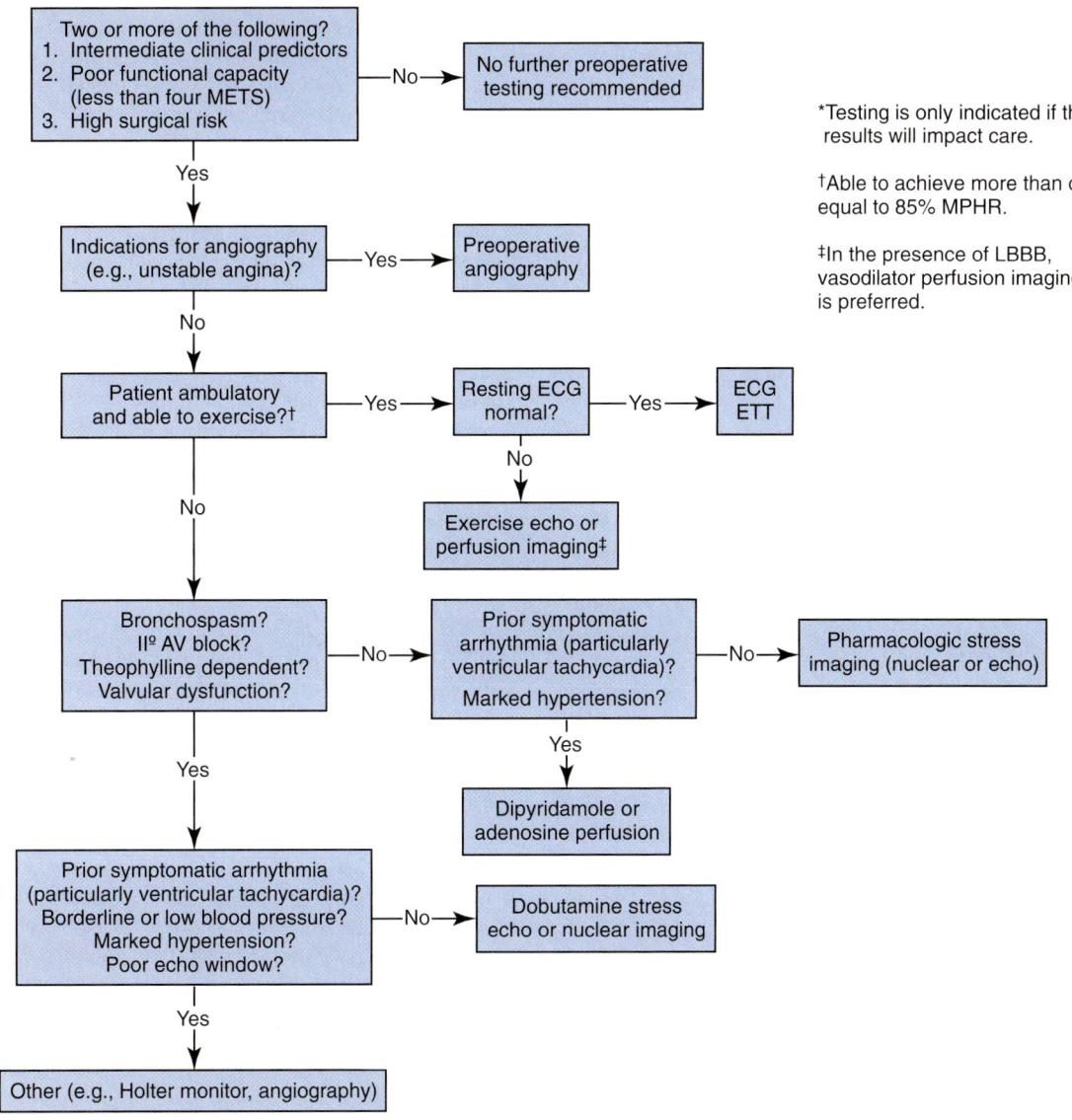

Fig. 27-2 ■ Supplemental preoperative evaluation: when and which test. Testing is indicated only if the results will have an impact on care. (From Eagle KA, Berger PB, Calkins H, et al: ACC/AHA guideline update for perioperative cardiovascular evaluation for noncardiac surgery-executive summary: a report of the American College of Cardiology/American Heart Association Task Force on Practice Guidelines [Committee to Update the 1996 Guidelines on Perioperative Cardiovascular Evaluation for Noncardiac Surgery], *J Am Coll Cardiol* 39:542-553, 2002.)

Figure 27-2 illustrates the decision-making process to provide the correct test for a specific patient.[5]

TREATMENT

"MEDICALLY OPTIMIZE"

It is essential for patients to be treated with optimal medical therapy. This is important pre- and postoperatively, as well as long-term. Optimal medical therapy should be personalized for each patient based on the specific cardiac conditions.[40]

BETA BLOCKERS

Patients with angina pectoris, known ischemia, previous MI, HF, hypertension, diabetes, or any combination of these conditions who already are on beta blockers should be continued with beta-blocker therapy in the perioperative setting.[40] The use of perioperative beta-blocker therapy has been proved in randomized controlled studies to reduce cardiac-related morbidity and, by extension, mortality in patients with known or highly suspected CAD who undergo high-risk surgery.[4] In addition, administration of beta blockers preoperatively has been proved to decrease the frequency of postoperative atrial fibrillation.[41-43] Thus, baseline cardiac risk is an important parameter in determining benefit of beta blockade. Beta blockers do benefit patients with high cardiovascular risk, while harm may occur to individuals in the low to moderate risk categories secondary to bradycardia and hypotension.[44] If beta blockers are initiated in the preoperative setting a "run-in" phase of at least seven days should be implemented.[45]

CALCIUM CHANNEL BLOCKERS

If patients have ongoing ischemia despite the use of beta blockers, calcium channel blockers may be used. There is also a benefit in terms of lowering blood pressure with this class of medications.

ASPIRIN

Individuals with angina pectoris, previous MI, and diabetes should be treated with aspirin. Most sources agree that aspirin should be withheld from 5 to 10 days before elective noncardiovascular surgery to prevent bleeding complications.[46] However, this can differ on a patient-to-patient basis as suggested by Madan and associates, who demonstrated minimal bleeding during and after minor oral surgery in patients who continued to take low-dose aspirin.[47]

STATINS

Treatment with a statin is generally considered optimal therapy for patients with a previous MI. This medication is usually part of a stable medical regimen and should be continued as soon as the patient may take medications by mouth.

NITRATES

This class of medications is relegated mainly to patients with chronic stable angina pectoris. If the angina is stable and nitrates are a part of the patient's normal medical regimen, they may be continued. There is a risk for hypotension in a patient who is hypovolemic. Patients taking this class of medications should be monitored closely.

PAIN MANAGEMENT

Most cardiac complications from noncardiac surgery occur postoperatively. This is at a time when increased stressors on the body can result in neurohormonal changes that can alter hemodynamics and the coagulation cascade. Although no studies definitively argue for analgesics and pain control as a preventive measure for postoperative cardiac events, they can blunt the stress response and are associated with lower pain scores and better patient satisfaction overall.[5]

OTHER RISK FACTORS

Patients who smoke should be counseled to stop tobacco use before surgery. This is to lessen not only hypertension and cardiac events but also pulmonary complications. Inotropic agents can increase the heart rate and myocardial oxygen consumption and should be avoided most of the time.

WHEN TO CALL A CARDIOLOGIST

There are reasonably defined guidelines for dealing with many postoperative cardiac scenarios. Many of them are successfully managed by noncardiologists in an emergency. However, in common practice, it is recommended and encouraged to call and consult a cardiologist for assistance in the following situations.

PULMONARY ARTERY CATHETERS

Existing evidence does not currently support the routine use of pulmonary artery catheters as standard of perioperative care.[5,15] However, with a capable physician and an experienced hospital staff, the information gained with this catheter can be extremely helpful, especially in a critical patient. The key is to attain the most benefit without harm. The American Society of Anesthesiologists has published practice parameters for the intraoperative use of pulmonary artery catheters.[48] This report also addresses the decision to place the catheter based on patient variables.

SURVEILLANCE FOR MYOCARDIAL INFARCTION

Perioperative MI can be detected by evaluating clinical symptoms, cardiac biomarkers, and left ventricular function by transthoracic echocardiography and serial ECGs. There is a body of evidence to support protocols to diagnose perioperative MI after noncardiac surgery. The least sensitive modality seems to be measurement of blood levels of myocardial-bound creatine kinase (CKMB), and the most sensitive is evaluation of new segmental wall motion abnormalities on transthoracic echocardiography.[5,15] The ACC/AHA recommendations incorporate CAD and risk into account. The guidelines affirm that in patients without known CAD, surveillance should be applied only to those who exhibit perioperative symptoms of cardiac decompensation. If a patient is known to have CAD, has high or intermediate clinical risk, and is undergoing high- or intermediate-risk surgery, baseline ECGs along with reevaluation directly after surgery and on a daily basis for two days following surgery are recommended.[5,15] Serum troponin assays have not been clearly validated but are part of the diagnostic approach for recognition of perioperative MI. Troponin may be sampled 24 hours postoperatively and again on day 4 or at hospital discharge, whichever event occurs earlier.[49] The degree of elevated troponin, existence or lack of changes on the ECG, hemodynamic instability, and clinical symptoms may assist in generating an accurate estimate of severity. A cardiologist should be consulted for further evaluation of the patient under such circumstances. [5,15]

MANAGEMENT OF ARRHYTHMIAS

Arrhythmias are very common postoperatively and are frequently caused by noncardiac factors such as hypoxia, infection, hypotension, or metabolic disturbances. Vagal maneuvers (Valsalva maneuver or carotid sinus massage) are quick and usually harmless first-line approaches in patients with sustained, regular narrow-complex tachycardia. Frequently, narrow-complex supraventricular arrhythmias are often due to atrioventricular nodal re-entrant tachycardia or atrioventricular reciprocating tachycardia. Intravenous adenosine is also an option to quickly slow down the rhythm but is mainly for diagnostic use to define the underlying rhythm disorder. Longer-acting agents such as beta blockers, calcium channel blockers, and antiarrhythmic agents are more optimal long-term treatments and may prevent recurrence.[15] If, however, the rhythm appears to be irregular or is causing hemodynamic instability, intravenous beta-blockers, calcium channel blockers, or even direct current cardioversion may need to be used, especially if the patient is symptomatic. An investigation into secondary causes of the arrhythmia should be launched and the causes corrected. Bradyarrhythmias are included in this scenario and are commonly the result of another issue such as overmedication, electrolyte derangements, hypoxia, or even ischemia. In an acute setting, atropine may resolve the problem. If the arrhythmia is due to sinus node dysfunction, temporary transcutaneous or transvenous pacing may be used, and a permanent pacemaker may need to be considered. Cardiac consultation should be considered in most of these situations. Premature ventricular contractions, even if very frequent, often do not require any treatment.[15]

IMPLANTABLE CARDIAC DEFIBRILLATORS

The use of electrocautery introduces radiofrequency current to cut or induce coagulation. There is a possibility of interaction between ICDs and pacemakers with electrocautery devices. If the surgical site on which the electrocautery device is used is too close to the implanted device, there is a higher risk of interaction. This communication is produced by electrical current and may cause derangements by inducing ICDs to fire, pacemakers to revert to a backup rate or to temporary or permanent inhibition, an increase in the pacing rate, or heat generation through a lead tip, which could cause myocardial injury. There are no formal guidelines on how to approach patients with these devices in the perioperative period, but with certain safety measures, the likelihood of adverse interactions may be reduced.[15]

All patients with devices who are undergoing surgery should have their ICD or pacemaker interrogated before and after surgery. This assessment should determine whether the patient is pacemaker-dependent, to check thresholds and battery status (if not done recently), and to ascertain whether the device is programmed in a rate-responsive setting. This feature should be inactivated before surgery.[15] Implantable cardiac defibrillators should also be inactivated during surgery. This may be achieved by either taping a magnet over the device, which suspends detection of arrhythmias without interrupting backup bradycardia pacing, or by programming the device to the off setting. The benefit of a magnet enables the surgeon to have very quick access to defibrillation with the patient's own device if a ventricular arrhythmia should occur. Uncomplicated removal of the magnet will allow the ICD to regain arrhythmia detection capability and deliver therapy when indicated. This approach prevents the delay in waiting for the cardiologist or the electrophysiology technician to return to reactivate the device. In either scenario, defibrillator pads should be in place while the defibrillator is inactivated with careful placement of the pads as far from the implanted device as possible and in a fashion likely to be perpendicular to the device leads.[15,50]

VALVULAR HEART DISEASE

A cardiac murmur detected before surgery is very common. It is important to classify and quantify which type of valvular heart disease is causing the murmur. The most threatening murmur to diagnose before surgery is aortic stenosis.[51] If the degree of aortic stenosis is severe, any non-urgent maxillofacial surgery should be postponed. If the surgery is elective, the patient needs to undergo aortic valve replacement surgery first. Occasionally, patients elect to refuse valve surgery and agree to accept higher-risk noncardiac surgery. In this setting, a patient with severe, unrepaired aortic stenosis has a 10% risk for mortality when undergoing noncardiac surgery.[15,52,53] In rare instances when the patient is not a candidate for aortic valve replacement, percutaneous balloon valvuloplasty may be a reasonable approach.[54]

Mitral stenosis is much less commonly seen since it is mostly associated with rheumatic heart disease. This valvular abnormality is important to distinguish because the diastolic filling period is compromised and the heart rate must be controlled. Although severe mitral valve stenosis can increase the likelihood of HF, there is no indication to correct the problem before noncardiac surgery. If the patient is to undergo high-risk surgery, balloon mitral valvuloplasty may be an alternative.[5,22]

MANAGEMENT RECOMMENDATIONS FOR CLINICAL CASES

CASE 1

Mr. H. was considered intermediate risk for intermediate-risk surgery. His history and physical examination showed that he was very active and participated in a weekly bowling league. His functional capacity was estimated to be 7 METs. Because his blood pressure was not at goal, beta-blocker therapy was started two weeks prior to surgery. With intermediate risk and good functional capacity, there is no further need to pursue cardiovascular testing. More notably, with a malignant tumor, there is an urgency to perform surgery without delay. Mr. H. was deemed stable for surgery and underwent surgery without complications.

CASE 2

Mrs. W. was evaluated by a cardiologist who considered her HF to be well compensated. She was also being maintained on optimal medical management. A magnet was taped over her ICD and she underwent semi-urgent surgery without complications. After surgery, the magnet was removed. Postoperatively, her ICD was checked to ensure that it was functioning properly. She had no postoperative events.

CASE 3

Mr. A. had transthoracic echocardiography performed several years before the present evaluation, and it was reasonable to reevaluate his aortic stenosis. A repeat study revealed no change in the severity of the aortic stenosis, and no symptoms of angina, syncope, or HF were detected on history and physical examination. He underwent a minor dental procedure without complications and is being evaluated by his cardiologist on an annual basis.

PEARLS AND PITFALLS

- The published guidelines, though straightforward and discrete, may not always fit the individual patient.
- In essence, the plan for cardiac testing or treatment should be the same for a patient undergoing surgery and one who is not. It is the timing that is dissimilar which is based on the urgency of the noncardiac surgery, patient-specific risk factors, and specific risks associated with the surgery.
- When unsure, it may be necessary to ask for cardiology consultation. Situations that may necessitate a consultation include the use of pulmonary artery catheters, surveillance for MI, management of arrhythmias, patients with ICDs, and the presence of valvular heart disease.
- An effective evaluation requires communication between all physicians providing care to the patient.[5]

REFERENCES

1. Mangano DT: Perioperative cardiac morbidity, *Anesthesiology* 72:153-184, 1990.
2. Medscape: *http://emedicine.medscape.com/article/285328-overview 7/10/09.*
3. Rudin AS, Fintel DJ: Preoperative cardiac evaluation. In Shields TW, editor: *General thoracic surgery*, ed 6, Philadelphia, 2005, Lippincott Williams & Wilkins, pp 345-356.
4. Karnath BM: Preoperative cardiac risk assessment, *Am Fam Physician* 66:1889-1896, 2002.
5. Eagle KA, Berger PB, Calkins H, et al. ACC/AHA guideline update for perioperative cardiovascular evaluation for noncardiac surgery—executive summary: a report of the American College of Cardiology/American Heart Association Task Force on Practice Guidelines (Committee to Update the 1996 Guidelines on Perioperative Cardiovascular Evaluation for Noncardiac Surgery), *J Am Coll Cardiol* 39:542-553, 2002.
6. Machala W, Szebla R: Effects of propofol induction on hemodynamics, *Anestezjol Intens Ter* 40:172-175, 2008.

7. O'Hara DA, Duff A, Berlin JA, et al: The effect of anesthetic technique on postoperative outcomes in hip fracture repair, *Anesthesiology* 92:947-957, 2000.

8. Leung JM, Goehner P, O'Kelly BF, et al: Isoflurane anesthesia and myocardial ischemia: comparative risk versus sufentanil anesthesia in patients undergoing coronary artery bypass graft surgery. The SPI (Study of Perioperative Ischemia) Research Group, *Anesthesiology* 74:838-847, 1991.

9. Baron JF, Bertrand M, Barre E, et al: Combined epidural and general anesthesia versus general anesthesia for abdominal aortic surgery, *Anesthesiology* 75:611-618, 1991.

10. Christopherson R, Beattie C, Frank SM, et al: Perioperative morbidity in patients randomized to epidural or general anesthesia for lower extremity vascular surgery: Perioperative Ischemia Randomized Anesthesia Trial Study Group, *Anesthesiology* 79:422-434, 1993.

11. Slogoff S, Keats AS: Randomized trial of primary anesthetic agents on outcome of coronary artery bypass operations, *Anesthesiology* 70:179-188, 1989.

12. Tuman KJ, McCarthy RJ, Spiess BD: Epidural anaesthesia and analgesia decreases postoperative hypercoagulability in high-risk vascular patients, *Anesth Analg* 70:S414, 1990.

13. Rodgers A, Walker N, Schug S, et al: Reduction of postoperative mortality and morbidity with epidural or spinal anesthesia: results from overview of randomised trials, *BMJ* 321:1493-1497, 2000.

14. Urwin SC, Parker MJ, Griffiths R: General versus regional anesthesia for hip fracture surgery: a meta-analysis of randomized trials, *Br J Anaesth* 84:450-455, 2000.

15. Fleisher LA, Beckman JA, Brown KA, et al: ACC/AHA guidelines on perioperative cardiovascular evaluation and care for noncardiac surgery: executive summary, *Circulation* 116:1971-1996, 2007.

16. Gerson MC, Hurst JM, Hertzberg VS, et al: Cardiac prognosis in noncardiac geriatric surgery, *Ann Intern Med* 103(6 Pt 1):832-833, 1985.

17. Fletcher GF, Balady G, Froelicher VF, et al: Exercise standards. A statement for healthcare professionals from the American Heart Association, *Circulation* 91:580-615, 1995.

18. Hlatky MA, Boineau RE, Higginbotham MB, et al: A brief self-administered questionnaire to determine functional capacity (the Duke Activity Status Index), *Am J Cardiol* 64:651-654, 1989.

19. Sutherland SE, Gazes PC, Keil JE, et al: Electrocardiographic abnormalities and 30-year mortality among white and black men of the Charleston Heart Study, *Circulation* 88:2685-2692, 1993.

20. Kannel WB, Gordon T, Offutt D: Left ventricular hypertrophy by electrocardiogram: prevalence, incidence, and mortality in the Framingham study, *Ann Intern Med* 71:89-105, 1969.

21. Tervahauta M, Pekkanen J, Punsar S, et al: Resting electrocardiographic abnormalities as predictors of coronary events and total mortality among elderly men, *Am J Med* 100:641-645, 1996.

22. Kreger BE, Cupples LA, Kannel WB: The electrocardiogram in prediction of sudden death: Framingham Study experience, *Am Heart J* 113:377-382, 1987.

23. Schein OD, Katz J, Bass EB, et al: The value of routine preoperative medical testing before cataract surgery. Study of Medical Testing for Cataract Surgery, *N Engl J Med* 342:168-175, 2000.

24. Kannel WB, Abbott RD: Incidence and prognosis of unrecognized myocardial infarction: an update on the Framingham study, *N Engl J Med* 311:1144-1147, 1984.

25. Crow RS, Prineas RJ, Hannan PJ, et al: Prognostic associations of Minnesota Code serial electrocardiographic change classification with coronary heart disease mortality in the Multiple Risk Intervention Trial, *Am J Cardiol* 80:138-144, 1997.

26. Kannel WB, Cobb J: Left ventricular hypertrophy and mortality: results from the Framingham Study, *Cardiology* 81:291-298, 1992.

27. Schneider JF, Thomas HE Jr, Kreger BE, et al: Newly acquired left bundle-branch block: the Framingham study, *Ann Intern Med* 90:303-310, 1979.

28. Rabkin SW, Mathewson FA, Tate RB: Natural history of left bundle-branch block, *Br Heart J* 43:164-169, 1980.

29. Chaitman BR: The changing role of the exercise electrocardiogram as a diagnostic and prognostic test for chronic ischemic heart disease, *J Am Coll Cardiol* 8:1195-1210, 1986.

30. Gianrossi R, Detrano R, Mulvihill D, et al: Exercise-induced ST depression in the diagnosis of coronary artery disease: a meta-analysis, *Circulation* 80:87-98, 1989.

31. Detrano R, Gianrossi R, Mulvihill D, et al: Exercise-induced ST segment depression in the diagnosis of multivessel coronary disease: a meta analysis, *J Am Coll Cardiol* 14:1501-1508, 1989.

32. Weiner DA, Ryan TJ, McCabe CH, et al: Prognostic importance of a clinical profile and exercise test in medically treated patients with coronary artery disease, *J Am Coll Cardiol* 3:772-779, 1984.

33. Shaw LJ, Eagle KA, Gersh BJ, et al: Meta-analysis of intravenous dipyridamole-thallium-201 imaging (1985 to 1994) and dobutamine echocardiography (1991 to 1994) for risk stratification before vascular surgery, *J Am Coll Cardiol* 27:787-798, 1996.

34. Dávila-Román VG, Waggoner AD, Sicard GA, et al: Dobutamine stress echocardiography predicts surgical outcome in patients with an aortic aneurysm and peripheral vascular disease, *J Am Coll Cardiol* 21:957-963, 1993.

35. Poldermans D, Arnese M, Fioretti PM, et al: Improved cardiac risk stratification in major

vascular surgery with dobutamine-atropine stress echocardiography, *J Am Coll Cardiol* 26:648-653, 1995.

36. Day SM, Younger JG, Karavite D, et al: Usefulness of hypotension during dobutamine echocardiography in predicting perioperative cardiac events, *Am J Cardiol* 85:478-483, 2000.

37. Bigatel DA, Franklin DP, Elmore JR, et al: Dobutamine stress echocardiography prior to aortic surgery: long-term cardiac outcome, *Ann Vasc Surg* 13:17-22, 1999.

38. Froehlich JB, Karavite D, Russman PL, et al: American College of Cardiology/American Heart Association preoperative assessment guidelines reduce resource utilization before aortic surgery, *J Vasc Surg* 36:758-763, 2002.

39. Kaluza GL, Joseph J, Lee JR, et al: Catastrophic outcomes of noncardiac surgery soon after coronary stenting, *J Am Coll Cardiol* 35:1288-1294, 2000.

40. Mukherjee D, Eagle K: Perioperative cardiac assessment for noncardiac surgery: eight steps to the best possible outcome, *Circulation* 107:2771, 2003.

41. Jakobsen CJ, Bille S, Ahlburg P, et al: Perioperative metoprolol reduces the frequency of atrial fibrillation after thoracotomy for lung resection, *J Cardiothorac Vasc Anesth* 11:746-751, 1997.

42. Mangano DT, Layug EL, Wallace A, et al: Effect of atenolol on mortality and cardiovascular morbidity after noncardiac surgery. Multicenter Study of Perioperative Ischemia Research Group [published erratum appears in *N Engl J Med* 1997;336:1039], *N Engl J Med* 335:1713-1720, 1996.

43. Poldermans D, Boersma E, Bax JJ, et al, for the Dutch Echocardiographic Cardiac Risk Evaluation Applying Stress Echocardiography Study Group: The effect of bisoprolol on perioperative mortality and myocardial infarction in high-risk patients undergoing vascular surgery, *N Engl J Med* 341:1789-1794, 1999.

44. Lindenauer PK, Pekow P, Wang K, et al.: Perioperative beta-blocker therapy and mortality after major noncardiac surgery. *N Engl J Med* 353:349-361, 2005.

45. Chopra V, Plaisance B, Cavusoglu E, et al.: Perioperative beta-blockers for major noncardiac surgery: primum non nocere. *Am J Med* 122:222-229, 2009.

46. Conti CR: Aspirin and elective surgical procedures [editorial], *Clin Cardiol* 15:709, 1992.

47. Madan GA, Madan SC, Madan G, et al: Minor oral surgery without stopping daily low-dose aspirin therapy: a study of 51 patients, *J Oral Maxillofac Surg* 63:1262-1265, 2005.

48. Practice guidelines for pulmonary artery catheterization: a report by the American Society of Anesthesiologists Task Force on Pulmonary Artery Catheterization, *Anesthesiology* 78:380-394, 1993.

49. Metzler H, Gries M, Rehak P, et al: Perioperative myocardial cell injury: the role of troponins, *Br J Anaesth* 78:386-390, 1997.

50. Stevenson WG, Chaitman BR, Ellenbogen KA, et al: Clinical assessment and management of patients with implanted cardioverter-defibrillators presenting to non-electrophysiologists, *Circulation* 110;3866-3869, 2004.

51. Goldman L, Caldera DL, Nussbaum SR, et al: Multifactorial index of cardiac risk in noncardiac surgical procedures, *N Engl J Med* 297:845-850, 1977.

52. Raymer K, Yang H: Patients with aortic stenosis: cardiac complications in noncardiac surgery, *Can J Anaesth* 45:855-859, 1998.

53. Torsher LC, Shub C, Rettke SR, et al: Risk of patients with severe aortic stenosis undergoing noncardiac surgery, *Am J Cardiol* 81:448-452, 1998.

54. Reyes VP, Raju BS, Wynne J, et al: Percutaneous balloon valvuloplasty compared with open surgical commissurotomy for mitral stenosis, *N Engl J Med* 331:961-967, 1994.

Chapter 28

Management of the Irradiated Patient

Martin I. Salgueiro, Mark R. Stevens

Management of head and neck cancer is a difficult but common challenge in the practice of oral and maxillofacial surgery. Radiotherapy is a proven modality for the treatment and palliation of head and neck malignancy.[1,2] Despite its benefit in the treatment of cancer, radiation has an immense potential for causing acute and chronic complications. Oral and maxillofacial surgeons and other dental specialists are not directly involved in the administration of radiotherapy, but they are often responsible for the prevention and treatment of adverse effects and complications resulting from it. Some of these complications are temporary and may resolve with time, and these are easy to manage; however, others, such as osteoradionecrosis (ORN), can be devastating and difficult to treat.

RADIATION PHYSIOLOGY

Radiation can be nonionizing and ionizing. Nonionizing radiation such as radio waves, microwaves, and light waves have little energy and do not have a therapeutic role in cancer treatment. Ionizing radiation has high energy. It forms ions as it passes through tissues by dislodging electrons from atoms.[3] Ionization results in cell death or irreversible damage to DNA with consequent loss of reproductive capabilities of the affected cells. It is this feature that makes ionizing radiation effective for the treatment of malignancy not only in the head and neck area but also in general.

The two main types of ionizing radiation are electromagnetic and particulate. Electromagnetic radiation comes from photons. Photons are elementary particles that have intrinsic properties of charge, mass, and spin, depending on the circumstances. Photons originating from the atomic nucleus produce gamma rays, and photons originating from electrons around the atomic nucleus produce x-rays. Particulate radiation includes electrons, protons, neutrons, and alpha and beta particles. The radiation source can be outside the body or implanted as radioactive seeds or needles (brachytherapy). The more common types of radiation used in the head and neck are high-energy photons, electrons, protons, and neutrons. Protons are the earliest type of radiation. Protons deposit most of their radiation energy in what is known as the Bragg peak.[4] The depth at which the Bragg peak occurs is energy-dependent and can be controlled to allow the maximum dose to be delivered to the target tumor with minimal damage to surrounding normal tissues. Proton radiation is available in just a few centers in the United States. Neutron beam radiation causes severe long-term complications and is used rarely for tumors resistant to other types of radiation. Intensity-modulated radiation therapy (IMRT) is a protocol in which multiple beams of radiation are delivered at different angles and intensities to target a tumor while minimizing radiation injury to the surrounding tissues. This technique requires tridimensional mapping of the tumor and careful positioning and immobilization of the patient during treatment.

The amount of radiation delivered to a target area is the radiation dose. The unit for measuring radiation is the gray (Gy). The amount of radiation in an abdominal radiograph is 1.4 milligray (mGy).[3] The typical radiation dose for the treatment of malignancies in the head and neck region ranges from 5000 to 7600 centigray (cGy) and averages around 7000 cGy.[5,6] The total dose is delivered in fractions, usually 200 cGy daily. Considerable research has been performed to define the most appropriate fractionation schedule.[7] Variations in protocol, called hypofractionation and hyperfractionation, deliver fewer but larger doses or smaller, more frequent doses. Fractionation is an important concept in radiotherapy. It provides normal tissue in the irradiated field the opportunity to heal between doses, thereby decreasing the amount of late complications. The presence of oxygen at the time of irradiation significantly enhances the effects of ionizing radiation in living tissues.[8] Tumors often have areas of hypoxia since uncontrolled rapid growth can compress blood vessels and reduce blood flow. Because of the high number of cells, tumors often outgrow their blood supply, which also results in areas of hypoxia.[9] Fractionation reduces the number of cells and the size of the tumor and allows reoxygenation, which directly increases the efficacy of radiation. Other variables affecting the sensitivity of cells to radiation include the type of cell and its stage in the reproductive cycle. Germinal and lymphoreticular cells are the most sensitive. Endothelial cells and fibroblasts have intermediate sensitivity. However, even reduced damage to these cell types may diminish the healing potential of tissues and result in late complications. Finally, muscle and nerve cells are the most resistant to the effects of ionizing radiation. Because tumor cells replicate at a rate faster than normal, they are more likely to be irradiated at a vulnerable time in their cell cycle,[5] and they therefore are the most sensitive to radiation therapy.

SIDE EFFECTS OF RADIATION THERAPY

The goal of radiotherapy in cancer treatment is eradication of every viable tumor cell with minimal damage to normal tissue. Unfortunately, it is not unexpected for cancer patients undergoing radiotherapy to suffer side effects resulting from damage to healthy tissue in the path of the radiation. The oral cavity and pharynx are covered with specialized mucosa that has rapid epithelial turnover and a rich vascularity to support it. The mandibular alveolus has a rapid bone cell turnover rate that can be 10 times that of long bones.[7] These features make this tissue susceptible to radiation-induced damage. Adverse effects can occur acutely or late. Acute adverse effects can cause significant discomfort to the patient. However, they are short term and generally resolve within weeks after completion of radiation therapy. The goal in management of these conditions is to provide immediate pain relief. Late adverse effects, such as ORN, xerostomia, and radiation-induced caries, cause significant morbidly and are much more difficult to treat. They also have a greater impact on quality of life and the distress level of cancer patients.[6]

RADIATION MUCOSITIS

Radiation-induced mucositis occurs in almost all patients undergoing radiotherapy for the treatment of head and neck cancer.[10,11] It is the result of repeated radiation insult to otherwise normal mucosa and usually develops within the first 2 weeks of treatment. The adverse clinical signs are evident by the second or third week. The early stage is characterized by a whitish discoloration caused by the lack of sufficient desquamation of keratin.[12] This evolves into a diffuse erythema with the presence of fibrinous exudates (Fig. 28-1).

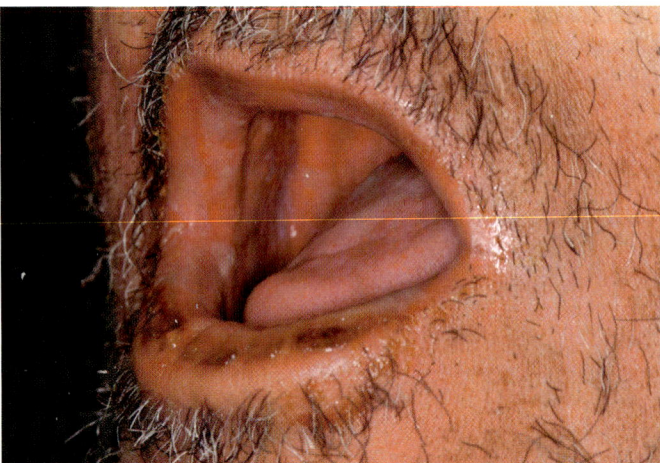

Fig. 28-1 ■ Radiation-induced mucositis with diffuse erythema and fibrinous exudates on the cheeks and lips.

The mucosa becomes friable and often ulcerated. Radiation-induced mucositis is a debilitating condition that produces a state of general discomfort. Burning pain, dysphagia, weight loss, and speech difficulties are some of the common complaints.[5,12,13] Rarely, radiation oncologists will agree to interrupt the treatment because of side effects; however, ulcerative mucositis is the major limitation to continuous, uninterrupted radiotherapy.[10,14]

Radiation-induced mucositis usually resolves within 3 to 4 weeks after completion of the last fraction. The treatment goals for these patients are prevention of opportunistic infection and pain control. It has been reported that 76% of head and neck cancer patients are found to be noncompliant with routine dental care and oral hygiene in pre-radiation consultation.[15] Ironically, adequate oral hygiene is a key factor in the prevention of infection resulting from bacterial colonization of ulcerated tissues. Traditional hygiene routines of tooth brushing and dental floss can be extremely painful. Therefore, antibiotic oral rinses play an important role in intraoral bacterial control. Chlorhexidine is a broad-spectrum topical antimicrobial agent that is widely prescribed by oral surgeons, other dental specialists, and general dentists. Use of 0.12% chlorhexidine oral rinse is recommended in patients with mild to severe radiation-induced mucositis.[5,6,16] Use of a chlorhexidine-soaked foam brush is an alternative for maintaining oral hygiene.[6] Viscous lidocaine 2% gel is usually helpful in controlling pain. Systemic analgesics, including nonsteroidal anti-inflammatory drugs and narcotics, are concomitantly prescribed when necessary. Antibiotics are indicated only in patients with secondary infection who have systemic manifestations such as fever or lymphadenopathy.

RADIATION DERMATITIS

Radiation-induced dermatitis usually occurs within 90 days of starting treatment.[17,18] Many of the skin changes are minor and reversible. The initial changes may be undetectable and can occur hours after exposure to radiation and fade within hours to days.[19] Apparent and sustained changes lasting for up to 2 weeks after completion of radiation therapy are most likely mediated by cytokines. They are described as a blanchable reactive pink hue with no other epidermal changes.[20] Cutaneous changes may be classified as acute, late, or chronic. The standard for evaluation of radiation-induced dermatitis is the National Cancer Institute's common toxicity criteria version 3.0. Grade 1 changes include mild or generalized erythema with pruritus, epilation, and depigmentation. Grade 2 changes occur after radiation doses higher than 4000 cGy.[21] At this stage persistent erythema may progress to loss of the epidermis limited to skin folds. This is more common in breast cancer patients because of the more pronounced skin folds. These changes usually peak 1 to 2 weeks after completing radiation therapy.[22] Epidermal regeneration is noted within 3 to 5 weeks, with complete healing taking place in 1 to 3 months.[12,18] When moist desquamation extends beyond the skin fold, it is classified as grade 3. Ulcer development, hemorrhage, and necrosis are considered grade 4 changes. As with radiation-induced mucositis, secondary infection is a common complication and thus skin care and hygiene are extremely important. Chronic radiation-induced dermatitis can appear months to years after radiotherapy. Manifestations include the following: textural changes, hyperpigmentation, hypopigmentation, telangiectasia, and fibrosis. Alopecia and decreased or absent sweating result from damage to hair follicles and sebaceous glands (Fig. 28-2). Some of these changes may improve and eventually normalize. Depending on variables such as the total dose, location, severity of the initial injury, skin type, and individual patient co-morbid conditions, they can be more severe or permanent.[22,23-26] The scalp is more tolerant of the effects of radiation than the face, neck, or chest are.[27] The treatment goals are pain

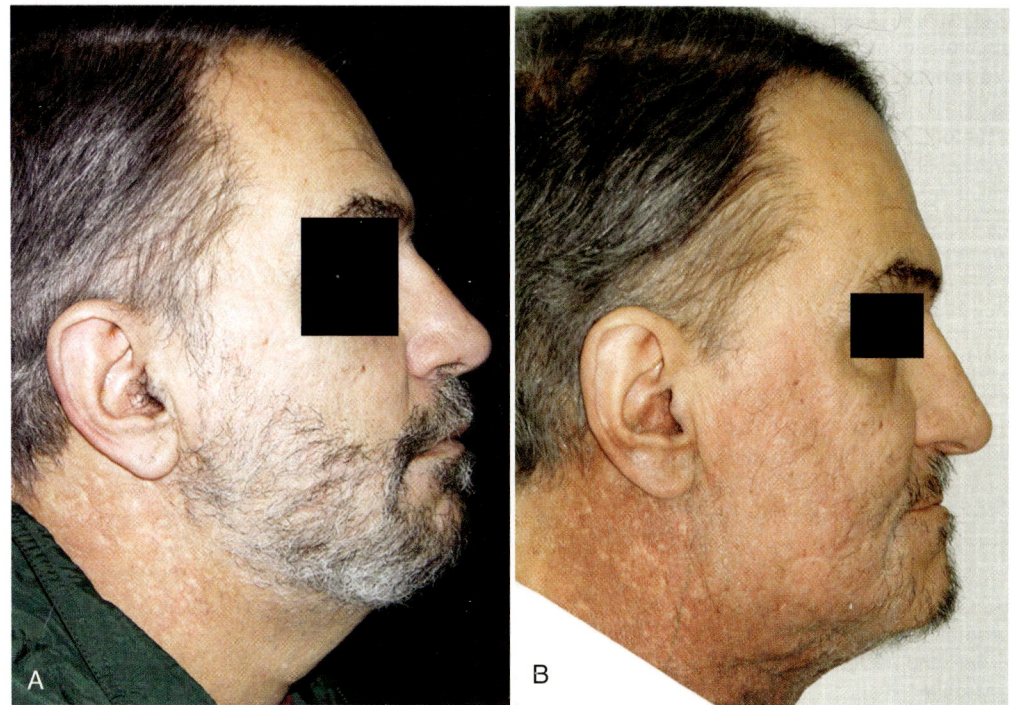

Fig. 28-2 ■ **A,** Patient before starting radiation therapy. **B,** Patient after radiation therapy. Notice the changes in skin color and loss of facial hair in the radiation field.

control, minimization of transepidermal water loss, and prevention of infection. Progression of erythema and dry desquamation to moist desquamation should be prevented.[18] Petrolatum-base emollients are commonly prescribed for the treatment of radiation-induced dermatitis. Non–petrolatum-based products with castor oil, balsam of Peru, trypsin, or aloe vera are also used.[18,28] Although the indication for topical steroids is controversial, they have likewise been used for the prevention and treatment of this condition. Pain control is achieved with oral analgesics. Topical and systemic antibiotics are indicated in the event of cutaneous infection.

XEROSTOMIA

A healthy adult produces about 1.5 liters of saliva per day. Saliva lubricates the oral mucosa and pharynx, facilitates speech and swallowing, and is involved in the control of oral flora. Saliva also aids in the digestion of food and buffering of acids produced by the fermentation of carbohydrates.[6] Radiation-induced xerostomia is a serious condition that significantly affects the quality of life of head and neck cancer patients. The slow turnover rate of glandular epithelium may provide salivary glands some degree of radio resistance. However, the ultimately decreased perfusion and destruction of the microvasculature often result in irreversible damage.[3,29] In addition to the normal complaint of dry mouth, xerostomia has multiple associated sequelae. Dysphagia, dysgeusia, dysosmia, pain, mucositis, and chewing and speech difficulty are some of the common complaints of patients with this condition.[30,31] Decreased or absent salivary flow promotes the proliferation of cariogenic bacteria such as *Streptococcus mutans* and *Lactobacillus* species.[3,31] Caries and periodontal disease can be directly related to radiation. The changes in oral flora are responsible for these conditions outside the field of radiation. Radiation doses higher than 3000 to 3500 cGy are associated with an increased risk for significant salivary gland dysfunction.[3,31,32] Doses lower than 2000 cGy may produce reversible damage. Marked irreversible and degenerative changes in

acinar cells and glandular ductal epithelium occur with radiation doses higher than 5000 cGy.[33]

Reduced salivary flow is seen in the first week of radiation therapy and may decrease to about 20% of baseline after 7 weeks.[33] Partial recovery may be possible within 12 to 18 months after treatment. The use of IMRT protocols can reduce the radiation dose delivered to the salivary glands and allow preservation of some gland function.[32,34] Two pharmaceutical agents have been advocated for the protection of salivary glands during treatment in an effort to minimize radiation injury. Pilocarpine (Salagen, MGI Pharma, Minneapolis, Minn) is a sialagogue that promotes salivation by stimulating muscarinic receptors on the salivary glands. Studies reported that a dose of 5 mg three to five times a day during radiation therapy did not prove to be effective in the preservation of salivary gland function.[35,36] The second agent is amifostine (Ethyol, MedImmune Oncology, Inc., Gaithersburg, Md). This drug has been approved by the U.S. Food and Drug Administration (FDA) for reduction of radiation-induced xerostomia. It is a sulfhydryl compound that has the ability to donate hydrogen ions to radiation-generated free oxygen radicals and thereby prevent oxidation damage. Amifostine has been shown to significantly reduce the incidence of acute and chronic radiation-induced xerostomia.[32,37,38] Furthermore it appears to offer selective protection to normal cells without affecting the efficacy of radiation in tumor treatment.[39,40] Amifostine is given daily 15 to 30 minutes before radiation therapy at a dose of 200 mg/m^2. Reported side effects are nausea, vomiting, hypotension, and local skin reaction at the injection site.[31,32,40] Another reported technique for prevention of xerostomia is surgical transfer of the submandibular gland to the submental space to place it outside the radiation field.[41,42]

It is common to see patients suffering from radiation-induced xerostomia with water bottles at all times. They require constant sipping to maintain the moisture of the oral mucosa. Salivary substitutes function as a temporary relief of discomfort by introducing moisture into the oral cavity[6]; however, they do not replace the antibacterial and immunologic protection of natural saliva.[43]

This population of patients also requires comprehensive dental care and close follow-up. Oral hygiene is a key factor in the prevention of caries and periodontal disease. Antimicrobial rinses (0.12% chlorhexidine) and topical fluoride application are recommended. Pilocarpine is approved by the FDA as a sialogogue agent; it is prescribed three times a day in doses of 5 to 10 mg. Increased salivary secretion occurs within 30 minutes after ingestion.[31,44] Treatment lasts for 8 to 12 weeks, and it may be used for longer periods as maintenance therapy.[45] Bethanechol (Urecholine, Odyssey Pharmaceuticals, East Hanover, NJ) is also used for the systemic treatment of xerostomia. It is given in doses of 25 to 50 mg three times a day.[46] It has been suggested that the use of sugarless gum and candy may stimulate residual gland function.[31] Sialogogue agents will increase salivary secretion by stimulating muscarinic receptors in viable residual gland tissue. Consequently, they are not effective when no salivary gland tissue survives radiation therapy.

TRISMUS

The cause of trismus in head and neck cancer patients is multifactorial. Limitation of mandibular range of motion can be a consequence of invasion of tumor into the masticatory muscles or the temporomandibular joint (TMJ), mechanical obstruction of the coronoid process by tumor growth, and scarring secondary to surgery.[47] Trismus is also seen in conjunction with ORN and usually improves after definitive treatment.[5] Radiation can also be directly associated with injury to tissues. Radiation-induced trismus has a reported incidence of 6% to 86%.[29] This wide range is explained by the multiple interpretations of how much limitation represents trismus. Other variables such as total radiation dose, type of radiation, location of the primary tumor, surgical procedures performed, and other individual patient factors can influence the incidence of trismus. It is very important for the clinician to identify the etiology before implementing therapy. Radiation-induced trismus is directly related to radiation damage to the masticatory muscles, TMJ, oral mucosa, and facial skin. Fibrosis of the oral mucosa, especially at the pterygomandibular raphe, anterior tonsillar pillar, and retromolar areas, can significantly restrict mandibular range of motion.[5] Trismus may compromise oral intake, speech, the ability to secure the airway (and thus increase the risk for aspiration), dental hygiene, and dental treatment.[29,47] Oromandibular dystonia, which is characterized by painful muscle contractions, cramps, and pain, has also been reported but is rare when compared with radiation-induced trismus.[29,48,49] Pain is reported in 15% to 30% of patients after radiation therapy.[50] It has been suggested that radiation doses greater than 5000 cGy to the TMJ and masticatory muscles are required to induce trismus.[47] The onset of trismus is usually seen early in the postradiation period, but it can develop 3 to 6 months after completion of therapy. The condition is progressive and can worsen with time for up to 9 months after onset.[29,47,51] Botulinum toxin A applied to each masseter muscle in a dose of 50 units has shown some value in the treatment of pain and oromandibular dystonia. However, it was ineffective in treating trismus.[49] Physical therapy (PT) with manual stretching exercises, tongue depressors, or mechanical devices such as the Therabite (Altos Medical, West Allis, Wisc) is a valuable tool in prevention and treatment of trismus. To be effective, PT must be initiated early after completion of radiation therapy and requires that patient compliance be maintained for several months afterward.[47,52]

Forced mouth-opening under general anesthesia is also used; however, it is less predictable and associated with increased risk for dentoalveolar and soft tissue trauma.[47] Some surgical options are available for patients with severe trismus or those who are not

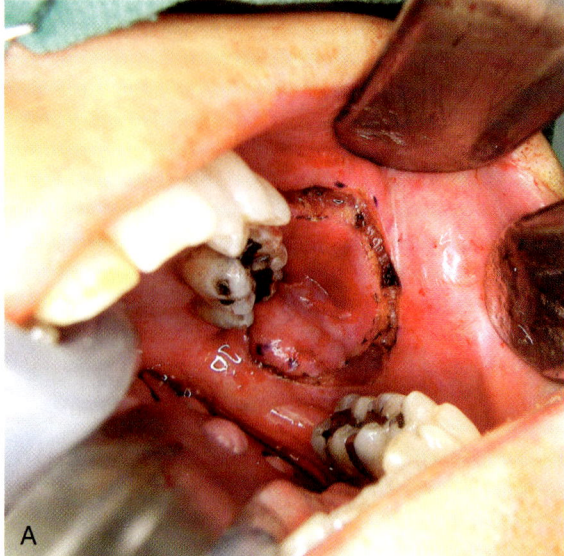

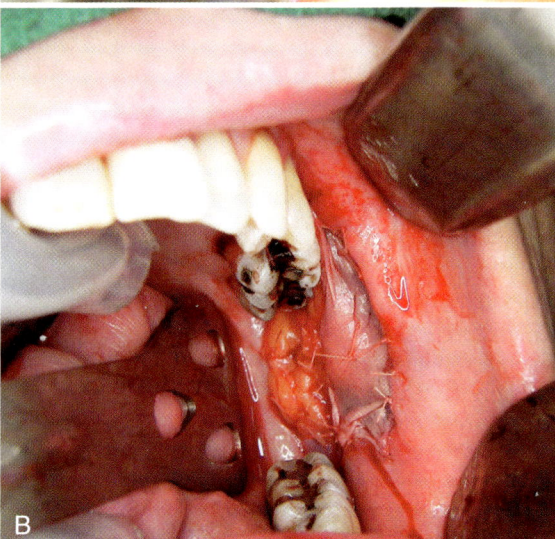

Fig. 28-3 ■ **A,** Excision of scar tissue from the cheek. **B,** Repair of the resulting defect with advancement of a fat pad and skin graft.

responsive to PT. If the trismus is due to scarring or fibrosis of the oral mucosa, excision of the specific affected tissues and grafting with a myocutaneous or free microvascular flap can be performed (Fig. 28-3). When the fibrosis is located at the masticatory muscles, surgical excision of tissue can compromise the blood supply to the mandible and induce ORN.[5] Coronoidectomy can significantly improve mandibular range of motion. The maximum interincisal opening 6 months to 1 year after surgery is usually less than what is initially obtained in the operating room or immediately postoperatively.[47] The use of adjutant PT at home helps maintain the results long-term.

DYSPHAGIA

Swallowing is a complex process that requires precise coordination of several muscle groups in the oral cavity, pharynx, larynx, and esophagus.[53] Normal swallowing has involuntary and voluntary components and is divided into four phases: oral preparation, oral, pharyngeal, and esophageal.[54] Dysphagia in the setting of head and neck cancer can be caused by tissue loss and scarring secondary to surgical excision and loss of sensation as a result of transection of nerves and muscles.[55] It can also be related to the size and location of the primary tumor. Many of the common sequelae of radiation therapy, such as trismus, rampant caries, xerostomia, and mucositis, can individually or in conjunction considerably affect swallowing. Dysphagia is often accompanied by odynophagia. It also appears as a late complication that is directly related to radiation damage to the structures involved in swallowing. Lymphedema, fibrosis and decreased contractility of the muscles of mastication, and loss of coordination and muscle strength, especially of the pharyngeal constrictors, adversely affect the harmony of the swallowing cycle. Hypopharyngeal and upper esophageal strictures are not uncommon and may require multiple dilation procedures to improve swallowing.[56] The use of feeding tubes for prolonged periods may result in muscular atrophy with subsequent dysphagia.[55,57]

Dysphagia increases the risk for aspiration. The cough reflex is usually ineffective or non-inexistent in almost half of affected patients.[58] Silent aspiration may result in aspiration pneumonia as a post-treatment complication of radiation therapy. Patients with tracheostomy tubes may also experience dysphagia and increased risk for aspiration. The most common methods for evaluation of swallowing function are the flexible endoscopic evaluation of swallowing (FEES) and the modified barium swallowing study (MBSS). FEES can easily be performed at bedside or in the office setting; however, it is useful only for evaluation of the pharyngeal phase of swallowing. Thus, many clinicians prefer MBSS over FEES.

Dysphagia and radiation have a dose-dependent relationship[59]; therefore, modifications in the treatment protocols aimed at reducing the dose given to healthy tissues may decrease the risk for and severity of dysphagia. Use of IMRT can reduce radiation injury not only to the pharyngeal musculature but also to the salivary glands.[32,34,60] Use of amifostine in the regimen previously described in an attempt to decrease salivary gland dysfunction is also valuable in the prevention of dysphagia.

The greatest incidence of swallowing disorders is seen 3 months after treatment. Significant improvement generally occurs in the following 12 months.[61] When required, rehabilitation is usually provided by the speech-language pathologist and consists of postural techniques, sensory techniques, motor exercises, swallowing maneuvers, and changes in diet. The majority of patients recover swallowing function over time without rehabilitation. It has been suggested that early intervention is superior to delayed intervention.[55]

RADIATION CARIES

Radiation-induced caries can be a direct consequence of radiation damage to the tooth structure or indirect damage as a result of xerostomia, changes in oral flora, deficient oral hygiene, and dietary changes. Salivary gland dysfunction with a consequent decrease in salivary flow has a dramatic impact on dental health. Decreases in secretory immunoglobulin A, changes in pH, decreased bicarbonate concentration with reduced buffering capacity, and changes in the oral flora have been reported in patients with radiation-induced xerostomia.[3,31,62] These changes are responsible for radiation-induced caries outside the field of radiation. Direct radiation damage to the teeth is due to pulpal necrosis and dentinal dehydration.[5] Radiation-induced caries usually occurs at the gingival margin, cusp tips, incisal borders, and dentine-enamel junction. It is manifested as hard black areas and resembles dentinogenesis imperfecta.[5]

It is important for the clinician to differentiate the concept of direct and indirect radiation-induced caries. Oral hygiene, prophylaxis, and topical fluoride may be effective in the treatment of indirect radiation-induced caries; however, they have no value in treating direct radiation-induced caries because it is a direct consequence of radiation damage to the tooth structure and is not

preventable. This mandates that any teeth planned to be or that were in the path of a significant radiation dose should be extracted before radiation therapy or early after it. The suggested high-risk dose for direct radiation-induced caries is 6000 cGy or higher.[5] It has been reported that 76% of head and neck cancer patients are noncompliant with dental care and oral hygiene.[63] Maintenance of adequate oral hygiene during and after radiation therapy can be extremely difficult and painful because of the mucositis, dermatitis, and trismus. Many of these patients have preexisting dental disease and will simultaneously benefit from multiple extractions despite the fact that they are scheduled for radiation therapy. Performing heroic dentistry to restore and save teeth in these cases will only delay extractions and increase the risk for ORN. Maintenance of oral hygiene is a key factor in the prevention of indirect radiation-induced caries. Periodic dental evaluation and treatment and topical fluoride application are usually effective and recommended.

MALNUTRITION

Multiple factors can be associated with malnutrition in head and neck cancer patients. Surgery and tumor bulk can certainly affect oral intake. However, many of these factors are directly or indirectly associated with radiotherapy. Xerostomia, trismus, dysphagia, odynophagia, direct or indirect radiation-induced caries, and mucositis can have a significant adverse effect on the nutritional status of patients. Malnutrition has been reported in 35% to 60% of head and neck cancer patients.[64,65] Ten percent weight loss is a factor predictive of postoperative complications, tumor recurrence, and mortality. Mortality rates can increase up to 30% with 20% weight loss and close to 100% when the weight loss is greater than 50%.[65,66] Assessment of nutritional status is important because it has a critical effect on wound healing and immune function. The estimated ideal body weight can be calculated with formulas. The Devine formula is the most popular; others, such as the Miller, Robinson, and Hamwi formulas, are variations of the Devine formula that include other variables and can be used as well. The serum albumin level is a good indicator of nutritional status. The half-life of albumin is approximately 20 days, and it is useful as a measure of chronic protein stores. Pre-albumin, however, has a half-life of 2 to 3 days and is an indicator of acute improvement or deterioration in nutritional status. Pre-albumin serum levels are evaluated twice a week to assess the efficacy of nutritional therapy. Total parenteral nutrition is commonly used for supplemental nutrition in patients unable to tolerate oral intake, but it is intended for short-term use and has been associated with venous thrombosis and sepsis. The preferred route for nutritional supplementation is the enteral route. It is delivered by nasogastric or gastrostomy tubes. Gastrostomy tubes are better tolerated and can be used for long-term nutritional support. They can be placed via open surgery or by percutaneous endoscopic gastrostomy (PEG). PEG is a quick and simple procedure that is often performed at bedside. Some clinicians advocate prophylactic placement of feeding tubes based on data supporting the fact that this may decrease weight loss.[55] Others are opposed to this practice because decreased use of the muscles of mastication and swallowing may cause atrophy and result in feeding tube dependency.[55,67] Consultation with a nutritionist is recommended to establish the nutritional needs of each individual patient.

OSTEORADIONECROSIS

ORN is one of the most devastating complications of radiation therapy. From its initial occurrence through the most advanced stage it often has a negative impact on the quality of life of head and neck cancer patients. The development of ORN is thought to be multifactorial. Variables such as primary site, T staging, proximity of the tumor to bone, dental health, dose and type of radiation, nutritional status, alcohol and tobacco use, and administration of adjunctive chemotherapy are among the commonly suggested risk factors for the development of ORN.[3,68,69] Recent assessment of these variables has suggested that the most important determinants for the development of ORN are radiation doses higher than 6600 cGy and nutritional status. Age, gender, alcohol and tobacco use, tumor stage, and adjutant use of chemotherapy appear to be associated with minimal risk in promoting ORN.[68] This study also suggested that the use of steroids and increased body mass index may decrease the risk for ORN. The onset of ORN most often occurs between 4 months and 2 years after radiation therapy; commonly developing during the first 6 to 12 months. The risk however, remains for life.[69,70] ORN is more common in the mandible than in any other bone of the head and neck. It may occur spontaneously or in relation to a traumatic event because the decreased vascularity is not able to support the increased metabolic needs of wound healing. Good oral hygiene is critical for maintenance of the remaining dentition and avoidance of the need for dental extraction and progression of periodontal disease. Prophylactic extraction of teeth planned to be in the path of a significant amount of radiation is critical in the prevention of ORN. The use of prophylactic and therapeutic hyperbaric oxygen (HBO) therapy is controversial. HBO has its advocates[71-73] and opponents[68-70,74]; however, it is still one of the most common therapies used today. When conservative therapies fail, resection with immediate or delayed reconstruction is the treatment of choice. Vascularized and nonvascularized grafts have been used successfully for reconstruction of the resulting defects. ORN is discussed further elsewhere in Chapter 59.

PEARLS AND PITFALLS

- Radiation-induced mucositis occurs in almost every patient undergoing radiation therapy. This debilitating condition will resolve within 3 to 4 weeks after completion of radiation therapy. Treatment should be focused on pain control, prevention of infection, and maintenance of an adequate oral diet.
- Sialogogue agents increase salivary secretion by stimulating muscarinic receptors in the salivary glands. They have a role in the treatment of xerostomia only if residual functional salivary gland tissue remains viable after radiation therapy.
- Direct radiation-induced caries is a direct consequence of radiation injury to dental tissues (pulp and dentin). It is not preventable, and teeth in the pathway of planned radiation doses of 6000 cGy or higher should be extracted.
- Most of the immediate side effects of radiation therapy impair or make oral intake difficult. Nutritional status and weight loss can significantly affect the outcome of head and neck cancer patients. Special attention should be placed on nutritional status to decrease complications and improve outcomes.

REFERENCES

1. Rosenthal DI, Machtay M: Radiation therapy for head and neck cancer. In Fonseca R, editor. *Oral and maxillofacial surgery*, Philadelphia, 2000, WB Saunders, pp 375-394.
2. Porter A, Aref A, Chodunsky Z, et al: A global strategy for radiotherapy. A WHO consultation, *Clin Oncol* 11:368-370, 1999.
3. Ferguson H, Stevens M: Advances in head and neck radiotherapy to the mandible, *Oral Maxillofac Surg Clin North Am* 19:553-563, 2007.
4. Chan A, Liebsch M: Proton radiation therapy for head and neck cancer, *J Surg Oncol* 97:697-700, 2008.
5. Marx RE, Stern D: *Oral and maxillofacial pathology: a rationale for diagnosis and treatment*, Carol Stream, IL, 2003, Quintessence, pp 375-394.
6. Carl W: Oral complications of local and systemic cancer treatment, *Curr Opin Oncol* 7:320-324, 1995.
7. Dixon RB, Tricker ND, Garetto LP: Bone turnover in elderly canine mandible and tibia [abstract], *J Dent Res* 76:2579, 1997.
8. Hall EJ: *Radiobiology for the radiologist*, ed 3, Philadelphia, 1997, JB Lippincott, pp 1040-1048.
9. Brown JM: Evidence for acutely hypoxic cells in mouse tumors and possible mechanism for regeneration, *Br J Radiol* 52:650-658, 1979.
10. Simoes A, Eduardo F, Luiz A, et al: Laser phototherapy as prophylaxis against head and neck radiotherapy-induced oral mucositis: comparison between low and high/low power lasers, *Lasers Surg Med* 41:264-270, 2009.
11. Scully C, Sonis S, Diz PD: Oral mucositis, *Oral Dis* 12:229-241, 2006.
12. Neville BW, Damm D, Allen CM, et al: *Oral & maxillofacial pathology*, ed 2, Philadelphia, 2002, WB Saunders, pp 253-284.
13. Keefe MD, Schubert MM, Elting SL, et al: Updated clinical practice guidelines for the prevention and treatment of mucositis, *Cancer* 109:820-831, 2007.
14. Sully C, Epstein BJ, Sonis S: Oral mucositis: a challenging complication of radiotherapy, chemotherapy and radiochemotherapy, I: pathogenesis and prophylaxis of mucositis, *Head Neck* 25:1057-1070, 2003.
15. Lockhard PB, Clark S: Pretherapy dental status of patients with malignant condition of the head and neck, *Oral Surg Oral Med Oral Pathol* 77:236-241, 1994.
16. Rutkauskas JS, Davis JW: Effects of chlorhexidine during immune-suppressive chemotherapy, *Oral Surg Oral Med Oral Pathol* 77:242-247, 1994.
17. DeLand MM, Weiss RA: Treatment of radiation-induced dermatitis with light-emitting diode (LED) photomodulation, *Lasers Surg Med* 39:164-168, 2007.
18. Hymes S, Storm E, Fife C: Radiation dermatitis: clinical presentation, pathophysiology, and treatment, *J Am Acad Dermatol* 54:28-46, 2006.
19. Simonen P, Hamilton C, Ferguson S, et al: Do inflammatory processes contribute to radiation-induced erythema observed in the skins of humans? *Radiother Oncol* 46:73-82, 1998.
20. Kupper TS: The activated keratinocyte: a model for inducible cytokine production by non–bone marrow–derived cells in cutaneous inflammatory and immune responses, *J Invest Dermatol* 94:146-150, 1990.
21. Mendelson FA, Divino CM, Reis ED, et al: Wound care after radiation therapy, *Adv Skin Care* 15:216-224, 2002.
22. Sfwat A, Bentzen SM, Turesson I, et al: Deterministic rather than stochastic factors explaining most of the variation in the expression of skin telangiectasia after radiotherapy, *Int J Radiat Oncol Biol Phys* 52:198-204, 2002.
23. Porock D, Kristjanson L, Nikoletti, S, et al: Predicting the severity of radiation skin reactions in women with breast cancer, *Oncol Nurs Forum* 25:1019-1029, 1998.
24. Hall EJ, Cox JD: Physical and biological bases of radiation therapy. In Cox JD, Ang KK, editors: *Radiation oncology*, St Louis, 2003, CV Mosby, pp 3-62.
25. Ross JG, Hussey DH, Mayr NA, et al: Acute and late reactions to radiation therapy in patients with collagen vascular diseases, *Cancer* 71:3744-3752, 1993.
26. Morris MM, Powell SN: Irradiation in the presence of collagen vascular disease: acute and late complications, *J Clin Oncol* 15:2728-2735, 1997.
27. Dutreix J: Human skin: early reactions in relation to dose and its time distribution, *Br J Radiol Suppl* 19:22-28, 1986.
28. Williams MS, Burk M, Loprinzi CL, et al: Phase III double blind evaluation of an aloe vera gel as prophylactic agent for radiation-induced skin toxicity, *Int J Radiat Oncol Biol Phys* 36:345-349, 1996.
29. Kent ML, Brennan TB, Noll JL, et al: Radiation-induced trismus in head and neck

cancer patients, *Support Care Cancer* 16:305-309, 2008.

30. Guchelaar HJ, Vermes A, Meerwaldt JH: Radiation-induced xerostomia: pathophysiology, clinical course and supportive treatment, *Support Cancer Care* 5:281-288, 1997.

31. Fischer DJ, Epstein JB: Management of patients who have undergone head and neck cancer therapy, *Dent Clin North Am* 52:39-60, 2008.

32. Rodrigues NA, Killion L, Hickey G, et al: A prospective study of salivary gland function in lymphoma patients receiving head and neck radiation, *Int J Radiat Oncol Biol Phys* 75:1079-1083, 2009.

33. Francen L, Funegard U, Ericson T, et al: Parotid gland function during and following radiotherapy of malignancies of the head and neck. A consecutive study of salivary flow and patient discomfort, *Eur J Cancer* 28:457-462, 1992.

34. Kam MK, Leung SF, Zee B, et al: Prospective randomized study of intensity-modulated radiotherapy on salivary gland function in early-stage nasopharyngeal carcinoma patients, *J Clin Oncol* 25:4873-4879, 2007.

35. Gornitsky M, Shenouda G, Sultanem K, et al: Double-blind randomized, placebo controlled study of pilocarpine to salvage salivary gland function during radiotherapy of patients with head and neck cancer, *Oral Surg Oral Med Oral Pathol Oral Radiol Endod* 98:45-52, 2004.

36. Warde P, O'Sullivan B, Aslanidis J, et al: A phase III placebo-controlled trial of oral pilocarpine in patients undergoing radiotherapy for head and neck cancer, *Int J Radiat Oncol Biol Phys* 54:9-13, 2002.

37. Brizel DM, Wasserman TH, Henke M, et al: Phase III randomized trial of amifostine as a radioprotector in head and neck cancer, *J Clin Oncol* 18:3339-3345, 2000.

38. Sasse AD, Clark LG, Sasse EC, et al: Amifostine reduces side effects and improves complete response rate during radiotherapy: results and meta-analysis, *Int J Radiat Oncol Biol Phys* 64:784-791, 2006.

39. Giatromanolaki A, Sivridis E, Maltezos E, et al: Down-regulation of intestinal-type alkaline phosphatase in the tumor vasculature and stroma provides a strong basis for explaining amifostine selectivity, *Semin Oncol* 29(6 Suppl 19):14-21, 2002.

40. Gosselin TK, Maunter B: Amifostine as radioprotectant, *Clin J Oncol Nurs* 6:175-177, 2002.

41. Jha N, Seikaly H, McGraw T, et al: Submandibular salivary gland transfer prevents radiation-induced xerostomia, *Int J Radiat Oncol Biol Phys* 46:7-11, 2000.

42. Seikaly H, Jha N, McGraw T, et al: Submandibular salivary gland transfer: a new method of preventing radiation induced xerostomia, *Laryngoscope* 111:347-352, 2001.

43. Visch LL, Gravenmade EJ, Schaub RM, et al: A double-blind crossover trial of CMC- and mucin-containing saliva substitutes, *Int J Oral Maxillofac Surg* 15:395-400, 1986.

44. Johnson JT, Ferreti GA, Nethery WJ, et al: Oral pilocarpine for post-irradiation xerostomia in patients with head and neck cancer, *N Engl J Med* 329:390-395, 1993.

45. Jacobs CD, van der Pas M: A multicenter maintenance study of oral pilocarpine tablets for radiation-induced xerostomia, *Oncology (Williston Park)* 10(Suppl 3):16-20, 1996.

46. Epstein JB, Bruchell JL, Emerton S, et al: A clinical trial of bethanechol in patients with xerostomia after radiation therapy, *Oral Surg Oral Med Oral Pathol* 77:610-614, 1994.

47. Bharny AD, Izzard M, Wood A, et al: Coronoidectomy for the treatment of trismus in head and neck cancer patients, *Laryngoscope* 117:1952-1956, 2007.

48. Van Daele DJ, Finnegan EM, Rodnitzky RL, et al: Head and neck muscle spasm after radiotherapy: management with botulinum toxin A injection, *Arch Otolaryngol Head Neck Surg* 128:956-959, 2002.

49. Hartl DM, Cohen M, Julieron M, et al: Botulinum toxin for radiation-induced facial pain and trismus, *Otolaryngol Head Neck Surg* 138:459-463, 2008.

50. List MA, Bilir SP: Functional outcomes in head and neck cancer, *Semin Radiat Oncol* 14:178-189, 2004.

51. Wang CJ, Huang EY, Hsu HC, et al: The degree and time course assessment of radiation induced trismus occurring after radiation therapy for nasopharyngeal cancer, *Laryngoscope* 115:1458-1460, 2005.

52. Buchbinder D, Currivan RB, Kaplan AJ, et al: Mobilization regimens for the prevention of jaw hypomobility in the radiated patient: a comparison of three different techniques, *J Oral Maxillofac Surg* 51:863-867, 1993.

53. Kendall K: Anatomy and physiology of deglutition. In Kendall LA, editor: *Dysphagia assessment and treatment planning*, San Diego, CA, 2008, Plural Publishing, pp 27-34.

54. Murray T, Carrau RL: Anatomy and function of the swallowing mechanism in clinical management of swallowing disorders. In Kendall LA, editor: *Dysphagia assessment and treatment planning*, San Diego, CA, 2008, Plural Publishing, pp 15-33.

55. Murohy BA, Gilberts J: Dysphagia in head and neck cancer patients treated with radiation: assessment, sequelae and rehabilitation, *Semin Radiat Oncol* 19:35-42, 2009.

56. Lee WT, Akst LM, Adelstein DJ, et al: Risk factors for hypopharyngeal/upper esophageal stricture after concurrent chemoradiation, *Head Neck* 28:808-812, 2006.

57. Lewin JS: Dysphagia after chemoradiation: prevention and treatment, *Int J Radiat Oncol Biol Phys* 69(2 Suppl):S86-87, 2007.

58. Nguyen NP, Duttan S, Alfierei A, et al: Aspiration occurrence during chemoradiation for head and neck cancer, *Anticancer Drugs* 3B:1669-1672, 2007.

59. Feng FY, Lyden TH, Haxer MJ, et al: Intensity-modulated radiotherapy of the head and neck cancer aiming to reduce dysphagia: early dose-effect relationship for swallowing structures, *Int J Radiat Oncol Biol Phys* 68:1289-1298, 2007.

60. Eisbruch A, Schwartz M, Rasch C, et al: Dysphagia and aspiration after chemoradiotherapy for head and neck cancer: which anatomic structures are affected and can be spared by IMRT? *Int J Radiat Biol Phys* 60:1425-1439, 2004.

61. Logemann JA, Pauloski BR, Rademaker AW, et al: Swallowing disorders in the first year after radiation and chemoradiation, *Head Neck* 30:148-158, 2008.

62. Keene HJ, Fleming TJ: Prevalence of caries-associated microflora after radiotherapy in patients with head and neck cancer, *Oral Surg Oral Med Oral Pathol* 64:421-426, 1987.

63. Lockhart PB, Clark S: Pretherapy dental status of patients with malignant conditions of the head and neck, *Oral Surg Oral Med Oral Pathol* 77:236-241, 1994.

64. Brookes GB: Nutritional status: a prognostic indicator in head and neck cancer, *Otolaryngol Head Neck Surg* 93:69-74, 1985.

65. Williams EF, Meguid MM: Nutritional concepts and considerations in head and neck surgery, *Head Neck* 11:393-399, 1989.

66. Arosarena OA: Perioperative management of the head and neck cancer patient, *J Oral Maxillofac Surg* 65:305-313, 2007.

67. Rosenthal DI, Eisbruch A: Prevention and treatment of dysphagia and aspiration after chemoradiation for head and neck cancer, *J Clin Ocol* 24:2636-2643, 2006.

68. Goldwaser BR, Cuang S, Kaban LB, et al: Risk factors assessment for the development of osteoradionecrosis, *J Oral Maxillofac Surg* 65:2311-2316, 2007.

69. Lyons A, Ghazali N: Osteoradionecrosis of the jaws: current understanding of its pathophysiology and treatment, *Br J Oral Maxillofac Surg* 46:653-660, 2008.

70. Clayman L: Clinical controversies in oral and maxillofacial surgery: part two. Management of dental extractions in irradiated jaws: a protocol without the use of hyperbaric oxygen therapy, *J Oral Maxillofac Surg* 45:104-111, 1997.

71. Marx RE: A new concept in the treatment of osteoradionecrosis, *J Oral Maxillofac Surg* 41:351-357, 1983.

72. Thorn JJ, Kallehave F, Westergaard P, et al: The effect of hyperbaric oxygen on irradiated oral tissues: transmucosal oxygen tension measurements, *J Oral Maxillofac Surg* 55:1103-1107, 1997.

73. Larsen P: Placement of dental implants in the irradiated mandible: a protocol involving adjunctive hyperbaric oxygen, *J Oral Maxillofac Surg* 55:967-971, 1997.

74. Maier A, Gaggl A, Klemen H, et al: Review of severe osteoradionecrosis treated by surgery alone or with postoperative hyperbaric oxygenation, *Br J Oral Maxillofac Surg* 38:173-176, 2000.

Chapter 29

Management of Trigeminal Nerve Injuries

Shahrokh C. Bagheri, Roger Albert Meyer

Injury to peripheral branches of the trigeminal nerve can arise from a wide variety of oral and maxillofacial surgical procedures or injuries, including dentoalveolar surgery, placement of dental implants, endodontic therapy, orthognathic surgical procedures, removal of benign or malignant tumors, and local anesthetic injections, as well as be a direct consequence of maxillofacial trauma or surgical interventions for repair of facial trauma.

The most commonly injured nerves in oral and maxillofacial surgery include the lingual nerve (LN) and inferior alveolar nerve (IAN) (Fig. 29-1). Injuries to these nerves produce decreased or lost sensation or painful sensations that interfere with appropriate sensory perception by the central nervous system (CNS). Loss or aberration of orofacial sensory input is detrimental to patients because of negative effects on speech, taste, swallowing, ability to maintain food and liquid competence, social interactions, playing of wind musical instruments, and pain perception. The majority of these injuries result in sensory changes that are temporary in nature and recover spontaneously with time. Although all nerves respond to injury with stereotypic pathophysiologic responses, genetic, hormonal, anatomic, physiologic, behavioral, or other factors may influence any individual nerve's recovery. Four factors are known to affect the rate and degree of peripheral sensory nerve recovery following injury age, state of general health, location of the injury, and type of injury.

The timing of surgical repair of a nerve injury remains a controversy. A consensus was reached and reported in 1992 by Alling and colleagues. Although there remains little scientific evidence to support these recommendations regarding the treatment of nerve injury, the timing of nerve repair surgery was originally based on the extensive experience of Seddon during and after World War II. During the ensuing years, the extensive clinical experience of oral and maxillofacial surgeons has validated the concepts of timing that were previously merely speculative. Based on this experience, Meyer and Ruggiero proposed specific timing guidelines. Because it is impossible to conduct valid prospective randomized clinical trials to compare early versus late repair, the surgeon is relegated to relying on retrospective cohort studies. This makes it difficult to know whether patients who undergo early repair would have improved (and to what degree) without surgical intervention.

Microsurgical operative management may be the most effective approach to restoring function in the subset of patients in whom significant LN or IAN sensory dysfunction has failed to resolve spontaneously after a reasonable interval of clinical observation. A number of outcome studies have explored the effects of microsurgical repair of the LN and IAN. Multiple studies have suggested no association between delayed repair and neurosensory outcome, whereas others, including our own work, strongly suggest improved outcomes with early repair. This controversy is primarily the result of the literature containing small case series with nonstandardized methods for evaluating outcomes, which makes comparison between studies problematic and their outcomes difficult to evaluate.

We retrospectively reviewed 222 LN and 186 IAN injuries that were observed for at least 1 year and demonstrated that microsurgical repair of LN and IAN injuries can result in sensory and functional improvement in patients who have surgical indications as determined by the history and standardized neurosensory testing (NST). The majority of operated patients do regain acceptable sensation and associated function as classified by the Medical Research Council (MRC) scale (Table 29-1). Relief of pain is also frequently a welcome benefit of surgical treatment. Microsurgical repair of an injured LN or IAN is a valid treatment for many patients. In our studies, the likelihood of recovery following nerve repair decreases progressively with time after injury and with increasing age of the patient.

Injuries to the IAN as a result of mandibular sagittal split ramus osteotomy (SSRO) deserve special attention and are distinguished by their anatomic and surgical complexity in comparison to third molar surgery. Since its introduction by Schuchardt and modification and popularization by Trauner and Obwegeser, SSRO has undergone multiple surgical refinements and instrument/equipment modifications to improve its results. SSRO is currently the most widely accepted method for surgical correction of mandibular skeletal abnormalities. Despite the versatility and numerous advantages of this procedure, neurosensory disturbances are common and are related to the surgical anatomy involved in this operation (Fig. 29-2). Postoperatively, transient or temporary changes in sensory function of the peripheral trigeminal nerve branches, most often the IAN but also including the LN, are an expected part of the patient's recovery as a result of these nerves' intimate proximity to the surgical site.

This chapter reviews the basics of microsurgical repair of the IAN and LN. Readers should refer to Suggested Readings for more in-depth information.

INCIDENCE/ETIOPATHOGENESIS

Although estimates vary, it is supported within the literature that a small number of patients who have sustained nerve injury experience permanent neurosensory dysfunction (NSD). The rate of permanent injury to the LN from third molar surgery ranges between 0.04% and 0.6%, whereas for the IAN it ranges between 0.1% and 1%. The incidence of persistent nerve impairment of the IAN 1 year after SSRO surgery in a recent systematic review was reported to be 12.8%. Spontaneous recovery of IAN function has been documented following SSRO, with the greatest improvement having been found in the first 3 months after injury. Numerous reports document sensory changes in the IAN after SSRO, but few have explored the incidence of temporary or permanent LN sensory alterations.

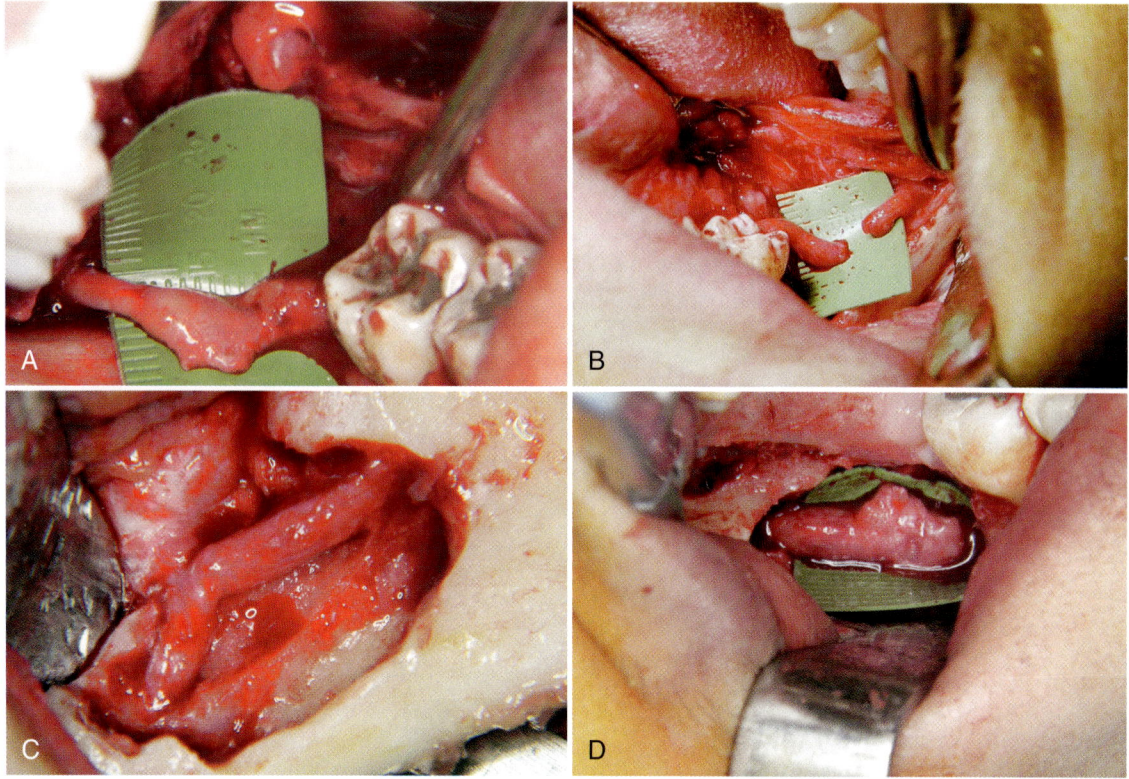

Fig. 29-1 ■ **A,** Large lingual nerve (LN) neuroma in continuity with a partial transection 6 months after third molar removal. The patient complained of pain and anesthesia of the right side of the tongue. **B,** Exposure of a transected LN after third molar surgery. **C,** Partial transection of the inferior alveolar nerve (IAN) during removal of a full bone-impacted third molar. The patient had pain and anesthesia of the right lower lip and gingiva. **D,** Neuroma in continuity of the IAN secondary to implant placement. The patient was evaluated 4 months after implant removal because of pain and numbness. (**A** and **B,** From Bagheri SC, Meyer RA, Khan HA, et al: A retrospective review of microsurgical repair of 222 lingual nerve injuries, *J Oral Maxillofac Surg* 68:715-723, 2010.)

TABLE 29-1	Medical Research Council Scale
GRADE*	**DESCRIPTION**
S0	No sensation
S1	Deep cutaneous pain in an autonomous zone
S2	Some superficial pain and touch sensation
S2+	Superficial pain and touch sensation plus hyperesthesia
S3	Superficial pain and touch sensation without hyperesthesia; static 2-point discrimination >15 mm
S3+	Same as S3 with good stimulus localization and static 2-point discrimination of 7-15 mm
S4	Same as S3 and static 2-point discrimination of 2-6 mm

*Grades S3, S3+, and S4 indicate useful sensory recovery.
Data from Birch R, Bonney G, Wynn-Parry CB: *Surgical disorders of the peripheral nerves*, Philadelphia, 1998, Churchill Livingstone, pp 405-414.

Fewer reports have mentioned LN changes after SSRO. Damage to the LN can be incapacitating to patients, who may experience tongue biting, difficulty masticating or tooth brushing, impaired phonation or swallowing, and loss or altered sense of taste because of paresthesia or dysesthesia in the tongue or lingual gingiva. Risk factors for LN injury during SSRO have not been emphasized previously. In our experience, the common mechanism of injury to the LN during SSRO occurs during the placement of bicortical superior border internal fixation screws. This may occur secondary to perforation of the lingual cortical bone of the mandible by the drill and inadvertent penetration of the unprotected LN or, less commonly, secondary to impalement of the LN by a fixation screw that extends beyond the limits of the bone (Fig. 29-3).

PATHOLOGIC ANATOMY

Anatomic drawings and descriptions that appear in textbooks are merely representations of average locations of the various human structures determined from observing literally hundreds of cadaver dissections. Therefore, the skeletal and soft tissue structures of the human head and neck may have significant variations from the accepted anatomic norms. The anatomy of the trigeminal nerve, as described in standard texts, is complex, but not necessarily accurate for a given patient. Perhaps variation in the position of the nerve or associated musculoskeletal structures contributes to the incidence of nerve injuries despite correct surgical techniques. In the largest known cadaver study, Behnia and associates looked at the anatomy of the LN in 669 nerves from 430 fresh cadavers. Measurements on each cadaver were made with a micrometer caliper to determine the horizontal and vertical position of the LN in the lower third molar region. In 94 cases (14.0%), the nerve was above the lingual crest, and in 1 case (0.15%), the nerve was in the retromolar pad region.

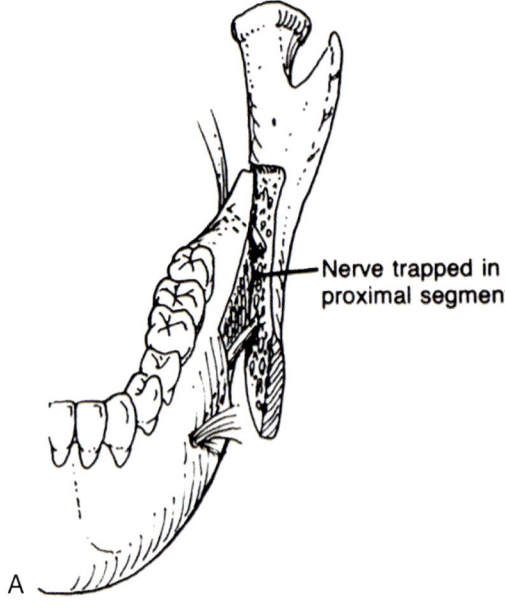

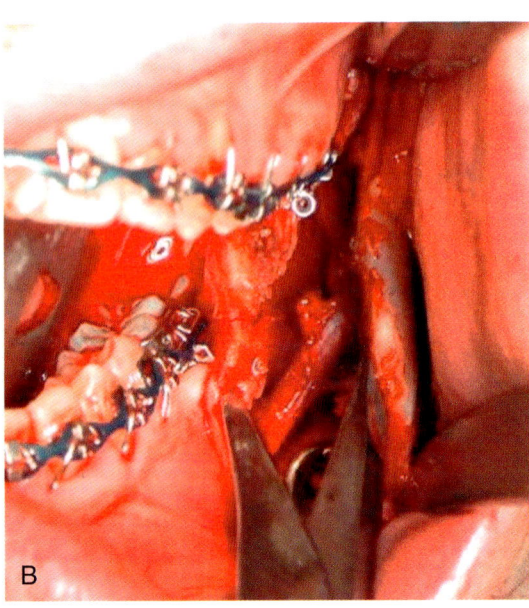

Fig. 29-2 ■ **A,** Diagrammatic representation of entrapment of the inferior alveolar nerve (IAN) within the cortex of the distal segment during mandibular sagittal split ramus osteotomy (SSRO). **B,** Exposure of an IAN injured during SSRO at the time of its subsequent repair. Note the lateral neuroma protruding from the superior surface of the nerve. (Microsurgical repair of the peripheral trigeminal nerves after mandibular sagittal split ramus osteotomy, *J Oral Maxillofac Surg* 68:2770-2782, 2010.)

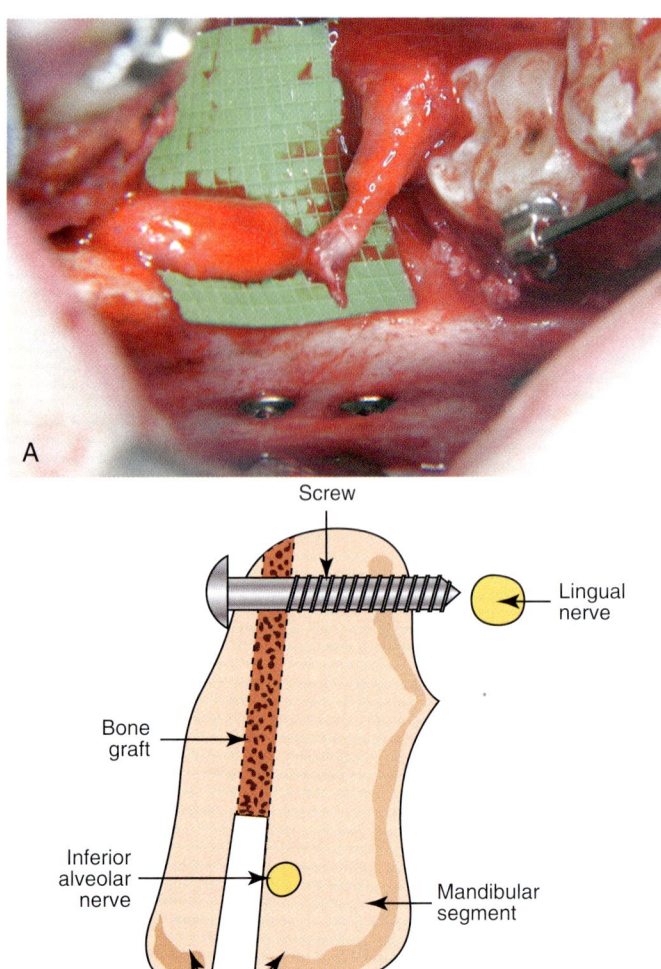

Fig. 29-3 ■ **A,** Nearly complete transection of the lingual nerve (LN) after mandibular sagittal split ramus osteotomy (SSRO). The patient was seen at 5 months with anesthesia of the right side of the tongue. Notice the position of the bicortical screws. **B,** Diagrammatic representation of a common mechanism of injury to the LN following SSRO caused by bicortical screw fixation of the superior border of the mandible. Injury to the nerve can occur as a result of direct injury by the drill or during placement of the screws (or both). (Microsurgical repair of the peripheral trigeminal nerves after mandibular sagittal split ramus osteotomy, *J Oral Maxillofac Surg* 68:2770-2782, 2010.)

In the remaining 574 cases (85.8%), the mean horizontal and vertical distances of the nerve to the lingual plate and lingual crest were 2.1 ± 1.1 mm and 3.0 ± 0.4 mm (range, 1.7 to 4.0 mm), respectively. In 149 cases (22.3%), the nerve was in direct contact with the lingual plate of the alveolar process. This study confirms the variable anatomy of the trigeminal nerve in the maxillofacial region.

Similarly, the position of the IAN has great variability. Although the nerve is known to traverse along an interosseous path from the mandibular foramen on the medial mandibular ramus to the mental foramen on the lateral mandibular body, its position within the mandible can have significant interosseous variation superoinferiorly or mediolaterally (or both) and in its relationship to the mandibular molar and premolar teeth (Fig. 29-4). In addition, the position of the nerve changes relative to the alveolar crest if the edentulous mandible undergoes resorption with age.

DIAGNOSTIC STUDIES

Because neurosensory function cannot be assessed directly, indirect clinical measures of sensation (e.g., temperature discernment, vibration, pinprick, light touch, two-point discrimination) are evaluated for representation of neurosensory function; there have been variable methods of determining these measures.

A modified MRC scale, originally developed for the upper extremities to grade and monitor brachial plexus injuries, has been adapted to assess the functional sensory recovery of trigeminal nerve injuries and make comparisons between studies possible (see Table 29-1). The MRC scale provides a global assessment of neurosensory

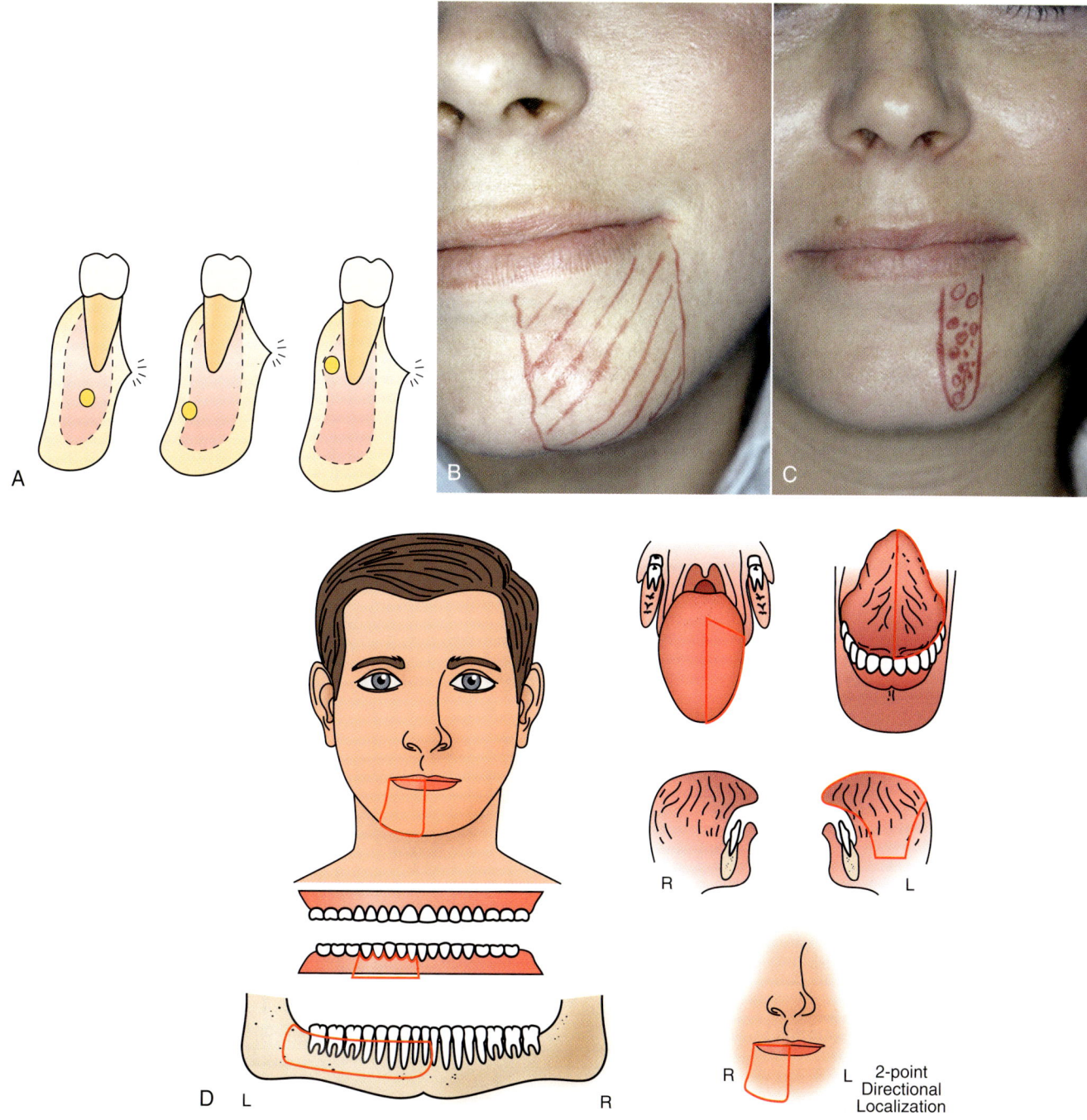

Fig. 29-4 ■ **A,** Diagrammatic representations of the inferior alveolar nerve (IAN) and its variations in interosseous anatomic location. **B,** Area of sensory dysfunction of the IAN in a patient 1 week following an SSRO procedure. There is complete anesthesia to neurosensory testing. **C,** Same patient 6 months postoperatively. The area of altered sensation has decreased in size, and there are now responses to painful stimuli and static light touch, findings indicative of significant recovery of sensory function. **D,** Diagrams that can be used to outline areas of altered sensation. (**B** to **D,** From Meyer RA, Bagheri SC: Clinical evaluation of peripheral trigeminal nerve injuries, *Atlas of oral and maxillofacial surgery clinics,* 2011.)

function by using a combination of measures. The scale ranges from a score of S0 (no improvement) to S4 (complete recovery). For peripheral nerve injuries, a score of S3 or higher has been defined as "useful sensory function" (USF). The advantages afforded by this scoring system are to (1) provide objective criteria for classification of results; (2) promote and develop common and accepted use of the scale in all disciplines in which peripheral nerve surgery is performed (i.e., hand surgery, plastic and reconstructive surgery,

neurosurgery, oral and maxillofacial surgery); and (3) enable comparison of data in various studies in the literature, even when the scale was not used originally by the study authors.

Documentation and mapping of the involved cranial nerve dermatomes on the patient's face and clinical photographs are helpful for monitoring and demonstrating changes over time in the affected area. Figure 29-4, *C,* shows a photograph of a patient's face with an outline of the affected area and a diagram for documentation.

TREATMENT/RECONSTRUCTIVE GOALS

The main goals of microsurgical repair of injured peripheral trigeminal nerves are improvement or restoration of sensory function and reduction or elimination of pain. In our review of 222 LN repairs, the majority of patients complained preoperatively of numbness (n = 122, 55.0%) or numbness with pain (n = 94, 42.3%). However, in our review of 186 IAN repairs, a greater number of patients complained of preoperative numbness with pain (n = 91, 48.9%) than numbness alone (n = 62, 33.3%).

Indications for surgery are dependent on the patient's chief complaint (pain, numbness), medical status, age, availability of microsurgical repair, and time since injury. Timely repair of peripheral nerve injuries has always been the sine qua non for successful recovery of nerve function. Delay in repair can result in centralization of pain or advanced wallerian degeneration of the distal nerve ending, thereby rendering it a poor candidate for microsurgical repair. Seddon's monumental experience with missile injuries to extremities during and after World War II compelled him to comment, "If a purely expectant policy is pursued, the most favorable time for operative intervention will always be missed … ," which is as pertinent today as it was more than 60 years ago. One of the authors (R.A.M.) had the opportunity to monitor 23 patients who were evaluated for IAN or LN injuries, initially had total anesthesia of the injured nerve on NST, refused surgical treatment, and were re-examined at regular intervals for 1 year or longer. None of these patients, all of whom were anesthetic and had no subjective symptoms of early recovery at 12 weeks following their nerve injury, eventually regained any significant spontaneous recovery of sensation in the distribution of the injured nerve. The so-called 12-week rule for an anesthetic patient has subsequently come to be regarded as the standard for timely decision making for a nerve injury patient who has unacceptable persistent total loss of sensory function. A patient who still has partial but unacceptable recovery of sensation at 3 months after nerve injury can be monitored at regular (1 to 2 month) intervals as long as the results of NST and subjective assessment of symptoms are improving at each visit. Once improvement ceases, it will not resume, and a treatment decision is made at that time, depending on the level of the sensory deficit on NST, the patient's subjective assessment of his status, and any associated functional impairment.

In patients who have suffered LN or IAN injury that remain anesthetic or have pain that is unacceptable beyond 3 months after injury, microsurgical consultation should be considered. We have developed a separate algorithm for the management of nerve injuries as a result of maxillofacial trauma and bilateral SSRO (Figs. 29-5 and 29-6) since the indication for repair is different from that for injuries incurred during third molar surgery.

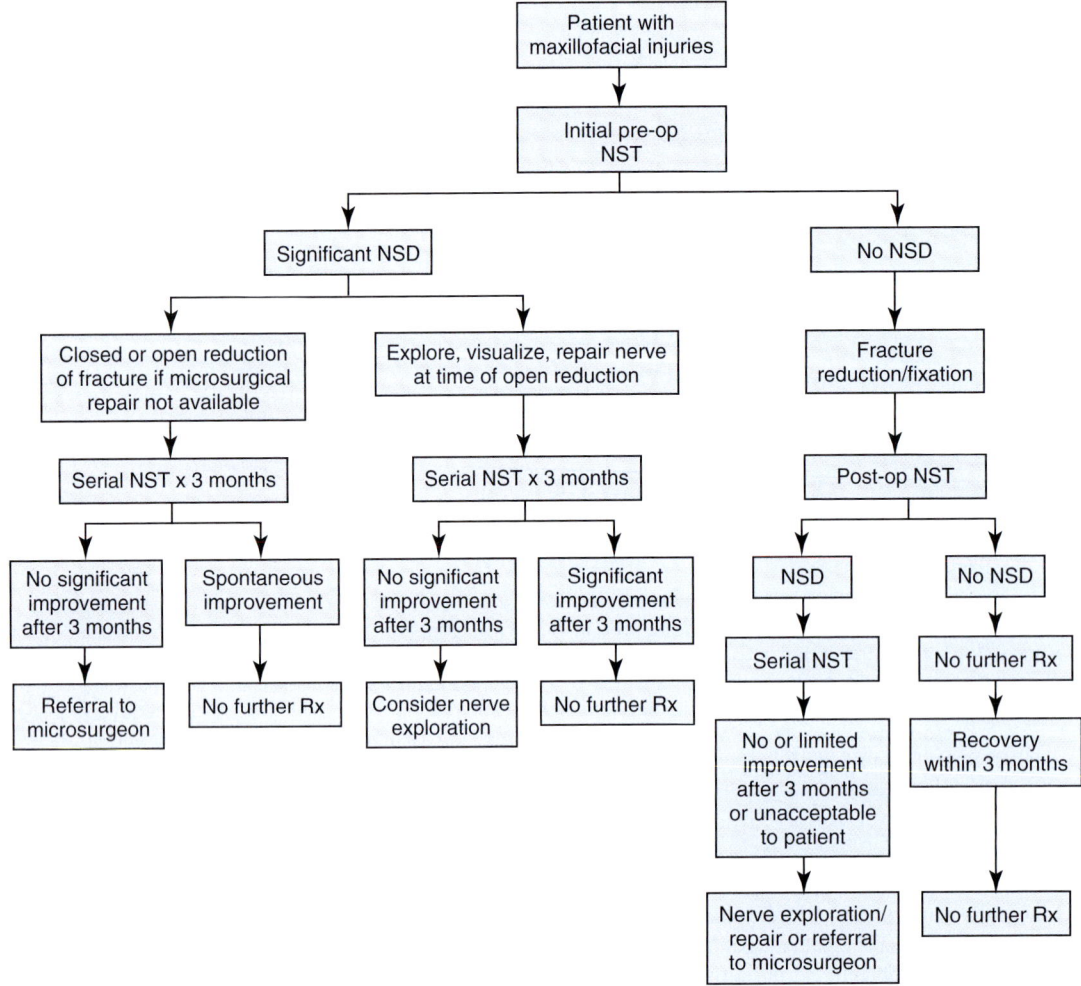

Fig. 29-5 ■ Algorithm for the evaluation and management of patients with maxillofacial injuries and associated peripheral trigeminal injuries. NSD, neurosensory dysfunction; NST, neurosensory testing; Rx, treatment. (From Bagheri SC, Meyer RA, Khan HA, et al: A retrospective review of microsurgical repair of 222 lingual nerve injuries, *J Oral Maxillofac Surg* 68:715-723, 2010.)

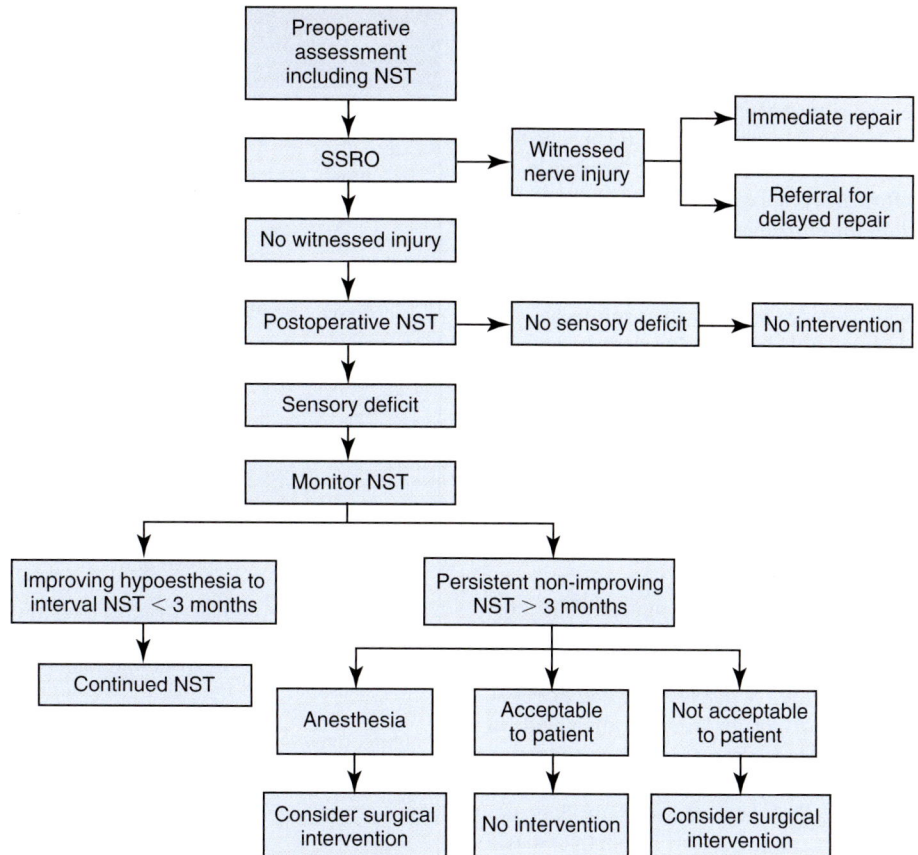

Fig. 29-6 ■ Algorithm for the evaluation and treatment of nerve injuries associated with sagittal split ramus osteotomy. (From Bagheri SC, Meyer, RA, Wallace J, et al: Microsurgical repair of the peripheral trigeminal nerves after mandibular sagittal split ramus osteotomy, *J Oral Maxillofac Surg* 68:2270-2282, 2010.)

The algorithm that we developed (see Fig. 29-5) is helpful in guiding clinicians during the evaluation and management of IAN and infraorbital nerve (ION) injuries associated with mandibular and mid-facial fractures, respectively. In all conscious patients with maxillofacial injuries, basic screening NST is performed. When no NSD of the IAN or ION is found, the facial injuries are repaired in the usual manner. Follow-up NST is done within the first postoperative week and then serially at 1, 2, and 3 months. If there is still no NSD at 3 months, no further evaluation is necessary. If the patient exhibits significant NSD 1 week after facial injury repair, follow-up NST is done serially for 3 months. If acceptable neurosensory recovery has not occurred by 3 months postoperatively, exploration and repair of the involved nerve by a microsurgeon **may** be considered.

In a patient with maxillofacial injuries and significant NSD, the fractures are repaired with additional considerations. If closed reduction is performed, manipulation is done gently to minimize additional trauma to the involved nerve. The patient is monitored postoperatively with serial NST. If the sensory deficit has not recovered to a level acceptable to the patient by 3 months after fracture reduction, the patient is referred to a microsurgeon for further evaluation.

If open reduction is performed and the nerve can be seen, it is first decompressed by enlarging the nerve canal (to compensate for possible postinjury osseous proliferation or edema of the nerve) and then repositioned or repaired (or both) accordingly as indicated. Care is taken to minimize the extent of manipulation of the fracture segments containing or adjacent to nerve canals (e.g., inferior alveolar canal, mental foramen, inferior orbital canal/foramen). If the surgeon elects to not repair an injured nerve (patient's condition too

critical as a result of other injuries or general health status, gross contamination of the injury area [e.g., battlefield wounds], surgeon lacking expertise in microsurgery), the nerve ends are tagged with fine nylon sutures. The extent and location of the nerve injury are mentioned in the operative report. After recovery from the facial injuries, the patient is referred to a microsurgeon for further evaluation and decision about the need to repair the nerve injury. Optimally, this will have occurred before 3 months has elapsed since the original injury.

Our algorithm (see Fig. 29-6) for the treatment of patients who sustain a nerve injury while undergoing SSRO is designed to aid clinicians in making timely decisions regarding evaluation and treatment of associated IAN and LN injuries. Preoperative evaluation with NST should be done routinely and any variations from normal documented in the patient's record. During the SSRO procedure, if a nerve injury is witnessed, the nerve can be repaired at that time provided that the attending surgeon has microsurgical skills. Lacking such skills, if the IAN is severed, the two ends are gently replaced in approximation into the inferior alveolar canal. If LN severance is observed (highly unlikely in our experience), the proximal and distal nerve stumps are placed in close proximity and tagged with fine sutures of non-reactive material (e.g., 4-0 or 6-0 nylon). A notation is made in the operative record regarding the location and nature of the injury, and the patient or family (or both) is informed following surgery. If the injured nerve has not been repaired, arrangements are made for referral to a microsurgeon for delayed repair. In most cases, the microsurgeon will elect to delay the repair for several weeks, if not 3 months. There are a number of reasons for such delay. In the early postoperative period, the inflammatory phase of healing creates a very vascular field with much bleeding, thus making hemostasis and visualization difficult. Early after injury the neural tissues are friable, which makes manipulation and suturing problematic. As the injury matures, the epineurium becomes thicker and easier to suture. Reoperation within the first few days after SSRO may disrupt osseous healing or cause secondary infection. The prognosis for neurosensory recovery after delayed repair (up to 3 months) is thought to be as good as that for immediate primary repair. There is also the possibility that the IAN injury will heal spontaneously because of the guidance and protection provided by the inferior alveolar canal. The LN, which resides totally within soft tissue, has no such protection, and a severed LN rarely, if ever recovers without timely surgical treatment. Early surgical treatment of an LN injury may preclude the formation of a proximal stump neuroma and be associated with a better outcome.

SPECIFIC TREATMENT AND TECHNIQUES

MICROSURGICAL TECHNIQUES

Specific surgical treatment is dependent on the diagnosis. The most commonly used classification, devised by Seddon in 1943, divides nerve injuries into three categories: neurapraxia, axonotmesis, and neurotmesis. Neurapraxia describes nerve damage, likened to a concussion, in which neither the nerve nor its sheath is disrupted. In such an injury there is temporary interruption of impulse conduction along the nerve fibers (axons), and complete recovery of nerve function takes place within 4 weeks. Wallerian degeneration does not occur and surgical intervention is not necessary. Axonotmesis is a more severe nerve injury characterized by disruption of the neuronal axon but maintenance of the myelin sheath. Wallerian degeneration occurs in the injured axons. There is prolonged loss of nerve function, and recovery does not begin until at least 5 weeks after injury. Recovery with regrowth of lost axons may take several months and may not be complete. In sensory nerve injuries, painful sensations (dysesthesias) may become persistent and troublesome. Surgical intervention may be indicated for improvement of sensation or relief of pain. In neurotmesis there is total, usually permanent disruption of neural transmission of impulses because of anatomic loss of continuity (complete transection) of the entire cross section of the nerve (not only all the axons but also the encapsulating connective tissues, endoneurium, perineurium, and epineurium) or because of pathophysiologic loss of the ability to conduct impulses secondary to replacement of a segment of the nerve with scar tissue as a result of stretching, ischemia, or exposure to a toxic substance. When the nerve has been transected, a neuroma often forms on the proximal nerve stump and is frequently the source of spontaneous or stimulus-induced pain. Recovery from neurotmesis is not generally possible unless surgical repair of the nerve is performed.

Table 29-2 presents a representative list of microneurosurgical procedures. Figure 29-7, *A* to *J*, shows various microsurgical operations. Although it is beyond the scope of this chapter to discuss all the techniques listed in Table 29-2, in our review of 222 LN repairs, the most commonly performed operation was excision of a proximal stump neuroma with neurorrhaphy ($n = 154$, 69.4%), followed by external decompression with internal neurolysis (EDIN) ($n = 29$, 13.1%). Nineteen patients (8.6%) underwent an autogenous nerve graft procedure (greater auricular nerve [GAN] or sural nerve [SN]) for reconstruction of a nerve gap. A collagen cuff was placed around the repair site in 8 (3.6%) patients (EDIN = 2, neurorrhaphy = 6). In our review of 186 IAN injuries, the most commonly performed operation was autogenous nerve grafting, followed by internal neurolysis ($n = 60$, 32.3%). Seventy-one (38.2%) autogenous nerve

TABLE 29-2	Representative List of Microneurosurgical Procedures
PROCEDURE	**DESCRIPTION**
External decompression	Removal of bone, soft tissue structures, and/or foreign material around the nerve
Internal neurolysis	Opening of the epineurium to inspect and decompress the nerve fascicles
Excision of neuroma	Removal of a neuroma associated with a nerve
Neurorrhaphy	Microsurgical anastomosis of a transected nerve
Nerve graft	Placement of a nerve graft (allogeneic or autogenous) for nerve reconstruction
Nerve sharing	Microsurgical anastomosis of a distal nerve to a different proximal nerve via an interposed nerve graft
"Guided" nerve regeneration	Placement of a conduit to guide axonal sprouting and regeneration across a nerve gap from proximal to distal portions of a nerve
Neurectomy	Microsurgical transection and removal of a segment of a peripheral nerve
Nerve capping	Covering of the proximal stump of a transected nerve with its epineurium to prevent neuroma formation
Nerve redirection	Redirection of a nerve's sensory innervation to a different anatomic location (usually adjacent muscle); generally done to prevent or minimize deafferentation

graft procedures (GAN or SN) were performed for reconstruction of a nerve gap. A synthetic nerve cuff of either collagen or polyglycolic acid was placed around the repair site in 19 (10.2%) patients.

Lingual Nerve Repair

Injuries to the LN secondary to third molar surgery are accessed via an intraoral incision. By using general nasotracheal intubation with hypotensive anesthesia, the LN can be approached through an incision in the buccal gingiva around the necks of the mandibular premolar and molar teeth, along with posterolateral extension from the last molar tooth into the retromolar pad to facilitate placement of self-retaining retractors. An incision in the lingual cervical gingiva followed by elevation of a lingual mucoperiosteal flap and careful dissection through the lingual periosteum will expose the LN. The nerve is exposed for several centimeters both proximal and distal to the area of injury. Based on intraoperative findings, appropriate repair is carried out under 2.5 to 5.0 magnification. Figure 29-8 demonstrates exposure of a transected LN and subsequent direct neurorrhaphy using 8-0 nylon after mobilization of the distal nerve from the floor of the mouth.

Inferior Alveolar Nerve Repair

The IAN has a long course; it branches from the mandibular nerve in the pterygomandibular space, travels anteriorly until it enters the mandibular foramen on the medial mandible, continues within the

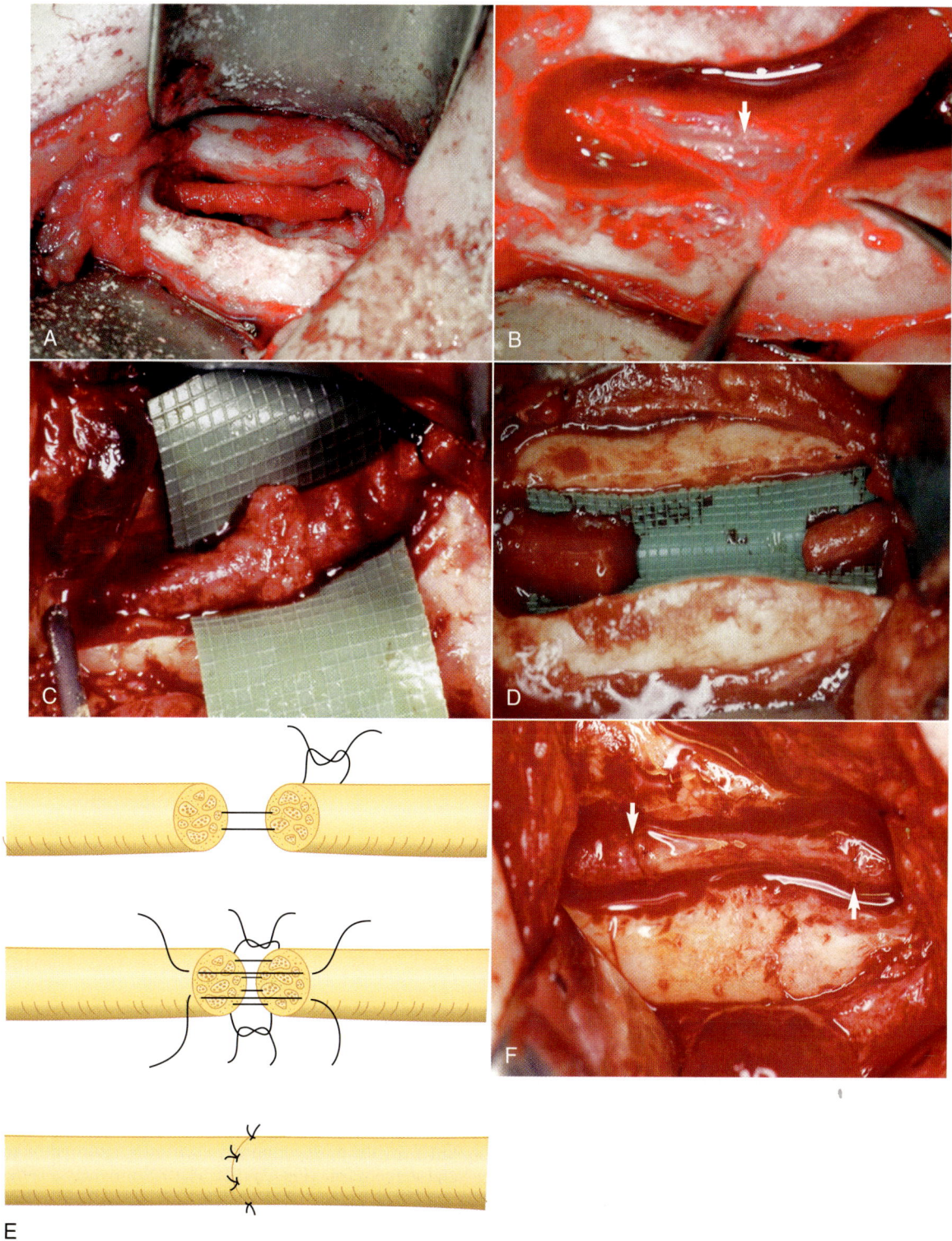

Fig. 29-7 ■ Microneurosurgical procedures. **A,** External decompression of the inferior alveolar nerve (IAN). **B,** Internal neurolysis of the IAN (*arrow*). **C,** Neuroma in continuity of the IAN. **D,** IAN after excision of a neuroma in continuity. **E,** Diagrammatic representation of direct neurorrhaphy. **F,** Sural nerve graft for IAN reconstruction (*arrows*).

inferior alveolar canal, and just before exiting at the mental foramen, divides into its two terminal branches, the incisive nerve and the mental nerve. Injuries to the nerve at the mandibular canal and more proximally in the pterygomandibular space are difficult to visualize and repair without performing a mandibular ramus osteotomy for additional access. Such operations are seldom done for nerve repair unless performed as part of tumor resection. The IAN at the area of the third molar can be accessed with both intraoral and transcutaneous incisions. The standard Risdon incision allows excellent access to the entire nerve from the area of the mandibular canal to the

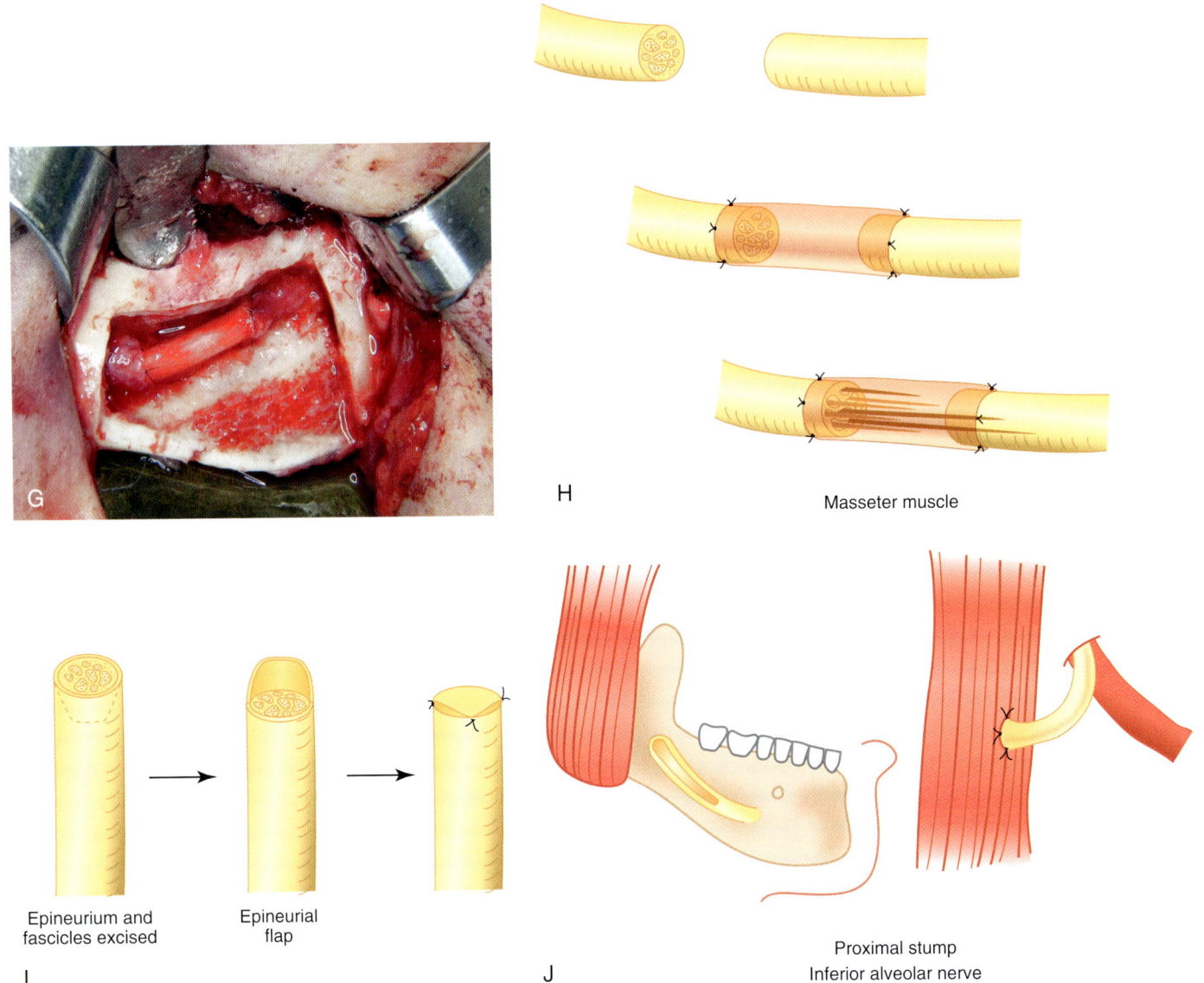

Fig. 29-7, cont'd ■ **G,** Decellularized human nerve graft (Axogen, Alachua, Fla.) for IAN reconstruction. **H,** Diagrammatic representation of guided tissue regeneration. **I,** Neurectomy and nerve capping. **J,** Nerve re-direction. (From Bagheri SC, Meyer RA: Management or mandibular nerve injuries from dental implants, *Atlas of Oral and Maxillofacial Surgery Clinics* 19(1):47-61, 2011.)

mental foramen. The main disadvantages of this access are scarring (especially in younger individuals who do not have a naturally visible neck crease) and a small possibility of injury to the marginal mandibular nerve (about 1% in our experience). Figure 29-9 shows photos of young patients with esthetically pleasing neck scars after IAN repair and harvesting of a GAN graft. The nerve can also be accessed intraorally via a variety of techniques, including a modified SSRO or removal of the external oblique ridge and superior lateral cortex (Fig. 29-10; see Fig. 29-1, *D*). The main disadvantage of the intraoral approach is reduced visibility and access. Though technically more difficult, successful nerve repair, including interpositional grafting, can be done via this approach (Fig. 29-11).

Nerve Grafts

The sine qua non of successful neurorrhaphy is to bring the proximal and distal stumps of a transected nerve together and suture them in this position without tension. When the surgeon is unable to accomplish this, reconstruction of the space between the two nerve stumps (the nerve gap) can be done with an interpositional nerve graft. Both autologous and allogeneic nerve grafts can be used. The SN and GAN are the most commonly used autogenous grafts for maxillofacial nerve repair (Fig. 29-12). The SN provides a better size match and longer length. Disadvantages of this graft are a vertical scar just posterior and superior to the lateral malleolus of the ankle, added operative time to access a distant surgical site, and associated donor site morbidity (anesthesia of the lateral aspect of the foot, temporary gait disturbance, pain; see Fig. 29-12, *C*). The GAN is easily harvested along its superficial course lateral to the sternocleidomastoid muscle approximately 6 cm inferior to the earlobe. The incision for harvesting the GAN is usually made in a natural skin crease in the lateral part of the neck, and an inconspicuous scar can be achieved by careful closure (see Fig. 29-9). The main disadvantages of using the GAN are its sometimes smaller (than the recipient IAN or LN) diameter, which can result in earlobe anesthesia, and the neck scar. The discrepancy in diameter can be overcome by placing a cable graft (Fig. 29-13).

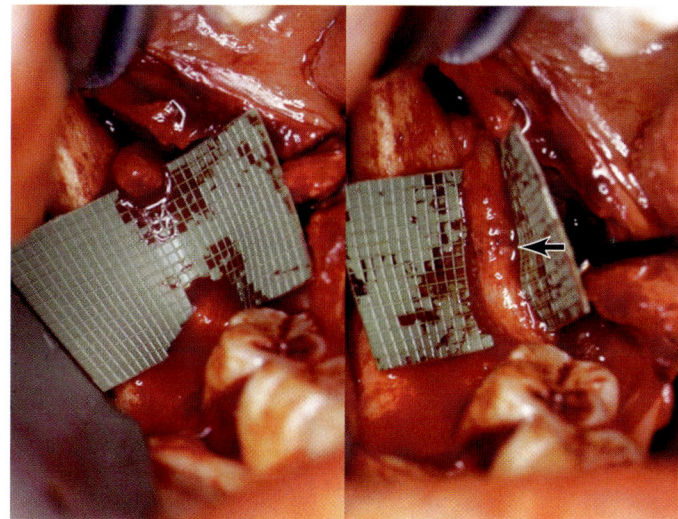

Fig. 29-8 ■ Exposure of a transected lingual nerve (LN) and subsequent direct neurorrhaphy with 8-0 nylon after mobilization of the distal nerve from the floor of the mouth. (From Bagheri SC, Meyer RA, Khan HA, et al: A retrospective review of microsurgical repair of 222 lingual nerve injuries, *J Oral Maxillofac Surg* 68:715-723, 2010.)

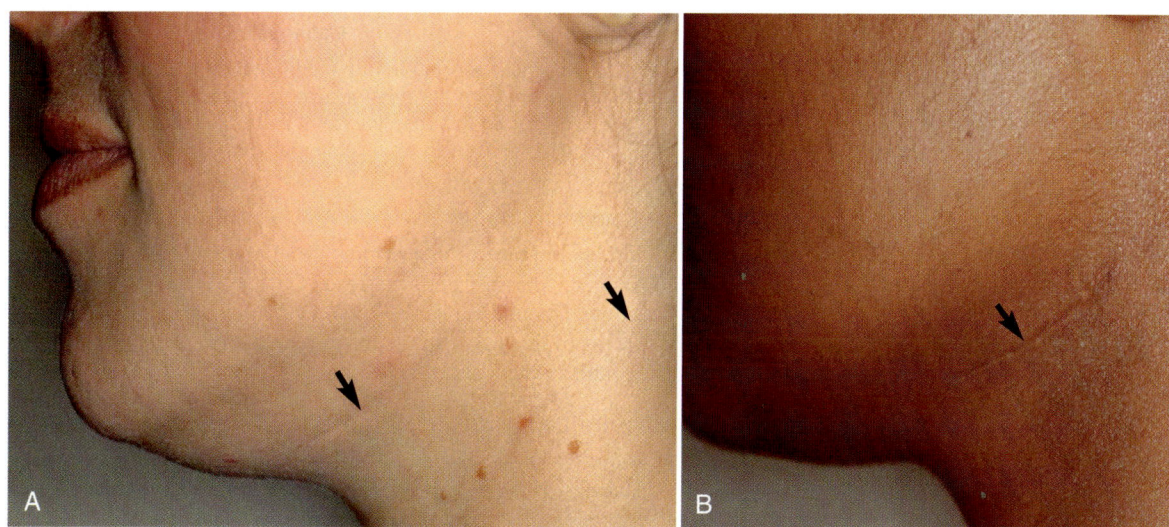

Fig. 29-9 ■ Careful plastic surgical closure of neck incisions after transcutaneous exposure of the inferior alveolar nerve (*left arrow*) and harvesting of an autogenous greater auricular nerve graft (*right arrow*). **A,** Eighteen-year-old white woman 12 months postoperatively. (From Bagheri SC, Meyer RA: Management or mandibular nerve injuries from dental implants, *Atlas of Oral and Maxillofacial Surgery Clinics* 19(1):47-61, 2011.) **B,** Twenty-one-year-old African-American woman at 13 months. The margins of the incision were injected with triamcinolone at the time of closure to reduce risk for the development of a hypertrophic scar or keloid.

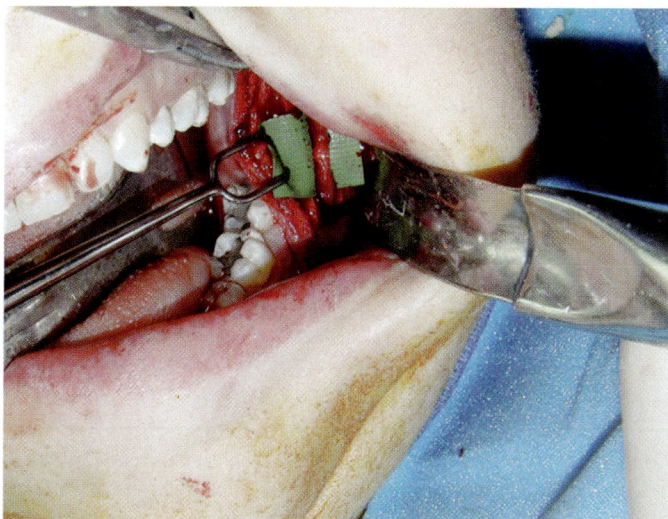

Fig. 29-10 ■ Exposure of the inferior alveolar nerve via an intraoral approach.

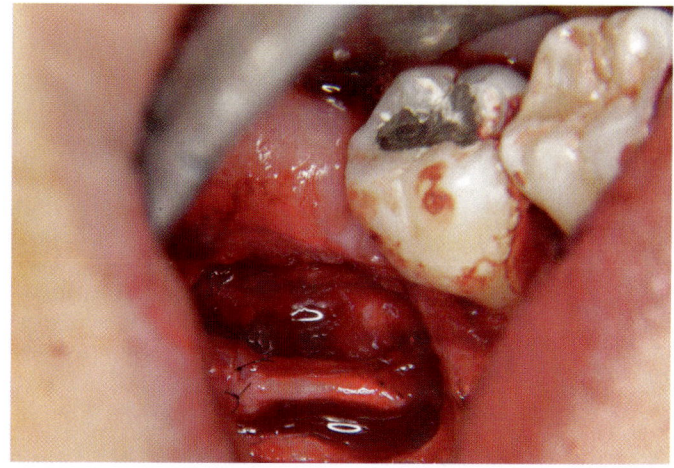

Fig. 29-11 ■ Reconstruction of the inferior alveolar nerve using the sural nerve via intraoral access. (From Bagheri SC, Meyer RA: Management or mandibular nerve injuries from dental implants, *Atlas of Oral and Maxillofacial Surgery Clinics* 19(1):47-61, 2011.)

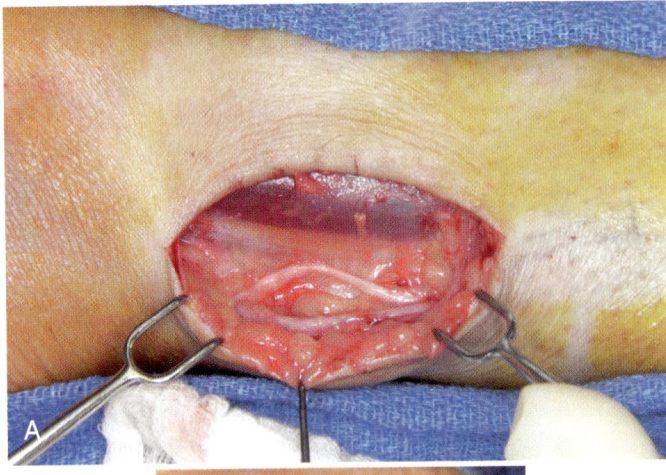

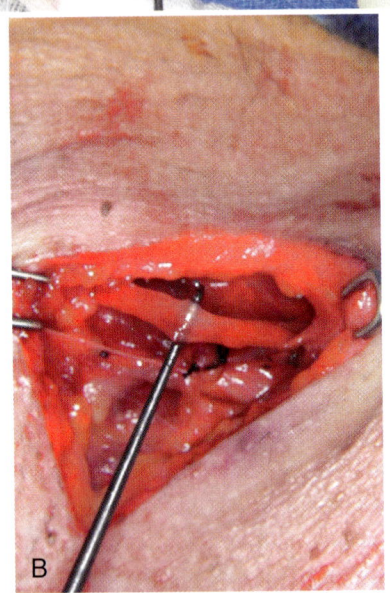

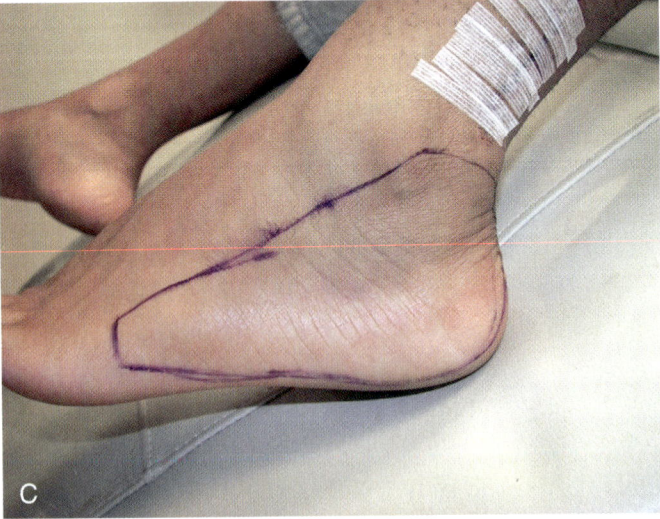

Fig. 29-12 ■ **A,** Sural nerve graft harvest. **B,** Greater auricular nerve harvest. **C,** Resulting area of anesthesia from harvest of the sural nerve. (From Bagheri SC, Meyer RA: Management or mandibular nerve injuries from dental implants, *Atlas of Oral and Maxillofacial Surgery Clinics* 19(1):47-61, 2011.)

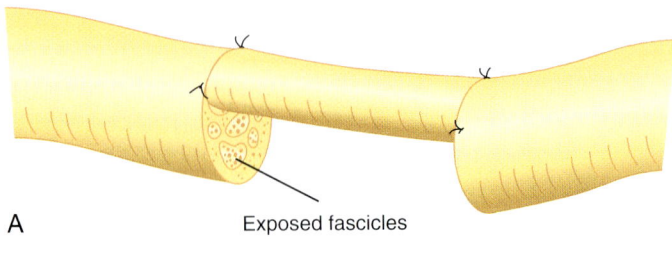

A   Exposed fascicles

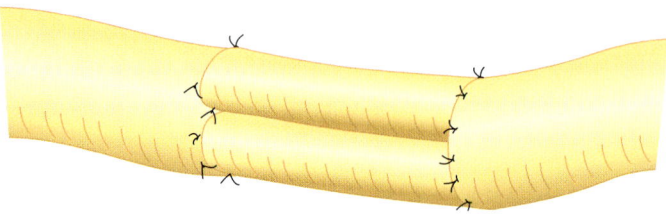

B   Cable graft

Fig. 29-13 ■ Representation of a cable graft. **A,** Note the discrepancy in diameter between the inferior alveolar nerve and greater auricular nerve (GAN) graft. **B,** When the GAN graft is smaller in diameter than the recipient nerve (as in **A**), a cable graft (two or more parallel strands of grafted nerve) is placed into the nerve gap.

As of the time of this writing, decellularized human nerve grafts (Axogen, Alachua, Fla.) are readily available for trigeminal nerve reconstruction (see Fig. 29-7, *G*). Ongoing studies to determine the success of this nerve in the maxillofacial area is pending, although the initial results are promising.

Nerve Cuff

When the nerve gap is short (<1.0 cm), the nerve might be repaired without nerve grafting by guided nerve regeneration. An entubulation procedure can be done with an autogenous vein (usually a vein adjacent to the surgical site such as the external jugular vein) or an alloplastic tube made of collagen or polyglycolic acid to bridge the nerve gap. The tube or vein is secured to the proximal and distal nerve stumps with fine sutures similar to those used for neurorrhaphy. Figure 29-14 shows drawings and a clinical photograph of entubulation. It is thought that the tube isolates the nerve gap, protects it from the ingrowth of scar tissue, and guides the new advancing axonal sprouts from the proximal nerve stump across the gap and into the distal nerve. Nerve gaps with a longer span (>1.0 cm) are probably best repaired with nerve grafting.

Nerve-Sharing Procedure

The proximal stump of the IAN or LN may be absent or impossible to locate because of the effects of missile injury, other trauma, infection, or anatomic variation and therefore unavailable for repair. If the distal limb of the nerve is visible and appears to be viable, the nerve can be reconstructed by a nerve-sharing procedure. An autogenous SN graft is harvested to create a connection between the proximal stump of the GAN and the viable IAN or LN distal stump (Fig. 29-15).

POSTOPERATIVE CARE/REHABILITATION

Younger individuals experience better functional recovery after peripheral nerve injury than adults do. Observations in human patients are limited, but clinical experience indicates that

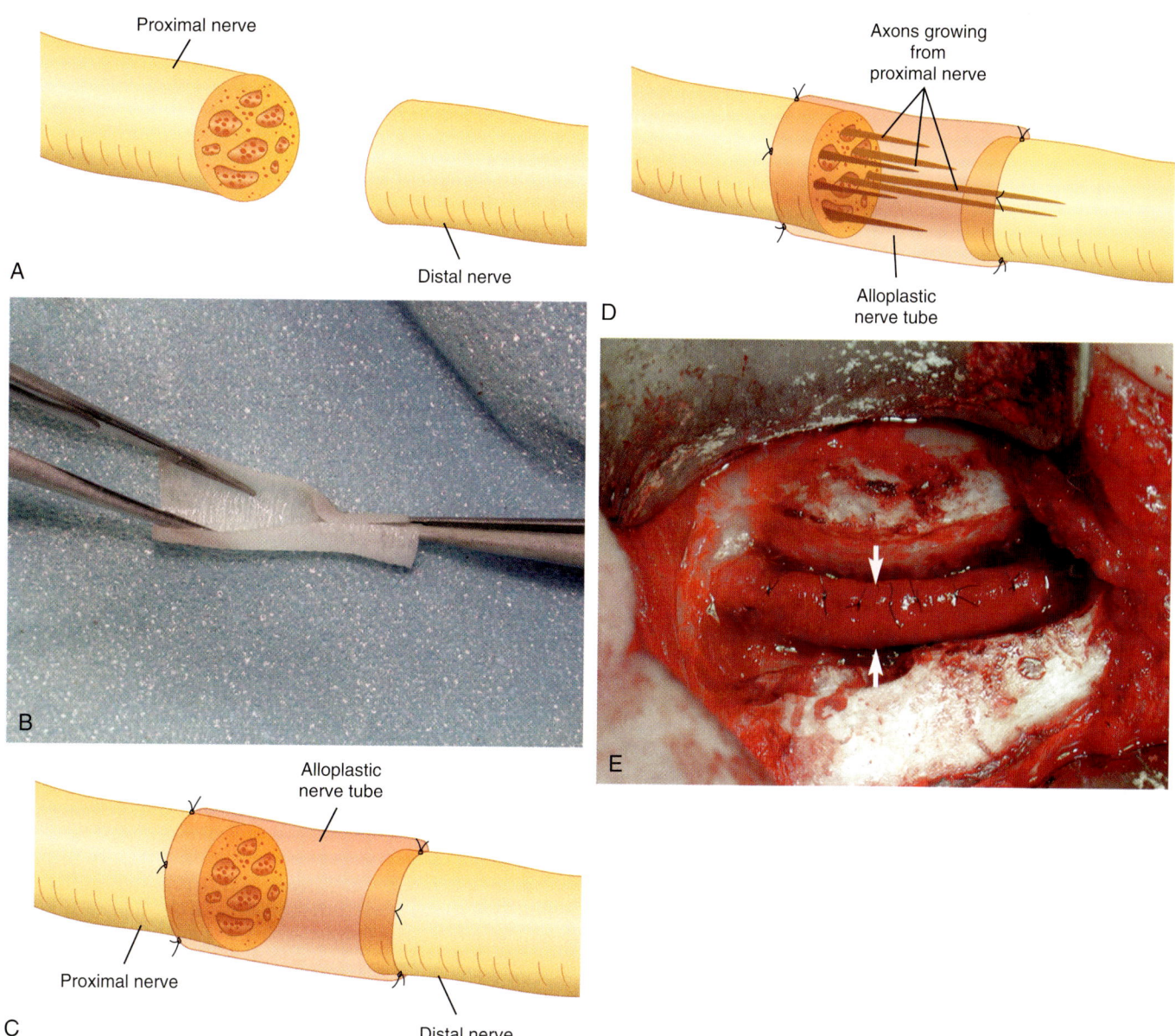

Fig. 29-14 ■ Guided nerve regeneration. **A,** Nerve stumps have been débrided and a significant gap exists. **B,** A collagen nerve sleeve is prepared. **C,** The alloplastic tube is sutured to the proximal and distal nerve stumps with fine sutures (8-0 or 10-0 nylon). **D,** Axonal growth from the proximal nerve stump is guided across the nerve gap by the tube. The axons enter endoneurial tubules of the distal nerve and continue their growth to sensory end-organs in the skin or mucosa. **E,** A collagen nerve tube is sutured to the inferior alveolar nerve.

regeneration is less efficient in later life. Aging influences several features of the peripheral nervous system. The results of experimental studies in animals, though sometimes variable, indicate a decline in regenerative capacity with age. Morphologic studies have found that aging is associated with loss of myelinated and unmyelinated nerve fibers, demyelination of myelinated fibers, decreased expression of the major myelin proteins, axonal atrophy, and reduced expression and impaired axonal transport of cytoskeletal proteins in the peripheral nerve. The effect of age on angiogenesis may also play a role in peripheral trigeminal nerve recovery. In a mouse model, Pola and co-workers found that the peripheral nerves of old and senescence-accelerated animals were unable to locally up-regulate vascular endothelial growth factor, a prototypic angiogenic cytokine, after injury and exhibited substantial deficits in

mounting an appropriate intraneural angiogenic response during nerve regeneration. Therefore, the ability of an injured nerve to recover to the level of USF is probably dependent in part on the patient's age and state of general health because these factors directly affect tissue healing.

Neuropsychological factors also influence the ability of older patients to recover successfully from a peripheral nerve injury following surgical repair. There is a need to learn new axonal connections with referral of sensory input to different areas of the CNS. Early in the recovery process, new axons are sparsely myelinated, which results in slower conduction time and makes interpretation more difficult for the CNS until accommodations can be achieved, a situation analogous to a baseball batter having to adjust to a change-up (dramatically slower-speed pitch). Although an older

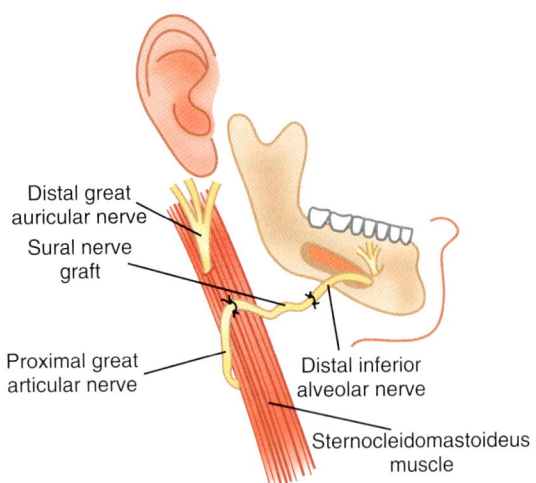

Fig. 29-15 ■ Nerve-sharing procedure. The proximal inferior alveolar nerve (IAN) is not available for reconstruction. An autogenous sural nerve (SN) graft is interposed between the proximal greater auricular nerve (GAN) and the viable distal IAN. After recovery, sensory input is transmitted from end-organs in the skin and oral tissues via the distal IAN, the bridging SN graft, and the proximal GAN via C2,3 to the central nervous system. Sensory re-education is helpful in rehabilitating the reinterpretation of input via new pathways and connections.

patient is slower to adapt to these changes imposed by recovery from a peripheral nerve injury, neuroplasticity (the concept that the brain has the capacity to adapt) is still viable even in advanced age. The concept of "sensory re-education," first developed by Wynn Parry for rehabilitation of hand and upper extremity injuries, has been adapted to the maxillofacial regions and shown to be successful in improving sensory function once responses to pain and static light touch have returned. The goals of sensory re-education for peripheral trigeminal nerve injuries are to improve or resolve synesthesia (failure to recognize the location of a stimulus), decrease hyperesthesia, improve recognition of the character and amplitude of stimuli (e.g., moving or stationary, sharp or dull, light or forceful application, size of the area of contact), and decrease subjective differences (e.g., numbness) between the affected area and the corresponding normal contralateral area. Following microneurosurgery, we generally recommend initiation of neurosensory exercises as soon as the area supplied by the repaired nerve begins to respond to painful stimuli and static light touch (usually within 3 to 6 months after surgery). Sensory re-education undoubtedly plays a role in a nerve-injured patient's ability to improve to the maximal level of sensory function over and above the USF level (from S3 to S3+ or S4).

RESULTS

The majority of patients who require microsurgical repair of IAN or LN injuries do regain acceptable sensation and associated function as classified by the MRC scale. Evaluation and management of IAN or LN dysfunction after SSRO remains a challenging clinical dilemma. Despite a considerable body of literature evaluating neurosensory recovery after orthognathic surgery, our understanding of the specific cause and predictability of the incidence of persistent sensory deficits or neuropathic pain after SSRO in a given individual patient remains inadequate.

Microsurgical repair of IAN and LN injuries resulting from SSRO can provide sensory and functional improvement in patients who have surgical indications as determined by the history and standardized NST. In our study we reviewed 54 SSRO patients who underwent microsurgical repair of IAN and LN injuries. The most commonly injured/repaired nerve was the IAN ($n = 39$). After a minimum 1-year follow-up, NST demonstrated that 8 nerves (14.8%) showed no sign of recovery, 19 nerves (35.2%) had regained USF, and 27 nerves (50%) showed full recovery as described by the MRC scale.

Approximately 8% to 66.7% of patients with mandibular fractures and 15% to 46% of patients with mid-facial fractures initially complain of NSD and associated orofacial dysfunction. Although estimates vary, it is clear that a proportion of patients who have sustained facial trauma have permanent NSD. In our study we reviewed the results of microsurgical repair of peripheral branches of the trigeminal nerve injured by maxillofacial trauma in 42 patients. Our results demonstrated a significant improvement (MRC score of S3 to S3+) or complete recovery (MRC score of S4) in 86% (36 of 42) of patients. These results compare favorably with microsurgical repair of peripheral trigeminal nerve injuries from other causes.

The clinical outcomes of microsurgical repair of the IAN or LN following elective oral surgery have frequently been reported in the literature. In our study of 222 LN injuries that were repaired by microsurgery, 191 were associated with removal of mandibular third molars. The overall success rate of nerve repair was 90% (MRC score of S3 to S4).

PEARLS AND PITFALLS

- Spontaneous recovery occurs in most, but not all patients. However, clinicians should not continue to expectantly monitor patients who are found to be anesthetic on NST beyond 3 months following injury or those who have severe, unacceptable (to the patient) hypoesthesia on NST beyond 4 months and are not improving. Such patients will not improve, and they should be referred promptly to a microsurgeon who can determine the need for timely surgical intervention. Further delay only compromises the chance for successful recovery of nerve function. LN injuries have a lower rate of spontaneous recovery.
- All nerve injuries should be documented and re-evaluated.
- Interval NST is essential.
- Injuries resolving within 1 month are indicative of neurapraxia and do not require treatment.
- Patients with painful sensation (anesthesia dolorosa, hyperpathia) should be considered for microsurgery, but only if anesthetic blockade of the suspected nerve produces good temporary pain relief. Other patients with painful nerve injuries may be treated nonsurgically (e.g., medications, counseling and behavior modification, physical therapy, support groups, multi-specialty pain clinic).
- An angry, uninformed, and neglected patient is a bad combination.
- Early surgical intervention produces the best results.
- Increasing patient age or poor medical status (e.g., diabetes mellitus, coronary heart or peripheral vascular disease, connective tissue diseases) compromises the success of microsurgical repair.
- Surgery is more likely to improve sensory deficits than to alleviate neuropathic pain.

BIBLIOGRAPHY

Alling CC, Schwartz E, Campbell RL, et al: Algorithm for diagnostic assessment and surgical treatment of traumatic trigeminal neuropathies and neuralgias, *Oral Maxillofac Surg Clin North Am* 4:555, 1992.

Bagheri SC, Meyer RA: Microsurgical repair of the long buccal nerve injuries in oral and maxillofacial surgery, abstract submitted for AAOMS 2010.

Bagheri SC, Meyer RA, Khan HA, et al: Microsurgical repair of peripheral trigeminal nerve injuries from maxillofacial trauma, *J Oral Maxillofac Surg*, 67:1791-1799, 2009.

Bagheri SC, Meyer RA, Khan HA, et al: A retrospective review of microsurgical repair of 222 lingual nerve injuries, *J Oral Maxillofac Surg* 68:715-723, 2010.

Bagheri SC, Meyer RA: Microsurgical repair of injuries to the inferior alveolar nerve associated with dental implants. In Steed MB: *Atlas of the oral and maxillofacial surgery Clinics of North America*, 2011.

Bagheri SC, Meyer, RA, Khan HA, et al: Microsurgical repair of the peripheral trigeminal nerves after mandibular sagittal split ramus osteotomy, *J Oral Maxillofac Surg* 68:2770-2782, 2010.

Bagheri SC, Meyer RA, Sung C, et al: A retrospective review of microsurgical repair of 186 inferior alveolar nerve injuries, *J Oral Maxillofac Surg* 68(9 Suppl 1):e27-e28, 2010.

Behnia H, Kheradvar A, Shahrokhi M: An anatomic study of the lingual nerve in the third molar region, *J Oral Maxillofac Surg* 58:649-651, discussion 652-653, 2000.

Birch R, Bonney G, Wynn Parry CB: *Surgical disorders of the peripheral nerves*, New York, 1998, Churchill Livingstone, pp 235-243.

Colella G, Cannavale R, Vicidomini A, et al: Neurosensory disturbance of the inferior alveolar nerve after bilateral sagittal split osteotomy: a systematic review, *J Oral Maxillofac Surg* 65:1707-1715, 2007.

Dodson TB, Kaban LB: Recommendations for management of trigeminal nerve defects based on a critical appraisal of the literature, *J Oral Maxillofac Surg* 55:1380-1386, discussion 1387, 1997.

Essick GK, Phillips C, Turvey TA, et al: Facial altered sensation and sensory impairment after orthognathic surgery, *Int J Oral Maxillofac Surg* 36:577-582, 2007.

Meyer RA: Protection of the lingual nerve during placement of rigid fixation after sagittal ramus osteotomy, *J Oral Maxillofac Surg* 48:1135, 1990.

Meyer RA: Applications of microneurosurgery to the repair of trigeminal nerve injuries, *Oral Maxillofac Surg Clin North Am* 4:405, 1992.

Meyer RA: Evaluation and management of neurologic complications. In: Kaban LB, Pogrel MA, Perrott DH, editors: *Complications in oral and maxillofacial surgery*, Philadelphia, 1997, WB Saunders, pp 69-88.

Meyer RA: Nerve harvesting procedures, *Atlas Oral Maxillofac Surg Clin North Am* 9:77-91, 2001.

Meyer RA: Surgical treatment of inferior alveolar nerve injuries associated with orthognathic surgery in the mandibular ramus. In: Bell WH, Guerrero CA, editors: *Distraction osteogenesis of the facial skeleton*, St Louis, 2007, Elsevier, pp 409-418.

Meyer RA, Bagheri SC: A bioabsorbable collagen nerve cuff (NeuraGen) for repair of lingual and inferior alveolar nerve injuries: a case series [letter], *J Oral Maxillofac Surg* 67:2550-2551, 2009.

Meyer RA, Rath EM: Sensory rehabilitation after trigeminal nerve injury or nerve repair, *Oral Maxillofac Surg Clin North Am* 13:365-376, 2001.

Meyer RA, Ruggiero SL: Guidelines for diagnosis and treatment of peripheral trigeminal nerve injuries, *Oral Maxillofac Surg Clin North Am* 13:383, 2001.

Pogrel MA: The results of microneurosurgery of the inferior alveolar and lingual nerve. *J Oral Maxillofac Surg* 60:485-489, 2002.

Pola R, Aprahamian TR, Bosch-Marce M, et al: Age-dependent VEGF expression and intraneural neovascularization during regeneration of peripheral nerves, *Neurobiol Aging* 25:1361-1368, 2004.

Seddon HJ: Three types of nerve injury, *Brain* 66:237-288, 1943.

Susarla S, Kaban L, Donoff RB, et al: Does early repair of lingual nerve injuries improve functional sensory recovery? *J Oral Maxillofac Surg* 65:1070-1076, 2007.

Wynn Parry CB: Brachial plexus injuries, *Br J Hosp Med* 32:130-132, 134-139, 1984.

Ziccardi V, Steinberg M: Timing of trigeminal nerve microsurgery: a review of the literature, *J Oral Maxillofac Surg* 65(7):1341-1345, 2007.

Zuniga JR, Meyer RA, Gregg JM, et al: The accuracy of clinical neurosensory testing for nerve injury diagnosis, *J Oral Maxillofac Surg* 56:2-8, 1998.

THE PAST

Oral and maxillofacial surgeons have been unique in providing anesthesia in combination with surgical care. The integration of intravenous sedation and anesthesia significantly increased the efficiency and convenience and improved the cost of minor surgical interventions. The profession has deep roots in the development of general anesthesia since 1846, with the contributions of William Morton and others beginning with the first demonstration of general anesthesia at the "ether dome" (see Chapter 1). Many of the local and general anesthetics of the past have been replaced with compounds that have improved safety (cardiopulmonary stability) and decreased side effects, which has contributed to the popularization of outpatient anesthesia. Anesthesia monitoring was entirely dependent on the astute and continuous clinical observations of the anesthesiologist, and only in the later part of the 20th century did adjunctive anesthesia monitoring technology (e.g., pulse oximetry, capnography, mechanical ventilation) add to the safety of office and hospital surgery.

THE PRESENT

The modern practice of anesthesia has expanded to routine office-based and hospital anesthesia, and its safety record is excellent. Presurgical cardiopulmonary risk assessment and enhanced monitoring have contributed considerably to current practice. The emergence of pain management as a subspecialty for treating chronic (and acute) pain has increased and added to the armamentarium of surgeons. In this section we include a chapter on nonsurgical management of facial pain in which new techniques and algorithms for addressing facial pain are elucidated. The current practice of anesthesia in oral and maxillofacial surgery has seen a trend toward increased office and outpatient surgical care and decreased inpatient hospital surgery. This trend is attributed in part to less invasive surgery, faster recovery, and smoother anesthesia, but it is also due to the financial forces and third-party payers that influence patient care.

THE FUTURE

The future of anesthesia care in oral and maxillofacial surgery will be enhanced further by an improved pharmacology and side effect profile of medications (decreased postoperative nausea, rapid onset, smooth emergence, cardiac and pulmonary stability). The delivery of local anesthetics by needle injection will be replaced by alternative noninvasive technology. Anesthesia monitoring will routinely include brain activity. All monitoring systems will be replaced by wireless technology. Cardiac monitors will become more accurate and unaffected by movement and artifacts. Real-time, noninvasive blood pressure monitoring will become standard. The operating rooms of the future will be equipped with advanced intraoperative imaging and monitoring to assist in both surgery and anesthesiology.

Chapter

30

Outpatient Intravenous Sedation for Oral Surgery

Harry Papadopoulos

Anesthesia has always been and will be one of the cornerstones of oral and maxillofacial surgery. Indeed, our success in this area has revolutionized the field of outpatient surgery by providing a safe environment where both the surgical procedure and the anesthesia can be provided uniquely by the same person. Our success has been well documented by multiple studies demonstrating the relatively low incidence of morbidity and mortality associated with our anesthesia services. This has been due to a variety of reasons, including advances made in the field of anesthesia itself and in the management of medically compromised patients, in addition to the development of strict criteria for the evaluation of patients requesting anesthesia and, more importantly, the ability to distinguish between patients who can undergo office anesthesia safely and who should be treated in a hospital setting. Moreover, few specialties are as introspective and self-critical with respect to patient safety as we are as a result of our extensive training in residency, state society office evaluations, and continuing education. This chapter reviews some basic principles and includes some of the recent advances made in office anesthesia, including monitoring, anesthetic agents, and combinations of anesthetics, as well as common complications.

PREOPERATIVE EVALUATION

The goal of every office procedure is to administer anesthesia and perform surgery safely and successfully. Quite succinctly, this means avoiding or minimizing morbidity and mortality while providing adequate patient comfort. Achievement of this goal starts with the preoperative evaluation. The value of the preoperative evaluation cannot be overstated, with the history and physical examination being its centerpiece. The preoperative evaluation is done in a systematic manner so that no pertinent information is missed and all information needed for planning and administering anesthesia is obtained. In addition, risk factors are identified that may alter the perioperative management of the patient and possibly the type of anesthetic given, if any. Most offices will use a health history

BOX 30-1	Respiratory and Cardiac Symptoms

Respiratory Symptoms	Cardiac Symptoms
Chest pain	Chest pain
Cough	Cyanosis
Cyanosis	Dependent edema
Dyspnea	Dyspnea
Hemoptysis	Fatigue
Sputum production	Hemoptysis
Wheezing	Irregularities in heart rhythm
	Syncope

TABLE 30-1	Common Medical Problems Requiring Laboratory Evaluation

MEDICAL CONDITION	REQUIRED LABS
Type 1 and 2 diabetes	Serum glucose, hemoglobin A_{1c}, serum electrolytes
Liver disease, coagulopathic disorders	Platelets, INR, PT, PTT
Kidney disease	Serum electrolytes
Blood disorders (e.g., anemia)	CBC

CBC, complete blood count; INR, international normalized ratio; PT, prothrombin time; PTT, partial thromboplastin time.

TABLE 30-2	American Society of Anesthesiologists Physical Status Classification

ASA I	A normal healthy patient
ASA II	A patient with mild systemic disease
ASA III	A patient with severe systemic disease
ASA IV	A patient with severe systemic disease that is a constant threat to life
ASA V	A moribund patient who is not expected to survive with or without surgery
ASA VI	A patient declared brain-dead whose organs are being removed for donor purposes

questionnaire as an initial screening tool. The purpose of this questionnaire is to help identify abnormalities in the health history that may need further investigation, as well as focus, when the practitioner initiates the formal history and physical examination. The questionnaire should be reviewed by the practitioner in the patient's presence to allow clarification of any questions that may arise.

A thorough history will not only provide information about any medical problems but also allow the oral and maxillofacial surgeon to assess their severity. In addition, information on the patient's past surgical history is obtained, including any adverse reactions to anesthetic agents; complications during surgery such as excessive bleeding; medications that the patient is taking, including herbals and other over-the-counter medications; allergies; and social history, including tobacco and alcohol use; as well as a family history, including any adverse reactions to anesthetic agents by a relative. Finally, a review of systems with a focus on the cardiac and respiratory systems is done. Indeed, most perioperative morbidity and mortality emanate from these two systems. A positive response to any of the symptoms in Box 30-1 should alert the practitioner to the possibility of underlying disease, diagnosed or undiagnosed. In addition, all patients should be asked about their exercise tolerance because it has been shown to predict long-term mortality, as well as short-term perioperative risks. Although it is beyond the scope of this chapter to review the significance of these symptoms, the practitioner is urged to know this information.

The physical examination is usually guided by the medical history, and once again special focus should be placed on the cardiac and respiratory systems. The basic principles of inspection, palpation, percussion, and auscultation, are followed. Any abnormality found on examination in either of these systems should alert the practitioner to the need for further studies, such as an electrocardiogram (ECG), echocardiogram, chest radiograph, or pulmonary function tests. For most outpatient anesthesia patients, routine laboratory studies do not add any value to the preoperative assessment. However, in select patients, laboratory data may add valuable information when determining whether the patient is a safe risk to undergo the procedure (Table 30-1). Although chest radiography is a relatively low-cost, low-risk means of screening or evaluating for cardiac and pulmonary disease, its efficacy in routine preoperative screening has been questioned. The practice guidelines of the American College of Radiology state that chest radiographs are indicated for evaluation of the signs and symptoms of the cardiac, respiratory, upper gastrointestinal, and thoracic musculoskeletal systems; follow-up of thoracic disease; monitoring of life support devices; surveillance studies required by public health law (i.e., active tuberculosis, occupational exposure); and preoperative assessment of patients with cardiorespiratory disease that may increase perioperative morbidity or mortality.

Although oral and maxillofacial surgeons are adequately trained in assessing a patient's risk related to anesthesia, in some instances a medical consultation may also be required to further clarify the extent and severity of any underlying conditions and anesthesia risk. Much has been written about assessing the risk for perioperative morbidity and mortality. In 1977, Goldman and co-authors published a landmark article that identified certain factors associated with perioperative morbidity. The usefulness of the Goldman criteria was that each factor was assigned a certain number of points based on its relative contribution to cardiac risk, thus allowing risk to be quantified. Therefore, the more points accumulated by the patient, the higher the risk for perioperative morbidity. Since Goldman and colleagues' article, others have modified the criteria or devised their own system of risk stratification. Regardless of the system used, there are known risk factors—because of their association with increased perioperative morbidity—that should make the practitioner reconsider administering office anesthesia. Such risk factors include decompensated heart failure, recent myocardial infarction (<6 months), unstable angina, presence of significant arrhythmias, severe valvular disease, and renal insufficiency. Advanced age, usually older than 70 years, has been reported as a risk factor in the literature. However, there does not seem to be uniform consensus on which age should be considered advanced. The simplest and arguably the most common classification used for assessing risk is the American Society of Anesthesiologists (ASA) Physical Status Classification System (Table 30-2). Patients who are ASA I and II are good candidates for office anesthesia, whereas those considered ASA III and IV are better suited for a hospital setting.

Oral and maxillofacial surgeons know all too well the potential pitfalls that exist when the area that we work in, mainly the mouth, is not only the surgical site but also the entrance to the airway.

TABLE 30-3	Pre-anesthesia NPO (Eating and Drinking) Guidelines
Clear liquids	2 hours
Nonhuman milk	6 hours
Light solid meal*	6 hours

*Large, fatty meals prolong gastric emptying and may require an increase in NPO time. Medical conditions such as obesity, diabetes, pregnancy, hiatal hernia, and gastroesophageal reflux disease may also prolong gastric emptying.
NPO, nil per os.

Factors that will make establishing an airway difficult, including adequate ventilation or a potentially difficult intubation, need to be noted. Such factors include limited mouth opening, large tongue size, retrognathic mandible, thyromental distance of less than 6 cm, and limited cervical spine mobility. In addition, the Mallampati classification should be used to assess the airway. For this classification the patient sits upright with the head in a neutral position, mouth open as wide as possible, and the tongue extended to the maximum. The practitioner then tries to visualize the hard palate, soft palate, uvula, and tonsillar pillars. In class I patients the hard palate, soft palate, uvula, and tonsillar pillars are all visible. In class II patients the hard palate, soft palate, and uvula are visible. In class III patients the hard palate and soft palate are visible. Finally, in class IV patients only the hard palate is visible. Needless to say, a patient who is Mallampati class I is relatively easy to intubate, whereas Mallampati class IV poses a difficult intubation. The presence of any of the aforementioned limiting factors, as well as a Mallampati classification of III or IV, should make the practitioner consider the comfort of a hospital operating room rather than office anesthesia.

The remainder of the preoperative evaluation should consist of discussing the anesthetic options; surgical options; the risks, benefits, and complications associated with the anesthesia and surgery; requirements for when to cease intake of food and drink (Table 30-3); escort requirements; and furthering the doctor-patient bond. This may be reinforced by allowing the patient time to express concerns and ask additional questions. The American Association of Oral and Maxillofacial Surgeons (AAOMS) has established standards for evaluating patients preoperatively before administration of an anesthetic.

PERIOPERATIVE MANAGEMENT OF COMMON MEDICAL PROBLEMS

The majority of patients undergoing oral and maxillofacial surgery in the office setting have few risk factors, if any, and good functional status. In addition, the oral and maxillofacial surgeon can take some comfort from the fact that the surgery usually performed is of low or intermediate risk, thus further diminishing the overall risk for an adverse perioperative event. For patients with advanced disease, however, it is imperative for the oral and maxillofacial surgeon to be able to identify those who are not candidates for office anesthesia, which is achieved by adequate history taking and physical examination.

CARDIAC DISEASE

According to the American Heart Association, in 2005 the overall death rate from cardiovascular disease was 278.9 per 100,000 in the United States. Although death rates declined by 26.4% in the

preceding 10-year period, cardiovascular disease remains a significant problem for most developed nations, including the United States. Therefore, it is not uncommon for the oral and maxillofacial surgeon to encounter patients with cardiac disease who desire office anesthesia for their procedure. Concern is minimal for a patient with stable cardiac disease but not for one with a recent myocardial infarction, unstable angina, decompensated heart failure, severe valvular disease, uncontrolled hypertension, or arrhythmias. Given the fact that approximately 46 million Americans do not have health insurance, it will be more likely that the oral and maxillofacial surgeon will encounter patients with unstable disease. In the hospital setting the anesthesiologist plays the central role in preoperative assessment. In the office setting, that role belongs to the oral and maxillofacial surgeon.

Several studies have demonstrated an increased incidence of reinfarction within 6 months of a myocardial infarction. It is for this reason and the potential for the development of arrhythmias that a history of myocardial infarction within the last 6 months has generally been regarded as a reason to postpone elective surgery. Some have made the case for postponement of elective surgery within the first 6 weeks after a myocardial infarction and that the risk after this period is based on the clinical manifestations of the disease. Regardless of whether one chooses to follow the 6-week or 6-month mantra, it is important to make sure that the patient is being managed in such a way that the risk for morbidity and mortality is being minimized. Rather than risk stratification, some authors argue for risk modification, which includes having the patient take beta blockers and statins. However, the role of coronary revascularization specifically to reduce perioperative cardiac morbidity in noncardiac surgery is unproven.

Similarly, the same risk modification is undertaken in patients who have stable angina, and office anesthesia is avoided in patients with unstable angina. Stable angina is characterized by chest pain precipitated by physical exertion or emotional stress. It is predictable with regard to precipitating factors, frequency, intensity, duration, and relieving factors. Stable angina is successfully relieved by rest or nitroglycerin given in 0.4-mg tablets or by sublingual spray repeated every 5 minutes if there is no relief of pain (provided that systolic blood pressure is >90 mm Hg). Lack of relief after three doses may indicate infarction and should lead to immediate activation of emergency medical services. In addition, any change in any of the aforementioned factors represents unstable angina or preinfarction angina. Anyone suspected of having acute myocardial infarction should receive morphine, oxygen, and non-enteric aspirin (MONA), in addition to nitroglycerin.

A patient with decompensated congestive heart failure will be found to have any or all of the symptoms in Box 30-1 on physical examination: elevated jugular venous pressure on inspection, hepatomegaly on palpation and percussion, pitting edema in the extremities, and the presence of a third heart sound (S_3) and pulmonary crackles on auscultation. Patients with these signs and symptoms are not candidates for office anesthesia, let alone any elective surgery, and should be referred for cardiac evaluation to determine the cause of the decompensation and to optimize their condition.

When a patient interview elicits a history of valvular disease, the two main concerns are the extent of cardiac disease and the possible need for antibiotic prophylaxis. Fortunately, in the United States it is uncommon for valvular disease to go unrepaired well into adulthood. When there is a history of valve repair, the possible presence of residual cardiac disease needs to be investigated. A recent echocardiogram may be helpful because it provides information on valvular function and the ejection fraction if the patient has concurrent heart failure. In 2007, the American Heart Association revised the recommendations for antibiotic prophylaxis. Patients with the following cardiac conditions require antibiotic prophylaxis for oral surgical procedures:

- Prosthetic cardiac valves
- Previous infective endocarditis
- Unrepaired cyanotic congenital heart disease
- Completely repaired congenital heart disease with prosthetic material or a device during the first 6 months after the procedure
- Repaired congenital heart disease with residual defects
- Cardiac transplant recipients with cardiac valvular disease

Patients with a history of hypertension should be encouraged to not cease taking their antihypertensive medications and continue taking them until and including the day of surgery. According to a 2002 report of the American College of Cardiology/American Heart Association, surgery should be delayed for patients whose blood pressure is higher than 180/110 mm Hg because the likelihood of myocardial ischemia is increased. Clinical judgment is clearly exercised in evaluating the patient regardless of blood pressure. Patients whose blood pressure is well controlled are less likely to have labile readings during the procedure. Certainly, factors such as anxiety, the effects of epinephrine in local anesthetics, pain, and hypercapnia can increase blood pressure intraoperatively. When blood pressure is unacceptably elevated, beta blockers such as esmolol and labetalol should be considered. Esmolol is a selective beta-1 blocker with a rapid onset (60 seconds) and short duration (10 to 20 minutes). The dosage is 0.5 to 1.0 mg/kg intravenously administered over a 30-second period for immediate control of tachycardia and hypertension, followed by an infusion of 150 µg/kg/min to a maximum of 300 µg/kg/min. Labetalol is a selective alpha-1 blocker and nonselective beta blocker. Therefore, it is contraindicated in patients with asthma. It is administered in a loading dose of 5 to 20 mg intravenously over a 2-minute period, followed by a 20- to 80-mg dose at 10-minute intervals or an infusion of 1 to 2 mg/min. The onset of action of labetalol is 5 minutes and its duration of action is 3 to 6 hours. For patients in whom beta blockers are contraindicated (i.e., asthmatics), hydralazine should be considered. The dosage of hydralazine is 5 to 25 mg intravenously. It takes effect in 5 minutes and its duration of action is 2 hours.

Treatment of blood pressure intraoperatively needs to be tempered by the fact that some of these patients require relatively high pressure to perfuse vital organs. Consequently, lowering blood pressure excessively may produce the same unwanted effects as excessive blood pressure does, an ischemic event. Treatment of hypotension is directed at the underlying cause. Therefore, if the patient is hypovolemic, a fluid bolus is given. If the cause is hypoxemia or hypercapnia (or both), the airway is secured while making sure that the patient is adequately oxygenated and ventilated. Sympathomimetic agents used in the management of hypotensive emergencies include ephedrine and phenylephrine. Ephedrine is both an alpha and beta receptor agonist. The dosage is 2.5 to 5 mg intravenously, which can be repeated until the blood pressure stabilizes. Its onset of action is 10 minutes, with a peak in 20 minutes and duration of action of 4 hours. Phenylephrine is an alpha agonist administered in 0.1-mg increments until the blood pressure is stabilized. Its effects are seen within 2 to 3 minutes and last for approximately 15 minutes. Epinephrine is used for hypotension secondary to anaphylaxis, bronchospasm, or cardiac arrest.

Patients with disturbances in cardiac rhythm may or may not be symptomatic. Indeed, the surgery and anesthesia itself may unmask an underlying arrhythmia and even exacerbate it by release of catecholamines from stress and hypoxia as a result of inadequate ventilation and lead to a decrease in cardiac output and an ischemic event.

Arrhythmias may also be exaggerated by the epinephrine present in local anesthetics and by the use of inhalational anesthetics. All patients with serious arrhythmias should have a 12-lead ECG performed and a cardiology consultation before any elective surgery. The most common arrhythmia in the oral surgical office is bradycardia secondary to a vasovagal reaction. Vasovagal reactions are triggered by anxiety and characterized by an initial rapid increase in heart rate, decrease in systolic pressure, and increase in diastolic pressure, followed by a decrease in the pulse rate. Patients are managed by placement in a reclined position with the legs elevated, administration of 100% oxygen, monitoring of vital signs, and administration of spirits of ammonia if needed.

In summary, the goal for patients with a history of cardiac disease should be to provide adequate oxygenation, maintain sufficient intravascular volume and control of blood pressure, and minimize pain and anxiety via proper sedation techniques. In addition, cardiac medications should not be discontinued. If patients are regularly scheduled to take their cardiac medication the morning of the procedure, they should be encouraged to continue to take it with a small sip of water.

DIABETES

Diabetes is the most commonly encountered endocrine disorder. Patients with diabetes are best scheduled for morning procedures. Management depends on the patient's metabolic control, the length of the procedure, and the likelihood of the patient having oral intake after the procedure. Traditionally, patients with type 1 diabetes who were to undergo relatively short procedures with office anesthesia were managed by administering a third to two thirds of their usual intermediate-acting insulin in the morning and withholding their regular insulin. Once intravenous access was established, glucose was given intravenously and the patients were monitored for hypoglycemia and hyperglycemia. During surgery, regular insulin was given subcutaneously to treat hyperglycemia while keeping blood glucose between 120 and 200 mg/dL. Patients were also encouraged to begin oral intake soon after surgery, usually within 3 hours. If oral intake was going to be restricted, the morning intermediate-acting insulin dose was decreased accordingly. For patients who use continuous subcutaneous insulin infusion, the basal rate is continued during surgery, with insulin boluses given as needed for hyperglycemia. Patients with type 2 diabetes who are to undergo office anesthesia should have their oral hypoglycemic agents discontinued the morning of surgery and restarted when adequate oral intake resumes. Metformin is an exception; it is discontinued 48 hours before surgery to protect against metformin-induced lactic acidosis. Perioperative blood glucose levels may be controlled with subcutaneous administration of regular insulin via a sliding scale.

Another anesthetic concern in diabetics is gastroparesis. Delayed gastric emptying as a result of diabetic gastroparesis can increase the risk for aspiration pneumonitis. Other patients at increased risk include those with hiatal hernia, obesity, and gastroesophageal reflux. Administration of prophylactic medications for the prevention of lung injury from aspiration of gastric contents is controversial. Medications used to prevent aspiration pneumonitis include H_2-receptor antagonists (e.g., ranitidine), metoclopramide, and non-particulate oral antacids (e.g., sodium citrate). H_2-receptor antagonists are effective in decreasing gastric acid secretion and raising pH. However, they do not affect acid already present in the stomach. Metoclopramide, a dopamine antagonist, reduces gastric volume by increasing gastric emptying and increases lower esophageal tone. It also has anti-emetic properties, which makes it a very useful drug in this patient population. Finally, non-particulate oral antacids raise pH but increase gastric volume. Aspiration pneumonitis is a life-threatening complication. Management includes aggressive suctioning and administration of 100% oxygen. If there is no improvement, activation of emergency medical services, intubation, and ventilation with positive pressure will be required.

ASTHMA

Asthma is an inflammatory disorder of the airways that causes episodic attacks of wheezing, shortness of breath, chest tightness, and coughing. The hallmark of asthma is airway hyperreactivity in response to a variety of stimuli, including pollen, dust, pollutants, exercise, exposure to cold, and viral infections. This reversible airway obstruction is the result of bronchial smooth muscle constriction or bronchospasm, edema, and increased mucus secretion. The severity of asthma is classified according to symptom frequency, nighttime symptoms, and forced expiratory volume in the first second (FEV_1) or the peak expiratory flow (PEF) rate (percentage of predicted and variability). In addition, valuable information regarding severity can be obtained by questioning the patient about the frequency of inhaler use; hospitalizations, including use of steroids and intubation; and visits to the emergency department. Assessment of severity will help determine whether the patient is a viable office anesthesia candidate. Suffice it to say, patients with intermittent (symptoms occurring less than once a week, brief exacerbations, nocturnal symptoms twice per month, FEV_1 or PEF 80% of predicted, PEF or FEV_1 variability less than 20%) and mild persistent (symptoms occurring more than once per week but less than once per day, exacerbations affecting activity and sleep, nocturnal symptoms more than twice per month, FEV_1 or PEF 80% of predicted, PEF or FEV_1 variability 20% to 30%) asthma are generally good candidates. Moderate persistent (symptoms occurring daily, exacerbations affecting activity and sleep, nocturnal symptoms more than once per week, daily use of an inhaled short-acting beta-2 agonist, FEV_1 or PEF 60% to 80% of predicted, PEF or FEV_1 variability greater than 30%) and severe persistent (symptoms occurring daily, frequent exacerbations, frequent nocturnal symptoms, limitations in physical activities, FEV_1 or PEF less than 60% of predicted, PEF or FEV_1 variability greater than 30%) are not good candidates.

All patients should have their lungs auscultated before the procedure. Audible wheezing should be treated with a beta-2 agonist by inhaler before proceeding with the planned procedure. Bronchospasm may occur intraoperatively. If the patient is awake, bronchospasm is managed by administering inhaled beta-2 agonist drugs as first-line treatment. If the patient is unable to cooperate, subcutaneous administration of 0.3 to 0.5 mg of a 1:1000 solution of epinephrine is the first choice. In both cases supplemental oxygen is given as well.

Children with a recent or current upper respiratory tract infection are susceptible to bronchospasm. A viral infection within 2 to 4 weeks places the child at an increased risk for perioperative pulmonary complications (laryngospasm, atelectasis, and hypoxemia). Therefore, elective surgery should be deferred until 3 weeks after the symptoms (runny nose with fever, cough, or sore throat) have resolved.

Laryngospasm is an involuntary spasm of the laryngeal musculature caused by sensory stimulation from pharyngeal secretions (i.e., blood, saliva) or foreign material. It usually occurs in patients who are in light planes of anesthesia or during extubation. Although it can occur in awake patients, this is less likely because these patients have the ability to clear secretions by coughing or swallowing. In partial laryngospasm a crowing sound is heard, and in complete laryngospasm no sound is heard. When laryngospasm is recognized, the oropharynx is suctioned and the patient is given gentle positive pressure ventilation with 100% oxygen by mask. If the partial laryngospasm persists and hypoxia develops, succinylcholine, 10 to 20 mg intravenously, is administered. Larger doses (20 to 40 mg) may be required for complete laryngospasm. In children who do not have intravenous access, succinylcholine, 4 mg/kg administered intramuscularly via a submental transcutaneous injection, will treat the laryngospasm.

RENAL INSUFFICIENCY

Patients with chronic renal insufficiency are at increased risk for perioperative morbidity and mortality. Electrolyte imbalances are a significant concern in these patients, in particular hyperkalemia. Consequently, patients with end-stage renal disease are encouraged to undergo dialysis the day before surgery. The oral and maxillofacial surgeon should request a set of blood electrolyte levels before the procedure. Fluid retention will necessitate judicious use of intravenous fluids. Intravenous access should be obtained in the extremity that does not have the shunt used for hemodialysis to avoid damage to it. Other considerations in these patients include anemia, platelet dysfunction secondary to uremia, and concomitant hypertension. In addition, certain drugs need to be avoided (penicillin, cephalosporins, nonsteroidal anti-inflammatory drugs), whereas others need to have their dosages decreased.

OBESITY

Obesity alone does not increase morbidity and mortality, but when it is severe, considerable morbidity and mortality can occur. The body mass index (BMI) is the ratio of body weight in kilograms to height in meters squared. This measurement is used by clinicians to define obesity from a quantitative standpoint. Therefore, a BMI lower than 25 kg/m^2 is considered normal. A BMI of 25 to 30 is overweight, and greater than 30 is obese. The excessive weight leads to restrictive effects on the thorax and diaphragm that decrease functional residual capacity and total lung capacity. As a result, obese patients are at risk for pulmonary complications such as atelectasis, bronchospasm, and pneumonia in the perioperative period. Further complicating matters, many may suffer from cardiovascular disease and obstructive sleep apnea (OSA). OSA is important as far as airway management and possible co-morbid conditions are concerned (systemic and pulmonary hypertension, polycythemia, arrhythmias, cor pulmonale). Therefore, short procedures with light sedation are encouraged, and deep sedation should be avoided in the office anesthesia setting. Consideration should also be given to performing procedures in a hospital setting for the morbidly obese.

CIGARETTE SMOKING

Cigarette smoking has multiple adverse effects on anesthesia. The carbon monoxide produced by smoking has 200 times greater affinity than oxygen for hemoglobin. This means that less oxygen will be carried by hemoglobin. As a result of this leftward shift in the oxygen dissociation curve, less oxygen will be delivered to peripheral tissues. In addition, carboxyhemoglobin is not detected by pulse oximetry, thereby producing a falsely high oxygen saturation reading. Nicotine, likewise present in cigarettes, is a potent vasoconstrictor and increases the heart rate, blood pressure, and peripheral vascular resistance. Smoking also impairs mucociliary clearance and promotes excessive mucus production, which increases the risk for postoperative pulmonary complications such as atelectasis, bronchospasm, and pneumonia. Cessation of smoking 24 hours before surgery decreases the likelihood of pulmonary complications and cardiac complications secondary to nicotine and carbon monoxide. From a surgical standpoint, deleterious effects of smoking on wound healing have been documented.

PREGNANCY

Mandatory pregnancy testing of all females of reproductive age is controversial. Concern arose from the teratogenic effects of certain drugs such as nitrous oxide and benzodiazepines in animal studies. Although these teratogenic effects are probably minimal in humans, pregnancy and lactation are relative contraindications to elective oral and maxillofacial surgery. When surgery cannot be deferred, consultation with the patient's obstetrician should be obtained and office surgery done under local anesthesia. Drugs used for office anesthesia will readily pass into breast milk and thus potentially harm the infant. However, there is less concern for drugs with a short half-life such as fentanyl, which pose minimal risk to the infant.

MONITORING

Monitoring is a necessity that provides many benefits. Not only does it give insight into how the patient is handling the procedure and anesthesia, but it also allows detection of emergencies that require an immediate response and it reveals trends that may indicate that a untoward event is going to occur, thereby allowing the practitioner time to prevent or treat the event. Finally, it allows us to evaluate the efficacy of the emergency treatment being rendered. Monitoring may be divided into two components: cardiac/circulation and respiratory.

Cardiac monitoring includes measurement of blood pressure and heart rate, as well as evaluation of rhythm. Heart rate and rhythm can be determined by palpation of a peripheral pulse or with a precordial stethoscope, a pulse oximeter, or an ECG. The precordial stethoscope is an excellent, noninvasive simple device that can provide important information on heart rate and rhythm, as well as respiration. The ECG is used to monitor heart rate and rhythm and detect acute ischemia. The most common ECG lead used in office anesthesia is lead II, which allows excellent monitoring for arrhythmias. Review of the management of the various arrhythmias is beyond the scope of this chapter; however, the practitioner must be current with advanced cardiac life support techniques. In the office setting, automated blood pressure devices are easy to use and accurate, but the cuff still needs to be positioned properly and the size needs to be appropriate for the patient's arm.

Respiratory monitoring can be further divided into ventilation and oxygenation. Monitoring of ventilation, more specifically the respiratory pattern, depth, and rate, can be accomplished with the precordial stethoscope, as well as by visual observation of chest excursion and movement of the reservoir bag on the gas machine. Oxygenation is monitored mainly by pulse oximetry, although observation of the color of mucous membranes and skin can still provide useful information.

The AAOMS has established guidelines for monitoring patients under sedation. For conscious sedation, the guidelines are:
1. Continuous monitoring of oxygen saturation by pulse oximetry
2. Measurement of heart rate and blood pressure at regular intervals
For deep sedation or general anesthesia, the guidelines are:
1. Continuous monitoring of ventilation and oxygenation with pulse oximetry and auscultation of breath sounds, along with at least one additional method of ventilator monitoring such as chest wall movement, observation of the reservoir bag, monitoring of patient color, or capnometry/capnography
2. Measurement of the heart rate and blood pressure at least every 5 minutes during anesthesia and at least every 10 minutes during the recovery period
3. Continuous monitoring of the ECG
4. Auscultation of heart sounds or palpation of a peripheral pulse
   Monitoring of patients under anesthesia continues to evolve. In recent years, consideration has been given to the addition of such modalities as capnography, capnometry, and bispectral analysis. By monitoring end-tidal CO_2 levels, capnography may allow earlier recognition of hypoxic events, before they becomes evident with the pulse oximeter. Although no one can dispute the benefits of pulse oximetry and indeed its usefulness has been documented in studies, it does have limitations. The relationship of PaO_2 and SaO_2 is defined by the oxygen-hemoglobin dissociation curve, but declining PaO_2 values may initially be undetected and not be reflected by changes in SaO_2. Therefore, adding capnography as an additional modality for monitoring ventilation may allow earlier detection of hypoventilation. Unfortunately, adequate studies documenting the absolute necessity for capnography in a non-intubated anesthesia patient have not been conducted. Limitations such as the accuracy of readings in an "open system" (e.g., in a non-intubated anesthesia patient) and cost have not made capnography part of the standard of care yet. To partially overcome the open-system problem, end-tidal CO_2 readings have been obtained from a nasal cannula, with one of the nasal prongs being used to administer oxygen and the other to read the end-tidal CO_2. However, as improvements in technology are made and costs are reduced, one can anticipate that capnography will become part of the everyday arsenal of office anesthesia. A capnometer provides a digital quantitative readout of the CO_2 concentration at a single point in time. Unlike capnography, which displays a continuous waveform of CO_2, capnometry provides individual measurements of inspired and end-tidal CO_2 concentrations. Like capnography, its popularity is increasing.

Monitoring the patient's level of consciousness allows the practitioner to measure the hypnotic effect of the anesthetic, thereby theoretically allowing more precise administration of the anesthetic and improved patient care. The bispectral index (BSI) is the most widely used level-of-consciousness monitor. It uses electroencephalography (EEG), a waveform that is a complex physiologic signal representing the sum of all brain activity produced by the cerebral cortex. Three electrodes are attached to the patient's forehead and connected to the BSI monitor. The EEG is recorded as a single number from 0 (no brain activity) to 100 (fully awake and cooperative) that represents the patient's level of consciousness. Usually, a BSI level of 70 to 80 is adequate for a proper level of sedation to produce little to no recall of surgical events. However, it should be noted that the BIS cannot be used to monitor the level of analgesia. Therefore, a patient who reacts to a painful stimulus but is in a normal range of sedation according to the BSI monitor probably needs more local anesthetic rather than sedative drugs. Thus, one of the biggest benefits of BSI has been a reduction in excessive or inadequate anesthetic effect, which has resulted in an overall decrease in the use of anesthetic agents and earlier recovery. However, BSI is not without disadvantages, including cost, artifacts, unpredictable data with various agents (nitrous oxide, ketamine), and uncertainty in terms of accuracy and reliability in patients with abnormal brain structure or central nervous system (CNS) disease.

It is important to note that monitoring alone cannot completely eliminate anesthetic complications. The oral and maxillofacial surgeon must be familiar with what is standard of care, as well as have knowledge of the adjunctive modalities available. However, these are no substitutes for good clinical skills and judgment since the goal is to ultimately improve patient care and minimize the frequency of adverse events.

DRUGS USED IN OFFICE-BASED DEEP SEDATION/GENERAL ANESTHESIA

From a pharmacologic perspective, delivery of intravenous deep sedation and general anesthesia has always been an evolving art form. Most oral surgeons use a combination of drugs in their office anesthesia regimens; however, it is important to realize that most of these drug combinations were developed over time. A look at the drugs most commonly used in oral surgery offices today illustrates this point. Meperidine (Demerol) was synthesized in 1939. Methohexital (Brevital) was introduced into clinical practice in 1957, with diazepam (Valium) following shortly thereafter in 1960. Fentanyl (Sublimaze) was introduced for clinical use in 1967, and midazolam (Versed) became part of oral surgery practice in the late 1970s. Propofol (Diprivan) was introduced into the United States in 1989. The newest opioid to be used in oral surgery practice, remifentanil (Ultiva), was developed in the late 1990s and is essentially a drug of the 21st century in terms of office-based oral surgery anesthesia practice.

Although the basic clinical effects of the drugs just cited were commonly known by practitioners when they began using them, thorough understanding of the drug's clinical effects lagged behind. For example, a model to explain how methohexital was distributed to various body compartments and how this distribution related to the clinical effects of the drug was published by Gillis and colleagues in 1976, 19 years after its introduction. The greater potency of midazolam than diazepam was not fully appreciated until well after midazolam was introduced into practice. Additionally, our understanding of the pharmacodynamics of anesthetic drugs grew with the advances in neuroscience and molecular biology that began to accelerate in the mid-1980s. Simply put, our understanding of which drugs to use for office-based deep sedation and general anesthesia has always been more developed than our knowledge of *how* to use the drugs.

To many, this act of practicing in the midst of evolving knowledge defines the art of anesthesia. Today, that art is less intuitive and much more scientific thanks to our deeper understanding of how anesthetic drugs work. Using history as our guide, this section reviews the evolution of anesthetic drugs commonly used for contemporary oral surgery office anesthesia, with notation of developments in clinical science that have occurred since their introduction into practice.

MEPERIDINE AND FENTANYL

The anesthetic properties of the early opioid meperidine were discovered indirectly, during an effort to develop an analogue of atropine. Like atropine, meperidine is associated with the production of dry mouth, increased heart rate, and other anticholinergic effects. The antisialagogue properties of this drug, along with its analgesic properties and short alpha half-life, made it well suited for oral surgery practice. Meperidine was initially combined with barbiturates as part of a balanced anesthetic technique in a number of medical and dental applications. This combination made sense from a pharmacologic standpoint since barbiturates have no appreciable intrinsic analgesia and increase the risk for laryngospasm when used as a sole agent. These shortcomings were overcome by the concurrent opiate action of meperidine in reducing airway reactivity. Barbiturate-opioid combinations were also used for mild to moderate degrees of sedation. An example of such a pairing is the Jorgenson technique, which combined meperidine, pentobarbital, and scopolamine. Side effects of meperidine include release of histamine and the production of a toxic, proconvulsant metabolite, normeperidine. These side effects limit the total dose of meperidine in an anesthetic technique and have an impact on the way that the drug is delivered.

The next phenylpiperidine opioid to be developed, fentanyl, provided better analgesia, fewer cardiovascular side effects, and a wider therapeutic index than noted with meperidine. In addition, fentanyl does not cause the release of histamine, does not produce active metabolites, and is estimated to be 100 to 300 times more potent than morphine (in contrast, meperidine is less potent than morphine). When compared with meperidine, fentanyl is more likely to cause respiratory depression, particularly when administered in combination with benzodiazepines or barbiturates. Careful titration of the drugs minimizes the incidence of clinically significant respiratory depression during deep sedation and general anesthesia. The use of fentanyl continues to the present day, largely because of its combination of high efficacy and low cost. Used by itself, fentanyl does not produce amnesia. It is nearly always used in combination with barbiturates, benzodiazepines, or other sedative and hypnotic agents.

Fentanyl is characterized by rapid distribution to the CNS, within 1 to 2 minutes of administration, with serum concentrations paralleling CNS concentrations after accounting for a 5-minute time lag between CNS and plasma concentrations. This time lag (termed *hysteresis*) is the basis for the recommendation to allow 3 to 5 minutes to pass between the intravenous administration of fentanyl and the beginning of oral surgical procedures. Co-administration of local anesthetic is associated with a similar time lag between intraoral injection and complete pulpal anesthesia, especially when operating on the mandible. This fact is easily overlooked in busy oral surgery practices, where surgery is begun almost immediately after the onset of sedation and administration of local anesthetic; unnecessary patient movement, discomfort, and the tendency to administer higher amounts of drug than needed during induction can occur when the time lag is not taken into account.

METHOHEXITAL

Methohexital is an ultrashort-acting barbiturate. Like other barbiturates, methohexital produces its anesthetic effects by binding to γ-aminobutyric acid A (GABA_A) receptors throughout the CNS. GABA is the major inhibitory neurotransmitter in the mammalian brain. The affinity of barbiturates to bind to GABA_A receptors correlates closely with their anesthetic potency. When first introduced into practice, methohexital was welcomed for its ability to produce rapid and profound unconsciousness while avoiding the prolonged postoperative recovery time associated with other intravenous barbiturates of that era, such as thiopental. The drug remains in use today despite the introduction of newer hypnotic agents with superior properties.

The distinguishing properties of methohexital are due to a specific structure-activity relationship: placement of a methyl group on the N3 nitrogen of the oxybarbiturate molecule. Barbiturates that include this structural characteristic also demonstrate proconvulsant activity and have been associated with the induction of seizures at high doses and in patients with undiagnosed epilepsy. The high pH of the drug solution renders aqueous solutions bacteriostatic. Aqueous methohexital solutions are stable for several days. The high alkalinity of methohexital solutions is associated with pain on intravenous injection, which occurs in approximately 5% of patients during induction. When using methohexital, practitioners are advised to use a large vein for intravenous cannulation to avoid burning. Other characteristics associated with methohexital include profound shivering during recovery and increased risk for laryngospasm during light anesthesia and surgical techniques with an open airway.

DIAZEPAM AND MIDAZOLAM

The popularity of these drugs, as well as other benzodiazepines, stems from the wide spectrum of desirable anesthetic effects that they produce and their dose-sparing effects when used in combination with other anesthetic drugs. Most benzodiazepines produce some degree of anterograde amnesia, anxiolysis, anticonvulsant action, sedation, and muscle relaxation. Individual benzodiazepines differ in their chemical properties, pharmacokinetic characteristics, and the degree to which they produce the characteristics just described. When compared with barbiturates, benzodiazepines produce superior anxiolysis and muscle relaxation at subhypnotic doses. This property allowed oral and maxillofacial surgeons to induce more effective and consistent minimal and moderate sedation (commonly termed "conscious sedation" before 2007). When used as a single agent, these drugs rarely cause cardiovascular or ventilatory depression; however, the use of benzodiazepines with other drugs, particularly opioids, can produce considerable respiratory depression. Overall, the therapeutic index of benzodiazepines is larger, thus making these drugs more "forgiving" than barbiturates.

Diazepam remains popular for its excellent anxiolytic properties and relative lack of mental impairment in comparison to midazolam. Concerns about the use of diazepam are often related to its irritating intravenous formulation, active metabolites, and long half-life. The lack of water solubility requires diazepam to be dissolved in organic solvents, thus precluding intramuscular injection and making the possibility of phlebitis a substantial concern during intravenous administration. After undergoing hepatic biotransformation, diazepam is converted to an active metabolite, desmethyldiazepam. Even though prolonged sedation is usually more likely in patients with chronic administration, recovery times after dental office sedation with midazolam are typically slow. In healthy volunteers, the beta half-life of diazepam is 21 to 37 hours.

Midazolam provides the same spectrum of effects as diazepam with two to three times the potency and a much shorter beta half-life (1.5 to 4 hours). It is a water-soluble, non-irritating solution that can be used for intramuscular injection, as well as for intravenous administration. The onset of effect after intramuscular injection occurs within 5 to 10 minutes, with a peak effect seen at 30 to 60 minutes. Midazolam is currently the most widely used benzodiazepine for parenteral sedation in medicine and dentistry today. Although it can be used alone or in combination, midazolam is most commonly combined with fentanyl or another opioid for the induction of moderate parenteral sedation.

PROPOFOL

Soon after its introduction into clinical practice in the late 1980s, propofol rapidly became the drug of choice for ambulatory surgery and office-based anesthesia. When compared with methohexital, propofol offers a comparable onset of action, excellent titratability, and more rapid and pleasant recovery. In addition, propofol also displays antiemetic properties, and the occurrence of postoperative nausea and vomiting (PONV), unrelated to the ingestion of blood from oral surgical wounds, is rare. The use of propofol is often reported to produce positive subjective experiences in patients ranging from euphoria to a sense of well-being. When compared with barbiturates, propofol is associated with fewer incidents of coughing, breath holding, and postoperative shivering. As with methohexital, variable degrees of hypotension and respiratory depression are seen with propofol, depending on the dose and rate of administration. Although the degree of hypotension is dependent on other drugs used and the physical status of the patient, deep sedation/general anesthesia is often associated with an approximately 20% drop in systolic blood pressure. Unlike methohexital, propofol must be used within 4 to 6 hours of being opened because of its ability to support bacterial growth. Although propofol produces pain on injection, particularly in small vessels, it is not typically associated with phlebitis or thrombosis.

REMIFENTANIL

The unique pharmacokinetic and pharmacodynamic properties of remifentanil make it arguably the best opioid available for balanced intravenous anesthesia in the oral surgery office. Though only slightly less potent than fentanyl, its latency (i.e., time between intravenous administration to peak effect) is only 1 to 2 minutes as opposed to the 4 to 6 minutes to peak effect noted after fentanyl administration. This clinically insignificant hysteresis provides the oral surgeon with the ability to begin local anesthetic administration faster, with less tendency to overdose. Offset is also rapid, with a context-sensitive half-time of 3 to 5 minutes, regardless of the length of the procedure. This is primarily due to the extrahepatic metabolism of remifentanil by non-specific plasma esterases to inactive metabolites. The time required for its concentration in blood to decrease by 80% is less than 15 minutes. When used in combination with propofol, many practitioners find that their patients wake up faster and are fit for discharge significantly sooner than with techniques using fentanyl and methohexital. The rapid offset of remifentanil's action also applies to its analgesic effects, and patients may experience postoperative pain very soon after recovery if local anesthesia has begun to wane. Augmentation of local anesthesia at the end of the procedure or administration of ketorolac (or both), as indicated, is a good strategy for circumventing this problem.

INTERMITTENT BOLUS VERSUS SYRINGE PUMP

Although short oral surgical procedures can often be conducted with an intermittent bolus anesthetic technique, the full utility of modern anesthetic drugs such as propofol and remifentanil cannot be appreciated without the use of a syringe infusion pump. Infusion pumps are to intravenous anesthesia what vaporizers are to anesthesia with inhaled agents. Propofol, midazolam, and remifentanil all display close correlation between serum drug levels and parallel drug concentrations at the site of drug action in the brain. This property, together with the short alpha half-life, allows the anesthesia provider to effectively adjust the level of anesthesia to the degree of intraoperative surgical stimulation. On converting from an intermittent bolus technique to an infusion pump technique, operators are often pleased by the consistency of the intraoperative anesthetic level and the lack of "peaks and troughs" characteristic of many intermediate bolus techniques. In fact, the use of potent, ultrashort-acting anesthetic drugs such as remifentanil without an infusion pump may lead to inconsistent depths of anesthesia, such as occurs with intermittent bolus techniques using older drugs that have less desirable pharmacokinetic properties.

DEFINITIONS

Volume of distribution (V_D): This theoretic "volume" is derived by dividing the dose of a drug administered to a patient by the concentration of that drug found in plasma at a given time.

$$\text{Volume of distribution} = \frac{\text{Dose of drug administered to the patient}}{\text{Concentration measured in plasma}}$$

A common source of confusion is to think of V_D as an actual volume (e.g., the volume in plasma or cerebrospinal fluid). This theoretic construct is simply a numerical index used to describe the extent of distribution of a drug into body tissue.

Clearance: Clearance is a theoretic "rate" expressed in units of volume per time that describes the ability of the body to remove a particular drug.

$$\text{Clearance} = \frac{\text{Rate of drug removal}}{\text{Concentration of drug in plasma}}$$

It is analogous to creatinine clearance, which describes the ability of the kidneys to remove creatinine.

It is important to note that clearance describes the intrinsic ability of the body to remove a drug from the body, not the actual rate of drug removal at any one time.

Half-life: Half-life is the time required for the concentration of a drug to fall to half its original value. This can be applied to either a compartment or the entire body. Applied to clinical anesthesia, the term *alpha half-life*, or *distribution half-life*, describes the time required for the concentration of the drug at the effect site (i.e., the brain) to fall by 50% as a result of redistribution to other tissues. The *elimination half-life* describes the time required for the total body concentration of a drug to be reduced by 50% as a result of elimination. Alpha half-life is often used to estimate how long a drug's primary anesthetic effect will be observed. The elimination half-life is used to estimate recovery and elimination. For example, the alpha half-life of diazepam is 3 to 10 minutes, whereas its elimination half-life is 20 to 30 hours.

Context-sensitive half-time: This term describes the time required for the concentration of a drug to fall by 50% after termination of a drug infusion of *a given length of time*. For most drugs, the context-sensitive half-time increases with the length of drug infusion. This reflects the effect of distribution of the drug to other tissues, the rate of biotransformation, the rate of elimination, and other factors. Context-sensitive half-times are valuable for estimation of the length of recovery and duration of residual effects in the postoperative period.

RECOVERY AND DISCHARGE

Ideally, the patient is fully alert and awake with return of vital signs to baseline at the conclusion of surgery. However, we all know too well that such is rarely the case and that each patient responds differently to anesthesia; therefore, all patients require postoperative monitoring. The length of the postoperative stay is influenced by not only the sedative drugs administered but also the type of surgery and any adverse events such as excessive pain, PONV, drowsiness, and any unexpected cardiorespiratory events. The recovery period is the period between the time when surgery has ended and there is no more administration of anesthetic and the time when the patient is ready for discharge. During the recovery period the patient is still being monitored. In fact, patients should be monitored until they are deemed ready for discharge. Supplemental oxygen is usually discontinued to see whether the patient can maintain oxygen saturation on room air. Discharge of the patient becomes the sole responsibility of the oral and maxillofacial surgeon, not the office staff. Various quantitative scoring systems have been developed to provide objective criteria for discharge. Although these systems may be useful, there is no substitute for a thorough clinical examination by the treating practitioner. Written as well as verbal postoperative instructions should be given not only to the patient but also to the patient's companion.

The greatest concerns of patients in the immediate postoperative period are pain control and PONV. Adequate dosing of an analgesic, usually opioids during the procedure, should assist in pain management and facilitate timely discharge with comfort. Patients may then begin their prescribed oral pain medications at home as needed. Infrequently, patients will have intolerable pain postoperatively, which will require attention. If the patient is awake and able to

BOX 30-2	**Causes of Postoperative Nausea and Vomiting (PONV)**

Medications (opioids, nitrous oxide, ketamine)
Pain
Early postoperative oral intake
Hypotension
Dehydration
Swallowing of blood

tolerate oral medications, an oral narcotic may be given, but oral medications may take time to work. Giving a small dose of fentanyl intravenously, 25 to 50 µg, can be effective in ameliorating postoperative pain. However, because of the respiratory effects of fentanyl and the need to monitor its effects, discharge will be delayed. Intravenous ketorolac does not have the sedative effects of opioids and provides excellent postoperative analgesia at doses of 15 to 30 mg, but some surgeons are concerned with its increased risk for increased bleeding or oozing. Ketorolac should be avoided in patients with a history of gastrointestinal ulcers or those whose kidney function is compromised. Finally, nalbuphine, a mixed agonist/antagonist opioid, has a good analgesic profile and less negative effects on respiration than fentanyl does. However, as with any intravenous drug, it does require a period (at least 30 minutes) of monitoring, which may possibly delay discharge.

PONV may be due to one factor or several factors (Box 30-2). Since PONV can contribute to delayed discharge, it may be prudent to identify patients who are at risk for it during the preoperative evaluation. Apfel and associates identified females, non-smokers, history of PONV, and the use of opioids as risk factors for PONV. Although not all patients will require prophylaxis for PONV, it should be considered in high-risk patients. Administering a single dose of dexamethasone, 8 mg intravenously at the beginning of a procedure, has been shown to be effective in preventing PONV. Serotonin 5-HT$_3$ antagonists have also been very useful in prevention of PONV. Ondansetron, 4 mg administered intravenously at the end of the procedure, seems most effective. The advantage of this class of medications has been avoidance of the side effects seen with traditional antiemetics such as prochlorperazine (extrapyramidal symptoms) or promethazine (drowsiness, dry mouth). Finally, propofol administered during the procedure has also been shown to reduce the incidence of PONV.

In recent years, OSA has received increased attention. Patients with OSA have an increased risk for adverse respiratory events perioperatively, especially if given with intravenous opioids. Many of these patients use continuous positive pressure airway devices at night and should be encouraged to bring them to the office, as well as use them postoperatively. The larger problem concerns patients with undiagnosed OSA. Indeed, the majority of them do not have the classic pickwickian appearance of obese males with short thick necks. Patients should be questioned regarding a history of loud snoring, excessive daytime sleepiness, morning headaches, nausea, depression, intellectual deterioration, and changes in personality. Patients suspected of having OSA should be encouraged to pursue evaluation and management because its long-term effects on health are well known (systemic and pulmonary hypertension, arrhythmias, polycythemia, cor pulmonale, and death). These patients should undergo brief procedures with conscious sedation. For longer procedures or those that require deeper sedation, a hospital setting should be considered.

PEARLS AND PITFALLS

- The purpose of the preoperative evaluation is to identify and modify factors that may lead to perioperative morbidity and mortality.
- Exercise tolerance is a good predictor of perioperative morbidity and mortality.
- Elective surgery should be deferred until 3 weeks after the resolution of symptoms in children with upper respiratory tract infections.
- Declining changes in arterial oxygenation may initially be undetected and not reflected by changes in pulse oximetry; therefore, the addition of capnography may allow earlier recognition of a hypoxic event.

- Knowledge of the advantages and disadvantages of the drugs available for anesthesia is absolutely necessary to allow the practitioner to use an effective balanced anesthesia technique safely in the office setting.
- Use of propofol during a procedure reduces the incidence of PONV.
- Patients with OSA may undergo short procedures and conscious sedation in the office setting; conversely, patients requiring long procedures or deep sedation should be treated in the hospital setting.

BIBLIOGRAPHY

American Association of Oral and Maxillofacial Surgeons: *Office anesthesia evaluation manual*, ed 7, Rosemont, Ill., 2006.

Bertin PM: Monitoring. In: Crowley KE, Sandler NA, editors: *Oral and maxillofacial surgery knowledge update*, vol 4, Rosemont, Ill., 2006, pp 21-29.

Goldman L, Caldera DL, Nussbaum SR, et al: Multifactorial index of cardiac risk in noncardiac surgical procedures, *N Engl J Med* 297:845-850, 1977.

Lee TH, Marcantonio ER, Mangione CM, et al: Derivation and prospective validation of a simple index for prediction of cardiac risk of major noncardiac surgery, *Circulation* 100:1043-1049, 1999.

Maddox TM: Preoperative cardiovascular evaluation for noncardiac surgery, *Mt Sinai J Med* 72:185-192, 2005.

Sarasin DS: Ambulatory anesthetic management of the patient with diabetes, *Oral Maxillofac Surg Clin North Am* 11:589-599, 1999.

Vezeau PJ: Anesthetic agent update. In: Fridrich KL, Burton RG, editors: *Oral and maxillofacial surgery knowledge update*, vol 3, Rosemont, Ill., 2001, pp 5-28.

Wilson W, Taubert KA, Gewitz M, et al: Prevention of infective endocarditis: guidelines from the American Heart Association: a guideline from the American Heart Association Rheumatic Fever, Endocarditis and Kawasaki Disease Committee, Council on Cardiovascular Disease in the Young, and the Council on Clinical Cardiology, Council on Cardiovascular Surgery and Anesthesia, and the Quality of Care and Outcomes Research Interdisciplinary Working Group, *Circulation* 116:1736-1754, 2007.

Yawn BP: Factors accounting for asthma variability: achieving optimal symptom control for individual patients, *Prim Care Respir J* 17:138-147, 2008.

Chapter 31

Nonsurgical Management of Facial Pain

Steven J. Scrivani, David A. Keith, Jennifer P. Bassiur, James A. Kraus, Noshir R. Mehta

Facial pain syndromes are common in clinical practice. Many of these syndromes are also unique, given the complex anatomy and specialized sensory innervation of the head, face, and neck, and thus can pose diagnostic challenges.

The common descriptive terms for craniofacial pain complaints are frequently misleading. To avoid confusion, clinicians should be familiar with the Diagnostic Classification for Head, Face, and Neck Pain Disorders of the International Headache Society (IHS), the "International Classification of Headache Disorders II" (Boxes 31-1 to 31-3).[1] Clinicians need to be able to distinguish among painful conditions that arise as a result of structural pathology of the oral and facial structures, temporomandibular joint (TMJ) disorders, myofascial pain disorders (MPDs), headache syndromes, and primary cranial neuralgias.

DIAGNOSTIC EVALUATION

Pain in the mouth or face is one of the most common symptoms seen in clinical practice. The majority of symptoms are related to dental disease, and in most cases the cause can readily be established, the problem dealt with expeditiously, and the pain eliminated. However, in a few patients, pain may be persistent and defy

---

BOX 31-1	International Classification of Headache Disorders II

14 Categories
- Primary headaches: 1-4
- Secondary headaches: 5-12
- Cranial neuralgias, central and primary facial pain, and other headache disorders: 13-14

From Headache Classification Subcommittee of the International Headache Society: The International Classification of Headache Disorders: 2nd edition, *Cephalalgia* 24(Suppl 1):9-160, 2004.

BOX 31-2	Headache or Facial Pain Attributed to Disorders of the Cranium, Neck, Eyes, Ears, Nose, Sinuses, Teeth, Mouth, or Other Facial or Cranial Structures (11.1-11.8)

11.1—Cranial bones
11.2—Neck
11.3—Eyes
11.4—Ears
11.5—Rhinosinusitis (sinus disorders)
11.6—Teeth, jaws, or related structures
11.7—TMJ disorders (TMD)
11.8—Other

TMD, temporomandibular disorder; TMJ, temporomandibular joint.
From Headache Classification Subcommittee of the International Headache Society: The International Classification of Headache Disorders: 2nd edition, *Cephalalgia* 24(Suppl 1):9-160, 2004.

BOX 31-3	Cranial Neuralgias, Central and Primary Facial Pain, and Other Headaches (13.1-13.19)

13.1—Trigeminal neuralgia
13.2—Glossopharyngeal neuralgia
13.8—Occipital neuralgia
13.12—Constant pain caused by compression, irritation, or distortion of cranial nerves or upper cervical roots by **structural lesions**
13.15—Head or facial pain attributed to herpes zoster
    Post-herpetic neuralgia
13.18—Central causes of facial pain
    Anesthesia dolorosa
    Central post-stroke pain
        Facial pain attributed to multiple sclerosis
        Persistent idiopathic facial pain
        Burning mouth syndrome

From Headache Classification Subcommittee of the International Headache Society: The International Classification of Headache Disorders: 2nd edition, *Cephalalgia* 24(Suppl 1):9-160, 2004.

---

attempts at treatment. Intractable oral and facial pain can be diagnostically challenging, given the many potential causes of pain, the anatomic complexity of the region, and the psychosocial importance of the face and mouth. A rigorous protocol for evaluating these patients includes a thorough history and an appropriate clinical examination.

A detailed history should always be obtained before examining the patient or ordering special tests or imaging studies because the history will establish a diagnosis in the majority of cases.

CHIEF COMPLAINT

The patient's description of the pain may provide clues to its cause. Primary neuralgias are frequently described as sharp and lancinating, secondary neuralgias have a burning quality, vascular headaches are throbbing, and muscle pain is described as a deep, dull ache. The patient may not be able to give all these descriptions at the first interview, and corroborating information from relatives and friends may be needed to build a general picture of the pain as it affects the patient. Each pain complaint should be listed in order of severity.

HISTORY OF PRESENT COMPLAINT

The intensity of the pain needs to be measured against the patient's own experience of pain, need for medication, and effect on lifestyle. For example, does the pain interfere with work, sleep, or social activities? How severe is it on a 10-point scale? Does it fluctuate over time? The origin of the pain should be determined by asking the patient to indicate the site of the pain or the site of its maximum intensity. Its anatomic distribution should be accurately traced in terms of local anatomy.

The patient should be encouraged to recall the events surrounding onset of the pain, even if it was several years ago. Any other instances of similar pain should be ascertained, even though the patient may not associate these events with the present problem. The time relationships of the pain should be clarified in terms of duration and frequency of attacks, as well as possible remissions.

Aggravating factors should be determined. Is the pain aggravated by the ingestion of specific foods or beverages; by lying down; during times of stress, talking, brushing the teeth, shaving, or applying make-up; or by other identifiable factors? In addition, relieving factors (e.g., lying down, sleeping, heat, and cold) are important clues.

The effects of previous treatments need to be clarified. Which medications have helped? Has surgery altered the nature of the pain? Has endodontic treatment or extraction affected the pain? Finally, the presence or absence of associated factors (e.g., swelling of the face, flushing, tearing, nasal congestion, or facial weakness) needs to be ascertained.

MEDICAL HISTORY

A careful medical history and detailed history of the pain should be taken. In particular, any trauma to the head, face, and mouth should be noted. Current and past medications, relevant family history, and the use of over-the-counter medications, supplements, and alternative or complementary therapies should be identified. Any jaw habits such as clenching, grinding, posturing the jaw, or gum chewing, including occupational or vocational habits (e.g., playing a wind instrument, scuba diving, and so on), need to be identified. A comprehensive psychosocial history is imperative for all patients with chronic pain disorders. The details of any pending or planned disability claims or litigation should be ascertained.

PHYSICAL EXAMINATION

The purpose of the physical examination is to discover any possible anatomic or physiologic basis for the pain; therefore, it is important to proceed systematically. Patients with facial pain should undergo a complete head and neck examination, not an examination directed by a presumed diagnosis.

NEUROLOGIC FUNCTION

The most important evaluations involve cranial nerves V (trigeminal) and VII (facial) and the upper cervical nerves (C2-4). The three divisions of the trigeminal nerve—supraorbital, infraorbital, and inferior alveolar nerves—supply the majority of sensation to the mouth and face. The skin distribution of all three divisions should be examined, as well as the intraoral distribution of the second and third divisions. Directional sense, two-point discrimination, and sensory perception with von Frey hairs (Semmes-Weinstein microfilaments) may help in making the diagnosis. Hot and cold sensitivity and taste may need to be tested in certain situations. Pain with pressure over the six foramina may indicate trigeminal involvement. The corneal and gag reflexes should be assessed. The size and strength of the masticatory muscles reflect the motor division of cranial nerve V. Facial nerve function can be assessed by asking the patient to whistle, purse the lips, smile, close the eyes, and frown.

Upper cervical nerve sensation can be assessed on the scalp for C2 and at the angle of the jaw and upper part of the neck for C3. Pressure over the mid-superior nuchal line directly affects the greater occipital nerve and may reproduce the headache in patients with occipital neuralgia.

Because of the overlap of cranial nerves V, VII, IX, and X and their convergence on the spinal trigeminal nucleus, a more detailed examination of these nerves may be necessary. Cranial nerve IV and VI palsies may indicate increased intracranial pressure.

MUSCLE FUNCTION

Pain in the masticatory muscles, face, posterior cervical spine, and upper part of the back (the suprascapular and pectoral girdle) is a common cause of head, face, and neck pain, so the neck, shoulder, and masticatory muscles should be assessed thoroughly. The size of the muscles can be assessed visually (e.g., temporal hollowing, masseteric hypertrophy). The muscles should be palpated, trigger points noted, and head and neck posture assessed. A more thorough evaluation of the masticatory muscles includes measuring the maximum interincisal opening and lateral and protrusive excursions. Tremors, deviations, and fasciculations should also be noted.

TEMPOROMANDIBULAR JOINT

The lateral pole of the mandibular condyle should be palpated for tenderness with the mouth open and closed. Coarse and fine crepitation should be noted and joint noises auscultated. Clicks and pops and their position in the opening or closing cycle should be observed. Determining whether they are eliminated by separating the teeth with a tongue blade or by posturing the jaw forward will help focus on the functional importance of these joint noises.

INTRAORAL EXAMINATION

Interdigitation of the maxillary and mandibular teeth should be evaluated when the mouth is closed (dental occlusion), as well as the state of the dentition and oral hygiene. Evidence of wear on the teeth, excessive toothbrush abrasion, or erosion of the palatal surfaces of the teeth from repetitive vomiting should be assessed. The health of the oropharyngeal mucosa should be recorded, as well as the moistness of the mucosa and pooling of saliva. The parotid and submandibular glands can be milked to evaluate the quality and quantity of saliva expressed. The tongue and soft palate should be centered midline and move freely and symmetrically. Excessive draping of the soft palate, as seen in sleep apnea, should be noted.

DIAGNOSTIC IMAGING

Periapical dental films and panoramic radiographs are inexpensive, are readily available, do not expose patients to excessive radiation, and offer detailed information about the teeth and jaws. Computed tomography (CT) can provide more detailed images of the bony structures of the jaws, TMJs, and base of the skull. Three-dimensional imaging can be helpful in some instances. Magnetic resonance imaging (MRI) is best for evaluating the soft tissues and can be used for assessing the deep oropharyngeal and nasopharyngeal anatomy and the internal anatomy of the TMJs. In addition, the brain can be evaluated with MRI, with and without gadolinium enhancement. MRI can also help determine whether the vasculature is impinging on the trigeminal ganglion, which can cause trigeminal neuralgia (TN).

A bone scan with technetium 99m will highlight areas of metabolic activity within the bone and can help identify areas of infection, tumor extension and continued growth, or degenerative change in the TMJ.

LABORATORY STUDIES

Routine blood tests include a complete blood count and differential to exclude anemia and blood dyscrasias. The erythrocyte sedimentation rate may be elevated in patients with temporal arteritis. Rheumatoid factor and Lyme titer may be helpful in evaluating TMJ disease.

COMMON FACIAL PAIN DISORDERS

As described earlier, the specialized structures of the head and face have a rich sensory innervation supplied by the trigeminal system, other cranial nerves, and the upper cervical roots. Consequently, pain is one of the most prominent symptoms of disease in this area. In most cases, the acute pain symptoms correlate closely with other signs and symptoms of disease. However, correlation between pain and symptoms may not be evident in a number of more complex, chronic pain problems, particularly those involving the craniofacial complex (Box 31-4).

TOOTH-RELATED DISORDERS (Table 31-1)

Tooth pulp has a specialized and possibly exclusively nociceptive innervation.[2] In contrast, periodontal tissues are innervated by a wide variety of sensory afferents.[2] Dental pain is usually well localized, and the quality of the pain can range from a dull ache to severe electric shocks, depending on the specific cause and extent of disease. Dental pain is typically provoked by thermal or mechanical stimulation of the damaged tooth. Clinical and radiographic findings

BOX 31-4	Common Craniofacial Pain Conditions

Dentoalveolar pathology
  Pulpal
  Periodontal
Odontogenic and non-odontogenic pathology
Trigeminal neuralgia and "equivalents"
Headache and neck pain
Temporomandibular disorders
Oral mucous membrane disease
Oral manifestations of systemic disease
Neuropathic pain (persistent idiopathic facial pain)
Burning mouth/tongue syndrome

TABLE 31-1	**Odontogenic Pain**			
DIAGNOSIS	**PULPITIS**	**PERIODONTAL**	**CRACKED TOOTH**	**DENTINAL**
Diagnostic features	Spontaneous and/or evoked deep/diffuse pain in compromised dental pulp. Pain may be sharp, throbbing, or dull	Localized deep continuous pain in compromised periodontium (e.g., gingiva, periodontal ligament) exacerbated by biting or chewing	Spontaneous or brief sharp pain in a tooth with a history of trauma or restorative work (e.g., crown, root canal)	Brief, sharp pain evoked by different kinds of stimuli to the dentin (e.g., hot or cold drinks)
Diagnostic evaluation	Look for deep caries and recent or extensive dental work. Pain provoked or exacerbated by percussion or thermal or electrical stimulation of affected tooth. Dental x-rays helpful (periapical)	Tooth percussion over compromised periodontium provokes pain. Look for inflammation or abscess (e.g., periodontitis). Apical dental x-rays helpful (bitewings, periapical)	Presence of tooth fracture may be detectable by x-ray. Percussion should elicit pain. Dental x-rays are helpful (periapical taken from different angles)	Exposed dentin or cementum caused by recession of periodontium. Possible erosion of dentinal structure. Cold stimulation reproduces pain
Treatment	Medication: NSAIDs, non-opiate analgesics Dentistry: remove carious lesion, tooth restoration, endodontic treatment, or tooth extraction	Medication: NSAIDs, non-opiate analgesics, antibiotics, mouthwashes Dentistry: drainage and débridement of periodontal pocket, scaling and root planing, periodontal surgery, endodontic treatment, or tooth extraction	Medication: NSAIDs, non-opiate analgesics Dentistry: depends on level of the tooth fracture-restoration; treatment, or extraction of the tooth	Medication: mouthwash (fluoride), desensitizing toothpaste Dentistry: fluoride or potassium salts, tooth restoration, endodontic treatment Patient education: diet, tooth-brushing force and frequency, proper toothpaste

NSAIDs, non-steroidal anti-inflammatory drugs.

of dental decay, tooth fracture, or abscess drainage may confirm the source of dental pain.

Dentinal pain is often evoked by stimuli and not well localized. It may result from areas of exposed dentin or defective restorations. Successful treatment involves the removal of any carious lesions and restoration of the tooth. In cases of exposed dentin sensitivity, treatment involves the use of desensitizing physical and chemical agents to decrease dentinal tubule permeability or decrease the sensitivity of dentinal neurons. Cervical hypersensitivity has also been managed successfully with the use of CO_2 and neodymium:yttrium-aluminum-garnet (Nd:YAG) lasers (see Table 31-1).

Pulpal pain, by contrast, is not stimulus-dependent, although it may be exacerbated by various stimuli (thermal, chemical, mechanical). When the patient describes the pain as mild to moderate and does not have a history of pain or pain on percussion, it is likely to be due to reversible pulpitis. Treatment is based on removal of the causative factor (e.g., caries), indirect pulp capping as necessary, and restoration of the tooth. When the described pain is moderate to severe or associated with a previous history of pain or with pain referral, it is most likely due to partial pulpal necrosis and irreversible pulpitis. Successful treatment consists of endodontic therapy or extraction (see Table 31-1).

Poorly localized pain in the orofacial region may also result from an incompletely fractured tooth. The typical pain of a cracked tooth is a sharp pain on biting and cold or hot hypersensitivity. However, patients may also complain of a more diffuse pain throughout the ipsilateral jaw, neck, ear, masticatory muscles, or TMJ. The diagnosis is based on the history and percussion or palpation of the individual cusps, transillumination of nonrestored or minimally restored teeth with fiberoptics, and probing of suspicious fissures, and it is confirmed by removal of restorations and direct inspection with or without staining. Treatment is dependent on the extent of the fracture (see Table 31-1).

Acute dental pain typically responds to local treatments (e.g., ice packs and reduced mechanical stimulation) or to systemic, non-steroidal anti-inflammatory drugs (NSAIDs). Opioid analgesics are also occasionally indicated, depending on the extent of objective pathology. Opioids should be used only short-term and in combination with NSAIDs. In many cases, treatment with antibiotic agents is appropriate and palliative until a definitive dental intervention is performed, as described earlier.

DISORDERS OF THE PERIODONTIUM (PERIODONTAL DISEASE)

Chronic periodontal disease is an immune-mediated inflammatory process initiated by pathogenic oral microorganisms[3] and resulting in either focal or generalized areas of destruction of the tooth-supporting structures and surrounding bone. Chronic periodontitis is not generally a chronically painful disorder. Typically, patients may notice gingival sensitivity and tenderness or gingival enlargement because of inflammation and bleeding with brushing or probing examination. There is loss of gingival attachment around the necks of teeth and soft tissue pocketing around the roots of teeth with loss of bone support, which may result in tooth sensitivity, tenderness, and mobility.

In patients with an acute infection in the periodontal tissues, tenderness to touch, erythema, and bleeding may be evident. An acute periodontal abscess may cause swelling and purulence (see Table 31-1). When inflammation or infection (i.e., acute pericoronitis) occurs in the soft tissue or bone around an erupting or partially erupted tooth (particularly third molars), similar signs and symptoms may be seen, with pain being a primary complaint.

The pain associated with periodontal disorders is likewise generally responsive to NSAIDs, opioid analgesic agents, or combination analgesic agents. An acute abscess may also have to be incised and drained. Areas of generalized periodontitis may be treated by tooth scaling and curettage of the gingival pocketing and, possibly, local or systemic antibiotic therapy.

ORAL MUCOUS MEMBRANE DISORDERS

Diseases of the oral mucosa are numerous and have a variety of local and systemic causes. Typically, these diseases are associated with pain and oral mucosal lesions, including vesicles, bullae, erosions, erythema, or red and white patches. Pain may be a symptom of the primary disease process, be secondary to an associated process (i.e., infection), or be related to damaged oral mucosa (i.e., mouth movements, chewing food, thermal, chemical) and is often treated with both systemic and local analgesic agents. Ulcerations of autoimmune etiology or unknown cause, such as aphthous ulcers, can be managed symptomatically with topical corticosteroids in an adherent vehicle for individual lesions. When multiple lesions are present, patients should use a solution containing corticosteroid with or without 2% viscous lidocaine.

DISORDERS OF THE MAXILLA AND MANDIBLE

Numerous disorders of the bony structure of the jaws may be associated with pain. These disorders are generally classified as being of odontogenic or non-odontogenic origin. Tumors may be benign or malignant (either primary or metastatic disease). Frequently, additional historical or examination findings warrant further evaluation (e.g., swelling, mass, discoloration, numbness, weakness, bleeding, drainage, tooth loss or mobility). Pain can be treated symptomatically until a definitive diagnosis is established and definitive therapy is initiated.

SALIVARY GLAND DISORDERS

Disorders of the three major pairs of salivary glands (parotid, submandibular, and sublingual) and the many hundreds of minor salivary glands in the mouth may also produce pain as a primary or associated symptom. These disorders are often accompanied by other signs and symptoms (including swelling, drainage, cervical adenopathy, or generalized signs of systemic infection), depending on the cause of the disorder. Disorders of the parotid gland can extend locally to produce otologic symptoms or cranial nerve (V, VII, or IX) involvement. Disorders of the submandibular gland may result in symptoms of impaired swallowing or impairment of cranial nerves V, IX, and XII.

BURNING MOUTH/TONGUE SYNDROME (ORAL BURNING)

See the section on neuropathic pain and Table 31-2.

OPHTHALMOLOGIC DISORDERS

Pain in and around the eye is a common problem. Most ophthalmologic conditions producing eye pain are associated with obvious ocular symptoms, signs, or histories that implicate the eye as the origin of pain. Several facial pain and headache syndromes have "eye pain" as the chief symptom. In addition, during the history

TABLE 31-2	**Trigeminal Neuropathic Pain Disorders**			
DIAGNOSIS	**TRIGEMINAL NEURALGIA**	**DEAFFERENTATION PAIN**	**ACUTE AND POST-HERPETIC NEURALGIA**	**BURNING MOUTH SYNDROME**
Diagnostic features	Brief severe lancinating pain evoked by mechanical stimulation of trigger zone (pain free between attacks). Usually unilateral, affects V2/V3 areas (rarely V1). Possible pain remission periods (for months/years)	Spontaneous or evoked pain with prolonged after-sensation following tactile stimulation. Trigger zone caused by surgery (tooth extraction) or trauma. Positive and negative descriptors (e.g., burning, nagging, boring)	Pain associated with herpetic lesions, usually in the V1 dermatome. Spontaneous pain (burning and tingling), but may be manifested as dull and aching. Occasional lancinating evoked pain	Constant burning pain of the mucous membranes, tongue, mouth, hard or soft palate, or lips. Usually affects women >50 years
Diagnostic evaluation	MRI for evidence of tumor or vasocompression of the trigeminal tract or root (cerebropontine angle). Rule out MS, especially in young adults	Etiologic factors such as trauma or surgery in the painful area. Order MRI if the area is intact to rule out peripheral or central lesions	Small cutaneous vesicles (AHN) or scarring (PHN), usually affecting V1. Loss of normal skin color. Corneal ulceration can occur. Sensory changes in affected area (e.g., hyperesthesia, dysesthesia)	Rule out salivary gland dysfunction (xerostomia) or tumor, Sjögren's syndrome, candidiasis, geographic or fissured tongue, chemical or mechanical irritation, nutrition, and menopause
Treatment	Medication: anticonvulsants (e.g., carbamazepine, gabapentin), antidepressants (e.g., amitriptyline, nortriptyline, desipramine), non-opiate analgesics, BTX. Combination of baclofen and anticonvulsants can produce good results. Surgery: microvascular decompression of trigeminal root, ablative surgeries (e.g., rhizotomy, Gamma Knife)	Medication: anticonvulsants (e.g., carbamazepine, gabapentin), antidepressants, non-opiate analgesics, topical agents (e.g., 5% lidocaine patches). Surgery: ablative surgeries (e.g., rhizotomy, Gamma Knife)	Medication: acyclovir (acute phase), anticonvulsants, antidepressants, non-opiate analgesics, topical agents (e.g., 5% lidocaine patches). Surgery: ablative surgeries (e.g., rhizotomy, Gamma Knife)	Medication: anticonvulsants, benzodiazepines, antidepressants, non-opiate analgesics, topical agents (e.g., lidocaine, mouthwashes). Cognitive-behavioral: biofeedback, relaxation, coping skills

AHN, acute herpetic neuralgia; BTX, botulinum toxin; MS, multiple sclerosis; PHN, post-herpetic neuralgia.

and physical examination, several signs and symptoms warn of more serious eye disease and even potentially life-threatening problems.

A complete ocular history should include any previous visual loss, ophthalmic diseases (e.g., corneal infections, uveitis, glaucoma), use of contact lenses, recent or remote ocular surgery, and ocular trauma. In addition to noting the specific features of the pain when taking the history for eye pain, such as the time of onset, severity, exacerbating and palliating factors, radiation, quality, duration, and frequency, the specific location of the pain should be ascertained (e.g., intraocular, retrobulbar, periocular, or frontal), as well as associated symptoms such as tearing, loss of vision, double vision, photophobia, and discharge.

Simple instruments are required to perform the basic eye examination, and a pain specialist can triage patients with eye pain and identify those who require formal ophthalmologic consultation. Such equipment includes a near vision card (Snellen card), a hand light, and a direct ophthalmoscope. The Snellen card is used to check visual acuity, which should be tested by using the patient's spectacle correction, and each eye should be tested individually. The pupil's response to light, the regularity of the pupil, and relative afferent papillary defects should be evaluated with a hand light. In addition, extraocular motility and the eyelids should be examined. A hand light should be used to assess the conjunctiva for chemosis, injections, and foreign bodies and the cornea for keratitis, foreign bodies, and lacerations. Evaluation of the optic nerve with a direct ophthalmoscope should be sufficient to exclude gross optic atrophy, funduscopic abnormalities, and papilledema.

Ocular and Orbital Causes of Eye Pain

The eye is rarely the source of head and facial pain localized to the periorbital structures without clinical signs such as red eye or symptoms such as decreased vision or a history of eye trauma. If findings on the basic eye history and examination are normal, an intraocular cause of the pain is less likely. However, in some ocular causes of eye pain, the eye is superficially normal. The clinician should be able to recognize the features of these uncommon causes of eye pain and make the necessary urgent or semi-urgent referral to an ophthalmologist.

In addition, a number of facial pain syndromes accompanied by prominent ophthalmologic signs and symptoms may be encountered by the oral and maxillofacial surgeon. The history and physical examination will define the differential diagnosis of these syndromes. Treatment of these disorders is specific to the disorder and may be part of the therapeutic spectrum of the oral and maxillofacial surgeon.

OTOLOGIC DISORDERS (Table 31-3)

Ear pain is a common complaint that may be due to otologic or non-otologic causes. The pain, often described as dull and aching with a stopped-up sensation, may be localized to the area around the ear or may spread to involve half or all of the head. It may also be referred to the vertex. Pain in the ear is as likely to be referred from other structures as it is to be stemming from the ear itself. If ear pain is not part of the orofacial pain complaint, it is highly unlikely that the ear is the pain source.

TABLE 31-3	Paranasal, Periocular, Periauricular, and Head and Neck Cancer Pain			
DIAGNOSIS	**PARANASAL SINUS PAIN**	**PERIOCULAR PAIN**	**PERIAURICULAR PAIN**	**HEAD AND NECK CANCER**
Diagnostic features	Bilateral or unilateral throbbing or pressure in the frontal area, pain exacerbated by leaning forward or palpation over the sinus	Pain or tenderness with or without eye movements, deep orbital pain, referred pain	Diffuse aching or sudden pain with or without aural discharge (e.g., otitis media)	Variety of symptoms. Pain may be due to tumor, nerve compression, secondary infection, secondary myofascial pain, deafferentation, radiotherapy, chemotherapy
Diagnostic evaluation	History of chronic allergies, frequent URIs, sinusitis, headaches of various types, sinus surgery. Refer to ENT for endoscopic and/or CT study (e.g., sinus opacification)	Examine the eyelids, lacrimal function, conjunctiva, sclera. Ophthalmoscopy and ophthalmology referral. Rule out primary headache, temporal arteritis, orbital pseudotumor	The area is innervated by multiple cranial and cervical nerves, so complete functional and structural examination necessary (e.g., inspect tympanic membrane, TMJ, and myofascia). CT and MRI invaluable for mastoiditis and cholesteatoma	Complete evaluation by multidisciplinary team, CT, MRI, endoscopy, biopsy, and surveillance. Treatment coordination by oncologist
Treatment	ENT evaluation/treatment. Medication: sinusitis—topical decongestants, systemic antibiotics; chronic sinus pain—NSAIDs, non-opiate analgesics, topical agents (lidocaine spray), anticonvulsants, antidepressants, BTX. Surgery	Proper ophthalmologic evaluation and treatment. Medication: NSAIDs, non-opiate analgesics, systemic antibiotics, topical corticosteroids, BTX across the forehead and glabellar areas in selected cases. Surgery	Proper ENT evaluation and treatment. Medication: NSAIDs, non-opiate analgesics, systemic antibiotics, topical corticosteroids, BTX in selected cases. Surgery	Oncologic evaluation and treatment. Medication: anticonvulsants, antidepressants, opiate or non-opiate analgesics, topical agents, muscle relaxants. Surgery: ablative surgeries

BTX, botulinum toxin; *CT*, computed tomography; *ENT*, ear, nose, and throat; *MRI*, magnetic resonance imaging; *NSAIDs*, non-steroidal anti-inflammatory drugs; TMJ, temporomandibular joint; URI, upper respiratory infection.

Primary otalgia arises from disease of the external or middle ear and is identified by inspection of the external ear and tympanic membrane. If the inspection reveals abnormal findings, otologic referral for comprehensive diagnosis and treatment would be appropriate. In the absence of local pathology, the pain is probably referred to the ear from another structure.

Sensory innervation of the ear involves cranial nerves V, VII, IX, and X, as well as C2 and C3. Pain referred to the ears (secondary otalgia) may originate in any structure with common innervations. Treatment of referred ear pain requires proper identification of the pain source.[9]

DISORDERS OF THE PARANASAL SINUSES
(see Table 31-3)

Sinus pain or "sinus headache" is another common complaint. Rhinosinusitis is inflammation of the nose or paranasal sinuses (or both) and is characterized by blockage or congestion, discharge, facial pain or pressure, loss of smell, or any combination of these symptoms. The inflammation is often due to allergy, infection, drugs, or hormones. Patients may also complain of sore throat, dysphonia, or coughing. The symptoms are frequently bilateral. Unilateral symptoms or associated bloody discharge may result from neoplasm and necessitates further evaluation and identification of the source of the pain. Immediate referral is necessary when any of the following symptoms are present: periorbital edema, a displaced globe, double vision, reduced visual acuity, or frontal swelling.

The American Academy of Otolaryngology–Head and Neck Surgery (AAO-HNS) recommends nasal endoscopy and CT of the paranasal sinuses for definitive diagnosis of rhinosinusitis, although most cases can be diagnosed clinically. The clinical findings must include two or more major factors or one major factor and two minor factors. These include chronic facial pressure of the maxillary region, headache, rhinorrhea, postnasal drip, decreased sense of smell, and dental pain. Classification of adult rhinosinusitis (acute, subacute, chronic, and acute exacerbations of chronic rhinitis) is important in providing appropriate treatment.

Acute sinusitis is assumed to be viral. Analgesics for pain relief, intranasal decongestants, and nasal irrigation with hypertonic saline can improve the symptoms but will not shorten their duration. If the symptoms worsen or do not improve within 7 days, the AAO-HNS guidelines suggest the addition of antibiotics and topical steroids. When the symptoms are severe or do not respond to treatment, appropriate referral must be considered.

Management of chronic rhinosinusitis is dependent on the underlying cause. The goal of treatment is elimination of infection and inflammation, removal of occlusion, and improvement of symptoms. Proper referral for evaluation and management is necessary. Patients who are refractory to conservative therapies may require surgery.

Chronic facial pain and headache are not generally thought to be due to chronic/recurrent sinus pathology and are probably another headache or facial pain syndrome. Recent consensus guidelines offer data to support this along with diagnostic and therapeutic recommendations for facial pain and headaches.[5]

TEMPORAL ARTERITIS

Orofacial pain may be vascular in origin. In giant cell arteritis (GCA), giant cells infiltrate the walls of the cranial arteries. In temporal arteritis, the superficial temporal artery is affected. Other arteries commonly affected by GCA include the maxillary, ophthalmic, and posterior ciliary arteries. It most commonly affects the elderly.

The involved artery may be enlarged and tender to palpation. Patients often complain of intense or deep headache that worsens on lying flat, malaise, weakness, and weight loss. Jaw claudication is a common finding that can mimic the much more common temporomandibular disorders. Occlusion of the optic artery may result in visual disturbances, including blindness. Laboratory studies reveal elevated erythrocyte sedimentation rates and C-reactive protein. Arterial biopsy is required for definitive diagnosis. Treatment with high-dose corticosteroid (40 to 60 mg/day) therapy should begin immediately, followed by referral for biopsy and long-term management. A delay in treatment may result in irreversible blindness. GCA is usually self-limited, but relapse does occur.

OTHER DISORDERS

Another vascular source of orofacial pain is carotid artery dissection. The pain is generally unilateral, and damage to the sympathetic plexus often results in unilateral Horner syndrome. Suspicion of carotid artery dissection necessitates immediate referral. Treatment includes the administration of anticoagulant or antiplatelet therapy or stent placement.

Orofacial pain may result from systemic disease, including connective tissue diseases, the diagnosis and treatment of which are beyond the scope of this text. However, it should be noted that appropriate diagnosis of underlying systemic disease, should it exist, is paramount in managing the associated symptoms.

TUMORS

Numerous intracranial and extracranial tumors can cause oral cavity, oropharyngeal, facial, and head pain as a primary initial symptom (see Table 31-3). Cancers of the upper aerodigestive tract, jaws, base of the skull, and neck may all be manifested as pain along with other associated signs and symptoms. In addition, numerous intracranial tumors and lesions (e.g., vascular malformations) can be accompanied by facial pain and headache. These are primarily tumors of the cerebellopontine angle; however, various primary brain neoplasms and metastatic disease have been associated with facial pain and headache. Headache and facial pain of unknown origin should warrant careful evaluation for an underlying occult tumor.[6-8]

Patients with facial pain or headache should undergo a comprehensive medical history and careful physical examination with particular attention directed to the cranial neurologic examination. Consideration should be given to obtaining appropriate imaging studies, including CT, MRI, and magnetic resonance angiography.

TEMPOROMANDIBULAR DISORDERS

Temporomandibular disorders are defined as a subgroup of craniofacial pain problems that involve the TMJ, masticatory muscles, and associated head and neck musculoskeletal structures. Patients with temporomandibular disorders most frequently have complaints of pain, limited or asymmetric mandibular motion, and TMJ sounds.[9,10] The pain or discomfort is often localized to the jaw, TMJ, and muscles of mastication. Common associated symptoms include ear pain and stuffiness, tinnitus, dizziness, neck pain, and headache. In some cases the onset is acute and the symptoms are mild and self-limited. In other patients, a chronic temporomandibular disorder with persistent pain in association with physical, behavioral, psychological, and psychosocial symptoms develops, similar to the findings in patients with chronic pain syndromes in other areas of the body[11-13] (e.g., arthritis, low back pain, chronic headache, fibromyalgia, and chronic regional pain syndrome [CRPS]), all requiring a coordinated interdisciplinary diagnostic and treatment approach.

Temporomandibular disorders are classified as one subtype of secondary headache disorder in the Classification of Headache Disorders II by the IHS (see Box 31-2).[1] The American Academy of Orofacial Pain has expanded on this IHS classification, as shown in Boxes 31-5 and 31-6.[14]

The prevalence among adults in the United States of at least one sign of temporomandibular disorders is reported to be 40% to 75%, and in those with at least one symptom, the prevalence is 33%.[13,15,16] TMJ sounds and deviation on opening the jaw occur in approximately 50% of otherwise asymptomatic persons and are considered within the range of normal and do not require treatment.[16] Other signs such as decreased mouth opening and occlusal changes occur in less than 5% of the general population.[17] Temporomandibular disorders are most commonly reported in young to middle-aged adults (20 to 50 years). The female-to-male ratio of patients seeking care has been reported to be 3:1 to as high as 9:1.[15,18] Despite the high prevalence of temporomandibular disorders, signs, and symptoms, only 5% to 10% of symptomatic people require treatment, given the wide spectrum of symptoms and the fact that the natural history of this disorder suggests that many patients (up to 40%) undergo spontaneous resolution of their symptoms.[13,19]

ETIOLOGY

In 1934, Dr. James Costen, an American otolaryngologist, evaluated 13 patients with pain in or near the ear, tinnitus, dizziness, a sensation of ear fullness, and difficulty swallowing.[13] He observed that these patients had many missing teeth and, as a result, their mandibles were over-closed. The patients seemed to improve when their missing teeth were replaced and the proper vertical dimension of the occlusion was restored. The malocclusion and improper jaw position were perceived to be the cause of both the "disturbed function of the temporomandibular joint" and the associated facial pain. Thereafter, the emphasis of treatment was on altering the affected patient's occlusion.

More recently, advances in the understanding of joint biomechanics, neuromuscular physiology, autoimmune and musculoskeletal disorders, psychological disorders, and pain mechanisms have resulted in changing concepts of the etiology of temporomandibular disorders. These disorders are now considered multifactorial in etiology, with biologic, behavioral, environmental, social, emotional, and cognitive factors alone or in combination contributing to the development of signs and symptoms of temporomandibular disorders.[14]

CLINICAL EVALUATION

Although temporomandibular disorders are a common cause of craniofacial pain, it is imperative for the clinician to obtain a comprehensive history, perform a careful physical examination, and obtain appropriate diagnostic studies to exclude other potentially serious disorders. The differential diagnosis should include odontogenic (caries, periodontal disease) and non-odontogenic causes of facial pain, primary or metastatic jaw tumors, intracranial and skull base tumors, disorders of other facial structures (including the salivary glands), primary and secondary headache syndromes, trigeminal neuropathic pain disorders, and systemic disease (cardiac, viral, autoimmune, diabetes, temporal arteritis).

The most common complaint of patients with temporomandibular disorders is unilateral facial pain. The pain may radiate to the ear, to the temporal and periorbital regions, to the angle of the mandible, and frequently to the posterior of the neck. The pain is usually reported as a dull, constant ache that is worse at certain times during the day. There can be bouts of more severe, sharp pain typically triggered by movements of the mandible. The pain may be present daily or intermittently, but many patients have pain-free intervals. Mandibular motion is generally limited, and attempts at active motion (chewing, talking, yawning) increase the pain. Patients frequently describe "locking" of the jaw, either in the closed mouth position with an inability to open it (most common) or in the open mouth position with an inability to close the jaw. These complaints are often worse in the morning, particularly in patients who clench or grind their teeth during sleep. Clenching, grinding of the teeth, and other nonfunctional, involuntary mandibular compensatory movements (so-called oral parafunctional habits) are common.

Along with limitation of motion, there is often deviation of the mandible to the affected side on opening and a "clicking" or "popping" noise in the joint. Although some of the aforementioned differential diagnoses can be accompanied by facial pain, temporomandibular disorders often have a stereotypic manifestation (as described earlier), which helps in the diagnostic process.

Physical examination should include observation and measurement of mandibular motion (maximal interincisal opening, lateral movements, protrusion), palpation of the muscles of mastication (masseter, temporalis, medial and lateral pterygoids) and the cervical musculature, and palpation or auscultation of the TMJ (or both), as well as examination of the oral cavity, dentition, occlusion, and salivary glands and inspection and palpation of the anterior and posterior aspect of the neck. Auscultation of the carotids and examination of the cranial nerves, with special attention directed to the trigeminal system, should also be part of the physical examination.

As already noted, noise in the TMJ on mandibular movement is frequently present in patients with temporomandibular disorders. However, noise alone is also a very common finding in completely asymptomatic people and may represent a range of normal rather than intra-articular pathology.[16-19] Muscle tenderness that produces pain or discomfort is generally found on both extraoral and intraoral palpation of the masticatory muscles. Tenderness may also be present in the anterior neck muscles (suprahyoid and sternocleidomastoid muscles), posterior cervical paraspinal muscles (semispinalis capitis, splenius capitis, and suboccipital muscles), and the upper shoulder muscles (trapezius and levator scapulae).[14,16] There may be mandibular hypomobility and deviation on opening. Finally, findings on the neurologic examination are typically normal, without any objective neurosensory or motor deficits of the trigeminal nerve or other focal cranial nerve abnormalities.

Diagnostic studies are performed to rule out other disorders and may include blood and serum inflammatory markers (to rule out autoimmune disorders and vasculitides), imaging, diagnostic nerve blocks, muscle trigger point injections, and dental models for maxillomandibular analysis.

IMAGING

The most important diagnostic advances have occurred in imaging techniques for the TMJ. The panoramic radiograph remains the most useful screening tool. Plain radiographs have almost completely been replaced by CT for evaluation of bone morphology and pathology of the joint, mandibular ramus, and condyle. Cone beam maxillofacial CT is a newer and faster technique with a radiation dose lower than that of conventional whole-body CT scans.[20] This technique provides thin-slice images in the axial, coronal, and sagittal planes that can be modified with an interactive viewing program to study all details of the maxillofacial skeleton. There is also a three-dimensional program for analysis before potential surgical procedures. CT provides fine, three-dimensional anatomic detail of the TMJ and surrounding skeleton.

MRI has replaced other imaging modalities for evaluation of soft tissue abnormalities of the joint and surrounding region. The anatomy of the joint and the position and structure of the intra-articular disc may be accurately visualized both at rest and in motion. The blood supply and vascularity of the condyle can be analyzed with MRI, and pathologic accumulation of fluid within and around the joint may be detected. Continuous cine-MRI allows evaluation of the joint structures during mandibular movement. In addition, investigators have demonstrated that in patients with intra-articular disc derangement disorders, there is poor correlation between signs and symptoms and displacement of the articular disc based on imaging studies alone.[21]

Skeletal scintigraphy is useful for evaluating developmental or growth abnormalities of the mandible but is not particularly helpful for the diagnosis of temporomandibular disorders.[22-25]

Arthroscopy is a minimally invasive surgical technique that allows direct visualization of the anatomy of the TMJ. Patients who have been treated with nonsurgical therapies for 3 to 6 months and continue to have persistent pain in the joint, decreased range of mandibular movement, and interference with normal daily activities (talking, chewing) may benefit from diagnostic or therapeutic arthroscopy, or both.[21,26-28] Synovitis, adhesions, cartilage degeneration, cartilage tears, loose bodies, disc degeneration, perforations, and capsular attachment tears can all be documented with arthroscopy.[28,29] Therapeutic surgical arthroscopy of the TMJ (as for other

joints) can eliminate cartilage and bone pathology, correct articular disc and ligament abnormalities, and remove true joint pathology (synovial chondromatosis, osteoarthritis).

MYOFASCIAL PAIN DISORDER
(Table 31-4)

MPD of the masticatory muscle system is the most common of all temporomandibular disorders. The vast majority of patients have facial pain, limitation of jaw motion, and muscle tenderness and stiffness, along with any number of associated complaints in the head, face, and neck region (described earlier). Imaging studies of the TMJs most commonly show no evidence of anatomic pathology. MPD can also be accompanied by myofascial trigger points, which are defined as a hyperirritable locus within a taut band of skeletal muscle that is located in muscular tissue or in its associated fascia or tendon. The spot is painful on compression and can evoke characteristic referred pain and autonomic phenomena.[39] Active trigger points may cause pain spontaneously or during movement. Latent trigger points are not usually painful but can create weakness and restriction of movement in a muscle.

Patients with MPD will generally respond to simple, noninvasive treatments (described in the following sections).

REASSURANCE/COUNSELING

It is important that the patient be counseled regarding the natural history and course of temporomandibular disorders, the role of stress and para-functional habits such as clenching and grinding of the teeth, the frequency of the problem in the population, and the self-limited nature of the disorder. As a health care professional, it is important to let the patient know that both the physical and emotional suffering associated with temporomandibular disorders is understood.

REST

Although it is not prudent to immobilize the mandible, the patient should be instructed to avoid extremes of mechanical movements (yawning, laughing, jaw clenching). Certain habits that may affect jaw function, such as chewing gum and biting fingernails or pencils, should be eliminated.

HEAT

Application of heat to the sides of the face by means of a heating pad, hot towel, or hot water bottle will be comforting and help relieve the muscle pain. More vigorous treatment may be achieved with ultrasound or short wave diathermy, which are widely available in physical therapy offices.[21,22]

MEDICATIONS

NSAIDs are often of value in the acute stage.[23-25] Treatment is usually administered for 10 to 14 days initially, at which time the patient should be reevaluated. Muscle relaxants are frequently used for acute episodes of pain but have not proved efficacious for chronic conditions.[23,28,29] Chronic opioid analgesic use should be avoided if at all possible.[23,27] Antidepressants have a long history of effectiveness for the treatment of chronic pain. Their use is often justified, especially when the pain and dysfunction are part of a complex of generalized muscle pain with signs and symptoms of depression.[30-36] Tricyclic antidepressants are the most widely used, and a bedtime-only schedule of 10 to 50 mg of nortriptyline, desipramine, or doxepin can be expected to alleviate the symptoms in 2 to 4 weeks.[30] Treatment, if successful, is maintained for 2 to 4

TABLE 31-4	Temporomandibular Disorders		
DIAGNOSIS	**TMJ ARTICULAR DISORDERS**	**MUSCLE DISORDERS**	**MYOFASCIAL DISORDERS**
Diagnostic features	Pain localized to the preauricular area during jaw function. Usually presence of painful click or crepitus during mouth opening. Limited opening (<35 mm), deviated or painful jaw movements	Tenderness of masticatory muscles. Dull, aching pain exacerbated by jaw function or palpation	Diffuse, dull, or aching pain affecting multiple groups of muscles of the head and neck region, as well as other parts of the body
Diagnostic evaluation	Internal derangement of the TMJ with abnormal function of the disc-condyle complex and/or degeneration of the joint surface. Palpation is painful. Possible joint swelling in acute phases. MRI, CT of the joint may rule out tumors and advanced degenerative stages	Tenderness during palpation of masticatory muscles and tendons. Possible limited range of jaw movement and during passive stretching examination. Can be associated with a parafunctional habit (bruxism—early morning pain)	Presence of trigger or tender points in one or more groups of muscles. Pain can radiate to distant areas with stimulation or not of the trigger points. Rule out presence of lupus erythematosus
Treatment	Patient education and self-care Medication: NSAIDs, non-opiate analgesics Physical therapy: exercise program Occlusal splints Oral maxillofacial surgery: arthrocentesis, arthroscopic surgery, open surgery	Patient education and self-care Medication: topical and systemic NSAIDs, non-opiate analgesics, muscle relaxants, antidepressants, (usually TCAs), anxiolytics, anticonvulsants, BTX, trigger point injections, vapocoolant spray Physical therapy: TENS, massage, exercise program Occlusal splints Cognitive-behavioral: biofeedback, relaxation, coping skills	Same as muscle disorders

BTX, botulinum toxin; *CT*, computed tomography; *MRI*, magnetic resonance imaging; *NSAIDs*, non-steroidal anti-inflammatory drugs; *TCAs*, tricyclic antidepressants; *TENS*, transcutaneous electrical nerve stimulation; *TMJ*, temporomandibular joint.

months and then tapered to a low maintenance dose. Recently, serotonin selective reuptake inhibitors have also been used as part of the treatment regimen.[23,25] However, some of these agents (fluoxetine and paroxetine) have now been implicated in producing increased masticatory muscle activity (bruxism), especially during sleep, and are not generally recommended.[37-40] The tricyclic antidepressants and some of the newer selective norepinephrine reuptake inhibitor antidepressants (e.g., duloxetine) can be recommended and show some efficacy. Anxiolytic agents, such as the benzodiazepines, are also commonly used.[23,27-29,41] Short-term use (a few weeks) of the long-acting benzodiazepines in low dose, typically at night, is recommended (diazepam, 2.5 to 5 mg, clonazepam, 0.5 mg). It is important that use of benzodiazepines be limited and patients be monitored frequently because of the potential for dependency.

JAW APPLIANCE THERAPY

Many types of intraoral orthotic jaw appliances are available for the treatment of temporomandibular disorders, and their multiplicity suggests that the optimal design has yet to be discovered. These devices are worn on the teeth and are usually made of processed, hard acrylic. They are designed to improve TMJ function by altering joint mechanics and increasing potential mobility, to improve function of the masticatory motor system while reducing abnormal muscle function, and to protect the teeth from jaw clenching and potential tooth fracture or attrition. It has been hypothesized that these devices may make patients more conscious of their oral parafunctional habits by altering the proprioceptive input and central motor system areas that initiate and regulate masticatory function ("oral central pattern generator").[42-44]

The most common appliance is one that is custom-made of hard acrylic and that fits over all the teeth in the dental arch (either upper or lower). Because of the difficulty in controlling for a study involving any type of appliance that is placed in the mouth, there have been few good randomized, controlled, and blinded studies of the long-term efficacy of these oral orthotic appliances. In a recent Cochrane Database review (2004), it was reported that there is insufficient evidence either for or against the use of oral appliance therapy.[48] However, with appropriate adjuvant therapies (as outlined earlier), these devices may play a role in alleviating the pain and dysfunction of temporomandibular disorders in 70% to 90% of patients.[45-48]

Malocclusion, loss of teeth, and tooth-to-tooth occlusal interference as a primary cause of TMJ and muscle symptoms are not well supported by the evidence.[49-52] However, as a general principle, maxillomandibular tooth-to-tooth interference and anterior-posterior jaw position discrepancies should be eliminated and missing teeth replaced in an effort to achieve optimal dental occlusion and masticatory function. In addition, the long-term efficacy of repositioning adult non-growing jaws via occlusal splints or functional appliances has not been proved by the data available.

BEHAVIORAL APPROACHES

Counseling, relaxation techniques, stress management, work pacing, guided imaging, biofeedback, cognitive therapy, and other behavioral modalities have all been reported as being helpful.[53-57] The 1996 National Institutes of Health Consensus Conference on Behavioral Medicine in the Management of Chronic Pain outlined techniques that are considered effective and the indications for using them.[58] The most important factor, however, is the therapeutic interaction (context effect) of the practitioner with the patient.

PHYSICAL MEDICINE

Manual manipulation, massage, ultrasound, and iontophoresis are helpful in reconditioning and retraining the masticatory and the other craniocervical muscles that are usually involved in temporomandibular disorders.[60-63] Passive motion has also been reported to be effective in rehabilitating some of the biochemical and biomechanical changes that occur in injured synovial joints, muscles, and periarticular tissues.[64,65] Several commercial jaw passive-motion devices (similar to those used for other joints in the body) are currently in use for temporomandibular disorders.

Treatment of myofascial trigger points includes spraying the involved muscle with ethyl chloride or fluoromethane followed by stretching, hot compresses, and range-of-motion exercises. Trigger point injections of procaine (0.5% solution in saline) or lidocaine (2% without epinephrine) have also commonly been used and more recently botulinum toxin (Botox), though not well studied.

INTRA-ARTICULAR DISC DERANGEMENT DISORDER (see Table 31-4)

Disc derangement disorder is defined as a temporomandibular disorder resulting from displacement of the TMJ disc from its normal position or deformation of the disc. It may lead to synovitis, pain, and limitation of motion.[4] The diagnosis is confirmed by the history, clinical examination, and MRI in the open and closed mouth positions. Diagnostic/therapeutic arthroscopy (as described earlier) may also be helpful in confirming the diagnosis and providing minimally invasive surgical manipulation, if necessary.[66,67]

Intra-articular disc derangements may include anterior displacement of the disc with reduction and anterior displacement without reduction.[4] Anterior displacement with reduction is defined as disc displacement in the closed mouth position that reduces (with a click) to the normal relationship at some time during opening. Reduction implies that to some extent, the disc is gliding normally with opening and translational movement. In these circumstances the patient complains of a click with a variable amount of pain on opening. Frequently, patients have no pain with this condition. The mandible deviates to the affected side on opening until the click occurs and then returns to the midline. This situation may worsen, and there may be intermittent locking of the disc.

Intermittent locking may progress over time to anterior disc displacement without reduction (closed lock).[4] This implies that the dislocated disc acts as a mechanical obstruction to opening and translation of the condyle. These patients have a marked decrease in mandibular opening on the affected side with a variable amount of pain. They feel that there is a mechanical obstruction in the joint to opening. Maximal opening may be limited to 20 to 25 mm with restricted movement to the contralateral side. There may also be a previous history of clicking with intermittent locking. MRI shows a displaced disc without reduction on opening (closed lock) and may also demonstrate degenerative changes in the condyle. In such cases, signs and symptoms of degenerative joint disease may also be present.[68]

Initial treatment of internal derangement consists of the same non-invasive therapies used for MPD: counseling, behavioral medicine, jaw appliances, heat, muscle relaxants, NSAIDs, physical therapy, and others. These strategies are often successful in patients with an anteriorly displaced disc with reduction (intermittent locking). In contrast, patients with a closed lock, especially one that is long standing, will most often require interventions such as intra-articular injection with steroids, arthrocentesis, or arthroscopy.[69,70] TMJ dislocation is also known as open lock when the condyle translates beyond the anterior eminence of the articular fossa with subsequent trapping in this open mouth position. Concomitant spasm of the elevator muscles results in subsequent trapping of the condyle anterior to the eminence in the open mouth position. Chronic hypertranslation can usually be managed by the subject physically manipulating the jaw. If the condition is chronic, the subject knows to relax the jaw-closing muscles and slip the condyle back into position. If the problem is related to trauma or to a sudden acute translation, the subluxation is considered to be an acute dislocation and requires medical intervention in which the muscles are relaxed with anesthetics or analgesics followed by manual manipulation of the joint with a downward and backward motion. Follow-up with anti-inflammatory medication, ice, and rest or a dental appliance may be necessary until the acute stage subsides.

OSTEOARTHRITIS

Osteoarthritis of the TMJ may result from trauma (acute or chronic), infection, metabolic disturbances, and previous joint surgery.[4] The patient complains of pain on moving the mandible, limited motion, and deviation of the jaw to the affected side. There may be acute tenderness on palpation of the joint. Joint sounds are described as grating, grinding, or crunching, but not as clicking or popping. Imaging studies typically reveal degenerative changes, remodeling, and loss of joint space.[71]

The features of degenerative disease of the TMJ are different from those of most other joints in the body. There is a strong predilection for females in the third or fourth decade. Only a few patients have generalized osteoarthritis. The natural course of the disease suggests that the pain and limitation may "burn themselves out" after as little as several months in some patients.[4,67,68] The majority of patients can be kept comfortable with the non-invasive techniques outlined earlier until remission.

In the acute phase, patients may require intra-articular injection of a long-acting corticosteroid (such as betamethasone) or hyaluronic acid.[69] Neither corticosteroids nor hyaluronic acid are recommended for long-term use and have equivocal data. These injection treatments are generally reserved for older patients and are limited to two or three injections separated by 4 to 6 weeks. In patients refractory to these techniques, surgery may be indicated to remove the loose fragments of bone (so-called joint mice) and reshape the condyle.

RHEUMATOID ARTHRITIS

Adults and children with rheumatoid arthritis may exhibit involvement of the TMJ. Fifty percent of children with juvenile rheumatoid arthritis have TMJ pain, swelling, or limitation of motion, alone or in combination.[72] There may be associated growth restriction of the jaw resulting in micrognathia and ankylosis. In adults with long-standing rheumatoid arthritis, TMJ symptoms may develop late in the course of the disease and patients may complain only when they have marked limitation of jaw motion. Other stigmata of rheumatoid arthritis will be evident. Findings on TMJ imaging vary depending on the stage of the disease, but ultimately, there is resorption of the condyle with shortening of the mandibular ramus-condyle unit and potential reduction of the joint space and hypomobility. Medical management along with alteration of TMJ biomechanics with the same modalities listed previously (physical medicine, jaw appliance, biobehavioral therapy) may be helpful initially. If medical management is not effective, surgical treatment may be necessary, similar to other joints in the body.

TRIGEMINAL NEURALGIA

TN is a well-recognized disorder characterized by sudden, unilateral lancinating attacks of severe, electric-like facial pain. Between attacks of intense momentary pain, most patients with TN are symptom-free and have normal findings on clinical examination.[55,56]

TN has an estimated incidence of 4 in 100,000, it is most common in patients older than 50 years and on the right side of the face, and women are affected slightly more often than men. Several lines of research support the view that TN results from a chronic partial nerve injury between the gasserian ganglion and the proximal trigeminal nerve root. However, despite recent advances in our understanding of trigeminal disorders, the basic pathophysiology of TN remains largely unknown.[57-63]

CLINICAL CLASSIFICATION

TN is a clinical syndrome; there is no laboratory test or radiographic study that can reliably confirm the diagnosis. Instead, the diagnosis of TN rests on a series of signs and symptoms that uniquely define the disorder and the clinician's ability to recognize that specific diagnostic pattern.

Although the major features of TN have been known for centuries, White and Sweet made a significant contribution by articulating diagnostic criteria for TN that were both precise and succinct. Their criteria rapidly gained popular clinical acceptance and are currently used by clinicians worldwide. White and Sweet emphasized five major clinical features that in their opinion established the diagnosis of TN[64]:

- The pain is paroxysmal.
- The pain may be provoked by light touch to the face (trigger zones).
- The pain is confined to the trigeminal distribution.
- The pain is unilateral.
- Findings on clinical sensory examination are normal.

Under the current IHS criteria, the International Classification of Headache Disorders II,[1] clinical cases of TN fall into two groups: "classic" (primary) and "symptomatic" (secondary) (see Boxes 31-3 and 31-4). "Classic TN" refers to the idiopathic syndrome, which means that the underlying cause of the disorder is not known. More than 90% of patients with TN fall into this category. "Symptomatic TN" identifies a group of patients who exhibit the clinical syndrome of TN as a symptom of another disease process. The most common disorders associated with symptomatic TN are multiple sclerosis and benign tumors in the region of the gasserian ganglion, trigeminal root, or cerebellopontine angle.

DIAGNOSTIC EVALUATION

The diagnosis of TN is based primarily on a clinical history consistent with the diagnostic criteria. However, the general physical and neurologic examinations are also very important. Imaging may prove valuable in patients with clinical findings that are not consistent with the classic diagnostic criteria.

The physical examination entails a thorough evaluation of the head and neck with special emphasis on the neurologic examination. Cranial nerve examination should be performed with particular attention to hearing and facial nerve abnormalities. In addition, clinical neurosensory testing of the trigeminal system should include light touch, sharp touch, temperature, direction, and two-point discrimination. Note should be taken of any trigger areas, and they should be appropriately mapped out. Aside from the trigger areas, when present, and minimal hypoalgesia or hypoesthesia in some patients, the results of neurologic examination are normal.

However, as many as 10% of patients meeting the clinical criteria for TN turn out to have symptomatic TN resulting from another primary underlying diagnosis, most commonly benign tumors or multiple sclerosis.[65,66] Most of these patients can be identified by a careful medical history and a pattern of more specific and different findings on examination and on MRI with special attention directed to the middle and posterior cranial fossa and brainstem.

MANAGEMENT

The current treatment of TN consists of medical and surgical therapies. Medical management includes pharmacologic and non-pharmacologic approaches, whereas surgical management consists of numerous peripheral and intracranial procedures. It is also important to emphasize that the current therapy suffers from a lack of rigorous clinical trials that might provide a scientific foundation for important clinical treatment decisions. Mathews and Scrivani developed an algorithm for the differential diagnosis and management of craniofacial pain disorders[66] (Fig. 31-1). This algorithm incorporates historical data, physical examination data, and some diagnostic testing to guide medical and surgical management strategies for patients with craniofacial pain.

Pharmacologic Therapy

The current first-line treatment is medical therapy with anticonvulsant/antiepileptic drugs (AEDs) such as phenytoin (Dilantin), carbamazepine (Tegretol), baclofen (Lioresal), clonazepam (Klonopin), gabapentin (Neurontin), lamotrigine (Lamictal), topiramate (Topamax), oxcarbazepine (Trileptal), tiagabine (Gabitril), levetiracetam (Keppra), or zonisamide (Zonegran), in single or combination regimens (Table 31-5).

Some of the AEDs have been carefully evaluated specifically for TN, whereas others have been evaluated for generalized neuropathic pain disorders. Specifically for TN, carbamazepine, clonazepam, baclofen, lamotrigine, tizanidine, and topiramate have been studied in randomized, placebo-controlled trials, whereas phenytoin, clonazepam, valproic acid, gabapentin, mexiletine, lamotrigine, and oxcarbazepine have been evaluated in uncontrolled, open-label or case series trials.

Pharmacologic therapy is effective for many patients; however, for some, these medications do not relieve the pain or they produce intolerable side effects with significant medical and functional morbidity. If medical therapy is unsuccessful or not tolerated, surgical treatment should be considered (see Fig 31-1).

TABLE 31-5	Pharmacologic Therapy	
	INITIAL	MAXIMUM
GBP	300 mg tid	2400-4800 mg
BAC	10 mg tid	60-80 mg
CLO	0.5 mg tid	4-8 mg
LTG	25 mg bid	300-600 mg
OXC	150-300 mg tid	1500-3000 mg
TOP	25 mg tid	100-300 mg
CBZ	100-300 mg tid	1200-2400 mg

BAC, baclofen; *CBZ*, carbamazepine; *CLO*, clonazepam; *GBP*, gabapentin; *LTG*, lamotrigine; *OXC*, oxcarbazepine; *TOP*, topiramate.

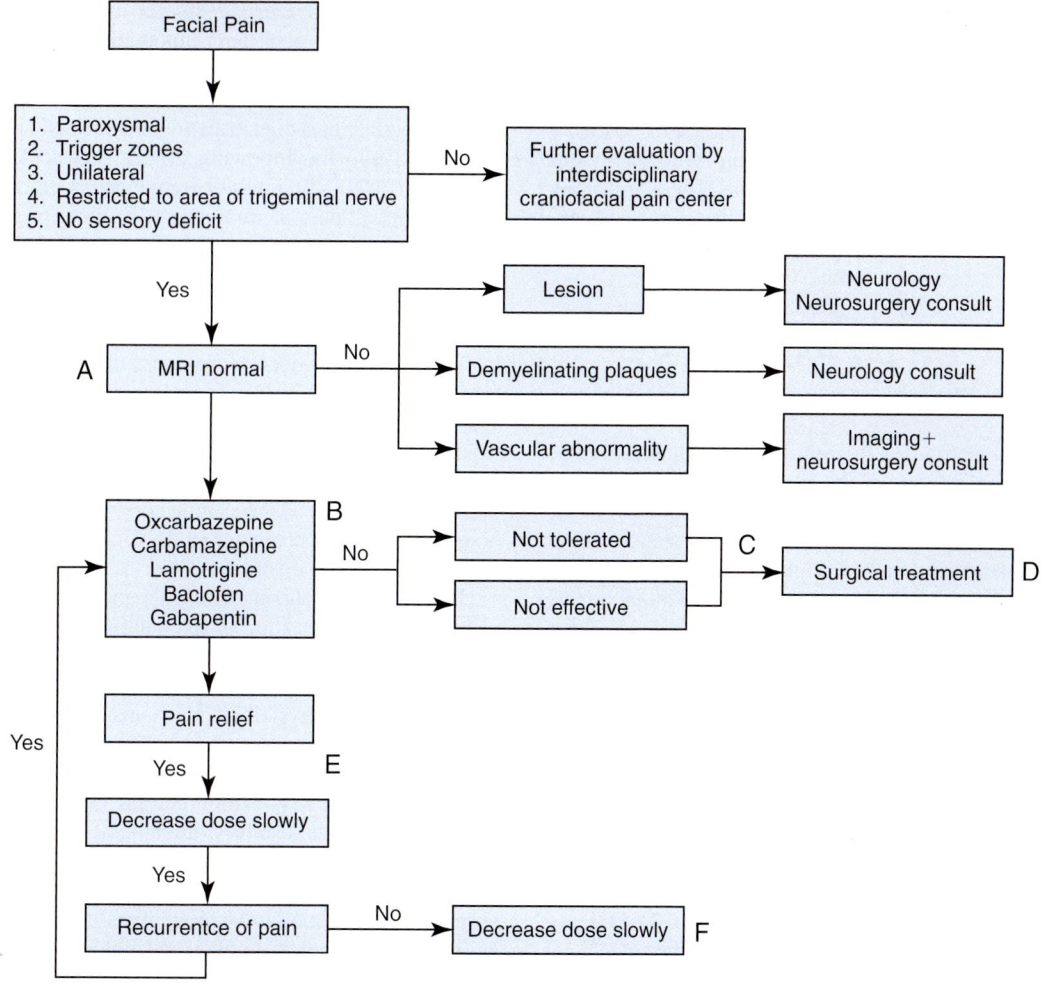

A MRI of the brain, brainstem and base of skull. Further diagnostic studies are performed when physical examination or MRI findings are abnormal.
B Medication is titrated progressively until pain is relieved or adverse effect(s) occur. Often a second AED is added early, if single therapy is ineffective.
C Drug allergy, idiosyncratic reaction, laboratory abnormalities, intolerable dangerous side effect, patient preference.
D Local anesthetic trigeminal nerve blocks are performed in some patients as part of a further diagnostic evaluation prior to surgical therapy.
E Dosages of medications can be tapered slowly if patient remains pain free after several weeks to months of pharmacotherapy.
F Further decrease in dosage of medication is predicated on the patients pain history. Many patients may need to be maintained on pharmacotherapy as preventive therapy.

Fig. 31-1 ■ Differential diagnosis and management of craniofacial pain disorders. (From Mathews ES, Scrivani SJ: Percutaneous stereotactic radiofrequency thermal rhizotomy for the treatment of trigeminal neuralgia, *Mt Sinai J Med* 67:288-299, 2000.)

Surgical Therapy

There are numerous surgical treatments of TN, yet several treatments are currently most commonly used. The surgical procedures currently commonly used for the treatment of TN include

1. Percutaneous stereotactic differential radiofrequency thermal rhizotomy
2. Posterior fossa exploration and microvascular decompression of the trigeminal root
3. Stereotactic radiosurgery—Gamma Knife radiosurgery or CyberKnife radiosurgery

Treatment of Acute Attacks

Occasionally, patients may initially be evaluated during acute attacks and exhibit frequent spontaneous or easily triggered high-intensity jolts of pain. In this situation, some form of acute intervention is warranted because the patient's functioning is generally severely affected by the pain attacks and, if it continues, the patient's ability to properly eat or drink may be altered. In such cases there has been some reported success with trigeminal division nerve blocks typically with a long-acting local anesthetic (bupivacaine). Occasionally, the application of a topical amide local anesthetic preparation (2%

to 5% lidocaine, EMLA [eutectic mixture of local anesthetics]) may be effective. However, there are few good data showing that the use of local anesthetics is consistently effective in stopping acute attacks or eliminating the recurrence of pain after the duration of action of the applied anesthetic has waned. Furthermore, some patients may benefit from the intravenous administration of fosphenytoin (Cerebyx), valproic acid (Depacon), or lidocaine. These infusions need to be performed in a carefully monitored setting with appropriate medical attention and emergency equipment available (outpatient surgical center or in the hospital).

NEUROPATHIC FACIAL PAIN
(see Box 31-4 and Table 31-2)

The International Association for the Study of Pain defines neuropathic pain as "pain initiated or caused by a primary lesion or dysfunction in the nervous system." Neuropathic pain syndromes result from pathology in the peripheral or central nervous system.[67] These disorders are particularly common in the head and neck, probably because of the dense and specialized sensory innervation in this region. When localized to the face and oral cavity, this painful disorder is described as neuropathic orofacial pain, which comprises a large array of painful trigeminal disorders. Unfortunately, these disorders have a great impact on the patient's life by interfering with important functions such as feeding and speech.

In the past, any facial pain disorder that did not have a definable cause was considered to be an idiopathic "atypical" facial pain syndrome. Over the years, many inappropriate "descriptive" diagnoses have been given to these disorders (atypical TN, atypical facial pain, atypical odontalgia, phantom tooth syndrome, and others). Under the current IHS classification[1] (see Box 31-6), these disorders are considered "central" causes of headache and facial pain and are classified as "persistent idiopathic facial pain."

There are several additional practical problems with classifying neuropathic pain syndromes[68,69]:

1. The perception of neuropathic pain is purely a subjective phenomenon that despite use of the most sophisticated equipment, cannot be measured.
2. There is rarely a diagnostic test that can confirm or refute the hypothesis of a nerve lesion or dysfunction.
3. The pain system is not static but can change in a dynamic and somewhat unpredictable fashion whenever the system is activated.
4. The signs and symptoms of neuropathic pain may change during the course of the disease and if it becomes chronic.
5. The requirement for diagnostic and classification validity and reliability has become more demanding.
6. Systematic reviews of treatment of neuropathic pain show that moderate pain relief can be achieved in approximately a third of patients regardless of the underlying disease/diagnosis or anatomy of such disease/diagnosis.

A form of neuropathic pain disorder, CRPS, may have similar features that can occur in the facial region.[70] CRPS refers to a syndrome characterized by constant pain, hyperesthesia, hyperalgesia, allodynia, or any combination of these symptoms. The pain is not typically limited to the territory of a particular nerve distribution, is often out of proportion to the stimulus applied to the area (if provoked), and is associated with autonomic-like epiphenomena (swelling, redness, warmth, sweating, conjunctival injection, nasal stuffiness, lacrimation). There are two types of CRPS: CRPS I, which is often not associated with any significant trauma or nerve injury, and CRPS II, which is typically associated with major nerve injury. Although the mechanisms for the pain and other symptoms are not fully understood, it appears that some "injury" to the peripheral nervous system is the common pathway to the pathophysiologic events.

For practical purposes, trigeminal neuropathic pain disorders can be divided into the following groups: (1) acute and postherpetic neuralgia (PHN), (2) a more heterogeneous group of neuralgic disorders termed "painful traumatic trigeminal neuropathy" (PTTN), and (3) burning mouth/tongue (oral burning) (see Table 31-2).

PAINFUL TRAUMATIC TRIGEMINAL NEUROPATHY

In a significant number of patients, chronic facial pain develops following trauma to sensory nerves in the craniocervical region.[71-73] Trauma to peripheral branches of the trigeminal nerve commonly results from disease, injury, or dental/surgical procedures. The peripheral nerve damage often causes transient or permanent sensory impairment and paresthesias in the distribution of the affected nerve branch. In a small percentage of these cases, the nerve injury results in a persistent pain disorder.

These cases are distinct from TN and usually grouped according to the nature and location of the painful nerve damage (neuralgia). Distinction between PTTN and TN is extremely important. First, the history, signs, and symptoms of PTTN differ from those of TN. Second, the pathophysiologic mechanism is probably different in the two syndromes. Third, the effective therapy and prognosis for PTTN and TN differ greatly.

Patients with PTTN exhibit chronic or recurrent pain in the area of the previous nerve injury, numbness, dysesthesias, and chronic burning sensations.[67,70,73] Diagnostic evaluations rule out any other cause of pain. Most cephalic neuralgias meet these general PTTN criteria, although individual clinical features vary depending on the specific syndrome. Common examples of cephalic neuralgias include PHN, inferior alveolar neuralgia following mandibular third molar extraction and other types of jaw surgery, and infraorbital neuralgia following maxillary trauma.

Patients with PTTN represent a significant clinical challenge since the symptoms of PTTN respond poorly, if at all, to the AEDs or surgical therapies commonly used for TN. Management of PTTN is the same as for other neuropathic pain disorders. An interdisciplinary approach is the most logical course. Pharmacologic therapy is often the mainstay of treatment, with first-line agents including tricyclic antidepressants, gabapentin, opioids, tramadol, and topical lidocaine.[68,70,74,75]

Recently, duloxetine and pregabalin have been approved for use in patients with neuropathic pain disorders. Other topical agents (ketamine, clonidine, capsaicin) have likewise been used with some efficacy.[75] Numerous other agents (AEDs, alpha agonists, benzodiazepines, ketamine) have also been used, but with very little data on efficacy. Electrical stimulation has been applied to peripheral nerves, as well as to the motor cortex, with few good data. Neuroablative procedures are also performed but are often not very successful and are fraught with many side effects. The role of surgical intervention in patients with neuropathic facial pain has not been fully understood.[76-79]

POSTHERPETIC NEURALGIA

PHN is a constant baseline burning, aching pain that is frequently accompanied by spontaneous, intermittent lancinating, jabbing bouts of pain. There is hyperesthesia or allodynia (or both) to mechanical and cold/warm stimuli. Sensory abnormalities are often present, such as itching, numbness, and tingling, along with sensory deficits (absent or diminished thermal, tactile sensations). Frequently, skin pigmentation changes, scarring, or both can be seen in the area of the acute lesions.

Herpes zoster (HZ) has a reported incidence of 2 to 3.4 per 1000 persons per year in the United States, mainly those older than 50 years.[80] The transition from HZ to PHN occurs immediately after the rash, or at about 1, 3, or 6 months after crusting of the skin lesions.[81] Approximately 8% of patients will have persistent pain at 1 month.[82] Of these, 42% to 66% will still have some pain after 12 months.[83] Depending on the definition applied, PHN will develop in 9% to 34% of all patients with HZ.[81] The most important risk factors for the development of PHN include age and the severity of acute pain and inflammation during HZ.[84]

Treatments are similar to those for other neuropathic pain disorders. There are numerous treatment algorithms that address several forms of pharmacologic therapies along with nerve blockade and topical agents.[85-87] Tricyclic antidepressants, AEDs, opioids, ketamine, and other neuropathic agents remain the primary pharmacologic therapy. There have been numerous reports of the efficacy of topical preparations for PHN, with lidocaine being the most effective. The efficacy of local injection therapy is still equivocal and controversial, but in individual cases it may be beneficial. Nonpharmacologic biobehavioral therapy may also provide some pain management.

BURNING MOUTH/TONGUE SYNDROME

Burning mouth/tongue syndrome (BMS) refers to oral burning pain, sometimes with dysesthetic qualities similar to those found in other neuropathic pain conditions but with the absence of any pathologic or medical findings that can account for the symptoms. The dorsal surface of the tongue, anterior portion of the palate, mucous membranes around the lips, vermilion of the lips, and gingival tissues are most commonly involved. Symptoms are generally bilateral. BMS has been found to be associated with jaw pain, jaw tightness, temporomandibular disorders, non-odontogenic tooth pain, craniocervical myofascial pain, and changes in taste, as well as other phantom oral sensations such as dry mouth, excessive saliva, phantom bite, and perceptions about the shape, size, and position of the teeth.[88,89]

BMS is a constant, burning, scalding pain sensation that often becomes progressively worse during the course of the day. It is frequently better with eating and with cold foods or liquids in the mouth. The pain rarely wakes the patient at night and is at its lowest intensity in the morning.[90] Patients frequently suffer from this constant, unremitting pain sensation and often have co-morbid psychological abnormalities, including anxiety and depression disorders.[91]

Based on association of the burning pain with frequent taste disturbances, it is believed that BMS could also be the clinical manifestation of taste damage with release of inhibition of the glossopharyngeal nerve (alterations in taste, touch, and pain) and the trigeminal nerve (alterations in touch and pain). Consistent with this model, severe taste damage has been found in many BMS patients.

Furthermore, it has also been suggested that incidentally, these patients were not limited by inhibition of the taste system. We have begun to speculate that alterations in taste and oral pain are not limited to BMS but can involve other orofacial pain complaints as well.[90,92] A hypothesis based on the taste pathways inhibiting other cranial nerves may explain why conditions such as BMS and other trigeminal neuropathic pain disorders can include sensory, motor, and sympathetic abnormalities.[90-92]

Current management of BMS includes pharmacologic therapy with the agents commonly used for other neuropathic pain disorders. Compounded topical agents (lidocaine, amitriptyline, gabapentin, capsaicin, ketamine, and clonazepam) are frequently used as in to other neuropathic pain disorders, yet there are virtually no data on efficacy.[93-95] In addition, biobehavioral therapies, stress reduction therapies, acupuncture, and physical medicine modalities are also potentially effective, as in the chronic neuropathic pain conditions.[96]

PEARLS AND PITFALLS

- The craniofacial region is an extremely complicated anatomic and physiologic region of the body.
- The differential diagnosis of craniofacial pain disorders is very broad and challenging.
- There is often a significant overlap of symptoms and signs in the craniofacial pain disorders.
- The diagnostic evaluation of craniofacial pain disorders must be comprehensive and is of paramount importance.
- A detailed physical examination of the entire craniofacial complex is mandatory for all patients, with particular attention paid to the cranial nerve neurologic examination.
- In addition, a detailed and focused psychosocial assessment is an essential part of the diagnostic evaluation.
- Structural pathology can often be responsible for what appears to be a common manifestation of a craniofacial pain disorder.
- Because temporomandibular disorders encompass a broad range of diagnostic subcategories, a more specific clinical diagnosis can aid in proper treatment.
- Neuropathic pain syndromes in the craniofacial region are common and difficult to diagnose and manage.
- Numerous unnecessary interventions and surgical procedures (dental and oral) should be avoided.
- Treatment of neuropathic craniofacial pain disorders is multimodality and based on other neuropathic pain disorders (e.g., CRPS).
- TN is a very specific diagnosis that should not be confused with other craniofacial pain syndromes.
- Treatment of TN is evidence based and typically either medical or surgical in nature.
- Interdisciplinary pain groups specializing in craniofacial pain disorders may be helpful in providing adjunctive evaluations for more complex diagnoses.

REFERENCES

1. Headache Classification Subcommittee of the International Headache Society: The International Classification of Headache Disorders: 2nd edition, *Cephalalgia* 24(Suppl 1):9-160, 2004.
2. Offenbacher S: Periodontal diseases: pathogenesis, *Ann Periodontol* 1:821-878, 1996.
3. Levine HL, Setzen M, Cady RK, et al: An otolaryngology, neurology, allergy, and primary care consensus on diagnosis and treatment of sinus headache, *Otolaryngol Head Neck Surg* 134:516-523, 2006.
4. Dworkin SF, Burgess JA: Orofacial pain of psychogenic origin: current concepts and classification, *J Am Dent Assoc* 115:565-571, 1987.
5. Parker MW, Holmes EK, Terezhalmy GT: Personality characteristics of patients with temporomandibular disorders: diagnostic and therapeutic implications, *J Orofac Pain* 7:337-334, 1993.

6. Solberg WK: Epidemiology, incidence and prevalence of temporomandibular disorders: a review. In: *The President's Conference on the Examination, Diagnosis and Management of Temporomandibular Disorders*, Chicago, 1983, American Dental Association, pp 30-39.

7. de Leeuw R: *Orofacial pain: guidelines for assessment, diagnosis and management*, ed 4, Chicago, 2008, Quintessence.

8. Schiffman E, Fricton JR: Epidemiology of TMJ and craniofacial pains. In Fricton JR, Kroening RJ, Hathaway KM, editors: *TMJ and craniofacial pain*, St Louis, 1988, Ishiro Euro America, pp 1-10.

9. Dworkin SF, Huggins KH, LeResche L, et al: Epidemiology of signs and symptoms of temporomandibular disorders: clinical signs in cases and controls, *J Am Dent Assoc* 120:273-281, 1990.

10. Wabeke KB, Spruijt RJ: *On temporomandibular joint sounds: dental and psychological studies [thesis]*. Amsterdam, 1994, University of Amsterdam, pp 91-103.

11. Huber NU, Hall EH: A comparison of the signs of temporomandibular joint dysfunction and occlusal discrepancies in a symptom-free population of men and women, *Oral Surg Oral Med Oral Pathol Oral Radiol Endod* 70:180-183, 1990.

12. Levitt SR, McKinney MW: Validating the TMJ scale in a national sample of 10,000 patients: demographic and epidemiologic characteristics, *J Orofac Pain* 8:25-34, 1994.

13. Costen JB: A syndrome of ear and sinus symptoms dependent upon disturbed function of the temporomandibular joint, *Ann Otol Rhinol Laryngol* 43:1-15, 1934.

14. Hashimoto K, Kawashima S, Kameoka S, et al: Comparison of image validity between cone beam computed tomography for dental use and multidetector row helical computed tomography, *Dentomaxillofac Radiol* 36: 465-471, 2007.

15. McCain JP, de la Rua H, Le Blanc WG: Correlation of clinical, radiographic, and arthroscopic findings in internal derangements of the TMJ. *J Oral Maxillofac Surg* 47:913-921, 1989.

16. Cisneros GJ, Kaban LB: Computerized skeletal scintigraphy for assessment of mandibular asymmetry, *J Oral Maxillofac Surg* 42:513-520, 1984.

17. Kaban LB, Cisneros GJ, Heyman S, et al: Assessment of mandibular growth by skeletal scintigraphy, *J Oral Maxillofac Surg* 40:18-22, 1982.

18. Cisneros G, Kaban LB: Computerized skeletal scintigraphy for assessment of mandibular asymmetry, *J Oral Maxillofac Surg* 42:513-520, 1984.

19. Pogrel MA: Quantitative assessment of isotope activity in the temporomandibular joint regions as a means of assessing unilateral condylar hypertrophy, *J Oral Maxillofac Surg* 60:15-17, 1985.

20. Malki GA, Zawawi KH, Melis M, et al: Prevalence of bruxism in children receiving treatment for attention deficit hyperactivity disorder: a pilot study, *J Clin Pediatr Dent* 29:63-67, 2004.

21. Lobbezoo F, van Denderen RJ, Verheij JG, et al: Reports of SSRI-associated bruxism in the family physician's office, *J Orofac Pain* 15:340-346, 2001.

22. Romanelli F, Adler DA, Bungay KM: Possible paroxetine-induced bruxism, *Ann Pharmacother* 30:1246-1248, 1996.

23. Singer E, Dionne R: A controlled evaluation of ibuprofen and diazepam for chronic orofacial muscle pain, *J Orofac Pain* 11:139-146, 1997.

24. Dao TT, Lavigne GJ: Oral splints: the crutches for temporomandibular disorders and bruxism? *Crit Rev Oral Biol Med* 9:345-361, 1998.

25. Fricton J: Myogenous temporomandibular disorders: diagnostic and management considerations, *Dent Clin North Am* 51:61-83, 2007.

26. Fricton J: Current evidence providing clarity in management of temporomandibular disorders: summary of a systematic review of randomized clinical trials for intra-oral appliances and occlusal therapies, *J Evid Based Dent Pract* 6:48-52, 2006.

27. Ekberg E, Nilner M: Treatment outcome of appliance therapy in temporomandibular disorder patients with myofascial pain after 6 and 12 months, *Acta Odontol Scand* 62:343-349, 2004.

28. Wassell RW, Adams N, Kelly PJ: The treatment of temporomandibular disorders with stabilizing splints in general dental practice: one-year follow-up, *J Am Dent Assoc* 137:1089-1098, quiz 1168-1169, 2006.

29. Al-Ani Z, Gray RJ, Davies SJ, et al: Stabilization splint therapy for the treatment of temporomandibular myofascial pain: a systematic review, *J Dent Educ* 69:1242-1250, 2005.

30. Al-Ani MZ, Davies SJ, Gray RJM, et al: Stabilization splint therapy for temporomandibular pain dysfunction, Cochrane Database Syst Rev 1:CD002778, 2004.

31. Seligman DA, Pullinger AG: Analysis of occlusal variables, dental attrition, and age for distinguishing healthy controls from female patients with intracapsular temporomandibular disorders, *J Prosthet Dent* 83:76-82, 2000.

32. Pullinger AG, Seligman DA: Quantification and validation of predictive values of occlusal variables in temporomandibular disorders using a multifactorial analysis. *J Prosthet Dent* 83:66-75, 2000.

33. Tsukiyama Y, Baba K, Clark GT: An evidence-based assessment of occlusal adjustment as a treatment for temporomandibular disorders, *J Prosthet Dent* 86:57-66, 2001.

34. Koh H, Robinson PG: Occlusal adjustment for treating and preventing temporomandibular joint disorders, *Cochrane Database Syst Rev* 1:CD003812, 2007.

35. Dworkin SF: The case for incorporating biobehavioral treatment into TMD management, *J Am Dent Assoc* 127:1607-1610, 1996.

36. Turk DC: Psychosocial and behavioral assessment of patients with temporomandibular disorders: diagnostic and treatment implications, *Oral Surg Oral Med Oral Pathol Oral Radiol Endod* 83:65-71, 1997.

37. Raphael KG, Klausner JJ, Nayak S, et al: Complementary and alternative therapy use by patients with myofascial temporomandibular disorders, *J Orofac Pain* 17:36-41, 2003.

38. Crider A, Glaros AG, Gevirtz RN: Efficacy of biofeedback-based treatments for temporomandibular disorders, *Appl Psychophysiol Biofeedback* 30:333-345, 2005.

39. Stowell AW, Gatchel RJ, Wildenstein L: Cost-effectiveness of treatments for temporomandibular disorders: biopsychosocial intervention versus treatment as usual, *J Am Dent Assoc* 138:202-208, 2007.

40. NIH Technology Assessment Panel: Integration of behavioral and relaxation approaches into the treatment of chronic pain and insomnia. Special communication, *JAMA* 276:313-318, 1996.

41. De Laat A, Stappaerts K, Papy S: Counseling and physical therapy as treatment for myofascial pain of the masticatory system, *J Orofac Pain* 17:42-49, 2003.

42. Venancio Rde A, Camparis CM, Lizarelli Rde F: Low intensity laser therapy in the treatment of temporomandibular disorders: a double-blind study, *J Oral Rehabil* 32:800-807, 2005.

43. McNeely ML, Armijo Olivo S, Magee DJ: A systematic review of the effectiveness of physical therapy interventions for temporomandibular disorders, *Phys Ther* 86:710-725, 2006.

44. Medlicott MS Harris SR: A systematic review of the effectiveness of exercise, manual therapy, electrotherapy, relaxation training, and biofeedback in the management of temporomandibular disorder, *Phys Ther* 86:955-973, 2006.

45. Craane B, De Laat A, Dijkstra PU, et al: Physical therapy for the management of patients with temporomandibular disorders and related pain, *Cochrane Database Syst Rev* 2:2007.

46. Israel HA, Syrop SB: The important role of motion in the rehabilitation of patients with mandibular hypomobility: a review of the literature, *Cranio* 15:74-83, 1997.

47. Horrell BM, Vogel LD, Israel HA: Passive motion therapy in temporomandibular joint disorders: the use of a new hydraulic device and case reports, *Compend Contin Educ Dent* 18:73-76, 1997.

48. Israel HA: Part 1: the use of arthroscopic surgery for the treatment of temporomandibular joint disorders, *J Oral Maxillofac Surg* 57:579-582, 1999.

49. Israel HA, Diamond B, Saed-Nejad F, et al: Osteoarthritis and synovitis as major pathoses of the temporomandibular joint: comparison of clinical diagnosis with arthroscopic morphology, *J Oral Maxillofac Surg* 56:1023-1027, 1998.

50. Dimitroulis G: The prevalence of osteoarthrosis in cases of advanced internal derangement of the temporomandibular joint: a clinical,

surgical and histological study, *Int J Oral Maxillofac Surg* 34:345-349, 2005.

51. Bjornland T, Gjaerum AA, Moystad O: Osteoarthritis of the temporomandibular joint: an evaluation of the effects and complications of corticosteroid injections compared with injection with sodium hyaluronate, *J Oral Rehabil* 34:583-589, 2007.

52. Koslin MG: Advanced arthroscopic surgery, *Oral Maxillofac Surg Clin North Am* 18:329-343, 2006.

53. Limchaichana N, Petersson A, Rohlin M: The efficacy of magnetic resonance imaging in the diagnosis of degenerative and inflammatory temporomandibular joint disorders: a systematic literature review, *Oral Surg Oral Med Oral Pathol Oral Radiol Endod* 102:521-536, 2006.

54. Kaban LB: Acquired abnormalities of the temporomandibular joint, juvenile rheumatoid arthritis. In: Kaban LB, Troulis MJ, editors: *Pediatric oral and maxillofacial surgery*, Philadelphia, 2004, WB Saunders, pp 372-375.

55. Etiology of trigeminal neuralgia [editorial], *JAMA* 194:553, 1965.

56. Adams CB: Trigeminal neuralgia: pathogenesis and treatment, *Br J Neurosurg* 11:493-495, 1997.

57. Anastasiades P: [Idiopathic neuralgia of the trigeminal nerve], *Stomatologia (Athenai)* 37:233-242, 1980.

58. Bayer DB, Stenger TG: Trigeminal neuralgia: an overview, *Oral Surg Oral Med Oral Pathol* 48:393-399, 1979.

59. Bowsher D: Trigeminal neuralgia: an anatomically oriented review, *Clin Anat* 10:409-415, 1997.

60. Brachmann F: [The etiology and pathogenesis of trigeminal neuralgia], *Zahnarztl Prax* 17:112-114, 1966.

61. Brito AJ: [Trigeminal neuralgia], *Acta Med Port* 12:187-193, 1999.

62. Canavero S, Bonicalzi V, Pagni CA: The riddle of trigeminal neuralgia, *Pain* 60:229-231, 1995.

63. Carney LR: Considerations on the cause and treatment of trigeminal neuralgia, *Neurology* 17:1143-1151, 1967.

64. White JC, Sweet WH: *Pain: its mechanisms and neurosurgical control*, Springfield, IL, 1955, Charles C Thomas.

65. Cheng TM, Cascino TL, Onofrio BM: Comprehensive study of diagnosis and treatment of trigeminal neuralgia secondary to tumors, *Neurology* 43:2298-2302, 1993.

66. Mathews ES, Scrivani SJ: Percutaneous stereotactic radiofrequency thermal rhizotomy for the treatment of trigeminal neuralgia, *Mt Sinai J Med* 67:288-299, 2000.

67. Merskey H, Bogduk N: *Classification of chronic pain: descriptions of chronic pain syndromes and definitions of pain terms*, 1994, IASP Press.

68. McQuay RH, Tramer M, Nye BA, et al: A systematic review of antidepressants in neuropathic pain, *Pain* 68:217-227, 1996.

69. Sindrup SH, Jensen TS: Efficacy of pharmacological treatments of neuropathic pain: an update and effect related to mechanism of drug actions, *Pain* 83:389-400, 1999.

70. Mellis M, Zawawi K, Badawi E, et al: Complex regional pain syndrome in the head and neck: a review of the literature, *J Orofac Pain* 16:93-104, 2002.

71. McFarland HR: Chronic traumatic trigeminal neuralgia, *South Med J* 75:814-816, 1982.

72. Sweet WH: Deafferentation pain after posterior rhizotomy, trauma to a limb and herpes zoster, *Neurosurgery* 15:928-932, 1984.

73. Gregg JM: Studies of traumatic neuralgias of the maxillofacial region: surgical pathology and neural mechanisms, *J Oral Maxillofac Surg* 48:228-237, 1990.

74. Dworkin RH, Backonja M, Rowbathan M, et al: Advances in neuropathic pain: diagnosis, mechanisms and treatment recommendations. Neurological review, *Arch Neurol* 60:1524-1534, 2003.

75. Dworkin RH, O'Connor AB, Backonja M, et al: Pharmacological management of neuropathic pain: evidence-based recommendations, *Pain* 132:237-251, 2007.

76. Taub E, Munz M, Tasker RR: Chronic electrical stimulation of the gasserian ganglion for the relief of pain in a series of 34 patients, *J Neurosurg* 86:197-202, 1997.

77. Nguyen JP, Lefaucher JP, Le Guerinel C, et al: Motor cortex stimulation in the treatment of central and neuropathic pain, *Arch Med Res* 31:263-265, 2000.

78. Tirakotai W, Riegel T, Sure U, et al: Image-guided motor cortex stimulation in patients with central pain, *Minim Invasive Neurosurg* 47:273-277, 2004.

79. Brown JA, Pilitsis JG: Motor cortex stimulation for central and neuropathic facial pain: a prospective study of 10 patients and observations of enhanced sensory and motor function during stimulation, *Neurosurgery* 56:290-297, discussion 290-297, 2005.

80. Donahue JG, Choo PW, Manson JE, et al: The incidence of herpes zoster. *Arch Intern Med* 155:1605-1609, 1995.

81. Dworkin RH, Portenoy RK: Pain and its persistence in herpes zoster, *Pain* 67:241-251, 1996.

82. Choo PW, Galil K, Donahue JG, et al: Risk factors for postherpetic neuralgia, *Arch Intern Med* 157:1217-1224, 1997.

83. Haanpaa M, Laippala P, Nurmikko T: Allodynia and pinprick hypesthesia in acute herpes zoster, and the development of postherpetic neuralgia, *J Pain Symptom Manage* 20:50-58, 2000.

84. Whitley RJ, Gnann JW: Herpes zoster: focus on treatment in older adults, *Antiviral Res* 44:145-154, 1999.

85. Watson CP: A new treatment for postherpetic neuralgia, *N Engl J Med* 343:1563-1565, 2000.

86. Bowsher D: The effects of pre-emptive treatment of postherpetic neuralgia with amitriptyline: a randomized, double-blind, placebo-controlled trial, *J Pain Symptom Manage* 13:327-331, 1997.

87. Watson CP: The treatment of postherpetic neuralgia, *Neurology* 45(12 Suppl 8):S58-S60, 1995.

88. Woda A, Pionchon P: A unified concept of idiopathic orofacial pain: clinical features, *J Orofac Pain* 13:172-184, 1999.

89. Woda A, Pionchon P: A unified concept of idiopathic orofacial pain: pathophysiologic features, *J Orofac Pain* 14:196-212, 2000.

90. Grushka M: Clinical features of burning mouth syndrome, *Oral Surg Oral Med Oral Pathol* 63:30-36, 1987.

91. Grushka M, Sessle BJ, Howley TP: Psychophysical assessment of tactile, pain and thermal sensory functions in burning mouth syndrome, *Pain* 28:169-184, 1987.

92. Grushka M, Bartoshuk LM, Chapo AK, et al: Oral pain: associated with damage to taste. Paper presented at the Proceedings of the 10th World Congress on Pain, San Diego, CA, 2002.

93. Grushka M, Epstein J, Mott A: An open-label, dose escalation pilot study of the effect of clonazepam in burning mouth syndrome, *Oral Surg Oral Med Oral Pathol Oral Radiol Endod* 86:557-561, 1998.

94. Ching V, Grushka M, Epstein JB: Clinical efficacy of titrated anticonvulsant analgesics on atypical odontalgia and burning mouth syndrome: retrospective study (in preparation).

95. Petruzzi M, Lauritano D, De Benedittis M, et al: Systemic capsicin for burning mouth syndrome: short-term results of a pilot study, *J Oral Pathol Med* 33:111-114, 2004.

96. Femiano F, Gombos F, Scully C: Burning mouth syndrome: open trial of psychotherapy alone, medication with alpha-lipoic acid (thioctic acid), and combination therapy, *Med Oral* 9:8-13, 2004.

BIBLIOGRAPHY

Cheng TM, Cascino TL, Onofrio BM: Comprehensive study of diagnosis and treatment of trigeminal neuralgia secondary to tumors, *Neurology* 43:2298-2302, 1993.

de Laat A, Stappaerts K, Papy S: Counseling and physical therapy as treatment for myofascial pain of the masticatory system, *J Orofac Pain* 17:42-49, 2003.

Denucci DJ, Dionne RA, Dubner R: Identifying a neurobiologic basis for drug therapy in TMDs, *J Am Dent Assoc* 127:581-593, 1996.

Dionne RA: Pharmacologic treatments for temporomandibular disorders, *Oral Surg Oral Med Oral Pathol Oral Radiol Endod* 83:134-142, 1997.

Fordyce WE: Pain and suffering, a reappraisal, *Am Psychol* 43:276-283, 1988.

Goldstein DJ, Lu Y, Detke MJ, et al: Duloxetine versus placebo in patients with painful diabetic neuropathy, *Pain* 116:109-118, 2005.

Herman CR, Schiffman EL, Look JO, et al: The effectiveness of adding pharmacologic treatment with clonazepam or cyclobenzaprine to patient education and self-care for the treatment of jaw pain upon awakening: a randomized clinical trial, *J Orofac Pain* 16:64-70, 2002.

Israel HA: Part I: the use of arthroscopic surgery for treatment of temporomandibular joint disorders, *J Oral Maxillofac Surg* 57:579-582, 1999.

Kerins C, Carlson D, McIntosh J, et al: A role for cyclooxygenase II inhibitors in modulating temporomandibular joint inflammation from a meal pattern analysis perspective, *J Oral Maxillofac Surg* 62:989-995, 2004.

Kishi Y: Paroxetine-induced bruxism effectively treated with tandospirone, *J Neuropsychiatry Clin Neurosci* 19:90-91, 2007.

List T, Axelsson S, Leijon G: Pharmacologic interventions in the treatment of temporomandibular disorders, atypical facial pain, and burning mouth syndrome. A qualitative systematic review, *J Orofac Pain* 17:301-310, 2003.

Maciewicz R, Mason P, Strassman A, et al: Organization of the trigeminal nociceptive pathways, *Semin Neurol* 8:255-264, 1988.

Mathews ES, Scrivani SJ: Percutaneous stereotactic radiofrequency thermal rhizotomy for the treatment of trigeminal neuralgia, *Mt Sinai J Med* 67:288-299, 2000.

Max MB, Lynch SA, Muir J, et al: Effects of desipramine, amitriptyline and fluoxetine on pain in diabetic neuropathy, *N Engl J Med* 326:1250-1256, 1992.

McCain JP, Sanders B, Koslin MG, et al: Temporomandibular joint arthroscopy: a 6-year multicenter retrospective study of 4,831 joints. *J Oral Maxillofac Surg* 50:926-930, 1992.

Nguyen M, Maciewicz R, Bouckoms A, et al: Facial pain in patients with cerebellopontine angle meningiomas, *Clin J Pain* 2:3-9, 1986.

Nitzan DW, Dolwick MF, Heft MW: Arthroscopic lavage and lysis of the temporomandibular joint: a change in perspective, *J Oral Maxillofac Surg* 48:798-801, discussion 802, 1990.

Okeson JP: *Bell's orofacial pains: the clinical management of orofacial pains*, ed 6, Chicago, 2004, Quintessence.

Onghena P, Van Houdenhove B: Antidepressant-induced analgesia in chronic nonmalignant pain: a meta-analysis of 39 placebo-controlled studies, *Pain* 49:205-219, 1992.

Perrott DH, Alborzi A, Kaban LB, et al: A prospective evaluation of the effectiveness of temporomandibular joint arthroscopy, *J Oral Maxillofac Surg* 48:1029-1032, 1990.

Rizzatti-Barbosa CM, Martinelli DA, Ambrosano GM, et al: Therapeutic response of benzodiazepine, orphenadrine citrate and occlusal splint association in TMD pain, *Cranio* 21:116-120, 2003.

Rowbotham MC, Goli V, Kunz NR, et al: Venlafaxine extended release in the treatment of painful diabetic neuropathy: a double-blind, placebo-controlled study, *Pain* 110:697-706, 2004.

Schutz TC, Andersen ML, Tufik S: Effects of COX-2 inhibitor in temporomandibular joint acute inflammation, *J Dent Res* 86:475-479, 2007.

Sindrup SH, Bach FW, Madsen C, et al: Venlafaxine versus imipramine in painful polyneuropathy: a randomized, controlled trial, *Neurology* 60:1284-1289, 2003.

Sullivan MD, Robinson JP: Antidepressant and anticonvulsant medication for chronic pain, *Phys Med Rehabil Clin N Am* 17:381-400, 2006.

Ta LE, Dionne RA: Treatment of painful temporomandibular joints with a cyclooxygenase-2 inhibitor: a randomized placebo-controlled comparison of celecoxib to naproxen, *Pain* 111:13-21, 2004.

Travell J, Rinzler SH: The myofascial genesis of pain, *Postgrad Med* 11:425-434, 1952.

Truelove E, Huggins KH, Mancl L, et al: The efficacy of traditional, low-cost and nonsplint therapies for temporomandibular disorder: a randomized controlled trial, *J Am Dent Assoc* 137:1099-1107, 2006.

Chapter **32**

The Pharmacology of Ketamine and Its Use in Outpatient Anesthesia

Christopher T. Kirkup, Jeffrey Bennett

Ketamine was initially introduced into clinical practice 40 years ago.[1] It was hoped that this new dissociative anesthetic would fulfill many of the ideal characteristics of an anesthetic drug, including analgesia and induction of loss of consciousness, while allowing a single-agent technique. Ketamine's side effects, as well as the introduction of newer intravenous induction agents, soon caused a decline in the use of this drug. Recently, however, there has been a resurgence in the use of ketamine as realization of its useful clinical applications has expanded beyond dissociative anesthesia.[2,3] Better understanding of the pharmacologic properties of ketamine has elucidated a number of clinical situations in which it is an ideal adjunctive or primary anesthetic agent. Such situations include intramuscular (IM) sedation of uncooperative patients, induction of anesthesia in patients with asthmatic disease, anesthetic management of patients in hemodynamic shock, and supplementation of regional or local anesthetic techniques. Newer studies are focusing on the neuroprotective effects of ketamine,[4-6] as well as preemptive analgesia and management of pain control in opioid-tolerant patients.[7-10] This chapter first examines the basic pharmacology of ketamine with a organ system approach, followed by a review of the useful clinical applications of ketamine in the outpatient anesthesia setting.

CLINICAL PHARMACOLOGY

PHARMACOKINETICS AND PHARMACODYNAMICS

Ketamine consists of a racemic mixture of two optical enantiomers, R(−) and S(+). The disposition of ketamine is similar to that of the short-acting barbiturates in that it has a rapid onset of effect, relatively short duration of action, and high lipid solubility. Peak plasma levels are achieved within 5 minutes following IM injection.[11] Ketamine is then distributed to highly perfused tissues, where levels four to five times those in plasma are achieved. The drug is then redistributed to vessel-poor tissues. The alpha elimination phase is several minutes, and the beta half-life is 2 to 3 hours. The major metabolic pathway involves N-demethylation by the cytochrome P-450 system to form the major metabolite norketamine. This metabolite appears to be a fifth to a third as potent as the original compound and may be involved in the prolonged analgesic effect of the drug.[12] Other anesthetic agents may alter the pharmacodynamics of ketamine. Diazepam, for example, has been shown to cause an increase in plasma levels of ketamine, as well as a decreased clearance rate.[13] Nitrous oxide has also been shown to reduce the amount of ketamine required to achieve surgical anesthesia, in addition to shortening the recovery period.[14]

MECHANISM OF ACTION

The binding of ketamine at receptors is complex and not fully understood. This drug interacts at multiple sites, including N-methyl-D-aspartate (NMDA) and non-NMDA glutamate receptors, nicotinic and muscarinic cholinergic receptors, and sodium, potassium, and calcium ion channels.[15-19] All these interactions may play a role in the clinical properties of ketamine; however, NMDA antagonism is primarily responsible for the analgesic, amnestic, and dissociative effects of the drug. The NMDA receptor is activated by the excitatory neurotransmitter glutamate. Ketamine binds to the phencyclidine receptor on the NMDA channel and inhibits glutamate stimulation of the channel noncompetitively. The S(+) enantiomer has three to four times the affinity as R(−) for the NMDA receptor. This difference correlates with the disparity observed in their analgesic and anesthetic effects.[20]

Ketamine also interacts with non-NMDA glutamate receptors as well. The effects are manifested through the glutamate–cyclic guanosine monophosphate–nitric oxide (NO) system. NO is known to be a central and peripheral transmitter involved in pain perception. Inhibition of NO synthase by ketamine is probably involved in its analgesic effects.[21]

Ketamine has also been shown to interact with nicotinic and muscarinic cholinergic receptors.[22,23] Because ketamine increases muscle tone by central mechanisms,[24] its inhibitory effect on nicotinic receptors in skeletal muscle is not apparent clinically but can be uncovered with muscle relaxants.[25]

CARDIOVASCULAR EFFECTS

Ketamine is a cardiovascular stimulant that induces increases in heart rate, blood pressure, and cardiac output.[26-28] Tweed and co-workers demonstrated a 33% increase in heart rate, 28% increase in blood pressure, and 29% increase in cardiac output.[26] Elucidation of the exact mechanisms of cardiovascular changes is difficult because they are probably the result of a complex interaction of direct drug effects on peripheral vessels, sympathetic stimulation, and modification of baroreceptor reflexes.[26] It was originally thought that the cardiostimulatory effects of ketamine were due to increased stimulation of the sympathetic nervous system with a concomitant increase in norepinephrine activity mediated by decreased baroreceptor control. Recent studies have demonstrated decreased sympathetic outflow when systemic blood pressure increases during ketamine anesthesia.[28] Sympathetic outflow was constant, however, when blood pressure was controlled with nitroprusside, thus indicating normal baroreceptor control in response to increased pressure with ketamine anesthesia. This study found increased plasma concentrations of both epinephrine and norepinephrine, even in patients with normalized blood pressure. It was concluded that ketamine has the effect of inhibiting catecholamine reuptake, thereby causing increased sympathetic tone locally in tissues.

Ketamine does not seem to have a significant effect on systemic vascular resistance.[29] This is due to its direct dilational effects on vascular smooth muscle in combination with sympathetically mediated vasoconstriction.[30] An early study indicated that there was no change in myocardial oxygen extraction with ketamine administration.[31] However, careful consideration should be given to the administration of ketamine to patients in whom coronary ischemia is a risk because increases in coronary blood flow through the vasodilatory effects of ketamine may be insufficient to meet the metabolic demands required by the increase in the rate-pressure product and cardiac work. Ketamine-induced cardiovascular stimulation and the rise in plasma free norepinephrine levels may be attenuated by premedication with diazepam or midazolam.[32]

It is well established that in the absence of autonomic control, ketamine has direct myocardial depressive properties. Critically ill or acutely traumatized patients may respond to ketamine with an unexpected drop in blood pressure because the sympathomimetic actions of ketamine are not balanced by the myocardial depressant and vasodilatory properties.[33-35] This effect may be exacerbated by the depressant effects of inhalational anesthetics.

RESPIRATORY EFFECTS

Clinical studies have demonstrated an increase in pulmonary compliance and a decrease in airway resistance and bronchospasm following the administration of ketamine. Maintenance of functional residual capacity also results with ketamine administration.[36-38] Propranolol mitigates the bronchodilation of epinephrine, but not that of ketamine, thus suggesting a mechanism other than beta-receptor interaction. This is probably due to its vagolytic and direct smooth muscle effects. Ketamine itself does not produce significant respiratory depression unless given as a rapid intravenous (IV) infusion. The respiratory response to carbon dioxide is maintained during ketamine anesthesia.[39] Additionally, ketamine appears to antagonize the opiate-induced depression of the respiratory drive.[40] These findings do not obviate the need for careful airway management during ketamine anesthesia. Both salivary and tracheal mucus secretion is increased by ketamine administration. Although retention of protective pharyngeal and laryngeal reflexes is reported, aspiration can occur following ketamine induction.[41,42]

CEREBRAL BLOOD FLOW AND INTRACRANIAL PRESSURE

Ketamine may have a protective role in the treatment of head-injured patients.[4-6] It antagonizes the excitatory amino acids at the NMDA receptor and may reduce the neuronal damage that occurs in patients with intracranial injury. Ketamine is infrequently used for the management of head-injured patients because of its detrimental effects on cerebral blood flow and intracranial pressure (ICP).[43-45] Newer studies outlining the use of ketamine in head-injury patients have been published[46-48] and suggest minimal effects on ICP and patient outcome when using specific multi-agent protocols. These preliminary studies suggest a role for ketamine in patients with intracranial injury, but further studies are warranted.

Ketamine was initially implicated in lowering the seizure threshold.[49] Current opinion is that ketamine possesses anticonvulsant activity and has been used clinically for the treatment of status epilepticus.[50]

CLINICAL APPLICATIONS

PROCEDURAL ANESTHESIA

A considerable amount of recent research on the use of ketamine for outpatient anesthesia is derived from the emergency medicine literature, particularly Green's group at Loma Linda, California.[51-54] They published a large review of the literature in 1990 as the popularity of using ketamine in the pediatric population was increasing.[51,52] Recently, the same group published an update of practice guidelines and a review of treatment recommendations.[54] This overview translates well to the management of outpatient oral and maxillofacial surgery patients, particularly the pediatric population.

Ketamine is unlike any other single anesthetic agent. This drug disconnects the thalamic and limbic systems to create a dissociative anesthetic state. This is achieved by simultaneous depression of the cortical and stimulation of the limbic systems. The result is a cataleptic state marked by potent analgesia, amnesia, and sedation with maintenance of cardiovascular stability and protective airway reflexes, as well as bronchodilation.[1,26,28,33,36,37,41] This unique combination of effects makes the agent very useful for painful procedures in patients in whom traditional anesthetic techniques would be very difficult or dangerous. The safety and efficacy of IM dosing make ketamine an ideal agent in the pediatric population or in patients with behavioral problems.

When used as a single agent, the dissociative state produced by ketamine does not have the continuum appreciated with other anesthetic agents.[52,55] The state either exists, or it does not. Once dissociation is achieved, further delivery of agent does not heighten the sedative or analgesic properties. Thus, the drug can be delivered as a single IM or IV bolus dose, with subsequent doses necessary only to maintain the dissociated state.

Because of the unique physiologic responses to ketamine, the sedated state can be called neither deep sedation nor general anesthesia. The patient is unable to respond to external stimuli but retains protective airway reflexes and maintains spontaneous ventilation. Green and Krauss define dissociative anesthesia as "a trancelike cataleptic state induced by the dissociative agent ketamine characterized by profound analgesia and amnesia, with retention of protective airway reflexes, spontaneous respirations, and cardiopulmonary stability."[53]

DOSING, ROUTE OF ADMINISTRATION, AND RECOVERY

Ketamine may be administered by the IM, IV, oral, rectal, or intranasal routes. Research studies support the safety and efficacy of these techniques, and thus the choice should be based on the clinical situation of the patient.[56,57] If IV access is available, it should be used to avoid the pain associated with IM injection. Once anesthesia has been achieved with an IM dose, it is prudent to establish vascular access, particularly if subsequent dosing is anticipated. IV access is also useful in adults for administration of additional agents in the event of unpleasant emergence reactions. A single IM or IV dose should provide approximately 20 minutes of an optimal level of anesthesia.[56,57] Because of the relative ease of titration with an IV technique when compared with other routes of administration, IV administration may provide more rapid recovery by limiting the amount of agent delivered to achieve the desired effect.

In its early use, a typical IM dose of ketamine was 15 mg/kg.[52] More recent studies suggest that 4 to 5 mg/kg should result in adequate anesthesia in most cases. In the event that this dose is ineffective, a full dose or half dose may be repeated in 10 minutes.[56]

The suggested IV dose to achieve adequate anesthesia is 1.5 mg/kg when used in a single-agent technique.[52,57] This may be supplemented with additional doses of 0.5 to 1 mg/kg until the desired state is achieved. It should be noted that although ketamine preserves spontaneous respiration, transient respiratory depression has been associated with rapid bolus dosing, and therefore IV dosing should be administered over a 60-second period.[52,57]

Oral ketamine has been shown to be a useful anesthetic technique. In the authors' opinion, the goal of oral ketamine is to establish a cataleptic state in a combative patient in whom IM injection or IV access cannot be achieved without risking injury to the health care provider. The effects of oral dosing are less predictable than those of parenteral routes, and a range of dosing from 3 to 10 mg/kg has been suggested.[58-62] As a single agent to achieve a dissociative state, 6 to 8 mg/kg is a reasonably efficacious dose.[58,60] The concomitant administration of additional oral premedications may necessitate adjustment in ketamine dosing.

The discussion of recovery after the administration of ketamine is complicated by the wide variety of reported anesthetic techniques, as well as the disparity in discharge criteria among reported studies. In some reports, the time to recovery from the onset of clinical effects ranged from 70 to 110 minutes after oral administration.[61,62] The addition of oral midazolam did not appear to significantly prolong the recovery period.[62] However, in another report, 20% of the patients were deeply sedated at 120 minutes with recovery taking up to 4 hours.[63] For IV and IM administration, similar ranges of 98 to 130 minutes are reported.[64-66] Evidence suggests that the combined administration of midazolam via these routes may prolong recovery periods.[66] A study comparing recovery following IM or IV ketamine and midazolam found equal effectiveness between the two groups, but a significantly longer recovery period with IV administration.[66]

Regardless of the duration of the recovery period, few adverse effects are associated with ketamine sedation, particularly when compared with other anesthetic techniques. A prospective study by Newman and colleagues compared outcomes of IM and IV ketamine anesthesia with other anesthetic techniques. Risk ratios of 0.68 and 0.86 were reported for ketamine and for ketamine with midazolam and atropine, respectively.[67]

EMERGENCE DELIRIUM

The emergence phenomena reported with ketamine have been well documented and include alterations in mood and body image, dissociative experiences, vivid dreams and illusions, and delirium.[68-71] The frequency of such reactions has been reported to be between 5% and 30%.[72,73] Emergence delirium occurs more frequently in patients older than 16 years, in female patients, in subjects who frequently dream, and with large IV doses of ketamine (>2 mg/kg or >40 mg/min).[74-76] A variety of agents have been suggested for premedication or simultaneous administration in an attempt to attenuate these effects. Benzodiazepines have been shown to decrease the sympathomimetic effects of ketamine.[77] This is believed to be related to the γ-aminobutyric acid (GABA)-mediated effects of these drugs. Since midazolam is pharmacokinetically similar to ketamine, it should be preferable for that purpose.[78] Because benzodiazepines may increase the recovery period following ketamine anesthesia and they appear to rapidly and consistently alleviate the emergence phenomena,[66] it may be prudent to use these agents only when necessary.

PREEMPTIVE ANALGESIA

Research suggests that activation of the NMDA receptor may be involved in the hyperalgesia after tissue injury, as well as the development to tolerance of opioids.[79] As an NMDA receptor antagonist, ketamine may prevent or reverse central sensitization to pain, thus decreasing postoperative pain, as well as enhancing opiate antinociception.[79-81] These analgesic effects are demonstrated at doses lower than those typically used to provide single-agent sedation with ketamine. Low-dose ketamine implies a dose of less than 2 mg/kg intramuscularly or 1 mg/kg intravenously. Research also suggests that there may be an even lower dose range that does not have intrinsic analgesic properties but may enhance pain control when used in combination with opioids.[82,83] As a sole analgesic agent, ketamine provides significant pain relief only at levels approaching the upper end of the low-dose range (1 mg/kg intravenously).[84]

Synergistic analgesic effects have been reported with the addition of low-dose ketamine to opioids.[82,85] Other studies indicate an additive effect.[86,87] This additive effect is probably due to the presynaptic opioid inhibition and afferent signal reduction in combination with postsynaptic NMDA blockade. Low-dose ketamine in combination with opioids may therefore be considered to be preventive of hyperalgesia rather than being purely analgesic.

SPECIAL PATIENT POPULATIONS: SCHIZOPHRENIA, AUTISM, AND DEPRESSIVE DISORDERS

Evidence suggests that the NMDA receptor is involved in the pathophysiology of schizophrenia. The administration of phencyclidine or ketamine has been reported to exacerbate the psychotic symptoms of the disease.[88] Ketamine has been used to elicit schizophrenic-like thought disorders in healthy volunteers.[89] For this reason, ketamine is often considered unsuitable for schizophrenic patients because it may induce psychotic emergence reactions in these patients. Although the use of ketamine certainly deserves careful consideration in this patient population, there is evidence that the drug may be used in combined-agent techniques without adverse outcomes.[90,91] Techniques using ketamine, fentanyl, and propofol have been reported with success. Even in light of these findings, more traditional anesthetic techniques may be prudent in this patient population.

The anesthetic management of autistic patients is challenging because they do not react well to changes in routine. For this reason, both oral and IM ketamine anesthetic techniques have proved useful in the management of these patients.[92,93] Traditional doses of 5 mg/kg intramuscularly or 6 to 8 mg/kg orally are suggested. There are no significant differences in the postoperative recovery of these patients. Even though precipitation of seizures in autistic patients is a concern, ketamine has been used for the treatment of seizures,[50] and no adverse events of seizure precipitation are reported in this group of patients. This technique also translates well to other patient populations in whom cooperation and excitability obviate the use of other induction methods.

The medical community is gaining an appreciation for the prevalence of depressive disorders. It is widely believed that as much as 10% of the population may be affected by these conditions. Current research indicates that the NMDA class of receptors is involved in the pathophysiology of major depression and the mechanism of action of antidepressant treatments.[94] Clinical trials have indicated that the administration of low-dose ketamine (0.5 mg/kg) has a significant antidepressant effect beyond the traditional clinical anesthetic effects of the drug.[95] Although further research in this area is certainly warranted, these findings suggest that ketamine is unlikely to exacerbate and may actually attenuate symptoms of depression postoperatively.

PEDIATRIC ANESTHETIC TECHNIQUES

Anesthesia and outpatient surgery can be an extremely stressful and even traumatic experience for pediatric patients. Ideally, outpatient anesthetic techniques should safely provide amnesia, analgesia, anxiolysis, immobility, and maintenance of cardiovascular and pulmonary function. An ideal agent exhibits ease of application, rapid onset, short duration of action, and lack of significant side effects. A wide variety of medications have been used for outpatient surgery and pediatric procedural anesthesia in the emergency department. Such medications include narcotics, benzodiazepines, barbiturates, antihistamines, propofol, chloral hydrate, and inhalational agents. One medication that has gained considerable acceptance as a pediatric anesthetic agent is ketamine. This drug comes as close as any to fulfilling the criteria for an ideal agent. It may be administered via a variety of routes, including oral, IM, IV, intranasal, and rectal.[96,97] Ketamine may be used effectively as a single-agent technique or in combination with many other anesthetic agents.

Although a tremendous variety of techniques have been reported to be successful, the combination of IM ketamine, a benzodiazepine, and anticholinergic medications seems to have widespread acceptance.[56,98] Pruitt and colleagues suggest dosing ketamine at 3 mg/kg, midazolam at 0.05 mg/kg, and glycopyrrolate at 0.005 mg/kg. Thirty percent of the patients who received this regimen had intermittent crying. A subsequent 1-mg/kg dose of ketamine was required in 14% of their patients. This regimen provides adequate sedation conditions for 30 minutes and a discharge time of 76 minutes from the initial injection. Midazolam seems to be the obvious choice of benzodiazepine because its pharmacokinetic profile is similar to that of ketamine. Midazolam also exhibited a better reduction in the incidence of unpleasant dreams than diazepam did.[99] Green and Johnson suggested a dose of 4 mg/kg of ketamine intramuscularly.[52] They found that this dose in conjunction with local anesthesia and mild restraint provided effective sedation and immobilization for minor emergency department procedures in approximately 97% of their patients. The working time for this dosing regimen was between 15 and 30 minutes with a mean recovery time of 82 minutes. Recovery with both techniques, however, was variable and could last several hours. For a brief surgical procedure, the surgeon may consider an IM dose of 2 to 3 mg/kg. Frequently, this dose is sufficient to alter the child's perception and allow completion of the procedure, although the practitioner will have to tolerate some movement and vocalization. The lower dose is advantageous in that it may expedite recovery and subsequent discharge. If the initial dose is insufficient, an additional IM injection may be given. Alternatively, the effect achieved from the initial injection will frequently allow the establishment of IV access, and anesthetic depth can be modified by titration of the IV medications.

Because salivation and tracheal and bronchial secretions are stimulated by ketamine, use of an anticholinergic medication is prudent to reduce the risk for aspiration. There does seem to be some variability in the choice of anticholinergic agent. Because of its quaternary amine structure, glycopyrrolate does not pass the blood-brain barrier as atropine and scopolamine do. Atropine and scopolamine can cause postoperative delirium secondary to their central effect. Glycopyrrolate also has a greater antisialagogue effect than atropine does, whereas atropine has a greater effect on the heart rate than glycopyrrolate does. Despite the ability of atropine to cross the blood-brain barrier, it has not been shown to increase the incidence of emergence phenomena. The change in heart rate may be greater with atropine.[100] Finally, consideration must be given to the route of anticholinergic administration. The peak effect of glycopyrrolate administered intramuscularly and intravenously is achieved in approximately 30 minutes and 1 minute, respectively.

Both techniques seem to be predictable and reliable. IV access is strongly recommended. This allows subsequent administration of medications with more rapid onset and ease of titration, as well as the administration of emergency medications should the need arise.

ADULT ANESTHETIC TECHNIQUES

The utility of ketamine in adult anesthetic techniques is different from that in the pediatric population. For outpatient anesthesia, ketamine is rarely used as a primary agent. Instead, it may be used as an adjunctive agent in multidrug techniques, which allows the exploitation of its unique properties as an anesthetic medication. The use of ketamine in monitored anesthesia care techniques is widely reported.[101-106] Ketamine may be administered during induction as a bolus dose, by continuous infusion, or as a combination of the two techniques. Typically, the drug is given in doses significantly lower than the single-agent anesthetic dose. Bolus doses ranging from 0.1 to 1.0 mg/kg in combination with propofol, midazolam, or both have been reported. When administered via continuous infusion, a ketamine-propofol 1:5 admixture has been reported to be safe and efficacious, with no subsequent delay in recovery.[107]

An additional indication for ketamine in an adult patient is a situation in which a satisfactory depth of anesthesia cannot be achieved, with the patient alternating between struggling and apnea. The administration of a bolus of ketamine will establish a dissociative state in which the patient becomes quiescent. Bolus doses between 0.1 and 0.5 mg/kg should effectively provide approximately 15 minutes of working time. Patient recovery from ketamine is different from that with either propofol or methohexital and occurs both more slowly and calmly. The patient movements observed may be robotic, and as these movements become more purposeful, incremental doses of ketamine may be administered to maintain the dissociated state.

The pharmacologic actions of ketamine make it useful in the anesthetic management of asthmatic patients. A 0.75-mg/kg dose of ketamine has been shown to provide relief of bronchospasm in patients who failed to respond to conventional therapy.[108] Additionally, the analgesic effects of ketamine may obviate the need for narcotic agents, which can cause bronchospasm in susceptible individuals.

Ketamine may not be appropriate in all clinical situations, and its use must be carefully considered when performing anesthesia in patients with poor cardiopulmonary reserve or decreased ability to tolerate labile cardiovascular parameters. When given in combination with propofol, ketamine may considerably reduce the drop in blood pressure observed during induction with propofol alone.[34,35] The doses of propofol used for ambulatory anesthesia in the oral and maxillofacial surgery office, however, do not usually result in significant cardiodepressant effects, and the balancing effect described earlier should not provide the benefit that would be seen in other situations. The inclusion of ketamine must be weighed against the risk for coronary ischemia in this patient population.

PEARLS AND PITFALLS

- Ketamine provides unique capabilities for selected situations in the anesthetic management of both pediatric and adult patients.
- Ketamine interacts at multiple sites, including NMDA and non-NMDA glutamate receptors, nicotinic and muscarinic cholinergic receptors, and sodium, potassium, and calcium ion channels.
- Ketamine can be administered by IM, IV, oral, rectal, or intranasal routes, and the choice should be based on the patient's clinical situation.
- The emergence phenomena reported with ketamine involve alterations in mood and body image, dissociative experiences, vivid dreams and illusions, and delirium.
- Ketamine is often considered unsuitable for schizophrenic patients because it may induce psychotic emergence reactions in these patients.
- Ketamine's pharmacologic actions make it useful in the anesthetic management of asthmatic patients.
- Careful consideration should be given when managing anesthesia in patients with poor cardiopulmonary reserve or decreased ability to tolerate labile cardiovascular parameters.

REFERENCES

1. Domino CF, Chodoff P, Corssen G: Pharmacologic effects of CI-581, a new dissociative anesthetic in man, *Clin Pharmacol Ther* 6:279-291, 1965.
2. Kors R, Durieux ME: Ketamine: teaching an old drug new tricks, *Anesth Analg* 87:1186-1193, 1998.
3. Raeder J: Ketamine, revival of a versatile intravenous anesthetic. In Vuyk J, Schraag S, editors: *Advances in modeling and clinical application of intravenous anesthesia*, New York 2003, Kluwer Academic/Plenum Publish, pp 269-277.
4. Hoffman WE, Pelligrino D, Werner C, et al: Ketamine decreases plasma catecholamines and improves neurologic outcome from incomplete cerebral ischemia in rats, *Anesthesiology* 76:755-762, 1992.
5. Shapira Y, Lam AM, Engl CC, et al: Therapeutic time window and dose response of the beneficial effects of ketamine in experimental head injury, *Stroke* 25:1637-1643, 1994.
6. Himmelseher S, Pfenninger E, Georgieff M: The effects of ketamine isomers on neuronal injury and regeneration in rat hippocampal neurons, *Anesth Analg* 83:505-512, 1996.
7. Bell RF: Low-dose subcutaneous ketamine infusion and morphine tolerance, *Pain* 83:101-103, 1999.
8. Haines DR, Gaines SP: Randomised controlled trials of oral ketamine in patients with chronic pain, *Pain* 83:283-287, 1999.
9. Suzuki M, Tsueda K, Lansing PS, et al: Small-dose ketamine enhances morphine-induced analgesia after outpatient anesthesia, *Anesth Analg* 89:98-103, 1999.
10. Fu ES, Migue R, Scharf JE: Preemptive ketamine decreases postoperative narcotic requirements in patients undergoing abdominal surgery, *Anesth Analg* 84:1086-1090, 1997.
11. Zsigmond EK, Domino EF: Ketamine—clinical pharmacology, pharmacokinetics, and current clinical uses, *Anesth Rev* 7:13-33, 1980.
12. Marietta MP, White PF, Pudwill CR, et al: Biodisposition of ketamine in the rat: self-induction of metabolism, *J Pharmacol Exp Ther* 196:536-544, 1976.
13. Lo JN, Cumming JF: Interaction between sedative premedicants and ketamine in man and in isolated perfused rat livers, *Anesthesiology* 43:307-312, 1975.

14. Wessels JV, Allen GW, Slogoff F: The effect of nitrous oxide on ketamine anesthesia, *Anesthesiology* 39:382-386, 1973.

15. Orser BA, Pennefather PS, MacDonald JF: Multiple mechanisms of ketamine blockade of *N*-methyl-D-aspartate receptors, *Anesthesiology* 86:903-917, 1997.

16. Reckziegel G, Friederich P, Urban BW: Ketamine effects on human neuronal Na^+ channels, *Eur J Anaesthesiol* 19:634-640, 2002.

17. Friederich P, Benzenberg D, Urban BW: Ketamine and propofol differentially inhibit human neuronal K^+ channels. *Eur Acad Anesthesiol* 18:177-183, 2001.

18. Wagner LE 2nd, Gingrich KJ, Kulli JC, et al: Ketamine blockade of voltage-gated sodium channels: evidence for a shared receptor site with local anesthetics, *Anesthesiology* 95:1406-1413, 2001.

19. Andoh T, Sasaki T, Okumura F, et al: Effects of ketamine stereoisomers on neuronal nicotinic acetylcholine receptors, *Anesthesiology* 91:A801, 1999.

20. White PF, Schüttler J, Shafer A, et al: Comparative pharmacology of the ketamine isomers. Studies in volunteers, *Br J Anaesth* 57:197-203, 1985.

21. Irifune M, Shimizu T, Fukuda T: Ketamine-induced anesthesia involves the *N*-methyl-D-aspartate receptor-channel complex in mice, *Brain Res* 569:1-9, 1992.

22. Durieux ME, Nietgen GW: Synergistic inhibition of muscarinic signaling by ketamine stereoisomers and the preservative benzethonium chloride, *Anesthesiology* 86:1326-1333, 1997.

23. Aronstam S, Narayanan L, Wegner DA: Ketamine inhibition of ligand binding to cholinergic receptors and ion channels, *Eur J Pharmacol* 78:367-370, 1982.

24. Kienbaum P, Heuter T, Pavlakovic G, et al: S(+)-ketamine increases muscle sympathetic activity and maintains the neural response to hypotensive challenges in humans, *Anesthesiology* 94:252-258, 2001.

25. Kress HG: Actions of ketamine not related to the NMDA and opiate receptors, *Anaesthesist* 43:S15-S24, 1994.

26. Tweed WA, Minuck M, Mymin D: Circulatory responses to ketamine anesthesia, *Anesthesiology* 37:613-619, 1972.

27. Kunst G, Martin E, Graf BM, et al: Actions of ketamine and its isomers on contractility and calcium transients in human myocardium, *Anesthesiology* 90:1363-1371, 1999.

28. Kienbaum P, Heuter T, Michel M, et al: Racemic ketamine decreases muscle sympathetic activity but maintains the neural response to hypotensive challenges in humans, *Anesthesiology* 92:94-101, 2000.

29. Liao JC, Kohentop DE, Buckley JJ: Dual effects of ketamine on the peripheral vasculature, *Anesthesiology* 51:S116, 1979.

30. Gooding JM, Dimicki AR, Tavakoil M: A physiologic analysis of cardiopulmonary responses to ketamine anesthesia in noncardiac patients, *Anesth Analg* 56:813-816, 1977.

31. Smith G, Thorburn J, Vance JP, et al: The effects of ketamine on canine coronary circulation, *Anaesthesia* 34:555-561, 1979.

32. Jackson AF, Dhadphale PR, Callaghan ML: Haemodynamic studies during induction of anesthesia for open-heart surgery using diazepam and ketamine, *Br J Anaesth* 50:375-377, 1978.

33. Waxman K, Shoemaker WC, Lippman M: Cardiovascular effects of anesthetic induction with ketamine, *Anesth Analg* 59:355-358, 1980.

34. Hoka S, Yamaura K, Takenaka T, et al: Propofol-induced increase in vascular capacitance is due to inhibition of sympathetic vasoconstrictive activity, *Anesthesiology* 89:1495-1500, 1998.

35. Furuya A, Matsukawa T, Ozaki M, et al: Intravenous ketamine attenuates arterial pressure changes during the induction of anesthesia with propofol, *Eur J Anaesthesiol* 18:8-92, 2001.

36. Huber FC, Reves JG, Gutierrez J, et al: Ketamine: its effects on airway resistance in man, *South Med J* 65:1176-1180, 1972.

37. Lundy PM, Gowdy CW, Colhoun EH: Tracheal smooth muscle relaxant effect of ketamine, *Br J Anaesth* 46:333-336, 1974.

38. Sato T, Matsuki A, Zsigmond E, et al: Ketamine relaxes airway smooth muscle contracted by endothelin, *Anesth Analg* 84:900-906, 1997.

39. Soliman MG, Brinale GF, Kuster G: Response to hypercapnia under ketamine anesthesia, *Can Anaesth Soc J* 22:486-494, 1975.

40. Persson J, Scheinin H, Hellstrom G, et al: Ketamine antagonizes alfentanil-induced hypoventilation in healthy male volunteers, *Acta Anaesthesiol Scand* 43:744-752, 1999.

41. Lanning CF, Harmel MH: Ketamine anesthesia, *Annu Rev Med* 26:137-141, 1975.

42. Taylor PA, Towey RM: Depression of laryngeal reflexes during ketamine anesthesia, *BMJ* 2:688-689, 1971.

43. Takeshita H, Okuda Y, Sari A: The effects of ketamine on cerebral circulation and metabolism in man, *Anesthesiology* 36:69-75, 1972.

44. Whyte SR, Shapiro HM, Turner P, et al: Ketamine-induced intracranial hypertension, *Anesthesiology* 36:174-176, 1972.

45. Schwedler M, Miletich DJ, Albrecht RF: Cerebral blood flow and metabolism following ketamine administration, *Can Anaesth Soc J* 29:222-226, 1982.

46. Langsjo J, Kaisti K, Aalto S, et al: Effects of subanesthetic doses of ketamine on regional cerebral blood flow, oxygen consumption, and blood volume in humans, *Anesthesiology* 99:614-623, 1999.

47. Bourgoin A, Albanese J, Wereszczynski N, et al: Safety of sedation with ketamine in severe head injury patients: comparison with sufentanil, *Crit Care Med* 31:711-717, 2003.

48. Sakai S, Cho S, Fukusaki M, et al: The effects of propofol with and without ketamine on human cerebral blood flow velocity and CO_2 response, *Anesth Analg* 90:377-382, 2000.

49. Ferrer-Allado T, Brechner VL, Dymond A, et al: Ketamine induced electroconvulsive phenomena in the human limbic and thalamic regions, *Anesthesiology* 38:333-334, 1973.

50. Seth RD, Gidal BE: Refractory status epilepticus: response to ketamine, *Neurology* 51:1755-1756, 1998.

51. Green SM, Nakamura R, Johnson NE: Ketamine sedation for pediatric procedure part 1: a prospective series, *Ann Emerg Med* 19:1024-1032, 1990.

52. Green SM, Johnson NE: Ketamine sedation for pediatric procedures: part 2, review and implications, *Ann Emerg Med* 19:1033-1046, 1990.

53. Green SM, Krauss B: Clinical practice guideline for emergency department ketamine dissociative sedation in children, *Ann Emerg Med* 44:460-471, 2004.

54. Green SM, Hummel C, Wittlake W, et al: What is the optimal dose of intramuscular ketamine for pediatric sedation? *Acad Emerg Med* 6:21-26, 1999.

55. Green SM, Hummel CB, Wittlake W: The semantics of ketamine, *Ann Emerg Med* 36:480-482, 2000.

56. Green SM, Rothrock SG, Lynch EL, et al: Intramuscular ketamine for pediatric sedation in the emergency department: safety profile with 1022 cases, *Ann Emerg Med* 31:688-697, 1998.

57. Green SM, Rothrock SG, Harris T, et al: Intravenous ketamine for pediatric sedation in the emergency department: safety profile with 156 cases, *Acad Emerg Med* 5:971-976, 1998.

58. Turhanoglu A, Kararmaz A, Kaya S, et al: Effects of different doses of oral ketamine for premedication in children, *Eur J Anaesthesiol* 20:56-60, 2003.

59. Kararmaz A, Kaya S, Turhanoglu S, et al: Oral ketamine premedication can prevent emergence agitation in children after desflurane anesthesia, *Paediatr Anaesth* 14:477-482, 2004.

60. Sullivan D, Wilson C, Webb M: A comparison of two oral ketamine-diazepam regimens for the sedation of anxious pediatric dental patients, *Pediatr Dent* 23:223-231, 2001.

61. Younge PA, Kendall JM: Sedation for children requiring wound repair: a randomized controlled double blind comparison of oral midazolam and oral ketamine, *Emerg Med J* 18:30-33, 2001.

62. Funk W, Jakob W, Riedl T, et al: Oral preanesthetic medication for children: double-blinded randomized study of a combination of midazolam and ketamine vs midazolam and ketamine alone, *Br J Anaesth* 84:335-340, 2002.

63. Alderson PJ, Lerman J: Oral premedication for paediatric ambulatory anesthesia: a comparison of midazolam and ketamine, *Can J Anaesth* 41:221-226, 1994.

64. Gloor A, Diller D, Gerber A: Ketamine for short ambulatory procedures in children: an audit, *Paediatr Anaesth* 11:533-539, 2001.

65. Acworth J, Purdie D, Clark R: Intravenous ketamine plus midazolam is superior to intranasal midazolam for emergency paediatric procedural sedation, *Emerg Med J* 18:39-45, 2001.

66. Sherwin TS, Green SM, Khan A, et al: Does adjunctive midazolam reduce recovery agitation after ketamine sedation for pediatric procedures? A randomized, double-blind, placebo-controlled trial, *Ann Emerg Med* 35:239-244, 2000.

67. Newman D, Azer M, Pitetti RD, et al: When is a patient safe for discharge after procedural sedation? The timing of adverse effect events in 1367 pediatric procedural sedations, *Ann Emerg Med* 42:627-635, 2003.

68. Perel A, Davidson JT: Recurrent hallucinations following ketamine, *Anaesthesia* 31:1081-1083, 1976.

69. Meyers EF, Charles P: Prolonged adverse reactions to ketamine in children, *Anesthesiology* 49:39-40, 1978.

70. Fine J, Finestone SC: Sensory disturbances following ketamine anesthesia—recurrent hallucinations, *Anesth Analg* 52:428-430, 1973.

71. White PF, Way WL, Trevor AJ: Ketamine—its pharmacology and therapeutic uses, *Anesthesiology* 56:119-136, 1982.

72. White PF, Ham J, Way WL: Pharmacology of ketamine isomers in surgical patients, *Anesthesiology* 52:231-239, 1980.

73. Krestow M: The effect of post-anesthetic dreaming on patient acceptance of ketamine anesthesia: a comparison with thiopentone–nitrous oxide anesthesia, *Can Anaesth Soc J* 21:385-389, 1974.

74. Heja P, Galloon S: A consideration of ketamine anesthesia dreams, *Can Anaesth Soc J* 22:100-105, 1975.

75. Bovill J, Coppel DL, Dundee J, et al: Current status of ketamine anesthesia, *Lancet* 1:1285-1288, 1971.

76. Dundee J, Bovill J, Clarke RS, et al: Problems with ketamine in adults, *Anaesthesia* 26:86, 1971.

77. White PF: Comparative evaluation of intravenous agents for rapid sequence induction: thiopental, ketamine, and midazolam, *Anesthesiology* 57:279-284, 1982.

78. Cartwright PD, Pingel SM: Midazolam and diazepam in ketamine anesthesia, *Anaesthesia* 39:439-442, 1984.

79. Mao J, Price D, Mayer D: Mechanisms of hyperalgesia and morphine tolerance: a current review of their possible interactions, *Pain* 62:259-274, 1995.

80. Schmid R, Sandler A, Katz J: Use and efficacy of low-dose ketamine in the management of acute postoperative pain: a review of current techniques and outcomes, *Pain* 82:111-125, 1999.

81. Subramaniam K, Subramaniam B, Steinbrook R: Ketamine as adjuvant analgesic to opioids: a qualitative and quantitative systematic review, *Anesth Analg* 99:482-495, 2004.

82. Chapman V, Dickinson A: The combination of NMDA antagonism and morphine produces profound antinociception in the rat dorsal horn, *Brain Res* 73:321-323, 1992.

83. Dickinson A: Combination therapy in analgesia: seeking synergy, *Curr Opin Anesthesiol* 6:861-865, 1993.

84. Jahangir S, Islam F, Aziz L: Ketamine infusion for postoperative analgesia in asthmatics: a comparison with intermittent meperidine, *Anesth Analg* 76:45-49, 1993.

85. Honoré P, Chapman V, Buritova J, et al: Concomitant administration of morphine and an N-methyl-D-aspartate receptor antagonist profoundly reduces inflammatory evoked spinal c-Fos expression, *Anesthesiology* 85:150-160, 1996.

86. Sethna N, Liu M, Gracely R, et al: Analgesic and cognitive effects of intravenous ketamine-alfentanil combinations versus either drug alone after intradermal capsaicin in normal subjects, *Anesth Analg* 86:1250-1256, 1998.

87. Suzuki M, Tsueda K, Lansing PS, et al: Small-dose ketamine enhances morphine-induced analgesia after outpatient surgery, *Anesth Analg* 89:98-103, 1999.

88. Malhotra A, Pinals D, Adler CM, et al: Ketamine-induced exacerbation of psychotic symptoms and cognitive impairment in neuroleptic-free schizophrenics, *Neuropsychopharmacology* 1:9-19, 1997.

89. Lahti A, Weiler M, Tamara Michaelidis BA, et al: Effects of ketamine in normal and schizophrenic volunteers, *Neuropsychopharmacology* 25:455-467, 2001.

90. Ishihara H, Kudo T, Murakawa T, et al: Uneventful total intravenous anesthesia with ketamine for schizophrenic surgical patients, *Eur J Anaesthesiol* 14:47-51, 1997.

91. Kudoh A, Katagai H, Takazawa T: Anesthesia with ketamine, propofol, and fentanyl decreases the frequency of postoperative psychosis emergence and confusion in schizophrenic patients, *J Clin Anesth* 14:107-110, 2002.

92. van der Walt J, Moran C: An audit of perioperative management of autistic children, *Paediatr Anaesth* 11:401-408, 2001.

93. Rainey L, van der Walt J: The anesthetic management of autistic children, *Anaesth Intensive Care* 26:682-686, 1998.

94. Skolnick P, Layer R, Popik P, et al: Adaptation of N-methyl-D-aspartate (NMDA) receptors following antidepressant treatment: implications for the pharmacotherapy of depression, *Pharmacopsychiatry* 29:23-26, 1996.

95. Berman R, Cappiello A, Anand A, et al: Antidepressant effects of ketamine in depressed patients, *Biol Psychiatry* 47:351-354, 2000.

96. Roelofse J, Shipton E, de la Harpe CJ, et al: Intranasal sufentanil/midazolam versus ketamine/midazolam for analgesia/sedation in the pediatric population prior to undergoing multiple dental extractions under general anesthesia: a prospective, double-blind, randomized comparison, *Anesth Prog* 51:113-121, 2004.

97. Green S, Kupperman N, Rothrock SG, et al: Predictors of adverse events with intramuscular ketamine sedation in children, *Ann Emerg Med* 35:35-42, 2000.

98. Pruitt J, Goldwasser M, Sabol SR, et al: Intramuscular ketamine, midazolam, and glycopyrrolate for pediatric sedation in the emergency department, *J Oral Maxillofac Surg* 53:13-17, discussion 18, 1995.

99. Cartwright PD, Pingel SM: Midazolam and diazepam in ketamine anesthesia. *Anaesthesia* 39:439-442, 1984.

100. Toft P, Rome UD: Glycopyrrolate compared with atropine in association with ketamine anesthesia, *Acta Anesthesiol Scand* 31:438-440, 1987.

101. Frizelle H, Duranteau J, Samii K: A comparison of propofol with a propofol-ketamine combination for sedation during spinal anesthesia, *Anesth Analg* 84:1318-1322, 1997.

102. Frey K, Sukhani R, Powlowski J, et al: Propofol versus propofol-ketamine sedation for retrobulbar nerve block: comparison of sedation quality, intraocular pressure changes, and recovery profiles, *Anesth Analg* 89:317-321, 1999.

103. Badrinath S, Avramov M, Shadrick M, et al: The use of a ketamine-propofol combination during monitored anesthesia care, *Anesth Analg* 90:858-862, 2000.

104. Vallejo M, Romeo R, Davis DJ, et al: Propofol-ketamine versus propofol-fentanyl for outpatient laparoscopy: comparison of postoperative nausea, emesis, analgesia, and recovery, *J Clin Anesth* 14:426-431, 2002.

105. Friedberg B: Propofol-ketamine technique: dissociative anesthesia for office surgery (a 5-year review of 1264 cases), *Aesthetic Plast Surg* 23:70-75, 1999.

106. Hui T, Short T, Hong W, et al: Additive interactions between propofol and ketamine when used for anesthesia induction in female patients, *Anesthesiology* 82:641-647, 1995.

107. Badrinath S, Avramov MN, Shadrick M, et al: Use of ketamine-propofol admixture during monitored anesthesia care, *Anesthesiology* 87:A10, 1997.

108. Sarma V: Use of ketamine in acute severe asthma, *Acta Anaesthesiol Scand* 36:106-107, 1992.

Chapter 33

Nerve Damage in Dentistry

M.A. Pogrel

Damage to the sensory nerves supplying the jaws can occur in a number of ways during the course of dental treatment. The nerves involved can be the maxillary division of the trigeminal nerve, terminating in the dental branches and the infraorbital nerve; the mandibular division of the trigeminal nerve, terminating in the lingual nerve; the inferior alveolar nerve and its branches; and the long buccal nerve. Most attention has been devoted to the inferior alveolar and lingual nerves, because these appear to be the nerves most commonly involved in routine dental treatment and the ones that cause patients the most problems. Injury to the maxillary nerve, in particular, is more likely to result from trauma, orthognathic surgery, or other major surgery.

Involvement of the inferior alveolar and lingual nerve can occur from a number of dental causes including:

1. Inferior alveolar nerve blocks
2. Root canal therapy
3. Dentoalveolar surgery including:
   - Implant placement
   - Tooth removal (principally third molars)
   - Periodontal surgery

INFERIOR ALVEOLAR NERVE BLOCKS

Although long-term injury has occasionally been described from other types of local anesthetic injection, it is most commonly described following an inferior alveolar nerve block. The true incidence is unknown, but permanent injury may occur in around 1 in 25,000 inferior alveolar nerve blocks.[1-8] When it occurs, most patients appear to recover fully, and it has been estimated that about 85% of patients will recover completely within 8 to 10 weeks, another 5% will recover over a longer period, and 10% will be permanently injured. The exact etiology of the injury is unknown because only about half of the patients are aware of the electric shock sensation when the injection is given; the lingual nerve is predominantly affected, and in a disproportionate number of the permanent cases, dysesthesia is the presenting factor, unlike traumatic nerve injuries. All local anesthetics appear to have the potential to cause this problem, and currently no therapy appears to be effective. In the small number of patients who have undergone surgical exploration, most frequently no injury is seen, and therefore no type of repair surgery has been possible. There is no evidence that any vitamin or other supplements are effective, and because of the high incidence of dysesthesia in these cases, referral to a pain center frequently occurs. Steroids are sometimes given in the early phases in an attempt to suppress any inflammatory component, but there is no evidence that this is successful, particularly because steroids normally cannot be started for at least 24 hours after the causative injections—patients rarely inform their dentist prior to this period. To be effective, steroids would need to be given in the very early inflammatory phase. Some advocates recommend that steroids be injected locally, or oral steroids can be utilized in the form of a Dosepak of either dexamethasone or methylprednisolone.

ROOT CANAL THERAPY

Injury to the inferior alveolar nerve can occur when root canal therapy is carried out on mandibular teeth posterior to the mental foramen (Fig. 33-1). It can be a purely mechanical injury with over-instrumentation through the apex of the tooth, but, in many cases, it represents a physicochemical injury from the sealant gaining access to the inferior alveolar nerve. All sealants currently in use appear to be neurotoxic, at least until they set.[9,10] They thus have the ability to cause physicochemical damage to the inferior alveolar nerve, should they penetrate the epineurium and come into contact with the fascicles. There does appear to be variation in the time needed to cause permanent nerve damage, which can vary from a few minutes to 2 or 3 days, depending on the root canal sealant used. Because all sealants are radiopaque, their proximity to the inferior alveolar canal can be visualized on post–root canal therapy radiographs. If on completion of root canal therapy, the postoperative radiograph indicates that sealant may have gained access to the inferior alveolar canal, the patient should be carefully monitored for evidence of nerve involvement. This may not always be apparent once the local anesthetic wears off, because sensation may be normal for 24 or even 36 hours before paresthesia develops, depending on the root canal sealant used. If there is any evidence of nerve involvement, the sooner the root canal sealant is removed from the canal, the better is the chance of nerve recovery.[11] Any surgery is normally carried out under general anesthesia, and, in most cases, it will require lateral decortication of the mandible, identification of the inferior alveolar canal, debridement of the canal and the epineurium itself, and careful replacement of the nerve in its canal after all sealant has been removed. If this is carried out within a short span of hours from when the damage becomes apparent, a good result can be anticipated.[9] If it is left longer than this, any nerve damage may well be permanent, and the only curative treatment would be to resect the permanently damaged segment of nerve and insert a graft of some kind, because the damage normally covers an area too extensive to be treated by direct anastomosis of the nerve ends.

DAMAGE FROM DENTOALVEOLAR SURGERY

DENTAL IMPLANTS

Implant placement in the mandible posterior to the mental foramen carries a risk of involvement of the inferior alveolar nerve, and, if this is felt to be at risk and one still wishes to insert implants, then three-dimensional scanning of the mandible (cone beam computed tomography [CBCT]), followed by careful planning and the use of

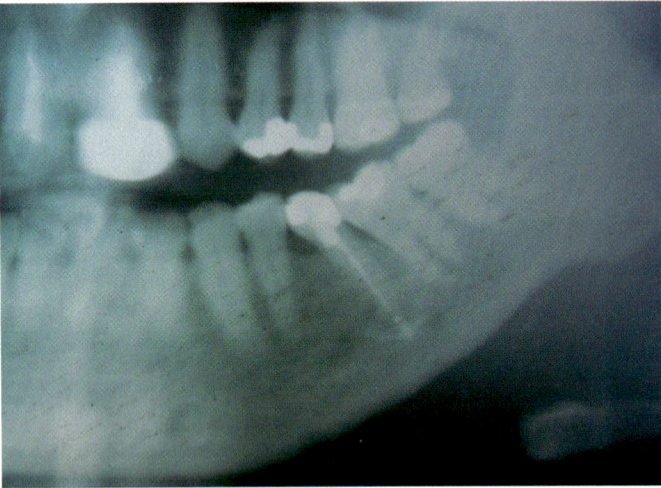

Fig. 33-1 ■ Root canal sealant in the inferior alveolar canal.

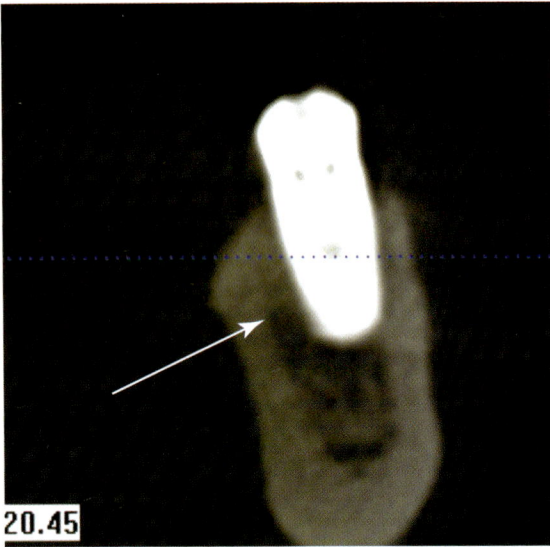

Fig. 33-2 ■ Cone beam CT scan of a dental implant in close proximity to the inferior alveolar nerve.

implant drills with a fixed and measured stop, may be indicated[12,13] (Fig. 33-2). When damage occurs, it is more likely due to the drilling process itself rather than the actual implant insertion so that withdrawal of the implant, if it is impinging on the nerve, is a sensible precaution but rarely relieves the symptoms if they were caused by the drilling process. Unfortunately, if the involvement is from the drilling, spontaneous recovery tends to be poor, because the area of damage can be fairly extensive. Surgery, however, equally does not give a very satisfactory result, because the damaged segment often has to be resected. Also, because of the extent of the damage, direct anastomosis is often not possible, meaning that a graft of some kind must be used with a subsequently lower success rate.

DENTAL EXTRACTIONS (MOST COMMONLY THIRD MOLARS)

The most common single cause of postoperative involvement of the inferior alveolar and lingual nerves results from removal of third molars.[14] A number of factors have been shown to be associated with a higher incidence of nerve involvement including[15]:

1. Full bony impaction.
2. Horizontal impaction.
3. The use of burs for bone removal.

4. Apices extending into or below the neurovascular bundle.
5. Clinical observation of the inferior alveolar bundle during surgery.
6. Excessive hemorrhage into the socket during surgery.
7. The age of the patient. It is possible that the incidence of nerve involvement is independent of age, but recovery occurs better at a younger age.
8. Injuries to the lingual nerve probably occur in cases where the lingual plate is not present to protect the lingual nerve. This can occur when either the lingual nerve is placed superior to the protective lingual plate or when the lingual plate is deficient either congenitally, due to chronic infection, or due to pathology such as a cyst or other process.

Newer imaging techniques, such as cone beam computerized tomography, can show in more detail the relationship of the inferior alveolar nerve to the third molar in three dimensions and can also show the thickness of the lingual plate of bone and the third molar's relationship to the lingual plate.[16,17] These images cannot, however, visualize the lingual nerve directly. Avoidance of injury to these nerves in relationship to third molar surgery can take on a number of forms: electing not to remove the teeth, if they are asymptomatic; removing pathologic tissue only, such as a dentigerous cyst, but leaving the third molar in place; removing the tooth and attempting an immediate repair if a nerve injury is visualized; carrying out a coronectomy where only the crown and coronal portion of the tooth's root is removed and the apical portion of the roots, in association with the inferior alveolar nerve, is retained.[18-20] Long-term results from many of these techniques are not yet available.

The use of lingual retraction remains controversial for protection of the lingual nerve during third molar removal, but advocates would state that although lingual nerve involvement can occur from the retraction alone, it is only transient, whereas nerve involvement in the absence of lingual retraction can be permanent.[21,22]

PERIODONTAL TREATMENT

The principal periodontal procedure that can be responsible for nerve injury is the so-called distal wedge procedure, which is carried out distal to a lower second molar in order to eliminate pocketing and nonkeratinized epithelium. In those patients for whom the lingual nerve runs superior to the lingual plate of bone (probably about 15% of patients),[23-26] the lingual nerve will be at risk during this procedure and can be damaged.[14,27]

NERVE EVALUATION PROTOCOL

If nerve damage occurs as a result of dental treatment, it is important to document and follow it to assess recovery. Spontaneous recovery can occur after most forms of nerve injury, but it is more frequent when a nerve is bruised or affected by hematoma or stretching rather than a partial or complete transection, and extensive injuries, such as those often caused by an implant-related drilling procedure, may have a lower incidence of spontaneous recovery. Evaluation should consist of both outlining the extent of the area involved and also testing within that area for the degree of nerve involvement. All tests are only semiobjective, in that they do rely on a cooperative patient able to give reproducible results. The area itself can be tested with the reverse end of a dental needle so that the patient can state when sensation changes, and, in this way, the area can be outlined. The outline can then be transferred to a drawing or can be photographed directly and stored in the patient's record. The degree of involvement can be tested with Von Frey hairs for quantity of sensation, with two-point discrimination for the quality of sensation, and for the ability to detect temperature changes and direction sense. When the lingual nerve is affected, the chorda tympani is also often affected, giving loss of taste or abnormal taste; taste-testing kits are available to evaluate the sense of taste. In general terms, patients are felt to have protective reflexes (can sense hot and cold foods that might harm them or can sense when they are biting the lip or tongue) when they have 30% of normal sensation or better.[28,29]

CRITERIA FOR POSSIBLE NERVE EXPLORATION AND SURGERY[29]

1. Following nerve damage from root canal sealant, the sooner the sealant is removed surgically the better. This is normally best performed by a lateral decortication of the mandible, and, ideally, it should be carried out within hours of identifying the problem. This can give a very high recovery rate.
2. When considering nerve injury from dental implants, if the implant appears to be impinging on the inferior alveolar canal, it should be withdrawn or replaced.
3. When there is a witnessed transection of the nerve (i.e., the dentist involved knows he or she has cut the nerve and can identify the injury), the sooner it is repaired, the better the result. Repairs carried out within a few hours of a witnessed injury carry a high success rate.
4. When a patient is still totally numb or has dysesthesia (unpleasant sensation) that does not improve after 8 weeks, consideration should be given to nerve exploration and repair at that time, because studies have shown that early repairs produce better results than late repairs.
5. When patients are 4 to 6 months postinjury and still do not have protective reflexes (less than 30% normal sensation), or have worsening dysesthesia, consideration should be given to surgical exploration and possible repair. A typical algorithm is shown below for nerve injuries caused by dentoalveolar surgery (Fig. 33-3).

NERVE EXPLORATION AND SURGERY

Currently, imaging cannot accurately identify the exact site or cause of the problem in most cases of nerve damage. Therefore, most surgical procedures are exploratory, in the first instance, in order to identify the nerve itself, identify the area of injury if possible, and devise a suitable treatment plan. When a nerve is compressed by scar tissue or bone spicules, for instance, decompression may give a satisfactory result. When the injury is more extensive and spontaneous recovery has not occurred, the injured area must be resected, and if the nerve can be adequately mobilized, a direct anastomosis is preferable. When direct anastomosis is not possible, a graft of some kind, which can be a nerve graft from a variety of sites or another autogenous graft, such as a vein has been used successfully to repair the inferior alveolar nerve, but not the lingual[30] or even freeze-dried muscle (can form a satisfactory interpositional nerve graft). To date, alloplastic grafts have not proved successful,[31,32] but an allograft may be possible. Overall, with good patient selection, nerve surgery can result in improvement in greater than 50% of the patients treated. However, complete cure and restoration to the premorbid condition is extremely unusual, and some residual deficit normally remains.[29]

When dysesthesia is the primary consideration or surgery is not successful, most patients must rely on medical therapy, and many are referred to a pain clinic to establish a successful protocol. Medications utilized include the nonsteroidal anti-inflammatory agents, narcotic analgesics, antiseizure medications (carbamazepine, phenytoin, valproic acid, gabapentin [Neurontin]), pregabalin (Lyrica), tricyclic antidepressants, alpha agonists such as clonidine, benzodiazepines such as clonazepam (Klonopin), local anesthetic analogs such as mexiletine and narcotic analgesics. Many patients end up on a cocktail of these medications to increase the efficiency and minimize side effects.[33]

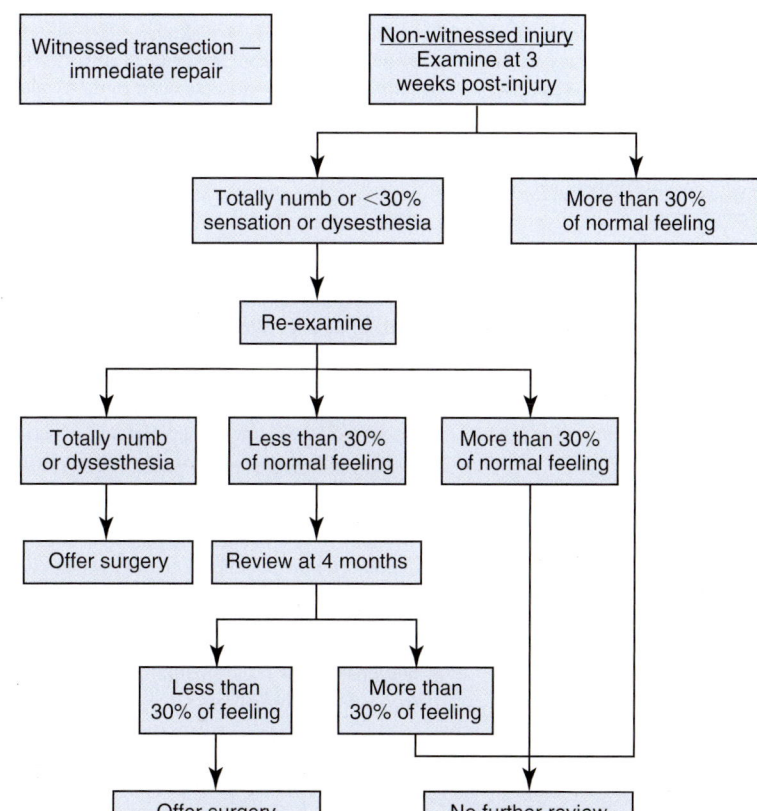

Fig. 33-3 ■ Typical algorithm for nerve injuries caused by dentoalveolar surgery. It is currently in use in the Department of Oral and Maxillofacial Surgery at the University of California, San Francisco.

PEARLS AND PITFALLS

- In up to 15% of cases, the lingual nerve can lie partially or totally superior to the crest of the lingual plate of the bone. Therefore, it is at risk in procedures carried out on the lingual side of the mandible.
- Cone beam computed tomography (CBCT) should be considered to determine the exact position and relationship of the inferior alveolar nerve when its position may determine the treatment plan.
- In general terms, if microneurosurgery is contemplated, early surgery gives better results than late surgery. The best results

with a witnessed transection are seen with surgery within a few days.
- The results of microneurosurgical repair of the lingual and inferior alveolar nerves overall are variable and not always successful.
- Early surgical exploration and debridement of root canal sealant around the inferior alveolar nerve may improve nerve function.
- Implants in contact with the inferior alveolar nerve and causing symptoms should be backed out or removed as soon as possible.

REFERENCES

1. Ehrenfeld M, Cornelius CP, Altenmuller E, et al: [Nerve injuries following nerve blocking in the pterygomandibular space]. *Dtsch Zahnarztl Z* 47(1):36-39, 1992.
2. Haas DA: Localized complications from local anesthesia. *J Calif Dent Assoc* 26(9):677-682, 1998.
3. Haas DA, Lennon D: A 21-year retrospective study of reports of paresthesia following local anesthetic administration. *J Can Dent Assoc* 61(4):319-320, 323-326, 329-330, 1995.
4. Harn SD, Durham TM: Incidence of lingual nerve trauma and postinjection complications in conventional mandibular block anesthesia. *J Am Dent Assoc* 121(4):519-523, 1990.
5. Krafft TC, Hickel R: Clinical investigation into the incidence of direct damage to the lingual nerve caused by local anaesthesia. *J Craniomaxillofac Surg* 22(5):294-296, 1994.
6. Pogrel MA, Bryan J, Regezi J: Nerve damage associated with inferior alveolar nerve blocks. *J Am Dent Assoc* 126(8):1150-1155, 1995.
7. Pogrel MA, Schmidt BL: Trigeminal nerve chemical neurotrauma from injectible materials. *J Oral Maxillofac Surg Clinic North Am* 13:247-253, 2001.
8. Pogrel MA, Thamby S: Permanent nerve involvement resulting from inferior alveolar nerve blocks. *J Am Dent Assoc* 131(7):901-907, 2000.
9. Pogrel MA: Neurotoxicity of available root sealant pastes. *Oral Surg Oral Med Oral Pathol Oral Radiol Endod* 98(4):385, 2004.
10. Scolozzi P, Lombardi T, Jaques B: Successful inferior alveolar nerve decompression for dysesthesia following endodontic treatment: report of 4 cases treated by mandibular sagittal osteotomy. *Oral Surg Oral Med Pathol Oral Radiol Endod* 97(5):625-631, 2004.
11. Pogrel MA: Damage to the inferior alveolar nerve as the result of root canal therapy. *J Am Dent Assoc* 138(1):65-69, 2007.
12. Hatcher DC, Dial C, Mayorga C: Cone beam CT for pre-surgical assessment of implant sites. *J Calif Dent Assoc* 31(11):825-833, 2003.

13. Sato S, Arai Y, Shinoda K, Ito K: Clinical application of a new cone-beam computerized tomography system to assess multiple two-dimensional images for the preoperative treatment planning of maxillary implants: case reports. *Quintessence Int* 35(7):525-528, 2004.
14. Pogrel MA, Thamby S: The etiology of altered sensation in the inferior alveolar, lingual, and mental nerves as a result of dental treatment. *J Calif Dent Assoc* 27(7):531, 534-538, 1999.
15. Kipp DP, Goldstein BH, Weiss WW Jr: Dysesthesia after mandibular third molar surgery: a retrospective study and analysis of 1,377 surgical procedures. *J Am Dent Assoc* 100(2):185-192, 1980.
16. Danforth RA, Peck J, Hall P: Cone beam volume tomography: an imaging option for diagnosis of complex mandibular third molar anatomical relationships. *J Calif Dent Assoc* 31(11):847-852, 2003.
17. Nakagawa Y, Kobayashi K, Ishii H, Mishima A, et al: Preoperative application of limited cone beam computerized tomography as an assessment tool before minor oral surgery. *Int J Oral Maxillofac Surg* 31(3):322-326, 2002.
18. O'Riordan BC: Coronectomy (intentional partial odontectomy of lower third molars). *Oral Surg Oral Med Oral Pathol Oral Radiol Endod* 98(3):274-280, 2004.
19. Pogrel MA, Lee JS, Muff DF: Coronectomy: a technique to protect the inferior alveolar nerve. *J Oral Maxillofac Surg* 62(12):1447-1452, 2004.
20. Renton T, Hankins M, Sproate C, McGurk M: A randomised controlled clinical trial to compare the incidence of injury to the inferior alveolar nerve as a result of coronectomy and removal of mandibular third molars. *Br J Oral Maxillofac Surg* 43(1):7-12, 2005.
21. Pogrel MA, Goldman KE: Lingual flap retraction for third molar removal. *J Oral Maxillofac Surg* 62(9):1125-1130, 2004.
22. Rood JP: Permanent damage to inferior alveolar and lingual nerves during the removal of impacted mandibular third molars. Comparison of two methods of bone removal. *Br Dent J* 172(3):108-110, 1992.

23. Behnia H, Kheradvar A, Shahrokhi M: An anatomic study of the lingual nerve in the third molar region. *J Oral Maxillofac Surg* 58(6):649-651, 2000; discussion 652-653.
24. Holzle FW, Wolff KD: Anatomic position of the lingual nerve in the mandibular third molar region with special consideration of an atrophied mandibular crest: an anatomical study. *Int J Oral Maxillofac Surg* 30(4):333-338, 2001.
25. Kiesselbach JE, Chamberlain JG: Clinical and anatomic observations on the relationship of the lingual nerve to the mandibular third molar region. *J Oral Maxillofac Surg* 42(9):565-567, 1984.
26. Pogrel MA, Renaut A, Schmidt B, Ammar A: The relationship of the lingual nerve to the mandibular third molar region: an anatomic study. *J Oral Maxillofac Surg* 53(10):1178-1181, 1995.
27. Hunt PR: Safety aspects of mandibular lingual surgery. *J Periodontol* 47(4):224-229, 1976.
28. Cadra M, Pogrel MA, Robert RC: Nerve evaluation protocol. Roseville, Calif, 2003, *California Association of Oral and Maxillofacial Surgeons.*
29. Pogrel MA: The results of microneurosurgery of the inferior alveolar and lingual nerve. *J Oral Maxillofac Surg* 60(5):485-489, 2002.
30. Pogrel MA, Maghen A: The use of autogenous vein grafts for inferior alveolar and lingual nerve reconstruction. *J Oral Maxillofac Surg* 59(9):985-988, 2001; discussion 988-993.
31. Pitta MC, Wolford LM, Mehra P, Hopkin J: Use of Gore-Tex tubing as a conduit for inferior alveolar and lingual nerve repair: experience with 6 cases. *J Oral Maxillofac Surg* 59(5):493-496, 2001; discussion 497.
32. Pogrel MA, McDonald AR, Kaban LB: Gore-Tex tubing as a conduit for repair of lingual and inferior alveolar nerve continuity defects: a preliminary report. *J Oral Maxillofac Surg* 56(3):319-321, 1998; discussion 321-322.
33. Gregg J: Medical management of traumatic neuropathies. *J Oral Maxillofac Surg Clinic North Am* 13:343-363, 2001.

THE PAST

The participation of oral and maxillofacial surgeons in facial trauma care has contributed to the expansion of the profession, eventually leading to the specialty's name change from oral surgery to oral maxillofacial surgery (OMFS). The frequent involvement of the dentoalveolar, maxillary, and mandibular segments and the importance of occlusion in facial trauma reconstruction demanded the expertise of surgeons familiar with dental and temporomandibular joint anatomy. Experience during wartime has significantly contributed to the evolution of the current management protocols. Facial trauma care of the past was more frequently based on closed reduction techniques and anatomic reduction using wire fixation with minimal access. The treatment of avulsed tissue as a result of trauma was difficult and based on local flaps and minimal bony, dental, or soft tissue reconstruction.

THE PRESENT

The current management of maxillofacial trauma has seen a tremendous change since the days of wire fixation. General trauma care has improved with the implementation of advanced trauma life support (ATLS), rapid patient transport, organized prehospital care, and the designation of trauma and burn centers. However, many regions of the United States remain relatively underserved, requiring patients to be airlifted to the nearest trauma center. The recognition of trauma as a significant "disease" contributing to major social and financial burden has allowed distribution of resources for trauma care. Oral and maxillofacial surgeons have

become a significant force in management of craniofacial trauma within the level I trauma centers of the United States.* Currently, the use of rigid and resorbable fixation and the integration of soft tissue and bone reconstruction have improved surgical care. The use of computed tomography (CT) scans and three-dimensional virtual diagnosis and reconstruction has become more common.

THE FUTURE

The future of oral and maxillofacial trauma care will evolve as the patterns of injury change with new technologic and public health safety measures, along with the changes in the transportation industry. However, and unfortunately, interpersonal violence and self-inflicted injuries will continue to be seen. Titanium rigid fixation plates are likely to be replaced by enhanced resorbable plates that will disappear shortly after a fracture heals, or, at any time, the click of a button will transmit an electromagnetic wave to the plate, initiating the rapid hydrolysis of the compound. Virtual holographic and three-dimensional intraoperative technology will be present in real time while positioning fracture segments. Minimally invasive techniques in conjunction with this technology will facilitate fracture repair and reconstruction. Ultrasound technology is likely to advance and be readily available for diagnostic imaging in most clinics. Oral and maxillofacial surgeons will become dominant players in facial trauma care. The necessity of a dental education for comprehensive facial trauma rehabilitation will be emphasized.

The Surgical Airway

Chapter **34**

Timothy Marx Osborn, Eric J. Dierks

HISTORY OF TRACHEOTOMY

Tracheotomy has been known for approximately 3500 years, with proponents and opponents arising at different times in history. Early references advising relief for choking persons by cutting open the trachea were made 3500 years ago by Homer and Alexander the Great.[1] For many years, the tracheotomy was considered a useless and dangerous procedure. In 1739, Heister described the operation in which he used a straight tube and trocar, and he remarked that the utility of this operation was widely neglected by modern surgeons.[2] Resolution of many of the highly debated issues surrounding the tracheotomy began with Chevalier Jackson, who advocated a long incision, avoidance of high cartilage dissection, slow and deliberate surgery, and cutting of the thyroid isthmus.[3] Today, the indications, techniques, and armamentarium for tracheotomy have evolved from thrusting a reed over the point of a sword into a choking soldier to the modern meticulous surgical procedure that

predictably bypasses the upper airway for a variety of indications, both emergent and nonemergent.[4]

INDICATIONS

The indications for tracheotomy fall in several general categories.
1. Need to bypass airway obstruction
2. Neck trauma
3. Subcutaneous emphysema that can lead to massive edema
4. Facial fractures
5. Airway edema (trauma, burns, infection, anaphylaxis, angioedema)

---

*Bagheri SC, Demassi M, Shahriari A, et al: Facial trauma coverage among level one trauma centers of the United States. *J Oral Maxillofac Surg* 66(5):963-967, 2008.

6. Need to provide a long-term route for mechanical ventilation
7. Pulmonary toilet (inadequate cough, secretion management, aspiration)
8. Extensive head and neck procedures
9. Severe sleep apnea

CONTRAINDICATIONS

There are no absolute contraindications to tracheotomy. However, there are instances, such as a high-riding innominate artery, goiter, or thyroid mass, that may alter the standard technique that may be employed. There are contraindications to percutaneous tracheotomy that will be discussed later.

TIMING OF TRACHEOTOMY

All surgeons involved in surgical procedures where general anesthesia is employed or where there is risk of airway loss should be prepared to secure a surgical airway. Preoperatively, the surgeon must consider the type of procedure and possible interventions and determine if a tracheotomy is necessary at the beginning of a procedure. Should there develop a potential for significant airway edema from the operation, tracheotomy can be reserved for the conclusion of the procedure, if determined to be necessary. Early tracheotomy may be beneficial in patients with severe craniomaxillofacial trauma or deep space neck infections.[5]

One of the most difficult decisions to make in the management of the mechanically ventilated patient is whether to continue translaryngeal intubation or to perform a tracheotomy. Reviews of the literature have concluded that there are not enough well-designed studies to establish guidelines regarding timing of tracheotomy. De Leyn et al concluded that in critically ill adult patients requiring prolonged mechanical ventilation, tracheotomy performed within the first week may shorten the duration of artificial ventilation and length of stay in the intensive care unit (ICU).[6] King and Moores suggest using Heffner's "anticipatory approach" (Fig. 34-1).[7]

Patients likely to be taken off the ventilator in 7 to 10 days should continue with endotracheal intubation, whereas those who are likely to require longer ventilatory support should be considered for tracheotomy. When the duration of intubation cannot be predicted, patients should be reevaluated daily. At the end of the day, the decision must be individualized, giving consideration to the patient's preferences and expected clinical course.

ELECTIVE ADULT TRACHEOTOMY: ANATOMY AND TECHNIQUE

Elective tracheotomy is preferably performed under general anesthesia in the operating room after the airway is secured with endotracheal intubation or laryngeal mask airway (LMA). A shoulder roll is placed, and the head is extended to make the tissues of the neck taut and to distract the trachea from the thorax. This distraction of the larynx and trachea increases the distance from the cricoid cartilage to the sternal notch, which facilitates the identification of these landmarks.

Once the field is prepared in a sterile fashion, local anesthesia is administered along the planned incision line. A 3- to 4-cm transverse incision is made between the medial borders of each sternocleidomastoid muscle at a level approximately half the distance between the cricoid cartilage and the sternal notch. Blunt dissection with gauze is used in the subcutaneous plane to facilitate identification and avoidance of the anterior jugular veins. This maneuver is much quicker than blunt or sharp dissection with instruments and is less likely to cause bleeding that may complicate the postoperative course. Once the subcutaneous layer is dissected, the cervical fascia is identified; Then the median raphe between the paramedian sternohyoid and sternothyroid muscles is identified and dissected with blunt hemostats. Retractors are then used to retract the strap muscles laterally. The operator and assistant alternate vertical and horizontal spreading down to the trachea, with repositioning of the retractors as dissection proceeds toward the trachea. It is imperative that the

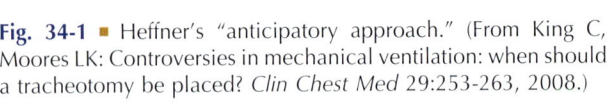

Fig. 34-1 ■ Heffner's "anticipatory approach." (From King C, Moores LK: Controversies in mechanical ventilation: when should a tracheotomy be placed? *Clin Chest Med* 29:253-263, 2008.)

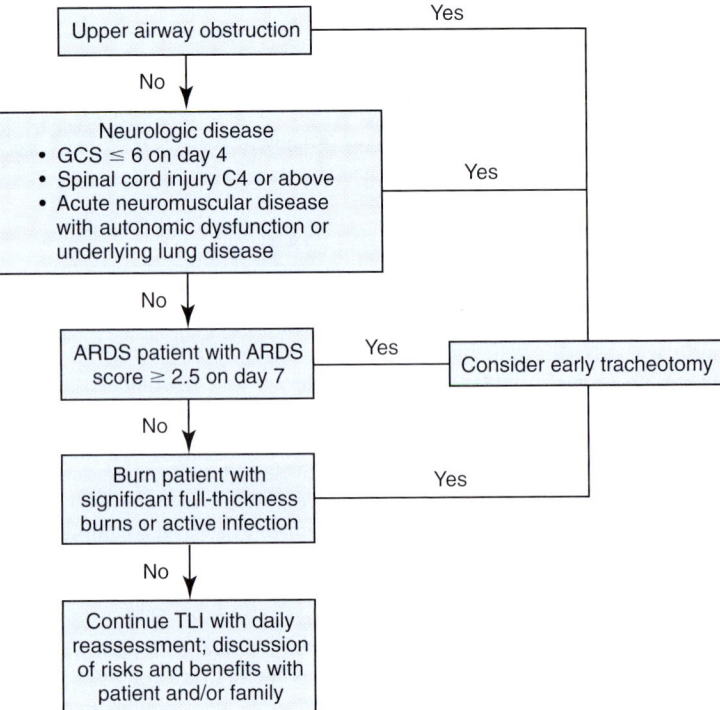

trachea be maintained in the midline and that the retraction does not pull the trachea out of the field of dissection.

Once past the strap muscles, the middle cervical fascia is sometimes identified with the thyroid isthmus overlying the trachea. It is usually possible to retract the thyroid superiorly out of the field. Rarely does the thyroid isthmus need to be divided, but if necessary, it can be suture ligated or cauterized. One must be sure that good hemostasis is achieved to prevent any postoperative issues with thyroid bleeding. Once the trachea is seen through the pretracheal fascia, a cricoid hook is placed, and the trachea is elevated into the surgical field. This is the most critical portion of the operation and helps to stabilize the trachea and facilitates visualization. The pretracheal fascia is dissected off the trachea to visualize the tracheal rings.

After visualizing the trachea, the surgeon can determine the size of tracheotomy tube needed for the airway, typically, a No. 8 for a man and a No. 6 for a woman. The tube must be tested by the scrub nurse and lubricated. At this point, the surgeon may elect to place stay sutures in the tracheal rings, which can be draped onto the chest skin. The authors do not use stay sutures on adult patients.

After alerting the anesthesiologist, a scalpel is used to make a tracheal incision of choice: a vertical incision through rings two, three, and occasionally four; a horizontal incision between rings two and three; or a T-shaped incision. One must be careful to avoid lacerating the posterior tracheal wall or cutting too far laterally and potentially injuring the recurrent laryngeal nerve. Once the trachea is entered, a tracheal dilator is placed and deployed to aid passage of the tracheal tube. With the cricoid hook still in place and with direct visualization of the trachea, the tracheal tube is inserted. The insertion stylet is removed, and the anesthesia tubing is connected. Once end-tidal CO_2 and breath sounds are confirmed, the cricoid hook can be removed and the tracheal tube flange secured to the skin with sutures. One can also use tracheal ties if no microvascular surgery has been performed or is planned in the neck. A portable chest radiograph is obtained immediately postoperatively to verify proper positioning, as well as to assess for hemopneumothorax.

COMPLICATIONS OF TRACHEOTOMY

Tracheotomy has a relatively low incidence of complications (roughly 15%), and most of these can be avoided by meticulous surgical technique and postoperative care. The complications can be defined by the interval from procedure to onset of complication(s) and stratified to the perioperative and postoperative periods. There is also a higher incidence of complications in those with medical or surgical comorbidities, such as in debilitated, obese, multiply injured, or burn patients. The most common complications are hemorrhage, tube obstruction, and tube displacement.[8,9]

PERIOPERATIVE COMPLICATIONS

Major hemorrhage during tracheotomy is uncommon and more frequently encountered in emergent tracheotomy. The incidence of operative and early hemorrhage is about 4%.[8,10] Bleeding sites include the superficial anterior jugular veins, the thyroid isthmus, and the thyroid ima artery. Deeper bleeding lateral to the trachea can arise from the lateral vascular arcade that nourishes the trachea.

Paratracheal or pretracheal placement of the tracheal tube can be a significant intraoperative complication if manual control of the airway is not maintained until end-tidal CO_2 is confirmed. The tracheal tube can sometimes follow a false passage anterior or lateral to the trachea. It is usually rapidly identified by lack of CO_2 and breath sounds. To prevent this, clean dissection down to the trachea should be assured, the trachea should be visualized, and the cricoid

hook should not be removed until verification of proper tube placement.

Pneumothorax is an uncommon complication and usually results from a difficult trachea or one with excessive lateral dissection, particularly in children. In cases where the airway is deviated due to infection, mass, or other etiology, the surgeon must be careful to avoid dissecting off course, inferiorly and laterally. A routine postoperative radiograph will detect a pneumothorax in most cases. Pneumothorax must be considered if ventilatory difficulty arises in a patient with a fresh tracheotomy; however, it is less likely than false passage or obstruction.

Other immediate complications include damage to adjacent structures, such as the esophagus or the recurrent laryngeal nerve (RLN). Damage to the RLN can be either by excessive lateral dissection, thermal injury from cautery, or from retraction injury. The esophagus may also be injured by overzealous incision into the trachea or excessive dissection, particularly if the trachea is being deviated by retraction or mass effect. Another potential complication is dissection made too far superiorly, with damage to the cricoid cartilage, particularly if a vertical tracheal incision is placed.

POSTOPERATIVE COMPLICATIONS

Postoperative complications occur during the first hours to days after surgery. Hemorrhage is the most common complication in the postoperative period as well. In the operating room, the patients are commonly hypotensive and do not have a cough. When they return to the normotensive state or become hypertensive postoperatively, they can experience either minor or major bleeding. Coughing postoperatively can precipitate bleeding. Bleeding usually responds to local measures, including local anesthesia with epinephrine, local packing, and/or direct pressure. One can also use adjuncts such as topical thrombin or tranexamic acid. Anticoagulated patients have their anticoagulants held prior to surgery, and bleeding can occur upon resumption of anticoagulation. This type of bleeding can also be managed with local measures as well as systemically by minimizing anticoagulation. The need for surgical exploration for postoperative hemorrhage is very rare, and, even when necessary, identification of a definitive source is frequently elusive.

Infection following tracheotomy is rare and most commonly occurs when the open wound is not vigilantly maintained. Dressings should be avoided, if possible, or changed frequently as they become saturated with blood and airway secretions. There can be pressure breakdown of wounds if there is excess pressure of the tracheal flange, particularly in obese patients. Foam dressings placed under the tracheal flange can be used to alleviate the pressure. When wound breakdown occurs, local wound care with packing can be used. The authors commonly use wet-to-dry packing soaked in 0.25% acetic acid solution to facilitate wound healing. Routine use of antibiotics is not recommended if wound care can be effectively done with local measures.

External granulation tissue around the tracheal tube can frequently develop following tracheotomy and has a tendency for troublesome bleeding. This can also occur following decannulation. Silver nitrate application will resolve most cases. Internal granulation tissue can develop insidiously and may require bronchoscopic and transtracheostomal removal and cautery. Tracheocutaneous fistula can also become a problem after decannulation and is more common in children than adults. In adults, layered closure with strap muscle interposition is necessary, whereas, in children, cauterization of the tract may stimulate closure.

Slow displacement of the tracheal tube out of the trachea into the peritracheal soft tissues can be a life-threatening complication of tracheotomy, particularly in the first few days after tracheotomy. It

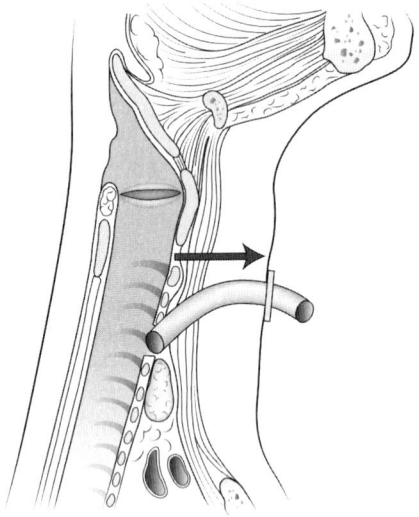

Fig. 34-2 ■ Slow displacement phenomenon type I: tracheal flange remains on the neck skin as tube slides out of trachea, often with catastrophic results. (From Dierks EJ: Tracheotomy: elective and emergent. *Oral Maxillofac Surg Clin North Am* 20(3):513-520, 2008.)

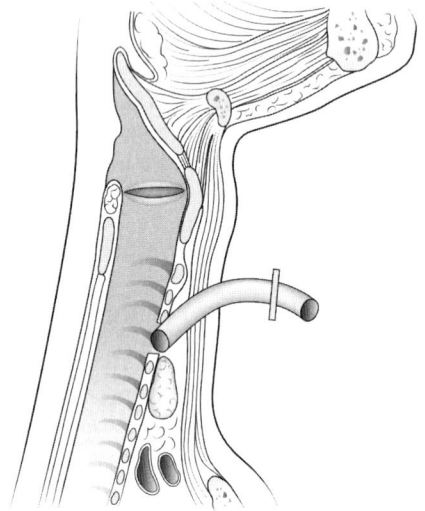

Fig. 34-3 ■ Slow displacement phenomenon type II: tracheal flange is elevated off skin of neck as patient is able to talk and breathe relatively normally. (From Dierks EJ: Tracheotomy: elective and emergent. *Oral Maxillofac Surg Clin North Am* 20(3):513-520, 2008.)

occurs in two forms.[11] Type I results from a progressive increase in the distance from the anterior tracheal wall to the neck skin, usually due to postoperative edema (Fig. 34-2). It occurs primarily in patients with thick or obese necks. As the tracheal tube nears complete dislodgement from the trachea, a suction catheter will become difficult to pass; however, ventilation is not yet compromised. If a suction catheter does not pass, immediate evaluation should be performed to confirm tracheal tube position. If the tracheal tube slips out completely, catastrophic airway obstruction can occur.

Type II displacement occurs in the absence of an increased distance from the anterior tracheal wall to the neck skin (Fig. 34-3). It is seen in patients with normal neck size and occurs later than type I displacement, often in patients ready for decannulation. Like type

I displacement, the hallmark is inability to pass a suction catheter. Visual inspection shows elevation of the tracheal tube flange off the skin. This occurs in patients with loose tracheal ties and no tracheal flange sutures. These patients are often able to breathe and phonate, and in these cases, the tracheal tube simply can be removed unless needed for other purposes.

Tracheo-innominate fistula (TIF) is a rare complication that can develop months after tracheotomy and is usually due to pressure erosion of the anterior tracheal wall by the tip or balloon of the tracheal tube. The erosion creeps in to the posterior wall of the innominate artery as it crosses over the trachea in the upper mediastinum. Oshinsky, in a cadaver study, found that the tip, cuff, or both were adjacent to a segment of the innominate artery when the tube was placed between the second and third tracheal rings.[12] TIF usually presents with a sentinel bleed, followed hours to weeks later by an exsanguinating hemorrhage that carries an 80% to 90% mortality.

TIF is best treated by prevention. Minimizing cuff pressure to achieve a seal for ventilation will prevent exceeding the capillary pressure of the tracheal mucosa. Proper fit of the tracheal tube will avoid pressure from the tip of the tube. If there is suspicion of tip impingement, a longer or shorter tube can be placed for a better fit. If there is a sentinel bleed, the cuff is inflated and the patient is evaluated for TIF. This can be done at bedside through bronchoscopy, but CT angiography is needed for definitive diagnosis. If there is a major bleed, the Utley maneuver involves opening the inferior aspect of the tracheal site to allow blunt finger dissection into the anterior mediastinum.[13] The anterior compression of the innominate artery against the undersurface of the sternum will diminish the hemorrhage until sternotomy can be performed.

Tracheal and subglottic stenoses are complications predisposed by previous prolonged endotracheal tube intubation, high tracheotomy/cricothyroidotomy, and trauma to the airway.[14] Circumferential mucosal ulcers develop from direct pressure, then deepen and lead to cartilage exposure, scarring, and subsequent stenosis. Stenosis at the level of the stoma is caused by an overly large stoma or excessive traction on the tracheotomy tube. Meticulous surgical technique, the use of flexible connectors to minimize traction, and use of high-volume, low-pressure cuffs help minimize the risk of stenosis. In Goldenberg's study of 1130 tracheotomies, there were 21 cases of tracheal stenosis, all of which occurred in patients who were intubated for more than 12 days.[8]

The degree and length of the stenosis dictate treatment. Small areas of subglottic or tracheal stenosis can be managed with a CO_2 laser or steroid injection. Fibrous stenosis can be managed with endoscopic excision or repeated endoscopic dilations. For lesions greater than 4 cm and hourglass stenoses resulting from loss of tracheal ring integrity, resection of the stenosis with end-to-end anastomosis can be performed (Fig. 34-4). Conservative management should be considered for all cases.

Tracheoesophageal fistula (TEF) is a rare complication (0.01% to 1% incidence) of tracheotomy with a 70% to 80% incidence of mortality.[15] TEF is thought to result from incidental damage to the posterior tracheal wall at the time of surgery or from pressure necrosis of the posterior tracheal wall from an ill-fitting tube or overinflated cuff, often coupled with a nasogastric tube in the esophagus. The diagnosis should be suspected clinically by coughing during eating, chronic coughing upon swallowing, recurrent aspiration, and pneumonia. Contrast swallow evaluation, methylene blue instillation into the esophagus with flexible fiberoptic evaluation, or a combination of modalities is diagnostic. Once the diagnosis is confirmed or cannot be ruled out, definitive surgical repair should be performed.

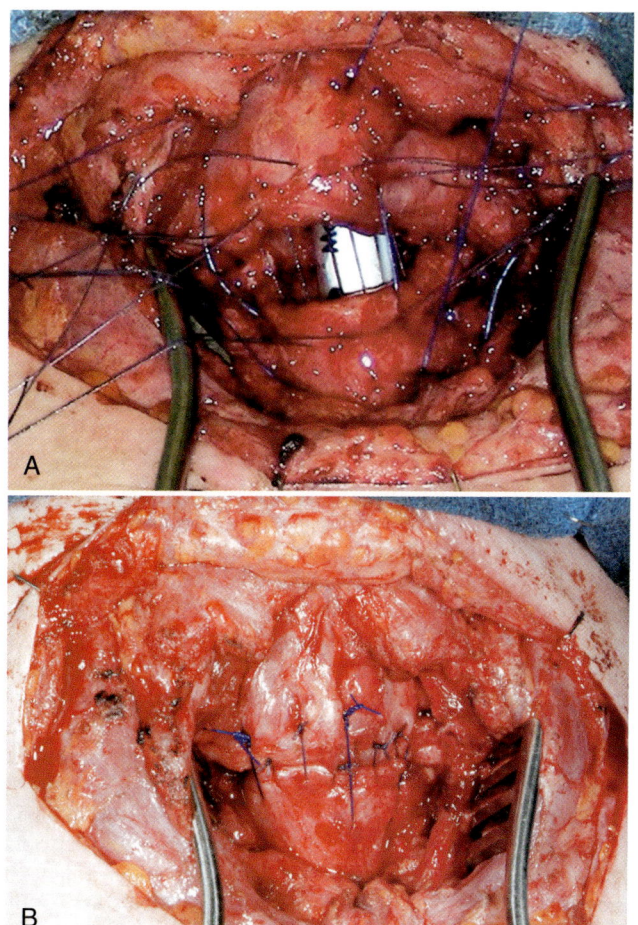

Fig. 34-4 ■ **A,** Tracheal sleeve resection of stenosis prior to anastomosis. **B,** Completed tracheal anastomosis.

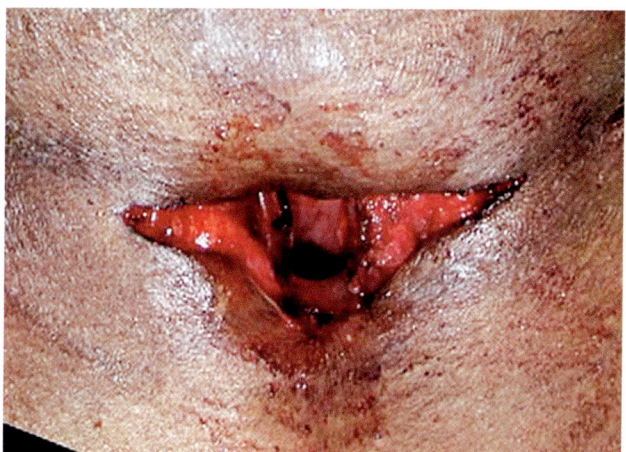

Fig. 34-5 ■ Tracheal stoma stands open and widely patent following obese tracheostomy. (From Dierks EJ: Tracheotomy: elective and emergent. *Oral Maxillofac Surg Clin North Am* 20(3):513-520, 2008.)

and a standard tracheotomy technique may be appropriate. In the truly obese neck, the increased distance from skin edge to anterior tracheal wall must be managed to avoid complications and potential catastrophe. Standard tracheal tubes are typically too short, so consideration should be given to the use of a specialized longer tracheal tube in the obese patient. Such tracheal tubes are referred to as having a *proximal* extension. If there is redundant tissue and excessive fat, a defatting tracheotomy may be indicated, and these procedures have been found to be safe and effective.[17] Formal division of the thyroid isthmus or resection of the isthmus facilitates tracheal stoma construction. Creation of a tracheal stoma through an inferiorly based tracheal flap (Bjork flap) combined with a superior skin flap will result in a tracheal stoma that stands open upon removal of the tracheal tube, which can prevent catastrophic airway loss (Fig. 34-5). This procedure could be referred to as a true "tracheostomy" because, like tracheostomal construction following laryngectomy, a permanent tracheal stoma is created.

SPECIAL CONSIDERATIONS

PEDIATRIC TRACHEOTOMY

The technique of pediatric tracheotomy differs from that of adult tracheotomy and is associated with a higher rate of complications. In children, the mobility of the trachea is more pronounced, making it more susceptible to deviation with retraction and displacement during surgery. The most feared complication is dissection toward the common carotid artery, which can be easily mistaken for the trachea. Aberrant dissection can also lead to the mediastinum resulting in hemopneumothorax. Children demonstrate smaller anatomic structures and decreased distances between landmarks. The greater elasticity of the cartilaginous tracheal rings allows more effective use of tracheal stay sutures. Stay sutures are more commonly used in children, considering the higher incidence of catastrophic airway loss with accidental decannulation.[16] In children, the size of the tracheal tube must be accurately matched, because the tracheal tubes are cuffless and rely on the fit for a seal. The surgeon must also carefully gauge the depth to avoid right mainstem bronchus intubation. Correct placement can be confirmed with chest radiograph as well as with auscultation of breath sounds.

TRACHEOTOMY IN THE OBESE PATIENT

The obese neck can present several potential problems when tracheotomy is planned. However, critical evaluation of the neck of an obese patient may show that the anterior neck is actually not obese,

PERCUTANEOUS DILATIONAL TRACHEOTOMY

Percutaneous dilational tracheotomy (PDT) is a technique based on the Seldinger dilational process that creates a tract for tracheal tube placement by serial dilation over a guidewire placed by percutaneous puncture. It was developed as a blind technique, although now it is most commonly performed with bronchoscopic guidance.[18] The main advantage of PDT is the ability to perform the procedure at the bedside in the ICU, thereby minimizing transport of critically ill patients and decreasing the cost of the procedure. This allows a shorter delay in the time between the decision for tracheotomy and the procedure. Other advantages include a small incision, less need for dissection, and fewer wound complications.[19] Disadvantages of PDT include bleeding, infection, and hypoxia. PDT is a closed procedure that can lead to paratracheal insertion and posterolateral tracheal wall laceration. One of the main disadvantages is that the PDT only allows for insertion of a single cannula tracheal tube that can increase the chance of mucous plugging.[20]

Table 34-1 compares the factors that favor percutaneous versus open tracheotomy. Unfavorable anatomy was identified as a restriction to the percutaneous technique, and the lack of palpable midline structures should direct the surgeon to perform an open

TABLE 34-1	Comparison of Dilational and Open Tracheotomy: Summary of Results
FAVORS PERCUTANEOUS TECHNIQUE	**FAVORS OPEN TECHNIQUE**
Wound infection ($P = .0002$)	Decannulation/obstruction ($P = .009$)
Unfavorable scarring ($P = .01$)	False passage ($P = .08$)
Cost-effectiveness ($P < .0001$)	Minor hemorrhage ($P = .77$)
Case length ($P < .0001$)	
Overall complications ($P = .05$)	
Major hemorrhage ($P = .17$)	
Subglottic stenosis ($P = .19$)	
Death ($P = .50$)	

From Higgins KM, Punthakee X: Meta-analysis comparison of open versus percutaneous tracheostomy. *Laryngoscope* 117:447-454, 2007.

procedure. It may be safer to perform open tracheotomy in emergency situations, in patients with malignancy at the site of the tracheotomy, in patients with obscured anatomy due to infection or mass effect, and in patients without cervical spine clearance or in obese patients.

EMERGENCY SURGICAL AIRWAY

Cricothyroidotomy has gained popularity as an emergency airway due to its straightforward nature and the fact that it can be performed quickly by those with minimal to no surgical training. Patients requiring emergency "crike" fall into one of two general categories: those whose cricothyroid membranes can be readily palpated and those who by virtue of obesity, edema, subcutaneous air, or blood cannot. In the former, cricothyroidotomy can be readily performed by stabilizing the cricoid with the nondominant hand while creating a transverse skin incision over the cricothyroid membrane. The surgeon will repalpate the cricothyroid membrane through the skin incision and make a second incision that enters the airway transversely through the membrane. In the latter category of patients, the surgeon may opt for a large vertical incision that allows a wider range of palpation of the membrane. Once palpated, the membrane is incised with a transverse incision. Once the airway is entered, it can be dilated by a finger or by twisting the back of the scalpel handle. A small endotracheal tube is placed. Once the patient has been stabilized after the emergent airway, consideration should be given to converting to a standard tracheotomy within 72 hours if intubation is still going to be required.[21] This approach potentially minimizes the trauma to the cricothyroid muscle and the articulation of the cricoid and thyroid cartilages, as well as the risk of subglottic stenosis.

In an emergent situation, the surgeon may also choose to perform tracheotomy if there is a temporary ability to ventilate the patient with a mask or laryngeal mask airway. One may also perform an emergent tracheotomy if the airway is lost during performance of an elective tracheotomy. Another emergency situation is that of reopening a tracheal site following decannulation if airway obstruction or loss of airway occurs. This is done by forcing a hemostat through the healing or healed tracheotomy wound or scar days to years after decannulation. In an emergency situation, any airway that can be placed regardless of collateral damage is a success.

ELECTIVE CRICOTHYROIDOTOMY

Cricothyroidotomy was condemned by Jackson in 1921, because it was associated with a high incidence of subglottic stenosis.[3] In 1976, two cardiothoracic surgeons published a paper highlighting their experience with 655 elective cricothyroidotomies among a population of elective thoracic surgery patients, stating simplicity and absence of cross contamination among median sternotomy patients, with a 6.1% complication rate.[22] After this, enthusiasm for elective cricothyroidotomy waxed and waned. It has been shown that the rate of complications of long-term cricothyroidotomy in trauma patients is no different than that in tracheotomy, with no cases of subglottic stenosis.[23] The authors refrain from elective cricothyroidotomy, because of the inability to use a large caliber tube, inability to use a double cannula tube, and reliability of elective tracheotomy at their institution.

Tracheotomy has emerged from the controversy surrounding its early history to become an important and commonly performed surgical procedure. As with all surgical interventions, it is not without risk, but its potential to benefit many patients has resulted in its widespread acceptance in modern surgery.

PEARLS AND PITFALLS

- Following placement of the tracheal tube, maintain the cricoid hook in position until ventilation and successful tracheal tube placement has been confirmed.
- Maintain a low threshold for utilizing extended-length tracheal tubes in obese patients or patients who otherwise have an increased distance from skin to trachea.
- The report from a bedside nurse that a suction catheter "hangs up" or is difficult to pass merits prompt attention, because it may signify the slow displacement phenomenon.
- If the tracheal cuff seems to require ever-increasing pressure to maintain a seal, consider replacing the tracheal tube with one of a different design or length to avoid tracheomalacia.
- In an emergency pediatric tracheotomy, the cervical structure that can be confused with the trachea is the common carotid artery.
- Obese patients who require tracheotomy often benefit from construction of a tracheal stoma with fat removal and creation of a Bjork flap.
- If landmarks cannot be palpated in emergency cricothyroidotomy, a large vertical skin incision will allow rapid and accurate identification of the cricothyroid membrane.

REFERENCES

1. Gordon BL: *The romance of medicine.* Philadelphia, 1947, FA Davis. p. 461.
2. Heister L: *General system of surgery,* vol 2, ed 8. London, 1768, Innys, p. 52.
3. Jackson C: Tracheotomy. *Laryngoscope* 19:285, 1909.
4. Frost EA: Tracing the tracheostomy. *Ann Otol Rhinol Laryngol* 85:618, 1976.
5. Potter JK, Herford AS, Ellis E 3rd: Tracheotomy versus endotracheal intubation for airway management in deep neck space infections. *J Oral Maxillofac Surg* 60:349-354, 2002.
6. De Leyn P, Bedert L, Delcroix M, et al: Tracheotomy: clinical review and guidelines. *Eur J Cardiothorac Surg* 32:412-421, 2007.
7. King C, Moores LK: Controversies in mechanical ventilation: when should a tracheotomy be placed? *Clin Chest Med* 29:253-263, 2008.
8. Goldenberg D, Ari EG, Golz A, et al: Tracheotomy complications: a retrospective study of 1130 cases. *Otolaryngol Head Neck Surg* 123:495-500, 2000.
9. Waldron J, Padgham NW, Hurley SE: Complications of emergency and elective tracheostomy. *Ann R Coll Surg Engl* 72:218-220, 1990.
10. Goldstein SI, Breda SD, Schneider KL: Surgical complications of bedside tracheotomy in an otolaryngology residency program. *Laryngoscope* 97:1407-1409, 1987.
11. Dierks EJ: Tracheotomy: elective and emergent. *Oral Maxillofac Surg Clin North Am* 20:513-520, 2008.
12. Oshinsky AE, Rubin JS, Gwozdz CS: The anatomical basis for post-tracheotomy innominate artery rupture. *Laryngoscope* 98:1061-1064, 1988.
13. Utley JR, Singer MM, Roe BB: Definitive management of innominate artery hemorrhage complicating tracheostomy. *JAMA* 4:577-579, 1972.
14. Esses BA, Jafek BW: Cricothyroidotomy: a decade of experience in Denver. *Ann Otol Rhinol Laryngol* 96:519-524, 1987.
15. Wood DE, Mathisen DJ: Late complications of tracheotomy. *Clin Chest Med* 12:597-609, 1991.
16. Carr MM, Poje CP, Kingston L, et al: Complications in pediatric tracheostomies. *Laryngoscope* 111:1925-1928, 2001.
17. Gross ND, Cohen JI, Andersen PE, Wax MK: Defatting tracheotomy in morbidly obese patients. *Laryngoscope* 112:1940-1944, 2002.
18. Ciaglia P, Firsching R, Syniec C: Elective percutaneous dilatational tracheostomy. A new simple bedside procedure; preliminary report. *Chest* 87:715-719, 1985.
19. Al-Ansari MA, Hijazi MH: Clinical review: percutaneous dilational tracheostomy. *Crit Care* 10:202, 2006.
20. Higgins KM, Punthakee X: Meta-analysis comparison of open versus percutaneous tracheostomy. *Laryngoscope* 117:447-454, 2007.
21. Heffner JE: Tracheotomy application and timing. *Clin Chest Med* 24:389-398, 2003.
22. Brantigan CO, Grow JB: Cricothyroidotomy: elective use in respiratory problems requiring tracheostomy. *J Thorac Cardiovasc Surg* 71:72-81, 1976.
23. Wright MJ, Greenberg DE, Hunt JP, et al: Surgical cricothyroidotomy in trauma patients. *South Med J* 96:465-467, 2003.

Chapter **35**

Traumatic Epistaxis

Michael M. Demo, Martin B. Steed

As the most anterior point of the face, the nose frequently lends itself to traumatic injury. Secondary to a rich vascular supply, the nasal complex is a common source of hemorrhage (epistaxis) in the trauma victim. Treatment of epistaxis is dictated by the etiology and the source of bleeding; thus knowledge of facial anatomy and a thorough physical evaluation of the patient will readily guide the proper treatment.

The incidence of severe hemorrhage resulting from maxillofacial trauma is rare, but is potentially life threatening. When maxillofacial injuries lead to life-threatening hemorrhage, the patient's airway, breathing, and circulation should be managed initially within the Advanced Trauma Life Support (ATLS) protocol.

Treatment of life-threatening nasal hemorrhage associated with post-traumatic craniofacial fracture is principally based on aggressive resuscitation combined with anterior and posterior nasal packing, which should be performed upon presentation in the emergency room or as soon as possible. Ardekian reported various treatment modalities for traumatic bleeding from the maxillofacial region, including nasal packing, reduction of fractures, arterial ligation, angiography, and selective embolization.

Because post-traumatic nasal bleeding frequently originates from lacerated arteries deep in the fractured facial skeleton and proximal to the nasal cavity, it is not always possible to attenuate bleeding by nasal packing alone. If nasal hemorrhage persists and blood pressure remains unstable after nasal packing, direct surgical ligation of the bleeding vessels or fixation of facial fractures is conventionally recommended. However, in the setting of multisystem trauma and shock, surgery to ligate the deep hemorrhaging nasal vessels may be too time-consuming and risky. In these cases, transarterial embolization (TAE) can offer an alternative to control hemorrhage. Early diagnosis and intervention of life-threatening hemorrhage is essential for a favorable outcome.

ETIOPATHOGENESIS/CAUSATIVE FACTORS

Epistaxis is the result of direct or indirect vascular injury within the nasal complex and its associated sinuses. Epistaxis may present as a result of tumors, orthognathic/cosmetic surgery, intubation, medications, arteriovenous malformations, and coagulopathies. However, in the setting of facial trauma, the more common etiologies are assault, motor vehicle collision (MVC), gunshot wounds, and athletic injuries. Identification of the etiology of epistaxis is crucial in managing the patient and providing appropriate treatment. With this in mind, epistaxis as a result of direct vascular injury may only need local measures to control the event, whereas, in the presence of a coagulopathy treatment, it will likely need systemic management in addition to local management.

DYSCRASIAS

Coagulopathies alone can cause significant epistaxis and must always be considered in the trauma victim when hemorrhage is disproportionate to the mechanism of injury. Anticoagulant medication or history of bleeding dyscrasias should always be determined and coagulation assays obtained when indicated. Reversal with appropriate medications, blood products, or coagulation factors may be necessary, in concert with local measures. All individuals with excessive epistaxis should be evaluated for dyscrasias and receive necessary fluid resuscitation and reversal early to prevent hemodynamic instability.

PSEUDOANEURYSM OF THE INTERNAL CAROTID ARTERY

An initially silent, but very serious consequence of maxillofacial injury is traumatic pseudoaneurysm of the internal carotid (TPICA). Initiated by blunt as well as penetrating trauma, pseudoaneurysms form when an artery has a partial transection. Resulting leakage of blood from the vessel forms a hematoma within the surrounding tissue. Tamponade from the hematoma slows bleeding and retains patency of the arterial lumen, preventing clinically significant hemorrhage. Complications from a pseudoaneurysm can manifest anywhere from days to months after the initial trauma, a direct consequence of a re-bleed of the injured vessel. Delayed hemorrhage from the pseudoaneurysm is due to hematoma resolution or tearing of the fibrous capsule wall that can form around the initial hematoma. A TPICA presents as varying degrees of neurologic deficits and hemorrhage, such as recurrent, often substantial epistaxis. TPICA rupture is associated with 30% to 50% mortality and, accordingly, must always be considered in patients with a history of trauma who present with recurrent epistaxis, especially with cranial nerve deficits. Brisk diagnosis and treatment, usually by arterial angiography and embolization, is imperative.

ARTERIAL ANATOMY

Comprehension of the nasal complex vascularity is essential for proper evaluation and treatment of epistaxis (Fig. 35-1). The arterial supply to the nasal fossa involves branches from both the external and internal carotid arteries. The external carotid artery contributes most of the arterial supply through the internal maxillary (sphenopalatine and greater palatine branches) and facial arteries (superior labial branch). A branch of the internal carotid artery, the ophthalmic artery, supplies the nasal fossa through the anterior and posterior ethmoidal arteries. The nasal blood supply can be considered to have three main sources with multiple anastomoses: the sphenopalatine (considered the primary source), the superior labial, and the ethmoidal arteries.

SPHENOPALATINE ARTERY

The sphenopalatine artery (SPA) serves as the major supply to the nasal fossa and enters the nasal cavity through the sphenopalatine foramen. The foramen is located on the posterior aspect of the lateral nasal wall posterior to the middle turbinate. The SPA most commonly splits into a septal and lateral branch just as it passes through the foramen. Alternatively, the SPA can have three or more branches and may split within the pterygopalatine fossa prior to entering the nasal fossa. These variations are important to consider when attempting surgical ligation.

SUPERIOR LABIAL ARTERY

The superior labial artery, arising from the facial artery, penetrates the orbicularis oris muscle at the level of the commissure and enters into the nasal osteum superficial to the depressor septi nasi muscle. It supplies the anterior portion of the septum and medial wall of the nasal vestibule through the septal branch.

ANTERIOR AND POSTERIOR ETHMOIDALS

The internal carotid arterial supply originates from the ophthalmic artery, entering the orbit along with the optic nerve through the optic canal. After the lacrimal artery divides off the ophthalmic artery, it continues along the superior and medial aspect of the orbit. The anterior and posterior ethmoidal arteries split off medially through the orbital wall into the ethmoid sinus, entering the nasal cavity superiorly through the cribriform plate (Fig. 35-2). The anterior and posterior ethmoidal arteries usually exit the orbit 24 mm and 36 mm posterior to the lacrimal crest, respectively, leaving the optic nerve only 6 mm behind the posterior ethmoidal arteries. These dimensions are important landmarks in order to avoid optic nerve injury when performing surgical ligation with any variation of the Lynch incision.

KIESSELBACH PLEXUS

The Kisselbach plexus, also known as the Little area, is a localized region of mucosa of the anteroinferior nasal septum. The plexus is principally supplied by branches and anastomoses of the sphenopalatine, superior labial, and anterior ethmoidal arteries and is the most common site of anterior epistaxis.

WOODRUFF PLEXUS

The Woodruff plexus is a network of anastomoses on the lateral nasal wall inferior to the posterior end of the inferior turbinate. Once thought to be the primary source of posterior epistaxis, it is now considered entirely venous and is thought to play a much less important role.

DIAGNOSTIC STUDIES

As for any emergent consult, a brief history of presenting illness, past medical/surgical history, allergies, and current medications should be assessed judiciously. Along with a simultaneous initial survey, the clinician should be able to assess the possible etiology (e.g., traumatic, pharmacologic, postsurgical), severity (amount, duration), and source (anterior or posterior) of the epistaxis.

This initial survey should dictate initial diagnostic studies. In the presence of a severe bleed, and any suspected posterior bleed, the

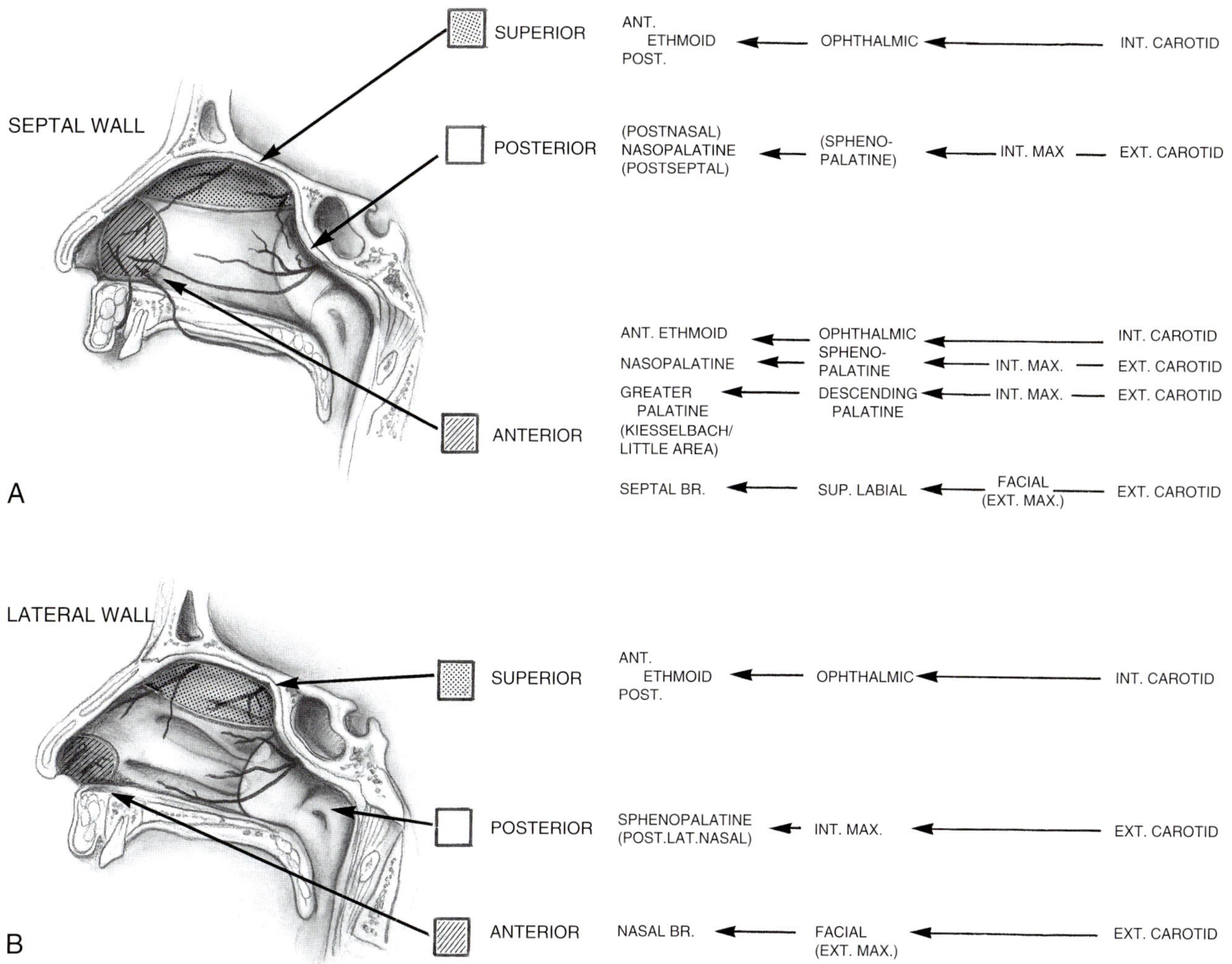

SEPTAL WALL

SUPERIOR	ANT. ETHMOID POST.	←	OPHTHALMIC	←	INT. CAROTID
POSTERIOR	(POSTNASAL) NASOPALATINE (POSTSEPTAL)	←	(SPHENO-PALATINE)	←	INT. MAX. ─ EXT. CAROTID

ANTERIOR	ANT. ETHMOID	←	OPHTHALMIC	←	INT. CAROTID
	NASOPALATINE	←	SPHENO-PALATINE	←	INT. MAX. ─ EXT. CAROTID
	GREATER PALATINE (KIESSELBACH/ LITTLE AREA)	←	DESCENDING PALATINE	←	INT. MAX. ─ EXT. CAROTID
	SEPTAL BR.	←	SUP. LABIAL	←	FACIAL (EXT. MAX.) ─ EXT. CAROTID

A

LATERAL WALL

SUPERIOR	ANT. ETHMOID POST.	←	OPHTHALMIC	←	INT. CAROTID
POSTERIOR	SPHENOPALATINE (POST.LAT.NASAL)	←	INT. MAX.	←	EXT. CAROTID
ANTERIOR	NASAL BR.	←	FACIAL (EXT. MAX.)	←	EXT. CAROTID

B

Fig. 35-1 ■ **A,** Anatomy of septal vessels. **B,** Anatomy of the vessels on lateral wall of nose. (From Lore JM, Medina JE: *An atlas of head and neck surgery,* ed 4. Philadelphia, 2005, Saunders.)

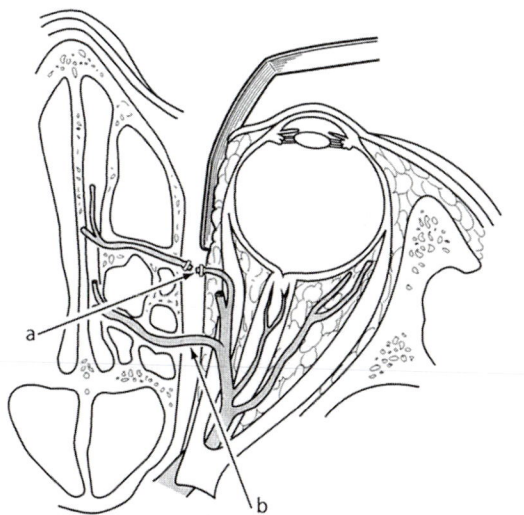

Fig. 35-2 ■ Anterior ethmoidal ligation. **A,** anterior ethmoid artery. **B,** posterior ethmoid artery. (From Viehweg TL, Roberson JB, Hudson JW: Epistaxis: diagnosis and treatment. *J Oral Maxillofac Surg* 64:511-518, 2006.)

clinician should establish intravenous (IV) access and consider a fluid bolus as well as laboratory tests, including, but not limited to, a complete blood count, coagulation panel, and platelet function assay. Direct inspection should be done only with the proper armamentarium, including a light source, suction, nasal speculum, and bayonet forceps. In cases of mild epistaxis, initial inspection can be performed without packing or a vasoconstrictor. This avoids temporarily hiding the offending vessel. Instead, consider a saline rinse and only use a vasoconstrictor and packing if initial visualization is impractical without attenuating the hemorrhage.

Epistaxis is typically classified as either anterior or posterior. Anterior epistaxis will present with the majority of hemorrhage exiting the nares; conversely, a true posterior epistaxis will primarily exit through the nasopharynx and can be visualized in the oropharynx, fairly easily distinguishing the two entities. These classifications do not have a defined anatomic dividing line between them; instead, the definition is an operational one. Anterior epistaxis has traditionally been defined as bleeding controlled through anterior rhinoscopy or anterior nasal packing, whereas posterior epistaxis is bleeding not easily visible anteriorly or that which is controlled only through posterior packing. Recent advances in endoscopy and endoscopic ligation/cauterization techniques blur the lines between these two divisions. It may be more appropriate to define anterior epistaxis as bleeding arising from the more anterior vessels (anterior

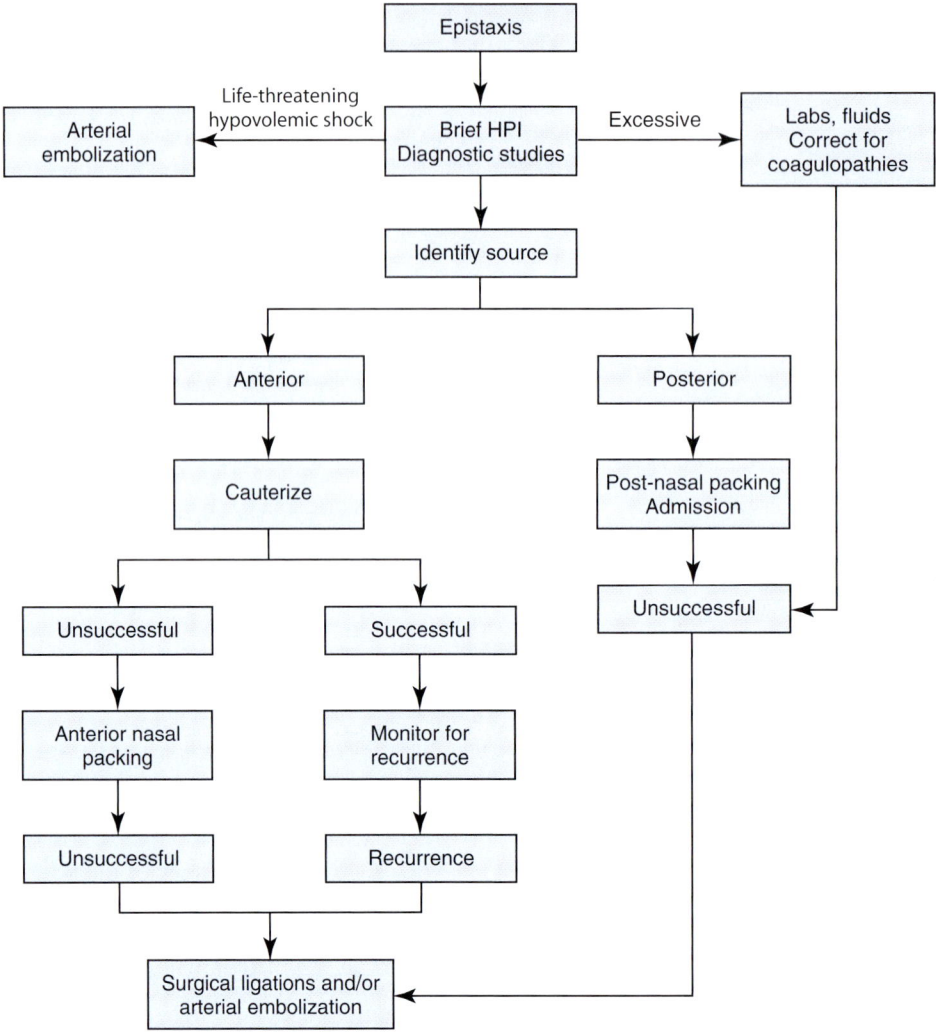

Fig. 35-3 ■ Traumatic epistaxis algorithm.

ethmoidal or superior labial) and posterior epistaxis as bleeding arising from the more posterior vessels (sphenopalatine branches). Although these definitions have a significant "gray area" because of anastomotic networks, such a classification helps define which treatment methods will be most successful.

Anterior epistaxis makes up 90% to 95% of all episodes of epistaxis. The great majority of these cases arise from the Kiesselbach plexus and tend to be more self-limiting and amenable to conservative treatment. Posterior epistaxis, due in part to location and access, tends to be more difficult to treat. In the face of posterior epistaxis and the high likelihood of sphenopalatine involvement, a V2 pterygopalatine ganglion block can vasoconstrict the sphenopalatine artery and enhance visualization. With the etiology, source, and severity of the epistaxis in mind from the diagnostic survey, the clinician is well prepared to initiate treatment.

TREATMENT GOALS

The treatment goal of traumatic epistaxis is immediate and sustained control of bleeding and site-specific hemostasis. The treatment of epistaxis has undergone significant changes in recent years. The days when patients underwent placement of an uncomfortable posterior nasal pack and spent several days on the surgical

ward, only to begin bleeding again upon removal, are close to past. More advanced packing devices, hemostatic agents, endoscopic approaches, and endovascular techniques have provided the surgeon with a variety of effective and better-tolerated treatment options. The goal remains the same but can now be accomplished with less discomfort, greater success, and perhaps better utilization of resources.

SPECIFIC TREATMENT AND TECHNIQUES

All trauma patients should be initially approached within the ATLS algorithm, and then a more focused algorithm for epistaxis is initiated (Fig. 35-3). For the patient who is hemodynamically stable, the same principles adhered to for a stable isolated facial trauma patient should be applied to one with idiopathic nasal bleeding. These principles include adequate preparation, proper instrumentation, inspection with direct visualization, and use of topically applied vasoconstrictor and anesthetic if necessary.

LOCAL MEASURES

After meticulous examination and inspection of the nasal cavity, local measures should be employed. Local measures include the application of topical vasoconstriction, which can be used prior to attempts at direct visualization. Oxymetazoline, the active ingredient of decongestants such as Afrin (Schering Plough Healthcare, Memphis, Tenn.), results in significant vasoconstriction and contraction of nasal mucosa. Anesthesia can be obtained in the awake facial trauma patient with local anesthesia injections or 4% topical lidocaine applied to cotton pledgets inserted into the nasal cavity for several minutes. Cocaine, in a 4% solution, provides both anesthetic and vasoconstrictive effects but may not be readily available in all emergency or operating rooms.

Cautery

If a discrete anterior source of bleeding has been adequately visualized, precise cautery can often provide definitive treatment. Cautery hemostasis can be either chemical (silver nitrate) or electrical (bipolar or hotwire) and should begin circumferentially around the bleeding site. Prolonged and deep electrical cautery of the septum should be avoided because perforation could result from injudicious force and poor visualization. Silver nitrate applicators can be utilized over the bleeding site with light but firm pressure for at least 5 seconds.

Nasal Packing

Nasal packing is often the next choice in the facial trauma setting for those nasal bleeds that are profuse or those in which visualization is inadequate for direct cautery. Nasal packing can consist of anterior nasal packing, posterior nasal packing, or a combination of both. The awake patient is ideally anesthetized prior to pack insertion. Various methods of nasal packing with a vast number of different materials have been advocated and used over time. Traditionally, packing was performed with ribbon gauze, usually coated with an antibiotic ointment or bismuth iodoform paraffin paste. Effective packing with gauze requires some training and can be a difficult process for the awake patient. Patients who have nasal packing should also be placed on systemic antibiotics, and packs with antibiotic ointment are recommended to prevent toxic shock syndrome (TSS). Considering no substantial evidence exists to demonstrate reduction in TSS with antibiotic prophylaxis, it is prudent to remove the packing within 5 days. Packs are generally left in for 1 to 5 days based on physician preference, response of the patient, risk factors, state of coagulopathy, and severity of initial bleed.

Proprietary types of nasal packs (Fig. 35-4) that are commonly used today include Merocel (Medtronic Xomed, Jacksonville, Fla.) and Rhino Rocket (Denver Splint Corp, Englewood, Colo.). These nasal packs are made from compressed hydroxylating polyvinyl acetate (PVA) that expands upon contact with liquid. The pack can

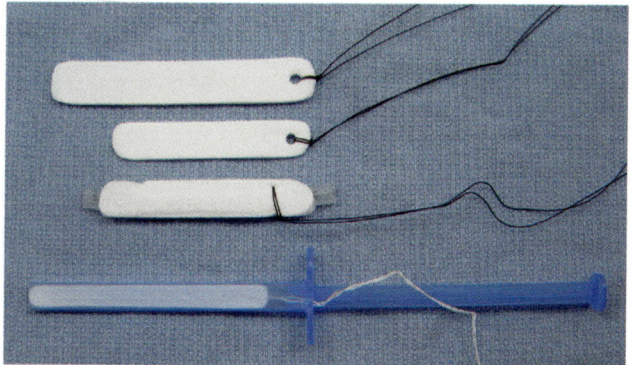

Fig. 35-4 ■ Nasal packing modalities. (From Viehweg TL, Roberson JB, Hudson JW et al: Epistaxis: diagnosis and treatment, *J Oral Maxillofac Surg* 64:511-518, 2006.)

be lubricated with an antibiotic ointment as well as viscous lidocaine for comfort. It is inserted into the nasal cavity with bayonet forceps and advanced posteriorly along the nasal floor with steady pressure until the entire packing is within the nose. The pack will expand upon contact with the blood in the nasal cavity and very rarely needs any additional saline for further expansion. It can be trimmed with scissors according to the patient's internal nasal anatomy.

Certain types of nasal packs possess an inflatable balloon. The Rapid Rhino (Applied Therapeutics, Tampa, Fla.) is composed of an inflatable balloon coated with a carboxymethylcellulose hydrocolloid compound, which acts as a platelet aggregator and also forms a lubricant upon contact with fluid. An advantage to the balloon packing is the ability to deflate the device before removal, allowing for inspection for re-bleeding as well as relatively atraumatic removal.

Similarly, Epistat (Medtronic Xomed) is a nasal catheter which can be inserted and then augmented as needed with iodoform gauze packing or nasal tampons as appropriate. The Epistat consists of one small, high-pressure, low-volume balloon designed to occlude the choanae posteriorly and a second, larger, low-pressure, high-volume balloon intended to fill the posterior nasal cavity. Appropriately placed, an Epistat can potentially control a posterior bleed. Posterior packing is not as commonly used as anterior packing and involves more risk. Posterior packs can be employed as an emergent temporizing procedure before other surgical or interventional therapy.

Alternatively, a large 16-F Foley catheter can be placed through the nose and passed to the posterior pharyngeal wall. Prior to placement, the catheter tip can be trimmed to avoid irritation and potential necrosis as it contacts the posterior pharyngeal wall. The balloon can then be inflated with appropriate volumes of saline (air-filled balloons tend to deflate over time) and the catheter pulled anteriorly to occlude the posterior choanae with the inflated balloons. The catheter can then be secured anteriorly with a large suture, an umbilical clip, or tied to a second contralaterally placed Foley, maintaining slight tension to prevent slippage of the inflated balloons into the oropharynx. Care should be taken to cushion the nostrils and columella from the secured catheters anteriorly. The nasal cavity can then be packed with a variety of material, including iodoform gauze or nasal tampons.

As with any posterior packing, adequate pressure is unlikely to be placed directly onto the bleeding site. Bleeding control actually comes from the resultant mucosal edema or from blood tamponaded within the posterior nose. Complications from anterior and posterior packs include ulcerations, septal perforation, sinusitis, synechiae, hypoxemia, and arrhythmias. Posterior packing can lead to alar, columellar, or palatal necrosis. The posterior pack may also cause apnea and hypoxia, with possible dysrhythmia. The apnea and hypoxia associated with posterior packing has previously been ascribed to stimulation of the nasopulmonary or "diving" reflex. Such a reflex pathway has never been firmly established and it is more likely that this phenomenon is a result of obstructive sleep apnea. Patients who have posterior packing should be admitted for inpatient observation, with continuous pulse oximetry and supplemental oxygen as needed. Additional care should be taken in individuals with a history of cardiopulmonary disease.

Hemostatic Compounds

The use of more easily applied and more favorably tolerated hemostatic compounds has been investigated in an attempt to avoid the discomfort associated with nasal packing. Antifibrinolytic agents, such as ε-amino caproic acid and tranexamic acid, have both been demonstrated to be effective, but their use has not been widespread.

Floseal (Baxter, Deerfield, Ill.) is a biodegradable hemostatic sealant composed of collagen-derived particles and topical bovine-derived thrombin, which is applied as a high viscosity gel. In a study of 70 patients with anterior epistaxis, Floseal was compared with standard packing (Merocel, Vaseline gauze, and Rhino Rocket) and was found to be significantly more effective and better tolerated than packing, and the patients were spared the discomfort of pack removal.

INVASIVE MEASURES

Surgical procedures and angiographic modalities for embolization have revolutionized the treatment of severe refractory epistaxis. Selective arterial embolization and surgical management remain reserved for patients with refractory or life-threatening bleeding

With widespread popularization of endoscopic sinus surgery and a greater understanding of local regional anatomy, endoscopic control of the sphenopalatine artery has been advocated as an effective alternative for the control of posterior epistaxis.

In general, the more proximal the ligation is from the bleeding vessel, the higher the failure rate that is clinically encountered secondary to anastomoses between circulations. This concept of ligation as close as possible to the bleeding point enables a ligation hierarchy to be developed for epistaxis, with the sphenopalatine being the ligation of choice (i.e., most distal), followed by internal maxillary and external carotid arteries. Given the position of the anterior ethmoidal artery, it is low in this hierarchy because of the secondary importance of the internal carotid-derived supply.

Sphenopalatine Artery Cautery or Ligation

Endoscopic nasal surgery, with cauterization or ligation of the sphenopalatine artery on its entry into the nasal cavity, has been shown to be effective and minimally invasive in treating and controlling intractable epistaxis (Fig. 35-5).

The sphenopalatine foramen is bounded superiorly by the body of the sphenoid, which closes the notch of the perpendicular plate of the palatine bone. The notch is bordered anteriorly by the orbital process (OP) of the palatine bone and posteriorly by the sphenoidal process (SP) of the palatine bone. The pterygopalatine space lies

lateral to the foramen. During surgery, a guide to the position of the foramen is a consistently present anatomic structure called the crista ethmoidalis of the palatine bone, which is positioned anterior and slightly superior to the neurovascular pedicle in most cases. Within the neurovascular pedicle are the sphenopalatine artery, vein, and the nasal palatine nerve (maxillary division of the trigeminal). It is not uncommon for the artery to divide before exiting the foramen, and a branch may exit posterior to the true foramen. Locating and exploring the bony foramen is thus vital to ensure that all branches are identified prior to ligation. The main artery branches form the septal, inferior turbinate, and middle turbinate arteries, which supply the majority of the nasal mucosa. The operation is performed under general anesthesia. Previously placed nasal packing is removed and topical vasoconstriction achieved using pledgets soaked in 1/1000 epinephrine. In most cases, an endoscopic middle meatal antrostomy is performed and enlarged posteriorly. If the middle meatus is wide, an antrostomy is avoided and access gained through a vertical incision in the posterior middle meatus. A mucoperiosteal flap is developed with a Freer elevator and dissected posteriorly, creating a mucosal tunnel under the sphenopalatine neurovascular bundle. The sphenopalatine artery trunk or branches are then identified just posterior to the crista ethmoidalis. The sphenopalatine artery is either clipped and/or diathermized with bipolar diathermy, either as a single emerging trunk or as its posterior lateral and posterior septal branches, depending upon the individual anatomy. The mucoperiosteal flap is repositioned, and the nasal cavity is usually left unpacked.

Embolization

Angiographic embolization for posterior epistaxis was first described in 1974. In this procedure, the artery is cannulated and contrast injected to demonstrate the bleeding area, which is then embolized with an agent. Common embolization targets include the internal maxillary artery (IMA) and facial artery. This requires skilled interventional radiologists, and some nasal packing materials may interfere with imaging, but high success rates have been achieved. Epistaxis refractory to initial treatment attempts, often cases of posterior bleeding, can be successfully treated by endovascular techniques. Because potential risks exist for inadvertent migration of

Fig. 35-5 ■ **A,** Vertical incision (*dashed line*) is made inferior to the posterior portion of the middle turbinate. **B,** Sphenopalatine artery is reached at its emergence from the sphenopalatine foramen by raising a mucoperiosteal flap backwards and upwards. **C,** Vascular clips are applied under direct vision choana; *arrow* indicates the sphenopalatine foramen. **D,** Mucoperiosteal flap is returned to its original position. *MT,* middle turbinate; *IT,* inferior turbinate. (From Voegels R, Thomé D, Iturralde P, Butugan O: Endoscopic ligature of the sphenopalatine artery for severe posterior epistaxis. *Otolaryngol Head Neck Surg* 124:464-467, 2001.)

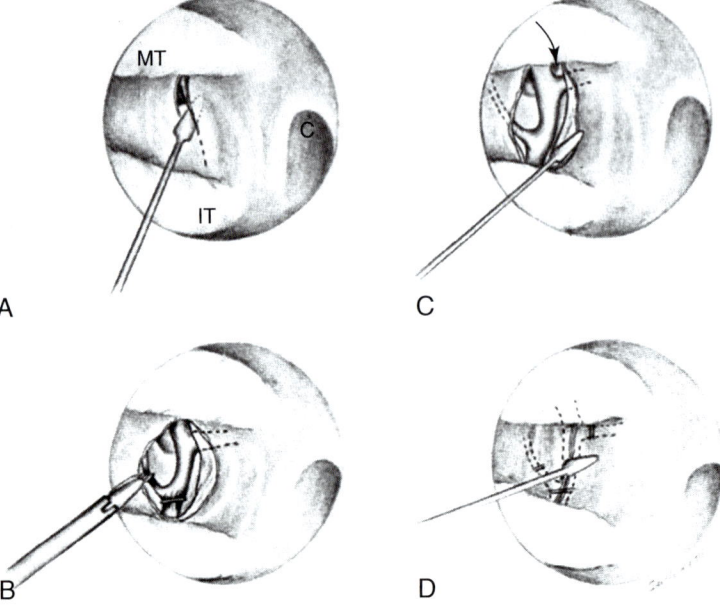

emboli through the abundant anastomoses between the external and internal carotid arteries, the application of transarterial embolization for traumatic nasal bleeding remains controversial. Because the techniques of coaxial microcatheterization and superselective embolization have improved dramatically, many authors now consider transarterial embolization to be a safe adjuvant method in the treatment of intractable post-traumatic nasal hemorrhage. Furthermore, early transarterial embolization performed in a preshock state has been demonstrated to be effective in decreasing necessary blood transfusion volume (Fig. 35-6).

Combined with endonasal packing, superselective embolization successfully stopped intractable post-traumatic nasal hemorrhage in 14 cases in a recent study, resulting in a survival rate of 78.6%. However, transarterial embolization and nasal packing failed to achieve hemostasis in three cases, which resulted in 100% mortality. Therefore, successful hemostasis of post-traumatic nasal hemorrhage by combined TAE and nasal packing significantly decreased deaths associated with profound hemorrhagic shock.

The protocol should include evaluation of the external carotid artery (ECA) to determine if the ECA or its branches are the source of bleeding. Digital subtraction angiography with road mapping is used to selectively guide the catheter to the region of interest that is typically the distal portion of the internal maxillary artery (Fig. 35-7). One must identify potentially dangerous anastomoses to the carotid siphon (such as the artery of the foramen rotundum) and ophthalmic artery to avoid the complications of stroke or blindness. The microcatheter is routinely advanced distal to branches with high potential for dangerous anastomoses collaterals, such as the middle meningeal, accessory meningeal, and superficial temporal arteries, to avoid nontarget embolization. Injection should not be performed too forcefully, because reflux into the ICA can occur. Control angiography is performed after embolization to assess the results.

Embolic materials frequently used for treatment of epistaxis include Gelfoam pieces (Upjohn, Kalamazoo, Mich.), polyvinyl alcohol particles, platinum coils, or a combination of materials. Polyvinyl alcohol particles (149 to 250 μm) are typically used. Platinum coils and Gelfoam pieces can be used to achieve proximal occlusion quickly. However, collateral formation and bleeding can occur after proximal occlusion. Additionally, Gelfoam

powder may embolize too distally and cause necrosis or cranial nerve palsy.

Failure of endovascular treatment of epistaxis is often related to continued bleeding from the ethmoidal branches of the ophthalmic artery (see Fig. 35-1). Embolization of these branches is

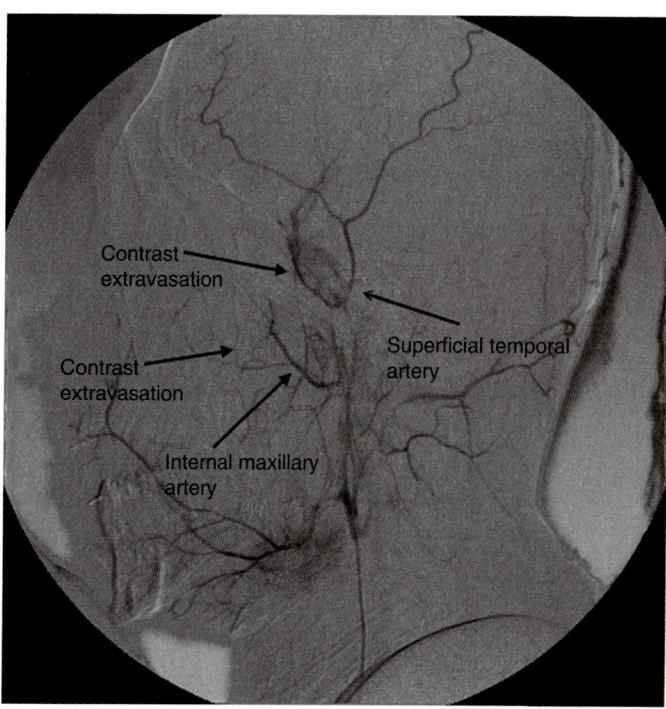

Fig. 35-6 ■ A 25-year-old patient with maxillofacial trauma complicated by life-threatening hemorrhage after a traffic accident. At the emergency department, massive epistaxis was noted. Nasal packing and blood transfusion were performed, but vital signs of the patient were still unstable. Cerebral angiography revealed contrast extravasation from the left superficial temporal and internal maxillary arteries of the left external carotid artery. After transarterial embolization was performed, the hemorrhage immediately stopped. (From Liu W, Yuan-Hao C, Hsieh C, et al: Transarterial embolization in the management of life-threatening hemorrhage after maxillofacial trauma: a case report and review of literature. *Am J Emerg Med* 26:516.e3-516.e5, 2008.)

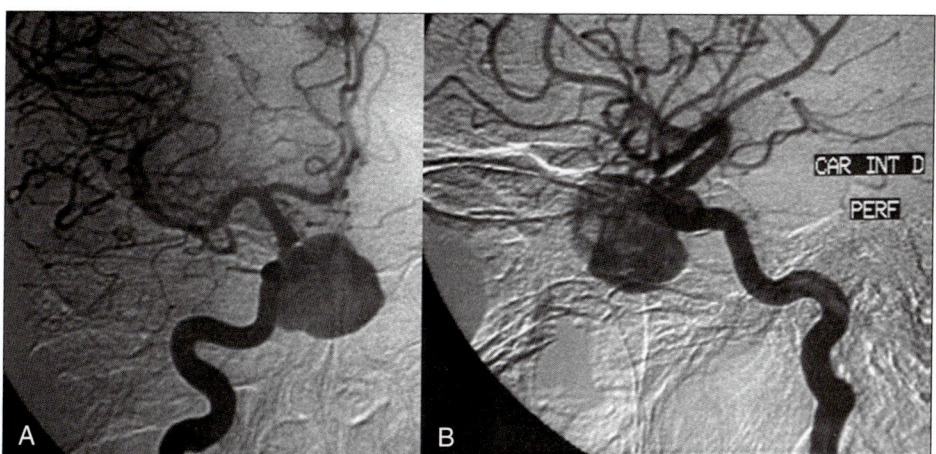

Fig. 35-7 ■ Digital subtraction angiography of a 22-year-old woman involved in a motor vehicle accident with facial and cranial blunt trauma 6 months earlier. On admission at another institution, she presented with nasal and oral bleeding (**A**). Anteroposterior view (**B**) of lateral angiography of the right internal carotid artery (ICA) demonstrating the cavernous segment giant pseudoaneurysm. (From Zanini MA, Tahara A, Santos GS, et al: Pseudoaneurysm of the internal carotid artery presenting with massive (recurrent) epistaxes: a life-threatening complication of craniofacial trauma. *Arq Neuropsiquiatr* [online] 66(2A):268-271, 2008.)

contraindicated, because ophthalmic artery embolization carries a high risk of blindness. However, the surgeon can ligate the anterior ethmoidal vessel as it perforates the medial wall of the orbit through variations of the Lynch incision. Complications from embolization include rebleeding, stroke, blindness, facial numbness, skin sloughing, carotid artery dissection, and hematoma formation.

POSTOPERATIVE CARE

Epistaxis can be chronic in nature and should be treated appropriately in the postoperative setting to avoid recurrence. Humidifiers and ocean nasal spray are encouraged to maintain a moist nasal mucosa. Nose blowing, sneezing through nose, and strenuous activity should be avoided, as well as nonsteroidal anti-inflammatory drugs (NSAIDS) and other medicines that mitigate coagulation.

PEARLS AND PITFALLS

- Identify life-threatening intractable traumatic epistaxis quickly and proceed with interventional radiology for embolization, or transfer the patient to a center with interventional capabilities.
- Consider coagulopathies in the presence of disproportionate hemorrhage and treat appropriately with fluid replacement and coagulation factors.
- Admit all patients with posterior packing to the hospital for observation.
- Reflex bradydysrhythmia can develop because of stimulation of the deep posterior oropharynx by the packing.
- Avoid overcauterization and bilateral cauterization of the nasal septum.
- Cauterization should only be utilized with direct visualization of the offending vessel.

BIBLIOGRAPHY

Abdelkeder M, Leong SC, White PS: Endoscopic control of the sphenopalatine artery for epistaxis: long-term results. *J Laryngol Otol* 121:759, 2007

Ardekian L, Samet N, Shoshani Y, Taicher S: Life-threatening bleeding following maxillofacial trauma, *J Craniomaxillofac Surg* 1993 21(8):336-338.

Frazee TA, Hauser MS: Non-surgical management of epistaxis. *J Oral Maxillofac Surg* 58:419, 2000.

Gifford TO, Orlandi RR: Epistaxis. *Otolaryngol Clin North Am* 41:525, 2008.

Koh E, Frazzini VI, Kagetsu NJ: Epistaxis: vascular anatomy, origins, and endovascular treatment. *Am J Radiol* 174:845, 2000.

Liao CC, Yu-Pao H, Chien-Tzung C, Yuan-Yun T: Transarterial embolization for intractable oronasal hemorrhage associated with craniofacial trauma: evaluation of prognostic factors. *J Trauma* 63:827, 2007.

Loughran S, Hilmi O, McGarry GW: Endoscopic sphenopalatine artery ligation—when, why and how to do it. *Clin Otolaryngol* 30:539, 2005.

Chapter **36**

Nasal Fractures

Tirbod Fattahi

The nasal complex is the most frequently fractured bone in the face in the adult patient. Due to its location on the face, less force is required to fracture the nasal complex than any other facial bone. Because of the frequency of injury, as well as complex topography and different components (bone, cartilage, mucosa, skin) of the nasal complex, appropriate management of the acutely injured nose is imperative in order to prevent adverse sequelae. The purpose of this chapter is to discuss the contemporary management of bony injuries to the nasal complex.

ETIOLOGY AND PATHOGENESIS

The most common etiologic factor for blunt nasal trauma is motor vehicle collisions followed by interpersonal injuries. The mechanism of injury is important in determining the nature of the deformity. Due to its projection, the bony complex is typically fractured in a lateral (outward) direction when the vector of the force is directly parallel to the nose. On the other hand, if the force is directed laterally to the nose (a right-handed punch to the left side of the nose), the nasal complex will then deviate away from the vector of force, with one nasal bone being medially displaced, while the other one will be laterally displaced. It is imperative to remember that the nasal septum will also be typically injured during blunt nasal trauma. The nasal septum must be appropriately reduced at the time of repair of the nasal bone; otherwise, the incidence of post-traumatic nasal deformity will significantly increase. It is also important to question the patient about the physical appearance of the nose and whether or not it is different than preinjury. Preexisting nasal bone and septal deviations should be acknowledged prior to any treatment planning.

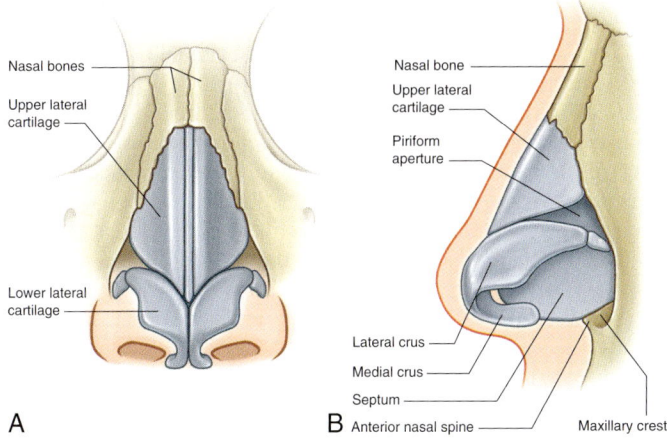

A

B

Fig. 36-1 ■ Frontal (**A**) and lateral (**B**) views of the nasal complex. Note the relationship between the nasal bones, upper lateral cartilages, and the frontal processes of the maxillary bone. (From Aston SJ, Steinbrech DS, Walden JL: *Aesthetic plastic surgery*. London, 2009, Saunders.)

PATHOLOGIC ANATOMY

The paired nasal bones are located between the nasofrontal suture cephalically and the upper lateral cartilages caudally. They are laterally bordered by the frontal processes of the maxillary bones. It is important to remember that the nasal bones overlap the cephalic portion of the upper lateral cartilages by 3 to 4 mm (Fig. 36-1). The nasal septum is composed of cartilage (anteriorly) and bone (posteriorly). The quadrangular portion of the nasal is the primary support mechanism of the nasal complex and is made of cartilage. The cartilage is thick posteriorly along the junction with the vomer and ethmoid bones, as well as along the maxillary crest (Fig. 36-2). Depending on the mechanism of injury, nasal bones and septum will be displaced along specific vectors. It is just as important to properly reduce a nasal septum as it is to reduce nasal bones. As the saying goes—"as the septum goes, so goes the nose."

DIAGNOSTIC STUDIES

The standard of care for mid- and upper face maxillofacial trauma radiography is computed tomography (CT) scan without contrast (Fig. 36-3). Nasal bone injuries, septal deviations, and fractures are clearly delineated by CT scanning. Although plain nasal radiographs are still utilized in some institutions, their value is limited. Photographs of the injured nose are helpful for documentation purposes as well as for pre- and postoperative comparison purposes.

RECONSTRUCTIVE GOALS

The goals of management of nasal bony injuries are to prevent development of a post-traumatic nasal deformity, to restore proper nasal air flow, to prevent cosmetic deformity, and to maintain proper nasal complex topography and projection. Restoration of the sense of smell is also important, although anosmia may occur following high-impact nasal and naso-orbital-ethmoidal injuries (see Chapter 42). It is important to remember that after 10 to 14 days, an adult nasal bone will begin to form a callus that may not be easily manipulated. Delay in the initial treatment of the acutely injured nose may require open reduction and bony osteotomy.

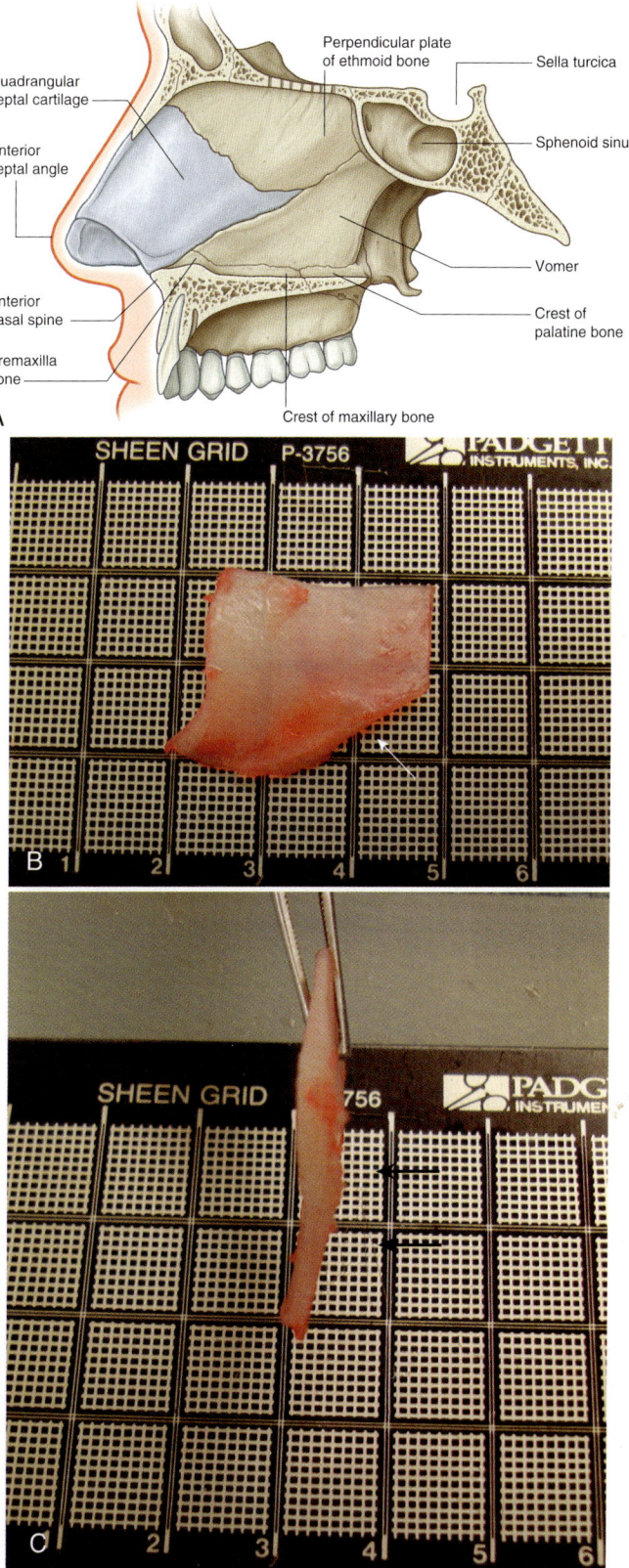

A

B

C

Fig. 36-2 ■ **A,** The nasal septum. Note relationship of the cartilaginous septum with the vomer bone (inferior) and ethmoid bone (superior). **B** and **C,** Harvested septum showing the thickened segment along the maxillary crest (*single arrow*) and along the bony attachment to the vomer and ethmoid (*double arrows*). (A, From Aston SJ, Steinbrech DS, Walden JL: *Aesthetic plastic surgery*. London, 2009, Saunders.)

SPECIFIC TREATMENT AND TECHNIQUES

Repair of nasal bone injuries can be done under local anesthesia, conscious sedation, or general anesthesia. However, the most efficient method, and perhaps the most comfortable route, is to perform the repair under general endotracheal intubation. Closed reduction of the nasal complex is still the most commonly performed maneuver for repair of the injured bony nose; however, the incidence of patients requiring a post-traumatic rhinoplasty following closed reduction can range from 9% to 62%. After the patient is intubated, a thorough manual examination of the nasal complex must be done. Crepitus, mobility, bony depressions, and asymmetries must be assessed and accounted for. Presence and/or absence of perinasal lacerations must also be confirmed. Intranasal exam is performed next. This can be accomplished by endoscopy or using a nasal

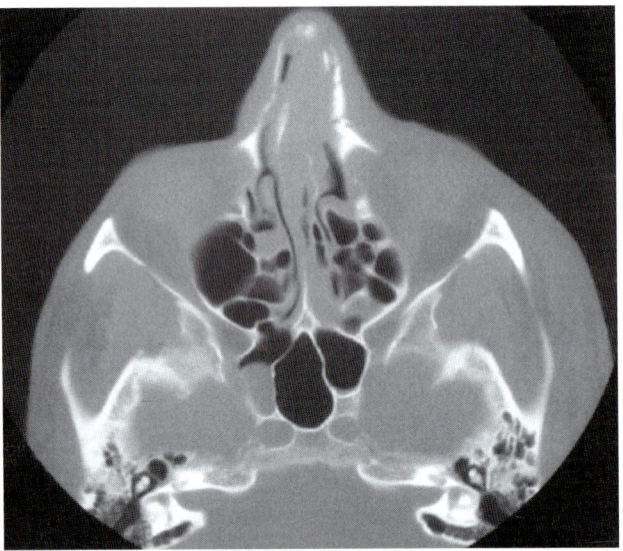

Fig. 36-3 ■ Bilateral comminuted nasal bone fractures and septal deviation following motor vehicle collision.

speculum and good lighting. Once the examination is completed, the nasal cavity is injected with a local anesthetic and a vasoconstrictor. The nasal cavity is then packed with cottonoid strips soaked in a vasoconstrictive solution. After waiting 10 to 15 minutes, the nasal cavity is examined again. The vasoconstriction significantly improves intranasal visualization. Using appropriate nasal reduction forceps, the nasal bones and the septum must be reduced in the appropriate vector (Fig. 36-4). The reduction must be maintained by intranasal packings and/or splints. If conventional methods to repair the nasal complex are not successful, the threshold for performing more extensive procedures, such as septoplasty (with or without harvest of cartilage) and bony osteotomies in the acute setting in order to "straighten" the nasal complex, should be rather low. The septum can simply be scored on its convex side to remove deviations. Although deviated septal cartilage can be removed at this time, it is more prudent to maintain all septal cartilage at the time of the initial repair in case a post-traumatic nasal deformity develops, at which point cartilage grafts from the septum become rather important reconstructive tools. If the nasal septum continues to deviate off of the anterior nasal spine (ANS), subperichondrial and subperiosteal dissections must be performed in the region of the ANS; the septum must be manually separated from the ANS and then reattached to it using sutures. This will ensure a midline caudal septum.

Bony vault deviation involving the nasal bones that are not reduced by closed reduction may require open reduction or osteotomies. The time interval from the initial injury to the time of repair (longer than 10 to 14 days) may impede closed reduction of nasal bones. In this situation, a transoral approach to the nasomaxillary buttresses, frontal processes of the maxilla, and the nasal bones may facilitate an open reduction with or without internal fixation. Endonasal or percutaneous lateral osteotomies to mobilize the bony nose can also be performed. Lateral nasal osteotomy is a powerful maneuver straightening the bony nasal vault. Again, consideration should be given to intranasal packing to maintain the mobilized bony segments. Use of external splints may also aid in elimination of dead space and maintenance of reduction (Fig. 36-5). Approaching the nasal bones through existing perinasal lacerations is also an acceptable approach. Open reduction, with or without fixation,

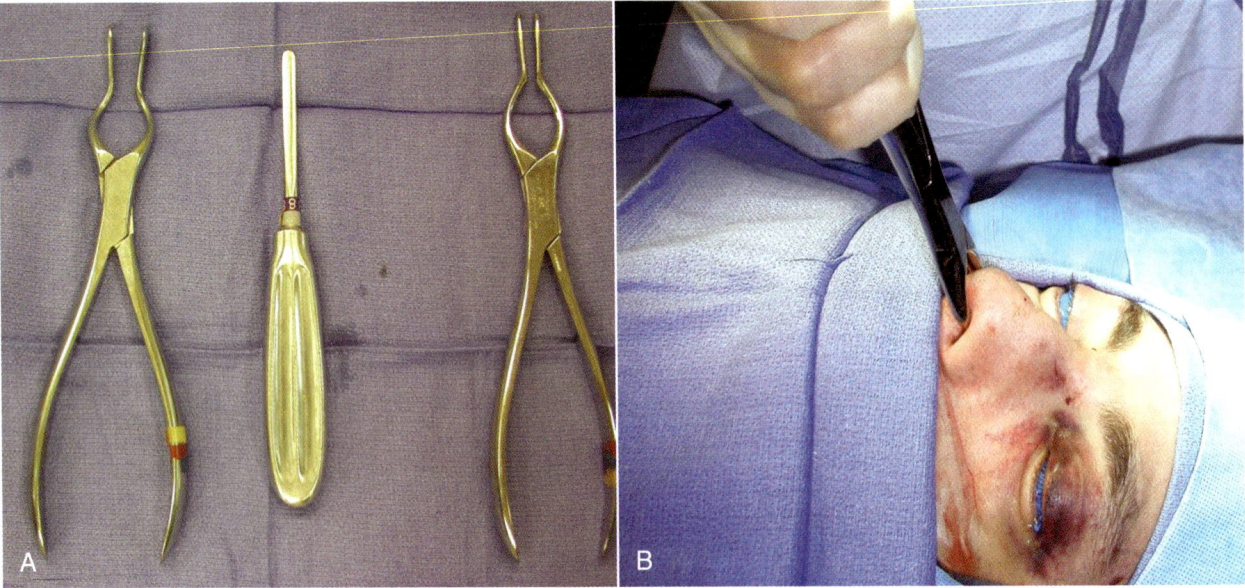

Fig. 36-4 ■ **A,** Commonly used instruments in the treatment of nasal fractures (from right to left): Walsham forceps, Boies elevator, Asch forceps. **B,** Asch forceps in use.

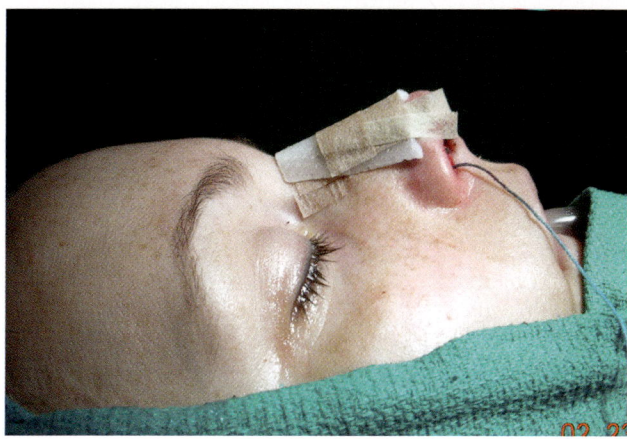

Fig. 36-5 ■ Typical external splint applied to the nasal dorsum.

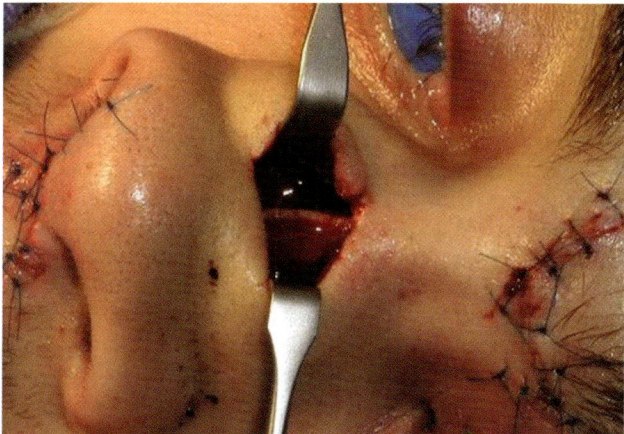

Fig. 36-6 ■ Access to the nasal complex through existing lacerations.

can be directly performed by this method and can be quite effective (Fig. 36-6).

POSTOPERATIVE CARE

Perioperative antibiotic therapy is indicated with nasal injuries. If nasal packings are used, consideration should be given to extending the duration of antibiotic coverage to decrease the incidence of toxic shock syndrome. All internal and external splints/packings are removed within the first week; if needed, a new external splint should be applied. Due to postoperative edema, all revision surgery, including post-traumatic rhinoplasty, should be delayed for several months unless the nasal complex is grossly deviated and malpositioned. Frequent postoperative follow-up is recommended to ensure proper functional and aesthetic outcome following the initial injury.

PEARLS AND PITFALLS

- Determine the appearance of the bony nose prior to the injury. Was it deviated preinjury?
- Try to reduce the nasal bone injuries within the first 10 to 14 days if possible.
- Discuss with the patient the incidence of patients who require a post-traumatic rhinoplasty following conventional repair of nasal bone injuries.
- The septum must be reduced at the initial time of repair; otherwise, the incidence of post-traumatic deformity will increase.
- Closed reduction of the acutely injured nose is still the most commonly employed method.
- The threshold for septoplasty in order to relieve deviation should be low.
- If closed reduction of the bony nasal complex is ineffective, open reduction and/or lateral nasal osteotomies should be routinely done.

BIBLIOGRAPHY

Chun K, Han SK, Kim SB, et al: Influence of nasal bone fracture and its reduction on the airway. *Head Neck Surg* 63:63-66, 2009.

Fattahi T, Steinberg B, Fernandes R, et al: Repair of nasal complex fractures and the need for secondary septo-rhinoplasty. *J Oral Maxillofac Surg* 64:1785-1789, 2006.

Fattahi T: Internal nasal valve: significance in nasal air flow. *J Oral Maxillofac Surg* 66:1921-1926, 2008.

Haug RH, Prather JL: The closed reduction of nasal fractures: an evaluation of the technique. *J Oral Maxillofac Surg* 49:1288-1292, 1991.

Hwang K, You SH, Kim SG, et al. Analysis of nasal bone fractures: a six-year study of 503 patients. *J Craniofac Surg* 17:261-264, 2006.

Low B, Massoomi N, Fattahi T: Three important considerations in posttraumatic rhinoplasty. *Am J Cosmetic Surg* 26:21-28, 2009.

Ziccardi VB, Braidy H: Management of nasal fractures. *Oral Maxillofac Surg North Am* 21:203-208, 2009.

Chapter 37

Mandibular Fractures

Stephen P.R. MacLeod

Fractures of the mandible are common. While diagnosis is usually straightforward, there are some occasions when signs and symptoms are subtle, particularly if there are associated injuries. Restoration of the occlusion is central to good outcomes. Both the presence and absence of teeth can complicate treatment. Early return to function is important to avoid complications of the temporomandibular joint apparatus and maximize patient satisfaction. This chapter will review the etiology, diagnosis, and management of fractures of the mandible, excluding fractures of the mandibular condyle, which will be covered elsewhere.

ETIOPATHOGENESIS

Fractures of the mandible can occur as the result of high-energy or low-energy trauma. In the presence of marked atrophy of the mandible, secondary to tooth loss or intrabony pathology (e.g., cysts, tumor), the causative trauma may not be noticed by the patient. In the case of high-energy trauma, the potential for other injuries must be remembered, particularly the cervical spine, upper airway, maxilla, and brain. Assessment and management of patients with mandibular injuries should always take place within the context of the Advanced Trauma Life Support (ATLS) principles established by the American College of Surgeons and accepted around the world.

PATHOLOGIC ANATOMY

The mandible is a U-shaped bone that articulates bilaterally with the temporal bones through the temporomandibular joints (TMJs). During function of the intact mandible, both TMJs have to move. When the mandible is fractured, the muscles acting on the mandible are able to displace the fragments in a horizontal and vertical plane. The forces generated give rise to areas of tension and compression as described by Champy (Figs. 37-1 and 37-2). An appreciation of the areas of tension and compression can be utilized to provide functionally stable fixation. The inferior alveolar nerve runs through the mandible from the lingula to the mental foramen and is at risk of damage both as the result of the injury and during fixation of the fracture. The position of the nerve changes with growth of the mandible and loss of alveolar bone secondary to tooth loss. Any altered sensation of the inferior alveolar nerve distribution must be noted at the time of the initial examination. The occlusion of the mandibular teeth with the maxillary teeth can be used as a guide to reduction of fractures. The teeth can also be used as a source of fixation (maxillomandibular fixation [MMF]). In the pediatric mandible, the presence of unerupted teeth can limit the placement of rigid fixation, and unerupted teeth can act as areas of weakness predisposed to fracture. This is particularly seen with unerupted third molars (wisdom teeth). With tooth loss, atrophy of the alveolar process can occur. If extreme,

this can dramatically reduce the bony volume of the mandible, making it susceptible to fracture from minimal trauma and making it difficult to apply fixation. The position of the branches of the facial nerve must be appreciated if a transcutaneous approach to repair is being considered.

DIAGNOSTIC STUDIES

A good clinical examination remains the mainstay of diagnosis of mandibular fractures. The patient should be evaluated for the presence of derangement of the occlusion, altered sensation of the inferior alveolar nerve distribution, and step-offs in the dentition.

While improved access to computed tomography (CT) scanning has increasingly led to this technique being adopted as the gold standard for assessment, most fractures can be diagnosed on panoramic (Panorex, Orthopantomogram) radiographs. Posteroanterior (PA) radiographs and reverse Towne radiographs can help to diagnose condylar injuries. Where CT facilities are unavailable, lower occlusal radiographs can show subtle fractures involving the lingual plate in the symphyseal region. Periapical films may be required for dentoalveolar fractures. The mechanisms of injury leading to mandibular fractures can also cause injuries to the cervical spine, and imaging of the cervical spine should be considered, particularly in patients with a history of altered consciousness or distracting injuries.

If available, previous dental models can be helpful in establishing the preinjury occlusion if there are multiple and/or comminuted fractures.

TREATMENT/RECONSTRUCTIVE GOALS

The goals of treatment of fractures of the mandible are:
1. Restoration of the preinjury occlusion
2. Early return of function
3. Acceptable cosmesis

In the dentate patient, restoration of the premorbid occlusion is crucial. Questioning of the patient about his preinjury occlusion is crucial, and dental models, if available in cases where the occlusion is not obvious, can be valuable in helping to determine the occlusion.

Reduction of the fractures may be open or closed. In closed reduction, the occlusion is used as an indirect guide to the adequacy of the reduction. Fixation of the fractures is usually required, although some undisplaced fractures may be managed conservatively, particularly in children. Fixation may be external or internal (Box 37-1).

An important concept in internal fixation of fractures is that of load-sharing versus load-bearing osteosynthesis. In load-sharing osteosynthesis, the interfragmentary fit of the fracture ends allows

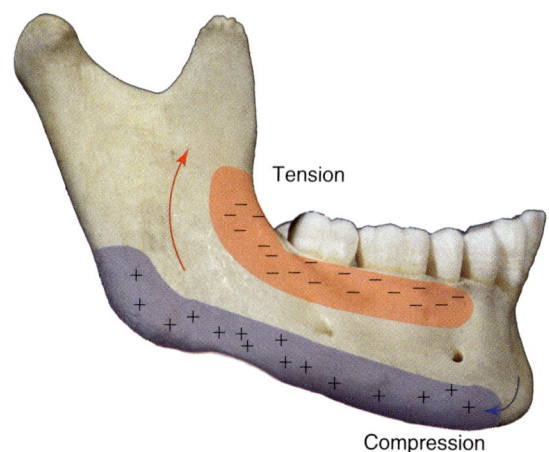

Fig. 37-1 ■ The areas of tension and compression of the mandible generated by the opposing muscle groups. (Adapted from Liebgott B: *The anatomical basis of dentistry*, ed 3, St. Louis, 2011, Mosby.)

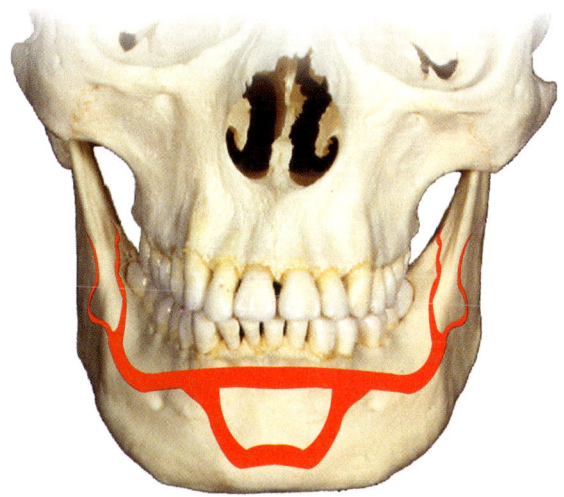

Fig. 37-2 ■ The lines of ideal osteosynthesis as described by Champy. (Adapted from Liebgott B: *The anatomical basis of dentistry*, ed 3, St. Louis, 2011, Mosby.)

BOX 37-1	External versus Internal Fixation
External Fixation	**Internal Fixation**
Arch bars with MMF	*Semirigid:*
Risdon cables with MMF	Mini-plates
Ivy loops, Ernst ligatures	Lag screw
with MMF	Bicortical positioning screws
External fixator	*Rigid:*
	Reconstruction plate and
	bicortical screws
	Locking reconstruction plate
	and bicortical screws

MMF, maxillomandibular fixation.

some buttressing of functional load across the fracture, and appropriately placed semirigid fixation, will resist movement across the fracture and allow bone healing to occur. In load-bearing osteosynthesis, there is insufficient or no buttressing possible across the fracture, and the fixation device must provide sufficiently rigid fixation of the fracture ends to prevent movement and provide a suitable environment for fracture healing to occur. This situation arises in

comminuted fractures, infected fractures, pathologic fractures, defect fractures, or fractures of the atrophic edentulous mandible. Failure to recognize the need for load-bearing osteosynthesis is a common cause of treatment failure. Load-bearing plates utilize bicortical screws to ensure maximal fixation. Ideally, three screws should be placed on each side of the fracture. Load-bearing plates may be locking or nonlocking. Locking plates have a thread that engages the plate and provides additional stability of the plate. The locking of the plate means that less-than-perfect contouring of the plate does not result in displacement of the fracture ends as the screws are tightened. The screws must, however, be placed parallel to the threads in the plate so that they can engage.

SPECIFIC TREATMENT AND TECHNIQUES

Most treatment of mandibular fractures requires general anesthesia. If treatment is being carried out under general anesthesia, nasal intubation is the route of choice to allow intraoperative assessment of the occlusion and the placement of MMF. If nasal intubation is not possible, alternative techniques, such as submental intubation or tracheostomy, may be necessary. It is occasionally possible to find sufficient space behind the last standing teeth for an armored oral tube to be placed and secured to the maxillary teeth while enabling the teeth to be brought into occlusion.

Parasymphyseal fractures can be treated with a variety of techniques, and treatment must be tailored to the particular characteristics of the fracture and patient circumstances. Simple parasymphyseal fractures can be managed closed with 4 to 6 weeks of MMF or with monocortical plates and screws placed along the lines of ideal osteosynthesis described by Champy (see Fig. 37-2). Typically, two plates are used to resist torsional forces, but if an arch bar has been placed, this can act as a tension band and the superior screw omitted. More rigid fixation of such fractures is required if there is a second fracture, such as a condylar or angle fracture, because monocortical fixation is not rigid enough to overcome splaying of the lingual aspect of the fracture due to muscle pull, which can lead to mandibular widening. If the fracture is situated near the midline fixation, using a lag screw technique can provide optimal fixation. The compression across the fracture provided by the screws effectively prevents mandibular widening. Adequate transoral exposure is required for the placement of lag screws or reconstruction plates, because it is necessary to visualize the lower border of the mandible. It may be necessary to skeletonize the mental nerve to allow adequate retraction and placement of hardware. Most noncomminuted parasymphyseal fractures can be approached transorally. The incision should be placed to allow the development of a mucosal muscle flap, which can allow for a watertight closure with resuspension of the mentalis muscle (Fig. 37-3). If there is difficulty restoring the occlusion and reducing the fracture, consideration must be given to the presence of an occult dentoalveolar fracture in the incisal region, because this is an occasional cause of nonreduction.

Fractures of the mandibular body can, similarly, be treated open or closed. Noncomminuted fractures can be approached transorally. If semirigid fixation is planned, load-sharing plates are used; a single plate as a tension band should be placed along the line of ideal osteosynthesis. Care must be taken to ensure that when screws are placed they do not violate tooth roots or the inferior alveolar canal. The drill bit should have a 6 to 8 mm stop to limit the depth that can be drilled. If a load-bearing plate is required, it often can be placed transorally below the level of the inferior alveolar canal, although a transbuccal trocar will be required to allow the screws to be placed in a bicortical manner perpendicular to the screw hole (Fig. 37-4).

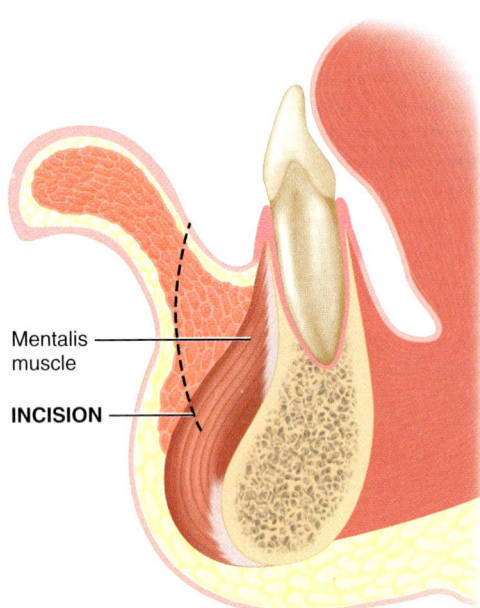

Fig. 37-3 ■ The transoral approach to the anterior mandible. Note the placement of the incision out toward the labial mucosa to provide an adequate cuff of soft tissue for closure.

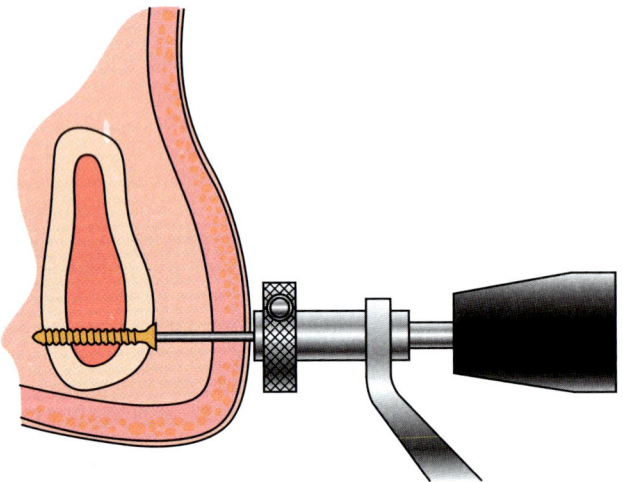

Fig. 37-4 ■ The use of the transbuccal trocar to allow placement of screws perpendicular to the plate below the inferior alveolar nerve.

Oblique fractures of the body may be suitable for fixation with lag screws utilizing a transbuccal trocar.

Fractures of the mandibular angle are rarely amenable to treatment using closed reduction with MMF, unless they are nondisplaced or buttressed by an unerupted wisdom tooth. Simple angle fractures can be approached and fixed transorally, placing a superior border plate in a monocortical manner as a tension band. If placing the plate entirely on the lateral aspect of the superior border, the screws will usually require placement using the transbuccal trocar. Typically, a 2-mm plate and screws are used, although work by Ellis has shown consistently good results with smaller plates. Management of wisdom teeth in the line of the fracture remains controversial. Regardless of whether or not the wisdom tooth is removed, the subsequent rate of plate removal is approximately 20%. It should be appreciated that often the wisdom tooth helps to buttress the fracture, and removal of the tooth may give rise to what is, in effect, a

defect fracture. Removal of bone to remove the wisdom tooth may compound the problem and reduce the bone available for placing screws. A pragmatic approach to management of the wisdom tooth in the line of the fracture is to consider removing it if it is obviously infected, broken, preventing reduction of the fracture, and easy to remove with no additional bone removal. In other circumstances, retain the wisdom tooth, with the patient being made aware that removal of the wisdom tooth and hardware will be required as an interval procedure after healing has occurred. If a transoral approach is used, the upper wisdom tooth should be evaluated to ensure it is not going to traumatize the mandibular mucosal flap. If such trauma appears likely, consideration should be given to removal of the upper wisdom tooth to help prevent wound breakdown. Placement of the proximal screws first enables the plate to be used as a "joystick" to manipulate the proximal fragment into a well-reduced position (Fig. 37-5, B). The masseter should only be reflected as far as is needed to ensure reduction and allow the placement of fixation. Excessive disruption of the pterygomasseteric sling reduces the compression at the lower border and may allow excessive splaying of the lower border. A small amount of splaying at the lower border on postoperative imaging is to be expected and will close down over the period of healing as the pterygomasseteric sling generates an area of compression at the lower border. Any comminution of fractures in the angle will preclude successful management using semirigid fixation, and load-bearing rigid fixation will be required. This is due to the relatively small area of bone contact available in the region of the angle. Such comminution must be carefully looked for both on the preoperative imaging and perioperatively. The possible need for conversion to a transcutaneous approach must be explained to the patient preoperatively

Fractures in children can usually be managed with a short period of MMF (2 to 3 weeks). The short clinical crowns of deciduous teeth and the presence of missing or partially erupted teeth can make the placement of arch bars or Ivy loops difficult. In such cases, the application of Risdon cables (Figs. 37-6 and 37-7) can be particularly helpful. Sagittal fractures can be reduced and held in position with circum-mandibular wires. Perfect reduction is not required because considerable growth and remodeling occurs, and this will adjust minor occlusal irregularities. If rigid fixation is felt to be necessary, then hardware removal should be planned after 3 to 6 months when healing has occurred, because appositional bone growth may result in the plate becoming embedded in the bone. Although the effect this has on mandibular growth is debated, such embedded plates can make subsequent procedures, such as orthognathic surgery, more complicated. To obviate the need for plate removal, some surgeons choose to use a resorbable plate and screw fixation. The plates can be difficult to contour and only provide semirigid (load-sharing) fixation.

Regardless of the method of treatment used for pediatric patients, long-term follow-up is essential to check for any growth disturbances.

Fractures of the atrophic edentulous mandible are best approached by a transcutaneous approach to allow the placement of rigid fixation with a large, locking reconstruction plate. Such rigid fixation is required to overcome the action of the suprahyoid depressors of the mandible, which can give rise to significant displacement (Fig. 37-8). Adequate fixation of atrophic mandibular fractures requires wide exposure so that the symphyseal and angle regions (the sites of bone stock) are capable of accommodating bicortical screws without splintering (Fig. 37-9). Thought should be given to primary bone grafting of atrophic fractures at the time of rigid fixation, because this provides a source of osteoprogenitor cells and provides improved bone volume for secondary implant restoration. Other

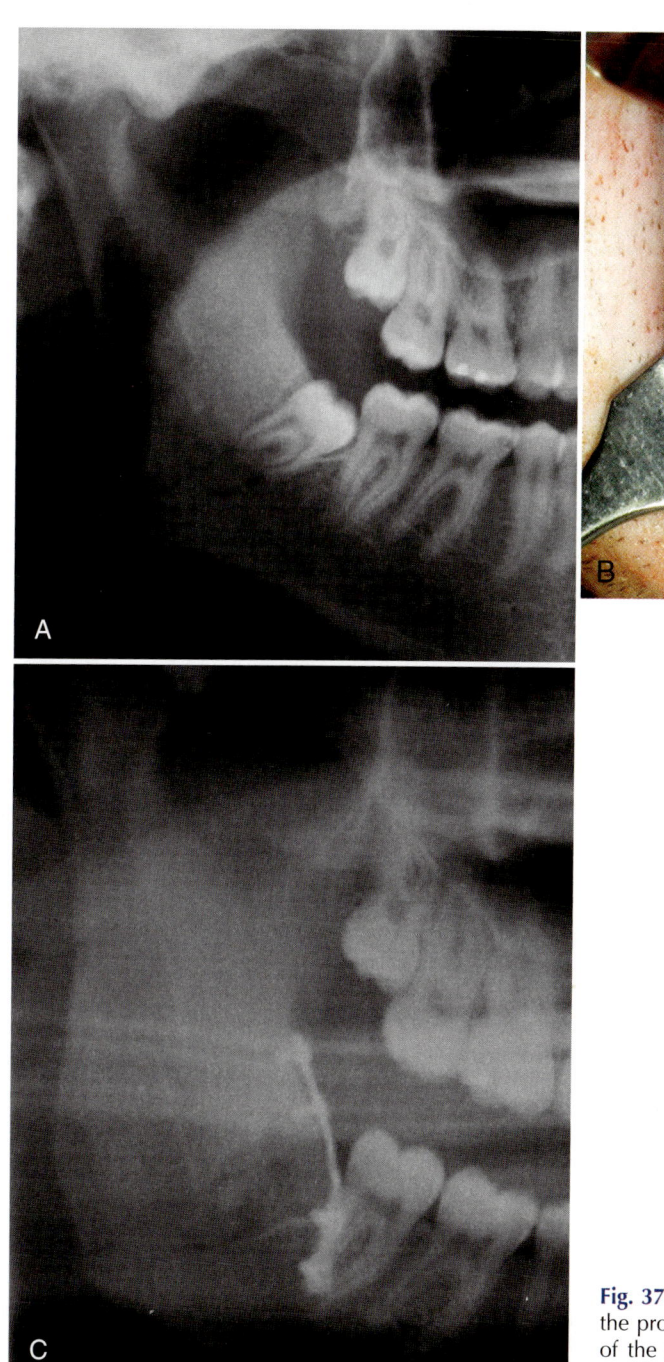

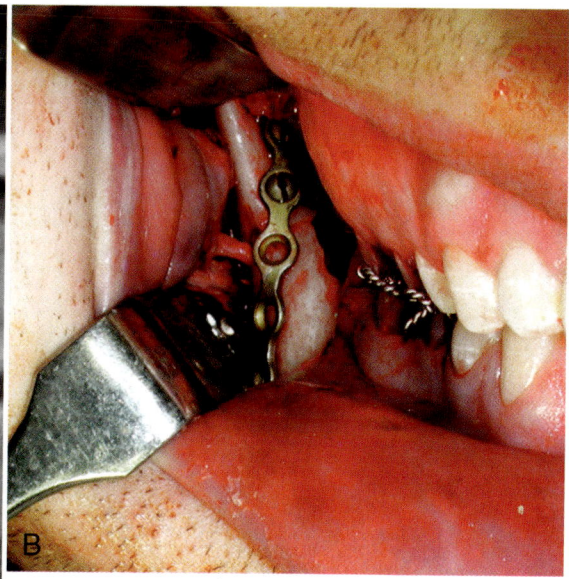

Fig. 37-5 ■ **A,** Preoperative Panorex. **B,** A superior border mini-plate in place with the proximal screws secured to allow the plate to act as a "joystick" for reduction of the proximal fragment. **C,** Postoperative Panorex showing the superior border miniplate in place.

techniques, such as the application of external fixation, MMF using Gunning splints, or modified dentures, have been used, but treatment may end up being very prolonged and is not predictable. In elderly patients, MMF can significantly reduce respiratory reserve and lead to excessive morbidity or even mortality. In the noncomminuted, nonatrophic (>20-mm thickness) mandible, transorally placed semi-rigid fixation can be considered.

Comminuted fractures require load-bearing osteosynthesis, usually by a transcutaneous approach. MMF has previously been used as a sole treatment modality, but in contemporary practice, the main use of MMF in comminuted fractures is the maintenance of the occlusal relationship while rigid fixation is applied. Having exposed the fractures and reestablished the occlusion, it may be helpful to "simplify" the fractures by fixing at least some of the

comminuted fragments with mini-plates and then spanning the area of comminution with a reconstruction plate (Fig. 37-10). It should be noted that the mini-plates are being used to aid reduction of the fractures and are not contributing to fixation. In select circumstances, external fixation can be used for the management of comminuted fractures.

Defect fractures, as classically seen in self-inflicted gunshot wounds, require rigid fixation. Replacement of the missing bone is ultimately required, because even rigid reconstruction plates will eventually fracture with prolonged function. Missing bone may be replaced with bone grafts or bone flaps, depending on the size of the defect and the quality of the soft tissue envelope. If cortical block grafts or bone flaps are used, these must be rigidly fixed to allow consolidation along the interface with the native mandible. Adequate

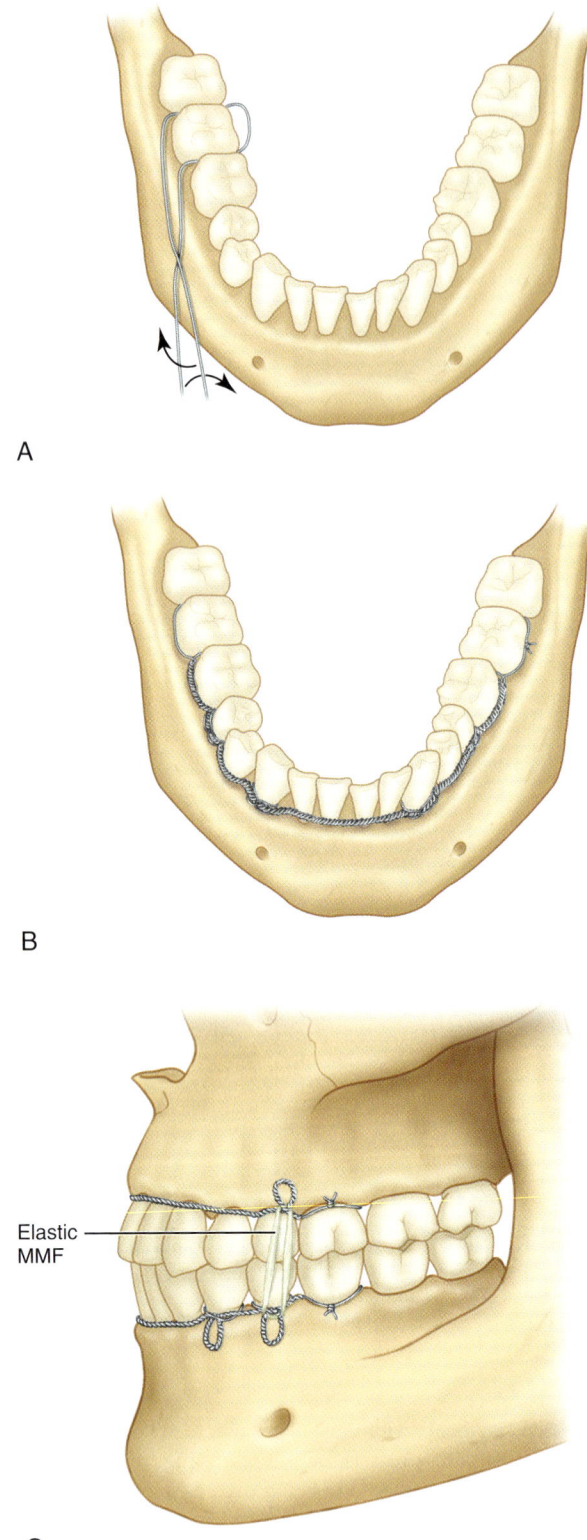

A

B

C

Fig. 37-6 ■ **A,** Risdon cable placement. A length of wire is placed through the most posterior contact and brought around the distal aspect of the most posterior tooth. The wire ends are then wrapped over to form a cable, passed through the most posterior contact on the opposite side, and secured. **B,** Risdon cable placement. The cable is secured to the teeth present, and the ends of the tie wire are formed into "rosettes" long enough to act as hooks for maxillomandibular fixation (MMF) elastics. **C,** Risdon cable in place with elastic MMF.

Elastic MMF

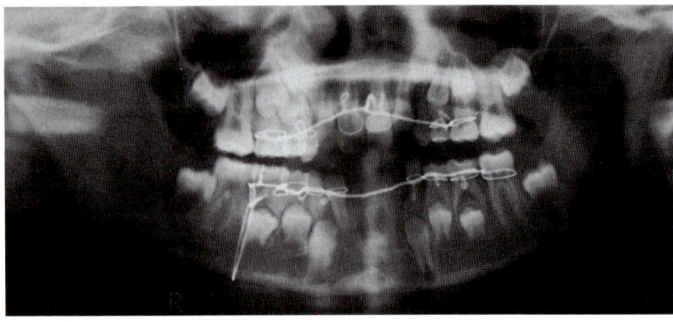

Fig. 37-7 ■ Radiograph of a pediatric patient in the mixed dentition with a sagittal fracture of the mandibular body. Risdon cables have been used for maxillomandibular fixation (MMF), and a circummandibular wire was placed to aid with reduction of the sagittal fracture.

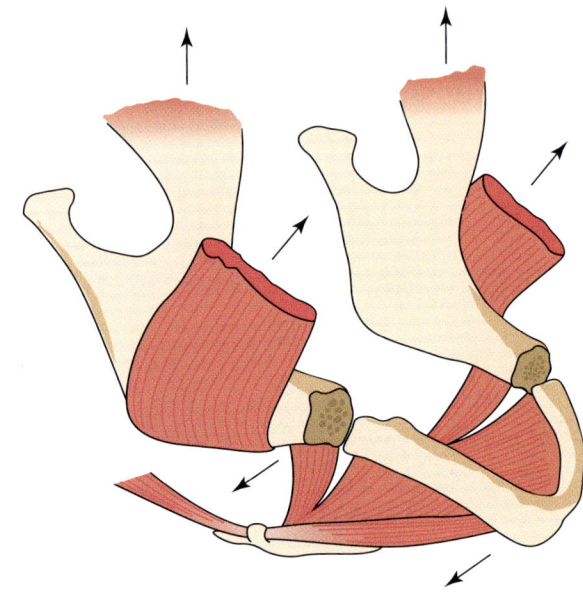

Fig. 37-8 ■ Opposing muscle groups can significantly displace atrophic mandibular fractures.

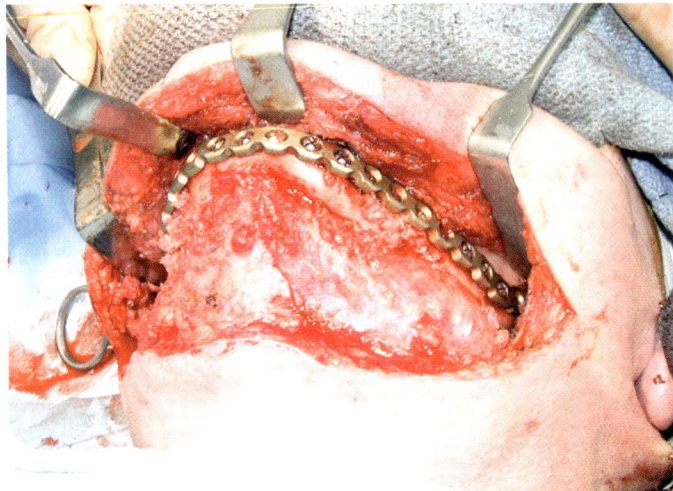

Fig. 37-9 ■ Wide transcutaneous exposure of an atrophic, edentulous, mandibular fracture to allow placement of rigid fixation with screw placement in the areas of maximal bone stock. Primary cancellous bone grafting has been performed.

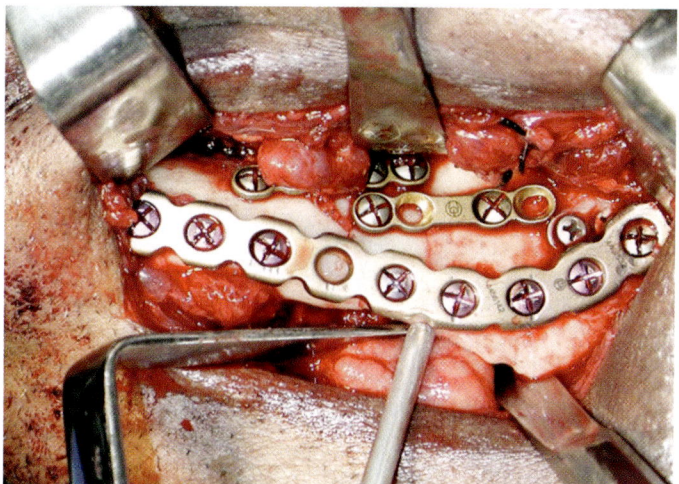

Fig. 37-10 ■ A comminuted fracture. Mini-plates have been used to simplify the fracture prior to the placement of rigid fixation.

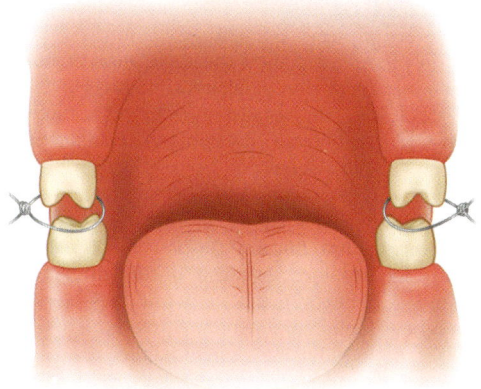

A

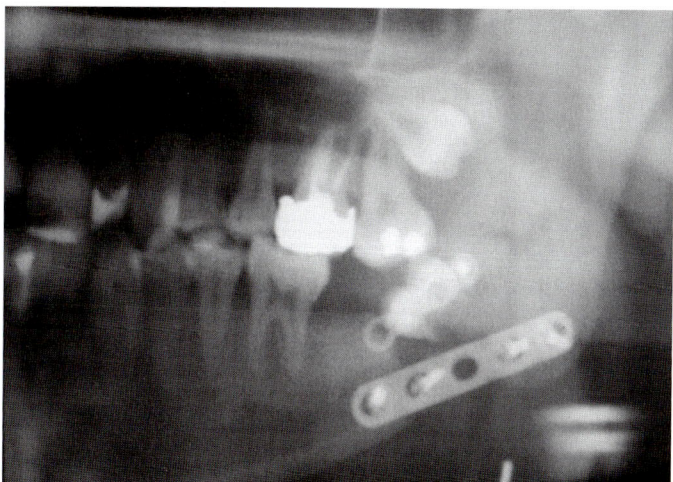

Fig. 37-11 ■ Radiograph showing inadequate fixation of an angle fracture allowing movement and secondary infection.

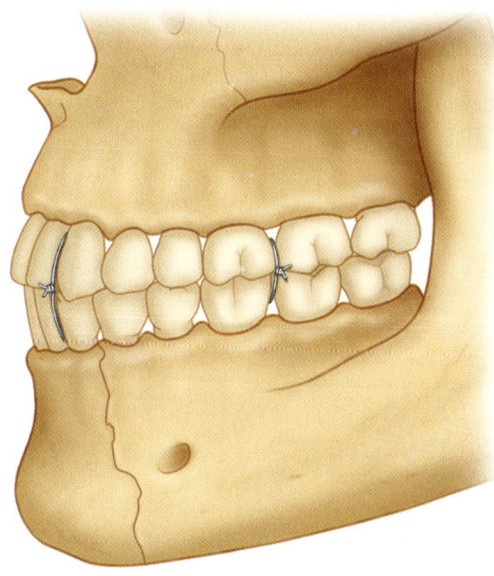

B

Fig. 37-12 ■ Technique of interdental wiring to provide temporary maxillomandibular fixation (MMF) prior to placement of rigid fixation when postoperative MMF will not be required.

fixation is vital, and the goal should be the placement of a minimum of three bicortical screws on each side of the fracture. External fixators can be used for stabilization of the fracture and prevention of soft tissue contraction in the unstable patient, but definitive repair with bone replacement will ultimately be required. Adequate soft tissue coverage of bone grafts is essential, and it may be necessary to recruit soft tissue into the region by means of a soft tissue flap.

Infected fractures are usually the result of delays in treatment or inadequate fixation (Fig. 37-11). Underlying host factors contributing to the fracture, such as uncontrolled diabetes or poor nutrition, should be sought and addressed prior to fracture fixation. In most cases, the infection is a secondary infection in an area of osteitis caused by mobility of the fracture, with the bone ends/fragments acting as a foreign body. True osteomyelitis in the area of the fracture is, mercifully, quite rare. Having ruled out osteomyelitis and optimized the patient, the infected fracture is best managed by rigid internal fixation and supported with peri-/postoperative antibiotics. Removal of the infected, nonvital bone may give rise to a defect fracture. Primary bone grafting of such defects has been shown to be predictably successful.

POSTOPERATIVE CARE

If MMF is left in place at the end of the procedure, care staff must be made aware of its location and how to remove it, should the patient have significant nausea/vomiting or airway compromise. Regardless of what form of fixation is used, patients must be reminded to pursue a soft, nonchew diet for several weeks as the fracture heals and gains strength. Excellent oral hygiene must be maintained to allow uneventful healing of intraoral wounds and prevent secondary healing. Although this can be done with simple mechanical measures, such as tooth brushing, an oral rinse such as chlorhexidine gluconate is commonly prescribed to reduce plaque loads until patients are comfortable to resume adequate oral hygiene measures. Although routinely used by many surgeons, the evidence base for postoperative antibiotic use is sparse.

PEARLS AND PITFALLS

- If MMF is only required to allow the application of internal fixation and the occlusion is obvious, with good contacts between adjacent teeth, the occlusion can be held quickly and securely with interdental wires placed between the contacts of adjacent mandibular teeth from buccal to lingual and from palatal to buccal between adjacent maxillary teeth (Fig. 37-12).
- If conservative management of a fracture is planned, careful follow-up is required because displacement can occur 7 to 10 days postinjury, and because postinflammatory osteolysis can lead to loss of interfragmentary fit and the potential for movement during even minimal function. A soft, nonchew diet must be strictly followed to prevent treatment failure.

- If multiple simple fractures are present, consideration must be given to placing more rigid fixation across one of the fractures, typically the more anterior fracture. This is because widening of the mandible can occur due to a "wish-boning" of the mandible during function. This can occur even if MMF is in place and leads to a scenario where the occlusion looks satisfactory but the mandible appears wide or swollen.
- When treating multiple fractures, the fractures in the tooth-bearing region should be repaired first to allow restoration of a normal mandibular arch form and occlusal relationship.

BIBLIOGRAPHY

Benson PD, Marshall MK, Engelstad ME, et al: The use of immediate bone grafting in reconstruction of clinically infected mandibular fractures: bone grafts in the presence of pus. *J Oral Maxillofac Surg* 64(1):122-126, 2006.

Champy M, Loddé JP, Schmitt R, et al: Mandibular osteosynthesis by miniature screwed plates via a buccal approach. *J Maxillofac Surg* 6(1):14-21, 1978.

Ellis E 3rd: Lag screw fixation of mandibular fractures. *J Craniomaxillofac Trauma* 3(1):16-26, 1997.

Ellis E 3rd: Management of fractures through the angle of the mandible. *Oral Maxillofac Surg Clin North Am* 21(2):163-174, 2009.

Herford AS, Ellis E 3rd: Use of a locking reconstruction bone plate/screw system for mandibular surgery. *J Oral Maxillofac Surg* 56(11):1261-1265, 1998.

Kushner GM, Tiwana PS: Fractures of the growing mandible. *Atlas Oral Maxillofacial Surg Clin North Am* 17:81-91, 2009.

Potter J, Ellis E 3rd: Treatment of mandibular angle fractures with a malleable noncompression miniplate. *J Oral Maxillofac Surg* 57(3):288-292, 1999; discussion 292-293.

Saubier S, Schön R, Otten JE, et al: The development of plate osteosynthesis for the treatment of fractures of the mandibular body—a literature review. *J Craniomaxillofac Surg* 36:(5):251-259, 2008.

Chapter **38**

Mandibular Subcondylar Fractures

Larry L. Cunningham, Jr., Aaron Sterling Card

The most common site of all mandibular fractures is the condylar or subcondylar region, where 9% to 45% of mandibular fractures occur.[1,2] The volume of debate about diagnosis and management of injuries to the temporomandibular joint (TMJ) sheds light on the difficulty associated with managing and repairing these complex injuries.[3-5]

ETIOPATHOGENESIS/CAUSATIVE FACTORS

The etiology of subcondylar fractures mirrors that of most facial trauma. In adults, the most common causes of subcondylar fractures of the mandible are motor vehicle accidents, interpersonal violence, work-related incidents, sporting accidents, and falls. In children, the most common causes are falls and bicycle accidents, although motor vehicle accidents also play an important role.[1,2,6]

PATHOLOGIC ANATOMY

Subcondylar fractures of the mandible are defined as fractures below the level of the most inferior point on the sigmoid notch (Fig. 38-1).[7] Depending on the circumstances, condylar neck fractures may be treated as subcondylar fractures; displacement and malocclusion in the setting of a long condylar neck (the ability to place at least two screws in the segment) would qualify. Historically, two systems have been developed for the classification of subcondylar fractures: the Lindahl system[8-11] and the MacLennan system[12]

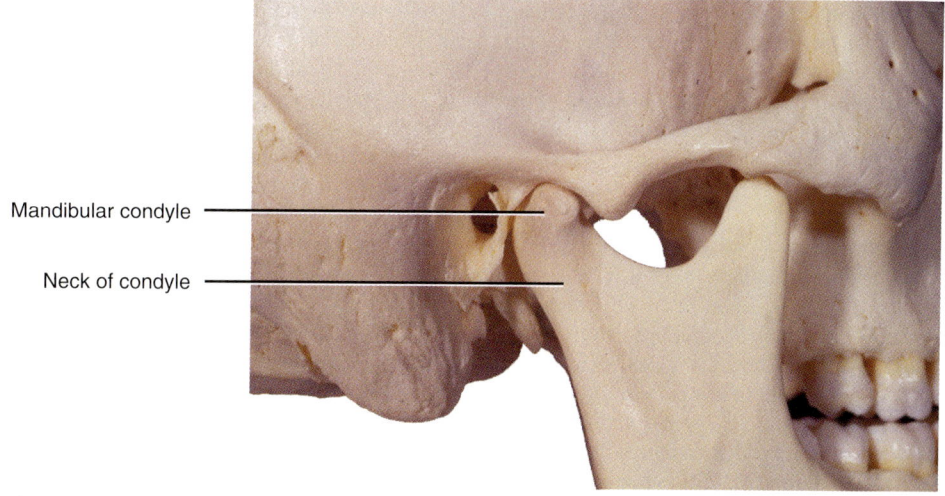

Mandibular condyle ——————

Neck of condyle ——————

Fig. 38-1 ■ Lateral view of bones of the temporomandibular joint. (From Liebgott B: *The anatomical basis of dentistry*, ed 3, St. Louis, 2011, Mosby.)

BOX 38-1	The Lindahl System[8-12]

The Lindahl system classifies subcondylar fractures according to their anatomic location and the specific relationship between the fractured condyle and the glenoid fossa. The anatomic location of the fracture is described first. The most superior fracture is in the condylar head, which means that the fracture probably lies in the capsule of the temporomandibular joint; the second is a fracture in the thin neck of the condyle. The most inferior fracture lies in the subcondylar region below the anatomic neck and extends to the inferior portion of the ramus.

Relationship of the condylar segment to the mandibular fragment:
1. Nondisplaced.
2. Deviated: angulation of the condylar head without dislocation of the fractured segments.
3. Displaced with medial or lateral overlap. The fractured condylar head lies either medial or lateral to the distal segment, with overlap. A medial position is more common because of the attachment and traction of the lateral pterygoid.

Relationship between the condylar head and the glenoid fossa:
1. Nondisplaced.
2. Displaced: the condylar head remains in the fossa, but the joint space is altered.
3. Dislocation. The condylar head lies completely outside the anatomic fossa. This position requires rupture of the capsule.

BOX 38-2	The MacLennan System[12]

Type I fracture, nondisplaced.
Type II fracture, deviated. Angulation without overlap or separation. Greenstick fractures are included in this category.
Type III fracture, displaced. This fracture displays overlap between the proximal and distal segments.
Type IV fracture, dislocated. The condylar head leaves the capsule and lies outside the glenoid fossa. The location could be medial, lateral, anterior, or posterior.

(Boxes 38-1 and 38-2). The main objectives of these classifications systems are to describe the relationship of the condyle to the glenoid fossa and the relationship between the fractured proximal and distal segments. The condylar head can remain in the fossa, can be dislocated out of the fossa either medially or laterally, or in rare cases can be dislocated into a fractured fossa. Fractured subcondylar segments can be nondisplaced (hairline fracture); alternatively, the proximal segment may be displaced either medially or laterally relative to the distal segment. Most of these fractures will be described as closed fractures unless they are associated with deep facial lacerations.

DIAGNOSTIC STUDIES

Panoramic radiographs and Towne projection radiographs are effective methods of evaluating the subcondylar region of the mandible. However, computed tomography (CT) is currently the state of the art for detecting subcondylar fractures of the mandible. Three-dimensional reconstructions of CT data offer the surgeon invaluable information about the position of the fractured segments, thereby allowing the most accurate planning of fracture management.[13]

TREATMENT/RECONSTRUCTIVE GOALS

The goals of treating any type of trauma are to restore pain-free, premorbid form and function. With respect to subcondylar fractures of the mandible, the goal is restoration or maintenance of facial symmetry and posterior mandibular height. Treatment should be completed without injury to the parotid gland or the facial nerve and, preferably, without obvious scarring. Ideal restoration of function after treatment of a subcondylar fracture includes re-establishment of maximum mandibular movements: a maximum incisal opening (MIO) of 40 mm without deviation, lateral excursive movements of greater than 5 mm to the right and left, and the absence of signs or symptoms of temporomandibular disorder.

SPECIFIC TREATMENT AND TECHNIQUES

SURGICAL ANATOMY TO CONSIDER

The facial nerve exits the skull from the stylomastoid foramen and passes obliquely inferiorly and laterally until it enters the parotid gland. The common facial divisions of the nerve are the temporal, zygomatic, buccal, marginal mandibular, and cervical divisions. The branches most at risk during a transfacial approach to the subcondylar region are the buccal and marginal mandibular branches; those most at risk during an approach to the TMJ or an intracapsular fracture are the zygomatic and temporal branches.

The confluence of the superficial temporal vein and the maxillary vein is called the retromandibular vein. This vascular structure can be the source of substantial bleeding deep to the ramus and the neck of the condyle because it descends just posterior to the ramus of the mandible through the parotid gland. This vein is lateral to the external carotid artery.

CLOSED MANAGEMENT

Closed management[3] is performed more than any other type of management because of its ease and long history of use. It is indicated for very specific subcondylar fractures, two of which are greenstick fractures in pediatric patients and nondisplaced fractures that do not "fall back"[7] under anesthesia in adults. In addition, closed management is indicated for the treatment of any patient who refuses surgery as an option. The technique can be applied variably: as a liquid diet (as in the situation with greenstick fractures in pediatric patients), as maxillomandibular fixation (MMF) with arch bars and wires, or as fixation with arch bars and elastic bands. Likewise, elastic bands may be used either in a light, guiding fashion or in a heavy fashion, in which case they are very similar to wire fixation.

Although closed management may still be commonplace, it cannot be considered the state of the art. It has even been shown that treatment by MMF may be associated with a higher incidence of temporomandibular dysfunction postoperatively than seen with other types of treatment and that closed treatment may not prevent further displacement of the fractured subcondylar segments.[14,15] However, closed management can avoid the risks associated with general anesthesia, facial nerve injury, parotid injury, and scarring and can also shorten the duration of soft tissue swelling after the injury.

OPEN REDUCTION WITH INTERNAL FIXATION

Indications

Zide and Kent presented the absolute and relative indications for open reduction of mandibular condylar fractures (Box 38-3).[16] Since their presentation of the clinical standard, many improvements have

been made in rigid internal fixation and endoscopic application to craniofacial fractures, and these improvements have allowed expanded indications for open reduction and internal fixation (ORIF) of subcondylar fractures.[10] More recent studies have focused on the complications associated with open and closed treatment of subcondylar fractures of the mandible (Box 38-4).[3,4,14,15,17-20]

The international principles guiding fracture management today include anatomic reduction of fractured segments, functionally stable internal fixation, and early mobilization; these principles have been well established in the dental literature.[21,22] The goal of fracture management is normal, pain-free function. As all surgeons know, the decision whether to operate is not always as clear as the guiding principles would suggest. Surgeons should discuss the following important points with the patient when deciding whether to open a subcondylar fracture: the severity of the fracture, the amount of disability that is likely to occur, the relative risks to important

---

BOX 38-3	**Zide and Kent's Indications for Open Reduction of Condylar Fractures[16]**

Absolute indications (pertain to children as well as to adults):
1. Displacement into the middle cranial fossa
2. Impossibility of obtaining adequate occlusion by closed reduction
3. Lateral extracapsular displacement of the condyle
4. Invasion by a foreign body (e.g., gunshot wound)

Relative indications:
1. Bilateral condylar fractures in an edentulous patient when a splint is unavailable or splinting is impossible because of atrophy of the alveolar ridge
2. Unilateral or bilateral condylar fractures for which splinting is not recommended for medical reasons or when adequate physiotherapy is impossible
3. Bilateral condylar fractures associated with comminuted midfacial fractures
4. Bilateral condylar fractures and associated gnathologic problems such as retrognathia or prognathism, open bite with periodontal problems or lack of posterior support, loss of multiple teeth and later need for elaborate reconstruction, bilateral fractures and unstable occlusion because of orthodontics, and unilateral condylar fracture with an unstable fracture base

---

BOX 38-4	**Considerations for Approach to Subcondylar Fractures**

In 2004, Edward Ellis III, DDS, gave a presentation at the Symposium on Management of Subcondylar Fractures; Historical Perspectives and New Horizons. He addressed the historical aspects of subcondylar fracture management and readdressed his indications for open surgical management in light of advancing techniques for stable internal fixation. He acknowledged the lack of universal agreement among surgeons with regard to management protocols, yet stated that most fractures may be managed satisfactorily with closed techniques. He summarized his indications for open treatment:
1. Displacement of the condyle into the middle cranial fossa (with or without fracture)
2. Lateral extracapsular displacement of the condyle (with or without fracture)
3. Impossibility of obtaining proper occlusion with closed techniques
4. Condylar fractures associated with comminuted fractures at or above Le Fort I

In addition, Ellis discussed the relative indications for open and closed management. He stated that surgeons, at their own discretion, may use either the open or closed method, depending on their own philosophy and experience. Factors to be considered when deciding between open and closed management include
1. Loss of ramus height beyond acceptable esthetic limits or loss of the posterior dentition that would ordinarily assist in maintaining height of the ramus
2. The skeletal age of the patient (Children's jaws can adapt to a new condylar position, or frank neocondylar synthesis may occur.)
3. Ability to attain stable fixation (If a fracture is located high on the condylar neck or in the capsule, nonsurgical management may be more appropriate. Some patients' medical condition may not be considered stable enough to allow them to undergo either open or closed management, or they may have a strong desire to avoid intermaxillary fixation and would therefore chose an alternative management method.)
4. Associated fractures, including bilateral condylar fractures, especially those that are displaced (Opening at least one fracture may improve occlusal outcomes.)
5. State of the patient's dentition (When dentition is incomplete, it may be impossible to maintain the position of the mandible when a new articulation is established. Open treatment may be the better option for preventing posterior vertical collapse or the need for additional splint fabrication to maintain stability.)

anatomic structures, the likelihood of scarring, and the patient's preferences. The patient should be made aware of the potential complications associated with subcondylar fractures, including changes in occlusion, pain and temporomandibular dysfunction, and possible alterations in the symmetry of the face.[4,7,15,18]

Transfacial approaches to the subcondylar region are favored because they allow direct access and visualization, thereby increasing the surgeon's ability to achieve anatomic reduction of the fracture. Surgical complications that are associated with open treatment of condylar process fractures and that lead to permanent dysfunction or deformity are generally uncommon.[17] However, some of these risks, such as facial nerve injury, sialocele, infection, and scarring, though uncommon, are serious and may be difficult to manage. Still, all of these approaches can be technically challenging, and learning curves should be expected. The most popular approaches are the submandibular approach and the retromandibular approach.[23] The senior author prefers the retromandibular approach for its proximity to the fracture site (Fig. 38-2).

The indications for endoscopically assisted ORIF of subcondylar fractures are the same as those for the open transfacial approaches. However, because the potential difficulty of the endoscopically assisted approach is considerably increased when comminuted fractures are present, its use may be contraindicated in such cases.[8]

The intraoral approach without the benefit of an endoscope was first reported by Jeter and co-authors. This approach reduced the risk for facial nerve damage and avoided the large facial scars associated with transfacial approaches; it also allowed the surgeon to accurately reduce and fixate the fracture while maintaining the patient's proper occlusion.[24] However, the difficulty associated with applying this technique without the advantage of an endoscope limited the number of patients who were able to benefit from open reduction of the condyle. The advantages of the endoscope have been described more recently and have furthered the argument for the endoscopic approach with intraoral access, an approach associated with minimal complications.[8,25] The technique has a steep learning curve, but the time required for applying this technique decreases after sufficient experience has been gained. Careful patient selection is essential.[13,26,27] The endoscopically assisted approach can allow restoration of the relationship between the condyle and the mandible and can re-establish function to a state that is as close as possible to the preinjury condition with minimal risk for facial nerve damage or facial scarring (Fig. 38-3).

Contraindications

High condylar neck fractures (i.e., those that leave a segment that is too short to accept two screws) and condylar head fractures should not be treated with ORIF. Displaced subcondylar fractures with

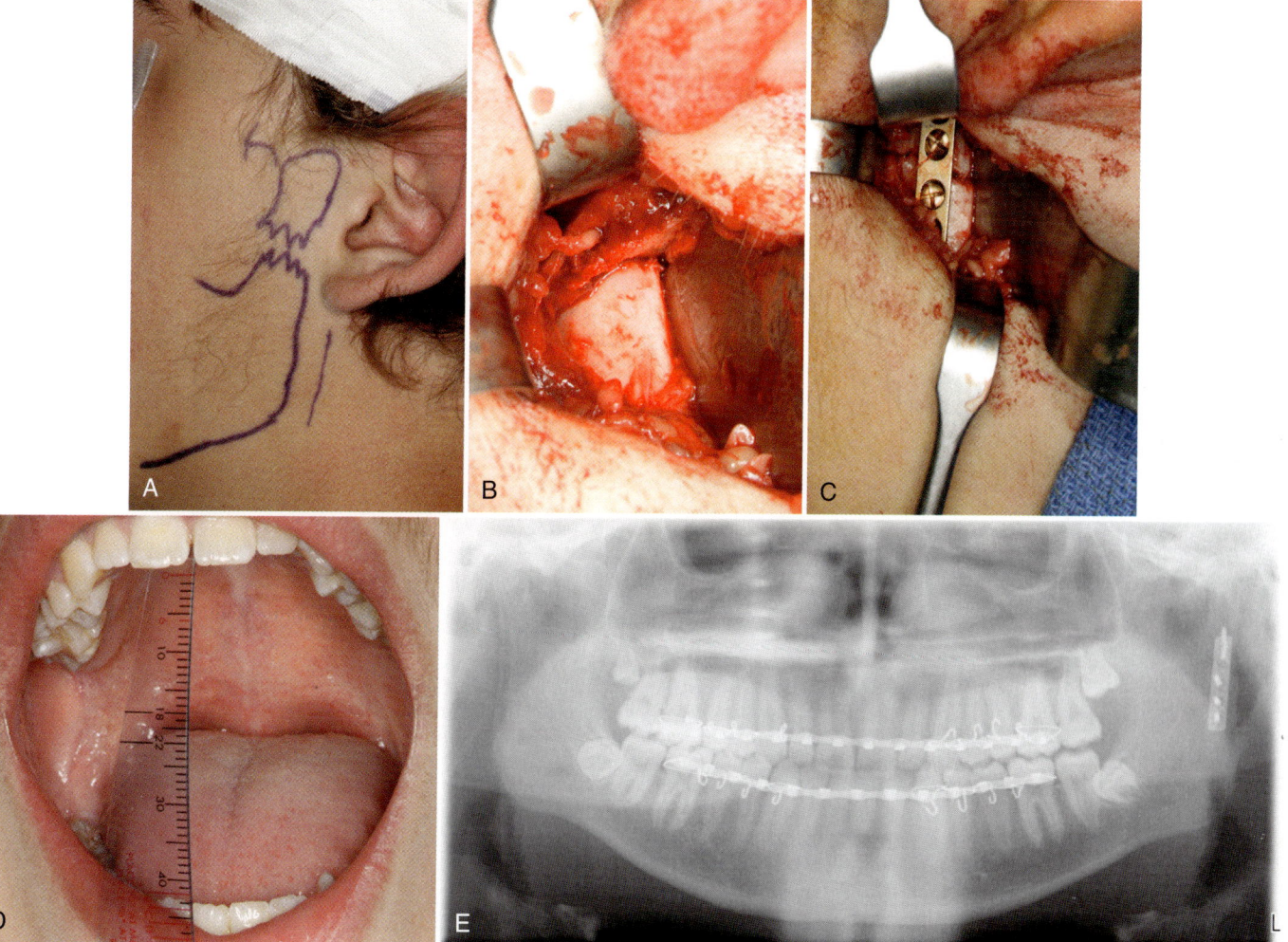

Fig. 38-2 ■ Extraoral approach to a mandibular subcondylar fracture via a retromandibular incision. **A,** Patient markings. **B,** Visualization of the fracture. The superior retractor allows visualization of the distal fractured stump of the proximal segment. **C,** Fixation plate in place after fracture reduction. **D,** Six weeks postoperatively with a maximum incisal opening of 40 mm. **E,** Postoperative panoramic radiograph.

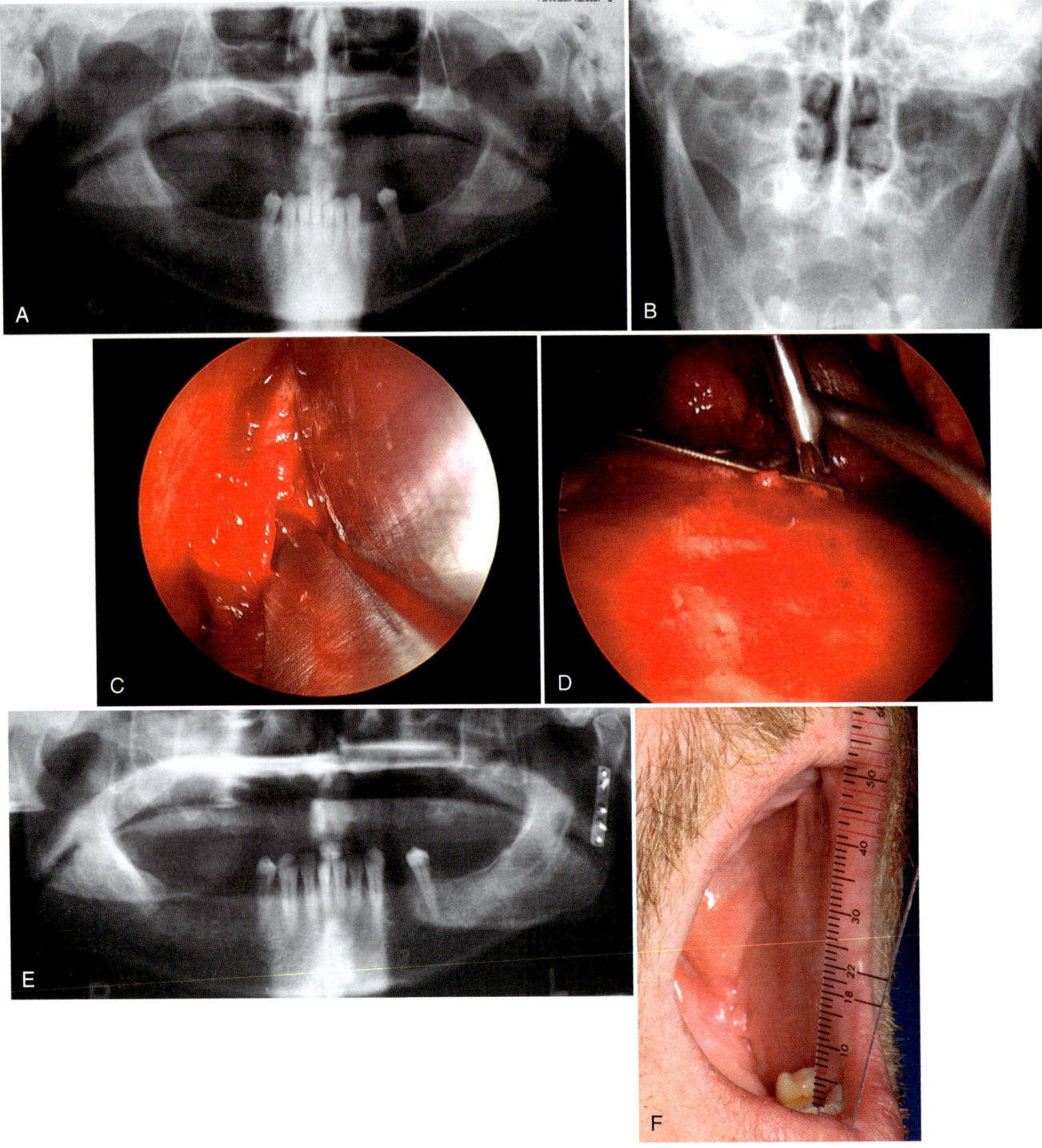

Fig. 38-3 ■ Endoscopically assisted approach to a mandibular subcondylar fracture. **A,** Preoperative panoramic radiograph. **B,** Preoperative Towne view showing significant lateral over-ride of the left subcondylar fracture. **C,** Endoscopic view of the distal fractured stump of the proximal segment. **D,** Endoscopic view of fixation placement. **E,** Postoperative panoramic radiograph. **F,** Postoperative maximum incisal opening of 50 mm to the maxillary edentulous ridge.

medial override of the proximal segment are the most difficult to reduce adequately with an endoscopically assisted approach. A surgical procedure is justified only when the condylar segments are displaced. Fractures that are unlikely to affect occlusion or facial height (greenstick fractures or medial pole fractures) should not be opened.[7]

POSTOPERATIVE CARE

Postoperative care after repair of subcondylar fractures should consist of the placement of light elastic bands for occlusal guidance; these bands should remain in place for 7 to 14 days. Generally, a full liquid diet is recommended for 3 days after surgery, followed by a soft mechanical diet for the next 3 to 4 weeks. Early mobilization of the joint is important so that ankylosis can be avoided. After an initial healing period of 2 weeks, patients are encouraged to begin their own physical therapy to increase MIO to the postoperative goal of 40 mm. Available commercial devices can assist in this rehabilitation; however, stacked tongue blades offer the patients an inexpensive and effective guide. Patients are encouraged to use tongue blades to assist in their rehabilitation four to five times during the day for a total of 30 minutes of stretching per day. In addition, they are asked to attempt to add one tongue blade to the stack every day or two until they achieve an MIO of 40 mm.

MANAGEMENT CONTROVERSY

Mobilization and rehabilitation are the keys in treating subcondylar fractures.[28] Management of subcondylar fractures is controversial because many of these fractures will heal with acceptable results after being treated by MMF. Avoidance of surgery certainly alleviates the risk for surgical complications. In addition, using shorter periods of MMF, 3 to 4 weeks rather than 6 weeks, creates less of a burden for the patient. Although MMF is faster and less expensive than ORIF,[29] it does not eliminate all complications and indeed may result in malocclusion, which requires a secondary surgical procedure, most often sagittal split osteotomy. Other potential complications associated with MMF are TMJ dysfunction, malocclusion, and altered facial symmetry.[4,14,15,18]

Although rigid internal fixation does not eliminate the importance of rehabilitation for increasing the patient's MIO, it is certainly associated with shorter convalescence, particularly for more difficult, severely displaced and dislocated fractures that cause substantial disturbances in occlusion, loss of ramal height, and facial asymmetry, as well as for multiple facial fractures. ORIF may also be the treatment of choice when MMF is not recommended, such as for patients with certain co-morbid conditions (learning disabilities, pulmonary diseases, seizure disorders).[18,30]

Ideally, surgeons would be adequately trained to provide alternative methods of care. When offered the option of surgery and rehabilitation or the option of any period of MMF, many patients choose the surgical procedure despite its potential risks.

FRACTURES IN CHILDREN

Subcondylar fractures in children are different from those in adults for a number of reasons. The presence of primary or mixed dentition, remaining growth potential, and the great capacity for the childhood condyle to remodel allow greater success of nonsurgical therapy in children than in adults. The general consensus is that nonsurgical management is the best option for children until they reach the age of 12 years, until there is a departure from mixed dentition, or until puberty begins.[3,8,16] Conservative treatment may consist of a liquid diet only or a brief period of MMF (1 to 2 weeks) with arch bars and heavy elastic bands. Following this short period of inactivity, active function and joint physiotherapy are important to reduce the formation of scar tissue and prevent TMJ fibrosis or ankylosis.[6]

ACKNOWLEDGMENT

The authors would like to thank Flo Witte for her expert editorial assistance.

PEARLS AND PITFALLS

- When subcondylar fractures are treated with MMF, close follow-up and rehabilitation are very important.
- Minor occlusal discrepancies after treatment can be treated with elastic bands or orthodontics and with vigilance in aiding the patient to achieve an MIO of 40 mm.
- Treating a patient with MMF when there is substantial overlap of the fractured segments or rotating the condylar segment during pretreatment imaging may be associated with a risk for malocclusion after treatment.
- When multiple fractures of the mandible are treated with ORIF of the subcondylar fracture, the mandible should be reduced and fixated in an anterior to posterior direction; the most anterior fracture should be plated first.
- MMF should not be in place when the subcondylar segment is reduced.
- MMF can be used before screw placement if the segments remain reduced.
- Endoscopic approaches are technique-sensitive, and the surgical instruments are unique.
- Surgeons should select early cases carefully so that they can familiarize themselves with the techniques.
- Fractures with lateral override are much easier to treat with endoscopic guidance, whereas medially displaced segments are more difficult to treat with this technique.
- The retromandibular approach to the subcondylar region is associated with a high risk for encountering the facial nerve.
- Blunt dissection through the parotid is mandatory, and the assistance of a nerve stimulator is recommended.

REFERENCES

1. Ellis E 3rd, Moos KF, el-Attar A: Ten years of mandibular fractures: an analysis of 2,137 cases, *Oral Surg Oral Med Oral Pathol* 59:120-129, 1985.
2. Haug RH, Prather J, Indresano AT: An epidemiologic survey of facial fractures and concomitant injuries, *J Oral Maxillofac Surg* 48:926-932, 1990.
3. Ellis E, Throckmorton GS: Treatment of mandibular condylar process fractures: biological considerations, *J Oral Maxillofac Surg* 63:115-134, 2005.
4. Ellis E 3rd, Simon P, Throckmorton GS: Occlusal results after open or closed treatment of fractures of the mandibular condylar process, *J Oral Maxillofac Surg* 58:260-268, 2000.
5. Nussbaum ML, Laskin DM, Best AM: Closed versus open reduction of mandibular condylar fractures in adults: a meta-analysis, *J Maxillofac Surg* 66:1087-1092, 2008.
6. Miller RI, McDonald DK: Remodeling of bilateral condylar fractures in a child, *J Maxillofac Surg* 44:1008-1010, 1986.
7. Ellis E 3rd: Method to determine when open treatment of condylar process fractures is not necessary, *J Oral Maxillofac Surg* 67:1685-1690, 2009.
8. Lindahl L, Hollender L: Condylar fractures of the mandible. II. A radiographic study of remodeling processes in the temporomandibular joint, *Int J Oral Surg* 6:153-165, 1977.
9. Lindahl L: Condylar fractures of the mandible. IV. Function of the masticatory system, *Int J Oral Surg* 6:195-203, 1977.
10. Lindahl L: Condylar fractures of the mandible. III. Positional changes of the chin, *Int J Oral Surg* 6:166-172, 1977.
11. Lindahl L: Condylar fractures of the mandible. I. Classification and relation to age, occlusion, and concomitant injuries of teeth and teeth-supporting structures, and fractures of the mandibular body, *Int J Oral Surg* 6:12-21, 1977.

12. MacLennan W: Consideration of 180 cases of typical fractures of the mandibular condylar process, *Br J Plast Surg* 5:122-128, 1952.

13. Kellman RM, Cienfuegos R: Endoscopic approaches to subcondylar fractures of the mandible, *Facial Plast Surg* 25:23-28, 2009.

14. Ellis E 3rd, Palmieri C, Throckmorton G: Further displacement of condylar process fractures after closed treatment, *J Oral Maxillofac Surg* 57:1307-1316, discussion 1316-1317, 1999.

15. Haug RH, Assael LA: Outcomes of open versus closed treatment of mandibular subcondylar fractures, *J Oral Maxillofac Surg* 59:370-375, discussion 375-376, 2001.

16. Zide MF, Kent JN: Indications for open reduction of mandibular condyle fractures, *J Oral Maxillofac Surg* 41:89-98, 1983.

17. Ellis E 3rd, McFadden D, Simon P, et al: Surgical complications with open treatment of mandibular condylar process fractures, *J Oral Maxillofac Surg* 58:950-958, 2000.

18. Ellis E 3rd, Throckmorton G: Facial symmetry after closed and open treatment of fractures of the mandibular condylar process, *J Oral Maxillofac Surg* 58:719-728, discussion 729-730, 2000.

19. Ellis E 3rd, Throckmorton GS: Bite forces after open or closed treatment of mandibular condylar process fractures, *J Oral Maxillofac Surg* 59:389-395, 2001.

20. Ellis E 3rd, Throckmorton GS, Palmieri C: Open treatment of condylar process fractures: assessment of adequacy of repositioning and maintenance of stability, *J Oral Maxillofac Surg* 58:27-35, discussion 35, 2000.

21. Greenberg AM, editor: *Craniomaxillofacial fractures: principles of internal fixation using the AO/ASIF technique*. New York, 1993, Springer-Verlag.

22. Prein J, editor: *Manual of internal fixation in the cranio-facial skeleton: techniques recommended by the AO/ASIF maxillofacial group*. New York, 1998, Springer-Verlag.

23. Chossegros C, Cheynet F, Blanc JL, et al: Short retromandibular approach of subcondylar fractures: clinical and radiologic long-term evaluation, *Oral Surg Oral Med Oral Pathol Oral Radiol Endod* 82:248-252, 1996.

24. Jeter TS, Van Sickels JE, Nishioka GJ: Intraoral open reduction with rigid internal fixation of mandibular subcondylar fractures, *J Oral Maxillofac Surg* 46:1113-1116, 1988.

25. Kellman RM: Endoscopically assisted repair of subcondylar fractures of the mandible: an evolving technique, *Arch Facial Plast Surg* 5:244-250, 2003.

26. Schmelzeisen R, Cienfuegos-Monroy R, Schon R et al: Patient benefit from endoscopically assisted fixation of condylar neck fractures—a randomized controlled trial, *J Oral Maxillofac Surg* 67:147-158, 2009.

27. Jensen T, Jensen J, Norholt SE et al: Open reduction and rigid internal fixation of mandibular condylar fractures by an intraoral approach: a long-term follow-up study of 15 patients, *J Oral Maxillofac Surg* 64:1771-1779, 2006.

28. Walker RV: Condylar fractures: nonsurgical management, *J Oral Maxillofac Surg* 52:1185, 1994.

29. Villarreal PM, Monje F, Junquera LM, et al: Mandibular condyle fractures: determinants of treatment and outcome, *J Oral Maxillofac Surg* 62:155-163, 2004.

30. Zachariades N, Mezitis M, Mourouzis C et al: Fractures of the mandibular condyle: a review of 466 cases. Literature review, reflections on treatment and proposals, *J Craniomaxillofac Surg* 34:421-432, 2006.

Chapter **39**

Orbital Fractures

R. Bryan Bell, Saif S. Al-Bustani

Optimal management of orbital fractures remains challenging and often enigmatic (Fig. 39-1). Orbital anatomy is complex, and various vital structures and highly specialized organs are bundled in a small space. A number of approaches exist and numerous materials are available for reconstruction. No individual approach and no single material is best suited for all patients. Primary repair offers injured patients their best chance at functional recovery. Complications related to the injury itself or to repair, such as persistent enophthalmos or ocular dysmotility, are difficult to predict in the acute setting and, once clinically manifested, are challenging to repair because of intraconal or extraconal fibrosis.

Several technologic advances have occurred in the last 3 decades that have had a significant impact on the management of patients with orbital injuries, including the following:

- Improved imaging modalities, such as high-resolution computed tomography (CT), which has resulted in a much greater ability to recognize, qualify, and quantify orbital injuries than was possible in the pre-CT scan era

- Refined alloplastic materials, which have largely replaced the once "gold standard" of calvarial bone grafts for use in the internal orbit

- Application of computer-aided design and computer-aided modeling (CAD/CAM) to maxillofacial surgery, which has provided a means to precisely analyze, segmentalize, and manipulate virtual images in advance of surgery to perform an ideal virtual reconstruction, as well as the construction of custom implants or guide stents

- The development of intraoperative navigation (frameless stereotaxy) and intraoperative CT scanners, which allow precise placement of implants or bone grafts, as well as confirmation of adequate reduction before leaving the operating room

- The application of minimally invasive, endoscopically assisted, transantral approaches to the orbits, which in selected cases obviates the need for a lower lid incision

This chapter is intended to provide readers with a rational approach to managing orbital injuries based on clinical and

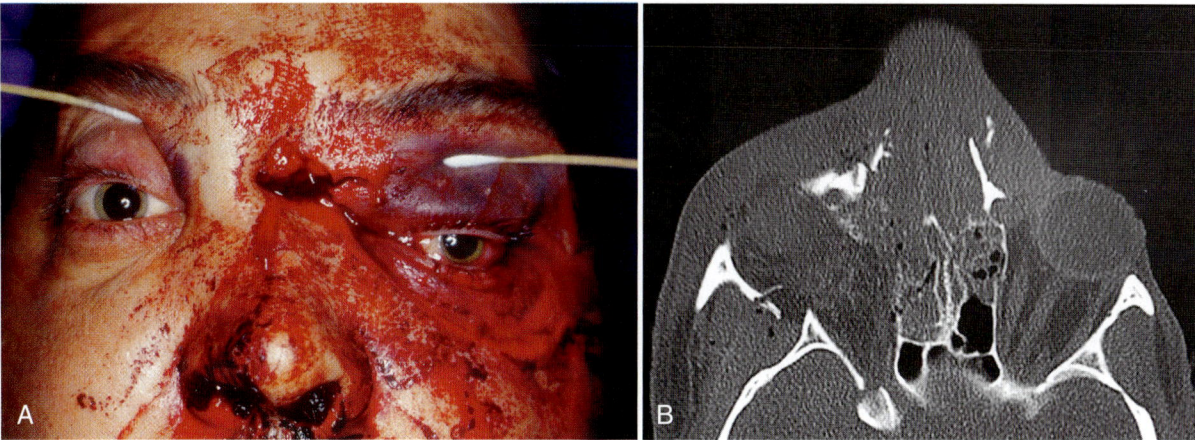

Fig. 39-1 ■ **A,** Severe mid-facial and orbital fractures resulting in orbital dystopia, telecanthus, and cranial neuropathy. **B,** Axial computed tomography scan.

radiographic findings and to review the currently available adjuncts that can be used to optimize treatment outcomes.

ETIOPATHOGENESIS

Data from a level I trauma registry have shown that the orbit is involved in approximately 47% of severely injured patients admitted to a trauma service.[1] The vast majority of these injuries occur as a result of blunt trauma, usually a motor vehicle collision or interpersonal violence, as well as sporting accidents, industrial accidents, and ground-level falls. Fractures involving the orbit may affect the internal orbit, the external orbital frame, or both (Figs. 39-2 to 39-5). For purposes of clarity and discussion, these fractures will be defined and discussed as follows:

- Orbitozygomaticomaxillary complex (OZMC) fractures
- Naso-orbito-ethmoid (NOE) fractures
- Internal orbital fractures (blowout, blow-in)
- Combined orbital fractures (shattered orbit).

Fractures of the internal orbit typically occur by one of two mechanisms. The first is through a force applied to the globe itself, which results in a sudden increase in intraorbital pressure that exerts an outward force against the internal orbital walls, the weakest of which fractures. This "hydraulic theory," popularized by Smith and Regan,[2] provides an explanation why most orbital blowout fractures occur just medial to the infraorbital canal. In other instances, however, the force is applied directly to the bone, often the zygomatic bone or the infraorbital rim, or both, which produces an orbital floor fracture through direct transmission of energy from the orbital rim to the floor and results in a compression-type fracture.[3] The orbital floor may fracture alone (termed pure blowout), or there may also be rim involvement (impure).

Once an internal orbital fracture occurs, the volume occupied by the soft tissue contents (the eye and adnexa) may expand or contract secondary to the direction of displacement of the orbital fracture (i.e., blow-in or blowout). Blow-in fractures typically occur on the orbital roof and are usually associated with high-velocity injuries involving the anterior skull base.[4] Blow-in fractures result in contraction of orbital volume and downward and forward displacement of the globe. Most blowout fractures, in contrast, occur on the inferior or inferomedial aspect of the orbit and result in volumetric expansion with displacement of the globe posteromedially and inferiorly.[5] Fracture displacement and orbital expansion or contraction

Internal Frame

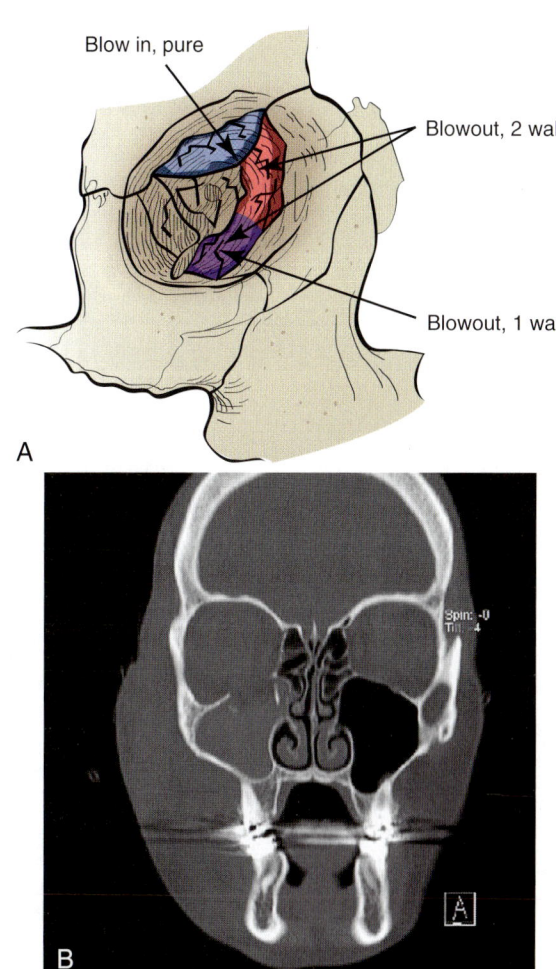

Fig. 39-2 ■ Type 1 fracture, internal frame. **A,** Type 1a, one-wall blowout; type 1b, two-wall blowout; type 1c, pure blow-in fracture of the orbital roof. **B,** Coronal CT scan of a type 1a fracture.

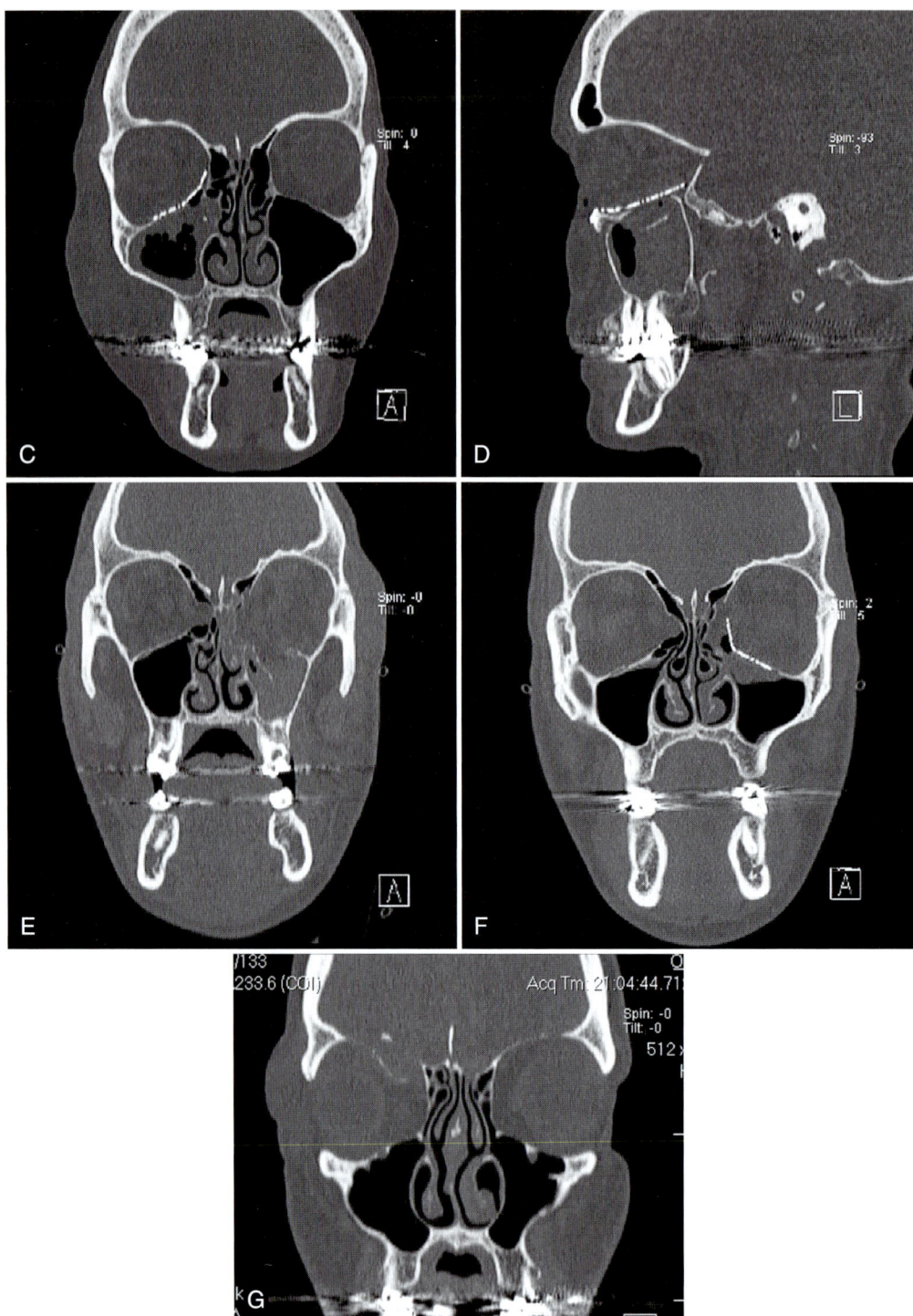

Fig. 39-2, cont'd ▪ **C,** Coronal CT scan of the patient in part **B** demonstrating optimal repair of single-wall defect. **D,** Sagittal CT scan of the patient in part **B** demonstrating restoration of the posterior antral bulge. **E,** Coronal CT scan of a type 1b, two-wall blowout. **F,** Coronal CT scan of the patient in part **E** demonstrating optimal restoration of the inferior and medial walls (medial/ethmoidal bulge). **G,** Coronal scan of a type 1c, pure blow-in fracture of the orbital roof (right side).

may lead to extraocular muscle imbalance and subjective diplopia, enophthalmos, or proptosis.

Extraocular muscle imbalance and diplopia are generally the result of muscle contusion. Less commonly, however, they can be the result of incarceration of either the extraocular muscle (e.g., inferior rectus muscle) or the soft tissue adjacent to the muscles,

cranial neuropathy (third, fourth, or fifth cranial nerves), or deviation of the visual axes. True entrapment in adult patients is very unusual. In children, however, blowout fractures may produce complete immobility of the ocular globe with enophthalmos (Fig. 39-6). Such severe loss of motion implies actual muscle incarceration, which is an indication for immediate orbital exploration with release of the

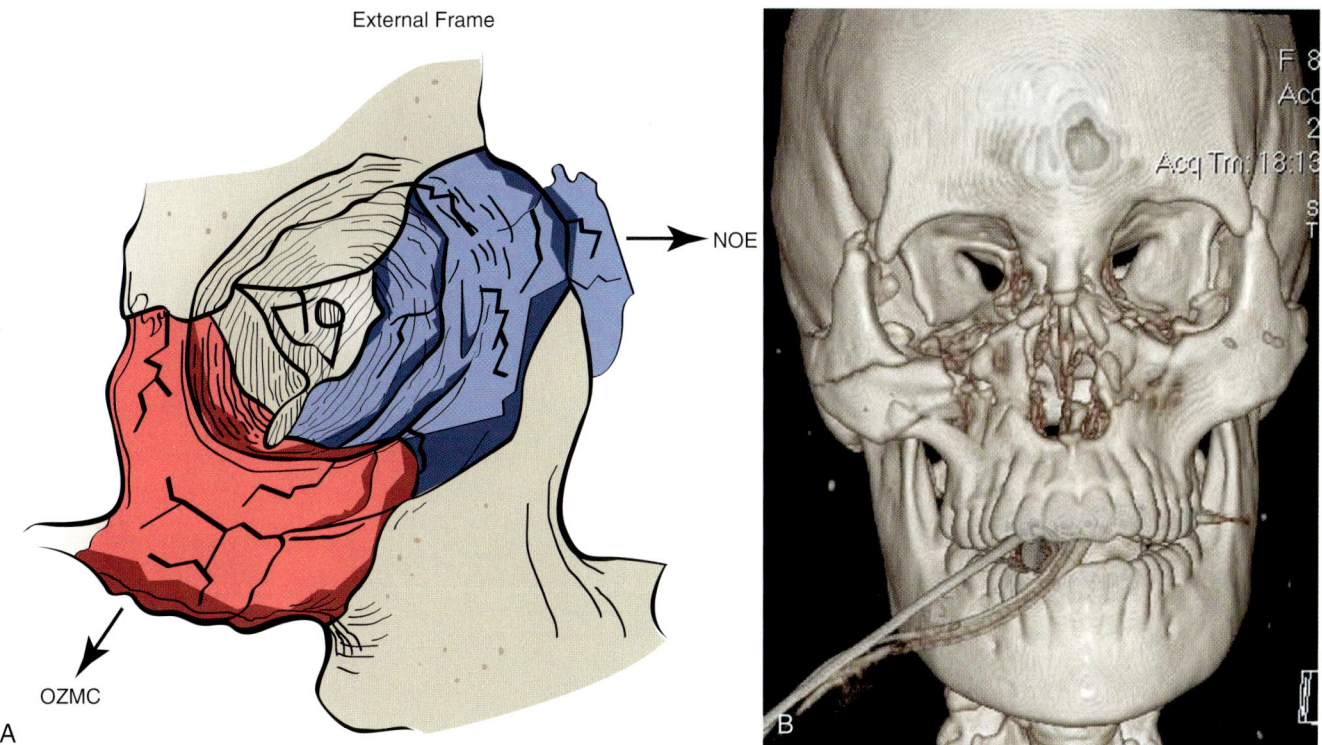

Fig. 39-3 ■ Type 2 fracture, external orbital frame. **A,** Type 2a, lateral frame, orbitozygomatico-maxillary fracture; type 2b, medial frame, naso-orbital-ethmoidal fracture. **B,** Three-dimensional CT scan demonstrating combined type 2a and type 2b fractures.

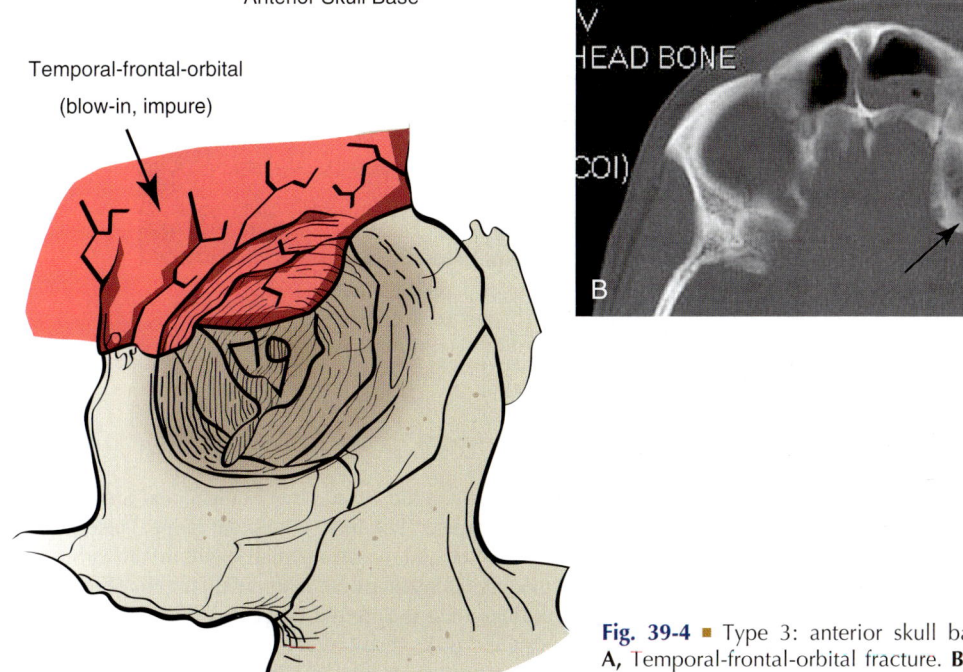

Fig. 39-4 ■ Type 3: anterior skull base fractures with orbital roof involvement. **A,** Temporal-frontal-orbital fracture. **B,** Axial CT scan of type 3, an impure orbital "blow-in" fracture. These fractures are associated with a high risk for disruption of the orbital apex and subsequent optic neuropathy.

entrapped extraocular muscle system. It is typically accompanied by pain on attempted rotation of the globe, nausea, and vomiting, all of which are unusual in adult patients with blowout fractures.

Enophthalmos is the second major potential complication of orbital injuries, the primary cause of which is an increase in orbital volume (Fig. 39-7). Other mechanisms for enophthalmos are

possible, including entrapment of extraocular muscles or periocular soft tissues, fat atrophy, or decrease in vitreous volume. For many years fat atrophy was thought to be a major etiologic factor in enophthalmos; however, studies by Manson and co-workers suggest that this is indeed not the case.[6] It has been shown that much of the globe support and position within the orbit is due to intramuscular

Combined (shattered orbit)

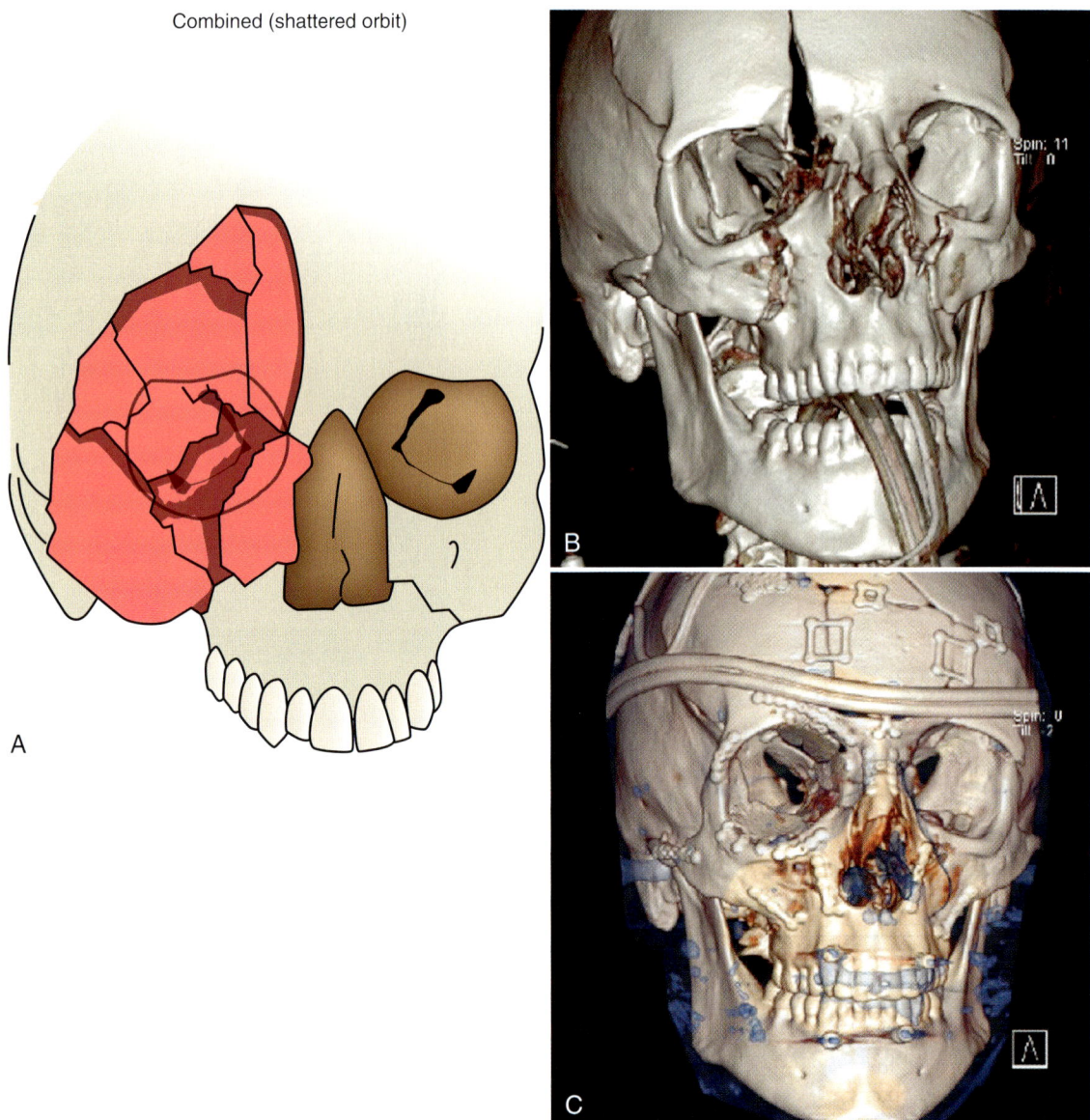

Fig. 39-5 ■ Type 4: combined orbital fracture (shattered orbit). **A,** Four-wall orbital fracture, including disruption of the anterior skull base and a combination of all previously described types. **B,** Three-dimensional CT scan of patient with a type 4 fracture. **C,** Three-dimensional scan following open reduction and internal fixation.

(intraconal) fat (Fig. 39-8). Fat is located in a primarily extraconal position in the anterior orbit; however, posteriorly, where it is needed, most of the fat is intraconal. It is thought that this intraconal fat is extruded into an extraconal location and that when combined with post-traumatic scarring, clinically significant enophthalmos can result.

PATHOLOGIC ANATOMY

In adult patients, orbital volume and external and internal morphology are remarkably consistent between individuals. The internal orbit is a cone-shaped pyramid with its apex oriented posteromedially and its base anterolaterally. The lateral orbital rim coincides with the midvertical axis of the globe. This relationship makes the lateral wall important in establishing correct anteroposterior position of the globe.

The internal orbit contains two critical bulges that are essential to restore when disrupted. The first "ethmoidal bulge," also termed the "key area," is located posteromedially within the orbit and results from medial extension of the ethmoidal air cells (Fig. 39-9). The second critical area, the "antral bulge," is located in the posteroinferior orbit and is the result of cranially oriented outpocketing of the maxillary antrum (Fig. 39-10). These outpocketings serve to support the anterior position of the globe. Failure to restore these critical bulges will predictably result in increased orbital volume and risk for enophthalmos.

Soft tissue support of globe position within the orbit is provided by interrelated suspensory ligaments and a network of orbital fat (Fig. 39-11). These ligaments include the medial and lateral canthal and check ligaments, the superior sling containing Whitnall's ligament, the inferior sling containing Lockwood's ligament, muscular sheaths and lacrimal ligaments, Tenon's capsule, and the

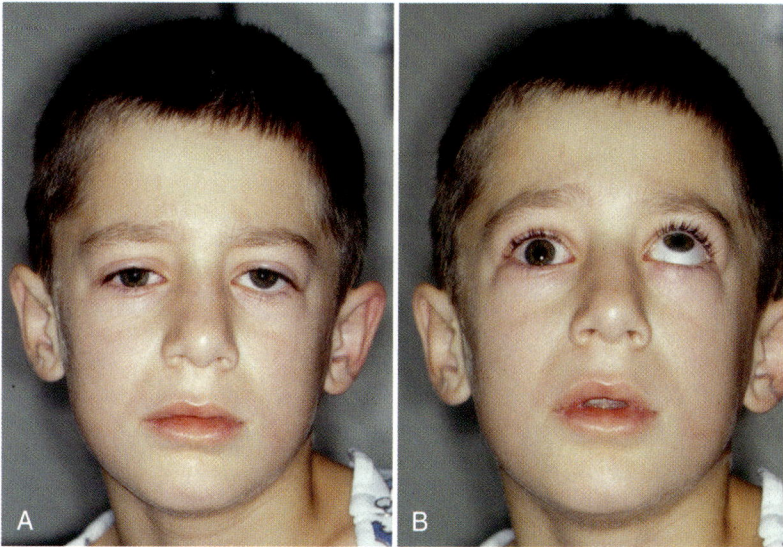

Fig. 39-6 ▪ Nine-year-old with a "trapdoor" blowout fracture of the orbital floor and entrapment of the inferior rectus muscle. This injury represents a surgical emergency; the orbit must be explored and the muscle released expeditiously. **A,** Frontal gaze. **B,** Upward gaze.

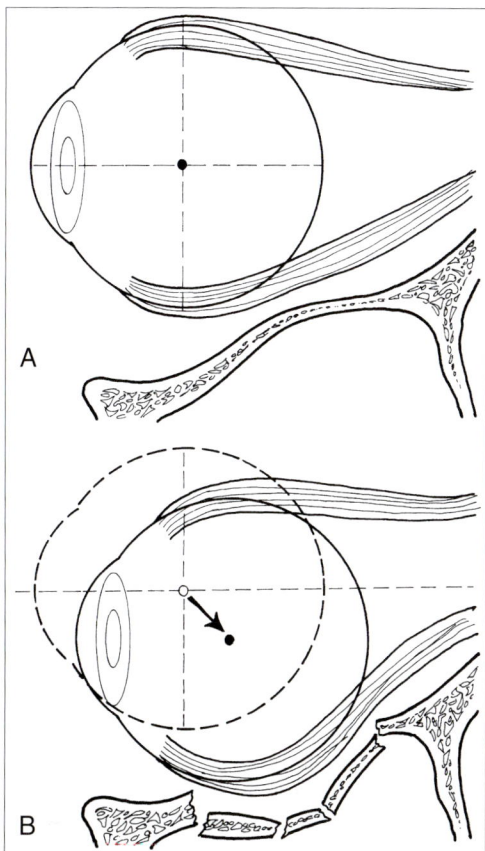

Fig. 39-7 ▪ Configuration of the fractured orbit. **A,** Normally, the orbital contents assume a conical shape with a mid-posterior bulge behind the globe. **B,** Spherical configuration in the post-traumatic orbit with a concave orbital floor resulting in enophthalmos and vertical dystopia. (From Albert DM, Miller JW: *Albert & Jakobiec's principles and practice of ophthalmology*, ed 3, Philadelphia, 2008, Saunders.)

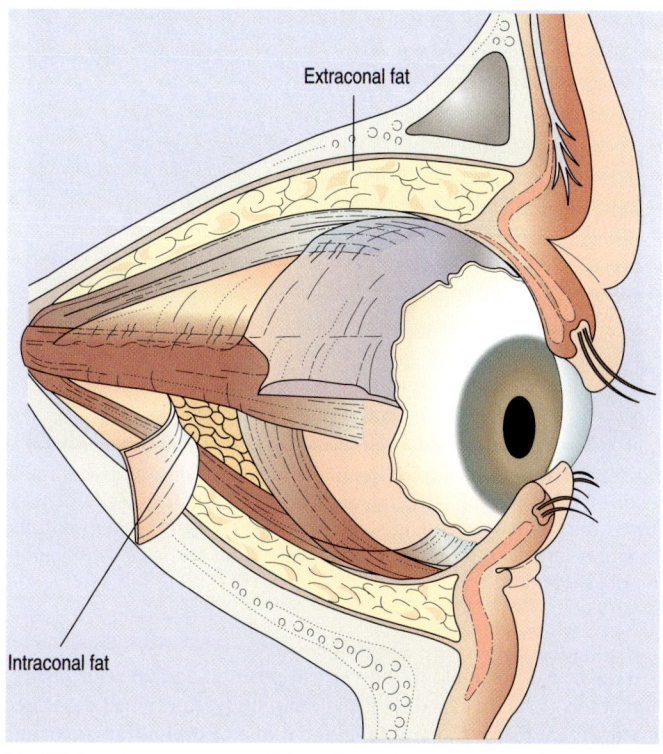

Fig. 39-8 ▪ Superior view of the orbit with transection of the superior and lateral muscle groups to demonstrate the major intraconal structures, including intraconal fat and extraconal fat. (Adapted from Yanoff M, Duker JS: *Ophthalmology*, ed 3, Philadelphia, 2009, Mosby.)

annulus of Zinn. Lockwood's ligament is essentially a fascial thickening at the inferior aspect of the orbit that provides support to the globe, even in the absence of an intact orbital floor. The extrinsic muscles that penetrate this ligament are encased in "tubular reflections" of the same fascia that creates muscle compartments. Orbital fat is thus characterized by its position relative to the extraocular muscle compartments as being either extramuscular (extraconal) or intramuscular (intraconal). As mentioned previously, intraconal fat

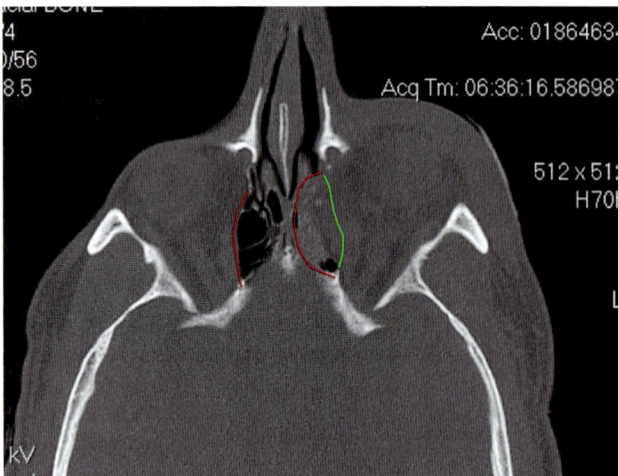

Fig. 39-9 ■ Factors leading to difficulty identifying and accurately reconstructing orbital bony landmarks. An axial CT scan demonstrates the normal posteromedial orbital bulge (*left, red*) and the common surgical error (*right, red*) of inadequate restoration of the posteromedial bulge. The *green line* represents the optimal orbital contour.

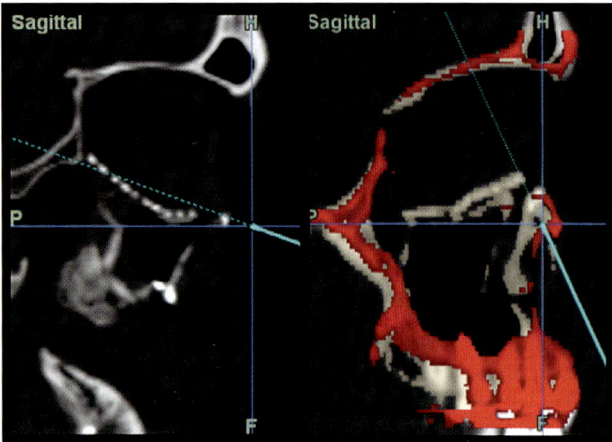

Fig. 39-10 ■ Factors leading to difficulty identifying and accurately reconstructing the orbital bony landmarks. A sagittal CT scan demonstrates the normal ascending slope of the posterior orbit (*left*) and the common surgical error (*right*) of inadequate restoration of the height of the posterior orbit.

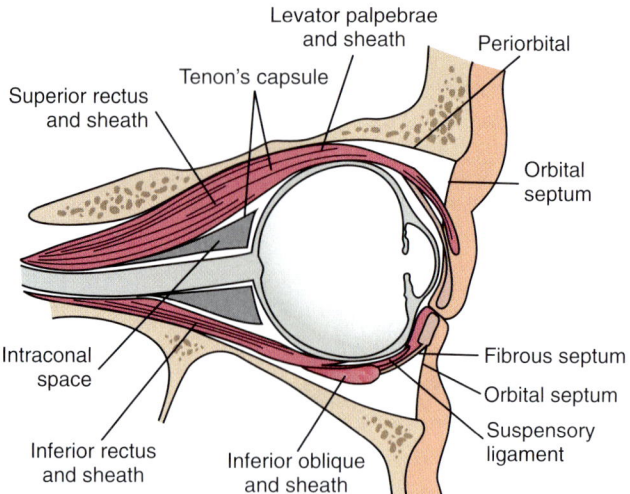

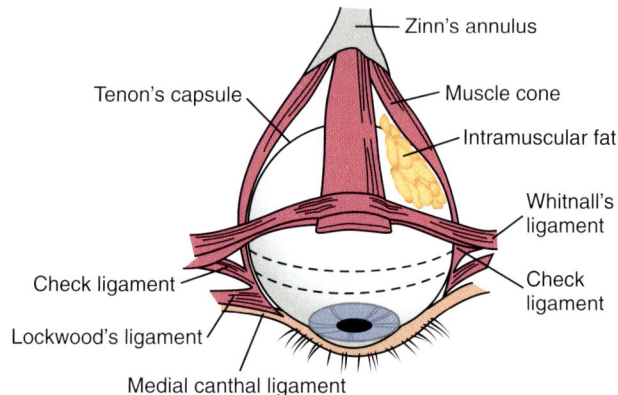

Fig. 39-11 ■ Tenon's capsule and the anterior orbital structures and septa.

is thought to contribute to the vertical position and anterior projection of the globe. In a landmark anatomic study, Koornneef described a connective tissue framework in the midst of orbital fat consisting of septa that anchor the globe and extraocular muscles to the orbital wall.[7] Thus, the globe receives its positional support from both structural soft tissue elements and the external and internal bony skeleton. Generally, a significant increase in orbital volume, caused by displacement or removal of one or more of the internal or external orbital walls, or a decrease in intraconal fat or globe volume will result in perceptible enophthalmos or ocular dysmotility.

It is clear that increased orbital volume alone has the potential to cause enophthalmos or ocular dysmotility in some, but not all patients; enophthalmos may become apparent weeks or months after injury; diplopia or ocular dysmotility can take weeks to resolve; surgical repair is necessary in some, but not all patients; and if indicated, surgical repair is optimally performed within the first 2 weeks after injury because of secondary scarring intraorbitally or

within Tenon's capsule. Therefore, the questions that need to be answered by the clinician are (1) which patients with orbital fractures will benefit from surgical repair (i.e., is there a quantitative volumetric or linear threshold that predicts functional or esthetic complications?) and (2) which patients can be safely observed?

DIAGNOSTIC STUDIES

High-speed helical CT with 1-mm cuts is the imaging study of choice for diagnosing and planning treatment of orbital fractures. Axial cuts alone are inadequate for thoroughly assessing orbital floor fractures since some areas of the floor measure less than 0.5 mm in thickness. It is essential to obtain and evaluate coronal and sagittal views. Sagittal reconstructions from axial data require less than 3-mm slice thickness to avoid a stepladder artifact. Axial images are used to provide information regarding the condition of the medial ethmoidal bulge and postoperative position of the implant relative to the anterior medial orbit and ethmoidal labyrinth. Sagittal images provide particularly useful information for assessing the preoperative condition of the antral bulge and postoperative position of an orbital implant relative to the optic foramen and posterior wall of the maxillary sinus. Coronal images provide excellent diagnostic information with regard to the inferior and medial aspect of the internal orbit and postoperative assessment of implant positioning relative to the maxillary and ethmoid sinuses. The routine use of plain films is no longer advocated.

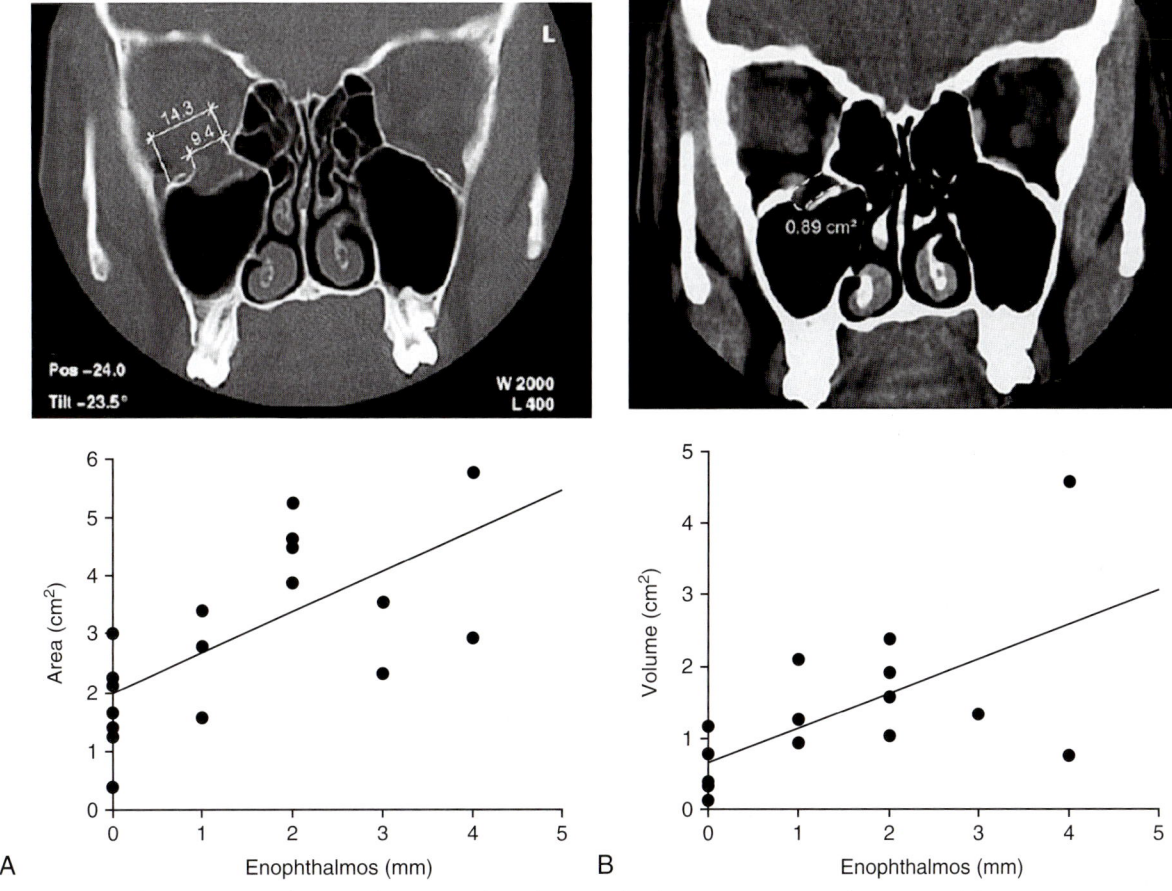

Fig. 39-12 ■ Evaluation of computer-based area and volume measurement from coronal CT scans in isolated blowout fractures of the orbital floor. (From Ploder O, Klug C, Voracek M, et al: Evaluation of computer-based area and volume measurement from coronal computed tomography scans in isolated blowout fractures of the orbital floor, *J Oral Maxillofac Surg* 60:1267-1272, 2002.)

Indirect CT evidence of orbital fractures includes an air-fluid level in the maxillary sinus or opacification of the ethmoidal sinuses, herniation of orbital fat or muscle through a fracture site, and orbital emphysema. A round and inferiorly displaced inferior rectus muscle seen on coronal CT is suggestive of inferior sling disruption and prolapse of the orbital contents with functional entrapment. In the authors' experience, this is an inconsistent finding.

CT has been used to correlate the volume of orbital expansion to the degree of enophthalmos in blowout fractures. It turns out that there is a linear relationship between increases in fracture area, volumetric soft tissue displacement, and enophthalmos. An increase in orbital volume of 1 cm^3 has been shown to correlate with 0.89 mm of enophthalmos.[8] This information has been used to predict the volume of reconstructive material grafted or implanted in a series of patients undergoing reconstruction for late enophthalmos.[9] In a more recent study, Ploder and co-workers found that the combination of an orbital floor area defect of 3.38 cm^2 and volumetric displacement of 1.62 cm^3 was associated with 2 mm of enophthalmos[10] (Fig. 39-12). By convention, 2 mm of enophthalmos is thought to be clinically detectable, and this has therefore been used by some authors as a threshold for undertaking repair of an orbital fracture.

Recently, intraoperative CT scanners, designed for use in neurosurgery, have found application in cranio-maxillofacial surgery. This concept began with fluoroscopic assessment of OZMC fractures. Modern intraoperative CT scanners, however, offer the surgeon an accurate three-dimensional representation of internal and external

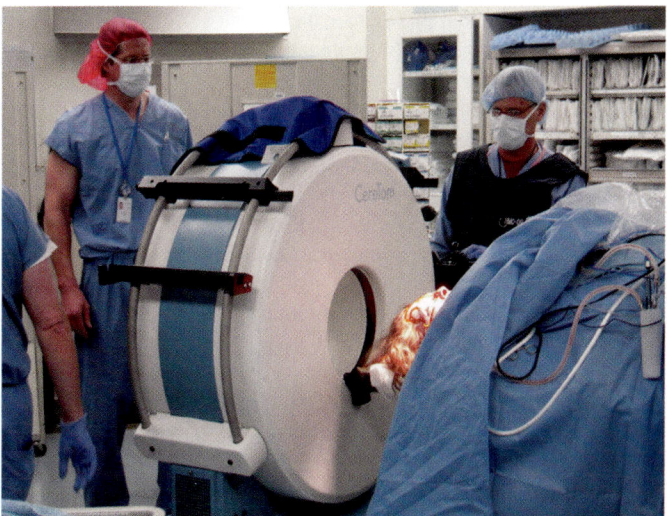

Fig. 39-13 ■ Intraoperative CT scanner.

bony anatomy that can provide intraoperative assessment of reduction, stabilization, and fixation of the segments, as well as the position of internal orbital implants (Fig. 39-13). In a recent study by Hoelzle and colleagues, 15% of a series of patients who underwent repair of OZMC fractures required revision when intraoperative

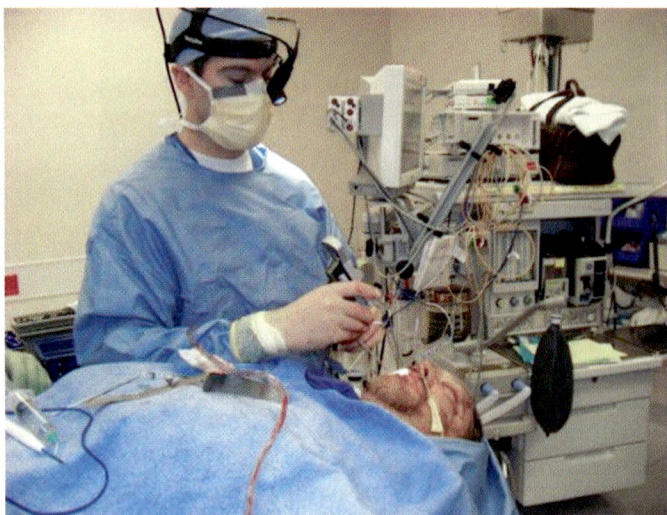

Fig. 39-14 ■ Intraoperative navigation (frameless stereotaxy).

scanning was used to assess reduction and implant position.[11] Furthermore, the use of intraoperative navigation systems (frameless stereotaxy) can be integrated with intraoperative CT scanning to provide optimal surgical guidance, which has particular benefit in the deep orbit and offers the potential for the most optimal outcomes in severely injured patients (Fig. 39-14).[12,13]

TREATMENT/RECONSTRUCTIVE GOALS

The goal of orbital reconstruction is to return the patient to form and function by restoring the external and internal orbital anatomy to its premorbid form and to repair or reposition entrapped or injured soft tissues. Various approaches, techniques, and materials are used to achieve these goals, and there is no universal acceptance of which approach, technique, or material is best in all instances.[14-24]

The senior author's general approach to orbital injuries involves a multistep assessment of whether the patient's injury will result in either a functional or esthetic problem. If the external orbital injury is such that an esthetic deformity such as cheek flattening will be clinically apparent, treatment is warranted. Once the external orbital frame is reduced into normal anatomic position and stabilized, rigid internal fixation is applied via the fewest approaches necessary. Internal orbital injuries are likewise assessed for ocular dysmotility or their potential to result in enophthalmos. If the orbital floor defect is greater than 3 cm^2 or volumetric displacement is greater than 1.5 cm^3 as demonstrated on CT, treatment of the internal orbit is deemed necessary. Furthermore, internal orbital disruptions posterior or medial (or both) to the equator of the globe are typically addressed unless the patient is completely devoid of symptoms.

In the authors' experience, most patients with low-velocity injuries involving the external orbital frame (e.g., bare-fisted assault or ground-level falls) can be adequately restored to form and function without exploration or treatment of the internal orbit. Conversely, most high-velocity injuries, such as those occurring in motor vehicle collisions, result in a displacement of energy that causes significant internal orbital disruption and necessitates repair of the internal orbit regardless of the level of displacement seen on CT. This selective approach to repair of the internal orbit takes into consideration the patient's subjective symptoms (e.g., blurred vision, diplopia), physical findings (e.g., entrapment of the inferior rectus muscle), limitation of extraocular muscle movement, radiographic findings (linear defect greater than 3.5 cm^2 and volumetric displacement greater

than 1.6 cm^3), and mechanism of injury (i.e., low velocity versus high velocity).

Complex, combined orbital fractures are some of the most challenging craniofacial injuries to manage. High-velocity trauma typically produces defects that affect two, three, or all four walls of the orbit. Such "shattered orbits" produce large volumetric increases intraorbitally, with massive herniation of periorbital contents into the surrounding anatomic spaces and occasional cranial neuropathies. Typically, these defects extend into the orbital cone and may involve the optic canal. Their complex patterns and loss of posterior support from the posteromedial and posteroinferior bulges make restoration of normal orbital anatomy challenging. Although refinements in surgical approaches and the development of new biologic materials have improved our ability to more predictably restore these patients' form and function, a significant number of these individuals will still require revision surgery despite the best efforts of an experienced surgeon.[15,17]

Four-wall fractures that involve the anterior skull base may require transcranial approaches, occasionally with the assistance of a neurosurgeon, and they often require management of the frontal sinus and occasionally the orbital apex. As the frontotemporal components are repositioned, the orbital roof must be restored with either titanium mesh or calvarial bone grafts and the anterior skull base lined to prevent leakage of cerebrospinal fluid.

When the entire orbit is disrupted and there are no posterior landmarks to guide the reconstruction, accurate positioning of bone grafts or titanium mesh becomes problematic. It is difficult to establish proper orbital contour, volume, and medial bulge projection, and there is a risk of encroachment on the orbital apex and optic nerve. Presurgical computer planning to virtually reconstruct the affected orbit or orbits, stereolithographic models to establish proper plate contour, and the use of intraoperative navigation to ensure accurate and safe positioning of the plate in a poorly visualized anatomic region afford even experienced surgeons greater confidence and predictability in treating fractures of the deep orbit.[25]

SPECIFIC TREATMENT AND TECHNIQUES

ORBITOZYGOMATICOMAXILLARY COMPLEX FRACTURES (OUTER ORBITAL FRAME)

Optimal management of OZMC fractures remains controversial. Although it is generally agreed that patients do not consistently require three- or four-point fixation, as has been advocated by authors in the past, there is still much confusion on which approach will offer adequate access for successful open reduction and internal fixation with minimal complications. In addition, no consensus has been reached regarding objective criteria for exploration and repair of the orbital floor.

The authors' approach to most OZMC fractures is a progressive technique that generally begins with an intraoral vestibular incision (Keen incision) to approach the maxillary buttress. Minimal to moderately displaced, low-velocity OZMC fractures can often be managed with simple one-point fixation at the maxillary buttress, provided that no significant intraorbital component exists. More commonly, moderately displaced fractures caused by both low- and high-velocity mechanisms can be managed with simple two-point fixation at the maxillary buttress via a Keen incision and at the zygomaticofrontal (ZF) suture via an upper lid blepharoplasty incision. If following reduction and stabilization with two-point fixation at the maxillary buttress and ZF suture the rotation of the OZMC is not adequately reduced or the infraorbital rim remains displaced, the transverse component of the orbital frame can be stabilized at the infraorbital rim via a transconjunctival incision. Skeletonization of the infraorbital rim is avoided if at all possible. However, if adequate height or width of the inferior orbital rim cannot be achieved, a 1.2 or 1.3 miniplate is placed along the infraorbital rim via either a transconjunctival or mid-lid incision.

Ellis and Kittidumkerng analyzed a series of patients with OZMC fractures with regard to the need for repair of the orbital floor or infraorbital rim.[26] Their indications for repair included increased orbital volume or comminution, as well as significant soft tissue prolapse. They found that internal orbital reconstruction was needed in only 44% of their series of patients. In patients who did require repair of the infraorbital rim or orbital floor, scleral show was associated with a lower eyelid incision in approximately 20% of the patients. In another study by Ellis and Reddy, the status of the internal orbit was analyzed after reduction in a series of patients who underwent repair of OZMC fractures but did not undergo orbital exploration.[27] Of these 65 patients, only 8 had minor, non–clinically significant increases in orbital volume. The residual defects became smaller with time.

The authors therefore prefer an approach similar to that of Shumrick and co-workers,[28] which involves selective management of the orbital rim and orbital floor in OZMC fractures based on clinical and radiographic findings. Such findings include persistent diplopia, enophthalmos, significant comminution at the orbital rim or displacement, displacement or comminution of greater than 50% of the orbital wall with herniation of orbital fat, combined orbital floor and medial wall defects with soft tissue displacement, and radiologic evidence of fracture or comminution of the body of the zygoma.

Numerous approaches to the orbit have been described, and although some have advantages over others, surgeons should generally use the approach with which they are most comfortable, that provides optimal cosmesis, and that results in minimal complications.[29-36] The authors' preferred approach for most isolated orbital fractures is a transconjunctival approach performed at the conjunctival fornix. Lateral canthotomy is not advised. Though once popular, the authors' experience is that lateral canthotomy combined with a transconjunctival incision for disarticulation of the lower lid often results in an unnatural appearance even when closed by an experienced surgeon. An isolated transconjunctival forniceal approach combined with upper lid blepharoplasty typically provides adequate access to the orbit for most applications.

Fractures that are the result of a high-velocity injury with severe fragmentation or comminution or those associated with pan-facial fractures are typically repaired with four-point stabilization. This includes a coronal approach to expose the zygomatic arch and reestablish facial/malar projection. Care must be taken to restore the arch to its normal flat contour rather than creating a rounded arch that will result in de-projection of the zygoma and widening of the face.

NASO-ORBITO-ETHMOID FRACTURE (MEDIAL ORBITAL FRAME)

Treatment of NOE fractures is one of the most challenging of all procedures in craniomaxillofacial surgery. Failure to adequately restore nasal projection, normal canthal width, and orbital volume will result in highly unfavorable functional or esthetic outcomes. Refer to Chapter 42 for a more comprehensive explanation of NOE fracture repair.

The authors typically approach these fractures via a coronal incision combined with a transcaruncular incision. Severe telescoping or combination of the nasal bones must be reduced, stabilized, and

fixated to reestablish normal nasal projection. Although strut calvarial bone grafts have been advocated for this purpose and are occasionally necessary, the authors find that adequate anatomic reduction of the nasal bones with stable fixation is often all that is necessary as long as the frontal bandeau is adequately restored. Once the internal orbital frame has been reduced and stabilized with miniplates and nasal projection reestablished, attention must be directed to management of the central fragment. Medial canthopexy is facilitated by using a commercially available titanium barbed wire. A thorough description of this technique is provided in Chapter 42.

FRACTURES OF THE INTERNAL ORBIT

The internal orbit is typically approached via a transconjunctival incision (Fig. 39-15). As stated previously, the incision is made at the conjunctival fornix with a fine needle-tipped Bovie. The incision is carried through conjunctiva and orbital fat to the orbital floor as a postseptal approach. Herniated soft tissue is teased back into the orbit from the maxillary sinus or ethmoid cavities and stabilized in place with a malleable retractor. Attention is then directed toward reestablishing normal orbital anatomy with particular attention paid to restoring the contours of the critical ethmoidal and antral bulges. Various materials are available to reconstruct the orbit, including autogenous bone, porous polyethylene (Medpor), and titanium mesh (Fig. 39-16). Our preference is to use titanium orbital plates for most routine fractures. Alternatively, porous polyethylene (Medpor) impregnated with titanium may be used. Porous polyethylene not impregnated with titanium is not advised because it is not radiographically apparent. Every effort is made to identify a stable posterior ledge within the orbit and restore the critical ethmoidal and antral bulges (Fig. 39-17).

Occasionally, one-wall isolated orbital floor fractures are of such significant volume that they cause symptoms and warrant treatment.

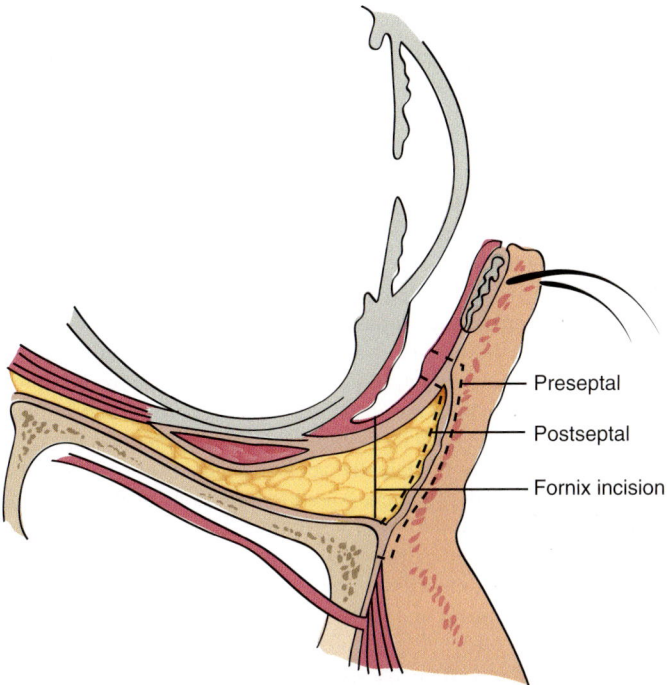

Fig. 39-15 ■ Transconjunctival fornix approach. A postseptal incision is made with a needle-tipped Bovie in the depth of the conjunctival fornix to lower the risk for postoperative entropion. (Modified from Myers EN: *Operative otolaryngology: head and neck surgery*, ed 2, Philadelphia, 2008, Saunders.)

Labels in figure: Preseptal / Postseptal / Fornix incision

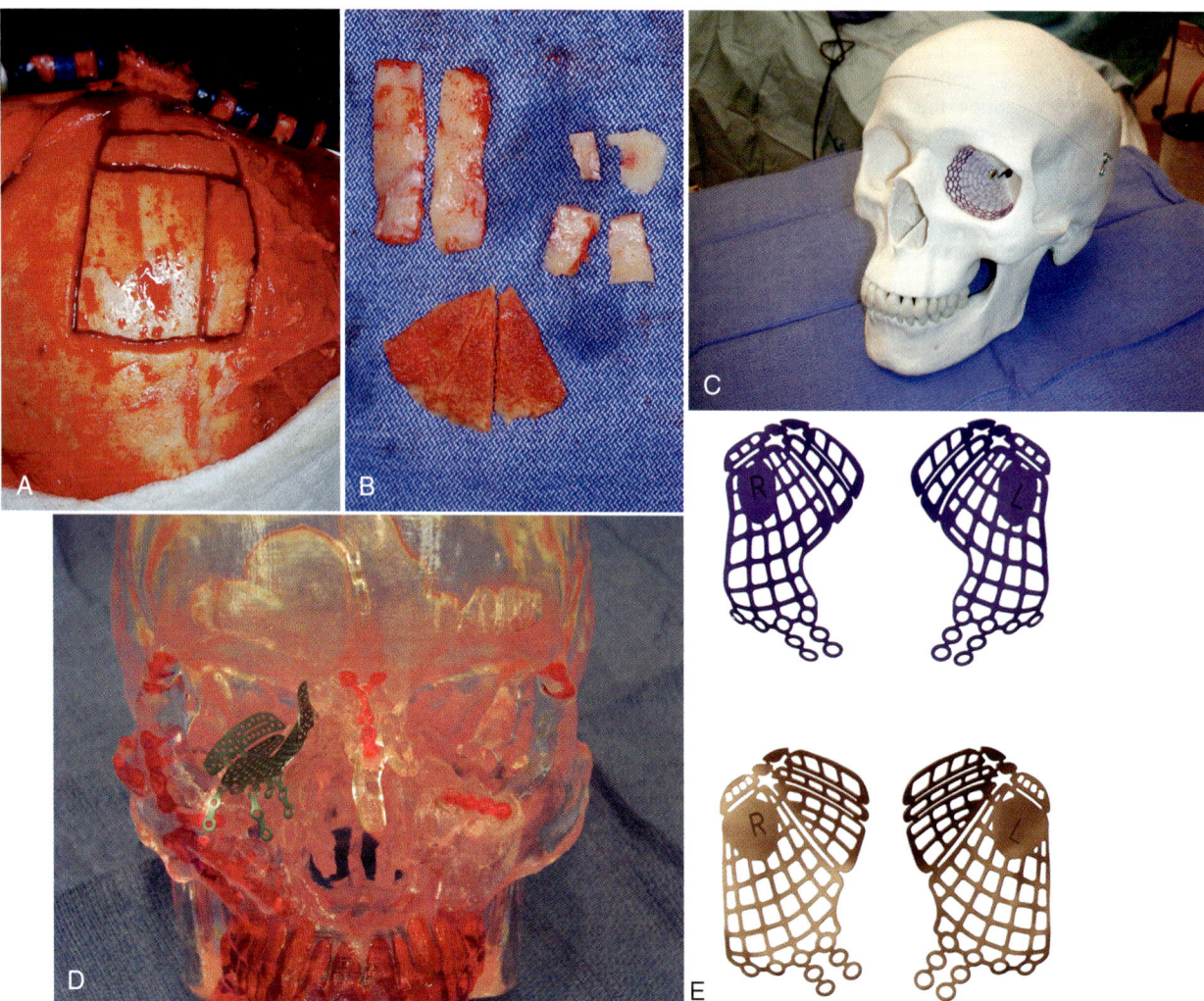

Fig. 39-16 ■ Options for reconstructing the internal orbit. **A,** Calvarial bone graft harvest. **B,** Split calvarial bone graft prepared for inset into the orbit. **C,** Porous polyethylene impregnated with titanium mesh (Medpor). The mesh is "pre-bent" on a stock plastic skull/orbital model. **D,** "Stock" titanium mesh "pre-bent" on a custom stereolithographic model (Stryker CMF). **E,** Preformed orbital implant based on a composite of normal orbits (Synthes).

An alternative to a lower lid/transconjunctival approach is endoscopically assisted transantral repair (Fig. 39-18). This technique is indicated only for one-wall orbital floor defects. A vestibular (Keen) incision is made in the depth of the mucobuccal fold and a full-thickness mucoperiosteal flap is reflected. A bone window is created with a rotary instrument placed in the maxillary antrum to provide access for instrumentation and endoscopic visualization. The prolapsed orbital contents are visualized endoscopically and repositioned back into the orbital cavity. The prolapsed contents are then supported by a titanium plate, the apex of which is inserted into the posterior ledge of the fracture. Anterior extensions of the plate are then brought through the antral window, and the plate is stabilized with at least two screws placed through the facial surface of the maxilla. The osteotomized antral wall is then repositioned and stabilized with miniplates and screws.

COMPLEX COMBINED ORBITAL FRACTURES (SHATTERED ORBIT)

Combined or complex orbital fractures are typically caused by high-velocity forces and are characterized by extension into the posterior third of the orbit with multiwall defects and a large internal increase in volume, massive herniation of periorbital contents into the surrounding anatomic spaces, and cranial neuropathies. These injuries are especially challenging to the reconstructive surgeon because of limited access, poor visualization, complex anatomy, and post-traumatic edema or scarring. These factors often lead to difficulty identifying and reconstructing the orbital bony landmarks, particularly the critical ethmoidal and antral bulges and the orbital apex.

Recently, preoperative computer-assisted planning along with virtual correction and construction of stereolithographic models has been combined with intraoperative navigation in an attempt to more accurately reconstruct the bony orbit and optimize treatment outcomes.[25] Gellrich and colleagues described the use of a navigation system for computer-assisted preoperative planning with virtual reconstruction to achieve symmetry of the orbits and intraoperative control of virtual contours in patients with unilateral post-traumatic orbital deformities.[12] Surgical procedures are preplanned with virtual correction by mirroring an individually defined three-dimensional segment of the unaffected side into the deformed side and thereby creating an ideal unilateral reconstruction. These computer models are then used intraoperatively as a virtual template to navigate the preplanned bony contours and globe projection (Fig. 39-19). A number of authors have subsequently refined these techniques by

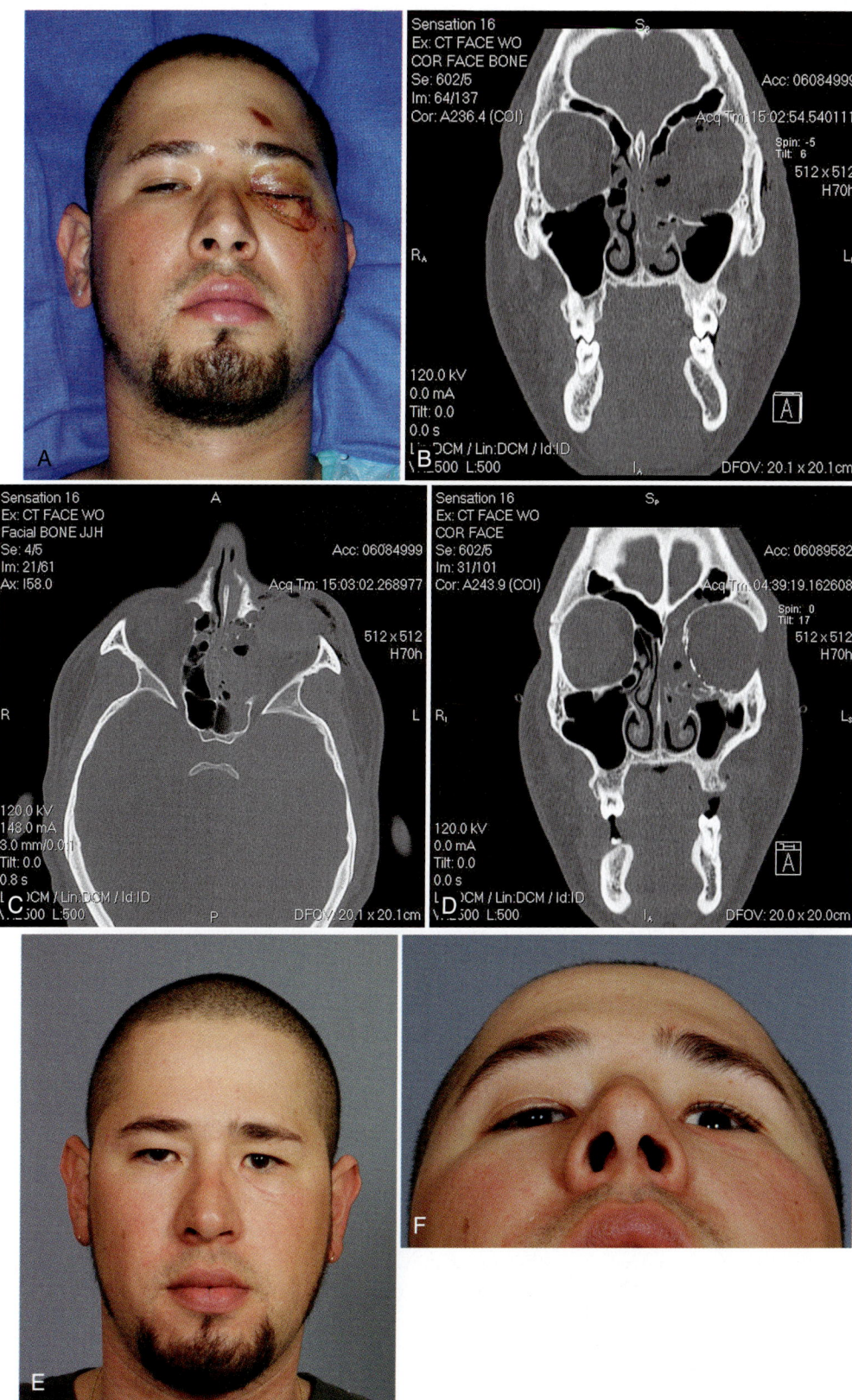

Fig. 39-17 ■ Twenty-three-year-old man involved in a motor vehicle collision and sustaining a severely displaced orbital blowout fracture involving the inferior and medial walls (type 1b). Repair was approached via a lower lid laceration, and the floor and medial wall were restored with porous polyethylene impregnated with titanium mesh. **A,** Preoperative appearance. **B,** Preoperative coronal CT scan. **C,** Preoperative axial CT scan. **D,** Postoperative coronal CT scan. **E,** Postoperative appearance. **F,** Postoperative appearance, worm's eye view.

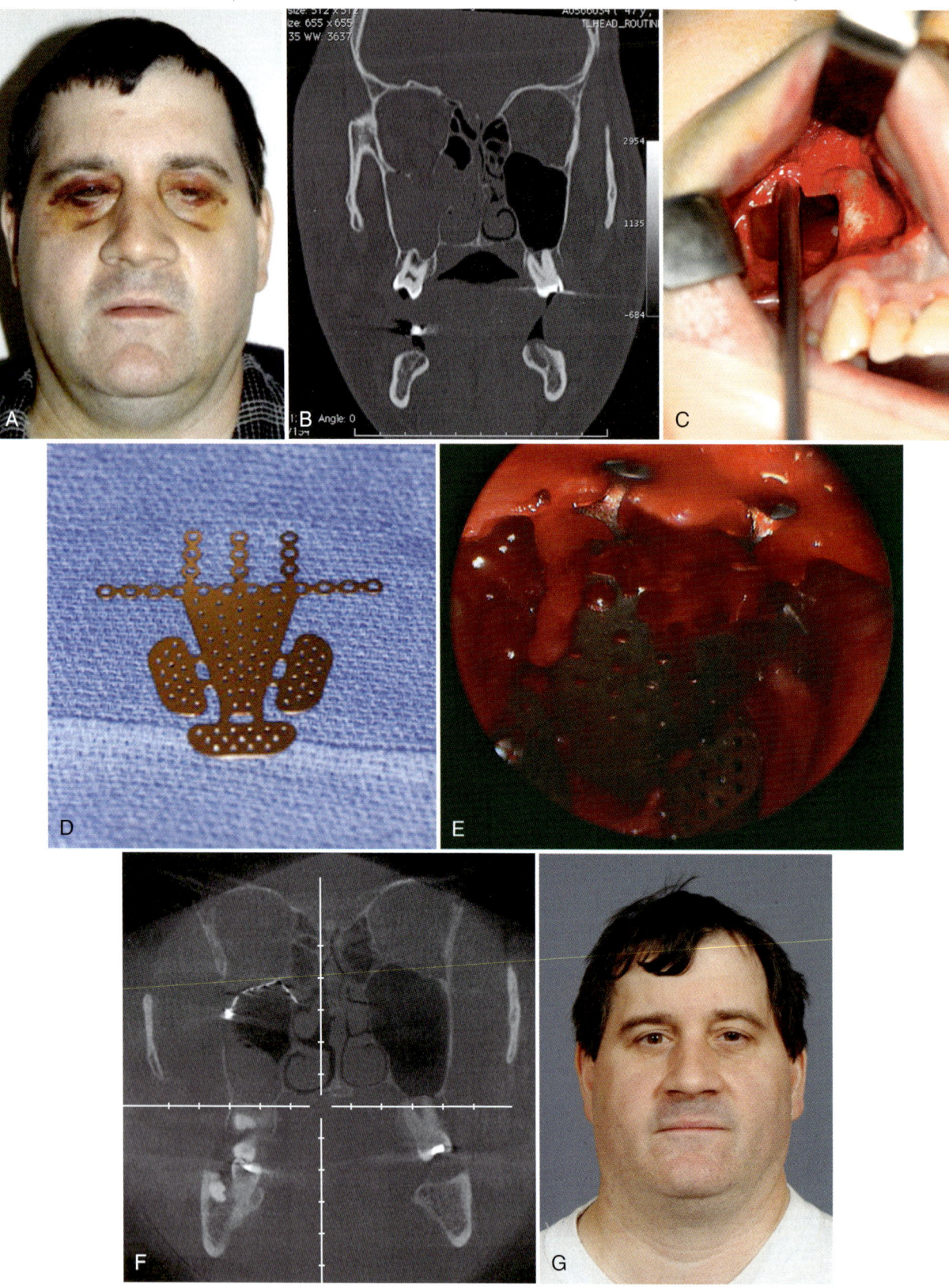

Fig. 39-18 ■ Fifty-three-year-old man involved in a motor vehicle collision and sustaining a right orbital blowout fracture involving the orbital floor with a displaced volume larger than 3 cm³ (type 1a). Repair was achieved via a transantral, endoscopic approach using a stock "angel" titanium plate (Synthes). **A,** Preoperative appearance. **B,** Preoperative coronal CT scan. **C,** Transantral approach with a 30-degree endoscope in place. **D,** "Angel" titanium plate (Synthes). **E,** Endoscopic view of the maxillary sinus roof/orbital floor with the implant in place and secured to the facial aspect of the anterior maxillary wall. **F,** Postoperative coronal cone beam image. **G,** Postoperative appearance.

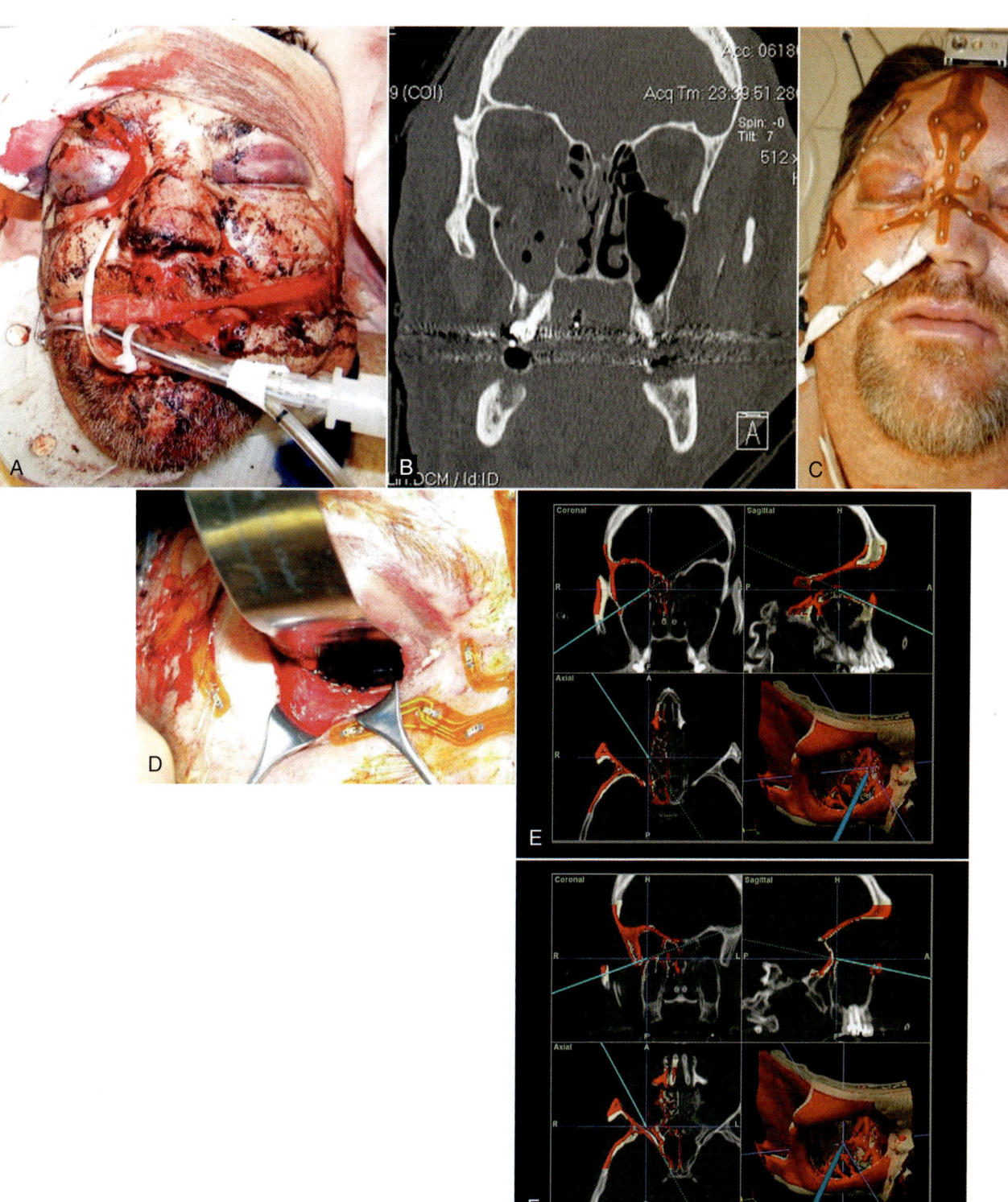

Fig. 39-19 ■ Fifty-one-year-old man involved in a high-speed motor vehicle collision who sustained a severely displaced right orbital blowout fracture with inferomedial displacement extending to the orbital apex and a massive increase in orbital volume (type 1b). Repair was facilitated by computer planning to mirror-image the unaffected side and was then performed with intraoperative navigation to ensure accurate and safe placement of the titanium plate. **A,** Preoperative appearance. **B,** Preoperative coronal CT image posterior. **C,** Facial mask with fiducial markers to enable registration before intraoperative navigation. **D,** Titanium implant placed via a lower lid approach. **E,** Intraoperative navigation images demonstrating a mirror image transferred from the affected side to the unaffected side (*red*) and accurate placement of the plate along the medial wall/ethmoidal bulge (*blue*). **F,** Navigated image with the implant placed at the posterosuperior aspect of the orbit (antral bulge).

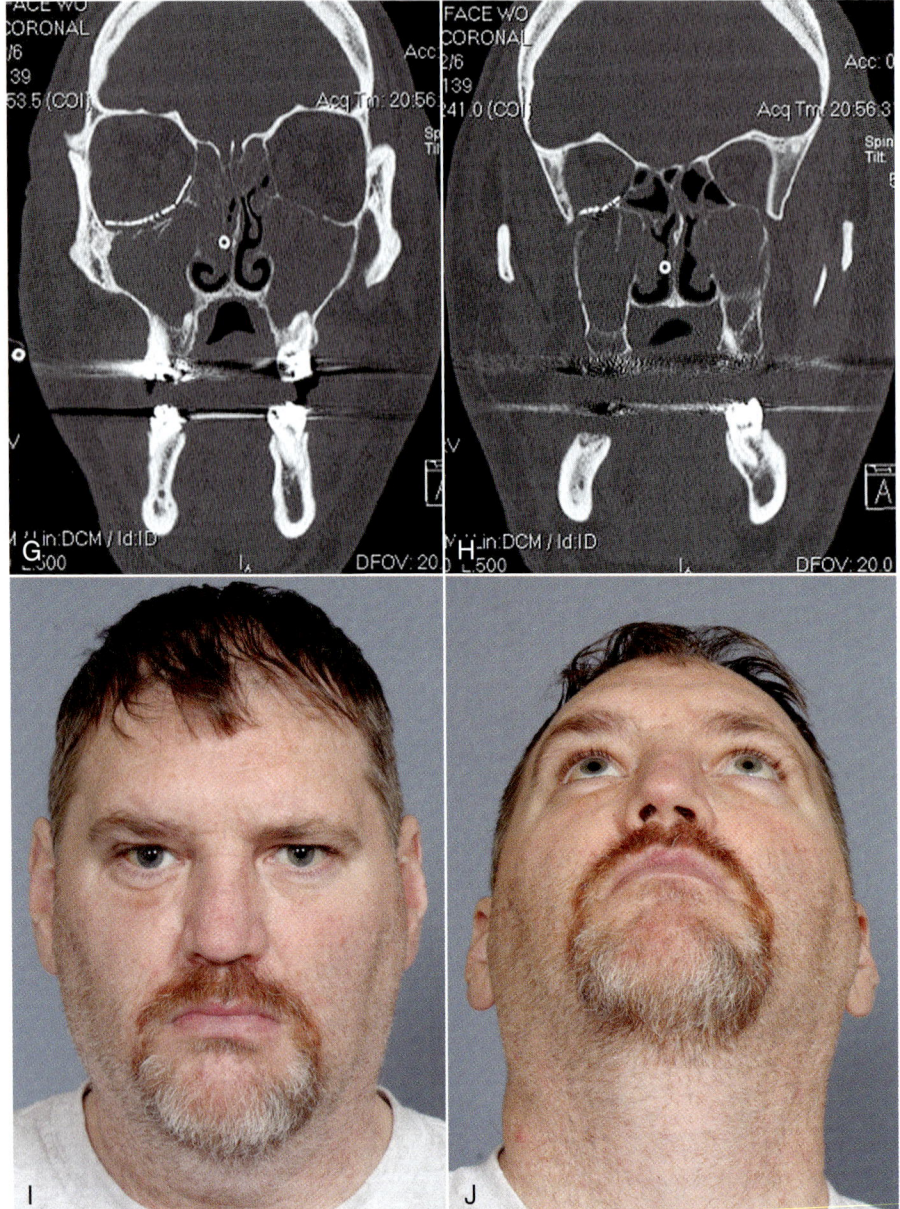

Fig. 39-19, cont'd ■ **G,** Postoperative coronal CT image. **H,** Postoperative coronal CT image, posterior. **I,** Postoperative appearance. **J,** Postoperative appearance, worm's eye view.

including customized preformed titanium mesh and point-to-point computer-assisted navigation based on stereolithographic models with navigation markers.[22,23,37]

Circumferential exposure of the orbit is often necessary for adequate reconstruction of these severe defects (Fig. 39-20). Such exposure is achieved with a coronal incision and mid–lower lid incision. The anterior cranial base is reduced and stabilized. The lateral external orbital component is then repositioned and stabilized with a miniplate at the ZF suture. Following this step, proper projection of the zygoma is achieved by reducing and stabilizing the zygomatic arch. The maxillary buttress is then stabilized via a transoral approach, and finally the infraorbital rim connects the lateral skeletal components to the medial NOE complex. Once the external orbital frame is reconstructed, attention is directed toward restoring the internal orbit as described previously. Calvarial bone grafts are occasionally needed for reconstruction of missing skeletal components of the external orbital frame, but their use in the internal orbit is now rarely needed in the acute setting (Fig. 39-21).

Presurgical planning using stereolithographic models to establish proper plate contour, as well as intraoperative navigation to ensure accurate and safe positioning of the plate in a poorly visualized anatomic region, provides even experienced surgeons greater confidence and predictability in treating fractures in the deep orbit.[25] In addition to navigating the orbital apex, computerized planning and pre-bent orbital plates have the potential to predictably restore the difficult-to-access posterior medial bulge region and antral bulge.

Recently, Metzger and associates described a semiautomatic procedure for individual preforming of titanium mesh for treatment of orbital fractures.[22] By using CT scan data, the topography of the orbital floor and wall structures was recalculated. After mirroring the unaffected side onto the affected side, the defect can be reconstructed virtually. Data for the individual virtual model of the orbital cavity are then sent to a template machine that reproduces the surface of the orbital floor and medial walls automatically. The titanium mesh can then be adjusted preoperatively for exact

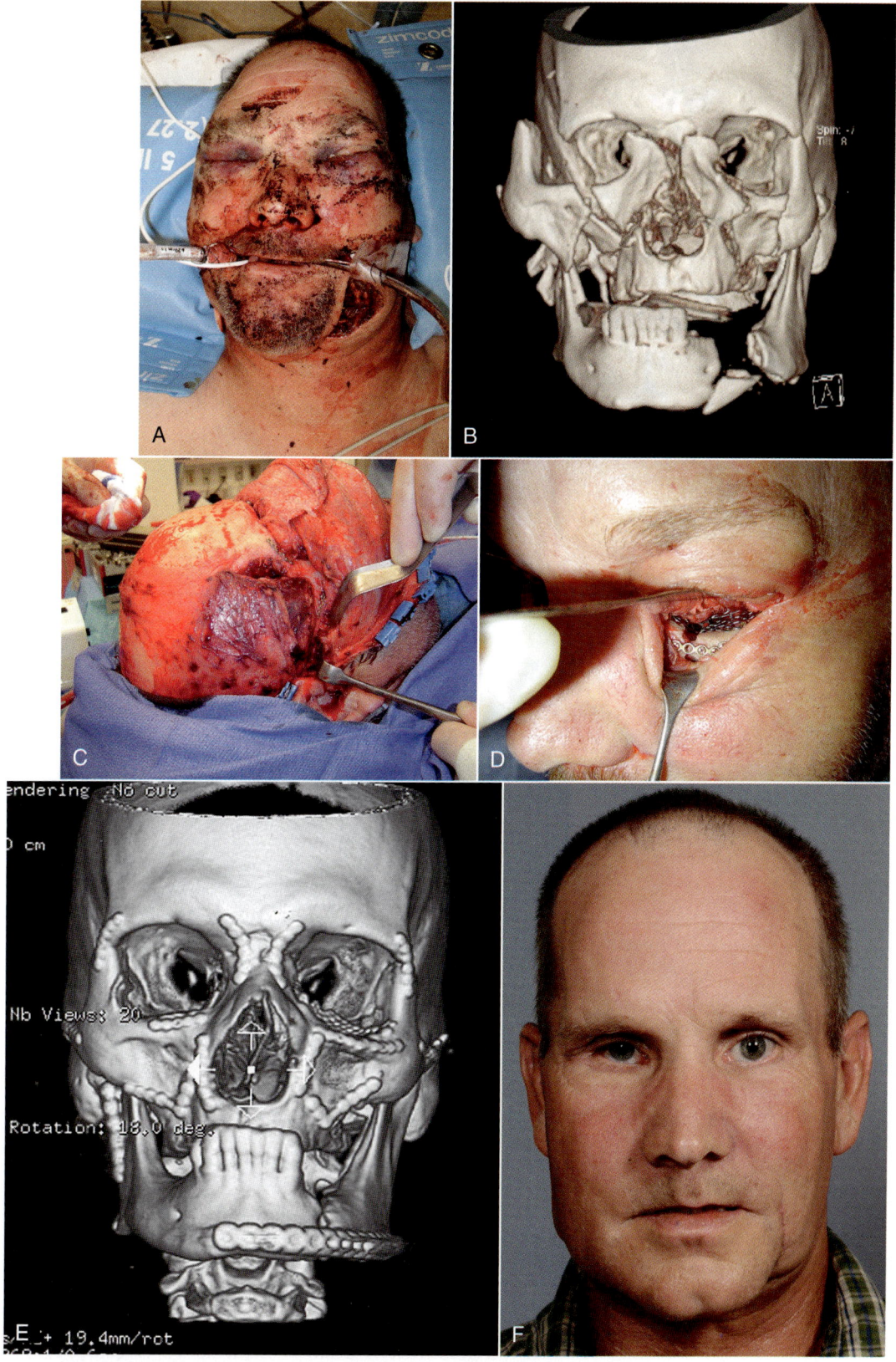

Fig. 39-20 ■ Forty-six-year-old man involved in a roll-over tractor accident and sustaining severely displaced pan-facial fractures, degloving lacerations extending into the oropharynx, and a massive increase in orbital volume (combined type 2 injury [a + b]). **A,** Preoperative appearance. **B,** Preoperative three-dimensional (3D) CT image. **C,** Coronal incision combined with a lower lid and transoral incision to facilitate circumferential exposure of the orbit and reduction and fixation of the external orbits. **D,** Titanium mesh used to reconstruct the internal orbit. **E,** Postoperative 3D CT image. **F,** Postoperative appearance.

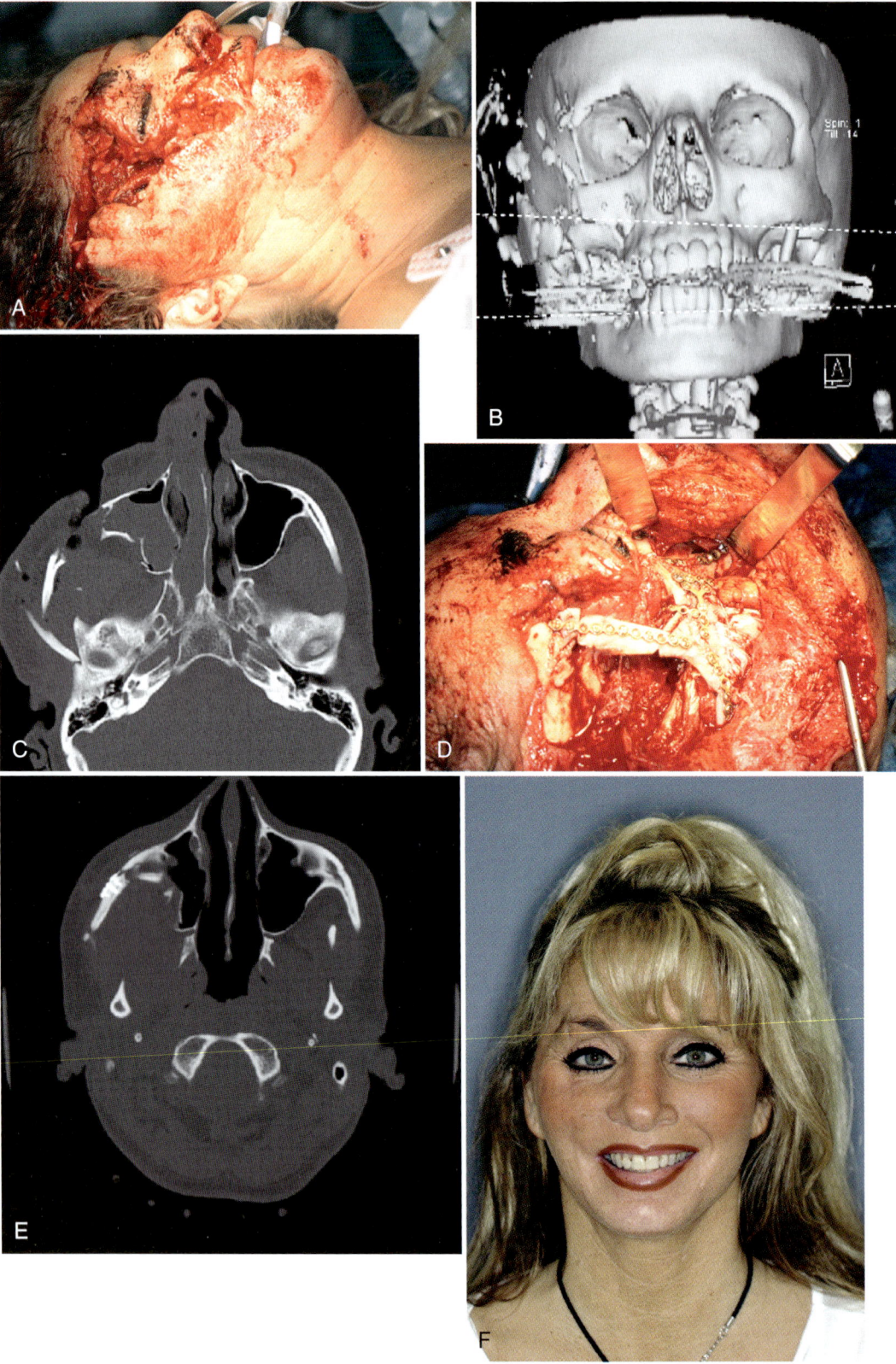

Fig. 39-21 ■ Thirty-one-year-old woman involved in a high-speed roll-over motor vehicle collision with ejection. She sustained severely displaced right orbitozygomatic fractures with avulsion of the lateral orbital rim and a massive increase in orbital volume (type 2a). Open reduction with internal fixation of the external frame was performed via a coronal approach combined with large lacerations. Calvarial bone grafts were harvested to restore the missing lateral orbital frame and internal orbital volume. **A,** Preoperative appearance. **B,** Preoperative three-dimensional CT image. **C,** Preoperative axial CT image—note the facial widening. **D,** Intraoperative open reduction and internal fixation of the orbital frame in addition to reconstruction with bone graft. **E,** Postoperative axial CT image—note the restoration of facial width/symmetry. **F,** Postoperative appearance.

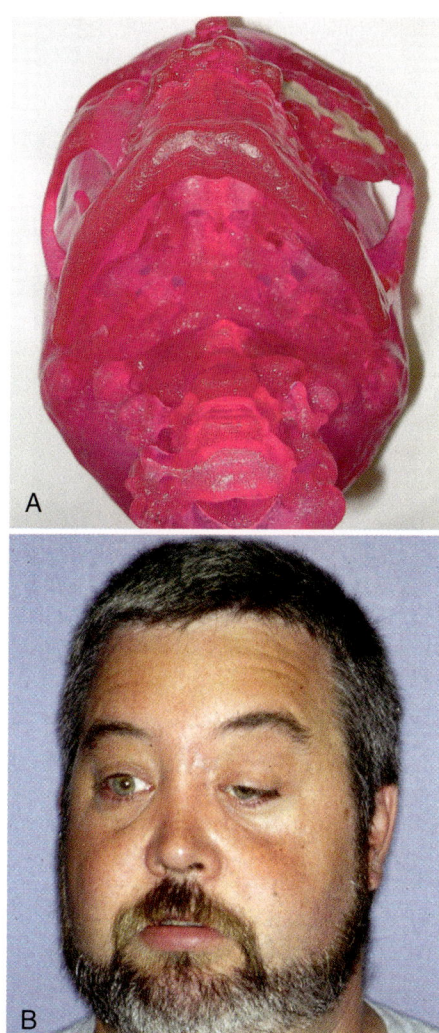

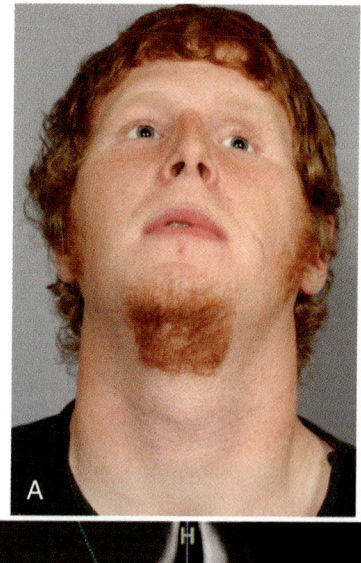

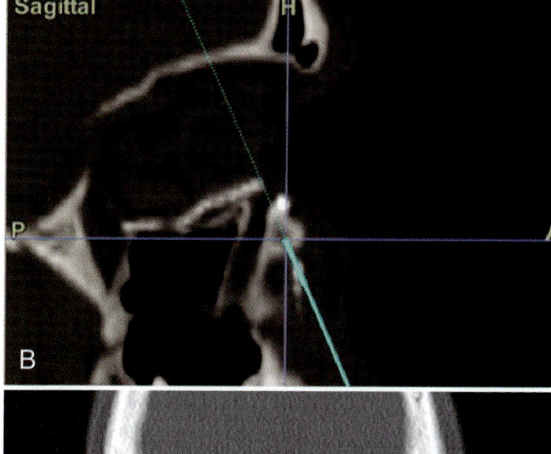

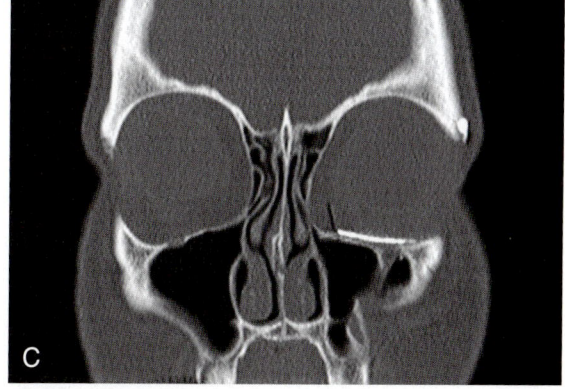

Fig. 39-22 ■ Importance of the zygoma for achieving normal facial width and symmetry. As facial/zygomatic projection decreases, facial width increases. **A,** Stereolithographic model of a patient following open reduction and internal fixation of severely comminuted facial factures with improperly restored projection of the zygoma. The zygoma should be "straight," not "arched," and is one of the most common mistakes made when restoring external orbital anatomy. **B,** Postoperative appearance—note the facial widening.

Fig. 39-23 ■ Importance of reconstructing the critical orbital bulges. **A,** Enophthalmos following inaccurate reconstruction of the medial ethmoidal and posterior antral bulges. **B,** Sagittal CT image demonstrating the common error of placing the orbital implant into the maxillary antrum along the posterior antral wall rather than superiorly in the orbit. **C,** Coronal CT image demonstrating lack of restoration of the medial bulge.

three-dimensional reconstruction, and an individually milled titanium implant is used with navigation to guarantee intraoperative placement of the preformed mesh. In the future, it is our opinion that custom plates such as these placed under intraoperative guidance with intraoperative CT confirmation will be the method of choice for repair of complex orbital injuries.

POSTOPERATIVE CARE

Application of ice to the affected or operative area for the first 48 hours and head elevation while sleeping are advised.[10] All patients are placed on sinus precautions preoperatively and for 2 weeks after repair. Oxymetazoline nasal spray is recommended for symptomatic relief in the immediate postoperative period for 2 to 3 days only. Also for symptomatic relief, pseudoephedrine hydrochloride is prescribed for 5 days. Severe chemosis must be treated with Lacri-Lube. If a coronal incision is used, a suction drain is placed for

24 hours. In patients in whom an intraoral incision is used, chlorhexidine mouth rinses are prescribed for 1 week. In the absence of lagophthalmos, no particular ophthalmic topical antibiotic is routinely prescribed.[38]

The use of steroids in the medical management of orbital fractures was reviewed in a prospective, randomized, double-blind study by Millman and colleagues.[39] All patients had diplopia and dysmotility. The treatment group received 1 mg/kg/day of prednisone for 10

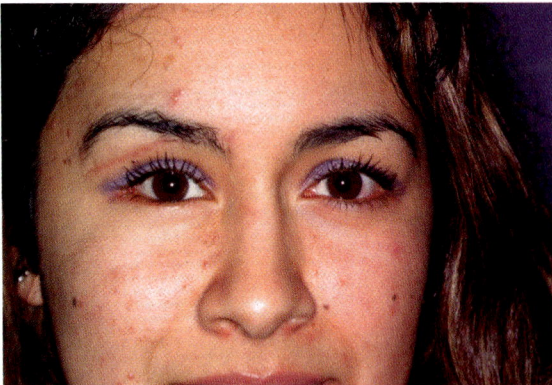

Fig. 39-24 ▪ Right lower lid entropion following a preseptal transconjunctival approach with lateral canthotomy. A postseptal, forniceal approach without lateral canthotomy has eliminated this complication in the authors' experience.

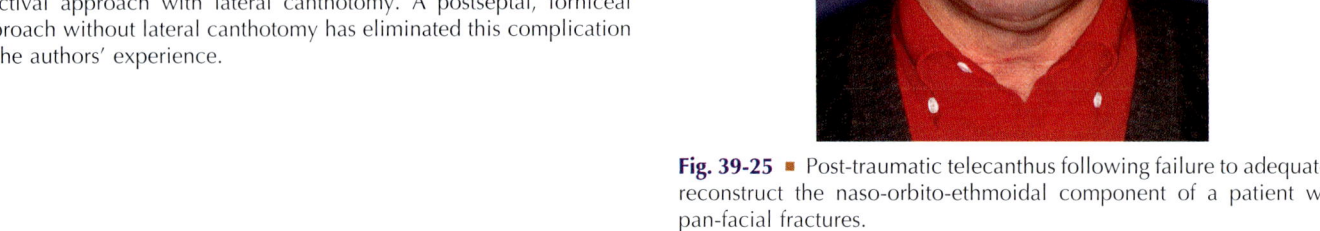

Fig. 39-25 ▪ Post-traumatic telecanthus following failure to adequately reconstruct the naso-orbito-ethmoidal component of a patient with pan-facial fractures.

days, with subsequent tapering over a 4-day period. Any residual dysmotility at the end of 2 weeks, with or without steroids, was treated surgically. The median follow-up period was 11 months. The mean time until resolution of dysmotility in patients without frank rectus entrapment was 4.4 days in the treatment group and 12.7 days in the placebo group. Less pain and disability were reported by the treatment group. Interestingly, enophthalmos was unveiled within 1 week in the treatment group versus 5 months in the placebo group, which allowed earlier surgical intervention in the treatment group. We recommend Solu-Medrol, 125 mg at surgery, as well as every 8 hours for 24 hours after admission. Depo-Medrol, 80 mg, is also given perioperatively.

PEARLS AND PITFALLS

- *Approach.* Approaches to the orbital floor should, in most cases, be achieved with a transconjunctival incision placed at the fornix. Previously popular, the preseptal approach is an elegant dissection; however, it has a tendency to cause ectropion, particularly if combined with lateral canthotomy. Lateral canthotomy is occasionally necessary, but care should be taken to resuspend the periorbital musculature and perform an accurate lateral canthopexy on closure. When wide access to the infraorbital rim is required, particularly in a post-traumatic patient in whom edema persists, a mid-lid incision is a predictable means of providing a good balance between cosmesis and minimization of the complications of increased scleral show or ectropion.

- *External Orbital Frame.* The most common error in reduction, stabilization, and fixation of external orbital fractures is inadequate restoration of malar projection. This is typically caused by creating an outward curve of the zygomatic arch facilitated by medial rotation of the zygomaticomaxillary complex. If a coronal incision is not performed, accurate rotation of the zygomaticomaxillary complex can be assessed by inspecting the sphenozygomatic suture region via an upper lid blepharoplasty approach. Failure to adequately flatten the zygomatic arch and achieve optimal rotation of the zygomaticomaxillary complex will result in flattening of the malar eminence and widening of the ipsilateral face (Fig. 39-22).

- *Internal Orbit.* The most common error related to internal orbital reconstruction is failure to adequately restore the critical orbital bulges at the posteroinferior (antral bulge) and posteromedial (ethmoidal bulge) aspects of the orbit. The typical error is that the surgeon places the orbital implant flush with the anterior portion of the orbit and it extends directly back to the posterior wall of the maxillary sinus (Fig. 39-23). A similar error is made in the medial orbit by inaccurately positioning the implant in the ethmoidal labyrinth. Radiographic assessment of accurate implant placement is essential. This can be provided either by postoperative CT in the axial, coronal, and sagittal views or by modern intraoperative CT scanning.

- *Soft Tissue Deformity.* Lower lid entropion or ectropion can be challenging and frustrating for both the surgeon and patient. The risk for entropion can be minimized by avoiding the use of lateral canthotomy combined with transconjunctival incisions (Fig. 39-24). Additionally, placement of the transconjunctival incision at the conjunctival fornix appears to minimize the risk for postoperative entropion. Ectropion can be avoided by performing a so-called mid-lid incision and avoiding the subciliary approach, which has a tendency to cause postoperative scarring and malposition. Finally, infraorbital or malar ptosis is almost unavoidable in some patients in whom the malar eminence and infraorbital rim are completely skeletonized. However, every effort should be made following reduction, stabilization, and fixation of the fractures to resuspend the infraorbital soft tissues to either bone or hardware.

- *Telecanthus.* Management of the medial canthus with a titanium barbed wire has been discussed previously. The importance of reestablishing the central component of NOE fractures is of paramount importance for achieving optimal functional and esthetic results (Fig. 39-25). In addition, it is important to avoid the unrecognized NOE fracture that occasionally accompanies fractures of the lateral orbit. In this instance, the operating surgeon will repair the OZMC component and neglect the NOE component, which results in unilateral telecanthus.

REFERENCES

1. Bell RB: The role of oral and maxillofacial surgery in the trauma care center, *J Oral Maxillofac Surg* 65:2544-2553, 2007.
2. Smith B, Regan WF: Blowout fracture of the orbit: mechanism and correction of internal orbital fracture, *Am J Ophthalmol* 44:733-739, 1957.
3. Fujino T: Experimental "blowout" fracture of the orbit, *Plast Reconstr Surg* 54:81-82, 1974.
4. Antonyshyn O, Gruss JS, Kassel EE: Blow-in fractures of the orbit, *Plast Reconstr Surg* 84:10-20, 1989.
5. Manson PN: Pure orbital blowout fracture: new concepts and importance of the medial orbital blowout fracture, *Plast Reconstr Surg* 104:878-882, 1999.
6 Manson PN, Clifford CM, Su CT, et al: Mechanisms of global support and post-traumatic enophthalmos: I. The anatomy of the ligament sling and its relation to intramuscular cone orbital fat, *Plast Reconstr Surg* 77:193-202, 1986.
7. Koornneef L: Current concepts on the management of orbital blow-out fractures, *Ann Plast Surg* 9:185-200, 1982.
8. Fan X, Li J, Zhu J, et al: Computer-assisted orbital volume measurement in the surgical correction of late enophthalmos caused by blowout fractures. *Ophthalmic Plast Reconstr Surg* 19:207-211, 2003.
9. Whitehouse RW, Batterbury M, Jackson A, et al: Prediction of enophthalmos by computed tomography after "blow out" orbital fracture, *Br J Ophthalmol* 78:618-620, 1994.
10. Ploder O, Klug C, Voracek M, et al: Evaluation of computer-based area and volume measurement from coronal computed tomography scans in isolated blowout fractures of the orbital floor, *J Oral Maxillofac Surg* 60:1267-1272, discussion 1273-1274, 2002.
11. Hoelzle F, Klein M, Schwerdtner O, et al: Intraoperative computed tomography with the mobile CT Tomoscan M during surgical treatment of orbital fractures, *Int J Oral Maxillofac Surg* 30:26-31, 2001.
12. Gellrich NC, Schramm A, Hammer B, et al: Computer-assisted secondary reconstruction of unilateral posttraumatic orbital deformity, *Plast Reconstr Surg* 110:1417-1429, 2002.
13. Eggers G, Kress B, Muhling J: Fully automated registration of intraoperative computed tomography image data for image-guided craniofacial surgery, *J Oral Maxillofac Surg* 66:1754-1760, 2008.

14. Converse JM, Smith B, Obear MF, et al: Orbital blowout fractures: a ten-year survey, *Plast Reconstr Surg* 39:20-36, 1967.
15. Kawamoto HK Jr: Late posttraumatic enophthalmos: a correctable deformity? *Plast Reconstr Surg* 69:423-432, 1982.
16. Manson PN, Grivas A, Rosenbaum A, et al: Studies on enophthalmos: II. The measurement of orbital injuries and their treatment by quantitative computed tomography, *Plast Reconstr Surg* 77:203-214, 1986.
17. Manson PN, Ruas EJ, Iliff NT: Deep orbital reconstruction for correction of post-traumatic enophthalmos, *Clin Plast Surg* 14:113-121, 1987.
18. Schon R, Metzger MC, Zizelmann C, et al: Individually preformed titanium mesh implants for a true-to-original repair of orbital fractures, *Int J Oral Maxillofac Surg* 35:990-995, 2006.
19. Glassman RD, Manson PN, Vanderkolk CA, et al: Rigid fixation of internal orbital fractures, *Plast Reconstr Surg* 86:1103-1109, discussion 1110-1111, 1990.
20. Romano JJ, Iliff NT, Manson PN: Use of Medpor porous polyethylcne implants in 140 patients with facial fractures, *J Craniofacial Surg* 4:142-147, 1993.
21. Ellis E 3rd, Tan Y: Assessment of internal orbital reconstructions for pure blowout fractures: cranial bone grafts versus titanium mesh, *J Oral Maxillofac Surg* 61:442-453, 2003.
22. Metzger MC, Schon R, Zizelmann C, et al: Semiautomatic procedure for individual preforming of titanium meshes for orbital fractures, *Plast Reconstr Surg* 119:969-976, 2007.
23. Metzger MC, Schon R, Weyer N, et al: Anatomical 3-dimensional pre-bent titanium implant for orbital floor fractures, *Ophthalmology* 113:1863-1868, 2006.
24. Scolozzi P, Momjian R, Heuberger J, et al: Accuracy and predictability in use of AO three-dimensionally preformed titanium mesh plates for posttraumatic orbital reconstruction: a pilot study, *J Craniofacial Surg* 20:1108-1113, 2009.
25. Bell RB, Markiewicz MR: Computer assisted planning, stereolithographic modeling, and intraoperative navigation for complex orbital reconstruction: a descriptive study on a preliminary cohort, *J Oral Maxillofac Surg* 67:2559-2570, 2009.
26. Ellis E 3rd, Kittidumkerng W: Analysis of treatment for isolated zygomaticomaxillary complex fractures, *J Oral Maxillofac Surg* 54:386-400, discussion 400-401, 1996.

27. Ellis E 3rd, Reddy L: Status of the internal orbit after reduction of zygomaticomaxillary complex fractures. *J Oral Maxillofac Surg* 62:275-283, 2004.
28. Shumrick KA, Kersten RC, Kulwin DR, et al: Criteria for selective management of the orbital rim and floor in zygomatic complex and midface fractures, *Arch Otolaryngol Head Neck Surg* 123:378-384, 1997.
29. Ellis E III, Zide MF: *Surgical approaches to the facial skeleton. Periorbital incisions*, ed 2, Philadelphia, 2006, Lippincott Williams & Wilkins, pp 7-78.
30. Holtmann B, Wray RC, Little AG: A randomized comparison of four incisions for orbital fractures, *Plast Reconstr Surg* 67:731-737, 1981.
31. Kushner GM: Surgical approaches to the infraorbital rim and orbital floor: the case for the transconjunctival approach, *J Oral Maxillofac Surg* 64:108-110, 2006.
32. Wilson S, Ellis E 3rd: Surgical approaches to the infraorbital rim and orbital floor: the case for the subtarsal approach, *J Oral Maxillofac Surg* 64:104-107, 2006.
33. Netscher DT, Patrinely JR, Peltier M, et al: Transconjunctival versus transcutaneous lower eyelid blepharoplasty: a prospective study, *Plast Reconstr Surg* 96:1053-1060, 1995.
34. Rohrich RJ, Janis JE, Adams WP Jr: Subciliary versus subtarsal approaches to orbitozygomatic fractures, *Plast Reconstr Surg* 111:1708-1174, 2003.
35. Baumann A, Ewers R: Transcaruncular approach for reconstruction of medial orbital wall fracture, *Int J Oral Maxillofac Surg* 29:264-267, 2000.
36. Lee CS, Yoon JS, Lee SY: Combined transconjunctival and transcaruncular approach for repair of large medial orbital wall fractures, *Arch Ophthalmol* 127:291-296, 2009.
37. Klug C, Schicho K, Ploder O, et al: Point to point computer assisted navigation for precise transfer of planned zygoma osteotomies from the stereolithographic model into reality, *J Oral Maxillofac Surg* 64:550-559, 2006.
38. Newlands C, Baggs PR, Kendrick R: Orbital trauma. Antibiotic prophylaxis needs to be given only in certain circumstances, *BMJ* 319:516-517, 1999.
39. Millman AL, Della Rocca RC, Spector S, et al: Steroids and orbital blowout fractures—a new systematic concept in medical management and surgical decision-making. *Adv Ophthalmic Plast Reconstr Surg* 6:291-300, 1987.

Zygomaticomaxillary Complex Fractures

Christopher John Haggerty, Nagi Demian, Jose M. Marchena

Fractures of the zygomaticomaxillary complex (ZMC) are the second most common of all facial fractures. Multiple fixation methods have been used over the years, including wire osteosynthesis, lag screw fixation, transfacial Kirschner wire fixation, titanium plate and screw fixation, and more recently, resorbable plating systems. Internal fixation with titanium plates and screws provides the most rigid fixation and thus greater immobility of the fractured segments. The degree of immobilization created with titanium plates and screws also allows fixation at fewer anatomic points.

Conceptually, the approach to ZMC fractures should depend on the type and mechanism of injury. Low-energy injuries typically result in minimal or no comminution, whereas high-energy injuries can cause extensive comminution of the segments and at the fracture lines. Early non-comminuted and minimally displaced fractures may be managed by reduction alone if the reduction is thought to be stable. Older, displaced, and minimally comminuted ZMC fractures are managed by open reduction and proper orientation of the ZMC in three dimensions. Plate fixation is carried out at the zygomaticofrontal suture area, zygomaticomaxillary buttress, and inferior orbital rim. High-energy injuries can result in significant comminution at the fracture interfaces and fragmentation of the supporting bony buttresses. These fractures tend to be unstable and thus require a certain degree of bony reconstruction of the zygoma and its supporting buttresses, orbit, or zygomatic arch.

Regardless of the approach or fixation pattern chosen, it is critical to understand that proper alignment of the zygomaticosphenoid suture and anatomic reduction of the zygomatic arch remain the most reliable indicator of proper reduction and orientation of the ZMC in three dimensions.

This chapter discusses the anatomy of ZMC fractures, important signs and symptoms, contemporary approaches to common fracture patterns, postoperative care, and potential complications.

ANATOMIC CONSIDERATIONS AND FRACTURE PATTERNS

The zygoma is a quadrangular-shaped bone that provides lateral anterior projection of the central part of the face. The zygoma articulates with the frontal, temporal, maxillary, and sphenoid bones at the zygomaticofrontal, zygomaticotemporal, zygomaticomaxillary, and zygomaticosphenoid sutures (Fig. 40-1, *A* and *B*). These articulating sutures are areas of weakness and are therefore the most commonly fractured sites. The zygomaticosphenoid suture and zygomatic arch are the key anatomic landmarks. Their geometric arrangement and spatial relationship to each other and to the zygoma and the remainder of the facial skeleton are such that when they are aligned, the entire zygomatic complex should be anatomically aligned in three dimensions (see Fig. 40-1, *A* and *B*). It is also important to understand that the zygoma forms major portions of the orbital floor and lateral wall. All zygomatic complex fractures therefore involve the orbit (Fig. 40-1, *C*). These areas are composed of thin bone and are consequently frequently fragmented and displaced. In fact, it has been estimated that ZMC fractures contribute to at least 76% of orbital fractures. Orbital floor or wall defects requiring bridging have been reported in up to 48% of ZMC fractures; however, there is certainly controversy on the severity of orbital floor disruption that would cause cosmetically apparent hypoglobus since anatomic reduction of the zygoma will frequently reduce the fractured orbital floor. Other areas of bony weakness are those containing a neurovascular bundle, such as the medial orbital rim at the level of the infraorbital foramen.

Sensory nerves associated with zygomatic complex fractures include the zygomatic, temporal, and facial branches of the second division of the trigeminal nerve as it passes through the body of the zygoma. The infraorbital nerve passes through the orbital floor and exits through the infraorbital foramen below the inferior orbital rim. Signs of nerve injury include paresthesia of the forehead, cheek, lateral part of the nose, upper lip, and anterior maxillary teeth. The infraorbital nerve is the most commonly affected, and it is has been estimated that approximately 95% of ZMC fractures involve the infraorbital canal and foramen. The reported incidence of posttraumatic, pretreatment infraorbital nerve sensory deficit ranges between 52% and 100%.

The position of the globe is largely due to the attachment of Lockwood's suspensory ligament and the attachment of the lateral canthal tendon to the lateral orbital wall. Lockwood's suspensory ligament largely determines the horizontal position of the globe and acts as a hammock to prevent inferior displacement of the globe in orbital blowout fractures. It attaches medially to the posterior aspect of the lacrimal bone and laterally to Whitnall's tubercle. Whitnall's tubercle is located within the lateral orbital rim 1 cm inferior to the zygomaticofrontal suture on the medial aspect of the frontal process of the maxilla. The lateral confluence of the orbicularis oculi muscle becomes the lateral canthal tendon, which attaches laterally to Whitnall's tubercle and suspends the lateral aspect of the globe. The lateral canthal tendon attaches 2 mm superior to the medial canthal tendon, which produces a slight lateral cephalic slant of the globe.

Key anatomic landmarks for ZMC fracture repair include the anterior and posterior ethmoidal arteries, the superior orbital fissure, and the optic canal. The anterior and posterior ethmoidal arteries are located two thirds of the way up the medial orbital wall within the frontoethmoidal suture line. The anterior ethmoidal foramen is 20 to 25 mm posterior to the medial orbital wall. The posterior ethmoidal foramen is situated an additional 10 mm posterior to the anterior ethmoidal foramen. The superior orbital fissure is located 35 mm posterior to the zygomaticofrontal suture and 40 mm

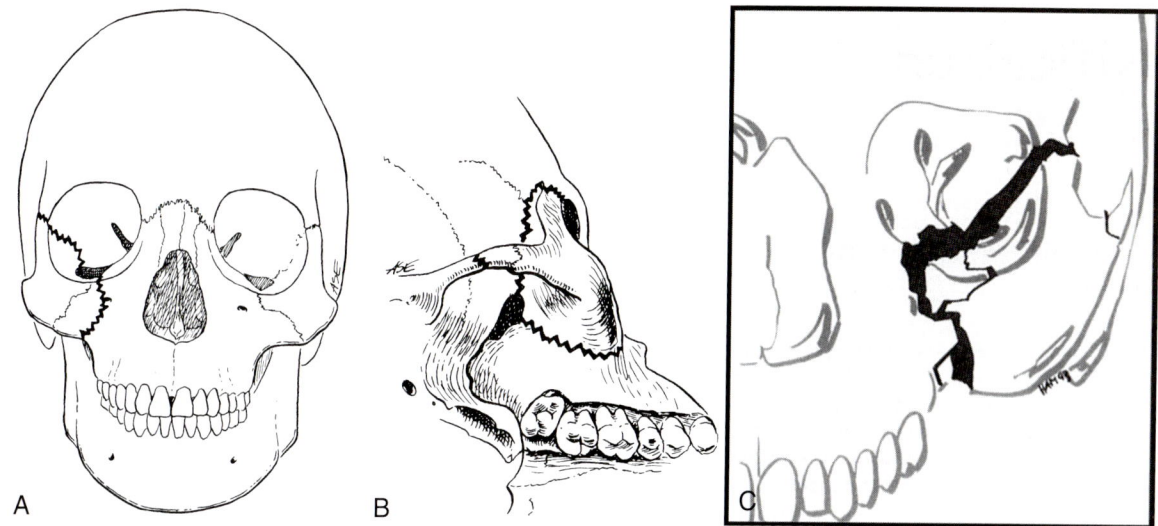

Fig. 40-1 ■ **A,** Anterior facial skeleton showing that the zygoma provides the anterior lateral projection of the face and the articulating sutures with the frontal, sphenoid, and maxillary bones. These sutures represent areas of weakness and are commonly fractured sites. **B,** Lateral aspect of the zygoma showing its spatial relationship and articulation with the sphenoid bone and with the temporal bone at the zygomatic arch. If the arch and the zygomaticosphenoid suture are aligned, the zygoma must be properly oriented in three dimensions. **C,** The zygoma forms major components of the orbital walls and frame. Zygomaticomaxillary complex fractures therefore invariably result in orbital fractures involving the orbital floor and wall, as well as the inferior and lateral orbital rims. (**A** and **B,** From Fonseca RJ, et al: *Oral and maxillofacial trauma*, vol 3, ed 3, St Louis, 2005, Saunders; **C,** from Hammer B: *Orbital fractures. Diagnosis, operative treatment, secondary corrections*, Seattle, 1995, Hegrefe & Hube.)

posterior to the supraorbital notch. The optic canal is 40 mm posterior to the infraorbital rim, 42 mm posterior to the anterior lacrimal crest, and 45 mm posterior to the supraorbital notch. Accepted safe dissection distances include 25 mm posterior to the inferior and lateral orbital rim and 30 mm posterior to the medial and superior orbital rims. This safe distance permits exploration and reconstruction of the orbit without damaging the contents of the optic canal or superior orbital fissure. However, it is important to remember that these safe distances are measured from intact orbital rims and that these measurements are not accurate in patients with significantly displaced or comminuted fractures.

Another important anatomic relationship for consideration when managing ZMC fractures is that of the temporal branch of the facial nerve. The temporal branch crosses the zygomatic arch approximately at its midpoint in a plane deep to the superficial temporal fascia and lateral to the periosteum. This important anatomic relationship is what dictates external approaches such as the Gillies approach and a coronal incision to access the zygomatic arch and outer orbital frame.

CLINICAL EXAMINATION

Patients who sustain facial trauma should be evaluated according to the advanced trauma life support protocol. Particular attention should be paid to concomitant maxillofacial injuries that may affect the airway, brain, and orbital contents. The examination is conducted with a cervical spine precaution protocol since the incidence of cervical spine injuries in patients with facial trauma has been reported to be as high as 3%. The examination should be detailed and systematic and should include evaluation of the cranial nerves, eyes, ears, and scalp. The face is then inspected and palpated for asymmetry caused by displaced fragments of the facial skeleton and

for areas of edema, ecchymosis, and lacerations. Patients with nondisplaced ZMC fractures may exhibit only soft tissue signs such as ecchymosis and edema overlying the fracture sites and conjunctival hemorrhage. Displaced fractures will generally cause ipsilateral facial flattening as a result of decreased anterior projection of the zygomatic body (Fig. 40-2). The zygomatic arch may be intact, fractured and depressed, or bowed out. Laterally displaced zygomatic fractures are less frequently encountered, and the majority are due to blast injuries or severe blunt trauma to the central aspect of the face and result in pan-facial fractures. Displaced ZMC and isolated zygomatic arch factures may also cause trismus as a result of spasm of the masseter muscle or mechanical impingement of the coronoid process against the displaced fragments.

The appearance of the periorbital area is typically also affected in displaced fractures. This is seen as a deformity of the palpebral fissure caused by displacement of fragments containing the attachment of the eyelids and the lateral canthal tendon (see Fig. 40-2, *A*). In fractures in which the orbital floor or orbital walls are displaced, the position of the globe is altered and it is usually seen as enophthalmos or hypoglobus. The globe typically becomes displaced posteriorly and inferiorly (Fig. 40-3). In the acute setting this may not be appreciated because of edema of the orbital contents. Herniation or entrapment of the orbital contents into orbital floor defects, as well as soft tissue contusion and edema, may lead to restricted movement of the globe.

Evaluation of the extraocular muscles is performed by finger tracking. A forced duction test will generally differentiate between mechanical entrapment and restriction secondary to edema or contusion. If restricted range of motion is detected, topical anesthesia is applied to the sclera and the forced duction test is performed by grasping the insertion of the rectus muscles at two simultaneous points with two pairs of Adson forceps. The rectus muscles are grasped 7 mm from the limbus, and the globe is rotated in

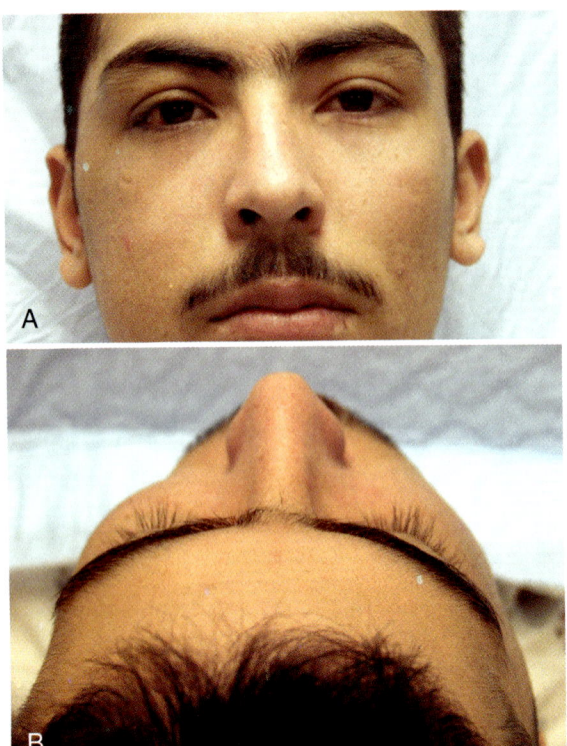

Fig. 40-2 ■ **A,** Typical appearance of a patient with a displaced fracture of the right zygomaticomaxillary complex. There is flattening in the area of the right malar eminence and inferior slanting of the right lower eyelid and palpebral fissure. **B,** Superior view of the same patient showing an obvious decreased projection of the fractured zygoma on the right. The zygoma is displaced posteriorly and nasally.

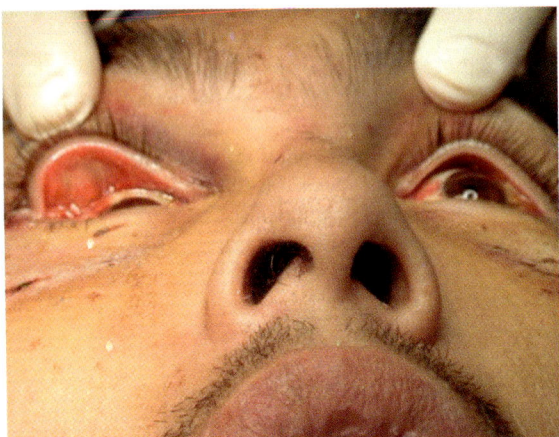

Fig. 40-3 ■ Enophthalmos in a patient with a displaced zygomaticomaxillary complex fracture complicated by a fracture and inferior dislocation of the orbital floor.

all directions. A positive forced duction test confirms soft tissue entrapment. A negative forced duction test with restricted extraocular movement indicates muscular hematoma or contusion or neurogenic causes of muscle paralysis.

An ophthalmology consultation should be considered if deemed necessary before surgical intervention and should include visual acuity and assessment of the status of the globe and retina, pupillary responses to light, visual field evaluation, and a funduscopic examination. Visual acuity examinations are performed with a Snellen chart at 20 feet or with a Near card at 16 inches from the patient.

Patients with glasses for correction of visual astigmatism should wear their glasses during the examination if possible. The pupils are examined for anisocoria and for afferent and efferent pupillary responses with a swinging light test. Visual fields are assessed by standing directly in front of the patient and testing one eye at a time. The patient should stare directly ahead while the examiner tests peripheral gaze with finger motion and finger counting at the extremes of the patient's visual fields. Extraocular muscle contusion or entrapment, as well as alteration in globe position, is commonly manifested as diplopia.

A funduscopic examination, if indicated, will assess for lens dislocation, vitreous hemorrhage, retinal detachment, and the presence of foreign bodies. Additional tests may include tonometry to indirectly measure intraocular pressure. Normal intraocular pressure is 10 to 20 mm Hg or symmetric readings. A slit-lamp examination will assess for irregularities in surface contour of the globe and cornea and can be used to rule out conjunctival chemosis, hemorrhage, foreign bodies, and hyphema. A cobalt blue light (Wood's lamp) with fluorescein dye is used to detect corneal abrasions and lacerations. The fluorescein dye pools at the site of an abrasion/laceration, and the cobalt blue light illuminates the dye by converting it to a bright green color.

Finally, an oral examination is also conducted and may show ecchymosis and crepitation at the zygomaticomaxillary interface. Dental occlusion and the integrity of the palate should also be evaluated. It is not uncommon to have concomitant maxillary fractures. If they are missed or left untreated, appropriate reduction of the ZMC and restoration of bite will not be possible, which will lead to a poor outcome.

IMAGING

A cervical spine series should be obtained as per hospital protocol. Computed tomography (CT) remains the "gold standard" modality for the evaluation of facial fractures. Scans in both the coronal and axial planes should be evaluated. For ZMC fractures, it is also useful to obtain sagittal cuts, as well as fine cuts through the orbit (Fig. 40-4, *A* to *C*). Both soft tissue and bone windows should be examined and particular attention paid to orbital volumetric changes, displacement of the globe, and herniation of orbital contents. Imaging software can be used to calculate the orbital volume of the fractured orbit for comparison with the uninjured side with a high degree of accuracy. Three-dimensional images reconstructed from two-dimensional CT scans may be used to obtain additional information on the spatial relationship of displaced and rotated ZMC fragments (Fig. 40-4, *D*). They are also useful as postoperative images to evaluate the accuracy of reduction and facial form and symmetry in complex cases. They should not be used as the sole diagnostic images because details of the fractures are lost as a result of volume averaging during processing of the digital data.

TREATMENT GOALS

The primary goals of surgical treatment of ZMC fractures are divided into two categories: (1) restoration of facial projection and facial symmetry and (2) restoration of orbital volume, globe position, and shape of the affected palpebral fissure (Fig. 40-5). Management, however, may range from observation for nondisplaced fractures to extensive reconstruction of the zygoma, orbital floor, orbital frame, and zygomatic arch for severe fractures. Treatment may also include concomitant management of associated and commonly seen maxillary or nasal fractures. The pattern and extent of exposure and plate fixation of the ZMC fracture ultimately

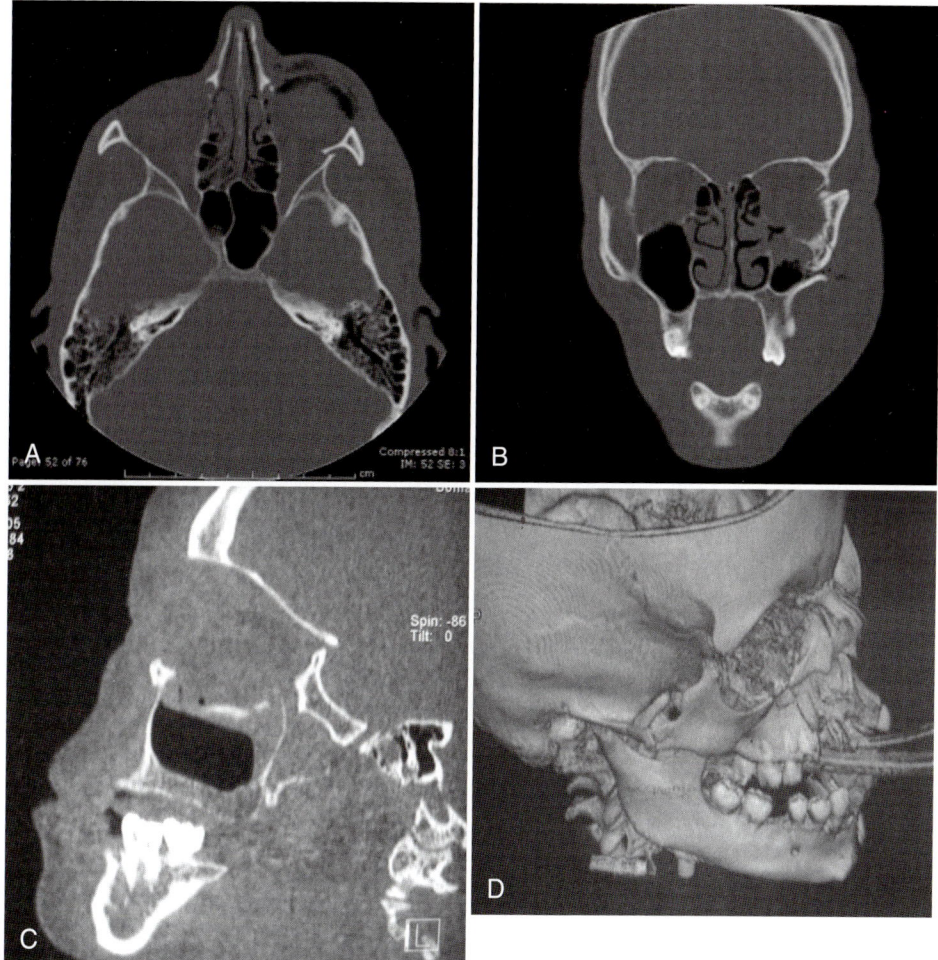

Fig. 40-4 ■ **A,** Axial computed tomographic (CT) scan showing separation at the zygomaticosphenoid suture. This finding is pathognomonic of zygomaticomaxillary complex (ZMC) fractures. **B,** Coronal CT scan of a patient with a medially displaced and inferiorly rotated ZMC fracture. There is separation at the zygomaticomaxillary buttress and frontozygomatic suture. The coronal image also shows the degree of orbital floor involvement. **C,** Sagittal cut showing a fractured and inferiorly displaced orbital floor. This leads to an increase in orbital volume and altered position of the globe. **D,** Three-dimensional reconstructed image showing the spatial relationship of the fragments. Though useful in evaluating the extent of the deformity, these images offer poor details of the fractured areas themselves and of critical structures encountered during surgery.

depend on the degree of comminution and stability of the ZMC and the presence of other associated fractures. It is recommended that surgery be delayed until the majority of the facial edema and conjunctival chemosis has resolved. All patients who sustain a ZMC fracture should undergo an eye examination. In patients requiring surgical treatment, preoperative examination is essential. The remainder of this section focuses on the management of isolated ZMC fractures. The importance of recognizing involvement of the orbit in these fractures and the role of the zygomaticosphenoid interface and zygomatic arch as guides to proper reduction of the ZMC are emphasized.

NON-DISPLACED FRACTURES

Non-displaced fractures confirmed by CT are managed nonsurgically and by serial observation. An analgesic, antibiotic, and decongestant are prescribed, and patients may be instructed to restrict their diet to liquids or soft foods to reduce the incidence of fracture displacement by the masseter muscle. The patient is monitored closely, and if fracture displacement and facial deformity develop, open reduction with internal fixation is indicated.

DISPLACED, MINIMALLY COMMINUTED FRACTURES

The vast majority of poor outcomes associated with the management of displaced ZMC fractures result from inadequate treatment. Insufficient exposure and reduction of the ZMC fragment and failure to restore orbital volume result in facial asymmetry and enophthalmos. More often than not, these problems are noticed weeks after surgical treatment. Depending on the accuracy of reduction and fracture stability, in the combined authors' experience displaced fractures are best managed by open reduction and fixation at two to three points. In the absence of comminution or instability at the zygomatic arch, reduction under direct visualization plus fixation at the frontozygomatic suture, zygomaticomaxillary buttress, and inferior orbital rim remains the best treatment option. Choosing this approach for displaced and rotated ZMC fractures offers several advantages. First, it allows superior reduction and orientation of the ZMC fragment in three dimensions by visualization and alignment at the zygomaticosphenoid interface. Second, it allows fixation at the zygomaticomaxillary buttress, which provides vertical support to the zygoma, stability against occlusal forces, and stability against

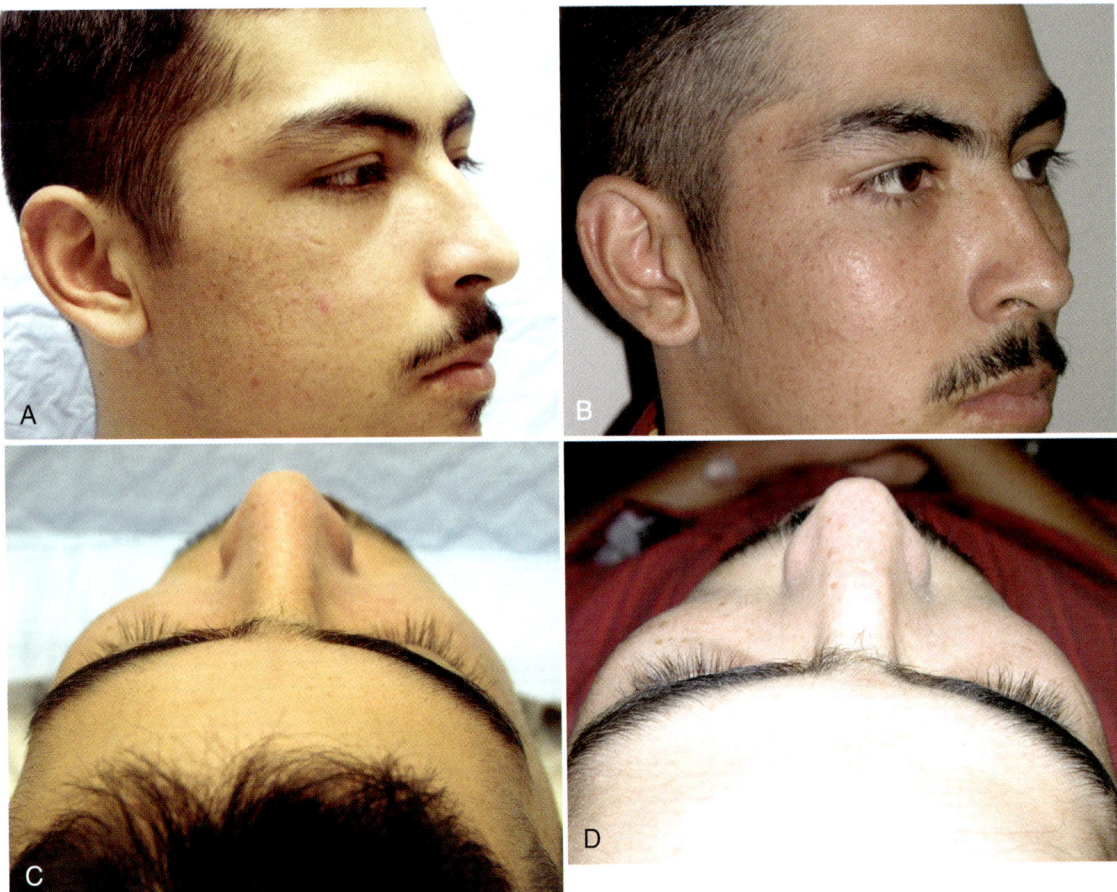

Fig. 40-5 ■ Preoperative (**A**) and postoperative (**B**) lateral photographs of a patient who underwent open reduction and fixation of a displaced fracture of the zygomaticomaxillary complex. There is great improvement in zygomatic projection, globe position, and the shape of the palpebral fissure. Preoperative (**C**) and postoperative (**D**) superior views of that same patient show great improvement in anterior malar projection.

inferior and medial rotation forces caused by the masseter muscle. Third, exposure and fixation at the infraorbital rim will allow simultaneous inspection of the orbital floor and, if necessary, bridging of defects. Accepted indications for orbital floor exploration include (1) herniation of orbital contents, (2) soft tissue entrapment with limitation of upward gaze, (3) severe displacement, (4) comminution, and (5) defect larger than 5 mm on CT. Indications for orbital floor/wall reconstruction are (1) enophthalmos, (2) defects larger than 5 to 10 mm, and (3) defects posterior to the axis of the globe.

Finally, after fixation at all three points, these fractures sites can be inspected for proper reduction intraoperatively before closure. Two-point fixation at the frontozygomatic suture and zygomaticomaxillary buttress is indicated when the following are present: (1) the fractures are minimally displaced, (2) the ZMC fracture remains stable after initial reduction with no palpable step deformity at the infraorbital rim, and (3) minimal changes in orbital volume and globe displacement are found on preoperative CT.

Open reduction and fixation of ZMC fractures should be carried out under general anesthesia. The frontozygomatic and zygomaticosphenoid sutures are exposed via a blepharoplasty incision in the supratarsal fold and subperiosteal dissection at the lateral supraorbital rim. The zygomaticomaxillary buttress is exposed via the standard oral vestibular access used for a Le Fort I osteotomy. Using a percutaneous stab incision, a bone hook or a Carroll-Girard screw is engaged at the body of the zygoma. The body of the zygoma is mobilized in a vector opposite the direction of displacement—typically forward, laterally, and upward. If necessary, the zygomatic

arch is also reduced via the intraoral approach. This may help in proper manipulation and rotation of the zygomatic complex into position. Alignment is confirmed at the zygomaticosphenoid interface and zygomaticomaxillary buttress. Traction on the bone hook is maintained and adjusted if necessary while fixation is carried out at the frontozygomatic suture first while maintaining alignment at the zygomaticosphenoid interface (Fig. 40-6, *A*). This is then followed by plating of the zygomaticomaxillary buttress with craniofacial miniplates (Fig. 40-6, *B*). If two-point fixation is planned, the infraorbital rim is palpated for the absence of a step deformity at the fracture site, the ZMC fragment is evaluated for stability, and a forced duction test for globe mobility is carried out before wound closure. If three-point fixation or orbital floor exploration/reconstruction is planned, the orbital rim and floor are accessed by combining an inferior fornix incision with lateral inferior cantholysis. This retroseptal approach provides good exposure of the orbital rim and floor and avoids the eyelid septum altogether. The cantholysis allows reduced tension on the eyelid during reduction and instrumentation. This combination therefore reduces the incidence of lid retraction or ectropion. If orbital fat is encountered, it is simply retracted out of the field with a malleable retractor. Any orbital contents herniated into the maxillary sinus are first carefully lifted back into the orbit with malleable retractors. Orbital floor defects are fully exposed via subperiosteal dissection until a sound bony ledge is encountered circumferentially. A transcaruncular extension of the conjunctival incision may be necessary to access and expose the nasal aspect of the defect. Once the defect is fully exposed, an

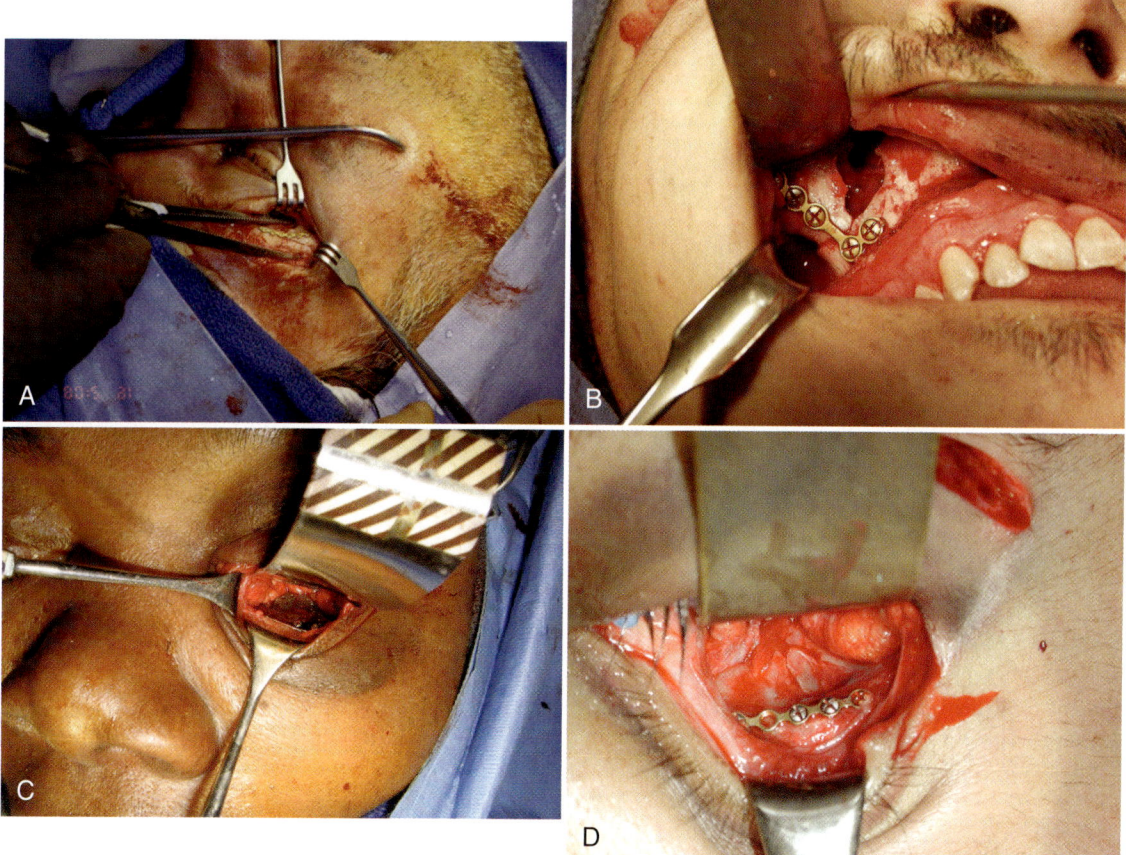

Fig. 40-6 ▪ **A,** Intraoperative photograph showing a bone hook engaged underneath the body of the zygoma. The zygoma is reduced and manipulated into position while visualizing the zygomaticosphenoid interface. Once the zygomaticosphenoid suture is aligned, the fragment is held in place with a bone clamp and the lateral rim is plated. **B,** After the zygomaticofrontal suture is plated, the zygomaticomaxillary buttress is addressed. It is recommended that alignment and stability at the zygomaticosphenoid interface and lateral rim be continually confirmed while plating the buttress. It may be necessary to maintain traction on the bone hook and keep the bone clamp in place at the lateral rim while plating the buttress. **C,** Photograph showing a retroseptal inferior forniceal incision to access the orbital floor. The orbital fat is retracted with a malleable retractor and the orbital floor plate is secured with screws at the inner aspect of the inferior orbital rim. **D,** Inferior forniceal access showing a miniplate secured at the inner aspect of the orbital rim. This is important to reduce the chance for adhesion of the hardware to the lower lid and the plate becoming palpable through the skin.

orbital floor plate is trimmed, contoured, and then gently placed over the defect while ensuring that the edges of the plate are resting on stable orbital floor bone. Failure to do so will result in displacement and mobility of the plate and problems with globe position. The plate is secured to the inner aspect of inferior orbital rim with two to three screws. It is important that the plates and implants be secured within the rim if possible to avoid palpability through the skin or scar and adhesion formation involving the eyelid (Fig. 40-6, *C* and *D*). A forced duction test for globe mobility is performed. The soft tissue over the malar eminence containing the lateral aspect of the lower eyelid is resuspended with a Vicryl suture and tacked to the lateral rim. The inferior lateral canthal ligament is reapproximated and tacked to the main canthal ligament with a subcuticular inverted 5.0 Vicryl suture. The orbicularis oculi and skin at the corner of the palpebral fissure are also meticulously aligned and reapproximated with fine sutures. As with any lower eyelid procedure, it is recommended that the lower eyelid be suspended superiorly with a suspension suture to reduce the incidence of ectropion. If needed, the zygomatic arch is immobilized with transcutaneous sutures suspended from and tied to a malleable finger splint (Fig. 40-7).

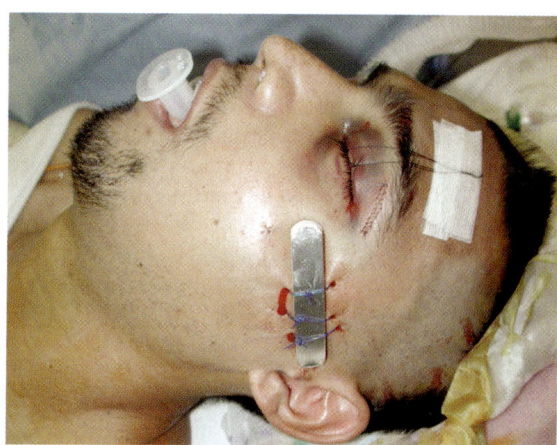

Fig. 40-7 ▪ Postoperative photograph showing stabilization of the zygomatic arch with transcutaneous Prolene sutures suspended and tied to a metallic finger splint. The lower eyelid is supported vertically with suspension sutures through the tarsal plate.

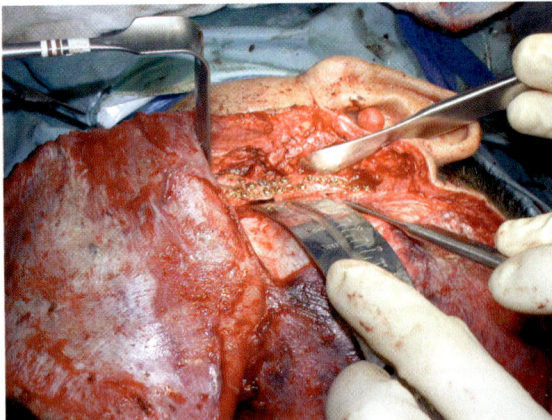

Fig. 40-8 ■ Reconstruction of the zygomatic arch via a coronal incision. This is the first step when reconstructing a comminuted and complex fracture of the zygomaticomaxillary complex. This step establishes the anterior projection of the body of the zygoma, which is then oriented in space by reducing the zygomaticosphenoid fracture line.

COMPLEX AND COMMINUTED FRACTURES

Treatment of complex ZMC fractures that are comminuted and unstable is different from the open reduction and fixation of non-comminuted fractures. These fractures may occur in isolation or in combination with severe frontal bone and Le Fort fractures. The critical concept here is that a fourth point of fixation at the zygomatic arch or reconstruction of the arch itself may be necessary for stability when there is comminution at the zygomaticomaxillary buttress or orbital rim. The zygomatic arch in essence is also used as a guide to reconstruction and orientation of the zygomatic complex in three dimensions by establishing and maintaining the anterior projection of the zygoma. In such cases, a coronal incision is needed to access the frontal bone, the upper and outer orbital frame, and the zygomatic arch. The central aspects of the frontal bone are reconstructed first. The zygomatic arch is then reduced and fixated. If severely comminuted, it is reconstructed with a calvarial bone graft and fixated to the zygoma (Fig. 40-8). Alignment at the zygomaticosphenoid interface is used as reference for proper alignment and orientation of the body of the zygoma to the frontal bone and reconstructed zygomatic arch. Once the zygomatic arch and outer orbital frame have been aligned, the orbital rim and orbital floor are then addressed as described previously. Any naso-orbito-ethmoid components are then addressed.

ISOLATED ZYGOMATIC ARCH FRACTURES

Depending on the nature of the traumatic event, isolated fractures of the zygomatic arch, body, or frontal process may occur. Zygomatic arch fractures are fairly common and are usually treated by open reduction via a transoral or transcutaneous approach. The transcutaneous Gillies incision approach is cleaner and fairly straightforward. The zygomatic arch is stabilized with transcutaneous 5-mm polyester fiber ligatures tied to a malleable finger splint (Fig. 40-9).

POSTOPERATIVE CARE

As soon as awakened from anesthesia, patients are evaluated for the presence of vision and the pupils are evaluated for size and reactivity. They are generally admitted for 24 hours to evaluate for potential ophthalmologic complications such as retrobulbar hematoma formation. Postoperative CT scans may be obtained at the discretion of the surgeon but are generally recommended for all complex cases

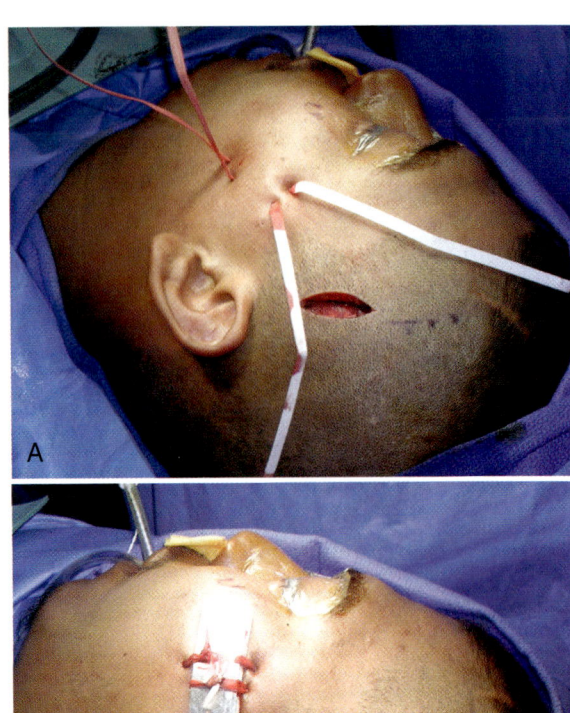

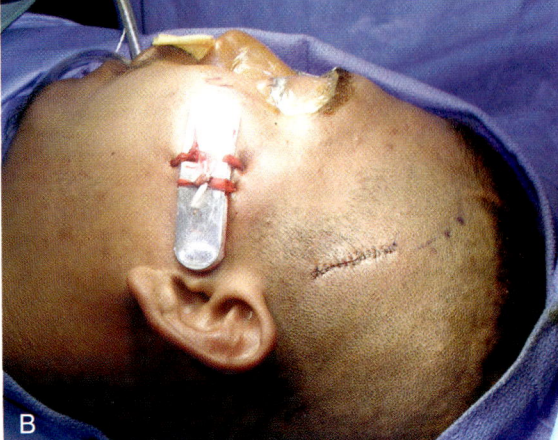

Fig. 40-9 ■ Reduction of a zygomatic arch fracture via a Gillies approach (**A**) and stabilization with transcutaneous polyester fiber ligatures tied to a malleable finger splint (**B**).

and for those in which orbital floor or wall defects were bridged with orbital floor plates or bone grafts (Fig. 40-10). Patients are discharged with prescriptions for antibiotics, analgesics, and decongestants and are scheduled for follow-up on days 3, 7, 14, 30, 60, and 90. During the follow-up period, patients are evaluated for possible wound infections, eyelid deformities, enophthalmos, diplopia, and the final cosmetic result.

Several postoperative complications are seen with treatment of ZMC fractures. Blindness immediately after surgery may indicate central retinal artery occlusion or impingement of the orbital apex contents by a bony fragment or orbital implant. This is managed by emergency return to the operating room. Another urgent complication that may lead to loss of vision is the formation of a retrobulbar hematoma. A retrobulbar hematoma can cause a compartment syndrome with compression of the central retinal artery. Compression of the central retinal artery causes ischemia of the optic nerve, which if not relieved urgently, will lead to permanent loss of vision. Symptoms include severe posterior orbital pain, globe proptosis, decreased extraocular movements, a tense globe on palpation, and decreased visual acuity. The diagnosis is based on clinical signs and symptoms. Treatment involves emergency lateral canthotomy, orbital decompression, evacuation of the posterior orbital hematoma, and placement of a Penrose drain.

Enophthalmos is a common postoperative complication associated with poor fracture reduction. Enophthalmos is due to posterior displacement of the globe because of an increase in orbital volume. This may be caused by rotation of the zygomatic complex or by

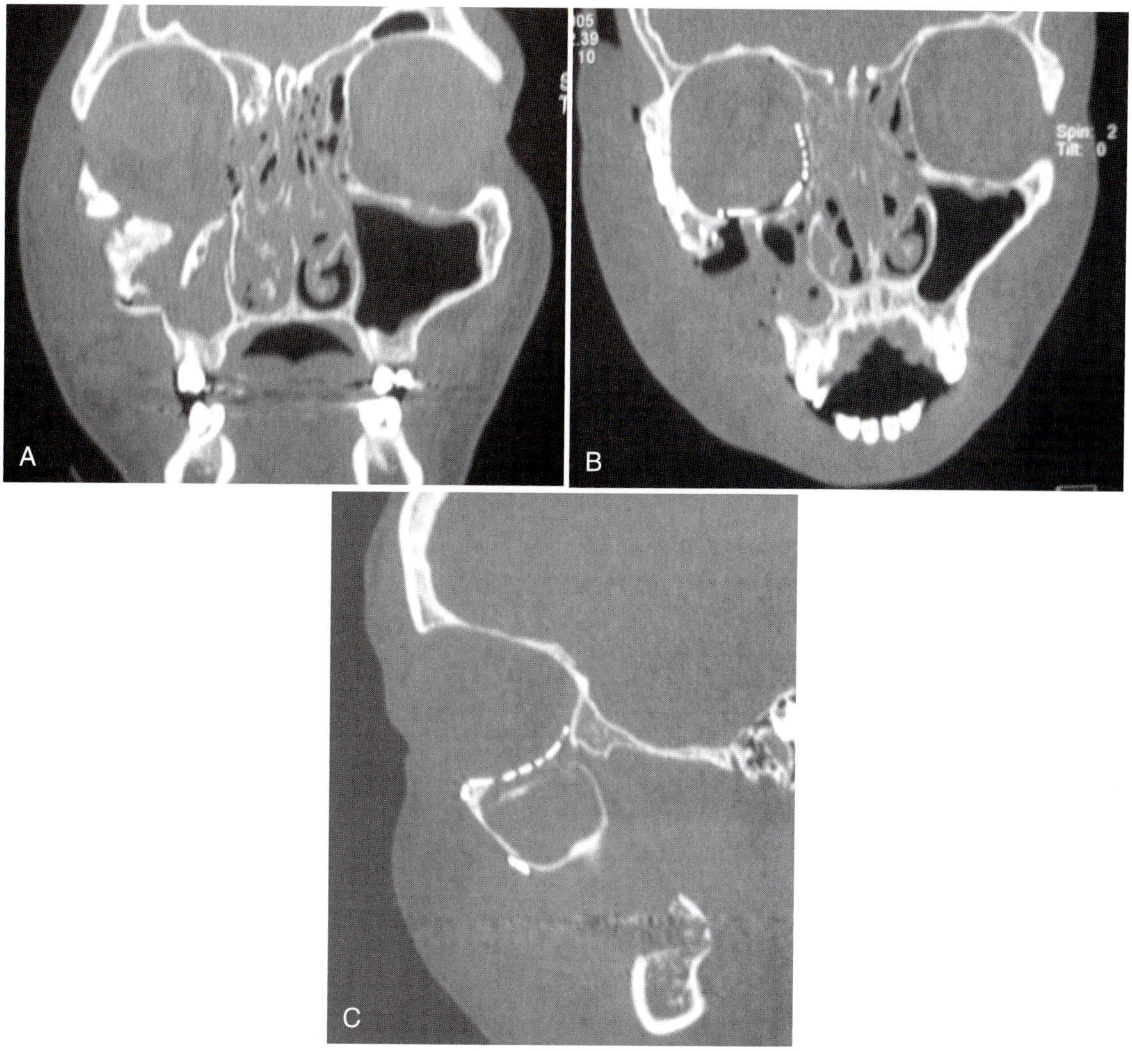

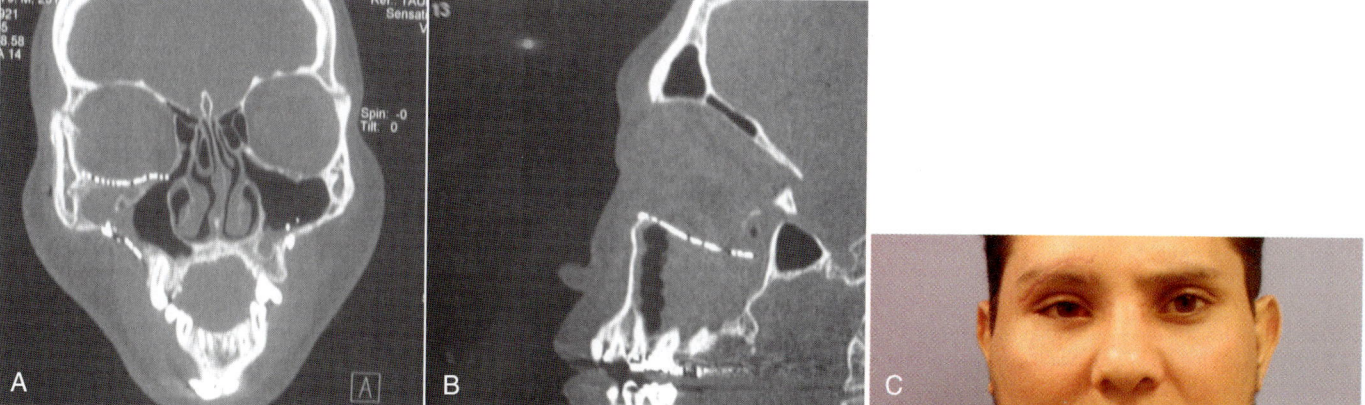

Fig. 40-10 ■ Preoperative (**A**) and postoperative (**B** and **C**) computed tomography (CT) scans of a patient who underwent open reduction of a zygomaticomaxillary complex fracture and orbital reconstruction. The orbital floor and medial wall defects are adequately bridged by a mesh plate that is correctly placed and supported by solid bone. Postoperative CT scans are valuable for evaluating the accuracy of fracture reduction, restoration of the orbital floor and volume, and the position of the orbital floor implant relative to the orbital apex.

Fig. 40-11 ■ Coronal (**A**) and sagittal (**B**) computed tomography scans of a patient with displacement of an orbital floor implant. This implant was not resting on solid bone. There is increased orbital volume and enophthalmos. **C,** Clinical photograph of that same patient showing significant enophthalmos.

displaced or missing segments of the orbital walls. Postoperative enophthalmos is due to inappropriate fracture reduction or inappropriate reconstruction of the internal orbit. Poor placement or displacement of the orbital floor implant by not resting it on stable remaining orbital floor results in increased orbital volume and enophthalmos (Fig. 40-11). Postoperative enophthalmos, if identified early and caused by improper treatment, is managed by removal of the fixation hardware and orbital floor implant followed by proper reduction of the fracture and bridging of the floor defect. If the fracture is deemed to have been properly treated and progressive enophthalmos is identified weeks after surgical treatment, it is due either to orbital soft tissue atrophy or scarring or to nonunion. If the patient is concerned about the cosmetic appearance or has diplopia, an orbital implant is used to elevate the globe and bring it forward. If the fracture was improperly reduced and has healed at the time of examination, a zygomatic complex osteotomy may be indicated. Alternatively, the use of zygoma contour augmentation implants along with an enophthalmos wedge implant is a less invasive approach.

Diplopia may also be encountered in the immediate postoperative period or later. Common causes of diplopia include postsurgical edema, hematoma formation, muscle contusion, or neurogenic causes. Diplopia as a result of edema, hematomas, and muscle contusions typically resolves within 14 days. Diplopia that does not resolve by 14 days and is associated with a negative forced duction test could indicate injury to the rectus muscles during surgery.

Cosmetic deformities attributable to ZMC surgery occur as a result of inadequate reduction of the fractured components or the development of palpebral fissure deformities. Inappropriate reduction results in a flattening or concavity of the malar area and the lateral and inferior orbital rims, particularly when visualized from a worm's eye view. Similarly, the zygomatic arch may be overcontoured or depressed. These deformities are best treated with facial implants if minor or with osteotomies if significant. Excessive retraction of the lower lid, violation of the orbital septum, or inappropriate canthopexy may result in ectropion or lid retraction, entropion, and increased scleral show requiring secondary corrective oculoplastic procedures.

Injury to the frontal branch of the facial nerve during exposure of the zygomatic arch or lateral orbital rim may lead to an inability to close the eye and paresis or paralysis of the frontalis, procerus, and corrugator muscles. If there is no resolution over time, an upper eyelid gold weight implant can be used to facilitate eye closure. Contralateral botulinum toxin injections may be used to mask the asymmetry of the appearance and movement of the upper part of the face.

Finally, many patients will have a transient or permanent postoperative infraorbital nerve sensory deficit. The reported incidence of an immediate postoperative sensory deficit approximates 55%, whereas that of a permanent deficit ranges between 15% and 46%. The current literature suggests that the incidence of infraorbital nerve sensory deficits is related to the degree of fracture displacement. The literature further suggests that fracture reduction within the first week after injury will reduce the incidence of a permanent sensory deficit.

PEARLS AND PITFALLS

- The surgeon must recognize that the approach to a ZMC fracture ultimately depends on the type and mechanism of injury and the degree of displacement and comminution.
- The majority of unfavorable outcomes relate to improper orientation of the zygomatic complex in three dimensions, which leads to failure to restore the facial contour.
- Exposure plus alignment of the zygomaticosphenoid suture during reduction and fixation of the zygomatic complex is a critical first step to ensure proper orientation of the ZMC fragment. Exposure plus reduction of the zygomaticofrontal suture and zygomaticosphenoid interface is therefore indicated in all cases of open reduction.
- It is recommended that exposure and fixation be carried out at the zygomaticomaxillary buttress in every case for stability reasons.
- Orbital floor reconstruction may be indicated in many displaced ZMC fractures.
- The surgeon must have a low threshold to bridge comminuted and unstable orbital floor fractures, especially those behind the axis of the globe. This will reduce the incidence of enophthalmos.
- When significant fracture comminution or instability is present, the zygomatic arch is used as a fourth point of fixation and as a guide to properly position the zygoma in the proper spatial relationship to the facial skeleton. In essence, if the zygomatic arch is reduced and the zygomaticosphenoid suture is aligned, the zygoma is properly oriented in space (see Fig. 40-1, B).
- The frontozygomatic suture is then fixated first, followed by the zygomaticomaxillary buttress and the orbital rim. Defects of the orbital floor and any fractures of the central part of the face are addressed last. This same sequence is followed when reconstructing the zygomatic complex during treatment of pan-facial fractures.
- The most common complications relate to poor cosmetic results and abnormalities in globe position.
- Poor reduction of the zygomatic complex is generally caused by inadequate exposure. Enophthalmos results from poor reduction (persistently increased orbital volume) or inadequate correction of orbital floor defects. Late enophthalmos may also result from scarring or atrophy of orbital soft tissues despite an adequate reconstruction.

BIBLIOGRAPHY

Bagheri SC, Meyer RA, Khan HA, et al: Microsurgical repair of peripheral trigeminal nerve injuries from maxillofacial trauma, *J Oral Maxillofac Surg* 67:1791-1799, 2009.

Bailey JS, Goldwasser MS: Management of zygomatic complex fractures. In Miloro M, editor, *Peterson's principles of oral and maxillofacial surgery*, Hamilton, 2004, BC Decker, pp 445-462.

Chang EL, Hatton MP, Bernardino CR, et al: Simplified repair of zygomatic fractures through a transconjunctival approach, *Ophthalmology* 112:1302-1309, 2005.

Chotkowski G, Eggleston TI, Buchbinder D: Lag screw fixation of a nonstable zygomatic complex fracture: a case report, *J Oral Maxillofac Surg* 55:183-185, 1997.

Ellis E, Kittidumkerng W: Analysis of treatment for isolated zygomaticomaxillary complex fractures, *J Oral Maxillofac Surg* 54:386-400, discussion 400-401, 1996.

Gruss JS, Van Wyck L, Phillips JH, et al: The importance of the zygomatic arch in complex midfacial fracture repair and correction of post-traumatic orbitozygomatic fracture deformities, *Plast Reconstr Surg* 85:878-890, 1990.

Hammer B: *Orbital fractures*, Göttingen, Germany, 2001, Hogrefer & Huber, pp 1-50.

Heiland M, Schulze D, Blake F, et al: Intraoperative imaging of zygomaticomaxillary complex fractures using a 3D C-arm system, *Int J Oral Maxillofac Surg* 34:369-375, 2005.

Hoelzle F, Klein M, Schwerdtner O, et al: Intraoperative computed tomography with the mobile CT Tomoscan M during surgical treatment of orbital fractures, *Int J Oral Maxillofac Surg* 30:26-31, 2001.

Hollier LH, Thornton J, Pazmino P, et al: The management of orbitozygomatic fractures,

Plast Reconstr Surg 111:2386-2392, quiz 2393, 2003.

Kushner GM: Surgical approaches to the infraorbital rim and orbital floor: the case for the transconjunctival approach, *J Oral Maxillofac Surg* 64:108-110, 2006.

Lieblich SE, Piecuch JF: Orbital-zygomatic trauma. In Kelly JP, editor: *Oral and maxillofacial surgery knowledge update,* vol 1, part II, Rosemont, Ill. 1995, AAOMS, pp 165-176.

Marchena JM, Johnson JV: Le Fort and palatal fractures. In Stewart MG, editor: *Head, neck, and face trauma,* New York, 2005, Thieme, pp 97-105

Mosgau-Schultze S, Erbe M, Rudolph D, et al: Prospective study on post-traumatic sensory disturbances of the inferior alveolar nerve and infraorbital nerve in mandibular and midfacial fractures, *J Craniomaxillofac Surg* 27:86-93, 1999

Ochs MW, Johns FR: Evaluation and management of periorbital and ocular injuries. In Piecuch JF, editor: *Oral and maxillofacial surgery knowledge update,* vol 2, Rosemont, Ill. 1998, AAOMS, pp 45-60.

Prein J: *Manual of internal fixation in the craniofacial skeleton,* New York, 1998, Springer-Verlag, pp 133-148.

Stanley RB: The zygomatic arch as a guide to reconstruction of comminuted malar fractures, *Arch Otolaryngol Head Neck Surg* 115:1459-1462, 1989.

Stewart MG: Zygomatic complex fractures. In Stewart MG, editor: *Head, neck, and face trauma,* New York, 2005, Thieme, pp 68-76.

Thurmuller P, Dodoson TB, Kaban LB: Nerve injuries associated with facial trauma: natural history, management, and outcomes of repair, *Oral Maxillofac Clin North Am* 13:283-293, 2001.

Wong MEK, Johnson JV: Management of midface injuries. In Fonseca R, Marciani R, Hendler B, editors: *Oral and maxillofacial surgery,* vol 3, Philadelphia, 2000, WB Saunders, pp 245-299.

Le Fort Fractures

Chapter 41

Zachary S. Peacock, Brian Thomas Bast

The mid-face is a complex anatomic region consisting of the maxilla and its multiple complex articulations with the adjacent upper and lower facial skeleton. The maxilla helps form the oral cavity, orbit, and nasal cavity; connects the cranial base with the occlusal plane; and allows proper anterior projection of the face. The maxilla along with the rest of the mid-face consists of multiple thickened buttresses running vertically, sagittally, and transversely that provide support for the underlying air-filled sinuses. The buttresses are protective against superior forces but are vulnerable to frontally and laterally directed forces.

René Le Fort famously characterized the types of fractures occurring in the mid-face with force directed anteriorly.[1-3] It is rare that fractures obey the classifications set forth by Le Fort. Classifications do, however, serve as a guide for systematic diagnosis and subsequent treatment (Fig. 41-1).

ETIOPATHOGENESIS/CAUSATIVE FACTORS

Le Fort fractures rarely occur in isolation but, instead, are frequently seen in conjunction with other facial fractures. Patients may also have lacerations and orthopedic or neurologic injuries. As with other facial fractures, they are most common in young men aged 16 to 40 years.[4]

PATHOLOGIC ANATOMY

Le Fort fractures involve multiple bones of the mid-face, including the maxilla, nasal bone, lacrimal bone, ethmoid, palatine bone, vomer, sphenoid, and zygoma. The maxilla is the largest bone involved in these fractures and actually consists of two bones that are fused at the midline and serve to attach the skull base to the lower part of the face. It has articulations with the frontal, lacrimal, nasal, inferior concha, vomer, sphenoid, ethmoid, palatine, and zygomatic bones. Each maxilla consists of a body and frontal, zygomatic, palatine, and alveolar processes. Through its articulations with the rest of the mid-face, the maxilla helps form three of the vertical buttresses of the face.[5] The nasomaxillary buttress includes the lateral piriform rim and, superiorly, the frontal process of the maxilla and the maxillary process of the frontal bone. The zygomaticomaxillary buttress runs from the frontal bone superiorly along the lateral orbital rim, including the zygoma and zygomatic process of the maxilla. The pterygomaxillary buttress includes the pterygoid plates of the sphenoid and maxillary tuberosity and establishes posterior facial height along with the mandibular condyle-ramus unit (Fig. 41-2, *A*). The horizontal buttresses are the frontal, zygomatic, maxillary, and mandibular buttresses. The frontal buttress consists of the superior orbital rim, and the zygomatic buttress consists of the zygomatic arch and body of the zygoma extending to the inferior orbital rim. The maxillary buttress consists of the palate at the level of the maxillary alveolus[5] (Fig. 41-2, *B*).

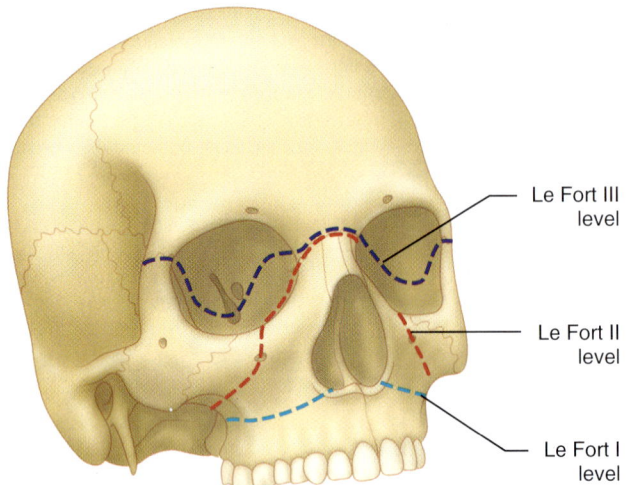

Fig. 41-1 ■ Classification of Le Fort fractures. (From Bagheri SC, Jo C: *Clinical review of oral and maxillofacial surgery*, St Louis, 2008, Mosby.)

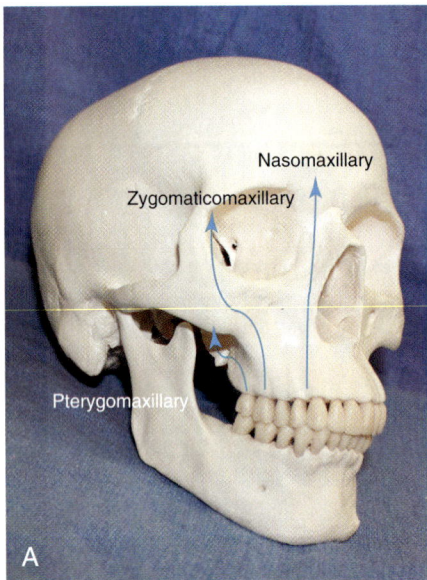

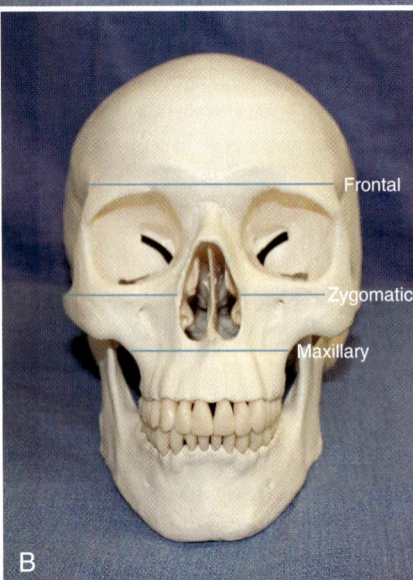

Fig. 41-2 ■ Vertical (**A**) and horizontal (**B**) buttresses of the mid-face.

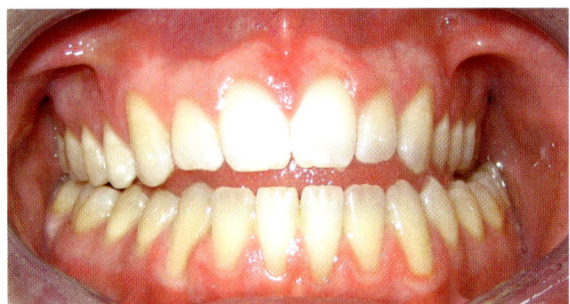

Fig. 41-3 ■ Anterior open bite in a patient with a Le Fort I fracture.

LE FORT CLASSIFICATIONS

LE FORT I

Le Fort I fractures result from a force directed above the dentoalveolar segment of the maxilla. The fracture generally courses from the piriform aperture posteriorly through the anterior and lateral wall of the maxillary sinus, the maxillary tuberosity, and the pterygoid plates. The fracture also often includes the nasal septum and it may disrupt the septal cartilage. The mobile segment includes the entire dentoalveolar segment and palate, including the palatine bone and the lower third of the pterygoid plates. The lateral and medial pterygoid muscles often remain attached to the pterygoid plates and maxillary tuberosity and pull the segment posteriorly and inferiorly. The patient may have an anterior open bite (Fig. 41-3).

LE FORT II

A Le Fort II fracture results from a somewhat more superior force directed at the nasal bones. The pyramidally shaped central mid-face is separated from the rest of the facial skeleton and skull base. The fracture line extends from the nasofrontal suture through the nasal and lacrimal bones to the zygomaticomaxillary suture along the orbital floor. The fracture then continues along the zygomaticomaxillary suture inferiorly to the maxillary tuberosity and through the pterygoid plates. The fractured segment includes the entire maxilla, the nasal bones, the medial third of the orbital rim, the nasal septum, the palatine bones, the dentoalveolar segment, and the inferior portion of the pterygoid plates.

LE FORT III

With a force directed at the level of the orbit, a Le Fort III fracture can occur and result in craniofacial disjunction. The fracture passes through the nasofrontal region along the medial orbit through the superior and inferior orbital fissures and then along the lateral orbital wall through the frontozygomatic suture. The fracture then extends through the zygomaticotemporal suture and inferiorly through the sphenoid bone and pterygomaxillary fissure. The zygoma, maxilla, palatine bones, and nasal bones, including the entire septum, are separated from the cranial base.

DIAGNOSIS

After initial resuscitation and stabilization of the trauma patient, a complete head and neck physical examination is performed as part of the secondary survey. The patient's head and neck are inspected for asymmetry, laceration, ecchymosis, and discharge from the nose or ears. For detection of mid-face fractures, the examiner should systematically and bimanually palpate the frontal bones, including

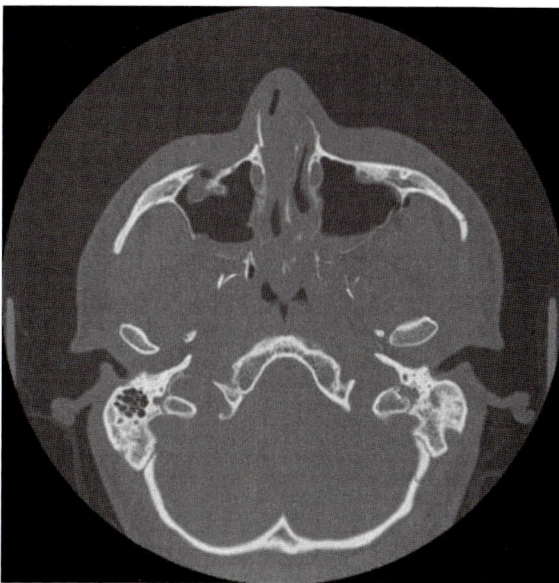

Fig. 41-4 ■ Axial computed tomography showing bilateral disruption of the pterygoid plates.

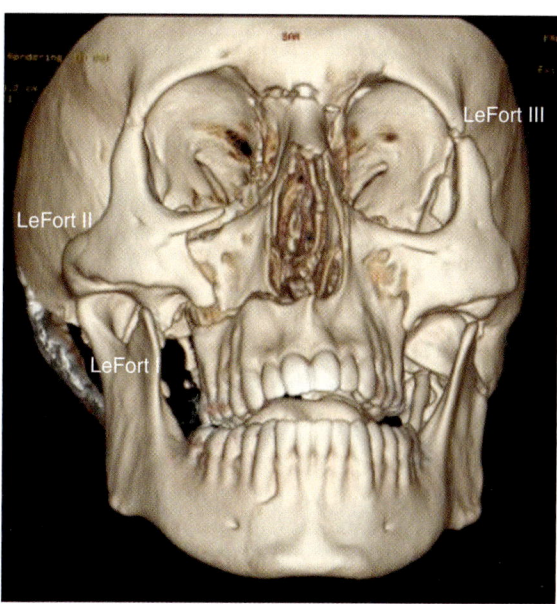

Fig. 41-5 ■ Radiographic characteristics of each Le Fort level fracture.

the supraorbital rims and the nasofrontal suture. Evaluation should then proceed along the lateral orbital rims and zygoma, including the zygomatic arch. The maximum incisal opening is noted, and the intraoral examination includes assessment of the maxillary vestibule, zygomaticomaxillary buttresses, and palate. The maxillary and mandibular arch should be evaluated for occlusal step-offs and malocclusions. One should assess for mobility of the maxilla at the three Le Fort levels by pulling forward on the anterior aspect of the alveolar process while palpating the nasal bridge and zygomaticofrontal sutures with the opposite hand.

Radiographs are obtained to confirm the clinical findings. Computed tomography (CT) is now the most frequently used technique for identifying fractures in the mid-face. A directed maxillofacial CT scan with fine cuts (1 mm or less) should be obtained. In addition to axial views, coronal and sagittal views are required to assess the orbits and nasoethmoid region.

Certain radiographic patterns are very helpful in properly diagnosing Le Fort fractures.[6] In all three levels of Le Fort fractures, a pterygoid plate fracture is seen. The finding of a pterygoid plate fracture unilaterally or bilaterally should alert the clinician to the possibility of a Le Fort fracture (Fig. 41-4). Each Le Fort fracture level has one unique fracture different from the other two levels. For Le Fort I, a fracture is seen through the lateral aspect of the piriform aperture. Only Le Fort II includes a fracture of the inferior orbital rim and zygomaticomaxillary buttress. Le Fort III fractures are the only level to contain fractures of the lateral orbital wall and zygomatic arch. Again, combinations of different levels bilaterally or even multiple levels on each side only complicate the radiographic diagnosis (Fig. 41-5). The high-energy injuries that result in Le Fort fractures often lead to fracture of the naso-orbito-ethmoid (NOE) region and zygomaticomaxillary complex on the contralateral side and should be closely evaluated radiographically. The palate should be analyzed in the axial plane for palatal fractures because they contribute to widening of the mid-face and complicate restoration of occlusion. Mandible fractures should be diagnosed since they often preclude stabilization of the maxillary segment to the lower part of the face. Recognition and proper diagnosis of the Le Fort

level on each side allow the clinician to decide on the extent of surgical access required.

TREATMENT/RECONSTRUCTIVE GOALS

Le Fort fractures result in both functional and cosmetic defects. The goals in treating mid-face fractures are to restore harmonious occlusion between the maxilla and mandible and reestablish mid-facial height and facial symmetry. To accomplish these objectives, one needs to systematically evaluate the extent of the fracture lines, the amount of displacement, and any horizontal or vertical loss of dimension.

INITIAL MANAGEMENT

Initial attention should be directed at securing the airway, as with any traumatic injury. Given the high vascularity of the mid-face, severe hemorrhage can often result. Most frequently, the branches of the maxillary artery are the cause of bleeding in Le Fort fractures. Bleeding is common from the nasal walls and septum and can generally be managed with the various types of nasal packing. Other areas of bleeding can also be managed with direct tamponade. Rarely, uncontrollable hemorrhage will necessitate angiography and embolization.[7,8] Other emergency conditions that can be seen with mid-face fractures include retrobulbar hemorrhage and septal hematoma, which should be addressed quickly as outlined elsewhere.

INCISIONS/APPROACHES

Le Fort I

Le Fort I fractures can generally be approached via maxillary vestibular incisions. Arch bars should be applied to the dentition when present. If difficulty arises in placing the patient in solid and reproducible occlusion, an occlusal splint should be fabricated from impressions of both arches. With palatal fractures, one may also need to fabricate a palatal splint to reproduce the premorbid width of the maxillary arch.

For isolated maxillary fractures at the Le Fort level, maxillo-mandibular fixation (MMF) should be applied and the maxilla manually reduced. The vertical buttresses of the maxilla should then be internally fixated with plates and screws. For bilateral fractures, it is recommended that 2.0-mm plates be applied to each nasomaxillary and zygomaticomaxillary buttress.[9]

If it is difficult to manually reduce the maxilla because of impaction and telescoping or because a significant amount of time has elapsed since the injury, Rowe or Hayton-Williams disimpaction forceps can be applied to free the maxillary segment before fixation.

In cases in which other fractures are present, consideration should be given to open reduction and internal fixation of the associated fractures first before fixation of the maxilla. When associated mandibular fractures are present, they should generally be addressed first because the mandible tends to allow better anatomic reduction. The anterior and lateral walls of the maxillary sinuses are often comminuted, and thus orientation of the maxilla in the sagittal and coronal planes can be difficult without a stable mandibular occlusion to refer to. Associated zygomaticomaxillary complex fractures should generally be secured to the stable upper craniofacial skeleton before securing the maxilla.[10]

As addressed later, bone defects after reduction of the maxilla should be grafted immediately. Loss of bony continuity of a severely comminuted anterior and lateral wall of the maxillary sinus will require grafting to prevent soft tissue prolapse and resultant facial scarring.[11]

Historically, a principal component of the treatment of Le Fort fractures was wire suspension to the zygoma or cranium to prevent elongation of the face. The thought was that the opening muscles of mastication would pull a maxilla treated by wires or MMF inferiorly and posteriorly and result in elongation of the face. Mid-face shortening because of telescoping or comminution of the maxilla is, however, usually the result of aggressive suspension wires.[12] Wire suspension has been replaced by rigid fixation for the treatment of mid-face fractures and is essentially no longer an issue.

Le Fort II

Occasionally, a Le Fort II fracture can be reduced with the use of Rowe disimpaction forceps and MMF. MMF for 4 weeks may be adequate for bony healing of stable fractures. More often, open reduction plus internal fixation is required to stabilize the fractures.

Exposure of a Le Fort II fracture can generally be accomplished with the combination of a maxillary buccal vestibule incision and any of the various approaches to the infraorbital rim, which are addressed in the chapter on orbital trauma. Occasionally, the nasofrontal suture needs to be exposed through bilateral Lynch incisions, open-sky approaches, or even bicoronally. Three- or four-point fixation can be accomplished at the zygomaticomaxillary suture and infraorbital rim, and 2.0-mm plates can be adapted to the zygomaticomaxillary buttress and 1.0- or 1.5-mm plates to the infraorbital rim.

Le Fort III

Treatment of the Le Fort III fracture involves breaking the injury into facial subunits. The approach can be simplified in this way and the injury can be thought of as bilateral zygomaticomaxillary complex fractures and a NOE fracture. A Le Fort III fracture rarely exists in isolation and is instead usually a component of "pan-facial" fractures. Many sequencing methods are advocated for reconstruction of pan-facial fractures and vary from "outside-in" to "bottom-up."[13]

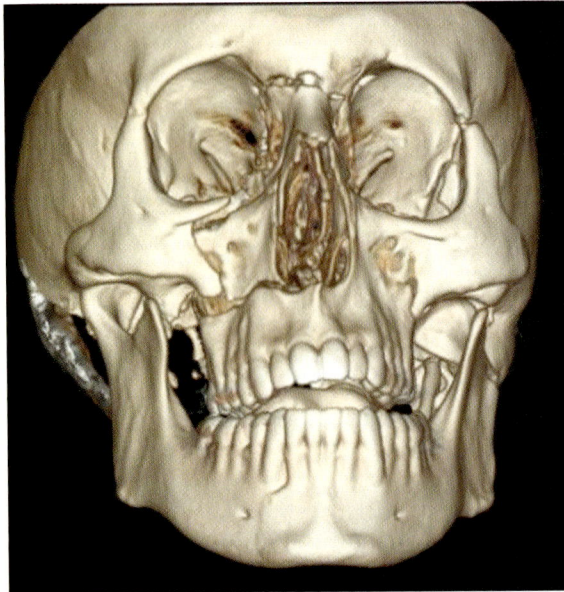

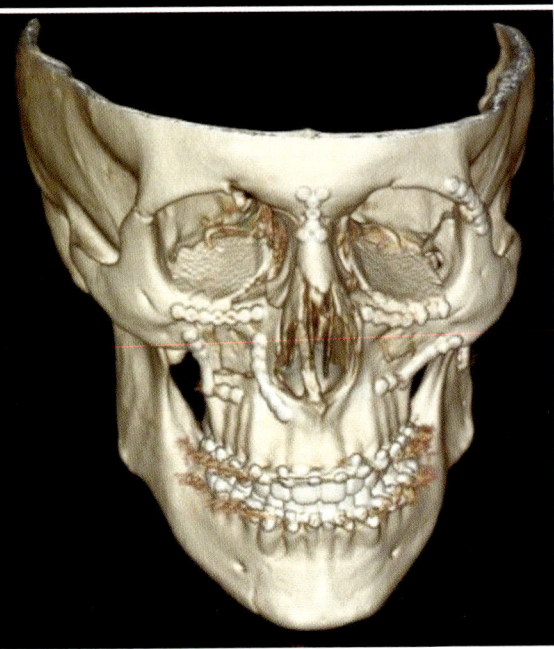

Fig. 41-6 ■ Multiple-level Le Fort fractures and bilateral orbital floor fractures.

A bicoronal incision is useful for exposure of the NOE region, the bilateral frontozygomatic sutures, and the lateral orbital rims. This can be combined with pre-auricular, lower lid, and maxillary vestibular incisions when necessary (Fig. 41-6).

SPECIFIC TREATMENT AND TECHNIQUES

PRIMARY BONE GRAFTING

Given the delicacy of the bones of the mid-face, comminution often results. Defects may remain in the orbital floor or in the lateral or anterior buttresses of the maxilla. To achieve adequate stability of the maxilla and prevent soft tissue deformities, primary bone grafting should be performed. The maxillary buttresses provide keys to maxillary reduction. The buttresses of the maxilla should be primarily bone-grafted when the pattern of fracture leads to loss or extreme instability. Large defects in the anterior or lateral wall of the maxilla can be bone-grafted or covered with titanium mesh to prevent soft tissue prolapse.[11,14] Cranial bone, rib, and iliac crest are all suitable for reconstruction of mid-face defects. The orbital floor, as addressed elsewhere, can be reconstructed with cranial bone, titanium, or other alloplastic material.

SOFT TISSUE CONSIDERATIONS

The soft tissue overlying the maxilla is a complex entity that circumscribes the orbit, nasal cavity, and mouth. The facial muscles allow diverse facial expressions. This soft tissue envelope is dependent on the underlying skeleton for its appearance and function. Frequently, the exposures required to adequately reduce and fixate the bones of the mid-face involve complete degloving of the overlying soft tissue. Significant deformities can result without proper management of the soft tissues despite excellent osseous reduction.[15]

The soft tissue must be closed in layers over an anatomically positioned skeleton and must be resuspended by fixation of the periosteum to the underlying skeleton. One should close the periosteum, fascia, muscle, and skin where incisions have been made. Complete degloving of tissues in the mid-face can result in soft tissue sag. The mucoperiosteal envelope must be resuspended to a solid structure such as the orbital rim or zygoma.[15]

CONCOMITANT LE FORT AND SUBCONDYLAR FRACTURES

If the patient suffers bilateral condylar fractures in addition to any level of Le Fort fracture, the vertical reference point of the lower part of the face is lost. Access to the often comminuted posterior maxilla is difficult, as is rigid fixation. Recreation of posterior facial height requires anatomic reduction of at least one of the mandibular condyles to provide a reference for subsequent positioning of the posterior maxilla. The retromandibular approach provides excellent exposure for reduction and fixation of subcondylar fractures (Fig. 41-7).

PALATAL FRACTURES

Concomitant fractures of the palate present additional challenges in the treatment of Le Fort fractures. They are found in 8% of Le Fort fractures and complicate the reestablishment of proper occlusion and width of the maxilla.[16] When a palatal fracture is diagnosed, it is important to obtain dental impressions to be able to properly assess the occlusion and perform model surgery. An acrylic palatal splint can be fabricated from the models and helps in determining the transverse width intraoperatively. In addition, application of arch bars will help serve as a "tension band" across the fracture but could lead to palatal and mesial tipping of the teeth and not reduction of the fracture, especially posteriorly. In some cases, application of rigid fixation directly to the hard palate is necessary. A longitudinal palatal incision in an anteroposterior direction or the use of an existing laceration allows exposure of the palate.[16] One must be careful to not compromise the blood supply to the palatal mucosa and remaining maxilla.

POSTOPERATIVE CARE

Antibiotics are used throughout the perioperative period. Antibiotics should provide both oral and sinus coverage. Perioperative steroids are also frequently administered. The first steroid dose is

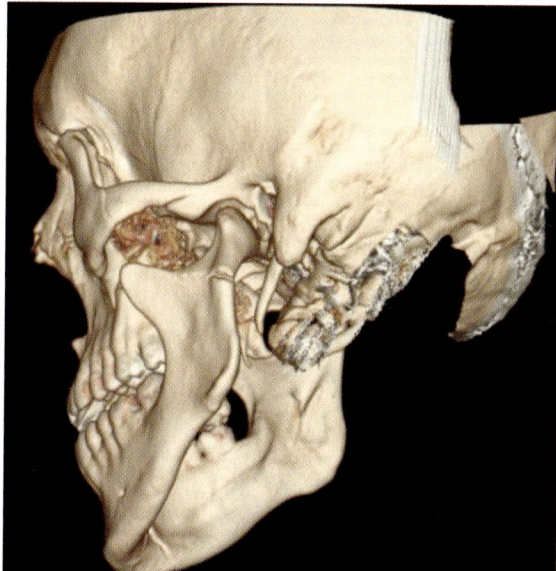

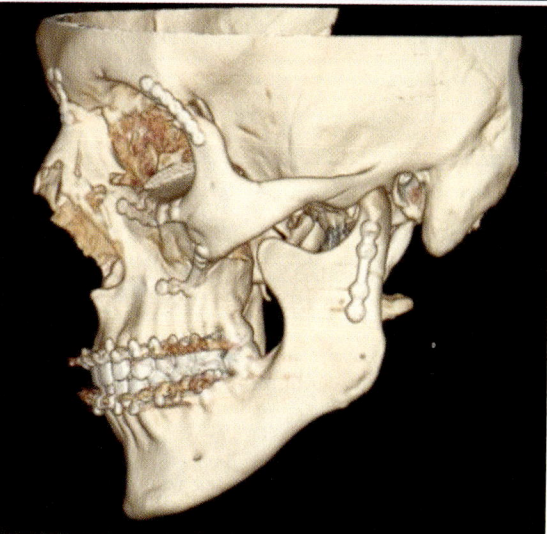

Fig. 41-7 ■ Mandibular subcondylar fractures in a patient with maxillary factures.

given immediately preoperatively and continued for 24 hours postoperatively. Patients may also benefit from nasal and sinus decongestants. MMF is generally maintained for a period of 2 to 4 weeks.

CONCLUSION

Maxillary fractures represent a complex group of facial injuries. Both mid-face form and function may be disrupted. Patients may have facial disfigurement, malocclusion, and pain. Oral and maxillofacial surgeons will always be involved in the evaluation and treatment of these injuries. Soft tissue and skeletal anatomy should be restored and patients should be returned to their preinjury occlusion. The severity of injury does have an impact on treatment outcomes. Advances in imaging and surgical technology will always aid in surgical care. A constant component for the best outcomes is the involvement of a well-trained, thoughtful surgeon.

PEARLS AND PITFALLS

- The mid-face connects the more stable frontal bone superiorly and the mandible inferiorly. Given its inherent weakness and position, the mid-face is considered a "dependent" structure.[15]
- Unfavorable outcomes in treating Le Fort fractures usually result from poor diagnosis, inadequate planning, lack of proper exposure, and inadequate fixation.
- Le Fort fractures of the various levels involve reconstruction of orbital volume and occlusion, which requires significant precision and accuracy of reduction and fixation to prevent enophthalmos and malocclusion.
- Malocclusion after maxillary fractures occurs in 8% to 20% of patients.[17-20] Those treated by closed reduction have the lowest rates of malocclusion, but they also are usually the least severe.[21]
- The fractured maxilla is secured to the mandible and then plated in the estimated vertical position, which is often complicated by comminution.
- Malocclusion occurs as a result of incorrect reduction and fixation during surgery because of inaccurate vertical positioning or poor seating of the condyles when applying MMF. In addition, malocclusion may result from failure to passively reposition the fractured maxilla because of inadequate mobility.[22]

- Frequently, strong disimpaction forces or even additional osteotomies must be created to allow passive positioning of the maxilla in relation to the mandible with the condyles correctly seated.[22]
- Other complications associated with Le Fort fractures include paresthesia of the infraorbital nerve, especially with Le Fort I and II fractures.
- Because of involvement of the orbital floor and rim with Le Fort II fractures and the zygomaticomaxillary complex with Le Fort III fractures, orbital dystopia and enophthalmos are possible complications, even after repair.
- Blindness is very rarely associated with Le Fort fractures[23,24] but can occur as a result of the primary injury mechanism or after reduction of the fracture.[25]
- Maxillary sinusitis is a relatively rare complication of fractures of the maxilla despite frequent comminution of the walls of the sinus.
- Other possible complications include dacryocystitis and epiphora, septal deviation, hematoma, synechiae, and various ocular injuries.
- Malunion or nonunion of the maxilla can occur as a result of delays in treatment and severe comminution without adequate bone grafting.[9]

REFERENCES

1. Le Fort R: Etude experimentale sur les fractures de la machoire superiore, *Rev Chir* 23:208-227, 1901.
2. Le Fort R: Etude experimentale sur les fractures de la machoire superiore, *Rev Chir* 23:360-379, 1901.
3. Le Fort R: Etude experimentale sur les fractures de la machoire superiore, *Rev Chir* 23:479-507, 1901.
4. Gassner R, Tuli T, Hächl O, et al: Craniomaxillofacial trauma in children: a review of 3,385 cases with 6,060 injuries in 10 years, *J Oral Maxillofac Surg* 62:399-407, 2004.
5. Manson PN, Hoopes JE, Su CT: Structural pillars of the facial skeleton: an approach to the management of Le Fort fractures, *Plast Reconstr Surg* 66:54-62, 1980.
6. Rhea JT, Novelline RA: How to simplify the CT diagnosis of Le Fort fractures, *AJR Am J Roentgenol* 184:1700-1705, 2005.
7. Borsa JJ, Fontaine AB, Eskridge JM, et al: Transcatheter arterial embolization for intractable epistaxis secondary to gunshot wounds, *J Vasc Interv Radiol* 10:297-302, 1999.
8. Ardekian L, Samet N, Shoshani Y, et al: Life-threatening bleeding following maxillofacial trauma, *J Craniomaxillofac Surg* 21:336-338, 1993.
9. Salin M, Smith BM: Diagnosis and treatment of midface fractures. In Fonseca RJ, et al, editors: *Oral and maxillofacial trauma*, vol 2, ed 3, St. Louis, 2005, CV Mosby, pp 643-691.
10. Cunningham L, Haug RH: Management of maxillary fractures. In Miloro M,

editor: *Peterson's principles of oral and maxillofacial surgery*, ed 2, Lewiston, 2004, BC Decker, pp 547-559.
11. Gruss JS, Phillips JH: Complex facial trauma: the evolving role of rigid fixation and immediate bone graft reconstruction, *Clin Plast Surg* 16:93-104, 1989.
12. Manson PN: Some thoughts on the classification and treatment of Le Fort fractures, *Ann Plast Surg* 17:356-363, 1986 .
13. Louis P: Management of panfacial fractures. In Miloro M, editor: *Peterson's principles of oral and maxillofacial surgery*, ed 2, Hamilton, Ontario, 2004, BC Decker.
14. Gruss JS, Mackinnon SE: Complex maxillary fractures: role of buttress reconstruction and immediate bone grafts, *Plast Reconstr Surg* 78:9-22, 1986.
15. Manson PN, Clark N, Robertson B, et al: Subunit principles in midface fractures: the importance of sagittal buttresses, soft-tissue reductions, and sequencing treatment of segmental fractures, *Plast Reconstr Surg* 103:1287-1306, quiz 1307, 1999.
16. Hendrickson M, Clark N, Manson PN, et al: Palatal fractures: classification, patterns, and treatment with rigid internal fixation, *Plast Reconstr Surg* 101:319-332, 1998.
17. Heimgartner-Candinas B, Heimgartner M, Jonutis A: Results of treatment of midfacial fractures. Indications for exploration and drainage of the maxillary sinuses, *J Maxillofac Surg* 6:293-301, 1978.
18. Steidler NE, Cook RM, Reade PC: Residual complications in patients with major middle third facial fractures, *Int J Oral Surg* 9:259-266, 1980.

19. Haug RH, Adams JM, Jordan RB: Comparison of the morbidity associated with maxillary fractures treated by maxillomandibular and rigid internal fixation, *Oral Surg Oral Med Oral Pathol Oral Radiol Endod* 80:629-637, 1995.
20. O'Sullivan ST, Snyder BJ, Moore MH, et al: Outcome measurement of the treatment of maxillary fractures: a prospective analysis of 100 consecutive cases, *Br J Plast Surg* 52:519-523, 1999.
21. Haug RH, Prather J, Bradrick JP, et al: The morbidity associated with fifty maxillary fractures treated by closed reduction, *Oral Surg Oral Med Oral Pathol* 73:659-663, 1992.
22. Ellis E: Passive repositioning of maxillary fractures: an occasional impossibility without osteotomy, *J Oral Maxillofac Surg* 62:1477-1485, 2004.
23. al-Qurainy IA, Stassen LF, Dutton GN, et al: The characteristics of midfacial fractures and the association with ocular injury: a prospective study, *Br J Oral Maxillofac Surg* 29:291-301, 1991.
24. Ashar A, Kovacs A, Khan S, et al: Blindness associated with midfacial fractures, *J Oral Maxillofac Surg* 56:1146-1150, discussion 1151, 1998.
25. Girotto JA, Gamble WB, Robertson B, et al: Blindness after reduction of facial fractures, *Plast Reconstr Surg* 102:1821-1834, 1998.

Chapter 42

Naso-Orbito-Ethmoid Fractures

Mark Engelstad

Humans recognize each other by the shape of the eyes and the middle third of the face.[1] For this reason, successful repair of the naso-orbito-ethmoid (NOE) region is difficult, and even minor shortcomings in the final result are recognizable to others. In addition, the NOE area contains several types of specialized tissues (bone, cartilage, sinus, tendon, and lacrimal and ocular tissues) and distinctive architectures that, once lost, are difficult for the surgeon to restore. The bone in this area is distinctly shaped, difficult to access, and covered by the thinnest soft tissue in the face.

A post-traumatic NOE deformity can have three key components: diminished nasal projection, increased intercanthal distance (telecanthus), and impaired nasofrontal or lacrimal drainage. The best outcomes following significant NOE injury are the result of accurate diagnosis and treatment of these three components.

ETIOPATHOGENESIS/CAUSATIVE FACTORS

The etiology of NOE trauma differs from that of mandibular and nasal trauma.[2] NOE injuries are the result of focused high-energy transfer to the intercanthal area. A motor vehicle accident is, for example, a more likely cause than interpersonal violence. The trauma surgeon should always remember that NOE injury is the result of significant energy transfer and that patients who have sustained considerable NOE trauma will often have associated cervical spine, ocular, or intracranial injuries.[3]

PATHOLOGIC ANATOMY AND EXAMINATION

The foundation of the NOE region is a paired set of midline facial buttresses that flow vertically from the piriform rim up to the frontal bar; these buttresses support nasal projection and attachment of the medial canthal tendon (MCT).

MEDIAL CANTHAL TENDON

It is helpful to conceptualize the MCT as the medial extent of a tarsal apparatus. The tarsal apparatus runs in the plane of the orbital septum and extends from the lateral canthus at Whitnall's tubercle, through the upper and lower tarsi, and into the MCT, where it attaches to the frontal process of the maxilla. The tarsal apparatus provides support to the eyelids and defines the normal almond shape of the palpebral fissure.

Before attaching to the frontal process of the maxilla, the MCT splits into anterior and posterior components, with the lacrimal sac between them. The superficial component attaches broadly to the anterior lacrimal crest, whereas the deep component of the MCT attaches along the posterior lacrimal crest. Restoration of this deep component after canthal detachment is critical for maintaining the proper shape and appearance of the eyelids; it *rounds* the eyelids against the medial aspect of the globe, thereby allowing normal lid function. When the MCT is repaired, its deep direction of attachment must be restored. The posterior component is also associated with a slip of orbicularis oculi called Horner's muscle; when Horner's muscle contracts, it assists movement of fluid through the lacrimal system (Fig. 42-1).

Direct blunt force to the NOE region buckles the medial orbital walls and fragments the thin nasal, lacrimal, ethmoid, and frontal bones. The nasal root can also telescope posteriorly into the ethmoid air cells as a single unit, lodge under the nasal process of the frontal bone, and obstruct nasofrontal outflow of the frontal sinus (Fig. 42-2). Frequently, NOE injury will be accompanied by an increased intercanthal distance (telecanthus) resulting from widening of the canthal-bearing bones, MCT detachment, or both.

A thorough examination will distinguish NOE injuries from an isolated nasal fracture. NOE injury has a distinctive appearance: a horizontally widened intercanthal region along with a vertically shortened nose that is flattened and widened with an upturned nasal tip. The deformity has a remarkably consistent appearance in patients (Fig. 42-3).

CLINICAL AND RADIOGRAPHIC ASSESSMENT

Thorough digital NOE examination for mobility, crepitus, and depressibility often yields the most information about the extent of NOE injury. The entire nose—or portions of it—may be digitally depressible. Formal preoperative ophthalmology consultation should be considered for a patient who has sustained enough force to fracture the orbital walls. Occult ocular injury may be present.

The status of the MCT attachment to bone can be assessed clinically by the "bowstring" test (Fig. 42-4): the lateral canthus is grasped and displaced laterally while observing and palpating the medial canthal area. Lateral displacement of the medial canthal area suggests a compromised bony attachment. This test can be difficult to interpret accurately, especially in the presence of acute edema and a conscious patient.

In the operating room, the status of the MCT can be assessed by placing an instrument in the nose under the bony MCT attachment while simultaneously palpating the area from the outside; manipulation of the instrument will help one understand the status of the MCT-bearing bone fragment.

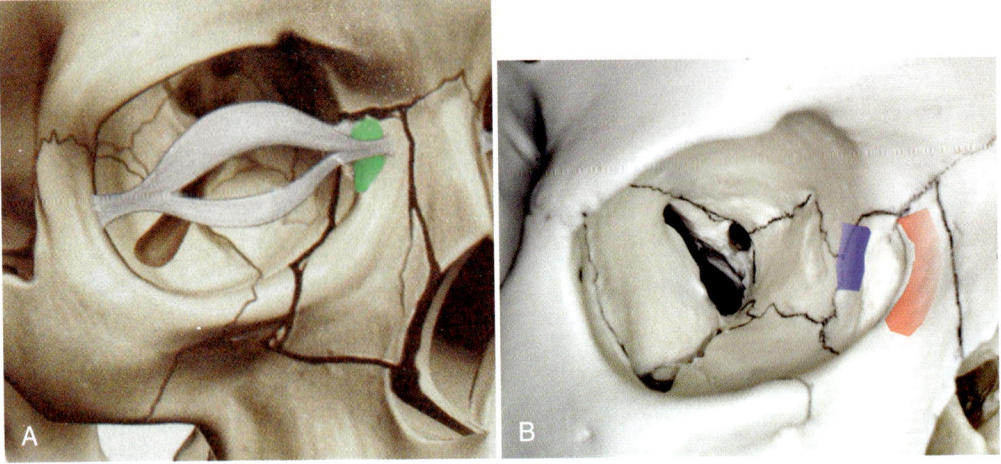

Fig. 42-1 ■ **A,** Tarsal apparatus extending from the lateral orbital wall to the frontal process of the maxilla. **B,** Areas of bony attachment of the deep (*blue*) and superficial (*red*) components of the medial canthal tendon.

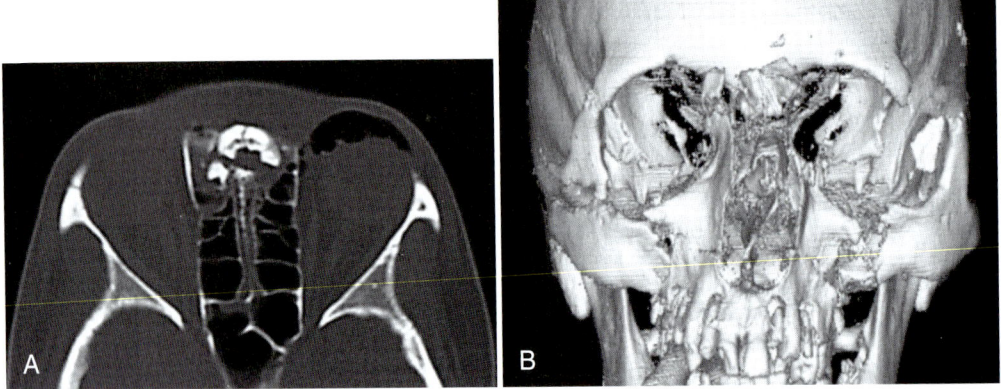

Fig. 42-2 ■ Axial computed tomography showing the nasal radix displaced posteriorly into the ethmoid air cells.

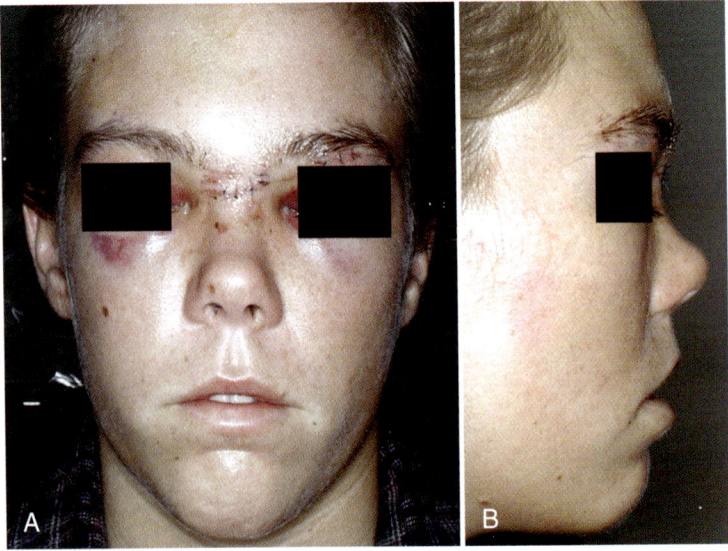

Fig. 42-3 ■ Five days following blunt naso-orbito-ethmoid (NOE) injury. This patient has a typical appearance following NOE injury. Note the telecanthus, depression of the nasal radix and dorsum, vertically shortened nose, and upturned nasal tip.

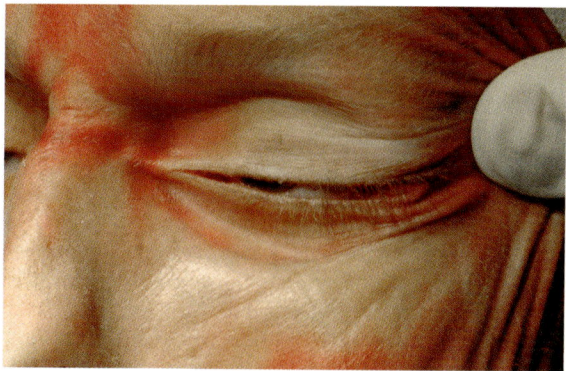

Fig. 42-4 ■ The "bowstring" test.

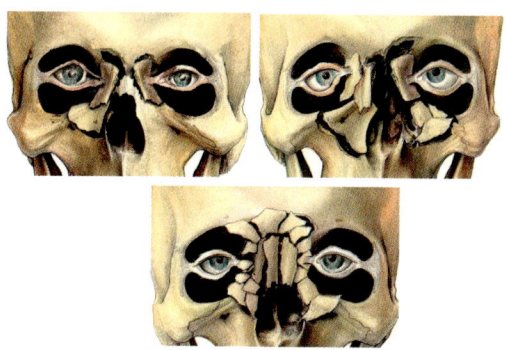

Fig. 42-5 ■ Classification of naso-orbito-ethmoid fractures. (From Fonseca RJ, et al: *Oral and maxillofacial surgery*, vol 2, ed 2. St Louis, 2009, WB Saunders.)

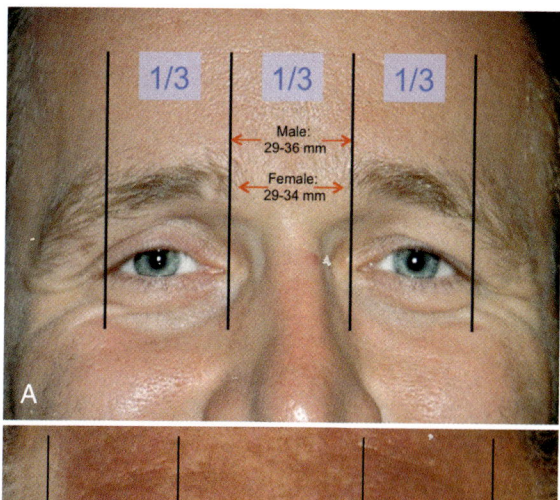

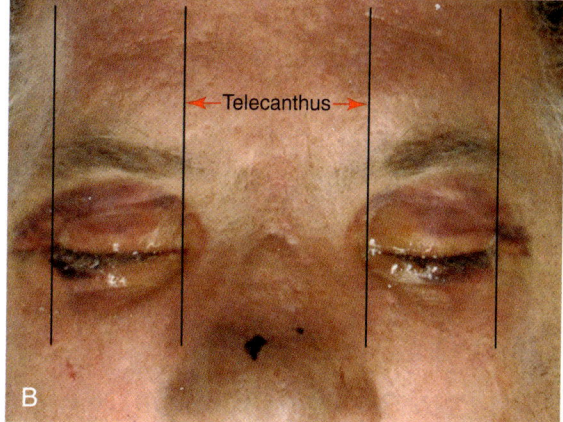

Fig. 42-6 ■ **A,** The normal intercanthal distance measured from one medial palpebral angle to the other. **B,** Telecanthus, or increased intercanthal distance.

DIAGNOSIS

CLASSIFICATION OF NASO-ORBITO-ETHMOID FRACTURES

Even though NOE trauma rarely resembles textbook diagrams, classifying the injury enhances both communication and treatment planning. The most widely used and therefore useful NOE injury classification scheme remains that developed by Markowitz and colleagues.[4] The status of the MCT, the canthal-bearing bone fragment, and the fracture pattern define a clinically useful classification system (Fig. 42-5). From type I to type III, the energy sustained from the injury increases.

- Type I: single-segment central fragment
- Type II: comminuted central fragment with fractures remaining external to the insertion of the MCT
- Type III: comminuted central fragment with fractures extending into bone bearing the canthal insertion

INTERCANTHAL DISTANCE

Increased intercanthal distance, called telecanthus, is one of the key deformities of NOE injuries. The normal intercanthal distance is approximately equal to the width of the palpebral aperture or half the interpupillary width. The distance, measured from one medial palpebral angle to the other, is approximately 29 to 34 mm in adult women and 29 to 36 mm in adult men, but it can vary considerably[5] (Fig. 42-6). An increase in intercanthal distance greater than 40 mm is strongly correlated with NOE injury requiring surgical treatment. However, accurate measurement is difficult in the presence of acute edema, and a surgical NOE treatment plan should not be based on a single measurement alone. Overall, intercanthal distance is less

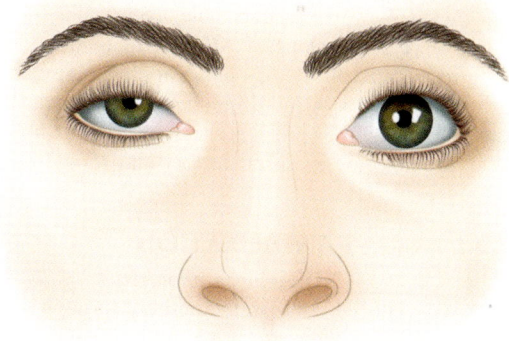

Fig. 42-7 ■ Left-sided palpebral aperture changes following unilateral medial canthal tendon detachment.

meaningful than the distance of each canthus from the facial midline; measuring each side independently helps diagnose unilateral injury.

REPAIR OF TELECANTHUS

Repair of telecanthus is one of the key components of NOE treatment. Telecanthus is caused by disruption of the MCT attachment, which slackens the entire tarsal apparatus. After disruption of the MCT, contraction of the orbicularis oculi muscle increases the intercanthal distance and causes lateral displacement and rounding of the medial palpebral fissure. Measuring the distance of each palpebral fissure to the facial midline will distinguish unilateral injury from bilateral injury (Fig. 42-7).

IMPAIRMENT OF NASOFRONTAL DRAINAGE

Assessment plus restoration of adequate frontal sinus drainage is another key component of NOE treatment. Rodriguez and co-workers demonstrated that nasofrontal obstruction is common with combined frontal sinus–NOE injury and that 99% of frontal sinus complications are a result of inadequate nasofrontal drainage.[6] Restoration of drainage is more likely when NOE projection is reestablished.

Historically, nasofrontal patency was assessed by injecting a fluid (saline, methylene blue, or fluorescein) into the nasofrontal duct and watching for its appearance in the nose. Definitive results of this test can be difficult to interpret in an acutely traumatized field. Assessment of the NOE injury for nasofrontal patency is more helpful preoperatively, during the treatment-planning phase. Modern-day fine-cut computed tomography (CT) in all three planes will demonstrate gross bony compromise of sinus outflow. Imaging alone is not entirely predictive of postoperative patency of the outflow tract, but it may be as predictive as invasive techniques.

When nasofrontal obstruction is a concern, postoperative CT a few months after treatment will reveal inadequate frontal sinus drainage. At that point, endoscopic frontal sinus surgery may reestablish sinus drainage.[7]

TREATMENT/RECONSTRUCTIVE GOALS

Success in repairing NOE injuries can vary, but the principles of treatment are constant: establish nasal projection and narrow the intercanthal distance.

TIMING OF NASO-ORBITO-ETHMOID REPAIR

There is general consensus that early repair of NOE injuries gives superior results.[8] Unless extreme, prolonged waiting for resolution of facial swelling is probably of little value. Trauma starts a cascade of inflammation, fibrosis, and healing. Surgery is a "second hit" of tissue injury. When repair is performed early rather than late, surgical inflammation may blend with the initial wound healing. What early repair means, however, is debatable. To the modern surgeon, the right time to perform a lengthy NOE repair is more dependent on operating room availability than on ideal physiology.

Achieving a satisfactory result from the primary repair is crucial. Secondary NOE repairs, as well as the scarring and fibrosis that follow them, are notoriously unsatisfactory and should be avoided if possible.

SURGICAL ACCESS AND FIXATION

A single-fragment, type I NOE injury *without superior displacement* can be accessed, reduced, and fixated entirely through a transoral approach. In these cases, the piriform and infraorbital rim alignment can be verified through the transoral approach, and a separate orbital incision is not required. A single plate along the piriform rim is usually adequate fixation for these injuries. If significant superior displacement of the type I fragment exists, accurate reduction may not be possible without additional access and fixation.

In type II and III NOE injuries, the goal of surgery is restoration of nasal projection and intercanthal distance. To achieve this objective, a coronal approach is generally necessary. Accessory approaches are also required, including a transconjunctival or subciliary incision for access to the infraorbital rim and orbital floor, as well as a transoral incision. There is little likelihood of achieving an acceptable outcome after a serious NOE injury without full surgical access. The coronal approach provides this and also allows cranial bone grafting for nasal dorsal struts or orbital wall defects. During dissection, close attention should be paid to the MCT and care taken to not detach it from its bony insertion.

Mid-facial degloving, which requires an extended transoral approach, has also been described for NOE repair,[9] but if orbital access for canthopexy or medial wall repair is needed, a coronal approach will still be necessary. A coronal approach, at its full extent, will provide access to the entire medial half of the orbit and most of the nasal dorsum.

Existing lacerations rarely provide adequate access for NOE reconstruction; enlargement of a facial laceration for NOE repair should be avoided when possible. Transcutaneous approaches, such as the gull wing, or "open sky," approach, also leave unacceptable facial scars that cannot be camouflaged.[10]

The size and position of bone plates for NOE repair are important. The skin overlying the medial orbital rim and lateral nasal bone area is quite thin. The presence of plates and screws can cause low-grade chronic inflammation of the overlying soft tissues, which is readily noticeable and difficult to resolve. Generally speaking, placement of plates, screws, and wires directly under the soft tissues in the MCT region should be minimized.

SEQUENCING OF NASO-ORBITO-ETHMOID REPAIR AND ASSOCIATED BONE INJURIES

NOE injury is often associated with significant orbital and frontal sinus trauma. Accurate reconstruction of the orbital walls is absolutely necessary for a successful outcome. Unless the normal orbital volume is restored, the result of NOE repair will be inadequate. Access to the deep orbit and orbital rims from the coronal approach is enhanced by canthal disruption. The nasal dorsum and radix can be reduced at any time, but once canthopexy is performed, visualization within the orbit is lost. For this reason, all associated facial buttress and orbital repairs should be accomplished before canthopexy. The proper sequence of steps for repair of NOE and associated injuries was described by Ellis.[11]

NASAL PROJECTION

Restoration of nasal length and dorsal projection is a key objective of NOE treatment. With a severe NOE injury, nasal dorsal strut grafting is often required to reestablish support for the entire nose. Definitive rhinoplasty can be done on a delayed basis if the nasal projection is excessive, but once the nose begins to heal in a collapsed and shortened state, regaining its premorbid length and projection is very difficult.

Nasal projection and telecanthus are inversely related: adequate projection of the nasal dorsum can mask telecanthus, whereas inadequate dorsal projection actually enhances the appearance of telecanthus. This phenomenon is called pseudo-telecanthus.

The dorsal nasal strut graft is cantilevered from stable frontal bone and placed in the subcutaneous plane, all the way down to the region of the nasal tip (Fig. 42-8). An endonasal approach to visualize the tip area and align the strut graft with the nasal cartilage can be helpful. To prevent shortening and provide support for the nasal cartilage and septum, the graft should span the length of the nasal dorsum.

A dorsal strut graft can be harvested from a variety of sites, but cranial bone is readily available and can be precisely contoured and stably fixated. Potter and colleagues have thoroughly described nasal management in patients after NOE injury.[12] Alloplastic materials are too often the source of chronic inflammation and should be avoided for nasal dorsum grafting.[13]

MEDIAL CANTHOPEXY

Except in the case of a gunshot wound or penetrating NOE trauma, the MCT is often left attached to some kind of central canthal-bearing bone fragment.[4,10] The size of the remaining

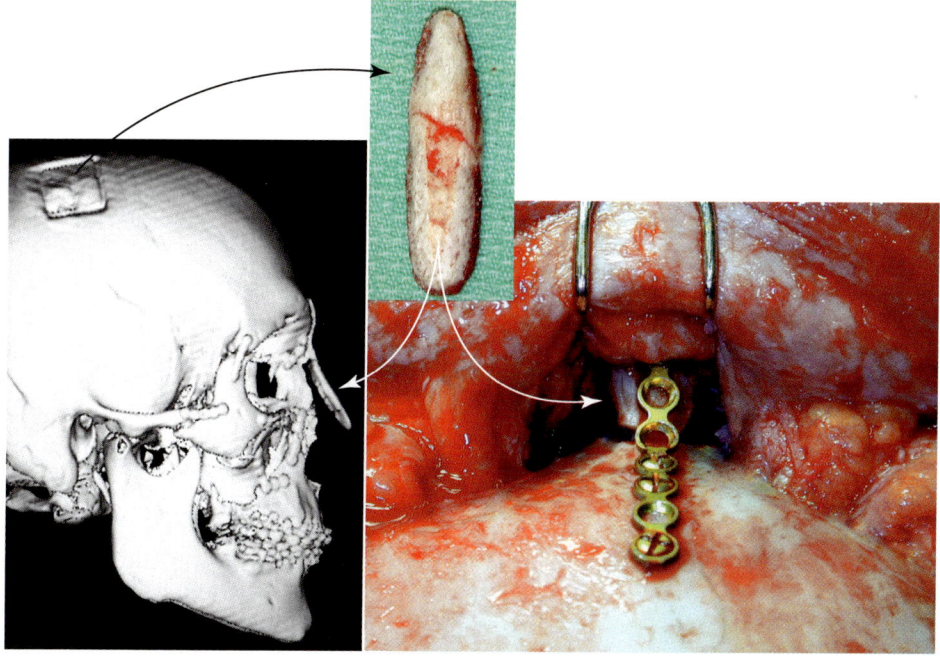

Fig. 42-8 ■ The outer table calvaria is contoured and then cantilevered from stable frontal bone to restore dorsal nasal stability, projection, and length. The plate may be placed superior or inferior to the bone graft. (Clinical images courtesy Gorman Louie, M.D.)

canthal-bearing bone fragment is critical. The surgeon will need to know whether it can be accurately positioned among the other fragments and whether it can be stabilized or fixated with the proper vector of reduction.

Reduction plus fixation of the canthal tendon–bearing bone fragment is the most direct way to restore intercanthal distance. If it is large enough to hold screws superiorly and inferiorly, internal fixation alone can stabilize the canthal-bearing fragment. If the central fragment is not large enough to be reliably reduced and fixated, the MCT itself should be identified, captured, and reduced to restore intercanthal distance. This is referred to as medial canthopexy. During medial canthopexy, the canthus should be directed to a point on the medial orbital wall that is slightly posterior and superior to the posterior lacrimal crest. This point is essential.

Medial canthopexy is one of the final steps in repair and is necessary only for severe NOE injuries. In these cases, the bone in the area of canthal attachment is often pulverized, with no stable bone left for canthal attachment or passage of a transnasal wire. Decreasing the intercanthal distance by simply wiring or suturing the canthi to one another will not achieve the correct posteriorly oriented medial canthal reduction necessary to restore normal appearance and function.

Traditionally, medial canthopexy is accomplished from the coronal approach by first identifying the MCT and then capturing it with wire or suture. Depending on the degree of trauma and presence of stable bone, the combination of transnasal wiring techniques and bone grafting of comminuted areas is used to reduce and stabilize the MCT. There is a body of literature that describes these techniques.[12,14] Successfully capturing the MCT or a small canthal-bearing bone fragment and then directing and stabilizing it in the proper vector are easier to diagram than to actually perform. In addition, finding and capturing the MCT can cause significant trauma to the delicate soft tissues of the NOE region.

External nasal bolsters and splints, even when transnasally wired, are poor substitutes for accurate *internal* reduction and stabilization.

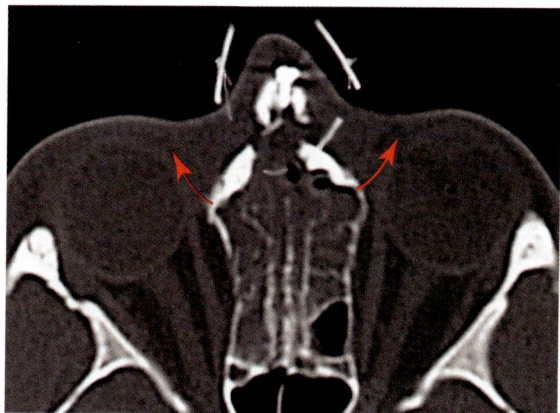

Fig. 42-9 ■ The use of transnasal wiring and bolsters to treat telecanthus actually causes widening of the bony medial canthal tendon insertion points, thereby making the telecanthus worse.

The postoperative axial CT scan in Figure 42-9 shows the possible result of using transnasal wire and external bolsters alone for MCT canthopexy. When the wires are applied anterior to the MCT, widening of the MCT insertion points and telecanthus can result. This is a well-known phenomenon.[12] It should also be noted that external bolsters do little to effect change at the depth of the MCT, where narrowing is most required.

CEREBROSPINAL FLUID RHINORRHEA

The absence of cerebrospinal fluid (CSF) rhinorrhea is also a goal of NOE reconstruction. When associated cribriform plate or anterior skull base fractures are present, CSF rhinorrhea is possible. The reduction of NOE fragments may stimulate CSF rhinorrhea from a previously undetectable dural injury. CSF rhinorrhea is usually self-limited but, when persistent, could require antibiotic therapy along with direct or endoscopic dural repair.

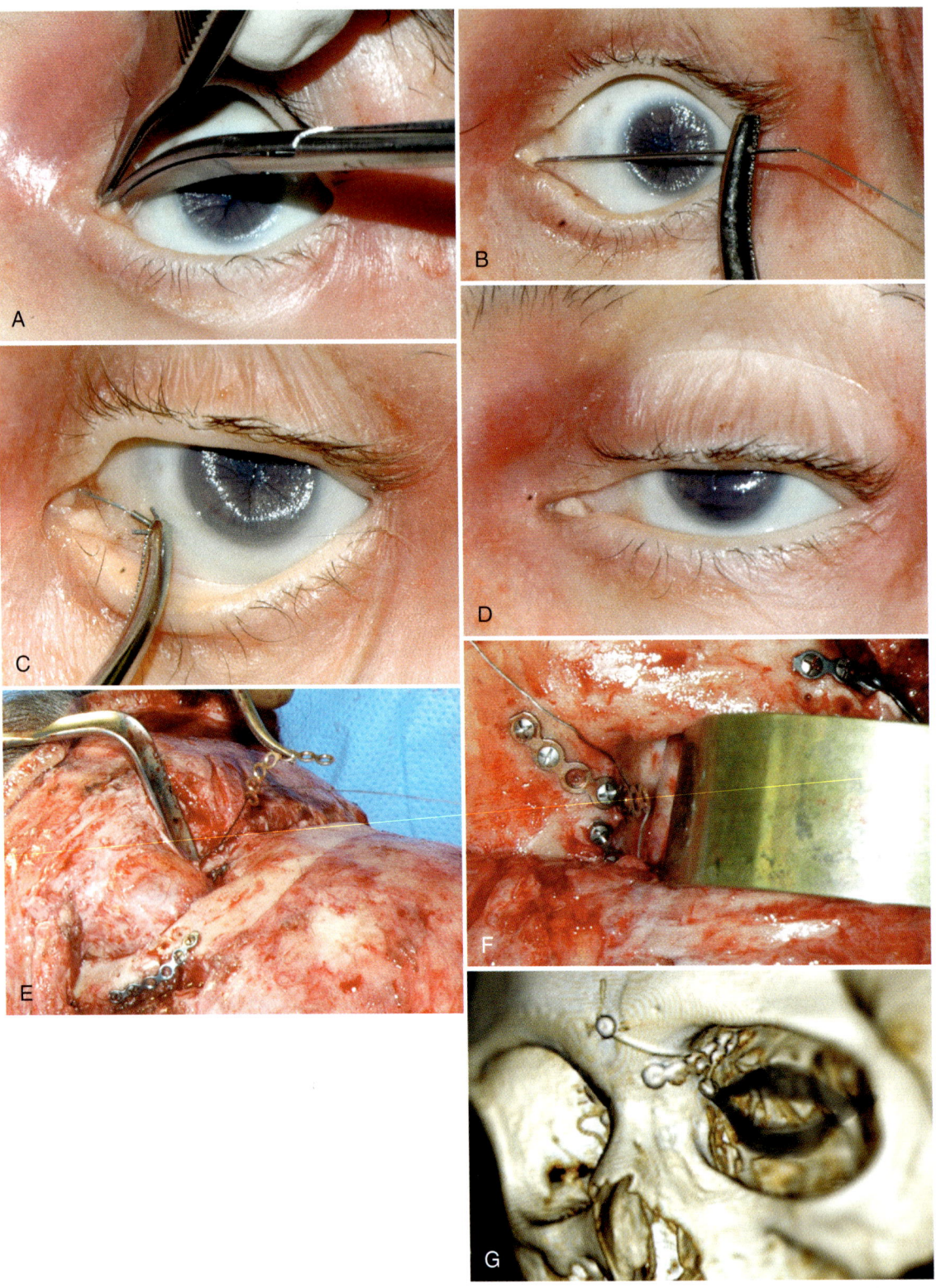

Fig. 42-10 ■ **A,** After a coronal approach, a small horizontal incision is made in the caruncle. **B,** The needle end of the canthal barb is passed through the caruncular incision and the medial canthal tendon (MCT). Special identification of the MCT is not required. The needle is then identified and pulled through from the deep side of the coronal flap. **C,** As it is pulled toward the caruncle, the canthal barb is guided into the incision in a horizontal orientation. **D,** The canthal barb is pulled into the incision and becomes engaged in the dense substance of the MCT. The barb is no longer visible. No closure of the caruncular incision is required. **E,** A thick miniplate is adapted to stable frontal bone and along the medial orbital wall. The most posterior hole of the plate is positioned slightly posterior and superior to the posterior lacrimal crest. The wire is then passed through the posterior plate hole. **F,** The miniplate is positioned and fixed to stable frontal bone. When the needle end of the wire is pulled, the barb will reduce the MCT toward the posterior plate hole and into an anatomically correct position, posterior and superior to the posterior lacrimal crest. The images demonstrate a unilateral technique. Alternatively, an awl could be used to create transnasal passage for the wire from the plate hole to the other orbit. **G,** The pulley configuration created by the canthal barb, wire, and plate can be visualized. After reduction of the MCT, the wire has been secured to a single frontal screw.

SPECIFIC TREATMENT AND TECHNIQUES

MEDIAL CANTHOPEXY WITH A CANTHAL BARB AND MINIPLATE

In this chapter the use of a canthal barb and miniplate to achieve anatomically correct medial canthopexy will be described. This technique is a minor modification of one previously described by B. Hammer (*Orbital fractures: Diagnosis, operative treatment, secondary corrections*, Hogrefe and Huber Publishers, 1995). Refer to the images in Figure 42-10 for illustration of the technique.

The technique requires a coronal approach and two simple implants. The first is a canthal barb, which is a micro-anchor–like device that becomes securely embedded within the MCT and can withstand the firm reduction tension required for canthopexy without pulling out. Commercially available barbs are attached to a length of wire or suture and needle. The second requirement is a titanium miniplate adapted to the contour of the frontal bone and medial orbital wall. The miniplate should be thick enough to resist deformation from the static tension required for medial canthopexy (see Fig. 42-10).

This canthal barb and plate technique has advantages over traditional transnasal wire canthopexy. First, surgical identification of the MCT is not necessary. In cadaver studies,[15] passage of the needle through the caruncle consistently engaged the canthal barb in dense medial canthal connective tissue without pulling through. Second, the presence of stable bone in the medial orbit for passage of the wire is not necessary. Instead, the plate, which can be positioned by the surgeon, provides the fulcrum and proper vector for canthal reduction. Third, a unilateral approach is possible. Transnasal wiring is not necessary and contralateral orbital dissection can be avoided.

As with any canthopexy technique, the MCT should be slightly over-reduced; it will predictably remodel and relax over the subsequent months (Fig. 42-11). Although bone at the medial wall is not required, grafting of the medial wall should be considered for extensive injuries.

POSTOPERATIVE CARE

Postoperative management of the NOE repair should include routine vision checks, especially if the orbit was involved. If nasal cartilage and septum were injured, temporary intranasal support with splinting can be valuable. Bilateral soft intranasal support, such as the Doyle splint, may be tolerated better than intranasal packing with gauze. Intranasal splinting for at least 2 weeks will help minimize synechiae and maintain patency; patients have difficulty tolerating splints much longer than this.

Partial resolution of NOE edema can take several weeks, and total resolution may take more than 6 months. The final result cannot be judged for at least 6 months. Some authors believe that several weeks of external nasal splinting minimizes edema and results in better final soft tissue contour.[12]

If the initial outcome is obviously substandard, secondary repair should not be delayed excessively.

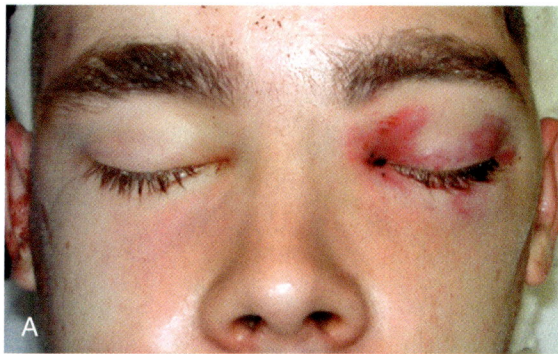
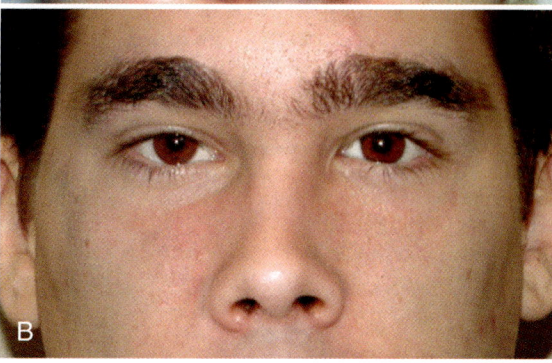

Fig. 42-11 ■ **A,** A gunshot has caused a unilateral type III naso-orbito-ethmoid injury with canthal disruption and left-sided telecanthus. **B,** One year after medial canthopexy with a canthal barb and miniplate technique.

PEARLS AND PITFALLS

- Good outcomes after NOE injuries depend on restoring nasal projection and narrowing the intercanthal distance and then allowing the delicate soft tissues to heal over the restored bony architecture with as little underlying hardware as possible.
- Inadequate projection of the nasal dorsum will create the illusion of telecanthus (pseudo-telecanthus), whereas a well-projected nasal dorsum will camouflage existing telecanthus.
- Lacrimal dysfunction is surprisingly rare following bony NOE injury.[16] Unless an obvious lacrimal injury is noted, such as a laceration through the medial third of the eyelid, routine lacrimal exploration or intubation does not diminish the incidence of postoperative epiphora and is not indicated.
- When performing medial canthopexy, the MCT should be reduced into a position slightly posterior and superior to the posterior lacrimal crest.
- During dissection, close attention should be paid to the MCT and care taken to not detach it from its bony insertion.
- The more hardware placed in the NOE region, the greater the potential for chronic inflammation from loose screws and plates. Piecing together every small fragment of bone with plates and screws is not necessary.
- Delayed or secondary repair of NOE injuries is associated with notoriously poor outcomes. The first operation is the best and only chance to achieve a great result.

REFERENCES

1. Keil MS: "I look in your eyes, honey": internal face features induce spatial frequency preference for human face processing, *PLoS Comput Biol* 5:e1000329, 2009.
2. Klenk G, Kovacs A: Etiology and patterns of facial fractures in the United Arab Emirates, *J Craniofac Surg* 14:78-84, 2003.
3. Lim LH, Lam LK, Moore MH, et al: Associated injuries in facial fractures: review of 839 patients, *Br J Plast Surg* 46:635-638, 1993.
4. Markowitz BL, Manson PN, Sargent L, et al: Management of the medial canthal tendon in nasoethmoid orbital fractures: the importance of the central fragment in classification and treatment, *Plast Reconstr Surg* 87:843-853, 1991.
5. Paskert JP, Manson PN, Iliff NT: Nasoethmoidal and orbital fractures, *Clin Plast Surg* 15:209-223, 1988.
6. Rodriguez ED, Stanwix MG, Nam AJ, et al: Twenty-six-year experience treating frontal sinus fractures: a novel algorithm based on anatomical fracture pattern and failure of conventional techniques, *Plast Reconstr Surg* 122:1850-1866, 2008.
7. Smith TL, Han JK, Loehrl TA, et al: Endoscopic management of the frontal recess in frontal sinus fractures: a shift in the paradigm? *Laryngoscope* 112:784-790, 2002.
8. Herford AS, Ying T, Brown B: Outcomes of severely comminuted (type III) nasoorbito-ethmoid fractures, *J Oral Maxillofac Surg* 63:1266-1277, 2005.
9. Cultrara A, Turk JB, Har-El G: Midfacial degloving approach for repair of naso-orbital-ethmoid and midfacial fractures, *Arch Facial Plast Surg* 6:133-135, 2004.
10. Cunningham LL, Haug RH: Management of fractures of the frontal sinus and the naso-orbito-ethmoid complex. In *Peterson's principles of oral and maxillofacial surgery*, vol 2, Philadelphia, 2004, BC Decker.
11. Ellis E 3rd: Sequencing treatment for naso-orbito-ethmoid fractures, *J Oral Maxillofac Surg* 51:543-558, 1993.
12. Sargent LA, Rogers GF: Nasoethmoid orbital fractures: diagnosis and management, *J Craniomaxillofac Trauma* 5:19-27, 1999.
13. Papadopoulos H, Salib NK: Management of naso-orbital-ethmoidal fractures, *Oral Maxillofac Surg Clin North Am* 21:221-225, vi, 2009.
14. Mustarde JC: Epicanthus and telecanthus, *Br J Plast Surg* 16:346-356, 1963.
15. Engelstad ME, Bastodkar P: Medial canthopexy with a canthal barb and plate technique, *J Craniofacial Trauma* (in press).
16. Becelli R, Renzi G, Mannino G, et al: Posttraumatic obstruction of lacrimal pathways: a retrospective analysis of 58 consecutive naso-orbitoethmoid fractures, *J Craniofac Surg* 15:29-33, 2004.

Chapter **43**

Frontal Sinus Fractures

Yoh Sawatari, Johanny Caceres

A frontal sinus fracture is a unique facial fracture that often requires complex management. The location of the frontal bone, which contains the frontal sinus, is adjacent to vital structures, including the brain and eyes. A frontal bone fracture often occurs concomitantly with fractures of the skull, orbital roof, and nose, and many times it is associated with Le Fort and naso-orbito-ethmoid (NOE) fractures.[1] In addition, management of a frontal sinus fracture is complicated by the presence of concomitant injuries, mucosal membranes, and the nasofrontal ducts. Evaluation of a patient with a frontal sinus fracture is similar to that for other facial fractures and involves clinical assessment, radiographic evaluation, and formulation of a treatment plan that allows appropriate management. Treatment of a frontal sinus fracture varies greatly because of variations in the fracture pattern. Minimally displaced anterior table fractures are straightforward and treatment is easily accomplished with an open or endoscopic approach. However, the most severely comminuted anterior and posterior fractures often require neurosurgical intervention, cranialization, sinus obliteration, obstruction of the nasofrontal ducts, and reconstruction of the anterior table. In addition to surgical management, follow-up care for patients sustaining a frontal sinus fracture is prolonged and critical. Complications, including osteomyelitis, mucocele, and mucopyocele formation, can cause severe discomfort for the patient and in the most severe state can lead to brain abscess and death. Meticulous preoperative and intraoperative evaluation will lead to accurate assessment of a frontal bone fracture, which will then subsequently lead to the appropriate treatment plan for the patient. Execution of management then becomes critical for the long-term health of the patient and reduction of complications.

ANATOMY

The anatomy of the frontal sinus is one of the most variable in the maxillofacial complex. The frontal sinus is a set of paired cavities in the frontal bone that communicate with the nasal cavity. Frontal sinuses are absent at birth, become well developed by age 6, and reach full size around 12 to 16 years, when they develop as the superior extension of the anterior ethmoidal sinus. Approximately 4% of the general population has absent frontal sinuses,[2] and the left and right aspects of the frontal sinus are usually asymmetric. The frontal sinus is generally separated by a bony septum and drains into the hiatus semilunaris of the middle meatus via the nasofrontal ducts. The presence of a well-defined nasofrontal duct is also variable, with an incidence limited to 15%, whereas in the remaining population the sinus drains via a large hole emptying into the frontal recess.[3] The typical size of a frontal sinus is $3.5 \times 2.5 \times 1.5$ cm, with significant variation. The floor of the frontal sinus forms the orbital roof, whereas the posterior wall separates the anterior cranial fossa from the sinus. The arterial blood supply to the sinus is provided by the supraorbital arteries off the ophthalmic artery and the anterior ethmoidal arteries. Venous drainage is derived from the arterial counterparts, with additional drainage provided by the diploic veins and sagittal sinus. Sensation to the forehead area is provided by the trigeminal nerve, specifically the supraorbital and supratrochlear nerves off the ophthalmic nerve. The supraorbital nerve supplies sensation to the skin from the forehead extending back to the lambdoidal suture of the scalp and the conjunctiva. The epithelial lining of the frontal sinus is consistent with respiratory epithelium. It is composed of pseudostratified ciliated and columnar epithelium with interspersed goblet cells. The mucin produced by goblet cells is effectively cleared by ciliary flow through the nasofrontal ducts.

EPIDEMIOLOGY

A frontal sinus fracture is a facial fracture that occurs mostly in adults. Although the frontal sinus begins development in utero and undergoes a secondary phase of pneumatization between 6 months and 2 years, it is not identifiable on radiographs until the age of 6.[4] The fact that frontal sinus fractures seldom occur in children and adolescents is consistent with this pattern of development. In the general population, the leading cause of a frontal sinus fracture is blunt trauma, with the majority occurring as a result of motor vehicle crashes.[2,5,6] When considering that the frontal bone can sustain between 800 and 2200 lb of force,[7] it is understandable that the incidence of frontal sinus fractures is lower than that of other facial fractures. Frontal sinus fractures account for 5% to 15% of all facial fractures,[8] and a third to half of all frontal sinus fractures are associated with other facial fractures, including orbital and NOE fractures.[9] Males sustain the majority of frontal sinus fractures, between 66% and 91%, and the peak age is between 20 and 30 years.[2,5,6] Of frontal sinus fractures, 43% to 61% had isolated anterior table involvement, 0.6% to 6% had isolated posterior table involvement, 19% to 51% had a combination of anterior and posterior involvement, and 2.5% to 25% had damage to the nasofrontal ducts.[6,10,11]

EVALUATION OF THE FRONTAL SINUS

The three components involved in frontal sinus management include the anterior table, posterior table, and nasofrontal ducts. Each component requires individual attention and can alter the extent of intervention required. Management begins with clinical examination and follows with radiographic evaluation. The clinical manifestations of a frontal sinus fracture vary greatly depending on its severity; however, the mechanisms of trauma, particularly motor vehicle crashes, warrant thorough evaluation of the facial skeleton. In any patient with altered mental status, an evaluation for possible skull fractures must be performed. Any lacerations, contusions, edema, and frontal or periorbital ecchymosis may be suggestive of frontal sinus injury. Additionally, if there is crepitus in the frontal, supraorbital, or nasofrontal areas, attention must be focused on the possibility of frontal sinus or nasofrontal duct injury. Finally, any patient with the aforementioned clinical findings should be evaluated for possible cerebrospinal fluid (CSF) leakage secondary to fractures of

the posterior table of the frontal sinus, cribriform plate, or fovea ethmoidalis.[12] CSF leakage has been documented to occur in as many as a third of all frontal sinus injuries.[13] The diagnosis of the CSF leakage can be made clinically by the ring test, or any fluid suggestive of CSF can be sent for analysis. In general, CSF fluid will have a higher concentration of chloride and a lower concentration of sodium than found in serum. However, the two most reliable tests for diagnosing CSF are beta$_2$-transferrin and beta-trace proteins. Beta$_2$-transferrin is a protein produced by neuraminidase activity in the brain, which is found only in CSF and perilymph. Beta-trace protein has higher predictive value, and the CSF-to-serum ratio of beta-trace protein is the highest of all CSF-specific proteins.[14] Therefore, any fluid with the presence of beta$_2$-transferrin or beta-trace protein is confirmatory of the presence of CSF.

The clinical examination must also include a neurologic examination because of the disproportionately high incidence of neurologic injury (50%) occurring concomitantly with a frontal sinus fracture.[9] Finally, ocular examination is necessary because of the proximity of the globe to the affected bone and the 25% incidence of ophthalmologic injury occurring concurrently with frontal sinus fractures.[9,15]

Once the clinical examination is completed, a radiographic examination is diagnostic for injuries to the frontal sinus and any other fractures often associated with the frontal sinus fracture. In past literature, authors have discussed the use of plain films; however, at the present time, any patient who sustains severe maxillofacial trauma will undergo non–contrast-enhanced facial computed tomography (CT). Facial CT is currently the most versatile diagnostic tool used to confirm the presence of a frontal sinus fracture. In addition, the severity of the fracture, concomitant fractures adjacent to the frontal sinus injury, and the presence of any foreign bodies can be evaluated effectively with CT.

The anterior table is more susceptible to fracture because of its anterior position. However, its cortex is far thicker than that of the posterior table, and it represents one of the horizontal buttresses of the maxillofacial complex. The general rule for management is well documented and states that any fracture of the anterior cortex greater than one cortex width requires intervention.[16] The rationale behind the one cortex width involves the resultant cosmetic deformity that develops because of displacement of the bone in a very conspicuous position on the face. Minimally displaced, isolated anterior table fractures do not usually cause any functional deficiencies. Anterior table fractures can occur in isolation or can extend from a concomitant NOE fracture or a Le Fort II or III fracture. Management of an anterior table fracture with regard to access, reduction, and fixation varies depending on its severity. For a minimally displaced anterior table fracture, conservative endoscopic management for reduction or recontouring has been reported.[17] If the anterior table fracture is severely comminuted or open, direct access to the bone is required (Fig. 43-1). Once generous access is established, visual assessment of the frontal sinus and evaluation of the nasofrontal duct can be performed. If the nasofrontal ducts are patent, the surgeon may proceed with the appropriate reduction and fixation of the anterior table fracture.

The second component of a frontal sinus fracture is the posterior table. The posterior table is thinner and provides less support; however, when fractured, it can lead to much more significant consequences. With the brain being directly adjacent to the posterior table, any force great enough to fracture the posterior table may lead to intracranial injury, including intracranial hematomas, contusions, dural tears, and a subsequent rise in intracranial pressure. The incidence of isolated posterior table involvement in a frontal sinus fracture is exceedingly rare, but when it occurs in combination with

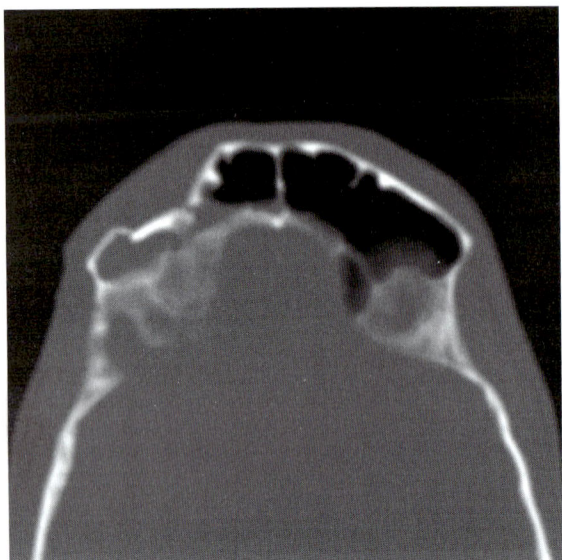

Fig. 43-1 ■ Displaced anterior table of a frontal sinus fracture.

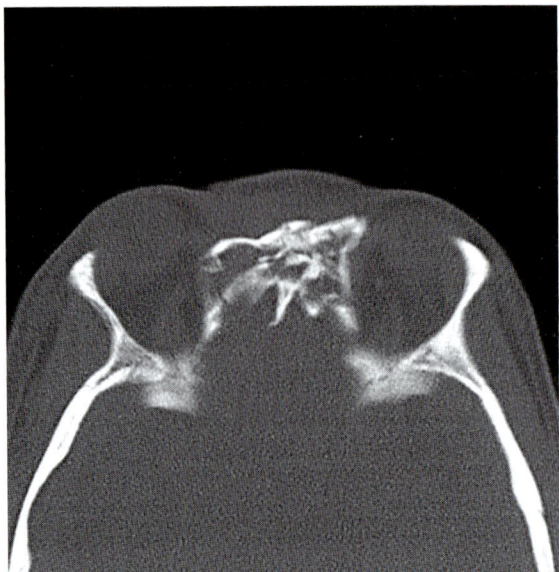

Fig. 43-3 ■ Concomitant comminuted naso-orbito-ethmoid fracture leading to an obstructed nasofrontal duct.

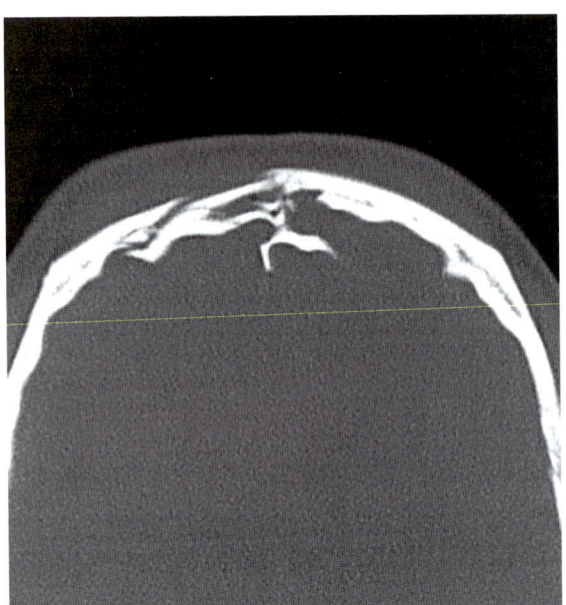

Fig. 43-2 ■ Displaced anterior and posterior tables in a patient with a frontal sinus fracture.

involvement of the anterior table, the incidence of intracranial injury and nasofrontal duct injury and the need for neurosurgical intervention increase significantly (Fig. 43-2). If the situation dictates, neurosurgical intervention is the highest priority for maintenance of the patient's life. Unlike isolated anterior table fractures, when the posterior table or the nasofrontal ducts are compromised, far more extensive surgical intervention is required. In the case of posterior table involvement in frontal sinus fractures, the determinant used for surgical intervention does not involve the displacement of a single cortical width, as for the anterior table. Reduction or débridement of a posterior table fracture is more influenced by neurosurgical need. If the patient has a significant dural tear with a persistent CSF leak, intracranial hemorrhage that necessitates evacuation, brain contusion with associated cerebral edema, and elevated intracranial pressure, craniotomy will be required to manage the injury to the

brain. This obligates removal of the posterior table, obliteration of the frontal sinus, and obliteration of the nasofrontal ducts.

The third component of a frontal sinus fracture is the nasofrontal duct. The frontal sinus, similar to other paranasal sinuses, is functional and has a lining of ciliated columnar epithelium. The ciliated epithelium is responsible for evacuation of the mucus produced by the goblet cells distributed within the epithelium. The mucosa of the frontal sinus is continuous with the ethmoidal air cells and the nasofrontal ducts. Cilia transport the mucus in a clockwise fashion through the frontal sinus, nasofrontal ducts, and hiatus semilunaris and eventually into the nose.[9] In the event that a patient's nasofrontal ducts are damaged, the mucus that is produced and circulated has no means of evacuation. In addition, with damage to the epithelium secondary to the fracture, drainage from goblet cells is also compromised and leads to potential mucocele or mucopyocele formation. When drainage of the nasofrontal ducts is compromised, the surgeon is obligated to open the frontal sinus and proceed with obstruction of the ducts and sinus. Nasofrontal duct patency is not usually affected by minimally displaced anterior table fractures. The most common cause of nasofrontal duct damage is concomitant injuries, including NOE and Le Fort fractures of the maxilla (Fig. 43-3). The nasal, ethmoid, lacrimal, maxillary, and frontal bones become comminuted and tear the sinus membrane and ductal epithelium, thereby obstructing the passage of mucus from the frontal sinus to the nose.

A variety of classification systems for fractures of the frontal sinus have appeared in the literature.[1,5,15] The main objective of classification systems for facial trauma has always involved transfer of information between providers and assistance in planning treatment and management. However, rather than using a classification system, with regard to the frontal sinus, it may be best to focus on the specific components of the frontal sinus, including the anterior table, posterior table, and nasofrontal ducts, as well as the need for neurosurgical intervention. Bell and co-workers have described a protocol for management of frontal sinus fractures emphasizing sinus preservation, based on the amount of displacement or communition of the anterior and/or posterior table, the integrity of the nasofrontal duct, and the neurologic status of the patient.[18-20] An algorithm for treatment is oftentimes more effective in delineating the necessary intervention (Fig. 43-4).

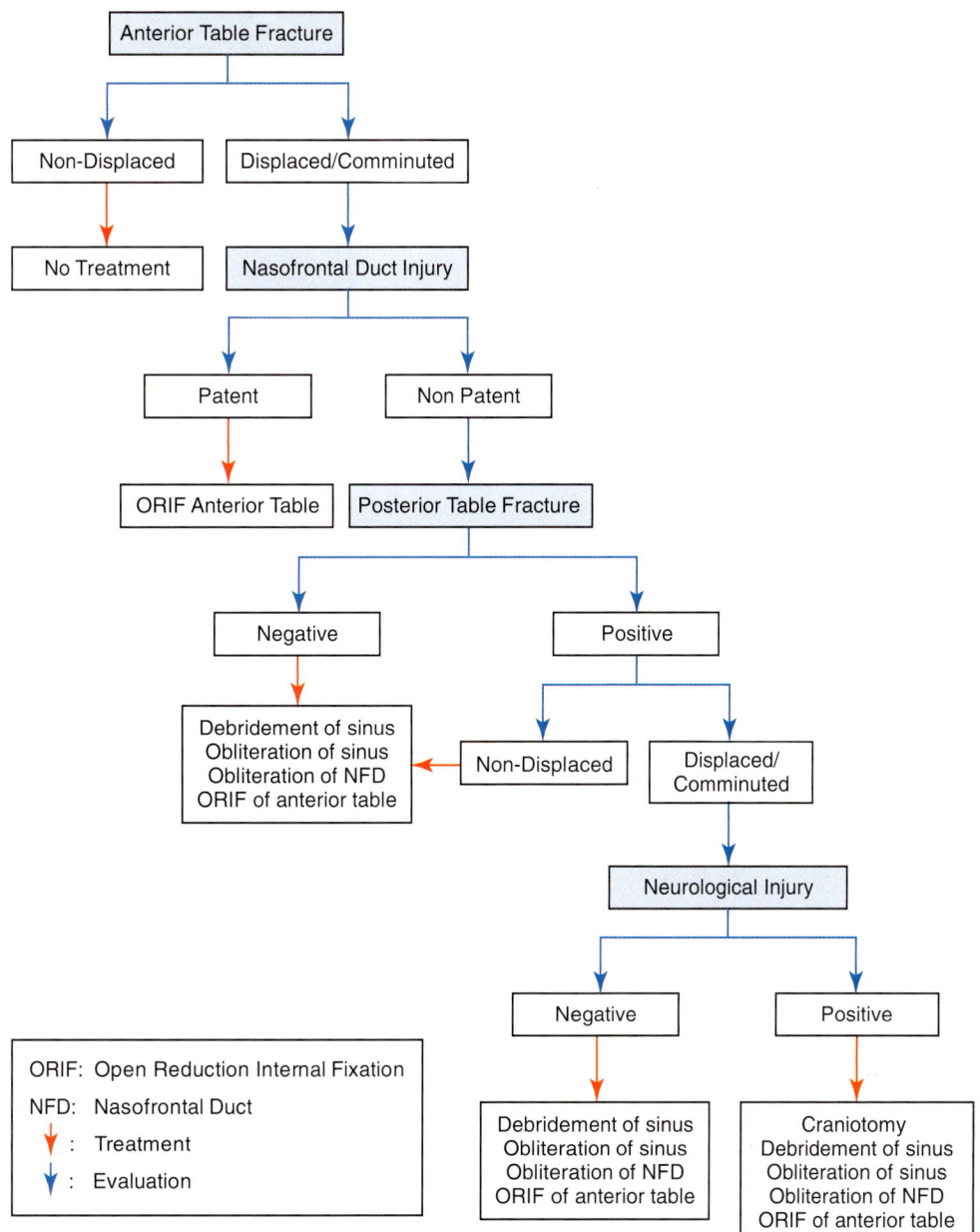

Fig. 43-4 ■ Algorithm used for the management of frontal sinus fractures.

TREATMENT OF THE FRONTAL SINUS

As with all facial fractures, the one critical aspect is access to the fracture. Generous access not only allows appropriate evaluation and management but also expedites surgical reduction and fixation. For isolated anterior table fractures, a preexisting laceration offering generous access is always the most ideal (Fig. 43-5); however, since the mechanism is usually blunt trauma in most instances, additional incisions for access need to be made. A coronal incision is the most versatile and cosmetic incision available to access all components of the frontal sinus, in addition to concomitant fractures, including NOE, Le Fort, and comminuted zygomaticomaxillary complex fractures. Additional incisions have been used, including the open-sky and Lynch incisions. However, such incisions usually leave significant scarring, and unless the patient has deep rhytides in the nasofrontal area, these incisions are very much discouraged. For anterior table frontal sinus fractures, once

dissection reaches the area of the fracture, the comminuted segments are reduced and fixated. Frequently, the comminution is severe and many of the segments are avulsed or significantly displaced during dissection. In these situations, fracture reduction mimics a complex jigsaw puzzle. If bone fragments are removed from the field, care must be taken to maintain their orientation. One useful technique involves placement of the segments on a sterile towel with labeling, whereas another technique involves placing marks on the bone segments so that adjacent pieces can be reoriented with each other (Fig. 43-6). If the surgeon haphazardly removes the bone, the reduction and fixation process often becomes prohibitively difficult. The actual fixation can be performed with low-profile miniplates or mesh (Fig. 43-7).

Although isolated posterior table frontal sinus fractures do occur, they are exceedingly rare. If the posterior table is fractured without any evidence of brain injury or dural tear, conservative management, including non-treatment, is recommended (Fig. 43-8). As mentioned

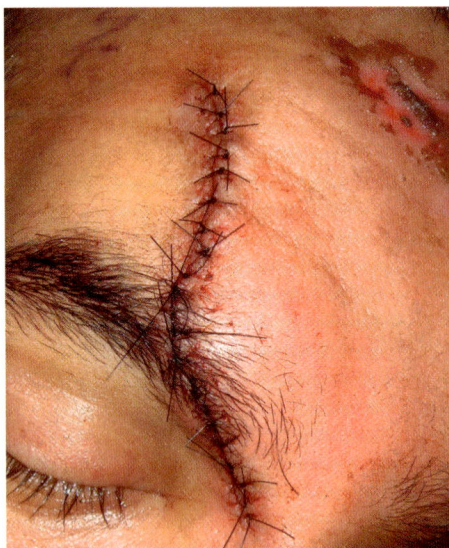

Fig. 43-5 ■ Access to the frontal sinus via an existing laceration.

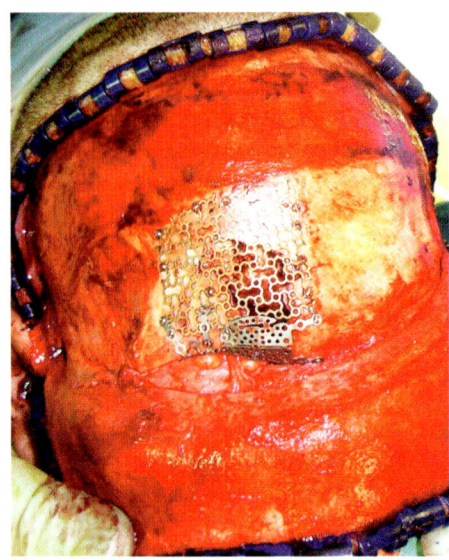

Fig. 43-7 ■ Reconstruction of the anterior table via coronal access with miniplates and mesh.

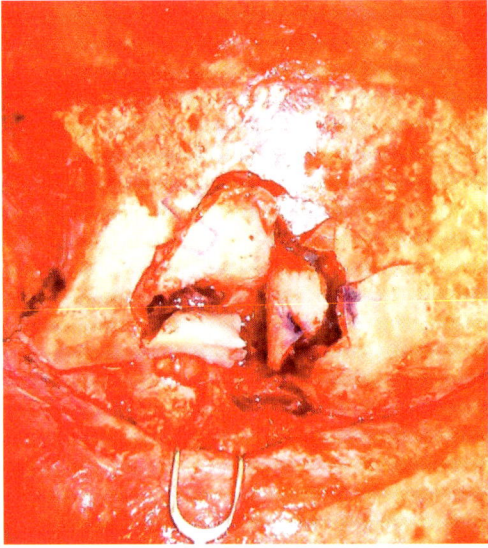

Fig. 43-6 ■ Bone segments marked for orientation after reflection via coronal access.

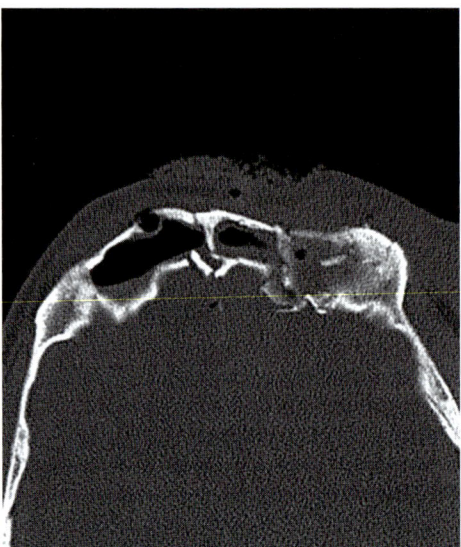

Fig. 43-8 ■ Minimally displaced posterior table frontal sinus fracture with no neurologic injury.

earlier, if the patient sustains an injury great enough to fracture the posterior table, in the majority of cases there will be a concomitant anterior table fracture. With the lack of intracranial injury, including dural tears, surgical intervention will be dictated by the previously mentioned rules for the anterior table, with treatment objectives being determined by displacement and the potential for cosmetic deformity.

For patients who sustain significant posterior table fractures leading to brain injury or patients with suspected or established nasofrontal duct injury, additional surgical procedures are required. For cases that involve anterior table fractures and nasofrontal duct injury, débridement of the sinus membrane and obliteration of the sinus and ducts must be performed. Care is taken to remove the bone segments of the anterior table to provide adequate access to the contents of the frontal sinus. At this point, confirmation of nasofrontal duct patency can be established. The nasofrontal ducts, located in the posteromedial aspect of the frontal sinus,

may be cannulated with an angiocatheter and methylene blue, sterile milk, fluorescein, or even saline injected.[21] This maneuver can clinically establish the patency of the nasofrontal ducts. If the ducts are not patent, the sinus membrane must be meticulously débrided. A curet can be used to remove the gross remnants of the sinus membrane with special attention to crevasses and areas adjacent to internal septa. Once thorough débridement has been completed, the next step involves the use of a burr for curettage of the bony cavity of the sinus. The frontal sinus has numerous canals within the bone, termed the foramina of Breschet, that contain invaginations of the sinus membrane.[22] One of the most important aspects of frontal sinus treatment involves débridement of the mucosa. Any residual mucosal tissue that remains may subsequently develop into a mucocele or mucopyocele. The incidence of these complications is exceedingly low; however, when they do occur, significant morbidity results, including brain abscess and even death.

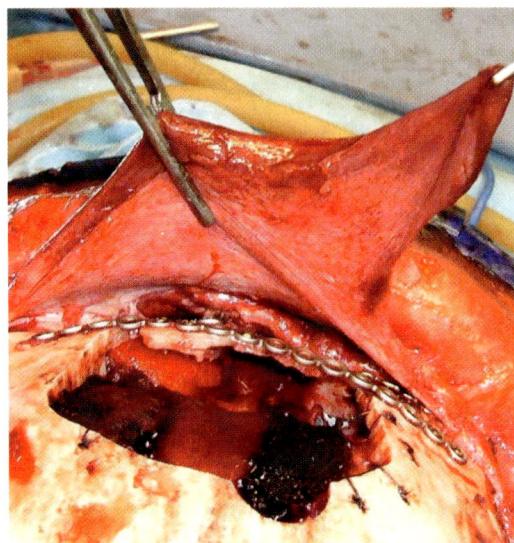

Fig. 43-9 ▪ Sinus obliteration using a pericranial flap after craniotomy.

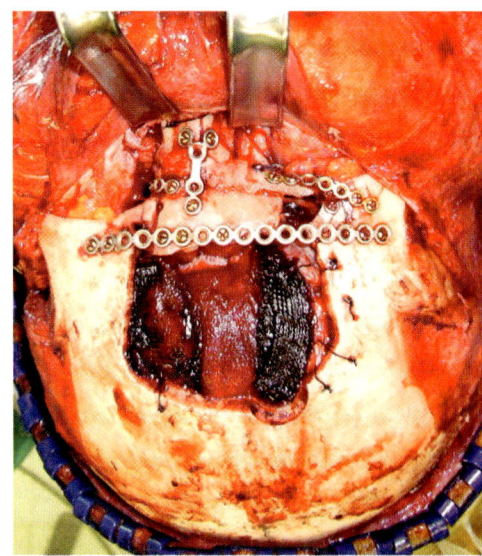

Fig. 43-10 ▪ Dural repair and reconstruction of the frontal bar after craniotomy.

After the sinus has been appropriately débrided, obliteration of the frontal sinus and the nasofrontal ducts is performed. There is great variability in the different materials that may be used for frontal sinus obliteration. The choice of material is based on surgeon experience and surgical convenience and includes pericranial flap, temporalis muscle, and most commonly, abdominal fat. The only recommendation generally made regarding the choice of material is avoidance of the use of alloplastic products, including hydroxyapatite and polymethylmethacrylate.[8] In general, the pericranial flap is both versatile and predictable and can easily be used for obliteration of the frontal sinus. A coronal flap provides surgical access, and a subgaleal flap is reflected to the supraorbital rims with care taken to avoid damage to the supraorbital and supratrochlear nerves. At this point an incision is made parallel to the coronal suture, and parallel incisions are made bilaterally along the temporal lines of fusion. Subperiosteal dissection proceeds anteriorly, and the pericranium is reflected to the supraorbital area. The reflected sheet of pericranium is then pedicled to the anterior skin flap. This sheet receives its blood supply from the supraorbital and supratrochlear arteries and can be manipulated to fill the dead space volume of the frontal sinus (Fig. 43-9). In addition to obliteration of the frontal sinus, it is also necessary to obliterate the nasofrontal ducts to prevent any nasal contaminants from migrating and entering the frontal sinus area. As for obliteration of the frontal sinus, a variety of materials may be used for this purpose, including abdominal fat, temporalis muscle, and bone fragments.[9] The obliteration procedures are then followed by reconstruction of the anterior table. If the original fragments of the anterior table bone can be used, they may be pieced together for reconstruction, and the skin flap is subsequently closed. If the fragments cannot be pieced together because of severe comminution or avulsion, the area can be reconstructed with autogenous bone or mesh.[23]

In the worst-case scenario when patient management requires cranialization, the posterior and anterior tables of the frontal sinus are removed. Removal allows the edematous brain to expand within the volume of the frontal sinus, thus decreasing intracranial pressure and further brain injury (Fig. 43-10). Once the cranialization is completed, the frontal sinus will be obliterated along with the nasofrontal ducts. The same protocol will be used as described for the management of a severely fractured posterior table fracture.

FOLLOW-UP

Diligent follow-up is then necessary as with any other postoperative patient. However, in the case of frontal sinus injury, the follow-up period is prolonged because of the incidence of delayed mucocele, mucopyocele, and brain abscess formation. Clinical examination is recommended weekly for the first postoperative month, then every 3 months for up to a year, and then every year for 5 years. After the initial 5 years, a follow-up examination should be performed every 5 years for life.[24] In addition, patients generally undergo follow-up CT scans at 1 week, 6 months, and 1 year. Additional CT evaluation is then required every year for 5 years after surgery or immediately when symptoms dictate.

COMPLICATIONS OF FRONTAL SINUS FRACTURES

Complications of frontal sinus fractures can be related to the injury or to the treatment. They can be cosmetic or functional and in some cases can be life-threatening.[6] Affected patients are at lifelong risk for complications, and the overall complication rate approaches 10% to 20%. Early complications occur during the first 4 to 6 months after trauma and include wound infection, CSF leaks, meningitis, pneumocephalus, sinusitis, and potentially death. Late complications generally occur after the 6-month period and include mucocele, mucopyocele, osteomyelitis, brain abscess, cosmetic deformity, and chronic pain.

EARLY COMPLICATIONS

Infections

Infections are not uncommon after facial trauma and occur more frequently than desired. As with any acute soft tissue or postoperative infection, identification of the cause of the infection is critical for management. For any infection to develop, two components are required: bacteria and a host site. As with any traumatic injury, bacteria are almost always introduced into the wound. The more important issue is whether the wound has a means of managing the bacteria. For frontal sinus fractures, bacteria can be introduced through an open wound or surgically during the access procedure, or they can migrate superiorly from the nose. The introduction is not as concerning as the means of evacuating the sinus. Therefore, as discussed earlier, one major component of a frontal sinus fracture is the nasofrontal duct. If the frontal sinus fracture or any concomitant NOE or Le Fort fracture causes obstruction of the nasofrontal duct, the frontal sinus is unable to circulate mucus and bacteria out of the sinus, which may in turn lead to an infection. Similarly, when evacuation is compromised, the collection may become secondarily infected and complicate fracture management in the event that a hematoma or seroma forms in the area of the fracture. Any collection that becomes infected can potentially progress to an epidural empyema. These infections may then lead to acute epidural or cerebral abscesses and meningitis via perforation through bone. Meningitis is a serious complication that occurs in approximately 5% to 10% of patients who sustain frontal sinus injuries.[25] Obliterative procedures will fail if the sinus mucosa is not meticulously removed from all internal aspects of the sinus with cutting burrs or if the nasal mucosa has migrated into the frontal sinus as a result of incomplete obstruction of the frontonasal duct. Finally, one additional source of infection involves residual non-vital bone or foreign bodies within the sinus cavity.

Management of a postoperative infection of the frontal sinus is essentially the same as for any other infection. It involves identification of the cause, aggressive surgical débridement of any potential nidus, drainage of any collections, and intravenous administration of antibiotics. In addition, CT imaging is very useful in the management of postoperative infections because of its versatility in identifying collections or possible foreign bodies. Revision of a frontal sinus obliteration that has failed requires identification of the cause of the failure, which may be retained mucosa in the frontal sinus, mucosal ingrowth from the nose or ethmoid sinuses, or the presence of granulation tissue in the dead space. If the infection involves a large portion of the obliterated sinus or failure is attributed to inadequate sealing of a frontonasal orifice, the entire obliteration must be revised. The problem with mucosal ingrowth can be even more serious if it occurs in a patient who has undergone a cranialization procedure that places the frontonasal orifices within the intracranial cavity.

Cerebrospinal Fluid Leaks

The risk for central nervous system infection is directly proportional to the presence of CSF and approaches 40%.[26] Therefore, diligent postoperative evaluation plus identification of any persistent CSF leak is essential. Similar to the preoperative evaluation, any fluid leaking from the nose postoperatively should be assessed for CSF. CSF leaks in the postoperative setting can most often be treated by bed rest, antibiotics, CSF diversion (lumbar drains to facilitate cessation of leakage), and occasionally extracranial ethmoid obliteration.[27]

Pneumocephalus

Pneumocephalus is the result of fracture of the posterior table in association with a dural tear. Small areas of pneumocephalus can be observed and allowed to resorb. Tension pneumocephalus results from accumulation of air in the subdural space under pressure and can cause a midline shift and compress the brain. The theory of accumulation involves air entering as CSF leaks out. The most common clinical manifestation of a patient with postoperative

pneumocephalus would be headache and possible changes in mental status. If the level of consciousness is not altered, the patient should lie flat and the process may resolve slowly or form a brain hygroma. Surgical decompression of tension pneumocephalus must be performed on an emergency basis if neurologic involvement is present. Wide-spectrum antibiotics and antiseizure medications should always be used in addition to the management of intracranial pressure.

LATE COMPLICATIONS

A mucocele is an expansile lesion of the sinus that becomes filled with fluid and continues to expand secondary to blockage of the nasofrontal duct; if and when it becomes infected, it is termed a mucopyocele. Mucoceles can appear up to 50 years after injury.[28] Frontal headaches, fullness in the forehead and upper eyelid region, diplopia, proptosis, nasal discharge, and obstruction are the most frequent clinical manifestations. If the mucocele is confined to the limits of the frontal sinus, the more common symptoms are headache and tenderness. If the mucocele expands and resorbs the inferior wall of the sinus, diplopia, proptosis, and disorders of ocular mobility may develop. Involvement of the posterior sinus wall may allow direct communication with the epidural and intracerebral space. The aggressive nature of mucoceles is believed to be related to several inflammatory components, including osteolytic mediators.[29,30] Disturbances in secretory transport, pathologic pneumatization, and atypical growth of mucosa caused by enhanced bone resorption are factors that contribute to mucocele formation.[29,31] Clinical and experimental evidence suggests that obstruction of the nasofrontal duct is a significant predisposing factor to the development of complications such as mucocele or mucopyocele formation.[32] An anaerobic environment may subsequently develop and cause frontal sinusitis, which may lead to osteomyelitis, meningitis, or brain abscess. Osteomyelitis of the frontal bone may occur either from compressive forces, from direct extension of infection from the frontal sinus into the surrounding marrow space, or even by way of the valveless diploic venous system. Finally, a pericranial abscess, or Pott's puffy tumor, is often associated with frontal bone obliteration or cranialization of the frontal sinus.

Poor Cosmetic Outcomes

Irregular forehead contours can usually be attributed to one or more of the following: (1) failure to recognize a fracture-dislocation that has produced a depression in the glabellar or medial supraorbital ridge area; (2) poor initial realignment or inadequate stabilization of displaced fragments that collapse with time across the forehead span; (3) cicatricial contracture of forehead skin that produces visible outlines of the fixation hardware or areas of less than ideal edge-to-edge reduction of bone fragments; and (4) loss of bone because of frontal sinus ablation, frontal sinusectomy, or craniectomy. Downward displacement of the globe can also occur and be caused by failure to restore the contour and level of the orbital projection of the frontal bone. The normal upward convexity of the roof is difficult to duplicate, and a reconstructed roof that seems to be at the correct level is often too flat, thereby pushing the globe inferiorly. Another cosmetic deformity can be caused by the lack of well-vascularized soft tissue coverage. Severe lacerations or contracture of forehead skin or scalp into large defects prevents camouflage of the bony irregularities and results in poor cosmesis of the forehead and scalp.

PEARLS AND PITFALLS

- Management of cosmetic deformities most often requires surgical intervention.
- The justification for corrective surgery is different from the necessity for management of osteomyelitis or mucopyocele.
- Most complications related to a frontal sinus fracture can be associated with significant morbidity; however, a poor cosmetic outcome

does not necessarily relate to the patient's well-being but to self-consciousness and societal acceptance.
- This type of surgical correction requires consideration of its benefits versus its potential complications.
- Management of cosmetic deformities often requires implant placement, rotational flaps, scar revision, and at worst, re-osteotomy.

REFERENCES

1. Tiwari P, Higuera S, Thornton J, et al: The management of frontal sinus fractures, *J Oral Maxillofac Surg* 63:1354-1360, 2005.
2. Helmy ES, Koh ML, Bays RA: Management of frontal sinus fractures: review of the literature and clinical update, *Oral Surg Oral Med Oral Pathol* 69:137-148, 1990.
3. Stanley RB: Fractures of the frontal sinus, *Clin Plast Surg* 16:115-123, 1989.
4. Chuang S, Dodson T: Evaluation and management of frontal sinus injuries. In Fonseca R, et al, editors: *Oral and maxillofacial trauma*, ed 3, St Louis, 2005, WB Saunders, pp 721-735.
5. Gonty AA, Marciani RD, Adornato DC: Management of frontal sinus fractures: a review of 33 cases, *J Oral Maxillofac Surg* 57:372-379, 1999.
6. Gerbino G, Roccia F, Benech A, et al: Analysis of 158 frontal sinus fractures: current surgical management and complications, *J Craniomaxillofac Surg* 28:133-139, 2000.
7. Lakhani RS, Shibuya TY, Mathog RH, et al: Titanium mesh repair of the severely comminuted frontal sinus fracture, *Arch Otolaryngol Head Neck Surg* 127:665-669, 2001.
8. Fattahi T, Johnson C, Steinberg B: Comparison of 2 preferred methods used for frontal sinus obliteration, *J Oral Maxillofac Surg* 63:487-491, 2005.
9. Manolidis S, Hollier L Jr: Management of frontal sinus fractures, *Plast Reconstr Surg* 120(6 Suppl 2):32S-48S, 2007.
10. Onishi K, Nakajima T, Yoshimura Y: Treatment and therapeutic devices in the management of frontal sinus fractures. Our experience with 42 cases, *J Craniomaxillofac Surg* 17:58-63, 1989.
11. Xie C, Mehendale N, Barrett D, et al: 30-year retrospective review of frontal sinus fractures: the Charity Hospital experience, *J Craniomaxillofac Trauma* 6:7-15, 2000.
12. Stanley RB Jr: Management of severe frontobasilar skull fractures, *Otolaryngol Clin North Am* 24:139-150, 1991.
13. Rohrich RJ, Hollier LH: Management of frontal sinus fractures: changing concepts, *Clin Plast Surg* 19:219-232, 1992.
14. Bachman G, Petereit H, Djenabi UC, et al: Predictive values of beta-trace protein by use of laser-nephelometry assay for the identification of cerebrospinal fluid, *Neurosurgery* 50:571-577, 2002.
15. Monolidis S: Frontal sinus injuries: associated injuries and surgical management of 93 patients, *J Oral Maxillofac Surg* 62:882-891, 2004.
16. Fattahi T: Management of frontal sinus fractures. In Fonseca R, et al, editors: *Oral and maxillofacial surgery*, ed 2, St Louis, 2008, WB Saunders, pp 256-269.
17. Strong EB, Buchalter GM, Moulthrop TH: Endoscopic repair of isolated anterior table frontal sinus fractures, *Arch Facial Plast Surg* 5:514-521, 2003.
18. Bell RB: Management of frontal sinus fractures, *Oral Maxillofac Surg Clin North Am* 21(2):227-242, 2009.
19. Bell RB, Chen J: Frontobasilar fractures: contemporary management, *Atlas Oral Maxillofac Surg Clin North Am* 18(2):181-196, 2010.
20. Bell RB, Dierks EJ, Brar P, et al: A protocol for the management of frontal sinus fractures emphasizing sinus preservation, *J Oral Maxillofac Surg* 65(5):825-839, 2007.
21. Cunningham L Jr, Haug R: Management of frontal sinus and naso-orbitoethmoid complex fractures. In Miloro M, Ghali G, Larsen P, et al, editors: *Peterson's principles of oral and maxillofacial surgery*, ed 2, Hamilton, Ontario, Canada, 2004, BC Decker, pp 491-507.
22. Mosher HP: A method of obliterating the naso-frontal duct and catheterizing the frontal sinus, *Laryngoscope* 21:946-947, 1911.
23. Montgomery WM: State-of-the-art for osteoplastic frontal sinus operation, *Otolaryngol Clin North Am* 34:167-177, 2001.
24. Haug RH, Cunningham LL: Management of fractures of the frontal bone and frontal sinus, *Select Readings Oral Maxillofac Surg* 10(6):1-32, 2002.
25. Neel HB, McDonald TJ, Facer GW: Modified Lynch procedure for chronic frontal sinus disease: rationale, technique, and long-term results, *Laryngoscope* 97:1274-1279, 1987.
26. Terrell JE: Primary sinus surgery. In Cummings CW, Frederickson JM, Harker LA, et al, editors: *Otolaryngology: head and neck surgery*, St. Louis, 1998, CV Mosby, pp 1145-1172.
27. Bell RB, Dierks EJ, Homer L, et al: Management of cerebrospinal fluid leaks associated with craniomaxillofacial trauma, *J Oral Maxillofac Surg* 62:676-684, 2004.
28. Mourouzis C, Evans BT, Shenouda E: Late presentation of a mucocele of the frontal sinus: 50 years post injury, *J Oral Maxillofac Surg* 66:1510-1513, 2008.
29. Constantinidis J, Steinhardt H, Schwerdtfeger K, et al: Therapy of invasive mucoceles of the frontal sinus, *Rhinology* 39:33-38, 2001.
30. Lund VJ, Henderson B, Song Y: Involvement of cytokines and vascular adhesion receptors in the pathology of fronto-ethmoidal mucoceles, *Acta Otolaryngol* 113:430-446, 1993.
31. Lund VJ, Wilson H, Meghji S, et al: Prostaglandin synthesis in the pathogenesis of fronto-ethmoidal mucoceles, *Acta Laryngol* 106:145-151, 1988.
32. Heller EM, Jacobs JB, Holliday RA: Evaluation of the frontonasal duct in frontal sinus fractures, *Head Neck* 11:46-50, 1989.

44

Pan-facial Trauma

Alan S. Herford

Treatment of complex pan-facial fractures can present unique challenges. Pan-facial trauma results in severe injury to the hard and soft tissues of the face and associated structures. These fractures are often comminuted and treatment must be individualized for each patient. These injuries are frequently complicated by concomitant injuries that can delay early repair. Inadequate early treatment often leads to secondary deformities that are difficult to treat. With the availability of detailed imaging, rigid fixation, primary bone grafting, proper sequencing, and soft tissue resuspension, outcomes can be optimized.

ETIOPATHOGENESIS/CAUSATIVE FACTORS

Patients with pan-facial fractures represent a small proportion of the overall patient population with facial fractures. Because of the force necessary to cause pan-facial injury, these patients often have other concomitant injuries.[1] Late complications can also occur with these fracture patterns.[2] Follmar and colleagues found that 53% of their patients had concomitant injuries, with intracranial injury or hemorrhage being the most common.[3] Mithani and co-authors reviewed 4786 patients treated for facial fractures and found that among all those with facial fractures, 461 (9.6%) also had cervical spine injuries and 2175 (45.4%) had associated head injuries.[4] Fractures of the upper part of the face were associated with an increased likelihood for mid to lower cervical spine injuries, severe intracranial injuries, and increased mortality rates. Bilateral mid-face injuries were associated with basilar skull fracture and death. Cranio-maxillofacial fractures are commonly associated with head and cervical spine injuries that involve predictable patterns of dispersion of force from the maxillofacial skeleton and transmission to the cranial vault and cervical spine. Concomitant injuries should be investigated closely with distinct types of facial fractures.

PATHOLOGIC ANATOMY

The anatomic patterns of fractures provide a useful framework for classifying these injuries. By categorizing the fracture patterns and highlighting the variables that may affect fracture management, surgeons can expand interpretation of the fracture pattern into a clinically useful diagnosis that affects fracture management.[5] Markowitz and associates described a useful classification system for naso-orbito-ethmoid (NOE) fractures based on the central bone fragment that provides attachment to the medial canthal tendon.[6]

The buttress system of the face absorbs and transmits forces and includes horizontal and vertical buttresses (Fig. 44-1). The vertical buttresses include the nasomaxillary (including the maxillary process of the frontal bone), zygomaticomaxillary, and pterygomaxillary buttresses and the posterior mandible (including the condyle and posterior mandibular ramus). In reconstructing pan-facial fractures, particular attention should be directed to restoring these buttresses to provide the most stable result. The pterygomaxillary buttress is not typically reconstructed because of difficulty accessing it.

DIAGNOSTIC STUDIES

Computed tomography (CT) has greatly added to the preoperative appreciation of the extent of fractures. It allows one to formulate a treatment plan, including surgical approaches and the sequencing of fracture repair. Axial, coronal, and sagittal views are helpful, as well as three-dimensional views, especially in patients with severely comminuted fractures (Fig. 44-2). Three-dimensional CT has not been shown to have increased accuracy for identifying mandibular fractures and is associated with decreased visualization of the soft tissues and deep internal architecture of the orbits. Two-dimensional CT more accurately displays injuries involving the paranasal sinuses, orbital walls, and soft tissues.[7] CT combined with navigation also provides the clinician with a technique that can optimize treatment.[8] Intraoperative CT allows more precise reduction of fractures and is especially useful for severe pan-facial fractures, as well as large orbital fractures.

TREATMENT/RECONSTRUCTIVE GOALS

The goals of treatment are to restore the face to as close to the pre-injury state as possible. This is accomplished by accurate reduction and fixation of the various fractures with special attention directed at restoring facial height, width, and projection. Treatment should focus on restoring both form and function while minimizing the need for secondary surgery.

SEQUENCE OF REDUCTION

Treatment of pan-facial fractures has changed significantly with the advent of rigid fixation, which allows more flexibility in the sequence of repair. The basic key to reconstruction is restoration of facial width, projection, and height. Much has been written about the sequencing of treatment of pan-facial fractures. There are two commonly advocated approaches, with variations, to sequencing of the treatment of pan-facial fractures, including sequences such as "top to bottom and outside-in" or "bottom to top to middle." Gruss and co-workers applied plate and screw fixation to pan-facial fractures in a "top-to-bottom" approach.[9] They advocate reconstruction of the outer facial frame beginning with the zygomatic arch, zygoma, and frontal bar. The inner facial frame (NOE complex) is reduced and stabilized, followed by the internal orbit. The maxilla (Le Fort I level) is then repositioned by aligning it with the now stabilized

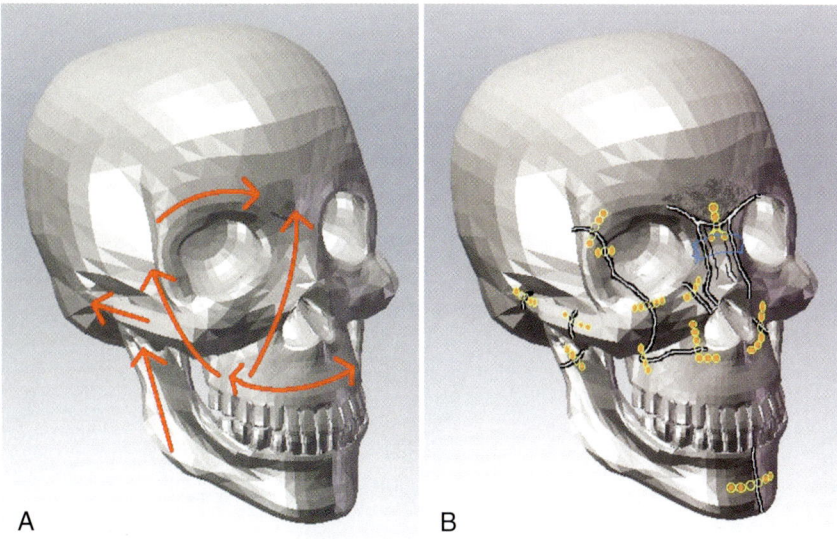

Fig. 44-1 ▪ Vertical and horizontal buttresses of the facial skeleton.

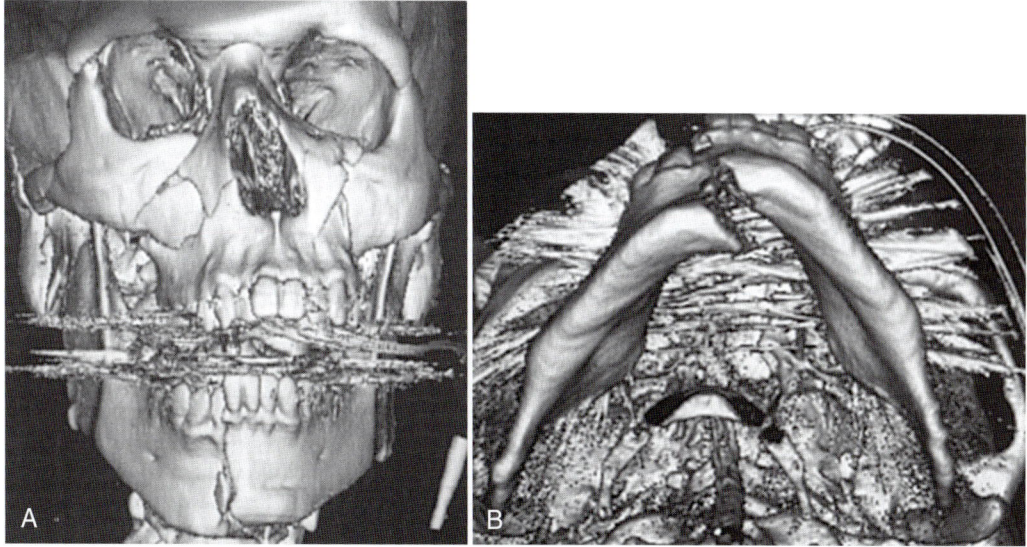

Fig. 44-2 ▪ Computed tomography scans revealing facial fractures. The scans help formulate a treatment plan.

mid-facial buttresses. Maxillomandibular fixation (MMF) is then used to restore the position of the mandible, which is fixated last. This approach does not require reduction and fixation of fractures involving the condylar region.

Others, such as Kelly and colleagues, advocate a "bottom-to-top-to-middle" approach.[10] This approach begins with reconstruction of the mandible, including subcondylar fractures, and placement of MMF. Once the maxillomandibular complex is reconstructed, the frontal and temporal regions are addressed. Naso-orbital fractures are reduced and stabilized. The outer facial frame is reconstructed beginning at the arch to restore facial projection. The internal orbit is reconstructed after the entire upper part of the face and the upper mid-face are repaired. Finally, reduction and fixation across the Le Fort I level are accomplished, with placement of bone grafts as necessary.

The exact sequence of exposure should be organized according to the clinical findings and fracture patterns of each individual patient. Principles to follow include exposure of multiple fractures

before fixation, fixation of fractures that are most stable and able to be anatomically reduced most precisely, and utilization of the occlusion to link the mandible to the lower mid-face. This author most commonly uses a bottom-up and outside-in approach based on these principles (Figs. 44-3 and 44-4). This is predicated on restoring the major vertical buttress in the lower part of the face by opening and fixating fractures involving the subcondylar region. However, if a condylar fracture is extremely comminuted or not conducive to open treatment, it will be necessary to rely on other areas for restoration of posterior facial height (Fig. 44-5). The author is in agreement with Paul Manson and associates, who suggested that "the exact order of treatment is not as important as the development of a plan that permits both flexibility and reproducibly accurate positioning of the various facial segments … any [order of treatment] is satisfactory if one understands the anatomy, goals, and procedures."[11]

The sequence of treatment of NOE fractures includes surgical exposure, identification of the medial canthal tendon/tendon-bearing bone fragment, reduction/reconstruction of the medial orbital rim,

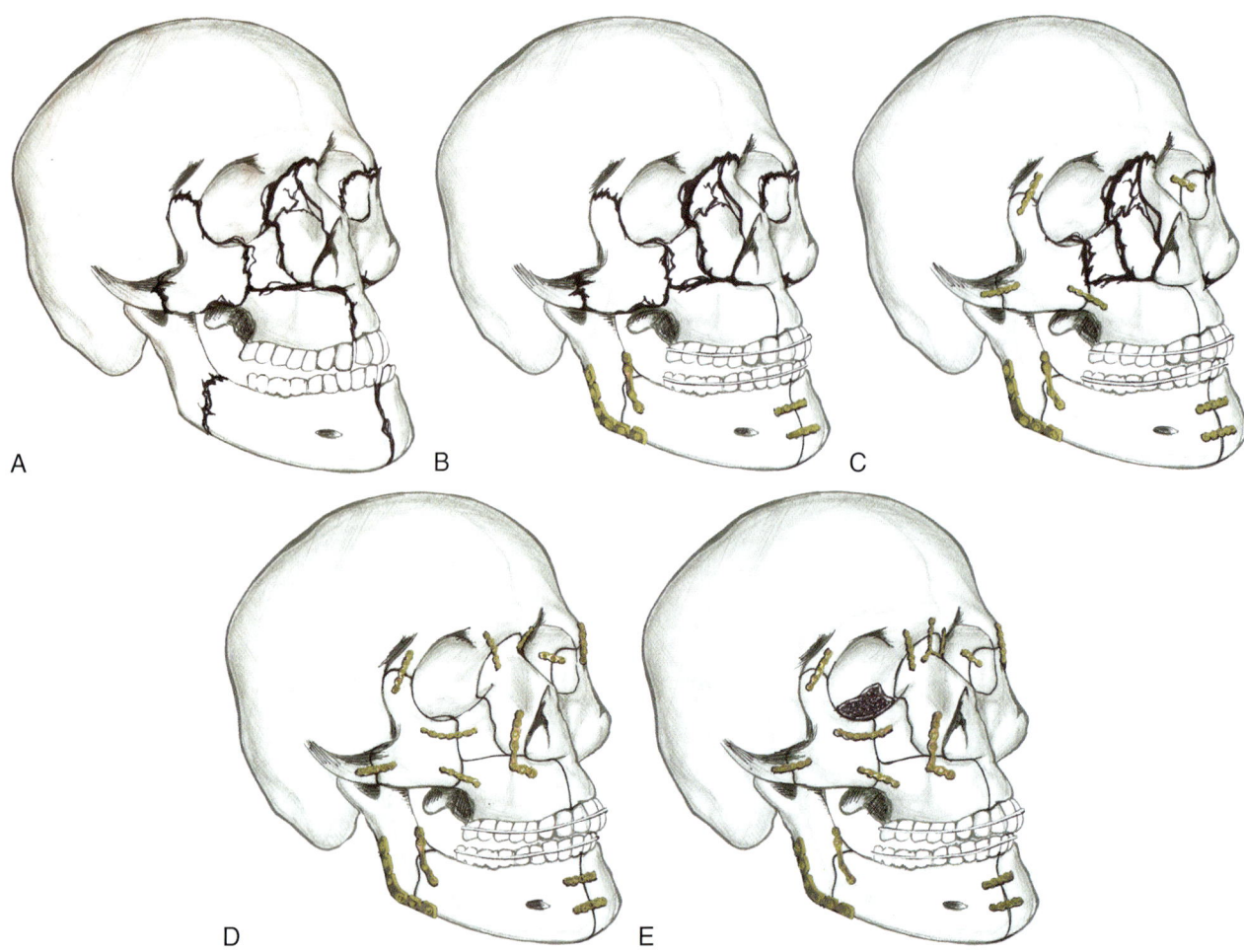

Fig. 44-3 ■ Sequencing of pan-facial treatment.

reconstruction of the medial orbital wall, transnasal canthopexy, reduction of septal fractures, reconstruction/augmentation of the nasal dorsum, and soft tissue adaptation.[12]

SPECIFIC TREATMENT AND TECHNIQUES

Reconstruction of the facial buttresses is important to achieve stable results.[11] When treating the NOE region in patients with pan-facial fractures, the importance of addressing the medial canthal tendon cannot be overemphasized.

The zygomatic arch provides a landmark useful in reestablishing facial projection.[12] It is especially helpful in edentulous patients and those with severe comminution. The zygomatic arch is typically more straight than the usual "arch." Inadequate reduction can lead to decreased facial projection and bowing of the arch with resultant facial fullness on the affected side.

The sphenozygomatic suture, along with the internal surface of the lateral orbital wall, provides a key landmark for reduction of zygomatic fractures. If the orbital roof and superior lateral orbit are intact, this suture can aid in proper positioning of the zygoma. Occasionally, it is necessary to place a small plate to maintain reduction of this important anatomic landmark.

Facial widening is common in patients with pan-facial fractures involving the mandible, especially those involving bilateral condylar fractures and fracture of a symphysis. It is important to visualize

the lingual border of the mandible while applying pressure on each side of the mandible to ensure adequate reduction and narrowing (Fig. 44-6). If inadequately reduced, the face will be widened postoperatively.

TIMING

Early treatment is associated with improved results. However, these fractures are frequently accompanied by other life-threatening injuries, treatment of which requires that management of facial fractures be delayed. If repair of extensive fractures is not accomplished before the onset of significant edema, it is often helpful to delay surgical intervention until some of the edema resolves, especially when using transconjunctival incisions to access the orbital floor and rim.

AIRWAY MANAGEMENT

Most dentate pan-facial fractures require intermaxillary fixation to support proper reduction of the fractures. It is frequently possible to wire the teeth together when the patient is orally intubated, with the orotracheal tube placed lateral to the teeth. It is helpful to wire the tube to the teeth to avoid inadvertent displacement during surgery. If the patient has extensive associated injuries, oral intubation is not possible, or prolonged intubation is required, a definitive surgical airway should be considered. This could include tracheostomy or submental tracheal intubation.[13]

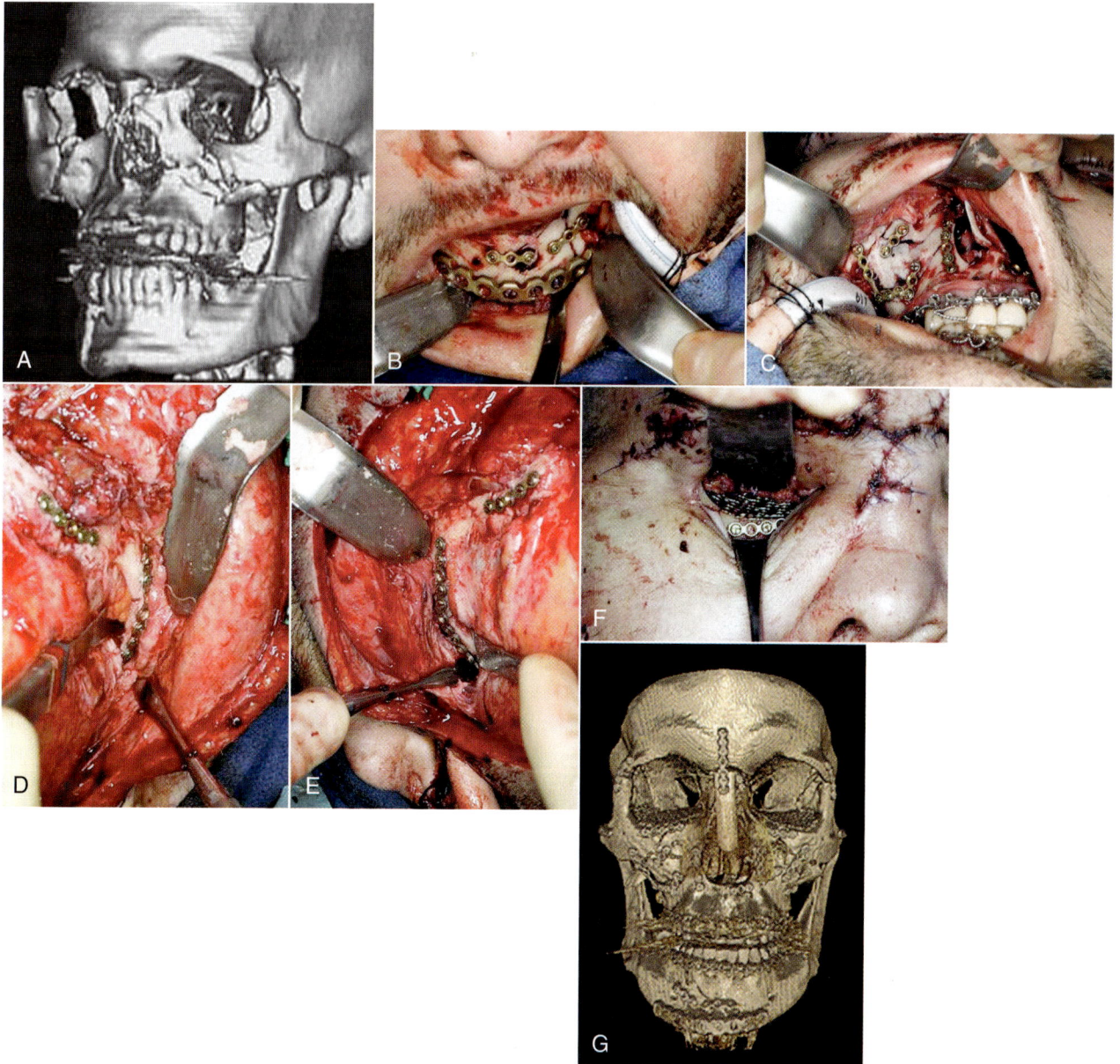

Fig. 44-4 ■ **A,** Pan-facial fractures. **B,** Repair of mandibular fractures to provide a stable base. **C,** Repair of mid-face fractures. Note that intraoperative maxillomandibular fixation is used. **D** and **E,** Reduction of the zygomatic arches to aid in reestablishing facial projection. **F,** Repair of the orbital fractures. **G,** Reestablishment of facial form with plate and screw fixation.

EXPOSURE AND FIXATION

Operative techniques for surgical exposure and reduction and fixation of fractures have evolved from standard facial incisions and wire fixation to complete exposure of the cranium and orbits via a coronal flap (Fig. 44-7). Craniofacial exposure techniques provide excellent visualization of the fractures. Typical incisions include intraoral vestibular incisions, lower eyelid incisions (transconjunctival, subciliary), and coronal incisions. Additional incisions may be required, such as submandibular or retromandibular incisions for certain mandibular fractures or exposure of the zygomatic arch through a coronal incision. Existing lacerations can occasionally be used but are not usually in ideal locations for exposure.

The choice of fixation depends on factors such as location and comminution of the fracture. When reconstructing fractures involving the facial buttresses, particularly those with missing bone, it is important to ensure adequate fixation to maintain the position of the bones. In areas that are under less force, such as the inferior orbital rim, smaller plates and screws are often used because larger ones can become palpable and may require removal. Titanium plates or resorbable plates can be used for pan-facial fractures. Fractures involving the mandible in adults frequently require stronger fixation with titanium. Improvement in resorbable technology has led to biodegradable systems with improved handling and sufficient mechanical stability for facial fractures.[14]

REPAIR OF THE NASOLACRIMAL APPARATUS

The incidence of nasolacrimal obstruction after open reduction of NOE fractures ranges from 5% to 21%.[6,15] If injury to the duct is suspected, an attempt can be made to place a silicone tube. However, if difficulty is encountered, further damage to the canaliculi should be avoided. Delayed assessment with possible secondary dacryocystorhinostomy can be performed if obstruction exists.

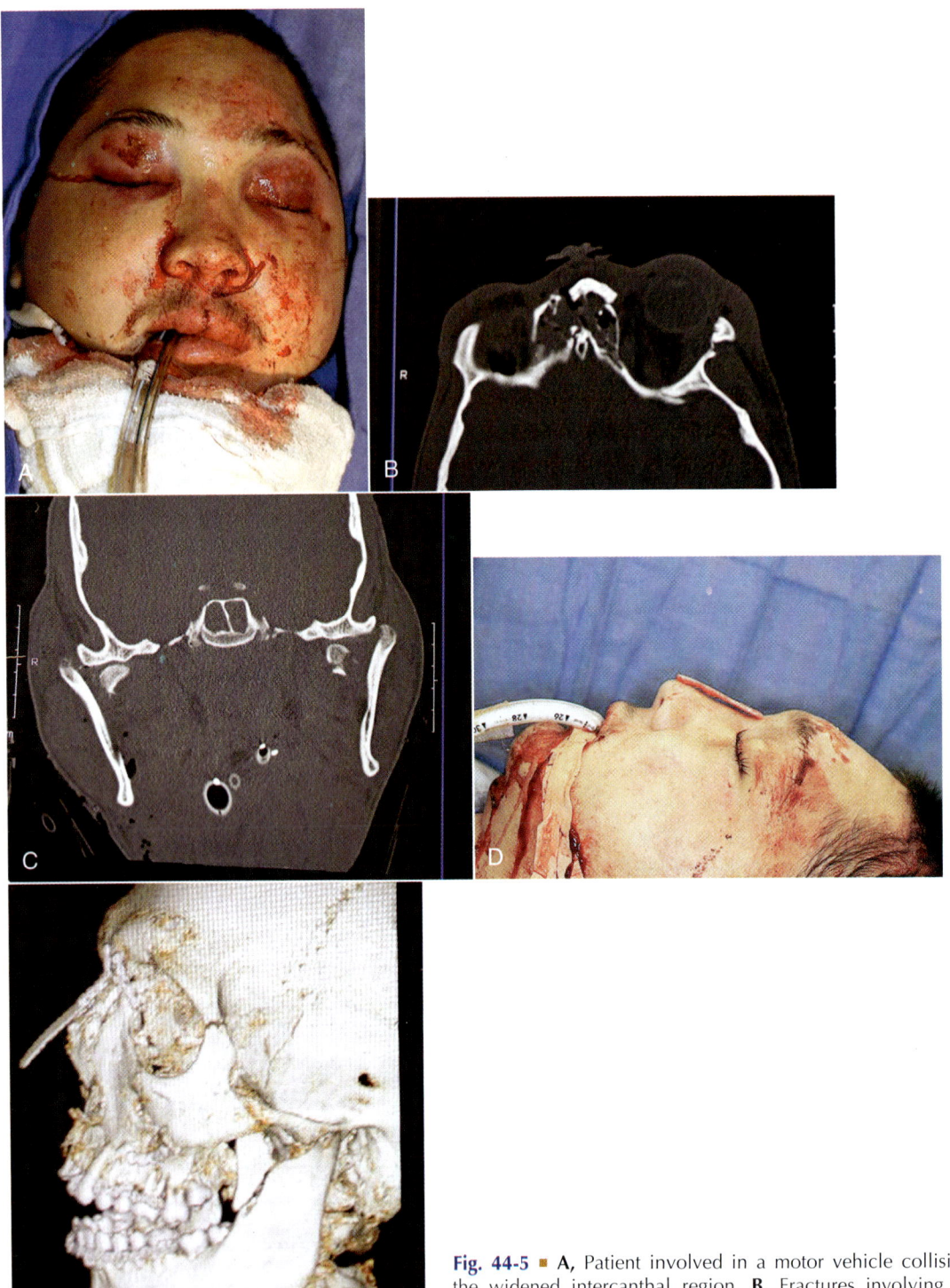

Fig. 44-5 ■ **A,** Patient involved in a motor vehicle collision with multiple fractures. Note the widened intercanthal region. **B,** Fractures involving the naso-orbito-ethmoid region. **C,** Comminuted fractures involving the condylar regions. Condylar fractures treated in closed fashion; mid-face fractures reduced to restore facial height. **D,** Bone graft harvested from the cranium to provide nasal support. **E,** Postoperative view of the reduced fractures.

PRIMARY BONE GRAFTING

Severely comminuted fractures involving the mid-face often require bone grafting, especially in the nasal region.[16] Reconstruction of the dorsum of the nose commonly requires placement of a cantilevered bone graft to prevent a postoperative "saddle" nose appearance. The need for grafting the nasal dorsum can frequently be determined at the time of surgery by palpating and determining the degree of support (Fig. 44-8). Bone harvested from the cranium works well for this area and is harvested through the coronal incision. Grafting promotes bone union, as well as minimizes secondary deformities.

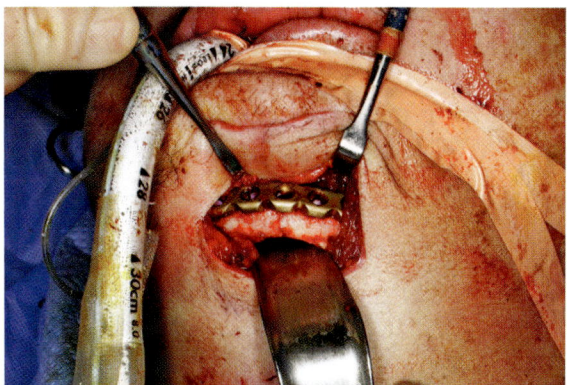

Fig. 44-6 ■ Visualization of the lingual portion of the mandible to achieve adequate reduction and avoid facial widening.

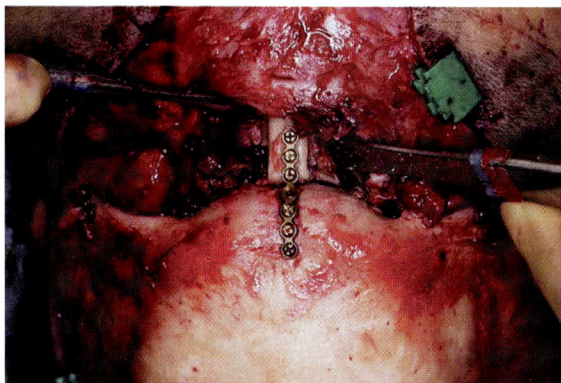

Fig. 44-7 ■ Coronal incision for exposure of upper facial fractures.

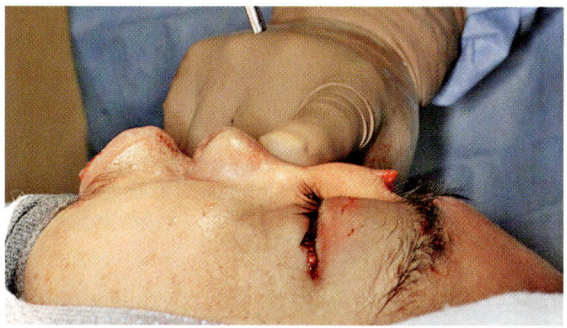

Fig. 44-8 ■ Palpation of the nasal vault after reduction of the naso-orbito-ethmoid portion. A graft is indicated if support is not adequate.

Orbital fractures may also be treated with cranial grafts, especially when a coronal incision is used.

SOFT TISSUE RESUSPENSION/READAPTATION

To avoid secondary defects such as temporal hollowing or lower eyelid teardrop deformities, it is important to resuspend the deep tissues on closing the incisions. When closing the coronal incision, the flap is resuspended to the temporalis fascia. When closing a lower eyelid incision, it is important to close the muscle over the plate because this helps prevent not only ectropion of the lower

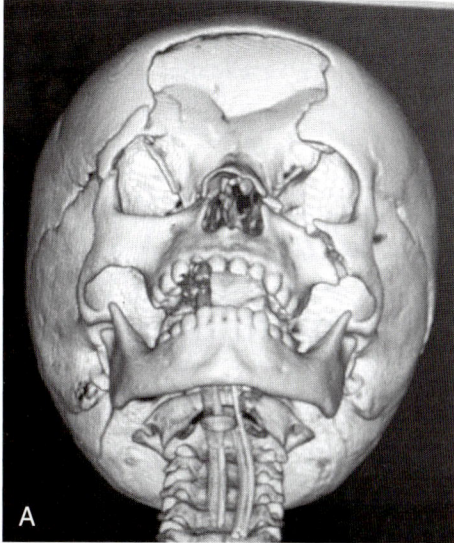

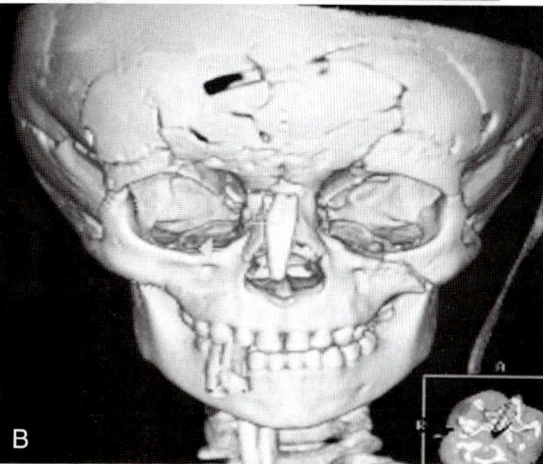

Fig. 44-9 ■ **A,** Pediatric patient with frontobasilar trauma. **B,** Reduction of the fractures with resorbable fixation.

eyelid but also a deformity caused by sagging of the tissue inferiorly over time.

PEDIATRIC FRACTURES

Pediatric fractures have traditionally been treated in closed fashion. However, in children with complex mid-facial and upper facial fractures, judicious use of rigid fixation has advantages over traditional techniques[17] (Fig. 44-9). Treatment of these fractures requires respect of the functional growth matrix and use of the least invasive surgical approach.[18] The need to provide fixation in these patients has led to the use of resorbable bone fixation. Because of the growth implications, these patients require long-term follow-up. A significant number of children may require reoperation for esthetic indications.[19]

SECONDARY (LATE) TREATMENT

Delayed reconstruction of pan-facial fractures is more challenging than primary treatment and often produces compromised results. CT and three-dimensional CT, model surgery, and occasionally three-dimensional models are often helpful for diagnosis and treatment.

In a series of patient presented by He and colleagues, only 64% were judged to have a good result.[20] Soft tissue problems, including lacerations and asymmetry, were frequently the factors that caused an unfavorable outcome.

POSTOPERATIVE CARE

Postoperative care should include elevation of the head to decrease the magnitude of postoperative edema. Antibiotics should be given postoperatively because the fractures involve the sinuses and oral cavity. Patients with dural tears should be observed for the resolution of any cerebrospinal fluid leaks. Ocular examinations should be performed to observe for any changes in visual status. Patients should be maintained on a soft diet immediately after surgery.

PEARLS AND PITFALLS

- Early treatment is optimal and often provides results superior to those of secondary treatment.
- Patients sustaining pan-facial fractures frequently have concomitant injuries that can delay early repair.
- Craniofacial exposure techniques provide excellent exposure for visualization and reduction of these fractures.
- Rigid fixation has revolutionized the way that these fractures are treated, with greatly improved results.
- Sequencing of pan-facial fractures should be individualized to specific facial fracture patterns while adhering to common principles (restoration of height, width, and projection).
- Intraoperative CT and surgical navigation provide enhanced treatment of severely comminuted and displaced fractures.

REFERENCES

1. Follmar KE, Debruijen M, Baccarani A, et al: Concomitant injuries in patients with panfacial fractures, *J Trauma* 63:831-835, 2007.
2. Newman F, Cillo JE: Late vascular complication associated with panfacial fractures, *J Oral Maxillofac Surg* 66:2374-2377, 2008.
3. Follmar KE, Debruijn M, Baccarani A, et al: Concomitant injuries in patients with panfacial fractures, *J Trauma* 63:831-835, 2007.
4. Mithani SK, St-Hilaire H, Brooke BS, et al: Predictable patterns of intracranial and cervical spine injury in craniomaxillofacial trauma: analysis of 4786 patients, *Plast Reconstr Surg* 123:1293-1301, 2009.
5. Fraioli RE, Branstetter BF 4th, Deleyiannis FW: Facial fractures: beyond Le Fort, *Otolaryngol Clin North Am* 41:51-76, 2008.
6. Markowitz BL, Manson PN, Sargent L, et al: Management of the medial canthal tendon in nasoethmoid orbital fractures: the importance of the central fragment in classification and treatment, *Plast Reconstr Surg* 87:843-853, 1991.
7. Mayer JJ, Wainwright DJ, Yeakley JW, et al: The role of three-dimensional computed tomography in the management of maxillofacial trauma, *J Trauma* 28:1043-1053, 1988.
8. Beumer HW, Puscas L: Computer modeling and navigation in maxillofacial surgery, *Curr Opin Otolaryngol Head Neck Surg* 17:270-273, 2009.
9. Gruss JS, Bubak PJ, Egbert MA: Craniofacial fractures: an algorithm to optimize results, *Clin Plast Surg* 19:195, 1992.
10. Kelly KJ, Manson PN, Vander Kolk CA, et al: Sequencing LeFort fracture treatment (organization of treatment for a panfacial fracture), *J Craniofacial Surg* 1:168-178, 1990.
11. Manson PN, Clark N, Robertson B, et al: Subunit principles in midface fractures: the importance of sagittal buttresses, soft tissue reductions, and sequencing treatment of segmental fractures, *Plast Reconstr Surg* 103:1287-1306, 1999.
12. Ellis E 3rd: Sequencing treatment for naso-orbito-ethmoid fractures, *J Oral Maxillofac Surg* 51:543-558, 1993.
13. Babu I, Sagtani A, Jain N, et al: Submental tracheal intubation in a case of panfacial trauma. *Kathmandu Univ Med J* 6:102-104, 2008
14. Reichwein A, Ashicho K, Moser D, et al: Clinical experiences with resorbable ultrasonic-guided, angle-stable osteosynthesis in the panfacial region, *J Oral Maxillofac Surg* 67:1211-1217, 2009.
15. Gruss JS: Naso-ethmoid-orbital fractures: classification and role of primary bone grafting, *Plast Reconstr Surg* 75:303-315, 1985.
16. Herford AS, Ying T, Brown B: Outcomes of severely comminuted (type III) nasoorbito-ethmoid fractures, *J Oral Maxillofac Surg* 63:1266-1277, 2005.
17. Koltai PJ, Rabkin D, Hoehn D: Rigid fixation of facial fractures in children, *J Craniomaxillofac Trauma* 1:32-42, 1995.
18. Clauser L, Dallera V, Sarti E, et al: Frontobasilar fractures in children, *Childs Nerv Syst* 20:168-175, 2004.
19. Burstein F, Cohen S, Hudgins R, et al: Frontal basilar trauma: classification and treatment, *Plast Reconstr Surg* 99:1314-1321, 1997.
20. He D, Zhang Y, Ellis E 3rd: Panfacial fractures; analysis of 33 cases treated late, *J Oral Maxillofac Surg* 65:2459-2465, 2005.

Management of Avulsive Gunshot Wounds to the Face

Amir H. Dorafshar, Eduardo D. Rodriguez

Ten percent of all non-fatal ballistic injuries involve the face. Management of these wounds is challenging because of the complex functional anatomy, mechanisms of injury, extensive composite tissue destruction, and uncertain prognosis. If not treated promptly and aggressively, tissue necrosis, infection, and scar contracture result. The approach to assessment and management of avulsive gunshot wounds to the face has changed in recent decades as our understanding of the mechanisms of tissue injury, diagnostic tools, and reconstructive options have improved.

ETIOPATHOGENESIS/CAUSATIVE FACTORS

Ballistic wounds are highly heterogeneous because of the complex interaction between the projectile and the tissues penetrated. Handguns, shotguns, and other firearms can produce different injury patterns. An understanding of the factors that determine the severity of ballistic wounds and how these factors are interrelated is critical for effective treatment of ballistic trauma. Wounds can generally be classified by the amount of energy imparted to create the wound. Projectile energy is calculated as kinetic energy according to the formula $KE = \frac{1}{2} mv^2$. Ballistic injuries are classified as low energy (speed <1200 ft/s) or high energy (speed >2000 ft/s). High-energy injuries have greater capacity for tissue damage and devascularization, although there are many other factors that determine actual wound severity and prognosis.

First, it should be noted that the kinetic energy equation simply estimates the *maximum* energy available—it does not calculate the energy *dissipated* within the target, which would be a much more complex mathematic function and would need to include not only projectile mass and velocity but also the size and shape of the projectile, its propensity for deformation and fragmentation, the amount of deflection of the projectile, and the exit velocity of the projectile. The shape of the projectile and its deflection (yaw, precession, and tumble) affect the amount of drag encountered while passing through tissues. Drag is a key mechanism of energy exchange. If the bullet deforms easily, it becomes wide and flat, thereby presenting a wider cross-sectional area and thus increasing drag. Fragmentation of the projectile increases yaw, deflection, and tissue drag and results in a larger wound. If the round passes completely through the body, whatever kinetic energy it retains reduces the maximum potential of the wound. To illustrate this point, it is useful to compare a shotgun with a rifle. Shotgun pellets travel at approximately 1200 ft/s, whereas rifled weaponry can fire high-velocity rounds well in excess of 2000 ft/s. A shotgun blast at close range, however, produces a more devastating wound than a high-velocity rifle at the same distance does. Shotgun pellets are soft with low mass and thus produce a wide wound with extensive soft tissue damage. Rifle ammunition is solid with hard tips or casings that resist deformation and fragmentation and consequently result in less tissue drag. This favors deep penetration with limited dissipation of energy. Handguns have a variety of munitions that produce variable wounding patterns. However, few handguns are capable of achieving greater than 1200 ft/s and therefore produce low-energy wounds with limited capacity for avulsion injuries and progressive necrosis.

PATHOLOGIC ANATOMY

Gunshot wounds may be classified into four major patterns of involvement: frontal cranium, orbit, lower mid-face, and mandible. Shotgun wounds, however, are best characterized by the region of tissue loss, with the patterns being (1) lateral mandible, (2) central face, (3) lateral mid-face and orbit, and (4) lateral cranium and orbit.

Ballistic wounds generally demonstrate the following features:

- *Penetration* is the maximum depth that the projectile reaches in tissues. It is affected by projectile momentum and drag of the tissues on the bullet.
- *Permanent cavity* refers to tissue destruction as a result of direct passage of the projectile and its fragments. It is determined by penetration, the cross-sectional area of the projectile, yaw, precession, and deformation.
- *Temporary cavity* is the transient radial deformation of tissues adjacent to the permanent cavity as the projectile passes by. In elastic soft tissues, the temporary cavity can be much larger than the permanent cavity. The quantity of damaged tissue is difficult to estimate. Mature bone, however, is capable of minimal elastic deformation before failure, and therefore bone in the region of the temporary cavity is usually fractured if the shock wave produced by the passing bullet is sufficient. The tendency for progressive necrosis to develop in the zone of tissue injury is difficult to predict, and this has significant implications for management.
- *Fragmentation*, if it occurs, enlarges the volume of injured tissue. Fragmentation is significantly increased if the projectile strikes hard or inflexible tissues such as bone.

DIAGNOSTIC STUDIES

A craniofacial protocol computed tomography (CT) scan with 1-mm cuts in the axial, sagittal, and coronal planes with three-dimensional remodeling is the diagnostic study of choice and can provide detailed information on both the soft and hard tissue extent of injury (Fig. 45-1). Furthermore, CT can be used to evaluate for possible concomitant cervical spine or vascular injuries. Plain films, such as the panoramic tomogram, are useful in relating the injuries to the occlusion. However, they are often plagued by superimposition artifact and poor clarity in the central region of the face/symphysis.

In addition, high-quality digital photographs of the face in the frontal, oblique, and side views with documentation of the site and

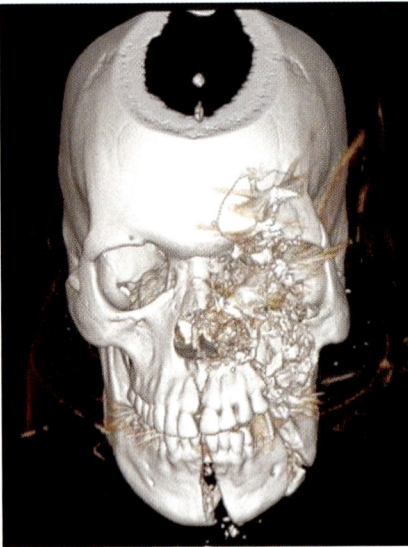

Fig. 45-1 ▪ Three-dimensional craniofacial computed tomography scan demonstrating an avulsive gunshot wound injury to the face on admission.

extent of injury, as well as pre-injury photographs, are important to assist in the reconstructive effort.

RECONSTRUCTIVE GOALS

The current philosophy of initial treatment is (1) serial inspection and débridement, (2) early reduction and fixation of bone, and (3) early definitive reconstruction, which may require recruitment of hard or soft tissue. Secondary revisions may be performed at a later stage if needed. This approach simplifies the procedures, reduces operating time, and lowers associated morbidity.

SPECIFIC TREATMENT AND TECHNIQUES

EMERGENCY MANAGEMENT AND TRIAGE

Initial management of any ballistic wound should follow the advanced trauma life support protocol. The airway should be addressed first and can be problematic to identify and secure. Normal anatomic landmarks can be distorted by edema, local tissue collapse because of loss of supporting bone, and hemorrhage. The best technique for airway management will depend on any concomitant cervical spine injury, the general condition of the patient, and the specifics of the maxillofacial injury. Orotracheal or nasotracheal intubation is always the preferred method of initial airway control, although nasal intubation should be avoided in patients with severe bleeding. Even though elective tracheostomy is often required in these patients, cricothyroidotomy is the most reliable surgical airway in the emergency setting, with future conversion to a formal tracheostomy in a controlled setting.

Control of hemorrhage should be addressed next. This can be challenging because fractured bones bleed substantially and vessels may be difficult to access. Pressure and packing should be used liberally, along with judicious ligation of obvious bleeding vessels. Ligation of vessels is best done in a controlled environment since blind clipping or clamping can easily damage vital facial nerve structures. Facial bleeding secondary to gunshot wounds usually occurs from branches of the external carotid artery, primarily the maxillary artery, followed by the facial and superficial temporal

arteries. When packing fails, selective arterial embolization by interventional radiology may be considered. Once the patient has been stabilized, the wound should be examined as discussed later in phase I.

PRINCIPLES OF MANAGEMENT

Contamination of wounds with projectile fragments and foreign bodies, as well as extensive zones of tissue necrosis and loss, predisposes all ballistic injuries to infection. In the past, attempts to initiate early reconstruction met with failure because of infection, fistulas, and unpredictable progressive tissue necrosis. Historically, treatment centered on initial débridement with prolonged observation and wound dressings. This method does not facilitate optimal functional and cosmetic outcomes. In particular, severe scarring and soft tissue contracture develop and make re-expansion of the soft tissue envelope extremely difficult if not impossible.

The modern approach centers on initial débridement with immediate open reduction and internal fixation of viable displaced bone, followed by serial inspection and débridement as the permanent zone of injury becomes apparent. The missing bony architecture is then reconstructed with either nonvascularized bone grafts or osseous free flaps to maintain the soft tissue envelope.

The surgeon's approach can be divided into three phases:

Phase I

In phase I, an ordered physical examination is performed to systematically assess the injury. The examination should proceed in a cephalocaudal manner and should evaluate first the extraoral injuries and then the intraoral injuries. It must accurately characterize both the soft and hard tissue. The first step is to try to determine the type of firearm and munition used. The entrance and exit wounds together give an estimate of the projectile's trajectory. If the patient is conscious, trigeminal and facial nerve function should be assessed. Starting from the scalp down to the face, soft tissue integrity should be evaluated. Careful assessment of the globe, vision, and extraocular movements is critical. Problems identified here may necessitate consultation with ophthalmology or neurosurgery (or both) and require a multidisciplinary approach. Inspection of the ears and otoscopy should be performed. Hemotympanum may indicate simple soft tissue damage or may be an early warning of more significant injury such as a skull base fracture.

Assessment of the hard tissue can be guided by evaluating each facial buttress—again starting high with the frontal bar, orbital rims, and nasomaxillary, zygomaticomaxillary, maxillary, and mandibular units while noting the status of the terminal alveolar processes. The stability of fractured bone units should be assessed manually. High-energy ballistic wounds produce comminuted, unstable injuries rather than large fracture segments. Finally, evaluation of occlusion should be undertaken. If conscious, the patient will provide the best information, but gross changes in interdigitation should be determined. Dental molds allow a more complete assessment.

Phase II

Phase II follows adequate assessment of the injury and begins with aggressive early débridement. Zones of obvious tissue devitalization and necrosis are removed, the wound is irrigated copiously, embedded debris is removed, and the remaining tissue is closed. The patient is then brought back to the operating room a few days later for a second look. It should be emphasized that this is *selective* débridement—only small pieces of devitalized bone and a narrow 1- to 2-mm margin of contused tissue should be removed. This process is repeated serially over the ensuing 3 to 4 days until no further necrosis is found.

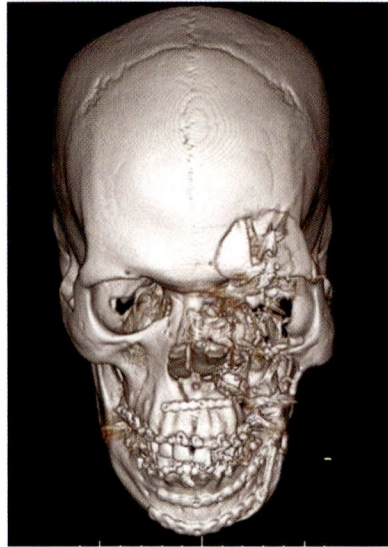

Fig. 45-2 ■ Three-dimensional craniofacial computed tomography scan following open reduction and internal fixation of fractured bone segments to achieve stable skeletal architecture and occlusion. Note that the postoperative course was complicated by necrosis of the left hemimaxillary dentoalveolar segment.

Phase III

Phase III is the reconstructive phase of management. The first and most important goal is to restore the occlusion by accurate reduction of the remaining dentoalveolar bone segments. The occlusal relationship and surrounding stable skeletal architecture are the foundation on which the facial buttresses are restored (Fig. 45-2). Small segments of missing bone surrounded by well-vascularized tissue are replaced with non-vascularized bone grafts, and segments larger than 6 cm are replaced with vascularized bone (Fig. 45-3). Following fracture stabilization, the internal mucosa and external skin envelope are closed. Watertight closure of the mucosa is essential for fracture healing. If primary closure is not possible, a pedicled or free flap is selected according to the size and location of the defect and the quality of surrounding tissues. When defects are large (>6 cm), free flaps are most useful and ideal if there is associated bone loss or large areas of dead space to be filled.

VASCULARIZED TISSUE OPTIONS

Ballistic trauma usually results in composite defects that include skin, mucosa, and bone. Three options are available for reconstructing large three-dimensional defects—prosthetic obturation, non-vascularized bone grafts with local tissue rearrangement, or composite free flaps. Obturators, particularly for large defects, are cumbersome and uncomfortable and lead to ongoing difficulties with phonation, mastication, and speech. If not properly fitted, the prosthesis can rub during insertion and removal and create raw tissue surfaces. Local tissue rearrangement with nonvascularized bone grafts is often not an option in ballistic trauma because the defect can be large and the surrounding tissue poorly vascularized. If vascularized tissue is not introduced, soft tissue contracture, bone graft resorption, and ultimately, loss of facial projection will result. Composite free tissue transfer delivers volume, fills dead space, seals fistulas, reestablishes the skeletal buttresses, and restores the soft tissue envelope in a single stage (Fig. 45-4). Donor site selection is guided by the type of tissue missing, donor site morbidity, ease of harvest, pedicle length, and finally, surgeon preference. Flap choice in ballistic trauma may be limited by a number of reasons.

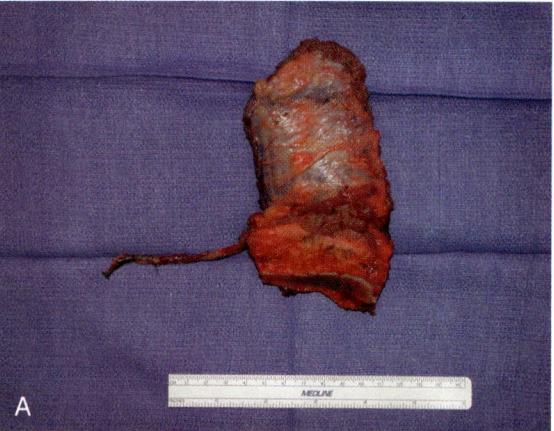

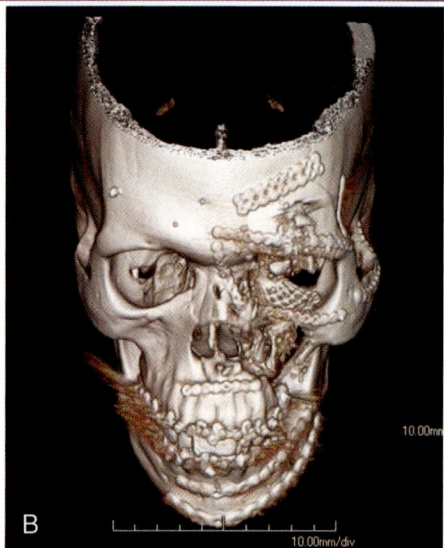

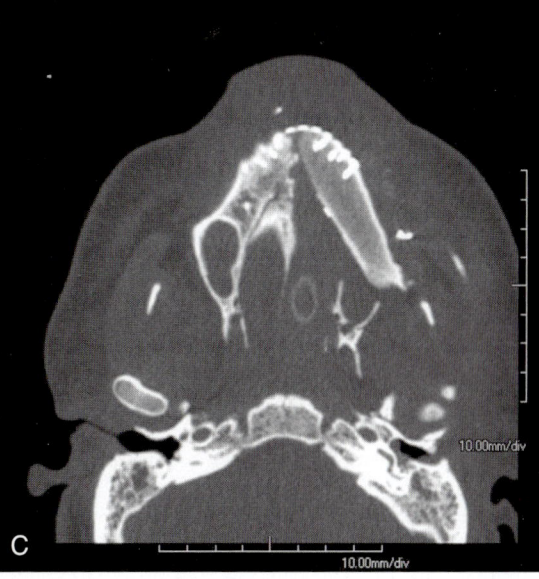

Fig. 45-3 ■ **A,** Deep circumflex iliac artery flap harvested for a type 1b left hemimaxillary defect. **B,** Three-dimensional craniofacial computed tomography (CT) scan following reconstruction of a type 1b left hemimaxillary defect with a vascularized iliac bone flap. Note that the iliac bone is plated to the remaining right hemimaxilla. **C,** Axial CT image of the maxilla demonstrating vascularized iliac bone fixed to the right hemimaxilla for reconstruction of a type 1b left hemimaxillary defect.

Potential donor sites may be eliminated because of concomitant injuries since victims of ballistic injury may have been shot multiple times or injured in a fall. Occasionally, some donor sites may be undamaged but nevertheless unavailable because of functional requirements. For example, use of the fibula in a patient with one functional lower limb is not recommended.

SOFT TISSUE

The ideal reconstruction of any facial defect, including ballistic ones, uses identical local tissues. This is certainly possible for small defects; however, for large defects in the face, free tissue transfer has become a routine method of reconstruction. The workhorse soft tissue free flaps for head and neck reconstruction remain the radial

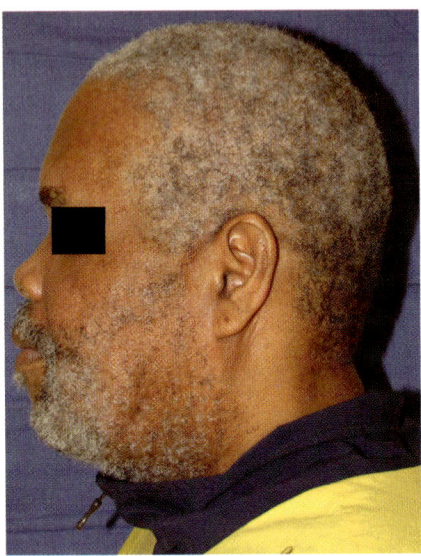

Fig. 45-4 ■ Photograph of the left profile of the patient in Figure 45-3 demonstrating satisfactory mid-face projection following a gunshot wound injury reconstructed with a vascularized iliac bone flap.

forearm and anterolateral thigh flaps. Free tissue transfer delivers adequate, well-vascularized volume to the defect. In a second stage the flap can be contoured, the skin paddle excised, and local tissues re-advanced to achieve better esthetic results.

HARD TISSUE

The goals of maxillary and mandibular reconstruction are to restore facial projection, separate the respiratory and digestive tracts, and provide a foundation for dental rehabilitation with osseointegrated implants. Composite vascularized bone flaps can achieve these goals in a single stage. The skin paddle provides volume and internal and external lining and obliterates fistulas, and the bone restores and maintains facial projection over time and provides a foundation for osseointegrated implants. Four bone sources can support osseointe-grated implants: the fibula, iliac, radius, and scapula. The authors prefer the iliac and fibula bone flaps because they have the best bone stock for osseointegrated implants and can be harvested simultane-ously by a second team. Selection of the fibula osteoseptocutaneous flap over the deep circumflex iliac artery (DCIA) flap is determined by the amount of bone and pedicle length required (Fig. 45-5). The fibula has a longer pedicle and predictable blood supply, which permits multiple osteotomies to achieve the appropriate contour. In the maxillary and orbital regions, the flexibility of the fibula flap is useful. For mandibular reconstructions, the fibula is significantly narrower than the height of the native mandible, thus making the DCIA flap attractive, particularly for defects that do not require multiple osteotomies for contouring.

DENTAL REHABILITATION

The development of osseointegrated dental implants has been a major advance in restorative dentistry. Previously, patients required either fixed prosthodontics, which requires intact adjacent teeth to serve as abutments for the prosthesis, or removable dentures, which are unstable and prone to complications. Osseointegrated implants provide rigid restoration without the need for preparation of the remaining sound teeth. Furthermore, the success rate and long-term

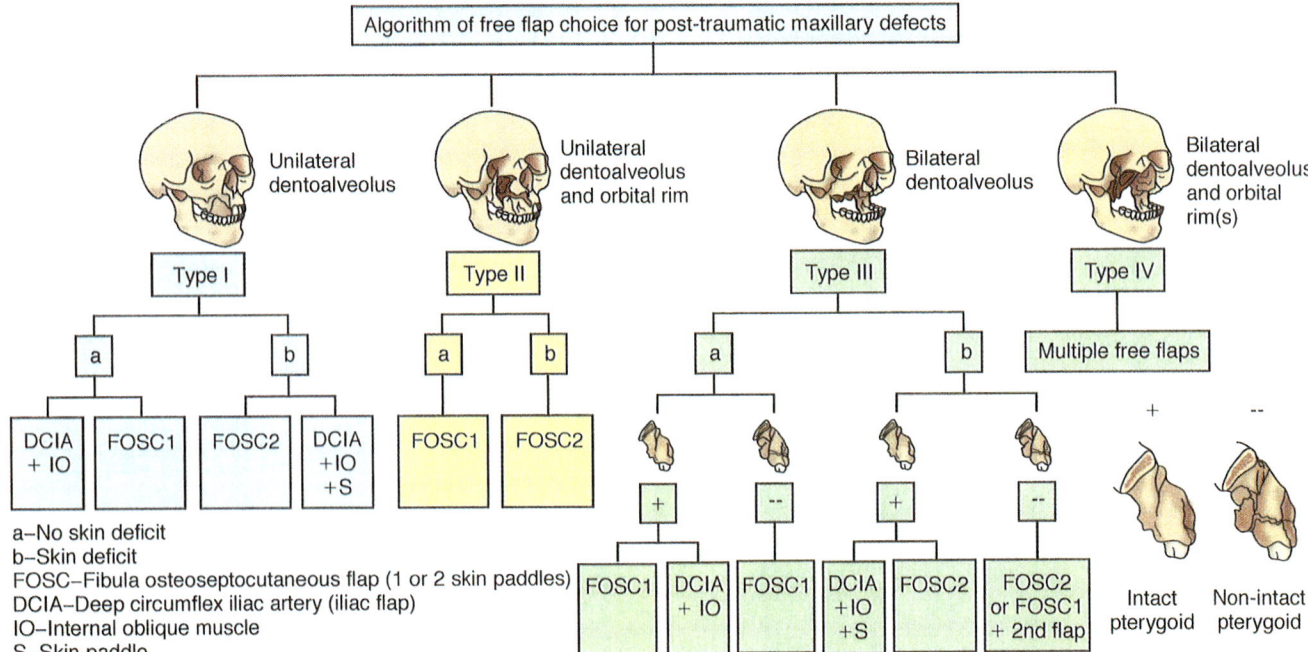

Fig. 45-5 ■ Algorithm to select a free flap for post-traumatic maxillary defects. (From Rodriguez ED, Martin M, Bluebond-Langner R, et al: Microsurgical reconstruction of posttraumatic high-energy maxillary defects: establishing the effectiveness of early reconstruction, *Plast Reconstr Surg* 120[7 Suppl 2]:103S-117S, 2007.)

durability of implant-based dental restorations are significantly greater than the alternative.

Placement of osseointegrated dental implants can be done in either a single-stage or multiple-stage procedure. After placement, most protocols call for at least 4 months of healing before the implant fixtures can be loaded with the final dental prosthesis. Some dental prostheses will resemble traditional dentures that can be removed by the patient for home maintenance, whereas others will be screwed or cemented in place and will require professional maintenance. In all cases, careful consultation with the restorative dentist and implant surgeon is essential to meet the predicted functional needs of the patient.

POSTOPERATIVE CARE

Postoperative care for these patients is best performed in an intensive care unit setting with specialized nursing. Airway management and tracheostomy care often have to be provided. Patients should have the head of the bed elevated to above 30 degrees in an attempt to minimize edema. Patients will frequently require moist saline-soaked gauze dressing changes on open wounds until definitive closure can be achieved. Compressive bandages should be avoided after adequate control of bleeding.

PEARLS AND PITFALLS

- Ballistic facial injuries represent a significant reconstructive challenge.
- Patients are often in critical condition with severe concomitant injuries that have to be evaluated and stabilized before reconstructive efforts.
- Multiple trips to the operating room followed by demanding and complex reconstructions may be necessary.
- Each case must be approached on its own merits, and no one-size-fits-all approach is possible if satisfactory outcomes are desired.
- Initial treatment should consist of serial inspection and débridement, early reduction and fixation of bone, and early definitive reconstruction, which may require recruitment of vascularized hard or soft tissue.
- Establishment of the occlusal relationship followed by preservation and stabilization of the remaining skeletal units and finally reconstruction of the soft tissue envelope leads to the best functional and esthetic outcomes.
- Subsequent reconstructive procedures are often necessary to perfect the esthetic and functional outcome.

BIBLIOGRAPHY

Clark N, Birely B, Manson PN, et al: High-energy ballistic and avulsive facial injuries: classification, patterns, and an algorithm for primary reconstruction, *Plast Reconstr Surg* 98:583-601, 1996.

Cunningham LL, Haug RH, Ford J: Firearm injuries to the maxillofacial region: an overview of current thoughts regarding demographics, pathophysiology, and management, *J Oral Maxillofac Surg* 61:932-942, 2003.

Robertson BC, Manson PN: High-energy ballistic and avulsive injuries. A management protocol for the next millennium, *Surg Clin North Am* 79(6):1489-1502, 1999.

Rodriguez ED, Martin M, Bluebond-Langner R, et al: Microsurgical reconstruction of posttraumatic high-energy maxillary defects: establishing the effectiveness of early reconstruction, *Plast Reconstr Surg* 120(7 Suppl 2):103S-117S, 2007.

Secondary Reconstruction of Post-traumatic Maxillomandibular Deformities

Chapter **46**

Rabie M. Shanti, Shahid R. Aziz

Treatment of maxillofacial trauma has evolved in the past 50 years as a result of technologic advances in diagnostic capabilities, improved rigid fixation techniques, and more specialized approaches to surgical training. Nonetheless, even in the hands of the most experienced surgeons, there is still the potential for the development of secondary morbidity, such as malunion, malocclusion, and temporomandibular joint (TMJ) dysfunction.[1] Therefore, management of patients with facial trauma requires that the clinician not only address the acute injuries but also be prepared to address any secondary morbidities should they arise. An understanding of the causes and management of post-traumatic deformities will allow the surgeon to reduce the likelihood of the development of these deformities.

The primary objective of this chapter is to address the initial assessment, treatment planning, and subsequent surgical correction of post-traumatic maxillomandibular skeletal deformities, particularly secondary (late) reconstruction of maxillofacial skeletal trauma.

ETIOPATHOGENESIS/CAUSATIVE FACTORS

Few reconstructive procedures are more challenging than the surgical repair of facial deformities secondary to trauma, and patients who suffer severe facial trauma may never function or appear as they did before the traumatic incident. This is in contrast to what is observed with congenital deformities, where any surgical intervention will result in major improvement and patient satisfaction. Nonetheless, although a plethora of literature exists on the epidemiology of facial trauma, unfortunately, very little is known about the epidemiology of post-traumatic maxillomandibular deformities caused by a myriad of local and systemic variables that contribute to these deformities.[2] Even though the incidence of post-traumatic maxillomandibular deformities is unknown, they are assumed to be relatively uncommon. Therefore, the best method for the prevention of most secondary post-traumatic maxillomandibular deformities is to perform appropriate treatment as soon as possible after injury.

As stated previously, the most common causes of post-traumatic maxillomandibular deformities include malunion, malposition, and nonunion of fractures because of an inadequate postoperative interocclusal relationship or bony reduction and fixation. In addition, secondary repair may be required in critically injured patients too unstable to undergo general anesthesia for primary repair of their facial injuries (neurologic instability, for example). Manson attributes malunion to poor visualization, telescoping of bone fragments, and in patients with mandibular fractures, rotation of the mandible in a lingual direction.[3] Ellis' group reviewed 33 cases of delayed treatment of pan-facial fractures in which most patients required delayed treatment because of severe brain injury (60% of patients); the others had associated injuries such as limb fractures.[4] Interestingly, all 33 patients had malocclusion and facial deformities, 20 (60%) had mouth opening limited to less than 30 mm, and 5 (15%) had ankylosis of the TMJ. The challenge in treating delayed cases is that it is believed that after a 3-week period, bone healing enters what is termed the "gray stage," during which the edges of bone fragments are undergoing resorption and remodeling, which can make achieving ideal bone reduction very difficult and can lead to malunion, nonunion, or even a bone defect.[4,5]

Other common causes of post-traumatic maxillomandibular malunion include the ever-controversial condylar fracture. This is a fracture whose management should be considered seriously, especially in the pediatric population and adults with a condylar head fracture, since the most commonly encountered hard tissue complication after sustaining facial trauma is TMJ dysfunction.[6] One such example is a bilateral condylar fracture, which when inadequately diagnosed or treated, can result in an open bite, trismus, or hypoplasia of the mandible, especially if it occurs in a pediatric patient (Fig. 46-1).

With regard to mid-face trauma, the most common cause of postoperative malocclusion after the treatment of mid-face trauma is maxillary widening or impaction when the transverse or anteroposterior dimensions (or both) were altered intraoperatively[6] (Fig. 46-2). In a patient with an impacted maxilla, the most common complaint is impaction of the nose.[6] Additionally, in the management of comminuted mid-face fractures, an oblique or tilted occlusal plane can easily develop.

PATHOLOGIC ANATOMY

Most post-traumatic facial deformities tend to involve either the maxilla or the mandible. Additionally, the mandible has been classically described as the esthetic and functional foundation of the lower part of the face.[7] The ultimate goals of secondary reconstruction of the anatomic regions of the mandible are aimed at reconstituting its three-dimensional shape while achieving excellent orofacial rehabilitation.

The goals of post-traumatic maxillary reconstruction are nearly the same as those for post-traumatic mandibular reconstruction but with additional anatomic structures such as the maxillary sinus and the horizontal and vertical facial buttresses. The maxilla is made up of six walls, with the superior, anterior, and inferior walls being the most significant in maxillary reconstruction. The inferior wall makes up the alveolus and is required for prosthodontic rehabilitation, the superior wall is part of the orbit and is required for orbital support, and the anterior wall determines cheek projection and makes a significant contribution to facial dimension in the sagittal plane. Facial disfigurement can result from lack of mid-face bony support because of a deficiency in maxillary buttress vertical support or a maxillary sagittal plane deficiency.

DIAGNOSTIC STUDIES

A thorough history and physical examination are critical for proper assessment of patients with post-traumatic deformities. The following data should be ascertained first: date of injury, mechanism of injury, and any associated injuries. The surgeon must rule out any associated intracranial, cervical spine, abdominal, or thoracic injuries, as well as any injury that would contraindicate the use of maxillomandibular fixation (MMF). Additionally, an assessment of trigeminal neurosensory function and visual function should always be carried out and documented because of the risk for compromise of these structures during traumatic incidents affecting the maxillofacial region. More focused diagnostics should consist of an analysis of facial esthetics, as well as more quantitative measurements (i.e., cephalometric image analysis). Similarly, mounted dental anatomic casts and study models are also another important component of a proper work-up of these patients. In addition, three-dimensional computed tomography (CT) and at times stereolithographic skull models can be quite useful in patients with more severe deformity, especially in providing an appreciation of the displaced skeletal structures (Fig. 46-3). Both have been shown to be useful in minimizing surgical approaches, saving operating time, providing a better understanding of the planes of the deformity, and even improving postoperative results in major facial reconstructive cases.[8] Three-dimensional CT and stereolithographic models can also be useful in planning surgery in patients with severe trauma when radiographic examination and cast analysis are impossible to obtain. Plain films are indicated only for cephalometric evaluation; aside from this, they provide minimal significant information.

Since the treatment of post-traumatic deformities is carried out in a non-acute manner, in most cases the surgeon can obtain pre-injury records (i.e., photographs, dental casts) indicating any pre-existing deformities or previous interventions. If there is associated dental trauma, an optimal treatment approach should consist of a multidisciplinary team that includes a maxillofacial prosthodontist and orthodontist. Both should be consulted before any surgical intervention is carried out to properly sequence the treatment in patients requiring any rehabilitation of the oral structures, especially in those with significant mandibular or maxillary defects that involve dentoalveolar structures. For instance, the prosthodontist is able to

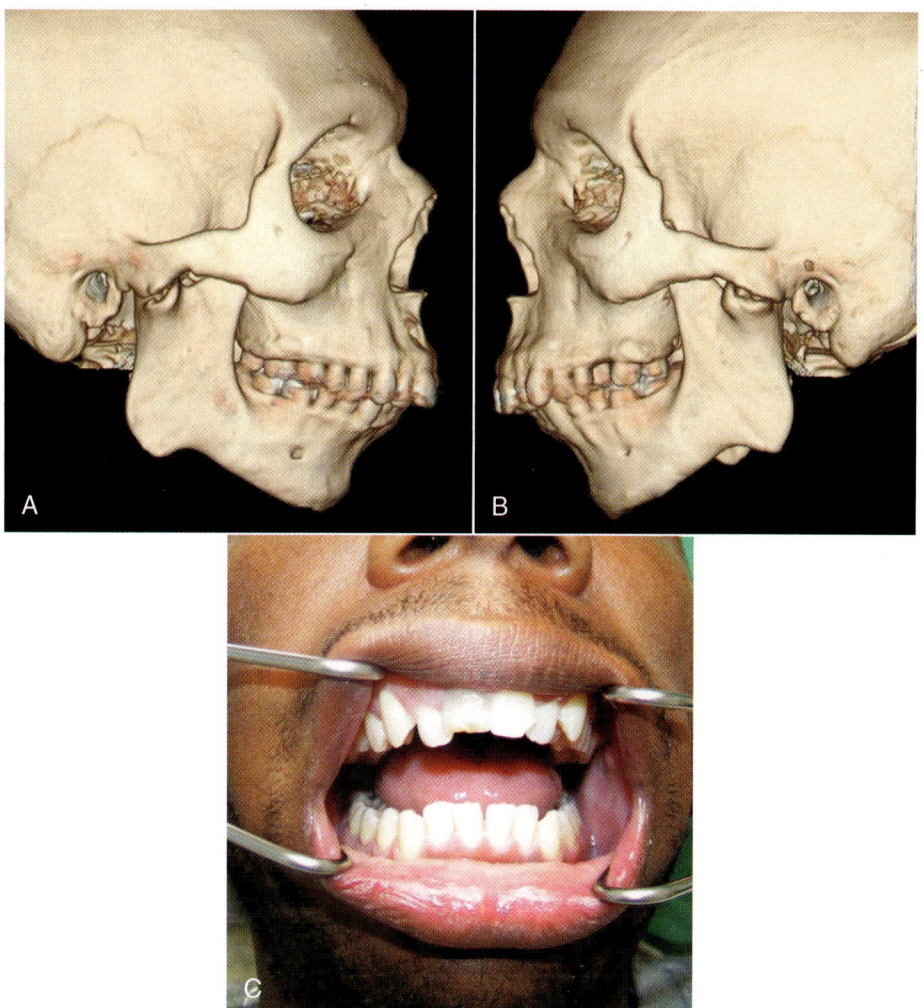

Fig. 46-1 ■ **A,** Twenty-five-year-old man 18 years after untreated bilateral condylar fractures that resulted in mandibular hypoplasia (retrognathia) and trismus. Three-dimensional computed tomography (CT) scan showing ankylosis of the right condyle. **B,** Three-dimensional CT scan showing ankylosis of the left condyle. **C,** Maximal incisal opening of 18 mm.

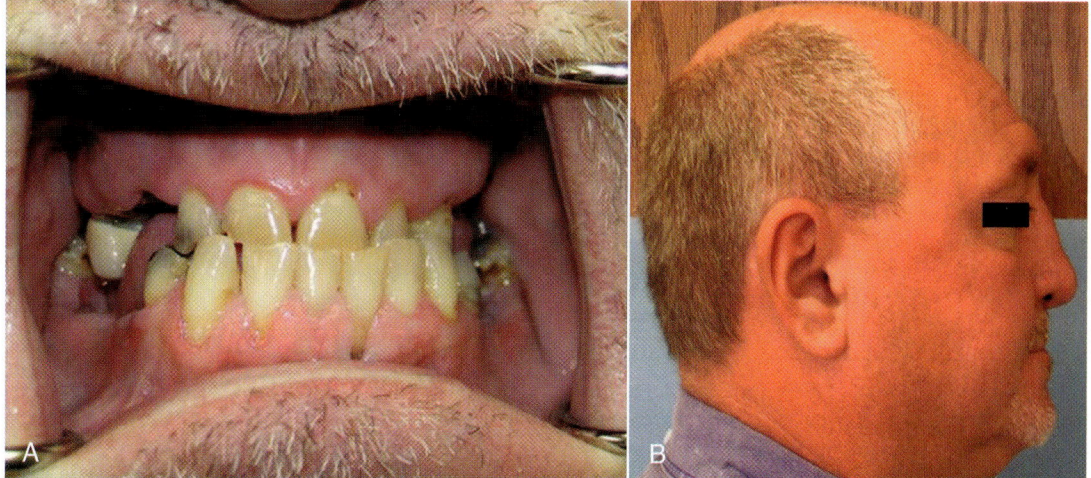

Fig. 46-2 ■ **A,** Fifty-three-year-old man 2 years after rigid fixation of a Le Fort I fracture. The maxilla was rigidly fixated in a posterior position, which created a class III malocclusion. **B,** Profile view demonstrating maxillary hypoplasia in the anteroposterior plane.

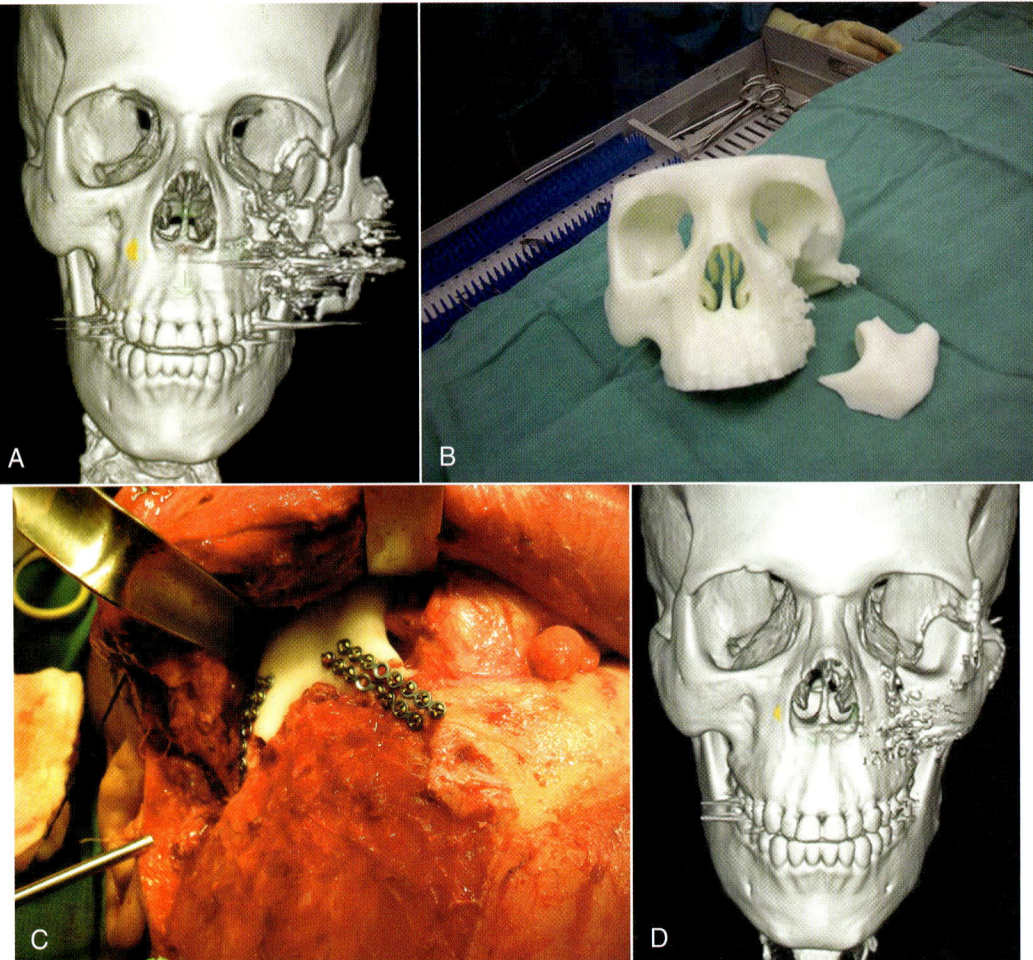

Fig. 46-3 ■ **A,** Eighteen-year-old man 1 month after a gunshot wound to his left zygoma that resulted in a comminuted fracture of the left zygomaticomaxillary complex. **B,** Stereolithographic model with a custom left zygomatic prosthesis. **C,** Débridement and placement of a prosthesis. **D,** Postoperative three-dimensional computed tomography scan. (Courtesy Dr. Talib Najjar.)

fabricate obturators, which are especially useful in enabling patients with maxillary defects to speak and swallow. Obturators can also provide temporary coverage to minimize contamination of the wound during the healing period. Successful reconstruction should restore facial projection and provide the foundation for a functional dental prosthesis. An orthodontic consultation is necessary in cases of malocclusion. This can be quite helpful since presurgical orthodontics can in certain cases negate the need for multisegment maxillary surgery[9] and allow a conventional Le Fort I osteotomy to be performed (Fig. 46-4). The aforementioned information gathered during the perioperative patient evaluation will allow proper diagnosis and surgical management of patients with post-traumatic deformities.

TREATMENT/RECONSTRUCTIVE GOALS

Post-traumatic maxillomandibular deformities present a complex challenge for the maxillofacial surgeon because these deformities can be difficult to manage nonoperatively and oftentimes require extensive surgical correction. When the surgeon is confronted with the situation of a patient requiring late correction of a post-traumatic maxillomandibular deformity, effort should be directed at understanding the circumstances and nature of the initial injury. Post-traumatic maxillomandibular deformities can be challenging to reconstruct because they involve several complex anatomic boundaries (i.e., dentoalveolar complex, TMJ, maxillary buttresses) and

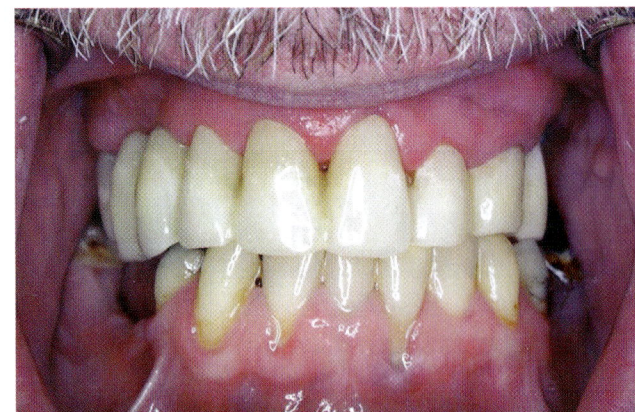

Fig. 46-4 ■ Same patient as in Figure 46-2 after Le Fort I advancement, orthodontics, and prosthetic reconstruction, which resulted in a class I occlusion.

any impairment or deficiency of these structures can result in significant functional and cosmetic deformity. Therefore, proper assessment of the severity of a post-traumatic patient's maxillomandibular deformity is critical, for this will determine the treatment options that will best address the patient's deformities. Secondary reconstruction of such deformities is an essential component in the care of a maxillofacial trauma patient since the maxillomandibular region is an important portion of the face because of multifaceted anatomic boundaries, the composite nature of tissues, its highly specific sensory and motor functions, and esthetic appearance. In short, the primary objective of secondary reconstruction of post-traumatic maxillomandibular deformities is to restore function and appearance. Furthermore, defects of the mandible can result in impaired speech, difficulty swallowing, deviation of the mandible during functional movements, poor control of salivary secretions, and cosmetic disfigurement.

In the authors' experience, one cannot overstress the need for clear communication with the patient. The patient's expectations should be assessed and the patient should participate in the decision-making process with realistic expectations. Although reestablishing the facial skeleton back to its pre-trauma anatomy and thereby restoring function and cosmesis is ideal, it is frequently impossible to achieve and, if possible, may require multiple surgeries. The primary difficulty is working in a soft tissue envelope that is often severely scarred down, thus limiting skeletal repositioning. The surgeon and the patient must be on the same page with regard to the goals of reconstruction, the number of surgeries potentially required, and the results that can realistically be expected. The ideal maxillomandibular reconstruction method must support the insertion of a prosthetic appliance (e.g., obturator, denture) or dental endosseous implants (or both), which represents the final phase of orofacial rehabilitation.

SPECIFIC TREATMENT AND TECHNIQUES

The aforementioned reconstructive goals should not only focus on restoring facial contour but also provide for the placement of dental endosseous implants, which are necessary for total oral rehabilitation. There is no set scheme for the treatment of post-traumatic maxillomandibular deformities. However, the majority of these deformities are treated with conventional osteotomies, bone grafting, or both. The majority of treatments are based on an amalgamation of the principles of trauma, orthognathic, and reconstructive surgery. It is also important to remember that surgery is not always the only option and that nonsurgical options should always be considered first. In certain clinical scenarios these options can address the patient's chief complaint. For example, a mild lateral open bite tends to resolve spontaneously, or canting of the maxillary or mandibular occlusal plane can often be treated with fixed partial dentures (e.g., crowns, bridge).

DEFECTS IN CONTINUITY

Defects caused by severe trauma such as gunshot wounds or injury by impalement often result in large defects accompanied by dysfunction (e.g., swallowing, control of saliva, mastication, speech) and disfigurement. Therefore, if these functional and cosmetic impairments are not addressed, the patient's quality of life will be adversely affected and significant morbidity will result. Prosthetic rehabilitation is one of the earliest reconstructive tools. It provides temporary closure of the defect during the healing period and, in patients with major defects, restores speech and swallowing; it also provides support for the lips and cheeks. Bone grafts play an important role in the correction of these defects. Bone grafts can be transplanted via one of the following techniques: (1) free bone grafts, (2) pedicled bone grafts, or (3) microvascular bone grafts. In determining which type of graft to use for reconstruction of a mandibular or maxillary defect the surgeon should consider the size, location, mechanism of injury, quality of the recipient site, and the presence of any medical co-morbid conditions. In a healthy patient with no associated soft tissue defects, a free bone graft (e.g., chin, retromolar area, rib, iliac crest, skull, tibia) is the graft of choice.

Pedicled and microvascular bone flaps are indicated for the reconstruction of large bone defects, bone defects with associated soft tissue loss, and poor-quality recipient area.[10]

MALUNION

Malunion is defined as bone healing in an improper position. In the maxillomandibular region, malunion can result in facial asymmetry, malocclusion, or both. Malocclusion is much more likely to occur. Usually, in less severe cases a patient can be guided into an acceptable maxillomandibular relationship with the use of nonoperative techniques such as occlusal equilibration or guiding elastics. However, if these conservative techniques fail, maxillary or mandibular osteotomies (or both) are indicated to achieve an optimal interocclusal relationship. The principles of orthognathic surgery with supportive orthodontic treatment are used to reproduce the initial fracture and reposition the mandible, maxilla, or both.[9] Similar to the management of a malpositioned zygoma in which osteotomies are performed along fracture lines, a similar approach is taken for maxillomandibular malunion.[9-12]

In the parasymphyseal and body regions, the fracture line is the ideal position for osteotomy. However, in cases of condylar malunion, reestablishing the condyles within the mandibular arch should be the first step, similar to the treatment of pan-facial fractures.[13] Additionally, with regard to malocclusion secondary to a healed unilateral condylar fracture and shortening of the ramus-condyle unit, surgeons recommend bilateral mandibular osteotomies (vertical ramus or sagittal split osteotomies) to correct the asymmetry caused by a condylar fracture.[6] Similar to defects in continuity, if gapping is present after osteotomy and repeat fixation, interpositional bone grafting should be considered. The advantages of interpositional bone grafts are that they provide a scaffold for secondary ossification, they act as mechanical stops to reduce the incidence of relapse, and they prevent soft tissue ingrowth/herniation into the osteotomy site.[14] Interpositional bone grafts are likely to be needed when osteotomies are performed at the site of fracture, for these osteotomies are usually irregular and often do not provide enough approximation of the fragments, which places the surgical site at risk for delayed healing. Correction of a severe open bite because of healed bilateral condylar fractures is a philosophic surgical dilemma. A Le Fort I osteotomy and ramus osteotomies are able to address the open bite; however, they both have their inherent advantages and disadvantages.[9] Even though closure of open-bite malocclusions can be achieved with a maxillary (Le Fort 1) procedure or a mandibular procedure, in the authors' experience, combined maxillary-mandibular osteotomies will often provide the most stable long-term result (Fig. 46-5).

As described previously, deformities from mid-face fractures almost always result in reversed overjet, open-bite, and cross-bite occlusal relationships because of posterior, superior, and transverse maxillary displacement.[9] Multisegmental osteotomies with interpositional bone grafts are usually needed to correct the malocclusion. A standard Le Fort I single osteotomy can be used; however, the complexity of the movements needed to correct the post-traumatic deformity generally require multisegmental osteotomies because of the presence of two or more occlusal planes. In addition, as mentioned earlier, presurgical orthodontics can negate the need for a multisegmental Le Fort I osteotomy.

Similar to the surgical correction of congenital maxillomandibular deformities, distraction osteogenesis has great potential in the treatment of maxillomandibular deformities. This technique is not routinely applied for the correction of post-traumatic deformities; however, its advantages include reduced operative time, less blood loss, and no requirement for MMF, rigid internal fixation, or bone grafting.[15-17]

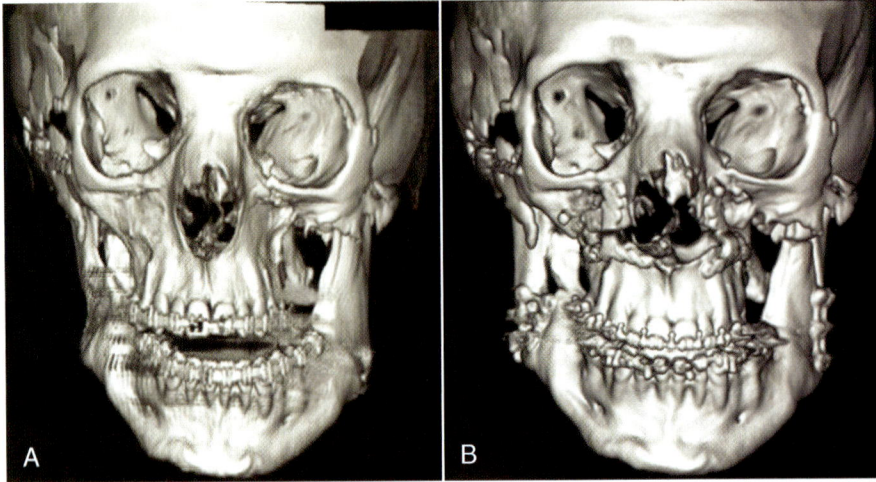

Fig. 46-5 ■ **A,** Seventeen-year-old 12 years after a gunshot wound to the face. As he grew, a significant open-bite malocclusion developed secondary to restricted growth of the maxilla. Preoperative three-dimensional computed tomography reveals an asymmetric and hypoplastic maxilla. **B,** Appearance after orthognathic surgery (Le Fort 1 osteotomy and bilateral vertical ramus osteotomies).

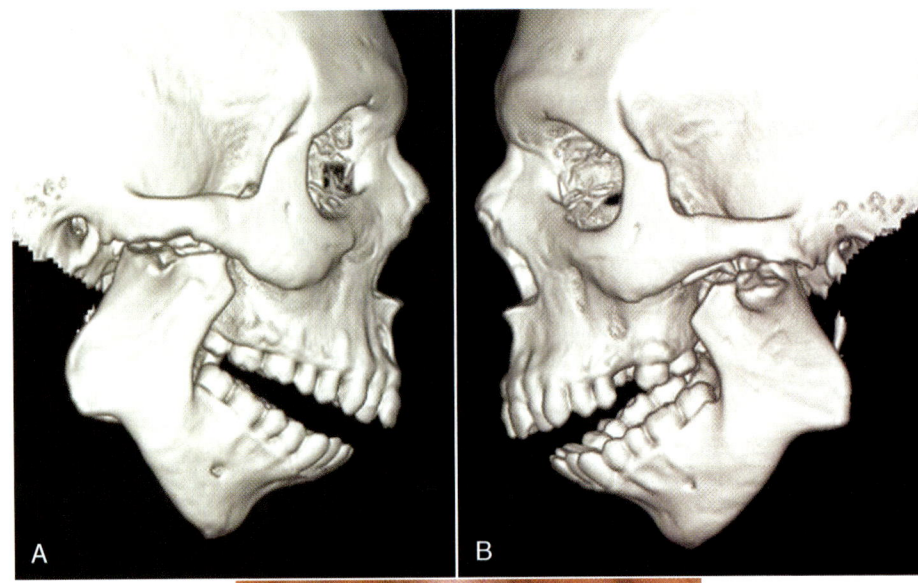

Fig. 46-6 ■ **A,** Three-dimensional computed tomography scan of the patient in Figure 46-4 after bilateral gap arthroplasties and bilateral coronoidectomies (right view). **B,** Left view. **C,** Maximal incisal opening of 45 mm.

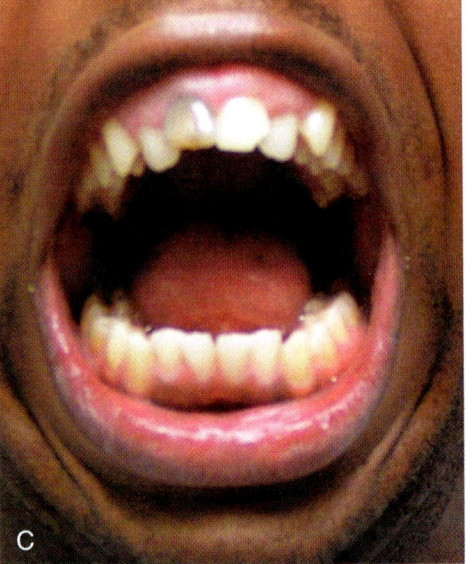

TEMPOROMANDIBULAR JOINT

A patient with TMJ involvement can have limited opening, a clicking or popping sound, joint stiffness, deviation of the jaw to one side on opening, pain on opening or closure of the jaw, or any combination of these findings. TMJ hypomobility or ankylosis can also result from TMJ injury or prolonged periods of MMF. TMJ noise without any other symptoms is not an indication for surgery. The goals of TMJ repair include achievement of a stable articulation and restoration of dental occlusion and facial form. Less invasive approaches such as physical therapy, medications (nonsteroidal anti-inflammatory drugs or muscle relaxants), and occlusal splints should always be the first-line treatment. Nonetheless, in some patients such approaches will fail and surgical interventions ranging from arthrocentesis to total TMJ reconstruction will be required. However, no matter what intervention is used, as stated earlier in this chapter, it is imperative to communicate to patients suffering from post-traumatic deformities that they might never return to their pre-injury state and that this will definitely be the case if they are not compliant with their postoperative physical therapy regimen (Fig. 46-6).

POSTOPERATIVE CARE

As with every maxillofacial surgical patient, the immediate postextubation concern is maintenance of patency of the airway, especially in patients undergoing MMF. At time of extubation in the operating room or recovery room, the surgeon should be prepared for the necessity of releasing the MMF on an emergency basis in the event of airway compromise and need for emergency re-intubation. In major facial reconstruction where airway compromise is a significant issue, the surgeon should discuss with the patient ahead of time the potential need for tracheostomy during surgery. It is the authors' preference that the patient be fully awake and responsive before extubation and able to breathe around the endotracheal tube cuff—this avoids airway emergencies. Additionally, a novice maxillofacial anesthesiologist may assume that the patient will be in severe pain once awake and may prefer to administer narcotics before extubation. It is our experience that if bupivacaine (Marcaine) local anesthetic trigeminal nerve blocks are used, the amount of postoperative pain is minimal. Therefore, educating the anesthesiologist in minimizing the use of narcotics in the immediate postoperative period to avoid airway compromise is warranted.

Postoperative care in the days following surgery should be focused on increasing adequate oral intake and ambulation. Patients will often need reassurance as well that the marked postoperative swelling will resolve over a 4- to 6-week period. Oral pain management should also be established. In the weeks following surgery, maintenance of oral hygiene, adequate oral intake, and prevention of infection are all essential.

PEARLS AND PITFALLS

- Knowledge of the causes of post-traumatic maxillomandibular deformities not only aids in treatment but may also allow their prevention.
- Obtaining three-dimensional images of the injured facial skeleton will provide optimal understanding of the traumatized anatomy, facilitate treatment planning, and provide an excellent resource for patient education.
- Severe anterior open bites are best addressed with a combined maxillary and mandibular approach.
- Proper communication with the patient is necessary to ensure that both the patient and surgeon have the same treatment goals and objectives and that realistic expectations are held by all involved.
- A multidisciplinary approach may provide the best outcome, especially when reconstruction includes dental rehabilitation. Working with prosthodontists and orthodontists to reconstruct the dentition is essential.
- At the end of the surgery before extubation, local anesthetic trigeminal nerve blocks should be used to minimize postoperative discomfort and narcotic use. The surgeon should also be prepared to release the MMF at extubation on an emergency basis if needed.

REFERENCES

1. Kearns GJ, Perrott DH, Kaban LB: Rigid fixation of mandibular fractures: does operator experience reduce complications? *J Oral Maxillofac Surg* 52:226-231, discussion 231-232, 1994.
2. Klotch DW, Futran ND: Considerations for reconstruction of the head and neck oncologic patient. In Greenberg A, Prein J, editors: *Craniomaxillofacial reconstructive and corrective bone surgery*, New York, 2006, Springer, pp 289-294.
3. Manson PN: Facial fractures. In Mathes S, editor: *Plastic surgery*, vol 3, Philadelphia, 2006, WB Saunders, pp 184-186.
4. He D, Zhang Y, Ellis E: Panfacial fractures: analysis of 33 cases treated late, *J Oral Maxillofac Surg* 65:2459-2465, 2007.
5. Carr RM, Mathog RH: Early and delayed repair of orbitozygomatic complex fractures, *J Oral Maxillofac Surg* 55:253-258, discussion 258-259, 1997.
6. Laine P, Kontio R, Salo A, et al: Secondary correction of malocclusion after treatment of maxillofacial trauma, *J Oral Maxillofac Surg* 62:1312-1320, 2004.
7. De Souza M, Oeltjen JC, Panthaki Z, et al: Posttraumatic mandibular deformities, *J Craniofac Surg* 18:912-916, 2007.
8. Kermer C, Lindner A, Friede I, et al: Preoperative stereolithographic model planning for primary reconstruction in craniomaxillofacial trauma surgery, *J Craniomaxillofac Surg* 26:136-139, 1998.
9. Becking AG, Zijderveld SA, Tuinzing DB: The surgical management of post-traumatic malocclusion, *Clin Plast Surg* 34:e37-e43, 2007.
10. Ehrenfeld M, Hagenmaier C: Autogenous bone grafts in maxillofacial reconstruction. In Greenberg A, Prein J: *Craniomaxillofacial reconstructive and corrective bone surgery*, New York, 2006, Springer, pp 295-309.
11. Perino KE, Zide MF, Kinnebrew MC: Late treatment of malunited malar fractures, *J Oral Maxillofac Surg* 42:20-34, 1984.
12. Roncevic R: Refractures of the zygomatic bone, *J Craniomaxillofac Surg* 16:160, 1988.
13. Tullio A, Sesenna E: Role of surgical reduction of condylar fractures in the management of panfacial fractures, *Br J Oral Maxillofac Surg* 38:472-476, 2000.
14. Lye KW, Deatherage JR, Waite PD: The use of demineralized bone matrix for grafting during Lefort I and chin osteotomies: techniques and complications, *J Oral Maxillofac Surg* 66:1580-1585, 2008.
15. Mitsukawa N, Satoh K, Morishita T, et al. Clinical application of distraction osteogenesis for traumatic maxillofacial deformities, *J Craniofac Surg* 17:431-437, 2006.
16. Steidler NE, Cook RM, Reade PC: Residual complications in patients with major middle third facial fractures, *Int J Oral Surg* 9:259-266, 1980.
17. Zachariades N, Papavassiliou D, Papademetrious J, et al: Neglected fractures of the facial skeleton, *J Maxillofac Surg* 12:36-40, 1984.

THE PAST

Head and neck surgery deals with the management of both benign and malignant pathologic conditions of the head and neck. The past has been characterized by radical operations that were performed without regard to the patient's quality of life or prognosis—whether good or bad. The tongue-jaw-neck operation was routinely performed for oral squamous cell carcinoma, and the patient was often left without any form of reconstruction. Radical neck dissection was performed for even the most superficial of tumors and resulted in unnecessary morbidity without a clear survival benefit.

THE PRESENT

Advances in diagnostic modalities, radiation delivery, chemotherapy, and ablative and reconstructive surgery have affected the contemporary management of patients with head and neck cancer. Changing philosophies that emphasize quality of life over quantity of life have resulted in a shift away from the radical, debilitating head and neck operations performed in years past to the more organ-sparing therapies of today. Operations for oral squamous cell carcinoma that once included routine segmental resection of the mandible and radical neck dissection with sacrifice of the sternocleidomastoid muscle, internal jugular vein, and spinal accessory nerve have largely been replaced by judicious composite resections and selective neck dissection based on known clinical and radiographic factors. Surgical resection of a large tumor that is technically resectable but will result in unacceptably high morbidity or dysfunction for the patient, without a significant survival benefit, is no longer advocated. Conversely, the development of microvascular free tissue transfer has significantly enhanced the surgeon's armamentarium for predictable reconstruction of ablative defects following oral cavity resections and has resulted in improved functional and esthetic outcomes for oral cancer patients. These technologic advances in surgery have been accompanied by novel chemotherapeutic regimens that are increasingly being incorporated into already well-established radiation therapy protocols using salivary gland–sparing intensity-modulated radiation therapy techniques. Similar emphasis on preservation of quality of life with respect to benign tumors is likewise gaining favor.

THE FUTURE

It is unlikely that there will be a cure for cancer in our lifetime. However, advances in molecular biology, cell signaling, immunomodulation, and angiogenesis will result in novel targeted therapies that will allow patients with cancer to live longer and healthier lives. Therapies will be tailored according to the biologic behavior of the tumor—whether benign or malignant—not just the histologic diagnosis. This will, in turn, be determined by pretreatment genetic/molecular/proteomic assessment so that the prescribed cure matches the patient's disease.

Chapter 47

Neck Mass: Diagnosis and Management

Deepak Kademani, Meredith August

Oral and maxillofacial surgeons are frequently involved in the management of patients with neck masses. It is therefore important for such surgeons to have a clear understanding of the etiology, pathogenesis, diagnostic evaluation, and treatment of cervical masses. One of the most important factors that help define a specific diagnosis is the patient's age. In general, three age groups need to be considered: pediatric (<15 years), young adults (16 to 40 years of age), and older adults (>40 years of age). Each of these age groups exhibits a certain relative frequency of disease occurrence, which can help the clinician develop an appropriate differential diagnosis[1,2] (Fig. 47-1).

It is important to note that the majority of neck masses in the young pediatric population are more commonly inflammatory and congenital rather than neoplastic.[3] In young adults, the rate of neoplasia begins to increase along with a relative decrease in congenital lesions. In patients older than 40 years, neoplasia is always the primary consideration in those in whom a neck mass of unknown origin develops.[4-6] The second important criterion in the diagnosis of a cervical mass is its location. Congenital, developmental, and traumatic neck masses are relatively consistent in their locations. Neoplasia, on the other hand, tends to vary in terms of anatomic location but is inclined to follow a systematic *pattern of lymphatic spread* from the primary oropharyngeal site. In 5% to 10% of patients, the primary source of the tumor is not readily apparent, and after a detailed, exhaustive physical examination coupled with imaging studies and directed biopsies of oropharyngeal tonsillar tissue, the pharyngeal walls, and the base of the tongue, approximately 1% to 2% remain carcinomas of unknown primary origin.[7,8] This chapter outlines a practical approach to the diagnosis and evaluation of adult patients with cervical neck masses.

DIAGNOSIS

HISTORY AND PHYSICAL EXAMINATION

The most important aspect in diagnosing a cervical neck mass is an accurate and detailed history and physical examination. Every patient with a neck mass should undergo a thorough examination of

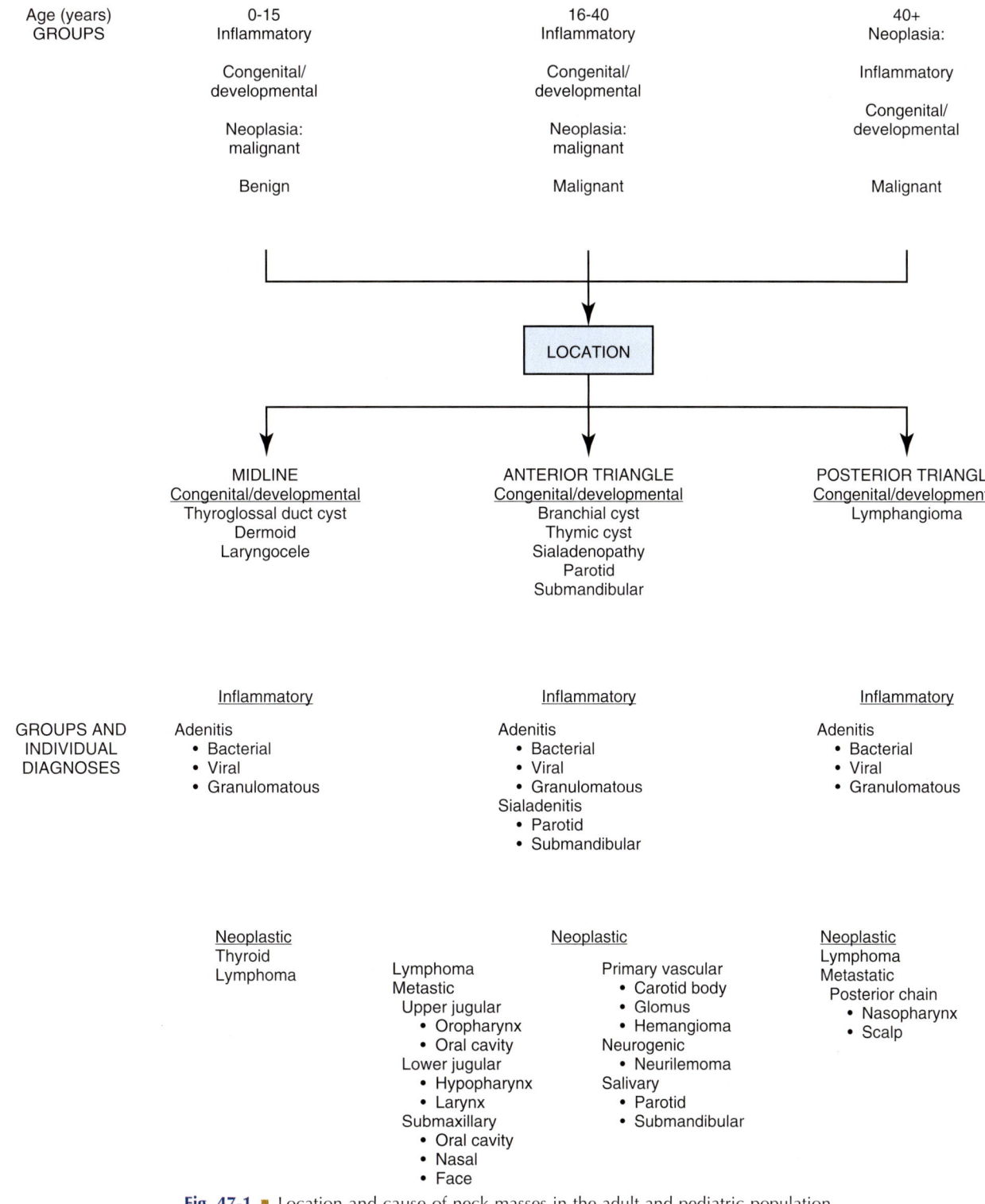

Fig. 47-1 ■ Location and cause of neck masses in the adult and pediatric population.

the entire head and neck with a detailed review of the time of development of the mass along with associated symptoms and any history of trauma, irradiation, and previous surgery. When conducting a physical examination, it is imperative for all mucosal surfaces of the oropharynx to be examined directly or by indirect mirror or fiber-optic visualization and to obtain a tissue diagnosis in a timely and orderly fashion so that an accurate diagnosis can be made. This is particularly important when the suspicion of malignancy is high.

Box 47-1 presents an algorithm for evaluation of a neck mass of unknown origin in an adult patient.

RELEVANT ANATOMY

Knowledge of the various lymphatic drainage routes within the head and neck allows the clinician to focus the examination and evaluation on specific oral mucosal sites within the head and neck

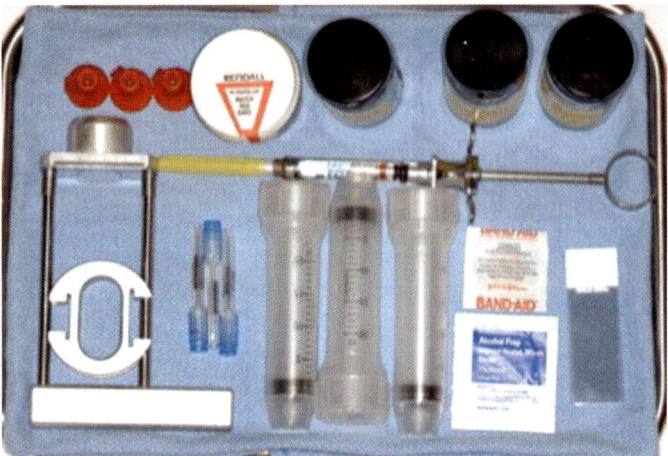

Fig. 47-2 ■ Typical instruments required for fine-needle aspiration.

BOX 47-1	Algorithm for Work-up of a Neck Mass in Adults

1. Thorough head and neck examination
   a. Direct and indirect visualization
   b. Digital palpation—neck and intraorally
2. Fine-needle aspiration
   a. Diagnostic? Benign? Removal
   b. Non-specific?
      (1) Repeat the head and neck examination
      (2) Endoscopy with biopsy
         (+) Diagnosis—treat based on the pathology
         (−) Diagnosis—open biopsy of the mass
   c. Diagnostic? Malignant?
      (1) Imaging study—computed tomography/magnetic resonance imaging/positron emission tomography
      (2) Endoscopy with guided biopsy
         (+) Malignancy—treat cancer
         (−) Open biopsy

BOX 47-2	First-Echelon Lymphatic Sites of Drainage of the Head and Neck

Occipital nodes
   Posterior scalp
Postauricular nodes
   Posterior scalp
   Mastoid
   Posterior auricle
Extraglandular parotid nodes
   Anterior scalp
Intraglandular parotid nodes
   Anterior scalp
   Temple
   Cheek/mid-face
Retropharyngeal nodes
   Posterior nasal cavity
   Sphenoid and ethmoid sinuses
   Hard palate
   Soft palate
   Nasopharynx
   Posterior pharyngeal wall
Level I-A (submental)
   Middle two thirds of the lower lip
   Anterior gingiva
   Anterior tongue
Level I-B (submandibular)
   Ipsilateral lower and upper lip
   Cheek
   Nose
   Medial canthus
   Oral cavity to the anterior tonsillar pillar
Levels II-A and II-B (upper jugular nodes)
   Oral cavity
   Nasal cavity
   Nasopharynx
   Oropharynx
   Hypopharynx
   Larynx
   Parotid gland
Level III (mid-jugular nodes)
   Oral cavity
   Oropharynx
   Nasopharynx
   Hypopharynx
   Larynx
Level IV (lower jugular nodes)
   Hypopharynx
   Thyroid
   Cervical esophagus
   Larynx
Level V-A (posterior triangle)
   Nasopharynx
   Oropharynx
   Skin of the posterior scalp and neck
Level V-B
   Aerodigestive tract malignancies
   Intra-abdominal metastasis
Level VI (anterior compartment delphian node)
   Thyroid gland
   Glottic and subglottic larynx
   Piriform sinus
   Cervical esophagus

(Box 47-2). If the neck mass is unilateral, the primary lesion should be sought in the ipsilateral mucosa or cutaneous sites. If the neck mass is bilateral, it is likely to be in a midline structure such as the base of the tongue, supraglottic larynx, or nasopharynx. Another potential explanation is that bilateral cervical lymphadenopathy can occur when a lateral lesion crosses the midline and violates the lymphatics in the contralateral neck. With lymphadenopathy involving the supraclavicular space and the lower deep lateral cervical chain in the lower portion of the posterior triangle, the primary lesion is often not within the aerodigestive tract, and the search for the primary tumor should be broadened to include pulmonary, breast, and intra-abdominal sources.

Fine-needle aspiration (FNA) of the mass should be considered as the first-line diagnostic tool when appropriate cytologic assessment can be performed in a timely fashion by an experienced cytopathologist (Fig. 47-2).

IMAGING STUDIES

Computed tomography (CT) of the neck has now become the standard of care for evaluating neck masses and providing detailed anatomic data, as well as for the identification of occult primary tumors. The puff cheek and modified Valsalva techniques can help open opposed mucosal surfaces in the oral cavity, oropharynx, and hypopharynx and allow easier detection of known mucosal primaries. CT and magnetic resonance imaging (MRI) have the highest specificity, 87% to 95%, for unknown primary head and neck tumors.[4,9] The most common sites for the origin of the primary tumor are the palatine tonsil (35%), base of the tongue (26%), lung (17%), and nasopharynx (9%), followed by a host of other subsites such as the esophagus, skin, and larynx, which contribute between 1% and 4%.[2,4,7,10] CT is helpful in delineating a cystic from a solid mass and can establish an accurate anatomic location within the neck when axial and coronal images are available. It is important to note that hypodensity within lymph nodes larger than 1.5 cm and loss of the traditional ovoid shape, as well as the presence of central areas of necrosis and nodal aggregation, are classic signs of metastatic carcinoma within a lymph node.[11]

MRI provides information similar to that obtained with CT. However, it can provide more detailed soft tissue visualization of the neck. T2-weighted images and fat suppression techniques have been helpful in looking for early mucosal disease as a cause of metastatic neck masses of unknown primary cause, particularly for detailed evaluation of the base of the tongue or the sinonasal tract.

Ultrasonography is useful for localization of a neck mass and differentiation of cystic from solid masses and is particularly helpful in differentiating congenital cysts from solid lymph nodes, glandular tumors, or vascular lesions.[12,13] Ultrasound may also be used as an image guidance technique for needle aspiration or core biopsy procedures.

Chest radiographs (posterior, anterior, and lateral views) allow the clinician to screen for primary lung neoplasms or lung metastases from primary head and neck malignancy or for the presence of mediastinal adenopathy.

If a suspicious lesion is found on chest radiography, further investigation with CT of the chest is appropriate. Plain chest radiography has a specificity and sensitivity of 73% and 80%, respectively, for evaluating pulmonary metastasis in patients with head and neck tumors.[10,11]

Positron emission tomography (PET) with ^{18}F-fluorodeoxyglucose is able to identify areas of hypermetabolism within the head and neck and is sensitive to lesions larger than 6 mm.[14-19] Though not currently standard therapy for the evaluation of head and neck cancer, PET is increasingly being used for disease surveillance and also for evaluation of patients with known primary head and neck tumors. PET is routinely becoming used for the evaluation of patients with occult primary tumors of the head and neck. The sensitivity and specificity of PET are reported in some studies to be 100% and 94%, respectively.[7,16] Positive and negative predictive values are 88.8% and 76.5%, respectively.[7,16] Newer technologies are now able to fuse the PET scan with the CT scan to further delineate the lesions. Waldeyer's ring is often difficult to interpret because of physiologic uptake in overlying structures such as lymphoid tissue and salivary glands.

PAN-ENDOSCOPY

Pan-endoscopy of the head and neck is an important diagnostic modality used to detect an occult primary mucosal lesion, as well as to identify synchronous primary tumors within the aerodigestive tract. The procedure begins with nasal endoscopy using a zero-degree rigid endoscope to examine the nasopharynx. Random, generous biopsy specimens are taken from the nasopharynx and subjected to histologic examination, which may include frozen section. Should this specimen be positive for a malignant process, the procedure is aborted because definitive treatment of nasopharyngeal carcinoma is radiation therapy and chemotherapy. If the results from the nasopharyngeal frozen section are negative, the evaluation

is advanced to examination and sampling of the oral cavity, oropharynx, hypopharynx, and larynx, along with inspection, palpation, and directed biopsy of the base of the tongue, tonsillar fossa, and posterior pharyngeal wall.

Controversy exists regarding the most appropriate mechanism for sampling the tonsil. This can include direct sampling of the tonsillar fossa or tonsillectomy to eliminate sampling error. Koch and associates reported a 10% rate of spread of metastatic carcinoma from a contralateral tonsil and therefore recommended bilateral tonsillectomy.[20] Bilateral tonsillectomy, however, is typically reserved for patients with bilateral metastatic cervical lymphadenopathy.[4,20,21] Once this is completed, rigid cervical esophagoscopy and bronchoscopy can be performed for evaluation of the remainder of the aerodigestive systems.

OPEN LYMPH NODE BIOPSY

FNA will be inconclusive in 25% of occult neck masses.[2,7,9] Despite repeated FNA, pan-endoscopy, imaging, and directed oropharyngeal biopsy, 1% to 2% of neck masses remain without a specific diagnosis.[7] In this situation, open lymph node biopsy can be performed. Traditional teaching recommends that it be performed via a transcervical incision that can be extended to allow completion neck dissection if necessary for the treatment of cervical metastasis.

Supplemental laboratory evaluation of patients with cervical neck masses is appropriate. Depending on the clinical impression and detailed history and physical examination, if an infectious lesion is suspected, further evaluation may include a complete blood count and sedimentation rate. Other diagnostic tests include a tuberculin skin test, an evaluation for coccidioidomycosis, histoplasmin serologic tests, monospot, toxoplasmosis test, Venereal Disease Research Laboratory (VDRL) serologic test for syphilis, and other appropriate viral and bacterial studies.

DIFFERENTIAL DIAGNOSIS

NEOPLASMS

Thyroid neoplasms, both benign and malignant, are a leading cause of anterior compartment neck masses in all age groups.

Thyromegaly

Lymph node metastasis is the initial symptom in about 15% of papillary carcinomas, is clinically present in 40% of patients with malignant thyroid nodules, and is seen histologically in up to 92% of patients on thorough microscopic examination of the neck dissection. Even though the majority of anterior neck masses are hyperplastic thyroid nodules, they must be proved to be benign.

Metastatic Squamous Cell Carcinoma

Neck mass in an adult patient should be considered metastatic squamous cell carcinoma until proven otherwise. Approximately 65% of patients with cancer of the oropharynx or hypopharynx will demonstrate cervical lymphadenopathy as the initial symptom prior to diagnosis. A high level of suspicion should be maintained when evaluating adult neck masses, even in the absence of identifiable upper aerodigestive tract lesions.

Lymphoma

Hodgkin or non-Hodgkin disease may be manifested as a solid cervical mass. It tends to typically occur in the pediatric and young adult population and accounts for up to 55% of all pediatric malignant tumors. As many as 80% of children with Hodgkin disease have a neck mass at diagnosis. Evaluation of a patient in whom a head and neck lymphoma is diagnosed consists of CT scans of the head, neck, chest, abdomen, and pelvis with a bone marrow biopsy. Because extranodal lymphomas may be associated with gastrointestinal and central nervous system involvement, additional radiographic evaluation is required.

Salivary Gland Tumors

Salivary gland neoplasms must be considered whenever an enlarging solid mass lies in front of the angle of the mandible or in the submandibular triangle. Benign salivary lesions are generally asymptomatic. However, the presence of rapid growth, pain, and cranial nerve VII involvement or skin fixation should suggest a malignant process. FNA may be performed before excisional biopsy if clinical suspicion is concerning for a malignant process. This approach allows a more detailed and appropriate presurgical consultation and planning of surgical resection.

Carotid Body and Glomus Tumors

In adults, carotid body and glomus vagale tumors occur in the upper anterior triangle in the region of the carotid bifurcation and are manifested as a pulsatile, compressible mass that rapidly refills on release and can be moved from side to side. A bruit is present, and in glomus vagale, the ipsilateral tonsil may pulsate and deviate toward the midline. The diagnosis is suggested by clinical suspicion and confirmed by angiography or CT. Small tumors can be resected in a subadventitial manner with the patient under hypotensive anesthesia. Larger glomus tumors (>6 cm) may require mandibular repositioning or preoperative embolization (or both) to limit blood loss at the time of surgery.

Neurogenic tumors (schwannomas and neurilemomas) are solid neurogenic tumors that may develop anywhere in the head and neck but occur most commonly in the parapharyngeal space and, on physical examination, are noted to cause medial tonsillar displacement. Tumors originating in the sympathetic chain may be associated with Horner syndrome.

Lipomas

Lipomas are ill-defined soft tissue masses that occur in various locations in the neck and usually in patients older than 35 years. They are asymptomatic and appear as a fat collection on imaging studies. Typically, the diagnosis is confirmed by excisional biopsy.

CONGENITAL AND DEVELOPMENTAL NECK MASSES

Epidermal and Sebaceous Cysts

Sebaceous and epidermal cysts are the most common congenital and developmental masses that occur in older patients. The key to preoperative diagnosis is that the overlying skin is typically dimpled. In fact, a sebaceous or epidermal cyst usually elevates the skin and moves with it. Pathologic examination is confirmed with complete excision of the mass. Dermoid cysts occur most commonly in younger patients and are frequently found in the midline. They enlarge slowly because of accumulation of the sebaceous content and are typically deep to the cervical fascia without being attached to the overlying skin, a feature that helps differentiate them from epidermal cysts.

Branchial Cleft Cysts

Branchial cleft cysts occur most commonly in late childhood or early adulthood. They frequently follow an upper respiratory tract infection and often appear initially as an inflammatory mass with symptoms of pain, swelling, tenderness, and fever. They are typically located in the anterior triangle of the neck. The more common branchial cleft cyst is a second branchial cleft cyst that occurs deep to and along the anterior edge of the sternocleidomastoid muscle. The less common first branchial cleft cyst occurs along the inferior mandible at the angle or just below the earlobe. FNA of these lesions typically yields a milky mucoid or brownish fluid that often contains cholesterol crystals. Treatment is initial control of local infection followed by surgical excision.

Thyroglossal Duct Cysts

Thyroglossal duct cysts are located in the midline of the neck and may be similar in findings to branchial cleft cysts. They often appear after respiratory tract infection. Physical examination documents vertical motion of the mass with swallowing of the tongue, and they are usually infrahyoid in location. A radionucleotide scan to determine whether the mass contains ectopic thyroid tissue is appropriate to exclude the presence of functioning thyroid tissue in thyroglossal duct cysts that on removal, would render the patient hypothyroid. The entire ductal tract can be removed with the midportion of the hyoid bar in a Sistrunk procedure.

Vascular Abnormalities

Hemangiomas and lymphangiomas represent true neoplasms of the vascular and lymphatic systems, respectively. They usually appear in infancy and are present at birth in more than 90% of cases. They generally progress during the first year of life (proliferative phase) and then slowly begin to involute by early adolescence. Typically, these lesions do not involve the facial skeleton and are soft tissue based. These lesions must be distinguished from vascular and lymphatic malformations, which are non-neoplastic collections of vascular tissue present at birth that grow commensally as the patient grows and do not undergo spontaneous involution. Though present at birth, they usually become clinically obvious later in life and may increase in size with hormonal, infectious, or traumatic stimuli. Kaban and Mullikan reported that unlike hemangiomas, vascular malformations affect the facial skeleton in 35% of cases.[22] A cervical lymphangioma is a fluctuant, diffuse soft mass, often with discrete margins. It may enlarge when upper respiratory tract infections are present and is believed to arise from incomplete development or obstruction of the normal lymphatic cysts. Transillumination along with physical appearance is characteristic. In keeping with the aforementioned vascular processes, these lesions are true lymphatic malformations and not lymphangiomas because they do not spontaneously involute.

UNKNOWN NECK MASS

If a detailed evaluation of the entire head and neck does not lead to a specific cause of a neck mass, this area must be approached with concern because the likelihood of malignancy is high (Fig. 47-3). An asymptomatic cervical mass is the initial symptom in approximately 12% of patients with head and neck cancers. This has been recognized since 1952 when Martin and Romieu, who stated that "an asymmetric enlargement of one or more of the cervical lymph nodes in an adult is almost always cancerous, and usually it is due to metastasis from a primary lesion in the mouth or oropharynx."[23] That principle remains valid today. It is important to note that an asymmetric, asymptomatic mass in an adult must be considered a malignancy until proved otherwise because approximately 30% of these lesions harbor some form of malignant process.[5,24] Approximately half to two thirds of patients with a neck mass in whom malignancy is subsequently diagnosed are found to have an obvious primary lesion in the head/neck on

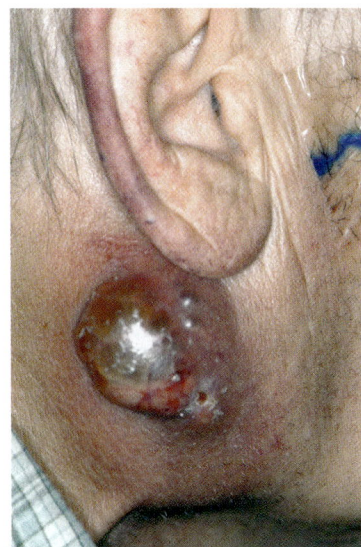

Fig. 47-3 ■ Patient with a large ulcerative neck mass of unknown primary origin.

either visual inspection or fiberoptic examination at the initial office evaluation.[25-27]

FNA is particularly useful in guiding therapy in adult patients and allowing differentiation between lymphoma and carcinoma. This distinction avoids endoscopy if lymphoma is either diagnosed or strongly suspected on FNA and allows histologic examination and flow cytometry. If the neck mass is FNA positive for carcinoma and a primary source is still elusive after repeated head and neck examination, pan-endoscopy is required with particular attention paid to the area being drained by the lymphatics and leading to the area of the neck mass.

Biopsies should be performed on any suspicious lesion, but when no mucosal lesions are found, random biopsies of the pharyngeal tonsils, base of the tongue, and posterior pharyngeal wall are appropriate (see earlier). The incidence of positive results of guided biopsy in patients with unknown primary tumors is approximately 20%. If repeated FNA provides an equivocal or negative result and the remainder of the head and neck examination remains negative, open excisional biopsy of the neck mass is the appropriate next step. This biopsy should be done through a traditional incision for performing neck dissection and should be done by a surgeon capable of performing completion neck dissection should it be required at the time of surgery. With contemporary imaging and diagnostic techniques as discussed, open biopsy for diagnosis is needed in less than 5% of all patients with neck masses.[18,26,28]

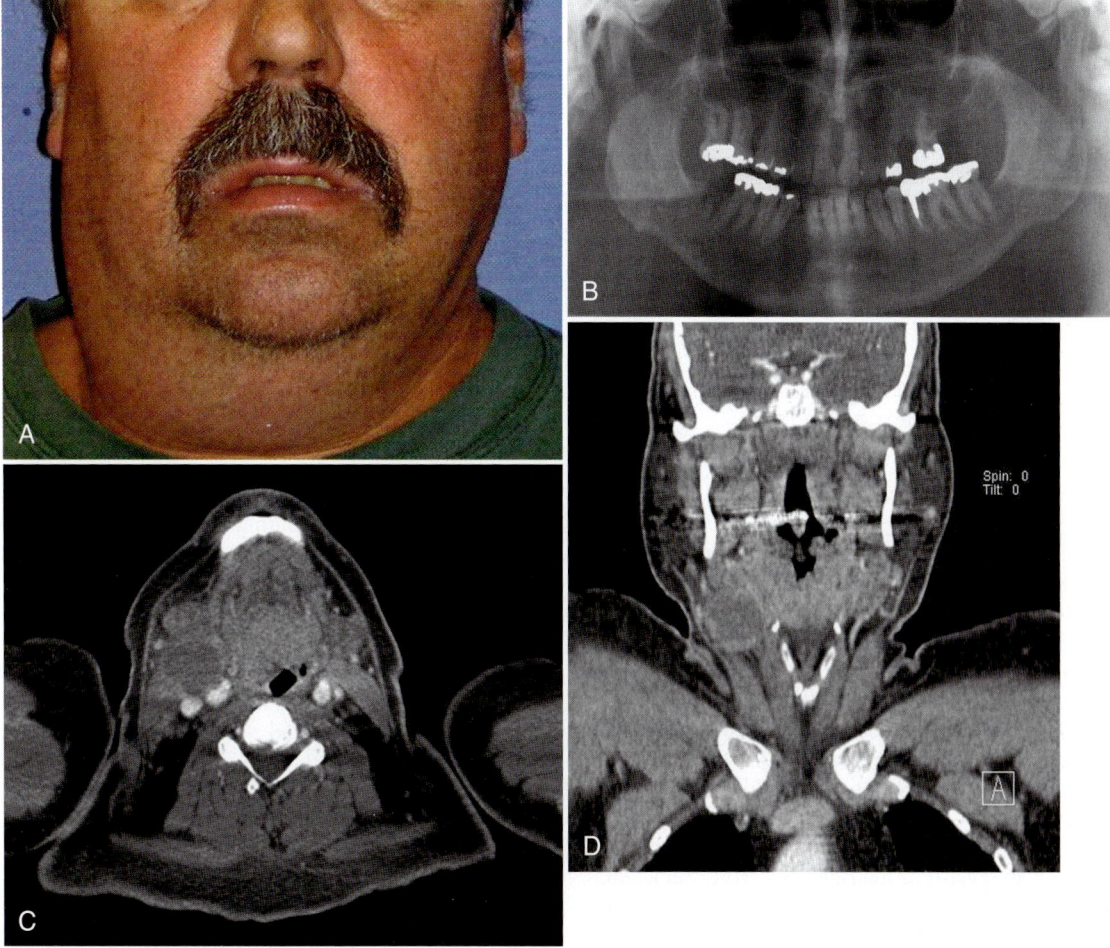

Fig. 47-4 ■ **A,** Clinical appearance of a 56-year-old man referred for evaluation of a right neck mass. **B,** A panoramic radiograph does not show any evidence of a specific cause. **C** and **D,** Contrast-enhanced computed tomography scans of a large cystic node in level II of the right side of the neck.

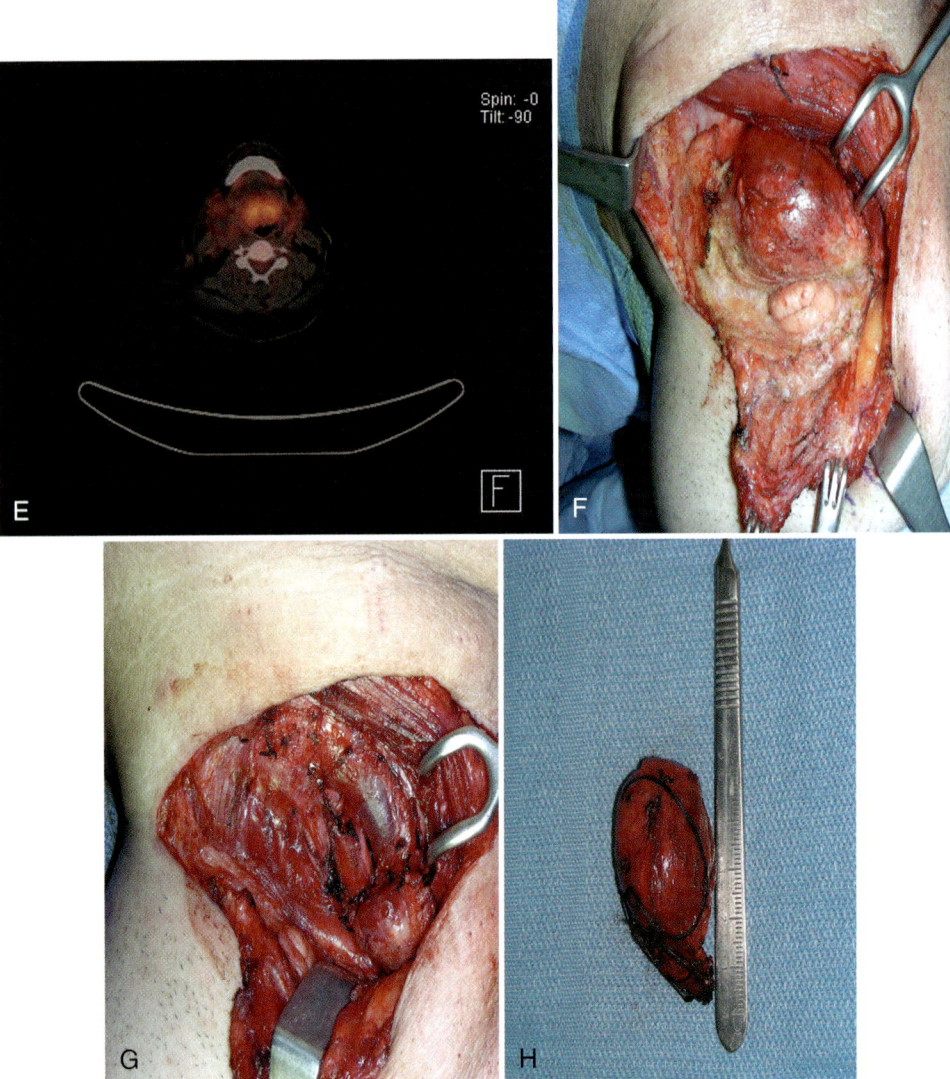

Fig. 47-4, cont'd ▪ **E,** Positron emission tomography scan. **F,** Intraoperative view of neck exploration and delineation of the mass. **G,** Intraoperative view showing the internal jugular vein and carotid artery after excision of the mass. **H,** Excision of a cystic mass confirmed the presence of a branchial cleft cyst.

CASE EXAMPLE

A 56-year-old man was referred for evaluation and consultation for a new-onset right lateral neck mass (Fig. 47-4, *A*). He was recently seen by a general dental and medical practitioner, who considered the neck mass to be associated with an odontogenic source. The patient did report fevers and chills on initial evaluation with a 5-lb weight loss during the past 3 months. He denied any further constitutional difficulties. Nasopharyngoscopy showed some slight fullness of the right base of the tongue and lingual tonsil. An orthopantogram showed a partially dentate maxilla and mandible without any clear odontogenic evidence of a potential source for the neck mass (Fig. 47-4, *B*). CT scans were obtained and showed a 4.5-cm unicystic mass in level II of the right side of the neck, adjacent to the bifurcation of the carotid artery, along with some associated compression of the internal jugular vein (Fig. 47-4, *C* and *D*). FNA was performed and showed purulence and the presence of atypical cells suggestive of malignancy. Based on these findings, a PET scan was obtained (Fig. 47-4, *E*). Areas of hypermetabolism were noted in the right lingual tonsil and base of the tongue, as well

as a mild area of uptake in the neck mass. The patient was subsequently taken to the operating room for formal examination under anesthesia, endoscopy, and direct biopsies (Fig. 47-4, *F*). The areas of hyperintensity on the PET scan were determined to be lymphoid hyperplasia without evidence of malignancy. Since the patient still did not have a tissue diagnosis, the neck mass was excised via a transcervical approach. It was intimately associated with the lateral wall of the external carotid artery (Fig. 47-4, *G*). The entire mass was removed en bloc and was preliminarily determined to be a branchial cleft cyst (Fig. 47-4, *H*) without evidence of malignancy by frozen section analysis. The final pathology was consistent with a branchial cleft cyst.

DISCUSSION

When a thorough diagnostic evaluation is undertaken as described, the primary tumor is located in the majority of cases. However, 1% to 2% of tumors remain elusive. During the evolution of the various diagnostic procedures, there is a 7% rate of diagnosis of a primary tumor site that was initially unknown. The 5-year disease-free survival rate is 35% in patients with detected primary tumors versus 70% to 90% in patients with unknown primaries. The survival rate decreases from 52% to 22% if the primary site is localized during the diagnostic work-up. There is a 7% rate of subsequent emergence of the primary tumor, which typically occurs within 2 years. When the primary site remains elusive, overall survival is better in patients treated by radiotherapy than by surgery alone, with survival rates of 34% to 64% and 22% to 44%, respectively. There are limited studies showing the effectiveness of additional chemotherapy in this patient cohort. Argiris and colleagues reported improved survival with concurrent chemoradiotherapy and an overall survival rate of 75%.[29] These results are promising but are difficult to interpret in the absence of significant prospective data, which are unavailable for primary tumors of unknown origin.

PEARLS AND PITFALLS

- As oral and maxillofacial surgeons, we will often evaluate patients with cervical neck masses. It is important for the practitioner to have detailed understanding of the possible causes and the importance of the patient's age and location of the mass in formulating a differential diagnosis.
- Having a well-designed diagnostic algorithm along with an index of suspicion based on the clinical history and location of the lesion will help guide the diagnostic steps necessary to obtain a diagnosis.
- The performance of endoscopy, FNA, and directed biopsies is important to establish a formal histologic diagnosis.
- On occasion, however, the diagnosis will remain elusive and requires the treating surgeon to obtain a complete specimen of the mass through an open biopsy approach.

REFERENCES

1. Jaffe B: Pediatric head and neck tumors: a study of 178 cases, *Laryngoscope* 83:1644-1651, 1973.
2. Altman E, Cadman E: An analysis of 1539 patients with cancer of unknown primary site, *Cancer* 57:120-124, 1986.
3. Jesse RH, Perez CA, Fletcher GH: Cervical lymph node metastasis: unknown primary cancer, *Cancer* 31:854-859, 1973.
4. Chepeha D, Koch W, Pitman K: Management of unknown primary tumor, *Head Neck* 25:499-504, 2003.
5. Jereczek-Fossa BA, Jassem J, Orecchia R: Cervical lymph node metastases of squamous cell carcinoma from an unknown primary, *Cancer Treat Rev* 30:153-164, 2004.
6. Weymuller E: Evaluation of a neck mass, *J Fam Pract* 1:1099-1106, 1980.
7. Gunthinas-Linhius O, Klussmann P, Dinh S, et al: Diagnostic workup and outcome of cervical metastasis from an unknown primary, *Acta Otolaryngol* 126:536-544, 2006.
8. Lindberg R: Distribution of cervical lymph node metastases from squamous cell carcinoma of the upper respiratory and digestive tracts, *Cancer* 9:1446-1449, 1972.
9. de Braud F, al-Sarraf M: Diagnosis and management of squamous cell carcinoma of unknown primary site of the neck, *Semin Oncol* 20:273-278, 1993.
10. Haas I, Hoffmann TK, Engers R, et al: Diagnostic strategies in cervical carcinoma of an unknown primary (CUP), *Eur Arch Otorhinolaryngol* 259:325-333, 2002.
11. Issing WJ, Taleban B, Tauber S: Diagnosis and management of carcinoma of unknown primary in the head and neck, *Eur Arch Otorhinolaryngol* 260:436-443, 2003.
12. Hainsworth JD, Greco FA: Treatment of patients with cancer of an unknown primary site, *N Engl J Med* 329:257-263, 1993.
13. Iganej S, Kagan R, Anderson P, et al: Metastatic squamous cell carcinoma of the neck from an unknown primary: management options and patterns of relapse. *Head Neck* 24:236-246, 2002.
14. Adams JR, O'Brien CJ: Unknown primary squamous cell carcinoma of the head and neck: a review of diagnosis, treatment and outcomes, *Asian J Surg* 25:188-193, 2002.
15. Hanasono MM, Kunda LD, Segall GM, et al: Uses and limitations of FDG positron emission tomography in patients with head and neck cancer, *Laryngoscope* 109:880-885, 1999.
16. Johansen J, Eigtved A, Buchwald C, et al: Implication of ^{18}F-fluoro-2-deoxy-D-glucose positron emission tomography on management of carcinoma of unknown primary in the head and neck: a Danish cohort study, *Laryngoscope* 112:2009-2014, 2002.
17. Jungehulsing M, Scheidhauer K, Damm M, et al: 2[F]-fluoro-2-deoxy-D-glucose positron emission tomography is a sensitive tool for the detection of occult primary cancer (carcinoma of unknown primary syndrome) with head and neck lymph node manifestation, *Otolaryngol Head Neck Surg* 123:294-301, 2000.
18. Miller F, Hussey D, Beeram M: Positron emission tomography in the management of unknown primary head and neck carcinoma, *Arch Otolaryngol Head Neck Surg* 131:626-629, 2005.
19. Schmidt M, Schmalenbach M, Jungehulsing M, et al: ^{18}F-FDG PET for detecting recurrent head and neck cancer, local lymph node involvement and distant metastases. Comparison of qualitative visual and semi-quantitative analysis, *Nucl Med* 43:91-101, quiz 102-104, 2004.
20. Koch W, Bhatti N, Williams M, et al: Oncologic rationale for bilateral tonsillectomy in head and neck squamous cell carcinoma of unknown source, *Otorhinolaryngol Head Neck Surg* 124:331-333, 2001.
21. Nieder C, Gregoire V, Ang KK: Cervical lymph node metastases from occult squamous cell carcinoma: cut down a tree to get an apple? *Int J Radiat Oncol Biol Phys* 50:727-733, 2001.
22. Kaban LB, Mullikan JB: Vascular anomalies of the maxillofacial region, *J Oral Maxillofac Surg* 44:203-213, 1986.
23. Martin H, Romieu C: The diagnostic significance of a "lump in the neck", *Postgrad Med* 11:491-500, 1952.
24. Koivunen P, Laranne J, Virtaniemi J, et al: Cervical metastasis of unknown origin: a series of 72 patients, *Acta Otolaryngol* 122:569-574, 2002.
25. Lee DJ, Rostock RA, Harris A, et al: Clinical evaluation of patients with metastatic squamous carcinoma of the neck with occult primary tumor, *South Med J* 79:979-983, 1986.
26. Nieder C, Ang KK: Cervical lymph node metastases from occult squamous cell carcinoma, *Curr Treat Options Oncol* 3:33-40, 2002.
27. Rades D, Kuhnel G, Wildfang I, et al: Localised disease in cancer of unknown primary (CUP): the value of positron emission tomography (PET) for individual therapeutic management, *Ann Oncol* 12:1605-1609, 2001.
28. Wong WL, Saunders M: The impact of FDG PET on the management of occult primary head and neck tumors, *Clin Oncol (R Coll Radiol)* 15:461-466, 2003.
29. Argiris A, Smith SM, Stenson K, et al: Concurrent chemoradiotherapy for N2 or N3 squamous cell carcinoma of the head and neck from an occult primary, *Ann Oncol* 14:1306-1311, 2003.

Keratocystic Odontogenic Tumor

M.A. Pogrel

A keratocystic odontogenic tumor (KOT) (formerly known as an odontogenic keratocyst) is a benign cystic tumor of dental origin that probably arises from primitive dental lamina, most commonly occurs in the posterior mandible, and almost certainly represents the lesion that used to be known as a primordial cyst.[1,2] It has a typical histologic appearance consisting of parakeratinization, a tumor lining five to six cells thick, and polarization of the basal layer on the basement membrane (Fig. 48-1). A KOT is thought to be benign, but locally aggressive.[3,4] An orthokeratinized version also occurs, but this is thought to represent a different lesion and not to be aggressive.[5,6] The parakeratinized version is normally quoted as having a recurrence rate varying from 25% to 60% following conservative management such as cystectomy or enucleation.[7,8] For this reason, alternative treatments have been actively pursued to decrease the recurrence rate but, at the same time, to not subject the patient to radical surgery with loss of teeth, bone, and nerves. The reason for recurrence of KOTs is uncertain. Some authorities believe that they are inherently more aggressive and have a higher mitotic index in the cyst lining,[8,9] others think that the lining is so friable that it is difficult not to leave small portions behind,[10] and still others believe that it is the presence of epithelial buds or daughter cysts projecting from the lesion that leads to recurrence. Alternative treatments that fall between cystectomy and radical resection are discussed in the following sections.

DECOMPRESSION OR MARSUPIALIZATION

Although these terms are used interchangeably, decompression technically denotes any treatment whereby the pressure is taken off the tumor by creation of a hole in the tumor from which it can drain. This can be a small opening into which a decompression tube can be placed (Fig. 48-2). Decompression is normally used as a means of decreasing the size of a KOT so that it can be enucleated later without risking additional teeth, the inferior alveolar nerve, or the integrity of the mandible.[11-13]

Marsupialization is a form of decompression that denotes the creation of a wider opening, which is often self-sustaining (Fig. 48-3), and this treatment can be performed for complete cure of the lesion.[14] Although KOT is an aggressive tumor, it does appear to respond successfully to marsupialization and can resolve totally following marsupialization, often over a period of 6 to 12 months (Fig. 48-4). Persistence and recurrences do occur, however, possibly from daughter cysts around the lining, and a personal report shows a 10% recurrence rate with marsupialization alone.[15] Histologic examination has shown that as the marsupialized tumor decreases in size, the lining differentiates from the typical appearance of a KOT to one more closely resembling oral mucosa.[14,16] Whether this occurs by metaplasia or overgrowth from the periphery remains unclear.

CYSTECTOMY WITH PERIPHERAL OSTECTOMY

There are essentially two techniques by which a rim of bone can be removed around a KOT in an attempt to eliminate any remnants of cystic lining and to remove any daughter cysts. In the first technique, en bloc resection is carried out whereby the tumor and a rim of bone are removed in continuity and the tumor itself is not separately removed.[17,18] In the second technique, the tumor is first enucleated, and a rim of bone approximately 1 mm in thickness is then removed all around the cystic cavity to eliminate any remnants of the lining or daughter cysts.[19] This rim of bone is normally removed with a large pineapple-type burr, and to ensure that bone removal is equal all around, the cavity can be stained with methylene blue or an alternative stain that reaches to a depth of around 1 mm, and then all the stained bone is removed with the burr. Conceptually, it is possible that if there are tumor remnants in this peripheral bone, a pineapple burr could drive them deeper into the bone rather than bringing them out, but this technique nevertheless appears to be successful and lowers the recurrence rate.

ENUCLEATION PLUS ADDITIONAL PHYSICOCHEMICAL MEANS TO REMOVE CYST REMNANTS OR DAUGHTER CYSTS IN THE PERIPHERAL BONE

There are two commonly advocated techniques to achieve this objective: one is to treat the peripheral bone with liquid nitrogen to kill any organic matter within the bone matrix around the lesion, and the other is to use Carnoy's solution to chemically fix any organic matter in the bone.

Liquid nitrogen sprayed into the cavity appears to kill any organic matter within about 1.5 mm of the cavity, which is appropriate for the management of a KOT.[20] A typical protocol will freeze the cavity for 1 minute and allow it to thaw spontaneously. This cycle is usually repeated three times. Once the liquid nitrogen boils off, it leaves the inorganic bone matrix present to act as a matrix for new bone formation. New bone formation can be accelerated by grafting the residual cavity with cancellous bone marrow, and this should be carried out for any tumor larger than 4 cm in diameter.[20,21] Liquid nitrogen treatment does temporarily significantly weaken the mandible; this weakness is maximal at 6 to 8 weeks, and pathologic fractures have been reported at this time.[21] Liquid nitrogen will affect the adjacent

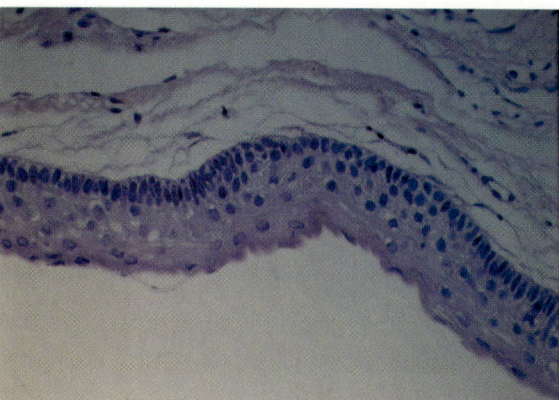

Fig. 48-1 ■ Histologic appearance of a typical keratocystic odontogenic tumor showing a tumor lining five to six cells in thickness with parakeratinization and polarization of the basal layer. (Hematoxylin-eosin stain, ×40.)

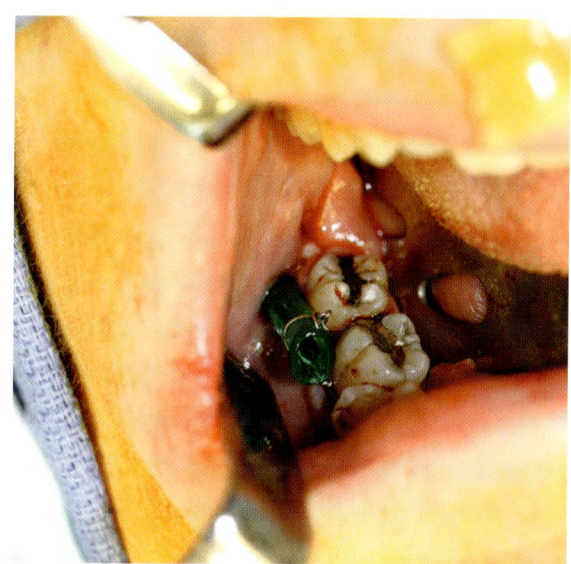

Fig. 48-2 ■ A keratocystic odontogenic tumor being decompressed by using the tubing from an intravenous giving set.

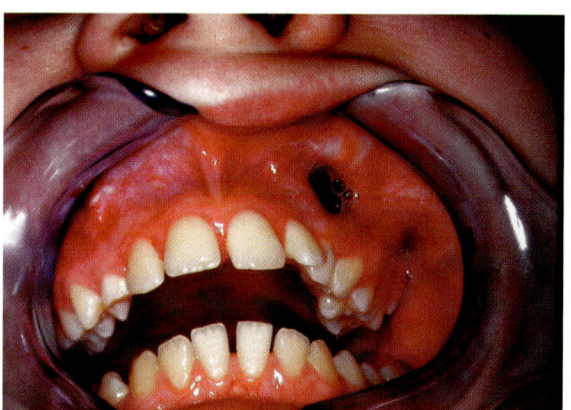

Fig. 48-3 ■ A keratocystic odontogenic tumor being marsupialized by means of a self-sustaining opening.

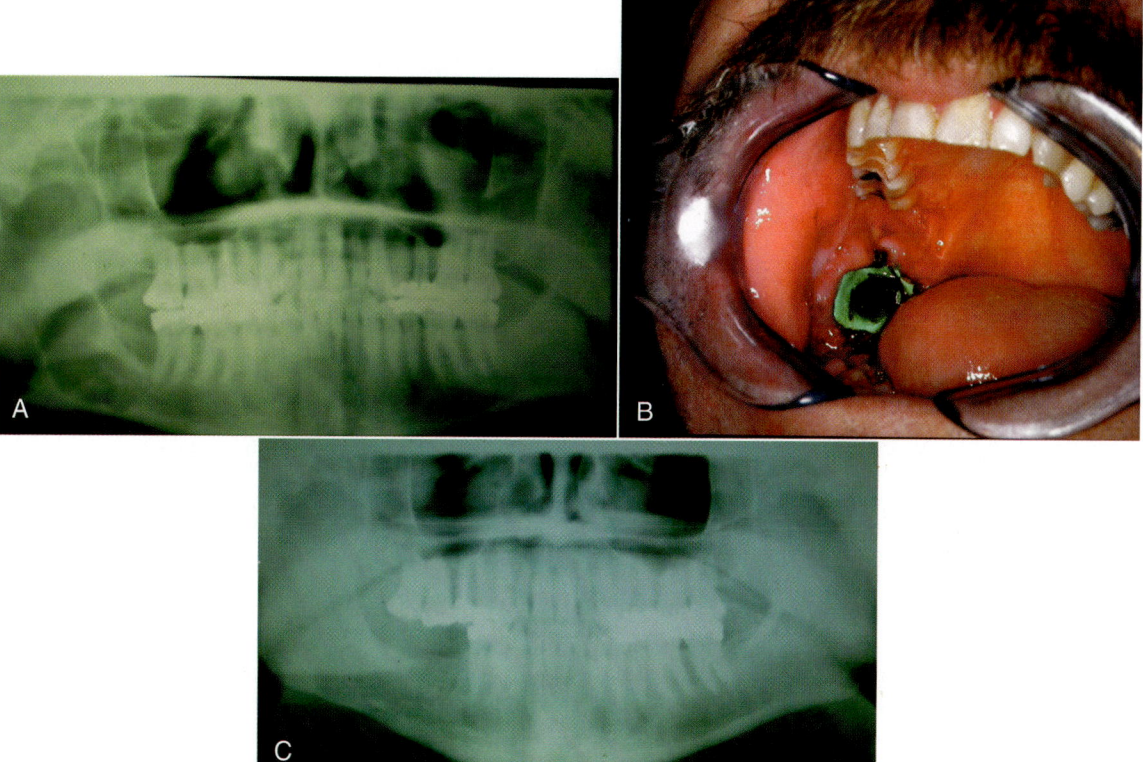

Fig. 48-4 ■ A keratocystic odontogenic tumor treated by marsupialization and decompression only. **A,** Preoperative photograph. Note the multilocular lesion in the right angle of the mandible and ascending ramus region. **B,** In the course of decomposition with a cut-down nasopharyngeal airway in place to keep the tumor open to drain. **C,** Radiographic appearance 2 years later. Note the complete bony in-filling of the lesion.

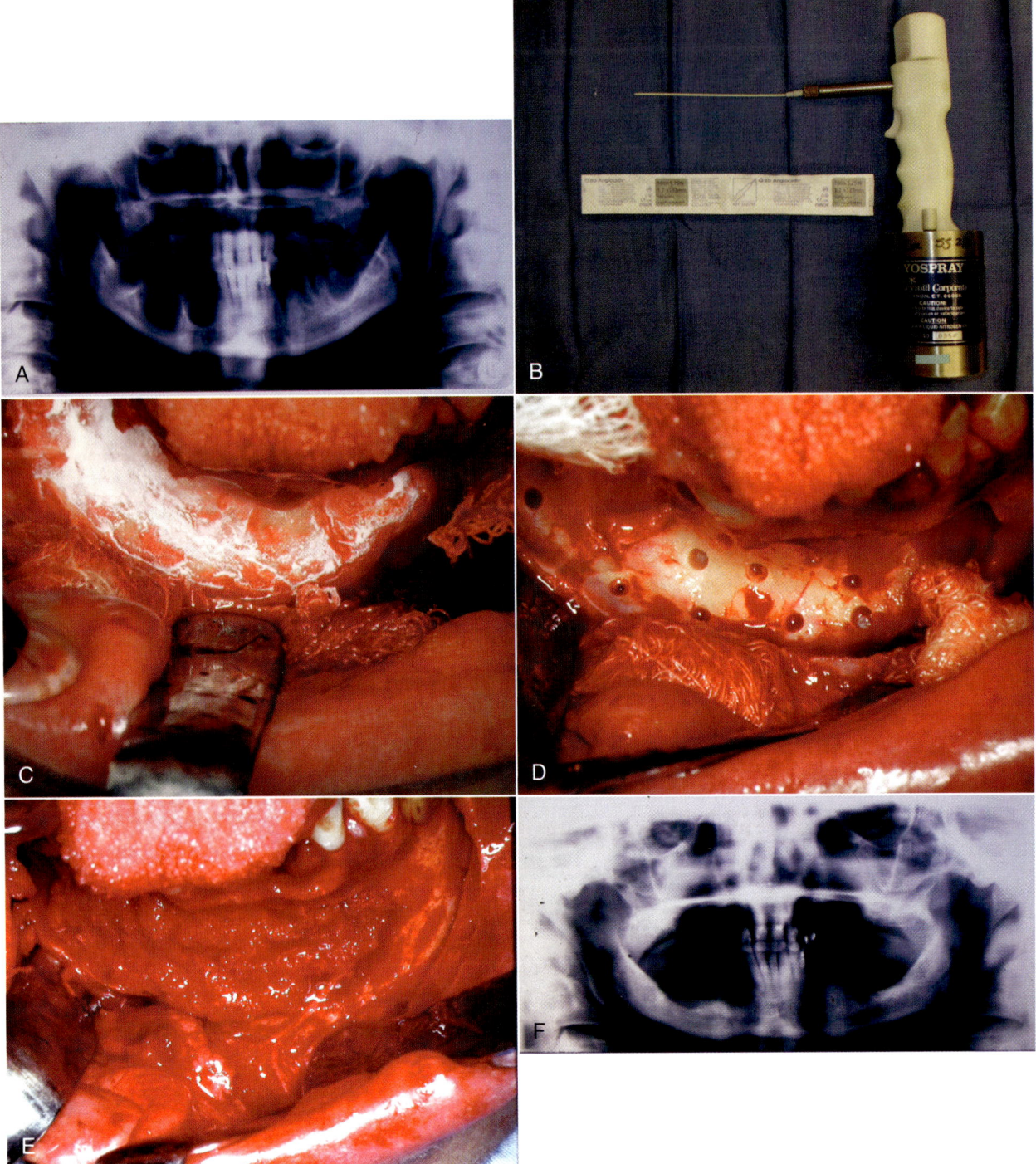

Fig. 48-5 ■ Multiple keratocystic odontogenic tumors. **A,** At initial evaluation. **B,** Liquid nitrogen spray apparatus with a flexible cannula to deliver the spray to the required region. **C,** Frost following liquid nitrogen cryospray. **D,** Following thawing and perforation, the tumor cavity can be bone-grafted. **E,** After bone grafting with a cancellous graft from the iliac crest. **F,** Appearance 1 year later with resolution of the lesions.

teeth but does not appear to cause long-term changes.[22] This technique is not applicable if the buccal or lingual plates are perforated since its use may cause soft tissue necrosis. If the inferior alveolar or lingual nerves are within the field of the liquid nitrogen treatment, they will be affected and paresthesia or anesthesia will result, although the axon sheath remains intact and new axon formation is usual, with most patients reporting recovery of sensation over a 3- to

6-month period.[23] The soft tissues must be protected from the liquid nitrogen, and meticulous soft tissue closure is essential. The recurrence rate appears to significantly decrease when KOTs are enucleated and the cavity treated with liquid nitrogen[24,25] (Fig. 48-5). The author has personally used this technique on 67 KOTs with 6 recurrences to date (1- to 25-year follow-up), which represents a 9% recurrence rate.

Carnoy's solution, which contains chloroform, ferric chloride, glacial acetic acid, and absolute alcohol,[26] is now difficult to obtain since the glacial acetic acid has to be handled in a high-volume fume cover and chloroform is technically classified as a carcinogen. In addition, most advocates of Carnoy's solution report that it should be mixed fresh to have the best effect and that stored Carnoy's solution is inappropriate.[27] If the KOT is enucleated, the residual cavity can be treated with Carnoy's solution applied with cotton-tipped swabs. Teeth and nerves should be avoided because permanent damage can be caused by Carnoy's solution. It does physically render the bone brown in color, and it is thought to be inappropriate to place a bone graft on top of this solution since it is difficult for the bone graft to become revascularized and the graft will fail. Thus,

healing following treatment with Carnoy's solution is often prolonged, but it does decrease the recurrence rate.[28-30]

All of the aforementioned techniques are applicable to the mandible and maxilla, provided that the maxillary sinus is not involved. If the sinus is involved, treatment can consist of conventional resection or marsupialization (into the oral cavity or the sinus). Liquid nitrogen cryotherapy or Carnoy's solution is not applicable to the sinus.

It is believed that any of the aforementioned treatments of KOT are acceptable as a means of avoiding sacrifice of teeth, bone, or nerves or the risk of loss of integrity of the mandible or maxilla. Treatments can also be combined, such as decompression followed by enucleation and treatment with liquid nitrogen cryotherapy.

REFERENCES

1. Pathology and genetics of head and neck tumours. In Barnes L, Eveson JW, Reichart P, et al, editors: *WHO classification of tumours series*, Geneva, 2005, World Health Organization.
2. Partridge M, Towers JF: The primordial cyst (odontogenic keratocyst): its tumour-like characteristics and behaviour, *Br J Oral Maxillofac Surg* 25:271-279, 1987.
3. Shear M: The aggressive nature of the odontogenic keratocyst: is it a benign cystic neoplasm? Part 3. Immunocytochemistry of cytokeratin and other epithelial cell markers, *Oral Oncol* 38:407-415, 2002.
4. Shear M: The aggressive nature of the odontogenic keratocyst: is it a benign cystic neoplasm? Part 2. Proliferation and genetic studies, *Oral Oncol* 38:323-331, 2002.
5. Crowley T, Kaugars GE, Gunsolley JC: Odontogenic keratocysts: a clinical and histologic comparison of the parakeratin and orthokeratin variants, *J Oral Maxillofac Surg* 50:22-26, 1992.
6. Wright JM: The odontogenic keratocyst: orthokeratinized variant, *Oral Surg Oral Med Oral Pathol* 51:609-618, 1981.
7. Bramley PA, Browne RM: Recurring odontogenic cysts, *Br J Oral Surg* 5:106-116, 1967.
8. Browne RM: The odontogenic keratocyst. Clinical aspects, *Br Dent J* 128:225-231, 1970.
9. Browne RM: The odontogenic keratocyst. Histological features and their correlation with clinical behaviour, *Br Dent J* 131:249-259, 1971.
10. Brady CL, Browne RM, Calverley BC, et al: Symposium on odontogenic epithelium, *Br J Oral Surg* 8:1-15, 1970.

11. Marker P, Brondum N, Clausen PP, et al: Treatment of large odontogenic keratocysts by decompression and later cystectomy: a long-term follow-up and a histologic study of 23 cases, *Oral Surg Oral Med Oral Pathol Oral Radiol Endod* 82:122-131, 1996.
12. Brondum N, Jensen VJ: Recurrence of keratocysts and decompression treatment. A long-term follow-up of forty-four cases, *Oral Surg Oral Med Oral Pathol* 72:265-269, 1991.
13. Tucker WM, Pleasants JE, MacComb WS: Decompression and secondary enucleation of a mandibular cyst: report of case, *J Oral Surg* 30:669-673, 1972.
14. Pogrel MA, Jordan RC: Marsupialization as a definitive treatment for the odontogenic keratocyst, *J Oral Maxillofac Surg* 62:651-655, discussion 655-656, 2004.
15. Pogrel MA: Decompression and marsupialization as definitive treatment for keratocysts—a partial retraction, *J Oral Maxillofac Surg* 65:362-363, 2007.
16. August M, Faquin WC, Troulis MJ, et al: Dedifferentiation of odontogenic keratocyst epithelium after cyst decompression, *J Oral Maxillofac Surg* 61:678-683, discussion 683-684, 2003.
17. Bramley P: The odontogenic keratocyst—an approach to treatment, *Int J Oral Surg* 3:337-341, 1974.
18. Bataineh AB, al Qudah M: Treatment of mandibular odontogenic keratocysts, *Oral Surg Oral Med Oral Pathol Oral Radiol Endod* 86:42-47, 1998.
19. Irvine GH, Bowerman JE: Mandibular keratocysts: surgical management, *Br J Oral Maxillofac Surg* 23:204-209, 1985.
20. Pogrel MA, Regezi JA, Fong B, et al: Effects of liquid nitrogen cryotherapy and bone

grafting on artificial bone defects in minipigs: a preliminary study, *Int J Oral Maxillofac Surg* 31:296-302, 2002.
21. Salmassy DA, Pogrel MA: Liquid nitrogen cryosurgery and immediate bone grafting in the management of aggressive primary jaw lesions, *J Oral Maxillofac Surg* 53:784-790, 1995.
22. Gordon NC, Laskin DM: The effects of local hypothermia on odontogenesis, *J Oral Surg* 37:235-244, 1979.
23. Schmidt BL, Pogrel MA: Neurosensory changes after liquid nitrogen cryotherapy, *J Oral Maxillofac Surg* 62:1183-1187, 2004.
24. Schmidt BL, Pogrel MA: The use of enucleation and liquid nitrogen cryotherapy in the management of odontogenic keratocysts, *J Oral Maxillofac Surg* 59:720-725, discussion 726-727, 2001.
25. Pogrel MA: The management of lesions of the jaws with liquid nitrogen cryotherapy, *J Calif Dent Assoc* 23:54-57, 1995.
26. Cutler E, Zollinger R: Sclerosing solution in the treatment of cysts and fistulae, *Am J Surg* 19:411-418, 1933.
27. Stoelinga PJ: Excision of the overlying, attached mucosa, in conjunction with cyst enucleation and treatment of the bony defect with Carnoy solution, *Oral Maxillofac Surg Clin North Am* 15:407-414, 2003.
28. Stoelinga PJ: Long-term follow-up on keratocysts treated according to a defined protocol, *Int J Oral Maxillofac Surg* 30:14-25, 2001.
29. Voorsmit RA, Stoelinga PJ, van Haelst UJ: The management of keratocysts, *J Maxillofac Surg* 9:228-236, 1981.
30. Voorsmit RA: The incredible keratocyst: a new approach to treatment, *Dtsch Zahnarztl Z* 40:641-644, 1985.

Chapter 49

Contemporary Treatment of Ameloblastoma

Deepak Kademani, David Michael Junck

Ameloblastoma is the most common benign tumor of the jaws, comprising approximately 10% of odontogenic tumors and 1% of all cysts and tumors.[1] Ameloblastoma was first described by Malassez in 1885.[2] Due to the historically high recurrence rates and potential for local destruction and locally uncontrollable disease, a thorough understanding of the pathogenesis and clinical behavior of ameloblastoma is imperative for the oral and maxillofacial surgeon. The treatment is based largely on the tumor biology, location, and extent of disease. Surgical management should primarily be focused on a curative intent with the least degree of associated morbidity. Surgeons have frequently struggled with this issue, due to the lack of standardized treatment for ameloblastoma and the variety of histologic variants described in the literature. This chapter will review the pathogenesis, clinical presentation, histology, and treatment for the contemporary management of ameloblastoma.

CLINICAL PRESENTATION/ PATHOGENESIS

The ameloblastoma arises from odontogenic ectoderm.[3] Malassez suggested that it arose from epithelial remnants of the developing root sheath.[2] However, the causes of ameloblastoma are largely unknown. Ameloblastoma is classically described as a benign locally aggressive tumor, but it has the ability for metastasis in rare situations. Presumptive factors causing local inflammation, such as tooth extraction, caries, infection, calculus, developing teeth, trauma, nutritional deficiencies, and viruses, have been investigated; however, no direct causative correlation exists.[4] Ameloblastoma is a slow-growing tumor that may take years before clinical presentation. The most common presenting symptom is painless swelling of the jaws (Fig. 49-1). Other symptoms include pain, loosening of teeth, malocclusion, and altered sensation. Many tumors are associated with unerupted teeth, which are often displaced from the tumor. Root resorption of adjacent teeth is frequently seen.[4] The majority of ameloblastomas, approximately 80%, arise in the mandible versus 20% in the maxilla.[2] Most mandibular tumors arise in the third molar region. There are three classic varieties of ameloblastoma: solid/multicystic, unicystic, and peripheral. The solid/multicystic and unicystic types have several histologic variants that can have different biologic behavior. In a review of 3677 cases, the solid/multicystic type comprises 92% of ameloblastomas, the unicystic type 6%, and the peripheral type accounts for 2%.[5]

CLASSIFICATION

SOLID/MULTICYSTIC

The solid/multicystic type is often termed the "conventional" ameloblastoma. It can be either a solid or multicystic lesion. It occurs equally in males and females. Commonly, it occurs in the third to seventh decade in life and is rarely seen in patients less than 20 years of age. The radiographic presentation is characterized as a multilocular radiolucency with a "soap bubble" or "honeycomb" appearance, although it may appear as a unilocular lesion (Fig. 49-2). Cortical expansion, resorption of adjacent teeth roots, and association with an unerupted tooth are common (Fig. 49-3). The radiographic margins appear irregular and scalloped, which may be seen with loss of the cortical bone margins. The histology of the solid/multicystic ameloblastoma is characterized by the presence of benign proliferation of odontogenic epithelium with stellate reticulum and varying composition of solid or cystic features. There are several variants of solid ameloblastoma from a histologic perspective that are important to recognize; however, these have limited impact on treatment decision making presently.

Follicular

The follicular pattern is the most common subtype of the solid/multicystic ameloblastoma. The tumor comprises epithelial islands that resemble an enamel organ in a background of fibrous connective tissue stroma. The epithelial islands consist of a single outer layer of tall columnar or cuboidal cells with nuclei located on the opposite pole to the basement membrane (reverse polarization) and resemble ameloblasts, and there is a central zone of cells that resemble stellate reticulum. Areas of cyst formation are frequently observed; these areas vary from large macroscopic cystic spaces to microcysts that result from degeneration within epithelial islands. (Fig. 49-4).

Plexiform

Plexiform ameloblastoma consists of larger sheets or long anastomosing cords of odontogenic epithelium. Similar to follicular ameloblastoma, the peripheral epithelial cells comprise ameloblast-like cells enclosing more loosely organized epithelial cells. Cyst formation is not common; however, if present, it is more likely due to degeneration of the connective tissue stroma (Fig. 49-5).

Granular Cell

In some cases, the neoplastic epithelial cells may show transformation to granular cells with eosinophilic granules in the cytoplasm, which are consistent with lysosomes. The term granular cell ameloblastoma should be reserved for those cases that show extensive presence of granular cells. Although initially suggested as a degenerative change in long-standing ameloblastomas, granular cells have been reported in younger patients and in clinically aggressive tumors.

Basal Cell

The basal cell type contains nests of basaloid cells without central stellate reticulum-like cells. This is the least common type of solid/multicystic ameloblastoma (Fig. 49-6).

Acanthomatous

The term acanthomatous ameloblastoma is used for those cases that show extensive squamous metaplasia and keratin production occurring in the central epithelial islands of the follicular ameloblastoma. Caution must be used to not confuse this histologic appearance with squamous cell carcinoma or squamous odontogenic tumor (Fig. 49-7).

Desmoplastic

Desmoplastic ameloblastoma is characterized by extensive stromal collagenization (desmoplasia) with small islands and cords of tumor cells[6] (Fig. 49-8).

Although there are many histologic subtypes of ameloblastoma, there does not appear to be a significant difference in clinical behavior.[4] However, Hong et al suggested that the follicular, granular cell,

and acanthomatous subtypes showed a higher recurrence rate, whereas the plexiform and desmoplastic patterns showed a lower rate of recurrence.[7] The desmoplastic type is the most recently identified form, first described by Eversole.[8] The incidence ranges from 0.9% to 12.1% and has a predilection for the anterior maxilla relative to the other types of solid/multicystic ameloblastomas.[6] Radiographic features are generally atypical of other ameloblastomas, being more characteristic of fibro-osseous lesions, including an indistinct radiographic border with radiolucent/radiopaque appearance and peripheral calcifications.[9] The maxilla is often more frequently involved with greater than 50% of desmoplastic ameloblastomas.[6,9] In a review of 80 cases of desmoplastic ameloblastoma by Beckley et al, the only reports of recurrence occurred when the tumor was treated with enucleation.[6] Due to the atypical radiographic appearance of the desmoplastic ameloblastoma, many are treated with enucleation initially. Upon histologic diagnosis, it is imperative that the tumor is resected with clear margins, due to the high recurrence rate with enucleation. There is insufficient evidence in the literature for varying treatment algorithms based on the histologic subtype; therefore, all solid/multicystic ameloblastomas require similar treatment to limit recurrence.[6,9]

UNICYSTIC

The clinical presentation of unicystic ameloblastomas varies from the solid/multicystic types. Age at presentation is typically less than for other forms of ameloblastoma, typically in the second and third decade of life. The unicystic ameloblastoma appears

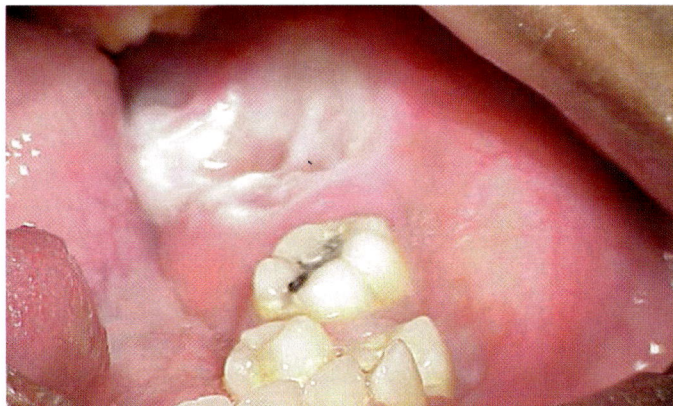

Fig. 49-1 ■ Expansile mass of the left posterior mandible. Mucosal changes consistent with hyperkeratosis due to the opposing dentition are seen.

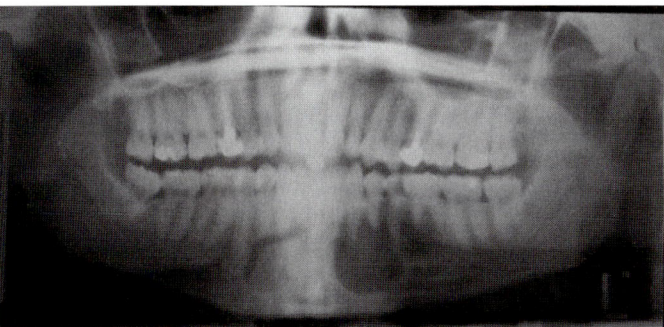

Fig. 49-2 ■ Multilocular radiolucency of the left body of the mandible represents solid/multicystic ameloblastoma. Marked resorption of roots of the first molar and first premolar is apparent.

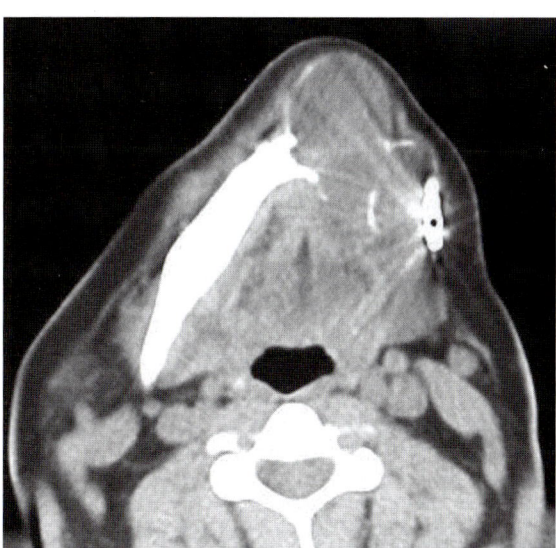

Fig. 49-3 ■ Axial computed tomography (CT) scan image of recurrent ameloblastoma. Significant expansion and disruption of the confines of the mandible are seen.

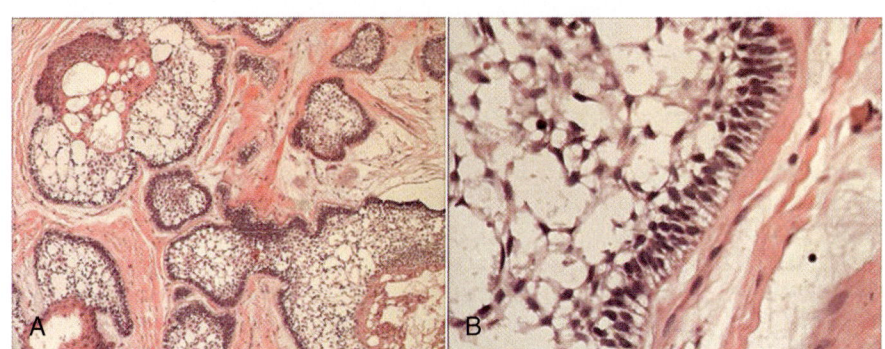

Fig. 49-4 ■ **A,** Ameloblastoma (follicular variant). Numerous neoplastic odontogenic islands featuring peripheral columnar cells with reverse polarization surrounding central zone of cells resembling stellate reticulum. **B,** Higher magnification that shows the reverse polarization of the peripheral columnar cells.

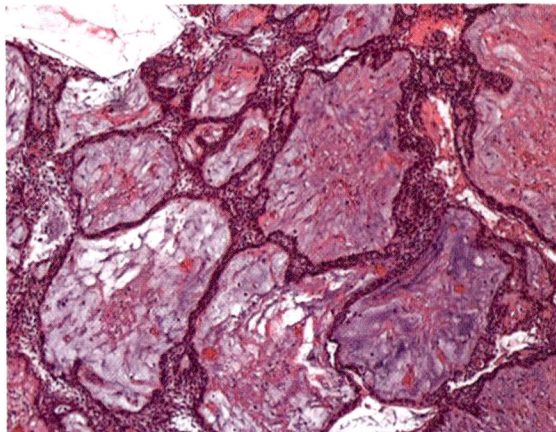

Fig. 49-5 ■ Ameloblastoma (plexiform variant). Pattern showing anastomosing cords of neoplastic odontogenic epithelium.

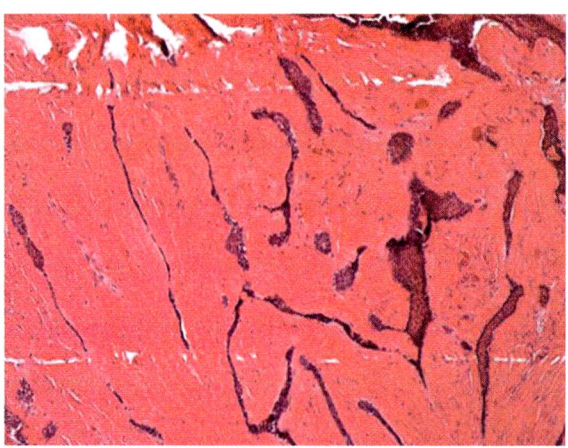

Fig. 49-8 ■ Ameloblastoma (desmoplastic variant). Dense connective tissue surrounding thin cords and islands of ameloblastoma.

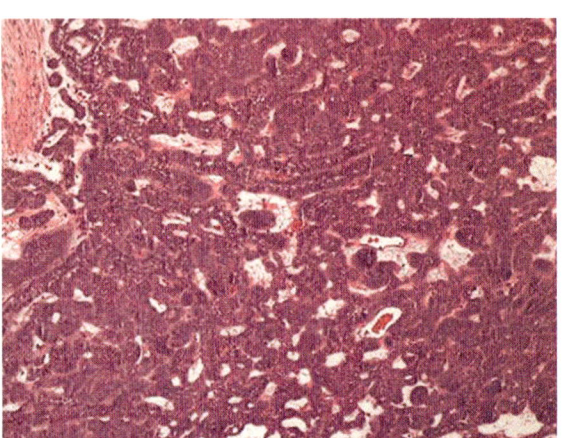

Fig. 49-6 ■ Ameloblastoma (basal cell variant). Neoplastic islands and cords featuring hyperchromatic cells that show peripheral palisading.

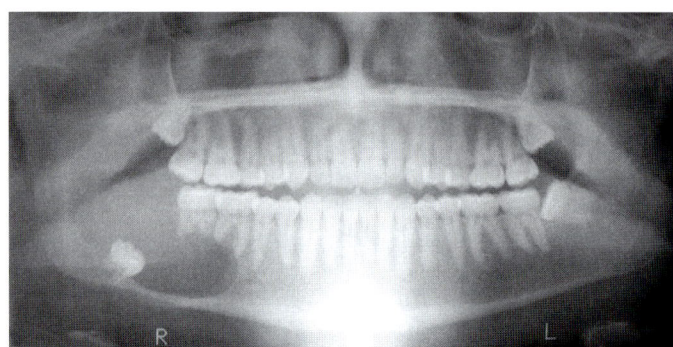

Fig. 49-9 ■ Large unilocular radiolucency of the posterior right mandible with displacement of the third molar to the inferior border and resorption of adjacent molar roots.

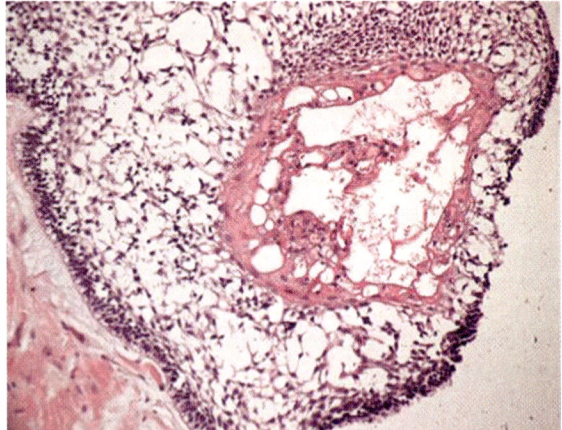

Fig. 49-7 ■ Ameloblastoma (acanthomatous variant). Neoplastic island of follicular ameloblastoma featuring central squamous differentiation.

radiographically, similar to the more common non-neoplastic dentigerous cyst (Fig. 49-9). Findings such as association with a crown of an impacted tooth, resorption of tooth roots, and cortical expansion may be seen (Fig. 49-10). In 1970, Vickers and Gorlin described three main histologic subtypes of unicystic ameloblastoma that have distinct clinical behavior: the luminal, intraluminal, and mural types.[10] Any form of unicystic ameloblastoma may arise within the

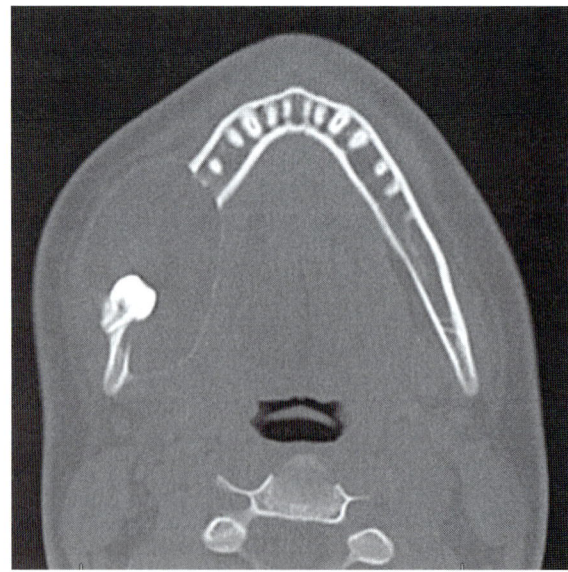

Fig. 49-10 ■ Axial computed tomography (CT) scan image of unicystic ameloblastoma of a 19-year-old male. Association with unerupted wisdom tooth that is displaced to the inferior border of the mandible. Expansion of both the medial and lateral cortices of the mandible is seen.

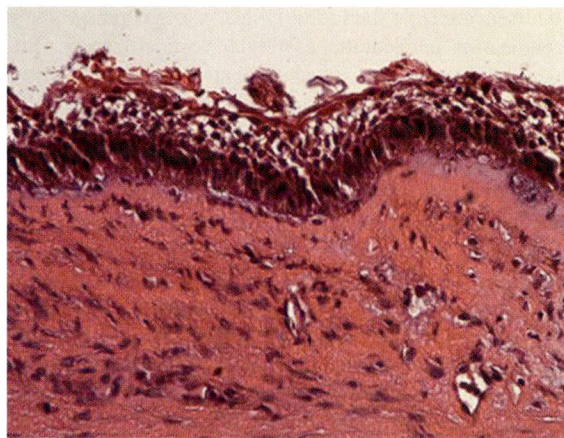

Fig. 49-11 ■ Unicystic ameloblastoma (luminal type). Cyst lined by odontogenic epithelium featuring hyperchromatic basal cells with stellate reticulum-like overlying epithelial cells.

lining of a dentigerous cyst, therefore changing the diagnosis to a unicystic ameloblastoma. The lining of a unicystic ameloblastoma may not be uniform, with portions of merely a dentigerous cystic lining to extensions of ameloblastoma beyond the confines of the cyst wall. The unicystic variants can be difficult to histologically differentiate from one another, unless the entire lesion can be evaluated.

Luminal

With the luminal type of unicystic ameloblastoma, the tumor is restricted to the luminal surface of the cyst. It contains a dense fibrous cyst wall that encapsulates the entire cystic tumor component, which consists of a columnar or cuboidal basal layer resembling ameloblasts with overlying cells that resemble stellate reticulum (Fig. 49-11).

Intraluminal

The intraluminal type is histologically similar to the luminal type, except that one or more extensions or islands of ameloblastoma project into the lumen. These extensions range from small to large in filling the cystic space. In certain cases, the luminal tumor extensions resemble the conventional plexiform ameloblastoma. These are referred to as plexiform unicystic ameloblastoma (Fig. 49-12).

Mural

The mural type of unicystic ameloblastoma is characterized by infiltration of the tumor islands into the fibrous connective tissue wall of the cyst. The ameloblastic extension could resemble both follicular or plexiform types of solid/multicystic ameloblastomas. The extent of infiltration into the connective tissue varies significantly, and therefore it is necessary to obtain several sections through the specimen so that mural invasion will not be missed (Fig. 49-13).

PERIPHERAL

The peripheral ameloblastoma comprises 2% to 10% of ameloblastomas.[11] The peripheral ameloblastoma is a tumor with the histologic characteristics of an intraosseous ameloblastoma, yet it occurs on the soft tissues covering the tooth-bearing aspect of the jaws.[12] It arises from epithelial rests from the periodontal ligament.[11] The peripheral ameloblastoma is characterized by a painless, firm, exophytic mass with a smooth surface without ulceration or induration. Its location is typically the attached gingiva or alveolar mucosa.[11] The clinical presentation may be indistinguishable from pyogenic granuloma, peripheral ossifying fibroma, peripheral giant cell

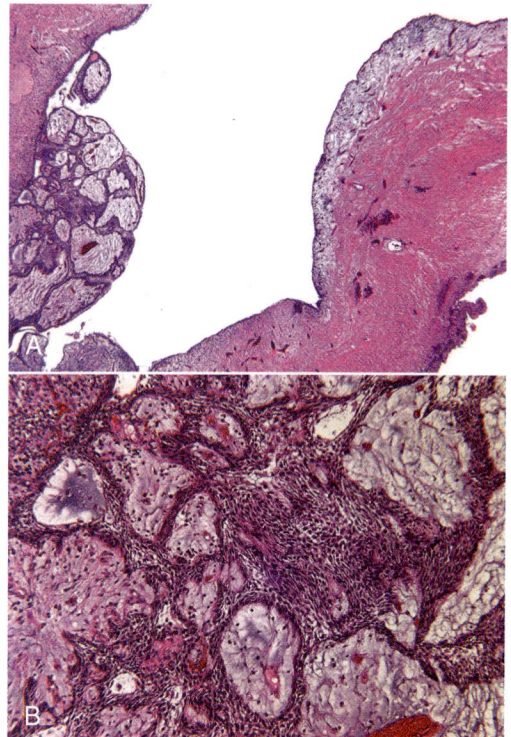

Fig. 49-12 ■ **A,** Unicystic ameloblastoma (intraluminal type). Notice the neoplastic mass developing from the cyst lining projecting into the lumen. **B,** Higher magnification of the intraluminal component.

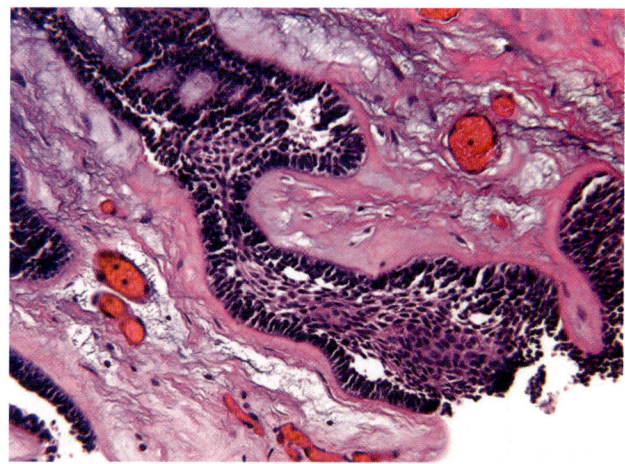

Fig. 49-13 ■ Unicystic ameloblastoma (mural type). Cystic component of ameloblastoma is observed along with neoplastic islands that have infiltrated the connective tissue wall.

granuloma, or peripheral odontogenic fibroma. There is typically no radiographic evidence of bony involvement. Some lesions can cause superficial pressure erosion of alveolar bone without invasion, causing the "cupping" or "saucerization" defect of the bone. The mandible is the predominant site of occurrence, comprising approximately 70% of the lesions.[11]

Histologically, peripheral ameloblastomas feature islands of neoplastic epithelial islands within the superficial connective tissue. The epithelial islands can resemble any of the histologic variants of solid/multicystic ameloblastomas, but the follicular and plexiform types are the most common. Almost half of the cases show contact of the neoplastic islands with the basal cell layer of the overlying surface epithelium.

TREATMENT

TREATMENT OF THE SOLID/MULTICYSTIC AMELOBLASTOMA

The goals of treatment of ameloblastoma should be with curative intent, while minimizing functional and esthetic consequences of ablative surgery. Historically, treatment has consisted of surgical resection with 1-cm tumor-free margins, but a variety of treatments based on clinical presentation, histologic type, and surgeon preference have been described.[13,14] Recurrence of ameloblastoma typically occurs within a decade from the initial presentation; however, there have been reports of tumor recurrence 30 years after initial treatment.[15]

Sehdev et al reported a 90% recurrence rate of the solid/multicystic ameloblastoma of the mandible when treated with curettage alone.[16] Marx et al showed that microscopic tumor cells can extend up to 8 mm beyond the radiographic extent of the lesion.[12] Therefore, resection with a safety margin of clinically normal-appearing bone is necessary. A review by Lau et al reported a recurrence rate of 3.6% surgical resection; this was corroborated by Hong et al, with a recurrence rate of 4.5% when treated with resection.[7,17] Therefore, the standard treatment of solid/multicystic ameloblastoma is surgical resection extending a minimum of 1 cm beyond the clinical extent of the tumor (Fig. 49-14).

UNICYSTIC AMELOBLASTOMAS

Historically, most unicystic ameloblastomas have been treated more "conservatively," due to a lower recurrence rate with enucleation compared with the solid/multicystic type. Additional treatments in conjunction with enucleation may be employed, including curettage, peripheral ostectomy, liquid nitrogen cryotherapy, and Carnoy solution. Lau et al reported a review of treatment of unicystic ameloblastoma, with a 30.5% recurrence rate with enucleation alone, 25% recurrence with marsupialization with subsequent enucleation and curettage, and 3.6% recurrence with marginal resection.[18] Although marsupialization has been described, it is generally not the preferred treatment modality, because it does not allow for examination of the entire lesion and is associated with a high risk of recurrence. Rosenstein et al reported a series of 21 unicystic ameloblastomas treated by enucleation and curettage, with a recurrence rate of 43%, 55% of which was of the mural type.[19] Overall, this resulted in a 64% recurrence rate of the mural type ameloblastoma when treated with enucleation and curettage. With marsupialization, the entire specimen is only evaluated on subsequent enucleation of the residual lesion. If at this time, histologic diagnosis of a mural type is made, then it is likely that ameloblastoma within the bone may exist at the periphery of the extent of the original lesion. The recurrences seen with enucleation are attributed to incomplete removal of the lining or extension of the tumor beyond the confines of the connective tissue capsule, which may occur with the mural type of unicystic ameloblastoma. Therefore, it can be concluded that recurrence of unicystic ameloblastomas with enucleation is largely due to mural invasion and microscopic extension of ameloblastoma into the surrounding cancellous bone. Unicystic ameloblastomas of the mural type should be treated in the same manner as the solid/multicystic type. Intraluminal or luminal unicystic ameloblastomas may be adequately treated with enucleation, given that the entire specimen is evaluated microscopically and the mural type is excluded.

Treatment of ameloblastoma in the pediatric population may require special considerations regarding the need to obtain local control and to balance the functional needs of the patient. Ameloblastomas in young patients, typically defined as 19 years old and younger, consist of approximately 10% to 15% of reported ameloblastomas, most of which are of the unicystic variant.[4] In Western countries, 76.5% were found to be unicystic in children.[20] Surgical treatment should not vary significantly from the adult patient with ameloblastoma.

TREATMENT OF THE PERIPHERAL AMELOBLASTOMA

The peripheral ameloblastoma does not typically behave as aggressively as its central counterpart, although rare malignant variants have been described.[11] Treatment consists of excision with clinically disease-free margins. If cupping or saucerization of alveolar bone is seen, the associated periosteum and/or bone should be excised. Recurrence rates of 16% to 19% are reported, and long-term follow-up is still imperative.[11]

SURGICAL TREATMENT AIDS AND ADJUNCTIVE THERAPIES

An intraoperative specimen radiograph may be used as an additional tool to ensure uninvolved margins in the resection. If bony margins appear close, the surgeon is able to remove additional bone immediately.[13] Additionally, intraoperative frozen section analysis of medullary bone may be used to evaluate margins.[13]

CRYOTHERAPY

Application of liquid nitrogen to the bony margins, as an adjunct to enucleation and curettage, may provide cellular devitalization within bone[21] up to 2 mm into surrounding bone. Application of liquid nitrogen cryotherapy may be used in areas where tumor-free margins are not easily achievable, such as the base of skull, the floor of the orbit, or at the time of enucleation of a luminal or intraluminal unicystic ameloblastoma.[22]

CHEMICAL FIXATION

The use of Carnoy solution has also been shown to be therapeutically beneficial. Based on the review by Lau et al of treatment of unicystic ameloblastoma, only 16% of all unicystic ameloblastomas recur with enucleation and application of Carnoy solution, although that review did not differentiate the subtypes of unicystic

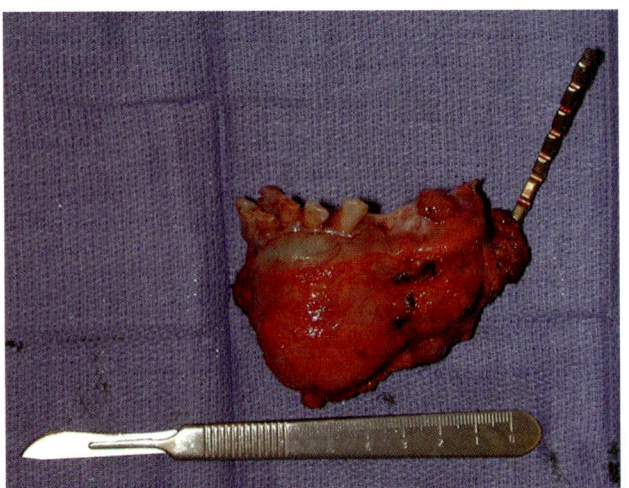

Fig. 49-14 ■ Specimen of resected recurrent ameloblastoma of the left mandible seen in Figure 49-3. (Courtesy Eric Dierks, DMD, MD, FACS.)

ameloblastomas.[18] Use of Carnoy solution may be more effective than enucleation alone for luminal and intraluminal types of unicystic ameloblastomas.

TREATMENT CONSIDERATIONS BASED ON ANATOMIC LOCATION

The location of the occurrence of ameloblastoma varies greatly, as does the treatment and clinical behavior. Approximately 80% of ameloblastomas occur in the mandible, compared with ≈20% in the maxilla.[2] Of those that occur in the maxilla, most are in the posterior maxilla. Only 2% of ameloblastomas occur in the anterior maxilla; in this location, the desmoplastic variant is the most common.[6] Due to the proximity of maxillary ameloblastomas to the orbit, paranasal sinuses, nasal cavity, and skull base, the locoregional extent of the tumor can be more difficult to control compared with the mandible. Due to the thin cortical bone of the maxilla, compared with the mandible, the tumor has the ability to penetrate the surrounding bone with earlier soft tissue extension. The maxillary ameloblastoma is more difficult to visualize clinically, and, on plain radiographs, this may prohibit early detection.[17] When planning treatment of ameloblastoma, imaging is imperative in order to view the tumor extension in three dimensions and to evaluate for cortical perforation and extraosseous extension of tumor.

SPECIAL CONSIDERATIONS FOR TREATMENT OF THE RECURRENT AMELOBLASTOMA

Many studies note recurrences within 5 years 50% of the time and the remainder within 10 years, but recurrence has been seen up to 30 years after the original treatment.[15] As noted, inadequate initial surgical treatment of ameloblastoma yields a high chance of local recurrence. Muller et al reported on 84 patients who underwent a total of 186 procedures for tumor clearance.[23] Many patients required multiple operations, more extensive surgery, greater difficulty in reconstruction, increased morbidity, and potential for mortality. Also, possibly there was increased chance of malignant change and metastasis.[24] A minimum follow-up period of 10 years is recommended, especially after treatment of a recurrent ameloblastoma. Only 80% of recurrent ameloblastomas are cured with resection.[16]

CONSIDERATIONS OF MALIGNANCY

There are two forms of malignant ameloblastoma. The term malignant ameloblastoma refers to a lesion with histologic similarity to conventional ameloblastoma, but it has metastasized. The ameloblastic carcinoma is a tumor that shows some features of ameloblastoma, but it has histologic features of malignancy. The ameloblastic carcinoma is considered a more aggressive lesion than conventional ameloblastoma.[25]

Malignant ameloblastoma is a lesion with the histologic appearance of a benign ameloblastoma that has metastasized. Metastasis is likely to be to the lung or regional lymph nodes primarily, along with reports of metastasis to liver, brain, bone, kidneys, and the gastrointestinal system.[26] The reported rate of metastasis of ameloblastoma is approximately 2%. The likelihood of metastasis is increased with large initial tumors, delay in treatment, recurrence, and primary mandibular tumors.[26] The treatment of malignant ameloblastoma is primarily surgical, because ameloblastoma is relatively resistant to irradiation.[27] Currently, no chemotherapeutic agent

has been efficacious for ameloblastoma. A screening examination is advised for patients diagnosed with ameloblastoma and a higher index of suspicion for those with recurrent ameloblastoma and those who develop clinical symptoms of pulmonary disease.[28]

Like ameloblastoma, ameloblastic carcinoma appears most frequently in the posterior mandible. Likewise, it presents most commonly as swelling. Pain, rapid growth, and trismus may also be found at presentation. The average age of presentation is approximately 30 years, with a reported range of 15 to 84 years. The majority of ameloblastic carcinomas were of the follicular and plexiform pattern.[25] In a review of 14 ameloblastic carcinomas by Hall et al, patients treated with surgical resection early in the course of treatment had an improved chance for cure and the fewest number of recurrences. In that series, 21.4% of the patients died of the disease.[25]

FOLLOW-UP CARE

Due to the slow-growing nature of the ameloblastoma, many recurrences occur after greater than 5 years, and as long as 30 years after the initial diagnosis. Tumor surveillance in asymptomatic patients should consist of clinical exams and orthopantomograms every 6 months for 1 year, then once per year for a minimum of 10 years. Routine use of computed tomography (CT) scans for monitoring of maxillary ameloblastomas is reasonable, due to anatomic overlap of structures in this region. Due to the potential for late recurrence with all types of ameloblastoma and the importance of long-term and vigorous follow-up, patients unable or unwilling to follow such recommendations may be candidates for initial radical resection, regardless of histologic variant of ameloblastoma, to minimize the risk of recurrence.

CONCLUSION

Ameloblastoma is a benign, locally aggressive tumor with several different histologic types. Treatment is based on the histology and clinical behavior and should be with curative intent. Debate continues in the literature regarding management of ameloblastoma. In general, solid/multicystic and mural unicystic variants of ameloblastoma or any recurrent tumors should be treated with surgical resection when feasible. Other unicystic variants of ameloblastoma can be considered for conservative management, such as enucleation and curettage with adjunctive therapies as first-line therapy, with the caveat that final treatment should be based on the complete histologic examination of the entire lesion. Resection must be considered a "conservative" treatment approach for many patients with ameloblastoma due to the greater likelihood for cure from the initial management and avoidance of often more complicated treatment necessary for management of recurrent disease.

PEARLS AND PITFALLS

- Initial surgical treatment of ameloblastoma gives the best chance for cure.
- Luminal and intraluminal variants of unicystic ameloblastoma may be amenable to enucleation and curettage with or without adjunctive therapies.
- Solid/multicystic and the mural type unicystic ameloblastoma require resection with a minimum of 1-cm margins.
- All patients with ameloblastoma should be followed for a minimum of 10 years, due to the potential for late recurrence.

REFERENCES

1. Vayvada H, et al: Surgical management of ameloblastoma in the mandible: segmental mandibulectomy and immediate reconstruction with free fibula or deep circumflex iliac artery flap (evaluation of the long-term esthetic and functional results). *J Oral Maxillofac Surg* 64(10):1532-1539, 2006.

2. Gorlin RJ: The pathology of ameloblastomas and its relationship to treatment. *Trans Int Conf Oral Surg* 230-553, 1970.

3. Zemann W, Feichtinger M, Kowatsch E, Kärcher H: Extensive ameloblastoma of the jaws: surgical management and immediate reconstruction using microvascular flaps. *Oral Surg Oral Med Oral Pathol Oral Radiol Endod* 103(2):190-196, 2007.

4. Kahn MA: Ameloblastoma in young persons: a clinicopathologic analysis and etiologic investigation. *Oral Surg Oral Med Oral Pathol* 67(6):706-715, 1989.

5. Reichart PA, Philipsen HP, Sonner S: Ameloblastoma: biological profile of 3677 cases. *Eur J Cancer B Oral Oncol* 31B(2):86-99, 1995.

6. Beckley ML, Farhood V, Helfend LK, Alijanian A: Desmoplastic ameloblastoma of the mandible: a case report and review of the literature. *J Oral Maxillofac Surg* 60(2):194-198, 2002.

7. Hong J, Yun PY, Chung IH, et al: Long-term follow up on recurrence of 305 ameloblastoma cases. *Int J Oral Maxillofac Surg* 36(4):283-288, 2007.

8. Eversole LR, Leider AS, Strub D: Radiographic characteristics of cystogenic ameloblastoma. *Oral Surg Oral Med Oral Pathol* 57(5):572-577, 1984.

9. Yoshimura Y, Saito H: Desmoplastic variant of ameloblastoma: report of a case and review of the literature. *J Oral Maxillofac Surg* 48(11):1231-1235, 1990.

10. Vickers RA, Gorlin RJ: Ameloblastoma: Delineation of early histopathologic features of neoplasia, *Cancer* 26(3):699-710, 1970.

11. Philipsen HP, Reichart PA, Nikai H, et al: Peripheral ameloblastoma: biological profile based on 160 cases from the literature. *Oral Oncol* 37(1):17-27, 2001.

12. Feinberg SE, Steinberg B: Surgical management of ameloblastoma. Current status of the literature. *Oral Surg Oral Med Oral Pathol Oral Radiol Endod* 81(4):383-388, 1996.

13. Carlson ER, Marx RE: The ameloblastoma: primary, curative surgical management. *J Oral Maxillofac Surg* 64(3):484-494, 2006.

14. Pogrel MA, Montes DM: Is there a role for enucleation in the management of ameloblastoma? *Int J Oral Maxillofac Surg* 38(8):807-812, 2009.

15. Hayward JR: Recurrent ameloblastoma 30 years after surgical treatment. *J Oral Surg* 31(5):368-370, 1973.

16. Sehdev MK, Huvos AG, Strong EW, et al: Proceedings: ameloblastoma of maxilla and mandible. *Cancer* 33(2):324-333, 1974.

17. Williams TP: Management of ameloblastoma: a changing perspective. *J Oral Maxillofac Surg* 51(10):1064-1070, 1993.

18. Lau SL, Samman N: Recurrence related to treatment modalities of unicystic ameloblastoma: a systematic review. *Int J Oral Maxillofac Surg* 35(8):681-690, 2006.

19. Rosenstein T, Pogrel MA, Smith RA, Regezi JA: Cystic ameloblastoma—behavior and treatment of 21 cases. *J Oral Maxillofac Surg* 59(11):1311-1316, 2001; discussion 1316-1318.

20. Ord RA, Blanchard RH Jr, Nikitakis NG, Sauk JJ: Ameloblastoma in children. *J Oral Maxillofac Surg* 60(7):762-770, 2002; discussion 770-771.

21. Sampson DE, Pogrel MA: Management of mandibular ameloblastoma: the clinical basis for a treatment algorithm. *J Oral Maxillofac Surg* 57(9):1074-1077, 1999; discussion 1078-1079.

22. Pogrel MA: The use of liquid nitrogen cryotherapy in the management of locally aggressive bone lesions. *J Oral Maxillofac Surg* 51(3):269-273, 1993; discussion 274.

23. Muller H, Slootweg PJ: The ameloblastoma, the controversial approach to therapy. *J Maxillofac Surg* 13(2):79-84, 1985.

24. Adekeye EO, Lavery KM: Recurrent ameloblastoma of the maxillo-facial region. Clinical features and treatment. *J Maxillofac Surg* 14(3):153-157, 1986.

25. Hall JM, Weathers DR, Unni KK: Ameloblastic carcinoma: an analysis of 14 cases. *Oral Surg Oral Med Oral Pathol Oral Radiol Endod* 103(6):799-807, 2007.

26. Cardoso A, Lazow SK, Solomon MP, et al: Metastatic ameloblastoma to the cervical lymph nodes: a case report and review of literature. *J Oral Maxillofac Surg* 67(6):1163-1166, 2009.

27. Goldwyn R, Constable J, Murray JE: Ameloblastoma of the jaw. A clinical study. *N Engl J Med* 269:126-129, 1963.

28. Witterick IJ, Parikh S, Mancer K, Gullane PJ: Malignant ameloblastoma. *Am J Otolaryngol* 17(2):122-126, 1996.

Chapter **50**

Jaw Cysts, Benign Odontogenic Tumors of the Jaws, and Fibro-osseous Diseases

Robert E. Marx

CYSTS OF THE JAWS

CORRECT TERMINOLOGY AND MECHANISM

A cyst is simply a pathologic cavity lined by epithelium. Therefore, some entities that may be referred to as "cysts" are not true cysts at all. An example of this is the so-called traumatic bone cyst, which is merely an empty cavity in the mandible and other bones as well,

and it is therefore better termed an idiopathic bone cavity. Another example is the so-called aneurysmal bone cyst, which is a blood-filled space within a central giant cell tumor and sometimes other tumors. Although it is a pathologic cavity, it is not lined by epithelium and therefore is also not a cyst.

All cysts of the jaws and facial region are developmental, that is, they arise from the proliferation of epithelial remnants left over from the development of a specific structure (e.g., tooth, thyroid glands, branchial pouches). Although some cysts, such as the apical periodontal cyst, are said to be "inflammatory cysts," they are actually developmental cysts, because they arise from epithelial rests. They are merely provoked to arise by the cytokines of inflammation. The development of a cyst begins with the proliferation of a developmental epithelial rest to a size of about 360 microns (0.36 mm). At that size, the center cells are too distant from the surrounding blood supply and break down. As further epithelial cellular proliferation occurs and the cytoplasmic content of the cells that have broken down accumulates, a hypertonic center space develops. This leads to imbibition of water by a diffusion gradient, resulting in the cystic fluid found in cysts. Because the cell membranes and nuclear membranes of the cells that broke down are high in cholesterol, it is not surprising that cholesterol clefts are found in many cyst walls. As the diffusion of water into the center space continues, the cyst lining becomes thinner, pressure builds, and the cyst expands to resorb bone or expand soft tissues. Because of the cyst expansion, the surrounding connective tissue becomes compressed, creating the third layer of a cyst. Therefore, a cyst contains the classic organization of three layers: a lumen, an epithelial lining, and a connective tissue wall.

ODONTOGENIC CYSTS

Apical Periodontal Cyst (Radicular Cyst)

The apical periodontal cyst is rarer than previously thought, because most apical radiolucencies diagnosed as a cyst represent chronic granulation tissue instead. Those apical radiolucencies that are actual cysts arise from the rests of Malassez, which are epithelial remnants from the development of the root via the Hertwig root sheath.

The treatment for this cyst is mostly tooth removal and curettage or root canal therapy.

Eruption Cyst

An eruption cyst is a type of dentigerous cyst formed when the stellate reticulum degenerates, leaving a cavity lined by the outer enamel epithelium before or during tooth eruption (Fig. 50-1). The cyst will appear as a bluish mucosal expansion as the tooth erupts and will most often burst, resulting in a "self-marsupialization" treatment. This is actually analogous to eruption of all teeth that erupt, with the outer enamel epithelium becoming fused to and part of the gingiva. In the rare case in which the cyst remains or is symptomatic, a surgical opening of the cyst (a marsupialization) is effective.

Dentigerous Cyst

Dentigerous cysts are cysts that, similar to the eruption cyst, arise when the stellate reticulum associated with the formation of the crown of the tooth breaks down. The epithelial lining is attached to

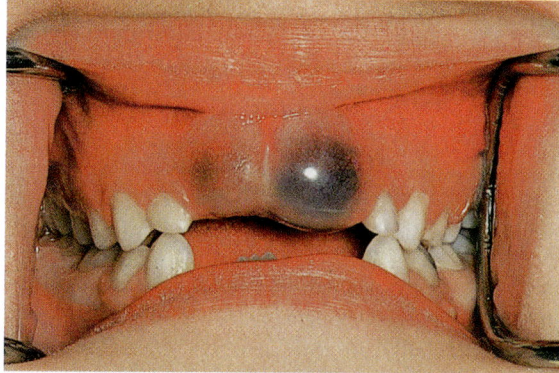

Fig. 50-1 ■ Eruption cyst.

the cemento-enamel junction, and the crown is in the lumen of the cyst (Fig. 50-2, *A*). The epithelial lining is squamous epithelium without a distinctive character, as is seen in the odontogenic keratocyst. The cyst can be very small, resembling a merely expanded dental follicular sac, or very large, displacing the associated tooth a great distance. The treatment is mostly enucleation with the removal of the associated tooth, which usually results in bone filling in the defect (Fig. 50-2, *B*).

Some surgeons prefer marsupialization. However, marsupialization requires a very compliant patient, often the need for a plug to keep the opening open, serial appointments thereafter, and often a secondary procedure to remove a remaining portion of the cyst (Fig. 50-3). With the lighting, retractors, and instruments available in the current armamentarium, there is less need for marsupialization. The remaining indications for marsupialization versus direct enucleation are (1) when the enucleation would realistically risk damage to adjunct structures, (2) when the anesthetic risk to the patient calls for a less extensive procedure, or (3) when an unerupted tooth can be brought into a functional position in the arch.

Odontogenic Keratocyst

The odontogenic keratocyst (OKC) is the most likely cyst to recur after treatment. It is also the most controversial cyst in both terminology and in treatment. The World Health Organization (WHO) has renamed the odontogenic keratocyst the odontogenic keratocystic tumor (OKT) based mostly on the finding of tumor markers *PCNA, K167,* and, specifically, mutations in the *PTCH* gene in the cystic epithelium. There is also a spectrum of cases in which a few cysts have attained a large destructive size mimicking the biology of an ameloblastoma (Fig. 50-4). However, the term OKT has not been generally accepted, because these same tumor markers may be seen variably in other cysts and in some inflammatory processes as well. Also, the vast majority of OKCs are not as clinically aggressive as those few that mimic an ameloblastoma. For the purpose of this book, the author will use the long-accepted term of odontogenic keratocyst, because it adheres to the definition of a cyst—a pathologic cavity lined by epithelium.

There are two types of OKCs: a dentigerous type and a primordial type. The dentigerous OKC may attain a large size and is associated with an impacted tooth but is usually less destructive and less recurrent. Its treatment is enucleation with removal of the associated tooth. The primordial type is unassociated with an impacted tooth and is often multilocular, more destructive, and seen to recur most often (Fig. 50-5). This is likely due to its origin from dental lamina rests (rests of Serres), which is a more primitive epithelial source than the reduced enamel epithelium of a dentigerous OKC.

The treatment of an OKC ranges from marsupialization, to enucleation, to enucleation with adjunctive treatment of the bony cavity, to resection. All of these treatments are valid, depending on the size, location, and locularity of the cyst, as well as the operator's experience. The basic and most common treatment is enucleation with or without adjunctive treatment of the bony cavity. If the operator prefers marsupialization, it is best applied to a unilocular OKC rather than a multilocular OKC, because not all of the compartments are likely to be decompressed. The treatment preferred by the author is wide access enucleation of the cyst in a single unit under general anesthesia without adjunctive treatment of the bony walls (Fig. 50-6). The rationale for this is that the most common reason for recurrence is a leftover portion of the cyst lining. If the cyst is removed in a single unit without shredding the cyst, the entire cyst is removed. Even if epithelial budding is seen in the cyst lining, a cyst removed in a single unit includes the wall of the cyst, which contains epithelial budding. A wide access with good lighting under

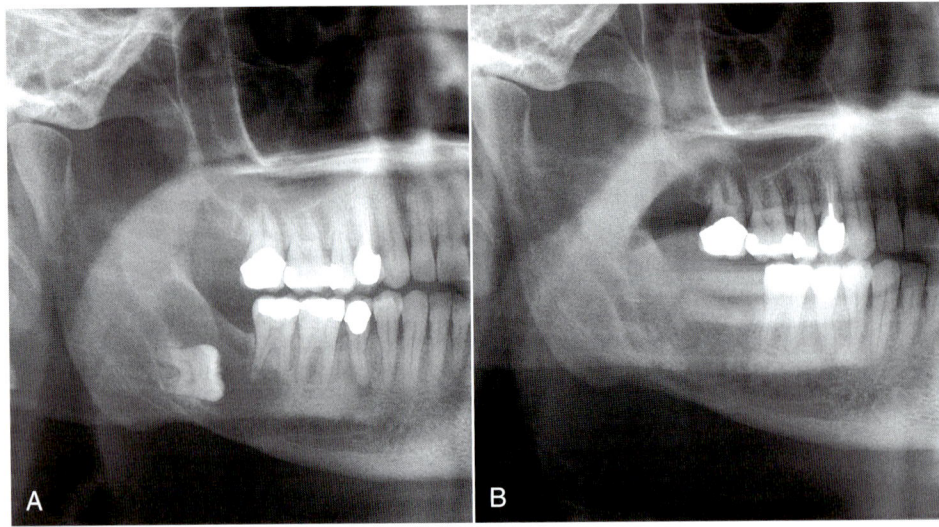

Fig. 50-2 ■ **A,** Dentigerous cyst. **B,** Bone regeneration after removal of the dentigerous cyst.

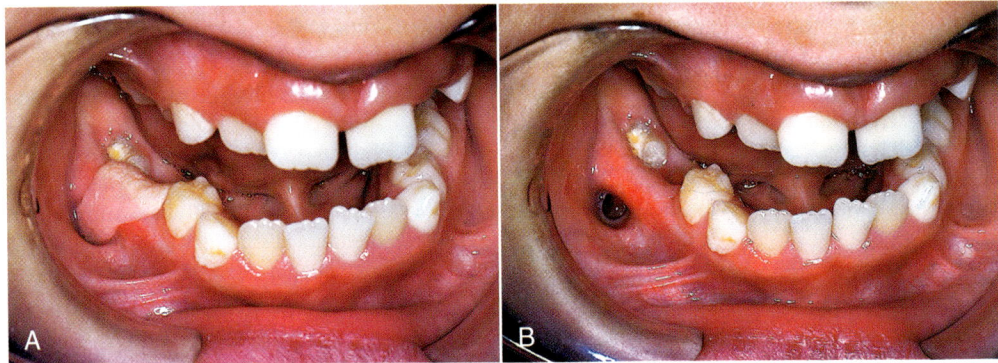

Fig. 50-3 ■ **A,** An acrylic plug is often required to maintain the opening of a marsupialization procedure. **B,** Marsupialized cyst with cyst lining confluent to oral mucosa.

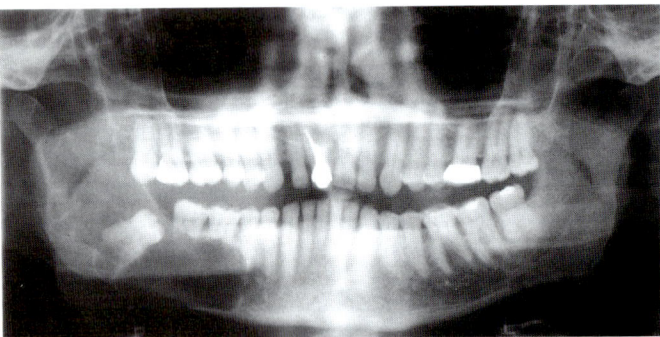

Fig. 50-4 ■ Large multilocular odontogenic keratocyst.

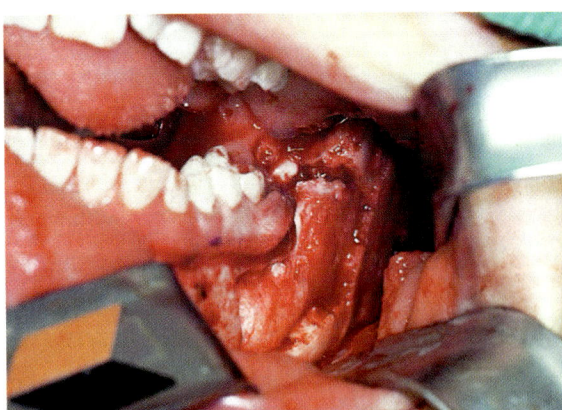

Fig. 50-6 ■ Wide-access decortication to directly visualize the cyst is the best approach to reduce recurrences from enucleation procedures.

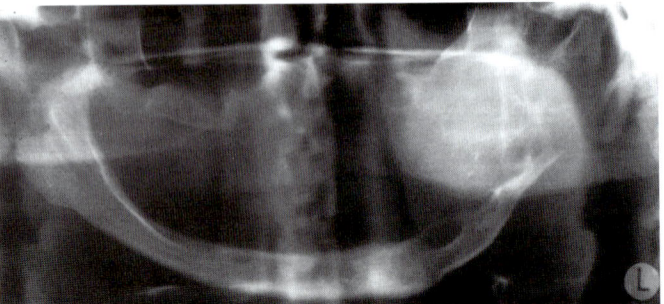

Fig. 50-5 ■ Large multilocular recurrent odontogenic keratocyst with a pathologic fracture.

general anesthesia promotes the visualization required to predictably remove the cyst in a single unit.

Adjunctive treatment of the bony walls includes cryotherapy, burring the bony walls, and use of Carnoy solution, among others. Although each has its advocates, these are all uncontrolled treatments where the depth of bone penetration or removal and the surface area covered is unknown. None has been found to statistically reduce the recurrence rate as compared with an enucleation without such treatment.

Resection is a valid option in OKC treatment in two instances—first, when the OKC is clinically and radiographically very aggressive and destructive (see Fig. 50-5). In such cases, a marsupialization is not likely to be effective, and an enucleation will leave so little native bone as to approach a continuity defect or tumor defect. The second instance is when previous treatments have resulted in two or more recurrences. Such resections are accomplished with 1-cm margins. Those in the mandible are mostly reconstructed with a titanium plate initially, followed by a bone graft later. Those in the maxilla are mostly treated with a primary closure initially and a bone graft later. The histopathology of the OKC is unique and specific. There is a corrugated parakeratinized surface facing the lumen, with an epithelial lining of 6 to 10 cells and an active deeply staining basal cell layer (Fig. 50-7). The production of keratin has no real meaning, because many other cysts will produce keratin as well.

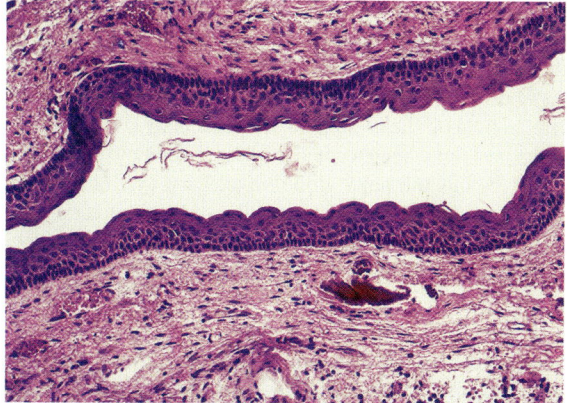

Fig. 50-7 ■ The histopathology of an odontogenic keratocyst is one of a corrugated parakeratinized lining surface, a 6- to 10-cell thickness, and a prominently stained basal cell layer. (Hematoxylin and eosin [H&E]; original magnification ×1.)

Lateral Periodontal Cyst

The lateral periodontal cyst is a unilocular cyst occurring most often between the bicuspid roots or between the roots of the canine and first bicuspid tooth. This cyst arises from the rests of Malassez. It usually remains less than 1.5 cm in diameter but is known to displace the roots of the teeth between which it occurs (Fig. 50-8, A).

The treatment of a lateral periodontal cyst is enucleation, which may be difficult due to the limited access between tooth roots. Occasionally, one or both associated teeth are removed in order to remove the entire cyst.

The histopathology of the lateral periodontal cyst is unique in having a thin 1- to 3-cell thickness lining with focal areas where the lining is thickened (Fig. 50-8, B). Because the odontogenic keratocyst may also manifest as a unilocular lesion between the roots of teeth, this unique histopathology needs to be confirmed.

Botryoid Odontogenic Cyst

Botryoid is Latin for "grapelike." Therefore, the botryoid odontogenic cyst is similar to the lateral periodontal cyst in location and size but is a multilocular cyst. It probably represents a multilocular variant of the lateral periodontal cyst, just as there is a multilocular ameloblastoma as a variant of a unilocular ameloblastoma. The histopathology of the botryoid odontogenic cyst is also a thin lining with focal areas of thickening, but it has multiseptated loculations (Fig. 50-9).

The treatment of the botryoid odontogenic cyst is enucleation. Due to the difficult access for removal from between roots and the thin multilocular epithelial lining, the botryoid odontogenic cyst is the second most common cyst to recur after treatment.

Calcifying Odontogenic Cyst

The calcifying odontogenic cyst is one of only two odontogenic cysts that have calcified material in their lining and therefore have some radiopacity to them. This cyst mostly occurs as a primordial cyst, but a few have also been found as a dentigerous cyst. The cyst is always unilocular and often shows a symmetrical half-moon radiolucency in its presentation, although the radiopacity more rarely may be spotted or sheetlike as well (Fig. 50-10, A).

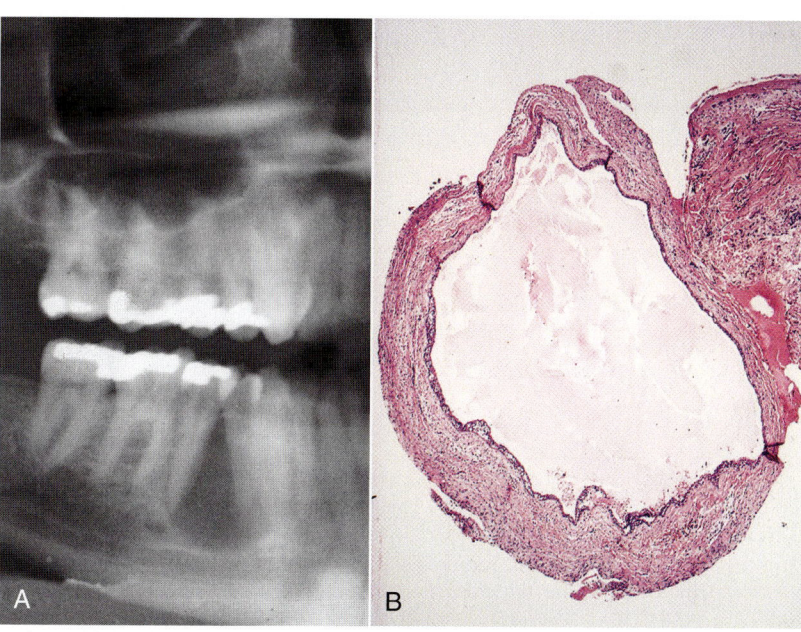

Fig. 50-8 ■ **A,** A lateral periodontal cyst will appear as a unilocular radiolucency, most often between the roots of bicuspid teeth. **B,** Lateral periodontal cyst with a thin unilocular lining. (H&E; original magnification ×1.)

The treatment is enucleation, which is facilitated by the thickness of the cyst lining and wall.

The unique histopathology is one of a thick multicellular epithelial lining that has focal areas of dystrophic calcification, keratinization, and enlarged pale cells called "ghost cells" (Fig. 50-10, *B*).

Adenomatoid Odontogenic Cyst

The adenomatoid odontogenic cyst is the second odontogenic cyst that may show calcifications in the epithelial lining. This cyst was termed an adenomatoid odontogenic tumor in the past. However, it is a true cyst with a lumen, a lining, and a connective tissue wall and is not a neoplasm. The confusion arose because the epithelial lining is usually very proliferative, causing an intraluminal tissue presence that resembles a tumor. The adenomatoid odontogenic cyst is always unilocular and always occurs anterior to the molars, mostly in the bicuspid and canine regions. It is more common in females versus males with a ratio of 2:1, in the maxilla versus the mandible, also with a ratio of 2:1, and it is associated with an unerupted tooth versus a primordial one. It occurs mostly in teenagers (Fig. 50-11).

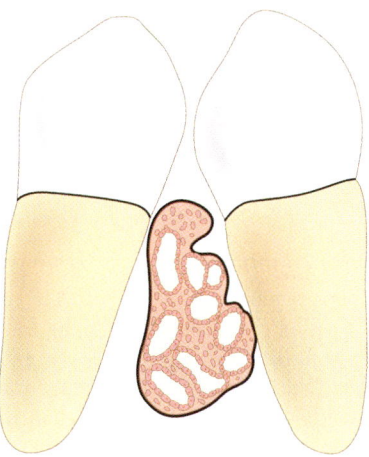

Fig. 50-9 ▪ A botryoid odontogenic cyst will appear as a multilocular variant of the lateral periodontal cyst. (From Marx RE, Stern D: *Oral and maxillofacial pathology: a rationale for diagnosis and treatment*, Hanover Park, Ill., 2002, Quintessence Publishing.)

The treatment is enucleation, which is also facilitated by the thick lining and wall of the cyst. Clinically, the unique feature of this cyst is that any associated tooth is entirely within the lumen of the cyst. This is because this cyst arises from proliferation of the Hertwig root sheath before it breaks up into epithelial rests of Malassez. Therefore, this cyst in not attached at the cementoenamel junction as is a dentigerous cyst, but it is attached at the apical or midroot level from the Hertwig root sheath (Fig. 50-12).

The unique histopathology of the adenomatoid odontogenic cyst is its thick lining with ductlike (adenomatoid) features that proliferate into the lumen (Fig. 50-13, *A*). It will also contain small flecks of calcified material, which are sometimes seen on radiographs and described with the term "driven-snow appearance" (Fig. 50-13, *B*). The ductlike structures are actually spherules of Hertwig epithelium, and the flecks of calcified material are dentinoid, which is what Hertwig epithelium induces in normal tooth root formation (Fig. 50-13, *C*).

NON-ODONTOGENIC CYSTS

Incisive Canal Cyst

The incisive canal cyst is a midline cyst of the anterior palate arising from the epithelial remnants of the sphenopalatine duct seen only in embryonic development. It may present as a buccal or palatal expansion with an oval or "heart-shaped" radiolucency (Fig. 50-14). Large ones in the past have been termed midline palatal cysts, a name since abandoned, as has the term globulomaxillary cyst because no epithelium existed between the premaxilla and the bilateral maxillary shelves or between the bilateral maxillary shelves.

The treatment is enucleation from either a lateral or palatal approach, depending on the direction of the greatest expansion. The histopathology will usually show a dual representation of squamous epithelium and respiratory epithelium in the lining, as well as nerves and small blood vessels, as part of the content of the incisive canal.

Branchial Cyst

The branchial cyst is thought to arise from entrapped pharyngeal pouch epithelium during development of the cervical chain of lymph nodes. Although branchial cysts can occur within the substance of the parotid in the preauricular area and in the supraclavicular area,

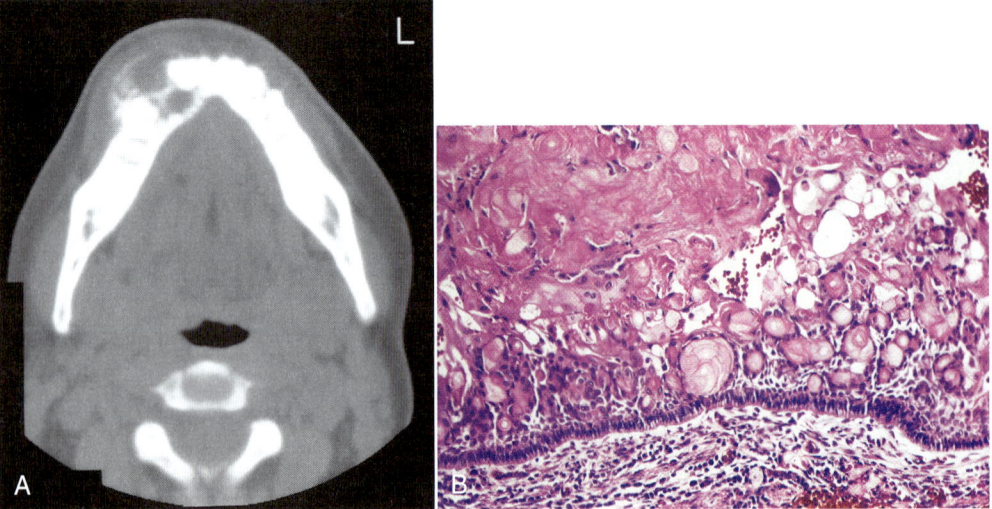

Fig. 50-10 ▪ **A,** A calcified odontogenic cyst with expansion and radiopacities. **B,** A calcified odontogenic cyst may show keratinized and calcified areas within the lining as well as clear "ghost" cells. (H&E; original magnification ×10.)

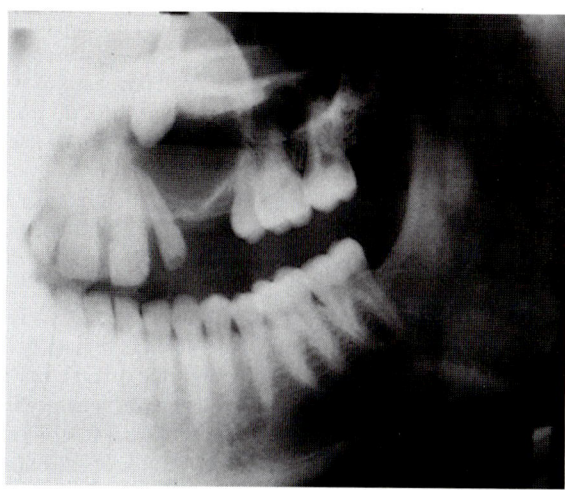

Fig. 50-11 ■ An adenomatoid odontogenic cyst will appear as a unilocular radiolucency that will encompass the entire tooth when it is associated with an impacted tooth.

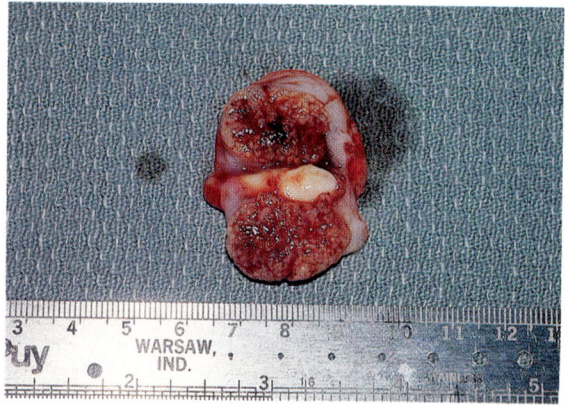

Fig. 50-12 ■ The gross open specimen of an adenomatoid odontogenic cyst will show a thick connective tissue wall, a proliferated lining growing into the lumen. The lining will be attached to the midroot level rather than at the cementoenamel junction, as is noted in a dentigerous cyst.

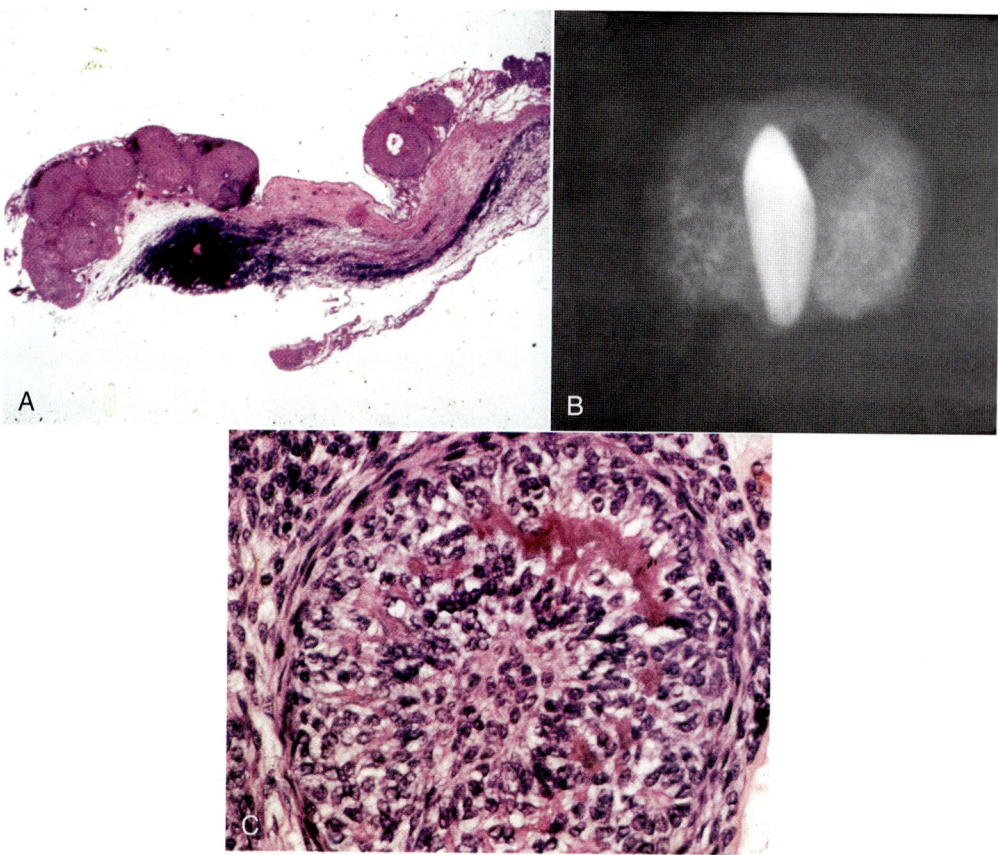

Fig. 50-13 ■ **A,** The low-power histopathology of an adenomatoid odontogenic cyst will identify ball-like proliferations of the lining extending into the lumen. (H&E; original magnification ×1.) **B,** A radiograph of the gross specimen of an adenomatoid odontogenic cyst will often show specks of a calcified product not seen in normal radiographs. **C,** The eosinophilic material seen in an adenomatoid odontogenic cyst is dentinoid. (H&E; original magnification ×40.)

90% occur at the level of the hyoid bone deep to the sternocleidomastoid muscle. The cyst most often occurs after an upper respiratory infection and emerges within 2 to 4 weeks to a significant size (Fig. 50-15, *A*). The cyst may be tender but is most often asymptomatic. A computed tomography (CT) scan is helpful in making a working diagnosis, if the aforementioned history and clinical presentation is present. The CT scan will show a spherical soft tissue mass with a hypodense center indicative of fluid and an even ring of encapsulated lining at the periphery (Fig. 50-15, *B*). Confirmation can be obtained by aspiration, in which case a thin chocolate-colored fluid may be aspirated (Fig. 50-15, *C*). The fluid is usually rich in lymphocytes and epithelium.

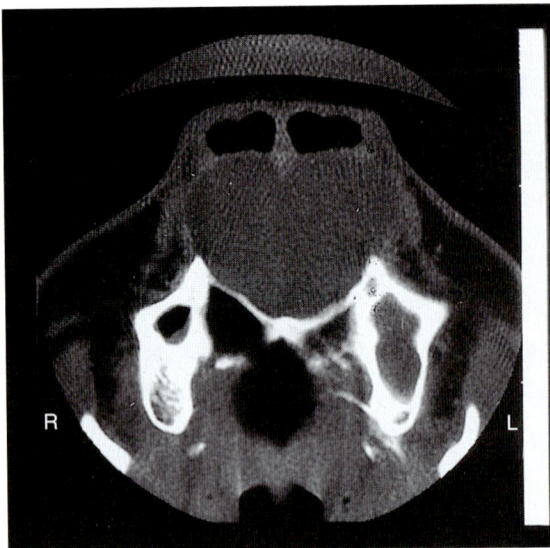

Fig. 50-14 ■ A nasopalatine duct cyst (incisive canal cyst) presents as a unilocular radiolucency in the midline of the maxilla. It is often said to be "heart shaped" as is seen here.

The treatment is a pericapsular dissection that is straightforward (Fig. 50-16, *A*). In about 85% of cases, the cyst will possess a tract that will course between the internal and external carotid arteries and on to the pharyngeal wall, confirming its origin from the pharyngeal pouches. In such cases, the tract is ligated just lateral to the bifurcation of the carotids (Fig. 50-16, *B*).

The histopathology will show a somewhat thin epithelial lining with a prominent lymphocyte collection in the wall of the cyst and, at times, germinal centers (Fig. 50-17).

Thyroglossal Tract Cyst

The thyroglossal tract cyst arises from epithelial remnants of the embryonic epithelium that invaginated from the tuberculum impar area of the tongue to eventually form the thyroid gland over the laryngeal cartilage surface. Similar to the branchial cyst, it usually arises 2 to 4 weeks after an upper respiratory tract infection and reaches a significant size rapidly. Most are asymptomatic, but some are mildly tender. About 85% are in the absolute midline, while 15% occur slightly off the midline (Fig. 50-18).

The treatment today is a modification of the original Sistrunk procedure. The cyst is approached through a horizontal incision across the midline of the neck. The cyst is usually found over the hyoid bone deep to the platysma muscle and superficial layer of the cervical fascia. The cyst will have a very thin lining; so, if the cyst is ruptured in the surgery, it will deflate and become difficult to remove. The author aspirates the thin cystic fluid, then connects a

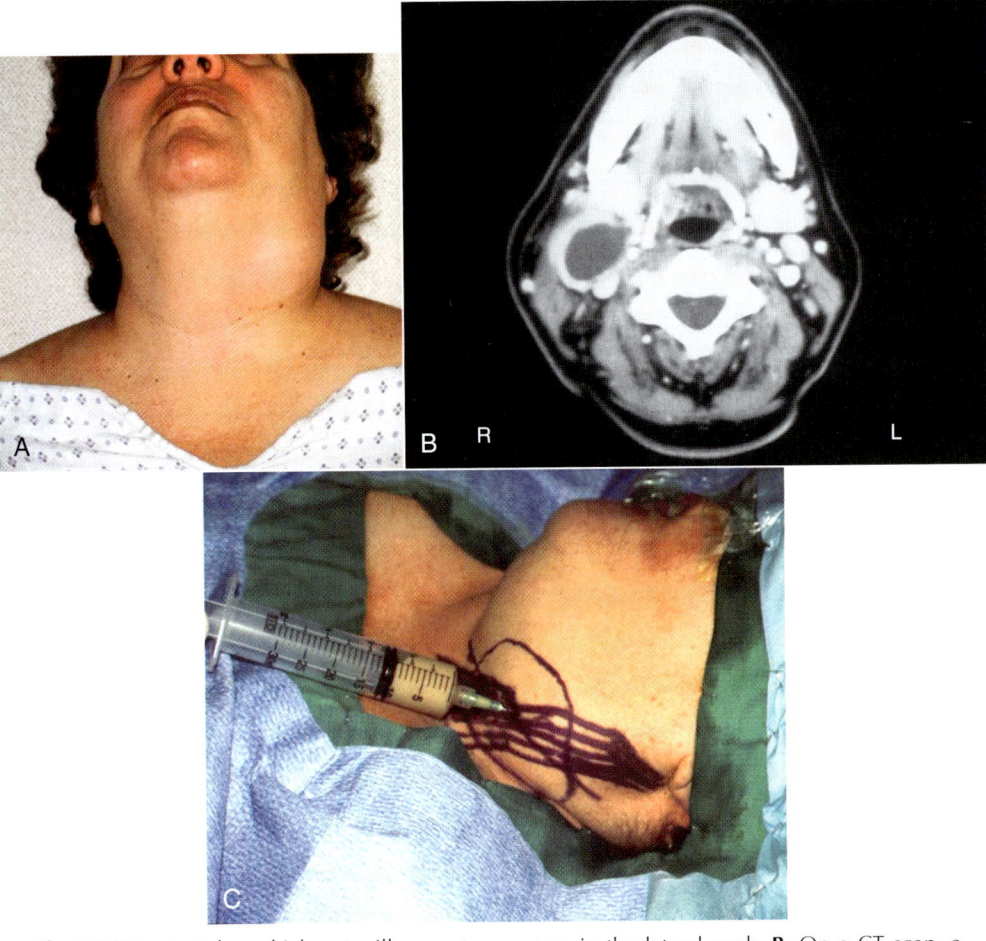

Fig. 50-15 ■ **A,** A branchial cyst will present as a mass in the lateral neck. **B,** On a CT scan, a branchial cyst will appear with a hypodense center, due to fluid in the lumen, and with a hyperdense periphery denoting the cyst lining and wall. **C,** Aspiration of a branchial cyst will often yield a chocolate-brown fluid.

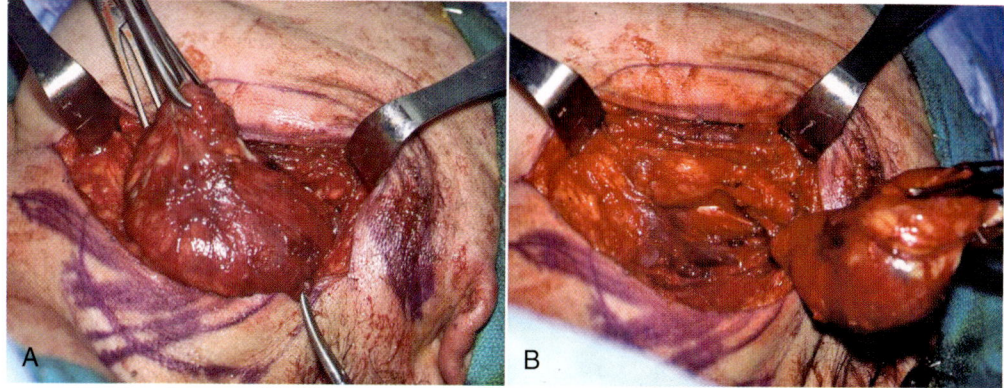

Fig. 50-16 ■ **A,** A branchial cyst is removed by a pericapsular dissection. **B,** About 85% of branchial cysts located at the level of the carotid bifurcation will have a tract coursing through the bifurcation.

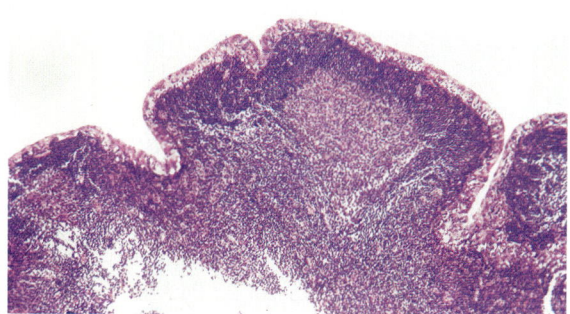

Fig. 50-17 ■ The histopathology of a branchial cyst will show a thin epithelial lining and lymphocytes/germinal centers in the cyst wall. (H&E, original magnification ×2.)

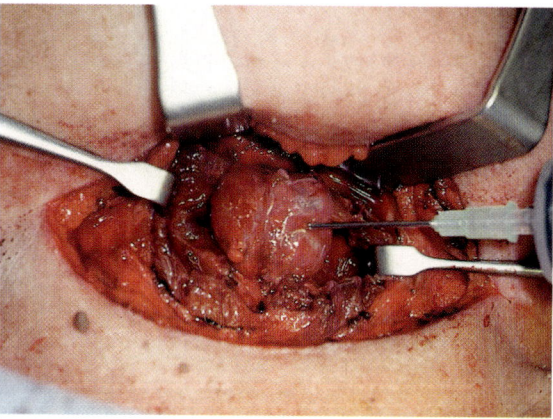

Fig. 50-19 ■ A thyroglossal tract cyst should be removed with a pericapsular excision. Injecting a rubbery consistency material into the lumen often assists the dissection.

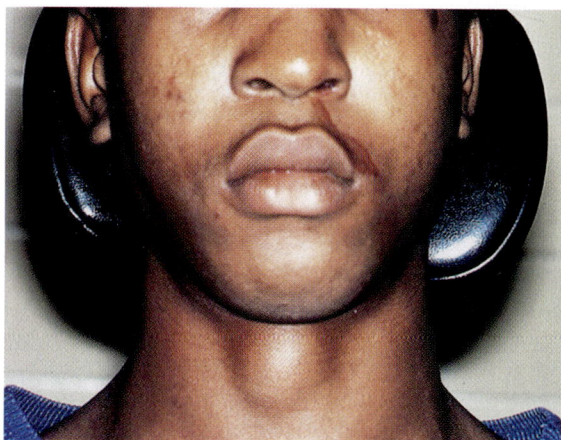

Fig. 50-18 ■ A thyroglossal tract cyst will occur in the midline or the paramidline area of the neck at the hyoid level.

syringe with impression material (Coe soft or alginate) and injects it into the lumen of the cyst (Fig. 50-19). Once the material sets, the cyst can be removed more easily with a pericapsular dissection. The cyst will always have a tract that goes through the body of the hyoid bone. Although the original Sistrunk procedure called for resection of the body of the hyoid bone, today the tract is transected at the hyoid surface, leaving the hyoid bone intact. No greater recurrences are seen with this less aggressive approach.

The histopathology will have a one- to three-cell epithelial lining, but the connective wall will have numerous areas of thyroid globulin and numerous capillaries and small blood vessels (Fig. 50-20).

Nasolabial Cyst

The nasolabial cyst is extremely rare. It is thought to arise from epithelial remnants of the nasolacrimal duct. The cyst will be located in the nasolabial crease as an expansion (Fig. 50-21). It may be found at the depth of the muscles of facial expression or deep to them, which can distinguish it clinically from epidermoid or dermoid cysts, which are superficial to this muscle level.

The treatment is a pericapsular excision through the nasolabial crease. An interoral approach may be used, if there is a clinical expansion of the oral mucosa.

The histopathology should identify respiratory epithelium in part or all of the cyst lining.

Epidermoid and Dermoid Cysts

Epidermoid and dermoid cysts most often occur in the floor of the mouth, within the tongue, or in the paramidline area of the neck with a tract to the midline. They are variable in size and can reach up to 10 cm in diameter (Fig. 50-22). They arise from entrapped epithelium in the midline.

The treatment for each is a soft tissue pericapsular excision, including the tract to the midline area (Fig. 50-23).

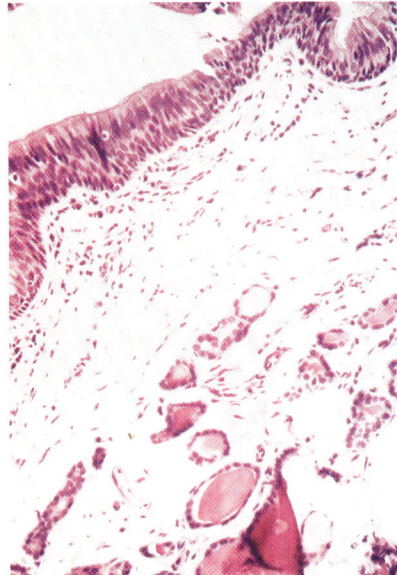

Fig. 50-20 ■ The histopathology of a thyroglossal tract cyst will show a thin epithelial lining and numerous thyroid globulin deposits in the cyst wall. (H&E; original magnification ×4.)

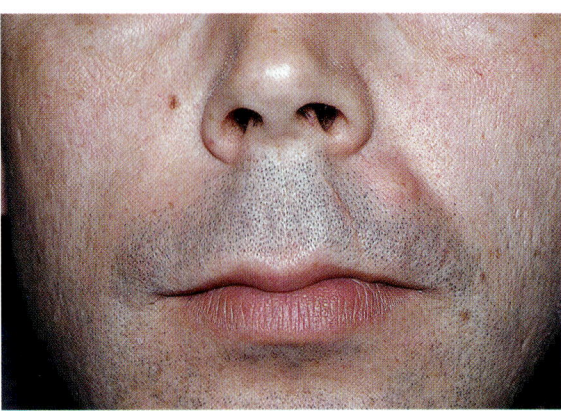

Fig. 50-21 ■ A nasolabial cyst will be found in the soft tissues deep to the muscles of facial expression.

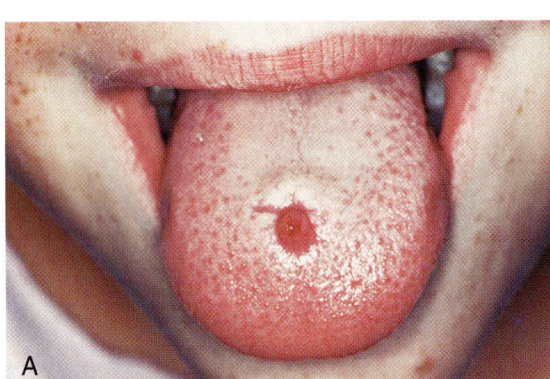

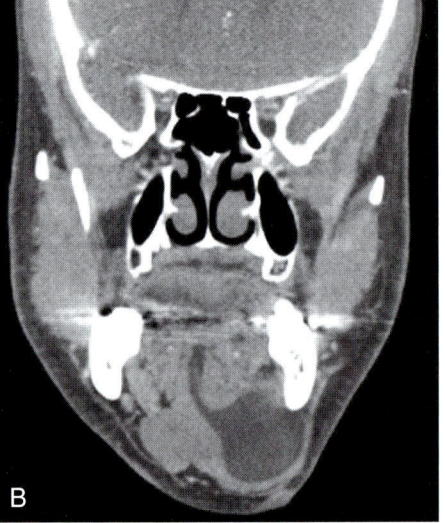

Fig. 50-22 ■ **A,** A dermoid cyst usually occurs in the midline or has a tract to the midline. **B,** This dermoid cyst developed laterally but had a tract to the midline.

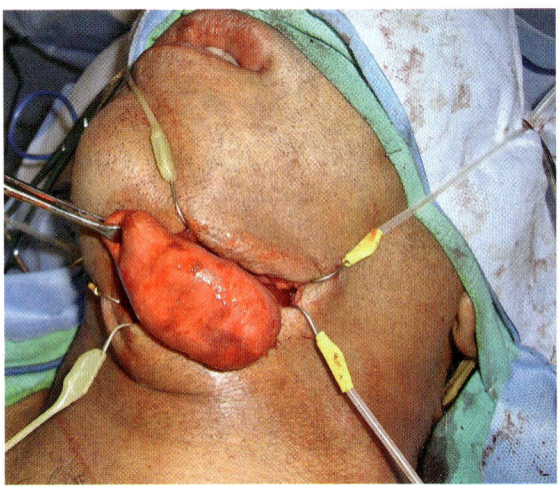

Fig. 50-23 ■ Some dermoid cysts become very large.

The epidermoid cyst may contain significant amounts of keratin (Fig. 50-24, *A*). It will have a nonspecific squamous epithelial lining and a connective tissue wall of collagen with no other structures (Fig. 50-24, *B*).

The dermoid cyst may also contain keratin and will also have a squamous epithelial lining. However, the connective tissue wall will contain any one of three possible adnexal structures: hair follicle epithelium, sebaceous glands, and sweat glands or ducts (Fig. 50-25). Usually, all three are present in a dermoid cyst.

Teratoid Cyst

Teratoid cysts are extremely rare in the oral cavity but are found more often in the ovary. Only extremely rare oral cases have been reported, mostly in the floor of the mouth and anterior mandible. These cysts are similar to the dermoid cyst but also include structures that arise from mesoderm, such as cartilage, bone, and even teeth with periodontal ligament structures (Fig. 50-26).

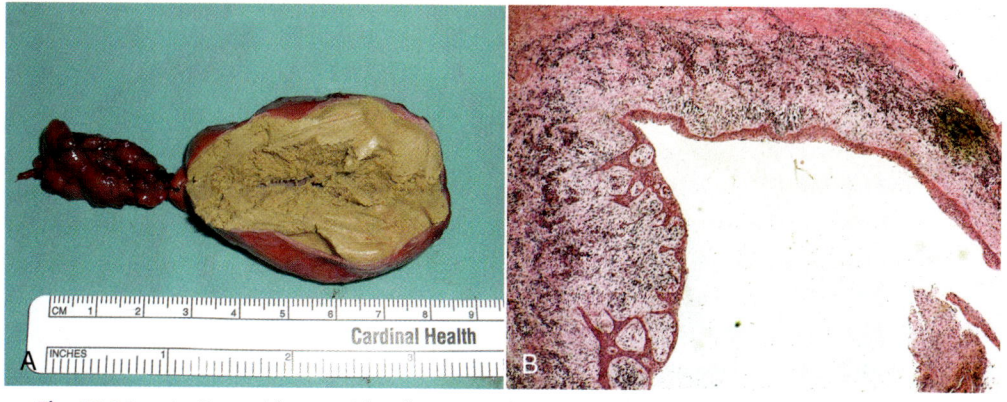

Fig. 50-24 ■ **A,** Dermoid cyst with a keratin and other proteinaceous material filling the lumen. **B,** If a cyst like those in Figures 50-22, *A* and 50-23 only has an epithelial lining, it is termed an epidermoid cyst. (H&E; original magnification ×2.)

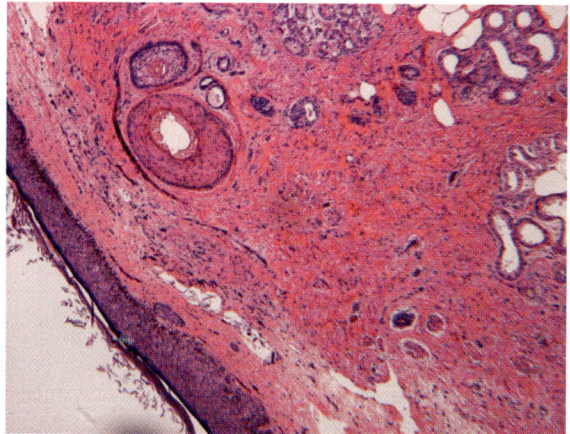

Fig. 50-25 ■ If a cyst like those in Figures 50-22, *A* and 50-23 has dermal structures, such as hair follicles, sebaceous glands, or sweat glands (adnexal structures) in the wall of the cyst, it is termed a dermoid cyst. (H&E; original magnification ×2.)

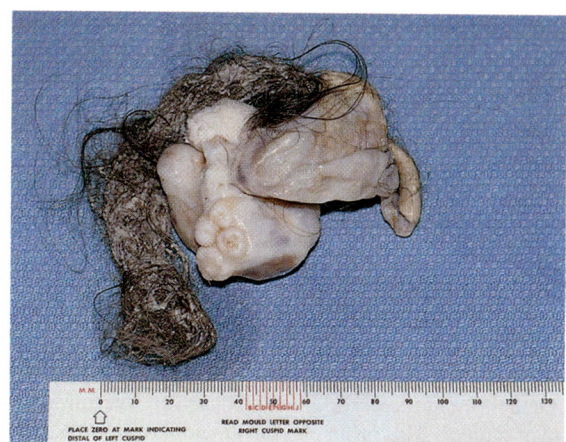

Fig. 50-26 ■ If a cyst contains structures from mesenchymal cells, such as cartilage, bone, or even teeth, it is termed a teratoid cyst.

Heterotopic Gastrointestinal Inclusion Cyst

The heterotopic gastrointestinal inclusion cyst is another extremely rare cyst that may occur in the oral cavity and is usually found in the floor of mouth and tongue. It is treated with a local excision and will show heterotopic gastric mucosal lining cells and sometimes intestinal cells and structures in the lining and wall of the cyst.

BENIGN ODONTOGENIC TUMORS

CORRECT TERMINOLOGY AND DEFINITIONS

Benign refers to a condition that is not life-threatening. Related to neoplasms, it refers to those neoplasms that do not metastasize. Benign odontogenic "tumors" are a group of cellular proliferations that are composed of hamartomas and true neoplasms. A hamartoma is a cellular proliferation of native tissue that reaches a certain size and then ceases growth. Related to odontogenic tumors, odontomas and the ameloblastic fibro-odontoma are examples of hamartomas. A benign neoplasm is a cellular proliferation of native tissue that continually grows but does not metastasize. The ameloblastoma and odontogenic myxoma are examples of true neoplasms. It should also be noted that although benign tumors do not metastasize to threaten life, they can and do reach extreme sizes (Fig. 50-27, *A*) if left untreated and can recur in dangerous anatomic spaces

if incompletely removed, thereby becoming life-threatening (Fig. 50-27, *B*).

AMELOBLASTOMA

The ameloblastoma is the prime example of a benign odontogenic neoplasm and is the most common odontogenic true neoplasm. It arises from any odontogenic epithelial source, that is, cyst epithelium, dental follicles, rests of Malassez, and rests of Serres. When it arises from cyst epithelium, it may proliferate into the lumen (intraluminal ameloblastoma) (Fig. 50-28, *A*), remain within the cyst lining (mural ameloblastoma) (Fig. 50-28, *B*), invade partially into the connective tissue wall (intramural ameloblastoma) (Fig. 50-28, *C*), invade through the full thickness of the connective tissue wall (transmural ameloblastoma) (Fig. 50-28, *D*), or invade through the cyst wall and into adjacent bone (invasive ameloblastoma) (Fig. 50-28, *E*). However, most ameloblastomas arise from epithelial sources other than cystic epithelium and are invasive from the outset. Therefore, the author recommends enucleation for the intraluminal, mural, and intramural ameloblastoma as a curative procedure, and resection for the transmural and invasive ameloblastomas.

The more common invasive ameloblastomas may present as a unilocular or multilocular radiolucency. The unilocular presentation has spawned the unfortunate term, "unicystic ameloblastoma," that

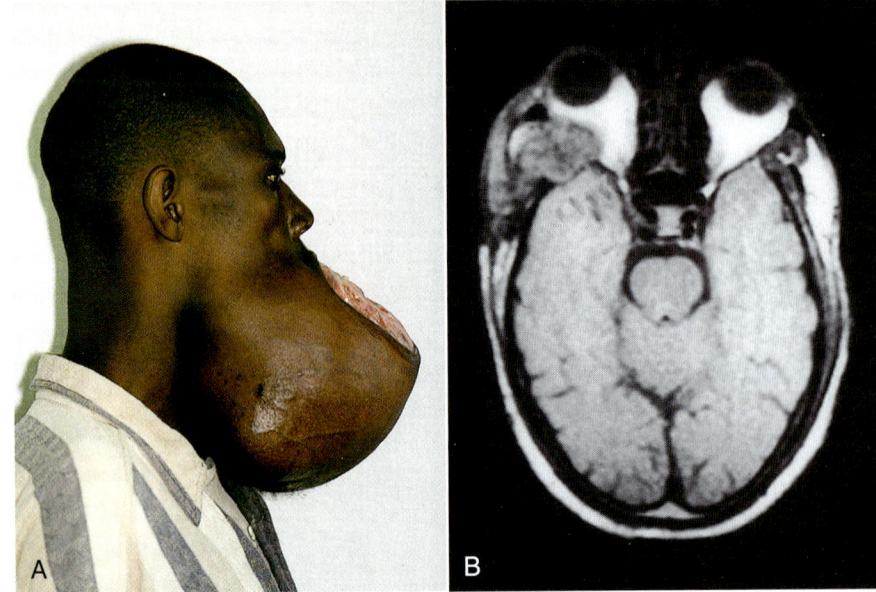

Fig. 50-27 ▪ **A,** Some ameloblastomas can reach an enormous size. **B,** Some ameloblastomas can extend into adjacent structures to be life-threatening, such as this one in the retro-orbital space, and it can cause a cerebrospinal fluid leak, as noted by the radiolucent streaks seen in the temporal lobe.

obscures the distinction between a cyst that has any one of the four patterns of ameloblastoma developing within a cyst or an invasive ameloblastoma that is just unilocular. It is a term that should be discarded.

The clinical and radiographic presentation suggestive of an ameloblastoma is confirmed by an incisional biopsy followed by a definitive surgery. The principles of ameloblastoma resection are 1-cm margins in bone and one layer of uninvolved soft tissue as a margin. Thus, if the ameloblastoma is small and is within the alveolar process, this principle may be satisfied with a peripheral resection. If not, a continuity resection is required. If the ameloblastoma resection with 1-cm margins does not allow 2 cm of residual condylar neck, then a disarticulation resection is indicated. Regarding soft tissue margins, with invasive ameloblastomas, which originate within the bone, the first anatomic barrier is the cortex. If the cortex has been resorbed by the tumor, the next anatomic barrier is the periosteum, recommending a supraperiosteal resection. If the periosteum is also breached by the ameloblastoma, then a cuff of adjacent tissue must be included (Fig. 50-29).

In the mandible, ameloblastomas are usually treated with a 1-cm margin continuity resection and the placement of a rigid titanium plate reconstruction. In some cases, where the oral communication is avoided or is easily closed, an immediate bone graft may be considered. However, most cases are reconstructed with a definitive bone graft 4 months or more after the resections to avoid the risk of infection from the oral microbial flora. In the maxilla, the defect is closed primarily with the preserved buccal and palatal mucosa for a later bone graft.

There are three histopathologic variants of the ameloblastoma that have significance. The most common pattern is the follicular pattern, where a nonspecific collagen stroma surrounds islands of columnar preameloblasts with reverse polarity. The islands of columnar preameloblasts surround stellate reticulum that may be seen to undergo a squamous metaplastic change or breakdown to form a cystic space (Fig. 50-30, *A*). This common evolution in the ameloblastoma gives rise to observed cystic spaces seen on gross examination (Fig. 50-30, *B*). The next most common pattern is the

plexiform pattern. In this pattern, the ameloblastoma follicular pattern seems to be turned inside out—that is, the preamelblasts are now surrounded by the stellate reticulum, and the latter cells surround the collagen stroma (Fig. 50-31). The plexiform pattern is thought to occur more frequently in maxillary ameloblastomas. The third pattern is known as the desmoplastic ameloblastoma, which has dense bands of collagen and focal areas of calcification in which strands of preameloblasts with reverse polarity exist (Fig. 50-32, *A*). This type of ameloblastoma is the only one that will appear partially radiopaque (Fig. 50-32, *B*).

EXTRAOSSEOUS AMELOBLASTOMA

On very rare occasions, a soft tissue mass with no emergence from bone or invasion into it shows the histopathology of an ameloblastoma. These growths are excised with a 5-mm cuff of surrounding mucosa followed by a primary closure.

ODONTOGENIC MYXOMA

The odontogenic myxoma arises from cells of the primitive dental pulp known as the dental papilla. It will clinically and radiographically present with an expansile multilocular radiolucency often described with the term "soap bubble" appearance (Fig. 50-33, *A*). Odontogenic myxomas do not arise from cysts; they are always invasive neoplasms.

Because a differential diagnosis of its usual presentation includes an ameloblastoma, an ameloblastic fibroma, a central giant cell tumor, an odontogenic keratocyst, and a central hemangioma of bone, an incisional biopsy to establish a definitive diagnosis is accomplished first.

The histopathology is one of a loose group of spindle cells with abundant extracellular matrix and strands of eosinophilic-staining collagen (Fig. 50-33, *B*). When the collagen strands are more numerous, some have named it a fibromyxoma. However, there is no difference in the biologic behavior.

The treatment is the same as that for an ameloblastoma. Thus, in the mandible, a resection is performed, observing 1-cm margins in bone and one uninvolved anatomic barrier against soft tissue. The

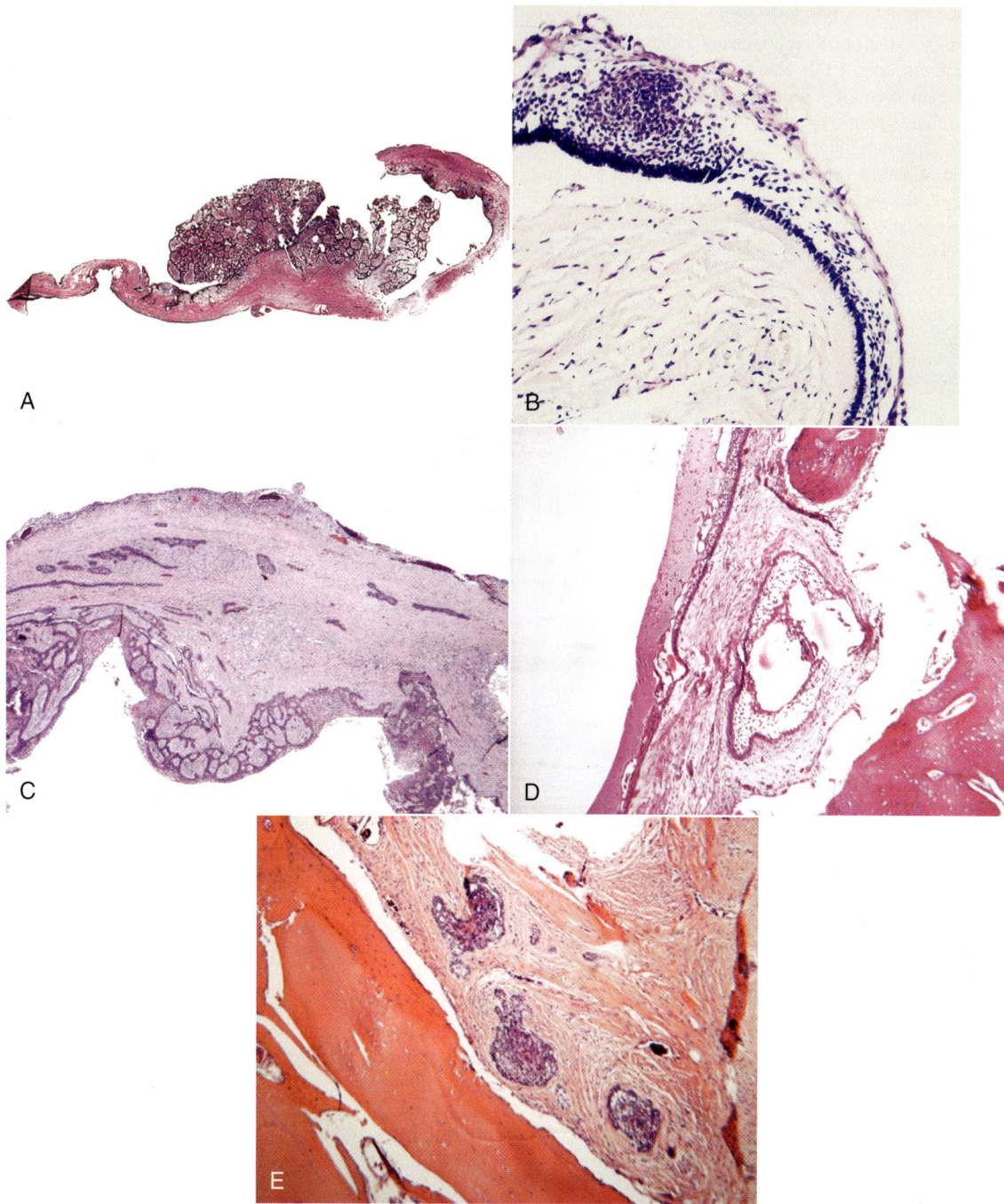

Fig. 50-28 ■ **A,** An intraluminal ameloblastoma. (H&E; original magnification ×1.) **B,** A mural ameloblastoma. (H&E; original magnification ×2.) **C,** An intramural ameloblastoma. (H&E; original magnification ×2.) **D,** A transmural ameloblastoma. (H&E; original magnification ×4.) **E,** An invasive ameloblastoma. (H&E; original magnification ×4.)

defect can be initially reconstructed with a titanium plate in preparation for a definitive bone graft later or an immediate bone graft in select cases. In the maxilla, a submucosal resection is the recommended curative approach, observing 1-cm margins in bone and one uninvolved anatomic layer against soft tissue, followed by a primary closure.

AMELOBLASTIC FIBROMA

The ameloblastic fibroma is a rare neoplasm that occurs mostly in children and teenagers. It is also radiolucent and expansile so that its clinical and radiographic pattern will be similar to an ameloblastoma and to an odontogenic myxoma (Fig. 50-34, *A*).

The histopathology of an ameloblastic fibroma is unique but is too often confused with that of an ameloblastoma. In the ameloblastic fibroma, the preameloblast island areas are smaller, and the surrounding connective tissue is not the eosinophilic-staining stromal collagen but a more blue-gray–staining cellular tissue without collagen production, representing odontogenic mesenchyme (Fig. 50-34, *B*).

The biologic behavior of an ameloblastic fibroma is also less invasive than that of an ameloblastoma. Smaller ones (less than 3 cm in size) may be treated with enucleation and curettage for cure. However, larger ones are often sufficiently destructive that a resection is the only option.

AMELOBLASTIC FIBROSARCOMA

Several of the benign odontogenic neoplasms have a malignant counterpart beyond the scope of this chapter. However, the ameloblastic fibroma is the one benign odontogenic tumor that undergoes either a malignant transformation over time or is malignant de novo more than any other. This malignant counterpart is usually low grade and may be subtle. Clinical clues to an ameloblastic fibroma are increased size, indistinct radiographic borders, more rapid growth, pain, or paresthesia (Fig. 50-35, *A*). Histopathologically, the malignant counterpart is the odontogenic mesenchyme, not the pre-ameloblasts, and is noted by the presence of mitotic figures in the odontogenic mesenchyme (Fig. 50-35, *B*). Because these sarcomas are usually low grade, they are mostly treated with a resection observing 1.5- to 2-cm margins. Chemotherapy and radiation therapy are not usually required.

CALCIFYING EPITHELIAL ODONTOGENIC TUMOR (PINDBORG TUMOR)

The calcifying epithelial odontogenic tumor (CEOT) is a very rare and very slow-growing neoplasm with a unique histopathology. It will present with a painless expansion but a mixed radiolucent-radiopaque appearance (Fig. 50-36, *A*).

The histopathology will show epithelial cells with prominent pleomorphism and a high nuclear to cytoplasmic ratio suggestive of a more aggressive behavior than this tumor is known for. The epithelium will often also show readily apparent intercellular bridges. Calcification with concentric rings will be seen throughout, as are pale-staining amorphic areas representing amyloid (Fig. 50-36, *B*). The amyloid may be identified more precisely by staining with either Congo red or the fluorescent stain thioflavin-T. Curative treatment for this tumor is similar to that for an ameloblastoma and odontogenic myxoma, that is, resection observing 1-cm margins and the same consideration for reconstruction.

AMELOBLASTIC FIBRO-ODONTOMA

This tumor is a hamartoma rather than a true neoplasm and represents a disturbed attempt at tooth formation. It mostly occurs in children and teenagers as a mixed radiolucent-radiopaque expansion or, at times, completely radiopaque expansion (Fig. 50-37, *A*).

The histopathology will have sections that represent an ameloblastic fibroma. However, within it will be dysplastic dentin seen as calcified areas with reversal lines mimicking bone but also obvious dentinal tubules and odontoblasts (Fig. 50-37, *B*).

The treatment is an enucleation in which the gritty and firm tissue mass readily separates from the surrounding bone.

ODONTOMA

The odontoma is the most common odontogenic tumor but not the most common odontogenic neoplasm, because it is another hamartoma rather than a true neoplasm. Like the ameloblastic fibro-odontoma, it represents a disturbed attempt at tooth formation. Traditionally, odontomas were separated into complex odontomas, in which an indistinct mass of mostly dentin exists (Fig. 50-38, *A*),

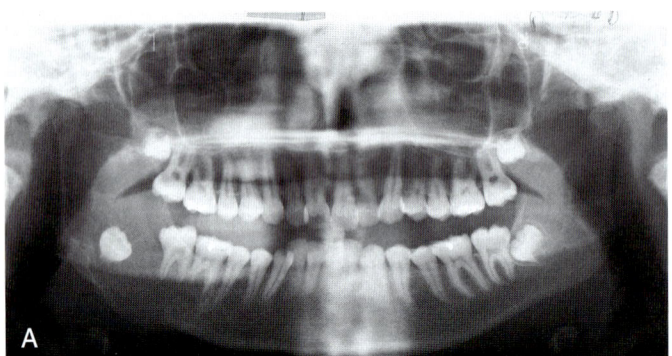

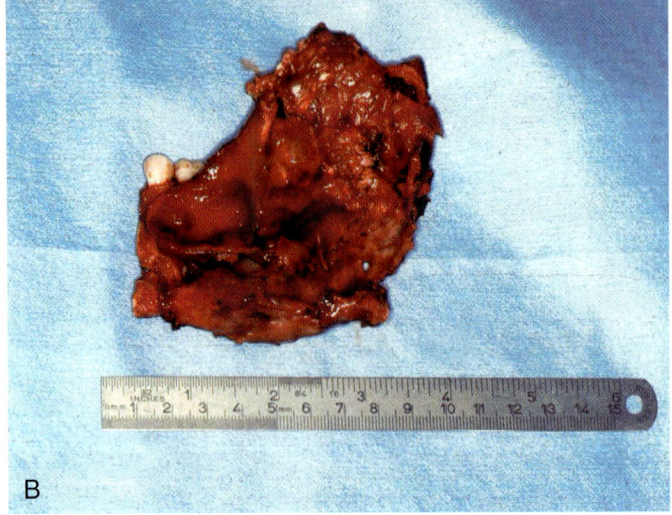

Fig. 50-29 ▪ A, Large ameloblastoma in right ramus of mandible. **B,** Resected specimen of an ameloblastoma, including periosteum and a cuff of a muscle due to tumor proliferating beyond the cortex and into the periosteum.

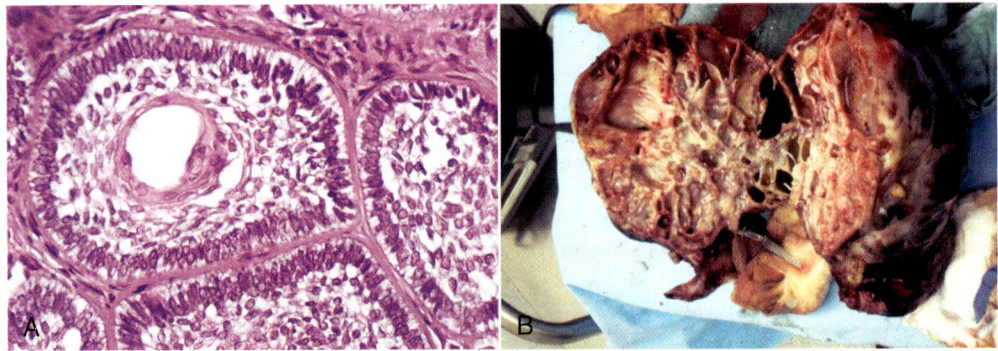

Fig. 50-30 ▪ A, Follicular pattern ameloblastoma with reverse polarization of the preameloblast nuclei and stellate reticulum. Note the beginning of a cystic space as the stellate reticulum breaks down. (H&E; original magnification ×10.) **B,** Gross specimen of a large ameloblastoma with multiple cystic spaces.

and a compound odontoma, in which multiple miniature teeth form (Fig. 50-38, *B*). This separation has little use other than as a mere academic exercise.

The treatment of both types of odontomas is enucleation, in which the calcified mass or multiple tooth-like structures readily separate from the surrounding bone.

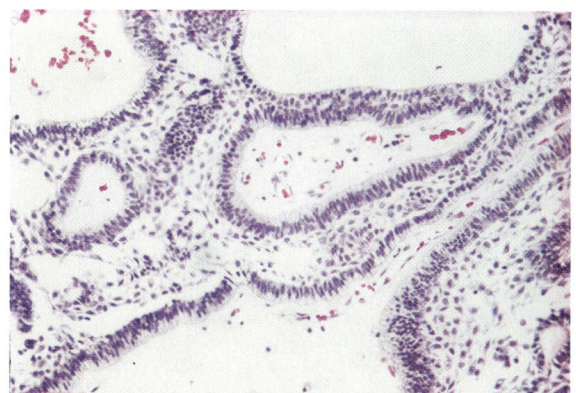

Fig. 50-31 ■ A plexiform pattern ameloblastoma with reverse polarization of the preameloblast nuclei but with stromal collagen surrounding the basal lamina. (H&E; original magnification ×10.)

CEMENTOBLASTOMA

The cementoblastoma is a rare very slow-growing but true neoplasm of cellular cementum. It occurs mostly in teenagers and young adults and is usually limited to the bicuspid and molar teeth in either jaw. There will be a slight expansion over the involved tooth root. There will also be a report from the patient of a constant deep ache within the expansion. However, the radiographic appearance is often pathognomic as a round radiopacity encompassing the apical half of the root and expanding outward (Fig. 50-39, *A*). The radiopacity will have a distinctive radiolucent rim mimicking a periodontal membrane space.

The treatment is removal of the involved tooth (Fig. 50-39, *B*). Despite the expansion of the tumor, a forceps extraction brings the tumor with it without difficulties. Root resection to remove the tumor and retain the crown has been a possibility advanced in the past. However, the tumor extends at least half way up the root and often into the furcation of multirooted teeth, leaving too little of remaining root support; therefore, this approach is not recommended. Today, the defect can be treated with alveolar socket grafting techniques, such as allogeneic bone grafts, local autogenous bone grafts, recombinant human bone morphogenetic protein-2 (rhBMP-2) grafts, or composites of these graft materials.

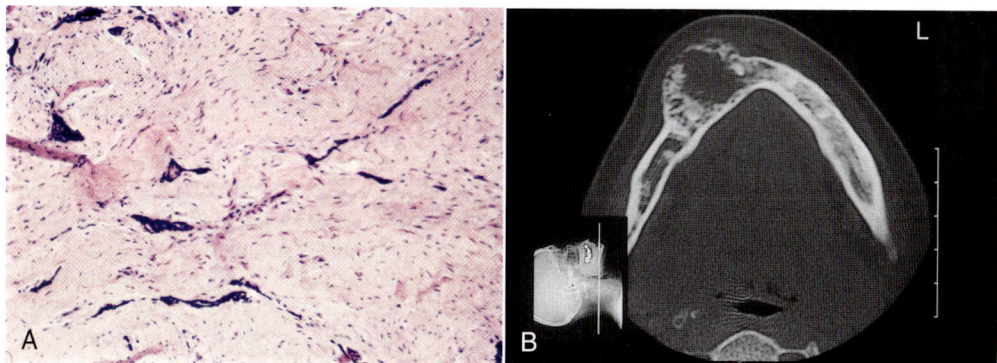

Fig. 50-32 ■ **A,** A desmoplastic ameloblastoma will show strands of preameloblast surrounded by dense stromal collagen. **B,** A desmoplastic ameloblastoma is the only ameloblastoma type that will show some radiopacity on radiographic films.

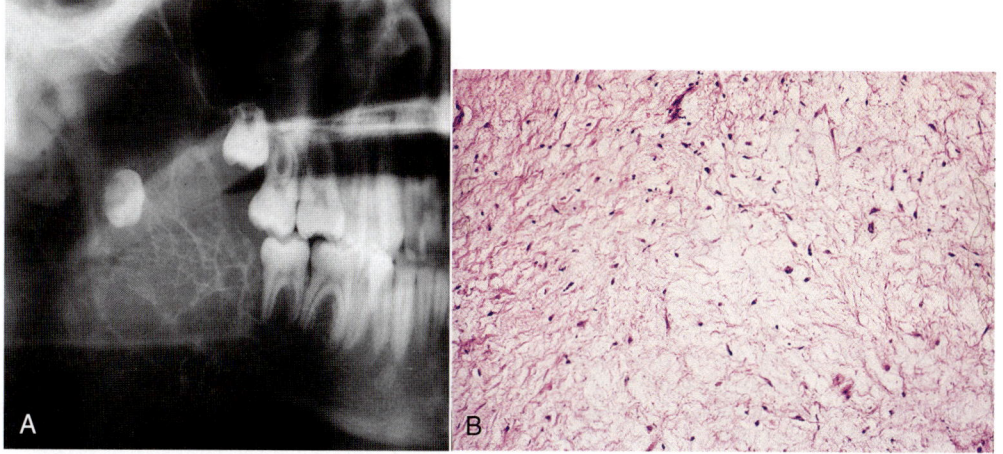

Fig. 50-33 ■ **A,** An odontogenic myxoma will frequently present as a fine "soap bubble" multilocular radiolucency. **B,** An odontogenic myxoma will have a sparse cellularity of odontogenic mesenchyme and a variable amount of collagen and rare islands of odontogenic epithelium. (H&E; original magnification ×2.)

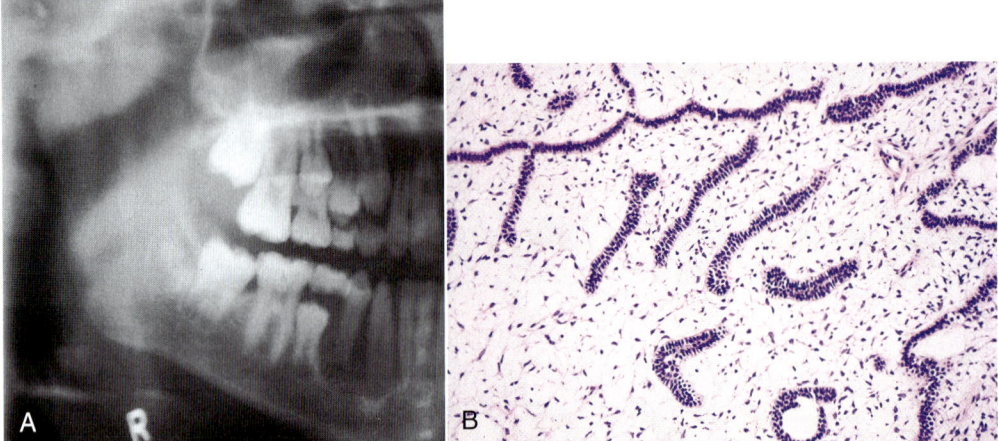

Fig. 50-34 ▪ **A,** A radiolucency in the canine/bicuspid area in an 11-year-old child should include an ameloblastic fibroma in the differential diagnosis. **B,** An ameloblastic fibroma will contain bluish-gray–staining cellular odontogenic mesenchyme and strands or islands of odontogenic epithelium. (H&E; original magnification ×4.)

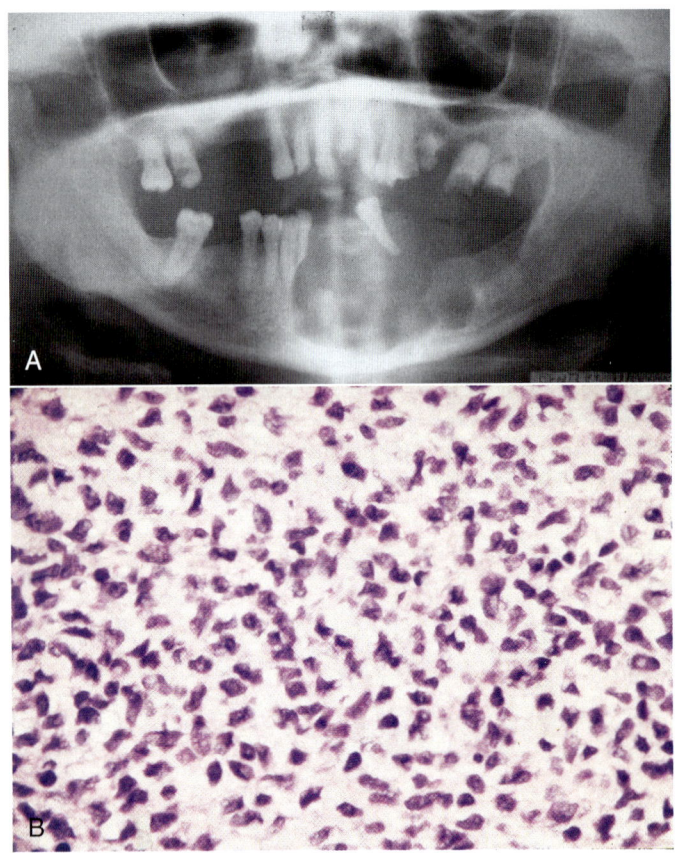

Fig. 50-35 ▪ **A,** The ameloblastic fibrosarcoma is the most common of the rare odontogenic malignant variants and will occur as a more destructive lesion in an older (adult range) age than the benign ameloblastic fibroma. **B,** The malignant part of the ameloblastic fibrosarcoma is the odontogenic mesenchyme (fibroma) portion seen as greater cellularity, larger and more pleomorphic nuclei, and rare mitotic figures. (H&E; original magnification ×10.)

FIBRO-OSSEOUS DISEASES

True fibro-osseous diseases are not neoplasms but disturbances in bone or connective tissue maturation or remodeling disturbances. They include fibrous dysplasia, cherubism, periapical dysplasia, and cemento-ossifying dysplasia.

FIBROUS DYSPLASIA

Fibrous dysplasia is caused by a gene deletion or gene mutation in the *GNAS-1* gene during embryogenesis. The protein product of the *GANS-1* gene has a pleiotropic effect, which means it has many effects depending on its time and location of action. If the normal *GANS-1* gene function is lost early in embryogenesis, the abnormal cell or cells will migrate to many locations in bone, in addition to several endocrine organs. This will result in the polyostotic form of fibrous dysplasia, together with café-au-lait spots and also precocious puberty, known as the McCune-Albright type (Fig. 50-40). If the normal *GANS-1* gene function is lost a little later in embryogenesis, the abnormal cells may migrate to several skeletal sites but not to endocrine organs, resulting in polyostotic fibrous dysplasia with café-au-lait spots but without precocious puberty, this is known as the Jaffe-Lichtenstein type. Then if the *GANS-1* gene function is lost just a short time later, the affected cells stay regional but may involve several adjacent bones, producing the craniofacial type of fibrous dysplasia (Fig. 50-41, *A*). Finally, if the *GANS-1* gene function is lost somewhat later, again the affected cells will remain localized in one site, producing the monostotic type of fibrous dysplasia (Fig. 50-41, *B*).

Although the cause of fibrous dysplasia occurs during embryogenesis, the clinical manifestation first becomes apparent between the ages of 5 and 15 years. It does not develop after the age of 20 years, a feature that distinguishes several cases from the bone neoplasm ossifying fibroma.

The diagnosis of fibrous dysplasia is less one of histopathology and more one of radiographic and CT scan features. The textbook description of woven bone without osteoblastic rimming is not seen in all cases or in all portions of a specimen. In many slides, a distinction between fibrous dysplasia and ossifying cannot be made with certainty.

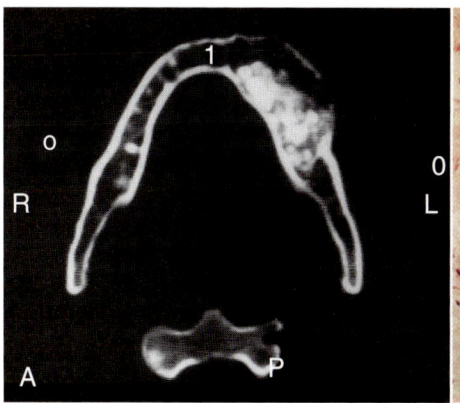
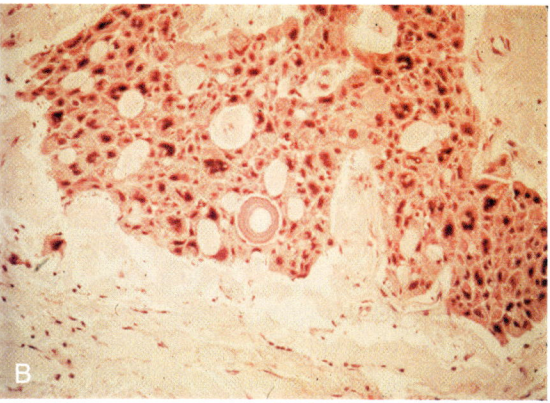

Fig. 50-36 ■ A, The calcified epithelial odontogenic tumor (Pindborg tumor) will present as a mixed radiolucent-radiopaque expansile mass. **B,** The unique histopathology of a calcified epithelial odontogenic tumor shows large epithelial cells with large bizarre nuclei and prominent intercellular bridges. There is also amyloid and some dystrophic calcifications. (H&E; original magnification ×2.)

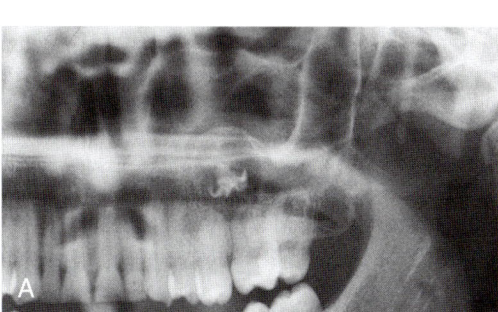
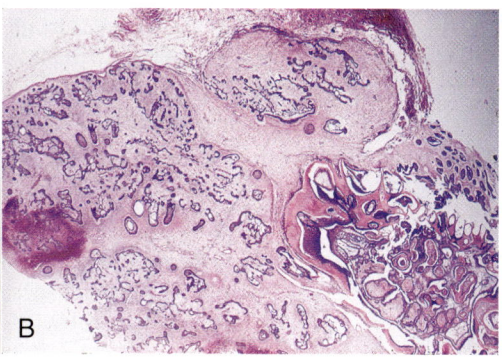

Fig. 50-37 ■ A, An ameloblastic fibro-odontoma will present as a mixed radiolucent-radiopaque lesion. **B,** An ameloblastic fibro-odontoma will have the histopathologic appearance of an ameloblastic fibroma with the addition of dysmorphic dentin. (H&E; original magnification ×1.)

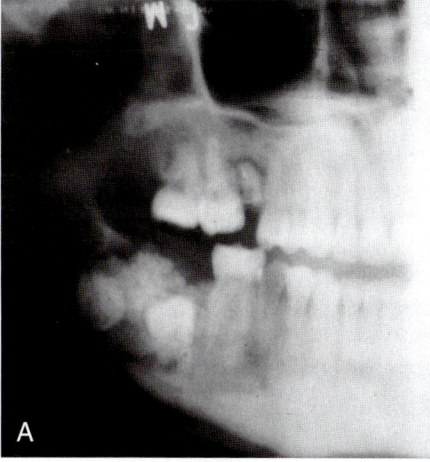
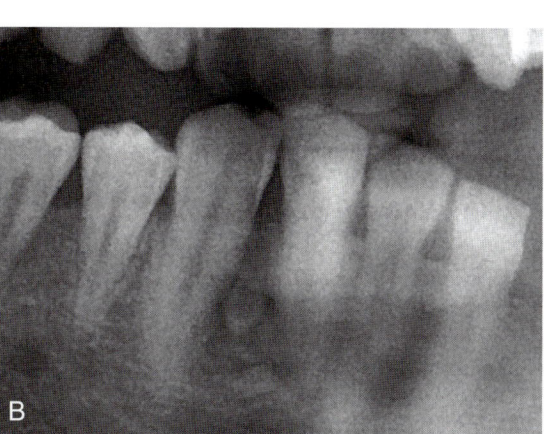

Fig. 50-38 ■ A, A complex odontoma presents as a diffuse radiopacity. **B,** A compound odontoma presents with the appearance of small tooth-like structures.

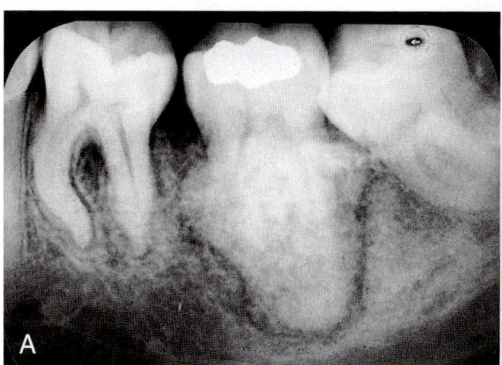
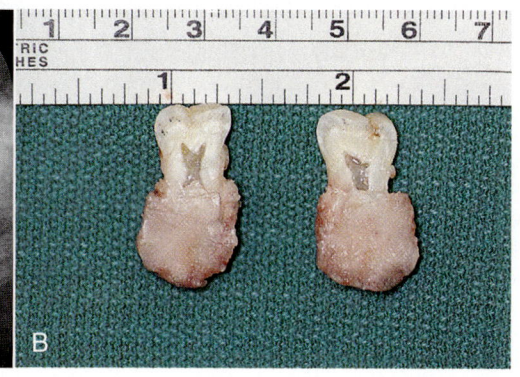

Fig. 50-39 ■ A, A cementoblastoma will form a bulbous radiopacity encompassing at least half of the root structure and bordered by a radiolucent band. **B,** A cut gross specimen of a cementoblastoma identifies its involvement with the entire root, in this case.

The diagnosis of fibrous dysplasia should note an expansion of bone that begins before the age of 20 years (Fig. 50-42, *A*). The radiograph and CT scan should show a diffuse hazy fusiform-shaped disturbance in the bone pattern, often described as having a "ground-glass appearance" (Fig. 50-42, *B*). This affected area will not be well demarcated from normal bone, and the cortices will be remodeled into the "ground-glass appearance" as well. This will distinguish it from an ossifying fibroma, which is spherical in shape and very well demarcated from normal bone (Fig. 50-43).

The treatment for fibrous dysplasia is generally no treatment, unless symptoms owing to nerve compression or ocular displacement causing visual changes or hearing problems warrant removal of the offending bone. Many patients and/or the family desire facial bone contouring, which is another indication for surgical intervention. In such cases, it is ideal to first accomplish this in the late teenage years, which is the period when facial bone growth ceases and the most stable long-term results will occur. Facial bone contouring at an earlier age will not stimulate excessive regrowth, as was once thought. However, the fibrous dysplasia will likely redevelop a facial contour expansion, because the fibrous dysplasia will grow at a rate faster than normal facial bone growth as it proceeds. Therefore, earlier facial contouring procedures should include an informed consent identifying the likely need for additional surgeries later.

CHERUBISM

Cherubism is an inherited autosomal dominant trait that also has a 40% sporadic occurrence (i.e., occurs as the first mutation in individuals with uninvolved parents and parents who are not carriers). Cherubism does not become apparent until age 2.5 to 4 years and will involve only the bones of the embryologically determined mandible or maxilla. Thus, in the most severe expression, it will cause a multilocular radiolucent expansion of the mandible that will spare the condyle, which does not develop by direction from Meckel cartilage. Cherubism will also involve the maxilla, including the middle turbinate, which is part of the embryologically determined maxilla, but it will spare the inferior turbinate, vomer, zygoma, and pterygoid plates, which are separate bones or parts of separate bones (Fig. 50-44).

There are three clinical expressions of cherubism. Type I cherubism only affects the bilateral rami and angles of the mandible and produces a minimal expansion (Fig. 50-45, *A*). Therefore, many cases go unnoticed or diagnosed as bilateral central giant cell tumors or other entities. Type II cherubism involves the bilateral rami and body of the mandible to the mental foramen area and the posterior maxilla to the bicuspid region (Fig. 50-45, *B*). This type does produce noticeable clinical expansion. Type III cherubism causes the greatest bilateral and symmetrical expansion of both the maxilla and mandible (Fig. 50-45, *C*). This form expands the maxilla and the maxillary bone's contribution to the orbital floor, causing a scleral show and the eyes to turn upward somewhat (see Fig. 50-44, *B*). This appearance of an upward gaze, together with symmetrical facial expansion, gives these individuals the look of the cherubs depicted in Renaissance art, hence the name cherubism.

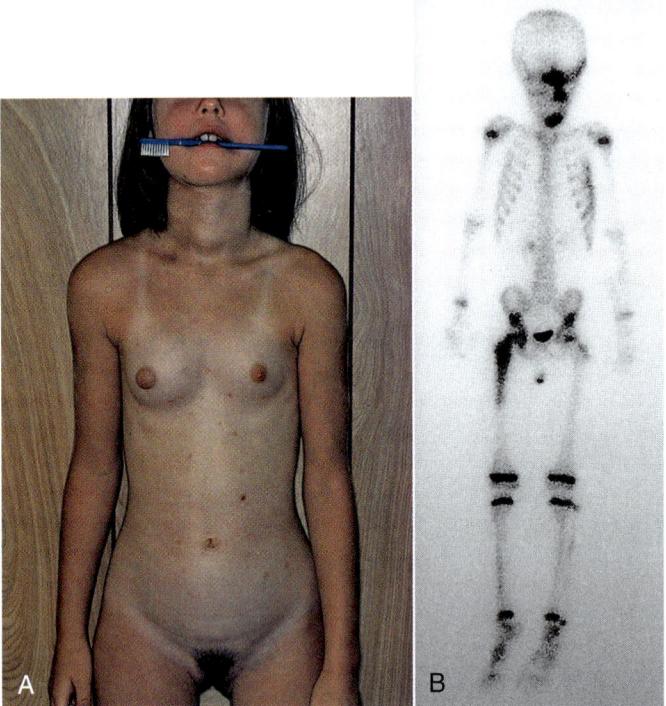

Fig. 50-40 ■ **A,** Polyostotic fibrous dysplasia of the McCune-Albright type will show precocious puberty and café-au-lait spots. **B,** A technetium 99m–methylene diphosphonate (MDP) scan shows several areas of abnormally high bone activity in polyostotic fibrous dysplasia.

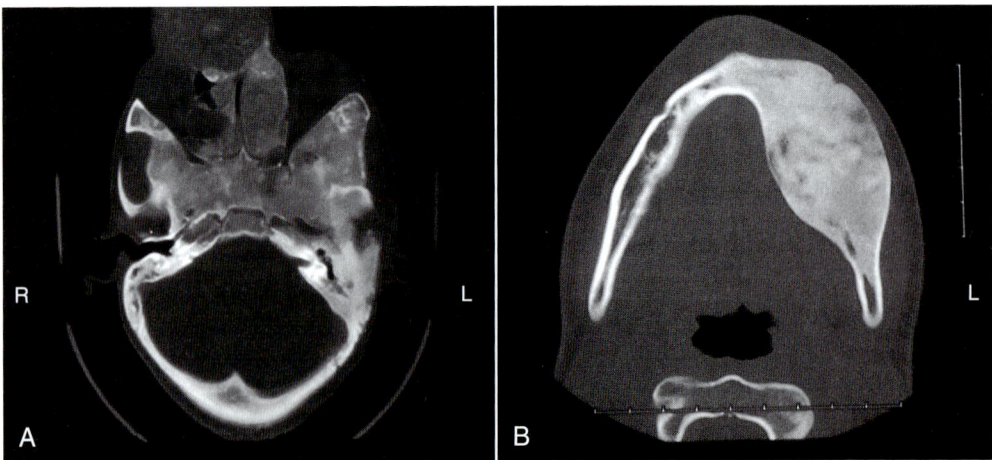

Fig. 50-41 ■ **A,** Craniofacial fibrous dysplasia involves contiguous bones of the face and/or base of skull. **B,** Monostotic fibrous dysplasia involves a single bone with a fusiform, poorly demarcated, ground-glass appearance.

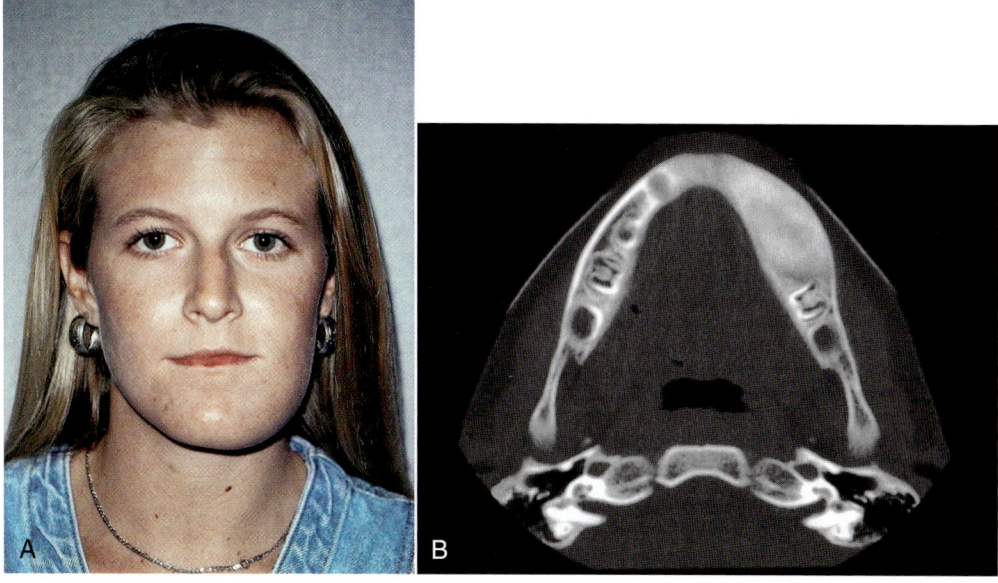

Fig. 50-42 ■ **A,** Monostotic fibrous dysplasia in a 17-year-old patient whose radiograph is seen in Figure 50-41, *B*. **B,** Fibrous dysplasia will radiographically appear with a ground-glass appearance that includes the cortex.

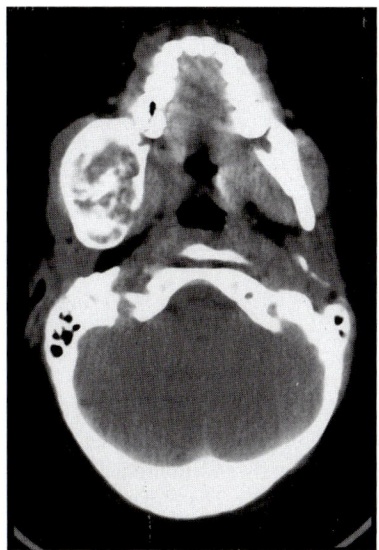

Fig. 50-43 ■ An ossifying fibroma will radiographically appear as a spherical or oval expansion with an expanded but identifiable cortex.

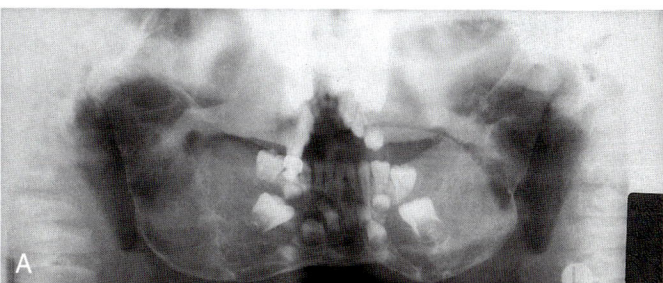

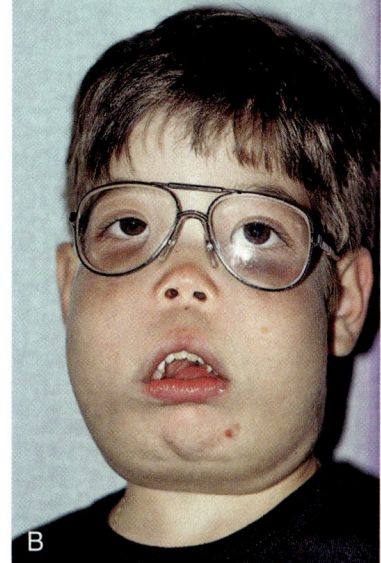

Fig. 50-44 ■ **A,** Type III cherubism involves the maxilla and mandible across the midline but spares the condyle. **B,** Type III cherubism with facial expansion and the eyes rotated superiorly, lending the term "eyes turned to heaven," thus resembling the cherubs of Renaissance art.

The natural course of cherubism is a slow expansion from about age 3 to 17 years, when the expansion usually ceases and an involution begins. In some cases, the expansion completely involutes within a few years to a normal facial contour, leaving nonexpanding radiolucencies in the jaws. In others, the expansion ceases, and the involution is slowed or does not occur at all. In these cases, recontouring at the age of 17 years, or thereafter, provides the best and most durable result.

If facial contouring surgery is planned, the surgeon should anticipate removing a significant amount of bone and be prepared for bleeding (Fig. 50-46). The cherubic tissue within the bone and the bone itself is extremely vascular. Preparation with typed and cross-matched blood for transfusion, as well as local hemostatic agents, such as bone wax, microfibular bovine collagen (Avitene; Davol,

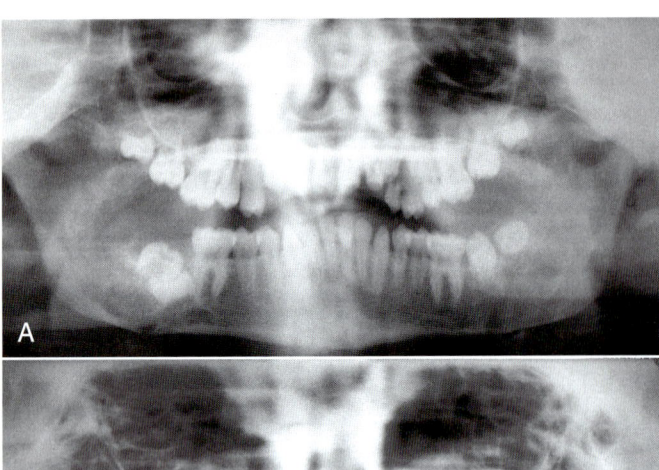

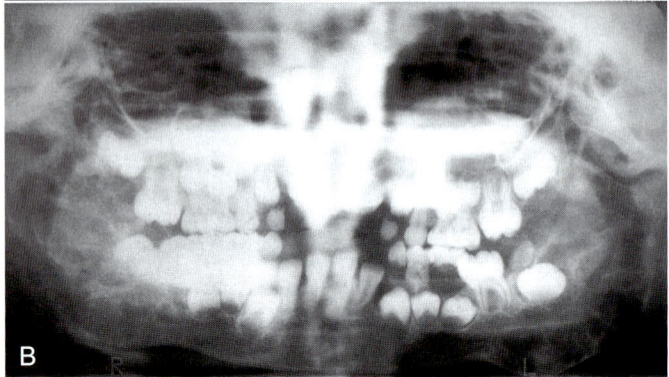

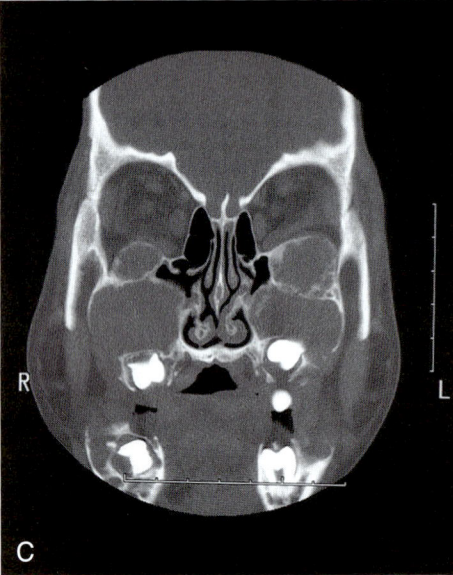

Fig. 50-45 ■ **A,** Type I cherubism is limited to the ramus and posterior mandible. **B,** Type II cherubism involves the bilateral mandible to the mental foramen and the posterior maxilla. **C,** The eyes turned toward the heavens in type III cherubism is due to expansion of the maxillary bone's contribution to the orbital floor.

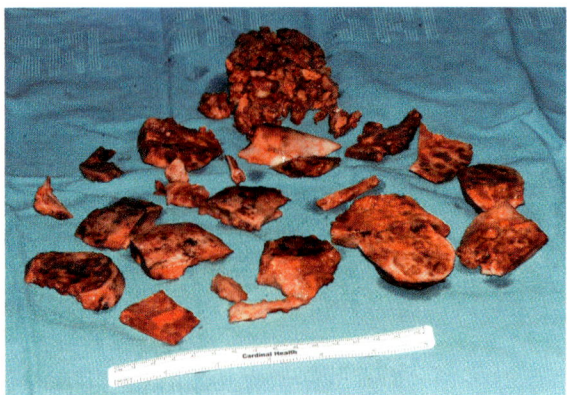

Fig. 50-46 ■ Contouring cherubism requires the removal of a significant amount of bone.

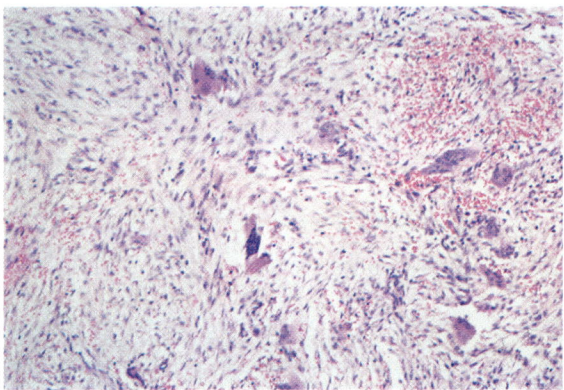

Fig. 50-47 ■ The histopathology of cherubism is not pathognomonic, because it will show a fibroblastic stroma and some multinucleated giant cells indistinguishable from a central giant cell tumor and or brown tumor of hyperparathyroidism. (H&E; original magnification ×2.)

Warwick, RI), Gelfoam (Pfizer, New York, NY), among others, should be readily available.

Genetic counseling is recommended, especially for a sporadic case, because the autosomal dominant trait will place three of four children at risk for developing cherubism.

The histopathology of cherubism may be undistinguishable from a central giant cell tumor. Therefore, the disease course, inheritance pattern, plain radiographs, and CT scans are the best diagnostic studies. The histopathology will show a fibrous stroma of immature

and young fibroblasts, producing minimal collagen along with extravasated red blood cells and multinucleated giant cells resembling osteoclasts (Fig. 50-47). There may be an eosinophilic deposit in a ring formation around small blood vessels as well. However, this is not seen in every specimen.

PERIAPICAL CEMENTAL DYSPLASIA

Periapical cemental dysplasia is a clinical/radiographic diagnosis seen most always in black women of African heritage who are in their midlife years (age 30 to 50). The lesions are usually asymptomatic and are incidental radiographic findings where radiolucencies, or mixed radiolucent-radiopaque, or completely radiopaque lesions are seen at the apices of the six mandibular anterior teeth. Followed over the years, there is an evolution of radiolucent to progressively more radiopaque quality (Fig. 50-48, *A*). The teeth associated with these are vital to pulp testing and are asymptomatic unless involved with caries or periodontal disease separately.

Few lesions are biopsied. However, the histopathology looks like dysplastic bone or cementum with irregular islands of bone cementum with reversal lines and a sparse cellular stroma resembling cementoblasts or osteoblasts (Fig. 50-48, *B*).

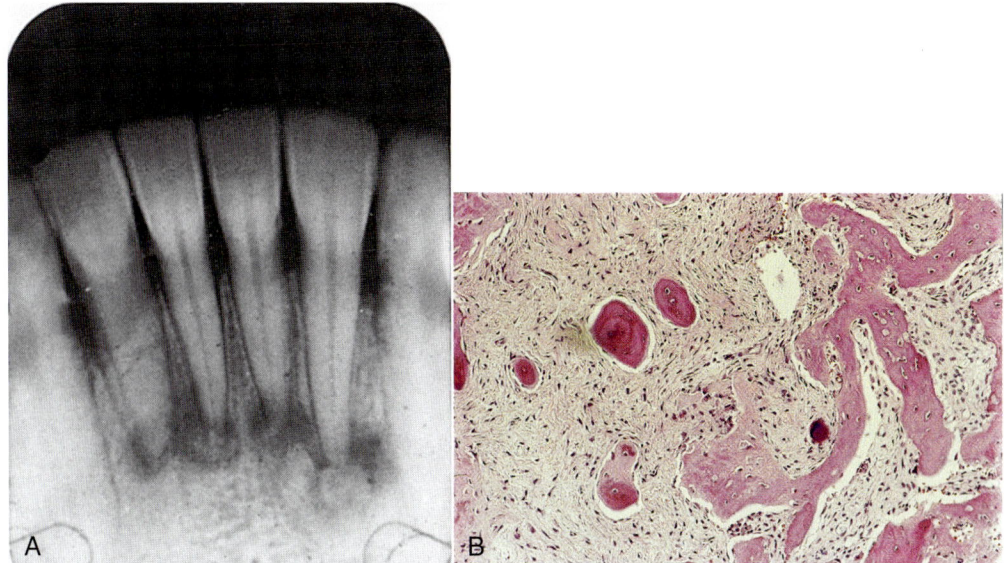

Fig. 50-48 ■ **A,** Periapical cemental dysplasia occurs in the anterior mandible with radiolucencies and radiopacities at the apex of the incisor teeth, usually in an adult of black African descent. **B,** Histopathology of a periapical cemental dysplasia will show a stromal proliferation of periodontal ligament fibroblasts and islands of bone/cementum. (H&E; original magnification ×4.)

Due to the racial focus of this condition, a genetic etiology has been suggested but remains unproven. No treatment is recommended, and root canal treatment should be discouraged because the teeth remain vital.

CEMENTO-OSSEOUS DYSPLASIA

Cemento-osseous dysplasia is similar to periapical cemental dysplasia in radiographic appearance and racial focus. However, the involvement of teeth and alveolar bone is not limited to the anterior mandibular teeth but is more widespread and may involve two to all four quadrants of the jaws and, hence in the past, was called florid osseous dysplasia. However, because it occurs only in the jaws and is limited to the alveolar bone (Fig. 50-49, *A*), similar to periapical cemental dysplasia, it is thought to be a defect in the remodeling of the bone-cementum-periodontal ligament complex.

Once again, this condition is diagnosed by its radiographic and clinical picture rather than histopathology. The rare histopathologic specimens show dense acellular mineralized bone with a hint of old reversal lines and no osteoblastic rimming (Fig. 50-49, *B*).

No treatment is required for asymptomatic cases. However, in cases where teeth have been removed in involved areas, the dense acellular bone may become exposed and then become secondarily infected and cause pain. In such cases, a debridement removing the dense bone down to the mandibular canal in the mandible, or to just below the sinus floor in the maxilla with a primary closure, usually resolves the exposed bone and symptoms. Because these patients are at risk for exposed bone and nonhealing extraction sockets, preventive dentistry aimed at avoiding the need for tooth removal(s) is recommended, as is root canal treatment rather than tooth removal if possible.

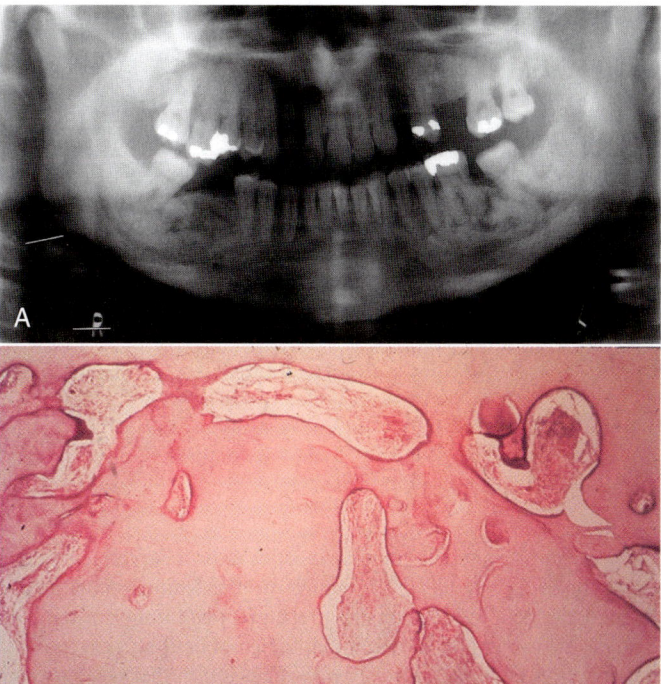

Fig. 50-49 ■ **A,** Cemento-osseous dysplasia also mostly occurs in adults of black African descent but involves posterior as well as anterior quadrants of alveolar bone, with mostly radiopaque masses. **B,** Histopathology of cemento-osseous dysplasia will show a poorly cellular mass of bone/cementum and a scant fibrous stroma.

- The basic treatment for odontogenic keratocysts remains enucleation and curettage. Select cases of large unilocular lesions may be treated by marsupialization, and large multilocular destructive ones or multiply recurrent lesions may be treated by resection.
- Use of the term odontogenic keratocystic tumor should not be used as a rationale to resect all cases of odontogenic keratocysts.
- Enucleation and curettage of ameloblastomas should be discouraged, because it is not curative and may actually seed tumor cells into the soft tissues.
- Branchial cysts and thyroglossal tract cysts often develop within 2 to 3 weeks after an upper respiratory tract infection.
- Odontogenic keratocysts mostly recur due to incomplete removal, whereby a small portion of the thin and friable lining is left behind. A smaller number recur as new cysts from activation of residual epithelial rests.
- Not all basal cell carcinomas in the basal cell nevus syndrome require removal. Although they may appear as carcinomas on histopathology, they do not behave as such.

- An ameloblastic fibrosarcoma histopathology may only show a mild to moderate number of mitotic figures. However, a suspicion for a de novo ameloblastic fibrosarcoma or one transformed from a benign ameloblastic fibroma may be raised by a larger lesion with a more destructive radiographic pattern.
- Ameloblastomas arising in the wall of a dentigerous cyst should be assessed relative to the depth of invasion into or through the connective wall of the cyst.
- Although a calcifying epithelial odontogenic tumor (CEOT) will contain cells with large pleomorphic nuclei resembling a malignant cytology, it remains a benign tumor.
- The adenomatoid odontogenic cyst (AOC) is a true cyst with a lumen, epithelial lining, and a connective tissue wall. It is not a true neoplasm. Therefore, the term adenomatoid odontogenic tumor (AOT) is inappropriate.
- Whereas fibrous dysplasia can be osseous, contoured without significant blood loss, cherubism is very vascular and is associated with a greater blood loss during an osseous contour procedure.
- Fibrous dysplasia is not hereditary, but cherubism occurs in an autosomal dominant pattern.

Chapter

51

The Central Giant Cell Granuloma

M.A. Pogrel

The central giant cell granuloma is felt to be a benign lesion that only occurs in the jaws, though similar lesions occur in the fingers and toes.[1] Its relationship to the giant cell tumor of the long bones is unknown, but it is felt that the giant cell tumor represents a more aggressive and possibly malignant lesion that rarely occurs in the jaws, if at all. Other authorities feel that these lesions represent a spectrum of disease from malignant to very benign. Central giant cell granulomas normally occur in the anterior part of the jaws (in areas where deciduous teeth were present) and normally occur in the second and third decades, although they have been noted in all decades of life. Histologically similar, or even identical, appearances may occur in hyperparathyroidism, cherubism, and aneurysmal bone cysts, which should normally be ruled out prior to establishing the diagnosis.

When the central giant cell granuloma was first identified as a distinct lesion (previously, it had been included in a group of lesions called "osteitis fibrosa cystica"), it was termed the reparative giant cell granuloma because it was felt to be a self-limiting lesion that would even heal.[2-4] It is difficult to ascertain the evidence on which this was based, but most authorities now feel that this is not a self-healing lesion and that it will progress if untreated. Worth, however, in the last edition of his textbook on radiology, followed a number of histologically proven central giant cell lesions of the jaws radiographically for many years with no other treatment than the biopsy, and he did show radiographically that some lesions did resolve.[5] The author of this chapter was also able to personally discuss this finding with Dr. Worth in 1978, when he did confirm that this had occurred.

The conventional treatment for the central giant cell granuloma is to establish the diagnosis histologically and to treat the lesions with aggressive curettage.[6] This is associated, however, with a recurrence rate of about 20%, and some authorities feel that there is a more aggressive variant of this lesion,[7,8] although all attempts to identify this histologically have been unsuccessful to date.[9-13] However, because of this recurrence rate, and even possible spontaneous regression,[5] alternative treatments have been suggested in an effort to either lower the recurrence rate or to avoid removal or damage to adjacent teeth, soft tissues, or the inferior alveolar and related nerves.

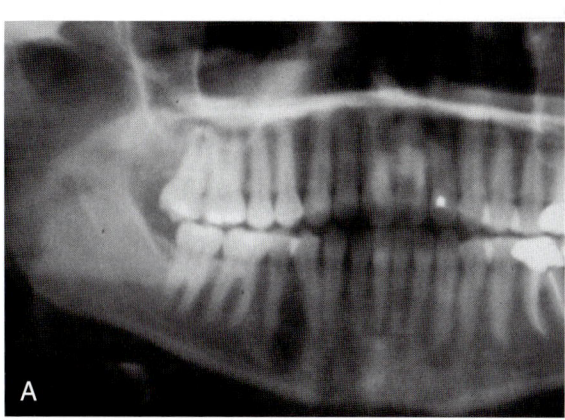
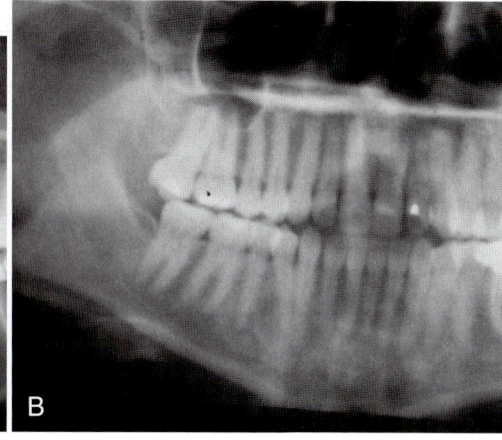

Fig. 51-1 ■ A biopsy-proven central giant cell granuloma in the bicuspid region of the right mandibular body involving the roots of the lower right bicuspids. **A,** On initial diagnosis. **B,** Six months after a course of six corticosteroid injections.

ALTERNATIVE MEDICAL TREATMENTS

INTRALESIONAL STEROID INJECTION

Intralesional steroid injection, an alternative treatment for the management of central giant cell granuloma, was first suggested in 1988.[14] The rationale at that time was that histologically these lesions have a superficial resemblance to the lesions of sarcoid, and because steroids are an effective treatment for sarcoid lesions, they were tried for the central giant cell granuloma. The protocol involves six injections with a 50% mixture of local anesthetic and triamcinolone 10 mg/mL at weekly intervals for six weeks. The protocol suggests the use of 2 cc of this solution for every 1 cc of lesion visible on a Panorex radiograph.[15] There are several reports in the literature on this technique, and most report variable success.[16,17] There are definitely cases in which this treatment has caused total resolution of the lesion, and even hypercalcification of the lesion as shown in Figure 51-1, but most authorities report about a 50% success rate. Most practitioners have examples of lesions that either stopped growing in size or partially calcified but still require curettage for the lesion as definitive treatment. It is possible that this treatment is more effective for smaller, unilocular, well-circumscribed lesions where the steroids can enter all parts of the lesion, rather than multilocular lesions where areas may be missed by the steroid injections.

SYSTEMIC CALCITONIN TREATMENT

Systemic calcitonin treatment was first advocated in 1993,[18] and the rationale for its use was that the central giant cell granuloma is histologically identical to the brown tumor of hyperparathyroidism. Although these patients do not have classic hyperparathyroidism, it was speculated that there may be a circulating related hormone that was causing these lesions. However, this hormone, if it exists, has not been identified. The mode of action of calcitonin in the management of central giant cell granulomas is therefore speculative. It may directly antagonize osteoclastic bone resorption, or it may act directly on other cell types in the lesion. Calcitonin receptors have been identified on the giant cells of the lesion.[19] However, immunohistochemical examination suggests that it is the stromal cell or fibroblast that is the etiologic cell of the central giant cell granuloma, and the giant cells themselves may be reactive.[12] The only form of calcitonin currently available in the United States is salmon calcitonin, and this can be administered subcutaneously or by nasal spray. The subcutaneous calcitonin is normally given as 100 units per day,

but this does cause nausea in a small number of younger patients, and, in that case, the dosage has been reduced temporarily to 50 units per day in these patients. The patients are monitored radiographically, and changes are not usually seen for about 9 months, and it normally takes 18 to 21 months for the lesions to resolve. The subcutaneous calcitonin is administered for this length of time. This treatment has been used for complete resolution of the lesion, and, to date, of 27 patients completed, all have resolved (Fig. 51-2), but there has been one noncompliant patient and one recurrence, which responded to a repeat course of calcitonin and has not recurred some 14 years later (Fig. 51-3).[20] Other authorities have used calcitonin for cure while others have used calcitonin to shrink the lesion, followed by curettage.[21-25] A further study reported primary treatment with curettage, followed by intranasal calcitonin to successfully prevent recurrence.[26] The intranasal calcitonin has a higher level of patient acceptance, but absorption is variable, and the results may therefore be more unpredictable.

Calcitonin treatment has also been attempted on the giant cell lesions of cherubism, Noonan syndrome, and multiple giant cell lesions associated with neurofibromatosis. In these cases, the lesions have not responded to calcitonin. The lesions of cherubism do not respond at all, and in Noonan syndrome and neurofibromatosis, the lesions stopped growing but did not regress, suggesting a different origin for these lesions. Now that the gene abnormalities in these conditions are being identified, it is obvious they represent different lesions, though histologically they may be identified to the central giant cell granuloma.[27-29]

INTERFERON-ALPHA

Assuming that the central giant cell granuloma is primarily a vascular lesion, interferon-alpha with its antiangiogenic properties has been utilized for the management of this lesion. The interferon-alpha is also given by subcutaneous injection and monitored by measurement of fibroblast growth factor in the urine. Dosages have commenced at 3 million units/m² of interferon-alpha per day, and the published protocol has been to carry out initial enucleation of the lesion followed by interferon–alpha treatment for 6 to 8 months to prevent recurrence.[30,31] In cases where it has been attempted to use interferon-alpha for complete cure or resolution without initial enucleation, often it has been of limited success due to only partial resolution and side effects. The side effects of interferon-alpha appear to be mainly fever, fatigue, and a flulike syndrome, which some patients have found quite debilitating.[32] Hospitalization may be necessary for some patients.

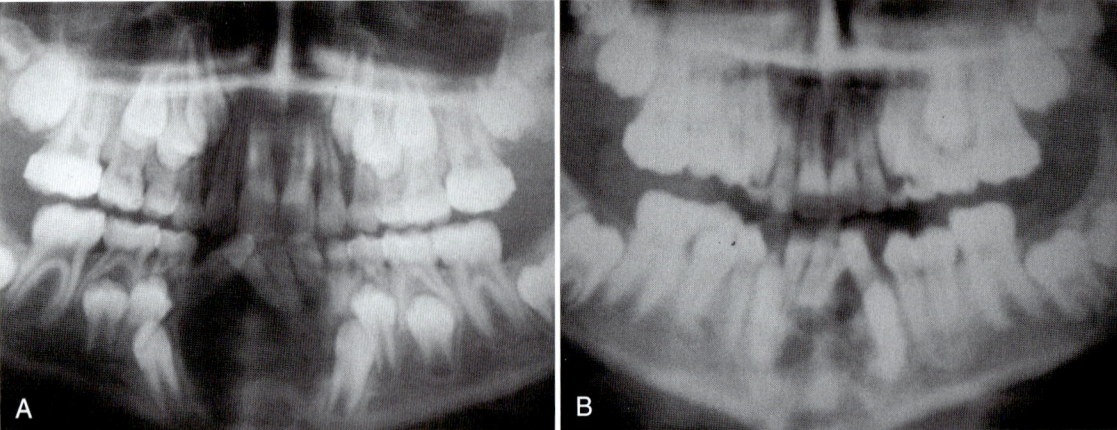

Fig. 51-2 ■ A biopsy-proven central giant cell granuloma of the anterior mandible causing displacement of teeth. **A,** On initial diagnosis. **B,** After 21 months of subcutaneous calcitonin therapy. Note calcification of the site of the lesion and movement of the affected teeth into the area previously occupied by the lesion.

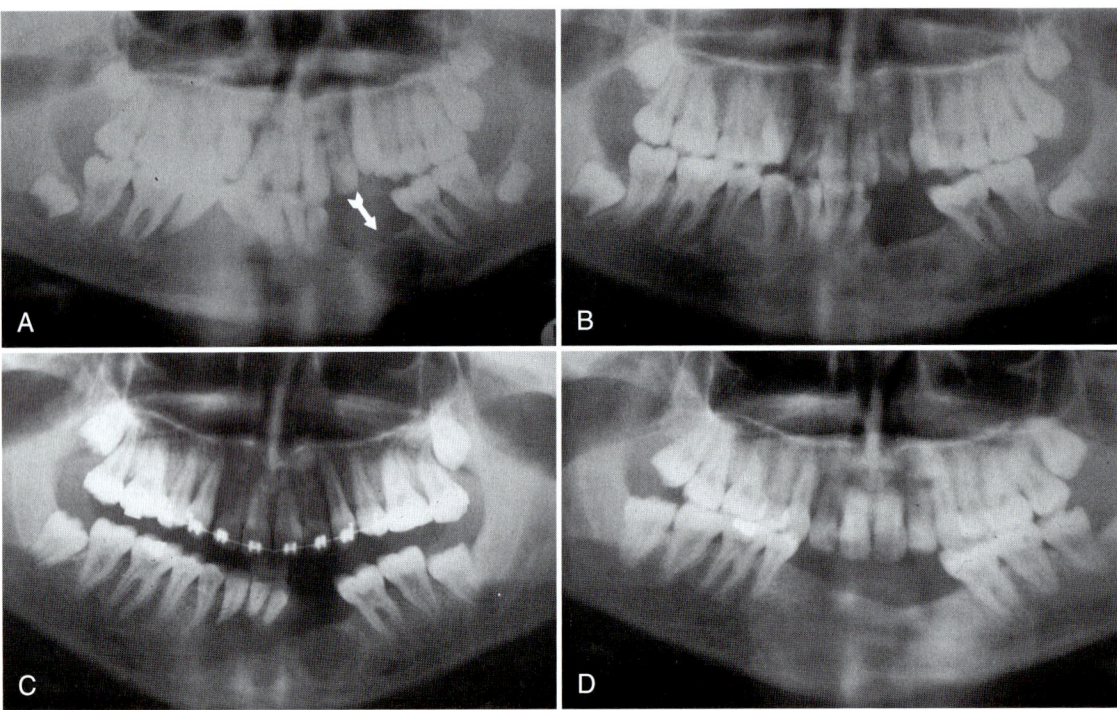

Fig. 51-3 ■ A 13-year-old patient with recurrent multiple central giant cell granulomas of the mandible in the absence of hyperparathyroidism or any other disease process that could cause multiple lesions. **A,** On initial referral with bilateral lesions of mandible and a pathologic fracture on the left. **B,** After 21 months of subcutaneous calcitonin, the mandibular fracture healed spontaneously. **C,** Appearance 2 years later showing a multilocular recurrence of the anterior mandible. **D,** Appearance 8 years later following removal of nonsalvageable lower anterior teeth and a repeated course of calcitonin.

PEARLS AND PITFALLS

- The histogenesis of the central giant cell granuloma remains controversial.
- The majority of patients respond well to local curettage, but there is a 15% to 25% recurrence rate.
- Interestingly, many patients also respond to nontraditional medical treatments.
- Nontraditional treatments include:

- Intralesional steroid injections
- Subcutaneous injections or nasal inhalation of calcitonin
- Subcutaneous injections of interferon-alpha
- These medical treatments all appear to cause resolution in many cases, though their means of action is largely unknown, which further complicates the debate on the true nature of these lesions.

REFERENCES

1. Yamaguchi T, Dorfman HD: Giant cell reparative granuloma: a comparative clinico-pathologic study of lesions in gnathic and extragnathic sites, *Int J Surg Pathol* 9(3):189-200, 2001.
2. Bernier JL: *The management of oral diseases*, St Louis, 1955, Mosby.
3. Bernier JL, Cahn LR: The peripheral giant cell reparative granuloma, *J Am Dent Assoc* 49(2):141-148, 1954.
4. Jaffe HL: Giant-cell reparative granuloma, traumatic bone cyst, and fibrous (fibro-osseous) dysplasia of the jawbones, *Oral Surg Oral Med Oral Pathol* 6(1):159-175, 1953.
5. Worth HM: *Principles and practice of oral radiology interpretation*, Chicago, 1963, Year Book Medical Publishers.
6. Stern M, Eisenbud L: Management of giant cell lesions of the jaws, *Oral Maxillofac Surg Clin North Am* 3:165, 1991.
7. Whitaker SB, Vigneswaran N, Budnick SD, Waldron CA: Giant cell lesions of the jaws: evaluation of nucleolar organizer regions in lesions of varying behavior, *J Oral Pathol Med* 22(9):402-405, 1993.
8. Chuong R, Kaban LB, Kozakewich H, Perez-Atayde A: Central giant cell lesions of the jaws: a clinicopathologic study, *J Oral Maxillofac Surg* 44(9):708-713, 1986.
9. Eckardt A, Pogrel MA, Kaban LB, et al: Central giant cell granulomas of the jaws. Nuclear DNA analysis using image cytometry, *Int J Oral Maxillofac Surg* 18(1):3-6, 1989.
10. Ficarra G, Kaban LB, Hansen LS: Central giant cell lesions of the mandible and maxilla: a clinicopathologic and cytometric study, *Oral Surg Oral Med Oral Pathol* 64(1):44-49, 1987.
11. Franklin CD, Craig GT, Smith CJ: Quantitative analysis of histological parameters in giant cell lesions of the jaws and long bones, *Histopathology* 3(6):511-522, 1979.
12. O'Malley M, Pogrel MA, Stewart JC, et al: Central giant cell granulomas of the jaws: phenotype and proliferation-associated markers, *J Oral Pathol Med* 26(4):159-163, 1997.
13. Regezi JA, Zarbo RJ, Lloyd RV: HLA-DR antigen detection in giant cell lesions, *J Oral Pathol* 15(8):434-438, 1986.
14. Jacoway JH, Howell FV, Terry BC: Central giant cell granuloma: an alternative to surgical therapy, *Oral Surg Oral Med Oral Pathol* 66:572, 1988.
15. Terry BC, Jacoway JR: Management of central giant cell lesions: an alternative to surgical therapy, *Oral Maxillofac Surg Clin North Am* 6:579, 1994.
16. Carlos R, Sedano HO: Intralesional corticosteroids as an alternative treatment for central giant cell granuloma, *Oral Surg Oral Med Oral Pathol Oral Radiol Endod* 93(2):161-166, 2002.
17. Kermer C, Millesi W, Watzke IM: Local injection of corticosteroids for central giant cell granuloma. A case report, *Int J Oral Maxillofac Surg* 23(6 Pt 1):366-368, 1994.
18. Harris M: Central giant cell granulomas of the jaws regress with calcitonin therapy, *Br J Oral Maxillofac Surg* 31(2):89-94, 1993.
19. Pogrel MA, Regezi JA, Harris ST, Goldring SR: Calcitonin treatment for central giant cell granulomas of the mandible: report of two cases, *J Oral Maxillofac Surg* 57(7):848-853, 1999.
20. Pogrel MA: Calcitonin therapy for central giant cell granuloma, *J Oral Maxillofac Surg* 61(6):649-653, 2003; discussion 53-54.
21. de Lange J, Rosenberg AJ, van den Akker HP, et al: Treatment of central giant cell granuloma of the jaw with calcitonin, *Int J Oral Maxillofac Surg* 28(5):372-376, 1999.
22. Lannon DA, Earley MJ: Cherubism and its charlatans, *Br J Plast Surg* 54(8):708-711, 2001.
23. O'Regan EM, Gibb DH, Odell EW: Rapid growth of giant cell granuloma in pregnancy treated with calcitonin, *Oral Surg Oral Med Oral Pathol Oral Radiol Endod* 92(5):532-538, 2001.
24. Penfold CN, Evans BT: Giant cell lesions complicating Paget's disease of bone and their response to calcitonin therapy, *Br J Oral Maxillofac Surg* 31(4):267, 1993.
25. Rosenberg AJ, Bosschaart AN, Jacobs JW, et al: [Calcitonin therapy in large or recurrent central giant cell granulomas of the lower jaw], *Ned Tijdschr Geneeskd* 141(7):335-339, 1997.
26. Beck-Mannagetta J, Krenkel C, Kassmann H, Prokop E: Ein Fortschritt in der Therapie des sentralen Riesenzellgranuloma: additive Verbreichung von Calcitonin Nasalspray, *Stomatolgie* 101(4):71-78, 2004.
27. Jongmans M, Otten B, Noordam K, van der Burgt I: Genetics and variation in phenotype in Noonan syndrome, *Horm Res* 62(Suppl 3):56-59, 2004.
28. Krammer U, Wimmer K, Wiesbauer P, et al: Neurofibromatosis 1: a novel NF1 mutation in an 11-year-old girl with a giant cell granuloma, *J Child Neurol* 18(5):371-373, 2003.
29. Ueki Y, Tiziani V, Santanna C, et al: Mutations in the gene encoding c-Abl-binding protein SH3BP2 cause cherubism, *Nat Genet* 2001 Jun;28(2):125-126.
30. Kaban LB, Mulliken JB, Ezekowitz RA, et al: Antiangiogenic therapy of a recurrent giant cell tumor of the mandible with interferon alfa-2a, *Pediatrics* 103(6 Pt 1):1145-1149, 1999.
31. Kaban LB, Troulis MJ, Ebb D, et al: Antiangiogenic therapy with interferon alpha for giant cell lesions of the jaws, *J Oral Maxillofac Surg* 60(10):1103-1111, 2002; discussion 1111-1113.
32. Dickerman JD: Interferon and giant cell tumors, *Pediatrics* 103(6 Pt 1):1282-1283, 1999.

Oral Squamous Cell Carcinoma: Epidemiology, Clinical and Radiographic Evaluation, and Staging

Brent B. Ward, Fayette C. Williams

EPIDEMIOLOGY

INCIDENCE

The global incidence of oral cancer has been estimated at 274,000 cases per year.[1] Approximately 126,000 deaths annually are attributed to oral cancer worldwide.[2] In the United States, 23,110 new cases and 5370 deaths are expected in 2009.[3] Squamous cell carcinoma is the predominant form of oral cancer and accounts for greater than 90% of malignant pathology.[4] Other forms include salivary gland tumors, mesenchymal tumors, lymphoma, and melanoma. Despite technologic advances in detection and treatment, survival rates for patients with oral cancer have shown minimal improvement over recent decades.

AGE

Oral cancer is predominantly a disease of older age. More than 92% of oral and pharyngeal cancers occur in individuals older than 40 years, with the average age being 63.[3] Its incidence increases until the age of 70 to 74 and then declines slightly.[5] A recent disturbing trend is the increase in oral cancer in younger adults in the United States and internationally.[6-9] A review from one large institution revealed an increase in tongue cancer from 4% to 18% in patients younger than 40 years between 1973 and 1995.[10] These patients ranged in age from 19 to 39 years; 59% were non-smokers, and 45% were non-drinkers. Assessment of 1973-2001 data from the Surveillance, Epidemiology and End Results (SEER) database revealed an increase in tongue cancer in young white men but a decrease in incidence in all other oral sites.[11] Even though it has been suggested that oral cancer is more aggressive in younger patients,[12-14] the evidence is conflicting. In a case-control study by Garavello and associates, young age was found to be an independent predictor of worse survival.[15] In contrast, two separate reviews of SEER data from 1973 to 2001 showed that younger patients had an overall higher 5-year survival rate for oral tongue cancer than older adults.[11,16] One meta-analysis found 3-year survival to be similar in patients younger than 40 and older than 40.[17] Atula and co-authors agreed that the prognosis for younger patients is similar to that for older patients.[18] A retrospective review of 76 patients by Manuel and colleagues found that patients younger than 45 years had similar outcomes and prognosis similar to older patients.[19]

GENDER

Once a predominantly male disease, females have experienced a steady rise in the incidence of oral cancer since the increase in female smokers began in the 1950s.[14,20-22] A Swedish group reported on 132 patients and concluded that females have a greater risk for oral cancer than men given the same quantity of tobacco use.[23] A report by Muscat and co-workers agreed that females are at higher risk than men who report the same number of pack-years of smoking.

Their study also noted that the percentage of non-smokers with oral cancer was significantly higher in females, especially in women older than 50 years.[24] This increased risk in older women was explored in a separate case-control study of 530 women with oral cancer. The authors suggested the possibility of a hormonal influence related to estrogen deficiency in postmenopausal women, although the data were not conclusive.[25] A 1995 review of SEER data revealed that women have higher risk than men for the development of second primary tumors of the head and neck, although the authors were unable to offer an explanation.[26] Conflicting data exist regarding how gender influences overall survival. In a review of cancer registry data from 1981 to 1998, an Italian study found that gender did not influence the prognosis for oral tongue cancer.[27] Arduino and colleagues conducted a retrospective review of 347 patients and found no difference in prognosis in terms of gender, although the minimum follow-up period was just 12 months.[28] A retrospective review of 193 patients older than 33 years found that survival was lower in men than in women for cancer of the tongue and floor of the mouth.[29] Similar findings showing a worse prognosis in men have been reported by Choi and colleagues,[30] Langdon and Rapidis,[31] Franco and co-authors,[32] and Funk and colleagues.[33]

RACE

African American men have the greatest risk for the development of oral cancer in the United States, whereas Hispanic men and women have the lowest risk. The incidence in whites is slightly higher than that in Asian Americans. The most striking disparity is the difference in both incidence and survival between African Americans and whites. Age-adjusted incidence rates for African American males are up to 20% higher than those for white males.[34] For all stages, whites have a relative 5-year survival rate of 61%, whereas only 36% of African Americans are alive after 5 years.[3] Reduced access to care has been suggested as one basis for this disparity because African Americans are more likely to lack health care coverage.[35] However, a large case-control study concluded that the higher oral cancer rates seen in African Americans can be attributed to increased alcohol and tobacco consumption.[36]

RISK FACTORS

Multiple factors have been associated with increased risk for oral cancer. Although the most compelling evidence implicates tobacco and alcohol, other associated factors, including viruses, nutritional deficiencies, previous upper aerodigestive malignancy, and immunocompromised status, have been proposed.

Population-based studies confirm the correlation between tobacco use and risk for oral cavity cancer.[37,38] Tobacco smoking is an independent risk factor with a relative risk of up to eight times that of non-smokers.[39] Oral cancer is twice as likely to develop in women as in men given the same amount of tobacco consumption.[24] It is thought that exposure to carcinogens leads to malignant transformation of cells. Even though smoking cessation is effective in reducing risk, former smokers still have higher risk than never smokers. Individuals who refrain from smoking for 1 to 9 years showed a 30% reduction in risk, whereas a 50% reduction in risk was noted for individuals who ceased smoking for more than 9 years.[37] Pipe and cigar smokers also have increased risk for oral cancer.

Smokeless tobacco's role in the development of oral cancer and its use as a smoking cessation tool have engendered a great deal of controversy. In 1981, Winn and co-authors reported a four-fold increase in risk in women users of smokeless tobacco.[40] However, a 1998 study reviewed statistics from West Virginia and found that the incidence and mortality of oral/pharyngeal cancer were less than the national average despite the remarkably heavy use of smokeless tobacco in this state.[41] Given this and other similar studies, transitioning smokers to smokeless tobacco has been advocated by some to lower the health risks associated with smoking. In a 2008 report, smokers who switched to smokeless tobacco were more than twice as likely to remain smoke free than were smokers who attempted cessation with traditional nicotine replacement products.[42] A recent meta-analysis of 89 studies (including 62 American and 18 Scandinavian studies) revealed only slight associations with oropharyngeal cancer, but the association disappeared for estimates published since 1990 and for alcohol-adjusted estimates.[43] Still, smokeless tobacco may not be without risk for other cancers, with a number of reports suggesting a possible association with esophageal, pancreatic, laryngeal, and renal cancer. In summary, although the overall health risks associated with smokeless tobacco are clearly significantly less than the risks with tobacco smoke,[44] patients should be advised that no tobacco product is considered completely safe at this time.[45] The National Cancer Institute continues to recommended that the public avoid all tobacco products, including smokeless tobacco.[46] A decision to use smokeless tobacco as a cessation method should take all these facts into consideration so that patients can act in an informed fashion regarding the risks and benefits of such an approach.

A final distinction should be made between smokeless tobacco manufactured in the United States and other forms used across the globe. Southeast Asia and India are known for heavy consumption of smokeless tobacco consisting of various combinations of betel nut and slaked lime. In addition to the high risk for the development of oral cancer, this habit has been associated with a significantly increased risk for leukoplakia, erythroplakia, and oral submucous fibrosis (a premalignant condition).[47] In one study the incidence of oral cavity cancer was 123-fold higher in individuals who smoked and chewed betel nut.[48] As a result, oral cavity cancer is one of the leading cancers in regions where this habit is practiced.

Alcohol is recognized as a distinct risk factor for the development of oral cancer, especially for consumers of dark liquors. The majority of patients in whom oral cancer develops are consumers of alcohol.[49] Lewin and colleagues demonstrated that low to moderate alcohol use does not increase the risk for oral cancer but high intake (>50 g) was an independent risk factor with a relative risk of 5.5. The study also noted that smoking had a synergistic effect with alcohol, with a relative risk of 22.1 versus a relative risk of 6.5 with smoking alone.[50] For consumers of very high levels of alcohol, risk for the development of oral cancer may be greater than that for smoking alone.[51]

Multiple viruses have been implicated in the etiology of oral cancer, including Epstein-Barr virus, herpes simplex viruses, retroviruses, and human papilloma viruses (HPVs). Human herpesvirus-8 is recognized as the most important pathogen in Kaposi sarcoma, although presence of the virus alone is not sufficient to cause malignancy.[52] Much of the recent research has focused on the link between HPV and upper aerodigestive malignancies. Patients with HPV-positive tumors have a significantly better prognosis than do those with HPV-negative tumors.[53] Although data for the role of HPV in the development of oropharyngeal carcinoma are clear, the role of HPV in oral cavity cancer is not as well defined. A 2001 study found HPV-16 to be present in oral cancer at a rate five times that in normal mucosa.[54] Over half of oral squamous cell carcinomas have been reported to harbor HPV.[55] However, direct causation has not been established, and the methodology of some studies has been questioned.[56,57] The literature shows a broad range of oral HPV prevalence in oral cavity cancer because of the multiple techniques used for detection of the virus, which vary in sensitivity.[58] Detection rates are also higher in samples taken from frozen tissue than from paraffin-embedded tissue.[55] These technical factors probably contribute to the wide range of reported prevalence rates, which makes causation difficult to establish.

Other factors are found in higher degrees in patients with oral cavity cancer, including poor diet and nutrition, poor oral hygiene, and ill-fitting oral prostheses. The chronic iron deficiency seen in patients with Plummer-Vinson syndrome has been associated with a higher incidence of oral and hypopharyngeal cancer.[59] A deficiency in vitamins A, C, and E has been associated with oral cancer.[60] Oral cancers have also been associated with low intake of fruits and vegetables, and a protective role may be afforded by diets high in fruits, vegetables, and fiber.[61,62] Poor oral hygiene as measured by caries and periodontal disease is noted more frequently in oral cancer patients.[63] A case-control study based in China found that poor oral hygiene was an independent risk factor for the development of oral cancer after controlling for smoking and alcohol.[64] A Swedish study reported that ill-fitting dentures were an independent risk factor for oral cancer,[23] whereas another study from the United States found no correlation.[65] Although an association between these factors and oral cancer is recognized, causality has not been established.

PATIENT EVALUATION

HISTORY

The pretreatment evaluation of all patients begins with a thorough history of the disease process, as well as a comprehensive past medical and surgical history. Specific focus should be placed on common problems in the oral cancer population, such as alcohol abuse, smoking, and malnutrition. The history should also review the functional capacity of the patient with regard to cardiopulmonary status. Patients with decreased cardiopulmonary reserve may benefit from preoperative medical consultation with their primary care physician. Finally, the history in oral cancer patients should note the level of home or family support available postoperatively. Lack of caregivers often requires the use of home nursing or postoperative placement in a skilled nursing facility.

The review of systems should search for symptoms of second primary tumors of the pharynx, esophagus, and lungs, which may be a useful guide for further clinical or radiologic examination. Typical red flag symptoms for second primaries include hoarseness, dysphagia, odynophagia, otalgia, stridor, and hemoptysis.

Physical capacity and performance status should be assessed before determining treatment. Various rating systems have been used in oncology patients to assess a patient's ability to conduct activities of daily living. The American Joint Committee on Cancer (AJCC) recommends recording the Karnofsky performance scale (KPS) along with standard staging data. This 100-point scale assesses performance status in 10-point increments to quantify physical capacity. Though not specific to head and neck cancer, the KPS has prognostic value in the general treatment of solid tumors.[66] Performance status was shown to predict overall survival in a series of more than 700 laryngeal cancer patients.[67] The author concluded that performance status probably reflected a patient's ability to resist the tumor.

PHYSICAL EXAMINATION

The physical examination should document a comprehensive assessment of the head and neck. Attention should be directed to the tumor's location, size, and relationship to adjacent anatomic structures. Bimanual palpation is useful to determine the extent of tumor in the floor of the mouth, buccal mucosa, and lips. Fixation to the mandible requires consideration of marginal versus segmental mandibulectomy. Proximity to the midline often guides the decision for unilateral versus bilateral neck dissection when indicated. Trismus or decreased tongue mobility may be an indication of invasion into deeper structures. Cranial nerve deficits suggest tumor involvement, which may increase suspicion for perineural spread. The status of the dentition should be assessed in patients in whom radiation therapy may be indicated because of the risk for xerostomia-related caries and osteoradionecrosis. Plans should be made for non-viable teeth to be removed at the time of surgery or before radiation therapy. Occasional difficulty is encountered in clinically determining the extent of the tumor in patients with trismus or pharyngeal extension. Although fiberoptic examination in the clinic may provide adequate visualization, direct laryngoscopy under general anesthesia is sometimes necessary before deciding on the final course of treatment. Biopsy of the primary tumor is required for histologic diagnosis and treatment planning.

Lymph nodes in the neck must be palpated carefully to assess for cervical metastasis or other abnormalities. The neck examination is performed by standing behind the patient and using both hands to evaluate for symmetry. The submandibular region is palpated with the fingers below the inferior border of the mandible. The examiner should not confuse the submandibular gland with lymphadenopathy. The sternocleidomastoid muscle is lifted between the thumb and fingers to palpate the jugular chain. The carotid bulb may be misinterpreted as a mass in thin patients, and feeling for a pulse will clarify any uncertainty. The supraclavicular and thyroid regions are palpated as well. Isolated supraclavicular adenopathy should raise suspicion for disease originating outside the head and neck region. The trachea is assessed with regard to the midline, and the larynx should elevate as the patient swallows. Palpable nodes should be evaluated for size, location, and fixation to skin or deeper structures.

The physical examination should also identify distant sites that may be used for reconstructive purposes. Ideal donor sites have healthy skin, adequate peripheral pulses, and should lack evidence of poor healing or chronic wounds. The Allen test is easily performed at the bedside if a radial forearm flap is anticipated. Scars from previous surgery should be noted because they may preclude the use of some donor sites. A pectoralis flap with a skin paddle is best avoided in patients who have previously undergone mastectomy, whereas axillary node dissection may render the latissimus flap unreliable. Previous abdominal procedures may prevent the use of a rectus flap.

NUTRITIONAL STATUS

Oral cancer patients commonly suffer from malnourishment related to pain, trismus, or dysfunction from their tumor. The high incidence of alcohol abuse in the oral cancer population further contributes to their nutritional compromise. Malnutrition has negative implications on immune function and wound healing, which may be exacerbated if postoperative radiation therapy is planned. Preoperative nutritional support in malnourished patients has been shown to improve complication rates and shorten hospital stays.[68] Surgical treatment or radiation therapy may further compromise the patient's ability to tolerate oral intake. Consideration should be given to placement of a gastrostomy tube in these patients, depending on the anticipated extent of surgery.

RADIOGRAPHIC ASSESSMENT

Pretreatment imaging is important for evaluation of the tumor's size and involvement of adjacent anatomic structures. Additional cervical staging and prognostic information is available with radiographic evaluation of regional and distant sites. Common imaging modalities include computed tomography (CT), magnetic resonance imaging (MRI), ultrasound (US), and positron emission tomography (PET). Each technique has its own set of indications and limitations that must be understood to optimize treatment planning and establish the prognosis. The two most common uses for radiographic studies are for staging the cervical lymphatics and evaluating the mandible for tumor invasion.

Radiologic criteria have been described for cervical nodal disease to characterize potentially positive nodes. Findings suggestive of nodal metastasis include enlarged size, rounder shape, and heterogeneity concerning for necrosis. Intranodal tumor necrosis is the most reliable criterion, but it is also a late sign. Therefore, nodal size and shape are the predictors commonly used in the assessment of palpably N0 necks.[69] Perhaps the most important role for neck imaging is to evaluate patients with no palpable nodes. Radiographic findings help determine whether elective neck treatment is necessary and to what extent.

Computed Tomography

CT is the imaging modality most commonly used for assessment of oral tumors.[70] Excellent bone detail, adequate soft tissue enhancement, and relatively low cost are advantages of CT for imaging the oral cavity. Debate exists among clinicians regarding the superiority of CT over MRI for the detection of cervical lymphadenopathy. A multi-institutional study of 211 patients found CT to perform only slightly better than MRI.[71] In practice, the modality used to image the primary tumor is also used to image the neck as an additional sequence. A disadvantage of CT is the artifact created by metallic dental restorations. This is particularly problematic when evaluating tumors at the level of the occlusal plane, such as the retromolar trigone or buccal mucosa. Additionally, irregular tooth sockets or periapical disease seen on CT may be confused with tumor invasion.[72]

Magnetic Resonance Imaging

Advantages of MRI include superior soft tissue detail and lack of ionizing radiation. However, MRI is more sensitive to motion artifact, is more expensive than CT, and can be difficult for patients who suffer from claustrophobia. Certain implants such as cardiac pacemakers and ferromagnetic aneurysm clips are absolute contraindications for MRI. For imaging of the cervical lymph nodes, the accuracy of MRI has been shown in multiple studies to be fairly equivalent to that of CT.[69] MRI is superior when there is concern for perineural invasion, skull base involvement, or intracranial spread.[73]

Positron Emission Tomography

Functional imaging with ^{18}F-fluorodeoxyglucose PET has been shown to be an effective tool in the diagnosis of head and neck cancer, although its role is still being defined. The integration of PET and CT technology is more accurate than either modality alone in the depiction of head and neck malignancies.[74] PET has shown promise in the evaluation of metastatic disease, tumor recurrence, and treatment response after chemotherapy or radiation therapy. Although some centers recommend that it be used routinely for staging advanced (T3 or T4) tumors, the high false-positive rate inherent with metabolic imaging is problematic. Even though studies have demonstrated the ability of PET to alter the staging of head and neck tumors,[75-77] it is still unclear whether this benefit outweighs the disadvantage of false-positive results in routine staging. The most widely accepted role for PET in patients with oral cancer is for the detection of recurrences.[78,79] Tissue beds are often scarred and irradiated and have postsurgical alterations in anatomy, which limits the utility of conventional imaging techniques and makes metabolic imaging more appealing. Although PET has shown improved sensitivity over conventional imaging techniques,[76,80,81] it is not accurate enough to preclude neck dissection in patients with no detectable cervical disease.[82-84] This limitation is due to the inadequate spatial resolution of PET, which results in an inability to detect micrometastases smaller than 5 mm in diameter.

Ultrasound

High-resolution diagnostic US is quick, non-invasive, and relatively inexpensive when compared with CT or MRI. Although US is used extensively for thyroid/parathyroid evaluation, it is of limited utility in the oral cavity. Orientation of the probe is restricted by the oral aperture. Bone does not transmit sound, which further decreases the utility of US. Evaluation of regional lymph nodes by US has been shown to be more accurate than palpation,[85-87] although this method has not been widely accepted. The greatest advantage of US involves the addition of fine-needle aspiration cytology, which greatly increases its efficacy and specificity.[88,89] Lymph nodes may be sampled immediately under ultrasound guidance.[90] Even though some authors report US to be superior to CT and MRI for the detection of cervical metastases,[91] others report no significant advantage.[92,93] Since US is highly technique-sensitive with a steep learning curve, this method has not gained wide acceptance.[94,95]

MANDIBULAR INVASION

The decision to resect the mandible deserves special consideration because of the functional sequelae and increased reconstructive complexity. Attention must be given to the appropriateness of marginal versus segmental resection when indicated. The inability to obtain reliable intraoperative frozen section analysis of bone places added emphasis on preoperative data. Although no single imaging technique accurately predicts invasion of tumor into the mandible, multiple modalities are available. Common techniques include CT, MRI, orthopantography, single-photon emission computed tomography (SPECT), conventional radionuclide scanning, and US.

CT is the most common method for assessment of mandibular invasion despite reports of variable efficacy. A prospective study by Close and colleagues examined 43 consecutive patients with CT preoperatively and compared the findings with the postoperative pathologic results.[96] The authors reported a sensitivity of 100% and a specificity of 97%. Similar findings were noted by Mukherji and co-workers using contrast-enhanced CT with 3-mm cuts.[97] However, other studies have produced less impressive results. Lane and associates analyzed preoperative CT data from 26 patients with retromolar trigone cancer.[98] They noted that CT was unable to identify bone invasion in 7 of 14 pathologically confirmed cases whereas it did detect bone invasion in 11 of 12 confirmed negative cases. The authors concluded that CT has limitations in the retromolar trigone region because of poor sensitivity (50%).

Cone beam computed tomography (CBCT) has experienced dramatic growth in recent years through the field of dental implantology. These machines are becoming increasingly available in dental offices and produce images of similar quality to conventional CT with lower cost and radiation exposure.[99,100] Only a handful of reports are available that address the utility of CBCT in identifying mandibular tumor invasion. In a 2007 report by Closmann and Schmidt, visualization of the extent of mandibular tumor involvement in three patients was better with CBCT than with MRI and Panorex.[101] Brockenbrough and colleagues reported on the use of CBCT in a series of 36 patients with oral cancer and suspicion of mandibular invasion.[102] The authors found a sensitivity of 95% and a specificity of 79%. Although no comparison was made with other imaging modalities, the authors concluded that CBCT was an accurate method for detecting mandibular invasion. At present, it is unclear whether CBCT technology will eventually play a greater role in assessing for bone invasion, especially given its inability to produce a contrast-enhanced soft tissue study. The majority of patients already require soft tissue imaging of the neck with CT or MRI for lymphatic staging, and the mandible is usually imaged in the same setting. For a separate CBCT to be worthwhile and routine, significant improvement in the detection of mandibular invasion will need to be demonstrated.

MRI offers the advantage of visualizing the marrow space of the mandible. Ator and co-workers reviewed data from 11 oral cancer patients and compared MRI with various conventional imaging methods.[103] They concluded that MRI was superior to CT in assessing mandibular invasion. A study from the Netherlands compared the accuracy of CT, MRI, and orthopantography in 29 patients. The authors noted that MRI demonstrated the highest sensitivity (94%) but had more false-positive results and often overestimated the extent of tumor invasion.[104] Brown and associates also noted the tendency for MRI to overestimate tumor invasion into the mandible.[105] The authors compared multiple modalities for their ability to predict mandibular invasion and found that MRI and bone scans overestimated the degree of invasion whereas CT and orthopantography underestimated the extent. A prospective study from Italy compared the findings on preoperative MRI with the histologic findings in surgical specimens from 43 patients who underwent marginal or segmental mandibulectomy.[106] For mandibular invasion, they found that the sensitivity of MRI was 93% with a specificity of 93% and a negative predictive value of 96%.

Nuclear imaging studies have demonstrated an impressive ability to detect mandibular invasion. SPECT has been shown in multiple studies to have high sensitivity, although its specificity is variable. Yamamoto and colleagues compared SPECT with CT and found the sensitivity and specificity of SPECT to be 100% and 88%, respectively, whereas that for CT was 45% and 95%.[107] Imola and co-workers compared SPECT with Panorex and CT in a prospective study of 38 patients.[108] The sensitivity of SPECT (95%) was significantly higher than that of CT (55%) and Panorex (50%), although its specificity was lower. Sensitivity for mandibular invasion has been shown to approach 100% in other studies as well.[109,110] A 2006 study from the Netherlands found a 100% sensitivity for SPECT in detecting mandibular invasion as determined by final histology.[111] The authors concluded that negative SPECT findings rule out mandibular invasion.

Panoramic and plain film radiography is less useful in the assessment of bone invasion. The lack of three-dimensional visualization is an inherent drawback when compared with other modalities such as CT and MRI. Early cortical erosion is easily missed on plain films. Panorex is most useful in planning osteotomies when marginal or segmental resection is indicated.

Of interest is the number of authors who place higher value on clinical examination than on radiographic assessment. Shaha reported that orthopantography and CT were not very useful in determining the need for marginal versus segmental mandibulectomy and that clinical examination was more reliable.[112] In a later report by the same author in which 66 patients with floor of the mouth cancer were reviewed, the decision to perform marginal mandibulectomy was based primarily on clinical judgment.[113] A review of imaging modalities by van den Brekel and colleagues concluded that no technique was sufficiently accurate in assessing mandibular invasion and that clinical examination should be the primary modality.[104] Werning and associates reviewed 222 patients who underwent marginal mandibulectomy over a 30-year period.[114] They found clinical examination to be more sensitive than radiologic modalities, although radiographic assessment had higher specificity. The authors concluded that combining clinical and radiographic assessment is more accurate than the use of either modality alone.

STAGING

Multiple staging systems are recognized internationally, but no single system is universally used.[115] Oral cavity tumors in the United States and much of Europe are staged with the TNM system, which has been formally adopted by the Union Internationale Contre le Cancre (UICC) and the AJCC. The purpose of staging is to group patients into statistical classifications that provide useful information on treatment and prognosis. Additionally, this standardized format facilitates research, assessment of outcomes, and communication among clinicians by establishing uniform reporting parameters. As a general rule, more advanced stage implies a worse prognosis. For oral cavity cancer, the TNM system used by the UICC and AJCC is only for squamous cell carcinoma and minor salivary gland cancers.[116]

Initial staging is performed by using all available clinical and radiographic data (cTNM). Final staging incorporates histopathologic data if surgery is performed (pTNM). The TNM system stages cancer purely on the anatomic extent of disease and does not account for the many biologic, molecular, or host characteristics that are known to influence prognosis.[117] The AJCC and UICC review new data every 6 to 8 years to revise the TNM criteria based on the most recent data. AJCC definitions for staging are presented in Box 52-1.

T STAGE

The primary tumor is evaluated for size and extent to determine the T stage. Size criteria generally place a primary tumor in the T1 to T3 categories, whereas invasion into bone or deeper structures will upstage a tumor to T4 regardless of size. It should be noted that the T stage criteria for oral cavity tumors are different from the T stage criteria described for tumors of the pharynx, larynx, paranasal sinuses, and thyroid gland. Although depth of invasion has been shown to be an important prognostic factor for some oral cavity subsites,[118-122] it is not included in the TNM system. An additional weakness is the lack of recognition of other prognostic indicators such as perineural invasion, vascular and lymphatic invasion, morphology (exophytic versus endophytic), and the nature of the tumor-host interface (infiltrative versus pushing).[116]

N STAGE

The cervical lymph nodes are assessed by palpation and imaging to document evidence of regional spread. Nodal presence, size, and location are recorded. N staging for oral cavity tumors is the same as for other head and neck sites except for the nasopharynx and thyroid.[123] Although size is incorporated into the N staging system,

---

| BOX 52-1 | AJCC Staging Definitions for Lip and Oral Cavity Cancer |

Primary Tumor (T)
- TX: Primary tumor cannot be assessed
- T0: No evidence of primary tumor
- Tis: Carcinoma in situ
- T1: Tumor no larger than 2 cm in greatest dimension
- T2: Tumor larger than 2 cm but no larger than 4 cm in greatest dimension
- T3: Tumor larger than 4 cm in greatest dimension
- T4: (lip) Tumor invades through cortical bone, inferior alveolar nerve, floor of mouth, or skin of face, i.e., chin or nose
- T4a: (oral cavity) Tumor invades adjacent structures (e.g., through cortical bone, into deep [extrinsic] muscle of tongue [genioglossus, hyoglossus, palatoglossus, and styloglossus], maxillary sinus, and skin of face)
- T4b: Tumor invades masticator space, pterygoid plates, or skull base and/or encases internal carotid artery

[Note: Superficial erosion alone of bone/tooth socket by gingival primary is not sufficient to classify a tumor as T4.]

Regional Lymph Nodes (N)
- NX: Regional lymph nodes cannot be assessed
- N0: No regional lymph node metastasis
- N1: Metastasis in a single ipsilateral lymph node, no larger than 3 cm in greatest dimension
- N2: Metastasis in a single ipsilateral lymph node, larger than 3 cm but no larger than 6 cm in greatest dimension; or in multiple ipsilateral lymph nodes, no larger than 6 cm in greatest dimension; or in bilateral or contralateral lymph nodes, no larger than 6 cm in greatest dimension
- N2a: Metastasis in a single ipsilateral lymph node larger than 3 cm but no larger than 6 cm in dimension
- N2b: Metastasis in multiple ipsilateral lymph nodes, no larger than 6 cm in greatest dimension
- N2c: Metastasis in bilateral or contralateral lymph nodes, no larger than 6 cm in greatest dimension
- N3: Metastasis in a lymph node larger than 6 cm in greatest dimension

During clinical evaluation, the actual size of the nodal mass should be measured and allowance made for intervening soft tissues. Most masses larger than 3 cm in diameter are not single nodes but are confluent nodes or tumors in soft tissues of the neck. The three stages of clinically positive nodes are N1, N2, and N3. Use of subgroups a, b, and c is not required but is recommended. Midline nodes are considered homolateral nodes.

Distant Metastasis (M)
- MX: Distant metastasis cannot be assessed
- M0: No distant metastasis
- M1: Distant metastasis

Used with the permission of the American Joint Committee on Cancer (AJCC), Chicago, Illinois. The original source for this material is *AJCC cancer staging manual*, ed 7, New York, 2010, Springer-Verlag, www.springer.com.

---

the classification does not include extracapsular spread or level of lymph node involvement, which are known negative prognostic factors.[124-126]

M STAGE

Metastatic disease refers to spread beyond the regional lymph node basin of the neck. M staging simply documents the presence or absence of metastatic disease. The lungs, bone, and liver are the

BOX 52-2   AJCC Stage Grouping

Stage 0
- Tis, N0, M0

Stage I
- T1, N0, M0
- Stage II
- T2, N0, M0

Stage III
- T3, N0, M0
- T1, N1, M0
- T2, N1, M0
- T3, N1, M0

Stage IVA
- T4a, N0, M0
- T4a, N1, M0
- T1, N2, M0
- T2, N2, M0
- T3, N2, M0
- T4a, N2, M0

Stage IVB
- Any T, N3, M0
- T4b, any N, M0

Stage IVC
- Any T, any N, M1

Used with the permission of the American Joint Committee on Cancer (AJCC), Chicago, Illinois. The original source for this material is *AJCC cancer staging manual*, ed 7, New York, 2010, Springer-Verlag, www.springer.com.

most common sites of distant metastasis from the oral cavity.[127,128] At present, metastatic spread of oral cancer is incurable. M staging criteria are the same for all head and neck sites.

AMERICAN JOINT COMMITTEE ON CANCER STAGE GROUPINGS

Since T and N staging criteria are site specific, the AJCC has formulated a uniform grouping to incorporate all head and neck sites except for tumors arising from the nasopharynx and

thyroid.[129] The classification follows a logical progression in that higher stage results in decreased survival. With stage grouping, statistical analysis is facilitated between head and neck sites with different TNM criteria. AJCC stage groupings are shown in Box 52-2.

PEARLS AND PITFALLS

- Oral cavity cancer affects more than a quarter of a million patients globally each year. Approximately 90% of these tumors are squamous cell carcinoma.
- Although multiple associations exist, tobacco and alcohol are the strongest risk factors for the development of oral cancer.
- Pretreatment clinical examination must include assessment of the size, location, and extent of the primary tumor, as well as palpation of the neck.
- Radiographic examination usually includes cross-sectional imaging of the neck and a chest x-ray or chest CT.
- The role of PET technology in the initial staging of oral cancer is not completely defined and is an area of ongoing research.
- Suspicion of mandibular invasion should be investigated thoroughly because of the increased morbidity and complexity involved in the reconstruction of segmental defects.
- Pretreatment staging allows the patient and clinician to understand the prognosis and formulate an optimal treatment plan.
- The AJCC/UICC TNM staging system is adequate for classifying the anatomic extent of oral cancers, but not all prognostic factors are included in this classification system.
- As our knowledge of the etiology, pretreatment evaluation, and staging of oral cancer advances, it is expected that patients will experience improvements in therapeutic outcomes.

REFERENCES

1. Parkin D: Global cancer statistics in the year 2000, *Lancet Oncol* 2:533-543, 2001.
2. Parkin DM, Bray F, Ferlay J, et al: Global cancer statistics, 2002. *CA Cancer J Clin* 55:74-108, 2005.
3. Horner MJ, Ries LAG, Krapcho M, et al, editors: SEER Cancer Statistics Review, 1975-2006, National Cancer Institute. Bethesda, MD, http://seer.cancer.gov/csr/1975_2006/, based on November 2008 SEER data submission, posted to the SEER web site, 2009.
4. McDowell J: An overview of epidemiology and common risk factors for oral squamous cell carcinoma, *Otolaryngol Clin North Am* 39:277-294, 2006.
5. Swango PA: Cancers of the oral cavity and pharynx in the United States: an epidemiologic overview, *J Public Health Dent* 56:309-318, 1996.
6. Chen JK, Eisenberg E, Krutchkoff DJ, et al: Changing trends in oral cancer in the United States, 1935 to 1985: a Connecticut study, *J Oral Maxillofac Surg* 49:1152-1158, 1991.
7. Macfarlane GJ, Boyle P, Scully C: Oral cancer in Scotland: changing incidence and mortality, *Br Med J (Clin Res Educ)* 305:1121-1123, 1992.
8. Shemen LJ, Klotz J, Schottenfeld D, et al: Increase of tongue cancer in young men, *JAMA* 252:1857-1857, 1984.
9. Schantz S, Yu G-P: Head and neck cancer incidence trends in young Americans, 1973-1997, with a special analysis for tongue cancer, *Arch Otolaryngol Head Neck Surg* 128:268-274, 2002.
10. Myers JN, Elkins T, Roberts D, et al: Squamous cell carcinoma of the tongue in young adults: increasing incidence and factors that predict treatment outcomes, *Otolaryngol Head Neck Surg* 122:44-51, 2000.
11. Shiboski C, Schmidt B, Jordan RCK: Tongue and tonsil carcinoma: increasing trends in the U.S. population ages 20-44 years, *Cancer* 103:1843-1849, 2005.
12. Sarkaria JN, Harari PM: Oral tongue cancer in young adults less than 40 years of age: rationale for aggressive therapy, *Head Neck* 16:107-111, 1994.
13. Jones JB, Lampe HB, Cheung HW: Carcinoma of the tongue in young patients, *J Otolaryngol* 18:105-108, 1989.
14. Prince S, Bailey BM: Squamous carcinoma of the tongue: review, *Br J Oral Maxillofac Surg* 37:164-174, 1999.
15. Garavello W, Spreafico R, Gaini R: Oral tongue cancer in young patients: a matched analysis, *Oral Oncol* 43:894-897, 2007.
16. Goldenberg D, Brooksby C, Hollenbeak C: Age as a determinant of outcomes for patients with oral cancer, *Oral Oncol* 45:e57-e61, 2009.
17. Pitman KT, Johnson JT, Wagner RL, et al: Cancer of the tongue in patients less than forty, *Head Neck* 22:297-302, 2000.
18. Atula S, Grénman R, Laippala P, et al: Cancer of the tongue in patients younger than 40 years, a distinct entity? *Arch Otolaryngol Head Neck Surg* 122:1313-1319, 1996.
19. Manuel S, Raghavan SK, Pandey M, et al: Survival in patients under 45 years with squamous cell carcinoma of the oral tongue, *Int J Oral Maxillofac Surg* 32:167-173, 2003.
20. McGregor GI, Davis N, Robins RE: Squamous cell carcinoma of the tongue and lower oral cavity in patients under 40 years of age, *Am J Surg* 146:88-92, 1983.
21. Davidson B: Epidemiology and etiology. In Shah J, editor: *Cancer of the head and neck. American Cancer Society atlas of clinical oncology.* Hamilton, Ontario, 2001, BC Decker, pp 1-18.
22. Callery CD, Spiro RH, Strong EW: Changing trends in the management of squamous carcinoma of the tongue, *Am J Surg* 148:449-454, 1984.
23. Rosenquist K: Risk factors in oral and oropharyngeal squamous cell carcinoma: a population-based case-control study in

southern Sweden, *Swed Dent J Suppl* 179:1-66, 2005.

24. Muscat JE, Richie JP Jr, Thompson S, et al: Gender differences in smoking and risk for oral cancer, *Cancer Res* 56:5192-5197, 1996.

25. Suba Z: Gender-related hormonal risk factors for oral cancer, *Pathol Oncol Res* 13:195-202, 2007.

26. Begg CB, Zhang ZF, Sun M, et al: Methodology for evaluating the incidence of second primary cancers with application to smoking-related cancers from the Surveillance, Epidemiology, and End Results (SEER) program, *Am J Epidemiol* 142:653-665, 1995.

27. Garavello W, Spreafico R, Somigliana E, et al: Prognostic influence of gender in patients with oral tongue cancer, *Otolaryngol Head Neck Surg* 138:768-771, 2008.

28. Arduino PG, Carrozzo M, Chiecchio A, et al: Clinical and histopathologic independent prognostic factors in oral squamous cell carcinoma: a retrospective study of 334 cases, *J Oral Maxillofac Surg* 66:1570-1579, 2008.

29. Pimenta Amaral TM, Da Silva Freire AR, Carvalho AL, et al: Predictive factors of occult metastasis and prognosis of clinical stages I and II squamous cell carcinoma of the tongue and floor of the mouth, *Oral Oncol* 40:780-786, 2004.

30. Choi KK, Kim MJ, Yun PY, et al: Independent prognostic factors of 861 cases of oral squamous cell carcinoma in Korean adults, *Oral Oncol* 42:208-217, 2006.

31. Langdon JD, Rapidis AD: Oral cancer and sex. Why do females do better? *J Maxillofac Surg* 7:177-181, 1979.

32. Franco EL, Dib LL, Pinto DS, et al: Race and gender influences on the survival of patients with mouth cancer, *J Clin Epidemiol* 46:37-46, 1993.

33. Funk GF, Karnell LH, Robinson RA, et al: Presentation, treatment, and outcome of oral cavity cancer: a National Cancer Data Base report, *Head Neck* 24:165-180, 2002.

34. Morse D, Kerr AR: Disparities in oral and pharyngeal cancer incidence, mortality and survival among black and white Americans, *J Am Dent Assoc* 137:203-212, 2006.

35. Parker SL, Davis KJ, Wingo PA, et al: Cancer statistics by race and ethnicity, *CA Cancer J Clin* 48:31-48, 1998.

36. Day GL, Blot WJ, Austin DF, et al: Racial differences in risk of oral and pharyngeal cancer: alcohol, tobacco, and other determinants, *J Natl Cancer Inst* 85:465-473, 1993.

37. Macfarlane GJ, Zheng T, Marshall JR, et al: Alcohol, tobacco, diet and the risk of oral cancer: a pooled analysis of three case-control studies, *Eur J Cancer Part B Oral Oncol* 31:181-187, 1995.

38. Tobacco and oral diseases—report of EU Working Group, 1999, *J Irish Dent Assoc* 46:12-19, 22, 2000.

39. Moreno-López LA, Esparza-Gómez GC, González-Navarro A, et al: Risk of oral cancer associated with tobacco smoking, alcohol consumption and oral hygiene: a case-control study in Madrid, Spain, *Oral Oncol* 36:170-174, 2000.

40. Winn DM, Blot WJ, Shy CM, et al: Snuff dipping and oral cancer among women in the southern United States, *N Engl J Med* 304:745-749, 1981.

41. Bouquot JE, Meckstroth RL: Oral cancer in a tobacco-chewing US population—no apparent increased incidence or mortality, *Oral Surg Oral Med Oral Pathol Oral Radiol Endod* 86:697-706, 1998.

42. Rodu B: Switching to smokeless tobacco as a smoking cessation method: evidence from the 2000 National Health Interview Survey, *Harm Reduct J* 5:18, 2008.

43. Lee PN, Hamling J: Systematic review of the relation between smokeless tobacco and cancer in Europe and North America, *BMC Cancer* 29:36, 2009.

44. Lee PN, Hamling J: The relation between smokeless tobacco and cancer in northern Europe and North America. A commentary on differences between the conclusions reached by two recent reviews, *BMC Cancer* 29:256, 2009.

45. Timberlake D, Zell J: Review of epidemiologic data on the debate over smokeless tobacco's role in harm reduction, *BMC Med* 7:61, 2009.

46. http://www.cancer.gov/cancertopics/factsheet/Tobacco/smokeless. Accessed March 15, 2010.

47. Jacob BJ, Straif K, Thomas G, et al: Betel quid without tobacco as a risk factor for oral precancers, *Oral Oncol* 40:697-704, 2004.

48. Ko YC, Huang YL, Lee CH, et al: Betel quid chewing, cigarette smoking and alcohol consumption related to oral cancer in Taiwan, *J Oral Pathol Med* 24:450-453, 1995.

49. Rothman K, Keller A: The effect of joint exposure to alcohol and tobacco on risk of cancer of the mouth and pharynx, *J Chronic Dis* 25:711-716, 1972.

50. Lewin F, Norell SE, Johansson H, et al: Smoking tobacco, oral snuff, and alcohol in the etiology of squamous cell carcinoma of the head and neck: a population-based case-referent study in Sweden, *Cancer* 82:1367-1375, 1998.

51. Brugere J, Guenel P, Leclerc A, et al: Differential effects of tobacco and alcohol in cancer of the larynx, pharynx, and mouth, *Cancer* 57:391-395, 1986.

52. Slots J: Oral viral infections of adults, *Periodontology* 49:60-86, 2000.

53. Sugiyama M, Bhawal UK, Kawamura M, et al: Human papillomavirus-16 in oral squamous cell carcinoma: clinical correlates and 5-year survival, *Br J Oral Maxillofac Surg* 45:116-122, 2007.

54. Miller CS, Johnstone BM: Human papillomavirus as a risk factor for oral squamous cell carcinoma: a meta-analysis, 1982-1997, *Oral Surg Oral Med Oral Pathol Oral Radiol Endod* 91:622-635, 2001.

55. Miller CS, White DK: Human papillomavirus expression in oral mucosa, premalignant conditions, and squamous cell carcinoma: a retrospective review of the literature, *Oral Surg Oral Med Oral Pathol Oral Radiol Endod* 82:57-68, 1996.

56. Boy S, Van Rensburg EJ, Engelbrecht S, et al: HPV detection in primary intra-oral squamous cell carcinomas—commensal, aetiological agent or contamination? *J Oral Pathol Med* 35:86-90, 2006.

57. Kansky AA, Seme K, Maver PJ, et al: Human papillomaviruses (HPV) in tissue specimens of oral squamous cell papillomas and normal oral mucosa, *Anticancer Res* 26(4B):3197-3201, 2006.

58. Termine N, Panzarella V, Falaschini S, et al: HPV in oral squamous cell carcinoma vs head and neck squamous cell carcinoma biopsies: a meta-analysis (1988-2007), *Ann Oncol* 19:1681-1690, 2008.

59. Larsson LG, Sandström A, Westling P: Relationship of Plummer-Vinson disease to cancer of the upper alimentary tract in Sweden, *Cancer Res* 35:3308-3316, 1975.

60. Mirvish SS: Effects of vitamins C and E on N-nitroso compound formation, carcinogenesis, and cancer, *Cancer* 58(8 Suppl):1842-1850, 1986.

61. Negri E, Franceschi S, Bosetti C, et al: Selected micronutrients and oral and pharyngeal cancer, *Int J Cancer* 86:122-127, 2000.

62. Levi F, Pasche C, La Vecchia C, et al: Food groups and risk of oral and pharyngeal cancer, *Int J Cancer* 77:705-709, 1998.

63. Talamini R, Vaccarella S, Barbone F, et al: Oral hygiene, dentition, sexual habits and risk of oral cancer, *Br J Cancer* 83:1238-1242, 2000.

64. Zheng TZ, Boyle P, Hu HF, et al: Dentition, oral hygiene, and risk of oral cancer: a case-control study in Beijing, People's Republic of China, *Cancer Causes Control* 1:235-241, 1990.

65. Gorsky M, Silverman S: Denture wearing and oral cancer, *J Prosthet Dent* 52:164-166, 1984.

66. De Boer MF, McCormick LK, Pruyn JF, et al: Physical and psychosocial correlates of head and neck cancer: a review of the literature, *Otolaryngol Head Neck Surg* 120:427-436, 1999.

67. Stell PM: Prognosis in laryngeal carcinoma: host factors, *Clin Otolaryngol Allied Sci* 15:111-119, 1990.

68. Flynn MB, Leightty FF: Preoperative outpatient nutritional support of patients with squamous cancer of the upper aerodigestive tract, *Am J Surg* 154:359-362, 1987.

69. Castelijns J, van den Brekel MWM, Imaging of lymphadenopathy in the neck, *Eur Radiol* 12:727-738, 2002.

70. Dillon WP, Harnsberger HR: The impact of radiologic imaging on staging of cancer of the head and neck, *Semin Oncol* 18:64-79, 1991.

71. Curtin HD, Ishwaran H, Mancuso AA, et al: Comparison of CT and MR imaging in staging of neck metastases, *Radiology* 207:123-130, 1998.

72. Genden EM, Rinaldo A, Jacobson A, et al: Management of mandibular invasion: when is a marginal mandibulectomy appropriate? *Oral Oncol* 41:776-782, 2005.

73. Ling FTK, Kountakis S: Advances in imaging of the paranasal sinuses, *Curr Allergy Asthma Rep* 6:502-507, 2006.

74. Branstetter BF 4th, Blodgett TM, Zimmer LA, et al: Head and neck malignancy: is PET/CT more accurate than PET or CT alone? *Radiology* 235:580-586, 2005.

75. Connell CA, Corry J, Milner AD, et al: Clinical impact of, and prognostic stratification by, F-18 FDG PET/CT in head and neck mucosal squamous cell carcinoma, *Head Neck* 29:986-995, 2007.

76. Ha PK, Hdeib A, Goldenberg D, et al: The role of positron emission tomography and computed tomography fusion in the management of early-stage and advanced-stage primary head and neck squamous cell carcinoma, *Arch Otolaryngol Head Neck Surg* 132:12-16, 2006.

77. Goerres GW, Schmid DT, Grätz KW, et al: Impact of whole body positron emission tomography on initial staging and therapy in patients with squamous cell carcinoma of the oral cavity, *Oral Oncol* 39:547-551, 2003.

78. Kao J, Vu HL, Genden EM, et al: The diagnostic and prognostic utility of positron emission tomography/computed tomography–based follow-up after radiotherapy for head and neck cancer, *Cancer* 115:4586-4594, 2009.

79. Schechter NR, Gillenwater AM, Byers RM, et al: Can positron emission tomography improve the quality of care for head-and-neck cancer patients? *Int J Radiat Oncol Biol Phys* 51:4-9, 2001.

80. Adams S, Baum RP, Stuckensen T, et al: Prospective comparison of ^{18}F-FDG PET with conventional imaging modalities (CT, MRI, US) in lymph node staging of head and neck cancer, *Eur J Nucl Med* 25:1255-1260, 1998.

81. Koshy M, Paulino AC, Howell R, et al: F-18 FDG PET-CT fusion in radiotherapy treatment planning for head and neck cancer, *Head Neck* 27:494-502, 2005.

82. Krabbe CA, Dijkstra PU, Pruim J, et al: FDG PET in oral and oropharyngeal cancer. Value for confirmation of N0 neck and detection of occult metastases, *Oral Oncol* 44:31-36, 2008.

83. Stoeckli SJ, Steinert H, Pfaltz M, et al: Is there a role for positron emission tomography with ^{18}F-fluorodeoxyglucose in the initial staging of nodal negative oral and oropharyngeal squamous cell carcinoma, *Head Neck* 24:345-349, 2002.

84. Pentenero M, Cistaro A, Brusa M, et al: Accuracy of ^{18}F-FDG-PET/CT for staging of oral squamous cell carcinoma, *Head Neck* 30:1488-1496, 2008.

85. Ishii J, Amagasa T, Tachibana T, et al: US and CT evaluation of cervical lymph node metastasis from oral cancer, *J Craniomaxillofac Surg* 19:123-127, 1991.

86. Prayer L, Winkelbauer H, Gritzmann N, et al: Sonography versus palpation in the detection of regional lymph-node metastases in patients with malignant melanoma, *Eur J Cancer* 26:827-830, 1990.

87. Baatenburg de Jong RJ, Rongen RJ, De Jong PC, et al: Screening for lymph nodes in the neck with ultrasound, *Clin Otolaryngol Allied Sci* 13:5-9, 1988.

88. Rottey S, Petrovic M, Bauters W, et al: Evaluation of metastatic lymph nodes in head and neck cancer: a comparative study between palpation, ultrasonography, ultrasound-guided fine needle aspiration cytology and computed tomography, *Acta Clin Belg* 61:236-241, 2006.

89. Baatenburg de Jong RJ, Rongen RJ, Laméris JS, et al: Metastatic neck disease. Palpation vs ultrasound examination, *Arch Otolaryngol Head Neck Surg* 115:689-690, 1989.

90. Atula TS, Grénman R, Varpula MJ, et al: Palpation, ultrasound, and ultrasound-guided fine-needle aspiration cytology in the assessment of cervical lymph node status in head and neck cancer patients, *Head Neck* 18:545-551, 1996.

91. Vassallo P, Edel G, Roos N, et al: In-vitro high-resolution ultrasonography of benign and malignant lymph nodes. A sonographic-pathologic correlation, *Invest Radiol* 28:698-705, 1993.

92. van den Brekel MW, Castelijns JA, Stel HV, et al: Modern imaging techniques and ultrasound-guided aspiration cytology for the assessment of neck node metastases: a prospective comparative study, *Eur Arch Otorhinolaryngol* 250:11-17, 1993.

93. Giancarlo T, Palmieri A, Giacomarra V, et al: Pre-operative evaluation of cervical adenopathies in tumours of the upper aerodigestive tract, *Anticancer Res* 18(4B):2805-2809, 1998.

94. Richards P, Peacock T: The role of ultrasound in the detection of cervical lymph node metastases in clinically N0 squamous cell carcinoma of the head and neck, *Cancer Imaging* 19:167-178, 2007.

95. Ng SH, Ko SF, Toh CH, et al: Imaging of neck metastases, *Chang Gung Med J* 29:119-129, 2006.

96. Close LG, Merkel M, Burns DK, et al: Computed tomography in the assessment of mandibular invasion by intraoral carcinoma, *Ann Otol Rhinol Laryngol* 95:383-388, 1986.

97. Mukherji SK, Isaacs DL, Creager A, et al: CT detection of mandibular invasion by squamous cell carcinoma of the oral cavity, *AJR Am J Roentgenol* 177:237-243, 2001.

98. Lane AP, Buckmire RA, Mukherji SK, et al: Use of computed tomography in the assessment of mandibular invasion in carcinoma of the retromolar trigone, *Otolaryngol Head Neck Surg* 122:673-677, 2000.

99. Roberts JA, Drage NA, Davies J, et al: Effective dose from cone beam CT examinations in dentistry, *Br J Radiol* 82:35-40, 2009.

100. Winter AA, Pollack AS, Frommer HH, et al: Cone beam volumetric tomography vs. medical CT scanners, *N Y State Dent J* 71:28-33, 2005.

101. Closmann J, Schmidt B: The use of cone beam computed tomography as an aid in evaluating and treatment planning for mandibular cancer, *J Oral Maxillofac Surg* 65:766-771, 2007.

102. Brockenbrough J, Petruzzelli G, Lomasney L: DentaScan as an accurate method of predicting mandibular invasion in patients with squamous cell carcinoma of the oral cavity, *Arch Otolaryngol Head Neck Surg* 129:113-117, 2003.

103. Ator GA, Abermayer E, Lufkin RB, et al: Evaluation of mandibular tumor invasion with magnetic resonance imaging, *Arch Otolaryngol Head Neck Surg* 116:454-459, 1990.

104. van den Brekel MW, Runne RW, Smeele LE, et al: Assessment of tumour invasion into the mandible: the value of different imaging techniques, *Eur Radiol* 8:1552-1557, 1998.

105. Brown JS, Griffith JF, Phelps PD, et al: A comparison of different imaging modalities and direct inspection after periosteal stripping in predicting the invasion of the mandible by oral squamous cell carcinoma, *Br J Oral Maxillofac Surg* 32:347-359, 1994.

106. Bolzoni A, Cappiello J, Piazza C, et al: Diagnostic accuracy of magnetic resonance imaging in the assessment of mandibular involvement in oral-oropharyngeal squamous cell carcinoma: a prospective study, *Arch Otolaryngol Head Neck Surg* 130:837-843, 2004.

107. Yamamoto Y, Nishiyama Y, Satoh K, et al: Dual-isotope SPECT using (99m)Tc-hydroxymethylene diphosphonate and (201)Tl-chloride to assess mandibular invasion by intraoral squamous cell carcinoma, *J Nucl Med* 43:1464-1468, 2002.

108. Imola MJ, Gapany M, Grund F, et al: Technetium 99m single positron emission computed tomography scanning for assessing mandible invasion in oral cavity cancer, *Laryngoscope* 111:373-381, 2001.

109. Zieron JO, Lauer I, Remmert S, et al: Single photon emission tomography: scintigraphy in the assessment of mandibular invasion by head and neck cancer, *Head Neck* 23:979-984, 2001.

110. Suzuki A, Togawa T, Kuyama J, et al: Evaluation of mandibular invasion by head and neck cancers using ^{99m}Tc-methylene diphosphonate or ^{99m}Tc-hydroxymethylene diphosphonate and ^{201}Tl chloride dual isotope single photon emission computed tomography, *Ann Nucl Med* 18:399-408, 2004.

111. Van Cann EM, Oyen WJ, Koole R, et al: Bone SPECT reduces the number of unnecessary mandibular resections in patients with squamous cell carcinoma, *Oral Oncol* 42:409-414, 2006.

112. Shaha AR: Preoperative evaluation of the mandible in patients with carcinoma of the floor of mouth, *Head Neck* 13:398-402, 1991.

113. Shaha AR: Marginal mandibulectomy for carcinoma of the floor of the mouth, *J Surg Oncol* 49:116-119, 1992.

114. Werning JW, Byers RM, Novas MA, et al: Preoperative assessment for and outcomes of mandibular conservation surgery, *Head Neck* 23:1024-1030, 2001.

115. Lydiatt WM, Shah JP, Hoffman HT: AJCC stage groupings for head and neck cancer: should we look at alternatives? A report of the Head and Neck Sites Task Force, *Head Neck* 23:607-612, 2001.

116. Patel S, Shah J: TNM staging of cancers of the head and neck: striving for uniformity among diversity, *CA Cancer J Clin* 55:242-258, 2005.

117. Manikantan K, Sayed SI, Syrigos KN, et al: Challenges for the future modifications of the TNM staging system for head and neck cancer: case for a new computational model? *Cancer Treat Rev* 35:639-644, 2009.

118. Fukano H, Matsuura H, Hasegawa Y, et al: Depth of invasion as a predictive factor for cervical lymph node metastasis in tongue carcinoma, *Head Neck* 19:205-210, 1997.

119. Warburton G, Nikitakis NG, Roberson P, et al: Histopathological and lymphangiogenic parameters in relation to lymph node metastasis in early stage oral squamous cell carcinoma, *J Oral Maxillofac Surg* 65:475-484, 2007.

120. Sparano A, Weinstein G, Chalian A, et al: Multivariate predictors of occult neck metastasis in early oral tongue cancer, *Otolaryngol Head Neck Surg* 131:472-476, 2004.

121. Keski-Säntti H, Atula T, Tikka J, et al: Predictive value of histopathologic parameters in early squamous cell carcinoma of oral tongue, *Oral Oncol* 43:1007-1013, 2007.

122. O-charoenrat P, Pillai G, Patel S, et al: Tumour thickness predicts cervical nodal metastases and survival in early oral tongue cancer, *Oral Oncol* 39:386-390, 2003.

123. van der Schroeff M, Baatenburg de Jong RJ: Staging and prognosis in head and neck cancer, *Oral Oncol* 45:356-360, 2009.

124. Stel PM, Morton RP, Singh SD: Cervical lymph node metastases: the significance of the level of the lymph node, *Clin l Oncol* 9:101-107, 1983.

125. Patel RS, Clark JR, Gao K, et al: Effectiveness of selective neck dissection in the treatment of the clinically positive neck, *Head Neck* 30:1231-1236, 2008.

126. Spiro RH, Alfonso AE, Farr HW, et al: Cervical node metastasis from epidermoid carcinoma of the oral cavity and oropharynx. A critical assessment of current staging, *Am J Surg* 128:562-567, 1974.

127. Younes RN, Gross JL, Silva JF, et al: Surgical treatment of lung metastases of head and neck tumors, *Am J Surg* 174:499-502, 1997.

128. Kowalski LP, Carvalho AL, Martins Priante AV, et al: Predictive factors for distant metastasis from oral and oropharyngeal squamous cell carcinoma, *Oral Oncol* 41:534-541, 2005.

129. American Joint Committee on Cancer: *AJCC cancer staging manual*, ed 6. New York, 2002, Springer-Verlag.

Chapter **53**

Oral Squamous Cell Carcinoma: Treatment

David L. Hirsch, Michael J. Spink

Malignant disease can affect the oral cavity, with the most common entity being squamous cell carcinoma (SCC). Immediate intervention is necessary for an acceptable prognosis. Early detection is the most advantageous factor in decreasing disease morbidity and mortality. The combined 5-year survival rate for early-stage tumors is between 60% and 80%, but patients initially seen with late-stage disease have less than a 50% survival rate at 5 years. Innovations in imaging and chemotherapy may alter treatment planning in certain cases, but biopsy of suspicious lesions and a thorough neck examination have remained the current diagnostic modality for nearly a hundred years of attempted progressive treatment.[1]

ETIOPATHOGENESIS/CAUSATIVE FACTORS

Etiologic risk factors for oral squamous cell carcinoma (OSCC) are usually dependent on patients' ethnicity and co-morbid conditions. The wide-ranging incidence of OSCC and cultural diversity throughout the world validate this fact, and the survival disparity in U.S. African Americans is exemplary. Diet, lifestyle, and available intoxicating luxuries also account for these differences.[2]

SUBSTANCE ABUSE

Long-term abuse of tobacco is the most common etiologic factor for OSCC. Alcohol, oral hygiene (specifically, polymicrobial supragingival plaque[3]), and nutritional deficits[4] are statistical complementary factors along with tobacco. The molecular mechanism for the initiation of cancer is believed to be a DNA insult from nitrosamine compounds and inhibition of repair from alcohol use. These factors account for nearly 75% of cases of OSCC worldwide. Individuals with greater than a 30 pack per year history of tobacco abuse have a four-fold greater propensity for the development of OSCC. Only smokers who have quit for more than 16 years have the same risk as non-smokers. Smokers who continue to smoke have a 40% chance for the development of a second primary. De novo detection of cancer in these patients could optimize survival and is being investigated with molecular markers. Presently, 23% of teens smoke in the United States.

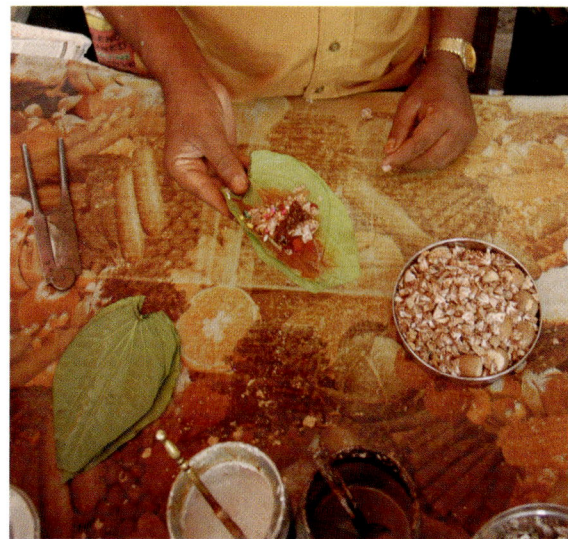

Fig. 53-1 ■ Areca nut and additives such as shell lime paste, coriander seed, cinnamon, cardamoms, and flavored dust create a "relish," which is then wrapped in betel leaf.

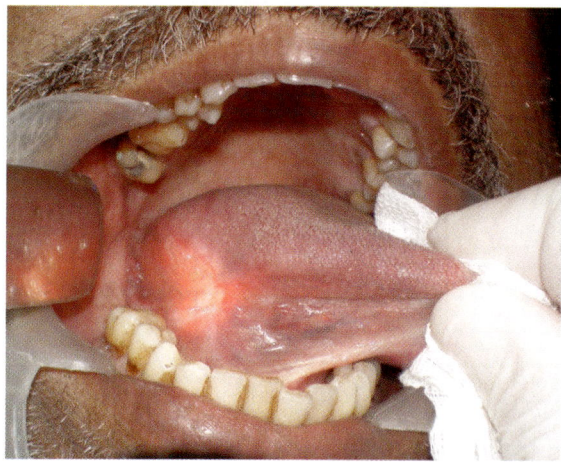

Fig. 53-2 ■ Posterolateral tongue recurrence beneath a radial forearm flap detected with the aid of anterior tongue retraction and digital palpation.

Many southern Asian populations chew *betel quid* (Fig. 53-1). The stimulant, socially acceptable as coffee, is associated with oral cancer with a predilection for the buccal mucosa in this subcontinent, thus hinting at a genetic predisposition. Recent studies suggest that targeting epidermal growth factor receptor (EGFR) may benefit patients with this habit because of overexpression of EGFR.[5] Many of these patients also have submucous fibrosis and, when combined with betel quid, yields an incidence of cancer from malignant transformation surpassing 7%.[6]

CO-MORBID CONDITIONS

Oral lichen planus, a leukoplakia and autoimmune inflammatory disease, does have the propensity to progress to malignancy. Other disease, such as Fanconi anemia, a genetic disorder with an increased incidence in patients with solid tumors, graft-versus-host disease in immunosuppressed patients, and syphilis are also prone to malignant conversion. All predispositions are a result of chronic inflammation and subsequent high cell turnover by immune-mediated cellular proliferation and attempted apoptosis—both known initiators of precancerous lesions.

ENVIRONMENT

Widespread knowledge of smoking's ill effects led to U.S. environmental protection laws forbidding smoking in many public spaces. Secondhand smoke was and, in some places, still is a ubiquitous insult. However, the likelihood of such governmental policy causing a decline in the statistical incidence of carcinoma cannot be known because of the latent onset of oral cancer. Other potential air pollutants, such as organic and inorganic particulates (e.g., nitrosamines, polycyclic aromatic hydrocarbons, and viruses), are associated with oral cancer in workplaces. Nonetheless, few regulations are instituted except for mandatory donning of safety masks to possibly decrease the transmission of airborne noxious particles.

UNKNOWN

A subset of cancer patients have no risk factors (i.e., never smoked and never drank).[7] This group is more often young women who are likely to be serologically positive for *human papillomavirus type 16* and to have early-stage carcinoma of the lateral border of the tongue

diagnosed. This population represented 18% of oral cancer patients in the United States, an increase from 4% in 1971. Short-term abuse—or the "binge" abuse of tobacco and alcohol that commonly exists in younger subcultures—may be accountable but has yet to be proved detrimental.

PATHOLOGIC ANATOMY

Spread of OSCC among anatomic planes can be cryptic, especially in recurrent cases. The oral cavity and thin, non-irradiated necks can easily be investigated for local occurrence and regional metastasis, respectively. However, some clinical disease manifestations do need extra attention because of either anatomic uniqueness or surgical access. This review of pathologic anatomy is for the oral oncologic surgeon and is by no means a comprehensive discussion. Furthermore, although the most common sites for oral cancer are the lateral aspect of the tongue and the floor of the mouth, the subunits in the following sections have unique surgical implications that require special attention.

COFFIN CORNER

The alveololingual sulcus, a "coffin corner" not unlike the blind niche found in the corner landing of a Victorian house stairwell, is a poorly accessed mucosal surface. Without the use of anterior retraction and digital palpation of the tongue, the region may be neglected (Fig. 53-2). This area should be thoroughly evaluated in patients with floor of the mouth or lateral tongue lesions. If cancer abuts the ramus, the surgeon should not hesitate to perform periosteal stripping by elevating the periosteum and then visually inspecting for macroinvasion.[8]

BONE INVASION

Lesions extending onto the maxillary and mandibular alveoli are highly susceptible to osseous invasion. Pathologists recognize two distinct patterns: (1) an invasive histology dotted with islands of bone and finger-like projections of abnormal epithelium that advance independently of the cancellous spaces and (2) an erosive type characterized by a broad advancing front projecting into the cancellous spaces with the aid of osteoclasts (e.g., verrucous carcinoma).

Invasion of OSCC into bone may occur from several routes: oral cavity occlusal route, mental or inferior alveolar foramen

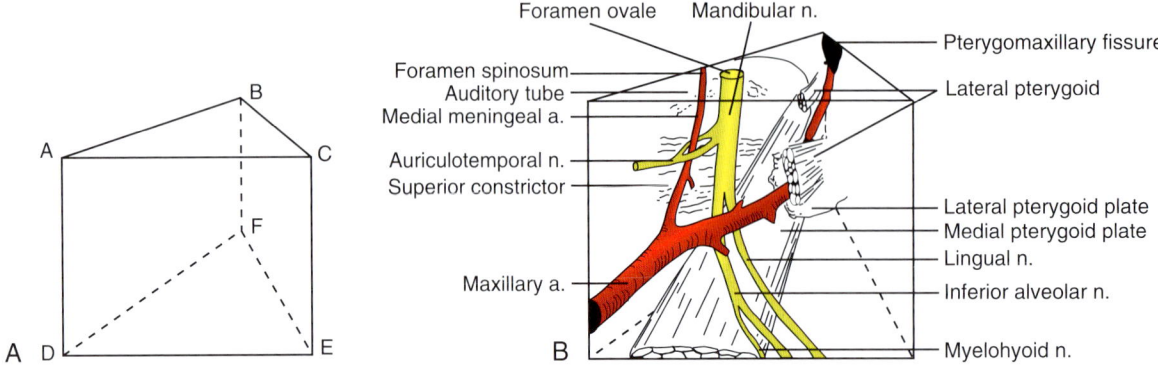

Fig. 53-3 ▪ Friedman wedge (**A**) and superimposed infratemporal fossa (**B**). *ABC*, superior plane—sphenoid–middle cranial fossa; *ABFD*, medial plane—styloid process and pterygoid hamulus; *ACED*, lateral plane—zygomatic arch and mandibular ramus; *AD*, posterior plane—mastoid process and styloid process; *BCEF*, anterior plane—posterior wall of the maxilla. (Adapted from Friedman WH, Katsantonis GP, Cooper MH, et al: Stylohamular dissection: a new method for en bloc resection of malignancies of the infratemporal fossa, *Laryngoscope* 91:1869-7189, 1981.)

(neurotrophic), secondary tumors in the neck through the lower border, cortical bone defects in an edentulous ridge, periodontal membrane in the dentate arch, and the attached gingiva. This incorrect paradigm led to more radical mandibular "rim" resection that included the inferior alveolar nerve for non-bulky tumors.

The greatest predilection is direct invasion, and remotely, neurotrophic-, marrow space–, or periodontal ligament–associated invasion is possible.[9] Computed tomography (CT) statistically misses 27% of these cases and is thus not considered a definitive evaluation. Therefore, periosteal stripping lends credence to the non-partisan and insidious spread of cancer to bone. Edentulous arches are not more susceptible than dentate ones but may lend themselves to more complicated reconstruction if a defect in continuity exists after resection.

PTERYGOPALATINE SPACE

Poor access and numerous vital structures may hinder isolation and prevent adequate resection of this retromaxillary region. Worthington previously documented the following passages as testaments to the area's obscure surgical difficulty[10]:

"An area seen with difficulty, round dark corners …" and "… the posterior section is carried out blind and by blunt leverage."*

"… critical margin in a cavity filled with blood within several millimetres of the internal carotid artery."†

The complexity of nerves, skull base, and multiple conduits necessitates accurate preoperative planning, which is best accomplished with the aid of magnetic resonance imaging (MRI) and positron emission tomography (PET). Diagrammatic representation of the fossa may assist in performing en bloc resection (Fig. 53-3).[11] The space's pathology or resected margins often originate from the antrum or buccal space. The buccal space and its extension (e.g., masseteric space, infratemporal fossa, middle cranial fossa) are extremely vulnerable in late-stage buccal OSCC, and preoperative imaging of radiographic changes in the infratemporal fossa should differentiate vascular insufficiency from extension of OSCC.

Attempting an "extended" maxillectomy by perioral resection (i.e., transpalatal or transantral approach) for OSCC extending into the pterygopalatine fossa is not possible because wide access must be gained to achieve negative margins and vascular hemostasis. Extirpation may be initiated from several other vantage points: transzygomatic, transcranial, transmandibular, facial translocation, or a combination of these techniques. The anterior transmandibular approach using the Dingman-Conley split lip, with or without marginal or segmental mandibulotomy for mandibular disease, provides proper exposure, whereas a Weber-Fergusson access, with subciliary or medial canthal extension if needed, is best suited for antral disease; a Barbosa design may be necessary for extensive antral disease.[12] The surgeon may modify skin incisions by using chevrons to take advantage of the relaxed skin tension lines of the face to achieve optimal esthetic outcomes.

SUBMANDIBULAR REGION

The submandibular gland (SMG) and its vessels and adjacent anatomy are responsible for the complexity of level IB.[13] The submandibular duct and hypoglossal and lingual nerves can easily be accessed with gentle downward traction of the SMG and ligation of the periglandular vessels. Recognition and isolation of these numerous vessels are important for prevention of postoperative oozing and selection of recipient vessels for microsurgical anastomosis. The SMG's primary arterial cascade is the facial and submental arteries, but there are variations from the external carotid, lingual, and deep lingual branches. Its main venous supply consists of the anterior facial, venae comitantes of the facial arteries, and gland hilum veins, but the external jugular veins, anterior jugular veins, and mental veins may be contributory.

FASCIA

Knowledge of the head and neck fascia and its spaces is essential, and it is a voluminous subject. The four layers of fascia consist of the superficial fascia and the superficial, middle, and deep layers of the deep cervical fascia. Its primary importance pertains to preservation of the marginal mandibular nerve and perifacial node dissection near the mandibular line (discussed in the following sections).

MARGINAL MANDIBULAR NERVE

This motor branch of the facial nerve to the lip depressor (*depressor anguli oris*) is a critical structure and can be injured during cervical access, perifacial node dissection, and elevation of lower cheek flaps. The nerve lies within or deep to the superficial layer of the deep cervical fascia. Almost 1 in 10 surgical patients will have at

*Crocket JD: Surgical approach to the back of the maxilla, *Br J Surg* 50:819-821, 1963.
†Dingman L, Conley J: Lateral approach to the pterygomaxillary region, *Ann Otol Rhinol Laryngol* 79:967, 1970.

least one branch of the marginal mandibular nerve located within 1 cm of the inferior border of the mandible lateral to the facial artery; medial to the facial artery, all rami are found above the inferior border of the mandible; and nearly all (95%) marginal mandibular nerves run superficial to the anterior facial and retromandibular veins.[14] To protect the nerve, all cervical incisions are made at least 2 cm caudal to the inferior border of the mandible, and all dissections are performed below the veins (Hayes-Martin maneuver).

CERVICAL LYMPHATICS

Henri Rouvière schematically described the lymphatic drainage of the head and neck as two concentric narrowing funnels draining caudally to the thoracic duct (left) and lymphatic duct (right). This paradigm is oversimplistic but is still taught in schools today. Regional metastases from the oral cavity often drain to Robbins levels I to III, hence the rationale for supraomohyoid neck dissection. Skip metastases are possible, and the tongue and soft palate are often discovered to have bilateral regional metastases on final pathologic evaluation. Table 53-1 illustrates the anatomic levels of the neck and their importance.

Predictable drainage of the oral cavity to the first echelon of the lymphatic basin does exist. However, as a result of data from large clinical outcome studies and the ability of lymphoscintigraphy to map sentinel nodes, surgeons now recognize that drainage can be on an individual basis. Skip metastases to level IV in lateral tongue SCC and retropharyngeal drainage of the soft palate follow this paradigm. Another *caveat lector* is that previously operated necks may have hitherto undiagnosed, nascent, or recurrent metastases. Therefore, lymphatic drainage can be unpredictable after surgery, and clinically positive (cN+) or negative (cN0) nodes with micrometastases may go undetected.

Radiologists combine nodal critical size and morphology to determine "suggestive" cervical adenopathy. Suspicion for regional metastases is high in the setting of OSCC if nodes display a central hypointensity consistent with central necrosis; if they are round and not kidney bean shaped, which represents expansion; if the surrounding fascial plane is obliterated, which signifies tissue necrosis or fixation; if their dimensions are greater than 15 mm at level II and greater than 10 mm elsewhere; or if a spiculated periphery indicative of extracapsular spread is present. This last characteristic is a significant poor prognostic indicator for OSCC.

PERIFACIAL NODE

The perifacial, perivascular, or supramandibular facial node lies just superior to the inferior mandibular bone margin near the antegonial notch where the facial artery and vein pass cephalad. Adjacent regional metastasis to the perifacial node is relatively highly likely if level Ib is positive—nearly 35% and 27% of node-positive and node-negative necks, respectively.[15] To gain access to the node, the superficial layer of the deep cervical fascia must be violated and dissection must proceed in a more superficial direction. Taking care to not damage the marginal mandibular nerve with this maneuver is imperative, and a risk/benefit decision must be made before dissection of occult disease.[16] Node-positive patients who require comprehensive neck dissection and have aggressive buccal and mandibular mucosal lesions should be candidates for perifacial node removal.

DIAGNOSTIC STUDIES

Modern imaging, though not essential for some early-stage cancers, often assists in treatment planning and may be a useful tool in postoperative surveillance.

ENDOSCOPY

Examination under anesthesia and direct laryngoscopy can be advantageous in investigating OSCC. Early-stage synchronous and metachronous distal secondary aerodigestive lesions may otherwise evade diagnostic imaging, although their rate may vary between 2.6% and 16%.[17,18] The sensitivity of flexible direct laryngoscopy is comparable to that of a rigid Hopkins lens in skilled hands. The assistance of topical analgesia, vasoconstriction, anxiolysis, and antisialagogues cannot be overstated. Bronchoscopy and esophagoscopy are essential in evaluating neck masses of unknown origin, but they may not be of added benefit when investigating primary OSCC, especially when symptomatic.[19]

PAN-TOMOGRAPHY

Pan-tomography may be the best imaging modality for evaluation of the alveolar process. As an initial investigation, pan-tomography is low-cost; provides a gestalt for pre-radiation dental prophylaxis, preoperative osseous ablation, and reconstruction planning; and gives hindsight when evaluating further imaging. Small anterior maxillary and mandibular arch lesions are better evaluated with an occlusal film because of cervical skeletal superimposition on pantomography. The surgeon should be aware that radiographic changes may not be evident until a third of the bone's density has been resorbed and that lingual cortical decortications may be masked by the mandible's bicortical thickness.

TABLE 53-1	Lymphatic Drainage of the Oral Cavity	
NECK REGION	**NODAL LEVEL**	**IMPORTANCE**
Submental triangle	Level Ia	Submental arteries as salvage for island flap
Submandibular triangle	Level Ib	Sentinel lymphatic basin for OSCC, node of Stahr
Para–internal jugular vein (infra–skull base to suprahyoid)	Level IIa	Sentinel lymphatic basin for most OSCC, jugulodigastric node (Küttner's node)
Posterior to the spinal accessory nerve	Level IIb	Dissect for N+ only (comprehensive ND only)
Para–internal jugular vein (infrahyoid to supracricoid)	Level III	Inferior extent of supraomohyoid ND, jugulo-omohyoid node (Poirier's node)
Para–internal jugular vein (infracricoid to supraclavicular)	Level IV	Possibly occult in lateral tongue cancer (extended ND only), Virchow's node*
Posterior triangle	Level V	Dissect for N+ neck (comprehensive ND only)
Perifacial node	Above superficial layer of deep cervical fascia	Risk for marginal mandibular nerve injury

*Left side only.
N+, node positive (pathologic neck); ND, neck dissection.

COMPUTED TOMOGRAPHY

CT is still the gold standard for evaluation and planning treatment of OSCC. It provides the possibility of high resolution of critical structures, three-dimensional image reconstruction, and comparable cost containment. Drawbacks of CT are its high-dose radiation, nephrotoxic dosing in patients with renal insufficiency, frequent hypersensitivity (allergy) to the contrast dye, and beam-hardening artifact with extensive amalgam restorations. Artifact can be minimized with open-mouth positioning, "puffed cheek" techniques, and postprocessing algorithms.[20]

MAGNETIC RESONANCE IMAGING

MRI may be an appropriate investigation in patients with tongue base or retromolar lesions and suspicion of perineural, extrinsic tongue muscle, oropharyngeal, soft palate, or skull base extension. Use of either T1-weighted non–contrast-enhanced/contrast-enhanced or fat-suppressed T2-weighted images is well suited for these purposes. Contrast-enhanced images have nearly comparable ability to detect cervical lymphadenopathy and may be optimal for N0 disease to determine tumor thickness in the tongue.[21] Its sensitivity and specificity for detection of OSCC are both 93%.[22] MRI may be plagued by motion artifact in uncooperative patients and is contraindicated in patients with pacemakers or vascular clips.

POSITRON EMISSION TOMOGRAPHY

PET has become a useful adjunct for diagnosing unknown primaries and regional and distant metastases at the time of staging, for salvage therapy, or for postoperative surveillance. Equivocal interpretation of findings on PET can be minimized by well-trained clinicians, and its expense is justified. Postsurgical inflammation and radiation-induced inflammation are the biggest culprits in causing its poor specificity. Other difficulties are carotid plaques, false-positive results with laryngeal activity such as talking, and false-negative results with hyperglycemia since serum glucose competes with the most common radioactive tracer, ^{18}F-fluorodeoxyglucose.

The benefit of PET in detecting regional or distant metastases in patients with initially advanced tumor size or in investigating or monitoring occult recurrent, secondary aerodigestive lesions is invaluable. Because OSCC patients are 10% more likely to have a second primary at initial evaluation and 22% more likely to have a second primary in 5 years, and because PET detects nearly 50% of unknown primaries that traditional imaging modalities miss, it is becoming more commonly used. The Mount Sinai Surveillance Protocol capitalizes on the specificity of PET by including a pretreatment scan, a 6-week postoperative scan, and one every 4 months for the first 2 years. Studies then continue every 6 months during the third and fourth years. This protocol minimizes the time until detection of cancer, which is most common within the first 2 years.

ULTRASOUND/FINE-NEEDLE ASPIRATION

Ultrasound (US) of the neck is often helpful for suspicious cervical masses in patients who have previously undergone surgery or for neck fields that have received high doses of radiation. Because of the efficacy of US when combined with fine-needle aspiration (FNA) in confirming the diagnosis, it is a practical alternative to CT in the hands of a well-versed FNA/US clinician; the sensitivity of FNA ranges between 77% and 95% and its specificity from 93% to 100%.[23] The most success with this combined modality is achieved for lymphadenopathy that exceeds 7 mm in level II and 6 mm elsewhere in the short-axis dimension.

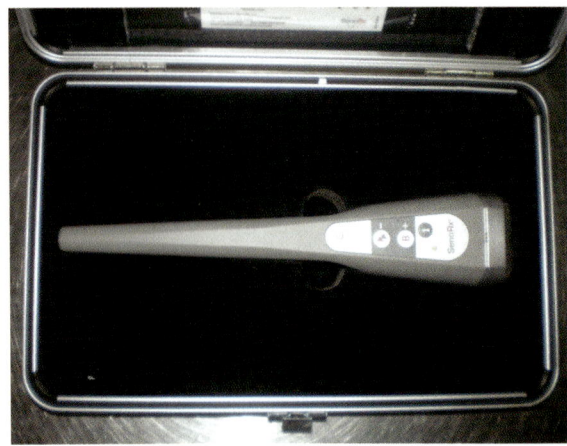

Fig. 53-4 ■ Geiger probe used in intraoperative sentinel lymph node biopsy.

LYMPHOSCINTIGRAPHY

Lymphoscintigraphy (LSG) is a procedural harbinger for detecting melanoma regional metastases, but it is gaining investigative confidence for staging OSCC in a cN0 neck. The first-echelon lymphatic basin is determined by injecting ^{99m}Tc-labeled sulfur colloid, a radioactive tracer, around the primary tumor and identifying intraoperative regional drainage with a sterilely covered Geiger probe to detect high gamma-radiation (Fig. 53-4). These isolated sentinel lymph nodes are dissected and sent as frozen sections. If the specimens are negative, neck dissection can be deferred; if positive, the surgeon should proceed with selective therapeutic supraomohyoid neck dissection. In essence, a "staging" neck dissection does not exist in this scenario.

If multilevel signals are detected on LSG, selective neck dissection may be a more appropriate surgical intervention than a non-"halstedian" approach, consistent with selective nodal vein "picking." Although LSG has a negative predictive value (the probability of not having disease when a test is negative) of nearly 100% with co-registration of CT to stereotactically localize micrometastases in cN0, a few patients' disease may elude all diagnostics for microscopic regional metastases.[24-26] LSG may show promise, but "scheduled" selective neck dissections are associated with much lower morbidity than comprehensive neck dissections in OSCC patients with delayed detected pN+ (pathologic node-positive neck dissection), which may rarely occur with LSG and sentinel node dissection.

TREATMENT/RECONSTRUCTIVE GOALS

The ablative surgeon's goal is to maximize tumor-free survival by wide local excision of the oral lesion and eradication of micrometastases and macrometastases, neck observation for lesions in their earliest stages (T1 lesions with a depth of invasion of less than 4 mm), neck dissection for staging when neck lymphadenopathy is not present (cN0) but regional metastasis is highly probable (any T lesion with a depth of invasion of greater than 4 mm), and comprehensive neck dissection in patients with palpable or radiographic lymphadenopathy (cN+). After achieving this oncologic objective, the reconstructive surgeon's focus is on maintaining orofacial function and cosmesis with the aid of the proverbial reconstructive ladder.

ACCESS

Maxillary access beyond a perioral approach via a vestibular or degloving incision may be achieved with upper lip incisions to create an "upper cheek" flap: the Weber-Fergusson or Diffenbach incision is a midline upper lip split through the center of the labial tubercle and philtrum that passes upward along the nose's lateral contour, the Altemir modification differs in that the inferior portion of the incision is lateral to the tubercle and along the philtral crest, an inferior transconjunctival forniceal extension is a Trotter modification, a superior extension has been described by Lynch, and a subciliary extension is credited to Crockett.[27]

Various lip incisions may gain additional access to the mandible directly or to the skull base inferiorly via the lower lip to create a "lower cheek" flap: the Roux-Trotter incision is a true midline lip split traditionally used in "commando procedures," the von Langenback or Robson (labiomental fold) incision is a corner lip or lateral lip-split approach most appropriate if previous radiation therapy and segmental mandibulectomy for anterior mandible SCC have deteriorated the lip's blood supply and the patient needs a second surgery on the remaining proximal mandible or maxillary extension, the McGregor incision is a cosmetic attempt to not violate the chin pad's convex contour, and the Hayter modification of the McGregor incision includes a chevron above the mental crease and may also include one on the vermilion of the lip itself.[28] The last of these designs provides the best cosmetic result.

MARGINS

Positive margins, or those that include OSCC, are the worst prognostic factor. To achieve a 5-mm pathologically clear margin, a 1-cm clinical margin must be resected. Wider margins may be needed because of the insidious ability of larger buccal OSCCs to spread to adjacent anatomic byways. Similarly, the surgeon should acknowledge the potential for floor of the mouth mucosal field cancerization—an abnormal entity of clonal expansion that may appear to migrate along the mucosal histologic margins. The process is actually multifocal, and the areas epitomize oral cancer's stepwise fashion toward malignancy, similar to colon cancer. The original dysplastic foci will aggregate with time and possible overlap with adjacent areas containing a lesser degree of dysplasia (Fig. 53-5). Frequently, only microscopic inspection of excised margins may depict adjacent foci. Either at histologic examination or with time, this margin can become malignant.[29] Careful evaluation of the tissue next to the surgical site plus verification of whether it appears to be suggestive of clinical or microscopic invasion is essential. Patients with specimen margins positive for p53 immunostaining, a laboratory method of labeling a tumor suppressor protein deleted early in the molecular pathogenesis of OSCC, are five times more likely to exhibit early recurrence.[30]

"Chasing" a dysplastic mucosal margin is surgically fruitless in patients with field cancerization. Such pursuit is worthy (i.e., improves disease-free survival in early-stage OSCC), however, when frozen sections are positive for mucosal malignancy, which has an investigative accuracy of 99%.[31] Skull base exploration for nerve infiltration by OSCC along the perineural lymphatics, though discouraging, has a moderate survival benefit.[32]

Regional nodal micrometastases, or those larger than 0.2 mm but smaller than 2 mm, can also be detected by protein-labeled polymerase chain reaction and may be prognostic of an adverse outcome.[33] Although ablative surgeons cannot presently use such in vivo staining for malignant resection, operative molecular targeting may be possible in the future.

CLASSIFICATION OF ABLATIVE OSSEOUS DEFECTS

Several descriptive nomenclatures for facial osseous defects have been devised. Knowledge of the commonly used classification systems is helpful when communicating by documentation in the event of recurrent disease, especially when the patient may seek treatment at a different hospital or the imaging is difficult to decipher. Collaborating reconstructive surgeons may have algorithmic plastic surgical approaches to ablative defects, but they may also lack the knowledge of when the use of implants and prostheses has potential in certain situations (e.g., zygomatic implants). Knowledge of this nomenclature will maximize communication and facilitate the best reconstructive result.

Maxillary defects have vertical (I, II, III) and horizontal (a, b, c) components of their dimensions. Numerous combinations can exist; for example, "class IIA" equates to a low hemimaxillectomy similar to a hemi–Le Fort designation. Vertical components progress with decreasing pillar support, whereas horizontal components progress with less remaining dentition (Fig. 53-6). When compared with "partial-structure," "infrastructure," and "suprastructure" maxillectomy, the designation may be cumbersome and not a function of prognosis (i.e., Ohngren's line). However, the combined taxonomy is descriptive in three dimensions and more informative to a referring reconstructive surgeon.

Mandibular resection may either be marginal, segmental, or hemimandibular (i.e., disarticulation). Jewer and colleagues described osseous segmental defects by their location, whether they cross the midline, or whether they include the condyle (Fig. 53-7).[34] Boyd and co-workers further incorporated the insight of classifying composite defects: "o" designates no defect, consistent with subperiosteal resection for intramedullary osseous pathology; "m" stands for mucosal resection; and "s" suggests a fistula from plate

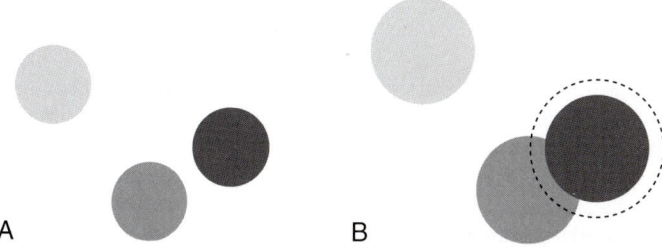

Fig. 53-5 ■ Field cancerization. **A,** Circles and darkness depict different degrees of dysplastic foci. **B,** As time passes, the dysplastic areas enlarge and may overlap. The dashed circle represents a biopsied field and shows the potential for inclusion of adjacent dysplastic foci.

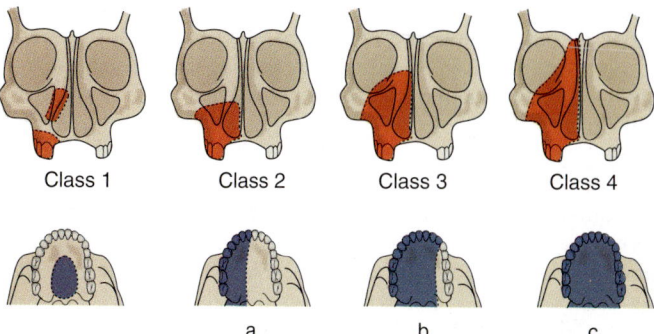

Class 1 Class 2 Class 3 Class 4

a b c

Fig. 53-6 ■ Maxillectomy classification. (Redrawn from Brown JS, Jones DC, Summerwill A, et al: Vascularized iliac crest with internal oblique arter maxillectomy, *Br J Oral Maxillofac Surg* 40(3):183-190, 2002.)

TABLE 53-2	Mandibular Resection			
CAWOOD-HOWELL		**NO BONE INVASION**	**EARLY INVASION**	**LATE INVASION**
Dentate or immediate postextraction (I-II)		Rim	Rim	Investigation*
Round or knife ridge (III-IV)		Rim	Investigation*	Segmental
Flat or depressed ridge (V-VI)		Investigation*	Segmental	Segmental

*Indeterminate resection scenarios may be best managed by intraoperative investigation (e.g., periosteal stripping, bone smear, or cytologic imprint) if gross epithelial growth is not seen in the cancellous space.
Adapted from Brown J, Chatterjee R, Lowe D, et al: A new guide to mandibular resection for oral squamous cell carcinoma based on the Cawood and Howell classification of the mandible, *Int J Oral Maxillofac Surg* 34:834-839, 2005.

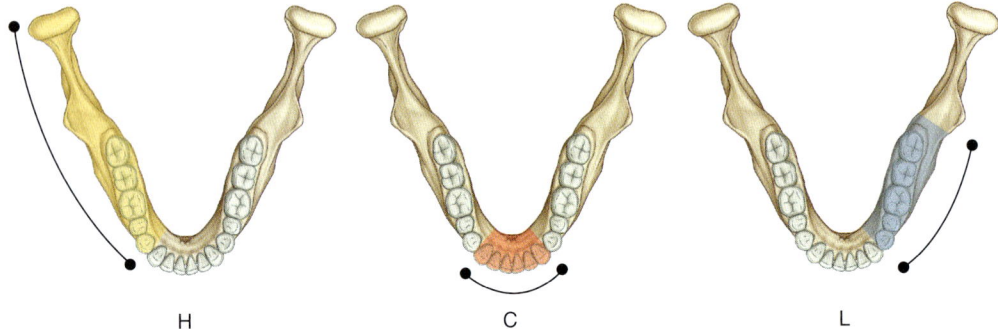

H   C   L

Fig. 53-7 ■ Mandibulectomy classification. "H" is a hemimandibular defect of any length extending from the condyle but not past the contralateral canine, "C" is a central segment defect involving the parasymphysis and isolated to a location between the canines, and "L" is lateral segment defect of the ramus or body that does not involve the condyle and does not extend past the contralateral canine. (Mandible illustration from Drake RL, Vogl W, Mitchell AWM: *Gray's anatomy for students*, Philadelphia, 2005, Churchill Livingstone.)

dehiscence, infection, or cancer with extraoral skin extension.[35] Therefore, a combination of a hard and soft tissue component, such as "LCLm," will equate to an angle-to-angle resection with only a mucosal defect.

Marginal resection is a method of retaining osseous continuity in mandibles that have cortical, not intramedullary OSCC invasion. The procedure should be not used in lieu of segmental resection if bone invasion is evident clinically, radiographically, or by smear, but it is appropriate for early-stage OSCC in a dentate, non-irradiated mandible.[36,37] When resecting non-irradiated edentulous mandibles, the design of the osteotomy should be based on imaging and be correlated with the mandible's residual osseous height while still using intraoperative cytologic smears in selected cases (Table 53-2).[38] A curvilinear design may be oriented horizontally ("rim") to include the coronoid process for SCC of the retromolar trigone and alveolar process (Fig. 53-8). Access can be attempted transbuccally with minimal iatrogenic cheek trauma with the aid of orthognathic and facial trauma instrumentation.[39] Otherwise, a postoperative iatrogenic or pathologic fracture is inevitable. Alternatively, SCC of the floor of the mouth can be resected with an oblique ("sagittal") osteotomy.

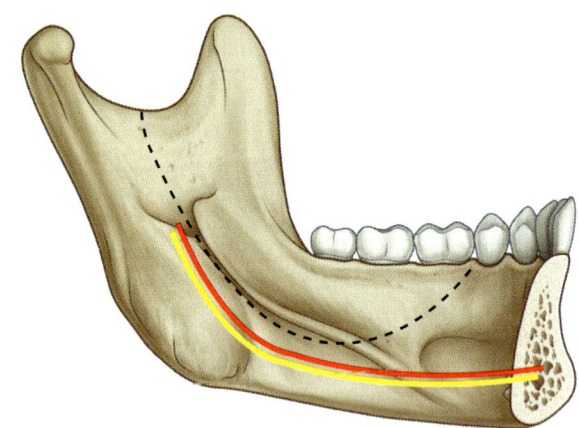

Fig. 53-8 ■ Marginal mandibulectomy above the inferior alveolar bundle (*yellow, red*) and including the coronoid process. (Mandible illustration from Drake RL, Vogl W, Mitchell AWM: *Gray's anatomy for students*, Philadelphia, 2005, Churchill Livingstone.)

NECK DISSECTION

Neck dissection is always indicated for palpable lymphadenopathy (N+) in necks not undergoing chemoradiation as a primary treatment modality and may be indicated for early OSCC without palpable cervical nodes (N0). The gold standard for evaluating subclinical disease (i.e., occult microscopic regional metastasis that evades physical examination and radiographic studies) is histologic analysis. Without mentioning LSG because at this time it is still an investigative procedure, a surgeon can use biopsy-proven tumor depth greater than 4 mm as the best predictor for positive subclinical

disease in patients with tongue lesions (Table 53-3).[40] Other risk factors for occult disease are poorly differentiated tumors, infiltrating invasive histologic types, lack of peritumor lymphocytic response, islands of tumor greater than 1 cm apart, and perineural invasion or angiolymphatic invasion. Tumors with a depth of 4 mm have a 30% likelihood of being associated with occult disease versus 7% for tumors with a depth of less than 4 mm. A rule of thumb is to dissect neck levels I through III in patients with OSCC when the likelihood of occult neck disease surpasses 20%.[41] An exception is lateral tongue SCC, which may also metastasize to level IV (21%)

TABLE 53-3	Management of Node-Negative Patients by Primary Anatomic Site		
SITE	**TONGUE, FLOOR OF MOUTH**	**BUCCAL, HARD AND SOFT PALATE**	**RETROMOLAR TRIGONE, ALVEOLUS**
Stage for prophylactic neck management	Tumor thickness >4 mm	Stage II	Stage II/III

TABLE 53-4	Neck Incisions			
	MODIFIED SCHOBINGER	**APRON**	**MCFEE**	**J**

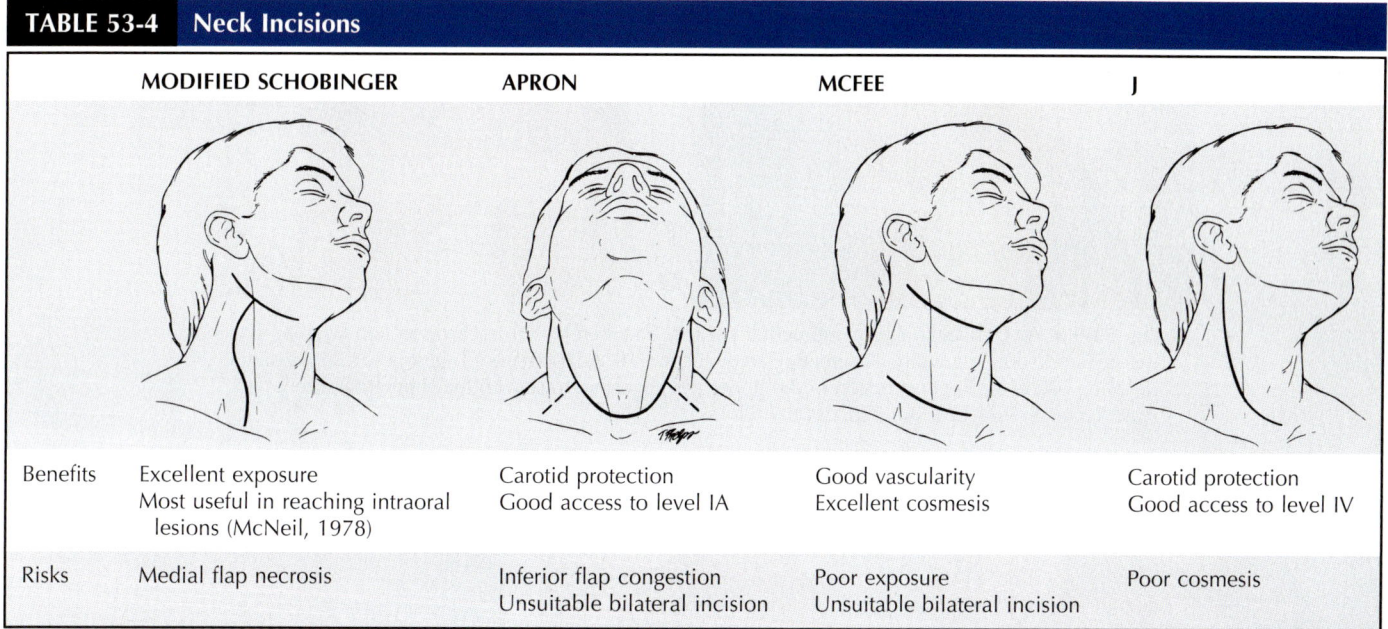

	MODIFIED SCHOBINGER	**APRON**	**MCFEE**	**J**
Benefits	Excellent exposure Most useful in reaching intraoral lesions (McNeil, 1978)	Carotid protection Good access to level IA	Good vascularity Excellent cosmesis	Carotid protection Good access to level IV
Risks	Medial flap necrosis	Inferior flap congestion Unsuitable bilateral incision	Poor exposure Unsuitable bilateral incision	Poor cosmesis

Data from Acar A, Dursun G, Aydin O, et al: J incision in neck dissections, *J Laryngol Otol* 112:55-60, 1998. (Images from Eisell D, Smith RV: *Complications in head and neck surgery*, ed 2, St. Louis, 2009, Mosby.)

and is best managed by dissecting levels I through IV since there is a possibility of skip metastasis within this region.[42]

The surgeon should be cognizant that neck dissection does not eliminate future disease and that postoperative conversion from highly probable (late-stage OSCC) in a pathologically confirmed N0 neck can take place as early as 3 months. Regional recurrence rates range from 2% to 4%, and the incidence of contralateral disease is as high as 5%. The rate of failure at level V nears 7%, but it generally likely when level IV is metastatic and it should therefore be included in the dissection in such instances. Level V failure is highest with lateral tongue disease, and early intervention with elective neck dissection improves disease-free survival in patients with tongue SCC.

Standard cervical flaps for access are based on the transverse cervical, superior thyroid, and facial arteries. Over the years, surgeons have created various neck incisions designed to achieve a balance between flap viability, carotid artery protection, planned tracheostomy, resurfacing, cosmesis, and surgical exposure.[43-46] The simple cervical and modified Schobinger incisions are the workhorse for selective and comprehensive neck dissections, respectively (Table 53-4).

RECONSTRUCTION

Postablative oral or orocutaneous defects have requirements of function and cosmesis. These necessities are fulfilled by a donor tissue's characteristics, whether it be bone, muscle, skin, or nerve. A "reconstructive ladder," or incremental stepwise approach of using a patient's tissue for reconstruction, epitomizes in hierarchical fashion a surgeon's thought process in reconstructing an ablative defect. Though not comprehensive, this section will accent a few novel

methods: the submental island flap (SIF), the facial artery musculomucosal (FAMM) flap, and technologic advances in fibular and radial forearm microvascular reconstruction.

The SIF is an ideal robust alternative to the sternocleidomastoid or nasolabial flap for small to moderate defects (e.g., T2N0M0 OSCC). Its harvest is ideal for an anterior mandibular marginal or floor of the mouth defect when primary closure is not possible and microvascular techniques are not an option (Fig. 53-9).[47] The reconstruction method is oncologically sound in an N0 patient and if level I is meticulously cleared but discouraged if the nodes are palpable or radiographically evident (N+).[48] The key to oncologic and flap viability success is dissection in the subplatysmal plane before neck dissection and preservation of the submental branch of the facial arteries—8-cm pedicle, 2-mm diameter.[49] The artery is identified on the superficial surface of the mylohyoid muscle and passes to the deep surface of the digastric muscle, but a Doppler probe can be helpful. To provide the highest viability, the anterior belly of the digastric muscle should be included in the submental myofasciocutaneous flap.

A FAMM flap is also an axial flap that may be appropriate for small to moderate ablative defects of the mucosa of the cheek, edentulous palate, alveolus, floor of the mouth, or vestibule when other "workhorse" flaps are not available (Fig. 53-10).[50-52] The flap may be superiorly based (retrograde flow) or inferiorly based (anterograde flow) to minimize pedicle torsion at the recipient site. Meticulous arterial dissection prevents iatrogenic injury to the superficial and proximal facial nerve branches supplying animation to the muscles of facial expression. Partial necrosis is not uncommon, but definitive revision because of flap failure is a rarer occurrence.

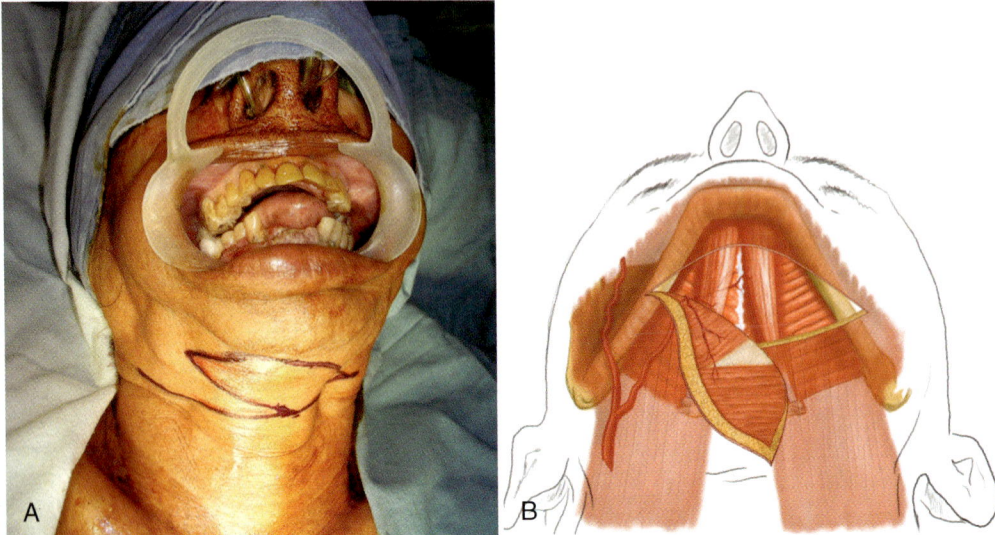

Fig. 53-9 ■ **A,** Delineation of a submental pedicle flap before N0 neck dissection by pinching excess skin to obtain primary closure. **B,** Flap dissection. (**B,** Adapted from Taghinia AH, Movassaghi K, Wang AX, et al: Reconstruction of the upper aerodigestive tract with the submental artery flap, *Plast Reconstr Surg* 123:562-570, 2009.)

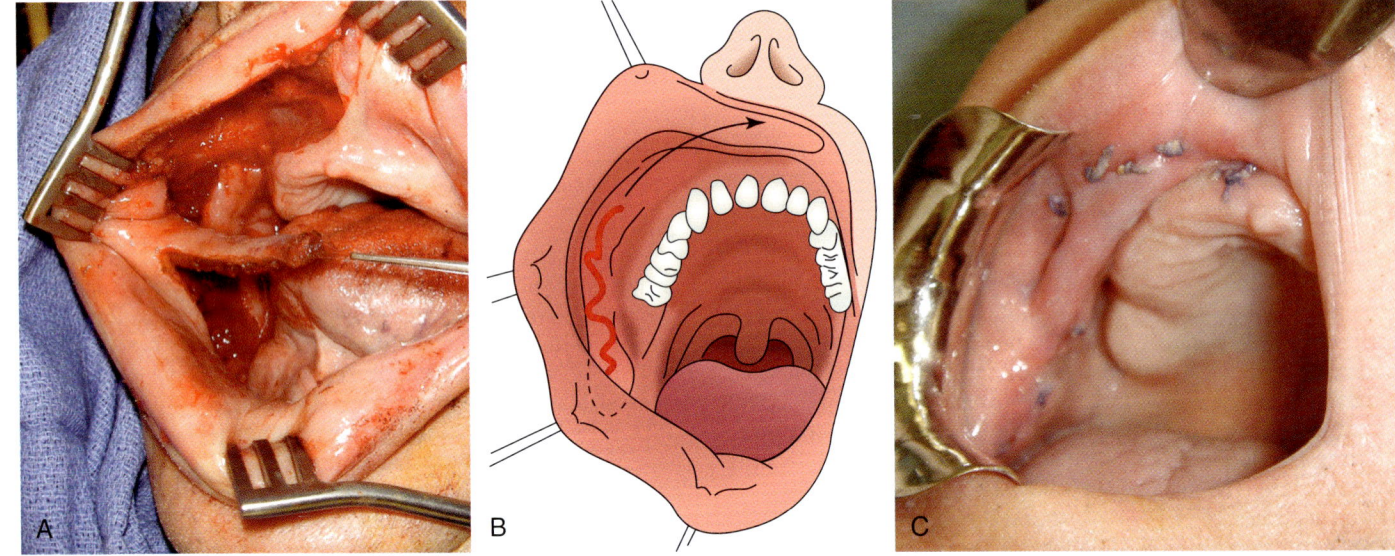

Fig. 53-10 ■ **A,** Facial artery–based musculomucosal flap before inset into the anterior maxillary vestibular ablative defect. **B,** Diagrammatic representation of facial artery–based musculomucosal flap, **C,** Postoperative appearance of patient in **A** following facial-artery based musculomucosal flap. (**B,** Redrawn from Pribaz JJ, Meara JG, Wright S, et al: Lip and vermilion reconstruction with the facial artery musculomucosal flap, *Plast Reconstr Surg* 105:864-872, 2000.)

Microvascular free flaps provide the best utility in healthy individuals with larger ablative defects. Their success rate nears 96%, with a re-exploration rate of 2% in skilled hands. After 2 weeks, an endothelium regenerate lines the microanastomosis. A critique of this reconstructive modality is poor cosmesis, specifically, skin color match and contour without revision.

The radial forearm flap (RFF) microvascular technique is a *true and tried* method for soft tissue requirements. With the advent of perforator flaps, large-volume soft tissue defects became well suited for the RFF's "big brother," the anterolateral thigh flap.[53] Similar to ballistic experiences from wars of the past that led to the development of reconstructive principles, the Bosnian War begat another flap—the "shape-modified method," or freestyle, radial forearm perforator flap (Fig. 53-11).[54,55] The technique's closure is ideal for

the delicate or dexterous hand needed for cosmesis and function, and its inset is amenable to a wide defect demanding pliability (e.g., cheek OSCC with extension to the oropharynx or floor of the mouth).

Mandibular or maxillary postablative defects are complex reconstructive dilemmas. If a mandibular body continuity defect is not restored (i.e., collapsing the defect), malocclusion, chin deviation, and tongue elevation will result, but recovery will be fast, with enhancement of speech and swallowing, unlike a bulky flap. This method may be adequate for a patient who may not tolerate a lengthy procedure. The sole use of a reconstruction plate to bridge an anterior mandibular continuity defect will probably result in wound dehiscence and exposure of the plate in the long-term after radiation therapy. Anterior segmental mandibular defects always necessitate reconstruction; otherwise, a crippling deformity will result from the ablation. Mandibular body continuity defects may be adequately restored with solely a reconstruction plate and pedicle flap (e.g., pectoralis major myocutaneous flap) to minimize operative time, monitor for recurrence, and decrease donor site morbidity. Fibular reconstruction offers good bone stock with the potential for placement of dental implants after definitive gross reconstruction and radiation therapy. Virtual planning, a method of using stereolithic models made from patients' imaging, can streamline treatment sequencing, decrease operative time, and theoretically determine a final "product" before making an incision in difficult cases (Fig. 53-12).[56] With or without an implant-supported prosthesis, referral to a prosthodontist before the operative procedure is advantageous to enhance quality of life.

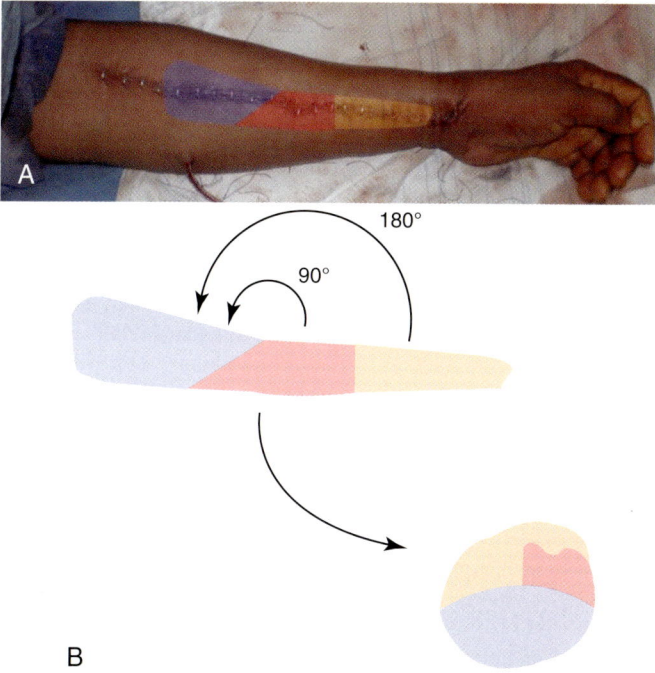

Fig. 53-11 ■ **A,** Primary closure of a radial forearm flap harvest site with a perforator flap indicated by the colored overlay. **B,** Diagrammatic representation of an exemplary freestyle geometry. (**B,** Adapted from Boyd J, Brain MD: Shape-modified method using the radial forearm perforator flap for reconstruction of soft-tissue defects of the scalp, *J Reconstr Microsurg* 21:21-24, 2005.)

SPECIFIC TREATMENT AND ADJUNCTIVE TECHNIQUES

Different ablative modalities other than surgery are available for definitive and combined treatment of OSCC. Some sole modalities are as equally efficacious as surgery, others are reserved for patients deferring surgery because of co-morbid conditions or choice, and combined treatments, whether neoadjuvant, adjuvant, or concomitant (concurrent with chemotherapy), are reserved for patients with late-stage disease or for clinical trial enrollment.

LASER

Light amplification by stimulation of emission of radiation (laser) does have a role in early-stage laryngeal ablation (i.e., transoral microsurgery).[57] Laser ablation does play an alternative non-diagnostic role in cases of suspected field oral cavity dysplasia. The neodymium:yttrium-aluminum-garnet (Nd:YAG) laser was evaluated in a 5-year follow-up for its ability to ablate premalignant and stage I OSCC.[58] However, nearly half the patients were lost to follow-up, and disease had recurred in a quarter of the patients with stage I at 5 years. Perhaps the best use of the laser is for the ablation of previously diagnosed field dysplasia without cancerous foci.

RADIATION

The primary indication for a 6-week (30 fractions) course of neck linear radiation therapy after surgery (>60 Gy; i.e., adjuvant) is extracapsular spread or multiple (more than three) metastatic nodes. Positive margins are an absolute indication for irradiation of the primary site but may best be managed by immediate re-excision in patients with negative margins. Perivascular emboli and perineural spread are relative indications for postoperative radiation therapy and may be considered if aggressive disease is suspected.

Hyperfractionation and accelerated fractionation are two alternative radiation regimens that are often used concurrently with chemotherapy. Patients with late-stage disease undergo these regimens either postoperatively or as palliation. Hyperfractionation increases

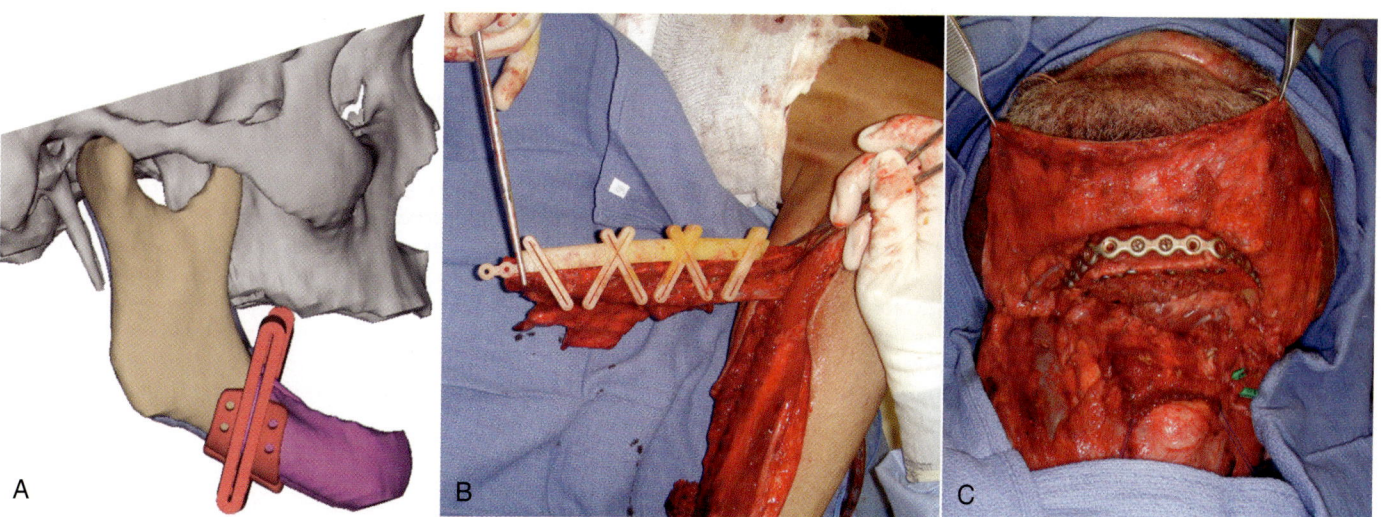

Fig. 53-12 ■ **A,** Virtual positional jig delineating the planned mandible osteotomy. **B,** In vivo fibula osteotomy at the donor site. **C,** Final reconstructive result.

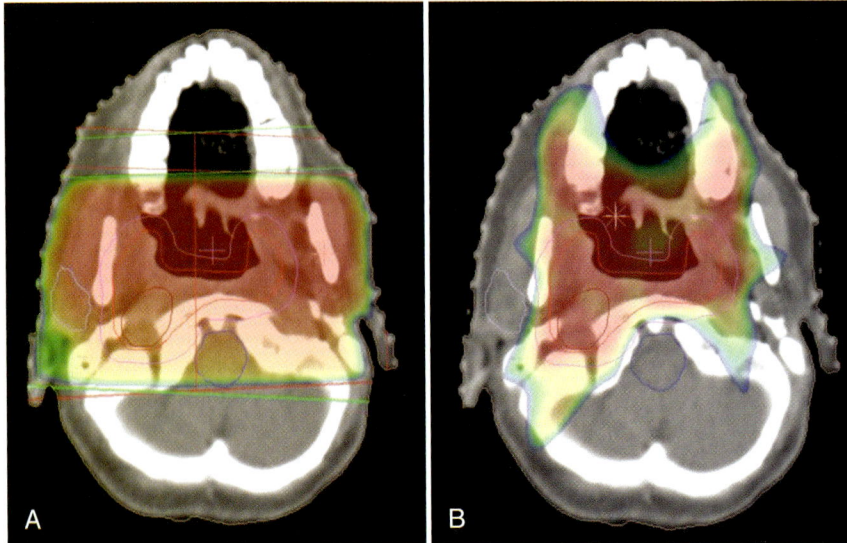

Fig. 53-13 ■ **A,** Oropharyngeal treatment planned with conventional radiotherapy. **B,** Parotid sparing with intensity-modulated radiotherapy.

the number of treatment intervals and lowers the individual dose while achieving the same cumulative dose, thereby preferentially sparing late-responding normal tissue. Accelerated fractionation is performed with the intent of eliminating tumor clonal proliferation by increasing the total radiation dose and decreasing the total treatment time. Both techniques show 10% to 15% improvement in local control but only modest improvement in survival.[59,60] The only subjective radiation-induced toxicity of these regimens was a more severe acute phase mucositis; long-term deficits were not detected.

Intensity-modulated radiation therapy takes advantage of multiple beams with custom multileaf collimation, three-dimensional conformational planning, and dose escalation. These properties minimize toxicity to organs (e.g., parotid, globe, and brain) and improve quality of life (Fig. 53-13). The mode of delivery is crucial in recurrent cases, in which osteoradionecrosis, radiation-induced tumors, and organ sparing (e.g., eyes and spinal cord) are a concern when the total dose exceeds 70 cGy.

CHEMOTHERAPY

Reserved for late-stage disease and recurrences (i.e., positive margins and extracapsular nodal spread), chemotherapy may be prescribed as a neoadjuvant (induction), adjuvant (after surgery), or concurrent (at the same time to increase radiosensitivity) modality.[61] The most common regimens are three cycles (days 1, 22, and 43) of cisplatin, 5-fluorouracil (5-FU), or both. If therapy is successful, the patient is designated a responder with complete tumor resolution or a partial responder with evident residual tumor. Only complete responders have an increased disease-free survival benefit with neoadjuvant therapy, but adjuvant therapy is under clinical investigation. However, all sequences of therapy, whether before or after surgery, fail to show locoregional control or a survival benefit. Evidence may exist to suggest that vital structures are spared by tumor down-staging and quality of life is improved by lessening surgical morbidity.

ORGAN PRESERVATION

Following in the footsteps of landmark randomized trials for laryngeal (organ) preservation, a group of oncologists have applied this knowledge to advanced-stage OSCC. Concurrent chemoradiation

protocols using bleomycin or peplomycin regimens may not be as successful as initial surgery when compared by stage, but complete responses do occur, and patients avoid resection.[62] The University of Michigan's methodology is one cycle of cisplatin and 5-FU before further chemoradiation therapy and salvage surgery; if the patient is a nonresponder, only salvage surgery is considered. The results suggest that complete responders have a survival benefit over partial responders. Therefore, organ preservation is possible.[63] For patients with nonresectable disease, concomitant surgery should always be considered.

IMMUNOTHERAPY

Cetuximab, an anti–epidermal growth factor receptor antibody and originally a treatment of metastatic colon cancer, is now indicated for the treatment of locally or regionally advanced head and neck SCC as a radiosensitizer or in conjunction with platinum-based chemotherapy in locally recurrent cases.

CHEMOPREVENTION

Although elimination of risk factors (e.g., tobacco and alcohol consumption) may be important for regression of dysplasia, certain vitamins, minerals, and anti-inflammatory agents may be chemopreventive. Retinoids are the most promising agent, but toxicities and reversible beneficial effects deter long-term therapy.

POSTOPERATIVE CARE

Postoperative care is just as crucial as treatment planning. Airway patency and flap survival are the greatest concerns beyond co-morbid conditions in the early period of the hospital stay. After this time, the need for inpatient and outpatient supportive care depends on patient homeostasis. Follow-up for recurrence and secondary prevention should be understood by the patient to be equally as important as surgical intervention.

EARLY

Intensive care is needed for the first 4 to 8 hours to provide invasive monitoring, vasoactive support, pain control, and if needed, airway patency with tracheotomy and ventilator support, as well as repetitive flap evaluation with the help of anesthesiologists and dedicated patient-skilled nursing. The duration of intensive care may differ, with short procedures involving minimal reconstruction or patients without co-morbid conditions generally having a shorter course of intensive care.

During first week, vigilant observation for flap survival is paramount. Anticoagulation protocols are numerous and contentious in their differences, similar to fluid management. Administration of blood products necessitates a delicate balance between cardiopulmonary status and volume resuscitation.

Though considered a convalescence period, the first 30 days after hospital discharge are also crucial for patient compliance. Diligent wound care, nutritional support, dental prophylaxis, and proper referral to medical and radiation oncology cannot be delayed.

LATE

Outpatient follow-up is especially important in the first 2 years after surgery. A rapport must be developed with the patient and family to ensure early detection of recurrence and second primaries. A follow-up protocol (Table 53-5) with appropriate non-invasive diagnostic studies provides the best surveillance of patients without overt signs and symptoms. PET is advantageous for detecting recurrent disease at the 6-month postoperative interval. US for questionable regional metastases is an inexpensive alternative if interpreted with

skill. Patients undergoing radiation therapy for high-risk disease benefit from investigation of thyroid-stimulating hormone since thyroid function declines. Dental prophylaxis and rehabilitation deter misadventures with osteoradionecrosis and improve function, respectively.

PEARLS AND PITFALLS

- Verrucous SCC and basaloid SCC are less and more aggressive, respectively, but should be treated in a similar manner.
- Neck observation is indicated for patients with N0 disease; also known as "watch and wait," observation is for future neck disease but should be avoided in patients with lesions greater than 4 mm in depth.
- The perifacial node deserves attention in all neck dissections for oral cavity malignancy. It is identified by palpating above the inferior aspect of the mandible during level IB dissection and violating the superficial layer of deep cervical fascia superficially near the marginal mandibular nerve.
- A pathologic report should dictate treatment, especially when used as a staging procedure. This information should never be equivocal when used for decision making.
- If a marginal mandibulectomy margin is positive, the patient should undergo repeated resection, not radiation therapy.
- A clinical subset of tongue carcinomas can be considerably tenacious. Such lesions should be treated aggressively with wide clear margins and extended (levels I to IV) neck dissection. If the surgical margin exhibits microscopic disease of even less than 5 mm (i.e., "close margin"), additional excision of the margin would be more prudent than radiation therapy for early-stage disease.
- Delay in detection is often possible in cases of recurrence because of disease hidden under bulky reconstructive flaps.
- The "lost to follow-up" period, or the first 24 months, is the most common time for recurrences and second primaries. The time during radiation therapy should not be used as an excuse to defer visits to the ablative surgeon.
- Postoperative airway management is paramount. Previous tracheotomy should not be a second guess.
- Clinicians should not be oblivious to patients' risk factors. Otherwise, recurrence is inevitable.

TABLE 53-5	Outpatient Surveillance
POSTOPERATIVE VISIT	**SCHEDULE**
0-3 months	Biweekly examination
3-12 months	Monthly examination
1-2 years	Examination every 2 months
2-4 years	Examination every 4 months
4-5 years	Examination every 6 months

REFERENCES

1. Neville BW, Day TA: Oral cancer and precancerous lesions, *CA Cancer J Clin* 52:195-215, 2002.
2. Shiu MN, Chen TH, Chang SH, et al: Risk factors for leukoplakia and malignant transformation to oral carcinoma: a leukoplakia cohort in Taiwan, *Br J Cancer* 82:1871-1874, 2000.
3. Bloching M, Reich W, Schubert J, et al: The influence of oral hygiene on salivary quality in the Ames test as a marker for genotoxic effects, *Oral Oncol* 43:933-939, 2007.
4. Enwonwu CO, Meeks VI: Bionutrition and oral cancer in humans, *Crit Rev Oral Biol Med* 6:5-17, 1995.
5. Chen IH, Chang JT, Liao CT, et al: Prognostic significance of EGFR and Her-2 in oral cavity cancer in betel quid prevalent areas on cancer prognosis, *Br J Cancer* 89:681-686, 2003.
6. Aziz SR: Oral submucous fibrosis: case report and review of diagnosis and treatment, *J Oral Maxillofac Surg* 66:2386-2389, 2008.

7. Dahlstrom KR, Little JA, Zafereo ME, et al: Squamous cell carcinoma of the head and neck in never smoker–never drinkers: a descriptive epidemiologic study, *Head Neck* 30:75-84, 2008.
8. Brown J: Mechanisms of cancer invasion of the mandible, *Curr Opin Otolaryngol Head Neck Surg* 11:96-102, 2003.
9. Brown JS, Lowe D, Kalavrezos N, et al: Patterns of invasion and routes of tumor entry into the mandible by oral squamous cell carcinoma, *Head Neck* 24:370-383, 2002.
10. Worthington P: The surgical approach to the pterygoid region, *Br J Oral Surg* 15:135-146, 1977.
11. Friedman WH, Katsantonis GP, Cooper MH, et al: Stylohamular dissection: a new method for en bloc reaction of malignancies of the infratemporal fossa, *Laryngoscope* 91:1869-1879, 1981.
12. Jian XC, Wang CX, Jiang CH: Surgical management of primary and secondary tumors in

the pterygopalatine fossa, *Otolaryngol Head Neck Surg* 132:90-94, 2005.
13. Li L, Gao XL, Song YZ, et al: Anatomy of arteries and veins of submandibular glands, *Chin Med J* 120:1179-1182, 2007.
14. Wang TM, Lin CL, Kuo KJ, et al: Surgical anatomy of the mandibular ramus of the facial nerve in Chinese adults, *Acta Anat* 142:126-131, 1991.
15. Lim YC, Lee JS, Choi EC: Perifacial lymph node metastasis in the submandibular triangle of patients with oral and oropharyngeal squamous cell carcinoma with clinically node-positive neck, *Laryngoscope* 116:2187-2190, 2006.
16. Lim YC, Kim JW, Koh YW, et al: Perivascular-submandibular lymph node metastasis in squamous cell carcinoma of the tongue and floor of mouth, *Eur J Surg Oncol* 30:692-698, 2004.
17. Davidson J, Gilbert R, Irish J, et al: The role of panendoscopy in the management of

mucosal head and neck malignancy—a prospective evaluation, *Head Neck* 22:449-454, discussion 454-455, 2000.

18. McGuirt WF: Panendoscopy as a screening examination for simultaneous primary tumors in head and neck cancer: a prospective sequential study and review of the literature, *Laryngoscopy* 92:569-576, 1982.

19. Benninger MS, Shariff A, Blazoff K: Symptom-directed selective endoscopy: long-term efficacy, *Arch Otolaryngol Head Neck Surg* 127:770-773, 2001.

20. Weissman JL, Carrau RL: "Puffed-cheek" CT improves evaluation of the oral cavity, *AJNR Am J Neuroradiol* 22:741-744, 2001.

21. Lam P, Au-Yeung K, Cheng P: Correlating MRI and histologic tumor thickness in the assessment of oral tongue cancer, *AJR Am J Roentgenol* 182:803-808, 2004.

22. Bolzoni A, Cappiello J, Piazza C, et al: Diagnostic accuracy of magnetic resonance imaging in the assessment of mandibular involvement in oral-oropharyngeal squamous cell carcinoma: a prospective study, *Arch Otolaryngol Head Neck Surg* 130:837-843, 2004.

23. Smallman LA, Young JA, Oates J: Fine needle aspiration cytology in the management of ENT patients, *J Laryngol Otol* 102:909-913, 1988.

24. Lopez R, Payoux P, Gantet P, et al: Multimodal image registration for localization of sentinel nodes in head and neck squamous cell carcinoma, *J Oral Maxillofac Surg* 62:1497-1504, 2004.

25. Stoeckli SJ: Sentinel node biopsy for oral and oropharyngeal squamous cell carcinoma of the head and neck, *Laryngoscope* 117:1539-1551, 2007.

26. Santaolalla F, Sanchez JM, Ereno C, et al: Non–sentinel node tumor invasion in oropharyngeal and oral cancer: risk of misdiagnosis of metastasis, *Acta Otolaryngol* 128:1159-1164, 2008.

27. Hayter JP, Vaughan ED, Brown JS: Aesthetic lip splits, *Br J Oral Maxillofac Surg* 34:432-435, 1996.

28. Rapidis AD, Valsamis S, Anterriotis DA, et al: Functional and aesthetic results of various lip-splitting incisions: a clinical analysis of 60 cases, *J Oral Maxillofac Surg* 59:1292-1296, 2001.

29. Slaughter DP, Southwick HW, Smejkal W: Field cancerization in oral stratified squamous epithelium; clinical implications of multicentric origin, *Cancer* 6:963-968, 1953.

30. Ball VA, Righi PD, Tejada E, et al: p53 immunostaining of surgical margins as a predictor of local recurrence in squamous cell carcinoma of the oral cavity and oropharynx, *Ear Nose Throat J* 76:818-823, 1997.

31. Ord RA, Aisner S: Accuracy of frozen sections in assessing margins in oral cancer resection, *J Oral Maxillofac Surg* 55:663-669, discussion 669-671, 1997.

32. Zupi A, Mangone GM, Piombino P, et al: Perineural invasion of the lower alveolar nerve by oral cancer: a follow-up study of 12 cases, *J Craniomaxillofac Surg* 26:318-321, 1998.

33. Ferlito A, Rinaldo A, Devaney KO, et al: Detection of lymph node micrometastases in patients with squamous carcinoma of the head and neck, *Eur Arch Otorhinolaryngol* 265:1147-1153, 2008.

34. Jewer DD, Boyd JB, Manktelow RT, et al: Orofacial and mandibular reconstruction with the iliac crest free flap: a review of 60 cases and a new method of classification, *Plast Reconstr Surg* 84:391-403, discussion 404-405, 1989.

35. Boyd JB, Gullane PJ, Rotstein LE, et al: Classification of mandibular defects, *Plast Reconstr Surg* 92:1266-1275, 1993.

36. Mukherji SK, Castelijns J, Castillo M: Squamous cell carcinoma of the oropharynx and oral cavity; how imaging makes a difference, *Semin Ultrasound CT MR* 19:463-475, 1998.

37. Munoz Guerra MF, Naval Gias L, Campo FR, et al: Marginal and segmental mandibulectomy in patients with oral cancer: a statistical analysis of 106 cases, *J Oral Maxillofac Surg* 61:1289-1296, 2003.

38. Brown J, Chatterjee R, Lowe D, et al: A new guide to mandibular resection for oral squamous cell carcinoma based on the Cawood and Howell classification of the mandible, *Int J Oral Maxillofac Surg* 34:834-839, 2005.

39. Hirsch DL, Dierks EJ: Use of a transbuccal technique for marginal mandibulectomy: a novel approach, *J Oral Maxillofac Surg* 65:1849-1851, 2007.

40. Alkureishi LW, Ross GL, Shoaib T, et al: Does tumor depth affect nodal upstaging in squamous cell carcinoma of the head and neck? *Laryngoscope* 118:629-634, 2008.

41. Weiss MH, Harrison LB, Isaacs RS: Use of decision analysis in planning a management strategy for the stage N0 neck, *Arch Otolaryngol Head Neck Surg* 120:699-702, 1994.

42. Shah JP, Candela FC, Poddar AK: The patterns of cervical lymph node metastases from squamous carcinoma of the oral cavity, *Cancer* 66:109-113, 1990.

43. McNeill R: Radical neck dissection: considerations in flat design, *J Laryngol Otol* 92:591-596, 1978.

44. Omura S, Bukawa H, Kawabe R, et al: Comparison between hockey stick and reversed hockey stick incision: gently curved single linear neck incisions for oral cancer, *Int J Oral Maxillofac Surg* 28:197-202, 1999.

45. Yii NW, Patel SG, Williamson P, et al: Use of apron flap incision for neck dissection, *Plast Reconstr Surg* 103:1655-1660, 1999.

46. Acar A, Dursun G, Aydin O, et al: J incision in neck dissections, *J Laryngol Otol* 112:55-60, 1998.

47. Taghinia AH, Movassaghi K, Wang AX, et al: Reconstruction of the upper aerodigestive tract with the submental artery flap, *Plast Reconstr Surg* 123:562-570, 2009.

48. Chow TL, Chan TT, Chow TK, et al: Reconstruction with submental flap for aggressive orofacial cancer, *Plast Reconstr Surg* 120:431-436, 2007.

49. Martin D, Pascal JF, Baudet J: The submental island flap: a new donor site. Anatomy and clinical applications as a free or pedicled flap, *Plast Reconstr Surg* 92:867-873, 1993.

50. Joshi A, Rajendraprasad JS, Shetty K: Reconstruction of intraoral defects using facial artery musculomucosal flap, *Br J Plast Surg* 58:1061-1066, 2005.

51. Hatoko M, Kuwahara M, Tanaka A, et al: Use of facial artery musculomucosal flap for closure of soft tissue defects of the mandibular vestibule, *Int J Oral Maxillofac Surg* 31:210-211, 2002.

52. Pribaz JJ, Meara JG, Wright S, et al: Lip and vermilion reconstruction with the facial artery musculomucosal flap, *Plast Reconstr Surg* 105:864-872, 2000.

53. Lyons AJ: Perforator flaps in head and neck surgery, *Int J Oral Maxillofac Surg* 35:199-207, 2006.

54. Mateev M, Beermanov K, Subanova L, et al: Reconstruction of soft tissue defects of the hand using the shape-modified radial forearm flap, *Scand J Plast Reconstr Surg Hand Surg* 38:228-231, 2004.

55. Boyd J, Brain MD: Shape-modified method using the radial forearm perforator flap for reconstruction of soft-tissue defects of the scalp, *J Reconstr Microsurg* 21:21-24, 2005.

56. Leiggener C, Messo E, Thor A, et al: A selective laser sintering guide for transferring a virtual plan to real time surgery in composite mandibular reconstruction with free fibula osseous flaps, *Int J Oral Maxillofac Surg* 38:187-192, 2009.

57. Cabanillas R, Rodrigo JP, Llorente JL, et al: Oncologic outcomes of transoral laser surgery of supraglottic carcinoma compared with a transcervical approach, *Head Neck* 30:750-755, 2008.

58. Tewari M, Rai P, Singh GB, et al: Long-term follow-up results of Nd:YAG laser treatment of premalignant and malignant (stage I) squamous cell carcinoma of the oral cavity, *J Surg Oncol* 95:281-285, 2007.

59. Nguyen LN, Ang KK: Radiotherapy for cancer of the head and neck: altered fractionation regimens, *Lancet Oncol* 3:693-701, 2002.

60. Bernier J, Bentzen SM: Altered fractionation and combined radiochemotherapy approaches: pioneering new opportunities in head and neck oncology, *Eur J Cancer* 39:560-571, 2003.

61. Cooper JS, Pajak TF, Forastiere AA, et al: Postoperative concurrent radiotherapy and chemotherapy for high-risk squamous-cell carcinoma of the head and neck, *N Engl J Med* 350:1937-1944, 2004.

62. Fuchihata H, Murakami S, Kubo K: Results of combined external irradiation and chemotherapy of bleomycin and peplomycin for squamous cell carcinomas of the lower gingival, *Int J Radiat Oncol Biol Phys* 29:705-709, 1994.

63. Urba S, Worden F, Carey T, et al: One cycle of induction chemotherapy (IC) to select for organ preservation for patients (PTS) with advanced squamous carcinoma of the oral cavity (SCCOC) [abstract 5555], *J Clin Oncol* 23(Suppl):513s, 2005.

Chapter 54

Oral Squamous Cell Carcinoma: Management of the Neck

Tuan Giang Bui, R. Bryan Bell

The status of the cervical lymph nodes is the most important prognostic factor in squamous cell carcinoma (SCC) of the head and neck, and the clinical significance of regional nodal metastases has long been recognized. The overall survival rate decreases by approximately 50% in patients with metastases to the cervical lymph nodes.[1,2] Despite the progress made in patient education and early detection of SCC of the oral cavity, approximately 40% of patients will initially be found to have evidence of regional nodal metastasis.[2] Therefore, management of the cervical lymphatics is an important component of the overall treatment of patients with head and neck cancer.

ANATOMY

The head and neck drain into an extensive network of cervical lymphatics, and earlier studies demonstrated that this drainage pattern usually occurs in a predictable manner for each site.[3,4] Knowledge of the anatomy of the regional lymphatic system is therefore important for clinicians treating patients with head and neck cancer. To facilitate communication among the various disciplines involved, the Head and Neck Service at the Memorial-Sloan Kettering Cancer Center proposed a system in which the cervical lymphatic system is divided into levels corresponding to certain clinical and radiographic landmarks. Further modifications of this system resulted in a widely accepted method of defining the levels of the cervical lymphatic network that is endorsed by the American Head and Neck Society and the American Academy of Otolaryngology[5-8] (Fig. 54-1, Box 54-1).

CLASSIFICATION OF NECK DISSECTIONS

Robbins and co-workers defined a classification system outlining the various types of neck dissection.[7]

RADICAL NECK DISSECTION

Radical neck dissection (RND) involves the en bloc removal of all ipsilateral lymph nodes from levels I through V, along with the ipsilateral spinal accessory nerve (SAN), internal jugular vein (IJV), and sternocleidomastoid muscle (SCM).

MODIFIED RADICAL NECK DISSECTION

When one or more non-lymphatic structures are preserved during the dissection, the procedure is termed a modified radical neck dissection (MRND). The basis for this modification is that the lymph node–containing tissues lie within the cervical fascial planes surrounding the SCM, IJV, and SAN and that these structures can be preserved if they are not involved with tumor by skeletonizing them during the dissection. MRND can be subclassified as follows: type I MRND preserves the SAN; type II MRND preserves the SAN and IJV; and type III MRND preserves the SAN, IJV, and SCM.

SELECTIVE NECK DISSECTION

In selective neck dissection (SND), one or more lymph node groups are preserved during cervical lymphadenectomy that are routinely removed with RND. The lymph node groups that are removed are dependent on the predictable patterns of metastases from the primary site. The levels of lymph nodes removed are identified (e.g., SND levels I to III).

EXTENDED NECK DISSECTION

With the removal of one or more lymph node groups or non-lymphatic structures, or both, that are not usually involved in RND, the procedure is termed extended neck dissection. Examples of lymph node groups include the parapharyngeal, paratracheal, and superior mediastinal nodes. Examples of non-lymphatic structures include the carotid artery, hypoglossal nerve, and paraspinal muscles.

MANAGEMENT OF NODE-POSITIVE NECKS

Oncologic principles dictate that the management of regional cervical nodal metastasis from head and neck cancer should involve removal of the diseased nodal groups and comprehensive clearance of all the remaining ipsilateral lymphatic groups.

RND was the initial form of comprehensive cervical lymphadenectomy and was popularized by Crile in 1906.[9] Further contributions by Martin[10] led to acceptance of RND as the standard operation for cervical lymphadenectomy in head and neck cancer, and it was the most common type of neck dissection performed until the 1960s. It has been proved to improve survival and is still considered the gold standard for management of metastasis to the cervical lymphatics.

However, because significant functional and cosmetic morbidity can be associated with removal of the SCM, IJV, and SAN,[11] modifications in RND were performed in the form of the MRND, as pioneered by Suarez, Bocca, Byers, and their colleagues.[12-15] Subsequent studies have demonstrated that MRND is as effective for regional control as RND in treating metastases to the cervical lymphatics in head and neck cancer.[16,17] MRND became the accepted standard for surgical management of cervical disease, although RND still has a role in cases in which the SAN, IJV, or SCM is involved.

Some surgeons advocate the use of SND even in the presence of nodal disease, although this contradicts the oncologic principles of en bloc excision of all ipsilateral cervical lymphatics. This remains a controversial topic. The reasoning for the use of SND in

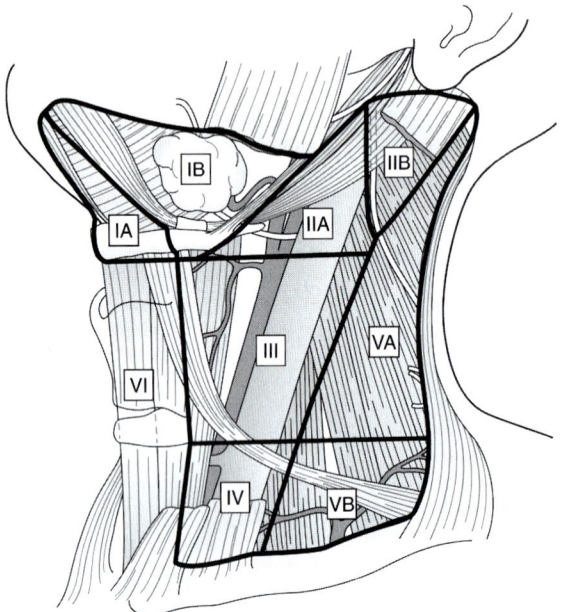

Fig. 54-1 ■ Levels and sublevels of the neck. (From Cheng A, Schmidt BL: Management of the N0 neck in oral squamous cell carcinoma, *Oral Maxillofac Surg Clin North Am* 20:477-497, 2008.)

node-positive necks is based on studies demonstrating the patterns of metastasis to the cervical lymphatics from various primary sites.[1,18] For instance, cancers originating from the oropharynx, hypopharynx, and larynx have a predilection to metastasize to levels II to IV. Oral cavity cancers have a tendency to metastasize to levels I to III. Furthermore, for oral cavity cancers that have spread to level I, II, or III, the risk for involvement of level IV increases from 3% to 17%; however, the risk for level V involvement increases from only 1% to 6%.[18] Therefore, for oral cavity cancers that have spread to the neck, surgical excision of levels I to IV will remove the majority of nodal metastases, and multiple studies have demonstrated good locoregional control rates with SND for node-positive necks.[17-21] Typically, SND of levels I to III is performed for oral cavity cancer and SND of levels II to IV for oropharyngeal, hypopharyngeal, and laryngeal cancer. If there is a suspicious node involved at the lowest level, it is recommended that the dissection be extended to include the next level. However, this may not apply to nodes involved in level IV because there is evidence that lymphatic flow does not occur from the jugular chain to the posterior triangle.[21] It is important to note that SND is not indicated in certain patients, specifically, those with massive adenopathy, clinical evidence of gross extracapsular spread, nodal fixation, previous neck surgery, or previous neck irradiation.[21]

Currently, MRND is the mainstay of surgical treatment of node-positive necks. However, there is evidence that the use of SND

<table>
<tr><td colspan="2">BOX 54-1   Division of the Cervical Lymphatic System into Levels Corresponding to Certain Clinical and Radiographic Landmarks</td></tr>
</table>

- Level I: Extends from the hyoid bone inferiorly to the inferior border of the mandible superiorly and bounded by the digastric muscle. The submental and submandibular nodes lie in this level. It is further subdivided into
  - Level Ia (submental group): Bounded by the anterior bellies of the digastric muscle and extends from the hyoid bone to the symphysis of the mandible.
  - Level Ib (submandibular group): Triangular area bounded by the posterior and anterior bellies of the digastric muscle and the body of the mandible. Includes the lymph nodes along the facial artery adjacent to the submandibular gland.
- Level II (upper jugular group): Contains nodes that surround the upper third of the internal jugular vein and the spinal accessory nerve. The jugulodigastric node lies here, which is the most common node for metastasis of squamous cell carcinoma of the oral cavity. This level can be subdivided based on the spinal accessory nerve:
  - Level IIa: Extends from the base of the skull superiorly to the hyoid bone (radiographic) or carotid bifurcation (clinical) inferiorly. It is bounded anteriorly by the lateral aspect of the sternohyoid muscle and posteriorly by a vertical plane defined by the course of the spinal accessory nerve.
  - Level IIb: Extends from the base of the skull superiorly to the hyoid bone (radiographic) or carotid bifurcation (clinical) inferiorly. It is bounded anteriorly by a vertical plane defined by the course of the spinal accessory nerve and posteriorly by the lateral edge of the sternocleidomastoid muscle.
- Level III (mid-jugular group): Contains nodes that encompass the middle third of the internal jugular vein. It is bounded superiorly by the hyoid bone (radiographic) or the carotid bifurcation (clinical) and inferiorly by the cricoid cartilage (radiographic) or the omohyoid muscle (clinical). Anteriorly, it extends to the lateral aspect of the sternohyoid muscle, and its posterior limit is the lateral edge of the sternocleidomastoid muscle. The juguloomohyoid node lies at this level.

- Level IV (lower jugular group): Contains nodes surrounding the inferior third of the internal jugular vein. It extends from the inferior border of level III to the clavicle. Anteriorly it is bounded by the lateral aspect of the sternohyoid muscle, and posteriorly it is bounded by the lateral edge of the sternocleidomastoid muscle. Of note, this level is rarely involved in oral cavity squamous cell carcinoma unless one of the higher-echelon nodes is involved ([1]).
- Level V (posterior triangle group): Contains nodes around the inferior portion of the spinal accessory nerve and transverse cervical vessels. Similar to level IV nodes, these nodes are not usually involved in oral cavity squamous cell carcinoma unless there is metastasis to the upper-echelon nodes ([1]). It can be subdivided into
  - Level Va: The superior border is the junction of the sternocleidomastoid and trapezius muscles. The inferior border is determined by a horizontal line drawn at the level of the cricoid cartilage. The anterior border is the lateral edge of the sternocleidomastoid muscle. Posteriorly, it extends to the medial aspect of the trapezius muscle.
  - Level Vb: The superior border is determined by a horizontal line drawn at the level of the cricoid cartilage. The clavicle represents the inferior border. The anterior border is the lateral edge of the sternocleidomastoid muscle. Posteriorly, it extends to the medial aspect of the trapezius muscle.
- Level VI (central compartment group): Extends from the hyoid bone superiorly to the suprasternal notch inferiorly. It lies between the medial borders of the carotid sheaths bilaterally. These nodes are rarely involved in oral cavity squamous cell carcinoma.
- Level VII (superior mediastinal group): Extends from the suprasternal notch to the innominate artery and includes the lymph nodes in the anterior superior mediastinum. Rarely involved in oral cavity squamous cell carcinoma.

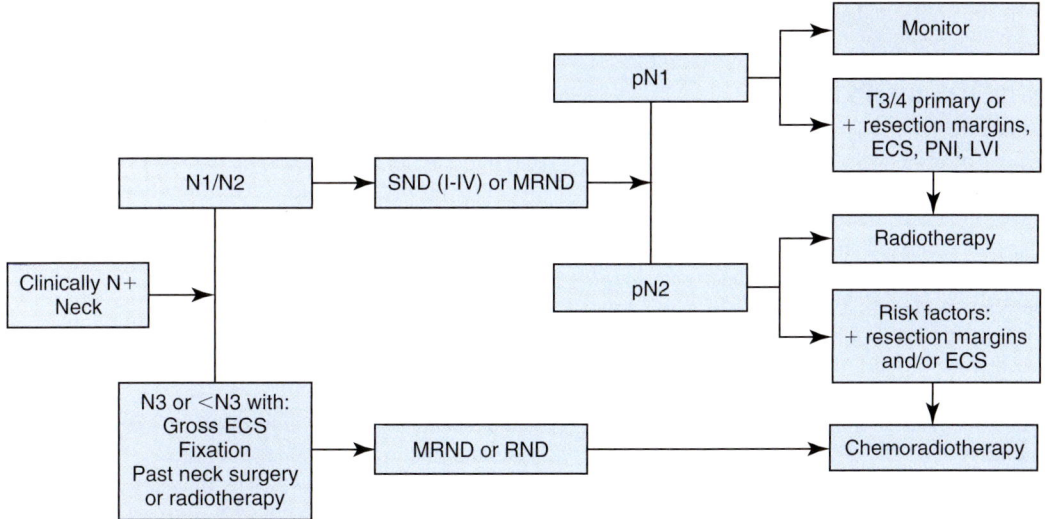

Fig. 54-2 ■ Management of clinically positive necks. (From Nikolarakos D, Bell RB: Management of the node-positive neck in oral cancer, *Oral Maxillofac Surg Clin North Am* 20:499-511, 2008.) *ECS,* Extracapsular spread; *PNI,* perineural invasion; *LVI,* lymphovascular invasion.

may be appropriate in select cases. A comprehensive review by Nikolarakos and co-authors discusses the management of node-positive necks in patients with oral SCC[22] (Fig. 54-2).

MANAGEMENT OF NODE-NEGATIVE NECKS

Treatment of a clinically node-negative neck (cN0) in a patient with oral SCC presents a significant dilemma to the head and neck oncologic surgeon. As mentioned previously, the presence of neck metastases reduces the 5-year survival rate by almost 50%. Studies have demonstrated that occult metastasis occurs in approximately 20% to 45% of patients who were clinically staged as N0.[23-27] This has led to the option of performing elective neck dissection (END) in patients with no clinical evidence of nodal metastases. However, this may lead to 55% to 80% of patients undergoing unnecessary neck dissections, along with the associated morbidity, particularly postoperative shoulder dysfunction. Therefore, accurate staging of the regional lymph nodes is important for prognostic and diagnostic purposes. Currently, the debate centers around determining which patients will benefit from elective treatment of a cN0 neck and which patients can be managed with a close observation, "wait-and-see" approach. This section discusses the various management issues and options currently available.

DIAGNOSTIC MODALITIES

The decision of when to electively treat a cN0 neck might be facilitated if there were an accurate, non-invasive method of determining the presence of occult nodal metastases.

The use of clinical examination alone to detect occult nodal metastasis has been proved to be inadequate, even by experienced clinicians. Studies evaluating the effectiveness of clinical palpation of the neck for nodal metastases have reported specificities and sensitivities ranging from 60% to 80%.[28] One study demonstrated the negative predictive value (NPV) of clinical examination to be only 55% in assessing for nodal metastasis from oral tongue cancer.[23]

Various anatomic imaging techniques have been used in an attempt to detect the 20% to 45% of cN0 necks that may harbor occult nodal metastases. The common techniques used are computed tomography (CT), magnetic resonance imaging (MRI), and ultrasound. However, the radiologic changes associated with nodal metastasis (e.g., central necrosis, cystic changes) are rarely seen in nodes with microscopic, occult disease. Furthermore, the orientation of the long axis of individual nodes is variable in different regions of the neck, thereby making it difficult to accurately identify their dimensions radiologically.[26] Therefore, distinguishing between a reactive lymph node and one that is infiltrated with tumor can be difficult.

Contrast-enhanced CT and MRI have been shown to produce similar results in assessing for occult nodal metastases, with sensitivities ranging from 56% to 85% and specificities from 47% to 95%.[29-32]

Ultrasound can be advantageous because it can readily be used to guide fine-needle aspiration biopsy (UGFNAB). However, for an N0 neck, studies have shown that the sensitivity of UGFNAB ranges from just 48% to 76%.[33-35] One study from a group advocating the use of UGFNAB along with the "wait-and-see" approach for the management of N0 necks found that lymph node metastasis developed in 21% of the patients during follow-up, with a salvage rate of 79% after therapeutic neck dissection and postoperative radiation therapy, for an overall regional control rate of 88%.[36] The disparity between the studies may be due to operator experience, with UGFNAB possibly requiring a high level of technical skill.

Positron emission tomography (PET) in combination with CT is a relatively new technology that is being used to evaluate patients with head and neck SCC. PET scans by themselves have been shown to be more sensitive than CT or MRI in identifying primary tumors and metastatic neck disease.[32] By combining PET with CT, the hope is to obtain better anatomic localization of the lesions[37] and thus improve the sensitivity of the study. However, a prospective study evaluating the use of PET/CT for detecting regional nodal metastasis in cN0 necks demonstrated a sensitivity for detection of disease of 67% and a specificity of 95%.[38] Based on the findings, the authors concluded that they do not recommend the use of PET/CT alone in the management of cN0 necks. Furthermore, the radiation exposure from PET/CT scans is associated with a small, but real risk for the development of a second cancer.[39]

Thus, although these modalities may be useful adjuncts in the diagnostic management of cN0 necks in patients with head and neck SCC, they are not sensitive enough to replace END for histopathologic staging as the gold standard for staging of head and neck SCC.

SENTINEL LYMPH NODE BIOPSY

Sentinel lymph node biopsy (SLNB) is described as an intermediate option for the management of cN0 necks, one that is between the close observation ("wait and see") and elective treatment groups.[40] It is potentially less morbid than neck dissection and can effectively stage the neck. SLNB is a concept based on the principle that cancers spread to regional lymph nodes in a predictable manner and that if the upper-echelon nodes can be identified and analyzed accurately, this will give valuable information regarding the status of the rest of the neck.[41] Radioactive tracers or blue dye (or both) is injected around the periphery of the primary tumor site, and with the use of lymphoscintigraphy and intraoperative gamma probes, the sentinel nodes are identified and harvested. These nodes then undergo comprehensive histopathologic analysis involving routine hematoxylin-eosin staining and immunohistochemistry, and the assumption is that if these nodes are negative for any tumor deposits, the rest of the neck is less likely to harbor any further metastases.[41]

The concept of SLNB was described in the 1960s, and its efficacy in the treatment of malignant melanoma and breast cancer has been well documented.[40-45] This tool has recently been applied to the management of cN0 necks in patients with head and neck SCC, and multiple pilot studies have demonstrated promising results.

A European prospective, multicenter trial investigated 227 patients who underwent SLNB alone or in conjunction with END.[46] These patients had T1/T2 SCC of the oral cavity or oropharynx and were clinically staged as N0. SLNB was successful in identifying a sentinel node in 93% of cases, with a rate of 83% for tumors of the floor of the mouth and 96% for all other sites. The difference may be due to the close proximity of tumors in the floor of the mouth to the draining nodes. An average of 2.8 nodes were identified per patient. Thirty-four percent of the cases were upstaged, and the sensitivity for the SLNB-alone group was 91%. They concluded, based on these preliminary results, that SLNB can be used alone to clinically stage N0 necks in most patients with T1/T2 SCC of the oral cavity and oropharynx, with those of the floor of the mouth being more difficult.

A subsequent North American prospective, multicenter trial investigated 140 patients with T1/T2 oral SCC and cN0 necks.[40] These patients underwent SLNB in conjunction with END. The average number of sentinel nodes harvested was three per patient. They found an overall NPV of 0.96 for SLNB, with no statistically significant difference between the various sites of the primary tumor. They did, however, find that the NPV was higher for T1 (NPV = 1) than for T2 (NPV = 0.94) tumors. They concluded that it may be reasonable to initiate clinical studies involving just SLNB and perform completion neck dissection only in patients with positive sentinel nodes.

A meta-analysis of 19 articles evaluating the effectiveness of SLNB in patients with head and neck SCC demonstrated an identification rate of 97.7% for sentinel nodes.[41] The overall sensitivity was 92.6%, and analysis of the potential outcomes (e.g., recurrence, death, disease-free survival) for SLNB versus END showed the cumulative payoff for the SLNB group to be about 1% lower than that for the END group.

Drawbacks of this method include subjecting patients to a second operation for formal therapeutic neck dissection if the sentinel nodes are found to harbor tumor deposits on histopathologic review. Furthermore, the close proximity of some primary tumors (e.g., floor of the mouth) to the upper-echelon nodes can make it difficult to identify the sentinel nodes in this region, with scatter from the primary tumor obscuring readings of the nodes by the gamma probe. In addition, some of the nodes may be small and not readily accessible.[47]

The use of SLNB can be a viable option for the management of cN0 necks in patients with early-stage SCC of the head and neck and may eventually prove to be the solution to the debate involving the close observation and elective treatment approaches. However, further studies are required to definitively demonstrate its clinical effectiveness, and a more standardized technique must be implemented among the various institutions.

PROGNOSTIC VARIABLES FOR NODAL METASTASIS

A retrospective cohort study of 105 patients with cN0 necks demonstrated that occult nodal metastasis occurred in 34% of the patients.[27] Tumor thickness was the only independent predictor of nodal metastases, with thin (≤5 mm) and thick (>5 mm) tumors having a 10% and 46% risk, respectively, for the development of nodal metastases ($P = .001$). Other variables, including the primary site, perineural invasion, lymphovascular invasion, histopathologic grading, and T stage, were not shown to independently predict nodal metastases on multivariate analysis. A thorough study by Yuen and colleagues evaluated multiple possible prognostic factors for nodal metastases in patients with oral tongue SCC and concluded that tumor thickness was the only independent predictor of nodal metastases.[48] Similarly, Warburton and co-workers found that tumor thickness is the only statistically significant independent predictor for nodal metastases in oral cavity SCC.[49]

Although tumor thickness has consistently been shown to be an independent risk factor for occult nodal metastasis, no uniform depth has been agreed on as the cutoff for prescribing elective neck treatment in patients with early-stage cancers, with the range of thickness in the literature being 1.5 to 8.0 mm.[27,48-54] There are many possible explanations for this discrepancy, such as variability in the method of measuring tumor thickness, the specimen fixation method used, or inaccurate sampling of the tumor by incisional biopsy.[49,50]

RADIATION VERSUS SURGERY

When the decision is made to electively treat a cN0 neck, options include radiation therapy or surgical lymphadenectomy. Although radiation therapy has been shown to be an effective modality for primary treatment of the neck,[55,56] surgery is still the preferred method of treatment in most instances.

One reason is that surgery allows histopathologic analysis of the nodes, thus leading to more accurate staging of the cancer and determination of potential further treatment requirements.

Another factor influencing the decision to choose either radiation therapy or surgery is the choice of treatment of the primary tumor. For instance, since radiation is usually chosen to treat cancers of the oropharynx, nasopharynx, hypopharynx, and larynx, it would make sense to also treat a cN0 neck with elective radiation therapy. However, for SCC of the oral cavity, surgery is usually the primary modality of treatment because of its lower morbidity and better control rates.[57,58] In these instances, END is generally performed concomitant with surgical resection of the primary cancer. Moreover, in cases in which microvascular free flap reconstruction of the residual primary defect is required, END can be performed since the neck will usually need to be accessed for microvascular anastomoses.

There is also the issue of recurrence, which for oral cavity SCC can be on the order of 4% to 6%.[59,60] Therefore, if radiation therapy is used as the initial primary treatment modality for early SCC of the oral cavity, this will exhaust its use in the event of future recurrence. Furthermore, surgical salvage for recurrent cancer in an irradiated field can be very challenging.

Radiation therapy also has potentially significant morbidity associated with the treatment, including osteoradionecrosis, mucositis, xerostomia, dysphagia, subcutaneous fibrosis, and poor wound healing.[61-63] This can lead to a more prolonged and difficult recovery than occurs with END.

Thus, for various reasons, the primary treatment of cN0 necks in patients with early-stage SCC of the oral cavity is surgical lymphadenectomy, although radiation therapy has its role in select cases.

ELECTIVE NECK DISSECTION

The question of what is the appropriate extent of neck dissection for cN0 necks has been studied extensively. As mentioned previously, MRND is currently the main form of neck dissection performed for node-positive necks. However, for cN0 necks, MRND may be too aggressive based on studies demonstrating the predictable manner of cervical metastatic lymphatic drainage for different subsites in the head and neck.[1,18] Specifically, SCC of the oral cavity tended to spread to levels I to III of the neck, with only 3% to 9% spreading to level IV and 1% level V.[1,18] Moreover, a positive node present in levels I to III increased the risk for spread to level IV by 17% and spread to level V by 6%. SCC in the oropharynx, hypopharynx, and larynx tended to metastasize to levels II to IV.[1,18] In addition, studies have demonstrated locoregional control rates for SND groups to be similar to those for MRND or RND groups.[17,19-21] The morbidity associated with neck dissection is less for SND than for MRND or RND, primarily as a result of sparing of the SAN during dissection.[64]

One study found that there was a 15% chance of "skip metastases" to level IV in oral cavity SCC and recommended that level IV be included in the neck dissection for these tumors,[15] although this has not been corroborated in other studies.

Therefore, the recommended extent of neck dissection in a cN0 neck is in the form of SND, namely, levels I to III for oral cavity SCC and levels II to IV for SCC of the oropharynx, hypopharynx, and larynx.

Some authors have advocated observation of cN0 necks. It appears, however, that patients in whom SCC recurs may have a worse prognosis than those whose cervical metastasis is identified at the time of surgical resection of the primary tumor. In the authors' opinion, there is currently sufficient evidence to warrant the use of SLNB as an alternative to "watch and wait" for even the smallest and most superficial of oral and oropharyngeal SCCs. Prospective, randomized controlled clinical trials are necessary, however, before widespread acceptance of SLNB as a stand-alone procedure for all cN0 necks.

Technique

The technique for type III MRND will be discussed here. MRND has come to replace RND as the standard neck dissection in most cases. Modifications to the MRND can be easily adapted in cases of RNDs or SNDs. Descriptions of the various forms of neck dissections are available in surgical textbooks or atlases.[65] The technique described here pertains to the authors' preferences, although there are multiple ways to perform MRND.

The patient is positioned supine on the operating table with the use of a Mayfield head holder. Slight hyperextension of the neck can make the dissection easier.

Several types of skin incisions have been described for neck dissections in oncologic procedures[13,65,66] (Fig. 54-3). The authors prefer to use a straight-line incision, which has been described previously[66] (Fig. 54-4). This incision allows adequate access to

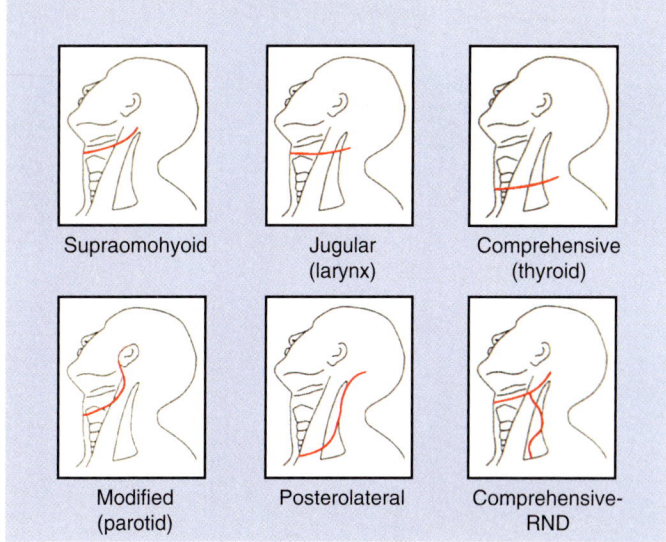

Fig. 54-3 ■ Common incisions for neck dissections. (From Shah JP, Patel SG: *Head and neck surgery and oncology*, ed 3, New York, 2003, Mosby.)

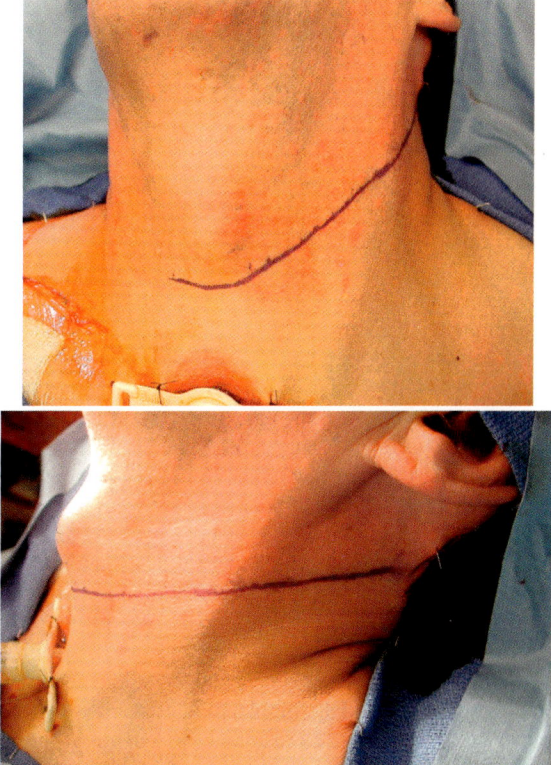

Fig. 54-4 ■ Straight-line neck incision placed 1 cm inferior to the thyroid lamina with a 1-cm paramedian extension into the contralateral neck. (From Kademani D, Dierks EJ: A straight-line incision for neck dissection: technical note, *J Oral Maxillofac Surg* 63:563-565, 2005.)

levels I to V. Various modifications of the incision are performed as needed, such as a lip-split technique to allow better access to the oral cavity.

The straight-line incision is performed in the mid-neck level, starting from the posterior neck hairline and extending across the midline for several centimeters at a level just superior to the cricoid cartilage. It is important to place the incision at least two to three fingerbreadths below the inferior border of the mandible to preserve

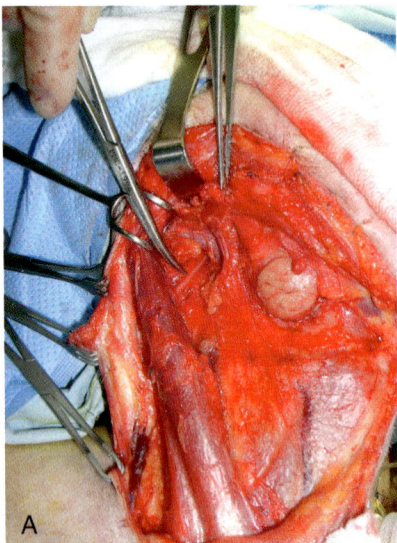 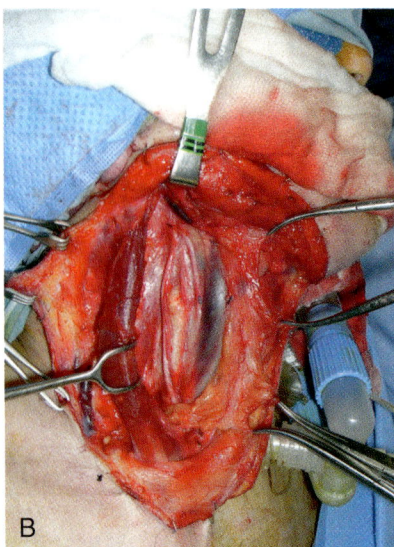 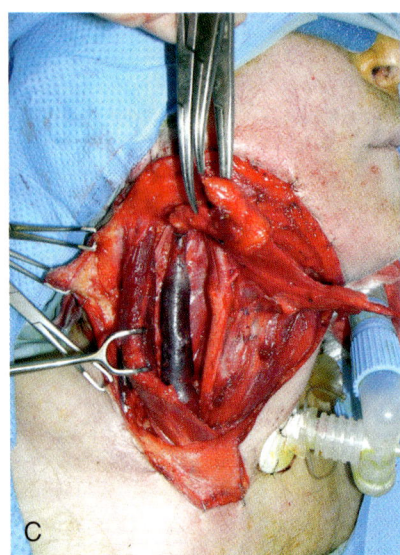

Fig. 54-5 ■ Modified radical neck dissection. **A,** Superficial layer of the deep cervical fascia elevated off the submandibular gland and medial dissection of the sternocleidomastoid muscle to identify the spinal accessory nerve. **B,** Dissection of fibroadipose tissues to visualize the carotid arteries, internal jugular vein, vagus nerve, and hypoglossal nerve (2 cm above the carotid bifurcation). **C,** Almost complete modified radical neck dissection with only the level I compartment remaining. The superior thyroid artery can be seen branching off the external carotid artery.

the marginal mandibular branch of the facial nerve. For a better cosmetic result, the incision can be placed along a natural skin crease.

The incision is made deep to the platysma muscle, and superior and inferior skin flaps are elevated in a subplatysmal plane toward the inferior border of the mandible and the clavicle, respectively. The platysma muscle is absent posteriorly, so dissection should proceed in a subcutaneous plane while staying superficial to the external jugular vein and greater auricular nerve. Care must be taken to not injure the SAN during elevation of the skin flaps posteriorly since the nerve exits the posterior aspect of the SCM in a subcutaneous plane. Maintaining the skin flaps under good tension perpendicular to the neck allows easier flap elevation.

Attention is then turned to protecting the marginal mandibular nerve. This nerve lies within the superficial layer of the deep cervical fascia and can be identified along its course, dissected free, and retracted superiorly. It can also be protected by elevating the superficial layer of the deep cervical fascia off the underlying submandibular gland, starting at a level approximately 2 cm below the inferior border of the mandible. Alternatively, the facial vein can be divided inferiorly and retracted cephalad. Dissection along the plane between the facial vein and the submandibular gland will protect the marginal mandibular nerve. Occasionally, at this point the prevascular nodes can be dissected free and sent off as a separate specimen since it may be difficult to keep them in continuity with the main specimen.

The fascia along the anterior border of the SCM is dissected along its length from the clavicle up to the mastoid process and is reflected medially. The external jugular vein may need to be divided. The fascial attachments of the SCM to the angle of the mandible are also divided. Dissection proceeds along the medial aspect of the SCM, with continued medial traction on the tissues. Tiny vessel branches to the SCM from the occipital and superior thyroid arteries may need to be divided. The SAN is identified by blunt spreading of tissue in the direction of the nerve's course, and it is dissected from its entry point to the SCM cephalad to the level of the posterior belly of the digastric muscle (Fig. 54-5, *A*). A decision must be made at this point whether to include nodes from level IIb. If they are to

be included in the dissection, the SAN must be carefully dissected free from the surrounding fibroadipose tissue. A vein retractor is used to gently retract the SAN, and the fibroadipose tissue from level IIb is dissected free and passed underneath the SAN to be included as part of the specimen.

Dissection now proceeds in the posterior triangle. Care must be taken to not injure the SAN as it exits the posterior edge of the SCM. With the SCM retracted laterally, the fibroadipose tissue is dissected from the underlying tissue while staying superficial to the posterior compartment muscles and associated deep cervical fascia. With the use of hemostats, the fibroadipose tissue is retracted medially. Attempts can be made to preserve the cervical plexus rootlets during this part of the dissection; however, they can be sacrificed without causing any long-term sequelae. Dissection proceeds in this area from the level of the clavicle up to the SAN, with continued retraction of the tissues in a medial direction.

Next, dissection proceeds along the IJV, from the level of the clavicle to the posterior belly of the digastric muscle. The omohyoid muscle is usually divided, but it can also be dissected free and retracted. Branches from the IJV are ligated and divided as needed. Again, the tissues are retracted medially as one specimen.

The dissection continues along the carotid artery. The hypoglossal nerve, along with its branch, the descendens hypoglossi, can be identified as it courses across the carotid arteries approximately 2 cm above the carotid bifurcation (Fig. 54-5, *B*). Careful dissection is performed superficial to the hypoglossal nerve. More cephalad, the dissection follows the digastric muscle, which lies superficial to the carotid artery. The superior thyroid artery is identified, and it can also serve as a guide for the plane of dissection. Inferiorly, the dissection proceeds up along the superior belly of the omohyoid muscle toward the submental triangle while staying superficial to the strap muscles.

The final step in the operation is dissection of the level I compartment (Fig. 54-5, *C*). The tissues are dissected off the anterior belly of the digastric muscle and mylohyoid muscle. Small vessels in the submental triangle will need to be identified and ligated. A right-angle retractor is placed at the posterior aspect of the mylohyoid muscle to retract it anteriorly while the submandibular gland is retracted inferiorly. This maneuver allows identification of the lingual nerve. At this point the submandibular duct is ligated and divided. The secretomotor fibers from the lingual nerve to the gland are transected, and its accompanying blood vessel is ligated and divided. The facial artery is then ligated and divided to allow final delivery of the specimen.

Of note, SND of levels I to III is commonly performed in patients with oral cavity cancers and cN0 necks. The technique for SND of levels I to III is similar to that described for MRND, with a few modifications. First, the skin incision may not have to be as large for SND as for MRND. Second, the SAN does not need to be dissected free and manipulated during SND since nodes from level IIb

are not generally included in the dissection. In addition, the cervical plexus rootlets are not usually transected in SND because there is no dissection of the posterior triangle. Finally, the omohyoid muscle is not transected as part of SND. All of these modifications can theoretically make SND less morbid than MRND.

RND and extended RND are rarely performed today. They are generally reserved as a salvage operation following failed multimodal therapy in patients with head and neck SCC. When indicated, the technique is often simpler than the previously described "functional neck dissections" because the SCM, IJV, and SAN are included in the dissection while moving inferior to superior as noted in Figure 54-6. Occasionally, as non-lymphatic structures are

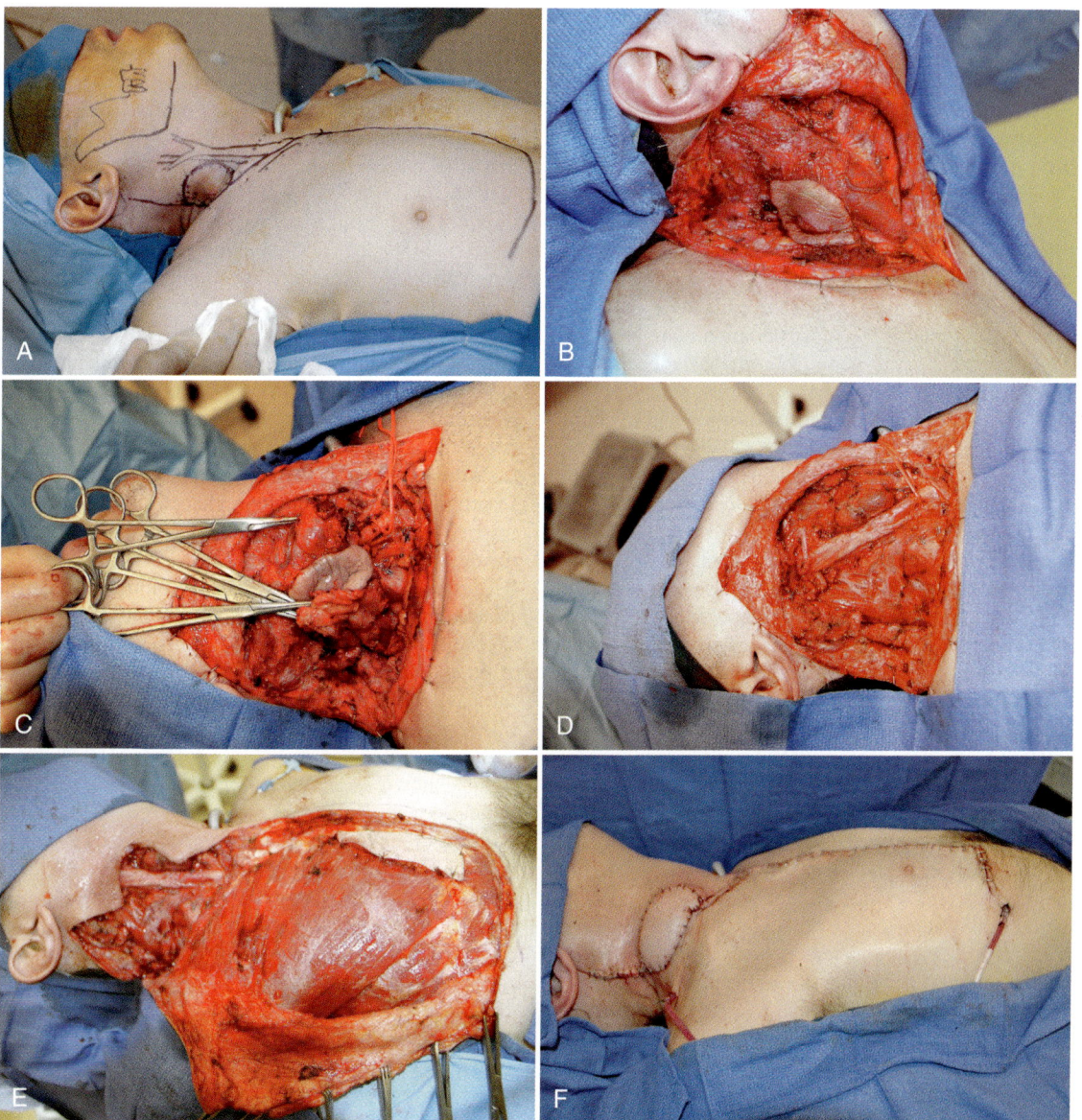

Fig. 54-6 ■ Extended radical neck dissection. **A,** Outline of the neck dissection to include sacrifice of the sternocleidomastoid muscle (SCM), spinal accessory nerve (SAN), and internal jugular vein (IJV), in addition to the skin of the neck. Because of the later non-lymphatic structure being included in the surgical salvage of this patient, the planned neck dissection is termed an "extended radical neck dissection," and soft tissue coverage with a pectoralis major myocutaneous flap is planned. **B,** The tumor-involved skin is included in the planned dissection as the flaps are developed in a subplatysmal plane. **C,** The fibroadipose lymphatic containing tissue from level IV is elevated off the carotid artery, along with the SCM and IJV. As the dissection proceeds cephalad, level V is included along with the SAN and levels I to III. **D,** Completed neck dissection with preservation of the hypoglossal nerve and carotid artery. **E,** Pectoralis major myocutaneous flap raised with a skin paddle corresponding to the cervical skin defect. **F,** Final closure.

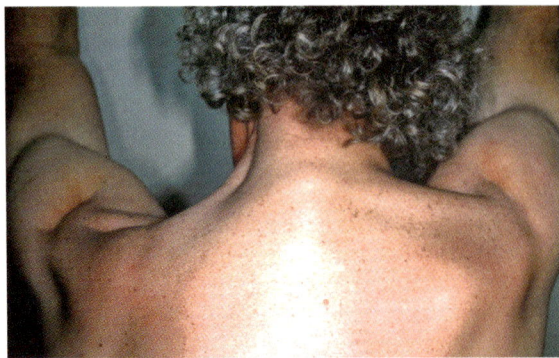

Fig. 54-7 ■ Injury to the spinal accessory nerve resulting in atrophy and contracture of the right trapezius muscle. (Courtesy Dr. Eric J. Dierks.)

sacrificed, soft tissue coverage with a pectoralis major myocutaneous flap or a microvascular free flap is advisable.

Complications

Fortunately, complications from neck dissections are relatively rare, especially since the inception of MRND and, more recently, SND. A brief review of some of the more common complications is presented here, and this topic has also previously been well summarized.[8]

Injury to the SAN can lead to shoulder dysfunction and result in the "shoulder syndrome," a condition characterized by shoulder pain, limitation of abduction, and scapular winging.[67] Studies have shown that the incidence of postoperative shoulder dysfunction is highest with RND and lowest with SND.[68,69] However, shoulder syndrome does not eventually develop in all patients in whom the SAN is sacrificed. Furthermore, preservation of the nerve does not guarantee that the patient will not have any shoulder dysfunction postoperatively. The extensive dissection and manipulation of the nerve can lead to significant postoperative morbidity. Patients should undergo a physiotherapy evaluation after neck dissection to determine whether any shoulder dysfunction is present and whether further rehabilitation is required (Fig. 54-7).

The hypoglossal nerve can also be injured during neck dissection, particularly in patients who have previously undergone neck irradiation or surgery because of extensive scarring and fibrosis of the soft tissues. The hypoglossal nerve can be inadvertently damaged during dissection around the carotid arteries. Immediate primary repair of the severed nerve can be attempted; however, most patients tolerate a unilateral hypoglossal nerve injury relatively well.

The marginal mandibular nerve can be damaged even though it had been appropriately protected by measures described earlier. Such injury is probably due to manual retraction of the nerve, which can lead to permanent dysfunction of the nerve, although more commonly the facial weakness is only temporary.

Injury to the lingual nerve usually occurs as a result of its involvement in the primary resection, but the nerve can also be injured at the time of dissection of the level I compartment if care is not taken to protect it. It is important to keep the lingual nerve in view at all times during removal of the contents in the submandibular triangle.

Much less common neurologic complications can involve injuries to the vagus nerve, phrenic nerve, brachial plexus, and cervical sympathetic chain. Damage to the vagus nerve can lead to unilateral vocal cord paresis and subsequent hoarseness. The vagus nerve is most at risk for injury during ligation of the IJV, and care must be taken to ensure that the IJV is circumferentially dissected before ligating it. Injuries to the phrenic nerve and brachial plexus are usually avoided since the dissection remains superficial to the deep cervical and prevertebral fascia. Horner syndrome can occur if the cervical sympathetic chain is damaged during dissection posterior to the carotid arteries, which is rarely indicated.

The thoracic duct lies posterior to the IJV deep in the left lower aspect of the neck. Extreme care must be taken during dissection of tissues in this area. If the IJV needs to be divided, it may be prudent to do so with a suture ligature. Injury to the thoracic duct is usually manifested as leakage of chyle, a cloudy white fluid, into the operative field. Maneuvers to increase intrathoracic pressure can confirm the presence of a chyle leak. If the injury is diagnosed intraoperatively, the duct can be oversewn with nonabsorbable suture, generally with the aid of loupes. Postoperatively, a chyle leak can be recognized as persistent drain output, drainage of milky fluid, or increased output of greater than 300 to 400 mL/day. The triglyceride content of the fluid can be compared with the serum value to confirm that it is indeed chyle. Initial attempts at management should be conservative and consist of a medium triglyceride diet, drainage of the fluid, and application of pressure. These conservative measures are generally adequate in treating most injuries to the thoracic duct. Surgical correction of persistent chyle leaks is usually difficult and frustrating to the surgeon. Preoperatively, the patient can be fed a diet rich in fat, such as cream, to increase chyle production and possibly help identify the leak intraoperatively. Attempts can be made to identify the area of the chyle leak in the wound bed and oversew the tissues; however, the use of vascularized tissues to cover the area offers the best chance of a successful outcome.

Wound infection usually occurs from an infected hematoma. Contributing factors include diabetes mellitus, immunocompromised status, preoperative radiotherapy, and communication with the oral cavity or pharynx.[70] The risk for postoperative infection can be reduced with the use of antibiotics postoperatively. First-generation cephalosporins or clindamycin given before the skin incision and continued for 24 hours postoperatively is the usual regimen. In cases of potential ongoing wound contamination, the antibiotics can be continued for more than 24 hours postoperatively.[8]

A disastrous complication is rupture of the carotid artery, commonly known as carotid blowout. Typically, this is preceded by a wound infection and necrosis of the overlying skin and is associated with an orocutaneous or pharyngocutaneous fistula.[70] A history of previous neck irradiation increases the risk for carotid blowout.[8] This complication can be prevented by coverage of the exposed carotid artery with vascularized tissue. In the event of carotid artery rupture, one should apply direct and constant pressure over the artery until emergency surgery in the operating room is commenced.[70]

SUMMARY

Management of the regional cervical lymphatics is an integral part of the treatment of cancers of the head and neck since the overall prognosis of patients depends on the extent of nodal involvement. Knowledge of the basic principles and techniques for managing the neck is imperative for all those involved in the care of these patients.

As our knowledge of SCC evolves, it is important to remain current on the newer concepts. Communication among the various disciplines is paramount while keeping in mind the goals of treatment: to improve survival and quality of life.

PEARLS AND PITFALLS

- Management of the lymph nodes of the neck is an important part of the overall treatment of head and neck cancers.
- Diagnostic imaging is a useful adjunct in management of the cervical lymph nodes.
- If possible, single-modality treatment of the primary tumor and neck is preferable (i.e., surgical lymphadenectomy of the neck if the primary tumor is to be resected).
- SLNB can be an intermediate option between the "wait and see" approach and surgical lymphadenectomy for a cN0 neck.
- Maintenance of one IJV is important to prevent postoperative swelling of the head and neck.
- Postoperative physical therapy can help prevent shoulder pain after neck dissection.
- Poor patient selection is a common cause of treatment failures in head and neck surgery.
- Inadequate perioperative nutritional status can have a negative impact on a patient's outcome.
- Lack of hemostasis can lead to hematoma formation and complicate postoperative healing.
- Failure to elevate skin flaps in a subplatysmal plane, especially in irradiated patients, can compromise their blood supply and lead to necrosis of the skin flaps.
- Failure to recognize and treat a major chyle leak can compromise a patient's recovery.
- Inadequate coverage of the carotid artery can lead to carotid blowout.

REFERENCES

1. Shah JP: Patterns of cervical lymph node metastasis from squamous carcinomas of the upper aerodigestive tract, *Am J Surg* 160:405-409, 1990.
2. Mendenhall WM, Million RR, Cassisi NJ: Elective neck irradiation in squamous cell carcinoma of the head and neck, *Head Neck Surg* 3:15-19, 1980.
3. Rouviere H: Lymphatic system of the head and neck. In Tobias MJ, editor. *Anatomy of the human lymphatic system*, Ann Arbor, MI, 1938, Edwards Brothers, pp 5-28.
4. Lindberg R: Distribution of cervical lymph node metastases from squamous cell carcinoma of the upper respiratory and digestive tracts, *Cancer* 29:1446-1449, 1972.
5. Robbins KT, Atkinson JL, Byers RM, et al: The use and misuse of neck dissection for head and neck cancer, *J Am Coll Surg* 193:91-102, 2001.
6. Pillsbury HC, Clark M: A rationale for therapy of the N0 neck. Joseph H. Ogura Lecture, *Laryngoscope* 107:1294-1315, 1997.
7. Robbins KT, Clayman G, Levine PA, et al: Neck dissection classification update, *Arch Otolaryngol Head Neck Surg* 128:751-758, 2002.
8. Holmes JD: Neck dissection: nomenclature, classification, and technique, *Oral Maxillofac Surg Clin North Am* 20:459-475, 2008.
9. Crile GW: Excision of cancer of the head and neck with special reference to the plane of dissection based upon one hundred thirty-two operations, *JAMA* 47:1780-1786, 1906.
10. Crile GW: Carcinoma of the jaws, tongue, cheek and lips, *Surg Gynecol Obstet* 36:159-162, 1923.
11. Short SO, Kaplan JN, Laramore GE, et al: Shoulder pain and function after neck dissection with or without preservation of the spinal accessory nerve, *Am J Surg* 148:478-482, 1984.
12. Ferlito A, Rinaldo A, Suarez O: Often-forgotten father of functional neck dissection (in the non–Spanish-speaking literature), *Laryngoscope* 114:1177-1188, 2004.
13. Bocca E, Pignataro O: A conservative technique in radical neck dissection, *Ann Otol Rhinol Laryngol* 76:975-987, 1967.

14. Suarez O: El problema de las metastasis linfaticas y alejadas del cancer de laringe e hipofaringe, *Rev Otorinolaringol* 23:83-99, 1963.
15. Byers RM, Weber RS, Andrews T, et al: Frequency and therapeutic implications of "skip metastases" in the neck from squamous carcinoma of the oral tongue, *Head Neck* 19:14-19, 1997.
16. Bocca E, Pignataro O, Oldini C, et al: Functional neck dissection: an evaluation and review of 843 cases, *Laryngoscope* 94:942-945, 1984.
17. Byers RM: Modified neck dissection. A study of 967 cases from 1970 to 1980, *Am J Surg* 150:414-421, 1985.
18. Shah JP, Candela FC, Poddar AK: The patterns of cervical lymph node metastases from squamous carcinoma of the oral cavity, *Cancer* 66:109-113, 1990.
19. Traynor SJ, Cohen JI, Gay J, et al: Selective neck dissection and the management of the node-positive neck, *Am J Surg* 172:654-657, 1996.
20. Ambrosch P, Kron M, Pradier O, et al: Efficacy of selective neck dissection: a review of 503 cases of elective and therapeutic treatment of the neck in squamous cell carcinoma of the upper aerodigestive tract, *Otolaryngol Head Neck Surg* 124:180-187, 2001.
21. Andersen PE, Warren F, Spiro J, et al: Results of selective neck dissection in the management of the node-positive neck, *Arch Otolaryngol Head Neck Surg* 128:1180-1184, 2002.
22. Nikolarakos D, Bell RB: Management of the node-positive neck in oral cancer, *Oral Maxillofac Surg Clin North Am* 20:499-511, 2008.
23. Byers RM, El-Nagger AK, Lee YY, et al: Can we detect or predict the presence of occult nodal metastases in patients with squamous carcinoma of the oral tongue? *Head Neck* 20:138-144, 1998.
24. Zbaren P, Nuyens M, Caversaccio M, et al: Elective neck dissection for carcinomas of the oral cavity: occult metastases, neck recurrences, and adjuvant treatment of pathologically positive necks, *Am J Surg* 191:756-760, 2006.

25. O'Brien CJ, Traynor SJ, McNeil E, et al: The use of clinical criteria alone in the management of the clinically negative neck among patients with squamous cell carcinoma of the oral cavity and oropharynx, *Arch Otolaryngol Head Neck Surg* 126:360-365, 2000.
26. Woolgar JA: Pathology of the N0 neck, *Br J Oral Maxillofac Surg* 37:205-209, 1999.
27. Clark JR, Naranjo N, Franklin JH, et al: Established prognostic variables in N0 oral carcinoma, *Otolaryngol Head Neck Surg* 135:748-753, 2006.
28. Takes RP: Staging of the neck in patients with head and neck squamous cell cancer: imaging techniques and biomarkers, *Oral Oncol* 40:656-667, 2004.
29. Adams S, Baum RP, Stuckensen T, et al: Prospective comparison of ^{18}F-FDG PET with conventional imaging modalities (CT, MRI, US) in lymph node staging of head and neck cancer, *Eur J Nucl Med* 25:1255-1260, 1998.
30. Di Martino E, Nowak B, Hassan HA, et al: Diagnosis and staging of head and neck cancer: a comparison of modern imaging modalities (positron emission tomography, computed tomography, color-coded duplex sonography) with panendoscopic and histopathologic findings, *Arch Otolaryngol Head Neck Surg* 126:1457-1461, 2000.
31. Hannah A, Scott AM, Tochon-Danguy H, et al: Evaluation of 18 F-fluorodeoxyglucose positron emission tomography and computed tomography with histopathologic correlation in the initial staging of head and neck cancer, *Ann Surg* 236:208-217, 2002.
32. Ng SH, Yen TC, Liao CT, et al: ^{18}F-FDG PET and CT/MRI in oral cavity squamous cell carcinoma: a prospective study of 124 patients with histologic correlation, *J Nucl Med* 46:1136-1143, 2005.
33. van den Brekel MW, Castelijns JA, Stel HV, et al: Occult metastatic neck disease: detection with US and US-guided fine-needle aspiration cytology, *Radiology* 180:457-461, 1991.
34. Takes RP, Righi P, Meeuwis CA, et al: The value of ultrasound with ultrasound-guided fine-needle aspiration biopsy compared to computed tomography in the detection of

regional metastases in the clinically negative neck, *Int J Radiat Oncol Biol Phys* 40:1027-1032, 1998.

35. Righi PD, Kopecky KK, Caldemeyer KS, et al: Comparison of ultrasound fine-needle aspiration and computed tomography in patients undergoing elective neck dissection, *Head Neck* 19:604-610, 1997.

36. Nieuwenhuis EJ, Castelijns JA, Pijpers R, et al: Wait-and-see policy for the N0 neck in early-stage oral and oropharyngeal squamous cell carcinoma using ultrasonography-guided cytology: is there a role for identification of the sentinel node? *Head Neck* 24:282-289, 2002.

37. Schoder H, Yeung HW, Gonen M, et al: Head and neck cancer: clinical usefulness and accuracy of PET/CT image fusion, *Radiology* 231:65-72, 2004.

38. Schoder H, Carlson DL, Kraus DH, et al: ^{18}F-FDG PET/CT for detecting nodal metastases in patients with oral cancer staged N0 by clinical examination and CT/MRI, *J Nucl Med* 47:755-762, 2006.

39. Wong WL, Batty V: Role of PET/CT in maxillo-facial surgery, *Br J Oral Maxillofac Surg* 47:259-267, 2009.

40. Civantos FJ, Zitsch RP, Schuller DE, et al: Sentinel lymph node biopsy accurately stages the regional lymph nodes for T1-T2 oral squamous cell carcinomas: results of a prospective multi-institutional trial, *J Clin Oncol* 28:1395-1400, 2008.

41. Paleri V, Rees G, Arullendran R, et al: Sentinel node biopsy in squamous cell cancer of the oral cavity and oral pharynx: a diagnostic meta-analysis, *Head Neck* 27:739-747, 2005.

42. Giuliano AE, Haigh PI, Brennan MB, et al: Prospective observational study of sentinel lymphadenectomy without further axillary dissection in patients with sentinel node–negative breast cancer, *J Clin Oncol* 18:2553-2559, 2000.

43. Morton DL, Wen DR, Wong JH, et al: Technical details of intraoperative lymphatic mapping for early stage melanoma, *Arch Surg* 127:392-399, 1992.

44. Morton DL, Thompson JF, Essner R, et al: Validation of the accuracy of intraoperative lymphatic mapping and sentinel lymphadenectomy for early-stage melanoma: a multicenter trial. Multicenter Selective Lymphadenectomy Trial Group, *Ann Surg* 230:453-463, 1999.

45. Essner R, Conforti A, Kelley MC, et al: Efficacy of lymphatic mapping, sentinel lymphadenectomy, and selective complete lymph node dissection as a therapeutic procedure for early-stage melanoma, *Ann Surg Oncol* 6:442-449, 1999.

46. Ross GL, Soutar DS, MacDonald DG, et al: Sentinel node biopsy in head and neck cancer: preliminary results of a multicenter trial, *Ann Surg Oncol* 11:690-696, 2004.

47. O'Brien CJ, Uren RF, Thompson JF, et al: Prediction of potential metastatic sites in cutaneous head and neck melanoma using lymphoscintigraphy, *Am J Surg* 170:461-466, 1995.

48. Yuen APW, Lam KY, Lam LK, et al: Prognostic factors of clinically stage I and II oral tongue carcinoma—a comparative study of stage, thickness, shape, growth pattern, invasive front malignancy grading, Martinez-Gimeno score, and pathologic features, *Head Neck* 24:513-520, 2002.

49. Warburton G, Nikitakis NG, Roberson P, et al: Histopathological and lymphangiogenic parameters in relation to lymph node metastasis in early stage oral squamous cell carcinoma, *J Oral Maxillofac Surg* 65:475-484, 2007.

50. Cheng A, Schmidt BL: Management of the N0 neck in oral squamous cell carcinoma, *Oral Maxillofac Surg Clin North Am* 20:477-497, 2008.

51. Mohit-Tabatabai MA, Sobel HJ, Rush BF, et al: Relation of thickness of floor of mouth stage I and II cancers to regional metastasis, *Am J Surg* 152:351-353, 1986.

52. Spiro RH, Huvos AG, Wong GY, et al: Predictive value of tumor thickness in squamous carcinoma confined to the tongue and floor of mouth, *Am J Surg* 152:345-350, 1986.

53. Jones KR, Lodge-Rigal RD, Reddick RL, et al: Prognostic factors in the recurrence of stage I and II squamous cell cancer of the oral cavity, *Arch Otolaryngol Head Neck Surg* 118:483-485, 1992.

54. O'Brien CJ, Lauer CS, Fredricks S, et al: Tumor thickness influences prognosis of T1 and T2 oral cavity cancer—but what thickness? *Head Neck* 25:937-945, 2003.

55. Mendenhall WM, Million RR, Cassisi NJ, et al: Elective neck irradiation in squamous-cell carcinoma of the head and neck, *Head Neck Surg* 3:15-20, 1980.

56. Spaulding CA, Korb LJ, Constable WC, et al: The influence of extent of neck treatment upon control of cervical lymphadenopathy in cancers of the oral tongue, *Int J Radiat Oncol Biol Phys* 21:577-581, 1991.

57. Wolfensberger M, Zbaeren P, Dulguerov P, et al: Surgical treatment of early oral carcinoma—results of a prospective controlled multicenter study, *Head Neck* 23:525-530, 2001.

58. Robertson AG, Soutar DS, Paul J, et al: Early closure of a randomized trial: surgery and postoperative radiotherapy versus radiotherapy in the management of intra-oral tumours, *Clin Oncol (R Coll Radiol)* 10:155-160, 1998.

59. Leon X, Quer M, Diez S, et al: Second neoplasm in patients with head and neck cancer, *Head Neck* 21:204-210, 1999.

60. Vikram B, Strong EW, Shah JP, et al: Second malignant neoplasms in patients successfully treated with multimodality treatment for advanced head and neck cancer, *Head Neck Surg* 6:736-737, 1984.

61. Rowell NP: Radiotherapy in the management of orofacial cancer. In Ward Booth P, Schendel SA, Hausamen J-E, editors: *Maxillofacial surgery*, vol 1, ed 2, St Louis, 2007, Churchill Livingstone, pp 331-351.

62. Denham JW, Peters LJ, Johansen J, et al: Do acute mucosal reactions lead to consequential late reactions in patients with head and neck cancer? *Radiother Oncol* 52:157-164, 1999.

63. Pauloski BR, Rademaker AW, Logemann JA, et al: Speech and swallowing in irradiated and nonirradiated postsurgical oral cancer patients, *Otolaryngol Head Neck Surg* 118:616-624, 1998.

64. Terrell JE, Welsh DE, Bradford CR, et al: Pain, quality of life, and spinal accessory nerve status after neck dissection, *Laryngoscope* 110:620-626, 2000.

65. Shah JP: *Head and neck surgery and oncology*, ed 3, New York, 2003, Elsevier.

66. Kademani D, Dierks EJ: A straight-line incision for neck dissection: technical note, *J Oral Maxillofac Surg* 63:563-565, 2005.

67. Nahum AM, Marmor M: A syndrome resulting from radical neck dissection, *Arch Otolaryngol* 74:82-86, 1961.

68. Chepeha DB, Taylor RJ, Chepeha JC, et al: Functional assessment using Constant's Shoulder Scale after modified radical and selective neck dissection, *Head Neck* 24:432-436, 2002.

69. Rogers SN, Ferlito A, Pellitteri PK, et al: Quality of life following neck dissections, *Acta Otolaryngol* 124:231-236, 2004.

70. Wengen DF, Donald PJ: Complications of radical neck dissection. In Shochley WW, Pillsbury HC III, editors: *The neck: diagnosis and surgery*, St Louis, 1994, CV Mosby, pp 483-509.

Indications for Adjuvant Chemotherapy and Radiation Therapy

Chapter 55

Robert Andrew Ord

Oral squamous cell carcinoma (OSCC) is a multidisciplinary disease, with surgery or radiation therapy used as a single modality for early disease (stage I and II) and combinations of surgery, radiation therapy, and chemotherapy used for stage III and IV disease. The exact role of chemotherapy is still being established, although its use is becoming more defined. Many chemotherapy trials have been flawed by not including a gold standard surgery arm or surgery plus radiation therapy arm and have compared different chemotherapeutic agents against each other; in addition, other variables are also frequently altered, such as the dose or fractionation method used for radiation therapy in each arm, thus making the results difficult to critically analyze. Moreover, because of the comparative rarity of OSCC, different head and neck sites have been lumped together in trials, which has made individual analysis for oral cavity cancer alone impossible. Despite these problems, we may consider the role of adjunctive chemotherapy with radiation therapy in three situations. First, it may be used as a definitive therapy in organ-sparing regimens. Second, it can be used for advanced locoregional or unresectable disease. Third, it can be used as combination adjuvant therapy after surgery in patients at high risk for failure.

In all three situations we must appreciate that the addition of chemotherapy will increase toxicity and therefore decrease the therapeutic index. Complications of therapy may prevent patients from completing adjuvant therapy of proven benefit, such as radiation therapy, so patient selection and experience in managing these aggressive protocols are essential to prevent excessive morbidity and mortality.

HISTORICAL PERSPECTIVE

In the 1990s to 2000 a number of large meta-analyses of chemotherapy trials were published[1-4] (Table 55-1). The conclusions from these studies were that neoadjuvant (induction) chemotherapy and adjuvant chemotherapy had no significant survival advantages over locoregional treatment alone. However, concurrent chemoradiation therapy was seen to confer a significant survival benefit over radiation therapy alone. These meta-analyses also showed an increase in both short- and long-term toxicity and demonstrated that the benefit from concurrent chemoradiation therapy was improved locoregional control with no significant effect on distant metastases. Thus, at the present time, concurrent chemoradiation therapy is the standard of care for the treatment of head and neck cancer.

DIAGNOSTIC STUDIES

Positron emission tomography (PET) may be helpful in staging or restaging cancer and planning radiation therapy.[5,6] This new imaging technique is useful for detecting recurrent disease, which computed tomography (CT) and magnetic resonance imaging have difficulty differentiating from scarring. In one series, treatment was changed in 38.7% of patients with recurrent head and neck cancer following PET/CT; 16.3% underwent major changes in therapy.[7] However, false-positive results in the area of the tonsils, base of the tongue, and oral tongue[8] are not uncommon. PET standard uptake values may also have prognostic value when they are very elevated.[9,10] The use of PET in deciding whether to perform neck dissection after chemoradiation therapy is discussed later in the chapter.

TREATMENT/GOALS

In discussing organ-sparing protocols it should be remembered that functional organ preservation is the goal. Preserving a mandible that later fractures and requires resection for osteoradionecrosis or preserving a tongue that cannot move because of fibrosis is not better than surgical resection and good reconstruction. In the unresectable/advanced locoregional disease category, definitions are complex, and different types of patient are often included in this category. Involvement of the internal carotid artery, spine, or brachial plexus may make a lesion surgically unresectable, but patients with large lesions that could be excised but only with gross functional morbidity are also often included in this cohort. Patients with resectable OSCC may be inoperable because of medical co-morbid conditions, and medically fit patients with resectable locoregional disease may not be candidates for extensive surgery if they already have distant metastases. Finally, when concurrent adjuvant chemoradiation therapy is used following surgery, an attempt is made to select patients who will benefit the most and will tolerate the extra toxicity.

In conventional fractionated radiation therapy, one fraction is given per day for 5 to 7 weeks up to a total dose of 65 to 70 Gy. Altered fractionation schedules to improve results include hyperfractionation and accelerated fractionation. Accelerated fractionation delivers the same total dose over a shorter period, either by giving more fractions per week or by giving twice-daily treatments during the final 12 days (concomitant boost). Hyperfractionation involves a higher total dose, but lower individual fractions are given twice per day to reduce acute toxicity. Intensity-modulated radiation therapy (IMRT) creates a very exact target volume that conforms to the three-dimensional structure of the tumor so that the tumor receives a higher dose with sparing of adjacent normal structures.

SPECIFIC TREATMENT AND TECHNIQUES

ORGAN-SPARING DEFINITIVE PRIMARY CHEMORADIATION THERAPY

Concurrent chemoradiation therapy protocols have been used as an alternative to surgery to spare important organs and preserve function. These protocols were initially used for laryngeal preservation,

TABLE 55-1	Large Meta-analyses of Chemotherapy Trials	
AUTHOR	**YEAR**	**NUMBER OF TRIALS**
Stell[1]	1992	28
Munro[2]	1995	54
El Sayed and Nelson[3]	1996	42
Pignon et al.[4]	2000	63

which is beyond the scope of this chapter. No trials have been specifically conducted for OSCC; however, this organ-sparing approach has been used for oropharyngeal primaries, especially base of the tongue and tonsil OSCC. Before data supporting the use of chemoradiation therapy, surgery and radiation were the mainstays of therapy.[11,12] In a randomized phase III trial of 226 patients with stage III and IV oropharyngeal SCC in which 70-Gy radiation alone was compared with 70-Gy radiation plus three cycles of carboplatin and fluorouracil, there was no statistical difference in severe late morbidity.[13,14] Overall survival, disease-free survival, and locoregional control rates at 5 years were 22% and 16%, 27% and 15%, and 48% and 25%, respectively, in favor of the chemoradiation arm. There was no change in the rate of distant metastases. The conclusions from this study were that chemoradiation therapy improves survival and locoregional control. Currently, the National Comprehensive Cancer Network (NCCN) guidelines for T3-T4a N0 or any N2 oropharyngeal SCC have chemoradiation therapy with a cisplatin-based regimen with or without planned neck dissection as their category 1 preferred treatment.[15] Evidence of the need for neck dissection in patients with N2 and N3 disease is contradictory in the literature. However, recent papers indicate that dissection is not indicated in patients with N2 disease who have a complete response following chemoradiation therapy.[16-18] In patients with residual nodes following chemoradiation therapy, published level I evidence supports PET scanning and observation of PET-negative necks while reserving neck dissection for PET-positive necks.[19]

In addition, identification of human papillomavirus (HPV) as an etiologic factor in a cohort of patients with tonsillar cancer. The subsequent findings of improved response and survival following radiation or chemoradiation therapy in prospective studies of these head and neck cancer patients[20] and in patients with OSCC associated with HPV[21] raises the possibility of using less aggressive protocols in patients with HPV-positive cancers in the future.

TREATMENT OF UNRESECTABLE/ADVANCED LOCOREGIONAL DISEASE

The majority of patients with head and neck cancer already have advanced disease at initial evaluation, and in surgically unresectable patients, the 5-year survival rate with radiation therapy alone is less than 25%.[22] Trials of altered fractionation resulted in improvement in locoregional control but no benefit in overall survival.[23,24] The publication of two large meta-analyses finally resolved the question of whether survival can be improved by altered fractionation. The first, with 6515 patients, showed not only improvement in locoregional control but also an overall survival benefit of 3.4% at 5 years, with 8% for hyperfractionation and only 2% for accelerated fractionation.[25] The second, with 10,225 patients, showed hyperfractionation to increase median survival by 14.2 months, which was highly significant. There was no benefit from accelerated radiotherapy. Also

in this trial, the addition of chemotherapy to all radiation regimens significantly improved absolute survival benefit 13% to 15% at 2 years. Concurrent chemotherapy with altered fractionation radiotherapy gave the most benefit.[26]

A meta-analysis by Pignon and colleagues involving 10,741 patients had previously shown that the greatest benefit from chemoradiation regimens was afforded by concurrent chemoradiation therapy, with an overall survival benefit of 8% at 5 years.[4] An update of this meta-analysis in which further trials were incorporated and the patient pool was increased to 16,000 confirmed a significant 8% increase in absolute overall survival and a 19% reduction in the risk for death with concurrent chemoradiation therapy.[27] Although this benefit is very similar to the results obtained with altered fractionation radiotherapy, concurrent chemoradiation therapy has become the standard of care in the United States. The current standard is the use of cisplatin (100 mg/m²) on days 1, 22, and 43. Although this results in better locoregional control and overall survival than conventional radiotherapy alone does, it does increase the toxicity. Whether the use of multiagent chemotherapy instead of a single agent has any benefit to justify the increased toxicity is unknown. The largest updated meta-analysis failed to show any benefit with multiple agents over cisplatin alone.[27]

CHEMORADIATION AS ADJUNCTIVE THERAPY AFTER SURGERY

The gold standard for treatment of advanced stage III and IV disease was surgery plus postoperative radiation therapy, although for patients with a single positive node without extracapsular spread (ECS), surgery alone without radiation therapy was considered sufficient. However, locoregional recurrence was frequently seen in patients with advanced disease, and it was questioned whether the addition of concurrent chemotherapy may improve the results. In view of the increased side effects and complications, there was a search to identify patients who may benefit the most, so-called targeted chemotherapy. In a paper examining rationales for postoperative radiation therapy, the argument for risk assessment by clusters was first proposed.[28] In this analysis, two or more positive nodes, ECS, or both were significantly associated with failure. In addition, combinations of two or more risk factors—oral primary, close/positive margins, perineural invasion, two or more nodes, nodes larger than 3 cm, delay longer than 6 weeks after surgery, and decreased patient performance status—increased the chance for local failure. In a further extension of this approach, analysis of Radiation Therapy Oncology Group (RTOG) data was undertaken to identify which histologic findings best defined high-risk postsurgical patients who would benefit from chemoradiation therapy.[29] As a result of this work, two major trials were established under the auspices of the European Organization for Research and Treatment of Cancer (EORTC) and the RTOG; the results, published in 2004, provided the first level I evidence for the benefit of chemoradiation therapy in postoperative high-risk patients.[30,31]

Both these landmark trials compared radiotherapy alone with a concurrent chemoradiation arm in postoperative patients considered to be at high risk for treatment failure. Overall, 750 patients were randomly allocated in the two trials. The criteria for "high-risk" patients were slightly different in the two trials. Both EORCT 22931 and RTOG 9501 included microscopically positive margins and ECS. The RTOG trial included two or more positive nodes, whereas the EORTC trial included stage III and IV, positive level IV and V nodes, vascular embolisms, and perineural invasion. Their findings were remarkably similar in favor of the chemoradiation arm (Table 55-2). Both reported significant improvement in locoregional control

TABLE 55-2	Findings with Concurrent Chemoradiation Therapy versus Radiation Therapy Alone	
OUTCOME	**EORTC 22931**	**RTOG 9501**
Locoregional failure	Significant	Significant
Disease-free survival	Significant	Significant
Overall survival	Significant	Not significant
Distant metastases	Not significant	Not significant
Acute toxicity	Significant	Significant

EORTC, European Organization for Research and Treatment of Cancer; RTOG, Radiation Therapy Oncology Group.

and disease-free survival. The EORTC trial showed a significant increase in overall survival not seen in the RTOG trial. As in previous trials, there was no effect on distant metastases. Both studies showed increased acute toxicity, although in the EORTC trial acute mucositis occurred less frequently. Late toxicities were not significantly different from those in the radiation-alone arm in either study.

The 2007 NCCN recommendations for adjuvant therapy were based on these results.[15] The NCCN classifies risk factors into major and minor. Minor risk factors are T3/4, N2/3 nodes, nodes at levels IV or V, and perineural/perivascular involvement. Major risk factors are positive margins and ECS. In patients with one node and no other risk factors, radiation therapy is optional. If fewer than two minor risk factors are identified, radiation therapy is recommended. If one or both major risk factors are present, chemoradiation therapy is the treatment of choice.

There are, however, two caveats to the 2007 "standard of practice." First, a recent Cochrane Database Systematic Review pointed out that although there is some evidence for the efficacy of chemoradiation therapy over radiation therapy alone after surgery, this has not been proved for specific sites such as the oral cavity since trials lump all head/neck sites together and that further subsite analysis needs to be undertaken.[32] Second, a more recent pooled analysis of EORCT 22931 and RTOG 9501 has shown only ECS and microscopically involved margins to be significant in both trials.[33,34] There was a trend in favor of chemoradiation therapy for some of the minor risk factors, but patients with two or more positive nodes and no ECS did not benefit from this treatment. Consequently, the 2008 NCCN guidelines recommended chemoradiation therapy as a category 1 preferred treatment only for patients with ECS and positive margins. In the case of other risk factors, radiation therapy alone or chemoradiation therapy is recommended.[35]

FUTURE DIRECTIONS

REDUCTION OF TOXICITY

The high rate of complications associated with intense multimodal regimens will reduce patient compliance. One review stated that "in most studies only half to two thirds of patients treated with high dose cisplatin based chemoradiation complete the planned three cycles."[33] This will become an increasingly relevant problem inasmuch as the National Cancer Database report on cancer of the head and neck showed a decrease in the use of radiation therapy alone in favor of chemotherapy-enhanced radiotherapy.[36] In radiation therapy, IMRT provides a way of directing more dosage to the tumor while

sparing adjacent tissues, such as the parotid gland. In addition, the use of drugs such as amifostine has been shown to reduce post–radiation therapy xerostomia.[37,38]

In chemotherapy, less toxic drugs need to be identified, perhaps the use of biologic agents (discussed later). Alternatively, targeting only high-risk patients for chemoradiation therapy or identifying patients in whom the intensity of treatment can be reduced (e.g., HPV-associated tumors) may be useful strategies. Patients more at risk for complications can also be identified. Older age, advanced T stage, laryngeal/hypopharyngeal primary sites, and neck dissection after concurrent chemoradiation therapy were all significant factors in one study.[39] It should also be noted that chemotherapy appears to confer less benefit in elderly patients,[27] so selection for intensive treatment in this cohort needs to be considered carefully. Perhaps in the future genetic markers or biologic markers may identify patients most likely to benefit from chemotherapy regimens. Delays or breaks in therapy caused by acute toxicity will increase the treatment package time (i.e., the total treatment time from surgery to the end of radiation therapy). A locoregional control rate of 76% was achieved with a treatment package time of 11 weeks and a control rate of 62% with 11 to 13 weeks, whereas longer than 13 weeks achieved only a 38% locoregional control rate in a recent randomized study.[40] This perhaps reflects tumor cells' ability to repopulate quickly.

NEOADJUVANT (INDUCTION) CHEMOTHERAPY

The gains made by the incorporation of concurrent chemoradiation therapy protocols in terms of disease-free, median, and overall survival have been achieved by an increase in locoregional control. It appears that cisplatin acts as a radiosensitizer to enhance the effectiveness of radiation therapy. However, 25% of patients in whom postoperative chemoradiation therapy fails now do so as a result of distant metastatic disease.[41] It has already discussed how earlier trials and meta-analyses failed to show an improvement in locoregional control with induction chemotherapy, which consequently had been replaced by the concept of concurrent chemoradiation therapy. Even when used for laryngeal preservation, the "nonsignificant negative effect for organ preservation indicates this procedure must remain investigational."[4] However, some neoadjuvant trials had previously shown shrinkage of the primary tumor and an effect on distant metastases, and there is now a push toward incorporating neoadjuvant chemotherapy into concurrent chemoradiation regimens in an attempt to improve overall success by reducing distant metastatic failure in addition to the improved locoregional benefits.[42,43] There has recently been great enthusiasm for the addition of taxanes to induction chemotherapy regimens; trials that incorporated taxanes have shown survival benefits over trials with induction chemotherapy arms not incorporating taxanes.[44,45] However, these taxane-based regimens have not been compared with concurrent chemoradiation therapy in any trial. In addition, the TAX 324 study showed no statistical difference in rates of distant metastases despite the fact that both induction chemotherapy arms (one with taxane and one without) were followed by concurrent chemoradiation therapy, which is the proposed new model.[45]

Although this theoretic approach may look attractive, it should be noted that there would be a further expected increase in toxicity, noncompliance, and lengthening of the package time. There are currently no trials that have compared this approach of induction chemotherapy plus concurrent chemoradiation therapy against the standard of care, concurrent chemoradiation therapy. The answer may be provided by three ongoing phase III trials, the Paradigm, Decide, and Italian trials, to see whether this approach makes any significant difference in survival.[22]

BIOLOGIC AGENTS

An alternative treatment to chemotherapy is the use of biologic agents such as cetuximab. Cetuximab is an anti–epidermal growth factor receptor monoclonal antibody. In a phase III study of 424 patients with locally advanced head and neck tumors who were randomized to radiation therapy only or radiation therapy plus cetuximab, the risk for death was decreased by 26% and the risk for locoregional progression by 32% with radiation therapy plus cetuximab.[46] In addition, locoregional control (14.9 versus 29.1 months), progression-free survival, and overall survival (29.3 versus 49 months) were significantly improved in the cetuximab arm. There was no decrease in the rate of distant metastases, and the only increased toxicity was associated with acne-form rashes and infusion reactions. However, Cooper cautions that judgment needs to be reserved at present for cetuximab.[47] He points out that this is only one trial, that 56% of the patients received concomitant boost-style accelerated radiotherapy, and that the beneficial effect was much less for laryngeal/hypopharyngeal than for oropharyngeal cancers, thus raising the possibility of an influence from HPV-associated cancers. There was also no chemoradiation arm in the trial, and how cetuximab compares with radiation therapy is unknown. This question may be answered by RTOG 0522, which will compare chemoradiation therapy with chemoradiation plus cetuximab. The possibility of using biologic agents with or instead of chemotherapy to add survival benefit and reduce toxicity is an exciting new dimension for the future.

PEARLS AND PITFALLS

- Concurrent chemoradiation therapy with single-agent cisplatin gives better results than radiation therapy alone in the primary treatment of T3/T4 and N2 oropharyngeal cancer, in advanced "unresectable" locoregional cancer, and as postoperative adjuvant therapy in patients at high risk for failure.
- Long-term analysis of the level I evidence for the use of concurrent chemoradiation therapy in postoperative patients at high risk for failure indicates that ECS and positive margins may be the only factors significantly affected.
- Acute toxicity is increased and patient compliance decreased by the addition of chemotherapy to radiation therapy, so careful patient selection is paramount.
- Concurrent chemoradiation therapy has no impact on distant metastases.
- Overall survival rates from hyperfractionated radiation therapy are equivalent to the effects of chemoradiation therapy in large meta-analyses.
- Although the use of neoadjuvant chemotherapy to improve survival was disproved in all meta-analyses of large trials, its use is currently being proposed in combination with concurrent chemoradiation therapy to reduce the incidence of distant metastases. There is at present no good scientific evidence that such an approach will give better results than concurrent chemoradiation therapy alone.
- Future directions include reduction of toxicity, development of biologic agents, and further trials to settle the question of the role of neoadjuvant chemotherapy.

REFERENCES

1. Stell PM: Adjuvant chemotherapy in head and neck cancer, *Semin Radiat Oncol* 2:195-205, 1992.
2. Munro AJ: An overview of randomized controlled trials of adjuvant chemotherapy in head and neck cancer, *Br J Cancer* 71:83-91 1995.
3. El-Sayed S, Nelson N: Adjuvant and adjunctive chemotherapy in the management of squamous cell carcinoma of the head and neck region. A meta-analysis of prospective and randomized trials, *J Clin Oncol* 14:838-847 1996.
4. Pignon JP, Bourhis J, Domenge C, et al: Chemotherapy added to loco-regional treatment for head and neck squamous cell carcinoma: three meta-analyses of updated individual data. MACH-NC Collaborative Group. Meta-Analysis of Chemotherapy on Head and Neck Cancer, *Lancet* 355:949-955, 2000.
5. Haddad RI, Shin DM: Recent advances in head and neck cancer, *N Engl J Med* 359:1143-1154, 2008.
6. Macmanus M, Nestle U, Rosenzweig KE, et al: Use of PET and PET/CT for radiation therapy planning: IAEA expert report 2006-2007, *Radiother Oncol* 91:85-94, 2009.
7. Pantavaidya GH, Agarwal JP, Deshpande MS, et al: PET-CT in recurrent head neck cancers: a study to evaluate impact on patient management, *J Surg Oncol* 100:401-403, 2009.
8. Ariji Y, Fuwa N, Kodaira T, et al: False positive positron emission tomography appearance with ^{18}F-fluorodeoxyglucose after

9. Liao CT, Chang JT, Wang HM, et al: Preoperative [^{18}F]fluorodeoxyglucose positron emission tomography standardized uptake value of lymph nodes predicts neck cancer control and survival rates in patients with oral cavity squamous cell carcinoma and pathologically positive lymph nodes, *Int J Radiat Oncol Biol Phys* 74:1054-1061, 2009.
10. Suzuki H, Hasegawa Y, Terada A, et al: FDG-PET predicts survival and distant metastasis in oral squamous cell carcinoma, *Oral Oncol* 45:569-573, 2009.
11. Genden EM, Ferlito A, Scully C, et al: Current management of tonsillar cancer, *Oral Oncol* 39:337-342, 2003.
12. Harrison LB, Ferlito A, Shaha AR, et al: Current philosophy on the management of cancer of the base of tongue, *Oral Oncol* 39:101-105, 2003.
13. Calais G, Alfonsi M, Bardet E, et al: Randomized trial of radiation therapy versus concomitant chemotherapy and radiation therapy for advanced-stage oropharynx carcinoma, *J Natl Cancer Inst* 91:2081-2086, 1999.
14. Denis F, Garaud P, Bardet E, et al: Final results of the 94-01 French Head and Neck Oncology and Radiotherapy Group randomized trial comparing radiotherapy alone with concomitant radiochemotherapy in advanced-stage oropharynx carcinoma, *J Clin Oncol* 22:69-76, 2004.

definitive radiotherapy for cancer of the mobile tongue, *Br J Radiol* 82:e3-e7, 2009.

15. National Comprehensive Cancer Network NCCN http://www.nccn.org/ Clinical Practice Guidelines in Oncology v.2. 2008 Cancer of the Head and Neck.
16. Rengan R, Pfister DG, Lee NY, et al: Long-term control rates after complete response to chemoradiation in patients with advanced head and neck cancer, *Am J Clin Oncol* 31:465-469, 2008.
17. Corry J, Peters L, Fisher R, et al: N2-N3 neck nodal control without planned neck dissection for clinical/radiologic complete responders—results of Trans Tasman Radiation Oncology Group Study 98.02, *Head Neck* 30:737-742, 2008.
18. Lau H, Phan T, Mackinnon J, et al: Absence of planned neck dissection for the N2-3 neck after chemoradiation for locally advanced squamous cell carcinoma of the head and neck, *Arch Otolaryngol Head Neck Surg* 134:257-261, 2008.
19. Porceddu SV, Jarmolowski E, Hicks RJ, et al: The role of positron emission tomography for the detection of disease in residual neck nodes after (chemo-radiotherapy in head and neck cancer, *Head Neck* 27:175-181, 2005.
20. Fakhry C, Westra WH, Li S, et al: Improved survival of patients with human papillomavirus–positive head and neck squamous cell carcinoma in a prospective clinical trial, *J Natl Cancer Inst* 100:261-269, 2008.
21. Chaturvedi AK, Engels EA, Anderson WF, et al: Incidence trends for human papillomavirus–related and –unrelated oral

squamous cell carcinomas in the United States, *J Clin Oncol* 26:612-619, 2008.

22. Culliney B, Birhan A, Young AV, et al: Management of locally advanced or unresectable head and neck cancer, *Oncology* 22:1152-1164, 2008.

23. Fu KK, Pajak TF, Trotti A, et al: A Radiation Therapy Oncology Group (RTOG) phase III randomized study to compare hyperfractionation and two variants of accelerated fractionation to standard fractionation radiotherapy for head and neck squamous cell carcinomas: first report of RTOG 9003, *Int J Radiat Oncol Biol Phys* 48:7-16, 2000.

24. Horiot JC, Le Fur R, N'Guyen T et al: Hyperfractionation versus conventional fractionation in oropharyngeal carcinoma: final analysis of a randomized trial of the EORTC cooperative group of radiotherapy, *Radiother Oncol* 25:231-241, 1992.

25. Bourhis J, Overgaard J, Audry H, et al, for the Meta-analysis of Radiotherapy in Carcinomas of the Head and Neck (MARCH) Collaborative Group: Hyperfractionated or accelerated radiotherapy in head and neck cancer; a meta-analysis, *Lancet* 368:843-854, 2006.

26. Budach W, Hehr T, Budach V, et al: A meta-analysis of hyperfractionated and accelerated radiotherapy and combined chemotherapy and radiotherapy regimes in unresected locally advanced squamous cell carcinoma of the head and neck, *BMC Cancer* 6:28, 2006.

27. Bourhis J, Amand C, Pignon JP, et al, for the MACH-NC Collaborative Group: Update of MACH-NC (Meta-analysis of Chemotherapy in Head and Neck Cancer) database focuses on concomitant chemoradiotherapy [abstract 5505], *Proc Am Soc Clin Oncol* 23:488, 2004.

28. Peters LJ, Goepfert H, Ang KK, et al Evaluation for the dose for postoperative radiation therapy of head and neck cancer: first report of a prospective randomized trial, *Int J Radiat Oncol Phys* 26:3-11, 1993.

29. Cooper JS, Pajak TF, Forstariere A, et al: Precisely defining high-risk operable head and neck tumors based on RTOG#85-03 and RTOG#88-24: targets for postoperative radiochemotherapy? *Head Neck* 20:588-594, 1998.

30. Bernier J, Domenge C, Ozsahin M, et al: Postoperative irradiation with or without concomitant chemotherapy for locally advanced head and neck cancer, *N Engl J Med* 350:1945-1952, 2004.

31. Cooper JS, Pajak TF, Forastiere AA, et al: Postoperative concurrent radiotherapy and chemotherapy for high risk squamous cell carcinoma of the head and neck, *N Engl J Med* 350:1937-1944, 2004.

32. Oliver RJ, Clarkson JE, Conway DI, et al: Interventions for the treatment of oral and oropharyngeal cancers: surgical treatment, *Cochrane Database Syst Rev* 17(4):CD006205. 2007.

33. Bernier J, Cooper JS, Pajak TF, et al Defining risk levels in locally advanced head and neck cancers: a comparative analysis of concurrent postoperative radiation plus chemotherapy trials of the EORTC (#22931) and RTOG (#9501), *Head Neck* 27:843-850, 2005.

34. Bernier J, Vermorken JB, Koch WM: Adjuvant therapy in patients with resected poor risk head and neck cancer, *J Clin Oncol* 24:2629-2634, 2006.

35. Bernier J, Pfister DG, Cooper JS: Adjuvant chemo- and radiotherapy for poor prognosis head and neck squamous cell carcinomas, *Crit Rev Oncol Hematol* 56:353-364, 2005.

36. Cooper JS, Porter K, Mallin K, et al: National Cancer Database report on cancer of the head and neck: 10-year outcome, *Head Neck* 31:748-758, 2009.

37. Anne PR, Machtay M, Rosenthal DI, et al: A phase II trial of subcutaneous amifostine and radiation therapy in patients with head and neck cancer, *Int J Radiat Oncol Biol Phys* 67:445-452, 2007.

38. Wasserman TH, Brizel DM, Henke M, et al: Influence of intravenous amifostine on xerostomia, tumor control and survival after radiotherapy for head and neck cancer: a 2-year follow up of a prospective, randomized phase III trial, *Int J Radiat Oncol Biol Phys* 15:985-990, 2005.

39. Machtay M, Moughan J, Trotti A, et al: Factors associated with severe late toxicity after concurrent chemoradiation for locally advanced head and neck cancer: an RTOG analysis, *J Clin Oncol* 26:3582-3589, 2008.

40. Ang KK, Trotti A, Brown BW, et al: Randomized trial addressing risk features and time factors of surgery plus radiotherapy in advanced head and neck cancer, *Int J Radiat Oncol Biol Phys* 51:571-578, 2001.

41. Bernier J, Bentzen SM: Head and neck cancer management. Which postoperative treatment best serves your patient? *Am Soc Clin Oncol Ed Book* 306-312, 2003.

42. Brizel DM, Vokes EE: Induction chemotherapy: to use or not to use? That is the question, *Semin Radiat Oncol* 19:11-16, 2009.

43. Gibson MK, Forastiere AA: Reassessment of the role of induction chemotherapy for head and neck cancer, *Lancet Oncol* 7:565-574, 2006.

44. Vermorken JB, Remenar E, van Herpen C, et al: Cisplatin, fluorouracil and docetaxel in unresectable head and neck cancer, *N Engl J Med* 357:1695-1704, 2007.

45. Posner MR, Hershock DM, Blajman CR, et al: Cisplatin and fluorouracil alone or with docetaxel in head and neck cancer, *N Engl J Med* 357:1705-1715, 2007.

46. Bonner JA, Harani PM, Giralt J, et al: Radiotherapy plus cetuximab for squamous cell carcinoma of the head and neck, *N Engl J Med* 354:567-578, 2006.

47. Cooper JS: The Culliney/Birhan/Young et al article reviewed, Rapidly growing options for advanced head and neck cancer, *Oncology* 22:1162-1164, 2008.

Salivary Gland Tumors: The Parotid Gland

Curtis Gregoire

Parotid gland tumors can be a challenging clinical entity to manage for the head and neck surgeon. Evaluation of these patients is no different from that for any other patient and should include a thorough history and physical examination followed by appropriate imaging when indicated and, ultimately, tissue biopsy to arrive at a diagnosis. Close collaboration between the referring physician, the head and neck surgeon, and the oncologist is required to ensure optimal patient care. Advances in microscopic diagnosis, imaging, and surgical techniques over the past decade have improved care for patients with salivary gland neoplasms.

ETIOPATHOGENESIS

Salivary gland tumors are rare in comparison to the overall incidence of tumors of the head and neck region. The overall incidence of salivary gland tumors varies around the world from approximately 0.4 to 13.5 cases per 100,000 people.[1] The parotid gland is the most common site of occurrence of salivary gland tumors, and in four large series published on primary epithelial salivary gland tumors,[2-5] the parotid gland accounted for 64% to 80% of all cases (Table 56-1).[6] Only 15% to 32% of these cases were malignant (Table 56-2). The most common benign parotid tumor is pleomorphic adenoma, and the most common malignant parotid tumor is mucoepidermoid carcinoma (Table 56-3).[7-9] Generally speaking, two thirds to three quarters of salivary gland tumors occur in the parotid and two thirds to three quarters of these tumors are benign.[6]

Very little is known about the etiology of salivary gland tumors (Box 56-1). The cause is thought to be multifactorial, and many factors have been suggested to play a role. One relationship often cited is between Epstein-Barr virus (and possible autoimmunity) and malignant lymphoepithelial tumors of the parotid. The strongest support for this contention comes from epidemiologic studies of the Eskimo population in Greenland. Merrick and colleagues found that the virus is normally present in the pharynx and salivary glands of this population and that the interrelationships of immunity, the virus, and the genetic composition of the host may all play a role in the malignant transformation of salivary gland epithelial cells.[10]

Dalpa and co-workers investigated the link between human herpesvirus 8 (HHV-8) and Warthin tumors.[11] They evaluated for the presence of HHV-8 in a series of Warthin tumors of the parotid gland and corresponding adjacent normal tissue. HHV-8 DNA was detected in 19 of 43 (44%) salivary gland tumor samples. Among the 15 cases with paired samples, 9 were HHV-8 positive for both samples, 4 were HHV-8 negative for both samples, and in 2 cases HHV-8 was detected only in the tumor specimens.[11] They concluded that HHV-8 is frequently detected in adenoid salivary neoplasms, thus suggesting a significant role of the virus in the etiopathogenesis of the disease.[11]

Vageli and associates examined the relationship between high-risk human papillomavirus (HPV) and parotid tumors.[12] They studied nine parotid lesions for HPV infection, including an oncocytoma, an acinic cell carcinoma, a high-grade adenocarcinoma, a low-grade polymorphous adenocarcinoma, a Warthin tumor, two pleomorphic adenomas, a lymphoepithelial cyst, and a lipoma of the parotid gland. DNA was extracted from formalin-fixed and paraffin-embedded tissue sections. HPV typing was carried out by multiplex polymerase chain reaction (PCR) for HPV genotypes 6, 11, 16, 18, and 33; positive samples were reconfirmed by PCR with specific primers for each type.[12] Quantitative real-time PCR for the high-risk HPV genotypes 16, 18, 31, 33, 35, 52, 58, and 67 was also performed to determine the viral load. Seven of the nine parotid lesions were HPV positive, whereas six of these seven had been infected by the HPV-16 or HPV-18 oncogenic types (or by both). A high viral load of the high-risk genotypes of HPV was found in the oncocytoma, in one of the pleomorphic adenomas, and in the Warthin tumor.[12] Finally, in situ PCR indicated that HPV-16 amplification occurred in the salivary gland tumors. Their results suggest possible involvement of the virus in the disease.[12]

An overwhelming body of literature supports the relationship between parotid tumors and ionizing radiation. Boukheris and colleagues evaluated the magnitude of the risk for the development of salivary gland tumors in patients who had undergone radiotherapy for Hodgkin lymphoma.[13] The risk for salivary gland carcinoma in 20,928 1-year survivors of Hodgkin lymphoma in whom the disease was diagnosed between 1973 and 2003 was evaluated in 11 population-based cancer registry areas of the Surveillance, Epidemiology and End Results (SEER) program.[13] Among 11,047 patients with Hodgkin lymphoma who received radiotherapy as part of their initial treatment, invasive salivary gland carcinoma subsequently developed in 21. The risk for radiation-related salivary gland carcinoma was highest in younger patients (age <20 years) with Hodgkin lymphoma and in 10-year survivors, with risks remaining elevated for at least 2 decades after irradiation.[13] Significant differences in risk by histologic type were observed, with a particularly high risk for the development of mucoepidermoid carcinoma and adenocarcinoma. They concluded that patients treated with radiotherapy experienced a significantly increased risk for salivary gland carcinoma, particularly when exposed at a young age or for at least 2 decades after exposure.[13]

Certain occupations have been shown to increase risk for the development of salivary gland tumors. Swanson and Burns assessed the risk for salivary gland cancers associated with diverse occupations and industries.[14] They carried out a population-based case-referent study using data from a SEER program cancer registry for patients and by telephone interview for patients and referents to evaluate workplace-associated risks for salivary gland cancer in black and white women and men.[14] They found significantly

TABLE 56-1	Sites of Occurrence of Primary Epithelial Salivary Gland Tumors				
		SITE OF OCCURRENCE			
AUTHOR	**NO. CASES**	**PAROTID**	**SUBMANDIBULAR**	**SUBLINGUAL**	**MINOR**
Ellis et al.[5]	13,749	64%	10%	0.3%	23%
Spiro[4]	2,807	70%	8%	Included with minor	22%
Seifert et al.[3]	2,579	80%	10%	1.0%	9%
Eveson and Cawson[2]	2,410	73%	11%	0.3%	14%

From Neville BW, Damm DD, Allen CM, et al: *Oral and maxillofacial pathology,* ed 3, St Louis, 2009, Saunders, p 474.

TABLE 56-2	Frequency of Malignant Salivary Tumors at Different Sites				
		PERCENTAGE OF MALIGNANT CASES			
AUTHOR	**NO. CASES**	**PAROTID**	**SUBMANDIBULAR**	**SUBLINGUAL**	**MINOR**
Ellis et al.[5]	13,749	32%	41%	70%	49%
Spiro[4]	2,807	25%	43%	Included with minor	82%
Seifert et al.[3]	2,579	20%	45%	90%	45%
Eveson and Cawson[2]	2,410	15%	37%	86%	46%

From Neville BW, Damm DD, Allen CM, et al: *Oral and maxillofacial pathology,* ed 3, St Louis, 2009, Saunders, p 474.

TABLE 56-3	Parotid Tumors				
	ELLIS ET AL.[5]	**EVESON AND CAWSON[2]**	**THACKRAY AND LUCAS[7]**	**ENEROTH[8]**	**FOOTE AND FRAZELL[9]**
Total number of cases	8,222	1,756	651	2,158	764
Benign Tumors					
Pleomorphic adenoma	53.0%	63.3%	72.0%	76.8%	58.5%
Warthin tumor	7.7%	14.0%	9.0%	4.7%	6.5%
Oncocytoma	1.9%	0.9%	0.6%	1.0%	0.1%
Basal cell adenoma	1.4%	—	—	—	—
Other	3.7%	7.1%	1.8%	—	0.7%
Total	67.7%	85.3%	83.4%	82.5%	65.8%
Malignant Tumors					
Mucoepidermoid carcinoma	9.6%	1.5%	2.3%	4.1%	11.8%
Acinic cell carcinoma	8.6%	2.5%	1.2%	3.1%	2.7%
Adenoid cystic carcinoma	2.0%	2.0%	3.3%	2.3%	2.1%
Malignant mixed tumor	2.5%	3.2%	4.1%	1.5%	6.0%
Squamous cell carcinoma	2.1%	1.1%	1.0%	0.3%	3.4%
Other	7.5%	4.4%	4.7%	6.3%	8.1%
Total	32.3%	14.7%	16.6%	17.5%	34.2%

From Neville BW, Damm DD, Allen CM, et al: *Oral and maxillofacial pathology,* ed 3, St Louis, 2009, Saunders, p 474.

| BOX 56-1 | Risk Factors of Parotid Tumors |

- Viral
  - Epstein-Barr virus
  - Human herpesvirus-8
  - Human papillomavirus
- Ionizing Radiation
- Occupation
  - Hairdresser
  - Asbestos mining
  - Plumber
  - Automobile manufacturing
- Oncogenes

elevated odds ratios in women employed as hairdressers and those working in beauty shops. They concluded that the risk for salivary gland cancer is elevated in women employed as hairdressers.[14]

Other occupations that have been shown to predispose one to the development of salivary gland tumors include asbestos mining,[15] manufacturing of rubber products,[16] plumbing,[17] and the automobile industry.[18]

The role of various oncogenes in salivary gland tumorigenesis has been investigated. Elledge reviewed the literature pertaining to individual oncogenes in which their role as diagnostic and prognostic markers and as potential targets for treatment was discussed.[19] He found articles pertaining to kit, PLAG1, Mect1-Maml2, HMGIC, HER2/neu, ras, c-fos, and Sox-4. All these studies were noted to be seminal small-scale studies with the potential for further research and eventual clinical application.[19] Elledge concluded that a wide variety of oncogenes have been implicated in salivary gland tumorigenesis, with evidence being confined to small murine or in vitro studies. He also concluded that there are possible roles for different oncogenes in therapeutics, prognosis, and management of specific salivary gland tumors.[19]

No association has been found between salivary gland tumors and smoking. Similarly, no association has been found between alcohol consumption and salivary gland neoplasms.

PATHOLOGIC ANATOMY

PAROTID GLAND

The parotid gland is the largest of three paired major salivary glands within the head and neck region. It is enclosed within a fascial capsule, the parotidomasseteric fascia, which is derived from the investing layer of the deep cervical fascia. This fascial covering is important from a surgical standpoint in that the overlying skin and subcutaneous tissue can easily be separated from it. The parotid lies within the confines of the parotid bed, which is located anteroinferior to the external acoustic canal. The apex of the parotid gland is posterior to the angle of the mandible, and its base is in close relation to the zygomatic arch. The parotid duct (Stensen duct) passes anteriorly, turns medially at the anterior border of the masseter, pierces the buccinators, and then enters the oral cavity through a small orifice opposite the second maxillary molar. The course of the duct is along a line extending from the base of the earlobe to the vermilion border of the upper lip.[3] Embedded within the substance of the parotid gland in a superficial to deep plane are the parotid plexus, the facial nerve and its branches, the retromandibular vein, and the external carotid artery. On the parotid sheath and within the gland are the parotid lymph nodes.[3]

Gregoire dissected a number of parotid glands from various mammals, including humans, and found that the parotid gland was divided into a deep and a superficial lobe with the facial nerve embedded between the two rather than penetrating the parenchyma.[3,20] The lateral or superficial lobe is the larger of the two. This is the anatomic basis of parotid surgery that allows preservation of the facial nerve. McWorther reported similar findings but also noted that the two lobes were joined by an isthmus that lies in the middle of the gland anterior to the division of the facial nerve.[3,21] Furthermore, he found that the two lobes are not always separated by a connective tissue layer.

FACIAL NERVE

The most crucial anatomic structure to identify and preserve during parotid surgery for benign and some malignant tumors is the facial nerve. The facial nerve has both sensory and motor components. It is the motor nerve to the muscles of facial expression and to the muscles of the scalp, external ear, buccinator, platysma, stapedius, stylohyoid, and posterior belly of the digastric.[22] It supplies special sensory taste to the anterior two thirds of the tongue and general sensation to parts of the external acoustic meatus, soft palate, and adjacent pharynx.[22] It also has a parasympathetic component that supplies secretomotor fibers for the submandibular, sublingual, lacrimal, nasal, and palatine glands.[22]

The facial nerve exits the stylomastoid foramen and gives off three branches before it bifurcates: a branch to the posterior belly of the digastric, the stylohyoid muscle, and the posterior auricular muscles. As it exits the stylomastoid foramen, the facial nerve passes anterior to the posterior belly of the digastric muscle and lateral to the styloid process, external carotid artery, and posterior facial vein and then runs anteriorly for approximately 2 cm before dividing into upper and lower divisions.[23] The nerve is approximately 3 mm in diameter at the point where it exits the stylomastoid foramen and bifurcates. The main trunk is invariably found where the tip of the mastoid process, cartilaginous auditory canal, and superior border of the posterior belly of the digastric muscle meet.[23] Within the parotid gland, it divides at the posterior border of the ramus of the mandible into two primary branches, the cervicofacial (vertically directed, longer and smaller) and the temporofacial (horizontally directed and larger).[23] Both divisions run through the substance of the gland and usually pass over the external jugular vein. After the nerve bifurcates, there are a variable number of tertiary limbs that communicate freely with each other in the periphery.[23] The temporofacial division lies between the superficial and deep lobes of the parotid gland and above the isthmus connecting the two lobes.[22]

Identification of the main trunk of the facial nerve (Fig. 56-1) is the key to safe and successful surgical management of benign and malignant tumors of the parotid gland when preservation of the nerve will not compromise sound oncologic principles. Many techniques have been described and used to identify the main trunk of the facial nerve. The most commonly described surgical landmarks include the tympanomastoid suture (TMS), the posterior belly of the digastric, the transverse process of the axis, the styloid process, and the tragal pointer. Most authors suggest that the TMS line is the most constant and consistent surgical landmark for identification of the main trunk of the facial nerve.[24-29] It is relatively easy to find and its position is constant. The position of the TMS relative to the main trunk of the facial nerve is very reliable because it leads directly to the stylomastoid foramen, where the nerve can be identified in an area that is not likely to be displaced.[30] On average, the facial nerve is located 2 to 4 mm deep to the medial end of the TMS line.[24]

The tragal pointer is another commonly used surgical landmark for identification of the main trunk of the facial nerve but has been

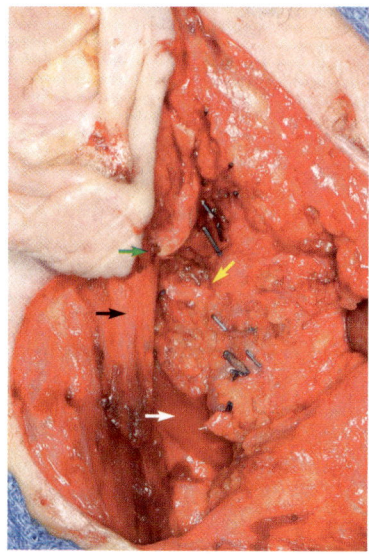

Fig. 56-1 ■ Superficial parotidectomy. Note the sternocleidomastoid (*black arrow*), the posterior belly of the digastric (*white arrow*), and the tragal pointer (*green arrow*). The main trunk of the facial nerve is indicated by the yellow arrow.

found to be somewhat variable in its position relative to the nerve and is therefore less reliable than other landmarks. On average, the nerve is located approximately 1 cm deep and anteroinferior to the tip of the tragal pointer.[24]

The two landmarks commonly cited as being the most reliable and accurate are the posterior belly of the digastric and the TMS line. Witt and colleagues compared the distance from the TMS and posterior belly of the digastric to the main trunk of the facial nerve in both cadavers and patients undergoing parotidectomy.[31] They found the mean distance from the TMS line to the facial nerve to be 1.8 mm (range, 0 to 4 mm) and from the posterior belly of the digastric to the facial nerve to be 12.4 mm (range, 7 to 17 mm) in cadavers.[31] They found the mean distance in live patients from the TMS and posterior belly of the digastric to the main trunk of the facial nerve to be 2.0 mm (range, 0 to 4 mm) and 10.7 mm (range, 5 to 14 mm), respectively.[31] They concluded that the TMS is a significantly closer surgical landmark than the posterior belly of the digastric in both cadaver and live dissections and recommend its use.[31]

Rea and associates had similar findings. They carried out cadaveric dissection of 52 facial halves and found the distance from the posterior belly of the digastric and TMS to the facial nerve to be 5.5 ± 2.1 mm and 2.5 ± 0.4 mm, respectively.[32]

In cases in which the main trunk of the facial nerve cannot be identified, a terminal branch of the nerve can be identified and dissected in retrograde fashion proximally to identify the main trunk. The marginal branch of the facial nerve is the most readily accessible branch for this technique and can normally be safely identified overlying the fascia of the submandibular gland and then traced back toward the main trunk.

DIAGNOSIS

In general, a definitive diagnosis is required for any mass involving the parotid gland before proceeding with surgery. The optimal method of arriving at a diagnosis is controversial at the present time. The most commonly described method for diagnosing a parotid gland mass is fine-needle aspiration (FNA) in conjunction with

imaging such as computed tomography (CT) or magnetic resonance imaging (MRI). Imaging is used to define the local relationships of the mass to adjacent structures and can often be used to differentiate benign from malignant tumors. The ability of FNA to distinguish malignant from benign is well established.[33]

Wong and Li investigated the exact role of FNA in the diagnostic evaluation of patients with parotid tumors.[34] They carried out a retrospective review of their 12-year experience in treating 186 consecutive patients. They reviewed the FNA results and final pathologic findings in all patients and found that FNA rendered the correct final pathologic condition in 54.3% of cases. They also found that it increased the rate of identification of malignancy to 64.5% versus 26% based solely on clinical signs.[34] Malignant FNA diagnoses (85.7%) and repeatedly inconclusive reports (25.7%) were associated with a higher incidence of malignancy. Wong and Li concluded that the results of FNA provide useful preoperative information and allow more reliable patient counseling, as well as a reduction in pathologic surprises on final pathology reports.[34] They suggested that because it increases the identification of malignant salivary gland neoplasms, it results in more aggressive surgical treatment and hence better tumor clearance.[34]

Zarben and colleagues analyzed and compared the value of FNA and frozen section (FS) analysis in the assessment of parotid gland tumors.[35] They performed a chart review and cross-sectional analysis and identified 110 parotid tumors for which both FNA and FS analysis were performed. Of the 110 parotid tumors, 68 malignancies and 42 benign tumors were analyzed and compared with the final histopathologic diagnosis. They found the accuracy, sensitivity, and specificity of FNA in detecting malignant tumors to be 79%, 74%, and 88%, respectively.[35] On FS analysis, they found the accuracy, sensitivity, and specificity in detecting malignant tumors to be 94%, 93%, and 95%, respectively. The histologic tumor type was correctly diagnosed by FNA and FS analysis in 27 of 42 (64%) and 39 of 42 (93%) benign tumors, respectively, and in 24 of 68 (35%) and 49 of 68 (72%) malignant neoplasms, respectively. Their results showed FS to be superior to FNA with regard to the diagnosis of malignancy and tumor typing. They also found that FNA can be useful in avoiding surgery, such as in patients with inflammatory lesions of the parotid, or in limiting surgery, such as in patients with benign tumors of the parotid.[35]

Both CT (Fig. 56-2) and MRI (Fig. 56-3) have been used for the assessment of parotid gland tumors, and both techniques have been shown to be valid modalities for this indication. However, MRI has been found to be superior to CT in localizing and defining tumor margins in several reports.[36-38] Barsotti and co-authors reported a case of pleomorphic adenoma of the parotid gland and compared the findings on CT and MRI.[39] They found that MRI was dramatically superior to CT for delineation of the tumor. They also noted that the tumor was not seen well on CT because it was isointense with the gland parenchyma.[39]

Two reports provide quantitative data on the ability of MRI to distinguish benign from malignant tumors of the parotid. Ikeda and colleagues published a paper on the usefulness of MRI in establishing the diagnosis of parotid pleomorphic adenoma.[40] T1- and T2-weighted MRI with and without contrast enhancement was performed in 82 patients with parotid tumors. Imaging findings in the 38 patients in whom surgery subsequently revealed pleomorphic adenoma were compared with findings in the 44 patients who had other types of tumor. They focused specifically on homogeneity, signal intensity, contrast enhancement, capsule thickness, lobulation, adenopathy, and infiltration of adjacent fat in the different types of tumors.[40] They found that a low-signal capsule on T2-weighted images and a lobulated contour characterized most pleomorphic

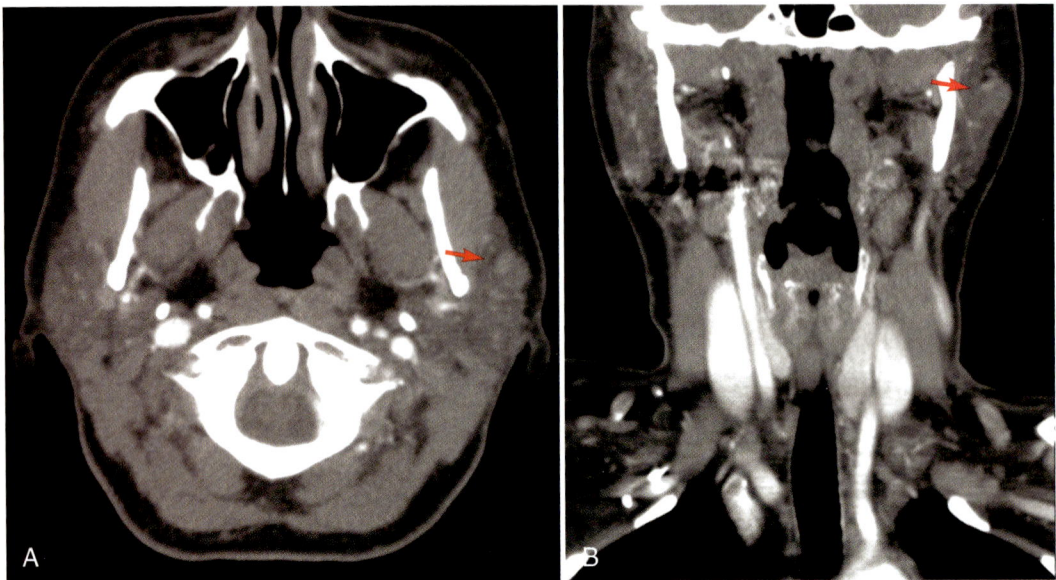

Fig. 56-2 ■ **A,** Computed tomographic axial image of a 1-cm left parotid tumor (*red arrow*). **B,** Coronal image of the same tumor (*red arrow*). Final histopathologic analysis demonstrated that the tumor was a pleomorphic adenoma.

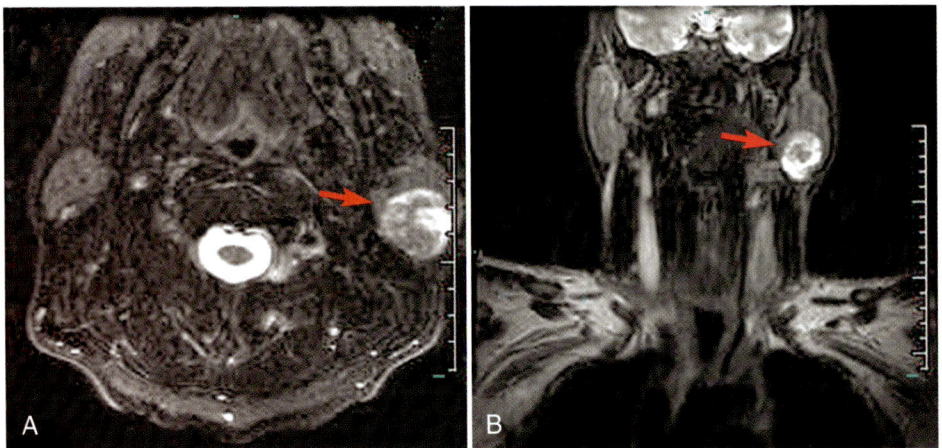

Fig. 56-3 ■ **A,** Magnetic resonance axial image of a 3-cm left parotid tumor (*red arrow*). **B,** Coronal image of the same tumor (*red arrow*). Final histopathologic analysis demonstrated pleomorphic adenoma. Note how easily the tumor can be delineated from the surrounding structures.

adenomas. The sensitivity of the first finding for pleomorphic adenoma was 82% with a specificity of 85%, a positive predictive value of 82%, and a negative predictive value of 84%. For the second finding, the sensitivity was 53% with a specificity of 84%, a positive predictive value of 74%, and a negative predictive value of 67%. They concluded that none of the signs evaluated had perfect sensitivity and specificity but that findings of a complete capsule, lobulated contour, or high T2 signal intensity on MRI have high predictive value for the diagnosis of pleomorphic adenoma.[40]

Okahara and associates examined the role of MRI in the diagnostic evaluation of parotid tumors. The purpose of their article was to illustrate the MRI features of parotid tumors and to correlate them with the pathologic findings.[41] They found marginal morphology, as well as ill-defined or infiltrative margins versus well-defined margins, to be most helpful on MRI in differentiating between a high-grade malignant tumor and a low-grade malignant tumor or benign tumor.[41] They also concluded that MRI can provide clues to the histology of pleomorphic adenoma, Warthin tumor,

monomorphic adenoma, low-grade mucoepidermoid carcinoma, and low-grade adenoid cystic carcinoma.[41]

Bartels and co-workers compared the value of FNA and imaging in the preoperative evaluation of parotid masses.[33] They established the sensitivity, specificity, and accuracy of imaging and FNA alone or in combination for distinguishing benign from malignant parotid tumors. They carried out a retrospective blinded review of preoperative imaging and FNA studies of patients with parotid masses and compared these results with the histologic findings after tumor excision. Forty-eight patients were identified (13 with CT, 35 with MRI).[33] Twenty-three (48%) of the lesions were malignant and 25 (52%) were benign. MRI, CT, and FNA misclassified 17%, 46%, and 21% of the lesions, respectively. They determined the sensitivity, specificity, and accuracy of these tests for detecting malignant lesions to be 88%, 77%, and 83% for MRI; 100%, 42%, and 69% for CT; and 83%, 86%, and 85% for FNA. None of these findings were found to be significantly different. They also found that combinations of imaging and FNA were not significantly better in

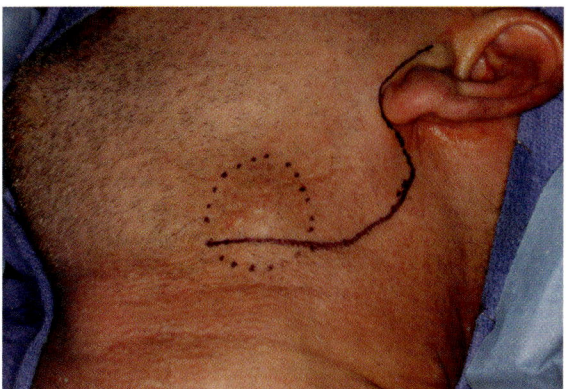

Fig. 56-4 ■ Surgical marking for a modified Blair incision.

detecting malignancy and that imaging and FNA were comparable in their ability to correctly identify malignant parotid lesions preoperatively. The authors suggested that combining these two modalities yields no advantage in terms of specificity, sensitivity, or accuracy of a malignant diagnosis.[33]

TREATMENT

Treatment of parotid tumors is based on proper preoperative assessment and diagnosis. The type of treatment is dictated by the specific diagnosis and can range from narrow local excision, as with extracapsular dissection, to total parotidectomy with sacrifice of the facial nerve and neck dissection.

Parotid tumors are most commonly accessed via the modified Blair incision (Fig. 56-4). This incision provides excellent access to the entire gland with minimal retraction of the skin flap required during dissection. The resultant scar is often inconspicuous because the majority of the incision can be camouflaged within a natural skin crease. In patients with benign pathology for whom cosmesis is of particular concern, a rhytidectomy incision can be used to access the gland. This approach provides very good access to the gland for dissection, but more aggressive retraction is often required. The resultant scar is almost imperceptible.

BENIGN TUMORS

Pleomorphic adenoma is the most common salivary gland tumor and accounts for approximately 80% of parotid tumors.[42] Complete or partial superficial parotidectomy with dissection and preservation of the facial nerve is the principal treatment used for the management of pleomorphic adenomas and other benign parotid tumors. However, there is evidence to support the more conservative approach of extracapsular dissection (Fig. 56-5). The main difference between partial superficial parotid resection and extracapsular parotid dissection is identification and dissection of the facial nerve and removal of a margin of uninvolved glandular tissue.[42] Several authors have shown that partial parotidectomy and extracapsular dissection of a benign pleomorphic adenoma can be performed with comparable rates of local recurrence.[42,43] However, Witt and Rejto compared extracapsular dissection with partial superficial parotidectomy with respect to tumor recurrence and transient and permanent facial nerve dysfunction.[44] They performed a literature review with statistical analysis of published series and found a significantly higher rate of recurrent pleomorphic adenoma and permanent facial

TABLE 56-4	TNM Classification of Major Salivary Gland Tumors	
CLASSIFICATION	**DESCRIPTION**	
Tumor Size		
TX	Primary tumor cannot be assessed	
T0	No tumor present	
T1	Tumor ≤2 cm without extraparenchymal extension	
T2	Tumor 2-4 cm without extraparenchymal extension	
T3	Tumor with extraparenchymal extension but without 7th nerve involvement and/or >4 cm	
T4a	Tumor invades the skin, mandible, ear canal, and/or facial nerve	
T4b	Tumor invades the skull base, pterygoid plates, and/or carotid artery	
Nodal Status		
NX	Lymph nodes cannot be assessed	
N0	No lymph node involvement	
N1	Metastasis to a single lymph node ≤3 cm	
N2	Metastasis to a single ipsilateral lymph node 3-6 cm; multiple ipsilateral, bilateral, or contralateral lymph nodes ≤6 cm	
N3	Metastasis in a lymph node >6 cm	
Metastasis		
MX	Unable to assess for distant metastasis	
M0	No distant metastasis	
M1	Distant metastasis	

Data from Edge SB, Byrd DR, Compton OC, et al: *AJCC cancer staging manual,* ed 7, New York, 2010, Springer.

nerve dysfunction and a lower rate of transient facial nerve dysfunction with extracapsular dissection than with partial superficial parotidectomy.[44]

MALIGNANT PAROTID TUMORS

Malignant parotid tumors are staged according to the TNM classification of the American Joint Committee on Cancer (Tables 56-4 and 56-5). Malignant tumors of the parotid gland are uncommon and represent about 0.5% of all cancers and less than 5% of tumors in the head and neck region.[45] Mucoepidermoid carcinoma is the most common tumor, followed by adenocarcinoma, mixed-type malignant tumor, adenoid cystic carcinoma, acinic cell carcinoma, undifferentiated carcinoma, and squamous cell carcinoma.[45]

The principal treatment of malignant tumors of the parotid gland is surgery with or without adjuvant therapy.[45] Surgery generally involves total parotidectomy with preservation of the facial nerve if sound oncologic principles are not violated. However, in cases in

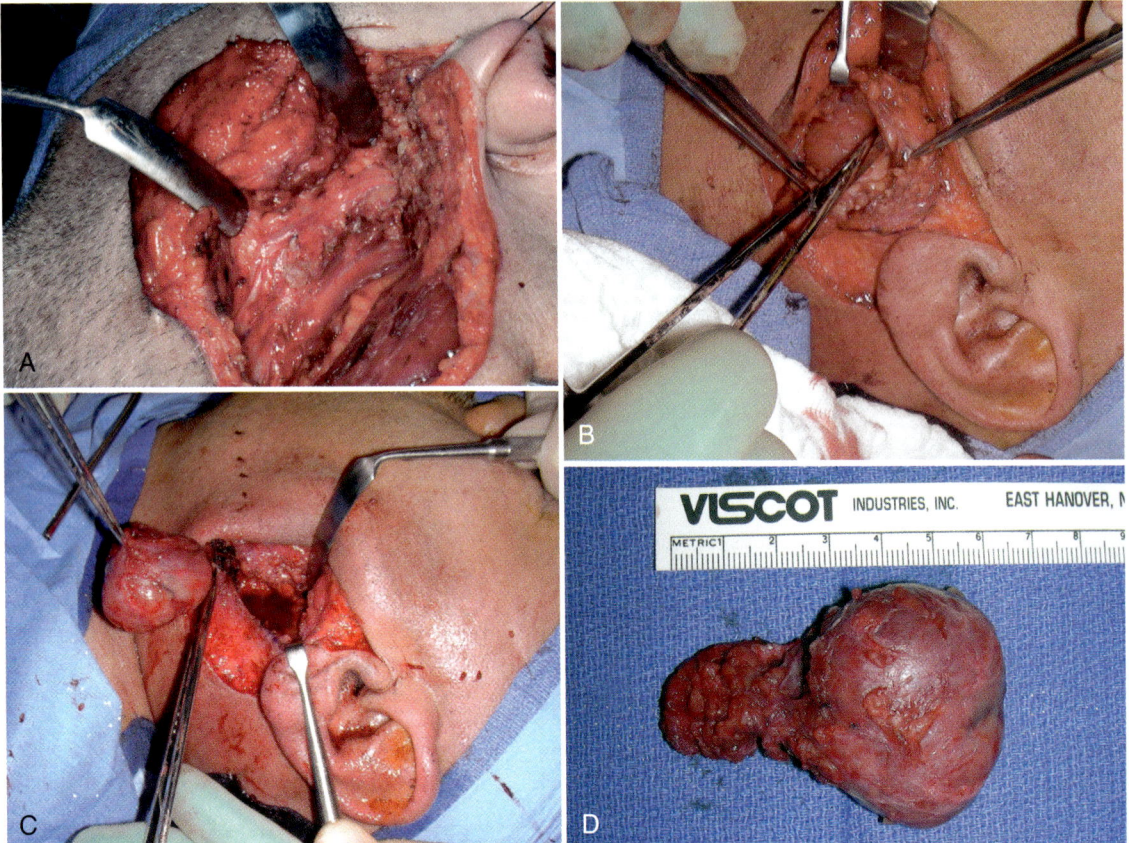

Fig. 56-5 ■ Extracapsular dissection. **A,** A skin flap is raised above the parotid capsule. **B,** The capsule is incised and a narrow rim of normal parotid tissue is removed around the periphery of the tumor. **C,** The tumor is delivered from the parotid bed. **D,** The final specimen.

TABLE 56-5	Staging for Major Salivary Gland Tumors
Stage I	T1N0M0
Stage II	T2N0M0
Stage III	T1N1M0
	T2N1M0
	T3N0M0
	T3N1M0
Stage IV	
Stage IVa	T1N2M0
	T2N2M0
	T3N3M0
	T4aN0M0
	T4aN1M0
	T4aN2M0
Stage IVb	Any T, N3M0
	T4bN0M0
Stage IVc	Any T, any N, M1

Data from Edge SB, Byrd DR, Compton OC, et al: *AJCC cancer staging manual,* ed 7, New York, 2010, Springer.

which the facial nerve is encased by tumor, it must be sacrificed to ensure complete tumor clearance. If the facial nerve is sacrificed, an attempt should be made to reconstruct it immediately with an interpositional nerve graft.[45] As for any oncologic surgical procedure, every reasonable attempt should be made to achieve negative resection margins at the time of ablative surgery. However, several studies have shown that despite negative margins, tumor will recur at the primary site in a significant number of patients.[46]

Factors that have been shown to be associated with more aggressive disease and poor outcomes include tumors with high-grade histology, locally or regionally advanced disease (T3, T4), positive margins, perineural/angiolymphatic invasion, facial nerve involvement/facial paralysis, and extraparotid/extracapsular extension.[46-56] Radiotherapy has been used as a complement to surgery both preoperatively and postoperatively for tumors that exhibit these characteristics.[45] Adenoid cystic carcinoma is associated with an extremely high likelihood of perineural invasion and spread. Consequently, most surgeons and oncologists recommend postoperative radiation therapy along the path of the nerve at risk for involvement.[46,57,58] With the advent of intensity-modulated radiation therapy, patients can receive postoperative radiation therapy without incurring many of the debilitating side effects associated with traditional radiotherapy. Postoperative radiotherapy has been shown to improve locoregional control in patients with advanced-stage salivary gland cancer; however, no prospective trials have demonstrated a beneficial effect on disease-free survival.[46,59-61]

A number of other adjuvant treatment modalities are being investigated at the present time. Adjuvant chemotherapy for salivary gland malignancies is reserved primarily for palliative treatment. At best, adjuvant chemotherapy may slow tumor progression and in some instances achieve a partial response.[62-64] Some of the chemotherapy trials have failed to demonstrate any activity against salivary gland malignancies, whereas others have shown some promise. In a small Italian series, Airoldi and colleagues were able to show that cisplatin-based concomitant chemoradiotherapy followed by adjuvant chemotherapy produced a 50% complete response rate in patients with advanced, unresectable, undifferentiated parotid carcinoma over a short-term follow-up period.[64] These same authors also demonstrated benefit with a combination of vinorelbine and cisplatin in patients with recurrent malignant salivary gland tumors in a separate trial.[65] Though not curative, single-agent therapy using cyclophosphamide, doxorubicin, 5-fluorouracil, or cisplatin has resulted in partial responses.[46,66-68] In general, the response rates achieved with combination therapy, most commonly cyclophosphamide, doxorubicin, and cisplatin, are higher than those with a single agent.[46,69-71]

Neutron beam radiotherapy has been used as adjuvant treatment of malignant salivary gland tumors (particularly adenoid cystic carcinoma) in the past several years, with promising results.[46] Neutron therapy was developed in a few centers in the United States and Europe from the 1930s to the 1980s, but no new facilities for external beam neutron radiotherapy have been scheduled in recent years.[72] Neutrons were the first hadrons used in clinical studies in centers equipped with a cyclotron, and several types of tumors were treated with controversial results. Phase III trials performed in the 1980s suggested that neutrons are indicated for specific tumor types, including salivary carcinomas.[63] During the past decade, neutron therapy has been limited to certain tumor sites (salivary glands, paranasal sinus, some bone and soft tissue sarcomas) because of the high risk for late damage to surrounding tissue.[72-75] This is attributable to the low spatial selectivity and high relative biologic effectiveness of neutrons. Grade 3 and 4 toxicity has been reported in patients undergoing neutron beam therapy, with significant complications such as osteoradionecrosis, central nervous system radionecrosis, optic neuritis/retinitis (blindness), and oral/pharyngeal cutaneous fistulas occurring in as many as 10% of patients.[46,74]

Comprehensive treatment of malignant parotid tumors requires definitive treatment of the primary tumor and consideration of treatment of the neck. Management of the neck may involve observation or neck dissection. The majority of these tumors have a low propensity for lymphatic spread.[76] With parotid tumors, management of the neck differs considerably from that of squamous carcinoma. Metastasis to the cervical regional nodal basins is uncommon with malignancy of the salivary glands in general, with less than 15% of parotid cancers demonstrating clinical evidence of nodal metastasis.[76,77] The incidence of lymph node metastases at the initial evaluation of patients with parotid carcinomas varies from 12.4% to 24%.[76] In reviewing the literature regarding neck dissection for malignant parotid tumors, it becomes evident that there is much controversy surrounding the topic. Most centers suggest elective neck dissection for patients with high-grade histology or large (>4 cm) tumors.[46,78,79] Bell and colleagues advocated comprehensive neck dissection for any node-positive neck, regardless of histology or site.[46] For patients with a clinically negative neck (N0), they advocated selective neck dissection for all patients with high-grade tumors, locally advanced disease, facial nerve paralysis/weakness, and advanced age.[46] They also suggested that there is probably little benefit from elective neck dissection in patients with N0 necks and small, low-grade tumors of the minor salivary glands.[46]

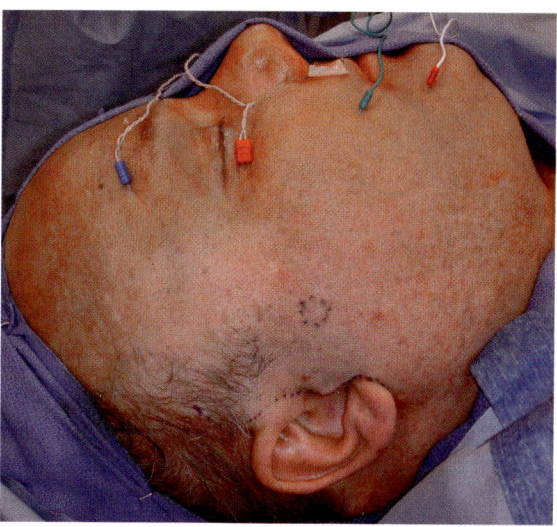

Fig. 56-6 ■ Facial nerve monitor.

COMPLICATIONS

Facial nerve injury is one of the most feared complications of parotid surgery because it results in both cosmetic and functional deficits and can lead to litigation against the surgeon. The incidence of temporary facial nerve deficit following parotid surgery has been reported to be in the range of 20% to 40% and that of permanent dysfunction in the range of 0% to 4%.[80-88] Passive electrophysiologic nerve monitoring (Fig. 56-6) is being used for various head and neck surgical procedures, including thyroidectomy, parathyroidectomy, and otologic and skull base procedures, in addition to parotidectomy. Nerve monitoring devices use needle electrodes placed on the skin to monitor electromyographic recordings from the facial muscles. Usually, four areas innervated by the facial nerve are monitored, the frontal, zygomatic, buccal, and marginal mandibular areas. The monitor alerts the surgeon when either active or passive nerve stimulation has occurred. Its use has increased in recent years for parotid surgery despite a paucity of evidence to support the contention that such monitoring reduces the incidence of temporary and permanent facial nerve injury.[89-91]

Frey syndrome, also known as gustatory sweating or auriculotemporal syndrome, is a well-documented complication of parotid surgery that is characterized by facial flushing and sweating.[92] It is thought to be the result of misdirected nerve regeneration in which the postganglionic parasympathetic fibers of the auriculotemporal nerve supplying the parotid gland regenerate and connect with severed distal sympathetic nerves that innervate subcutaneous sweat glands. When salivation is stimulated, the nerves now stimulate sweat glands in the distribution area of the auriculotemporal nerve.[92] A recent study suggests that it may be one of the most unpleasant long-term complications of parotid surgery.[93] The incidence of Frey syndrome following parotidectomy is highly variable and has been reported to range from 2.6% to 97.6%.[92] A number of measures can be taken to prevent the development of Frey syndrome, including autologous adipose tissue, temporal fascia, fascia lata femoris, and sternocleidomastoid myocutaneous flaps and allogeneic dermal matrix grafts.[92] The latter has been shown to be associated with a significant reduction in the incidence of Frey syndrome and produces excellent cosmetic results without the need for an additional donor site.[94] Frey syndrome can be managed safely and effectively following parotidectomy with injections of botulinum toxin.[95]

PEARLS AND PITFALLS

- Salivary gland tumors are rare when compared with the overall incidence of tumors of the head and neck region. The parotid gland is the most common site of occurrence.
- The facial nerve is the most crucial anatomic structure to identify and preserve during parotid surgery for benign and some malignant tumors because it has both sensory and motor components.
- Commonly described surgical landmarks used to identify the main trunk of the facial nerve include the TMS, the posterior belly of the digastric, the transverse process of the axis, the styloid process, and the tragal pointer.
- The TMS line is usually considered the most constant and consistent surgical landmark for identification of the main trunk of the facial nerve.
- A definitive diagnosis is necessary for any mass involving the parotid gland before proceeding with surgery, but the best method for making a diagnosis is controversial.

- FNA with imaging such as CT or MRI is the most common method for diagnosing a parotid gland mass.
- The principal treatment of pleomorphic adenoma (the most common salivary gland tumor) is complete or partial superficial parotidectomy with dissection and preservation of the facial nerve.
- Treatment of malignant tumors of the parotid gland is usually total parotidectomy with preservation of the facial nerve if sound oncologic principles are not violated.
- If the facial nerve is encased by tumor, it must be sacrificed to ensure complete tumor clearance. An attempt should be made to reconstruct it immediately with an interpositional nerve graft.
- A number of adjuvant treatment therapies are being investigated, including chemotherapy and neutron beam radiotherapy.
- Facial nerve injury is one of the most serious complications of parotid surgery because it causes cosmetic and functional deficits.

REFERENCES

1. Ellis GL, Auclair PL: *Tumors of the salivary glands*, Washington, DC, 1996, Armed Forces Institute of Pathology.
2. Eveson JW, Cawson RA: Salivary gland tumours: a review of 2410 cases with particular reference to histological types, site, age, and sex distribution, *J Pathol* 146:51-58, 1985.
3. Seifert G, Miehlke A, Haubrich J: Diseases of the salivary glands. In Seifert G: *Pathology-diagnosis-treatment-facial nerve surgery*, New York, 1986, George Thieme Verlag.
4. Spiro RH: Salivary neoplasms: overview of a 35-year experience with 2,807 patients, *Head Neck Surg* 8:177-184, 1986.
5. Ellis GL, Auclair PL, Gnepp OR: *Surgical pathology of the salivary glands*, Philadelphia, 1991, WB Saunders.
6. Neville BW, Damm DD, Allen CM, et al: *Oral and maxillofacial pathology*, ed 3, St Louis, 2009, WB Saunders.
7. Thackray AC, Lucas RB: Tumors of the major salivary glands. In *Atlas of tumor pathology*, 2nd series, vol. 10, Washington, DC, 1974, Armed Forces Institute of Pathology.
8. Eneroth CM: Salivary gland tumors in the parotid gland, submandibular gland, and the palate region, *Cancer* 27:1415-1418, 1971.
9. Foote FW, Frazell EL: Tumors of the major salivary glands, *Cancer* 6:1065-1113, 1953.
10. Merrick Y, Albeck H, Nielsen NH, et al: Familial clustering of salivary gland carcinoma in Greenland, *Cancer* 57:2097-2102, 1986.
11. Dalpa E, Gourvas V, Baritaki S, et al: High prevalence of human herpes virus 8 (HHV-8) in patients with Warthin's tumors of the salivary gland, *J Clin Virol* 42:182-185, 2008.
12. Vageli D, Sourvinos G, Ioannou M, et al: High-risk human papillomavirus (HPV) in parotid lesions, *Int J Biol Markers* 22:239-244, 2007.
13. Boukheris H, Ron E, Dores GM, et al: Risk of radiation-related salivary gland carcinomas among survivors of Hodgkin lymphoma: a population-based analysis, *Cancer* 113:3153-3159, 2008.
14. Swanson GM, Burns PB: Cancers of the salivary gland: workplace risks among women and men, *Ann Epidemiol* 7:369-374, 1997.
15. Graham S, Blanchet M, Rohrer T: Cancer in asbestos-mining and other areas of Quebec, *J Natl Cancer Inst* 59:1139-1145, 1977.
16. Mancuso TF, Brennan MJ: Epidemiological considerations of cancer of the gallbladder, bile ducts and salivary glands in the rubber industry, *J Occup Med* 12:333-341, 1970.
17. Milham S Jr: Cancer mortality pattern associated with exposure to metals, *Ann N Y Acad Sci* 271:243-249, 1976.
18. Swanson GM, Belle SH: Cancer morbidity among woodworkers in the U.S. automotive industry, *J Occup Med* 24:315-319, 1982.
19. Elledge R: Current concepts in research related to oncogenes implicated in salivary gland tumourigenesis: a review of the literature, *Oral Dis* 15:249-254, 2009.
20. Gregoire R: Le nerf facialet la parotid, *J Anat (Paris)* 48:437-447, 1912.
21. McWorther G: The relations of the superficial and deep lobe of the parotid gland to the ducts and facial nerve, *Anat Rec* 12:149-154, 1917.
22. Proctor B: The extratemporal facial nerve, *Otolaryngol Head Neck Surg* 92:537-545, 1984.
23. May M: The facial nerve, *Am J Otol* 4:269, 1983.
24. Witt R: *Salivary gland diseases: surgical and medical management*, New York, 2005, Thieme.
25. De Ru JA, Van Benthem PPG, Bleys RLAW, et al: Landmarks for parotid surgery, *J Laryngol Otol* 115:122-125, 2001.
26. De Ru JA, Bleys RLAW, Van Benthem PPG, et al: Preoperative determination of the location of parotid gland tumours by analysis of the position of the facial nerve, *J Oral Maxillofac Surg* 59:525-528, 2001.
27. Bron LP, O'Brien CJ: Facial nerve function after parotidectomy, *Arch Otolaryngol Head Neck Surg* 123:1091-1096, 1997.
28. Browne HJ: Exposure of the facial nerve, *Br J Surg* 75:724-725, 1988.
29. Nishida M, Matsuura H: A landmark for facial nerve identification during parotid surgery, *J Oral Maxillofac Surg* 51:451-453, 1993.
30. Pather N, Osman M: Landmarks of the facial nerve: implications for parotidectomy, *Surg Radiol Anat* 28:170-175, 2006.
31. Witt RL, Weinstein GS, Rejto LK: Tympanomastoid suture and digastric muscle in cadaver and live parotidectomy, *Laryngoscope* 115:574-577, 2005.
32. Rea PM, McGarry G, Shaw-Dunn J: The precision of four commonly used surgical landmarks for locating the facial nerve in anterograde parotidectomy in humans, *Ann Anat* 192:27-32, 2010.
33. Bartels S, Talbot JM, DiTomasso J, et al: The relative value of fine-needle aspiration and imaging in the preoperative evaluation of parotid masses, *Head Neck* 22:781-786, 2000.
34. Wong DS, Li GK: The role of fine-needle aspiration cytology in the management of parotid tumors: a critical clinical appraisal, *Head Neck* 22:469-473, 2000.
35. Zbaren P, Guelat D, Loosli H, et al: Parotid tumors: fine-needle aspiration and/or frozen section, *Otolaryngol Head Neck Surg* 139:811-815, 2008.
36. Som PM, Shugar JM, Sacher M, et al: Benign and malignant parotid pleomorphic adenomas: CT and MR studies, *J Comput Assist Tomogr* 12:65-69, 1988.
37. Mirich DR, McArdle CB, Kulkarni MV: Benign pleomorphic adenomas of the salivary glands: surface coil MR imaging versus CT, *J Comput Assist Tomogr* 11:620-623, 1987.
38. Teresi LM, Lufkin RB, Wortham DG, et al: Parotid masses: MR imaging, *Radiology* 163:405-409, 1987.
39. Barsotti JB, Westesson PL, Coniglio JU: Superiority of magnetic resonance over computed tomography for imaging parotid tumor, *Ann Otol Rhinol Laryngol* 103:737-740, 1994.

40. Ikeda K, Katoh T, Ha-Kawa SK, et al: The usefulness of MR in establishing the diagnosis of parotid pleomorphic adenoma, *AJNR Am J Neuroradiol* 17:555-559, 1996.

41. Okahara M, Kiyosue H, Hori Y, et al: Parotid tumors: MR imaging with pathological correlation, *Eur Radiol* 13(Suppl 4):L25-L33, 2003.

42. Salama AR, Ord RA: Clinical implications of the neck in salivary gland disease, *Oral Maxillofac Surg Clin North Am* 20:445-458, 2008.

43. Smith SL, Komisar A: Limited parotidectomy: the role of extracapsular dissection in parotid gland neoplasms, *Laryngoscope* 117:1163-1167, 2007.

44. Witt RL, Rejto L: Pleomorphic adenoma: extracapsular dissection versus partial superficial parotidectomy with facial nerve dissection, *Del Med J* 81:119-125, 2009.

45. Cederblad L, Johansson S, Enblad G, et al: Cancer of the parotid gland; long-term follow-up. A single centre experience on recurrence and survival, *Acta Oncol* 48:549-555, 2009.

46. Bell RB, Dierks EJ, Homer L, et al: Management and outcome of patients with malignant salivary gland tumors, *J Oral Maxillofac Surg* 63:917-928, 2005.

47. Spiro RH, Armstrong J, Harrison L, et al: Carcinoma of major salivary glands, *Arch Otolaryngol Head Neck Surg* 155:316-321, 1989.

48. Calearo C, Pastore A, Storchi OF, et al: Parotid gland carcinoma: analysis of prognostic factors, *Ann Otol Rhinol Laryngol* 107:969-973, 1998.

49. Hocwald E, Karkmaz H, Yoo G, et al: Prognostic factors in major salivary gland cancer, *Laryngoscope* 111:1434-1439, 2001.

50. Witten J, Hybert F, Hansen HS: Treatment of malignant tumors in the parotid glands, *Cancer* 65:2515-2520, 1990.

51. O'Brien CJ, Soong SJ, Herrera GA, et al: Malignant salivary tumors: analysis of prognostic factors and survival, *Head Neck Surg* 9:82-89, 1986.

52. Beckhardt RN, Weber RS, Zane R, et al: Minor salivary gland tumors of the palate: clinical and pathologic correlates of outcome, *Laryngoscope* 105:1155-1160, 1995.

53. Jansisyanont P, Blanchaert RH, Ord RA: Intraoral minor salivary gland neoplasm: a single institution experience of 80 cases, *Int J Oral Maxillofac Surg* 31:257-261, 2002.

54. Kane W, McCaffrey RV, Olsen KD, et al: Primary parotid malignancies: a clinical and pathologic review, *Arch Otolarygnol Head Neck Surg* 117:307-315, 1991.

55. Renehan AG, Gleave EN, Slevin NJ, et al: Clinico-pathological and treatment-related factors influencing survival in parotid cancer, *Br J Cancer* 80:1296-1300, 1999.

56. Poulsen MG, Pratt GR, Kynaston B, et al: Prognostic variables in malignant epithelial tumors of the parotid, *Int J Radiat Oncol Biol Phys* 23:327-332, 1992.

57. Le QT, Birdwell S, Terris DJ, et al: Postoperative irradiation of minor salivary gland malignancies of the head and neck, *Radiother Oncol* 52:165-171, 1999.

58. Avery CM, Moody AB, McKinna FE, et al: Combined treatment of adenoid cystic carcinoma of the salivary glands, *Int J Oral Maxillofac Surg* 29:277-279, 2000.

59. Armstrong JG, Harrison L, Sprio RH, et al: Malignant tumors of major salivary gland origin. A matched pair analysis of the role of combined surgery and postoperative radiotherapy, *Arch Otolaryngol Head Neck Surg* 116:290-293, 1990.

60. North CA, Lee DJ, Piantoadosi S, et al: Carcinoma of the major salivary glands treated by surgery or surgery plus postoperative radiotherapy, *Int J Radiat Oncol Biol Phys* 18:1319-1326, 1990.

61. Garden AS, el-Nagger AK, Morrison WH, et al: Postoperative radiotherapy for malignant tumors of the parotid gland, *Int J Radiat Oncol Biol Phys* 37:79-85, 1997.

62. Scianna JM, Petruzzelli GJ: Contemporary management of tumors of the salivary glands, *Curr Oncol Rep* 9:134-138, 2007.

63. Gedlicka C, Schull B, Formanek M, et al: Mitoxantrone and cisplatin in recurrent and/or metastatic salivary gland malignancies, *Anticancer Drugs* 13:491-495, 2002.

64. Airoldi M, Fornari G, Pedani F, et al: Paclitaxel and carboplatin for recurrent salivary gland malignancies, *Anticancer Res* 20:3781-3783, 2000.

65. Airoldi M, Pedani F, Succo G, et al: Phase II randomized trial comparing vinorelbine versus vinorelbine plus cisplatin in patients with recurrent salivary gland malignancies, *Cancer* 91:541-547, 2001.

66. Licitra L, Marchini S, Spinazze S, et al: Cisplatin in advanced salivary gland carcinoma. A phase II study of 25 patients, *Cancer* 68:1874-1877, 1991.

67. Jones AS, Phillips DE, Cook JA, et al: A randomized phase II trial of epirubicin and 5-fluorouracil versus cisplatinum in the palliation of advanced and recurrent malignant tumour of the salivary glands, *Br J Cancer* 37:112-114, 1993.

68. Rentscheler R, Burgess MA, Byers R: Chemotherapy for malignant salivary gland neoplasm: a 25 year review of M.D. Anderson Hospital experience, *Cancer* 40:619-624, 1977.

69. Triozzi PL, Brantely A, Fisher S, et al: 5-Fluorouracil, cyclophosphamide, and vincristine for adenoid cystic carcinoma of the head and neck, *Cancer* 59:887-890, 1987.

70. Posner MR, Ervin TJ, Weichselbaum RR, et al: Chemotherapy of advanced salivary gland neoplasms, *Cancer* 50:2261-2264, 1982.

71. Vennok AP, Tseng A, Meyers FJ, et al: Cisplatin, doxorubicin and 5-fluorouracil chemotherapy for salivary gland malignancies: a pilot study of the Northern California Oncology Group, *J Clin Oncol* 5:951-955, 1987.

72. Jereczek-Fossa BA, Krengli M, Orecchia R: Particle beam radiotherapy for head and neck tumors: radiobiological basis and clinical experience, *Head Neck* 28:750-760, 2006.

73. Wambersie A, Richard F, Breteau N: Development of fast neutron therapy worldwide, *Acta Oncol* 33:261-274, 1994.

74. Laramore GE: The use of neutrons in cancer therapy: a historical perspective through the modern era, *Semin Oncol* 24:672-685, 1997.

75. Maor MN, Errington RD, Caplan RJ, et al: Fast-neutron therapy in advanced head and neck cancer: a collaborative international randomized trial, *Int J Radiat Oncol Biol Phys* 32:599-604, 1995.

76. Ferlito A, Pellitteri PK, Robbins KT, et al: Management of the neck in cancer of the major salivary glands, thyroid and parathyroid glands, *Acta Otolaryngol* 122:673-678, 2002.

77. Armstrong JG, Harrison LB, Thaler HT, et al: The indications for elective treatment of the neck in cancer of the major salivary glands, *Cancer* 69:615-619, 1992.

78. Harrison LB, Armstrong JG, Thaler HT, et al: The indications for elective treatment of the neck in cancer of the major salivary glands, *Cancer* 69:615-619, 1992.

79. Medina J: Neck dissection in the treatment of cancer of major salivary glands, *Otolaryngol Clin North Am* 31:815-822, 1998.

80. Eisele DW, Wang SJ, Orloff LA: Electrophysiologic facial nerve monitoring during parotidectomy, *Head Neck* 32:399-405, 2010.

81. Nouraei SA, Ismail Y, Ferguson MS, et al: Analysis of complications following surgical treatment of benign parotid disease, *Aust N Z J Surg* 73:134-138, 2008.

82. Upton DC, McNamar JP, Connor NP, et al: Parotidectomy: ten-year review of 237 cases at a single institution, *Otolaryngol Head Neck Surg* 136:788-792, 2007.

83. Gaillard C, Perie S, Susini B, et al: Facial nerve dysfunction after parotidectomy: the role of local factors, *Laryngoscope* 115:287-291, 2005.

84. Guntinas-Lichius O, Klussmann JP, Wittekindt C, et al: Parotidectomy for benign disease at a university teaching hospital: outcome of 963 operations, *Laryngoscope* 116:534-540, 2006.

85. Witt RL: Facial nerve function after partial superficial parotidectomy: an 11-year review (1987-1997), *Otolaryngol Head Neck Surg* 121:210-213, 1999.

86. Bron LP, O'Brien CJ: Facial nerve function after parotidectomy, *Arch Otolaryngol Head Neck Surg* 123:1091-1096, 1997.

87. Leverstein H, van der Wal JE, Tiwari RM, et al: Surgical management of 246 previously untreated pleomorphic adenomas of the parotid gland, *Br J Surg* 84:399-403, 1997.

88. Laccourreye H, Laccourreye O, Cauchois R, et al: Total conservative parotidectomy for primary benign pleomorphic adenoma of the parotid gland: a 25-year experience with 229 patients, *Laryngoscope* 104:1487-1494, 1994.

89. Terrell JE, Kileny PR, Yian C, et al: Clinical outcome of continuous facial nerve monitoring during primary parotidectomy, *Arch Otolaryngol Head Neck Surg* 157:1081-1087, 1997.

90. Witt RL: Facial nerve monitoring in parotid surgery: the standard of care? *Otolaryngol Head Neck Surg* 119:468-470, 1998.
91. Dulguerov P, Marchal F, Lehmann W: Postparotidectomy facial nerve paralysis: possible etiologic factors and results with routine facial monitoring, *Laryngoscope* 109:754-762, 1999.
92. Laccourreye L, Muscatelo B, Bonan C, et al: Botulinum toxin type A for Frey's syndrome: a preliminary prospective study, *Ann Otol Rhinol Laryngol* 107:52-55, 1998.
93. Baek CH, Chung MK, Jeong HS, et al: Questionnaire evaluation of sequelae over 5 years after parotidectomy for benign diseases, *J Plast Reconstr Aesthet Surg* 62:633-638, 2009.
94. Ye WM, Zhu HG, Zheng JW, et al: Use of allogenic acellular dermal matrix in prevention of Frey's syndrome after parotidectomy, *Br J Oral Maxillofac Surg* 46:649-652, 2008.
95. Martos Díaz P, Bances del Castillo R, Mancha de la Plata M, et al: Clinical results in the management of Frey's syndrome with injections of botulinum toxin, *Med Oral Patol Oral Cir Bucal* 13:E248-E252, 2008.

Chapter

57

Minor Salivary Gland Tumors

Antonia Kolokythas, Michael Miloro

Minor salivary gland tumors form a heterogeneous group of lesions in the head and neck because of their unique composition and ubiquitous distribution throughout the oropharynx, nasopharynx, and hypopharynx. It has been estimated that there are approximately 500 to 1000 lobules of minor salivary gland tissue dispersed throughout the oral mucosal and submucosal tissues of the lips, floor of mouth, hard and soft palates, tonsillar pillars, buccal mucosa, and tongue. These minor salivary gland lobules typically begin development in utero during the third month of gestation. As a group, salivary gland neoplasms constitute less than 3% of all head and neck tumors, but because of their remarkable structural variability, behavior, and presentation, these tumors remain an area of great clinical and research interest, while debate regarding assessment and management continues among clinicians.

ETIOPATHOGENESIS/CAUSATIVE FACTORS

The salivary gland primordia arise as buds of proliferative epithelium from the primitive stomodeum (oral cavity) that is partly ectodermal and partly endodermal in origin, and this is responsible for the diversity seen in minor gland neoplasms. The two cells of origin for the majority of the salivary gland parenchymal neoplasms are the intercalated cell, a stem or reserve excretory cell within the salivary duct system, and the myoepithelial cell.[1,2] The etiologic factors responsible for the development of salivary gland tumors are poorly understood, and only rarely there is an antecedent disease that predisposes to their development. However, controversy exists regarding the incidence of salivary gland tumors in patients with breast cancer, because studies have shown either increased incidence or no association, whereas radiation treatment primarily for benign conditions has been implicated in 11.3% of cases.[3,4] Approximately 25%

of all salivary gland tumors are found in the minor salivary glands, and 50% of these tumors are malignant.[1]

PATHOLOGIC ANATOMY

Usually the minor salivary glands are not clinically evident, although salivary lobules often can be palpated in the lips. For the most part, the gland lobules are 1 to 5 mm in size and separated from one another by a connective tissue stroma, but glands in the posterior hard palate tend to be more numerous and confluent. Most salivary gland lobules have individual excretory ducts that open directly into the oral cavity, but the ductal orifices are not usually visually perceptible in the normal oral mucosa. Minor salivary glands are mostly mucous type exocrine glands with the exception of those located around the circumvallate papillae and the lateral tongue that are serous in composition. The minor glands are mostly nonencapsulated and lie in close approximation with the structures around them such as the muscles of the tongue and lips. This intramuscular, nonencapsulated morphology is a factor to be considered in the histologic evaluation of invasive growth and malignancy in minor salivary gland neoplasms.[1,5] Lymphatic drainage of the minor salivary gland is site specific and closely follows the lymphatic drainage of each particular site.[6]

The glands can be grouped into vestibular, palatine, and lingual based on location in the oral cavity, and each group consists of contiguous subgroups. The vestibular glands include the labial, buccal, and retromolar subgroups, whereas the palatine group consists of the hard and soft palate and glossopalatine glands. Based on their distribution over the body of the tongue, the lingual glands are located anteriorly, posteriorly, over the faucial area, known as deep posterior groups, or within the lingual sulcus or sublingual groups.[5]

The ratio of benign to malignant neoplasms is 1.1 : 1 and most, roughly 50-60%, originate from the palatine group at the junction

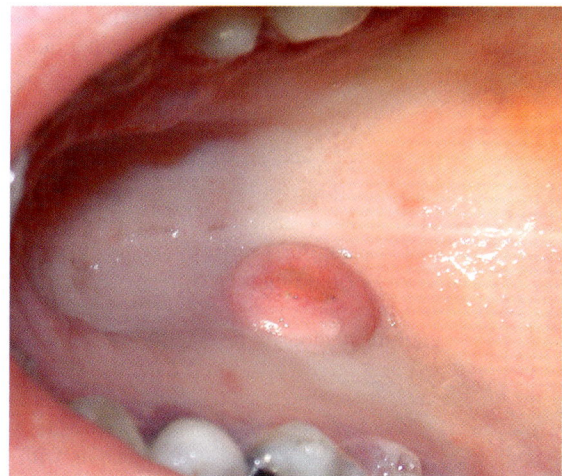

Fig. 57-1 ■ Pleomorphic adenoma (PA) of the hard palate.

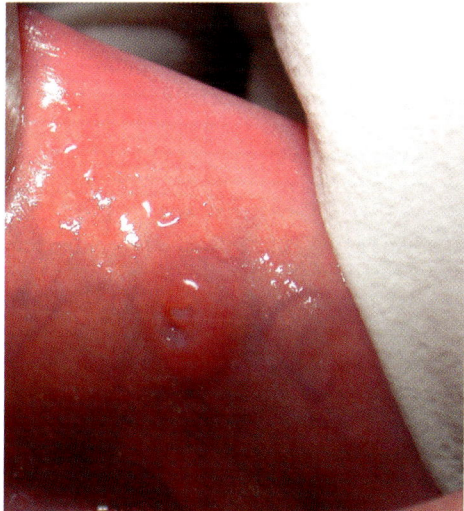

Fig. 57-2 ■ Inverted ductal papilloma (lip).

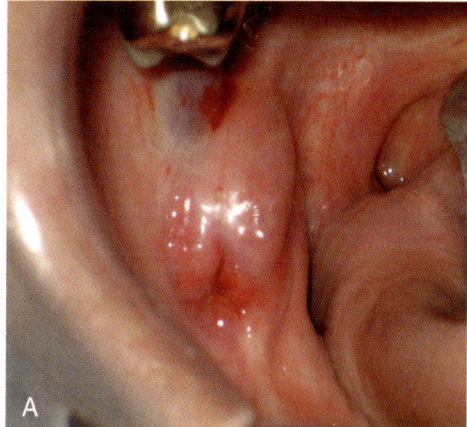

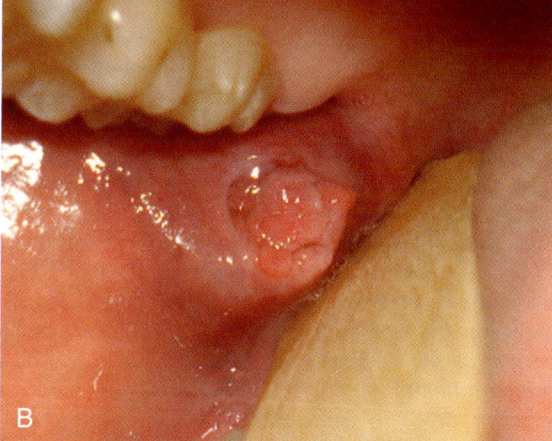

Fig. 57-3 ■ **A,** Low-grade mucoepidermoid carcinoma (MECA). **B,** Intermediate-grade mucoepidermoid carcinoma (MECA).

TABLE 57-1	Distribution of Minor Salivary Gland Neoplasms in Descending Frequency (RMF: Retromolar Fossa)
SITE BENIGN	**SITE MALIGNANT**
Palate	Palate
Upper lip	Buccal mucosa/RMF
Buccal mucosa/RMF	Tongue
Lower lip	Floor of mouth
Tongue	Other/not specified
Floor of mouth	Upper lip
Other/not specified	Lower lip

of the hard and the soft palates. The predominance of the pleomorphic adenoma (PA) (Fig. 57-1) in the benign category and adenoid cystic carcinoma (ACC) among the malignant tumors is consistent throughout the reported case series regarding these tumors. Terminal duct adenocarcinomas and mucoepidermoid carcinomas (MECA) (intermediate or low grade) are the second most common low-grade neoplasm groups to demonstrate a strong predilection for the palate.[5,7-10]

Among the vestibular glands, most benign neoplasms occur in the upper lip (84.5%) with monomorphic adenomas (inverted ductal papilloma [Fig. 57-2] and sialadenoma papilliferum) occurring more commonly than pleomorphic adenomas.

Although the lower lip is a less frequently involved site (15.5%), the majority of these neoplasms are malignant (93.8%). Once again, ACC and MECA, followed by acinic cell carcinomas, are the malignant tumors most likely to be found in this anatomic site.[11-13] Although the retromolar fossa (RMF) contains only scattered minor salivary glands, it is a relatively common site of origin for MECA, which may or may not involve the underlying bone (Fig. 57-3). Finally, the base of the tongue is the site of predilection for malignant minor salivary gland tumors, whereas benign tumors (which are very rare) favor the middle and anterior portions of the tongue. ACC and MECA account for roughly two thirds of the malignant

neoplasms in this anatomic site. The distribution of occurrence for benign and malignant neoplasms is shown in Table 57-1.

DIAGNOSTIC STUDIES

Various diagnostic techniques—including sialography, radionucleotide scanning, ultrasonography, computed tomography scanning, and magnetic resonance imaging—are available as adjunctive studies useful in the assessment of salivary gland disorders. Most of these modalities are useful only for the major salivary glands, specifically the parotid and submandibular glands. Computed tomography (CT) and magnetic resonance imaging (MRI) are the preferred diagnostic techniques for evaluation of minor salivary gland pathology. A CT scan with contrast is easily obtained, is cost effective, and may provide valuable information regarding potential bony involvement and differentiation between inflammatory and neoplastic processes. The limitations of CT scanning include dental restoration artifacts and the inability to evaluate for perineural invasion (PNI); therefore, MRI is considered by many clinicians to be the imaging study of choice.[14,15] Since the introduction of gadolinium and the marked improvement in the resolution of the images obtained by contemporary equipment, MRI is considered equal, if not superior, to contrast-enhanced CT scans.[16] In addition, MRI permits evaluation of PNI, which is a critical factor in treatment planning of certain neoplasms, such as adenoid cystic carcinoma.[15,17]

Although studies have demonstrated a correlation between findings on CT and MRI and histopathologic findings that assist in differentiation between benign and malignant processes, a histologic tissue diagnosis is mandatory for appropriate multidisciplinary treatment planning.[16] Fine-needle aspiration biopsy (FNAB) for cytologic examination has gained popularity with increased experience among institutions in performing as well as interpreting the FNAB, and recent studies have reported sensitivity and specificity of 84.8-93.7%, with an overall accuracy of 91.1%.[15,18] FNAB is valuable in the diagnosis of salivary gland neoplasms of the major salivary glands, but it has limited to no value for minor gland pathology because of the small size of the minor glands, as well as the fact that open biopsy is easily performed via transoral access for lesions in the oral cavity and oropharynx.

Both the first (1972) and second edition (1991) of the World Health Organization's (WHO) histologic classification of the salivary gland neoplasms are based on the histologic features observed with the conventional light microscope.[2,19,20] Immunohistochemistry, cytophotometry, molecular and cytogenic studies, and electron microscopy are all recognized as being very useful in the identification of specific neoplasms, differentiation among a variety of salivary gland tumors, as well as an assessment of their behavioral characteristics.

Specific substance identification—such as S-100 protein for cells of neural origin; actin and myosin for identification of myoepithelial cells; cytokeratin stains for differentiation among lymphoma, melanoma, and undifferentiated carcinoma; amylase levels for different variants of acinic cell carcinoma; and carcinoembryonic antigen (CEA) or thyroglobulin for distinction among primary clear cell tumors and metastatic thyroid carcinoma—is made possible with immunocytochemistry.[2,19,21-23] More recently, beta-6 Integrin, tenascin-C, and MMP-1 (matrix metalloproteinase-1), which are invasion-related proteins, frequently overexpressed in many human malignancies, were identified in three salivary gland tumor groups (ACC, polymorphous low-grade adenocarcinoma [PLGA], and PA).[24] Although cytophotometry does not provide additional diagnostic information for all salivary gland tumors, a statistical correlation between DNA content (ploidy and S-phase fractions) and biologic aggressiveness of MECA, ACC, myoepithelioma, and some adenocarcinomas not otherwise specified has been demonstrated experimentally.[25-27]

Determination of overexpression of oncoproteins, oncogenes, and proliferative markers, as well as identification of specific structural genetic aberrations, has been associated with poorer prognosis, independent of other known prognostic indicators.[2,25,26,28-35] The clinical application of these techniques has yet to be determined. Finally, electron microscopy (EM) can be beneficial in providing diagnostic information that may not be obtained with other studies, although distinguishing between benign and malignant tumors is not possible with EM.[36,37]

TREATMENT/RECONSTRUCTIVE GOALS

Treatment for salivary gland tumors has not changed dramatically over the past several decades, and surgery remains the primary treatment modality of choice. For benign tumors, such as PA, that account for the majority of the minor salivary gland tumors, wide local excision with 5-mm margins to ensure adequate margins is considered the preferred method of treatment. The periosteum is usually not involved and serves as a good anatomic barrier, so it should be left intact in managing hard palate and retromolar fossa benign tumors.[2,15,37,38] For low-grade malignancies such as low-grade MECA and PLGA (Fig. 57-4), wide local excision with 1-cm margins, or excision to the next anatomic barrier, should provide for adequate resection and clear margins. For high-grade malignancies that invade surrounding structures, or cases of adenoid cystic carcinoma of the hard palate with a high risk of neural involvement, in addition to wide local excision with 1-cm margins and excision to the next anatomic barrier (following the basic principles of oncologic surgery), perioperative biopsy of nerve tissue in the vicinity of the tumor at risk for tumor invasion is considered to be necessary. When clear evidence of nodal involvement is present or for intrabony malignancies of the mandible, neck dissection is indicated.

Removal of the "at risk" or involved levels of the cervical nodes should be done based on the known patterns of drainage for each anatomic site.[15,38] For advanced tumors with extension into the paranasal sinuses, nasopharynx, or with evidence of perineural invasion, surgery alone may not be adequate to ensure clear margins and therefore adjuvant postoperative radiation therapy should be considered.[15,39] The role of conventional radiotherapy as the primary treatment option for minor salivary gland malignancies remains controversial because there is a paucity of prospective randomized trials, although some studies indicate that local regional control rates are unacceptably poor at 25%.[40] The current practice of combined surgery and radiation therapy is based on the presence of significant adverse prognostic factors associated with high-grade malignancies such as perineural or bony invasion, or the presence of positive margins following resection surgery. In addition, combined therapy has been shown to be useful in cases amenable to palliative therapy alone.[41] Most recently, the efficacy of fast neutron radiotherapy for

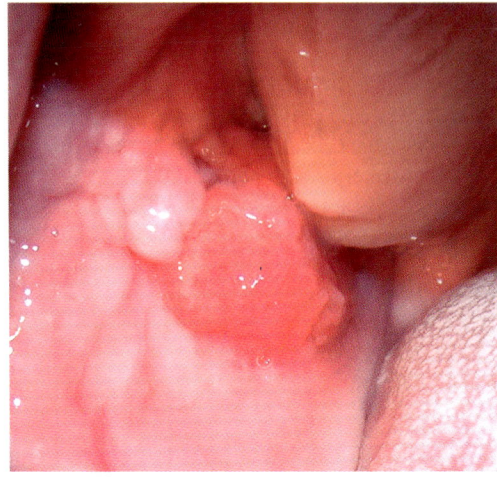

Fig. 57-4 ■ Polymorphous low-grade adenocarcinoma (PLGA).

the treatment of salivary gland tumors has been evaluated, and there is increasing evidence that this may be effective in treatment cases with gross residual disease following resection or for recurrent tumors. Excellent local and regional control rates were reported in cases in which fast neutron radiotherapy regimens were used for postresection surgery "maintenance" when no evidence of residual disease was present.[42-44]

Perhaps one of the most significant major advances in the management of minor salivary gland tumors has been the reconstruction option available currently with the wide utilization of free tissue transfer techniques. Traditionally, ablative defects involving the palate or the maxilla are "reconstructed" with the insertion of obturator prostheses for assistance with speech and swallowing, while ignoring the hard and soft tissue defects. Midface and maxillary reconstruction remains a surgical challenge even for the experienced head and neck surgeon, and it is difficult to achieve consistently good or excellent results. The primary reconstructive objective remains the replacement of missing tissue with similar tissue, and free tissue transfer offers the unique ability to predictably accomplish this goal. Restoration of form and function is of paramount importance and can be achieved with microvascular flaps that allow for replacement of hard or soft tissues. Rehabilitation can be achieved with osteocutaneous flaps when indicated, which can provide the required substructures for support of dental implants and subsequent implant-retained prostheses. Fibula, deep circumflex iliac artery, scapular system, and radial forearm flaps are most commonly used for head and neck reconstruction based on the location as well as the residual defect and hard and soft tissues required following ablative surgery.[45] Primary closure with the use of local and regional flaps remains a valuable option for small defects that cause minimal functional and aesthetic deficits and for individuals with significant co-morbid conditions classifying these patients poor surgical candidates.

NEW DIRECTIONS IN MANAGEMENT

Unlike squamous cell carcinoma involving the head and neck, adjuvant chemoradiotherapy has limited or no role in the overall management of localized salivary gland malignancies. However, in cases of nonresectable lesions, locally advanced tumors, or distant metastatic disease (commonly associated with aggressive histologic diagnoses, such as ACC, high-grade MECA, and salivary duct carcinoma), systemic therapy may become an option, and adjuvant radiation therapy is often recommended.[46] Traditional chemotherapeutic agents and combination regimens with antitumor activity have only shown modest efficacy in the management of minor salivary gland neoplasms and have no impact on survival rates. Therefore, the minimal improvement in clinical response achieved with combination versus monotherapy regimens cannot justify the associated increased morbidity and toxicity of the treatment protocols.[47-50] As expected, the alteration of the expression of molecular markers in cancer has heightened interest specifically in salivary gland malignancies, and novel agents directed at these targets have been incorporated in recent study protocols. The focus has been directed toward c-kit, vascular endothelial growth factor/receptor (VEGF/VEGFR), epidermal growth factor receptor (EGFR), nerve growth factor (NGF), and Her-2/neu, as these are overexpressed in high-grade malignancies.[51-55] What remains unclear from the available in vitro and in vivo studies is whether these phenomena correlate with patient outcomes. Results from phase I and II studies with inhibitors for these markers are somewhat difficult to interpret because these tumors are rare, so adequate subject numbers and response to treatment are unclear in such indolent disease

processes.[46] The most promising target at the present time appears to be the dual targeting with Lapatinib against EGFR and Her-2/neu because of the potential cross-talk between the two tyrosine kinase receptors. In one study, tumor stabilization was noted in 75% of the subjects with adenoid cystic carcinoma versus 47% in the non-ACC group; further, the 6-month stable clinical disease was noted to be higher than historically identified.[56] Future directions in chemotherapeutic indications for salivary gland tumor treatment require further investigation and molecular profiling of these specific malignancies, as well as the development of multitarget chemotherapy agents.

POSTOPERATIVE CARE

Benign minor salivary gland pathology, managed appropriately, does not usually present significant challenges with regard to the need for additional therapy. In general, follow-up care is individualized based on the subsite of salivary glands involved, the type of surgery performed, and the subsequent reconstructive techniques utilized. Maxillary obturator prostheses usually require frequent initial adjustments until the final prosthetic appliance is fabricated, usually by a maxillofacial prosthodontist, when available. In the

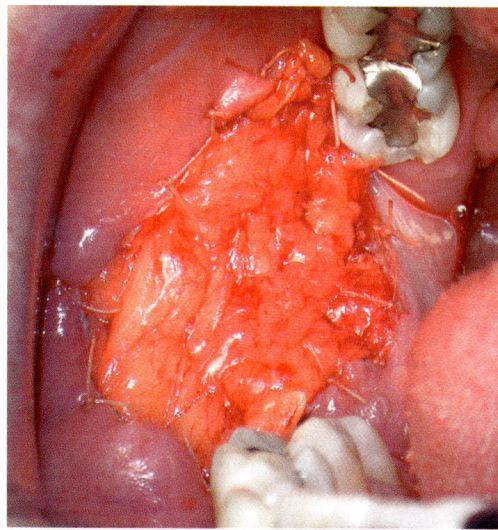

Fig. 57-5 ■ Buccal fat pad flap for reconstruction post resection.

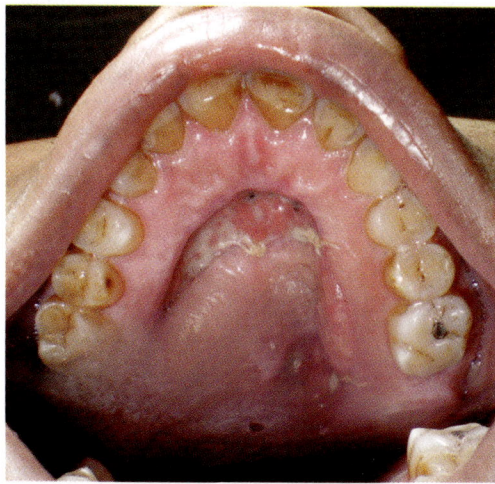

Fig. 57-6 ■ Palatal flap for reconstruction of palatal defect 2 weeks postoperatively.

postoperative period, the wounds should be inspected carefully and frequently for appropriate healing, especially in this patient population with compromised immune function and co-morbidities, and sutures may be removed at the appropriate time periods based on the anatomic site involved.

Consistent with basic oncologic principles, regularly scheduled interim posttreatment follow-up visits and local and regional surveillance for tumor recurrence should be standardized when managing patients with malignant tumors. Of paramount importance is the incorporation of regular surveillance for distant metastases in cases of high-grade malignancies. For example, cases of ACC with a predilection for neurotropism have the risk of proximal spread because of perineural invasion and skip metastasis, as well as pulmonary involvement; therefore, assessment of these distant sites is of primary importance in the short- and long-term patient postsurgical assessment.

Periodic imaging with MRI scanning is of primary importance, as well as annual chest x-ray imaging, and or chest CT scanning. Periodic comparison of imaging studies over time for evaluation of disease stability or progression is the primary goal of follow-up care and guides the decision-making process and the future need for intervention. It should be noted that these are malignancies with indolent courses and that treatment failures increase with increased survival time, unlike other types of cancers.[5,6,15]

PEARLS AND PITFALLS

- The relative rarity, histologic diversity, and subtle histologic differences among these variably behaving minor salivary gland tumors can occasionally cause diagnostic dilemmas and may lead to difficulties in treatment planning and management. The clinician must have a high index of suspicion based on a careful consideration of the patient signs and symptoms, as well as a detailed clinical examination with appropriate radiographic imaging in order to appropriately diagnose and manage these neoplasms.

- Adequate biopsy specimens must be obtained with an appropriate technique following basic surgical principles, with recognition of the subsequent surgical plan in order to avoid a misdiagnosis or a delay in diagnosis and treatment. Regarding histopathology, there must be a low threshold for obtaining additional specialty pathologic consultations or utilizing special staining techniques for further investigation if there is uncertainty in the microscopic diagnosis.

- Also important are a strict adherence to oncologic principles and an in-depth understanding of specific tumor behavior and characteristics when treating minor salivary gland tumors. For example, the lack of capsule found in pleomorphic adenomas, the tendency of ACC to result in skip metastasis and spread via perineural invasion, or the risk of high grade MECA to present with lymph node involvement or resemble squamous cell carcinoma histologically are some of the unique characteristics of salivary gland tumors that require careful treatment planning and appropriate follow-up. Malignant salivary gland tumors should be routinely presented and discussed at a multidisciplinary head and neck tumor board so the expertise from various specialty groups, with diverse knowledge and experience, will allow for an exchange of ideas and the utilization of the most up-to-date treatment protocols available. The surgical team should be familiar and proficient with the variety of reconstructive options and available rehabilitation following complex intraoral resection surgery in order to provide the patient with acceptable restoration of form and function.

  For example, in cases of buccal or RMF neoplasms, innovative utilization of local tissues such as the buccal fat pad flap (Fig. 57-5) or a variety of palatal flaps (Fig. 57-6) for palatal tumors can be invaluable for reconstruction of residual defects. Similarly, the expertise of a maxillofacial prosthodontist is very helpful in the planning and restoration of masticatory function and facial cosmesis, with the ultimate goal of improvement of quality of life. Quality of life is a critical outcome measure in head and neck cancer management, including salivary gland tumors, mainly because of the inability to improve survival, especially in cases of advanced disease. As with oral cancer, treatment for salivary gland neoplasms has not drastically changed over the past several decades. Surgery remains, for the most part, the treatment modality most commonly offered, with the addition of radiation therapy when indicated. The focus on patient care has shifted toward preservation of form and function via the careful selection of appropriate reconstruction techniques.

- It should be noted that chronic pain and difficulties with mastication, swallowing, and speech all negatively influence function and adversely impact on quality of life. In general, studies have demonstrated that improved function following resection is most appropriately achieved with the utilization of free tissue composite flaps that correct bone continuity and soft tissue defects and can support dental implants and future dental prostheses. Both patient subjective perception of improved quality of life and objectively measured health-related quality of life indicators have been demonstrated in multiple studies in the head and neck cancer literature.[57-60]

- Chronic pain issues from the temporomandibular joint and muscles of mastication are unique to the management of oral cavity neoplasms, including salivary gland tumors. In addition to some of the potential neurologic complications associated with head and neck surgery and the specific type and location of the tumor, as well as possible functional limitations, these factors certainly impact poorly on activities of daily living and contribute to an overall poor quality of life for these patients. Finally, facial disfigurement, scarring, speech impairment, the inability to control secretions, loss of taste, the need for removable prosthetic appliances, and difficulties with mastication may have serious psychological impact on these patients.

- The surgical oncologic principles that ensure adequate tumor resection in order to prevent recurrence or limit metastasis should be combined with the basic principles of hard and soft tissue reconstruction that will provide the most successful long-term outcomes regarding form and function in order to ensure an acceptable quality of life.

REFERENCES

1. Regezi JA, Sciubba JJ, Jordan R: In Regezi JA, editor: *Oral pathology clinicopathologic correlations*, vol 1, St. Louis, 2003, Saunders.
2. Thawley SE: In Thawley SE, editor: *Comprehensive management of head and neck tumors*, vol 2, Philadelphia, 1999, W.B. Saunders.
3. Abbey LM, Schwab BH, Landau GC: Incidence of second primary breast cancer among patients with a first primary salivary gland tumor, *Cancer* 54:1943, 1984.
4. Spitz MR: Incidence of salivary gland cancer in United States relative to radiation exposure, *Head Neck Surg* 10:305, 1988.
5. Shah JP, Johnson NW, Batsakis JG: In Shah JP, editor: *Oral cancer*, vol 1, London, 2003, Martin Dunitz Taylor & Francis Group.
6. Harrison LR, Sessions R, Hong W: In Harrison LB, editor: *Head and neck cancer: a multidisciplinary approach*, vol 1, Philadelphia, 2004, Lippincott Williams & Wilkins.

7. Goldblatt LI: Salivary gland tumors of the tongue: analysis of 55 new cases and review of the literature, *Cancer* 60:74-81, 1987.

8. Waldron CA: Tumors of the intraoral salivary glands: a demographic and histologic study of 426 cases, *Oral Surg Oral Med Oral Pathol* 66:323-333, 1988.

9. Ito FA: Salivary gland tumors in the Brazilian population: a retrospective study of 496 cases, *Int J Oral Maxillofac Surg* 34(5):533-536, 2005.

10. Pires F: Intraoral minor salivary gland tumors: a clinicopathological study of 546 cases, *Oral Oncol* 43(5):463-470, 2009.

11. Neville BW: Labial salivary gland tumors, *Cancer* 61:2113-2116, 1988.

12. Batsakis J: Oral monomorphic adenomas, *Ann Otol Rhinol Laryngol* 100:348-350, 1991.

13. Brannon RB: Ductal papillomas of the salivary gland origin: a report of 19 cases and a review of the literature, *Oral Surg Oral Med Oral Pathol* 92:68-77, 2001.

14. Kaneda T: Imaging tumors of the minor salivary glands, *Oral Surg Oral Med Oral Pathol* 78(3):385-390, 1994.

15. Calzada GG, Hanna EY: In Cummings CW, editor: *Benign neoplasms of the salivary glands*, ed 5, St. Louis, 2010, Mosby.

16. Yabuuchi H: Salivary gland tumors: a diagnostic value of gadolinium-enhanced dynamic MR imaging with histopathologic correlation, *Radiology* 226:345-354, 2002.

17. Yousem DM: Major salivary gland imaging, *Radiology* 216:19-29, 2000.

18. Costas A: Fine needle aspiration biopsy (FNAB) for lesions of the salivary glands, *Br J Oral Maxillofacial Surg* 38:539-542, 2000.

19. Seifert G, Sobin SL: The World Health Organization's histological classification of salivary gland tumors: a commentary on the second edition, *Cancer* 70(2):379-385, 1992.

20. Seifert G, Sobin SL: Histologic classification of salivary gland tumors. In *International histologic classification of tumors*, Berlin, 1991, Springer-Verlag.

21. Mori M, Ninomiya NT, Okada Y: Myoepithelioma and myoepithelial adenomas of salivary gland origin: immunohistochemical evaluation of filament proteins, *Path Res Pract* 184, 1989.

22. Williams SB, Ellis GL, Auclair PL: Immunohistochemical analysis of basal cell adenocarcinoma, *Oral Surg Oral Med Oral Pathol* 75, 1993.

23. Hellquist HB, et al: Bcl-2 immunoreactivity in salivary gland neoplasms is unrelated to the expression of mRNA for natural killer cell stimulatory cytokines interleukin (IL)-2 and IL-12, *Virchows Arch* 429(2-3):149-158, 1996.

24. Westernoff TH, et al: Beta-6 Integrin, tenascin-C, and MMP-1 expression in salivary gland neoplasms, *Oral Oncol* 41(2):170-174, 2005.

25. Timon CI, et al: Acinic cell carcinoma of salivary glands: prognostic relevance of DNA flow cytometry and nucleolar organizer regions, *Arch Otolaryngol Head Neck Surg* 120, 1994.

26. Stenman G, et al: Adenoid cystic carcinoma: a third type of human salivary gland neoplasms characterized cytogenetically by reciprocal translocations, *Anticancer Res* 2(1-2):11-15, 1982.

27. Pinto AE, et al: Objective biologic parameters and their clinical relevance in assessing salivary gland neoplasms, *Adv Anat Pathol* 7(5):294-306, 2000.

28. Maruya S, et al: Gene expression screening of salivary gland neoplasms: molecular markers of potential histogenetic and clinical significance, *J Mol Diagn* 6(3):180-190, 2004.

29. Maruya S, et al: Differential expression of p63 isotypes (DeltaN and TA) in salivary gland neoplasms: biological and diagnostic implications, *Hum Pathol* 36(7):821-827, 2005.

30. Marques YM, et al: Mdm2, p53, p21 and pAKT protein pathways in benign neoplasms of the salivary gland, *Oral Oncol* 44(9):903-908, 2008.

31. Jordan R, et al: Demonstration of c-erbB-2 oncogene overexpression in salivary gland neoplasms by in situ hybridization, *J Oral Pathol Med* 23(5):226-231, 1994.

32. Honjo N, et al: Comprehensive loss of heterozygosity analysis and identification of a novel hotspot at 3p21 in salivary gland neoplasms, *Otolaryngol Head Neck Surg* 137(1):119-125, 2007.

33. Giannoni C, et al: c-erbB-2/neu oncogene and Ki-67 analysis in the assessment of palatal salivary gland neoplasms, *Otolaryngol Head Neck Surg* 112(3):391-398, 1995.

34. El-Naggar AK, et al: Chromosomal and DNA ploidy characterization of salivary gland neoplasms by combined FISH and flow cytometry, *Hum Pathol* 28(8):881-886, 1997.

35. Edwards PC, Bhuiya T, Kelsch RD: Assessment of p63 expression in the salivary gland neoplasms adenoid cystic carcinoma, polymorphous low-grade adenocarcinoma, and basal cell and canalicular adenomas, *Oral Surg Oral Med Oral Pathol Oral Radiol Endod* 97(5):613-619, 2004.

36. Dardick I: A role for electron microscopy in salivary gland neoplasms, *Ultrastruct Pathol* 9(1-2):151-161, 1985.

37. Batsakis JG: The pathology of head and neck tumors: Salivary glands: Part I, *Head Neck Surg* 1:59, 1978.

38. Ord RA: Salivary gland disease and tumors. In Miloro M, editor: *Peterson's principles of oral and maxillofacial surgery*, ed 2, vol 1, Hamilton, Ontario, 2004, BC Decker.

39. Sadeghi A: Minor salivary gland tumors of the head and neck: treatment strategies and prognosis, *Am J Hematol Oncol* 16(1):3-12, 1993.

40. Laramore GE: Radiotherapy as a primary treatment for malignant salivary gland neoplasms. In Johnson DM, editor, *Head and neck cancer*, New Year, 1993, Elsevier Science.

41. Garden A: Postoperative radiation therapy for malignant tumors of minor salivary glands: outcomes and patterns of failure, *Cancer* 73:2563, 1994.

42. Douglas JGL: Treatment of locally advanced adenoid cystic carcinoma of the head and neck with neutron radiotherapy, *Int J Radiat Oncol Biol Phys* 46:551-557, 2000.

43. Douglas JGK: Treatment of salivary gland neoplasms with fast neutron radiotherapy, *Arch Otolaryngol Head Neck Surg* 129:944-948, 2003.

44. Douglas JG, Silbergeld DL, Laramore GE: Gamma knife stereotactic radiosurgical boost for patients treated primarily with neutron radiotherapy for salivary gland neoplasms, *Stereotact Funct Neurosurg* 82(2-3):84-89, 2004.

45. Fernandes, R: Reconstruction of maxillary defects with the radial forearm free flap. In Tirbod Fattahi RF, editor: *Atlas of Oral and Maxillofacial Surgery Clinics of North America: maxillary reconstruction*, Philadelphia, 2007, W.B. Saunders.

46. Mehra, R, Cohen, RB: New agents in the treatment of malignancies of the salivary and thyroid glands, *Hematol Oncol Clin North Am* 22:1279-1295, 2008.

47. Licitra L, Marchini S, Spinazze S, et al: Cisplatin in advanced salivary gland carcinoma. A phase II study of 25 patients, *Cancer* 68(9):1874-1847, 1991.

48. Airoldi M, Pedani F, Succo G, et al: Phase II randomized trial comparing vinorelbine versus vinorelbine plus cisplatin in patients with recurrent salivary gland malignancies, *Cancer* 91(3):541-547, 2001.

49. Airoldi M, Fornari G, Pedani F: Paclitaxel and carboplatin for recurrent salivary gland malignancies, *Anticancer Res* 20(5C):3781-3783, 2000.

50. Gilbert J, Li Y, Pinto HA, et al: Phase II trial of taxol in salivary gland malignancies (E 1394): a trial of the Eastern Cooperative Oncology Group, *Head Neck* 28(3):197-204, 2006.

51. Edwards P, Bhuiya T, Kelsch RD: C-kit expression in the salivary gland neoplasms adenoid cystic carcinoma, polymorphous low grade adenocarcinoma and monomorphic adenoma, *Oral Surg Oral Med Oral Pathol* 95(5):586-593, 2003.

52. Adreadis D, Epivatianos A, Poulopoulos A, et al: Detection of C-KIT (CD 117) molecule in benign and malignant salivary gland tumors, *Oral Oncol* 42(1):57-65, 2006.

53. Lequerica-Fernandez P, Astudilo A, de Vicente IC: Expression of vascular endothelial growth factor of salivary gland carcinomas correlates with lymph node metastasis, *Anticancer Res* 27(5B):3661-3666, 2007.

54. Zhang J, Peng B: In vitro angiogenesis and expression of nuclear factor kappaB and VEGF in high and low metastasis cell lines of salivary gland adenoid cystic carcinoma, *BMC Cancer* 7:95-101, 2007.

55. Wang L, Sun Y, Jiang L, et al: Nerve growth factor and Tyrosine kinase A in human salivary adenoid cystic carcinoma: expression patterns and effects on in vitro invasive behavior, *J Oral Maxillofac Surg* 64(4):636-641, 2006.

56. Agulnik M, Cohen EW, Cohen RB, et al: Phase II study of lapatinib in recurrent or

metastatic epidermal growth factor and/or erbB2 expressing adenoid cystic carcinoma and non adenoid cystic carcinoma malignant tumors of the salivary glands, *J Clin Oncol* 25(25):3978-3984, 2007.

57. Urken ML: Oromandibular reconstruction using microvascular composite free flaps,

Arch Otolaryngol Head Neck Surg 117:733-744, 1991.

58. Urken ML: Functional evaluation following microvascular oromandibular reconstruction of the oral cancer patient: a comparative study of reconstructed and nonreconstructed patients, *Laryngoscope* 101:935-950, 1991.

59. Vaughan, E: An analysis of morbidity following major head and neck surgery with particular reference to mouth function, *J Max Fac Surg* 10:129, 1982.

60. Rogers SN: Health related quality of life and clinical function after primary surgery for oral cancer, *Br J Oral Max Surg* 40:11-18, 2002.

Chapter **58**

Management of Head and Neck Sarcoma

Rafael A. Madero-Visbal, Thomas D. Shellenberger

Sarcomas of the head and neck are a heterogeneous group of malignancies that display a spectrum of clinical behavior from slow growing to locally aggressive and regionally destructive lesions with the potential for systemic metastases. Like sarcomas of other sites of origin, those arising in the head and neck constitute a diverse array of histologic types with variable biologic behavior. Sarcoma affects a multiplicity of subsites within the head and neck, each with unique anatomic implications on form and function. Although sarcomas are uncommon malignancies overall, these tumors occur even less commonly in the head and neck region; only about 10% of primary tumors arise from this region. Therefore, treatment recommendations are drawn from the results of multi-institutional trials representing small subgroups of patients with head and neck sarcoma and from the few retrospective series from single institutions. Together, these factors contribute to the formidable challenge posed by these malignancies for the surgeon, the radiation oncologist, and the medical oncologist managing sarcomas in the head and neck region.

ETIOPATHOGENESIS/CAUSATIVE FACTORS

Approximately 9% of soft tissue sarcomas in adults originate in the head and neck, whereas most arise in an extremity (59%), the trunk (19%), or the retroperitoneum (15%).[1] Like sarcoma in general, head and neck sarcoma occurs in a wide range of age groups, though most often in children, adolescents, and young adults. Indeed, in children, as many as 35% of rhabdomyosarcomas arise in the head and neck.[2] Sarcomas are very rare among head and neck neoplasms, representing only 1% of all primary tumors located within the head and neck region.[3] The majority of head and neck sarcomas arise sporadically in patients without identifiable predisposing genetic risk factors, and exposure to a known environmental carcinogen can be identified in less than 10% of patients with head and neck sarcomas.[4]

PATHOLOGIC ANATOMY

Considering the preponderance of benign soft tissue masses and the relative frequency of cervical metastases from squamous cell carcinoma of the upper aerodigestive tract, a diagnosis of sarcoma is rare in the head and neck. Moreover, the nonspecific nature of presenting symptoms, sometimes brought to attention by antecedent trauma, typically fails to raise the suspicion of sarcoma, resulting in delay in diagnosis. Together, these factors contribute to the difficulty in diagnosing sarcoma at most head and neck sites. A minority of patients develop tumors at subsites that produce symptoms early and allow earlier detection. The subsite of origin determines the clinical presentation and subsequent diagnostic evaluation of patients with sarcoma of the head and neck.

Among 1161 patients evaluated with sarcoma of the head and neck at the University of Texas M. D. Anderson Cancer Center between 1970 and 2004 (Table 58-1), the most frequent subsites of origin included the scalp or face (30%) and the sinonasal tract or anteromedial skull base (31%). The parotid gland or neck accounted for 19% of these tumors and the upper aerodigestive tract (oral cavity, oro/hypopharynx, and larynx) for 18%; sarcomas arising from the ear or posterolateral skull base were exceedingly rare (only 1%).

Like soft tissue sarcomas of the extremity and trunk, those arising in the neck commonly present as a painless mass. Although a frequent presentation of head and neck sarcoma, a solitary neck mass is only rarely diagnosed as a primary soft tissue sarcoma. Although the presentation of a patient with a painless neck mass raises a broad range of diagnostic possibilities, the clinical setting alone can often narrow the differential diagnosis. Tumors of the neck can impinge on vital structures, causing dysphagia, hoarseness, and even dyspnea. Physical examination typically reveals a subcutaneous mass with possible distortion or destruction of adjacent structures. Associated signs and symptoms of pain and fixation to deep structures are ominous. Like painless masses arising in the neck, those in the parotid region do not frequently raise suspicion of sarcoma on differential diagnosis. Sarcoma of the scalp and face may present with

TABLE 58-1   Head and Neck Sarcomas at the University of Texas M. D. Anderson Cancer Center (1970-2004)

HISTOLOGIC TYPE	NO.	%	SCALP AND FACE	SITE OF ORIGIN SINONASAL TRACT ANTEROMEDIAL SKULL BASE	EAR POSTEROLATERAL SKULL BASE	UPPER AERODIGESTIVE TRACT	PAROTID AND NECK
Bony							
Osteosarcoma	173	14.9	0	95	1	76	1
Cartilaginous							
Chondrosarcoma	75	6.5	1	50	0	22	2
Fibrous							
Malignant fibrous Histiocytoma	111	9.6	37	24	3	13	34
Fibrosarcoma	42	3.6	13	15	0	7	7
Dermatofibrosarcoma protuberans	60	5.2	48	0	1	0	11
Muscular							
Rhabdomyosarcoma	150	12.9	21	82	4	29	14
Leiomyosarcoma	33	2.8	7	8	0	8	10
Vascular							
Angiosarcoma	135	11.6	115	5	3	3	9
Hemangiopericytoma	23	2.0	6	8	0	2	7
Neural							
Neurogenic sarcoma	59	5.1	20	6	0	1	32
Fatty							
Liposarcoma	28	2.4	7	3	0	4	14
Histogenesis unclear							
Synovial sarcoma	46	4.0	11	3	0	11	21
Ewing's sarcoma	13	1.1	4	5	0	0	4
Alveolar soft part sarcoma	6	0.5	1	3	0	1	1
Unclassified	207	17.8	58	56	2	32	59
Head and neck sarcoma (Totals)	1161	100	349	363	14	209	226

From Shellenberger TD, Sturgis EM: Sarcoma: special situations: head and neck. In Pollock RE, Curley SA, Ross MI, Perrier ND, editors: *Advanced therapy in surgical oncology*, Philadelphia, 2007, BC Decker.

skin and soft tissue manifestations that suggest the pathologic type. For instance, erythematous or violaceous macular lesions, which are often described as a spreading bruise, suggest angiosarcoma, whereas a raised, sclerotic, reddish blue plaquelike nodule is associated with dermatofibrosarcoma protuberans.

DIAGNOSTIC STUDIES

Imaging studies augment the physical examination with a more accurate assessment of the size and location of tumors in the head and neck.[5] Imaging studies also delineate bony involvement, intracranial extension, and regional nodal disease. High-resolution computed tomography (CT) and magnetic resonance imaging (MRI) scans are the studies of choice in nearly all cases. CT scanning is rapid and presents fewer problems with motion artifact than MRI. CT also offers greater sensitivity for bony abnormalities, another advantage of this modality. Furthermore, CT imaging is less expensive than MRI. MRI, however, offers much better soft tissue resolution and is therefore better able to evaluate the primary lesion, perineural extension, dural involvement, bone marrow replacement, and orbital invasion. Multiplanar imaging also provides more accurate views of the tumor and adjacent structures. Other advantages of MRI are the lack of exposure to radiation and iodinated contrast material. Because of the unique qualities of CT and MRI, they can often be used in a complementary fashion, especially for surgical planning for skull base tumors. Imaging characteristics can differentiate between various histologic entities to predict specific pathologic features that assist in diagnosis. For example, osteosarcoma classically causes the radial periosteal and extracortical bone deposition that produce a sunburst appearance on plain radiographs or CT scan.

Upon completion of imaging studies, a biopsy should be performed to establish a definitive tissue diagnosis and histologic classification for optimal planning of therapy, regardless of how strongly the history, physical findings, and radiographic studies suggest sarcoma. Whereas an initial biopsy can be done with simple fine-needle aspiration, core needle biopsies provide adequate tissue to accurately subtype the tumor. Nevertheless, some institutions and pathologists prefer an open biopsy. When an open approach is required, the technique should be carefully considered to avoid contamination of uninvolved adjacent fascial compartments. Complete surgical excision is preferred over incisional biopsy for small masses in the neck or parotid. Incisional biopsy should be reserved for cases in children and for large masses when dysfunction or disfigurement might result from complete surgical resection. The incision for any biopsy should be oriented to easily incorporate future definitive surgical approaches. Moreover, the extent of tissue dissection and tumor resection should be limited to achieve only the goals of obtaining representative tissue. All specimens from current and previous biopsies, along with clinical and radiographic features, must be reviewed by a pathologist with experience in sarcoma subtyping. Special immunohistochemical stains and cytogenetic studies can greatly assist in identifying the tissue of origin. Because few centers have extensive experience in sarcoma evaluation, a second opinion from an outside facility can aid in resolving any diagnostic dilemmas.

Sarcomas are classified pathologically by tissue of origin to aid in determining prognosis and optimal treatment strategies. Head and neck sarcomas arise from bony or soft tissue elements depending on the mesenchymal cells from which they are derived. Among our series of patients with head and neck sarcomas at the University of Texas M. D. Anderson Cancer Center, most tumors, approximately 80%, were of the soft tissue type, and only 20% were of bony or cartilaginous origin (see Table 58-1). The most common subtypes of sarcoma found within the head and neck region are osteosarcoma, pleomorphic sarcoma (malignant fibrous histiocytoma), angiosarcoma, and rhabdomyosarcoma.

TREATMENT/RECONSTRUCTIVE GOALS

The treatment approach toward sarcoma of the head and neck is determined by the tumor type, location, and grade, along with consideration of patient age and performance status. The treatment goals are determined by resectability. Surgery alone or combined with adjuvant radiotherapy is the mainstay of treatment for sarcomas of the head and neck. A multimodal approach offers improved local control in the management of head and neck sarcoma, especially for those lesions with high histologic grade or anatomic limitations to en bloc resection. An optimal approach is best planned in a multidisciplinary setting with consideration for the timing and sequence of modes of therapy, reconstructive strategies, and plans for rehabilitation. In parallel with limb-sparing surgical approaches permitted by multimodal therapy for extremity sarcomas, functional organ preservation has emerged in the treatment strategies for head and neck sarcoma.

SPECIFIC TREATMENT AND TECHNIQUES

SURGERY

Surgical resection with wide margins, alone or combined with adjuvant radiotherapy, provides the best chance for cure of head and neck sarcoma in the absence of metastatic disease. The unique anatomic considerations of the head and neck allow smaller tumors to involve critical neurovascular structures, limiting complete en bloc resection, with implications for both local control and survival. Therefore, the operation should be planned by an experienced surgical team with the expertise of specialized radiologists and pathologists. Moreover, consultation with neurologic, ophthalmologic, and plastic surgeons is often warranted.

Surgery for sarcoma of the head and neck should follow the same sound oncologic principles applied to sarcoma operations at other sites. The conduct of surgery for sarcoma of any site of origin is dictated by a growth pattern in which centrifugal expansion occurs with infiltration along tissue planes formed by fascia, muscle, and bone. Compressed tissue surrounding the enlarging mass forms a pseudocapsule that is penetrated by malignant cells extending a considerable distance from gross tumor.[26] Therefore, excision along involved planes leaves extracapsular microscopic disease in situ at the circumference of the resection margin, leading to the possibility of multicentric recurrence, and such extracapsular enucleation of sarcoma carries a local recurrence rate of up to 90%.[27] Conversely, complete excision may be accomplished by limiting dissection to uninvolved tissue planes and resecting the tumor en bloc with wide (2 to 3 cm) margins—including, when possible, at least one uninvolved tissue plane circumferentially. The resection may include skin, subcutaneous tissue, and soft tissue or bone adjacent to the tumor. Any incisions and tracts of a previous biopsy should be excised en bloc with the specimen. Major neurovascular structures should be widely exposed proximally and distally to allow meticulous assessment of the perineural or adventitial planes in determining resectability. The resected specimen margins are carefully inked for pathologic assessment of microscopic clearance. Residual disease is a powerful predictor of local recurrence and disease-related mortality.

Surgery for sarcoma of the head and neck combines these oncologic principles with basic tenets that apply to surgical procedures at each subsite. Though guided by similar sound oncologic principles, surgery in the head and neck poses additional challenges because of the unique anatomic considerations of the site. Operations for sarcoma of the head and neck vary with the subsite of tumor. The primary surgical goal, however, remains the same as that for sarcomas at other sites—complete en bloc excision.

Sarcomas presenting as a mass in the neck often arise from tissue within the fascial compartment of the neck. Tumors may be contained within the fascial compartment or expand to involve superficial or deep structures. Complete resection is attained more easily for soft tissue sarcomas of the neck than for those arising at other head and neck sites. The primary goal of en bloc resection can usually be achieved by neck dissections defined by the boundaries of uninvolved structures. When the mass is contained within a fascial compartment, the mass can be removed by excision of the involved compartment and its structures by modifications of standard oncologic neck dissection. Such an approach adheres to the oncologic principles of compartment dissection of the neck defined by tissue planes rather than the goal of complete lymphadenectomy. Neck wounds can typically be closed primarily. When primary closure places undue tension on wound edges, however, larger skin defects can occasionally be closed with local rotation flaps or split thickness skin grafts. Larger defects and those requiring bulk are best handled by pedicled myocutaneous flaps from pectoralis major and trapezius muscle donor sites. These more complex reconstructive options should also be considered to abrogate the potential risk for complications related to preoperative radiotherapy or subsequent postoperative radiotherapy.

Sarcomas may arise as a mass in the parotid gland. For tumors arising in the superficial lobe of the parotid gland, superficial parotidectomy can be performed with preservation of the facial nerve. Those tumors arising from the deep lobe often present as a parapharyngeal space mass and may be excised by a transcervical approach. Tumors involving both the superficial and deep lobes of the parotid often present with facial paralysis and require radical parotidectomy, sacrificing the facial nerve to obtain complete resection. Moreover, mastoidectomy may be required to obtain negative surgical margins.

Wide local excision is the initial step in treatment for the majority of soft tissue sarcomas of the scalp and face. The ability to achieve clear surgical margins is hampered, however, by the propensity for radial spread (particularly for angiosarcoma) and the desire to preserve form and function. For most lesions of the scalp and some of the face, the procedure of choice is wide local excision down to bone, including the periosteum, with meticulous frozen sections to ensure negative margins. For scalp tumors with bony involvement of the calvarium, craniectomy is required. For lesions overlying the parotid gland, the excision is extended to include superficial parotidectomy with facial nerve dissection to preserve the main trunk and uninvolved branches. With eyelid involvement, total lid resection may be required, whereas extension beyond the periorbita or orbital septum may require orbital exenteration for complete resection. Although conservative surgery followed by adjuvant therapy may preserve a globe, the implications of incomplete resection on survival must be considered. Extension of tumor to the bony and cartilaginous structures of the midface may require maxillectomy and rhinectomy for adequate resection. Perineural spread of tumor along major cranial nerve branches is an ominous sign, often limiting complete resection owing to skull base involvement and the unreliability of frozen section assessment of involved nerves. Although such perineural extension is common for other head and neck histologic types (squamous cell carcinoma and adenoid cystic carcinoma), it is rare for sarcomas of the head and neck.

The approach to reconstruction of defects resulting from surgical resection of soft tissue sarcoma of the scalp and face is determined by the size and complexity of the defect. Options vary from simple primary closure to more advanced techniques such as microvascular free-tissue transfer. The primary reconstructive goals are to restore form by providing coverage of exposed bone and preventing radiotherapy-associated complications. Additional goals include restoration of eyelid function, oral competence, and a patent nasal airway. Well-executed reconstruction is critical to maximizing form, function, and quality of life. Primary closure with local rotation or advancement flaps is often adequate for facial soft tissue defects. Scalp defects more commonly require split-thickness skin graft coverage. For defects widely exposing cortical bone, removal of the outer table can provide a well-vascularized medullary bone surface capable of supporting a skin graft. Larger defects resulting from resection of facial bones and overlying soft tissue often require microvascular free flap reconstruction. Moreover, prostheses may be invaluable in restoring facial form and oronasal separation after orbital exenteration, total rhinectomy, or maxillectomy without major loss of skin and soft tissue. For sarcomas of the upper aerodigestive tract, more classic procedures such as laryngectomy or mandibulectomy may be required.

RADIOTHERAPY

The rationale for adjuvant radiation in the management of head and neck soft tissue sarcoma in adults has stemmed from the results of limb-sparing surgery combined with postoperative radiotherapy for extremity sarcoma. Indeed, that approach offers improved functional results and local control rates similar to those of radical amputation without compromising overall survival.[28] Although adjuvant radiation therapy for management of the extremity sarcoma is supported by randomized trials and large institutional series, patients with head and neck sarcoma were either excluded or insufficient in number to allow meaningful subgroup analysis. Moreover, no similar studies focusing on the treatment of head and neck sarcoma are available to define the optimal role of radiation therapy. Therefore, support for the use of adjuvant radiation therapy for the head and neck soft tissue sarcoma is largely empirical, extrapolated from the experience at other sites of origin or based on retrospective reviews of head and neck series.

The need for adjuvant local therapy is strongly supported by the high rate of local recurrence linked to the difficulty in obtaining microscopically negative margins after resection of tumors in close proximity to vital structures within the head and neck region. Bentz et al. reported a series of adult soft tissue sarcomas of the head and neck from Memorial Sloan-Kettering Cancer Center in which final pathologic findings demonstrated positive margins in 42% of patients overall and 63% of patients presenting after prior treatment.[29] A high rate of local recurrence was attributed to the predominance of patients treated with surgery alone (77%) and, more important, demonstrated a close relationship between local recurrence and survival. Thus, adjuvant radiotherapy appears to improve local control rates with the potential of increasing disease-free survival.

Our standard approach administers adjuvant radiotherapy after surgery for head and neck soft tissue sarcoma in patients with high-grade and some intermediate-grade tumors of any size. Only patients with small (<5 cm), previously untreated, low-grade tumors resected with negative microscopic margins may be considered adequately treated by wide local excision alone. External beam therapy is delivered postoperatively to total doses similar to those employed in sarcoma of the extremity, 60 to 70 Gy in standard fractions over 4 to 6 weeks.

Brachytherapy is an alternative approach to adjuvant radiotherapy in patients with head and neck soft tissue sarcoma, involving placement of multiple catheters within the tumor resection bed to deliver iridium. Brachytherapy offers the theoretical advantage of delivering an adequate dose of ionizing radiation to the surgical bed while sparing adjacent vital structures of the head and neck region based on the radiobiology of the inverse square law. The utility of brachytherapy in head and neck sites can be inferred from the report of Harrison et al. of a prospective trial in which surgery plus adjuvant brachytherapy improved local control rate to 90% from 65% with surgery alone for completely resected high-grade sarcomas of the extremities and trunk.[30]

Like the mode of radiotherapy, the optimal timing of radiotherapy has not been determined. Preoperative radiotherapy offers several theoretic advantages over postoperative radiotherapy.[31] First, radiation therapy delivered early in the course of a multidisciplinary approach can improve planning and ensure that treatment is delivered without the delays imposed by perioperative complications. Second, a lower total dose of radiation can be delivered to a smaller field of tumor that may have greater tissue oxygenation. Finally, preoperative radiation can result in a tumor response that facilitates surgical resectability. A randomized trial of soft tissue sarcoma of the extremities found a higher rate of wound complications in patients treated with preoperative radiation (35%) than patients treated with postoperative radiation (17%), with similarly high rates of local control and progression-free survival.[32] Nonetheless, wound healing complications in the head and neck may be offset by a generally better regional blood supply and more frequent use of primary reconstruction with vascularized tissue.[33]

Preoperative radiation may also be justified in selected patients whose soft tissue sarcoma of the head and neck has been deemed unresectable or inoperable, if conservative resection can offer palliation. De Paoli et al. reported the use of preoperative radiation therapy prior to resection of skull base sarcomas that had been considered unresectable. In each of seven patients, an initially inoperable tumor was conservatively resected in order to preserve function or maximize palliation.[34]

CHEMOTHERAPY

Despite adequate local tumor control with surgery and radiotherapy, mortality from head and neck sarcoma occurs from distant metastasis, most commonly to lungs. Thus, the goals of chemotherapy for sarcoma have been directed toward systemic control in an attempt to prolong disease-free survival. Such efforts have been approached with therapeutic, adjuvant, and palliative intentions. The use of traditional generic approaches to chemotherapy belies the heterogeneity of soft tissue sarcomas in that chemosensitivity varies according to the tumor subtype.[35] Head and neck sarcomas range according to histologic subtype from highly responsive to universally resistant to cytotoxic chemotherapy. The likelihood of a response is further influenced by tumor grade, the patient's age and performance status, and the timing of metastatic disease.[35] Therefore, major obstacles to the use of adjuvant chemotherapy have been the risks of toxicity in patients who are unlikely to respond to therapy and the difficulty in identifying patients who are most likely to benefit from therapy.

The use of postoperative chemotherapy for head and neck soft tissue sarcoma bears a burden of proof similar to that for localized, resectable soft tissue sarcoma of other sites. A lack of benefit from adjuvant chemotherapy for head and neck sarcoma may be implied from the Sarcoma Meta-analysis Collaboration, which evaluated 14 trials of doxorubicin-based adjuvant chemotherapy, several of which included head and neck sites.[36] Thus, there is still no conclusive evidence for the use of adjuvant chemotherapy following resection for patients with head and neck soft tissue sarcoma.

Findings of the European Organisation for Research and Treatment of Cancer (EORTC) trial in 468 soft tissue sarcoma patients comparing an adjuvant regimen of CYVADIC (cyclophosphamide, vincristine, doxorubicin, and dacarbazine) with no chemotherapy carry implications in the treatment of head and neck soft tissue sarcoma.[37] Relapse-free survival rate was significantly increased (56% versus 43% for controls) and local recurrence rate significantly reduced (17% versus 31%) by adjuvant chemotherapy despite similar rates of distant metastasis and overall survival. The reduction in local recurrence rate was apparent only in head and neck and trunk tumors but not in extremity tumors. Thus, these findings suggest a potential for adjuvant chemotherapy to improve local control in high-risk disease sites such as the head and neck, where radical surgery and radiation are less feasible.

Preoperative chemotherapy for head and neck sarcoma offers several of the same theoretical advantages proposed for chemotherapy at other disease sites and for preoperative radiotherapy.[38] First, delivering systemic therapy earlier in the disease course may be more effective against smaller tumor burdens of micrometastatic disease. Second, induction therapy may result in a response that improves the likelihood of complete resection with negative margins

that might not be possible otherwise. Another advantage is the ability to assess a tumor response in situ by radiologic imaging and pathologically after resection and thus tailor subsequent treatment approaches while providing additional prognostic information. The feasibility of surgery after neoadjuvant chemotherapy has been demonstrated by Meric et al. in a retrospective review of 309 patients who underwent surgery for extremity or retroperitoneal/visceral soft tissue sarcoma.[38] Patients who received neoadjuvant chemotherapy had no increase in early or delayed surgical complications compared to those who underwent surgery without neoadjuvant therapy.

Although preoperative chemoradiation strategies have been investigated in the treatment of extremity and retroperitoneal soft tissue sarcomas since the early 1990s, similar approaches for head and neck tumors have been less studied. Such strategies are based primarily on maximizing local control while preserving function and secondarily on early treatment of potential micrometastatic disease. The rationale is directed toward prolonging recurrence-free or even overall survival in selected patients. Pisters and colleagues cite the promise of future investigation supported by (1) the favorable response rates and acceptable toxicity profiles in preliminary reports of extended-duration chemotherapy with concurrent radiation., (2) local control rates in excess of 95% with concurrent (intravenous or intra-arterial) doxorubicin-based chemoradiation for locally advanced soft tissue sarcoma, and (3) favorable preliminary survival data from RTOG 95-14.[39] This multi-institutional phase II trial has shown a 2-year actuarial overall survival rate of 95% among 66 patients with high-risk extremity sarcoma treated by preoperative sequential chemotherapy and split-course radiation.[40] Furthermore, novel approaches to radiosensitization—including doxorubicin-, gemcitabine-, idoxuridine-, razoxane-, and ifosfamide-based regimens—have shown promise in selected patients with soft tissue sarcomas of various sites. Though limited by the local complications of intra-arterial delivery to tumors of the head and neck, chemotherapy with doxorubicin-based regimens delivered by intravenous routes and combined with concurrent or sequential radiation may offer similar promise. Furthermore, the comparability of response rates between head and neck and extremity sites of soft tissue sarcoma warrants the inclusion of patients with head and neck tumors in future multi-institutional trials.

POSTOPERATIVE CARE

The major objectives for surveillance after curative therapy for head and neck sarcoma parallel those outlined by Patel and colleagues for soft tissue sarcoma: (1) early identification of curable recurrences and reversible/treatable complications of therapy, (2) identification of second primary tumors, and, increasingly, (3) reassurance of the patient. These objectives are met by careful consideration of prognostic factors and patterns of recurrence.[41]

After curative therapy for head and neck sarcoma, the major determinant of survival is the control of local and distant recurrence. In contrast to patients with a primary tumor of the extremity or trunk, patients with head and neck sarcoma have a greater tendency toward local recurrence rather than distant metastases. In series reported by Weber[3] and by Tran,[42] the lung was the most common site of distant metastasis, and the majority of local recurrences occur within 2 years of treatment. Whereas patients with isolated local recurrence have had 5- and 10-year disease-specific survival rates of 51% and 48%, respectively, the rates for patients with distant relapse are dismal at 16% and 10%.[41] Nonetheless, the overall 5-, 10-, and 15-year disease-specific survival rates of 27%, 22%, and 19%, respectively, for patients after first relapse attest that a small group of patients can be long-term survivors.[41] Surveillance strategies should thus attempt to identify favorable subsets of these patients with resectable recurrences.

We monitor patients who have undergone curative therapy for head and neck soft tissue sarcoma with history, physical exam, chest x-ray, and cross-sectional imaging every 3 to 4 months for the first 2 years, every 4 to 6 months for the next 2 years, and every 6 to 12 months for the fifth year. Laboratory tests may include a complete blood count, electrolytes, liver function tests, and creatinine at each follow-up visit. Cross-sectional imaging, especially for surgical sites difficult to examine clinically, may be performed by CT alone or by MRI. Ultrasonography provides an additional means of surveillance and offers the advantage of fine-needle aspiration biopsy to aid in the evaluation of suspect findings. Although its role in surveillance after therapy for sarcoma remains to be defined, positron emission tomography (PET) scanning offers promise in differentiating recurrent disease from postoperative scar tissue in selected cases.

PEARLS AND PITFALLS

- Osteosarcoma is a primary malignancy of osteoblastic tissue that is defined by the direct formation of bone or osteoid by tumor cells.
- About 10% of osteosarcomas occur in the head and neck region,[5] although these malignancies accounted for 15% of head and neck sarcomas in our series (see Table 58-1).
- Patients typically present in the third or fourth decade of life, some 10 to 15 years older on average than those presenting with osteosarcoma of the long bones.
- The mandible and maxilla are the sites most frequently affected in the head and neck region, followed by bones of the skull.
- At least one third of osteosarcomas of the head and neck are of low histologic grade, perhaps explaining their lower potential for distant metastasis compared with primary tumors of other sites.[6]
- Malignant fibrous histiocytoma, also known as pleomorphic sarcoma, the most common histologic subtype of soft tissue sarcoma overall,[7] represents a significant proportion of head and neck sarcomas (14% of head and neck soft tissue sarcomas in our series) (see Table 58-1).
- With the increased accuracy of ultrastructural and immunohistochemical subtyping, the diagnosis of malignant fibrous histiocytoma currently includes tumors of a broadened range of cellular origins.
- In the head and neck region, these lesions present as subcutaneous or submucosal lesions in the parotid, sinonasal tract, or upper aerodigestive tract, and rarely in bone.
- Angiosarcoma is a malignancy of vascular endothelial cell origin that, while rare, occurs in the head and neck region in about 50% of cases.[8]
- These lesions classically present as bruiselike macules and plaques on the forehead and scalp of elderly white men.[9]
- Immunohistochemical markers such as CD31, CD34, factor VIII, and von Willebrand factor aid in the histologic classification.[10-12]
- Rhabdomyosarcoma, though rarely affecting adults, represents the most common form of sarcoma in children and arises in the head and neck region in about 40% of cases.[13]
- Unlike other types of soft tissue sarcoma, these tumors carry significant potential for metastasis to regional lymph nodes in the neck.
- A thorough investigation is warranted, since as many as 23% of patients harbor disease at distant sites.[14-17]
- The current American Joint Committee on Cancer (AJCC) staging system for soft tissue sarcoma is based on histologic grade, tumor size and depth, and the presence of regional nodal or distant metastasis.[18]
- Although the staging system is optimally designed for staging extremity tumors, a major limitation is its lack of consideration for anatomic and histologic heterogeneity among soft tissue sarcomas. These concerns apply especially to head and neck sites where primary tumors are relatively smaller at presentation but commonly lie deep to the deep fascia.
- For adult soft tissue sarcomas of all sites, size (>5 cm), high-grade, local extension (to skin, major neurovascular structures, or bone), and positive surgical margins have been linked in multivariate analysis to increased rates of local recurrence and distant failure, and decreased disease-specific survival.[19,20]
- Most series have reported a correlation between tumor size (>5 cm) and high histologic grade and decreased disease-specific survival.[3,21-23]
- A few studies have evaluated the impact of local tumor extent on outcome. Farhood and colleagues found a univariate association of bony involvement with decreased overall survival,[24] whereas LeVay and colleagues demonstrated by multivariate analysis that local extent predicts rates of local recurrence, distant metastases, and disease-free survival.[25] In five studies, surgical margin status was linked to both local control and survival, and two of these confirmed the association in multivariate analyses.[19,21]
- The strongest prognostic factors for sarcoma of the head and neck appear to include tumor size, local extent, grade, and margin status, and these factors provide a basis for comparing results of treatment strategies and for determining the role of adjuvant therapies.

REFERENCES

1. DeVita VT Jr, Hellman S, Rosenberg SA: Sarcomas of the soft tissues and bone. In DeVita VT Jr, Hellman S, Rosenberg SA, editors: *Cancer: principles and practice of oncology,* ed 6, Philadelphia, 2005, Lippincott Williams & Wilkins, pp 1841-1891.
2. Lawrence W Jr, Anderson JR, Gehan EA, Maurer H: Pretreatment TNM staging of childhood rhabdomyosarcoma: a report of the Intergroup Rhabdomyosarcoma Study Group. Children's Cancer Study Group. Pediatric Oncology Group, *Cancer* 80:1165-1170, 1997.
3. Weber RS, Benjamin RS, Peters LJ, et al: Soft tissue sarcomas of the head and neck in adolescents and adults, *Am J Surg* 152:386-392, 1986.
4. McClay EF: Epidemiology of bone and soft tissue sarcomas, *Semin Oncol* 16:264-272, 1989.
5. Potter BO, Sturgis EM: Sarcomas of the head and neck, *Surg Oncol Clin N Am* 12:379-417, 2003.
6. O'Sullivan B, Audet N, Catton C, Gullane P: Soft tissue and bone sarcomas of the head and neck. In Harrison LB, Sessions RB, Hong WK, editors: *Head and neck cancer: a multidisciplinary approach,* ed 2, Philadelphia, 2003, Lippincott Williams & Wilkins, pp 786-824.
7. Enzinger FM: Malignant fibrous histiocytoma 20 years after Staout, *Am J Surg Pathol* 10(Suppl 1):43-53, 1986.
8. Lydiatt WM, Shaha AR, Shah JP: Angiosarcoma of the head and neck, *Am J Surg* 168:451-454, 1994.
9. Morrison WH, Byers RM, Garden AS, et al: Cutaneous angiosarcoma of the head and neck: a therapeutic dilemma, *Cancer* 76:319-327, 1995.
10. Mark RJ, Tran LM, Sercarz J, et al: Angiosarcoma of the head and neck: the UCLA experience 1955 through 1990, *Arch Otolaryngol Head Neck Surg* 119:973-978, 1993.

11. Loos BM, Wieneke JA, Thompson LD: Laryngeal angiosarcoma: a clinicopathologic study of five cases with a review of the literature, *Laryngoscope* 111:1197-1202, 2001.

12. Aust MR, Olsen KD, Lewis JE, et al: Angiosarcomas of the head and neck: clinical and pathologic characteristics, *Ann Otol Rhinol Laryngol* 106:943-951, 1997.

13. Callender TA, Weber RS, Janjan N, et al: Rhabdomyosarcoma of the nose and paranasal sinuses in adults and children, *Otolaryngol Head Neck Surg* 112:252-257, 1995.

14. Nayar RC, Prudhomme F, Parise O, et al: Rhabdomyosarcoma of the head and neck in adults: a study of 26 patients, *Laryngoscope* 103:1362-1366, 1993.

15. Kraus DH, Saenz NC, Gollamudi S, et al: Pediatric rhabdomyosarcoma of the head and neck, *Am J Surg* 174:556-560, 1997.

16. Anderson GJ, Toth GK, Gibbons WA: Protein engineering of the IgE receptor and its subunits by solid-phase synthesis and spectroscopy, *Biochem Soc Trans* 10:1306-1307, 1990.

17. Feldman BA: Rhabdomyosarcoma of the head and neck, *Laryngoscope* 92:424-440, 1982.

18. Green FL, Page DL, Flemming FD, et al: Soft tissue sarcoma. In Page DL, editor: *American Joint Committee on Cancer: cancer staging manual*, ed 6, New York, 2002, Springer, pp 221-226.

19. LeVay J, O'Sullivan B, Catton C, et al: Outcome and prognostic factors in soft tissue sarcoma in the adult, *Int J Radiat Oncol Biol Phys* 27:1091-1099, 1993.

20. Cakir S, Dincbas FO, Uzel O: Multivariate analysis of prognostic factors in 75 patients with soft tissue sarcoma, *Radiother Oncol* 37:10-16, 1995.

21. Kraus DH, Dubner S, Harrison LB, et al: Prognostic factors for recurrence and survival in head and neck soft tissue sarcomas, *Cancer* 74:697-702, 1994.

22. Wanebo HJ, Koness RJ, MacFarlane JK, et al: Head and neck sarcoma: report of the Head and Neck Sarcoma Registry. Society of Head and Neck Surgeons Committee on Research, *Head Neck* 14:1-17, 1992.

23. Greager JA, Patel MK, Briele HA, et al: Soft tissue sarcomas of the adult head and neck, *Cancer* 56:820-824, 1985.

24. Farhood AI, Hajdu SI, Shiu MH, Strong EW: Soft tissue sarcomas of the head and neck in adults, *Am J Surg* 160:365-369, 1990.

25. LeVay J, O'Sullivan B, Catton C, et al: An assessment of prognostic factors in soft-tissue sarcoma of the head and neck, *Arch Otolaryngol Head Neck Surg* 120:981-986, 1994.

26. Bowden L, Booher RJ: The principles and technique of resection of soft parts form sarcoma, *Surgery* 44:963-976, 1958.

27. Enneking WK, In Enneking WK, editor: *Musculoskeletal tumor surgery*, New York, 1958, Churchill Livingstone, pp 1-23.

28. Yang JC, Chang AE, Baker AR, et al: Randomized prospective study of the benefit of adjuvant radiation therapy in the treatment of soft tissue sarcomas of the extremity, *J Clin Oncol* 16:197-203, 1998.

29. Bentz BG, Singh B, Woodruff J, et al: Head and neck soft tissue sarcomas: a multivariate analysis of outcomes, *Ann Surg Oncol* 11:619-628, 2004.

30. Harrison LB, Franzese F, Gaynor JJ, Brennan MF: Long-term results of a prospective randomized trial of adjuvant brachytherapy in the management of completely resected soft tissue sarcomas of the extremity and superficial trunk, *Int J Radiat Oncol Biol Phys* 27:259-265, 1993.

31. Cormier JN, Pollock RE: Soft tissue sarcomas, *CA Cancer J Clin* 54:94-109, 2004.

32. O'Sullivan B, Davis AM, Turcotte R, et al: Preoperative versus postoperative radiotherapy in soft-tissue sarcoma of the limbs: a randomized trial, *Lancet* 359:2235-2241, 2002.

33. O'Sullivan B, Gullane P, Irish J, et al: Preoperative radiotherapy for adult head and neck soft tissue sarcoma: assessment of wound complication rates and cancer outcome in a prospective series, *World J Surg* 27:875-883, 2003.

34. De Paoli A, Bertola G, Boz G, et al: Radiation therapy and conservative surgery for soft tissue sarcomas of the extremities, torso and head and neck, *Ann Oncol* (3 Suppl 2):S97-S101, 1992.

35. Clark MA, Fisher C, Judson I, Thomas JM: Soft-tissue sarcomas in adults, *N Engl J Med* 353:701-711, 2005.

36. Adjuvant chemotherapy for localised resectable soft-tissue sarcoma of adults: meta-analysis of individual data. Sarcoma Meta-analysis Collaboration, *Lancet* 350:1647-1654, 1997.

37. Bramwell V, Rouesse J, Steward W, et al: Adjuvant CYVADIC chemotherapy for adult soft tissue sarcoma–reduced local recurrence but no improvement in survival: a study of the European Organization for Research and Treatment of Cancer Soft Tissue and Bone Sarcoma Group, *J Clin Oncol* 12(6):1137-1149, 1994.

38. Meric F, Milas M, Hunt KK, et al: Impact of neoadjuvant chemotherapy on postoperative morbidity in soft tissue sarcomas, *J Clin Oncol* 18:3378-3383, 2000.

39. Pisters PW, Ballo MT, Patel SR: Preoperative chemoradiation treatment strategies for localized sarcoma, *Ann Surg Oncol* 9:535-542, 2002.

40. Kraybill WG, Spiro IJ, Harris JA, et al: Radiation Therapy Oncology (RTOG) 95-14: a phase II study of neoadjuvant chemotherapy and radiation therapy in high risk, high grade, soft tissue sarcoma of the extremities and body wall: a preliminary report, *Proc Am Soc Clin Oncol* 20:348a, 2001.

41. Patel SR, Zagars GK, Pisters PW: The follow-up of adult soft-tissue sarcomas, *Semin Oncol* 30:413-416, 2003.

42. Tran LM, Mark R, Meier R, et al: Sarcomas of the head and neck: prognostic factors and treatment strategies, *Cancer* 70:169-177, 1992.

Chapter 59

Osteoradionecrosis

Kevin Arce

Treatment of head and neck malignancies has evolved since the mid-1980s. Advances in surgical techniques, chemotherapeutic options, and radiation techniques have improved locoregional disease control and survival. Radiation therapy is used as the primary therapy for early stage malignancies, as adjuvant treatment following ablative surgery for advanced carcinomas and in patients with unresectable, locally advanced carcinomas, concurrent chemoradiotherapy has become the primary treatment modality.

In radiation therapy, the normal tissue tolerance is the dose-limiting factor for treatment of a malignancy. Mucosa, salivary gland tissue, skin, bone, and cartilage each have their own dose sensitivities and response to radiation-induced trauma. The side effects of radiation therapy are divided into acute and late toxicities, with each having an impact on the patient's quality of life. Acute side effects include mucositis, xerostomia, pain, dermatitis, and dysgeusia, and late radiation-induced side effects include xerostomia, dysphagia, and skin fibrosis. Radiation-associated skeletal injuries differ in the adult and pediatric populations. In the pediatric population, the concerns center mostly on growth and development, whereas for the adult population it is the development of necrosis and pathologic fractures.[1,2]

Osteoradionecrosis (ORN) was first described in 1922 by Regaud,[3] and it remains a serious complication of radiation therapy. Patients afflicted with ORN in the head and neck region can experience pain, dysesthesia, trismus, orocutaneous fistula, and the late development of pathologic fractures. Utilizing data from pooled studies of head and neck radiated patients conducted between 1968 and 1992, Clayman reported a crude rate for ORN of 5.4%.[4] More recently, Wahl estimated the incidence to be 3% when utilizing data from studies performed between 1997 and 2004.[5] This current decline in ORN incidence appears to be multifactorial. The multidisciplinary care of head and neck cancer patients has provided for dental screening and preventive care to be instituted prior to the start of definitive therapy. This helps identify dental risk factors and addresses current and potential oral health problems for the radiation-therapy patient. The use of the more uniformly absorbed megavoltage radiation instead of kilovoltage therapy with its higher bone absorption, advances in 3D radiation planning, dose delivery monitoring, and computer-controlled delivery have resulted in 3D conformal radiation therapy and intensity-modulated radiation therapy (IMRT), which limit the radiation dose to surrounding normal tissue and associated treatment side effects.[6,7]

DEFINITION

Osteoradionecrosis has also been referred to as radiation osteitis, radio-osteonecrosis, radiation osteomyelitis, and postradiation osteonecrosis. There is currently no standardized clinical definition for ORN. Case series utilize different temporal and size criteria of chronic bone exposure in a radiated field when defining mandibular ORN. It has been defined as bone in the radiation field exposed for at least 2 months in the absence of local neoplastic disease[8] and an area greater than 1 cm of exposed bone in a field of irradiation that has failed to show any evidence of healing for at least 6 months.[9] The most commonly used definition is that of exposed, devitalized bone in a radiated field without healing for 3 months without any evidence of tumor recurrence.[10]

PATHOPHYSIOLOGY

Bones are resistant to high radiation doses as long as the overlying soft tissue remains intact. In 1938, Watson and Scarborough described three crucial factors in the development of ORN: exposure to radiotherapy above a critical dose, local injury, and the development of an infection.[11] In 1960, Gowgiel[12] used the *Macacus rhesus* monkey as an animal model to study the disease pathogenesis, total radiation dose needed for development of ORN, and the difference in disease incidence between the maxilla and mandible. His observations were that development of ORN was a result of direct damage to the osteocytes and that the vascular changes noted histologically played a role in disease progression. These vascular changes were found predominantly in the field of radiation and consisted of thickening of the arteriolar walls that resembled those seen in arteriosclerosis. The intima and media changes could be evident as early as $1\frac{1}{2}$ weeks after completion of therapy, with complete occlusion observed within 5 to 7 weeks postradiation therapy. Gowgiel hypothesized that the difference in incidence of ORN between the maxilla and mandible centered on the vascular supply, with the maxilla having a rich vascular plexus when compared to the single inferior alveolar vessel for the mandible.

In 1970, Meyer described the triad of radiation, trauma, and infection for the pathogenesis of ORN.[13] Tissue injury provided the entry of oral bacteria to a compromised bed, which led to the development of an infection and necrosis. Marx, in 1983, examined several bone specimens to determine the pathogenesis of ORN.[9] Bacteria were only identified superficially in the ORN specimens, and the conclusion was that organisms played a minor role in the pathophysiology of ORN and were not the causative agent but rather contaminants. Marx then characterized ORN as a wound healing complication and not an infectious process. In the radiated tissue, the hypovascular, hypoxic, and hypocellular environment would hinder a normal healing response to trauma and a chronic, nonhealing wound then develop. This became the theory of the pathophysiology of ORN for decades. It also served as the foundation for the use of hyperbaric oxygen therapy in the prevention and management of ORN because of its mechanism of action and its effect on radiated hard and soft tissue.

Molecular advances have allowed for a better understanding of the pathogenesis of osteoradionecrosis and the complexity of wound healing after radiation therapy.[14,15] Osteoradionecrosis is now considered to be a late effect of radiation induced fibroatrophic process.[16,17] Each fraction of radiation therapy represents a series of small tissue insults produced by a burst of free radicals. The process of inflammation and regeneration is altered by the influence of cytokines and growth factors on fibroblasts and the associated extracellular matrix deposition. Histopathologically, radiation-induced fibrosis is divided into three phases. In the *prefibrotic phase*, which is often asymptomatic, there are signs of chronic inflammation evident. The second phase is that of *organized fibrosis*, where there are areas of active fibrosis with a high concentration of myofibroblasts within a poorly organized matrix. These areas are adjacent to regions of aging fibroblasts in a poorly cellular, fibrotic, and dense sclerotic matrix. In the late *fibroatrophic phase*, retractile fibrosis and gradual loss of parenchymal cells takes place.[16,17] The ability of radiated tissue to repair itself after an insult is then compromised by these cellular changes and can lead to the development of necrosis in susceptible individuals.

RISK FACTORS

Multiple risk factors are associated with the development of mandibular ORN. These factors can be divided into treatment-dependent factors (radiation therapy factors and tumor-related factors) and patient-dependent factors.[18,19] Among the radiation therapy factors, the type of radiation, its total dose, fractionation, and field have all been correlated with the development of ORN. The higher the total radiation dose, the higher the risk of ORN because of the tissue trauma that is sustained. Although a radiation dose of less than 60 Gy is associated with less risk of ORN, it is still not a negligible risk.[5,20-22] In hyperfractionated radiation therapy, the total dose of radiation is divided into small doses and treatments are given more than once a day. This allows for total dose escalation to increase the rate of tumor control while limiting an increase in late complications. Conflicting data exist regarding the relationship of dose fractionation and the risk of ORN.[23] A randomized, multicenter trial comparing continuous, hyperfractionated, accelerated radiotherapy (CHART) to conventional radiotherapy in 918 head and neck cancer patients found a 0.4% overall incidence of ORN in the CHART group compared to 1.4% for conventional radiotherapy.[24] Niewald et al. showed in a retrospective analysis of 168 oral cavity carcinoma patients that ORN occurred in 8.6% of the patients treated conventionally when compared to 22.9% in those treated with hyperfractionation.[25]

Tumors close to the mandible and those located in the tonsillar and retromolar trigone region appear to carry a higher risk of ORN.[22,26,27] The treatment of these sites with radiation therapy places the posterior mandible where the buccal cortex appears to be more susceptible to the development of ORN in the treatment field.[22,28] Mandibular surgery is, at times, required because of the extent of the tumor invasion or because its location calls for a wider access for proper oncologic surgery. The need for a mandibulotomy or mandibulectomy has also been correlated with a higher risk of ORN.[21,29]

Patient age, dental status, oral hygiene, and use of tobacco have all been identified as risk factors for the development of ORN.[8,18,30-32] In head and neck cancer patients, smoking cessation becomes an integral part of posttreatment surveillance, as it is not only associated with higher incidence of locoregional failure and development of a second primary tumor but also with osteoradionecrosis. A longitudinal study of the oral health of head and neck cancer patients found that patients who developed ORN experienced worsening of their periodontal status after completion of radiation therapy.[18] The presence of greater than 60% alveolar bone loss, high dental plaque score, and pocket depths greater than 5 mm showed a strong correlation with the development of ORN.

In patients with head and neck carcinomas, nutritional status has been identified as a prognostic factor. Goldwaser et al.[33] also identified it as a risk factor for ORN. In a retrospective cohort study of 82 head and neck cancer patients, they observed that the risk of ORN decreased by 50% in patients with normal BMI and by 43% in patients with a BMI between 25 and 29.9. Also, the use of steroid therapy before or after radiation treatment reduced the risk of ORN by 96%. This finding appears to support the current radiation-induced fibroatrophic process theory for ORN, as the anti-inflammatory effects of steroid therapy would limit the initial inflammatory phase of radiation therapy.

Trauma associated with dentoalveolar surgery after radiation therapy has always been considered one of the major risk factors for ORN.[34] Despite the presence of spontaneous cases of ORN, most of ORN cases reported are preceded by tooth extractions. Utilizing pooled studies since 1986, Wahl estimated the incidence of ORN for preradiation extractions and postradiation extractions to be 3.0-3.2% and 3.1-3.5%, respectively.[5] A 10-year single institution review of 405 patients who underwent extractions prior, during, and postradiation therapy showed an overall ORN incidence of 0.7%. Of the three ORN cases reported, two were associated with preradiation extraction and one with postradiation extractions, and no cases were identified in the treatment group where extractions were performed during therapy.[35] Sulaiman et al. reported on 951 extractions performed on 187 patients, with 41.18% performed before radiation therapy and 57.22% after radiation therapy.[36] They reported four cases of ORN with two patients having extractions prior to radiation therapy and two within 21 days of completion of therapy. In 2007, Chang et al. analyzed the impact of dental status and preradiation extractions on the risk of ORN in a study population of 413 patients who underwent radiation therapy for treatment of oropharyngeal carcinomas.[37] Of those patients that developed ORN, 54% of them had preradiation extractions and 16% postradiation extractions. The conventional wisdom has been that preradiation extractions reduce the risk of ORN. These large retrospective studies certainly question the empirical practice of extraction of teeth as a preventive measure. Extraction of dentition should be based on the periodontal status of the tooth, the tumor-related prognosis, and the radiation field and dose planned. Also, the practice of indiscriminant extractions has an impact on the patient's quality of life. Lost dentition can lead to a limited amount of functional teeth and an associated decrease in masticatory efficiency, especially in those cases where financial considerations limit restorative options.[38]

The role of actinomyces in the pathogenesis of osteoradionecrosis has been brought into question.[39-43] It was thought that the presence of actinomyces and other microorganisms constituted a surface contaminant and an opportunistic infection in a susceptible, local environment.[9] Actinomyces are gram-positive, non–spore-forming anaerobic or microaerophilic rods and a common mucosal inhabitant in the oral cavity. Through the use of DNA-DNA hybridization techniques, scanning, and transmission electron microscopy and polymerase chain reaction (PCR) techniques, actinomyces and other anaerobic bacteria have been identified deep in ORN specimens. Actinomyces have been shown to induce bone resorption[44,45] and could be a prognostic factor in ORN, as some authors have shown that their culture in bone specimens could lead to prolonged treatment and worst outcome.[41-43] The role of microorganisms in the disease pathogenesis or treatment response is to be determined, but careful consideration needs to be given to instituting an effective antibiotic therapy strategy when there are clinical signs of infection in conjunction with necrosis.

DIAGNOSTIC STUDIES

The diagnosis of mandibular osteoradionecrosis remains primarily based on the clinical signs and symptoms present. Imaging studies allow for the confirmation of radiographic signs of necrosis and assessment of disease severity for treatment decisions and to rule out a malignant process, such as tumor recurrence or metastatic disease. The clinical changes associated with radiation therapy have a tendency to diminish the otherwise distinct radiographic features of a tumor and may be mistaken for residual or recurrent disease in some situations.[46] A masslike effect could be present in the masseter and pterygoid muscles as manifested by an abnormal T2 signal intensity and soft tissue enhancement and thickening on magnetic resonance imaging.[47] These soft tissue changes could also be visible on computed tomography, where swelling and enhancement could be found localized or diffusely around the areas of necrosis, making radiographic interpretation challenging.[48]

The radiographic findings of ORN are not specific and are found in other conditions such as osteomyelitis and bisphosphonate-related osteonecrosis of the jaws. Panorex x-rays are a good screening modality but tend to underestimate the extent of the disease[48,49] (Fig. 59-1, A). The use of computed tomography (CT) scans provides three-dimensional evaluation and better determination of the extent of necrosis to help guide management strategies. One is also able to rule out a malignant process with the use of one imaging modality. Among the osseous abnormalities found in plain films and CT, there is thinning of cortical bone, periodontal ligament widening, osteolysis, sclerosis, and sequestration[49] (Fig. 59-1, B and C). Loss of bone marrow trabeculation can be seen on CT examination in addition to the predilection of the buccal cortex in manifesting radiographic changes. Air can also be present in advanced cases where an orocutaneous fistula is present.[48]

Magnetic resonance imaging (MRI) is a valuable diagnostic modality utilized in the management of ORN. It can depict early bone marrow changes prior to clinical manifestation of the disease, and the distortion resulting from dental artifacts is low. When ORN is present, bone marrow edema is depicted in MRI as reduced signal intensity in T1-weighted images and increased signal intensity in T2-weighted images when compared to normal.[50] During treatment planning, these signal changes could be utilized for presurgical determination of the extent of necrosis, the surgical margins required, and, therefore, the reconstructive options to be considered. Functional imaging modalities also allow for means of visualizing osteoblastic and inflammatory activity in the bone. The use of classic bone scintigraphy in the diagnostic evaluation of ORN is limited by its spatial resolution and lack of specificity. In the evaluation of a patient with ORN, an increase in uptake could be representative of tumor infiltration or inflammation associated with a localized infection of dental origin.[50] F-18 fluorodeoxyglucose (FDG) and F-18 positron emission tomography (PET) scans have been proposed as a possible tool for the assessment of disease severity in BRONJ patients because of the increase in tracer uptake in areas of inflammatory activity.[51] Tracer activity has been correlated with prognosis in the management of head and neck carcinomas, and although no information is available on its use in ORN at this time, the use of PET/CT scans could help guide treatment decisions and predict outcomes in the future.

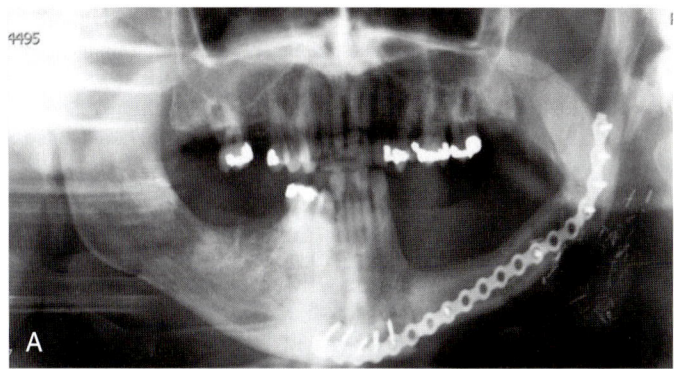

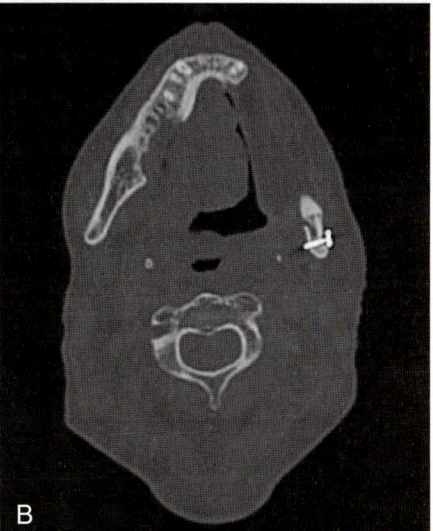

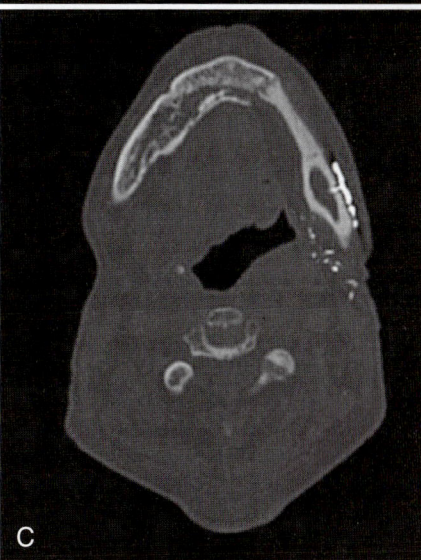

Fig. 59-1 ■ **A,** Panoramic x-ray of patient with history of left mandibular ORN treated with a segmental mandibulectomy and free fibula flap. **B,** CT scan demonstrating osteolysis and sclerosis in the right mandibular body region. **C,** CT scan showing extension of radiographic signs of necrosis to the anterior mandible with osteolysis, sclerosis and sequestration.

DISEASE STAGING

Disease staging allows for comparison of outcome studies; it also helps guide treatment strategies and estimate prognosis. Acute and late adverse events of radiotherapy are rated, utilizing different scales. In the case of osteoradionecrosis, the lack of a uniform staging system makes comparison of the efficacy of an intervention between trials difficult. The current systems utilize a variety of criteria that could include radiographic findings, treatment response, disease progression, and the extent of necrosis.[22,52-55] There is also a Radiation Therapy Oncology Group (RTOG) scoring criteria for bone morbidity and a comprehensive system, the Late Effects Normal Tissue Task Force subjective, objective, management, and analytic (LENT/SOMA) score,[56] developed between European Organization for Research and Treatment of Cancer (EORTC) and the RTOG, which utilizes subjective and objective criteria in conjunction with radiographic findings and therapeutic interventions as part of the scoring system (Tables 59-1 to 59-8).

TREATMENT

ORN can occur at any time after radiation therapy, with most cases developing within the first 3 years of completion of therapy.[57] Despite a body of literature available on the management of mandibular osteoradionecrosis, there still exists a division as to what are the most appropriate therapeutic modalities and the role and timing of hyperbaric oxygen therapy (HBO) as adjuvant therapy. The use of HBO in radiation therapy dates back to the 1960s when it was described as an adjunct to help overcome radio-resistance in hypoxic tumor cells.[58,59] There is some evidence that hyperbaric oxygen therapy improves local tumor control and survival in head and neck cancer patients, but the advent of orally administered radiosensitizing agents, the technical difficulties of administering radiation therapy in a hyperbaric chamber, and the inconclusive data available as to its effectiveness led to its abandonment in the management of malignancies in the 1980s.[60]

TABLE 59-1   Glanzmann and Gratz Classification System[22]

GRADE EVENT

1 Bone exposure without signs of infection and persistent for at least 3 months

2 Bone exposure with signs of infection or sequester and without the signs of grades 3-5

3 Bone necrosis treated with mandibular resection with a satisfactory result

4 Bone necrosis with persistent problems despite mandibular resection

5 Death resulting from osteoradionecrosis

TABLE 59-2   Schwartz and Kagan Classification System[73]

STAGE EVENT

I Superficial involvement only with the necrotic bone confined to the exposed cortical bone. Soft tissue ulceration is minimal.

II Localized involvement with only a portion of the cortical and medullary bone being necrotic.

III Diffuse, full thickness involvement of the mandible including the lower border.
Pathologic fracture may occur.
Division A: Soft tissue ulceration is minimal.
Division B: Soft-tissue necrosis, including orocutaneous fistulation.

TABLE 59-3   Notani et al. Classification System[55]

GRADE EVENT

I ORN confined to the alveolar bone

II ORN limited to the alveolar bone and or mandible above the level of mandibular alveolar canal

III ORN that extended to the level of the mandibular alveolar canal and ORN with a skin fistula or a pathologic fracture

---

TABLE 59-4   Store and Boysen Classification System[54]

STAGE EVENT

0 Mucosal defects only

1 Radiologic evidence of necrotic bone with intact mucosa

2 Positive radiologic findings with denuded bone intraorally

3 Clinically exposed bone, verified by imaging techniques, along with skin fistula and infection

---

TABLE 59-5   Epstein et al. Classification System[52]

STAGE EVENT

I Resolved, healed
  Ia No pathologic fracture
  Ib Pathologic fracture

II Chronic, persistent, nonprogressive
  IIa No pathologic fracture
  IIb Pathologic fracture

III Active, progressive
  IIIa No pathologic fracture
  IIIb Pathologic fracture

TABLE 59-6   RTOG/EORTC Late Radiation Morbidity Scoring Schema

SCORE BONE MORBIDITY

0 None

1 Asymptomatic, no growth retardation, reduced bone density

2 Moderate pain or tenderness, growth retardation, irregular bone sclerosis

3 Severe pain or tenderness, complete arrest of bone growth, dense bone sclerosis

4 Necrosis, spontaneous fracture

Data from http://www.rtog.org/ResearchAssociates/AdverseEventReporting/RTOGEORTCLateRadiationMorbidityScoringSchema.aspx

TABLE 59-7	LENT/SOMA Scale[56]			
	GRADE 1	**GRADE 2**	**GRADE 3**	**GRADE 4**
Subjective				
Pain	Occasional, minimal	Intermittent and tolerable	Persistent and intense	Refractory and excruciating
Mastication	Difficulty with solids	Difficulty with soft foods		
Denture use		Loose dentures	Inability to use dentures	
Trismus	Noted but not measurable	Preventing normal eating	Difficulty eating	Inadequate oral intake
Objective				
Exposed bone		≤2 cm	>2 cm or limited sequestration	Fracture
Trismus		1 cm-2 cm opening	0.5 cm-1 cm opening	<0.5 cm opening
Management				
Pain	Occasional non-narcotic	Regular non-narcotic	Regular narcotic	Surgical intervention or resection
Exposed bone		Antibiotics	Debridement, HBO therapy	Resection
Trismus and mastication		Soft diet	Liquid diet, antibiotics, muscle relaxants	NG tube, gastrostomy
Analytic				
Mandibular radiograph	Questionable changes or none	Osteoporosis (radiolucent) Osteosclerosis (radiodense)	Sequestra	Fracture
Panograph x-rays/CT	Assessment of necrosis progression			

The 9 SOM parameters are scored 0 to 4 (0 = no toxicity), scores total and divided by 9.

TABLE 59-8	Marx Osteoradionecrosis Protocol[9]

STAGE EVENT

I Patients receive 30 sessions of HBO at 2.4 ATA for 90 minutes. Patients that respond to HBO treatment alone are classified as stage I responders and undergo additional 10 sessions and allowed to continue healing process.

II Patients who have not improved after initial 30 HBO sessions and require transoral debridement with primary wound closure. Patients receive 10 additional HBO sessions.

III Stage I or II nonresponders or those patients who present with pathologic fracture, cutaneous fistula, or osteolysis involving inferior border of the mandible. Patients undergo segmental resection, stabilization of segments, and 10 postsurgical HBO sessions followed by delayed reconstruction.

HBO has been advocated as a treatment modality for osteoradionecrosis, usually in conjunction with surgery, as well as a preventive measure when a surgical procedure is required in the radiated head and neck patient. Hyperbaric oxygen therapy increases oxygen supply in hypoxic tissue, stimulating fibroblast proliferation and angiogenesis. It can also be bactericidal or bacteriostatic to anaerobic bacterial species. The role of hyperbaric oxygen therapy in the management and prevention of ORN remains controversial to date.[61,62] There is conflicting evidence as to its effectiveness and the role it should play in the treatment protocol of ORN.[63-67] Randomized controlled trials provide the highest level of evidence of the efficacy of an intervention, and in the case of HBO therapy and ORN, there is a paucity of trials available to draw definitive conclusions. Systematic reviews have shown that the majority of studies available are retrospective in nature, consist mostly of case series, and lack a control group and definitive end-points.[62,68-71]

The use of HBO as a preventive measure prior to dentoalveolar surgery was evaluated by Marx and colleagues in 1985[72] in a randomized trial where they compared hyperbaric oxygen to systemic antibiotics in the prevention of ORN. The study group consisted of 74 previously radiated patients who required extraction of indicated teeth. They found an incidence of ORN of 5.4% in the HBO group as compared with 29.9% in the antibiotic group. Since this initial trial, no other randomized trials have been conducted on HBO as a preventive intervention for ORN. Although it has been advocated for routine preoperative management of the postradiation surgical patient, there is insufficient evidence to support its routine use at this time as a preventive measure.[5,36,73]

Three randomized trials have evaluated the use of HBO therapy in the management of osteoradionecrosis. Marx reported on the use of HBO therapy on 104 patients requiring hemimandibular reconstruction and 160 patients requiring major soft tissue surgery or flaps postradiation therapy.[74,75] Patients were subjected to 20 preoperative HBO sessions at 2.4 atmospheres absolute (ATA) for 90 minutes daily 5 days a week, followed by 10 sessions postoperatively. There was better outcome in the HBO group in terms of mucosal coverage, bony continuity, and wound dehiscence. However, these two trials were published in a book chapter and had no information regarding randomization scheme, allocation concealment, control group intervention, or clearly defined outcomes. A randomized, double-blind, placebo-controlled trial was conducted in 12 centers in Paris to assess the efficacy and safety of HBO therapy in patients with osteoradionecrosis.[76] Patients were randomized to receive preoperatively 30 hyperbaric oxygen therapy sessions at 2.4 ATA for 90 minutes or placebo and 10 additional hyperbaric oxygen therapy dives or placebo postoperatively. Placebo consisted of a gas containing 9% oxygen at 2.4 ATA, which is equivalent to breathing 21% oxygen at surface pressure. The primary outcome was a 1-year ORN recovery rate that was defined as (1) absence of pain, (2) absence of any area of bone exposure, (3) stabilization or regression of radiographic findings, and (4) absence of the following: fracture, bone necrosis to the inferior border of the mandible, cutaneous fistula, or need for a surgical intervention in patients who did not initially require one. A sample size of 222 patients was to be recruited in order to detect a difference with HBO therapy of at least 20%. After enrolling 68 patients, 37 in the HBO group and 31 in the placebo group, the trial was stopped by the independent data safety monitoring board because of the lack of superiority in the HBO therapy arm, with failure to stop osteoradionecrosis progression or improvement in pain.

Not only should the efficacy of HBO therapy be considered but also its cost utility. The average 90-minute hyperbaric oxygen treatment in the United States has been estimated to cost between $300 and $400, with the total cost of 30 to 40 sessions being between $9000 and $16,000.[77] This is without taking into consideration patient's travel cost and lost wages given the amount of chambers available in the United States, which would require a number of patients to travel extensively for therapy.[5] Hyperbaric oxygen treatment also has its complications. Patients may experience a reduction in visual acuity secondary to conformational changes in the lens, claustrophobia, and seizures resulting from oxygen toxicity.[71] There are also pressure-related adverse events, such as barotraumatic otitis and pneumothorax, with most episodes of barotrauma being mild and not requiring therapy to be stopped as these patients are easily treated or recover spontaneously.[70]

The angiogenic effect of HBO therapy raises the concern of growth promotion of residual tumors in cancer patients. There are clinical case reports of rapid progression of tumor growths after HBO therapy.[78,79] However, the causality between HBO therapy and tumor growth has not been definitively established. Animal studies have failed to show changes in the tumor microenvironment that could lead to growth promotion as a result of HBO therapy.[80] The risk of cancer recurrence with the use of HBO in the management of late radiation complications in head and neck patients with a history of recurrence successfully salvaged was recently evaluated.[81] Eleven patients successfully salvaged after loco-regional recurrence and who later developed tissue necrosis for which HBO and surgery was utilized for management were matched by primary cancer subsite, initial cancer stage, age, and gender to a group of successfully salvaged recurrent head and neck cancer patients. The incidence of cancer re-recurrences and survival were the primary outcomes of interest in this study. Their findings were that there was a higher incidence of loco-regional failure in the HBO therapy group, a faster recurrence rate than in the non-HBO group, and unusual location for recurrence given the location of the primary tumor. Although this retrospective study consisted of a small number of cases and there are no other published reports on this patient population to date, the benefits of HBO therapy for management of ORN might need to be carefully considered in patients with a history of recurrence successfully salvaged.

The treatment of ORN depends the disease severity at the time of presentation. Treatment strategies for early disease rely on conservative measures that consist of local irrigation, avoidance of irritants, antibiotics, and minor debridement/sequestrectomy. This treatment appears to be effective when there is evidence both clinically and radiographically of a minimal amount of necrotic bone. Conservative measures have been estimated to result in healing in approximately 50% of cases without the adjunctive use of hyperbaric oxygen therapy.[82,83] While this is the case, the treatment can be protracted and several months of therapy can take place before clinical improvement occurs.[68]

In patients with advanced mandibular osteoradionecrosis, where there is evidence of pathologic fracture, oro-cutaneous fistula, full-thickness necrosis of bone, or intractable pain, a more radical mode of therapy is often necessary (Fig. 59-2, A). This usually entails segmental mandibulectomy with reconstruction of the defect (Fig. 59-2, B). Reconstruction options for the restoration of mandibular continuity after ablative surgery for osteoradionecrosis include the use of pedicled soft tissue flaps, reconstruction plates, secondary reconstruction with corticocancellous bone grafts, and microvascular composite free tissue transfer. This represents a surgical challenge, as the late effects of radiation therapy alter the tissue environment in such a way that the soft tissue manipulation is often difficult, thus limiting dissection and passive primary wound closure (Fig. 59-3). Immediate reconstruction with vascularized free tissue transfer has grown in favor over the use of delayed nonvascularized reconstruction in conjunction with HBO therapy[84] in most major centers because of its ability to remove necrotic tissue and restore mastication, deglutition, speech, and oral competence in a single stage[85] (Fig. 59-4).

Surgical access through a transcervical approach provides adequate exposure for the resection and reconstruction. However, care should be taken to minimize the risk of neck skin necrosis by elevating a skin access flap in a subplatysmal plane with adequate thickness and length in order to maintain its vascularity.[86] The extent of mandibular resection is determined according to clinical and radiographic criteria. The presence of active bleeding from the resection margins is often utilized as a measure of the adequacy of resection. This bleeding assessment could be difficult, especially in the ramus and subcondylar region where there is a dense cortical bone and small amount of bone marrow present. This difficulty is illustrated by the fact that a recent series of ORN patients demonstrated that up to 25% of treated patients have recurrent or persistent osteoradionecrosis.[87]

The fibula, scapula, iliac crest, and osteocutaneous radial forearm free flap are all composite flaps that could be utilized for mandibular reconstruction. The fibula free flap offers many advantages and has therefore become the workhorse in microvascular mandibular reconstruction. One can obtain sufficient bone length for reconstruction of an array of defect sizes, and in most instances it provides an adequate vascular pedicle length (Fig. 59-5). This is important in irradiated necks where the inability to identify adequate recipient vessels in the ipsilateral neck might require the use of the contralateral neck. Multiple osteotomies can be performed on the fibula to provide adequate facial contours, and the reconstruction of the mandibular condyle in cases where it is incorporated into the surgical

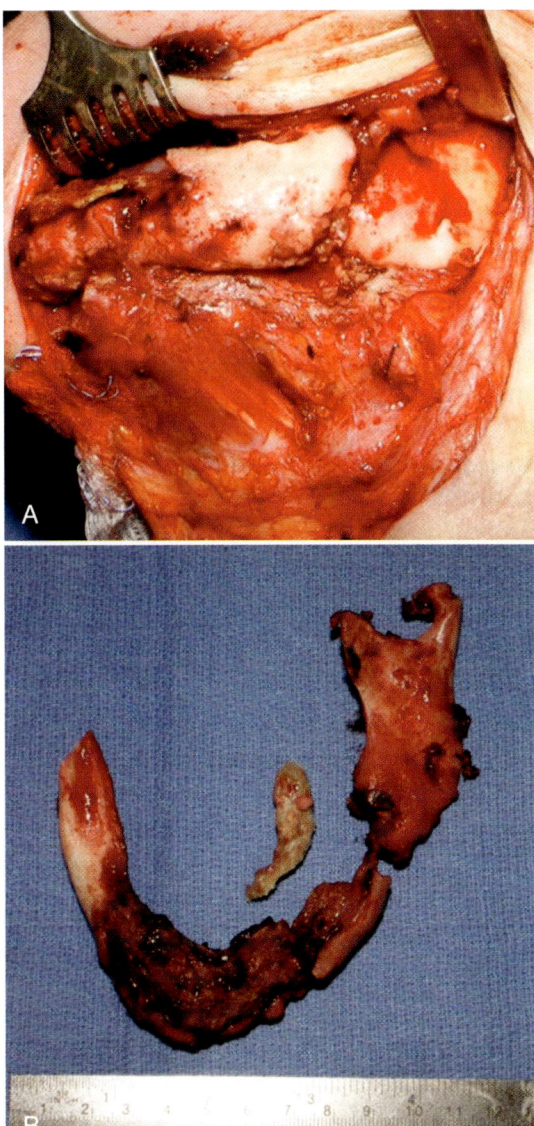

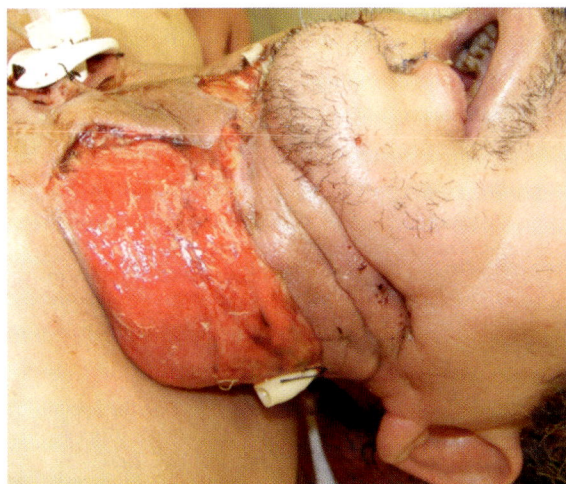

Fig. 59-2 ■ **A,** Extensive osteoradionecrosis leading to pathologic fracture and development of orocutaneous fistula and intractable pain clinically. **B,** Near total segmental mandibulectomy specimen.

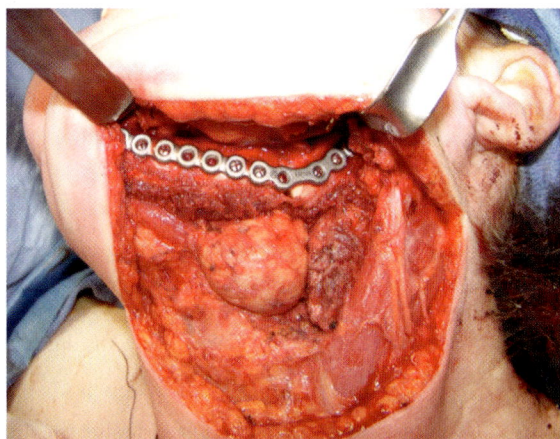

Fig. 59-4 ■ Free fibula flap composite reconstruction of mandibular body segmental defect.

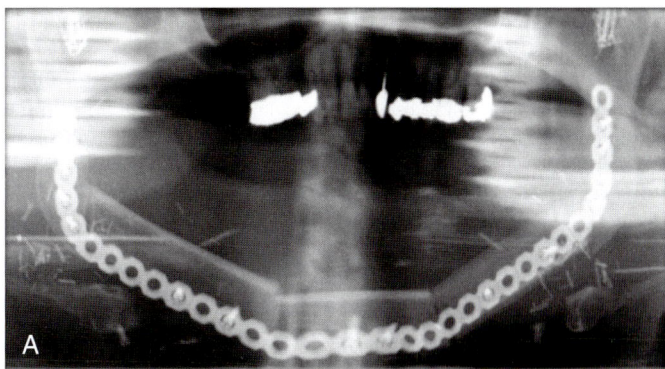

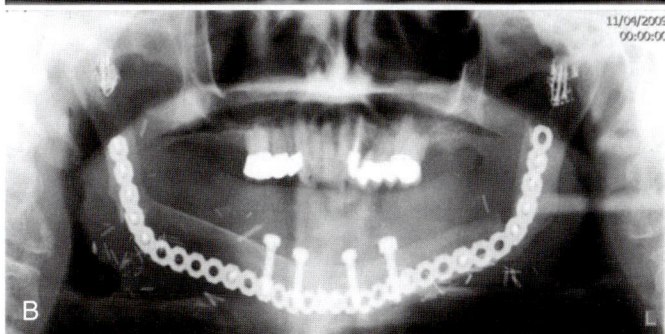

Fig. 59-5 ■ **A,** Mandibular angle-to-angle composite defect reconstructed with a free fibula flap. **B,** Placement of four endosseous implants for fabrication of mandibular fixed prosthesis in order to achieve full functional rehabilitation.

Fig. 59-3 ■ Pectoralis major flap rotated to left neck to aid in coverage of great vessels and closure of neck wound, which could not be closed primarily because of fibrosis present.

plan could be accomplished without the need of a prosthetic implant.[88,89] However, not all patients are candidates for reconstruction with a free fibula flap. Those with a history of previous trauma, surgical procedures to the lower extremities, or severe peripheral vascular disease might not be suitable candidates for a fibula flap. In those cases, other microvascular reconstruction options include the use of the scapula, iliac crest, and osteocutaneous radial forearm free flap. The scapula flap provides three separate vascular axes that allow the design of two skin paddles and one bone paddle, making it useful in the reconstruction of through-and-through defects. However, the skin paddle of the scapula flap could be quite bulky for the defect present, as could be the case of the iliac crest flap. The osteocutaneous radial forearm free flap (OCRFFF) can provide bony continuity of segmental mandibular defects and a thin, pliable skin paddle for oral mucosal defects in a predictable fashion and with fewer donor site complications when compared to the free fibula flap.[90,91] The quality of bone stock for subsequent implant rehabilitation could be inadequate when the OCRFFF is utilized and would require the use of grafting techniques if there are future prosthetic considerations. In patients who have a poor prognosis and with a lateral defect, reconstruction with a reconstruction plate and a soft tissue flap, such as anterolateral thigh or radial forearm flap, can offer an expedient way of providing well-vascularized tissue for primary wound closure while curtailing the complications associated with a longer and more complex composite reconstruction. This can provide an improvement in the quality of life for this selective group of patients by eliminating pain and necrotic tissue while still providing adequate function.

The use of microvascular reconstruction in the management of advanced ORN has been shown to provide excellent disease resolution.[86,87,92-98] However, careful consideration still needs to be given to the surgical intervention of ORN patients, as there is a significant risk of morbidity associated with ORN surgery. In recent studies of microvascular reconstruction of mandibular ORN defects, the wound complication rates have been in the range of 24-55%.[86,87,92-94] In some series, the rate of flap loss has also been higher for ORN patients in comparison to other microvascular reconstructions in the head and neck region,[86,95,96] with predictive factors of complication other than exposure to radiation therapy still elusive.

The radiation-induced fibrosis theory as pathogenesis for ORN has led to the use of antioxidants and antifibrotic drugs for management of patients. There have been encouraging preliminary results in the use of pentoxifylline and vitamin E with clodronate in the management of osteoradionecrosis patients.[99-101] A recent phase II trial on 54 patients with refractory ORN who were treated with pentoxifylline and vitamin E with clodronate combination showed this drug combination to be safe and effective.[101] There was clinical improvement in the amount of bone exposure with complete resolution in the 16 patients followed long term and with no disease recurrence after cessation of therapy. Two thirds of the patients underwent chairside sequestrectomy during follow-up visits, and no major surgical interventions were required. Although there were several study limitations, which include the number of patients lost to follow-up, this could represent a predictable and effective management strategy of refractory ORN cases that would need to be confirmed by large clinical trials.

CONCLUSION

Osteoradionecrosis continues to be a debilitating and challenging late adverse event of radiation therapy. The complex interaction of radiation, tumor, and patient-related factors may account for the variety of clinical presentations and response to therapy. Molecular advances have allowed for a better understanding of the pathogenesis of ORN and the design of targeted therapy with encouraging preliminary results for disease treatment and as a possible preventive strategy.[102] The use of molecular targeting agents to improve tumor radioresponse[103] and the technologic advances in radiation therapy delivery[104,105] will continue to improve the preventive strategies for late adverse events while maintaining adequate tumor control and survival in head and neck cancer patients.

PEARLS AND PITFALLS

- Osteoradionecrosis continues to be a serious late adverse event of radiation therapy with significant impact on the patient's quality of life after successful treatment of a malignancy.
- Prevention is of utmost importance in the management strategy of osteoradionecrosis. The proper oral evaluation and management of patients prior, during, and after radiation therapy plays a vital role in reducing acute and late complications of therapy. Treatment alternatives for xerostomia and caries prevention help maintain an oral environment that preserves teeth vitality and periodontium support in order to minimize the risk of trauma secondary to extraction of nonrestorable dentition.
- Treatment of mandibular osteoradionecrosis is dependent on the amount of necrosis present at the time of evaluation. Conservative treatment strategies appear to have success in the cure and arrest of disease progression in a number of patients, with a smaller patient population developing advanced disease.
- Resection and mandibular reconstruction of advanced disease presents a surgical challenge because of the high wound complication rate and the need for transfer of vascularized tissue in the majority of patients. Antibiotic therapy is required in patients with clinical signs of infection, and the presence of bacteria appears to have an impact on treatment response and disease progression.
- Targeted therapy for ORN with bisphosphonates, antioxidants, and antifibrotic drugs appears to be a reliable and safe treatment strategy that awaits validation in larger clinical trials.

REFERENCES

1. Krasin MJ, Constine LS, Friedman DL, Marks LB: Radiation-related treatment Effects across the age spectrum: differences and similarities or what the old and young can learn from each other, *Semin Radiat Oncol* 20(1):21-29, 2010.
2. Mitchell MJ, Logan P: Radiation-induced changes in bone, *RadioGraphics* 18:1125-1136, 1998.
3. Regaud C: Sur la sensibilite du tissue osseux normal vis-a-vis des rayons X et gamma et sur la mecanisme de l'osteoradionecrose, *CR Soc Biol (Paris)* 87:929-932, 1922.
4. Clayman L: Management of dental extractions in irradiated jaws: a protocol without hyperbaric oxygen therapy, *J Oral Maxillofac Surg* 55:275-281, 1997.
5. Wahl M: Osteoradionecrosis prevention myths, *Inter J Radiat Oncol Bio Phys* 64(3):661-669, 2006.
6. Bhide SA, Nutting CM: Advances in radiotherapy for head and neck cancer, *Oral Oncol* 46(6):439-441, 2010.
7. Brahme A: Recent advances in light ion radiation therapy, *Int J Radiat Oncol Biol Phys* 58:603-616, 2004.
8. Beumer J, Silverman S, Benak SB: Hard and soft tissue necroses following radiation therapy for oral cancer, *J Prosthet Dent* 27:640-644, 1972.
9. Marx RE: Osteoradionecrosis: a new concept of its pathophysiology, *J Oral Maxillofac Surg* 41:283-288, 1983.
10. Widmark G, Sagme S, Heikel P: Osteoradionecrosis of the jaws, *Int J Oral Maxillofac Surg* 18:302-306, 1989.
11. Watson WL, Scarborough JE: Osteoradionecrosis in intraoral cancer, *Am J Roengenol* 40:524-534, 1938
12. Gowgiel J: Experimental radio-osteonecrosis of the jaws, *J Dent Res* 39:176-197, 1960.
13. Meyer I: Infectious diseases of the jaws, *J Oral Surg* 28:17-26, 1970.
14. Denham JW, Hauer-Jensen M: The radiotherapeutic injury: a complex "wound," *Radiother Oncol* 63:129-145, 2002.
15. Rodemann HP, Bamberg M: Cellular basis of radiation-induced fibrosis, *Radiother Oncol* 35:83-90, 1995.
16. Delanian S, Lefaix J: Current management for late normal tissue injury: radiation-induced fibrosis and necrosis, *Semin Radia Oncol* 17(2):99-107, 2007.
17. Delanian S, Lefaix J: The radiation-induced fibroatrophic process: therapeutic perspective via the antioxidant pathway, *Radiother Oncol* 73(2):119-131, 2005.
18. Katsura K, Sasai K, Sato K, et al: Relationship between oral health status and development of osteoradionecrosis of the mandible: a retrospective longitudinal study, *Oral Surg,*

Oral Med, Oral Pathol, Oral Radiol, Endod 105(6):731-738, 2008.

19. Jereczek-Fossa BA, Orecchia R: Radiotherapy-induced mandibular bone complications, *Cancer Treat Rev* 28:65-74, 2002.

20. Morrish RB, Chan E, Silverman S, et al: Osteonecrosis in patients irradiated for head and neck carcinoma, *Cancer* 47(8):1980-1983, 1981.

21. Lee IJ, Koom WS, Lee CG, et al: Risk factors and dose–effect relationship for mandibular osteoradionecrosis in oral and oropharyngeal cancer patients, *Int J Radiat Oncol Biol Phy* 75(4):1084-1091, 2009.

22. Glanzmann C, Gratz KW: Radionecrosis of the mandibula: a retrospective analysis of the incidence and risk factors, *Radiother Oncol* 36:94-1001, 1995.

23. Beck-Bornholdt H-P, Dubben H-H, Liertz-Petersen C, Willers H: Hyperfractionation: where do we stand? *Radiother Oncol* 46:1-21, 1997.

24. Dische S, Saunders M, Barrett A, et al: A randomised multicentre trial of CHART versus conventional radiotherapy in head and neck cancer, *Radiother Oncol* 44:123-136, 1997.

25. Niewald M, Barbie O, Schnabel K, Engel M, et al: Risk factors and dose-effect relationship for osteoradionecrosis after hyperfractionated and conventionally fractionated radiotherapy for oral cancer, *Br J Radiol* 69:847-851, 1996.

26. Murray C, Henson J, Daly T, Zimmerman S: Radiation necrosis of the mandible: a 10 year study. Part I: factors influencing the onset of necrosis, *Int J Radiat Oncol Biol Phys* 6:543-548, 1980.

27. Murray C, Henson J, Zimmerman S: Radiation necrosis of the mandible: a 10 year study. Part II: dental factors, onset, duration and management of necrosis, *Int J Radiat Oncol Biol Phys* 6:549-553, 1980.

28. Bras J. de Jonge HK, van Merkesteyn JP: Osteoradionecrosis of the mandible: pathogenesis, *Am J Otolaryngol* 11:244-250, 1990.

29. Reuther T, Schuster T, Mende U, Kübler A: Osteoradionecrosis of the jaws as a side effect of radiotherapy of head and neck tumour patients—a report of a thirty year retrospective review, *Int J Oral Maxillofac Surg* 32(3):289-295, 2003.

30. Murray CG, Daly TE, Zimmerman S: The relationship between dental disease and radiation necrosis of the mandible, *Oral Surg, Oral Med, Oral Pathol, Oral Radiol, Endod* 49:99-104, 1980.

31. Kluth EV, Jain PR, Stuchell RN, Frich JC: A study of factors contributing to the development of osteoradionecrosis of the jaws, *J Prosthet Dent* 59:194-201, 1988.

32. Shimizutani K, Inoue T, Inoue T, Yoshioka Y et al: Late complications after high-dose-rate interstitial brachytherapy for tongue cancer, *Oral Radiol* 21(1):1-5, 2005.

33. Goldwaser B, Chuang S, Kaban L, August M: Risk factor assessment for the development of osteoradionecrosis, *J Oral Maxillofac Surg* 65(11):2311-2316, 2007.

34. Koga DH, Salvajoli JV, Alves FA: Dental extractions and radiotherapy in head and neck oncology: review of the literature, *Oral Diseases* 14(1):40-44, 2007.

35. Koga D, Salvajoli J, Kowalski L: Dental extractions related to head and neck radiotherapy: ten-year experience of a single institution, *Oral Surg, Oral Med, Oral Pathol, Oral Radiol, Endod* 105(5):e1-e6, 2008.

36. Sulaiman F, Huryn JM, Zlotolow IM: Dental extractions in the irradiated head and neck patient: a retrospective analysis of memorial sloan-kettering cancer center protocols, criteria, and end results, *J Oral Maxillofac Surg* 61(10):1123-1131, 2003.

37. Chang DT, Sandow PR, Morris CG, et al: Do pre-irradiation dental extractions reduce the risk of osteoradionecrosis of the mandible? *Head Neck* 29(6):528-536, 2007.

38. Allison PJ, Locker D, Feine JS: The relationship between dental status and health-related quality of life in upper aerodigestive tract cancer patients, *Oral Oncol* 35:138-143, 1999.

39. Store G, Eribe E, Olsen I: DNA-DNA hybridization demonstrates multiple bacteria in osteoradionecrosis, *Int J Oral Maxillofac Surg* 34(2):193-196, 2005.

40. Store G, Olsen I: Scanning and transmission electron microscopy demonstrates bacteria in osteoradionecrosis, *Int J Oral Maxillofac Surg* 34(7):777-781, 2005.

41. Hansen T, Kunkel M, Kirkpatrick C, Weber A: Actinomyces in infected osteoradionecrosis—underestimated? *Hum Pathol* 37(1):61-67, 2006.

42. Hansen T, Wagner W, Kirkpatrick C, Kunkel M: Infected osteoradionecrosis of the mandible: follow-up study suggests deterioration in outcome for patients with Actinomyces-positive bone biopsies, *Int J Oral Maxillofac Surg* 35(11):1001-1004, 2006.

43. Curi MM, Dib LL, Kowalski LP, et al: Opportunistic actinomycosis in osteoradionecrosis of the jaws in patients affected by head and neck cancer: incidence and clinical significance, *Oral Oncol* 36:294-299, 2000.

44. Nair SP, Meghji S, Wilson M, et al: Bacterially induced bone destruction: mechanisms and misconceptions, *Infect Immun* 64:2371-2380, 1996.

45. Garant P: Light and electron microscopic observations of osteoclastic alveolar bone resorption in rats monoinfected with Actinomyces naeslundi, *J Periodontol* 47:717-723, 1976.

46. Glastonbury CM, Parker EE, Hoang JK: The postradiation neck: evaluating response to treatment and recognizing complications, *AJR* 195(2):W164-W171, 2010.

47. Chong J, Hinckley LK, Ginsberg LE: Masticator space abnormalities associated with mandibular osteoradionecrosis: MR and CT findings in five patients, *AJNR* 21:175-178, 2000.

48. Hermans R, Fossion E, Ioannides C, et al: CT findings in osteoradionecrosis of the mandible, *Skeletal Radiol* 25:31-36, 1996.

49. Store G, Larhiem T: Mandibular osteoradionecrosis: a comparison of computed tomography with panoramic radiography, *Dentomaxillofac Radiol* 28:295-300, 1999.

50. Bachmann G, Röler R, Klett R, et al: The role of magnetic resonance imaging and scintigraphy in the diagnosis of pathologic changes of the mandible after radiation therapy, *Int J Oral Maxillofac Surg* 25:189-195, 1996.

51. Wilde F, Steinhoff K, Frerich B, et al: Positron-emission tomography imaging in the diagnosis of bisphosphonate-related osteonecrosis of the jaw, *Oral Surg, Oral Med, Oral Pathol, Oral Radiol, Endod* 107:412-419, 2009.

52. Epstein JB, Wong FLW, Stevenson-Moore P: Osteoradionecrosis: clinical experience and a proposal for classification, *J Oral Maxillofac Surg* 45:104-110, 1987.

53. Cooper JS, Fu K, Marks J, Silverman S: Late effects of radiation therapy in the head and neck region, *Int J Radiat Oncol Biol Phys* 31:1141-1164, 1995.

54. Store G, Boysen M: Mandibular osteoradionecrosis: clinical behaviour and diagnostic aspects, *Clin Otolaryngol* 25:378-384, 2000.

55. Notani K-i, Yamazaki Y, Kitada H, et al: Management of mandibular osteoradionecrosis corresponding to the severity of osteoradionecrosis and the method of radiotherapy, *Head Neck* 25(3):181-186, 2003.

56. Lent Soma Scales for all anatomic sites, *Int J Radiat Oncol Biol Phys* 31:1049-1091, 1995.

57. Thorn J, Hansen H, Specht L, Bastholt L: Osteoradionecrosis of the jaws: clinical characteristics and relation to the field of irradiation, *J Oral Maxillofac Surg* 58(10):1088-1093, 2000.

58. Gray LH, Conger AD, Ebert M, et al: The concentration of oxygen dissolved in tissues at the time of irradiation as a factor in radiotherapy, *Br J Radiol* 126:638-648, 1953.

59. Churchill-Davidson I: The oxygen effect in radiotherapy, *Oncology* 20:18-29, 1966.

60. Bennett M, Feldmeier J, Smee R, Milross C: Hyperbaric oxygenation for tumour sensitisation to radiotherapy: a systematic review of randomised controlled trials, *Cancer Treat Rev* 34(7):577-591, 2008.

61. Freiberger JJ, Feldmeier J: Evidence supporting the use of hyperbaric oxygen in the treatment of osteoradionecrosis of the jaw, *J Oral Maxillofac Surg* 68:1903-1906, 2010.

62. Bessereau J, Annane D: Treatment of osteoradionecrosis of the jaw: The case against the use of hyperbaric oxygen, *J Oral Maxillofac Surg* 68:1907-1910, 2010.

63. Freiberger JJ, Yoo DS, de Lisle Dear G, et al: MultiModality surgical and hyperbaric management of mandibular osteoradionecrosis, *Intl J Radiat Oncol Biol Phys* 75(3):717-724, 2009.

64. Maier A, Gaggl A, Klemen H, et al: Review of severe osteoradionecrosis treated by surgery alone or surgery with postoperative hyperbaric oxygenation, *Br J Oral Maxillofac Surg* 38(3):173-176, 2000.

65. Bui Q, Lieber M, Withers H, et al: The efficacy of hyperbaric oxygen therapy in the treatment of radiation-induced late side effects, *Int J Radiat Oncol Biol Phys* 60(3):871-878, 2004.

66. Dsouza J, Goru J, Goru S, et al: The influence of hyperbaric oxygen on the outcome of patients treated for osteoradionecrosis: 8 year study, *Intl J Oral Maxillofac Surg* 36(9):783-787, 2007.

67. Aitasalo K, Niinikoski J, Grenman R, Virolainen E: A modified protocol for early treatment of osteomyelitis and osteoradionecrosis of the mandible, *Head Neck* 20:411-417, 1997.

68. Pasquier D: Hyperbaric oxygen therapy in the treatment of radio-induced lesions in normal tissues: a literature review, *Radiother Oncol* 72(1):1-13, 2004.

69. Spiegelberg L, Djasim UM, van Neck HW, et al: Hyperbaric oxygen therapy in the management of radiation-induced injury in the head and neck region: a review of the literature, *J Oral Maxillofac Surg* 68(8):1732-1739, 2010.

70. Bennett MH, Feldmeier J, Hampson N, et al: Hyperbaric oxygen therapy for late radiation tissue injury, *Cochrane Database Syst Rev* (2), 2009.

71. Wang C, Schwaitzberg S, Berliner E, et al: Hyperbaric oxygen for treating wounds: a systematic review of the literature, *Arch Surg* 138:272-279, 2003.

72. Marx RE, Johnson RP, Kline SN: Prevention of osteoradionecrosis: a randomized prospective clinical trial of hyperbaric oxygen versus penicillin, *J Am Dent Assoc* 111:49-54, 1985.

73. Schwartz HC, Kagan R: Osteoradionecrosis of the mandible: scientific basis for clinical staging, *Am J Clin Oncol* 25:168-171, 2002.

74. Marx RE: Bony reconstruction of the jaw. In Kindwall EP, Whelan HT, editors: *Hyperbaric medicine practice*, ed 2, Flagstaff, AZ, 1999, Best Publishing, pp 460-463.

75. Marx RE: Soft tissue flaps. In Kindwall EP, Whelan HT, editors: *Hyperbaric medicine practice*, ed 2, Flagstaff, AZ, 1999, Best Publishing, pp 464-468.

76. Annane D, Depondt J, Aubert P, et al: Hyperbaric oxygen therapy for radionecrosis of the jaw: a randomized, placebo-controlled, double-blind trial from the ORN96 study group, *J Clin Oncol* 22(24):4893-4900, 2004.

77. Tibbles PM, Edelsberg JS: Hyperbaric oxygen therapy, *N Engl J Med* 334:1642-1648, 1996.

78. Bradfield JJ, Kinsella J, Mader JT, Bridges EW: Rapid progression of head and neck squamous carcinoma after hyperbaric oxygenation, *Otolaryngol Head Neck Surg* 114:793-797, 1996.

79. Wang PH, Yuan CC, Lai CR, et al: Rapid progression of squamous cell carcinoma of the cervix after hyperbaric oxygenation, *Eur J Obstet Gynecol Reprod Biol* 82:89-91, 1999.

80. Shi Y, Lee CS, Wu J, et al: Effects of hyperbaric oxygen exposure on experimental head and neck tumor growth, oxygenation, and vasculature, *Head Neck* 27(5):362-369, 2005.

81. Lin H-Y, Ku C-H, Liu D-W, et al: Hyperbaric oxygen therapy for late radiation-associated tissue necroses: is it safe in patients with locoregionally recurrent and then successfully salvaged head-and-neck cancers? *Int J Radiat Oncol Biol Phys* 74(4):1077-1082, 2009.

82. Wong JK, Wood RE, McLean M: Conservative management of osteoradionecrosis, *Oral Surg, Oral Med, Oral Pathol, Oral Radiol, Endod* 84:16-21, 1997.

83. Epstein J, van der Meij E, McKenzie M, et al: Postradiation osteonecrosis of the mandible: a long-term follow-up study, *Oral Surg, Oral Med, Oral Pathol, Oral Radiol, Endod* 83:657-662, 1997.

84. Peleg M, Lopez EA: The treatment of osteoradionecrosis of the mandible: the case for hyperbaric oxygen and bone graft reconstruction, *J Oral Maxillofac Surg* 64:956-960, 2006.

85. Buchbinder D, Sthilaire H: The use of free tissue transfer in advanced osteoradionecrosis of the mandible, *J Oral Maxillofac Surg* 64(6):961-964, 2006.

86. Hirsch D, Bell R, Dierks E, et al: Analysis of microvascular free flaps for reconstruction of advanced mandibular osteoradionecrosis: a retrospective cohort study, *J Oral Maxillofac Surg* 66(12):2545-2556, 2008.

87. Suh JD, Blackwell KE, Sercarz JA, et al: Disease relapse after segmental resection and free flap reconstruction for mandibular osteoradionecrosis, *Otolaryngol Head Neck Surg* 142(4):586-591, 2010.

88. Wax MK, Winslow C, Hansen J, et al: A retrospective analysis of temporomandibular joint reconstruction with free fibula microvascular flap, *Laryngoscope* 110:977-981, 2000.

89. González-García R, Naval-Gias L, Rodríguez-Campo FJ, et al: Vascularized fibular flap for reconstruction of the condyle after mandibular ablation, *J Oral Maxillofac Surg* 66:1133-1137, 2008.

90. Kim JH, Rosenthal E, Ellis T, Wax MK: Radial forearm osteocutaneous free flap in maxillofacial and oromandibular reconstructions. *Laryngoscope* 115:1697-1701, 2005.

91. Virgin FW, Iseli T, Iseli CE, et al: Functional outcomes of fibula and osteocutaneous forearm free flap reconstruction for segmental mandibular defects, *Laryngoscope* 120:663-667, 2010.

92. Gal TJ, Yueh B, Futran ND: Influence of prior hyperbaric oxygen therapy in complications following microvascular reconstruction for advanced osteoradionecrosis, *Arch Otolaryngol Head Neck Surg* 129:72-76, 2003.

93. Alam DS, Nuara M, Christian J: Analysis of outcomes of vascularized flap reconstruction in patients with advanced mandibular osteoradionecrosis, *Otolaryngol Head Neck Surg* 141:196-201, 2009.

94. Curi M, Oliveiradossantos M, Feher O, et al: Management of extensive osteoradionecrosis of the mandible with radical resection and immediate microvascular reconstruction, *J Oral Maxillofac Surg* 65(3):434-438, 2007.

95. Cannady SB, Dean N, Kroeker A, et al: Free flap reconstruction for osteoradionecrosis of the jaws—outcomes and predictive factors for success, *Head Neck* 33:424-428, 2011.

96. Chang DW, Oh HK, Robb GL, Miller MJ: Management of advanced mandibular osteoradionecrosis with free flap reconstruction, *Head Neck* 23:830-835, 2001.

97. Ioannides C, Fosssion E, Boeckx W, et al: Surgical management of the osteoradionecrotic mandible with free vascularised composite flaps, *J Craniomaxillofac Surg* 22:330-334, 1994.

98. Shaha AR, Cordeiro PG, Hidalgo DA, et al: Resection and immediate microvascular reconstruction in the management of osteoradionecrosis of the mandible, *Head Neck* 19:406-411, 1997.

99. Delanian S, Depondt J, Lefaix J-L: Major healing of refractory mandible osteoradionecrosis after treatment combining pentoxifylline and tocopherol: a phase II trial, *Head Neck* 27(2):114-123, 2005.

100. Delanian S, Balla-Mekias S, Lefaix J-L: Striking regression of chronic radiotherapy damage in a clinical trial of combined pentoxifylline and tocopherol, *J Clin Oncol* 17:3283-3290, 1999.

101. Delanian S, Chatel C, Porcher R, et al: Complete restoration of refractory mandibular osteoradionecrosis by prolonged treatment with a pentoxifylline-tocopherol-clodronate combination (PENTOCLO): a phase II trial, *Int J Radiat Oncol Biol Phys* 80(3):832-839, 2010.

102. Lyons A, Ghazali N: Osteoradionecrosis of the jaws: current understanding of its pathophysiology and treatment, *Br J Oral Maxillofac Surg* 46:653-660, 2008.

103. Milas L, Mason KA, Liao Z, Ang KK: Chemoradiotherapy: emerging treatment improvement strategies, *Head Neck* 25(2):152-167, 2003.

104. Gomez DR, Zhung JE, Gomez J, et al: Intensity-modulated radiotherapy in postoperative treatment of oral cavity cancers, *Int J Radiat Oncol Biol Phys* 73(4):1096-1103, 2009.

105. Ben-David M, Diamante M, Radawski J, et al: Lack of osteoradionecrosis of the mandible after intensity-modulated radiotherapy for head and neck cancer: likely contributions of both dental care and improved dose distributions, *Int J Radiat Oncol BiolPhys* 68(2):396-402, 2007.

THE PAST

Maxillofacial reconstructive surgery deals with the restoration of missing or deformed anatomy, such as bone, skin, mucosa, muscle, and nerve. Experiences in World War I and World War II resulted in unprecedented advances in maxillofacial reconstructive surgery such as the use of nonvascularized bone grafts, interdental wire fixation, skin grafts, and "tubed" pedicled soft tissue flaps. By the end of World War II, advances in surgical technique, advances in anesthesiology, and the advent of penicillin led to improvements in morbidity and mortality and made reconstructive surgery a common reality. Despite these improvements in clinical care, treatment times were excessively long and were plagued by high rates of complications and bone graft failure unless performed in a staged manner.

THE PRESENT

The contemporary maxillofacial surgeon has in his or her arsenal a wide range of soft tissue, bone and composite flaps—both pedicled and free—that afford a much greater degree of predictability than in years past. Autogenous and allogeneic grafts can be used to restore skin, mucosa, and nerves in an effective manner. In addition, treatment times for restoring a patient to form and function is shorter. Composite tissue defects involving the maxillomandibular skeleton may be restored to premorbid form, and function may be returned through successful dental implant supported rehabilitation. The controversy of whether or not to perform a staged or immediate reconstruction is largely dead, as most patients can be reconstructed in a single operation and only a few patients need undergo multiple reconstructive procedures.

THE FUTURE

Microvascular techniques will continue to improve, as customized, "designer" flaps evolve for evermore niche purposes. The recently successful attempts at facial allotransplantation will spark expanded interest and intense study, which will in turn be facilitated by improved immunosuppression solutions. Tissue engineering/regenerative medicine—currently an emerging multidisciplinary field involving biology, medicine, and engineering—will revolutionize the ways we restore, maintain, or enhance tissue and organ function. In addition to having a therapeutic application, where the tissue is either grown in a patient or outside the patient and transplanted, tissue engineering may have diagnostic applications whereby the tissue is made in vitro and used for testing drug metabolism and uptake, toxicity, and pathogenicity.

Chapter 60

Mandibular Reconstruction

Jason K. Potter

Reconstruction of the mandible is by definition restoring form and function to the mandibular bone and its dentition as well as its investing soft tissue envelope. This may be accomplished by a wide variety of procedures depending on, among other things, the etiology and extent of the deformity. Restoring form and function for a congenital deformity is obviously approached in a much different manner than a composite segmental defect acquired as a result of a cancer operation. Recognizing that there are too numerous techniques suitable for each potential clinical situation to discuss in this chapter, it will therefore focus on the most common, namely, reconstruction of acquired segmental defects of the mandible with nonvascularized grafts or vascularized bone flaps.

ETIOPATHOGENESIS/CAUSATIVE FACTORS

Acquired segmental defects of the mandible are most commonly secondary to ablative tumor therapy or avulsive traumatic injury. Other less common causes include inflammatory or infectious conditions that result in devitalization of the mandibular bone requiring its debridement. Segmental defects secondary to tumor therapy may result from the management of aggressive benign tumors arising within the mandible such as ameloblastoma or myxoma or from malignancies (carcinomas/sarcomas) arising in the associated soft tissue envelope that invade or extend to the mandible. Management of oral squamous cell carcinoma is the most common malignancy resulting in acquired segmental defects of the mandible.

Avulsive segmental wounds most commonly arise from high-velocity injuries such as firearms, industrial accidents, and occasionally motor vehicle collisions. Fortunately, most traumatic injuries to the jaws do not result in segmental defects because of the lower kinetic energies associated with the injury. Kinetic energy (KE = mv^2) increases dramatically as the speed of the missile or the speed of impact increases, resulting in comminution of bone, destruction of the soft tissue envelope, and devitalization of large areas of bone and soft tissue. The extent of devitalization from high-velocity injuries may not be completely apparent at the time of presentation. The astute clinician will recognize the potential for extensive tissue loss in these patients and utilize wound care and temporary stabilization of the wound until all tissue loss has had opportunity to declare itself prior to definitive reconstruction.

Inflammatory conditions that result in devitalization of mandibular bone can be quite destructive. Osteoradionecrosis and bisphosphonate osteonecrosis represent two of the most common etiologies and may present with or without an associated acute osteomyelitis of the involved bone. Osteoradionecrosis results from a profound hypovascularity of the bone secondary to radiotherapy, whereas bisphosphonate osteonecrosis results from dysfunction of the osteoclasts caused most commonly by intravenous bisphosphonate therapy. The management of these specific etiologies is beyond the scope of this chapter; however, in the author's experience, large segmental defects resulting from either process are amenable to reconstruction with vascularized fibular bone grafts.

PATHOLOGIC ANATOMY/ CLASSIFICATION OF DEFECTS

The location of the mandibular defect has a direct implication to management. Complex classification schemes have been proposed to help guide therapy based on bony, soft tissue, and neurologic deficits.[1] The author prefers a simplified approach based on the position of the defect relative to the mandibular anatomy. This scheme divides the mandible into functional segments consisting of the symphysis (anterior) unit, the body (lateral) unit, the ramus-condyle (posterior) unit, and the alveolus (Box 60-1).

Each of these sites has variable physiologic factors that result in different functional deficits when lost as a result of tumor ablation or traumatic disruption. Each region is also subject to significantly different forces (torsion, tension, compression) acting across the defect during function. Furthermore, numerous studies have evaluated failure rates for various techniques for mandibular reconstruction and identified differences based on the location of the defect. Consequently, reconstruction of each anatomic unit demands an individualized approach based on factors related to the patient, the reconstructive procedure, and the disease process. The impact of defect location and consideration of reconstructive technique will be further discussed later in the text.

A second factor for consideration is the importance of the soft tissue envelope. Evaluation of the soft tissue envelope should consider both the quality of the tissues and the quantity of tissue remaining or removed. Kazanjian in 1952 identified four essential factors for successful bone grafting, the first two of which were (1) implantation into healthy tissue and (2) good blood supply in the recipient area. Wounds that lack healthy soft tissue because of extensive trauma to the tissues or large volume loss of soft tissue as a result of resection are poor candidates for immediate nonvascular bone grafting. Likewise, wounds that are hypovascular due to radiotherapy or extensive scarring will provide poor wound beds for successful nonvascular bone grafting. In these situations, transfer of healthy vascularized tissue is essential for successful reconstruction.

BOX 60-1	Classification of Mandibular Defects

Alveolar defects. Loss of alveolar segment without loss of mandibular continuity.
Anterior defects. Segmental defect incorporating the region of the mandibular symphysis or extending from cuspid to cuspid.
Lateral defects. Segmental defect involving the mandibular body region or extending from the mandibular cuspid to the retromolar region.
Posterior defects. Segmental defects involving the ramus and mandibular angle with or without loss of the condylar process.

Complication rates for mandibular reconstruction have shown a tendency to increase with the increasing soft tissue resection.[2] Loss of a significant volume of tissue precludes immediate nonvascular bone grafting in most situations. Failure rates with immediate nonvascular bone grafting techniques have been reported as high as 50% in such situations. Therefore, when a segmental defect is associated with extensive loss of soft tissues, immediate reconstruction with vascularized tissue transfer or delayed reconstruction should be considered.

DIAGNOSTIC STUDIES

Diagnostic studies to assess the ability of the patient to tolerate the proposed operation or the extent of malignant disease are beyond the scope of this chapter. Diagnostic studies pertinent to mandibular reconstruction include preoperative imaging of the mandible, computer-generated models or surgical guides (tactile medical imaging), and preoperative vascular studies specific to various reconstructive techniques.

Preoperative computed tomography (CT) of the mandible is critical to establishing the anticipated defect. Plain radiographs may be useful adjuncts to clinical evaluation but lack sufficient detail alone to establish the extent of disease. CT imaging allows evaluation of disease within the marrow space and can better evaluate cortical erosions that may otherwise be missed with plain radiographs. Axial and coronal scans are the minimal requirement and may be combined with sagittal images or three-dimensional reconstructions as needed to further define the extent of tumor involvement. Magnetic resonance imaging (MRI) may be useful as an additional study to identify extension along the inferior alveolar for certain tumor biologies. Because of its poor detail of osseous anatomy, MRI is not routinely utilized alone.

Tactile medical imaging is the display, in physical form, of anatomic data derived from medical imaging studies. Stereolithography and 3D printing represent the two main technologies for tactile medical models. Stereolithography utilizes laser photopolymerization of a liquid polymer to create an accurate, durable, translucent and sterilizable model of the patient's skeletal anatomy (Fig. 60-1, *A*), whereas 3-D printing utilizes an inkjet-based printing method to create a skeletal model by injection of liquid into a plaster powder (Fig. 60-1, *B*). Three-dimensional printing models are accurate and opaque, but they are fragile and not sterilizable. Both allow hands-on study and treatment planning, but the stereolithographic models may also be used intraoperatively to assist with prebending of surgical fixation systems, model surgery, and shaping of bone grafts (Fig. 60-2).

Current technology also allows for virtual treatment planning and surgery for the creation of surgical guides from computer-based images (Fig. 60-3).[3,4] Intraoperative use of these guides has been shown to improve accuracy of osteotomies and decrease operative time.[5]

Preoperative vascular studies are at times necessary to delineate the recipient (neck) or donor (flap) vascular anatomy prior to free tissue transfer. The head and neck cancer patient may have unclear vascular anatomy to serve as recipient vessels for free tissue transfer, especially in the multiply operated neck. Preoperative angiogram of the head and neck can identify the presence or lack thereof of arterial structures suitable for microsurgery and can also identify the status of the internal jugular vein. Patients with vessel-depleted necks may require vein grafting or creation of a vascular loop from distant vessels. This information can be critical in the decision process and preparation in such patients and ultimately make the difference in a successful reconstruction.[6] Preoperative assessment of donor vessels

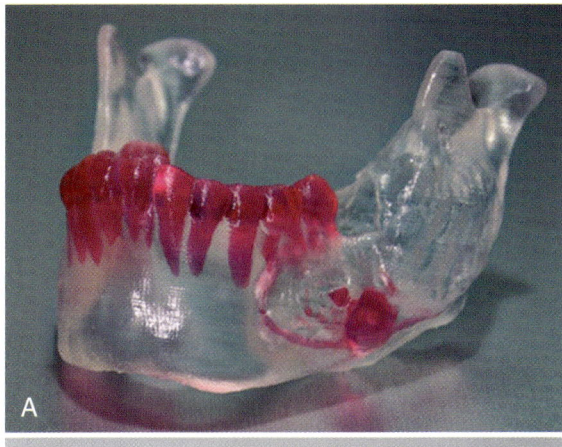

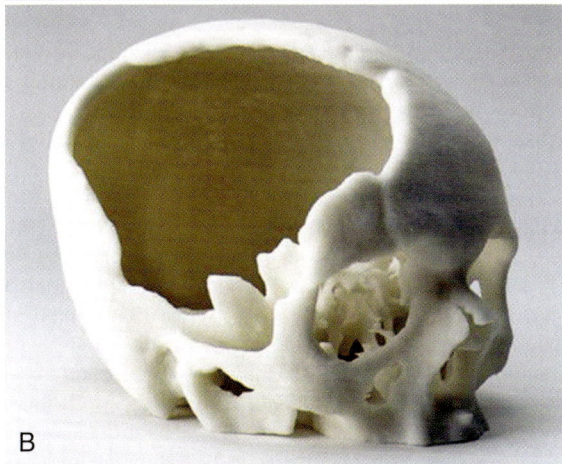

Fig. 60-1 ■ **A,** Stereolithographic model of mandible. **B,** Three-dimensional printing model of skull. (Courtesy of Medical Modeling Inc., Golden, Colo.)

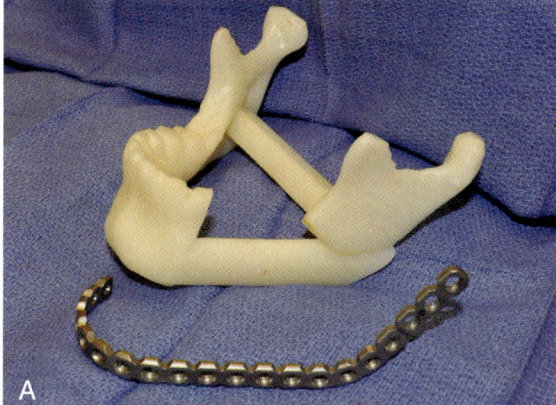

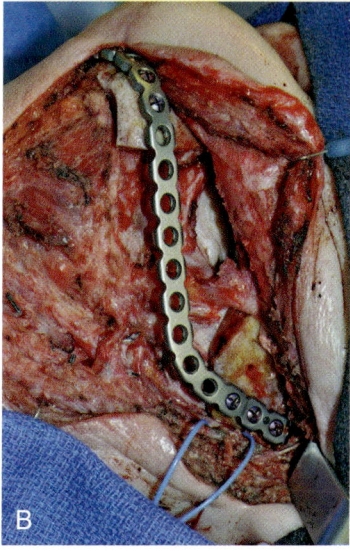

Fig. 60-2 ■ **A,** Stereolithographic model of mandibular reconstruction and prebent reconstruction plate. **B,** Plate secured to mandibular remnants with accurate reestablishment of jaw relations.

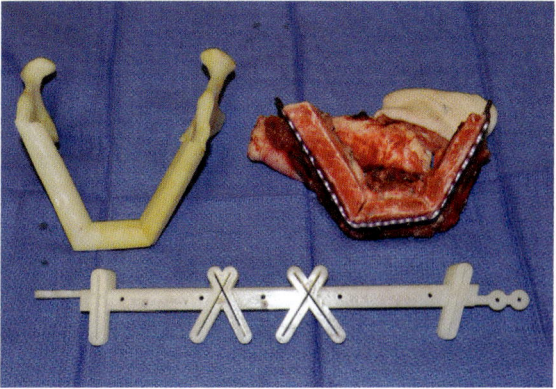

Fig. 60-3 ■ Surgical guides created from CT data and stereolithographic models.

is helpful in certain situations as well. Some patients may demonstrate surgical scars from prior surgery that may have disrupted the potential donor vessels. An example would be patients with lateral thoracotomy scars or low transverse abdominal scars that are being considered for latissimus dorsi or rectus abdominis muscle transfer respectively. Preoperative angiography can confirm the patency of the donor vessels. Probably the most common use of preoperative angiography of donor vessels is associated with fibula transfer. Two clinical situations that are critical to identify in patients considered for fibula transfer are the presence of inadequate vascularity of the leg to allow harvest of the peroneal artery and the presence of a dominant peroneal artery system. Both conditions can result in ischemia of the foot and are contraindications to the harvest of the fibular flap. Studies have demonstrated that dominant peroneal systems are present in approximately 5-10% of the population.[7] Peripheral vascular disease resulting in compromised vascularity of the lower extremity is common in the elderly, tobacco-using population characteristic of head and neck cancer patients. Screening of potential candidates with lower extremity pulse exams can identify patients needing preoperative lower extremity angiography. Patients with normal lower extremity pulse exams, in general, do not require preoperative angiography.[8]

TREATMENT/RECONSTRUCTIVE GOALS

The goal of mandibular reconstruction is the restoration of form and function of the mandibular apparatus. Specifically, this requires reestablishing an acceptable appearance and mandibular continuity,

maintaining a pain-free mandibular range of motion and relatively normal soft tissue relationships within the oral cavity to facilitate speech and deglutination, and providing a foundation on which to reconstruct the dentition.

Treatment options for reconstruction of segmental defects of the mandible include collapse of the defect, mandibular reconstruction plates (MRP) with or without soft tissue flaps (no osseous reconstruction), nonvascularized bone grafts, and vascularized bone flaps.

Choice of technique is influenced by several factors including (1) surgeon training/preference, (2) location of defect, (3) length of bony defect, (4) extent of oral mucosal or facial skin loss, (5) quality/vascularity of the wound bed, and (6) patient medical comorbidities.

TIMING OF RECONSTRUCTION

The ideal timing of mandibular reconstruction has been widely debated, especially in patients with malignant disease. Historically, proponents of a delayed or staged approach advocated a period of observation to monitor the patient for development of recurrent disease or to establish histologically clear bony margins prior to reconstruction. Today, however, it is widely accepted that immediate reconstruction may be performed without risk for a delayed diagnosis of recurrent disease.[9] Prior to microsurgical techniques, delayed reconstruction was critical to allow maturation of the wound bed for nonvascular bone grafting. Lawson et al. reported their results with immediate and delayed reconstruction utilizing corticocancellous grafts.[10] They reported a 90% success rate with delayed reconstruction, compared to 46% with immediate reconstruction when using nonvascularized bone grafts. Subsequent reports have demonstrated successful use of delayed, nonvascular bone grafts in select patients, and indeed nonvascular grafts are still frequently utilized today.[11-13] There are, however, strong arguments for the utilization of immediate vascularized bone flaps for most segmental mandibular defects compared to delayed reconstruction with nonvascular bone grafts. These include both patient factors and treatment/technical factors. The literature supports that delayed reconstruction of segmental defects of the mandible requires temporary stabilization of the mandibular remnants with mandibular reconstruction plates (MRP) with or without soft tissue flaps; temporary stabilization with MRP/myocutaneous flaps is associated with high complication rates especially in the anterior region; MRP failures can occur within 18 months with mean time to failure reported as early as 6 to 8 months; and complication rates for nonvascular bone grafts are greater for defects larger than 6 cm compared to vascularized bone flaps.

Immediate reconstruction has several other advantages over delayed reconstruction for mandibular reconstruction. Health-related quality of life (QOL) studies have demonstrated that immediate reconstruction significantly improves QOL and that most patients prefer immediate reconstruction.[14-17] Furthermore, Boyd reported that patients who underwent reconstruction with vascularized bone flaps experienced an average of 4 days life lost for secondary procedures,[18] compared to 35 days for patients who underwent plate and soft tissue flaps.

SURGEON TRAINING/PREFERENCE

The choice of any surgical procedure is affected by the training and skill level of the surgeon. In every specialty of medicine, new techniques or improvements of existing techniques are occurring at rapid pace. A thorough understanding of the available literature regarding techniques, complication rates, and indications and contraindications should guide the surgeon through the choice of available procedures. Although every surgeon may not be comfortable or adept with every technique, it is the responsibility of every surgeon to be familiar with the most current therapies and seek consultation or referral when in the best interest of the patient.

COLLAPSE THE DEFECT

The simplest technique for mandibular reconstruction is actually no reconstruction at all. Collapse of the mandibular segments and wound closure is rarely performed today but is acceptable for some patients with defects of the ramus-condyle and lateral body units. A characteristic deformity is created with deviation of the chin to the affected side and elevation of the tongue on the affected side. With appropriate physical therapy, reasonable mandibular function is maintained. The effect on speech and swallowing depends on the amount of soft tissue resected and the relationship of the remaining intraoral soft tissues following wound closure. Collapse of the defect should be reserved for select patients with significant medical comorbidities or extremely poor prognosis.

LOCATION OF DEFECT AND MANDIBULAR RECONSTRUCTION PLATES (MRPs)

As previously mentioned, the location of the segmental defect affects the complication rate of the technique. This is most important when considering reconstruction with a MRP with or without a soft tissue flap or a delayed, nonvascularized osseous reconstruction where the patient will require temporary stabilization with a MRP. In these situations, reconstruction of defects of the anterior region demonstrates high complication rates.

Spiessel in 1976 was the first to report bridging a tumor defect with a reconstruction plate. However, Schmoker was the first to propose reconstruction of mandibular defects with a reconstruction plate without osseous reconstruction.[19] This concept had many early advocates through the 1980s because of its ease, lack of a second surgical donor site, the quickness for which it could be performed, and a concern for high recurrence rates. By the 1990s, many authors reported high complication rates (Fig. 60-4) with MRPs, especially in the anterior region. Kim and Donoff reported their experience with 41 plates in 37 patients.[20] They divided the study into three groups based on location of the defect. Defects of the anterior mandible had a 52% failure rate compared to 12.5% for the body segment and 7.7% for the condyle-ramus unit. The overall wound dehiscence rate was 17%. Other authors reported high complication rates for lateral defects and overall outcome.[21,22] To combat the high rate of extrusion, several authors proposed the use of soft tissue flaps in conjunction with MRPs. Cordieri and Hildalgo reported their experience with soft tissue coverage of mandibular reconstruction plates for mandibular reconstruction in 14 patients; 9 patients underwent pectoralis muscle flaps and 5 underwent soft tissue free flaps for defects of the anterior mandible.[23] The pectoralis group had a 44%

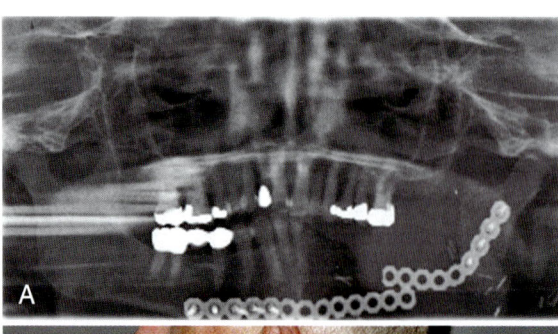
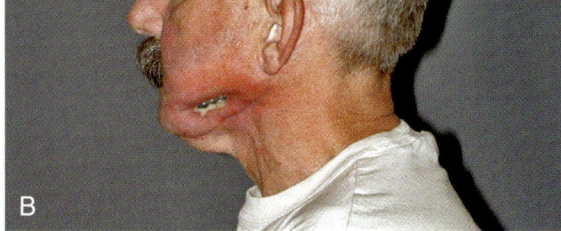

Fig. 60-4 ■ Complications of mandibular reconstruction plates. **A,** Plate fracture. **B,** Plate exposure.

extrusion rate, compared to 0% for the free flap group. They hypothesized the difference was due to tethering and tension on the pectoralis flap caused by the limitations of its reach by the nature of its pedicle attachment. Wei and colleagues reported their experience with reconstruction of composite segmental defects of the mandible utilizing MRPs and soft tissue flaps in 80 patients.[24] The overall complication rate was 69%, with plate exposure occurring in 46%. Seventy-eight percent underwent a second reconstructive procedure. Extrusion rates have also been shown to be higher in irradiated tissues.[25-27] In the author's experience, reconstructions of anterior defects and larger lateral defects with soft tissue flaps (free or pedicled) have high rates of extrusion, especially in the irradiated patient. This is likely due to the narrow profile of the plates providing poor support of the soft tissues, in association with contracture of the soft tissue envelope creating pressure necrosis. MRPs with or without soft flaps are doomed to failure in the anterior region. Reconstruction of the mandible with MRPs or temporization with MRPs in anticipation of delayed nonvascular bone grafts should be reserved for smaller defects of the lateral or posterior units in patients not requiring radiotherapy and considered poor candidates for vascularized bone flaps.

ANTERIOR DEFECTS

Defects in this region represent the most difficult to reconstruct for many reasons. The symphysis has multiple forces acting across the region depending on the mandibular function. Both compressive and tensile forces are present as well as torsional forces placing significant stress on any construct. The curved shape of the symphysis tends to be more difficult to re-create compared to the relative straight segments of the posterior and lateral regions. Its shape may influence the appearance of the lip and vertical height of the lower face. The symphysis also serves as the site for attachment of the suprahyoid and tongue musculature. When nonosseous reconstructions are performed in this region, the force of these muscle attachments is essentially conferred to the soft tissue envelope. This results in increased pressure of the soft tissues against the reconstruction plates and the opportunity for pressure necrosis of the overlying tissue with subsequent hardware exposure. As previously mentioned, anterior defects reconstructed with reconstruction plates and soft tissue flaps have been shown to be at high risk of failure.[22,28] Although vascularized bone flaps may have some limitations in contouring, the high failure rates associated with MRPs in the anterior region (without immediate osseous reconstruction) make them the procedure of choice for the anterior region.

LATERAL DEFECTS

Lateral defects characteristically are less complicated to reconstruct. They are relatively straight, do not have as significant muscle attachments, demonstrate lower complication rates compared to anterior defects, and in general have less impact on facial form. Lateral defects smaller than 6 cm and associated with benign disease are candidates for nonvascular bone grafting in patients not desiring immediate reconstruction. Lateral defects 6 cm and larger, associated with larger soft tissue loss, and having a history or need for radiation therapy should be reconstructed with vascularized bone flaps. Two important considerations present themselves when planning reconstruction with dental rehabilitation of lateral defects: the lateral and vertical position of the osseous construct. The normal mandibular body contour tends to be wider than the position of the alveolar bone. Therefore, when planning the contour of reconstruction plates and the position of the bone graft or flap there is often a

balance between placing the bone in a location to recreate the ideal facial contour versus a location that is ideal or at least usable for dental implants. Vertical position of bone flaps must also be considered. Fibula bone flaps have a much lower profile compared to the dentate mandible. Setting the reconstruction plate and the bone flap at the inferior border will recreate the most ideal jawline but may create a significant prosthetic challenge when one considers the location of the bone in relation to the occlusal platform. In the edentulous mandible, the fibula is an excellent size match and vertical height does not usually pose a problem.

POSTERIOR DEFECTS

Posterior defects, similar to lateral defects, involve a relatively straight segment of the mandible and are therefore less complicated to reconstruct unless involving the condylar process. They can impact facial form, including posterior vertical height of the mandible, and may create a more significant impact on mandibular range of motion because of the relationship with the temporomandibular joint and muscles of mastication. Posterior defects do represent a region that is amenable to allowing collapse of the defect without reconstruction when dictated by the patient's clinical situation. Depending on local and patient factors such as volume of tissue loss, disease process, status of the temporomandibular joint, and radiation therapy defects of the posterior unit may be reconstructed with costochondral/corticancellous grafts, alloplastic prostheses, or vascular bone flaps. Alloplastic joint prostheses probably do not have a role for true segmental defects involving the posterior unit and should be reserved for isolated loss of the condylar process in the absence of radiation therapy and significant tissue loss. Marx and colleagues reported the successful use of reconstruction plates with condylar prostheses for defects of the posterior unit including the condylar process.[29] Complications including plate fracture and erosion into the glenoid fossa have been reported (Fig. 60-5) and should limit their application to temporary stabilization prior to reconstruction of the mandible but should not be considered a definitive reconstruction of the condylar process. Preservation of the condylar process when oncologically feasible has positive effects on mandibular function. The condyle may be stabilized to the mandibular construct with internal fixation systems when adequate condylar structure is present or with wire fixation for smaller segments. Potter and Dierks have proposed an algorithm for vascularized reconstruction of the mandibular condyle and posterior segment defects that includes the condylar process.[30]

VASCULARIZED BONE FLAPS VS. NONVASCULAR BONE GRAFTS/ IMPORTANCE OF DEFECT LENGTH OF THE BONY DEFECT

Probably no other topic in mandibular reconstruction has generated as much discussion as that of vascular bone flaps versus nonvascular bone grafts. Both procedures have strong advocates. Marx has stated that "microvascular bone-periosteal flaps … do not represent a true advance in jaw reconstruction."[31] He has proposed that nonvascular bone grafts provide more adequate bone volume, improved continuity, better arch form, better alveolar bone height, and endosseous implant success. Success rates for nonvascularized bone grafts have been reported from 38-100%,[17,32-34] and similarly failure rates have been reported from 20-81%.[10,11,13,32,35-51] Most of these studies represent retrospective observations. August et al. reported several factors

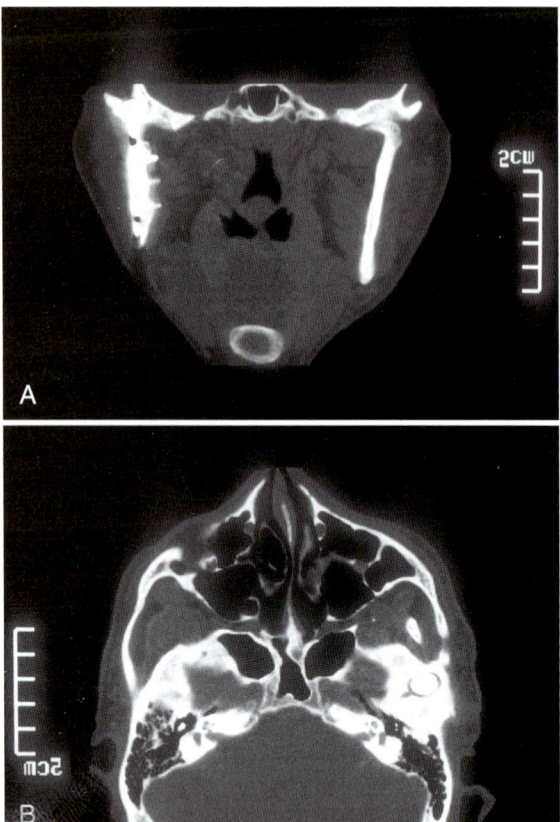

Fig. 60-5 ■ CT images demonstrating erosion of mandibular reconstruction plate with condylar prosthesis into temporal bone.

TABLE 60-1	Parameters Statistically Associated with Bone Graft Outcome	
VARIABLE		**P**
Graft Failure within 1 Year (Univariate Analysis)		
1. Length of mandibular defect		.028
2. Estimated blood loss		.021
3. Days on postoperative antibiotics		.048
4. Postoperative recipient site complications		.009
Graft Failure within 1 Year (Multivariate Analysis)		
1. Estimate blood loss		.018
2. Postoperative recipient site complications		.010
Bone Graft Survival Time (Univariate Analysis)		
1. Length of mandibular defect		.018
2. Use of sternocleidomastoid flap		.018
3. Duration of suction drainage		.002
4. Intraoral communication		.006
5. Estimated blood loss		.003
6. Days on postoperative antibiotics		.009
7. Postoperative recipient site complications		.012
Graft Survival Time (Multivariate Analysis)		
1. Use of sternocleidomastoid flap		.001
2. Duration of suction drainage		.001
3. Postoperative recipient site complications		.013
4. Malignant disease		.006

From August M, Tompach P, Chang YC, Kaban LB: Factors influencing the long-term outcome of mandibular reconstruction, *J Oral Maxillofac Surg* 58:731, 2000.

affecting the outcome of mandibular reconstruction including length of the mandibular defect, timing of reconstruction, radiotherapy, postoperative recipient site complications, malignant diagnosis, and intraoral communication (Table 60-1).[50] Several studies have compared nonvascualrized bone grafts and vascularized bone flaps and demonstrated the benefits of vascularized bone flaps. Pogrel et al. compared vascularized bone flaps to nonvascular bone grafts for reconstruction of mandibular continuity defects.[49] Thirty-nine patients underwent vascularized bone flaps, and 29 underwent nonvascular bone grafts. Vascularized bone flaps demonstrated a 95% success rate compared to 76% for nonvascular bone grafts. When evaluating for length of defect, the nonvascular bone grafts failed 17% of the time for defects less than 6 cm and 75% for defects greater than 6 cm. They concluded that vascularized bone flaps were the treatment of choice for defects greater than 6 cm and in the presence of irradiated tissues. Foster performed an outcome analysis for vascularized bone flaps and nonvascular bone grafts comparing primary bone union and endosseous implant success.[48] Forty-nine patients underwent vascular bone flaps (VBF), and 26 underwent nonvascular bone grafts (NVBG). Forty-five percent of VBF patients received radiotherapy compared to 11% for NVBG. Vascular bone flaps achieved a higher incidence of union (96% versus 69%; $p < .0005$) in a fewer number of procedures (1.1 versus 2.3; $p < .001$), and the endosseous implant success rate was significantly greater in the vascular bone flap group (99% versus 82%; $p < .0001$) despite a higher prevalence of radiotherapy. Many other reports have documented the high success rate of vascularized bone flaps as well. An additional benefit to vascular bone flaps is the ability to include variable amounts of vascularized soft tissue, a characteristic that is extremely useful in the face of extensive soft tissue resection and irradiated wound beds (Fig. 60-6). In the author's opinion based on the previous discussion, vascular bone flaps provide a highly successful means of immediate reconstruction of the mandible useful in most clinical situations. Nonvascular bone grafts should be reserved for lateral or posterior lateral defects smaller than 6 cm without extensive soft tissue loss in patients who have not or will not receive radiotherapy.

QUALITY/VASCULARITY OF THE WOUND BED

Radiotherapy is another important consideration when selecting the type of osseous reconstruction. Nonvascular grafts demonstrate higher failure rates in an irradiated wound bed.[49] Regional muscle flaps have been proposed to provide a vascular wound bed to support nonvascular bone grafting and to help prevent MRP extrusion[21,23,52] in patients with extensive tissue loss or requiring radiotherapy. Although regional muscle flaps represented an important advance in mandibular reconstruction to improve the success of nonvascular grafts prior to predictable free tissue transfer techniques, they do not represent the state of the art of current techniques. Regional muscle transfer results in an unsightly bulge in the neck because of the

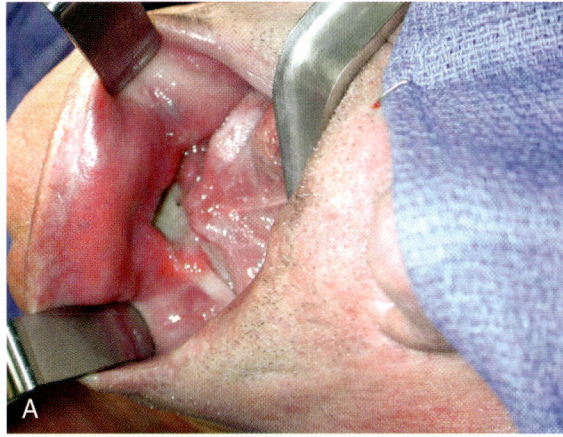

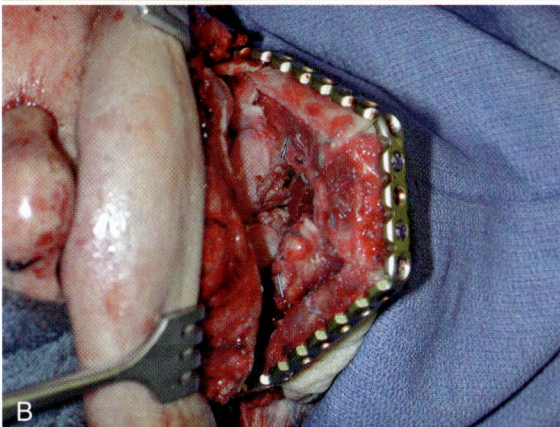

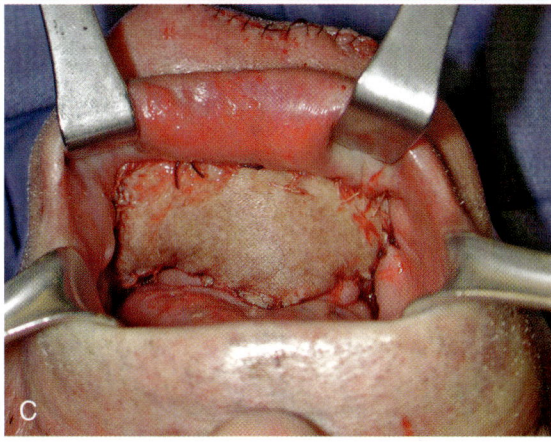

Fig. 60-6 ▪ **A,** Ameloblastic carcinoma of anterior mandible with involvement of oral mucosa. **B,** Vascularized fibula flap for immediate reconstruction of anterior mandibular segmental defect. **C,** Soft tissue component of osteocutaneous fibula flap provides vascularized soft tissue for intraoral lining reconstruction.

requirement of maintaining its vascular pedicle, which is objectionable to most patients. Furthermore, extrusion rates of MRPs have been shown to remain high despite the use of regional musculocutaneous flaps or soft tissue free flaps, especially in the anterior region.[23,28] If regional muscle transfer is performed prior to radiotherapy, the wound bed is subject to the same hypovascular effects of radiation. This leads to potential graft failure in two ways. First and most obvious is the risk for graft failure, or resorption in the hypovascular wound bed resulting in inadequate volume of the graft. Second, wound healing complications are increased in the radiated wound, which can lead to wound dehiscence and graft exposure with

subsequent failure.[50] Vascularized bone grafts in contrast have been shown to have high success rates in all regions of the mandible, tolerate radiotherapy, have the potential to proceed to a healed wound following exposure, and lead to fewer secondary procedures.

SPECIFIC TREATMENT AND TECHNIQUES

Nonvascularized Bone Grafts

The ilium represents the most common site for harvest of cancellous and corticocancellous tissue for nonvascular bone grafting of segmental mandibular defects. Although other sites are available for nonvascular bone graft harvest, they do not provide sufficient graft volume for most segmental defects. Two approaches for iliac crest bone graft (ICBG) harvest are available depending on the volume of graft needed for reconstruction: the anterior approach and the posterior approach.

The anterior approach may provide up to 50 cc of bone material and has the advantage of being obtained from the supine position. Both cortical and cancellous material may be harvested. The graft may be harvested from either the lateral or the medial aspect of the anterior ilium. The anteromedial approach has the advantage of avoiding the stripping of the gluteus medius, minimus, and tensor fascia lata muscles from their attachments to the iliac crest. This tends to result in less gait disturbance than the anterolateral approach,[53] which requires elevation of the iliacus muscle from the medial cortex of the ilium. The posterior approach requires the patient to be positioned prone, essentially precluding simultaneous harvest, and requires a position change during surgery. It can provide up to 90 cc of graft material and is therefore useful for larger defects. Marx and Morales have also suggested that the posterior approach results in less postoperative gait disturbance compared to the anterolateral approach.[54]

TECHNIQUE FOR ILIAC CREST BONE GRAFT HARVEST

Anterior Approach

The anatomic landmarks (Fig. 60-7, *A*) for the anterior approach include the iliac crest and the anterior superior iliac spine (ASIS). A knowledge of the regional (lateral cutaneous branch of subcostal nerve (T12), lateral cutaneous branch of iliohypogastric nerve, and lateral femoral cutaneous nerve) sensory nerves and their relation to the ASIS help to prevent their inadvertent injury. The patient is placed in the supine position and a hip roll is placed on the ipsilateral side during patient positioning to improve access to the area. The anterolateral hip region is prepared and draped sterilely with subsequent placement of an iodine adhesive dressing. The landmarks are placed on the superficial surface with a surgical marker. The location of the incision is approximately 2 cm posterior to the ASIS and 2 cm below the iliac crest. The proposed incision site is infiltrated with several milliliters of local anesthetic with epinephrine for hemostasis. Incision is performed with a 10-blade scalpel, and subcutaneous dissection is continued through the superficial fascia to the level of the investing fascia of the external oblique and tensor fascia lata/gluteus medius muscles. At the iliac crest, these fascia structures form a white tendinous attachment that is devoid of muscle. The fascia and periosteum is divided at this location to minimize injury to the muscles. In growing children, preservation of the cartilaginous cap of the iliac crest is important for potential growth considerations. In this situation, the fascial/periosteal incision may be moved slightly superiorly to include a very small cuff of external oblique

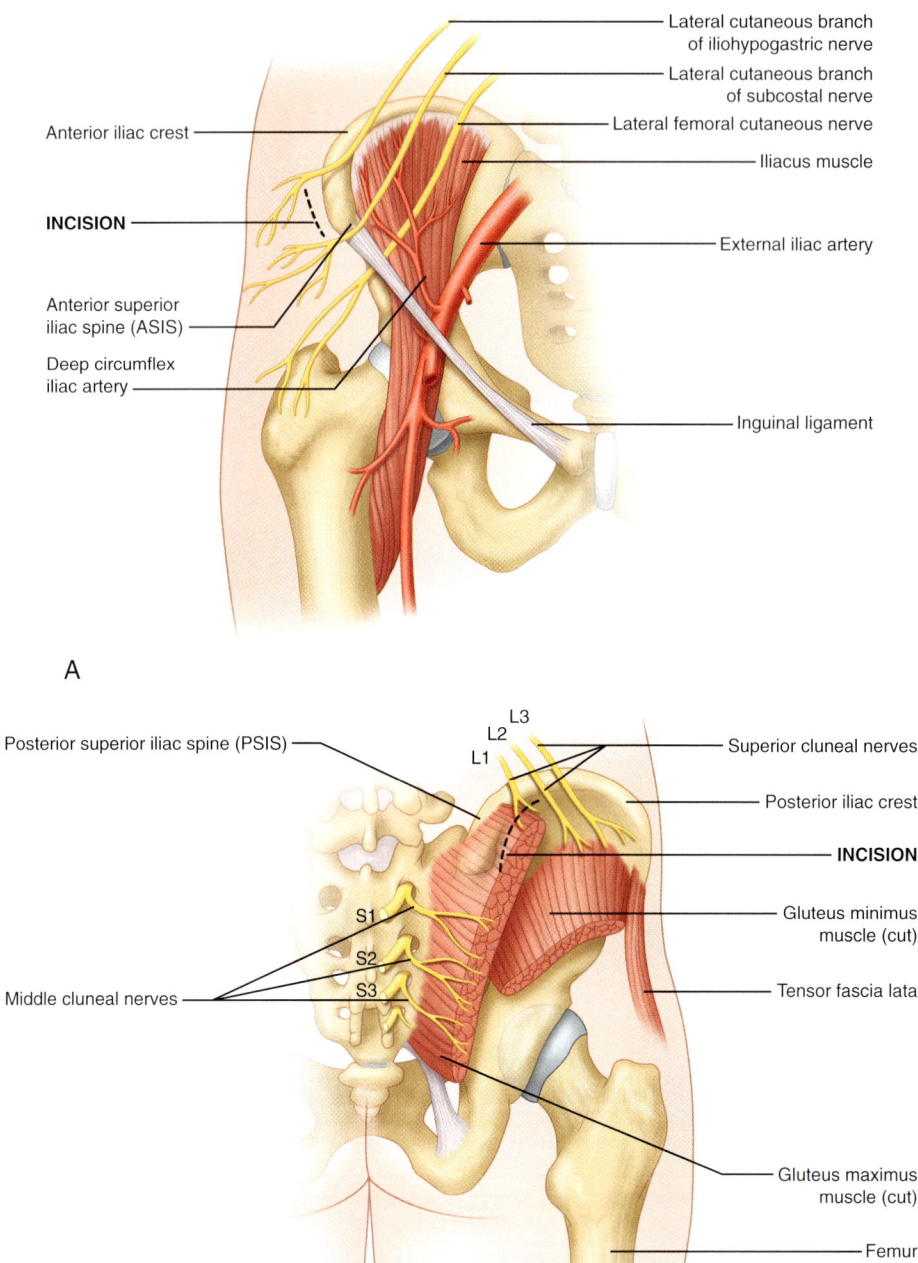

A

B

Fig. 60-7 ■ Regional anatomy for iliac crest bone graft harvest. **A,** Anterior ilium. **B,** Posterior ilium. (From Bagheri SC, Jo C: *Clinical review of oral and maxillofacial surgery*, St. Louis, Mo., 2008, Mosby.)

muscle and to leave the cartilaginous cap undisturbed. The skin and subcutaneous tissues may be retracted anteriorly and posteriorly to allow a greater length of incision in the periosteal layer than in the skin. This can significantly improve surgical access with a smaller skin incision. Sharp dissection or use of monopolar cautery can facilitate the release of the attachment over the iliac crest. Careful subperiosteal dissection proceeds widely over the medial or lateral cortex depending on the clinical situation. Wide elevation of the periosteum facilitates surgical access. The author prefers a medial approach to minimize gait disturbance. Following medial dissection, a Taylor retractor is placed to facilitate retraction of the iliacus muscle and visualization of the medial cortex. A determination of

the required graft volume is marked on the medial cortex. Osteotomies of the medial cortex (monocortical) and iliac crest (partial thickness) are completed with a reciprocating saw and straight osteotomes. If a cortical graft is to be harvested, the inferior osteotomy is completed with curved osteotomes. If a cortical graft is not required, a cortical window is created by way of a greenstick fracture at the inferior extent of the harvest site. Under direct visualization, the medial cortex is carefully elevated with straight osteotomes and placed in storage media (blood aspirated from the wound) on the back table or retracted medially if being preserved. Cancellous bone is then harvested with bone gouges and curettes and similarly stored on the back table. The wound is irrigated with copious sterile saline. Hemostasis is assured with cautery, judicious use of bone wax, or hemostatic dressings (Gelfoam) as needed. If a cortical window was performed, the medial cortex is compressed back into place. The wound is then closed in layers with reconstruction of the periosteal, superficial fascial, dermal, and epidermal layers. Suction drains are usually not necessary.

Posterior Approach

The anatomic landmarks (Fig. 60-7, *B*) for the posterior approach include the spinous processes and the posterior superior iliac crest. The regional nerves of importance include the superior and middle cluneal nerves (L1-S3). The patient is placed in the prone position with slight flexion and a hip roll is placed. The posterolateral hip region is prepared and draped sterilely with subsequent placement of an iodine adhesive dressing. The landmarks are marked on the superficial surface with a surgical marker. The incision is located overlying the posterior iliac crest. The proposed incision site is infiltrated with several milliliters of local anesthetic with epinephrine for hemostasis. Incision is performed with a 10-blade scalpel, and subcutaneous dissection is continued through the superficial fascia and fibroadipose tissue to the level of the investing fascia of the external oblique/paraspinous muscles and tensor fascia lata/gluteus maximus muscles. The white tendinous insertion is identified and the fascia and periosteum are incised in this location to avoid dividing muscle fibers. Subperiosteal dissection is performed widely, being careful to avoid the sacroiliac ligament. Bone is harvested similar to the anterior approach. The wound is irrigated, hemostasis assured, and closed in a layered fashion as previously described.

TECHNIQUE FOR GRAFTING SEGMENTAL DEFECTS

Reconstruction of the segmental defect is performed in a delayed fashion and utilizing a "two-team approach" when possible. One team prepares the recipient site while the other harvests the graft material. This is obviously not possible with posterior iliac crest harvest techniques. The mandible is approached via an extraoral, submandibular incision located in a prominent skin crease. The incision proceeds through the skin, subcutaneous tissue, and platysma musculature. The flap is then elevated in the subplatysmal plane. The superficial layer of the deep cervical fascia is incised horizontally, allowing elevation of a fascial flap to protect the marginal mandibular branch of the facial nerve, and blunt dissection proceeds toward the inferior border of the mandible. The marginal mandibular branch of the facial nerve travels deep to the platysma and superficial to the facial vein. It may be located up to 2 cm below the inferior border of the mandible posterior to the anterior border of the masseter. Anterior to this point, the nerve is found superior to the inferior border. Care must be taken to protect the marginal branch to prevent paresis of the lower lip depressors. The periosteum is incised along the inferior border of the proximal and distal mandibular segments, allowing elevation of the periosteum and exposure of the mandibular remnants. Scar tissue is excised deep to the mandibular reconstruction plate with extreme caution to protect the integrity of the oral mucosa (Fig. 60-8, *A*).

The graft material is prepared for implantation. If cortical bone has been harvested, it may be cut into particulate matter with rongeurs or double-action scissors. The cancellous bone is likewise cut into smaller particles with scissors. The graft material may now be compacted into 10-cc syringes to increase its cellular density. The graft material is then carefully transferred to the recipient site. Several options are available to assist with shaping a neo-mandible

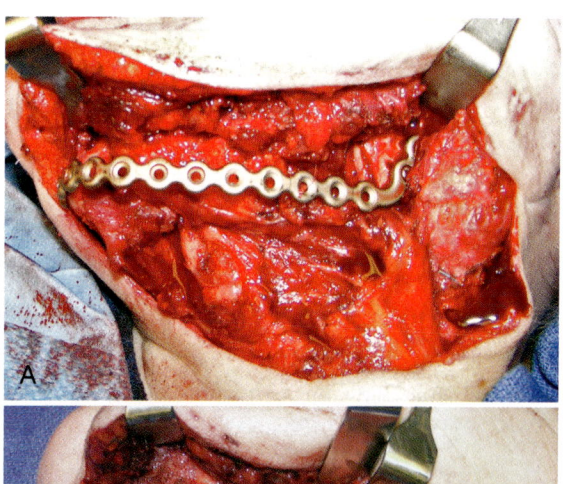

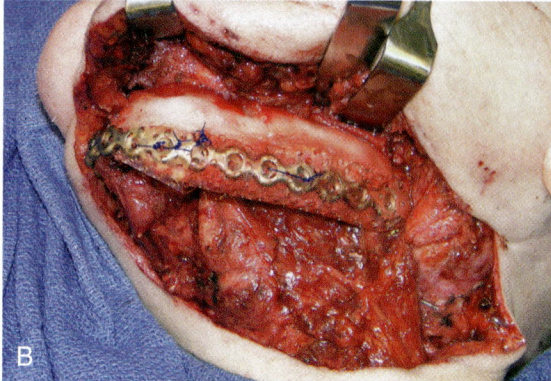

Fig. 60-8 ■ A, Lateral mandibular segmental defect with MRP exposed and healthy wound bed. **B,** Resorbable mesh crib placed and filled with corticocancellous graft material for delayed reconstruction of defect.

with the graft material. Cadaveric mandibular cribs, biodegradable mesh cribs, or cancellous blocks may be placed into the defect and secured to the reconstruction plate (Fig. 60-8, *B*). These assist in condensing and confining the graft material to the defect site and are especially helpful for larger defects. Layered closure of the periosteum (if possible), platysma, dermis, and epidermis is then performed over closed suction drains.

PECTORALIS MAJOR MYOCUTANEOUS FLAP

Pectoralis muscle flaps are planned on the ipsilateral chest wall (Fig. 60-9, *A*). The pectoralis major is a type V muscle having a dominant pedicle (pectoral branch of the thoracoacromial artery) and several minor pedicles (perforators of the internal mammary and intercostal arteries). Regional transfer for mandibular reconstruction is based on its dominant pedicle. The origin of the pedicle emerges from under the clavicle near its midpoint. The cutaneous territory of the pectoralis major is located between the parasternal line and anterior axillary line and extends from the clavicle to the sixth intercostal space. The skin paddle is designed along the sternal or costal border depending on the size and location of the defect. The most consistent perforators are located within 3 to 4 cm of midline. Reach of the flap should be confirmed prior to incision utilizing a suture held with forceps at the location of the pedicle and extending to the distal extent of the skin paddle, which is then transposed to the farthest point of the defect simulating the arc of rotation. This helps to prevent inadequate reach and excessive tension of the flap.

Standard landmarks for the pectoralis flap are the clavicle superiorly, sternum medially, and the anterior axillary fold laterally. The skin paddle is incised with a 10-blade scalpel. The subcutaneous dissection should bevel away from the skin paddle to maximize

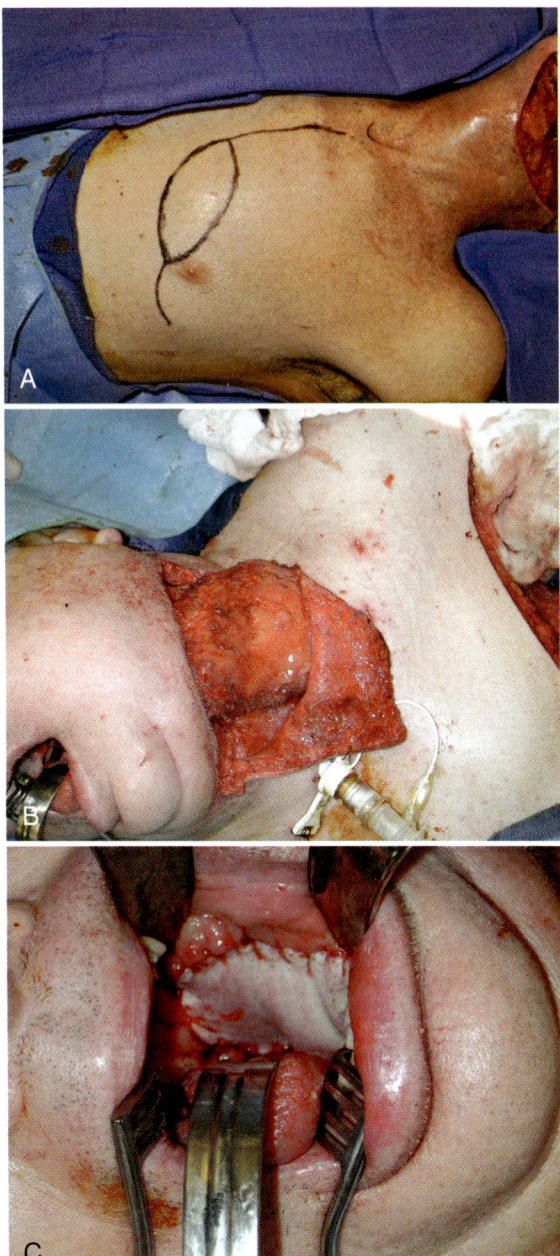

Fig. 60-9 ■ **A,** Designing pectoralis major myocutaneous flap for mandible reconstruction. **B,** Pectoralis muscle transposed through subcutaneous tunnel for head and neck reconstruction. **C,** Pectoralis muscle inset into oral cavity.

upper chest for transposition of the flap (Fig. 60-9, *B*). Care is taken to ensure a wide berth for compression free passage of the flap. The flap is transposed through the tunnel and inset (Fig. 60-9, *C*). The donor site is closed in layers over closed suction drains.

VASCULARIZED BONE FLAPS

Several vascularized bone flaps have been reported for mandibular reconstruction, including the radial forearm osteocutaneous flap, scapular osteocutaneous flap, fibular osteocutaneous flap, and the deep circumflex iliac artery osteocutaneous flap (iliac crest). In the author's opinion, the radial forearm flap has inadequate bone stock in most patients for reconstruction of the mandible; positioning requirements for the scapular flap generally preclude harvest in a simultaneous two-team approach significantly extending the length of surgery, and these flaps therefore have limited application for mandibular reconstruction. The deep circumflex iliac artery (DCIA), although providing excellent bone stock, creates significant donor site morbidity and may have excessive soft tissue thickness for intraoral reconstruction in the obese population. The fibula provides adequate bone stock for total mandibular reconstruction, may include one or two skin paddles for simultaneous intraoral and extraoral soft tissue reconstruction, and is the author's preference for most mandibular reconstructions when not contraindicated.

Reconstruction of the mandible with vascularized bone flaps is facilitated by using a two-team approach to minimize operating time. The ablative team performs the mandibular resection and neck dissection if indicated, while the microvascular team harvests and prepares the bone flap for transfer. Stabilization of the remaining proximal and distal mandibular bone segments with a mandibular reconstruction plate may be performed by either team; however, it should be coordinated so that the shape and position of the plate coincides with the reconstructive plan if placed by the ablative team, and appropriate means are available to reestablish correct jaw relations if placed by the microvascular team after creation of the continuity defect. Several techniques are available for reestablishing correct jaw relations: the plate may be bent in situ and holes predrilled (when oncologically feasible), the plate may be prebent based on stereolithographic models, or the jaws may be wired into maxillomandibular fixation and the plate adapted to the proximal and distal segments. The reconstruction plate is then secured ideally with a minimum three bicortical fixation screws in each segment. The bone flap is then fashioned to fill the segmental defect utilizing closing wedge osteotomies to create necessary contours and to ensure intimate approximation to the native mandibular segments. The skin paddle is inset as appropriate and the microvascular anastomoses are completed.

DEEP CIRCUMFLEX ILIAC ARTERY COMPOSITE FLAP (DCIA)

The DCIA composite flap consists of the anterior iliac crest extending posteriorly from the ASIS and includes the overlying skin and optionally the internal oblique muscle. The dominant pedicle is the deep circumflex iliac artery arising from the external iliac artery. It courses laterally from its origin following the curvature of the iliac crest. Standard landmarks for elevation of the flap are the ASIS, pubic tubercle, and the iliac crest. The skin territory is located over the anterior iliac crest, extending from the ASIS to the posterior axillary line. A skin paddle approximately 12 × 6 cm and a bone segment 8 × 18 cm may be harvested.

The patient is positioned in the supine position, and the ipsilateral buttock is elevated slightly with placement of a beanbag or hip roll to facilitate flap dissection. The anterolateral hip region is prepared

blood supply. Elevation of the flap is usually possible through the incision of the skin paddle with or without extension of the incision. The anterior skin flap is elevated off the pectoralis major muscle. The lateral border of the muscle is identified and the subpectoral plane is entered. Monopolar cautery is utilized to release the muscle attachment along the inferior costal and sternal margins. Large medial perforators should be divided and ligated to prevent untoward bleeding. The muscle is mobilized proximally toward the vascular pedicle. The pedicle is visualized on the deep surface of the muscle at the junction of the lateral and middle thirds of the clavicle. The humeral attachment is carefully divided lateral to the pedicle location. Complete release of all attachments should extend up to the clavicle to maximize the arc of rotation. A tunnel is then created in the subcutaneous plane from the neck wound onto the

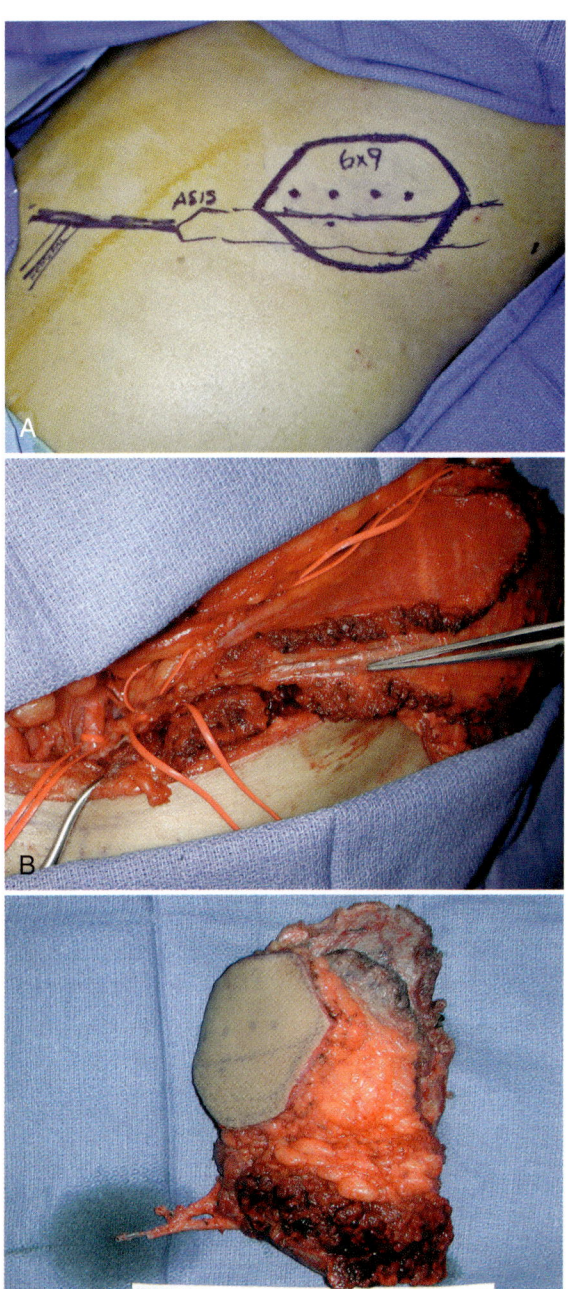

Fig. 60-10 ■ **A**, Landmarks for elevation of DCIA composite flap. **B**, DCIA pedicle. **C**, DCIA osteomyocutaneous flap. Note bulk of soft tissue possible with this flap.

The internal oblique and transversus abdominis muscle are divided following the course of the DCIA to the ASIS. The skin paddle is then elevated to within 3 to 4 cm of the iliac crest and the EO, internal oblique (IO), and transversus abdominis muscles are incised resulting in a 2 to 3 cm cuff of muscle included with the flap. Alternatively a wider cuff of internal oblique muscle may be included for intraoral lining when the skin paddle is needed for extraoral reconstruction. At the level of the ASIS, the ascending branch of the DCIA is identified and divided. Dissection proceeds laterally along the course of the pedicle as it travels along the iliac crest to the planned posterior extent of the flap (Fig. 60-10, *B*). The vascular pedicle is divided and ligated at the distal extent of the flap. The iliac fascia and iliacus muscle are then divided inferior to the vascular pedicle, allowing visualization of the periosteum of the ilium. The posterolateral skin incision is completed and subcutaneous dissection proceeds to the investing fascia of the gluteus medius and tensor fascia lata (TFL). These muscles are then divided from their origin along the iliac crest. Periosteal elevators are utilized to dissect the gluteus medius and TFL from the lateral cortex of the ilium. Medial retraction of the peritoneal contents is performed, and a reciprocating saw is then utilized to perform the osteotomies at the desired locations and complete elevation of the flap. The ASIS should be preserved when possible. When ready for transfer, the DCIA pedicle is divided and ligated at its origin from the external iliac system and the artery is flushed with heparinized saline. The flap is taken to the recipient site and inset prior to microvascular anastomosis.

Proper closure of the donor site is critical to avoid abdominal wall hernia. The wound is irrigated with copious sterile saline and hemostasis is assured. Closed suction drains are placed. The iliacus muscle and fascia are sutured to the transversalis muscle and fascia. The IO and EO muscles are then sutured to the gluteus medius and TFL muscles. The inguinal ligament is repaired. The author prefers to reinforce the abdominal wall repair with a Prolene mesh onlay secured under tension with nonresorbable suture. The superficial fascia, dermis, and epidermis are then repaired in a layered fashion.

FIBULA FLAP

The fibula flap may be elevated as an osteocutaneous or osseous-only flap. The dominant pedicle is the peroneal artery and vein, which travel along the medial aspect of the fibula. Standard landmarks for elevation of the fibula flap are the fibula head, lateral malleolus, and posterolateral intermuscular septum. The skin territory is centered over the posterolateral intermuscular septum and extends from approximately 6 cm below the proximal end of the fibula to approximately 8 cm from its distal end. Separate skin paddles may be elevated within the skin territory based on identified perforators to facilitate the simultaneous reconstruction of extensive soft tissue defects (Fig. 60-11). The osseous component extends from a point 4 cm below the proximal end of the fibula to a point 6 cm proximal to the lateral malleolus. A segment of bone measuring up to 40 cm (depending on patient height) may be harvested in the adult patient.

The patient is positioned in the supine position and the lower extremity is circumferentially prepped and draped sterilely. To facilitate dissection, the leg should be elevated on a stack of towels to allow the tissues to fall away from the fibula, and the leg (knee) should be able to be placed in a flexed position or internally rotated as needed. The posterolateral septum is visualized by placing lateral pressure on the posterior compartment muscles. A Doppler ultrasound is utilized to identify septocutaneous perforators at the junction of the middle and distal thirds of the leg. A skin paddle corresponding to the soft tissue needs is then designed about these

and draped sterilely. The skin paddle is designed according to the anticipated soft tissue defect (Fig. 60-10, *A*). The skin incision is made along the anteromedial border of the skin island with a 10-blade scalpel and continued through the subcutaneous tissue beveling away to the level of the external oblique (EO) aponeurosis. A linear extension of the incision is performed from the anterior tip of the skin paddle over the location of the inguinal ligament. The EO muscle is split just superior and parallel to the inguinal ligament up to the ASIS. The lateral cutaneous nerve is identified and protected just proximal to the ASIS. Medial retraction of the spermatic cord allows identification of the external iliac artery and vein. The DCIA emerges from the lateral aspect of the external iliac artery. The DCIA vessels are carefully dissected along their course laterally.

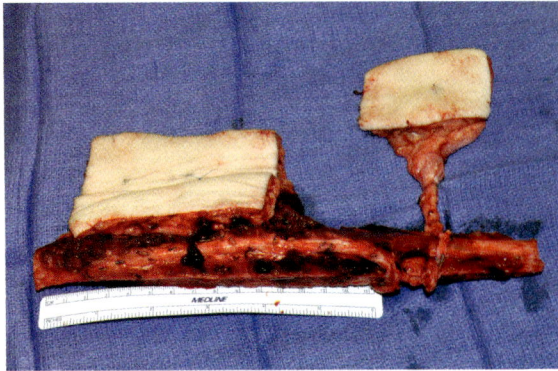

Fig. 60-11 ■ Multiple soft tissue paddles based on perforator anatomy may be harvested with fibula flap when needed for extensive soft tissue defects.

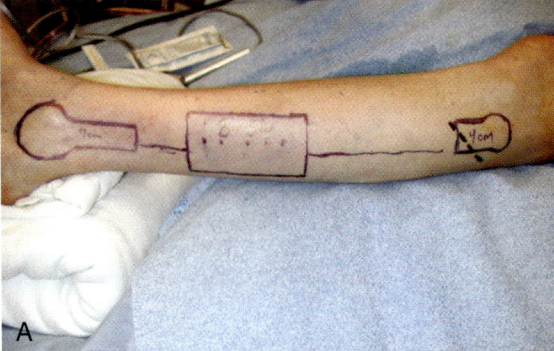

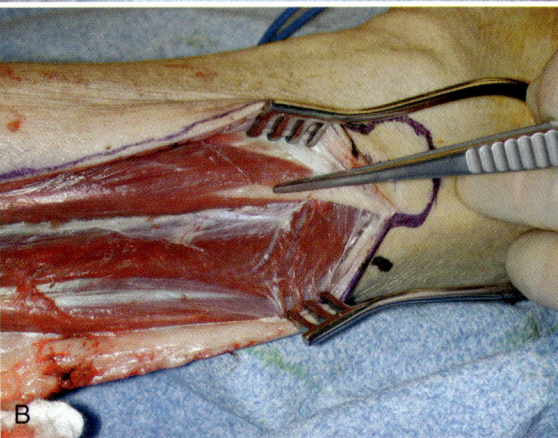

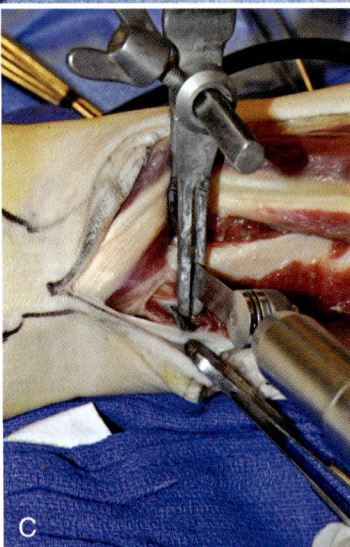

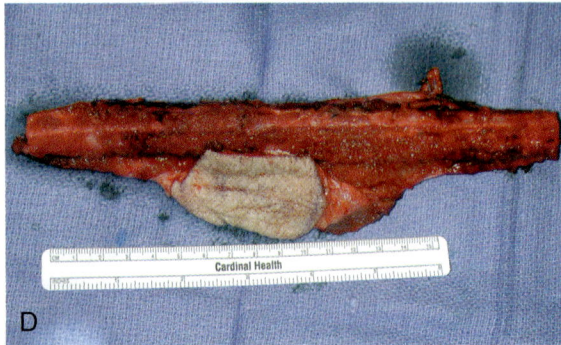

Fig. 60-12 ■ Harvest of fibula flap. **A,** Skin markings. **B,** Identification of deep peroneal nerve. **C,** Completion of osteotomies. **D,** Harvested flap.

perforators, centered over the septum (Fig. 60-12, *A*). The extremity is exsanguinated with an Esmarch dressing and tourniquet inflated. Incision around the skin paddle and along the access incision is performed with a 10-blade scalpel. Subcutaneous dissection continues to the investing fascia of the leg. The fascia along the anterior edge of the skin paddle is incised and carefully elevated with blunt finger dissection to the level of the intermuscular septum. Septocutaneous perforators are identified, marked, and protected. The peroneus longus and brevis are then elevated from the lateral aspect of the fibula with sharp scissor dissection. The deep peroneal nerve is identified as it crosses just below the head of the fibula and is protected throughout the dissection (Fig. 60-12, *B*). The extensor digitorum longus and extensor hallucis longus are then released along the anterior edge of the fibula revealing the interosseous septum. Proximal and distal osteotomies are now performed, taking care to protect the underlying vascular pedicle, especially at the proximal site (Fig. 60-12, *C*). Osteotomies are performed at locations 4 cm distal to the fibula head and at least 6 cm proximal to the lateral malleolus to maintain ligamentous integrity at these attachments. After completion of the osteotomies, the peroneal artery and vena comitantes are divided and ligated at the distal osteotomy, the interosseous membrane is released with scissors, and the fibula is now free to roll laterally facilitating dissection of the pedicle. The tibialis posterior is divided along its attachment, exposing the peroneal artery and vena comitantes. The posterior skin paddle is carefully elevated to the septum. Musculocutaneous perforators may be identified and preserved at this point. A narrow cuff of soleus and flexor hallucis longus muscles may be included to protect these perforators adjacent to the skin paddle. Dissection of the pedicle is now completed in a distal to proximal direction. Care is taken to identify the posterior tibial neurovascular bundle as the dissection proceeds proximally. The tourniquet is released, hemostasis achieved, and the flap allowed to reperfuse while the recipient site is readied for tissue transfer.

The flap is harvested with division and ligation of the peroneal artery and vena comitantes distal to their takeoff from the tibioperoneal trunk (Fig. 60-12, *D*). The flap is flushed with heparinized saline. Templates are utilized to determine the length of bone segments. Proximally, the pedicle is carefully dissected from the fibula in the subperiosteal plane to the level of the proximal osteotomy. Similar dissection is performed distally. Osteotomies are performed with sagittal or reciprocating saws and the unneeded bone is discarded. If multiple bone segments are required, closing wedge osteotomies are performed (see Fig. 60-3). In the location of the wedge osteotomies, limited subperiosteal dissection is performed only over the bone to be discarded, the pedicle is carefully retracted for protection, and the osteotomies completed. The flap is then inset into the segmental defect and secured to the reconstruction plate with two screws per segment. Soft tissue inset is completed prior to microsurgery when feasible.

Closure of the donor site is performed in a layered fashion over closed suction drains. Skin paddle defects wider than 6 cm generally require skin grafting. When performing primary closure, careful attention must be given to the wound tension to prevent a compartment syndrome. When in doubt, perform a skin graft.

POSTOPERATIVE CARE

Postoperative care is catered to each patient individually. Free flap patients are frequently admitted to the intensive care unit postoperatively for flap monitoring and supportive care; however, nonmicrovascular reconstructions are evaluated on a case-by-case basis for care in the intensive care unit. In one study, postoperative medical morbidities occurred in approximately 40% of patients over age 70 undergoing complex reconstructive surgery.[55] All patients undergoing head and neck reconstruction should have a thorough evaluation for postoperative upper airway edema and every effort made to provide a secure airway. Postoperative endotracheal intubation or tracheotomy may be necessary. Careful and frequent assessment of the patient's cardiovascular status is important to ensure adequate volume status and perfusion of vital organs and tissue transfers. Free flap monitoring is performed hourly the first 48 to 72 hours. Most free flap failures secondary to anastomotic thrombosis occur in the first 24 to 36 hours. No single technique for flap monitoring is considered the single most accurate. The flaps should be monitored for failure of the arterial and venous systems. Doppler ultrasound is an effective method for monitoring arterial (and sometimes venous)

flow within larger vessels within the flap. Color monitoring provides an effective means for assessing venous obstruction and the microcirculation. Capillary refill should be visible in adequately perfused flaps, and any evidence of venous congestion should prompt a more thorough assessment of anastomotic patency. Patients are monitored closely for evidence of infection or wound healing issues.

PEARLS AND PITFALLS

- Nonvascular bone grafts are ideally reserved for lateral and posterior defects smaller than 6 cm.
- Nonvascular bone grafts should be placed in a delayed fashion with techniques to maximize cellular density of grafts.
- Soft tissue flaps (free or pedicled) can be utilized to support nonvascular bone grafts when necessary in poor quality wound beds.
- The fibula is arguably the most useful vascularized bone flap for mandibular reconstruction.
- Preoperative vascular studies should be performed when abnormal pulses are identified on physical examination of the legs.
- The distal 6 to 8 cm of the fibula should not be harvested to prevent instability of the ankle
- The deep peroneal nerve must be identified proximally and protected to prevent injury.
- The DCIA composite flap provides excellent bone stock but the soft tissue component can be bulky.
- Meticulous layered closure, reinforced with alloplastic mesh, is essential to prevent abdominal wall hernia.
- Nonvascular bone grafts and vascular bone flaps will both support osteointegrated implants when adequate bone volume is transferred.

REFERENCES

1. Urken ML, Weinberg H, Vickery C, et al: Oromandibular reconstruction using microvascular composite free flaps, *Arch Otolaryngol Head Neck Surg* 117:733, 1991.
2. Arden RL: Volume-length impact of lateral jaw resections on complication rates, *Arch Otolaryn* 125:68, 1990.
3. Hirsch DL, Garfein ES, Christensen AM, et al: Use of computer-aided design and computer-aided manufacturing to produce orthognathically ideal surgical outcomes: a paradigm shift in head and neck reconstruction, *J Oral Maxillofac Surg* 67(10):2115-2122, 2009.
4. Bell RB, Weimer KA, Dierks EJ, et al: Computer planning and intraoperative navigation for palato-maxillary and mandibular reconstruction with fibular free flaps, *J Oral Maxillofac Surg* 69(3):724-732, 2011.
5. Garfein E, Hirsch D, Levine J: *CAD-CAM Mandible reconstruction: decreased operative time, increased accuracy.* Presented at the American Society of Reconstructive Microsurgeons Annual Meeting, 2010.
6. Potter JK, Osborn, TM: Preparation of the neck for microsurgical reconstruction of the head and neck, *Oral Maxillofacial Surg Clin N Am* 20:521-526, 2008.
7. Kim D, Orron D, Skillman JJ: Surgical significance of popliteal arterial variants: a

unified angiographic classification, *Ann Surg* 210(6):776, 1989.
8. Lutz BS, Wei FC, Ng SH, et al: Routine donor leg angiography before vascularized free fibula transplantation is not necessary: a prospective study in 120 clinical cases, *Plas Recon Surg* 103(1):121-127, 1999.
9. Schusterman MA, Harris SW, Raymond AK, Goepfert H: Immediate free flap mandibular reconstruction: significance of adequate surgical margins, *Head Neck* 15:204, 1993.
10. Lawson W, Loscalzo LJ, Baek SM, et al: Experience with immediate and delayed mandibular reconstruction, *Laryngoscope* 92:5, 1982.
11. Marx RE, Ames JR: The use of hyperbaric oxygen therapy in bony reconstruction of the irradiated and tissue deficient patient, *J Oral Maxillofac Surg* 40:410, 1982.
12. Marx RE: Mandibular reconstruction, *J Oral Maxillofac Surg* 51:466, 1993.
13. Carlson ER, Monteleone K: An analysis of inadvertent perforations of mucosa and skin concurrent with mandibular reconstruction, *J Oral Maxillofac Surg* 62:1103, 2004.
14. Cordeiro PG, Hidalgo DA: Conceptual considerations in mandibular reconstruction, *Clin Plast Surg* 22:61, 1995.

15. Baker A, McMahon J, Parmar S: Immediate reconstruction of continuity defects of the mandible after tumor surgery, *J Oral Maxillofac Surg* 59:1333, 2001.
16. Netscher DT, Meade RA, Goodman CM, et al: Quality of life and disease specific functional status following microvascular reconstruction for advanced (T3 and T4) oropharyngeal cancers, *Plast Reconstr Surg* 105:1628, 2000.
17. Weymuller EA, Yueh B, Deleyiannis FWB, et al: Quality of life in patients with head and neck cancer, *Arch Otolaryngol Head Neck Surg* 126:329, 2000.
18. Boyd JB, Mullholland RS, Davidson J, et al: The free flap and plate in oromandibular reconstruction: long-term review and indications, *Plast Reconstr Surg* 95:1018, 1995.
19. Schmoker RR: Mandibular reconstruction using a special plate: animal experiments and clinical application, *J Maxillofacial Surg* 11:99, 1983.
20. Kim MR, Donoff RB: Critical analysis of mandibular reconstruction using AO plates, *J Oral Maxillofac Surg* 50:1152, 1992.
21. Blackwell KE, Buchbinder D, Urken ML: Lateral mandibular reconstruction using soft tissue free flaps and plates, *Arch Otolaryngol Head Neck Surg* 122:672, 1996.

22. Ueyama Y, Naitoh R, Yamagata A, Matsumura T: Analysis of reconstruction of mandibular defects using single stainless steel AO reconstruction plates, *J Oral Maxillofac Surg* 54:858, 1996.

23. Cordiero PG, Hidalgo DA: Soft tissue coverage of mandibular reconstruction plates, *Head Neck* 16:112, 1994.

24. Wei FC, Celik N, Yang WG, et al: Complications after reconstruction by plate and soft tissue free flap in composite mandibular defects and secondary salvage reconstruction with osteocutaneous flap, *Plast Reconstr Surg* 112:37, 2003.

25. Ryu JK, Stern RL, Robinson MG, et al: Mandibular reconstruction using a titanium plate: the impact of radiation therapy on plate preservation, *Int J Radiat Oncol Biol Phys* 32:627, 1995.

26. Raveh Y, Stich H, Sutter F, Greiner R: New concepts in the reconstruction of mandibular defects following tumor resection, *J Oral Maxillofac Surg* 41:3, 1983.

27. Yi Z, Jian GZ, Guang YY, et al: Reconstruction plates to bridge mandibular defects: a clinical and experimental investigation in biomechanical aspects, *Int J Oral Maxillofac Surg* 28:445, 1999.

28. Schusterman MA, Reece RP, Kroll SS, Weldon ME: Use of the AO plate for mandibular reconstruction in cancer patients, *Plas Recon Surg* 88:588-593, 1991.

29. Marx RE, Cillo JE, Broumand V, Ulloa JJ: outcome analysis of mandibular condylar replacements in tumor and trauma reconstruction: a prospective analysis of 131 cases with long-term follow-up, *J Oral Maxillofac Surg* 66(12):2515-2523, 2008.

30. Potter JK, Dierks EJ: Microvascular options for reconstruction of the mandibular condyle, *Semin Plast Surg* 22(3):156-160, 2008.

31. Marx RE: Current advances in reconstruction of the mandible in head and neck cancer surgery, *Semin Surg Oncol* 7(1):47-57, 1991.

32. Adamo AR, Szal RL: Timing, results and complications of mandibular reconstructive surgery, *J Oral Surg* 37:755, 1979.

33. Donoff RB, May JW: Microvascular mandibular reconstruction, *J Oral Maxillofac Surg* 40:122, 1982.

34. Tidstrom KD, Keller EE: Reconstruction of mandibular discontinuity with autogenous iliac bone grafting: report of 34 consecutive patients, *J Oral Maxillofac Surg* 48:336, 1990.

35. Mowlem R: Cancellous chip bone grafts: report of 75 cases, *Lancet* 2:746, 1944.

36. Blocker TG, Weiss LR: Use of cancellous bone in the repair of defects about the jaws, *Ann Surg* 123:622, 1946.

37. Obwegeser HL: Simultaneous resection and reconstruction of parts of the mandible via the intraoral route in patients with and without gross infections, *J Oral Surg* 21:703, 1966.

38. Boyne PJ, Zarem H: Osseous reconstruction of the resected mandible, *Am J Surg* 132:149, 1976.

39. Bromberg BE, Song NC, Craig GT: Split rib mandibular reconstruction, *Plast Reconstr Surg* 50:357, 1972.

40. Millard DR, Deane M, Garst W: Bending an iliac bone graft for anterior mandibular arch repair, *Plast Reconstr Surg* 48:600, 1972.

41. Brown RG, Vasconez LD, Jurkiewicz MJ: Reconstruction of the central mandible with a single block of iliac bone, *Br J Plast Surg* 29:191, 1976.

42. Adekeye EO: Reconstruction of mandibular defects by autogenous bone grafts: review of 37 cases, *J Oral Surg* 36:125, 1978.

43. Kudo K, Fujioka Y: Review of bone grafting for reconstruction of discontinuity defects of the mandible, *J Oral Surg* 36:791, 1978.

44. Weaver AW, Smith DB: Frozen autogenous mandibular stent-graft for immediate reconstruction in oral cancer surgery, *Am J Surg* 126:505, 1973.

45. Salyer KS, Newsom HT, Holmes R, et al: Mandibular reconstruction, *Am J Surg* 134:461, 1977.

46. Giordano A, Brady D, Foster C, et al: Particulate cancellous marrow crib graft reconstruction of mandibular defects, *Laryngoscope* 90:2027, 1980.

47. Margolis IB, Smith RL, Davis WC: Reconstruction of defects of the mandible, *Plas Reconstr Surg* 79:638, 1976.

48. Foster RD, Anthony JP, Sharma A, Pogrel MA: Vascularized bone flaps versus nonvascularized bone grafts for mandibular reconstruction: an outcome analysis of primary bony union and endosseous implant success, *Head Neck* 21:66, 1999.

49. Pogrel MA, Podlesh S, Anthony JP, Alexander JA: Comparison of vascularized and nonvascularized bone grafts for reconstruction of mandibular continuity defects, *J Oral Maxillofac Surg* 55:1200, 1997.

50. August M, Tompach P, Chang YC, Kaban LB: Factors influencing the long-term outcome of mandibular reconstruction, *J Oral Maxillofac Surg* 58:731, 2000.

51. Troulis MJ, Williams WB, Kaban LB: Staged protocol for resection skeletal reconstruction and oral rehabilitation of children with jaw tumors, *J Oral Maxillofac Surg* 62:335, 2004.

52. Mariani PB, Kowalski LP, Magrin J: Reconstruction of large defects postmandibulectomy for oral cancer using plates and myocutaneous flaps: a long term follow up, *Int J Oral Maxillofac Surg* 35:427-432, 2006.

53. Keller EE, Triplett WW: Iliac bone grafting: review of 160 consecutive cases, *J Oral Maxillofac Surg* 45:11-14, 1987.

54. Marx RE, Morales MJ: Morbidity from bone harvest in major jaw reconstruction: a randomized trial comparing the lateral anterior and posterior approaches to the ilium, *J Oral Maxillofac Surg* 48:196, 1988.

55. Howard MA, Cordiero PG, Disa J, et al: Free tissue transfer in the elderly: incidence of perioperative complications following microsurgical reconstruction of 197 septuagenarians and octogenarians, *Plas Reconstr Surg* 116(6):1659, 2005.

Chapter 61

Palato-Maxillary Reconstruction

Dimitrios Nikolarakos, Jason K. Potter

Maxillary defects are associated with a wide spectrum of deformities that may be as simple as an oral-antral fistula or as complex as a total maxillectomy. They can be some of the most technically challenging deformities to reconstruct because of the complicated three-dimensional anatomy of the region and the multitude of functions that are directly affected by loss of tissue in this region. Maxillary defects can also have a devastating effect on the patient's facial esthetics. Successful maxillary reconstruction is therefore accomplished through a goal-oriented approach that uses many different techniques that can be applied to each individual patient's situation.

ETIOPATHOGENESIS/CAUSATIVE FACTORS

Complex maxillary defects most commonly arise from ablative tumor surgery or avulsive, high-energy trauma. Over the last several decades, advances in the management and stabilization of critically injured patients, especially in the military setting, have resulted in patients surviving devastating wounds of the mid-face. Although survival rates of patients treated for oral mucosal carcinoma involving the maxilla have remained essentially unchanged during that time, our ability to diagnose and image the extent of and excise both benign and malignant tumors involving the maxilla and skull base has improved. Major advances and refinements in reconstructive surgical techniques now allow the expectation of reasonable return of form and certain functions in these patients and a quality of life that justifies the extent of surgery.[1]

PATHOLOGIC ANATOMY

The maxillary bones contribute significantly to the esthetics and critical functions of the mid-facial skeleton. They are anatomically related to the globe, sinonasal complex, dentoalveolar complex, and oral cavity. Resection of mid-facial structures (both soft and hard tissue) during ablative tumor surgery results in loss of mid-facial support of the lip, cheek, and periorbital soft tissue, which has an obvious impact on facial esthetics (Fig. 61-1). Furthermore, the loss of palatal competence, creation of oronasal and oroantral fistulas, and loss of dentoalveolar segments and bony support for the eye result in impairments in vision, breathing, speech, and deglutition. The culmination of these effects is a significant negative impact on the quality of life of patients if left unrestored.

CLASSIFICATION OF DEFECTS

A number of classifications have been proposed for maxillary defects. The one favored by the authors is that of Brown and colleagues.[2] It has been found to be useful in communicating the anticipated defect and for guiding treatment planning. The major determinant of class is the vertical extent of the defect from the alveolus. Subdivisions within each class delineate the horizontal extent of the defect (Fig. 61-2).

VERTICAL COMPONENT

Class 1—Maxillectomy with no oroantral fistula: removal of alveolar bone without resulting in an oronasal or oroantral fistula. Resections of the ethmoid and frontal sinus cavities or removal of the lateral nasal wall would fit into this part of the classification. Included in this group is the removal of only palatal bone, which will inevitably result in an oronasal fistula but leaves the dental-bearing portion of the maxilla intact.

Class 2—Low maxillectomy: the alveolus and antral walls are resected but not the orbital floor or rim.

Class 3—High maxillectomy, including resection of the floor of the orbit with or without the periorbita and with or without skull base resection.

Class 4—Radical maxillectomy plus orbital exenteration with or without resection of the anterior skull base.

HORIZONTAL COMPONENT

a. Unilateral resection of the alveolar maxilla and hard palate—resection of half or less of the alveolar bone and hard palate and not involving the nasal septum or crossing the midline

b. Bilateral resection of the alveolar maxilla and hard palate—includes a smaller resection that crosses the midline of the alveolar bone, including the nasal septum

c. Removal of the entire alveolar maxilla and hard palate

PREOPERATIVE ASSESSMENT AND DIAGNOSTIC STUDIES

From a reconstructive point of view, the preoperative assessment of a patient should include a thorough history, physical examination, and appropriate imaging with the aim of

- Identifying medical problems that would limit the patient's capacity to withstand the proposed operation
- Predicting the final configuration of the defect and resultant reconstructive requirements
- Identifying conditions that may have a negative impact on the outcome of the proposed reconstructive surgery

Medical conditions that will have an impact on the patient's general fitness for surgery are outside the scope of this chapter. Conditions that may directly affect reconstruction and must be elicited include but are not limited to peripheral vascular disease, diabetes mellitus, deep vein thrombosis, coagulopathies, immune deficiencies, previous surgery or radiotherapy, and traumatic injuries.

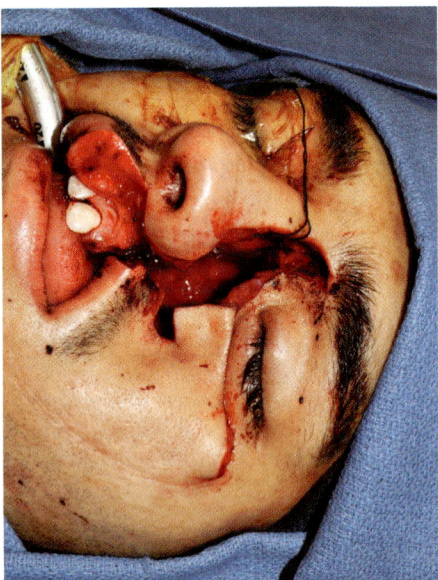

Fig. 61-1 ■ Note the loss of support for the globe, cheek, and nasal base following class III maxillectomy.

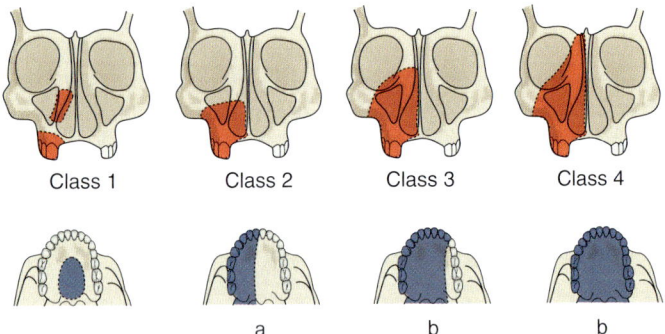

Class 1   Class 2   Class 3   Class 4

a   b   b

Fig. 61-2 ■ Classification of maxillary defects. (Redrawn from Brown JS, Jones DC, Summerwill A, et al: Vascularized iliac crest with internal oblique arter maxillectomy, *Br J Oral Maxillofac Surg* 40(3):183-190, 2002.)

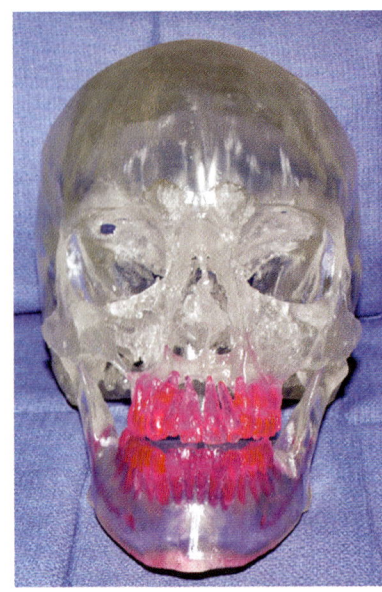

Fig. 61-3 ■ Stereolithographic model.

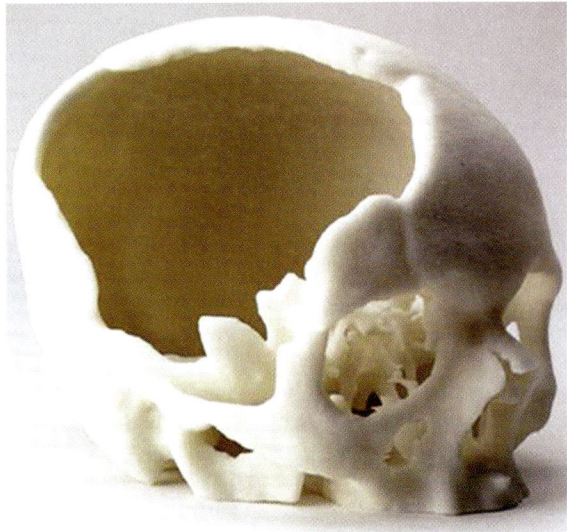

Fig. 61-4 ■ Three-dimensional printing model. (Courtesy Medical Modeling Inc., Golden, Colo.)

Diagnostic studies pertinent to maxillary reconstruction include preoperative imaging of the maxillofacial region, computer-generated models or surgical guides (tactile medical imaging), and preoperative vascular studies specific to the various reconstructive techniques.

Computed tomography (CT) of the mid-face is essential for establishing the anticipated ablative defect and the probable reconstructive requirements. Axial and coronal scans are the minimum recommended and may be combined with sagittal images or three-dimensional reconstructions, as needed, to further define the extent of tumor involvement. CT is ideal for defining bone involvement in the mid-facial skeleton, whereas magnetic resonance imaging (MRI) is useful for identifying soft tissue involvement, such as the orbital adnexa when CT demonstrates destruction of the orbital floor or medial orbital wall, or for differentiating soft tissue masses within the sinuses from inflammatory collections.

Tactile medical imaging is the display, in physical form, of anatomic data derived from imaging studies. Stereolithography and three-dimensional printing are the two main technologies for tactile medical models. Stereolithography involves laser photopolymerization of a liquid polymer to create an accurate, durable, translucent and sterilizable model of the patient's skeletal anatomy (Fig. 61-3),

whereas three-dimensional printing uses an ink jet–based printing method to create a skeletal model by injection of liquid into a plaster powder (Fig. 61-4). Three-dimensional printing models are accurate and opaque but are fragile and cannot be sterilized. Both these techniques allow hands-on study and surgical planning. Stereolithographic models can also be used intraoperatively to assist in pre-bending of surgical fixation systems and implants, model surgery, and shaping of bone grafts.

Current technology also allows preoperative virtual treatment planning and surgery. Surgical stents can be fashioned from these computer-based treatment plans to guide osteotomies and the placement of pre-bent fixation devices or implants (Fig. 61-5).[3] Intraoperative use of these guides has been shown to improve the accuracy of the resultant osteotomies and decrease operative time.[4]

Preoperative physical examination is critical for identifying impediments to microvascular surgery in the neck and for determining the suitability of the soft and hard tissues of potential free tissue

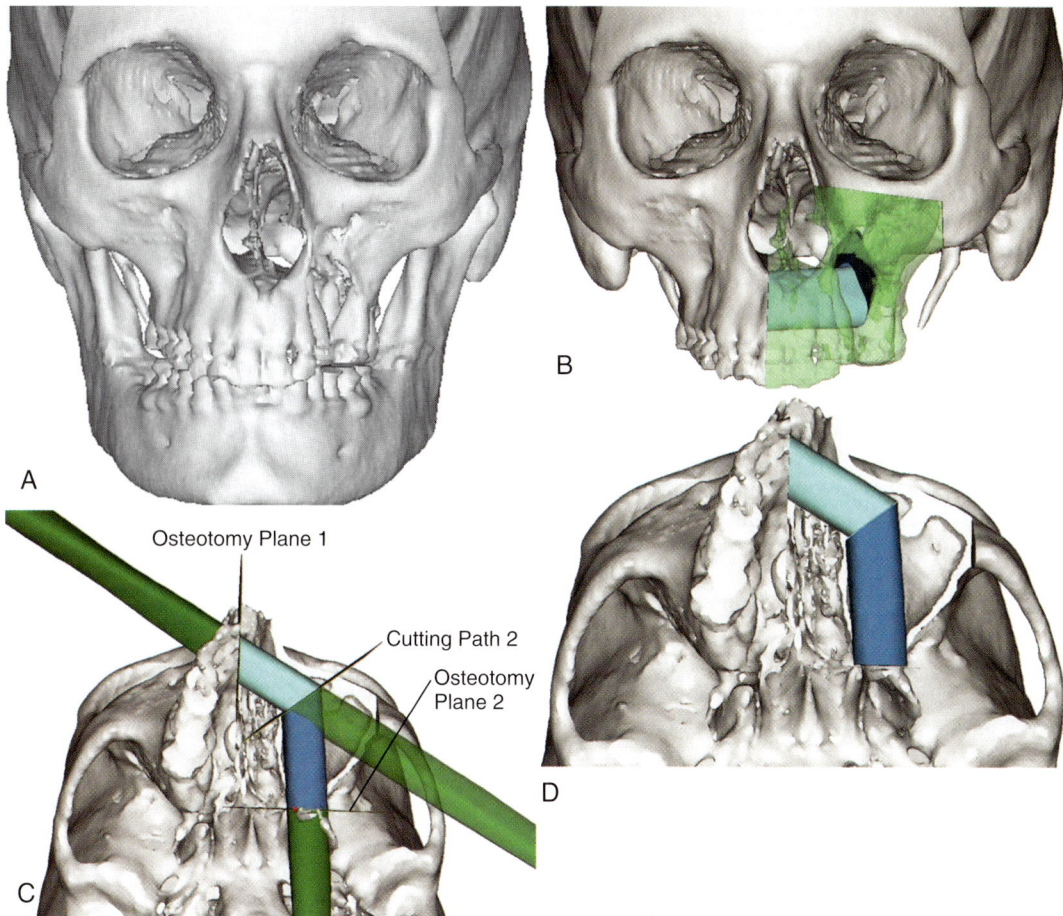

Fig. 61-5 ■ Virtual surgical treatment planning for hemimaxillectomy and immediate reconstruction with an osteocutaneous fibula flap. **A,** Three-dimensional preoperative image. Note the destruction of bone in the left side of the maxilla. **B,** Planned hemimaxillectomy. **C,** Planning fibula osteotomies. **D,** Final fibula orientation/reconstruction.

donor sites. Carefully selected vascular studies are necessary to identify the presence and quality of recipient or donor vessels.

Patients with head and neck cancer may have altered vascular anatomy, especially those with multiply operated necks. Physical examination and appropriately selected angiography of the head and neck (either CT or femoral) can help identify the presence or absence of arterial structures suitable for microsurgery. They can also confirm the status of the internal jugular vein. Patients with vessel-depleted necks may require vein grafting or the creation of a vascular loop from more distant vessels. This information is critical in planning treatment and preparing such patients and ultimately has an impact on the success of the reconstructive effort.[5]

Potential donor sites should be thoroughly examined with regard to the quality and quantity of hard and soft tissues. The skin surface may reveal evidence of underlying macrovascular or microvascular disease, such as ulceration, loss of hair, or sclerotic changes. Excessive subcutaneous fat may limit the suitability of certain donor sites. This is most often encountered in the abdominal wall when contemplating the rectus abdominis and deep circumflex iliac artery (DCIA)-based flaps and in the lateral aspect of the thigh when considering the anterolateral thigh (ALT) flap.

Estimation of the pedicle length required is critical because the maxilla is distant from most recipient vessels in the neck, which must be taken into account when selecting the free flap. Although published accounts of the average pedicle lengths that can be harvested for specific flaps are helpful, clinical evaluation of the patient is essential to avoid the added complexity that accompanies vein grafting.

Physical examination may also demonstrate surgical scars from previous surgery that may have disrupted the potential donor vessels. Examples include patients with lateral thoracotomy scars or low transverse abdominal scars who are being considered for latissimus dorsi or rectus abdominis transfer, respectively. Previous inguinal hernia repair or non-vascularized bone harvest from the iliac crest may result in alterations in the vascular territory usually supplied by the deep circumflex iliac artery.

The Allen test is the most useful clinical evaluation of the radial forearm donor site. The radial and ulnar arteries are simultaneously occluded with digital pressure while the patient opens and closes the fist to exsanguinate the palmar arch. The ulnar artery is then released and the palm examined for return of perfusion. The palm should become pink within 7 seconds, which confirms adequacy of the ulnar artery to perfuse the entire hand. Delays of more than 7 seconds should prompt testing of the contralateral hand or color flow Doppler ultrasound studies to map the vasculature of the hand.

Vascular studies can be helpful in confirming the patency of specific donor vessels, and these techniques are most commonly used in association with free fibular transfer. Two situations must be identified in patients being considered for fibula flaps:

1. The presence of significant atherosclerotic disease involving the anterior and posterior tibial arteries, which would result in compromised vascularity of the foot following harvest of the peroneal artery
2. The presence of a dominant peroneal artery (peroneus magnus), a condition associated with congenital hypoplasia or aplasia of the tibialis posterior or anterior

Both these conditions will result in critical ischemia of the foot on harvesting of the peroneal artery and are contraindications to use of a fibula free flap. Dominant peroneal systems are present in 1% of the population.[6] Peripheral vascular disease of the lower extremity is common in the elderly and in those who use tobacco, both characteristics of the majority of head and neck cancer patients.

Young and fit patients with normal lower extremity pulses can be investigated with color flow Doppler. These studies are usually readily available, are non-invasive, and involve no radiation dose. They will confirm the presence of triple-vessel runoff to the foot and detect gross atherosclerotic disease.[7,8] Patients with abnormal pulses or those at high risk for vascular disease are further investigated with lower limb angiography. CT, MRI, and femoral angiography are equally reliable in identifying tibioperoneal anatomy and the extent of atherosclerotic disease. MRI, however, has the advantages of no radiation dosage, no insult by contrast material, and the ability to image septocutaneous perforators down to 1 mm in diameter.[9,10] The choice of investigation depends on patient factors and the availability of local resources.

TREATMENT/RECONSTRUCTIVE GOALS

AIMS OF RECONSTRUCTION

- Achieve healed surgical wound
- Restoration of facial contours and esthetics
- Separation of the sinonasal cavity from the oral cavity and restoration of palatal competence required for speech and deglutition
- Maintenance of globe position within the orbit or obliteration of the orbital cavity in cases of exenteration
- Restoration of the dentition for masticatory function
- Restoration of the patient's body image and sense of wholeness

The plethora of reconstructive options available is testament to the difficulty of adequately achieving these goals. No single technique is available that meets all the goals in every case. This is the net result of

- The anatomic variability of the defects created by extirpative surgery
- The variable patient co-morbid conditions, which have an impact on
  - Their ability to tolerate lengthy surgical procedures
  - The availability of quality vessels required for free tissue transfer
  - Their coordination and dexterity, which are required for the care of oral prostheses
- The negative impact of adjuvant radiotherapy on
  - The bone quality required for dental implants
  - Maintenance of the existing dentition
  - Quality of saliva required for deglutition
  - Mouth opening required for the care of oral prostheses

The reconstructive surgeon must balance all these factors, the advantages and disadvantages of the various reconstructive techniques, and the patient's own wishes when selecting the most appropriate option for that individual.

SPECIFIC TREATMENT AND TECHNIQUES

RECONSTRUCTIVE LADDER

The general principles of reconstruction apply in the decision-making process when managing any maxillofacial wound:

- Use the simplest method available that will achieve the desired goals.
- Replace like tissues with like.
- Use vascularized tissue when the recipient site has compromised vascularity.
- Plan for possible failure of the primary reconstruction.

The reconstructive ladder helps the surgeon choose the appropriate technique. The levels of the ladder with respect to maxillary reconstruction from the lowest rung to the top are:

- Healing by secondary intention with or without a split-thickness skin graft. This technique entails the use of a prosthesis to fill the residual cavity and restore local form and function.
- Local and regional flaps for small defects that are amenable to rehabilitation with soft tissue. These wounds are generally limited in size and do not require bone to restore function. Techniques include, but are not limited to buccal advancement flaps, palatal rotation flaps, tongue flaps, buccal fat pad advancement, facial artery myomucosal flaps, nasolabial flaps, temporalis flaps, temporal-parietal-galeal flaps, and latissimus dorsi flaps.
- Free tissue transfer. These can be soft tissue only (radial forearm fasciocutaneous, latissimus dorsi, ALT, and rectus abdominis flaps) or bone containing (radial forearm osteocutaneous, fibular osteocutaneous, DCIA-based iliac crest, and scapula flaps). The benefits of these techniques lie in the quality, quantity, and geometric adaptability of the tissue that can be transferred.

PROSTHETIC VERSUS BIOLOGIC RECONSTRUCTION

Prosthetic obturation of maxillectomy defects has historically been the workhorse of reconstructive efforts for maxillary defects. The technique has many advantages that still make it a useful part of the surgeon's armamentarium:

- *Often well tolerated by patients.* Small palatal and alveolar defects are especially amenable. The presence of natural dentition in good condition improves retention and patient comfort. Retention can be enhanced by the placement of dental implants in the remaining alveolus or by the use of zygomatic implants.
- *Shorter operating time.* Immediate reconstruction of the defect following maxillectomy, especially with free tissue transfer, adds significantly to the complexity and potential morbidity of the procedure, which may not be tolerated by patients in poor general health.
- *Availability of surgical skills and local facilities.* Sophisticated reconstructive techniques require both specialized training and equipment. Prosthetic rehabilitation is inexpensive and can be achieved by dentally trained surgeons or prosthetists.
- *Allows staging of the reconstruction.* The prosthesis can be used as an interim reconstruction while awaiting the final pathology report. This is particularly useful when the pathologic diagnosis or the resection margins are in doubt.
- *Allows tumor surveillance.* Inspection of the cavity for early detection of recurrence is a commonly cited reason to opt for prosthetic rather than biologic reconstruction. Current imaging techniques have eliminated the need for visual surveillance of maxillectomy defects because they can accurately assess the resection site. Arguably, recurrence is most likely to occur near

the base of skull and is unlikely to be amenable to further treatment. Surveillance is therefore not a strong justification for delaying definitive reconstruction.

- *Biologic reconstruction rarely recreates the preexisting anatomy of the oral cavity*, in particular, the vestibule–alveolar ridge anatomy, which is essential for the retention of standard dental prostheses. Frequently, the soft tissue of the reconstruction forms a flat, springy surface extending from the hard palate to the buccal mucosa. In an edentulous patient, a standard denture cannot be retained. If dental implants are not an option, for whatever reason, the patient may be condemned to remain unrestored dentally. This loss of function, along with postradiotherapy xerostomia and loss of taste, can have a devastating impact on patients' oral intake and quality of life.

Obturator rehabilitation, however, is not without its own problems. Many of the disadvantages have a negative impact on quality of life and can outweigh the perceived benefits of this technique.

- One of the aims of reconstruction is reestablishment of the patient's sense of wholeness. Although the prosthesis can mask the resection defect, the patient can remain conscious of it. The need for frequent removal of the device for cleaning, reliance on it for adequate speech and swallowing, leakage, and oronasal regurgitation are constant reminders of the disfigurement. In some cases this can lead to significant psychological distress that has an impact on body image and the way that patients interact with their family and the wider community.
- As discussed previously, care of the prosthesis mandates that it be removed regularly for cleaning of the device and the maxillectomy cavity. This requires a degree of manual dexterity and coordination, which some in this population group do not possess. Additionally, postsurgical trismus, preexisting arthritis affecting the wrists and fingers, decreased proprioception, and vision deficits can further compromise the patient's ability to care for the obturator.
- Comfort, stability, and retention of the obturator are dependent on the geometry of the cavity, the presence of retentive surfaces, and the quality and distribution of the remaining dentition. These are negatively affected by increasing size of the defect (both vertically and horizontally), loss of the zygomatic prominence, and postoperative radiotherapy. The residual cavity collapses rapidly once the obturator is removed. Reinsertion of the obturator can become difficult or impossible if it is delayed.
- Esthetics becomes compromised with involvement of the orbital floor (essential for globe position), orbital contents, nasal complex, or anterior maxilla (essential for nasal projection and lip support). Cutaneous defects of the cheek or upper lip mandate some form of soft tissue reconstruction. This can be incorporated into biologic reconstruction of the defect or combined with prosthetic reconstruction.

Rogers and co-workers compared the impact of obturator reconstruction versus free flaps on quality of life.[1] They found associations between the size of the maxillectomy defect and the domains of recreation, physical functioning, and overall quality of life. Though not statistically significant, obturator patients appear to be more concerned about their appearance, have more pain and soreness in their mouth, are more aware of their upper teeth, are more self-conscious and less satisfied with their upper dentures, and are less satisfied with function. These findings have been supported by yet to be published research by the authors of this chapter.

It is the authors' philosophy that primary biologic reconstruction should be recommended in most instances, unless specific contraindications to this approach are identified.

RECONSTRUCTION BY DEFECT TYPE

Class 1 Defects

These defects are the simplest to repair. The only functional requirement is separation of the nasal and oral cavities. This can readily be achieved with soft tissue alone.

Smaller defects can be closed with local tissue in the form of palatal rotation flaps based on one of the greater palatine vessels. Almost all the palatal mucoperiosteum can be raised on one pedicle and rotated up to 180 degrees. The exposed donor site can be left to heal by secondary intention. The authors routinely use a healing plate covered with periodontal dressing material for improved patient comfort. This can be retained with clasps on the native dentition or fixed with screws into the remaining palate. It is removed after 10 to 14 days.

The tongue is another local source of tissue. It is a limited tissue stock, and is therefore most useful for the repair of small defects, especially those that are refractory to previous local repair. Various designs for these flaps have been described, but all are based on a random pattern of vascular supply and require a second stage, 14 days later, to separate the base of the flap from the tongue. This technique relies on tension-free closure and intermaxillary fixation to limit movement of the tongue during the healing phase.

The buccal fat pad is the well-vascularized lining of the masticator space that separates the muscles of mastication. It can be harvested through a maxillary vestibular incision and used to close small defects (Fig. 61-6). If the dentition interferes with insetting of the flap or a more central defect is being repaired, the flap can be passed through the maxillary sinus. The flap mucosalizes within 2 to 3 weeks and therefore does not require skin grafting.

Larger defects can be repaired with temporalis or temporal-parietal-galeal flaps (Fig. 61-7). These flaps can be passed through the maxillary sinus to reach a more central defect. Bilateral flaps can be used if a single flap does not reach across the entire defect. Both mucosalize without the need for skin grafting.

The temporalis muscle can be harvested in its entirety or be split coronally or sagittally, while being mindful of the vascular pedicle, to reduce the hollowing defect caused by complete harvest. The arc of rotation can be improved by temporarily removing the zygomatic arch and passing the pedicle on its medial surface. This flap should not be used if the vascular pedicle is compromised following ligation of the ipsilateral external carotid, maxillary, or superficial temporal arteries.

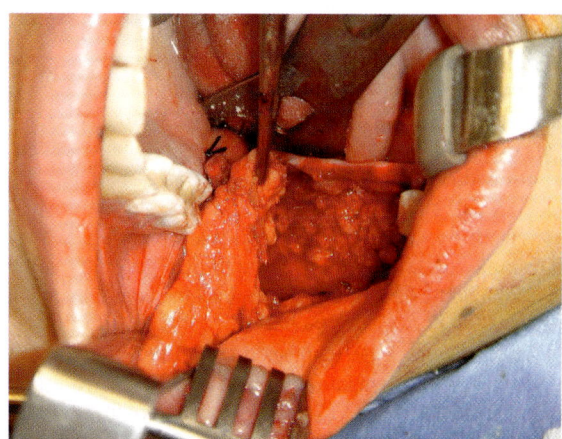

Fig. 61-6 ■ Buccal fat pad flap for intraoral reconstruction.

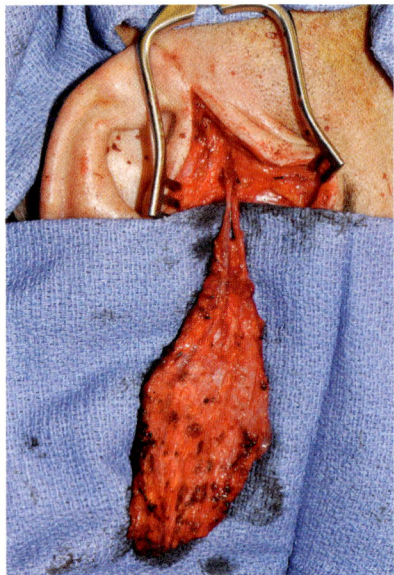

Fig. 61-7 ■ Temporoparietal fascia flap. This flap may be pedicled or harvested as a free flap.

Class 2 Defects

These are the most common postablative defects that the reconstructive surgeon is required to manage in the maxilla. Apart from the need to separate the oral and nasal cavities, the functional requirements of the reconstruction depend on the position of the defect, its horizontal extent, and the condition of the remaining dentition.

Posterolateral defects (distal to the canine) may be managed with an obturator or soft tissue—only flaps, especially if the remaining dentition is adequate to support a prosthesis. Bone reconstruction is favored when the patient desires rehabilitation with dental implants and when reconstructing anterior, b or c class II defect subtypes, which are difficult to prosthetically obdurate.

Soft tissue can be rotated in with locoregional flaps. Free tissue transfer, however, has largely superseded these flaps. The workhorse soft tissue–only flaps for reconstruction of these defects are the radial forearm (Fig. 61-8) and ALT (Fig. 61-9) free flaps. Both these flaps provide thin, pliable skin paddles and good-caliber vessels. The ALT flap is somewhat disadvantaged by its shorter pedicle length and thicker subcutaneous layer of fat in more obese patients.

When inset, these flaps have a tendency to hang down into the oral cavity. This can interfere with the existing dentition, alter speech, and compromise swallowing. With time, the surgical edema resolves, the subcutaneous fat atrophies, and a flat platform is left across the surgical defect (Fig. 61-10).

When the existing dentition is inadequate to support a prosthesis or implants are planned for dental rehabilitation, bone-containing flaps are ideal for reconstruction. The most commonly used flap is the fibula osteocutaneous free flap (Fig. 61-11). It has excellent bone stock (both width, height, length, and bone quality), a long vascular pedicle, and a thin, pliable skin paddle. The flap is occasionally disadvantaged by atherosclerotic disease affecting the pedicle vessels, a bulky muscular cuff, and the limited geometry achievable with the skin paddle tethered to the bone by the lateral intermuscular septum.

The fibula bone can be suspended from the residual zygomatic bone and fixed to the remaining maxilla anteriorly. Wider, subtype b and c defects require closing osteotomies to fashion the neo-alveolus. It is important to reconstruct any infraorbital/anterior maxillary wall defect not filled by the fibula to prevent an unnatural

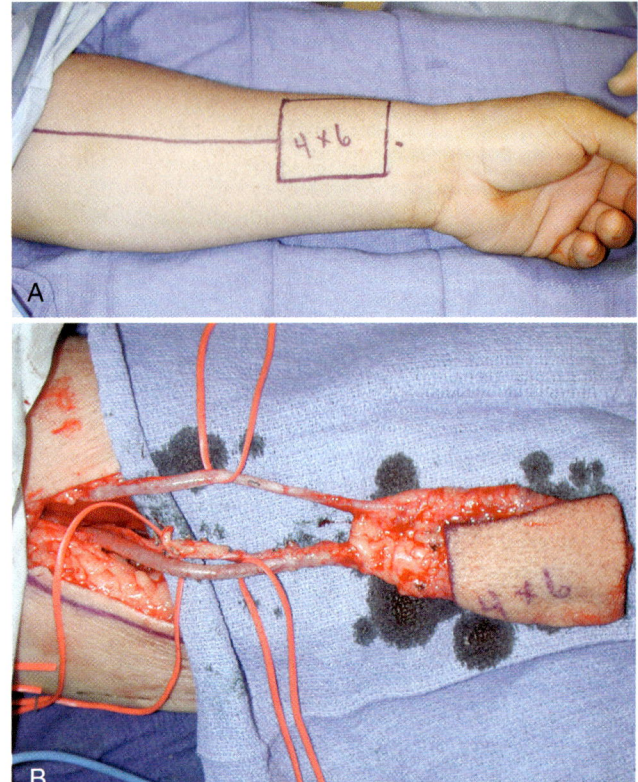

Fig. 61-8 ■ Radial forearm flap. **A,** Skin markings. **B,** Elevated flap.

depression from forming in the skin of the cheek in this area. This can readily be achieved with free cortical bone harvested from the unused portion of the fibula.

Alternative bone-containing flaps include the radial forearm osteocutaneous free flap (Fig. 61-12) and the subscapular system of free flaps.

The radial forearm flap has limited bone stock, with only 40% of the diameter of the radius able to be safely harvested and a length limited to around 10 cm. This bone is not suitable for implants but is very useful:

- When a strut of bone is required to maintain nasal and upper lip projection following anterior maxillectomies.
- To reduce the sagging effect of soft tissues when reconstructing more posterior defects. The skin is suspended by its attachment to the radial bone at the level of the neoalveolar crest.

The practice of prophylactic plating of the remaining radius has significantly reduced the rate of postoperative fracture of this bone. The donor site defect is well tolerated and does not impede the patient's mobility as a fibula flap does. It represents an excellent reconstructive option in elderly patients and for those with advanced atherosclerotic disease affecting the lower extremity.[11]

The scapula and parascapular free flaps, based on the subscapular artery and its branches, become increasingly attractive options with increasing vertical and horizontal extent of the maxillary defects or involvement of overlying skin. The greatest advantages of these flaps are the amount of soft tissue that can be harvested (both skin and muscle) and the variety of geometry achievable, with the bony and soft tissue components able to be rotated independently on individual vascular pedicles.

In the setting of class 2 defects, the scapula free flap has been most widely described for the reconstruction of subtypes b and c. The tip of the scapula anatomically resembles the hard palate and

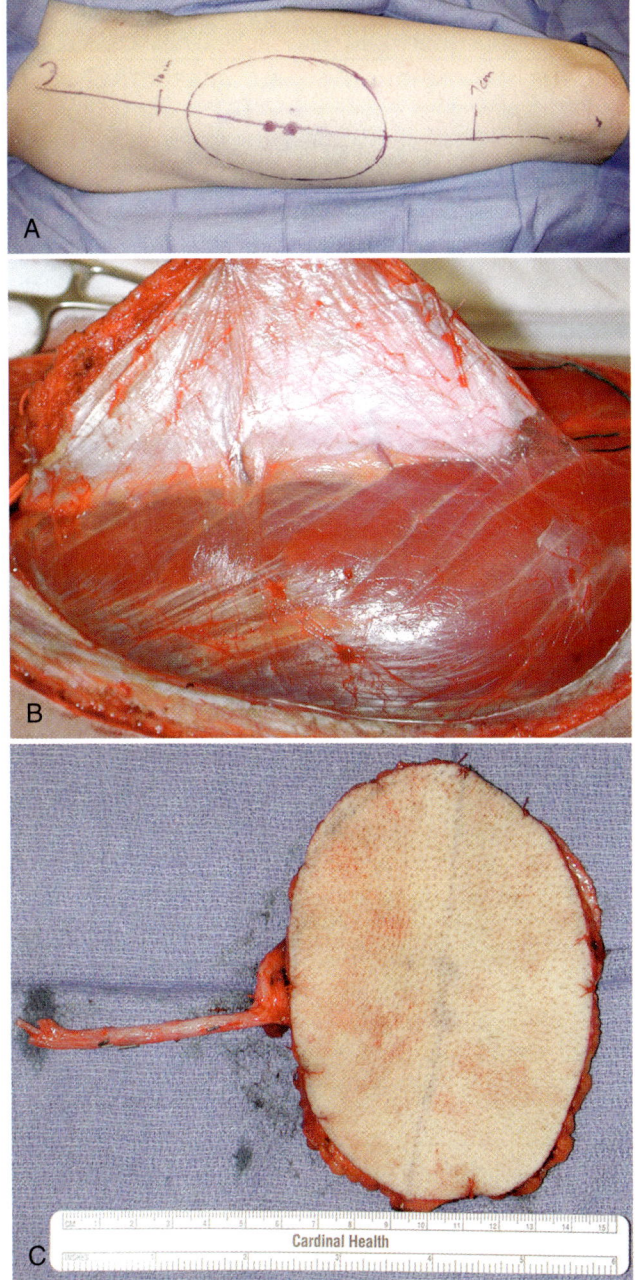

Fig. 61-9 ■ Anterolateral thigh flap. **A,** Skin markings. **B,** Musculocutaneous perforators to the skin paddle. **C,** Flap harvested.

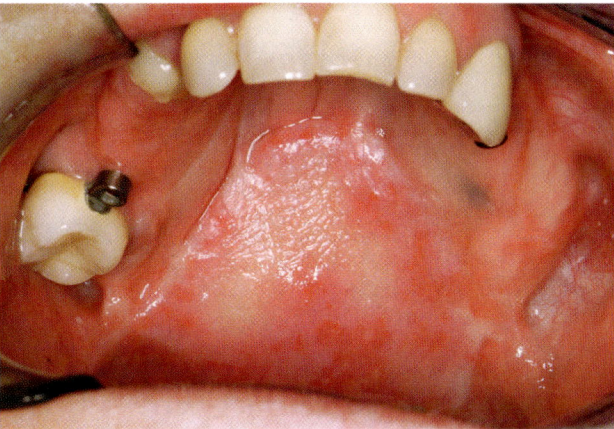

Fig. 61-10 ■ One-year appearance of a radial forearm free flap to reconstruct a class I maxillary defect of the palate. Note the excellent contour after resolution of the edema.

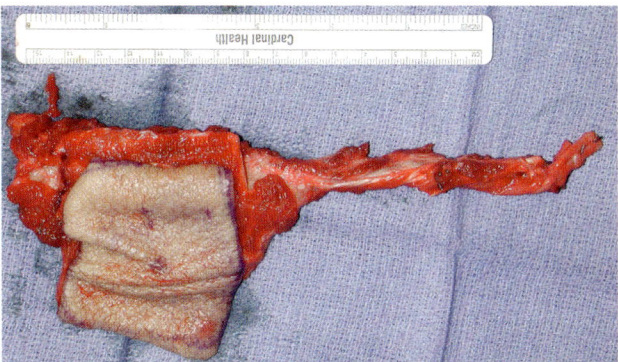

Fig. 61-11 ■ Fibula osteocutaneous free flap.

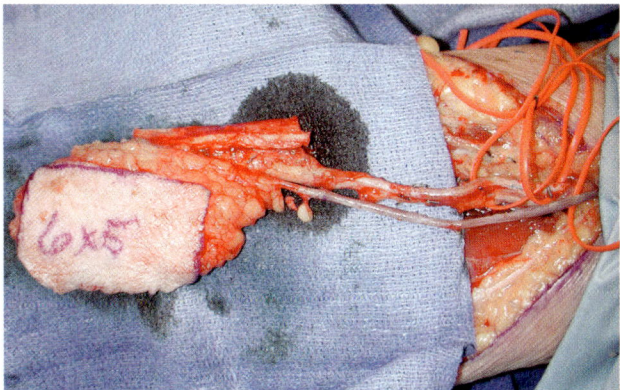

Fig. 61-12 ■ Radial forearm osteocutaneous free flap. Note the small volume of bone characteristic of this flap.

edentulous alveolar ridge. It can therefore be used to reconstruct wide, cross-arch, or complete low maxillectomy defects. The bone is relatively thin when used in this fashion, thus limiting its usefulness for dental implant rehabilitation. The need to turn the patient prohibits simultaneous ablative surgery and flap harvesting and increases anesthetic risks for the patient. When large soft tissue volumes are required for reconstruction, the authors prefer to harvest two free flaps from the supine position instead of harvesting capsular flaps. Osteocutaneous fibula, radial forearm, and ALT flaps may all be harvested simultaneously with the resection and in general allow completion of the procedure in a more timely fashion when compared with scapular flaps, which requires changes in patient positioning.

Class 3 and 4 Defects

Class 3 (Fig. 61-13) and class 4 (Fig. 61-14) defects are less commonly encountered but are far more challenging to reconstruct. The demands on the reconstruction increase as the geometry of the defect becomes more complex. The large number of reported techniques for reconstructing these defects bears testament to this fact. There is no one method or flap that will be ideal for every occasion. Each case must be evaluated independently and the reconstructive goals defined early. In general, the reconstructive goals for class 3 and 4 defects are to maintain support for the globe, nasal base, and cheek

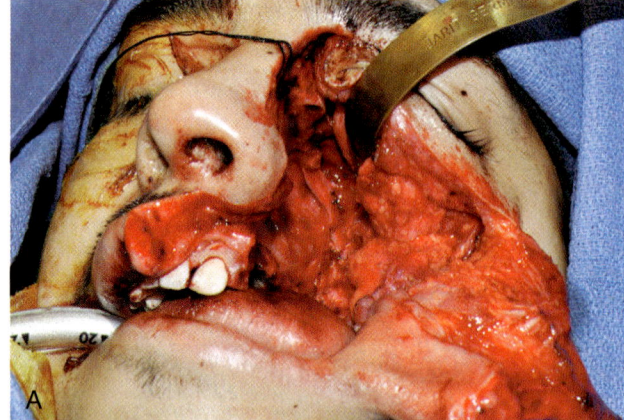

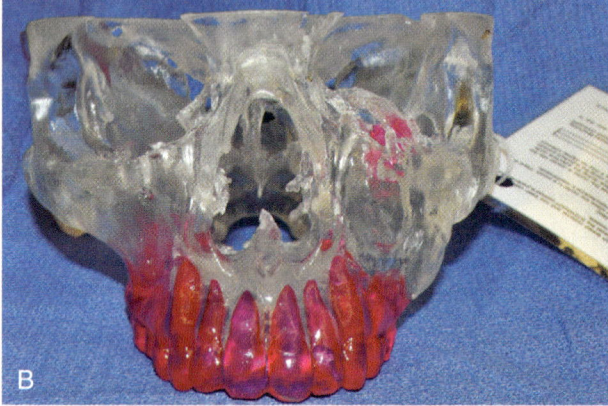

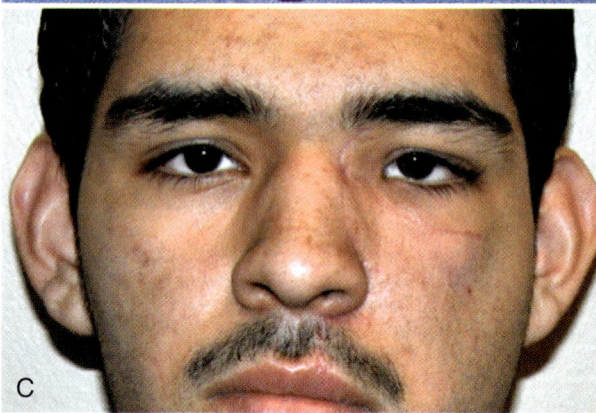

TABLE 61-1   Subunits Lost, Reconstructive Goals and Options

SUBUNIT LOST	RECONSTRUCTIVE GOALS	RECONSTRUCTIVE OPTIONS
Alveolar bone and palatal shelf	Separate the oral and nasal cavities Provide a platform against which the tongue can initiate swallowing and create sounds Provide a base for dental rehabilitation	Bone-containing free flaps: RFFF Fibula Scapula DCIA
Orbital floor	Support the globe	Free flap plus free bone graft Composite free flap: RFFF Fibula Scapula DCIA
Orbital contents	Obliterate the orbital cavity	Soft tissue free flaps: Rectus abdominis Latissimus dorsi Radial forearm Composite free flap: Scapula Radial forearm
Cranial base	Separate the cranial and nasal cavities	Soft tissue free flaps: Rectus abdominis Latissimus dorsi RFFF
Facial skin	Replace facial skin	Multiple-component free flaps: Subscapular system flap Second fasciocutaneous free flaps: RFFF ALT

ALT, anterolateral thigh; *DCIA,* deep circumflex iliac artery; *RFFF,* radial forearm free flap.

Fig. 61-13 ■ Class III maxillary defect following resection of ameloblastoma. **A,** Class III maxillectomy defect with loss of the orbital walls but preservation of the orbital adnexa. **B,** Stereolithographic model demonstrating expansive tumor encroaching into the orbit. Note the impacted tooth (*pink*) near the orbital floor. The model was sterilized and used intraoperatively to contour cranial bone grafts for orbital wall reconstruction. **C,** Three-month follow-up. Note the excellent symmetry and globe position.

contours. This may be achieved by reconstruction of skeletal support and soft tissue coverage or obliteration of the defect with large-volume soft tissue flaps such as the rectus abdominis or ALT flaps harvested with muscle.

It is not possible to provide a prescriptive approach to the reconstruction of these patients. When evaluating the individual defect, it is useful to define the subunits lost because they will determine the goals to be achieved and help guide the best choice of reconstruction to meet these goals (Table 61-1). On occasion, multiple flaps may be required to adequately meet these goals.

ALGORITHM FOR RECONSTRUCTION BASED ON PATIENTS' DESIRES FOR DENTAL REHABILITATION

Advances in reconstructive surgery over the last 30 years have resulted in the development of many highly predictable and dependable tissue transfer techniques. There has been a paradigm shift away from prosthetic obturator rehabilitation to the routine use of biologic reconstruction. It is, however, no longer satisfactory for reconstructive surgeons to define success as a maxillary defect filled with healthy hard and soft tissues. Reconstructive goals now need to reflect the patient's desires to maximize function and esthetics.

Anecdotally, one of the most common complaints that patients have following cancer surgery and reconstruction is the negative impact on their ability to chew because of the loss of teeth and the psychological impact that this has on their socialization and, ultimately, their quality of life. By identifying these concerns and

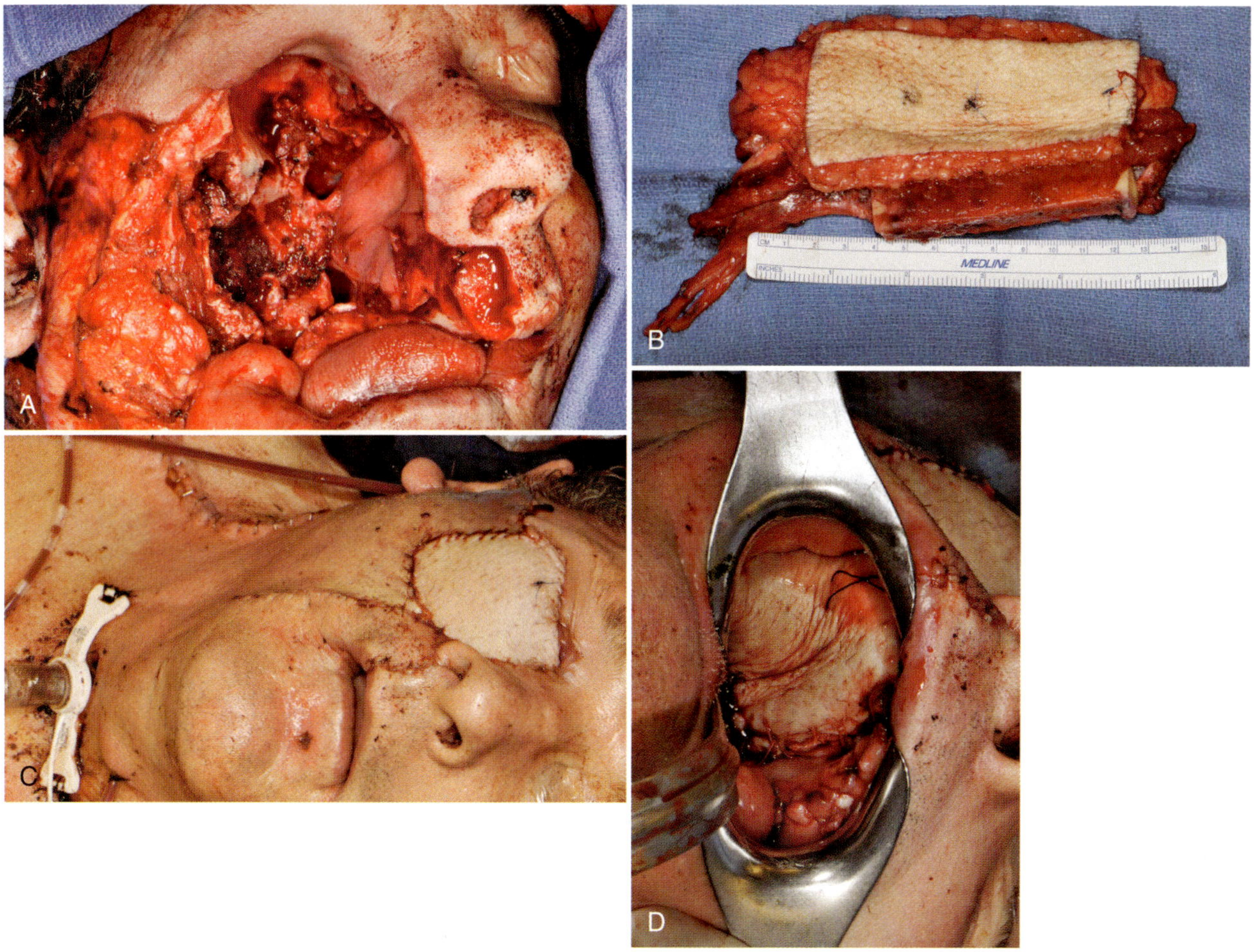

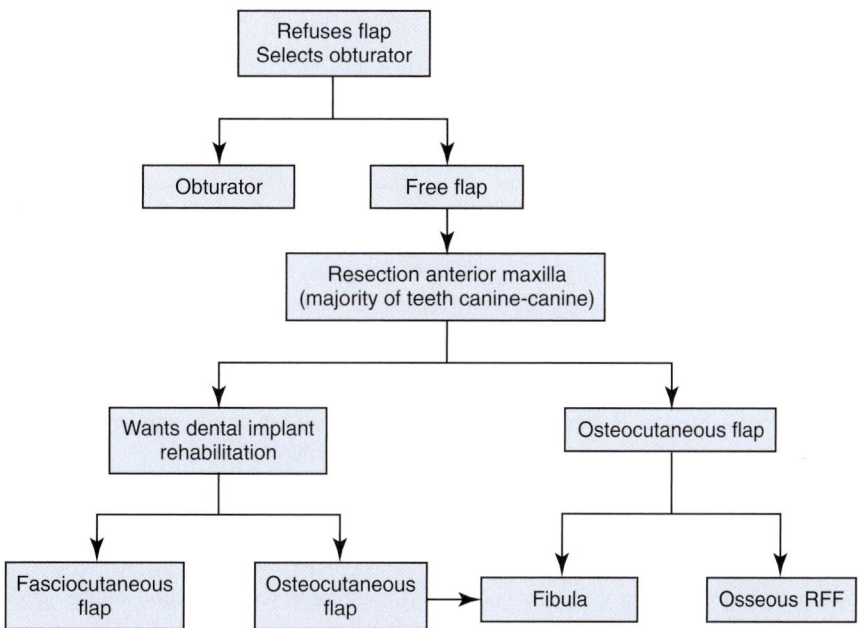

Fig. 61-14 ■ Class IV maxillectomy with orbital exenteration defect following resection of extensive squamous cell carcinoma of the maxillary sinus. **A,** Class IV maxillectomy defect. **B,** Fibula osteocutaneous flap. **C,** Reestablishment of facial contours and skeletal support. **D,** Soft tissue coverage provided for intraoral and facial soft tissue defects.

Fig. 61-15 ■ Algorithm for reconstruction of class II maxillectomy defects.

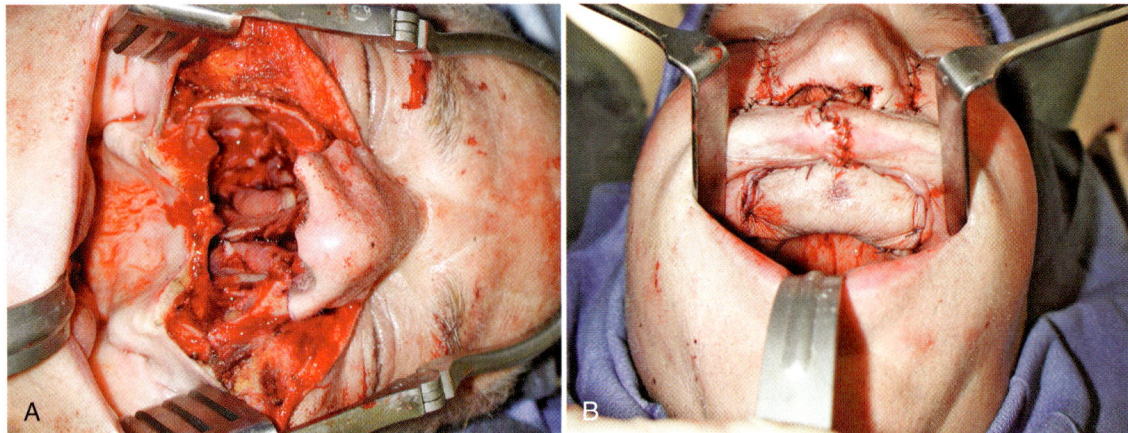

Fig. 61-16 ■ **A,** Class II defect of the anterior maxilla. **B,** Osteocutaneous fibula flap to restore nasal support and provide bone for later dental implant rehabilitation.

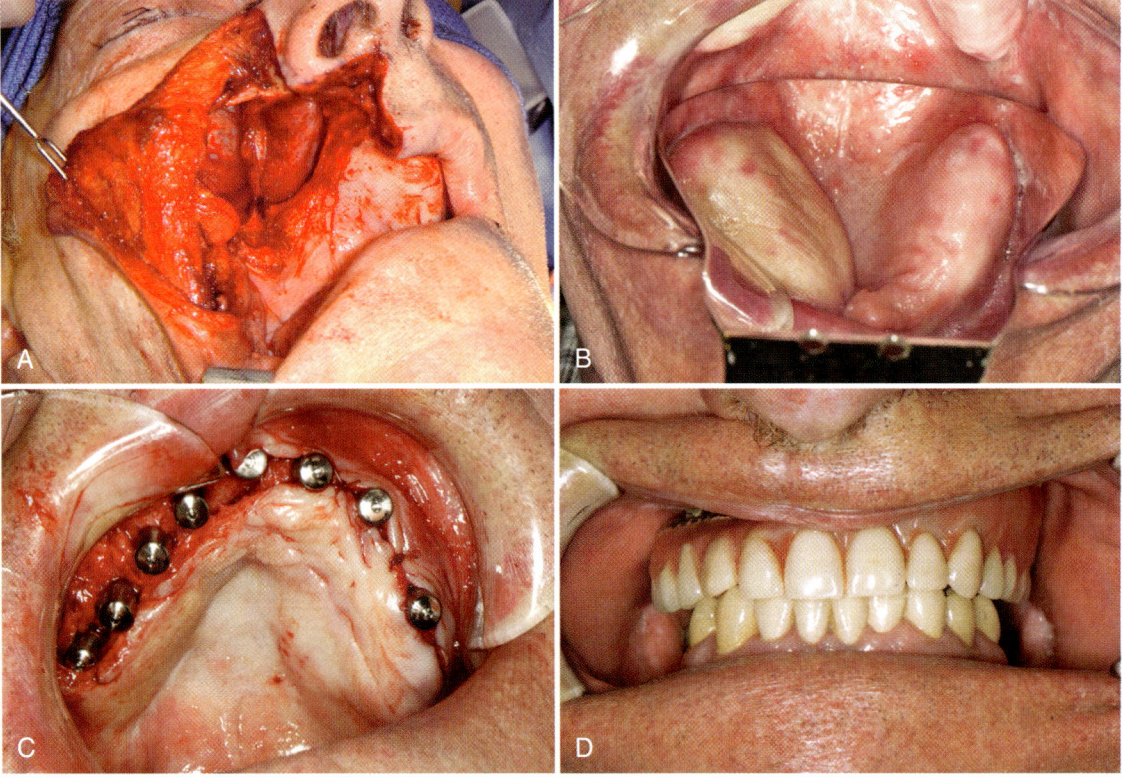

Fig. 61-17 ■ **A,** Class II defect of the lateral portion of the maxilla. A fibula flap was selected because of the patient's desire for dental implants. **B,** Healed flap. **C,** Dental implants placed in the fibula bone and maxillary remnant. **D,** Final prosthesis.

desires early, the surgeon can select the reconstructive technique that will maximize the potential dental rehabilitation. Factors that must be considered include the following:

- The patient's desire for rehabilitation
- Availability of the skills, resources, and finances required for the desired dental rehabilitation
- The timing and impact of adjuvant therapies on the suitability of dental rehabilitation techniques, especially the effect of radiotherapy on dental implant and denture techniques

- The quality, quantity, and location of residual native hard tissues that may need to be supplemented or enhanced to support dental rehabilitation

Figure 61-15 presents a simplified algorithm that can guide the reconstructive decision-making process for the most common maxillary defects encountered—class 2 defects.

The first step is to identify the patient's desire and suitability for biologic reconstruction of the proposed or existing maxillary defect.

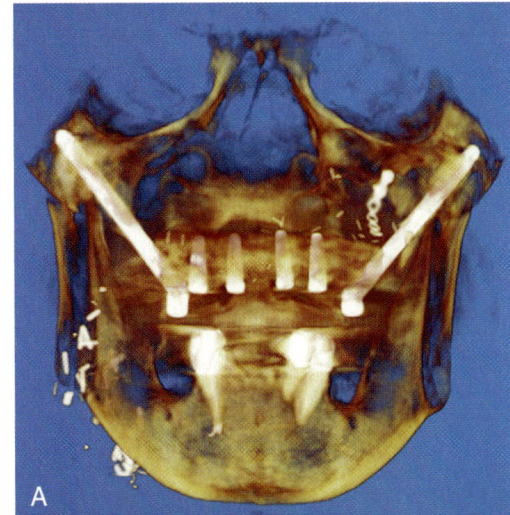

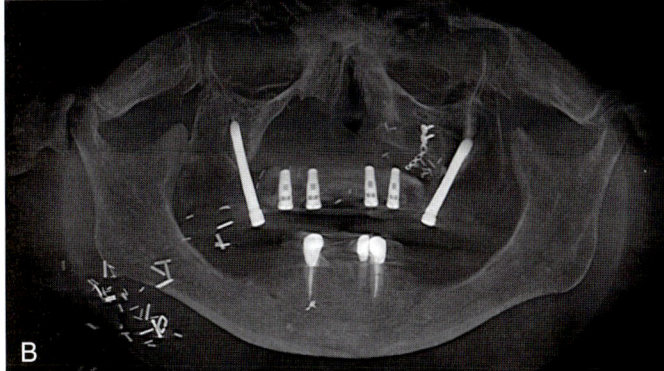

Fig. 61-18 ■ Placement of zygomatic implants in conjunction with traditional dental implants within the fibula bone flap. **A,** Three-dimensional cone beam computed tomography image. **B,** Panoramic radiograph.

If the defect involves the anterior maxilla, an osseous free flap is required to adequately reconstruct the projection of the mid-face, upper lip, and nose (Fig. 61-16). Additionally, it will provide a platform for a denture or dental implants. The choice of osseous flap will depend on the patient's desire and suitability for dental implants. If implants are a realistic option, the fibula flap is selected because it provides adequate bone height and pedicle length to reach the defect site. Otherwise, the osseous radial forearm flap is selected because it is generally the less morbid procedure.

When the defect is purely lateral, the patient's desire and suitability for dental implants will again guide the choice of flap (Fig. 61-17). When implants are to be used, an osseous flap is selected. The fibula flap is the most popular choice in this situation because of adequate bone stock and pedicle length and the ability to be harvested simultaneously. If no implants are to be used, a simple fasciocutaneous flap is selected.

Zygomatic implants are useful in patients who have lost significant maxillary bone for traditional dental implantation (Fig. 61-18). They can be placed at the time of primary reconstruction or secondarily. Zygomatic implants can provide cross-arch support to supplement the natural dentition on the contralateral side and can be placed through an open defect or a fasciocutaneous flap regardless of the presence of a neoalveolus.

PEARLS AND PITFALLS

- Management of complex maxillofacial defects should be attempted within a multidisciplinary team, which can bring together the many elements required to maximize the patient's reconstructive outcome.
- Preoperative planning with particular attention to the probable defect geometry and consideration of the reconstructive goals and the desires of the patient will help the surgeon select and execute the reconstructive technique that best balances all these needs.
- Reconstruction of maxillary defects can be achieved with either autologous tissue reconstruction or prostheses (obturation).
- Age should not be considered a contraindication to free flap reconstruction. Frequently, the elderly are the patients who benefit the most because they may not have the dexterity and mouth opening to manage a prosthetic obturator. Biologic reconstruction can have a significant impact on quality of life for these patients.
- Poor tumor biology is not a contraindication to free flap reconstruction. The benefit of improved quality of life outweighs the physician's desire to inspect the postresection cavity. Recurrences in this area carry a grim prognosis and salvage is rarely feasible.
- Pedicle length should always be maximized when harvesting free flaps for maxillary reconstruction. Vein grafting is occasionally necessary.
- Osseointegrated implants can be an important adjunct to the reconstructive effort. They can be in the form of traditional dental implants, zygomatic implants to support an oral prosthesis, or craniofacial implants for an extraoral prosthesis.
- Be wary of patients with unrealistic expectations. All patients should be thoroughly counseled about what is achievable and in what time frame.
- Prosthetic obturators can be very effective, but with larger defects, they may have an unsatisfactory seal and result in poor speech, excessive leakage of fluid, and difficulty managing the device. Adjuvant radiotherapy and chemotherapy increase the difficulty in achieving a successful prosthesis.
- Occasionally, larger defects can be challenging to reconstruct, and the results can be suboptimal if one technique is used to meet all the patient's requirements. It may be better to choose two simple flaps rather than one larger, potentially more complex flap to meet the subunit demands.
- Failure to reconstruct the anterior wall of the maxilla between the alveolus and orbital rim will lead to noticeable facial hollowing, which is difficult to correct secondarily. A little extra time adding bone graft to this area will avoid this unsightly complication. Support for facial soft tissues can be restored with bulky soft tissue flaps (rectus/ALT), especially if the defect is large or the cranial cavity is breached. Soft tissue–only flaps will, however, variably contract over time without underlying osseous reconstruction of the skeletal buttresses.
- Respect the recipient tissue bed and be wary of previously irradiated patients. Facial wounds in these patients have a high propensity to break down. Reconstruct these patients with free flaps, which bring vital vascularity with them. Non-vascular bone grafts require restoration of a healthy wound bed. If these types of grafts are to be used, consider staging the reconstruction or recruiting adjacent non-irradiated tissue to maximize the health of the wound bed.

REFERENCES

1. Rogers SN, Lowe D, McNally D, et al: Health-related quality of life after maxillectomy: a comparison between prosthetic obturation and free flap, *J Oral Maxillofac Surg* 61:174-181, 2003.
2. Brown JS, Rogers SN, McNally DN, et al: A modified classification for the maxillectomy defect, *Head Neck* 22:17-26, 2000.
3. Bell RB, Weimer KA, Dierks EJ, et al: Computer planning and intraoperative navigation for palato-maxillary and mandibular reconstruction with fibular free flaps, *J Oral Maxillofac Surg* 69(3):724-732, 2011.
4. Hirsch DL, Garfein ES, Christensen AM, et al: Use of computer-aided design and computer-aided manufacturing to produce orthognathically ideal surgical outcomes: a paradigm shift in head and neck reconstruction, *J Oral Maxillofac Surg* 67:2115-2122, 2009.
5. Potter JK, Osborn TM: Preparation of the neck for microvascular reconstruction of the head and neck, *Oral Maxillofac Surg Clin North Am* 20:521-526, 2008.
6. Day CP, Orme R: Popliteal artery branching patterns—an angiographic study, *Clin Radiol* 61:696-699, 2006.
7. Smith RB, Thomas RD, Funk GF: Fibula free flaps: the role of angiography in patients with abnormal results on preoperative color flow Doppler studies, *Arch Otolaryngol Head Neck Surg* 129:712-715, 2003.
8. Whitley SP, Sandhu S, Cardozo A: Preoperative vascular assessment of the lower limb for harvest of a fibular flap: the views of vascular surgeons in the United Kingdom, *Br J Oral Maxillofac Surg* 42:307-310, 2004.
9. Fukaya E, Grossman RF, Saloner D, et al: Magnetic resonance angiography for free fibula flap transfer, *J Reconstr Microsurg* 23:205-211, 2007.
10. Fukaya E, Saloner D, Leon P, et al: Magnetic resonance angiography to evaluate septocutaneous perforators in free fibula flap transfer, *J Plast Reconstr Aesthet Surg* 63:1099-1104, 2010.
11. Avery CM: Review of the radial free flap: still evolving or facing extinction? Part two: osteocutaneous radial free flap, *Br J Oral Maxillofac Surg* 48:253-260, 2010.

Chapter

62

Contemporary Methods in Tongue Reconstruction

Phillip Pirgousis, Rui Fernandes

Like many specialized organs in the head and neck region, the tongue is perhaps the most critical in terms of function, thus making its loss as a result of disease central to functional reconstruction and optimal speech and swallowing rehabilitation.

The tongue is enveloped by mucosa that contains mucous and serous glands, special taste sensory end-organs, and general sensory end-organs. Anatomically, it is composed of extrinsic and intrinsic muscles, all of which are paramount in its ability to perform the complex synchronized movements needed for speech articulation, manipulation of food boluses, and deglutition. There are four paired extrinsic tongue muscles: the genioglossus, hyoglossus, palatoglossus, and styloglossus. The intrinsic muscles consist of an ill-defined network of fiber bundles. The nerve supply is derived from four cranial nerves, the hypoglossal, vagus, lingual, and glossopharyngeal nerves. It is obvious from this anatomy that the specialized tissues in the tongue that control its complex motor and sensory activity make it a far more difficult structure to duplicate than the less specialized and adynamic tissues surrounding it, including the floor of the mouth, cheek, and mandible.

Contemporary tongue reconstruction is now considered to involve more than satisfactory wound healing and flap survival. The complex neuromuscular coordination involved in speech and deglutition is increasingly understood, and impairment in any of these components can result in dysphagia, aspiration, or poorly comprehensible speech. It should be the goal of every reconstructive surgeon to restore function to as close as possible to the preoperative state, which will also translate into significant improvements in patients' quality of life.

PATHOLOGIC ANATOMY/ CLASSIFICATION OF DEFECTS

The tongue can arbitrarily be divided into the anterior two thirds, which is essentially the mobile tongue, and the posterior third and tongue base, which is the less mobile component. This division is defined by the circumvallate papillae. Furthermore, quantification of ablative defects based on the volume of tissue lost can be divided into longitudinal quarters. Such classification systems are important for uniform reporting of results and, to a lesser degree, for planning appropriate reconstruction. Although division of the tongue in this fashion is useful for descriptive and classification purposes, denervation of the remnant tongue is more important than the volume of tongue resected with respect to ultimate functional outcome.

Ablative defects consisting of less than half the tongue are generally referred to as partial glossectomy defects. Hemiglossectomy results from resection of half the tongue, whereas resections of more than half or all of the tongue are referred to as subtotal or total glossectomy defects. Defining defect volume as just described allows the surgeon to anticipate the type of reconstruction necessary in each instance.

TREATMENT/RECONSTRUCTIVE GOALS

The aims of tongue reconstruction are to achieve wound closure or coverage while minimizing complications and optimizing articulation and deglutition. Although primary wound closure and avoidance of wound complications were major concerns historically for most degrees of tongue defects, contemporary reconstructive surgery rarely fails to attain these basic objectives. However, restoration of optimal articulation and deglutition remain serious challenges for all reconstructive surgeons.

Furthermore, many studies have now confirmed that good functional reconstruction of the tongue provides significant objective and subjective improvements in quality of life.

Despite the method of reconstruction, the ability of the patient to articulate intelligibly and swallow is directly proportional to the amount of tongue resected. Important differences exist in instances in which primary closure as opposed to flap repair is used for tongue reconstruction. Flap tissue, though necessary for large defects, has demonstrably inferior outcomes in terms of speech and swallowing. This is probably a result of the introduction of adynamic bulky flap tissue, which somewhat impairs the function of the remaining tongue. Hence, it is preferable when possible to close partial glossectomy defects primarily.

For larger defects in which primary closure is not possible, it is critical to restore bulk to the tongue and, most importantly, preserve mobility of the remaining tongue. If possible, restoration of sensation to the flap, though variable, may help facilitate speech and swallowing rehabilitation.

Preservation of tongue mobility in patients with large defects in which adjacent tissues such as the floor of the mouth, mandible, and retromolar trigone are also involved can be achieved by independent reconstruction of these units with respect to the tongue defect.

The importance of replacement of tissue volume is of greater concern for subtotal and total glossectomy defects, with or without involvement of the tongue base. In such instances, sufficient tongue bulk in the midline is helpful in directing food and liquids toward the piriform sinuses. The critical role of the tongue base in swallowing is two-fold. The first piston-like action drives the food bolus through the oropharynx and creates positive pressure in the upper pharynx. This requires a competent palate and pharyngeal constrictor muscles and an adequate dynamic tongue base. It becomes apparent in extensive resections involving these additional structures that patients frequently fail to regain swallowing ability and remain dependent on percutaneous gastrostomy tubes for nutrition. The second pump is created by elevation of the larynx and opening of the piriformis, which causes negative pressure and suction action in the hypopharynx.

Finally, a controversial yet important consideration in reconstruction of large tongue defects is restoration of sensation. Kapur and colleagues in 1990 demonstrated the detrimental effects of regional oral anesthesia on mastication. Hence, the use of sensate flaps for reconstruction of the oral tongue may improve manipulation of the food bolus; however, the adynamic nature of flap tissue may offset this benefit. Restoration of sensation at the tongue base has not conclusively been shown to improve the swallowing reflex.

RECONSTRUCTIVE TECHNIQUES

PARTIAL GLOSSECTOMY DEFECTS

Facial Artery Musculomucosal Flap/Buccinator Flap

The buccinator flap, first described by Bozola and co-authors in 1989, and the facial artery musculomucosal (FAMM) flap, described by Pribaz in 1992, are useful intraoral pedicled axial-pattern musculomucosal flaps. The buccinator flap is based on the buccal artery, a terminal branch of the internal maxillary artery, whereas the FAMM flap is based on the facial artery. Both flaps provide excellent, reliable, and easily accessible reconstructive options for moderate-sized tongue defects. They have a rich vascular supply with a relatively constant anatomic course. Their mucosal nature provides a better surface for relining tongue defects than skin flaps do. Both flaps are easy to raise and their donor sites can be closed primarily with minimal morbidity.

Their limitations include a restricted arc of rotation and the necessity of remaining pedicled for 3 weeks before division of the pedicle, which invariably requires a second procedure.

Submental Artery Island Flap

The submental artery island flap (Fig. 62-1) was first described by Martin and colleagues in 1992. Since then, many other reports in the literature have confirmed its versatile use in head and neck reconstruction, and it is an excellent option for reconstruction of

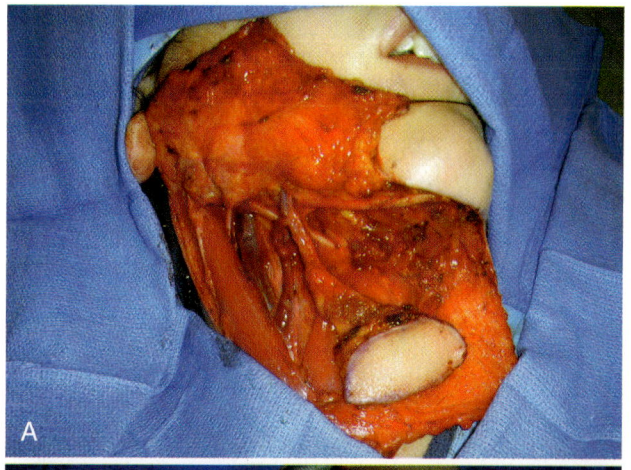
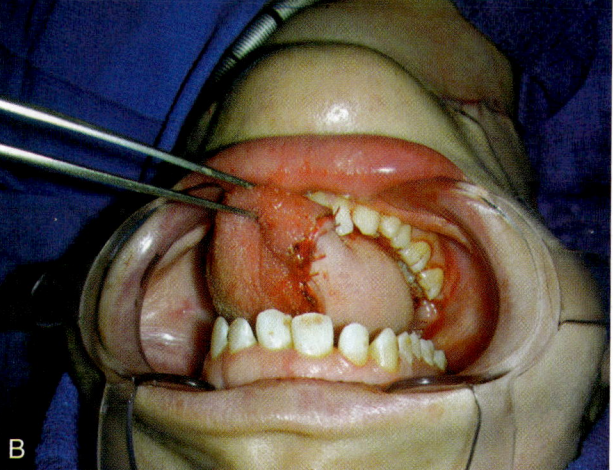

Fig. 62-1 ▪ Submental island flap (SIF). **A,** Harvested SIF before transfer into the oral cavity. **B,** Tongue reconstruction with the SIF.

partial glossectomy defects. Its advantages include reasonable flap thickness, tissue pliability, and versatility in design. Its close proximity to the tongue makes it an excellent choice for pedicled flap reconstruction, and the location of the donor site is cosmetically pleasing and frequently allows primary closure. Interestingly, Martin also described its use as a free flap.

The submental artery is a well-defined and consistent branch of the facial artery; it arises deep to the submandibular gland, passes forward and medially across the mylohyoid muscle, either superficial or deep to the digastric muscle, and terminates behind the mandibular symphysis over the anterior belly of the digastric. Along its course, the submental artery gives off several cutaneous branches that pierce the platysma to supply a broad cutaneous distribution of the upper ipsilateral neck extending to the contralateral neck. This allows a large flap to be raised from mandibular angle to mandibular angle, with width being limited by the flaccidity of neck skin in allowing direct closure. Its broad arc of rotation enables easy transfer into tongue defects.

The patient is positioned with the neck extended and the skin flap outlined in the midline submental region. Maximum flap width is determined by a pinch test to allow primary closure. The flap is raised in a distal to proximal direction in the subplatysmal plane, superficial to the contralateral anterior belly of the digastric, but deep to the ipsilateral digastric and superficial to the mylohyoid muscle. Inclusion of the digastric muscle adds a margin of safety to the vascularity of the skin island. The flap is separated from the submandibular gland until the facial vessels become apparent, and the facial pedicle is dissected proximally until adequate pedicle length is achieved. The marginal mandibular branch of the facial nerve, as well as the venous drainage, should be identified and preserved. The isolated flap is now tunneled between the mylohyoid muscle into the oral cavity for inset into the tongue defect.

HEMIGLOSSECTOMY DEFECTS

Fasciocutaneous Radial Forearm Free Flap

The radial forearm free flap (Fig. 62-2) continues to find widespread use for the reconstruction of substantial glossectomy defects. Since its initial description in 1978 in the Chinese literature and later more comprehensively by Yang and associates in 1981 and Song and co-workers in 1982, this flap remains the workhorse flap for a variety of head and neck defects.

The fasciocutaneous radial forearm free flap has many advantages, including consistent vascular anatomy, ease of harvest, excellent pliability, thinness, a long and high-caliber vascular pedicle, and relatively low donor site morbidity. Its disadvantages include perfusion deficits in the hand, unesthetic donor site location, potential functional hand deficits, and poor skin graft take, with a reported incidence of 30% to 50%.

The radial artery, which forms the deep palmar arch of the hand, is located in the intermuscular septum between the brachioradialis and flexor carpi radialis muscles. During its course in the flexor surface of the forearm it gives off 9 to 17 branches to the forearm fascia concentrated particularly in its distal third. These branches form a rich fascial plexus that provides perfusion to the entire forearm skin. Venous drainage of the forearm flap is via the paired venae comitantes or the superficial venous system, commonly the cephalic vein.

Before raising the flap, an Allen test must be performed to assess the adequacy of collateral circulation via the ulnar and interosseous arteries, especially to the thumb. The nondominant arm is typically chosen. Following standard skin preparation and sterile draping, the arm is exsanguinated and a sterile tourniquet inflated to around

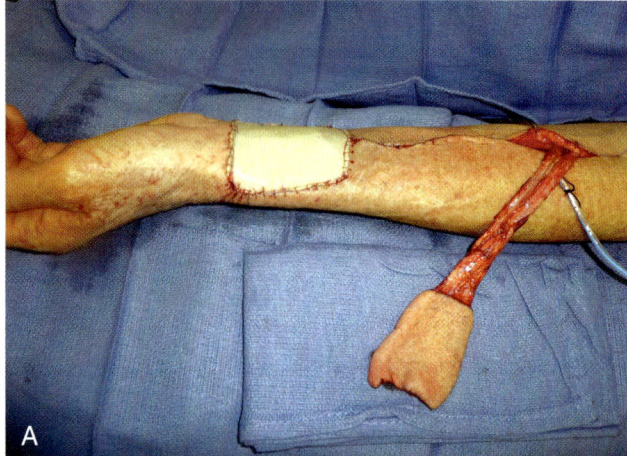

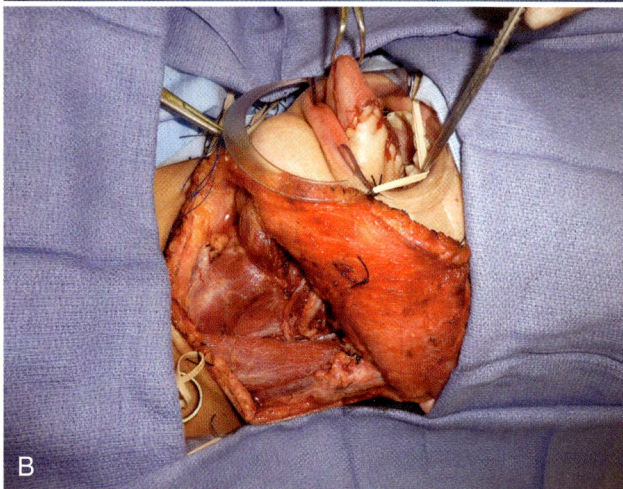

Fig. 62-2 ■ Radial forearm free flap (RFFF). **A,** Harvest of an RFFF for tongue reconstruction before takedown and transfer of the flap. **B,** Inset of the RFFF to reconstruct a hemi-tongue defect.

250 mm Hg. The desired dimensions of the skin paddle are outlined, with the distal flap border placed a minimum of 3 cm proximal to the flexor crease of the wrist. The flap is raised in an ulnar to radial direction in a subfascial plane while leaving the paratenon covering the flexor tendons. After identifying the radial pedicle at the wrist, the distal end is ligated and divided. A wavy-line incision extending to the antecubital fossa enables exposure of the proximal pedicle, and division at its origin from the brachial artery is performed before transfer of the flap to the tongue defect. The vessels are prepared with the aid of the operating microscope before anastomosis, frequently to the facial vessels with 9-0 nylon sutures.

Fasciocutaneous Lateral Arm Free Flap

The lateral arm flap (Fig. 62-3) was first introduced in 1982 by Song and co-workers as an alternative flap to the more popular radial forearm flap. Subsequent reports have further elucidated and expanded its use for the reconstruction of various head and neck defects. The lateral arm flap shares many of the desired qualities of the radial forearm flap, but its texture and favorable skin quality and color match, combined with its more esthetic donor site location, have earned it increasing popularity.

For tongue reconstruction, its adequate bulk, thinness, and pliability allow it to conform well to the shape of the defect. This flap also has a reliable vascular supply with good skin perfusion, an

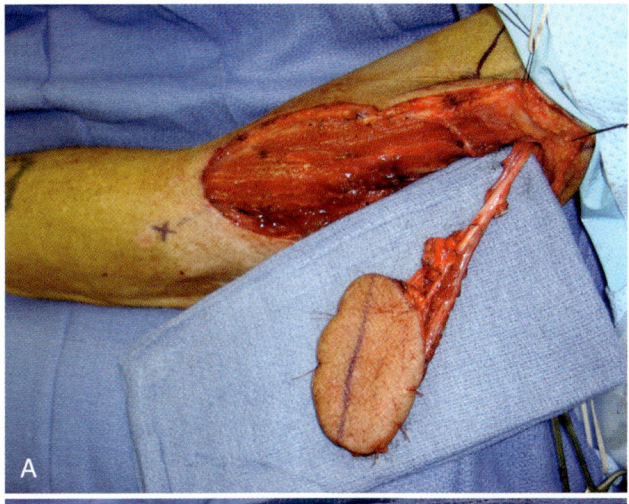

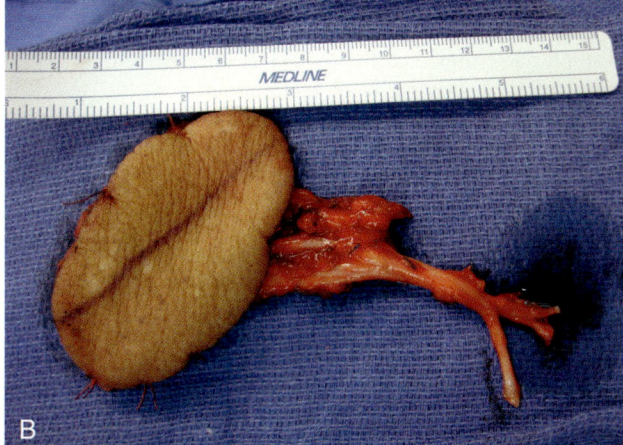

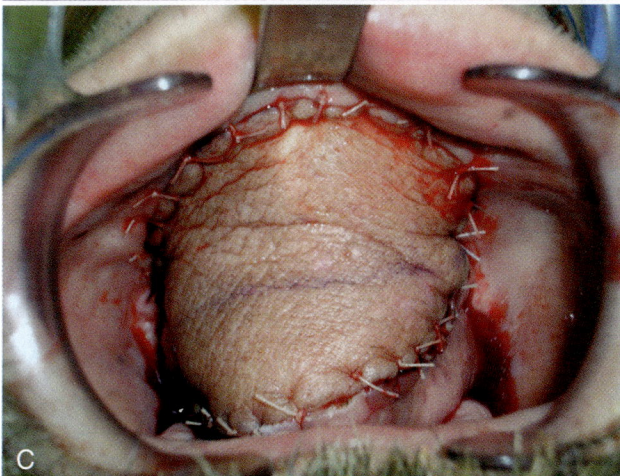

Fig. 62-3 ▪ Lateral arm flap. **A,** Lateral arm flap harvest before take-down. **B,** Flap before transfer to the oral cavity. **C,** Reconstructed tongue and floor of the mouth with a lateral arm flap.

vascular pedicle follows the radial nerve toward the spiral groove of the humerus. Venous drainage of the lateral arm skin is via the paired venae comitantes that follow the posterior radial collateral artery. The option of a sensate flap is possible if the posterior cutaneous nerve of the arm is harvested during flap elevation.

Pertinent landmarks for raising this flap are the deltoid insertion into the humerus, the lateral humeral epicondyle, and the lateral intermuscular septum, which lies on a line connecting these points. The desired skin island dimensions are outlined and centered on the intermuscular septum; however, flap width is limited by the ability to close the wound primarily. This feature, combined with the shorter pedicle length and smaller-caliber vessels, is its main limitation.

Following standard skin preparation and draping, the arm is placed in the flexed position with the wrist resting on the patient's abdomen to expose the lateral aspect of the upper part of the arm. The desired skin paddle dimensions are outlined and incisions are deepened to the brachial fascia. Once through this fascia, a posterior approach is used with dissection proceeding anteriorly toward the intermuscular septum to eventually reveal the vascular pedicle coursing inferiorly. After its identification, combined anterior and posterior dissection allows isolation and protection of the pedicle, with division of the brachial fascia off the underlying humerus permitting mobilization of the pedicle. The distal end of the pedicle is ligated and divided, and the pedicle is traced proximally to its origin at the spiral groove, where it is divided.

Microvascular anastomosis is once again performed with 10-0 nylon sutures under the operating microscope. Caliber mismatch of donor and recipient vessels is more of an issue with this flap because of the small-caliber vessels, which are commonly 1 mm or less in diameter.

SUBTOTAL/TOTAL GLOSSECTOMY DEFECTS

Anterolateral Thigh Flap

The anterolateral thigh (ALT) flap (Fig. 62-4) was first reported in 1984 by Song and co-authors as a septocutaneous perforator–based flap. Subsequent descriptions have since detailed its widespread applications, with the largest series to date published by Wei and colleagues in 2002, in which they reported their experience with 672 ALT flaps over a 5-year period.

The recent popularity of the ALT flap for head and neck reconstruction relates to its versatility of harvest; it can be raised as a subcutaneous, fasciocutaneous, myocutaneous, or adipofascial flap, depending on the demands and site of the ablative defect.

The abundance of tissue available from this donor site makes the ALT flap a well-suited reconstructive option for large tongue defects. Several studies have reported on speech and swallowing outcomes after reconstruction with the ALT flap for subtotal and total glossectomy. In such defects, improved speech intelligibility is achieved by restoring adequate flap bulk anteriorly to enable better contact between the neo-tongue and soft palate. The ALT flap meets this criterion comfortably. Furthermore, the aim of reconstruction after subtotal and total glossectomy should be to completely rehabilitate patients to full swallowing competency on their normal diet with no or minimal aspiration. Much emphasis is placed on restoring tongue volume, form, and when possible, sensation. Some authors claim that attempts to maintain flap innervation are crucial for preserving overall symmetry of the neo-tongue, which aids swallowing.

Sensate flaps remain a highly controversial topic, with advocates claiming that improved perception of the food bolus will produce superior swallowing outcomes through better oral bolus control, whereas others dispute this phenomenon and claim that ensuring

esthetically pleasing donor site, no impairment in perfusion of the distal upper extremity, and minimal donor site morbidity with donor defects commonly being closed primarily, thus avoiding skin grafts.

The vascularity of the lateral arm flap is based on septocutaneous branches arising from the posterior radial collateral artery, which originates from the profunda brachii artery. The cutaneous branches reach the skin via the lateral intermuscular septum, between the biceps and lateral head of the triceps muscles. Proximally, the

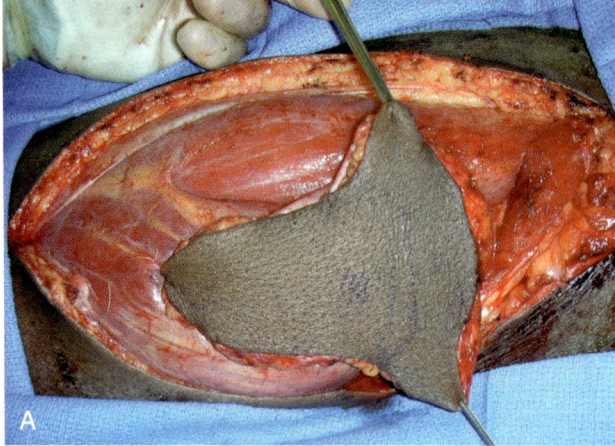

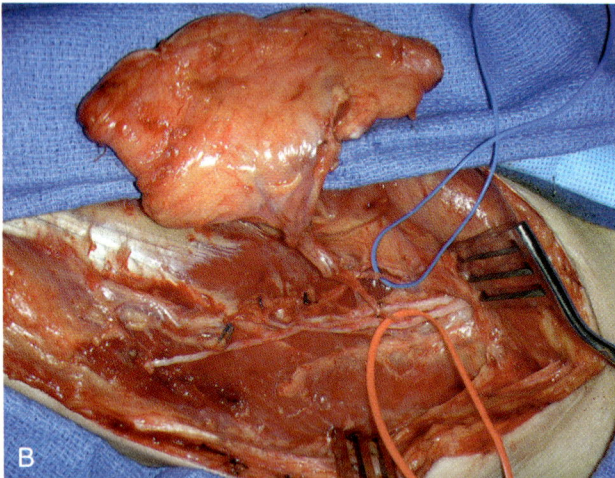

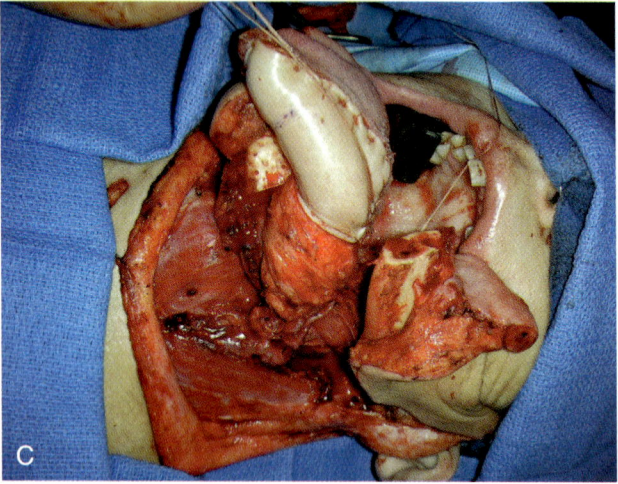

Fig. 62-4 ■ Anterolateral thigh (ALT) flap. **A,** ALT flap harvest for reconstruction of a total tongue defect. **B,** ALT flap in situ before harvest and transfer. **C,** ALT flap reconstruction of a hemi-tongue defect.

adequate mobility and recreating the original form of the tongue play a greater role in swallowing rehabilitation.

The ALT flap is supplied by septocutaneous (20% of cases) and septomyocutaneous (80% of cases) perforators arising from the descending branch of the lateral circumflex femoral artery. The descending branch travels inferiorly in the intermuscular septum between the rectus femoris and vastus lateralis muscles and gives rise to numerous perforators to the lateral thigh skin along its course.

The dominant sensory nerve supplying the area is the lateral femoral cutaneous nerve, a branch of the lumbar plexus, which passes through the thigh toward the fascia lata. This nerve may be harvested with the flap if sensory reinnervation is attempted. Its venous drainage is via paired venae comitantes.

Flap raising begins with delineation of relevant landmarks, including the anterior superior iliac spine and the upper lateral border of the patella. A line joining these points corresponds to the intermuscular septum underneath, and a 2-cm radius of skin around the midpoint of this line represents the area with the highest consistency and concentration of skin perforators. These are confirmed with Doppler and marked on the overlying skin, and the desired skin island is centered over these lines.

The incision begins on the medial aspect of the skin island and is extended superiorly and inferiorly and then deepened to the level of the deep fascia. At this point a thicker suprafascial or thinner subfascial flap can be developed, the former being a more tedious dissection. One continues to dissect toward the intermuscular septum from a medial approach while taking care to identify and preserve the Doppler-determined perforators. Once encountered, these perforators are traced proximally to their origin from the descending branch, at which time complete exposure of the intermuscular space is achieved by medial retraction of the rectus femoris. The pedicle is then dissected in retrograde fashion after completion of the lateral skin paddle incision. Where myocutaneous perforators are present, a small cuff of vastus lateralis surrounding the pedicle may be taken, thereby avoiding time-consuming intramuscular dissection and potential vessel trauma and kinking. After the origin of the descending branch from the profunda femoris is exposed, the pedicle can be ligated, divided, and transferred to the tongue defect with the pedicle tunneled into the neck for anastomosis.

Latissimus Dorsi Free Flap

The latissimus dorsi free flap (Fig. 62-5) was the first musculocutaneous flap described in the literature (by Tansini in 1896) for chest wall reconstruction after mastectomy; it remains a routinely used flap today in breast surgery. Its first reported use as a pedicled flap in the head and neck was by Quillen and co-workers in 1978, with Watson and associates performing the first successful microvascular transfer in 1979.

The latissimus dorsi free flap remains a popular flap in head and neck reconstruction, especially for large-volume defects, because of the abundance of donor tissue available, excellent length and caliber of the neurovascular pedicle, ease of harvest, anatomic consistency, and minimal donor site morbidity. Its use is ideally suited for cases of subtotal and total glossectomy when replacement of volume is critical, particularly in the anterior and anterolateral aspects of the neo-tongue to optimize the chance for successful swallowing rehabilitation and intelligible speech, a finding supported by many studies. Its major drawback is the necessity to turn the patient laterally intraoperatively, thus preventing a simultaneous two-team approach.

The latissimus dorsi is a broad flat muscle that covers a large area of the lower part of the back. It arises from the spinous processes of the lower six thoracic vertebrae, the thoracolumbar fascia, and the fascia of the iliac crest laterally. It inserts into the medial surface of the humerus to allow adduction, internal rotation, and extension of the arm during function.

The dominant vascular supply to this flap is via the thoracodorsal artery and vein, themselves being terminal branches of the subscapular artery and vein. Additional musculocutaneous perforators are located along its anterior border and distally from the segmental intercostal arteries. This anatomic appearance is consistent with

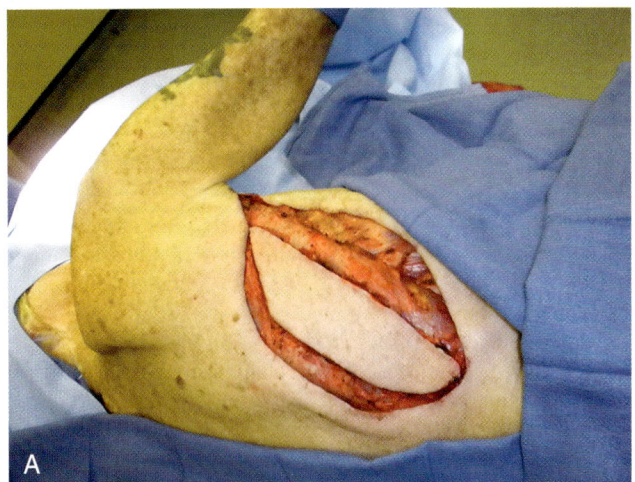

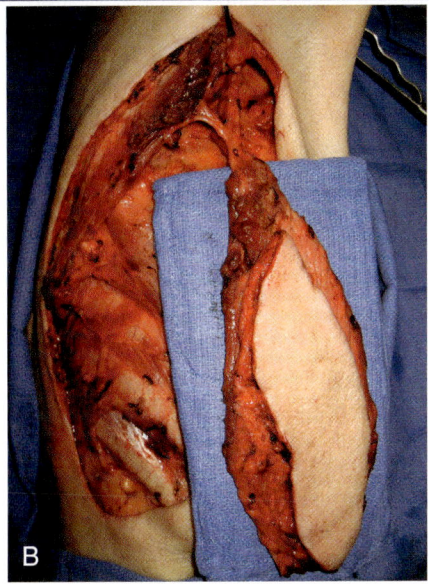

Fig. 62-5 ■ Latissimus flap. **A,** Harvest of a large latissimus flap. **B,** Mobilized latissimus flap with a dissected vascular pedicle before takedown and transfer.

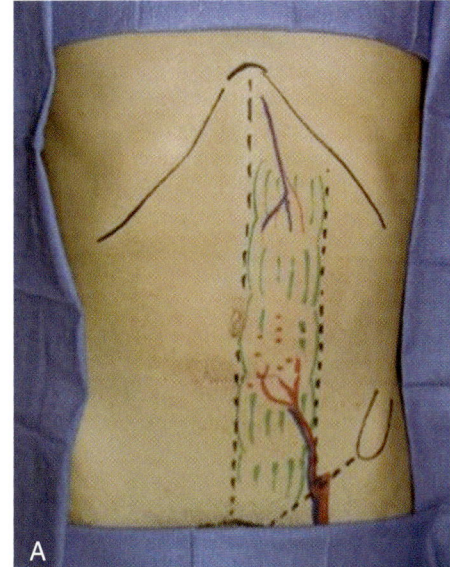

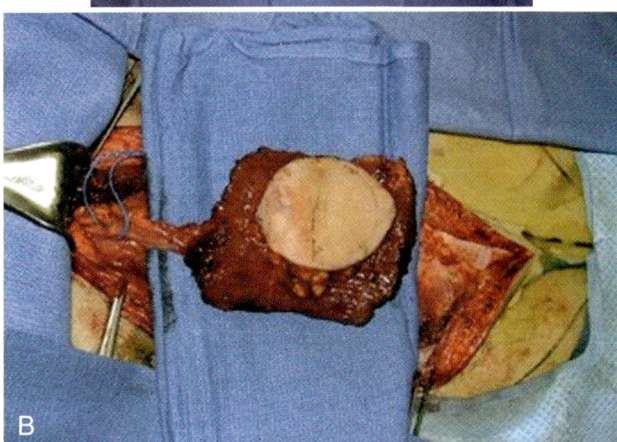

Fig. 62-6 ■ Rectus abdominis flap. **A,** Skin markings before harvest of a rectus abdominis flap. **B,** Harvested rectus flap before transfer to the oral cavity.

little variation. Its motor supply is via the thoracodorsal nerve, a useful nerve to harvest, which when anastomosed to a motor nerve in the head and neck prevents muscle atrophy and contracture of the flap.

Harvesting of a latissimus flap mandates positioning the patient in the lateral decubitus position with a pad supporting the head and neck on the contralateral side to prevent potential brachial plexus injury. The ipsilateral arm, shoulder, and back must be included in the preparation and draping of the operative field to allow uninhibited movement of the upper limb and unhindered access to the axilla.

The skin island should ideally be centered over the proximal two thirds of the muscle and within its anterior edge to ensure adequate skin perfusion from the underlying perforators. The skin incision proximal to the skin paddle is made 4 to 5 cm behind its anterior border and extended into the axilla. One then begins by incising the outlined skin paddle and continuing the incision into the axilla. Once through skin and subcutaneous fat, the plane of dissection is deepened until the anterior border of the muscle is identified and exposed along its entire anterior edge. One may encounter a prominent vessel supplying the serratus anterior muscle, which if traced proximally will lead directly to the thoracodorsal pedicle. Division of the

inferior extent of the muscle allows mobilization of the undersurface of the myocutaneous unit and, when combined with anterior dissection, will reveal the thoracodorsal pedicle coursing beneath the muscle and permit safe dissection of it cranially toward the axilla. Depending on the desired pedicle length, the thoracodorsal vessels are traced into the axilla until the circumflex scapula branch is seen. At this point the muscle overlying the pedicle proximally may be carefully divided, followed by ligation and division of the pedicle itself, and transferred to the tongue defect for inset and vessel anastomosis. Primary closure of the donor site over a suction drain is usually always achieved.

Rectus Abdominis Free Flap

Brown and colleagues in 1975 are credited with the first description of the use of cutaneous abdominal flaps (Fig. 62-6) based on perforators of the rectus abdominis muscle. This myocutaneous flap has assumed a central role in head and neck reconstruction because of its ease of harvest, long vascular pedicle, anatomic consistency, and tremendous reliability.

For tongue reconstruction it has assumed a pivotal role as the workhorse flap for subtotal and total glossectomy. Its bulk is suited to large extirpative defects in which replacement of volume is required. In tongue reconstruction, apart from restoring bulk to the site, it recontours well to the floor of the mouth, provides good coverage of the lingual mandible, and introduces stable, vascularized tissue that can withstand radiotherapy well. In addition, the favorable donor site position enables simultaneous tumor ablation and flap harvest, which significantly reduces operative time.

From a functional standpoint, reported results with regard to speech and swallowing outcomes are inconsistent. Although some studies report good uniform results, the experience of others is mixed, with a cohort of patients having poor speech intelligibility, swallowing dysfunction and aspiration necessitating dependence on gastrostomy, and problematic drooling.

The rectus abdominis flap is most commonly harvested as a myocutaneous flap with skin, subcutaneous fat, fascia, and muscle components. Advocates of this flap also recommend harvest of its innervating nerves, which appears to reduce denervation atrophy. Skin flap designs vary enormously, and the flap can be tailored to any defect. A more cephalad position of the skin island can also add significant length to the pedicle.

Like the ALT flap, a common limiting factor for the use of this flap in the Western population is a large body habitus because an excessive subcutaneous fat component may prove problematic for some defects.

Placement of the skin island, commonly in the para-umbilical region, allows capture of the greatest concentration of musculocutaneous perforators located in a zone 2 cm above and 3 cm below the umbilicus. The blood supply to the rectus abdominis is from the continuation of the internal mammary artery superiorly via the deep superior epigastric artery and vein and inferiorly from the deep inferior epigastric artery and vein. The two blood supplies meet in the midline to form a concentrated plexus. The mixed sensory and motor nerve supply is derived from the lower six intercostal nerves traversing in the plane between the transversus abdominis and internal oblique muscles.

Following design of the intended skin island, pertinent landmarks are outlined over the anterior abdominal wall, including the position of the palpable femoral vessels, costal margin, iliac crest, linea alba, and linea semilunaris. The deep inferior epigastric pedicle courses on the undersurface of the rectus abdominis. Flap harvest begins with an incision in the cephalad portion of the skin island and deepened down to the level of the anterior rectus sheath. The anterior sheath is then incised to reveal the rectus muscle, which is then exposed across its full width. Division of the cephalad portion of the muscle is performed with appropriate hemostasis to mobilize the upper aspect. The remaining skin paddle outline is completed with an incision down to the level of the muscle. The caudal aspect of the rectus is now exposed by a continuing inferior incision to allow longitudinal opening of the anterior rectus sheath. The skin paddle and underlying rectus muscle are then elevated off the posterior sheath carefully in a cephalad to caudal direction until the deep inferior epigastric pedicle is visualized so that the rectus muscle can be entered laterally. This will now define the inferior extent of the harvested rectus muscle, and attention can then be diverted to dissection of the pedicle proximally to its origin from the iliac vessels. Ligation and transection of the pedicle are performed to complete harvesting of the flap.

The donor site is closed over a suction drain. Insertion of mesh to restore the anterior rectus sheath defect is frequently performed to prevent ventral wall herniation, although this practice remains controversial.

POSTOPERATIVE CARE

All patients following ablative or reconstructive surgery for diseases of the tongue, most commonly malignancy, require a minimum standard of postoperative care, which varies little between head and neck surgery units.

Postoperative care in such patients is divided into general and specific issues, with specific care being further divided into that related to the donor and recipient sites.

General postoperative care of any head and neck surgery patient begins immediately after surgery. Most patients following any volume of tongue resection require varying lengths of postoperative monitoring and hospital stay consistent with the complexity of their surgery. Patient monitoring after tongue resection is important and consists of close observation for tongue swelling, bleeding, and any associated airway distress; such monitoring may take place in an intensive care environment or in a specialized head and neck surgery ward.

Other aspects of care common to every surgical patient involve commencement of appropriate prophylactic antibiotics, relevant prophylaxis for deep vein thrombosis, and intravenous fluid replacement and maintenance.

Specific to patients who have undergone any head and neck surgery is consideration of alternative methods of feeding and nutritional supplementation. In most cases it is common practice to keep patients fasted postoperatively for variable lengths of time to avoid contamination of the oral/pharyngeal reconstruction site. Nasoenteric or gastrostomy feeding is initiated early after surgery to avoid detrimental catabolic states.

Specific postoperative care issues following large tongue resections involve standard tracheostomy care. Nursing care is necessary to ensure that tracheostomy tubes are secure, wounds remain clean and dry, and pulmonary toilet with regular tracheal suctioning takes place to avoid respiratory sepsis. Chest physiotherapy may be necessary to help patients with mobilization and clearance of secretions.

The oral environment—and specifically the flap—is kept clean by gentle débridement with chlorhexidine-soaked swabs.

When a microvascular flap has been used for tongue reconstruction, regular flap observation is critical for early detection of threatened viability. Flap observation with note of skin color, temperature, capillary refill, and bleeding on pinprick is universal. In addition, Doppler assessment to confirm flap perfusion is routine in some units.

Speech and swallowing therapy assessment is vital in patients after significant tongue resections to determine safe commencement of oral feeding and identify patients with aspiration.

Individual donor sites also have specific care requirements pertinent to each donor site. Generally, each donor site should be kept clean and dressed and then inspected in 5 to 7 days, at which time sutures or skin staples may require removal. Suction drains are maintained and removed when there is minimal discharge.

PEARLS AND PITFALLS

- Outcomes following tongue reconstruction vary and are directly proportional to the volume of tongue resected and the method of reconstruction used.
- Small tongue defects that are closed primarily or with local flaps have better functional outcomes and quality-of-life scores than do larger defects. As the amount of tongue removed increases, the impact on speech and swallowing becomes more obvious and measurable. This trend has been confirmed by many studies.
- As the size of the defect increases, replacement of the missing tongue volume necessitates free tissue transfer. The reconstructive objective in these circumstances is restoration of form closely resembling the natural tongue and maintenance of good tongue mobility. Prevention of tongue restriction and tethering is core to establishing optimal speech intelligibility and return to an oral diet.
- After subtotal and total glossectomy, functional outcomes are influenced by both the type of reconstruction and the attention given to recreation of a neo-tongue during flap inset. Adjunctive procedures, including laryngeal suspension, epiglottic laryngoplasty, and innervation of flaps, have also been shown in various reports to improve outcomes and prevent complications.
- The addition of flap innervation in tongue reconstruction to restore sensation has shown variable outcomes. More important in cases of subtotal and total glossectomy is the use of innervated flaps to prevent flap contracture secondary to muscle atrophy. Anastomosis of the motor nerve innervating the flap to a recipient motor nerve in the head and neck site has proved effective and translates to better speech and swallowing rehabilitation and quality of life.

BIBLIOGRAPHY

Bokhari WA, Wong SJ: Tongue reconstruction: recent advances, *Curr Opin Otolaryngol Head Neck Surg* 15:202-207, 2007.

Bozola AR, Gasques JA, Carriquiry CE, Cardoso de Oliveira M: The buccinators musculomucosal flap: anatomic study and clinical application, *Plast Reconstr Surg* 84(2):250-257, 1989.

Brandt K, Khouri R: The lateral arm/proximal forearm flap, *Plast Reconstr Surg* 92:1137-1143, 1993.

Brown RG, Vasconez LO, Jurkiewicz MJ: Transverse abdominal flaps and the deep epigastric arcade, *Plast Reconstr Surg* 55(4):416-421, 1975.

Chana JS, Wei FC: A review of the advantages of the anterolateral thigh flap in head and neck reconstruction, *Br J Plast Surg* 57:603-609, 2004.

Haddock NT, DeLacure MD, Saadeh PB: Functional reconstruction of glossectomy defects: the vertical rectus abdominis myocutaneous neotongue, *J Reconstr Microsurg* 24:343-350, 2008.

Kapur KK, Garrett NR, Fischer E: Effects of anaesthesia of human oral structures on masticatory performance and food particle size distribution, *Arch Oral Biol* 35:397-403, 1990.

Magrin J, Kowalski LP, Sabóia M, et al: Major glossectomy: end results of 106 cases, *Eur J Cancer B Oral Oncol* 32B:407-412, 1996.

Martin D, Pascal JF, Baudet J, et al: The submental island flap: a new donor site. Anatomy and clinical applications as a free or pedicled flap, *Plast Reconstr Surg* 92:867-873, 1993.

Matsui Y, Shirota T, Yamashita Y, et al: Analyses of speech intelligibility in patients after glossectomy and reconstruction with fasciocutaneous/myocutaneous flaps, *Int J Oral Maxillofac Surg* 38:339-345, 2009.

Pribaz J, Stephens W, Crespo L, Gifford G: A new intraoral flap: facial artery musculomucosal (FAMM) flap, *Plast Reconstr Surg* 90(3):421-429, 1992.

Quillen CG, Shearin JC Jr., Georgiade NG: Use of the latissimus dorsi myocutaneous island flap for reconstruction in the head and neck area: case report, *Plast Reconstr Surg* 62(1):113-117, 1978.

Sabri AN, Sniezek J, Burkey BB: Sensate free flaps, *Operative Techniques Otolaryngol Head Neck Surg* 11:195-197, 2000.

Song R, Gao Y, Song Y, et al: the forearm flap, *Clin Plast Surg* 9(1):21-26, 1982.

Song R, Song Y, Yu Y, et al: The upper arm free flap, *Clin Plast Surg* 9(1):27-35, 1982.

Tansini I: Nuovo process per l'amputazione della mammilla per cancre, *Reforma Med* 12:3-5, 1896.

Vaughan ED: The radial forearm free flap in orofacial reconstruction. Personal experience in 120 consecutive cases, *J Craniomaxillofac Surg* 18:2-7, 1990.

Vural E, Suen JY: The submental island flap in head and neck reconstruction, *Head Neck* 22:572-578, 2000.

Watson JS, Craig RD, Orton CI: The free latissimus dorsi myocutaneous flap, *Plast Reconstr Surg* 64(3):299-305, 1979.

Wei FC, Jain V, Celik N, et al: Have we found and ideal soft-tissue flap? An experience with 672 anterolateral thigh flaps, *Plast Reconstr Surg* 109(7):2219-2226, discussion 2227-2230, 2002.

Yanai C, Kikutani T, Adachi M, et al: Functional outcome after total and subtotal glossectomy with free flap reconstruction, *Head Neck* 30:909-918, 2008.

Yang G, Chen B, Gao Y: Forearm free skin flap transplantation, *Nat Med J China* 61:139, 1981.

Zhao Z, Zhang Z, Li Y, et al: The musculomucosal island flap for partial tongue reconstruction, *J Am Coll Surg* 196:753-760, 2003.

Lip Cancer—Ablative and Reconstructive Surgery

Eric R. Carlson, Andres Guerra

Lip cancer is one of the more common cancers of the head and neck region and should be one of the most curable because of its ability to be detected in the early stages. In general terms, its prognosis is quite favorable, with 5-year survival statistics exceeding 90% in most reports. Some lip cancers have been observed to exhibit aggressive behavior, however, with recurrence or mortality noted in up to 15% of cases. Lymph node metastases seem to occur in 5% to 20% of patients, and the overall incidence is quoted at 10%. The frequency of lip cancer varies internationally, with an incidence of 30% of all cases of oral cancer in certain regions. In the United States the incidence of lip cancer is 1.8 per 100,000 population.

Lip cancer is occasionally described as being one of the *oral* cancers. These authors choose to consider lip cancer as one of the facial *skin* cancers for anatomic and logistic reasons. Anatomically, the most common location for lip cancer is the vermilion or mucocutaneous junction. In general, the behavior of cancer of the lip is similar to that of skin cancer rather than oral mucosal cancer in terms of both survival and lymph node metastases. Finally, the most frequently identified carcinogen of the most common lower lip cancer, squamous cell carcinoma, is ultraviolet radiation, as is the case for the most common type of upper lip cancer, basal cell carcinoma. For these reasons, lip cancer should be considered a skin cancer rather than an oral cancer.

Approximately 90% of cases of lip cancer occur on the lower lip, with nearly 7% of cases occurring on the upper lip and the remainder located at the commissure. Squamous cell carcinoma is clearly the most common histologic variant, with basal cell carcinoma, melanoma, and minor salivary gland cancers of mucosal origin constituting the other histologic variants. The latter diagnosis is certainly an exception to the previous statement that lip cancer should be considered a skin cancer rather than an oral cancer. When they occur, minor salivary gland neoplasms are most commonly seen within the mucosa of the upper lip, and the overwhelming majority of these tumors are benign. Approximately 95% of lip cancers occur in men, typically those older than 50 years. The most common age range at diagnosis is 54 to 65 years, although these cancers will occasionally occur in patients younger than 30 years.

ETIOPATHOGENESIS/CAUSATIVE FACTORS

The etiology of lip cancer is probably best described as multifactorial and perhaps poorly understood, as is the case with many human cancers. Approximately a third of lip cancers are associated with excessive sun exposure in patients with outdoor occupations. Most tumors originate on the exposed vermilion of the lower lip. Lip cancer is seen commonly in patients with second primary skin malignancies. Like other head and neck skin cancers, these patients may have light complexions, freckles, blue eyes, and fair-colored hair. The lower lip is at higher risk for skin cancer than the upper lip because of the prominence of the lower lip. This anatomic feature accounts for the discrepancy between the incidence of upper and lower lip cancers. The prevalence of lip cancer is at least 10 times higher in whites than in those with darker skin, and it is very rare in black people.

Other risk factors for lip cancer include the traditional carcinogens for head and neck cancer such as cigarette and pipe smoking, lip trauma, and immunosuppression. Although these risk factors may be related to the development of lip cancer, the overwhelming anecdotal evidence points to prolonged and cumulative sun exposure as the most significant carcinogen involved in the development of melanoma and non-melanoma lip cancers.

PATHOLOGIC ANATOMY

The upper lip is formed embryologically by fusion of the lateral maxillary processes and a central nasofrontal process. Because of anatomic separation of the lateral segments, contralateral lymphatic cervical metastases are quite rare from upper lip cancers. This anatomic feature is in contradistinction to the lower lip, which forms by the fusion of two lateral mandibular processes in the midline. Lower lip cancers, therefore, are at higher risk for contralateral metastasis. The blood supply to the lips is derived from the superior and inferior labial arteries.

Lymphatic drainage of the lips follows a predictable course of metastatic dissemination. Lymph node metastases related to lip cancer occur in fewer than 10% of patients with cancer of the lower lip and in up to 20% of patients with cancer of the upper lip and commissure. Cancers of the lateral aspect of the upper lip preferentially metastasize to the buccal, periparotid, and preauricular region overlying the body of the mandible. Secondary metastases will occur to the cervical lymph nodes in the submandibular triangle. Cancers of the lower lip preferentially drain into the cervical lymph nodes of the submental and submandibular triangles of level I cervical lymph nodes. Subsequent metastases can occur in level II and III lymph nodes. Dissemination to level IV and V lymph nodes is quite rare, although when cervical metastases do occur from lower lip cancers, bilateral level I metastases are not uncommon.

The sensory nerve distribution of the upper and lower lips is provided by the maxillary and mandibular divisions of the trigeminal nerve, respectively. The neurosensory innervation of the lower lip is of significance in the evaluation of patients with lower lip cancer, specifically with regard to obtaining a screening panoramic radiograph to rule out mandibular involvement by the cancer as a result of perineural spread (Fig. 63-1).

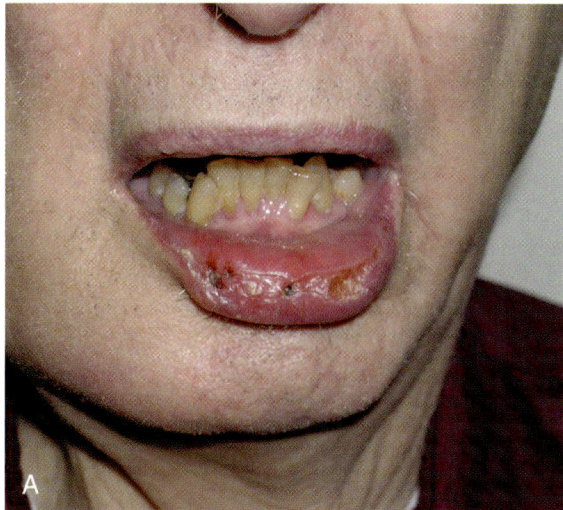

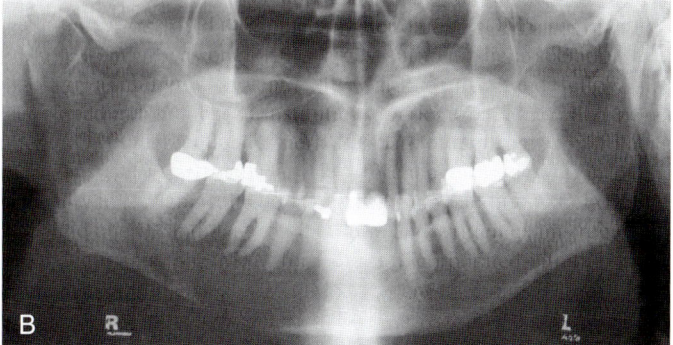

Fig. 63-1 ■ **A,** Biopsy-proven squamous cell carcinoma of the lower lip in an 85-year-old man. This cancer shows a flat ulcer rather than an elevated mass. **B,** The utility of obtaining a panoramic radiograph in patients with lower lip cancer is noted in this image, which shows significant bone erosion in the right mandible by virtue of perineural spread of the cancer.

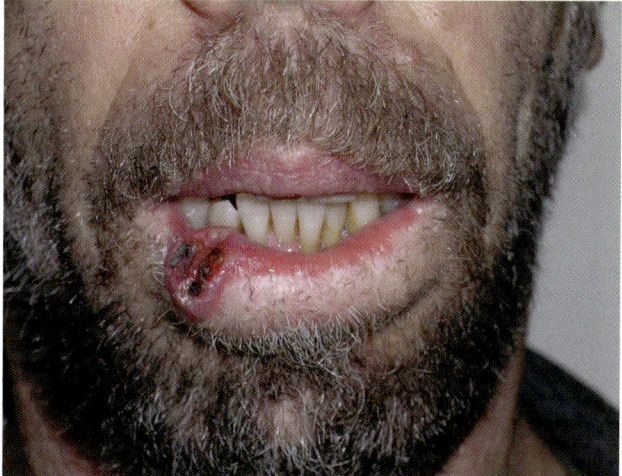

Fig. 63-2 ■ This lower lip cancer has formed a mass.

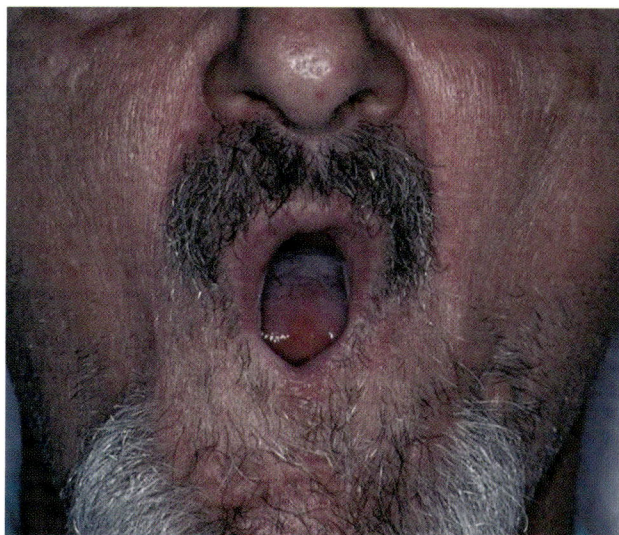

Fig. 63-3 ■ This patient underwent wedge excision of extensive cancer of his lower lip with primary closure. The result is profound microstomia. This result of this patient's surgery is a testimony to the need to offer flap reconstruction to patients undergoing removal of large lower lip cancers to avoid microstomia.

DIAGNOSTIC STUDIES

The history, physical examination, and incisional biopsy are the most valuable tools in establishing a diagnosis of lip cancer. A history of a non-healing crusted lesion of the lip that persists for several months is typical. Physical examination will reveal an area of crusting and surrounding induration or a mass, depending on the chronicity of the cancer (Fig. 63-2). The incisional biopsy should be performed within the center of the lesion to establish the diagnosis. Once the diagnosis has been made, it is most important to obtain a panoramic radiograph to investigate for a widened mental foramen or erosion of the mandible, which could occur by perineural spread of a lower lip cancer (see Fig. 63-1). In general terms, special imaging studies such as computed tomography (CT), magnetic resonance imaging, and positron emission tomography (PET/CT) are not required to assist in ablative surgery associated with a lip cancer when clinical neck examination does not reveal suspicious adenopathy (N0). When the neck is classified as N+, however, special imaging studies, particularly PET/CT, are indicated. This is especially the case when unilateral adenopathy exists in association with a lower lip cancer and PET/CT will provide images of the contralateral neck. Distant metastases are identified in less than 2% of patients at the time of initial evaluation of a previously untreated lip carcinoma. In preparation for ablative surgery performed in an operating room setting, routine blood work, an electrocardiogram, and chest radiographs are obtained according to standards set by the surgeon's operating room and attending anesthesiologists.

TREATMENT/RECONSTRUCTIVE GOALS

Management of lip cancer should include the objectives of proper ablation of the patient's cancer and functionally and esthetically acceptable immediate biologic reconstruction of the lip. To this end, lip cancer is unique in that there is no ability to negotiate for delayed biologic reconstruction. This statement represents a departure from the management of some head and neck cancers, where alloplastic reconstruction of the mandible with a bone plate can take place while performing delayed biologic reconstructive surgery of a segmental defect. Lip cancer must be managed with immediate soft tissue reconstruction. In so doing, the reconstruction must be performed in a manner that avoids microstomia (Fig. 63-3). Soft tissue flaps, as may be used in these reconstructions, may be categorized according to their blood supply. Three flap patterns are recognized:

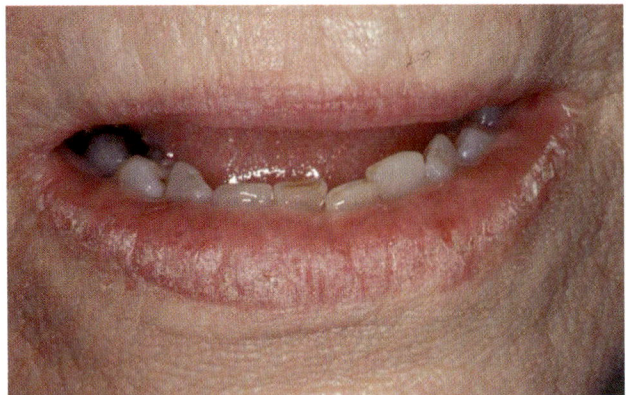

Fig. 63-4 ■ Actinic keratosis of the lower lip. The lip is white and dry.

random-pattern, axial-pattern, and microvascular free flaps. Random-pattern flaps are those in which specific pedicles are not identified or necessarily preserved within the flap. By contrast, an axial-pattern flap is one in which the pedicle is identified and intentionally preserved within the flap that is rotated into the recipient tissue bed. Axial-pattern flaps for head and neck reconstruction may be local or regional according to their anatomic site of origin, whereas axial- and random-pattern flaps for lip reconstruction are distinctly local in nature. Finally, microvascular flaps involve distant soft tissue transfers in which arterial and venous anastomoses are required for flap viability.

Any discussion of cancer undoubtedly warrants a discussion of pre-cancer. The most common pre-cancer of the lower lip is actinic keratosis (Fig. 63-4). Actinic keratosis results from damage to the lower lip by ultraviolet radiation. It is named for the white color of the vermilion of the lower lip that is affected by actinic keratosis. The lip is also characteristically dry in its appearance. Ulcerations may be present, but a mass is not noted in patients with actinic keratosis. Histologic evaluation of actinic keratosis may reveal signs of dysplasia or carcinoma in situ. When a mass is present, a diagnosis of invasive cancer is almost certain to be established through the required incisional biopsy. Actinic keratosis is a clinical diagnosis that does not require preoperative incisional biopsy but certainly necessitates histologic confirmation at the time of excision.

SPECIFIC TREATMENT AND TECHNIQUES

Ablative and reconstructive surgery of the lips is performed in an operating room setting with nasoendotracheal intubation. Oral intubation may distort the anatomy of the lips and therefore alter the geometry of the reconstruction.

VERMILIONECTOMY (LIP SHAVE) AND MUCOSAL ADVANCEMENT FLAP

Vermilionectomy, also known as a lip shave, is indicated for the management of actinic keratosis with or without dysplasia. In addition, micro-invasive squamous cell carcinoma may be managed successfully with vermilionectomy, provided that excision of the cancer is accomplished with a negative deep margin in the vermilionectomy. Frankly invasive cancer based on incisional biopsy represents a contraindication to vermilionectomy. The vermilionectomy must be performed from commissure to commissure because of the diffuse nature of lower lip actinic keratosis. In addition, the cosmetic result of a mucosal advancement flap is enhanced by complete lower lip mucosal reconstruction. Partial vermilionectomy with an isolated

mucosal advancement flap will create a stark color difference in the reconstruction that will be esthetically unacceptable. Following vermilionectomy and frozen section analysis of the specimen, the remaining lower lip mucosa is undermined and advanced in uniform fashion to permit closure in a single layer without undue tension and with a smooth contour (Fig. 63-5).

WEDGE EXCISION AND PRIMARY CLOSURE

Invasive cancers of the upper and lower lips require full-thickness excision and immediate reconstruction, depending on the magnitude of the excision. When the excision involves up to a third of the lower lip, wedge excision may be performed with linear primary closure (Fig. 63-6). Some authors have recommended wedge excision and primary closure for defects measuring up to half the lower lip. Perhaps the most important factor in using this technique is the laxity of the remaining tissues of the lower lip and face. An older patient with relatively greater tissue redundancy may be able to undergo primary closure of a relatively large defect that would require local flap reconstruction in a younger patient with less laxity of the surrounding soft tissues. One contraindication to wedge excision and primary closure is extension of the lip cancer to the oral commissure. The wedge excision should not cross the labiomental fold since hypertrophic scars tend to occur in this location.

BLOCK EXCISION WITH KARAPANDZIC FLAP RECONSTRUCTION

Cancer excisions involving between half and two thirds of the upper or lower lips cannot be reconstructed with primary closure without introducing microstomia. In these circumstances, local flap reconstruction is required. In fact, the surgeon may wish to implement local flap reconstruction of the lower lip when excising less than half of it. The Karapandzic flap is such a reconstruction (Fig. 63-7). These flaps were originally described in 1974 and based on the facial artery. Block excision of the lip is designed to accommodate the Karapandzic flap reconstruction. Following excision of the lip cancer and frozen section analysis of the margins of the specimen, the flap design is accomplished. In so doing, assessment is made of the need for bilateral flaps. As the magnitude of the excision increases, the need for bilateral Karapandzic flaps also increases, particularly in cases in which the excision crosses the midline of the lower lip. The relaxed skin tension lines of the nasolabial folds are used for development of the flaps. These flaps are created through skin and muscle but do not communicate with the oral cavity. When an upper lip cancer is excised, the reconstruction is accomplished with *reverse* Karapandzic flaps (Fig. 63-8). As discussed previously, some small cancers may be excised and reconstruction performed with Karapandzic flaps in younger patients who do not have acceptable surrounding soft tissue laxity to permit closure primarily. If any doubt exists about the possibility of postoperative microstomia, the surgeon should excise the lip cancer and perform reconstruction with a local flap as opposed to wedge excision with primary closure. As with wedge excision, Karapandzic flap reconstruction is contraindicated when the commissure is excised with the specimen.

WEDGE EXCISION WITH AN ABBE FLAP OR ABBE-ESTLANDER FLAP RECONSTRUCTION

The Abbe flap was originally reported by several authors in the 19th century before Abbe's description, after which the technique took his name. The flap is a two-staged procedure that represents a cross-transfer of full-thickness tissue from one lip to the other and is limited in the amount of tissue that it can reconstruct. When used to

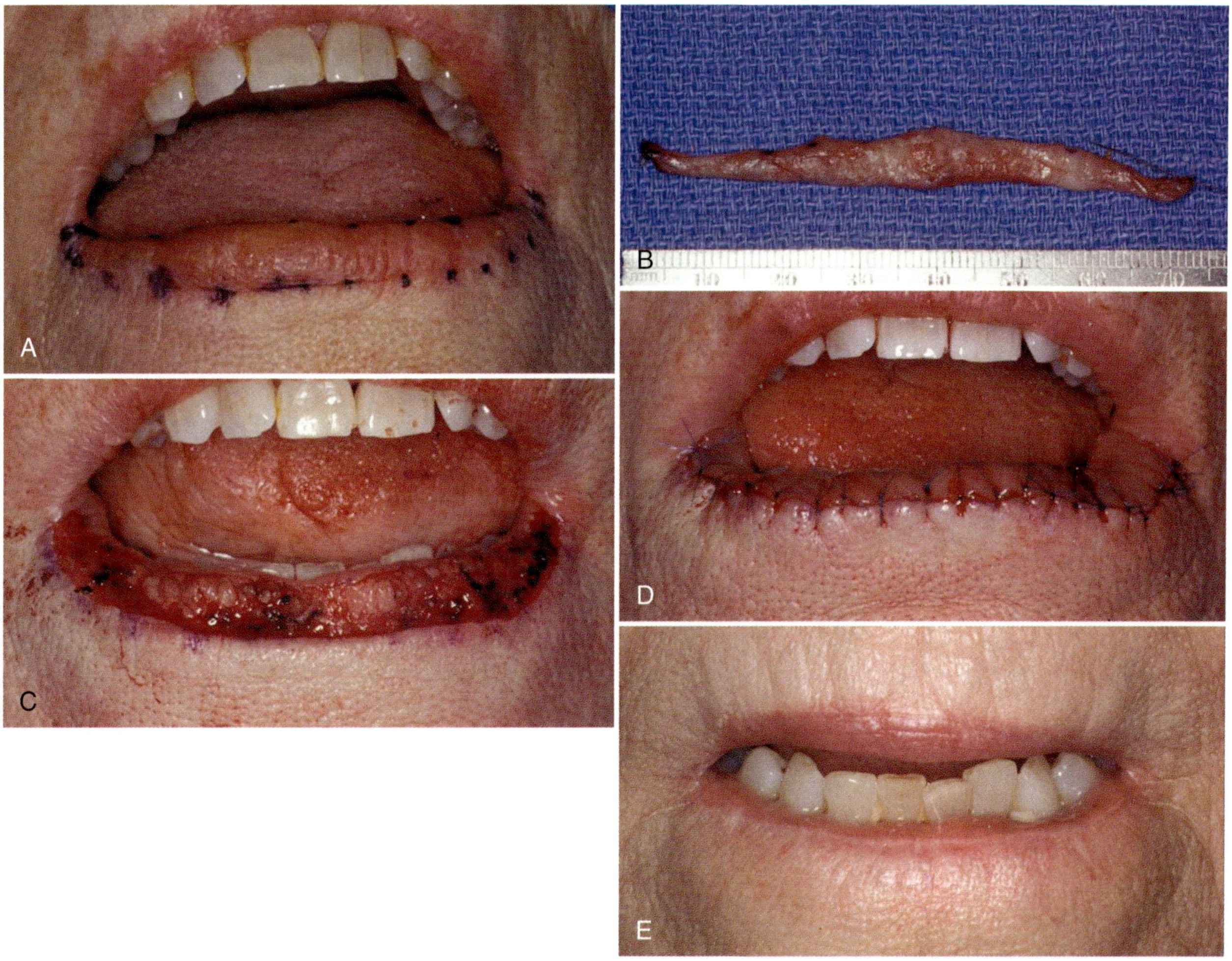

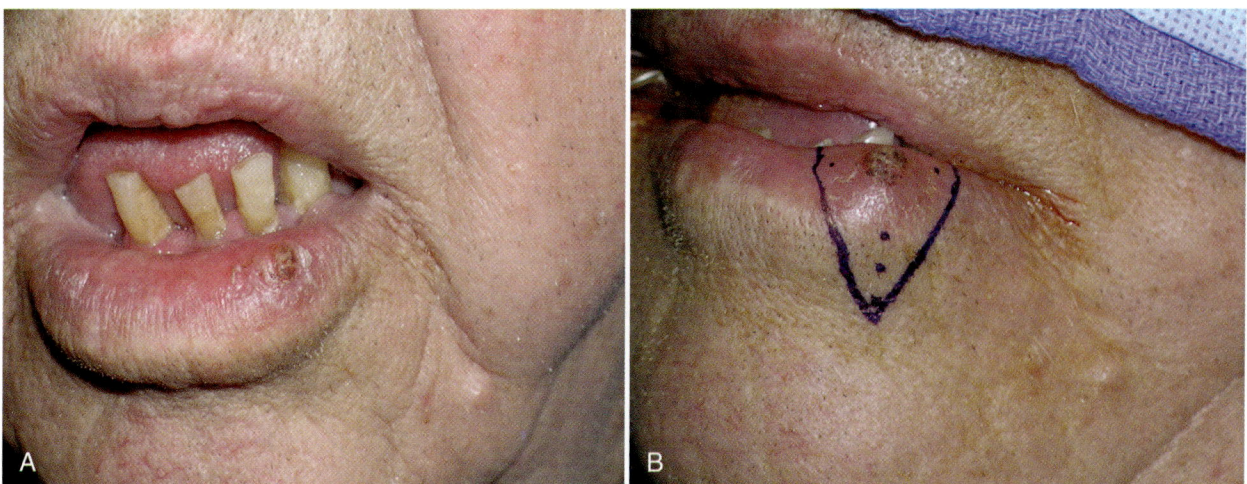

Fig. 63-5 ■ **A,** A vermilionectomy (lip shave) is demarcated that will excise the entire vermilion. **B,** The specimen is examined histologically for dysplasia and the presence of invasive squamous cell carcinoma. **C,** The defect is noted. Care is taken to preserve the anatomic location of the terminal portions of the mental nerves. **D,** The lower lip mucosa is undermined, advanced, and closed primarily in single-layer fashion. **E,** Result of this patient's vermilionectomy 1 year postoperatively.

Fig. 63-6 ■ **A,** This biopsy-proven squamous cell carcinoma of the lower lip is able to be managed by wedge excision with primary closure since the cancer occupies approximately a third of the lower lip. **B,** The wedge excision is demarcated with a skin-marking pen. Note that the commissure is preserved in the excision, the inferior aspect of the excision does not cross the mentolabial fold, and the dimensions of the excision do not exceed a third of the lower lip. All three issues must be observed when performing a wedge excision.

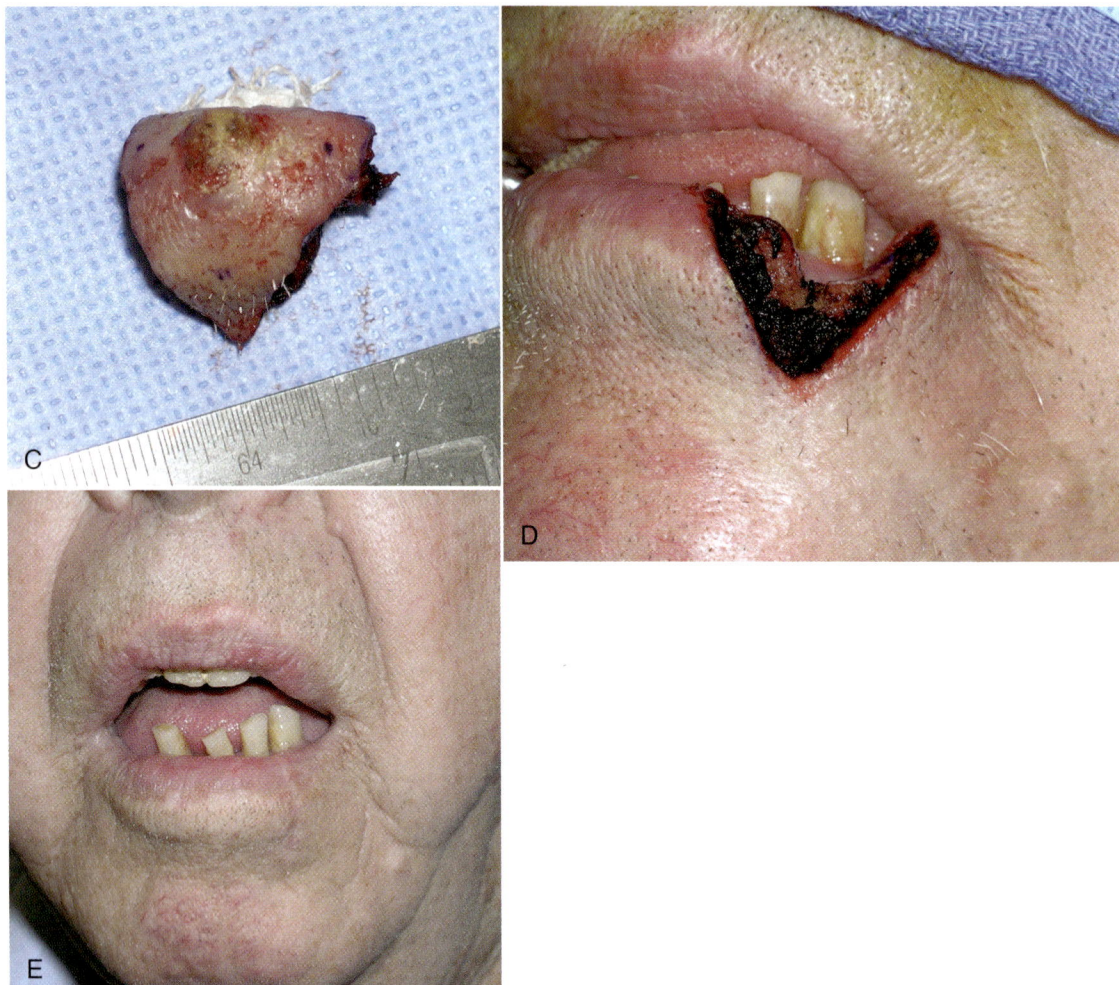

Fig. 63-6, cont'd ▪ **C,** The specimen is examined by frozen section for complete excision. **D,** The resultant defect is noted. **E,** Result of this patient's wedge excision 1 year postoperatively.

reconstruct an upper lip defect, a flap consisting of a quarter of the lower lip is used to reconstruct as much as a third of the upper lip (Fig. 63-9). The height of the defect and the height of the flap must coincide. The flap is based on the labial artery in the vermilion of the lip. Advantages of the Abbe flap include acceptable skin texture and color match with the surrounding tissue of the recipient tissue bed. Following primary closure, the pedicle crosses the oral stoma and may be severed in 2 to 3 weeks. The Abbe-Estlander flap was originally designed to reconstruct defects near the oral commissure (Fig. 63-10). The medial pedicle of the flap is used to reconstruct the commissure.

BLOCK EXCISION WITH THE WEBSTER MODIFICATION OF BERNARD CHEILOPLASTY

Defects created by excision of cancer involving more than two thirds of the lower lip may be reconstructed with the Webster modification of the Bernard cheiloplasty. First described in 1960, this technique is random pattern in nature and requires the development of Burow's triangles in its implementation (Fig. 63-11). Burow's triangles are designed so that the medial vertical limb is incorporated into the nasolabial fold. The width of the base of the triangle is designed so that the distance from the oral commissure to the lateral portion of the base equals half the width of lip tissue excised. This type of reconstruction is suitable for restoration of the lower lip when neck

dissection is not being performed. Laxity of the buccal region, as occurs in older patients, is required to advance bilateral cheek tissue into the reconstruction. The Webster modification of the Bernard cheiloplasty is particularly suited to reconstruction of the oral commissure and should be considered first in such circumstances.

EXCISION WITH FREE MICROVASCULAR FLAP RECONSTRUCTION

Defects created by excision of cancer of the entire lower lip and adjacent facial soft tissues may be reconstructed with a distant flap. When neck dissection is planned as part of such cancer surgery and the carotid artery and internal jugular vein will be dissected and preserved, reconstruction involving microvascular anastomosis is most appropriate (Fig. 63-12). The radial forearm free flap is a fasciocutaneous flap based on the radial artery and vein and the venae comitantes. The soft tissue is relatively thin and well suited for full-thickness lower lip defects when skin and mucosa must be reconstructed. The large available skin paddle from the forearm permits reconstruction of large defects involving the entire lower lip and surrounding facial skin that would not be able to be reconstructed with the local flaps previously reviewed in this chapter. In addition, the skin paddle can be centered over the palmaris longus tendon and the skin folded over this tendon to provide internal and external skin lining. The two ends of the palmaris longus tendon can

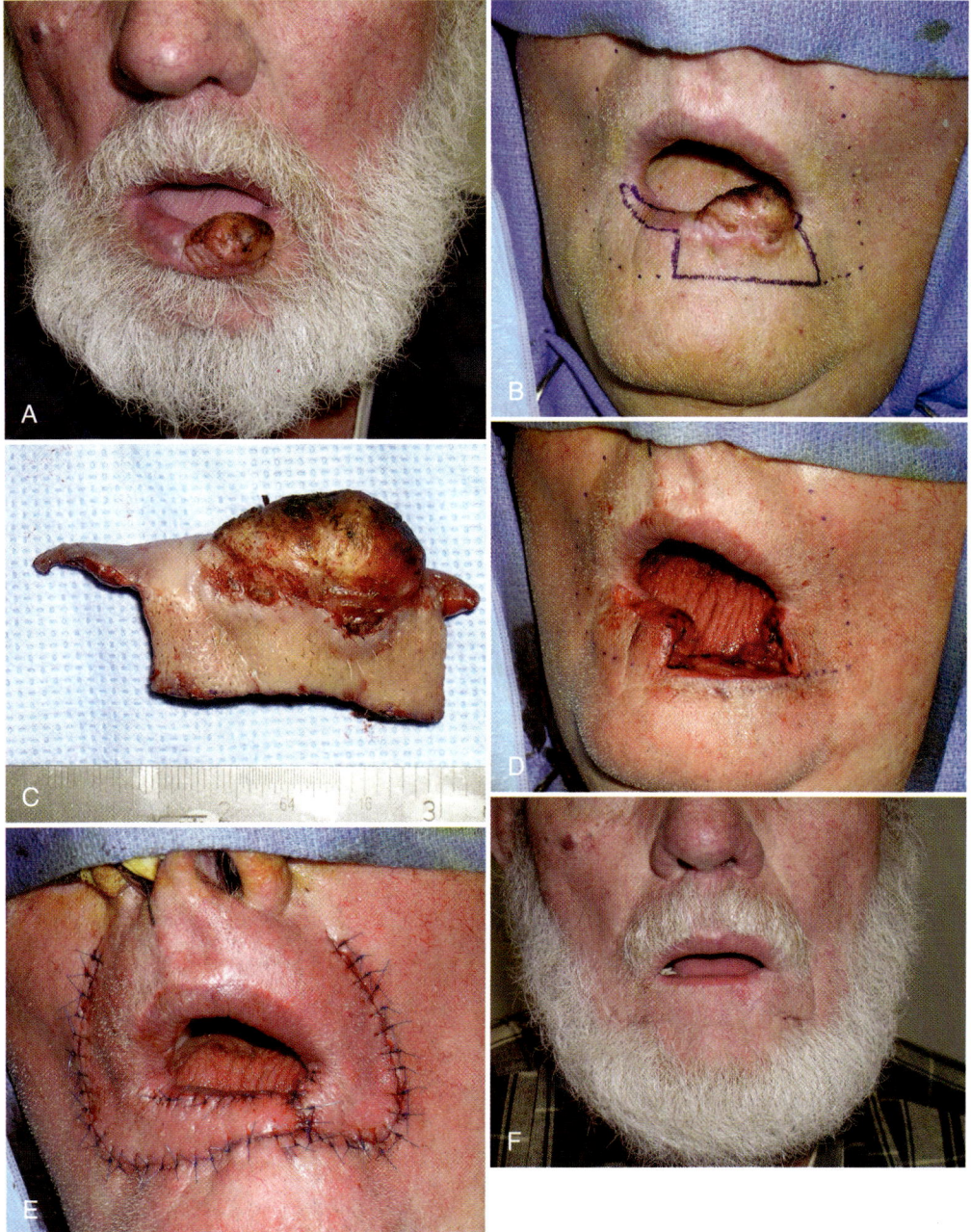

Fig. 63-7 ■ **A,** This large, biopsy-proven squamous cell carcinoma occupies approximately half of the lower lip. Consequently, wedge excision and primary closure cannot be performed because it would probably result in microstomia. The vermilion shows diffuse actinic keratosis. **B,** A block excision and vermilionectomy are outlined. This excision design will permit reconstruction with Karapandzic flaps as outlined. **C,** The specimen should be examined for adequacy of excision with frozen sections. **D,** The resultant defect of the lower lip is noted. **E,** Reconstruction is performed with Karapandzic flaps and a mucosal advancement flap. **F,** One-year postoperative result.

be attached to the remaining orbicularis oris muscle to suspend and support the reconstruction.

POSTOPERATIVE CARE

Postoperative care of patients undergoing ablative and reconstructive surgery for lip cancer typically involves suture line care and effective oral hygiene by the patient. Sutures and neck drains in the event of neck dissection are most commonly removed 1 week postoperatively. The lip specimen must be thoroughly evaluated histologically for perineural/intraneural invasion by the cancer (Fig. 63-13). When perineural/intraneural invasion is present, postoperative radiation therapy is indicated and should be initiated by 6 to 8 weeks postoperatively. In these circumstances, patients should be monitored indefinitely because of the high likelihood of recurrent disease and their inherently poor prognosis. There is reasonable medical justification for providing long-term follow-up for the remainder of patients who have undergone surgery for lip cancer, despite a good prognosis, to detect an unlikely focus of recurrent disease associated with the lip cancer.

Text continued on p. 526

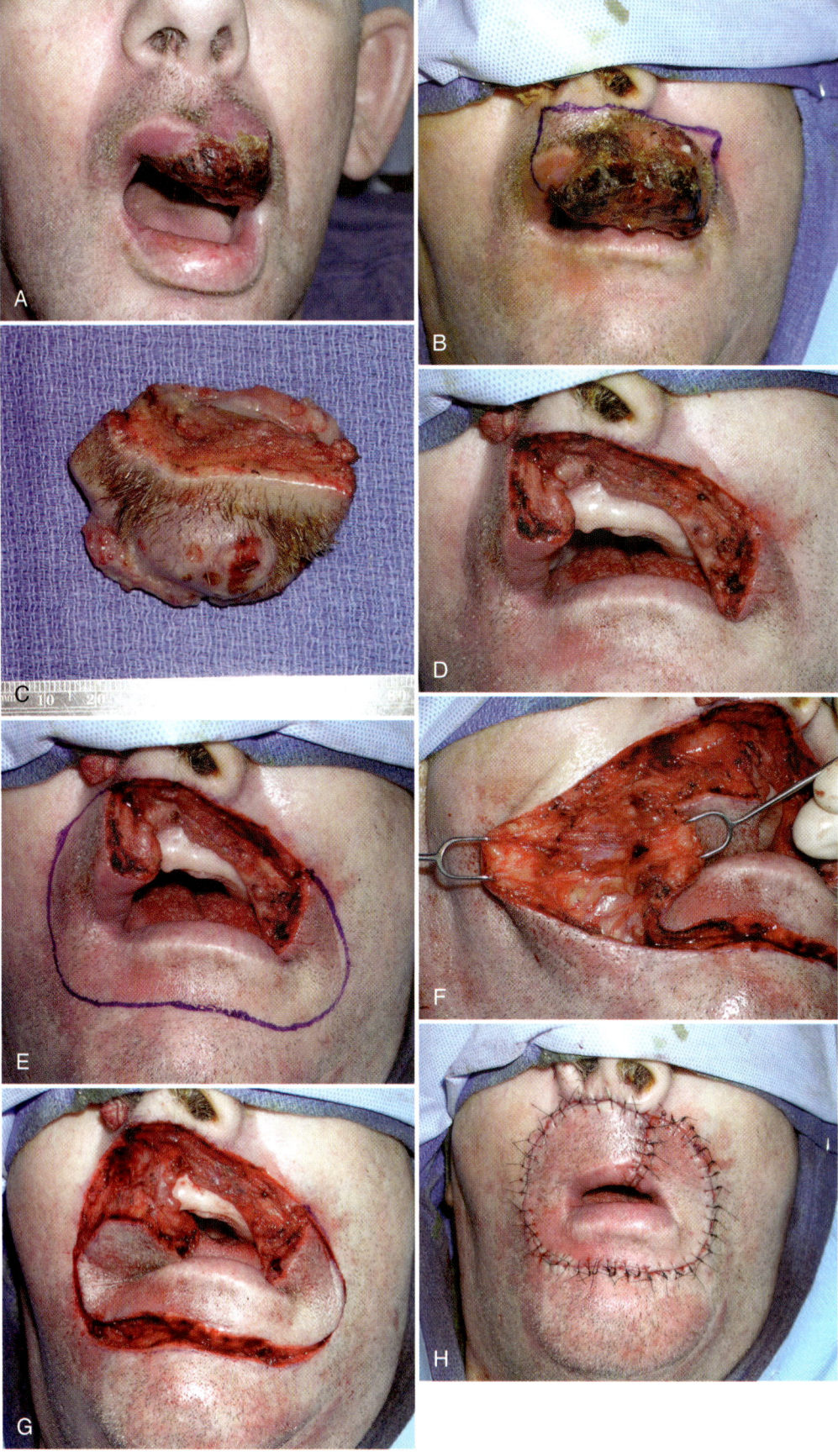

Fig. 63-8 ■ **A,** A large squamous cell carcinoma occupying approximately two thirds of the upper lip. **B,** A block excision is outlined with the intention of performing immediate reconstruction. **C,** The specimen is submitted for frozen section analysis of the margins. **D,** The resultant defect. **E,** Reconstruction is performed with *reverse* Karapandzic flaps. **F,** The facial arteries are preserved bilaterally such that axial-pattern flaps are realized. **G,** The *reverse* Karapandzic flaps are prepared for advancement and closure. **H,** Closure is accomplished in anatomic layers.

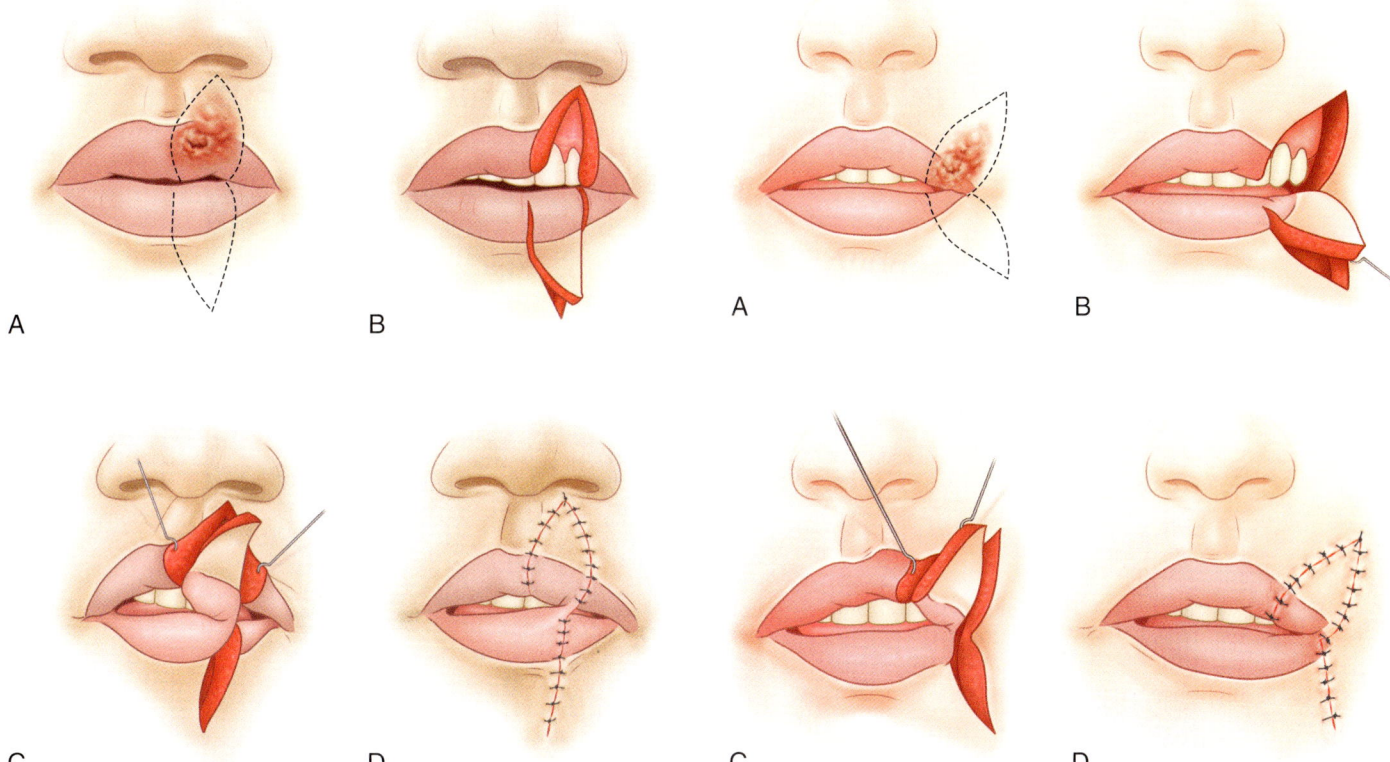

Fig. 63-9 ■ Diagrammatic representation of excision of an upper lip cancer and immediate reconstruction with an Abbe flap from the lower lip based on the inferior labial artery. The pedicle noted in part **D** is cut at approximately 2 to 3 weeks postoperatively.

Fig. 63-10 ■ Diagrammatic representation of excision of an upper lip cancer, including the commissure, with immediate reconstruction using an Abbe-Estlander flap from the lower lip based on the inferior labial artery. The pedicle noted in part **D** is cut at approximately 2 to 3 weeks postoperatively.

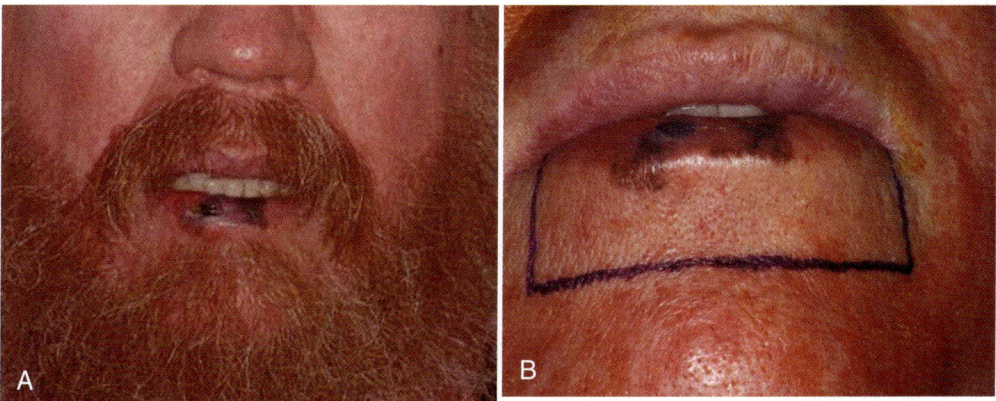

Fig. 63-11 ■ **A,** A nodular melanoma is present in the lower lip. **B,** The outline for cancer excision includes nearly the entire lower lip.

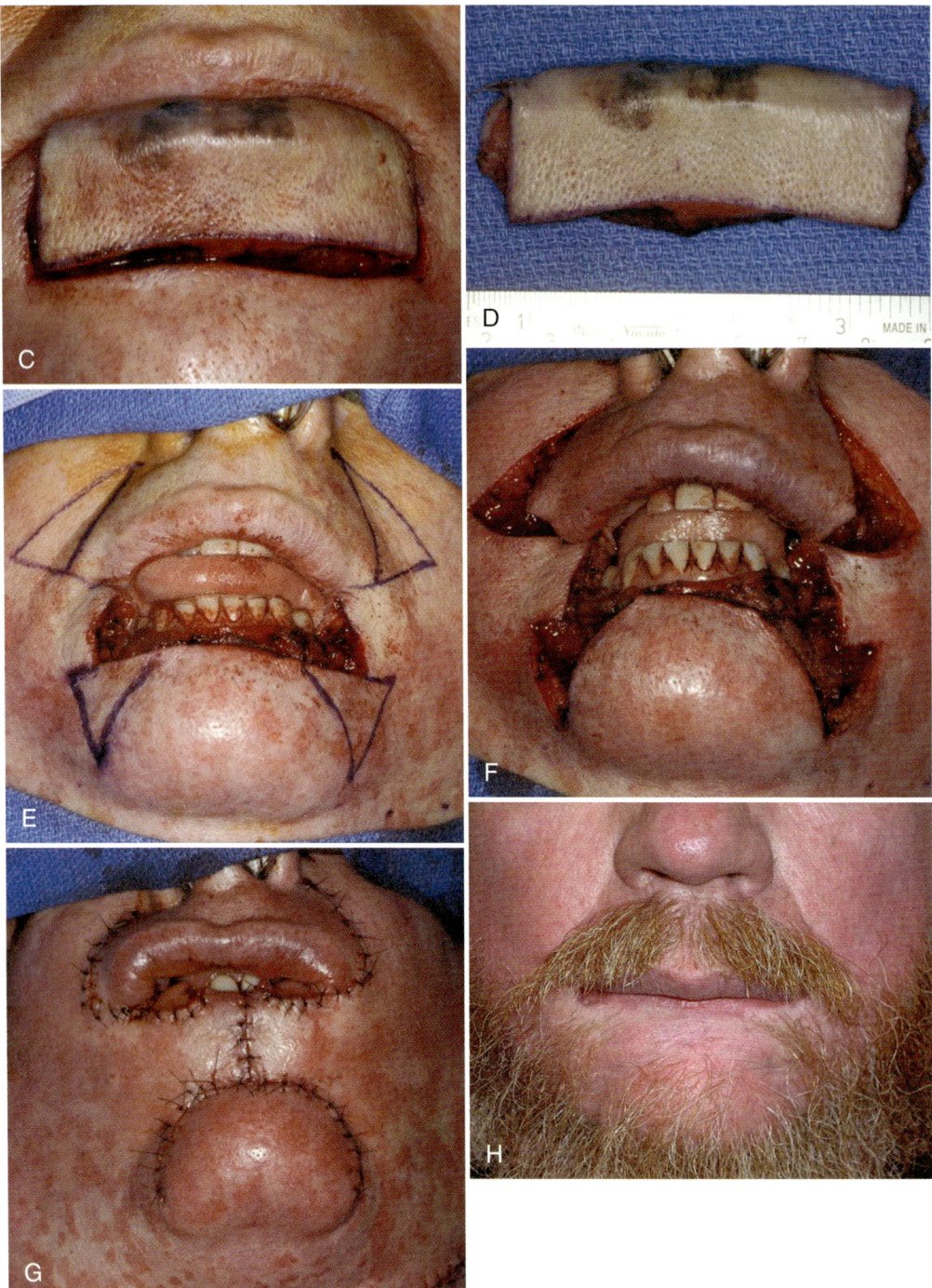

Fig. 63-11, cont'd ■ C, The excision is completed. **D,** The specimen is submitted for routine frozen section and permanent section analysis using immunostains (S-100, HMB-45). **E** and **F,** Reconstruction of this lower lip defect is accomplished with the Webster modification of the Bernard cheiloplasty and Burow's triangles. **G,** Closure is accomplished in anatomic layers. **H,** The 2-year postoperative result.

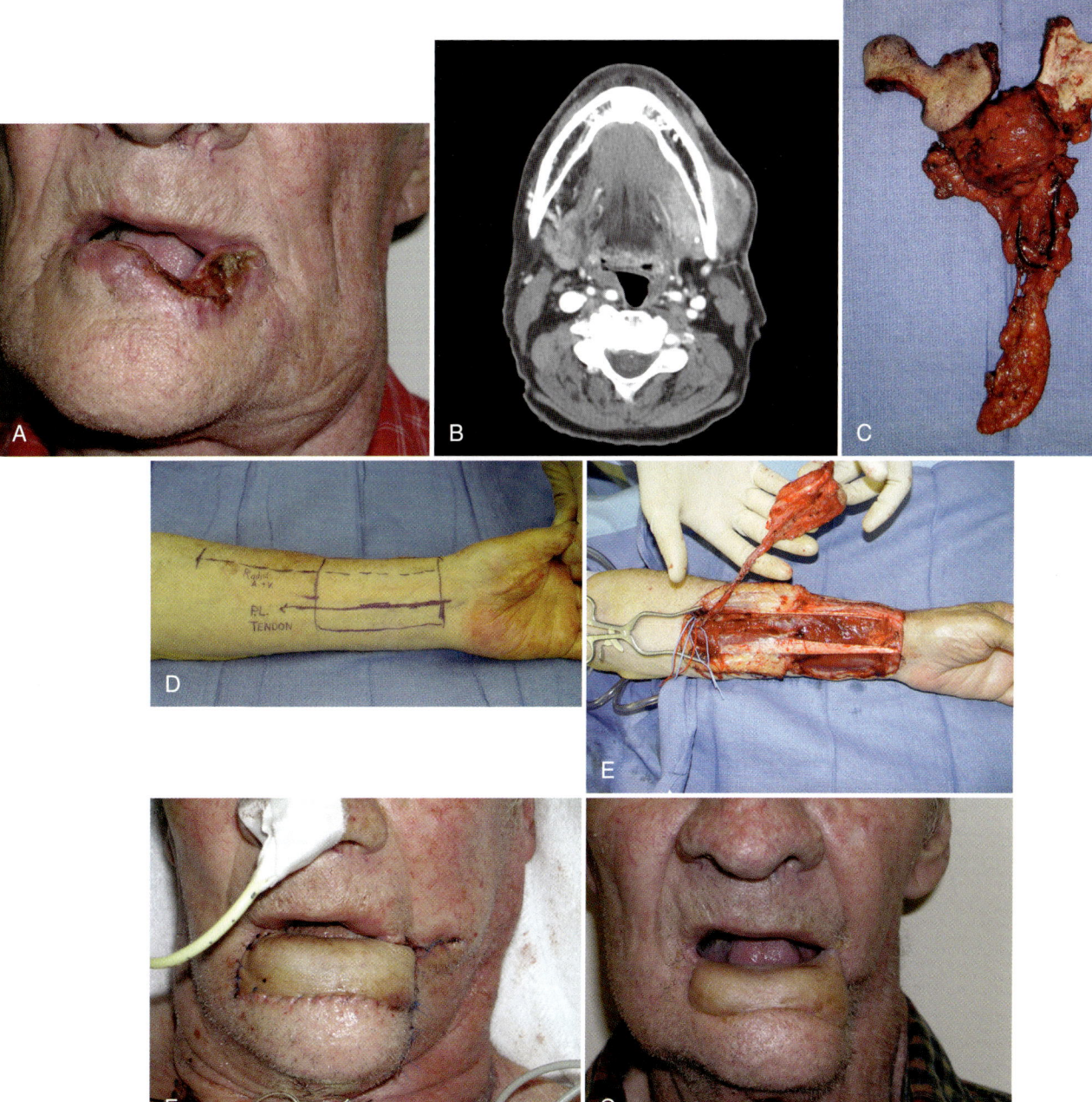

Fig. 63-12 ■ **A,** A large cancer is present in the lower lip. Also evident is left level I cervical metastatic disease. **B,** Computed tomography scan demonstrating metastatic nodal disease in the left side of the patient's neck. Because the surgical treatment plan consisted of complete removal of the lower lip, mandibular resection, and neck dissection, it was also decided that reconstruction with a radial forearm free flap would be appropriate in this case. **C,** The specimen from this surgery. **D,** The outline for harvest of a radial forearm free flap for lower lip reconstruction. The palmaris longus (PL) tendon was included to suspend the flap for more anatomic reconstruction of the lower lip. **E,** The flap was based on the radial artery and veins. **F,** Placement of the flap in the recipient tissue bed. **G,** The flap provides acceptable reconstruction of the lower lip as noted 2 years postoperatively.

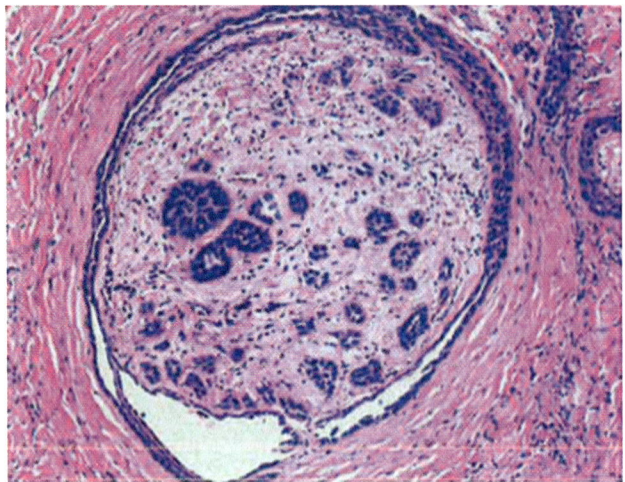

Fig. 63-13 ■ The patient's (from Fig. 63-1) specimen showed extensive perineural and intraneural invasion as noted in this histomicrograph. Accordingly, postoperative radiation therapy was administered.

BIBLIOGRAPHY

Esclamado RM, Krause CJ: Lip cancer. In Bailey BJ, editor: *Head and neck surgery—otolaryngology*, ed 2, Philadelphia, 1998, Lippincott-Raven, pp 1509-1521.

Hasson O: Squamous cell carcinoma of the lower lip, *J Oral Maxillofac Surg* 66:1259-1262, 2008.

Heller KS, Shah JP: Carcinoma of the lip, *Am J Surg* 138:600-603, 1979.

Herrera E, Bosch RJ, Barrera MV: Reconstruction of the lower lip: Bernard technique and its variants, *Dermatol Surg* 34:648-655, 2008.

Karapandzic M: Reconstruction of lip defects by local arterial flaps, *Br J Plast Surg* 27:93-97, 1974.

Regezi JA, Sciubba JJ, Jordan RCK, editors: *Oral pathology—clinical pathologic correlations*, ed 5, St Louis, 2008, WB Saunders, pp 21-71.

Renner G: Reconstruction of the lip. In Baker SR, Swanson NA, editors: *Local flaps in facial reconstruction*, St Louis, 1995, CV Mosby, pp 345-396.

Salgarelli AC, Sartorelli F, Cangiano A, et al: Treatment of lower lip cancer: an experience of 48 cases, *Int J Oral Maxillofac Surg* 34:27-32, 2005.

Shah JP, Patel SG, editors: *Head and neck surgery and oncology*, ed 3, Edinburgh, 2003, CV Mosby, pp 149-172.

Sykes JW, Ghali GE: Lip cancer. In Miloro M, Ghali GE, Larsen P, et al, editors: *Peterson's principles of oral and maxillofacial surgery*, ed 2, Hamilton, Ontario, 2004, BC Decker, pp 659-669.

Teichgraeber JF, Larson DL: Some oncologic considerations in the treatment of lip cancer, *Otolaryngol Head Neck Surg* 98:589-592, 1988.

Webster RC, Coffey RJ, Kelleher RE: Total and partial reconstruction of the lower lip with innervated muscle-bearing flaps, *Plast Reconstr Surg* 25:360-371, 1960.

Zide BM: Deformities of the lips and cheeks. In McCarthy JG, editor: *Plastic surgery*, Philadelphia, 1990, WB Saunders, pp 2009-2056.

Zitsch RP, Park CW, Renner GJ, et al: Outcome analysis for lip carcinoma, *Otolaryngol Head Neck Surg* 113:589-596, 1995.

The Temporalis System of Flaps in Head and Neck Reconstruction: Temporoparietal Fascia and Temporalis Muscle Flaps

Chapter 64

Jon D. Holmes

Because of its unique blood supply, the temporal area provides a tripartite system of flaps for reconstruction. Two of these, the temporoparietal (TP) fascia and temporalis flaps, are most commonly used for reconstructing defects in the head and neck because of their proximity, reliability, and adaptability. Both are described here, including their indications, anatomy, and flap-harvesting technique, along with contraindications and potential complications.

ETIOPATHOGENESIS/CAUSATIVE FACTORS

Composite defects of the maxillofacial region requiring regional tissue transfer most commonly result from oncologic resection. The resultant defects often lead to communication between the oral, nasal, sinus, and rarely, cranial contents. In addition, avulsive traumatic injuries can result in defects too large for coverage with local advancement flaps. Finally, recalcitrant oral-antral and oral-nasal communications from previous cleft palate or dentoalveolar misadventures that have failed previous attempts at closure may require regional flaps for closure. Although obturation with a prosthesis is possible, patients are often unwilling or unable to accept management with a prosthesis. Even if prosthetic obturation is planned, flaps may be indicated. For example, flaps may be used to offer support to the globe in cases of loss of the orbital floor, to cover the bone of the orbit following orbital exenteration, or to seal off communication with the cranial vault. See further discussion later under specific indications and contraindications.

ANATOMY

An understanding of the anatomic layers of the temporal area is critical for proper flap development. The nomenclature describing the various fascial layers in this area is often confusing because of inconsistencies in use. For example, some authors refer to the temporalis muscle fascia as the deep temporal fascia and the TP fascia as the superficial temporal fascia. For consistency, the terminology used here to describe the five layers of the scalp in the temporal area from superficial to deep include skin and subcutaneous fat, TP fascia, loose areolar tissue, temporalis muscular fascia, and temporalis muscle (Fig. 64-1). Beneath the temporalis muscle lies the pericranium.

The TP fascia is the continuation of the superficial musculoaponeurotic system (SMAS) above the zygoma. Superiorly, it becomes the galea aponeurotica at the temporal line. Superficial to the TP fascia is subcutaneous tissue, which varies in thickness. In addition, above the temporal line, dense fibrous connections exist between the dermis and the TP fascia. Beneath the TP fascia is a loose areolar

tissue plane that separates it from the firm, glistening temporalis muscular fascia. This areolar tissue plane is avascular and allows mobility of the scalp over the deeper layers.

The temporalis fascia attaches superiorly along the superior temporal line and covers the temporalis muscle. Approximately 2 cm above the zygomatic arch at the line of fusion the temporalis muscle fascia divides into the superficial layer of the temporal fascia and the deep layer of the temporalis fascia, between which lies the temporal fat pad. Inferiorly, the deep layer of the temporalis fascia blends with the periosteum of the zygomatic arch and extends inferiorly as the fascia overlying the masseter muscle. The temporalis fascia fuses to the pericranium above the temporal line.

Of critical importance to raising of flaps in the temporal region is the relationship of the facial nerve, specifically the frontal branches, which are at risk during flap development and inset. The frontal branch courses on the undersurface of the TP fascia approximately 1.5 cm lateral to the orbital rim. It crosses the zygomatic arch an average of 2 cm (range, 0.8 to 3.5 cm) anterior to the external auditory canal.

The vascular pedicle of the TP fascia flap is the superficial temporal artery arising from the external carotid system and the associated superficial temporal vein. The TP fascia also receives contributions from the occipital, postauricular, supraorbital, and supratrochlear vessels via multiple anastomotic connections. Division of these vessels during development of the flap, however, does not compromise it. The superficial temporal artery tends to run within the fascia, whereas the vein usually lies more superficially on the outer surface of the fascia and posterior to the artery. The artery typically divides into anterior and posterior branches approximately 3 cm above the tragus or 1 cm above the superior helix. The auriculotemporal nerve lies posterior to the vessels and is usually easily preserved during flap harvest.

The temporalis fascia is supplied primarily by the middle temporal artery, which branches from the superficial temporal artery just superior to the zygomatic arch. Preservation of this branch allows the development of a separate layer of fascia. This attribute is most commonly exploited along with the TP fascial flap to sandwich cartilage grafts.

The temporalis muscle is supplied by two dominant pedicles, the anterior and posterior deep temporal arteries, which arise from the internal maxillary artery and their associated veins. In addition, the most posterior aspect of the muscle receives its blood supply from the middle temporal artery. The two dominant pedicles allow development of a bilobed flap. Because of the small contribution of the middle temporal artery to the posterior aspect of the muscle, the muscle is generally divided in a one-third anterior and two-thirds posterior design. This allows the posterior limb to be supplied by

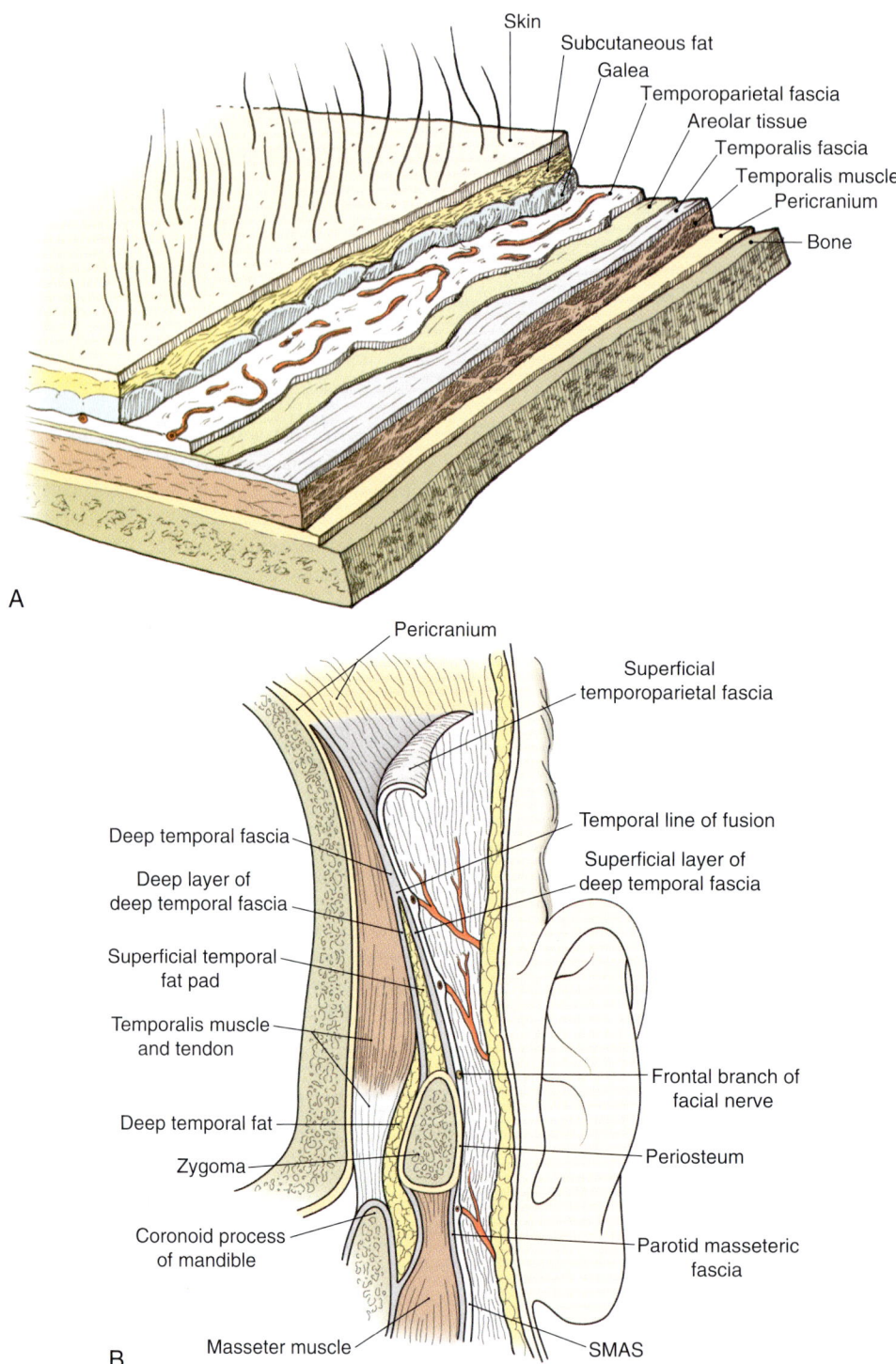

Fig. 64-1 ■ Lateral (**A**) and sagittal (**B**) views demonstrating the fascial layers and anatomic relationships of the temporal regions. (From Baker SR: *Local flaps in facial reconstruction*, ed 2, St Louis, 2007, Mosby.) *SMAS,* superficial musculoaponeurotic system.

the posterior temporal artery. The anterior and posterior temporal arteries enter on the deep, inferior surface and course between the muscle and periosteum, thus making their preservation easier when approached from a superior direction (see the later discussion on surgical technique). Though superficial to the periosteum, from a practical standpoint the vessels are intimate with the bone and may actually groove it. For this reason it is critical to raise the muscle from the bone in a subperiosteal plane.

DIAGNOSTIC STUDIES

TEMPOROPARIETAL FASCIA FLAP

When considering the TP fascia flap, inspection of the temporal area should be undertaken with attention paid to previous surgical scars in the area that may have interrupted the superficial temporal vessels. A familial history or clinical findings consistent with male pattern baldness should be noted because it is a relative contraindication to use of the TP flap (see later). Doppler can be used to outline the course of the superficial temporal artery preoperatively.

TEMPORALIS FLAP

Likewise, when a temporalis flap is considered, the area should be examined for evidence of previous surgery. Since the blood supply to the muscle enters on its deep surface, it is unlikely that it has been compromised unless the patient has previously undergone surgical approaches to the infratemporal fossa or lateral skull base approaches. Evidence of temporal wasting can be a clue to a compromised temporalis. In addition, having patients clench their teeth preoperatively can give some idea regarding the size of the muscle and its viability.

INDICATIONS (TREATMENT/ RECONSTRUCTIVE GOALS)

TEMPOROPARIETAL FASCIA FLAP

The TP fascia provides highly vascularized, thin tissue with excellent draping characteristics up to approximately 12×12 cm. It can be harvested with hair-bearing skin or will consistently take a skin graft. The TP fascia can be used as a pedicled flap or free tissue transfer. Pedicled, it can reach the orbit, malar region, and proximal part of the mandible. Split-thickness skin grafts applied to the bony orbit following exenteration are often too thin and frequently become excoriated, whereas the bulk of muscle flaps placed into the orbit often preclude the creation of a natural-appearing prosthesis. Lining the bony orbit with TP fascia covered with a split-thickness skin graft creates a more durable lining that is not too bulky to accept a prosthesis. The TP fascia can also be used to cover free cranial bone grafts placed in the mid-face. This is especially useful in covering the side of the bone exposed to the paranasal sinuses to improve mucosalization. Vascularized bone-containing flaps can also be developed if preferred. If the middle temporal artery is taken along with the pedicle, the temporalis muscular fascia can be harvested as a separate layer and, along with the TP fascia, can be used to envelop grafts of cartilage or bone.

The TP fascia can also function as reliable soft tissue filler. It can be used to cover the parotid bed following parotidectomy to decrease the incidence of gustatory sweating (Frey syndrome) and to prevent some of the soft tissue depression following parotidectomy. It is often used to mitigate some of the temporal depression following harvest of a temporalis muscle flap.

The thinness and draping characteristics of the TP fascial flap make it useful for auricular reconstruction. It can cover an auricle that has been denuded of perichondrium by cancer excision or trauma. A split- or full-thickness skin graft can then be placed reliably. TP fascia can also be used to cover cartilage frameworks created for reconstruction of the auricle. Placement of a small suction drain will aid in conforming the fascia to the underlying framework, and it can be covered with a skin graft. Transfer of hair to the brow or upper lip can be accomplished by taking an island of hair-bearing skin with the TP fascia.

The TP fascia flap also provides an excellent means of dealing with recalcitrant oral-antral and oral-nasal fistulas. Multiple previous attempts at closure have often exhausted other sources of pedicled flaps such as the buccal fat and palate. TP fascia will reliably mucosalize when placed into these defects. Consideration can be given to covering the site with a surgical stent while mucosalization

is occurring as long as no pressure is put on the flap. Similarly, TP fascia can be used to cover large areas of the maxillary alveolus and palate denuded during the excision of extensive squamous or verrucoid cancers in which the periosteum is sacrificed over a large area. Covering the bone in these cases leads to more rapid mucosalization and increased comfort.

TEMPORALIS FLAP

The temporalis flap can be raised as a myofascial, myo-osseous, or myocutaneous flap. Dimensions vary by body habitus and sex, but it easily provides approximately 10 cm along its anterior border, 12 cm along its posterior border, and 14 cm along its superior border. Its typical thickness is 4 to 8 mm. The temporalis flap can also be used to obliterate the orbit following exenteration, but it is best used in this situation if there is a need for the bulk provided by muscle, for example, to act as a barrier to intracranial communication. The coronoid process can be pedicled on the temporalis muscle and brought medially when the coronoid is plated. This provides support for the globe or a prosthesis when the floor has been excised. Vascularized cranial bone can also be included with a temporalis muscle flap to reconstruct the malar or maxillary regions. The temporalis muscle and fascia can be used to close a maxillectomy defect in patients unable to tolerate an obturator. Bilateral flaps can be used to close bilateral maxillectomy defects. Small temporalis muscle flaps can be developed for reconstruction of the temporomandibular joint. Placement of the muscle as an interpositional flap in cases of gap arthroplasty can be especially useful in patients with recurrent ankylosis.

By far one of the more common uses of the temporalis flap is for facial reanimation following the loss of facial nerve function. A bilobed flap can be developed and the anterior limb passed subcutaneously and secured to the commissure. If length is a problem, an interpositional graft of fascia lata or Gore-Tex (W.L. Gore & Associates, Inc., Flagstaff, Ariz.) can be used. Alternatively, dissection of the flap can be accomplished superiorly to include the pericranium and galea (see the section on technique later). The posterior limb is then used to obliterate the anterior portion of the temporal defect.

CONTRAINDICATIONS

The most important consideration when harvesting a TP or temporalis flap is previous surgery in the area. Preauricular and coronal incisions commonly involve sacrifice of the superficial temporal artery, and the presence of a scar here necessitates further evaluation, including Doppler studies (see earlier). Lateral skull base approaches, infratemporal fossa resections, and less commonly, maxillectomy can damage the deep temporal arteries and should be considered. Previous radiation therapy in the area is a relative contraindication to the TP fascial flap, especially if a temporalis muscle flap is planned. Harvest of the TP fascia and temporalis muscle in these cases will most likely lead to necrosis of the overlying soft tissue. Male pattern baldness leaves a significant visible scar from harvest of either flap, and patients should be counseled accordingly.

Patients should also be counseled about the difficulty of wearing a prosthesis following obliteration of maxillectomy defects with the temporalis muscle flap. Similarly, closure of large oral-antral or oral-nasal fistulas with the TP fascia flap can make wearing a complete denture difficult because of the resultant scar band crossing the vestibule. In both cases, further reconstructive efforts will usually be necessary to enable patients to wear a prosthesis.

SURGICAL TECHNIQUE (SPECIFIC TREATMENT AND TECHNIQUES)

The TP fascia flap can be developed as a filler to mitigate the temporal hollowing associated with use of the temporalis flap. Here we will describe development of the TP fascial flap in that context with the understanding that either can be developed alone.

Harvest of the flaps is aided by the use of a Mayfield head rest. Preoperative shaving is not necessary, but the use of rubber hair bands or clips may help if the patient has long hair. Oral or nasal intubation is used, depending on the location of the recipient site. If nasal intubation is used, the endotracheal tube can be secured to the naris with suture and secured along the opposite side of the head. If oral intubation is used, the tube can be brought inferiorly along the chest. Paralysis should be avoided so that a nerve stimulator may be used if needed. Loupe magnification, though not absolutely necessary, is recommended to aid in identification of the correct plane of dissection and the frontal branch of the facial nerve. Bipolar and needle tip monopolar cautery should be available. The entire face should be included in the preparation and draping so that landmarks are visible. The external auditory canal should be protected with sterile cotton saturated with mineral oil.

Initially, Doppler can be used to mark the course of the superficial temporal artery and vein. The temporal line can also be marked preoperatively. The temporalis muscle inserts at the inferior temporal line. The superior temporal line serves as a demarcation of the TP fascia below and the galea aponeurotica above. At the superior temporal line the temporalis fascia blends with the periosteum covering the calvaria. The temporalis muscle inserts along the inferior temporal line. The course of the frontal branch of the facial nerve can be marked along a line extending from a point 0.5 cm below the tragus to a point 1.5 cm above the lateral brow. Dissection should remain posterior to this line.

An incision is outlined and extended superiorly along a preauricular crease to the root of the helix. Here, it is best to direct the incision slightly posteriorly to avoid carrying it directly over the course of the superficial temporal vessels. In addition, the dominant venous outflow can also course posterior to the artery, and carrying the temporal extension of the incision posteriorly aids in avoiding it. A Y extension superiorly can aid in access. Bilateral flaps can be elevated through a coronal incision.

The incision is carried through the skin into a plane just deep to the hair follicles. The vein runs along the superficial aspect of the TP fascia, whereas the artery follows a tortuous course deep to the vein within the fascia. Establishment of a correct plane early in the dissection is critical to avoid damage to the pedicle. Beginning the dissection approximately 2 cm above the auricle is recommended. Here, the hair follicles are easily identified, and the dermis is not as adherent to the TP fascia as it is along and above the temporal line, where fibrous septa firmly connect the dermis to the fascia. Dissection of the skin flaps is tedious and becomes more so as the dissection proceeds superiorly, especially if an extended flap is planned and necessitates dissection above the temporal line. In addition, the dissection becomes more superficial superiorly, and care is taken to remain at the level of the hair follicles while maintaining enough thickness to decrease the risk for alopecia. Once developed, the skin flaps should be covered and kept moist.

At this point the vascular pedicles are evident, and an appropriately sized flap can be outlined (Fig. 64-2, *A*). As noted previously, the course of the frontal branch of the facial nerve delineates the anterior extent of the flap. It can often be identified coursing deep to the TP fascia. The anterior branch of the superficial temporal artery usually requires ligation at the anterior extent of the flap while

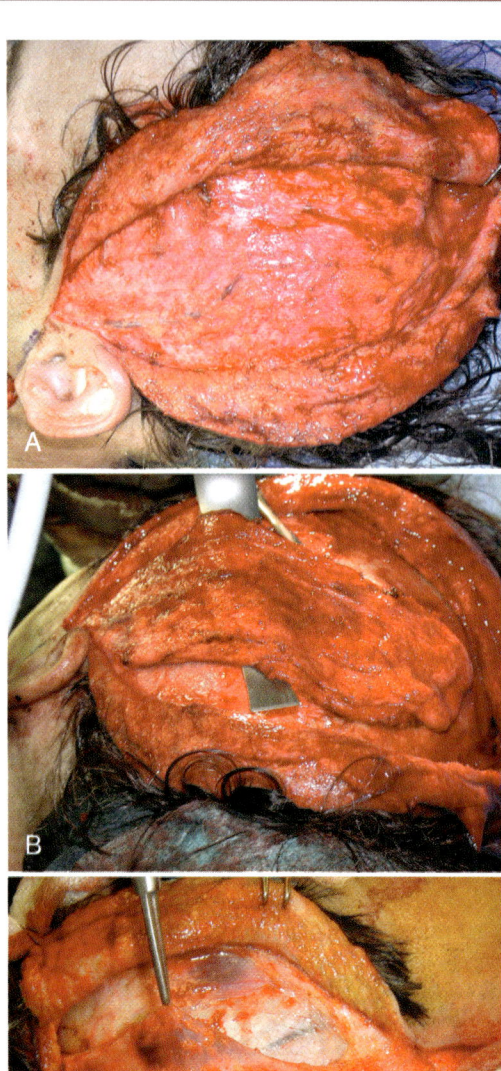

Fig. 64-2 ■ **A,** Temporoparietal (TP) fascia exposed following elevation of the skin flaps. **B,** Elevation of the TP fascia from the temporalis fascia. **C,** Demonstration of the TP fascia and underlying temporalis fascia. Note the separate vascular pedicles to the TP fascia (superficial temporal artery) and temporalis fascia (middle temporal artery).

remaining posterior to the course of the frontal branch of the facial nerve. The TP fascia is incised along the superior temporal line, which usually serves as the superior extent of the flap. It should be noted, however, that extending the harvest to the midline to include the galea is possible to add bulk. If harvesting an extended flap above the temporal line containing the galea, it is often easier to elevate the TP fascia off the temporalis muscular fascia. Next, the galea is elevated off the pericranium. Finally, the two are connected by incising the dense attachments along the temporal line. If sharp dissection is attempted from a superior direction without first elevating the TP fascia off the temporal fascia, it is possible to enter the wrong plane deep to the temporalis muscular fascia. Once the TP fascia is incised, the medial dissection begins. The avascular plane containing the loose areolar tissue that separates the TP fascia from the underlying temporalis muscular fascia makes this dissection simple. The TP fascia can be swept off the dense temporalis fascia with a periosteal elevator (Fig. 64-2, *B*). As noted previously, the temporalis muscle fascia can be developed as a separate layer by including the take-off of the middle temporal artery from the superficial temporal artery (Fig. 64-2, *C*). This branching occurs just above the zygomatic arch. The pedicle length of the superficial temporal vessels is limited as the root of the helix is approached. Just inferior to this, it dives deep into the parotid, thus making dissection of it very difficult without identification and isolation of the facial nerve. If it is used as a free flap, the pedicle is typically divided at the root of the helix.

If an isolated TP fascia flap is needed intraorally, a generous tunnel should be created for passage of it. Although division of the zygomatic arch adds somewhat to pedicle length and decreases the risk for venous congestion, it is not usually necessary if the tunnel is large enough. Creation of a tunnel is usually accomplished by passing a large clamp from the oral cavity defect superiorly to exit at the root of the zygomatic arch. Blunt dissection will avoid damage to the frontal branch of the facial nerve. The tunnel should not constrict the pedicle because constriction will invariably lead to venous congestion.

If a skin graft is placed over the fascia, care should be taken when tacking the graft to the flap to not pierce or compress the main pedicle. Likewise, if a surgical stent is placed over the flap, it should not compress the flap. Prolonged flap edema is not uncommon and should be taken into consideration, especially if the flap is used for coverage of an auricular reconstruction.

At this point the temporalis muscle and its overlying muscular fascia (if not previously developed as a separate flap, see earlier) are exposed (see Fig. 64-2, *B*). It should be noted that if the TP flap is not needed, elevation of the skin flaps to expose the muscle should take place in a plane directly on the temporalis muscular fascia. Elevation of the TP fascia with the skin flaps lessens the risk for damage to the frontal branch of the facial nerve and decreases the risk for skin necrosis and alopecia. Dissection typically begins by incising the temporalis fascia from the root of the zygoma and extending it 45 degrees superiorly into the temporal fat pad, which lies between the superficial layer of the temporalis fascia and the deep layer of the temporalis fascia. Reflection of this layer forward in this plane protects the frontal branch of the facial nerve if it has not already been identified and protected while raising a TP fascial flap. Subperiosteal dissection is carried along the zygomatic arch for a distance of approximately 2 cm if an osteotomy of the arch is planned to allow passage of the flap underneath the arch. Although it is possible to pass the muscle under the arch without an osteotomy in some cases, traction on the muscle can put undue tension on the flap, and removing the arch allows easier passage. A small titanium plate can be contoured before the osteotomy to allow easy replacement. Passage over the arch is possible as well but decreases the arc of rotation by 3 to 4 cm and also leads to some cosmetic deformity because the bulk of the muscle lies lateral to the arch in a subcutaneous plane.

At this point the fascia can be swept from the muscle with relative ease. Some surgeons prefer to leave the fascia on the muscle to improve retention of sutures. In addition, the fascia can be left attached to the muscle along the superior edge to allow extended reach for facial reanimation.

Following exposure of the muscle, Doppler can be used to identify the anterior and posterior branches of the deep temporal arteries. This is more important if there is a plan to develop two separate (anterior and posterior) flaps. Usually, it is best to develop the anterior third of the muscle based on the anterior branch and the posterior two thirds on the posterior branch.

The muscle is detached from the inferior temporal line. If the temporalis fascia is raised with the flap, it must be detached from the superior temporal line first. At this point a periosteal elevator is used to carefully detach the deep aspect of the muscle from the skull. Care should be exercised as the zygomatic arch is approached because the vascular pedicles typically enter the muscle along the deep aspect at its inferior third. If the skull is grooved by the vascular pedicles, careful dissection directly on the bone is needed to preserve them. The temporalis muscular fascia should be incised along its attachment to the zygomatic arch to allow complete rotation.

Once freed, the muscle can be passed under the arch if necessary into the oral cavity, or an osteotomy can be performed as described earlier. Passage is best accomplished by placing heavy traction sutures into the muscle or fascia if it was taken. A clamp can be passed from the oral cavity underneath the arch and used to gently tease the flap into position. Additional length can be gained by carefully performing an osteotomy of the coronoid process. It is not necessary to remove the coronoid process from its attachments to the temporalis. In fact, the bone can be used to reconstruct a portion of the missing maxilla. When reconstructing a maxillary defect, it is best to elevate the palatal mucosa from the bone edge and place a series of holes in the bone. Fixing sutures can then be placed through the muscle or fascia into these holes to anchor the flap. The residual mucosal edge can then be laid back over this suture line and tacked to the muscle.

Techniques to deal with the donor site defect are varied. A variety of alloplasts can be used to fill the defect, but autogenous tissue is best given the artificial feel of the implants and the risk for extrusion. If only the anterior portion of the muscle is used, the posterior portion can be rotated anteriorly to fill the more visible defect along the lateral orbital rim. Similarly, a TP fascial flap can be developed at the outset of harvest of the temporalis muscle, folded, and secured to fill the anterior portion of the defect.

BONE-CONTAINING FLAPS

Both the temporalis and TP fascial flaps can be harvested as myo-osseous and osteofascial flaps, respectively. The TP fascial flap can be used to carry split calvarial bone from the parietal skull just superior to the temporal line. The temporalis muscle can be designed to carry calvarial bone or the coronoid process and a variable amount of ascending ramus. Even though full-thickness cranial bone has been carried with these flaps, most often split calvarial bone is used.

Harvest of a bone-containing TP fascial flap is performed in a similar manner as a TP fascial flap with the exception of carrying the incision further toward the midline. A generous cuff of fascia and periosteum (pericranium) should be harvested around the perimeter of the proposed bone segment (Fig. 64-3, *A*). Care must be taken to not strip this cuff from the bone segment during flap harvest and manipulation. Once the area of osteotomy is isolated, beveled cuts are made through the outer table at the superior, anterior, and posterior edges. Placement of a malleable, ribbon-type retractor or lighted retractor allows access to make the cut along the inferior edge without disturbing the fascia. Thin osteotomes can then be used to complete the harvest in an identical fashion to harvest of cranial bone grafts (Fig. 64-3, *B*). Bleeding from the inner aspect of the bone confirms that this is an osseous flap and not a graft. Holes can be drilled along the bone margin and the fascia secured to the bone with absorbable suture. The excess fascia harvested around the perimeter can be used to wrap the bone segment after fixation. Care should be taken, however, to not interpose fascia between bone edges and thus preclude osseous union with the recipient site.

The temporalis myo-osseous flap is used when increased bulk is necessary. Harvest is identical in most respects to the technique described earlier for the TP osseofascial flap. Indeed, most authors

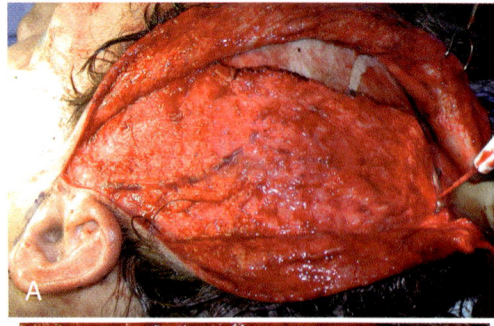

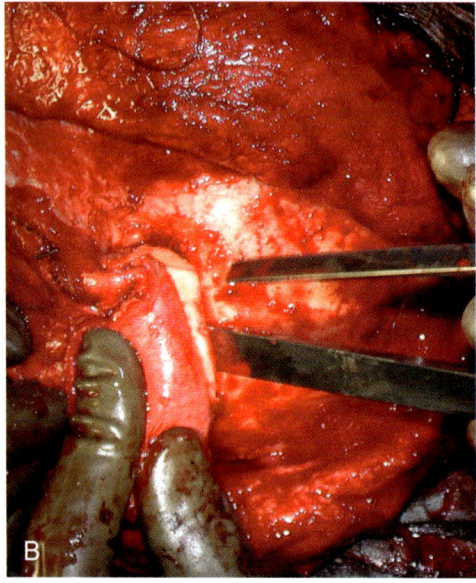

Fig. 64-3 ▪ **A,** Cutting of the pericranium should be done some distance from the proposed bone cuts. **B,** Small osteotomes are used to separate the outer cortex of cranium. Note the care taken to prevent shearing of fascia from the bone.

describe development of the temporalis flap with the overlying TP fascia and galea aponeurotica when carrying a bone segment. At a minimum, the temporalis muscular fascia should be harvested with the muscle. Again, the pericranium is incised some distance away from the proposed osteotomy for the bone segment. Release along the temporal line is carried out carefully to prevent tearing.

Aside from cranial bone, the temporalis can also be used to develop a bone-containing flap involving the coronoid process. This flap is developed by making an intraoral incision to access the coronoid process, or access can often be gained through a maxillectomy defect if one has been performed. The coronoid process along with a variable amount of ascending ramus is harvested while leaving the superior attachments of the temporalis and taking care to not damage the vascular pedicle along the deep surface of the temporalis. Sectioning of the coronoid process provides bone as well as increases the arc of rotation of the temporalis muscle flap. Alternatively, the temporalis can be left attached superiorly, and the coronoid process and its attached temporalis muscle can be swung medially and rigidly fixed to give support to the globe or the mid-face (see indications earlier).

POSTOPERATIVE CARE

Closure is performed over a suction drain with 3-0 resorbable subcutaneous sutures and surgical staples. A light head dressing can be applied but is not necessary. If a head wrap is used, care should be taken to not compress the pedicle, especially in the case of a TP fascia flap. The head of the bed should be elevated to decrease flap edema, which is more common with the TP fascia flap. Some authors suggest that eyeglasses be modified to ensure that pressure is not placed on the pedicle. Trismus is not uncommon with either the TP fascial or temporalis muscle flap but resolves early with function. Patients are allowed to shampoo their hair lightly with a mild soap after 48 to 72 hours. Chlorhexidine rinses are used perioperatively. Patients should be advised that formation of a fibrinous layer, which often spontaneously exfoliates after the temporalis muscle flap mucosalizes, is common when used to reconstruct intraoral defects. Patients may be alarmed and think that the flap itself has been lost if not forewarned. In cases of facial reanimation, physical therapy is instituted early to improve appearance and decrease dyskinesis.

COMPLICATIONS

Both the TP fascia and the temporalis muscle flaps have a robust blood supply and flap loss is rare. It is probably more common with the TP flap and if the temporalis muscle is split into anterior and posterior segments. Protection of the superficial temporal artery is predicated on knowledge of its location and beginning the dissection in the correct area (see earlier). In addition, dissection of the pedicle inferior to the root of the helix should be avoided. Here, the pedicle becomes more medial and is lost within the parotid gland, thus increasing the risk for damage to it and the facial nerve. Given their protected location, damage to the deep temporal arteries is less common, and subsequent loss of the temporalis muscle flap is less common still. If splitting of the muscle is contemplated, Doppler can be used to aid in identification of the two branches. Aside from vascular compromise, more common complications of both flaps are issues related to the donor site.

Alopecia along the area of subcutaneous dissection is not uncommon during harvest of the TP fascia flap and usually occurs within 2 to 3 cm of the incision line. Skin loss in the area of subcutaneous dissection is also a risk. Typically, the areas are small and heal by secondary intention. Prevention is achieved by paying strict attention to the level of dissection just beneath the hair follicles, judicious use of bipolar cautery, and gentle handling of skin flaps, including keeping them moist. In either case, serial excision of the affected areas may be necessary. Avoidance of hematoma is paramount. If a bone flap is harvested, bone wax may be necessary to stop bleeding from the cancellous surface of the donor site. Alopecia is less common when the temporalis muscle flap alone is developed, but the resultant temporal hollowing is potentially the greatest drawback to use of the flap. A variety of techniques have been used to deal with the defect, including TP fascia flaps as discussed earlier, alloplasts, and flap splitting. Alloplasts are the most commonly used technique, but they are not without difficulty. The flap is often used in a clean-contaminated environment, and contamination of the implant is a consideration. In addition, implants lack a natural feel and can become exposed.

Potential for injury to the facial nerve exists with both flaps. Adherence to the techniques discussed earlier can mitigate the risk for facial nerve transection, but retraction alone can lead to neurapraxia. Eye taping and lubrication are recommended while the nerve recovers. If recovery is prolonged, eyelid rehabilitation with either a gold or titanium weight is indicated. Lower branches of the facial nerve are also at risk during the development of tunnels for passage of the flaps. Injury to the auriculotemporal nerve is less common but is a risk. Finally, the location of the parotid duct should be considered when developing and insetting either flap to avoid transection or, more commonly, compression.

PEARLS AND PITFALLS

- Avoid harvesting both TP fascia and temporalis flaps when the area has previously undergone radiation treatment.
- Consider previous preauricular or coronal flaps a relative contraindication to the TP fascia flap.
- Begin harvesting the TP fascia flap approximately 2 cm above the auricle where the tissue planes are easiest to identify.
- Stay just deep to the hair follicles and protect the skin flaps to decrease the risk for alopecia and skin loss.

- Avoid the facial nerve by staying posterior to a line from 0.5 cm below the tragus to 1.5 cm above the lateral brow. Anterior to this line, dissection must be deep to the TP fascia.
- Dissect the temporalis muscle from the underlying bone in a subperiosteal plane to avoid injury to the deep temporal vessels.
- Place holes in the palatal bone for securing the flaps.

BIBLIOGRAPHY

Abubaker AO, Abouzgia MB: The temporalis muscle flap in reconstruction of intraoral defects: an appraisal of the technique, *Oral Surg Oral Med Oral Pathol Oral Radiol Endod* 94:24-30, 2000.

Bradley P, Brockbank J: The temporalis muscle in oral reconstruction: a cadaveric, animal and clinical study, *J Maxillofac Surg* 9:139-145, 1981.

Cheney ML: Temporalis. In Urken ML, editor: *Atlas of regional and free flaps for head and neck reconstruction*, New York, 1995, Raven Press, p 65.

Cheney ML: Temporoparietal fascia. In Urken ML, editor: *Atlas of regional and free flaps for head and neck reconstruction*, New York, 1995, Raven Press, p 197.

Cheney ML, Varvares MA, Nadol JB Jr: The temporoparietal fascial flap in head and neck reconstruction, *Arch Otolaryngol Head Neck Surg* 119:618-623, 1993.

Dallan I, Lenzi R, Sellari-Franceschini S, et al: Temporalis myofascial flap in maxillary reconstruction: an anatomical study and clinical application, *J Craniomaxillofac Surg* 37:96-101, 2009.

Eldaly A, Magdy EA, Nour YA, et al: Temporalis myofascial flap for primary cranial base reconstruction after tumor resection, *Skull Base* 18:253-263, 2008.

Kelly JP: The use of flaps for reconstruction in oral and maxillofacial surgery, *Selected Readings Oral Maxillofac Surg* 2(7):10, 1993.

Lettieri S: Frontal branch of the facial nerve: galeal temporal relationship, *Aesthet Surg J* 28:143-146, 2008.

Lutcavage GJ, Schaberg SJ: Reconstruction of maxillary defects, *Selected Readings Oral Maxillofac Surg* 5(6):10, 1996.

McGregor IA: The temporal flap in intra-oral cancer: its use in repairing the post-excisional defect, *Br J Plast Surg* 16:318-335, 1963.

Stuzin JM, Wagstrom L, Kawamoto HK, et al: Anatomy of the frontal branch of the facial nerve: the significance of the temporal fat pad, *J Plast Reconstr Surg* 83:265-271, 1989.

Tolhurst DE, Carstens MH, Greco RJ, et al: The surgical anatomy of the scalp, *J Plast Reconstr Surg* 87:603-612, discussion 613-614, 1991.

Ward BB: Temporalis system in maxillary reconstruction: temporalis muscle and temporoparietal galea flaps, *Atlas Oral Maxillofac Surg Clin North Am* 15:33-42, 2007.

Bisphosphonates and Bisphosphonate-Induced Osteonecrosis of the Jaws

Chapter **65**

Robert E. Marx

Though a bisphosphonate, etidronate (Didronel) was introduced in the 1980s mostly for the treatment of Paget disease and bony ankylosis; it was not until the early 2000s that cases of exposed bone in the jaws, now known as bisphosphonate-induced osteonecrosis of the jaws (BIONJ) (Fig. 65-1), became evident. This was largely the result of the introduction of the vastly more potent intravenous bisphosphonates pamidronate (Aredia) and zoledronate (Zometa) for the treatment of hypercalcemia of malignancy and stabilization of metastatic malignancies in bone, as well as the oral bisphosphonate alendronate (Fosamax) for the treatment of osteoporosis. It was available in 1995 but did not become popular until 1999. The increased potency was due to pharmacologic restructuring of the basic bisphosphonate molecule in which nitrogen-containing side chains were added to the backbone carbon.

Today, seven bisphosphonates are currently available in the United States: etidronate (Didronel), tiludronate (Skelid), risedronate (Actonel), alendronate (Fosamax), ibandronate (Boniva), pamidronate (Aredia), and zoledronate (Zometa, 4 mg intravenously once monthly, and Reclast, 5 mg intravenously once every 1 to 2 years). All except etidronate and tiludronate have a nitrogen-containing side chain, which makes all of them much more potent than either etidronate or tiludronate. Alendronate and pamidronate

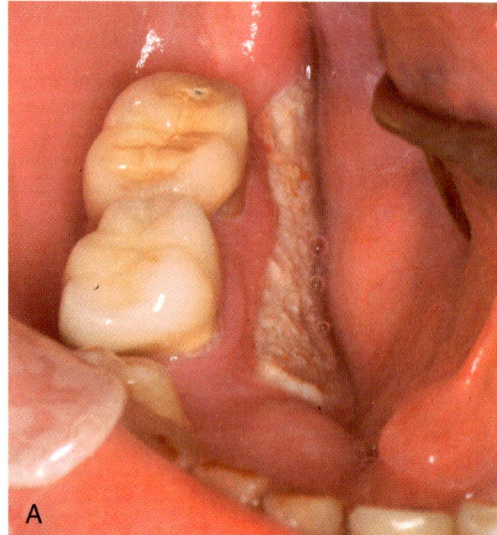

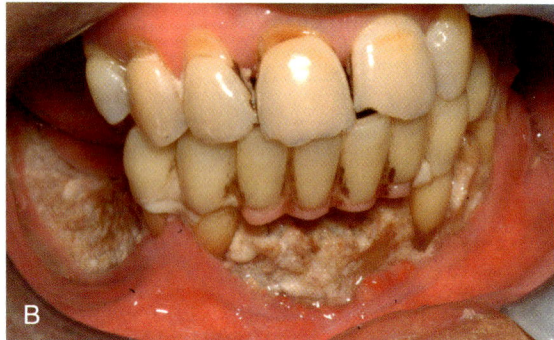

Fig. 65-1 ■ **A,** Bisphosphonate-induced osteonecrosis caused by the oral bisphosphonate alendronate (Fosamax). **B,** Bisphosphonate-induced osteonecrosis caused by the intravenous bisphosphonate zoledronate (Zometa).

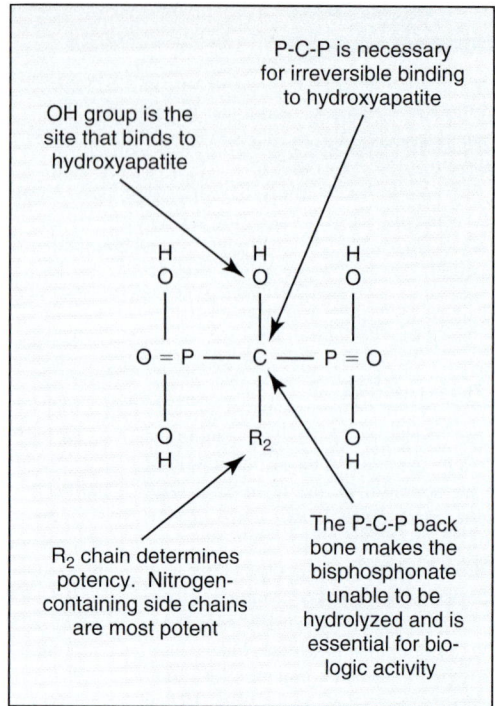

Fig. 65-2 ■ Chemistry of bisphosphonates.

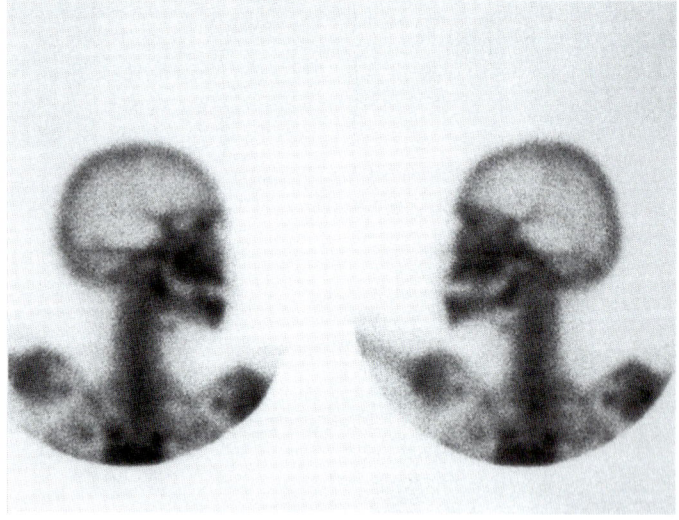

Fig. 65-3 ■ Diphosphonates such as technetium Tc 99m diphosphonate used in diagnostic bone scans have increased uptake in the jaws.

are 5000 times more potent than etidronate, and zoledronate is 10,000 times more potent than etidronate. Only bisphosphonates with a nitrogen-containing side chain cause BIONJ.

BISPHOSPHONATE CHEMISTRY AND PHARMACOLOGY

The basic bisphosphonate molecule is shown in Figure 65-2. The phosphate components impart an affinity for bone from the systemic circulation in the same way that diagnostic technetium Tc 99m methylene diphosphonate bone scan radionuclides collect in more active areas of bone turnover (Fig. 65-3). The backbone carbon provides strong binding to hydroxyapatite in bone, which is made even more irreversible with the addition of an OH group on the backbone carbon. The binding site on the backbone carbon atom opposite this OH group is the site for the nitrogen-containing side chains that confer potency. The result is a bisphosphonate molecule that is irreversibly bound to bone and cannot be metabolized by the human body. Its half-life in bone has been found to be longer than 11 years. The only way that it can be removed from bone is by osteoclastic resorption, which in turn causes apoptosis (cell death) of the osteoclast.

Intravenous administration of a bisphosphonate results in renal clearance of 30% to 40% of the drug. The remaining 60% to 70% becomes bound to bone with a half-life of 11 years. Therefore, some renal toxicity, as well as BIONJ, has been reported with intravenous

bisphosphonates. Oral administration of a bisphosphonate results in only 0.64% of the dose actually being absorbed into the systemic circulation, 30% to 40% of which is cleared in the kidneys. The result is that renal toxicity is not seen with oral bisphosphonates, but frequent severe esophagitis and even rare esophageal cancers have been reported with oral bisphosphonates, presumably because of residual non-absorbed bisphosphonate in contact with the esophageal mucosa. Related to oral bisphosphonates, intravenous bisphosphonates have 140 times the bone bioavailability. The result is that clinical BIONJ caused by intravenous bisphosphonates appears much sooner, is generally more severe, and is less responsive to discontinuation of use of the drug (Fig. 65-4).

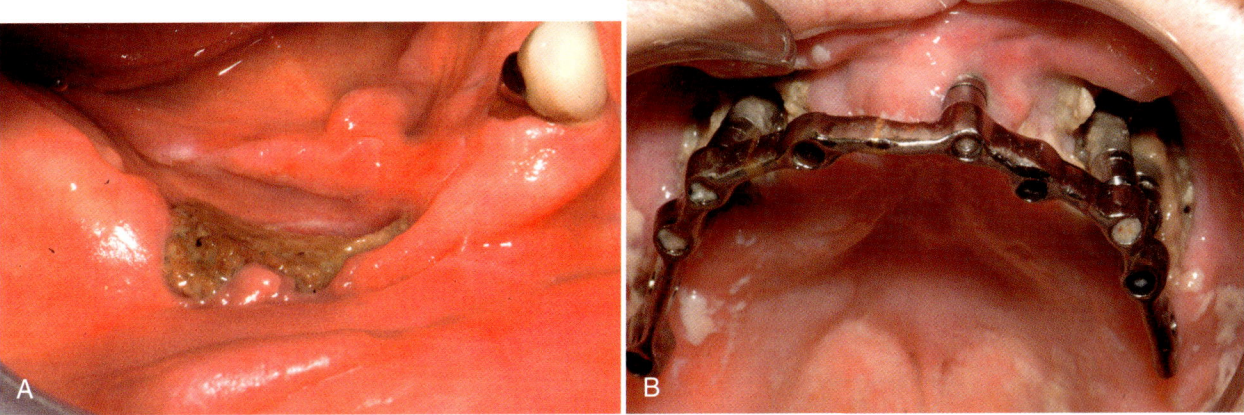

Fig. 65-4 ■ Oral bisphosphonate–induced osteonecrosis (**A**) is generally less extensive and severe than that caused by an intravenous bisphosphonate–induced osteonecrosis (**B**), which is more severe and extensive. (See also Fig. 65-1.)

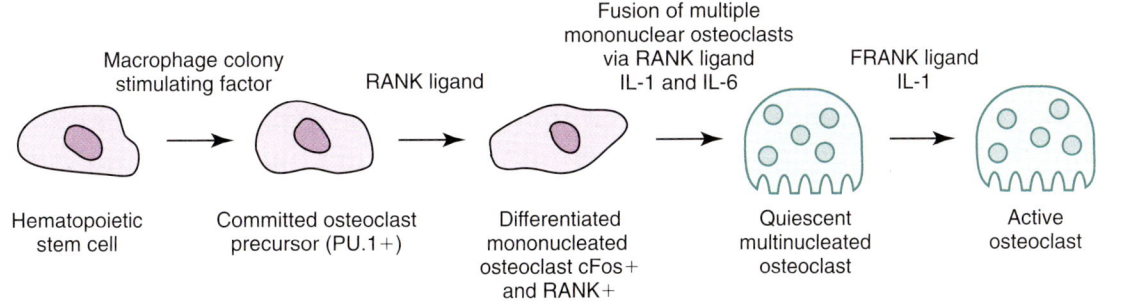

Fig. 65-5 ■ Osteoclasts arise from bone marrow precursor cells and mature in response to serial cytokines. (From Marx RE: *Oral & intravenous bisphosphonate–induced osteonecrosis of the jaws: history, etiology, prevention, and treatment*, ed 2, Hanover Park, IL, 2011, Quintessence.)

MECHANISM OF ACTION AND PATHOLOGY

THE BONE-REMODELING CYCLE

The target of both the therapeutic and adverse effects of bisphosphonates is the osteoclast. Osteoclasts are multinucleated cells that arise from mononuclear bone marrow precursors in a series of maturation steps involving macrophage colony-stimulating factor, receptor activator of nuclear factor κB ligand (RANKL), interleukin-1, and interleukin-6 (Fig. 65-5) into a mature but quiescent osteoclast with a life span of only 14 days. In the normal state, RANKL activates quiescent osteoclasts to actively resorb bone. However, normal bone secretes osteoprotegerin, which competitively inhibits RANKL. Therefore, young healthy bone is not resorbed and the overall skeleton remains stable. However, osteocytes that live for about 180 days become old, and their secretion of osteoprotegerin drops, which allows RANKL to cause resorption of only this old or dead bone (Fig. 65-6). Therefore, evolution has created a mechanism of identifying and eliminating weak and structurally unsound older bone. It has also created a mechanism to replace it with new, more elastic and structurally more supportive bone. That is, during the resorption process, bone morphogenetic protein (BMP) and insulin-like growth factors I and II (IGF-I and IGF-II), which were placed in the bone matrix by osteoblasts at the time of bone formation, are released. These growth and differentiation factors stimulate new bone formation to replace the resorbed bone, thus renewing bone and maintaining skeletal mass and strength (Fig. 65-7).

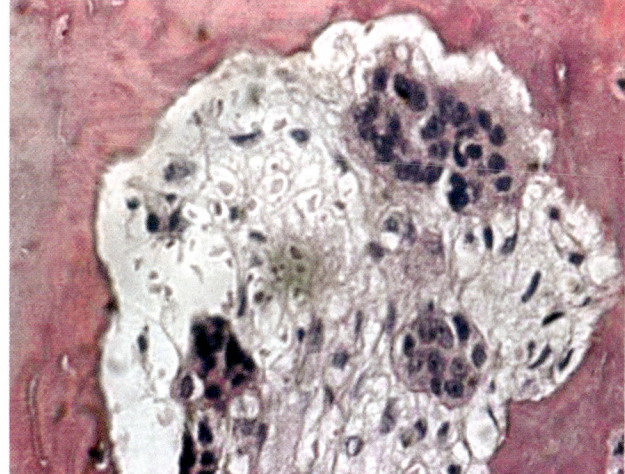

Fig. 65-6 ■ Once RANKL levels exceed the osteoprotegerin levels produced by osteocytes, osteoclastic resorption begins and initiates resorption—a new bone apposition cycle.

STRATEGIES IN BISPHOSPHONATE THERAPEUTICS

Most cancers do not resorb bone by themselves. Instead, they secrete RANKL and RANKL-like substances that locally activate osteoclasts to resorb bone for them. The cancer merely proliferates into the resorbed space. Hence, metastatic cancer deposits accumulate in bone and weaken it to the point of a pathologic fracture, which

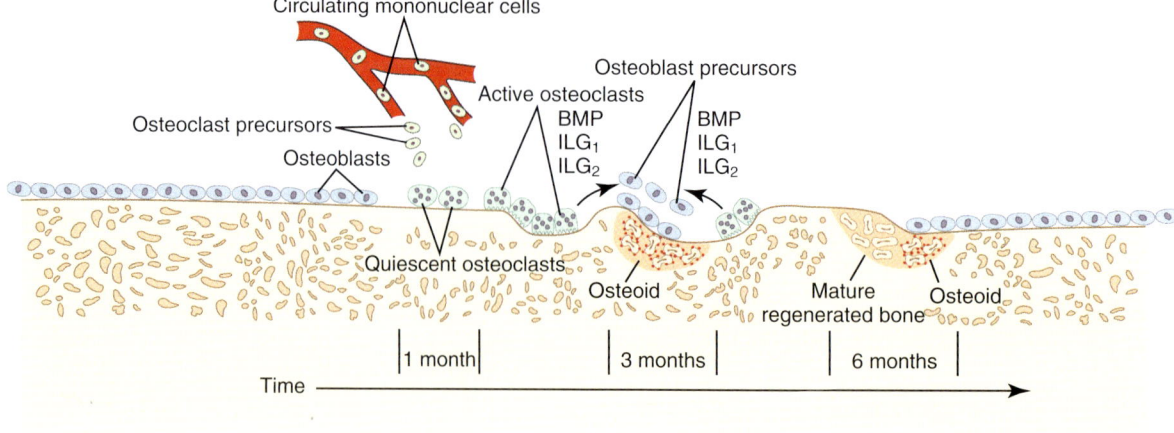

Fig. 65-7 ■ Osteoclasts release bone morphogenetic protein (BMP) and insulin-like growth factors (IGFs) to stimulate new bone formation and maintain skeletal mass. (From Marx RE: *Oral & intravenous bisphosphonate-induced osteonecrosis of the jaws: history, etiology, prevention, and treatment*, ed 2, Hanover Park, IL, 2011, Quintessence.)

causes pain and morbidity. In many cancers, excessive bone resorption results in hypercalcemia, whereas in others (notably small cell carcinoma of the lung), a parathyroid hormone–like peptide is secreted that induces osteoclastic bone resorption and subsequent hypercalcemia. By literally killing off osteoclasts with bisphosphonates, the cancer cannot resorb bone and calcium levels are returned to normal, thereby sparing patients the pain and disability of pathologic fractures and the symptoms of hypercalcemia, such as mental confusion and constipation.

In the treatment of osteoporosis with oral bisphosphonates, their interruption of bone renewal results in greater density of bone by the accumulation of older and more mineralized bone. This is measured by dual-energy x-ray absorptiometry (DEXA). However, although DEXA measures increased bone mineral density, which adds bone strength and resistance to fracturing up to a point, repeated use of an oral bisphosphonate builds up old and more brittle bone, which may actually fracture more easily. Long-bone fractures caused by the use of alendronate for longer than 6 years has already been reported in the literature, and prospective randomized double-blind studies have shown that the therapeutic effects of alendronate cease after 5 years of use. Coupled with the knowledge that the incidence of BIONJ increases and clinical severity worsens after 3 years, the editor of *The Journal of the American Medical Association* stated in the journal that "alendronate—five years of a good thing is enough."

PATHOPHYSIOLOGY OF BISPHOSPHONATE-INDUCED OSTEONECROSIS OF THE JAWS

BIONJ always begins in the alveolar bone or in the surface bone of mandibular or maxillary tori. This is due to the more rapid turnover rate of these bony areas than that found in any other part of the adult skeleton. It is sometimes seen as sclerosis of the lamina dura and widening of the periodontal ligament space because this bone remodels in response to occlusal forces (Fig. 65-8). Since the molar areas have a wider occlusal table and compressive forces are greater on the molars, there is a higher incidence of BIONJ in the molar regions. Even in edentulous patients the target area remains alveolar bone because of compressive forces from denture wearing on the alveolar crest or around dental implants that are loaded for denture function.

Essentially, bisphosphonates prevent the normal renewal of bone in the lamina dura and the edentulous alveolar crest, which results

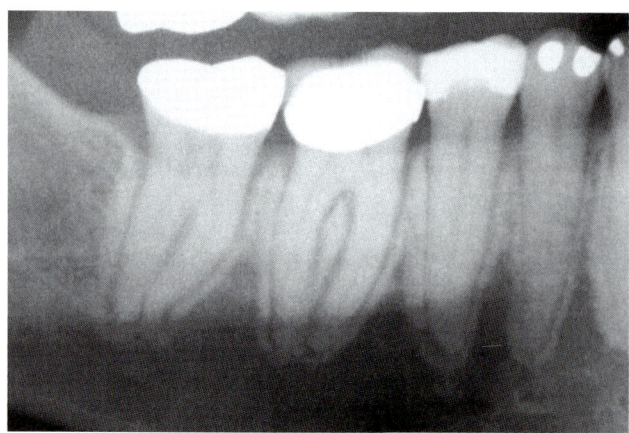

Fig. 65-8 ■ Bisphosphonates retain old non-renewed bone more so in areas of active bone remodeling such as the lamina dura, which may show signs of sclerosis as an indicator.

in retention of old bone that dies off and is not replaced. Such necrotic bone fails to support the blood supply of the overlying mucosa and therefore results in loss of mucosa and bone exposure. The exposed bone in turn may be colonized by microorganisms and give rise to pain from an inflammatory reaction around the colonized area on the bone surface and secondary infection of the surrounding soft tissues. In some cases the microorganism invades into the bone and produces secondary osteomyelitis. The exposed bone by itself is not painful; it is necrotic and absent of blood vessels and nerves. It is only when secondary infection of the soft tissues or, more rarely, the bone occurs that the condition becomes painful.

CLINICAL DISEASE: PREVENTION AND TREATMENT

INTRAVENOUS BISPHOSPHONATE–INDUCED OSTEONECROSIS

Because of the extreme potency of pamidronate and zoledronate and their direct access to bone via the intravenous route, risk for the development of BIONJ begins at about the third dose and increases

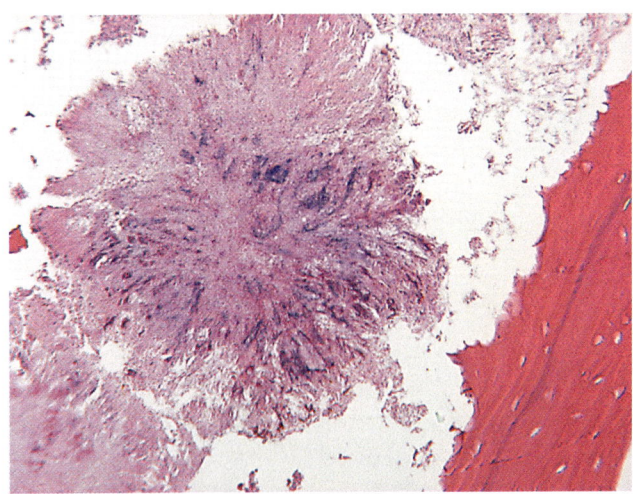

Fig. 65-9 ■ Colony of *Actinomyces* organisms on the surface of exposed necrotic bone in a patient with bisphosphonate-induced osteonecrosis.

with subsequent doses. Co-morbid conditions such as the cancer itself, chemotherapy, and steroids do not cause BIONJ by themselves or even together. However, they may cause it to develop sooner and with more severity. This is illustrated by our prospective analysis of 180 consecutive cases of exposed bone seen in the Oral and Maxillofacial Surgery Service at the University of Miami Miller School of Medicine in patients with no radiation exposure of the jaws between 2003 and 2009. All 180 cases (100%) occurred in individuals who had taken a bisphosphonate, whereas only 50 (27.8%) patients had taken steroids ($P = .001$), 49 (27.2%) had undergone chemotherapy ($P = .001$), 20 (11.1%) had taken antihypertensive drugs ($P = .001$), and 11 (6.1%) had taken any other single class of drugs ($P = .001$) (Fig. 65-9). In addition, during the same period, 25 patients with osteomyelitis were seen, but only 1 (4.0%; $P = 0.001$) had exposed bone.

Intravenous BIONJ may be manifested as spontaneous bone exposure (25%), but 75% of cases are initiated by some type of trauma that increases the remodeling rate of alveolar bone. Tooth removal accounts for the initiation of about 38%; active periodontitis, 22%; periodontal surgery, 11%; and dental implant placement, 4%. This knowledge provides a basis for prevention and restorative strategies focused around the concept of preventive dentistry to reduce the need for tooth removal, periodontal surgery, and other surgically invasive procedures involving bone once the patient is being treated with an intravenous bisphosphonate. Recommendations for prevention are structured into two time frames.

RECOMMENDATIONS FOR PREVENTION BEFORE THE PATIENT BEGINS INTRAVENOUS BISPHOSPHONATE THERAPY

- Removal of unsalvageable teeth
- Dental prophylaxis with instruction in plaque control by a dental hygienist
- Periodontal therapy if indicated
- Restoration of teeth with caries
- Replacement of missing teeth with fixed bridgework, removable partial dentures, or full dentures without placing new implants
- Maintenance of existing implants as one would a natural tooth

Dental practitioners should develop a close working relationship with medical oncologists to support their care of cancer patients.

Because of its life-threatening potential, cancer therapy has greater priority than does the prevention or treatment of BIONJ. Therefore, close communication with medical oncologists is in the patient's best interest. We request deferment of the onset of intravenous bisphosphonate therapy for 2 months to allow sufficient time to accomplish these preventive measures. Most oncologists concur and defer their bisphosphonate treatment. If an oncologist believes that immediate intravenous bisphosphonate therapy is indicated, the practitioner has up to 2 months after the first dose to carry out these preventive measures before significant risk begins.

RECOMMENDATIONS FOR PREVENTION BY PERFORMING DENTAL TREATMENT DURING INTRAVENOUS BISPHOSPHONATE THERAPY

- Avoid or work around invasive surgeries involving bone (e.g., tooth removal, periodontal surgery, apicoectomy, dental implants, torus removal).
- Treat caries and restore all teeth requiring restorative procedures. Restorations, crowns, bridgework, and removable partial and full dentures are safe at any time, as are non-surgical root canal treatments. If necessary, one should perform a root canal procedure on a non-restorable tooth, amputate the crown, and restore it with a post and core crown or leave the root in place for an overdenture concept.
- Perform prophylaxis and scaling.
- Splint mobile teeth.

If an extraction is unavoidable, such as because of significant mobility, a vertical root fracture, or other causes, informed consent concerning risk for BIONJ should be obtained.

TREATMENT OF INTRAVENOUS BISPHOSPHONATE–INDUCED OSTEONECROSIS

The definition of BIONJ is "exposed non-healing bone in the mandible or maxilla that persists for more than 8 weeks in a person who received a systemic bisphosphonate but has not undergone local radiation to the jaws." Some patients will have asymptomatic exposed bone (31%), which indicates that secondary infection is not present. However, 69% will have exposed bone and pain indicative of a secondary infection. Individuals may also have draining oral or cutaneous fistulas, mobile teeth, sinus infections, and pathologic fractures. The most common microorganism seen in patients with BIONJ is *Actinomyces*, with *Moraxella*, *Veillonella*, and *Eikenella* also frequently being found (see Fig. 65-9). Therefore, penicillin is the drug of choice to treat such secondary infections, and clindamycin is not indicated for patients with BIONJ because these organisms are either resistant or are poorly susceptible to clindamycin.

Staging of both intravenous and oral BIONJ cases is disputed among different organization position papers. Most falsely use pain as a criterion. Since pain is due to secondary infection and is unrelated to the objective severity or extent of the disease, this author does not use pain as a criterion but the clinical surface area and the radiographic picture instead as follows:

Stage I: One quadrant or less of exposed bone without osteolysis beyond the alveolus or extension into the maxillary sinus

Stage II: Two or more quadrants with exposed bone without evidence of osteolysis beyond the alveolus or extension into the maxillary sinus

Stage III: Any occurrence of osteolysis beyond the alveolus or a pathologic fracture.

Treatment of patients with stage I, stage II, and selective stage III disease is centered around control of pain and maintenance of function. Other than rounding sharp edges of bone that abrade the tongue, attempts at localized débridement have been mostly ineffective and have actually resulted in a larger area of exposed bone and are thus not recommended. Surgeries must be extensive and take the form of alveolectomies or continuity resections to resolve intravenous BIONJ, which may create a functional loss or disability worse than the existing dead bone. In addition, such patients with cancer are often at serious risk for complications during anesthesia, and their potential bone donor sites may contain cancer, thus making reconstruction afterward in these patients problematic. Therefore, control of pain, limitation of secondary infection, and extension of the exposed bone are the primary goals. This is achieved with 0.12% chlorhexidine (Peridex), 15-mL oral swish and spitting three times daily as the baseline treatment. Penicillin VK, 500 mg by mouth four times daily, is the antibiotic of choice to control the pain associated with secondary infection initially and is restarted during exacerbations. If the patient is allergic to penicillin, doxycycline, 100 mg once daily, levofloxacin (Levaquin), 500 mg, and azithromycin, 500 mg once daily, are reasonable alternatives. However, one must limit levofloxacin to no more than 14 days because of the risk for tendon rupture and azithromycin to no more than 14 days because of elevations in liver enzyme levels. In patients who have a minimal response to either of these antibiotic regimens or have frequent exacerbations, adding metronidazole, 500 mg three times daily for 10 days, to these antibiotics will usually resolve the secondary infection. Stage III patients who have a pathologic fracture or experience repeated exacerbations are candidates for resection. In the maxilla, such resections often become hemi-maxillectomies with thorough débridement of the infected sinus membrane. The resultant defect may be closed immediately with a buccal fat pad transfer if the defect is small or with a temporalis muscle flap if the defect is sufficiently large (Fig. 65-10). Otherwise, the resultant oral-antral-nasal communication will require a maxillary obturator prosthesis (Fig. 65-11).

In the mandible, such surgeries most often take the form of a continuity resection. The margins of the continuity resection may be difficult to anticipate. However, recalling that BIONJ starts in alveolar bone and that areas of greatest occlusal force are at the greatest risk, one can usually plan a resection with adequate margins. That is, resection to the ramus or condyles will result in a less than involved proximal margin, and resection to edentulous areas or to areas where the bone about the incisors and canines is not radiographically involved will usually result in an adequate distal margin (Fig. 65-12). A titanium reconstruction plate should be placed and secured to the intact mandible based on the anticipated resection margins and bicortical screws placed into tapped screw holes for the best long-term stability. This is necessary because a reconstruction plate will probably be the only definitive reconstruction that one can offer. Therefore, one should also plan to place at least four screws in each segment to provide maximum stability. As a final check of the adequacy of the margins, the resection edges should contain some residual soft marrow, bleeding of which indicates viable bone (see Fig. 65-12, C). In most cases a soft tissue flap is not required. This is in contrast to most cases of osteoradionecrosis (ORN) because radiation damages and reduces the blood supply to both bone and soft tissues. Bisphosphonate-induced osteonecrosis targets only the bone directly. The soft tissue effects are due to secondary infection. Therefore, it is only in patients with long-standing BIONJ and secondary infection that sufficient soft tissue is lost to require a soft tissue flap (Fig. 65-13). This fundamental contrast between ORN, which is a radiation-induced injury to the blood vessels and stem cells in bone, as well as to adjacent soft tissues, in which an oxygen gradient deficit is created, and BIONJ, which is a specific

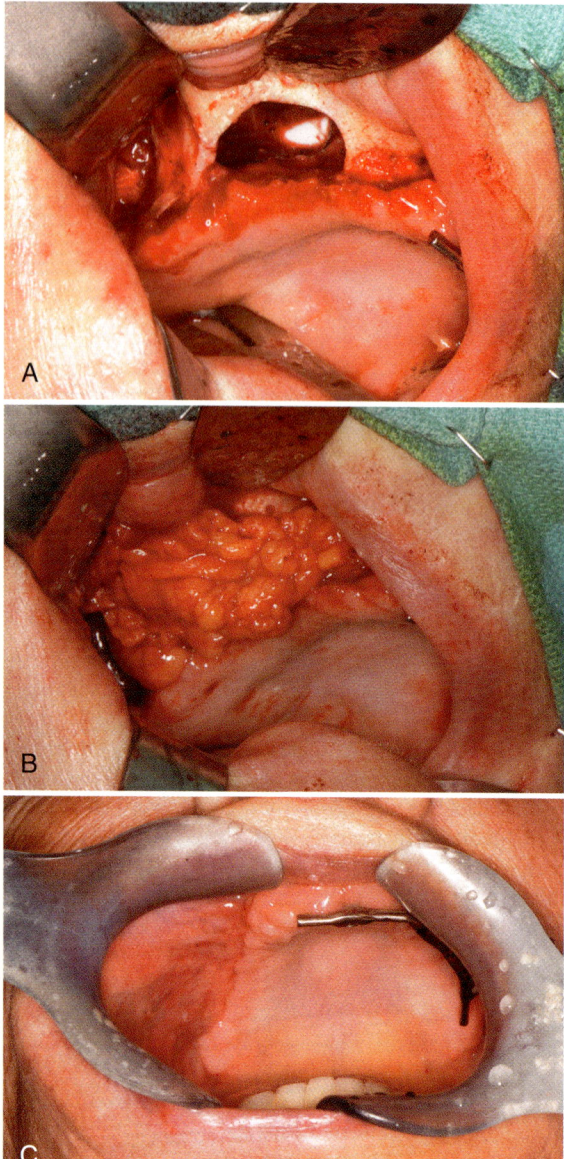

Fig. 65-10 ■ **A,** Defect of the maxilla caused by an intravenous bisphosphonate. **B,** Advancement of a pedicled buccal fat pad is useful to obliterate the dead space and bring vascular tissue into the area. **C,** Healed maxilla after débridement and buccal fat pad transfer.

drug-induced cellular toxicity that occurs only in bone, is also why hyperbaric oxygen, though of great effectiveness for ORN, is of no therapeutic value for BIONJ.

In cases of BIONJ that require resection (20% to 30%), the resection usually resolves the disease. As long as the resection does not create a worse functional loss or deformity, it is a useful treatment of selected stage III cases and selected refractory cases.

In monitoring the healing of patients after resection it is often noted that new bone partially regenerates in the defect from the retained periosteum (see Fig. 65-13, A). This observation underscores the selective toxicity of bisphosphonates on osteoclasts and sparing of osteoblasts in the periosteum, which do not come into direct contact with bisphosphonates because they do not resorb bone.

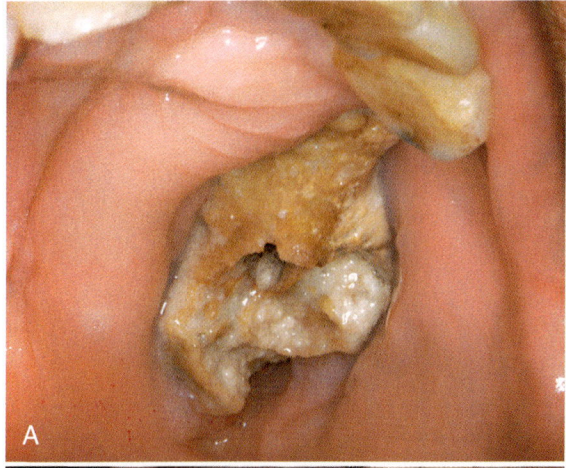

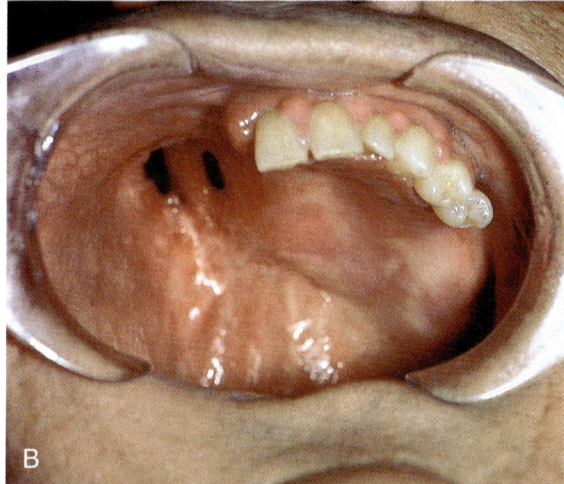

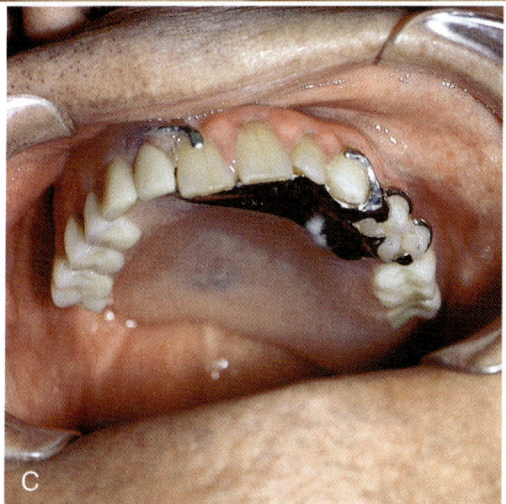

Fig. 65-11 ■ **A,** Intravenous bisphosphonate–induced osteonecrosis of the maxilla. **B,** Resultant defect from resection of necrotic bone. **C,** A maxillary obturator prosthesis is required to manage the oral-antral-nasal defect resulting from surgery.

ORAL BISPHOSPHONATE–INDUCED OSTEONECROSIS OF THE JAWS

The osteoporosis market is worth $10 billion per year. Thus, big drug companies are very competitive and attempt to gain and maintain a large market share. Merck (Whitehouse Station, NJ), the manufacturer of Fosamax, made $3.2 billion per year in the

mid-2000s before their patent expired, but it still earns $1.3 billion per year. It commanded the biggest market share because it doubled the dose of alendronate over that of the competitors risedronate (Actonel) and ibandronate (Boniva), yet all of these drugs are equally absorbed and equally potent. The result is that alendronate accounts for more than 95% of all BIONJ cases caused by oral bisphosphonates. Novartis Pharmaceutical Company (Basel, Switzerland) introduced zoledronate, 5 mg intravenously once yearly, in 2007 for the indication of osteoporosis to capture their share of the osteoporosis marketplace. Zoledronate is the same drug that this company uses for cancer metastasis and hypercalcemia of malignancy at 4 mg intravenously once monthly. Changing the dose or the frequency of a drug allows companies to use it for a different indication and with a different name. In just 2 years on the market, cases of BIONJ caused by Reclast are occurring.

In the clinical setting, alendronate is the drug at greatest risk for causing BIONJ. As stated earlier, oral BIONJ cases are less common, less severe, and more amenable to localized surgery than intravenous BIONJ cases are. Nevertheless, stage III cases, which are usually associated with use for longer than 6 years and require resection, are also seen. Although some cases occur after only 1 or 2 years of alendronate use, most develop after 3 years of use and the severity increases thereafter.

RECOMMENDATIONS FOR PREVENTION BEFORE THE PATIENT BEGINS THERAPY WITH AN ORAL BISPHOSPHONATE

The same commonsense preventive and restorative dentistry as outlined for patients before receiving an intravenous bisphosphonate applies to those about to begin or have just begun treatment with an oral bisphosphonate. However, in the case of oral bisphosphonate use, there is more time for the dentition and oral health to be optimized because of more gradual accumulation of oral bisphosphonates into bone.

RECOMMENDATIONS FOR PREVENTION BY PERFORMING DENTAL TREATMENT DURING ORAL BISPHOSPHONATE THERAPY

As stated for patients receiving intravenous bisphosphonate therapy, non-surgical dental procedures such as restorative dentistry, dental prophylaxis, scaling, and prosthodontic care are safe at all times. It is surgical trauma, the constant inflammatory disease of periodontitis, and traumatic occlusion that place patients at greater risk for the development of oral BIONJ. The commonality of all three is that the stress for more constant bone remodeling is suppressed and may be over-suppressed by the oral bisphosphonates. However, because bone accumulation is slower and less extensive than with intravenous bisphosphonates, alveolar bone can recover with temporary discontinuation of the drug, referred to as a "drug holiday." During a drug holiday, the bone marrow, which was less affected by oral bisphosphonate toxicity that it would have been by an intravenous bisphosphonate, is able to repopulate much of the lost osteoclasts. The return of osteoclast activity restores bone renewal capacity and allows healing. This can be measured to an approximate degree by the morning fasting serum C-terminal telopeptide (CTX) test.

The CTX test measures an octapeptide fragment of a branching chain in bone collagen that is released during osteoclastic bone resorption. It is an index of osteoclastic activity and was used in most of the original research studies on the therapeutic effects of oral bisphosphonates, as well as that of Reclast. It is a limited study that is not accurate in patients with active cancer, those who have

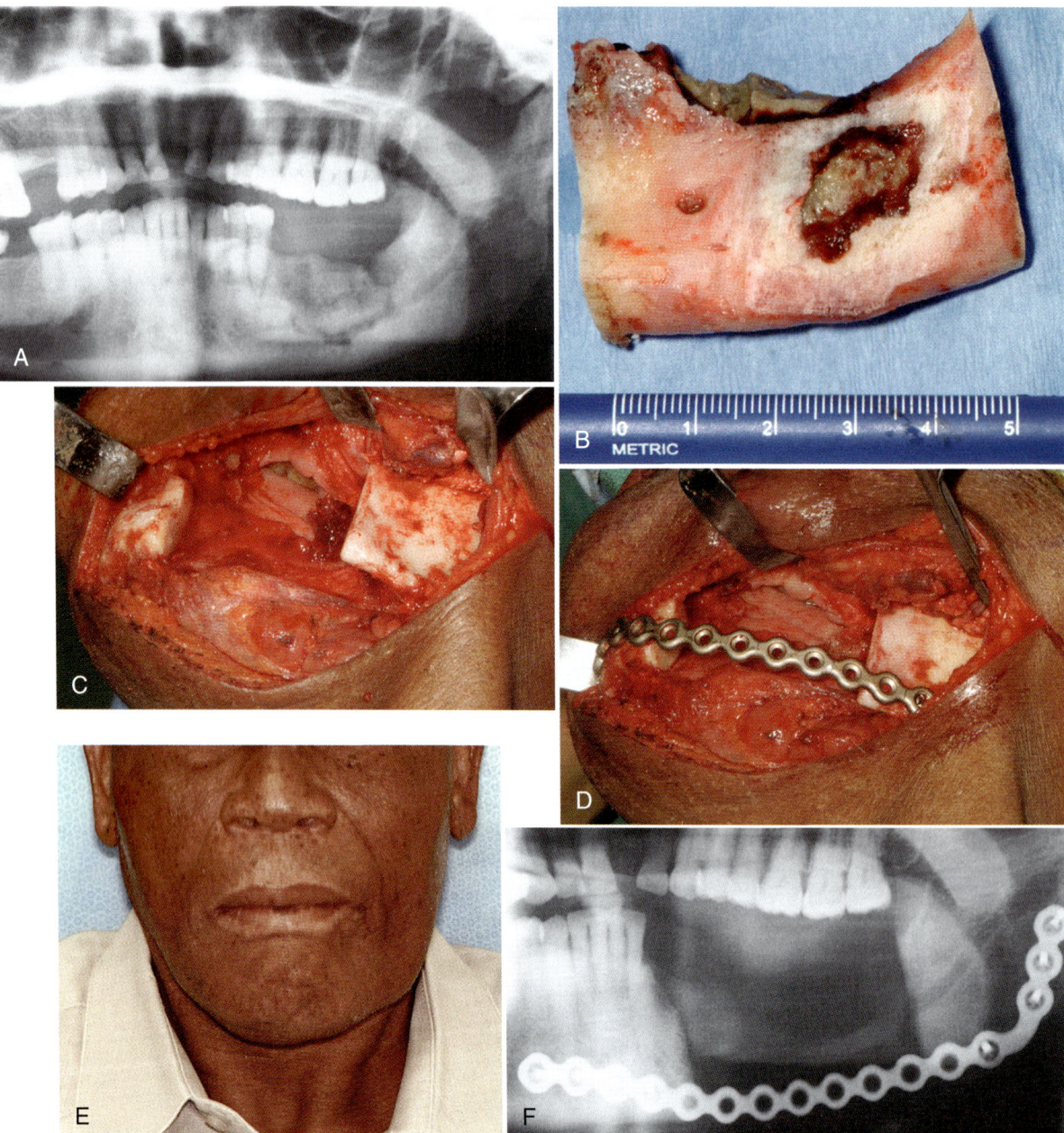

Fig. 65-12 ■ **A,** Stage III intravenous bisphosphonate–induced osteonecrosis with osteolysis of the inferior border caused by Zometa. **B,** Five-centimeter resection specimen. **C,** Consequent defect in continuity and oral opening as a result of resection for intravenous bisphosphonate–induced osteonecrosis. **D,** Resection defect reconstructed with a rigid titanium plate. **E,** Postresection photograph showing maintenance of facial contours and lip position after surgery. **F,** Three-year follow-up after resection showing a stable titanium plate. Note the new bone regenerated at the superior edge of the defect. This results from retained periosteum and indicates that bisphosphonate toxicity does not directly extend to osteoblasts.

taken either prednisone or methotrexate, or those who are currently taking raloxifene (Evista). Therefore, it is of limited use in intravenous bisphosphonate–treated patients with a malignancy and in most rheumatoid patients because of their exposure to prednisone and methotrexate. However, for more than 90% of women with osteopenia or osteoporosis, CTX values correlate closely with risk for oral BIONJ and with disease activity if they have exposed bone.

In individuals who require an oral surgical procedure and have taken an oral bisphosphonate or are currently taking an oral bisphosphonate, the author obtains a baseline CTX value. Since most oral bisphosphonates are taken once each week, the best results are

obtained if the morning fasting blood is drawn 5 days after the weekly dose. Values lower than 100 pg/mL are concerning and represent a significant risk for the development of BIONJ. Values between 101 and 150 pg/mL are less concerning and represent a mild to moderate risk. That is, minimally traumatic procedures can be performed but more extensive procedures should be deferred. Values above 150 pg/mL have been found to allow normal healing after any oral surgical procedures.

If elective surgery is planned, a drug holiday is recommended from the prescribing physician. Such drug holidays will result in a gradual improvement in CTX values over a period of 6 to 9 months.

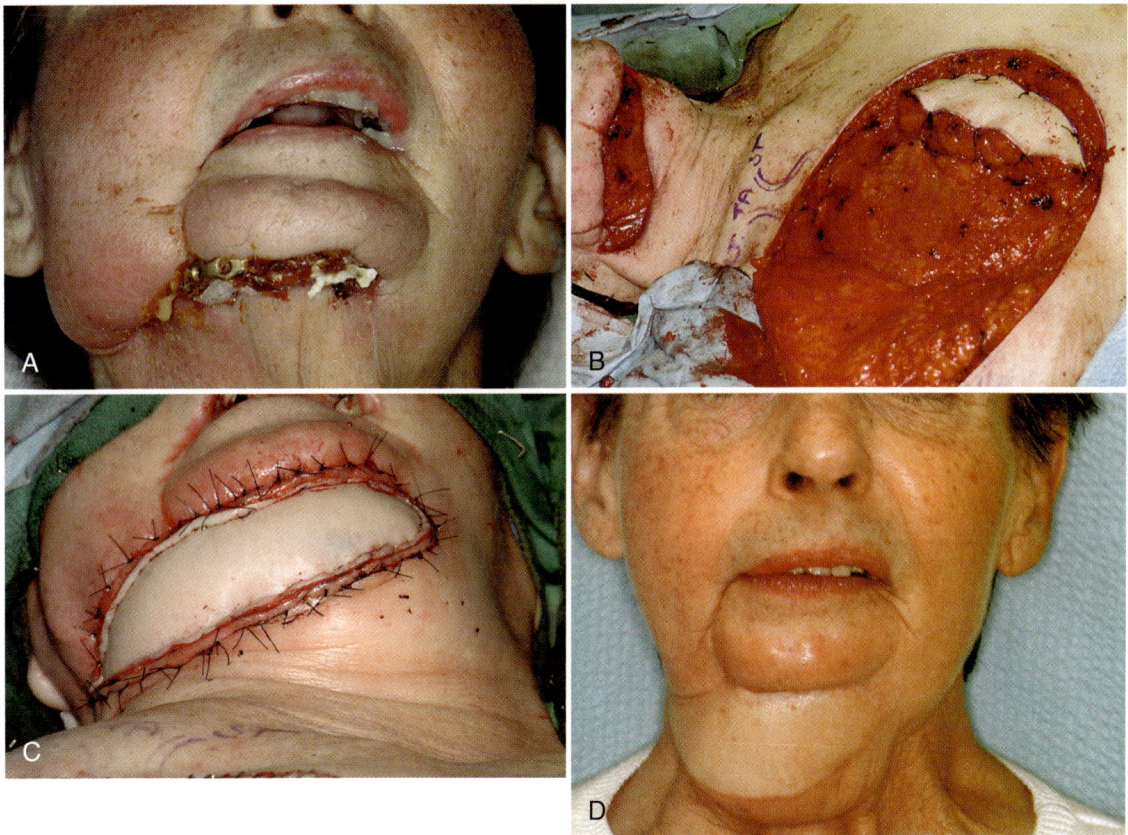

Fig. 65-13 ■ **A,** Intravenous bisphosphonate–induced osteonecrosis with significant loss of skin as a result of secondary infection. **B,** A pectoralis major myocutaneous flap was required to replace the lost skin and subcutaneous tissue. **C,** Skin paddle of the pectoralis major myocutaneous flap sutured into the defect. **D,** Resolved intravenous bisphosphonate–induced osteonecrosis and secondary infection with replacement of lost soft tissue.

Ideally, the surgery can be performed when the CTX value exceeds 150 pg/mL or stabilizes above 100 pg/mL with no further increase. The drug holiday is extended for 2 months after the surgery, which allows sufficient time for bone healing to occur before restarting a bisphosphonate.

Drug holidays are usually agreed to and implemented by the prescribing physician for several reasons. First, the physician has the opportunity to restart a bisphosphonate 2 months after the oral surgery procedure. Second, alternative osteoporosis treatments that do not pose the same risk as a bisphosphonate may be used during the drug holiday. Such alternatives include calcium and vitamin D, raloxifene (Evista), salmon calcitonin (Miacalcin) and rh1-34PTH (Forteo). Third, a sentinel study by Black and colleagues showed that discontinuation of alendronate for 5 years does not result in worsening of osteoporosis as indicated by osteoporosis-related fractures. Therefore, drug holidays for even several years are safe and effective.

TREATMENT RECOMMENDATIONS FOR ORAL BISPHOSPHONATE–INDUCED OSTEONECROSIS OF THE JAWS

The exposed bone caused by the use of an oral bisphosphonate is non-vital, as is the exposed bone caused by the use of an intravenous bisphosphonate (see Figs 65-1 and 65-4). However, because of the more gradual accumulation of an oral bisphosphonate into bone, the bone marrow had been able to repopulate and maintain the osteoclast precursor population. Therefore, during a drug holiday, the bone marrow recovers and increases the population of osteoclasts, which begin to resorb the non-viable bone and separate it from the viable bone. In some cases in which the amount of non-viable exposed bone is small, it is completely resorbed and the area heals (Fig. 65-14). In other cases the non-viable bone is separated as a sequestrum and sloughed off or can be removed in a straightforward office procedure that leads to healing (Fig. 65-15). In advanced cases in which the amount of non-viable bone is great, the return of osteoclast function is still incapable of complete resorption or a sequestration process, thus indicating the need for more aggressive débridement or resection (Fig. 65-16).

In each situation, CTX values usually increase with the drug holiday. When the CTX value exceeds 150 pg/mL, we have found that débridement surgeries, often conducted in the office setting, heal without further exposed bone. In many cases a clear line of demarcation between non-viable and viable bone can be seen and guide the débridement (Fig. 65-17; also see Fig. 65-15, *B*). In cases in which resection is indicated, a CTX value greater than 150 pg/ mL has also been associated with uncomplicated healing.

Localized defects resulting from débridement surgery may be grafted with either autogenous bone grafts or bone-regenerative grafts consisting of recombinant human BMP (rhBMP-2)/acellular collagen sponge (rhBMP-2/ACS) combined with particulate freeze-dried bone allograft and platelet-rich plasma (Fig. 65-18). In addition, once oral BIONJ has been resolved, the residual bone can receive and predictably osseointegrate dental implants (Fig. 65-19).

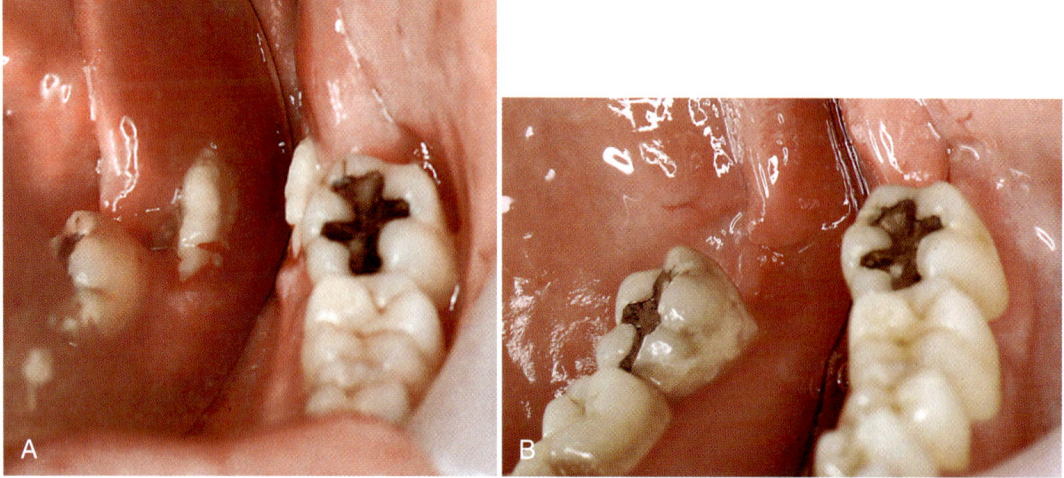

Fig. 65-14 ■ **A,** Oral bisphosphonate–induced osteonecrosis caused by Fosamax before a drug holiday. **B,** The exposed bone sloughed and the mucosa healed after a 6-month drug holiday and rising CTX values.

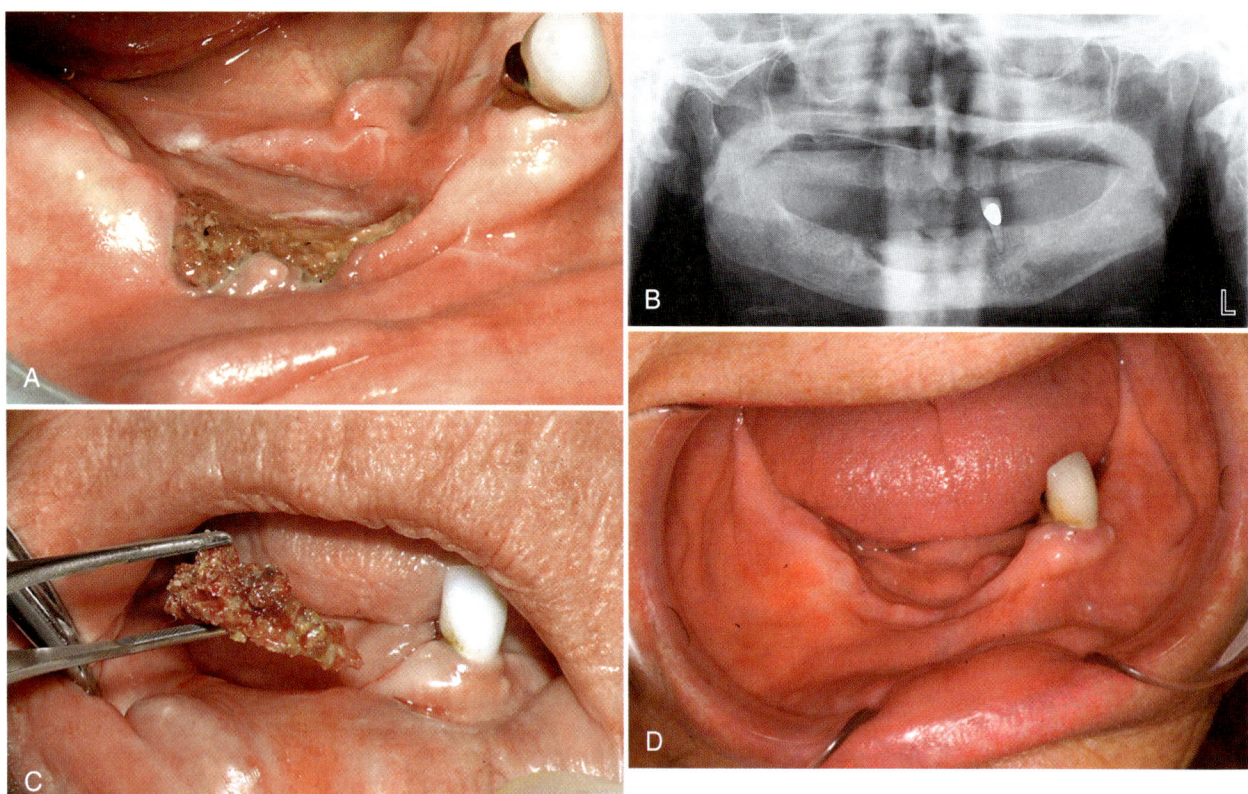

Fig. 65-15 ■ **A,** Oral bisphosphonate–induced osteonecrosis caused by Fosamax before a drug holiday. **B,** Panoramic film showing a sequestrum and involucrum after a 6-month drug holiday and rising CTX values. **C,** This patient required only office-based local débridement to resolve the exposed bone. **D,** Healed bone and mucosa as a result of the drug holiday and local débridement accomplished after the drug holiday.

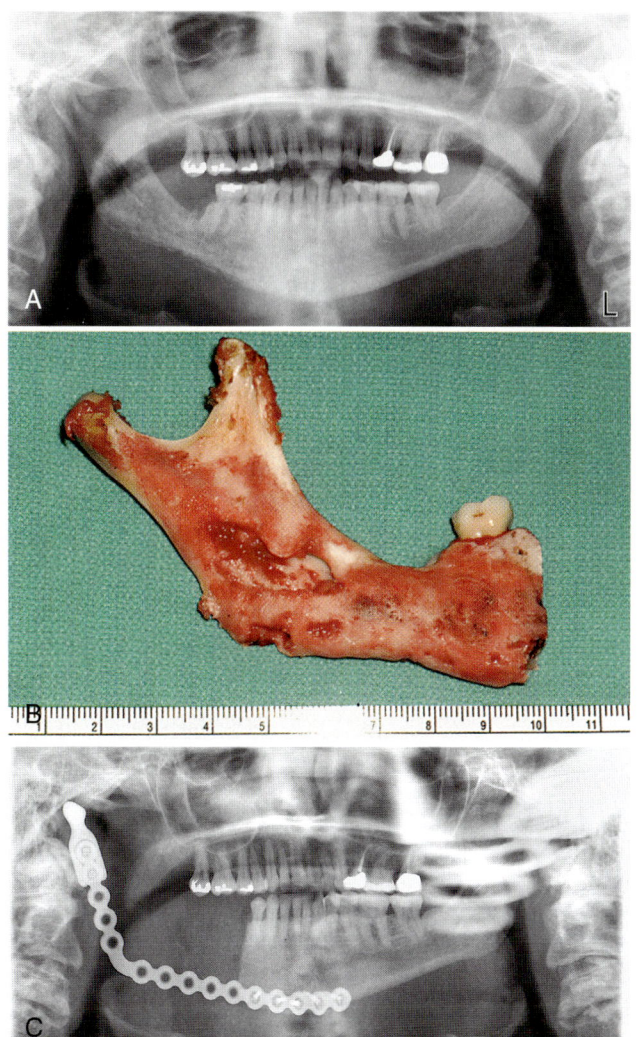

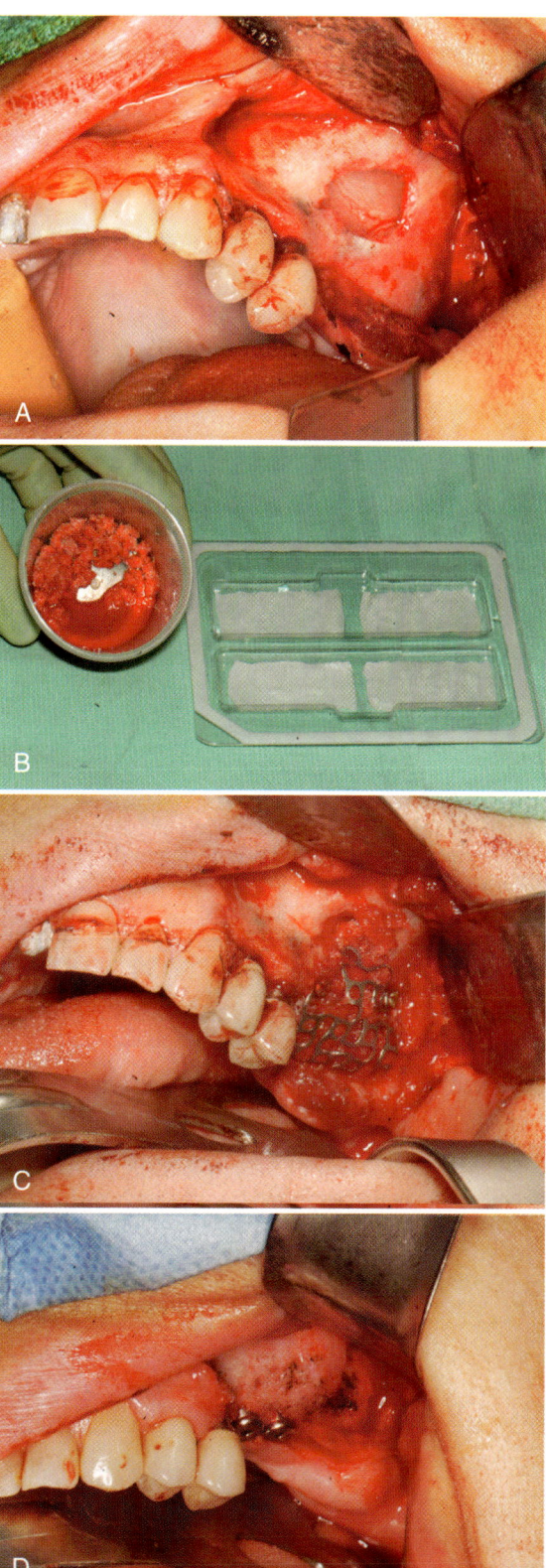

Fig. 65-16 ■ **A,** Stage III oral bisphosphonate–induced osteonecrosis after extraction of tooth No. 31 in a patient with a 10-year exposure to Fosamax. **B,** The extensive bone involvement caused by 10-year exposure to Fosamax required a disarticulation hemi-mandibulectomy. **C,** The defect resulting from the resection required a titanium plate with a condylar replacement.

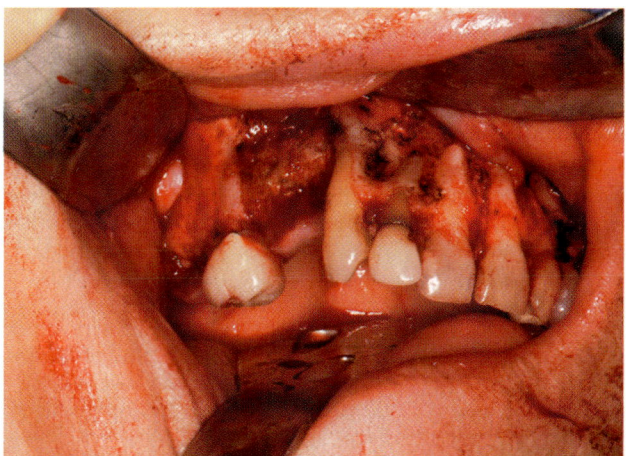

Fig. 65-17 ■ A line of demarcation between necrotic bone and viable bone is seen after a 9-month drug holiday in this patient with oral bisphosphonate–induced osteonecrosis.

Fig. 65-18 ■ **A,** Maxillary defect resulting from débridement of oral bisphosphonate–induced osteonecrosis. **B,** Regeneration of many bone defects caused by oral bisphosphonate–induced osteonecrosis can be accomplished by using recombinant human bone morphogenetic protein (rhBMP), mineralized freeze-dried allogeneic bone (MFDAB), and platelet-rich plasma (PRP) (rhBMP-MFDAB-PRP). **C,** The graft is usually contained within a titanium mesh. **D,** Complete regeneration of bone from a rhBMP-2–CCFDAB-PRP graft with dental implants in place.

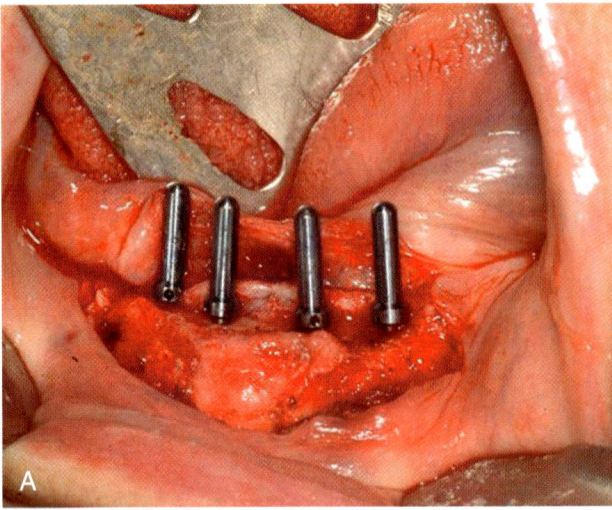
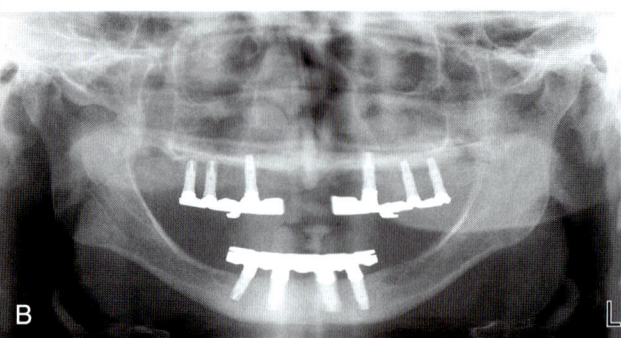

Fig. 65-19 ■ A and **B,** Patients with resolved oral bisphosphonate–induced osteonecrosis can undergo dental implant rehabilitation if the drug holiday continues.

PEARLS AND PITFALLS

- Office-based local débridement for intravenous bisphosphonate induced osteonecrosis of the jaws (BIONJ) often results in further exposed bone and worsening of the condition.
- Since 0.12% chlorhexidine and intermittent courses of antibiotics are able to control secondary infection and pain in most cases, a policy of resection for all patients rather than selected patients with intravenous bisphosphonate–induced osteonecrosis results in irreversible excessive morbidity that is not necessary.
- The presence of infection and osteolysis is a secondary infection of necrotic bone caused by the bisphosphonate. It is not a primary osteomyelitis.
- The CTX test is reliable only in patients with uncomplicated osteopenia and osteoporosis. In cancer patients receiving an intravenous bisphosphonate or in patients who received steroids or methotrexate together with an oral bisphosphonate, the CTX test is unreliable.
- Alendronate (Fosamax) is the more worrisome oral bisphosphonate and has caused the most cases of oral bisphosphonate–induced osteonecrosis, mainly because it is marketed at twice the equivalent dose of other oral bisphosphonates.
- Although oral bisphosphonate–induced osteonecrosis is generally less severe than that caused by intravenous bisphosphonates, some cases of long-term oral bisphosphonate use result in extensive bone exposure and pathologic fractures and require resection.
- Avoidance of trauma to alveolar bone, such as occurs with tooth extractions, implant placement, and periodontal surgery, remains the best method for preventing intravenous bisphosphonate–induced osteonecrosis.
- Alveolar bone surgery such as tooth extractions, implant placement, and periodontal surgery can be accomplished safely in patients with a history of oral bisphosphonate use if they have been on a drug holiday for 9 months or more or have a serum CTX value of 150 pg/mL or greater.
- Drug holidays from intravenous antibiotics do not reduce the risk for bisphosphonate-induced osteonecrosis, as occurs with drug holidays from oral bisphosphonates, because of the greater bone accumulation with the intravenous route.
- Dental professionals should not have patients discontinue use of an intravenous bisphosphonate. It is the decision of the medical oncologist. Control of cancer is always more important than the bisphosphonate-induced osteonecrosis.
- Also, dental professionals should not have patients discontinue use of an oral bisphosphonate. It is the responsibility and decision of the prescribing physician. The dental professional should request a drug holiday from the prescribing physician.

BIBLIOGRAPHY

Advisory Task Force on Bisphosphonate-Related Osteonecrosis of the Jaws: American Association of Oral and Maxillofacial Surgeons position paper on bisphosphonate-related osteonecrosis of the jaws, *J Oral Maxillofac Surg* 65:369-376, 2007.

Black DM, Delmas PD, Eastell R, et al, for the HORIZON Pivotal Fracture Trial: Once-yearly zoledronic acid for treatment of postmenopausal osteoporosis, *N Engl J Med* 356:1809-1822, 2007.

Black DM, Schwartz AV, Ensrud KE, et al, for the FLEX Research Group: Effects of continuing or stopping alendronate after 5 years of treatment, *JAMA* 296:2927-2938, 2006.

Bone HG, Hosking D, Devogelaer JP, et al, for the Alendronate Phase III Osteoporosis Treatment Study Group: Ten years' experience with alendronate for osteoporosis in postmenopausal women, *N Engl J Med* 350:1189-1199, 2004.

Colón-Emeric CS: Ten vs. five years of bisphosphonate treatment for post menopausal osteoporosis: enough of a good thing, *JAMA* 296:2968-2969, 2006.

Dental management of patients receiving oral bisphosphonate therapy. Expert Panel Recommendations, *J Am Dent Assoc* 134:1144-1152, 2006.

Ensrud KE, Barrett-Connor EL, Schwartz A, et al, for the Fracture Intervention Trial Long-Term Extension Research Group: Randomized trial of effect of alendronate continuation versus discontinuation in women with low BMD: results from the Fracture Intervention Trial Long-Term Extension, *J Bone Miner Res* 19:1259-1269, 2004.

Khosla S, Burr D, Cauley J, et al, for the American Society for Bone and Mineral Research: Bisphosphonate-associated osteonecrosis of the jaw: report of a task force of the American Society for Bone and Mineral Research, *J Bone Miner Res* 22:1479-1491, 2007.

Kunchur R, Need A, Hughes T, et al: Clinical investigation of C-terminal cross-linking telopeptide test in prevention and management of bisphosphonate-associated osteonecrosis of the jaws, *J Oral Maxillofac Surg* 67:1167-1173, 2009.

Kwon YD, Kim DY, Ohe JY, et al: Correlation between serum C-terminal cross-linking telopeptide of type I collagen and staging of oral bisphosphonate–related osteonecrosis of the jaws, *J Oral Maxillofac Surg* 67:2644-2648, 2009.

Lasseter KC, Porros AG, Denker A, et al: Pharmacokinetic considerations in determining the terminal elimination half lives of bisphosphonates, *Clin Drug Invest* 25:107-114, 2005.

Lenart BA, Lorich DG, Lane JM: Atypical fractures of the femoral diaphysis in postmenopausal women taking alendronate, *N Engl J Med* 358:1304-1306, 2008.

Martin TJ, Gill V: Bisphosphonates—mechanism of action. Experimental and clinical pharmacology, *Auctr Preser* 23:130, 2000.

Marx RE: Pamidronate (Aredia) and zoledronate (Zometa) induce avascular necrosis of the jaws. A growing epidemic, *J Oral Maxillofac Surg* 61:1115-1117, 2003.

Marx RE, Cillo JE Jr, Ulloa JJ: Oral bisphosphonate-induced osteonecrosis: risk factors, prediction of risk using serum CTX testing, prevention, and treatment, *J Oral Maxillofac Surg* 65:2397-2410, 2007.

Neviaser AS, Lane JM, Lenart BA, et al: Low-energy femoral shaft fractures associated with alendronate use, *J Orthop Trauma* 22:346-350, 2008.

Ribeiro A, DeVault KR, Wolfe JT 3rd, et al: Alendronate-associated esophagitis: endoscopic and pathologic features, *Gastrointest Endosc* 47:525-528, 1998.

Rogers MJ, Frith JC, Luckman SP, et al: Molecular mechanisms of action of bisphosphonates, *Bone* 24(5 Suppl):73S-79S, 1999.

Rosen HN, Moses AC, Garber J, et al: Serum CTX: a new marker of bone resorption that shows treatment effect more often than other markers because of low coefficient of variability and large changes with bisphosphonate therapy, *Calcif Tissue Int* 66:100-103, 2000.

Ruggiero SL, Mehrota B, Rosenberg TJ, et al: Osteonecrosis of the jaws associated with the use of bisphosphonates: a review of 63 cases, *J Oral Maxillofac Surg* 62:527-534, 2004.

Russell RG, Croucher PI, Rogers MJ: Bisphosphonates: pharmacology, mechanisms of action and clinical uses, *Osteoporos Int* 9(Suppl 2):S66-S80, 1999.

Spiegel A: How a bone disease grew to fit the prescription. NPR. http://www.npr.org/templates/story/story.php?storyid=121609815.

Wysowski DK: Reports of esophageal cancer with oral bisphosphonate use, *N Engl J Med* 360:89-90, 2009.

Maxillofacial Reconstruction Using Cancellous Cellular Marrow Grafts

Chapter **66**

Robert E. Marx

Bone regeneration using cancellous cellular marrow grafts has been the mainstay for oral and maxillofacial surgeons simply because they produce the most bone in the correct arch form and are best able to support functional needs. Even though most oral and maxillofacial surgeons today use such cancellous cellular marrow grafts, many other head and neck surgeons use microvascular fibula grafts. Each has its advocates and its own set of advantages and disadvantages.

A free vascular fibula graft has the advantage of being useful for immediate reconstruction in the presence of an oral communication and is capable of bringing soft tissue along with bone. However, the fibula is too small and straight to conform to the arch form of the mandible or maxilla, and because of its strictly cortical nature and low profile, it does not hold dental implants well after functional loading (Fig. 66-1). In addition, the length of surgery, the need for postoperative intensive care unit (ICU) management, the morbidity of leg and foot paresthesia (Fig. 66-2), and weakness of the great toe have always been its major disadvantages. It is also a graft that may be lost as a result of failure of the vascular anastomosis.

A cancellous marrow graft, in contrast, has the disadvantage of being prone to infection because of oral communications and is unable to be used for the reconstruction of soft tissue loss at the same time, thus necessitating delayed, yet definitive reconstruction.

Its advantages are that it predictably regenerates bone of greater height, width, and arch form than a fibula graft does (Fig. 66-3) and it has an excellent track record of implant osseointegration in which implants can be placed into more ideal position for functional loading (Fig. 66-4). Cancellous marrow grafting is a less lengthy surgical procedure, does not usually require postoperative ICU stay, and is associated with much less and a more reversible donor site morbidity.

BIOLOGY OF BONE REGENERATION GRAFTS

Whereas in a microvascular bone transfer a preformed bone is moved from one anatomic site to another site (the leg to the jaws in this case), a cancellous cellular marrow graft regenerates a new remodeling bone that is sized and shaped to the needs of the recipient site. Regeneration of bone relies on the classic tissue-engineering triangle of cells (in this case mesenchymal stem cells and osteoprogenitor cells), a signal (growth factors such as bone morphogenetic protein [BMP], insulin-like growth factor [IGF], and transforming growth factor-β [TGF-β]), and a matrix (a scaffold) for bone development (Fig. 66-5). An autogenous cancellous marrow

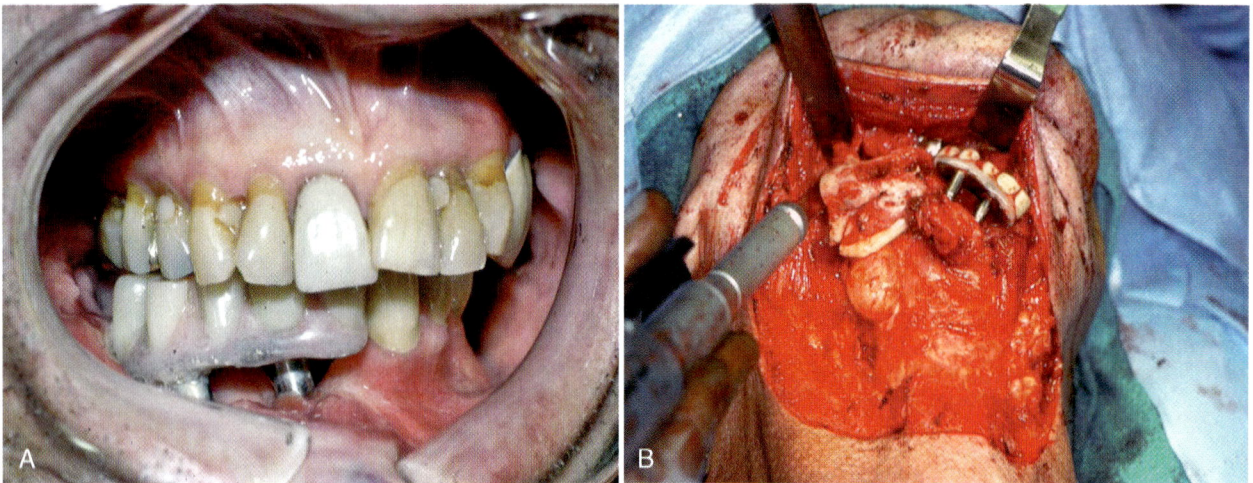

Fig. 66-1 ▪ Dental implants placed into fibula grafts often fail because of deficient bone height and an inappropriate crown-root ratio.

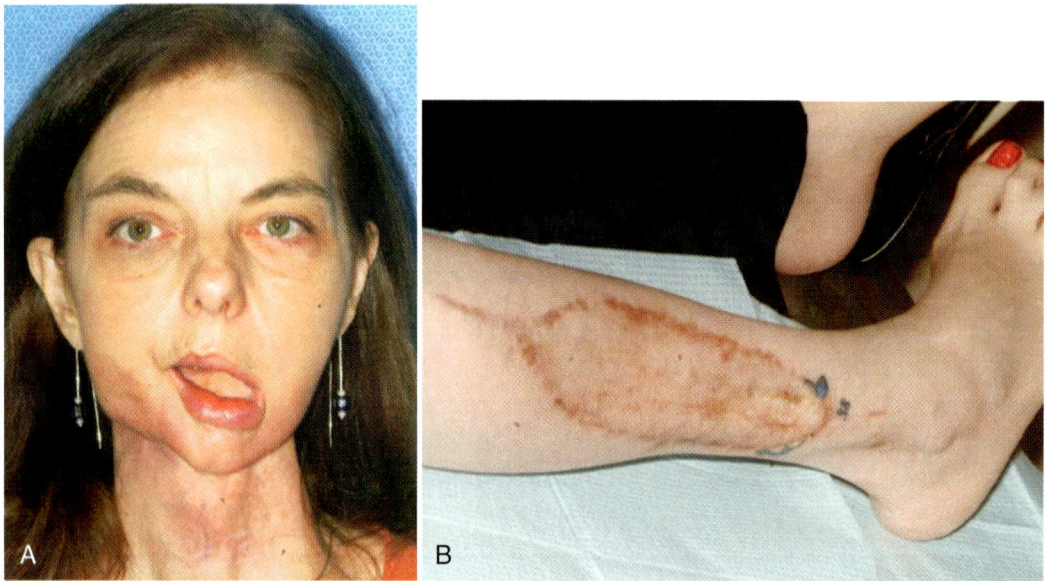

Fig. 66-2 ▪ Fibula grafts result in high functional and cosmetic morbidity in both the recipient and donor sites.

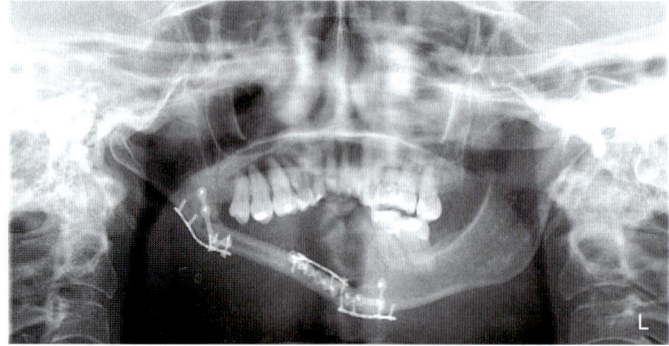

Fig. 66-3 ▪ Fibula graft with deficient bone height and contour inappropriate for dental rehabilitation.

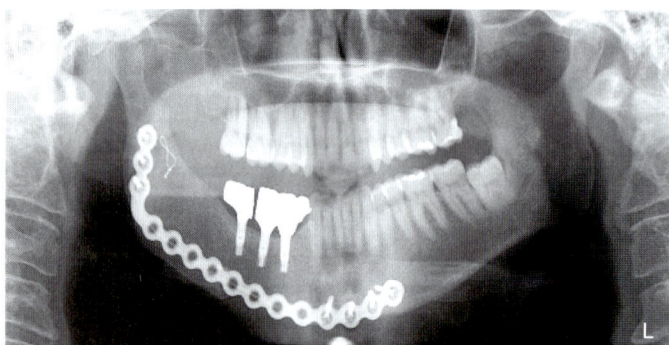

Fig. 66-4 ▪ Cancellous cellular marrow graft with ideal bone height and contour for function and dental rehabilitation.

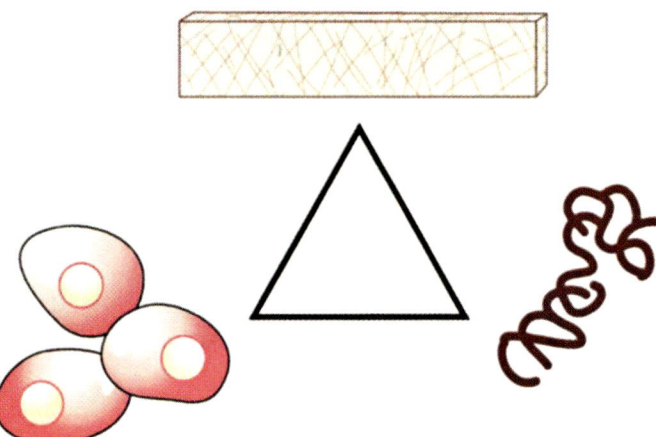

Fig. 66-5 ■ Bone regeneration requires the presence of all three components of the tissue-engineering triangle: cells, signal, and a matrix.

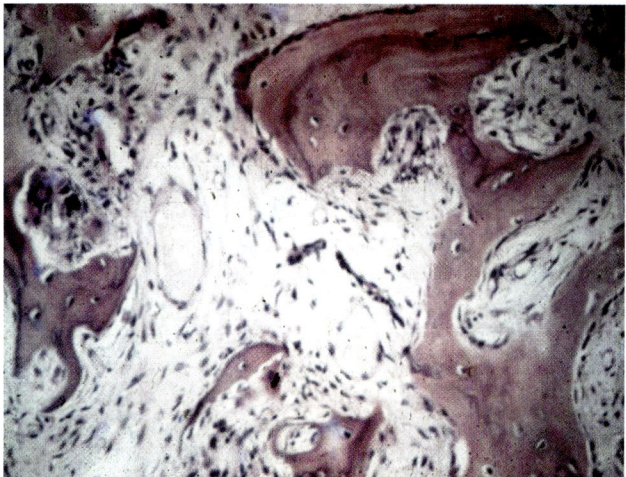

Fig. 66-6 ■ Cancellous cellular bone marrow contains stromal stem cells, endosteal osteoblasts, and hematopoietic stem cells, as well as mineralized trabecular bone containing osteocytes.

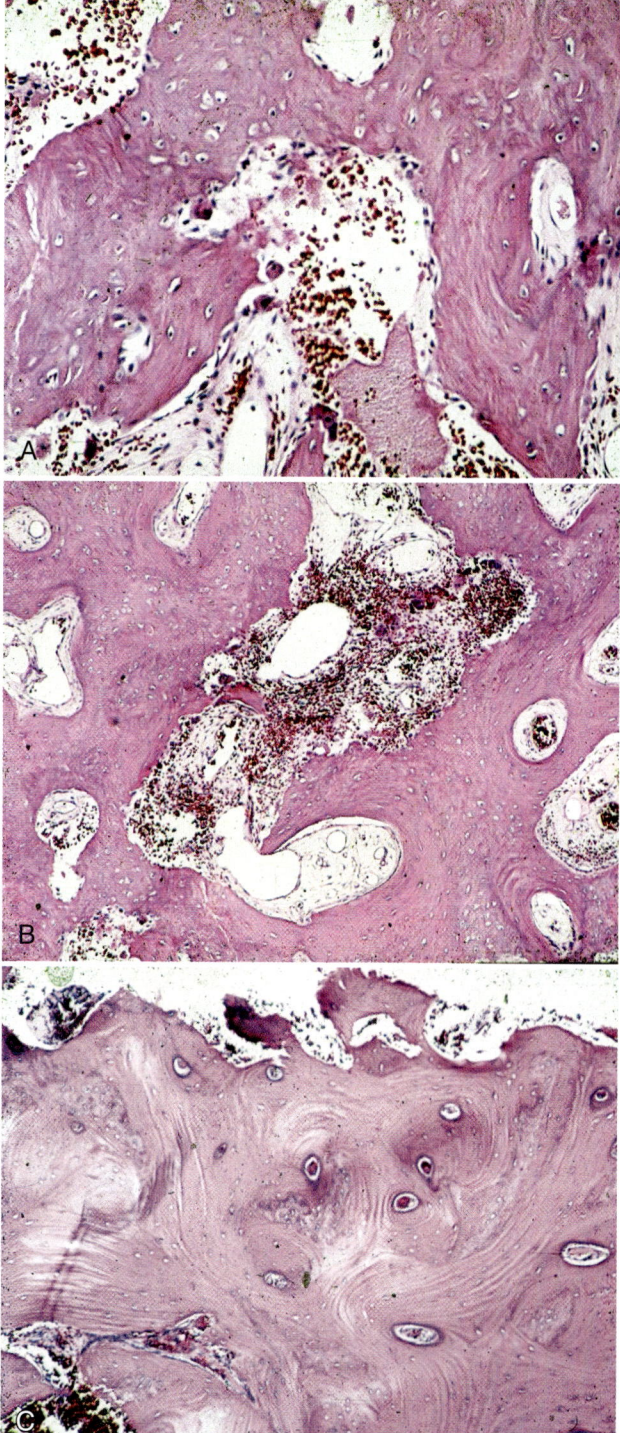

Fig. 66-7 ■ Physiology and biochemistry of a cancellous cellular marrow graft on day 1 (**A**), day 7 (**B**), and day 14 (**C**).

graft contains all three components of this tissue-engineering triangle, which is why it is referred to as the "gold standard." At the time of this writing, the three portions of this triangle have been put together separately to regenerate functionally useful bone in patients without using any autogenous bone source. This new biotechnology is discussed later in this chapter.

In the routinely used cancellous marrow graft, trabecular bone from the donor site that has surface osteoblasts, osteoprogenitor cells, and mesenchymal stem cells (Fig. 66-6) is placed into the recipient site along with the blood clot inherent in all wounds. The platelets within the blood clot degranulate and liberate seven growth factors (platelet-derived growth factors AA, BB, and AB; TGF-β1 and TGF-β2, vascular endothelial growth factor, and epithelial growth factor) into the local environment (Fig. 66-7, *A*). These growth factors initiate the proliferation of osteoprogenitor cells, osteoblasts, and mesenchymal stem cells, as well as capillary ingrowth. After 7 days the platelets are depleted, but by that time, wound-healing macrophages have migrated into the hypoxic environment of the wound and continue the secretion of growth factors (Fig. 66-7, *B*). By days 14 to 20 the graft is completely revascularized and osteoid production has started (Fig. 66-7, *C*). Because of

the fragile state of the graft for these first 21 days, graft site immobility is crucial and can be achieved with maxillo-mandibular fixation, titanium plates and mesh, membranes, and other means, depending on the size and location of the graft.

As a result of the nutrients derived from capillary ingrowth, significant osteoid production occurs, consolidates the graft into a single unit, and fuses it to the host bone from the third to the sixth weeks. At this time any fixation or stabilizing device can be released

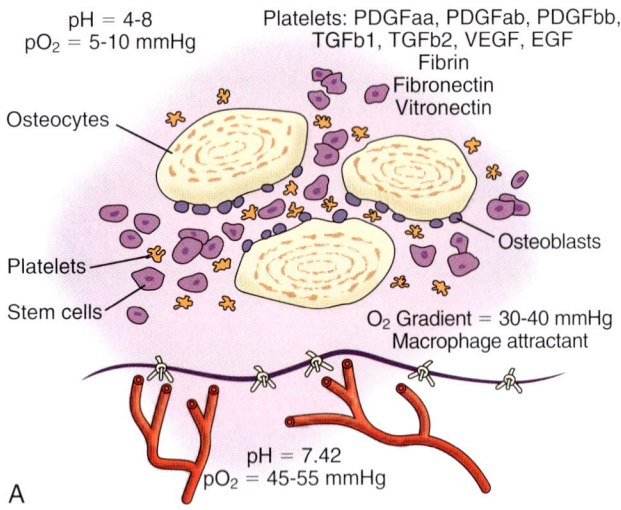

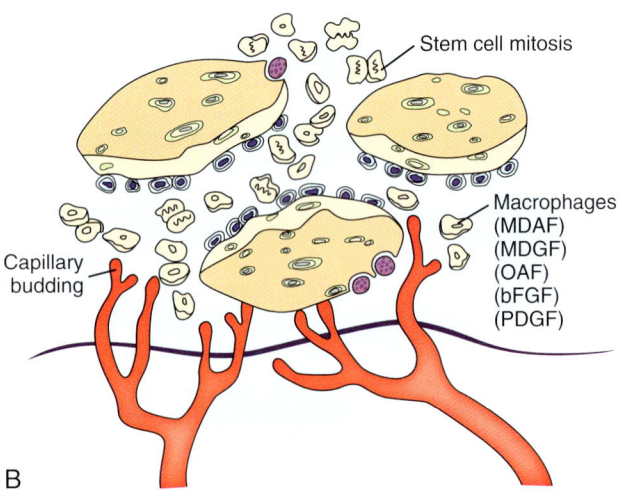

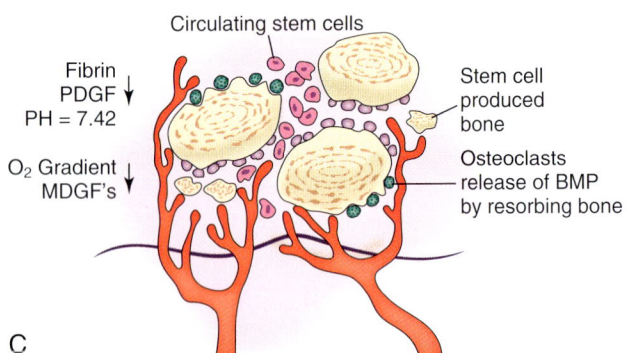

Fig. 66-8 ■ *A,* Bone regeneration begins with the formation of cellular osteoid. *B,* The initial osteoid is resorbed and replaced with a less cellular and more mature bone with lamellar architecture. *C,* A mature bone graft contains mostly lamellar bone with haversian systems and interconnecting Volkmann canals.

and light function begun. After 6 weeks the graft is set but contains immature bone that will undergo the normal physiologic resorption–new bone apposition–remodeling cycle (Fig. 66-8) to create a more mature and mineralized bone, which by 6 months can receive dental implants or support conventional dentures (Fig. 66-9).

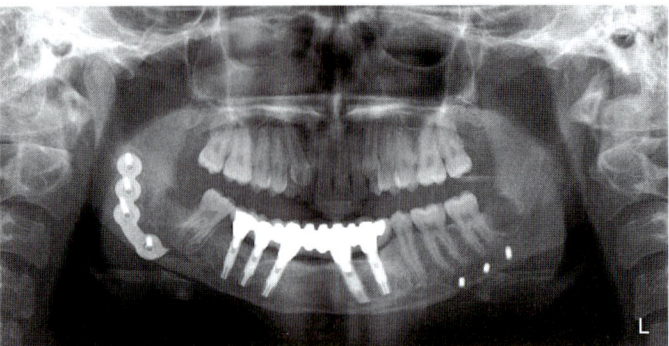

Fig. 66-9 ■ A bone graft should be able to accept dental implants.

TECHNIQUES FOR GRAFTING MANDIBULAR CONTINUITY DEFECTS

The three important clinical scenarios involved in reconstructing mandibular continuity defects are (1) a hemimandibular defect with a proximal and distal native bone edge, (2) a hemimandibular defect with a missing condyle but with a distal native bone edge, and (3) a defect that may be of varying size and crosses the midline but has a right and left proximal bone edge. The commonality of each case is that autogenous cancellous marrow usually harvested from the posterior ilium is the graft material and that crib containment must be planned. The containment may be a crib of either various allogeneic bone segments (split ribs, ilium forms, or hollowed-out mandibular cribs), titanium mesh cribs, or titanium plates with soft tissue sutured directly to the plate or used together with allogeneic bone cribs or titanium mesh cribs.

The variability in each case involves the location of the defect and the quality and quantity of the soft tissue. In patients with soft tissue deficiency because of tumor surgery or radiation-induced fibrosis, it is best to add soft tissue with a flap suited to the size of the defect 3 months in advance of the bone graft. In patients who have received radiation therapy, the site should be improved by using the standard protocol of hyperbaric oxygen: 30 sessions of 100% oxygen at a pressure of 2.4 atm for 90 minutes each session.

HEMIMANDIBULAR DEFECT WITH A PROXIMAL AND DISTAL BONE EDGE

The incision is best placed in the neck within a natural skin fold, within a previous surgical scar, or parallel to the inferior border of the mandible and 3 cm below it (Fig. 66-10, *A*). The plane of dissection to the mandible should be deep to the superficial layer of the deep cervical fascia to preserve the marginal mandibular branch of the facial nerve. The periosteum of each native bone edge needs to be thoroughly reflected for 3 to 4 cm from the edge of the defect (Fig. 66-10, *B*). If a titanium plate is in place from the ablative surgery, it should be removed and the band of plate scar excised. To complete development of the tissue bed, scar tissue needs to be released to the level of the submucosa without perforation into the mouth. This may be facilitated by either palpating the maxillary teeth through the mucosa to gain an appreciation of the thickness of the tissue or by placing a gloved finger in the mouth to guide the dissection and then changing the glove when this maneuver is completed.

The graft material is then compacted with amalgam pluggers or Penfield bone packers beginning at each bone segment and working toward the center while being sure to pack the graft material to the height of the dissected recipient tissue (Fig. 66-10, *C*). Whatever

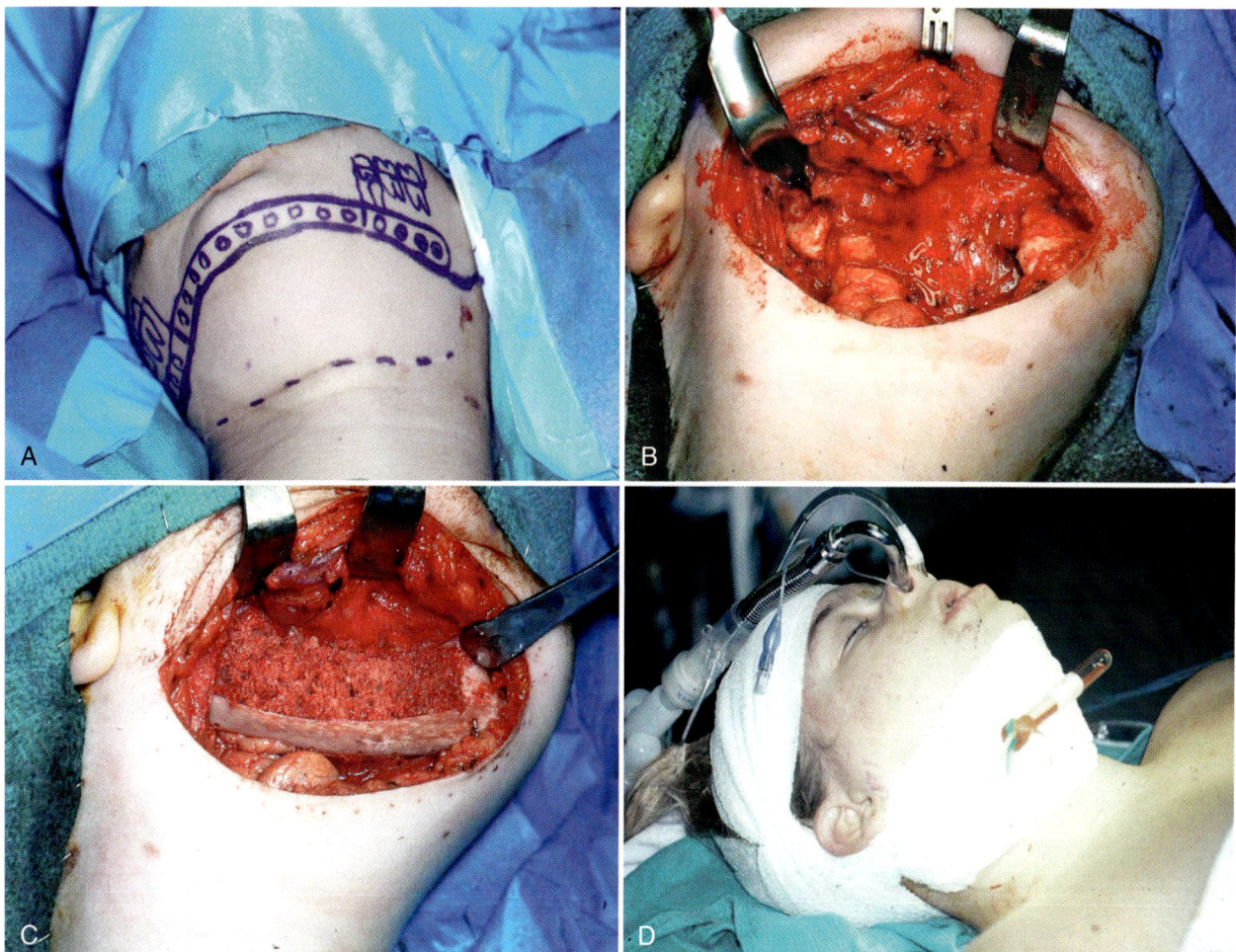

Fig. 66-10 ■ **A,** The incision should be placed within a natural skin fold in the neck or parallel to the inferior border and 3 cm inferior to it. **B,** The recipient site is developed so that each bone end is exposed and oral communication is avoided. **C,** The graft should be densely packed within the recipient site and in contact with each bone end. **D,** A pressure dressing to collapse dead space is recommended.

crib is used, rigid titanium plate, titanium mesh, allogeneic bone, or combinations, the surgeon should suture the fascia of the neck to the crib so that the graft does not become displaced into the neck. This is followed by closure of the periosteum, fascia/platysma, subcutaneous tissue, and skin. The author usually places a non-suction drain (Penrose drain) between the periosteum and fascia/platysma, followed by a pressure dressing (Fig. 66-10, *D*).

HEMIMANDIBULAR DEFECT WITH A MISSING CONDYLE

This defect is grafted with the techniques described for a hemimandibular defect with both proximal and distal bone segments except for the development of a condylar articulation. There are several ways that a condylar articulation can be created. The first is to also harvest a rib for use in the costochondral articulation and as part of the containment crib if it is secured to the inferior border (Fig. 66-11, *A*). The second is to use an allogeneic mandibulare crib in which the condyle is hollowed out (Fig. 66-11, *B*). The cancellous cellular marrow graft is then packed into the hollowed-out mandible, as well as the hollowed-out condyle (Fig. 66-11, *C*). A third is to use a titanium plate with an allogeneic ramus and condyle affixed to it, which is once again hollowed out to receive cancellous cellular

marrow (Fig. 66-11, *D*). A fourth is to use a titanium plate with a titanium condyle and place the cancellous marrow lingual to the plate but no higher than the mid-ramus (Fig. 66-11, *E*). The titanium condyle would be the permanent articulation and the bone graft itself would be the reconstruction that would allow dental rehabilitation. Because of the past poor experience with total temporomandibular joint (TMJ) prostheses in patients with temporomandibular dysfunction (TMD), this approach may be thought to be risky. However, the use of titanium condyles that articulate against a native disc or soft tissue interface in the fossa in tumor patients rather than TMD patients has a proven track record of stable and uncomplicated function and is the author's preferred approach in this situation.

CONTINUITY DEFECTS THAT CROSSES THE MIDLINE

For continuity defects that cross the midline, the curvature of this area must be re-established and the chin point placed in the midline. The soft tissue dissection is in the same plane as the previous two graft approaches. In this case the challenge is to develop a crib containment that will comply with the curvature and midline requirements. For defects between the two mental foramina, the author

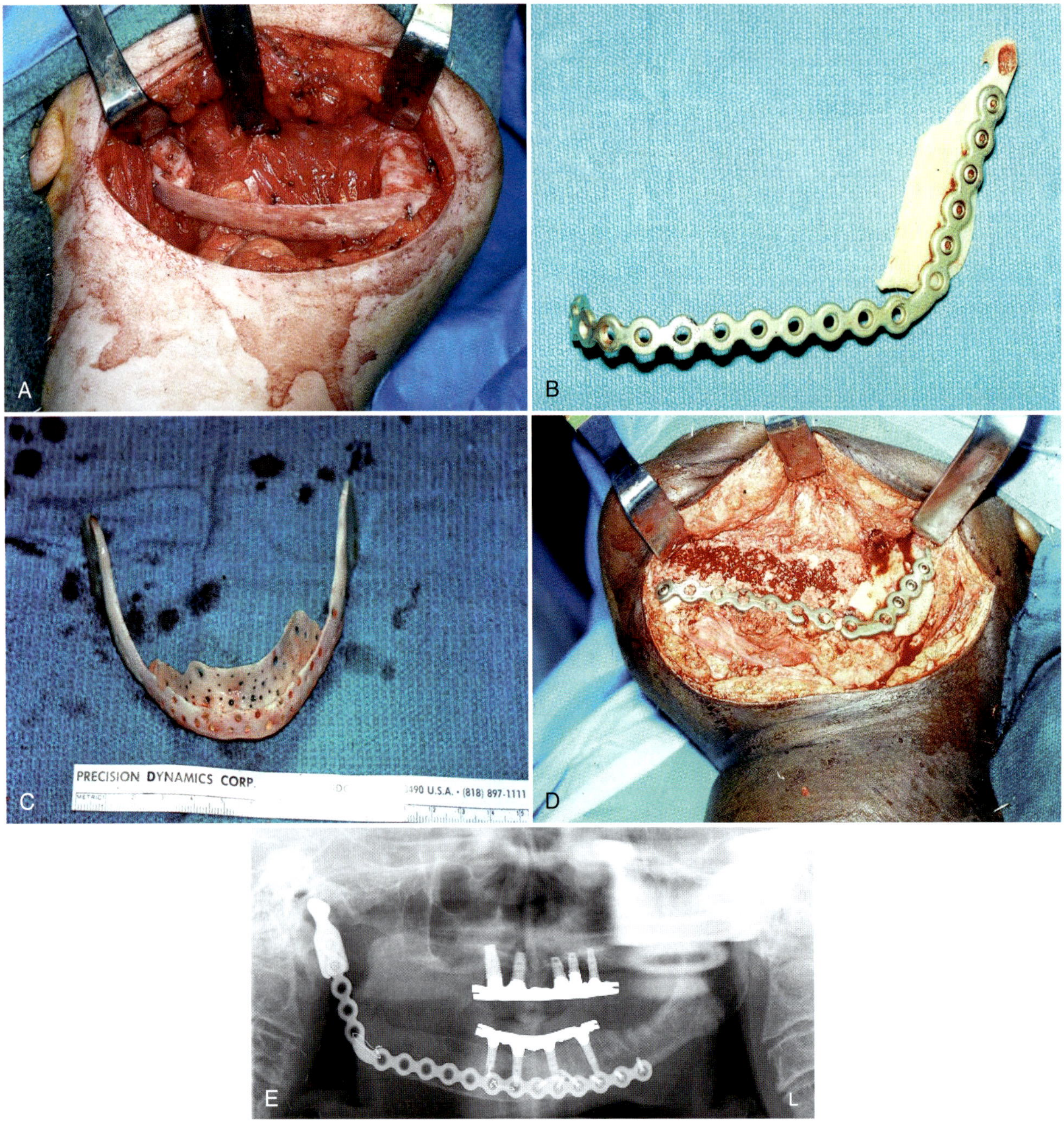

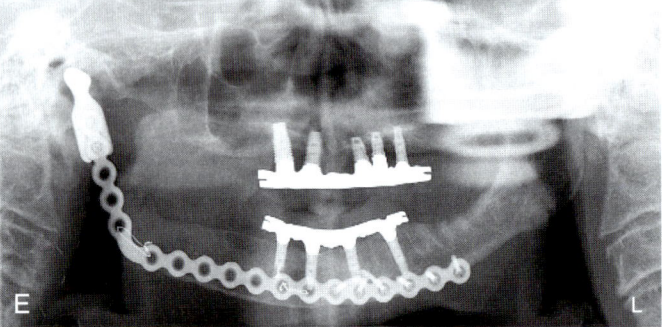

Fig. 66-11 ■ **A,** An allogeneic split rib serves well as a resorbable crib containment. **B,** An allogeneic mandible with a hollowed-out condyle packed with autogenous cancellous marrow is one way to create an articulation. **C,** An allogeneic mandible hollowed out and with a reduced lingual cortex serves as an excellent crib containment for large mandibular cancellous marrow grafts. **D,** Combining a titanium plate and an allogeneic ramus with a hollowed-out condyle is another way to create an articulation of the graft. **E,** A titanium plate with its metal condyle supporting a graft to the mid-ramus level is still another option to construct an articulation graft.

prefers to split an allogeneic rib lengthwise and thin each cortex by removing the adherent cancellous bone so that each piece can be bent without breaking. The inner rib cortex is planned so that it recapitulates the lingual cortex of the mandible and the outer rib cortex, the buccal cortex of the mandible (Fig. 66-12, *A*). They may be secured with a single bicortical mattress wire to create a matrix band construction in which the cancellous cellular marrow is placed in between (Fig. 66-12, *B* to *F*).

For continuity defects that extend past the mental foramen on one side or the other or for total mandibular reconstruction, the author prefers the use of either an allogeneic mandible or a full rigid titanium reconstruction plate as a crib containment. If an allogeneic mandible is used, it is hollowed out in a "J" shape with the lowest cortical containment on the lingual side because of the greater revascularization from the this side and packed with the cancellous cellular marrow (Fig. 66-13, *A*). Burr holes are also placed through the

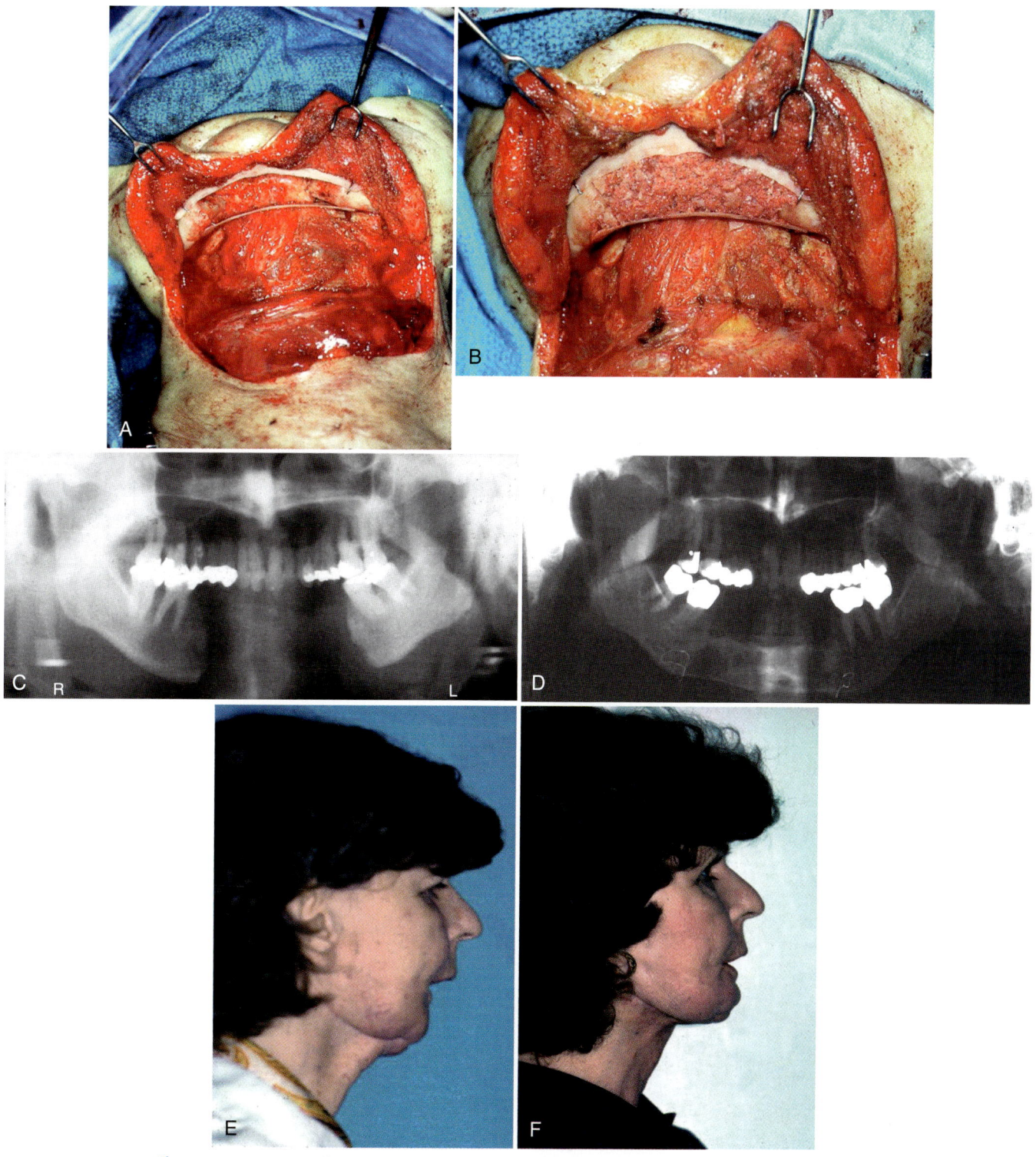

Fig. 66-12 ■ **A,** Two allogeneic split-rib segments fashioned in this manner can help in reconstruction of the anterior mandible. **B,** Packing the cancellous acellular marrow graft between the rib segments allows one to condense the maximum amount of graft material. **C,** Panoramic film before graft placement. **D,** Panoramic film of the mature graft. **E,** Profile before the graft. **F,** Profile after the graft.

inferior border to accommodate suturing the neck fascia to the inferior border of the crib (Fig. 66-13, *B*). If a rigid titanium plate is used, the fascia is sutured to the holes in the plate, which will also help contain the cancellous cellular marrow graft.

For continuity defects that cross the midline and in which some residual occlusion is present, it is wise to achieve maxillo-mandibular

fixation as best as possible. If no residual tooth contact is present, stability relies on the rigidity of the allogeneic crib or the rigid titanium plate and restrictive bandaging for 3 weeks. Despite the frequent inability to achieve maxillo-mandibular fixation in such cases, bone regeneration usually proceeds undisturbed because of the loss of opening and closing power from the muscle attachments

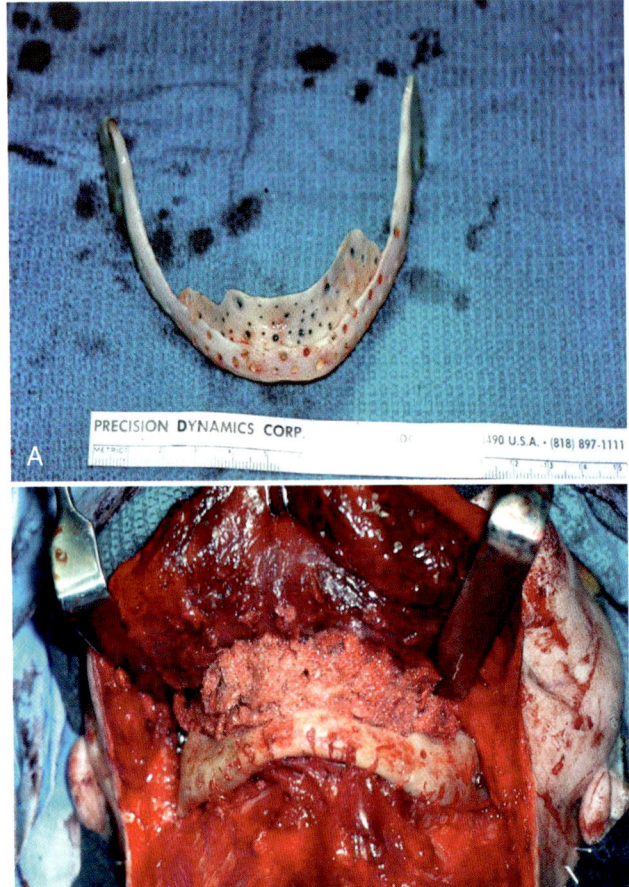

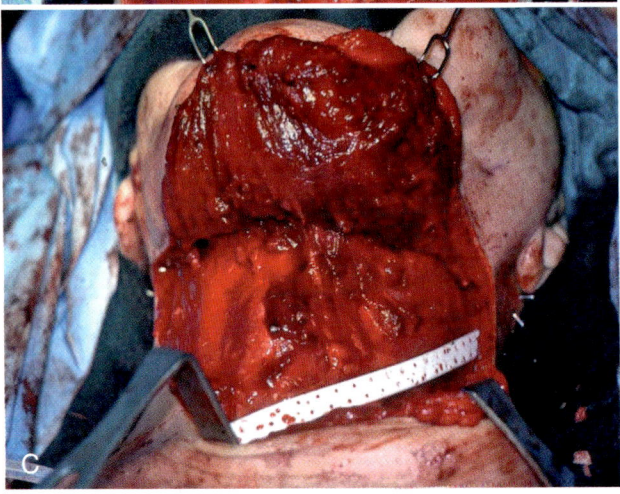

Fig. 66-13 ■ **A,** Hollowed-out allogeneic mandible for a large mandibular defect. **B,** Hollowed-out allogeneic mandible packed with cancellous cellular marrow. **C,** Suturing the deep tissues of the neck to the inferior border eliminated dead space.

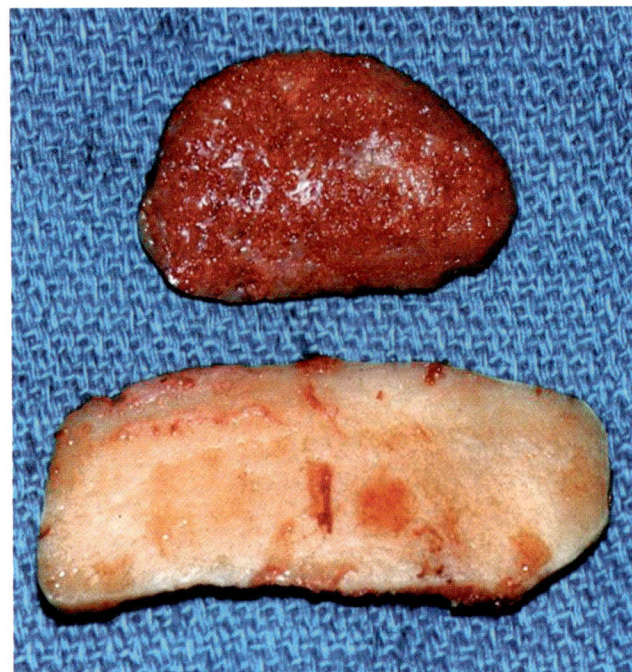

Fig. 66-14 ■ Cranial bone grafts have natural concave/convex contours suitable for mid-face grafting.

MAXILLARY RECONSTRUCTION

There are two primary indications for maxillary reconstruction: the less common indication is to restore facial contour and the more common indication is to reconstruct the alveolar process for the purpose of dental rehabilitation.

To restore facial contours, the best outcome is achieved with a cranial bone graft. This is not technically a cancellous cellular marrow graft but is a cortical cancellous marrow graft. Cranial bone grafts, particularly from parietal bone, are preferred because their convex contour is similar to that of the anterior wall of the maxilla and the lateral wall of the zygoma (Fig. 66-14). They are also preferred because they maintain their size and shape better than do grafts from other harvest sites. This is thought to be due to similar embryologic derivation as the maxilla, with both being directed from the neural crest. In addition, earlier revascularization by virtue of its numerous diploetic channels also incorporates the graft faster.

The approach is usually achieved via a modified Weber-Ferguson incision that does not split the lip. The incision creates a pocket within the cheek between the mucosa on the deep side and the skin on the superficial side (Fig. 66-15, *A*). The block graft is then shaped to allow fixation to the infraorbital rim, if still present superiorly, or otherwise to the nasal bones medial-superiorly, the midline alveolar bone medial-inferiorly, and the zygoma laterally (Fig. 66-15, *B*). At times, a dermal fat graft can be overlaid to achieve a softer texture (Fig. 66-15, *C*). However, this approach usually restores a symmetric contour to the infraorbital maxillary mid-face area (Fig. 66-15, *D* and *E*).

To regenerate alveolar bone in the maxilla for support of denture function with or without implants, any oral-antral or oral-nasal communication must be reconstructed first. Small to medium-sized defects posterior to the first bicuspid tooth are generally closed with a buccal fat pad transfer, which has an excellent blood supply and becomes mucosalized over a period of 6 weeks. Larger

that are not present in such defects. To this end, the surgeon should make every effort to suture the anterior digastric muscles, as well as the closing muscle, to the graft crib so that these muscle can reattach to the graft as it regenerates bone, thereby restoring as much opening and closing function as possible (Fig. 66-13, *C*).

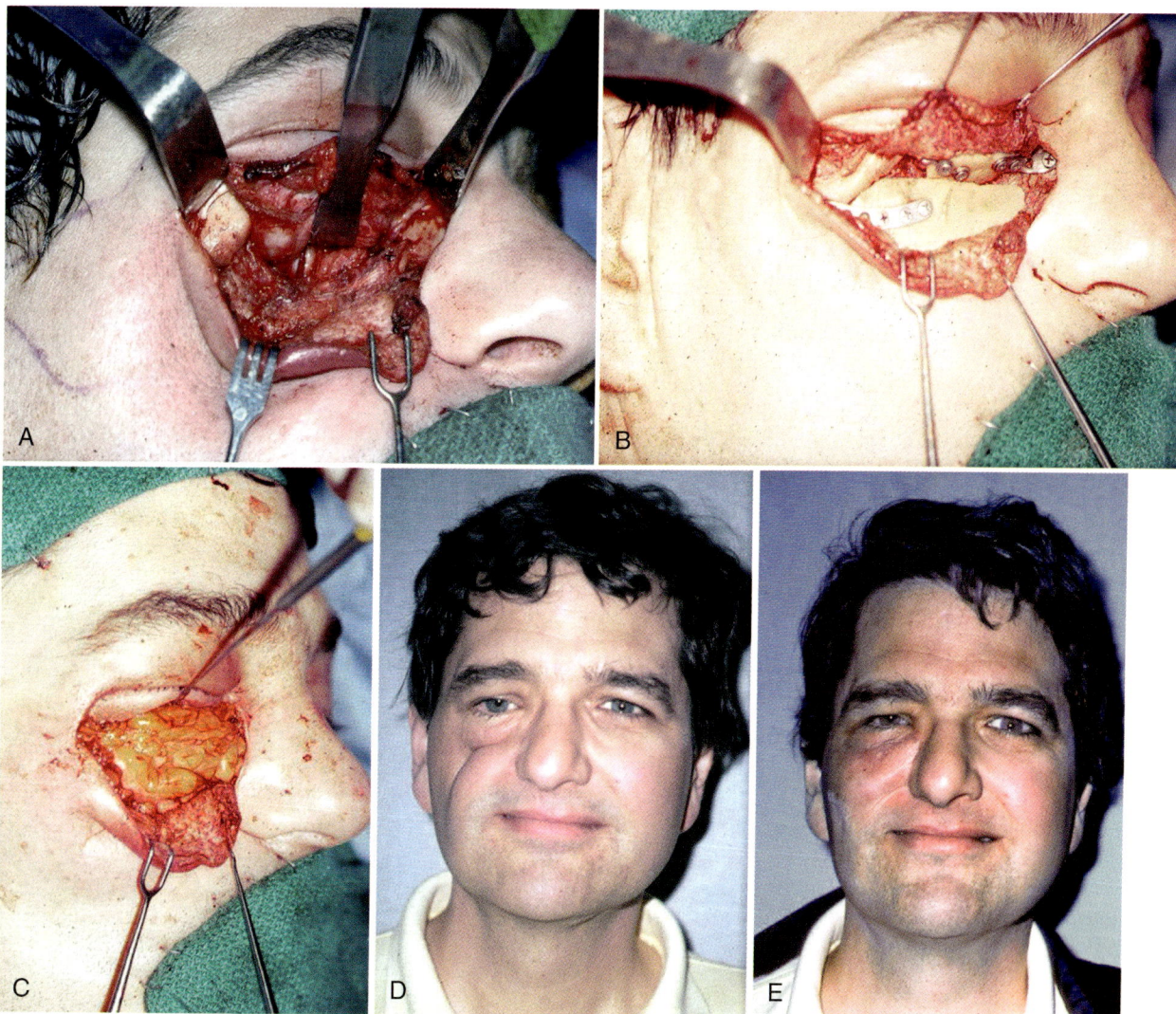

Fig. 66-15 ■ **A,** Weber-Ferguson approach for placing a mid-face orbital graft from the cranium. **B,** Fixation of cranial bone grafts to the orbital floor and anterior maxilla. **C,** A dermal fat graft adds soft tissue texture over a graft. **D,** Facial view before cranial bone and dermal fat grafting. **E,** Facial view after cranial bone and dermal fat grafting.

defects extending to the midline area may be closed with a split temporalis muscle flap, which also has an excellent blood supply and mucosalizes over a 6-week period, or with a free vascular soft tissue flap.

A mid-crestal incision is made over the affected area. If the bony walls of the maxilla are intact, a full-thickness buccal mucoperiosteal flap is reflected, as is a palatal flap, to expose as much bone surface as possible (Fig. 66-16, *A*). This situation amounts to an extensive horizontal and vertical ridge augmentation. If soft tissue closure was performed to correct an oral-antral fistula before the bone graft surgery or there are defects with no bony wall separating the maxillary sinus or nasal cavity, a split-thickness flap with a soft tissue base is raised over these areas. A full-thickness flap is raised over areas that have a bony base. In these cases the author prefers a titanium mesh crib because of its ability to maintain the necessary arch form as well as space for bone regeneration, and its rigidity (Fig. 66-16, *B*). Resorbable cribs are preferred by others, but the concern that resorption by-products will inhibit bone regeneration remains. There are insufficient data to recommend such cribs at this

time. All residual scar and periosteum should be removed from the maxillary bone surface so that the graft contacts host bone directly. This can be achieved by roughing up the surface with a burr or a curet. Drilling burr holes to enter the marrow space is unnecessary. The cancellous cellular marrow is then compacted into the crib as though it were impression material in an impression tray (Fig. 66-16, *C*). The titanium crib and graft are then placed and secured with monocortical screws.

In such cases, closure of the soft tissue is crucial. To achieve tension-free closure, extensive undermining of the buccal mucosa and an everted mattress closure to the palatal flap are necessary. Over-closure with interrupted sutures or a running suture can also be added to the mattress closure (Fig. 66-16, *D*).

Mesh exposure does occur (Fig. 66-16, *E*). If the titanium mesh becomes exposed in the first 10 days, the graft will suffer some bone loss or even complete loss as a result of secondary infection. This is due to the fact that the graft has not sufficiently revascularized at that time. It also underscores the importance of tension-free closure. If the mesh becomes exposed after the 10th postoperative day,

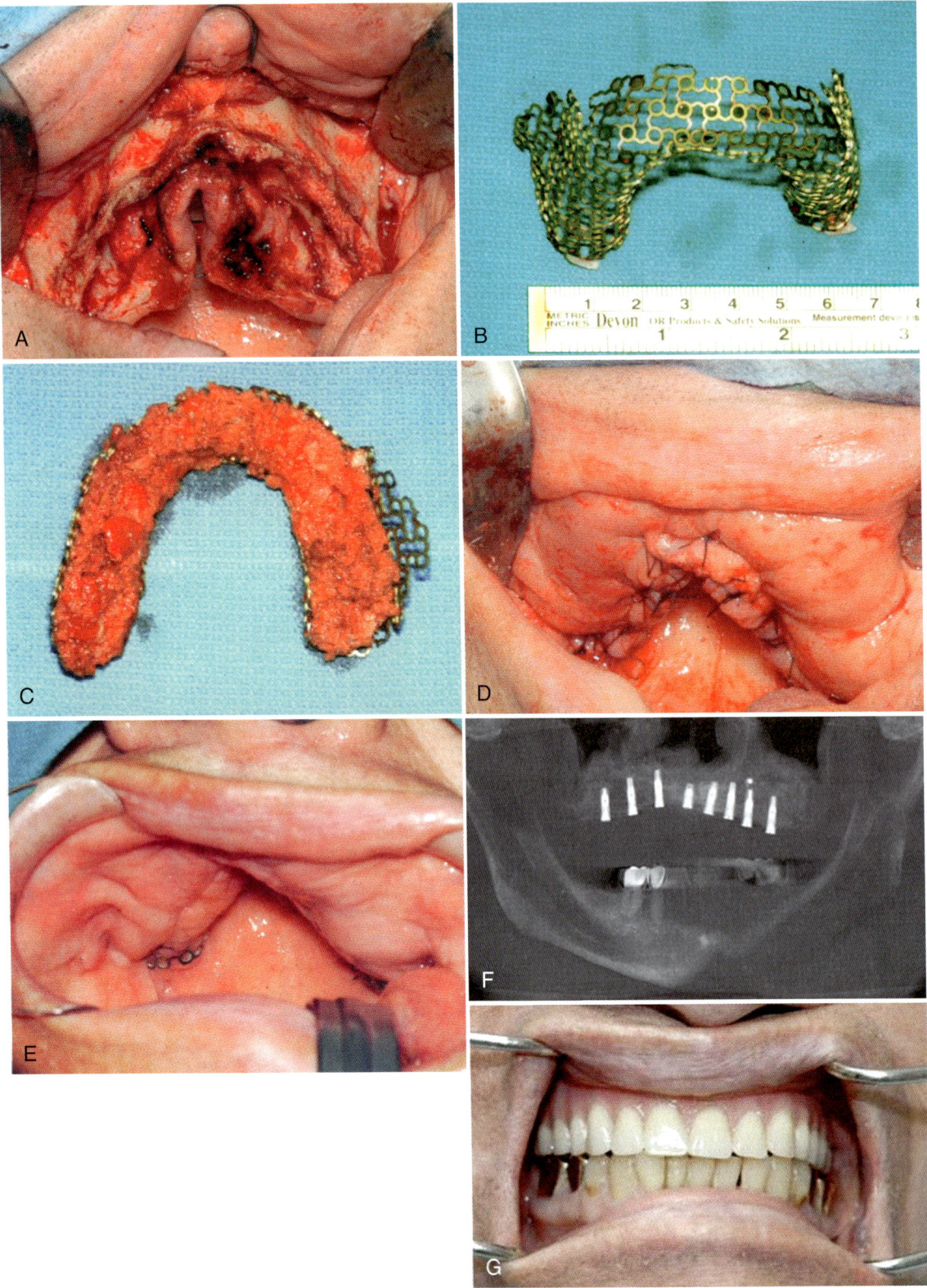

Fig. 66-16 ■ **A,** Knife-edged ridge with vertical maxillary deficiency. **B,** Titanium mesh crib used to contain the graft material. **C,** Cancellous cellular marrow graft within a titanium mesh crib. **D,** Significant undermining of the mucosa is necessary to achieve tension-free closure. **E,** Mesh exposure occurred 1 month after graft placement but did not inhibit bone regeneration. **F,** Radiograph of regenerated bone and dental implants. **G,** Implant-retained prosthesis.

the graft has already revascularized and can resist infection and mucosalize over the graft but under the mesh. The graft usually suffers no loss, and no further treatment is required.

Such grafts have been extremely successful in regenerating bone. However, because of the presence of the titanium crib, a second surgery to remove the mesh and often to perform vestibuloplasty or place dental implants becomes necessary (Fig. 66-16, *F* and *G*).

USING RECOMBINANT BONE MORPHOGENETIC PROTEIN AS AN ALTERNATIVE TO AUTOGENOUS CANCELLOUS CELLULAR MARROW

Recombinant human BMP in an acellular collagen sponge (rhBMP-2/ACS [Infuse]) is approved by the Food and Drug Administration for bone regeneration in extraction socket grafting and maxillary sinus augmentation grafting, as well as for the orthopedic indications of lumbar spinal fusion and fresh tibial fractures. However, numerous oral and maxillofacial surgeons have used rhBMP-2/ACS in advanced applications, also called "off-label" use, with great success and elimination of donor site morbidity.

In the tissue-engineering triangle, rhBMP-2/ACS serves as the signal for bone regeneration, and if the surgeon supplies a suitable matrix and a source of osteocompetent cells, bone regeneration takes place without the use of autogenous bone harvesting.

The author has used rhBMP-2/ACS extensively as an alternative to autogenous bone and discovered that the ACS is a great binder of the protein and releases it over a 21-day period in an ideal fashion, but it is an inadequate matrix. Therefore, for use in maxillary ridge augmentations and continuity defects of 6 cm or less, crushed cancellous freeze-dried allogeneic bone (ccFDAB) and platelet-rich plasma (PRP) are added to the rhBMP-2/ACS to achieve predictable bone regeneration. In this application, the ccFDAB acts as an improved matrix, and the PRP adds to the matrix with its three cell adhesion molecules, fibrin, fibronectin, and vitronectin, and amplifies the rhBMP-2/ACS signaling effect with its own growth factors (stromal derived activation factor-1 alpha (SDAF-1α). In these situations the source of cells is the host bone surface onto which this composite is applied, as well as the stem cells and osteoprogenitor cells (CD44+, CD90+, and CD105+ cells) that are present within the PRP.

When using this biotechnology, the lyophilized rhBMP-2 powder must be allowed to solubilize in the sterile water provided in the Infuse packaging for 5 minutes. The resultant clear liquid is then dripped onto the ACS and allowed to bind to the collagen for 15 minutes (Fig. 66-17, *A*). Approximately 93% of the rhBMP-2 binds to the ACS within 15 minutes. It should be cautioned that the rhBMP-2/ACS preparation should be used within 2 hours to avoid the sponge drying out and possible inactivation of the protein. The rhBMP-2/ACS preparation is next cut into 1-cm squares and then added to the ccFDAB-PRP composite and mixed thoroughly (Fig. 66-17, *B*). It can then be placed in the recipient site as one would place an autogenous cancellous cellular marrow graft (Fig. 66-17, *C*).

For continuity defects of the mandible larger than 6 cm and total maxillary ridge reconstruction in a patient who has not received radiation therapy, the chemotactic effect of the rhBMP-2/ACS is insufficient to attract and proliferate the number of osteocompetent cells to predictably regenerate bone in such large defects.

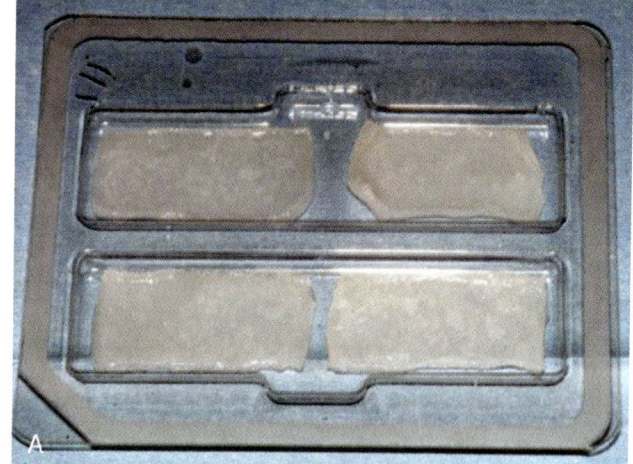

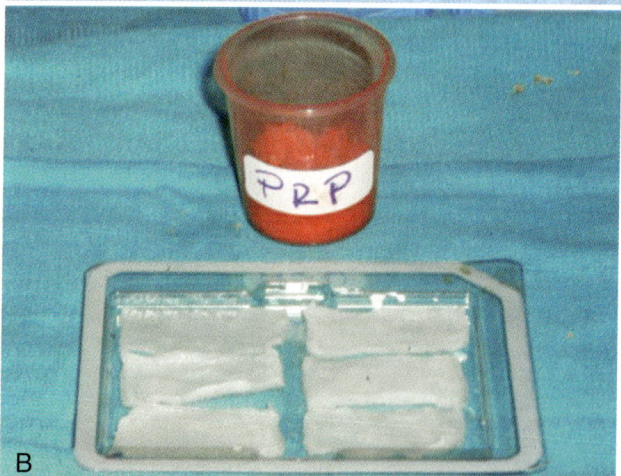

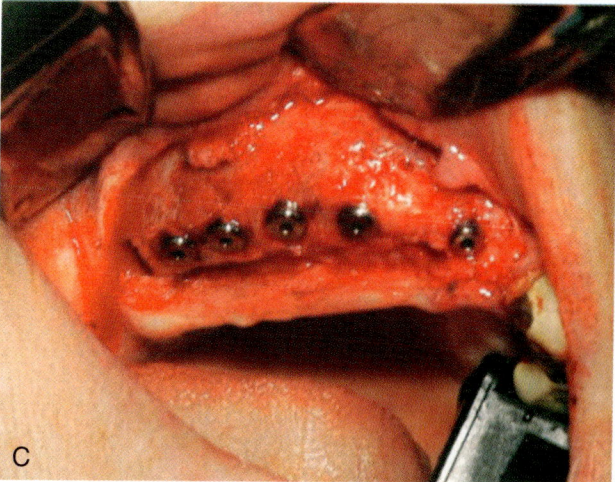

Fig. 66-17 ▪ **A,** Ninety- three percent of recombinant human bone morphogenetic protein-2 (rhBMP-2) binds to the acellular collagen sponge (ACS) in 15 minutes. **B,** Composite graft of rhBMP-2/ACS, crushed cancellous freeze-dried allogeneic bone (ccFDAB), and platelet-rich plasma (PRP). **C,** Bone regeneration outcome of the composite graft.

To compensate for this limitation, the author uses bone marrow aspirated from the anterior ilium and concentrated in the SmartPReP Device (Harvest Technologies Corp., Plymouth, Mass.), which is the same device used to prepare PRP (Fig. 66-18, *A*). Ten milliliters of bone marrow concentrate (known as bone marrow aspirate

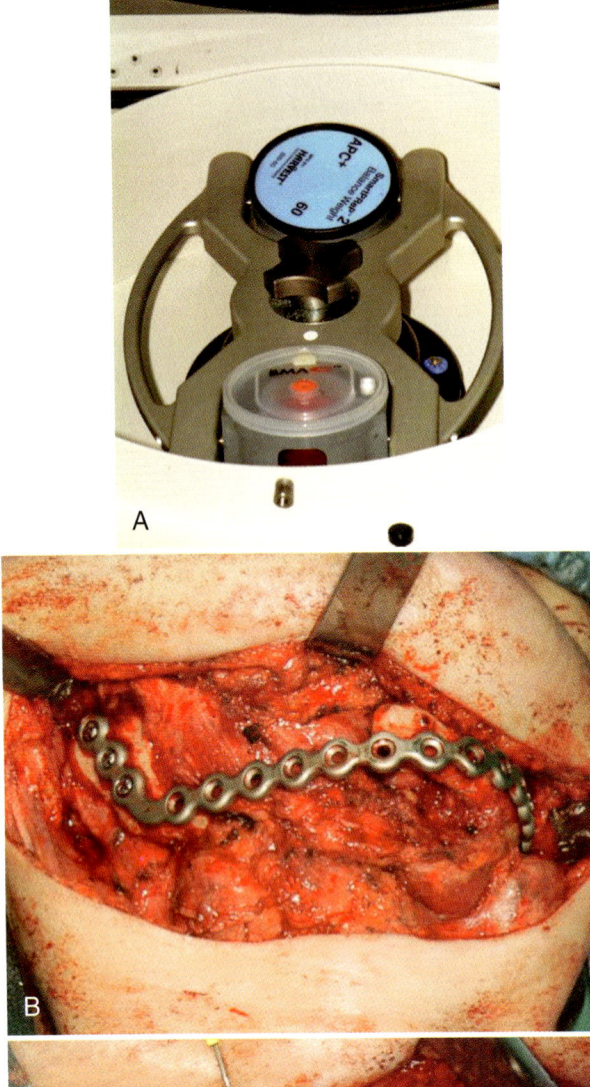

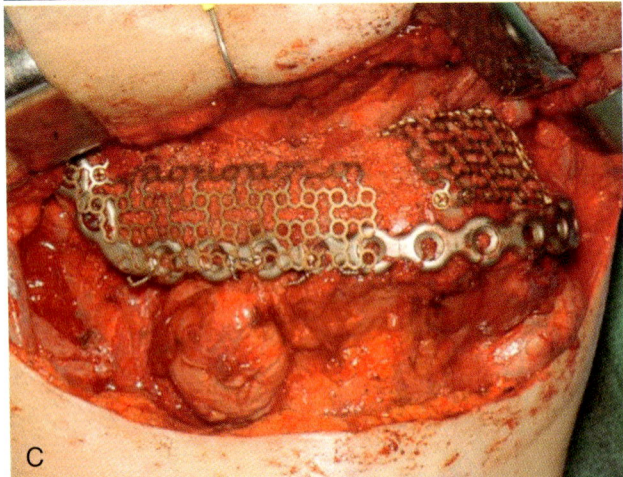

Fig. 66-18 ■ **A,** The Harvest Technologies automatic double-spin centrifugation device prepares both platelet-rich plasma (PRP) from peripheral blood and bone marrow aspirate concentrates (BMACs) from bone marrow. **B,** Large continuity defect of the mandible. **C,** Graft of BMAC, ccFDAB, and rhBMP-2/ACS in place.

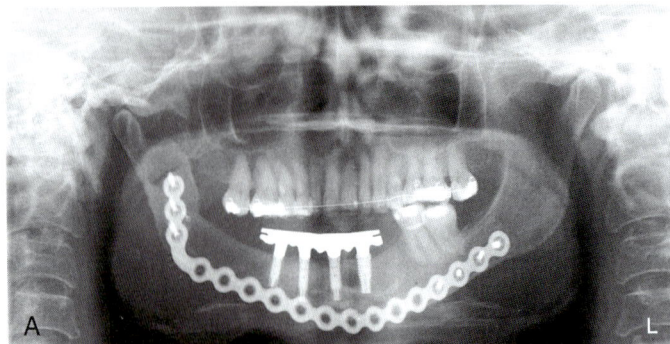

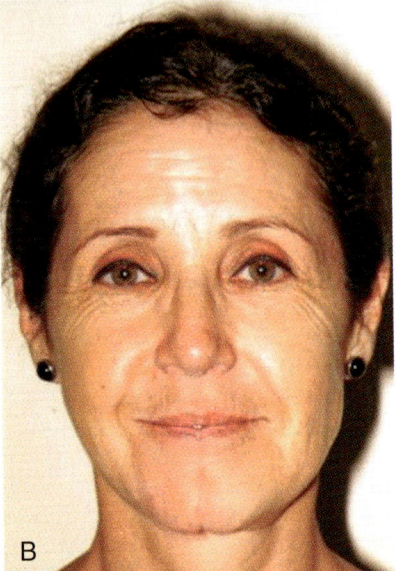

Fig. 66-19 ■ **A,** Graft outcome of the continuity defect seen in Figure 66-18, B, grafted with BMAC, rhBMP-2/ACS, and ccFDAB. **B,** Result of reconstructing the continuity defect in Figure 66-18 without autogenous bone.

concentrate [BMAC]) has been assayed to contain 1.6×10^9 total nucleated marrow cells and 2.5×10^6 CD44$^+$, CD90$^+$, and CD105$^+$ osteoprogenitor cells. The addition of BMAC along with PRP to the rhBMP-2/ACS and ccFDAB adds the number of mesenchymal stem cells/osteoprogenitor cells needed to regenerate bone, as well as the cell adhesion molecules of PRP, in this very large but non-irradiated defect (Fig. 66-18, B and C).

Continuity defects in irradiated tissue remain the most difficult challenge in bone regeneration. Although hyperbaric oxygen is required and improves the recipient tissue by capillary neoangiogenesis, it does not restore the stem cell and osteoprogenitor cell populations. In such cases, some autogenous cancellous cellular marrow is required but much less than needed when rhBMP-2/ACS–ccFDAB-BMAC is not used. In such regeneratively compromised patients, the author uses 50% autogenous cancellous marrow, 50% ccFDAB together with 12 mg of rhBMP-2/ACS per hemimandible, and 10 mL of BMAC to achieve the most predictable reconstruction in this group with the least donor site morbidity (Fig. 66-19).

The technique of obtaining BMAC is straightforward and readily learned. To harvest bone marrow, 20 mL of a solution of 2,000 units of heparin/mL is prepared and used to coat the aspiration trocar and aspiration syringes. A collection bag for the aspirated marrow must

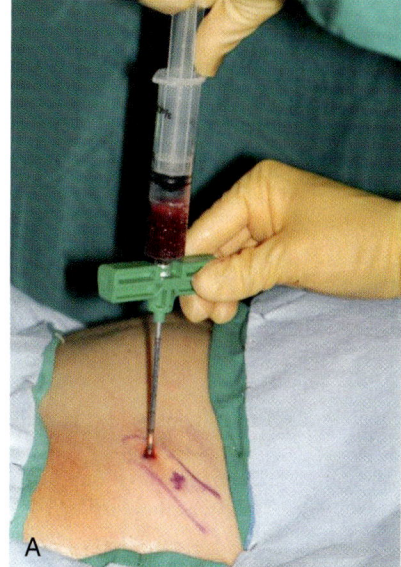

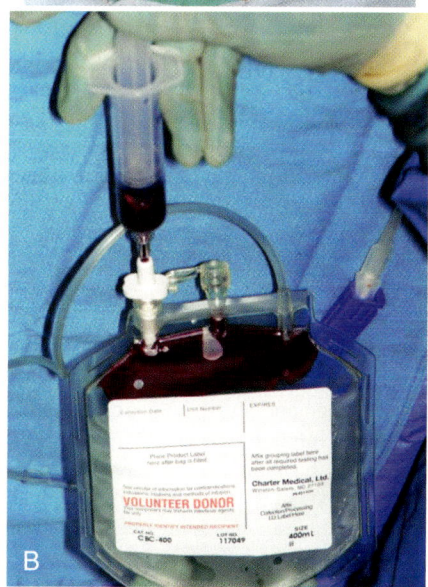

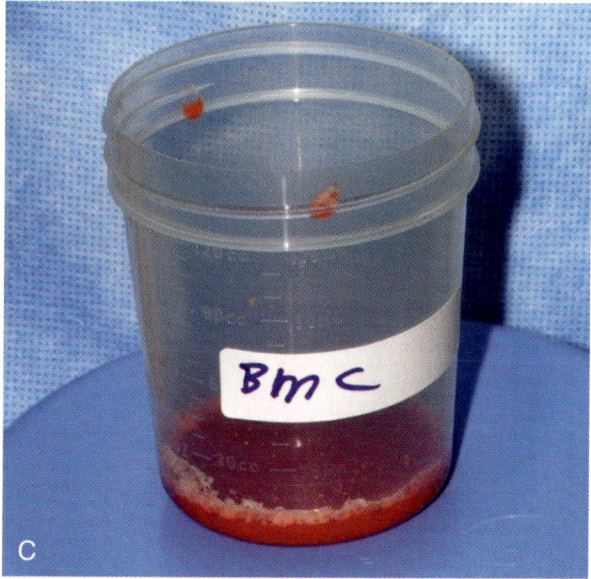

also be prepared by injecting 4 mL of anticoagulant citrate dextrose-A (ACD-A) into the bag.

Two small "stab" incisions are made about 2 cm apart over the crest of each anterior ilium, and blunt dissection is carried down to the bone with a hemostat. In sequence, a heparin-coated bone trocar within a hollow sleeve is inserted into the marrow space between the cortices with a wrist rotation motion and hand pressure. Once firmly within the marrow space, a heparin-coated 20-mL syringe is attached to the Luer-Lock connector on the trocar. Withdrawing the plunger will aspirate bone marrow, which will appear much the same as blood (Fig. 66-20, *A*). To maximize the yield of stem cells and osteoprogenitor cells, the syringe is slowly rotated 360 degrees while aspirating 5 mL of marrow, at which time the trocar sleeve is withdrawn or inserted another 5 mm for another 5-mL aspiration while rotating the syringe 360 degrees until 15 mL of bone marrow is obtained in each syringe. Using four separate aspiration sites will yield 60 mL of bone marrow aspirate, which is placed in the collection bag with the ACD-A. Once 60 mL of bone marrow has been obtained, it is withdrawn, placed in the specially designed canister, and concentrated with the same centrifugation parameters used to concentrate PRP (Fig. 66-20, *B* and *C*). As with PRP, the bone marrow plasma fraction is aspirated as a cell-poor fraction, and the remaining cell-rich 10-mL fraction is what is used and contains the concentrated osteoprogenitor cells and bone marrow mesenchymal stem cells.

PEARLS AND PITFALLS

- Although growth factors, hyperbaric oxygen, and microvascular techniques are valuable, the three keys to successful bone grafting are infection- and contamination-free tissue, graft stability, and a vascular soft tissue bed.
- The limitations of a microvascular fibula graft are its small size, brittleness, and straight morphology.
- Bone regeneration occurs in three stages: a biochemical–cellular proliferation phase, an osteoid synthesis phase, and a resorption-remodeling-maturation phase.
- Suturing soft tissues directly to the graft and application of a pressure dressing are two recommended maneuvers that decrease dead space around a graft.
- Cranial bone grafts are preferred for mid-face and orbital reconstruction because of their similar embryology and earlier revascularization.
- Early oral exposure of titanium mesh often leads to graft infection. Late exposure of titanium mesh does not.
- rhBMP-2 must be used with the ACS because it will bind to the collagen and be released over the ensuing 14 to 21 days.
- Continuity defects of the mandible 6 cm or smaller in a non-irradiated patient can be grafted without autogenous bone by using a composite graft of rhBMP-2/ACS, BMAC, and crushed cancellous allogeneic bone.
- The critical requirement for all ridge augmentation grafts is tension-free closure, which may require extensive undermining to achieve.
- Condensing or tightly packing an autogenous cancellous marrow graft is recommended to increase the cellular density of osteoblasts and osteoprogenitor cells that will regenerate new bone.

Fig. 66-20 ■ Bone marrow aspirates (BMAs) (**A**) are placed in a collection bag (**B**) containing 4 mL of ACD-A until 60 mL is obtained. **C**, Sixty milliliters of BMA is centrifuged to obtain 10 mL of BMAC containing 902×10^6 total nucleated cells and 8×10^6 CD44$^+$ osteoprogenitor (stem) cells.

67 Ear Reconstruction

Shawn A. McClure, Steven P. Best

With the importance of cosmetic appearance in today's society, the ears are often overlooked until a traumatic event leads to an acquired deformity. Because the long-term psychological effects of the disfigurement can be devastating, the ability to correct these injuries can have a life-changing effect on the patient. The surgeon not only must be prepared to treat the initial injury but must also be familiar with the continued pathogenesis of injury and its treatment to provide the best overall care for the patient.

ETIOPATHOGENESIS/CAUSATIVE FACTORS

Because of the prominent and exposed position of the ears in the maxillofacial region they routinely experience trauma. Increasing the likelihood of trauma to the ears is the natural inclination to turn one's face away from impending trauma, thus escalating the severity and incidence of damage. Violent altercations, motor vehicle accidents, thermal insults, and other sources of trauma can cause a vast array of injuries. Steffin and colleagues reviewed 56 publications including 74 cases of auricular avulsion and found that more than a third were caused by bites from humans and animals.

After the initial reconstruction, postoperative care can be challenging because of potential complications unique to this area of the maxillofacial region. These potential challenges in surgical repair of the auricle extend beyond trauma and include sequelae from elective cosmetic surgery, pathologic resection, body piercing, and infection.

PATHOLOGIC ANATOMY

The external ear consists of the auricle, external acoustic meatus, and tympanic membrane, which function together to receive and transmit sound waves to the middle ear. The auricle is traditionally broken down into subunits (Fig. 67-1). The avascular cartilage providing the semi-rigid configuration of the auricle is a primary concern in the treatment and postoperative management of an ear injury.

Symmetry of the ears in both their location and proportion is critical for pleasant esthetics. Normal adult ear height is between 5.5 and 6.6 cm, and its width is approximately 55% of the height. Lateral projection of the ear from the head should be between 1.5 and 2 cm.

As with most soft tissue of the maxillofacial region, the ears have a plentiful and unique blood supply. Ascending anteriorly, the superficial temporal artery can provide a combination of one to three branches to the ear. The upper branch supplies the superior auricle, the middle branch ends at the tragus, and finally, a lower branch supplies the lobule. The posterior auricular artery courses between the meatal cartilage and mastoid and provides branches to the upper and middle auricle.

The skin of the ear and perichondrium is supplied by a vast array of arterioles and venules, whereas the cartilage is avascular and relies on the perichondrium for diffusion of oxygen and removal of metabolic waste. Shearing forces from blunt trauma may cause tearing of the perichondrium with bleeding into the space between the avascular cartilage and perichondrium. This bleeding or extravasation of serous fluid can become trapped beneath the perichondrium and prevent the metabolically necessary transport, and damage to the cartilage is likely to occur. Damage can occur in the form of necrosis of the cartilage and make further reconstruction difficult.

Another possible outcome of a collection beneath the perichondrium is a "cauliflower ear," an unsightly thickening of the ear formed by fibrosis and the creation of new, haphazard cartilage. Incision plus drainage of the collection is only one part of the treatment; occlusive dressings are required to prevent recurrence. Hematoma and seroma also increase the risk for development of an infection, which can also cause permanent damage to the structure of the auricular cartilage and leave the patient with a disfigured ear after resolution of the infection.

The risk for keloid formation on the ear is higher than in other areas of the body. This can present further complications with any procedure involving the ear, including repair of traumatic injury. Prevention and treatment of keloids are discussed in more detail later in the text.

DIAGNOSTIC STUDIES

Most evaluations of an acute ear injury will occur in the emergency department. As with any trauma, the principles of advanced trauma life support should be followed when indicated. Computed tomography of the head may be necessary if the consultant suspects an intracranial injury. Evaluation of an injury to the ear begins with assessment of the auricle and other external ear landmarks. Otoscopic examination of the tympanic membrane and the ear canal should be performed before treatment. Hearing assessment should also be performed before definitive care.

RECONSTRUCTIVE GOALS

Reconstruction of the ear presents the surgeon with unique challenges not encountered elsewhere in the maxillofacial region. The anatomy of the ear, with its relatively thin layer of skin overlying the perichondrium and avascular cartilage, tends to increase the risk for poor surgical outcomes. An understanding of the pathogenesis of complications in ear reconstruction is necessary to prevent a poor surgical result. As mentioned previously, bilateral symmetry and correct proportion of the anatomic features of the ear are equally

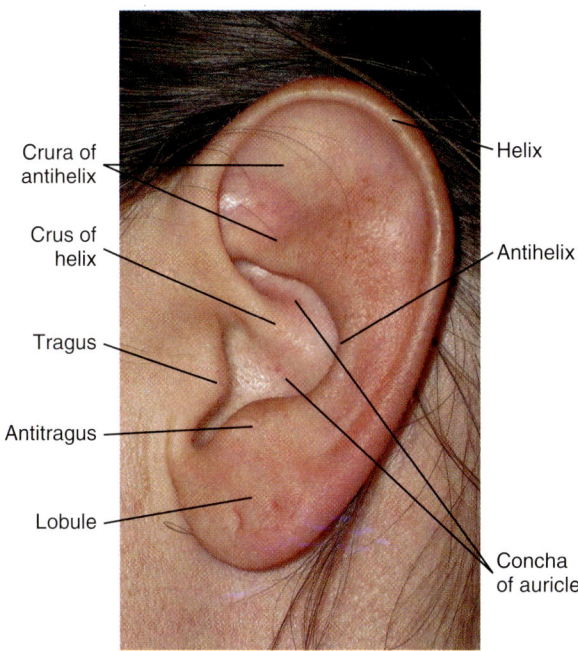

Crura of
antihelix

Crus of
helix

Tragus

Antitragus

Lobule

Helix

Antihelix

Concha
of auricle

Fig. 67-1 ■ Basic anatomy of the auricle.

important considerations in ear reconstruction to achieve the best esthetic results.

TRAUMA

There are various and challenging techniques to repair trauma to the ear. It is not the author's intent to cover every existing method for reconstruction of the ear but just to inform readers of an assortment of techniques that they may include in their surgical armamentarium. The initial step is to categorize the wound. Once categorized, the treatment with the best surgical outcome may be used. When considering trauma to the auricle, the wounds are classified as laceration, extended laceration, partial avulsion, and total avulsion.

LACERATIONS

Ear lacerations are usually easily treated in the emergency department under local anesthesia. The general principles of wound repair are the same for the ear as they are elsewhere on the face. First is copious irrigation and débridement. The ear is then repaired with 6-0 non-absorbable monofilament sutures through the skin in correct anatomic position. When repairing lacerations there is usually no need for sutures in the cartilage of the auricle.

EXTENDED LACERATIONS

An extended laceration is defined as any large laceration that has greatly disrupted the anatomy of the external ear and yet enough tissue remains attached to provide the displaced segment with a blood supply. Again, the general principles of wound repair are followed. It is essential for the bridge of tissue to remain attached. Because the soft tissue of the ear is so vascular, pedicles of skin with a small base tend to survive better here than elsewhere in the body. The segments are approximated in correct anatomic position and sutured with 6-0 non-absorbable monofilament suture through the skin. Sutures are placed within the auricular cartilage only when deemed necessary and are kept to a minimum. Too many sutures through the avascular cartilage may lead to devitalization of that particular region of the cartilage. Sutures through the cartilage have a tendency to erode through the thin overlying tissue and cause

unsightly markings, as well as being a nidus for infection. If sutures do erode through the skin, they must be removed with minimal damage to the overlying skin.

Although the arterial supply to the ear is generous, venous outflow is questionable in a recent injury, especially avulsions. Large extended lacerations with a minimal bridge of tissue may be accompanied by the development of venous congestion. Leech therapy or any other anticoagulation techniques may be needed in the postoperative period.

PARTIAL AVULSION

Acute traumatic avulsion of auricular tissue can range from very small defects to full avulsions. The type of reconstruction depends on the size of the defect and the region of the helix affected. Acquired defects of the superior auricle no larger than 2 cm can be repaired primarily by advancing the helix in both directions. As described by Antia and Buch, the entire helix is freed from the scapha, and incisions are made in the helical sulcus and cartilage to advance the two flaps and retain the anatomic contour of the superior helix (Fig. 67-2).

Middle auricle defects 2 cm or smaller can again be closed primarily with the help of Burrow triangles to allow approximation of tissue without tension. Lower third auricular defects are difficult to repair because of their lack of cartilaginous support. Various techniques have been described to repair a traumatically missing earlobe. Local skin flaps as reported by Converse and Brent and even a combination cartilage and skin flap have been described.

Larger defects will need increasingly complex reconstructive techniques to achieve esthetic acceptance. If the avulsion is large enough, microvascular anastomosis may be achieved, although it is very rare for partial avulsions to have recipient vessels sufficient for the anastomosis. Depending on the amount of cartilage lost, a variety of techniques involving local skin flaps, contralateral conchal cartilage, and rib cartilage can be used (Fig. 67-3).

Techniques such as the "pocket principle" should be used with caution or not at all. After dermabrading the anterior and posterior ear segment, it is placed into a retroauricular pocket and the dermabraded skin allowed to reepithelialize over the ear cartilage within the pocket. After 3 weeks the segment is released from the mastoid skin. Some authors believe that the cartilage of the ear is too thin and delicate to retain sufficient shape against the forces of scar contracture. Not only can the cartilage not be used in this situation, but useful retroauricular skin may now not be available for secondary reconstruction.

There are few anecdotal case reports of success in suturing the avulsed segment as a composite graft. Generally, this will result in failure, but it serves two functions. First, the patient believes that there has been an "attempt" to salvage the ear segment. Second, the retroauricular skin is not damaged by attachment of the composite graft and may be used for secondary reconstruction. By and large, reconstruction of a large avulsed ear segment is usually achieved through secondary reconstruction with rib cartilage (Fig. 67-4) and a temporoparietal flap. The rib cartilage graft contains sufficient strength to maintain its shape through the healing process and scar contracture.

FULL AVULSION

Every attempt should be made to perform microvascular replantation of an avulsed ear. Over the years there has been an increase in success when using microvascular techniques in this scenario. Ideally, arterial inflow and venous outflow should be anastomosed with the superficial temporal vessels. Microvascular attempts at ear replantation have even been successful with no venous outflow, just

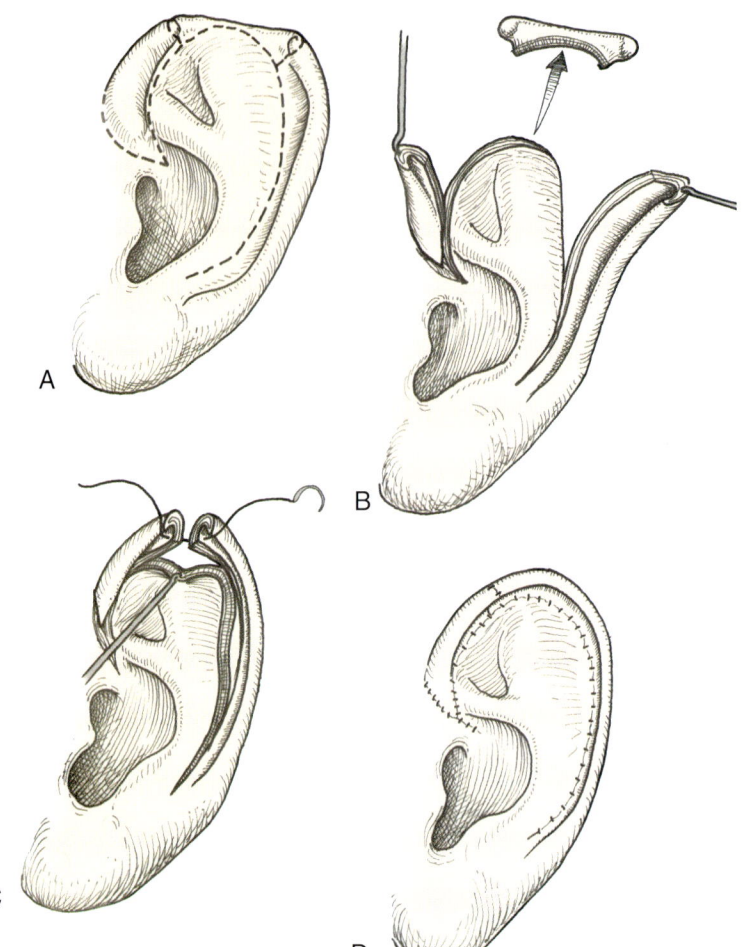

Fig. 67-2 ▪ Auricular chondrocutaneous composite flaps. **A,** Helical defect. Broken lines indicate incisions through skin and cartilage. **B,** Island advancement flap consisting of the helical root advanced on a medial soft tissue pedicle. The remaining helix is pedicled on the earlobe. **C,** Flaps advanced. **D,** Wound closure. (From Baker SR: *Local flaps in facial reconstruction*, ed 2, St Louis, 2007, Mosby.)

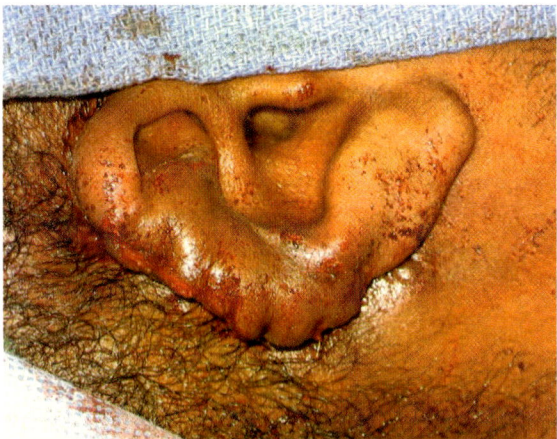

Fig. 67-3 ▪ Partial avulsion of the most lateral portion of the auricle, including the cartilage. The remaining auricle was then grafted with contralateral conchal cartilage and closed in a "pocket" technique. At this point the pocket has been released with primary closure of the newly formed helix.

arterial inflow. Regardless of whether the venous outflow is patent, leech therapy is needed to treat the impending venous congestion. Petrolatum gauze is placed in the external ear canal to prevent migration of a leech into the middle ear. Leeches are placed three to four times a day about 20 minutes per leech. They generally fall off once finished. Constant monitoring of the patient's hemoglobin

and hematocrit is necessary, with transfusion of packed red blood cells as needed. If the attempt at microvascular replantation fails, a rib cartilage graft is placed secondarily (Fig. 67-5).

EAR PROSTHESIS

Prosthetic reconstruction may be considered when the skin overlying the mastoid region is unusable. The primary example is radiation therapy after tumor ablation. The patient must be capable of maintaining the prosthesis and the soft tissue to which the prosthesis will attach. The most popular is a silicone prosthesis, which is usually attached with an adhesive. Newer adhesives have increased strength, thus making detachment of the prosthesis from the skin more difficult. Another alternative to adhesives is an osseointegrated implant-retained prosthesis. Although these prostheses avoid the hassle of applying and cleaning adhesives, meticulous hygiene must be practiced. The tissue surrounding the implant can become inflamed and require discontinuation of the prosthesis until the symptoms resolve. Prosthetic reconstruction is contraindicated in children. Besides the meticulous hygiene needed to maintain the prosthesis, the prosthesis is removable and may result in the child having psychosocial problems.

DRESSINGS

Most ear lacerations occur in the pinna, which is also the portion of the ear that is most susceptible to hematoma formation. If the patient is being admitted to the hospital with other injuries, the ear can be closely monitored for hematoma formation. Otherwise, an occlusive

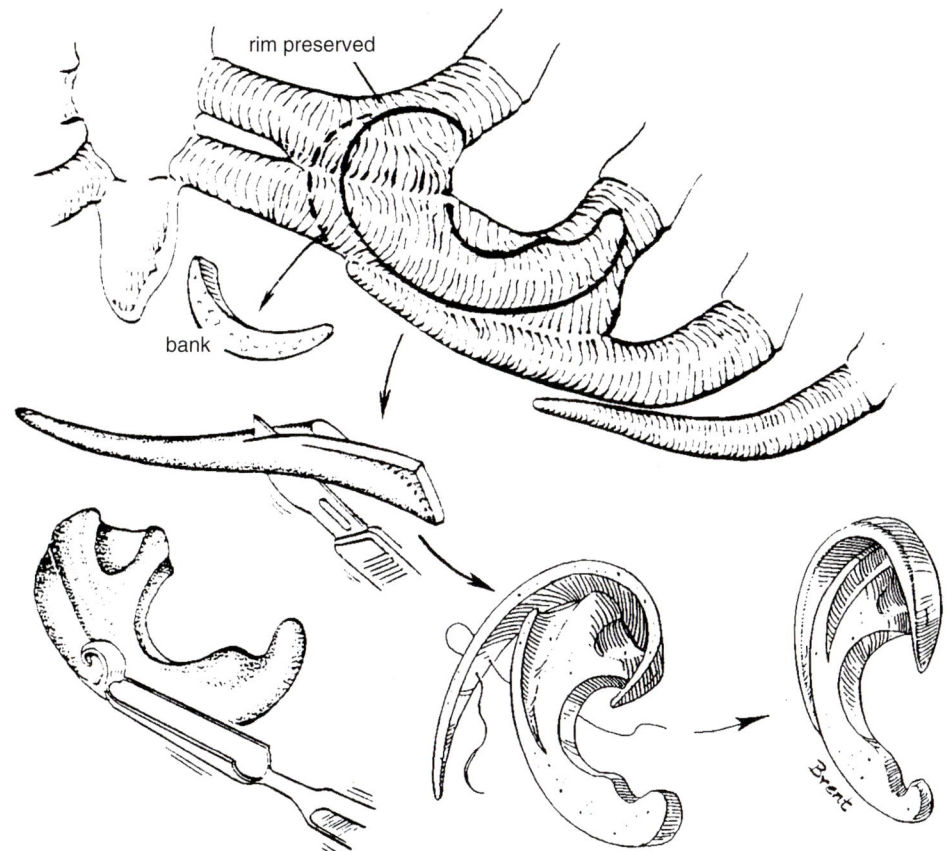

rim preserved

bank

Fig. 67-4 ■ Harvest of rib cartilage for fabrication of the ear framework. (From Brent B: Ear reconstruction. In Mathes SJ, editor: *Plastic surgery*, vol 3, ed 2, Philadelphia, 2006, Saunders.)

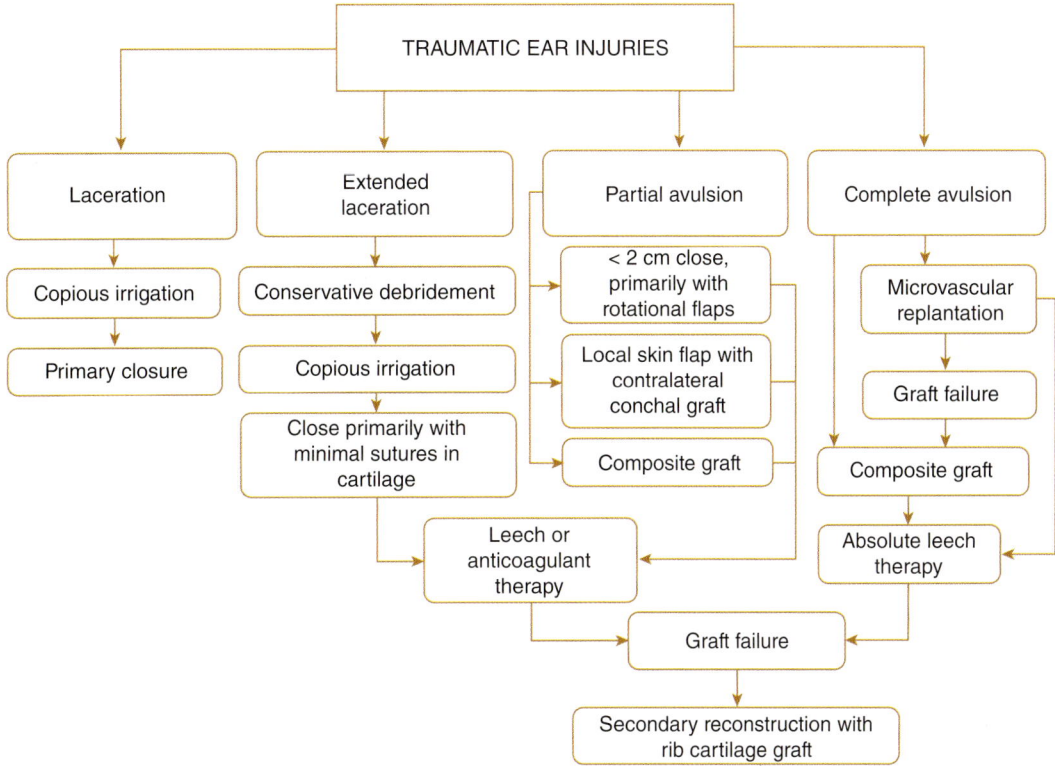

TRAUMATIC EAR INJURIES

Laceration	Extended laceration	Partial avulsion	Complete avulsion

Laceration → Copious irrigation → Primary closure

Extended laceration → Conservative debridement → Copious irrigation → Close primarily with minimal sutures in cartilage

Partial avulsion → < 2 cm close, primarily with rotational flaps / Local skin flap with contralateral conchal graft / Composite graft

Complete avulsion → Microvascular replantation → Graft failure → Composite graft → Absolute leech therapy

Leech or anticoagulant therapy

Graft failure

Secondary reconstruction with rib cartilage graft

Fig. 67-5 ■ Categorization and treatment of ear injuries.

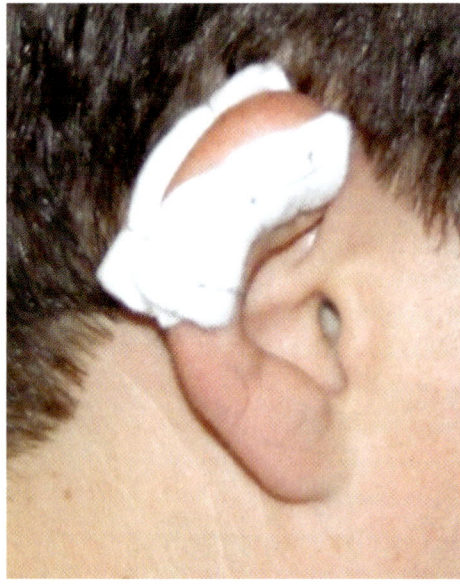

Fig. 67-6 ▪ Through-and-through suture through the pinna with a cotton roll bolster to maintain contact of the soft tissue with the cartilage on both sides of the ear.

dressing will be necessary. Different types of dressings are available, and appropriate selection depends on the injury.

The simplest dressing to place is a through-and-through suture through the pinna with gauze or cotton roll bolsters to maintain contact of the soft tissue with the cartilage on both sides of the ear (Fig. 67-6). This dressing works well in the area of the conchal bowl or between the helix and antihelix. The bolsters are adapted to both sides of the ear and must be placed exactly opposite each other. The bolsters are held in place while a non-resorbable monofilament suture is passed through the ear, around each bolster, and tied down. If the area of concern is not localized to these areas, another dressing should be considered.

When stellate, multiple, or long lacerations occur over the ear, larger areas of compression will be needed. Antibiotic-impregnated petrolatum gauze is often readily available in the emergency department. It can be folded over itself and easily trimmed and molded to fit within the conchal bowl to provide relief for the antihelix. Another piece of antibiotic-impregnated petrolatum gauze can then be formed to fit behind the ear over the mastoid to support the ear in its appropriate position in relation to the head. Fluff in the form of 4 × 4 gauze is then placed over the antibiotic-saturated petrolatum gauze and the head wrapped with gauze cling to compress the dressing without covering the contralateral ear. Antibiotic coverage is necessary not only for the laceration itself but also for otitis media/externa prophylaxis while the dressing is in place.

The polyvinylsiloxane (PVS) mold method is similar in principle to the antibiotic-impregnated petrolatum gauze dressing (Fig. 67-7). The PVS mold provides more intimate adaptation with the tissue, but most hospitals do not stock the necessary materials. PVS may become embedded by the sutures and make removal of the dressing almost impossible without causing more tissue damage. To prevent this complication, PVS should be injected after the ear is covered with well-adapted antibiotic ointment–coated gauze. A cotton ball must also be carefully placed in the external auditory meatus to prevent flow of material into the canal; the cotton is removed after the PVS has solidified and before the ear is completely dressed. Support between the mastoid and posterior ear should be provided

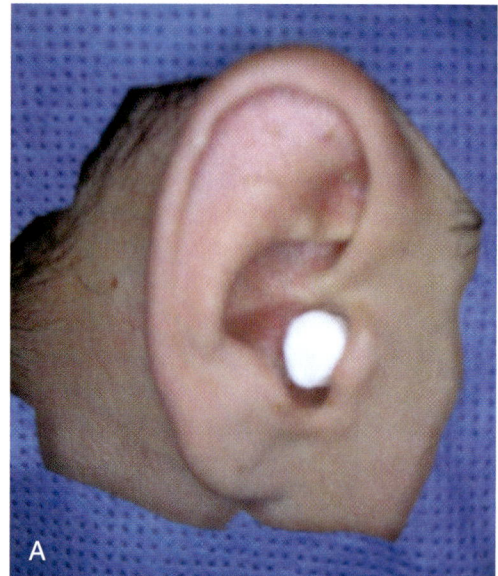

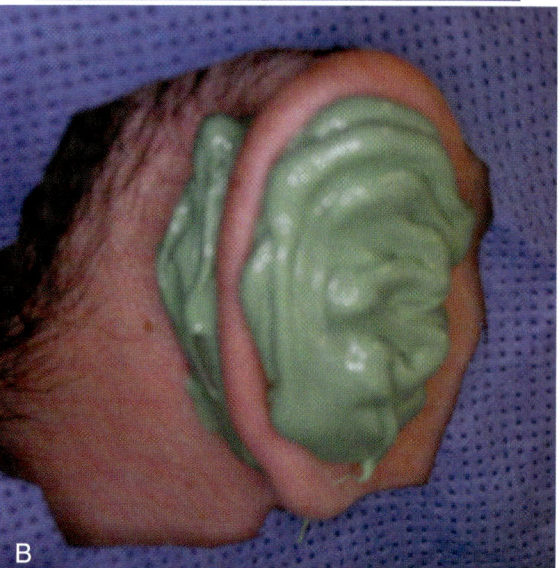

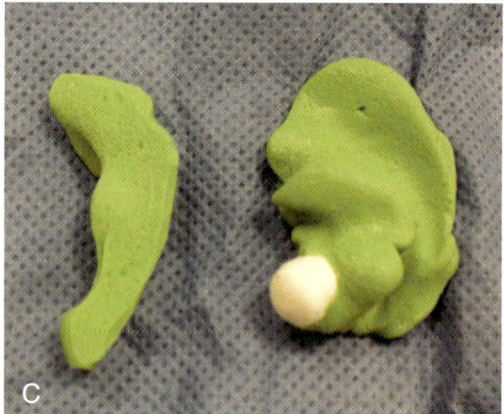

Fig. 67-7 ▪ **A,** On a non-lacerated ear (a sutured ear requires placement of a protective barrier of petrolatum gauze), a small section of cotton roll should be placed in the external canal to prevent flow of polyvinylsiloxane (PVS) into the canal. **B,** PVS is allowed to set within the auricle and in the posterior auricular area to provide support and compression. **C,** Completed compression dressings.

by packed gauze or, preferentially, another PVS mold, followed by a gauze cling head wrap to maintain pressure. Again, antibiotic prophylaxis must be considered when the canal is occluded.

ANIMAL BITES

As discussed earlier, human and animal bites are common sources of auricular injury. In general, the injury is repaired in the same manner as lacerations of the ear. Although microorganisms vary between animal and human bites, antibiotic coverage is similar. Cat bites are far more likely than dog bites to become infected. The first-line choice of antibiotic is oral amoxicillin-clavulanate. In penicillin-allergic patients with human bites, oral clindamycin is an appropriate choice with or without trimethoprim-sulfamethoxazole. Infections from animal bites are caused by *Pasteurella multocida* about 25% of the time, which is resistant to clindamycin; a more appropriate antibiotic in a penicillin-allergic patient with an animal bite is cefuroxime.

PIERCINGS

In many cultures worldwide, piercing of the ears for decorative purposes is common. Complications from piercing can arise as a result of traumatic removal of the earring and subsequent tearing of the soft tissues or as a result of the piercing procedure itself in the form of keloid formation or infection during the healing process.

The anatomic location of the piercing also plays a part in the pathogenesis of these complications. Infections arising from a lobe piercing, if treated early, tend to be associated with fewer complications than do infections arising from higher on the auricle. Piercings in this region are more likely to result in a deformity of the auricle. Piercings involving penetration of the relatively avascular auricular cartilage lend themselves to bacterial proliferation through a thinly epithelialized tract. The resultant auricular chondritis often causes structural collapse of the auricle, a dramatic deformity that persists after the infection resolves.

Patients with an infection from a high piercing usually have a full-blown infection requiring incision and drainage and frequently intravenous antibiotics. Material for culture can be collected at the time of incision and drainage. Nonetheless, approximately 95% of auricular infections are due to *Pseudomonas aeruginosa*. First-line treatment consists of ciprofloxacin or imipenem-cilastatin.

KELOIDS

PATHOGENESIS

The term *keloid* is often used erroneously when referring to a hypertrophic scar. By definition, a hypertrophic scar is always contained within the site and size of the original wound. Keloids are areas of hypertrophy that extend beyond the boundaries of the original wound and will frequently recur after surgical excision.

An in-depth discussion of the pathogenesis of keloid formation is beyond the scope of this text. It will suffice to know that the process of keloid formation involves loss of control of normal healing mechanisms. This loss of control consists of a combination of cell proliferation and abnormal apoptosis.

Keloid formation is more frequent in darker-skinned races. The ears are one of the more common locations for keloid formation in the maxillofacial region. These facts should be taken into account when planning any procedures on the ears from simple piercing to complete reconstruction.

SURGICAL EXCISION OF KELOIDS

Surgical excision as a sole treatment of keloids has been shown to be largely ineffective in the long term. Recurrence rates following excision alone range from 45% to 100%. Combining surgical excision with an adjuvant form of therapy can reduce recurrence rates to below 50%.

Excision can easily be carried out under local anesthesia in the clinic setting. The surgical site should be prepared and the patient anesthetized. Donkor recommended performing the excision intralesionally rather than extralesionally and thereby avoiding induction of an inflammatory response in the unaffected skin. Should the keloid recur, the larger margins of an extralesional excision may result in a larger keloid. The bulk of the keloid should be excised while leaving a small margin of keloid, which will be closed primarily following undermining of the skin. Once hemostasis is ensured, closure can be completed with 6-0 non-resorbable monofilament suture. Some may prefer to use a fast-absorbing gut suture; however, this tends to enhance the inflammatory response, which increases the likelihood of recurrence. Sutures should be removed in 10 to 14 days. Postoperative dressings are dependent on the location of the excision.

INTRALESIONAL CORTICOSTEROID INJECTION

The aim of intralesional injection of corticosteroids is two-fold: first, to inhibit the excess collagen production, and second, to inhibit the action of collagenase inhibitors. This therapy is the first line in treating most keloids because it is less invasive than other treatments and has fewer side effects. Adverse reactions from corticosteroid injection include hypopigmentation, atrophy of skin, and less commonly, a cushingoid effect from systemic absorption. Shaffer and colleagues' review of five studies found that although up to 70% of keloids respond to intralesional steroid injection, the recurrence rate is rather high.

Triamcinolone acetonide is available in multidose vials with varying concentration. It is provided as a suspension, and it may be necessary to dilute the suspension with normal saline. Some practitioners prefer to use lidocaine without epinephrine to eliminate the burning sensation associated with delivery; however, a study comparing the discomfort from injection of normal saline and buffered lidocaine showed no significant difference between the two. Most practitioners use corticosteroid monotherapy at a dose of 40 mg/mL every 4 weeks with at least four doses. The treatment may be carried out longer for more persistent keloids, but it is recommended that surgical excision be considered if corticosteroid monotherapy fails to resolve the keloid.

A small 1- or 3-mL syringe is used with a 27- or 30-gauge needle. The skin is prepared with alcohol and the needle is advanced into the lesion with care to avoid subcutaneous tissue and injection into the mid-dermis. Significant resistance is felt when injecting into the mid-dermis. Injection will also cause a wheal and blanching reaction on the skin. The needle can be withdrawn and other areas of the lesion injected as necessity dictates.

EXCISION OF THE KELOID WITH INJECTION OF CORTICOSTEROID

Combining surgical excision with postoperative intralesional corticosteroid injection reduces the rate of recurrence found with either treatment alone. Intraoperative injections are a point of controversy; although intraoperative corticosteroids suppress the inflammatory response that leads to keloid formation, they also inhibit the inflammation that promotes wound healing. The result will be a prolonged

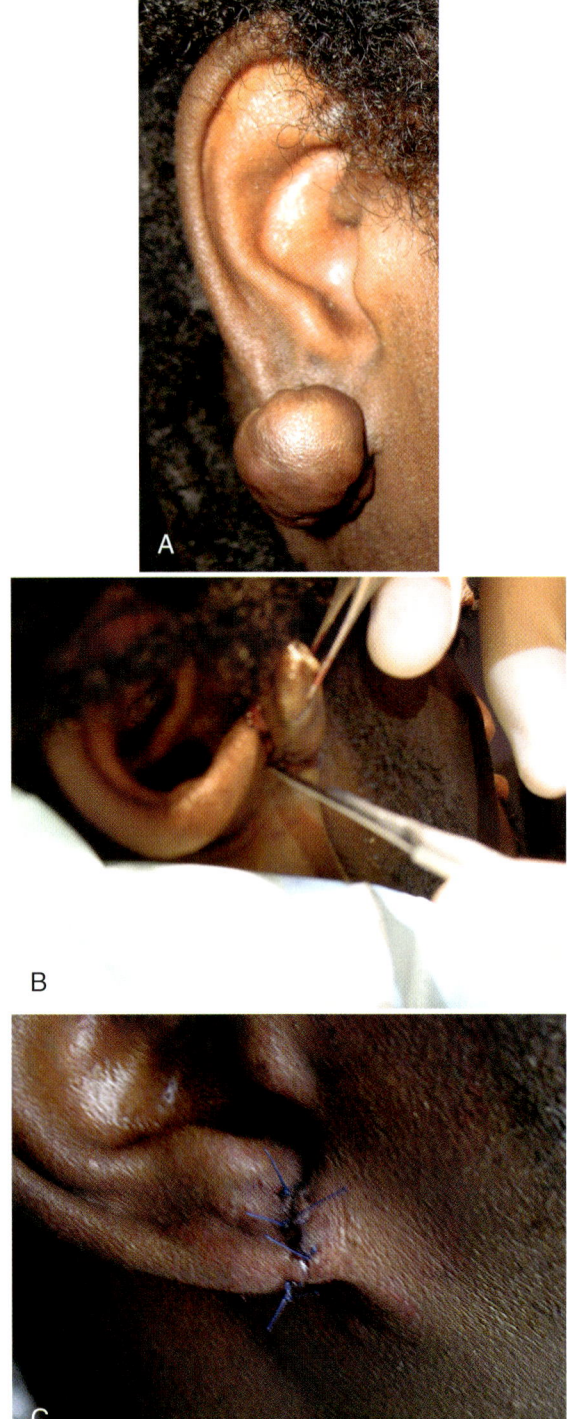

Fig. 67-8 ■ **A,** An earlobe keloid developed after routine ear piercing. **B,** Surgical excision of the keloid with care to leave a small cuff of keloid. **C,** Primary closure. At this point injection of triamcinolone should be withheld because it can inhibit initial healing. Steroids can be injected at the suture removal appointment.

healing period, and thus intraoperative injections should be avoided (Fig. 67-8).

When the patient returns for suture removal 10 to 14 days postoperatively, the excision site can be cleaned and intralesional corticosteroids can be injected into the residual lesion. The injection should be repeated every month for two to three more doses and

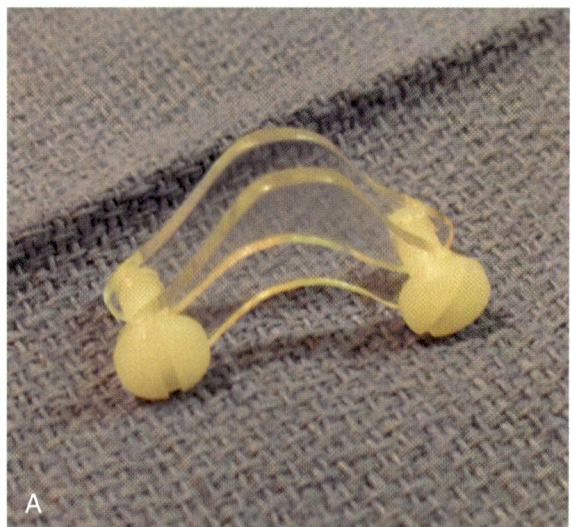

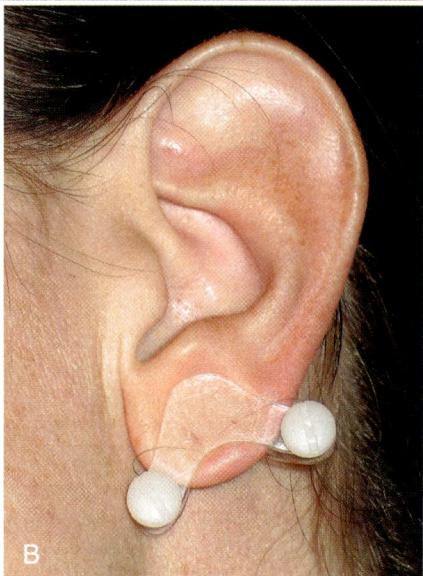

Fig. 67-9 ■ **A,** Pressure earrings fabricated from acrylic plates. **B,** Pressure earrings in use by the patient for prevention of earlobe keloid.

carried out in similar fashion as corticosteroid monotherapy. The dosage of triamcinolone should not exceed 40 mg per visit.

PRESSURE EARRINGS

Pressure earrings prevent keloid formation by occluding blood vessels, which results in hypoxia and eventually degeneration of fibroblasts and cell breakdown. Pressure earrings can be used alone or in conjunction with intralesional injections, surgical excision, or a combination of treatments. Pressure therapy should be maintained for 6 continuous months with the patient wearing the device at night if tolerated. This therapy is limited to the lobule only.

If pressure therapy is used as an adjunct to excision, therapy begins following removal of the sutures 10 to 14 days postoperatively. The patient is then fitted with pressure earrings, several types of which exist. Prefabricated pressure earrings disguised as jewelry can be obtained from several sources. These types are not usually amenable to customization.

Another option is fabrication of customized acrylic splints that consist of two thin plates of acrylic attached with screws on either end that when tightened, compress the lobe between the two plates (Fig. 67-9). This system allows more control over the level of compression exerted on the lobe, but it does not resemble normal earrings and is more noticeable.

KELOID EXCISION WITH ADJUVANT EXTERNAL BEAM RADIATION THERAPY OR HIGH-DOSE-RATE BRACHYTHERAPY

Single-fraction external beam radiotherapy following surgical excision has been suggested to be successful in the treatment of ear keloids. Based on a study by Ragoowansi and co-workers, the risk for development of a radiation-induced malignancy is estimated to be 1 in 1,348 (0.07%). It has been postulated that high-dose-rate brachytherapy offers a reduction in this risk because the dose and treatment field are smaller. On the other hand, conventional external beam radiation consists of orthoradiation, which has much lower voltage than the treatment used for most malignancies.

Brachytherapy involves placement of a catheter through the skin on either side of the lesion at the time of surgical excision before closure of the skin. Once closure is completed, the patient is sent to the radiation oncology department. According to the prescribed treatment plan, an iridium-192 source is passed by the machine through the catheter and back with stops programmed to deliver the appropriate dose of radiation to the surrounding tissue. This is done again on postoperative days 2 and 3, with the patient receiving fractions of 500 cGy per visit. After the third visit the catheter is removed and the wounds dressed.

Although proponents of both methods of adjuvant radiation therapy will extol their virtue of low dosage or small field, neither can deny a small risk for future malignancy. This risk can cause some patients to defer radiation as an adjunctive treatment.

AURICULAR CHONDRITIS

Auricular chondritis can be due to a variety of causes, such as previous surgery, trauma, and piercings. Generally, treatment is the same. The stage of disease is the first consideration. Early disease is characterized by erythema, non-fluctuant edema, and tenderness. These cases usually resolve with the use of oral antibiotics and leave little or no residual damage. More extensive disease characterized by fluctuance requires immediate incision and drainage, sometimes with judicious débridement of affected tissue followed by parenteral antibiotics. A specimen should be taken at the time of drainage for culture and sensitivity testing.

Pseudomonas aeruginosa is the most common microbiologic agent involved in auricular infection. First-line antibiotic coverage consists of ciprofloxacin or imipenem-cilastatin. Kishore retrospectively reviewed 61 patients with auricular chondritis of varying causes. It was found that the antibiotic sensitivity of *P. aeruginosa* did vary, thus illustrating the need for culture and sensitivity testing at the time of incision and drainage.

When incision plus drainage is warranted, an occlusive dressing is necessary postoperatively to prevent reaccumulation of fluid. This is crucial to avoid further destruction of the cartilage and the resultant deformity.

THERMAL INJURIES

As noted previously, the location of the auricles with their outward extension from the head predisposes them to injury. This is most evident in thermal injuries involving the head and neck. When auricular burn injuries occur, the damage is usually severe and complete loss of the auricle is not uncommon. Initial treatment consists of débridement, local wound care, and the application of antibiotic effective against *P. aeruginosa*. The patient must be monitored meticulously for the development of chondritis.

Smaller portions of the auricle lost to thermal damage can be reconstructed in the same manner as an avulsion. If damage to the ear and surrounding skin is severe, skin grafting can be used to cover the defect.

Frostbite, like thermal injury, is particularly devastating when the auricle is affected. The thin soft tissue covering the cartilage can easily be lost as a result of frostbite. Initial treatment consists of rapid rewarming of the affected tissue. This is a painful process and therefore appropriate analgesia should be provided. Moist heat is preferred because dry heat is difficult to regulate. Manipulation of the ears should be avoided; rubbing the ear during rewarming is contraindicated since this can exacerbate the damage. During the postinjury period bullae often form, and drainage should be avoided because this can provide an opportunity for infection. Use of prophylactic antibiotics in patients with frostbite injury involving the ear is controversial, but given the susceptibility of the auricle to infection, antibiotic coverage is reasonable. Areas of necrosis that arise must be débrided as they develop and repair performed.

PEARLS AND PITFALLS

- The avascular cartilage can predispose the ear to complications and deformities. Prevention of chondritis with antibiotics and appropriate dressings is crucial.
- Ninety-five percent of cases of chondritis are caused by *P. aeruginosa*.
- When reconstructing large avulsions, care should be taken to maintain the retro-auricular skin for secondary reconstruction. The "pocket principle" must be used with caution because it may prevent use of this tissue in the future.
- Leech and anticoagulant therapy should be considered for lacerations in which venous outflow is a concern. It is mandatory following all avulsion repairs.
- Occlusive dressings are an important adjunct to prevent future complications.
- Postrepair follow-up must consider monitoring for keloid formation so that intervention can be initiated promptly.

BIBLIOGRAPHY

Antia NH, Buch VI: Chondrocutaneous advancement flap for the marginal defect of the ear, *Plast Reconstr Surg* 39:472-477, 1967.

Gilbert DN, Moellering RC Jr, Eliopoulos GM, et al: *The Sanford guide to antimicrobial therapy 2008*, ed 38, Sperryville, VA, 2008, Antimicrobial Therapy, Inc.

Kind GM: Microvascular ear replantation, *Clin Plast Surg* 29:233-248, 2002.

Lugo-Janer G, Padial M, Sanchez JL: Less painful alternatives for local anesthesia, *J Dermatol Surg Oncol* 19:237-240, 1993.

Margulis A, Bauer B, Alizadeh K: Ear reconstruction after auricular chondritis secondary to ear piercing, *Plast Reconstr Surg* 111:891-877, discussion 898, 2003.

Punjabi AP, Haug RH, Jordan RB: Management of injuries to the auricle, *J Oral Maxillofac Surg* 55:732-739, 1997.

Ragoowansi R, Cornes PGS, Moss AL, et al: Treatment of keloids by surgical excision and immediate post-operative single-fraction radiotherapy, *Plast Reconstr Surg* 111:1853-1859, 2003.

Savion Y, Sela M: Prefabricated pressure earring for earlobe keloids, *J Prosthet Dent* 99:406-407, 2008.

Shaffer JJ, Taylor SC, Cook-Bolden F: Keloidal scars: a review with a critical look at

therapeutic options, *J Am Acad Dermatol* 46(2 Suppl):S63-S97, 2002.

Steffen A, Katzbagh R, Klaiber S: Comparison of ear reattachment methods: a review of 25 years since Pennington, *Plast Reconstr Surg* 118:1358-1364, 2006.

Thorne C: Otoplasty and ear reconstruction. In Thorne C, et al, editors: *Grabb and Smith's*

plastic surgery, ed 6. Philadelphia, 2006, Lippincott Williams & Wilkins.

Vachiramon A, Bamber MA: A U-loop pressure clip for earlobe keloid, *J Prosthet Dent* 92: 389-391, 2004.

Chapter

68

The Pectoralis Major Myocutaneous Flap

Dale A. Baur, Michael P. Horan, Juan C. Rodriguez

Large maxillofacial defects secondary to trauma or cancer ablation frequently pose a challenge for the reconstructive surgeon. These defects often cannot be closed without excessive tension and obliteration of normal anatomy. Various surgical methods have been developed to restore soft tissue bulk and recreate form and function. One of the earliest methods described involved development of the pectoralis major (PM) myocutaneous flap, which was first used by Dr. Stephan Ariyan in the late 1970s for reconstruction of ablative surgical defects in patients with head and neck cancer.[1] Since then, it has been extensively used in the context of head and neck reconstructive surgery to reliably repair large soft tissue deficits associated with continuity defects in the mandible, floor of the mouth, and related orofacial structures.[2-6] The design of this axial-pattern flap is versatile in that it can be used to provide coverage of both mucosal and cutaneous defects simultaneously.[5] The flap provides protection for neurovascular structures in the neck and reinforces tissue with compromised vascularity or at increased risk for dehiscence and breakdown (e.g., irradiated tissue, diabetic patients).[6,7] A variation of the flap, the myofascial flap, lacks the associated skin paddle and can be used to effectively close smaller mucosal defects and provide soft tissue bulk.

With recent advances in microvascular surgery, free flap procedures have assumed a more dominant role in the reconstruction of head and neck defects. Free fibula grafts are now used frequently for the reconstruction of large mandibular continuity defects.[8] However, these procedures require great expertise and extensive time to perform, whereas the PM flap is easy to develop and can be performed quickly. One of the many variants of the originally described PM myocutaneous flap incorporates an osseous component (e.g., rib) that remains pedicled to the flap.[9-12] Thus, more than 30 years after its inception, the PM flap continues to be a robust, versatile flap design used extensively in head and neck reconstructive surgery.[13]

TREATMENT/RECONSTRUCTIVE GOALS

INDICATIONS

The PM myocutaneous flap should be considered in any patient with a soft tissue defect involving the oral cavity or associated cutaneous structures. This flap is ideally used to reconstruct defects involving the mandible, floor of the mouth, upper part of the neck, and lower third of the face.[14] The flap also provides undamaged, well-vascularized tissue for defects secondary to osteoradionecrosis. For surgeons who perform non-vascularized secondary bone grafts, the flap provides a generous soft tissue envelope. Advantages of the PM flap are numerous. They include the capability of customizing the skin paddle to the size of the defect, a reliable vascular supply, the ability to easily close the donor site, and technical ease in elevating the flap. While evaluating the patient, it is important to assess the extent of the defect and determine the amount of mucosal or cutaneous soft tissue coverage needed. Whether this is a viable option is dependent on a number of factors, including the patient's anatomy and flap design and inset.[15] In general, the superior "absolute" limits for flap rotation extraorally and intraorally are the zygomatic arch and the superior aspect of the tonsillar pillar, respectively. If a smaller defect is anticipated, a myofascial flap may be used without the associated skin paddle.

CONTRAINDICATIONS

There are relatively few contraindications to reconstruction with the PM flap. That being said, the reconstructive surgeon must consider the following situations. If the dimension of the defect is too large or the defect extends outside the reach of the flap, other techniques for reconstruction should be considered. This technique should also be used with caution in patients who have previously sustained trauma to the chest wall or undergone chest surgery (e.g., mastectomy, implants, pacemakers, compromising scars, burns, previous subclavian puncture, or MEDport use) because the anatomy of the approach to the PM is likely to be altered and the muscle itself may have a compromised vascular supply and exhibit fibrosis and contracture. In patients with the Poland anomaly, a congenital condition with an incidence of 1 in 10,000 to 100,000, this procedure is an absolute contraindication since the PM muscle is underdeveloped or absent.

PREOPERATIVE CONSIDERATIONS

Rotation of the flap from the chest to the orofacial defect will result in an asymmetric chest deformity and, in females, breast asymmetry and may cause excessive bulking at the site of the defect and the ipsilateral neck. Use of this flap will inherently weaken the patent's shoulder and arm on the ipsilateral side, thereby potentially resulting in disability during the postoperative period,[16] although this is normally well tolerated in most patients. As with many surgical procedures in this region, use of the PM flap carries with it a risk for infection, hematoma formation, seroma formation, hemothorax, and pneumothorax. Other disadvantages inherent in using the PM flap for reconstruction include skin color mismatch at the recipient site, limited range of rotation when used for maxillary defects, hair growth when the flap is placed intraorally because the adnexal structures in the skin are left intact, and altered external chest morphology and breast asymmetry in females. If the patient experiences complications in the postoperative period, extensive wound care may be necessary.[17] Furthermore, additional surgical procedures may be necessary to salvage the flap or to provide adequate wound closure.

SURGICAL ANATOMY

The fan-shaped PM muscle is situated deep to the subcutaneous connective tissue in the anterior chest wall (Fig. 68-1). In female patients, the breast and associated glandular tissue overlie the majority of the muscle. The muscle itself has two heads, the clavicular and sternocostal. These heads are recognized as the origins of the PM muscle. The clavicular head attaches superomedially to the medial half of the anterior aspect of the clavicle. The sternocostal head attaches inferomedially to the anterior surface of the sternum and the superior aspect of the costal cartilages of the first six ribs. Inferiorly, the muscle originates from the aponeurosis of the external oblique muscle. In addition, the pectoralis muscle fascia inferiorly is confluent with the rectus abdominis muscle fascia. Superolaterally, the PM muscle inserts onto the head of the proximal end of the humerus at the intertubercular groove. The PM muscle is a major structural component of the anterior wall of the axilla and contributes to the formation of the anterior axillary fold. The summative action of the two heads of the PM muscle is to adduct and medially rotate the humerus. Once the muscle flap has been elevated, arm function is typically compensated by the latissimus dorsi muscle. Deep to the PM muscle are the pectoralis minor muscle, the subclavius muscle, the serratus anterior muscle, and the intercostal muscles. The PM muscle is surrounded by a layer of fascia, which facilitates dissection.

VASCULAR SUPPLY OF THE PECTORALIS MAJOR

The pectoral branch of the thoracoacromial artery provides the main vascular supply to the PM muscle once elevated (see Fig. 68-1). The pectoral branch of the artery courses obliquely and parallel to a line between the acromion process and xiphoid process. The thoracoacromial artery is the first branch of the axillary artery. It arises from the axillary artery deep to the clavicle. The pectoral branch of the thoracoacromial artery is one of four main branches (the others include the deltoid, acromial, and clavicular branches) (Fig. 68-2). As the thoracoacromial artery branches off the axillary artery, it penetrates the clavipectoral fascia (Fig. 68-3) and courses deep to the pectoralis muscle, at which point it enters the muscle from its deep surface and branches intramuscularly (see Fig. 68-2). Vascular supply to the elevated PM muscle flap is also provided by the lateral thoracic artery, albeit to a lesser extent. Maintenance of the integrity of this vessel improves viability. The superior thoracic artery also contributes a negligible amount. The aforementioned arteries are accompanied by their venae comitantes.

Parasternal perforators from the internal mammary artery provide vascularity to the medial aspect of the PM muscle while the muscle is in situ. During elevation of the flap, these vessels are often transected. However, care should be taken to maintain the integrity of the first and second perforators because they supply the skin used in the deltopectoral flap. Maintenance of this blood supply is

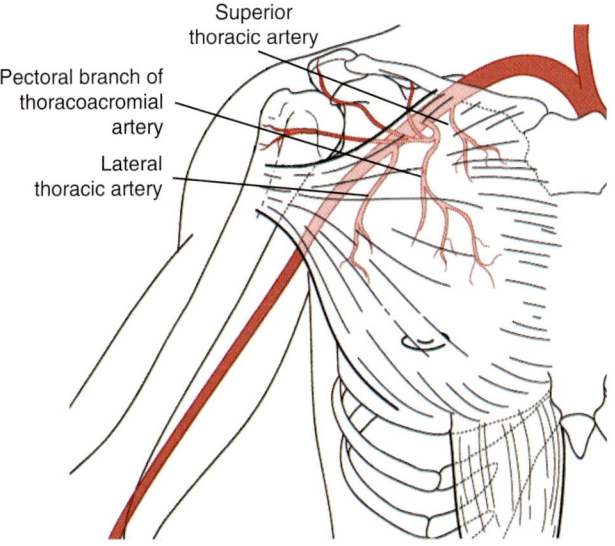

Fig. 68-1 ■ Relationship of muscle and vascular supply. Note the origins at the clavicle, sternum, and ribs. The muscle inserts at the humerus. (Courtesy Jordan Mastrodonato, Fort Gordon, Ga.)

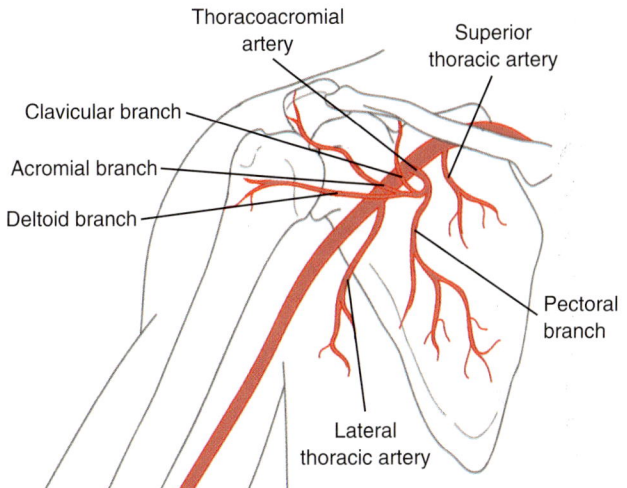

Fig. 68-2 ■ Blood supply to the pectoralis major muscle. (Courtesy Jordan Mastrodonato, Fort Gordon, Ga.)

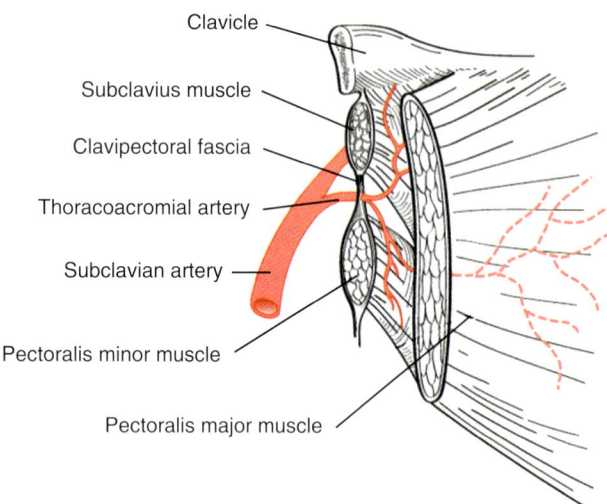

Fig. 68-3 ■ Thoracoacromial artery penetrating the clavipectoral fascia. (Courtesy Jordan Mastrodonato, Fort Gordon, Ga.)

important should a salvage procedure be required, although the deltopectoral flap is rarely used today.[18]

INNERVATION OF THE PECTORALIS MAJOR

Both the lateral and medial pectoral nerves, nerves that are branches of the brachial plexus, provide motor innervation to the PM muscle. The lateral pectoral nerve arises from the lateral cord of the brachial plexus and is composed of branches of C5, C6, and C7. It provides control of the clavicular head and cross-innervates the sternocostal head of the muscle. The medial pectoral nerve arises from the medial cord of the brachial plexus and is composed of branches of C8 and T1. A few branches transect the pectoralis minor muscle and enter the PM to provide motor control of the sternocostal head of the muscle. These nerves are transected as they are encountered in the surgical dissection. The benefit of doing so is two-fold: it improves the arc of rotation of the flap, and denervation of the flap causes the muscle to atrophy, thereby debulking the flap over time.[19]

SURGICAL TECHNIQUE

Surgical landmarks are identified, including the ipsilateral clavicle, the ipsilateral sternal border, the xiphoid process of the sternum, and the humeral insertion of the PM muscle (see Fig. 68-1). The approximate size and location of the skin paddle should be outlined after the recipient site has been prepared. In general, the skin paddle is located inferomedial to the nipple, along the border of the pectoralis muscle at its insertion on the lateral border of the sternum. To a great extent, the location of the skin paddle depends on the size and location of the defect to be reconstructed. Flaps with up to 400 cm² of skin have been reported in the literature. Theoretically, the skin overlying any part of the PM muscle can be used for this purpose.

While designing the flap, the arc of rotation needs to be verified. The arc of rotation can be extended by placing the skin paddle slightly inferior to the most inferior extent of the muscle and extending the skin paddle onto the rectus fascia. However, this distal skin over the rectus fascia is more of a random-pattern flap and is not as reliable. After the recipient site has been appropriately prepared, the initial incision is designed. Three types of incisions have been reported in the literature, namely, an oblique incision, lateral incision, and medial incision.

The oblique incision is best suited for a male patient and provides excellent visualization. The incision begins 8 to 10 cm inferior to the lateral portion of the clavicle and proceeds in a medial/inferior direction (Fig. 68-4, A). The incision is made with a scalpel, and then cautery is used to deepen the incision while leaving the pectoralis muscle fascia intact. Dissection is continued medially and laterally to expose the full extent of the PM muscle (Fig. 68-4, B). When developing the skin paddle, care is taken to not undermine the paddle by diverging away from the skin as the incision is deepened. To avoid shearing the delicate myocutaneous vascular perforators supplying the skin paddle, the skin paddle is sutured to the underlying muscle fascia (Fig. 68-4, C). These sutures can be removed later if necessary to facilitate suturing the skin paddle to the recipient site.

The lateral incision is best suited for female patients because there is less distortion of the breast. The superior/lateral starting point for the incision is the same as for the oblique incision; however, the incision is carried inferiorly and gently curves into the inframammary crease (Fig. 68-5, A). Once this incision is developed, the dissection proceeds in the same manner as with the oblique incision.

The medial incision (Fig. 68-5, B) is much shorter and results in a more cosmetic outcome in both male and female patients. Access is limited, and it is therefore technically more difficult to perform. The dissection is facilitated with the use of lighted retractors.

Once the recipient site has been prepared and the size of the defect is apparent, development of the PM flap begins by designing the appropriate size of skin paddle and verifying the arc of rotation. As mentioned previously, care should be taken to not extend the skin paddle too far inferiorly onto the rectus fascia because this skin is not as reliable as a result of the random-pattern blood supply of this segment of skin. The surgeon can select the incision type in accordance with the patient's needs. The first key step, regardless of incision design, is to develop a plane of dissection just superficial to the PM fascia and expose the superficial aspect of the PM (see Fig. 68-4, B). The proposed skin paddle is isolated and sutured to the underlying PM fascia.

At this point, elevation of the flap begins inferiorly by incising through the rectus fascia while staying superficial to the rectus muscle (see Fig. 68-4, C). The origins of the PM muscle are released from the ribs and sternum by electrocautery. The dissection plane deep to the PM muscle is avascular and easily developed once the attachments to the ribs are released. The surgeon should avoid violating the intercostal muscles and leave the pectoralis minor muscle intact. Some authors recommend leaving a 1-cm cuff of PM muscle attached to the sternum.

As the dissection proceeds superiorly, attempts should be made to visually identify the vessels on the undersurface of the muscle. The vascular pedicle is usually located on the medial aspect of the pectoralis minor muscle. A Doppler probe can be used to help locate the vessels (Fig. 68-6, A). Dissection on the inferior portion of the PM muscle proceeds to the clavicle, with care taken to not dissect deep to the clavicle. For most defects of the oral cavity, the humeral insertion of the PM muscle will need to be released for better mobility and an improved arc of rotation. This insertion is best released slowly and incrementally while keeping the vascular pedicle in full view (Fig. 68-6, B). As the dissection proceeds, one should attempt to avoid the cephalic vein in this region.

Once the PM flap has been fully elevated (Fig. 68-7, A), a tunnel is developed in the neck in a plane deep to the platysma muscle for passage of the PM flap to the defect (Fig. 68-7, B). This tunnel is extended superiorly to the defect, above the clavicle, and into the anterolateral aspect of the neck. Extension of the flap through the neck into the oral cavity is dependent on the location of the defect.

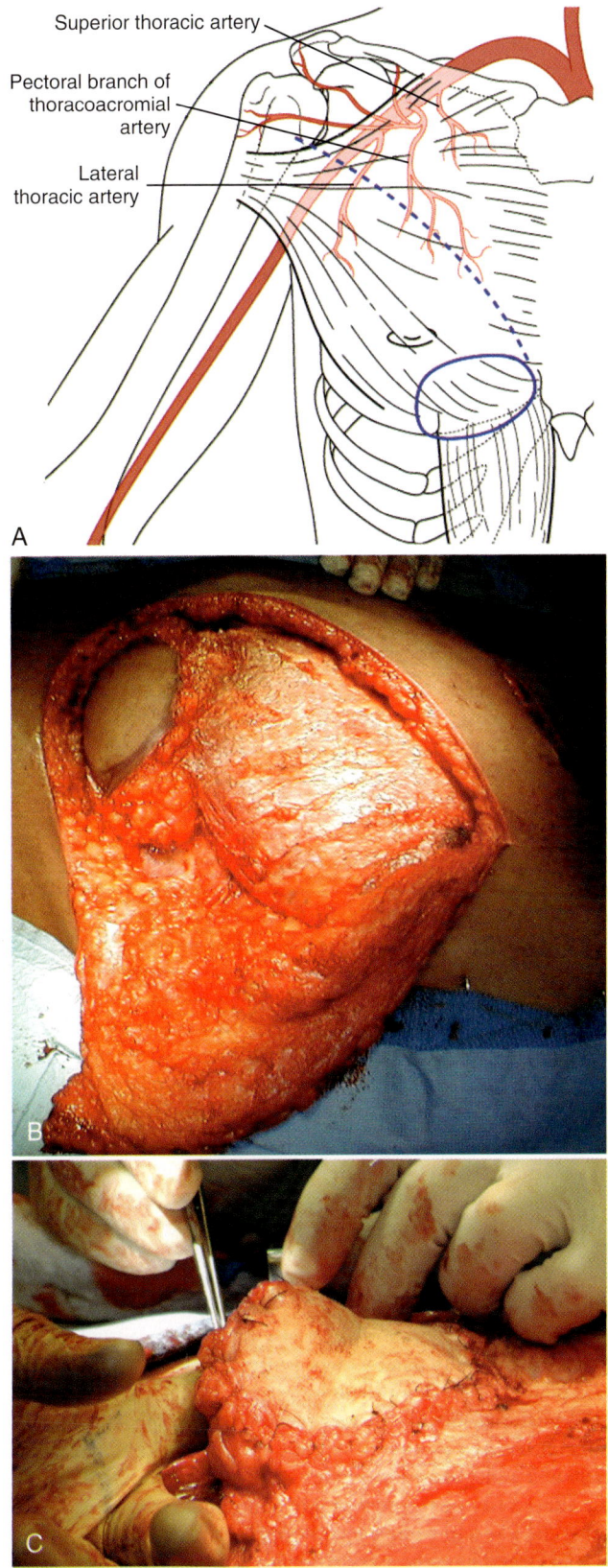

Fig. 68-4 ▪ A, Incision design and skin paddle demonstrated using an oblique incision. B, The entire superficial extent of the muscle with associated skin paddle is exposed and ready to be elevated. C, Elevation of the flap has begun from the inferior aspect. Note how the skin paddle has been sutured to the muscle fascia to prevent shearing of the delicate myocutaneous perforators. (A, Courtesy Jordan Mastrodonato, Fort Gordon, Ga.)

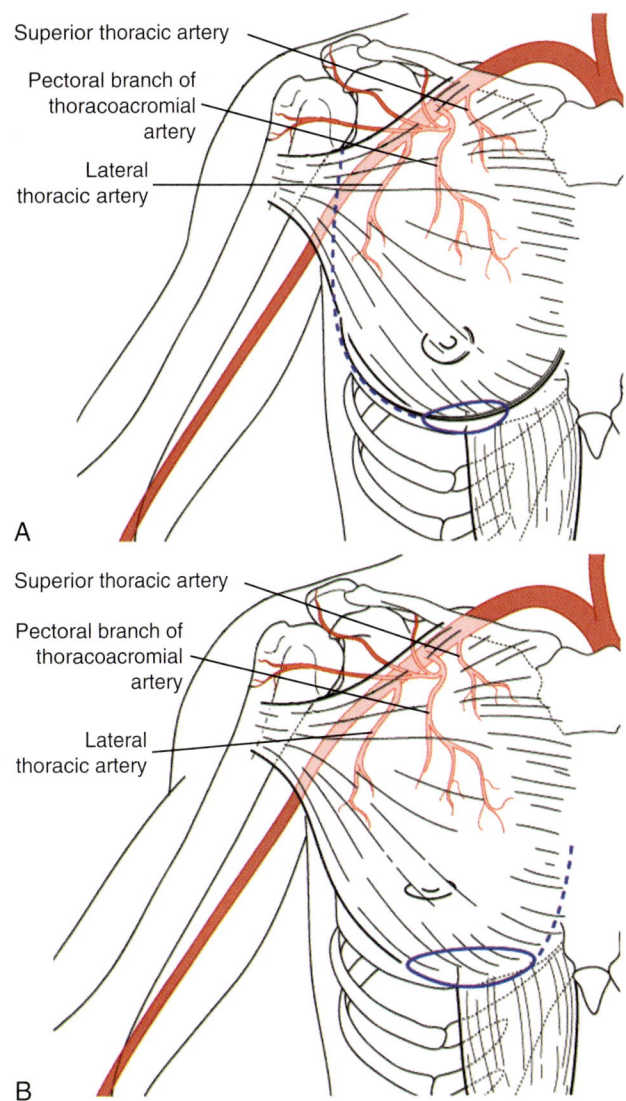

Fig. 68-5 ▪ A, Incision and skin paddle design with a lateral approach, best suited for female patients. B, Incision and skin paddle design with a medial approach. (Courtesy Jordan Mastrodonato, Fort Gordon, Ga.)

A general rule is that to avoid compression of the flap, the surgeon should be able to pass four fingers comfortably through the tunnel that will serve as passage for the flap. An additional incision (Fig. 68-7, C) made over the clavicle can be used to facilitate passage of the flap into the defect. If the surgeon attempts to "squeeze" the flap and skin paddle into a tunnel that is too small or is too rough with the skin paddle during placement, there is a high likelihood that the delicate myocutaneous perforators will be damaged and result in skin loss. It is also important to be sure that the flap pedicle is neither twisted nor kinked, which can lead to failure.

Once the flap is extended to the defect, vascular perfusion and patency of the vessels are assessed. This can be done by visualizing flap color and capillary refill by Doppler perfusion or pinprick testing. If none of these positive signs are present, the flap should be returned to its original position and be re-evaluated to ensure adequate blood flow to the skin paddle. Before closure, suction drains should be positioned so that they provide adequate drainage of the surgical site but do not overlie the flap pedicle. Once adequate

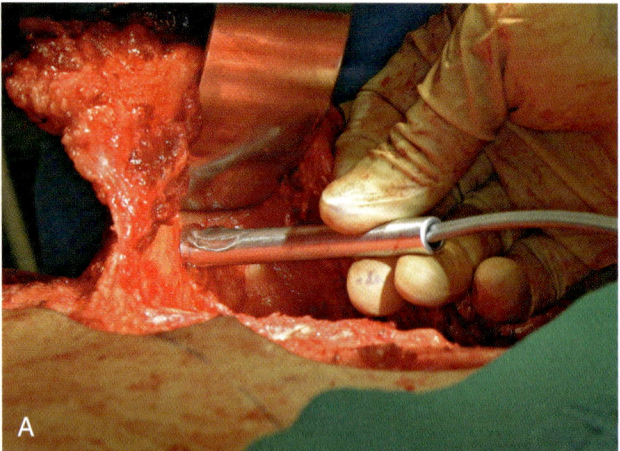

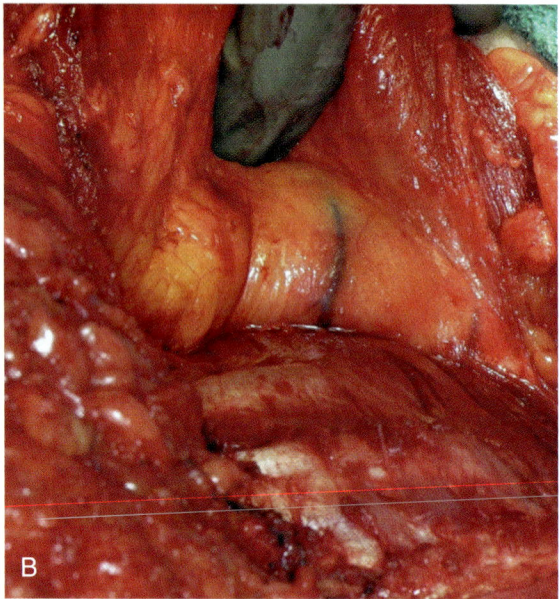

Fig. 68-6 ■ **A,** A Doppler probe is used to identify and verify patent arterial flow. **B,** The flap has been elevated off the chest wall. Note the nutrient vessel visible on the undersurface of the flap.

perfusion is ensured, the flap is sutured in place to reconstruct the defect (Fig. 68-7, *D*).

Attention is then turned to closure of the chest. Undermining of the surrounding tissue usually provides adequate mobility of the tissue for primary closure. Once again, closure is performed in a layered, tension-free fashion (Fig. 68-7, *E*). In the rare event that primary closure cannot be achieved, a split-thickness skin graft should be used.

POSTOPERATIVE CARE

Drains with suction are placed to avoid hematoma formation during the postoperative period and should be maintained until output is less than 30 mL in a 24-hour period. Antibiotic ointment is placed over the skin incisions and standard dressing is used. Pressure dressings on the neck should be avoided because they may compromise perfusion of the flap pedicle. It is recommended that a feeding tube be maintained for 7 to 10 days if the flap lines the oral cavity to allow adequate closure and protect the suture line.

Range-of-movement exercises may be initiated safely as early as 3 to 4 days after surgery.

COMPLICATIONS

To minimize complications, it is important to be able to identify preoperative risk factors that have been associated with poor outcomes. These preoperative risk factors, identified by Shah,[6] include age older than 70 years, female gender, obesity, uncontrolled systemic disease, oral cavity defects, poor nutritional status, and albumin concentration less than 4 g/dL. Unfortunately, many of the patients who require reconstruction have one or more of the aforementioned risk factors. Thus, it is up to the surgeon to weigh the risk for potential postoperative complications against the benefit of using this flap design for reconstruction.

Cordova and associates divided potential postoperative complications into those related to the recipient site and those related to the donor site.[12] Of those related to the recipient site, the most common included postoperative infection, hematoma, seroma, surgical site dehiscence, fistula formation, flap congestion, and flap necrosis.[20-22] Unfortunately, if blood flow to the flap is compromised, little can be done to salvage it. Hyperbaric oxygen therapy has been suggested but shown to be quite ineffective in this regard. Once blood flow to the flap is disrupted, necrosis ensues shortly thereafter. Salvage typically requires aggressive débridement of the necrotic tissue and the use of regional salvage flaps or microvascular free flaps. That being said, the overall rate of partial flap necrosis has been reported to be 14% (defined as greater than 50% loss of the skin paddle) and that of total flap necrosis reported to be 1%.[23] It has been noted in the literature that excessively small skin paddles may lack a sufficient number of myocutaneous perforators for survival; in these cases, consideration should be given to the use of a myofascial flap. The surgeon should judiciously use electrocautery when in close proximity to the skin paddle because there is a risk for retrograde thrombosis. Over time, the skin paddle eventually looks more mucosa-like in appearance (Fig. 68-8).

Complications are not limited to just the recipient site. Of those related to the donor site, Cordova and colleagues stated that the most important complications include bleeding, hematoma, wound dehiscence, seroma, and distortion of the breast in female patients.[12] Incision design is especially important in patients with a previous sternotomy. If an oblique incision is used, there is the potential for skin sloughing in the narrow isthmus of skin between incisions at the inferior aspect of the sternum. This donor site complication can be avoided by leaving a 1-cm cuff of PM muscle attached to the sternum or by incorporating the sternotomy incision into the flap design.

In patients in whom a reconstruction plate is used on the mandible for a continuity defect, there is often confusion on which side of the plate the PM flap should be placed. For defects in the body/ramus area, one should consider placing the flap pedicle medial to the reconstruction plate unless there is a high likelihood that the patient will undergo postoperative radiation therapy. In this instance, if the skin overlying the plate is thin, consideration may be given to placing the PM flap pedicle lateral to the plate to help reinforce the tissue and avoid future skin breakdown and plate exposure. However, the surgeon needs to be aware that the pedicle could be compressed between the reconstruction plate and the soft tissue and result in skin necrosis. For mandibular continuity defects in the symphysis area, the flap is best placed lateral to the plate. This allows the surgeon to reattach the suprahyoid muscles to the reconstruction plate, thereby preventing the tongue from prolapsing and obstructing the airway.

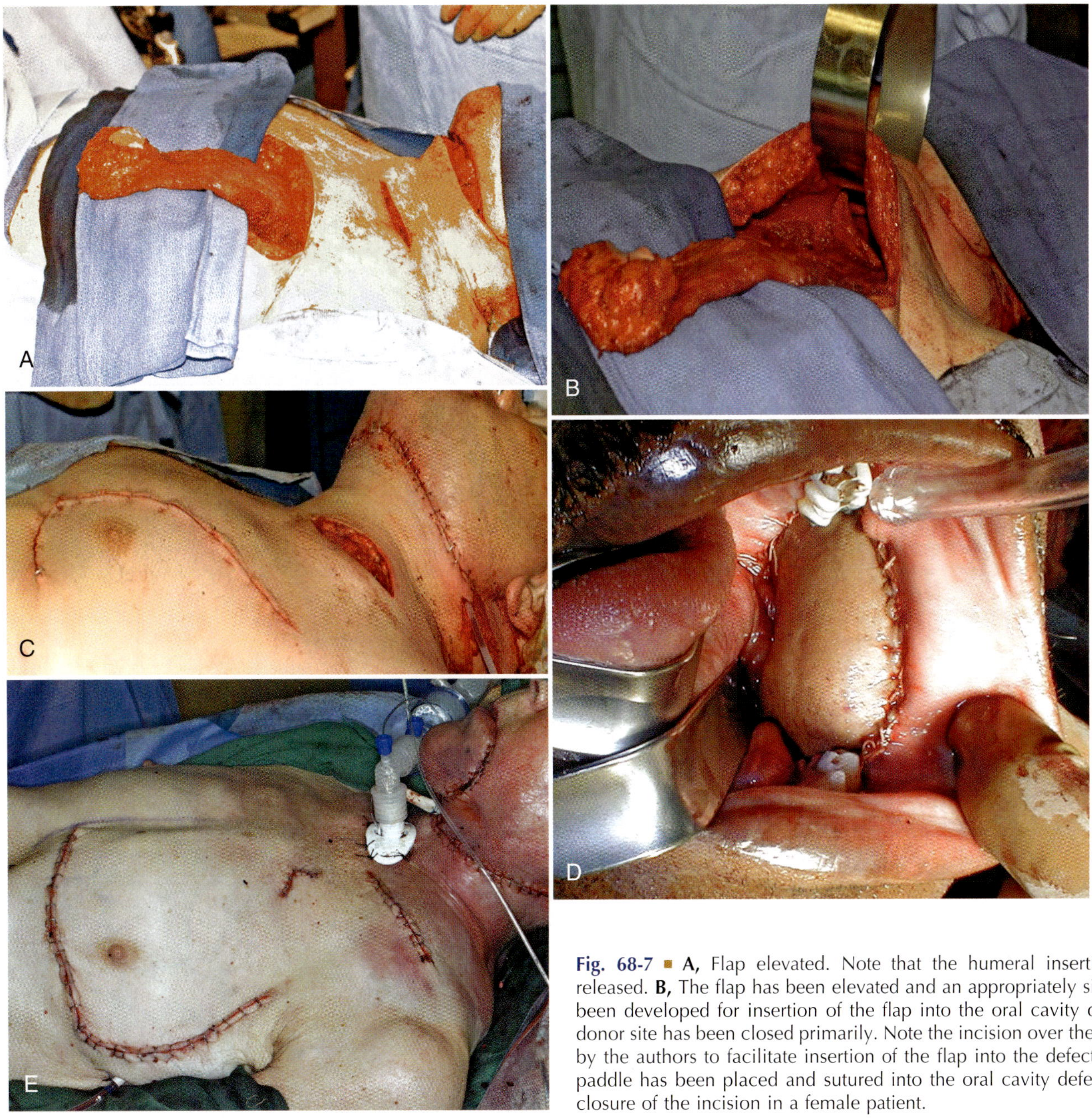

Fig. 68-7 ■ **A,** Flap elevated. Note that the humeral insertion has been released. **B,** The flap has been elevated and an appropriately size tunnel has been developed for insertion of the flap into the oral cavity defect. **C,** The donor site has been closed primarily. Note the incision over the clavicle used by the authors to facilitate insertion of the flap into the defect. **D,** The skin paddle has been placed and sutured into the oral cavity defect. **E,** Primary closure of the incision in a female patient.

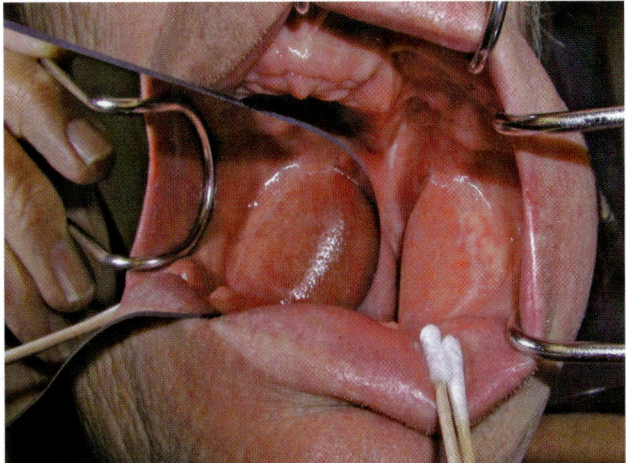

Fig. 68-8 ■ View of the flap 1 year postoperatively.

PEARLS AND PITFALLS

- The PM myocutaneous flap is a robust, versatile flap design that has been used effectively for decades in the reconstruction of oral and maxillofacial defects related to pathologic ablative surgery and trauma.
- Even with recent advances in microvascular surgery, free flap surgical procedures are more labor intensive and time consuming.
- With relatively few complications and high overall success rates, the PM flap continues to have a significant role in the reconstruction of head and neck defects.

REFERENCES

1. Ariyan S: The pectoralis major myocutaneous flap. A versatile flap for reconstruction in the head and neck, *Plast Reconstr Surg* 63:73-81, 1979.
2. Arlyan S, Cuono CB: Use of the pectoralis major myocutaneous flap for reconstruction of large cervical, facial or cranial defects, *Am J Surg* 140:503-506, 1980.
3. Phillips JG, Postlethwaite K, Peckitt N: The pectoralis major muscle flap without skin in intra-oral reconstruction, *Br J Oral Maxillofac Surg* 26:479-485, 1988.
4. Ord RA, Avery BS: Side-by-side double paddle pectoralis major flap for cheek defects, *Br J Oral Maxillofac Surg* 27:177-185, 1989.
5. Haers PE, Gratz KW, Sailer HF: The bilobed myocutaneous pectoralis major flap in closure of combined intra- and extraoral defects, *Int J Oral Maxillofac Surg* 23:214-218, 1994.
6. Carlson ER, Layne JM: The pectoralis major myocutaneous flap for reconstruction of soft-tissue oncologic defects, *Atlas Oral Maxillofac Surg Clin North Am* 5:15-35, 1997.
7. Moloy PJ: Reconstruction of intermediate sized mucosal defects with the pectoralis major myofascial flap, *J Otolaryngol* 18:32-35, 1989.
8. de Bree R, Reith R, Quak JJ, et al: Free radial forearm flap versus pectoralis major myocutaneous flap reconstruction of oral and oropharyngeal defects: a cost analysis, *Clin Otolaryngol* 32:275-282, 2007.
9. Jones NF, Sommerlad BC: Reconstruction of the zygoma, temporo-mandibular joint and mandible using a compound pectoralis major osteo-muscular flap, *Br J Plast Surg* 36:491-497, 1983.
10. Lam KH, Wei WI, Siu KF: The pectoralis major costomyocutaneous flap for mandibular reconstruction, *Plast Reconstr Surg* 73:904-910, 1984.
11. Savant D, Bhathena H, Kavarana N: The pectoralis major osteomyocutaneous flap in mandibular reconstruction, *Br J Plast Surg* 49:191, 1996.
12. Cordova SW, Bailey JS, Terezides AG: Pectoralis major myocutaneous flap reconstruction of the mandible, *Atlas Oral Maxillofac Surg Clin North Am* 14:171-178, 2006.
13. Milenovic A, Virag M, Uglesic V, et al: The pectoralis major flap in head and neck reconstruction: first 500 patients, *J Craniomaxillofac Surg* 34:340-343, 2006.
14. Brusati R, Collini M, Bozzetti A, et al: The pectoralis major myocutaneous flap. Experience in 100 consecutive cases, *J Craniomaxillofac Surg* 16:35-39, 1988.
15. Marx RE, Smith BR: An improved technique for development of the pectoralis major myocutaneous flap, *J Oral Maxillofac Surg* 48:1168-1180, 1990.
16. Merve A, Mitra I, Swindell R, et al: Shoulder morbidity after pectoralis major flap reconstruction for head and neck cancer, *Head Neck* 31:1470-1476, 2009.
17. Wadwongtham W, Isipradit P, Supanakorn S: The pectoralis major myocutaneous flap: applications and complications in head and neck reconstruction, *J Med Assoc Thai* 87(Suppl 2):S95-S99, 2004.
18. Varghese BT: Pectoralis major flap perfusion, *J Plast Reconstr Aesthet Surg* 63:e183, 2010.
19. Corten EM, Schellekens PP, Bleys RL, et al: The nerve supply to the clavicular part of the pectoralis major muscle: an anatomical study and clinical application of the function-preserving pectoralis major island flap, *Plast Reconstr Surg* 112:969-975, 2003.
20. Mehta S, Sarkar S, Karavana N, et al: Complications of the pectoralis major myocutaneous flap in the oral cavity: a prospective evaluation of 220 cases, *Plast Reconstr Surg* 98:31-37, 1996.
21. Cunha-Gomes D, Choudhari C, Kavarana NM: Vascular compromise of the pectoralis major musculocutaneous flap in head and neck reconstruction, *Ann Plast Surg* 51:450-454, 2003.
22. Ethunandan M, Ansell M, Mellor TK, et al: Skin necrosis of a pectoralis major myocutaneous flap, caused by methicillin-resistant *Staphylococcus aureus*, *Br J Oral Maxillofac Surg* 42:38-40, 2004.
23. Ferri T, Bacchi G, Baccui A, et al: The pectoralis major myocutaneous flap in head and neck reconstructive surgery: 16 years of experience, *Acta Biomed Ateneo Parmense* 70:13-17, 1999.

Chapter

69

Radial Forearm Free Flap

Brian M. Woo, D. David Kim

The radial forearm fasciocutaneous flap was first described by Yang and colleagues in the Chinese literature in 1981[1] and was coined the "Chinese flap." It later became popularized as the "workhorse" for head and neck reconstruction by Soutar and co-workers in the 1980s because of its reliability and flexibility in design.[2-4]

INDICATIONS

The thin and pliable skin of the volar aspect of the forearm, as well as its rich vascularity and long pedicle, has made it a nearly ideal donor site for reconstruction of defects in the head and neck and for oral defects. It has been reported in the literature for reconstruction of defects in the floor of the mouth, tongue, buccal mucosa, hard palate, soft palate, skull base, pharynx, larynx, lips, orbit, and skin.[2,3,5-17] It is most ideal for the reconstruction of oral defects requiring thin, mobile tissue, such as in the floor of the mouth, tongue, and soft palate. Based on the radial artery, venae comitantes, and cephalic vein, the flap can be designed to include bone (partial-thickness radius), tendon (palmaris longus), muscle (brachioradialis), and nerve, as well as the skin and fascia.[4,17-19] Nearly the entire skin of the forearm (from the flexor crease of the wrist to the antecubital fossa and nearly the entire circumference, except for a small strip on the ulnar aspect of the forearm) can be raised with the flap. The shape and overall dimensions can be tailored to the clinical situation. Bilobed, dual cutaneous paddle, fascia only, and folded and tubed flaps have been designed and successfully used for different reconstructive needs.[6,11,12,14,20,21]

ANATOMY

The hand and lower part of the arm receive their blood supply from the radial and ulnar branches of the brachial artery. The radial artery terminates in the deep palmar arch and the ulnar artery in the superficial palmar arch. Because harvesting of the radial forearm flap requires complete disruption of the radial artery, the hand and digits will be totally reliant on the ulnar artery for their blood supply. The blood supply to the third, fourth, and fifth digits is normally provided by the ulnar artery, so perfusion to the thumb and index finger is at greatest risk when harvesting this flap. For ischemia of the thumb or index finger to occur, two anatomic variations must be present. First, the superficial palmar arch must lack branches to the thumb and index finger. Second, the superficial and deep palmar arches must completely lack communicating branches. In a cadaver study, Coleman and Anson found that the superficial arch supplied all four fingers and the thumb in 77.3% of cases; however, a combination of the two arterial anomalies that would put the thumb and index finger at risk for ischemia was present in 12% of specimens.[22] An aberrant radial artery and aberrant courses of the radial artery have also been reported and may lead to inaccurate results on Allen test.[23-26] Anomalies of the ulnar artery have also been reported.[27] The skin of the forearm is supplied by septocutaneous and musculocutaneous perforators arising from the radial, ulnar, anterior, and posterior interosseous arteries.[28] The lateral intermuscular septum separates the brachioradialis and flexor carpi radialis muscles in the forearm. Within the lateral intermuscular septum runs the radial artery and its two venae comitantes, and it gives off most of the fascial branches to the skin of the forearm. The radial artery also sends branches to the muscles of the flexor compartment, the palmaris longus tendon, and the radial nerve. Because the lateral intermuscular septum is attached to the distal end of the radius, it also supplies branches to the periosteum, thus giving the option of harvesting a segment of vascularized bone.[29] The length of the arterial pedicle is limited by the recurrent radial artery, the first major branch of the radial artery after it arises from the brachial artery. Venous drainage for the radial forearm flap is via the deeper paired venae comitantes that run with the radial artery in the intermuscular septum and from larger superficial veins, such as the cephalic vein. The veins that accompany the fascial branches of the radial artery to the skin of the forearm drain via the paired venae comitantes. There are multiple communications between the venae comitantes and the superficial veins of the forearm, thus allowing either of these venous systems to be used for the venous anastomosis. Unlike the arterial pedicle, the cephalic vein may be harvested along its entire course to its junction with the subclavian vein. Cutaneous innervation of the forearm is derived from the medial, lateral, and posterior antebrachial cutaneous nerves. The lateral antebrachial cutaneous nerve is the main sensory nerve to the harvested forearm skin and travels with the cephalic vein in the upper part of the forearm. The radial nerve is a mixed motor and sensory nerve. It provides motor innervation for the majority of the muscles of the extensor compartment, as well as the abductor pollicis longus and brevis. It provides sensory innervation for portions of the upper part of the arm and the dorsum of the forearm via the posterior antebrachial cutaneous nerve. The superficial branch of the radial nerve encountered in the wrist during flap harvest provides sensation to the dorsum of the hand, the thumb, and the index and middle fingers.

WORK-UP/DIAGNOSTIC TESTS AND IMAGING

As with any presurgical evaluation, a thorough history and physical examination should be performed, including elicitation of the presence of any co-morbid disease states. If applicable, a head and neck cancer work-up should include a complete blood count; comprehensive metabolic panel, including liver function tests; prothrombin time, partial thromboplastin time, and international normalized ratio; and chest radiograph, applicable computed tomography scans, stereolithographic models, and a Panorex radiograph. Along with preoperative imaging, the physical examination should evaluate for the estimated size of the defect, the location of the lesion, and the tissues to be resected (skin, mucosa, muscle, bone, etc.) to aid in flap selection. Hypercoagulable states are the only true contraindications to microvascular free tissue transfer.[30] This includes diseases such as polycythemia, thrombocytosis, and possibly sickle cell anemia (Box 69-1). Patients taking antiestrogen medications and hormone therapy such as tamoxifen for breast cancer should have the use of these drugs discontinued before surgery because of their known thrombogenic activity.[31] For similar reasons, as well as decreased flap perfusion and impaired wound healing, smokers should be encouraged to stop smoking at least 1 week before surgery. The history and physical examination should also evaluate the patient for prior trauma to the forearm and previous indwelling

BOX 69-1	Hypercoagulable States

Inherited
- Antithrombin III deficiency
- Protein C deficiency
- Protein S deficiency
- Activated protein C resistance
- Factor V Leiden
- Dysfibrinogenemia
- Plasminogen activator deficiency
- Plasminogen deficiency
- Factor XII deficiency
- Polycythemia
- Thrombocytosis
- Sickle cell anemia
- Heparin cofactor II deficiency

Acquired
- Prolonged immobilization
- Pregnancy
- Surgery/trauma
- Oral contraceptives/antiestrogens
- Homocystinuria
- Vitamin K deficiency
- Disseminated intravascular coagulation
- Smoking
- Nephrotic syndrome
- L-Asparaginase
- Diabetes mellitus
- Hyperlipidemia
- Malignancy
- Lupus anticoagulant
- Anticardiolipin antibody

radial artery catheters. The Allen test is the most important preoperative evaluation to determine the adequacy of circulation to the hand via the ulnar artery. The Allen test is performed by simultaneously occluding the radial and ulnar arteries while the hand is alternately opened and closed, thus causing the hand to become pale from mechanical exsanguination. The hand is then opened to a relaxed position before ceasing compression of the ulnar artery. The fingers should not be held in a hyperextended position because this can cause them to remain pale and yield a false-positive result. Release of the ulnar artery should result in a blush or reperfusion of the hand within 15 to 20 seconds. Special attention should be paid to the thumb and index finger. With a result beyond 15 to 20 seconds, a radial forearm flap should not be performed. In dark-skinned individuals in whom it is difficult to visualize the blush or reperfusion, it is often helpful to evaluate the nail bed instead by compressing and releasing the fingernail. Sometimes it is also helpful to apply a pulse oximeter to the thumb to assess waveform changes and alterations in oxygen saturation when the radial and ulnar arteries are occluded and when the ulnar artery is released. An accurate Allen test result is necessary for avoiding potential ischemic complications after flap harvest. If the result of the Allen test is equivocal or difficult to interpret, radial artery mapping can objectively determine the pattern of flow and reversal of flow following occlusion of the radial artery.

TREATMENT AND RECONSTRUCTIVE GOALS

The treatment and reconstructive goals of the radial forearm flap include provision of soft tissue closure and replacement of resected oral cavity soft tissue, along with restoration of adequate function (e.g., speech, mastication, oral continence) and cosmesis to enable the patient to enjoy a reasonable quality of life. Foremost of the advantages of microvascular free tissue transfer is the ability to tailor the donor flap to the specific needs of the ablative site. As mentioned previously, the thin pliable skin of the radial forearm fasciocutaneous flap makes it ideal for the reconstruction of partial defects of the tongue, floor of the mouth, and soft palate. Flap design and orientation should be thoroughly thought out and performed with care because the three-dimensional nature of oral cavity reconstruction can be complex. For example, soft palate reconstruction with the radial forearm flap may require that the skin paddle be folded for adequate reconstruction, thus making positioning and orientation of the vascular pedicle of paramount importance.

TECHNIQUE (Fig. 69-1)

Once the design of the skin paddle is confirmed and marked out, the arm is exsanguinated with an Esmarch bandage and a tourniquet inflated to 250 mm Hg. Flap elevation is begun at the distal-most aspect of the skin paddle. An incision through skin, subcutaneous fat, and fascia allows identification of the distal radial artery and cephalic vein, which are ligated and transected. The superficial branches of the radial nerve will also be encountered at this time and may be preserved or sacrificed depending on the surgeon's preference. The longitudinal borders of the skin paddle can now be incised through skin and subcutaneous tissue down through the fascia of the brachioradialis muscle radially and the flexor muscles on the ulnar side. This dissection continues in the subfascial plane to the lateral intermuscular septum between the brachioradialis and flexor carpi radialis. Care must be taken to leave a thin film

of paratenon on the tendons of the wrist flexors or wound complications as a result of skin graft failure will be a problem. At this point the proximal portion of the skin paddle can be incised. Care must be taken to avoid injury to the cephalic vein as it emerges from the flap in the subcutaneous fat. A linear incision is then made from the proximal portion of the skin paddle to the antecubital fossa to facilitate dissection of the vascular pedicle from between the brachioradialis and flexor carpi radialis. This incision is then undermined in the subcutaneous plane laterally and medially. Completion of dissection of the cephalic vein can be performed at this stage to the appropriate length and in a circumferential fashion. Finally, the flap can be elevated in a distal to proximal direction to carefully dissect the radial artery and its venae comitantes. Vascular clips will be necessary to control the numerous branches to the surrounding musculature and radial bone. The fascia of the brachioradialis will need to be incised along its length to facilitate proximal dissection of the radial artery. The proximal extent of this dissection is limited by the radial recurrent artery near the antecubital fossa. Once the dissection is complete, the tourniquet is deflated and the flap reperfused for a period of at least 20 minutes. During this time, hemostasis can be achieved with cautery and hemoclips, and final preparation of the recipient site can be performed. After the flap has been allowed to reperfuse, the flap can be harvested by using hemoclips at the desired pedicle length. A suction drain is placed, and the wound is closed in layers with absorbable suture in the deep tissue to reapproximate the divided fascia, as well as in the subdermal layer. Primary closure of the proximal linear incision is easily achieved and may also be possible for the area of the skin paddle. However, the skin paddle area usually requires coverage with a skin graft to avoid excessive tension. Either a split- or full-thickness skin graft may be used and inset with resorbable suture. The graft should be perforated to allow seepage of fluid during healing. This graft should be compressed to the recipient bed with petrolatum gauze, gauze, and cast padding and supported by a plaster splint fabricated to the volar aspect of the lower part of the arm and hand while keeping the wrist, hand, and fingers moderately extended. The splint should be left in place for 7 days to prevent sheer forces on the skin graft. Before placing the final dressing with an elastic wrap, perfusion to the index finger and thumb should be verified by checking capillary refill. The flap should be inset and the microvascular anastomosis carried out promptly to minimize ischemia time. The radial artery is usually a good size match to many recipient arteries in the head and neck, including the facial, superior thyroid, and transverse cervical arteries. The cephalic vein also has excellent caliber and can be matched to the external jugular or facial veins. Thus, this flap has been described as a "macro-microvascular flap." The decision to use both the cephalic vein and the venae comitantes should be made on a case-by-case basis. Although the flap is well known to survive with drainage from either the superficial or deep venous systems, many surgeons perform more than one venous anastomosis when adequate recipient veins are present. The superficial veins are usually chosen over the venae comitantes when only one venous anastomosis is to be performed because of their larger caliber and thicker vessel walls.

POSTOPERATIVE CARE/MONITORING/ COMPLICATIONS

Protocols for postoperative management of patients undergoing microvascular free tissue transfer vary by institution and are based on surgeon preference, personal experience, and possibly

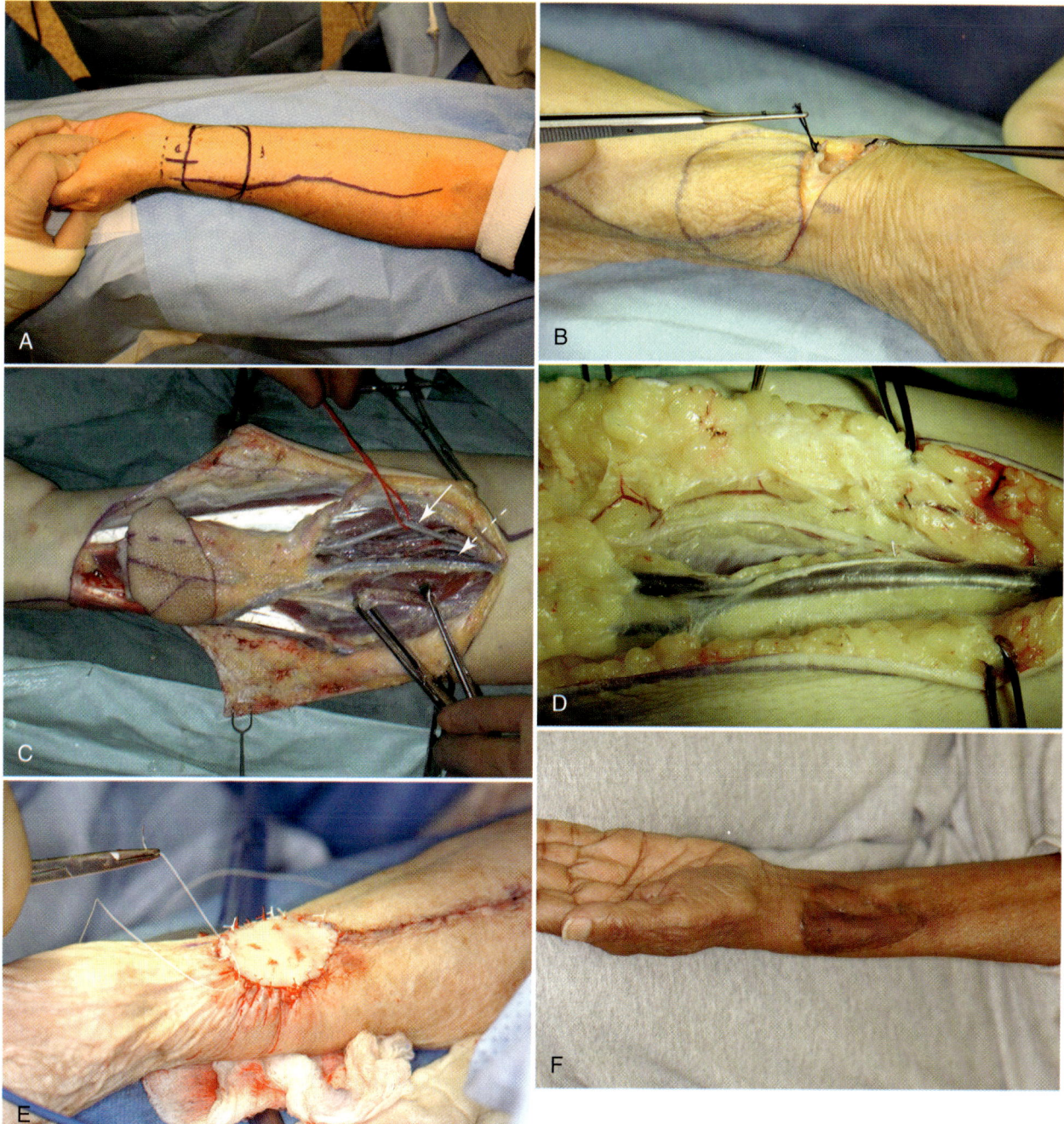

Fig. 69-1 ■ **A,** The design of the skin paddle is marked while trying to center the radial vessels in the skin paddle. The radial artery is drawn out at the distal aspect of the skin paddle between the tendons of the brachioradialis and flexor carpi radialis muscles. The course of the cephalic vein is also drawn out. Note the flexor crease marked by the dashed line. When designing the skin paddle it is helpful to make the distal incision of the skin paddle further up the forearm a centimeter or more proximal to the flexor crease to avoid the palmar carpal ligament (volar carpal ligament) and the flexor retinaculum during the dissection; however, this will slightly shorten the length of the pedicle. **B,** Ligation of the radial artery and its two accompanying venae comitantes. **C,** Completed dissection showing the radial artery in the vessel loop (*solid arrow*) and the cephalic vein (*broken arrow*). Note the two Allis clamps retracting the brachioradialis muscle. **D,** Exposure of the cephalic vein in the proximal part of the forearm. Note the lateral antebrachial cutaneous nerve traveling with the cephalic vein. **E,** Full-thickness skin graft being sutured in place to reconstruct the skin paddle defect. **F,** Healed skin graft.

superstition. Scientific evidence of the efficacy of postoperative management is lacking. At the authors' institution the patient is initially admitted to the intensive care unit for the first 48 to 72 hours for monitoring of the flap. Pressure on the microvascular pedicle should be avoided at all times. Therefore, circumferential ties or straps around the neck such as tracheostomy ties and straps for oxygen tents should be avoided because they can easily compress the vascular pedicle. Kinking and undue tension on the vessels should also be avoided. The position of the neck that optimizes vessel geometry should be strictly maintained during the immediate postoperative period. This can be achieved by using postoperative sedation with ventilatory support. A paralytic agent can also be added if needed. Typically, patients are kept sedated with a fentanyl and midazolam drip overnight and weaned within the first 24 hours if they are cooperative and understand the importance of maintaining their neck in a neutral position or the position that optimizes vessel geometry. Postoperatively, patients are given intravenous fluids at the regular maintenance rate for their weight in kilograms and boluses administered as indicated. Hemodynamics should be maintained as close to normal limits as possible. Avoidance of extreme hypertension or hypotension is crucial to prevent hematoma formation while maintaining perfusion of the flap. A balance between the oxygen-carrying capacity of blood and blood viscosity must also be achieved. Although little scientific evidence exists, a hematocrit of 28% to 30% is generally accepted as the desired goal for the immediate postoperative period, and consideration should be given to transfusion of packed red blood cells to maintain this hematocrit level, especially if the patient has a history of cardiovascular disease.[32,33] Many modalities for monitoring flaps have been described, but clinical examination of the flap's skin paddle remains the "gold standard." The parameters evaluated include color, capillary refill, flap turgor, and warmth. The frequency of serial postoperative flap evaluations also varies by institution, from every hour to once every 4 hours. Typically, the flap should be evaluated every 2 hours postoperatively. The frequency is based on the fact that the time between the onset of a thrombotic event and its recognition may be critical to salvage of the flap.[34] In pig skin flaps, this critical time is 7 hours.[35] After 8 to 12 hours it may not be possible to re-establish the flap's circulation.[36] A helpful adjunct to the clinical examination is the pinprick test. After puncturing the center of the skin paddle with a 25-gauge needle, the rapidity, color, and amount of blood return are evaluated. A healthy flap will bleed bright red blood within 1 to 3 seconds. Rapid return of dark-colored blood combined with an ecchymotic skin paddle suggests venous insufficiency. No blood return with a flap cool to touch suggests arterial thrombosis. The next most commonly used modality in postoperative flap monitoring is the Doppler probe, handheld or implantable. The practical utilization of the Doppler probe is mainly for confirmation of arterial flow, but its ability to monitor venous outflow has been proposed.[37,38] Observance of a change in the character of the "phases" of the Doppler signal may help the clinician identify impending failure of a flap. However, because thrombotic complications are usually venous in nature, the utility of this modality is severely limited. The Cook-Swartz implantable Doppler probe was originally designed to monitor venous outflow, but a high number of false-positive results culminating in unnecessary flap exploration have been reported.[38] Usefulness of the Cook-Swartz implantable Doppler probe for monitoring arterial flow has been shown, especially for buried flaps. However, when it is used to monitor arterial flow, it has been shown to be unable to detect venous thrombosis.[38] It should also be kept in mind that Doppler signals obtained near the anastomotic site may be unreliable because of the proximity of the carotid arteries. Other adjunctive modalities that have been

described include tissue PO_2 monitoring, tissue pH, pulse oximetry, photoplethysmography, and laser Doppler flowmeters.[39-44] Each of these modalities have their own advantages and disadvantages, but none have made their way into mainstream microsurgical monitoring. Most recently, laser-assisted indocyanine green fluorescent dye angiography (the SPY system) has been used intraoperatively to evaluate free tissue transfers because it allows visualization of the microsurgical anastomoses and confirmation of arterial inflow, venous outflow, and flap perfusion throughout the flap tissues. The SPY system also shows promise for identification of perforators before committing to flap design, for evaluation of perfusion once the flap is raised, for preoperative evaluation of vascular anatomy, and for postoperative flap monitoring.[39] Like flap monitoring, institutions vary on which pharmacologic agent they use for the prevention of thrombosis in patients undergoing microvascular surgery; selection usually reflects individual practitioner experience or retrospective case studies. Postoperatively, it is the authors' practice to administer aspirin, 325 mg orally, via nasogastric tube or rectally. Aspirin acetylates cyclooxygenase and inhibits the production of arachidonic acid metabolites, including thromboxane and prostacyclin. Thromboxane A_2 is a potent vasoconstrictor and platelet-activating agent produced by platelet cyclooxygenase. Prostacyclin, in contrast, is derived from endothelial cyclooxygenase and is a potent vasodilator and inhibitor of platelet aggregation.[45] Low doses of aspirin (1 to 5 mg/kg) are theorized to preferentially inhibit thromboxane but not prostacyclin production.[46] In an animal model, low-dose aspirin inhibited venous thrombosis and improved microcirculatory perfusion.[47] Rare side effects include bleeding, gastritis, and renal failure and should be considered when administering aspirin to elderly patients. The other main pharmacologic agents used for prevention of thrombosis in microvascular surgery are heparin and dextran. The heparin family of molecules acts by binding to and inducing a conformational change in antithrombin III in which antithrombin III is changed from a slow inhibitor of coagulation to a more rapid one. It is the inhibition of thrombin (factor IIa) and other factors in the coagulation cascade (XIIa, XIa, IXa, and Xa) that results in the anticoagulant effect seen with heparin.[48] Arterial thrombi usually form in areas of high or disrupted flow or in sites of atherosclerotic plaque rupture and consist mainly of platelet aggregates bound together by thin fibrin strands, thus being dependent on the action of platelets and the coagulation cascade. Venous thrombi, however, may be more reliant on the coagulation cascade because they form in areas of blood stasis and consist mostly of red blood cells and fibrin rather than platelets.[45] Consequently, it has been suggested that heparin may be more effective than antiplatelet agents such as aspirin in preventing arterial and venous thrombi.[46,49] In a study involving rats, inhibition of the platelet aggregation pathway did not improve vessel patency because fibrin alone can form a thrombus without platelet aggregation. A therapeutic level of heparin in the rats was more effective in preventing arterial and venous thrombi than antiplatelet agents were.[49] Despite these findings, the systemic use of heparin immediately postoperatively in patients undergoing microvascular surgery is generally limited to a few institutions or is reserved for salvaging a threatened flap. This is probably due to fear of hemorrhagic complications such as hematoma formation or donor site bleeding. Dextran is a polysaccharide synthesized from sucrose by *Leuconostoc mesenteroides* that is generally used in its low-molecular-weight form (40,000 daltons—dextran 40). Its mechanism of action is not completely understood, but proposed actions include (1) increasing the electronegativity of platelets and endothelium, which results in decreased platelet aggregation; (2) increasing fibrin degradation by modifying its structure; (3) inhibition of alpha-2 antiplasmin with subsequent plasminogen activation; (4) decreasing amounts of factor VIII and von Willebrand factor; and (5) altering the rheologic properties of blood by acting as a volume expander.[45] Dextran has potential antigenicity, and cases of anaphylaxis and cardiac arrest have been reported.[50-54] It is recommended that a test dose of 20 mL be given before continuous infusion; however, despite a test dose with hapten (dextran 1), serious reactions may still occur.[50,52] The infusion is generally administered at a rate of 25 to 50 mL/h for 5 days postoperatively, and it can be initiated immediately preoperatively, just before release of the microvascular clamps, or immediately postoperatively. It is discontinued after 5 days without tapering.[55] Dextran has been associated with noncardiogenic pulmonary edema and acute respiratory distress syndrome. Other systemic complications that have been associated with the use of dextran include myocardial infarction, congestive heart failure, pulmonary edema, pleural effusion, pneumonia, acute hypotension, hypoxia, coagulopathy, and anemia.[56] Despite the high reported success rates of microvascular free tissue transfer, numerous perioperative complications have been reported[57-70] (Box 69-2; Fig. 69-2).

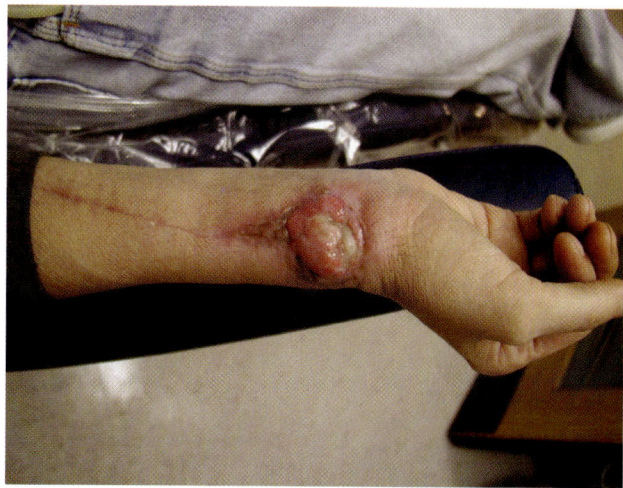

Fig. 69-2 ■ Postoperative complication from skin graft failure and formation of excessive granulation tissue.

BOX 69-2   Complications Associated with the Radial Forearm Free Flap

Perioperative surgical/reconstructive complications of the radial forearm free flap that have been described in the literature include
- Venous thrombosis/arterial thrombosis
- Venous congestion
- Wound infection
- Salivary fistula
- Seroma
- Cervical hematoma
- Partial free flap necrosis
- Total free flap necrosis
- Hardware extrusion
- Carotid artery rupture
- Donor site complications (infection, skin graft failure, radius fracture if bone is harvested, abnormal sensation, decreased grip strength, ischemic hand)

Perioperative medical complications in patients being treated with a radial forearm free flap that have been described in the literature include
- Myocardial infarction
- Cerebrovascular accident
- Deep vein thrombosis
- Congestive heart failure/pulmonary edema
- Pneumonia/atelectasis
- Acute respiratory distress syndrome
- Pneumothorax
- Arrhythmia
- Gastrointestinal hemorrhage/perforation
- Liver failure
- Change in mental status
- Mortality

PEARLS AND PITFALLS

- For defects requiring small skin paddles, it has been found that the distal cephalic vein will often be located outside the authors' designed skin paddle, so it is important to make sure that the distal cephalic vein is incorporated with a cuff of fascia beyond the vein when dissecting the flap in a subfascial plane to the lateral intermuscular septum. To facilitate this dissection it is helpful to make the linear incision from the proximal portion of the skin paddle to the antecubital fossa early and raise the skin and subcutaneous tissue flaps laterally and medially for exposure of the superficial venous system and the course of the cephalic vein from the proximal portion of the skin paddle to the antecubital fossa. By exposing the superficial veins early, the surgeon can also inspect the cephalic vein for any areas of stenosis along its course caused by previous venipunctures and indwelling venous catheters. If there is an area of stenosis along the course of the cephalic vein, it may be possible for the surgeon to incorporate other superficial veins in the flap harvest that drain into the cephalic vein proximal to the area of stenosis. If this is not possible, the forearm flap may be harvested based solely on the venae comitantes for its venous drainage.
- Sometimes it is also beneficial to include a cuff of fascia and subcutaneous tissue around the vascular pedicle when harvesting to provide additional padding for the pedicle as it passes through the tunnel created from the maxilla or mandible into the neck.
- When designing the skin paddle it is also helpful to make the distal incision of the skin paddle further up the forearm a centimeter or more proximal to the flexor crease to avoid the palmar carpal ligament (volar carpal ligament) and the flexor retinaculum during the dissection; however, this will slightly shorten the length of the pedicle.
- Instead of using a split-thickness skin graft for covering the skin paddle defect, the authors have found at their institution that a full-thickness skin graft harvested from the inner aspect of the upper part of the arm results in less secondary contracture and better cosmesis. This technique also results in a well-hidden scar in this location. No problems have been encountered with skin graft take as long as enough paratenon is preserved.
- One thing to avoid is placing excessive tension on the skin of the skin paddle during harvesting, which could result in separation of the skin from its underlying fascia.
- When raising the skin paddle it is also important to make sure that one dissects in a plane deep to the radial artery and the venae comitantes because it is easy to become disoriented and raise the skin paddle without incorporating the radial artery and the venae comitantes.

REFERENCES

1. Yang G, Chen B, Gao Y, et al: Forearm free skin flap transplantation, *Natl Med J China* 61:139-142, 1981.
2. Soutar DS, McGregor IA: The radial forearm flap in intraoral reconstruction: the experience of 60 consecutive cases, *Plast Reconstr Surg* 78:1-8, 1986.
3. Soutar DS, Scheker LR, Tanner NSB, et al: The radial forearm flap: a versatile method for intraoral reconstruction, *Br J Plast Surg* 36:1-8, 1983.
4. Soutar DS, Widdowson WP: Immediate reconstruction of the mandible using a vascularized segment of radius, *Head Neck* 8:232-246, 1986.
5. Baird W, Wornmom I, Culbertson J: Forehead reconstruction with a modified radial forearm flap: a case report, *J Reconstr Microsurg* 4:363-367, 1988.
6. Boorman JG, Green MF: A split Chinese forearm flap for simultaneous oral lining and skin cover, *Br J Plast Surg* 39:179-182, 1986.
7. Chantrain G, Deraemaecker R, Andry G, et al: Wide vertical hemipharyngolaryngectomy with immediate glottic and pharyngeal reconstruction using a radial forearm free flap: preliminary results, *Laryngoscope* 101:869-875, 1991.
8. Chircarelli Z, Ariyan S, Cuono C: Free radial forearm flap versatility for the head and neck and lower extremity, *J Reconstr Microsurg* 2:221-228, 1986.
9. Chircarelli Z, Ariyan S, Cuono C: Single stage repair of complex scalp and cranial defects with the free radial forearm flap, *Plast Reconstr Surg* 77:577-585, 1986.
10. Hagen R: Laryngoplasty with a radialis pedicle flap from the forearm: a surgical procedure for voice rehabilitation after total laryngectomy, *Am J Otolaryngol* 11:85-89, 1990.
11. Harii K, Ebihara S, Ono I, et al: Pharyngoesophageal reconstruction using a fabricated forearm free flap, *Plast Reconstr Surg* 75:463-476, 1985.
12. Hatoko M, Harashina T, Inoue T, et al: Reconstruction of palate with radial forearm flap: a report of 3 cases, *Br J Plast Surg* 43:350-354, 1990.
13. Kawashima T, Harii K, Ono I, et al: Intraoral and oropharyngeal reconstruction using a deepithelialized forearm flap, *Head Neck* 11:358-363, 1989.
14. Martin IC, Brown AE: Free vascularized fascial flap in oral cavity reconstruction, *Head Neck* 16:45-50, 1994.
15. Sadove R, Luce E, McGrath P: Reconstruction of the lower lip and chin with the composite radial forearm–palmaris longus free flap, *Plast Reconstr Surg* 88:209-214, 1991.
16. Tahara S, Susuki T: Eye socket reconstruction with free radial forearm flap, *Ann Plast Surg* 23:112-116, 1989.
17. Takada K, Sugata T, Yoshiga K, et al: Total upper lip reconstruction using a free radial forearm flap incorporating the brachioradialis muscle: report of a case, *J Oral Maxillofac Surg* 45:959-962, 1987.
18. Reid CD, Moss ALH: One stage repair with vascularized tendon grafts in a dorsal hand injury using the "Chinese" forearm flap, *Br J Plast Surg* 36:473-479, 1983.
19. Taylor GI, Ham FJ: The free vascularized nerve graft. A further experimental and clinical application of microvascular techniques, *Plast Reconstr Surg* 57:413-426, 1976.
20. Urken ML, Biller HF: A new bilobed design for the sensate radial forearm flap to preserve tongue mobility following significant glossectomy, *Arch Otolaryngol Head Neck Surg* 120:26-31, 1994.
21. Bhathena HM, Kavarana NM: Bipaddled retrograde radial extended forearm flap with microarterial anastomoses for reconstruction in oral cancer, *Br J Plast Surg* 41:354-357, 1988.
22. Coleman T, Anson B: Arterial patterns in the hand based upon a study of 650 specimens, *Surg Gynecol Obstet* 113:409-424, 1961.
23. Hedén P, Gylbert L: Anomaly of the radial artery encountered during elevation of the radial forearm flap, *J Microsurg* 6:139-141, 1990.
24. Loetzke HH, Kleinau W: [Simultaneous occurrence of the Aa. brachialis superficialis, radialis and antebrachialis dorsalis superficialis, as well as their branches,] *Anat Anz* 122:137-141, 1968.
25. Otsuka T, Terauchi M: An anomaly of the radial artery—relevance for the forearm flap, *Br J Plast Surg* 44:390-391, 1991.
26. Small J, Miller R: The radial artery forearm flap: an anomaly of the radial artery, *Br J Plast Surg* 38:501-503, 1985.
27. Fatah M, Nancarrow J, Murray D: Raising the radial artery forearm flap: the superficial ulnar artery "trap," *Br J Plast Surg* 38:394-395, 1985.
28. Lamberty BGH, Cormack GC: The forearm angiosomes, *Br J Plast Surg* 35:420-429, 1982.
29. Cormack G, Duncan MJ, Lamberty B: The blood supply of the bone component of the compound osteocutaneous radial artery forearm flap: an anatomical study, *Br J Plast Surg* 39:173-175, 1986.
30. Ayala C, Blackwell KE: Protein C deficiency in microvascular head and neck reconstruction, *Laryngoscope* 109:259-265, 1999.
31. Peverill RE: Hormone therapy and venous thromboembolism, *Best Pract Res Clin Endocrinol Metab* 17:149-164, 2003.
32. Carson J, Duff A, Poses R, et al: Effect of anaemia and cardiovascular disease on surgical mortality and morbidity, *Lancet* 348:1055-1060, 1996.
33. Djamali A, Becker Y, Simmons W, et al: Increasing hematocrit reduces early posttransplant cardiovascular risk in diabetic transplant recipients, *Transplantation* 76:816-820, 2003.
34. Hidalgo DA, Jones CS: The role of emergent exploration in free tissue transfer: a review of 150 consecutive cases, *Plast Reconstr Surg* 86:592-601, 1990.
35. Kerrigan CL, Zelt RG, Daniel RK: Secondary critical ischemia time of experimental skin flaps, *Plast Reconstr Surg* 74:522-526, 1984.
36. May JW Jr, Chait LA, O'Brien BM, et al: The no-reflow phenomenon in experimental free flaps, *Plast Reconstr Surg* 61:256-267, 1978.
37. Jones NF: Intraoperative and postoperative monitoring of microsurgical free tissue transfers, *Clin Plast Surg* 19:783-797, 1992.
38. Guillemaud J, Seikaly H, Cote D, et al: The implantable Cook-Swartz Doppler probe for postoperative monitoring in head and neck free flap reconstruction, *Arch Otolaryngol Head Neck Surg* 134:729-734, 2008.
39. Achauer BM, Black KS: Transcutaneous oxygen and flaps, *Plast Reconstr Surg* 74:721-722, 1984.
40. Dunn RM, Kaplan IB, Moncoll J, et al: Experimental and clinical use of pH monitoring of free tissue transfers, *Ann Plast Surg* 31:539-545, 1993.
41. Menick FJ: The pulse oximetry in free muscle flap surgery. "A microvascular surgeon's sleep aid," *J Reconstr Microsurg* 4:331-334, 1998.
42. Harrison DH, Firling M, Mott G: Experience in monitoring the circulation in free flap transfers, *Plast Reconstr Surg* 68:543-555, 1981.
43. Goldberg J, Sepka RS, Perona BP, et al: Laser Doppler blood flow measurements of common cutaneous donor sites for reconstructive surgery, *Plast Reconstr Surg* 85:581-586, 1990.
44. Yuen JC, Feng Z: Monitoring free flaps using laser Doppler flowmeter: 5 year experience, *Plast Reconstr Surg* 105:55-61, 2000.
45. Conrad MH, Adams WP: Pharmacologic optimization of microsurgery in the new millennium, *Plast Reconstr Surg* 108:2008-2096, quiz 2097, 2001.
46. Peter FW, Steinau HU, Homann HH, et al: Aspirin and microvascular surgery: an update, *Plast Reconstr Surg* 112:1368-1370, 2003.
47. Peter FW, Franken RJPM, Wang WZ, et al: Effect of low dose aspirin on thrombus formation at arterial and venous microanastomoses and on the tissue microcirculation, *Plast Reconstr Surg* 99:1112-1121, 1997.
48. Rosenberg RD: Actions and interactions of antithrombin and heparin, *N Engl J Med* 292:146-151, 1975.
49. Khouri RK, Cooley BC, Kenna DM, et al: Thrombosis of microvascular anastomoses in traumatized vessels: fibrin versus platelets, *Plast Reconstr Surg* 86:110-117, 1990.
50. Renck H, Ljungström KG, Rosenberg B, et al: Prevention of dextran-induced anaphylactic reactions by hapten inhibition: II. A comparison of the effects of 20 ml Dextran 1, 15% administered either admixed or before dextran 70 or dextran 40, *Acta Chir Scand* 149:349-353, 1983.
51. Michelson E: Anaphylactic reaction to dextrans, *N Engl J Med* 278:552, 1968.
52. Berg E, Fasting S, Sellevold O: Serious complications with dextran 70 despite hapten prophylaxis: is it best avoided prior to delivery? *Anaesthesia* 46:1033-1035, 1991.
53. Krenzelok E, Parker W: Dextran 40 anaphylaxis, *Anesth Analg* 54:736-738, 1975.

54. Maddi V, Wyso E, Zinner E: Dextran anaphylaxis, *Angiology* 20:243-248, 1969.

55. Johnson P, Barker J: Thrombosis and antithrombotic therapy in microvascular surgery, *Clin Plast Surg* 19:799-807, 1992.

56. Disa J, Polvora V, Pusic A, et al: Dextran related complications in head and neck microsurgery: do the benefits outweigh the risk? A prospective randomized analysis, *Plast Reconstr Surg* 112:1534-1539, 2003.

57. Suh JD, Sercarz JA, Abemayor E, et al: Analysis of outcome and complications in 400 cases of microvascular head and neck reconstruction, *Arch Otolaryngol Head Neck Surg* 130:962-966, 2004.

58. Serletti JM, Higgins JP, Moran S, et al: Factors affecting outcome in free-tissue transfer in the elderly, *Plast Reconstr Surg* 106:66-70, 2000.

59. Choi S, Schwartz DL, Farwell DG, et al: Radiation therapy does not impact local complication rates after free flap reconstruction for head and neck cancer, *Arch Otolaryngol Head Neck Surg* 130:1308-1312, 2004.

60. Singh B, Cordeiro PG, Santamaria E, et al: Factors associated with complications in microvascular reconstruction of head and neck defects, *Plast Reconstr Surg* 103:403-411, 1999.

61. Kroll SS, Schusterman MA, Reece GP, et al: Choice of flap and incidence of free flap success, *Plast Reconstr Surg* 98:459-463, 1996.

62. Khouri RK, Cooley BC, Kunselman AR, et al: A prospective study of microvascular free-flap surgery and outcome, *Plast Reconstr Surg* 102:711-721, 1998.

63. Blackwell K: Unsurpassed reliability of free flaps for head and neck reconstruction, *Arch Otolaryngol Head Neck Surg* 125:295-299, 1999.

64. Urken ML, Weinberg H, Buchbinder D, et al: Microvascular free flaps in and head and neck reconstruction, *Arch Otolaryngol Head Neck Surg* 120:633-640, 1994.

65. Shaari CM, Buchbinder D, Constantino PD, et al: Complications of microvascular head and neck surgery in the elderly, *Arch Otolaryngol Head Neck Surg* 124:407-411, 1998.

66. Chen CM, Lin GT, Fu YC, et al: Complications of free radial forearm flap transfers for head and neck reconstruction, *Oral Surg Oral Med Oral Pathol Oral Radiol Endod* 99:671-676, 2005.

67. Jones B, O'Brien C: Acute ischemia of the hand resulting from elevation of a radial forearm flap, *Br J Plast Surg* 38:396-397, 1985.

68. Hallock G: Complication of the free flap donor site from a community hospital perspective, *J Reconstr Microsurg* 7:331-334, 1991.

69. Pestana I, Coan B, Erdmann D, et al: Early experience with fluorescent angiography in free-tissue transfer reconstruction, *Plast Reconstr Surg* 123:1239-1244, 2009.

70. Kim D, Ghali G: Microvascular free tissue reconstruction of the oral cavity, *Selected Readings Oral Maxillofac Surg* 12(4), 2004.

Fibula Free Flap and Mandibular Reconstruction

Chapter **70**

Phillip Pirgousis, Rui Fernandes

HISTORY

The first case of microvascular bone transfer of a vascularized myoosseous segment of fibula to treat a post-traumatic tibial defect was reported by Taylor and co-workers in 1975. All cases that followed did not include a skin paddle.

Description of the harvesting technique for this composite fibula flap by Gilbert in 1981 via the lateral approach allowed direct visualization of the perforating cutaneous branches of the peroneal artery and provided the basis for safe inclusion of a skin paddle with the bone flap.

Hidalgo in 1989 performed the first mandibular reconstruction with a segment of fibula by using multiple defined osteotomies to reproduce the shape of almost an entire mandible. Since then the fibula free flap has enjoyed much popularity for mandibular reconstruction and has continued to undergo technical developments. Variable skin paddle positions relative to the bone, harvesting of two separate skin paddles for reconstruction of composite through-and-through defects of the face, the use of sensate skin islands, and the "double-barreled" fibula flap to improve restoration of bone height have all been described.

SURGICAL ANATOMY

The fibula is a long thin non–weight-bearing bone of the lower extremity. It has a tubular shape with a thick circumference of cortical bone providing it with significant inherent strength. Approximately 22 to 25 cm of bone may be harvested while preserving 6 to 7 cm of bone proximally and distally to maintain integrity and functional stability of both the knee and ankle joints, respectively. An additional limitation of proximal dissection is the common peroneal nerve, which wraps around the neck of the fibula.

The fibula can be harvested as a free osseous or free osteoseptocutaneous flap. The inclusion of an overlying skin paddle is possible because septocutaneous or musculocutaneous perforators from the peroneal artery and vein provide a viable blood supply to this area of skin.

The peroneal artery and vein represent the dominant blood supply and vascular pedicle for the fibula osteocutaneous flap. Classically, the popliteal artery divides into the anterior and posterior tibial arteries below the knee, with the latter vessel subsequently giving rise to the peroneal artery. The peroneal artery and its paired venae comitantes descend in the lower part of the leg between the flexor hallucis longus and tibialis posterior muscles as they course toward the foot.

The peroneal artery via a nutrient medullary artery, along with multiple periosteal feeding vessels, provides a rich endosteal vascular supply to the fibula. The vascular supply to the skin over the fibula arises from numerous fasciocutaneous perforators running in the posterior crural septum. Their position and course may be highly variable. The amount of skin that can be harvested is usually limited by the ability to primarily close the defect, although skin grafting of the donor site defect is also frequently performed successfully.

The sensory supply to the skin over the lateral aspect of the calf is derived from the lateral sural cutaneous nerve, a branch of the common peroneal nerve, arising within or above the popliteal fossa. When harvested as part of the osteocutaneous fibula flap it can provide variable sensation to the accompanying skin paddle.

PATHOLOGIC ANATOMY

Hypoplasia or complete absence of the fibula with replacement solely by a fibrous band is a rare phenomenon that is clinically apparent as a shortened leg and abnormally bowed tibia.

Anatomic variations in the vasculature supplying the lower part of the leg and foot are of greater relevance and concern when using the fibula free flap for bony reconstruction. Normally, the peroneal artery contributes minimally to the vascular supply of the foot, with the dominant supply being provided by the anterior and posterior tibial vessels. In 10% of cases, these two normally dominant vessels may be significantly attenuated or individually absent. In such circumstances, the primary vascular supply is derived from the peroneal artery (peroneal arteria magna), and sacrifice of it will result in limb-threatening ischemia of the foot.

DIAGNOSTIC STUDIES

The goal of preoperative arteriography with respect to the free fibula flap is to identify patients in whom harvest of this flap would result in either a non-viable flap or compromised extremity. Though controversial, it is generally thought by most reconstructive surgeons that angiography for imaging of the lower limb vessels is the "gold standard" for preoperative assessment of patients. However, it is still routine practice in many centers to rely solely on preoperative clinical assessment.

Non-invasive clinical assessment begins with a thorough patient history and general physical examination. Claudication with walking should alert the clinician to underlying occlusive arterial disease. A more detailed examination of the perfusion status of the lower part of the leg and foot is performed to look for signs of limb deformity, previous surgery, or trauma. Stigmata of peripheral arterial or venous vascular disease include skin pallor or cyanosis, ulceration, cool skin temperature, sparse hair growth, and thickened nail beds. Palpation of the popliteal, posterior tibial, and dorsalis pedis pulses is mandatory. Questionable or absent pulses should be investigated further with Doppler flow assessment.

Conventional angiography, computed tomographic angiography, or magnetic resonance angiography, though more invasive, provide superior anatomic detail and functional assessment of the adequacy of limb perfusion and quality of the donor vessels (Fig. 70-1).

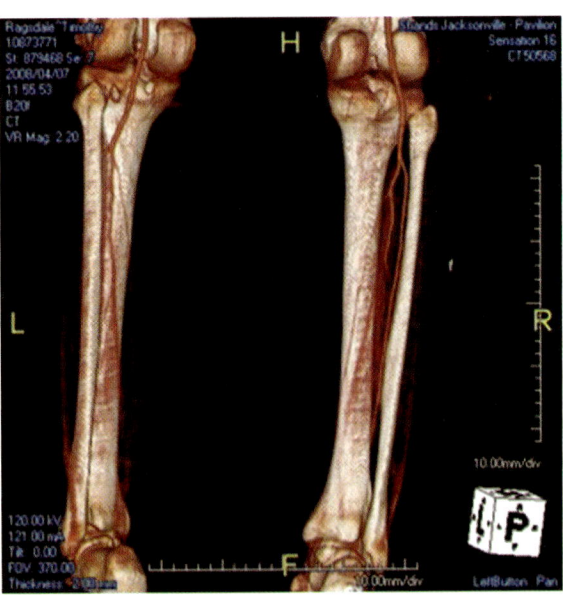

Fig. 70-1 ■ Computed tomographic angiography depicting the lower extremity vasculature and patency of the vessels before harvesting a fibula free flap.

Angiographic findings precluding use of the fibula as a reconstructive donor site can be either congenital or acquired. Congenital conditions include peroneal arteria magna. Acquired conditions include a history of lower limb trauma and peripheral vascular disease, both of which can significantly diminish the vascularity of the lower extremity. Kim and co-workers in 1989 reviewed a large series of lower extremity angiograms and identified numerous vascular anomalies. In their patients, hypoplasia or absence of the anterior tibial artery was noted in 4%, hypoplasia or absence of the posterior tibial artery was seen in 2%, and a dominant peroneal supply to the lower limb was present in 7%. Congenital absence of the peroneal vessels was estimated to occur in 0.1% of the population by Lippert and Pabst in 1985.

Finally, routine use of preoperative angiography must be weighed against the risk for associated complications, including arterial occlusion, aortic dissection, renal failure, nerve injury, intimal damage, hematoma, and anaphylaxis, which occur at an incidence as high as 5%.

Aside from the donor site, equal attention must be given to the recipient site in question. The site and size of the anticipated mandibular defect can often be evaluated clinically and radiologically with a plain panoramic radiograph or computed tomography scan. Knowledge of the nature of the mandibular pathology is important with respect to any concomitant neck surgery required. Knowledge of the extent of neck surgery for malignant disease is paramount to the reconstructive surgeon with regard to adequate availability of recipient vessels for microvascular anastomosis. This issue is even more important in patients with previous neck surgery, specifically previous neck dissection, in which sacrifice of typical recipient vessels was warranted for clearance of disease. In such cases, neck angiography may also be necessary to define the availability, position, and caliber of possible recipient vessels.

TREATMENT/RECONSTRUCTIVE GOALS

The aims of mandibular reconstruction are numerous and clearly demonstrate the important structural, functional, and esthetic significance that the mandible plays in the orofacial complex. Attention to plus restoration of each of these crucial parameters has a great impact on patients' psychosocial state and quality of life.

The mandible is a critical component of the facial complex and stomatognathic system and forms the key structure in the lower third of the face. More importantly, it is intimately involved in daily functions such as mastication, speech, swallowing, and respiration. Esthetically, it supports the lower lip and chin and delineates the facial complex from the neck. It is thus obvious that any attempts at mandibular reconstruction mandate attention to each of these vital functions.

The fibula free flap is a versatile flap well suited to mandibular reconstruction. Its excellent bone stability and soft tissue component allow reconstruction of complex composite defects. With up to 25 cm of bone able to be harvested, reconstruction of an entire mandible is possible. Its dense bony cortex and profuse periosteal blood supply enable multiple bony osteotomies to be performed for close reproduction of the contour of the native mandible, and its adequate bone stock and innate strength readily support osseointegrated implants for oral rehabilitation. Additionally, reconstruction of mandibular defects re-establishes the floor of the mouth and allows subsequent resuspension of the tongue to the neo-mandible, an important determinant of optimal speech, swallowing, and respiratory outcomes.

FLAP HARVEST AND INSETTING TECHNIQUES

The fibula free flap can be harvested as an osseous or osteocutaneous flap. The latter is described first because the former does not require preservation of cutaneous perforator vessels.

The patient is positioned supine on the operating table with the hip and knee slightly flexed and internally rotated and maintained in that position. The entire lower extremity is prepared and draped in standard fashion with circumferential exposure up to the groin. The sole of the foot is supported with a sandbag or a 1-L saline bag. Pertinent landmarks such as the head of the fibula, lateral malleolus, and peroneal nerve are outlined on the skin. A vertical mark joining the proximal and distal ends of the fibula represents the intermuscular septum. The necessary skin island is outlined over the junction of the middle and lower thirds of the fibula to capture septocutaneous perforators of the largest possible caliber. Doppler examination will frequently reliably aid in identifying these perforators and ensure that the skin island is centered over the perforators. A sterile tourniquet is applied, the lower extremity is exsanguinated, and the tourniquet is inflated to 350 mm Hg.

The incision begins at the anterior margin of the skin island and is extended proximally and distally to within 6 cm of the fibular head and lateral malleolus, respectively, to a level below the superficial fascia (Fig. 70-2). Subfascial dissection in the lateral compartment proceeds toward the intermuscular septum, where attention focuses on identifying and ensuring incorporation of the relevant perforators. Exposure and anterior retraction of the peroneus longus and brevis muscles allow dissection of these muscles off the fibula directed toward the anterior crural septum. An incision through the anterior crural septum provides entry into the anterior compartment for exposure of the anterior tibial vessels and deep peroneal nerve beneath, which are preserved and gently retracted anteriorly. One then encounters the interosseous membrane, which is incised to reveal the tibialis posterior muscle and its typical chevron-appearing fibers. Further dissection through this muscle will reveal the peroneal vessels lying beneath and running close to the medial aspect of the fibula. Attention now focuses on proximal and distal exposure

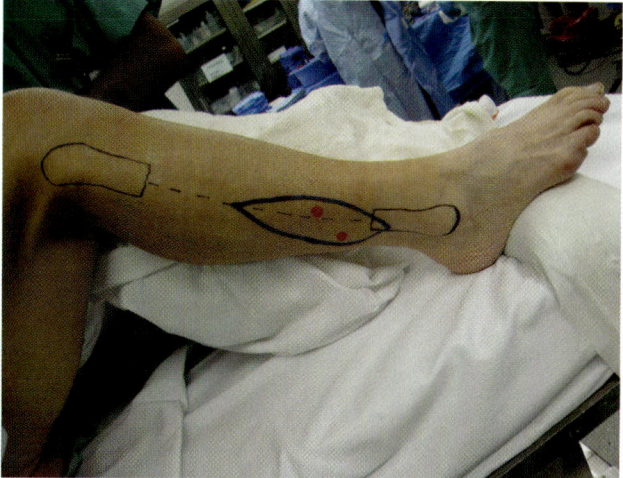

Fig. 70-2 ■ Markings for harvesting of a fibula osseocutaneous free flap. Note that approximately 6 to 8 cm of bone is preserved both distally and proximally to maintain stability of the ankle and knee.

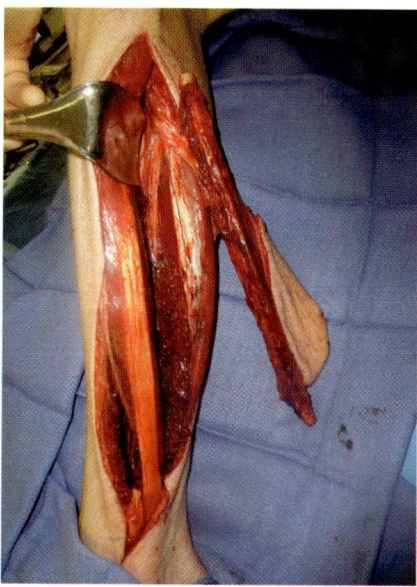

Fig. 70-3 ■ Dissection of the vascular pedicle of the fibula flap before takedown of the flap.

of the fibula via subperiosteal dissection 6 cm below the fibular head and 8 cm proximal to the lateral malleolus, where with the aid of curved periosteal elevators to protect the peroneal vessels immediately deep to the fibula, appropriate osteotomies can be made with the oscillating saw and a 1-cm segment of fibula removed. The pedicle can now be ligated and divided distally, and the fibula is able to be rotated laterally to enable easier and safer dissection of the pedicle in a distal to proximal fashion (Fig. 70-3). On reaching the tibioperoneal trunk the peroneal artery and venae comitantes are isolated. The posterior incision of the skin island can now be performed down to the soleus muscle, where it is optional to include a small cuff of soleus and flexor hallucis longus in cases in which musculocutaneous perforators are encountered. With the composite flap now isolated on its pedicle, the tourniquet is deflated and hemostasis of the donor bed is achieved. The flap is allowed to reperfuse for at least 30 minutes before division of the pedicle and transfer to the head and neck recipient site.

In instances in which a bone-only flap is required, one need only make a linear skin incision without inclusion of a skin island, with

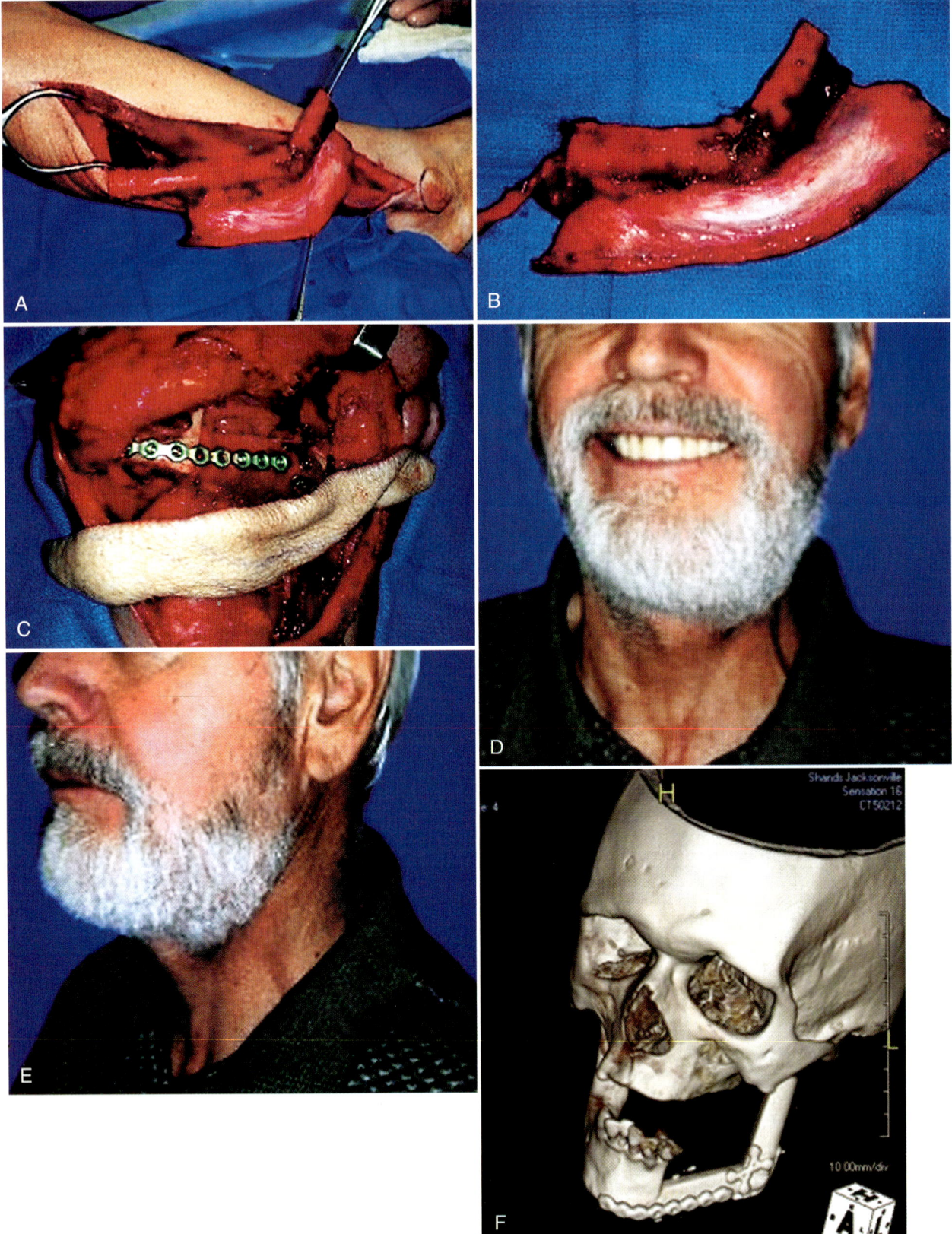

Fig. 70-4 ■ **A,** In situ osteotomy of a fibula osseocutaneous flap to reconstruct a hemimandibular defect including the condyle. **B,** Flap after takedown. **C,** Inset of the flap into the defect. **D,** Postoperative profile view of the patient. **E,** Postoperative frontal view of the patient after reconstruction of a hemimandibular defect with a vascularized fibula. **F,** Three-dimensional computed tomographic view of the reconstructed mandible.

dissection directed toward the intermuscular septum, where the remainder of the flap harvest technique proceeds as described earlier.

Closure of the donor site is performed with loose approximation of muscles and suturing of the flexor hallucis longus to tibialis posterior to optimize postoperative great toe flexion. A suction drain is placed and secured. A split-thickness skin graft harvested from the thigh is sutured to the skin paddle donor defect, followed by the application of a bolster and posterior splint. While the patient is non-ambulatory, leg elevation is advised to minimize dependent edema. The cast and bolster are removed after 7 days, at which time ambulation may commence.

Following division of the pedicle, the flap is transferred to the prepared recipient site. Preparation of the fibula at this stage is dependent on the site of the mandibular defect. For reconstruction of straight segments, fibula preparation is minimal, often with no osteotomies required. For defects in which osteotomies are required to reproduce the mandibular contour, one or more osteotomies may be necessary (Fig. 70-4). A variety of methods and techniques have been described to aid the surgeon in this task. Regardless of the method used, the ultimate aim is efficiency and accuracy in closing osteotomies so that the mandibular contour is reproduced and flap ischemia time is minimized. Additionally, it is important to achieve maximum bone contact at the interface between the fibula segments and between the fibula and native mandible. The osteotomized fibula is then secured to a pre-adapted reconstruction plate with fixation screws and subsequently fixed in situ to the native mandibular defect. The skin paddle, if raised as part of the flap, is loosely sutured to the margins of the soft tissue defect, with the vascular pedicle tunneled into the neck in preparation for microvascular anastomosis. An operating microscope is used for anastomosis of the peroneal vessels to the recipient artery and vein in the neck.

POSTOPERATIVE CARE

Patients frequently remain immobile for the first 5 to 7 days. While bed bound, the lower extremity should remain elevated to aid venous drainage and reduce postoperative edema, and antithrombotic therapy with heparin is commenced immediately after surgery and continued until discharge. This period of immobilization is more important in patients in whom a skin island has also been harvested to maximize the chance of successful take of the skin graft.

At 5 to 7 days when the splint is removed, assisted mobilization can begin with the help of a physical therapist.

Suction drains can be removed once drainage is minimal, ideally less than 20 mL over a 24-hour period.

The skin graft donor and recipient sites are typically assessed about 7 days postoperatively.

Resumption of normal activities can recommence 4 to 6 weeks after surgery.

PEARLS AND PITFALLS

- The most devastating complication of fibula flap transfer is lack of adequate collateral circulation to the foot and irreversible ischemia. Thorough preoperative assessment both clinically and radiologically can avoid this problem.
- Likewise, an equally serious complication is complete flap loss, the incidence of which is reported to be about 5% in most series. The incidence of skin flap loss in osteoseptocutaneous flaps is approximately 5% to 10%, and the loss may be complete or partial. This is a result of inadequate incorporation of skin perforators during harvest of the skin island. Preoperative Doppler identification of skin perforators and careful dissection of them can avoid this problem. Alternatively, when the quality or caliber of such skin perforators is doubtful, reports have shown that problematic skin loss can be avoided by incorporation of a cuff of underlying soleus and flexor hallucis longus muscles.
- Other reported functional deficits in the donor site include weakness in dorsiflexion of the great toe, which results from either injury to branches of the peroneal nerve or scarring of the flexor hallucis longus muscle; chronic pain; and weakness on ambulation and gait disturbance as a result of knee or ankle instability.
- Neurologic injury involving the common peroneal nerve can produce an equinovarus deformity and anesthesia along the anterolateral aspect of the leg and dorsum of the foot.
- Infection, hematoma, and incomplete take of skin grafts are also possible but uncommon donor site complications.

BIBLIOGRAPHY

Chen ZW, Yan W: The study and clinical application of the osteocutaneous flap of fibula, *Microsurgery* 4(1):11-16, 1983.

Cordeiro PG, Disa JJ, Hidalgo DA, et al: Reconstruction of the mandible with osseous free flaps: a 10-year experience in 150 consecutive patients, *Plast Reconstr Surg* 104: 1314-1320, 1999.

Garrett A, Ducic Y, Athre RS, et al: Evaluation of fibula free flap donor site morbidity, *Am J Otolaryngol* 27:29-32, 2006.

Gilbert A: Free vascularized bone grafts, *Int Surg* 66(1):27-31, 1981.

Hidalgo DA: Fibula free flap: a new method of mandible reconstruction, *Plast Reconstr Surg* 84(1):71-79, 1989.

Hidalgo DA, Pusic AL: Free flap mandibular reconstruction: a 10-year follow-up study, *Plast Reconstr Surg* 110:438-449, 2002.

Kim D, Orron DE, Skillman JJ: Surgical significance of popliteal artery variants. A unified angiographic classification, *Ann Surg* 210: 776-781, 1989.

Lippert H, Pabst R: *Arterial variations in man: classification and frequency*, New York, 1985, JF Bergman Verlag, pp 60-63.

Smith RB, Thomas RD, Funk GF: Fibula free flaps, *Arch Otolaryngol Head Neck Surg* 129:712-715, 2003.

Taylor GI, Miller DH, Ham FJ: The free vascularized bone graft. A clinical extension of microvascular techniques, *Plast Reconstr Surg* 55:533-544, 1975.

Chapter 71

Anterolateral Thigh Flap

Joshua Eli Lubek, Stephen L. Engroff

The anterolateral thigh flap was first introduced by Song and colleagues in 1984 as a septocutaneous perforator–based flap.[1] Advantages of this flap include long pedicle length, large vessel diameter, large skin paddle, two-team approach, and minimal donor site morbidity. Though originally presented as a septocutaneous flap, it is now known that the anterolateral thigh anatomy is quite variable, with the majority of patients having musculocutaneous perforators. Nonetheless, the anterolateral thigh flap has become one of the most popular soft tissue flaps and serves as a "workhorse" in oral and maxillofacial reconstruction with greater than a 90% success rate.[2-4]

ANATOMY

The anterolateral thigh flap is well known for variability in its vascular anatomy. It most often receives its blood supply from perforating vessels of the descending branch of the lateral circumflex femoral artery (Fig. 71-1). The artery is quite robust with a mean diameter of 1.5 to 2.5 mm. Its paired venae comitantes usually have a diameter ranging from 1.8 to 3 mm. The artery travels inferiorly in the intermuscular space between the vastus lateralis and the rectus femoris muscles (Fig. 71-2). Several perforator vessels then supply the skin of the lateral aspect of the thigh, with the dominant perforator usually being centered along a midpoint between an imaginary line drawn from the anterior superior iliac spine to the lateral aspect of the patella.[4,5] Although Song and associates originally described the flap as a septocutaneous perforator flap, based on anatomic dissection it is now known that the majority of the perforator vessels (80%) are musculocutaneous and travel through the vastus lateralis.

There are two common anatomic variations through which the musculocutaneous perforators traverse the vastus lateralis muscle. The more usual one involves a short course of approximately 3 to 5 cm through the muscle with origin from the descending branch of the lateral circumflex femoral artery. The second, less common variant of the musculocutaneous perforator involves an intramuscular course of approximately 6 to 7 cm, parallel to the vastus lateralis and branching from the transverse branch of the lateral circumflex artery or the lateral circumflex artery itself.[5-7] In reviewing 37 consecutive anterolateral thigh flaps, Shieh and co-workers noted that the more common musculocutaneous course occurred in 57% of patients, with an intramuscular perforator length of 5 cm and a mobile pedicle length of 12 cm. A musculocutaneous course arising directly off the lateral circumflex artery occurred in 27% of patients, with an intramuscular perforator length of 7 cm and a mobile pedicle length of 11 cm.[8] In a recent review of 89 consecutive anterolateral thigh flaps, Wong and associates described an oblique artery and associated paired venae comitantes, previously unnamed, traveling between the descending and transverse branches of the lateral circumflex femoral artery. This distinct artery was present in 35% of patients and had a mean diameter of 1.5 mm and pedicle length of 12 cm. The oblique branch was usually accompanied by the motor nerve to the vastus lateralis.[9] Other vascular patterns do exist, including vessels arising independently from the profunda femoris or the trunk of the femoral artery, both of which occur less than 2% of the time.[6] Absence of perforators has also been reported in 1% to 5% of patients.[6,9]

The quadriceps musculature is composed of four muscles: the rectus femoris, the vastus lateralis, the vastus intermedius, and the vastus medialis. It is responsible for both knee extension via concentric contraction and knee deceleration via eccentric muscle contraction. The quadriceps femoris converges into the quadriceps tendon, which both attaches to and stabilizes the patella. The vastus lateralis muscle is the largest of the quadriceps muscles. It is innervated by motor nerves traveling within the intermuscular septum between the rectus femoris and vastus lateralis. These motor nerve branches, derived from the femoral nerve, are often intimately associated with the vascular pedicle of the anterolateral thigh flap.[10,11] A review of 36 cadaveric thighs by Rozen and co-workers demonstrated four to seven motor nerve branches passing through the main vascular pedicle or between perforators in 31% of patients.[12]

The anterolateral thigh flap derives its sensory innervation from the lateral femoral cutaneous nerve as it enters the thigh deep to the inguinal ligament just inferior to the anterior superior iliac spine. This nerve then divides into a larger anterior branch, which provides sensation to the anterolateral aspect of the thigh, and a smaller posterior nerve branch.[13]

DIAGNOSTIC STUDIES

The greatest concentration of reliable perforators is located within a 3-cm radius at the midpoint between an imaginary line drawn from the anterior superior iliac spine to the ipsilateral lateral patella. Traditionally, no advanced studies have been required other than to preoperatively perform Doppler flowmetry and mark the skin perforators before making any incision.[7] Various studies have reported that acoustic Doppler flowmetry has a 40% concordance rate with the intraoperative findings whereas color Doppler, though time consuming and ultrasonographer dependent, has a 96% to 100% positive predictive value.[14,15] Frequently, one can make an incision along the pre-drawn line and carefully reflect the skin and fascia laterally until a perforator is identified. The flap can then be centered over this perforator. Computed tomographic angiography has also been used to assess perforator availability when selecting the anterolateral thigh as a possible flap donor site.[16,17] Ribuffo and colleagues were able to determine perforator location and size and identify the septal/musculocutaneous pathway with computed tomographic angiography. The authors noted that all of the flaps survived and that

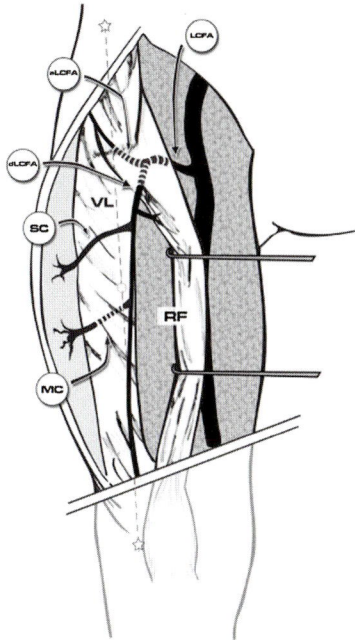

Fig. 71-1 ■ Anatomy of the anterolateral thigh flap and descending branch of the lateral circumflex femoral pedicle. aLCFA, ascending lateral circumflex femoral artery; dLCFA, descending lateral circumflex femoral artery; LCFA, lateral circumflex femoral artery; MC, musculocutaneous perforator; RF, rectus femoris muscle; SC, septocutaneous perforator; VL, vastus lateralis muscle. (From Mäkitie AA, Beasley NJP, Neligan PC, et al: Head and neck reconstruction with anterolateral thigh flap, *Otolaryngol Head Neck Surg* 129:547-555, 2003.)

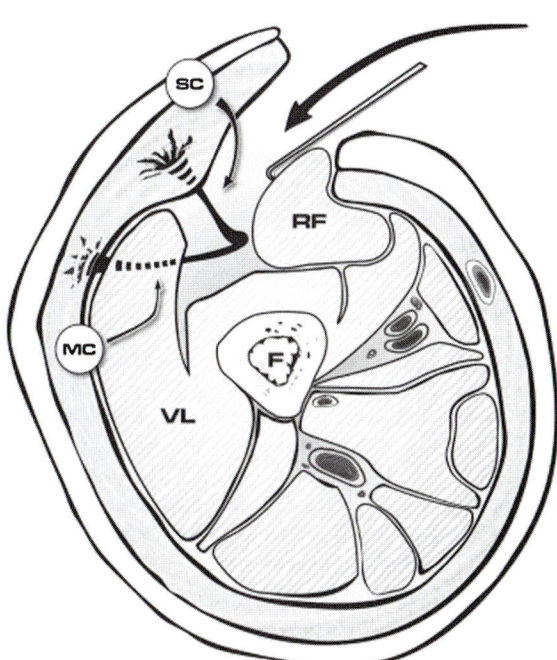

Fig. 71-2 ■ Cross section of the thigh. The descending branch of the lateral circumflex femoral artery is situated between the vastus lateralis and rectus femoris muscles. F, femur; MC, musculocutaneous perforator; RF, rectus femoris muscle; SC, septocutaneous perforator; VL, vastus lateralis muscle. (From Mäkitie AA, Beasley NJP, Neligan PC, et al: Head and neck reconstruction with anterolateral thigh flap, *Otolaryngol Head Neck Surg* 129:547-555, 2003.)

preoperative imaging anatomy coincided with the operative findings. Disadvantages of the study included absence of a control group (handheld Doppler identification of perforators), cost of the imaging, and exposure of the patient to radiation.[16] Preoperative angiography for the purpose of identifying significant vascular disease in the descending branch of the lateral circumflex femoral artery is unnecessary and of low yield because of the low incidence of atherosclerosis in this vessel.[15,18]

Clinical examination is also of importance because previous surgeries on the thigh, including vascular bypass procedures, exclude the use of this flap. Large body habitus and excessive subcutaneous fat make both dissection and flap inset difficult.[13]

TREATMENT/RECONSTRUCTIVE GOALS

The anterolateral thigh flap is ideally suited for reconstruction in the oral and maxillofacial region. It can be used for large soft tissue defects both extraorally and intraorally (Figs. 71-3 and 71-4).[2,3,19] It can be harvested as either a fasciocutaneous or a musculocutaneous flap, depending on the amount of soft tissue required. A true chimeric flap can also be elevated by combining the anterolateral thigh fasciocutaneous flap with the rectus femoris, vastus lateralis, and tensor fasciae latae. The flap is able to be thinned primarily in patients with excessive subcutaneous fat.[5,20] The vascular pedicle is generally of good caliber and length, thus facilitating vessel

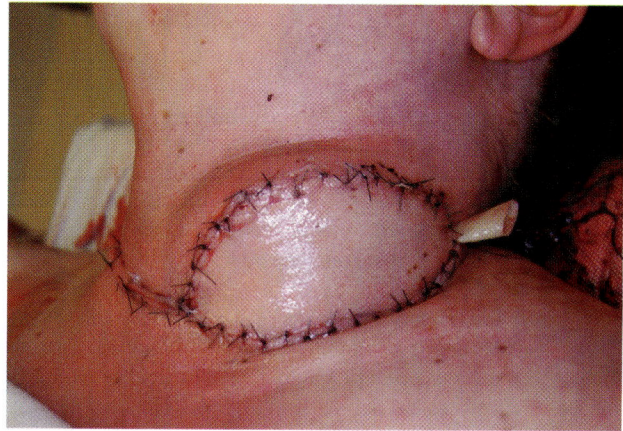

Fig. 71-3 ■ Anterolateral thigh flap used for reconstruction of a defect in the neck caused by ablation of metastatic carcinoma.

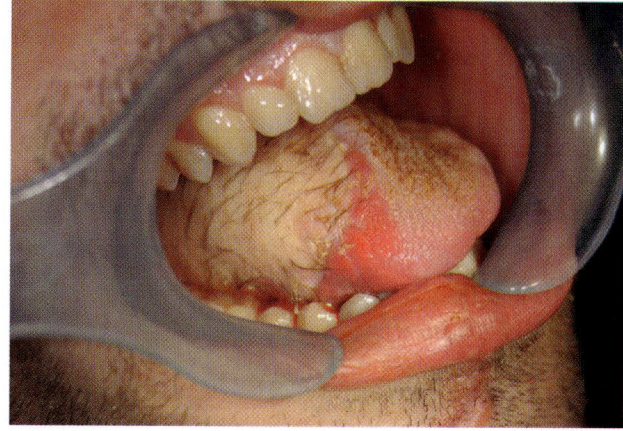

Fig. 71-4 ■ Postoperative photograph of an anterolateral thigh flap for reconstruction of a right hemiglossectomy defect.

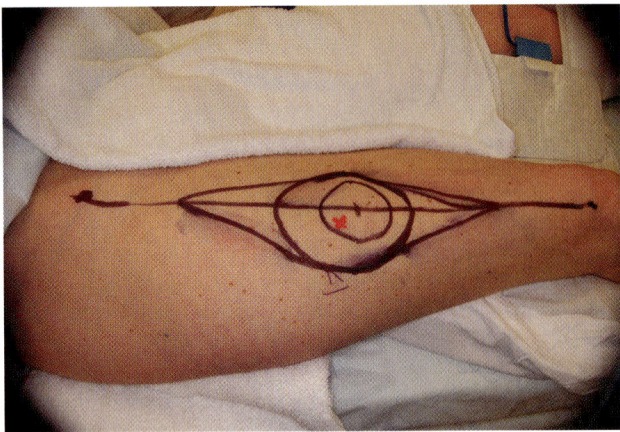

Fig. 71-5 ■ Skin paddle outlined.

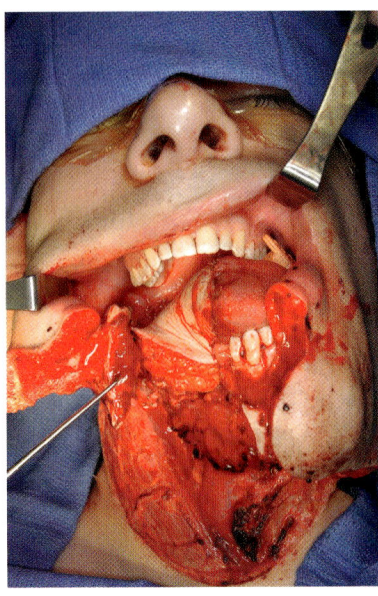

Fig. 71-6 ■ Intraoperative photograph of an anterolateral thigh flap inset for a hemiglossectomy defect.

anastomosis. A sensate flap based on the lateral femoral cutaneous nerve can be elevated if so desired. There is minimal donor site morbidity, and the anterolateral thigh flap can be raised in a two-team approach, which decreases surgery and anesthesia time.[5,21]

TECHNIQUE

The patient is placed in a supine position and a line is drawn from the anterior superior iliac spine to the superolateral patella. A 3-cm circle is outlined about the midpoint along this line, and the main perforator, located within this circle, is identified with Doppler ultrasound. The skin paddle is then outlined based on the identified perforator or perforators to a maximum width of 20 cm and length of 30 cm (Fig. 71-5).[22] The skin incision is initially placed on the medial aspect of the designed flap. This allows identification and protection of a skin perforator situated laterally. If a fasciocutaneous flap is desired, the incision is carried down through the deep fascia to expose the underlying musculature. The fasciocutaneous flap is retracted laterally and the dominant perforator identified. To harvest a thin flap via a suprafascial technique, dissection proceeds in the plane between the fascia and subcutaneous tissue while carefully identifying the perforator to the skin. After medial dissection in a suprafascial or subfascial plane, one can easily determine the course of the perforator either as a musculocutaneous vessel through the vastus lateralis or as a septocutaneous perforator traveling within the intermuscular septum of the rectus femoris and vastus lateralis muscles. If a perforator is not identified, options include (1) harvest of a tensor fasciae latae thigh flap based on a more superior perforator, (2) harvest of an anterior medial thigh flap using a more medial perforator, (3) conversion to a vastus lateralis muscle flap with or without a skin graft, or (4) selection of a different flap site.[23] The vascular pedicle can now be visualized in the intermuscular septum by gentle medial retraction of the rectus femoris muscle. The course of the perforator should at this time be identified by carefully unroofing the muscle or septum over the perforator and tracing the vessel proximally to its origin at the main vascular pedicle.[3,24] As intramuscular dissection proceeds, any small branches to the muscle are ligated as the musculocutaneous perforator is isolated. A small cuff of muscle can be left around the pedicle in patients with musculocutaneous perforators. A 5-cm cuff of fascia should also be left around the perforator if suprafascial dissection is performed to avoid kinking and disrupting the vasculature to the subdermal plexus. The lateral aspect of the skin paddle can now be elevated in a suprafascial or subfascial plane. Once again, care must be taken to avoid inadvertently damaging the perforator as the flap is lifted from the lateral aspect. The vascular pedicle can now be ligated distal to the origin of the perforator and traced proximally, with branches into neighboring muscles being ligated until the usual origin at the lateral circumflex femoral artery is visualized. One should also try to preserve the motor branches to the vastus lateralis traveling with the vascular pedicle, if possible. If two cutaneous perforators are available, the flap can be used to provide both intraoral and extraoral coverage. Once the recipient site is prepared, the pedicle of the anterolateral thigh flap can be divided at its origin and transferred to the maxillofacial region (Figs. 71-6 and 71-7).[2,5]

In situations requiring excessive tissue bulk, a musculocutaneous flap may be desired. There is no need to dissect any intramuscular or septocutaneous perforators in these cases. The section of vastus lateralis through which the perforators travel is included, with ligation of intramuscular branches as necessary. The pedicle is then dissected in the usual fashion.

The thigh donor site is generally closed in layers—superficial fascia, subcutaneous tissue, and skin. Reapproximation of the muscle can be difficult because it has a tendency to not hold suture well. Closure of the deep fascia can also create a problem related to thigh compression and compartment syndrome. Donor site defects less than 8 cm in width can usually be closed without the need for skin grafting.[4] This can be extended, depending on the laxity of the skin and the amount of subcutaneous tissue remaining. If there is any concern that primary closure will create excessive wound tension, skin grafting should be performed.

POSTOPERATIVE CARE

Postoperative monitoring of a non-buried anterolateral thigh flap involves evaluation of flap color, temperature, capillary refill, bleeding, and audible Doppler signal. This can easily be accomplished by both nursing staff and surgical trainees. It is important to understand that intraoral flaps do not lose heat and therefore surface temperature monitoring has little application for intraoral flaps. Buried flaps

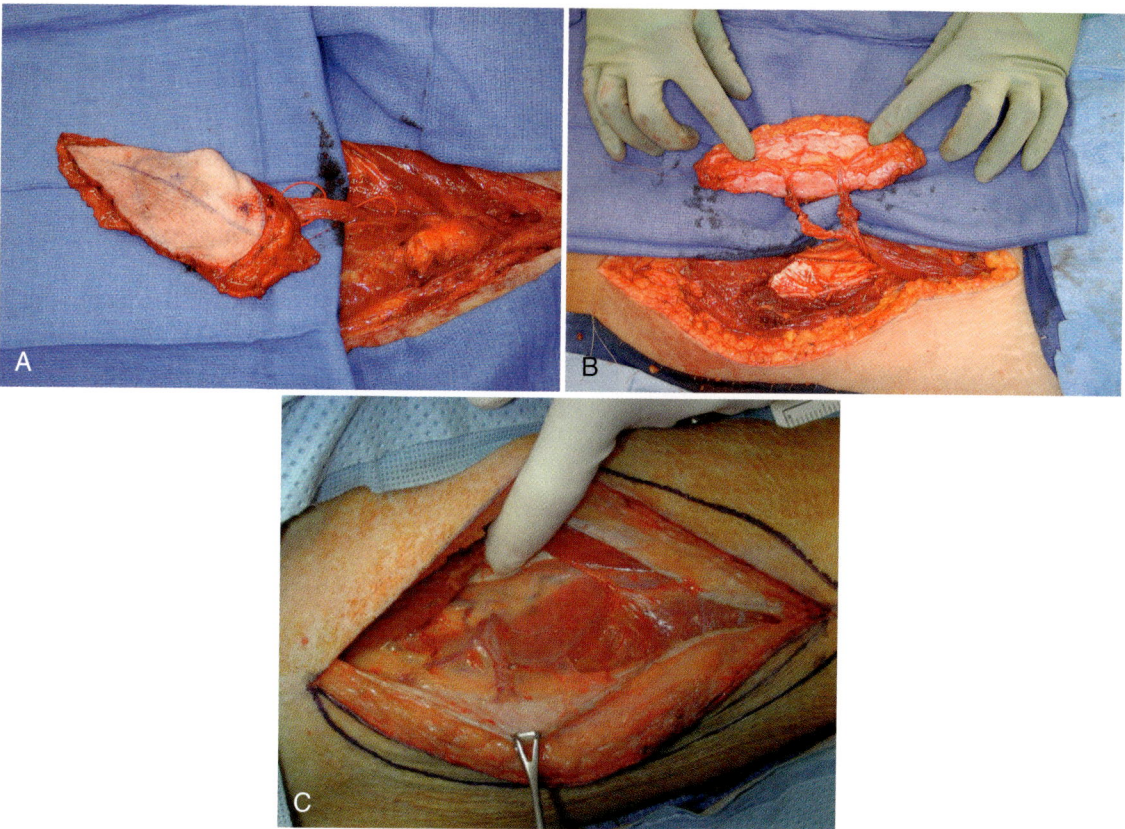

Fig. 71-7 ■ **A,** Anterolateral thigh flap in situ, vessel loop identifying the descending branch of the lateral circumflex femoral artery. **B,** Anterolateral thigh flap with two musculocutaneous perforator vessels. The motor branch of the femoral nerve to the vastus lateralis can need be visualized traveling with the pedicle. **C,** Septocutaneous perforator identified within the septum between the vastus lateralis and rectus femoris muscles. (Courtesy Dr. John Cacccamese, University of Maryland.)

present a more difficult challenge, including an inability to visualize color and capillary refill and unreliable Doppler signal because of the proximity of the carotid arteries and internal jugular veins. It is also possible to be deceived by a continuous arterial Doppler sound despite the presence of an occluded vein. Methods of monitoring buried anterolateral thigh flaps include implantable Doppler devices, measurement of tissue oxygen tension, and externalization of a portion of the flap either by de-epithelialization or division of the flap if a second perforator is available.[25,26] Early detection of vascular compromise is essential to prevent the "no-reflow" phenomenon, which will occur within 8 to 12 hours of ischemia. As with all microvascular free tissue transfers, the majority of failures occur on the venous side and generally within the first 72 hours following anastomosis.[27,28] Based on this knowledge, many microsurgical units have protocols in place such as flap checks every 1 to 2 hours for the first 24 hours, followed by flap monitoring every 2 to 4 hours for the next 48 hours.

Most patients do not complain of esthetic issues at the donor site, especially when primary closure is achieved. Kimata and associates evaluated 32 donor sites that were closed primarily and reported that 87.5% of patients were satisfied with their postoperative thigh appearance. Of patients who were dissatisfied, the majority were female. Patients should also be made aware that they will have some degree of sensory deficit along the distribution of the medial branch of the lateral cutaneous nerve of the thigh.[29] Various kinetic studies have evaluated and demonstrated minimal impairment of postoperative thigh function.[10,11] Kuo and co-workers evaluated donor site function using an objective kinetic communicator. They showed no

significant difference in isometric power and isokinetic peak torque ratio between the donor site and normal thigh. Patients did have mild weakness on knee extension when compared with the non-donor thigh on isokinetic concentric contraction (knee extension). All the patients in their study did resume daily ambulation without any difficulty.[11] In the study by Kimata and colleagues, the donor site was assessed by both subjective and manual muscle testing. They found that morbidity was related to the amount of damage to the vastus lateralis. Patients complained of weakness and fatigue but were still able to perform normal daily activities with normal range of motion at the knee and hip. Patients did have more difficulty navigating stairs than walking on level ground.[29] Staples or sutures are usually removed between postoperative days 10 and 14. Patients ambulate with assistance beginning on the third postoperative day and generally start physical therapy within 1 to 2 weeks following surgery when possible. Hair growth is not usually a concern in female patients or those receiving postoperative radiotherapy. If it does become an esthetic concern, standard methods of hair removal are available and painless, especially with insensate anterolateral thigh flaps. As stated previously, donor site defects greater than 8 to 10 cm in width usually require a skin graft. This will help prevent the complications of wound dehiscence, delayed healing, unsightly scars, and distal deep venous thrombosis or the possibility of a thigh compartment syndrome. Early symptoms of thigh compartment syndrome include excessive pain and a swollen, tense thigh. Addison and co-authors reported two cases of compartment syndrome following previous anterolateral thigh flap harvest with primary donor site closures of 10 and 12 cm.[30]

PEARLS AND PITFALLS

- The majority of the cutaneous perforators to the anterolateral thigh flap are located in a 3-cm radius at the midpoint along a line drawn from the anterior superior iliac crest to the superolateral patella.
- The anatomy of the anterolateral thigh flap is quite variable, with the majority of perforators being musculocutaneous and originating from the descending branch of the lateral circumflex femoral artery.
- The surgeon should be familiar with the anatomy and have the ability to elevate the tensor fasciae latae musculocutaneous flap and the anteromedial thigh flap in situations in which difficulties arise with the anterolateral thigh flap.
- Large body habitus and excessive subcutaneous tissue increase the difficulty of flap harvest and inset. In these situations the surgeon can thin the flap by suprafascial dissection. At least 3 to 5 cm of fascia should surround the perforator to both protect and avoid kinking the perforator. Excessive thinning of subcutaneous tissue

to a thickness of less than 5 mm increases the risk for marginal flap necrosis.
- Meticulous attention should be directed to hemostasis because the perforator vessels are extremely small and can be at risk for compression/venous occlusion.
- Small postablative defects and thick anterolateral thigh flaps can cause constriction of the perforator/subdermal plexus and lead to vascular congestion and, ultimately, flap failure. Flap selection is essential; smaller defects may be better suited for flaps such as the thinner radial free forearm flap.
- Proper orientation of the flap is necessary to avoid twisting of the perforator. This can easily be accomplished with orientation sutures and should be done before transfer of the flap to the head and neck region.
- One should consider skin-grafting donor site defects larger than 8 cm or in situations in which excessive wound tension is noted during skin closure.

REFERENCES

1. Song YG, Chen GZ, Song YL: The free thigh flap: a new free flap concept based on the septocutaneous artery, *Br J Plast Surg* 37:149-159, 1984.
2. Makitie AA, Beasley NJP, Neligan PC, et al: Head and neck reconstruction with anterolateral thigh flap, *Otolaryngol Head Neck Surg* 129:547-555, 2003.
3. Wei FC, Jain V, Celik N, et al: Have we found an ideal soft-tissue flap? An experience with 672 anterolateral thigh flaps, *Plast Reconstr Surg* 109:2219-2226, 2002.
4. Wolff KD, Kesting M, Thurmuller P, et al: The anterolateral thigh as a universal donor site for soft tissue reconstruction in maxillofacial surgery, *J Craniomaxillofac Surg* 34:323-331, 2006.
5. Kimata Y, Uchiyama K, Ebihara S, et al: Versatility of the free anterolateral thigh flap for reconstruction of head and neck defects, *Arch Otolaryngol Head Neck Surg* 123:1325-1331, 1997.
6. Kimata Y, Uchiyama K, Ebihara S, et al: Anatomic variations and technical problems of the anterolateral thigh flap: a report of 74 cases, *Plast Reconstr Surg* 102:1517-1523, 1998.
7. Da-Chuan X, Shi-zhen Z, Ji-ming K, et al: Applied anatomy of the anterolateral femoral flap, *Plast Reconstr Surg* 82:305-310, 1988.
8. Shieh SJ, Chiu HY, Yu JC, et al: Free anterolateral thigh flap for reconstruction of head and neck defects following cancer ablation, *Plast Reconstr Surg* 105:2349-2357, 2000.
9. Wong CH, Wei FC, Fu B, et al: Alternative vascular pedicle of the anterolateral thigh flap: the oblique branch of the lateral circumflex femoral artery, *Plast Reconstr Surg* 123:571-577, 2009.
10. Tsuji N, Suga H, Uda K, et al: Functional evaluation of anterolateral thigh flap donor sites: isokinetic torque comparisons for knee function, *Microsurgery* 28:233-237, 2008.
11. Kuo YR, Jeng SF, Kuo MH, et al: Free anterolateral thigh flap for extremity reconstruction:

clinical experience and functional assessment of donor site, *Plast Reconstr Surg* 107:1766-1771, 2001.
12. Rozen WM, le Roux CM, Ashton MW, et al: The unfavorable anatomy of vastus lateralis motor nerves: a cause of donor-site morbidity after anterolateral thigh flap harvest, *Plast Reconstr Surg* 123:1505-1508, 2009.
13. Lin DT, Coppit GL, Burkey BB: Use of the anterolateral thigh flap for reconstruction of the head and neck, *Curr Opin Otolaryngol Head Neck Surg* 12:300-304, 2004.
14. Iida H, Ohashi I, Kishimoto S, et al: Preoperative assessment of anterolateral thigh flap cutaneous perforators by colour Doppler flowmetry, *Br J Plast Surg* 56:21-25, 2003.
15. Halvorson EG, Taylor HOB, Orgill DP: Patency of the descending branch of the lateral circumflex femoral artery in patients with vascular disease, *Plast Reconstr Surg* 121:121-129, 2008.
16. Ribuffo D, Atzeni M, Saba L, et al: Angio computed tomography preoperative evaluation for anterolateral thigh flap harvesting, *Ann Plast Surg* 62:368-371, 2009.
17. Rozen WM, Ashton MW, Pan WR et al: Anatomical variations in the harvest of anterolateral thigh flap perforators: a cadaveric and clinical study, *Microsurgery* 29:16-23, 2009.
18. Hage JJ, Woerdeman LAE: Lower limb necrosis after use of the anterolateral thigh flap: is preoperative angiography indicated? *Ann Plast Surg* 52:315-318, 2004.
19. de Vicente JC, de Villalain L, Torre A, et al: Microvascular free tissue transfer for tongue reconstruction after hemiglossectomy: a functional assessment of radial forearm versus anterolateral thigh flap, *J Oral Maxillofac Surg* 66:2270-2275, 2008.
20. Ross GL, Dunn R, Kirkpatrick CE, et al: To thin or not to thin: the use of the anterolateral thigh flap in the reconstruction of intraoral defects, *Br J Plast Surg* 56:409-413, 2003.

21. Kuo YR, Jeng SF, Kuo MH, et al: Versatility of the free anterolateral thigh flap for reconstruction of soft-tissue defects: review of 140 cases, *Ann Plast Surg* 48:161-166, 2002.
22. Saint-Cyr M, Schaverien M, Wong C, et al: The extended anterolateral thigh flap: anatomical basis and clinical experience, *Plast Reconstr Surg* 123:1245-1255, 2009.
23. Hsieh CH, Yang JCS, Chen CC, et al: Alternative reconstructive choices for anterolateral thigh flap dissection in cases in which no sizable skin perforator is available, *Head Neck* 31:571-575, 2009.
24. Wong CH, Kao HK, Fu B, et al: A cautionary point in the harvest of the anterolateral thigh myocutaneous flap, *Ann Plast Surg* 62:637-639, 2009.
25. Spyropolou GA, Kuo YR, Chien CY et al: Buried anterolateral thigh flap for pharyngoesophageal reconstruction: our method for monitoring, *Head Neck* 31:882-887, 2009.
26. Abdel-Galil K, Mitchell D: Post-operative monitoring of microsurgical free tissue transfer for head and neck reconstruction: a systematic review of current techniques—Part I. Non-invasive techniques, *Br J Oral Maxillofac Surg* 47:351-355, 2009.
27. Chen KT, Mardini S, Chuang DCC, et al: Timing of presentation of the first signs of vascular compromise dictates the salvage outcome of free flap transfers, *Plast Reconstr Surg* 120:187-195, 2007.
28. Carroll WR, Esclamado RM: Ischemia/reperfusion injury in microvascular surgery, *Head Neck* 22:700-713, 2000.
29. Kimata Y, Uchiyama K, Ebihara S, et al: Anterolateral thigh flap donor-site complications and morbidity, *Plast Reconstr Surg* 106:584-589, 2000.
30. Addison PD, Lannon D, Neligan PC: Compartment syndrome after closure of the anterolateral thigh flap donor site: a report of two cases, *Ann Plast Surg* 60:635-638, 2008.

Deep Circumflex Iliac Artery Free Flap

Chapter 72

Stephen L. Engroff, Joshua Eli Lubek

The iliac crest has been used for graft reconstruction of the maxillofacial region for many decades. It was not until 1979 that a reliable vascular supply to the anterior ilium was elucidated by Taylor and co-workers,[1] and this flap was routinely used for microvascular free tissue transfer. It has since been applied to reconstruction of the mandible and maxilla and used as a composite flap for complex defects of the face. The vascular anatomy is reliable, and success rates are high.

ANATOMY

The deep circumflex iliac artery (DCIA) (Fig. 72-1) originates from the lateral portion of the external iliac artery just above the inguinal ligament. It is a robust artery that is generally 2 to 3 mm in diameter. The DCIA ascends parallel to the inguinal ligament to a point medial to the anterior superior iliac spine (ASIS) and then penetrates the transversalis fascia and continues its course along the medial lip of the iliac crest between the iliacus and transversus abdominis muscles. The main course of the artery serves the bone of the iliac crest through periosteal and endosteal branches. The bone supplied extends from the ASIS to the sacroiliac joint. Perforating vessels to the surrounding soft tissues are somewhat variable. In the majority of patients (70% to 80%), a large (1 mm) single vessel termed the ascending branch originates from the DCIA and serves the internal oblique muscle. A minority of individuals have multiple perforating vessels serving the muscular layers of the abdominal wall rather than a well-defined ascending branch. On rare occasions (1%), the ascending branch will directly join the external iliac artery. In these situations, if one desires to use the internal oblique muscle as part of the reconstruction, a separate anastomosis of this vessel will also need to be performed, as well as the DCIA. Perforating vessels to the skin arise 6 to 9 cm posterior to the ASIS and 2 to 3 cm medial to the crest. One dominant perforator or several smaller ones are required for reliable vascular supply to the skin. These skin perforators arise from branches that perforate all three muscular layers of the abdominal wall (transversus abdominis, internal oblique, and external oblique).

Venous drainage of the flap generally follows the arterial anatomy. Accompanying the smaller arteries are paired venae comitantes. These vessels usually combine to form a single deep circumflex iliac vein several centimeters above the external iliac vein, which provides a 3- to 5-mm vein for venous anastomosis. Occasionally, the venae comitantes will not join, thus making two venous anastomoses advisable.

The motor nerves to the muscles of the abdominal wall are segmental and arise from the lower thoracic and upper lumbar levels. They are not generally suitable for providing dynamic muscular reinnervation to a flap. The lateral femoral cutaneous nerve provides sensation to the lateral thigh skin. It courses in the fascia above the iliacus muscle medial to the ASIS. Its course relative to the DCIA is variable. When it is deep to the vascular pedicle, it can usually be preserved without much difficulty. Occasionally, it will be found superficial to the vessels and requires division. Patients should be informed preoperatively about the resulting sensory disturbance. The surgeon should be aware that the femoral nerve runs with the external iliac artery and vein as they pass under the inguinal ligament. Although it will not generally be visualized during dissection, placement of sutures in this area during closure could potentially place it at risk.

The muscular anatomy in this area is primarily related to the layers of the abdominal wall. In addition, the iliacus muscle runs along the medial aspect of the ilium. The flexors of the hip attach along the lateral ilium and the sartorius tendon to the ASIS.

DIAGNOSTIC STUDIES

The iliac artery is prone to atherosclerotic changes, but the DCIA is relatively immune. Therefore, preoperative vascular imaging studies are not usually recommended. Preoperative pencil Doppler ultrasonography is used to locate perforating vessels to the skin medial to the iliac crest when a skin paddle is required for composite reconstruction. Previous surgeries such as appendectomy and repair of an inguinal hernia can affect the vascular anatomy and should be taken into consideration when present. An alternative flap should be selected for patients who have previously undergone vascular bypass surgery in the inguinal region.

TREATMENT/RECONSTRUCTION GOALS

The DCIA free flap is a reconstructive option with many potential applications. A significant limitation of using the DCIA flap involves the length of bone available. It will generally restore the hemimandible or the symphyseal region well, but the fibula may be a better option for more extensive mandibular defects. The contour of the ilium matches the lateral mandibular shape well. Closing osteotomies along the medial aspect of the flap will allow reconstruction of the symphysis, but care must be taken to avoid injury to the vessels. An L-shaped extension along the anterior bone margin below the ASIS or posteriorly in the ilium will allow the formation of a new mandibular angle and increase the functional length of bone available (Fig. 72-2). When smaller lengths of bone are needed, preservation of 3 cm of bone at the ASIS will improve the patient's postoperative function and serve to lengthen the vascular pedicle. If less than 3 cm of bone is left at the ASIS, the risk for fracture postoperatively is high.

Applications of the DCIA flap for reconstruction of maxillary defects have been developed. Brown has reported use of the DCIA flap for reconstruction of the infrastructure and central and larger maxillectomy defects, including those with orbital exenteration.[2] The bone receives implants well to facilitate dental rehabilitation. The internal oblique muscle can be used to close the oral-nasal fistula with thin tissue that will mucosalize. It will support the orbital contents and can be used to reconstruct the orbital floor.

Vascular pedicle length is generally 5 to 7 cm from the external iliac vessels to the ASIS. When the flap is taken posterior to the ASIS, the pedicle is effectively lengthened. Care needs to be exercised during preoperative assessment of the patient to accurately plan the flap inset, geometry of the pedicle, and source vessels. The surgeon should be prepared to use a vein graft if increased pedicle length is needed for tension-free anastomosis. An alternative to vein grafting has recently been described.[3] The descending branch of the circumflex femoral artery and its venae comitantes (the vascular

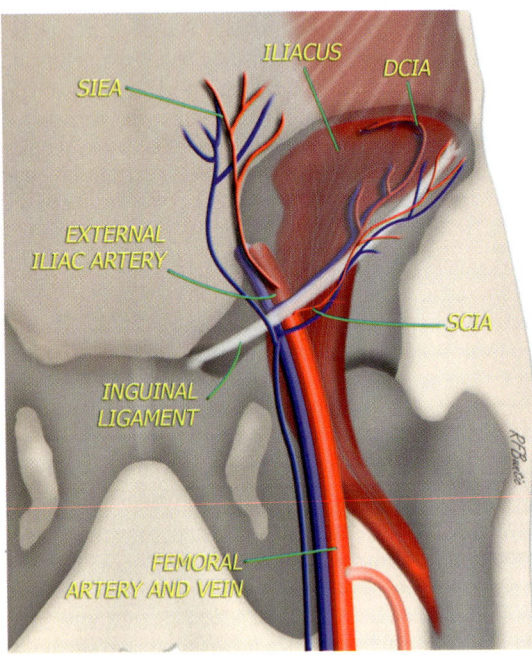

Fig. 72-1 ■ Vascular anatomy of the deep circumflex iliac artery (DCIA). (© 2001-2010 Rudolf F. Buntic, MD, *www.microsurgeon.org*.)

pedicle for the anterolateral thigh flap) can be used as an interposition graft. This has the advantage of using an arterial graft and a venous graft of similar caliber that are accessible in the same operative field. For mandibular reconstruction, the facial and superior thyroid vessels are frequently the vessels of choice. The thicker iliac crest is often positioned at the alveolar ridge because the wider bone easily accepts endosseous implants. An alternative orientation with the crest at the inferior border of the mandible will produce more usable length and flexibility of the vessels. This orientation of the flap is still acceptable for implant placement and future dental rehabilitation of the patient.

The soft tissue component of the flap is an important consideration. This flap has several potential soft tissue modifications that are helpful, depending on the defect to be reconstructed and the body habitus of the patient. All but the thinnest of patients will have a very bulky soft tissue component of the flap when the skin is included. For through-and-through defects of the tongue/mandible/facial skin, the flap can be fashioned with the internal oblique muscle to provide oral lining and the skin flap positioned on the face. Use of the skin for oral lining will result in an overly bulky flap in all but the largest of defects, even in thin patients. One must also remember that the skin paddle is quite adherent to the bone and that its limited arc of rotation may make soft tissue reconstruction difficult. Therefore, when oral lining is the only soft tissue deficiency, the muscular component is a superior option. Large mucosal defects can be covered by using the entire internal oblique muscle based on a large ascending branch, which provides a muscle paddle of up to 8 × 15 cm. This will mucosalize with some contraction. Such contraction can be beneficial, however, when covering the mandible or the palate because it replicates the attached mucosa.

When using this flap for maxillary reconstruction, some particular issues should be considered. First, the vascular pedicle may be inadequate to reach deep into the neck. The use of vein grafts should be considered, or alternative source vessels such as the superficial temporal vessels should be selected. Second, the orientation of the bone at the orbital rim is in a different plane from the alveolar ridge. Proper restoration of facial form will require the bone flap to be aligned with the orbital rim and zygoma, whereas acceptable dental rehabilitation will require the flap to extend from the native alveolus to the pterygoid plates.

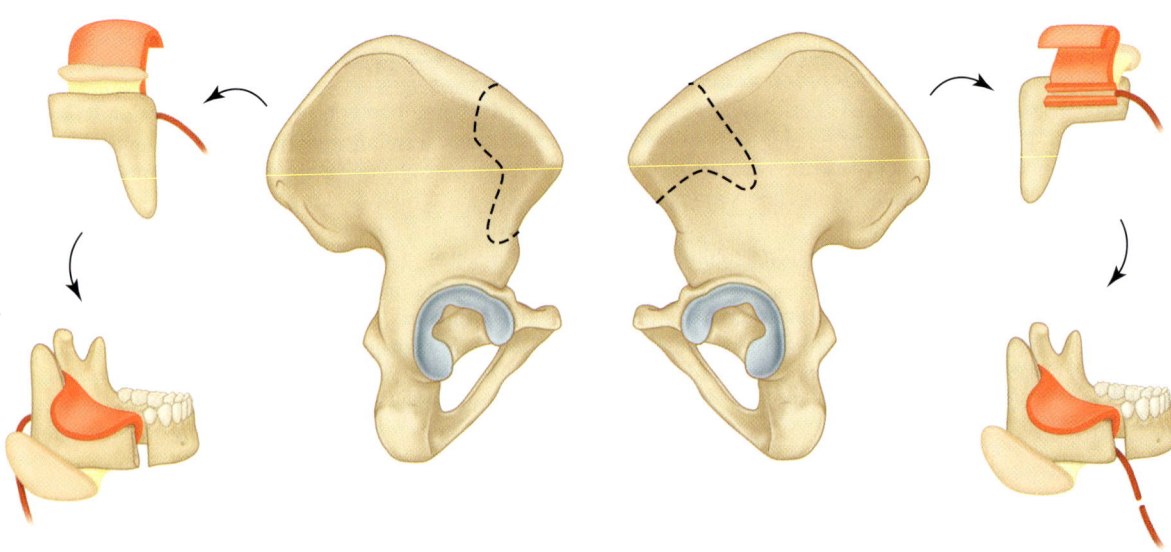

Fig. 72-2 ■ Orientation of the deep circumflex iliac artery flap for right hemimandibular reconstruction. Use of the right iliac crest will place the vascular pedicle posteriorly, and use of the left iliac crest will place the vascular pedicle anteriorly.

TECHNIQUE

The DCIA free flap is amenable to a two-team approach. The ipsilateral hip is elevated slightly. The surface landmarks of the ASIS, pubic tubercle, and inguinal ligament are marked out, as well as the outline of the iliac crest. When a skin flap is required, the ellipse of skin starts at the ASIS and is centered 2 to 3 cm medial to the crest. The distal end of the skin island is generally pointing at the tip of the scapula. A handheld Doppler is used to identify the perforators and ensure that they are centered in the skin paddle. Skin flaps of up to 20 × 10 cm have been used successfully for oromandibular reconstruction. If an osteomuscular flap is required, the incision extends from the area of the inguinal ligament along the medial portion of the ilium. The skin is incised along the medial portion of the paddle to expose the external oblique muscle. The skin can be elevated from the muscle, but care needs to be taken to preserve the skin perforators when a skin paddle is needed. A cuff of external oblique, internal oblique, and transversus abdominis muscles must be included to preserve the vascular supply to the skin. The external oblique muscle and fascia are divided parallel to the fibers and just medial to the crest to expose the internal oblique muscle. The external oblique is then elevated from the internal oblique up to the costal margin if necessary. A flap of internal oblique muscle is marked as required for the defect and incised. As the internal oblique is elevated from the transversus abdominis muscle, the ascending branch is identified and protected. The transversus muscle is divided medial to the vessels. In this area the pre-peritoneal fat should be protected and care taken to avoid injury to the abdominal contents. Following the ascending branch downward will identify the DCIA if it has not already been isolated. The iliacus muscle can be identified, and generally the lateral femoral cutaneous nerve is also isolated and preserved when possible. The vessels can now be dissected down to the external iliac vessels. Medially, a 2-cm cuff of iliacus muscle should remain attached to the iliac crest to protect the vascular pedicle. Laterally, the hip flexors can be elevated from the bone in a subperiosteal plane. The territory of bone to be harvested can now be delineated.

A reciprocating saw is then used to create the osteotomy. The vessels and the abdominal contents must be carefully protected. Once the bone cuts are completed, the flap is mobilized on its vascular source. The flap can then be taken and passed to the head and neck field.

Closure of the wound is done carefully. Sutures should not be allowed to injure the bowel or the femoral nerve. Secure closure is required to avoid the development of an incisional hernia. Frequently, burr holes are made in the medial cortex of the ilium to secure the transversalis fascia, transversus abdominis, and iliacus muscles to the bone with permanent suture. Bone wax may be needed to control marrow bleeding. Secure closure of the external oblique is completed, drains placed, and the remaining soft tissues closed per surgeon preference.

POSTOPERATIVE CARE

Flap monitoring is done per institution protocol for any microvascular free flap. There is a low risk of failure, but the majority of flap failures will occur within the first 48 to 72 hours and are related to venous obstruction. When identified early, a number of these flaps can be salvaged with prompt re-exploration.

Anticoagulation for the flaps in the postoperative period is also non-standard and should conform to the institution's usual routine. Anticoagulation may not be required at all. Our routine is to use low-dose aspirin in most patients. Higher-risk flaps (patients with tobacco use, estrogen replacement therapy, and large composite flaps with longer ischemia time) may warrant low-dose heparin.

Management of the donor site is important. Bed rest is generally prescribed for 2 to 3 days, with progressive mobilization thereafter. Physiologic ileus is common and patients should have their diets advanced slowly once bowel sounds and flatus are appreciated. Frequently, nasogastric tubes are placed peri-operatively. Stool softeners should be prescribed as well. Physical therapy and an abdominal binder are often helpful. Stairs are usually navigated at 3 weeks postoperatively, and lifting objects heavier than 5 lb or excessive straining should be avoided for 3 months to help prevent hernia formation. Patients should also be made aware that they may have a contour deformity in the hip region, especially in thinner patients.

Postoperative bleeding from the donor site may not be readily determined on clinical examination because retroperitoneal collections may develop. Therefore, close monitoring of the hematocrit is necessary. Computed tomography may be necessary to visualize the inguinal/pelvic region. Management of postoperative retroperitoneal bleeding may include observation, blood transfusion, or formal angiography and embolization.

PEARLS AND PITFALLS

- Careful closure of the donor site is required to avoid hernia—consider non-resorbable mesh if the integrity of the tissues is poor.
- Evaluate patients with any previous surgery for possible interruption of the vascular supply to the flap.
- Incorporating skin into the flap will create a very thick flap, even in thin persons.
- Carefully take the flap geometry and vessel length into account in the preoperative plan.
- Extreme care must be taken when performing closing osteotomies to avoid injury to the pedicle situated on the medial aspect of the ilium.
- Leaving less than 3 cm of bone behind the ASIS is associated with risk for a fracture postoperatively.

REFERENCES

1. Taylor GI, Townsend P, Corlett R: Superiority of the deep circumflex iliac vessels as the supply for free groin flaps: experimental work, *Plast Reconstr Surg* 64:595-604, 1979.

2. Brown JS: Deep circumflex iliac artery free flap with internal oblique muscle as a new method of immediate reconstruction of maxillectomy defect, *Head Neck* 18:412-421, 1996.

3. Bianchi B, Copelli C, Ferrari S, et al: Anterolateral thigh flap pedicle for interposition artery and vein grafts in head and neck reconstruction: a case report, *Microsurgery* 29: 136-137, 2009.

Chapter 73

Implant-Assisted Prosthetic Reconstruction after Tumor Ablation

Devin Joseph Okay, Daniel Buchbinder

MAXILLOMANDIBULAR DEFECTS

The primary objective of prosthetic rehabilitation is to restore and improve speech and swallowing function. Esthetic considerations are equally important after tumor ablation when structures that lend support to facial projection and symmetry are extirpated in the surgery. The goals of reconstruction may vary in different patients as a result of the need to achieve a balance between the components of the defect, co-morbid conditions affecting surgical reconstruction, and patient motivation. Contemporary management of patients with head and neck cancer integrates surgical reconstructive techniques with prosthetic rehabilitation to optimize function and esthetics.[1-3] Microvascular free tissue transfer for surgical reconstruction has been revolutionary in addressing the functional deficits present after ablative surgery of large tumors. The biology of the disease and the wound-healing properties of the recipient site after previous therapy are taken into account to determine a plan for reconstruction. If bone is to be part of the reconstructive effort, a method of fixation to ensure flap stability is needed until bony union takes place. Major advancements in surgical reconstructive techniques and new approaches to maxillomandibular defects have effectively provided a more conventional setting for prosthetic reconstruction of the dentoalveolar arch and surrounding structures. Composite free flaps from the fibula, iliac crest, and scapula regions are designed and harvested to address loss of tissue volume for restoration of mandibular continuity and to separate the oral from the sinonasal cavity.[4-6]

Preservation of tongue motion and restoration of tongue volume are critical in achieving a favorable functional outcome if the tumor extends to the tongue or floor of the mouth. Soft tissue defects involving the overlying skin or mucosal defects involving the lip or cheek, as well as any sensory and motor nerve deficits, will define which reconstructive option is best for functional recovery. Vascularized bone free flaps (VBFFs) from the fibula or iliac crest provide good to excellent bone volume and the quality required by the underlying bone for osseointegration and the application of prosthetics.[7] VBFFs will either restore discontinuity of the mandible or re-establish a stable base for the maxilla. Bone harvested from a distant donor site with its own blood supply presents additional strategies for osseointegration and prosthetic rehabilitation when reconstructing defects caused by the ablative treatment of benign and malignant tumors. Among such strategies is use of the vascular bed for osseointegration before radiation therapy. Placement of implants in the immediate surgical setting will shorten the overall treatment time until definitive prosthetic restoration can be accomplished. Once the bone is secured to the reconstruction plate and anastomosis of the recipient vessels is completed, implant placement is performed. After primary implant placement, the restorative team must allow 12 to 16 weeks for osseointegration and undisturbed

healing.[8,9] When a patient has completed radiation therapy after reconstruction and primary implant placement, the fixtures are uncovered once the soft tissue reaction has subsided. Soft tissue modifications can also be performed at this time, such as flap debulking or vestibuloplasty procedures. A surgical stent can be used and screwed into the implants for healing purposes before definitive prosthetic rehabilitation. Primary implant placement is helpful in developing a comprehensive approach to ablative surgery, subsequent reconstruction, and prosthodontic rehabilitation with adjunctive radiation therapy. This also holds true for placement of implants into native bone at the time of tumor resection to optimize function without surgical reconstructive procedures. This strategy circumvents the need for treatment with hyperbaric oxygen in patients requiring radiation therapy.[10,11] In addition, primary implant placement will minimize time with an unstable prosthesis and compromised function in an edentulous patient, especially edentulous maxillectomy patients (Fig. 73-1). As the defect enlarges, side effects such as hypernasal speech and nasal regurgitation of food are frequently encountered with an unstable prosthesis.[12,13]

PROSTHETIC DESIGN CONSIDERATIONS

The decision for fixed versus removable prosthetic restorations is dependent on clinical factors such as the availability of bone, the number and position of implants to assist or support restorations, maintenance of hygiene, and manual dexterity. Palatal obturators for maxillectomy patients or palatal augmentation prostheses to restore lingual-palatal contact for glossectomy patients are removable. If tumor surveillance is also a consideration, a removable prosthesis is indicated.

In addition to these clinical factors, other considerations such as comfort and psychosocial implications affect prosthetic design. When addressing reconstruction of the dental arch with osseointegrated prostheses, our preference is to provide patients with a fixed implant-supported restoration. In patients in whom the remaining arch is edentulous and lateral mandibular reconstruction is being performed, the implants should be placed in the anterior native mandible. This is an ideal location for placement of fixtures in patients undergoing lateral jaw resection for posterior alveolar, floor of the mouth/lateral tongue, or tonsillar primary tumors because this area is usually spared during radiation therapy. Placement of a minimum of four or five implants with the greatest anterior-posterior spread possible to minimize cantilever forces on the distal extension of the prosthesis and posterior placement of the distal implant on the contralateral side are potentially limited by the mental nerve and foramina. This landmark must be identified and care taken to avoid injury to the mental nerve.

These restorations are retained by screws when the prosthesis is retrievable as opposed to a cemented restoration. This design

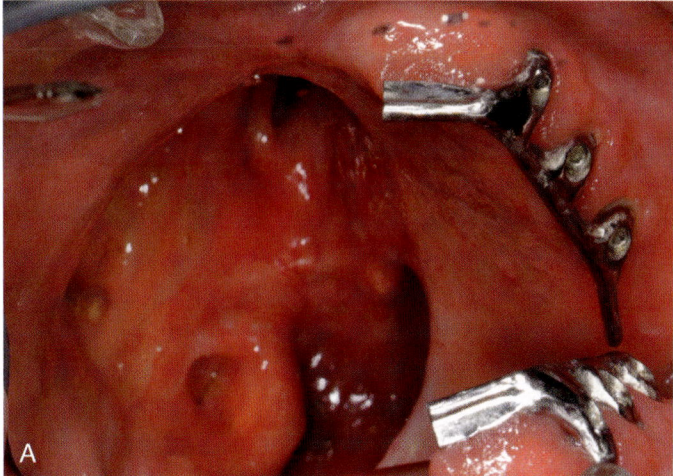

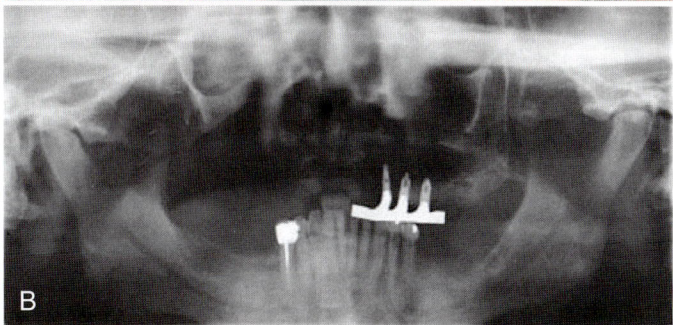

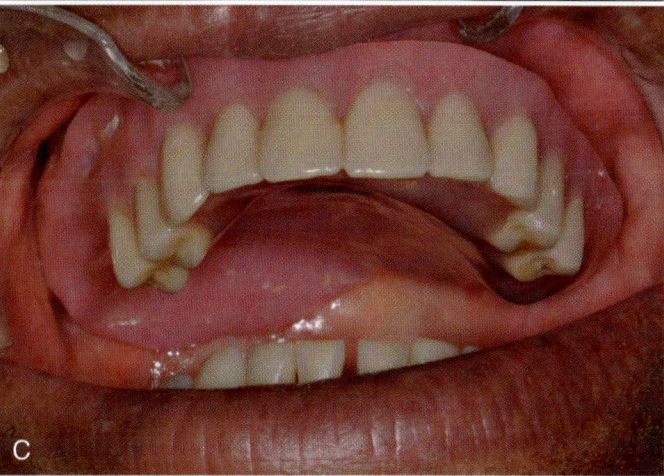

Fig. 73-1 ■ Sixty-three-year-old man in whom poorly differentiated squamous cell carcinoma of the right maxilla was diagnosed. The patient underwent maxillectomy, primary implant placement, and radiation treatment. Prosthetic reconstruction is accomplished with a bar framework (**A** and **B**) and obturator (**C**).

consideration is an important factor in cases in which direct visualization of tissue is necessary. There are also issues of maintenance. Composite free flaps can use muscle for lining the oral cavity, and on occasion, peri-implant mucosa requires surgical débridement of hyperplastic inflammatory tissue. In addition, because of a lack of innervation of the free flap, muscle will atrophy over time and require secondary impressions and relining procedures to prevent food debris from collecting under the prosthesis.

MANAGING THE HEIGHT OF THE FIBULA

The advantages of the fibula free flap have made it a "workhorse" flap for reconstruction of mandibular discontinuity defects. The length of bone that can be harvested is excellent for reconstruction

of the inferior border of the mandible and restoration of symmetry to the lower third of the face. The low donor site morbidity and the ability of a second surgical team to harvest the fibula free flap simultaneously also contribute to its favorable characteristics. Additionally, there is good to excellent bone stock for osseointegration. Because of the bicortical nature of the fibula, it possesses approximately 12 mm of bone height for endosteal implants.[14] Use of the fibula versus the iliac crest can present a geometric challenge for prosthetic reconstruction. As mentioned, the fibula is best positioned so that it reproduces the contours of the outline of the lower third of the face. This may lead to an intraoral discrepancy in height with the native mandible. Additionally, the dental arch lies lingually above the reconstruction so that implants can be positioned facial to the dental arch and the occlusal plane. There are surgical techniques to overcome this discrepancy in height. One is to position the fibula more superiorly and use the reconstruction plating system to reproduce the contours of the inferior border. Another is the "double-barrel" technique in which the fibula is folded to increase the height of the fibula free flap.[15] We have found that the height discrepancy can also be addressed through prosthetic design. The use of a bar framework designed to sit lingual to the implants can overcome the discrepancy in height and facial position. An implant-assisted removable overdenture can be constructed in a manner that promotes lip and cheek competence. The overdenture will have small fenestrations at the base of the facial flange to overcome the facial position of the implants. Resistance to cantilever forces is possible as a result of the bicortical nature of the fibula (Fig. 73-2).

These concepts can also be applied to a screw-retained fixed restoration in a dentate patient by using a cast mesostructure-superstructure design. The mesostructure is milled so that the support for the implant is centralized over the mandibular neo-ridge and the corresponding superstructure acts as a fixed partial denture that is set with screws into the mesostructure (Fig. 73-3).

The contours of the mandibular prosthesis can provide support to the lower lip for restoration of projection and symmetry of the mouth. The loss of motor function from the marginal mandibular branch of the facial nerve as a result of ablative procedures can be ameliorated with this means of lip support.

PALATOMAXILLARY RECONSTRUCTION

Surgical reconstruction of palatomaxillary defects has evolved over the past decade and emerged as a viable option for patients undergoing resection of large tumors. Although surgical closure of large palatomaxillary defects can also provide closure of the oral cavity, problems are encountered when large soft tissue flaps occupy the functional space over the tongue and are not amenable to dental reconstruction. The use of VBFFs to reconstruct large palatomaxillary defects provides surgical closure and restores the stable base of the hard palate above the alveolar process.[16] As with mandibular reconstruction, it allows the placement of dental implants for prosthetic rehabilitation. This approach optimizes function and addresses the shortcomings of an obturator. Even though an obturator can be used for successful restoration and remains a standard for prosthetic rehabilitation, as defects get larger, nasal escape can compromise speech and swallowing. Because these side effects also have implications for comfort and psychosocial interaction, surgical reconstruction of palatomaxillary defects is an excellent alternative approach to optimal functional rehabilitation.[17,18]

Our classification system essentially addresses the size and location of palatomaxillary defects and considers the biomechanical properties that contribute to prosthetic instability and compromised function.[19] The remaining dental arch and palatal shelf, as well as other components involved in anatomic retention, such as scar band

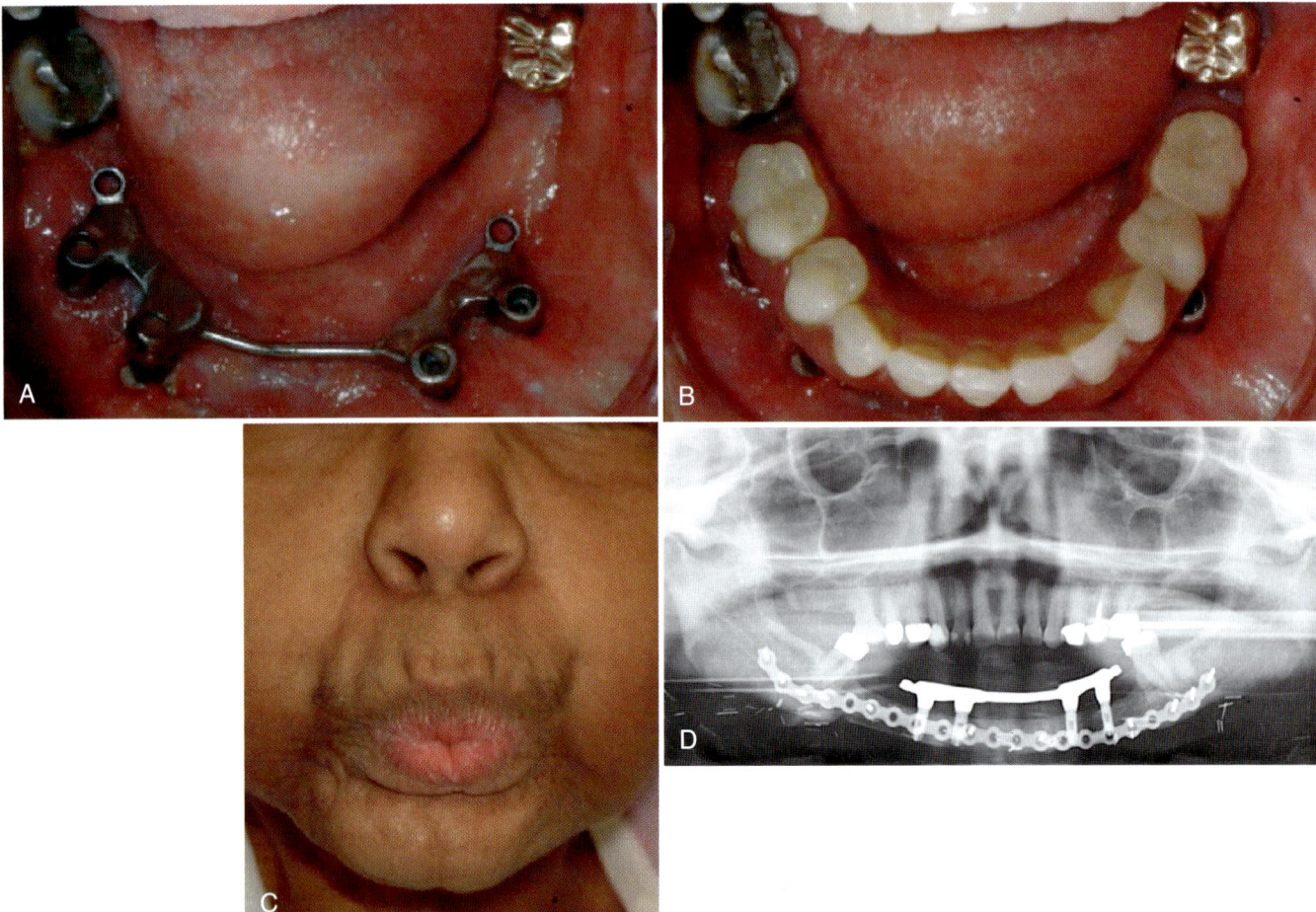

Fig. 73-2 ■ Sixty-five-year old-woman in whom adenocarcinoma of the floor of the mouth and ventral surface of the tongue was diagnosed. **A,** She underwent fibula free flap reconstruction of the mandible with osseointegrated implants and a lingual cantilevered bar framework. **B,** Implant position in relation to the facial flange of the removable overdenture. **C,** This design promotes lip and cheek competence. **D,** Panoramic view.

formation with a split-thickness skin graft (STSG), have been useful prognostic factors in treatment algorithms and, in particular, the indications for VBFF reconstruction. As the remaining dental arch shortens and the palatal surface decreases, prosthetic instability is more likely to occur (Fig. 73-4). Three categories of defects describe the horizontal nature of palatal defects. If an orbital defect is accompanied by a maxillectomy defect, surgical reconstruction should address the separation of the combined defects separately. Maxillectomy defects have the subscripts "o" for orbital floor and "z" for zygoma to address these areas in the restorative decision-making process. A class I defect is a subtotal maxillectomy defect in which there is loss of the posterior alveolus to the canine tooth. This type of defect has sufficient remaining retentive and stabilizing components. Class I defects are therefore amenable to either prosthetic obturation or surgical reconstruction with a radial forearm free flap or palatal island flap. The remaining dental arch and palate are used to provide restoration of the dental arch with a tissue-borne prosthesis. Implants in the remaining native maxilla are necessary if the dentition is hopeless or the patient is edentulous. A class II defect is a hemimaxillectomy defect extending to the midline. In class II defects, the increased size of the defect and loss of the ipsilateral canine and molar dentition make the use of a VBFF reconstruction important if the surgeon decides to not use a prosthetic obturator. A class III defect extends beyond the midline. The defect involves both canines and the ipsilateral molar dentition and results

in a bilateral defect with a poor prosthodontic prognosis (Fig. 73-5). As the maxillectomy defect increases in size and the remaining dentition and palate decreases in size, a VBFF is preferred over a fasciocutaneous free flap. Osseointegration and prosthodontic rehabilitation can restore dentoalveolar structures and occlusal contact to optimize speech and swallowing functions. Once again, a fixed-implant restoration is the authors' preference in this situation. Treatment planning involves more implants rather than a minimum number for support of a restoration. In the event of implant failure, prosthetic success can still be achieved with a shorter restoration of the dental arch or an implant-assisted overdenture without added time or surgery.

COMPUTER PLANNING

Computer planning software and computer-aided design have ushered in a new way of thinking and new approaches to implant-assisted prosthetic reconstruction. Rapid prototyping is an automated process in which construction is accomplished with a three-dimensional printer, stereolithography machines, and laser-driven polymerization or sintering devices. Advanced digital technology can create accurate models from three-dimensional imaging data or can be applied to the fabrication of surgical templates with the aid of software programs. The software programs allow the use of virtual surgery for preoperative planning, and these data are then

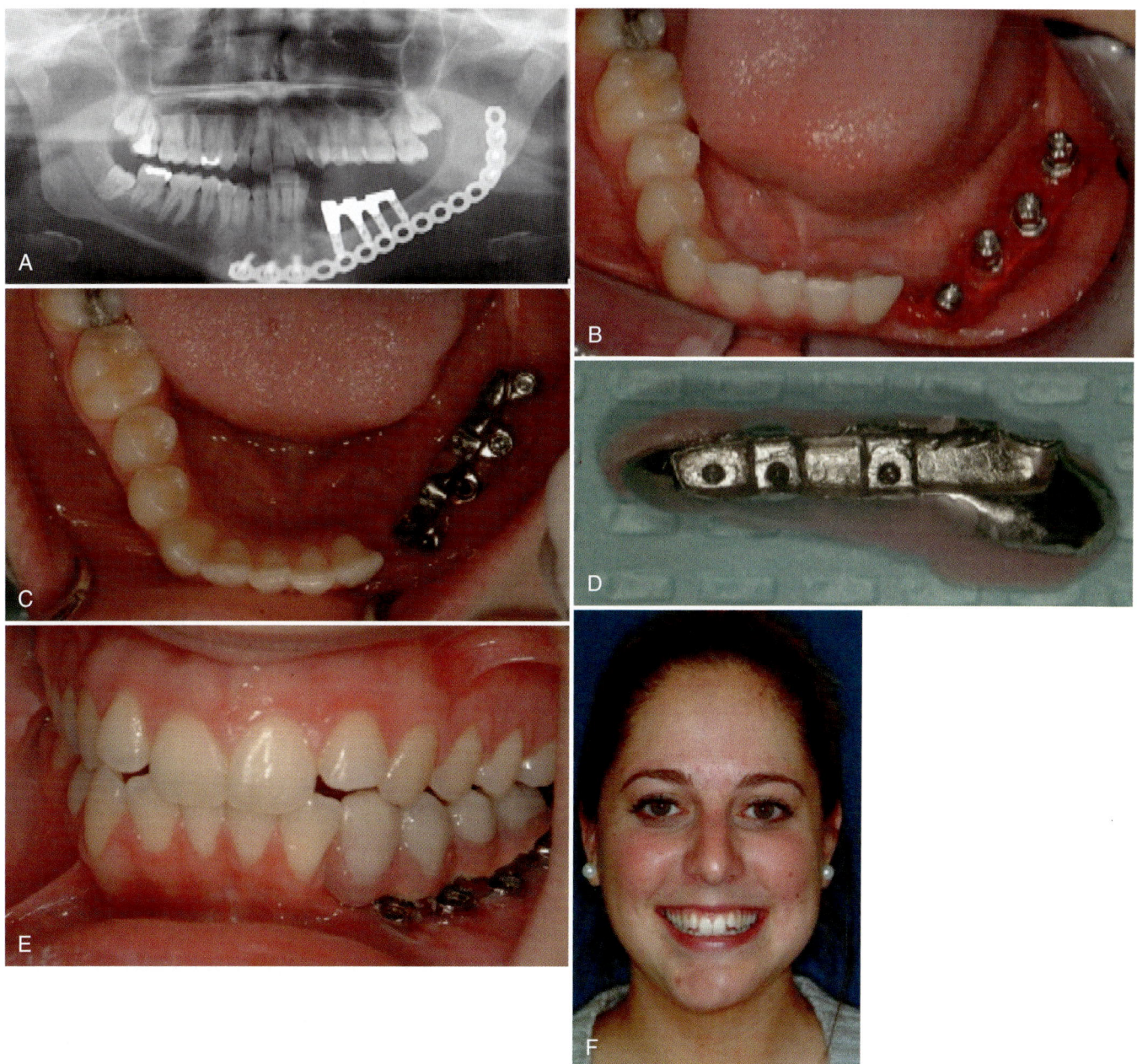

Fig. 73-3 ■ A, Twenty-one-year-old woman after resection of a benign tumor of the left mandible and reconstruction with cortical cancellous iliac crest free grafts and platelet-rich plasma (**B**). Implants are indexed with polymer resin before making the impression. The cast mesostructure is cantilevered lingually (**A** and **C**) so that the corresponding superstructure replaces the dentition in a normal occlusal relationship (**D** and **E**). **F,** Esthetic restoration respecting the symmetry of the lower third of the face.

translated to surgery via the template. For implant placement, this approach is prosthetically driven and computed tomography (CT) studies are obtained with a radiographic scanning appliance. The appliance is fabricated from a mixture of polymethylmethacrylate and barium sulfate so that the position of the dentition and their surfaces are captured in the CT scan. The scanning appliance is fabricated from the duplication of a diagnostic wax-up or interim prosthesis. Three-dimensional simulation software provides the panoramic, axial, and horizontal planes for performing accurate virtual placement of the implant with selected dimensions and sizes according to bone availability.[20] The implants are positioned so that they avoid vital structures and safety is ensured (Fig. 73-6). The angulation of the fixtures is such that their screw access is confined to the occlusal surface, which is desirable for a screw-retained

restoration, rather than perforating esthetic facial surfaces. Prosthetic design considerations are part of the computer planning stage because the tooth position is visualized. A computer-aided manufactured surgical template is fabricated by a process involving stereo-lithography and rapid prototyping techniques. CT-derived implant surgical templates can be designed so that they are supported by a tooth, mucosa, or bone. Confidence in the accuracy and position of the implants also allows them to be placed without raising soft tissue off the periosteum. A tooth-supported surgical template has clinical significance in free flap reconstruction because the subperiosteal blood supply does not need to be disturbed with this transmucosal approach. In addition, postoperative tenderness, pain, and swelling can be minimized with this less invasive surgery.[21] If the angulation and position of the implants are accurate, a restoration can be

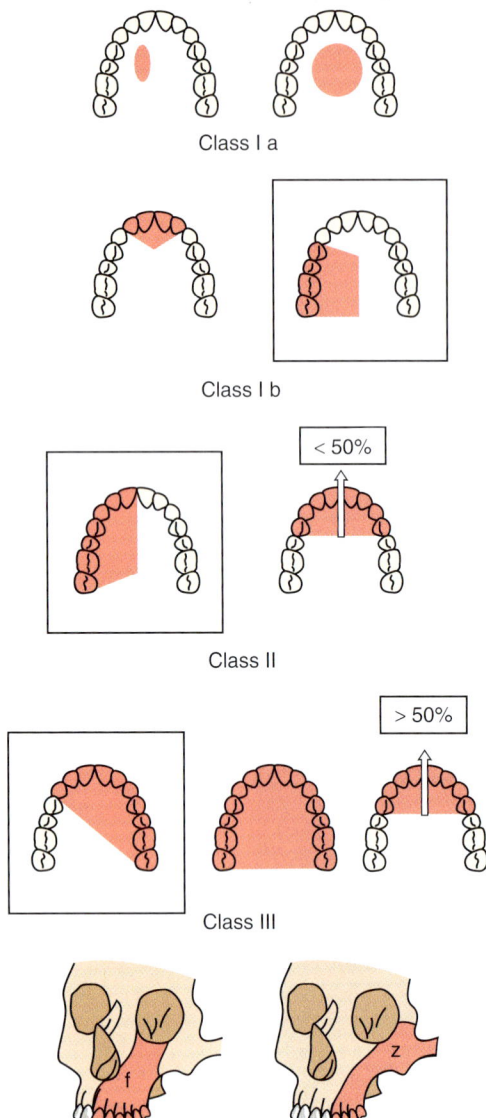

Class I a

Class I b

< 50%

Class II

> 50%

Class III

Fig. 73-4 ■ Classification of surgical reconstruction of palatomaxillary defects. Separate subscripts for extension of the defect to the floor of the orbit (f) and zygoma (z) should be addressed through surgical reconstruction. The defects are classified to assist in selecting the appropriate soft tissue (class I) and vascularized bone free flap reconstruction (class II, III). (Redrawn from Okay DJ, Genden E, Buchbinder D, et al: Prosthetic guidelines for surgical reconstruction of the maxilla: a classification of defects, *J Prosthet Dent* 86:352-363, 2001.)

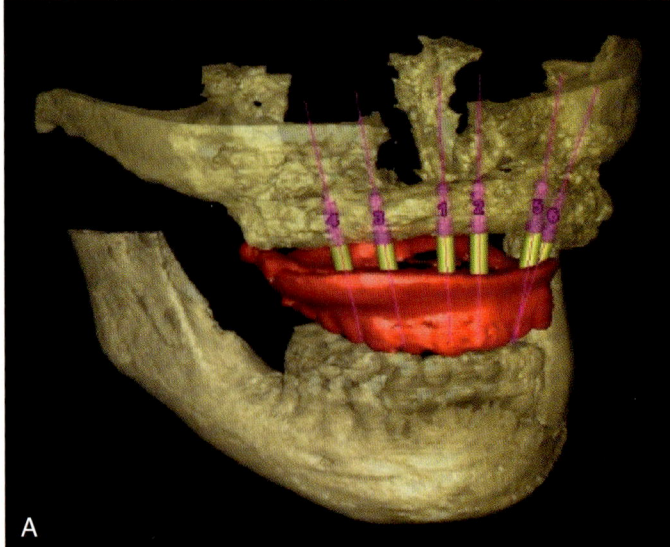

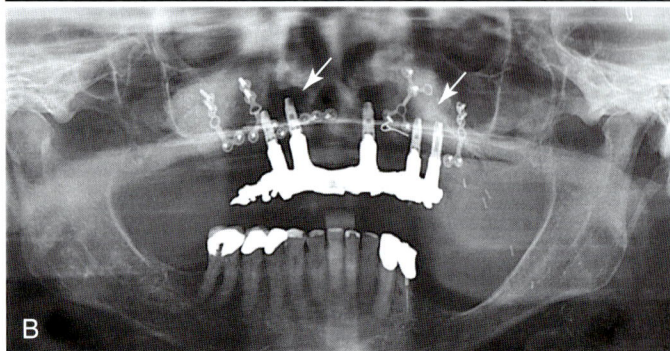

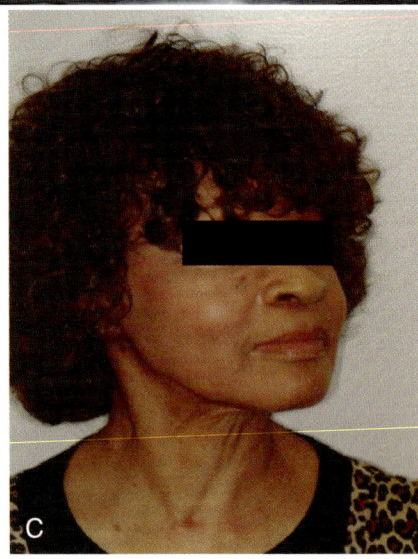

Fig. 73-5 ■ Seventy-four-year-old woman after fibula free flap reconstruction of the maxilla (class III). **A,** Three-dimensional reconstruction of the computer-generated plan for implant placement shows the radiographic scanning appliance and angulation of the implants. Identification of the plating system and screws in the planning stage facilitates placement of the implant with a bone-supported surgical template. **B,** Cast framework of the fixed implant restoration in place. **C,** Restoration of symmetry and projection of the mid-face.

fabricated immediately and used for prosthetic reconstruction, provided that the restoration is protected from any occlusal force and the primary implant stability exceeds 20 Ncm.[22-27] This procedure can be performed because of the absence of a bloody field and predetermined orientation of the angulation of the implant to the denture teeth. Patient selection is critical for success; those with questionable bone quality or availability should be avoided (Fig. 73-7).

Computer planning has been helpful and impressive as a means of facilitating implant surgery and reconstructive techniques. In our clinical setting, its use is considered routine for prosthetic restorations and VBFF surgical reconstruction of maxillomandibular defects. In some patients, the position of the vascular pedicle may not be conducive to primary placement, and thus secondary implant placement may be more beneficial. In the absence of postoperative radiation therapy, secondary placement of implants with computer

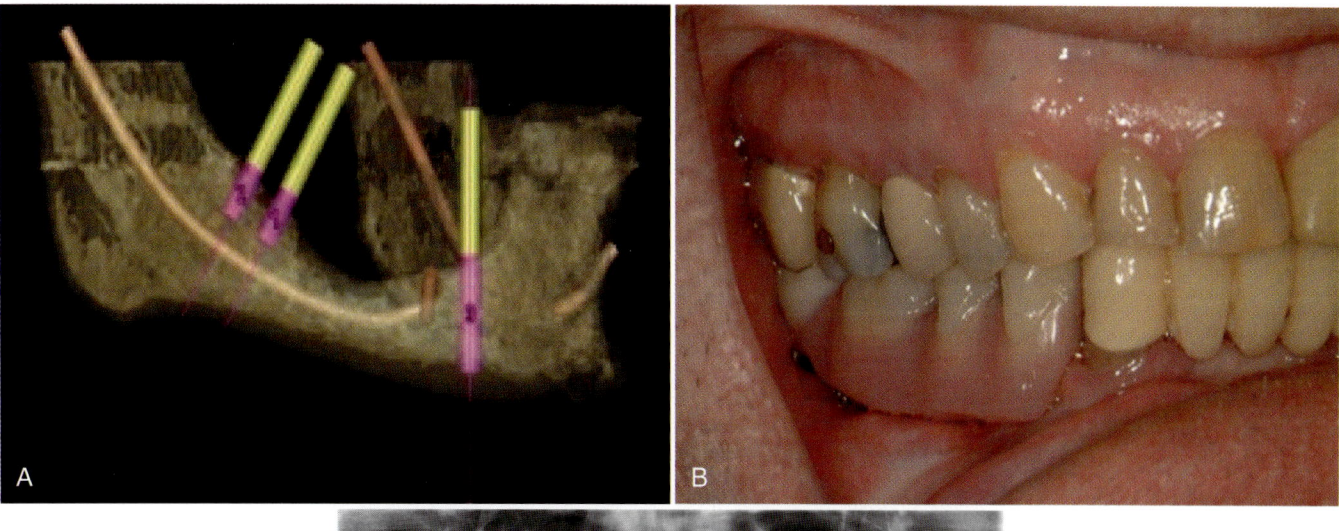

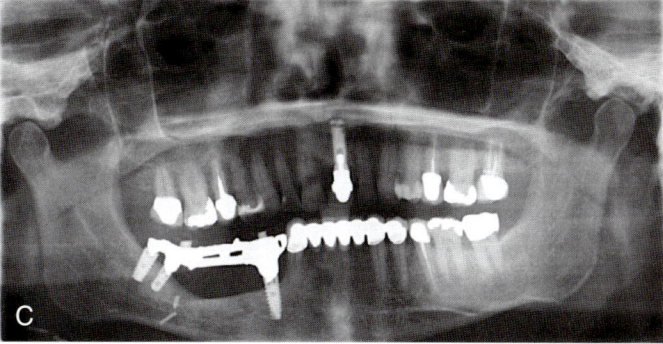

Fig. 73-6 ■ Eighty-year-old man after right marginal mandibulectomy for squamous cell carcinoma of the gingiva. Computer planning (**A**) identifies the inferior alveolar canal for osseointegration and a fixed screw-retained restoration (**B** and **C**).

planning is a progressive approach toward prosthetic reconstruction. The accuracy provided by computer planning can be exploited 4 to 6 weeks after VBFF reconstruction. Soft tissue modification or debulking procedures can be performed at the time of implant placement as well. Reconstruction plating systems can be avoided with virtual implant surgery, or a decision can be made to remove plating structures that may interfere with placing a sufficient number of implants for a fixed restoration. In this situation, implant surgery is performed once bony union of the VBFF osteotomies is established, approximately 8 weeks after surgical reconstruction, and a bone-supported CT-derived surgical template is used.

CRANIOFACIAL PROSTHETICS

The desirability of prosthetic reconstruction, whether it be auricular, orbital, or nasal, should be determined at the early stages of treatment planning and communicated thoughtfully to the patient so that the use of prosthetics versus surgical reconstruction with the patient's own tissue can be determined. There is always the option to not treat the defect with a prosthesis because of its artificial or foreign nature. There is also the prospect of rejecting surgery if multiple procedures are necessary for reconstruction. Surgical reconstruction of the external ear and nose has limitations, however, and when addressing subtotal defects in these areas, patients are likely to accept asymmetric results with native tissue over a prosthetic solution. It is for this reason that subtotal defects of the nose are not as frequently evaluated for prosthetic reconstruction. Patients who undergo orbital exenteration may choose to not have the orbit reconstructed because of the static nature of a prosthesis in replacing a dynamic organ.

Pre-prosthetic surgery can enhance prosthetic restorations. Interdisciplinary planning and preparation of the defect for prosthetic reconstruction will save time for patients. This includes the use of craniofacial implants for auricular, nasal, and orbital defects, in addition to the general principles applied to facial sites. The bone margins should be smoothed and unsupported tissue remnants removed. Tissue transfer with fasciocutaneous free flaps or a pedicled flap to repair a defect is limited by the space for prosthetic material.

Craniofacial implants allow prosthetic reconstructions to be more effective than adhesive-retained prosthetics. The implants are placed in an atraumatic protocol. Their design is suited for the facial skeleton. The fixtures are 3 or 4 mm in length and 3.75 mm in width and have a wide flange at the head of the implant for support and stability. Use of a drill guide and the flange design prevent inadvertent injury to the dura.[28,29] Predictable placement is achieved with implants in the temporal bone for auricular prosthetics. Implants in the orbital rim or nasion/glabella of the frontal bone have been associated with higher failure rates because of less vascular bone in these areas.[30-34] Craniofacial implants benefit from the hyperbaric oxygen protocol in patients who have undergone radiotherapy for treatment of cancer.[11] Coordination of primary implant placement can greatly diminish overall treatment time for implant-assisted prosthetic reconstruction.

Reproducible orientation of the prosthesis by the use of implant bars or magnets contributes to margins that are well adapted. The prosthesis is fabricated from silicone polymer materials, and oil-based pigments and nylon flocking provide its intrinsic and extrinsic characteristics. An esthetic result improves

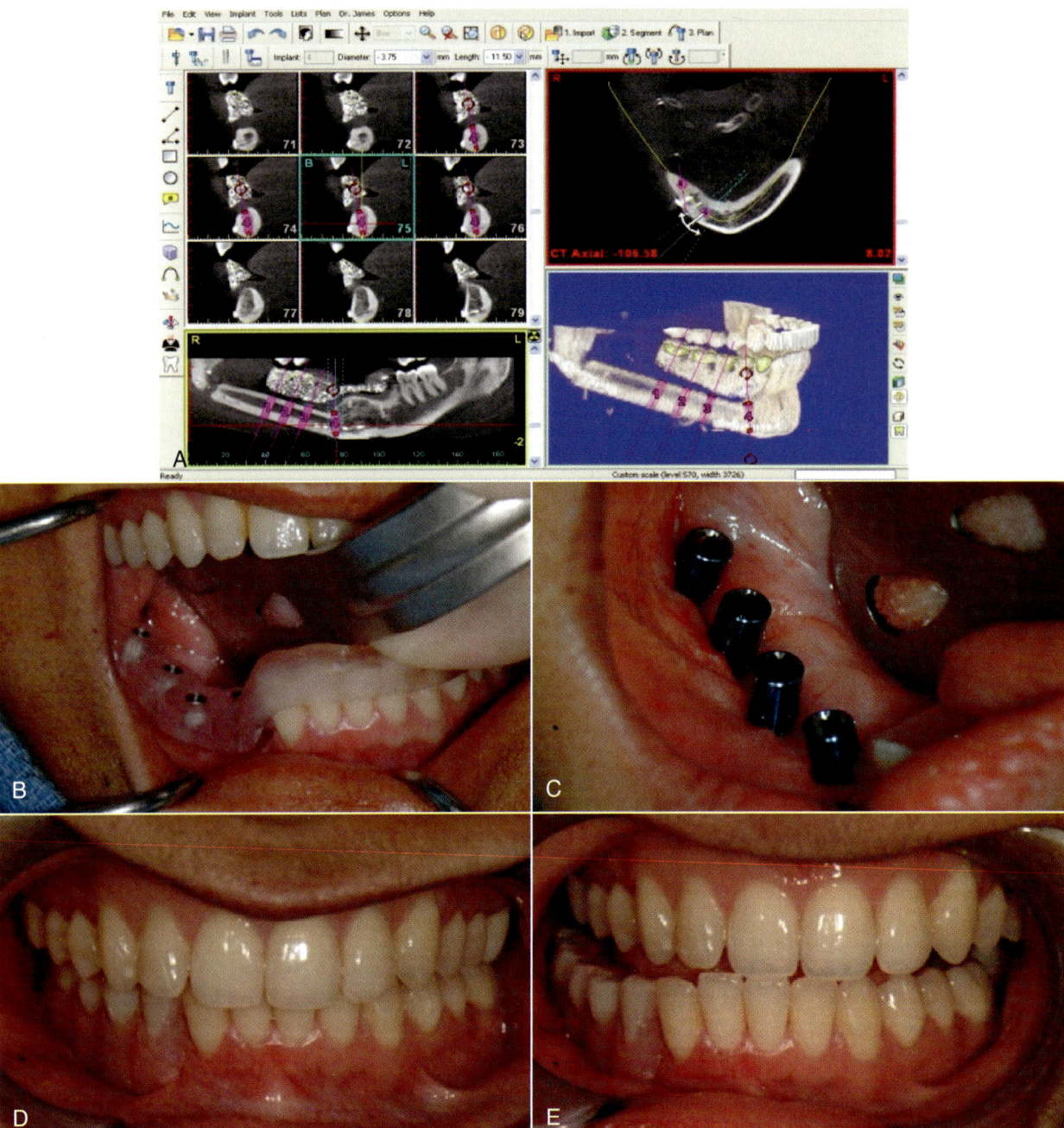

Fig. 73-7 ■ Computer planning for a 26-year-old with fibula free flap reconstruction of the right mandible for malignant squamous cell carcinoma. **A,** Implants are planned with a radiographic scanning appliance. **B,** Computed tomography–derived surgical template supported in place by a tooth. **C,** Implants placed via a transmucosal approach. **D** and **E,** Immediate restoration screw retained with no occlusal contact at the maximum intercuspation and excursive movement of the mandible.

the likelihood of a successful restoration, acceptable patient appearance, and improved quality of life. Techniques using a urethane line prosthesis may further enhance the appearance of margins by making them as thin as possible while possessing good tear strength.[35]

A satisfactory outcome is achieved by careful planning of the number, position, and angulation of the implants. Craniofacial implants eliminate the adverse skin reactions associated with adhesives and will improve hygiene and maintenance. However, careful maintenance by the patient and follow-up are necessary to prevent skin reactions around the implant.[36] Patient education

with specific instructions for hygiene and maintenance will help minimize problems with peri-implant inflammation. The silicone polymer materials used for facial prostheses do have limited longevity. Ultraviolet light, patient handling, staining, tearing, and fatigue contribute to discoloration and failure of a prosthesis.[37]

Implant-assisted craniofacial prosthetics are a reliable treatment option for the restoration of defects related to congenital disorders, trauma, and ablative surgery. However, aftercare is necessary and a new prosthesis may be required within a few years.[38]

Further descriptions and recommendations are outlined in the following sections for auricular, nasal, and orbital defects.

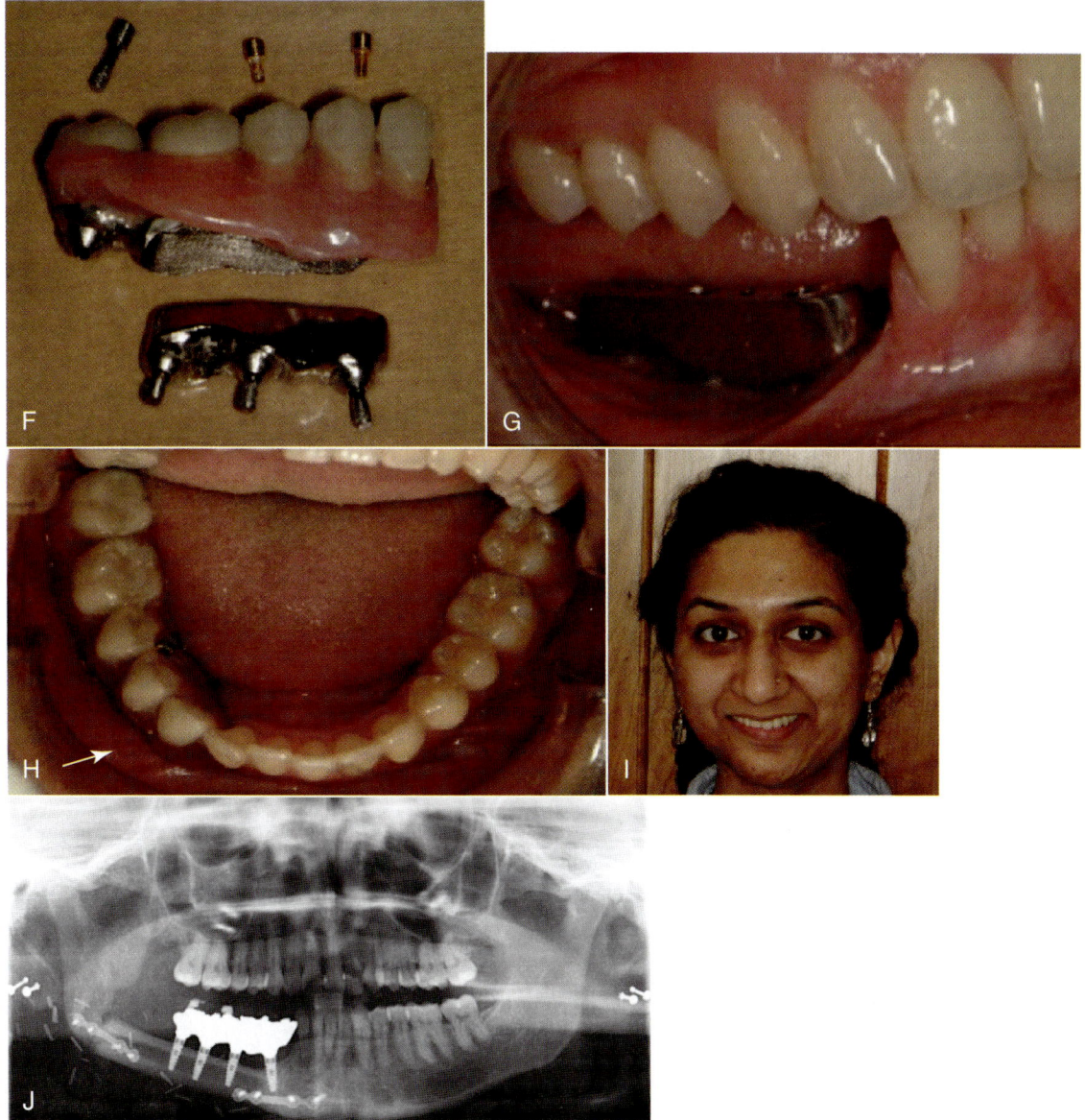

Fig. 73-7, cont'd ▪ **F** and **G**, Definitive restoration using a cast mesostructure to negotiate the difference in height. **H** and **I**, Superstructure in place with facial contour to support the lower lip after loss of the marginal mandibular branch of the facial nerve. **J**, Panoramic view of the definitive restoration in place.

AURICULAR

After ablative procedures resulting in subtotal and total defects are performed, an STSG can be used to help close the defect and create a firm tissue bed for prosthetic reconstruction. If the tragus can be maintained, it will help camouflage the prosthetic margins. Two implants are recommended because of high osseointegration success rates. A bar framework is frequently used for retentive purposes. Proper connection to the prosthesis takes multiple visits and involves procedures to obtain an accurate sectional moulage and master cast.[39] A sculpture for the prosthesis can be improved with the use of medical models and rapid prototyping techniques.[40-45] Computer software with segmentation, mirroring, and subtraction applications allows reproduction of the contours on the contralateral side to the defect. Application of advanced digital technology is effective for the fabrication of auricular prosthetics. Implant placement can be planned with software, and a CT-derived surgical template can be

fabricated. Examination of the temporal bone under the internal aspect of the helix is helpful for planning the prosthetic reconstruction (Fig. 73-8).

NASAL

Patients who undergo total rhinectomy can be reconstructed with an implant-assisted nasal prosthesis. All bone margins should be smoothed and rounded at the conclusion of the ablative procedure. If possible, the anterior nasal spine should be spared. Normal lip position can be maintained by placing an STSG along the inferior aspect of the defect. An implant can be placed at the superior aspect of the defect. The nasal bones need to be removed for access to implantable bone. Implants can also be placed in the maxilla along the nasal sill; however, one implant can suffice for reconstruction. Either a bar framework or magnet can be used. A cantilevered bar can be used for reconstruction because of the absence of excessive

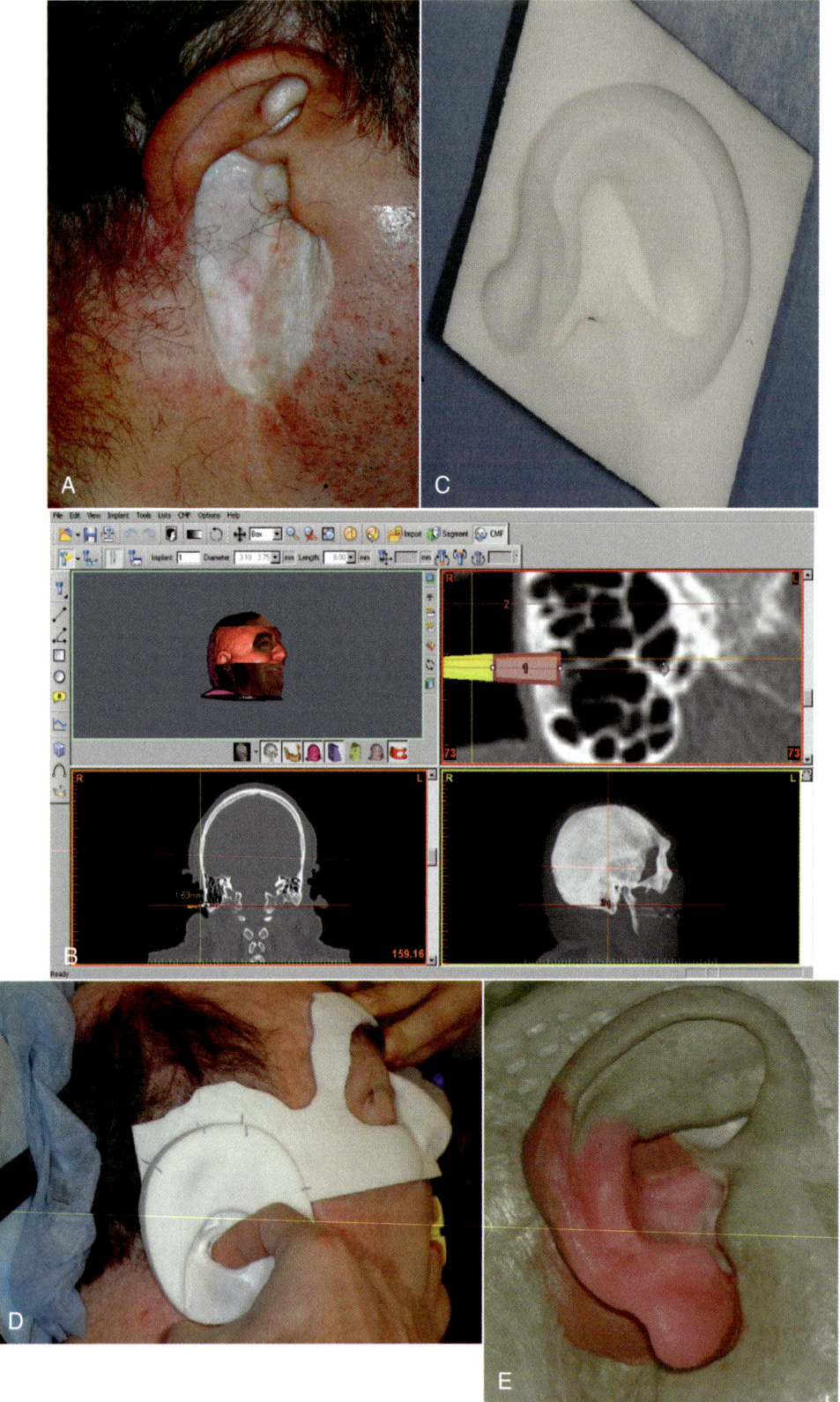

Fig. 73-8 ■ Sixty-six-year-old man after subtotal resection of a basal cell carcinoma. **A,** A split-thickness skin graft is in place and the tragus is intact. **B,** Computer planning for placement of the implant and prosthetic reconstruction of the right auricular defect. **C** and **D,** Surgical template and medical model fabricated with stereolithography and rapid prototyping techniques. **E,** Sculpture completed before investment into stone molds and processing with silicone polymer material.

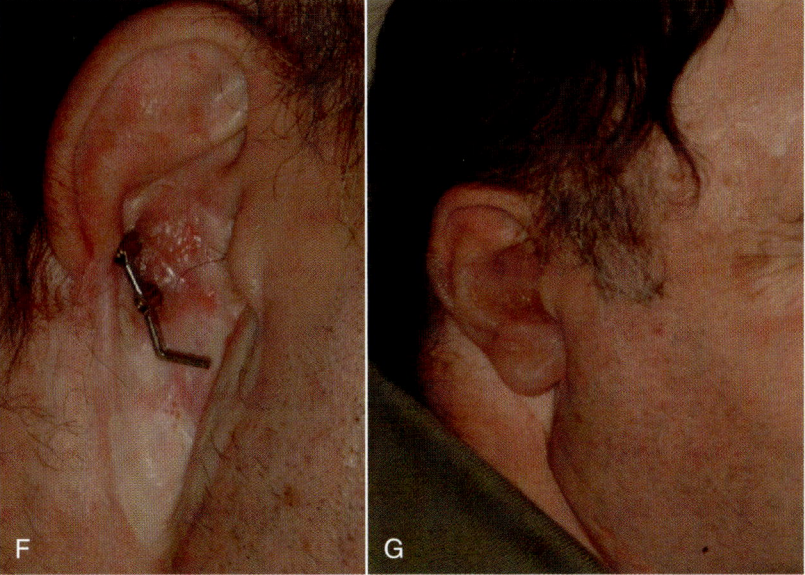

Fig. 73-8, cont'd ■ **F,** Cast titanium bar in place to retain the prosthetic reconstruction. **G,** Implant-assisted prosthetic reconstruction of the subtotal auricular defect.

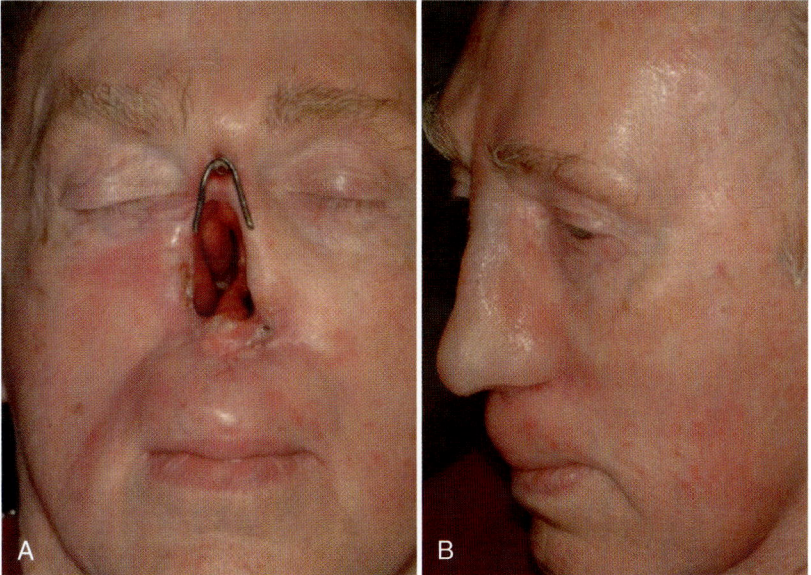

Fig. 73-9 ■ Seventy-three-year-old man in whom recurrent squamous cell carcinoma was diagnosed. The patient underwent total rhinectomy. Implant placement occurs before radiation therapy. **A,** One implant in the nasion/glabella is secured with a bar framework. The silicone prosthesis is clipped into place. **B,** This reproducibility of the position of the prosthesis improves adaptation of the margins and esthetics.

loading force. Nasal prostheses are fabricated "hollow" to maintain the airway. Their form can be well captured in the sculpture of the prosthesis and the superior margins hidden underneath eyeglasses (Fig. 73-9).

ORBIT

Attention to not overbulk the surgical site is important if a facial prosthesis is planned. An STSG can be used to line the defect. Orbital defects with bony structures intact can have an STSG placed to line the cavity. This allows the prosthesis to contact the tissue at the depth of the defect. Radiation status may prevent the use of an STSG in favor of a fasciocutaneous flap. Reconstruction of the orbit

is indicated to improve the appearance of the prosthesis and minimize the defect extending into the face.

Two or three implants in the superior lateral border of the orbit are sufficient for an orbital prosthesis. Magnetic attachments are commonly used to overcome the conflicting paths of the implants along the perimeter of the orbit (Fig. 73-10). During fabrication of the prosthesis, conjugation of the pupils from the ocular component is critical for appearance. The ocular component is fabricated from acrylic resin and connected to an acrylic resin framework with magnets on the tissue surface. Hours of labor are needed for orbital prosthetic reconstruction because of technical, coloring, and clinical considerations.

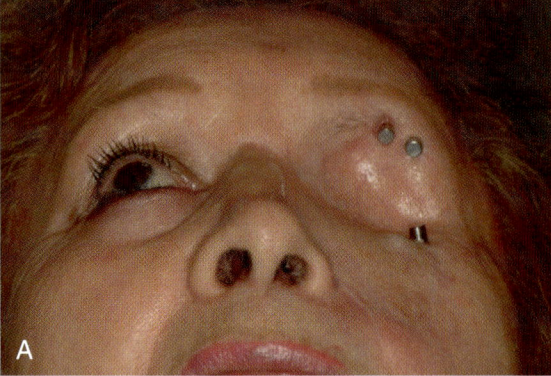

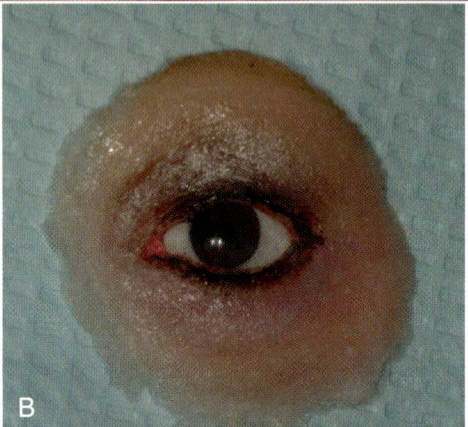

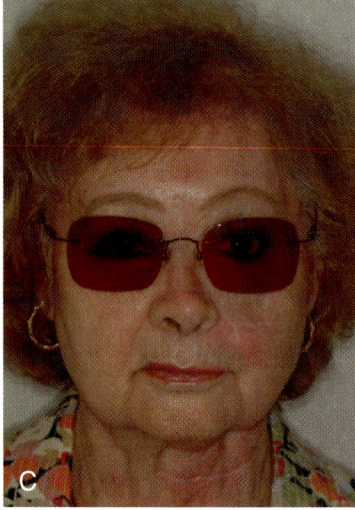

Fig. 73-10 ■ Eighty-two-year-old woman with squamous cell carcinoma extending from the left orbit to the nasal cavity and inferior orbital rim. Radial forearm free flap reconstruction with calvarial bone grafts was performed for dorsal nose projection. Primary implant placement takes advantage of the vascularity before radiation therapy. Magnetic abutments in place (**A**) for retention of the orbital prosthesis (**B**). **C,** Tinted eyeglasses used to camouflage the margins and static nature of the prosthetic reconstruction.

PEARLS AND PITFALLS

- The primary objective of prosthetic rehabilitation is to restore and improve speech and swallowing function. Contemporary management of patients with head and neck cancer involves the integration of surgical reconstructive techniques using vascularized, bone-containing flaps with prosthetic rehabilitation to optimize function and esthetics.
- Preservation of tongue motion and restoration of tongue volume are critical to achieve a favorable functional outcome if the tumor extends to the tongue or floor of the mouth. Soft tissue defects involving the overlying skin or mucosal defects involving the lip or cheek, as well as sensory and motor nerve deficits, must be taken into account when deciding on the best reconstructive option that will result in an acceptable level of functional recovery.
- Placement of implants in the immediate surgical setting will shorten the overall treatment time for definitive prosthetic restoration and take advantage of the well-vascularized bed for osseointegration before radiation therapy.
- The decision for fixed versus removable prosthetic restorations is dependent on clinical factors such as the availability of bone, the number and position of implants to assist or support restorations, maintenance of hygiene, and manual dexterity. Palatal obturators for maxillectomy patients or palatal augmentation prostheses to restore lingual-palatal contact for glossectomy patients are usually removable appliances. If tumor surveillance is also a consideration, a removable prosthesis may be indicated.
- Management of the discrepancy in height between the native mandible and fibula can be challenging. Surgical techniques to overcome this height discrepancy include positioning the fibula more superiorly and using a reconstruction plating system to reproduce the contours of the inferior border. Another option is the "double-barrel" technique in which the fibula is folded to increase the height of the fibula free flap. We have found that that the discrepancy in height can also be addressed through prosthetic design by using a cast mesostructure-superstructure design. A milled mesostructure is used to make up some of the height deficiency and to ensure that support for the implant is centralized over the mandibular neo-ridge, and the corresponding superstructure acts as a fixed partial denture that is set with screws into the mesostructure.
- The contours of the mandibular prosthesis can provide support to the lower lip for restoration of projection and symmetry of the mouth. The loss of motor function from the marginal mandibular branch of the facial nerve as a result of ablative procedures can be ameliorated with this means of lip support.
- The use of vascularized bone free flaps to reconstruct large palatomaxillary defects provides surgical closure and restores a stable infrastructure (alveolar process) to allow placement of dental implants for prosthetic rehabilitation. This approach optimizes function and addresses the shortcomings of an obturator.
- Craniofacial implants allow prosthetic reconstruction to be more effective than adhesive-retained prosthetics. Implant-assisted craniofacial prosthetics are a reliable treatment option for the restoration of defects related to congenital disorders, trauma, and ablative surgery.
- Computer planning software and computer-aided design have ushered in a new way of thinking that has resulted in a prosthetically driven approach to implant-assisted postablative functional reconstruction.

REFERENCES

1. Urken ML, Buchbinder D, Weinberg H, et al: Functional evaluation following microvascular oromandibular reconstruction of the oral cancer patient: a comparative study of reconstructed and nonreconstructed patients, *Laryngoscope* 101:935-950, 1991.

2. Leung AC, Cheung LK: Dental implants in reconstructed jaws: patients' evaluation of functional and quality-of-life outcomes,

Int J Oral Maxillofac Implants 18:127-134, 2003.

3. Schmelzeisen R, Neukam FW, Shirota T, et al: Postoperative function after implant insertion in vascularized bone grafts in maxilla and mandible, *Plast Reconstr Surg* 97:719-725, 1996.

4. Urken ML, Bridger AG, Zur KB: The scapular osteofasciocutaneous flap: a 12 year experience, *Arch Otolaryngol Head Neck Surg* 127:862-869, 2001.

5. Hidalgo DA: Fibula free flap; a new method for mandible reconstruction, *Plast Reconstr Surg* 84:71-79, 1989.

6. Genden EM, Okay D, Buchbinder D, et al: Iliac crest internal oblique osteomusculocutaneous free-flap reconstruction of the postablative palatomaxillary defect, *Otolaryngol Head Neck Surg* 127:854-861, 2001.

7. Frodel JL, Funk GF, Capper DT, et al: Osseointegrated implants: a comparative study of bone thickness in four vascularized bone flaps, *Plast Reconstr Surg* 92:449-455, 1993.

8. Brånemark PI: Osseointegration and its experimental background, *J Prosthet Dent* 50:399-410, 1983.

9. Urken ML, Buchbinder D, Weinberg H, et al: Primary placement of osseointegrated implants in microvascular mandibular reconstruction, *Otolaryngol Head Neck Surg* 101: 56-73, 1989.

10. Marx RE: A new concept in the treatment of osteoradionecrosis, *J Oral Maxillofac Surg* 41:351-357, 1983.

11. Granstrom G, Jacobsson M, Tjellstrom A: Titanium implants in irradiated tissue: benefits from hyperbaric oxygen, *Int J Oral Maxillofac Surg* 7:15-35, 1992.

12. Rieger J, Wolfaardt J, Jha N, et al: Maxillary obturators: the relationship between patient satisfaction and speech outcome, *Head Neck* 25:895-903, 2003.

13. Rieger J, Wolfaardt J, Seikaly H, et al: Speech outcomes in patients rehabilitated with maxillary obturator prostheses after maxillectomy: a prospective study, *Int J Prosthodont* 15:139-144, 2002.

14. Moscoso JF, Keller J, Genden E, et al: Vascularized bone flaps in oromandibular reconstruction. A comparative anatomic study of bone stock from various donor sites to assess suitability for enosseous dental implants, *Arch Otolaryngol Head Neck Surg* 120:36-43, 1994.

15. Bahr W, Stoll P, Wachter R: Use of the "double barrel" free vascularized fibula for mandible reconstruction, *J Oral Maxillofac Surg* 56:38-44, 1998.

16. Brown J: Deep circumflex iliac artery free flap with internal oblique muscle as a new method of immediate reconstruction of the maxillectomy defect, *Head Neck* 18:412-421, 1996.

17. Genden E, Wallace D, Okay D, et al: Reconstruction of the hard palate using the radial forearm free flap: indications and outcomes, *Head Neck* 26:808-814, 2004.

18. Genden EM, Okay D, Stepp MT, et al: Comparison of functional and quality of life outcomes in patients with and without palatomaxillary reconstruction: a preliminary report, *Arch Otolaryngol Head Neck Surg* 129:775-780, 2003.

19. Okay DJ, Genden E, Buchbinder D, et al: Prosthodontic guidelines for surgical reconstruction of the maxilla: a classification system of defects, *J Prosthet Dent* 86:352-363, 2001.

20. DiGiacomo GA, Cury PR, de Arajo N, et al: Clinical application of stereolithographic surgical guides for implant placement: preliminary results, *J Periodontol* 76:503-507, 2005.

21. Nkenke E, Eitner S, Radespiel-Tröger M, et al: Patient-centered outcomes comparing transmucosal implant placement with an open approach in the maxilla: a prospective, non-randomized pilot study, *Clin Oral Implants Res* 18:197-203, 2007.

22. Luongo G, Di Raimondo R, Fillippini P, et al: Early loading of sandblasted, acid etched implants in the posterior maxilla and mandible: a 1 year follow-up report from a multi-center 3 year prospective study, *Int J Oral Maxillofac Implants* 20:84-91, 2005.

23. Vanden Bogaerde L, Peddretti G, Dellacasa P, et al: Early function of splinted implants in maxillas and posterior mandibles using Brånemark Ti Unite implants: an 18-month prospective clinical multicenter study, *Clin Implant Dent Relat Res* 6:121-129, 2004.

24. Cornelini R, Cangini F, Covani U, et al: Immediate loading of implants with 3 unit fixed partial dentures: 12 month clinical study, *Int J Oral Maxilofac Implants* 21:914-918, 2006.

25. Schincaglia G, Marzola R, Scapoli C, et al: Immediate loading of dental implants supporting fixed partial dentures in the posterior mandible: a randomized controlled split mouth study—machined versus titanium oxide implant surface, *Int J Oral Maxillofac Implants* 22:35-46, 2007.

26. Ormianer Z, Paiti A, Shifman A: Survival of immediately loaded implants in deficient alveolar bone sites augmented with beta-tricalcium phosphate, *Implant Dent* 15:395-403, 2006.

27. Del Fabbreo M, Testori T, Francettti L, et al: Systemic review of survival rates for immediately loaded dental implants, *Int J Periodontics Restorative Dent* 26:249-263, 2006.

28. Parel SM, Holt R, Brånemark P-I, et al: Osseointegration and facial prosthetics, *Int J Oral Maxillofac Implants* 1:27-29, 1986.

29. Parel S, Tjellström A: The United States and Swedish experience with osseointegration and facial prostheses, *Int J Oral Maxillofac Implants* 6:75-79, 1991.

30. Jacobsson M, Tjellström A, Fine L, et al: Retrospective study of osseointegrated skin-penetrating titanium fixture used for retaining facial prostheses, *Int J Oral Maxillofac Implants* 7:523-528, 1992.

31. Wolfaardt JF, Wilkes GH, Parel SM, et al: Craniofacial osseointegration: the Canadian experience, *Int J Oral Maxillofac Implants* 8:197-204, 1993.

32. Roumanas E, Nishimura RD, Beumer J, et al: Craniofacial defects and osseointegrated implants: six-year follow-up report on the success rates of craniofacial implants at UCLA, *Int J Oral Maxillofac Implants* 9:579-585, 1994.

33. Nishimura RD, Roumanas E, Moy PK, et al: Osseointegrated implants and orbital defects: U.C.L.A. experience, *J Prosthet Dent* 79:304-309, 1998.

34. Nishimura RD, Roumanas E, Moy PK, et al: Nasal defects and osseointegrated implants: UCLA experience, *J Prosthet Dent* 76:579-602, 1996.

35. Udagama A: Urethane-lined silicone facial prostheses, *J Prosthet Dent* 58:351-354, 1987.

36. Holgers KM, Tjellström A, Bjursten LM, et al: Soft tissue reactions around percutaneous implants: a clinical study on skin-penetrating titanium implants used for bone-anchored auricular prostheses, *Int Oral Maxillofac Implants* 2:225-228, 1987.

37. Andres CJ, Haug SP, Munoz CA, et al: Effects of environmental factors on maxillofacial elastomers. Part I—literature review, *J Prosthet Dent* 68:327-330, 1992.

38. Visser A, Raghoebar GM, van Oort RP, et al: Fate of implant-retained craniofacial prostheses: life span and aftercare, *Int J Oral Maxillofac Implants* 23:89-98, 2008.

39. Wolfaardt JF, Coss P, Levesque R: Craniofacial osseointegration: technique of bar and acrylic resin substructure construction for auricular prostheses, *J Prosthet Dent* 76:603-607, 1996.

40. Sykes LM, Parrott AM, Owen CP, et al: Applications of rapid prototyping technology in maxillofacial prosthetics, *Int J Prosthodont* 17:454-459, 2004.

41. Jiao T, Zhang F, Huang X, et al: Design and fabrication of auricular prostheses by CAD/CAM system, *Int J Prosthodont* 17:460-463, 2004.

42. Subburaj K, Nair C, Rajesh S, et al: Rapid development of auricular prosthesis using CAD and rapid prototyping technologies, *Int J Oral Maxillofac Surg* 36:938-943, 2007.

43. Runte C, Dirksen D, Deleré H, et al: Optical data acquisition for computer-assisted design of facial prostheses, *Int J Prosthodont* 15:129-132, 2002.

44. Cheah CM, Chua CK, Tan KH: Integration of laser surface digitizing with CAD/CAM techniques for developing facial prostheses. Part 2: development of molding techniques for casting prosthetic parts, *Int J Prothodont* 16:543-548, 2003.

45. Eggbeer D, Bibb R, Evans P: Toward identifying specification requirements for digital bone-anchored prosthesis design incorporating substructure fabrication: a pilot study, *Int J Prosthodont* 19:258-263, 2006.

THE PAST

During much of the second half of the twentieth century, most dentofacial deformities were managed by repositioning the mandible alone, regardless of the location of the deformity (maxilla or mandible), via transcervical approaches, and utilizing skeletal wires and long periods of maxillo-mandibular fixation to achieve bony healing. Even as maxillary surgery became more wide spread and the biological basis of all orthognathic procedures was developed, treatment was characterized by unpredictable movements and skeletal instability in both the long and short term.

THE PRESENT

Advances in rigid internal fixation are primarily responsible for the high level of predictability and skeletal stability that is associated with modern orthognathic surgical procedures. Procedures of the maxilla, mandible, and chin are often combined with each other based upon the individual deformity and are performed on an outpatient basis, and are virtually always performed via a transoral approach. Postoperative recovery and a rapid return to function is facilitated by avoiding long periods of maxillo-mandibular fixation. As five decades of experience has been elucidated, combined surgical and orthodontic techniques have been refined, so as to optimize the functional and esthetic outcomes and minimize morbidity.

THE FUTURE

Persistent problems with long orthodontic treatment times, difficulties with controlling tooth movements, and inaccuracies in analytical model surgery will be vastly improved in the near future. Modern techniques that combine the use of plates and screws to achieve skeletal orthodontic anchorage will be refined, their efficacy established, and indications defined. Orthognathic surgical procedures will be planned using three-dimensional computer programs based upon cone beam computed tomography imaging. The virtual plan will be transferred to the patient using computer-aided design/computer aided modeling (CAD/CAM) splints and guide stents, which will completely replace the plaster casts and analytic model surgery used today. Finally, currently available titanium plates and screws will be replaced by biodegradable fixation devices that provide adequate rigidity to achieve bony union, and then resorb.

Chapter

74

Computer-Aided Surgical Simulation for Orthognathic Surgery

James J. Xia, Jaime Gateno, John F. Teichgraeber

The success of orthognathic surgery depends not only on the technical aspects of the operation but, also, to a larger extent, on the formulation of a precise surgical plan.[1-10] Over the last 50 years, while there have been significant improvements in the technical aspects of surgery, that is, rigid fixation, resorbable materials, distraction osteogenesis, minimally invasive approaches, among others, the planning methods have mostly remained unchanged.[3,4,6,10] Unfortunately, there are a number of problems with the current planning methods. Each one of these problems can result in a bad surgical outcome. In isolation, these problems may seem trivial, but, when added together, the results can be devastating.

PROBLEMS WITH TRADITIONAL PLANNING METHODS FOR PLANNING ORTHOGNATHIC SURGERY

In orthognathic surgery, surgical planning involves a series of logical steps. These steps include (1) data gathering, (2) diagnosis and quantification of the condition, (3) establishment of a preliminary surgical plan, (4) surgical simulation, (5) establishment of the final surgical plan, and (6) transfer of the plan to the patient.

The traditional planning methods for orthognathic surgery follow a basic sequence. Data is gathered from a multitude of different sources. These include the physical examination, medical photographs, x-rays (e.g., cephalogram, orthopantomogram), computed tomography (CT) scans, and mounted stone dental models.[1,2] Each of these sources provides a portion of the whole data set that is needed for successful planning. In practice, a surgeon evaluates each of these data sources in a sequential manner and creates a complete three-dimensional (3D) mental picture of the condition.

The next step in the planning process is the diagnosis and quantification of deformity. In orthognathic surgery, an important part of this process is the cephalometric analysis.[1,11] This is done by tracing the bony outlines and soft tissue profiles of a cephalogram. The angles, distances, and relationships are measured between selected landmarks. These measurements help surgeons to diagnose and quantify the problems.

After the surgeon has formulated the diagnosis, in the third step, he or she develops a preliminary plan. In many instances, the surgeon will also develop alternative plans. To test the feasibility of the preliminary plan(s), the surgeon simulates the planned surgery. In orthognathic surgery, this is accomplished by completing prediction tracings and dental model surgery.[1,2] Prediction tracings are made by tracing the silhouette of the facial bones from a two-dimensional cephalogram onto a piece of acetate paper. These tracings are then cut and moved to evaluate possible outcomes. Dental model surgery is done on stone dental models that have been mounted on an articulator. An articulator is a mechanical device that reproduces the positions of the mandible in relation to the maxilla. Dental model surgery is performed by physically cutting the models and moving them to the desired position.

After the simulation has been completed, in the fourth step, the surgeon formulates the final surgical plan. The final step in the planning process is to transfer the surgical plan to the patient at the time of surgery. In orthognathic surgery, the surgical plan is transferred to the patient using surgical splints and selected measurements. The surgical splints are plastic wafers that are placed between the teeth at the time of surgery. They relate a cut jaw segment to an uncut one. Prior to surgery, the splints are fabricated on the stone dental models on which the surgery has been simulated.

There are a number of problems with the traditional planning system. These include:

1. The various data sources use different coordinate systems. The physical examination and the medical photographs are taken with the patient's head oriented to the neutral head posture (NHP). The cephalogram is oriented to the Frankfurt horizontal (FH) plane, and the articulated dental models are oriented to the axis-orbital plane.[12] On average, these planes differ from each other by 8 degrees.[12] Currently, most surgeons are unaware of this problem and fail to account for these differences. This problem alone can be responsible for a 15% difference in maxillary projection between planned and actual outcomes.[12]

2. With the traditional method, surgeons are never able to visualize the whole data set in three dimensions.[3-5,10,13,14] As stated above, the surgeons have to create this picture in their minds. This causes problems in communicating with the other members of the treatment team. As would be expected, it is impossible to ensure that all involved have the same picture.

3. The cephalometric analysis is in two dimensions. Therefore, it only measures structures in a single plane. It may be appropriate for patients with symmetrical deformities but is grossly inadequate for patients with asymmetrical conditions.[3,8] It has been calculated that 34% of patients with dentofacial deformities have asymmetrical conditions.[15]

4. The orientation of dental models mounted on an articulator is often inaccurate. The occlusal plane inclination of models mounted on a semiadjustable articulator is, on average, 8 degrees too steep.[12,16] In addition, there are design flaws in the current devices used to orient the dental models on an articulator (i.e., the facebow). A patient can easily tilt the facebow during the registration process, creating an inaccurate recording of the occlusal cant (roll of the upper jaw). An inaccurate initial model position will always create an inaccurate plan.[16]

5. The stone dental models do not depict the surrounding bones. Dental model surgery is done for two purposes. The first is to establish the occlusion and the second is to reorient the models to ensure that the bones are placed in the ideal position at surgery. Because stone dental models do not depict the surrounding bones, the surgeon is unable to visualize the effects of the model position on the facial skeleton.[5,6,17] Therefore, the attainment of the ideal bone position becomes a random event.[4,6,7] In our opinion, this problem is the largest source of error.

6. Prediction tracing and model surgery are two separate processes that are inaccurate and time consuming.[3,18,19] Currently, an experienced surgeon spends 3 to 5 hours completing these steps.[20]

7. Some surgeons use CT-based rapid prototyping models to plan complex surgeries.[13] The drawbacks to these rapid prototyping models are that they are costly (models range in price from $400 to $2500), they are unable to simulate different iterations of a given plan on a single model (i.e., once the model is cut, the cut cannot be undone), and they fail to render the teeth with the precision necessary for surgical planning.[3,4,10]

8. The fabrication of splints is time consuming. A busy surgeon performs several of these operations per week, and many patients require two splints. The fabrication of each splint may take an additional hour.[2,20]

COMPUTER-AIDED SURGICAL SIMULATION (CASS) FOR ORTHOGNATHIC SURGERY

It is clear that many compromised surgical outcomes are the result of deficient planning. The need to improve the traditional surgical planning methods has led our group to develop a 3D computer-aided surgical simulation (CASS) system to plan craniomaxillofacial surgeries. The ultimate goal of CASS is to completely eliminate the problems associated with the traditional surgical planning methods. Using this CASS system, all the patient information (clinical examination, clinical photographs, cephalogram, dental models, and CT images) is merged into a single data set that is oriented in a unique 3D coordinate system, the NHP. In addition, the patient's anatomic structures (the bones, teeth, and soft tissues) are rendered three dimensionally and can be visualized from any arbitrary viewpoint. CASS also eliminates the inaccurate facebow transfer by digitally incorporating dental models into the bone models using fiducial markers. Furthermore, the prediction tracing, dental model surgery, and CT model surgery are merged into a single virtual process. Surgeons can perform "virtual surgery" and create a 3D prediction of the patient's surgical outcomes, as if they are performing surgery in the operating room. Finally, the surgical splints and templates are designed and fabricated in the computer using computer-aided design and computer-aided manufacturing (CAD/CAM) techniques.

Our CASS system incorporates three distinctive features and innovations: (1) multiple imaging modalities are used to create an accurate model of the craniofacial skeleton, (2) special techniques are employed to orient the computerized bone model in the NHP, and (3) CAD/CAM techniques are used to fabricate accurate surgical splints and templates to transfer the surgical plan to the operating room. We have used this system in maxillofacial surgery,[9,21-23] craniofacial surgery,[24] trauma, and distraction osteogenesis.[24-26] In addition, we have also documented the clinical feasibility,[4,10] the accuracy,[27] and the cost-effectiveness[20] of this system. Our CASS planning protocol for orthognathic surgery is presented step-by-step as follows.

STEP 1: PHYSICAL EXAMINATION AND ANTHROPOMETRIC MEASUREMENTS

A complete physical examination and anthropometric measurements are essential in the clinical decision-making process.[1,28,29] These approaches are the only way to obtain information regarding the quality of the tissues and their dynamic deformation with function (see Pearls and Pitfalls section for details). During the physical examination, critical areas of concern should be head orientation, incisor show at rest and with smiling, midline deviations, and any dystopia.

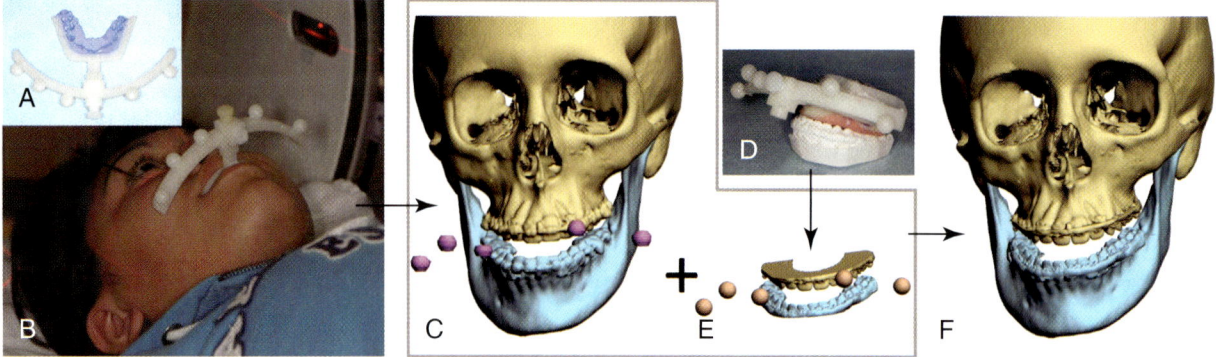

Fig. 74-1 ■ Creation of the computerized composite skull model. **A,** Facebow with fiducial markers is attached to the bite-jig. **B,** The patient is biting on the bite-jig and facebow during computed (CT) scan. **C,** Three separate but correlated computer models are reconstructed: a midface, a mandibular, and a fiducial-marker model. **D,** The bite-jig and facebow is placed between the upper and lower plaster dental models during the scanning process. **E,** Three separate but correlated computer models are also reconstructed: an upper digital dental, a lower digital dental, and a fiducial-marker model. **F,** By aligning the fiducial markers, the digital dental models are incorporated into the 3D CT skull model. The computerized composite skull model is thus created. It simultaneously displays an accurate rendition of both the bony structures and the teeth. (From Xia JJ, Gateno J, Teichgraeber JF: New clinical protocol to evaluate craniomaxillofacial deformity and plan surgical correction, *J Oral Maxillofac Surg* 67(10):2093-2106, 2009.)

STEP 2: CREATION OF A COMPUTERIZED COMPOSITE SKULL MODEL

A composite skull model is a computerized 3D model that is an accurate rendition of the soft tissues, bones, and teeth. Although CT scans have been successfully used to visualize the soft tissues and bones, they have not been used for surgical simulation, because CT does not render the teeth with the accuracy that is necessary for surgical planning. To solve this problem, the authors developed a composite skull model by incorporating accurate digital dental models into a 3D CT model of the face.[17,30] This was done by merging two separate digital data sets: the digital dental models and the 3D CT. The separate data sets are merged by using fiducial markers (common reference points). The fiducial markers used in this protocol are spheres that are part of a specially designed facebow (Medical Modeling Inc., Golden, Colo.). The facebow is attached to a bite registration that is placed between the patient's maxillary and mandibular dental arches and between the stone models before they are scanned (Fig. 74-1).

There are four steps in the process of creating a composite skull model: (1) create a bite registration, (2) create 3D CT models of the craniomaxillofacial skeleton, (3) create a set of digital dental models, and (4) merge the digital dental models into the patient's CT models.

The first step is to fabricate a bite registration. The main purpose of the bite registration is to relate the fiducial markers to the teeth, but it is also used to maintain the mandible in centric relation (CR) during scanning. For this purpose, a special bite fork has been designed that is placed buccally to the teeth. It is composed of a plastic frame with a layer of paper that holds the bite registration material (Fig. 74-2, *A*). The bite fork has an anterior attachment for the removable facebow (Fig. 74-2, *B*). It is necessary to use a dimensionally stable, rigid, bite registration material, for instance, LuxaBite (Chemisch-Pharmazeutische Fabrik GmbH, Hamburg, Germany) to prevent the deformation and distortion of the bite registration. This material sets rigidly and can be carved with a bur (Fig. 74-3). In order to make the actual registration, the material is first placed over the paper underside of the bite fork, and an impression is taken of occlusal surfaces of the maxillary teeth. After the material has

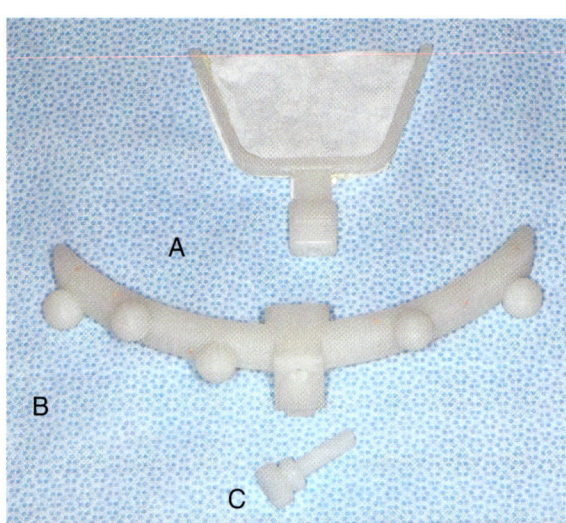

Fig. 74-2 ■ A special bite fork is composed of a plastic frame with a layer of paper that holds the bite registration material (**A**). It has an anterior attachment for the removable facebow (**B**) through a nylon screw (**C**).

hardened and the paper backing is removed, additional material is added on the mandibular side of the fork. The mandibular bite registration is captured in CR (Fig. 74-4). Once the bite registration is created, it is attached to the facebow (see Fig. 74-1, *A*).

The second step is to create 3D CT models of the craniomaxillofacial skeleton. A CT scan of the patient's craniofacial skeleton is obtained with the bite-registration–facebow assembly in place (see Fig. 74-1, *B*). The CT scan is completed using the standard scanning algorithm, matrix of 512×512 at 0.625-mm slice thickness, 25-cm or less field-of-view (FOV), 0-degree gantry tilt, and 1:1 pitch. Once the CT scan is obtained, it is segmented, and three separate but correlated computer models are generated: a midface, a mandibular, and a fiducial-marker model (see Fig. 74-1, *C*).

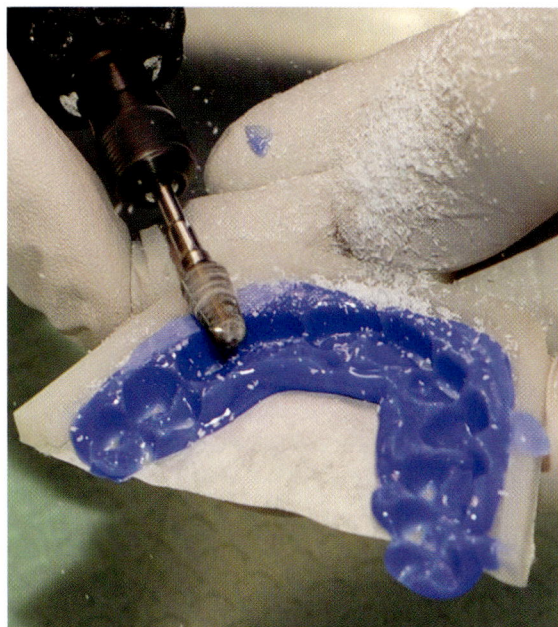

Fig. 74-3 ■ The bite registration material sets rigidly and can be carved with a bur.

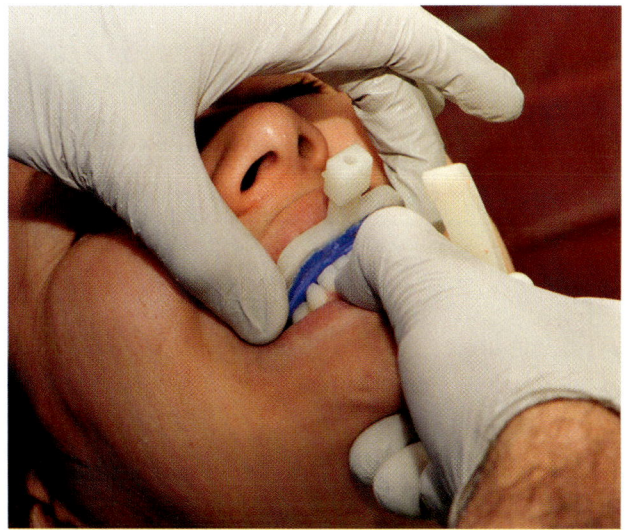

Fig. 74-4 ■ It is critical to capture the mandibular bite registration in centric relation (CR).

The third step is to create a set of digital dental models. First, dental impressions are taken of the upper and lower teeth. The impressions are poured with a special dimensionally stable and laser-friendly stone, for instance, Diamond Die (Hi-Tec Dental Products Inc, Greenback, Tenn.). The stone dental models are then placed on the bite-registration–facebow assembly and mounted on a custom jig that keeps the relationship between the models unaltered during scanning. The models are then scanned using a surface laser scanner (resolution: 0.1 mm or higher). An alternative is to scan the models with a micro-CT scanner (resolution: 7 μm to 75 μm) (see Fig. 74-1, *D*). After scanning, the data is segmented generating three separate but correlated computer models: an upper digital dental, a lower digital dental, and a fiducial-marker model (see Fig. 74-1, *E*).

The final step is to merge the digital dental models into the patient's CT models. After the 3D CT models and the digital dental models are obtained, the teeth on the 3D CT model are removed, leaving the fiducial markers in place. The maxillary and the mandibular digital dental models with their corresponding fiducial markers are imported into the CT skull model. By aligning the fiducial markers, the digital dental models are incorporated into the 3D CT skull model. The fiducial markers are then marked hidden. This results in a computerized composite skull model that simultaneously displays an accurate rendition of the bones and the teeth (see Fig. 74-1, *F*).[4,10,17,30,31]

STEP 3: REORIENTATION OF THE COMPOSITE SKULL MODEL TO THE NEUTRAL HEAD POSTURE

An important prerequisite for accurate planning is to orient the 3D composite skull model to the NHP in the computer. In order to capture a patient's NHP, a digital orientation sensor is attached to the facebow that was used to create a composite skull model. With the patient in the NHP, the pitch, roll, and yaw of the face are recorded.[32-34]

The recorded information is then used to reorient the composite skull model in the computer. A digital replica (CAD model) of the digital orientation sensor–face-bow assembly is registered (i.e., superimposed) to the fiducial markers of the composite skull model, and the two objects are attached to each other. Afterward, the recorded pitch, roll, and yaw are applied to the center of the CAD model of the digital orientation sensor, reorienting the composite skull model to the NHP (Fig. 74-5).

STEP 4: ANALYSIS AND QUANTIFICATION OF THE DEFORMITY

In CASS, the analysis and quantification of the deformity is completed in both two and three dimensions. Initially, to facilitate this task, a unique 3D reference system is constructed for the composite skull model. The reference system has its origin at the soft tissue nasion and consists of three orthogonal planes: sagittal, coronal, and axial. In the reference system, the sagittal plane is the patient's true midsagittal plane. Once the composite model is positioned in the 3D reference system, the user digitizes the selected cephalometric landmarks and chooses the desired analysis.

In the 3D analysis, we first examine the anatomic structures for symmetry. To examine the symmetry of the maxilla, we have developed a method based on the work of Grayson.[35-37] In this method, a triangular spline is created on the maxillary dentition by digitizing three landmarks: the maxillary dental midline and two corresponding landmarks on the right and left molars (usually the mesiobuccal cusp of the maxillary right and left first molars, Fig. 74-6). The software reads the x, y, and z coordinates of each vertex of the triangle to automatically calculate the pitch, roll, and yaw of the maxilla as well as the maxillary midline deviation. The pitch represents the maxillary occlusal plane inclination, while the roll and yaw represent the occlusal cant and the horizontal rotation. In some instances, because of the difficulty interpreting some 3D data and the unavailability of the 3D normative data, we still use a conventional 2D analysis, in which all the 3D landmarks are projected onto the midsagittal plane. Bilateral landmarks are averaged in the anteroposterior and vertical axes. In this mode, we make decisions regarding anteroposterior projection, vertical position, and inclinations of the occlusal plane and mandibular plane (pitch).

In addition to the 2D and 3D measurements, the CASS system is also able to perform volumetric measurements. These

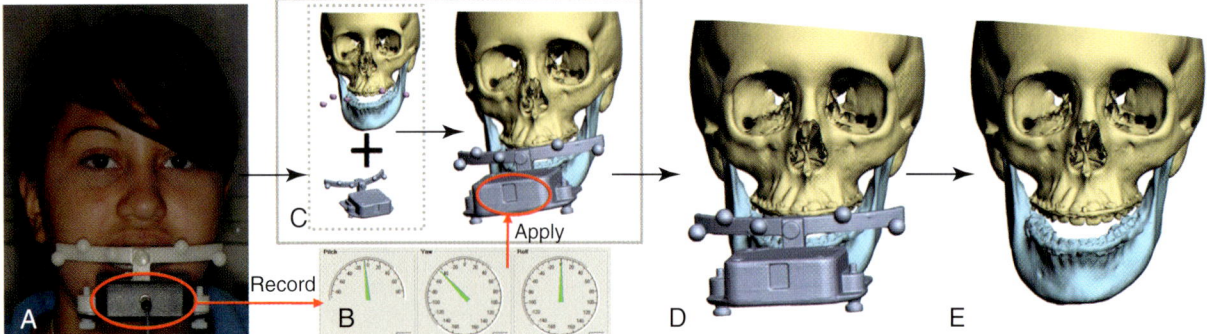

Fig. 74-5 ■ Orientation of the composite skull model to the neutral head posture (NHP) using the digital orientation sensor method. **A,** A digital orientation sensor is attached to the bite-jig and facebow. **B,** The pitch, roll, and yaw of the digital orientation sensor are recorded. **C,** In the computer, a digital replica (computer-aided design [CAD] model) of the orientation sensor is registered to the composite skull model (by the fiducial markers) and the two objects are attached to each other. **D,** The recorded pitch, roll, and yaw are applied to the center of the CAD model of the digital orientation sensor, reorienting the composite skull model to the NHP. **E,** After the composite skull is oriented to the NHP, the gyroscope replica is marked hidden. (From Xia JJ, Gateno J, Teichgraeber JF: New clinical protocol to evaluate craniomaxillofacial deformity and plan surgical correction, *J Oral Maxillofac Surg* 67(10):2093-2106, 2009.)

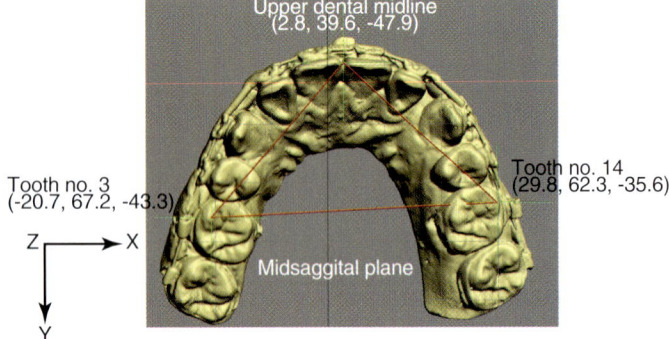

Fig. 74-6 ■ In the triangle method, a triangular spline is created on the maxillary dentition by digitizing three landmarks: (1) the dental midline, (2) the mesiobuccal cusp of the maxillary right first molar, and (3) the mesiobuccal cusp of the maxillary left first molar. The software reads the x, y, and z coordinates of each vertex of the triangle to automatically calculate the pitch, roll, and yaw of the maxilla as well as the maxillary midline deviation. The pitch represents the maxillary occlusal plane, while the roll and yaw represent the occlusal cant and the horizontal discrepancy. (From Xia JJ, Gateno J, Teichgraeber JF: New clinical protocol to evaluate craniomaxillofacial deformity and plan surgical correction, *J Oral Maxillofac Surg* 67(10):2093-2106, 2009.)

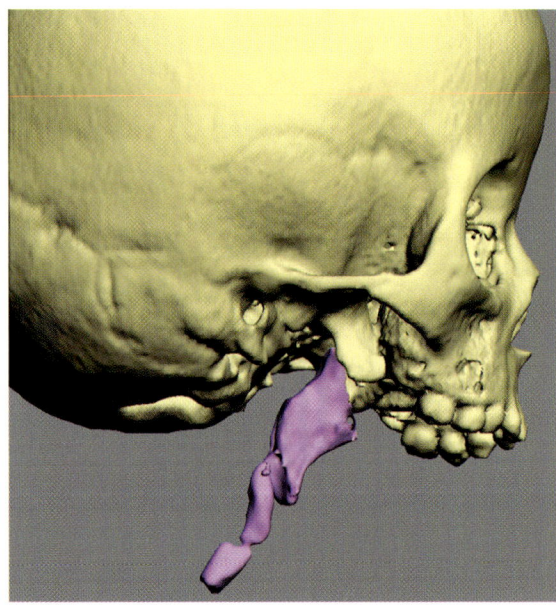

Fig. 74-7 ■ Volumetric measurements are used to measure the size of the airway and orbital volumes. (From Xia JJ, Gateno J, Teichgraeber JF: New clinical protocol to evaluate craniomaxillofacial deformity and plan surgical correction, *J Oral Maxillofac Surg* 67(10):2093-2106, 2009.)

measurements have proven to be useful in the quantification of airway and orbital volumes (Fig. 74-7).

STEP 5: SIMULATION OF SURGERY IN THE COMPUTER

Any type of osteotomy can be simulated in this CASS system, for instance, Le Fort I, sagittal split, and genioplasty, among others. After the bones are osteotomized, the user can move and rotate the bony segments to the desired position. In patients requiring bimaxillary surgery, the maxillary surgery is usually simulated first. The maxilla is first repositioned to symmetry. The triangular spline used to quantify the maxillary asymmetry is "attached" to the maxilla so that any movement of the triangle is automatically transferred to the maxilla. The software reads the x, y, and z coordinates of the triangle vertices and calculates the discrepancy between right and left. It then automatically moves the upper dental midline to the midsagittal plane, and rotates the triangle to symmetry (0 degrees of roll, 0 degrees of yaw, and balanced pitch, Fig. 74-8). This triangular method works especially well when the dental arch itself is symmetrical. If the dental arch is asymmetrical, the user's intervention may be required to move/rotate the maxilla to the most balanced position. After the asymmetry of the maxilla is corrected, the maxillary pitch (occlusal plane inclination) is adjusted, and the maxilla is moved anteroposteriorly and superoinferiorly to the desired position based on the cephalometric analysis and clinical measurements.

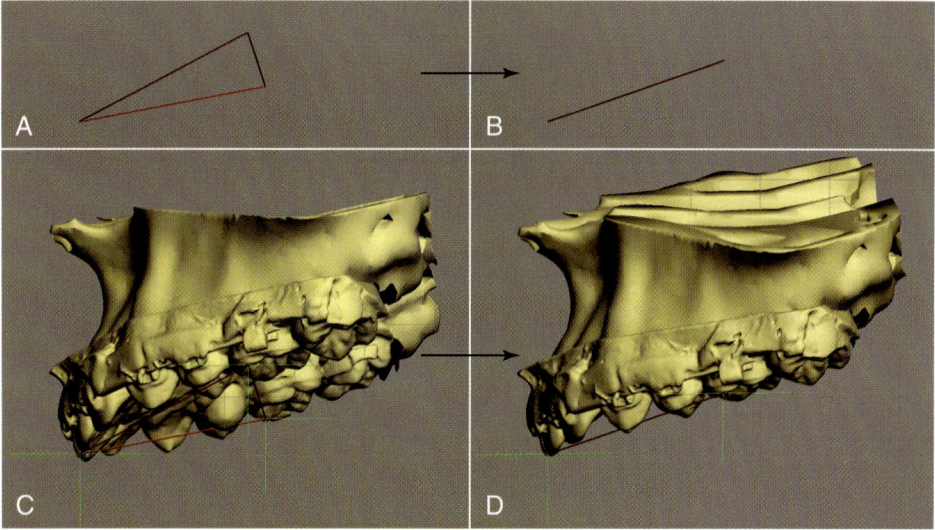

Fig. 74-8 ▪ The triangular spline used to quantify the maxillary asymmetry is "glued" to the maxilla. **A** and **B,** The computer reads the x, y, and z coordinates of the triangle vertices and moves them to symmetry (0 degree of roll, 0 degree of yaw). **C** and **D,** The movement of the triangle is automatically transferred to the maxilla. (From Xia JJ, Gateno J, Teichgraeber JF: New clinical protocol to evaluate craniomaxillofacial deformity and plan surgical correction, *J Oral Maxillofac Surg* 67(10):2093-2106, 2009.)

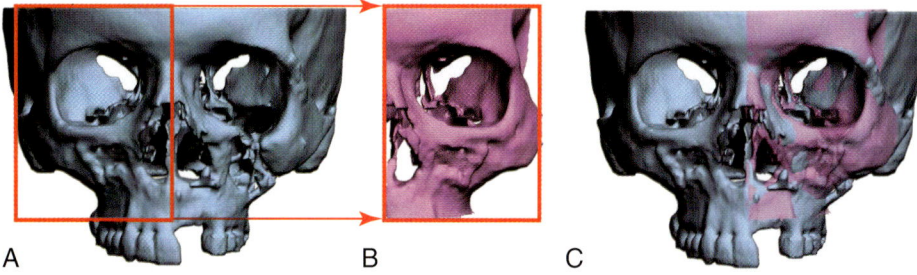

Fig. 74-9 ▪ In the mirror-image routine, one half of the face is selected (**A**), copied (**B**) and flipped (mirror-imaged), and superimposed onto the contralateral side (**C**). (From Xia JJ, Gateno J, Teichgraeber JF: New clinical protocol to evaluate craniomaxillofacial deformity and plan surgical correction, *J Oral Maxillofac Surg* 67(10):2093-2106, 2009.)

After the maxilla is placed in its final position, the distal segment of the mandible is moved to maximal intercuspation (MI). Unfortunately, in the computer, the establishment of MI is difficult. It is almost impossible to be certain that what is seen in the computer truly represents the best possible alignment. To ensure that the digital final occlusion is at its correct MI, the stone models are first physically positioned in MI (final occlusion) and then scanned in this position. This second set of digital models is used to guide the precise placement of the distal mandible into MI. Once the distal segment is in position, the proximal segments of the mandible are aligned. If necessary, a genioplasty can also be simulated.

In some instances, the repositioning of the osteotomized segments is not sufficient to recreate facial symmetry. This is due to the fact that in many patients with facial asymmetries, the bones are not only asymmetrically displaced but also differ in size and shape from one side to the other. Therefore, it is necessary to reevaluate the symmetry after the simulation of the jaw movements. To help with this, a mirror-imaging tool is used. With it, one half of the face is selected, copied, mirror-imaged (flipped), and superimposed on the contralateral side (Fig. 74-9). The differences between the two sides are then calculated using a *Boolean* operation. Based on this

information, the surgeon may decide to add volume (grafting), remove volume (ostectomy), or adjust the position of the segments (camouflage).

STEP 6: TRANSFER OF THE COMPUTERIZED PLAN TO THE PATIENT

After the surgical plan is finalized, it is necessary to transfer the plan to the patient at the time of the surgery. Surgical dental splints or surgical templates can be created for this purpose. Surgical dental splints are used to reposition dentate bony segments, while surgical templates are used to reposition nondentate ones. The surgical dental splints are created by inserting a digital wafer between the maxillary and mandibular dental arches. A *Boolean* operation is then performed, resulting in a digital surgical splint (Fig. 74-10, *A*). The surgical templates record the 3D surface geometry of the area of interest so that they fit on the bone in a unique position (Fig. 74-10, *B*). The system can export the digital splints and templates in "stl" format. These are fabricated using a rapid prototyping machine (Figs. 74-10, *C* and *D*), and are subsequently used at the time of surgery (Figs. 74-10, *E* and *F*).

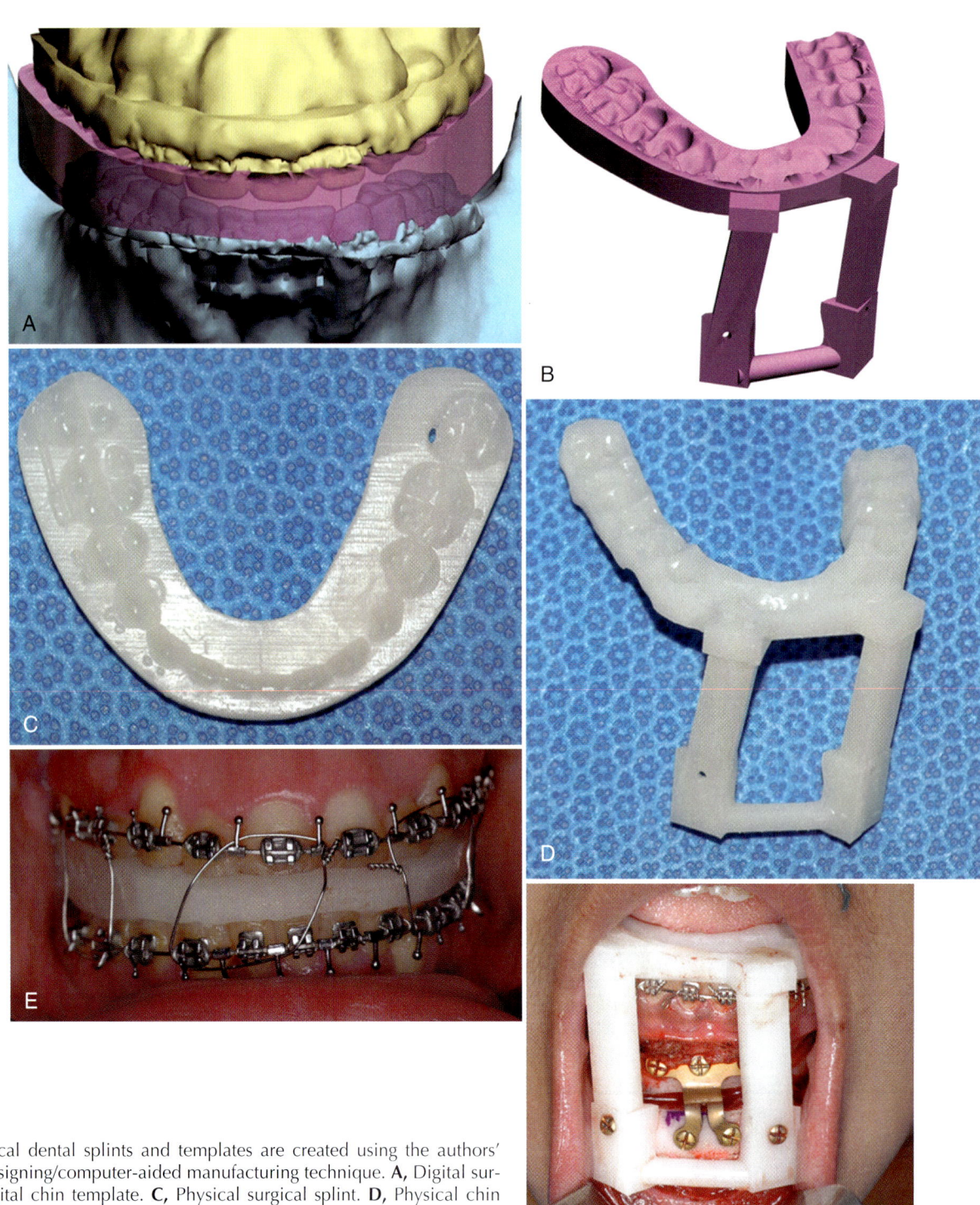

Fig. 74-10 ■ Surgical dental splints and templates are created using the authors' computer-aided designing/computer-aided manufacturing technique. **A,** Digital surgical splint. **B,** Digital chin template. **C,** Physical surgical splint. **D,** Physical chin template. **E,** The use of physical surgical splint at the time of the surgery. **F,** The use of physical chin template at the time of the surgery. (From Xia JJ, Gateno J, Teichgraeber JF: New clinical protocol to evaluate craniomaxillofacial deformity and plan surgical correction, *J Oral Maxillofac Surg* 67(10):2093-2106, 2009.)

TREATMENT OUTCOMES OF USING THE CASS PLANNING SYSTEM

STUDY 1: ACCURACY OF THE CASS SYSTEM

We have completed a study to determine the accuracy of the CASS system by comparing planned outcomes developed in CASS with actual surgical outcomes. In this study, 25 patients requiring double-jaw orthognathic surgery were enrolled. The surgical plan was developed using the CASS system. This plan was transferred to the patient at the time of surgery using CAD/CAM surgical splints and templates. A postoperative CT scan was obtained within 6 weeks of surgery. The actual outcomes were compared with the planned outcomes by superimposing postoperative 3D models of the cranio-facial skeleton to a 3D model depicting the planned outcome (Fig. 74-11). The method of superimposition was developed and validated in a previous study.[27] The linear and angular differences between models were calculated.

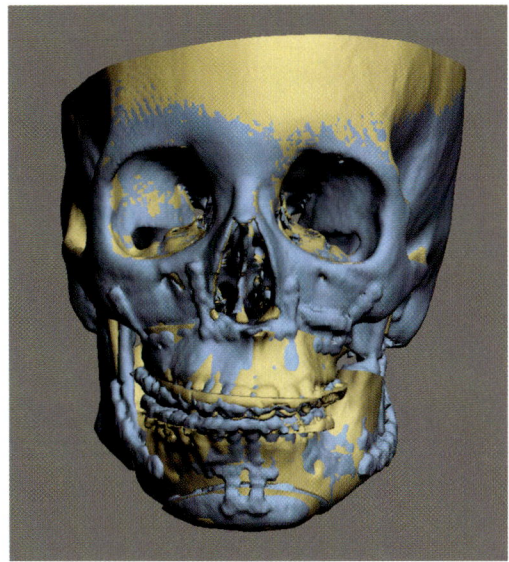

Fig. 74-11 ■ The actual outcomes were compared with the planned outcomes by superimposing postoperative 3D models *(blue)* of the craniofacial skeleton to a 3D model depicting the planned outcome *(yellow)*.

The statistical analyses included paired *t*-tests, two-way mixed intraclass correlation coefficients (absolute agreement definition), and the Bland and Altman method for assessing measurement agreement.[38] Based on previous studies, we determined, a priori, that linear differences of less than 2 mm in each direction and angular differences of less than 4 degrees were not clinically significant.[39-42]

The results showed that the mean linear difference between the planned and the actual outcomes was within 0.5 mm and that the standard deviation (SD) was within 1 mm (Table 74-1). The mean angular difference was within 0.5 degrees, and the SD was within 1.5 degrees (Table 74-2). The paired *t*-test showed no statistically significant differences between the planned and actual surgical outcomes. The intraclass correlation coefficients were greater than 0.75, indicating a high degree of absolute agreement between the planned and actual outcomes. The Bland and Altman method showed that the measurement agreement of linear differences between the planned and actual outcomes, in each dimension, were within ±2 mm (see Table 74-1), and that the angular differences in pitch, roll, and yaw between the planned and actual outcomes were within ±3 degrees (see Table 74-2). In conclusion, this study confirmed the accuracy of the CASS system for orthognathic surgery.

| TABLE 74-1 | Linear Differences between the Planned and the Actual Outcomes |

	X				Y				Z			
	MEAN	SD	LOW	HIGH	MEAN	SD	LOW	HIGH	MEAN	SD	LOW	HIGH
Maxilla												
Tooth 16	−0.30	0.76	(−1.80	1.19)	0.29	0.79	(−1.26	1.84)	0.14	0.57	(−0.98	1.26)
Upper Midline	−0.10	0.59	(−1.25	1.06)	0.26	0.55	(−0.82	1.35)	−0.10	0.62	(−1.31	1.11)
Tooth 26	−0.43	0.72	(−1.84	0.98)	0.54	0.65	(−0.74	1.82)	0.24	0.60	(−0.93	1.41)
Mandible												
Tooth 46	−0.40	0.74	(−1.85	1.04)	0.33	0.68	(−1.01	1.67)	0.00	0.67	(−1.31	1.31)
Lower Midline	−0.05	0.64	(−1.30	1.20)	0.36	0.62	(−0.85	1.57)	−0.09	0.50	(−1.07	0.89)
Tooth 36	0.05	0.73	(−1.39	1.48)	0.44	0.79	(−1.11	1.99)	−0.08	0.63	(−1.32	1.16)
Chin												
Point 1	0.07	0.82	(−1.53	1.66)	0.39	0.65	(−0.89	1.67)	−0.06	0.79	(−1.60	1.49)
Pogonion	0.00	0.99	(−1.93	1.94)	0.43	0.56	(−0.66	1.53)	−0.02	0.68	(−1.35	1.32)
Pont 2	−0.05	0.98	(−1.97	1.86)	0.22	0.79	(−1.32	1.76)	0.26	0.57	(−0.85	1.38)

| TABLE 74-2 | Angular Differences between the Planned and the Actual Outcomes |

	PITCH				ROLL				YAW			
	MEAN	SD	LOW	HIGH	MEAN	SD	LOW	HIGH	MEAN	SD	LOW	HIGH
Maxilla	0.48	1.27	(−2.00	2.96)	0.10	0.70	(−1.27	1.46)	0.28	1.21	(−2.10	2.65)
Mandible	0.10	1.48	(−2.80	3.00)	−0.11	0.91	(−1.89	1.67)	0.08	1.02	(−1.92	2.08)
Chin	0.41	1.30	(−2.14	2.96)	0.28	1.18	(−2.04	2.59)	−0.26	0.84	(−1.90	1.38)

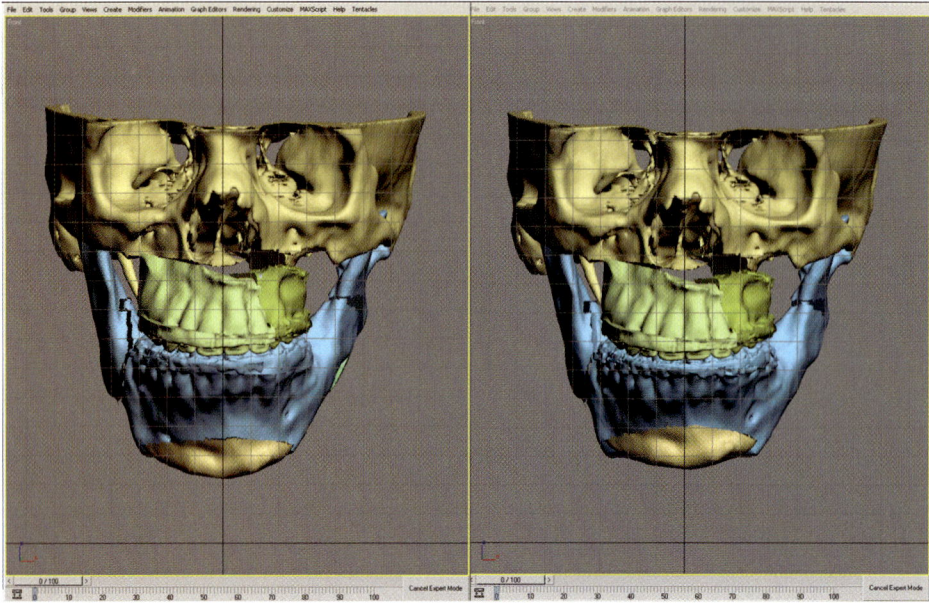

Fig. 74-12 ■ During the evaluation, the two 3D models of the same patient were placed side by side on a 24-inch high-resolution screen.

STUDY 2: COMPARISON OF SURGICAL OUTCOMES ACHIEVED WITH CASS AND TRADITIONAL METHODS

We have completed another study to compare the surgical outcome achieved with CASS with the ones achieved using the traditional planning methods. The records of 12 consecutive patients who underwent double-jaw orthognathic surgery were used for this study. Two virtual surgeries were performed on the 3D computer models of each patient: one following the plan reached by the CASS method (experimental group) and the other one following the plan reached by the traditional method (control group).

First, the surgeon planned the surgery using the CASS method, and, at least a year later, the same surgeon planned the second virtual surgery using the traditional planning methods. We felt that the 1-year interval of "wash-out memory" would adequately prevent undue influence on the surgical plan from CASS. Finally, the outcomes achieved with the two different plans were evaluated and compared by two experienced craniomaxillofacial (CMF) surgeons, who were not involved in either the surgical planning or the virtual surgery.

During the evaluation, the two 3D models of the same patient were placed side by side on a 24-inch high-resolution screen (Fig. 74-12). Blinded to the planning methods, the examiner evaluated each pair of the 3D models using a visual analogy scale (VAS, range of 0 to 10); a score of "10" entailed the best outcome, while a score of "0" entailed the worst. The primary outcome variable was the overall CMF skeletal harmony. The secondary outcome variables were maxillary midline, cant, yaw, and occlusal plane correction; mandibular symmetry, proximal/distal segment placement; and chin position and projection in all three dimensions. After the evaluation, the surgical planning methods were unblinded. The VAS scores determined by the two evaluators were paired. A two-way mixed intraclass correlation coefficient (absolute agreement definition) was performed to detect the consistency of the measurements between the two evaluators. The result showed that the intraclass correlation coefficient was 0.83 (95% confidence interval [CI]: 0.77, 0.88, $P < 0.01$), indicating that the measurements between the two evaluators were highly consistent. The VAS scores determined by the

two evaluators were then averaged and paired for the two planning methods.

Finally, the VAS score for each evaluation was paired, and the differences (CASS vs. traditional) were calculated. The data was initially screened and its distribution was normally shaped. The paired t-test (for primary outcome variable) and analysis of variance (ANOVA) for repeated measures (for the secondary outcome variables) were used to detect whether there was a statistically significant difference between the two planning methods.

The results showed that the overall CMF skeletal harmony achieved with the CASS method was statistically significantly better than the one achieved with the traditional methods ($P < .01$). In addition, the maxillary and mandibular outcomes achieved with the CASS method were also statistically significantly better than the outcome achieved with the traditional methods ($P < .01$). The computation of within-subject contrast showed the outcome achieved with CASS was significantly better in each measurement. Finally, because only three patients required a genioplasty, we could not perform statistical analyses on outcomes measures for this type of surgery. However, there was a trend that the genioplasty achieved by CASS was better than the genioplasty achieved by the traditional planning methods (mean difference of VAS score: 3.0 antero-posteriorly, 3.0 horizontally, and 3.5 vertically). During the evaluation, both evaluators found that the outcome difference between the two planning methods was greater in those patients with more severe or asymmetrical deformity. The outcome difference was less pronounced in those patients with mild and symmetrical deformities. In conclusion, this study confirmed that the surgical outcome achieved with the CASS method is significantly better than the outcome achieved with the traditional planning methods.

IMPORTANCE OF NEUTRAL HEAD POSTURE

An important prerequisite for accurate planning is to orientate the 3D composite skull model to a reference position. In 2D cephalometry, the reference planes are usually the Frankfort horizontal (FH) plane and sella-nasion plane. However, many patients with CMF

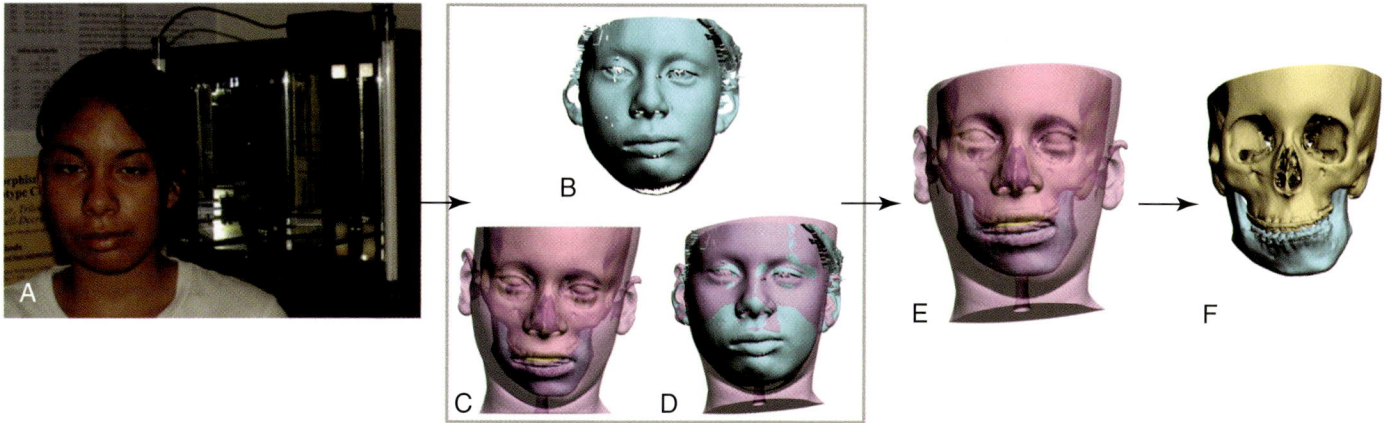

Fig. 74-13 ■ Orientation of the composite skull model to the neutral head posture (NHP) using the laser scanner method. **A,** The surface geometry of the facial soft tissue is captured while the patient is sitting on a calibrated chair at the center of the laser scanner. **B,** Captured surface geometry (scanned image) of the facial soft tissue. **C,** In the computer, a soft tissues model is rendered, and the composite model is "glued" to the soft tissue model. **D,** The soft tissue model is aligned to the NHP by matching it to the scanned image. **E,** Both soft tissue and composite skull models are thus oriented to the NHP. **F,** The composite skull model is in the NHP after the soft tissue is hidden. (From Xia JJ, Gateno J, Teichgraeber JF: New clinical protocol to evaluate craniomaxillofacial deformity and plan surgical correction, *J Oral Maxillofac Surg* 67(10):2093-2106, 2009.)

deformities have significant asymmetries of the upper face and skull base. Common intracranial cephalometric landmarks and planes often cannot be used to orient the composite skull model. The use of the neutral head posture obviates the need for intracranial landmarks and provides a reproducible reference framework. NHP can be either self-balanced or physician-manipulated head orientation.

Currently, there is still a question of how to record the NHP and transfer it to the 3D model. The simplest method is to visualize the 3D model in the computer and to orient it to a balanced position based on the user's best estimate. Although it is not the patient's true NHP, this method may approximate the NHP if the craniofacial structures are symmetrical. However, when the upper face and skull base have significant asymmetries, this method is inadequate. It is the authors' opinion that NHP should be recorded directly on the patient.

It is also questionable that the NHP be recorded during the CT scanning. When a medical CT scanner is used for scanning, the patient is scanned in the supine position. Therefore, it is impossible to place the patient's head in NHP during scanning. If a cone beam computed tomography (CBCT) scanner is used, the patient is in a sitting or standing position. A chin rest is required to stabilize the patient's head, ensuring the quality of CT images, because the shortest acquisition time is 5 seconds.[43] While it is possible to position the patient's head in NHP without the chin rest, the quality of CT images may be compromised. Clearly, there is a need for a technique that records the patient's NHP and accurately transfers it to the 3D model.

Our laboratory has developed two techniques to reorient the composite CT model to the NHP. The first one uses a calibrated 3D laser surface scanner, and the second one, described in detail in the previous section, uses a digital orientation sensor. In both methods, the NHP is established using the modified Molhave method.[44] While in an isolated standing position, the patient faces a blank wall at a distance of 2 meters. The patient is then asked to establish the NHP by flexing and extending her head and then balancing in a position of comfort while looking straight ahead without a specific focus. If a patient has difficulties with establishing self-balanced head

orientation, a physician can manually establish a balanced head orientation for the patient.

The method that uses a calibrated laser surface scanner captures the surface geometry of the facial soft tissues while the patient is in NHP. During the scanning, the patient is seated on a calibrated chair at the center of the scanner. The scanner creates an accurately oriented 3D image of the face. The soft tissues of the composite model are then rendered and the model is aligned to NHP by matching its soft tissues to the scanned image (Fig. 74-13).[4,10]

The method that uses the digital orientation sensor has the advantages of cost and convenience. The cost of the digital orientation sensor is a hundred times less than the cost of the laser scanner. Moreover, it is portable and requires little maintenance. For these reasons, we have adopted this technique in our clinical practice.

IMPORTANCE OF PHYSICAL EXAMINATION

With the new computer simulation technology, we are able to create 3D models of the face that incorporate accurate renditions of the teeth, the skeleton, and the soft tissues. Moreover, these models can be placed in a certain reference head orientation, that is, the neutral head posture (NHP). From this, one may infer that the value of the physical examination in the clinical decision-making process will become diminished. In our experience, this is far from true. Although, these models can capture the anatomy in great detail, they are static and only present the status of the tissues at the time when the image was captured. The physical examination still provides us with extremely valuable dynamic information that cannot be obtained from any other source. To illustrate this, we will discuss several pitfalls that can be encountered by relaying only on the static images.

The first example is one of a patient with significant mandibular laterognathia (lateral chin deviation) (Fig. 74-14, *A*). On assessing the alignment of the maxillary dental midline, we have discovered that in some of these patients the relationship of the maxillary dental midline to the upper lip varies depending on the mediolateral

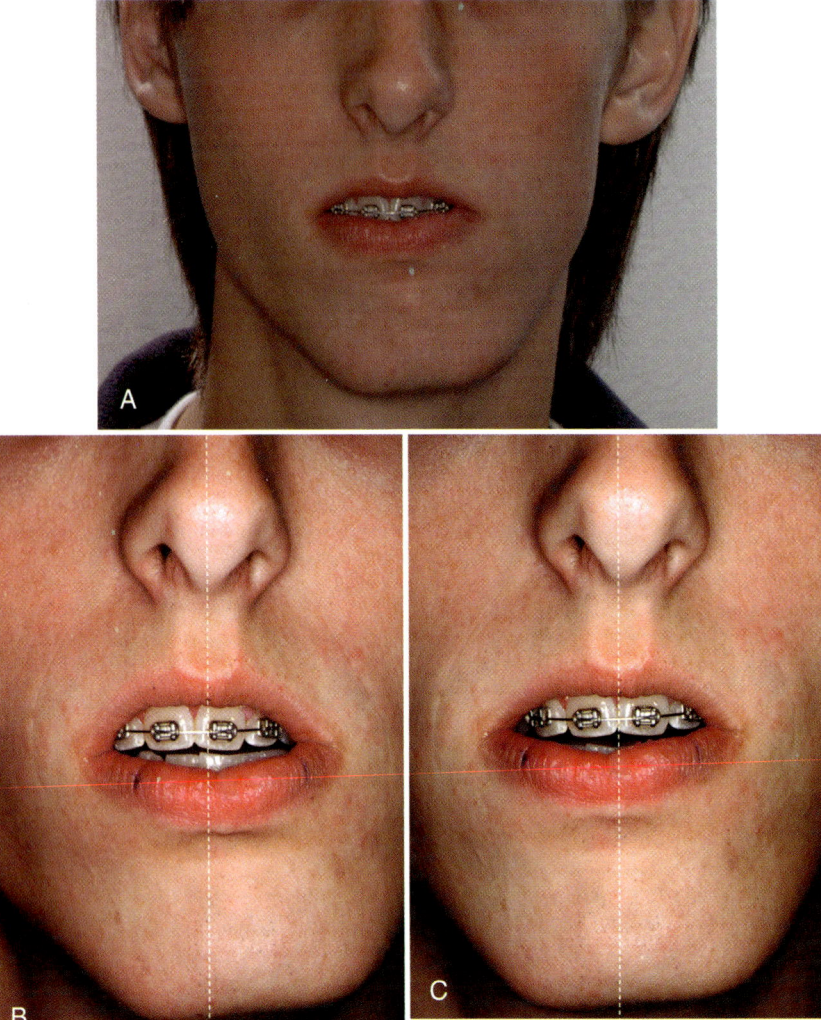

Fig. 74-14 ■ The maxillary dental midline deviation changes depending on different mandibular position. **A,** A patient with significant mandibular laterognathia (lateral chin deviation). **B,** The maxillary dental midline seems to be deviated opposite to the chin deviation while the patient is in centric relation. **C,** The maxillary dental midline is no longer deviated after we have asked the patient to move his chin to the midline, simulating correction of the mandibular asymmetry. (From Xia JJ, Gateno J, Teichgraeber JF: New clinical protocol to evaluate craniomaxillofacial deformity and plan surgical correction, *J Oral Maxillofac Surg* 67(10):2093-2106, 2009.)

position of the chin. During the physical examination, we first measured the transverse alignment of the maxillary dental midline to the middle of the upper lip while the patient was in centric relation. In this position, the maxillary dental midline seemed to be deviated opposite the chin deviation (Fig. 74-14, *B*). We then measured the same alignment after we had asked the patient to move his chin to the midline simulating the correction of the mandibular asymmetry. In this position, the maxillary dental midline is no longer deviated (Fig. 74-14, *C*). What happened here is that the lateral displacement of the mandible was producing a deformation of the upper lip by dragging it to the side of the chin deviation. When the chin was moved to the midline, the upper lip regained its normal shape. The pitfall here is that if this dynamic deformation is not taken into account, the surgeon will "correct" a maxillary dental midline deviation that is nonexistent. Obviously, this will create and unwanted outcome. Therefore, we recommend that the decision of correcting a maxillary midline deviation should be based on physical examination, rather than the study images.

Another example of a possible pitfall of simply relying on static images is the assessment of the amount of maxillary incisal show. The amount of incisal show varies with the patient's position. It tends to decrease when the patient changes position from supine, to sitting, and to standing (Fig. 74-15, *A*). If the CT scan is done on a medical scanner, it is done with the patient in the supine position. In this case, the amount of incisal show may seem excessive, when it is not (Fig. 74-15, *B*). If the scan is done with a cone-beam CT scanner, it is usually done with the patient sitting or standing. In this case, the amount of incisal show seems to more accurately reflect the actual amount. However, one has to remember another issue regarding the measurement of the incisal show on an acquired static image—the uncertainty of the functional state of the lips. Ideally, the upper and lower lips should be in repose during the measurement. However, the functional state of the lips is questionable unless the surgeon is present during the scanning. Strained lips will produce an inaccurate determination of the incisal show. In addition, the CT and CBCT images are usually acquired when the patient is biting in

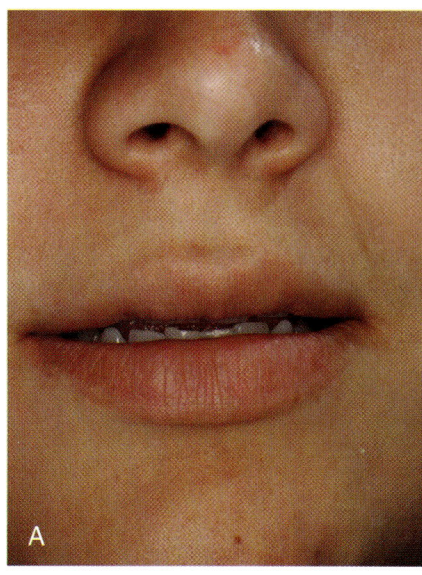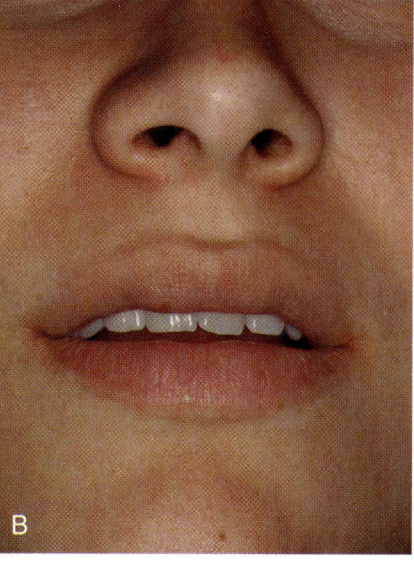

Fig. 74-15 ▪ The amount of maxillary incisor show may vary with the patient's position. **A,** Incisor show with subject in standing position. **B,** Incisor show with the same subject in supine position. (From Xia JJ, Gateno J, Teichgraeber JF: New clinical protocol to evaluate craniomaxillofacial deformity and plan surgical correction, *J Oral Maxillofac Surg* 67(10):2093-2106, 2009.)

occlusion. Therefore, it is best to determine this parameter clinically during the physical exam rather than relying on the computer images. During the physical exam, this parameter should be measured with the patient standing in front of the surgeon. The decision on how much to change the amount of incisal show should not be based solely on the amount of show at rest. Other important issues should also be taken into account. These include the amount of gingival show during smiling, the presence of delayed passive eruption, or the presence of attrition. Finally, clinical measurements of the occlusal cant, degree of dystopia, and ear position also serve to verify that the composite skull model is correctly oriented in the 3D coordinate system.

IMPORTANCE OF BITE REGISTRATION TO BE DONE IN CENTRIC RELATION

For surgical planning, it is critical that the bite registration is captured in centric relation. It serves as a reference and foundation for the entire process of orthognathic surgery. Failure to capture the occlusion in centric relation will cause either an unwanted outcome or an inaccurate plan.

In the scenario of a single-jaw mandibular surgery, failure to accurately capture CR does not influence the final outcome. This is because the final position for the distal mandible is dictated by the maxilla. Nonetheless, failure to accurately capture CR produces an inaccurate surgical plan. This is because the planned surgical movements at the level of the osteotomies and the actual movements will be different.

In the scenario of a single-jaw maxillary surgery, failure to accurately capture CR results in a maxilla and mandible that are more retruded than planned. During this type of surgery, the maxilla is first osteotomized and then wired to the mandible in maximum intercuspation. Afterward, the maxilla and mandible are rotated together to the planned vertical dimension. This maneuver is always done with the mandible in CR. If the imaging studies used for planning are acquired with the mandible in a forward position (i.e., not in the most retruded position, CR), the surgeon will plan the maxillary position based on this erroneous mandibular position. These positions will differ from the actual positions at the time of surgery, which, as stated before, will be more retruded.

In the scenario of a double-jaw surgery, failure to accurately capture CR may result in different outcomes depending on which jaw is osteotomized first. If the mandible is osteotomized first, the final surgical outcome will not differ from the planned outcome, but the planned mandibular movements at the level of the osteotomies will be different from the actual movements. If the maxilla is osteotomized first, both the maxilla and the mandible will be placed in a more retruded position than planned. The reason for this is the same as for the single-jaw maxillary surgery.

PEARLS AND PITFALLS

- The success of orthognathic surgery depends not only on the technical aspects of the operation, but also, to a larger extent, on the formulation of a precise surgical plan.
- There are a number of problems with the traditional planning methods. Although in isolation these problems may seem trivial, when added together, the results can be significant.
- CASS completely eliminates the problems associated with the traditional surgical planning methods.
- Using CASS, all the patient information (clinical examination, clinical photographs, cephalogram, dental models, and CT images) can be merged into a single data set that is oriented in a unique 3D coordinate system (the NHP); the patient's 3D anatomic structures (the bones, the teeth, and the soft tissues) can be accurately rendered; surgeons can perform "virtual surgery" and create a 3D prediction of the patient's surgical outcomes, as if they are performing surgery in the operating room; and finally, the computerized surgical plan can be transferred to the patient at the time of the surgery using computer-generated surgical splints and templates.
- Fabricating the bite-jig in CR is extremely important for CASS. It serves as a reference and foundation for the entire process of orthognathic surgery. Failure to capture the occlusion in CR will cause either an unwanted outcome or an inaccurate plan.
- The physical examination is also extremely important in the clinical decision-making process in CASS. It provides us with extremely valuable dynamic information that cannot be obtained from any other source.
- Recording the patient's NHP and orienting the 3D composite skull model is an important prerequisite for accurate CASS planning.

REFERENCES

1. Bell WH (ed): *Surgical correction of dentofacial deformities*. Philadelphia, 1980, WB Saunders.

2. Bell WH (ed): *Modern practice in orthognathic and reconstructive surgery*. Philadelphia, 1992, WB Saunders.

3. Bell WH, Guerrero CA (eds): *Distraction osteogenesis of the facial skeleton*, ed 1. Hamilton, Ontario, Canada, 2006, BC Decker.

4. Gateno J, Xia JJ, Teichgraeber JF, et al: Clinical feasibility of computer-aided surgical simulation (CASS) in the treatment of complex cranio-maxillofacial deformities, *J Oral Maxillofac Surg* 65:728, 2007.

5. Santler G: 3-D COSMOS: a new 3-D model based computerised operation simulation and navigation system. *J Maxillofac Surg* 28:287, 2000.

6. Swennen GR, Barth EL, Eulzer C, et al: The use of a new 3D splint and double CT scan procedure to obtain an accurate anatomic virtual augmented model of the skull, *Int J Oral Maxillofac Surg* 36:146, 2007.

7. Swennen GR, Mommaerts MY, Abeloos J, et al: The use of a wax bite wafer and a double computed tomography scan procedure to obtain a three-dimensional augmented virtual skull model, *J Craniofac Surg* 18:533, 2007.

8. Troulis MJ, Everett P, Seldin EB, et al: Development of a three-dimensional treatment planning system based on computed tomographic data, *Int J Oral Maxillofac Surg* 31:349, 2002.

9. Xia J, Ip HH, Samman N, et al: Computer-assisted three-dimensional surgical planning and simulation: 3D virtual osteotomy, *Int J Oral Maxillofac Surg* 29:11, 2000.

10. Xia JJ, Gateno J, Teichgraeber JF: Three-dimensional computer-aided surgical simulation for maxillofacial surgery, *Atlas Oral Maxillofac Surg Clin North Am* 13:25, 2005.

11. Proffit WR, Fields HW Jr, Ackerman JL, et al: *Contemporary orthodontics*, ed 3. St Louis, 2000, Mosby.

12. Gateno J, Forrest KK, Camp B: A comparison of 3 methods of face-bow transfer recording: implications for orthognathic surgery, *J Oral Maxillofac Surg* 59:635, 2001.

13. Santler G, Karcher H, Gaggl A, et al: Stereolithography versus milled three-dimensional models: comparison of production method, indication, and accuracy, *Comput Aided Surg* 3:248, 1998.

14. English JD, Peltomaki T, Pham-Litschel K: *Mosby's orthodontic review*, ed 1. St Louis, 2008, Mosby.

15. Severt TR, Proffit WR: The prevalence of facial asymmetry in the dentofacial deformities population at the University of North Carolina, *Int J Adult Orthodon Orthognath Surg* 12:171, 1997.

16. Ellis E 3rd, Tharanon W, Gambrell K: Accuracy of face-bow transfer: effect on surgical prediction and postsurgical result, *J Oral Maxillofac Surg* 50:562, 1992.

17. Gateno J, Xia J, Teichgraeber JF, et al: A new technique for the creation of a computerized composite skull model, *J Oral Maxillofac Surg* 61:222, 2003.

18. Swennen GR, Schutyser F: Three-dimensional cephalometry: spiral multi-slice vs cone-beam computed tomography, *Am J Orthod Dentofacial Orthop* 130:410, 2006.

19. Swennen GR, Schutyser F, Barth EL, et al: A new method of 3-D cephalometry Part I: the anatomic Cartesian 3-D reference system, *J Craniofac Surg* 17:314, 2006.

20. Xia JJ, Phillips CV, Gateno J, et al: Cost-effectiveness analysis for computer-aided surgical simulation in complex cranio-maxillofacial surgery, *J Oral Maxillofac Surg* 64:1780, 2006.

21. Xia J, Samman N, Yeung RW, et al: Three-dimensional virtual reality surgical planning and simulation workbench for orthognathic surgery, *Int J Adult Orthodon Orthognath Surg* 15:265, 2000.

22. Xia J, Samman N, Yeung RW, et al: Computer-assisted three-dimensional surgical planing and simulation. 3D soft tissue planning and prediction, *Int J Oral Maxillofac Surg* 29:250, 2000.

23. Xia J, Ip HH, Samman N, et al: Three-dimensional virtual-reality surgical planning and soft-tissue prediction for orthognathic surgery, *IEEE Trans Inf Technol Biomed* 5:97, 2001.

24. Gateno J, Teichgraeber JF, Xia JJ: Three-dimensional surgical planning for maxillary and midface distraction osteogenesis, *J Craniofac Surg* 14:833, 2003.

25. Gateno J, Teichgraeber JF, Aguilar E: Computer planning for distraction osteogenesis, *Plast Reconstr Surg* 105:873, 2000.

26. Gateno J, Allen ME, Teichgraeber JF, et al: An in vitro study of the accuracy of a new protocol for planning distraction osteogenesis of the mandible, *J Oral Maxillofac Surg* 58:985, 2000.

27. Xia JJ, Gateno J, Teichgraeber JF, et al: Accuracy of the computer-aided surgical simulation (CASS) system in the treatment of patients with complex craniomaxillofacial deformity: a pilot study, *J Oral Maxillofac Surg* 65:248, 2007.

28. Epker BN, Stella JP, Fish LC (eds): *Dentofacial deformities*. St Louis, 1995, Mosby.

29. Nelson CL, Spagnoli DB (eds): *Oral and maxillofacial surgery knowledge update, vol 1, part II. Orthognathic surgery sections*. Rosemont, Ill, 1995, American Association of Oral and Maxillofacial Surgeons.

30. Gateno J, Teichgraeber JF, Xia J: *Method and apparatus for fabricating orthognathic surgical splints (US Patent 6,671,539), in USPTO Patent Full-Text and Image Database*. Washington, DC, 2003, US Patent and Trademark Office.

31. Gateno J, Xia J, Teichgraeber JF, et al: The precision of computer-generated surgical splints, *J Oral Maxillofac Surg* 61:814, 2003.

32. Schatz EC: *A new technique for recording natural head position in three dimensions [MS thesis]*. Houston, Tex, Orthodontics, University of Texas Health Science Center at Houston, 2006.

33. Weiskircher MN: *Accuracy of a new technique for recording natural head position in three dimensions [MS thesis]*. Houston, Tex, Orthodontics, University of Texas Health Science Center at Houston, 2007.

34. Xia JJ, Gateno J, Schatz EC, et al: *Accuracy of a new technique for recording natural head position in three dimensions*. 90th Annual Meeting of American Association of Oral and Maxillofacial Surgeons, Sept 16-20, 2008, Seattle, Wash.

35. Grayson B, Cutting C, Bookstein FL, et al: The three-dimensional cephalogram: theory, technique, and clinical application, *Am J Orthod Dentofacial Orthop* 94:327, 1988.

36. Grayson BH, LaBatto FA, Kolber AB, et al: Basilar multiplane cephalometric analysis, *Am J Orthod* 88:503, 1985.

37. Grayson BH, McCarthy JG, Bookstein F: Analysis of craniofacial asymmetry by multiplane cephalometry, *Am J Orthod* 84:217, 1983.

38. Bland JM, Altman DG: Statistical methods for assessing agreement between two methods of clinical measurement, *Lancet* 1:307, 1986.

39. Donatsky O, Bjorn-Jorgensen J, Holmqvist-Larsen M, et al: Computerized cephalometric evaluation of orthognathic surgical precision and stability in relation to maxillary superior repositioning combined with mandibular advancement or setback, *J Oral Maxillofac Surg* 55:1071, 1997.

40. Ong TK, Banks RJ, Hildreth AJ: Surgical accuracy in Le Fort I maxillary osteotomies, *Br J Oral Maxillofac Surg* 39:96, 2001.

41. Tng TT, Chan TC, Hagg U, et al: Validity of cephalometric landmarks. An experimental study on human skulls, *Eur J Orthod* 16:110, 1994.

42. Padwa BL, Kaiser MO, Kaban LB: Occlusal cant in the frontal plane as a reflection of facial asymmetry, *J Oral Maxillofac Surg* 55:811, 1997.

43. Next generation i-CAT specifications. Available at http://www.imagingsciences.com/pro_iCAT_NextGen_specs.htm. Accessed Feb 26, 2009.

44. Moorrees CF: Natural head position—a revival. *Am J Orthod Dentofacial Orthop* 105:512, 1994.

Chapter 75

Mandibular Deficiency: Bilateral Sagittal Split Osteotomy

Jessica J. Lee

Mandibular osteotomy is the most commonly used surgical procedure for correction of dentofacial deformities, particularly mandibular deficiency. Although there are numerous technical variations, sagittal split osteotomy is the technique most familiar and widely used by oral and maxillofacial surgeons. The purpose of this chapter is to provide a practical guide for surgeons in treatment planning and performing the bilateral sagittal split osteotomy (BSSO) for mandibular advancement.

ANATOMIC CONSIDERATION

The mandible is surrounded by a rich network of vascular and neural structures. Potential hemorrhage, although rare, may occur when the soft tissue is not properly retracted and the vessels located within the periosteal envelope are violated, such as maxillary, facial, and retromandibular vessels and their tributaries. Aside from the vascular structure surrounding the mandible, there is essentially one major anatomic structure of which surgeons must be aware in performing BSSO—the inferior alveolar (IA) nerve. Avoiding damage to the IA nerve is a major surgical goal, although postoperative neurosensory disturbance is an expected sequela of this technique and its avoidance is nearly impossible. Consistency in well-defined criteria for neurosensory deficit in the literature is sketchy at best. However, it would be misleading to say that the patients' neurosensory recovery following BSSO would return to 100% of the baseline before surgery, because there are many instances where this is not the case. The clinical implications of neurosensory disturbances following BSSO will be discussed further in the latter part of this chapter, but the anatomic relationship of the IA canal to the buccal cortex of the mandible has been shown to be a factor in the development of neurosensory disturbance after BSSO. The IA canal that comes in contact with the buccal cortical bone has a significantly greater incidence of neurosensory disturbance than the IA canal that does not contact the buccal cortex, and it is also significantly more likely that altered sensation will be present 1 year after surgery. Contrary to the conventional wisdom, manipulation of the IA nerve does not consistently result in nerve dysfunction based on sensory-evoked potential, but the nerve conduction is clearly disturbed in cases with nerve laceration. Short mandibular height and the location of the mandibular canal near the inferior border of the mandible may increase the risk of IA nerve injury.

DIAGNOSTIC STUDIES

Lateral cephalometric and panoramic radiographs are routine diagnostic imaging necessary for surgical planning. Cone beam computed tomography (CT) is gaining popularity in orthognathic surgery, and although it can be a valuable adjunct to plain films in diagnosing jaw asymmetry and condylar abnormalities, routine use can be inhibitive in terms of cost to the patient.

Condylar morphology, position of the IA nerve, presence of impacted third molars, differential silhouettes of the inferior border of the mandible suggesting skeletal asymmetry, and steepness of the mandibular plane angle are some of the crucial checkpoints that must be evaluated on the plain films or CT images if they are available.

MODEL SURGERY CHECKLIST

In setting up the models for mandibular advancement, one has to check for the following:
1. Presence of nonfunctional maxillary second molar following mandibular advancement.
2. Incisor and canine relationship after simulated mandibular advancement.
3. Presence of the curve of Spee. If the curve of Spee is to be leveled postoperatively, then 0.5 to 1 mm extra overjet should be built into the final set-up, because the lower incisors will move forward during postoperative leveling of the curve of Spee.
4. Extent of the curve of Wilson (if there is a residual dental compensation evidenced by buccal tipping of the maxillary molars and lingual tipping of the mandibular molars) (see the section Adjunctive Technique: Midline Osteotomy).
5. Presence of residual bicuspid extraction spaces. Sometimes, the orthodontist was not able to fully close the extraction spaces prior to surgery; one must then consider use of a temporary anchorage device for protraction of posterior segment for extraction space closure, or for overcorrection to an end-to-end incisor relationship to account for postoperative retraction of the lower incisors to close the extraction space.

SURGICAL TECHNIQUE

The incision is made over the anterior portion of the vertical ramus, extending to the mesial aspect of the first molar. Subperiosteal dissection is carried down to the inferior border of the mandible, and a lateral channel retractor is placed. The exposure should be limited posteriorly to preserve the blood supply to the proximal segment. A forked retractor is used to strip the temporalis attachment superiorly, at least to the level of the sigmoid notch to ensure adequate access for the medial cut. Posteromedially, the periosteum must be reflected to the medial flare of the condylar neck. Inferiorly, the medial cortex is exposed to immediately above the lingula, and a medial channel retractor is placed.

A long bur is used to make a horizontal bone cut through the medial cortex of the ramus, just above the lingula. The medial cut should be approximately halfway into the ramus, and the surgeon must be able to look straight down to the cup of the medial channel retractor. The vertical cut is made through the buccal cortex, distal to the second molar or further anteriorly if a greater advancement is necessary. The cut must be made perpendicular to the inferior border and just through the lateral cortex, because the IA nerve is typically located just medial to the lateral cortex. The vertical and horizontal cuts are connected in the sagittal plane using a short-taper fissure bur or saw blade, just into the cancellous bone. In younger patients with a tendency for slower split, the sagittal bone cut is made a little deeper to facilitate the split propagating through the marrow space. If a third molar is present and is completely impacted, then the cut should be made through the entire mesiodistal width of the crown so that the crown will split into two halves as the mandibular split progresses.

Next, a curved osteotome is used to make sure that the medial cortical split is completed. A fine straight osteotome is tapped into the sagittal cut. A spreader and a narrow osteotome are used to gently lift the lateral cortex, and the osteotome is used to step along the connecting cut to ensure that the split stays close to the lateral cortex. Caution must be taken to visualize the IA nerve as soon as possible, because it is easy to lose sight of the nerve as the lateral cortex is split off from the medial cortex. Once the split is complete, the periosteal attachment of the medial pterygoid is stripped off the proximal segment to allow tension-free movement between the proximal and distal segment. A groove can be made with an acrylic bur in the inner aspect of the proximal segment to accommodate the IA nerve and decrease the chance of nerve compression as the proximal and distal segments are approximated and fixated.

In the case of a "bad split," measures must be taken to correct the unfavorable split if possible. If there is a buccal cortex fracture, the fractured segment must be fixated with plates and monocortical screws to reestablish the continuity of the proximal segment. If there is a lingual cortex fracture, a bicortical fixation is necessary to secure both cortices, because it is typically not easy to plate the lingual cortex. If the split goes superiorly to the condyle, either the condyle must be fixated or the patient must be placed in maxillomandibular fixation and the procedure aborted. The condyle must be allowed to heal for at least 12 months before proceeding with mandibular osteotomy again, and computed tomography may be a better method of assessing condylar healing than plain films. Caution should be exercised when evaluating condylar healing solely based on a plain film, because it may give a false sense of security when taking the patient back to the operating room for reoperation. Patients may not display symptoms and signs of condylar dysfunction and may mask the incomplete healing of the condyle, resulting in an unstable condylar segment and potential distortion of condylar guidance during BSSO fixation.

A prefabricated surgical splint is inserted and maxillomandibular fixation wires are placed. Fixation techniques are variable depending on the surgeon's preference, either monocortical plates and screws and/or bicortical screws, either transorally or transbuccally. Following the release of maxillomandibular fixation wires, occlusion must be confirmed, and condylar seating must be checked by applying gentle posterior–superior pressure at the labiomental fold. If the mandibular midline shifts to one side, the side toward which the mandibular midline is shifting must be released and fixated again, because the condyle drops back and the dental midline shifts toward the side where the condyle was not seated properly. Incisions are closed with a resorbable running suture. Drains and pressure bandages are not necessary.

ADJUNCTIVE TECHNIQUE: MIDLINE OSTEOTOMY

Transverse problems in dentofacial deformity are one of the most underdiagnosed and unrecognized issues that can compromise the final results after orthodontic and orthognathic surgical treatments.

Often, a transverse problem is not recognized until after the surgical correction is done, making it difficult, if not impossible, to obtain an adequate buccal overjet in the posterior region that is stable long term.

Clinical scenarios in which transverse problems can be problematic are:

- A constricted maxillary arch (absolute transverse deficiency)
- A secondary posterior crossbite following mandibular advancement (relative transverse discrepancy)

Constricted Maxillary Arch

In this scenario, a two- or multipiece segmental LeFort I osteotomy would normally be the mainstream treatment depending on the degree of arch constriction, if there are other concomitant vertical, horizontal, or anterior–posterior discrepancies of the maxilla. However, if the transverse problem is the only issue with the maxilla and the mandibular advancement is warranted, then the mandibular midline osteotomy can be considered as an adjunctive procedure to BSSO.

Advantages are obvious in that surgery can be limited to one jaw, which has significant financial implications for the patient and implications for the difference in postoperative care necessary for one-jaw versus two-jaw surgery. As illustrated in the surgical technique section, the mandibular midline osteotomy adds very little to the operating time and can be performed in conjunction with the horizontal osteotomy (genioplasty) of the chin.

Secondary Posterior Crossbite with Mandibular Advancement

When the patient presents to the surgeon's office ready for surgery, progress models should be taken to assess the final arch relationship. When the casts are held in Class I canine relationship, it will become apparent if there is a buccal crossbite in the molar area as the surgeon simulates the mandibular advancement. If the orthodontist has appropriately decompensated by uprighting the posterior molars and leveling the curve of Wilson, then the true extent of transverse discrepancy can be visualized. This is best evaluated by viewing the models from the back and visualizing the second molar buccal overjet (Fig. 75-1). If there is a posterior crossbite or a cusp-to-cusp relationship, the surgeon then has to either consider a surgical posterior maxillary expansion to correct this problem, accept the transverse discrepancy as is, or make a more rational choice to consider the mandibular constriction. The surgeon may consider deferring surgery and request that the orthodontist do a further posterior dental expansion by tipping the maxillary molars buccally and mandibular molars lingually; however, this can prolong the treatment time, and these types of dental movements may not be stable long term. It also presents cusp interferences as the mandible is advanced, due to the inferior and buccal rotation of the maxillary palatal cusps. Posterior crossbite after orthognathic surgery is not an easy problem to correct orthodontically; it would require an extensive dental compensation, and the end results would be an unstable occlusal relationship bound to relapse.

TRANSVERSE CORRECTION IN CLASS II MANDIBULAR DEFICIENCY

Mandibular advancement tends to aggravate transverse discrepancies as the wider posterior molar segment is brought forward to occlude with the narrower portion of the maxillary arch. Minor discrepancies can be corrected with buccal and lingual crown torque

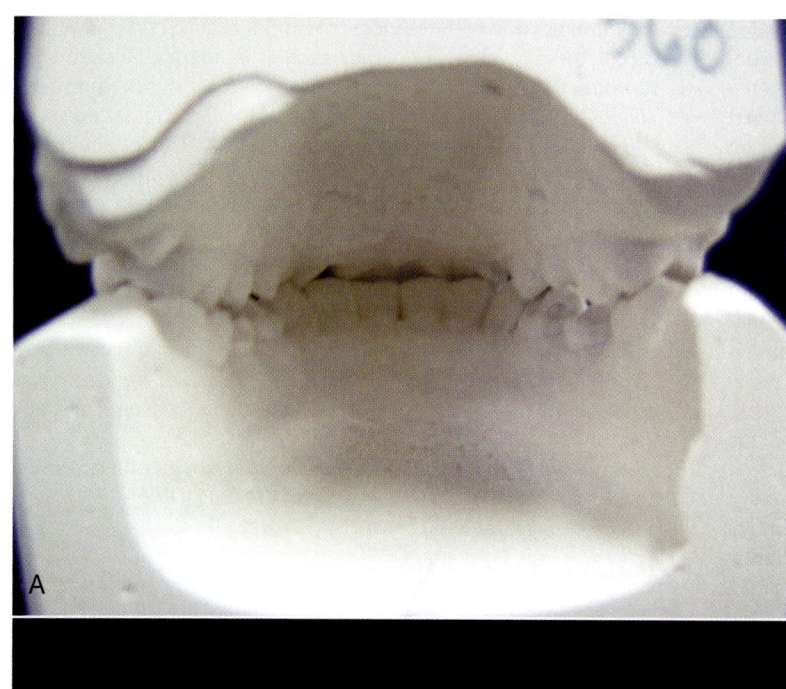

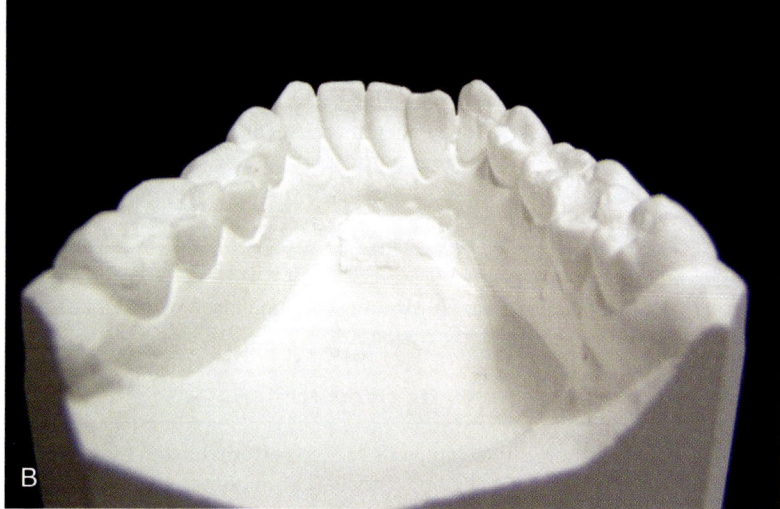

Fig. 75-1 ■ Note the curve of Wilson and lingual inclination of the mandibular molars in the lower arch. Orthodontist must decompensate and upright the lower molars. The posterior buccal overjet is best evaluated by viewing the models from the back.

of the maxillary and mandibular molars, respectively. Dental tipping tends to introduce cusp interferences, because the maxillary palatal cusps are rotated buccally and inferiorly. Such movement tends to result in a dental relapse following surgery, and it should be eliminated prior to surgical correction. This clinical dilemma has led to a search for an alternative procedure that is more stable than a segmental maxillary osteotomy.

Similar to the two-piece LeFort I widening, the magnitude of mandibular constriction increases progressively from anterior to posterior, with the greatest constriction occurring in the second molar area. Five-year follow-up shows no statistically significant relapse between the canines and first molars, but a statistically significant relapse of 0.6 mm in the second molar. However, this was clinically insignificant, because there was no incidence of posterior crossbite at the latest follow-up. The maximum, stable mandibular constriction observed is approximately 10 mm, which is comparable to the surgically assisted rapid palatal expansion (up to 14 mm expansion) and the segmental LeFort I expansion (up to 15 mm), but the latter procedures have significantly higher relapse rates of 40% to 50%, with the degree of relapse directly proportional to the magnitude of surgical expansion.

Mandibular midline or symphysis osteotomy is not a brand-new concept and has been used in oral and maxillofacial surgery. Earlier variations of mandibular midline or symphysis osteotomy have been reported in the literature. Historically, it has been a workhorse in oncologic procedures in which a superb surgical access to the oral and pharyngeal tumors was gained by performing the mandibular midline split. There have been few reports in the literature in which mandibular symphyseal ostectomies were used for surgical correction of various dentofacial deformities, such as mandibular prognathism and asymmetry. Current modification of the mandibular midline osteotomy with the advent of rigid fixation has provided a stable and practical method of correcting the transverse discrepancies.

There are several questions raised by surgeons and orthodontists about the long-term implications of this procedure, particularly the potential adverse effects on periodontal attachment of central incisors in the line of osteotomy and temporomandibular joints. Postoperative periapical radiographs showed good bone healing without an evidence of periodontal defect. Pocket depths, gingival attachment level, gingival bleeding index, and plaque depths were measured following mandibular midline osteotomies.

The periodontal tissue at the interdental osteotomy site responded favorably to the constriction when compared with the control site, which implies that the gingival attachment is not disrupted by the osteotomy cut. A 5-year periodontal evaluation at the interdental osteotomy site again confirmed that there was no adverse effect on the periodontal tissues.

Transverse constriction in the mandible may raise a concern for alteration in condylar position and potential adverse influence on the temporomandibular joint. It is well known that a temporomandibular joint dysfunction may occur in a minority of patients who underwent orthognathic surgery, which is thought to be secondary to the condylar displacement in the transverse dimension. Computed tomography of the condylar position after orthognathic surgery traditionally showed apparent changes, but the clinical implications of these changes are controversial. Therefore, it is logical to investigate the clinical outcome of the midline osteotomy for constriction. Does it cause the transverse displacement of the proximal segment, and if so, does it manifest as clinical symptoms and signs? Contrary to the theoretical assumption, temporomandibular joint (TMJ) examinations did not reveal any changes in joint pain and noises at 5-month follow-up. A 5-year follow-up study showed that the patients who underwent midline constriction with mandibular advancement reported no significant difference in temporomandibular joint function compared with those who underwent mandibular advancement alone. There was no difference between the two groups in the amount of maximum mouth opening and jaw range of motion, which were found to be within the normal limits. Likewise, a question may be raised that, although there are no clinical symptoms, there may be a change in intercondylar width and angulation with the midline constriction. Interestingly, submentovertex radiographs of the patients who underwent mandibular advancement with constriction, in fact, showed less but statistically significant change in intercondylar width and angulation than did the mandibular advancement–only group.

There are practical advantages of mandibular midline osteotomy for patients. Surgery cost is significantly reduced compared with a two-jaw surgery, and the duration of recovery and patient downtime from work after surgery are substantially reduced. In this age of cost containment and limited third-party reimbursement, patients are often left with the decision to abandon the surgical option altogether, due to the high cost of orthognathic surgery. If a surgical procedure can fulfill the treatment objectives with less invasive surgery at a reasonable cost, then an adjunctive procedure, such as the midline osteotomy, would provide the patients with better overall surgical care. Moreover, it would reduce the total treatment time for postsurgical orthodontic treatment and improve the final occlusal outcome.

PREOPERATIVE CHECKLIST

- Take progress models.
- Put the casts into Class I canine relationship and assess the molar cusp relationship (Fig. 75-2).
- If no surgical treatment is planned in the maxilla and there is an end-to-end cusp relationship or buccal crossbite, plan for midline constriction. Make sure that the vertical inclinations of the mandibular second molars are upright without dental compensation and lingual tipping.
- Check the width of interseptal bone between lower central incisors on the radiograph. Typically, there is very little bone between the incisors, but this is rarely a problem as long as there is more than 1 mm of bone between the roots of the incisors.

- Communication with orthodontist is critical. The curve of Wilson needs to be leveled and molars should be oriented upright prior to surgery. Any dental compensation needs to be eliminated. There will be a minor lingual torque of the mandibular posterior segments following the midline constriction. This effect can be exacerbated by the preexisting lingual crown torque caused by the orthodontic mechanics for correcting posterior crossbite, which will introduce a built-in instability postoperatively.
- Consult with orthodontist to place a constricting arch wire in the lower arch within 1 week or less prior to surgery. Rectangular arch wires have enough memory such that if they are not narrowed just before surgery, they will cause dental movements, and this may contribute to the skeletal relapse of the transverse correction. This can be done at the time of surgical hook placement.
- Keep in mind that mandibular constrictions greater than 10 mm, measured at the second molars, tend to be unstable.

MODEL SURGERY

Mark a vertical line on the back of the mandibular cast, corresponding to the central groove of the second molars. Measure and record the transverse distance between these two lines.

Section the cast between the central incisors until the palatal cusps of maxillary second molars occlude into the central fossa of the mandibular second molars. Secure the cast with sticky wax. Complete the model surgery for splint fabrication.

SURGICAL INSTRUMENTS

- Oscillating saw blade
- Reciprocating saw if planning for simultaneous genioplasty,
- 10-mm fine straight osteotome

SURGICAL TECHNIQUE

Standard surgical technique is used to perform bilateral sagittal split osteotomy as described previously. The midline cut is made following the completion of sagittal split osteotomies and placement of maxillomandibular fixation with the surgical splint in place. Wires are tightened just enough to provide a stable means of maxillomandibular fixation while the midline osteotomy is performed, but it is not necessary to completely tighten the wires at this point. Next, a vestibular canine-to-canine incision is made 2 to 3 mm below the mucogingival junction. Minimal subperiosteal dissection is carried out, leaving the mentalis attachment mostly intact. Next, the oscillating saw is used to make a bicortical midline cut starting from the inferior border of the mandible to the midpoint between the apices of the central incisors (Fig. 75-3). To ensure a safe distance from the root apices, the tip of the saw blade should be at least 3 mm away from the root apices. The cut is continued only through the buccal cortex up to the attached gingiva. Inferiorly, the cuts through the buccal and lingual cortices are completed, and the fine straight osteotome is wedged into the midline cut, and with a gentle rotational movement, the two halves of the mandible are mobilized. If the cuts were completely through the cortices, it is not necessary to tap the osteotome with a mallet, and gentle finger pressure is all that is needed. A No. 9 periosteal elevator is used to push the posterior segments lingually, and the teeth should fit into the splint. Maxillomandibular wires are then tightened. The arch wire is not cut, because it is the continuity of arch wire that ensures stability of the osteotomized segments. A 4-hole 2-mm straight plate is adapted to fit across the osteotomy site passively. Rarely, two plates may be

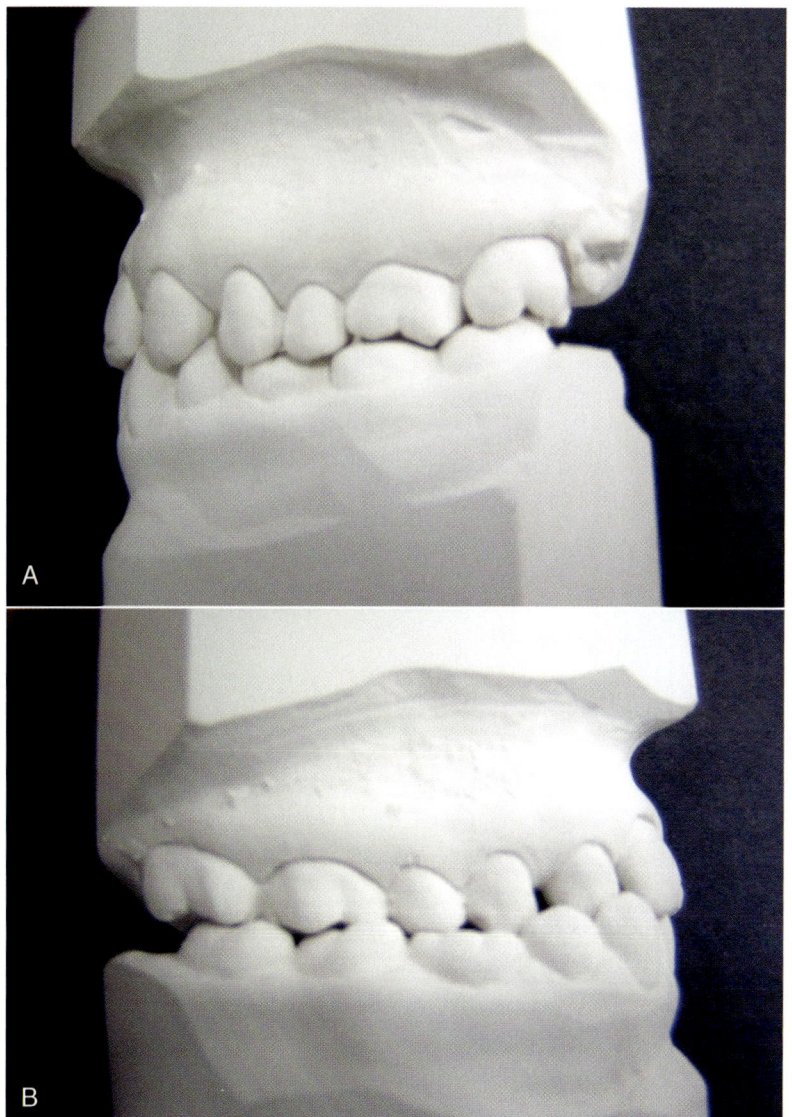

A

B

Fig. 75-2 ■ Placing the casts into Class I canine relationship reveals the inherent posterior transverse discrepancy between the maxillary and mandibular arches.

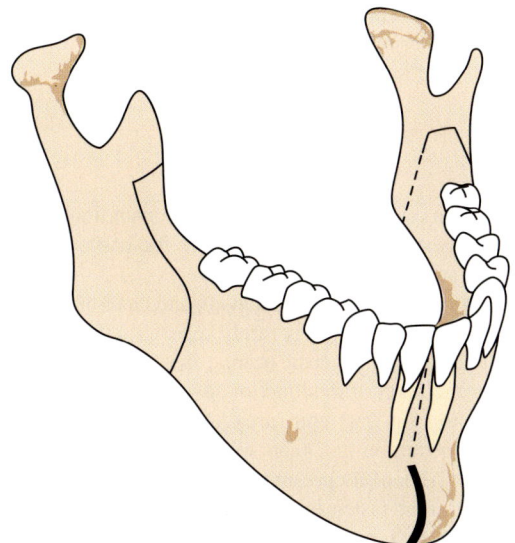

Fig. 75-3 ■ A bicortical midline cut starting from the inferior border of the mandible to the midpoint between the apices of the central incisors.

used for fixation over the midline osteotomy in cases where a correction of a large tranverse discrepancy in excess of 8 mm is required or the bone is soft with minimal cortical thickness. 2.0 bicortical screws are drilled in place; the wound is irrigated and closed with resorbable sutures. Finally, the fixation of sagittal split osteotomies is completed as described previously (Fig. 75-4).

If a horizontal osteotomy of the chin (advancement genioplasty) is planned, a monocortical, midline cut is made 2 to 3 mm away from the apices of the central incisors in the buccal cortex only. A horizontal osteotomy cut is made with a reciprocating saw inferior to the mental foramina, and the chin segment is separated. The midline cut is completed from the inferior aspect of the midline cut made previously, and care is taken to avoid the roots of central incisors. Similarly, the fine straight osteotome is twisted in the midline cut to separate the two segments of the mandible, and maxillomandibular wires are tightened. Chin segment is advanced and a No. 2 round bur is used to create three countersink holes. A long drill is used to drill the holes from the chin segment to the native mandible. Bicortical screws, measuring 12 to 16 mm are placed depending on the bone thickness, and it is important to place these screws passively as positional screws. The wound is irrigated and closed using the resorbable sutures (Fig. 75-5).

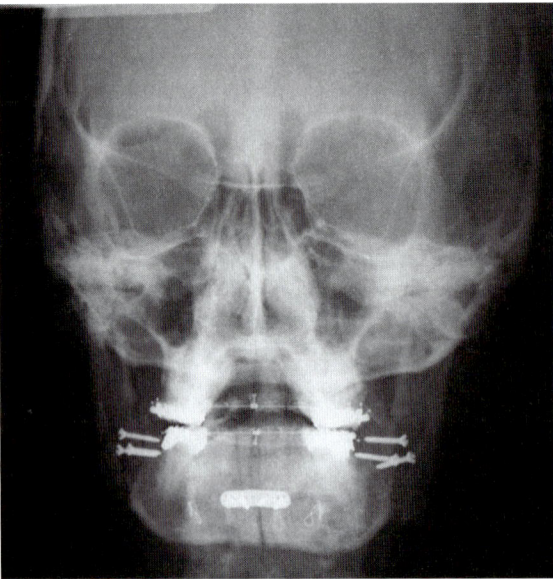

Fig. 75-4 ■ A 4-hole 2-mm straight plate adapted to fit across the osteotomy site. Two-millimeter diameter bicortical screws are drilled in place.

POSTOPERATIVE CARE

Postoperative care following mandibular osteotomy is not different from any other oral and maxillofacial surgery procedures. Applying an ice pack to the face, head elevation, pressure dressing, bedside suction, analgesia, and intravenous (IV) steroid during the postoperative period may alleviate patient discomfort and facilitate discharge. A postoperative antiemetic regimen is most commonly administered by an intravenous route, but a transdermal patch for motion sickness (i.e., scopolamine) may be useful in decreasing postoperative nausea refractory to IV antiemetics.

CLINICAL IMPLICATIONS OF BILATERAL SAGITTAL SPLIT OSTEOTOMY

NEUROSENSORY DISTURBANCES

The most common nerve dysfunction following BSSO lies with the IA nerve. Neurosensory recovery, in general, may take up to a year or longer. Patient age, degree of mandibular movement, actual nerve damage during surgery, and quality of the split have been identified as some of the predictors for IA nerve dysfunction following BSSO. The incidence of nerve dysfunction recorded postoperatively ranges widely, from 22% to 78% after 1 year post-BSSO. Systematic review of neurosensory disturbance following BSSO is difficult, due to the variability in documentation methods and lack of standardization in postoperative assessment for nerve dysfunction, but there are a few interesting findings that are worthy of discussion.

It is suggested in the literature that older patients have greater sensory losses than younger patients, in general, and large advancements and addition of a genioplasty in older populations appear to increase the risk of long-term neurosensory deficit. Fortunately, a long-term, complete sensory loss is very rare, and patients seem to adapt to a mild neurosensory deficit and report sensory function returning to be close to the baseline at 1 year after BSSO. From the technical standpoint, the surgeon's experience and the extent of soft

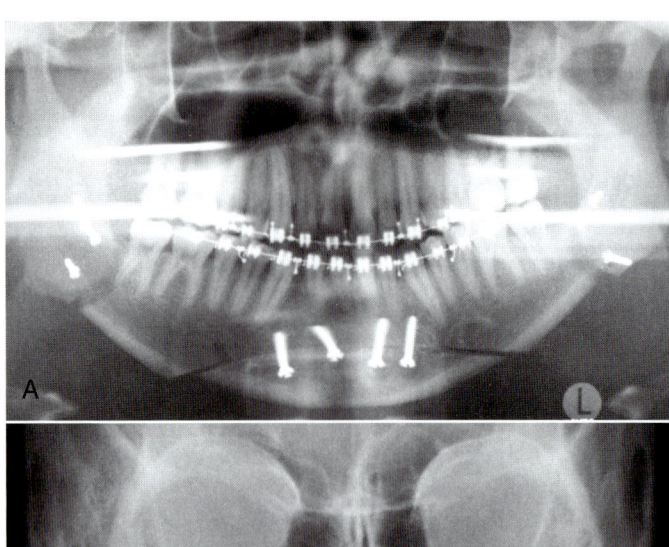

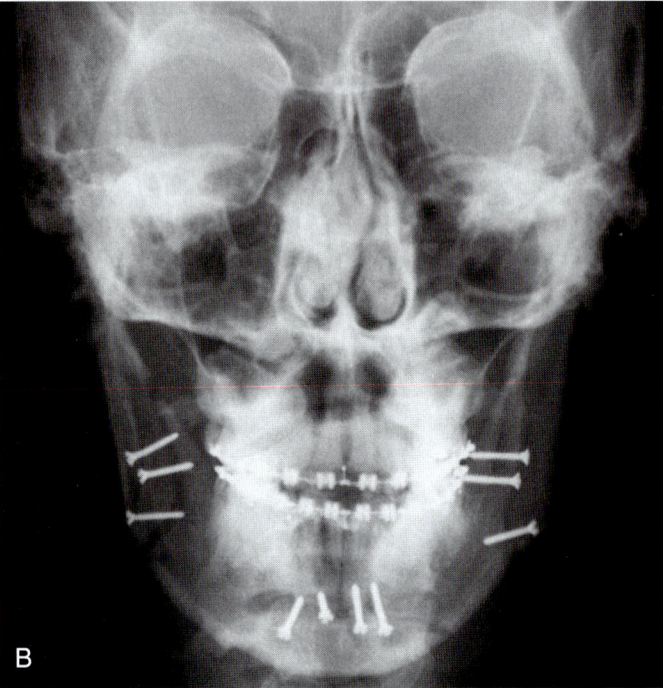

Fig. 75-5 ■ Horizontal osteotomy of the chin (advancement genioplasty). **A,** Horizontal osteotomy cut made with a reciprocating saw inferior to the mental foramina, and the chin segment is separated. The midline cut is completed from the inferior aspect of the midline cut made previously. **B,** Chin segment is advanced, and three countersink holes are created using No. 2 round bur. Bicortical screws measuring 12 to 16 mm are placed.

tissue dissection on the medial aspect of the mandibular ramus have also been suggested as being responsible for nerve dysfunction of the lower lip and chin after BSSO.

Alteration in perceived taste intensity and taste-quality identification on the localized tongue is rarely reported after BSSO, but the incidence is not zero. When it occurs, it is very difficult to objectively assess the level of dysfunction, even more so than the altered sensation in the lip and chin area. After BSSO, perceived taste intensity of the tongue has been shown to decrease for some taste perceptions to 72% of its presurgery value. Correct quality identifications of different tastes may also decrease to 75% after BSSO, compared with 96% presurgery and at 6 months postsurgery. The lingual taste function, reduced at 1 to 2 months after BSSO, is likely due to the impaired chorda tympani nerve function, but fortunately appears to return approximately 6 months after the surgery.

Relapse

Surgical relapse is an unfavorable but sometimes inevitable consequence of BSSO. In the literature, there are potential factors which may contribute to the surgical relapse following BSSO: high mandibular plane angle, type of rigid fixation, degree of mandibular advancement, and condylar position within the glenoid fossa, to mention a few.

When comparing the postoperative changes in high-angle and low-angle Class II patients after BSSO advancement with rigid fixation, few studies suggest that the high mandibular plane angle contributes to relapse following BSSO. The high mandibular plane angle is defined by some as a mandibular plane angle of 43.0 degrees (±4.0 degrees) or greater. It has been demonstrated that the high-angle patients tend to have a different pattern of surgical and postoperative changes. High-angle patients tend to be associated with both a higher frequency and a greater magnitude of horizontal relapse. While 95% of the total relapse takes place during the first 2 months after surgery in the low-angle group, high-angle patients demonstrate a more continuous relapse pattern, which may occur late in the follow-up period. It is a widely accepted theory that perioperative surgical increase in the mandibular plane angle and posterior facial height contribute to the relapse following BSSO, but there is lack of convincing evidence that this is the primary etiologic factor for relapse. In fact, the etiology behind the BSSO relapse appears to be multifactorial in nature and not exclusively due to the increase in posterior facial height.

The type of fixation may play a role in surgical stability following BSSO advancement. When comparing intermaxillary fixation and rigid fixation, the majority of studies indicate improved stability with rigid fixation. In those cases where the relapse occurred with rigid fixation, condylar displacement, condylar torquing, and improper seating of condyle are possible causes of postoperative relapse in both the horizontal and vertical dimensions. In one study, the short-term relapse for bicortical screws was 1.5% to 32.7%, for miniplates 1.5% to 18.0%, and for bioresorbable bicortical screws 10.4% to 17.4% at point B. The long-term relapse for bicortical screws was 2.0% to 50.3%, and for miniplates 1.5% to 8.9% at point B. Bicortical screws, regardless of material, do not appear to be different in terms of skeletal stability when compared with miniplates in the short term. This study demonstrates that the etiology of relapse is multifactorial, including the proper seating of the condyles, the amount of advancement, the soft tissue and muscles, the mandibular plane angle, the remaining growth and remodeling, the skill of the surgeon, and the preoperative age of patients. Patients with a low mandibular plane angle have increased vertical relapse, whereas patients with a high mandibular plane angle have more horizontal relapse. Advancements in the range of 6 to 7 mm or more predispose to horizontal relapse.

In comparing two groups of patients who underwent BSSO with either wire or rigid fixations, the final position of the condyle does not differ much. The condyles in both groups tend to move posteriorly and superiorly after BSSO advancement. No single factor could be identified to account for this change. It is suggested that a change in mechanical load may have resulted in remodeling and adaptation of the condyles, more so than how the condyles were positioned intraoperatively.

To preserve the preoperative position of the mandibular condyle during BSSO, in the past few years, several authors have proposed using condylar positioning devices, based on the assumption that accurate mandibular condyle repositioning is important in obtaining stable skeletal and occlusal results, and to prevent the onset of temporomandibular disorders. Condylar positioning devices lead to longer operating times, surgeons must keep the intermaxillary fixation as stable as possible during the application, and a high degree of precision is required in the construction of a surgical splint. Therefore, there is no scientific justification to support the routine use of condylar positioning devices in mandibular osteotomies.

The intraoperative diagnosis of an unfavorable condylar position is critical. The manual positioning of the condyle is the easiest way, but it requires a pair of experienced hands to properly seat the condyles, and this is not error-proof in all cases. Muscle tone is important in maintaining a contact between the condylar head and glenoid fossa within the temporomandibular joint. The patient under general anesthesia tends have a condylar position posterior to the one in the awake state. Under general anesthesia, the condyle may be distracted inferiorly, and this may result in condylar sag. So-called intraoperative awakening, or purposeful decrease in the depth of anesthesia in an attempt to duplicate the patient's muscle tone close to the awake state, is used by some surgeons and may be useful with those patients for whom the intraoperative condyle repositioning does not capture the patient's natural, physiologic condylar position in the awake state. However, there is no scientific evidence to support routine use of the "intraoperative lightening" in all BSSO advancement cases. In fact, malocclusion may not be noted during the operation while the patient is under any level of anesthesia, but it may become apparent when the patient fully awakes from the anesthesia, up to 12 to 24 hours later. Therefore, intraoperative recognition of condylar sag or improper condylar seating and prompt correction is the best treatment strategy.

TEMPOROMANDIBULAR JOINT DYSFUNCTION

The potential effects of orthognathic surgery on signs and symptoms of temporomandibular joint disorder are still controversial. Surgeons performing BSSO must be aware of the potential implication of BSSO advancement on the onset and progression of temporomandibular disorders in patients with Class II malocclusion. There is a small but statistically significant improvement in the reported symptoms of muscle pain from before BSSO to after surgery. The number of patients with clicking upon opening typically decreases, but the number of patients with fine crepitus may increase several years after surgery, indicating further condylar remodeling. Interestingly, counterclockwise rotation of the mandible appears to be associated with more muscle tenderness, especially in patients undergoing greater BSSO advancements. The combination of long advancement with counterclockwise rotation may be associated with increased joint symptoms, although these symptoms tend to decline over the 2-year follow-up period, suggesting that the degree of advancement and mandibular rotation are not necessarily the risk factors for developing temporomandibular joint disorder in patients without preexisting conditions and that normal temporomandibular joints adapt well to the biologic changes occurring in the condyle following BSSO advancement.

COMPLICATIONS OF BILATERAL SAGITTAL SPLIT OSTEOTOMY

Postoperative complications may include bleeding, infection, IA nerve damage, reoperation due to fixation failure or condylar malposition, unfavorable split, weakness of the facial nerve, and nonunion at the site of osteotomy that requires bone graft, osteomyelitis, and anesthesia-related complications.

The use of antibiotic prophylaxis in relation to the infection rate in orthognathic surgery is a complex issue. The orthognathic surgery–related complication rate is reported to be less than 10%,

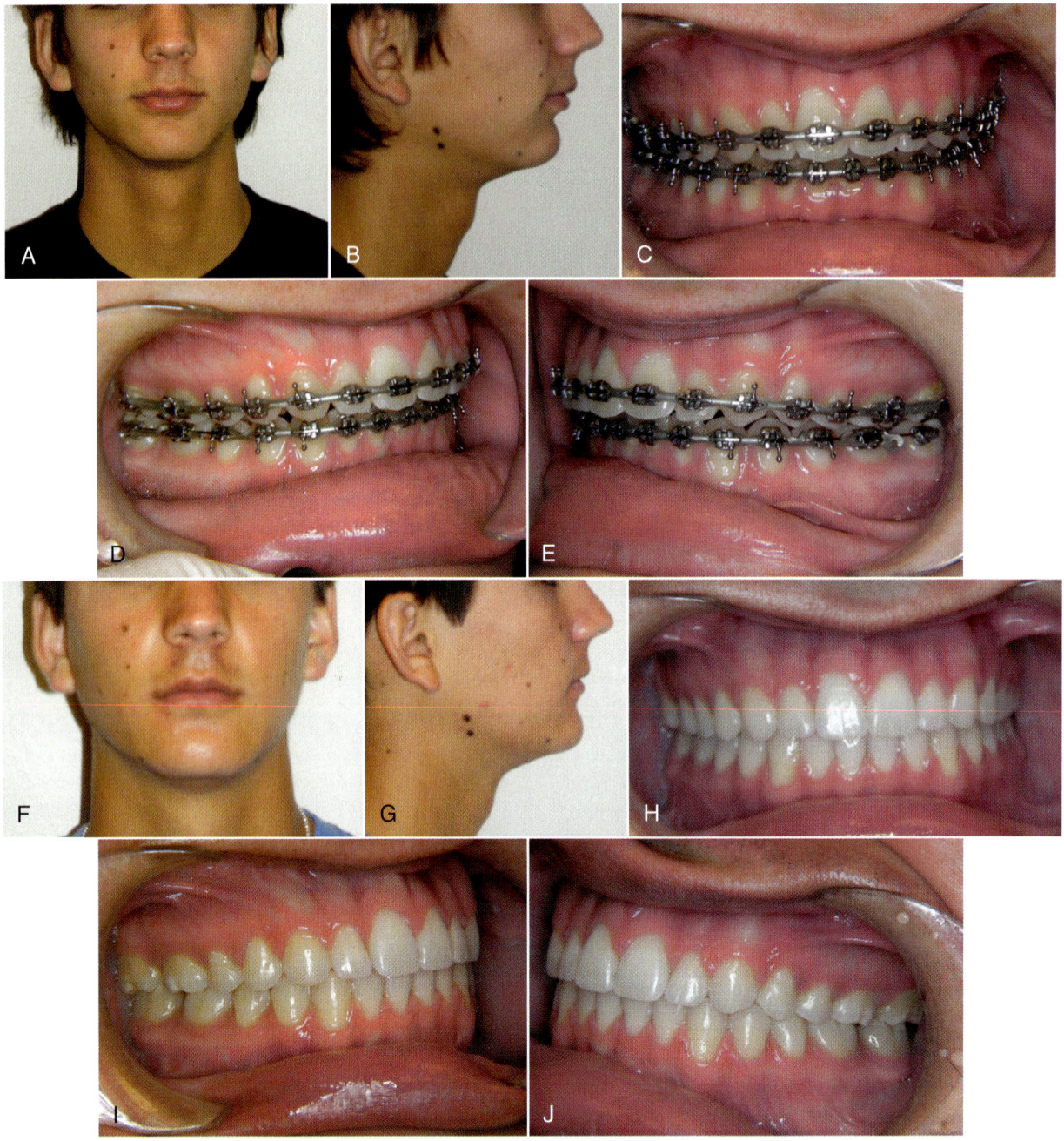

Fig. 75-6 ■ Bilateral sagittal split osteotomy advancement on a 17-year-old male with Class II mandibular deficiency. Midline osteotomy was performed in conjunction with BSSO to address the transverse discrepancy. **A** to **E**, Preoperative facial (**A** and **B**) and intraoral (**C** to **E**) photos. **F** to **J**, Postoperative facial (**F** and **G**) and intraoral (**H** to **J**) photos.

with greater than 50% of the complications related to postoperative infection, although the overall prevalence of infection after BSSO is relatively low given the complexity of the procedure performed in the intraoral environment. In one study, patients who received a single preoperative dose of antibiotics had a significantly higher infection rate (17.3%) than those who also received postoperative antibiotics for various durations. A preoperative dose of prophylactic antibiotics together with at least 2 days of postoperative doses has been shown to be useful in reducing the infection rate compared with a single dose of prophylactic antibiotics.

Complications with rigid fixation may include early loosening of fixation, hardware exposure, skeletal instability or early relapses,

persistent nerve impairments, infection, and scar formation. The use of transbuccal, bicortical screws for stabilization of bony segments have a removal rate of less than 3%, mainly due to hardware infection.

CASE STUDY

A 17-year-old male with Class II mandibular deficiency underwent BSSO advancement. Note the tight buccal overjet in the molar region, which would be aggravated by mandibular advancement. Midline osteotomy was performed in conjunction with BSSO to address the transverse discrepancy (Fig. 75-6).

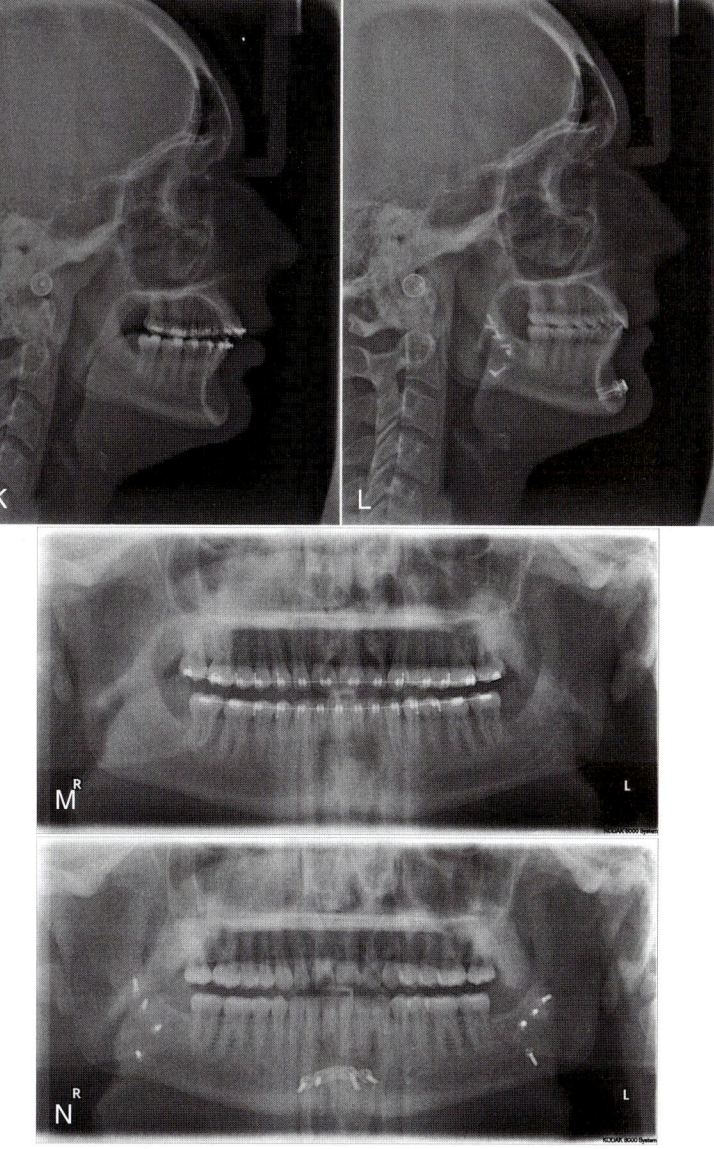

Fig. 75-6, cont'd ■ Before (**K**) and after (**L**) cephalometric views. Before (**M**) and after (**N**) panoramic views.

PEARLS AND PITFALLS

- If there is a buccal cortex fracture, the fractured segment must be fixated with plates and screws to reestablish the continuity of the proximal segment.
- If there is a lingual cortex fracture, a bicortical fixation is necessary to secure both cortices, because it is typically not easy to plate the lingual cortex.
- If the split goes superiorly to the condyle, either the condyle must be fixated or the patient must be placed in maxillomandibular fixation and the procedure aborted. The condyle must be allowed to heal for at least 9 to 12 months before proceeding with mandibular osteotomy again.

- Improper seating of the condyle must be recognized and managed intraoperatively.
- Mandibular midline osteotomy is a procedure that should be a part of the oral and maxillofacial surgeon's armamentarium. Excellent long-term stability, decreased operating time and morbidity compared with two-jaw surgery, and also reduced surgical cost and better treatment outcome for patients are some of the rationales for using this technique.

BIBLIOGRAPHY

Alexander CD, Bloomquist DS, Wallen TR: Stability of mandibular constriction with a symphyseal osteotomy, *Am J Orthod Dentofac Orthop* 103:15, 1993.

Becelli R, Fini G, Renzi G, et al: Complications of bicortical screw fixation observed in 482 mandibular sagittal osteotomies, *J Craniofac Surg* 15:64, 2004.

Bouwman JP, Husak A, Putnam GD, et al: Screw fixation following bilateral sagittal ramus osteotomy for mandibular advancement—complications in 700 consecutive cases, *Br J Oral Maxillofac Surg* 33:231, 1995.

Bouwman JP, Tuinzing DB, Kostense PJ, et al: The value of long-term follow-up of mandibular advancement surgery in patients with a low to normal mandibular plane angle, *Mund Kiefer Gesichtschir* 1:311, 1997.

Chow LK, Singh B, Chiu WK, Samman N: Prevalence of postoperative complications after orthognathic surgery: a 15-year review, *J Oral Maxillofac Surg* 65:984, 2007.

Frey DR, Hatch JP, Van Sickels JE, et al: Alteration of the mandibular plane during sagittal split advancement: short- and long-term stability, *Oral Surg Oral Med Oral Pathol Oral Radiol Endod* 104:160, 2007.

Frey DR, Hatch JP, Van Sickels JE, et al: Effects of surgical mandibular advancement and rotation on signs and symptoms of temporomandibular disorder: a 2-year follow-up study, *Am J Orthod Dentofacial Orthop* 133:490, 2008.

Gent JF, Shafer DM, Frank ME: The effect of orthognathic surgery on taste function on the palate and tongue, *J Oral Maxillofac Surg* 61:766, 2003.

Gerressen M, Stockbrink G, Riediger D, Ghassemi A: Skeletal stability following BSSO with and without condylar positioning device, *J Oral Maxillofac Surg* 65:1297, 2007.

Joondeph DR: Condylar changes and TMJ function associated with mandibular osteotomy for constriction, *Am J Orthod Dentofacial Orthop* (in press).

Joss CU, Vassalli IM: Stability after bilateral sagittal split osteotomy advancement surgery with rigid internal fixation: a systematic review, *J Oral Maxillofac Surg* 67:301, 2009.

Mobarak KA, Espeland L, Krogstad O, Lyberg T: Mandibular advancement surgery in high-angle and low-angle Class II patients: different long-term skeletal responses, *Am J Orthod Dentofacial Orthop* 119:368, 2001.

Politi M, Toro Costa F, Polini F, Robiony M: Intraoperative awakening of the patient during orthognathic surgery: a method to prevent the condylar sag, *J Oral Maxillofac Surg* 65:109, 2007.

Precious DS, Lung KE, Pynn BR, Goodday RH: Presence of impacted teeth as a determining factor of unfavorable splits in 1256 sagittal-split osteotomies, *Oral Surg Oral Med Oral Pathol Oral Radiol Endod* 85:362, 1998.

Reyneke JP, Ferretti C: Intraoperative diagnosis of condylar sag after bilateral sagittal split ramus osteotomy, *Br J Oral Maxillofac Surg* 40:285, 2002.

Rodrigues-Garcia RC, Sakai S, Rugh JD, et al: Effects of major Class II occlusal corrections on temporomandibular signs and symptoms, *J Orofac Pain* 12:185, 1998.

Teltzrow T, Kramer FJ, Schulze A, et al: Perioperative complications following sagittal split osteotomy of the mandible, *J Craniomaxillofac Surg* 33:307, 2005.

Van Sickels JE, Hatch JP, Dolce C, et al: Effects of age, amount of advancement, and genioplasty on neurosensory disturbance after a bilateral sagittal split osteotomy, *J Oral Maxillofac Surg* 60:1012, 2002.

Van Sickels JE, Tiner BD, Keeling SD, et al: Condylar position with rigid fixation vs. wire osteosynthesis of a sagittal split advancement, *J Oral Maxillofac Surg* 57:31, 1999.

Westermark A, Bystedt H, von Konow L: Inferior alveolar nerve function after sagittal split osteotomy of the mandible: correlation with degree of intraoperative nerve encounter and other variables in 496 operations, *Br J Oral Maxillofac Surg* 56:429, 1998.

White CS, Dolwick MF: Prevalence and variance of temporomandibular dysfunction in orthognathic surgery patients, *Int J Adult Orthod Orthognath Surg* 7:7, 1992.

Yamamoto R, Nakamura A, Ohno K, Michi KI: Relationship of the mandibular canal to the lateral cortex of the mandibular ramus as a factor in the development of neurosensory disturbance after bilateral sagittal split osteotomy, *J Oral Maxillofac Surg* 60:490, 2002.

Yip L, Korczak P: Clinical audit on the incidence of inferior alveolar nerve dysfunction following mandibular sagittal split osteotomies at the Derby Royal Infirmary, England, *Int J Adult Orthodon Orthognath Surg* 16:266, 2001.

Ylikontiola L, Kinnunen J, Oikarinen K: Factors affecting neurosensory disturbance after mandibular bilateral sagittal split osteotomy, *J Oral Maxillofac Surg* 58:1234, 2000.

Chapter

76

Maxillary Deficiency: Le Fort I Osteotomy

Vincent James Perciaccante

The term **maxillary deficiency** can be applied to deficiencies or hypoplasias of the maxilla in the transverse, anteroposterior (AP), and vertical dimensions. These deficiencies rarely occur in isolation and often present in some combination with each other and/or other skeletal abnormalities. For example, a patient could have a vertical maxillary hyperplasia, or excess, and nonetheless have a transverse deficiency. For sake of discussion in this chapter, we will focus on the discrepancies individually, with the understanding that their treatments may be combined with each other or other treatments.

When looking at the hierarchy of stability, the treatments of many maxillary deficiencies fall lower on the hierarchy of stability, specifically with regard to downgrafting of the maxilla and treatment of transverse discrepancy. Various techniques can be employed in an effort to mitigate this inherent instability. In this chapter, we will discuss surgically assisted rapid palatal expansion (SARPE), segmental Le Fort osteotomy, maxillary downgrafting with autogenous or bone alloplasts and donor bone (with the choice of material being open to personal preference), geometric osteotomies for downward movement without need for downgrafting, as well as straightforward maxillary advancement. The management of cleft patients and the use of distraction osteogenesis are covered elsewhere in this book.

ETIOPATHOGENESIS/CAUSATIVE FACTORS

As with most skeletofacial deformities, maxillary deficiency is multifactorial. It can be congenital (syndromic), developmental (from variations in magnitude, direction, and timing of facial growth or as a result of a habit such as thumb sucking), traumatic (either in the absolute deformity or growth disturbance as a result of trauma), or iatrogenic in nature (such as secondary to cleft repair). Though the typical complaint of a Class III patient is that their "lower jaw is too big," some degree of maxillary skeletal deficiency, without mandibular prognathism or excess, is present in as many as 75% of patients with Class III malocclusions. Transverse deficiency often is seen with maxillary AP deficiency. It has also been reported that 30% of all adult patients seeking orthodontic treatment for a dentofacial deformity have a component of transverse maxillary deficiency.

PATHOLOGIC ANATOMY

The most significant issue regarding pathologic anatomy in patients with maxillary deficiencies is the quality and quantity of the bone of the maxilla. It is a frequent finding for the bone of the anterior maxillary wall to be extremely thin in AP deficiency, in particular, and apertognathia may be present, though that is not the topic of this chapter. In both AP and transverse deficiency, there is typically crowding of the maxillary dentition, which often results in flaring of the maxillary incisors. This compensation can camouflage the appearance of the degree of the underlying skeletal deformity.

DIAGNOSTIC STUDIES

An important "diagnostic study" in the treatment of dentofacial deformities is consultation with an orthodontist. Typically, at the time of evaluation by the surgeon, a patient has had an initial consultation with an orthodontist, because patients usually seek out orthodontic consultation first, and the orthodontist refers them for surgical evaluation. Once evaluations have been completed by both professionals, they must confer to align treatment goals, establish estimated timelines, sequence, and phases of treatment.

For evaluation and treatment planning, routine panoramic radiographs as well as cephalometric radiographs and tracings are necessary. Panoramic radiographs are evaluated for presence or absence of teeth, impacted teeth, periodontal status, root relationships, bone pathology, or osseous temporomandibular joint pathology. Multitudes of cephalometric analyses exist. To evaluate maxillary deficiency, the cephalometric measurements that can be used include measurements to assess (1) AP position (sella-nasion-A-point [SNA], Pt A to Na perpendicular, Co-Pt), (2) vertical position (nasion to anterior nasal spine [ANS], ANS to Me, upper facial height [UFH]/lower anterior facial height [LAFH] ratio, AFH, posterior facial height [PFH], PFH/AFH ratio, U1-ANS), and (3) intermaxillary relationships (A point nasion B point [ANB] and Wits). The Wits analysis is used to establish the apical base relationship between the maxillary and the mandibular arches as measured along the occlusal plane. The Wits measurement is established by drawing a line from A point and B point, which proceeds perpendicular to the occlusal plane. If the B point line intersects the occlusal plane posterior to the A point line the Wits measurement is positive. If the B point line intersects the occlusal plane anterior to the A point line the Wits measurement is negative. The millimeter distance between the lines is the Wits measurement. Zero to plus one millimeter Wits is considered ideal.

Clinical database measurements, mounted models/model surgery, and clinical photographs are also used in this stage of treatment planning. Computerized tomography may be helpful in evaluation and planning but is not routinely performed at this time.

TREATMENT/RECONSTRUCTIVE GOALS

The goal of any orthognathic surgery is to establish proper function and esthetics through establishment (and maintenance) of the appropriate form and position of the jaws, a Class I occlusion with appropriate buccal-lingual relationship and appropriate overlap and overjet with aesthetic vertical and soft tissue relationships. As stated earlier, the surgical correction of vertical and transverse maxillary deficiencies, in particular, are less stable procedures and therefore a major treatment goal includes mitigation of this inherent instability.

SPECIFIC TREATMENTS AND TECHNIQUES

ANTERIOR REPOSITIONING

The basic technique for Le Fort I osteotomy is as follows.

Local anesthetic with vasoconstrictor is injected into the maxillary mucobuccal fold prior to preparing and draping the patient. This allows time for the vasoconstrictor to take effect during scrubbing, preparation, and draping and prevents wasting time under general anesthesia without progress being made. A circumvestibular incision is made by incising horizontally through the buccolabial mucoperiosteum above the attached gingiva at the level of the maxillary teeth apices.

The incision extends from first molar to first molar. The parotid papilla must be identified and protected. As the cut is carried deeper, an effort must be made to remain inferiorly. The incision is made higher posteriorly and lowers anteriorly to avoid perforation into the nasal cavity.

Usually the incision is made as a hemivestibular incision with subperiosteal dissection and exposure of each side individually. Subperiosteal dissection begins at the piriform rim and is carried superiorly and laterally along the anterior maxilla, exposing the infraorbital nerve as it exits the foramen. Posterior dissection, as it is carried behind the zygomatic buttress, must be tunneled inferiorly toward the mucogingival junction with maintenance of the subperiosteal plane, as it is carried back toward the pterygomaxillary fissure, to avoid vascular structures or exposure of the buccal fat pad. A toe-out retractor is placed behind the buttress and does not usually require being held. Dissection inside the piriform rim is started with a Woodson elevator and must be carried posteriorly with a Freer or periosteal elevator, including along the nasal floor (Fig. 76-1, A to C). Adequate elevation of this tissue is critical to prevent damage to it during the remainder of the procedure. Reference marks are made with a fissure bur for the purpose of vertical measurement.

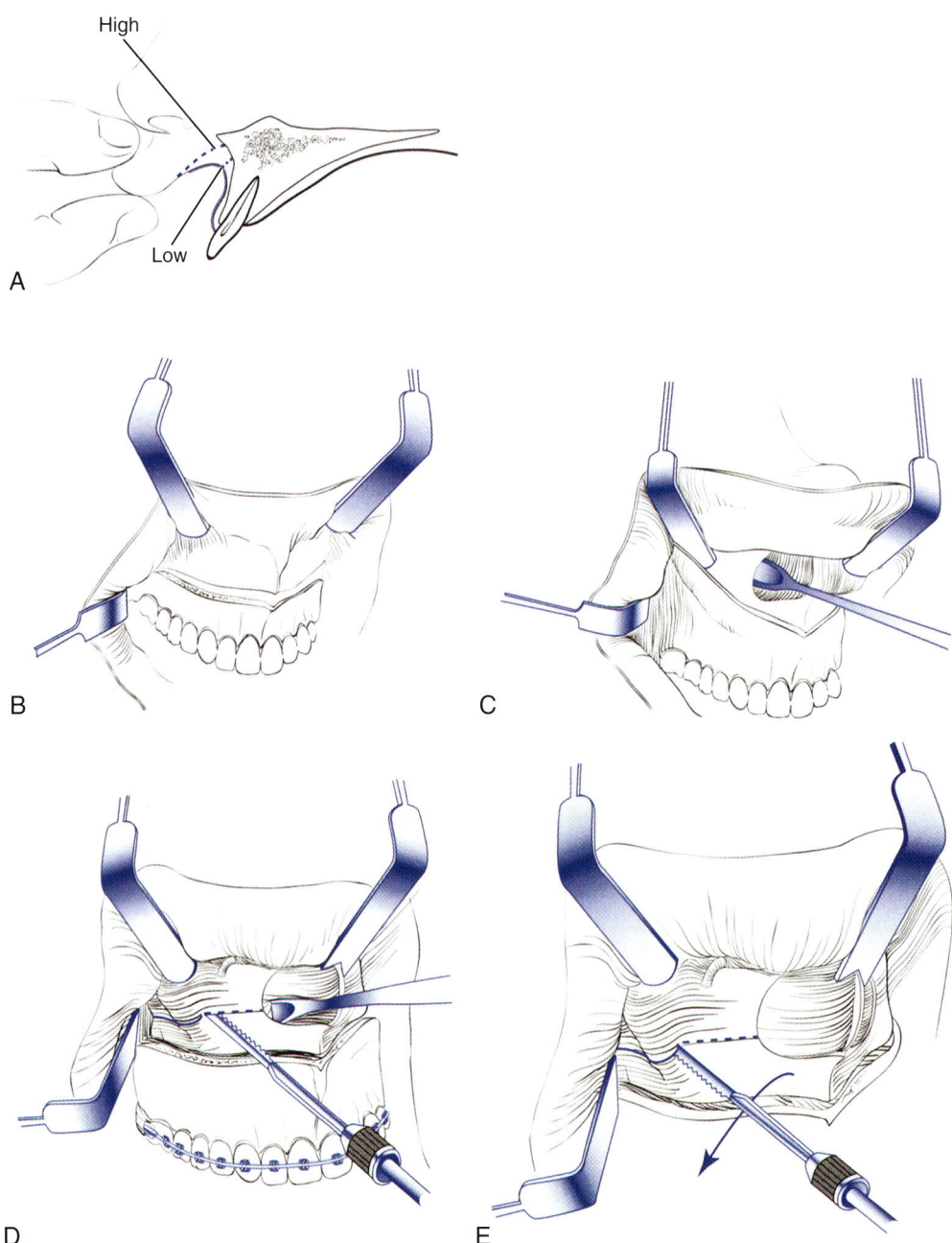

Fig. 76-1 ■ **A,** The soft tissue incision for maxillary surgery. **B,** The circumvestibular incision extends from the area of the first molar to the same location on the opposite side. **C,** The nasal mucosa is elevated beginning on the superolateral surface of the piriform rim. **D,** Lateral wall osteotomy is begun at the greatest convexity of the buttress and brought forward to the piriform rim with a periosteal elevator protecting the nasal mucosa and the endotracheal tube. **E,** The saw is then turned inside out, and the osteotomy from the buttress to the pterygomaxillary junction is made angling downward as it goes posteriorly.

A reciprocating saw is used to make a horizontal osteotomy from the maxillary buttress to the piriform rim in the area above the apices of the teeth. The saw is turned around and an inside out cut is made behind the buttress (Fig. 76-1, *D* and *E*). Exactly the same procedure is carried out on the opposite side. A guarded osteotome is driven along the lateral nasal wall to a depth of approximately 20 mm to stop short of the descending palatine arteries. The nasal septum is separated from the nasal crest of the maxilla using a septal osteotome (Fig. 76-1, *F*). As it is driven posteriorly, care must be taken to direct it slightly inferiorly and maintain it in the midline. As the osteotome reaches the vomer, it will have a tendency to ride

superiorly. The pterygoid plates are separated with a small, sharp osteotome (Fig. 76-1, *G*). This will sharply separate the pterygomaxillary junction in a controlled manner, rather than use of a broader more blunt osteotome, which can cause fracture. This osteotome, as well as spatula osteotomes used later, is sharpened before every procedure. The osteotome is directed as anteriorly, inferiorly, and medially as possible, with a finger placed palatally for palpation of complete separation.

Once the completeness of these osteotomies is ensured, the maxilla is downfractured with moderate pressure on the anterior maxilla with the sharp end of a Senn retractor. As the maxilla is

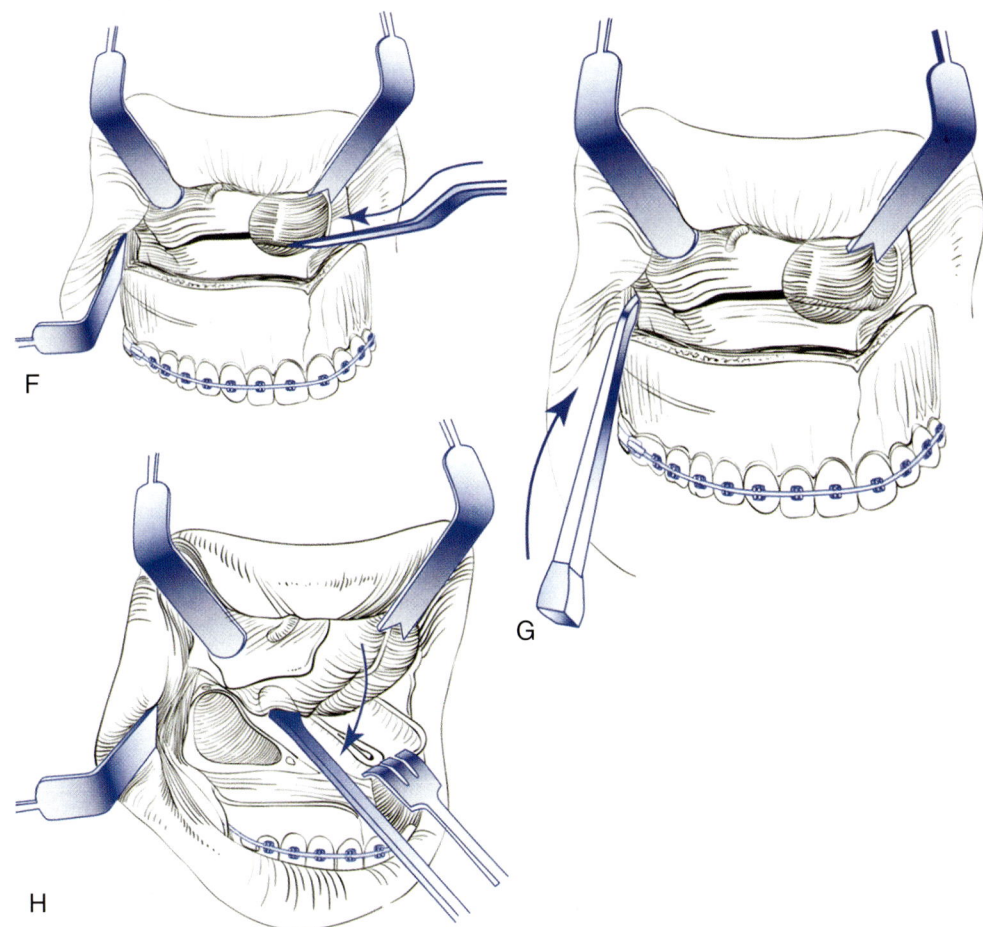

Fig. 76-1, cont'd ▪ **F,** Separation of the nasal septum from the septal crest of the maxilla with a special osteotome. **G,** Pterygomaxillary separation with a small sharp curved osteotome directed medially. **H,** Downfracturing is accomplished with a sharp-toothed Senn retractor with simultaneous elevation of the nasal mucoperiosteum. (From Miloro M (ed). Peterson's principles of oral and maxillofacial surgery, ed 2. Shelton, Conn, 2004, PMPH-USA. Reprinted with permission.)

downfractured, the nasal mucoperiosteum is elevated posteriorly to the posterior edge of the hard palate (Fig. 76-1, *H*).

Often, the key feature in anterior repositioning of the maxilla is adequate mobilization. After downfracturing, the author routinely performs ligation and division of the descending palatine arteries (DPA). The blood flow to the distal segment of the maxilla has been shown to have no significant difference before and after ligation of the arteries. Ligation of the arteries decreases blood loss, allows removal of areas of potential bony interferences, frees a potential point of tethering mobility, and eliminates unintended or unrecognized damage of the DPA. He has not experienced an ischemic event as a result of dividing the DPA, even in segmental surgery. Prior to ligation, bony irregularities in the perpendicular plate of the palatine bone around the neurovascular bundle are carefully removed with a rongeur and a Woodson elevator (Fig. 76-2, *A*).

Mobilization of the maxilla can be performed in numerous ways. My preference is to either place a J stripper through the osteotomy and around the posterior hard palate and place traction, or place a Seldon retractor or Tessier retromaxillary levers behind the buttresses on either side and place forward pressure (Fig. 76-2, *B*). To ensure that the maxilla is adequately mobilized, the oral surgical splint is placed on the mandible, and the maxilla is demonstrated to be able to easily reach its necessary position in the splint and, in fact, exceed its necessary position in the splint, with traction on the

arch wire with an Adson forceps. It is not possible to place heavy force for anterior traction with the Adson forceps, and therefore, if the appropriate position can be reached with this technique, the maxilla is well mobilized.

The maxilla is wired to the mandible using the prefabricated oral surgical split. The maxillomandibular complex is rotated, with care taken to seat the condyles. Bony interferences are removed until the desired vertical position is reached. The maxilla is secured in place using plates in the piriform and buttress regions bilaterally. Typically, 2.0- or 1.5-mm plates and screws are used (Fig. 76-2, *C*). The plates must be bent so that they are passive before placement of screws. The intermaxillary fixation is released and the occlusion is checked.

For more significant advancements, prebent plates can be used to secure the maxilla. These prebent plates are annealed after they are formed, and therefore the stresses of bending have been removed, increasing their strength and resistance to deformation.

Straight osteotomies tend to be inclined forward to avoid the cuspid tooth root. A stepped osteotomy can be designed to accommodate the planned moves according to preference (Fig. 76-3, *A* and *B*). When grafting is used, the steps provide better sites for grafting than the pterygomaxillary fissure.

The wounds are closed with 3-0 chromic gut suture. Alar base cinch suturing and V-Y closure may be used to control soft tissue esthetics. Contouring of the anterior nasal spine (ANS) is also

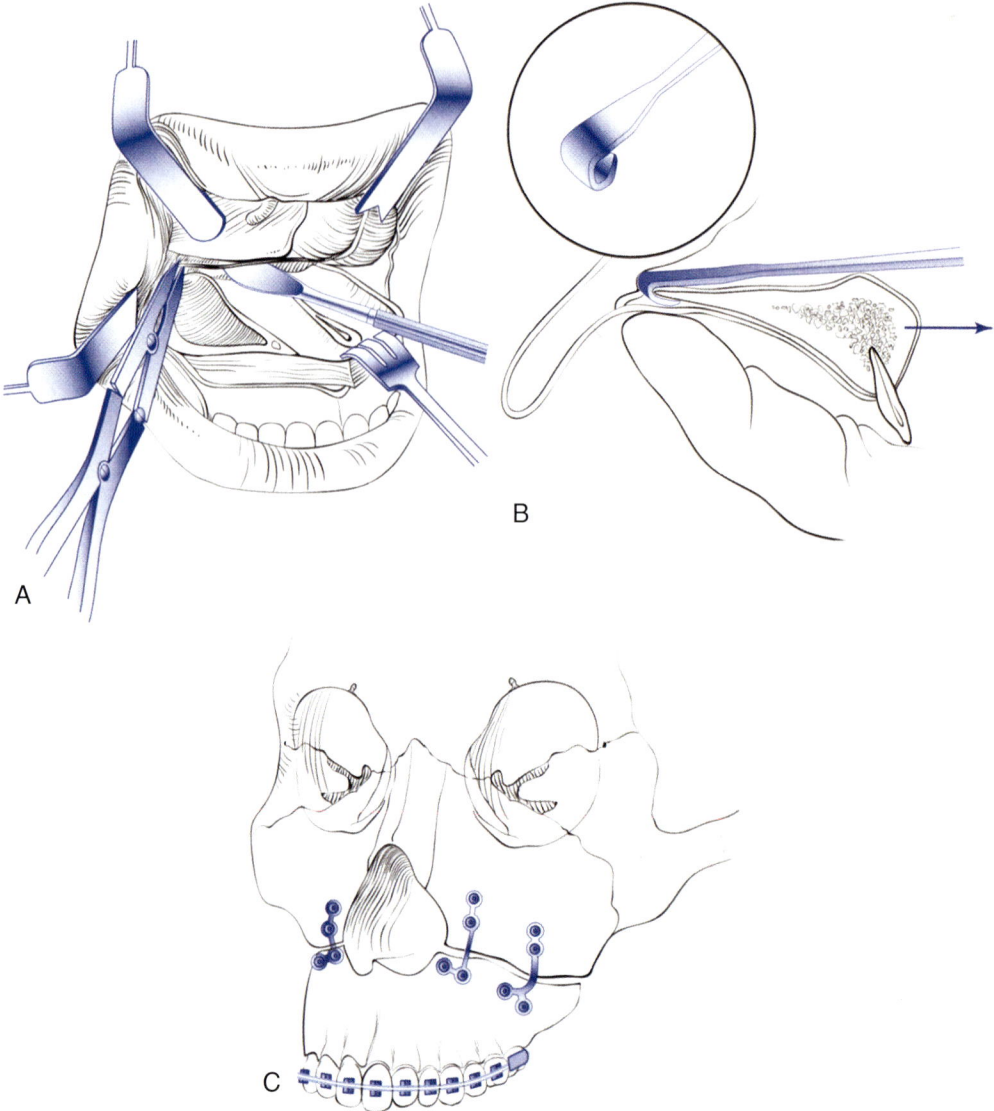

Fig. 76-2 ■ **A,** Complete removal of bone around the perpendicular plate of the palatine bone. The descending palatine artery is isolated, ligated, and divided. **B,** Mobilization of the maxilla with a J stripper. **C,** Bone plating encompasses a wide variety of plates and screws, ranging from very rigid to very malleable. Generally, 2.0-mm plates are used in the piriform rims and either 2.0- or 1.5-mm plates in the buttresses. (From Miloro M (ed). Peterson's principles of oral and maxillofacial surgery, ed 2. Shelton, Conn, 2004, PMPH-USA. Reprinted with permission.)

helpful in this regard. The nasal septum is secured to the ANS prior to closure (Fig. 76-3, *C*).

INFERIOR POSITIONING

Inferior positioning of the maxilla is the second most unstable move. When there is a need for performing inferior positioning of the maxilla, typically to allow a more esthetic amount of tooth show and/or to lengthen a brachiocephalic face, it often occurs with anterior repositioning of the maxilla. In a situation where the maxilla is moving down and forward, performance of a geometrically shaped cut often allows for good bone-to-bone contact and stability without the need for placement of a graft. This can be performed by making the osteotomy in the anterior and lateral maxillary wall in a "Z-" (or "M-") shaped osteotomy. The angle of the osteotomy is dictated by the ratio between the inferior position and the anterior position. For example, if the maxilla is being repositioned 4 mm inferiorly and

4 mm anteriorly, this is a 1 : 1 relationship, and therefore the angled osteotomy is performed at approximately 45 degrees from the horizontal. The apex of the anterior portion of the Z (M) usually occurs just below the infraorbital nerve. It is carried anterior inferiorly to the piriform rim and posteriorly to the area of the buttress (Fig. 76-4, *A* to *D*). This is usually performed with a reciprocating saw. The cut behind the buttress will often be more easily performed with a 701 fissure bur. If, for the sake of argument, more inferior positioning is desired than anterior positioning, the cut can be made more steeply and, if less, in a more shallow manner. The geometric portion of the osteotomy can be done only anteriorly or only posteriorly, depending on any rotation desired with the inferior positioning (Fig. 76-4, *E* and *F*).

In instances where pure inferior positioning is required, grafting may be necessary to allow adequate bone-to-bone contact for healing and stability. In these instances, autogenous bone, such as iliac crest;

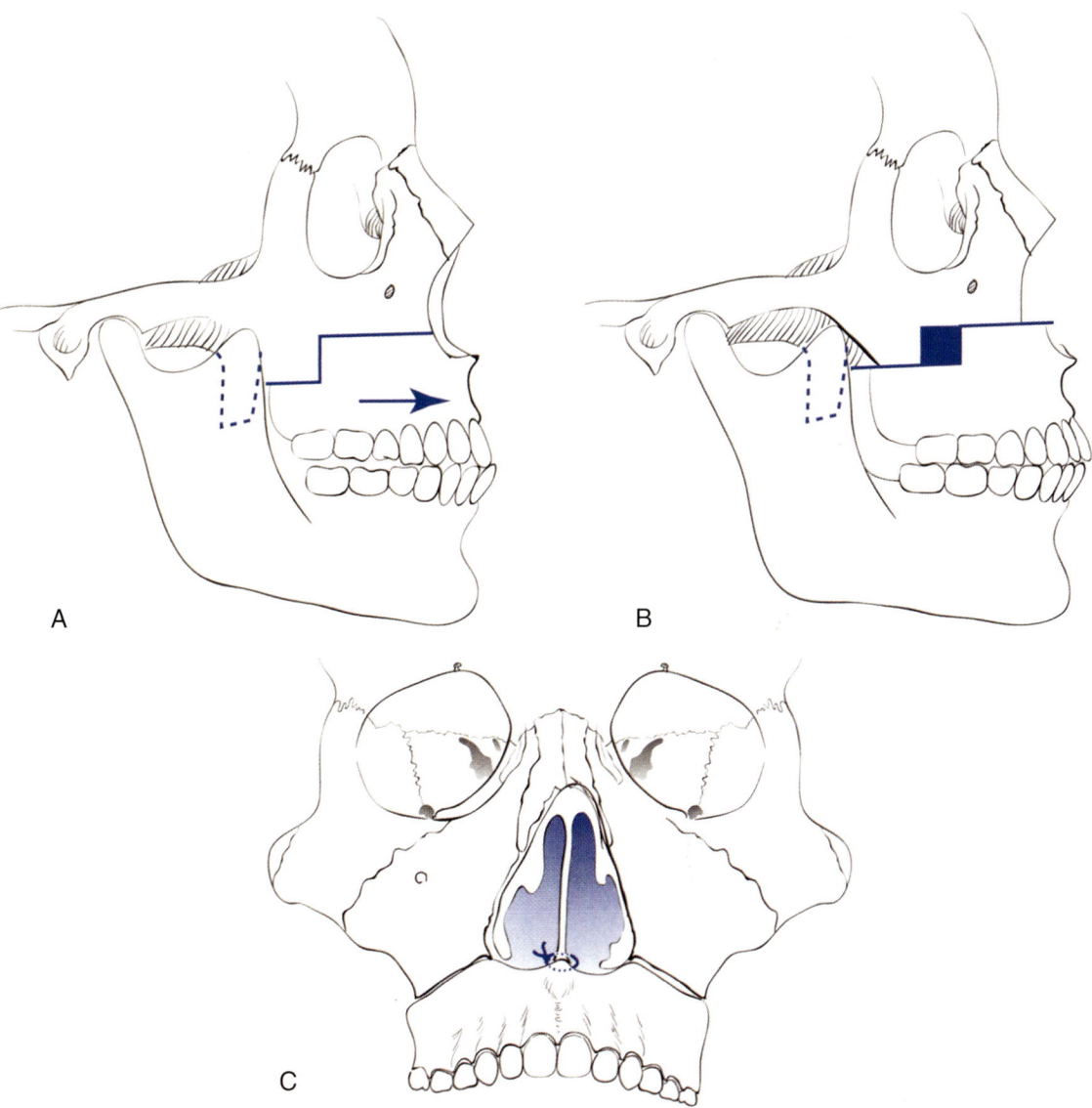

A

B

C

Fig. 76-3 ■ An alternative method for advancement is to create a step (**A**) in the buttress and place a bone graft (**B**) in the step after repositioning. **C,** To avoid septal deviation, the cartilaginous septum should be sutured to the anterior nasal spine. (From Miloro M (ed), *Peterson's principles of oral and maxillofacial surgery,* ed 2. Shelton, Conn, 2004, PMPH-USA. Reprinted with permission.)

banked bone, such as a freeze dried fibula; or alloplast, such as hydroxyapatite, can be used. Typically, the author would use the freeze dried fibula to prevent a need for an additional surgical site, additional surgical time, donor site pain, and morbidity. The segment of freeze dried bone is cut to the desired size and mortised to fit around the superior segment and inferior fragment. The graft is usually placed in four positions, at the buttresses and the piriform rims bilaterally. The need for two or four segments is dictated by the actual bone-to-bone contact and geometry of the inferior positioning. The graft can be secured with plates, screws, or wires. Wires may be necessary in the frequent situation where this bone is paper thin. A hole is drilled in the center of the graft and in the inferior and superior sides of the cut. A 28-gauge wire is used in a fashion similar to an Ivy loop to secure the graft in place (Fig. 76-5). The maxilla is secured in place using titanium fixation plates in the normal fashion. Plates of size 2.0 or 1.5 mm can be used according

to preference, but particularly an inferior positioning situation; 2.0 plates are preferred.

TRANSVERSE DEFICIENCY

The least stable orthognathic procedure is widening of the maxilla. In general, the author has a preference for the SARPE procedure versus segmental Le Fort, though neither is appropriate for all situations and both have their place. SARPE is distraction osteogenesis of the maxilla in a transverse plane. The benefits of its use are gradual callous distraction that allows the soft tissues to accommodate and greater long-term stability. Therefore, the reasons for preference of the SARPE procedure include ease of the surgical procedure versus the segmental Le Fort, the ability to perform the surgeries without need for retained occlusal or palatal splints, the ability for ultimately greater expansion, increased stability, and lower morbidity. Drawbacks of the SARPE procedure are pointed

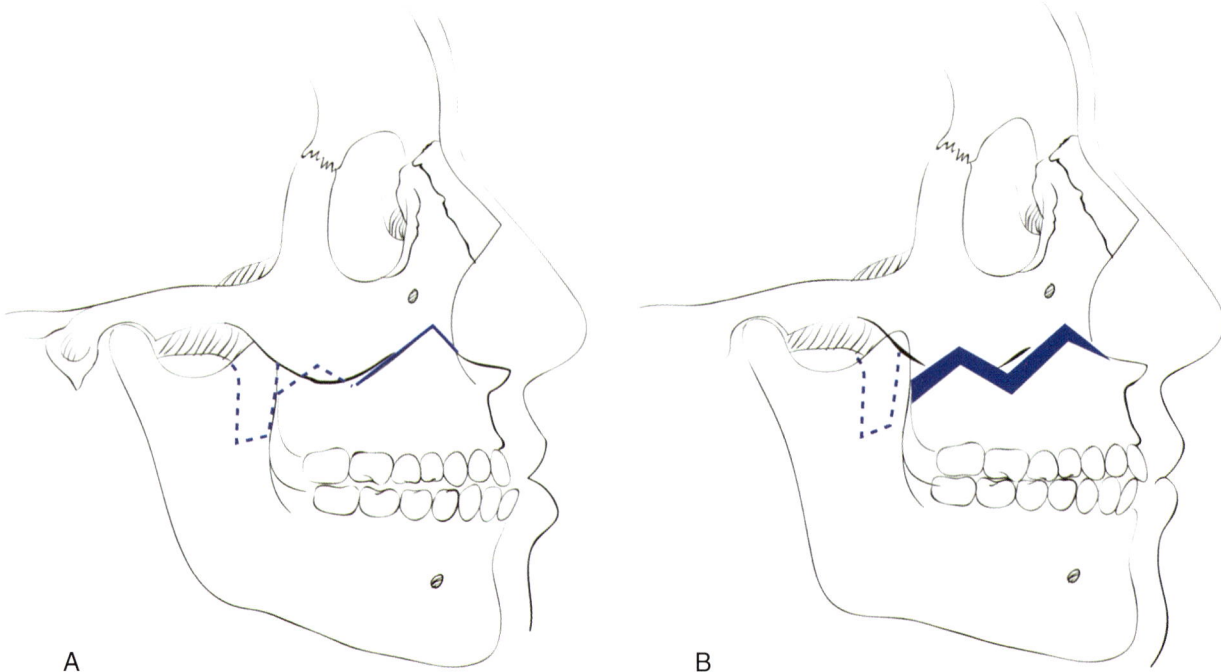

Fig. 76-4 ■ **A,** A Z-shaped osteotomy can be designed in the lateral walls of the piriform rims and the buttresses so that the maxilla may be moved downward and forward (**B**) without loss of all bony contact.

out primarily regarding the fact that, except in cases of isolated transverse deficiency, it involves two surgical procedures. It is my feeling that though two surgical procedures may be performed, they are cumulatively less difficult for the patient and the operator for the aforementioned benefits of the procedure.

When both expansion and repositioning of the maxilla are necessary, the two options are stage I SARPE followed by stage II single-piece Le Fort or a one-stage segmental Le Fort osteotomy. Factors to consider in making this determination include arch length discrepancy, arch morphology, vertical dimension, and ectopic eruption of posterior teeth.

In summary, SARPE increases arch circumference to permit alignment of crowded teeth without extraction of premolars or flaring of incisors. SARPE also will allow changing the arch morphology with anterior flattening of the characteristic tapering arch form seen in transverse deficiency, which also would require extraction in the case of a segmental Le Fort. When a multiplane occlusion is present in the vertical dimension, use of a three- or four-piece Le Fort to level the arch and simultaneously correct the transverse deficiency is indicated. Lastly, if there is ectopic eruption or extrusion of teeth that exceeds orthodontic correction, a segmental Le Fort would be indicated for correction.

SURGICALLY ASSISTED RAPID PALATAL EXPANSION

SARPE can be performed as an outpatient procedure in the operating room under full general anesthetic or in an office setting under total intravenous (IV) general anesthetic or IV sedation. The choice of the setting may depend upon the aggressiveness with which the maxilla is mobilized, surgeon and patient comfort levels, and the ability to manage potential intraoperative bleeding. If wisdom teeth are present, they can be removed at the time of the SARPE

procedure, with adequate time for healing prior to the opportunity to perform definitive orthognathic surgery.

The expansion device, usually a Hyrax, is fashioned by the orthodontist and placed prior to the time of the surgical procedure. Incisions made in performing a SARPE involve horizontal vestibular incisions in the posterior area and a vertical incision in the maxillary buccal alveolar gingiva and mucosa, in the midline (Fig. 76-6, *A*). The vestibular incision is made in the bicuspid area, with subperiosteal tunneling performed from the pterygoid maxillary fissure to the piriform rims bilaterally. The nasal mucosa is dissected free from the inside of the piriform rim, retracted medially, and protected throughout. A reciprocating saw is used to make a horizontal osteotomy from the maxillary buttress to the piriform rim in the area above the apices of the teeth. The saw is turned around, and an inside-out cut is made behind the buttress. After performing this bilaterally, a cement spatula osteotome is driven transgingivally into the mucosa, beginning at the area of the crest of the ridge and moving superiorly to the area of the anterior nasal spine. The surgeon places a finger on the inside of the palate in the anterior region, palpating as the osteotome goes through the alveolar bone and stopping before it harms the palatal tissue. At the height of the palate, the osteotome is driven back parallel to the palate for a distance of approximately 1.5 cm to open the midpalatal suture (Fig. 76-6, *B* to *E*).

The author also prefers to perform pterygomaxillary disjunction and separation of the nasal septum. The degree of mobilization necessary for adequate separation and stability of SARPE is an issue that has been of significant debate in the literature. These procedures are not absolutely necessary, and descriptions exist which do not involve these separations. Adequate separation and stability have been shown without septal or pterygoid separation, and for many years this was the technique the author has employed. I have become more aggressive with separation and mobilization over the years, because the decreased resistance appears to lead to less patient

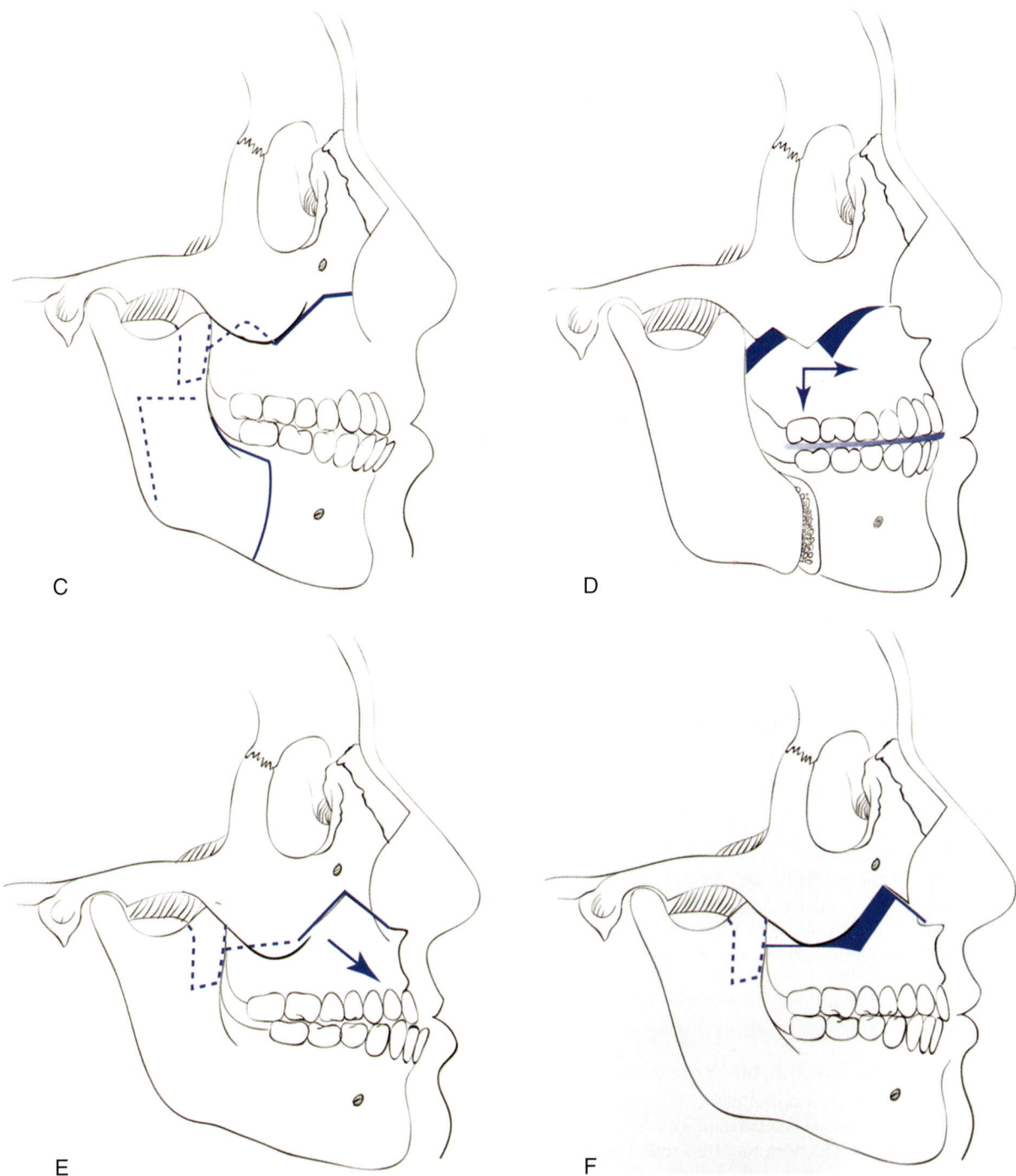

Fig. 76-4, cont'd ■ **C,** Z osteotomy with the posterior cut steeper than the anterior one to increase posterior facial height and (**D**) to rotate the maxilla downward and forward with adjustment to the occlusal plane. **E,** Z osteotomy with the posterior cut shallower than the anterior one to increase anterior facial height and (**F**) to rotate the maxilla down in front and adjust the occlusal plane to a steeper angle. (From Miloro M, editor, *Peterson's principles of oral and maxillofacial surgery,* ed 2. Shelton, Conn, 2004, PMPH-USA. Reprinted with permission.)

discomfort upon activation, decreased risk of septal deviation, and, theoretically, decreased risk of aberrant fractures caused by forces against unreleased articulations.

At this point, the independent mobility of the segments is confirmed. The Hyrax device is activated to ensure independent mobility and usually backed down to a 0.5- to 1-mm gap (Fig. 76-6, *F*). The wounds are then closed with chromic gut suture. The patient is

discharged and is seen for follow-up in approximately 5 to 7 days. At that time, assuming the soft tissue is healing properly, activation is begun. Activation could range from 1 to 2 turns per day, depending on the patient's age. Each turn is equivalent to 0.25 mm of expansion (0.20 mm on some devices). The author's preference is prefer to have the patient return to the orthodontist prior to reaching the suspected amount of necessary widening. It is incumbent upon

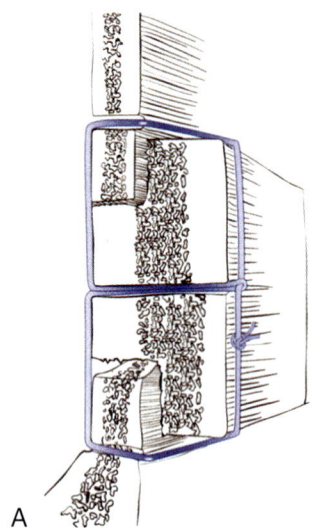
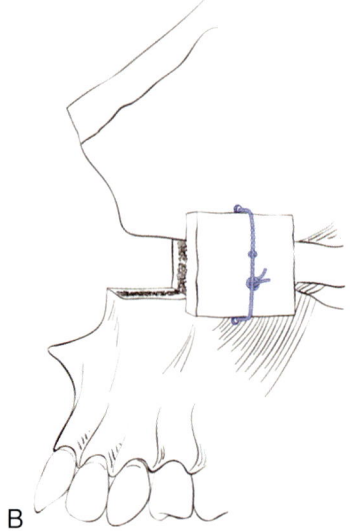

Fig. 76-5 ■ **A,** A single hole is placed in the middle of the bone graft, and a loop of 28-gauge stainless steel wire is placed through the hole from inside out. The two ends are divided, with one placed through the superior cranial base wall and the other through the inferior maxillary segment. Finally, one end is passed through the loop and twisted to the other, much like an Ivy loop. **B,** Bone graft shown in place. (From Miloro M (ed). Peterson's principles of oral and maxillofacial surgery, ed 2. Shelton, Conn, 2004, PMPH-USA. Reprinted with permission.)

the surgeon to indicate the time for beginning the turning and widening procedure and incumbent upon the orthodontist to determine when enough turns and widening have occurred.

Often, the patient is not in full orthodontic appliances at this time. At some point afterward, the central incisors tend to begin to drift medially together on their own. They tend to do this in a faster fashion without orthodontic appliances, with tipping of the crowns centrally, and then orthodontic appliances can be placed to bring the roots upright. If orthodontic appliances are present, segmentalization of the arch wire is necessary at the time of the surgery. Also of note, it is important that the patient or surgeon bring the activation key to the operating room (to be used), and then the surgeon retains the activation key until the postoperative visit when instruction on turning is performed.

SEGMENTAL LE FORT OSTEOTOMY

Segmentalization of the maxilla can be performed in a 2-, 3-, or 4-piece osteotomy. It can be done symmetrically or asymmetrically. Preoperative model surgery will determine the most appropriate design.

In addition to gaining width, segmentalization allows for vertical changes and adjustment of the angulations of the posterior maxillary segments. The most common sites for segmentalization are between the central incisors, the canines and lateral incisors, or the canine and premolar teeth. The need for additional intercanine width will be a determining factor in this decision.

Conservative tunneling from the standard circumvestibular incision can be made inferiorly to the alveolar crest on the buccal surface of the maxilla with a Woodson elevator. The interdental osteotomy is made with a thin cement spatula osteotome, palpating palatally prior to performing the horizontal osteotomy while the maxilla is still stable (Fig. 76-7). Osseous exposure requirements at the alveolar crest level are minimal when using these thin osteotomes. The osteotomy can be carried superiorly to the level of the planned horizontal maxillary osteotomy. After downfracturing and

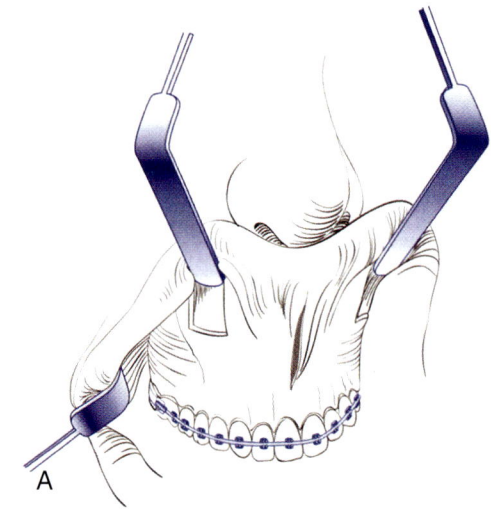

Fig. 76-6 ■ Surgically assisted rapid palatal expansion. **A,** Bilateral vestibular incisions are made from the first premolar to the second molar, shown with a midline vertical incision.

complete mobilization of the maxilla, segmentalization of the palate can be completed. Bilateral parasagittal segmentalization is preferred, because the palatal soft tissue is thicker lateral to the midline and the bone is thinner, decreasing the chance of perforation. A rounded tip bur, such as a Steiger or 1703 bur, is used. These parasagittal cuts are connected to the interdental cuts in the area of the incisive canal (see Fig. 76-7, *B*). The orthodontic arch wire must be cut at the interdental osteotomy sites to properly mobilize the segments. Conservative and careful elevation of the mucoperiosteum along these cuts may aid in soft tissue relaxation to allow mobilization. The teeth are wired to the prefabricated oral surgical

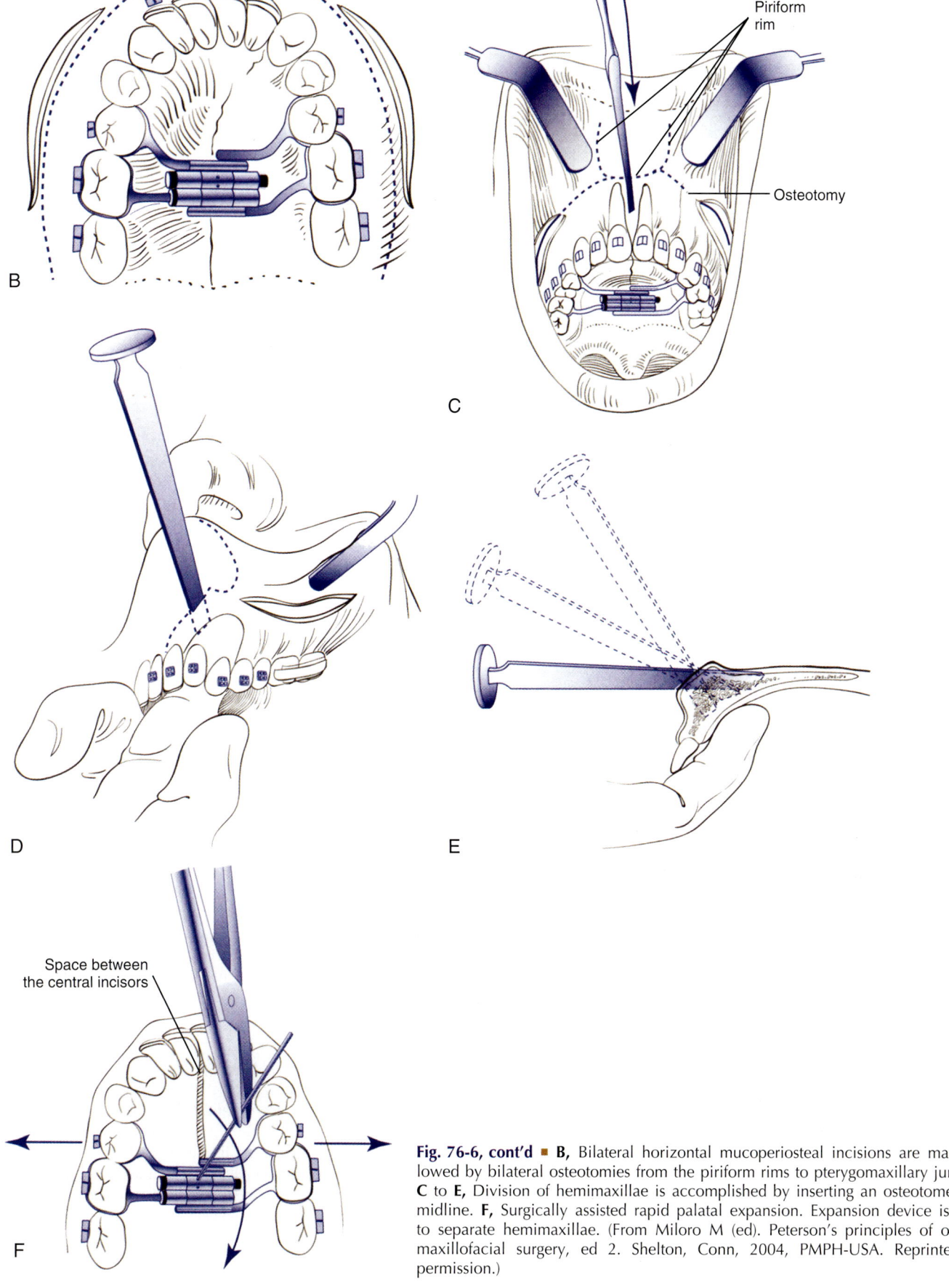

B

C

Piriform rim

Osteotomy

D

E

Space between the central incisors

F

Fig. 76-6, cont'd ▪ B, Bilateral horizontal mucoperiosteal incisions are made, followed by bilateral osteotomies from the piriform rims to pterygomaxillary junctions. **C to E,** Division of hemimaxillae is accomplished by inserting an osteotome in the midline. **F,** Surgically assisted rapid palatal expansion. Expansion device is turned to separate hemimaxillae. (From Miloro M (ed). Peterson's principles of oral and maxillofacial surgery, ed 2. Shelton, Conn, 2004, PMPH-USA. Reprinted with permission.)

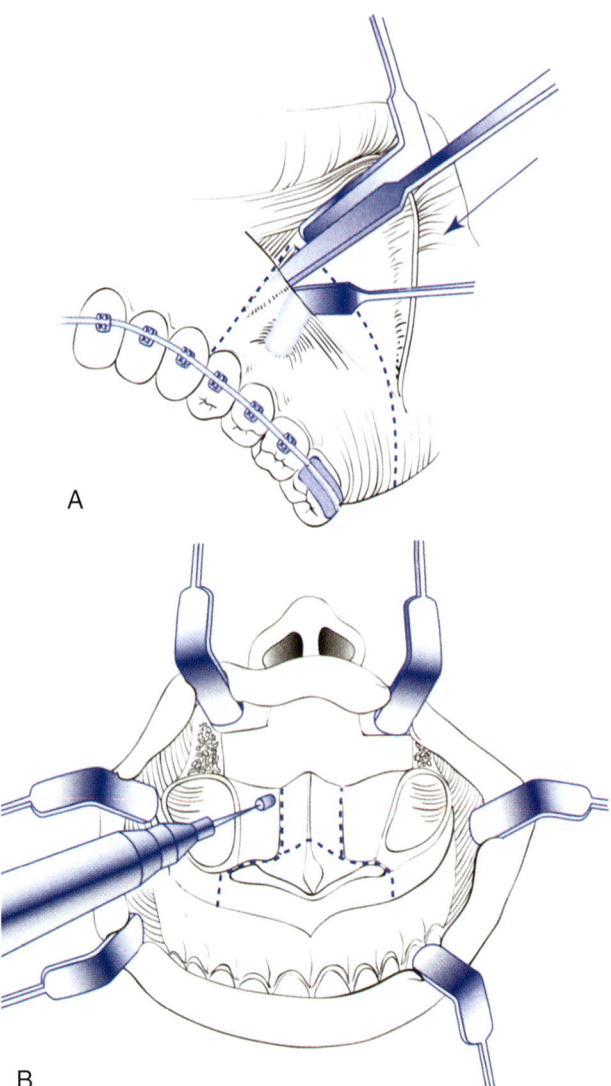

Fig. 76-7 ▪ **A,** Posterior maxillary osteotomy. Horizontal vestibular incision with tunneling access to the interdental papilla. The *dashed line* marks horizontal and interdental osteotomies. **B,** Following down-fracturing, the maxilla is segmentalized with a rounded end-cutting bur, such as a Steiger bur, by making two parasagittal cuts that join across the midline and connect with the interdental osteotomies. (From Miloro M (ed). Peterson's principles of oral and maxillofacial surgery, ed 2. Shelton, Conn, 2004, PMPH-USA. Reprinted with permission.)

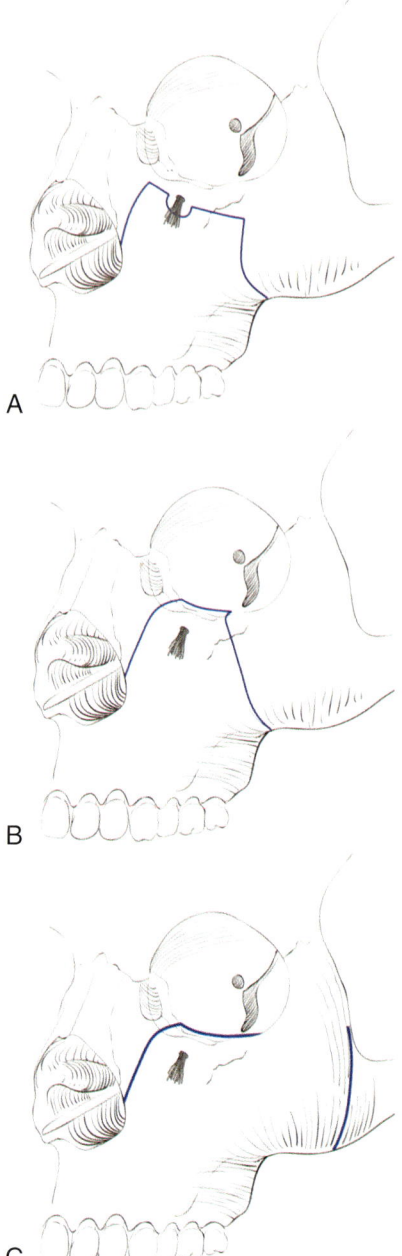

Fig. 76-8 ▪ Modified Le Fort I osteotomy. **A,** High Le Fort I below the infraorbital rims. **B,** Quadrangular Le Fort I extending into the orbital floor. **C,** Quadrangular Le Fort I including the lateral orbital rim and zygoma. (From Miloro M (ed). Peterson's principles of oral and maxillofacial surgery, ed 2. Shelton, Conn, 2004, PMPH-USA. Reprinted with permission.)

splint. This splint can be an occlusal coverage or palatal coverage split. A palatal strap is usually desired on an occlusal coverage splint to add rigidity. Ideally, plate and screw fixation will include all segments and also span the interdental cuts. At times, particularly when segmentalization occurs between the lateral incisors and the canines, the anterior segment may only be fixated to the splint. Bone removed during the maxillary osteotomy or osseous coagulum collected from a mandibular osteotomy can be grafted to the interdental sites prior to closure. If grafting of the palatal defect is desired, it must be performed prior to fixation of the maxilla.

MODIFIED LE FORT OSTEOTOMIES

Some degree of malar and or infraorbital hypoplasia is often present with other maxillary deficiency. Modified Le Fort I (high, extended quadrangular), II, and III can be used to correct these deficiencies (Fig. 76-8). These osteotomies are limited regarding the ability for expansion and for more complicated rotational and torquing movements. Except in cases of syndromic patients, augmentation with porous polyethylene or silicone implants to the malar, infraorbital, lateral orbital, and paranasal regions is simpler, less invasive, and provides excellent results.

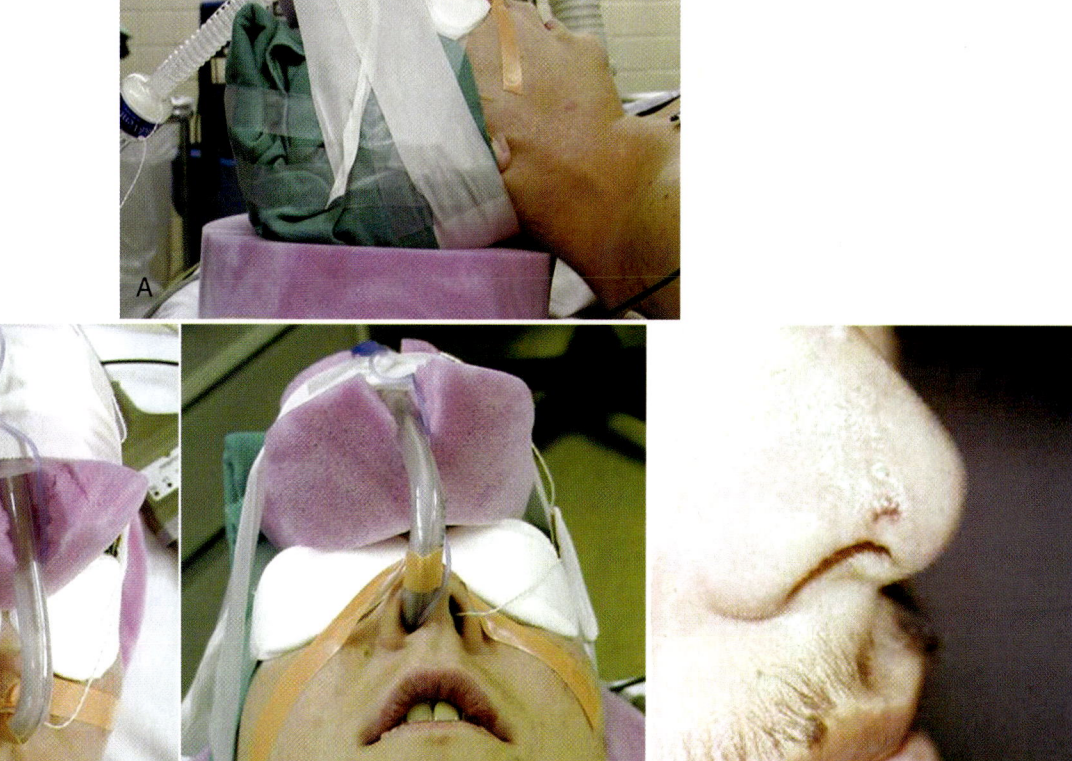

Fig. 76-9 ■ **A,** Tube secured to prevent dislodgement during surgery. **B** and **C,** Minimal distortion of the nose and upper lip due to the position of the tube. **D,** Example of necrosis caused by undue stress.

POSTOPERATIVE CARE

Antibiotics are generally not needed beyond perioperative dosing. Short-term use of nasal saline spray, decongestant sprays, and pills are beneficial for patient comfort. Intravenous dexamethasone, which is given preoperatively, is repeated 6 hours later for inpatients, and 80 mg of intramuscular methylprednisolone is administered prior to discharge. Patients undergoing maxillary surgery must be counseled preoperatively regarding general sinus precautions, including no nose blowing and open mouth sneezing, without an effort to stifle the sneeze. Some mild intermittent nose bleeding is expected postoperatively, particularly with change of position when, for instance, a patient gets out of bed to go to the bathroom. Patients should also be counseled that palatal numbness immediately postoperative gives a sensation of "something" being in the back of the throat and swallowing feels funny. The swallowing action is unaltered and will occur just as preoperatively, though the sensation is not as one is accustomed. Patients accept this very well, when they are told ahead of time to expect it.

The duration of time that a splint remains in place will vary depending on the amount and type of movement made by the segments and the adequacy of the fixation, including all of the segments. This could be as little as 3 and as much as 8 weeks. The patient must see the orthodontist immediately upon removal of the splint to have a continuous arch wire placed.

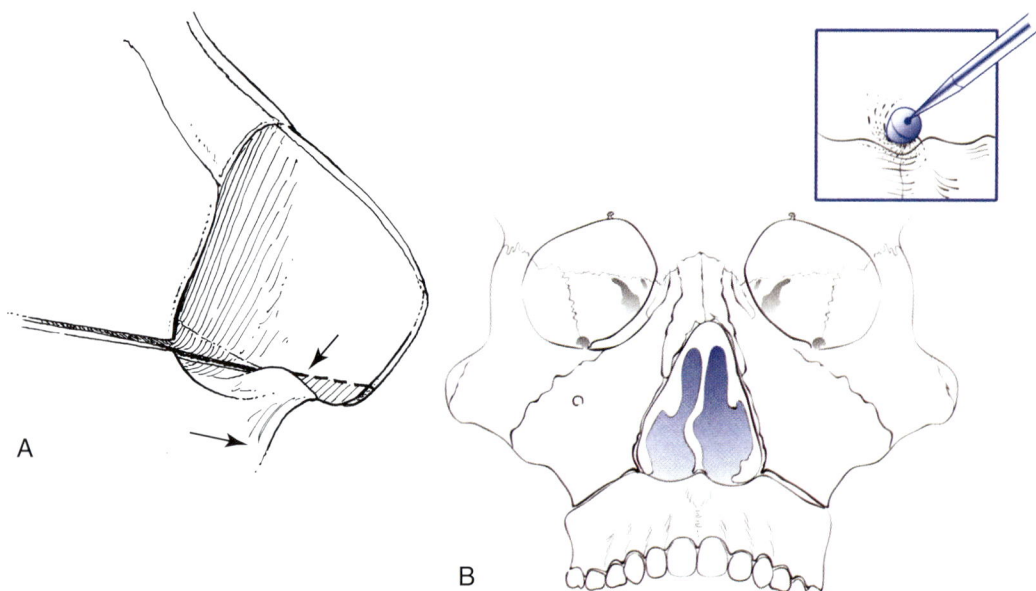

Fig. 76-10 ■ **A,** The septal crest of the maxilla rises from the tip of the anterior nasal (ANS) to a more superior level before falling inferiorly in the posterior region. The septal cartilage follows this undulating course. Therefore, there is septal cartilage over the ANS that will be buckled by the most prominent part of the maxilla as it is advanced, even if the maxilla is not superiorly reposi-tioned. **B,** Pure horizontal advancement of the maxilla will buckle the septum unless adequate bony and cartilaginous relief is provided. (**B,** From Miloro M (ed). Peterson's principles of oral and maxillofacial surgery, ed 2. Shelton, Conn, 2004, PMPH-USA. Reprinted with permission.)

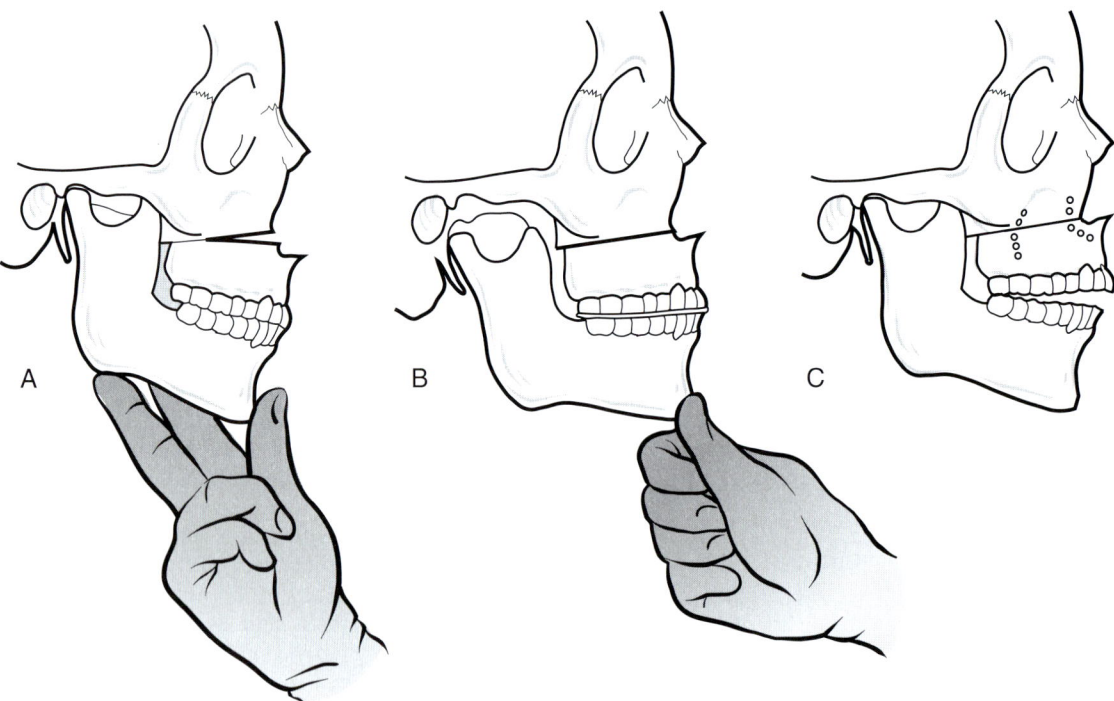

Fig. 76-11 ■ **A,** The proper method for condylar seating at the time of maxillary positioning prior to fixation. Posterior prematurities are best appreciated with this method. **B,** Pressure on the chin to push the anterior aspect of the maxillary osteotomy together may rotate the condyles inferiorly and posteriorly while maxillary fixation is applied. **C,** Upon release of intermaxillary fixation, the condyles may return to the fosse, and an open bite may appear. Unfortunately, this open bite may not appear immediately, especially if postoperative elastics are used to "guide" the occlusion. (From Bays RA: Complications of orthognathic surgery. In Kaban LB, Pogrel MA, Perrot DH (eds): Complications in oral and maxillofacial surgery. Philadelphia, 1997, Saunders.)

PEARLS AND PITFALLS

Anesthesia
- Maxillary orthognathic surgery is typically done with hypotensive anesthesia.
- Maintenance of a mean arterial pressure of approximately 60 mm Hg, as well as patient positioning in a lawn chair position, is useful in managing blood loss during downfracturing.
- Because downfracturing usually occurs early in the surgical procedures, it is critical that the anesthesia staff is aware of these needs ahead of time so that they can quickly get the blood pressure to 60 mm Hg, for reduction of the overall blood loss.

Nasoendotracheal Tube
- Management of the nasoendotracheal tube used during orthognathic surgery is very important.
  1. The tube must be adequately secured to prevent dislodgement during the frequent changes in head position that occur during orthognathic surgery (Fig. 76-9, *A*).
  2. The tube position must be such that the minimal distortion of the nose and upper lip occurs (Fig. 76-9, *B* and *C*).
  3. The tube must not cause undue stress upon the ala of the nose, or in a long case, necrosis of the alar rim could occur (Fig. 76-9, *D*).

Nasal Septum
- Care must be taken to ensure that the nasal septum is not buckled or displaced with repositioning of the maxilla, particularly in maxillary advancement.
- The most anterior inferior portion of the caudal septum extends below the height of the anterior nasal spine as it courses anteriorly to it and when the maxilla is advanced. Even without any impaction, there is an interference that will occur (Fig. 76-10, *A*).
- Osseous recontouring of the nasal crest of the maxilla and/or resection of a portion of the caudal extent of the cartilaginous septum is recommended to prevent interference (Fig. 76-10, *B*). Placement of a suture through the anterior nasal spine and cartilaginous septum to prevent its displacement upon removal of the nasoendotracheal tube is beneficial (Fig. 76-3, *C*).

Proper Positioning
- Proper positioning can be difficult in isolated maxillary surgery, usually due to unrecognized posterior bony interferences.
- With an unrecognized posterior interference and inadequate effort or improper seating of the condyles, the maxilla can rotate around this interference, resulting in an anterior open bite after release of intermaxillary fixation. Care must be taken to ensure that the maxillomandibular complex is rotated with pressure seating the condyles in the fossa (Fig. 76-11).
- Looking for the posterior interferences and eliminating them will result in the intended postoperative occlusion. Prior to any attempt to position the maxilla, effort is devoted to removing bone in the most likely areas of potential posterior interference, that being the area posterior to the second molar and along the perpendicular process of the palatine bone.
- Whether or not there is a potential for interference in the area of the pterygoid plates, per se, depends upon the surgical move. This is much less likely with advancement than it is with other moves such as impaction.
- It is often easiest to adapt the plates for fixation with Le Fort osteotomy and initially secure them only to the inferior fragment. Once all the plates are properly bent and secured to the inferior fragment, the maxillomandibular complex and condyles can be positioned with great care, and the shape and bending of the plates critically evaluated and secured to the superior fragment in succession while the maxillomandibular complex is held in position.

BIBLIOGRAPHY

Bailey LJ, White RP, Proffit WR, Turvey TA: Segmental LeFort I osteotomy for management of transverse maxillary deficiency. *J Oral Maxillofac Surg* 55:728-731, 1997.

Bays RA, Greco JM: Surgically assisted rapid palatal expansion: an outpatient technique with long-term stability. *J Oral Maxillofac Surg* 50(2):110-113, 1992; discussion 114-115.

Costa F, Robiony M, Politi M: Stability of Le Fort I osteotomy in maxillary inferior repositioning: review of the literature. *Int J Adult Orthodon Orthognath Surg* 15(3):197-204, 2000.

Ellis E, McNamara JA: Components of adult Class III malocclusion. *J Oral Maxillofac Surg* 42:295-305, 1984.

Lanigan DT, Mintz SM: Complications of surgically assisted rapid palatal expansion: review of the literature and report of a case. *J Oral Maxillofac Surg* 60:104-110, 2002.

Perciaccante VJ, Bays RA: Maxillary orthognathic surgery. In Miloro M, Larsen P, Ghali G, Waite P (eds): *Peterson's principles of oral and maxillofacial surgery*, ed 2. Hamilton, Ontario, Canada, 2004, BC Decker.

Proffit WR, Turvey TA, Phillips C: Orthognathic surgery: a hierarchy of stability. *Int J Adult Orthodon Orthognath Surg* 11(3):191-204, 1996.

Reyneke JP, Masureik CJ: Treatment of maxillary deficiency by a Le Fort I downsliding technique. *J Oral Maxillofac Surg* 43:914-916, 1985.

Reyneke JP: *Essentials of orthognathic surgery*. Hanover Park, Ill, 2003, Quintessence Publishing.

Silverstein K, Quinn PD: Surgically-assisted rapid palatal expansion for management of transverse maxillary deficiency. *J Oral Maxillofac Surg* 55:725-727, 1997.

Vandersea BA, Ruvo AT, Frost DE: Maxillary transverse deficiency—surgical alternatives to management. *Oral Maxillofacial Surg Clin N Am* 19:351-368, 2007.

Chapter 77

Maxillary Deficiency: Transverse Plane Discrepancies

Rafael E. Alcalde, Dale S. Bloomquist, Don Joondeph

Modern orthognathic surgery has gone through different paradigm shifts since its origins. Research and technologic advances have influenced diagnosis, planning, and treatment, which has allowed surgical orthodontics to advance from a skeletal and functional paradigm to a soft tissue and facial esthetics paradigm in the 1990s.[1] The latest shift is toward increased efficiency, decreased operating time, and ambulatory procedures that allow lower cost while keeping the highest standards regarding skeletal, functional, and soft tissue esthetic outcomes.

Increased efficiency, patient access to care, and affordability can be achieved by avoiding unnecessarily complex surgeries. This, in combination with constant communication between the members of the interdisciplinary team and the use of simple and effective procedures in office surgical suites or ambulatory surgery centers, will allow us to reduce costly operating room time and minimize the need for prolonged postoperative admission.

Discrepancies in the transverse plane are commonly diagnosed as isolated problems or as part of complex dentofacial deformities with a prevalence ranging from 10% to 15% in adolescents and up to 30% in adults.[2-5] The most common transverse problems complicating the treatment of patients with dentofacial deformities are transverse maxillary deficiency and transverse mandibular excess. Transverse maxillary excess and transverse mandibular deficiency, though reported, are less frequent.

Correction of transverse problems in non-growing patients is a somewhat controversial subject in both the orthodontic and surgical literature. In patients with maxillary transverse deficiency, conventional orthodontic expansion is limited by the buccal cortical bone of the maxilla and by the lingual bone of the mandible. The orthodontist can compensate in some of these patients by using buccal crown torque in the maxillary posterior dentition or lingual crown torque in the mandible. Frequently, this type of compensation is unstable and may create functional interference.[6] Oral and maxillofacial surgeons, in contrast, have traditionally been managing transverse problems with surgery on the maxilla via either surgically assisted rapid palatal expansion (SARPE)[7-11] or segmental Le Fort I osteotomy.[12,13] Use of a midline osteotomy for mandibular constriction has more recently been suggested for patients with wide mandibular arches who are undergoing concomitant bilateral ramus osteotomies. Although research on the results achieved with these surgical procedures has consistently shown acceptable stability on long-term follow-up, most studies are limited by either the number of patients studied or the length of follow-up (or by both).[14,15]

This chapter emphasizes the diagnosis, indications, biologic foundation, limitations, stability, effects on facial esthetics, and postoperative care of each treatment alternative for discrepancies in the transverse plane.

ETIOPATHOGENESIS

The etiology of transverse maxillary and mandibular problems has been related to genetic factors, environmental influences, or a combination of these factors. The most common transverse problems are maxillary deficiency, mandibular excess, or a combination of both.

In children, maxillary constriction is manifested as a narrow palatal vault and unilateral or bilateral posterior crossbite. Appropriate orthodontic correction of this transverse skeletal discrepancy requires orthopedic maxillary expansion, which is possible only in patients who are still growing. The younger the child, the more effective the skeletal expansion; dental tipping is minimized and sutural distraction histogenesis is maximized. For this reason, orthopedic maxillary expansion is usually accomplished as part of a phase I treatment before puberty. At this stage, maxillary expansion removes the premature contacts that induce lateral functional shifts caused by the transverse discrepancy. When left untreated, these functional shifts can result in progressive and permanent mandibular skeletal asymmetry.[6]

Rapid palatal expansion with a jackscrew appliance has been used reliably for more than 125 years in skeletally immature individuals. Even in the current practice of orthodontics, the most commonly used fixed expansion orthopedic appliances are tooth borne. Therefore, unwanted dentoalveolar movement should be expected to represent about 50% of the total expansion. This leads to a long-term loss of about 30% of the total arch expansion even after appropriate retention, thus confirming the need for overexpansion.[16]

Multiple studies have reported on the age and process of closure of the mid-palatal suture. Most authors agree that mid-palatal suture growth continues until at least the age of 16 to 18, with a great deal of variation found among individuals. However, difficulty separating the maxillas in postpubertal individuals is not due just to complete fusion of the mid-palatal suture but also to the numerous mechanical interlocking that takes place in the circum-maxillary suture system once the patient stops growing and the sutures become non-functional. Because of these changes in adolescent and older patients, orthopedic expansion results in more dentoalveolar than skeletal movement, thereby increasing the risk for excessive dental tipping in the posterior segments, gingival recession, reduced alveolar bone height on the buccal root surfaces, lack of occlusal stability, and eventually relapse.[6] Therefore, in mature patients undergoing orthodontic consultation for transverse discrepancies, diagnosis and treatment should be undertaken jointly by the orthodontist and surgeon.

ANATOMY

Unilateral and bilateral crossbites, proclined and crowded teeth, narrow and tapered arches with the maxillary alveolar processes tipped outward, arch-length discrepancy, noticeable buccal corridors,

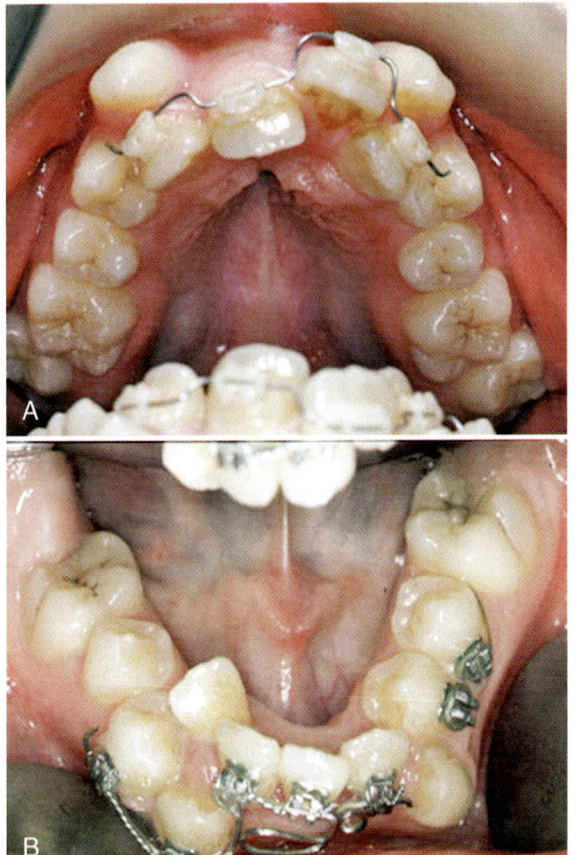

Fig. 77-1 ■ Clinical intraoral photographs showing tapered dental arches and severe crowding associated with transverse deficiency.

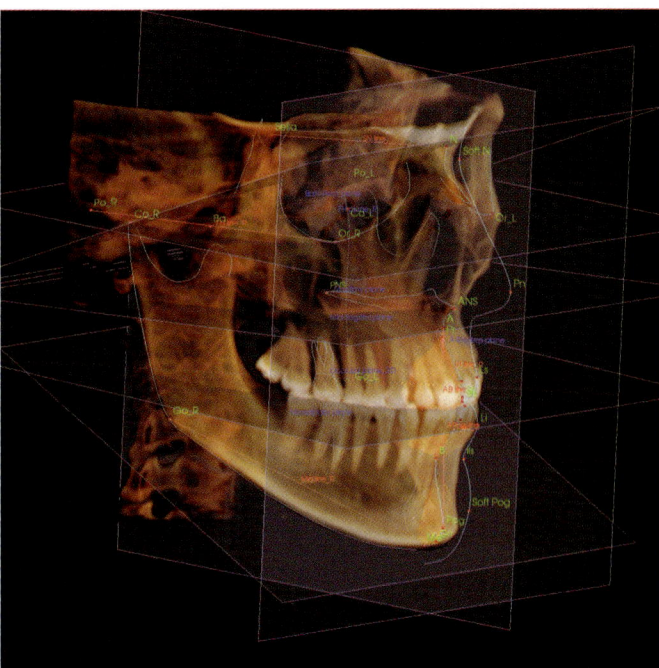

Fig. 77-2 ■ Facial three-dimensional computed tomography scan displaying the x-, y-, and z-axes. (Courtesy Anatomage, San Jose, CA.)

and a deep palate are clinical hallmarks of skeletal transverse maxillary deficiency (Fig. 77-1). Although excessive buccal corridors or negative space, defined as the space between the commissure and the buccal surfaces of the maxillary dentition during a full smile, may be due to a narrow maxilla, it can also be affected by the anteroposterior (AP) and vertical position of the maxilla relative to the lip drape. Crossbites with a wide palatal vault and maxillary alveolar processes tipped inward are commonly seen in patients with dental maxillary deficiency. Posterior crossbites with a three-dimensionally well-positioned maxilla, adequate upper incisor display, and the absence of buccal corridors and dental crowding are usually diagnosed as mandibular transverse excess. This is frequently seen in patients with mandibular AP deficiency and confirmed when models are positioned in class I occlusion.

DIAGNOSTIC STUDIES

Diagnostic studies use standard orthodontic records, which include cephalograms, models, orthodontic setups, and cephalometric analysis. The use of three-dimensional (3D) measurements with cone beam computed tomography (CBCT) is becoming more common and is of specific interest in the diagnosis and treatment planning of patients with transverse discrepancies and facial asymmetry.

To make an accurate diagnosis of a transverse discrepancy, the dental and skeletal components of the discrepancy need to be delineated. Models and orthodontic setups have commonly been used to evaluate these discrepancies. The first step includes leveling and alignment of the dentition over the basal bone to determine whether the discrepancy is an isolated dental problem. This is followed by analysis of models placed in class I canine occlusion to determine whether the transverse problem is absolute or whether it is a relative transverse deficiency or excess secondary to an AP discrepancy.

At this point, the presence and severity of the transverse discrepancy at the canine and molar levels must be determined. This is extremely important in establishing which orthodontic or surgical procedure (or both) will be indicated based on the pattern of expansion needed.

Ricketts proposed analysis with a transverse plane PA cephalogram to determine the presence of transverse skeletal dysplasia.[17] The clinical application of earlier two-dimensional analyses was made difficult by imaging limitations such as the superimposition of anatomic structures, magnification, and the lack of reproducible measurements on PA cephalograms as a result of major changes induced by head positioning, even when standardized techniques were used.[18]

Adaptation of these and other analyses to the more readily available CBCT will allow greater accuracy in the diagnosis of these deformities. The third dimension missing from the cephalometric radiograph is the transverse plane or x-axis in the 3D coordinate system. The advent of CBCT and 3D software has made it possible for the orthodontist and surgeon to visualize, evaluate, and simulate hard and soft tissue changes in all three dimensions of the craniofacial structure (Fig. 77-2).[18-20]

TREATMENT/RECONSTRUCTIVE GOALS

- An adequate transverse relationship improves dentofacial esthetics and periodontal health and increases long-term orthodontic stability. Transverse skeletal dysplasia is a risk factor for maxillary buccal gingival recession and periodontal disease.
- Improved smile esthetics is the main soft tissue effect of transverse skeletal correction.

SPECIFIC TREATMENT AND TECHNIQUES

LE FORT I SEGMENTAL OSTEOTOMY

Background

In 1972, Steinhauser reported a one-stage surgical procedure for expansion of the maxilla. The midline split could be performed on the posterior maxilla, anterior maxilla, or total maxilla. He thought widening the total maxilla to be technically difficult, however, because of the need to bone-graft the midline gap. To facilitate the procedure, palatal incisions were added to the buccal approach. Intermaxillary fixation was maintained for 4 to 6 weeks, and a retention plate was worn for 6 months to assist in stabilization of the transverse repositioning and to aid in consolidation of the bone graft. West and Epker described the application of Schuchardt's two-stage (1959) and Kufner's single-stage (1970) posterior maxillary osteotomies for correction of unilateral and bilateral posterior crossbite in patients whose mid-palatal suture was closed. With this technique, maxillary expansion became a one-stage osteotomy that separated the alveolus from the palate. Bell and Turvey reported the results of segmental maxillary surgery performed on 10 patients with a posterior crossbite. Segments were mobilized and positioned into a preoperatively determined occlusal relationship with a surgical splint and stabilized with wire fixation and intermaxillary fixation for 6 to 8 weeks. In 1985 in a series of 104 patients undergoing maxillary osteotomy, Turvey pointed out that transverse maxillary deficiency is seldom the only maxillary deformity, and he therefore recommended that a multisegment maxilla be created to correct the hypoplastic maxilla in all three planes of space.[12,21-23]

Technique

Before surgery, orthodontic decompensation, leveling, and alignment should be achieved. Sufficient room between the dental roots should exist at the planned interdental osteotomy sites to minimize any damage to periodontal tissue.

Fabrication of two surgical splints, a palatal splint and an occlusal splint, minimizes intraoperative time. Maxillary segmentation for correction of the transverse deficiency is done on completion of the total maxillary osteotomy and down-fracture. Para-midline sagittal or horseshoe osteotomies are ideal when no changes in the maxillary occlusal plane are needed for the following reasons:

- It allows two separate areas of soft tissue expansion in the posterior maxilla to minimize tension, which can prevent expansion or induce relapse.
- The lateral palatal soft tissues are thicker, which minimizes the possibility of perforation or rupture of tissue. It improves the anatomy since most of these patients have a deep and narrow palatal vault preoperatively, and the palate will not only be wider but will also become less deep by lowering the central portion.

The lateral para-midline osteotomy and interdental cuts can be made with a small side-cutting bur or with a saw. Fine spatula osteotomes are also sometimes used to finish the cuts. In all cases a finger is placed on the palate to decrease the chance of soft tissue damage, as well as to ensure that the osteotomy is completed. Minimal soft tissue dissection at the interdental osteotomy sites is of upmost importance to preserve the blood supply to the dentoalveolar structures (Fig. 77-3). The segments are mobilized with finger pressure, and a palatal splint without occlusal coverage is inserted.[24] This palatal splint, which is held in place with wires or ball clasps, is constructed with acrylic and abuts the palatal surfaces of the upper teeth. The splint will stabilize the transverse change intraoperatively, and postoperatively it will be maintained for a period

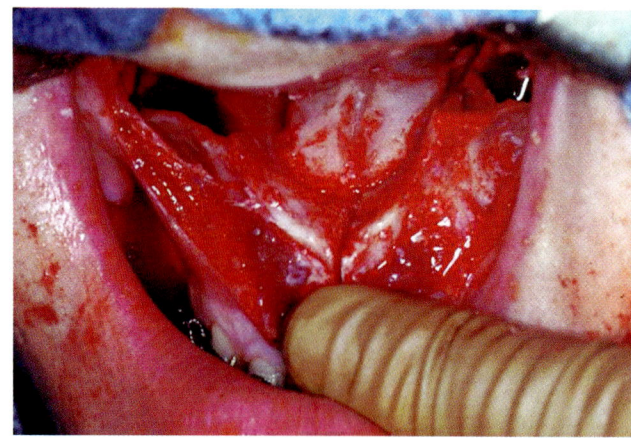

Fig. 77-3 ■ Palatal view after maxillary down-fracture with osteotomy cuts in a horseshoe pattern.

of 6 to 10 weeks, at which point it can be replaced by an orthodontic transpalatal appliance. Lack of occlusal coverage allows placement of an occlusal splint for AP and vertical repositioning of the maxilla. The occlusal splint is removed before the patient leaves the operating room to facilitate oral hygiene and avoid the discomfort that occurs with wiring the classic occlusal splint to the upper dentition. Grafting with autogenous bone, allogeneic bone, or hydroxyapatite, as well as plate and screw fixation across the palatal osteotomy gap, has been described, but there are no adequate data on long-term stability in support of one technique over the other.

Finally, the maxilla is put into its normal relationship with the mandible and placed in intermaxillary fixation. The maxilla is passively repositioned and secured with bone plates and screws, after which the intermaxillary fixation is removed and the occlusion confirmed. The soft tissue is closed carefully to minimize shortening of the lip, which often requires the use of an alar base cinch and V-Y closure to maximize paranasal and upper lip esthetics.

Pattern of Expansion

The multisegment Le Fort I osteotomy allows repositioning of the maxilla in all three dimensions, and correction of the transverse problem can be performed simultaneously with maxillary AP and vertical repositioning. When a maxilla is widened with the osteotomy made between the central incisors, the segments rotate outward with one or two axes of rotation at the incisal level, and the greatest surgical change occurs at the level of the second molars, which allows more intermolar than intercanine expansion.

Soft Tissue Esthetics

Soft tissue changes associated with Le Fort I osteotomies include upturning of the nose, increased exposure of the nares, increased width of the alar cartilage, shortening of the columella, shortening of the upper lip, and possibly loss of exposed vermilion and upper lip curl.[25] These changes may be positive or negative, depending on the presurgical facial esthetic characteristics of the patient. In most patients with maxillary hypoplasia, the Le Fort I osteotomy with advancement and inferior repositioning of the maxilla will result in positive changes by improving the acute nasolabial angle and providing support for the paranasal soft tissues. However, its effects on the facial esthetics of patients with a short upper lip, thin vermilion border, and upturned nasal tip can be disastrous, even when soft tissue closure such as the alar cinch and V-Y closure are used to minimize these potential negative effects.

Stability

Segmental osteotomy for maxillary expansion is at the bottom of the hierarchy of stability as reported by Phillips and co-authors, with a relapse rate of 49% at the second molars and a more clinically significant 29% incidence of crossbite at the end of orthodontic treatment.[13] Studies on maxillary expansion using rigid fixation give us a better idea of the stability of this procedure at the present time. To improve transverse stability, it is recommended that expansions greater than 10 mm be avoided and that overexpansion be built into the occlusal splint, which is maintained for 6 to 10 weeks and replaced with a transpalatal arch or any other orthodontic appliance to assist in maintenance of intermolar width during healing and postsurgical orthodontic treatment.

SURGICALLY ASSISTED RAPID PALATAL EXPANSION

Background

Kole in 1959 was the first to discuss corticotomy for the treatment of adults with maxillary constriction; the lateral maxillary wall was cut 1 cm above the apices, and a palatal incision was used to make a horizontal cut into the maxillary antrum. This was followed by the insertion of a dental-borne expansion device 8 weeks later. In the same year, Converse and Horowitz described three different surgical-orthodontic techniques.

1. Osteotomy through the entire mandibular or maxillary bone thickness
2. Dentoalveolar osteotomy in which the body is left intact but the teeth and their supporting structures are moved segmentally into a planned position
3. Cortical osteotomy or corticotomy to achieve displacement of the dentoalveolar segments more rapidly than with orthodontics alone, especially for maxillary expansion

Lines reintroduced corticotomy for adult rapid maxillary expansion in 1975. He reported making lateral incisions at the depth of the vestibule from the canine to the tuberosity and cutting the cortical plate from the piriform aperture to the zygomatic buttress. A palatal incision is made from behind the incisive papilla to the end of the hard palate with a burr. The expansion device is cemented 2 to 3 weeks postoperatively to allow healing and revascularization. This author extended the midline interdental bony cut to the piriform rim instead of using the interdental corticotomy described by Kole. Lines also suggested that because of the short duration and uneventful postoperative course, this procedure can be performed in an outpatient visit with local anesthesia and premedication. From this report two different groups of procedures have developed: SARPE originally and surgically facilitated orthodontic treatment (SFOT) more recently. The latter involves three different techniques that can be used alone or in combination, depending on the correction needed: a corticotomy-facilitated technique (with or without bone grafting), dentoalveolar distraction osteogenesis, and skeletal anchorage devices. SFOT is primarily indicated for dental movement, closure of extraction sites, and opening of implant sites, but it is also used for arch development and correction of dentoalveolar transverse discrepancies. Bell and Epker (1976) reported 15 patients who underwent SARPE under local anesthesia. Lateral maxillary bone cuts, pterygomaxillary disjunction, and interdental midline osteotomy were performed in all patients. Parasagittal palatal osteotomies were performed only in those with unilateral posterior crossbite. In the same year Kennedy and colleagues showed in their animal study that lateral maxillary osteotomies are key in achieving maxillary expansion.[23,26-30]

Key factors to be considered in maxillary expansion include the extent of the arch length discrepancy, arch form, magnitude of the arch deficiency, smile esthetics, and vertical as well as AP position of the maxilla.

To determine the target expansion, it is advantageous to decompensate the lower arch by removing the curve of Wilson before proceeding with maxillary expansion or by doing a pretreatment orthodontic setup.

Technique

SARPE is usually done before placement of full fixed orthodontic appliances on the upper dentition since in most cases a tooth-borne distraction device is used (Hyrax, Haas, or any other jackscrew device). It is important that the upper molars and bicuspids, which are being used as anchors for the palatal device, be intact and not have recently been subjected to orthodontic forces. This is not necessary if a bone-borne distraction device is used. The palatal expander is fabricated and adapted by the orthodontist before the scheduled procedure, and a trial fitting must be done to avoid difficulty placing the expander during surgery.

The procedure is usually done as an outpatient procedure with intravenous sedation or general anesthesia in the office or surgical center. After local anesthetic with epinephrine is infiltrated at the surgical sites, incisions are made bilaterally at the depth of the vestibule from the first molar area to the distal aspect of the canine. The mucoperiosteum is elevated and the maxillary bone exposed from the pterygomaxillary fissure through a subperiosteal tunnel to the piriform aperture. After identifying the infraorbital nerve, an osteotomy is performed horizontally at least 5 mm above the apices of the upper teeth from the piriform aperture to the pterygomaxillary fissure. The pterygoid plates are not separated from the maxilla. A single incision is made at the palatal midline, and bilateral mucoperiosteal flaps are elevated to allow parasagittal osteotomies to be performed at each side of the nasal septum to reduce areas of resistance, which can cause unwanted asymmetric maxillary expansion. These osteotomies are usually done with a burr or a saw and they extend from the posterior hard palate to the incisive foramen. Anteriorly, the maxilla is separated by malleting a spatula osteotome between the central incisors at a level below the anterior nasal spine (Fig. 77-4).

The surgical sites are irrigated and sutured. After the palatal expander is cemented by the surgeon, the screw is activated immediately just enough to confirm completion of the osteotomies.

An anterior nasal package, ice packs, or a pressure bandage can be applied for a day. Antibiotics, analgesic drugs, and an oroantral regimen should be prescribed. Activation of 1 mm/day then starts on postoperative day 3 to reduce the possibility of soft tissue dehiscence.

Pattern of Expansion

Maxillary expansion sometimes occurs more at the anterior maxilla than in the molar region. This allows an increase in arch length by creating a midline diastema (Fig. 77-5).

Soft Tissue Esthetics

Facial esthetics improves as a result of a widened smile and a reduction in buccal corridors. Soft tissue changes, similar to those with a multisegment Le Fort I procedure, are related to the extension of soft tissue dissection. The aforementioned technique minimizes soft tissue dissection in the esthetic zone since the vestibular incisions extend only from the first molar to the canine region and the midline dissection is limited to the bony cut site at the lateral aspect of the piriform rim. Palatal incisions and pterygomaxillary disjunctions

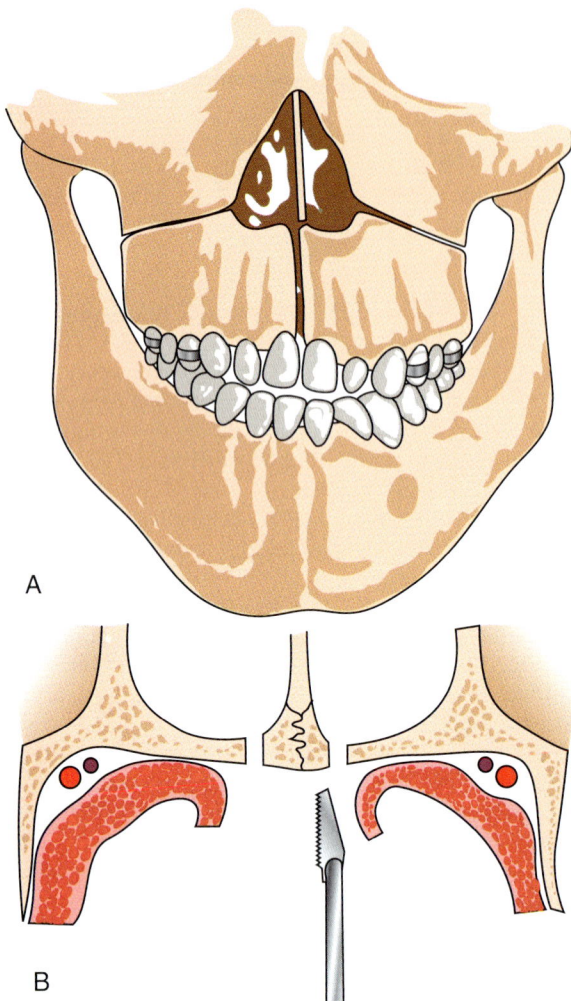

Fig. 77-4 ▪ **A,** Frontal view showing osteotomies for surgically assisted rapid palatal expansion. **B,** Palatal cross section showing bilateral osteotomies at each side of the nasal septum.

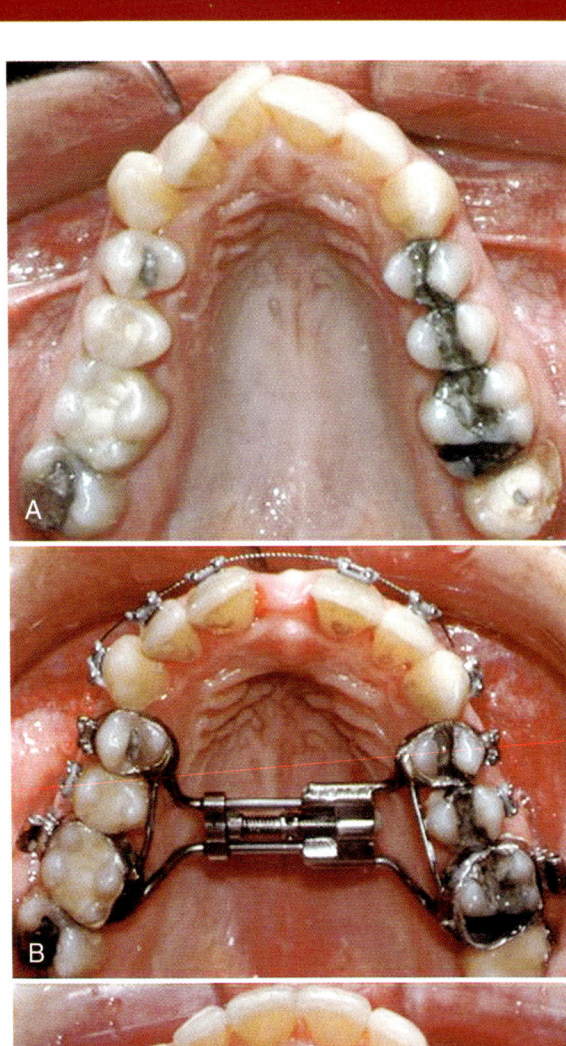

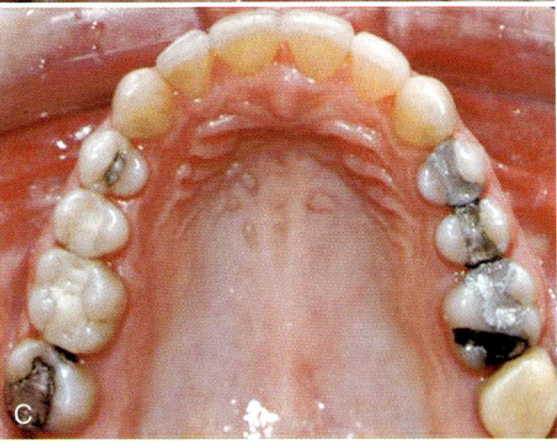

Fig. 77-5 ▪ **A,** Palatal view showing a narrow maxilla before surgery and orthodontic treatment. **B,** Maxilla during expansion with the Hyrax device. **C,** Expanded maxilla after removal of the orthodontic appliances.

have no effect on esthetics as long as maxillary down-fracture is not performed. A factor that needs to be taken into consideration is the potential loss of upper lip support caused by uprighting or retracting the upper incisors as a result of closure of the space following expansion. It is important to exercise good torque control during orthodontic postsurgical closure of the space to maintain upper lip support and lip curl.

Stability

Rea and colleagues presented a systematic review of the literature on SARPE done by two examiners through an exhaustive MEDLINE computer search to identify all studies involving maxillary surgery in the English literature from 1970 to 2001.[31] A total of 45 of 4,983 studies were identified as human clinical trials reporting SARPE. Five studies met the strict inclusion and exclusion criteria (Box 77-1).

All studies were retrospective non-randomized trials without a control group and with sample sizes ranging from 10 to 30 subjects. In all five studies, osteotomies were done at the lateral wall of the maxilla and mid-palate and also included pterygomaxillary release (Table 77-1).

Canine and molar expansion was reviewed (Tables 77-2 and 77-3). The mean canine relapse rate was between 8% and 25%, and the mean molar relapse rate was 9% to 22%. SARPE has been found

to be a relatively simple procedure that produces predictable and stable increases in maxillary width; when overcorrection is considered, it should not be planned to be more than 25% of the intended expansion.[31]

MANDIBULAR CONSTRICTION

Background

Mandibular constriction is a valuable adjunctive surgical procedure for dealing with transverse problems whenever bilateral sagittal osteotomies are to be performed. Although there have been other

TABLE 77-1	Included Studies				
STUDY	PATIENTS	AGE (YR)	GENDER	FOLLOW-UP (MO)	OSTEOTOMIES
Pogrel, 1992	12	16-32	M: 4/F: 8	12	Bilateral zygomatic buttress, mid-palate
Bays, 1992	19	15-40	M: 3/F: 16	12-48	Bilateral zygomatic buttress, mid-palate
Stromberg, 1995	20	18-59	M: 11/F: 9	12-42	Bilateral zygomatic buttress, palate × 2
Northway, 1997	23	16-38	M: 6/F: 17	12	Bilateral zygomatic buttress, palate × 2
Berger, 1998	28	13-35	M: 12/F: 16	12	Bilateral zygomatic buttress, mid-palate pterygoid release

TABLE 77-2	Results of Canine Data		
STUDY	PATIENTS	EXPANSION (MM)	RELAPSE (MM)
Pogrel, 1992	12	N/A	N/A
Bays, 1992	19	4.5 ± 3.28	*0.39 ± 0.79
Stromberg, 1995	20	5.0 ± 2.2	*0.76 ± 0.95
Northway, 1997	23	3.74 ± 0.45	0.41 ± 0.5
Berger, 1998	28	4.84 ± 0.89	1.12 ± 0.77
Weighted total	90	3.99 ± 2.08	*0.48 ± 1.26 (8%-25%)

*No relapse.

TABLE 77-3	Results of Molar Data		
STUDY	PATIENTS	EXPANSION (MM)	RELAPSE (MM)
Pogrel, 1992	12	7.5	0.88 ± 0.48
Bays, 1992	19	5.28 ± 2.68	*0.45 ± 0.69
Stromberg, 1995	20	8.3 ± 2.6	*1.2 ± 1.3
Northway, 1997	23	4.16 ± 0.96	0.35 ± 0.6
Berger, 1998	28	5.78 ± 1.03	1.01+/−0.56
Weighted total	90	6.11 ± 2.64	*0.78 ± 1.1 (9%-22%)

*No relapse.

BOX 77-1	Inclusion and Exclusion Criteria for Surgically Assisted Rapid Palatal Expansion

Inclusion Criteria
- Human clinical trials
- Sample size of 10 or more patients
  - Expansion and relapse measured on study models
  - Tooth-borne appliance
- At least 12-month follow-up after surgically assisted rapid palatal expansion

Exclusion Criteria
- Non-surgical maxillary expansion
- Clinical trials using segmental Le Fort I expansion
- Patients with cleft lip and palate
- Patients with craniofacial syndrome

reviews of symphyseal ostectomies, the first known discussion of midline osteotomy was published in 1976. This initial report was included in a description of the surgical techniques used in a patient in whom widening of the mandible was necessary. However, the technique was described in more detail by Brusati and co-authors, who reported use of this osteotomy for mandibular constriction. Alexander and associates were the first to describe stabilization of the mandibular midline osteotomy with rigid internal fixation. This article reviewed stability with a single plate placed across the osteotomy.[14,15,32]

Mandibular midline osteotomy is generally indicated in patients who require a mandibular ramus osteotomy and have no other maxillary discrepancy. It is much easier to treat the transverse problem with a simple mandibular midline osteotomy, thereby avoiding a segmental Le Fort I osteotomy. This frequently occurs in patients with mandibular retrognathia who began treatment with a normal molar buccal overjet, and because they have a tapered arch form or a severe AP discrepancy, a transverse deficiency develops secondary to the mandibular advancement. Traditionally, orthodontists have compensated in adults by altering the axial inclinations of the molars and, less often, by bodily moving the teeth. Either type of dental movement can be a problem when advancing the mandible. Tipping the maxillary posterior teeth buccally or the mandibular teeth lingually can result in cusp interference for the surgeon. This problem can be compounded by instability caused by the orthodontist's attempts at narrowing the posterior mandibular arch or expanding the posterior maxillary arch. If no attempt is made at correcting this kind of transverse discrepancy before surgery, the surgeon has three treatment options besides performing a mandibular midline osteotomy: adding a maxillary segmental osteotomy with expansion, performing SARPE, or leaving the patient with a posterior crossbite or an end-to-end cusp relationship.

One of the biggest advantages of mandibular midline osteotomy for constriction is that the decision to surgically correct a transverse discrepancy can be deferred to presurgical evaluation when the dentition is fully decompensated. In addition, mandibular constriction can be added to the treatment plan with almost no impact on the patient because of the minimal additional surgical time and cost. Use of the mandibular midline osteotomy saves the patient from needing to undergo maxillary surgery, as well as significantly reduces surgical costs. Finally, less time is required by the orthodontist in attempting to compensate for any transverse discrepancies that may exist between the maxilla and the mandible (Fig. 77-6).[33]

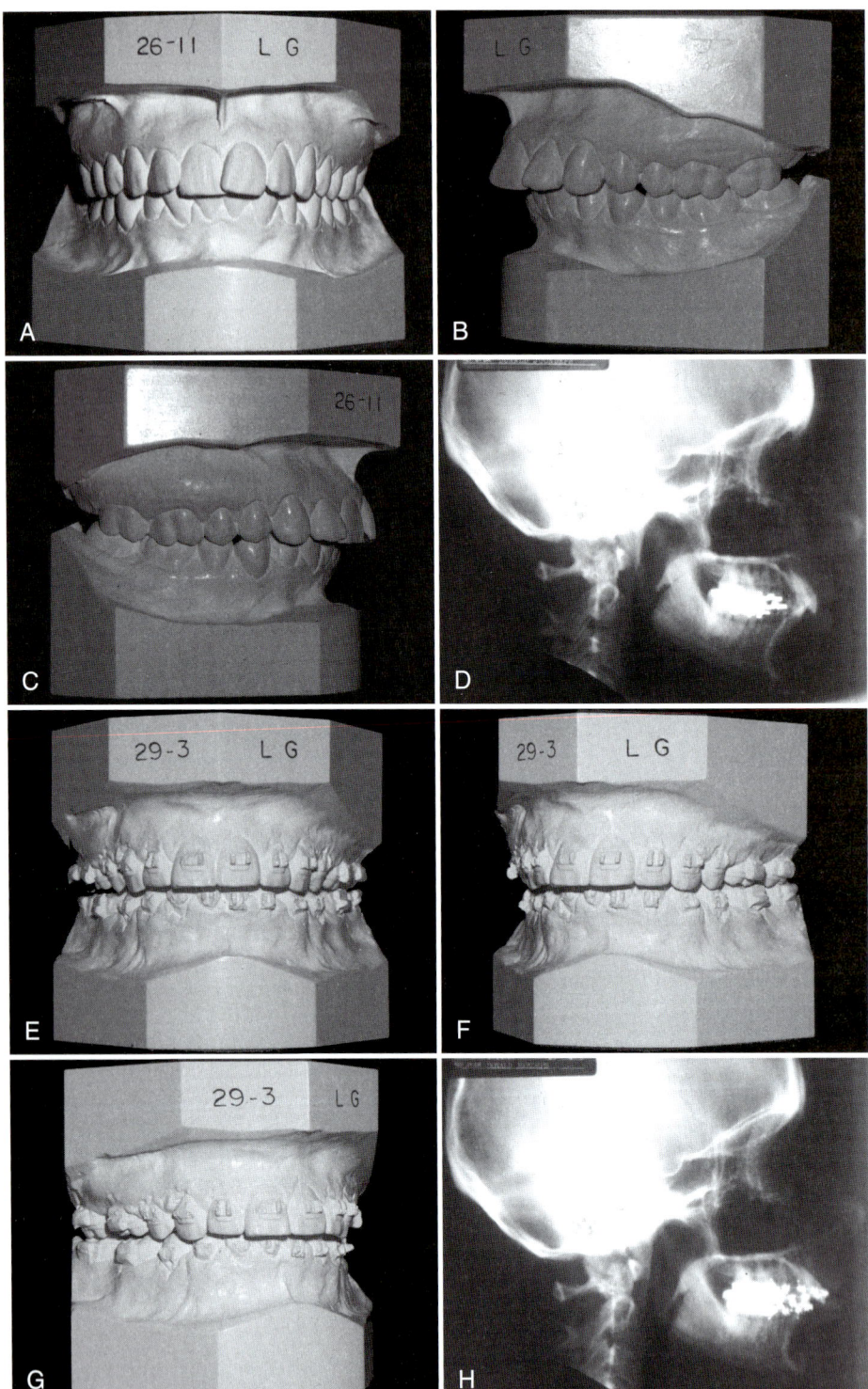

Fig. 77-6 ■ Initial models (**A** to **C**) and a lateral cephalogram (**D**) show class II malocclusion. Presurgical models (**E** to **G**) and a lateral cephalogram (**H**) show increased overjet after extraction of the lower first bicuspids and closure of the space to maximize mandibular advancement.

Technique

The surgical technique for mandibular narrowing is always done in conjunction with mandibular bilateral sagittal split osteotomies. The midline cut is made after the sagittal splits are completed, and the mandible is placed in intermaxillary fixation with an occlusal splint. Fixing the occlusion at this time stabilizes the mandible during the osteotomy. A 1.5-cm incision is made below the attached tissue but generally not into the lip. A sagittal saw is used to make a bicortical cut from the inferior border of the mandible to a point midway between the apices of the central incisors. The cut is then continued only through the buccal cortex up to the attached gingiva. A fine osteotome is twisted in the cut to achieve final splitting of the mandible. Based on postoperative peri-apical films, this last fracture line travels up the periodontal ligament space of one of the incisors. The two mandibular body segments are then fully seated into the surgical splint, and the intermaxillary fixation is tightened. A four-hole 2-mm

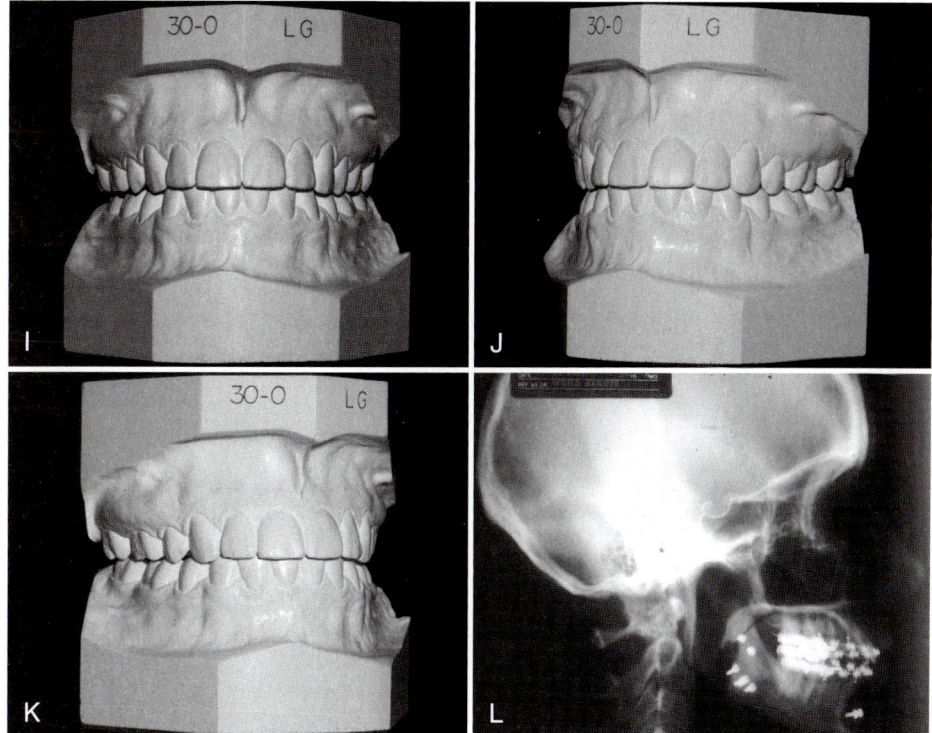

Fig. 77-6, cont'd ■ **I** to **K,** Final models and a lateral cephalogram (**L**) after mandibular advancement combined with mandibular constriction.

plate is contoured to fit passively across the osteotomy site and secured with bicortical screws. The use of bicortical screws was driven by some early problems with unexpected transverse relapse in patients with relatively small constrictions measuring 4 to 6 mm. Rigid fixation of the bilateral sagittal split is then completed, and the intermaxillary wires are removed to check the occlusion. Two plates are rarely used for fixation of the midline osteotomy—when correction of a large transverse discrepancy (8 to 10 mm) is required or there is "soft bone" with minimal cortical thickness. The orthodontic arch wire is not cut at the midline during this procedure because we have found that continuity of the wire adds to the stability of the osteotomy. This technique is completely different from mandibular intercanine narrowing with midline ostectomy in that removal of symphyseal bone is not necessary (Fig. 77-7).

Pattern of Expansion

The amount of mandibular constriction has been shown to be statistically significant and occurs progressively from the anterior to the posterior aspect of the arch. There is minimal change in intercanine width, with most of the constriction taking place across the second molars.[34]

Soft Tissue Esthetics

The transverse soft tissue response is 60% of the narrowing at the posterior mandible; however, these changes are not noticed by patients since they are minimal and their perception is distracted by the more noticeable AP and vertical changes associated with the mandibular advancement.[35]

Stability

The orthodontist can aid stability by not trying to make any significant transverse corrections other than uprighting the molars and reducing the curve of Wilson before surgery. Finally, it has been found that large rectangular arch wires have sufficient memory that

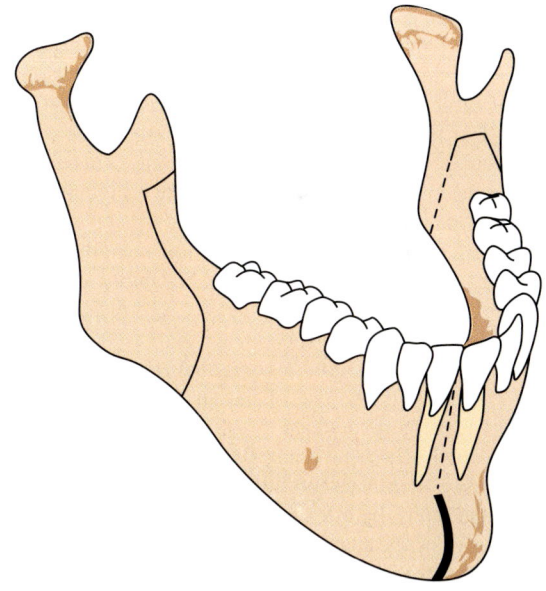

Fig. 77-7 ■ Bilateral sagittal split and midline osteotomies.

if not narrowed just before surgery, they will cause dental and possibly skeletal relapse of the transverse correction. The orthodontist will usually schedule an appointment with the patient 1 to 2 days before surgery to place surgical hooks on the arch wire, as well as to narrow the arch wire the amount of the anticipated constriction. In this short time before surgery, no significant dental movement takes place that will cause difficulty fitting the surgical splint at the time of surgery. It needs to be emphasized that as in all surgeries to correct transverse discrepancies, close cooperation with the

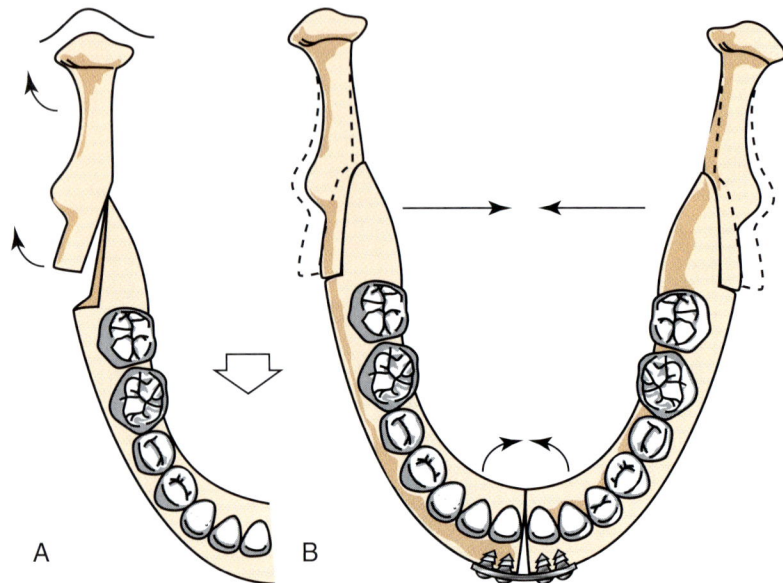

Fig. 77-8 ■ **A,** Condylar rotation during mandibular advancement caused by lateral displacement of the proximal segment. **B,** Example of how mandibular constriction reduces condylar rotation induced by mandibular advancement.

orthodontist is essential to minimize relapse. If the orthodontist attempts to correct the transverse discrepancy in adult patients before surgery, there is a poor chance of a long-term successful result because of the instability of the dental compensations. The best results are achieved when the orthodontist uprights the posterior teeth before surgery by removing the curve of Wilson. It has been determined that there is minor lingual torquing of the mandibular posterior segments during the midline osteotomy. This effect, when added to lingual crown torquing caused by the orthodontic mechanics, can result in an unstable correction.

It has been reported that narrowing the mandible more than 10 mm at the second molars results in instability. Although two plates have been used in these situations, significant relapse has occurred.

In his master's thesis, Pitts investigated the stability of mandibular constriction with the use of plaster casts.[34] His study group had undergone surgery at least 5 years earlier, and he noted a small but statistically significant 0.6-mm relapse at the second molars; however, there were no instances of crossbite at follow-up. Other than the study by Alexander and associates,[15] a significant difficulty in any of the maxillary or mandibular research has been reliance on measuring the transverse corrections with plaster models. Obviously, any changes in torque made by the orthodontic appliances after surgery can affect these results. Probably, the best way to assess the stability of any type of transverse correction would be evaluation of posterior occlusion after there has been a sufficient time during which no orthodontic appliances or retainers have been used.

Five years after orthodontic treatment, no statistically significant relapse was found from the canines through the first molars, but there was a relapse of 0.6 mm in second molar width as mentioned earlier. Although this relapse was statistically significant, the author concluded that the small amount of change was not clinically significant, especially in the absence of crossbite or end-to-end occlusion at the end of orthodontic treatment and at the 5-year follow-up.[15,34]

Effects on the Temporomandibular Joint

Patient self-reports designed to elicit information about temporomandibular joint function 3 to 4 years after treatment in a study by Joondeph and Bloomquist showed no significant differences when comparing patients who underwent midline constriction with mandibular advancement with those who underwent mandibular advancement alone.[33] Long-term patient examination also found no differences between the two groups in the extent of maximum opening and range of motion, both of which were within normal limits. It is not surprising that patients undergoing midline constriction do not have a higher likelihood of temporomandibular dysfunction. A study comparing submentovertex radiographs to measure condylar rotation and lateral movement in 20 consecutive patients showed that mandibular advancement and constriction actually resulted in less change in condylar angulation and width, especially at the medial pole, as a result of surgery than did mandibular advancement alone. The subjective reports of temporomandibular joint symptoms from both groups of patients were not significantly different. Joondeph and Bloomquist's findings from evaluating the effects of sagittal split alone on the temporomandibular joint were similar to what has been reported by other authors (Fig. 77-8).[35]

Periodontal Effects

In 5-year postsurgical periodontal evaluations of both the midline osteotomy site and the mandibular anterior incision site, no differences were found in pocket depth, attachment loss, or recession when compared with other mandibular anterior sites in the same patient.

POSTOPERATIVE CARE

There is no difference in the postoperative care of patients after a normal sagittal split since intermaxillary fixation is not needed. If the orthodontist has not narrowed the mandibular arch wire before surgery, it needs to be done as soon as practical after surgery.

PEARLS AND PITFALLS

Discrepancies in maxillo-mandibular width may be manifested as three different patterns. Selection of the surgical procedure for each pattern will be determined by the location (intercanine, intermolar, or both) of the deficiency, the magnitude of the discrepancy, Bolton analysis, the pattern and limits of expansion or constriction, stability, and effects on facial esthetics.

Narrow Maxilla with a Normal Mandible

- Maxillary intercanine deficiency: SARPE.
  - Indication: isolated transverse maxillary skeletal deficiencies; if maxillary or mandibular repositioning is needed, a second surgery will be required. Simultaneous anterior or inferior maxillary repositioning (or both) can be achieved by distraction osteogenesis with application of the floating bone concept.
  - Usually performed before orthodontic decompensation.
  - Range of expansion of 5 to 15 mm.
  - Increases arch length for correction of an arch length deficiency with minimal esthetic impact, except for improvement in smile esthetics. Mild increases in alar width may be seen.
  - Maxillary expansion is the same or larger at the anterior maxilla than at the molar region, thereby creating a maxillary midline diastema.
  - The limitations of the soft tissue–induced expansion of the multisegment Le Fort I osteotomy do not apply to this technique.
- Maxillary intermolar deficiency: segmental Le Fort I.
  - Indication: maxillary expansion when simultaneous AP or vertical repositioning (or both) is necessary. This procedure can be done alone or combined with mandibular osteotomies.
  - It is usually performed after orthodontic decompensation of the maxillary arch is completed, which can be challenging, especially in patients with significant dental crowding.
  - The amount of expansion is usually restricted by the soft tissues at the osteotomy sites.
  - More posterior than anterior maxillary expansion is achieved since the axis of rotation is at the upper dental midline for a two-piece maxilla.
  - The Le Fort I procedure has considerable esthetic impact as described previously.
  - Overcorrection is indicated to compensate for relapse-induced posterior crossbite at the end of treatment.
- Pitfall: segmental Le Fort I osteotomies with expansions of up to 15 mm have been reported, but expansions greater than 10 mm at the posterior maxilla may be associated with relapse postoperatively.

Wide Mandible with Normal Maxilla

- Mandibular intermolar excess: mandibular constriction.
  - Indication: mainly for patients with mandibular transverse excess (<10 mm) who have ideal maxillary position and smile esthetics or whose facial esthetics are likely to be negatively affected by the soft tissue changes associated with Le Fort I osteotomy. This technique is commonly used in patients with an absolute transverse discrepancy as a result of mandibular advancement.
  - The decision to surgically correct a transverse discrepancy can be deferred to the presurgical evaluation when the dentition is fully decompensated.
  - There are minimal risks and morbidity, which saves the patient from undergoing additional maxillary surgery with increased operating time and cost.
  - It decreases the transverse mandibular dimensions mainly at the posterior mandible, with the dental midline as the axis of constriction producing negligible soft tissue impact.
  - Mandibular constriction ranging from 3 to 10 mm has been reported.
- Pitfall: although this procedure has excellent long-term stability, relapse has been noted with constrictions greater than 10 mm at the second molars.
- Mandibular intercanine excess.
  - It is rarely treated surgically because it is usually diagnosed as a discrepancy in tooth size and treated orthodontically.

Narrow Maxilla with a Wide Mandible (Severe Transverse Maxillomandibular Discrepancy >10 mm)

- A combination of the aforementioned techniques is indicated to minimize postoperative relapse.

Summary

- The sparse literature on surgical correction of transverse discrepancies is a consequence of less than ideal tools to diagnose and evaluate treatment outcomes. Better-designed studies will take place with the development of new 3D imagery. This will then lead to more accurate diagnosis and treatment of dentofacial transverse problems. As presented in this chapter, each treatment option has its indications, and therefore all three procedures should be routine in the practice of any surgeon providing orthognathic surgery.

REFERENCES

1. Sarver DM, Profitt WR, Ackerman JL: Evaluation of facial soft tissues. In Profitt WR, White RP Jr, Sarver DM, editors: *Contemporary treatment of dentofacial deformity*, St. Louis, 2003, CV Mosby.
2. Kelly JE, Harvey CR: *An assessment of the occlusion of the teeth of youths 12-17 years*, U.S. Public Health Service Publication No 77:164, Government Printing Office, 1977.
3. McLain JB, Steedle JR, Vig PS: Face height and dental relationships in 1600 children: a survey, *J Dent Res* 62:308-313, 1983.
4. Bell WH: *Surgical correction of dentofacial deformities: new concepts*, Philadelphia, 1985, WB Saunders, pp 2-3.
5. Proffit WR, Phillips C, Dann C IV: Who seeks surgical-orthodontic treatment? *Int J Adult Orthod Orthognath Surg* 3:153-160, 1990.
6. Kluemper GT, Spalding PM: Realities of craniofacial growth modification, *Atlas Oral Maxillofac Surg Clin North Am* 9:23-57, 2001.
7. Bays RA, Greco JM: Surgically assisted rapid palatal expansion: an outpatient technique with long term stability, *J Oral Maxillofac Surg* 50:110-113, discussion 114-115, 1992.
8. Pogrel MA, Kaban LB, Vargervik K, et al: Surgically assisted rapid maxillary expansion in adults, *Int J Adult Orthod Orthognath Surg* 7:37-41, 1992.
9. Stromberg C, Holm J: Surgically assisted, rapid maxillary expansion in adults. A retrospective long-term follow-up study, *J Craniomaxillofac Surg* 23:222-227, 1995.
10. Northway WM, Meade JB Jr: Surgically assisted rapid maxillary expansion: a comparison of technique, response, and stability, *Angle Orthod* 67:309-320, 1997.
11. Berger JL, Pangrazio-Kulbersh V, Borgula T, et al: Stability of orthopedic and surgically assisted rapid palatal expansion over time, *Am J Orthod Dentofacial Orthop* 114:638-645. 1998.
12. Turvey TA: Maxillary expansion: a surgical technique based on surgical-orthodontic treatment objectives and anatomical considerations, *J Maxillofac Surg* 13:51-58, 1985.
13. Phillips C, Medland W, Fields H Jr, et al: Stability of surgical maxillary expansion, *Int J Adult Orthodont Orthognath Surg* 7:139-146, 1992.
14. Brusati R, Sesenna E, Mannucci N, et al: The midline mandibular osteotomy-ostectomy in the correction of dentofacial deformities, *Int*

J Adult Orthodon Orthognath Surg 2:37-50, 1987.

15. Alexander CD, Bloomquist DS, Wallen TR: Stability of mandibular constriction with a symphyseal osteotomy, *Am J Orthod Dentofacial Orthop* 103:15-23, 1993.

16. Krebs AA: Rapid expansion of midpalatal suture studied by means of fixed appliance: an implant study over a 7 year period. *Trans Eur Orthod Soc* 40:131-142, 1964.

17. Ricketts RM: Perspectives in the clinical application of cephalometrics, the first fifty years, *Angle Orthod* 51:115-150, 1981.

18. Ludlow JB, Gubler M, Cevidanes L, et al: Precision of cephalometric landmark identification: cone-beam computed tomography vs conventional cephalometric views, *Am J Orthod Dentofacial Orthop* 136:312.e1-312e10, discussion 312-313, 2009.

19. Swennen RJ, Schutyser F: Three-dimensional cephalometry: spiral multi-slice vs. cone-beam computed tomography, *Am J Orthod Dentofacial Orthop* 130:410-416, 2006.

20. Park SH, Yu HS, Kim KD, et al: A proposal for a new analysis of craniofacial morphology by 3-dimensional computed tomography, *Am J Orthod Dentofacial Orthop* 129:600.e23-600.e34. 2006.

21. Steinhauser EW: Midline splitting of the maxilla for correction of malocclusion, *J Oral Surg* 30:413-422, 1972.

22. West RA, Epker BN: Posterior maxillary surgery: its place in the treatment of dentofacial deformities, *J Oral Surg* 30:562-563, 1972.

23. Bell WH, Epker BN: Surgical-orthodontic expansion of the maxilla, *Am J Orthod* 70:517-528, 1976.

24. Reinkingh MR, Rosenberg A: Palatal surgical splint for transverse stability of LeFort I osteotomies: a technical note, *Int J Oral Maxillofac Surg* 25:105-106, 1996.

25. Betts N, Dowd K: Soft tissue changes associated with orthognathic surgery, *Atlas Oral Maxillofac Surg Clin North Am* 8:13-38, 2000.

26. Kole H: Surgical operations on the alveolar ridge to correct occlusal abnormalities, *Oral Surg* 12:515-529, 1959.

27. Converse JM, Horowitz SL: The surgical-orthodontic approach to the treatment of dentofacial deformities, *Am J Orthod* 55:217-243, 1969.

28. Lines PA: Adult rapid maxillary expansion with corticotomy, *Am J Orthod* 67:44-56, 1975.

29. Roblee R, Bolding S, Landers J: *Surgically facilitated orthodontic therapy: a new tool for optimal interdisciplinary results*, Philadelphia, 2009, WB Saunders.

30. Kennedy JE, Bell WH, Kimbrough OL, et al: Osteotomy as an adjunct to rapid maxillary expansion, *Am J Orthod* 70:123-137, 1976.

31. Rea A, Alcalde RE, Bloomquist D, et al: *Systematic review of surgically assisted rapid maxillary expansion*, Chicago, September 2002, 84th Annual Meeting of the American Association of Oral and Maxillofacial Surgeons.

32. Plumpton S: Surgical correction of unilateral mandibular prognathism by intra-oral ostectomy of the symphysis, *Br J Plast Surg* 20:70-77, 1967.

33. Joondeph D, Bloomquist D: Mandibular midline osteotomy for constriction, *Am J Orthod Dentofacial Orthop* 126:268-270, 2004.

34. Pitts AL: Mandibular midline osteotomy: stability, periodontal status, TMJ function [master's thesis], Seattle, 1996, University of Washington.

35. Alcalde RE: Soft tissue changes associated with mandibular constriction with midline osteotomy, *J Oral Maxillofac Surg* 60:72, 2002.

Chapter

78

Mandibular Orthognathic Surgery: Vertical Ramus Osteotomy vs. Sagittal Split Osteotomy

Shahid R. Aziz, Steven M. Roser

Treatment of maxillofacial skeletal deformities, particularly mandibular deformities, has developed into an art, as well as science. The two "workhorse" osteotomies that maxillofacial surgeons use to treat mandibular deformities are the sagittal split osteotomy (SSO) and the vertical ramus osteotomy (VRO). Both osteotomies are typically performed via an intraoral approach. However, VRO is limited to mandibular setback procedures for the treatment of mandibular prognathia or to mandibular advancement of 2 mm or less. Bilateral SSOs can be used to treat mandibular prognathia or retrognathia (mandibular setback or advancement). In addition, mandibular asymmetries can be treated via bilateral SSOs or a combination of unilateral VRO and contralateral SSO.

HISTORICAL PERSPECTIVE

The origins of mandibular orthognathic surgery lie along the banks of the Ohio River, where a Wheeling, West Virginia, surgeon named Simon Hullihen performed the first documented bilateral mandibular osteotomy to treat a skeletal open bite in 1848.[1] Further development of mandibular orthognathic surgery followed with Vilray Blair designing the "St. Louis operation," which consisted of bilateral body ostectomies to treat mandibular prognathism in 1897. Multiple mandibular osteotomy designs were developed by American and European surgeons to correct a malpositioned mandible, all of which required extraoral incisions, as well as sacrifice of the mandibular nerve. VRO was first developed at Walter Reed Medical Center by

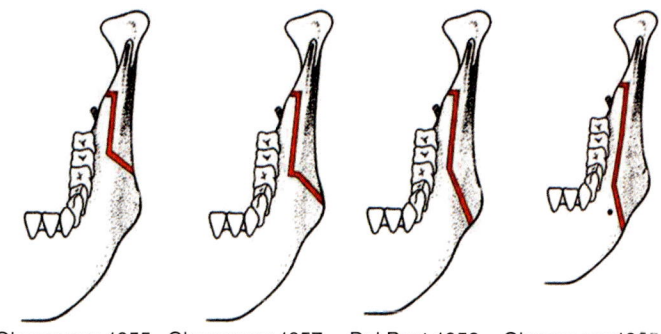

Obwegeser 1955   Obwegeser 1957   Dal Pont 1958   Obwegeser 1968

Fig. 78-1 ■ Evolution of the sagittal split osteotomy. (Modified from Obwegeser HL: Orthognathic surgery and a tale of how three procedures came to be: a letter to the next generations of surgeons, *Clin Plast Surg* 34:331-355, 2007.)

Jack Caldwell and George Letterman in 1954.[2] It was originally a procedure performed from an extraoral approach and used to treat mandibular prognathism. Its novelty lay in that it was an osteotomy that minimized injury to the mandibular nerve. In 1970, Jon Kent and Ed Hinds (from the University of Texas-Houston) designed an intraoral 90-degree saw for osteotomizing the ascending ramus of the mandible from a purely intraoral approach.[3] During the 1970s and 1980s, David Hall (from Vanderbilt University) further refined the VRO procedure and demonstrated that it could be used to treat not only mandibular prognathism but also mild mandibular retrognathia (advancement of 2 mm or less). In addition, Hall and McKenna championed VRO as a treatment of temporomandibular joint dysfunction.[4]

SSO has a more complex history, with its origins in Europe. Hugo Obwegeser first developed this approach. He felt compelled to design a new mandibular osteotomy because he "wanted an osteotomy that could be performed transorally only, avoiding a skin incision, and which would produce broad contacting bone surfaces, even after the repositioning."[5] Consequently, he designed the SSO after studying cadaver mandibles and determining that this procedure could be done transorally. The first case was performed on a prognathic/edentulous 27-year-old woman on February 17, 1953, under local anesthesia. The initial osteotomy was different from the current SSO procedure in that it was limited to the ramus only. Over the next 30 years, multiple modifications by Obwegeser and others were suggested (Fig. 78-1). The original SSO was extended to include the buccal cortex of the mandibular body in the area of the second molar to provide more stability and increased bone-to-bone contact. Although the Italian surgeon G. Dal Pont is credited in the literature with this modification (the "Dal Pont modification"), Obwegeser noted in subsequent publications that this was actually a modification that he performed with Dal Pont as his assistant; Dal Pont went ahead and published this modification without Obwegeser's knowledge or inclusion. The Dal Pont modification of the SSO is the most common one currently performed. Although these original osteotomies were secured with wire osteosynthesis, today's SSO includes rigid fixation.

PATHOLOGIC ANATOMY

The surgical anatomy for SSO and VRO is similar because both procedures are completed in the posterior mandible. Both osteotomies are done via a transoral technique through an incision in the posterior mandibular vestibule. The dissection differs, however.

Dissection for VRO is limited to exposing the lateral ramus, from gonial angle to sigmoid notch. Dissection on the medial aspect of the ascending ramus is avoided to maintain muscle attachment. Detaching the lateral soft tissue attachments of the ascending ramus but maintaining the medial attachments is important in that this dissection technique allows muscular support of the proximal (condylar) segment of the VRO. If lateral and medial dissection of the ascending ramus is performed, the proximal segment may sag inferiorly from lack of muscular support and result in poor positioning of the condyle in the glenoid fossa. This in turn may cause malocclusion postoperatively once the maxillo-mandibular fixation (MMF) is released.

Dissection for SSO is the opposite technique—the medial aspect of the ascending ramus is dissected and exposed and the lateral ramus attachments are maintained. The medial dissection is performed to permit visualization of the mandibular nerve passing into the mandible, and a saw or drill is used to create the medial ramus SSO corticotomy.

Other pertinent anatomic landmarks include the sigmoid notch in both procedures. When completing the superior aspect of the osteotomy during VRO, visualization of the sigmoid notch and the Bauer retractor will permit better control of the saw so that one can avoid dropping the saw blade into the area medial to the notch where the internal maxillary artery (IMA) is located. Visualization of the sigmoid notch during the medial dissection while performing the SSO allows accurate placement of the saw or drill when performing the medial cortical osteotomy. Exposure and identification of the posterior border of the ramus will permit the operator to keep the osteotomy 5 mm anterior to the border. Identification of the antilingula on the lateral aspect of the ascending ramus when scoring the ramus for the VRO helps locate the position on the medial aspect of the ramus through which the mandibular nerve passes from the foramen to the mandible. Cadaver studies have shown that placing the VRO 5 mm posterior to the antilingula minimizes injury to the mandibular nerve.[6] During SSO, visualization of the lingula (or at least observation of the insertion of the mandibular nerve into the mandible) is important to ensure that the medial SSO osteotomy is performed without injury to nerves or vessels. Visualization of the depression on the medial aspect of the ramus posterior to the area where the mandibular nerve passes into the mandible helps in identifying the posterior limit of the medial osteotomy.

DIAGNOSTIC STUDIES

When preparing for mandibular orthognathic surgery, preoperative imaging is essential. Although plain films (panoramic radiograph, lateral cephalogram, anteroposterior cephalogram) are the basic minimum requirement in planning surgical treatment, computed tomography (CT) with three-dimensional (3D) volumetric rendering is evolving into the "gold standard" in maxillofacial imaging for orthognathic surgery. Identification of asymmetries and anatomic anomalies will permit proper selection of orthognathic procedures. Specific to mandibular osteotomies, 3D CT allows realistic visualization of the lingula and antilingula. This in turn permits more precise planning of the osteotomies (Fig. 78-2). In addition, being able to visualize the size of the coronoid processes via 3D CT is helpful in planning treatment in that a large coronoid process can limit the amount of mandibular setback with a VRO and consequently require coronoidectomies to adequately mobilize the mandible. Routine 3D visualization of the location of the course of the mandibular nerve will greatly assist in reducing the incidence of nerve injury that occurs during SSO.

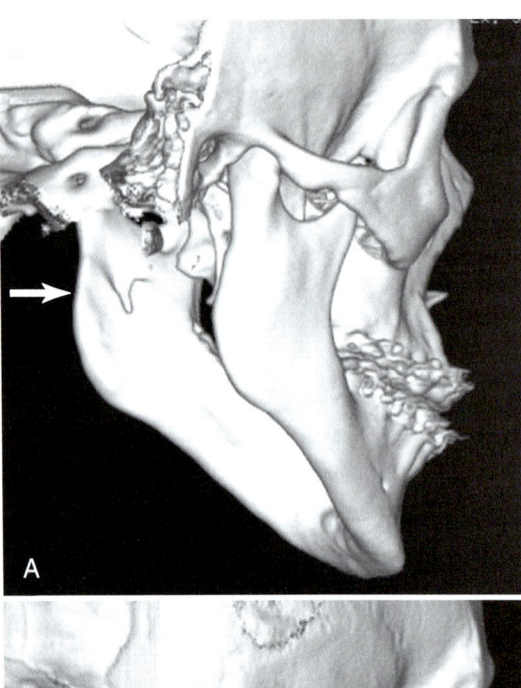

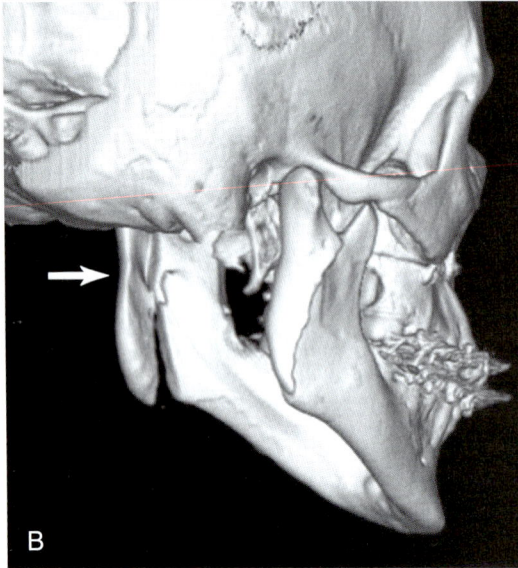

Fig. 78-2 ■ **A,** Three-dimensional (3D) maxillofacial computed tomography (CT) allows excellent visualization of the lingual position on the medial ascending ramus of the mandible (*arrow*). **B,** 3D CT in same patient immediately after surgery with the vertical ramus osteotomy just posterior to the lingual position (*arrow*).

CT scans are easier to obtain in the immediate postoperative period than plain films are and are far more helpful. The patient does not have to stand, and CT can be done on a fast scanner in less than 15 seconds. It is the authors' opinion that within a short time, preoperative planning for orthognathic surgery will routinely be done with virtual surgery software and that intraoperative CT scanning will be routine when necessary to position the maxilla or mandible. Assessment of outcomes will be far more accurate with CT.

INDICATIONS AND TREATMENT GOALS

The primary indication for VRO is the treatment of mandibular prognathism. VRO can be used for anterior jaw repositioning of 2 mm or less. SSO is more versatile in that it allows movement of the mandible posteriorly and anteriorly. Contraindications to SSO

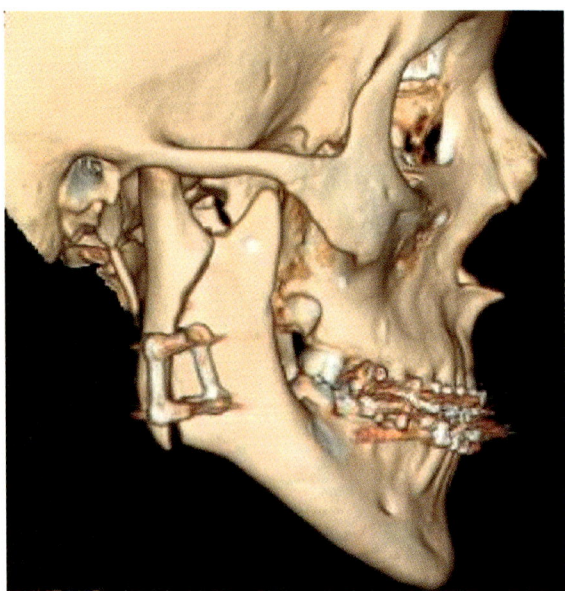

Fig. 78-3 ■ Rigid fixation of a vertical ramus osteotomy.

include the presence of unerupted second molars, a severely narrow anteroposterior or mediolateral dimension of the ramus with no medullary bone between the buccal and lingual cortices, and significant mandibular asymmetry.[7]

The main differences in the treatment of mandibular prognathism via SSO and VRO include the following:

1. Technical—SSO is a technically more challenging surgical procedure with more opportunity for intraoperative and postoperative complications. The most common complications involve fractures of the proximal or distal segments in unplanned/unfavorable locations. Most of these "bad splits" can be repaired with little impact on outcome, but they take time and may require a period of MMF to allow healing.
2. Rigid fixation—SSO is rigidly fixated. VRO is typically not rigidly fixated because access to the overlapped proximal and distal segments is limited. However some operators routinely rigid fixate the VRO (Fig. 78-3). If not rigidly secured, 3 weeks of MMF is recommended.
3. Neurologic damage—because the mandibular nerve lies centrally in the SSO, its risk for injury is far greater than with VRO. The incidence of inferior alveolar nerve injury associated with VRO is 1% as compared with up to 15% to 85% with SSO.[8]
4. Removal of wisdom teeth—though not recommended because of the potential for increased complications, removal of impacted third molars during a VRO procedure has less impact on the procedure than removal of molars does on SSO. Although third molar removal can be accomplished during SSO, there is increased risk for unfavorable splitting of the ramus when an impacted third molar is present. It is recommended that impacted wisdom teeth be removed 6 to 12 months before either procedure.

Outcome studies comparing VRO and SSO for the treatment of mandibular prognathism demonstrate similarly low rates of relapse.[9] Variables associated with relapse include the amount of setback, condylar displacement, clockwise rotation of the proximal segment, mode of fixation, and growth. Significant mandibular setback (>10 mm) may require anterior movement of the maxilla combined with mandibular retrusion to reduce the risk for relapse.

SPECIFIC TREATMENT AND TECHNIQUES

VERICAL RAMUS OSTEOTOMY

The approach for VRO is via an intraoral technique. The incision starts on the anterior border of the ramus 1 cm posterior to the third molar region and sweeps forward into the buccal vestibule while leaving an adequate cuff of mucosa superiorly to allow easy closure. The anterior extent of the incision is to the area adjacent to the first molar. The course of the incision in the retromolar area must be kept buccal to prevent injury to the lingual nerve and to be able to access the incision margins with the patient in fixation. Dissection of the lateral ramus is started by detaching the insertion of the temporalis muscle on the anterior border of the ramus. The Hargis anterior border stripper is recommended. The temporalis should be stripped to the tip of the coronoid process. This allows release of tissues to access the lateral ramus and also to minimize relapse by the action of the temporalis on the distal segment. The dissection then proceeds to stripping the lateral border of the ramus and identifying the sigmoid notch and the posterior border of the ramus. Care must be taken to not strip on the medial aspect of the posterior border (area of the retromandibular vein) or at the inferior border because of attachment of the medial pterygoid muscle, which should be left intact to prevent sagging of the proximal segment (condylar sag). Landmarks to be identified at this time are the sigmoid notch, the posterior border of the ramus, the angle, and the inferior border of the mandible to the anterior aspect of the antegonial notch. Identifying the area of the antilingula, a bump on the lateral cortex, helps localize the point of entry of the mandibular nerve into the medial ramus. Bauer retractors are placed in the sigmoid notch superiorly and at the antegonial notch inferiorly. Use of fiberoptic Bauer retractors is also helpful for illuminating the surgical cavity and maximizing visualization (Fig. 78-4). Additionally, a posterior border retractor, the Merrill-LeVasseur retractor, can be used as well.

Once the surgical cavity is adequately exposed and illuminated, the VRO saw is used. The VRO saw typically comes in two blade sizes—7- and 12-mm length—and is angled to permit the operator to create the osteotomy at a bias away from the neurovascular bundle. The vast majority of osteotomies can be completed with the 7-mm blade. A score mark is placed 5 mm behind the antilingula and checked with a dental mirror. If there is not a prominent antilingula, the osteotomy can be started by placing the saw 5 to 7 mm anterior to the posterior border in the mid-ramus area. The osteotomy is scored from a position posterior to the antilingula, inferior to the posterior aspect of the antegonial notch, and superior to the midportion of the sigmoid notch. Once the score mark has been completed and determined to be in an acceptable position, the osteotomy can be started at the antilingula and walked down the lateral ramus to the antegonial angle with the aid of a Bauer retractor. Once the inferior aspect of the ramus osteotomy has been completed, the VRO saw is then walked back up the ramus superiorly. After the saw has passed the antilingula, it should be directed slightly anteriorly to complete the osteotomy into the sigmoid notch. Care should be taken to not run the saw into the contents of the sigmoid notch, specifically the masseteric artery or the IMA. Injury to the masseteric artery close to its takeoff from the IMA or injury to the IMA itself can cause significant bleeding that is impossible to control locally and may require embolization. Injury to the masseteric artery 1 to 2 cm away from its takeoff from the IMA can usually be controlled by pressure. By completing the osteotomy at the superior aspect last, if bleeding does occur, the osteotomy can be completed quickly and more effective pressure applied.

Once bilateral VROs are completed, the mandible should be passively positioned posteriorly and placed into the predetermined final occlusal relationship. If difficulty is encountered in setting the mandible posteriorly, there may be interference in the form of the coronoid process being trapped under the zygomatic arch. If this is the case, coronoidotomies may be required. Other areas of bone interference include the medial aspect of the proximal segment of the osteotomy and the edges of the proximal and distal segments in the sigmoid notch area. Trimming of the bone with a burr is usually required.

In thinner patients, the inferior aspect of the proximal segment will be palpable through the skin as sharp projections.

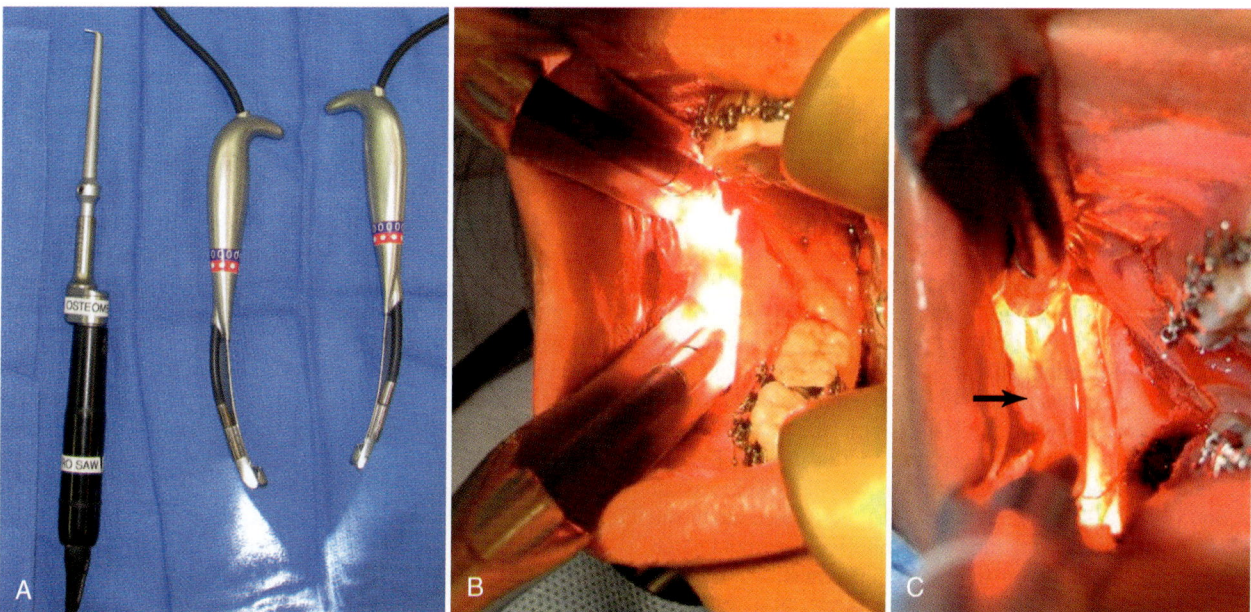

Fig. 78-4 ■ **A,** Fiberoptic Bauer retractors and vertical ramus osteotomy (VRO) saw (7-mm blade). **B,** Surgical cavity illuminated by fiberoptic Bauer retractors. **C,** VRO in the illuminated surgical cavity completed, with the proximal segment lateralized.

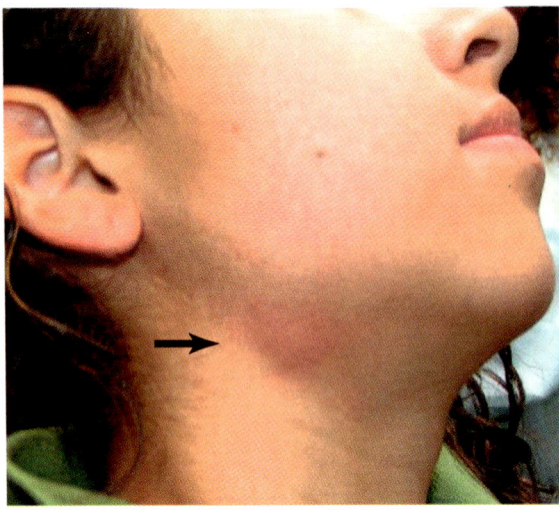

Fig. 78-5 ■ Four months after vertical ramus osteotomy (VRO), the patient has pain, edema, and erythema as a result of necrosis of the inferior point of the proximal segment of the VRO.

In this situation it is advisable to have the most inferior 5 mm of the proximal segment removed with a bur. Leaving the sharp ends of the proximal segments may cause some discomfort for the patient, as well as the potential for the area to become necrotic and infected weeks to months after surgery (Fig. 78-5). After the mandible has been set back and the ideal occlusion achieved, the mandible is wired to the maxilla. Once MMF is completed, the proximal segments of the osteotomies should be checked to ensure that they are laterally positioned with adequate bone overlap and contact and the vertical position of the proximal segment determined. If the proximal segment can be pushed superiorly more than 2 to 3 mm, condylar sag is present and must be addressed. Management of condylar sag requires fixation to hold the proximal segment in a more superior position with a 1.5-mm L-shaped plate, bisegment screws, and a screw/wire technique (Figs. 78-6 and 78-7). The incision is closed in a single layer with combinations of interrupted sutures in the posterior aspect of the incision and a running suture anteriorly. One should always remember to remove the throat pack before the patient is placed in MMF.

SAGITTAL SPLIT OSTEOTOMY

The incision for SSO typically extends 1 cm up on the anterior ramus and continues inferiorly along the external oblique ridge into the mandibular vestibule to the mesial side of the first molar, often with a vertical release. Subperiosteal dissection is carried to the inferior border for exposure of the lateral body of the mandible in the molar region. Identification of the mental foramen in the short segment of the mandible is helpful to prevent injury to the mental nerve, particularly if fixation will include a monocortical plate. The anterior border of the ramus is stripped of the temporalis attachment to the tip of the coronoid with the Hargis ramus stripper. The dissection is carried to the tip of the coronoid, and an angled Kokher clamp is attached to the coronoid and clamped to the towel to assist in retraction of the tissues. Dissection is also performed along the medial aspect of the ascending ramus to identify the sigmoid notch and the postlingual depression in the medial ramus. The lingula should be identified. This may be difficult in some cases, so it may be helpful to take a small curved hemostat and run it along the medial-superior aspect of the ascending ramus until the sigmoid notch is felt. The lingula is often 10 to 15 mm inferior to the sigmoid

notch. If this does not allow identification of the lingula, completion of the medial ramus corticotomy at the level of the maxillary occlusal plane will often ensure that the corticotomy is superior to the lingula. Before beginning the medial ramus corticotomy, the authors have found it helpful to use a small pineapple-shaped burr to remove/bevel the medial aspect of the external oblique ridge at the level of the medial corticotomy to provide improved visualization of the medial ramus (Fig. 78-8, *A*).

The medial ramus corticotomy is completed with either a thin reciprocating saw or a Lindemann burr. It is important during this procedure to have the retractor on the medial ramus securely in place to allow the best visualization possible and protection of the neurovascular bundle from the back of the saw blade or bur. In addition, the surgeon must realize that this is a corticotomy only, with the bone cut only through the medial cortex of the ramus and stopping once medullary bleeding is encountered. If a reciprocating saw is used, the saw is turned and carried inferiorly along the anterior border of the ramus while keeping it parallel to the buccal cortex. The saw is then carried along the external oblique ridge to a point short of the planned vertical buccal cortical osteotomy. The course of the mandibular nerve in the retromolar area in particular must be determined by preoperative imaging so that the operator knows how deep the saw blade or bur can be inserted. The coronoid retractor is removed and a toe-out retractor or a channel retractor is placed at the planned base of the buccal osteotomy at the inferior border of the mandible. The buccal osteotomy is performed, and the inferior border is osteotomized by tipping the handle of the saw outward and wrapping the tip of the saw around the inferior border while making sure that the osteotomy is through the inferior border of the cortex. On completion of the buccal osteotomy, the horizontal osteotomy is performed by connecting the three cortical osteotomies. If burs are to be used, a 1.0-mm tapered fissure bur is used to mark out the remaining portion of the SSO, which extends from the anterior end of the medial corticotomy and down the external oblique ridge to the lateral body of the mandible and the planned point of the buccal osteotomy. The anterior osteotomy can be performed with either a burr or a reciprocating saw. The vertical buccal corticotomy is completed to the inferior border of the mandible with a 2.1-mm fissure burr. Regardless of whether burs or a reciprocating saw is used, an oscillating saw may be helpful to start the split at the inferior border of the mandible (Fig. 78-8, *B*). There are three areas that often prevent one from making an easy split and require attention at this point—the junction between the medial ramus corticotomy and the corticotomy along the external oblique ridge, the junction between the vertical corticotomy and the horizontal body corticotomy, and the inferior border of the mandible. These areas should be checked for completion of the osteotomy and continuity with the other osteotomies. A trough of bone created along the distal edge of the buccal osteotomy can be fashioned to allow a fine osteotome to be tapped down the buccal cut to start the split at this margin. At this point a series of osteotomes are used to complete the sagittal split. It is preferable to start with thin spatula osteotomes initially and then progress to larger/thicker osteotomes. The osteotomes should be used throughout the entire length of the SSO. Once the SSO segment appears to be mobile, two Smith separators are placed in the horizontal corticotomy in the body of the mandible. A Smith spreader is then placed in the vertical corticotomy. In a controlled fashion, the separators and spreader are engaged until the split is completed (frequently a "pop" is heard). As the SSO is spread apart, the surgeon should visualize the mandibular nerve in the body of the mandible to ensure that it is along the medial aspect (distal segment) of the split. If it is not, the nerve may need to be freed from the bony canal and gently repositioned medially. After the SSO is completed, a

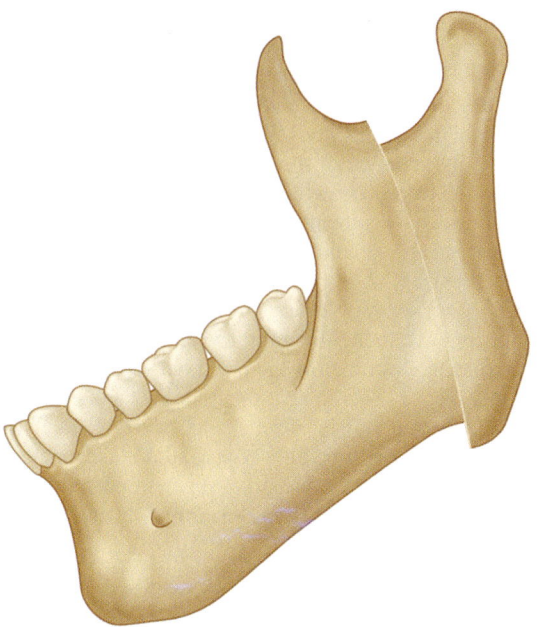

A. Proximal segment has sagged inferiorly.

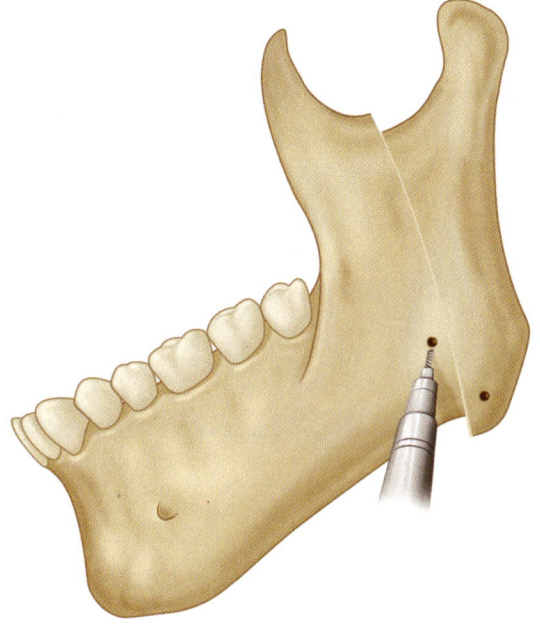

B. Hole already placed in proximal segment. Hole in ramus at 45° angle. The distance superior to the proximal hole is the distance estimated to elevate proximal segment into fossa.

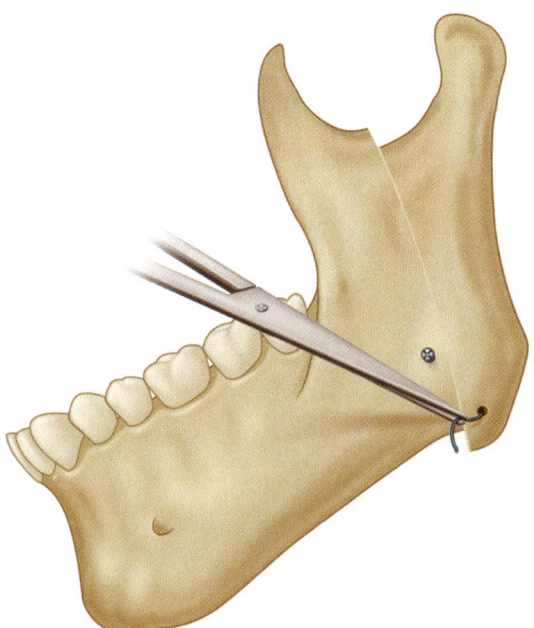

C. 26g wire placed in proximal hole and tied around 2.0 screw placed in distal segment.

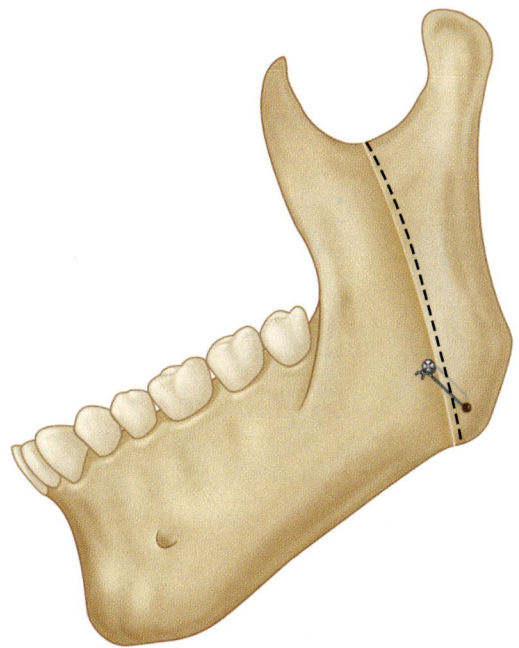

D. Tightened to achieve elevation and overlap.

Fig. 78-6 ■ Correction of condylar sag. **A,** Proximal segment has sagged inferiorly. **B,** Hole already placed in proximal segment. Hole in ramus at 45-degree angle. The distance superior to the proximal hole is the distance estimated to elevate proximal segment into the fossa. **C,** 26-gauge wire placed in proximal hole and tied around 2.0 screw placed in distal segment. **D,** Tightened to achieve elevation and overlap.

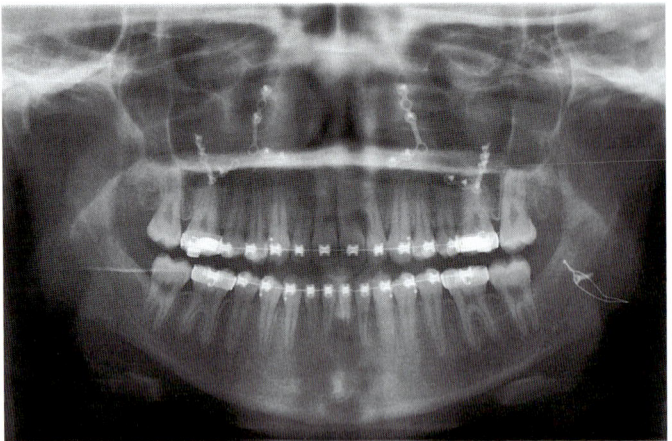

Fig. 78-7 ■ Screw/wire fixation placed intraoperatively to correct condylar sag in the proximal segment. This fixation can be removed in the office after healing.

clamp should be placed on the proximal segment and the segment mobilized to remove the remaining medial pterygoid muscle attachments (Fig. 78-8, *C*). Once the SSO is completed bilaterally, the mandible should be repositioned into its planned position. If the distal segment is being moved forward symmetrically, there is no need for bone removal. If the mandible is to be repositioned posteriorly or rotated, bone will need to be trimmed from either the proximal or distal segment to allow adaption of the segments. Once the tooth-bearing segment of the mandible is repositioned and MMF performed, the SSO is rigidly fixated. At this point the condyle requires proper seating. A variety of techniques have been described. The authors have found it helpful to make a small purchase point in the anterosuperior corner of the proximal segment to allow a crane pick to be placed. This in turn then allows the surgeon to push the proximal segment posteriorly and superiorly to seat the condyle while pushing medially to allow maximum bone contact (Fig. 78-8, *D*). The key is to seat the proximal segment posteriorly and superiorly. Rigid fixation is completed at this point with either three to

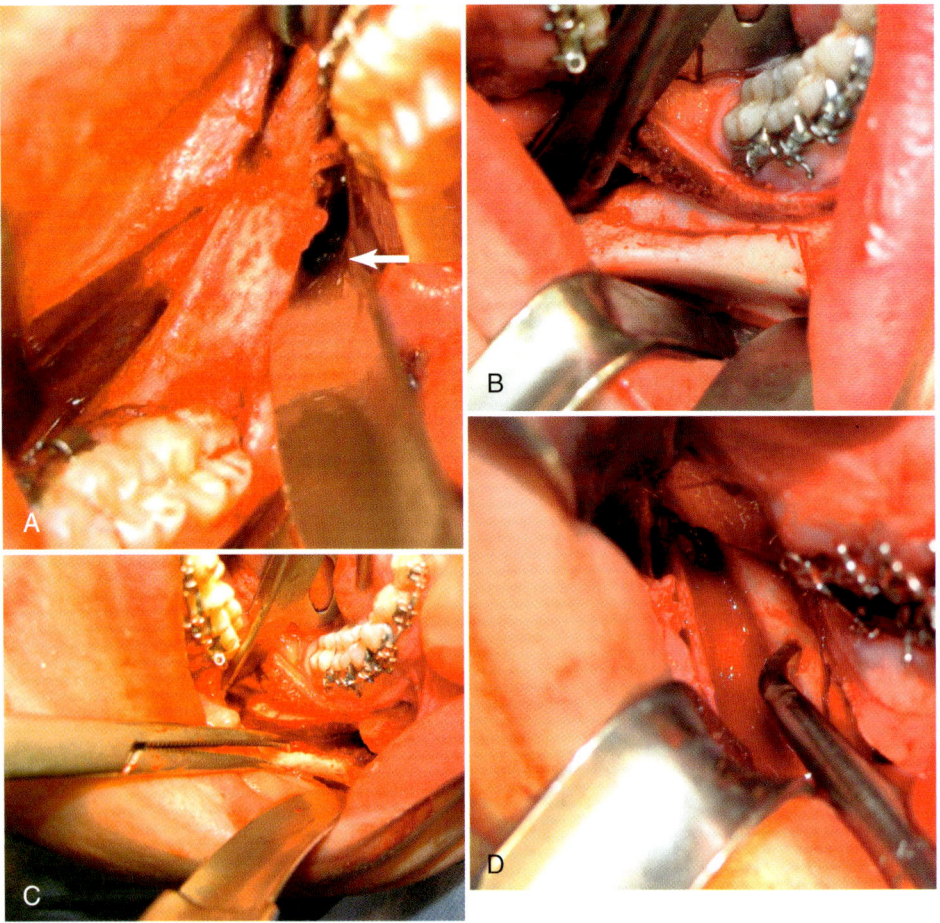

Fig. 78-8 ■ **A,** Small notch made along the medial aspect of the external oblique ridge. **B,** Outline of the sagittal split osteotomy (SSO). **C,** Clamp mobilizing the SSO. **D,** Crane pick for pushing the proximal segment of the SSO to the distal segment, as well as seating the condyle.

four bicortical screws or a combination of a buccal monocortical plate and bicortical screws. Once rigid fixation has been carried out bilaterally, the MMF should be removed and the occlusion checked to be sure that it is reproducible and acceptable. If not, the rigid fixation needs to be removed and the condyles reseated again, with replacement of the rigid fixation. If a combination of plate/bicortical screws is used, the plate is placed first on both sides. The MMF is released. If the occlusion is not reproducible, the two screws from the proximal segment are removed with the patient back in fixation and the plate used as a handle to reposition the proximal segment. At the end of surgery the patient may be placed in MMF if there is any concern regarding the stability of the rigid fixation.

POSTOPERATIVE CARE

As with any maxillofacial surgical patient, protection of the airway is the primary concern at extubation. Before extubation the patient should be fully awake and able to follow commands. In patients placed into wire/elastic MMF, the team should be prepared to remove the wires on an emergency basis if desaturation occurs, which means having wire cutters immediately available, and the peri-operative team should know how to release the patient's fixation. The first 24 hours postoperatively are critical. An intensive care unit or step-down bed may be the best situation for the patient, depending on the resources and setup available at the local institution. After the 24-hour postoperative period, the patient is allowed to increase oral intake, as well as ambulate. A preoperative dose of antibiotics is recommended. It is the surgeon's preference how long the antibiotics should be continued postoperatively. It appears that steroids do assist in minimizing postoperative swelling and that their use is standard for orthognathic surgery. There is little evidence to support postoperative steroid therapy beyond the first 24 hours. On discharge, the patient should receive oral antibiotics, pain medication, and dietary and oral hygiene instructions. It is recommended that patients receive detailed preoperative and postoperative dietary instruction, particularly if a postoperative period of MMF is planned. Three weeks of MMF usually translates to a 10- to 15-lb weight loss. This is usually tolerated by teenagers but can be onerous for adult orthognathic patients and lead to a period of postoperative depression. Weekly office visits for 6 weeks after surgery is recommended, with a 2-week interval possible at the 4- or 5-week mark. VRO patients are typically kept in MMF for 3 weeks, followed by a period of 2 to 3 weeks of guiding elastics. This is similar for SSO patients who are in MMF. For SSO patients in elastics immediately after surgery, physical therapy can typically commence 2 weeks after surgery; for patients in MMF, physical therapy can commence when the MMF is removed. Without 3 to 4 weeks of daily range-of-motion exercises, permanent restriction of movement can occur. SSO patients routinely have more restriction of movement and need to exercise more vigorously than do VRO patients. Postoperative radiographs are important to verify occlusion, rigid fixation, and condylar position. CT scans with 3D reconstruction are recommended on the next day. Modern scanners are very fast, with only seconds to a minute required to complete a maxillofacial scan (Fig. 78-9). In addition to the speed, the patient does not have to stand but can lie supine for the scan, which makes it much easier than plain films.

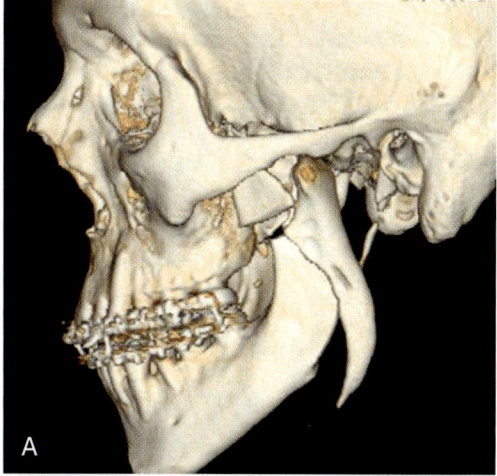
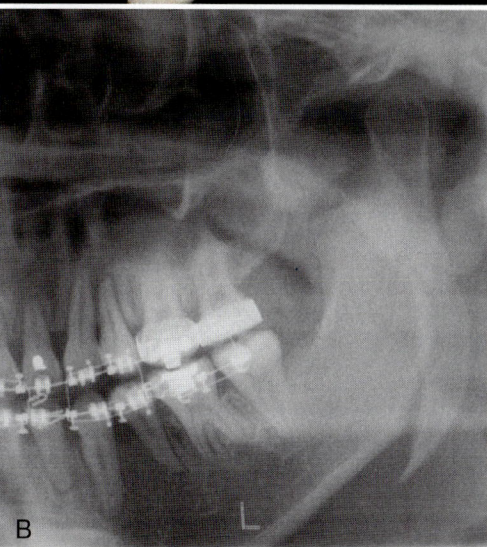
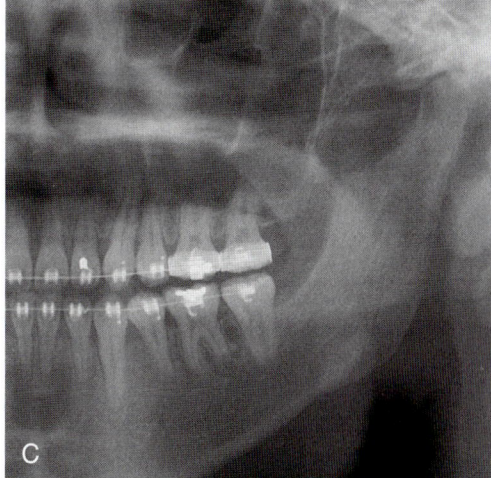

Fig. 78-9 ■ **A,** Three-dimensional computed tomography of the vertical ramus osteotomy immediately after surgery demonstrates dislocation of the left condyle anterior to the articular eminence. A decision was made to observe the patient to see whether muscle pull would reduce the condyle without surgical intervention. **B,** Four days after surgery, the condyle is now reducing. **C,** Six months after surgery, the condyle is well positioned in the glenoid fossa.

PEARLS AND PITFALLS

Vertical Ramus Osteotomy

- VRO is used for setbacks and minor (2-mm) advancements.
- Be sure to keep the incision lateral to allow closure with patient in MMF.
- Fiberoptic retractors allow improved visualization.
- Remove the inferior tip of the proximal segments.
- Obtain 3D CT scans preoperatively for better surgical planning, including localization of the mandibular canal and the position of the segment postoperatively.
- During lateral ramus dissection, leave as much medial pterygoid attachment as possible to avoid condylar sag.
- Osteotomy should be performed 5 to 7 mm anterior to the posterior border to avoid the mandibular neurovascular bundle and ensure the maximum amount of medial pterygoid muscle attachment on the proximal segment.
- After the patient is placed into MMF, always ensure that proximal segments are lateralized.

- Remember to remove the throat pack before MMF is placed.
- MMF is maintained for 3 weeks, with an additional 3 weeks of physical therapy with elastics.

Sagittal Split Osteotomy

- 3D CT should be used for preoperative treatment planning.
- A pineapple-shaped bur is used to create a notch on the medial aspect of the external oblique ridge to visualize the lingula.
- Split corticotomies are performed with a series of osteotomes of increasing width.
- Patience is needed when making the split.
- As the split is separating, identify the mandibular nerve and ensure that it is in the medial aspect of the split; if not, it may need to be repositioned.
- The proximal segment should be pushed posteriorly and superiorly to seat the condyle in the fossa.

REFERENCES

1. Aziz SR: Simon P. Hullihen and the origin of orthognathic surgery, *J Oral Maxillofac Surg* 62:1303-1307, 2004.
2. Caldwell, JB, Letterman GS: Vertical osteotomy in the mandibular rami for the correction of prognathism, *J Oral Surg (Chic)* 12:185-202, 1954.
3. Hebert JM, Kent JN, Hinds EC: Correction of prognathism by an intraoral vertical subcondylar osteotomy, *J Oral Surg* 28:651-653, 1970.
4. Hall HD, McKenna S: Further refinement and evaluation of the intraoral vertical ramus osteotomy, *J Oral Maxillofac Surg* 45:684-688, 1987.
5. Obwegeser HL: Orthognathic surgery and a tale of how three procedures came to be: a letter to the next generations of surgeons, *Clin Plast Surg* 34:331-355, 2007.
6. Aziz SR, Dorfman B, Ziccardi VB, et al: Accuracy of using the antilingula as a sole determinant of vertical ramus osteotomy position, *J Oral Maxillofac Surg* 65:859-862, 2007.
7. Wolford L: The sagittal split ramus osteotomy as the preferred treatment for mandibular prognathism, *J Oral Maxillofac Surg* 58:310-312, 2000.
8. Ghali GE, Sikes JW: Intraoral vertical ramus osteotomy as the preferred treatment for mandibular prognathism, *J Oral Maxillofac Surg* 58:313-315, 2000.
9. Yoshioka I, Khanal A, Tominaga K, et al: Vertical ramus versus sagittal split osteotomies: comparison of stability after mandibular setback, *J Oral Maxillofac Surg* 66:1138-1144, 2008.

Chapter

79

Distraction Osteogenesis

Marianela Gonzalez, Cesar A. Guerrero, Michael P. Ding

Since 1976, distraction osteogenesis (DO) has been performed in a single direction, in this case to increase the maxillary arch and allow correction of anterior crowding, to avoid premolar extractions, and to promote wider smiles. DO leads to the formation of bone and soft tissue across the surgical site, which may allow a more predictable and stable result in patients after orthognathic surgery. Extreme surgical moves and feared complications such as surgical relapse as a result of osseous defects and restrictive soft tissue may be more predictably avoided with the selective use of DO combined with conventional orthognathic surgery. DO is another tool in the surgeon's armamentarium for the management of patients undergoing orthognathic surgery.

ETIOPATHOGENESIS/CAUSATIVE FACTORS

Maxillofacial skeletal deformities and their associated etiopathogenesis have been thoroughly described in the literature. Not only have congenital syndromes been associated with craniofacial

Distraction Osteogenesis 659

dysplasia, but acquired causes such as skeletal deformities as a result of trauma or pathologic resection are also often encountered in patients undergoing maxillofacial surgery. Perfect surgical interventions have been ruined after surgery because of poor orthodontic understanding of the biology of DO. The distraction appliance needs to stay in place for at least 3 months for consolidation and be replaced by screws and plates; for transverse maxillary movement, a transpalatal bar is fixed to the first or second molars in the maxilla for the remainder of the orthodontic treatment. The heavily keratinized palatal mucosa has been stretched and will return to its original dimension unless a strong transpalatal bar is maintained in position until complete mineralization takes place in the maxillary midline, from the alveolar ridge to the palatine bone. Many orthodontists do not understand this situation, and immediate transverse relapse ensues. Consequently, cross-arch elastics are used to incline the teeth toward the buccal mucosa, which creates heavy forces that can move the teeth out of the alveolar ridge and produce periodontal problems at a later stage. Some just accept the posterior crossbite and blame it on the surgery or an "unstable surgical procedure."

DIAGNOSTIC STUDIES

For the treatment of simultaneous maxillo-mandibular discrepancies and skeletal deformities, analysis of each patient should include not only a thorough clinical examination but also radiographic images (lateral cephalometric, posteroanterior, and a panoramic radiograph) and determination of available space versus the required space, inclination of the incisors (incisal mandibular plane angle [IMPA] of 90 degrees), presence of a deep bite or a marked curve of Spee, intermolar width, and the size and shape of the incisors. In certain cases in which complicated bimaxillary movements are planned, stereolithographic models are helpful in the presurgical phase of planning to assist the surgeon in planning the vector of movement and pre-bending hardware. Along with the clinical and radiographic information, occlusograms from study models are important in evaluating patients.

TREATMENT/RECONSTRUCTIVE GOALS

Developments in technology and instrumentation have permitted surgeons to perform interventions for making changes in the three dimensions of space. The surgical procedure is based on the combination of conventional orthognathic surgery and selective DO; for the maxilla, a down-fractured Le Fort I osteotomy could be combined with increasing the transverse dimension either anteriorly or posteriorly with the aid of distraction and semi-rigid fixation. Orthodontists play a major role in the presurgical and postsurgical phases in that the mandible must have ideal tooth positioning, the Hyrax appliance needs to be cemented 2 to 3 days before the surgery, and all brackets and second molar bands need to be in place. No transverse corrections are to be performed in the maxilla before surgery. Either a nitinol or a 0.014-mm arch is fixed to the maxillary brackets, and the canines and premolars must have hooks for use of elastics after surgery.

Patients with ideal anterior smile width, no anterior crowding, and a bilateral crossbite may benefit from posterior maxillary widening while keeping the anterior maxillary width intact. The occlusogram has been an excellent analytic tool for evaluating and calculating the exact amount of millimeters needed in the anterior and posterior maxilla for expansion. Photocopies of the dental models are used to draw diagrams of the teeth on acetate paper. Acetate copies of the maxilla and mandible are overlaid on one another and measurements are made at the canines, premolars, and

molars in the transverse dimension. The proper cuspid and molar relationships in a class I position are calculated, measured, and planned for surgery.

Bolton analysis is also necessary to identify the anterior dental mass and to compare the maxillary and mandibular anterior dimensions to obtain a perfect overjet and over bite, coincident midlines, and proper interdigitation. This analysis indicates the need for extraction of a lower incisor, dental stripping, and opening diastemas to be filled with dental resin or to change the inclination of the incisors to obtain an adequate fit. The space required is also calculated in the dental models. A Koesling setup in which every tooth is cut off the dental model and fixed in the ideal position with wax helps identify the different variables involved.

There are clinical situations in which posterior maxillary width is ideal with respect to posterior mandibular width but there is a major crowding situation anteriorly and the maxilla has a triangular shape. Anterior mandibular widening would benefit the patient in terms of avoiding premolar extractions, obtaining better spacing for easier orthodontic treatment, and creating a wider smile.

The indications for mandibular widening are a narrow V-shaped mandible, severe mandibular crowding to avoid dental extractions, a scissors bite (Brodie syndrome), maxillo-mandibular transverse deficiency (tunnel smile, crocodile bite), impacted anterior teeth to allow natural or forced eruption, retreatment after bicuspid extractions, and congenital missing teeth. Indications for lengthening of the mandibular body include major mandibular advancements (>8 mm), temporomandibular joint (TMJ) degenerative joint disease as a precondition, sleep apnea (if the baseline problem is severe mandibular deficiency), inadequate mandibular anatomy to perform a conventional bilateral sagittal split osteotomy (BSSO), secondary mandibular advancements (relapse of the mandibular advancement after conventional BSSO), and severe mandibular deformities in children.

Vertical lengthening of the ramus is another consideration when treating skeletal deformities, and there are many variables involved in the diagnosis and treatment planning to solve all of the growth and consequent asymmetry problems when using this technique. The most common use of vertical distraction of the ramus is for type I and II craniofacial microsomia and ankylosis. Distraction during growth, though challenging, can address some of the soft and hard tissue issues that these patients have. Prediction of growth on the opposite side and vector control, however, remain difficult. A very critical piece of information about ramus lengthening is that distraction of the ramus will push the ramus against an intact joint and the pterygomasseteric sling will become stretched. This creates a vertical force on the condylar head against the glenoid fossa that compresses the intracapsular structures. The ultimate consequence may be unpredictable resorption, remodeling, or adaptation of the TMJ. These types of pressure can cause the cartilage surfaces to be flattened and thereby put pressure on the synovial spaces. Most authors who perform vertical distraction of the ramus during growth suggest that the patient may need secondary surgery when growth is complete because of some of these concerns. When treating patients with ankylosis, the vertical ramus lengthening procedure is performed before releasing the ankylosis, so the gap arthroplasty is performed 6 months after consolidation, followed by physiotherapy.

SPECIFIC TREATMENT AND TECHNIQUES

MANDIBULAR ANTEROPOSTERIOR DISTRACTION

Indications for mandibular lengthening include major advancements, TMJ degenerative disease as a precondition, sleep apnea (if the baseline problem is severe mandibular deficiency), inadequate

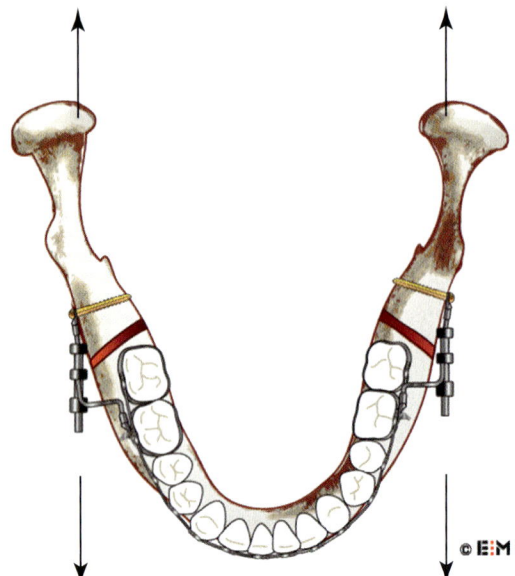

Fig. 79-1 ■ Adequate position of the distractor for mandibular antero-posterior distraction (see text for detailed description).

mandibular anatomy for conventional BSSO, secondary mandibular advancements (relapse of the mandibular advancements by BSSO), and severe deformities in children.

Adequate positioning of the distractors is fundamental to achieve the correct distraction vector; obviously, the possibility of changing the distraction vector after surgery is sometimes required for an ideal functional-esthetic outcome. Preferably, minimal changes should be needed at the end of the activation phase to achieve adequate occlusion.

Additionally, because the natural shape of the mandible is transversely wider in its posterior aspect and narrower in its anterior aspect, the distractor appliances need to be adjusted by creating a 5- to 8-mm step in the anterior fixation plates so that the distractor's screw can be placed parallel to the axis of distraction. If this is underestimated, the reciprocal forces exerted on the mandible by the appliance will advance the mandible by moving the proximal segment not only posteriorly but also laterally and exert very detrimental forces on the TMJ, which will cause pain, dysfunction, and damage to the joints. In addition, there will be lateral torque force against the condyle, loosening of the screws, and bending of the appliance as the muscle forces bend the device. This situation is overcome with the use of heavy class II elastics, 6 oz per side, during the activation and consolidation period (Fig. 79-1).

For bilateral mandibular lengthening, the right appliance must be parallel to the left one. If the occlusion is unstable when the activation period is finished, occlusal masticatory forces will cause instability in the appliance, movement of the distraction chamber, and weakening of the callus.

A 2.5-cm full-thickness incision is made over the external oblique line and extended inferiorly over the alveolar ridge to the position of the first molar. Meticulous subperiosteal tunneling is performed with a periosteal elevator to expose the alveolar ridge and the buccal cortex down to the inferior border of the mandible between the second and third molars, where a small channel retractor is placed to protect the soft tissues during the osteotomy. The periosteum, muscles, and soft tissues are detached minimally to maintain the best blood supply to the area. With the channel retractor in position, a reciprocating saw is used to section the inferior border of the mandible bicortically at a 45-degree angle to increase the bone

surfaces up to approximately 3 mm away from the inferior alveolar nerve and continuing only on the lateral cortex superiorly (Fig. 79-2, A to C).

A periosteal elevator is placed between the lingual soft tissues and the mandible to guard against injury to the lingual nerve while the alveolar area is sectioned bicortically from the top toward an area 3 to 5 mm short of the inferior alveolar nerve with the saw upside down and at a 45-degree angle. At this point there is just 6 mm of uncut bone around the mandibular nerve; the inferior, superior, and lateral cortices have been osteotomized, but the mandible is still rigid.

Before completing the osteotomy, the mucoperiosteal flap is repositioned and maintained in place with horizontal mattress sutures while leaving a small opening at the top of the incision (Fig. 79-2, D). The distractors are secured transmucosally over the mandible with bicortical screws; the anterior superior arm might be secured with a 0.024-inch wire around the teeth and supported by acrylic to make it rigid.

Once the distractor is well fixated with bicortical screws, the appliance is activated 2 mm to create tension on the incomplete fracture line, and a chisel osteotome is placed between the proximal and distal segments at the superior border of the mandible through the small incision left open. A torque movement is applied to the chisel to complete the mandibular osteotomy (Fig. 79-2, E to G).

After the bone fragments have been separated with the chisel, a single mattress suture is used to close the remnant of the wound and ensure primary closure over the osteotomy, eliminate contamination of the distraction chamber, and provide periosteal integrity (Fig. 79-3).

Commonly, a transverse mandibular deficiency is also present; for minimal discrepancies between the upper and lower arches, orthodontic movements at the molar level would allow an adequate relationship between the arches. In patients with moderate or severe deficiencies, maxillo-mandibular widening by DO should be indicated in the same surgical procedure (Fig. 79-4).

Combined Transverse, Anteroposterior, and Vertical Maxillary Movements

The patient is properly prepared orthodontically; ideally, a Hyrax appliance is constructed and cemented, well above the equator of the teeth, to ensure rigidity and prevent expulsion during surgery or postsurgical activation. All braces and second molars bands are installed before surgery.

After induction of general anesthesia and nasoendotracheal intubation, a Le Fort I osteotomy is performed. Reference lines are well marked to objectively measure the planned three-dimensional maxillary movement and the final positioning with semi-rigid fixation. After an incision is made from first premolar to first premolar, a tunnel is created to access the posterior maxilla, and an Obwegeser turn-out retractor is placed under the periosteum. The infraorbital nerve is protected with two Obwegeser turn-in retractors medial and lateral to the nerve. A periosteal elevator is used to separate the nasal mucosa and protect the lachrymal duct exit under the inferior turbinate. The osteotomies are performed according to the surgical plan to make the vertical and anteroposterior changes. Once the lateral osteotomies are finalized, a spatula osteotome (Barros chisel) is used to section the medial sinus walls, and no effort is made to invade the soft tissues behind the posterior wall, just weakening of the bone to allow an easy well-delineated down-fracture. An additional incision is made in the tuberosity area in a horizontal fashion to position the curved osteotome transversely so that the palatine bone at the tuberosity site can be accessed. This second incision ensures better

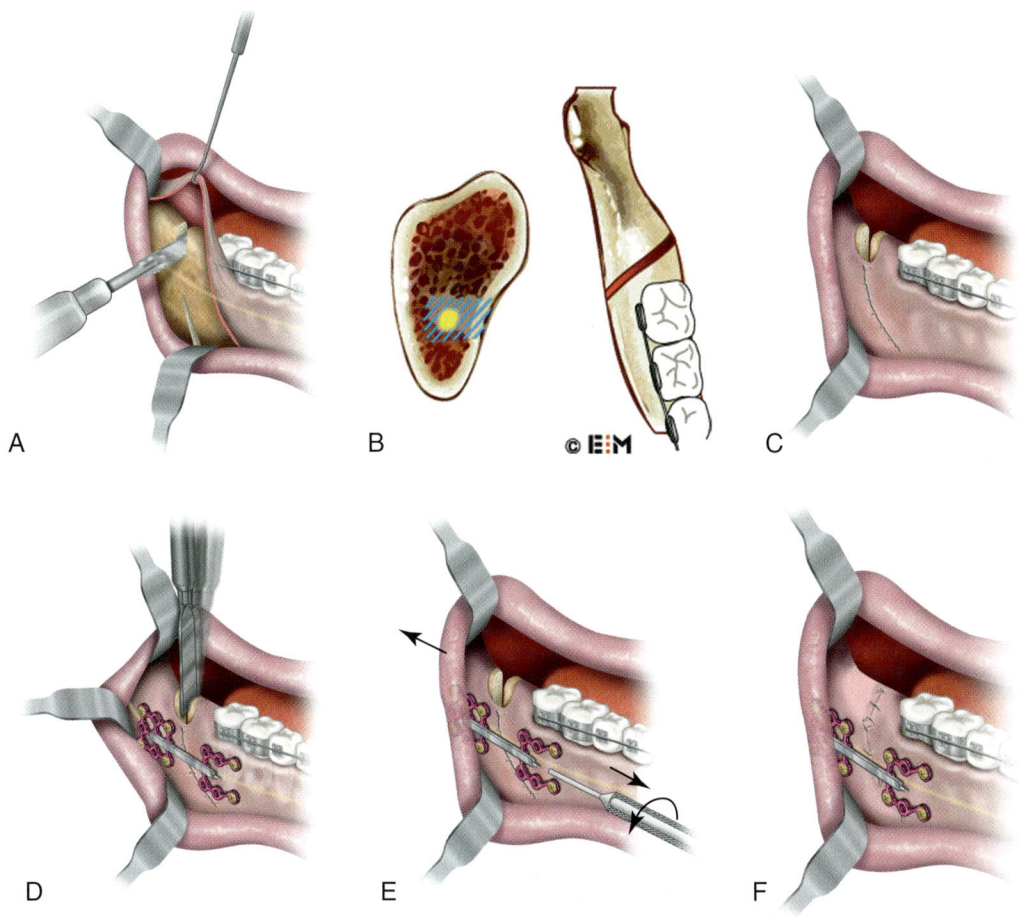

Fig. 79-2 ■ Bilateral mandibular lengthening and mandibular anteroposterior distraction (see text for detailed description). (**D** and **F,** From Gonzalez M, Egbert M, Guerrero CA: Vertical and horizontal mandibular lengthening of the ramus and body, *Atlas Oral Maxillofac Surg Clin North Am* 16:215-236, 2008.)

buccal vascularity to the maxilla and prevents rupturing the mucosa as the curved chisel inclines and reaches the palatine bone. The nasal mucosa is elevated and the septum separated with a ball chisel.

At this point the maxilla is manually down-fractured slowly and progressively, with detachment of any nasal mucosa still attached to the posterior maxilla. Any excess of bone is removed with rongeurs, and the nasal septum and turbinates are treated if necessary. The anterior palatine arteries are meticulously maintained if possible, and again, no instruments or suction tip are manipulated behind the intact periosteum in the posterior maxilla. The pterygoid plates are left intact since the levator and tensor palatine muscles are attached to this anatomic structure. All major bleeding during this surgical procedure has been attributed to the anterior palatine artery or branches of the internal maxillary artery.

The maxilla is then sectioned anteroposteriorly with a reciprocating saw starting in the palatine bone area and proceeding anteriorly off the midline. The soft tissue is left 5 to 6 mm thicker in this area than in the midline in an attempt to prevent the formation of an oronasal fistula. As the osteotomy reaches the alveolar bone, the interdental cut must be performed at a point where the dental roots are anatomically separated. The soft tissues are carefully elevated and a 701 burr is used to section just the outer cortex between the roots. Finally, a spatula osteotome is used to complete the cut toward the palate, with the surgeon's finger in the palatal region to palpate the osteotome so that perforation of the soft tissues is avoided. The Rodriguez-Hyrax appliance is then activated

approximately 2 mm. The importance of rigidity of the appliance and having it well cemented to the teeth is evident at this moment. Of note, after down-fracture, the orthodontic arch wire is sectioned at the osteotomy site.

An interdental splint is then placed and intermaxillary fixation performed; one anterior box and two bilaterally in the posterior region are enough to ensure adequate fixation. The inferior aspect of the zygoma body is exposed and a 703 burr is used to make a hole to pass a 0.024-inch wire, which is fixed to the first or second molar tube bilaterally. If the band does not have a tube to insert the wire, an Ivy loop is placed between the first and second molars and the maxilla is placed in the planned position according to the reference lines. A 0.7- or 0.8-mm-thick flexible plate is secured to the piriform rim with either four or six screws. A step equal to the preplanned expansion in millimeters is created in the plate. The amount of widening is divided between the two piriform plates and transferred to the maxilla. As the device is activated, the tension in the plate disappears.

The intermaxillary fixation and interdental splint are then removed. The position of the maxilla is evaluated in three dimensions; the canines and molars should be in class I occlusion with symmetric posterior contact and coincident dental midlines. The posterior suspension wires can be adjusted to ensure bilateral molar contact.

The wounds are closed in layers after first placing heavy internal nasal sutures to reduce nasal width. A second layer is placed to

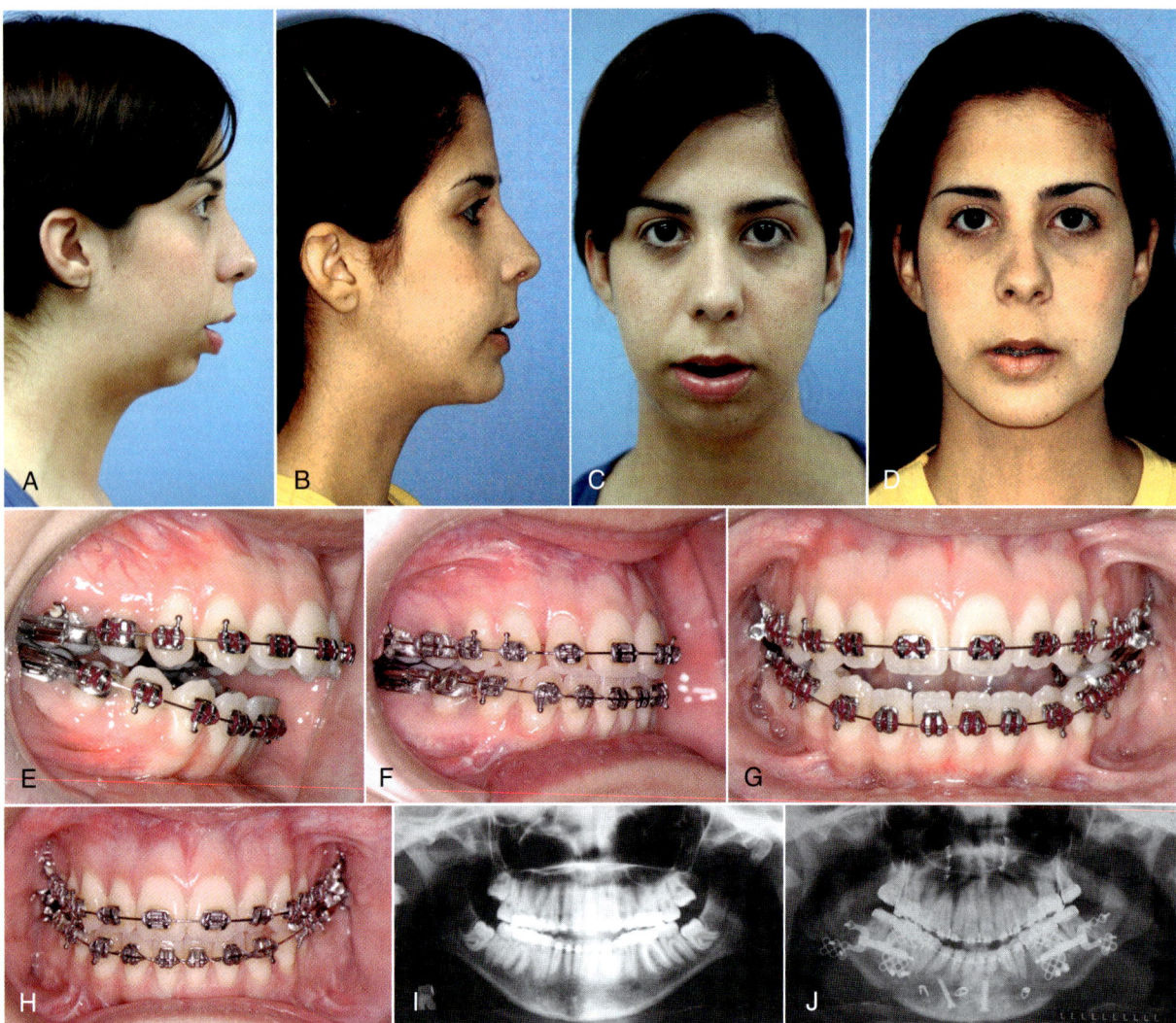

Fig. 79-3 ■ Simultaneous conventional maxillary Le Fort I advancement of 3 mm with posterior clockwise impaction of 6 mm, mandibular advancement by distraction osteogenesis of 12 mm, and advancement genioplasty of 6 mm. Mandibular distractors remained in place for 3 months. The total orthodontic/surgical treatment time was 14 months. Preoperative facial views, profile (**A**) and frontal (**C**), and intraoral views, right (**E**) and frontal (**G**). Postoperative facial views, profile (**B**) and frontal (**D**), and intraoral views, right (**F**) and frontal (**H**). Preoperative (**I**) and postoperative (3 months after surgery) (**J**) panoramic views.

Fig. 79-4 ■ Simultaneous left high condylectomy of 5 mm, maxillary Le Fort I osteotomy for 6-mm impaction on the left side and 3-mm impaction on the right side, maxillo-mandibular transverse distraction, and three-dimensional genioplasty correction (3-mm advancement, 3-mm correction of the symphyseal midline to the right, and 3-mm vertical reduction of the right side). The distractors remained in place for 3 months. The total orthodontic/surgical treatment time was 2 years and 7 months. Preoperative frontal facial view (**A**) and intraoral views, frontal (**C**), maxillary occlusal (**E**), and mandibular occlusal (**F**). Postoperative facial views (2 years and 7 months after surgery), frontal facial view (**B**) and intraoral views, frontal (**D**), maxillary occlusal (**G**), and mandibular occlusal (**H**). **I,** An intraoral palatal distractor was placed by the orthodontist 48 hours before surgery. An intraoperative view shows the Le Fort I osteotomy with the maxilla sectioned in two pieces in the midline. **J,** An intraoral lingual distractor was placed by the orthodontist 48 hours before surgery. An intraoperative view shows the symphyseal osteotomy between the canine and the lateral incisor. An advancement genioplasty was performed and fixed with wires. **K,** Intraoral buccal distractor and symphyseal osteotomy away from the midline because of lack of space between the central incisors. If the technique does not involve genioplasty, the osteotomy needs to be finished in the midline to avoid symphyseal asymmetries. Preoperative (**L**), 7-day postoperative (**M**), and 3-year postoperative panoramic views (**N**). (**K,** From Gonzalez M, Guerrero CA: Intra-arch distraction, *Atlas Oral Maxillofac Surg Clin North Am* 16:169-183, 2008.)

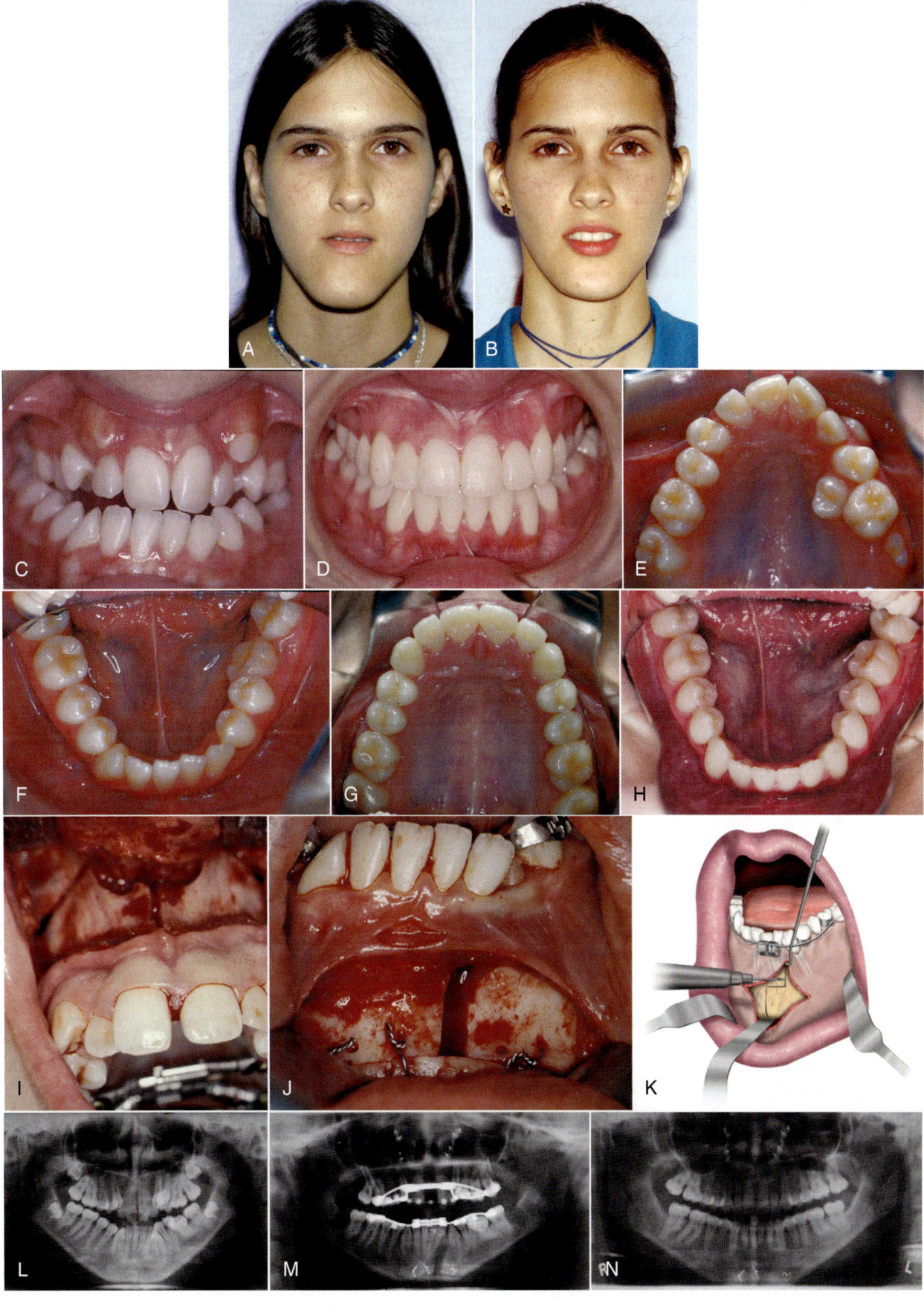

approximate the soft tissues toward the midline. Finally, a V-Y mucosa closure is performed to obtain adequate nasal width and hyperprojection of the vermilion.

After a latency period, activation is commenced 7 days later at a rate of 1 mm/day until the ideal width is achieved. No overexpansion is necessary, and at that moment acrylic is placed over the screw to obtain extra rigidity. The patient can then be advanced to a soft diet.

The suspension wires are removed 2 months after surgery and the nasal alae are evaluated. If the distance has increased after surgery or is in need of reduction, the Weir method is performed at the time of removal of the suspension wires. The Hyrax appliance is removed by the orthodontist 3 months after consolidation, and a transpalatal bar is installed at that appointment and kept in place for the remainder of the orthodontic treatment (Fig. 79-5).

Three-Dimensional Movement with Anterior Maxillary Widening and Maintenance of Posterior Width

There are clinical situations in which posterior maxillary width is ideal with respect to posterior mandibular width but there is a major crowding situation anteriorly, and the maxilla has a triangular shape. Anterior mandibular widening would benefit the patient in terms of avoiding premolar extractions, obtaining better spacing for easier orthodontic treatment, and creating a wider smile.

A similar occlusogram analysis is performed to calculate the exact amount of millimeters needed to widen the maxilla anteriorly. Bolton analysis needs to be performed, as well as a Koesling setup.

The patient is referred for surgery with no distraction device. The mandibular orthodontics must be advanced to alignment, leveling, and ideal central incisor positioning to the IMPA. Rectangular arch wire fixation with welded copper pins so that intermaxillary elastics can be worn postsurgically is advised. All brackets and bands need to be placed, including bands on the second molars. The second molars are not leveled in class II or III cases because the lack of tooth contact avoids excessive overloading, bone instability, and patient discomfort once the maxilla is placed in a class I relationship.

Under NET general anesthesia, the surgical procedure is similar to that described up to the moment of midline osteotomy. Once the maxilla is separated with the spatula osteotome, a bone-anchored distractor or a buccal mono-arm screw is fixed to the premolars and molars, similar to the one popularized for the mandible. To maintain the intermolar distance with no variation, either a transpalatal bar, intermolar wire (0.024-inch wires between both first molars), or transmucosal plate in the posterior maxilla is needed.

The appliance is activated up to 2 mm during surgery, and the maxilla is fixed with two semi-rigid 0.7- or 0.8-mm plates at the piriform rim. The same wound closure and surgical protocol are then performed (Fig. 79-6).

Three-Dimensional Movement with Posterior Maxillary Widening and Maintenance of Anterior Width

Patients with an ideal anterior smile width, no anterior crowding, and a bilateral crossbite may benefit from posterior maxillary widening while keeping the anterior maxillary width intact.

The occlusogram has been an excellent analytic tool to evaluate and calculate the exact amount of millimeters needed in the anterior and posterior maxilla for expansion. Photocopies of the dental models are used to draw diagrams of the teeth on acetate paper. Acetate copies of the maxilla and mandible are overlaid on one another and measurements are made at the canines, premolars, and molars in the transverse dimension. The proper cuspid and molar relationships in a class I position are calculated, measured, and planned for surgery.

Bolton analysis is also necessary to identify the anterior dental mass and to compare the maxillary and mandibular anterior dimensions to obtain a perfect overjet, over bite, coincident midlines, and proper interdigitation. This analysis indicates the need for extraction of a lower incisor, dental stripping, and opening diastemas to be filled with dental resin or to change the inclination of the incisors to obtain an adequate fit. The required space is also calculated in the dental models. A Koesling setup in which every tooth is cut off the dental model and fixed in the ideal position with wax helps identify the different variables involved.

The Hyrax appliance is a single-armed device that spans from first molar to first molar. If the patient is undergoing surgery with a regular Hyrax welded to the premolars and molars, the surgeon should section the anterior arm as it reaches the premolar bands. Finger pressure is applied to the body of the appliance during sectioning to avoid expulsion secondary to fracturing of the cement because of the vibration. Complete brackets and bands need to be in place, and the orthodontic arch is not sectioned in the midline.

The surgical intervention is similar to the previous case up to the point of completing the midline osteotomy. At this time a four-hole, 0.8-mm anterior plate is fixed to the anterior maxilla above the level of the teeth. It is secured with 2.0-mm, 12-mm-long screws while maintaining both segments at the same level. In addition, a Bridle 0.024-inch wire is passed around the four incisors and tightened until there is no diastema between the central incisors. Once again, the orthodontic arch is not sectioned. This surgical step transforms a two-piece maxilla into a single piece; two suspension wires and two anterior plates are used for fixation. The DO protocol is also similar. The Bridle wire is removed along with the suspension wires 60 days after surgery (Fig. 79-7).

MAXILLARY ANTEROPOSTERIOR DISTRACTION IN PATIENTS WITH CLEFT LIP AND PALATE

A high Le Fort I osteotomy is used to advance the mid-face. The osteotomy is carried out medially and above the infraorbital nerve to divide the malar process. Two widely curved osteotomies are placed behind the maxillary tuberosities to displace the malar-maxillary complex. The posterior arms of the distractors are fixed to the malar bone, and the two anterior arms are wired to the teeth or fixed with screws transmucosally, depending on the level of the osteotomy. For cases in which the appliance is buried under the mucosa, a flexible connector is attached to the distractor activation head to facilitate activation.

In cleft patients there is a need for maxillary stability. First, an anterior wire is placed from one side of the lateral incisor, passes up through the nasal dorsum, and emerges to the other side of the lateral incisor to provide premaxillary stability; second, a surgical splint is placed on the palatal side; and third, one plate is placed from one side of the tuberosity to the other side and fixed with three screws in each segment to unify the maxillary process. After the fixation protocol, bone graft is placed in the alveolar cleft. During surgery, 2 mm of activation is initiated after all appliances are in place. The incisions are closed with suture in different layers, nasal and mucosa (Fig. 79-8).

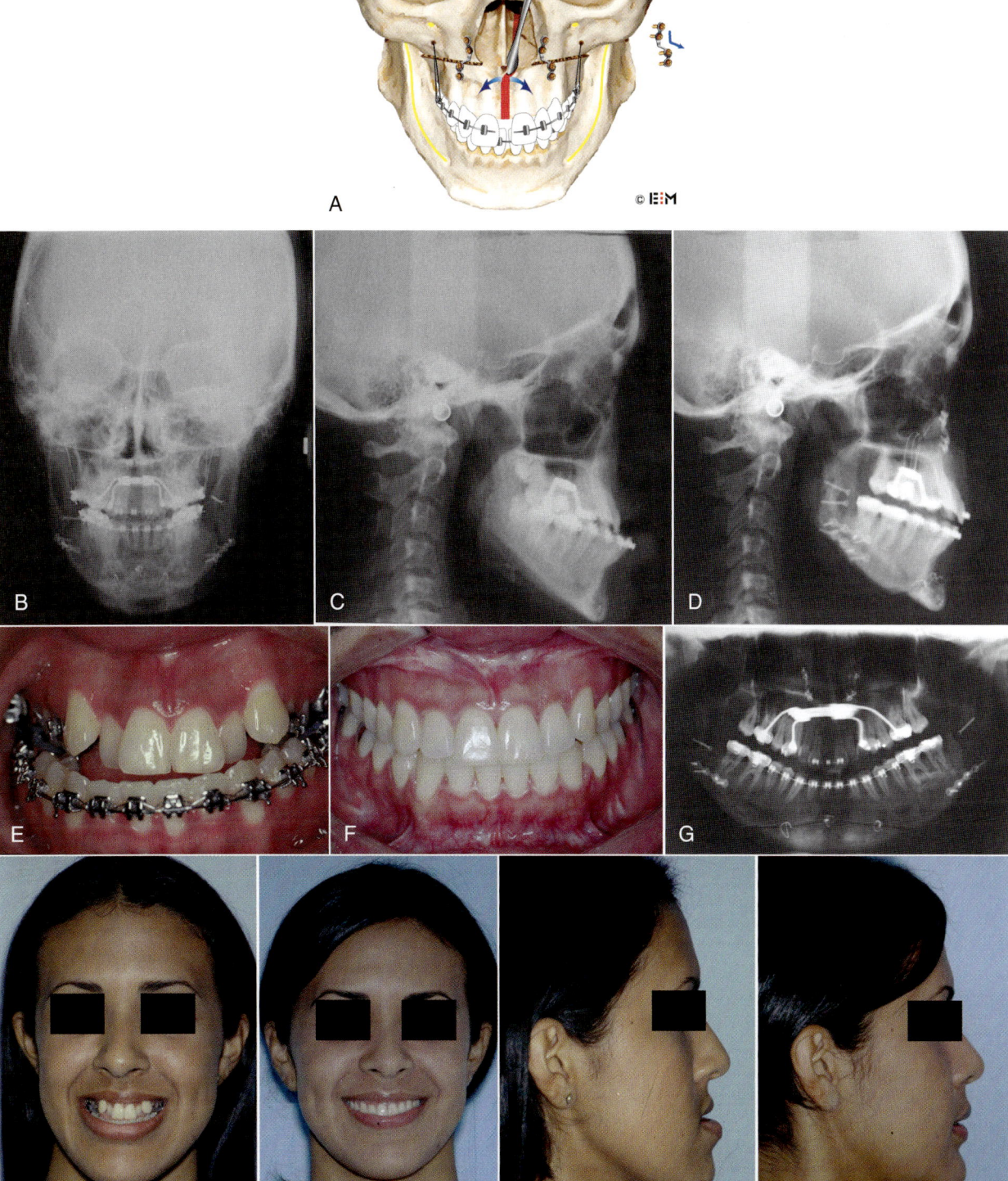

Fig. 79-5 ■ Simultaneous maxillary vertical reduction of 4 mm, advancement of 4 mm, and intra-oral maxillary transverse distraction of 7 mm at the premolar level. Bilateral mandibular sagittal split osteotomies to achieve a 7-mm setback and advancement genioplasty of 6 mm were performed. The distractor remained in place for 3 months. The total orthodontic/surgical treatment time was 1 year and 11 months. **A,** Simultaneous Le Fort I osteotomy in two pieces with midline distraction via a palatal distractor. Two posterior suspension wires and two pre-bent 2.0-mm plates with the estimated transverse widening were used. **B,** Posteroanterior cephalic radiograph after maxillary distraction was completed. **C,** Preoperative cephalic radiograph. **D,** Postoperative cephalic radiograph during the distraction consolidation period. Preoperative frontal intraoral (**E**), facial frontal (**H**), and profile (**J**) views. **G,** Panoramic radiograph during the distraction consolidation period. Two-year postoperative intraoral frontal (**F**), facial frontal (**I**), and profile (**K**) views.

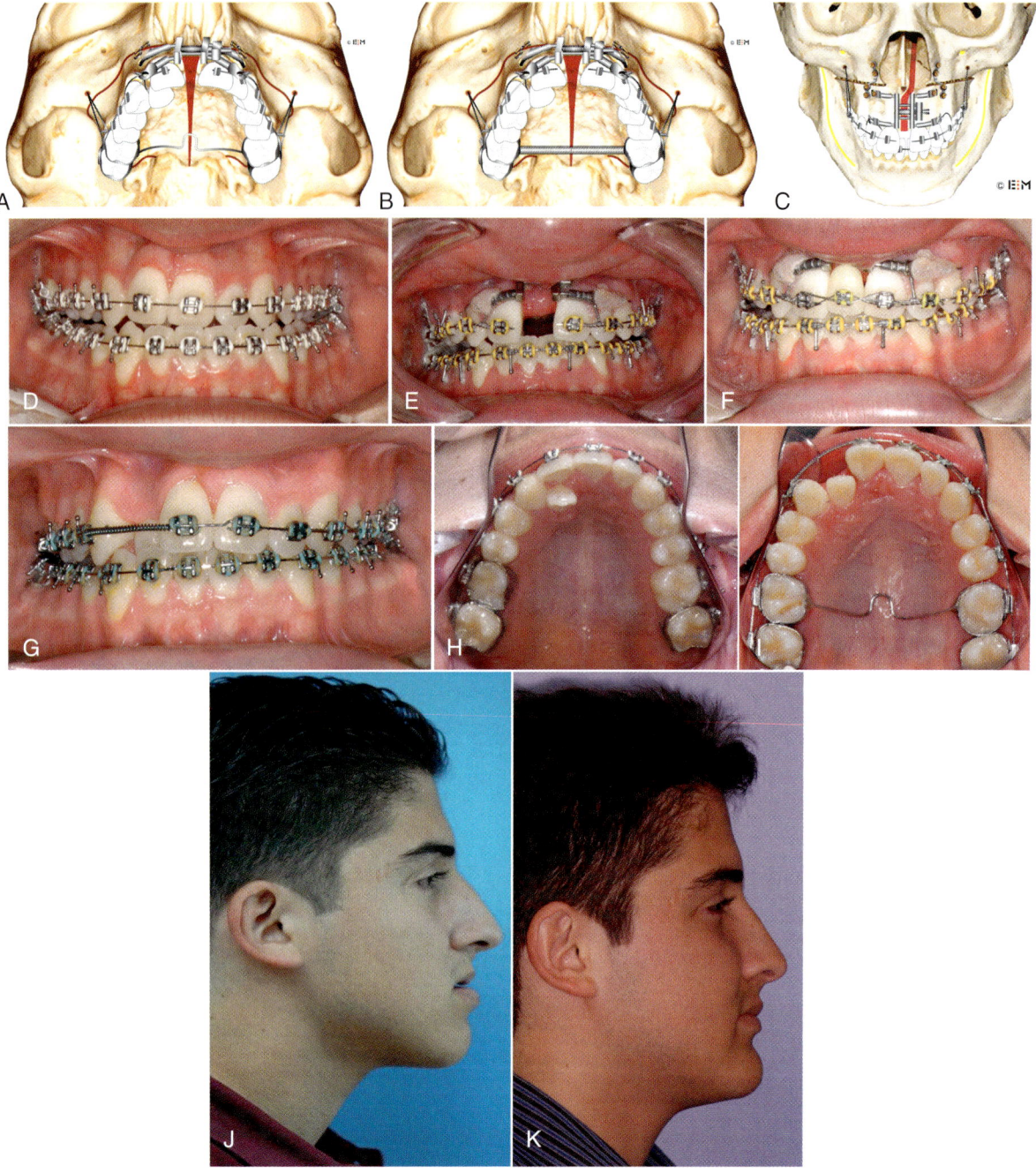

Fig. 79-6 ■ Simultaneous maxillary advancement of 5 mm, selective anterior maxillary distraction of 7 mm, sagittal split osteotomy on the right side for a 3-mm setback, advancement genioplasty of 4 mm, and 4-mm correction to the right of the symphyseal midline. The distractor remained in place for 2 months and 2 weeks. The total orthodontic/surgical treatment at the present time is 18 months. **A,** Le Fort I osteotomy in two pieces maintained in one piece with a buccal tooth-borne/bone-borne appliance, suspension wires, and pre-bent 2.0-mm bone plates with the distraction amount calculated. **B,** Occlusal view with a palatal bar attached to the molar bands to maintain the posterior transverse dimension during distraction and avoid distraction of the posterior maxilla, which will create a crossbite. **C,** More rigid palatal bar placed by the orthodontist to remain in place for the consolidation period. **D,** Preoperative frontal intraoral view. **E,** Intraoral frontal view at the end of anterior distraction. **F,** Intraoral frontal view during the consolidation period. An acrylic tooth is added as a central incisor in the midline of the orthodontic arch to maintain the space and cosmesis. **G,** Intraoral frontal view while the orthodontist is closing the space in the midline by reducing the size of the acrylic incisor and moving the lateral incisor into the arch. **H,** Preoperative intraoral occlusal view with the lateral incisor completely blocked in the palate. **I,** Occlusal intraoral view with the incisor in the correct position after combined orthodontics and distraction for 18 months of treatment. Facial profile views: preoperative (**J**) and 18 months after treatment (**K**).

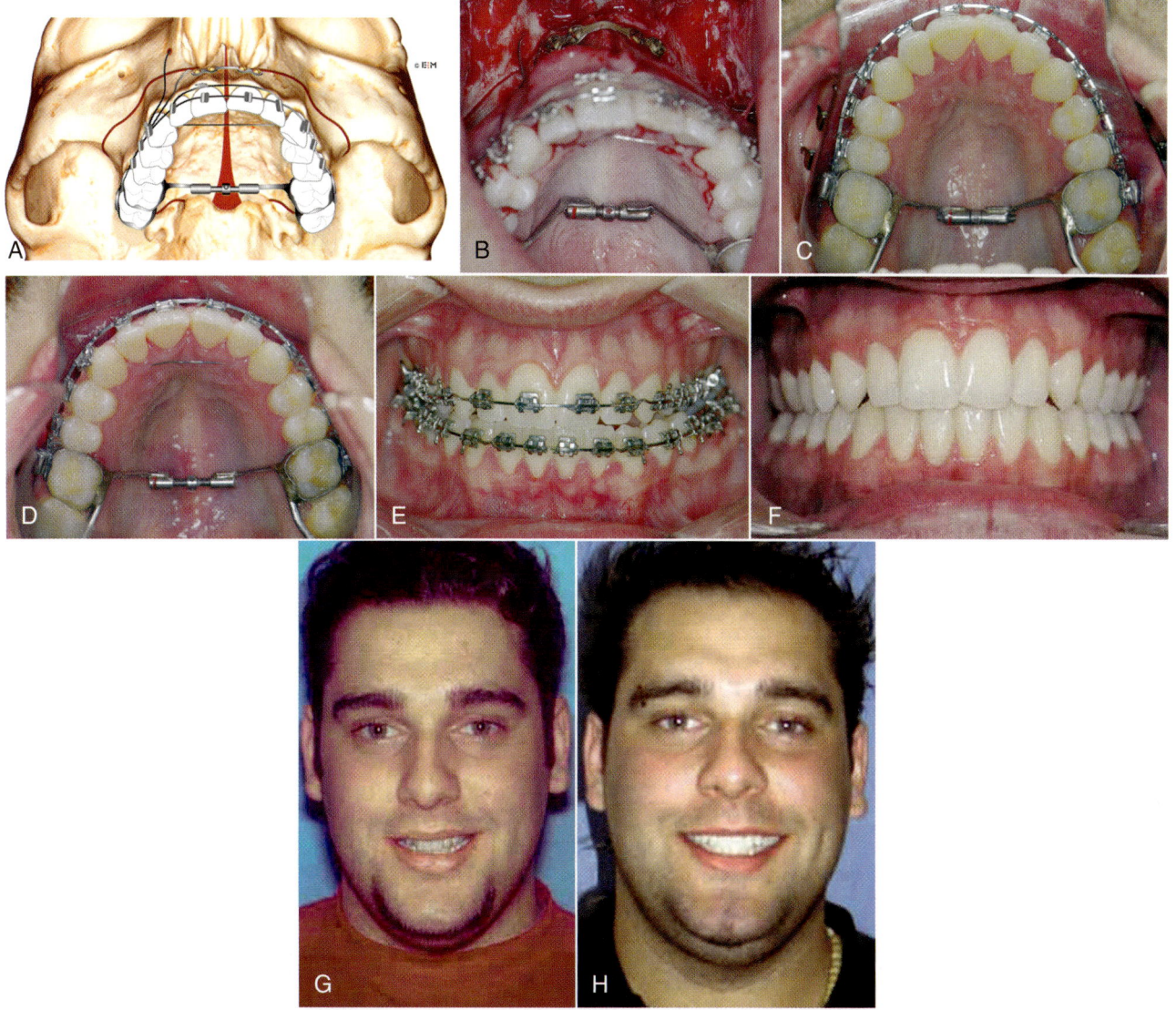

Fig. 79-7 ■ Le Fort I with midline osteotomy for selective posterior maxillary transverse distraction of 14 mm. The distractor remained in place for 3 months. The total orthodontic/surgical treatment time was 1 year. **A,** Occlusal view with a palatal distractor in a four-hole, 0.8-mm plate with 2.0-mm bicortical screws at the nasal spine to prevent distraction of the anterior maxilla. **B,** Intraoperative view with the palatal distractor placed by the orthodontist 48 hours before surgery. The Le Fort I osteotomy is fixed with wires, and the anterior nasal spine plate controls transverse movement of the anterior maxilla to avoid an anterior crossbite. Intraoral occlusal view: immediately after surgery (**C**) and during distraction (**D**). Intraoral frontal views: before surgery (**E**) and with the posterior transverse problem corrected at the 2 year follow-up (**F**). Frontal facial views: preoperative (**G**) and 2 years after treatment (**H**).

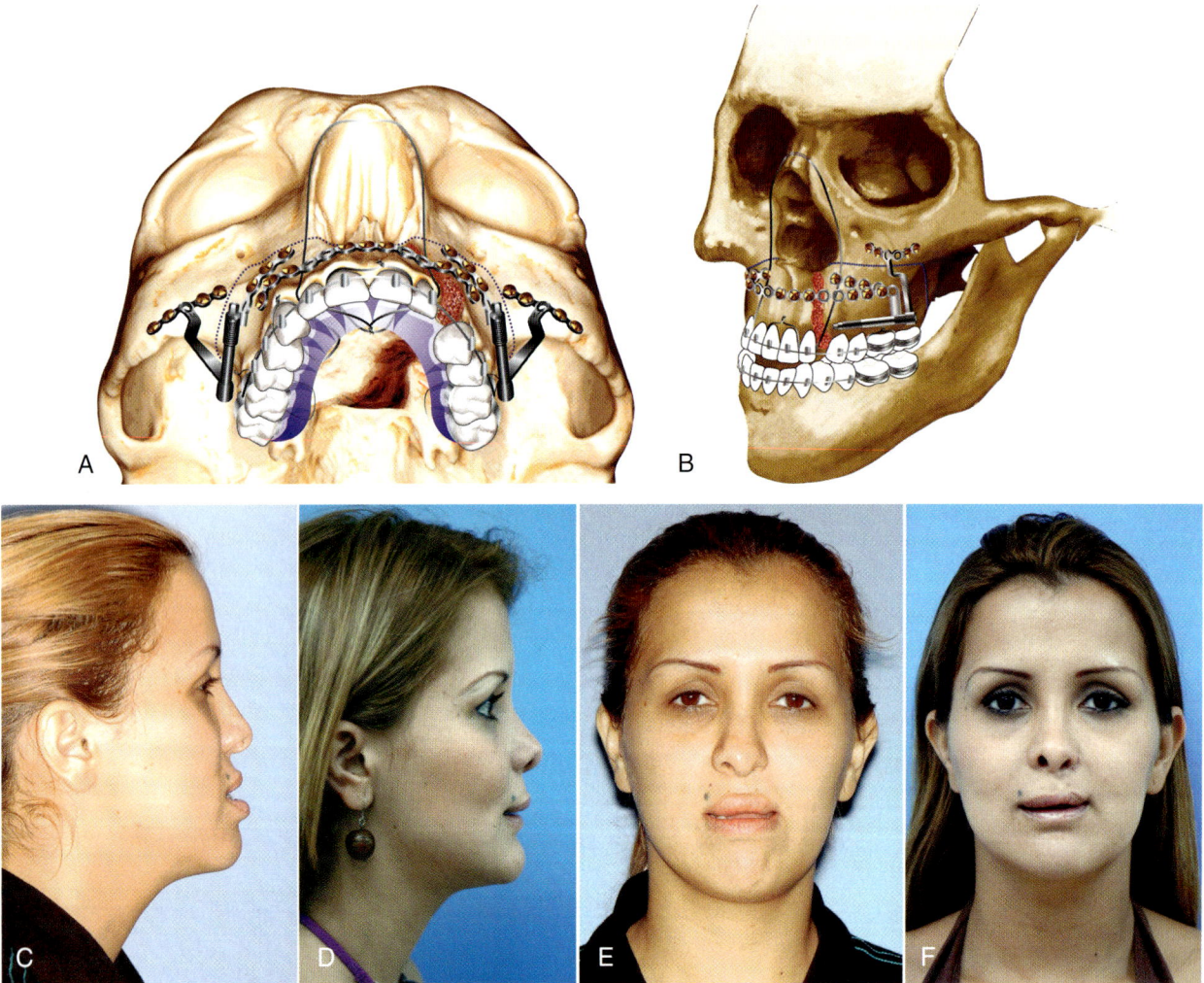

Fig. 79-8 ■ Simultaneous Le Fort I osteotomy to achieve 9-mm maxillary advancement by distraction osteogenesis, segmental osteotomies to close the space of No. 3, extraction of the first mandibular premolars, subapical osteotomy setback to close the spaces of the mandibular first premolars, alveolar bone grafting, cheiloplasty, and rhinoplasty. A dental implant was placed in a second stage in the No. 9 area. The maxillary distractors remained in place for 3 months. The total orthodontic/surgical treatment time was 28 months. **A** and **B**, See text for a detailed description. Preoperative facial views: profile (**C**) and frontal (**E**) views. After an orthodontic/surgical treatment time of 28 months: facial profile (**D**) and frontal (**F**) views.

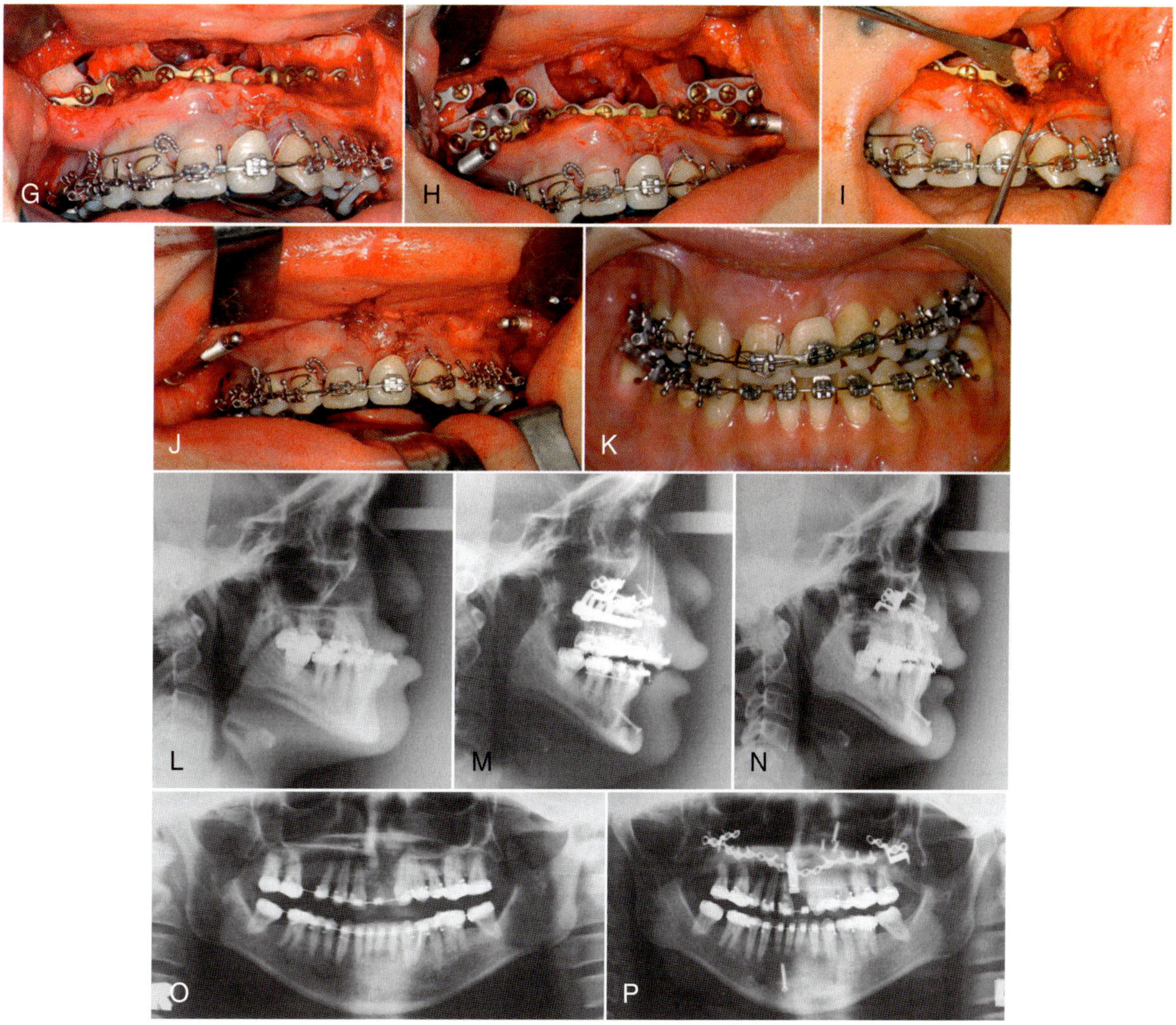

Fig. 79-8, cont'd ■ **G,** Reinforced miniplate across the entire maxilla to convert the two-piece cleft maxilla into one piece, as well as a palatal splint. **H,** The two intraoral maxillary distractors for maxillary advancement. **I,** Alveolar bone graft on the cleft area for better cosmetic results. **J,** Closure of the Le Fort I incision. The active part of the distractors is exposed for activation, and the bodies of the distractors are located submucosally. **K,** Intraoral frontal view of the occlusion after surgery. Cephalic radiographic views: preoperatively (**L**), immediately after surgery (**M**), and after the distractors were removed (3 months after surgery) (**N**). Panoramic views: preoperatively (**O**) and 6 months after surgery with an implant in the No. 9 area (**P**).

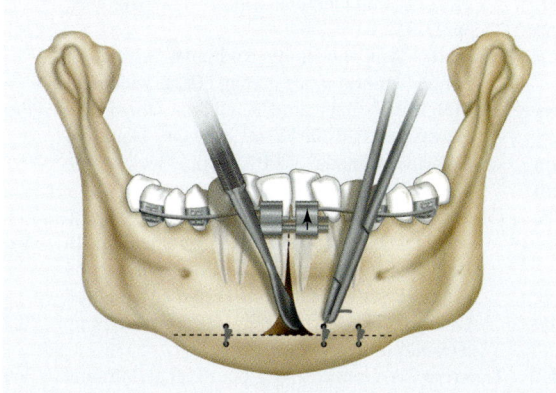

Fig. 79-9 ■ Mandibular widening and genioplasty performed simultaneously. A periosteal elevator is kept in between the two halves of the mandible so that an acute widening at the basal bone is achieved while the wires are tightened. (From Gonzalez M, Guerrero CA: Intra-arch distraction, *Atlas Oral Maxillofac Surg Clin North Am* 16:169-183, 2008.)

POSTOPERATIVE CARE

At the end of distraction, acrylic is placed over the distractor rod and patients are advanced from a liquid to a soft diet. At this time the orthodontist also adds a cosmetic acrylic tooth to the orthodontic arch to prevent the teeth from "walking" into the immature distraction area when distraction is performed to gain transverse space, either for the maxilla or the mandible. After consolidation is achieved, all the appliances are removed; 3 months of consolidation is required for each centimeter of distraction. The patient is sent back to the orthodontist to continue treatment. For transverse cases, the acrylic tooth that was in the distraction area is ground 0.5 mm from each interproximal surface (1 mm) each month to progressively close the distraction gap and finish the orthodontic treatment. The occlusion is carefully finished, and standard retention is indicated when needed.

PEARLS AND PITFALLS

- The distractors should be removed after proper consolidation has occurred; premature removal of the distractors will result in a complete relapse.
- The consolidation process involves different primary variables: the age of the patient, the amount of movement, and quality and quantity of bone available for distraction. Other variables are infection as a result of bad oral hygiene, inadequate stability during consolidation, poor patient selection, and some systemic diseases.
- All osteotomies designed for distraction are complete osteotomies and not greenstick fractures.
- When an osteotomy is performed in between teeth, 1.5 mm of bone should be preserved on both sides to avoid periodontal injury and promote bone formation from both sides.
- When symphyseal distraction is planned for increasing the transverse dimension, the osteotomy should be performed in the midline; if there is no space between the central incisors or the orthodontist did not move the roots to create space, the osteotomy should start in the midline at the inferior border of the mandible and finish in between the incisors with more space to avoid facial asymmetry.

- When planning mandibular lengthening, the presence of impacted third molars should be considered; extractions are performed 6 months before the mandibular lengthening procedure to allow good bone formation distal to the second molars.
- After consolidation is completed, the distractors can be removed under intravenous sedation. For the maxilla, the distractor can be sectioned distal to the distraction rod and the posterior plate left behind; it is not necessary to make a big incision for this procedure. For the mandible, since the distractor is fixated transmucosally, there is no need for a new incision; removal of the screws and wires is sufficient to release the distractor. Perhaps a mattress suture will be required to close the small wound at the point where the distractor exits the maxilla.
- When mandibular widening and genioplasty are needed, the procedure can be performed at the same time if one takes into consideration that fixation of the genioplasty cannot be rigid, the use of wires is indicated, and a periosteal elevator is kept in place between the two halves of the mandible to obtain acute widening at the basal bone while tightening the wires. The wire fixation should be flexible enough to allow transverse widening (Fig. 79-9).

BIBLIOGRAPHY

Bell WH: Revascularization and bone healing after anterior maxillary osteotomy: a study using adult rhesus monkey, *J Oral Surg* 27:249-255, 1969.

Bell WH, Epker BN: Surgical-orthodontic expansion of the maxilla, *Am J Orthod* 70:517-528, 1976.

Bell WH, Gonzalez M, Samchukov ML, et al: Intraoral widening and lengthening of the mandible in baboons by distraction osteogenesis, *J Oral Maxillofac Surg* 57:548-562, 1999.

Bell WH, Harper RP, Gonzalez M, et al: Distraction osteogenesis to widen the mandible, *Br J Oral Maxillofac Surg* 35:11-19, 1997.

Bell WH, Pinto L, Chu S, et al: Simultaneous correction of three-dimensional maxillary deformity by the Le Fort I osteotomy and distraction osteogenesis technique. In Bell WH, Guerrero CA, editors: *Distraction osteogenesis of the facial skeleton*, Hamilton, Ontario, Canada, 2007, BC Decker, pp 233-260.

Gonzalez M, Guerrero CA: Intra-arch distraction, *Atlas Oral Maxillofac Surg Clin North Am* 16:169-183, 2008.

Guerrero C: Rapid mandibular expansion, *Rev Venez Ortod* 48:1-2, 1990.

Guerrero CA, Bell WH: Intraoral distraction. In McCarthy JG, editor: *Distraction of the craniofacial skeleton*, New York, 1999, Springer, pp 219-248.

Guerrero CA, Bell WH, Gonzalez M, et al: Intraoral distraction osteogenesis. In Fonseca RJ, editor: *Oral and maxillofacial surgery*, Philadelphia, 2000, WB Saunders, pp 359-402.

Guerrero CA, Contasti G: Transverse mandibular deficiency. In Bell WH, editor: *Modern practice in orthognathic and reconstructive surgery*, Philadelphia, 1992, WB Saunders, pp 23-83.

Guerrero CA, Contasti GI, Rodriguez AM, et al: Surgical orthodontics in mandibular widening. In Bell WH, Guerrero CA, editors. *Distraction osteogenesis of the facial skeleton*, Hamilton Ontario, Canada, 2007, BC Decker, pp 153-165.

Guerrero CA, Figueroa F, Bell WH, et al: Surgical orthodontics in mandibular lengthening. In Bell WH, Guerrero CA, editors. *Distraction osteogenesis of the facial skeleton*, Hamilton Ontario, Canada, 2007, BC Decker, pp 373-388.

Guerrero CA, Gonzalez M, Lopez P, et al: Intraoral distraction osteogenesis. In Fonseca RJ, editor: *Oral and maxillofacial surgery*, Philadelphia, 2008, WB Saunders, pp 338-363.

Little RM, Riedel RA, Artun J: An evaluation of changes in mandibular anterior alignment from 10 to 20 years post-retention, *Am J Orthod Dentofacial Orthop* 93:423-428, 1988.

Little RM, Wallen TR, Riedel RA: Stability and relapse of mandibular anterior alignment–first premolar extraction cases treated by traditional edgewise orthodontics, *Am J Orthod* 80:349-365, 1981.

Proffit WR, Ackerman JL: Diagnosis and treatment planning in orthodontics. In Graber TM, Vanarsdall RL, editors: *Orthodontics: current principles and techniques*, ed 2, St Louis, 1994, Mosby–Year Book, pp 3-95.

Proffit WR, White RP: The need for surgical-orthodontic treatment. In Proffit WR, White RP, editors: *Surgical orthodontic treatment*, ed 3, St Louis, 1991, Mosby–Year Book, pp 2-33.

Vanarsdall RL: Periodontal/orthodontic interrelationships. In Graber TM, Vanarsdall RL, editors: *Orthodontics: current principles and techniques*, ed 2, St Louis, 1994, Mosby–Year Book, p 719.

Van Sickels LE, Richardson DA: Stability of orthognathic surgery: a review of rigid fixation, *Br J Oral Maxillofacial Surg* 34:279-285, 1996.

Mandibular Asymmetry: Diagnosis and Treatment Considerations

Chapter 80

Brian B. Farrell, Myron R. Tucker

Facial asymmetry is a typical finding in the majority of individuals. When present, it is most often located in the lower third of the face.[1] Consequently, correction of dentofacial deformities frequently involves the management of asymmetry. This is important to note when planning for orthognathic surgery in that patients are able to appreciate correction of their asymmetry more so than the change in profile achieved with surgery. When evaluating mandibular asymmetry, deviation of the chin is more easily recognized than a discrepancy involving the angles of the mandible. Therefore, surgical correction may involve only genioplasty to correct chin position, with maintenance of asymmetry of the mandibular angles being acceptable.

Long-standing skeletal asymmetry can lead to dental compensation and soft tissue changes. Some degree of abnormality in each dimension will occur as a result of warping, bending, or distortion of both the hard and soft tissues. A three-dimensional (3D) perspective is required when evaluating facial asymmetry. The terms *roll*, *pitch*, and *yaw* have been used to describe rotation of the dental arches in patients with asymmetry. Roll is frontal cant of the occlusal plane, whereas pitch is the angle of occlusion in a sagittal dimension and yaw is rotation of the arch of the maxilla and mandible to the cranial base. The midlines may be on the central axis, but excessive yaw creates increased fullness on one side of the face with the converse appearing flat. The shift in arch form creates full tooth show to the commissure and a void in the opposite buccal corridor.

Earlier surgical intervention may be aimed at correcting the cause of the asymmetry to prevent continued exacerbation of the deformity. A stable asymmetric deformity allows definitive management of the malocclusion with conventional osteotomies. Although subtle asymmetries may be corrected by routine orthodontic preparation and orthognathic surgery, complex asymmetries involve detailed treatment planning, increased orthodontic effort, and more extensive surgery to achieve satisfactory functional and esthetic results.

MANDIBULAR ASYMMETRY

DEFICIENCIES

Deviation of the mandible can result from either deficiency or excess. In the case of mandibular deficiency, the mandible will deviate to the affected side secondary to decreased growth, degenerative changes, or trauma. Decreased growth often occurs as a result of a congenital or developmental anomaly. Hemifacial microsomia and Parry-Romberg syndrome are two such examples that are characterized by decreased hard and soft tissue growth resulting in asymmetry.

Acquired anomalies such as osteoarthritis and progressive rheumatoid arthritis may cause degeneration of the condyle and result in collapse of mandibular length through resorption of the condyle.

Such remodeling creates loss of height with decreased projection of the remaining mandible. The loss of vertical dimension typically results in an open bite on the contralateral side as the dentition fulcrums on the affected side.

Trauma to the mandibular condyle is an acquired defect to consider when evaluating facial asymmetry. Fractures involving the condyle and neck can decrease ramus height and create deviation of the mandible. Return of sound functioning following injury to the condyle is the most important principle in acute management, whether it be by open or closed reduction. Failure to establish range of motion can lead to progressive degenerative changes or restricted growth in an immature individual since translation of the condyle is responsible for growth in the mandible.[2] Limited movement of the condyle within the fossa will result in restricted growth and lead to progressive asymmetry of the mandible.[3]

EXCESSIVE GROWTH

Mandibular asymmetry may also result from excess growth. Increased unilateral growth often causes deviation of the skeletal and dental midline away from the affected side. Unilateral prognathism results in deviation in a horizontal vector. This simple excessive growth creates a class III malocclusion of the canine and molar on the affected side. Unilateral condylar hyperplasia is classified as either hemimandibular elongation or hemimandibular hyperplasia.[4,5]

Hemimandibular Elongation

Hemimandibular elongation is associated with lengthening of the condyle and ramus. The affected side of the mandible is longer than the normal side but is not associated with prognathism. The progressive changes produced by overgrowth of the condyle result in deviation of the chin. Enlargement of the condyle is not evident, and despite the elongation, the height of the face on the affected and unaffected sides is similar. Minimal distortion of the remaining mandible and overlying soft tissue occurs with hemimandibular elongation. A midline discrepancy is evident secondary to the excessive unilateral growth, and a crossbite relationship can develop on the contralateral side as the mandible deviates laterally. Subtle compensation of the arches can occur with the elongation, although the arch forms are generally well aligned.

The radiographic findings accompanying hemimandibular elongation can be subtle. The panoramic radiograph may illustrate dental and skeletal deviation with respect to the midline structures of the maxilla (nasal crest and septum). Elongation of the condyle and ramus may be identified in pronounced cases. Lateral cephalometric films will demonstrate superimposition of the dentition and inferior borders of the lower jaw as the elongation is expressed horizontally. The posteroanterior (PA) cephalometric image is the most diagnostic plain film for identification of hemimandibular elongation. The

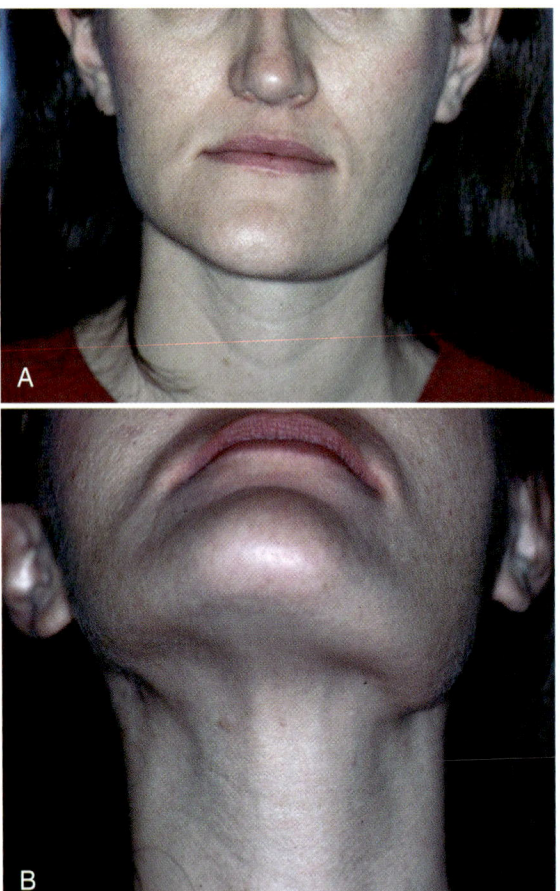

Fig. 80-1 ■ Asymmetry associated with hemimandibular hyperplasia. The increased vertical growth creates disparity at the inferior borders of the mandible. The skewed appearance is exacerbated by the decreased facial height on the unaffected side.

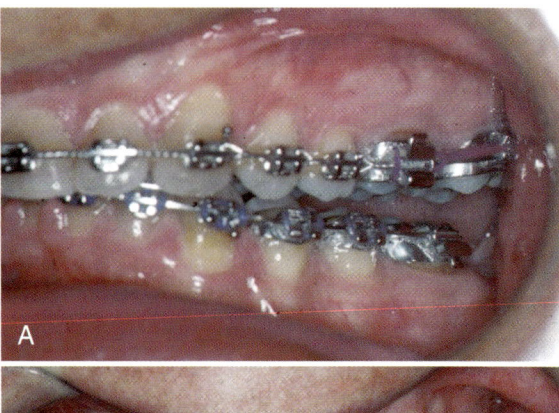

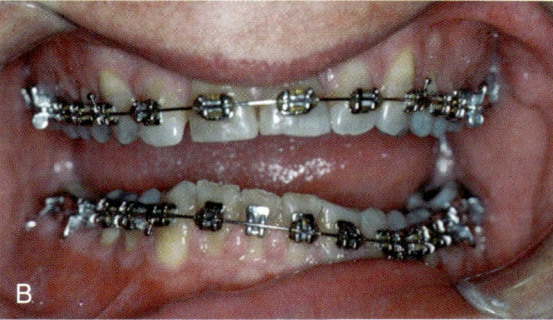

Fig. 80-2 ■ Occlusal influence of hemimandibular hyperplasia. The increased vertical growth creates displacement of the mandibular dentition and results in an open bite and accentuated curve of Spee.

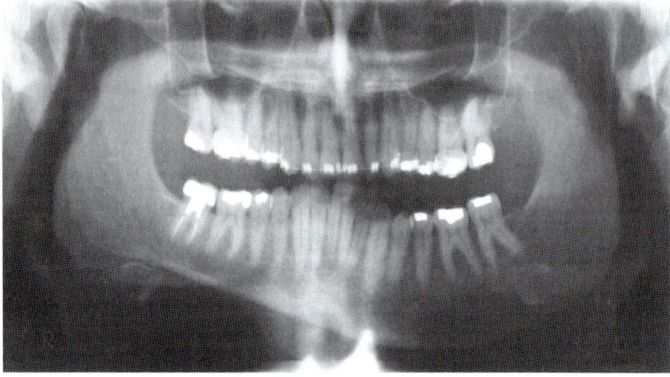

Fig. 80-3 ■ Panorex film illustrating unilateral enlargement of the mandible involving the condyle, ramus, and body associated with hemimandibular hyperplasia. The downward bowing of the inferior border is a result of the increased vertical growth. The compensatory changes in occlusion are noted with an accentuated curve of Spee in the mandibular arch. Supra-eruption of the maxillary dentition is not evident.

image provides skeletal assessment of the asymmetry since chin deviation, midline shift, and contrasting length of the mandibular rami are visualized.

Hemimandibular Hyperplasia

Hemimandibular hyperplasia is enlargement of one side of the mandible involving the condyle, neck, ramus, and body. A pronounced vertical discrepancy of the mandible is evident clinically as the increased growth creates downward bowing. The opposite half of the mandible is affected by the unilateral hyperplasia as the inferior border is rotated laterally and upward. The result is a distorted facial appearance created by increased length on the affected side with decreased height on the normal side (Fig. 80-1). The skeletal asymmetry results in soft tissue distortion, with an oblique appearance created by the commissure of the lip similarly being displaced inferiorly.

The dentition is affected by the increased vertical growth of the mandible. An accentuated curve of Spee develops on the ipsilateral side as downward growth of the mandible drags the teeth inferiorly (Fig. 80-2). The rapid vertical development typically creates an open bite because compensatory maxillary growth cannot keep pace. Development of the hyperplasia before puberty may allow the development of a canted occlusal plane if not controlled with a functional hybrid appliance. Hemimandibular hyperplasia is typically identified following the adolescent growth spurt as a result of continued

growth of the affected mandible after growth on the opposite side has ceased.

Unilateral enlargement of the body, ramus, and condyle is seen radiographically on a panoramic film (Fig. 80-3). A dramatic increase in bone volume is noted with hemimandibular hyperplasia. The appearance of the inferior border of the mandible is characteristic, with the affected side illustrating the downward bowing and the opposite side possessing a straighter slope running from the angle to the symphysis. The rounded angle is accentuated as the broad curvature extends from the ramus to the body. The body of the mandible opposite the hyperplasia possesses a flattened and thinned shape, as though it is being stretched by the overgrowth. The contrast between the enlarged, thickened, rounded hyperplastic half and

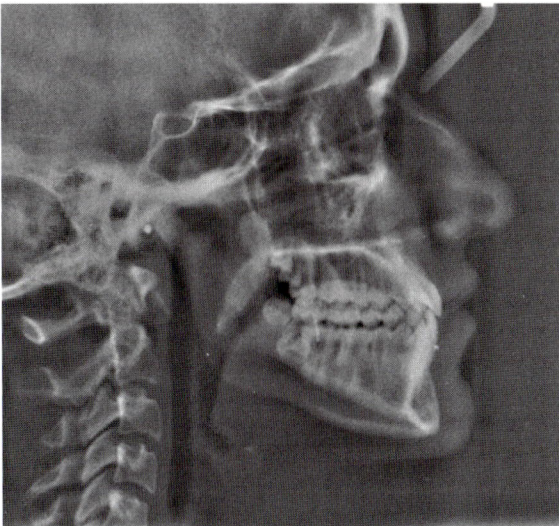

Fig. 80-4 ■ Lateral cephalometric film illustrating the lack of superimposition of the dentition and inferior border of the mandible. The vertical discrepancy between the right and left sides creates the appearance of multiple rows of teeth and distinct inferior borders. A radiographic artifact based on head positioning can create the appearance of asymmetry.

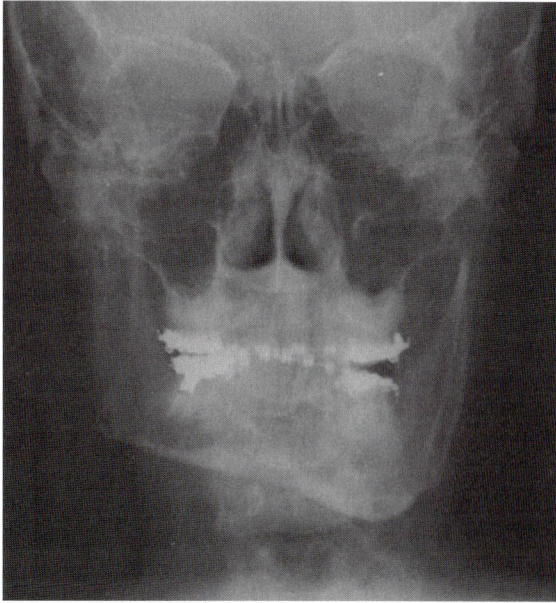

Fig. 80-5 ■ Posteroanterior cephalometric film demonstrating excessive vertical growth of the mandible as a result of hemimandibular hyperplasia. Lateral flaring of the mandible opposite the overgrowth results in decreased lower facial height, which accentuates the asymmetry and discrepancy within the face. The open-bite malocclusion is caused by downward growth of the mandible.

the shortened, thinned, straight side exacerbates the warped contrast of the asymmetry.

A lateral cephalometric film will illustrate failure of the dentition and inferior borders of the mandible to superimpose as a single entity as a result of the vertical disparity (Fig. 80-4). The increased vertical growth evident skeletally is typically greater than that appreciated in the occlusion. This information is valuable in guiding surgical treatment in that management of the occlusion by traditional mandibular ramus surgery will require additional correction via inferior border recontouring or augmentation efforts on the opposite side.

DIAGNOSIS

The examination should detail the dentofacial deformity and the influence of asymmetry on the skeleton, dentition, and soft tissue. The changes directly associated with the asymmetry should be noted, in addition to effects that are the result of skeletal and dental compensation.

Imaging plays a valuable role in assessing skeletal asymmetry. Plain films, including a Panorex, lateral cephalogram, PA cephalogram, and submental vertex image, aid in characterizing the anatomic changes associated with the asymmetry and are valuable resources for planning treatment. Severe asymmetries may warrant additional imaging studies, including computed tomography (CT) and 3D reconstructions. The detailed imaging improves visualization of the condyle, where the source of the asymmetry typically arises.

Panoramic radiographs provide an opportunity to evaluate the condylar architecture and discrepancies within the ramus or body of the mandible. One must be aware, however, that distortion of the image may occur as a result of inappropriate positioning in the radiographic unit and create the impression of an enlarged mandible. Staff experience in obtaining routine panoramic films makes the likelihood of an artifact slim. An imaging artifact can be excluded if the size of the mandibular molars is comparable on the affected and unaffected sides.

The lateral cephalometric film is a mainstay in preparing for orthognathic surgery. Simple unilateral prognathism or hemimandibular elongation isolated to a horizontal plane is not readily identified on the lateral image, however. Vertical asymmetries are depicted as superimposition of distinct inferior borders and an occlusal plane discrepancy with multiple rows of teeth. The difference in the inferior borders is often greater than that noted in the occlusal plane, thus indicating the potential need for recontouring of the inferior border in addition to ramus surgery to correct the occlusion. Caution is also necessary to avoid radiographic artifact with the lateral cephalometric image. Clinicians should be mindful that individuals may have ear canals at varying heights creating the misperception of asymmetry. Finally, periodic interpretation of lateral cephalographic tracings will also aid in determining the timing of surgical intervention, whether it be related to documenting skeletal maturity or progressive change.

The PA cephalometric film will generally highlight the skeletal discrepancy in both its horizontal and vertical dimensions (Fig. 80-5). The positioning of the mandibular dental midline against the opposing arch and the central skeletal axis of the mandible will be illustrated. Corresponding dental and skeletal midline asymmetry may allow surgical correction to be isolated to ramus osteotomies. The addition of an anterior segmental osteotomy of the inferior border to further correct chin positioning may be warranted if the imaging illustrates greater skeletal deviation than noted dentally. The PA cephalometric film allows interpretation of any dental compensation attributed to the asymmetry in the transverse plane, similar to incisor angulation on a lateral cephalometric image. The transverse orientation of the teeth as a result of natural and orthodontic efforts can be appreciated as the dentition attempts to keep up with the skeletal skewing.

The submental vertex image helps identify anatomic characteristics associated with the asymmetry. The bowing and warping of the mandible as a result of asymmetric growth can be visualized for both

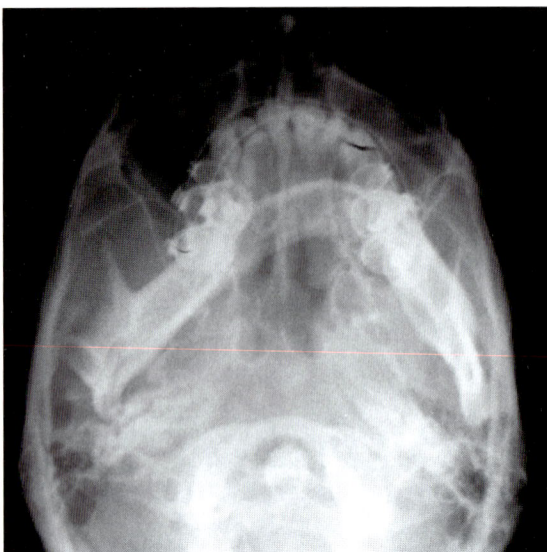

Fig. 80-6 ■ Submental vertex film illustrating the disparity of the mandible as a result of an asymmetric deformity. The divergent nature of the right ramus favors setback via a vertical ramus osteotomy, whereas the left is best managed with a sagittal ramus osteotomy.

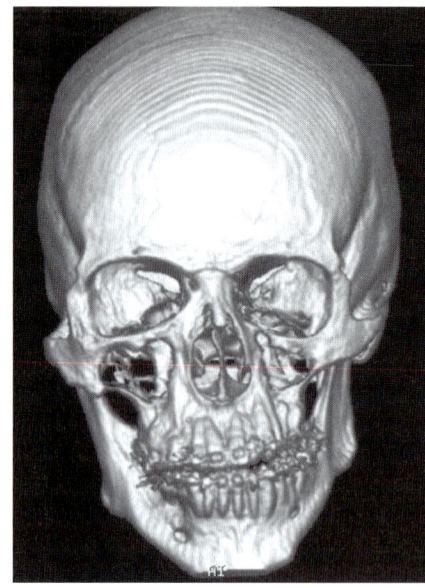

Fig. 80-7 ■ Three-dimensional reconstructed computed tomography scan of a patient with facial asymmetry. The distortion of the mandible is more clearly defined than on plain films. The detailed imaging aids in understanding the extent of the asymmetry in multiple dimensions and serves as a guide for treatment planning. Thinning of the left ramus mediolaterally will require modification of the sagittal ramus osteotomy during correction of the deformity. (From Hupp JR, Ellis E, Tucker MR: *Contemporary oral and maxillofacial surgery*, ed 5, St. Louis, 2008, Mosby.)

diagnostic and treatment considerations. The submental vertex film (Fig. 80-6) aids in selection of osteotomy design for mandibular setback based on the shape of the ramus. A U-shaped mandible is best suited for a sagittal osteotomy, whereas a vertical ramus osteotomy is recommended with a divergent V-shaped ramus. A divergent ramus allows passive positioning of the condylar segment lateral to the mandible on a setback. Performance of sagittal osteotomy on a flared V-shaped mandible will create segment interference and lateral displacement of the proximal segments following mandibular repositioning.

CT provides extensive information on dentofacial deformities. The images provided in a CT scan help augment information gathered through examination and plain films. The ability to view an asymmetry in multiple dimensions helps in understanding the anatomic distortion that has occurred. The capacity to distinguish alterations in the architecture of the ramus and body of the mandible on both the affected and unaffected sides aids in identifying possible challenges that may exist intraoperatively. The improved visualization of the condyle helps one understand the cause of the mandibular asymmetry, such as excessive growth or condylar remodeling. In addition, imaging may reveal previously unidentified injuries to the condyle not readily discernible on plain films.

Reconstructed CT images provide perspective on the deformity and the influence that the asymmetry has on the skeletal and dental elements. 3D reconstructed images can illustrate the anatomic changes on the affected side and associated compensation (Fig. 80-7). The visual representation provides an opportunity to demonstrate the deformity to the patient, as well as the necessary movements required to produce symmetry. Continuing advancements in radiology and CT afford the opportunity to develop treatment predictions and create templates for surgical guidance.

Stereolithographic models may be obtained from the reconstructed images to gain additional insight into the deformity. The model allows a reference for calculating the movements necessary to achieve symmetry. The decision to perform additional surgery consisting of resection or augmentation of the inferior border in the body or angle may be guided by the anatomic reproduction. The stereolithographic model can also be used for model surgery to assist

in planning the need for additional skeletal correction of any bony asymmetry that may persist after addressing the malocclusion.

Diagnostic stone models of the dentition record the skeletal malocclusion that exists as a result of asymmetric mandibular growth. The variation in arch form and compensation within both the mandibular and maxillary arches can be assessed. Horizontal asymmetry of the mandible will result in lingual tipping of the dentition as the bone deviates laterally from the central axis. The maxillary arch will flare laterally to compensate for the skeletal change in the mandible. Progress models provide an indication of the orthodontic decompensation, as well as arch compatibility for correction of the malocclusion. Mounted diagnostic models are valuable when attempting to determine the status of the asymmetry. Progression of the asymmetry can be plotted through records of the occlusion. Persistent changes in the occlusion over an interval (12 to 18 months) indicate continued progression of the asymmetry, and surgery should be delayed until stability can be confirmed. An occlusal record with minimal change in an individual who has achieved skeletal maturity is probably an indication that surgical treatment may proceed.

Imaging to evaluate progression of the asymmetry is accomplished through a nuclear medicine bone scan. A technetium-99m bone scan is frequently used to determine metabolic activity in the condyles (Fig. 80-8). The bone scan is sensitive to increased activity but is not specific for degeneration or excessive growth. The imaging study serves as a guide for determining the status of the asymmetry for planning treatment.[6] Increased uptake of the labeled marker on the affected side indicates activity and probably continued progression of the asymmetry. The presence of increased uptake may warrant delaying surgical correction until stability of the asymmetry can be documented. Activity on the scan with persistent worsening of the deformity may indicate that earlier surgical efforts are necessary to address the source of the excessive growth at the head of the condyle or to stabilize a degenerative process.

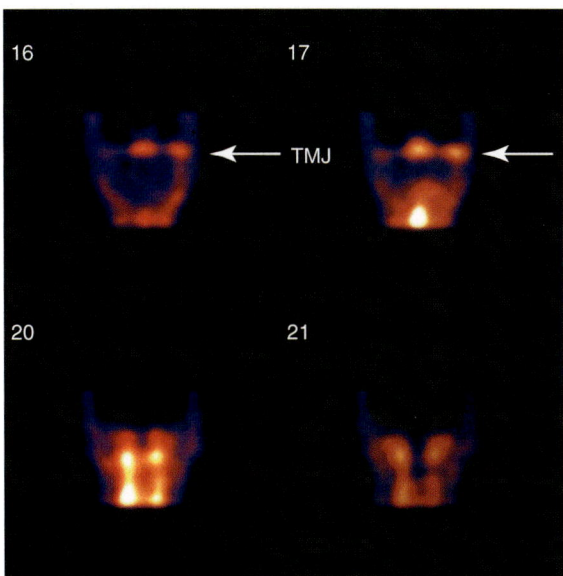

Fig. 80-8 ■ Technetium-99m bone scan. A nuclear medicine bone scan evaluates metabolic activity in the condyles. The bone scan is sensitive to increased activity and serves as a guide for determining the stability of the asymmetry.

TREATMENT

SURGICAL PLANNING

Determination of stability is the initial step in managing an asymmetric dentofacial deformity. The presence of a deformity requires a thorough history to help establish the nature and progression of the asymmetry. The opportunity to label the asymmetry as stable or progressive based on the interview is an early indicator of the timing of treatment. Acute changes will probably require more diagnostic effort than will deviation that has been "like this for years." The information gathered through examination and imaging creates an initial reference to which additional studies may be compared. The decision to delay or initiate surgery is derived from recall examinations and repeated imaging illustrating either pronounced or minimal change, respectively. Surgery is best delayed until progression of the asymmetry has ceased and stability has been documented through periodic monitoring. Stability is typically established by documenting the absence of change in the dentition and bone over an extended time. A period ranging from 6 months to several years may be warranted to monitor for continued change based on the history of the deformity.

Delaying the initiation of comprehensive orthodontic treatment should be considered until progression of the deformity has ceased, although early interceptive orthodontics may be necessary to prevent compensatory changes in the dentition. Functional appliances are used to limit the extent of the asymmetry, encourage growth, and prevent compensatory changes in the maxilla. Orthodontic efforts to control compensation in the maxilla may allow surgical intervention to be isolated to the mandible. A presurgical orthodontic phase focused on alignment and coordination of arch form provides additional time for monitoring the stability of the asymmetry.

Conventional ramus surgery performed during progressive changes within the condyle will probably result in a compromised outcome. Any symmetry obtained following correction of the deformity will be influenced by continued growth or degeneration. Relapse of the advanced osteotomy may occur with persistent loss of vertical ramus height in patients with active condylar degeneration. Degenerative changes within the condyle should be stabilized by conservative efforts to limit the remodeling before surgery to correct the malocclusion. Continued lengthening at the head of the condyle in cases of excessive growth will result in return of the deformity.

The dynamic changes creating the asymmetry may warrant either a "wait it out" approach with continued monitoring or early surgical intervention focused on the underlying cause. In patients requiring the latter, intracapsular surgery may be necessary to correct asymmetries that stem from deficient or excessive growth. Deviation of the mandible from deficient growth is the result of restricted translation of the condyle. Addressing the functional ankylosis through intra-articular surgery is the goal of early intervention in a growing individual to improve the chance for favorable growth and limit the severity of the resultant deformity.[2] Following surgery, functional appliances are then implemented to aid in modifying growth by repositioning of the mandible once range of motion has returned.

In a growing patient, recontouring of the condyle or condylectomy with reconstruction via a costochondral graft may be required to return range of motion and improve the chance for more favorable growth. In contrast, reconstruction with a total joint prosthesis may be a treatment option in a skeletally mature patient for elimination of joint pathology and establishment of symmetry.

Condylar surgery may be necessary even when the deformity is not progressive. An enlarged condyle may restrict translation, compromise growth, and further exacerbate the asymmetry.

Intervention on the condyle may be required to prevent continued excessive proliferation of an asymmetry that stems from overgrowth. In this situation, partial condylectomy should be considered. This procedure involves eliminating the growth center of the mandible by removing the head of the condyle (approximately 5 mm). Once the condyle has been reduced, mandibular growth should cease, thereby creating a static situation in which one can plan correction of the residual asymmetry.

Traditional model surgery can be used to transfer the workup to the operating room for correction of an asymmetric skeletal malocclusion. The absence of compensation within the maxillary arch will allow a template for repositioning the asymmetric mandible in isolated lower jaw surgery. A semi-adjustable articulator can be used to plan surgical movements involving the maxilla and mandible for correction of multidimensional deformities. A model table is used to calculate measurements completed after diagnostic mounting and repositioning of the models to quantify both the existing deformity and movements required to achieve correction of the malocclusion. Fabrication of an intermediate splint transfers the desired skeletal movements intraoperatively to create a symmetric reference. Surgery in the opposite arch addresses the residual asymmetry and finalizes the occlusion as it is repositioned to the stabilized symmetrical reference established with the initial osteotomy. An error that occurs within the process of conventional model surgery (inaccurate face bow or bite registration, improper mounting, inadequate references, inexact movements) may result in failure to correct the asymmetry. Surgery may be completed without difficulty but the result may be compromised even prior to entering the operating room as the anticipated plan is skewed based on improper surgical workup.

Advances in imaging technology and three-dimensional analyses have improved the precision in surgical correction of complex dentofacial deformities (Fig. 80-9). Reconstructed images used initially to enhance the appreciation of the multidimensional nature of deformities can be applied to the surgical workup. Laser scanning of diagnostic models enhances the occlusal anatomy currently limited with present CT scan modalities. The fine details of

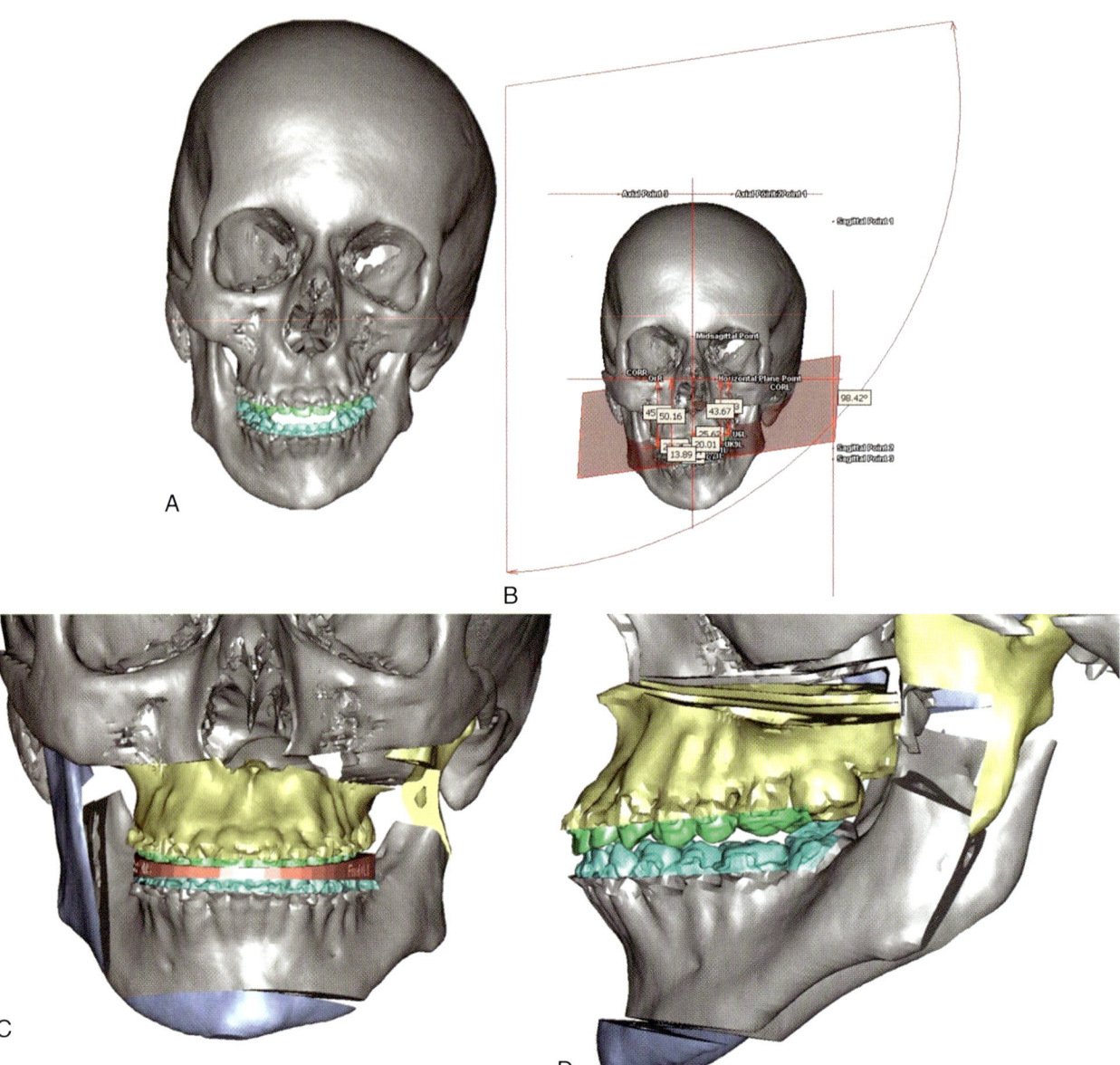

Fig. 80-9 ■ Three-dimensional imaging and virtual planning. **A,** Imaging will allow an improved perspective on the multidimensional nature of an asymmetric dentofacial deformity to aid in diagnosis and planning of surgical correction. The detail of the occlusal anatomy is input into the CT scan with laser scanning of the dental casts to accurately depict the malocclusion. **B,** Skeletal cephalometric analysis to skeletal references will quantify the deformity and assist in planning the necessary movements required to correct the asymmetry. **C and D,** Computer-simulated osteotomies (right, through a sagittal ramus osteotomy and left an inverted L) establish the final occlusion and symmetry. Virtual planning will illustrate potential interferences with anticipated segment positioning and limited bone contact at the osteotomy site that will require grafting. Three dimensional planning will depict that additional measures (anterior segmental osteotomy of the inferior border) are required to establish skeletal symmetry not obtained through conventional ramus osteotomies. (Courtesy of Dr. R. Bryan Bell.)

the occlusion are input into the 3D data to generate a computer rendering of the skeletal deformity and malocclusion. Imaging software permits virtual osteotomies to be created that can be manipulated and repositioned according to the anticipated surgical plan. The intended movement of the mandible or maxilla respectively can be inspected in all planes (e.g., cant, yaw, etc.) to gauge symmetry and to skeletal reference points and modified accordingly. The simulation may provide valuable anatomic information that can aid in surgical preparation through an improved understanding of the

movements required to address the deformity and subsequently applied intraoperatively. The virtual osteotomy may illustrate an interference with repositioning of segments, a gap at an osteotomy site that may necessitate bone grafting, or persistent skeletal asymmetry that will require additional efforts despite correction of the malocclusion.

Transfer of the virtual plan established through computer simulation to the operating room is possible through fabrication of a milled occlusal splint. The CAD CAM wafer is prepared to the occlusal

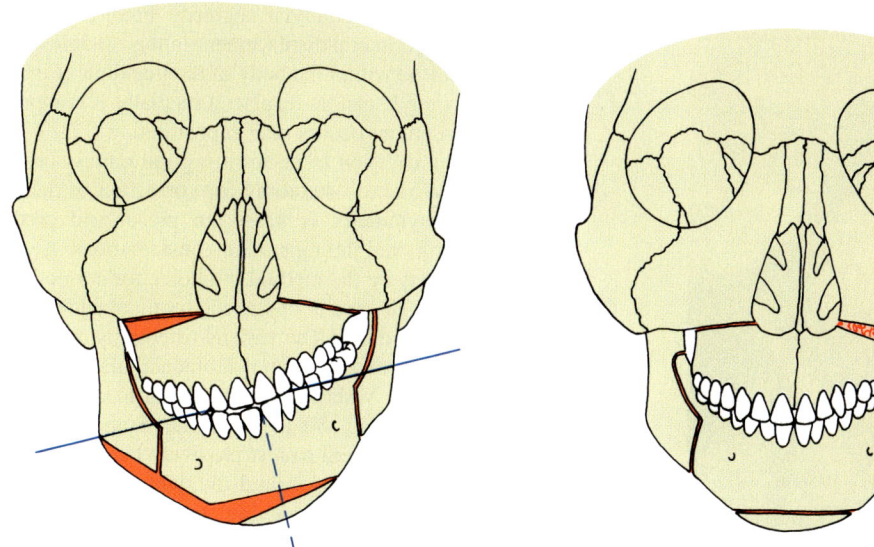

Fig. 80-10 ■ Correction of the deformity associated with hemimandibular hyperplasia. Leveling of the occlusal plane and management of the skeletal asymmetry require extensive surgery on the maxilla and mandible. Differential repositioning of the maxilla, unequal movement in the ramus osteotomies, resection of the inferior border, and asymmetric wedge resection of the chin are necessary to create symmetry. The movements needed for correction of the asymmetry are determined through imaging studies and three-dimensional model surgery. (From Hupp JR, Ellis E, Tucker MR: *Contemporary oral and maxillofacial surgery*, ed 5, St. Louis, 2008, Mosby.)

relationship that has been created through computer simulation of the virtually repositioned jaw against the unaltered arch. The splint is processed and delivered to the surgeon bypassing the typical laboratory steps required with traditional model surgery. The final splint used to set the occlusion after mobilizing the second osteotomy, whether on the maxilla or mandible, can be milled from the completed virtual plan or traditional model surgery on diagnostic casts.

The execution of the planned surgery through computer simulation will translate to a surgeon possessing a greater understanding of the deformity, knowledge of the skeletal movements necessary to correct the asymmetry, and confidence in the outcome delivering satisfactory results. Virtual planning with computer simulation will continue to evolve and can improve the accuracy of surgical treatment for complex dentofacial asymmetry.

SURGICAL CORRECTION OF ASYMMETRIES

Correction of the malocclusion that results from mandibular asymmetry is accomplished through conventional osteotomies. Isolation of the deformity to the mandible establishes the maxilla as the reference for repositioning. Sound orthodontic preparation is vital to create arch form and alignment in the maxilla and mandible, respectively. Positioning the teeth ideally within the arches will unmask the skeletal discrepancy and make the malocclusion more pronounced. Completing decompensation to the fullest extent provides the opportunity to maximize the surgical movement for correction of the underlying asymmetry. Persistence of the asymmetry after correction of the malocclusion can result from a skeletal discrepancy more extensive than that seen in the dentition. Severe deformities may require additional recontouring or osteotomies to correct asymmetry that is not completely resolved with surgical intervention for the occlusion (Fig. 80-10).

The versatility of sagittal ramus osteotomy for correction of mandibular deficiency or excess enables the technique to be the primary procedure for the management of mandibular asymmetry. The osteotomy can be used for correction of asymmetries ranging

from mild to severe. It can also be used when the asymmetry will require unequal movements at the osteotomy sites. Deviation of the mandible resulting from deficiency will require greater advancement on the affected side to provide skeletal symmetry and approximation of the dental midlines. Surgery aimed at correction of mandibular hyperplasia with asymmetry may ultimately result in a net advancement on the unaffected side as the excessive side is reduced and the symphysis is rotated toward the central axis of the face.

Distorted anatomy of the mandible may increase the complexity of the osteotomy. Thinning of the ramus mediolaterally with warping of the body and severe asymmetry may prevent performance of a traditional osteotomy. The initial superior cut on the lingual aspect of the mandible requires greater vertical or downward orientation than does a typical oblique tangential cut into the retrolingual depression (Fig. 80-11). Frequently, however, the most technique-sensitive aspect of the osteotomy involves the inferior border cut. The displaced inferior border requires more soft tissue reflection to allow better visualization and access. The inferior border may be "rolled under" in cases of elongation, thereby increasing the difficulty of ensuring a proper cut through the inferior border. This is an important point because the incidence of unfavorable fractures increases without a sound osteotomy through the inferior border.

The skeletal variation found in patients with mandibular asymmetry may also alter the position of the inferior alveolar nerve as it courses through the mandibular canal. Elongation and thinning of the mandible can position the canal closer to the superior border of the ramus and posterior body and make the nerve susceptible to injury from traditional placement of the saw or burr. This is especially evident during the inferior border cut since extra effort is required to ensure a sound split.

Once the asymmetric mandible is split, alignment and fixation of the osteotomies will be more complex than that of traditional orthognathic surgery. Alignment of the inferior borders during reorientation of the segments remains the focus to ensure stability of the

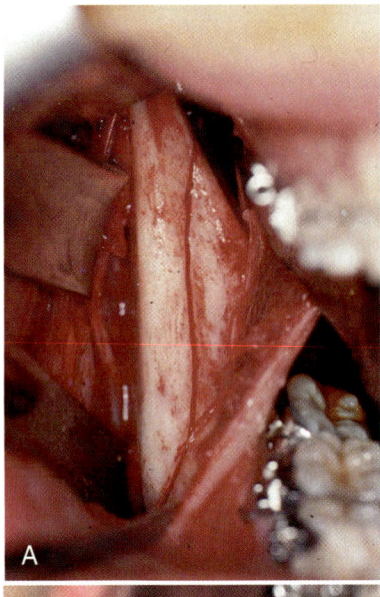
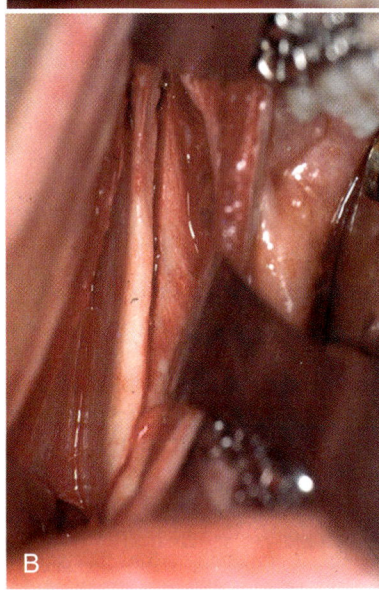

Fig. 80-11 ■ The altered anatomy created by the asymmetry requires modification of the traditional ramus osteotomy. Because of the thin nature of the ramus, the osteotomy must be performed superiorly into the shallow retrolingular depression through to the body of the mandible to take a more vertical orientation. The osteotomy through the inferior border can also become more complex as a result of the asymmetric growth.

correction. Movement in multiple directions occurs because the segments can have different rotational and vertical changes. Rotation of the asymmetric deformity can result in lateral flaring of the distal segment. The vertical changes can also create a superior border discrepancy, similar to that noted on mandibular setbacks managed with sagittal ramus surgery. Reduction of the superior border may be necessary to aid in visualization during fixation. This reduction will also help avoid periodontal issues distal to the last molar.

Additional technical considerations may be required to orient the proximal and distal segments. Recontouring of the segments may be necessary to ensure passive positioning of the proximal segment. Failure to relieve any bony interference may displace or torque the condyle within the fossa and potentially lead to pain and dysfunction postoperatively.[7] Reduction of interference should be completed on the proximal and laterally displaced distal segment to eliminate

flaring of the condylar segment. Failure to eliminate interference will cause lateral displacement of the condyle once bicortical screws are placed within the body of the mandible (Fig. 80-12). In addition, the condyle can be displaced medially if compression of the proximal segment occurs after repositioning (Fig. 80-13).

The decision to perform sagittal ramus surgery versus transoral vertical ramus osteotomy for correction of mandibular hyperplasia with asymmetry is based on presurgical predictions, review of imaging, and intraoperative considerations. A vertical ramus osteotomy may be the method of choice for correction of the asymmetry based on the extent of setback required and the underlying anatomy of the mandible.[8] The vertical osteotomy may be performed through a transoral or an extraoral submandibular approach. The presence of a divergent V-shaped ramus is best managed with a vertical ramus procedure (Fig. 80-14). The flared anatomy allows the proximal condylar segment to rest passively lateral to the repositioned distal segment. Ensuring sound overlap of the proximal and distal segments is vital to achieving stability and fixation at the osteotomy. The proximal segment can be rotated subtly, but a vertical ramus osteotomy is not feasible if the setback is minimal. Passive repositioning of the segments is necessary to prevent displacement of the condyle. Any interference between the segments is managed with a recontouring burr to reduce the bony irregularities on both surfaces (lingual to the proximal segment and facial to the distal segment) simultaneously. Rigid fixation can be applied through percutaneous access after gentle seating of the condyle.

Skeletal asymmetry may persist after orthognathic surgery aimed at correcting a malocclusion. Deviation of the chin is often a concern for patients and may persist after sagittal or vertical ramus osteotomy. Increased awareness of the deformity in the frontal plane warrants additional surgical effort to ensure that the results are esthetically acceptable. As mentioned, correction of dental asymmetry through midline approximation may not overcome the underlying skeletal discrepancy. Additional correction via genioplasty may be required to achieve skeletal symmetry of the chin. Imaging studies help establish a surgical treatment plan for reorienting the chin. Subtle overprojection or irregularities may be reduced by recontouring with rotary instruments or reciprocating rasps. One should exercise caution, however, to avoid recontouring through the cortex because remodeling of medullary bone may be unpredictable and the overlying soft tissue drape may become uneven. For chin asymmetries in which recontouring will not suffice, genioplasty provides the opportunity to correct residual asymmetry in multiple planes. The sliding osteotomy can be repositioned inferiorly under the mandible to establish symmetry not achieved with conventional ramus surgery. Correction of a vertical discrepancy may require an asymmetric wedge resection to level the anterior mandible. Liberal soft tissue dissection to expose the anterior mandible is performed within the boundaries of the mental foramen. Reflection posterior to the mental nerve is important to avoid the creation of a short osteotomy. Scoring of the cortex is done before performing the osteotomy to establish a reference for anticipated movements. The bony symmetry can be evaluated following stabilization by visual inspection and palpation over the "wings" of the osteotomy. The soft tissue can be returned over the bony reorientation to gauge the expected form and contours.

Resection of the inferior border is necessary to correct the downward displacement of the mandible evident in hemimandibular hyperplasia (Fig. 80-15). Generous soft tissue reflection is necessary to help in visualization of the skeletal deformity. Exposure of the bone allows intraoperative comparison of the affected and unaffected sides referenced to the treatment plan established through the preoperative evaluation. It is very infrequent that an asymmetry is overcorrected. Resection of the inferior border is best managed in

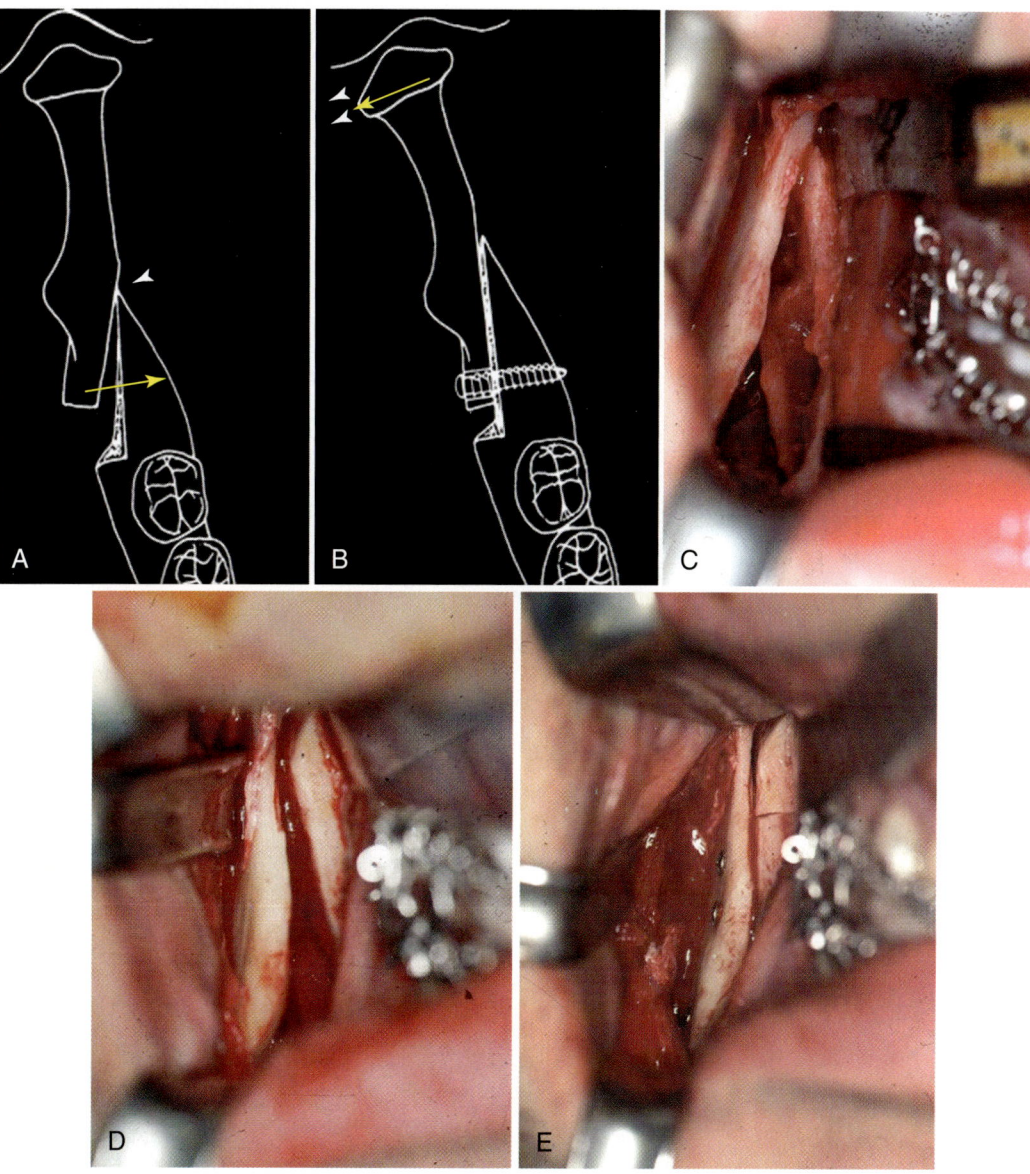

Fig. 80-12 ■ Displacement of the distal segment creates interference at the osteotomy. The interference (*arrow*) will prevent passive repositioning of the proximal segment. Placement of fixation will result in displacement of the condyle laterally. Passive seating of the proximal segment is prevented by interference by the distal segment. Fixation will create lateral displacement of the condyle as the proximal segment fulcrums off the interference. Fixation is performed once passive positioning of the segments is achieved through elimination of the interference.

conjunction with the sagittal ramus osteotomy before establishing fixation. Consideration should be given to extending the Dalpont cut of the sagittal osteotomy as anteriorly as possible to allow visualization of the nerve before osteotomy of the inferior border. Resection of the proximal segment is performed by rotating the segment superiorly while stabilizing it with an instrument. Rotation provides improved visualization of the inferior border to the angle for resection with a reciprocating saw. Management of bone removal from the inferior aspect of the distal segment depends on the proximity of the inferior alveolar nerve. The resection can be completed without lateralization of the nerve if the required bone removal does not encroach on the path of the mandibular canal. The need for substantial bone removal from the inferior border typically requires exposure of the inferior alveolar nerve within the distal segment.

The nerve is identified at the mental foramen and a corticotomy is performed posteriorly for lateralization of the nerve. The course of the nerve within the remaining distal segment is readily identified through the sagittal osteotomy. The nerve can then be reflected superiorly for completion of the inferior border resection on the distal segment. The ample exposure of the mandible provided by reflection of the soft tissue allows the osteotomy on the distal segment to be completed from the angle to the chin. Recontouring of the mandible with rotary burrs or reciprocating rasps may be required to eliminate irregularities.

Augmentation of the mandible may be necessary for a deformity that creates decreased facial height. The vertical discrepancy associated with hemimandibular hyperplasia may require resection of the inferior border on the affected side with simultaneous augmentation

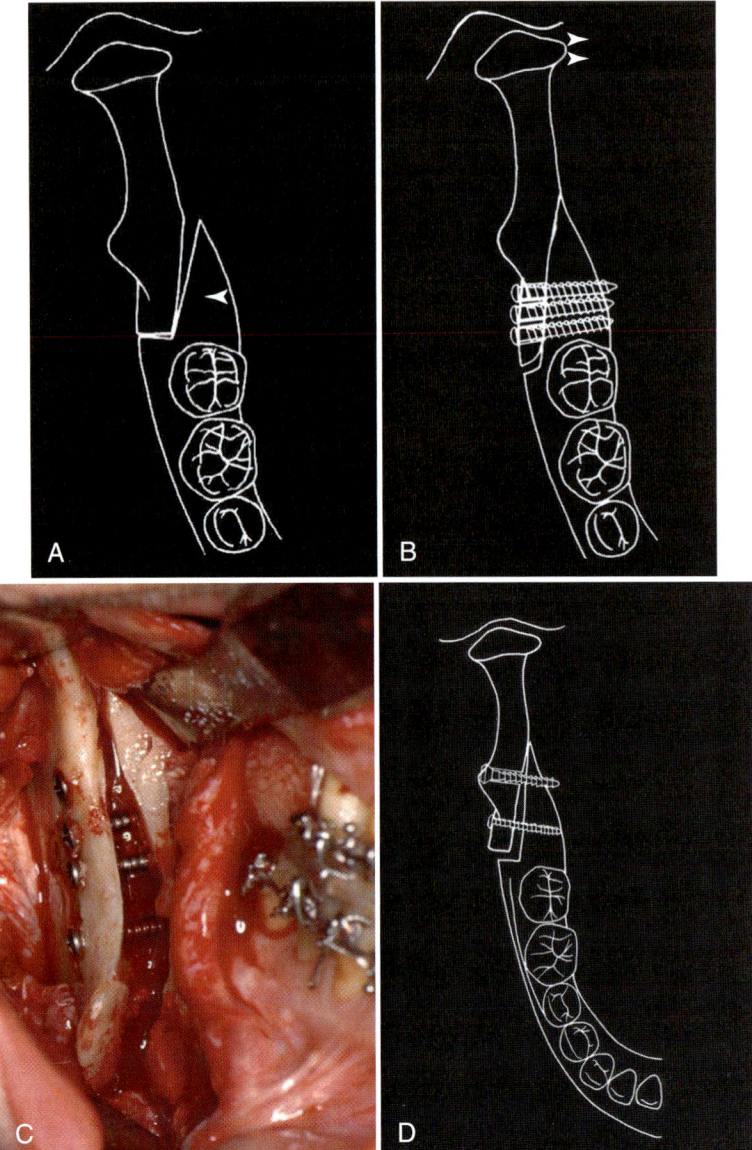

Fig. 80-13 ■ The condyle can be displaced medially with fixation. Positional screws or a bone shim may be necessary to eliminate torque on the proximal segment. Use of a lag screw in an area of sound bone contact is encouraged to ensure rigidity at the osteotomy because tightening of the positional screw may be the head of the screw against the lateral cortex and not necessarily engaging the distal segment.

on the unaffected, yet distorted side. Bone may be obtained through resection of the hyperplastic inferior border or harvesting of corticocancellous bone from the hip. The graft can be secured to the inferior border of the shortened side with rigid fixation. The stability of the augmentation is difficult to predict under the influence of the soft tissue. Resorption and subsequent remodeling of the augmentation with autogenous bone cannot be calculated. Implants may provide improved rigidity under the influence of the soft tissue and pterygomasseteric sling but possess potential limitations as a result of being a foreign body, causing restriction of mobility, or creating palpable steps.

Two-jaw surgery may be required if compensation in the maxilla has arisen as a result of deviation of the mandible. Rapidly progressive vertical changes in the mandible may create an open bite on the affected side or, if left unattended, a canted occlusal plane as the

maxillary teeth supra-erupt. Early interceptive orthodontics may prevent a response in the maxilla to the progressive deformity in the mandible. Correction of the canted occlusal plane requires surgery on the maxilla, in addition to surgery on the deformity within the mandibular arch. The vertical changes in the maxilla will require asymmetric repositioning to level the occlusal plane. The maxillary osteotomy must address the traditional focus of vertical repositioning established with exposure of the incisors at rest. Leveling of the occlusal plane may require superior repositioning on the affected side or down-grafting on the unaffected side. The principles of stability with orthognathic movement of the maxilla must be taken into account to ensure a sound stable final result. Superior repositioning of a Le Fort osteotomy possesses much greater stability than does inferior repositioning, which resides at the opposite end of the stability hierarchy.[9]

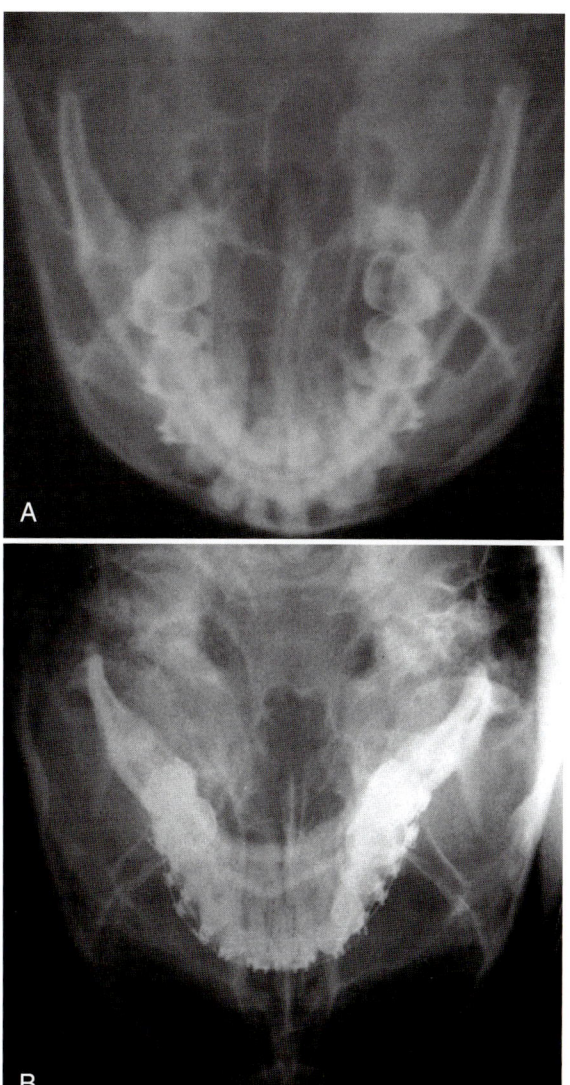

Fig. 80-14 ■ Mandibular ramus anatomy for mandibular setback. A submental vertex (SMV) radiograph illustrates parallel orientation of the ramus mimicking a U shape. The anatomy of the mandible favors sagittal ramus osteotomy. SMV radiography depicts a divergent ramus (V shaped) best suited for mandibular setback via vertical ramus osteotomy as the proximal segment telescopes lateral to the repositioned mandible.

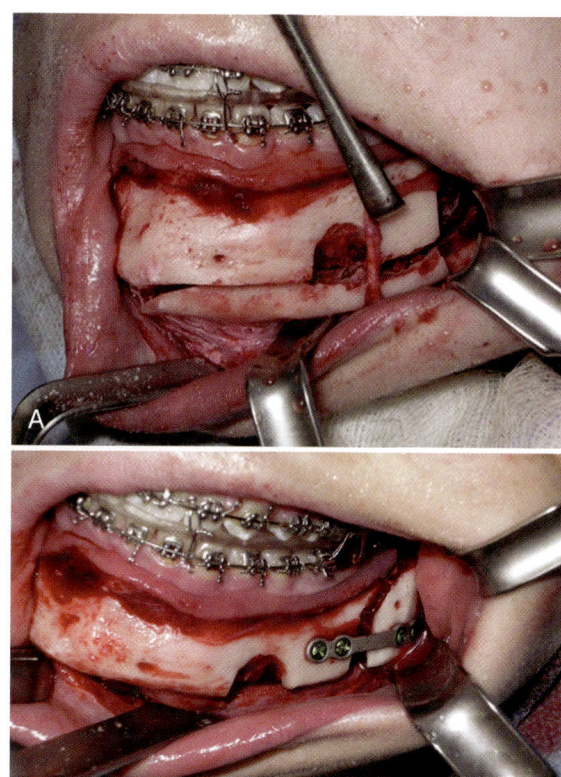

Fig. 80-15 ■ Generous exposure is necessary for visualization and access to correct the skeletal deformity. Resection of the inferior border is completed after lateralizing the inferior alveolar nerve from the distal segment.

POSTOPERATIVE CARE

Postoperative care following surgical intervention to correct asymmetric dentofacial deformities is similar to that for conventional orthognathic surgery. A tape dressing is frequently placed after closure to help the soft tissue drape against the bony correction on the chin. Next, a compression dressing is used for several days to eliminate dead space. Significant postoperative swelling may occur, so the edema should be expected to mask the bony correction for weeks. Even though the final bony and soft tissue changes are typically not apparent for an extended time, correction of the asymmetry is generally appreciated early in the postoperative period.

Neuromuscular reprogramming is important postoperatively after correction of an asymmetric malocclusion. Elastic guidance is frequently required to overcome memory within the muscles following surgery. The guidance elastics aid in education of the mind and muscles to the newly established occlusion. The residual soft tissue influence will frequently deviate the mandible until reprogramming is accomplished.

CASE REVIEWS—DENTOFACIAL DEFORMITY WITH ASYMMETRY

MANDIBULAR HYPERPLASIA WITH ASYMMETRY AND MAXILLARY COMPENSATION

Unilateral prognathism creates horizontal deviation of the lower third of the face to the left. A subtle cant of the occlusal plane is evident with increased gingival exposure on the right during animation (Fig. 80-16, *A*). Orthodontic decompensation achieves sound arch form and alignment with the mandibular midline to the left. A PA cephalometric film illustrates the skeletal asymmetry with deviation of the mandible and canting of the occlusal plane (Fig. 80-16, *B*).

A facial view following correction of asymmetric dentofacial deformity highlights improved symmetry and esthetics with animation (Fig. 80-16, *D*). After treatment, occlusion with solid coupling and stability was achieved (Fig. 80-16, *E*). A PA cephalometric film illustrates the symmetry achieved through conventional maxillary and mandibular surgery (Fig. 80-16, *F*). Additional measures (genioplasty) were not necessary to achieve symmetry because the dental and skeletal asymmetry were coincident.

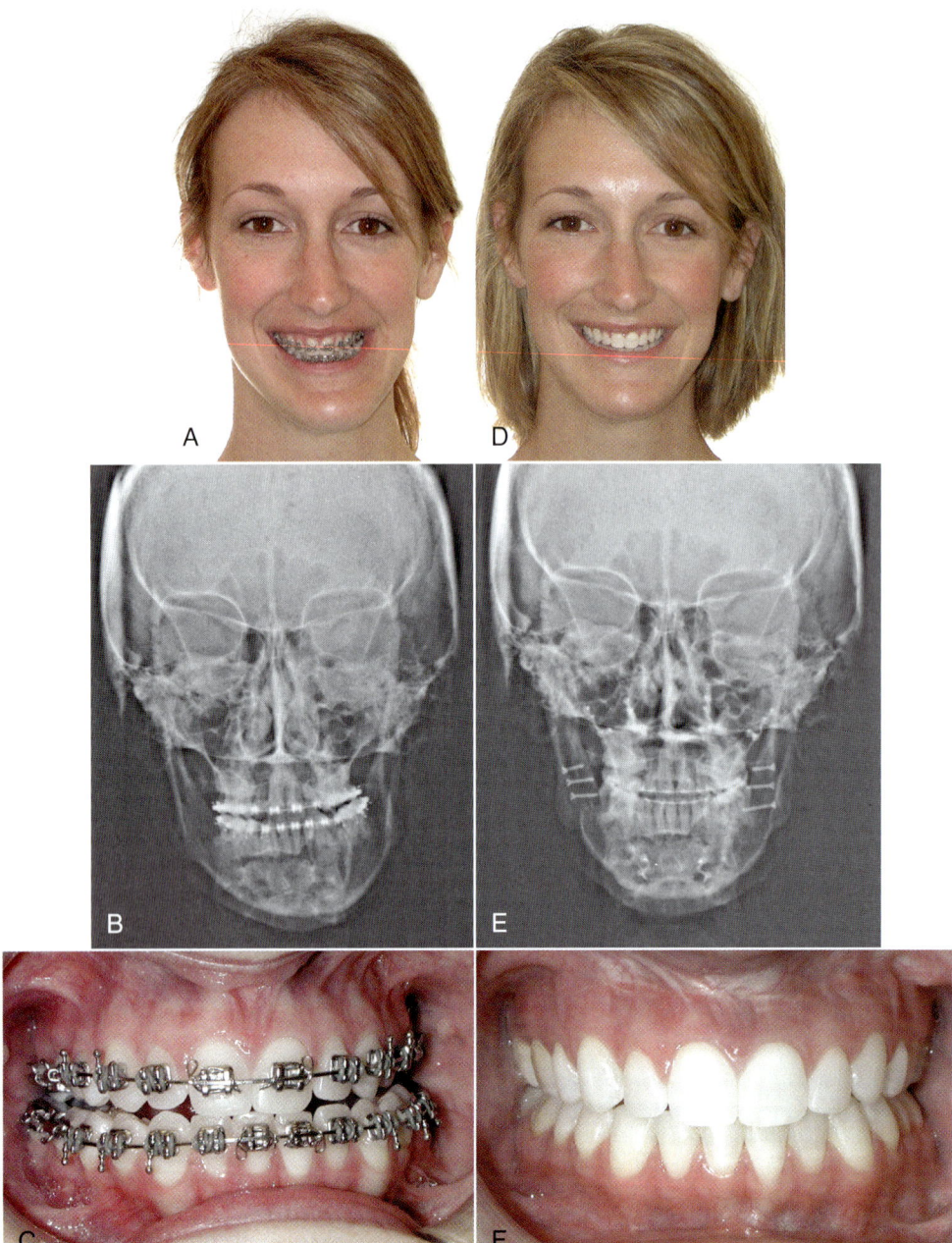

Fig. 80-16 ■ Pretreatment photographs. **A,** Unilateral prognathism causing horizontal deviation to the left in the lower third of the face. **B,** Posteroanterior (PA) cephalometric film showing the skeletal asymmetry with deviation of the mandible and canting of the occlusal plane. **C,** Subtle cant of the occlusal plane is evident with increased gingival exposure on the right during animation. **D,** Post-treatment photograph showing improved symmetry and esthetics with animation. **E,** PA cephalometric film showing the symmetry achieved with conventional maxillary and mandibular surgery. **F,** Post-treatment occlusion with solid coupling and stability. (From Hupp JR, Ellis E, Tucker MR: *Contemporary oral and maxillofacial surgery*, ed 5, St. Louis, 2008, Mosby.)

ASYMMETRIC DENTOFACIAL DEFORMITY

The examination and PA cephalometric film illustrate deviation of the mandible to the left with compensation of the maxillary arch toward the skeletal asymmetry (Fig. 80-17, *A* and *B*). The image allows reference of the dental to the skeletal midline to aid in planning the surgical correction. The addition of an anterior segmental osteotomy may be necessary if the skeletal asymmetry is more pronounced than the dental discrepancy.

Midline deviation and unilateral crossbite with mandibular hyperplasia and asymmetry are apparent (Fig. 80-17, *C* to *E*). Compensation in the maxillary arch is evident as flaring of the teeth laterally in an effort to control the skeletal discrepancy.

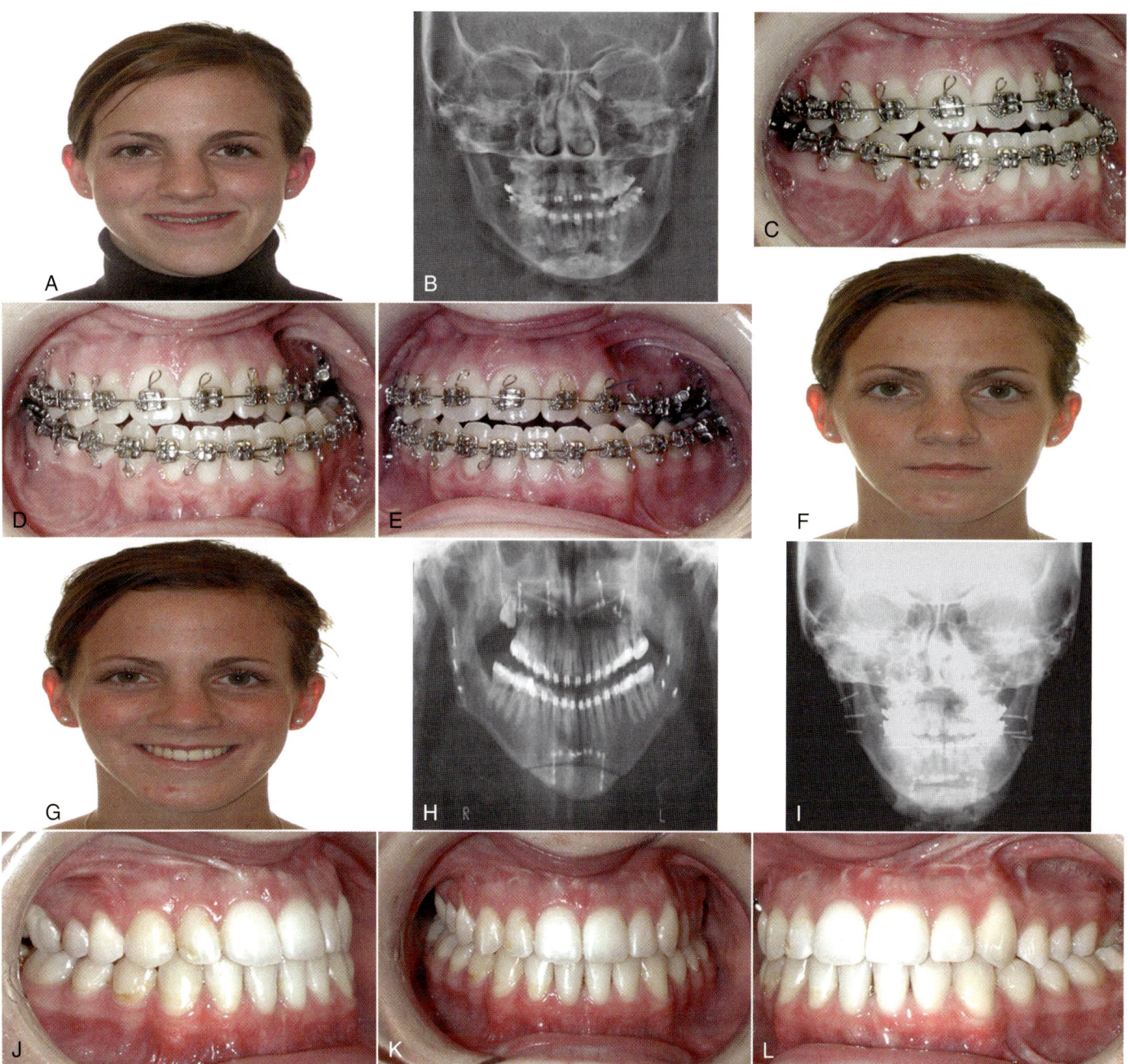

Fig. 80-17 ■ Pretreatment photographs. **A** and **B,** A facial photograph (**A**) and posteroanterior (PA) cephalometric film (**B**) show deviation of the mandible to the left with compensation of the maxillary arch toward the skeletal asymmetry. **C** to **E,** Intraoral photographs showing midline deviation and unilateral crossbite with mandibular hyperplasia and asymmetry. **F** and **G,** Post-treatment facial photographs show good facial esthetics. **H,** Panorex radiograph illustrating the surgical correction. **I,** PA cephalometric film showing improved symmetry of the skeletal and dental elements. **J** to **L,** Intraoral photographs showing the final occlusion with good midline approximation, anterior coupling, and posterior interdigitation.

Correction of asymmetry establishes good facial esthetics (Fig. 80-17, *F* and *G*), and the final occlusion has good midline approximation, anterior coupling, and posterior interdigitation.

A postoperative Panorex view illustrates the surgical correction (Fig. 80-17, *H*). The anatomic characteristics of the mandible and the rotational movement necessary for correction of the asymmetry dictated performance of a vertical ramus osteotomy with setback on the right and net advancement via sagittal ramus osteotomy on the left. Additional correction of asymmetry in the chin required a sliding anterior segmental osteotomy. A midline vertical segmental osteotomy was performed simultaneously in the mandible to narrow the arch form and limit interference from the distal segment within the ramus. A PA cephalometric film illustrates improved symmetry of the skeletal and dental elements (Fig. 80-17, *I*). Figure 80-17, *J* to *L*, shows the final results.

PEARLS AND PITFALLS

- Correction of asymmetric dentofacial deformities involves thorough data collection, imaging studies, treatment planning, and a broad understanding of orthognathic surgical techniques.
- The timing of surgical intervention depends on the stability of the asymmetry.
- Early intervention may be necessary to improve growth potential from restricted movement or to eliminate progressive asymmetry.
- Late surgical correction may be considered once the dynamic changes causing the asymmetry have ceased.
- In either situation, a mandibular osteotomy alone may not completely resolve the skeletal asymmetry. Adjunctive procedures such as genioplasty and inferior border resection may be required to establish facial symmetry.
- Advances in imaging technology and three-dimensional analyses have improved the accuracy of asymmetry correction through computer simulation and transfer of the virtual plan to the operating room through milled splints.
- Asymmetric dentofacial deformities managed with thoughtful preparation and technique will result in functional and esthetic success.

REFERENCES

1. Severt TR, Proffit WR: The prevalence of facial asymmetry in the dentofacial deformities population at the University of North Carolina, *Int J Adult Orthodon Orthognath Surg* 12:171-176, 1997.
2. Proffit WR, Turvey TA: Dentofacial asymmetry. In Proffit WR, White RA Jr, Sarver DM, editors: *Contemporary treatment of dentofacial deformity*, St Louis, 2003, CV Mosby.
3. Proffit WR, Vig KWL, Turvey TA: Fractures of the mandible condyle: frequently an unsuspected cause of facial asymmetry, *Am J Orthod* 78:1-24, 1980.
4. Obwegeser HL, Maked MS: Hemimandibular hyperplasia–hemimandibular elongation, *J Maxillofac Surg* 14:183, 1986.
5. Obwegeser HL: *Mandibular growth anomalies*, Berlin, 2001, Springer-Verlag.
6. Robinson PD, Harris K, Coghlan KC, et al: Bone scans and the timing of treatment for condylar hyperplasia, *Int J Oral Maxillofac Surg* 19:243-246, 1990.
7. Tucker MR, Frost DE, Terry BC: Mandibular surgery. In Tucker MR, White RA Jr, Terry BC, et al, editors: *Rigid fixation for maxillofacial surgery*, Philadelphia, 1991, JB Lippincott.
8. Hall HD, Chase DC, Payor LG: Evaluation and realignment of the intraoral vertical subcondylar osteotomy, *J Oral Surg* 33:333-341, 1975.
9. Proffit WR, Turvey TA, Phillips C: Orthognathic surgery: a hierarchy of stability, *Int J Adult Orthodon Orthognath Surg* 11:191-204, 1996.

Chapter **81**

Mandibular Asymmetry: Condylar Elongation/Hypertrophy

Felice O'Ryan

Unilateral condylar hyperplasia (CH) is an uncommon pathologic entity with a wide spectrum of clinical manifestations that results from the overgrowth of one condyle. Lack of consistent terminology has contributed to the confusion with this diagnosis, but the common underlying feature is hypertrophy or hyperplasia of the mandibular condyle. Depending on the age at onset, and rapidity, and duration of the condylar growth, facial asymmetry and, associated malocclusions are common. CH is usually self-limited, and after cessation of growth, orthognathic surgery may be needed to correct the resultant asymmetry. Condylectomy is indicated if growth is rapid and causes functional or psychosocial problems. The purpose of this chapter is to review the etiopathogenesis, pathologic anatomy, diagnostic studies, and treatment options for correction of unilateral CH and its associated manifestations.

ETIOPATHOGENESIS

CH is a rare disorder characterized by excessive unilateral growth of the mandibular condyle. Although the precise etiology is uncertain, it is generally agreed that one of two processes occur: either excess growth of one condyle or continued unilateral condylar growth after completion of skeletal growth.[1-4] Trauma, infection, hormonal disturbances, and a genetic predisposition have been implicated in the pathogenesis of CH.[5,6] Common to all cases of CH, the pathology occurs within the temporomandibular joint (TMJ). Manifestations of CH are not limited to the mandible and may involve the maxilla and even the orbits. Malocclusion is common, and TMJ pain and dysfunction may also be seen. CH has been described in all ethnicities and both sexes with a slight female predilection.[3,7-10]

Although the onset of CH can vary widely, it generally begins in early adolescence and ceases in the second and third decades; though condylar growth has been found to continue into the 50s and 60s.[11-13] Histologic analysis of affected condyles has shown increased width of the overlying fibrocartilaginous layer with undifferentiated germinating mesenchymal cells, islands of chondrocytes in the subchondral bone, and large masses of hyaline cartilage.[7,14-16] Once the hyperplastic growth has ceased, the histologic appearance of the condyle is normal.[1]

The spectrum of facial asymmetry associated with CH depends on three factors: (1) age at onset, (2) duration, and (3) degree of abnormal growth. Obwegeser and Makek categorized CH into three groups based on the primary direction of mandibular growth (vertical or horizontal).[17] They described hemimandibular hyperplasia as asymmetric enlargement of the condylar head and neck, mandibular ramus, and body up to the symphysis with elongation and bowing of the inferior border of the mandible. In cases of early onset, compensatory vertical maxillary growth can result in canting of the occlusal plane. In contrast, if condylar growth was rapid, an open bite on the affected side could also be seen. The second group, described as hemimandibular elongation, was characterized by lateral deviation of the mandible and chin without vertical lengthening of the ramus. The third category was a combination of the two. With the advent of three-dimensional imaging, it appears likely that CH represents a continuum with varying degrees of both vertical and horizontal growth components.[18,19]

PATHOLOGIC ANATOMY

The pathologic anatomy of CH is ascertained from the clinical examination, supporting imaging studies, and history of the asymmetry (Table 81-1). Progression of the asymmetry is often slow and may not be clinically apparent to the patient until clinical signs of TMJ dysfunction or malocclusion are noted.

CLINICAL EXAMINATION

The most salient information is obtained from clinical evaluation with the patient in repose and animation. Anatomic components are assessed from the frontal, oblique, and profile views, with additional views obtained as needed. Evaluation of the patient from the basal (worm's eye) and cranial (bird's eye) views can provide additional information about the location, magnitude, and three-dimensional characterization of the asymmetry. Examination of the patient during dynamic function, while speaking and smiling, provides additional information about the soft tissue response to the asymmetry.

Clinical examination begins with the upper third of the face. Varying degrees of orbital dystopia may be seen in patients with CH, depending on the magnitude of the asymmetric growth and the age at which the growth began. Patients with hemimandibular hyperplasia can have associated orbital dystopia because of distortion of the middle and anterior cranial fossae (Fig. 81-1). The level of the orbits is important to consider in planning treatment because the interorbital line, a line drawn tangent to the supraorbital rims, is commonly used as the horizontal reference for measuring maxillary occlusal cant.[20]

Examination of the mid-face and maxilla, in repose and smiling, will further reveal associated maxillary asymmetries, which occur in up to 50% of patients with CH.[10] The maxillary dental midline should be noted. Malar and maxillary asymmetry (projection and yaw) are best assessed from the basal view. Determination of the cant of the labial commissures and occlusal plane is aided by having the patient bite on a tongue blade (Fig. 81-2). This provides a useful horizontal reference plane and can help determine the degree and location of the asymmetry. Smile analysis provides important

TABLE 81-1	Differential Diagnosis of Mandibular Asymmetry		
DIAGNOSIS	**ONSET**	**CLINICAL FINDINGS**	**IMAGING FINDINGS**
Condylar hyperplasia	13-30 years	Elongation or enlargement of the hemimandible Mandibular asymmetry away from the affected side Malocclusion (crossbite/open bite) Slowly progressive	Enlargement of the condylar head and elongation of the condylar neck Scintigraphy positive or negative
Condylar tumors: osteochondroma, osteoma, chondroma, osteoblastoma	40.5 years	Elongation or enlargement of the hemimandible Mandibular asymmetry toward the contralateral side Malocclusion (crossbite/open bite) Slowly progressive	"Mushroom-shaped" mass associated with the condylar head Scintigraphy positive
Torticollis	Congenital	Mass/band of SCM Head deviated toward the affected side Variable presence of malocclusion Not progressive	Normal condylar shape/size Scintigraphy negative
Condylar hypoplasia/ degeneration	1st-6th decades	Shortening of the ipsilateral hemimandible Mandibular asymmetry toward the affected side Malocclusion (premature contact on the affected side) Slowly progressive	Degenerative changes in the condylar head Scintigraphy positive or negative (consistent with DJD)
Condylar fracture	Any	Shortening of the ipsilateral hemimandible Mandibular asymmetry toward the affected side Acute	Evidence of fracture (acute) Degenerative changes in the condylar head (old) Scintigraphy negative
Craniofacial syndromes: hemifacial microsomia, hypomelanosis of Ito	Congenital	Shortening of the ipsilateral hemimandible Mandibular asymmetry toward the affected side Slowly progressive	Variable degrees of DJD to absence of the condyle Scintigraphy negative

DJD, Degenerative joint disease; *SCM,* sternocleidomastoid muscle.

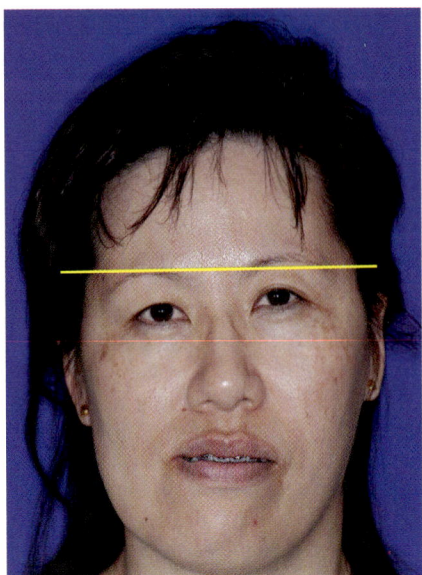

Fig. 81-1 ■ Orbital dystopia associated with hemimandibular hyperplasia.

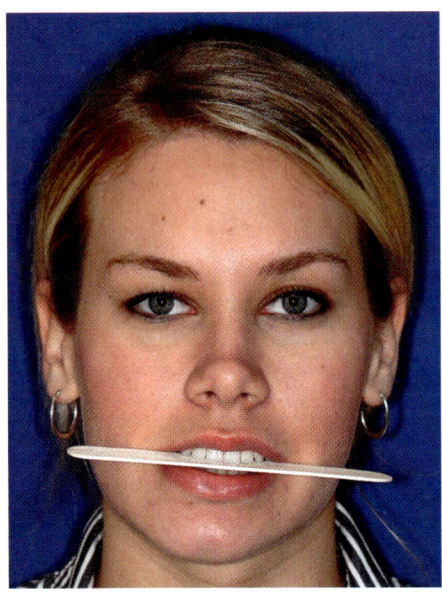

Fig. 81-2 ■ Patient biting on a tongue blade to determine the cant of the labial commissures and occlusal plane.

information about the location and appearance of the asymmetry during dynamic function. A posed smile is voluntary and reproducible.[21,22] Asymmetric function of the lips during smiling should be differentiated from skeletal asymmetry. Characteristics of an attractive smile, more so for females than males, include absence of visible buccal corridors, adequate exposure of the maxillary teeth, and gingival display above the incisors and premolars. There should be approximately 2 to 3 mm of gingival exposure above the premolars.[23] The amount of gingival display in patients with accompanying maxillary asymmetries is important in determining whether the deficient side should be down-grafted or the elongated side should be impacted (Fig. 81-3).

Condylar hyperplasia is most evident in the lower third of the face, where abnormal chin shape and position are obvious (Fig.

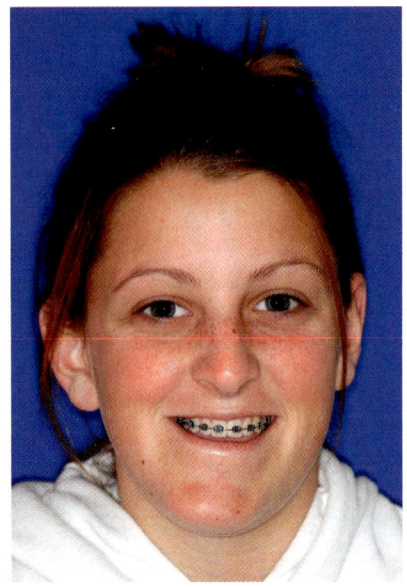

Fig. 81-3 ■ The amount of gingival display in patients with maxillary asymmetries is important in determining whether the deficient side should be downgrafted or the elongated side should be impacted.

81-4, *A* and *B*). Bowing of the inferior border of the mandible and deficient width and projection of the mandibular angle are features commonly seen in these cases. Right and left oblique views will further disclose the difference between the mandibular angles (Fig. 81-4, *C* and *D*). Patients should be queried about which side they believe is more attractive.

A class III malocclusion is frequently associated with CH and midline deviation away from the affected side. A posterior open bite may be present (also on the affected side), and dental compensations consisting of lingual tipping of the mandibular premolars and molars on the contralateral side are common.

TMJ range of motion in patients with CH is largely normal, but approximately 25% complain of pain and dysfunction.[10,17] Pain and dysfunction are commonly seen in the contralateral TMJ, probably because of compression from growth of the affected joint.

DIAGNOSTIC STUDIES

Plain films, including lateral and posteroanterior cephalograms and panoramic radiographs, demonstrate the characteristic findings of condylar elongation or enlargement (or both), deviation of the mandibular midline, and asymmetry of the mandibular body. The mandibular ramus is vertically longer than on the unaffected side with increased dentoalveolar height and displacement of the inferior alveolar nerve toward the inferior border (Fig. 81-5, *A* and *B*). (There is often compensatory maxillary growth on the affected side with increased alveolar height below the sinus floor.) Bowing of the inferior border of the mandible can also be seen as two distinct inferior mandibular borders on the lateral cephalometric radiograph (Fig. 81-5, *C*).

Uniform enlargement of the condylar head and neck and proportional enlargement of the glenoid fossa are common findings seen on TMJ tomograms and computed tomography (CT) scans[10] (Fig. 81-6). Osteochondroma, in contrast, when present in the TMJ, often has a distinctly different appearance and is seen as a globular mass projecting from a relatively normal condyle[24] (Fig. 81-7).

Three-dimensional CT scans are helpful in visualizing and quantifying the location and extent of the asymmetry (Fig. 81-8).

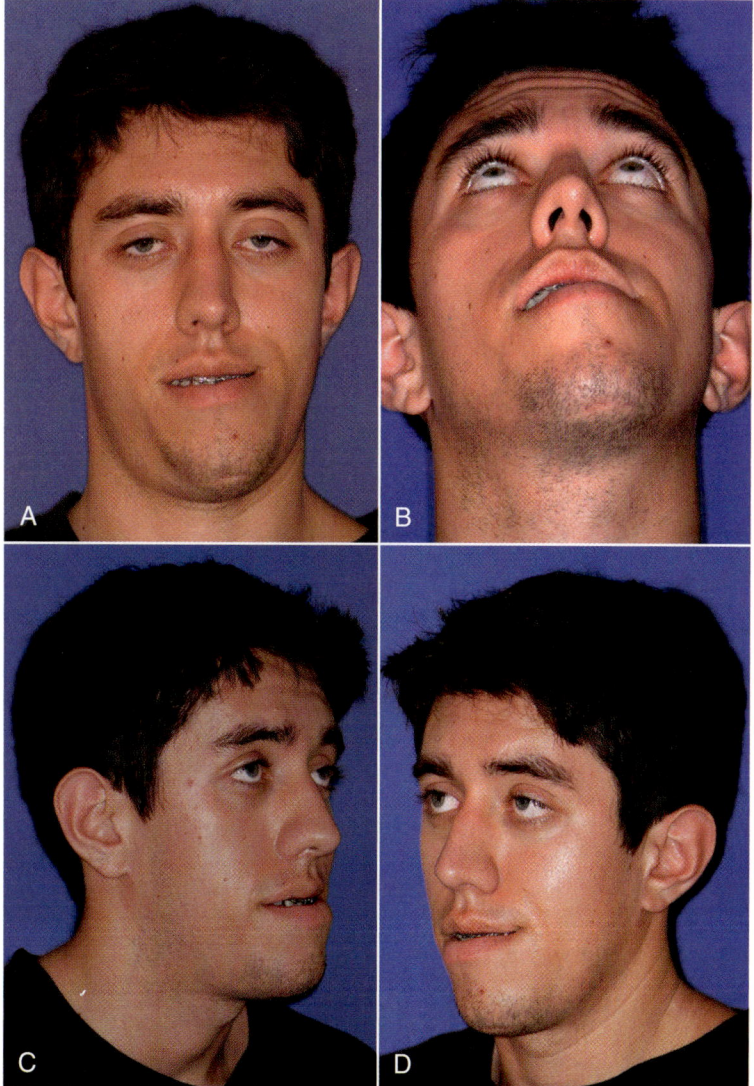

Fig. 81-4 ■ **A** and **B,** Obvious abnormal chin shape and position as a result of condylar hyperplasia. **C** and **D,** Oblique views further demonstrating the difference between the mandibular angles.

Radionuclide imaging, including bone scintigraphy, is useful in determining whether there is active condylar growth. Bone scintigraphy, usually with the ligand methylene diphosphonate, has been used widely in patients with CH and can demonstrate relative activity of one side versus the other but does not provide quantitative information about the amount of condylar growth.[11-13,16] Positron emission tomography is more useful for quantifying bone metabolism and may be used more commonly in the future.[25,26]

TREATMENT/RECONSTRUCTIVE GOALS

The goals of treatment are to restore facial symmetry, correct the associated malocclusion, and do so in a manner that will provide a stable result without continued condylar growth. Decisions about when and where to operate are predicated on the patient's age and complaints and the growth status of the affected condyle. Patients referred for treatment as adults with long-standing stable asymmetry and unchanged occlusion are best treated by orthognathic surgery with the condyle left intact. In adults with ongoing CH, positive scintigraphic findings, and progressive asymmetry and malocclusion, resection of the affected condyle is indicated.

Management decisions in children and adolescents are more difficult because of the certainty of continued, but unpredictable pathologic condylar growth. Definitive treatment may be postponed until growth has ceased, or in those with significant asymmetric growth causing functional or psychosocial problems, condylectomy can be performed, and correction of the residual malocclusion and asymmetry can be accomplished after the completion of skeletal growth.

It is important to remember that CH often causes distortion of the entire facial skeleton in three dimensions and that achieving acceptable symmetry with a single operation is often not possible. Furthermore, it can be difficult to make accurate judgments about facial symmetry intraoperatively when the patient's face is swollen. In such cases we routinely perform secondary correction, especially mandibular angle augmentation and straightening genioplasty, approximately 6 months later after the edema has resolved.

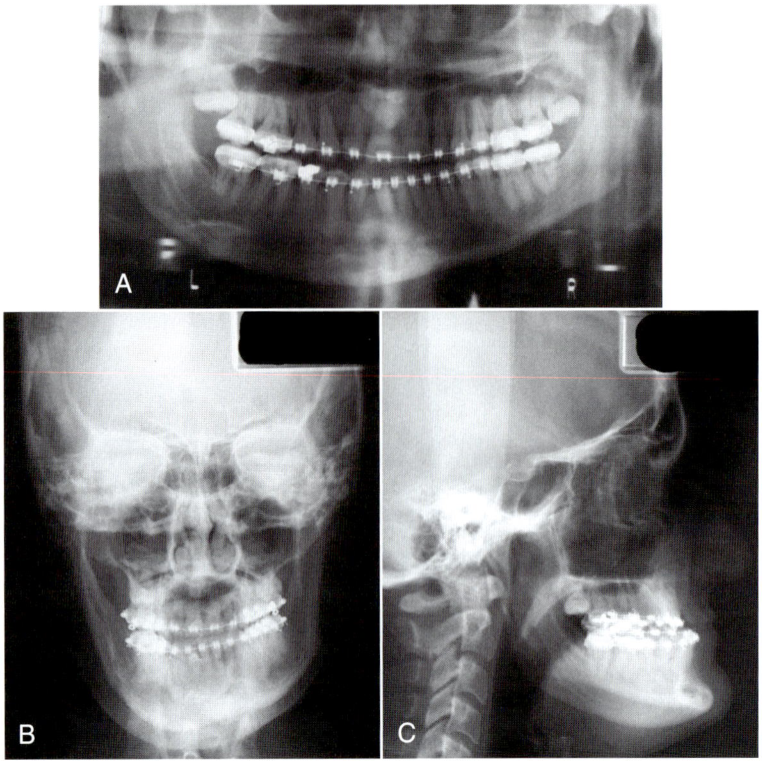

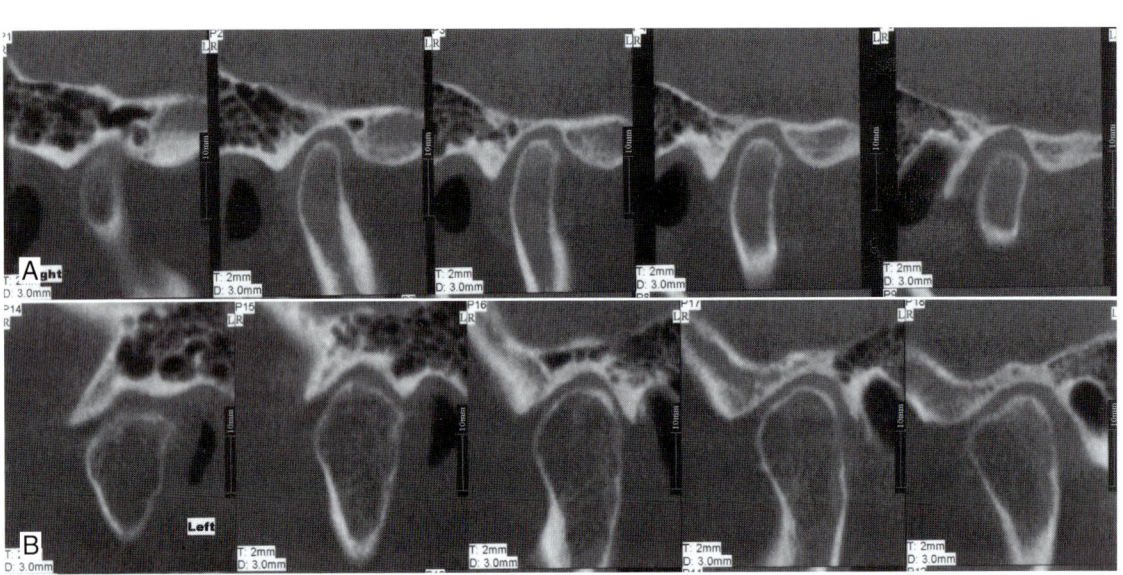

Fig. 81-5 ■ Panoramic (**A**) and cephalometric (**B**) radiographs show a mandibular ramus vertically longer than the unaffected side with increased dentoalveolar height and displacement of the inferior alveolar nerve toward the inferior border. **C,** Lateral cephalometric radiograph showing bowing of the inferior border of the mandible and two distinct inferior mandibular borders.

Fig. 81-6 ■ Computed tomography scans of the temporomandibular joint showing enlargement of the condylar head and neck (**A**) and proportional enlargement of the glenoid fossa (**B**).

SPECIFIC TREATMENT AND TECHNIQUES

CONDYLAR HYPERPLASIA IN AN ASYMPTOMATIC ADULT TREATED BY ORTHOGNATHIC SURGERY

A 44-year-old woman was referred by her orthodontist for correction of a long-standing facial asymmetry that began in her teens (Fig. 81-9, *A*). In addition to orbital dystopia, elongation of the left mandibular body with deviation of the mandible to the right was noted. A class III malocclusion on the left with deviation of the midline to the right and tipping of the mandibular right posterior teeth was present. Plain films and TMJ tomograms demonstrated the maxillary and mandibular asymmetry and symmetric enlargement of the left mandibular condylar head and neck and glenoid fossa (Fig. 81-9, *B* to *D*). Orthognathic surgery consisted of Le Fort I osteotomy with impaction of the left maxilla and bilateral sagittal ramus osteotomies with rotation and shortening of the left side and advancement of the right side. The final postoperative facial views and radiographs demonstrate improved symmetry with residual chin deviation for which the patient declined correction (Fig. 81-9, *J* to *O*).

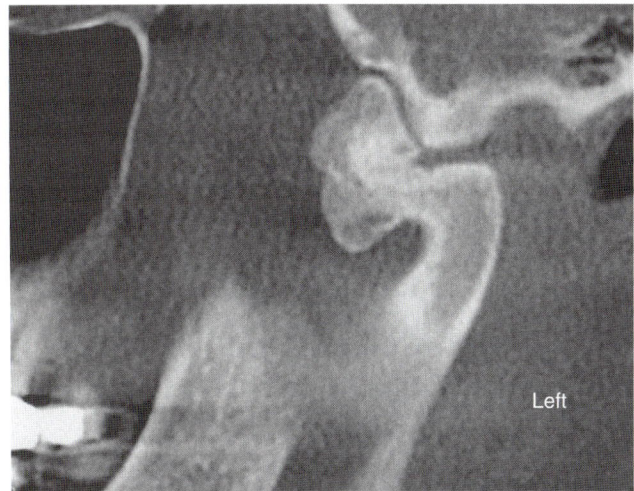

Fig. 81-7 ▪ Tomogram of the temporomandibular joint showing an osteochondroma.

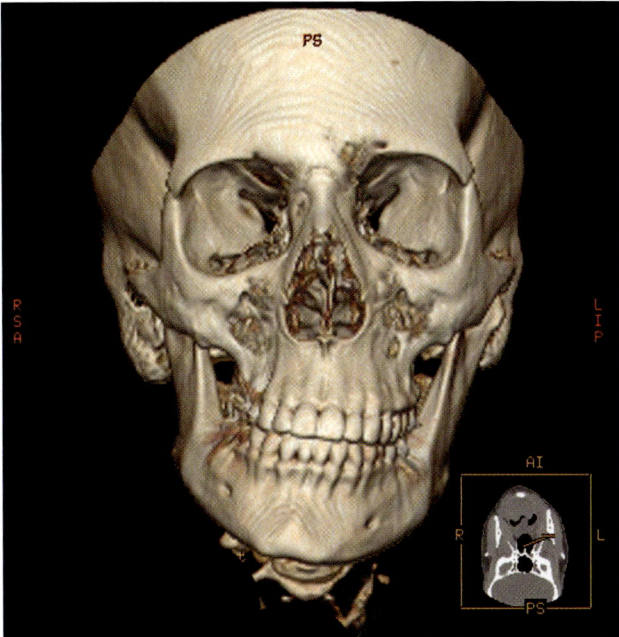

Fig. 81-8 ▪ Computed tomography scan demonstrating the location and extent of the asymmetry.

CONDYLAR HYPERPLASIA TREATED BY CONDYLECTOMY AND ORTHOGNATHIC SURGERY

A 15-year-old girl was evaluated for progressive development of facial asymmetry, class III malocclusion with midline deviation and an open bite on the affected side, and worsening contralateral TMJ pain and dysfunction (Fig. 81-10, *A* to *F*). The onset of menses occurred at 11.5 years of age, and her general skeletal growth was completed by the age of 14. Plain films demonstrated the asymmetry along with uniform enlargement of the left mandibular condyle, bowing of the inferior border of the mandible, and deviation of the mandible to the right (Fig. 81-10, *G* to *I*). ^{99m}Tc scintigraphy was positive in the left mandibular condyle (Fig. 81-10, *J* and *K*). Because of her functional complaints, a two-stage approach (left condylectomy in one stage and separate orthognathic

surgery) was undertaken. TMJ tomograms 8 months following condylectomy demonstrate complete removal of the growth center with formation of a cortical outline over the condylar head (Fig. 81-10, *L* to *N*).

Orthognathic surgery consisted of LeFort I osteotomy and bilateral sagittal split ramus osteotomies. Based on her smile esthetics, leveling of the maxillary occlusal plane was accomplished by downgrafting the right side and impacting the left side. Correction of the mandibular asymmetry with sagittal ramus osteotomies rather than vertical ramus osteotomies was done because lengthening on the right side was planned with harvesting of bone from the proximal segment on the left side for use as an interpositional bone graft in the maxilla. The final postoperative results are seen 3 years later (Fig. 81-10, *O* to *Q*).

CONDYLAR HYPERPLASIA TREATED BY ORTHOGNATHIC SURGERY AND SECONDARY MANDIBULAR AUGMENTATION

Complex asymmetries with rotation and deviation of the mid-face, maxilla, and mandible are often evident in patients with CH. As discussed earlier, the best results in such cases can be achieved with a staged approach consisting of correction of the major maxillary and mandibular asymmetries and "fine-tuning" done secondarily. A 19-year-old man was referred for correction of a maxillomandibular asymmetry. The asymmetry was first noted when he was 8 years of age and continued through puberty; it ceased when his skeletal growth was complete. At the initial evaluation he had no TMJ symptoms and thought that his occlusion was stable. Clinical examination demonstrated asymmetric maxillary hypoplasia with a downward cant on the right and less maxillary projection on the left, mandibular asymmetry with deviation of the chin to the left, elongation of the right mandible, and deficiency of the left mandibular angle. An asymmetric class III malocclusion was present with a left crossbite (Fig. 81-11, *A* to *G*). Imaging demonstrated maxillary and mandibular asymmetry and right condylar elongation, with negative findings on ^{99m}Tc scintigraphy (Fig. 81-11, *H* to *J*). Surgical treatment consisted of a LeFort I osteotomy with differential impaction and advancement of the left side and bilateral sagittal ramus osteotomies with planned augmentation of the left mandibular ramus secondarily. One year following the initial surgery he returned for Medpor (Stryker CMF, Newnan, Ga) augmentation of the left ramus (Fig. 81-11, *K* to *M*). A 2.5-year follow-up is seen in Fig. 81-11, *N* to *Q*.

PEARLS AND PITFALLS

- Obtain a proper history to decide whether the asymmetry is congenital or acquired.
- Ascertain the cause of the asymmetry—condylar hyperplasia, condylar tumor, or degeneration of the contralateral condyle.
- Assess growth activity by monitoring the occlusion, comparing serial cephalometric radiographs, or performing bone scintigraphy, if indicated.
- Determine whether a condylectomy is indicated—rapid growth causing functional or psychosocial problems—or whether treatment of the malocclusion and facial asymmetry can be accomplished without joint surgery.
- Characterize the facial asymmetry and be willing to perform secondary surgery for correction of residual asymmetries, especially those in the chin and mandibular angle.

Text continued on p. 695

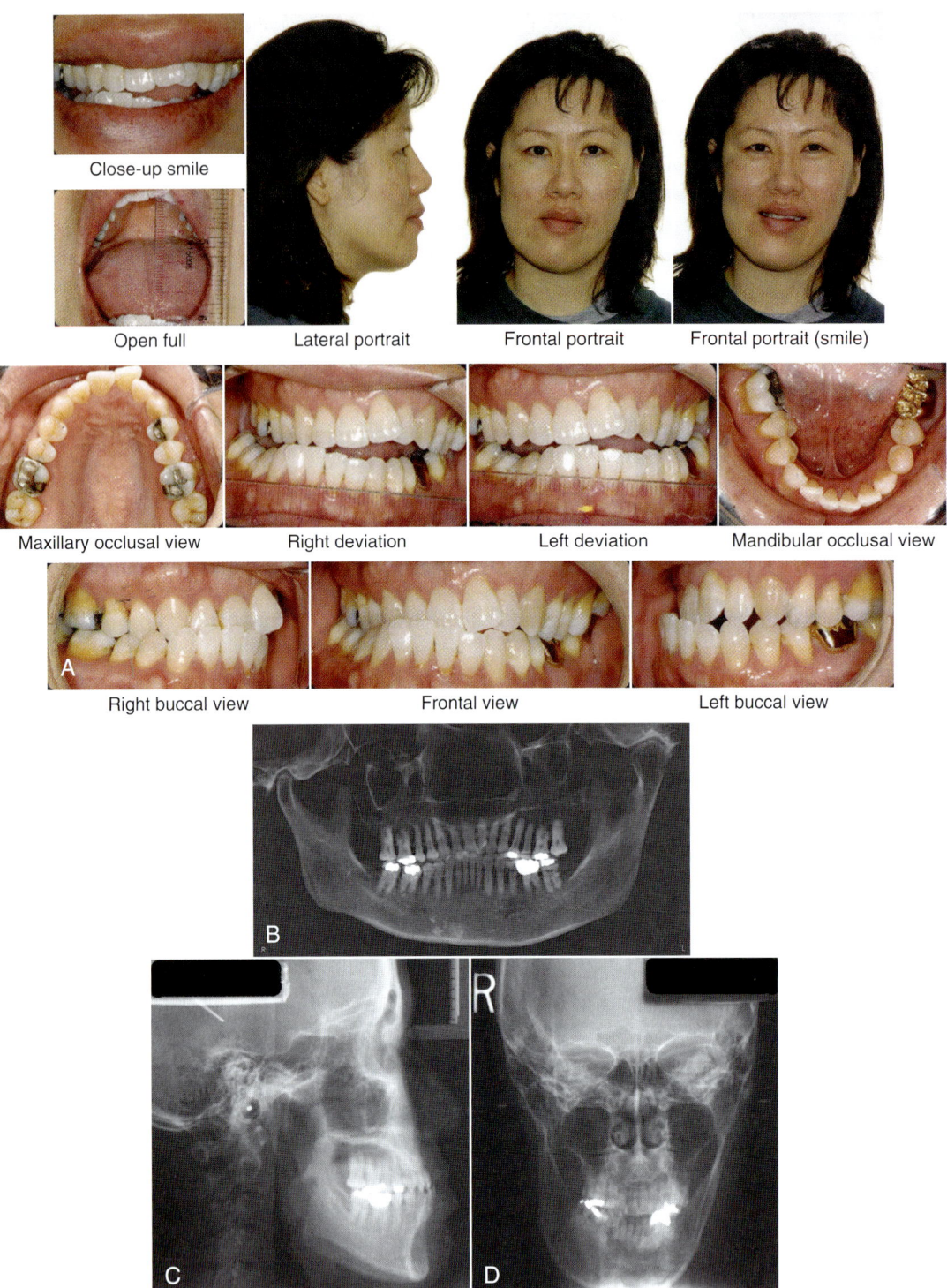

Close-up smile

Open full   Lateral portrait   Frontal portrait   Frontal portrait (smile)

Maxillary occlusal view   Right deviation   Left deviation   Mandibular occlusal view

Right buccal view   Frontal view   Left buccal view

Fig. 81-9 ■ **A,** Pretreatment facial and intraoral photographs showing facial asymmetry. Radiographic views (**B** to **D**) show maxillary and mandibular asymmetry and symmetric enlargement of the left mandibular condylar head and neck and glenoid fossa.

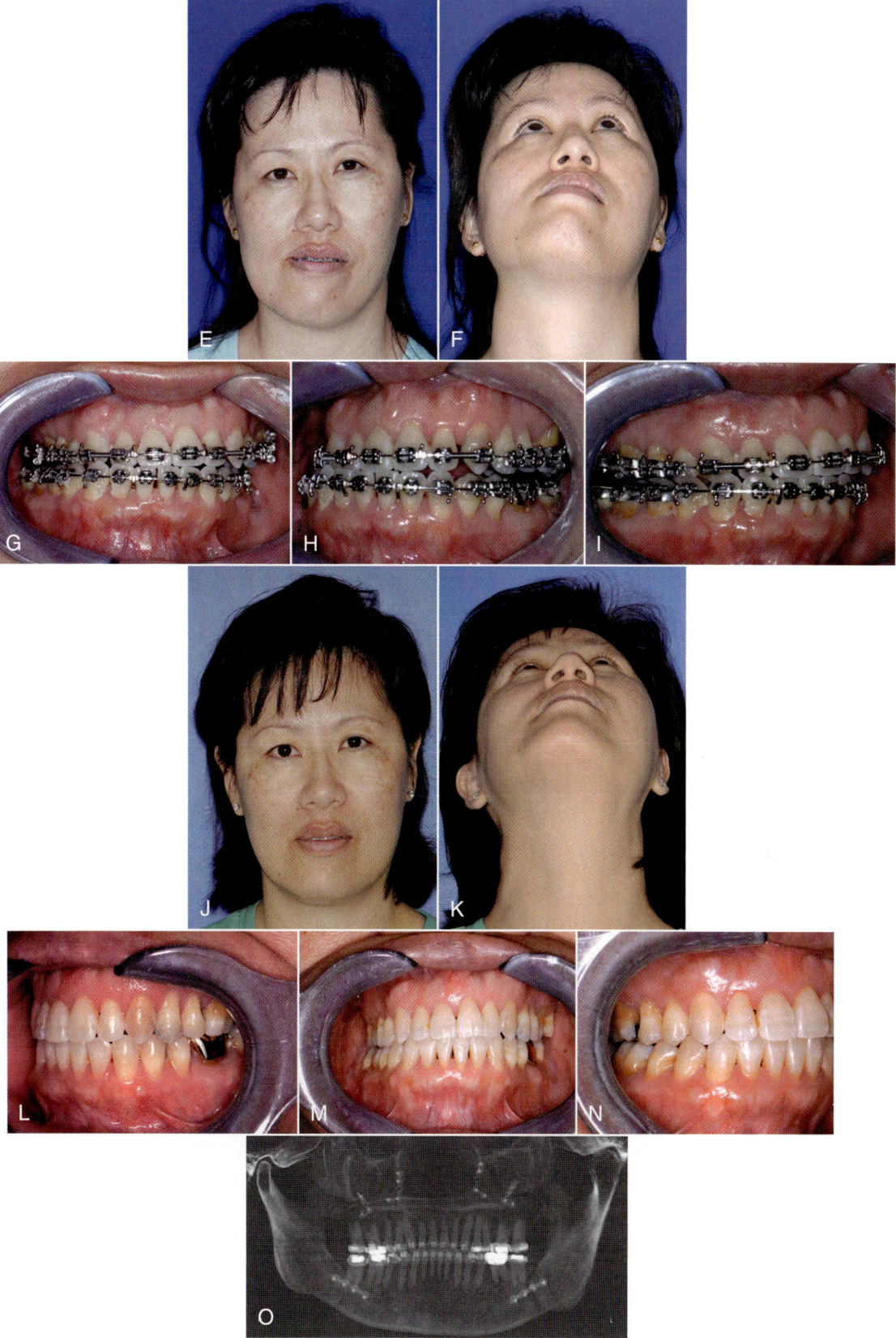

Fig. 81-9, cont'd ■ **E** to **I,** Pretreatment facial (**E** and **F**) and intraoral (**G** to **I**) photographs. Postoperative facial (**J** and **K**), intraoral (**L** to **N**), and radiographic (**O**) views demonstrated improved symmetry with residual chin deviation.

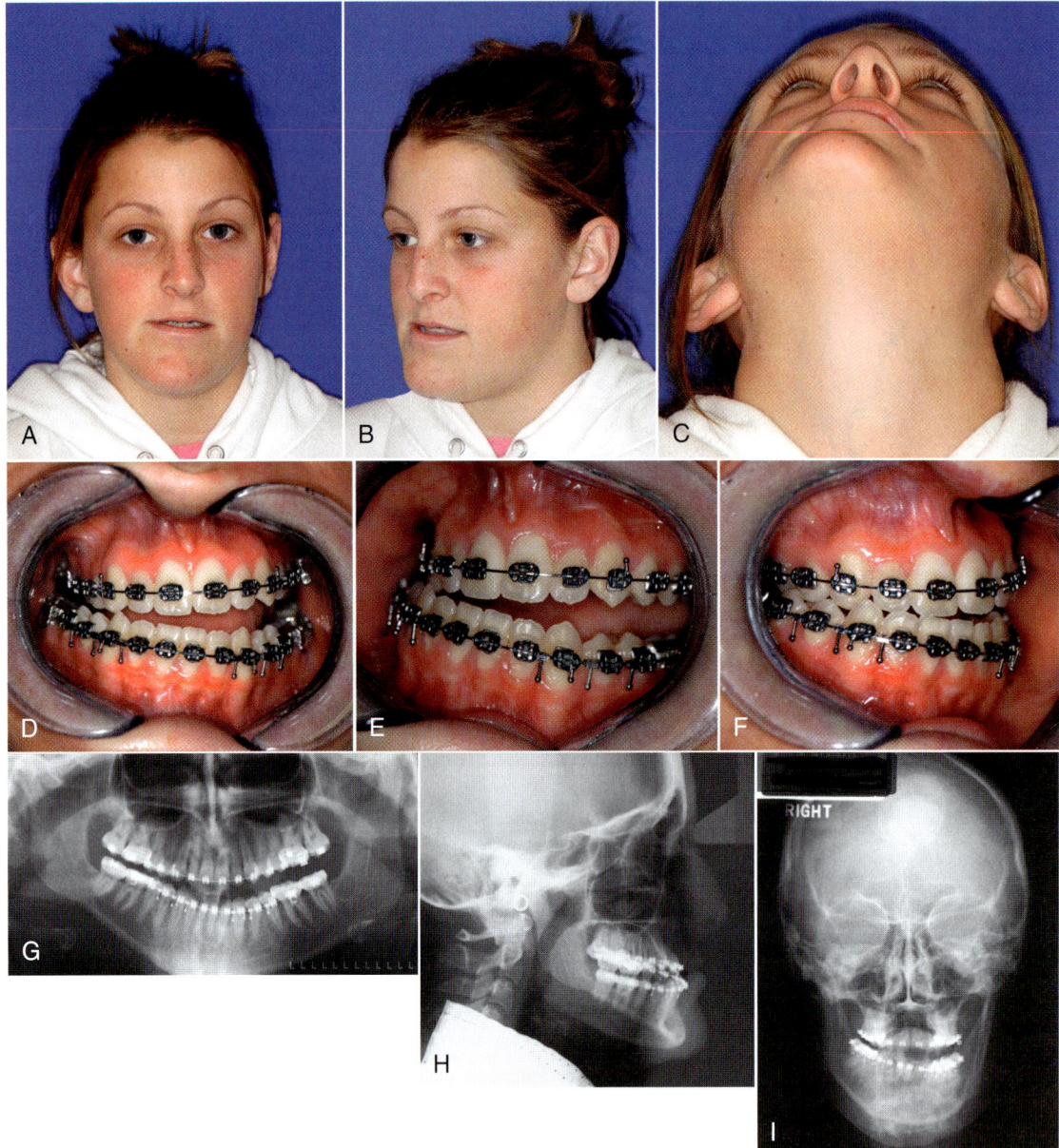

Fig. 81-10 ■ Facial (**A** to **C**) and intraoral (**D** to **F**) views showing progressive development of facial asymmetry, class III malocclusion with midline deviation, and an open bite on the affected side. The patient was evaluated because of worsening contralateral temporomandibular joint (TMJ) pain and dysfunction. **G** to **I,** Radiographic views show asymmetry with uniform enlargement of the left mandibular condyle, bowing of the inferior border of the mandible, and deviation of the mandible to the right.

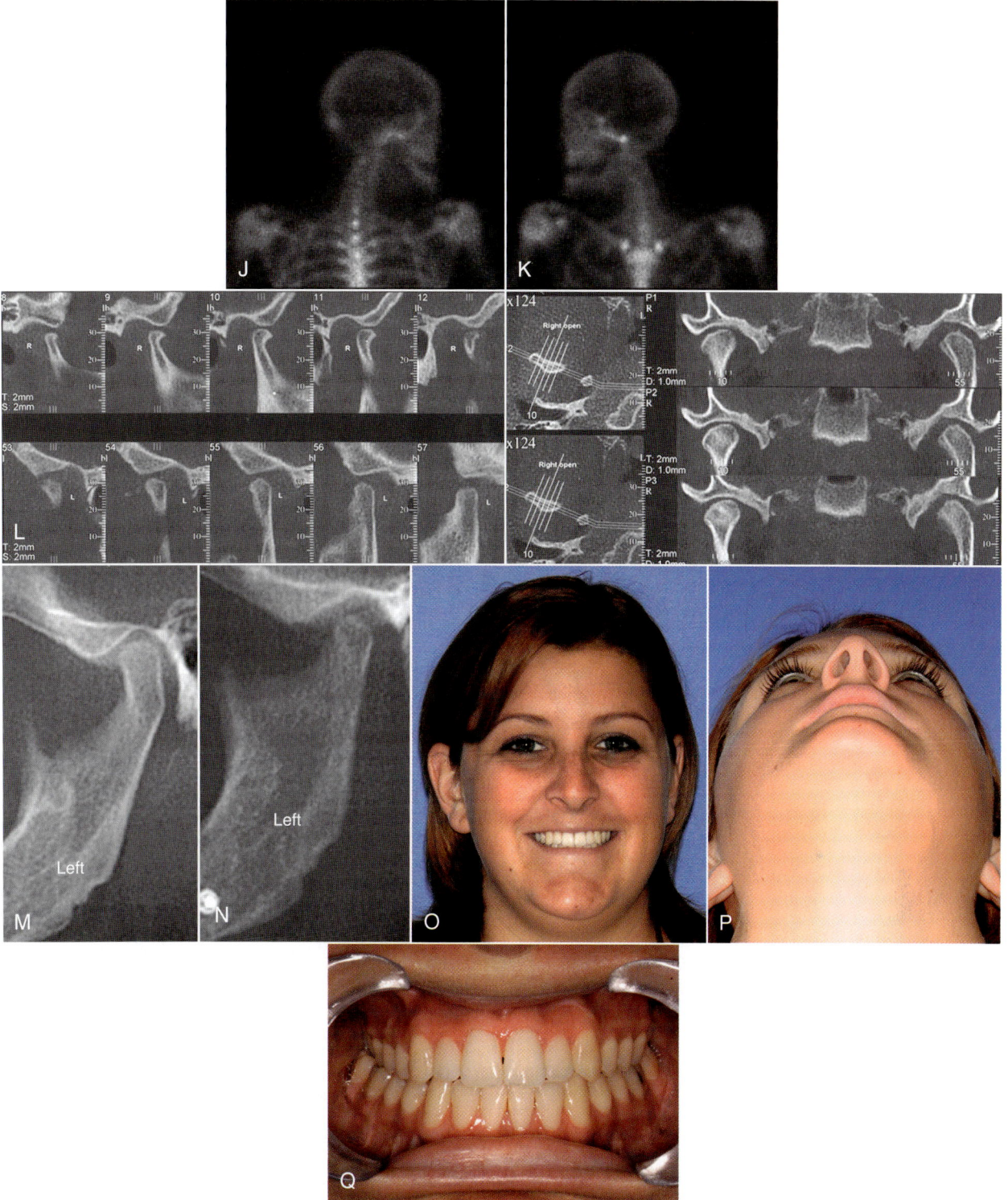

Fig. 81-10, cont'd ■ **J** and **K,** ^{99m}Tc scintigraphy of the left mandibular condyle. **L** to **N,** TMJ tomograms 8 months after condylectomy show complete removal of the growth center with the formation of a cortical outline over the condylar head. **O** to **Q,** Appearance 3 years after treatment.

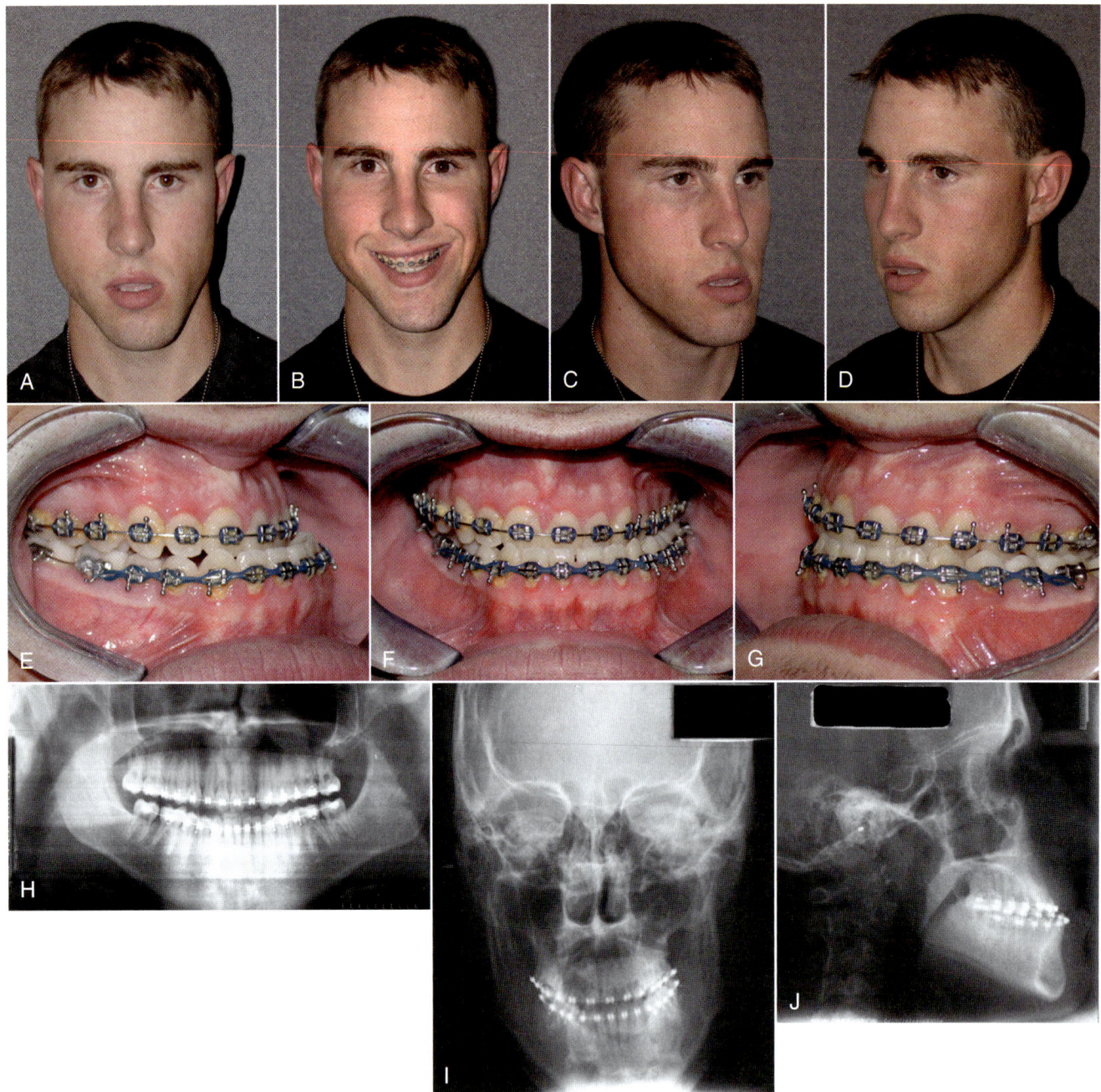

Fig. 81-11 ■ Facial (**A** to **D**) and intraoral (**E** to **G**) views showing asymmetric maxillary hypoplasia with a downward cant on the right and less maxillary projection on the left, mandibular asymmetry with deviation of the chin to the left, elongation of the right mandible, and deficiency of the left mandibular angle. An asymmetric class III malocclusion was present with a left crossbite. **H** to **J,** Radiographic views showing maxillary and mandibular asymmetry and right condylar elongation with negative findings on ^{99m}Tc scintigraphy.

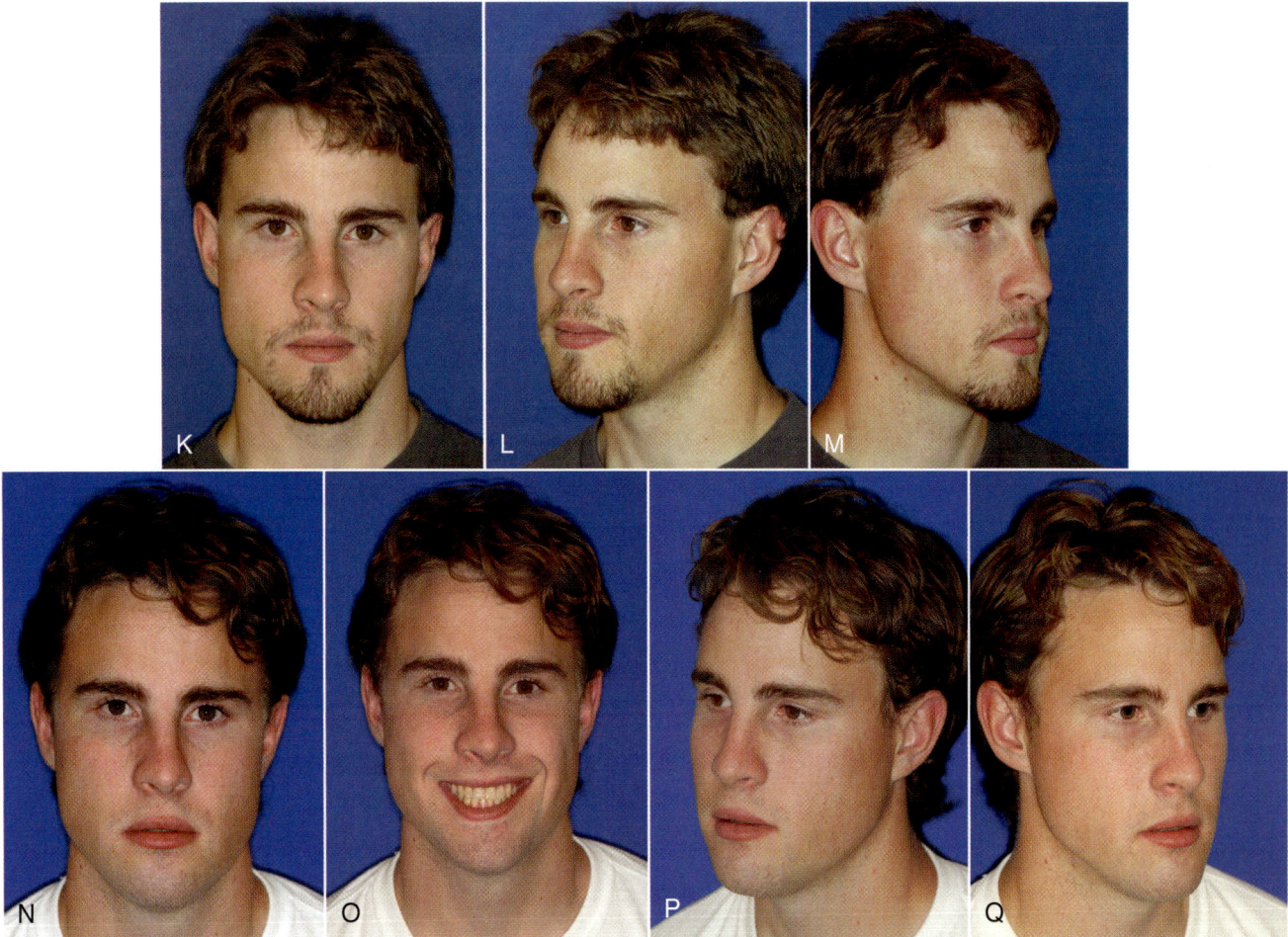

Fig. 81-11, cont'd ■ **K** to **M,** One year after the initial surgery and after Medpor augmentation of the left ramus. **N** to **Q,** Two and a half years after Medpor augmentation.

REFERENCES

1. Norman JE, Painter DM: Hyperplasia of the mandibular condyle. A historical review of important early cases with a presentation and analysis of twelve patients, *J Maxillofac Surg* 8:161-175, 1980.

2. Hovell JH: Condylar hyperplasia, *Br J Oral Surg* 47:105-111, 1963.

3. Bruce RA, Hayward JR: Condylar hyperplasia and mandibular asymmetry: a review, *J Oral Surg* 26:281-290, 1968.

4. Oberg T, Fajers CM, Lysell G, et al: Unilateral hyperplasia of the mandibular condylar process. A histological, microradiographic and autoradiographic examination of one case, *Acta Odontol Scand* 20:485-504, 1962.

5. Slootweg PJ, Muller H: Condylar hyperplasia: a clinic-pathological analysis of 22 cases, *J Maxillofac Surg* 14:209-214, 1986.

6. Yang J, Lingnelli JL, Ruprecht A: Mirror-image condylar hyperplasia in two siblings, *Oral Sur Oral Med Oral Pathol Oral Radiol Endod* 97:281-285, 2004.

7. Gray RJ, Sloan P, Quayle AA, et al: Histopathological and scintigraphic features of condylar hyperplasia, *Int J Oral Maxillofac Surg* 19:65-71, 1990.

8. Blomquist K, Hogeman KE: Benign unilateral hyperplasia of the mandibular condyle: report of eight cases, *Acta Chir Scand* 126:414-426, 1963.

9. Henderson MJ, Wastie JL, Bromige M, et al: Technetium-99m bone scintigraphy and mandibular condylar hyperplasia, *Clin Radiol* 41:411-414, 1990.

10. Nitzan DW, Katsnelson A, Bermanis I, et al: The clinical characteristics of condylar hyperplasia: experience with 61 patients, *J Oral Maxillofac Surg* 66:312-318, 2008.

11. Matteson SR, Proffit WR, Terry BC, et al: Bone scanning with 99m-technectium phosphate to assess condylar hyperplasia: report of two cases, *Oral Sur Oral Med Oral Pathol Oral Radiol Endod* 60:356-367, 1985.

12. Hodder SC, Rees JL, Oliver TB, et al: SPECT bone scintigraphy in the diagnosis and management of mandibular condylar hyperplasia, *Br J Oral Maxillofac Surg* 38:87-93, 2000.

13. Murray IP, Ford JC: Tc-99m medronate scintigraphy in mandibular condylar hyperplasia, *Clin Nucl Med* 7:474-475, 1982.

14. Luz JG, de Rezende JR, Jaeger RG, et al: Microanatomic features of unilateral condylar hyperplasia, *Bull Group Int Rech Sci Stomatol Odontol* 37:87-92, 1994.

15. Eales E, Jones ML, Sugar AW: Condylar hyperplasia causing progressive facial asymmetry during orthodontic treatment: a case report, *Int J Paediatr Dent* 3:145-150, 1993.

16. Gray RJ, Horner K, Testa HJ, et al: Condylar hyperplasia: correlation of histological and scintigraphic features, *Dentomaxillofac Radiol* 23:103-107, 1994.

17. Obwegeser HL, Makek MS: Hemimandibular hyperplasia–hemimandibular elongation, *J Maxillofac Surg* 14:183-208, 1986.

18. Mutoh Y, Ohashi Y, Uchimaya N, et al: Three-dimensional analysis of condylar hyperplasia with computed tomography, *J Craniomaxillofac Surg* 19:49-55, 1991.

19. Kwon TG, Park HS, Ryoo HM, et al: A comparison of craniofacial morphology in patients

with and without facial asymmetry—a three-dimensional analysis with computed tomography, *Int J Oral Maxillofac Surg* 35:43-48, 2006.

20. Susarla SM, Dodson TB, Kaban LB: Measurement and interpretation of a maxillary occlusal cant in the frontal plane, *J Oral Maxillofac Surg* 66:2498-2502, 2008.

21. Ackerman JL, Ackerman MB, Brensinger CM, et al: A morphometric analysis of the posed smile, *Clin Orthod Res* 1:2-11, 1998.

22. Ackerman MB, Ackerman JL: Smile analysis and design in the digital era, *J Clin Orthod* 36:221-236, 2002.

23. Van Der Geld P, Oosterveld P, Berge SJ, et al: Tooth display and lip position during spontaneous and posed smiling in adults, *Acta Odontol Scand* 66:207-213, 2008.

24. Avinash K, Rajagopal K, Ramakrishnaiah R, et al: Computed tomographic features of mandibular osteochondroma, *Dentomaxillofac Radiol* 36:434-436, 2007.

25. Piert M, Zittel R, Becker GA, et al: Assessment of porcine bone metabolism by dynamic [18F]fluoride ion PET. Correlation with bone histomorphometry, *J Nucl Med* 42:1091-1100, 2001.

26. Saridin CP, Raijmakers PGHM, Kloet RW, et al: No signs of metabolic hyperactivity in patients with unilateral condylar hyperactivity: an in vivo positron emission tomography study, *J Oral Maxillofac Surg* 67:576-581, 2009.

Chapter

82

Mandibular Asymmetry: Temporomandibular Joint Degeneration

Larry M. Wolford

Facial asymmetry can occur in all three planes of space: vertical, transverse, and anteroposterior (AP) and usually in combinations of these. Facial asymmetry can involve one or more of the following four anatomic areas: dentoalveolar, skeletal, soft tissues, and the temporomandibular joint (TMJ). Possible causative factors for facial asymmetry include genetics, birth molding, congenital and developmental deformities, abnormal growth, tumors or other pathology of facial structures and jaws, TMJ pathology, trauma, neurologic or neuromuscular disorders/pathology, and iatrogenic injury, among others. A comprehensive diagnosis, including identification of the causative factors, as well as an inclusive treatment plan that will provide optimal treatment outcomes, can be achieved through a thorough and complete workup including history, clinical, radiographic, and dental model analysis as well as MRI, CT scan, cone beam imaging, and the like when indicated.

Traditionally, facial asymmetry has been classified as either overdevelopment or underdevelopment of the facial structures. Because of the complexities and etiologies of facial asymmetries, a comprehensive classification may be impossible. Hundreds of known syndromes can cause facial asymmetry,[1] so a discussion of all of them is beyond the scope of this chapter. This chapter focuses instead on the most common types of facial asymmetries, the diagnoses, evidence-based treatment, surgical options, and treatment outcomes.

Facial asymmetry is usually the least at the cranial base level and increases at lower levels of the face, with the mandible and chin commonly exhibiting the greatest asymmetry. Exceptions include cranial and craniofacial deformities such as plagiocephaly, unilateral

craniosynostosis, orbital dystopia, and tumors involving the cranium and midface. In most facial asymmetry cases, cranial base structures can be used as the base reference for determining the type and extent of the asymmetry affecting the midface and jaw structures (Fig. 82-1). The presence of orbital dystopia, unequal pupillary heights, or unequal ear heights will make the assessment more challenging. Detailed methodology of the author's comprehensive patient analysis and treatment planning has previously been published,[2,3] with specifics for facial asymmetry,[4] and will not be reiterated here.

TMJ AND FACIAL ASYMMETRY

TMJ disorders and pathology are common causative factors for, or the result of, facial asymmetries. Certain TMJ pathologies can produce a progressive worsening of the facial asymmetry and malocclusion, from minimal change to 4 to 5 mm or more per year depending on the nature of the pathology. Other TMJ conditions may only cause pain or dysfunction without worsening facial asymmetry, but may still need to be addressed for optimal pain relief, stability, and good functional and esthetic treatment outcomes. Condylar underdevelopment or condylar resorption can cause the mandible and face to be smaller on one side and shift toward that side. On the other hand, a unilateral condyle enlargement can cause overdevelopment of the mandible and associated structures, causing facial asymmetry. Performing orthognathic surgery *only* and ignoring the TMJ pathology during treatment or failure to render proper TMJ management for the specific pathology could result in the asymmetry and malocclusion redeveloping with worsening TMJ-associated symptoms including jaw dysfunction and pain.[5,6] The TMJs should always be evaluated in patients with facial asymmetry to determine if they are the etiologic factor, a problem that has developed because of facial asymmetry, a coexisting pretreatment condition, or normal and healthy joints.

Figures 82-1, 82-2, 82-3, 82-4, 85-5, 82-7C and D, 82-9, 82-10, 82-11, 82-12A to E, 82-13, 82-24, 82-25, 82-26 From Fonseca RJ, Marciani RD, Turvey TA: Oral and maxillofacial surgery, vol 3, ed 2, St Louis, Saunders, 2009.

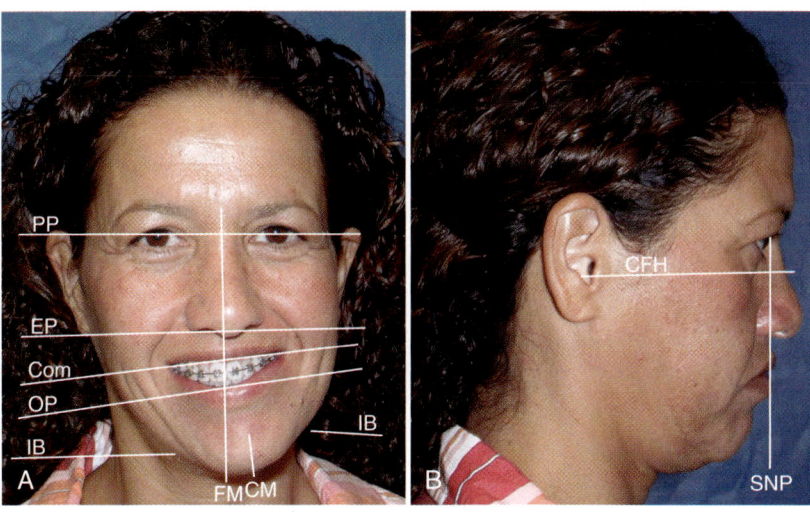

Fig. 82-1 ■ **A,** The pupillary and ear planes can usually be used as horizontal references. A perpendicular plane through nasion can be helpful in assessing the left to right facial asymmetry. The asymmetry is usually the least at the cranial base area and the worst at the mandible and chin area as seen in this 45-year-old female with a right mandibular condylar osteochondroma. PP, Pupillary plane; EP, Ear plane; Com, Commissure plane; OP, Occlusal plane; IB, Inferior border of mandible; FM, Facial Midline plane; and CM, Chin midline. **B,** The profile view is helpful to assess AP and vertical facial imbalance as well as to aid in the determination of etiology of the asymmetry. CFH, Clinical Frankfort horizontal plane; SNP, Subnasale perpendicular plane. (From Fonseca RJ, Marciani RD, Turvey TA: *Oral and maxillofacial surgery,* ed 2, vol 3, St. Louis, 2009, Saunders.)

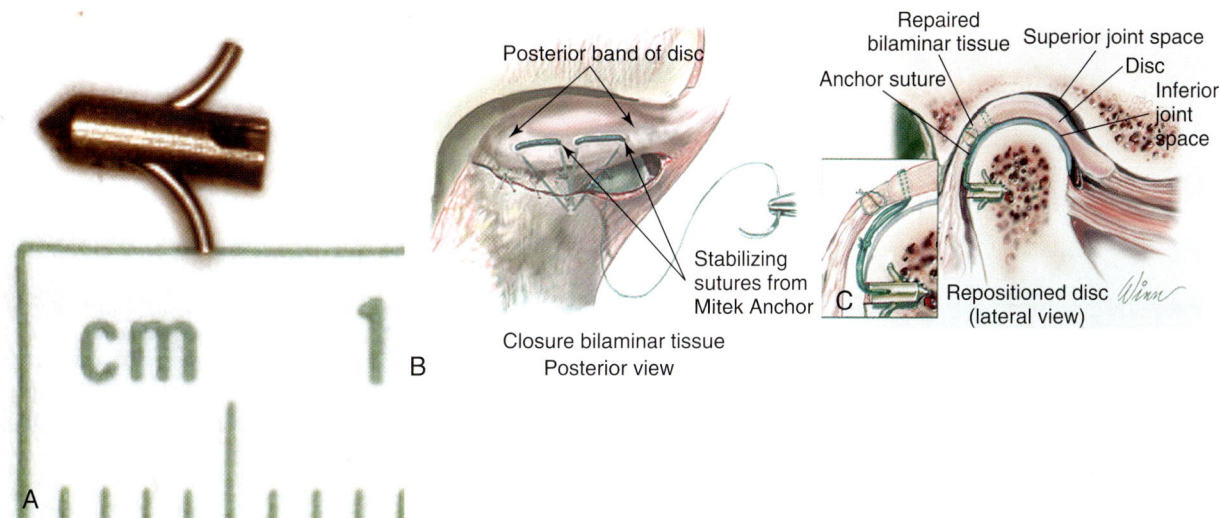

Fig. 82-2 ■ **A,** A common TMJ disorder is an anteriorly displaced articular disc. **B,** Posterior view of the condyle. The Mitek anchor is inserted in the posterior head of the condyle, 8 mm below the top and lateral to the midsagittal plane. Two 0-Ethibond sutures (Ethicon Inc., Summerville, New Jersey) supported by the anchor are passed through the posterior aspect of the posterior band of the disc to secure the disc in the proper position. **C,** Sagittal view. The anchor is in place with the artificial ligaments secured, stabilizing the disc into position. (From Fonseca RJ, Marciani RD, Turvey TA: *Oral and maxillofacial surgery,* ed 2, vol 3, St. Louis, 2009, Saunders.)

NUMBER AND TYPE OF PREVIOUS SURGERIES

The number of previous surgeries, particularly to the TMJ, may dictate the TMJ surgical procedure options. For example, patients with articular disc dislocation, with 0 to 1 previous TMJ surgeries, and without significant other joint or systemic disease involvement may benefit from articular disc repositioning and ligament repair with Mitek anchors (Mitek Products Inc., Westwood, Mass) to achieve a stable treatment outcome (Fig. 82-2).[7-9]

A patient with two or more previous TMJ surgeries will have a high failure rate if autogenous tissues are used for the TMJ reconstruction.[10,11] A patient-fitted TMJ total joint prosthesis, such as the TMJ Concepts system (TMJ Concepts Inc., Ventura, Calif) will have a much higher rate of success (see Fig. 82-13, *B*). End-stage TMJ conditions, such as connective tissue/autoimmune diseases, severe arthritis, ankylosis, severe TMJ damage from trauma, and failed TMJ alloplastic implants, will get the most predictable results with patient-fitted total joint prostheses[11-21] and fat grafts packed around the articulating components of the prostheses.[22-24]

AGE FOR SURGICAL INTERVENTION

Some facial asymmetry conditions may get worse with growth and development. Predictability of results and limiting correction of the jaw and TMJ-related deformities to one major operation can usually best be achieved by waiting until growth is relatively complete. Although there are individual variations, females usually have the majority of their facial growth (98%) complete by the age of 15 years and males by the age of 17 to 18 years. Performing surgery at earlier ages may result in the need for additional surgery at a later time to correct asymmetry and malocclusion that may develop during the completion of growth. There are definite indications for early surgery, such as ankylosis, growth center transplants (i.e., sternoclavicular or rib grafts), masticatory dysfunction, tumor

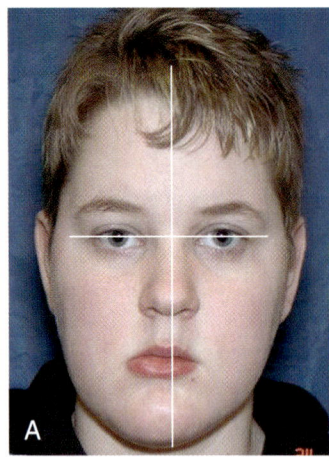
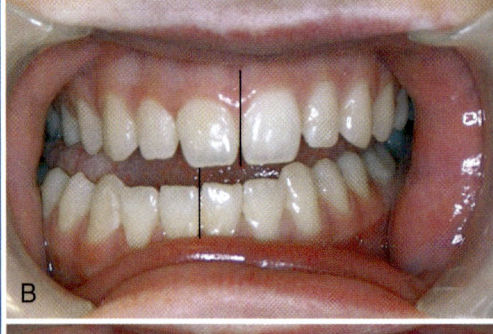
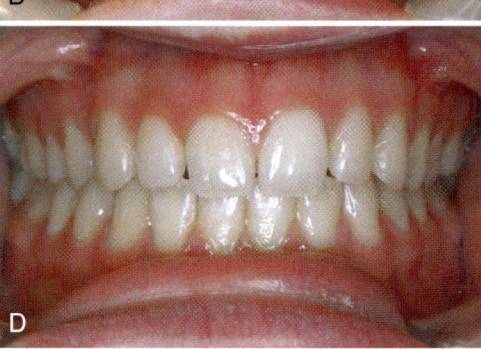
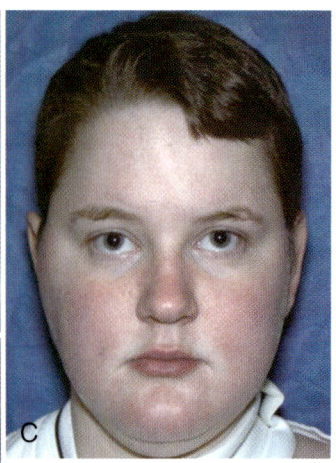

Fig. 82-3 ■ **A,** A 16-year-old female with Ehlers-Danlos syndrome has unilateral left muscular hyperdystonia causing a transverse shift of the mandible toward the right with the left condyle postured forward in the fossa. **B,** The occlusion will shift into a contralateral crossbite and usually into a class III occlusion with a posterior open bite on the ipsilateral side. **C,** The patient is seen 1 year after a unilateral left double Mitek anchor condylar plication technique.[53] **D,** The occlusion is stable and functional. (From Fonseca RJ, Marciani RD, Turvey TA: *Oral and maxillofacial surgery,* ed 2, vol 3, St. Louis, 2009, Saunders.)

removal, and airway obstruction. Wolford et al. have published reports on maxillary and mandibular surgery and the effects on growth, with guidelines for age when considering surgical intervention.[25,26]

For simplicity, facial asymmetry can be divided into four categories: (1) pseudo-asymmetry, (2) nonpathologic facial asymmetry, (3) unilateral overdevelopment, and (4) unilateral underdevelopment/degeneration.

PSEUDO-ASYMMETRY

Some patients may have pseudo-asymmetry where the mandible is postured asymmetrically toward one side with one condyle displaced forward relative to the centric relation position in the fossa, usually caused by occlusal interferences, neuromuscular dysfunction, habitual posturing, condylar dislocation, and the like (Fig. 82-3, *A, B*). Pseudo-asymmetry can also be caused by temporary unilateral facial swelling as a result of conditions such as facial trauma or infection, where the asymmetry resolves as the swelling dissipates. The most common pseudo-asymmetry conditions are discussed next.

MALOCCLUSION

Malocclusion may be the result of occlusal interferences in a TMJ centric relation position causing the mandible to shift toward one side for a better or more comfortable occlusal fit with one condyle postured forward in the fossa. These patients will exhibit a facial asymmetry with the mandible and chin shifted toward the contralateral side. Intraorally, there will be a class III occlusion on the side where the condyle is postured forward and a crossbite on the contralateral side. The facial, occlusal, and imaging appearance will be similar to the patient in Fig. 82-3, *A, B*. These patients may be asymptomatic, but some may experience muscle or TMJ pain and

headaches. The mandible can usually be shifted into a TMJ centric relation position with elimination of the facial asymmetry, but occlusal interferences may be present. Imaging will demonstrate a unilateral condyle postured forward in the fossa, similar to Fig. 82-4, *A.* Orthodontics and when indicated orthognathic surgery will usually correct the malocclusion.

NEUROMUSCULAR DYSFUNCTION (DYSTONIA)

A unilateral neuromuscular hyperfunction commonly involves the lateral pterygoid muscle, although other muscles can be contributory. The stimulus may be derived from malocclusion, neuromuscular disorder, myofascial pain, myositis, muscle spasm, reflex splinting, psychogenic origin, nutritional and electrolyte imbalances, drug induced, and so on. The onset is usually relatively sudden with muscle dysfunction on one side that displaces one condyle forward in the fossa and shifts the mandible off toward the opposite side, creating facial asymmetry (see Figs. 82-3, *A, B* and 82-4, *A*). These patients often experience pain, class III occlusal relation on the involved side, crossbite on the opposite side, and decreased range of motion. The mandible can usually be positioned into a TMJ centric relation position eliminating the facial asymmetry, but it likely won't stay there until the etiologic factors are resolved and muscles relaxed. Effective treatment methods may include muscle relaxants, ant-seizure medications, physical therapy, psychological intervention, eminoplasty, eminectomy, myotomy, Botox injections, Mitek anchor technique (Fig. 82-3, *C, D*), and so on.[27,28]

CONDYLAR DISLOCATION

Condylar dislocation occurs when the ligaments that normally keep the condyle within a normal functional range are ineffective because of laxity (i.e., cutis laxa, Ehlers-Danlos syndrome), stretched, torn, herniated, or degenerated. Condylar hypermobility or muscle dysfunction pulls the condyle anterior to the articular eminence where

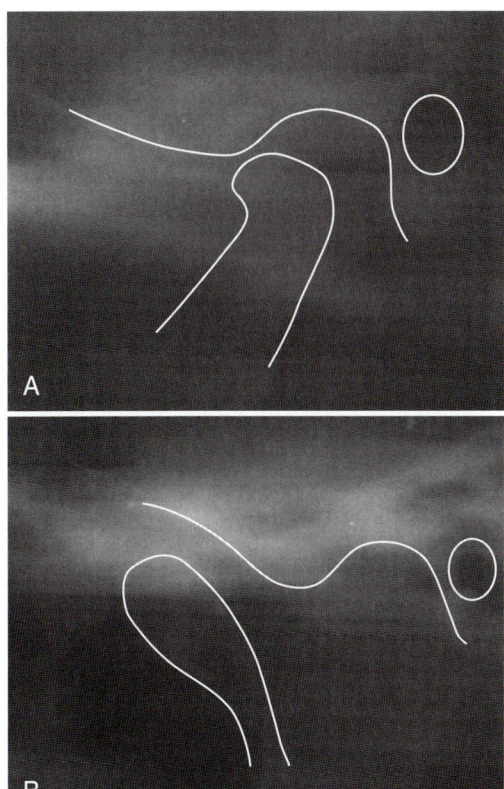

Fig. 82-4 ▪ **A,** The condyle on the ipsilateral side will be positioned forward in the fossa. **B,** Unilateral condylar dislocation may present a similar clinical picture as Fig. 82-3, **A-B** but with a more exaggerated asymmetry, and the condyle will be positioned anterior to the articular eminence. (From Fonseca RJ, Marciani RD, Turvey TA: *Oral and maxillofacial surgery,* ed 2, vol 3, St. Louis, 2009, Saunders.)

it may become locked. A unilateral anteriorly dislocated condyle shifts the mandible toward the opposite side. This can be a sudden onset or a chronic occurring condition, creating a significant functional impairment, facial deformity, malocclusion, and pain. The malocclusion will present as a class III relation on the involved side and a crossbite on the opposite side. The clinical appearance will be similar but more exaggerated compared to the patient in Fig. 82-3, *A*, *B*. Reduction and placing the condyle in a TMJ centric relation position will eliminate the facial asymmetry.

Radiographic imaging will show a unilateral condyle dislocated anterior to the articular eminence (Fig. 82-4, *B*). The dislocated condyle may reduce spontaneously or require physical manipulation back into the fossa. Medications, myotomy, eminectomy, eminoplasty, augmentation of eminence, sclerosing agents, Botox injection, and Mitek anchor technique are treatments that have been advocated to manage this condition when it is recurrent.[27,28]

INFECTION

Unilateral facial swelling can be caused by a bacterial or viral infection of dental structures, bones, soft tissues, glands, spaces, implanted devices, or foreign bodies. A unilateral infection usually presents with facial swelling, relatively quick onset, pain, induration, erythema, febrile, purulence, malaise, and increased white blood cell count.

Radiographic imaging such as MRI, CT scan, cone beam, or other imaging technology usually shows evidence of dental, bone, soft tissue, gland, implant, or foreign body involvement.

Treatment may include incision and drainage; culture and sensitivity; debridement and removal of infected teeth, hard and soft

tissue structures, devices, or foreign bodies; irrigation; and antibiotics and other medications or therapy as indicated. With proper treatment, resolution of the infection and asymmetry should be expected.

NONPATHOLOGIC FACIAL ASYMMETRY

Nonpathologic, nonsyndrome developmental facial asymmetry most commonly occurs as a result of genetics, intrauterine molding, or natural growth variance. The asymmetry is usually present at birth, but it may not be identified until later depending on the severity of the deformity. Growth usually maintains the asymmetry and does not get significantly worse. The occlusion (although it can be class I, II, or III) remains relatively constant. The extent of the deformity stops at completion of growth providing no TMJ pathology develops during the growth process. These deformities are usually less severe in degree of asymmetry and symptoms as compared to those that involve TMJ pathology. Some cases may demonstrate an asymmetry involving just the dental alveolus with the rest of the face being relatively symmetric.

Lateral and AP cephalometric radiographic analysis may show vertical asymmetry at the occlusal plane and mandibular inferior border and ramus. TMJ condyles may be relatively equal in size and shape without evidence of TMJ pathology or one condyle may be somewhat smaller but the proportion between the condyles should remain constant during growth. Orthodontics and orthognathic surgery may be required to correct skeletal and occlusal imbalances. Surgical treatment should be delayed until facial growth is essentially complete, particularly if maxillary surgery is required. Unilateral facial augmentation of hard or soft tissues may be necessary to optimize the treatment results.

DENTOALVEOLAR ASYMMETRY

Dentoalveolar asymmetry can involve the alveolar bone, teeth, and gingiva. Missing, unerupted, or ankylosed teeth, partial anodontia, unilateral alveolar or palatal clefts, radiation, tumor involvement, and abnormal growth, among other factors, can contribute to asymmetry. Ankylosed teeth can be induced by genetics, trauma, inflammation, excessive orthodontic forces, and so on as the catalyst for the bone to root fusion causing an adverse effect on dentoalveolar growth and development. Unilateral dentoalveolar asymmetry can include unilateral crossbite, buccal or lingual (Fig. 82-5, *A*); unilateral open bite or deep bite; transverse cant in the occlusal plane; AP, vertical, or transverse dental arch asymmetry; and so on.

Orthodontics is usually a necessary part of treatment and in some cases can correct the asymmetry. However, dentoalveolar surgery and orthognathic surgery may also be required, as well as restorative dentistry to obtain the best results (Fig. 82-5, *B*). Ankylosed teeth will act as an anchor, and if the involved tooth is out of alignment and tied into the orthodontic arch wire, the adjacent teeth will be displaced toward the malaligned ankylosed tooth. Treatment options for ankylosed teeth include luxating the ankylosed tooth (teeth) and immediate orthodontics or distraction, crowning, extraction with replacement, or osteotomies with single tooth or multiple teeth segments for repositioning or distraction. Dental implants and restorative dentistry can restore missing, decayed, and deformed teeth.

OVERDEVELOPMENT

Unilateral overdevelopment of the face can cause significant facial asymmetry, with the most common conditions including (1) condylar hyperplasia, (2) unilateral muscle hyperplasia, (3) tumors, and (4) neurologic and neuromuscular disorders. As each of these

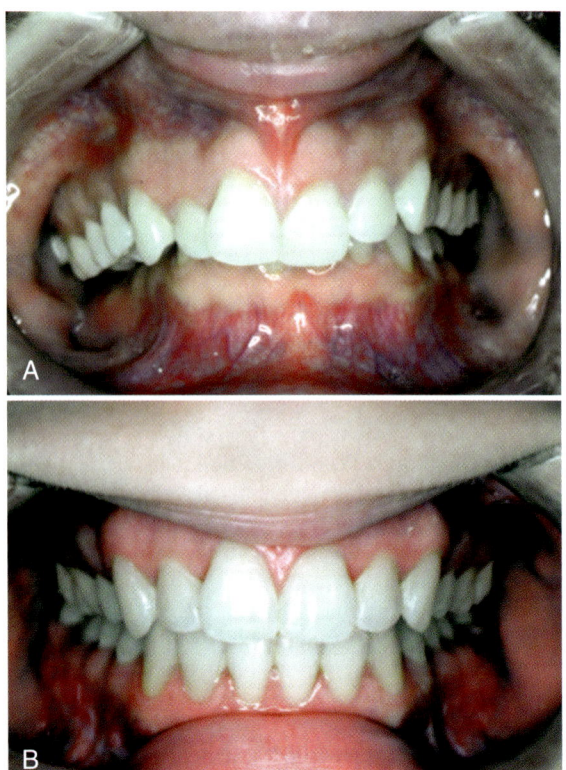

Fig. 82-5 ■ **A,** A dentoalveolar asymmetry deformity is seen in a 15-year-old female with a full right side buccal crossbite, as well as vertical and transverse asymmetry of the maxillary and mandibular dentoalveolus. **B,** The symmetric occlusion is seen after treatment following orthodontics and orthognathic surgery including bilateral mandibular ramus osteotomies, multiple maxillary osteotomies, and mandibular anterior and right posterior subapical osteotomies. (From Fonseca RJ, Marciani RD, Turvey TA: *Oral and maxillofacial surgery,* ed 2, vol 3, St. Louis, 2009, Saunders.)

pathologic conditions requires specific treatment protocols, it is important to have an accurate diagnosis.

Condylar hyperplasia (CH) refers to enlargement or overgrowth of the mandibular condyle. Several etiologies cause CH. Wolford has developed a simple classification system based on the specific pathology and rate of occurrence. CH type 1 refers to an accelerated and often prolonged overgrowth of the "normal" growth center of the condyle. CH type 1A refers to the bilateral condition, as it is the most commonly occurring form of CH, and CH type 1B refers to the unilateral form of the pathology. CH type 2 refers to the most common benign unilateral tumors, with CH type 2A designating osteochondromas and CH type 2B referring to osteomas. CH type 3 refers to any other pathology that causes condylar enlargement, with CH type 3A being other benign tumors and CH type 3B referring to malignant tumors.

CONDYLAR HYPERPLASIA (CH TYPE 1)

CH type 1 is a pathologic condition affecting the "normal" condylar growth center, causing an accelerated and prolonged overdevelopment of the mandible and creating mandibular prognathism and esthetic deformity (Fig. 82-6, *A-F*). CH type 1 usually begins during the pubertal growth phase, and the mandible can continue to grow at an accelerated rate but the growth is self-limiting and usually stops when affected individuals are in their mid-20s.[29-31] These patients usually begin with a class I skeletal and occlusal relationship and develop into a class III relationship, or start as class III but develop a worse class III relationship as the mandible grows

predominantly in a horizontal direction, although sometimes there can be a vertical growth vector. Asymmetry of the mandible can occur by unilateral (CH type 1B) or bilateral CH (CH type 1A) where one condyle grows faster than the opposite side. In this situation, the mandible becomes deviated toward the contralateral side; there is a class III occlusion on the ipsilateral side and a crossbite on the contralateral side; the mandible, mandibular dental midline, and chin are shifted toward the contralateral side; the mandible continues to grow asymmetrically beyond the normal growth years but usually will complete its development when these individuals are in their mid-20s. Disc displacement may occur on the "normal" contralateral side from increased joint loading created by the ipsilateral CH.

Although the condyle usually retains a relatively normal architecture, there is an increased length of the condylar head, neck, and mandibular body (Fig. 82-7, *A*). The normal pubertal growth rate from condylion to point B in females is a mean of 1.6 mm per year, with 98% of growth complete by the age of 15 years. Males grow at a mean rate of 2.2 mm per year, with 98% of growth complete by the age of 17 to 18 years.[25,26,32] The identification of sex hormone receptors in and around the TMJ and the pubertal onset of CH type 1 are strongly suggestive of a hormonal influence in the etiology. However, trauma, infection, heredity, intrauterine factors, and hypervascularity, have also been implicated as causative factors. Approximately one third of bilateral CH cases have a familial history.[33]

Histologic observations of CH type 1 condyles may appear similar to normal bony architecture, but in some cases the proliferative layer may demonstrate greater thickness in some areas and less in others; however cartilage-producing cells may be prevalent at its lower border. In normal condyles, the formation of cartilage from the proliferative layer and the replacement of cartilage by bone cease by approximately 20 years of age. The marrow cavity is entirely occluded from the remaining cartilage by the closure of the bone plate. The inability of this plate to close in the presence of an active proliferative cartilage layer may be a major etiologic factor in CH type 1.

Bone scans may not be of value in diagnosing CH type 1 because the growth rate is slow and continuous so there may not be much differentiation in the amount of isotope uptake compared to a normal joint. MRI may show a displaced articular disc on the contralateral side and sometimes on the ipsilateral side. Serial radiographs (lateral cephalograms, cephalometric TMJ tomograms), dental models, and clinical evaluations are usually the most advantageous methods to determine if the growth process is still active.

Treatment of this deformity varies depending on whether the growth is still active. If jaw growth has stopped, orthognathic surgical procedures can usually be performed to correct the asymmetry and malocclusion. However, if the patient is still a teenager or even in his or her early 20s, the growth process can be active and progressive. If there is confirmed active growth, then there are two predictable treatment options. The most predictable option is to perform a high condylectomy, removing 4 to 5 mm of the top of the condylar head on the involved side (both sides for bilateral CH), reposition the articular disc over the remaining condyle using the Mitek anchor technique (Fig. 82-7, *C, D*), and perform the appropriate orthognathic surgery to correct the associated dentofacial deformity (Fig. 82-7, *B*).[30,31] This can be done in one operation or divided into two operations, but the TMJ surgery must be performed first. This is a highly predictable treatment that will stop mandibular growth with long-term stable functional and esthetic outcomes (Fig. 82-6, *G-L*).[30,31] The recommended age for unilateral CH surgery is 15 years for females and 17 years for males. Performing a unilateral high condylectomy earlier will result in arresting the growth on the

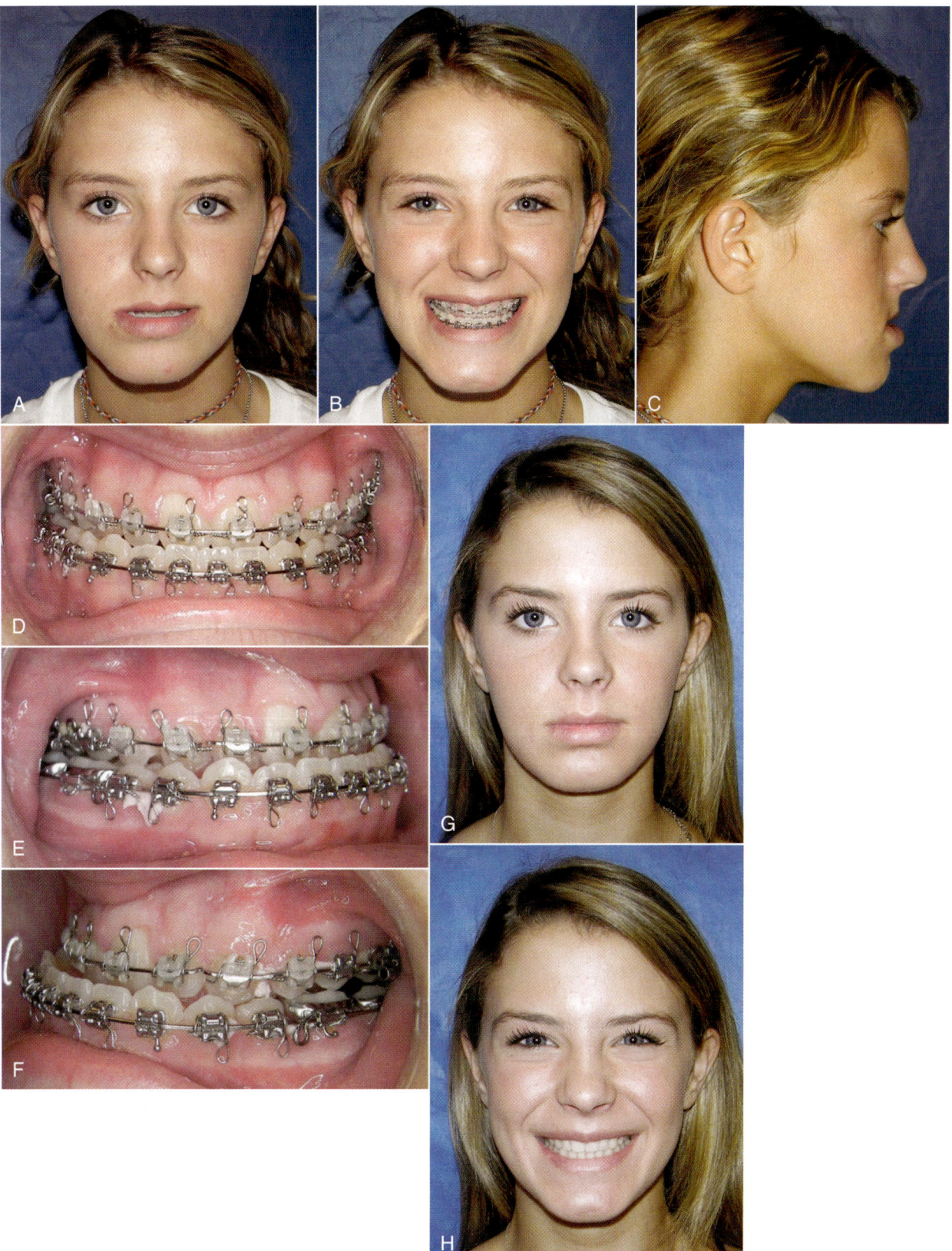

Fig. 82-6 ■ **A-F,** A 14-year-old female presents with active CH type 1A with the left side growing faster than the right side creating a progressive shift of the mandible toward the right side, class III occlusion that was greater on the left side, with a right posterior crossbite and apparent facial asymmetry. **G-L,** The patient 2 years after surgery demonstrating good facial balance and stability with elimination of the condylar hyperplastic growth pathology by the bilateral high condylectomies and double jaw orthognathic surgery performed in one operation.

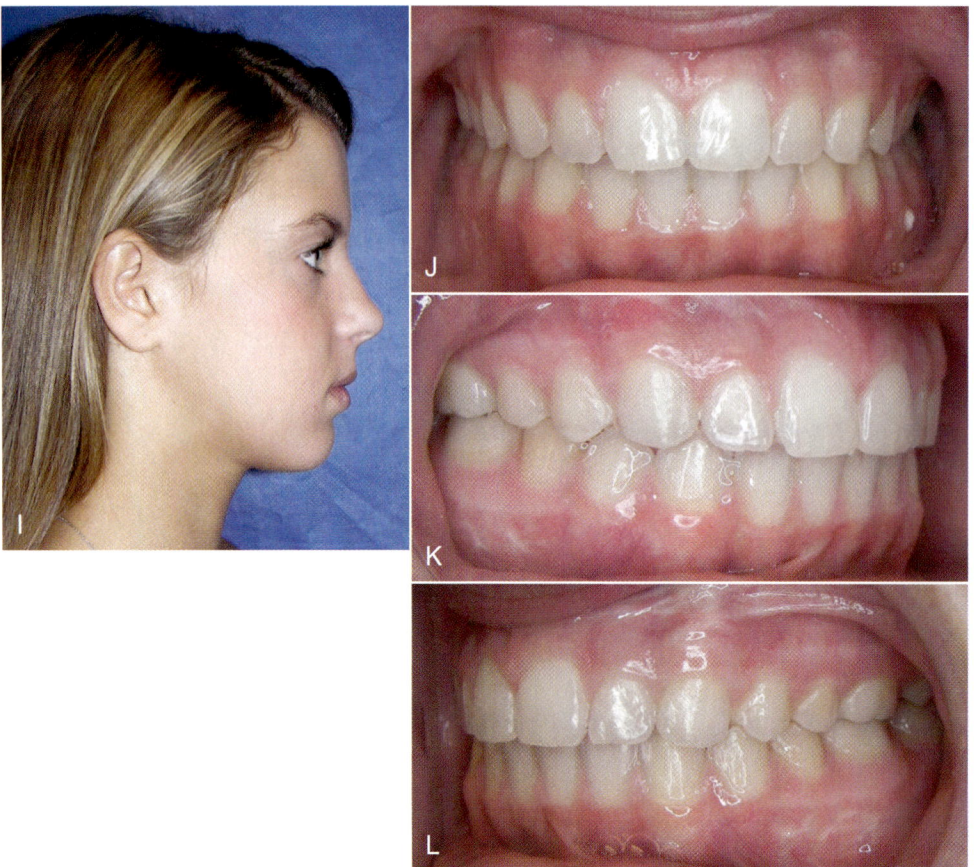

Fig. 82-6, cont'd.

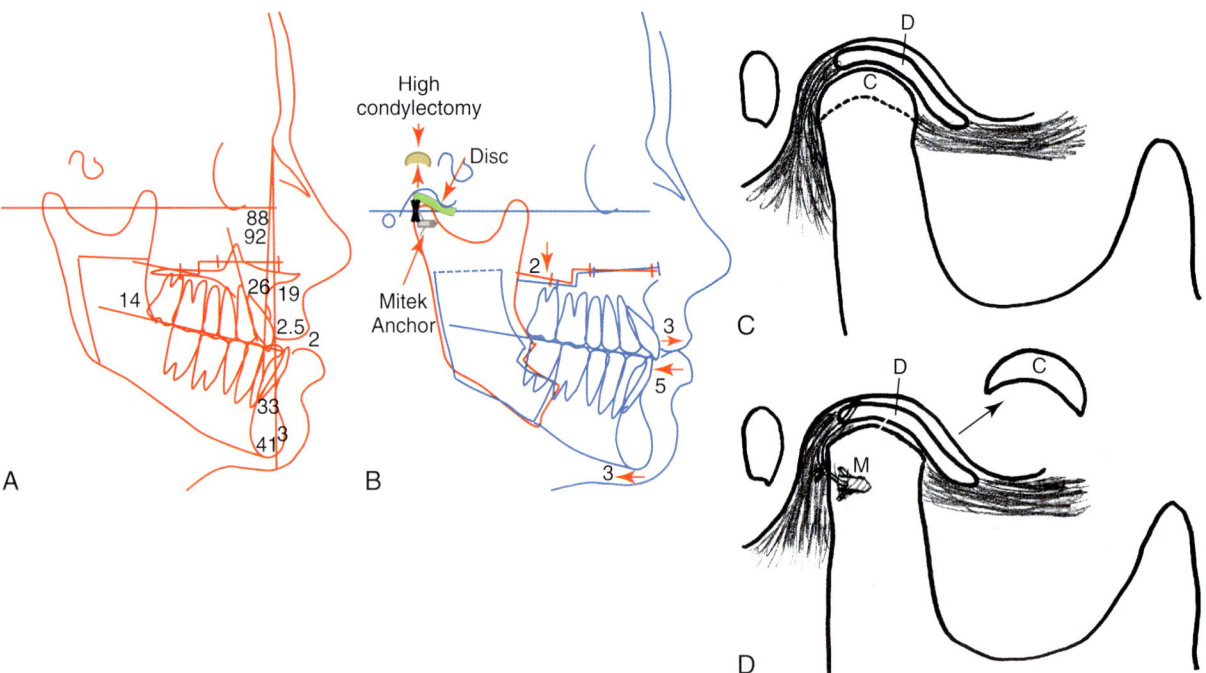

Fig. 82-7 ■ **A,** The cephalometric analysis of the patient in Fig. 82-6 demonstrates mandibular prognathism and elongated condylar heads and necks, consistent with condylar hyperplasia. She has a skeletal and occlusal class III relationship and a high occlusal plane angle. Her deformity was getting progressively worse with increasing facial asymmetry. **B,** The treatment plan consisted of bilateral high condylectomies with disc repositioning with Mitek anchors, bilateral mandibular sagittal split osteotomies, and multiple maxillary osteotomies. **C** and **D,** Treatment of active condylar hyperplasia includes high condylectomy removing the top 4 to 5 mm of the condyle with articular disc repositioning that will predictably stop the mandibular AP growth. The Mitek anchor (*M*) can be used to stabilize the articular disc. *C,* condyle. *D,* disc. (**C** and **D,** From Fonseca RJ, Marciani RD, Turvey TA: *Oral and maxillofacial surgery,* ed 2, vol 3, St. Louis, 2009, Saunders.)

CH side, but the normal side can continue to grow until normal cessation occurs, with the potential of causing asymmetry by the mandible shifting toward the original CH side.

The second option is to delay surgery until growth is complete. However, because these cases often continue to grow into the individual's mid-20s, the surgery would be delayed until it is confirmed that the growth has stopped. The longer the abnormal growth is allowed to proceed, the worse the facial deformity, asymmetry, and dental compensations will become, affecting both the hard and soft tissues. This may increase the difficulties in obtaining an optimal functional and esthetic result, as well as adversely affect the patient's psychosocial development.

MANDIBULAR CONDYLAR HYPERPLASIA TYPE 2: OSTEOCHONDROMA OR OSTEOMA

These benign tumors can occur in the mandibular condyle at any age, causing unilateral enlargement and deformity of the condyle and mandible and creating significant facial asymmetry.[34,35] These conditions have also been termed hemimandibular hyperplasia and hemimandibular elongation.[36] Osteochondromas (CH type 2A) have a proliferation of islands of cartilage and bone within the condylar head, creating the enlargement and often osteophytic outgrowths from the condyle. Osteomas (CH type 2B) are the overproliferation of bone within the condyle causing enlargement, but histologically they may appear as normal bone. In both of these conditions, the neck of the condyle usually increases in diameter as a response to the enlargement of the condylar head. The vertical height of the ipsilateral mandibular ramus and body increases as a result of the increased height of the condylar head and neck, with vertical alveolar bone growth as a natural response for the eruption of teeth trying to close the ipsilateral lateral open bite that commonly develops (Figs. 82-8, *A-F*, and 82-9, *A*). Additional features of CH type 2A and B include increased chin asymmetry vertically and transversely; ipsilateral lateral open bite particularly in more rapid-growing pathology; compensatory ipsilateral maxillary down growth; transverse cant in the occlusal plane; and sometimes TMJ clicking, popping, pain, and headaches, if the contralateral side has arthritic changes and a displaced articular disc from the functional overload caused by the ipsilateral pathology.

The highly predictable treatment protocol for CH type 2 includes performing an ipsilateral low condylectomy (Fig. 82-9, *B*); reshaping the remaining condylar neck to function as the new condyle; repositioning the articular disc over the remaining condylar neck and repositioning the articular disc on the contralateral side, if displaced, with the Mitek anchor technique; performing orthognathic surgery to correct the maxillary and mandibular asymmetries; and performing an inferior border ostectomy on the ipsilateral side if indicated, with preservation of the inferior alveolar nerve, to reestablish vertical balance of the mandible (Fig. 82-8, *G-L*).[34] This treatment approach will allow removal of the tumor yet still use the enlarged condylar neck as the new condyle. Other treatment considerations include condylar replacement with a total joint prosthesis or autogenous tissues such as sternoclavicular or rib grafts, free bone grafts, and pedicled osseous grafts.[35,37]

MUSCLE HYPERTROPHY

Excessive unilateral hyperfunction of the muscles of mastication can result in hyperplasia and enlargement of the masseter or temporalis muscles. The mandible may develop an outward curvature of the angle created by the constant tension of the hyperfunctioning masseter muscle. Patients with this condition often have a history of clenching/bruxism and stress. Repetitive unilateral clenching builds up the muscle causing the enlargement, although commonly this condition occurs bilaterally. When this condition occurs unilaterally, it will demonstrate unilateral masseteric or temporalis muscle enlargement with increased soft tissue volume of the face in the involved muscle areas. Having the patient clench will usually show significant enlargement of the involved muscle as compared to the contralateral side.

PA cephalogram may show outward curvature on the angle of the mandible on the ipsilateral side. MRI and CT scan will show enlargement of the involved muscles compared to the opposite side. Treatment can include muscle relaxants, antiseizure medications, biofeedback therapy, Botox injection, muscle resection, bone recontouring, and so on.

NEUROMUSCULAR DISORDERS

The most common unilateral facial neuromuscular disorders involve adverse effects on the facial nerve, cranial nerve (CN) VII, resulting in partial or complete unilateral facial paralysis that can create an increased soft tissue thickening. These conditions include CN VII trauma, Bell's palsy, Ramsey-Hunt syndrome, Möbius syndrome, middle ear or mastoid infections, tumors, cerebral vascular accidents, and bacterial or viral infections affecting the facial nerve (Fig. 82-10). Bell's palsy is commonly caused by an immune or viral disorder creating swelling and subsequent compression of the CN VII as it passes through the temporal bone resulting in ischemia and paresis.[38] Surgical trauma to CN VII or its branches can also occur as a result of extraoral approaches for tumor removal, orthognathic surgery, trauma, TMJ surgery, and so on. Clinical features include usually a sudden onset; unilateral facial paralysis, partial or complete; possibly increased fullness of the soft tissues on the ipsilateral side likely related to loss of muscle tone and decreased function of the lymphatic system; and an asymmetric smile. The condition may or may not resolve (see Fig. 82-10).

Standard x-rays, tomograms, CT scans, and MRI exams may show pathologic conditions such as cranial base fractures, infections, or tumors that may be causative factors for some of these disorders but will not be particularly beneficial for immune, viral, or congenital causes. If the nerve is stretched, bruised, or compressed from trauma or surgery, without irreversible damage, then the neuromuscular disorder should eventually resolve. For some of these conditions (e.g., Bell's palsy, Ramsey-Hunt, and Möbius syndrome), there is no treatment that will predictably provide significant improvement with return of normal function. Steroids can be used with a relatively quick onset of the facial paralysis. Eye lubrication and eye patching may be indicated to prevent ocular damage. In severe cases, a tarsorrhaphy may be indicated. If physical impingement is present, then surgical decompression of CN VII may be warranted. Transection or crush injuries to the nerve may require surgical repair or reconstruction, including nerve grafting, cross-face nerve grafting, nerve crossover, neuromuscular grafts, and muscle or fascia slings.[39]

TUMOR

Tumors are benign or malignant pathology affecting bone or soft tissues. Tumors usually have a relatively slow development, firm enlargement, and are not painful until advanced. If numbness, paralysis, or significant pain develops, regardless of whether there is facial enlargement, then malignancy must be strongly considered. Unilateral facial enlargement (Fig. 82-11, *A, B*) occurs with expansile hard or soft tissue tumors (i.e., fibrous dysplasia, Paget's disease of bone, Sturge-Weber syndrome, neurofibromatosis, ameloblastoma, lymphangioma, hemangioma, or any other type of expansile tumor or pathology).

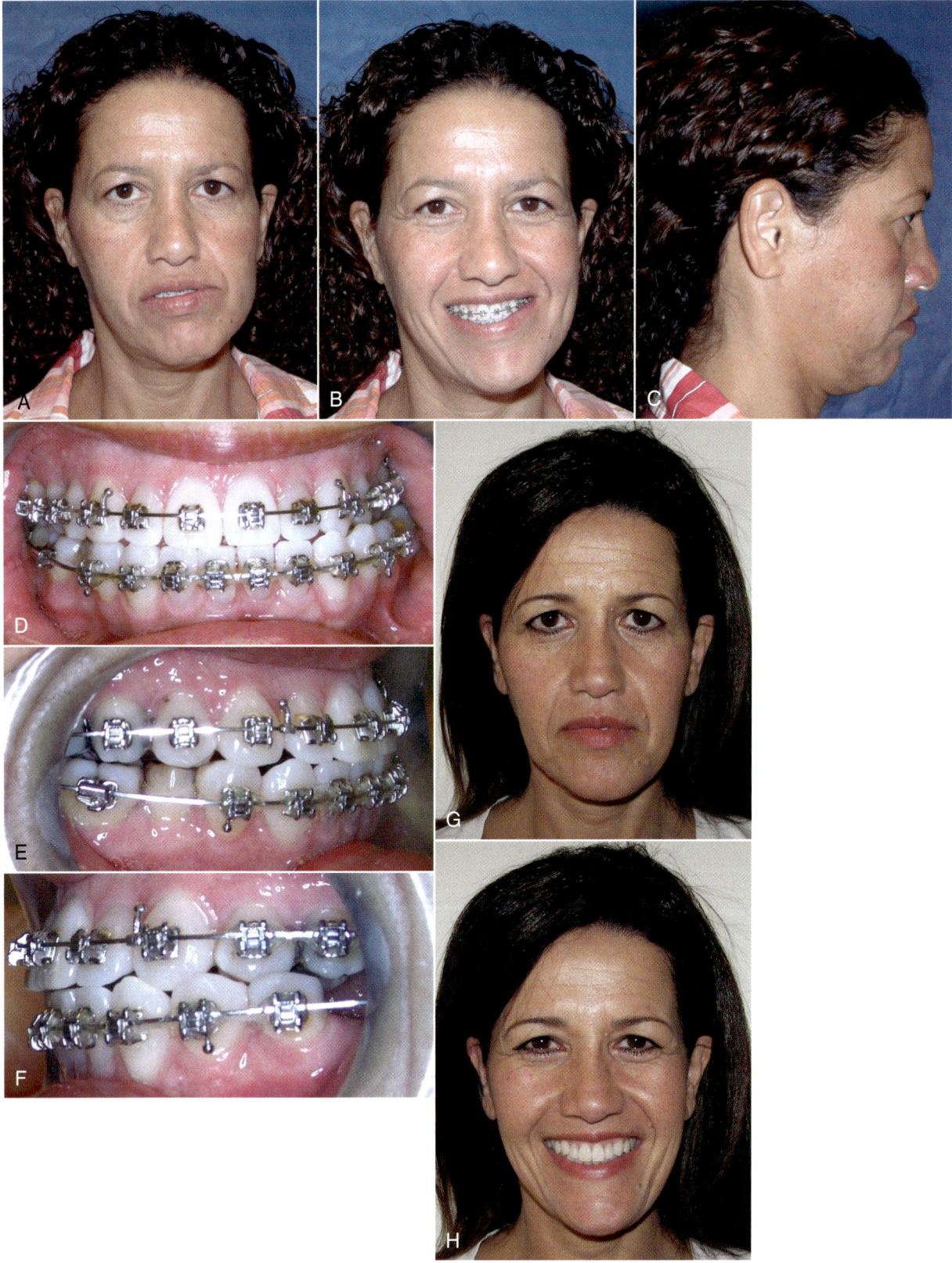

Fig. 82-8 ■ **A-F,** A 45-year-old female had a right-sided mandibular condylar osteochondroma causing severe vertical elongation of the right side of the face and transverse facial asymmetry. She has a posterior open bite tendency on the right side. **G-L,** The patient had a right low condylectomy, articular disc repositioning, multiple maxillary osteotomies, bilateral mandibular ramus osteotomies, and right inferior border ostectomy. She is seen at a 4 ½ year follow-up with no recurrence of the pathology and good facial balance and occlusion.

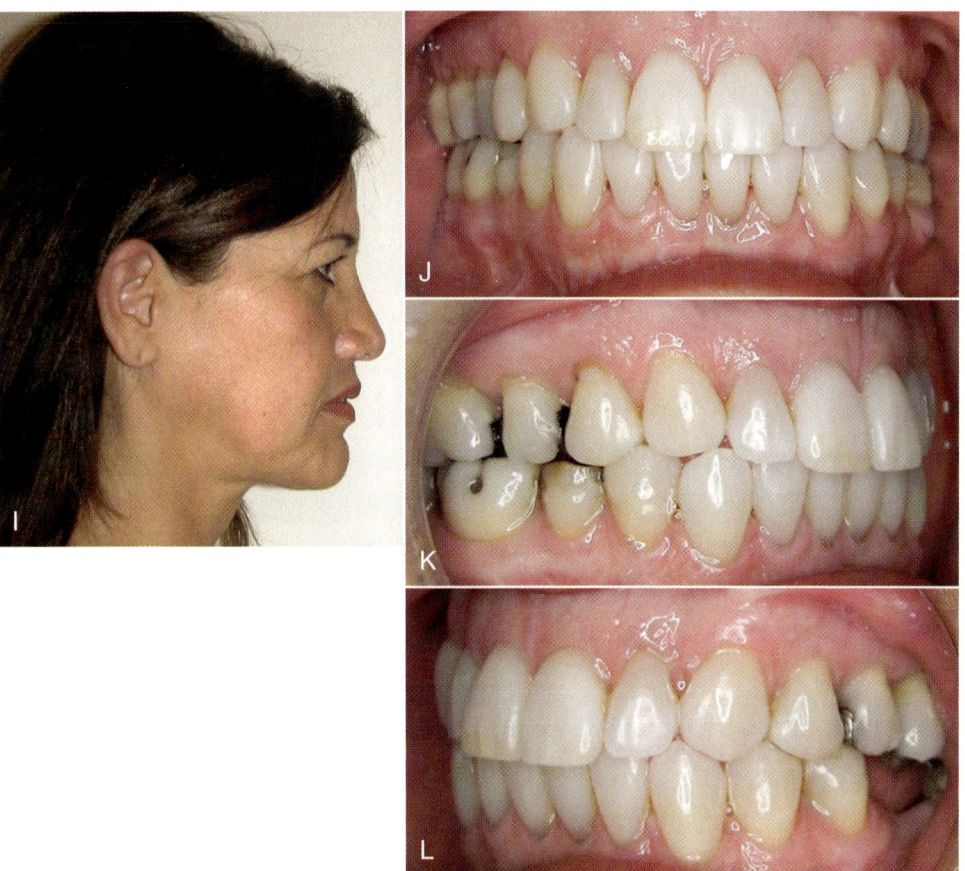

Fig. 82-8, cont'd.

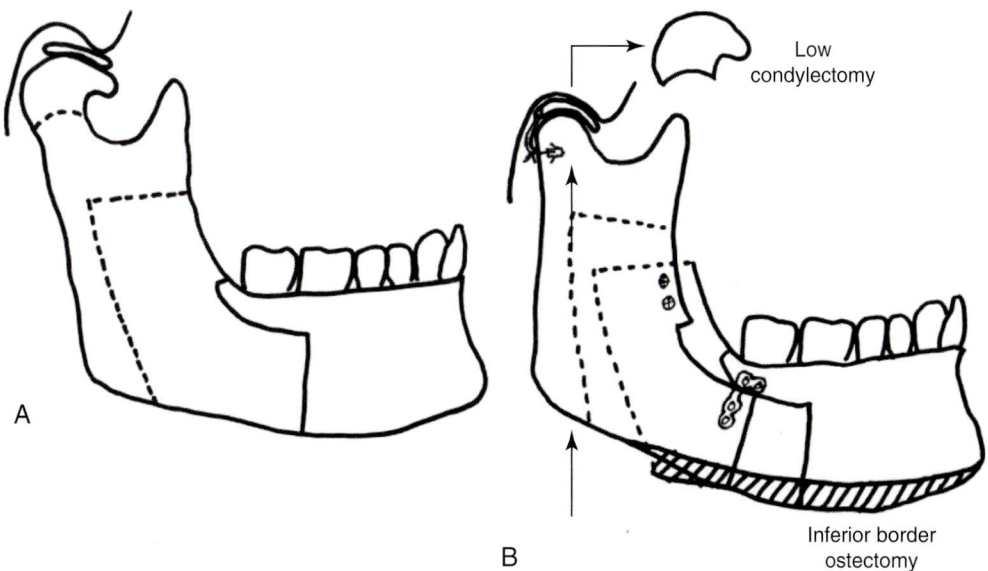

Fig. 82-9 ■ A, The right condyle and vertical height of the mandible are considerably larger than the left side. B, A low condylectomy with articular disc repositioning will predictably stop the pathologic growth process of an osteochondroma or osteoma and shorten the vertical height of the mandible on the ipsilateral side. Orthognathic surgery can be done at the same operation, usually requiring maxillary and mandibular osteotomies. An ipsilateral inferior border ostectomy will reestablish vertical symmetry of the body height. (From Fonseca RJ, Marciani RD, Turvey TA: *Oral and maxillofacial surgery*, ed 2, vol 3, St. Louis, 2009, Saunders.)

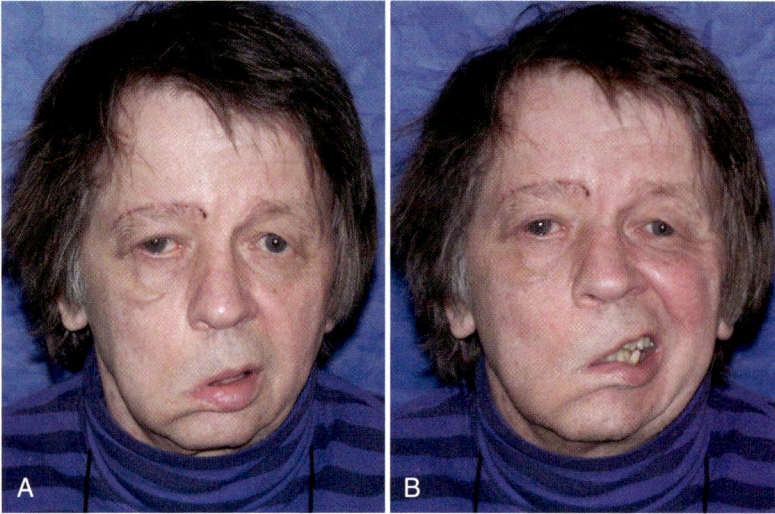

Fig. 82-10 ■ **A,** A 58-year-old man who suffered a stroke 1 year earlier, paralyzing the right side of his face. He has increased soft tissue fullness because of loss of muscle tone and decreased function of the lymphatic system. **B,** Smiling exaggerates the asymmetry. (From Fonseca RJ, Marciani RD, Turvey TA: *Oral and maxillofacial surgery,* ed 2, vol 3, St. Louis, 2009, Saunders.)

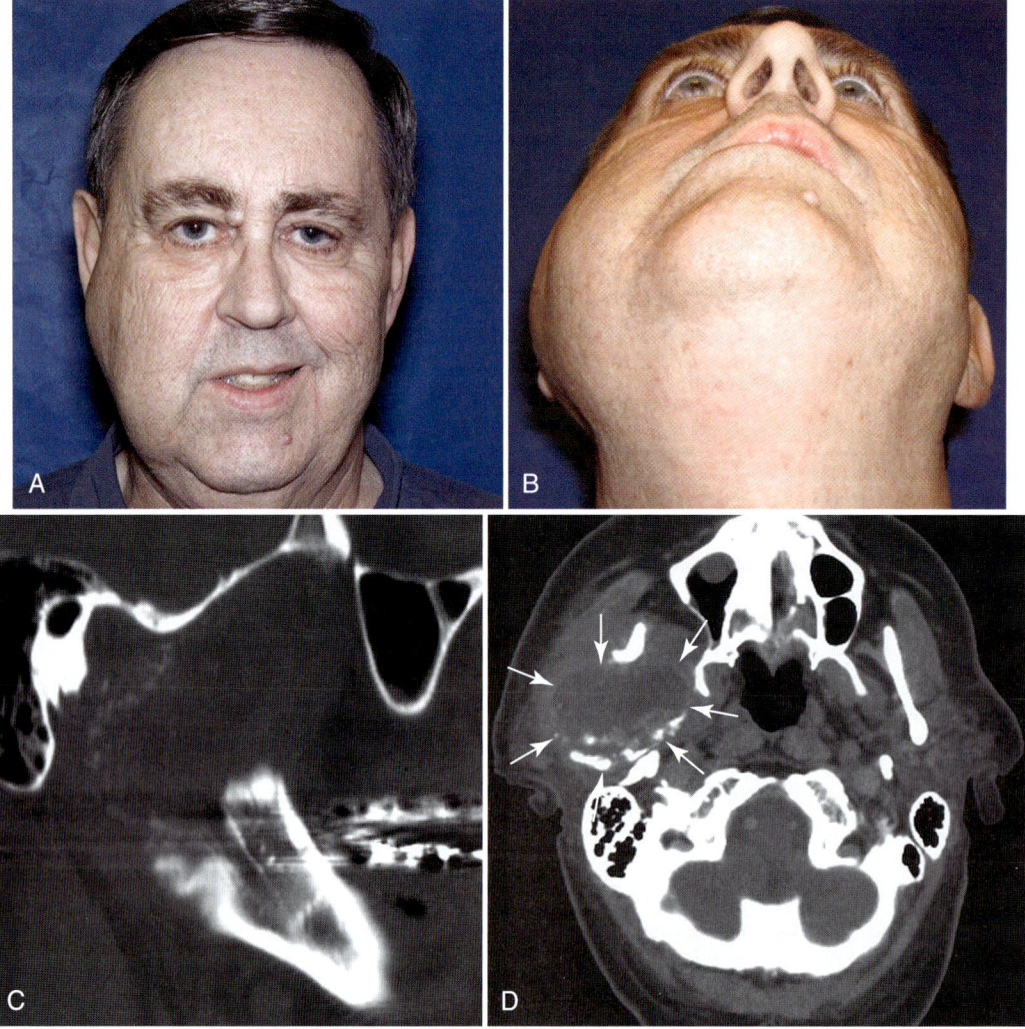

Fig. 82-11 ■ **A and B,** A 56-year-old man developed a progressive right-sided facial swelling over the past year. He complained of pain and was beginning to develop facial nerve paralysis. **C,** Radiographic evaluation revealed significant bony destruction of the right mandibular condyle and ramus. **D,** Arrows outline the tumor on the axial film. He was diagnosed with a metastatic carcinoma. (From Fonseca RJ, Marciani RD, Turvey TA: *Oral and maxillofacial surgery,* ed 2, vol 3, St. Louis, 2009, Saunders.)

Radiographs will usually show bone destruction or deposition when the skeletal structures are involved (Fig. 82-11, *C, D*). MRI, CT scans, and bone scans may show bone or soft tissue involvement. Treatment will depend on the nature and extent of the pathology, benign or malignant, structures involved, age of patient, and other medical conditions present, as well as other factors. In most cases, treatment may include removal of the tumor or pathologic process with appropriate adjunctive treatment for the specific pathologic process. Treatment planning should include consideration for jaw or TMJ reconstruction when indicated.

UNILATERAL FACIAL UNDERDEVELOPMENT OR DEGENERATION

The most common causes of unilateral facial underdevelopment or degeneration include the following:

- Acquired: that is, trauma, infection, ankylosis, iatrogenic (e.g., tumor resection, radiation, unstable orthognathic procedure, adverse surgical event, etc.), failed TMJ alloplastic implants such as Proplast/Teflon devices (Vitek Inc., Houston, Tex, USA) and Silastic (Dow-Corning Inc., Midland, Mich.), failed autogenous tissue grafts, and so on
- Congenital deformities (i.e., unilateral cleft lip and palate, hemifacial microsomia, Treacher-Collins)
- Adolescent internal condylar resorption (AICR)
- TMJ reactive (inflammatory) arthritis
- Connective tissue/autoimmune diseases

TRAUMA

Traumatic injuries usually develop facial asymmetry as a result of unilateral condylar or subcondylar fractures, multiple mandibular or midfacial fractures that are inadequately reduced. The mandible is more commonly involved compared to the midface. Patients with a unilateral displaced subcondylar fracture may exhibit the following: mandible deviated toward the affected side, pain and jaw dysfunction, deficient growth on the affected side when occurring in growing patients, class II skeletal and occlusal relationships, premature contact and crossbite on the ipsilateral side, open bite tendency anteriorly and on the contralateral side, and chin shifted toward the ipsilateral side (Fig. 82-12, *A-E*).

Imaging may show evidence of a subcondylar fracture with the condyle malpositioned downward, forward, and medial to the fossa with decreased vertical ramus/condyle length (Fig. 82-13, *A*). At the initial presentation of the trauma, the options for treating facial fractures are open reduction, closed reduction, or no treatment. The amount of displacement and the condition of the fracture(s) will affect the treatment. When identified early, fractures may be best treated by open reduction for moderate to significantly displaced segments or closed reduction for minimally displaced segments to achieve a symmetric face, stable occlusion, and good growth potential in growing patients. If the condylar segment is not significantly displaced, it may be upright and grow relatively normally with conservative, nonsurgical management. If the condyle is minimally to moderately displaced, still salvageable along with its articular disc but already healed, then it is possible that orthognathic surgery could realign the jaw structures properly. If the condyle is severely deformed and nonsalvageable, then reconstruction of the TMJ and mandible may be indicated using a total joint prosthesis (Figs. 82-13, *B*, and 82-12, *F-J*), sternoclavicular or rib graft. If a unilateral condylar or subcondylar fracture occurs during the growth years, a significant asymmetry can develop that also can involve the maxilla with the development of a transverse occlusal cant and class II occlusion with an increased occlusal plane angle. Open reduction of displaced subcondylar fractures in growing patients may circumvent the potential growth issues.

IATROGENIC FACIAL ASYMMETRY

These conditions can occur as a result of tumor resection without immediate reconstruction; surgical misadventures as in orthognathic surgery, TMJ surgery, or trauma surgery (inadequate reduction of facial fractures, soft tissue injuries); radiation therapy in growing patients; facial nerve damage associated with previous surgery; and so on. Clinical features will depend on the nature of the iatrogenic insult.

Imaging features will also depend on the nature of the iatrogenic insult, but they could involve the TMJ, bone, teeth, and soft tissues of the head and neck area. Treatment will depend on the nature of the deformity and the necessary procedures to correct and reestablish facial symmetry. Surgical misadventures in orthognathic, TMJ, and trauma surgery as well as secondary reconstruction following tumor resection or radiation therapy and the like may require osteotomies, bone grafting, hard and soft tissue augmentation or grafting, flap procedures, TMJ surgery, dental implants, restorative dentistry, and similar treatments to achieve optimal outcomes.

TMJ ANKYLOSIS

TMJ ankylosis usually develops as a result of trauma, inflammation, sepsis, or systemic diseases.[40] Fibrous ankylosis usually allows some rotational jaw opening but no translation. Bony ankylosis is caused by bony fusion or by reactive or heterotopic bone formation between or around the condyle and fossa, causing severely limited jaw function as well as oral hygiene and nutritional problems. When this condition occurs during the growing years, it can severely affect jaw growth and development. In unilateral ankylosis, the other joint will continue to grow but may be retarded in its true growth potential. The common clinical and radiographic characteristics of unilateral TMJ ankylosis, particularly when occurring in children, include decreased jaw mobility and function, decreased growth on the involved side, facial asymmetry with the mandible shifted toward the ipsilateral side, retruded mandible, decreased vertical height of the maxilla and mandible on the ipsilateral side, usually a class II occlusion and crossbite tendency on the ipsilateral side, transverse cant in the occlusal plane (Fig. 82-14, *A-F*), evidence of bony ankylosis between the condyle and the fossa, and decreased oropharyngeal airway (Fig. 82-15, *A, B*).

The most predictable treatment for the ankylosed TMJ patient includes release of the ankylosed joint; removal of the heterotopic and reactive bone with thorough debridement of the TMJ and adjacent areas; reconstruction of the TMJ (and if indicated, advancement of the mandible) with a patient-fitted total joint prosthesis (TMJ Concepts system) (Fig. 82-15, *C*); ipsilateral coronoidotomy or coronoidectomy if the ramus is significantly advanced or vertically lengthened with the prosthesis; autogenous fat graft (harvested from the abdomen or buttock) packed around the prosthesis in the TMJ area; additional orthognathic surgery if indicated, including a ramus osteotomy on the contralateral side and maxillary osteotomies; and any additional adjunctive procedures indicated (genioplasty, rhinoplasty, turbinectomies, septoplasty, etc.) (Fig. 82-14, *G-L*).[11-21] In these cases it is absolutely necessary that fat grafts be packed around the articulating parts of the prosthesis to prevent the reoccurrence of heterotopic and reactive bone as well as to minimize fibrosis development.[22-24] Orthodontics can be performed presurgery in some cases by using bonded brackets on the teeth. In some cases

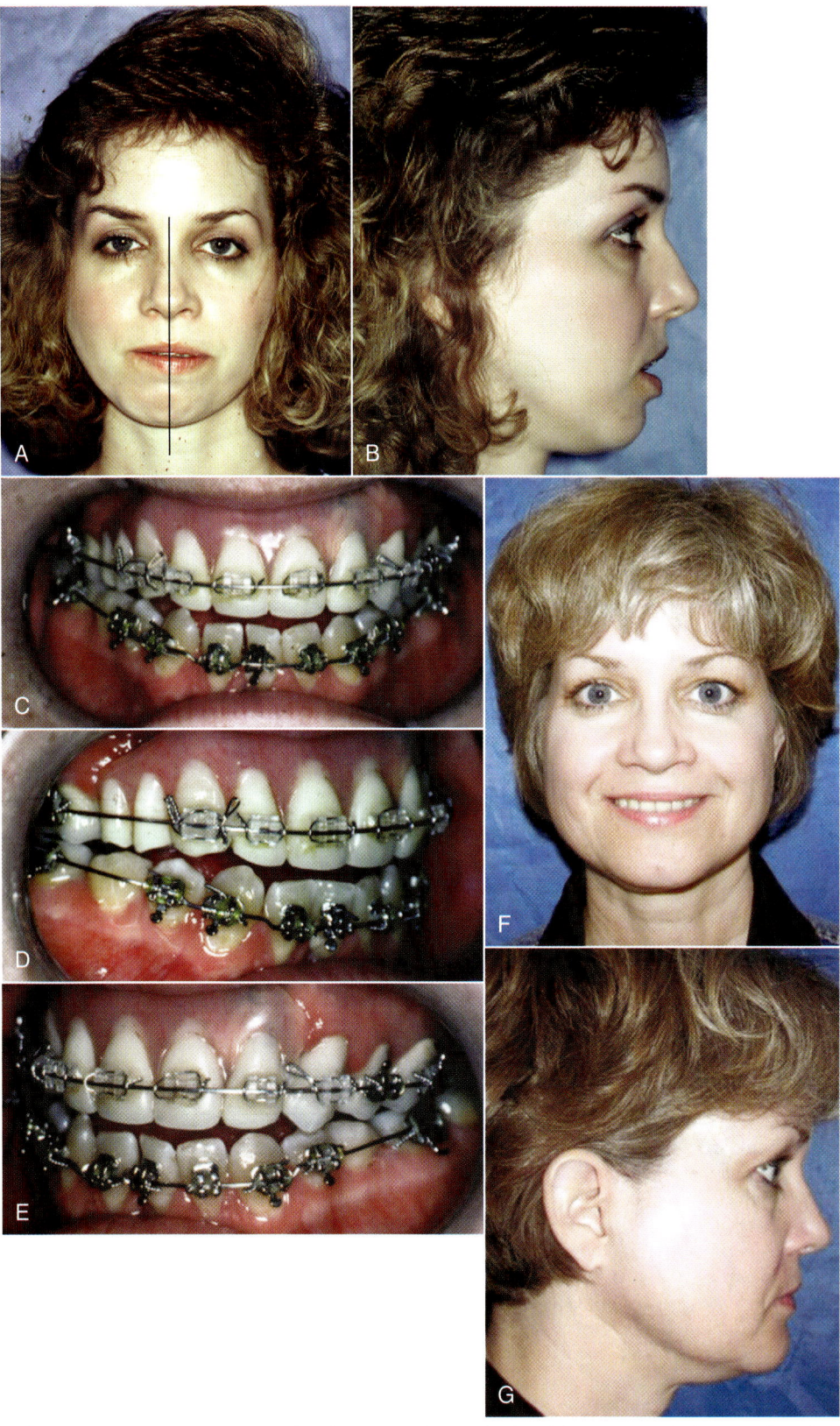

Fig. 82-12 ▪ **A-E,** A 27-year old-female sustained multiple facial fractures, including a right sub-condylar fracture with significant displacement, 4 years earlier. She lost most of her maxillary teeth, but they had been replaced with implants and prosthesis. She had severe pain, significant malocclusion, and facial asymmetry. **F-J,** The patient was treated with a TMJ Concepts total joint prosthesis to reconstruct the right TMJ and advance the mandible 14 mm. She had a unilateral left sagittal split osteotomy to advance that side and multiple maxillary osteotomies. She is seen 18 years postsurgery showing good facial symmetry and occlusion and remains pain-free. (**A-E,** From Fonseca RJ, Marciani RD, Turvey TA: *Oral and maxillofacial surgery,* ed 2, vol 3, St. Louis, 2009, Saunders.)

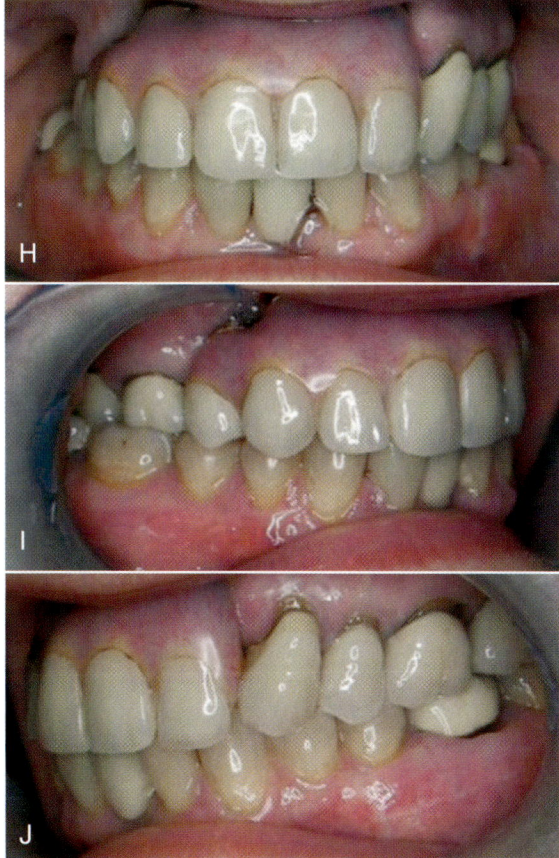

Fig. 82-12, cont'd.

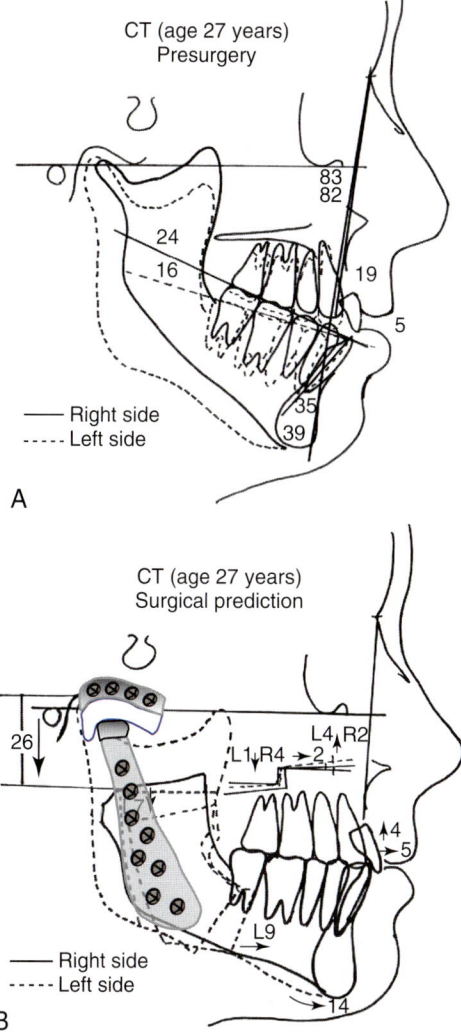

Fig. 82-13 ▪ **A,** Pretreatment lateral cephalometric tracing demonstrates the shortening of the right ramus secondary to the malunion of the subcondylar fracture and the AP mandibular deficiency. **B,** The surgical prediction tracing demonstrates the planned surgical movements to reestablish good facial symmetry and occlusion, reconstruct the right TMJ, and eliminate her severe pain and headaches. The right ramus was lengthened 26 mm with the TMJ Concepts total joint prosthesis. A left mandibular ramus sagittal split osteotomy and maxillary osteotomies were performed at the same surgery. (From Fonseca RJ, Marciani RD, Turvey TA: *Oral and maxillofacial surgery*, ed 2, vol 3, St. Louis, 2009, Saunders.)

it may be necessary to reconstruct the TMJ first, followed by secondary orthognathic surgery.

Other techniques that have been advocated for reconstruction of TMJ ankylosis include using autogenous tissues such as temporal fascia and muscle flaps, dermis-fat grafts rib grafts, sternoclavicular grafts, vertical sliding osteotomy, and so on.[40,41] The total joint prosthesis with a fat graft packed around it is a superior technique relative to prevention of reankylosis, provides jaw and occlusion stability, improves function, and eliminates or decreases pain. When treating young growing patients (10 years or older), the patient-fitted total joint prosthesis may still be the best option to eliminate the ankylosis. However, because there would be no growth potential on the ipsilateral side of the mandible (there is also no growth potential with a bony ankylosis), orthognathic surgery will likely be necessary but can be delayed until the patient has most of the facial growth complete (females age 15 years, males age 17 to 18 years). Then double jaw orthognathic surgery can be performed, including a ramus sagittal split on the side of the prosthesis to reposition the jaws into the best alignment, or the ipsilateral side can be advanced by repositioning the mandibular component of the prosthesis or fabricating a new, longer mandibular component.

HEMIFACIAL MICROSOMIA (HFM)

HFM is only one of hundreds of syndromes that can cause facial asymmetry, but it is one of the more common syndromes seen. It is also known as Goldenhar's syndrome, oculo-auriculo-vertebral spectrum, and branchial arch syndrome. HFM is present at birth, occurs sporadically in most cases, and can be considered as a nonspecific symptom complex that is etiologically and pathogenetically heterogeneous. Extreme variability of expression is characteristic of this disorder.[1] The condition usually occurs unilaterally but can occur bilaterally. Clinical and radiographic features of HFM usually include unilateral hypoplasia or aplasia of the mandible and condyle as well as hypoplasia of the maxilla, zygomatico-orbital complex, and temporal bone; decreased ipsilateral facial height; retruded chin deviated toward the ipsilateral side; eye, ear, and vertebral anomalies; class II malocclusion; premature contact on the ipsilateral side; transverse cant in the occlusal plane and skeletal structures; hypoeruption of the teeth on the ipsilateral side; significant soft tissue deficiency on the involved side affecting muscles, subcutaneous tissues, and skin volume, and a decreased oropharyngeal airway (Figs. 82-16, *A-F* and 82-17, *A*). With growth, the facial deformity, asymmetry, and malocclusion worsen.

The age at treatment can affect the treatment protocol. For instance, a hemifacial microsomia patient that is 6 to 12 years old with absence of the TMJ may benefit from a growth center

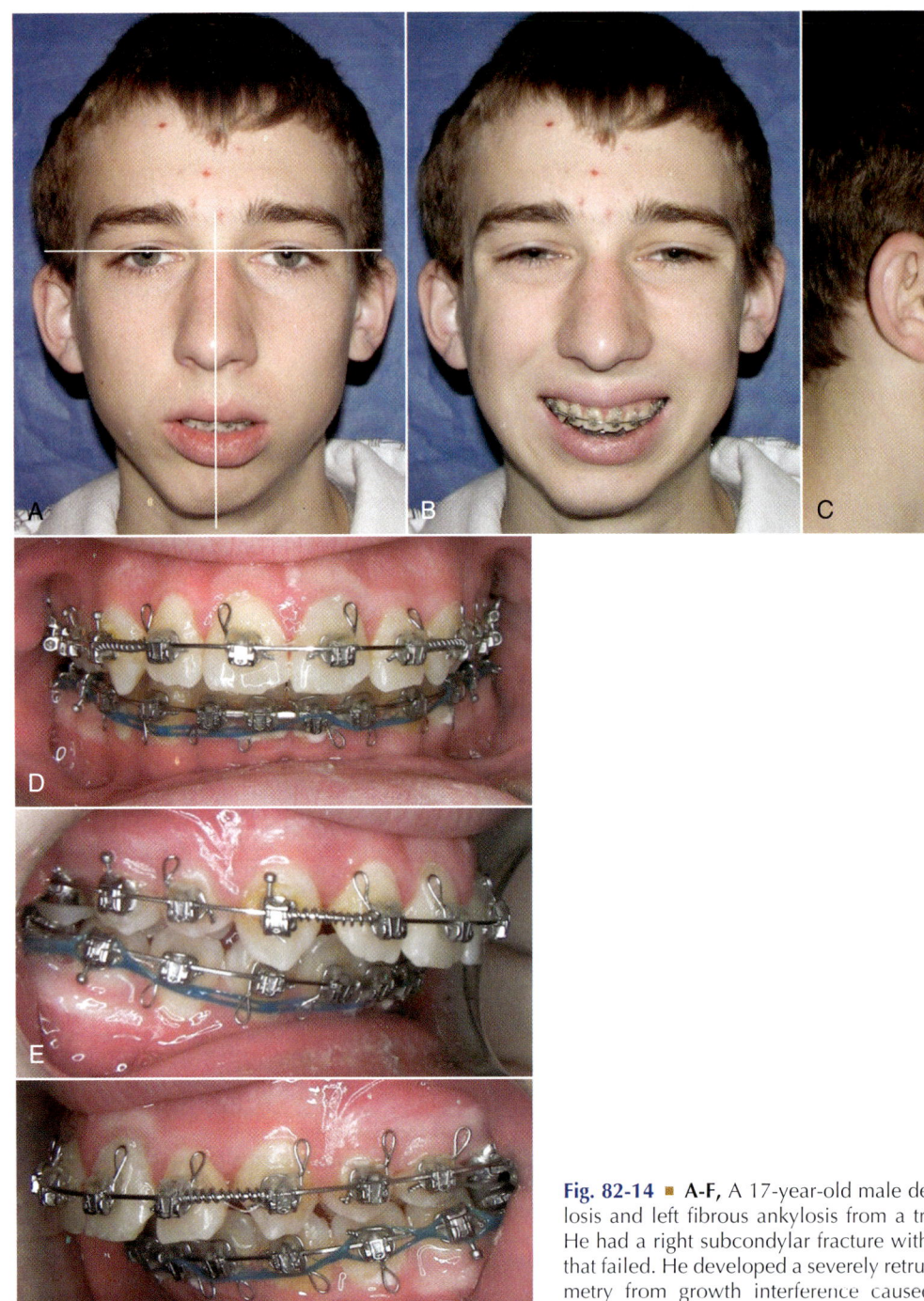

Fig. 82-14 ■ **A-F,** A 17-year-old male developed right TMJ bony anky-losis and left fibrous ankylosis from a traumatic injury at 8 years old. He had a right subcondylar fracture with an attempted open reduction that failed. He developed a severely retruded mandible and facial asym-metry from growth interference caused by the ankylosis; the right condyle was worse than the left side. He has a class II occlusion with a transverse cant.

transplant, using a sternoclavicular graft[42] or rib graft. The author has found rib grafts to be unpredictable relative to growth and stabil-ity. Sternoclavicular grafts tend to have better growth potential similar to normal TMJ growth. Rib grafts may overgrow or not grow at all. Orthognathic surgery may be necessary at a later age (follow-ing completion of growth) to maximize the functional and esthetic results. Teenage or older patients with significant deformity of the condyle and ramus may have a much better outcome using a patient-fitted TMJ total joint prosthesis (TMJ Concepts system) to advance and lengthen the ramus on the ipsilateral side (Fig. 82-17, C).[11-15,19,20] Deferring treatment until the patient is closer to completion of

facial growth (females 15 years old, males 17 to 18 years old) will help minimize subsequent contralateral normal growth effect on the treatment outcome. A mandibular ramus sagittal split osteotomy can be performed on the contralateral side and the indicated maxil-lary osteotomies completed as well as any other adjunctive proce-dures (genioplasty, rhinoplasty, turbinectomies, nasoseptoplasty) (Figs. 82-16, G-L, and 82-17, B). Additional reconstruction may be necessary using bone grafts, synthetic bone, alloplastic implants to build up the residual deformed skeletal structures. Soft tissue recon-structed using fat grafts, tissue flaps, free vascularized grafts may be necessary to fill out the soft tissue defects.

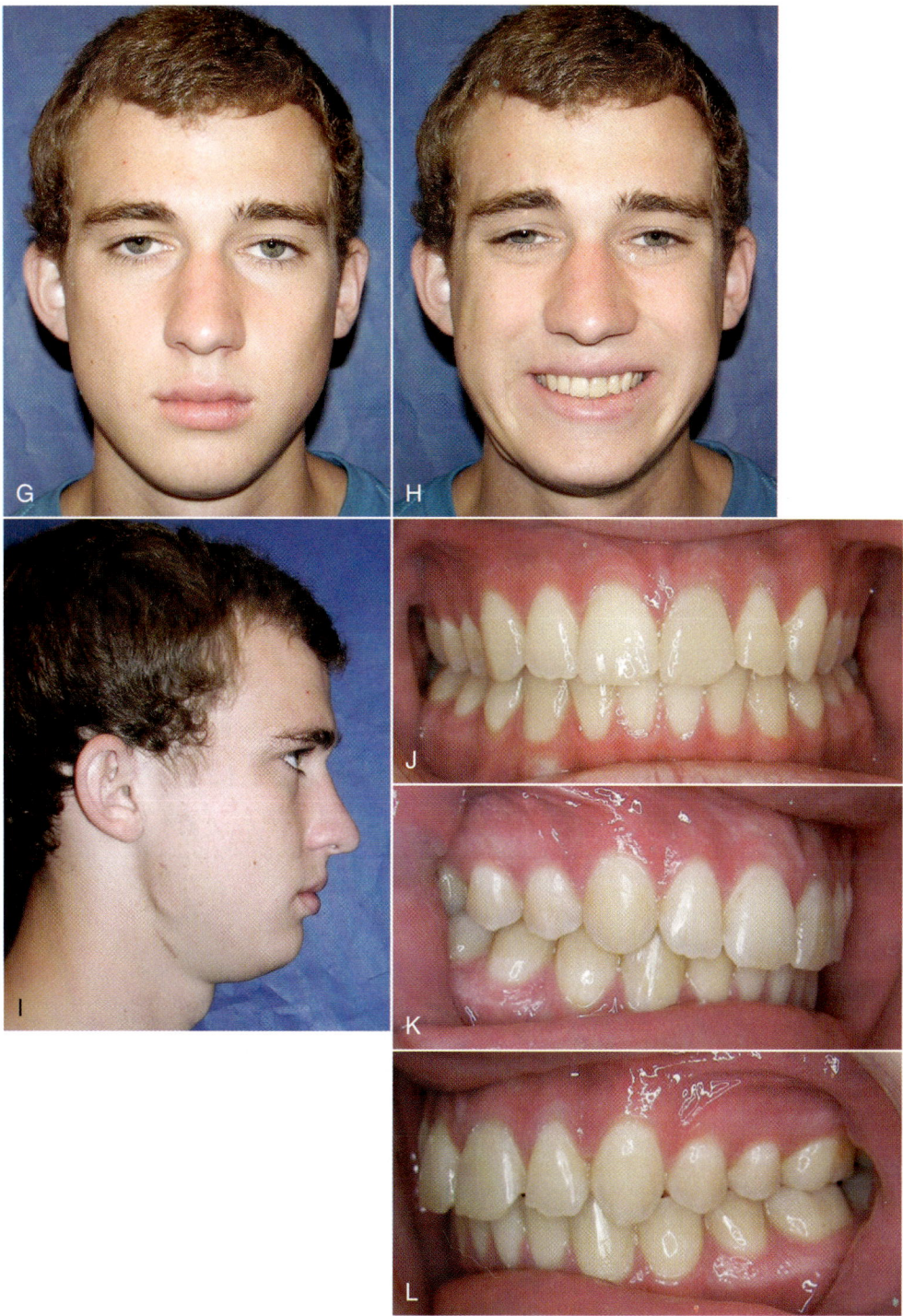

Fig. 82-14, cont'd ■ **G-L,** The patient 20 months after bilateral TMJ reconstruction and mandibular advancement with a TMJ Concepts total joint prosthesis, multiple maxillary osteotomies and genioplasty. He has an improved facial balance and good jaw function (52 mm opening) without pain.

ADOLESCENT INTERNAL CONDYLAR RESORPTION (AICR)

AICR, formerly referred to as idiopathic condylar resorption,[43-46] is one of the most common TMJ conditions affecting teenage females. AICR has also been called cheerleader syndrome, idiopathic condylysis, condylar atrophy, and progressive condylar resorption. This TMJ pathology occurs with a 9:1 female-to-male ratio, has no apparent genetic etiology, and rarely develops after the age of 16 years.[43,44]

Specific clinical characteristics of AICR include predominately teenage females, age of onset range from 11 to 15 years old, high occlusal plane angle and mandibular plane angle (Dolichocephalic) facial morphology, and predominance of class II skeletal and occlusal relationship with or without open bite (Fig. 82-18, *A-F*); TMJ symptoms could include clicking, popping, TMJ pain, headaches,

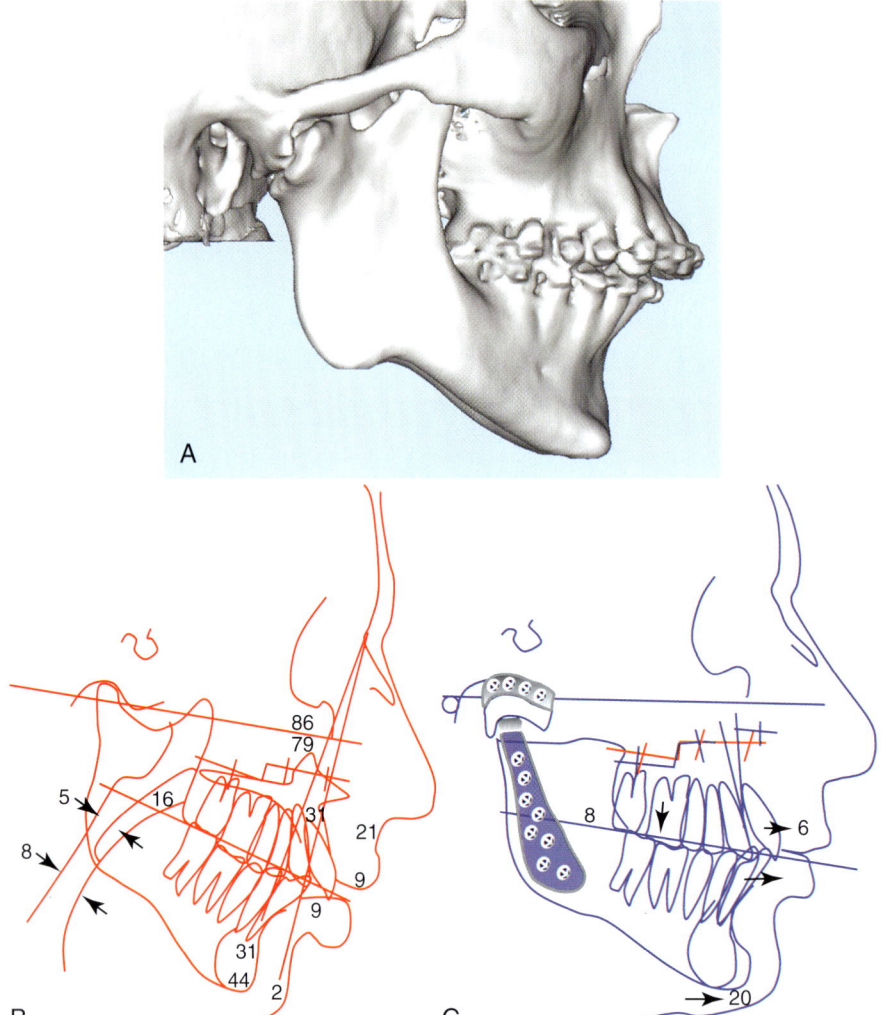

Fig. 82-15 ■ **A,** A 3D stereo lithographic model demonstrates the magnitude of the right TMJ ankylosis. **B,** Cephalometric analysis shows the retruded mandible and maxilla, skeletal and occlusal class II relation, high occlusal plane angle, and decreased oropharyngeal airway. **C,** A prediction tracing shows the planned surgery with the mandible being advanced forward 20 mm with a counterclockwise rotation and rami lengthened using bilateral patient-fitted TMJ Concepts total joint prostheses, bilateral TMJ fat grafts to prevent heterotopic bone formation harvested from the abdomen, as well as multiple maxillary osteotomies, bilateral coronoidotomies, genioplasty, and partial inferior turbinectomies.

myofascial pain, earaches, tinnitus, vertigo; no other joints areinvolved.[43-46] AICR rarely occurs in low occlusal and mandibular plane angle (Brachiocephalic) facial types or in class III skeletal relationships. When it occurs unilaterally or one side has greater condylar resorption than the other, additional characteristics include mandible deviated toward the affected side; progressive worsening facial deformity and occlusion, although occurring at a slow rate (the average rate of condylar resorption is 1.5 mm per year); premature contact on the ipsilateral side; and the possible development of an anterior and contralateral open bite (see Fig. 82-18, *A-F*).[43,44] Twenty-five percent of AICR patients have no symptoms including no noises, joint pain, or headaches.[43,44] Because this condition occurs only in teenagers, condylar resorption that is initiated in late teens or at a later age is not AICR and may need a different treatment approach.

The strong predilection of AICR for teenage females in their pubertal growth phase supports a theory of hormonal mediation. The author's hypothesis for the progression of this disease is that female hormones mediate biochemical changes within the TMJ, causing hyperplasia of the synovial tissues that stimulate the production of destructive substrates that initiate breakdown of the ligaments that normally stabilize the articular disc to the condyle. The disc becomes anteriorly displaced. The hyperplastic synovial tissue then surrounds the head of the condyle. The substrates penetrate through the outer surface of the condyle and cause thinning of the cortical bone and breakdown of the subcortical bone, causing the condyle to slowly collapses in all three planes of space without clinically apparent destruction of the fibrocartilage on the condylar head and roof of the fossa, unlike the arthritides, where the fibrocartilage and cortical bone are destroyed by an inflammatory connective tissue or autoimmune disease process. AICR can progress for a while and then may go into remission or proceed until the entire condylar head has resorbed. In cases where it goes into remission, excessive joint loading (e.g., parafunctional habits, trauma, orthodontics,

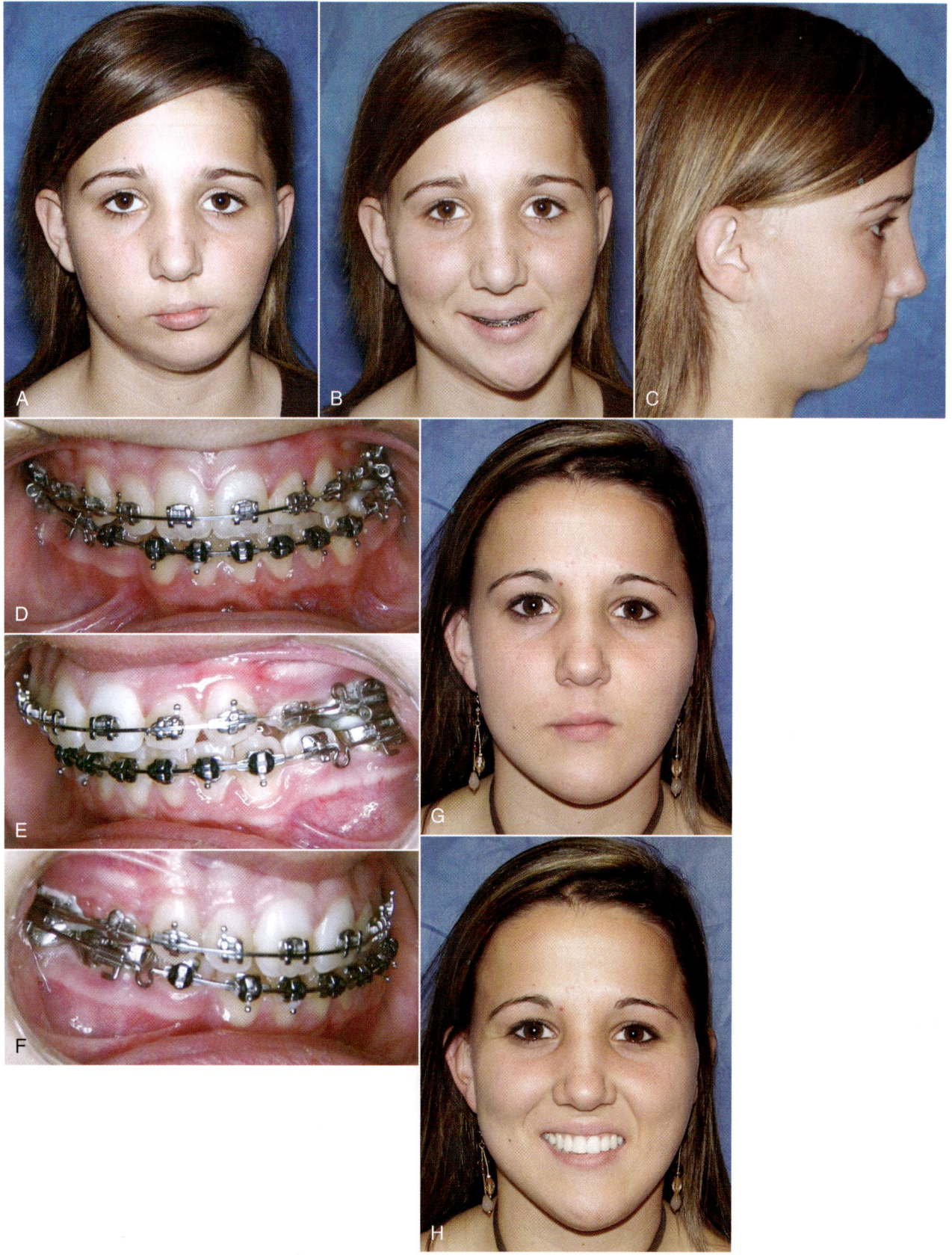

Fig. 82-16 ■ **A-F,** A 14-year-old female was born with left-sided hemifacial microsomia. She was absent the left mandibular condyle and the ramus was hypoplastic. She had significant transverse asymmetry, retruded mandible, and class II occlusion. **G-L,** The patient 2 years after surgery for left TMJ reconstruction and mandibular advancement in a counterclockwise direction with a TMJ Concepts patient-fitted total joint prosthesis, advancement of the right mandible with a ramus sagittal split osteotomy, multiple maxillary osteotomies, a fat graft around the left total joint prosthesis, and bilateral turbinectomies to improve her airway. Facial symmetry is very good, the patient is pain free, and there is an incisal opening of 42 mm.

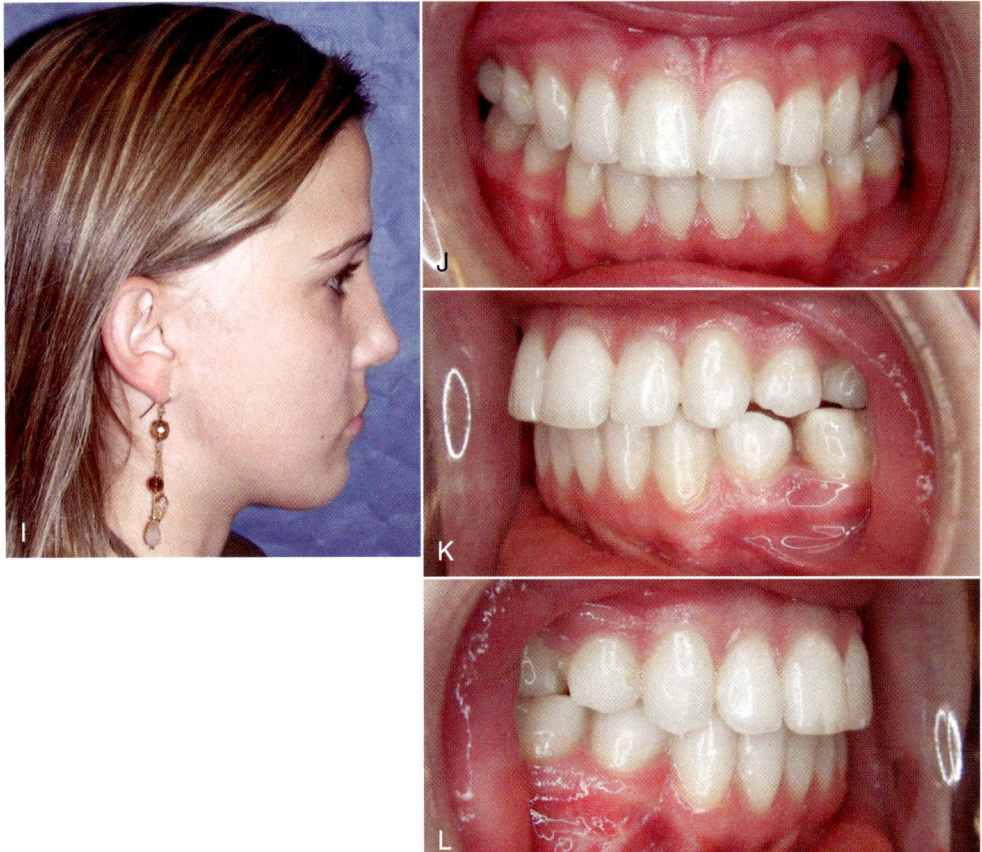

Fig. 82-16, cont'd.

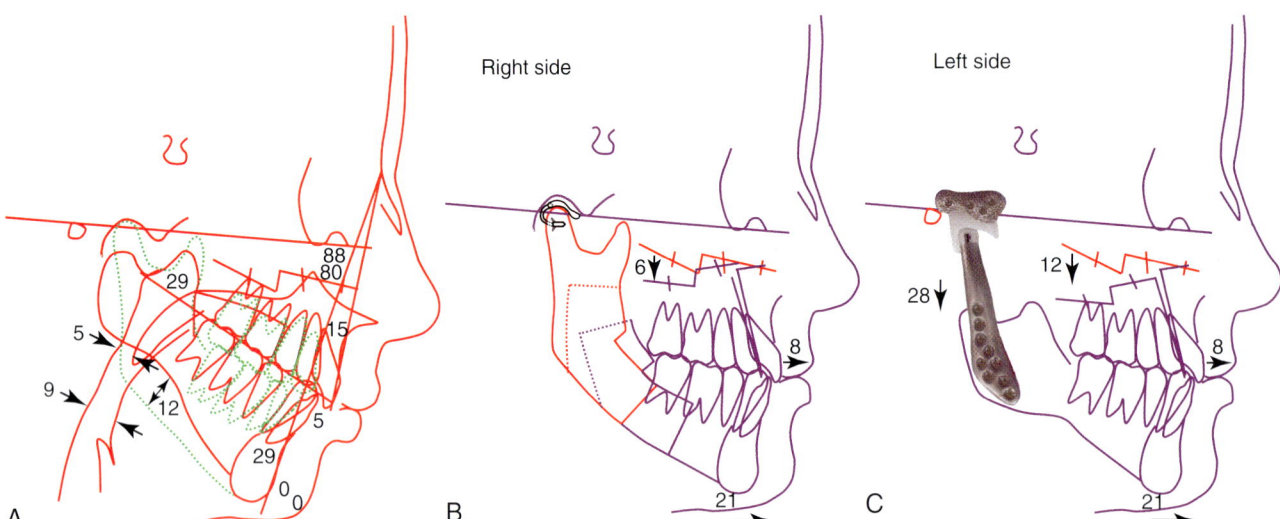

Fig. 82-17 ■ **A,** The cephalometric analysis demonstrates the retruded mandible and maxilla, vertical facial asymmetry, high occlusal plane angle, skeletal and occlusal class II relation, and a decreased oropharyngeal airway. **B,** The prediction tracing shows the right TMJ had an anteriorly displaced disc repaired with the Mitek anchor technique. A right ramus sagittal split osteotomy was used to advance the mandible and the maxilla was down-grafted 6 mm posteriorly. **C,** The prediction tracing shows the left TMJ reconstructed and mandible advanced in a counterclockwise rotation with a patient-fitted TMJ Concepts total joint prosthesis as well as a right mandible ramus sagittal split osteotomy and multiple maxillary osteotomies with the posterior down-grafted 12 mm. Pogonion advanced 21 mm.

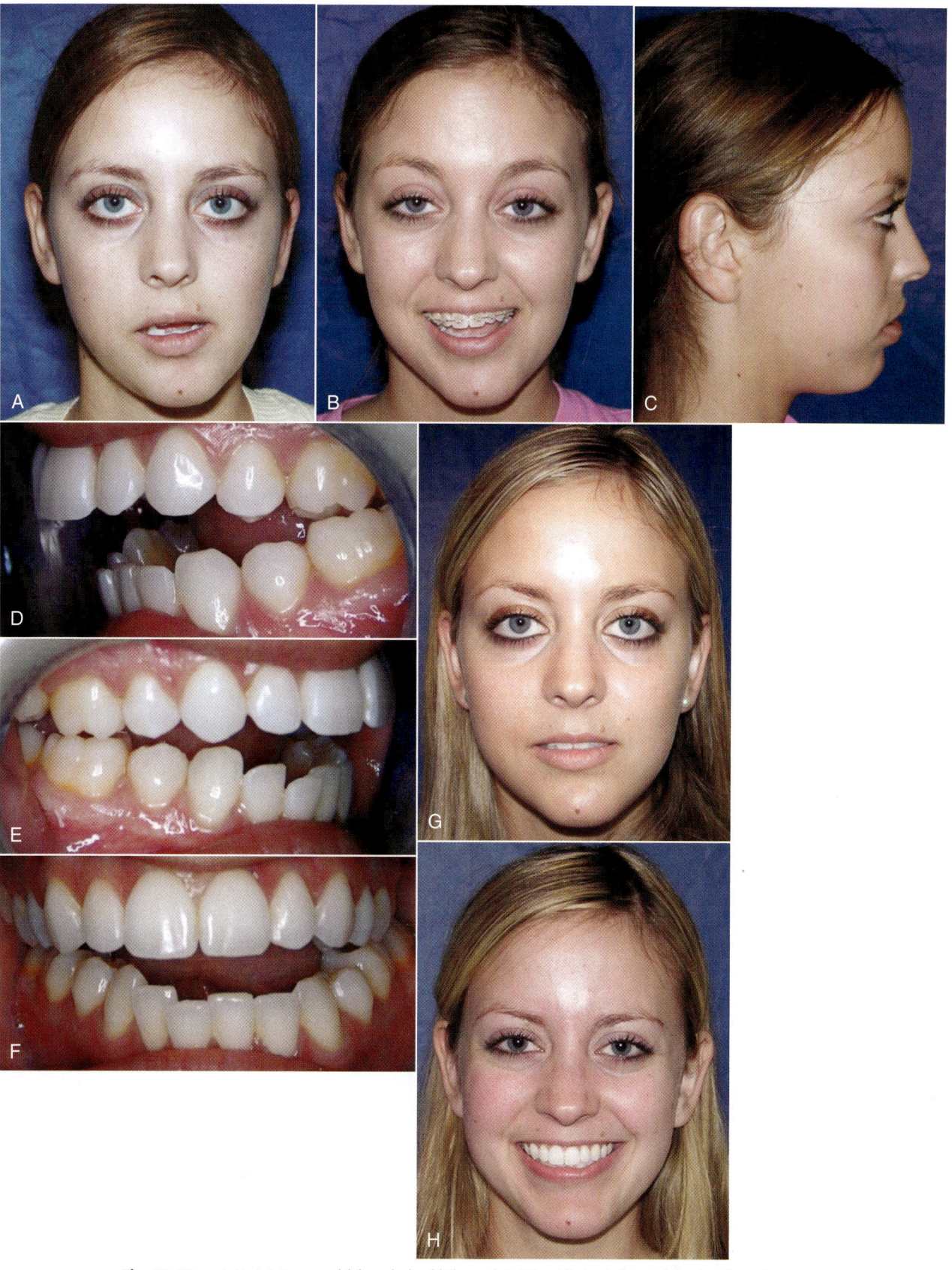

Fig. 82-18 ■ **A-F,** A 16-year-old female had bilateral AICR with the left condyle significantly more resorbed and progressive than the right side. The occlusion was class II open bite with a transverse cant in the occlusion and significant facial asymmetry. The onset of the TMJ pathology began at age 12 years. She had been treated with splint therapy for 4 years tempt continued condylar resorption. **G-L,** The patient 2 years after treatment for bilateral TMJ disc repositioning with Mitek anchors, bilateral mandibular ramus osteotomies with counterclockwise rotation and advancement, and maxillary osteotomies. A predictable and stable result was achieved using the specific protocol for this TMJ pathology.

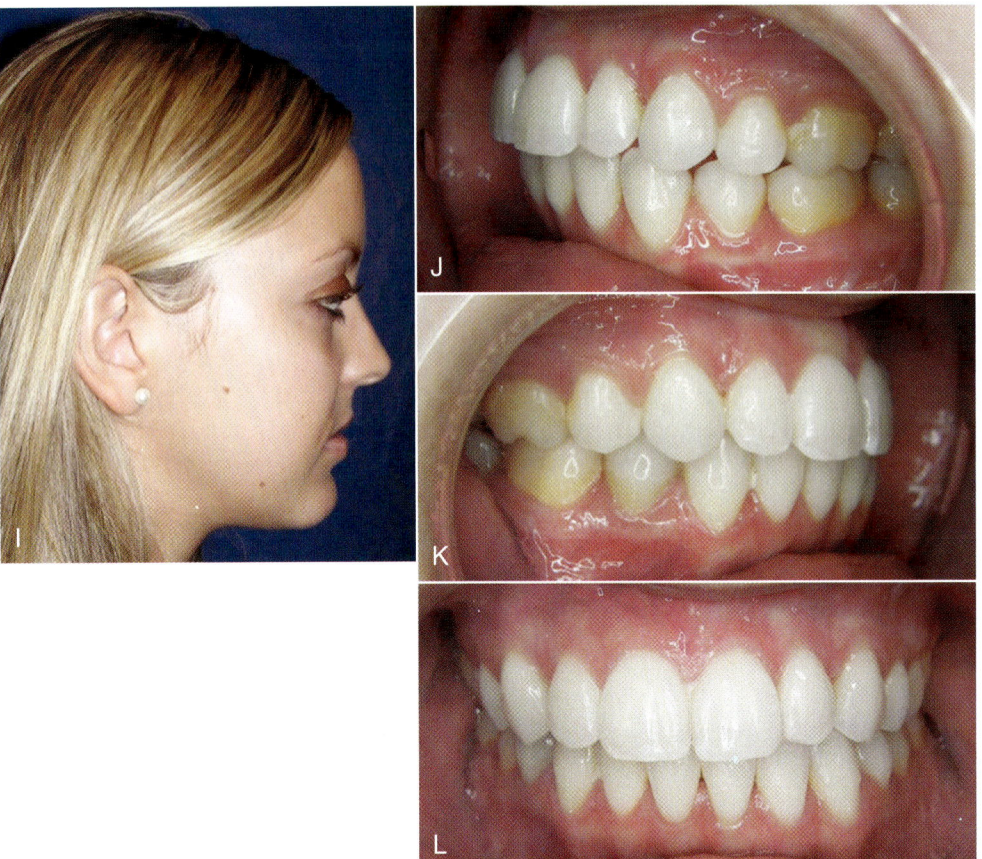

Fig. 82-18, cont'd.

orthognathic surgery, etc.) can reinitiate the resorption process later in life. Although this condition usually occurs bilaterally, it can occur unilaterally or occur at a more rapid rate on one side, causing asymmetry.

MRI features include a small condyle on the affected side compared to a normal condyle; decreased vertical height of the ramus and condyle on the involved side; and articular disc anteriorly displaced with amorphous-appearing tissue surrounding the condyle, with or without an increased joint space (Fig. 82-19). The lateral cephalogram shows the classic class II skeletal and occlusal relation, anterior open bite, and high occlusal plane angulation (Fig. 82-20, A).

The highly predictable and stable protocol for treating AICR includes removing the bilaminar tissue surrounding the condyle, repositioning the articular disc and stabilizing it to the condyle with a Mitek anchor, and performing the indicated orthognathic surgery (Fig. 82-20, B).[43,44,47] This treatment method stops the disease process and allows the orthognathic surgery to be done during the same operation. The orthognathic surgery usually requires double jaw surgery with counterclockwise rotation of the maxillo-mandibular complex to achieve optimal results (Figs. 82-18 G-L, and see Fig. 82-20, B). In growing patients, this approach not only stops the condylar resorption, but mandibular growth will begin again.[43,44,47] In cases where the disc is nonsalvageable because of severe deformation/degeneration or there is severe condylar resorption, then total joint prostheses may be the best treatment method

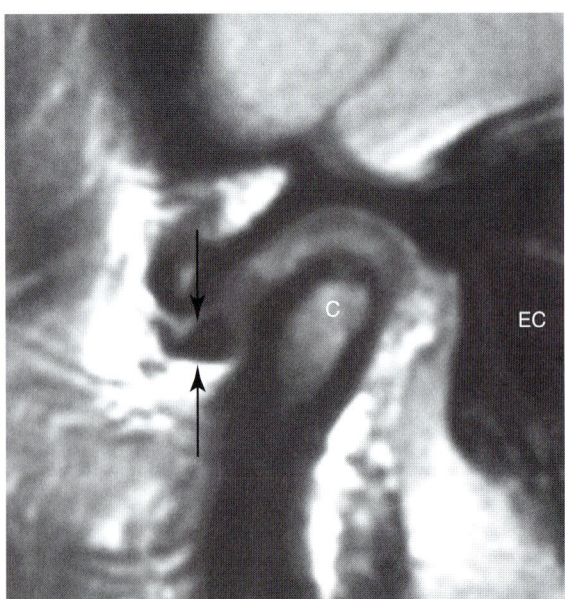

Fig. 82-19 ■ MRI shows a condyle that lost vertical dimension with decreased condylar volume, increased bilaminar tissue thickness, and anteriorly displaced articular disc; classic for AICR. The arrows point to the disc, *C,* condyle. *EC,* ear canal.

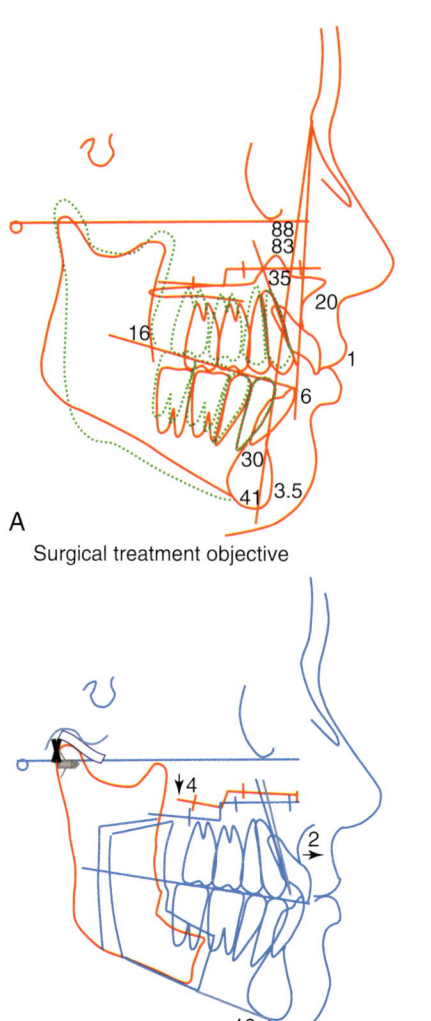

Fig. 82-20 ■ **A,** Cephalometric tracing shows a retruded mandible, class II skeletal and occlusal relation, and large anterior open bite. **B,** The prediction tracing shows the intended treatment of bilateral TMJ articular disc repositioning with Mitek anchors, bilateral mandibular ramus, and multiple maxillary osteotomies to advance the maxillomandibular complex with a counterclockwise rotation.

where the TMJ can be reconstructed and the mandible advanced in a counterclockwise direction with the prostheses, along with maxillary osteotomies.[19-21]

REACTIVE ARTHRITIS

Reactive arthritis usually involves bacterial or viral microorganisms within the tissues of the TMJ that stimulate the production of substrates that cause breakdown of the joint structures and pain. Although this condition can occur at any age, it is more commonly seen in the late teens up through the 4th decade. These predominately female patients usually demonstrate a displaced articular disc as part of the mechanism to develop the reactive arthritis. We have shown that bacteria are commonly found in the TMJs when the discs are displaced.[48-53] These bacteria include Chlamydia and Mycoplasma species and have been found in the bilaminar tissues in 70% of patients with displaced discs in the TMJs. This could be the etiology or simply a contributing factor to the pathologic process. It is known

that these bacteria produce cytokines substance P, tissue necrosis factor, and similar pain mediators.[54] There may be a genetic predisposition to susceptibility to TMJ disorders and pathology as well as increased susceptibility to these bacteria.[55]

Although this condition commonly occurs bilaterally, it can occur unilaterally where the following features may be observed: the mandible deviation toward the ipsilateral side; progressive worsening skeletal and occlusal deformity, although it may occur at a slow rate; class II occlusion and crossbite as well as premature contact of the occlusion on the ipsilateral side; an anterior and contralateral open bite relationship; common associated TMJ symptoms including clicking, popping, crepitus, TMJ pain, headaches, myofascial pain, jaw dysfunction, earaches, tinnitus, and vertigo; and other joints may be involved (Fig. 82-21, *A-F*).

Imaging features include arthritic condyle on the affected side compared to a normal condyle with loss of vertical dimension; possible erosion with loss of the fibrocartilage covering on the articular surface of the condyle and fossa; decreased vertical height of the ramus and condyle on the ipsilateral side; and a possible retruded and asymmetric mandible. MRI will often show the articular disc anteriorly displaced with joint effusion and inflammation present (Figs. 82-22, *A, B,* and 82-23, *A*).

Treatment depends on the length of time that the pathology has been present, the amount of destruction to the disc and condyle at the time of surgery, and the presence of other joint involvement (polyarthritis), or other related systemic conditions. If the TMJ condition is identified within the first 4 years of the onset of the disc dislocation, the destruction is not significant, and no other joints or systemic conditions are present; then repositioning the articular disc with the Mitek anchor technique may work well, preserving the normal anatomic structures (see Fig. 82-3).[7-9,47] The orthognathic surgery can be done when the joint repair is performed (Figs. 82-21, *G-L*, and 82-23, *B*) or as a separate procedure. If there is significant destruction of the condyle and the disc is not salvageable or multiple other joints are involved, then the most predictable procedure is the total joint prosthesis (TMJ Concepts system) to reconstruct the condyle as well as reposition the mandible to its proper position (Fig. 82-23, *C*).[11-21] Fat grafts packed around the total joint prosthesis will be an important component to help prevent fibrous tissue and heterotopic bone from forming.[22-24]

CONNECTIVE TISSUE/AUTOIMMUNE DISEASES (CT/AI)

CT/AI diseases that can affect the TMJs include rheumatoid arthritis, juvenile rheumatoid arthritis, psoriatic arthritis, ankylosing spondylitis, Sjogren's syndrome, systemic lupus erythematosus, scleroderma, and mixed connective tissue disease. The triggers and precise pathophysiology are unknown for most of these disorders. Multiple systems are usually involved. Joint damage may be mediated by cytokines, chemokines, and metalloproteases. Peripheral joints are usually symmetrically inflamed, resulting in progressive destruction of articular structures.[56] Facial asymmetry can occur with unilateral involvement or if one TMJ is more severely affected than the other, causing greater unilateral condylar resorption.

Clinical features when occurring unilaterally or when one TMJ is affected greater than the other side include deviation of the mandible toward the ipsilateral side; progressive worsening facial and occlusal deformity; class II occlusion, crossbite tendency and premature contact on the ipsilateral side; commonly the development of an anterior and contralateral open bite relationship; TMJ symptoms, which could include clicking, popping, crepitus, TMJ pain,

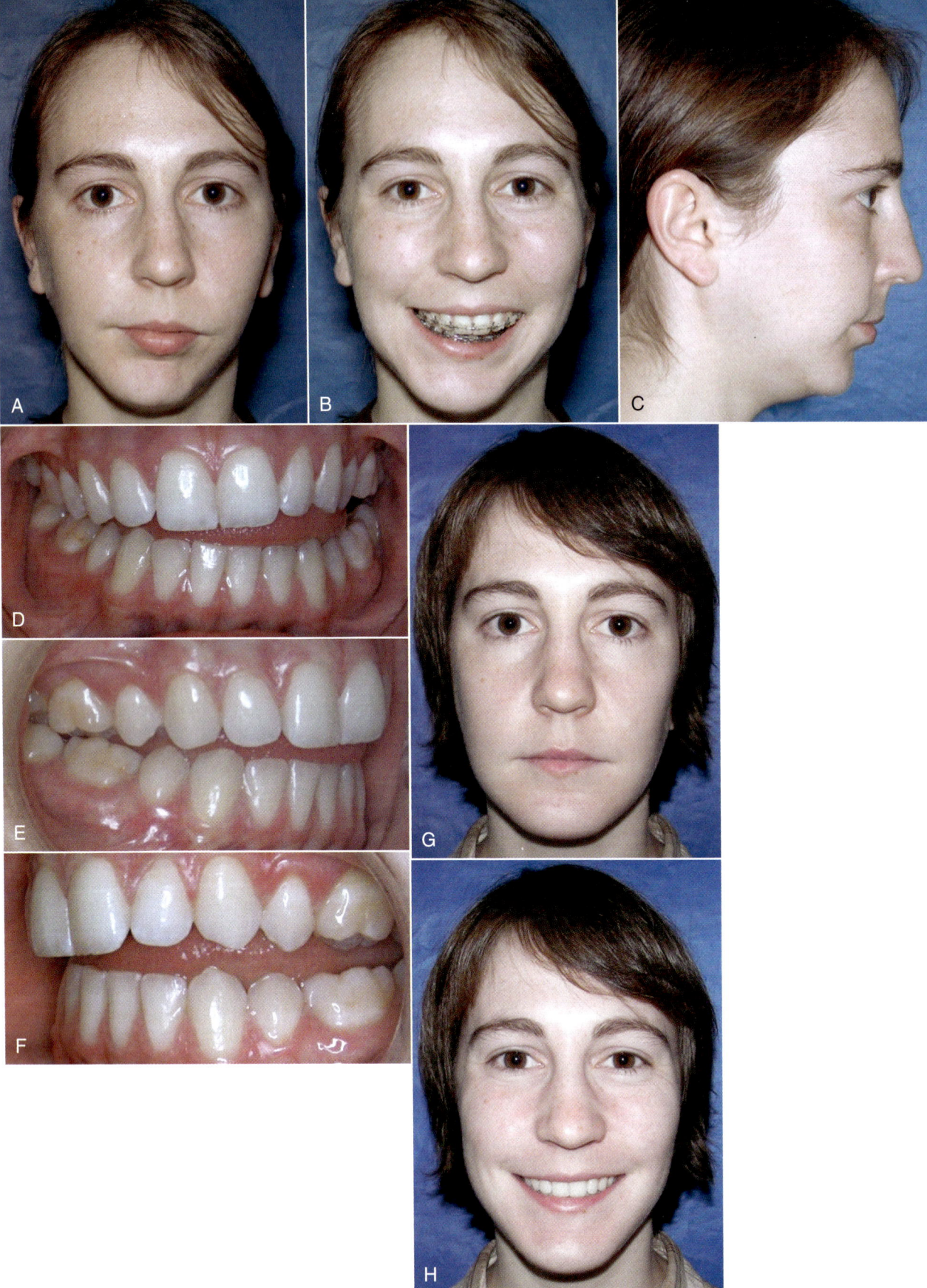

Fig. 82-21 ■ **A-F,** A 27-year-old female had a good orthodontic result until about 4 years ago when her bite began undergoing major changes. She developed a significant malocclusion, pain, and sleep apnea. She has a retruded mandible, a high occlusal angulation facial morphology, and significant facial asymmetry. She had bilateral TMJ pain, worse on the right side but clicking only on the left. **G-L,** The patient 1 year following surgery with good facial balance, occlusion, and function, pain free, with elimination of her sleep apnea.

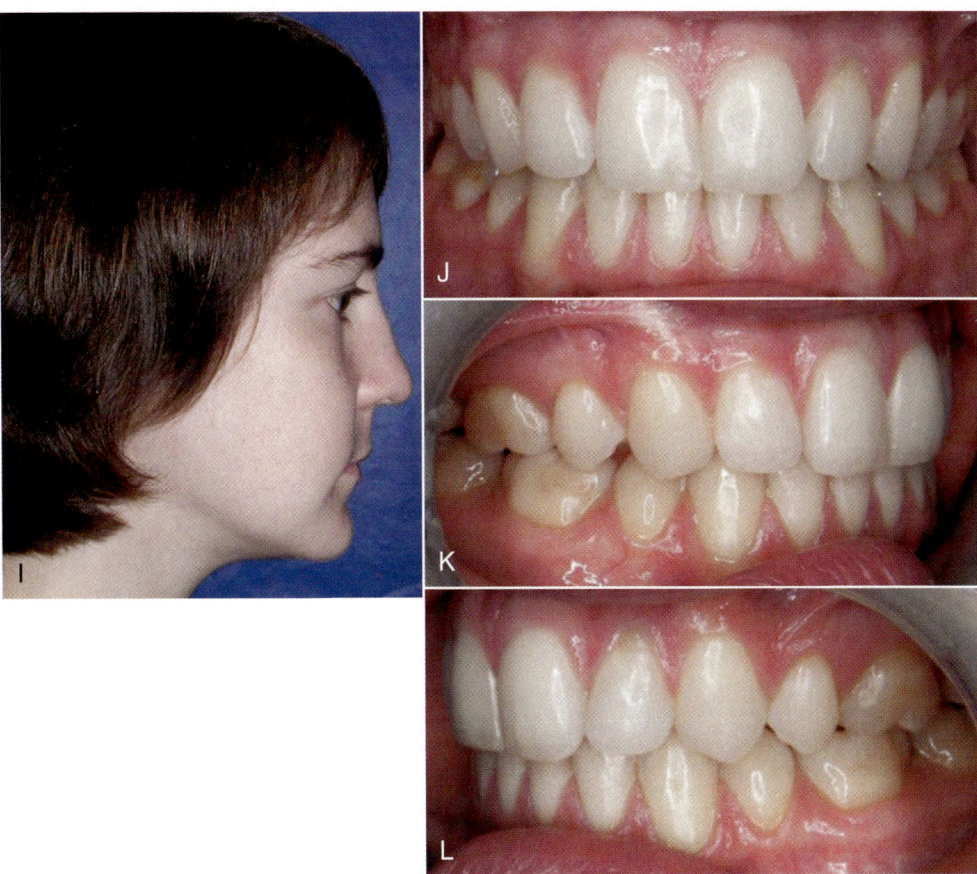

Fig. 82-21, cont'd.

headaches, myofascial pain, earaches, tinnitus, and vertigo; jaw and jaw joint dysfunction; and the involvement of other joints and systems (Fig. 82-24, *A-F*).

Radiographic and MRI features when occurring unilaterally or when one side resorbs at a faster rate than the other side include condylar loss of vertical dimension; significant mediolaterally narrowing that may become broad in the AP direction; an articular disc that may be in position but surrounded by a pannus (reactive tissue) that eventually destroys the disc but also causes condylar and articular eminence resorption (Fig. 82-25); in more severe cases, a condylar stump that may function beneath the remaining articular eminence; and decreased vertical height of the ramus and condyle. The mandible becomes progressively retruded with development of a class II occlusion and an anterior open bite (Fig. 82-26, *A*).

The most predictable treatment for the TMJ affected by CT/AI diseases includes reconstruction of the TMJ (and if indicated, advancement of the mandible) with a patient-fitted total joint prosthesis (TMJ Concepts system),[11-21] an ipsilateral coronoidotomy or coronoidectomy if the ramus is significantly advanced or vertically lengthened with the prosthesis, an autogenous fat graft packed around the prosthesis in the articulation area,[22-24] additional orthognathic surgery if indicated including sagittal split osteotomy on the opposite ramus if there is no TMJ pathology in the contralateral joint, maxillary osteotomies (Figs. 82-24, *G-L*, and 82-26, *B*), and any additional adjunctive procedures indicated (e.g., genioplasty,

rhinoplasty, turbinectomies, septoplasty). Because an inflammatory process is a factor in these diseases, reactive or heterotopic bone will tend to form around the prostheses. Therefore, it is necessary that fat grafts (harvested from the abdomen or buttock) be packed around the articulating parts of the prostheses to prevent the reoccurrence of heterotopic and reactive bone as well as to minimize scar tissue formation.[22-24] Orthognathic surgery can be performed at the same time as the TMJ is reconstructed or performed at a later surgery. Other techniques that have been advocated for TMJ reconstruction in the CT/AI diseases include using autogenous tissues such as temporal fascia and muscle flaps, rib grafts, sternoclavicular grafts, vertical sliding osteotomy, and so on. However, the disease process that created the original TMJ pathology can attack the autogenous tissues used in the TMJ reconstruction, causing failure of the grafts. The total joint prosthesis with a fat graft packed around it is a superior technique relative to elimination of the disease process in the TMJ; this approach also improves both function and esthetics and eliminates or decreases pain. When treating young growing patients (10 years or older), the total joint prosthesis may still be the best option to eliminate the disease process. However, because there would be no growth potential on the involved side of the mandible, orthognathic surgery may be necessary but can be delayed until most of the patient's facial growth is complete. Then double jaw surgery can be performed, including the sagittal split on the side of the prosthesis to reposition the jaws into the best alignment, or

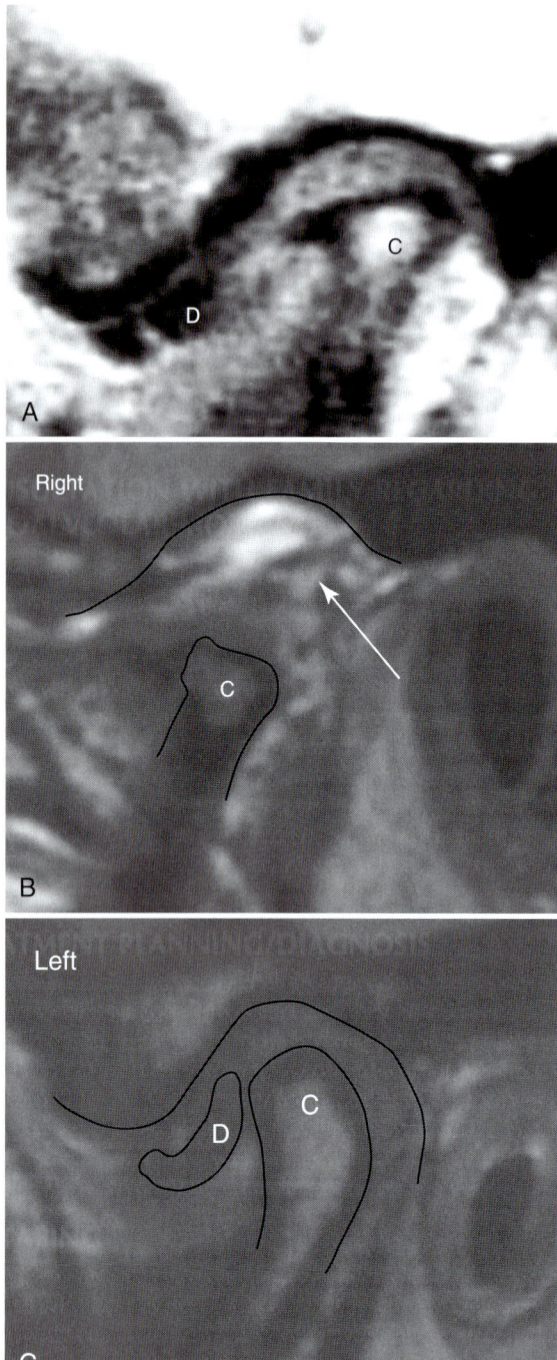

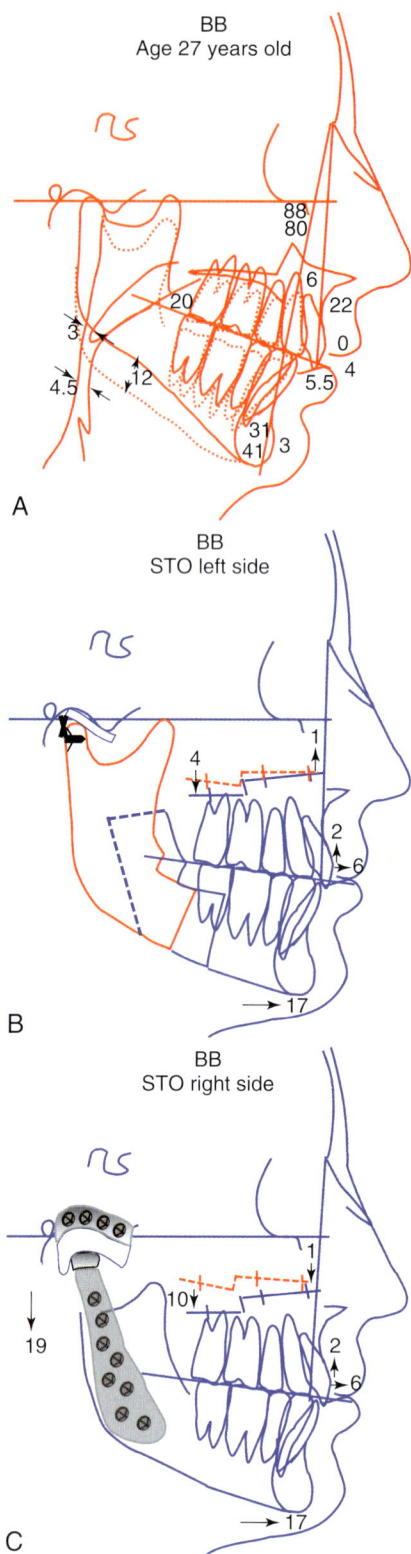

Fig. 82-22 ▪ A, An MRI of reactive arthritis will show degenerative changes in the bone and articular disc with the disc frequently anteriorly displaced. The black "C" marks the condyle and the white "D" indicates the disc anteriorly displaced. **B,** In more aggressive forms of reactive arthritis, such as in the patient in Fig. 82-21, there can be significant destruction of the condyle and disc and the presence of inflammatory tissue within the joint *(arrow)*. There is no identifiable disc tissue in the right TMJ. The articular eminence is partially eroded. **C,** The left TMJ of the patient in Fig. 82-21 has an anteriorly displaced disc. In facial asymmetry patients, it is common to see displaced articular discs in the "normal" TMJ, opposite the obviously pathologic joint.

Fig. 82-23 ▪ A, The lateral cephalogram for the patient in Fig. 82-21 demonstrates the significant deformity with retruded mandible, open bite, high occlusal plane angulation, vertical asymmetry at the occlusal plane, and inferior border of the mandible, and decreased oropharyngeal airway. **B,** The prediction tracing shows the surgical changes to be achieved. On the left side the disc will be repositioned with a Mitek anchor, mandible advanced with a ramus sagittal split osteotomy, and maxillary osteotomies. **C,** The right TMJ is reconstructed and mandible advanced with a TMJ Concepts total joint prosthesis, right coronoidotomy, right TMJ fat graft harvested from the abdomen, and maxillary osteotomies. Pogonion advanced 17 mm.

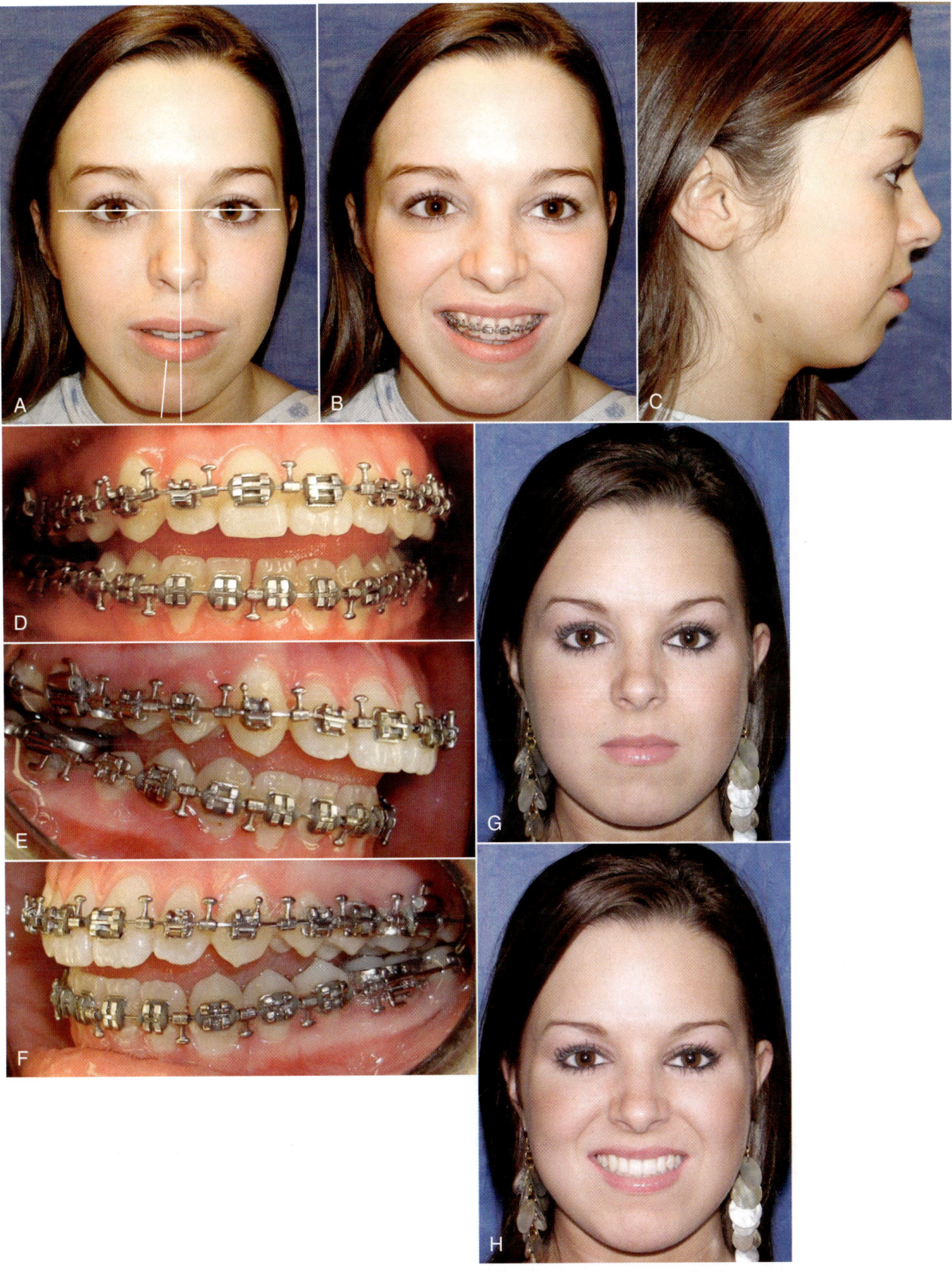

Fig. 82-24 ■ **A-F,** A 16-year-old female with bilateral TMJ juvenile rheumatoid arthritis (JRA) with greater condylar resorption of the right side. Other joints and systemic systems were involved. She had facial asymmetry, retruded mandible, and a malocclusion that was class II with a crossbite on the ipsilateral side and open bite anteriorly and on the left side. **G-L,** Patient 2 years after treatment following orthodontics and surgery that included bilateral TMJ reconstruction and mandibular advancement with TMJ Concepts total joint prosthesis, a fat graft packed around the articulating part of the prosthesis, bilateral coronoidectomy, and maxillary osteotomies. (From Fonseca RJ, Marciani RD, Turvey TA: *Oral and maxillofacial surgery,* ed 2, vol 3, St. Louis, 2009, Saunders.)

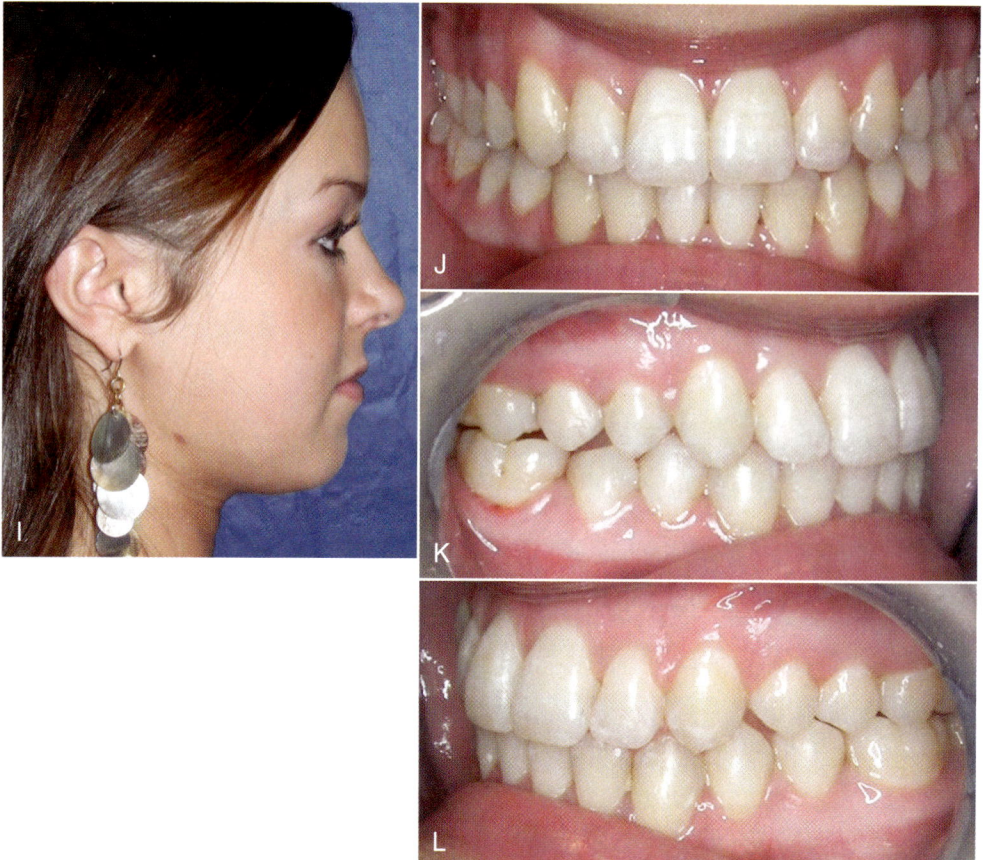

Fig. 82-24, cont'd.

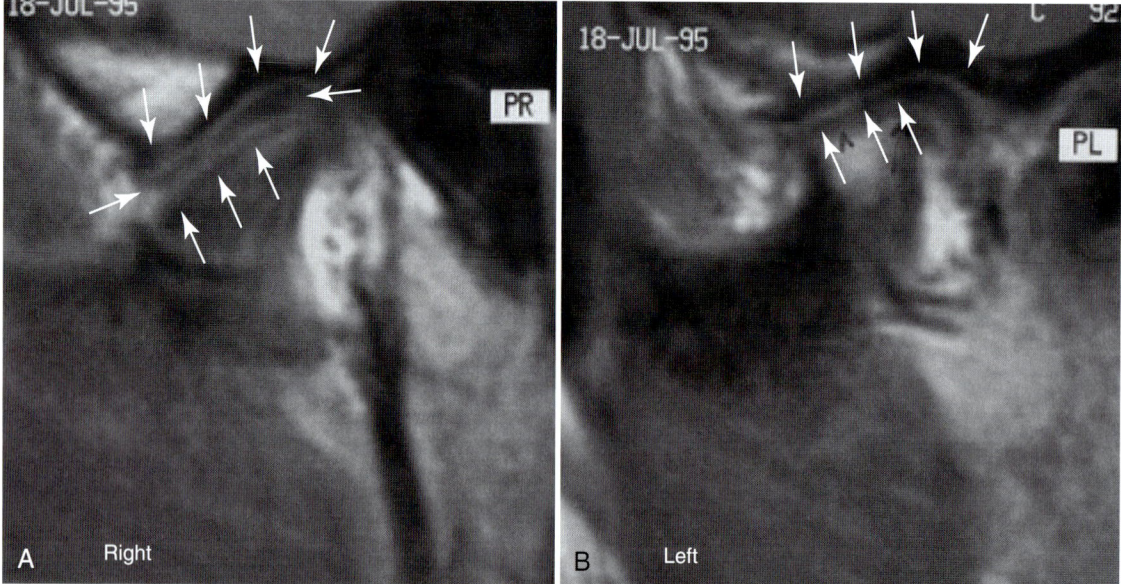

Fig. 82-25 ■ A and **B,** MRI of AI/CT diseases may demonstrate significant bone resorption, but sometimes increased AP dimension of the condyle as a result of bone deposition (white arrows outline the condyle and fossa margins). The articular disc in normal position but surrounded by a pannus of reactive tissue (grayish tissue surrounding the disc) that is the causative factor in condylar and articular eminence resorption and degeneration of the articular disc. (From Fonseca RJ, Marciani RD, Turvey TA: *Oral and maxillofacial surgery,* ed 2, vol 3, St. Louis, 2009, Saunders.)

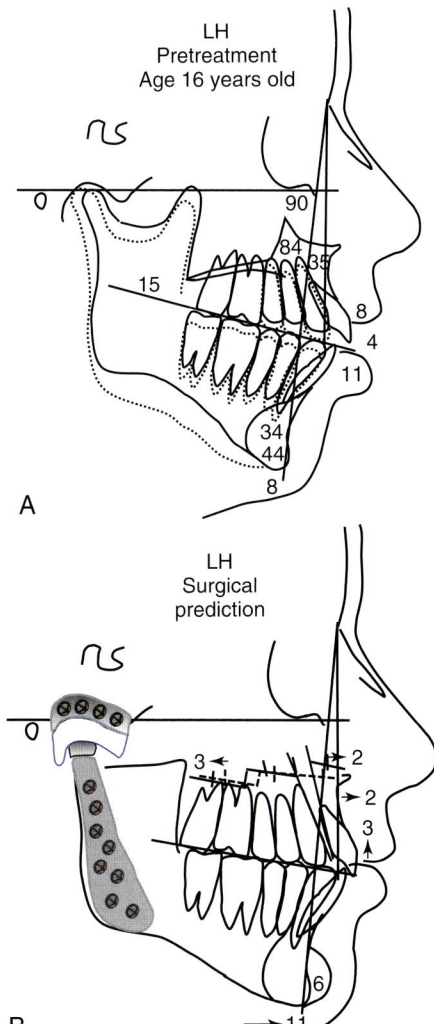

LH
Pretreatment
Age 16 years old

A

LH
Surgical
prediction

B

Fig. 82-26 ■ **A,** The cephalometric tracing of the patient in Fig. 82-24 shows the vertical differences of the inferior border of the mandible and occlusal plane, as well as the retruded mandible and posterior maxillary vertical hypoplasia. **B,** The prediction tracing shows the surgical changes including TMJ reconstruction and mandibular advancement with TMJ Concepts total joint prostheses and multiple maxillary osteotomies with counterclockwise rotation of the maxillomandibular complex. Pogonion advanced 11 mm. (From Fonseca RJ, Marciani RD, Turvey TA: *Oral and maxillofacial surgery,* ed 2, vol 3, St. Louis, 2009, Saunders.)

to reposition the mandibular component of the prosthesis, or to manufacture a new mandibular component to allow advancement of the mandible on the involved side.

CONCLUSION

There are numerous etiologies for facial asymmetry as discussed in this chapter. Accurate diagnosis of the causative factors and associated hard and soft tissue involvement is paramount to develop a comprehensive treatment plan to achieve optimal results for patients.

- Facial asymmetry commonly involves TMJ pathology or disorders. Therefore, the TMJs should always be evaluated (whether symptomatic or asymptomatic) to determine if the TMJs are the etiologic factor, a problem that developed because of facial asymmetry, a coexisting pretreatment condition, or that the joints are normal and healthy. Progressive worsening facial asymmetry usually indicates that TMJ pathology is present with one condyle either resorbing or growing.
- An orthognathic surgery patient that initially had a good treatment result but subsequently develops facial asymmetry probably had a presurgical unrecognized and untreated TMJ pathologic condition. In this situation, TMJ surgical intervention as well as possible repeat orthognathic surgery may be indicated to achieve a quality stable result and pain-free outcome.
- A TMJ that is "silent" during function can have pathology such as nonreducing disc; medial, lateral, or posteriorly displaced disc; anteriorly displaced disc with very early reduction (preclick position); AICR; or connective tissue/autoimmune diseases. Do not ignore the TMJs just because they are "silent" or nonpainful in patients requiring orthognathic surgery. These are the joints that may cause major postorthognathic surgical problems relative to stability and pain for patients if TMJ pathology is present.
- MRI is a valuable tool in determining most TMJ pathologies. The best diagnostic views include closed coronal, closed and open sagittal, and dynamic. However, a CT scan will be more beneficial for TMJ ankylosis, multiply operated joints, or failed alloplastic implants or autogenous tissues such as rib grafts and sternoclavicular grafts.
- When TMJ and orthognathic conditions coexist, then open TMJ surgery should be done first, followed by the orthognathic surgery at one operation or separated into two. Failure to treat TMJ pathology will likely result in continued pathologic changes within the TMJs, resulting in redevelopment of the facial asymmetry, malocclusion, and a high probability of increased pain and TMJ dysfunction.
- A Mitek anchor is a predictable method to stabilize a salvageable disc in the correct anatomic position. It is important to minimize soft tissue dissection off the condylar head when performing this technique to maximize blood flow to the condyle and prevent avascular changes that can occur from aggressive reflection of soft tissue off the condyle. Repositioning discs within the first 4 years of disc displacement with the Mitek anchor technique provides the best results. After 4 years, the natural progression of degeneration may decrease outcome predictability.
- Patients with two or more previous TMJ surgeries, connective tissue autoimmune diseases, advanced reactive arthritis or osteoarthritis, ankylosis, absence of the TMJ as in hemifacial microsomia, failed TMJ alloplastic implants or autogenous grafts, severe trauma, or other end-stage TMJ conditions will usually have better outcomes with patient-fitted TMJ total joint prostheses.
- Fat grafts are a key element in the successful outcome of total joint prostheses as they can inhibit the development of heterotopic bone and fibrosis. Fat grafts should be harvested just prior to placement and packed around all four sides of the articulating portion of the prostheses: medial, anterior, posterior, and lateral. If autogenous TMJ reconstruction is used such as rib or sternoclavicular grafts, packing fat grafts around the articulating area will help prevent heterotopic bone formation and minimize fibrosis.

REFERENCES

1. Gorlin RJ, Cohen MM Jr, Hemekam RCM: *Syndromes of the head and neck*, ed 4, Oxford, United Kingdom, 2001, Oxford University Press, pp 405-408, 790-797.
2. Wolford LM, Fields RT Jr.: Diagnosis and treatment planning for orthognathic surgery. In Betts N, Turvey T, editors: *Oral and maxillofacial surgery*, vol 2 (Fonseca RJ, editor), Chapter 2, St. Louis, 2000, Saunders, pp. 24-55.
3. Wolford LM, Fields RT: Surgical planning. In Booth PW, Schendel SA, Hausamen JE, editors: *Maxillofacial surgery*, vol 2, Chapter 73, Edinburgh, 1999, Churchill Livingstone, pp. 1205-1257.
4. Wolford LM: Facial asymmetry: diagnosis and treatment considerations. In Fonseca RJ, Marciani RD, Turvey TA, editors: *Oral and maxillofacial surgery*, ed 2, vol III, Chapter 13, St. Louis, 2008, Saunders, pp. 272-315.
5. Wolford LM, Reiche-Fischel O, Mehra P: Changes in TMJ dysfunction after orthognathic surgery, *J Oral Maxillofac Surg* 61:655-660, 2003.
6. Fuselier C, Wolford LM, Pitta M, Talwar R: Condylar changes after orthognathic surgery with untreated TMJ internal derangement, *J Oral Maxillofac Surg* 56(Suppl 4):61, 1998.
7. Wolford LM, Cottrell DA, Karras SC: *Mitek mini anchor in maxillofacial surgery. Proceedings of SMST-94, the First International Conference on Shape Memory and Superelastic Technologies*, Monterey, CA, 1995, MIAS: 477-482.
8. Wolford LM, Karras SC, Mehra P: Concomitant temporomandibular joint and orthognathic surgery: a preliminary report, *J Oral Maxillofac Surg* 60:356-362, 2002.
9. Mehra P, Wolford LM: The Mitek mini anchor for TMJ disc repositioning: surgical technique and results, *Int J Oral Maxillofac Surg* 30:497-503, 2001.
10. Badrick JP, Indresano AT: Failure rates of repetitive temporomandibular joint surgical procedures. Presented at the American Association of Oral and Maxillofacial Surgeons 74th Annual Meeting, Scientific Poster Session III held in Honolulu, HI, September 1992 (abstr).
11. Wolford LM, Cottrell DA, Henry CH: Temporomandibular joint reconstruction of the complex patient with the Techmedica custom-made total joint prosthesis, *J Oral Maxillofac Surg* 52:2-10, 1994.
12. Mehra P, Wolford LM: Custom-made TMJ reconstruction and simultaneous mandibular advancement in autoimmune/connective tissue diseases, *J Oral Maxillofac Surg* 58(Suppl 1):95, 2000.
13. Wolford LM, Pitta MC, Reiche-Fischel O, Franco PF: TMJ concepts/techmedica custom-made TMJ total joint prosthesis: 5-year follow-up, *Int J Oral Maxillofac Surg* 32:268-274, 2003.
14. Wolford LM: Temporomandibular joint devices: treatment factors and outcomes, *Oral Surg Oral Med Oral Pathol Oral Radiol Endod* 83:143-149, 1997.
15. Wolford LM, Mehra P: Custom-made total joint prostheses for temporomandibular joint reconstruction, *Bayl Univ Med Cent Proc* 13:135-138, 2000.
16. Mercuri LG, Wolford LM, Sanders B, et al: Custom CAD/CAM total temporomandibular joint reconstruction system: preliminary multicenter report, *J Oral Maxillofac Surg* 53:106-115, 1995.
17. Mercuri LG: The TMJ concepts patient fitted total temporomandibular joint reconstruction prosthesis, *Oral Maxillofac Clin N Am* 12:73-91, 2000.
18. Mercuri LG, Wolford LM, Sanders B, et al: Long-term follow-up of the CAD/CAM patient fitted total temporomandibular joint reconstruction system, *J Oral Maxillofac Surg* 60:1440-1448, 2002.
19. Coleta KE, Wolford LM, Goncalves JR, et al: Maxillo-mandibular counter-clockwise rotation and mandibular advancement with TMJ concepts total joint prostheses: part I—skeletal and dental stability, *Int J Oral Maxillofac Surg* Feb;38(2):126-138, 2009.
20. Coleta KE, Wolford LM, Goncalves JR, et al: Maxillo-mandibular counter-clockwise rotation and mandibular advancement with TMJ concepts total joint prostheses: part II—airway changes and stability, *Int J Oral Maxillofac Surg* Mar;38(3):228-235, 2009.
21. Pinto LP, Wolford LM, Buschang PH et al: Maxillo-mandibular counter-clockwise rotation and mandibular advancement with TMJ concepts total joint prostheses: part III—pain and dysfunction outcomes, *Int J Oral Maxillofac Surg* Apr;38(4):326-331, 2009.
22. Wolford LM, Karras SC: Autologous fat transplantation around temporomandibular joint total joint prostheses: preliminary treatment outcomes, *J Oral Maxillofac Surg* 55:245-251, 1997.
23. Morales-Ryan CA, Wolford LM: The use of autologous fat grafts in the temporomandibular joint reconstruction, *J Oral Maxillofac Surg* 59(8 [Suppl 1]):121, 2001.
24. Mercuri LG, Ali FA, Woolson R: Outcomes of total alloplastic replacement with periarticular autogenous fat grafting for management of reankylosis of the temporomandibular joint, *J Oral Maxillofac Surg* Sep;66(9):1794-1803, 2008.
25. Wolford LM, Karras SC, Mehra P: Considerations for orthognathic surgery during growth, part 1: mandibular deformities, *Am J Orthod Dentofac Orthop* 119:95-101, 2001.
26. Wolford LM, Karras SC, Mehra P: Considerations for orthognathic surgery during growth, part 2: maxillary deformities, *Am J Orthod Dentofac Orthop*, 119:102-105, 2001.
27. Merrill RG: Mandibular dislocation and hypermobility, *Oral Maxillofac Surg Clinics No Am: Disorders of the TMJ II: Arthrotomy* 1: 399-413, 1989.
28. Wolford LM, Pitta MC, Mehra P: Mitek anchors for treatment of chronic mandibular dislocation, *O Surg O Med O Pathol O Radiol Endod* 92(5):495-498, 2001.
29. Wolford LM, LeBanc J: Condylectomy to arrest disproportionate mandibular growth. Abstract presentation at the American Cleft Palate Association Meeting, New York, 1986.
30. Wolford LM, Mehra P, Reiche-Fischel O, et al: Efficacy of high condylectomy for management of condylar hyperplasia, *Am J Orthod Dentofacial Orthop* 121(2):136-151, 2002.
31. Garcia-Morales P, Wolford LM, Mehra P, et al: Efficacy of high condylectomy for management of condylar hyperplasia, *J Oral Maxillofac Surg* 59(8) [Suppl 1]:106, 2001.
32. Riolo ML, Moyers RE, McNamara JA, Hunter WS: *An atlas of craniofacial growth.* Ann Arbor, 1974, Center for Human Growth and Development, University of Michigan.
33. Gottlieb OP: Hyperplasia of the mandibular condyle, *J Oral Surg* 9:118-135, 1951.
34. Wolford LM, Mehra P, Franco P: Use of conservative condylectomy for treatment of osteochondroma of the mandibular condyle, *J Oral Maxillofac Surg* 60:262, 2002.
35. Adzuki T, Schroth G, Laeng RH, et al: Osteochondroma of the mandibular condyle, *J Oral Maxillofac Surg* 54:495-500, 1996.
36. Obwegeser HL, Makek MS: Hemimandibular hyperplasia-hemimandibular elongation, *J Maxillofac Surg* 14:183-208, 1986.
37. Karras SC, Wolford LM, Cottrell DA: Concurrent osteochondroma of the mandibular condyle and ipsilateral cranial base resulting in temporomandibular joint ankylosis: report of a case and review of the literature, *J Oral Maxillofac Surg* 54:640-646, 1996.
38. Beers MH, Porter RS, Jones TV, et al: *The Merck manual of diagnosis and therapy*, ed 18, Whitehouse Station, NJ, 2006, Merck Research Laboratories, pp 1875-1877, 259-272.
39. Baker DC: Facial paralysis. In McCarthy JG, editor: *Plastic surgery*, vol 3, Philadelphia, 1990, Saunders, pp 2237-2319.
40. Tompach P, Dodson TB, Kaban LB: Autogenous temporomandibular joint replacement. In *Fonseca oral and maxillofacial surgery: temporomandibular disorders*, Philadelphia, 2000, Saunders, pp 301-315.
41. Dimitroulis G: The use of dermis grafts after discectomy for internal derangement of the temporomandibular joint, *J Oral Maxillofacial Surg* 63:173-178, 2005.
42. Wolford LM, Cottrell DA, Henry CH: Sternoclavicular grafts for temporomandibular joint reconstruction, *J Oral Maxillofac Surg* 52:119-128, 1994.
43. Wolford LM, Cardenas L: Idiopathic condylar resorption: diagnosis, treatment protocol, and outcomes, *Am J Orthod Dentofac Orthop* 116:667-676, 1999.
44. Wolford LM: Idiopathic condylar resorption of the temporomandibular joint in teenage

girls (cheerleaders syndrome), *Baylor Univ Med Cent Proc* 14:246-252, 2001.

45. Morales-Ryan CA, Garcia-Morales P, Wolford LM: Idiopathic condylar resorption: outcome assessment of TMJ disc repositioning and orthognathic surgery, *J Oral Maxillofac Surg* 60:(8 [Suppl 1]):53, 2002.

46. Wolford LM: Concomitant temporomandibular joint and orthognathic surgery, *J Oral Maxillofac Surg* 61:1198-1204, 2003.

47. Goncalves JR, Cassano DS, Wolford LM, et al: Postsurgical stability of counterclockwise maxillomandibular advancement surgery: effect of articular disc repositioning, *J Oral Maxillofac Surg* Apr;66(4):724-738, 2008.

48. Henry CH, Hudson AP, Gerard HC, et al: Identification of chlamydia trachomatis in the human temporomandibular joint, *J Oral Maxillofac Surg* 57: 683-688, 1999.

49. Henry CH, Hughes CV, Gerard HC, et al: Reactive arthritis: preliminary microbiologic analysis of the human temporomandibular joint, *J Oral Maxillofac Surg* 58:1137-1142, 2000.

50. Henry CH, Pitta MC, Wolford LM: Frequency of chlamydial antibodies in patients with internal derangement of the temporomandibular joint, *Oral Surg Oral Med Oral Pathol Oral Radiol Endod* 91:287-292, 2001.

51. Wolford LM, Gerard HC, Henry CH, Hudson AP: Chlamydia psittaci infection may be involved in development of temporomandibular joint dysfunction, *J Oral Maxillofac Surg* 59(Suppl 1):30, 2001.

52. Hudson AP, Henry C, Wolford L, Gerard HC: Chlamydia psittaci infection may influence development of temporomandibular joint dysfunction, *J Arthritis & Rheumatism* 43:S174, 2000.

53. Wolford LM, Henry CH, Goncalves JR: TMJ and systemic effects associated with chlamydia psittaci, *J Oral Maxillofac Surg* 62(Suppl 1):50-51, 2004.

54. Henry CH, Wolford LM: Substance P and mast cells: preliminary histologic analysis of the human temporomandibular joint, *Oral Surg Oral Med Oral Pathol Oral Radiol Endod* 92:384-389, 2001.

55. Henry CH, Nikaein A, Wolford LM: Analysis of human leukocyte antigens in patients with internal derangement of the temporomandibular joint, *J Oral Maxillofac Surg* 60:778-783, 2002.

56. Mehra P, Wolford LM, Baran S, Cassano DS: Single-stage comprehensive surgical treatment of the rheumatoid arthritis temporomandibular joint patient, *J Oral Maxillofac Surg* Sep;67(9):1859-1872, 2009.

THE PAST

The care of the pediatric patient is complicated by the different physiology, anatomy, patient/parent–doctor relationships and the difficulties in communication and cooperation. This will remain relatively unchanged despite any advances in science and medicine. Many of these distinctions were not emphasized in training programs. In the past, the role of oral and maxillofacial surgery (OMFS) in the pediatric arena was mostly related to the elimination of odontogenic infection and basic oral trauma. Graduating surgeons had minimal exposure to complex pediatric surgical care and had no formalized training. The specialty had little or no involvement in the treatment of pediatric maxillofacial trauma or craniofacial congenital deformities. The anatomic restriction of the profession to the oral cavity was even more restricted when treating the pediatric patient.

THE PRESENT

Children are not just smaller adults. The marked distinction in anatomy and physiology has been further acknowledged along with the significant implications in surgical care. Although the specialty has placed more emphasis on training surgeons for pediatric care, the complexity of many craniofacial disorders and anomalies is overwhelming for the core training of most surgeons. The publication of the first textbook of *Pediatric Oral and Maxillofacial Surgery* by Leonard B. Kaban in 1990 is likely the birth of this subspecialty, and formal recognition in this arena as part of OMFS. It also demonstrates the previous void in the literature and the much needed advancement. Currently there are only a few postresidency fellowship training programs in the United States that focus on pediatric craniofacial surgery. There is increasing interest in many oral and maxillofacial surgeons to participate in cleft lip and palate repair, including established mission trips to underserved areas of the world. The increasing number of children's hospitals and pediatric wards is evidence of the greater need for this discipline in all aspects of surgery, medicine, and dentistry.

THE FUTURE

The future of pediatric oral and maxillofacial surgery will involve the formal establishment of a subspecialty that requires training beyond the core OMFS residency, not unlike general surgery and the subsequent development of pediatric general surgery as a separate specialty in the 1940s. Pediatric craniofacial surgery may develop and evolve into a subspecialty where the training is available to several specialties that meet the training standards. Further insight into the human genome and stem cell research will dramatically change the treatment of many acquired and congenital disorders using gene therapy and genetic engineering for pediatric and adult care. Medical genetics will become a prerequisite for all premedical and dental education. Oral and maxillofacial surgeons with advanced training will become more recognized as essential elements of the craniofacial surgical teams contributing to both soft and hard tissue reconstructive surgery. Advances in imaging and prenatal care may increasingly expand the involvement of surgeons during the intrauterine period.

Chapter

83

Cleft Lip and Palate: Timing and Approaches to Reconstruction

Radhika Chigurupati

Clefts of the lip and palate are the most common craniofacial birth defects, next only to congenital heart defects and clubfoot.[1] This condition has significant psychosocial ramifications and should be managed appropriately to avoid unnecessary anxiety and exhaustion of the patient and family members. It is a treatable condition that can result in a good outcome when interdisciplinary care is provided by a team of specialists in a timely fashion from birth to adolescence. A cleft team generally includes a pediatrician, nurse practitioner, speech pathologist, pediatric dentist, orthodontist, social worker, geneticist, and surgeons with expertise in oral and maxillofacial surgery/plastic surgery and pediatric otolaryngology. The timing of various surgical interventions has been a subject of debate. This is particularly true for palate, nose, and alveolar cleft repair because of the concern about the impact of surgery on facial growth and development. The timing of surgical and nonsurgical interventions should ideally coincide with the physical, cognitive, and psychological development of the child, rather than merely chronological age. In reality, however, treatment is often dictated by socioeconomic factors, access to cleft care centers, the nutritional status of the child, and associated medical conditions.[2] An economic evaluation of the impact of treating cleft lip and palate disorders revealed the immense gain for the individual and society.[3] The ultimate goal of treatment is to achieve normality in speech, overall appearance, physical and psychological development, allowing the individual to be confident and successful in life. This chapter presents current evidence and rationale for timing and approaches to diagnosis and management of the child with a cleft deformity, from prenatal period to adolescence (Box 83 1).

BOX 83-1	Sequence of Interdisciplinary Care of Cleft Patient

Prenatal
Diagnosis and parental counseling

0 to 6 Months after Birth
General assessment and genetics evaluation
Evaluation of airway, feeding, swallowing, and hearing
Infant presurgical orthopedics
Cleft lip repair

6 Months to 2 Years
Cleft palate repair
Grommets/ear tubes
Assess oral sensory motor development and speech

Pre-school: 3 to 5 Years
Evaluation of primary dentition
Speech assessment and therapy
Nasolabial revision if indicated

Childhood: 6 to 12 Years
Correction of velopharyngeal insufficiency
Orthodontic treatment (phase I)
Monitor facial growth and development of permanent dentition
Alveolar cleft repair

Adolescence: 13 to 19 Years
Orthodontic treatment (phase II)
Orthognathic surgery for correction of maxillary hypoplasia
Revision of secondary lip and nasal deformities
Replacement of missing teeth
Genetic counseling

BOX 83-2	Epidemiology of Oral Clefts

Distribution of Oral Clefts
Cleft lip and palate: 46%
Cleft palate only: 33%
Cleft lip only: 21%

Cleft Lip with or without Palate (CL/P)
Average birth prevalence: 1:700
More common in males
Unilateral > bilateral
Left side > right side
Association with other anomalies: 10%

Cleft Palate Only (CP)
Average birth prevalence: 1:2000
More common in females
Association with other anomalies: 50-60%

Some Syndromes Associated with CL/P
Fetal alcohol syndrome
Down syndrome
Van der Woude syndrome
Ectrodactyly-ectodermal dysplasia-clefting syndrome
Popliteal pterygium syndromes
Opitz syndrome
Craniofacial microsomia

Some Syndromes Associated with CP
Down syndrome
22q deletion syndromes: DiGeorge syndrome, Shprintzen syndrome
Stickler syndrome
Treacher Collins syndrome
Apert syndrome
De Lange syndrome

EPIDEMIOLOGY

Clefts of lip and palate are the most common congenital facial defects, with an incidence ranging from 1:500 to 1:2000 live births. Cleft lip with or without cleft palate (CL/P) shows considerable variation among various ethnic groups, with Native Americans and Asians (1:500) clearly at a higher risk in comparison to whites (1:1000) and those of African descent (1:2000). In contrast, clefts of palate only (CP) have lower incidence (1:2000) and a more homogeneous distribution across all populations compared to CL/P.[4-9] About half of the oral clefts involve both lip and palate (46%), a third involve only the palate (33%), and a fifth are clefts of lip alone (21%). Clefts of lip with or without palate (CL/P) are more often unilateral than bilateral and more common in males than females. The unilateral defects occur more often on the left side than right side. Clefts of lip occur in the ratio of 6:3:1 for unilateral left, unilateral right, and bilateral.[10] Cleft palate, on the other hand, is more common in females and more often associated with other developmental anomalies. Clefts may be classified as syndromic or isolated depending on the presence or absence of other developmental anomalies. Syndromic association is more common in CP (50%), whereas the majority of CL/P (80%) are isolated.[10,11] Oral clefts are a common presentation in many syndromes; some of the more common syndromes associated with cleft lip and palate, include Van der Woude, Down, orofacial digital, Opitz, and fetal alcohol syndrome (Box 83-2).[12,13] The triad of micrognathia, glossoptosis, and airway obstruction (Pierre Robin sequence) may sometimes be present in both syndromic and nonsyndromic children with cleft palate. The most common syndromic presentations of Pierre Robin sequence are Stickler's syndrome, velocardiofacial (VCF) syndrome, and Treacher-Collins syndrome.[14]

BOX 83-3	Etiology of Cleft Lip and Palate

Estimated Contributions of Identified Genes to CL/P
IRF 6 (Interferon regulatory factor 6): 12%
FGFs (Fibroblast growth factors): 3%
MSX1(Msh homeobox 1): 2%
Private mutations in candidate genes: 6%

Contribution of Environmental Factors to CL/P
Maternal smoking
Maternal folate deficiency
Maternal diabetes
Maternal drug use: alcohol, steroids, phenytoin sodium

Data from Vieira AR: Unraveling human cleft lip and palate research, *J Dent Res* Feb;87(2):119-125, 2008.

ETIOLOGY AND GENETICS

Nonsyndromic CL/P is a complex trait with a multifactorial etiology that results from a combination of genetic and environmental factors (Box 83-3).[15] Research to identify candidate genes and loci responsible for clefting in recent years suggests that anywhere from 3 to

14 genes contribute to cleft lip and palate.[16-18] For nonsyndromic cleft lip and palate, candidate genes and loci have been identified on chromosomes 1, 2, 4, 6, 11, 14, 17, and 19.[19-21] Clues from mendelian forms of clefting disorders such as Van der Woude syndrome, which is an autosomal dominant condition, have facilitated the mapping of genes responsible for nonsyndromic cleft lip and palate.[22] Using this model, Zucchero et al. have shown that DNA-sequence variants associated with the gene IRF6 (interferon regulatory factor 6) are major contributors (12%) to CL/P.[23] The genes IRF6 and MSX-1 and FGFR1 account for about 15% of all nonsyndromic cleft lip and palate.[24] The genes contributing to cleft palate are different. Aberrant TGF-b3 signaling plays a role in the pathogenesis of cleft palate. Mutations in other genes TBX22, FGFR1, and P63 also contribute to syndromic clefts of the palate.[24]

Environmental factors that contribute to the etiology of facial clefting disorders can be divided into four groups: drugs, chemicals, maternal metabolic imbalances, and maternal infections. Cigarette smoking during pregnancy,[25-27] maternal exposure to alcohol and teratogenic medications such as retinoids, corticosteroids, and anticonvulsants (phenytoin and valproic acid),[19] low dietary intake of B-complex vitamins, and folic acid deficiency during the periconceptional period can cause clefting disorders.[28,29] Co-sanguinous marriages, maternal diabetes, and obesity have also been linked to an increased risk of orofacial clefts.[30] Less consistent associations have been found between clefts and maternal viral infections such as rubella and varicella.[31] Studies conducted to determine the risk of clefting disorders show that every parent has about a 0.14% (1 : 700) chance of having a child with CL/P and a 0.04% (1 : 2000) chance of having a child with CP. The risk of recurrence of a cleft condition is determined by a number of factors including the number of family members with clefts, their relationship to family members with clefts, race, sex, and the type and severity of cleft of the affected individuals. Studies show that the recurrence risk for first-degree relatives is about 3.3% for cleft lip with or without palate, and for isolated cleft palate it is 2%.[32] Once parents have a child with a cleft, the risk of having a second child with a cleft is about 2-5%, and after two affected children that risk rises to 9-12%.[13,33] In twins with cleft lip and palate and those with isolated cleft of palate, the concordance is far greater for monozygotic twins (43%) than for dizygotic twins (5%).[30,31] Parents and young adults should be counseled appropriately by a geneticist so that they are in a better position to make decisions about future pregnancies.

EMBRYOLOGY

The embryo undergoes rapid changes in shape and growth between 4 and 8 weeks as the brain expands and the six branchial arches are formed. The first two branchial arches are primarily responsible for the development of the face and cranium. The development of the face begins from the neural crest ectomesenchyme that forms five prominences: the frontonasal process and paired maxillary and mandibular processes surrounding a central depression. During the 5th and 6th weeks, the bilateral maxillary processes derived from first brachial arch fuse with the medial nasal process to form the upper lip, alveolus, and primary palate. The lateral nasal process forms the alar structures of the nose. The mandibular processes form the lower lip and jaw (Fig. 83-1).[34] This process of formation of facial structures is the consequence of events such as cell proliferation, cell differentiation, cell adhesion, and apoptosis. The processes of the neural crest cells are directed by molecular signals that are controlled by an array of genes. These include fibroblast growth factors (FGFs), sonic hedgehog (SHH), bone morphogenic proteins (BMPs), members of the transforming growth factor beta (TGF-b)

superfamily, and other transcription factors. Failure or error in any of these cellular mechanisms can disrupt the fusion of the medial nasal process with the lateral nasal process and maxillary process, thus causing orofacial clefts. The severity of the cleft is proportionate to the failure of penetration by the neuroectoderm.[4,18]

The formation of the secondary palate is embryologically different and begins during the 6th week after conception, from the two palatal shelves, which extend from the internal aspect of the maxillary processes. During the 8th week, these bilateral maxillary palatal shelves, after ascending to an appropriate position above the tongue, fuse with each other and the primary palate. A disruption in the fusion of these embryonic components can occur because of a delay in elevation of the palatal shelves from vertical to horizontal, defective shelf fusion, or postfusion rupture resulting in a cleft of the secondary palate (Fig. 83-2).[34]

SEQUENCE OF INTERDISCIPLINARY MANAGEMENT OF CHILD WITH A CLEFT DEFORMITY

PRENATAL PERIOD

Diagnosis and Counseling

Sophisticated high-resolution 3D ultrasonography has facilitated the diagnosis of a higher percentage of craniofacial anomalies before birth (Fig. 83-3). However, the majority of orofacial clefts are still detected postnatally. In the United States, about 25-30% of clefts of the lip with or without the palate are diagnosed before birth. Clefts of the lip with or without the palate can be diagnosed prenatally with a transabdominal ultrasound at 16 to 20 weeks of pregnancy and sometimes as early as 11 weeks with a transvaginal ultrasound. Clefts of the palate alone are rarely seen on ultrasound. Johnson et al. showed that the frequencies of prenatal diagnosis for cleft lip and palate, cleft lip only, and cleft palate only were 33.3%, 20.3%, and 0.3%, respectively.[35,36] Several factors may influence the accuracy of ultrasound studies: the sophistication of the scanning equipment, the experience and skill of the sonographer, the number of weeks into pregnancy, the position of the baby while scanning, the amount of amniotic fluid, the maternal body structure, and the severity of the cleft. The accuracy of prenatal ultrasound diagnosis of cleft lip alone is in the range of 75-81%. Higher detection rates in some studies may be attributable to the routine inclusion of specific views of the fetal face, namely tangential and transverse, during a routine anomaly scan. The position of the fetal head (ideally occipitoposterior) enables satisfactory views in the desired planes.[36,37] Premaxillary protrusion is an important clue to the presence of a complete cleft lip and cleft palate and may be more conspicuous than the cleft itself. The presence of a paranasal echogenic mass favors the presence of a bilateral cleft lip and cleft palate. A recent study showed that fetal MRI allows more detailed prenatal evaluation of the upper lip and palate than sonograms. The main advantage is that the secondary palate, which is rarely evaluated adequately on sonograms, is visible on MRI, which will enable a prospective diagnosis of clefts of secondary palate.[37,38] Prenatal diagnosis and parental counseling may help families to be better prepared and provide an opportunity for possible chromosomal studies to look for other malformations. The main disadvantage of prenatal diagnosis is the anxiety, the emotional disturbance for the mother, and the inability to correct it prenatally. The capability of such tests raises both ethical and psychological issues such as the dilemma of termination of birth. Physicians and surgeons have to inform parents that cleft lip and palate in the

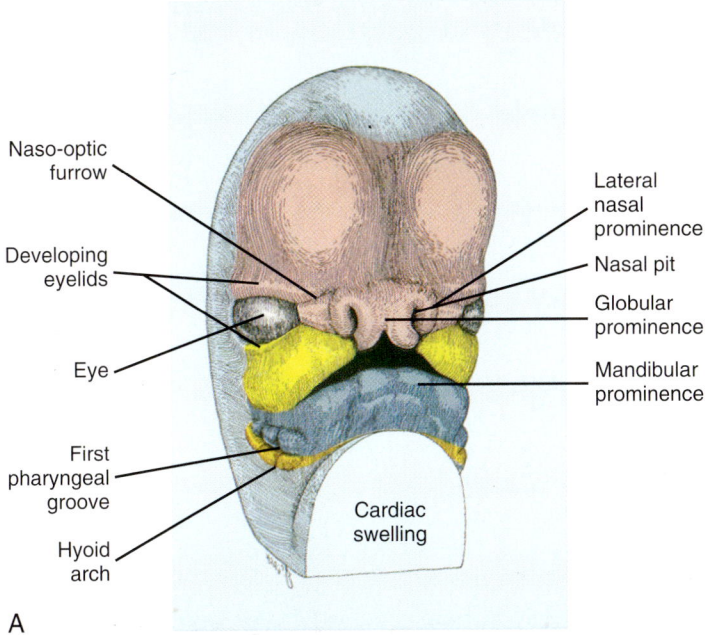

Naso-optic
furrow

Developing
eyelids

Eye

First
pharyngeal
groove

Hyoid
arch

Lateral
nasal
prominence

Nasal pit

Globular
prominence

Mandibular
prominence

Cardiac
swelling

A

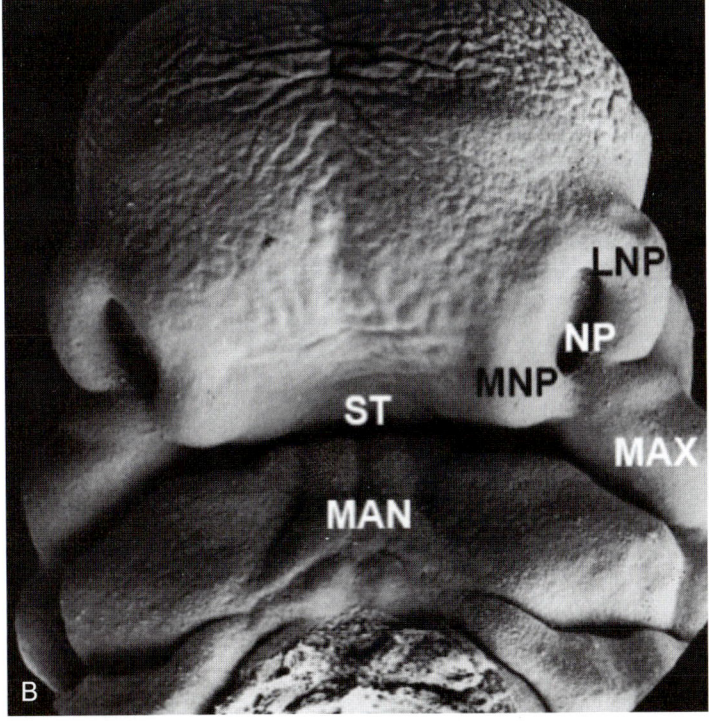

LNP

NP

MNP

ST

MAX

MAN

B

Fig. 83-1 ■ **A,** Embryonic development of the face, 6th week. **B,** Electron microscopy showing the development of the face of a 37-day-old human embryo. The nasal pit (NP) is surrounded by the medial nasal process (MNP) and lateral nasal process (LNP) and maxillary process (MAX). (**A,** From Avery JK, Chiego DJ: *Essentials of oral histology and embryology: a clinical approach,* ed 3, St. Louis, 2006, Elsevier. **B,** From Hinrichsen K: The early development of morphology and patterns of the face in the human embryo, *Adv Anat Embryol Cell Biol* 98:1-79, 1985.)

absence of other major systemic anomalies is a treatable, non-life-threatening condition. Jones presented an algorithm for prenatal diagnosis of cleft lip and palate and strategies for counseling parents.[39] The cleft team can discuss feeding issues, determine the timing of lip and palate surgery, and help establish contact with support groups for the family. Parents seem to be affected more by the manner in which the diagnosis is presented than the timing of the diagnosis.[40] Although the benefits of fetal healing have been well documented, at this time there is no indication for intrauterine repair of the cleft lip deformity as the risk of fetal surgery is far too high both for the fetus and mother for correction of this non-life-threatening condition.

0 TO 6 MONTHS AFTER BIRTH

General Assessment

Every child born with a cleft of lip or palate should be thoroughly assessed by a neonatologist or pediatrician soon after birth (Box 83-4). If the child is delivered in a nonmedical facility or a small hospital, he or she should be referred to a tertiary hospital with specialists or a craniofacial team for further evaluation. A complete physical examination including the necessary diagnostic tests should be carried out to check for airway anomalies or other associated cardiovascular, renal, and musculoskeletal abnormalities. The possibility of syndromic association should be considered, particularly

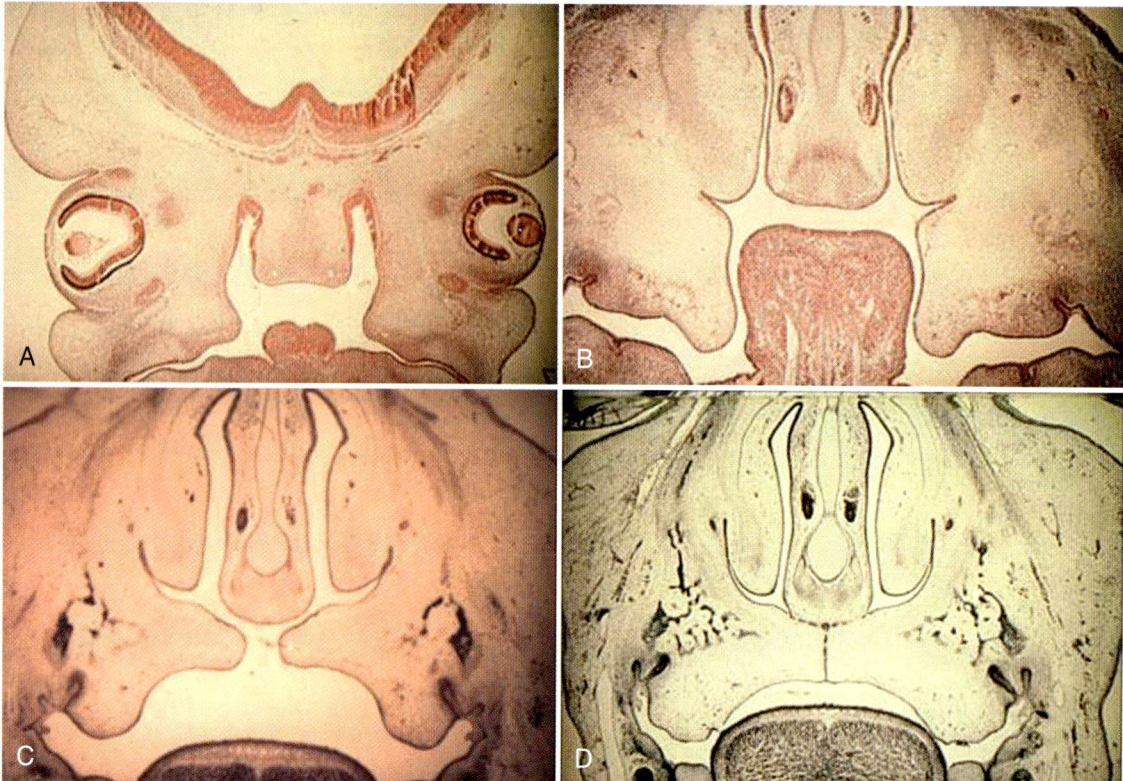

Fig. 83-2 ■ Coronal scanning electron microscopy photos of a human embryo showing the stages of formation of the palate between 8 and 9 weeks. **A,** Development of the palate showing palatal shelves and tongue position. **B,** The vertical orientation of the palatal shelves on either side of the tongue. **C,** Palatal shelves elevate. **D,** Palatal shelves fuse with each other and the nasal septum in the midline. (From Chigurupati R, Heggie A, Bonanthaya K: Cleft lip and palate: an overview. In Anderson L, Kahnberg K, Pogrel MA: *Oral and maxillofacial surgery*, Hoboken, N.J., 2011, Wiley and Sons.)

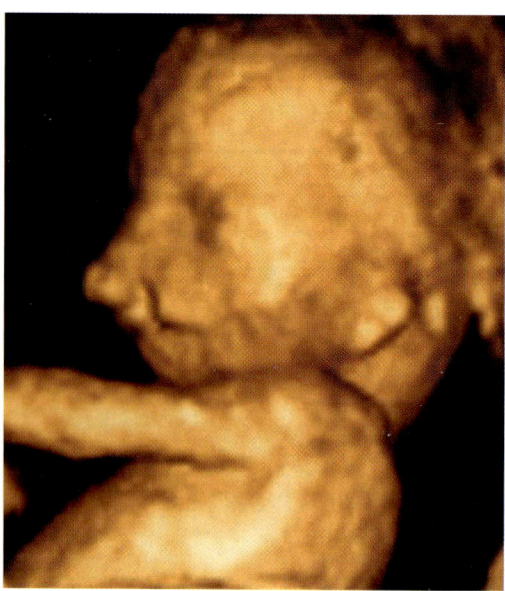

Fig. 83-3 ■ A 3D-rendered ultrasound image at 17 weeks showing the bilateral cleft lip and palate with premaxillary protrusion. (From Nyberg DA, Hyett J, Johnson J, Sourter V: First-trimester screening, *Ultrasound Clin* Apr;1(2):231-255, 2006.)

BOX 83-4	Evaluation of a Newborn Child with a Cleft Deformity

1. Assess breathing and look for signs of airway obstruction.
2. Evaluate ability to feed and provide parental counseling for feeding.
3. Assess nutritional intake, weight gain, and growth.
4. Assess for concomitant anomalies (e.g., cardiac/renal/pulmonary/musculoskeletal).
5. Assess syndromic association and request appropriate genetic testing.
6. Perform craniofacial examination including head shape and circumference, ears, eyes, nose, jaws, and oral cavity.
7. Evaluate severity and type of cleft defect, width of cleft, position of alveolar segments and premaxilla, as well as nasal deformity.
8. Assess need for presurgical orthopedics and type of appliance necessary.
9. Prepare child and parents for surgical repair of cleft lip.

in children with cleft palate (Fig. 83-4). Parents should receive proper counseling for nutrition, and feeding should be initiated immediately.

Airway Evaluation

Infants are obligate nasal breathers. Concomitant anomalies of the upper and lower airway are common in children with craniofacial birth defects. Assessment of the airway should be a priority for a

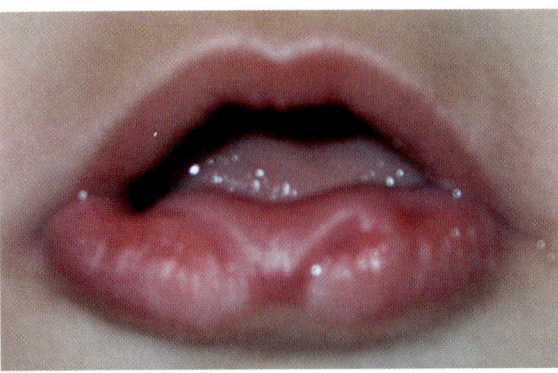

Fig. 83-4 ■ In Van der Woude syndrome, lower lip pits are an associated anomaly, along with cleft lip and palate.

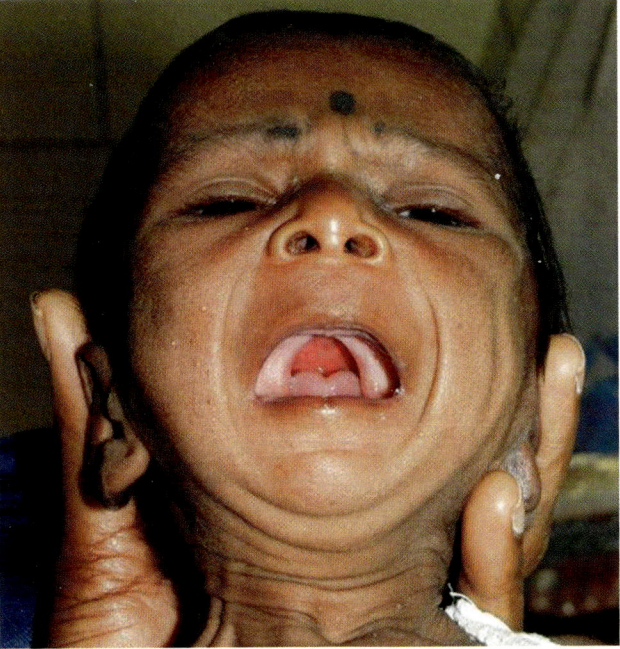

Fig. 83-5 ■ Child with Pierre Robin Sequence (PRS), showing signs of increased respiratory effort as a result of micrognathia, glossoptosis, and upper airway obstruction.

newborn with a cleft deformity. Children born with a cleft of the palate may have associated micrognathia, glossoptosis, and airway obstruction (Fig. 83-5). In these children, one should look for signs of increased effort while breathing, stridor, difficulty in feeding, weight loss, and failure to thrive. Parents should be informed to watch for an abnormal breathing pattern or respiratory distress, particularly during upper respiratory tract infection. If there are signs of obstruction, a pediatric otolaryngologist should be consulted to perform an endoscopic evaluation of the upper and lower airways to look for any possible cause of obstruction. In the upper airway, the patency of nares, choanae, jaw size and position, as well as tongue position in relation to the cleft of the palate, should be assessed. Examination of the lower airway to detect laryngotracheal anomalies such as tracheomalacia, laryngeal clefts, and stenosis is necessary.

Feeding and Nutrition

Children with cleft deformities have difficulty feeding because of their inability to create a proper seal around the nipple of the bottle or breast. Feeding is not a major problem when the cleft involves only the lip. Despite the problems with maintaining sucking pressures, the swallowing mechanisms in children with cleft palate are usually normal. Therefore, if the milk or formula can reach the oropharynx, the natural swallowing reflexes can move it into the esophagus. Babies with isolated clefts of the lip or palate can usually feed by mouth with some adjustments to bottle-feeding techniques. Tube feeding is rarely required. Initially, some children with cleft palate may show some discoordination of the "breathe, suck, swallow" reflex, resulting in nasal regurgitation of feeds or intermittent choking spells. These episodes often are self-limited, and the infant soon learns to prevent nasal regurgitation and coordinate swallowing. Placing the infant in an upright position during feeding may reduce the occurrence of nasal regurgitation. The strategies that have been developed to feed infants with clefts of the palate are designed to overcome the lack of negative pressure during sucking. These include, but are not limited to, cross-cut fissured feeding nipples or squeezable soft bottles that can deliver more milk under less pressure. Studies show that the use of a passive palatal feeding appliance does not improve growth outcomes of children with cleft lip and palate.[41,42] The team nurse should provide the parents with information on feeding during prenatal counseling or immediately after birth. The goal is to provide adequate nutrition to satisfy the caloric requirements for growth and prepare the child for timely surgical repair of lip and palate during the first year after birth.

Hearing and Early Speech Evaluation

An audiology assessment is recommended soon after birth to check for hearing abnormalities. In children with cleft palate it is best to perform this hearing screening within the first few days of life, when the middle ear is well aerated and the child has not yet developed effusion. The screening test is most useful during this effusion-free period. These children also exhibit a higher frequency of otitis media because of eustachian tube dysfunction prior to palate repair. This can contribute to conductive hearing loss and sometimes speech and language delay.[41,43] Insertion of pressure-equalizing tubes (grommets) at the time of palate repair is recommended to avoid middle ear ventilation disorders.[42,44] Although not as common as conductive hearing loss, sensorineural hearing deficits exist within the cleft population, and they have an effect on speech perception and clarity, as well as auditory comprehension skills. An initial speech evaluation no later than 6 months after birth is recommended for children with cleft palate.

Presurgical Orthopedics

The benefits of presurgical orthopedics include better alignment of the alveolar segments, premaxilla, tension-free approximation of the cleft lip edges, and improvement of nostril symmetry as well as shape. McNeill and Burston introduced presurgical orthopedics in 1950 to align the collapsed maxillary alveolar segments prior to lip surgery using a palatal acrylic appliance. In 1975, Latham and Georgiade subsequently described the use of an active pin retained device to expand the collapsed lateral maxillary segments and retract the premaxilla in complete bilateral clefts and to achieve symmetry of the alveolar arch in complete unilateral clefts (Fig. 83-6).[44-46] These early techniques focused on the alveolar and premaxillary segments but did not address the deformity of the nasal cartilage.

More recently, Grayson and others (1993), showed that gentle application of presurgical orthopedic forces to mold the alveolar segments and the nostrils within 3 months has shown some benefits in correction of the nasal deformity in children with complete bilateral cleft lip and palate and wide unilateral clefts. Nasoalveolar molding (NAM) increases the surface area of the nasal mucosal lining and helps to elongate and upright the columella, and improves

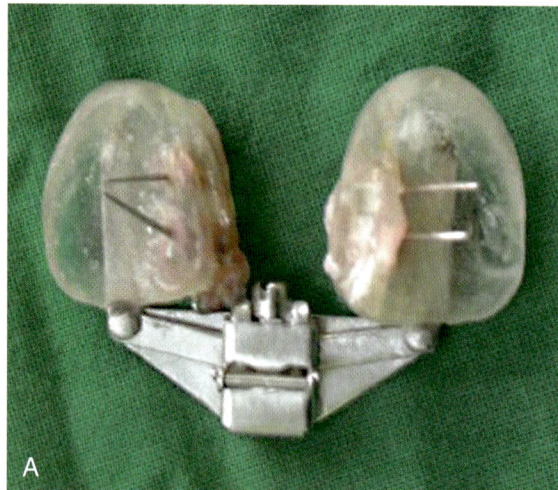

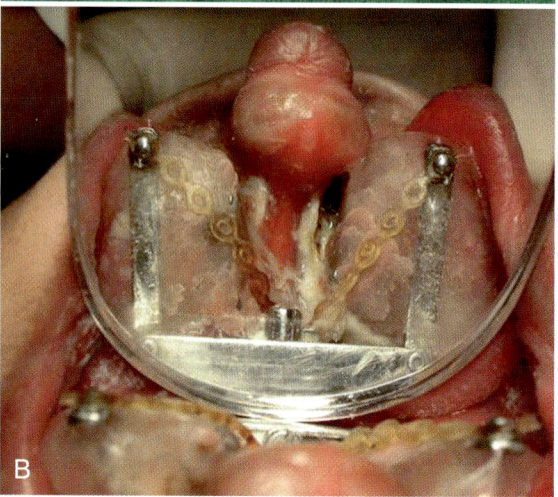

Fig. 83-6 ■ Latham device used to achieve better position of pre-maxilla and alveolar segments in a bilateral cleft palate. (Courtesy Dr. Hirji Adenwalla, Charles Pinto Cleft Center, Jubilee Mission Hospital, Kerala, India.)

nostril symmetry. This preoperative expansion of the nasal lining allows suturing of interdomal cartilages without tension and decreases widening of the nose.[47-51] This technique also allows better position of the alveolar segments, facilitates gingivoperiosteoplasty at the time of lip repair, and may prevent the need for secondary bone grafting in select cases (Fig. 83-7). In recent years, several centers have reported the adoption of the nasoalveolar molding technique to improve the outcomes of lip and nose repair, especially in complete bilateral clefts of the lip and palate, but there is a wide variation in the availability of expertise and cost of treatment.[52] It is important to evaluate these recent studies critically for their overall clinical and cost effectiveness.[53] Consideration should be given to other cost-effective and simple techniques of nonsurgical lip adhesion, such as lip taping (Fig. 83-8) prior to surgical repair, which have been used in the past in infants with wide clefts.

Cleft Lip Repair

Timing of Cleft Lip Repair The timing for primary lip repair is usually between 3 to 6 months after birth, but it can be performed slightly earlier or later depending on the associated medical conditions and nutritional status of child. Most craniofacial centers around the world follow the rule of tens, which implies that the infant should be at least 10 weeks of age, weigh at least 10 pounds, and have at least 10 gm/100 ml of hemoglobin to withstand the surgical and anesthetic stress. In general, surgery is indicated when the infant is adequately nourished, when he or she has been thoroughly evaluated for other concomitant systemic anomalies, and when respiratory control mechanisms are mature. Ziak et al. reported that the most common reasons for delay in lip repair are prematurity, hypoxia, respiratory tract infections such as recurrent bronchopulmonary pneumonia, and anemia.[52,54] In general, most centers prefer to perform the unilateral lip repair when the infant is aged 3 to 4 months. Some centers have advocated lip repair in the early neonatal period, with a theoretical benefit in the scar appearance and nasal cartilage adaptability, thus minimizing the nasal deformity. However, it appears that the main advantage in performing lip repair in this early neonatal period versus at 3 months of age is the psychological benefit and satisfaction expressed by mothers with no added benefit in terms of success of surgical outcome.[53,55] By the time the baby is 3 months old, the tissue of the lip is more full and the lip elements are larger and better defined, which allows meticulous reconstruction and the child is better able to withstand the stress of surgery and anesthesia.[54,56]

One Stage vs. Two-Stage Lip Repair Primary lip repair can be staged by performing a lip adhesion initially followed by a definitive cheiloplasty.[57] A surgical lip adhesion may be preferred as an initial surgical procedure within 6 to 8 weeks after birth as it helps to mold the alveolar segments and decreases the width of the cleft, thereby facilitating the definitive repair without tension at a later date. Good approximation of the alveolar segments also allows the surgeon to perform a gingivoperiosteoplasty at the time of definitive cheiloplasty. However, this may not be the case always, as the molded lesser segment can collapse. The disadvantages of converting the complete cleft lip to an incomplete one by lip adhesion are the need for an extra operation and the possibility of removal of more tissue at the time of definitive lip repair. Nonsurgical orthopedic techniques during the first 6 to 8 weeks after birth, as described earlier with presurgical orthopedics, can produce good alignment of the alveolar segments.

Evolution and Surgical Principles of Unilateral Cleft Lip and Nose Repair (Box 83-5) Several surgeons, including Rose (1891), Thompson (1912), Blair (1930), Le Mesurier (1949), Tennison and Randall (1952), and Skoog (1974), have contributed to the evolution of cleft lip repair, but the most popular technique was introduced by Millard (1955) who described the rotation-advancement concept.[58-60] Today, various modifications of the Millard advancement rotation technique, an extremely versatile procedure, are used to repair the unilateral cleft lip deformity. In Millard's technique, the medial flap is rotated downward to achieve length, while the lateral flap is advanced. The advantage of this technique is that the suture line lies on the recreated philtral column and incision allows easy access for primary rhinoplasty to reposition the nasal septum, lower lateral cartilage, and alar base. It is a versatile technique and enables the surgeon to modify or adjust while operating, depending on the physical characteristics of the cleft.[61] The main disadvantage is that the inexperienced surgeon requires good surgical judgment during the operation, as it is not based on exact measurements. Inadequate rotation and advancement is a common error that can produce suboptimal results.[62] On the other hand, the triangular flap technique described by Tennison and Randall is based on exact measurements, can be reproduced well, and is used more easily in wide clefts of the lip. Despite inherent variations in different techniques, there are some similarities that form the guiding principles in surgical repair of the unilateral cleft lip deformity.

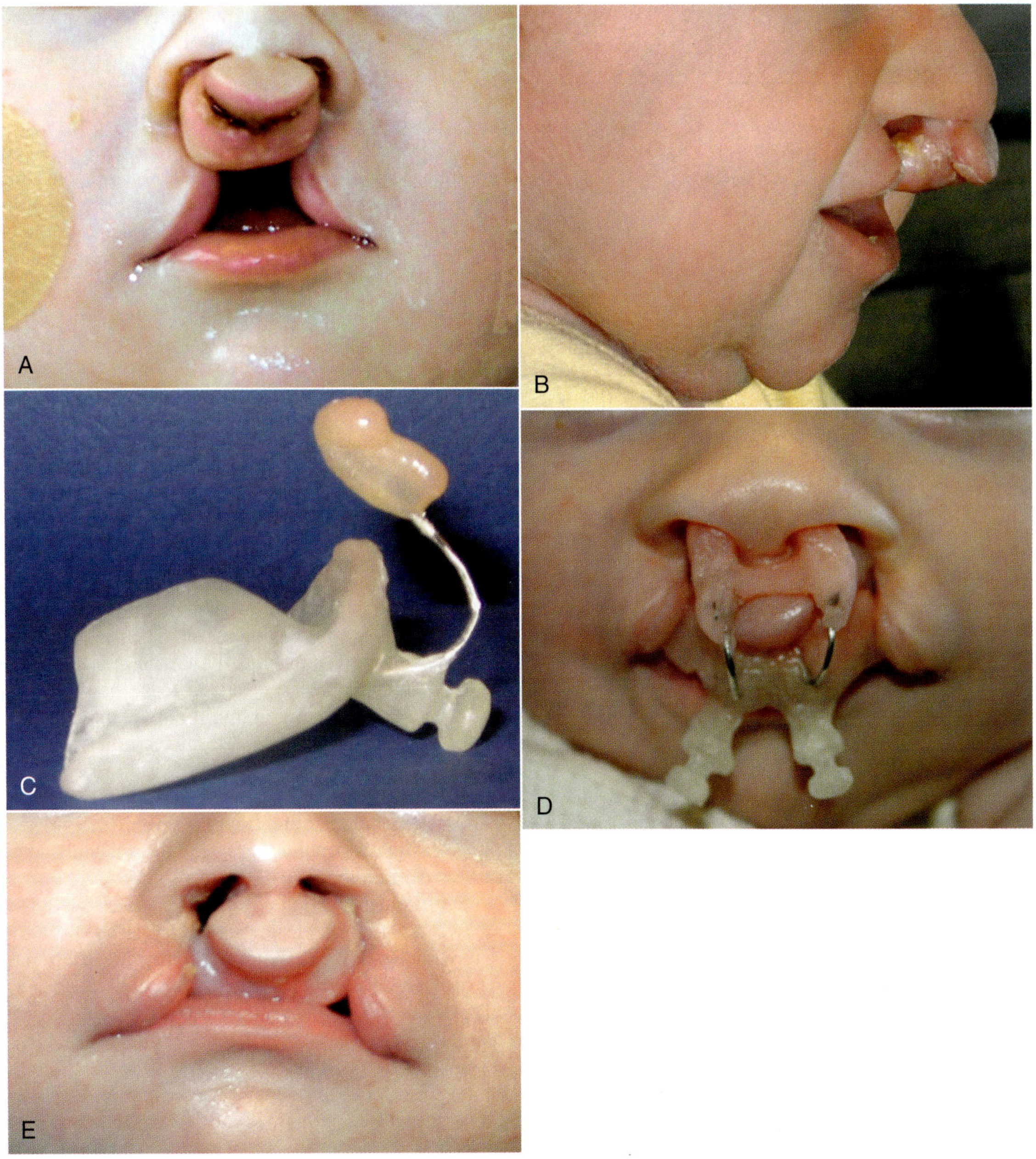

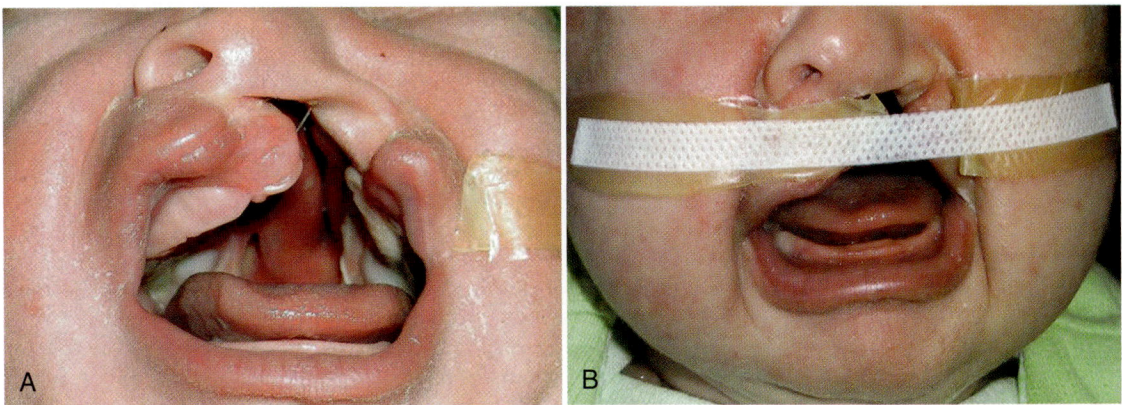

Fig. 83-7 ■ Child with BCLP managed by nasoalveolar molding before surgical lip repair. Prominent premaxilla (**A** and **B**) before nasoalveolar molding. Appliance for nasoalveolar molding (**C**) and appliance in use (**D**). **E,** The position of premaxilla after nasoalveolar molding. (Courtesy Dr. Snehlata Oberoi, UCSF Center for Craniofacial Anomalies, San Francisco.)

Fig. 83-8 ■ Child with a wide UCLP (**A**) being managed by lip taping (**B**) to decrease width of cleft prior to primary lip repair.

BOX 83-5   Surgical Principles of Unilateral and Bilateral Cleft Lip Repair

Unilateral

Rotation and lengthening of shortened vertical height of medial lip element

Advancement of tissue flap from lateral to medial

Alignment and approximation of orbicularis oris

Maintenance of Cupid's bow and creating a philtral column on cleft side

Alignment of alveolar segments and restoration of continuity if possible

Primary repair of the collapsed alar cartilages and nasal septum

Bilateral

Managing the premaxilla by nasoalveolar molding prior to lip repair

Establishing symmetry by simultaneous bilateral repair

Creating appropriate design and width of prolabial flap (narrow and biconcave)

Reconstructing Cupid's bow and tubercle from lateral lip elements

Establishing continuity of orbicularis oris muscle beneath the prolabium

Maintaining a vestibule between lip and alveolar segments

Creating columella and tip by repositioning lower lateral cartilages with interdomal sutures

Repositioning and cinching alar base

The basic principles and goals of unilateral cleft lip repair are to achieve symmetry, proper alignment, and continuity of the orbicularis oris muscle and creation of a philtral column on the affected side.[63-65] Proper approximation of the orbicularis muscle with mattress sutures will improve the prominence of the philtral column on the cleft side. If the alveolar ridges are in a favorable position a gingivoperiosteoplasty may be performed simultaneously. In the unilateral deformity, the normal side serves as a guide to identify the key points and to plan the incisions on the cleft side. The correction of the nasal deformity at the time of primary lip repair has been well documented with long-term outcomes.[66,67] It is important to mobilize the collapsed lower lateral cartilage from the overlying skin by wide dissection and undermining. The cartilage and deviated nasal septum should be anatomically repositioned and fixed with sutures to create a symmetric nostril shape[68] (Fig. 83-9).

Evolution and Surgical Principles of Bilateral Cleft Lip and Nose Repair (see Box 83-5)

Complete bilateral clefts of lip (Fig. 83-10) are rare, accounting for only 10% of cleft lips; therefore, the experience in treating these deformities is limited. Bilateral cleft lip repair is much more challenging and the results are often less satisfactory than that of unilateral cleft lip. The anatomic abnormalities that make this deformity so difficult to repair are the absence of muscle in the prolabial segment resulting in lack of philtral dimple, philtral columns, white roll margin, the median tubercle, the angular peaks, and the typical Cupid's bow. The premaxilla is protuberant and sometimes deviated to one side, making tension-free approximation of muscle and cleft margins difficult. The orbicularis oris muscle, which is in the lateral lip elements, inserts at the alar base on each side. The accompanying nasal deformity consists of a columella that is abnormally short, a wide nasal tip, and a flared alar base as a result of the malpositioned splayed alar cartilages.[69]

The evolution of repair of the bilateral cleft lip over the years has shown that it is best to repair both sides of the cleft lip at the same time. In many centers today, primary nasal correction is performed along with the repair of the lip. The observation that the alar cartilages are splayed and rotated caudally was important in the evolution of primary rhinoplasty in cleft lip repair. The fear of growth interference when nasal cartilage is manipulated during primary repair has been one of the reasons for delaying nasal repair. For many years forked flaps were used to lengthen the columella, but McComb and Mulliken emphasized the importance of early repositioning of the alar cartilages and unraveled the problem of the short columella and broad nasal tip in the bilateral cleft lip. McComb, after reviewing his initial work over a period of 15 years, found that the nostril shape was still abnormal, the tip remained broad, and the columella was long after repair of the lip.[70,71]

The basic principles guiding repair of the bilateral cleft lip deformity are maintaining symmetry, establishing muscle continuity, designing the prolabial flap to achieve appropriate philtral width and shape, forming a Cupid's bow and median tubercle from the lateral labial tissue, and, finally, repositioning the alar cartilages to construct the nasal tip and columella. The principles outlined here are those of the Mulliken simultaneous lip and nose repair.[69] Nasoalveolar molding prior to bilateral cleft lip repair is useful when the premaxillary segment is protuberant or deviated. Symmetry can be best achieved by performing repair of both sides simultaneously. The prolabial flap should be designed to be narrow and biconcave to avoid an abnormally wide philtrum as the child grows. The mucosa of the prolabium can be used to increase the vestibular depth. The prolabium has a very narrow strip of vermilion, and hence the lateral lip vermilion flaps are often necessary to reconstruct the central portion or the tubercle and Cupid's bow. In a complete bilateral cleft, the prolabium is devoid of muscle fibers. Establishing continuity of muscle beneath the skin of the prolabium is the only way to reconstruct a normal functioning lip. The muscle fibers that are inserted at the alar base on each side should be released and reoriented to be approximated in the midline with vertical mattress sutures. A sulcular incision bilaterally beneath the lateral lip elements is essential to mobilize the lip by wide subperiosteal dissection to achieve tension-less closure.[64] The lower lateral cartilages should be mobilized adequately from the overlying skin by wide dissection and undermining. These cartilage domes can be approached by combining rim incisions with the prolabial flap. The nasal tip and columella can be created by anatomically repositioning and fixing them with interdomal mattress sutures.[72]

FROM 6 MONTHS TO 2 YEARS

Timing and Principles of Cleft Palate Repair

The goals of palate repair are to normalize speech by surgical approximation and realignment of the aberrant attachments of the palatal muscles and to seal the communication between the oral and nasal cavities.

Timing of Repair

The timing of palate repair to achieve optimal speech with minimal facial growth disturbance has been one of the more debated topics in cleft literature. Historically, cleft repair of the hard palate was delayed to minimize impairment of maxillofacial growth. It is now well accepted and evidence in the literature shows that speech outcomes are better when soft and hard palate repair is completed before speech development.[43,73,74] Palate surgery is therefore timed according to the infant's speech development rather than chronologic age. For most children developing normally, this is around 9 to 12 months. The majority of the surgeons repair the palate

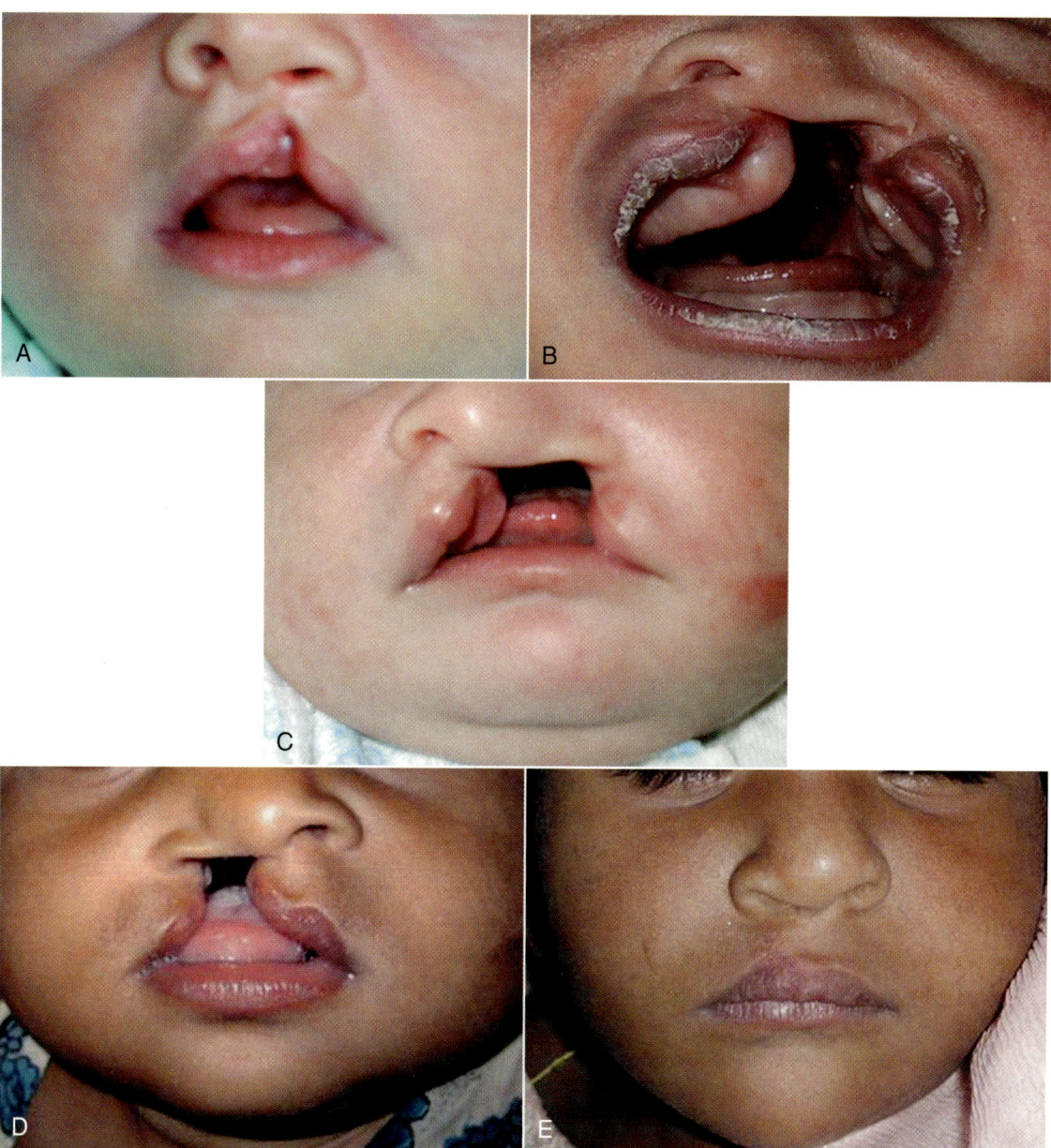

Fig. 83-9 ■ Variations of unilateral cleft lip and palate. **A,** Incomplete left unilateral cleft lip. **B** and **C,** Complete left unilateral cleft lip and palate. **D** and **E,** Complete right unilateral cleft lip and palate before (**D**) and after (**E**) repair. (**D, E,** Courtesy Dr. Krishnamurthy Bonanthaya, Cleft Center, Mahavir Jain Hospital, Bangalore, India.)

(i.e., hard and soft palate) in one stage before the child is 12 months old.[74] Some recommend a two-stage repair with soft palate repair as early as 3 to 6 months at the time of primary lip repair and hard palate by 12 to 15 months of age.[43] Children with cleft palate often have other systemic anomalies, and it may be necessary to modify the timing of repair in the presence of co-morbidities, particularly airway anomalies. Repair of the palate may be delayed up to 14 to 16 months if there are concerns of airway obstruction. Premature babies and infants with micrognathia are at increased risk for postoperative episodes of apnea after palate repair.[43]

The muscles of the soft palate that help with the function of speech and swallowing include the levator palatini, tensor palatini, palatopharyngeus, palatoglossus, and musculus uvulae. The soft palate in a noncleft individual acts as a muscular valve that can lift superiorly and posteriorly to oppose the pharyngeal wall and achieve velopharyngeal closure during speech. In a child with an unrepaired cleft, the soft palate cannot function as a muscular valve because of the abnormal orientation and attachment of the muscles, primarily the levator palatini. The bundles of the levator on each side are longitudinally directed to insert into the posterior edge of the palatine bone instead of joining in the midline in a transverse orientation and inserting into the palatine aponeurosis[75] (Fig. 83-11). In addition, the sphincter action of the palatoglossus, palatopharyngeus, and superior constrictor muscles at the oropharyngeal aperture is compromised, leading to velopharyngeal insufficiency.[76] The tensor palatini muscle fibers that control the opening of the eustachian tube and aerate the middle ear do not function optimally, often leading to chronic otitis media.

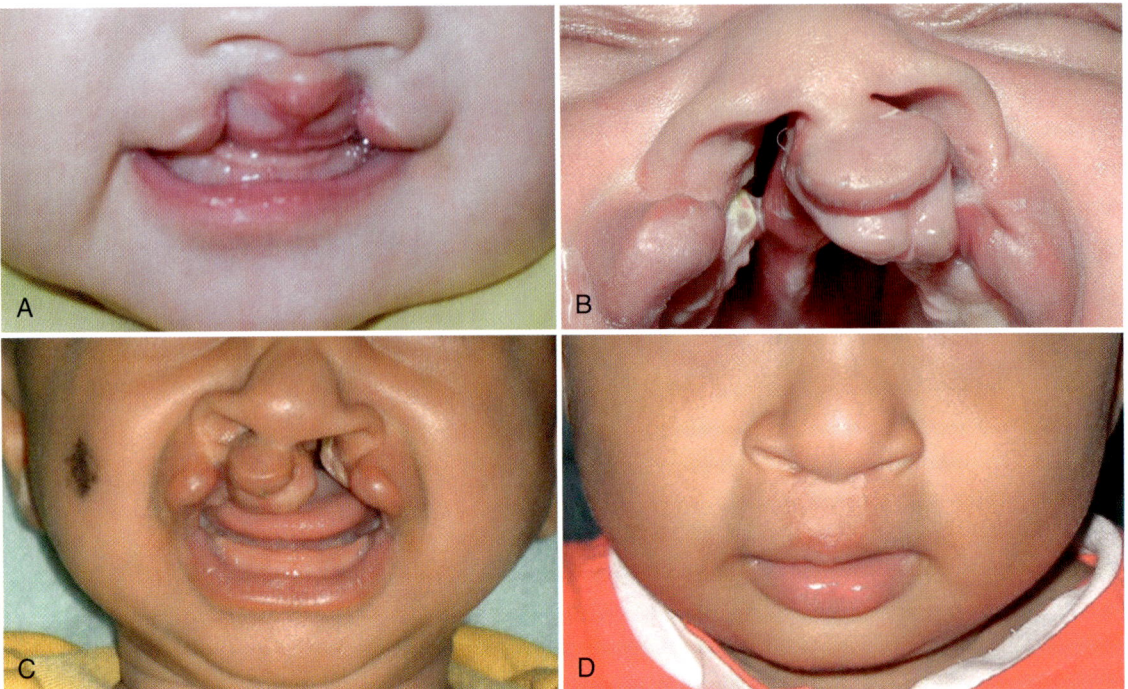

Fig. 83-10 ■ Variations of bilateral cleft lip and palate. **A,** Incomplete bilateral cleft lip. **B,** Complete bilateral cleft lip and palate. **C** and **D,** Complete BCLP before (**C**) and after (**D**) repair. (**C** and **D,** Courtesy Dr. Krishnamurthy Bonanthaya, Cleft Center, Mahavir Jain Hospital, Bangalore, India.)

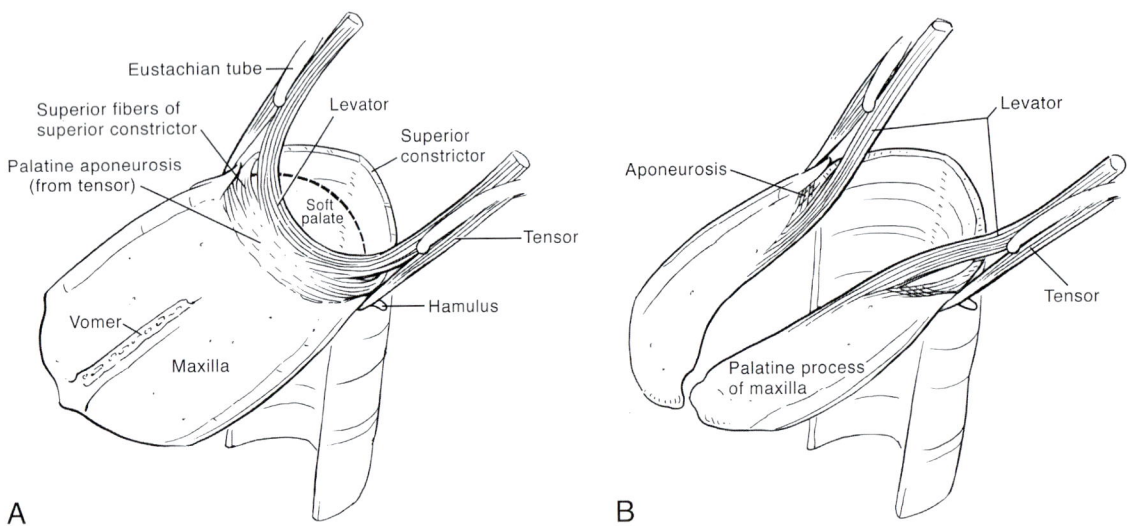

Fig. 83-11 ■ Muscles of palate in normal (**A**) and cleft (**B**) individuals. (From Sadove AM, van Aalst JA, Culp JA: Cleft palate repair: art and issues, *Clin Plast Surg* Apr;31(2):231-241, 2004.)

Evolution and Principles of Cleft Palate Repair As early as 1760, a French dentist, Le Monnier, first attempted repair of a cleft palate. Since then several other surgeons, including Philbert Roux, Carl Ferdinad Von Graefe, and Johann Dieffenbach, have described techniques to repair the palate. Von Langenbeck first described the use of pedicled mucoperiosteal flaps for closure of the cleft palate.[77] Braithwaite in 1968 emphasized the importance of the levator palatini muscle in cleft palate repair and Kriens, in 1969, introduced the concept of an anatomic approach to veloplasty by restoring the levator sling in cleft palate surgery.[78,79] The main principle of cleft palate repair is to detach and retropose the abnormal insertion of the levator palatini and join the muscles of both halves of the soft palate in the midline at the junction of the middle and posterior third of the soft palate in order to achieve proper elevation of the soft palate.[79] In the hard palate, the most important principle is to reflect mucoperiosteal flaps based on the grater palatine arteries that emerge from the greater palatine foramen bilaterally at the posterolateral area of the hard palate.

The choice of surgical technique depends of the type of cleft (Fig. 83-12). For the cleft of the secondary palate, a Von Langenbeck repair can be used. In this technique, bilateral relaxing incisions are made, and the mucoperiosteum is elevated to complete the stripping and closure of nasal layer, muscle, and oral layers.[80] The Veau-Wardwill-Kilner (V-Y pushback) technique (named after Victor

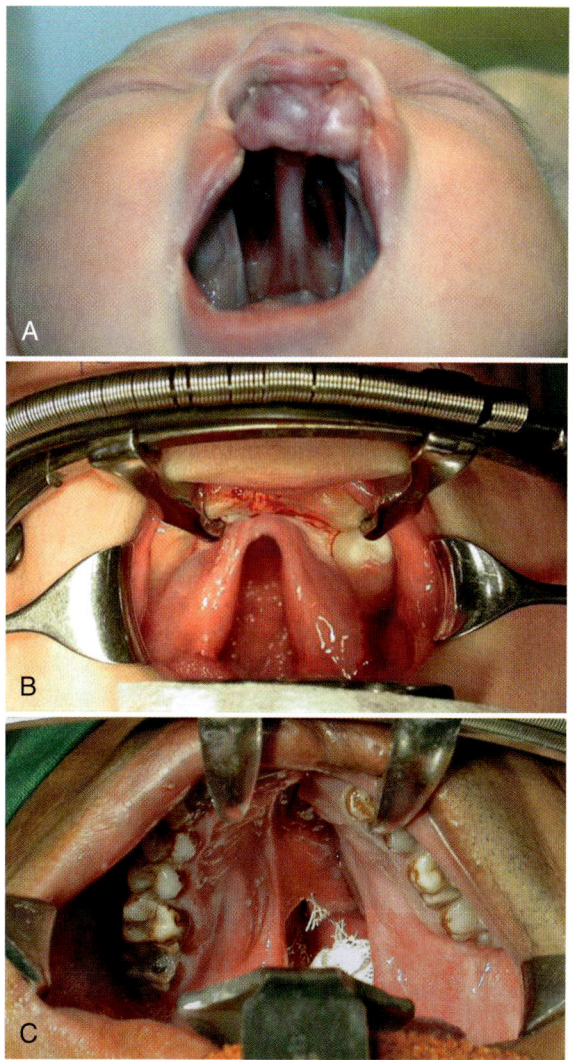

Fig. 83-12 ▪ Variations of cleft palate. **A,** Bilateral unrepaired cleft palate showing nasal septum and premaxilla. **B,** Cleft of secondary palate only. **C,** Unilateral unrepaired cleft of palate in an adult.

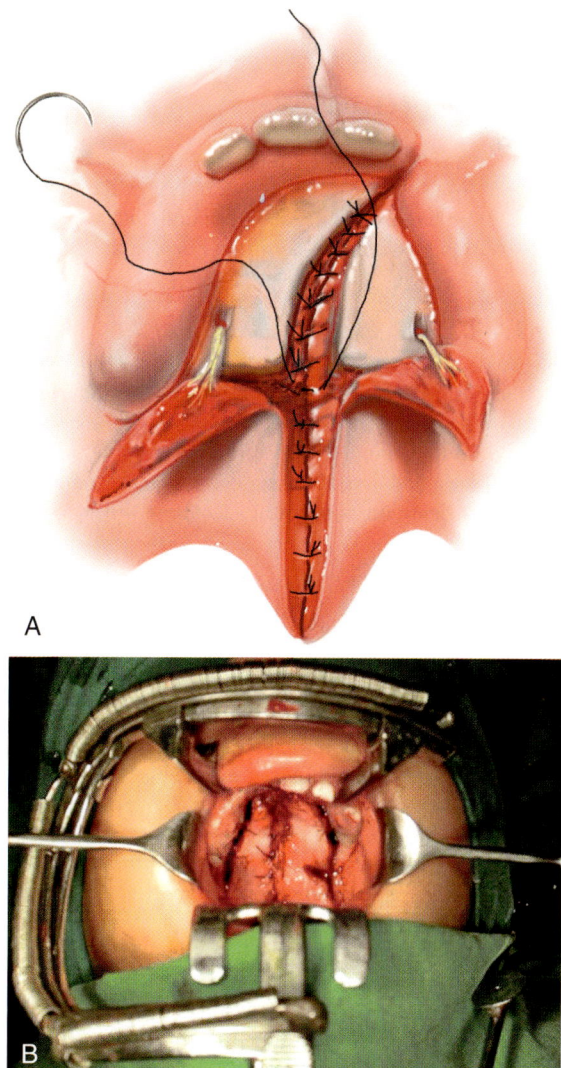

Fig. 83-13 ▪ **A,** Two-flap palatoplasty. **B,** Clinical photo showing repaired unilateral cleft palate. (**A,** From Posnick J: *Craniofacial and maxillofacial surgery in children and young adults,* Philadelphia, 2000, Saunders. **B,** Courtesy Dr. Hirji Adenwallah, Charles Pinto Cleft Center, Jubilee Mission Hospital, Bangalore, India.)

Veau, William Wardwill, and Thomas Kilner) is used less often for repair of the cleft of the secondary palate. In this technique, the oral mucosa is divided anteriorly, which may lengthen the palate but leaves areas of exposed bone in the anterior hard palate that can potentially cause maxillary growth disturbances.[81] Dr. Leonard Furlow, Jr., introduced double reversing Furlow Z-plasty in 1978.[68,82] This technique uses two reversed Z-plasties of the oral and nasal mucosa to repair the cleft. The advantages are restoration of normal anatomic position of the levator palatini in the middle and posterior third of soft palate and an increase in soft palate length. The more commonly used technique for complete clefts of the palate is the two flap palatoplasty as described by Bardach[68,83] (Fig. 83-13). The edges of the cleft are incised from the alveolus to the base of the uvula and bilateral full thickness pedicled mucoperiosteal flaps are reflected. The levator palatini muscle is released and dissected to be repositioned horizontally and sutured. More radical dissection and repositioning of the levator palatini has been shown to influence velar function.[84] Bilateral releasing incisions are made to decrease the tension in the midline. Complications of palatoplasty include postoperative bleeding, airway obstruction, wound dehiscence, and

fistula formation. Care should be taken to achieve adequate intra-operative hemostasis, and careful postoperative monitoring is essential to avoid airway obstruction.[74]

Insertion of Tympanostomy Ear Tubes/Grommets

At the time of the primary palatoplasty, the ears should be inspected. If there is evidence of serous otitis, a myringotomy is performed and fluid aspirated with the placement of grommets or ventilating tubes in the myringotomy incisions. Eustachian tube dysfunction can cause middle ear effusions and associated conductive hearing loss. Surgical placement of tympanostomy tubes (or pressure equalizing tubes, or PETs) is the currently recommended treatment to relieve the middle ear fluid. The tube functions by allowing air to enter the middle ear through the hole in the tube, preventing fluid buildup and reducing conductive hearing loss due to the fluid. The timing of tube placement varies between otolaryngologists, with most being placed at the time of cleft palate repair. Hearing tests are recommended following the tympanostomy tube placement to confirm normalization of hearing.[43,75]

PRESCHOOL (3 TO 5 YEARS)

Lip and Nose Revision

Early lip and nose revision is rarely necessary in the child with a unilateral cleft lip but may be needed in a child with a bilateral cleft lip. Typically, this procedure is performed before the child goes to school.

Dental Evaluation: Primary Dentition

The primary dentition in children with clefts is generally complete. A family dentist or pediatric dentist should see the child in the first 18 months to 2 years. The parent should be given instructions on helping the child to maintain good oral hygiene, preserve the health of gingival tissues, and avoid nursing caries. The maintenance of a healthy primary dentition is necessary to allow timely eruption of the permanent teeth.

Speech Assessment

Children with palatal clefts are at risk for a wide range of speech problems related to resonance, articulation, phonation, learning, and language delay. These speech abnormalities in children with cleft palate can be caused by velopharyngeal insufficiency, oronasal fistula, weak lip pressure, abnormal tongue pressure, malpositioned teeth, abnormal jaw relationship, neuromuscular dysfunction, and conductive or sensorineural hearing loss. It is important to identify and associate the cause with the effect. Assessment of speech should begin as early as 6 months and be monitored throughout adolescence. Assessment of speech for velopharyngeal insufficiency has to be both clinical and instrumental. Clinical assessment of resonance characteristics is best performed as a child's articulatory repertoire develops. Noninstrumental testing utilizing visualization of airflow with a reflecting mirror and nasal pinching often assists with the prediction of velopharyngeal function during speech. If deficits are identified, then further assessment using nasoendoscopy to assess posterior and lateral pharyngeal wall motion or videofluoroscopy is indicated. Nasopharyngoscopy helps the surgeon to make a decision regarding the need for surgical intervention. Small-diameter pediatric flexible endoscopes with good light source and topical anesthetic for nasal mucosa will help children become more compliant with this procedure.[85,86]

Correction of Velopharyngeal Insufficiency

Typically, velopharyngeal insufficiency (VPI) refers to the inability of the soft palate and the posterior and lateral pharyngeal walls to come together to create a seal during speech production. The timing of correction depends on when this condition is recognized. It would be better to correct it before the child is of school age to ensure proper school performance. Studies show that the need for surgical correction of velopharyngeal incompetence ranges from 4-30%.[69,85] The most effective method for correction of VPI is controversial but the choice of the procedure depends on the cause and where the abnormality is found, whether on the lateral or posterior pharyngeal wall.[70,86] A posterior flap pharyngoplasty is indicated when there is limited or a lack of posterior wall motion. The flap may be superiorly or inferiorly based. A superiorly based flap with the base at the level of the tubercle of the atlas and insertion into the soft palate is more popular than the inferiorly based flap. A lateral pharyngoplasty is advocated for managing decreased lateral wall motion by creating a dynamic sphincter to control the size of the pharyngeal orifice. Orticochea first described this method, and Jackson modified it.[87,88]

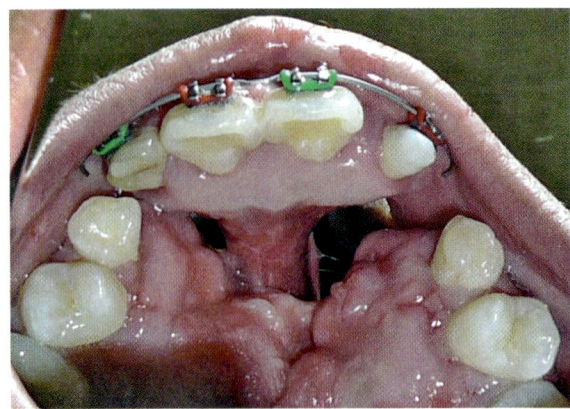

Fig. 83-14 ■ Large palatal oronasal fistula with lack of adequate soft tissue.

Correction Oronasal Fistulae

One of the complications of primary cleft palate repair is failure of healing or breakdown of wound, resulting in oronasal (ON) fistulae (Fig. 83-14). Fistulae can occur at any location in the hard or soft palate. The reports on incidence of fistula formation are variable and range anywhere from 2-43%. Incidence of ON fistulae depends on several variables including experience of the surgeon, age at the time of repair, and, less often, the type of repair and severity of cleft deformity. The most significant variable seems to be the experience of the operating surgeon.[73,74,89-91]

The technique for repair of the fistula depends on its size, anatomic location (anterior or posterior part of the palate), and previous surgical scar. Palatal mucoperiosteal flaps, tongue flaps based laterally or anteriorly, buccal musculomucosal flaps based on the facial artery, or a temporalis flap can be used to close fistulae (Fig. 83-15). More recently, interpositional grafts made of acellular dermis have been used to achieve tension-free closure of ON fistulae.[75,92] It is important to have at least a two-layered closure without tension and maintain good blood supply to the flap in order to achieve a watertight seal of the defect. Almost all of the fistulae can be repaired by local pedicled flaps as described here. However, occasionally a free vascularized flap may help to close a scarred palate with a large defect.

CHILDHOOD (6 TO 12 YEARS)

Phase I Orthodontic Treatment (Box 83-6)

The goal of orthodontic treatment in this phase is to monitor facial growth and eruption of permanent teeth and to expand maxillary cleft segments in preparation for repair of the alveolar cleft. In the early mixed dentition phase (6 to 9 years), the maxillary central incisors adjacent to the cleft often erupt ectopically. Other common dental findings include presence of supernumerary or malformed teeth, enamel hypoplasia of teeth adjacent to cleft, and congenital absence of teeth, mainly maxillary lateral incisors in the line of the cleft and sometimes premolars. Children with complete clefts of lip and palate often develop a posterior and anterior crossbite. The crossbite is asymmetric in the unilateral clefts, affecting mainly the lesser segment or cleft side. In the bilateral clefts, there is collapse of both lateral segments with a bilateral posterior crossbite and protrusion of the premaxilla. Adequate expansion of the maxillary arch with proper position of the alveolar segments is necessary prior to alveolar bone grafting. This can be achieved by using a quad helix or a screw expansion device that will allow greater expansion in the anterior maxillary arch (Fig. 83-16). Appliances with gentle forces

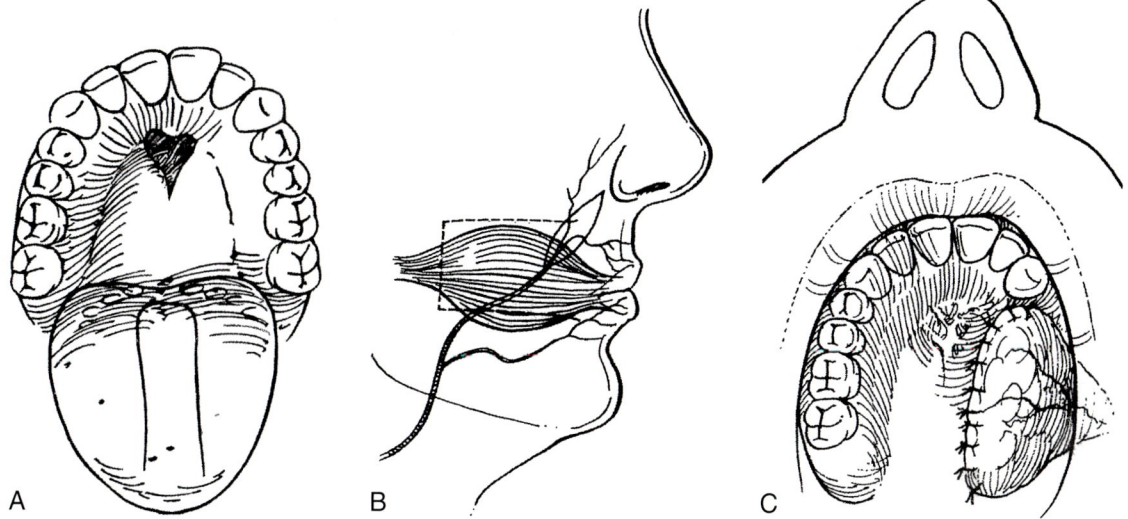

Fig. 83-15 ■ **A,** Tongue flap for closure of palatal fistulae (anteriorly based design). **B** and **C,** Facial artery myomucosal (FAMM) flap for closure of palatal fistulae. (From Assael LA: Maxillary intraoral reconstruction with regional flaps, *Atlas Oral Maxillofac Surg Clin North Am* 3(1):63-73, 1995.)

BOX 83-6	Orthodontic Management in Cleft Individuals

Age: 2 to 10 weeks
Treatment: Presurgical orthopedics

Age: 6 to 10 years
Treatment: Phase I orthodontics
- Begin maxillary expansion and removal of supernumerary teeth for alveolar bone grafting
- Align premaxillary segment in bilateral cleft lip and palate prior to bone grafting
- Monitor facial growth and consider maxillary protraction when indicated

Age: 10 to 14 years
Treatment:
- Maintain maxillary expansion and alignment of teeth
- Monitor facial growth and eruption of permanent teeth, particularly those in the line of the cleft
- Consider maxillary distraction if maxillary deficiency is severe

Age: 14 to 18 years
Treatment: Phase II orthodontics
- Begin orthodontic treatment with full fixed appliances to align teeth
- Prepare for orthognathic surgery when indicated
- Extract teeth if arch is crowded
- Decide whether to replace/substitute the absent maxillary lateral incisor

should also be used to correct the malpositioned central incisors prior to alveolar cleft repair. An appliance is required to maintain the expanded maxillary arch form during and after repair of the alveolar cleft.

Assessment of Facial Growth

Monitoring facial growth during childhood and early mixed dentition helps to identify early signs of maxillary hypoplasia and assess need for orthodontic or surgical intervention. Maxillary growth may be restricted in vertical, transverse, and anteroposterior dimensions in children with complete cleft lip and palate (Fig. 83-17).[93,94] Children with signs of severe deficiency may benefit from maxillary protraction during early mixed dentition phase (6 to 9 years). A reverse pull headgear may be considered to protract the maxilla. This is an effective treatment modality but requires considerable compliance on the part of the patient. There is some uncertainty in predicting the outcome of early maxillary protraction because of the difficulty in anticipating future lower jaw growth.[95]

Alveolar Cleft Repair

The timing, source of bone, surgical technique, perioperative management, and outcome of bone grafting have all been studied and debated extensively over the years. The terms *primary bone grafting* (2 to 5 years), *secondary bone grafting* (7 to 11 years), and late *secondary bone grafting* (14 to 18 years) have been based on age at which alveolar cleft repair is performed.[96,97] The majority of the centers use secondary alveolar bone grafting in the mixed dentition phase between the ages of 7 and 11 years after maxillary expansion. Typically, this coincides with one-half to two-thirds root development of the maxillary canine or lateral incisor (if present) in the line of the cleft. The primary goal of alveolar cleft repair is to establish bony continuity of the maxillary alveolar ridge, provide bone support for the teeth adjacent to the cleft, and seal the communication between the nose and oral cavity when there is a patent oronasal fistula (Fig. 83-18). A successful alveolar bone graft should facilitate eruption and orthodontic movement of teeth in the line of the cleft (most often the maxillary canine), maintain health of periodontium of teeth adjacent to the cleft, provide alar base support, and improve nasal symmetry (Fig. 83-19).[79,80,98,99] Completion of the maxillary expansion prior to grafting provides adequate access to the cleft defect and aligns the cleft segments better. The gold standard for the grafting material has been particulate corticocancellous bone marrow harvested from the iliac crest, which was first described by Boyne and Sands.[81,100] Although other sites that have been described including rib, symphysis, calvarium, and tibia,[82] the iliac crest is the most commonly used donor site. More recently the use of bone growth factors such as recombinant human bone morphogenic protein-2 (rhBMP-2) has been shown to be effective in grafting the defect.

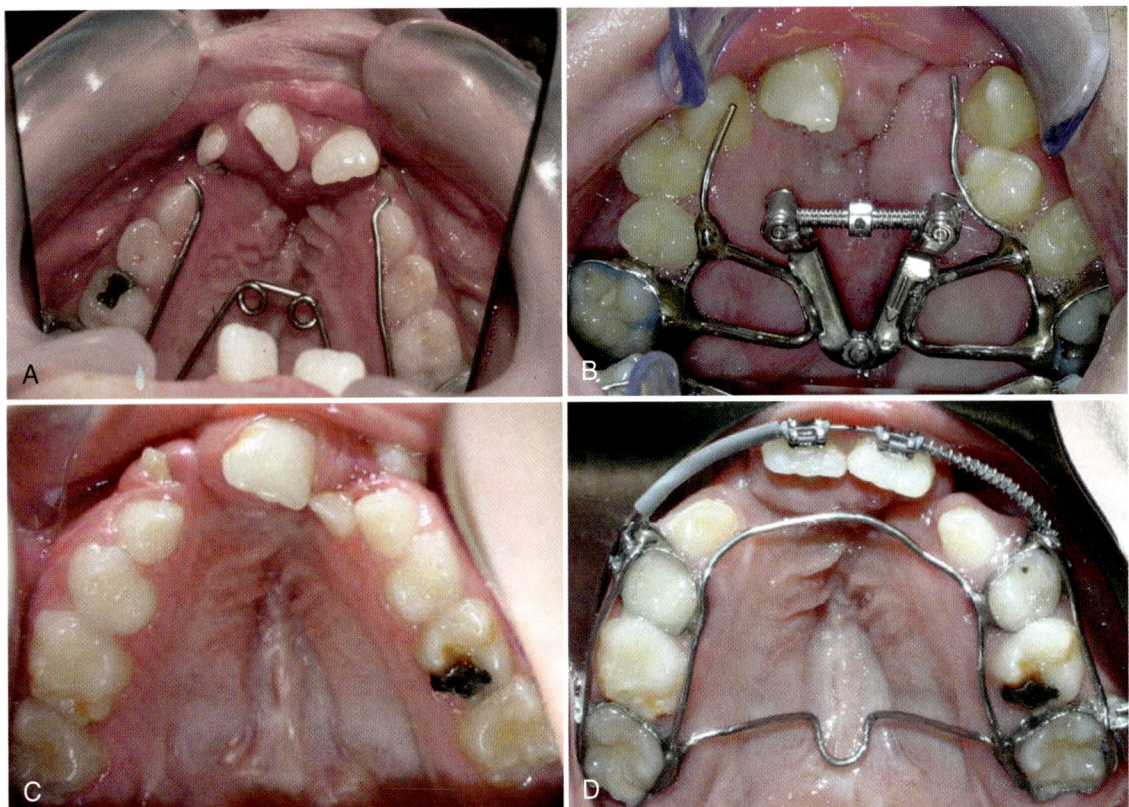

Fig. 83-16 ■ Expansion of the maxillary arch. **A,** Quadhelix-maxillary expansion device for expansion in a bilateral cleft palate. **B,** Fanscrew-shaped device allows greater anterior maxillary expansion. **C** and **D,** A case of bilateral cleft before (**C**) and after expansion (**D**) maintaining arch width and ready for alveolar cleft repair.

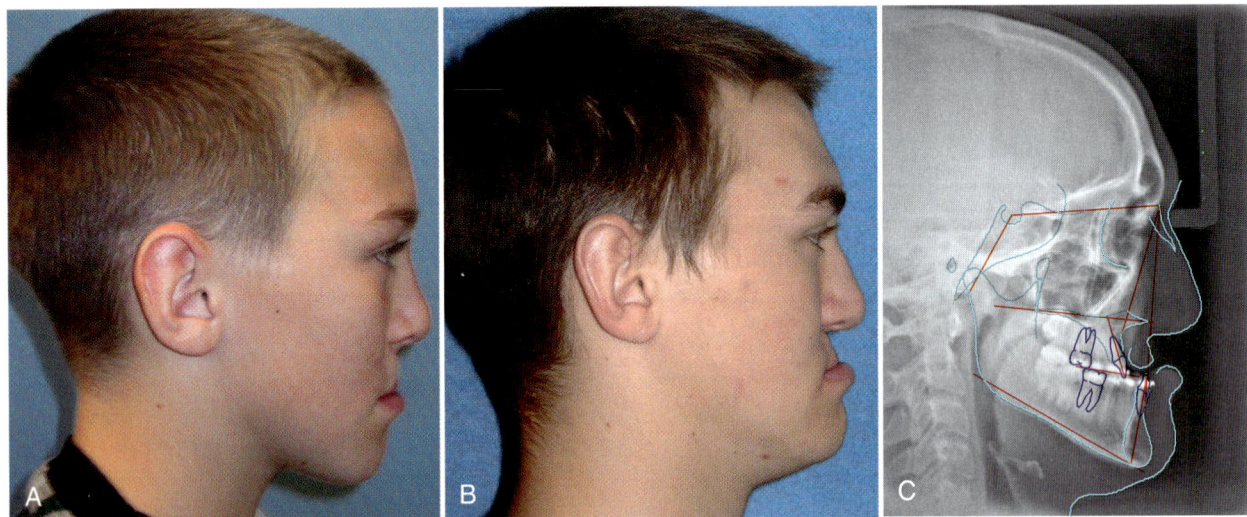

Fig. 83-17 ■ Facial growth in a child with BCLP showing maxillary deficiency. **A,** 9-year-old child with a unilateral cleft lip and palate. The signs of maxillary deficiency are apparent in profile view. **B,** The severe deficiency of the maxilla in anteroposterior and vertical dimensions and its relative position to the mandible is seen at age 15. **C,** Lateral cephalometric radiograph showing severe maxillary deficiency.

BMP-2 is a growth factor that promotes differentiation of pluripotential cells into cells that can form new bone in the defect. This eliminates donor site morbidity and minimizes hospital stay and postoperative pain and discomfort.[83-85,101-103] Gingivoperiosteoplasty performed at the time of primary lip repair may seal the oronasal communication but does not always preclude the need for a bone graft. Some studies show that at least 40-50% of these patients require bone grafting in the future.[86-88,104-106] More recently, Meazzini et al. showed that patients who had a gingivoperiosteoplasty at the time of primary repair did not require bone grafting at a later date;

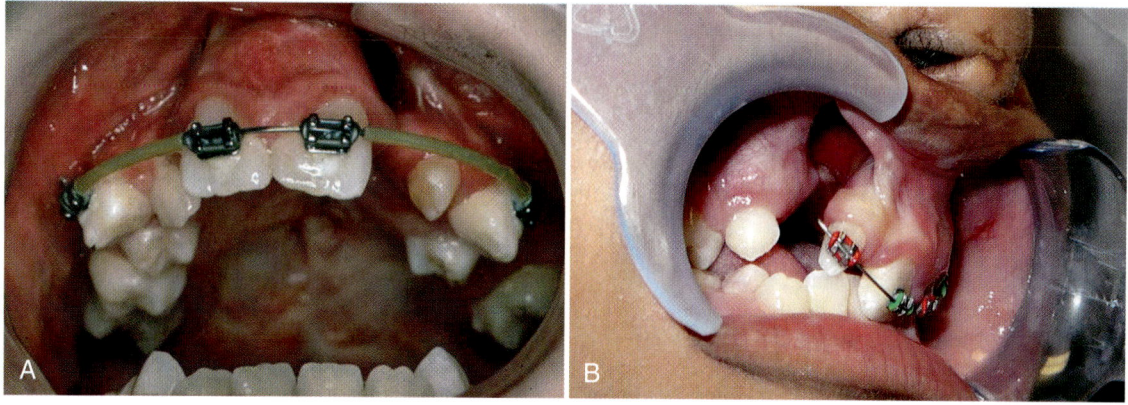

Fig. 83-18 ■ Large labial oronasal fistula in an individual with bilateral cleft lip and palate.

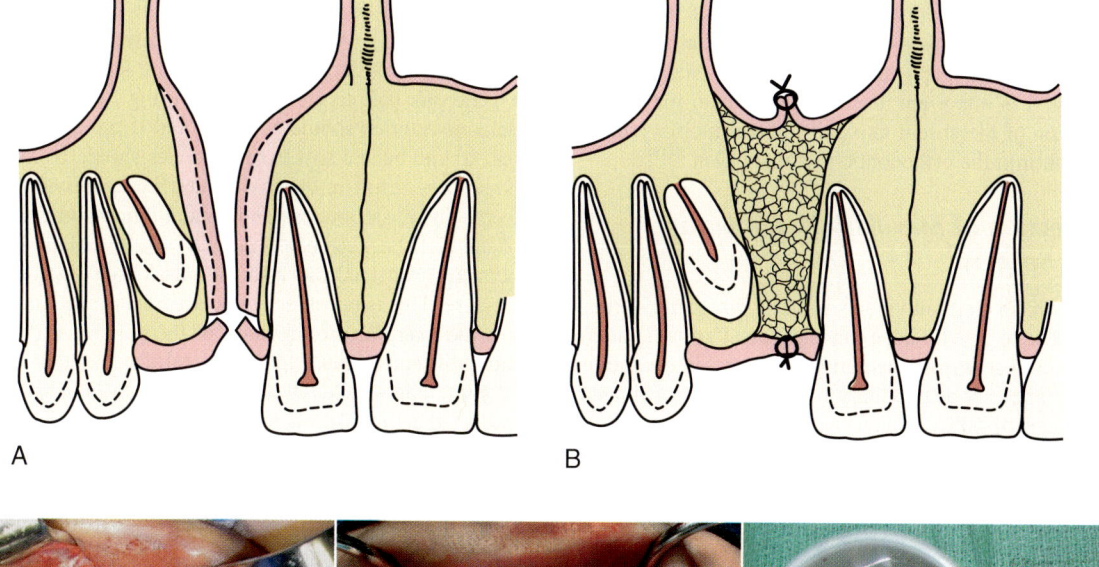

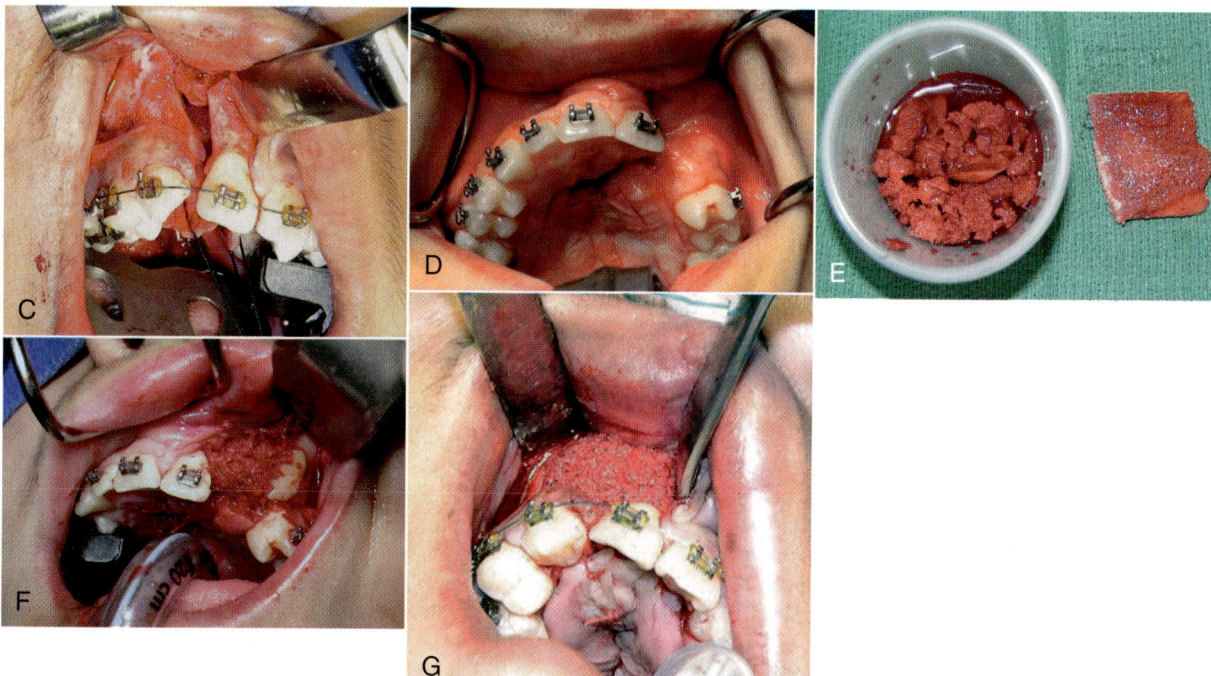

Fig. 83-19 ■ Alveolar cleft repair. **A** and **B,** Technique for alveolar bone grafting. **C,** Unrepaired alveolar cleft defect in an older child with permanent dentition. **D,** Exposed bony cleft margin after reflection of the oral mucosa and closure of oronasal fistula. **E,** Corticocancellous bone harvested (typically from the anterior iliac crest). **F** and **G,** Bone packed into the cleft defect after exposure of the cleft. (**A** and **B,** From Hupp JR, Ellis E, Tucker M: *Contemporary oral and maxillofacial surgery,* ed 5, St. Louis, 2008, Mosby.)

however, they reported a greater need for surgical correction of maxillary hypoplasia.[89,107]

ADOLESCENCE (13 TO 19 YEARS)

Phase II Orthodontic Treatment

Phase II orthodontic treatment (see Box 83-6) for a cleft patient consists of maintaining maxillary arch width after repair of the alveolar cleft, monitoring eruption of permanent teeth adjacent to the grafted cleft site, and aligning permanent teeth with full fixed appliances. Orthodontic treatment should be timed appropriately based on the need for orthognathic surgery, the individual's growth potential, ability to cooperate, and ability to maintain oral hygiene. When surgery is indicated, orthodontic treatment timing should be coordinated with growth completion, which is around age 15 to 16 years for females and 17 to 19 years for males. Although the timing of surgical correction is typically after completion of mandibular growth, early surgical maxillary advancement can be considered before growth for psychological reasons or to minimize a severe skeletal deformity. It is important to integrate the plan for replacement or substitution of the absent maxillary lateral incisor and any other missing teeth into the orthodontic treatment plan.[90,108]

Surgical Correction of Maxillary Hypoplasia/Orthognathic Surgery

Maxillary hypoplasia in cleft individuals is partly due to the intrinsic deformity, partly due to genetic inheritance of facial growth pattern, and partly the result of scar from the multiple surgical interventions. Regardless of the etiology of maxillary hypoplasia, approximately 25% (reported range 14-50%) of cleft individuals undergo surgical correction of this maxillary deficiency.[94,109] The criteria for surgical necessity can be subjective and vary from surgeon to surgeon. The need to improve midface projection, correct the occlusion, increase nasal tip support, and nasolabial angle and improve lip competence are some of the indications for surgical correction of maxillary hypoplasia. The degree of hypoplasia and the need for surgical intervention have been shown to be higher with an increase in severity of the cleft.[91,94]

Surgical correction of maxillary hypoplasia can be performed by conventional orthognathic surgery or distraction osteogenesis (Fig. 83-20). Since the early 2000s, distraction osteogenesis of the facial skeleton has become popular because of the ability to perform large maxillary advancement without the need for bone grafting.[110] Staged maxillary advancement remains a predictable option for patients, but the ability to produce large advancements using distraction is attractive in those with marked retrusion. In others, a combined maxillary advancement and mandibular reduction can be performed to correct severe deformities after completion of growth.

A meta-analysis of literature from 1996 to 2003 by Cheung et al. on cleft maxillary osteotomy and distraction osteogenesis showed most patients who underwent conventional maxillary osteotomies were older (16 to 20 years) compared to those who had distraction (11 to 15 years).[111] The mean advancement for both groups was similar but larger maximum advancement was achieved in the distraction group. The most commonly used system was the rigid external distractor (RED) device. They subsequently conducted a randomized, controlled study comparing maxillary distraction and orthognathic surgery in 29 nongrowing cleft patients. Intraoral distractors were used in 15 patients in the distraction group and routine miniplate fixation for the 14 patients in the orthognathic surgery group. Clinical morbidity and stability was assessed using a questionnaire and lateral cephalometric tracings, respectively. It was found that there was no significant difference in the clinical morbidities, but the maxillary movement in the distraction group was more stable than with orthognathic repositioning. Skeletal relapse was evident in the first 3 months following conventional cleft maxillary advancement.[111,112]

Orthognathic surgery in the cleft patient is much more challenging than for the noncleft patient. Starting from anesthetic management to surgical postoperative care, several modifications are necessary for orthognathic surgery in the cleft individual. The presence of a deviated nasal septum or a pharyngeal flap may necessitate the use of a fiberoptic assisted intubation technique, or it may be necessary to pass the endotracheal tube over a more rigid tube or catheter. The vascularity of the labial and palatal mucoperiosteal tissues is invariably affected by previous surgical procedures for lip and palate repair. Drommer and Luhr demonstrated with the use of angiography that the greater palatine arteries were significantly smaller in 10 of 24 sides in 12 cleft patients prior to maxillary advancement.[113] When surgical incisions are made to provide access for maxillary osteotomies, care should be taken to maintain a generous soft tissue pedicle. During down-fracture, the greater palatine arteries should be preserved if possible, and trauma to the palatal and buccal soft tissue pedicles should be avoided. Failure to do so may result in the loss of attached gingival tissues, bone, and teeth. The nasal mucosa and palatal mucosa are fused in the region of the cleft because of the primary palate repair. This tissue should be sharply incised close to the nasal floor just prior to the down-fracture. This is necessary to down-fracture and to adequately mobilize the maxilla. Mobilization of the maxilla after down-fracture is more difficult because of the palatal scar tissue or a pharyngeal flap. In some cases, release or division of the pharyngeal flap may be indicated to reposition the maxilla into the desired position. The primary palatal repair often results in more bone formation and stronger union at the pterygomaxillary junction. Use of a curved chisel to osteotomize directly through the maxillary tuberosities rather than the dense bone of the pterygomaxillary junction is helpful to complete this posterior osteotomy. Complete mobilization to achieve sufficient advancement requires progressive, careful stretching, as the scarred soft tissues are less compliant.

The maxillary deficiency in the vertical, transverse, and sagittal dimensions makes bone grafting a necessity for cleft maxillary osteotomies performed by conventional orthognathic surgery. The presence of a persistent oronasal fistula and alveolar cleft defect, requires careful soft tissue closure and bone grafting. The maxilla can separate into two segments during the down-fracture and mobilization, even when the alveolar cleft site has been previously grafted. Corticocancellous bone harvested from the anterior iliac crest can be used to graft the residual alveolar cleft defect, bridge the gap at the osteotomy site after anterior and inferior repositioning of the maxilla, and augment the deficient area at the piriform rim on the cleft side (Fig. 83-21).

Rigid fixation with plates and screws has to be performed carefully, as the quantity and quality of bone may be poor. When there is deficiency of the midface and malar region, adjunctive procedures, such as zygomatic osteotomies or a modified Le Fort I osteotomy, can enhance cheek prominence and facial contours. The soft tissue of the upper lip may be tight with a shallow vestibular depth and deficient vermilion show that may become worse following maxillary advancement. When closing the incision, incorporating a "V-Y" design to minimize lip shortening should be considered.

Postoperative stability after maxillary osteotomy is less favorable in the cleft than in the noncleft patient. Relapse in the cleft individual is mainly due to the inability to mobilize the maxilla adequately.

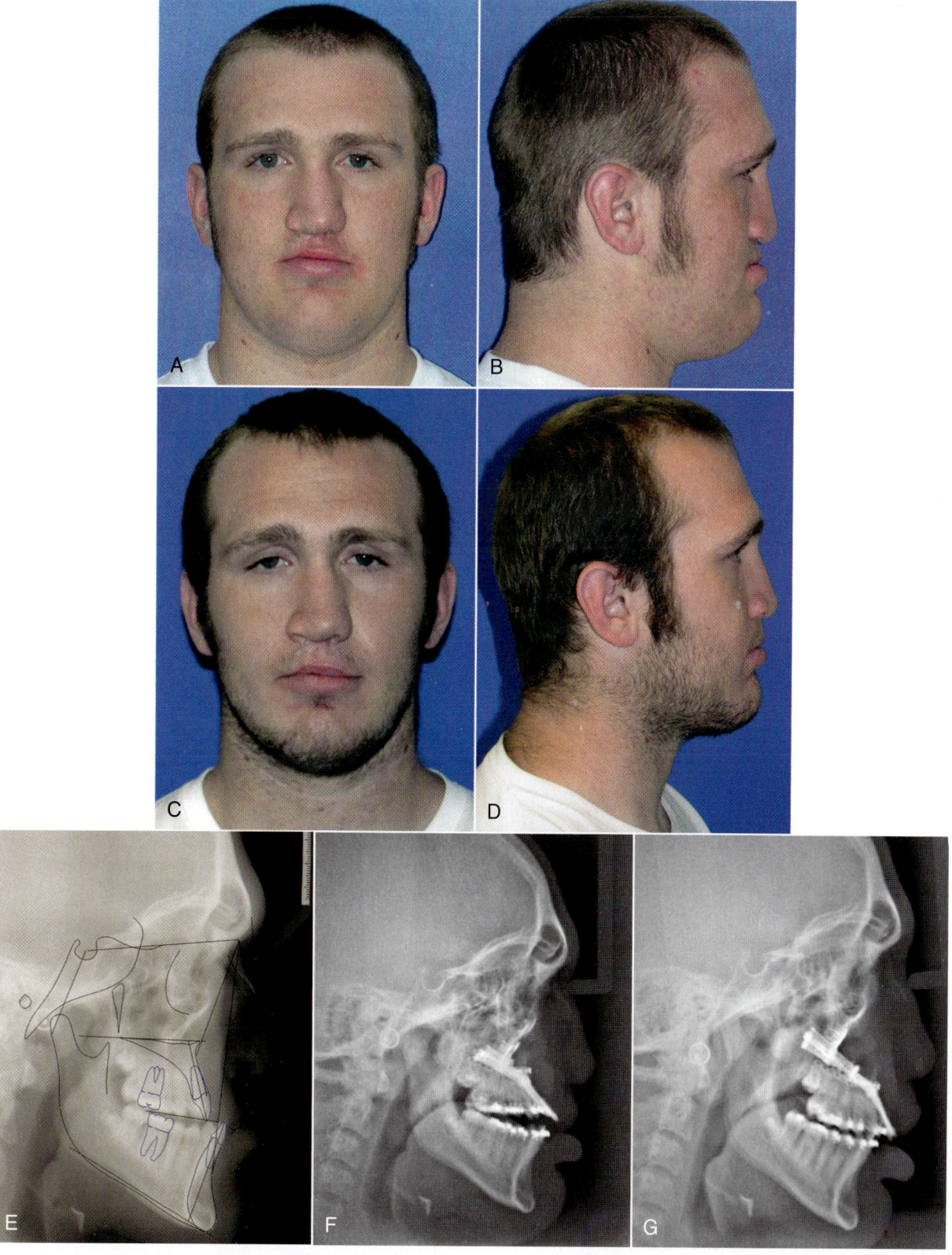

Fig. 83-20 ■ Maxillary hypoplasia correction with distraction. Predistraction frontal (**A**) and profile (**B**) views. Postdistraction frontal (**C**) and profile (**D**) views (1 year). Lateral predistraction (**E**), during treatment (**F**) and immediate postdistraction (**G**) cephalometric radiographs.

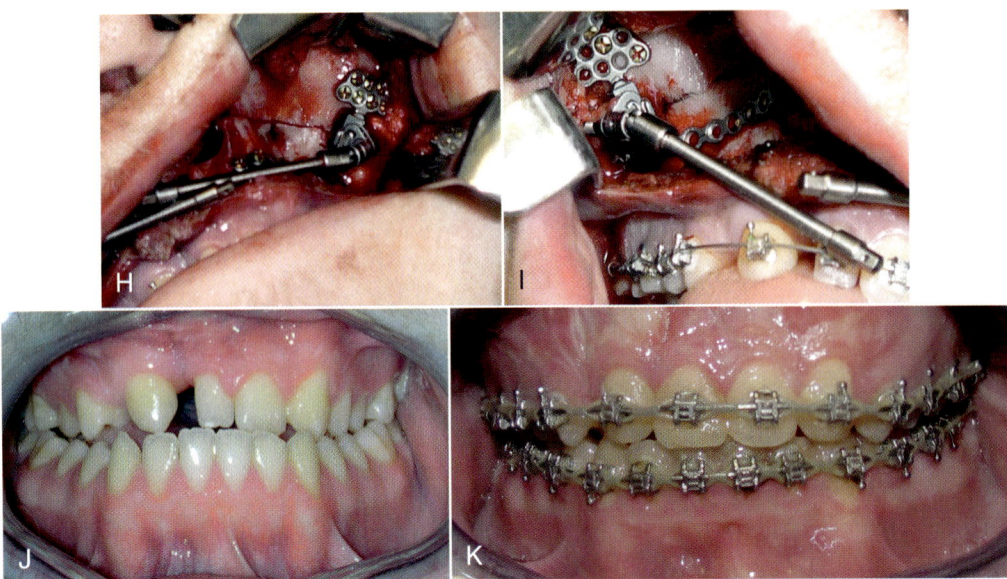

Fig. 83-20, cont'd ▪ **H** and **I,** Distractions in place. Occlusion before (**J**) and 1 year after (**K**) treatment.

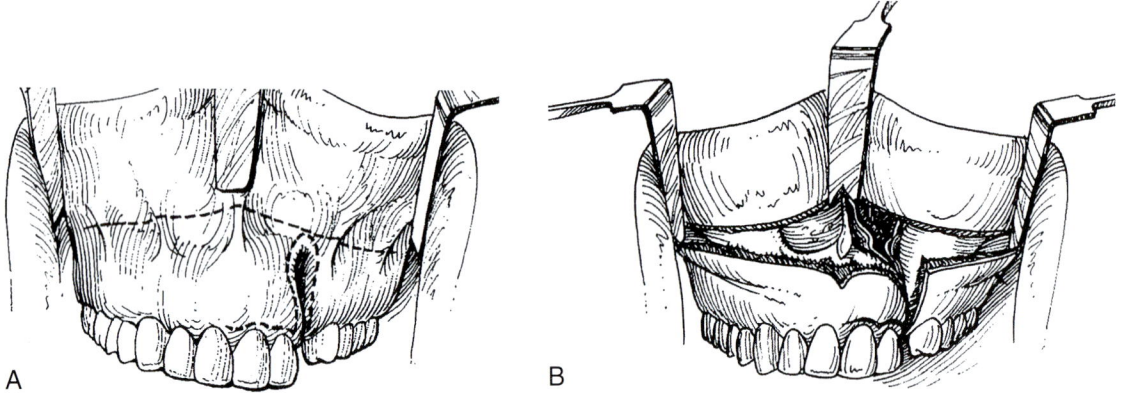

Fig. 83-21 ▪ Le Fort I osteotomy in unilateral cleft lip and palate deformity. **A,** Incisors design with simultaneous grafting of the cleft maxilla. **B,** Exposure of the greater and lesser maxillary segments. (From Assael LA: Maxillary intraoral reconstruction with regional flaps, *Atlas Oral Maxillofac Surg Clin North Am* 3(1):63-73, 1995.)

The tight scarred soft tissue envelope of the palate and upper lip limit the ability to mobilize and achieve the desired movement. Despite bone grafting and rigid internal fixation, relapse in the sagittal and vertical dimensions after maxillary osteotomy has been reported in several studies.[114-116] The predictability of VPI after conventional orthognathic surgery is based on premorbid speech quality. If there is moderate to severe velopharyngeal insufficiency prior to maxillary advancement, it is more likely that individuals will need a postsurgical pharyngeal flap or pharyngoplasty. It is therefore important that these patients are thoroughly assessed for VPI prior to cleft maxillary surgery.[117]

Secondary Correction of Lip and Nasal Deformities

Residual lip and nose deformities can be corrected at anytime; however, one must keep in mind that multiple revisions will cause increased scar formation in the young child. If there is no strong psychological or functional indication such as nasal obstruction, then definitive correction of secondary lip and nose deformities can be performed after skeletal correction of maxillary hypoplasia, and completion of orthodontic treatment can take place when the patient is between 16 and 20 years of age. The position of the nasal tip is influenced by surgical advancement of the maxilla, and similarly the position of the upper lip and nasolabial angle are determined by the inclination of the incisors after orthodontic treatment. Therefore, final correction of lip and nose to achieve balanced facial esthetics can be performed in the final phase of treatment.[94,95,118,119]

Secondary Cheiloplasty

The severity of the cleft deformity can be defined by the extent of disruption at the vermilion-cutaneous junction and has been classified as minor-form, microform, and mini-microform cleft lip. These anatomic descriptions help to determine the type of nasolabial repair and also correlate with type and frequency of revision necessary after the initial repair.[120] Notching or mismatch at the vermillion-cutaneous junction can be corrected by realignment, small triangular flaps, or a "Z-plasty" procedure. A poorly defined tubercle can be corrected by a "V-Y" advancement. It is important to differentiate and maintain the zone of wet and dry mucosa when correcting these deformities. Vertical shortening of the lip after a Millard repair is due to underestimation of the vertical height and inadequate rotation of lip on the noncleft side at the time of primary repair. Shortening of the lip can also result from severe scar contracture. Correction of a prominent scar with inadequate lip length and compromised muscle function requires a full thickness revision where all three layers (skin, muscle, and mucosa) have to be cleanly dissected and meticulously repaired.

In the case of a poorly repaired bilateral cleft lip, the deformity can present as a tight upper lip with poorly defined philtral columns and Cupid's bow, a short and wide prolabium with deficiency of vermillion in the center, unsightly scars, exposed wet mucosa, and a shallow labial sulcus (Fig. 83-22). Deficiency of the labial sulcus can be corrected by releasing the scar and performing a Z-plasty. In the case of a tight upper lip, an Abbe flap can be used successfully for reconstruction of the upper lip deformity. This is an axial pattern flap based on the labial artery, consisting of vermilion, mucosa, skin,

and muscle from the lower lip described by Abbe in 1898. The advantages of this flap are that it carries the dimple from the lower lip to form a philtral dimple in the Cupid's bow and the scars give a semblance of philtral columns.

Cleft Septo-Rhinoplasty

Secondary revisions of cleft-related nasal deformities should aim to improve tip projection and support, as well as symmetry of the alar cartilages. Simultaneous correction of septal deviation and reduction of hypertrophied turbinates will also improve the nasal airway.[97,121] Total correction of the cleft nasal deformity is best approached by an open rhinoplasty under direct vision. Wide exposure provides access for mobilization and repair of the collapsed and deformed alar cartilages. For unilateral cleft nasal deformity, an open rhinoplasty approach can be performed using a trans-columellar incision combined with rim incisions. Complete degloving of the lower lateral cartilages and dissection to the cartilaginous septum enable a full septoplasty with relocation of the caudal septum and the harvesting of cartilage grafts if indicated. Dorsal reduction is commonly undertaken with lateral nasal bone osteotomies to restore the bony vault. Additionally, stiffening the columella by a cartilage strut is necessary to provide tip projection, support, and symmetry of the nasal tip. Reshaping the deficient lateral crus may require a batten graft, and alar base repositioning may be required to improve nostril symmetry.[122,123] In a bilateral cleft nasal deformity, the goal is to stretch the nasal tip, to dissect and approximate the lower lateral cartilages to achieve a more triangular inferior nasal shape. The short columella is the main problem in the bilateral cleft. The columella can be lengthened by "V-Y" advancement or it can be constructed by using the entire prolabium of the upper lip. The defect

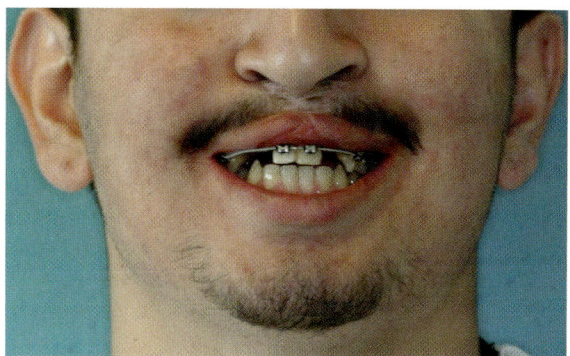

Fig. 83-22 ■ Secondary lip deformity. Vermilion is mismatched and scar is poor after bilateral lip repair.

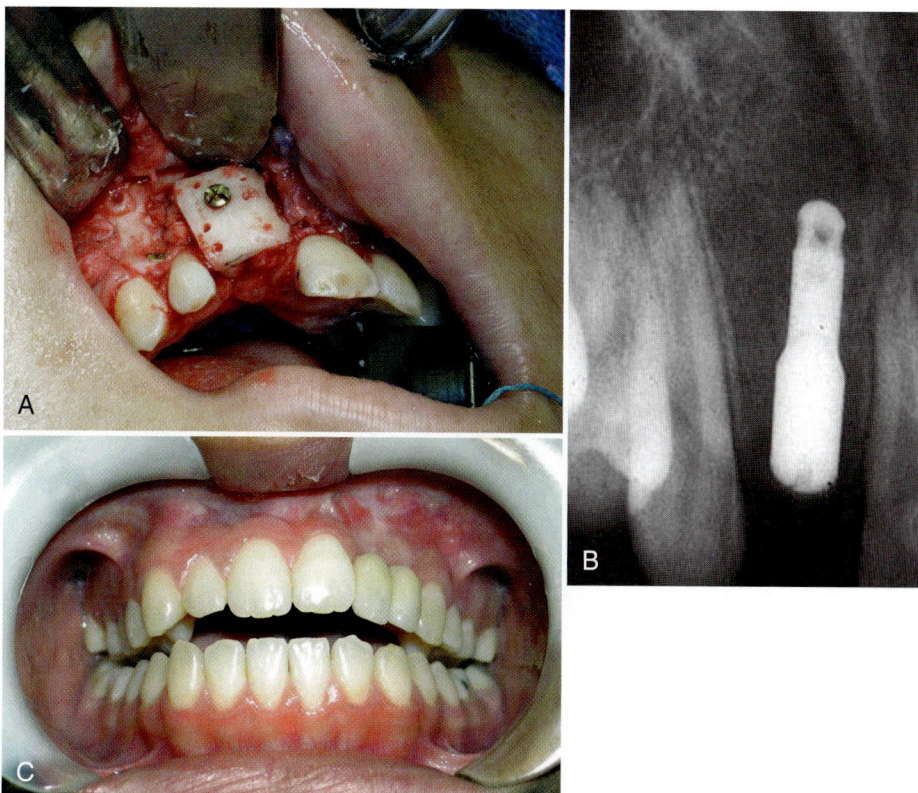

Fig. 83-23 ■ Replacement of missing teeth. **A,** Alveolar ridge augmentation with a cortical bone onlay is often necessary to increase width and height before placement of an implant, in the grafted cleft site. **B,** Radiograph showing missing lateral incisor replaced with an endosseous implant. **C,** Restored implant replacing lateral incisor in maxillary arch.

Fig. 83-24 ■ Zygomaticus implant with obturator. Female patient with inadequate cleft care during childhood presented with an unrepaired bilateral cleft palate, poor unintelligible speech, early loss of teeth and ability to chew, atrophy of premaxilla, poor upper lip support, and severe midface deficiency in AP and vertical dimensions. The patient was rehabilitated with an obturator prosthesis to provide the best possible functional and esthetic result. Pretreatment frontal (**A**) and profile (**B**) views. Postoperative frontal (**C**) and profile (**D**) views. **E,** AP cephalometric radiograph showing the implants in the zygoma and mandible. **F** to **H,** The cleft defect was obturated (**F**) and the teeth were replaced with a Zygomaticus implant retained prosthesis (**G**) to achieve a functional occlusion (**H**).

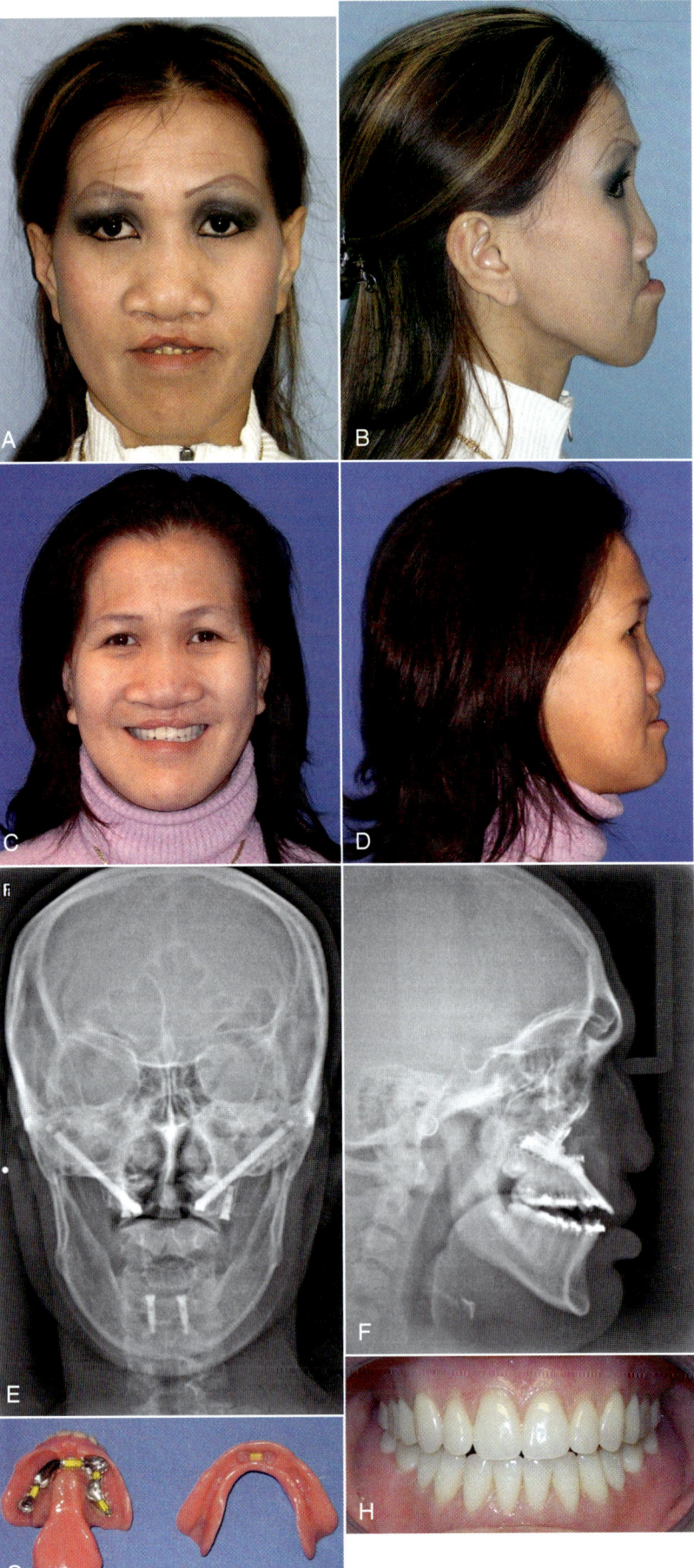

in the central part of the upper lip can be constructed by an Abbe flap. This technique allows simultaneous correction of lip and nasal deformity, but it may sometimes cause undesirable scarring.[124]

Replacement of Teeth in the Line of the Cleft

Replacement of congenitally missing teeth is usually the final step in rehabilitation of the cleft patient. The maxillary lateral incisor is the most commonly missing or malformed tooth (50-75% of unilateral clefts) in the line cleft. It can be managed either by closing the space and substituting the adjacent canine in its position or by opening space and replacing it with a fixed or removable prosthesis. The need to replace missing teeth should be assessed at the beginning of phase II orthodontic treatment; however, definitive replacement of the tooth is performed after completion of growth, secondary surgical procedures, and orthodontic treatment. Substitution of the lateral incisor with the adjacent canine is cost-effective and feasible in selective cases, when there are no other missing teeth in the arch.[125] The main disadvantage is loss of arch length and a decrease in the transverse dimension of the maxillary arch. It can also be unesthetic because of the asymmetry in tooth size and shape in the unilateral cleft deformity where there is one missing lateral incisor. Replacement of congenitally missing teeth with an implant-retained crown is recommended when canine substitution is not feasible. The main disadvantages are the need for additional surgical intervention to augment the bone, when there is inadequate alveolar bone for placement of an implant, and the cost of treatment. Even though the alveolar cleft may have been previously grafted, bone height and width may be inadequate for implant placement at the time of tooth replacement.[126] Additional augmentation can be performed with cortical bone harvested from the ramus or symphysis of the mandible to provide adequate bone height and width about 4 to 6 months prior to implant placement[127] (Fig. 83-23). Our experience at the center for cleft and craniofacial anomalies at the University of California has shown that the success of implants in grafted unilateral clefts is better than in bilateral clefts. In the bilateral cases, very often the periodontal health of the adjacent central incisors is compromised, in addition to absent lateral incisors, making it very difficult to augment the alveolar bone. Longer implants—those at least 13 mm—reportedly have a higher survival rate compared to shorter implants. Other implant parameters such as surface characteristics and diameter do not seem to influence significantly the longevity of implants placed into grafted alveolar clefts.[128,129] Use of teeth-supported fixed prosthetic restorations such as a bridge across the unrepaired alveolar cleft segments should be avoided as movement of the cleft segments results in failure of the prosthesis and loss of abutment teeth. Occasionally, it may be better to replace the missing teeth with a removable prosthesis to achieve a better esthetic and functional outcome. This is the case when there is severe atrophy of the maxilla with missing teeth, lack of adequate soft tissue, absent premaxilla with poor upper lip support, and an unrepaired cleft palate (Fig. 83-24).[130]

PEARLS AND PITFALLS

- CLP has significant psychosocial ramifications. Parents should be counseled appropriately that this is a treatable condition in the absence of other life threatening systemic anomalies.
- The treatment outcomes are best, when care is provided by an interdisciplinary team of specialists. Operator experience has a significant impact on the outcomes of both lip and palate surgery.
- Specialists should provide adequate and timely information about the condition regarding necessary staged surgical and non surgical interventions to alleviate anxiety of the parents and family members.
- The impact of surgical procedures on speech, facial growth and appearance should be closely monitored. Staging of treatment with minimal number of procedures and good surgical technique is essential to decrease scar formation and the associated complications.
- Surgical interventions during the first year after birth and early childhood should basically address function (speech) and psychosocial concerns.
- The procedures in late childhood and adolescence should address occlusion, aesthetics and psychosocial concerns. They should be timed according to the child's facial growth and eruption status of teeth, emotional maturity, and ability to cope with treatment.
- The ultimate goal of treatment should be to achieve intelligible speech and normal appearance with good balance of facial skeleton, soft tissues, and occlusion, with the aim to help the child to develop into a confident young adult.

REFERENCES

1. Bale J, Stoll B, Lucas A: *Reducing birth defects: meeting the challenge in the developing world*, Washington DC, 2003, National Academies Press.
2. Mulliken JB: The changing faces of children with cleft lip and palate, *N Engl J Med* 351(8):745-747, 2004.
3. Corlew DS: Estimation of impact of surgical disease through economic modeling of cleft lip and palate care, *World J Surg* 34(3):391-396, 2010.
4. Marazita ML, Mooney MP: Current concepts in the embryology and genetics of cleft lip and cleft palate, *Clin Plast Surg* 31(2):125-140, 2004.
5. Mossey P: Epidemiology underpinning research in the aetiology of orofacial clefts, *Orthod Craniofac Res* 10(3):114-120, 2007.
6. Forrester MB, Merz RD: Descriptive epidemiology of oral clefts in a multiethnic population, Hawaii, 1986-2000, *Cleft Palate Craniofac J* 41(6):622-628, 2004.
7. Cooper ME, Ratay JS, Marazita ML: Asian oral-facial cleft birth prevalence, *Cleft Palate Craniofac J* 43(5):580-589, 2006.
8. Melnick M, et al: Cleft lip palate: an overview of the literature and an analysis of Danish cases born between 1941 and 1968, *Am J Med Genet* 6(1):83-97, 1980.
9. Vanderas AP: Incidence of cleft lip, cleft palate, and cleft lip and palate among races: a review, *Cleft Palate J* 24(3):216-225, 1987.
10. Cohen MM, Jr: Syndromes with cleft lip and cleft palate, *Cleft Palate J* 15(4):306-328, 1978.
11. Hagberg C, Larson O, Milerad J: Incidence of cleft lip and palate and risks of additional malformations, *Cleft Palate Craniofac J* 35(1):40-45, 1998.
12. Jones MC: Facial clefting. Etiology and developmental pathogenesis, *Clin Plast Surg* 20(4):599-606, 1993.
13. Jones MC: The genetics of cleft lip and palate, in Cleft Lip and Palate: Information for families, Cleft Palate Foundation, 2001, Chapel Hill. pp. 4-8.
14. Cohen MM, Jr: The Robin anomalad—its nonspecificity and associated syndromes, *J Oral Surg* 34(7):587-593, 1976.
15. Cobourne MT: The complex genetics of cleft lip and palate, *Eur J Orthod* 26(1):7-16, 2004.
16. Schliekelman P, Slatkin M: Multiplex relative risk and estimation of the number of loci underlying an inherited disease, *Am J Hum Genet* 71(6):1369-1385, 2002.
17. Blanton SH, et al: Nonsyndromic cleft lip and palate: four chromosomal regions of interest, *Am J Med Genet A* 125A(1):28-37, 2004.

18. Murray JC: Gene/environment causes of cleft lip and/or palate, *Clin Genet* 61(4):248-256, 2002.

19. Eppley BL, et al: The spectrum of orofacial clefting, *Plast Reconstr Surg* 115(7):101e-114e, 2005.

20. Jugessur A, Murray JC: Orofacial clefting: recent insights into a complex trait, *Curr Opin Genet Dev* 15(3):270-278, 2005.

21. Vieira AR, et al: Medical sequencing of candidate genes for nonsyndromic cleft lip and palate, *PLoS Genet* 1(6):e64, 2005.

22. Stanier P, Moore GE: Genetics of cleft lip and palate: syndromic genes contribute to the incidence of non-syndromic clefts, *Hum Mol Genet* 13 Spec No 1:R73-R81, 2004.

23. Zuccchero TM, et al: Interferon regulatory factor 6 (IRF6) gene variants and the risk of isolated cleft lip or palate, *N Engl J Med* 351(8):769-780, 2004.

24. Vieira AR: Unraveling human cleft lip and palate research, *J Dent Res* 87(2):119-125, 2008.

25. Kallen K: Maternal smoking and orofacial clefts, *Cleft Palate Craniofac J* 34(1):11-16, 1997.

26. Little J, Cardy A, Munger RG: Tobacco smoking and oral clefts: a meta-analysis, *Bull World Health Organ* 82(3):213-218, 2004.

27. Meyer KA, et al: Smoking and the risk of oral clefts: exploring the impact of study designs, *Epidemiology* 15(6):671-678, 2004.

28. Yazdy MM, Honein MA, Xing J: Reduction in orofacial clefts following folic acid fortification of the U.S. grain supply, *Birth Defects Res A Clin Mol Teratol* 79(1):16-23, 2007.

29. Wilcox AJ, et al: Folic acid supplements and risk of facial clefts: national population based case-control study, *BMJ* 334(7591):464, 2007.

30. Mossey PA, Davies JA, Little J: Prevention of orofacial clefts: does pregnancy planning have a role? *Cleft Palate Craniofac J* 44(3):244-250, 2007.

31. Cohen MM: Etiology and pathogenesis of orofacial clefting, *Oral Maxillofac Surg Clin North Am* 12(3):379-397, 2000.

32. Fraser FC: The genetics of cleft lip and cleft palate, *Am J Hum Genet* 22(3):336-352, 1970.

33. Mitchell LE, Risch N: Correlates of genetic risk for non-syndromic cleft lip with or without cleft palate, *Clin Genet* 43(5):255-260, 1993.

34. Sperber GH, et al: *Craniofacial development*, Hamilton, Ont.; vol vi, London, 2001, B.C. Decker, pp. 220.

35. Johnson CY, et al: Prenatal diagnosis of orofacial clefts, National Birth Defects Prevention Study, 1998-2004, *Prenat Diagn* 29(9):833-839, 2009.

36. Mulliken JB, Benacerraf BR: Prenatal diagnosis of cleft lip: what the sonologist needs to tell the surgeon, *J Ultrasound Med* 20(11):1159-1164, 2001.

37. Wayne C, et al: Sensitivity and accuracy of routine antenatal ultrasound screening for isolated facial clefts, *Br J Radiol* 75(895):584-589, 2002.

38. Stroustrup Smith A, et al: Prenatal diagnosis of cleft lip and cleft palate using MRI, *AJR Am J Roentgenol* 183(1):229-235, 2004.

39. Jones MC: Prenatal diagnosis of cleft lip and palate: detection rates, accuracy of ultrasonography, associated anomalies, and strategies for counseling, *Cleft Palate Craniofac J* 39(2):169-173, 2002.

40. Strauss RP: Beyond easy answers: prenatal diagnosis and counseling during pregnancy, *Cleft Palate Craniofac J* 39(2):164-168, 2002.

41. Prahl C, et al: Presurgical orthopedics and satisfaction in motherhood: a randomized clinical trial (Dutchcleft), *Cleft Palate Craniofac J* 45(3):284-288, 2008.

42. Glenny, AM, et al: Feeding interventions for growth and development in infants with cleft lip, cleft palate or cleft lip and palate. *Cochrane Database Syst Rev* 2004(3):CD003315.

43. Rohrich RJ, et al: Timing of hard palatal closure: a critical long-term analysis, *Plast Reconstr Surg* 98(2):236-246, 1996.

44. Lous J, et al: Grommets (ventilation tubes) for hearing loss associated with otitis media with effusion in children. *Cochrane Database Syst Rev* 2005(1):CD001801.

45. Millard DR, Jr, et al: A discussion of presurgical orthodontics in patients with clefts, *Cleft Palate J* 25(4):403-412, 1988.

46. Berkowitz S, Mejia M, Bystrik A: A comparison of the effects of the Latham-Millard procedure with those of a conservative treatment approach for dental occlusion and facial aesthetics in unilateral and bilateral complete cleft lip and palate: part I. Dental occlusion, *Plast Reconstr Surg* 113(1):1-18, 2004.

47. Spengler AL, et al: Presurgical nasoalveolar molding therapy for the treatment of bilateral cleft lip and palate: A preliminary study, *Cleft Palate Craniofac J* 43(3):321-328, 2006.

48. Grayson BH, Cutting CB: Presurgical nasoalveolar orthopedic molding in primary correction of the nose, lip, and alveolus of infants born with unilateral and bilateral clefts, *Cleft Palate Craniofac J* 38(3):193-198, 2001.

49. Grayson BH, Shetye PR: Presurgical nasoalveolar moulding treatment in cleft lip and palate patients, *Indian J Plast Surg* 42 Suppl:S56-S61, 2009.

50. Liou EJ, Subramanian M, Chen PK: Progressive changes of columella length and nasal growth after nasoalveolar molding in bilateral cleft patients: a 3-year follow-up study, *Plast Reconstr Surg* 119(2):642-648, 2007.

51. Barillas I, et al: Nasoalveolar molding improves long-term nasal symmetry in complete unilateral cleft lip-cleft palate patients, *Plast Reconstr Surg* 123(3):1002-1006, 2009.

52. Da Silveira AC, et al: Modified nasal alveolar molding appliance for management of cleft lip defect, *J Craniofac Surg* 14(5):700-703, 2003.

53. Weinfeld AB, et al: International trends in the treatment of cleft lip and palate, *Clin Plast Surg* 32(1):19-23, vii, 2005.

54. Ziak P, et al: Timing of primary lip repair in cleft patients according to surgical treatment protocol, *Bratisl Lek Listy* 111(3):160-162, 2010.

55. McHeik JN, Levard G: [Neonatal cleft lip repair: psychological impact on mothers], *Arch Pediatr* 13(4):346-351, 2006.

56. Goodacre TE, et al: Does repairing a cleft lip neonatally have any effect on the longer-term attractiveness of the repair? *Cleft Palate Craniofac J* 41(6):603-608, 2004.

57. Tatum SA: Two-stage unilateral cleft lip repair, *Facial Plast Surg* 23(2):91-99, 2007.

58. Achauer BM, et al: Plastic surgery: indications, operations, and outcomes. In Kolk CAV, editor: *Craniomaxillofacial, Cleft and Pediatric surgery*, St. Louis, 2000, Mosby, 5 v. (xl, 2887).

59. Demke JC, Tatum SA: Analysis and evolution of rotation principles in unilateral cleft lip repair, *J Plast Reconstr Aesthet Surg* 64(3):313-318, 2011.

60. Lazarus DD, et al: Repair of unilateral cleft lip: a comparison of five techniques, *Ann Plast Surg* 41(6):587-594, 1998.

61. Millard D: *Cleft craft: The evolution of its surgery*. Vol. 1, The unilateral Deformity, Boston, 1977, Little, Brown.

62. Ray RM: Unilateral cleft lip repair by rotation/advancement: potential errors and how to avoid them, *Facial Plast Surg* 23(2):87-90, 2007.

63. Randall P, Whitaker LA, LaRossa D: The importance of muscle reconstruction in primary and secondary cleft lip repair, *Plast Reconstr Surg* 54(3):316-323, 1974.

64. Delaire J: Theoretical principles and technique of functional closure of the lip and nasal aperture, *J Maxillofac Surg* 6(2):109-116, 1978.

65. Schendel SA: Unilateral cleft lip repair–state of the art, *Cleft Palate Craniofac J* 37(4):335-341, 2000.

66. Millard DR, Jr, Morovic CG: Primary unilateral cleft nose correction: a 10-year follow-up, *Plast Reconstr Surg* 102(5):1331-1338, 1998.

67. McComb HK, Coghlan BA: Primary repair of the unilateral cleft lip nose: completion of a longitudinal study, *Cleft Palate Craniofac J* 33(1):23-30; discussion 30-1, 1996.

68. Salyer KE, Genecov ER, Genecov DG: Unilateral cleft lip-nose repair–long-term outcome, *Clin Plast Surg* 31(2):191-208, 2004.

69. Mulliken JB: Bilateral cleft lip. *Clin Plast Surg* 31(2):209-220, 2004.

70. McComb H: Primary repair of the bilateral cleft lip nose: a 4-year review, *Plast Reconstr Surg* 94(1):37-47; discussion 48-50, 1994.

71. McComb H: Primary repair of the bilateral cleft lip nose: a 15-year review and a new treatment plan, *Plast Reconstr Surg* 86(5):882-889; discussion 890-3, 1990.

72. Hardesty RA, Afifi GY: Bilateral Cleft lip in plastic surgery: indications, operations and outcomes. In Aucher BM, Eriksson E, editors: *Craniomaxillofacial, Cleft. and Pediatric Surgery*, ed 1, Vol 2, St. Louis, 2000, Mosby.

73. Dorf DS, Curtin JW: Early cleft palate repair and speech outcome, *Plast Reconstr Surg* 70(1):74-81, 1982.

74. van Aalst JA, Kolappa KK, Sadove M: MOC-PSSM CME article: Nonsyndromic cleft palate, *Plast Reconstr Surg* 121(1 Suppl):1-14, 2008.

75. Vacher C, Pavy B, Ascherman J: Musculature of the soft palate: clinico-anatomic correlations and therapeutic implications in the treatment of cleft palates, *Cleft Palate Craniofac J* 34(3):189-194, 1997.

76. Kriens O: Anatomy of the velopharyngeal area in cleft palate, *Clin Plast Surg* 2(2):261-288, 1975.

77. William Y, Hoffman DLM: Cleft Palate repair. In Mathes S J, editor: *Vol. Pediatric Plastic Surgery*, ed 2, Philadelphia, 2006, Saunders Elsevier, pp. 249-270.

78. Braithwaite F, Maurice DG: The importance of the levator palati muscle in cleft palate closure, *Br J Plast Surg* 21(1):60-62, 1968.

79. Kriens OB: An anatomical approach to veloplasty, *Plast Reconstr Surg* 43(1):29-41, 1969.

80. Trier WC: Primary palatoplasty, *Clin Plast Surg* 12(4):659-675, 1985.

81. Heliovaara A, Ranta R: One-stage closure of isolated cleft palate with the Veau-Wardill-Kilner V to Y pushback procedure or the Cronin modification. III. Comparison of lateral craniofacial morphology, *Acta Odontol Scand* 51(5):313-321, 1993.

82. Furlow LT, Jr: Cleft palate repair by double opposing Z-plasty, *Plast Reconstr Surg* 78(6):724-738, 1986.

83. Bardach J: Two-flap palatoplasty: Bardach's technique, *Oper Tech Plast Surg* 2(4):211-214, 1995.

84. Sommerlad BC: A technique for cleft palate repair, *Plast Reconstr Surg* 112(6):1542-1548, 2003.

85. Markus A, Watts R: Cleft Palate Speech, *Oral Maxillofac Surg Clin North Am* 12(3):481-498, 2000.

86. Marsh JL: The evaluation and management of velopharyngeal dysfunction, *Clin Plast Surg* 31(2):261-269, 2004.

87. Orticochea M: Results of the dynamic muscle sphincter operation in cleft palates, *Br J Plast Surg* 23(2):108-114, 1970.

88. Jackson I, Rogers A: Velopharyngeal Insufficiency, *Curr Ther Plastic Surg* 475-481, 2006.

89. Muzaffar AR, et al: Incidence of cleft palate fistula: an institutional experience with two-stage palatal repair, *Plast Reconstr Surg* 108(6):1515-1518, 2001.

90. Emory RE, Jr, et al: Fistula formation and repair after palatal closure: an institutional perspective, *Plast Reconstr Surg* 99(6):1535-1538, 1997.

91. Inman DS, et al: Oro-nasal fistula development and velopharyngeal insufficiency following primary cleft palate surgery–an audit of 148 children born between 1985 and 1997, *Br J Plast Surg* 58(8):1051-1054, 2005.

92. Kirschner RE, et al: Repair of oronasal fistulae with acellular dermal matrices, *Plast Reconstr Surg* 118(6):1431-1440, 2006.

93. Narula JK, Ross RB: Facial growth in children with complete bilateral cleft lip and palate, *Cleft Palate J* 7:239-248, 1970.

94. Goode PM, Mulliken JB, Padwa BL: Frequency of Le Fort I osteotomy after repaired cleft lip and palate or cleft palate, *Cleft Palate Craniofac J* 44(4):396-401, 2007.

95. Tindlund RS: Skeletal response to maxillary protraction in patients with cleft lip and palate before age 10 years, *Cleft Palate Craniofac J* 31(4):295-308, 1994.

96. Eppley BL: Alveolar cleft bone grafting (Part I): Primary bone grafting, *J Oral Maxillofac Surg* 54(1):74-82, 1996.

97. Ochs MW: Alveolar cleft bone grafting (Part II): Secondary bone grafting, *J Oral Maxillofac Surg* 54(1):83-88, 1996.

98. Bergland O, et al: Secondary bone grafting and orthodontic treatment in patients with bilateral complete clefts of the lip and palate, *Ann Plast Surg* 17(6):460-474, 1986.

99. da Silva Filho OG, et al: Secondary bone graft and eruption of the permanent canine in patients with alveolar clefts: literature review and case report, *Angle Orthod* 70(2):174-178, 2000.

100. Boyne PJ: Autogenous cancellous bone and marrow transplants, *Clin Orthop Relat Res* 73:199-209, 1970.

101. Dickinson BP, et al: Reduced morbidity and improved healing with bone morphogenic protein-2 in older patients with alveolar cleft defects, *Plast Reconstr Surg* 121(1):209-217, 2008.

102. Chin M, et al: Repair of alveolar clefts with recombinant human bone morphogenetic protein (rhBMP-2) in patients with clefts, *J Craniofac Surg* 16(5):778-789, 2005.

103. Herford AS, et al: Bone morphogenetic protein-induced repair of the premaxillary cleft, *J Oral Maxillofac Surg* 65(11):2136-2141, 2007.

104. Santiago PE, et al: Reduced need for alveolar bone grafting by presurgical orthopedics and primary gingivoperiosteoplasty, *Cleft Palate Craniofac J* 35(1):77-80, 1998.

105. Sato Y, et al: Success rate of gingivoperiosteoplasty with and without secondary bone grafts compared with secondary alveolar bone grafts alone, *Plast Reconstr Surg* 121(4):1356-1367; discussion 1368-9, 2008.

106. Matic DB, Power SM: The effects of gingivoperiosteoplasty following alveolar molding with a pin-retained Latham appliance versus secondary bone grafting on midfacial growth in patients with unilateral clefts, *Plast Reconstr Surg* 122(3):863-870; discussion 871-873, 2008.

107. Meazzini MC, et al: Early Secondary gingivo-alveolo-plasty in the treatment of unilateral cleft lip and palate patients: 20 years experience, *J Craniomaxillofac Surg* 38(3):185-191, 2010.

108. Evans CA: Orthodontic treatment for patients with clefts, *Clin Plast Surg* 31(2):271-290, 2004.

109. Oberoi S, Chigurupati R, Vargervik K: Morphologic and management characteristics of individuals with unilateral cleft lip and palate who required maxillary advancement, *Cleft Palate Craniofac J* 45(1):42-49, 2008.

110. Wong GB, Ciminello FS, Padwa BL: Distraction osteogenesis of the cleft maxilla, *Facial Plast Surg* 24(4):467-471, 2008.

111. Cheung LK, Chua HD: A meta-analysis of cleft maxillary osteotomy and distraction osteogenesis, *Int J Oral Maxillofac Surg* 35(1):14-24, 2006.

112. Cheung LK, Chua HD, Hagg MB: Cleft maxillary distraction versus orthognathic surgery: clinical morbidities and surgical relapse, *Plast Reconstr Surg* 118(4):996-1008; discussion 1009, 2006.

113. Drommer R: Selective angiographic studies prior to Le Fort I osteotomy in patients with cleft lip and palate, *J Maxillofac Surg* 7(4):264-270, 1979.

114. Posnick JC, Dagys AP: Skeletal stability and relapse patterns after Le Fort I maxillary osteotomy fixed with miniplates: the unilateral cleft lip and palate deformity, *Plast Reconstr Surg* 94(7):924-932, 1994.

115. Posnick JC, Taylor M: Skeletal stability and relapse patterns after Le Fort I osteotomy using miniplate fixation in patients with isolated cleft palate, *Plast Reconstr Surg* 94(1):51-58; discussion 59-60, 1994.

116. Cheung LK, et al: The 3-dimensional stability of maxillary osteotomies in cleft palate patients with residual alveolar clefts, *Br J Oral Maxillofac Surg* 32(1):6-12, 1994.

117. Phillips JH, et al: Predictors of velopharyngeal insufficiency in cleft palate orthognathic surgery, *Plast Reconstr Surg* 115(3):681-686, 2005.

118. Stal S, Hollier L: Correction of secondary deformities of the cleft lip nose, *Plast Reconstr Surg* 109(4):1386-1392; quiz 1393, 2002.

119. Stal S, Hollier L: Correction of secondary cleft lip deformities, *Plast Reconstr Surg* 109(5):1672-1681; quiz 1682, 2002.

120. Yuzuriha S, Mulliken JB: Minor-form, microform, and mini-microform cleft lip: anatomical features, operative techniques, and revisions, *Plast Reconstr Surg* 122(5):1485-1493, 2008.

121. Huffman WC, Lierle DM: Studies on the pathologic anatomy of the unilateral harelip nose, *Plast Reconstr Surg (1946)* 4(3):225-234, 1949.

122. Guyuron B: MOC-PS(SM) CME article: late cleft lip nasal deformity, *Plast Reconstr Surg* 121(4 Suppl):1-11, 2008.

123. Balaji SM: One-stage correction of severe nasal deformity associated with a unilateral cleft lip, *Scand J Plast Reconstr Surg Hand Surg* 37(6):332-338, 2003.

124. Lo LJ, Kane AA, Chen YR: Simultaneous reconstruction of the secondary bilateral cleft lip and nasal deformity: Abbe flap revisited, *Plast Reconstr Surg* 112(5):1219-1227, 2003.

125. Cassolato SF, et al: Treatment of dental anomalies in children with complete unilateral cleft lip and palate at SickKids hospital,

Toronto, *Cleft Palate Craniofac J* 46(2):166-172, 2009.

126. Kearns G, et al: Placement of endosseous implants in grafted alveolar clefts, *Cleft Palate Craniofac J* 34(6):520-525, 1997.

127. Cune MS, Meijer GJ, Koole R: Anterior tooth replacement with implants in grafted alveolar cleft sites: a case series, *Clin Oral Implants Res* 15(5):616-624, 2004.

128. Pena WA, et al: The role of endosseous implants in the management of alveolar

clefts, *Pediatr Dent* 31(4):329-333, 2009.

129. Kramer FJ, et al: Dental implants in patients with orofacial clefts: a long-term follow-up study, *Int J Oral Maxillofac Surg* 34(7):715-721, 2005.

130. Pham AV, et al: Rehabilitation of a patient with cleft lip and palate with an extremely edentulous atrophied posterior maxilla using zygomatic implants: case report, *Cleft Palate Craniofac J* 41(5):571-574, 2004.

Chapter 84

Cleft Lip and Palate: Nasoalveolar Molding

Judah S. Garfinkle, Barry H. Grayson

The desire for presurgical management of the cleft lip and palate (CLP) deformity can be traced back several centuries. The goal was to presurgically mitigate the severity of the deformity in hopes of achieving a superior surgical outcome. Most attempts at presurgical management only addressed the alveolar deformity. Until nasoalveolar molding (NAM) was introduced, the nasal deformity that was associated with cleft lip and palate was addressed entirely by surgical means.

This chapter will present the role of NAM in optimizing the primary surgical repair of the nose, lip, and alveolus in infants born with unilateral cleft lip and palate (UCLP) and bilateral cleft lip and palate (BCLP). This chapter will primarily apply to nonsyndromic cleft lip and palate, although NAM can be used to treat certain syndromic cleft cases. Although the principles of treatments are similar for patients with UCLP and BCLP, there are also unique features to each group that deserve specific attention.

ETIOPATHOGENESIS/CAUSATIVE FACTORS

The cleft lip results from failure of the medial nasal and maxillary processes to fuse between the 4th to the 6th week of fetal development. Clefting of the palate results when the left and right palatal processes fail to elevate and fuse in the midline between the 8th to the 12th week of fetal development.

It is generally accepted that the majority of clefts are a product of both a genetic susceptibility and an environmental insult to the developing fetus. Progress has been made in the genetic determination of clefting and regarding issues related to prenatal care.

PATHOLOGIC ANATOMY

Clefting of the lip and palate can occur in combination, as an isolated deformity, or as part of a syndrome, and can affect either one (unilateral) or both sides (bilateral) of the face. The severity of each cleft is variable as well and can be either a complete cleft or an incomplete cleft. The classic descriptions below are offered for complete UCLP and BCLP.

UNILATERAL CLEFT LIP AND PALATE

In UCLP, the alveolus is asymmetrically divided into two pieces: the greater alveolar segment (including the premaxilla) and the lesser alveolar segment (on the cleft side). With the greater alveolar segment protruded anteriorly and deviated to the noncleft side, the medial and lateral insertions of the cleft side nasal alar cartilage and the lip segments are drawn apart, resulting in the classic UCLP deformities. Perhaps one of the most disfiguring components of the UCLP deformity (and most challenging to repair) is the prolapsed cleft side alar cartilage, which is often under tension from the malpositioned medial and lateral points of insertion (Fig. 84-1).

BILATERAL CLEFT LIP AND PALATE

In BCLP, the alveolar ridge is divided into three segments. The premaxillary segment is often positioned outside the mouth. There are two lateral (or posterior) alveolar segments located intraorally. The lip is also divided into three parts. The prolabium appears to originate from the tip of the nose, because the columella is severely deficient. The lateral lip segments are located significantly behind the anteriorly protruding premaxilla and prolabium. This results in a widened nasal tip and nasal base, as the lateral points of insertion of

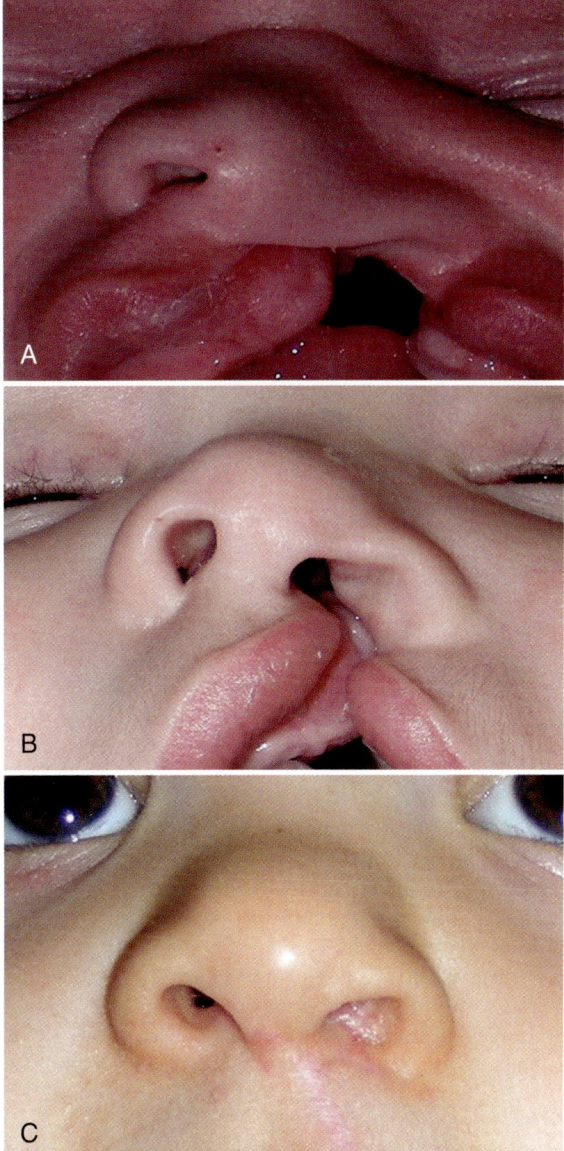

Fig. 84-1 ■ **A,** Infant with UCLP. Note the prolapsed alar cartilage on the cleft side, depressed nasal tip, wide gap between the lip segments, and deviation of the nose toward the noncleft side. **B,** Following NAM, note improved nasal symmetry, nasal tip projection, and approximation of the lip segments. **C,** Seven months following primary surgery.

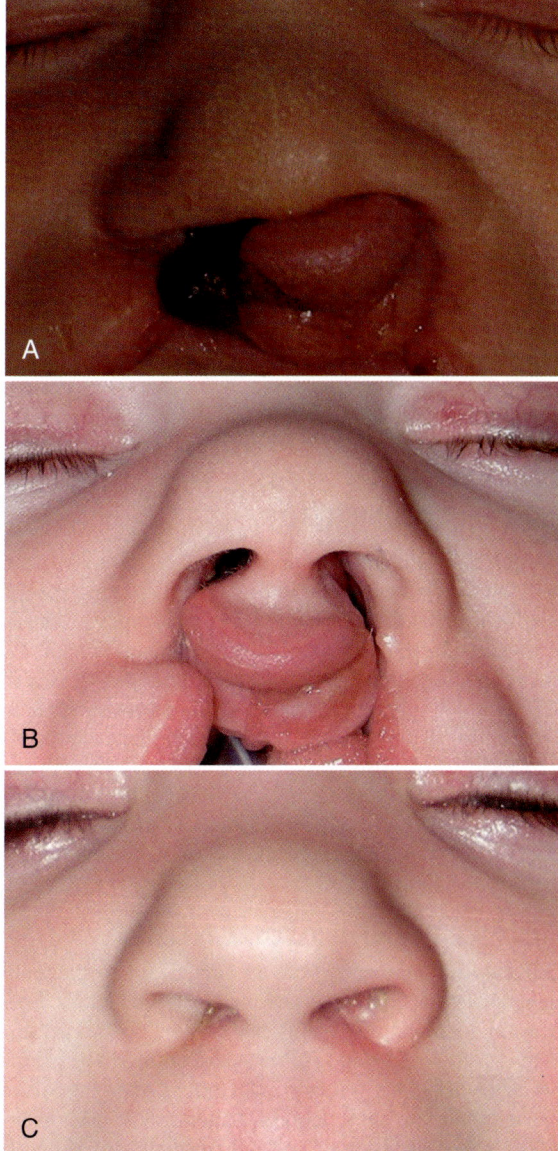

Fig. 84-2 ■ **A,** Infant with BCLP. Note the extraoral position of the premaxilla, deficient columella, and wide nasal tip and alar base. **B,** Following NAM, note the increased length of columella, increased projection of nasal tip, and approximation of the alveolar and lip segments. **C,** Nine months following primary surgery.

the alar wings are tethered posteriorly with the lips and as the nasal tip is drawn forward with the premaxilla and prolabium (Fig. 84-2).

DIAGNOSTIC STUDIES

ULTRASONOGRAPHY

At the 20-week structural ultrasonogram that most women have, it is possible to observe most clefts of the lip and palate.

DIRECT EXAMINATION OF CLEFT TYPE

Ultimately, it is the surgeon's decision to include NAM in the treatment protocol if he or she feels a superior primary outcome could be achieved following its use. Then it is up to the orthodontist (or whoever is performing the NAM) to determine if the presurgical result desired by the surgeon can be achieved. At this point, NAM

is presented to the family as a treatment alternative and discussed in detail as described later.

Clefting of the nose, lip, alveolus, and palate can have variable presentation. While NAM is appropriate for most cleft types, its use is not indicated in all of them. For example, isolated palatal clefts do not benefit from NAM, because the alveolar ridge is intact and nasal morphology is not affected. On the other hand, partial lip clefts with intact or notched alveolar ridges but with significant nasal deformity can benefit from NAM.

TREATMENT/RECONSTRUCTIVE GOALS

The rationale for performing NAM is to reduce the severity of the initial cleft deformity prior to the primary surgery. In this way, the optimal outcome may be achieved, leading to (1) normalized social interaction at the earliest stage of development possible by reducing the stigmata of living with a cleft, (2) reduction in the need for costly surgical revisions, and (3) a decrease in the cost and burden of cleft rehabilitation on the patient, family, and society.

Specifically, in UCLP, the treatment goals are to (1) reduce the alveolar gap, (2) bring the lip segments into passive contact, (3) increase the surface area of the nasal mucosal lining, (4) reduce nasal septum deviation, and (5) to achieve symmetry between the lower lateral alar cartilages.

In BCLP, the treatment goals are to (1) position the premaxilla in the midline and between the lateral alveolar segments, (2) bring the lip segments into passive contact, (3) increase the surface area of the nasal mucosal lining, (4) increase nasal tip projection, and (5) perform nonsurgical columella elongation.

SPECIFIC TREATMENT AND TECHNIQUES

CONSULTATION WITH FAMILY REGARDING NASOALVEOLAR MOLDING

NAM requires considerable time and energy from both the cleft team and the family undergoing the treatment. To ensure NAM is a good fit for each individual family, a comprehensive consultation should be performed with each family, explaining the commitment that they will need to make to have a successful outcome with NAM. Use of pictures in a photo album or by a computer slide show can be quite helpful. Using a toy doll fitted with the face tapes and a modified plate can be instructive as well. Drawing attention to the weekly visits and responsibilities with the taping is vital. This is time well spent, because it ensures that the treatment goals and expectations for the family are clear and helps them to decide whether to pursue NAM.

TREATMENT PLANNING/DIAGNOSIS

After careful examination by both the surgeon and orthodontist, the treatment goals are confirmed and ancillary procedures identified. On occasion, there may be a tooth bud erupted on the margin of the cleft. This is often removed to allow complete approximation of the alveolar segments. This primary tooth bud is often not surrounded by bone and therefore not functional. In addition, if a Simonart band (soft tissue bridge) is observed and anticipated to inhibit the alveolar molding, it is surgically separated.

LIP TAPING

Placing tapes across the cleft lip gap in both UCLP and BCLP prior to NAM can not only achieve reduction in the alveolar cleft width, but in addition, it provides the caregiver(s) a chance to handle/manage the tapes and is a good test to make sure there is satisfactory commitment and cooperation for NAM treatment.

In UCLP, two Steri-Strips are connected with an orthodontic elastic between them and is placed under tension from cheek to cheek (Fig. 84-3, A) For BCLP cases, a special pad is created by wrapping a hydrocolloid bandage around a Steri-Strip, flanked by a Steri-Strip and orthodontic elastic on each side. The pad is placed at the junction of the columella and prolabium to begin premaxillary retraction. Base tapes should be used on the cheeks to reduce skin irritation (Fig. 84-3, B).

MAXILLARY AND NASAL IMPRESSION

The impression of the maxillary arch is taken with an infant impression tray loaded with a heavy-bodied impression material (Coltene Rapid Soft Putty, ISO 4823, type 0, made of polysiloxane, condensation type; Alstaetten, Switzerland). The infant is swaddled and held upside down. The impression tray is seated with positive pressure.

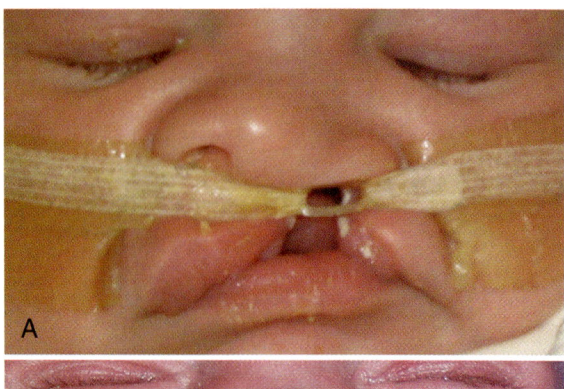
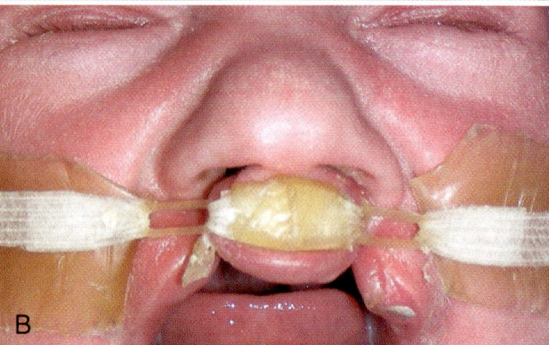

Fig. 84-3 ■ A, Pre-NAM lip taping to begin molding of the greater alveolar segment. B, Pre-NAM lip taping to begin retraction of the premaxilla.

The airway is observed and maintained by holding the tongue superiorly with the handle of a mouth mirror. After removal of the impression, an oral examination is performed to ensure no material broke off. One of the advantages to using the putty material is that it does not tear as easily as alginate does. An impression of the nose is captured with a light-bodied material (Memosil 2, vinyl polysiloxane; Heraeus Kulzer, Hanau, Germany). Care is taken to include the medial canthi in the impression for registration points.

APPLIANCE FABRICATION

The maxillary and nasal impressions are poured up with dental stone and allowed to set completely. The maxillary impression is prepared to serve as the template for construction of the intraoral plate. Preparation includes trimming, blocking out undercuts, and coating with a separating material to prevent the acrylic from sticking to the dental stone. Both self-cure acrylic and 2-mm thick Biocryl (Great Lakes Orthodontics, Tonowanda, NY) can produce an excellent device. In some BCLP cases in which the premaxilla is deviated to one side, the premaxillary segment of the dental cast can be repositioned a few millimeters toward the midline prior to appliance fabrication (or manually repositioned during the impression), which will result in a more symmetrical NAM plate and ease the process of premaxillary centering. Ensuring that the material across the cleft gap is built to the same vertical dimension as the rest of the maxillary arch will facilitate adjustment of the device.

APPLIANCE DELIVERY

The caregivers are instructed to have the infant a bit hungry during the appointment in which the appliance will be delivered. In this way, once the plate is inserted, the infant will be motivated to feed.

Although each device is fabricated from a unique maxillary cast, further customization of the appliance is required during the initial fitting with the baby. Hold it in place with superiorly directed pressure to evaluate the vestibular extension and relationship with the maxillary frenal attachments. To honor the dynamics of the soft tissues and molding action of the device, reduce the buccal extensions to provide for approximately 2 mm of space between the height of the vestibule and all frenal attachments. Intraoral sores most frequently develop in these areas. Confirm that the plate is uniformly thick to ensure adequate strength and resistance to cracking. The plate is delivered with minimal molding activation to ensure a good fit and to allow the baby to adjust for the first week.

A hole of approximately 5 mm in diameter is made through the palatal surface. This hole provides a continuous flow of air should the posterior border of the plate lose retention and rotate down toward the tongue.

The location of the retention button(s) is determined while the plate is seated in the mouth. For the UCLP device, one button is placed on the labial aspect between the lip segments. The button is placed slightly toward the greater segment, anticipating its gradual migration toward the noncleft side as the alveolar cleft narrows. The BCLP device has two retention buttons, each placed in the gap between prolabium and lateral lip segments. The buttons can be prefabricated and attached to the labial aspect of the molding plate. The button(s) should be approximately 10 mm long from the surface of the device, which is usually adequate to ensure clearance of the lips by the tapes and elastics (described later) and to create an appropriate force vector to optimize retention of the plate to the palate and alveolar segments. The button should be placed at approximately 30 degrees to the occlusal plane. A too steep or shallow angle may compromise retention (Fig. 84-4).

An adjustment period for both the infant and caregivers is to be expected and may last from 1 to 3 days. This may include disruption to any pattern established for both feeding and sleeping. Assuming the plate is fitting well, the infant (and caregivers) should adapt quite well.

TAPING TECHNIQUES

The intraoral portion of the NAM device is retained in the mouth primarily from a series of tapes originating from the cheeks. The bottom layer, or base tape, is a hydrocolloid type bandage (e.g., DuoDerm, extra thin; Bristol-Myers Squibb, New York, NY) that serves as a barrier between the retention tapes and the cheeks to minimize tissue irritation. They are placed bilaterally at an angle just below the eyes, with the more medial portion angled inferiorly. The retention tapes are fashioned out of a ¼-inch Steri-Strip wrapped around an orthodontic elastic at one end (¼-inch or ³⁄₁₆-inch, 4.5 oz). The elastic then engages the button that extends anteriorly from the intraoral plate (Fig. 84-5). To optimize the alveolar retraction force, the elastic should be stretched to approximately two times its resting diameter. The retention tapes are changed daily, whereas the base tapes can last up to a week.

In UCLP, addition of a cross-cheek tape may facilitate alveolar gap closure. While manually approximating the cheeks, this ¼-inch Steri-Strip tape is stretched across the cleft, anchored onto a base tape on each cheek. Following placement of the cross-cheek tape, the NAM device is placed in the mouth, and the NAM device retention tapes are attached.

In BCLP, a prolabial tape can be used to assist with the nonsurgical columella elongation. Two elastics are knotted and embedded into a piece of Steri-Strip shaped to fit onto the prolabium. Each end of the elastic is attached to the retention button on its respective side. The application of a tissue adhesive (e.g., Mastisol; Eloquest Healthcare, Ferndale, Mich) to the prolabium greatly facilitates retention of this tape (Fig. 84-6).

ALVEOLAR MOLDING

The first step in NAM is to address the alveolar deformity. This step is crucial to create some laxity of the tethered alar cartilage prior to initiating nasal molding. Reducing the width of the alveolar cleft to approximately 5 mm is suggested prior to adding the nasal stent. Alveolar molding is achieved through two mechanisms: (1) gentle forces delivered to the alveolar segments by the orthodontic elastics attached to the molding plate and (2) reciprocal additions and subtractions of hard and soft acrylic to the molding plate. All additions and subtractions are done in 0.5- to 1.0-mm increments.

Alveolar molding in UCLP is aimed at slowly providing normal curvature to the extended and protrusive greater alveolar segment. The projecting premaxillary portion of the greater alveolar segment is retracted into the mouth while allowing the lesser alveolar segment to remain in its place. Small amounts of hard acrylic are removed from the lining of the molding plate surrounding the anterior surface of the lesser alveolar segment to allow the greater

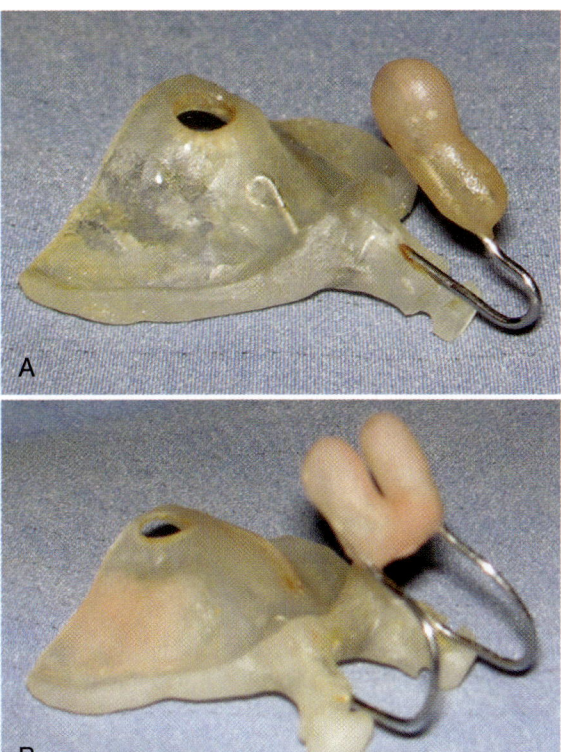

Fig. 84-4 ■ **A,** UCLP NAM device consisting of an intraoral molding plate and wire armature that supports the intranasal stent. **B,** BCLP NAM device consisting of an intraoral molding plate and a pair of intranasal stents supported by two wire armatures. There is a columella band connecting the two intranasal stents.

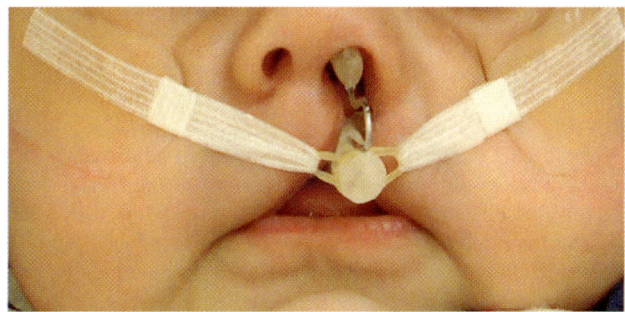

Fig. 84-5 ■ NAM taping. Note the position of base tapes and Steri-Strips.

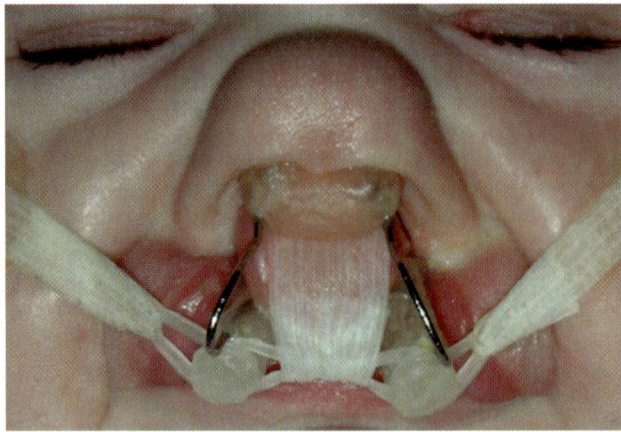

Fig. 84-6 ■ Prolabial taping. The downward pull on the prolabium by this tape is partly responsible for the increase in length of the columella.

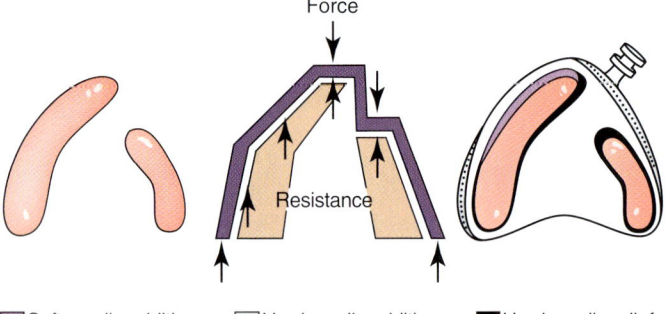

☐ Soft acrylic additions   ☷ Hard acrylic additions   ■ Hard acrylic relief

Fig. 84-7 ■ UCLP biomechanics. (Redrawn from Losee JE: *Comprehensive cleft care*, New York, 2009, McGraw-Hill.)

segment to be retracted under the elastic force delivered to the plate from the tapes. To maintain adequate thickness of the plate, it will be necessary to periodically add hard acrylic to the external surfaces of the plate prior to the sequential subtractions of material from the internal surfaces. Reduction in the cleft width is also achieved by removal of hard acrylic located in the alveolar cleft and addition of soft acrylic on the internal aspect of the plate around the labial/buccal aspect of the greater segment. This is done in balance with reduction of an equal amount of hard acrylic on the palatal side of the greater segment to ensure the full labiopalatal dimension of the alveolar ridge is maintained (Fig. 84-7).

In BCLP, alveolar molding is aimed at centering and retracting the protrusive premaxilla into position between the lateral alveolar segments. Sometimes, the posterior alveolar segments are expanded or narrowed to attain a good fit with the width of the retracting premaxilla. In order for the retraction of the premaxilla to occur, it is necessary to remove acrylic from the anterior and buccal portions of the internal aspect of the molding plate around the lateral alveolar segments. Adding increments of soft acrylic on the internal aspect of the plate labial to the premaxilla and removing hard acrylic from between the alveolar clefts serves to further reduce the alveolar cleft width (Fig. 84-8).

In both UCLP and BCLP, the recommended adjustments of the molding plate result in its gradual posterior drift and impingement upon the glossopalatine arch or soft tissue fauces. Thus, the posterior border of the molding plate should be gradually reduced to prevent irritation of these tissues and interference with the retraction of the molding plate and associated anatomic structures.

The transverse dimension of the plate should be gradually increased at the rate of approximately 1 mm per month to keep up

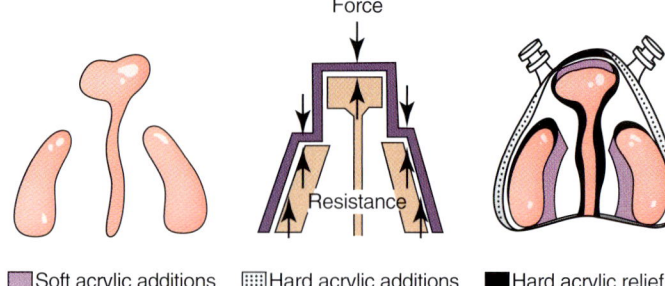

☐ Soft acrylic additions   ☷ Hard acrylic additions   ■ Hard acrylic relief

Fig. 84-8 ■ BCLP biomechanics. The three primary ways that molding forces are generated are (1) application of the elastic retention tapes, resulting in a posteriorly directed force to tissue surfaces contacting the inside of the NAM device; (2) reciprocal additions and subtractions of acrylic are made to the NAM appliance; and (3) the reaction to pushing forward on the nasal tip is pushing back on the projecting alveolar processes. (Redrawn from Losee JE: *Comprehensive cleft care*, New York, 2009, McGraw-Hill.)

with normal increase in the transverse arch width of the maxillary alveolar processes.

ADDITION OF NASAL STENT

Once the alveolar gap(s) is/are reduced to approximately 5 mm, nasal molding can begin. A short section of utility wax can be used to fashion a template for the nasal stent wire by bending it in a "U" shape with both open ends pointed toward the infant. The bottom leg is placed along the retention button, and the top is positioned to fit into the nasal aperture. This wax form serves as a template for the construction of the nasal stent. A 0.036-inch diameter stainless steel wire is bent to emulate the curvature and length of the wax template and to intimately fit within an acrylic channel created on the existing molding plate. The channel is created with a narrow-diameter acrylic cutting bur. Care is taken to not perforate the molding plate. The wire originates in a small loop (to improve retention in the acrylic) on the anterior inferior aspect of the molding plate. It wraps around the retention button(s) at the point where the buttons join the molding plate, extends along the top of the button, gradually curves back toward the molding plate in a "swan neck" bend, and terminates in a series of bends resulting in an "R" shape that will serve as the intranasal portion of the nasal stent. This carefully formed wire is then embedded within the molding plate by adding hard acrylic to fill in the channel and lock the wire into place. A shell of hard acrylic is also added to the "R"-shaped bends, which gives the nasal stent the classic "kidney bean" shape. The intranasal portion of the nasal stent is now coated with a thin layer of PermaSoft (Perma Laboratories, Millersburg, Ohio). Using a bird beak and a three-prong pliers, the nasal stent is carefully positioned in the nostril along the side of the columella and the nostril apex is slightly elevated. The caregivers are educated about the nasal molding process and care of the child and the appliance. A small amount of lubricant may be applied to the surface of the nasal stent to facilitate insertion and to prevent irritation from friction. Upon delivery, mild tissue blanching at the nostril apex and support of the nasal tip should be seen. The blanching should dissipate after a few minutes. Excessive pressure will result in breakdown of the nasal tissues and should be avoided.

NASAL MOLDING

The form of the nasal stent is specific and dictated by the function that it serves. There are two lobes to the nasal stent. The superior lobe is used to project the nasal tip forward, increase nasal protrusion, and expand the nasal mucosal lining. The inferior lobe defines

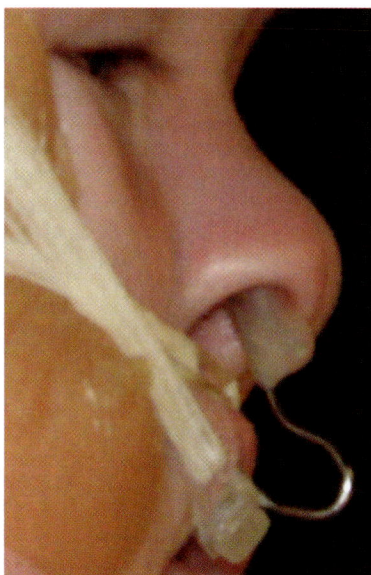

Fig. 84-9 ■ UCLP nasal stent in nose. Note the position of superior and inferior lobes. The superior lobe achieves forward projection of the nasal tip and molding of the lower lateral nasal cartilages. The lower lobe lifts the nostril apex.

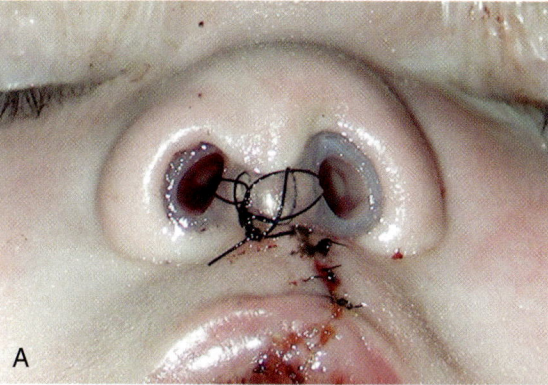

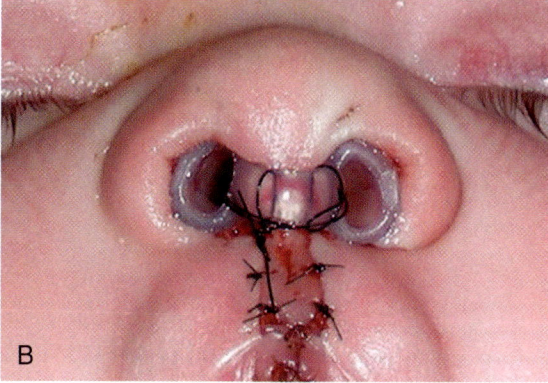

Fig. 84-10 ■ **A,** UCLP postprimary surgery with nasal stent retainer. **B,** BCLP postprimary surgery with nasal stent retainer.

the nostril apex and, in BCLP, contributes to the nonsurgical elongation of the columella (Fig. 84-9). At each subsequent NAM adjustment appointment, the nasal stent can be activated by adding increments of PermaSoft or bending the wire along its length to achieve the desired molding effect on the nose. Bending the wire close to the nasal stent results in a change in orientation of the lobes of the nasal stent, whereas bending the wire closer to the molding plate has a greater effect on modifying the overall height of the nasal stent. Each addition of PermaSoft should show no edges or sharp elevations, to minimize the chances of mucosal irritation or the risk of developing a sore on the nasal lining.

Nasal molding in BCLP has some unique features that distinguish it from nasal molding in UCLP. Two nasal stents are used in BCLP cases. These stents can be formed from a single wire. To facilitate nonsurgical columella elongation, the two nasal stents are connected by a horizontal band of PermaSoft (when 2 to 3 mm of columella is formed) and subsequently increased in height to achieve the desired tissue expansion (see Fig. 84-6).

The goal for nasal molding should be to achieve overcorrection of nasal tip projection, because some postsurgical relapse can be anticipated.

POSTOPERATIVE CARE

Following delivery of the molding plate, a 1- to 3-day adjustment period for both the infant and the caregivers is to be expected while each adapts to life with NAM. It is normal for any patterns that have formed to be disrupted, including those associated with feeding and sleeping. Assuming the device is appropriately adjusted, new patterns will soon be established, and life with NAM will become the norm for the family. Appointments for adjustment of the NAM appliance should be performed every 1 to 2 weeks. Treatment is usually completed within 4 to 5 months. While an intraoral examination is performed at every follow-up visit, it is important for the caregivers to do this daily as the plate is removed for cleaning.

Following the primary surgical repair, use of a postoperative nasal stent would be helpful in reducing relapse (Fig. 84-10).

PEARLS AND PITFALLS

- Careful focus on adequate relief around all frenal attachments and movable mucosa will minimize the risk of creating an intraoral sore.
- If retention of the plate is compromised (1) alter the length and/or angle of the retention button, (2) change the angle/tension of the tapes, and/or (3) consider using a very small amount of denture adhesive (e.g., Fixodent).
- If the baby learns how to express the plate with the tongue, adding a bell-shaped curve extension anchored off the posterior border of the plate can help to prevent displacement.
- NAM can be used effectively in the treatment of incomplete clefts for correction of prolapsed alar cartilage and deficient columella length.
- Anecdotally, parents often report improved feeding ability of the infant with the NAM appliance.
- On occasion, it may not be possible to completely close the alveolar cleft due to deviation of the nasal septum against the inferior nasal turbinate or, perhaps, from a more extensive deficiency of alveolar tissue.
- Compression of the labiopalatal dimension of the greater alveolar segment can occur if reciprocal additions and subtractions of material are not made appropriately.
- The greater alveolar segment can appear to be displaced superiorly along the cleft margins. When this is the case, it can be repositioned inferiorly by the addition of PermaSoft to the inferior aspect of the nasal stent. This will very gradually push the upturned edge of the alveolar segments downward to achieve leveling of the alveolar occlusal plane.
- If the NAM device needs to be removed in between adjustment appointments, caregivers should be instructed to use a crosscheek tape until the next visit.

BIBLIOGRAPHY

Barillas I, Dec W, Warren SM, et al: Nasoalveolar molding improves long-term nasal symmetry in complete unilateral cleft lip-cleft palate patients. *Plast Reconstr Surg* 123(3):1002-1006, 2009.

Cutting C, Grayson B, Brecht L, et al: Presurgical columellar elongation and primary retrograde nasal reconstruction in one-stage bilateral cleft lip and nose repair. *Plast Reconstr Surg* 101(3):630-639, 1998.

Garfinkle JS, King T, Grayson, BH, et al: A 12-year anthropometric evaluation of the nose in bilateral cleft lip and palate patients following nasoalveolar molding and cutting bilateral cleft lip and nose reconstruction, *Plast Reconstr Surg* 127(4):1659-1667, 2011.

Grayson BH, Maull D: Nasoalveolar molding for infants born with clefts of the lip, alveolus, and palate [review]. *Clin Plast Surg* 31(2):149-158, vii, 2004 .

Grayson BH, Santiago PE, Brecht LE, Cutting CB: Presurgical nasoalveolar molding in infants with cleft lip and palate. *Cleft Palate Craniofac J* 36(6):486-498, 1999.

Lee CT, Garfinkle JS, Warren SM, et al: Nasoalveolar molding improves appearance of children with bilateral cleft lip-cleft palate. *Plast Reconstr Surg* 122(4):1131-1137, 2008.

Liou EJ, Subramanian M, Chen PK: Progressive changes of columella length and nasal growth after nasoalveolar molding in bilateral cleft patients: a 3-year follow-up study. *Plast Reconstr Surg* 119(2):642-648, 2007.

Chapter

85

Cleft Lip and Palate: Primary Cleft Lip Repair

Bernard J. Costello, Ramon L. Ruiz

The comprehensive treatment of cleft lip and palate deformities requires thoughtful consideration of the anatomic complexities of the deformity and the delicate balance between intervention and growth. Comprehensive and coordinated care from infancy through adolescence is essential to achieve the best outcome, and surgeons with formal training and experience in all the phases of care must be actively involved in the planning and treatment. Specific goals of surgical care for children born with cleft lip and palate include the following:

- Normalized esthetic appearance of the lip and nose
- Intact primary and secondary palate
- Normal speech, language, and hearing
- Nasal airway patency
- Class I occlusion with normal masticatory function
- Good dental and periodontal health
- Normal psychosocial development

Successful management of the child born with a cleft lip and palate requires coordinated care provided by a number of different specialties, including oral and maxillofacial surgery, otolaryngology, plastic surgery, genetics and dysmorphology, speech-language pathology, orthodontics, pediatric dentistry, and prosthodontics. In most cases, care of patients with congenital clefts has become a subspecialty area of clinical practice within these different professions. In addition to the primary cleft repairs in infancy, treatment plans routinely involve multiple treatment interventions to achieve the above goals staged throughout childhood. Because care is provided over the entire course of the child's development, long-term follow-up is essential under the care of these different health care providers.

The formation of interdisciplinary cleft palate teams has served two key objectives of successful cleft care: (1) coordinated care provided by the necessary disciplines and (2) continuity of care with close-interval follow-up of the patient throughout periods of active growth and ongoing stages of reconstruction. The best outcomes are achieved when the team's care is centered on the patient, family, and community rather than a particular surgeon, specialty, or hospital. Healthy team dynamics and optimal patient care are achieved when all members are active participants, when team protocols and referral patterns are equitable, and when the needs of the child are placed above the needs of the team or individual members.

The surgical reconstruction of clefts requires that the surgeon undertaking this important work maintain a cognitive understanding of the complex malformation itself, the varied operative techniques used, facial growth considerations, and the psychosocial health of the patient and family. This chapter presents the overall staged reconstructive approach for repair of cleft lip and palate from infancy through the time of skeletal maturity, as well as a discussion of the surgical procedures involved in cleft lip and palate repair.

GENETICS AND ETIOLOGY

Clefts of the upper lip and palate are the most common major congenital craniofacial abnormality and are present in approximately 1 in 600 live births. Although inheritance may play a role, cleft lip and palate is often not considered a single-gene disease. Instead, clefts are thought to be of a multifactorial etiology with a number of potential contributing factors. These factors may include chemical exposures, radiation, maternal hypoxia, teratogenic drugs, nutritional deficiencies, physical obstruction, and genetic influences. One prevailing theory relates the process of clefting as a point when multiple factors come together to raise the individual above a threshold, at which time the mechanism of fusion fails. Multiple genes recently have been implicated in the etiology of clefting. Some of these genes include the *MSX*, *LHX*, *goosecoid*, and *DLX* genes. Additional disturbances in growth factors or their receptors that may be involved in the failure of fusion include fibroblast growth factor, transforming growth factor, platelet-derived growth factor, and epidermal growth factor.

Clefts of the lip occur more commonly in males than in females. In addition, left-sided cleft lips are more common than right-sided cleft lips, and unilateral cleft lips are more common than bilateral cleft lips. Bilateral clefts of the lip are most often associated with clefting of both the primary and secondary palates. Cleft palate alone is seen in approximately 1 in 2000 live births, an incidence similar in all racial groups. Significant differences in the prevalence of clefts exist when specific populations are examined.

In the majority of cases, unilateral cleft lip and palate is an isolated nonsyndromic birth defect not associated with any other major anomalies. By comparison, a much greater proportion of patients with an isolated cleft palate have an associated syndrome or sequence. Some of the more common syndromes seen in this group include Stickler, van der Woude, and DiGeorge syndromes. Early diagnosis is important because functional issues may arise early in life and go unnoticed. For example, patients with an isolated cleft palate should be evaluated early by an experienced pediatric ophthalmologist to evaluate the possibility of Stickler syndrome. Patients with Stickler syndrome may have ocular abnormalities that lead to retinal detachment. In an otherwise healthy-appearing child, these findings may be difficult to diagnose, so early visual loss may go unnoticed. In many cases, long-term genetic follow-up is necessary to make a definitive diagnosis and provide genetic counseling.

CLASSIFICATION

The typical classification system used clinically to describe standard clefts of the lip and palate is based on careful anatomic description. Clefts can be unilateral or bilateral; microform, incomplete, or complete; and may involve the lip, nose, primary palate, and/or secondary palates (Figs. 85-1 and 85-2). The presentation of clefts is

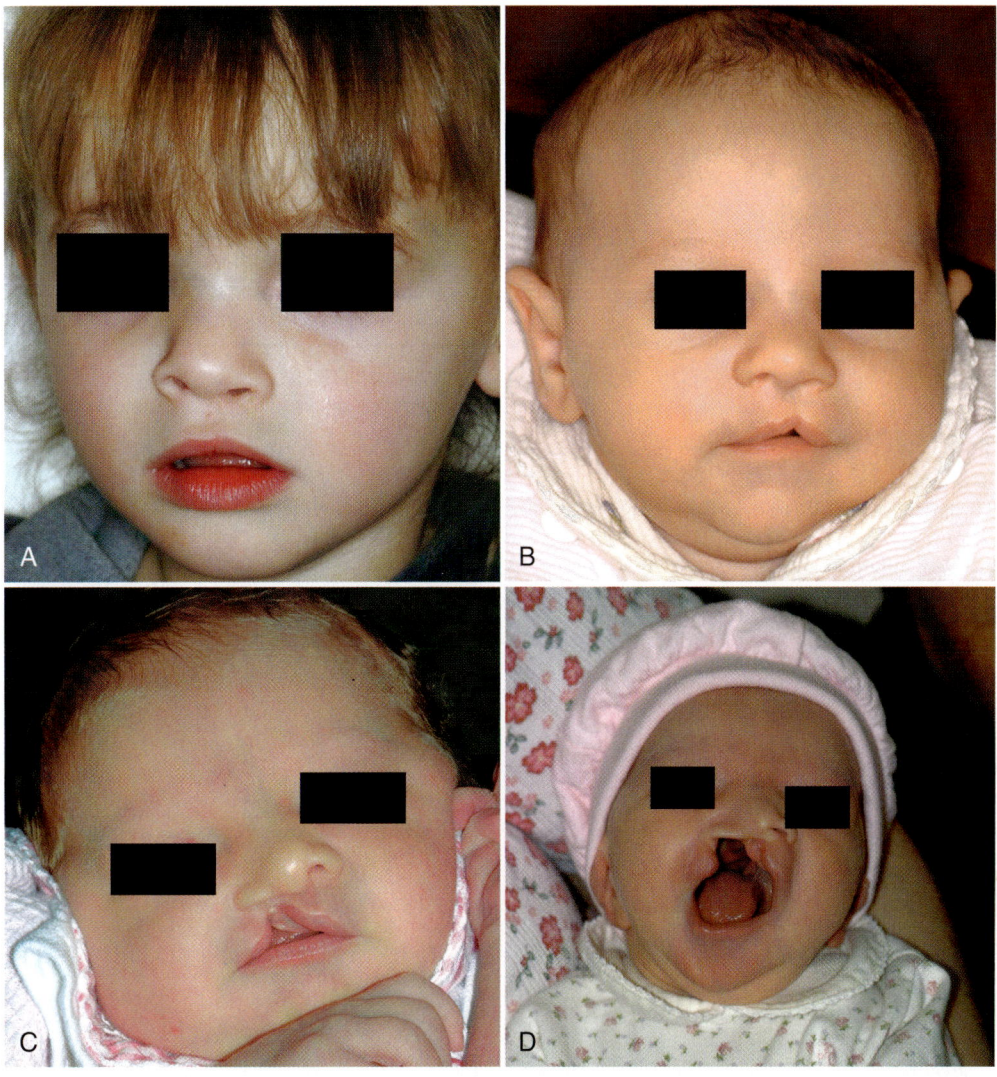

Fig. 85-1 ■ Cleft lips come in a variety of configurations; each repair must be customized to establish the most normal morphology. **A,** Microform left unilateral cleft lip only, not requiring primary repair. **B,** Minor left incomplete unilateral cleft lip only. **C,** Left incomplete unilateral cleft lip and palate with a Simonarts band. **D,** Wide left complete unilateral cleft lip and palate. (From Myers EN: *Operative otolaryngology: head and neck surgery*, ed 2. Philadelphia, 2008, Saunders.)

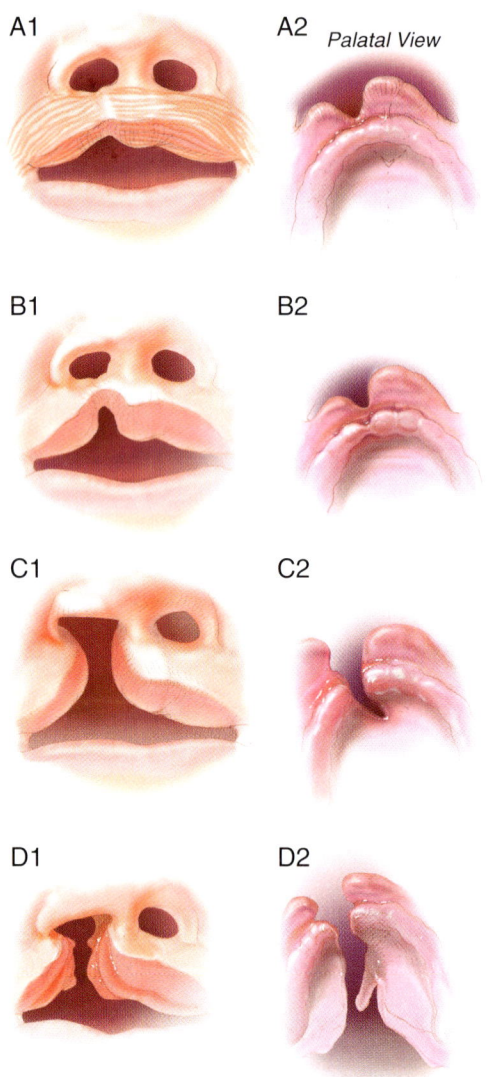

Palatal View

extremely variable, and the individual repairs are custom-tailored to achieve the best symmetry and balance. More severe facial clefting is most commonly described by using Paul Tessier's orbitocentric system of numbering (Fig. 85-3). Other systems are based on embryologic fusion planes, but are these are cumbersome to use in routine clinical practice.

PRENATAL COUNSELING

Recent advances in imaging have revolutionized prenatal care and maternal-fetal medicine. Currently ultrasound images of clefts of the lip can be visualized at about 16 weeks. Diagnostic images of the palate are more difficult to acquire, making the correct prenatal diagnosis of a cleft palate less predictable. Anterior palatal structures may be visualized using sagittal and coronal views, but this currently requires the latest technology and a skilled ultrasonographer with experience performing this type of study.

TREATMENT PLANNING AND TIMING

The timing of cleft lip and palate repair is controversial. Despite a number of meaningful advancements in the care of patients with cleft lip and palate, a lack of consensus exists regarding the timing and specific techniques used during each stage of cleft reconstruction. Surgeons must continue to balance the functional needs, aesthetic concerns, and the issue of ongoing growth carefully when deciding how and when to intervene. In no other type of surgical problem is the issue of the effect of early surgery on growth more apparent than in the treatment of cleft lip and palate deformities. Understanding the growth and development of the craniofacial skeleton is critical to the treatment planning process.

Each stage of surgical reconstruction and the suggested timing based on the patient's age are presented in Table 85-1. Special considerations may alter the sequencing or timing of the various procedures based on individual functional or esthetic needs. Significant

Fig. 85-2 ■ There is significant variation in the configuration and severity of the unilateral cleft lip and nasal deformity. The surgical repair is tailored to the specific dysmorphology of each patient. Approximately 75% of all unilateral cleft lip defects, including microform and incomplete cases, will also have a defect of the underlying skeletal structures of the maxilla and alveolus. **A1** and **A2,** Microform cleft lip. **B1** and **B2,** When repair is indicated, these defects require excision of the hypoplastic tissue within the cleft (incomplete fusion), dissection of the appropriate layers for reapproximation, and mirror-image reconstruction with the contralateral side. Incomplete cleft lip deformities may have a short noncleft vertical height, and the nasal deformity may be relatively mild. **C1** and **C2,** Complete unilateral clefts of the lip without a cleft palate will exhibit the significantly rotated and flattened lower lateral cartilage, hypoplastic vermilion and white roll tissue, as well as even shorter vertical height along the noncleft margin medially. The anterior palate cleft can exhibit more separation and shows involvement up to the incisive foramen, which is the embryologic division point between the primary and secondary palate. **D1** and **D2,** The complete unilateral cleft lip and palate typically presents as a wider defect with larger separation at the alveolus. The nasal deformity may be more severe, and the vertical mismatch between the lateral and medial segments may be more significant. The septum may or may not be attached to the contralateral palatal shelf (unilateral or bilateral cleft palate). (From Costello BJ, Ruiz FL: Unilateral cleft lip and nasal repair: the rotation—advancement flap technique atlas of the oral and maxillofacial surgery clinics. 17(2):103-116, 2009.)

TABLE 85-1	Staged Reconstruction of Cleft Lip and Palate Deformities
PROCEDURE	**TIME FRAME**
Cleft lip repair	After 10 weeks
Cleft palate repair	Age 9 to 18 months
Pharyngeal flap or pharyngoplasty	Age 3 to 5 years or later based on speech development
Maxillary/alveolar reconstruction with bone grafting	Age 6 to 9 years based on dental development
Cleft orthognathic surgery	Age 14 to 16 years in girls, 16 to 18 years in boys
Cleft rhinoplasty	After age 5 years but preferably at skeletal maturity, after orthognathic surgery when possible.
Cleft lip revision	Any time once initial remodeling and scar maturation is complete but best performed after age 5 years

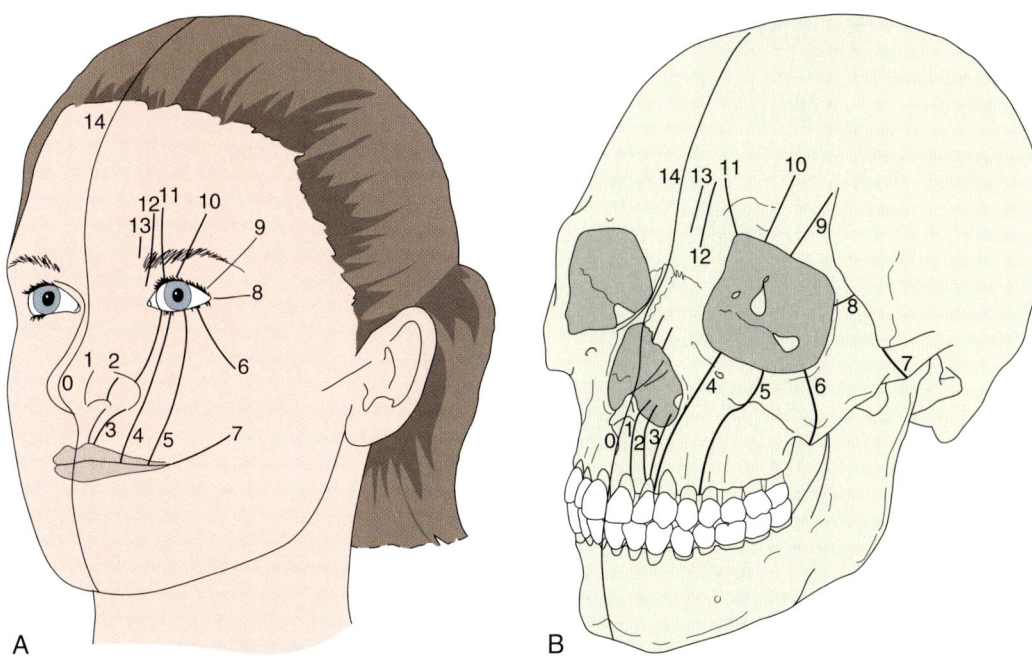

Fig. 85-3 ■ **A** and **B,** Complex facial clefts can be classified according to Tessier's original orbito-centric system of numbering. Clefts may involve all tissue planes, including skin, mucosa, bone, teeth, muscle, brain, peripheral nerve, and other specialized tissues. (From Myers EN: *Operative otolaryngology: head and neck surgery*, ed 2, Philadelphia, 2008, Saunders.)

differences exist worldwide regarding the timing of different repairs. Currently, the timing of repair cannot be guided by truly definitive outcome research or level I evidence.

Cleft lip repair generally is undertaken at some point after 10 weeks of age. Waiting until the child is 10 to 12 weeks of age allows enough time for a complete medical evaluation of the patient so that any associated congenital defects affecting other organ systems (e.g., cardiac or renal anomalies) may be uncovered. The surgical procedure itself may be easier when the child is slightly larger and the anatomic landmarks are more prominent and well defined. Historically, the anesthetic risk–related data suggested that the safest time for surgery in this population of infants could be outlined simply by using the "rule of 10s." This referred to delaying lip repair until the child was at least 10 weeks old, 10 pounds in weight, and with a minimum hemoglobin level of 10 mg/dL. Today, more sophisticated pediatric anesthetic techniques, advances in intraoperative monitoring, and improved anesthetic agents have all resulted in the ability to provide safe general anesthesia much earlier in life. Despite this ability, no measurable benefit exists to performing lip repair before 3 months of age.

As with the timing of other interventions, lip and nasal revision is best performed after the majority of growth is complete. Most of the lip and nasal growth is complete after age 5 years. Lip revision may be considered just before school begins, at approximately 5 years of age or later. However, this may be performed earlier if the deformity is severe. Nasal revision is performed after age 5 years, because most of the nasal growth is complete by this time. If orthognathic reconstruction is likely, rhinoplasty is best performed after orthognathic surgery, because maxillary advancement improves many characteristics of nasal support. However, when nasal deformity is particularly severe, rhinoplasty can be considered earlier even if orthognathic surgery is expected. Multiple early revisions of the lip or nose should be avoided so that excess scarring does not potentially impair ongoing growth.

PRESURGICAL TAPING AND PRESURGICAL ORTHOPEDICS

Facial taping with elastic devices may be used for application of selective external pressure and may improve lip and nasal position before the lip repair procedure. In the authors' opinions, these techniques often have greater impact in cases of wide bilateral cleft lip and palate in which manipulation of the premaxillary segment may make primary repair technically easier. Although one of the basic surgical tenets of wound repair is to close wounds under minimal tension, attempts at improving the arrangement of the segments by using taping methods have not shown a measurable improvement.

Some surgeons prefer presurgical orthopedic (PSO) appliances rather than lip taping to achieve similar goals. PSO appliances are composed of a custom-made acrylic base plate that provides improved anchorage in the molding of lip, nasal, and alveolar structures during the presurgical phase of treatment. Frequent appointments are necessary to monitor the anatomic changes and periodic appliance adjustment.

In their current state of technical refinement, minimal high-level and convincing evidence exists that any of the PSOs offer an improved outcome regarding esthetics, function, or growth in patients with cleft lip and palate. Coupled with the fact that appliances are time-consuming and have a high cost of fabrication and utilization, advocating their uniform use is difficult. As with other interventions considered for patients with clefts, costly and unproven interventions should be avoided, although they may prove to be helpful in select cases. A subset of more severe clefts appears to benefit from the devices.

LIP ADHESION

Some surgeons attempt to surgically approximate the segments of the cleft lip prior to definitive lip repair in an attempt to achieve a better relationship of both the lip structures and the dental arches.

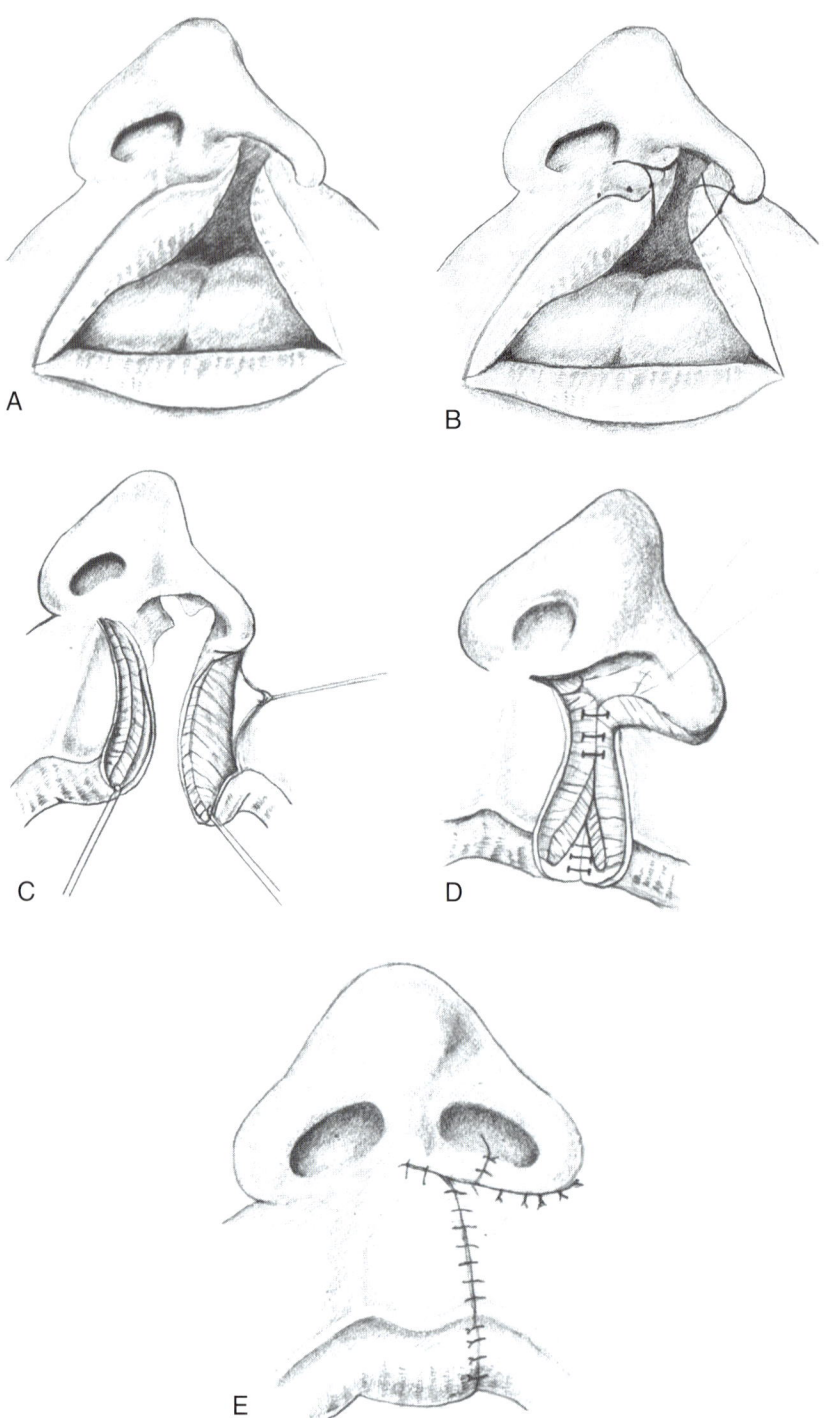

Fig. 85-4 ▪ **A,** Complete unilateral cleft of the lip, highlighting the hypoplastic tissue in the cleft site not used in the reconstruction. Note the nasal deformities typical in the unilateral cleft, including displaced lower lateral nasal cartilages, deviated anterior septum, and nasal floor clefting. **B,** The typical markings for the authors' preferred repair, highlighting the need to excise the hypoplastic tissue and approximate good vermilion and white roll tissue for the repair. **C,** Once the hypoplastic tissue has been excised, the three layers of tissue are dissected (skin, muscle, and mucosa). Completely freeing the orbicularis oris from its abnormal insertions on the anterior nasal spine area and lateral ala is important. Nasal flaps also are incorporated into the dissection to repair the nasal floor (not shown). **D,** The orbicularis oris muscle is approximated with multiple interrupted sutures, and the vermillion border/white roll complex is reconstructed. The nasal floor and mucosal flaps are approximated. **E,** The lateral flap is advanced, and the medial segment is rotated downward to create a healing scar line that will resemble the natural philtral column on the opposite side. The incision lines are hidden in natural contours and folds of the nose and lip. (From Fonseca RJ, Marciani RD, Turvey TA: *Oral and maxillofacial surgery,* vol 3, ed 2, St Louis, 2009, Saunders.)

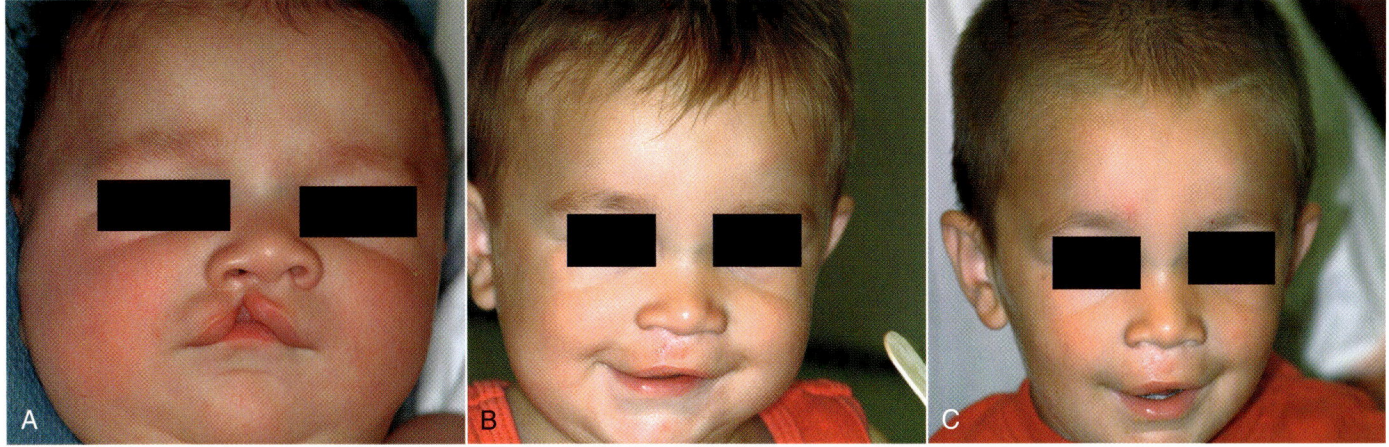

Fig. 85-5 ▪ **A,** Three-month-old child with a right-sided incomplete unilateral cleft lip. Note the short philtrum near the midline that must be rotated downward to avoid notching and improve symmetry. **B,** Nine-month-old boy after the rotation-advancement repair of his cleft lip and nasal deformities. **C,** The same child as in (**B**) 2½ years after his cleft lip and nasal repairs. (From Myers EN: *Operative otolaryngology: head and neck surgery,* ed 2, Philadelphia, 2008, Saunders.)

This is achieved by advancing small flaps of tissue across the cleft site. While some surgeons advocate the use of this technique in wide bilateral clefts, it is rarely performed in unilateral cases. The lip adhesion is usually completed at 3 months of age. In most cases, this will convert a wide complete cleft into a wide incomplete cleft, because the scar will eventually be excised from the cleft site, re-creating a similar wide deformity. The definitive lip repair is then completed 3 to 9 months later by excising the scar and reapproximating the remaining lip structures. Furthermore, at the second procedure, there is usually less supple tissue to work with when performing the definitive repair. As with most endeavors in cleft surgery, repeated early interventions tend to complicate later refinements due to excessive scarring. In general, adequate mobilization of the flaps in one stage will make tension-free skin closure possible in most every case without the need for taping, presurgical orthopedic appliances, and/or lip adhesion.

PRIMARY UNILATERAL CLEFT LIP REPAIR

Unilateral clefts of the lip and nose present with a high degree of variability; thus, each repair design is unique (see Figs. 85-1 and 85-2). The repair technique preferred by the authors for cleft lip and nasal deformities is shown in Figures 85-4 and 85-5. The basic premise of the repair is to create a three-layered closure of skin, muscle, and mucosa that approximates normal tissue and excises hypoplastic tissue at the cleft margins. Critical to the process is the reconstruction of the orbicularis oris and the surrounding musculature into a continuous sphincter and functional unit. The Millard rotation advancement technique has the advantage of allowing each of the incision lines to fall within the natural contours of the lip and nose.

Primary nasal reconstruction may be considered at the time of lip repair to reposition the displaced lower lateral cartilages and alar tissues. Several techniques are advocated, and considerable variation exists regarding the exact nasal reconstruction performed by each surgeon. The primary nasal repair may be achieved by releasing the alar base, augmenting the area with allogeneic dermal grafts, or even performing a formal open rhinoplasty. Given that lip repair is performed at such an early point in growth and development, the authors prefer minimal surgical dissection, because of the effects of scarring on the subsequent growth of these tissues. McComb described a technique that has become popular; it consists of

dissecting the lower lateral cartilages free from the alar base and the surrounding attachments through an alar crease incision. This allows the nose to be bolstered and/or stented from within the nostril to improve symmetry.

PRIMARY BILATERAL LIP REPAIR

Bilateral cleft lip repair can be one of the most challenging technical procedures performed in children with clefts. The lack of quality tissue present and the widely displaced segments are major challenges to achieving exceptional results, but superior technique and complete mobilization of the tissue flaps usually yields excellent aesthetic results (Figs. 85-6 and 85-7). In addition, the columella may be quite short in length, and the premaxillary segment may be significantly rotated. Adequate mobilization of the segments and attention to the details of using only appropriately developed tissue will yield excellent results even in the face of significant asymmetry. Some surgeons have used techniques to lengthen the columella surgically and preserve hypoplastic tissue with banked fork flaps. Early and aggressive tissue flaps in the nostril and columella areas do not look natural after significant growth has occurred and result in abnormal tissue contours. The authors prefer a primary nasal reconstruction that can be performed in a similar fashion to the technique described by McComb. This allows release and repositioning of the lower lateral cartilages and alar base on both sides without aggressive degloving of the entire nasal complex. Other open rhinoplasty techniques that use direct incision on the nasal tip or prolabial unwinding techniques have been suggested.

CONCLUSION

The comprehensive care of patients with clefts requires an interdisciplinary approach that demands precise surgical execution of the various procedures necessary to effectively treat cleft deformities. Cleft lip and nose reconstruction has come a long way since the initial straight-line repairs and early modifications of Z-plasty techniques. Still, clear evidence-based literature that sorts out the differences between repair techniques is lacking. Surgeons are left to use their own experience and training when deciding which repair technique is best for a particular patient. Excellent results can be achieved using any number of variations of the rotation-advancement technique for unilateral cleft lip and nose repair.

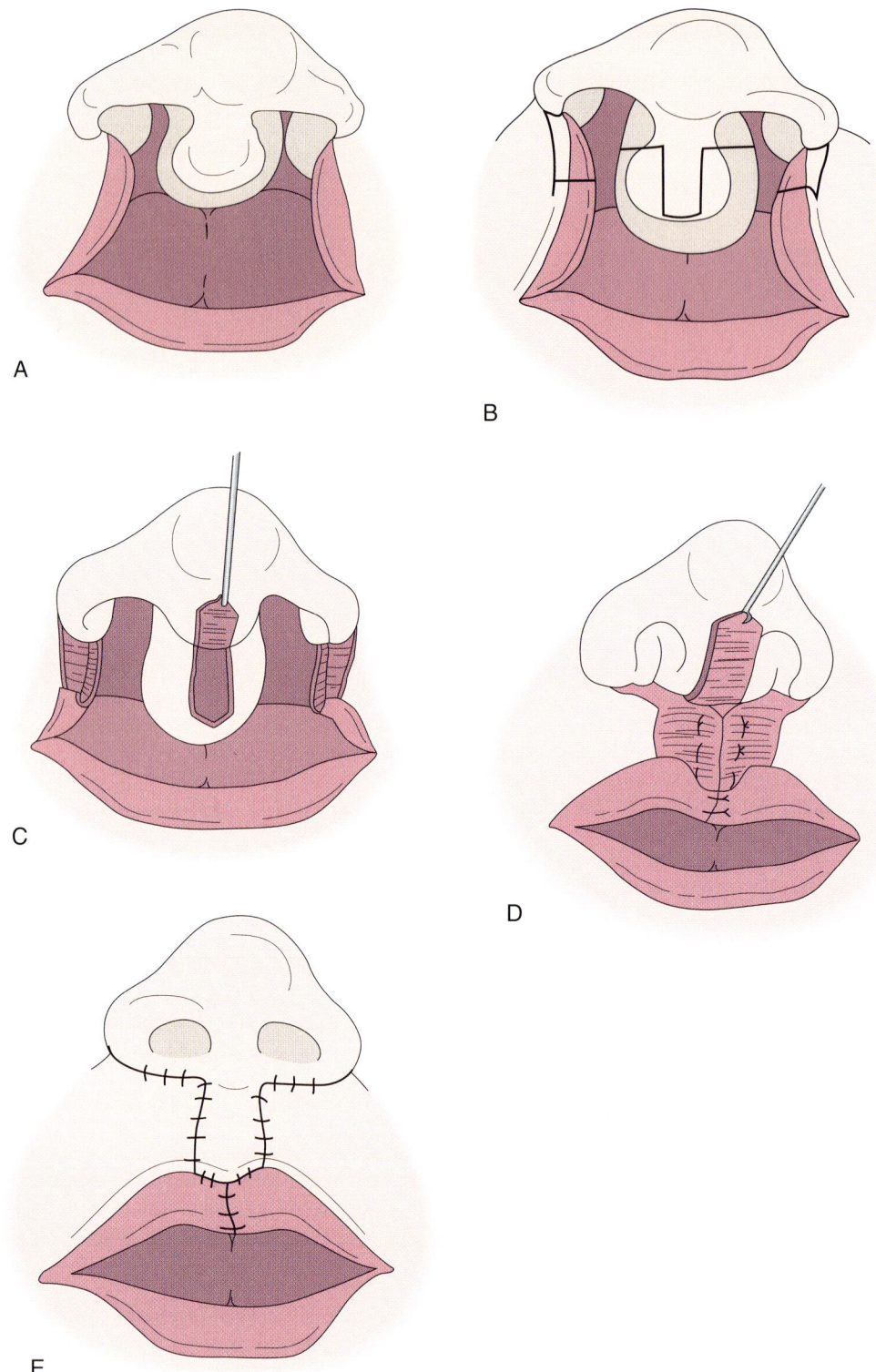

Fig. 85-6 ■ **A,** The bilateral cleft of the lip and maxilla shown is complete and highlights the nature of hypoplastic tissue along the cleft edges. The importance of the nasal deformity is evident in the shorter columella and disrupted nasal complexes. **B,** Markings of the authors' preferred repair, with an emphasis on excision of hypoplastic tissue and approximating more normal tissue with the advancement flaps. **C,** A new philtrum is created by excising the lateral hypoplastic tissue and elevating the philtrum superiorly. In addition, the lateral advancement flaps are dissected into three distinct layers (skin, muscle, and mucosa). Nasal floor reconstruction also occurs in conjunction with these advancement flaps. **D,** The orbicularis oris musculature is approximated in the midline with multiple interrupted and/or mattress sutures. This is a critical step in the total reconstruction of the functional lip. No musculature is present in the premaxillary segment, which must be brought to the midline from each lateral advancement flap. The nasal floor flaps are sutured at this time as well. The new vermilion border is reconstructed in the midline with good white roll tissue advanced from the lateral flaps. **E,** The final approximation of the skin and mucosal tissues is performed, leaving the healing incision lines in natural contours of the lip and nose. (From Myers EN: *Operative otolaryngology: head and neck surgery,* ed 2, Philadelphia, 2008, Saunders.)

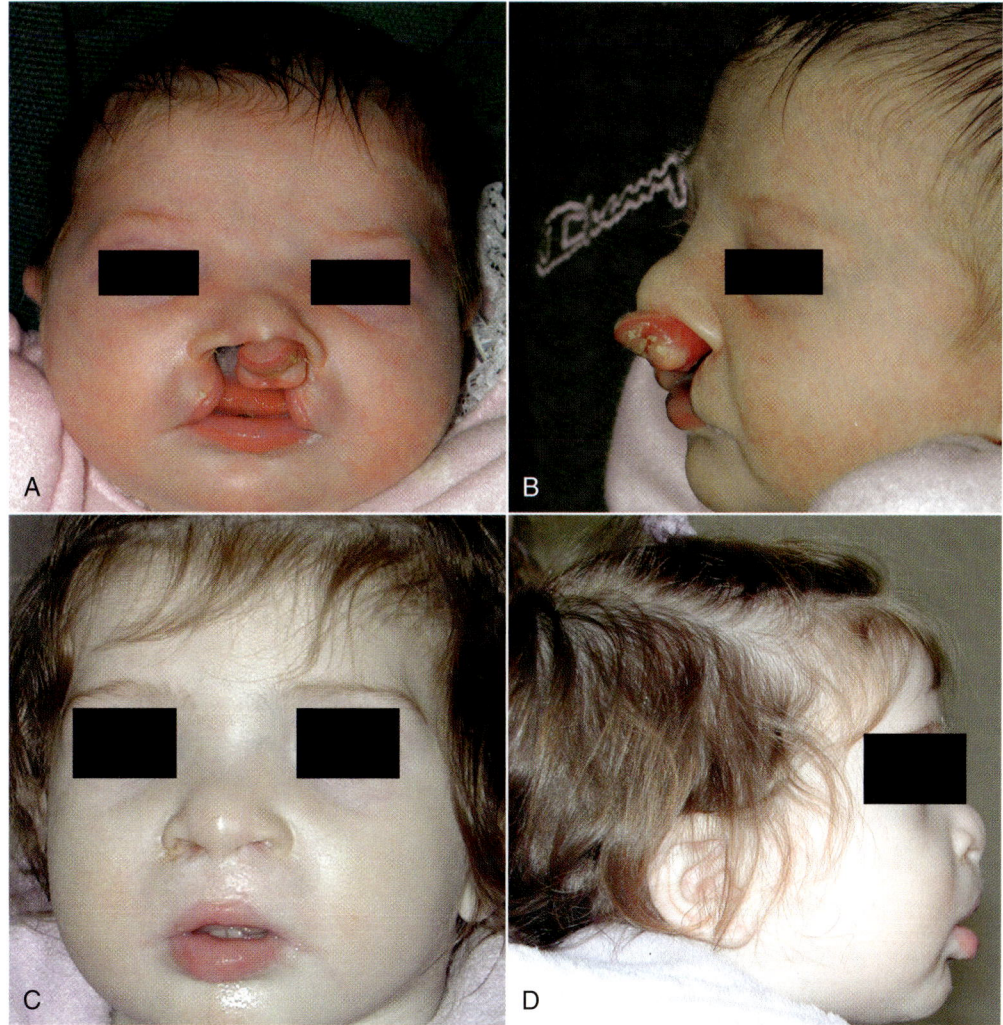

Fig. 85-7 ■ **A** and **B,** Presurgical appearance of a bilateral cleft lip and palate with impressive asymmetry and rotation of the premaxillary segment. Note the significant nasal asymmetry and bunching of the orbicularis oris laterally. **C** and **D,** The same child at 14 months of age after repair of cleft lip and palate. (From Myers EN: *Operative otolaryngology: head and neck surgery*, ed 2, Philadelphia, 2008, Saunders.)

PEARLS AND PITFALLS

- Marking the key landmarks is important for obtaining the best result, and the temptation to keep hypoplastic tissue should be discouraged.
- Nasoalveolar molding appliances may be helpful in reapproximating the segments to allow easier surgical repair, and they may improve the esthetic result of the lip and nose.
- A three-layered closure is the key to both functional and esthetic repair of the lip.
- Some nasal asymmetry is expected in wide unilateral clefts, but this can be minimized by conservative primary nasal reconstruction.
- Nasal bolsters or silicone nasal stents can be used to help mold the nose in the postoperative period.
- Arm restraints may be used for the first 2 weeks to help avoid injury to the lip repair, but they should be removed occasionally to allow range of motion of the arms.

- To optimize the skeletal base, lip revision and rhinoplasty may be best performed after orthognathic surgery is complete.
- A common pitfall is to incompletely reconstruct the musculature of the lip or palate.
- Careful wound care is necessary, because some bolsters used to help mold the nose may cause pressure necrosis of the columella or nasal base if placed too tightly or kept in place for too long.
- Cleft lip reconstructions should incorporate a careful muscular reconstruction, and, if incomplete, will yield less than ideal results. Some surgeons consider it exceptionally important to reconstruct the perinasal musculature as a key component of lip and nose repair.

BIBLIOGRAPHY

American Cleft Palate-Craniofacial Association: Parameters for the evaluation and treatment of patients with cleft lip/palate or other craniofacial anomalies. *Cleft Palate Craniofac J* 30(Suppl 1):4, 1993.

Berkowitz S: The comparison of treatment results in complete cleft lip/palate using conservative approach vs. Millard-Latham PSOT procedure. *Semin Orthod* 2:169, 1996.

Millard DR: *Cleft craft*, vol 1. Boston, 1976, Little, Brown.

Posnick JC: The staging of cleft lip and palate reconstruction: infancy through adolescence. In Posnick JC (ed): *Craniofacial and maxillofacial surgery in children and young adults*. Philadelphia, 2000, WB Saunders, pp 785-826.

Prahl C, Kuijpers-Jagman AM, Van'tHof MA, et al: A randomized prospective clinical trial of the effect of infant orthopedics in unilateral cleft lip and palate: prevention of collapse of the alveolar segments (Dutch cleft). *Cleft Palate Craniofac J* 40:337-342, 2003.

Shaw WC, Asher-McDade C, Brattstrom V, et al: A six-center international study of treatment outcome in patients with clefts of the lip and palate. Part 5. General discussion and conclusions. *Cleft Palate Craniofac J* 29:413-418, 1992.

Shaw WC, Semb G: Current approaches to the orthodontic management of cleft lip and palate. *J R Soc Med* 83:30-33, 1990.

Tessier P: Anatomical classification of facial, cranio-facial, and latero-facial clefts. *J Maxillofac Surg* 4:69-92, 1976.

Chapter

86

Cleft Lip and Palate: Primary Cleft Palate Repair

Paul S. Tiwana, Matthew J. Madsen

Facial clefting is one of the most common congenital defects identified in human development. Isolated cleft palate occurs in about 1 in 1000 births.[1] It presents a myriad of challenges to both the patient and those involved in his or her orofacial habilitation. The medical, surgical, and psychologic impact requires a team approach to achieve the best overall result. The surgical management of cleft palate is not simply correcting an anatomic aberration; rather, it requires an understanding of the delicate balance between growth, speech development, and surgical timing, in addition to good surgical technique. This must also take into account the child's health and medical management. Interval follow-ups by the interdisciplinary cleft team are necessary to meet the goals of correcting the initial deformity, as well as staging the reconstruction at later phases of growth to optimize care.

Challenges to the child born with a cleft palate are numerous. Newborns with cleft palate potentially have difficulty feeding, because of their inability to obtain an oral seal. This can result in failure to thrive, which, if unchecked, can have severe consequences for the long term. In addition, speech remains a paramount issue. A number of children will develop velopharyngeal insufficiency, despite a serious surgical effort directed at meticulous palatal repair within an appropriate time frame to help mitigate the deleterious effects of the cleft on speech. When the primary palate (anterior to the incisive foramen) is affected, bone graft construction of the maxilla and orthodontic assistance become necessary. Lastly, the impact of these cumulative staged interventions can have a negative effect on maxillary growth, necessitating further surgical care.

ETIOPATHOGENESIS/CAUSATIVE FACTORS

Normal palatogenesis starts during the 5th week of gestation when the nasal placodes invaginate to form nasal pits. Ridges of tissue form on the lateral portion of the nasal pits, which become tissue processes that begin to migrate. During a period of 2 weeks (approximately 5 to 7 weeks gestation), these tissues migrate to form the structures anterior to the incisive foramen. This includes the prolabium (the middle portion of the upper lip), the premaxilla, as well as portions of the nose. The primary palate is formed by the end of the 6th week of gestation. The secondary palate then begins to form at approximately 6 weeks. This is when the medial nasal process, the lateral nasal process, and the maxillary process migrate and fuse. The fusion of the palatine shelves occurs at the 7th week, with the shelves first meeting just behind the incisive foramen. Fusion continues in an anterior-posterior direction, ending at the uvula. Fusion also occurs in a superior direction, with the hard palate fusing to the vomer of the nasal septum at approximately the 9th week. This complete process continues until about the 12th week of gestation.[2]

Palatal clefting may occur when the processes that form the palatal shelves are disrupted either in their migration or fusion medially. Clefting of the secondary palate results from failure of the maxillary process to fuse with the secondary palatal shelves. Although the exact mechanism is unknown, there appears to be a complex interaction between molecular pathway defects, genetic causes, and environmental exposure to drugs and teratogens occurring together as in utero insults.[3-6] The complexity of these interactions leads to a variety of clefts on physical examination.

A multitude of molecular studies and signaling pathways in animal models help us to understand the etiopathogenesis of facial clefting. A comprehensive review of these pathways will not be addressed in this chapter; however, some pathways merit discussion. Fibroblast growth factor-R1 (FGF-R1) and fibroblast growth factor-R2 (FGF-R2) are expressed specifically in the epithelium of the developing palatal shelves from the time of the outgrowth from the maxillary process through completion of fusion.[7] In murine models, it has been demonstrated that by truncating FGF receptor subtypes, there is a change in epithelial–mesenchymal interactions, and the receptor signaling pathways alone are sufficient for cleft formation.[8]

Other signaling molecules include the transforming growth factors, which have biologic cellular activities that control adhesion, proliferation, differentiation, and epithelial–mesenchymal transformation.[9] Mutated transforming growth factor (TGF-β3) in mice has shown a consistent cleft palate phenotype.[10,11]

Aside from molecules that signal epithelial migration, there are also signals that induce apoptosis, an element of palatogenesis that has also been extensively studied. In palate formation, apoptosis is thought to facilitate adherence, or touching, of the opposing epithelium to form a midpalatal seam.[12-14] Studies have shown that intershelf distance increases in an inverse relationship between the number of epithelial cells undergoing apoptosis as the palatal edges migrate and the number of cells transforming into mesenchymal cells during palate fusion.[15] Currently, it is unknown whether the balance between cell death and cell transformation is caused by the inadequate migration of the palatal shelves or if, in fact, it is the cause of the delay. Nonetheless, both apoptosis and epithelial–mesenchymal transformation appear to be necessary for normal palate formation, because clefting occurs in the absence of either one.

Another proposed theory is that deforming forces guide morphogenesis. There are various tissues in the embryo growing at different rates, which may induce stress and strain forces. These mechanical forces may in turn translate into the molecular cues for cell differentiation, migration, death, and transformation. This rationale is used to explain the cause of Pierre Robin sequence, where there is a decrease in the amniotic fluid index causing more external pressure on the fetal chin; this in turn prevents the tongue from relaxing to the floor of the mouth. The presence of the tongue between the palatal shelves prevents fusion.

There are an estimated 300 syndromes that include some form of cleft palate in their presentation; thus, genetic consultation should always be obtained.[16] Some of the more common syndromes that are associated with clefts are velocardiofacial syndrome, Stickler syndrome, Van der Woude syndrome, and Pierre Robin sequence. Nonsyndromic causes include drugs, such as dilantin and corticosteroids, retinoids in high doses (vitamin A), hypoxia, and alcohol.[17] The nonsyndromic causes are far more common, but isolated cleft palate is more frequently associated with syndromic involvement.

PATHOLOGIC ANATOMY

A developmentally intact palate serves two purposes. First, the hard palate serves as a structural component of the face, dividing the oropharynx from the nasopharynx. Second, the soft palate has a functional component where the musculature, including the tensor veli palatini, levator veli palatini, superior pharyngeal constrictor, muscularis uvulae, palatopharyngeus, and palatoglossus, forms a dynamic valve called the velopharyngeal sphincter, which is raised during speech and swallowing to divide the nose from the mouth. The levator veli palatini fuses to form a "sling" that is primarily responsible for elevation of the palate.[18] The palatoglossus and palatopharyngeus originate from the midline of the palate and insert into the tongue and pharyngeal walls, respectively.

Clefting alters the normal hard and soft tissue anatomy. This changes the normal physiologic relationship between the upper and lower lip, the tongue with the palate, and the soft palate with the pharyngeal walls. The end result is that there is alteration in speech valves, airway patency, feeding, and, iatrogenically, growth. The velar mechanism that is formed by the aponeurosis, or meeting of the tensor veli and levator veli palatini, is disrupted. This results in inadequate closure of the velopharyngeal orifice during speech and swallowing.[19] Also, both muscles originate from the eustachian tube. The tensor veli palatini muscle acts as the primary dilator of the eustachian tube and may aerate the middle ear to prevent recurrent otitis media and hearing loss.[20] Palatal clefting disrupts muscle insertion and function, resulting in inadequate valve closure. Velopharyngeal insufficiency (VPI) becomes obvious in patients with unrepaired clefts. Even after repair, it must continue to be monitored, because patients with repaired clefts often merit secondary procedures to correct the valve incompetence as speech develops.

Classification schemes for cleft palate are usually anatomically based. This may include complete or incomplete, unilateral or bilateral, as well as the submucous cleft and bifid uvula. The incomplete cleft may involve the soft palate, the hard palate, or both up to the incisive foramen. The terms unilateral or bilateral are used to describe clefting of the secondary palate. A unilateral cleft occurs when one of the palatal shelves has fused with the vomer while the other shelf has failed to migrate and fuse completely. A submucous cleft implies that there is occult clefting of the musculature beneath the oral mucosa. This is the result of separation of the soft palate musculature that has been previously described. It is the most common type of posterior palatal cleft.[21] The natural history of this cleft type often involves its discovery when the child develops velopharyngeal incompetence, manifested as hypernasal speech.[22] It is important to note that not all submucous cleft palates require repair.

DIAGNOSTIC STUDIES

When a child is born with a cleft, there are a number of physical findings that require evaluation. Although the diagnosis of cleft lip and palate is primarily one that is solely based on a thorough, routine examination at birth, there are a number of other studies that can be done to supplement the diagnosis as well as determine the timing for repair. The first studies may occur before birth when cleft lip diagnosis by ultrasound examination is commonplace; however, diagnosis of cleft palate using ultrasonography is not as reliable. The author prefers that mothers with a fetus diagnosed with orofacial cleft by ultrasonography see the cleft surgeon prior to delivery.

Diagnosis of VPD can be aided by video fluoroscopy, which demonstrates ineffective pharyngeal wall function as well as oronasal patency. Nasoendoscopic guided–speech assessment also evaluates lateral motion of the pharyngeal walls, soft palate function, and the adenoid pad, and it is preferred.

TREATMENT/RECONSTRUCTIVE GOALS

The primary goal of cleft palate repair is to restore the function of the palate, one of the most important functions being the development of normal speech. In addition to an intact palate without fistula

- Restoration of palatal form, an intact hard and soft palate with no fistulae
- Provision of mechanism for normal speech development
- Improved feeding and/or nutritional status
- Improved oral and/or nasal function
- Elimination of need for prosthetic appliances
- Separate oral and nasal cavities
- Improved eustachian tube and middle ear function
- Provide for improved dental management
- Optimization of the psychologic impact on patient and family
- Limited period of disability
- Improved social and psychologic development
- Limited adverse maxillofacial growth and development
- Minimal scar formation
- Appropriate understanding by patient (family) of treatment options and acceptance of treatment plan
- Appropriate understanding and acceptance by patient (family) of favorable outcomes and known risks and complications
- Absence of infection

*Adapted from American Association of Oral and Maxillofacial Surgeons: Parameters of care: clinical practice guidelines for oral and maxillofacial surgery (AAOMS ParCare 07 Ver 4.0), *J Oral Maxillofac Surg* 32(Suppl):238-245, 2007.

formation, speech quality remains a significant measure by which the surgeon can determine surgical outcome.

Despite a number of techniques to reconstruct cleft palate structural and functional deficiencies, there remains some controversy regarding the timing and surgical approach. Outcomes are limited to reports from operator experience and small sample sizes, with a lack of definitive data from prospective studies, although large-sample prospective studies, such as the Eurocleft study, are ongoing and promising. Current thinking is that the repair of the cleft palate should correspond with the development of speech needs, with maxillary growth as a consideration. Multiple procedures with attendant scarring can restrict maxillary growth, resulting in the need for further corrective surgery later in life. So, the question of timing still remains and essentially is divided into three philosophies.

Early timing, when surgical repair occurs before 6 months, has essentially been abandoned, due to surgical risks and comorbidities. Traditional timing with single-stage closure of the oronasal communication and establishing a competent velopharyngeal sphincter at 6 to 12 months of age reduces compensatory speech patterns and the potential risk for maxillary growth alteration. This time frame is largely accepted as the best time to balance surgical morbidity with speech development. Repair after 18 months of age increases the risk of speech disturbance. This approach has largely been abandoned with the exception of a few centers that may stage the soft and hard palate repair or when other overall medical concerns delay closure of the palate. The reconstructive goals are the same and are summarized in Box 86-1.

SPECIFIC TREATMENT AND TECHNIQUES

Descriptions of attempts of palatal repair can be encountered prior to the mid-1800s, most of which entailed attempts to reposition the cleft using bandages or simple surgical techniques. By the early 20th century, the goal in cleft palate repair was no longer simple closure of the hard and soft palate but included lengthening the palate to improve speech in the cleft patient. There are three main techniques, with variations: the von Langenbeck, Furlow Z-plasty, and Bardach two-flap technique. There is debate regarding the optimal technique, with each method having its theoretical advantages and limitations.

VON LANGENBECK

One of the first palatoplasty procedures was described by Bernhard von Langenbeck in the mid-1800s (Fig. 86-1).[23] The von Langenbeck palatoplasty involves relaxing incisions along the lateral edge of the hard palate, starting anteriorly near the palatomaxillary suture line, running posteriorly just medial to the alveolar ridge, and ending lateral to the hamulus, about 1 cm posterior to the greater tuberosity of the alveolus. The mucosa along the edges of the cleft is also incised. The entire mucoperiosteum is then raised from the oral surface of the hard palate; care is taken to preserve the two neurovascular pedicles—the greater palatine pedicle posteriorly and the incisive pedicle anteriorly. Bipedicled mucoperiosteal flaps are created on both sides of the cleft. The nasal side of the cleft is closed first, using redundant mucoperiosteum from the incision along the cleft edge. Then the bipedicled flaps are approximated to cover the oral surface of the cleft.[24]

The Furlow technique (Fig. 86-2) essentially consists of repairing palatal clefts using Z-plasties of the oral and nasal mucosa.[25] The theoretical advantage is that the soft palate may be lengthened while preventing longitudinal scar contracture and palatal shortening. The posteriorly based myomucosal flaps reapproximate the palatal musculature, reconstructing the levator sling.

The essential components of the Furlow Z-plasty include oral- and nasal-based mucosal and muscle flaps that are designed as Z-plasty flaps on one side and then reversed in configuration on the underlying side. The incisions are planned with the limbs of the Z forming a 60-degree angle. Care must be taken when dissecting the oral mucosa from the nasal mucosa, as well as when identifying the muscle layers. The oral flaps are retracted laterally to reveal the underlying nasal layer. Once the flaps have been adequately mobilized, closure may commence. This begins first by closing the nasal layer. Vomer flaps may be used for closure of the nasal side. Attention is then directed to tacking the nasal mucosa to the junction of hard palate. The second, opposite nasal flap of mucosa and muscle is transposed and sutured along the anterior flap. Oral flaps are then repositioned, keeping in mind that the anteromedial should be closed in a similar manner opposite the nasal flap.

BARDACH TWO-FLAP PALATOPLASTY

The Bardach two-flap palatoplasty technique (Figs. 86-3 and 86-4) was developed with the objective of having a one-stage procedure to close the entire palatal cleft.[26] The procedure as named is a two-flap technique where the oral and nasal mucosae are incised bilaterally from the uvula anteriorly to the leading edge of the cleft. A second incision is made on each palatal shelf near the level where the alveolar mucosa meets the palatal mucosa. These incisions course posteriorly from the leading edge of the cleft toward the hamular notch where releasing incisions are carried behind the maxillary tuberosity. A full-thickness mucoperiosteal flap is elevated on each side of the cleft, which preserves the palatal neurovascular bundle. The soft palate musculature is then released from the attachment to the palatal bones. At this point, systematic closure of the wound edges begins with closure of the nasal mucosa in a running or interrupted fashion starting from the incisive foramen and working toward the hard–soft palate junction. Closure of the nasal mucosa is completed by closing from the uvula and working forward to the hard–soft palate junction. The soft palate musculature is then sutured back to the midline. The oral mucosa is closed from the uvula forward to the incisive foramen, using care not to place the cleft edges in too much tension.

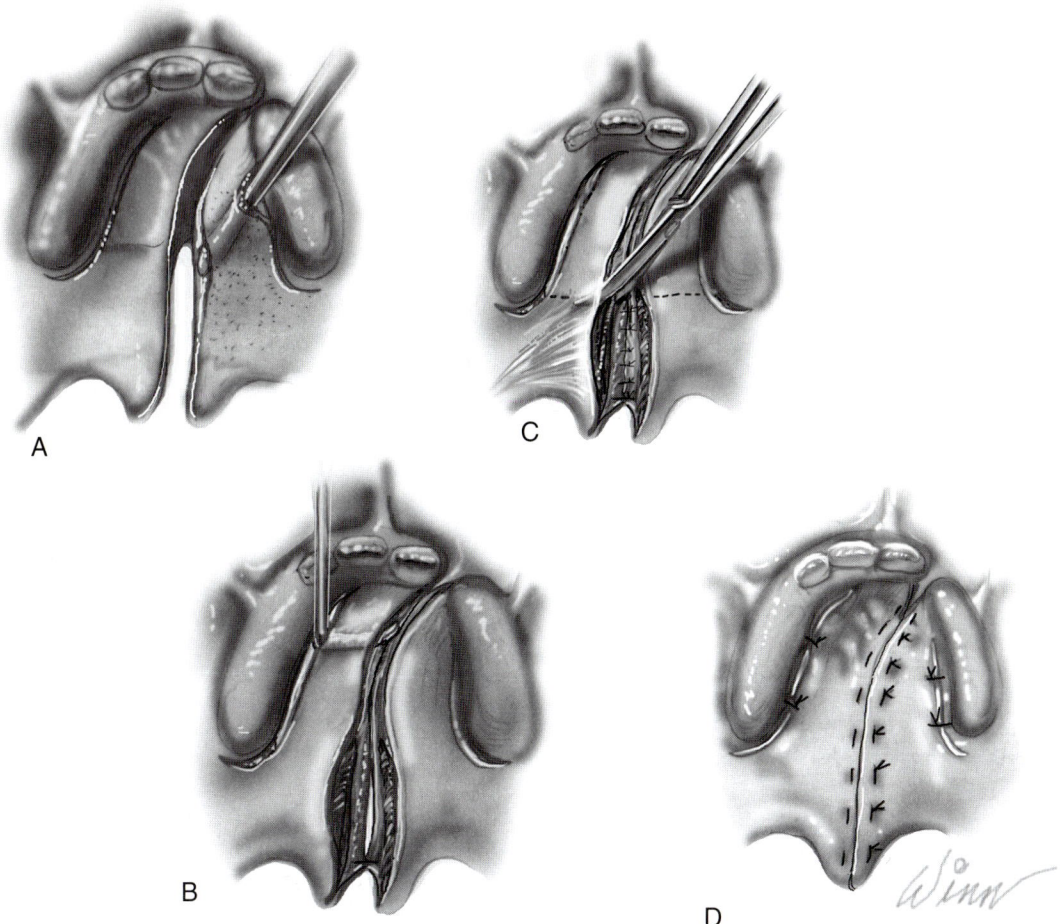

Fig. 86-1 ■ Von Langenback palatoplasty. (From Posnick JC: *Craniofacial and maxillofacial surgery in children and young adults. Cleft lip and palate: infancy through adolescence*, Philadelphia, 2000, Saunders.)

POSTOPERATIVE CARE

Postoperative care is important in contributing to the overall goals of developing an improved speech mechanism, improving oral and/or nasal function, and improving swallowing. Normal feeding can resume as soon as the infant is stable, with the exception that active sucking is to be avoided for at least 2 weeks. This is essential to allow soft tissue healing and can be assisted by the use of a cleft palate bottle/feeder with a one-way valve. Elbow immobilizers may be used, but some surgeons argue that they are not necessary. Generally, perioperative corticosteroids and antibiotics are given to help minimize the postoperative swelling and infection. Regular follow-up appointments should be scheduled, with the first being 1 week after surgery.

Special attention must be directed to the postoperative period. Immediate postoperative risks include breakdown of the repair due to tension, palatal ischemia, secondary pressure, secondary trauma, or bleeding. Any failure of healing may result in the formation of an oronasal fistula. If it does occur, it most commonly forms at the junction of the hard and soft palate (Fig. 86-5). The risks of fistula development relate to the type of palate repair, surgical experience, cleft width, cleft type, and even age at closure. A number of papers exist that attempt to provide an answer to the rates of fistula formation experienced in the postoperative period; however, it is difficult to determine with accuracy the actual rates, because of the variance of study design and techniques employed.[28] Other long-term complications include midface growth deficiency, velopharyngeal incompetence, recurrent fistula, and sleep apnea.

PEARLS AND PITFALLS

- It is important to understand the three-dimensional anatomy and complex interplay between growth and function (speech).
- Meticulous, gentle technique usually yields the best result, regardless of specific surgical approach.
- There must be a two-layer tension-free, watertight closure.
- Allogeneic dermal films placed across areas of tension—for example, between the hard and soft palate junction—before final closure may help prevent dehiscence and fistula formation.
- Early cleft palate repair (before 1 year of age) results in better speech.
- Operating too early (before 6 months) or waiting too long (after 18 months) should be avoided.
- Tearing the nasal mucosa during dissection.
- Revision surgery for velopharyngeal dysfunction is necessary twice as often in patients with isolated cleft palate than in those with clefts of the lip and palate.
- Inexperience.
- The initial width of the cleft is harder to close and results in a greater likelihood of fistula.
- Extensive undermining of the mucoperiosteum results in growth restriction of the maxilla.

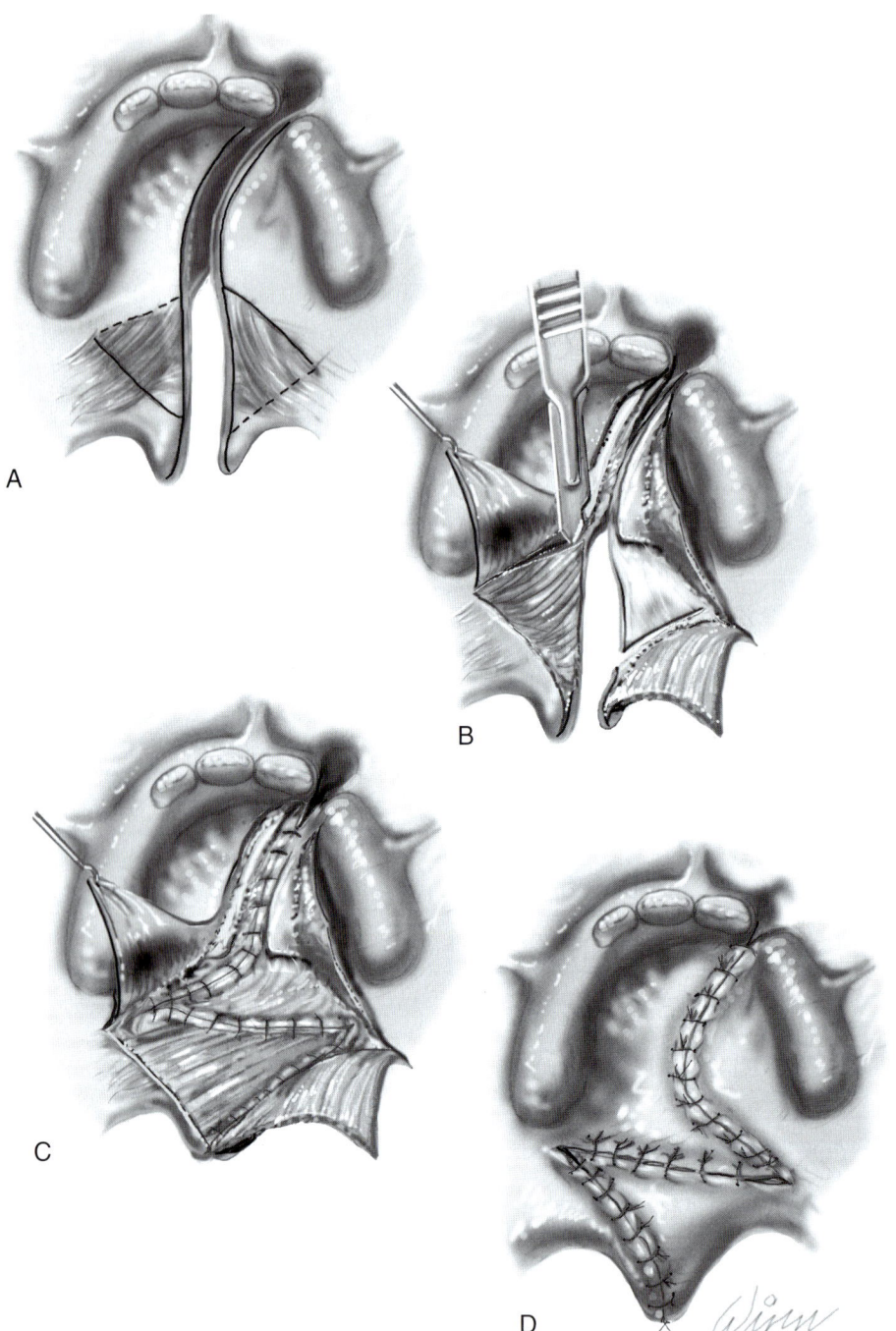

Fig. 86-2 ■ The Furlow Z-plasty. (From Posnick JC: *Craniofacial and maxillofacial surgery in children and young adults. Cleft lip and palate: infancy through adolescence*, Philadelphia, 2000, Saunders.)

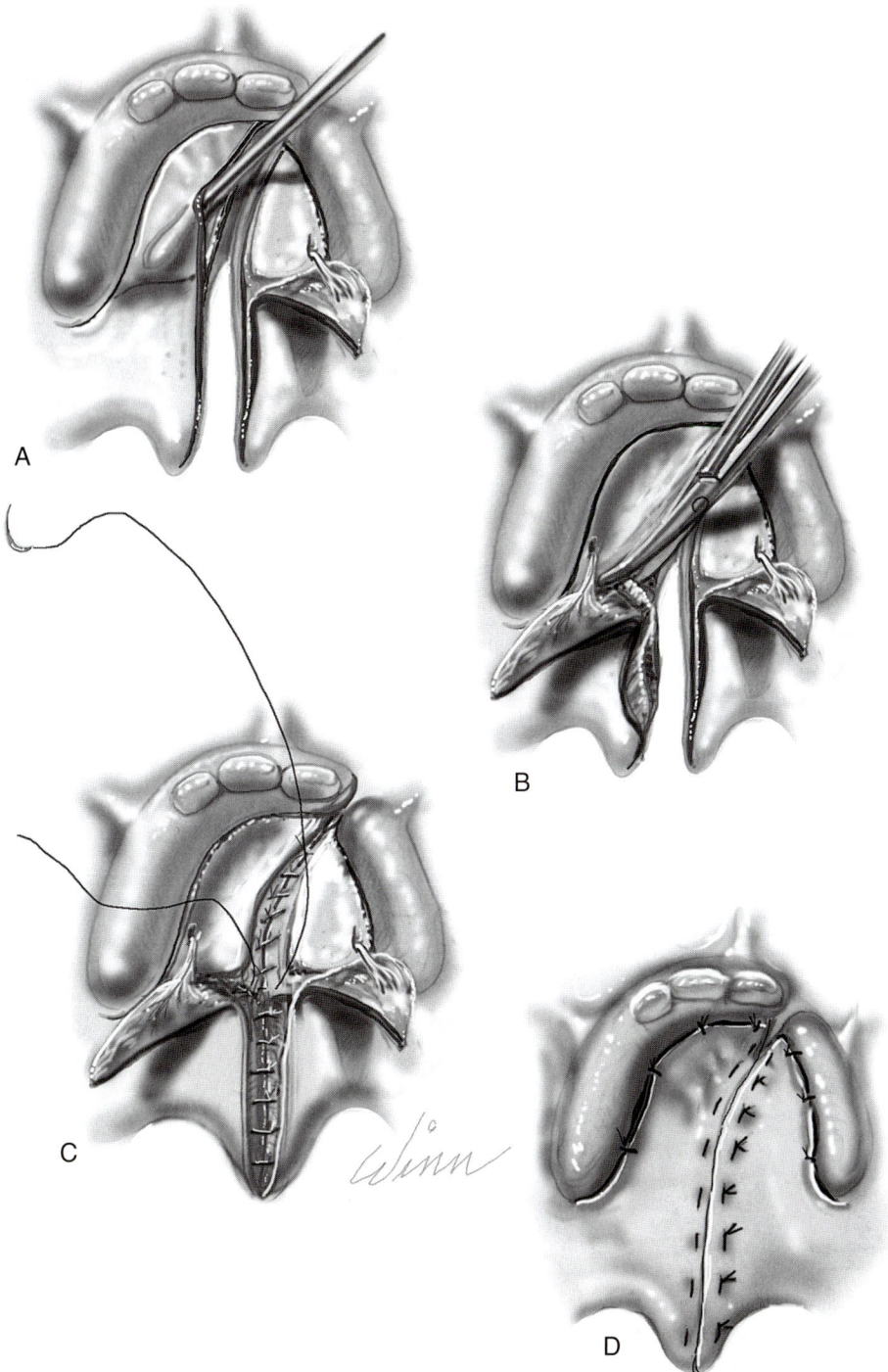

Fig. 86-3 ■ The Bardach two-flap palatoplasty. **A,** Intraoperative view of two-flap palate palatoplasty incisions marked out. **B,** Intraoperative view demonstrating dissection of two-flap palatoplasty. **C,** Intraoperative view of nasal mucosa repair with dissected overlying axial flaps. **D,** Intraoperative view of transposed mucosal flaps now repaired. (**A,** From Posnick JC: *Craniofacial and maxillofacial surgery in children and young adults. Cleft lip and palate: infancy through adolescence.* Philadelphia, 2000, Saunders.)

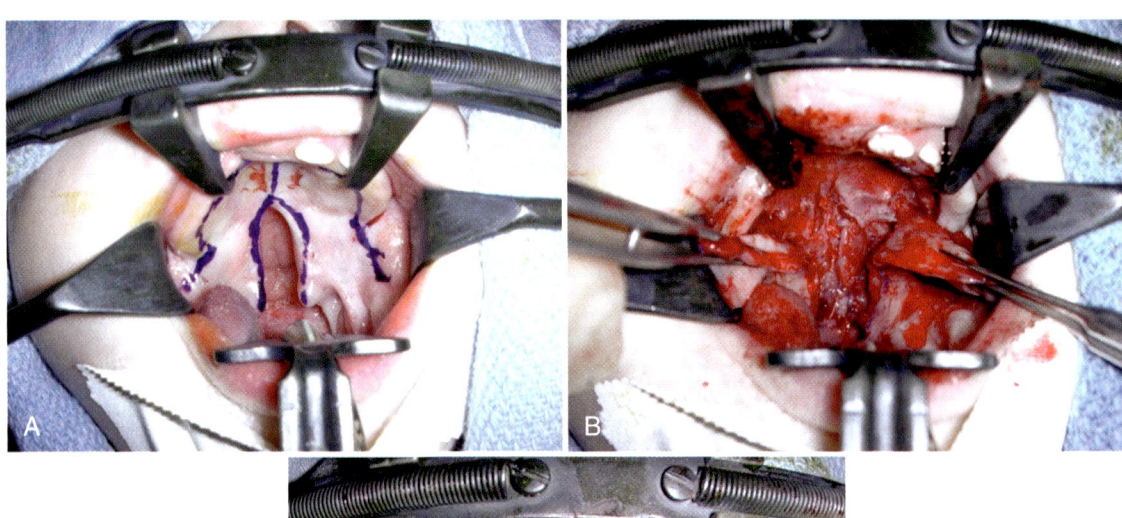

Fig. 86-4 ▪ Bardach two-flap palatoplasty. **A,** Preoperative outline. **B,** Intraoperative dissection. **C,** Closure.

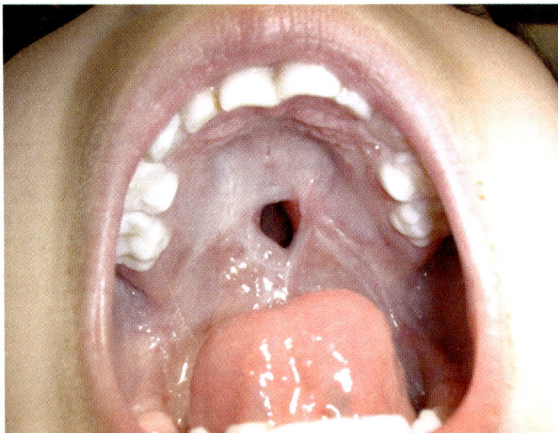

Fig. 86-5 ▪ Fistula development postoperatively. Note position at the hard and soft palate junction.

REFERENCES

1. Gorlin RJ, Cohen MM Jr, Hennekam RCM: *Syndromes of the head and neck*, ed 4. New York, 2001, Oxford University Press, pp 850-853.
2. Marks MW, Marks C: Cleft lip and palate. In Marks MW, Marks C (eds): *Fundamentals of plastic surgery*. Philadelphia, 1997, WB Saunders, pp 156-173.
3. Romitti PA, Lidral AC, Munger RG, et al: Candidate genes for nonsyndromic cleft lip and palate and maternal cigarette smoking and alcohol consumption: evaluation of genotype-environment interactions from a population-based case-control study of orofacial clefts. *Teratology* 59:39, 1999.
4. Maestri NE, Beaty TH, Hetmanski J, et al: Application of transmission disequilibrium tests to nonsyndromic oral clefts: including candidate genes and environmental exposures in the models. *Am J Med Genet* 73:337, 1997.
5. Lidral AC, Murray JC, Buetow KH, et al: Studies of the candidate genes TGFB2, MSX1, TGFA, and TGFB3 in the etiology of cleft lip and palate in the Philippines. *Cleft Palate Craniofac J* 34:1, 1997.
6. Hwang SJ, Beaty TH, Panny SR, et al: Association study of transforming growth factor alpha (TGF alpha) TaqI polymorphism and oral clefts: indication of gene-environment interaction in a population-based sample of

infants with birth defects. *Am J Epidemiol* 141:629, 1995.

7. Lee S, Crisera CA, Erfani S, et al: Immunolocalization of fibroblast growth factor receptors 1 and 2 in mouse palate development. *Plast Reconstr Surg* 107:1776, 2001.

8. Crisera C, Teng E, Wasson K, et al: Formation of in vitro murine cleft palate by abrogation of fibroblast growth factor signaling. *Plast Reconstr Surg* 121:1, 2007.

9. Roberts AB, Sporn MB: The transforming growth factor. In Sporn MB, Roberts AB (eds): *Peptide growth factors and their receptors: handbook of experimental pharmacology.* Heidelberg, 1990, Springer-Verlag, pp 419-472.

10. Koo S, Cunningham M, Arabshahi B, et al: The transforming growth factor-3 knock-out mouse: an animal model for cleft palate. *Plast Reconstr Surg* 108:938, 2001.

11. Proetzel G, Pawlowski SA, Wiles MV, et al: Transforming growth factor-3 is required for secondary palate fusion. *Nat Genet* 11:409, 1995.

12. Ferguson MW, Honig LS: Epithelial-mesenchymal interactions during vertebrate palatogenesis. In Zimmerman EF (ed): *Current topics in developmental biology, vol 19. Palate development: normal and abnormal, cellular and molecular aspects.* New York, 1984, Academic Press, pp 137-164.

13. Taniguchi K, Sato N, Uchiyama Y: Apoptosis and heterophagy of medial edge epithelial cells of the secondary palatine shelves during fusion. *Arch Histol Cytol* 58:191, 1995.

14. Martinez-Alvarez C, Tudela C, Perez-Miguelsanz J, et al: Medial edge epithelial cell fate during palatal fusion. *Dev Biol* 220:343, 2000.

15. Erfani S, Maldonado TS, Crisera CA, et al: An in vitro mouse model of cleft palate: defining a critical inter-shelf distance necessary for palatal clefting. *Plast Reconstr Surg* 108:403, 2001.

16. Strong EB, Buckmiller LM: Management of the cleft palate. *Fac Plast Surg Clin North Am* 9:15-25, 2001.

17. Witt PD, Marsh JL: Cleft palate deformities. In Bentz M (ed): *Pediatric plastic surgery.* New York, 1998, Appleton and Lange, pp 93-105.

18. Kuehn DP, Folkins JW, Cutting CB: Relationships between muscle activity and velar position. *Cleft Palate J* 19:25, 1982.

19. Kuehn DP, Folkins JW, Cutting CB: Relationships between muscle activity and velar position. *Cleft Palate J* 19:25, 1982.

20. Honjo I, Okazaki N, Kumazawa T: Experimental study of the eustachian tube function with regard to its related muscles. *Acta Otolaryngol (Stockh)* 87:84, 1979.

21. Gosain AK, Conley SF, Marks S, Larson DL: Submucous cleft palate: diagnostic methods and outcomes of surgical treatment. *Plast Reconstr Surg* 97:1497-1507, 1996.

22. Weatherley-White RCA, Sakura CY, Brenner LD, et al: Submucous cleft palate: its incidence, natural history and indications for treatment. *Plast Reconstr Surg* 49:297-304, 1972.

23. von Langenbeck, B: Die Uranoplastik mittelst Ablösung des mucös-periostalen Gaumenüberzuges. *Arch Klin Chir* 2:205, 1861.

24. Sadove M, van Aalst JA, Culp JA: Cleft palate repair: art and issues. *Clin Plastic Surg* 31:231-241, 2004.

25. Furlow LT Jr: Cleft palate repair: preliminary report on lengthening and muscle transportation by Z-Plasty. Presented at the Annual Meeting of the Southeastern Society of Plastic and Reconstructive Surgeons, May 16, 1978, Boca Raton, Fla.

26. Bardach J, Nosal P: *Geometry of the two-flap palatoplasty. Surgical techniques in cleft lip and palate.* St Louis, 1987, Mosby-Year Book, pp 192-197.

27. American Association of Oral and Maxillofacial Surgeons: Parameters of care: clinical practice guidelines for oral and maxillofacial surgery (AAOMS ParCare 07 Ver 4.0). *J Oral Maxillofac Surg* 32(Suppl):238-245, 2007.

28. Cohen SR, Kalinowski J, LaRossa D, Randall P: Cleft palate fistulas: a multivariate statistical analysis of prevalence, etiology, and surgical management. *Plast Reconstr Surg* 87:1041, 1991.

Cleft Lip and Palate: Bone Graft Reconstruction of the Cleft Maxilla

Chapter **87**

Gregory J. MacKay

Cleft lip and palate deformities are the second most frequently occurring congenital anomalies. In both the unilateral and bilateral complete cleft lip and palate deformity, there is a bony deficiency of the maxilla. The degree of hypoplasia of the maxilla is usually proportionate to the severity of the cleft lip deformity. In the incomplete cleft lip patient, there is usually minimal or no deformity of the maxilla. This is in contrast to the typical cleft lip and palate patient with maxillary alveolar bone involvement. In the unilateral complete cleft, there are varying degrees of hypoplasia of the maxilla on the cleft side, usually associated with a malpositioned maxillary segment and an absent or malformed lateral incisor (Fig. 87-1, *A*). In the bilateral cleft patient, the bony maxillary deformity is usually symmetrical and relative to the position of the premaxilla (Fig. 87-1, *B*). Clefts of the alveolar process of the maxilla inhibit the eruption and maintenance of the permanent dentition and can affect facial growth and symmetry. The key to treatment of cleft lip and palate patients with maxillary deformities is early diagnosis of the skeletal and dental involvement and combined surgical and orthodontic care.

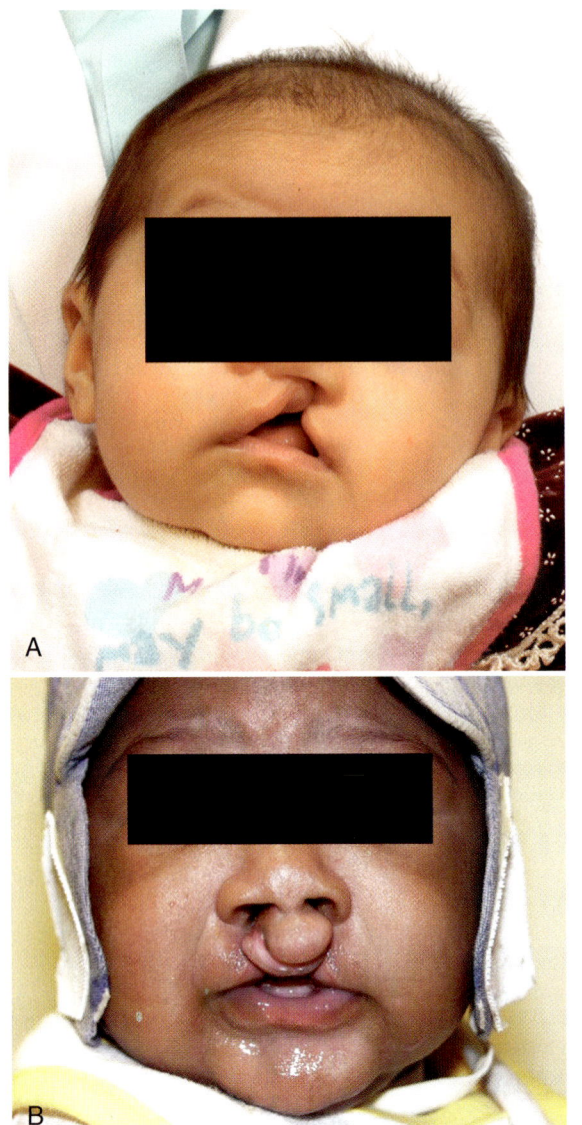

Fig. 87-1 ■ **A,** Unilateral cleft lip and palate deformity. **B,** Bilateral cleft lip and palate deformity.

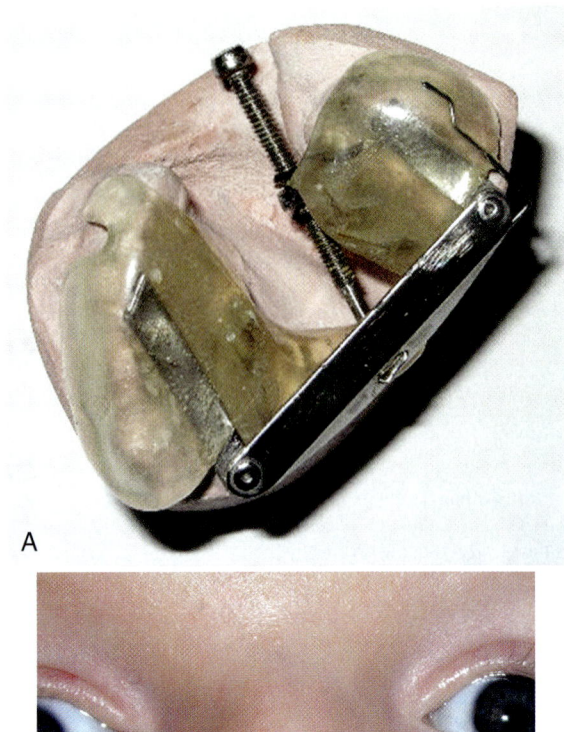

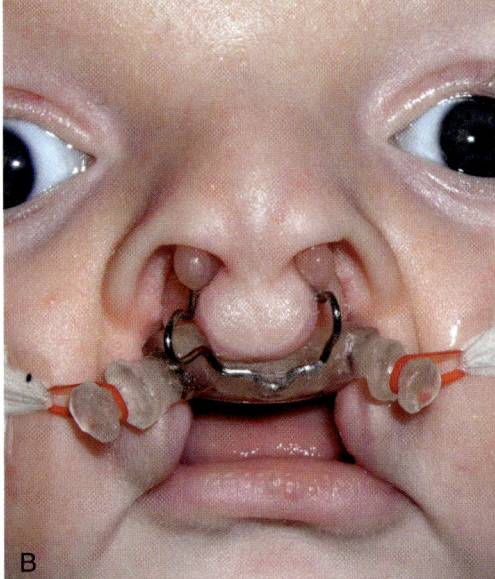

Fig. 87-2 ■ **A,** Latham pinned appliance. **B,** Passive nasal-alveolar molding appliance (Courtesy Michael Granger, DMD, Children's Hospital, Atlanta.)

ALVEOLAR CLEFTS

EARLY TREATMENT

Early management of the cleft patient with a maxillary deformity will often involve presurgical orthopedics to realign the maxillary segments. Alignment of the maxillary segments will allow easier repair of the cleft lip and nasal deformity. Either active traction devices, such as the Latham pinned appliance (Fig. 87-2, *A*), or passive molding appliances (Fig. 87-2, *B*) can be used.[1,2] Presurgical orthopedics is often initiated within the first few months of life to promote alignment of the maxillary segments prior to closure of the cleft lip. If the alveolar segments are brought to within 2 mm of each other, some cleft surgeons will advocate performing a gingivoperiosteoplasty as part of the primary lip and palate repair. This procedure can result in bony bridging across the alveolar cleft and obviate the need for delayed secondary alveolar bone grafting, but it is still

controversial whether this may also result in decreased maxillary growth.[3-5]

Early primary grafting of the alveolar cleft defect with rib grafts, performed at the time of initial lip repair, was initially thought to be beneficial in that it might correct the alveolar defect early and minimize the extent of the maxillary deformity. Unfortunately, this "early"-phase bone grafting has been associated with reports of moderate to severe long-term maxillary growth restriction.[6]

DELAYED TREATMENT (MIXED DENTITION PHASE)

Delayed secondary bone grafting in the mixed dentition phase (between 7 and 10 years of age) after initial cleft lip and palate closure is considered the more accepted time period for bone grafting of alveolar defects. Bone grafting should be completed prior to eruption of the permanent canine through the cleft site so that appropriate support for the erupting teeth around the cleft is present. In addition to providing support for the erupting teeth, the bone graft will also provide additional support for the alar base and pyriform aperture as well as minimize perialveolar fistula development. Delaying the bone grafting until the mixed dentition phase allows for increased maxillary growth in both the transverse and horizontal planes. Numerous studies have demonstrated the advantages of delayed secondary alveolar bone grafting both from an occlusal and periodontal standpoint.[7]

TREATMENT CONSIDERATIONS

ORTHODONTIC/DENTAL TREATMENT

In the mixed dentition phase the goal of orthodontic care is to align the maxillary arch in preparation for the bone graft. This usually involves expansion of the arch in a transverse diameter and results in opening up the alveolar cleft to some degree. A lingual expansion device, such as a quadhelix, is most often used (Fig. 87-3). Meticulous dental care addresses treatment of any periodontal disease and/or extraction of any aberrant teeth to prepare the cleft site for bone grafting. Significant periodontal disease at the time of bone grafting can result in postoperative infection, further resulting in loss of the graft.

SURGICAL TECHNIQUE FOR BONE GRAFTING

Several donor sites are available for obtaining bone for grafting into the alveolar cleft, including rib, cranial bone, mandibular symphysis, and iliac crest. The iliac crest is the most widely used for harvesting cancellous bone, which has been shown to have the greatest viability when grafted into alveolar cleft defects. The iliac crest also has adequate volume to harvest for either a unilateral or bilateral alveolar cleft. The cranium can also provide adequate bone for an alveolar cleft and can be readily harvested with the use of a Hudson brace.

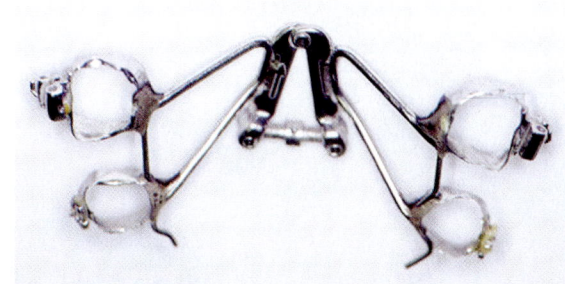

Fig. 87-3 ■ Quadhelix expansion device for palate. (Courtesy Michael Granger, DMD, Children's Hospital, Atlanta.)

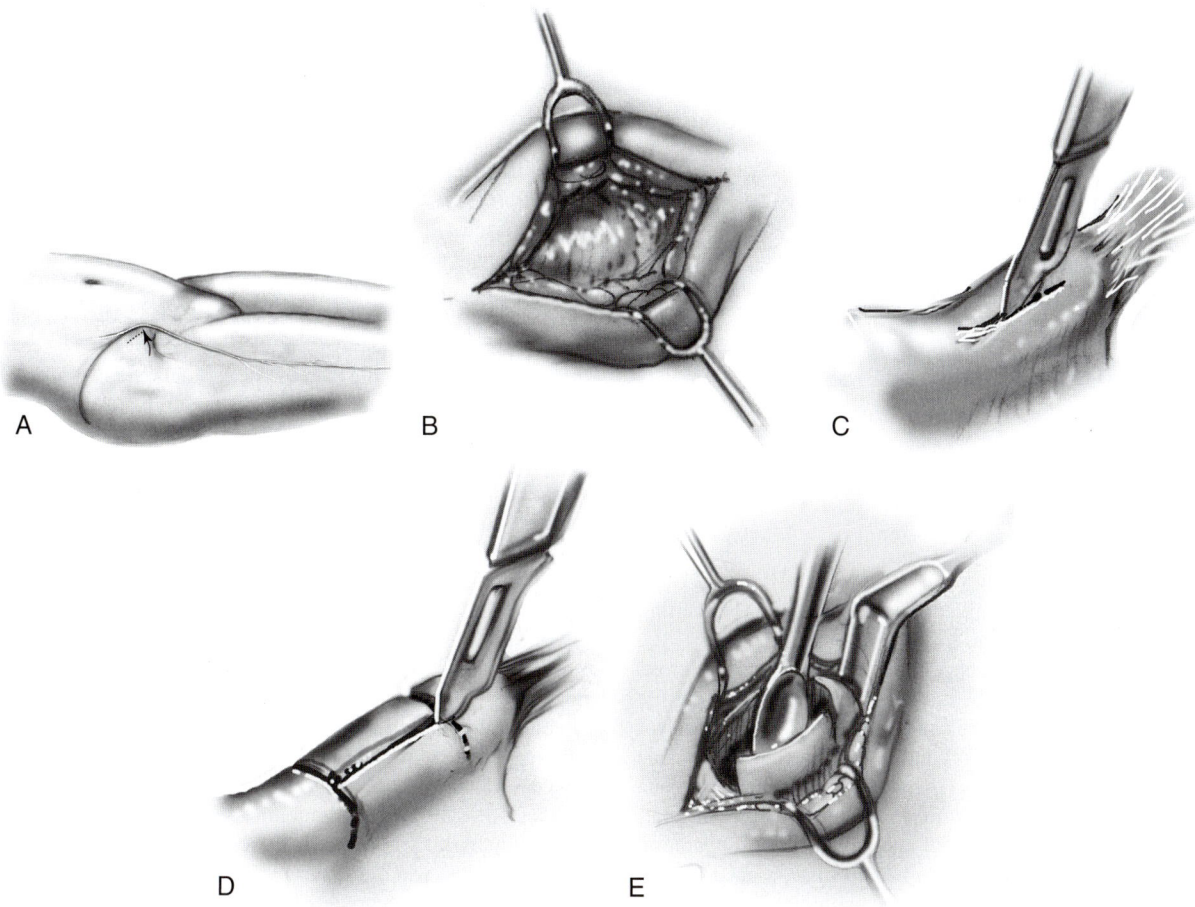

Fig. 87-4 ■ **A** to **G,** Bone harvested from iliac crest with open technique. (From Posnick JC: *Craniofacial and maxillofacial surgery in children and young adults*, Philadelphia, 2000, Saunders.)

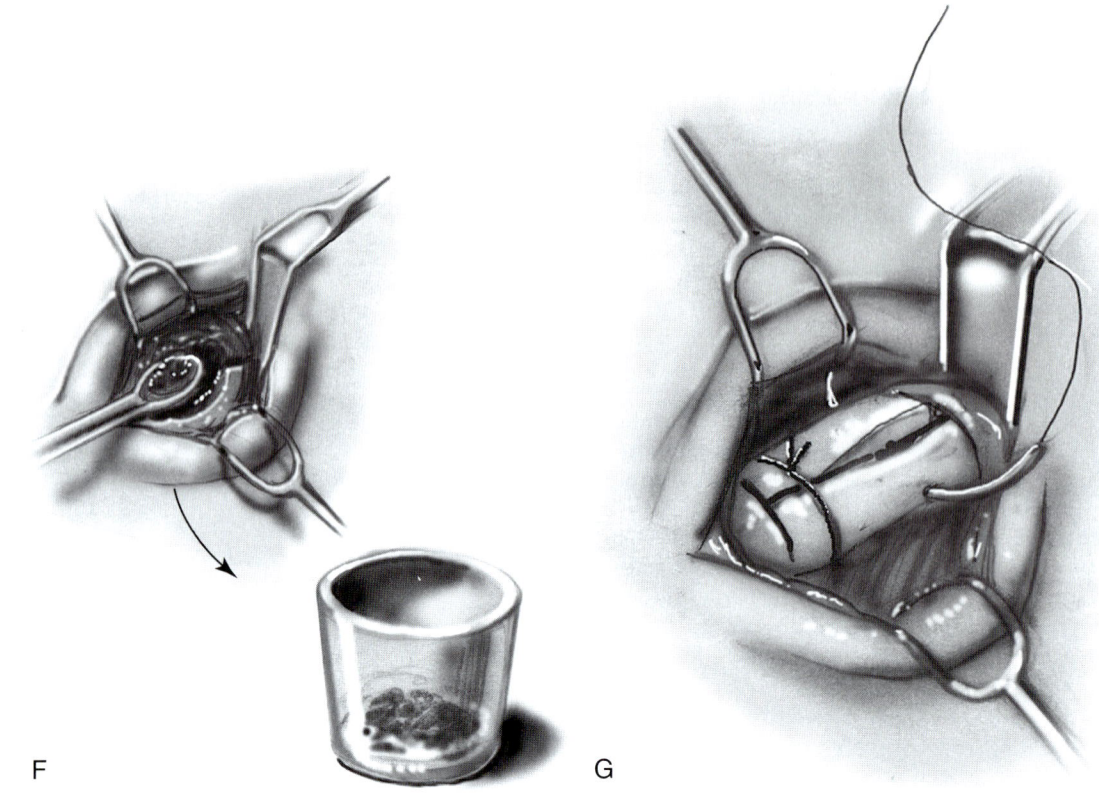

F   G

Fig. 87-4, cont'd.

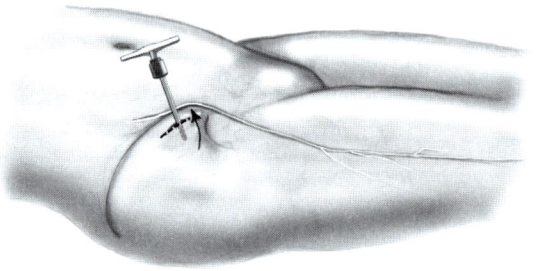

Fig. 87-5 ■ Bone harvested from iliac crest with "quick draw" bone harvester. (Adapted from Posnick JC: *Craniofacial and maxillofacial surgery in children and young adults*, Philadelphia, 2000, Saunders.)

The mandibular symphysis can provide adequate bone for grafting but usually only in small amounts.[8]

The authors' choice is to use cancellous bone from the iliac crest. Iliac crest cancellous bone can be harvested either by splitting the cartilaginous cap and removing the cancellous bone with curettes or by using a bone harvester (Figs. 87-4 and 87-5). Once adequate bone is harvested, the alveolar cleft site is prepared for grafting. Complete exposure of the alveolar cleft deformity, whether unilateral or bilateral, is obtained by elevation of labial and palatal flaps. Separation of the nasal and oral mucosa is necessary so that the nasal lining can be closed. Once the nasal lining has been completely closed, the cancellous bone can be packed into the entire cleft defect. The labial and palatal flaps can then be advanced and closed over the bone graft (Fig. 87-6). The elevation of the labial and palatal flaps is the most difficult part of the surgical procedure and requires meticulous dissection, because there is often previously scarred and somewhat friable tissue along the cleft.

POSTOPERATIVE CARE

Postoperative care of the patient after alveolar bone grafting involves a liquid diet for the first few days. The diet is advanced to a puree-diet that is maintained for 3 to 4 weeks. Oral hygiene is important, and routine oral rinse with Peridex three times per day for the first week, followed by gentle brushing with a soft tooth brush beginning the second week is recommended. Sports and strenuous activity are limited for 4 to 6 weeks to prevent potential injury to the hip donor site.

RESULTS AND COMPLICATIONS

Alveolar bone grafting in the mixed dentition phase allows the canine teeth to migrate and erupt through the cancellous bone. Success rates with bone grafting are generally reported at 90% to 95%.[9] Postsurgical orthodontic care usually involves maxillary arch support and guidance of the erupting canine into position. Complications, when they arise, are most often the result of inadequate soft tissue coverage of the bone graft leading to exposure. These complications are usually minor and can be managed by continued soft diet, oral hygiene, and antibiotics.

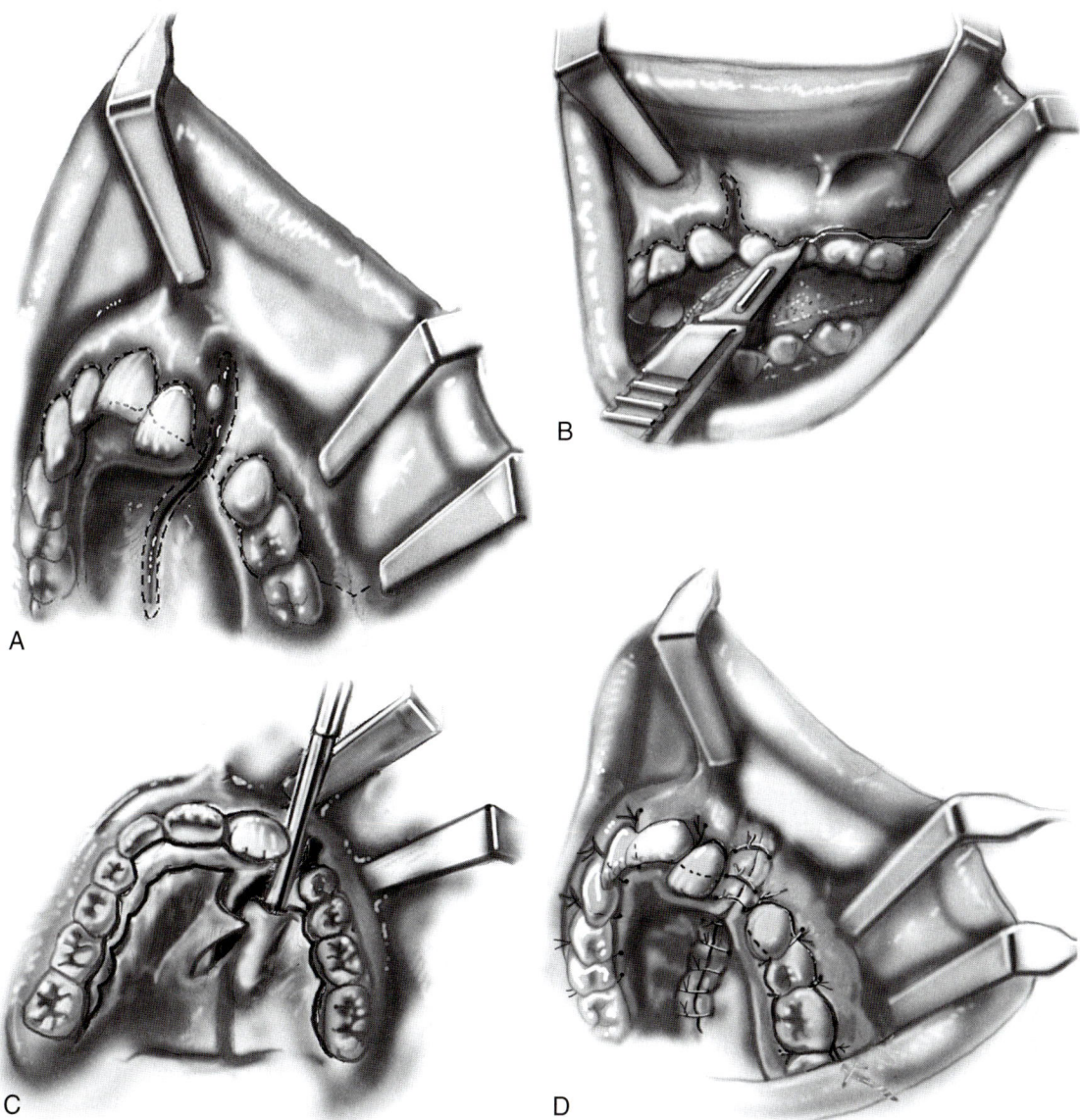

Fig. 87-6 ■ **A,** Alveolar cleft deformity. **B** to **D,** Surgical exposure for alveolar cleft repair. (From Posnick JC: *Craniofacial and maxillofacial surgery in children and young adults,* Philadelphia, 2000, Saunders.)

PEARLS AND PITFALLS

- From the cleft surgeon's standpoint, it is important to work closely with an orthodontist familiar with the needs of cleft patients.
- A clearly defined treatment plan prior to and following bone grafting is essential.
- Following placement of the bone graft, stabilizing the maxillary arch with an orthodontic appliance is often helpful and should be placed after the incisions have healed.
- There is often a moderate amount of scar tissue in and around the cleft deformity, and blood flow to the gingival flaps may be somewhat compromised.

- If the alveolar cleft deformity is quite large, a secondary bone grafting procedure may be necessary later, and this should be discussed in the treatment plan.
- In bilateral cleft deformities, it may be necessary to obtain cancellous bone from both hips. .
- Appropriate postoperative dental x-rays at 6 to 12 months will give the best information for evaluating the "take" of the bone graft.

REFERENCES

1. Millard DR Jr, Latham RA: Improved primary surgical and dental treatment of clefts. *Plast Reconstr Surg* 86:856-871, 1990.
2. Sato Y, Grayson BH, Garfinkel JS, et al: Success rate of gingivoperiosteoplasty with and without secondary bone grafts compared with secondary alveolar bone grafts alone. *Plast Reconstr Surg* 121:1356-1367, 2008.
3. Santiago PE, Grayson BH, Cutting CB, et al: Reduced need for alveolar bone grafting by presurgical orthopedics and primary gingivo-periosteoplasty. *Cleft Palate Craniofac J* 35:77-80, 1997.
4. Power S, Matic DB: Gingivoperiosteoplasty following alveolar molding with a Latham appliance versus secondary bone grafting: the effects on bone production and midfacial growth in patients with bilateral clefts. *Plast Reconstr Surg* 124:573-581, 2009.
5. Matic DB, Power SM: Evaluating the success of gingivoperiosteoplasty versus secondary bone grafting in patients with unilateral clefts. *Plast Reconstr Surg* 121:1343-1353, 2008; discussion 1368-1369.
6. Ross RB: Treatment variables affecting facial growth in complete unilateral cleft lip and palate: an overview of treatment and facial growth. *Cleft Palate J* 24:5-77, 1987.
7. Bergland O, Semb G, Abyholm FE: Elimination of the residual alveolar cleft by secondary bone grafting and subsequent orthodontic treatment. *Cleft Palate J* 23:175-205, 1986.
8. LaRossa D, Buchmann S, Rothkopf DM, et al: A comparison of iliac and cranial bone in secondary grafting of alveolar clefts. *Plast Reconstr Surg* 96:789-797, 1995.
9. Kortebein MJ, Nelson CL, Sadove AM: Retrospective analysis of 135 secondary alveolar cleft grafts using iliac or calvarial gone. *J Oral Maxillofac Surg* 49:493-498, 1991.

Chapter

88

Cleft Lip and Palate: Orthognathic Surgery

David S. Precious

Improvement in the results of correction of maxillofacial deformities by orthodontic treatment and orthognathic surgery has been dramatic over the past 30 years. The vast majority of treated patients show improved occlusion and esthetics, but it must be stressed that unless symmetry and balance characterize relevant muscles, the predictability of long-term changes in bone and soft tissue is variable, irrespective of the method used to move bones.

In cleft lip/palate (CLP) patients, aberrations in craniofacial morphology and growth have often been attributed to the technique and timing of primary lip and palate surgery. This attribution overlooks the influence of inherent growth tendencies, such as those resulting from variation in cranial base morphology, irrespective of the technique and timing of cleft surgery (Fig. 88-1). Thus, when evaluating the results of surgical treatment in CLP patients, cranial base morphology should be included as one influential factor in dental/skeletal relationships.

Orthognathic surgery is often thought of only in terms of osteotomies. This perception probably arises because orthognathic surgery is unsurpassed in its applicability for correcting certain dentofacial deformities, such as vertical maxillary excess. Orthognathic surgery, though, is much broader than just osteotomies; it is a constellation of procedures that permits differential alteration and repositioning of bone, cartilage, muscle, teeth, gingiva, mucosa, and skin. Development of the midface is both hierarchical and integrated. The development of muscles precedes that of bones. The bones of the midface develop under the influence and at the direction of the enveloping muscles. In other words, muscles are shaping bones.

A good example of muscles controlling bones is what happens in utero with cleft lip and palate. The distortion of the bones is already present when the baby is born. This is muscle distortion of bone, and in the case of cleft lip and palate, all of the cheek muscles and lip-nose muscles, acting through the breach, combine to distort the face. Early orthognathic surgery is muscle surgery. In this case, early orthognathic surgery seeks to achieve differential alteration in repositioning of cartilage, muscle, mucosa, gingiva, and skin. Once this has been accomplished, the bones will follow.

Accordingly, the cleft surgeon obviously must master the surgical techniques that best meet the needs of the patient at given ages. Moreover, he or she must also be a physiologist, particularly in knowing and using, to the benefit of patients, all of the details of the development of the facial skeleton, the quality of which, at the end of growth, essentially determines the quality of the surgical result and the ultimate need for and execution of orthognathic surgery in patients with cleft lip and palate.

ETIOPATHOGENESIS, CAUSATIVE FACTORS, AND PATHOLOGIC ANATOMY

The major subdivisions of the human skull are the desmocranium (skull proper), chondrocranium (cartilaginous base of the skull and the sense capsules), and viscerocranium (maxillofacial and mandibular skeleton). The major functional skeletal units of the maxilla consist of dermal (membrane) bones that develop directly

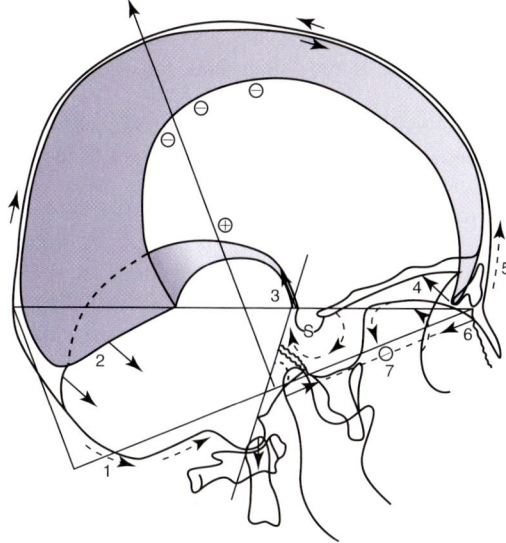

Fig. 88-1 ■ Cranial base patterns can predispose an individual to certain growth patterns, for example, as the sphenoidal angle *(S)* opens the glenoid fossa it is relatively more posteriorly positioned in the cranium, which tends to predispose to Class II morphology. Similar predisposition occurs as the anterior cranial angle closes. The inverse of these two changes tends to predispose the individual to Class III morphology.

(intramembranously) in embryonic mesenchyme without the involvement of a cartilaginous model or precursor.

The osteoblasts and osteocytes that form the maxillofacial skeleton do not arise in situ but, rather, arise from cells that are initially associated with the developing neural tube. These cells, the neural crest cells, must therefore migrate to their final site in the developing embryo.

During the formation of the primary neural axis, a special population of cells, the neural crest cells, can be found in the folds of the developing neural tube. As the neural folds close over, these cells break free of the neuroepithelium, undergo a morphologic transformation from an epithelial organization (as part of the continuous sheet of cells of the neural tube) to a mesenchymal (loose meshwork) organization, and begin to migrate from the neural tube toward the future facial primordia.

The skeletogenic capability of the neural crest has been determined both by following labeled cells in vivo as they differentiate into chondroblasts, osteoblasts, and odontoblasts (dentine is also a neural crest derivative) and by culturing or grafting neural crest–derived mesenchyme along with an appropriate inducer of chondrogenesis or osteogenesis. How future skeletogenic neural crest cells localize appropriately along the developing neural tube remains largely unknown.

Although the human maxillofacial skeleton lies completely within the territory of neural crest–derived structures, much of the skull roof does not; it arises from mesodermally derived mesenchyme that forms in situ.

Neither neural crest– nor mesodermally derived mesenchyme self-differentiates into osteoblasts, chondroblasts, or odontoblasts; rather, they have to be induced to differentiate. These particular inductions are known as epithelial–mesenchymal interactions, because the inducing tissue is an epithelium and the responding tissue is mesenchyme. Most skeletogenic inductions are matrix-mediated and are therefore time dependent.

Once differentiation has been initiated by one or more epithelial–mesenchymal interactions, other factors regulate subsequent

development and growth of the maxillofacial complex. Individual elements or regions do not develop and grow at the same rate. Such regional differences imply that development and growth are not regulated globally. Even factors such as hormones that circulate throughout the developing embryo can only act upon cells that possess the appropriate receptors.

Evidence for differences in local environments within the embryo comes from the concept of functional matrices. During late embryonic life, the development and growth of the cranium is influenced by the expanding and growing brain, that of the mandible and palate by the growing tongue, and the maxillofacial region by the expanding eye and growing nasal septum. Postnatally, these functional matrices are replaced by growing muscles, ligaments, and erupting teeth. The same elements of the head and face are therefore subject to regulation by different factors at different times during pre- and postnatal development.

Adjacent skeletal units, even though controlled by different functional matrices, influence one another because they are adjacent, begin their development at different times, develop and grow at different rates, and respond to different controls. Thus, the cranium grows fast and early to keep pace with the early and rapidly growing brain while the mandible and maxilla grow slowly and late, their rates being more in tune with general somatic growth than with brain growth. The influence of cranial growth on facial growth is because of timing, structure, and function. Because the cranium grows to keep pace with the rapid and early growth of the brain, it especially influences growth of the upper third of the face, which, accordingly, displays the fastest rate of facial growth and complete growth first (around 12 years of age). The remainder of the maxillofacial region is less affected by brain growth and, accordingly, grows more slowly and for a longer time, growth not being completed until the late teens or early twenties.

DIAGNOSIS, RECONSTRUCTIVE GOALS, AND TREATMENT

The use of cephalometrics has become a specialized part of the evaluation of patients with craniofacial deformities, permitting the clinician to systematically describe discrepancies in the maxilla, mandible, dentoalveolus, and soft tissue mask of the face. The relationships of points, lines, and angles measured on the conventional cephalometric radiograph are useful diagnostic aids to the extent that they are based on statistical means from which deviations have clinical significance. Conventional cephalometry does not stress pathophysiologic principles, nor do conventional cephalometric analyses include cranial analysis, because the conventional lateral cephalometric radiograph does not include an image of all of the cranial osseous structures.

Delaire has advocated the use of the architectural and structural craniofacial analysis that was conceived to account for all of the architectural and structural craniofacial information available on the lateral skull radiograph. This includes all of the head and its associated soft tissue: nose, lips, scalp, larynx, pharynx, and the neck, including the first three or four cervical vertebrae (Fig. 88-2). All of these structures can be assessed, to a greater or lesser degree, in a cephalic context by the use of the architectural and structural craniofacial analysis of Delaire. The analysis is composed of two distinct phases. The lines of craniofacial balance, which allow us to view objectively and quantify the variations of equilibrium between the patient being examined and the "normal" patient in his or her peer group, represents the "architectural analysis" (Fig. 88-3, *A*). Direct study of the cephalometric radiograph of the osseous

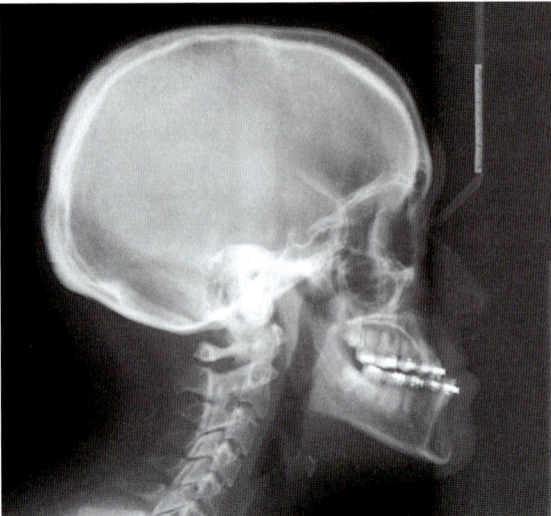

Fig. 88-2 ■ Lateral cephalometric image that includes all of the head and its associated soft tissue: nose, lips, scalp, larynx, pharynx, and the neck, including the first three or four cervical vertebra.

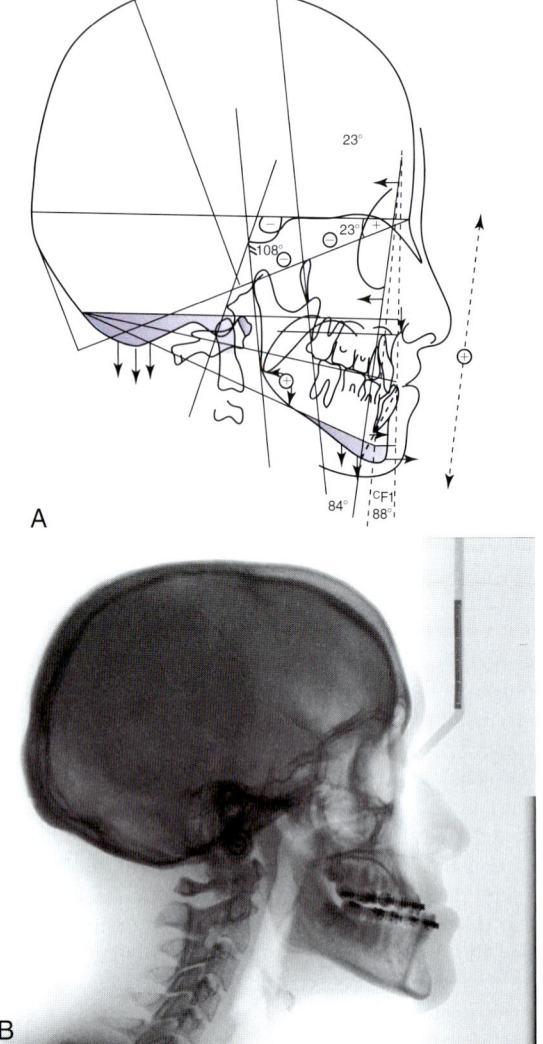

Fig. 88-3 ■ **A,** Architectural analysis of Delaire using lines of cranio-facial balance, which allow the surgeon to view objectively and quantify the variations of equilibrium between the patient being examined and the "normal" patient in his or her peer group. **B,** Structural analysis of Delaire reveals the osseous and soft tissue structures of the patient.

structures—their dimensions; degree of ossification, trabeculation, and cortication (external contour); and neighboring soft tissues (both superficial and deep)—represents the "structural analysis" (Fig. 88-3, *B*).

The analysis requires a lateral cephalometric radiograph of high quality, showing clearly the hard and soft tissues of the whole head and neck region. It should be taken with the patient staring into infinity, the mandible closed in centric relation, and the lips in repose (see Fig. 88-2).

There are six operations which constitute the basic skill set necessary to effectively manage patients with cleft lip and palate.
1. Primary functional cheilorhinoplasty and primary veloplasty
2. Palatoplasty
3. Alveolar bone graft
4. Maxillary osteotomy with secondary functional cheilorhinoplasty
5. Mandibular osteotomy
6. Functional genioplasty

PRIMARY FUNCTIONAL CHEILORHINOPLASTY AND PRIMARY VELOPLASTY

Surgical correction of cleft lip remains an elusive problem, principally because the fundamental surgical problem is not clearly conceptualized. This failure to accurately define the problem is attributable to the fact that the relevant anatomy is complex, poorly understood, and frequently erroneously described. Meaningful correction of cleft lip can be achieved only when the surgeon is fully appreciative of both normal and pathologic spatial relationships *and* functions of the anatomic elements, particularly the muscular elements that cause the deformity. The treatment goal, therefore, is to obtain anatomic functional balance between the soft tissues and the skeleton.

To reestablish a "normal" situation and dimension of the mucocutaneous elements in primary closure of labiomaxillary clefts, it is necessary to achieve good position of the skin of the floor and sill of the nostril, obtain good height of the skin of the cleft side, re-create good form and continuity of the white roll of the lip, establish equal vermilion height on both sides of the cleft and on both sides of the middle of the lip, and excise abnormal mucosa from both sides of the cleft.

To achieve good positioning of the skin of the floor and the sill of the nostril, it is absolutely imperative to respect the cutaneous areas and their individual characteristics relative to the skin of the lip. By definition, this rules out all those incisions that intrude on these areas, notably, those that enter the nostril, curving either inside or outside of the ala and extending to the columellar base. This also rules out all cutaneous excision in the upper part of the lip. The best incisions in the upper part of the lip, therefore, are those that pass exactly between the skin of the nose and that of the lip, and that stop laterally at the external border of the alar base and medially below the border of the columella (Fig. 88-4).

Accordingly, at the end of the primary lip operation, the surgeon must have achieved (1) a straight nasal septum positioned in the facial midline, (2) symmetrical reconstruction of the nasolabial muscles, (3) absence of vestibular oral nasal communication, and (4) a functional, patent nostril on the cleft side (Fig. 88-5).

PALATOPLASTY

Velopalatine clefts are associated with divided, separated, displaced, hypotrophic, and sometimes hypoplastic muscles of the soft palate. The tongue and floor of the mouth are abnormally low, and the pterygoid processes are displaced laterally. The palatoglossus

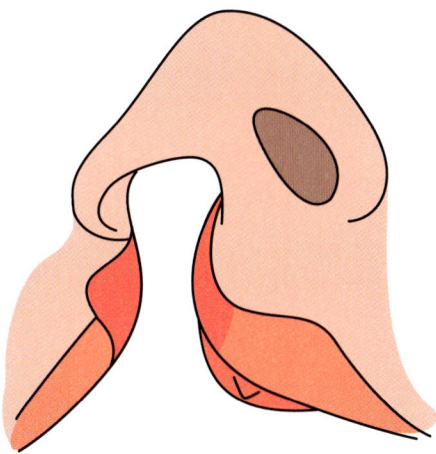

Fig. 88-4 ■ The best incisions in the upper part of the lip are those that pass exactly between the skin of the nose and that of the lip and stop laterally at the external border of the alar base and medially below the border of the columella.

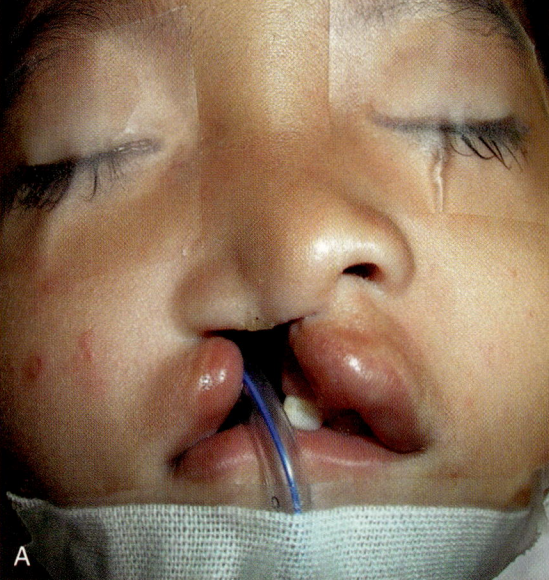

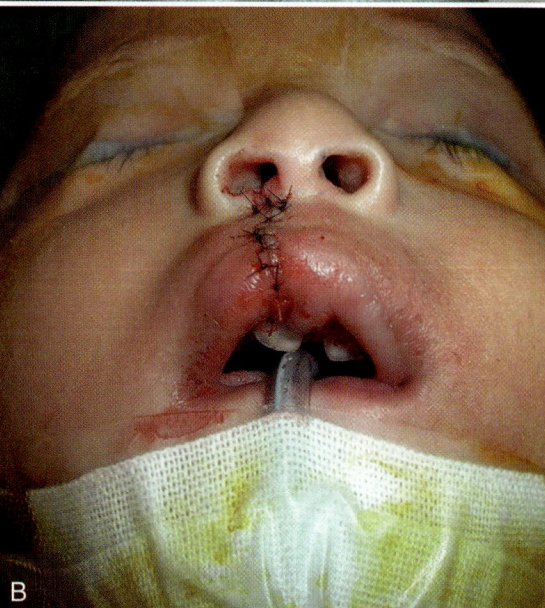

Fig. 88-5 ■ **A,** Immediate presurgical muscle-induced facial distortion. **B,** Facial distortion corrected "orthognathically" by achieving a straight nasal septum positioned in the facial midline, symmetrical reconstruction of the nasolabial muscles, absence of vestibular oral nasal communication, and a functional patent nostril on the cleft side.

muscles are retracted laterally, and the levator veli palatini and palatopharyngeus muscles are displaced both laterally and superiorly. Because of the low position of the tongue, the tip can engage the posterior part of the cleft, thus exaggerating the lateral displacement of the pterygoid muscles and widening of the cleft.

The unwanted effects of either poor or incomplete reconstruction of the soft palate include hypotony, hypotrophy, and retraction of the soft palate and its anterior pillar, which lead to atrophy and sclerosis. As a consequence of an unfavorable tongue position, there is a tendency to mandibular protrusion and maxillary retrusion. Good reconstruction of the soft palate, therefore, should reconstitute the posterosuperior parts of the soft palate, particularly the levator veli palatini muscle. This reconstruction permits the soft palate to assume relatively normal functions of phonation, deglutition, and tongue position, all of which optimize skeletal morphogenesis in an orthognathic manner.

Whether the global deformity is due to true hypoplasia, hypofunction, and attendant hypodevelopment or a combination of both, the principal surgical goal is the same: to establish good function through careful muscle reconstruction, which, in turn, will permit optimum subsequent growth and development of the facial skeleton. This principle is important, both in primary and secondary cleft corrections, because good function is prerequisite to good facial esthetics.

There are three rather distinct regions of mucoperiosteum that cover the palate (Fig. 88-6).

It is the thick maxillary mucoperiosteum, so important in the transverse and vertical growth of the palate, with which the surgeon must take special care in surgery of the hard palate. In total bilateral cleft palate, it is the palatine part that is missing, but the gingival and maxillary regions are usually, essentially normal. This explains why in unoperated bilateral cleft palate, with the exception of the vomer and the palatine shelves themselves, development of the palatal vault is almost normal. In classic palatorrhaphy techniques, large widely undermined flaps of the maxillary region are swung medially to cover the defect of the palatine part, thus leaving bilateral donor areas of exposed bone that eventually undergo wound contraction and scarring. From its new position, the displaced maxillary mucoperiosteum cannot play its important role in transverse and vertical growth of the palatal vault. Furthermore, because this tissue is thick (rather than the thin palatine mucoperiosteum that is

normally situated here), there is a "filling in" effect, which further compromises the depth of the palatal vault. The nasal fossae, normally under the influence of the palatine region of mucoperiosteum, do not fully develop their transverse dimension, which, in turn, can affect nasal airway patency. In classic palatorrhaphy, it is also common to obtain the nasal layer of the two-layer closure by the use of flaps of vomerine mucosa. This establishes an insufficient vertical dimension of the maxilla and, therefore, also of the nasal fossae; the net result favors a vertically deficient, retrodisplaced maxilla and overclosure of the mandible.

From these observations, it seems prudent for the surgeon to attempt to avoid medial transposition of maxillary mucoperiosteal flaps, exposed areas of bone at completion of the operation, and fixation of the vomer to the palate by use of vomerine mucosa to establish the nasal plane in two-plane closures. Staging of the

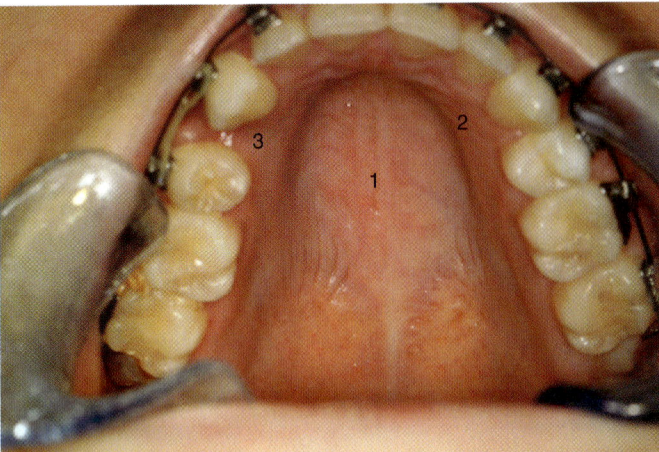

Fig. 88-6 ■ There are three rather distinct regions of mucoperiosteum that covers the palate: (1) palatine, the thin, smooth lining that covers the middle and posterior parts of the vault, corresponding roughly to the dimensions of the overlying nasal floor; (2) maxillary, the thick lining that has rugae and is rich in blood vessels, nerves, and connective tissue covering that part of the palate between the palatine and gingival regions; and (3) gingival, the palatal gingiva that is intimately related to the maxillary dentoalveolus.

surgical procedures based on variation of the individual case should be planned such that it is possible to respect the principles of anatomy and physiology of the three regions of mucoperiosteum that cover the palate.

In complete cleft lip and palate, the soft palate is closed at the same time as the cleft lip at about 3 to 5 months of age. The surgical goal is to establish both continuity and function of the muscles of the soft palate. Adequate length of the soft palate can be achieved without either complex, multiple Z-plasties or microsurgical techniques. Incisions are made on the margins of the cleft of the soft palate, slightly favoring the nasal side. To obtain the best exposure of the levator muscle, which is retracted toward the nasal side, a small triangle of mucosa is excised from the nasal surface of the divided velum on both sides. Reconstitution of the levator veli palate, as well as the palatopharyngeus and palatoglossus muscles, is prerequisite to obtaining adequate soft palate length. Mucosal incisions are made on both sides to allow exposure of the hamular process, which is not fractured by design. Adequate soft tissue mobilization can easily be realized by meticulous muscle dissection. The tensor palati and superficial portion of the palatopharyngeus muscles are freed from the posterior border of the palate so that their orientation from longitudinal to transverse can be accomplished. Muscle reconstruction, including the palatoglossus, establishes a functional sphincter of the soft palate. No vomer flap is employed.

Following closure of the soft palate and the cleft lip, there is now function both anteriorly and posteriorly, which causes the distance between the hamular processes, tuberosities, and the divided hard palate to dramatically diminish by the age of about 12 months. At this time, the residual hard palate cleft can be closed, very often without the use of lateral palatal incisions (Fig. 88-7). Again, no vomer flap is used because the nasal side of the cleft is closed using nasal mucosa situated below the inferior border of the vomer. Isolated cleft palate, both hard and soft, is treated at about 9 months of age. The same fundamental principles are employed in revision surgery to obtain lengthening and improved function of the soft palate.

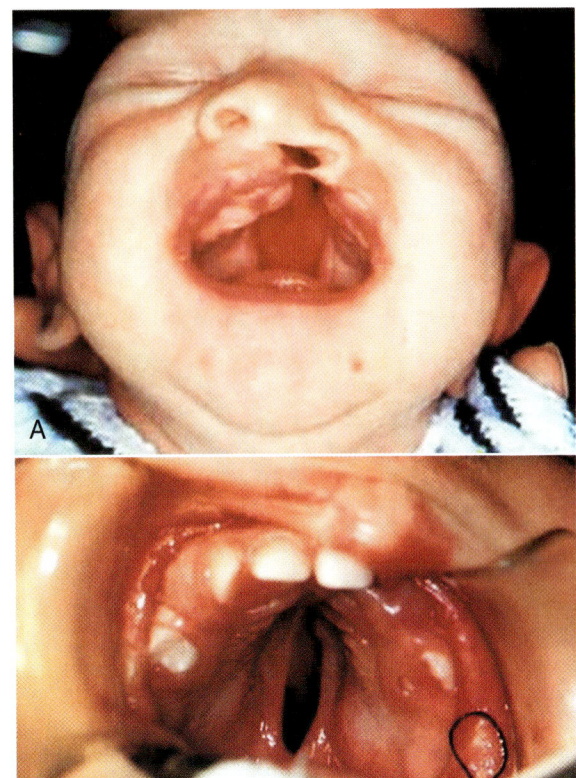

Fig. 88-7 ■ **A,** Wide cleft palate in newborn infant. **B,** Following closure of the soft palate and the cleft lip, there is now function both anteriorly and posteriorly, which causes the distance between the hamular processes, tuberosities, and the divided hard palate to dramatically diminish by the age of about 12 months. At this time, the residual hard palate cleft can be closed, very often without the use of lateral palatal incisions.

ALVEOLAR BONE GRAFT

When the timing of alveolar bone grafting is based on the eruptive progress of the permanent maxillary canine teeth, the surgical procedure is, by definition, delayed until the late mixed dentition. This treatment strategy overlooks both the crown length and the periodontal condition of the maxillary permanent incisors adjacent to the cleft defect.

The goals of alveolar bone grafts are

- closure of vestibular and palatal oral nasal fistulae.
- to provide adequate bone stock for the permanent maxillary central incisor, lateral incisor, and canine teeth.
- to establish the nasal skeletal base.
- to provide a suitable bony architecture on which to perform symmetrical nasolabial muscle reconstruction.
- to establish a functional floor of nose and nasal airway on the cleft side.
- to provide adequate bone stock for placement of an osseointegrated dental implant.

Grafting is usually performed when the maxillary permanent incisor teeth are visible in the mouth but not yet fully erupted. Simultaneous secondary functional cheilorhinoplasty is performed if there is muscular dysfunction of the lip as determined by deviation of the nasal septum to the noncleft side, presence of vestibular oral nasal fistula, and/or inability of the child to symmetrically project the lips. Total palatal reconstruction is carried out if there are palatal

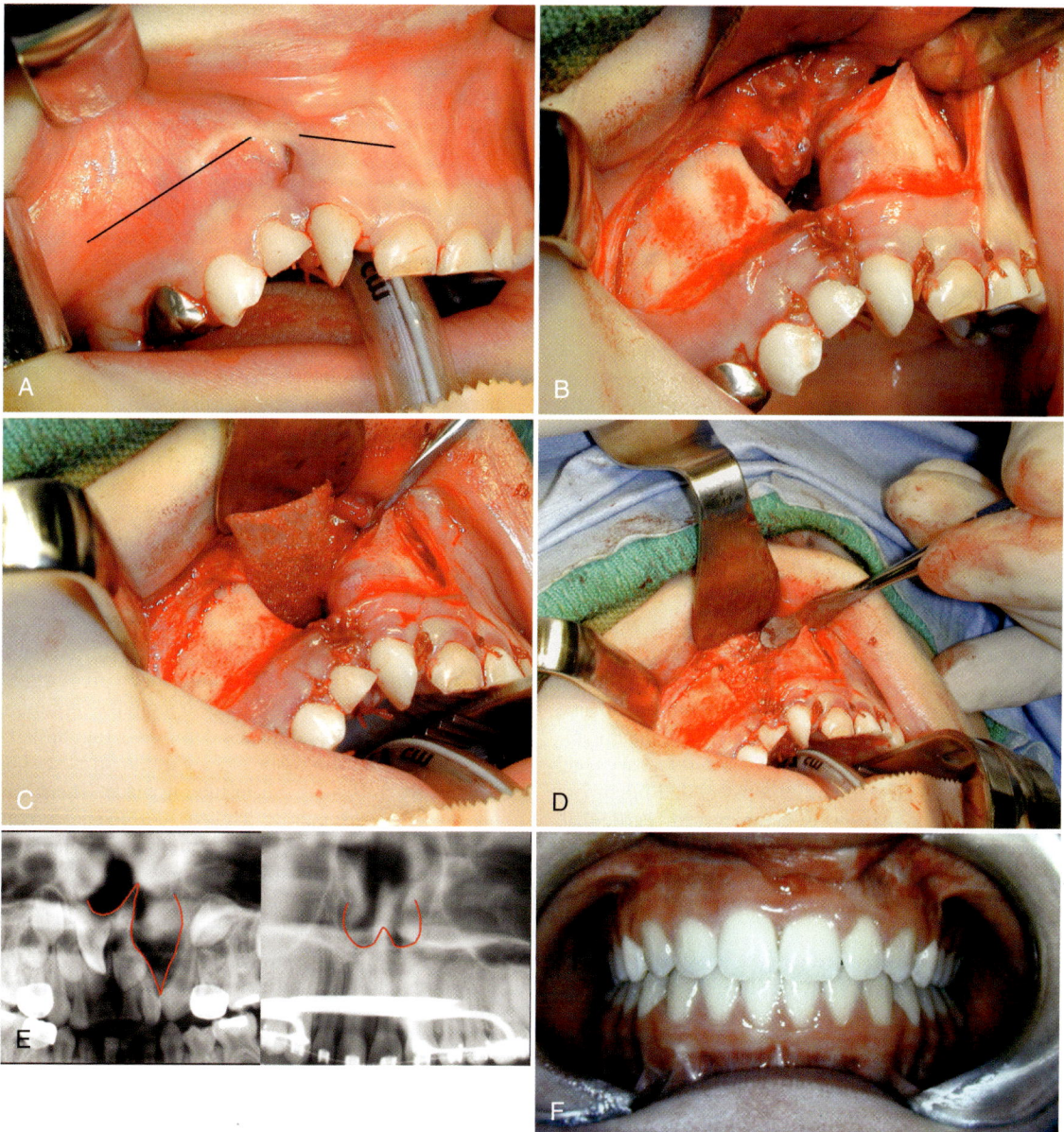

Fig. 88-8 ■ **A,** Lateral and medial mucoperiosteal incision design used to define and expose the cleft alveolus. **B,** Wide exposure of the relevant structures permits meticulous reconstruction of the nasal floor and attached labial gingival, both of which, when properly repaired, contribute to the orthognathic context. **C,** The cortical side of the thin bone sheet is placed toward the nasal mucosa to enhance stability of the newly constructed nasal floor. **D,** The greatest possible density of particulate marrow is placed in the defect, filling all dimensions. **E,** Symmetry of the nasal skeletal base is always improved after this type of grafting. **F,** When alveolar bone grafts are performed at about 6 years of age, good symmetry of the clinical crowns of the central incisors almost always results.

fistulae or distorted palatal anatomy resulting from inaccurate and inadequate primary surgery. Except in the most severe cases, the bone graft procedure is carried out *prior to* orthodontic expansion, which is usually initiated about 8 to 12 weeks *after* grafting. This allows the arch expansion to be accomplished concomitant with a type of distraction osteogenesis, accompanied by appropriate palatal mucosa expansion.

The procedure begins with infiltration of 2% lidocaine with 1/100,000 epinephrine into both the palatal mucoperiosteum and the vestibular sulcus on both sides of the cleft. Full-thickness mucoperiosteal palatal flaps are developed on both sides of the palatal aspect of the cleft using incisions extending from the tuberosity region,

around the cervical portion of the teeth to meet at the cleft in the anterior maxilla. This broad dissection allows accurate definition of the palatal-nasal defect and its contiguous nasal mucosa.

A horizontal incision is then made on the vestibular side about 5 mm above the attached gingiva and extended medially to a point just short of the margin of the fistula if present, but, in any case, just short of the bony margin of the cleft defect (Fig. 88-8, *A*). The lateral aspect of the maxilla is widely exposed to include the lateral aspect of the cleft from the existing alveolar bone margin to a point on the lateral aspect of the pyriform aperture equal in height to that of the infraorbital foramen. This dissection is carried on the inner aspect of the maxilla in the nasal aspect such that a vertical sheet of nasal mucosa is developed that is continuous with the palatal dissection already carried out. On the medial aspect of the cleft, a similar horizontal vestibular incision is made that permits complete exposure of the lateral nasal margin of the noncleft nostril, the anterior nasal spine, and the medial margin of the cleft alveolus. The nasal mucosa on the medial aspect of the cleft is then developed such that this dissection too is continuous with the palatal dissection. A small vertical incision then is made in the attached gingiva so that the entire cleft alveolar defect is now clearly visible.

The palatal mucosa is reconstructed, from posterior to anterior, using interrupted mattress sutures to ensure as perfect palatal mucosal anatomy as possible. The reconstructed palatal mucosa is left as a large single palatal flap until the nasal reconstruction is completed. From the vestibular side, the nasal mucosa is now reconstructed such that the height of the nasal floor is equal to or slightly superior to that on the noncleft side. This is a very important technical point, because unless there is adequate space for bone between the palatal and nasal layers, long-term bone stock quantity will be insufficient. Part of the nasal mucosal suturing is carried out through the access created by delaying the final suturing of the palate. Meticulous attention to detail in suturing the nasal mucosa is important so that a smooth and even mucosal layer presents to what will be the roof of the bone graft (Fig. 88-8, *B*).

A thin piece of cortical bone is fashioned to snugly fit in the nostril defect, dividing the graft from the nasal mucosa at a height slightly above the nostril floor on the noncleft side. The cortical side of this piece of bone is placed against the nasal mucosa, the medullary side thus facing the graft (Fig. 88-8, *C*). A nasopharyngeal airway is now placed in the nose to ensure a patent and functional airway while the particulate marrow is being placed. Particulate marrow is packed into the defect with pressure. As much bone as possible is placed into the confines of the defect, paying particular attention to the alveolar margin of the cleft in the region of the erupting teeth (Fig. 88-8, *D*).

The vertical incision in the attached gingiva is closed such that the reconstructed gingiva is resting on newly grafted bone. The palatal flap is then returned to its ideal position and sutured in place around the necks of the teeth and at the anterior aspect over the graft. The vestibular horizontal incisions are closed so that the resulting vestibular depth is not diminished. The procedure is very similar when carried out in conjunction with secondary functional cheilorhinoplasty. At the end of the operation, only palatal mucosa is on the palate, only nasal mucosa forms the nasal floor, attached gingiva (not alveolar mucosa or any other foreign tissue) covers the teeth and the graft at the alveolar margin, and the maxillary vestibule is lined only by alveolar mucosa. This strict anatomical geography is critical to the long-term success of the operation. No splints are used, but the patient is placed on a soft diet for about 1 week after surgery.

Alveolar bone grafts that are performed just prior to or very soon after the beginning of eruption of the maxillary permanent central incisor contralateral to the cleft provide good nasal floor symmetry (Fig. 88-8, *E*) and almost normal symmetry of clinical crown length of the two erupted permanent maxillary central incisors (Fig. 88-8, *F*).

MAXILLARY OSTEOTOMY

The maxillary osteotomy of preference is usually the Le Fort I type, but the clinician should be aware of the applicability of the modified Le Fort III or maxillomalar osteotomy when there is deficiency in the anterior projection of the malar aspect of the face.

The approach to the maxilla for the Le Fort I osteotomy is similar to that described by Bell, with several modifications. The horizontal

incision is kept very low such that only a few millimeters of unattached mucosa remain on the inferior segment. This modification, when combined with very wide subperiosteal exposure, particularly on the cleft side, allows maximum advancement of soft tissue toward the midline. We invariably use a superior step in the zygomatic region of the maxilla to enhance the accuracy of intraoral spatial orientation, to provide solid bone for application of rigid fixation devices, and to maximize bony contact of the bony fragments (Fig. 88-9, *A*). We do not use a chisel to separate the maxilla from the pterygoid plates; rather, we employ a Tessier spreader to exert downward pressure on the posterior aspect of the maxilla, which results in a clean and easy pterygomaxillary separation. The maxilla is then oriented on the mandible using an intermaxillary occlusal splint, which is initially ligated to the maxillary arch. Contoured miniplates are used to fixate the maxilla in its planned (slightly overcorrected) position. The reverse step in the osteotomy design permits use of posterior wire osseous fixation, which "locks in" the bony segments and reduces the cost of the fixation (Fig. 88-9, *B*).

Concomitant mandibular surgery, which is necessary occasionally, can be performed more easily if the anesthetist changes the oral tube to a nasal tube. Alternatively, an armored oral endotracheal tube can be used such that it exits the mouth on the noncleft side through the buccal space from behind the occlusal splint.

Revision secondary cheilorhinoplasty can be carried out at the same time as a Le Fort I osteotomy, which gives direct access to the nasal septum and affords the surgeon the optimum moment to correct the septal deviation and deformity (Fig. 88-9, *C*). Whichever sequence is used, soft tissue closure of the lip-nose should be carried out with an oral-endotracheal tube in place. There are three important muscles and muscle groups that must be reconstructed to achieve symmetry and good function of the upper lip. The lateral nasal muscle must be identified and sutured with nonresorbable material to the base of the cartilaginous nasal septum near the anterior nasal spine. The levator muscles of the lip must be identified and sutured to the nasal septum anterior to the position chosen for the lateral nasal muscle. Finally, the pyramidal portion of the orbicularis oris muscle must be identified and sutured to the most anterior portion of the nasal septum such that the upper lip is somewhat like a circus tent, with the central pole being the anterior nasal spine and septum. If this reconstruction is carried out meticulously, good eversion and protrusion of the lip should be possible after surgery (Figs. 88-9, *D* to *F* and 88-10).

MANDIBULAR OSTEOTOMY

Mandibular surgery is sometimes required in patients with cleft lip and palate. In general, with few exceptions, impacted third molars should be removed concomitant with sagittal split (SSO) osteotomies for patients having mandibular orthognathic surgery, because doing so limits risk, is cost efficient, minimizes unwanted postsurgical consequences, and provides a reliable, deft means by which planned surgery can be accomplished.

Surgical technique is important when performing removal of impacted third molars concomitant with SSO. Our preferred SSO technique, when impacted third molars are present, employs cuts that are performed through the greater sagittal length of the impacted third molar tooth during the sagittal osteotomy (Fig. 88-11, *A*).

The sagittal-split is initiated with a flat blade spatula, followed by the use of Smith and Tessier spreaders, respectively. No malleting with a chisel is used in any case. Completion of the split is accomplished superoinferiorly, not anteroposteriorly, because the last point of osseous resistance (Fig. 88-11, *B*) is usually encountered on the lingual cortex below the entrance of the inferior alveolar nerve

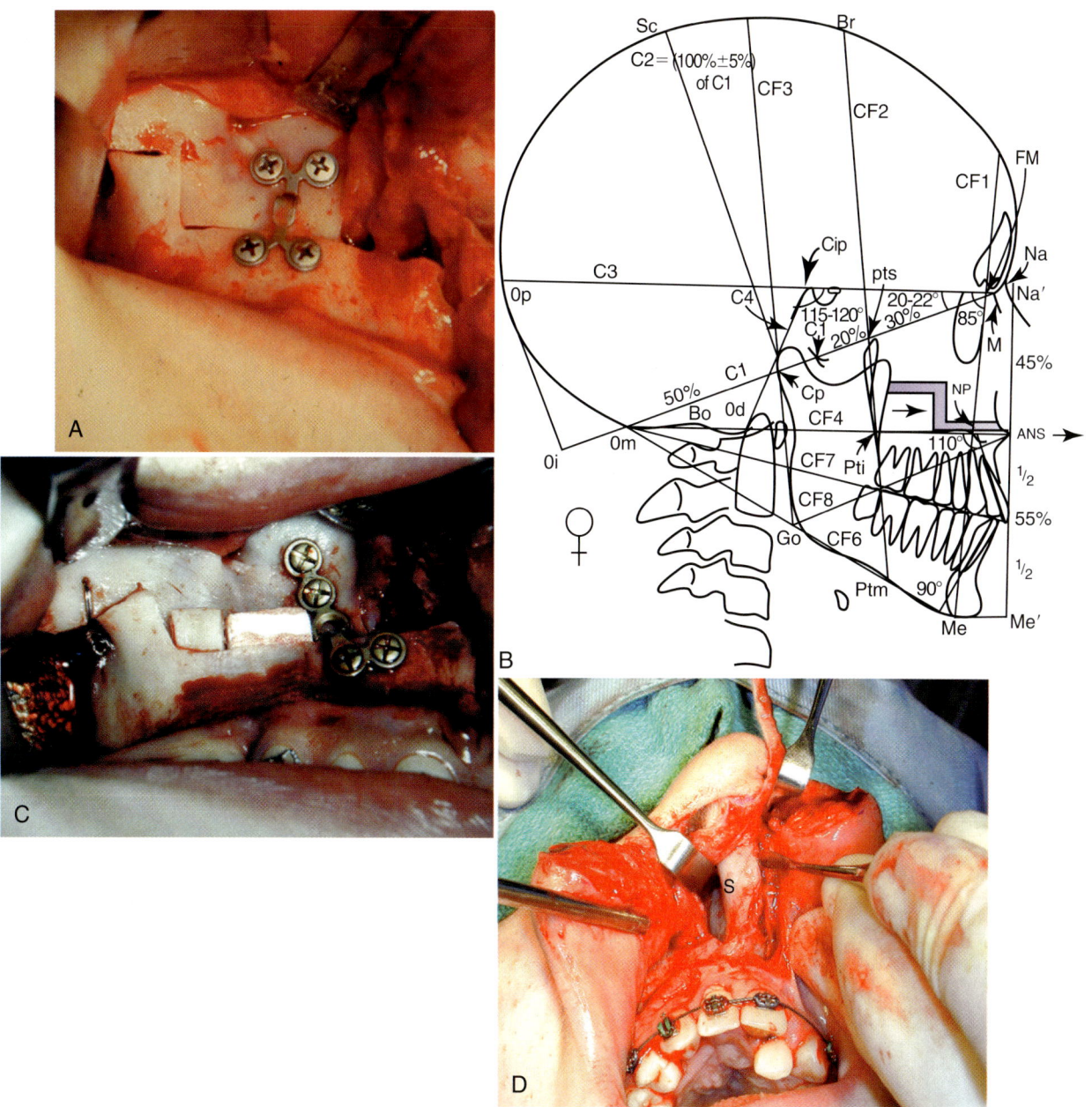

Fig. 88-9 ■ **A** and **B,** A superior ("reverse") step in the zygomatic region of the maxilla enhances the accuracy of intraoral spatial orientation, provides solid bone for application of rigid fixation devices, and maximizes contact of the bony fragments. **C,** Posterior wires combined with anterior plate and screw fixation can reduce the cost of the fixation devices used to stabilize the maxilla. **D,** LeFort I osteotomy concomitant with secondary functional cheilorhinoplasty gives unsurpassed access to the deviated and distorted nasal septum so commonly found in patients with inadequately repaired cleft lip and palate.

(IAN). Fixation is accomplished using plate and unicortical screw fixation of the osteotomy sites (Fig. 88-11, *C*).

Although, as early as 1986, Epker recommended that "impacted third molars be generally removed at the time of orthognathic surgery to avoid an additional operative procedure," there remained a body of opinion (which to some extent still persists) that the presence of third molars at the time of orthognathic surgery would contribute to a higher incidence of unwanted fracture with SSO. This has not proved to be the case.

FUNCTIONAL GENIOPLASTY

The term functional genioplasty, at first blush, seems to represent something of a paradox because, in the past, surgery on the chin has been thought of primarily in the context of cosmesis. In man, changes in form produce attendant changes in function; the functional genioplasty is an example of an operation that can bring about a beneficial change in function by altering the position and form of the chin and its associated myocutaneous structures.

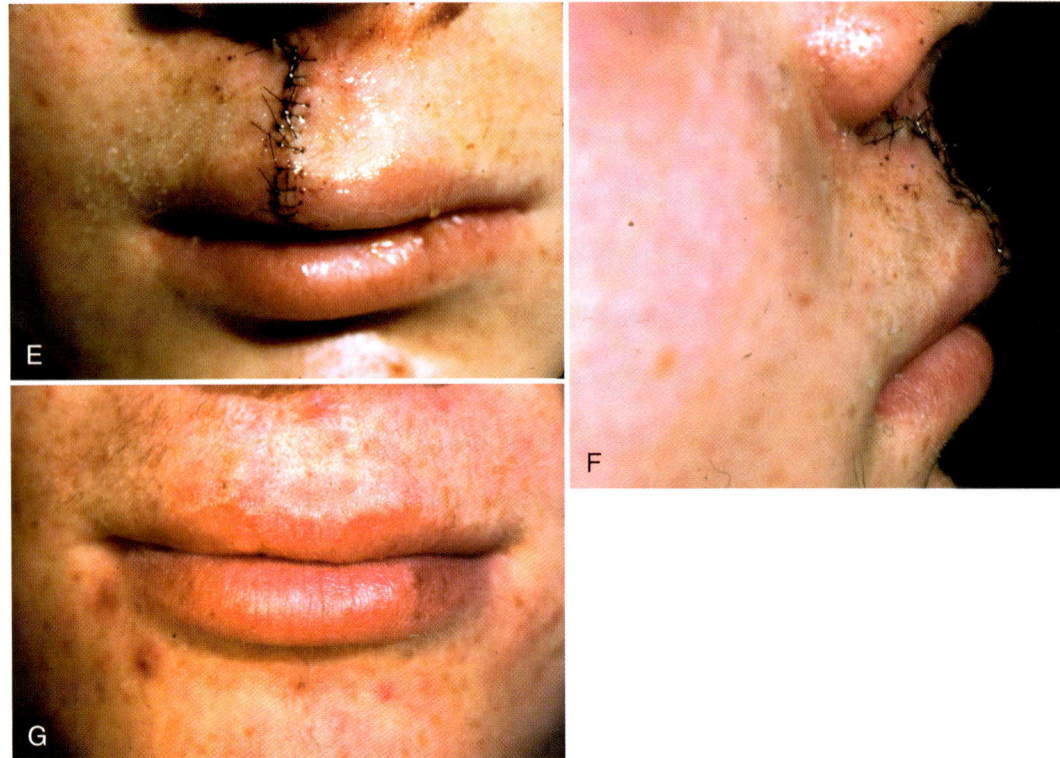

Fig. 88-9, cont'd ■ Frontal (**E**) and lateral (**F**) views of a 19-year-old male patient 2 days after LeFort I osteotomy and secondary functional cheilorhinoplasty. Note good symmetry and projection of the lip. **G,** Patient 24 months after surgery demonstrating preservation of good symmetry achieved at surgery.

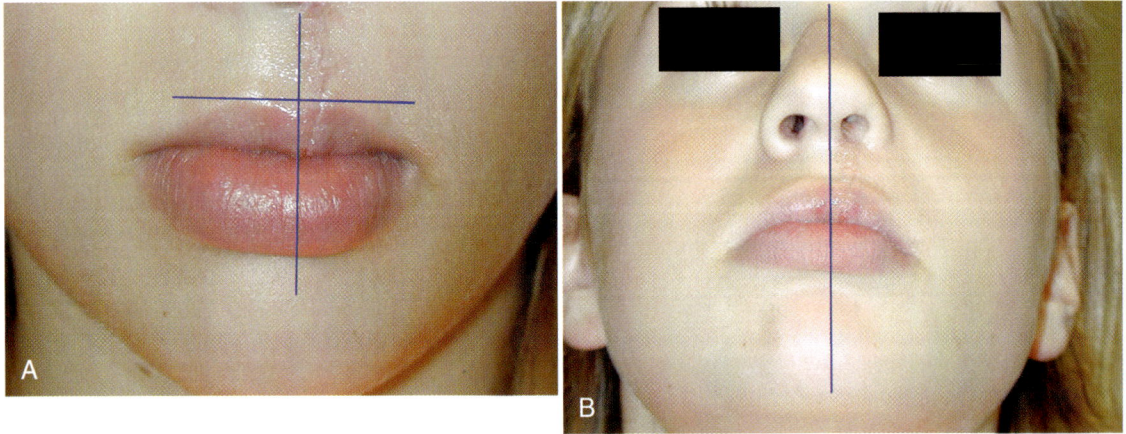

Fig. 88-10 ■ **A,** Frontal view of a 20-year-old female patient 3 weeks after Le Fort I osteotomy and secondary functional cheilorhinoplasty showing good symmetry of the summits of the cupid's bow. **B,** Good coincidence of all of the midline structures of the face 3 weeks after surgery.

The indications for functional genioplasty are vertical excess of the lower anterior facial height in which the following clinical signs and radiographic findings are present:

- Lip incompetence when the lips are in repose and existence of a normal relationship of the maxillary incisor tooth to the upper lip.
- Open-mouth posture with interposition of the tongue between the teeth.
- Elevation of the mental soft tissues in order to obtain lip closure.

- Thinning of the alveolar bone overlying the facial surfaces of the roots of the anterior mandibular teeth.
- Flattening of the contour of the anterior surface of the soft tissue profile of the chin.
- Residual and associated deformities or cleft lip–cleft palate, particularly in the case of the insufficient cheiloplasty where the upper lip is too short (Fig. 88-12, *A* and *B*). The superior repositioning of the mental osseous and myocutaneous tissues can aid in both achievement of lip competence and development of the upper lip.

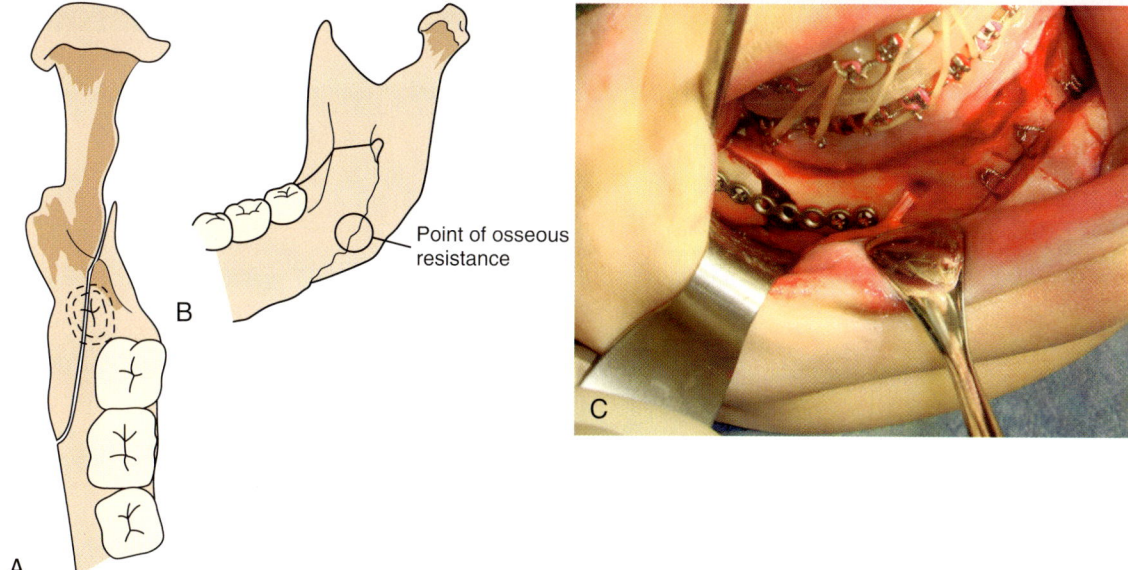

Fig. 88-11 ▪ **A,** Sagittal osteotomy (SO) technique when impacted third molars are present employs cuts that are performed through the greater sagittal length of the impacted third molar tooth during the sagittal osteotomy. **B,** Completion of the split from "top to bottom" (rather than from "front to back") because the last point of osseous resistance is usually encountered on the lingual cortex below the entrance of the inferior alveolar nerve (IAN). This technique allows identification of the IAN very early in the bone-splitting process. **C,** When genioplasty is combined with split-sagittal osteotomy (SSO), we use a complete circummandibular incision for improved access and surgical accuracy.

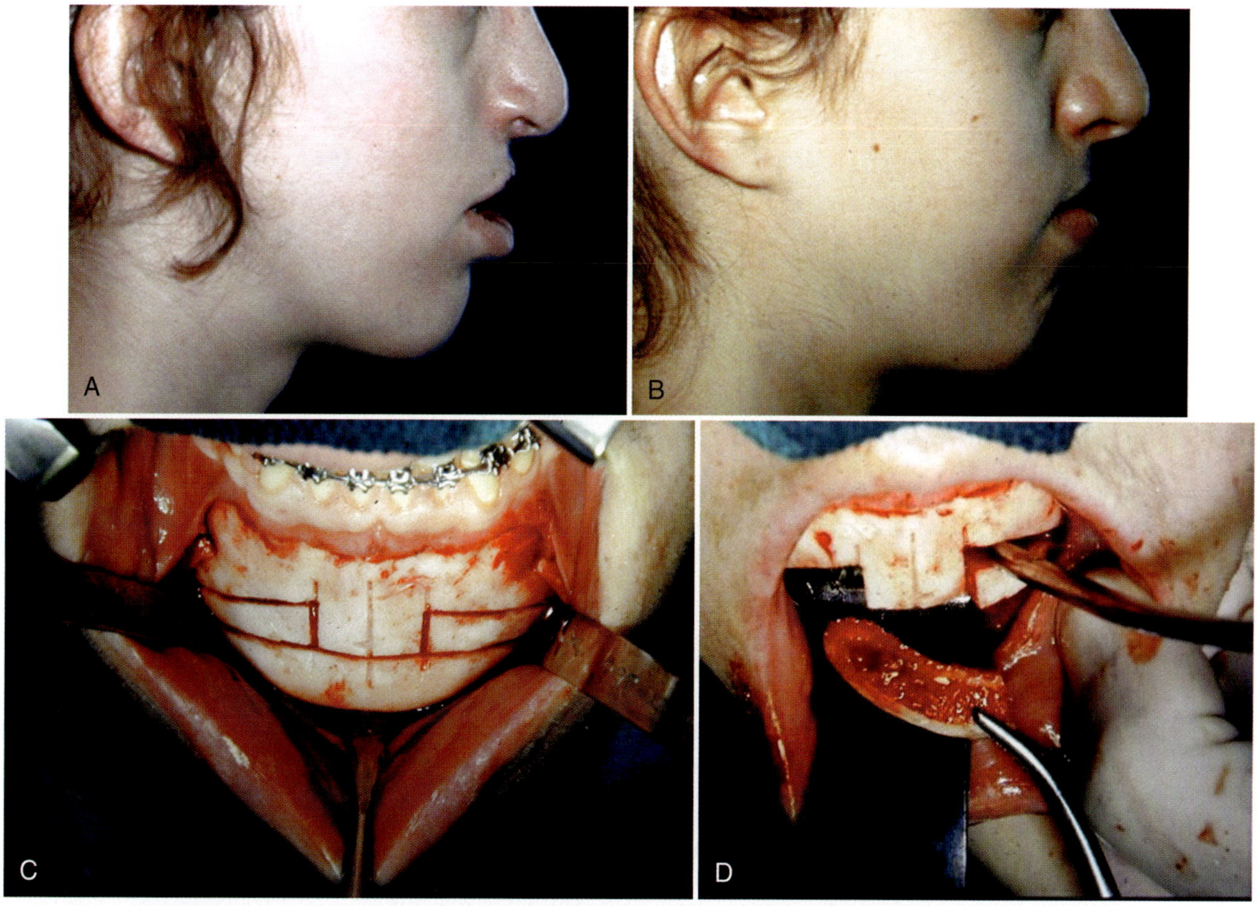

Fig. 88-12 ▪ **A,** Residual, associated deformities of cleft lip–cleft palate, particularly in the case of the insufficient cheiloplasty where the upper lip is too short, thus contributing further to anterior mandibular excess and lip incompetence. **B,** Hyperactivity of the mentalis and other muscles to attempt to achieve lip closure. **C,** The horizontal osteotomy of the anterior mandible, with construction by segmental ostectomies of a superior tenon and an inferior lingual mortise. **D,** The resected fragments are wedge shaped by design and provide excellent, small, bicortical grafts for defects caused by segmental osteotomy in the maxilla.

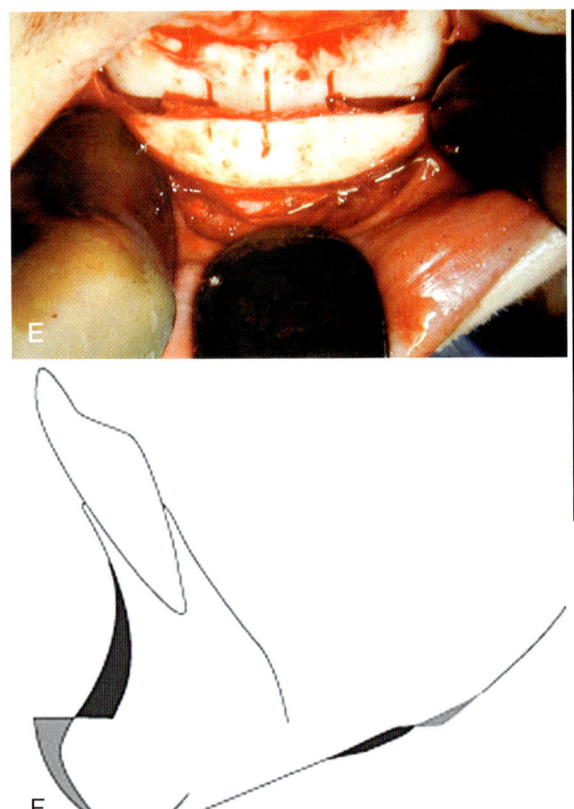

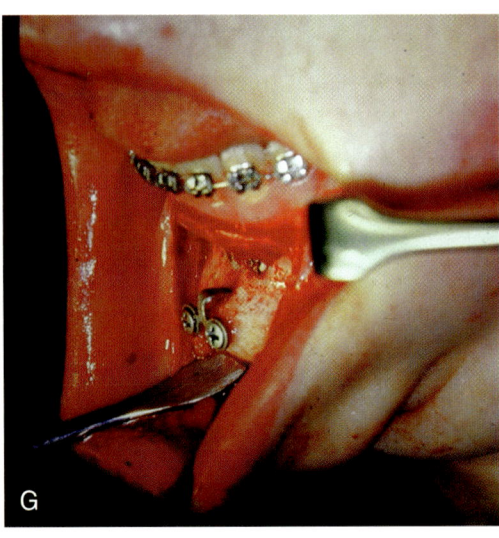

Fig. 88-12, cont'd ▪ **E,** The inferior fragment of the chin is both advanced and superiorly repositioned by fitting the mortise on the tenon. **F,** The specific pattern of bone apposition and resorption observed after functional genioplasty forms the basis for our proposal that the maxillofacial surgeon should attempt to place fixation devices in areas of future bone apposition. *Shaded* areas represent bone resorption, while *black* areas represent bone apposition at approximately 1 year after genioplasty. **G,** In cases where the fixation device was situated in a region of bone loss, the metal was externalized from the bone, and where the metal was placed in a region of bony apposition, it was buried by new bone.

The actual surgical procedure consists of a horizontal osteotomy of the anterior mandible, with construction by segmental ostectomies of a superior tenon and an inferior lingual mortise (Fig. 88-12, *C*). The resected fragments are wedge shaped by design (Fig. 88-12, *D*) and thus are perfectly suited to placement as bone grafts in other surgical sites (e.g., in the bony defects created by multisegment Le Fort osteotomy of the maxilla).

The functional genioplasty can be carried out as soon as the mandibular permanent cuspid teeth have erupted. The procedure is performed with the patient under general anesthesia through a mandibular labial vestibular incision, which is extended from one premolar area to the other, after infiltration of local anesthesia with a 1:100,000 solution of epinephrine. The anterior aspect of the mandible is exposed by subperiosteal dissection, which stops at the inferior border, thereby preserving as much as possible the insertions of the labiomental muscles. Specifically, these muscles include the mentalis, depressor anguli oris, depressor labii inferioris, and part of the orbicularis oris.

The osteotomy cuts are outlined with a small bur. The height of the vertical arms of the tenon corresponds to the magnitude of the predetermined bony resection. The inferior horizontal osteotomy is then completed with a reciprocating saw, after which the bicortical tenon is constructed by resecting lateral wedge-shaped pieces of bone (see Fig. 88-12, *D*). A mortise is now cut in the midsuperior portion of the lingual aspect of the inferior bony fragment. The depth of the mortise is the difference between the amount of predetermined chin advancement and the thickness of the inferior bony fragment. The inferior fragment is then both advanced and superiorly repositioned by fitting the mortise on the tenon (Fig. 88-12, *E*).

Although there can be considerable adaptation of the suprahyoid muscles to change in length, stretching of the suprahyoid musculature as a result of mandibular advancement surgery is a major factor leading to skeletal relapse. Because a substantial part of the suprahyoid group of muscles remains undisturbed and attached to the lingual aspect of the tenon, these fibers are not stretched when the inferior bony segment is advanced, and thus one would expect the stability of the surgical result to be enhanced. Fixation is accomplished by transosseous wires that are placed to create a direction of pull such that the anterior inferior mortise is brought into good apposition with the superior and now posterior tenon. Watertight closure of the vestibular incision is accomplished with 3-0 polyglycolic acid sutures, after which a pressure dressing is placed on the skin overlying the mental tissues for 5 days.

It is important to stress the simplicity of this technique. Morbidity is minimal, and there is a very low incidence of alteration in mental nerve function associated with this procedure, which we have used to the patient's benefit as an important aid in achieving bilabial contact in patients who suffer from residual deformities associated with labiopalatine clefts.

We examined the pattern of osseous change in the chin after genioplasty in two groups of selected, representative patients; one group had rigid fixation, and the other had wire osteosynthesis. The specific pattern of bone apposition and resorption observed after functional genioplasty (Fig. 88-12, *F*) forms the basis for our proposal that the maxillofacial surgeon should attempt to place fixation devices in areas of future bone apposition, because in cases where the metal was situated in a region of bone loss, the metal was externalized from the bone, and where the metal was placed in a region of bony apposition, it was buried by new bone (Fig. 88-12, *G*).

SUMMARY

Orthognathic surgery for patients with cleft lip and palate should be provided at various stages throughout the patient's life. Early, primary orthognathic surgery should establish symmetrical, functional muscular balance so that there will be a beneficial influence on subsequent growth (Fig. 88-13). Orthognathic surgery performed in adolescence or adulthood should correct the maxillofacial deformity extant at the time. We should not interpret the need for orthognathic surgery as failure of the primary procedures; rather, we should celebrate the fact that we can perform accurate, safe orthognathic surgery for the benefit of the patients who need it (Fig. 88-14).

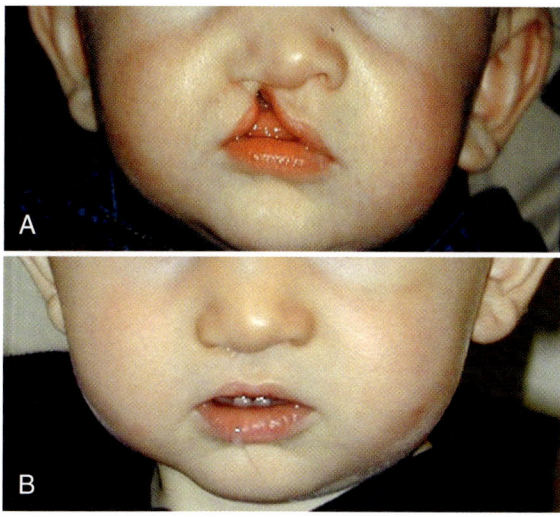

Fig. 88-13 ■ Early primary orthognathic surgery (**A**) should establish symmetrical, functional, and muscular balance (**B**) so that there will be a beneficial influence on subsequent growth.

PEARLS AND PITFALLS

- Orthognathic surgery includes primary surgical procedures for cleft lip and palate, because they influence the balance and symmetry of facial structures in an orthognathic context.
- Primary functional cheilorhinoplasty should be performed concomitantly with primary functional veloplasty at about 6 months of age.
- Primary palatoplasty should be performed at about 1 year of age.
- If needed, alveolar bone grafts and fistulae closure should be performed at about 5½ to 6 years of age.
- Orthodontic expansion of the maxillary arch should be carried out after the alveolar bone graft.
- The entire cranium should be visible on the cephalometric image.
- Le Fort I osteotomy to advance the retruded maxilla can include a "reverse step" to enhance bone overlap of the advanced maxillary position.
- Impacted third molars should be removed at the same time as sagittal split osteotomy of the mandibular ramus.
- Genioplasty for both cleft and noncleft patients is a functional procedure.
- When performing functional genioplasty, the maxillofacial surgeon should attempt to place fixation devices in areas of future bone apposition.

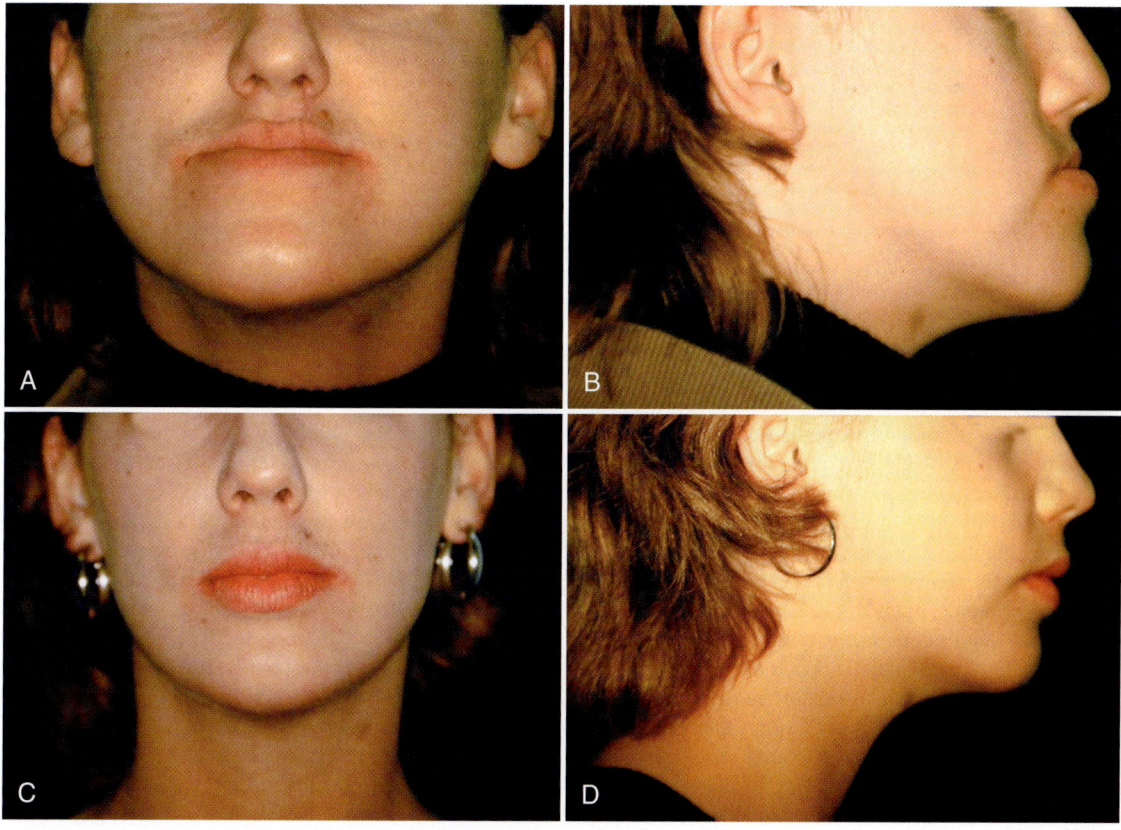

Fig. 88-14 ■ Orthognathic surgery performed in adulthood (**A** and **B**) should correct the maxillofacial deformity extant at the time (**C** and **D**).

BIBLIOGRAPHY

Delaire J, Precious D: Influence of the nasal septum on maxillonasal growth in patients with congenital labiomaxillary cleft. *Cleft Palate J* 23:270-277, 1986.

Delaire J: Fentes labiales congenitales. In Levignac J (ed): *Chirurgie des levres*. Paris, 1991, Masson, pp 41-80.

Delaire J, Precious D: Surgical considerations of mucocutaneous anomalies in cleft lip. *Scand J Plast Reconstr Surg* 23:55-72, 1989.

Delaire J, Precious D, Gordeef A: The advantage of wide subperiosteal exposure in primary surgical correction of labial-maxillary clefts. *Scand J Plast Reconstr Surg* 22:147-151, 1988.

Epker BN, Fish LC: *Dentofacial deformities. Integrated orthodontic and surgical correction*, vol 1, St. Louis, 1986, Mosby.

Hall BK: *Developmental and cellular skeletal biology*. New York, 1978, Academic Press.

Hall BK: The embryonic development of bone. *Amer Sci* 76(2):174-178, 1988.

Mooney MP, Siegel MI, Kimes KR, Todhunter J: Development of the orbicularis oris muscle in normal and cleft lip and palate human fetuses using three-dimensional computer reconstruction. *Plast Reconstr Surg* 81:336-345, 1988.

Moss ML: The functional matrix. In Krauss BS, Riedel RA (eds): *Vistas in orthodontics*. Philadelphia, 1962, Lea and Febiger.

Precious DS: The use of rigid fixation for cleft lip and palate deformities. In Gruss JG, Manson P, Yaremchuk M (eds): *Rigid fixation of the craniomaxillofacial skeleton*. Boston, 1992, Year Book Medical, pp 486-499.

Precious DS: Genioplasty. In Fonseca RJ (ed): *Oral and maxillofacial surgery*, vol 2, ed 2, New York, 2008, Elsevier.

Precious DS: A new reliable method for alveolar bone grafting at about 6 years of age. *J Oral Maxillofac Surg* 67:2045-2053, 2009.

Precious DS: Primary unilateral cleft lip/nose repair via the Delaire technique. In Ghali G

(ed): *Atlas of the Oral and Maxillofacial Clinics of North America*, vol 17. Philadelphia, 2009, Elsevier, pp 125-135.

Precious DS, Delaire J: Balanced facial growth. *Oral Surg Oral Med Oral Path* 63:637-650, 1987.

Precious DS, Delaire J: Surgical considerations in patients with cleft deformities. In WH Bell (ed): *Modern practice in orthognathic and reconstructive surgery*, vol 1, chapter 14. Philadelphia, 1992, WB Saunders.

Precious DS, Delaire J: Clinical observations of cleft lip and palate. *Oral Surg Oral Med Oral Pathol* 75:141-151, 1993.

Precious DS, Farrell L, Lung K, Terris G: *Early secondary grafting of alveolar clefts. 8th International Congress on Cleft Palate and Related Craniofacial Anomalies Transactions*. September 7-12, 1997, Singapore, pp 259-263.

Chapter

89

Cleft Lip and Palate: Prosthetic Rehabilitation in the Growing Cleft Patient

Betsy K. Davis

Rehabilitation of the cleft lip and palate patient populations requires a multidisciplinary team of craniofacial surgeons, oral and maxillofacial surgeons, orthodontists, pediatric dentists, restorative dentists, and speech and swallowing pathologists.[1] Treatment of these patients during the growing years requires an understanding of craniofacial growth and its effect on the timing of implant placement. Although not documented as intensively in the literature, there are the psychological and functional deficiencies associated with this patient population. In years past, many of these patients experienced problems with shyness, depression, social isolation, fighting, and impulsive behavior.[2,3] The functional deficits of a decreased vertical dimension of occlusion, decreased facial support, temporomandibular joint symptoms, lack of functional occlusion, altered speech, poor esthetics, lack of a normal smile, and altered anatomy in the lower third of the face contributed to a feeling of being different from other children.[3] With the recent advances in both medical and dental technologies, this patient population can now be rehabilitated to a near normal appearance (Fig. 89-1).

TREATMENT AND RESTORATIVE GOALS

Prosthodontics originally played a much greater role with this patient population (Fig. 89-2). For example, speech bulb prostheses (Fig. 89-3, *A*), obturators, and palatal lift prostheses (Fig. 89-3, *B*) were used in the past as definitive treatment. Now, they are rarely used and, if used at all, only as an interim measure. For the growing cleft palate child, most velopharyngeal discrepancies are managed surgically with a palatal push-back and closure procedure at 9 to 18 months, followed by a superiorly placed pharyngeal flap at 3 to 7 years. Today, a prosthesis is made only for patients with failed attempts following pharyngeal surgery. The prosthesis is used to correct the resulting hypernasality and inadequate speech. In addition, a prosthesis may also be used in those situations in which the cleft is confined to the secondary palate. In cases of velopharyngeal insufficiency in which the surgically repaired soft palate is too short and does not make contact with the pharyngeal walls during function, a prosthesis allows proper nasal airflow, resulting in normal

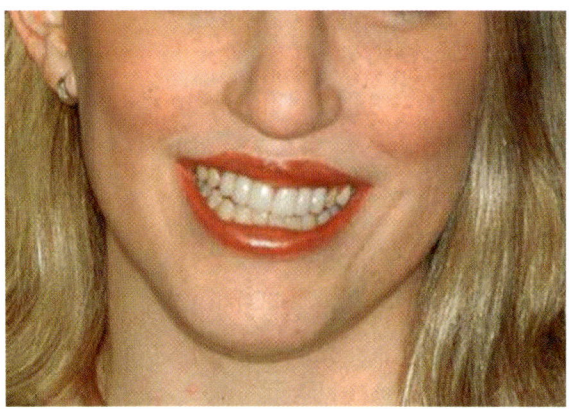

Fig. 89-1 ■ An example of a patient with bilateral cleft lip and palate who had surgical repair followed by placement of an endosseous screw-retained lateral incisor.

speech and prevention of nasal regurgitation while eating. Its purpose is to seal the nasal cavity from the oropharynx during bodily functions of eating and speaking. In cases of velopharyngeal incompetency in which the surgically repaired soft palate is of adequate length but of inadequate mobility to elevate to achieve velopharyngeal closure, the palatal lift prosthesis elevates the soft palate, contributing to normal speech. For this prosthesis to be most effective and to prevent the opposing downward muscle force of the soft palate, retention is most important. This prosthesis requires clasping multiple teeth for adequate retention. In those situations in which surgical repair was unsuccessful or an oronasal fistula is present, an obturator prosthesis may be necessary as an interim measure.[4] One significant advancement in the care of the infant cleft lip and palate patient has been nasoalveolar molding. This prosthesis is used prior to cleft lip repair to bring in the alveolar arches and to elongate the columella (Fig. 89-4).

Currently, the greatest prosthetic issue facing the growing cleft palate patient is treatment for the edentulous alveolar cleft and missing teeth.[1,5,6] It is important to remember that jaw growth and

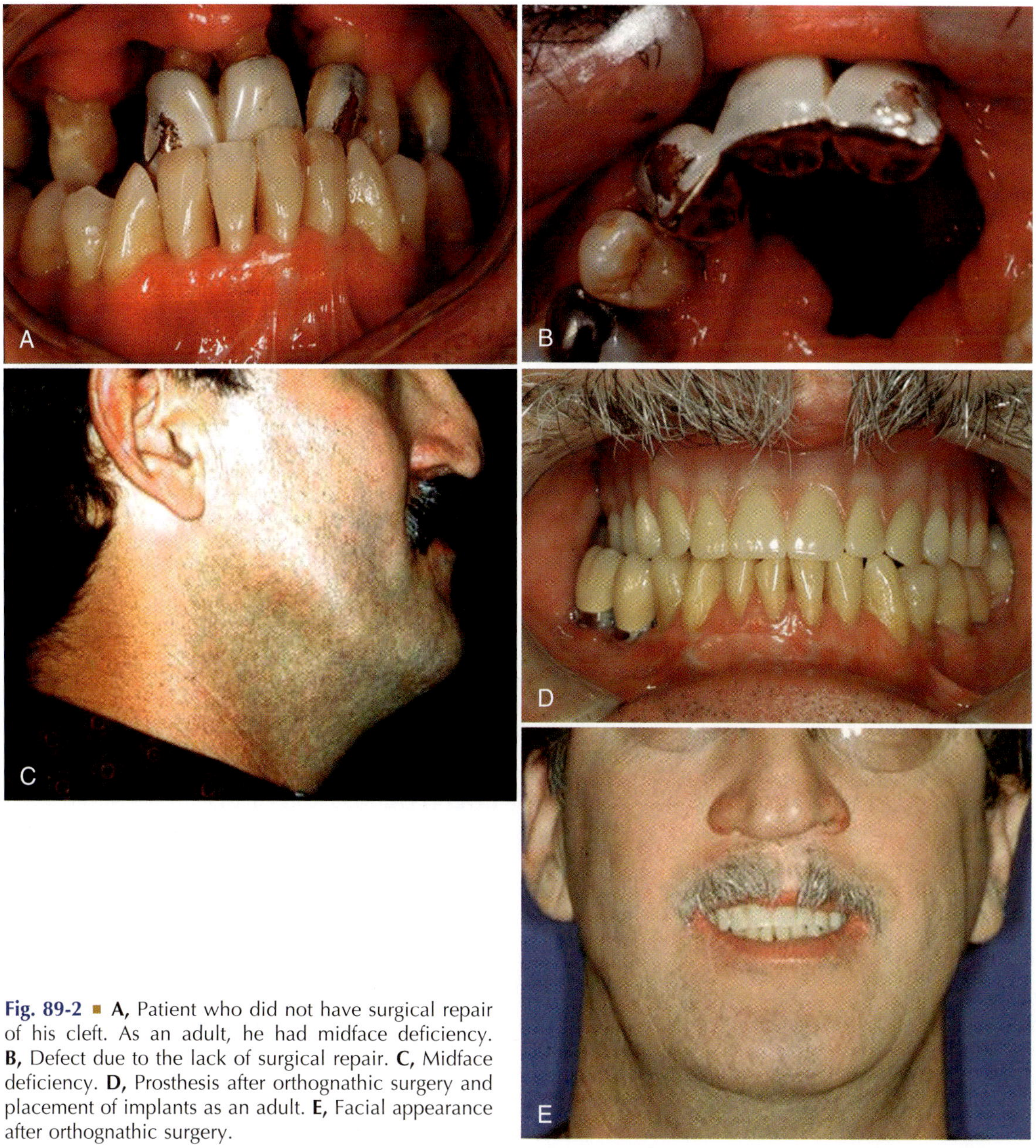

Fig. 89-2 ■ **A,** Patient who did not have surgical repair of his cleft. As an adult, he had midface deficiency. **B,** Defect due to the lack of surgical repair. **C,** Midface deficiency. **D,** Prosthesis after orthognathic surgery and placement of implants as an adult. **E,** Facial appearance after orthognathic surgery.

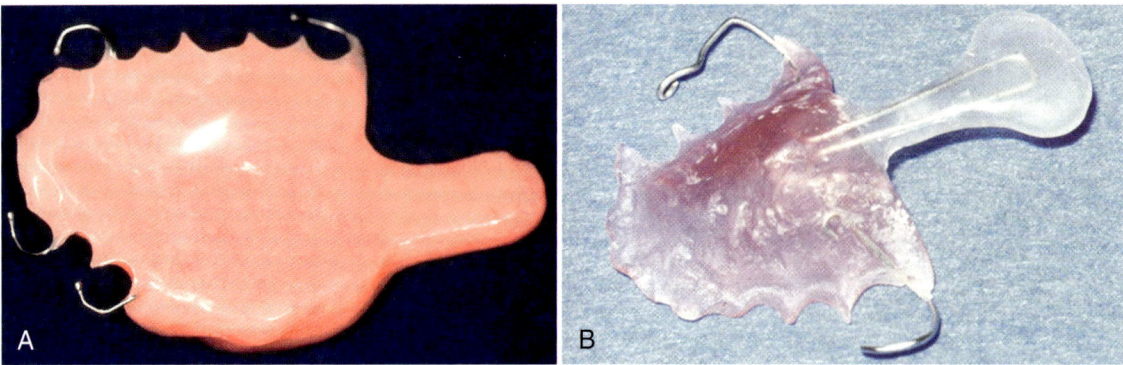

Fig. 89-3 ■ **A,** Speech bulb prosthesis. **B,** Palatal lift prosthesis. (**B,** From Flint PW, Haughey BH, Lund VJ: *Cummings otolaryngology head and neck surgery*, ed 5, Philadelphia, 2010, Mosby.)

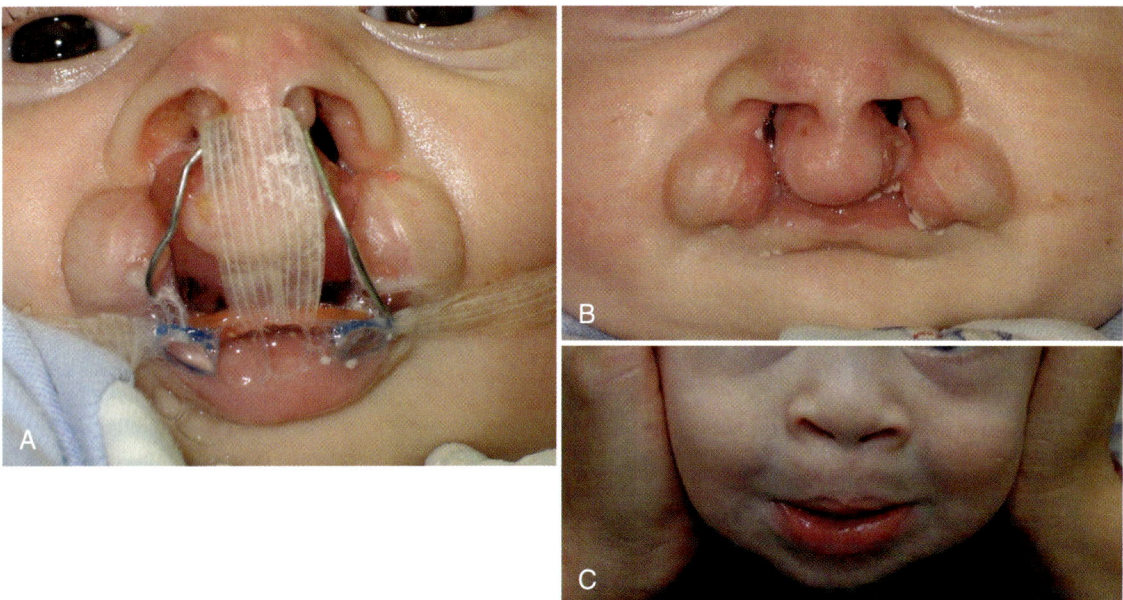

Fig. 89-4 ■ **A,** Nasoalveolar molding appliance. **B,** The purpose of the appliance is to bring the alveolar arches in and elongate the columella. **C,** The result of nasoalveolar molding.

dentoalveolar development do not follow normal patterns of growth. The prosthetic needs of the growing cleft child during the primary dentition state are minimal. Usually, jaw relationships, occlusion, and individual teeth remain relatively stable. In cases of severe tooth decay and tooth loss, the occlusion and jaw relationship may vary during growth. On the other hand, with the mixed dentition stage, there is a discrepancy between the maxillary and mandibular arches with respect to size. Definitive prosthodontic care is usually one of the last treatments needed and is recommended after the completion of craniofacial growth, usually after 18 years of age.

TREATMENT TECHNIQUES

HYPODONTIA

Hypodontia has been reported to occur approximately 10 times more frequently on the cleft side in this patient population.[5,6] Ranta found a positive association between hypodontia and cleft severity, with the incidence of hypodontia increasing strongly with the cleft's severity.[7] Bohn reported a prevalence of tooth agenesis of 46% in the cleft area,[8] whereas Slayton et al reported an incidence of 48%

for missing lateral incisors for this patient population.[9] Shapira et al found a 77% incidence of hypodontia in nonsyndromic cleft children.[5] The tooth most commonly missing is the permanent maxillary lateral incisor (74% incidence) followed by the maxillary and mandibular second premolars.[5,6] Prosthetic treatment of implant prosthetics and fixed prosthetics are more commonly used to address these functional deficits.

EDENTULOUS CLEFT SITE

Although the lip and nose are satisfactorily repaired, inadequate bony contour, maxillary retrognathism, and hypodontia contribute to the severity of the facial deformity.[10] Hence, addressing the closure of the edentulous cleft site with bone grafting is critically important.[10-13] The objectives of bone grafting include providing bony support to the adjacent teeth, facilitating prosthetic restoration, providing bony matrix for tooth eruption into the cleft site, stabilizing the segments, elevating the alar base, eliminating the oronasal fistula, and providing adequate bone volume for implant placement.[14-16] Bone grafting is necessary in 30% to 40% of cleft palate patients.[11-13] It has been reported that the best results are achieved if the graft was done between the ages of 9 to 11 before

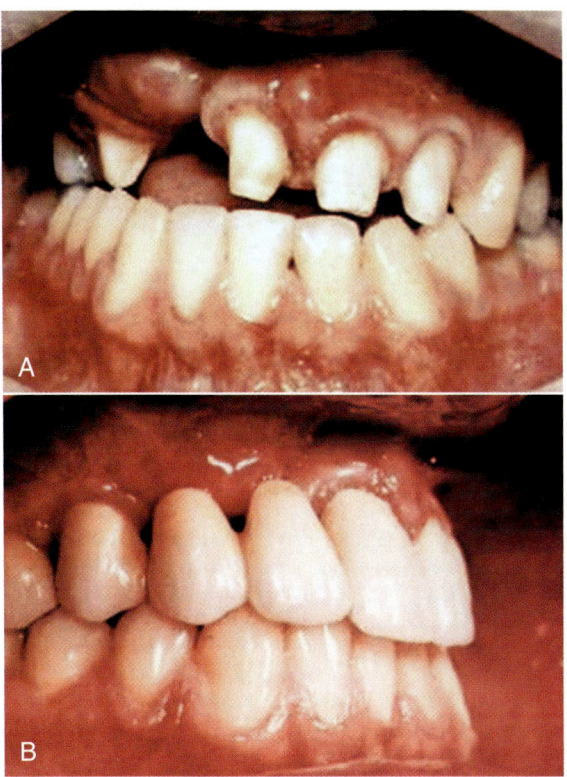

Fig. 89-5 ■ **A,** Fixed prosthesis used as a definitive prosthesis for a cleft palate patient. **B,** The definitive treatment of a fixed prosthesis.

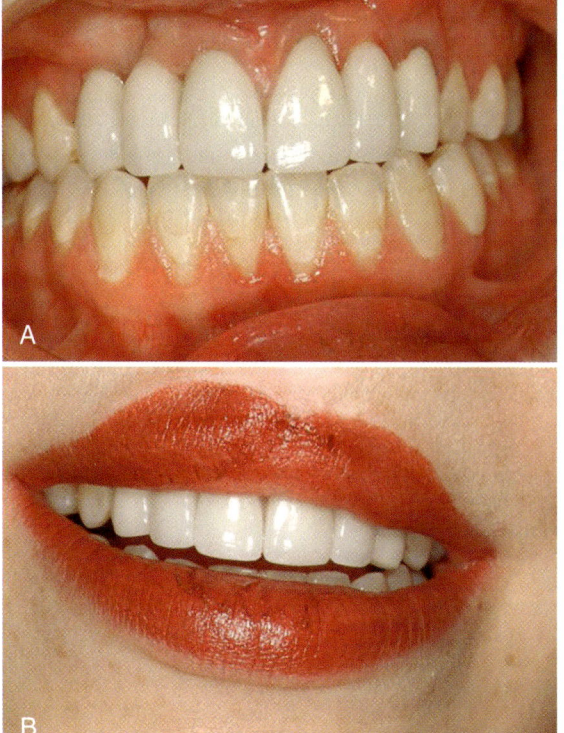

Fig. 89-6 ■ **A,** Definitive treatment of an implant crown and fixed prosthesis. **B,** The resulting smile.

the eruption of the canines.[17-21] Grafting allows the cleft to be restored either with orthodontics, conventional prosthodontics of either a removable partial denture or a fixed prosthesis, or implant prosthesis.[4,14,22]

Orthodontic management with or without orthognathic surgery guides the cuspid tooth into the lateral position.[13,17,20,23,24] This treatment will also require either a porcelain veneer or recontouring of the cuspid tooth into the shape of the lateral incisor. In addition, the premolar may have to be recontoured into the shape of the cuspid or will require placement of a porcelain veneer. In those instances in which the lateral incisor is malformed or having a "peg"-like appearance, a veneer of either porcelain or composite may be necessary.[4,22,25] It has been reported in the literature that positioning the cuspid tooth into the lateral incisor position may predispose the patient to occlusal dysfunction, as well as transversal discrepancy problems and poor aesthetics.[25,26] If grafting is not accomplished until after eruption of the canines, orthodontic closure is reduced to 72%, with an increase of 28% for prosthetic treatment.[11,20]

Conventional prosthodontics of either a removable partial denture or a fixed prosthesis may be used as a form of tooth replacement. In most instances, the orthodontist will incorporate a lateral incisor pontic tooth with the braces or the retainer. If a removable partial denture is used, it is usually used as a temporary measure only. It may have to be used as a definitive measure if there are multiple missing teeth with a long edentulous span that cannot be restored with fixed prosthesis or implant prosthesis. Most removable prostheses can cause tissue irritation. The known movement of the prosthesis contributes to decreased functions of speech and chewing and may contribute to a feeling of anxiety in the growing child. Rehabilitation of the cleft site with a fixed partial denture prosthesis or a resin-bonded prosthesis is another option (Fig. 89-5). With the

advent of dental implants, fixed and removable prosthesis are not commonly used as a definitive treatment option.[4,14]

The option that is probably most documented in the literature is the use of an implant prosthesis in the grafted alveolar cleft[14,22] (Fig. 89-6). Pena et al found that grafting the site with autologous bone had the highest success rates and is considered the gold standard.[14] Most studies recommend grafting of the cleft between the ages of 9 and 11 years.[14,17-21] This will allow space for the implant. The two critical factors for implant success are the timing of implant placement and implant type.[14]

It has been well documented that implants with a length of 13 mm have a higher survival rate than shorter implants in the grafted alveolar clefts.[14,26-28] Also, implant diameter and surface characteristics may affect implant survival success.[14] Implants placed immediately after bone grafting have been shown to have a high rate of failure due to lack of stability.[14,22,26-28] Numerous studies report that the most important factor in implant success or failure is the timing of secondary bone grafting and implant placement.[14,22,26-28] Most studies recommend a two-stage procedure of grafting and implant placement, with the ideal time of implant placement being 6 months later.[1,14,22,26] The work of Kearns et al showed a 90% success rate in the two-stage procedure, with an average follow-up between implantation and subsequent follow-up of 39.1 months,[22] whereas Hartel et al reported a success rate of 96%, with an average follow-up of 28 months.[29] Matsui et al reported a success rate of 99% for the two-stage procedure, with an average follow-up of 60 months.[26] Longer wait times of greater than 6 months contributed to a loss of interdental alveolar bone height and thickness.[14] If the graft is placed between the ages of 8 and 11 years, an implant should not be placed 6 months later, because the implant performs as an ankylosed tooth and may not be at the ideal location after craniofacial growth is complete. Therefore, if the graft is done between the ages of 8 and 11 years, it is recommended that the alveolus is regrafted at 15 to 17 years of age, with implant placement 6 months later.[14]

CONCLUSION

Although the role of prosthodontics in the growing cleft child has diminished, the resulting discoveries in surgical reconstruction and nasoalveolar molding have transformed the treatment so functional and aesthetic results are optimized.

REFERENCES

1. Dempf R, Teltzrow T, Kramer FJ, Hausamen JE, et al: Alveolar bone grafting in patients with complete clefts: a comparative study between secondary and tertiary bone grafting. *Cleft Palate Craniofac J* 39(1):18-25, 2002.
2. Endriga MC, Kapp-Simon KA: Psychological issues in craniofacial care: state of the art. *Cleft Palate Craniofac J* 36:3-11, 1999.
3. Hickey AJ, Salter M: Prosthodontic and psychological factors in treating patients with congenital and craniofacial defects. *J Prosthet Dent* 95(5):392-396, 2006.
4. Reisberg D: Dental and prosthodontic care for patients with cleft or craniofacial conditions. *Cleft Palate Craniofac J* 37(6):534-537, 2000.
5. Shapira Y, Lubit E, Kuftinec MM: Congenitally missing second premolars in cleft lip and cleft palate children. *Am J Orthod Dentofac Orthop* 115:396-400, 1999.
6. Oberoi S, Vargervik K: Hypoplasia and hypodontia in Van der Woude syndrome. *Cleft Palate Craniofac J* 42:459-466, 2005.
7. Ranta R: A review of tooth formation in children with cleft lip/palate. *Am J Orthod Dentofac Orthop* 90:11-18, 1986.
8. Bohn A: Dental abnormalities in harelip and cleft palate. *Acta Odont Scand* 21:1-109, 1963.
9. Slayton RL, Williams L, Murray JC, et al: Genetic association studies of cleft lip and/or palate with hypodontia outside the cleft region. *Cleft Palate Craniofac J* 2003;40:274-279.
10. Bergland O, Semb G, Aryholm F: Elimination of the residual alveolar cleft by secondary bone grafting and subsequent orthodontic treatment. *Cleft Palate J* 23:175-204, 1986.
11. Duskova M, Kotova M, Sedlakova K, et al: Bone reconstruction of the maxillary alveolus for subsequent insertion of a dental implant in patients with cleft lip and palate. *J Craniofac Surg* 18(3):630-638, 2007.
12. McCarthy J: *Plastic surgery*, vol 4, *Cleft lip and palate and craniofacial anomalies*. Philadelphia, 1990, Elsevier.
13. Boyne P, Sands N: Combined orthodontic-surgical management of residual palato-alveolar cleft defects. *Am J Orthod* 70:20-37, 1976.
14. Pena WA, Vargervik K, Sharma A, Oberoi S: The role of endosseous implant in the management of alveolar clefts. *Pediatr Dent* 31(4):329-333, 2009.
15. Isono H, Kaida K, Hamada Y, et al: The reconstruction of bilateral clefts using endosseous implants after bone grafting. *Am J Orthod Dentofac Orthop* 121:403-410, 2002.
16. Hogan L, Shand JM, Heggie AA, Kilpatrick N: Canine eruption into grafted alveolar clefts: a retrospective study. *Aust Dent J* 48:119-124, 2003.
17. Jia YL, Fu MK, Ma L: Long-term outcome of secondary alveolar bone grafting in patients with various types of clefts. *Br J Oral Maxillofac Surg* 44:308-312, 2006.
18. Enemark H, Sindet-Pedersen S, Bundgaard M: Long-term results after secondary bone grafting of the alveolar clefts. *J Oral Maxillofac Surg* 45:913-919, 1987.
19. Hall DH, Posnick JC: Early results of secondary bone grafts in 106 alveolar clefts. *J Oral Maxillofac Surg* 41:289-294, 1983.
20. Bergland O, Semb G, Abyholm F: Elimination of the residual alveolar clefts by secondary bone grafting and subsequent orthodontic treatment. *Cleft Palate J* 23:175-205, 1986.
21. Jia YL, James DR, Mars M: Bilateral alveolar bone grafting: a report of 55 consecutively-treated patients. *Eur J Orthod* 20:299-307, 1998.
22. Kearns G, Perrott DH, Sharma A, et al: Placement of endosseous implants in grafted alveolar clefts. *Cleft Palate Craniofac J* 34(6):520-525, 1997.
23. Amanat N, Langdon JD: Secondary alveolar bone grafting in clefts of the lip and palate. *J Craniomaxillofac Surg* 19:7-14, 1991.
24. Johanson B, Ohlsson A, Friede H, Ahlgren J: A follow-up study of cleft lip and palate patients treated with orthodontics, secondary bone grafting and prosthetic rehabilitation. *Scand J Plastic Reconstr Surg* 8:121-135, 1974.
25. D'Amico A: The canine teeth—normal functional relationship of the natural teeth in man. *J South Calif Dent Assoc* 26:127-142, 1958.
26. Matsui Y, Ohno K, Nishimura K, et al: Long-term study of dental implants placed into alveolar cleft sites. *Cleft Palate Craniofac J* 44(4):444-447, 2007.
27. Kramer FJ, Baethge C, Swennen G, et al: Dental implants in patients with orofacial clefts: a long-term followup study. *Int J Oral Maxillofac Surg* 34:715-721, 2005.
28. Takahashi T, Fukuda M, Yamaguchi T, Kochi S: Use of endosseous implants for dental reconstruction of patients with grafted alveolar clefts. *J Oral Maxillofac Surg* 55:576-583, 1997.
29. Hartel J, Pogl C, Henkel K, Gundlach K: Dental implants in alveolar cleft patients: a retrospective study. *J Craniomaxillofac Surg* 27:354-357, 1999.

Chapter 90

Nonsyndromic Single Suture Craniosynostosis

Pat Ricalde

Craniosynostosis is a congenital defect resulting in the premature fusion of one or more cranial sutures. There are eight bones that make up the human cranium. In infancy, they are separated from each other by fibrous tissue junctions called sutures. Sutures undergo ossification during postnatal development and distinguish an adult from an infant skull (Fig. 90-1). If sutures fuse prenatally, brain growth cannot occur perpendicular to the fused suture. Growth will occur parallel to the suture, causing a potential cosmetic and functional deterioration. Although craniosynostosis occurs in about 1 in 2000 live births, its etiology is still widely unknown. It has a similar prevalence to those affected with colorectal cancer (1 per 1,800) but is certainly not as well known to the general population, nor is its research as well funded. The sagittal suture is the most commonly involved cranial suture, followed by the coronal and the metopic. Lambdoid synostosis is the rarest.

ETIOLOGY

The mineralization of the cranial vault begins around 13 weeks' gestation from several ossification centers. At around 18 weeks, the bone edges meet and sutures are induced. The suture is two plates of bone separated by a narrow space of immature, rapidly dividing osteogenic stem cells. Some of these differentiate to osteoblasts and create new bone. The skull initially enlarges by sutural expansion, with deposition of bone matrix along suture margins. This is particularly important during infancy, when the brain and skull grow exponentially, reaching 80% of adult size by 1 year of age. After this, the rate of skull growth significantly tapers off, the skull thickens, and the sutures become firmer with ossification. Skull growth continues but now relies on the much slower process of resorption and deposition that has been described by Enlow. At this point, the ongoing growth of the brain stimulates resorption of bone from the inner cortex of the cranium and deposition of bone to the outer cortex. When one or more sutures prematurely fuse, the harmonious patterns of skull growth change. These changes were described by Virchow in 1851. He suggested that skull growth is restricted in a plane perpendicular to the affected prematurely fused suture and compensates at the open sutures. Thus, growth occurs parallel to the closed suture. This theory persists today as the main one explaining the observed clinical changes.

It is believed that both genetic and environmental factors contribute to craniosynostosis. Abnormal mechanical forces have been suggested as a predisposing factor. Family history of associated anomalies suggests a genetic link. Over 100 syndromes have been described as associated with craniosynostosis. Many different mutations of six principal genes, *MSX2, FGFR1, FGFR2, FGFR3, FBN1,* and *TWIST,* have craniosynostosis as a primary clinical feature.

DIAGNOSIS

Patients with craniosynostosis classically present with a misshapen head, which can easily be mistaken for simple deformational molding. Craniosynostosis is present at the time of birth. Because of the natural changes that occur in an infant's craniofacial morphology during the first few months of life, the shape of the skull can appear to worsen with time. Deformational molding, on the other hand, will tend to improve with time. Because craniosynostosis is a true malformation of the skull, traditional treatments for deformational molding (including repositioning techniques and cranial molding appliances) will not be effective in true craniosynostosis.

The distinction of craniosynostosis from deformational molding is imperative. The diagnosis of craniosynostosis is usually a clinical one. Careful history, along with clinical examination by a competent practitioner, is usually satisfactory. Each type of suture closure causes a typical and recognizable cranial malformation. There have been many reports of misdiagnosis, which were unfortunately brought to light by the Wall Street Journal in 1996 after the Centers for Disease Control (CDC) was called out to investigate a 400% increase in incidence of craniosynostosis in the Colorado region. Many patients had unnecessary surgery, which led to the careful review and publication of the clinical differences between the two conditions by Huang et al.

CRANIOSYNOSTOSIS SYNDROMES

METOPIC CRANIOSYNOSTOSIS

Metopic synostosis typically causes a narrow forehead, bulging biparietal areas, a ridge over the metopic suture, and recessed lateral orbital rims. Patients can have apparent or true hypotelorism. Their overall cranial morphology is trigonocephalic. Up to a third of these patients will be syndromic, and many of these syndromic patients will have developmental delays.

UNICORONAL CRANIOSYNOSTOSIS

Patients with unicoronal synostosis typically develop a plagiocephalic cranial morphology. On the affected side, there is a flattened forehead, elevation of the supraorbital rim, widening of the palpebral fissure, a recessed lateral orbital rim, and deviation of the nasal radix toward the fused suture. The orbit on the involved side is small, and the globe is proptotic. The chin point can be deviated toward the opposite side, and the posterior cranial vault is rarely symmetrical due to compensatory changes. There is usually a palpable ridge over the fused suture.

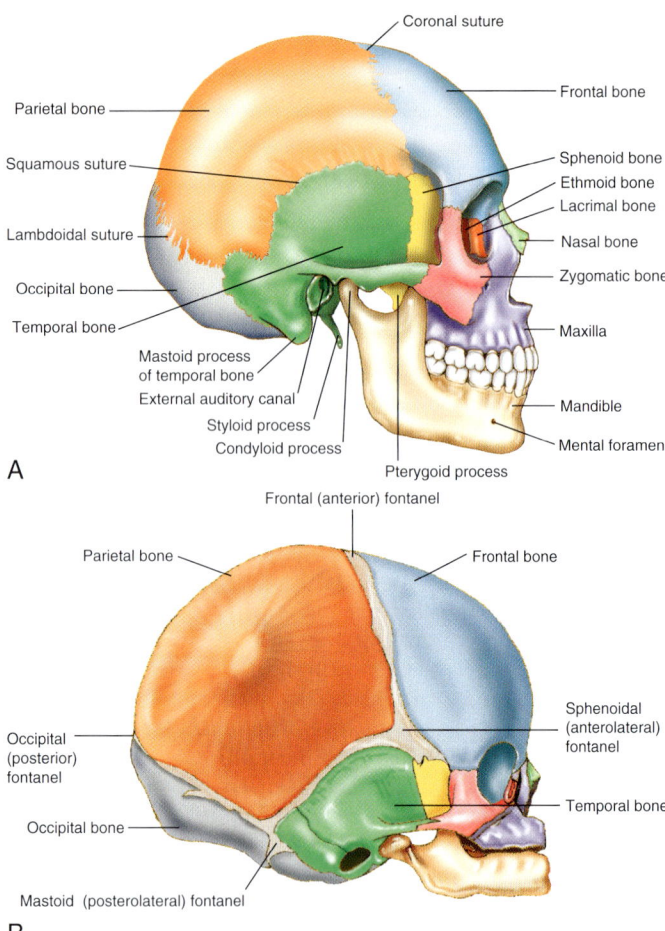

A

B

Fig. 90-1 ■ Adult (**A**) and infant (**B**) skull anatomy. (From Sanders MJ: Mosby's paramedic textbook, ed 3. St Louis, 2007, Mosby.)

SAGITTAL CRANIOSYNOSTOSIS

Sagittal synostosis typically results in a scaphocephalic (keel-shaped) head. The bitemporal and biparietal dimensions are narrow, the forehead bossed, and the occipital region is prominent. There is sometimes an occipital shelf. A ridge is often palpable over the fused suture. These head shapes are most likely to be confused with the deformational molding that takes place in babies with prolonged hospital stays, for instance, premature infants.

LAMBDOID CRANIOSYNOSTOSIS

Lambdoid synostosis is quite rare—1 in 30,000 births. The presentation can be most difficult to distinguish from deformational molding, because the head shape typically is plagiocephalic. The vertical ear position from an occipital view reveals inferior displacement on the affected side. There may be a ridge over the fused suture and posterior displacement of the ear toward the ipsilateral side. The head shape from a vertex view has been described as trapezoidal. Often there is an associated head tilt. With positional plagiocephaly, the head shape is rhomboidal, or like a parallelogram.

Isolated squamosal, cranial base, or facial craniosynostosis are exceedingly rare. Red flags that should raise suspicion for cranio-synostosis are enumerated in Box 90-1.

NATURAL HISTORY

Because the fusion occurs prenatally, the abnormal cranial morphology is present at the time of birth. However, this can appear to worsen over the first several months as the baby grows, develops

---

BOX 90-1   "Red Flags" during Assessment That May Indicate Craniosynostosis

- Misshapen head present at birth
- Early repositioning techniques do not improve the abnormal head shape
- Ridging over the suture
- Small, displaced, or absent fontanel
- Trapezoid head shape from vertex view
- Inferiorly displaced ear from occipital view
- Orbital involvement—wide palpebral fissure
- Other—abnormal bulges, facial asymmetry, associated with developmental delays, severity of case

---

better tone, and begins to redistribute some of the initial deformational soft tissue changes that occur during the birthing process. The infant brain is rapidly expanding against this area of constriction where the fusion has occurred. This rapid expansion is the stimulus to the skull to grow and makes the deformation more obvious. If left untreated, negative neurologic consequences may develop. In general, single suture synostosis should not cause cerebral damage. This is a very difficult to study, and because of ethical dilemmas, many questions about this condition will likely never be answered. In 1982, Renier et al. published a landmark study describing placement of epidural pressure catheters in 92 patients with cranio-synostosis. They found that 14% of patients with single suture craniosynostosis developed an elevation of intracranial pressure, compared with 42% of patients with multiple sutures involved. Increased intracranial pressure can lead to various neurologic compromises, such as developmental delays, headaches, irritability, behavioral changes, decreased vision, and cognitive delays. True symptoms related to increased intracranial pressure in patients with single-suture craniosynostosis have rarely been reported prior to the age of 1 and (in some cases) can reemerge after cranial vault expansion. These are often insidious findings, can be difficult to detect, and can be irreversible.

Hydrocephalus is not commonly associated with nonsyndromic single suture craniosynostosis, but may occur independently and not necessarily as a consequence of the condition. Ophthalmologic changes, however, can be a direct effect of craniosynostosis. Papilledema, optic nerve atrophy, loss of vision, exophthalmos, orbital dystopia, ptosis, strabismus, corneal erosions, or ulcers are all potential risks.

IMAGING

The diagnosis is primarily a clinical one. Imaging studies can confirm the diagnosis of craniosynostosis but may not be necessary and can expose the patient to significant radiation. Plain films can reveal the absence of an open suture or calcification along the suture edge. This calcification can however be seen with secondary synostosis. Craniosynostosis can also be identified using computed tomography (CT) with three-dimensional (3D) reconstruction. The use of imaging studies should be carefully selected, because they are sometimes also used for surgical planning. Therefore, if cranio-synostosis is suspected, it is prudent to make a referral to the treating surgeon and allow him or her to order the study. It is also helpful to avoid the use of outdated and improper terminology when describing this condition. Terms such as fibrous synostosis, suture dysfunction, and impending synostosis are misleading. This may be confusing to parents and health care providers and can result in inappropriate treatment.

Careful consideration should be employed prior to radiographic exposure of the pediatric patient. Awareness of the potential harm to the developing eyes and brain has led to a national "image gently" campaign, and some interest has surfaced regarding the use of ultrasonography for diagnosis.

TREATMENT TIMING

Surgery for craniosynostosis has evolved over the years. Initial reports described removing the affected suture by a "strip craniectomy." The goal was to decompress the brain and allow for its continued normal growth to correct the cranial deformity. Results were frequently unsatisfactory, probably because the surgery was not adequate to allow for the necessary cranial remodeling prior to the reossification of the bony segments. In an infant, reossification can occur quickly, even before the cranial shape has a chance to remold. Attempts to delay ossification with Zenker solution or Silastic strips were attempted. While strip craniectomies are still done endoscopically, external molding devices are used to accelerate natural shaping. Some began performing "extended strip craniectomies," where biparietal osteotomies were created to allow further cranial expansion. Many variations of the operation were developed, because there was no single procedure that gave consistently good results. After Paul Tessier developed the modern methods of craniofacial surgery employed today, these techniques were transferred to the management of craniosynostosis, and cranial vault reconstruction (CVR) evolved. The evolution has led to the understanding that both the timing of surgery and the techniques employed are equally important in patient outcomes.

There are two indications for operating on patients with craniosynostosis: functional and cosmetic. Nonsyndromic single suture craniosynostosis is not by itself associated with cognitive delay. Chronic increased intracranial pressure is. A certain percentage (about 15%) of children with nonsyndromic single suture craniosynostosis will have increased intracranial pressure. The infant's brain is protected by the rapid ability of the skull to expand. With multiple suture synostoses, this protection is compromised. Ideally, surgery is performed prior to the development of effects of increased intracranial pressure. Surgery is usually done within the first year of life. Secondly, esthetic concerns must be acknowledged. The goal is to correct the cranial malformation in one surgery so that risks are minimized and the results are long lasting. Operating on skeletally immature structures always demands the careful consideration of growth alteration and its effects.

Although there remains controversy in the literature regarding the ideal time to operate, the theoretical advantage of operating "early" (prior to 6 months) to prevent the deleterious effects of increased intracranial pressure has not been well assessed with outcome studies. Most who advocate this approach have inadequate sample sizes, follow-up, or present cases using subjective methods. One retrospective study looked at 296 patients and found that calvarial growth was abnormal after all surgeries, with a tendency toward recurrence of the primary deformity. Growth, however, was less diminished in procedures performed in older infants. This coincides with numerous studies that have looked at other growing craniofacial structures, and show that the most predictable results with the lowest long-term relapse occur when surgery is accomplished at or near growth cessation. Posnick et al looked at the issue of timing of surgery versus surgical outcomes in patients with craniosynostosis who were treated with CVR between the ages of 9 and 11 months. Standard measurements from CT scans were compared with age-matched normative values. They determined that long-term predictable results could be achieved. So, in effect, there is a delicate

balance between maximum functional and maximum aesthetic benefits that must be considered when planning for surgery.

BOX 90-2	General Treatment of Craniosynostosis Involving Forehead/Orbits (Coronal and Metopic)

- Preparation of the patient includes placement of two large intravenous catheters and an arterial line.
- Bilateral tarsorrhaphies are placed and the eyes draped in the field, if periorbital work is being done
- Bicoronal postauricular incision through skin, galea, and pericranium is accomplished while maintaining meticulous hemostasis.
- Fronto-orbital osteotomies are created.
- Orbital bandeau is separated through the nasofrontal junction, including the entire lateral orbital rim if affected.
- Temporal extension is accomplished as needed.
- Reconstruction using rigid fixation (resorbable or metal plates and screws).
- Layered closure with careful reapproximation of skin edges.

TREATMENT TECHNIQUE

The standardized surgical approach to cranial vault reconstruction is to remove the dysmorphic units, reshape and reconstruct the segments, and replace them in a rigid fashion. The exact placement of the osteotomies depends on the severity and type of the malformation. The approach is different for sagittal synostosis and for coronal or metopic synostosis (Box 90-2).

CASE EXAMPLES
Sagittal Craniosynostosis

The case is of an otherwise healthy boy born with sagittal craniosynostosis. At the age of 6 months, he underwent posterior cranial vault reconstruction (Fig. 90-2).

Metopic Craniosynostosis

The case is of an otherwise healthy boy born with metopic craniosynostosis. At the age of 9 months, he underwent anterior cranial vault reconstruction (Fig. 90-3).

Unicoronal Craniosynostosis

The case is of an otherwise healthy girl born with unicoronal craniosynostosis. At the age of 12 months, she underwent anterior cranial vault reconstruction (Fig. 90-4).

SPECIAL CONSIDERATIONS
RE-FUSION VERSUS REOSSIFICATION

It is important to distinguish the known, theorized, and unknown aspects of this condition. For example, it is known that when sutures fuse prior to birth, the patient has craniosynostosis. Fusion after surgery, however, is a theoretical condition and is actually poorly documented in the scientific literature. This secondary synostosis may occur in a child with severe hydrocephalus, macrocephaly, and cerebral damage or hydranencephaly who is shunted and has overlapping sutures. With time in this scenario, the overlapping sutures may fuse. The topic is often discussed, and the terminology is easy to confuse. Some argue that if a suture was never present, how could

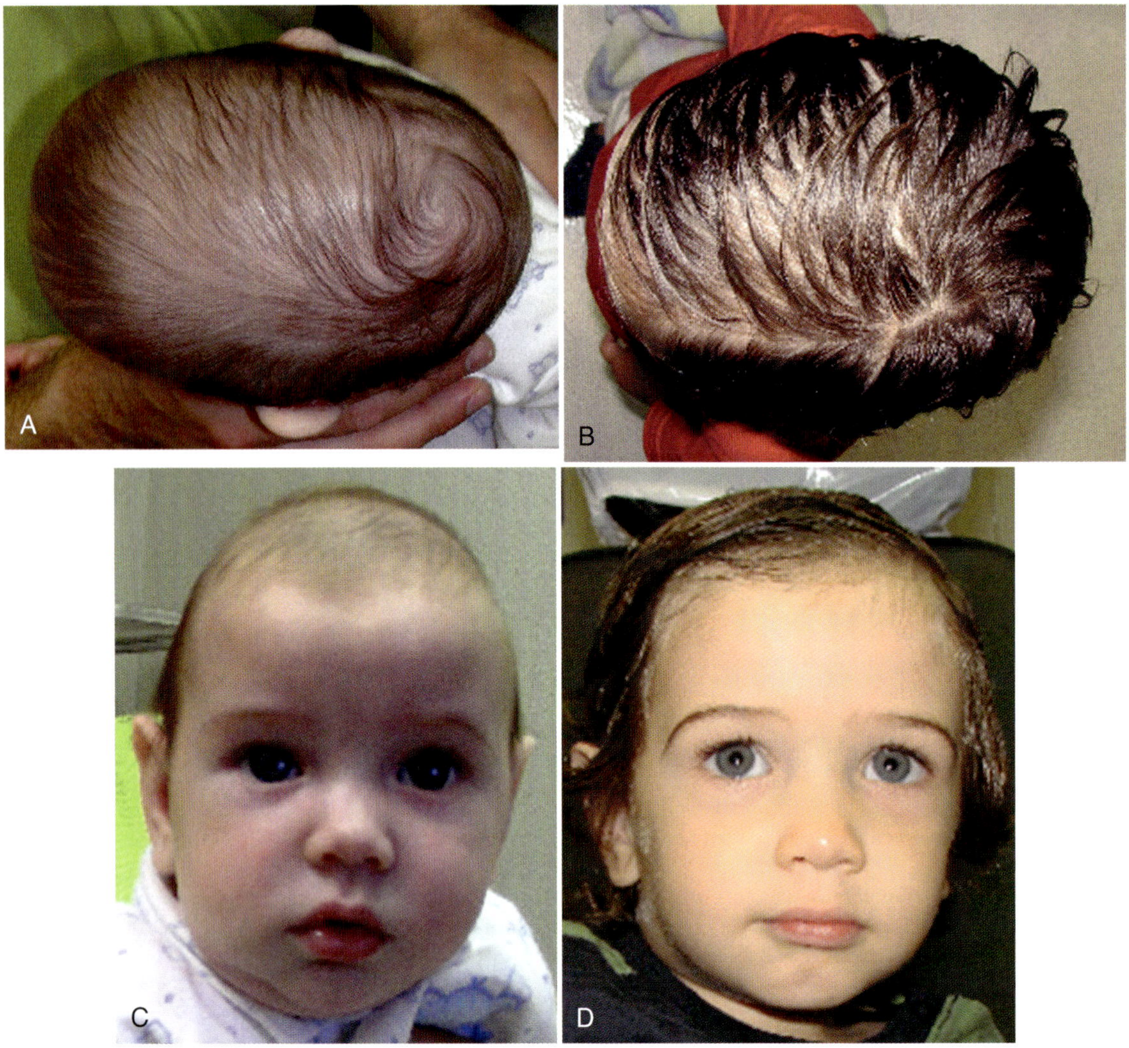

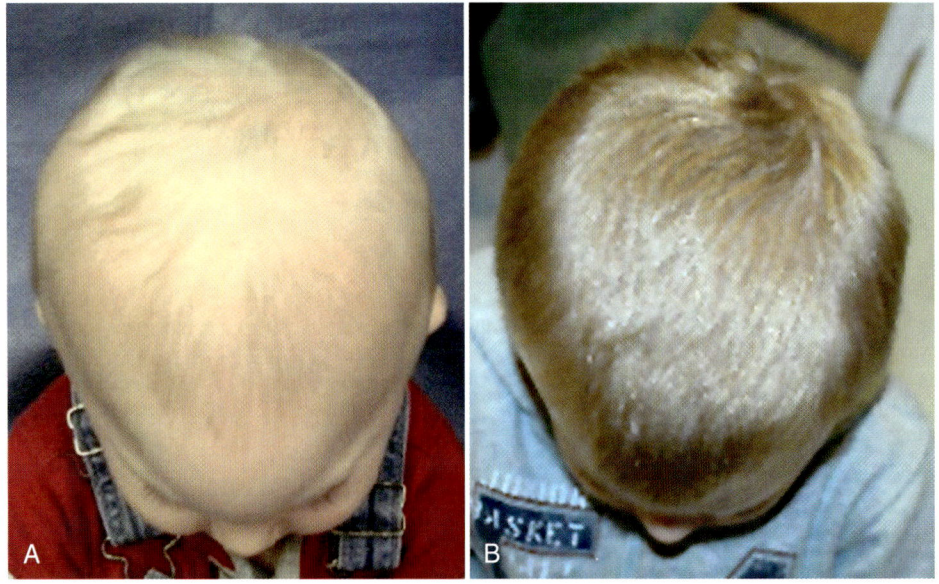

Fig. 90-2 ■ Sagittal synostosis. **A** and **B,** Top of head before and after treatment. **C** and **D,** Frontal view before and after treatment.

Fig. 90-3 ■ Metopic synostosis. **A** and **B,** Top of head before and after treatment.

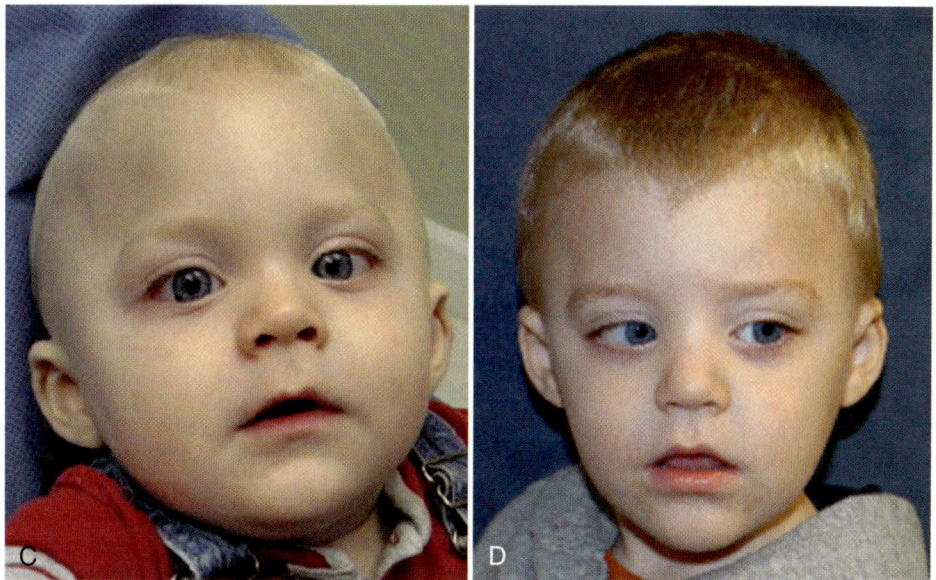

Fig. 90-3, cont'd ■ **C** and **D,** Frontal view before and after treatment.

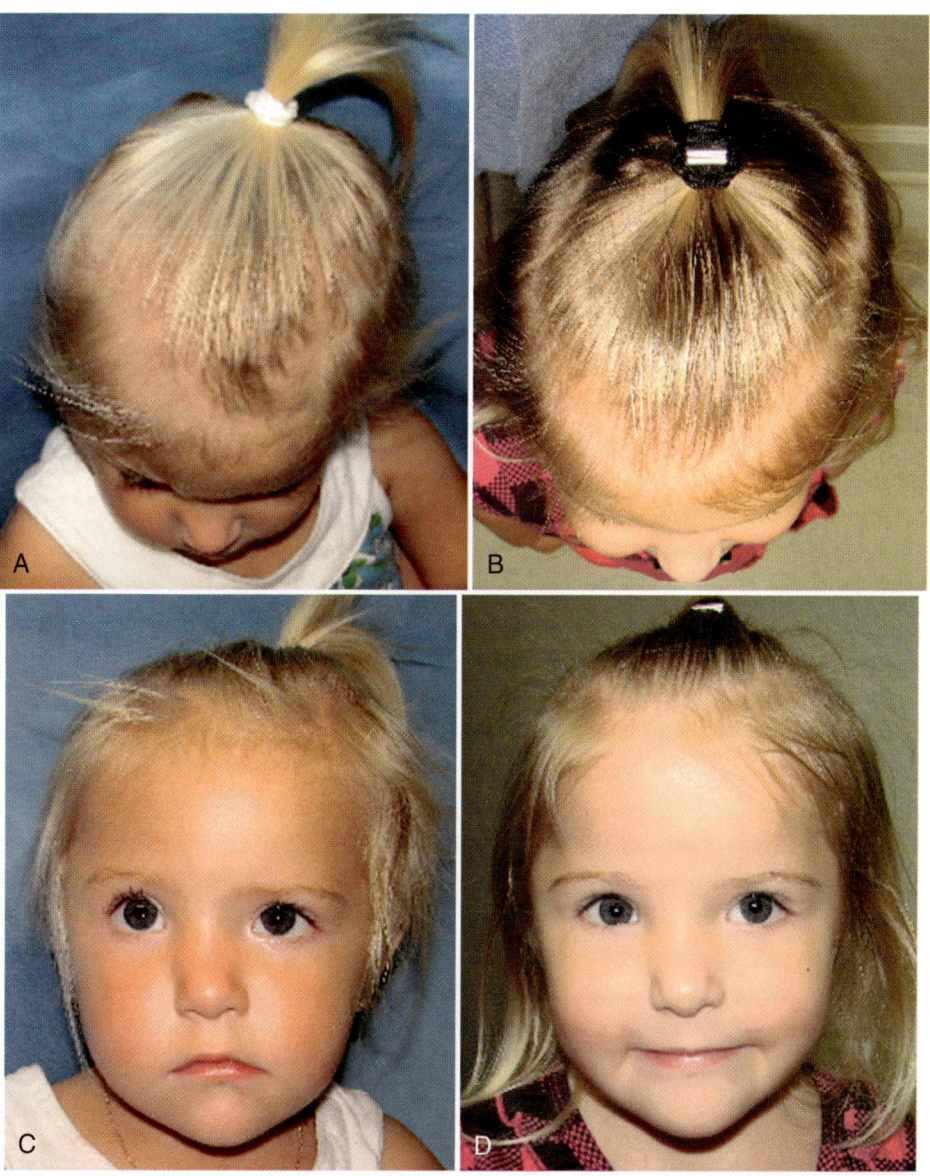

Fig. 90-4 ■ Unicoronal synostosis. **A** and **B,** Top of head before and after treatment. **C** and **D,** Frontal view before and after treatment.

it re-fuse. And how can we prove that the suture has re-fused, rather than the more common (more likely) scenario—that relapse has occurred? It is better to use the term *reossification*, rather than *refusion*, when cranial sutures are noted to be fused following an operation for craniosynostosis.

ENDOSCOPIC VERSUS TRADITIONAL TREATMENT

It is important to understand that the terms *endoscopic surgery* or *minimally invasive surgery* do not define the two critical components in determining the potential outcome of surgery (timing and technique). With endoscopic surgery, a smaller incision (or two) is made, and the endoscopy is essentially used as a light source to assist in surgery. The timing of surgery and the actual techniques performed are far more important in outcome assessments than whether an endoscope was used to assist the surgeon. Endoscopic surgery for craniosynostosis has become a heavily marketed and discussed topic. It became popular in the late 1990s when a series of articles were published on the topic. Those publications have been heavily criticized due to their lack of scientific format, generalizations ("all patients had excellent results"), and notable paucity of objective measurements or medical-quality photographs. Nevertheless, claims of performing surgical repair using minimally invasive techniques with less blood loss and decreased length of hospital stay are attractive. Upon review of the published data regarding endoscopic surgery for the management of craniosynostosis, the actual technique that was initially employed was a strip craniectomy. Although documentation is sparse, it appears that history has repeated itself. As in the early 1900s, early relapse has been a problem. Modifications were employed (as they were 100 years ago) by extending the craniectomies to improve results. This was followed by another modification, the addition of a cranial orthotic device for about a year postsurgery, to try remolding the head shape and to improve the less-than-desirable cosmesis from the surgery alone. Although these procedures have been employed for many years, outcome studies are still not available. This author believes that eventually a clear role for the endoscopic treatment of this condition will surface. It will likely be most beneficial for the management of "mild" sagittal and lambdoid craniosynostosis, with minimal or no facial concerns. The forehead and periorbital region do not improve with a helmet.

RIGID INTERNAL FIXATION: METAL VERSUS RESORBABLE IMPLANTS

Plate and screw internal fixation has been a major advance in the management of craniomaxillofacial deformities. Its use is firmly established as a device to assist bone healing and to achieve 3D morphologic changes in the craniomaxillofacial skeleton. Concerns over the placement of metallic internal fixation in the immature (growing) skeleton have been raised. Although there are no reports in the literature that the metallic implants have caused "major"

deleterious effects (e.g., stroke, seizure, intracranial bleeds, neurologic compromise), the observed translocation of hardware in association with ongoing cranial growth has resulted in the development of resorbable internal fixation as an alternative. The disadvantages of these resorbable implants are the decreased strength as compared with their metallic counterparts and the prolonged resorption times. There seems to be a direct inverse relationship between strength and resorption rates. Presumably, stronger plates allow better morphologic results with less relapse.

TEAM APPROACH TO THERAPY: A NEW STANDARD OF CARE

Historically, the management of craniosynostosis has been by a neurosurgeon working alone or in conjunction with a general plastic surgeon. Since the development of formal craniofacial training programs, neurosurgeons and craniofacial surgeons working together as part of a craniofacial team have emerged and set a new standard of care for the management of these patients. These teams can include a developmental specialist, psychologist, dentist, orthodontist, otolaryngologist, geneticist, speech/physical/occupational therapist, audiologist, ophthalmologist, and social worker, among others. The advantage of the team approach to therapy is multifold. Each discipline has an opportunity to examine the patient and prepare the parents with short- and long-term goals. There is dialogue among the practitioners, which can stimulate new ideas and management strategies, especially for complex treatment plans. Coordination of care is much more streamlined, saving the patient/parent multiple doctor visits, tests, radiation exposure, cost, time away from work and school, and, most importantly, the "sick kid" mentality.

PEARLS AND PITFALLS

- Nonsyndromic single suture craniosynostosis typically presents as a misshapen head with various degrees of severity.
- It is imperative that craniosynostosis is distinguished from deformational molding. Ideally, this is accomplished in one procedure, to minimize risks.
- The surgeon has one opportunity to meet these goals, because once the pediatric cranium has been operated on, its growth and development are altered.
- Ill-timed approaches to management cannot be reversed; thus, new techniques should be examined carefully using prospective trials with a control group and a thorough informed consent process through an institutional review board.
- A craniofacial team with a focus on streamlining care and minimizing interventions should follow these patients.

BIBLIOGRAPHY

Arnaud E, Renier D: Pediatric craniofacial osteosynthesis and distraction using an ultrasonic-assisted pinned resorbable system: a prospective report with a minimum 30 months' follow-up. *J Craniofac Surg* 20(6): 2081-2086, 2009.

Barone CM, Jimenez DF: Endoscopic craniectomy for early correction of craniosynostosis. *Plast Reconstr Surg* 104(7):1965-1973, 1999; discussion 1974-1975.

Cartwright CC, Jimenez DF, Barone CM, Baker L: Endoscopic strip craniectomy: a minimally invasive treatment for early correction of craniosynostosis. *J Neurosci Nurs* 35(3):130-138, 2003.

Currarino G: Premature closure of the frontozygomatic suture: unusual frontoorbital dysplasia mimicking unilateral coronal synostosis.

AJNR Am J Neuroradiol 6(4):643-646, 1985.

Enlow DH: *Handbook of craniofacial growth,* Philadelphia, 1990, Saunders.

Faber HK, Towne EB: Early craniectomy as preventive measure in oxycephaly and allied conditions with special reference to the prevention of blindness. *Am J Med Sci* 173:701, 1927.

Fearon JA, Ruotolo RA, Kolar JC: Single sutural craniosynostoses: surgical outcomes and long-term growth. *Plast Reconstr Surg* 123(2):635-642, 2009.

French LR, Jackson IT, Melton LJ 3rd: A population-based study of craniosynostosis. *J Clin Epidemiol* 43(1):69-73, 1990.

Huang MH, Mouradian WE, Cohen SR, Gruss JS: The differential diagnosis of abnormal head shapes: separating craniosynostosis from positional deformities and normal variants. *Cleft Palate Craniofac J* 35(3):204-211, 1998.

Jimenez DF, Barone CM: Endoscopic craniectomy for early surgical correction of sagittal craniosynostosis. *J Neurosurg* 88(1):77-81, 1998.

Jimenez DF, Barone CM: Endoscopy-assisted wide-vertex craniectomy, "barrel-stave" osteotomies, and postoperative helmet molding therapy in the early management of sagittal suture craniosynostosis. *Neurosurg Focus* 9(3):e2, 2000.

Jimenez DF, Barone CM, Argamaso RV, et al: Asterion region synostosis. *Cleft Palate Craniofac J* 31(2):136-141, 1994.

Jimenez DF, Barone CM, Cartwright CC, Baker L: Early management of craniosynostosis using endoscopic-assisted strip craniectomies and cranial orthotic molding therapy. *Pediatrics* 110(1 Pt 1):97-104, 2002.

Jimenez DF, Barone CM, McGee ME, et al: Endoscopy-assisted wide-vertex craniectomy, barrel stave osteotomies, and postoperative helmet molding therapy in the management of sagittal suture craniosynostosis. *J Neurosurg* 100(Suppl 5 Pediatrics):407-417, 2004.

Kohan E, Wexler A, Cahan L, et al: Sagittal synostotic twins: reverse pi procedure for scaphocephaly correction gives superior result compared to endoscopic repair followed by helmet therapy. *J Craniofac Surg* 19(6):1453-1458, 2008.

Lane LC: Pioneer craniectomy for relief of mental imbecility due to premature sutural closure and microcephalus. *JAMA* 18:49, 1892.

Lannelongue M: De la craniectomie dans la microcephalie. *Compte Rendu Acad Sci* 110:1382, 1890.

Marchac D, Renier D: Treatment of craniosynostosis in infancy. *Clin Plast Surg* 14(1):61-72, 1987.

McCarthy JG, Glasberg SB, Cutting CB, et al: Sagittal craniosynostosis outcome assessment for two methods and timings of intervention. *Plast Reconstr Surg* 103(6):1574-1584, 1999.

Posnick JC, Armstrong D, Bite U: Metopic and sagittal synostosis: intracranial volume measurements prior to and after cranio-orbital reshaping in childhood. *Plast Reconstr Surg* 96(2):299-309, 1995; discussion 310-315.

Posnick JC, Lin KY, Chen P, Armstrong D: Sagittal synostosis: quantitative assessment of presenting deformity and surgical results based on CT scans. *Plast Reconstr Surg* 92(6):1015-1024, 1993; discussion 1225-1226.

Pyle J, Glazier S, Couture D, et al: Spring-assisted surgery—a surgeon's manual for the manufacture and utilization of springs in craniofacial surgery. *J Craniofac Surg* 20(6):1962-1968, 2009.

Renier D, Sainte-Rose C, Marchac D, Hirsch JF: Intracranial pressure in craniostenosis. *J Neurosurg* 57(3):370-377, 1982.

Sanchez-Lara PA, Carmichael SL, Graham JM Jr, et al: National Birth Defects Prevention Study. Fetal constraint as a potential risk factor for craniosynostosis. *Am J Med Genet A* 152A(2):394-400, 2010.

Tellado MG, Lema A: Coronal suturectomy through minimal incisions and distraction osteogenesis are enough without other craniotomies for the treatment of plagiocephaly due to coronal synostosis. *J Craniofac Surg* 20(6):1975-1977, 2009.

Virchow R: Ueber den Cretinismus, namentlich in Franken, und über pathologische Schädelformen. *Verh Physikalisch Med Ges Würzburg* 2:230-271, 1851.

Whitaker LA, Bartlett SP, Schut L, Bruce D: Craniosynostosis: an analysis of the timing, treatment, and complications in 164 consecutive patients. *Plast Reconstr Surg* 80(2):195-212, 1987.

Wisoff J, Zide BM: Twenty-year experience with early surgery for craniosynostosis: I. Isolated craniofacial synostosis—results and unsolved problems. *Plast Reconstr Surg* 96(2):272-283, 1995.

Craniofacial Dysostosis Syndromes

Chapter 91

Jeffrey C. Posnick, Ramon L. Ruiz, Paul S. Tiwana

Cranial vault sutures are a form of bone articulation in which the margins of the bones are connected by a thin layer of fibrous tissue. The cranial vault of an infant is composed of six major sutural areas and several minor sutures, which serve two critical functions during the postnatal period. Initially, the sutures allow head deformation during vaginal delivery as part of the birthing process. Later, during an infant's postnatal development, cranial vault sutures facilitate head expansion to accommodate propulsive brain growth. Only a small amount of pressure (5 mm Hg) from the growing brain is required to stimulate bone deposition at the margins of a cranial bone. Under normal conditions, brain volume will triple within the first year of life, and by 2 years of age, cranial capacity is four times that at birth. Under normal circumstances, closure of the cranial vault sutures occurs earlier than closure of the membranous facial bone sutures, which often remain patent until adulthood.

The term *craniosynostosis* is defined as premature fusion of a cranial vault suture. With rare exception, this is an intrauterine event. Virchow, in 1851, coined the term *craniosynostosis* and formulated the classic theory known as Virchow's law. This states that premature fusion of a cranial vault suture (craniosynostosis) inhibits normal skull growth perpendicular to the fused suture and that compensatory growth occurs at the open sutures. The general direction of growth after synostosis is parallel to the fused suture.

The term *craniofacial dysostosis* is used in a general way to describe syndromic forms of craniosynostosis. These disorders are characterized by sutural involvement that not only includes the cranial vault but also extends into the skull base and mid-facial skeletal structures. Craniofacial dysostosis syndromes have been described by Carpenter, Apert, Crouzon, Saethre and Chotzen, and Pfeiffer. Although the cranial vault and cranial base are thought to be the regions of primary involvement, there is also significant impact on mid-facial growth and development. In addition to cranial vault dysmorphology, patients with these inherited conditions exhibit a characteristic "total mid-face" deficiency that is syndrome specific and must be addressed as part of a staged reconstructive approach.

FUNCTIONAL CONSIDERATIONS

RESTRICTED BRAIN GROWTH AND INTRACRANIAL PRESSURE

If the rapid brain growth that normally occurs during infancy is to proceed unhindered, the cranial vault and base sutures must remain open and expand during the phases of rapid growth, with marginal ossification taking place. In craniosynostosis, premature fusion of the suture or sutures causes limited and abnormal skeletal expansion in the presence of continued brain growth. Depending on the number and location of prematurely fused sutures, growth of the brain may be restricted. In addition, abnormal cranial vault and mid-facial morphology occurs. If surgical release of the affected sutures and reshaping to restore a more normal intracranial volume and configuration are not performed, decreased cognitive and behavioral function is likely to be the end result.

Elevated intracranial pressure (ICP) is the most serious functional problem associated with premature fusion of sutures. Radiographic findings that may suggest elevated ICP include a "beaten-copper" appearance along the inner table of the cranial vault seen on plain radiographs and loss of brain cisternae observed on computed tomography (CT). Though suggestive of increased ICP, these are considered soft radiographic findings.

Increased ICP is most likely to affect patients with great disparity between brain growth and intracranial capacity and may occur in as many as 42% of untreated children in whom more than one suture is affected. Unfortunately, there is no absolute agreement on what levels of ICP are normal at any given age in infancy and early childhood.

The clinical signs and symptoms related to elevated ICP may have a slow onset and be difficult to recognize in the pediatric population. Although standardized CT allows indirect measurement of intracranial volume, it is not yet possible to use these studies to make judgments on those who require craniotomy for decompression. Careful neurosurgical and pediatric ophthalmologic evaluation is a critical component of the data-gathering process required to formulate definitive treatment plans in patients with craniosynostosis.

VISION

Untreated craniosynostosis with elevated ICP will cause papilledema and eventually optic nerve atrophy and result in partial or complete blindness. If the orbits are shallow (exorbitism) and the eyes are proptotic (exophthalmos), as occurs in the craniofacial dysostosis syndromes, the cornea may be exposed and abrasions or ulcerations could occur. An eyeball extending outside a shallow orbit is also at risk for trauma. If the orbits are extremely shallow, herniation of the globe itself may occur and necessitate emergency reduction followed by tarsorrhaphy or urgent orbital decompression.

Some forms of craniofacial dysostosis result in a marked degree of orbital hypertelorism that may compromise visual acuity and restrict binocular vision. Divergent or convergent non-paralytic strabismus or exotropia occurs frequently and should be considered during the diagnostic evaluation. This may be the result of congenital anomalies of the extraocular muscles themselves. Paralytic or non-paralytic unilateral or bilateral upper eyelid ptosis also occurs with greater frequency than in the general population.

HYDROCEPHALUS

Hydrocephalus affects as many as 10% of patients with a craniofacial dysostosis syndrome. Although the cause is often not clear, hydrocephalus may be secondary to generalized cranial base stenosis with constriction of all the cranial base foramina, which has an impact on the patient's cerebral venous drainage and cerebrospinal fluid (CSF) flow dynamics. Hydrocephalus may be identified with the help of CT or magnetic resonance imaging to document progressively enlarging ventricles. Difficulty exists in interpreting the ventricular findings seen on CT, especially when the skull and cranial base are brachycephalic. The skeletal dysmorphology present in a child with severe cranial dysmorphology related to craniosynostosis may translate into an abnormal ventricular shape that is not necessarily related to abnormal CSF flow. Serial imaging and clinical correlation are indicated, and a great deal of clinical judgment is often required in making these assessments.

EFFECTS OF MID-FACE DEFICIENCY ON THE AIRWAY

All newborn infants are obligate nasal breathers. Many infants born with a craniofacial dysostosis syndrome have moderate to severe hypoplasia of the mid-face as a component of their malformation. They will have diminished nasal and nasopharyngeal space with resulting increased nasal airway resistance (obstruction). Affected children are thus forced to breathe through the mouth. For a newborn infant to ingest food through the mouth requires sucking from a nipple to achieve negative pressure, as well as an intact swallowing mechanism. A neonate with severe mid-face hypoplasia will experience diminished nasal airflow and be unable to accomplish this task and breathe through the nose at the same time. Complicating this clinical picture may be an elongated and ptotic palate and enlarged tonsils and adenoids. A compromised infant expends significant energy respiring, and this may push the child into a catabolic state (negative nitrogen balance). Failure to thrive results unless either nasogastric tube feeding is instituted or a feeding gastrostomy tube is placed. Evaluation by a pediatrician, pediatric otolaryngologist, and feeding specialist with craniofacial experience can help distinguish minor feeding difficulties from those requiring more aggressive treatment.

Sleep apnea of either central or obstructive origin may also be present. If the apnea is found to be secondary to upper airway obstruction based on a formal sleep study, a tracheostomy may be indicated. In rare situations, "early" mid-face advancement is useful to improve the airway and allow tracheostomy decannulation. Central apnea may occur as a result of poorly treated intracranial hypertension, as well as other contributing factors. If so, the condition may improve by reducing ICP to a normal range through cranio-orbital or posterior cranial vault decompression/expansion.

DENTITION AND OCCLUSION

The incidence of dental and oral anomalies is higher in children with craniofacial dysostosis syndromes than in the general population. In Apert syndrome in particular, the palate is high and constricted in width. The incidence of isolated cleft palate in patients with Apert syndrome approaches 30%. Clefting of the secondary palate may be submucous, incomplete, or complete. Confusion has arisen over whether the oral malformations and absence of teeth that are often characteristic of these conditions are a result of congenital or iatrogenic factors (e.g., injury to dental follicles associated with early mid-face surgery). The mid-facial hypoplasia seen in children with craniofacial dysostosis syndromes often results in limited maxillary alveolar bone to house a full complement of teeth. The result is severe crowding, which often requires serial extractions to address the problem. An Angle class III skeletal relationship in combination with an anterior open bite deformity is typical.

MORPHOLOGIC CONSIDERATIONS

GENERAL

Examination of the patient's entire craniofacial region should be meticulous and systematic. The skeleton and soft tissues are assessed in a standard fashion to identify all normal and abnormal anatomy. Specific findings tend to occur with particular malformations, but each patient is unique. Achievement of symmetry and normal proportions and reconstruction of specific esthetic units are essential to recreate an unobtrusive face in a child born with one of the craniofacial dysostosis syndromes.

FRONTO-FOREHEAD ESTHETIC UNIT

The fronto-forehead region is dysmorphic in an infant with craniofacial dysostosis. Establishing normal position of the forehead is critical to achieve overall facial symmetry and balance. The forehead may be considered as two separate esthetic components: the supraorbital ridge–lateral orbital rim region and the superior forehead. The supraorbital ridge–lateral orbital rim region includes the glabella and supraorbital rim and extends inferiorly down each frontozygomatic suture toward the infraorbital rim and posteriorly along each temporoparietal region. The morphology and position of the supraorbital ridge–lateral orbital rim region are key elements of upper facial esthetics. In a normal forehead, at the level of the frontonasal suture an angle ranging from 90 to 110 degrees is formed by the supraorbital ridge and the nasal bones when viewed in profile. Additionally, the eyebrows, which overlie the supraorbital ridge, should be anterior to the cornea. When the supraorbital ridge is viewed from above, the rim should arc posteriorly to achieve a gentle 90-degree angle at the temporal fossa with the central point of the arc at the level of each frontozygomatic suture. The superior forehead component, about 1.0 to 1.5 cm up from the supraorbital rim, should have a gentle posterior curve of about 60 degrees and level out at the coronal suture region when seen in profile.

ORBITO-NASO-ZYGOMATIC ESTHETIC UNIT

In the craniofacial dysostosis syndromes, the orbito-naso-zygomatic regional deformity is a reflection of the cranial base malformation. For example, in Crouzon syndrome, when bilateral coronal suture synostosis is combined with skull base and mid-facial deficiency, the orbito-naso-zygomatic region will be dysmorphic and consistent with a short (anteroposterior) and wide (transverse) anterior cranial base. In Apert syndrome, the nasal bones, orbits, and zygomas, like the anterior cranial base, are transversely wide and horizontally short (retruded), thereby resulting in a shallow hyperteloric upper mid-face (zygomas, orbits, and nose). Advancing the mid-face without simultaneously addressing the increased transverse width will not adequately correct the dysmorphology

MAXILLARY-NASAL BASE ESTHETIC UNIT

In a patient with craniofacial dysostosis and mid-face deficiency, the upper anterior portion of the face (nasion to maxillary incisor) is vertically short, and there is a lack of horizontal (anteroposterior) projection of the midface. These findings may be confirmed by cephalometric analysis, which indicates an SNA angle below the mean value and a short upper anterior facial height (nasion to anterior nasal spine). The width of the maxilla in the dentoalveolar region is generally constricted with a high arched palate. To normalize the maxillary-nasal base region, multidirectional surgical expansion and reshaping are generally required. The maxillary lip-to-tooth relationship and occlusion are normalized through Le Fort I osteotomy and orthodontic treatment as part of the staged reconstruction.

SURGICAL MANAGEMENT

GENERAL CONSIDERATIONS

Philosophy Regarding Timing of Intervention

In considering the timing and type of intervention, experienced surgeons will take several biologic realities into account: the natural course of the malformation (i.e., is the dysmorphology associated with progressively worsening Crouzon syndrome or is it a nonprogressive craniofacial deformity?), the tendency toward restricted growth of an operated-on bone (esthetic unit) that has not yet reached maturity (i.e., we know that operating on the palate of a child born with a cleft in infancy will cause scarring and later result in maxillary hypoplasia in a significant percentage of individuals), and the uncertain relationship between the underlying growing viscera (i.e., brain or eyes) and the congenitally affected and surgically altered skeleton (i.e., if the cranial vault is not surgically decompressed/expanded by 1 year of life in a patient with a syndrome, will brain compression occur?).

In attempting to limit functional impairment and also achieve long-term ideal facial esthetics, an essential question that the surgeon must ask is, "*during the course of craniofacial development, does the operated-on facial skeleton of a child with craniofacial dysostosis tend to grow abnormally and result in further distortions and dysmorphology, or are the initial positive skeletal changes (achieved at surgery) maintained during ongoing growth?*" Unfortunately, the theory that craniofacial procedures carried out early in infancy will "unlock growth" has not been documented through the scientific method.

Management of Intracranial Dead Space

Management of dead space during cranial vault/cranial base expansion is critical to limit complications. Dead space within the cranial vault after cranial expansion at the time of reconstruction is managed by gentle handling of the tissues, achievement of good hemostasis, closure of tissue layers, placement of bone grafts, and obliteration (of dead space) with soft tissue flaps/grafts.

Expansion of the cranial vault with forward advancement of the anterior cranial base, orbits, and mid-face results in both extradural (retrofrontal) dead space and communication of the anterior fossa with the nasal cavity. The anterior cranial vault dead space and communication of the frontal fossa with the nasal cavity across the anterior skull base may result in hematoma formation, leakage of CSF, infection, and fistula formation. Management of this expanded space in the anterior cranial fossa following frontofacial or forehead advancement remains controversial. Relatively rapid filling of the expanded intracranial space by the frontal lobes has been documented in infants and young children when the expansion remains in a physiologic range. This observation supports the conservative management of dead space in younger patients. More gradual and less complete filling is thought to occur in older children and adults. If so, this may be particularly troublesome when the anterior fossa dead space communicates directly with the nasal cavity (e.g., after monobloc advancement, facial bipartition, intracranial Le Fort III). If possible, closing off (sealing) the nasal cavity from the cranial fossa at the time of surgery is preferred. Insertion of a pericranial flap can help separate the cavities and at the same time obliterate dead space. The use of fibrin glue to seal the anterior cranial base also provides a temporary repair between the cavities and allows time for reepithelialization of the nasal mucosa. Until the torn nasopharyngeal mucosa heals, communication between the nasal cavity and cranial fossa poses the potential for leakage (air, fluid, bacteria) and nasocranial fistula formation. To prevent these complications, postoperative endotracheal intubation may be extended for 3 to 5 days or bilateral nasopharyngeal airways can be placed after extubation (or both). In addition, sinus precautions and restriction of nose blowing further limit reflux (nose to cranial fossa) of air and fluid during the postoperative period. All these maneuvers are aimed at avoiding a pressure gradient and will facilitate sealing of the intracranial cavity from the upper aerodigestive tract. When forehead procedures are performed and aerated frontal sinuses are present, management consists of either cranialization or obliteration.

When a patient with craniofacial dysostosis is to undergo intracranial volume expansion as part of the craniofacial procedure and also requires management of hydrocephalus, the potential for problems increases. Complications may arise from excessive CSF drainage (overshunting). With "overshunting" there is decreased brain volume and dead space remains. Fronto-orbital advancement or cranial vault expansion procedures (or both) should be carefully staged with ventriculoperitoneal (VP) shunting procedures. Ultimately, the decision regarding sequencing and shunting is based on the patient's neurologic findings and the neurosurgeon's judgment. In a patient with a VP shunt in place before surgery, careful neurosurgical evaluation, including CT of the ventricular system, is carried out to confirm that the shunt is functioning appropriately.

When feasible, after mid-face advancement the anterior skull base is reconstructed (i.e., bone grafts) to facilitate healing across the skull base and thereby limit CSF leakage and prevent fistula formation.

CROUZON SYNDROME

STAGING OF RECONSTRUCTION FOR CROUZON SYNDROME

Primary Cranio-orbital Decompression: Reshaping in Infancy

The initial treatment of any craniofacial dysostosis syndrome generally requires bilateral release of the coronal sutures with decompression, simultaneous anterior cranial vault and upper orbital osteotomies, and reshaping and advancement (Fig. 91-1). The authors' preference is to carry this surgery out when the child is 9 to 11 months of age unless clear signs of increased ICP are identified earlier in life. Reshaping of the upper three quarters of the orbital

rims and supraorbital ridges is geared to decrease bitemporal and anterior cranial base width, with simultaneous horizontal advancement performed to increase the anteroposterior dimension. This also increases the depth of the upper orbits, with some improvement in eye proptosis. The overlying forehead is then reconstructed according to morphologic needs. A degree of overcorrection is preferred at the level of the supraorbital ridge when the procedure is carried out in infancy. In our opinion, by allowing additional growth to occur (waiting until the child is 9 to 11 months old), the reconstructed cranial vault and upper orbital shape are better maintained with less need for repeat craniotomy procedures but without risking compression of the underlying brain.

The goals at this stage are to provide increased intracranial space in the anterior cranial vault for the brain; increased orbital volume, which allows the eyes to be positioned more normally for better protection from exposure; and improved morphology of the forehead and upper orbits.

A postauricular coronal (scalp) incision is made, and the anterior flap is elevated along with the temporalis muscle in the subperiosteal plane. Bilateral circumferential periorbital dissection follows, with detachment of the lateral canthi but preservation of the medial canthi and nasolacrimal apparatus to the medial orbital walls. The subperiosteal dissection is continued down the lateral and infraorbital rims to include the anterior aspect of the maxilla and zygomatic buttress. The neurosurgeon then completes the craniotomy to remove the dysmorphic anterior cranial vault. With retraction of the frontal and temporal lobes of the brain (remaining anterior to each olfactory bulb), safe direct visualization of the anterior cranial base and orbits is possible.

The orbital osteotomies are then completed across the orbital roof and superior aspect of the medial orbital wall, laterally through the lateral orbital wall and inferiorly just into the inferior orbital fissure. The three-quarters orbital osteotomy units, with their tenon extensions, are removed from the field. The orbital units are reshaped and re-inset into a preferred position. Orbital depth is thereby increased, and global proptosis is reduced. Fixation is generally achieved with 28-gauge interosseous wires at each infraorbital rim and with plates and screws at the tenon extensions and frontonasal regions.

The removed calvaria is cut into segments, which are placed individually to achieve a more normally configured anterior cranial vault. The goal of reshaping is to narrow the anterior cranial base and orbital width slightly and provide more forward projection and overall normal morphology.

Repeat Craniotomy for Additional Cranial Vault Expansion and Reshaping in Young Children

After the initial suture release, decompression and reshaping are carried out during infancy; the child is observed clinically at intervals by the craniofacial surgeon, pediatric neurosurgeon, pediatric ophthalmologist, and developmental specialist and undergoes periodic CT. Should signs of increased ICP develop, urgent brain decompression with cranial vault expansion and reshaping is performed. When increased ICP is suspected, the location of brain compression influences the region of the skull for which further expansion and reshaping is planned.

If the brain compression is judged to be anterior, further anterior cranial vault and upper orbital osteotomies with reshaping and advancement are carried out. The technique is similar to that described previously. If the problem is posterior compression, expansion of the posterior cranial vault, with the patient in the prone position, is required.

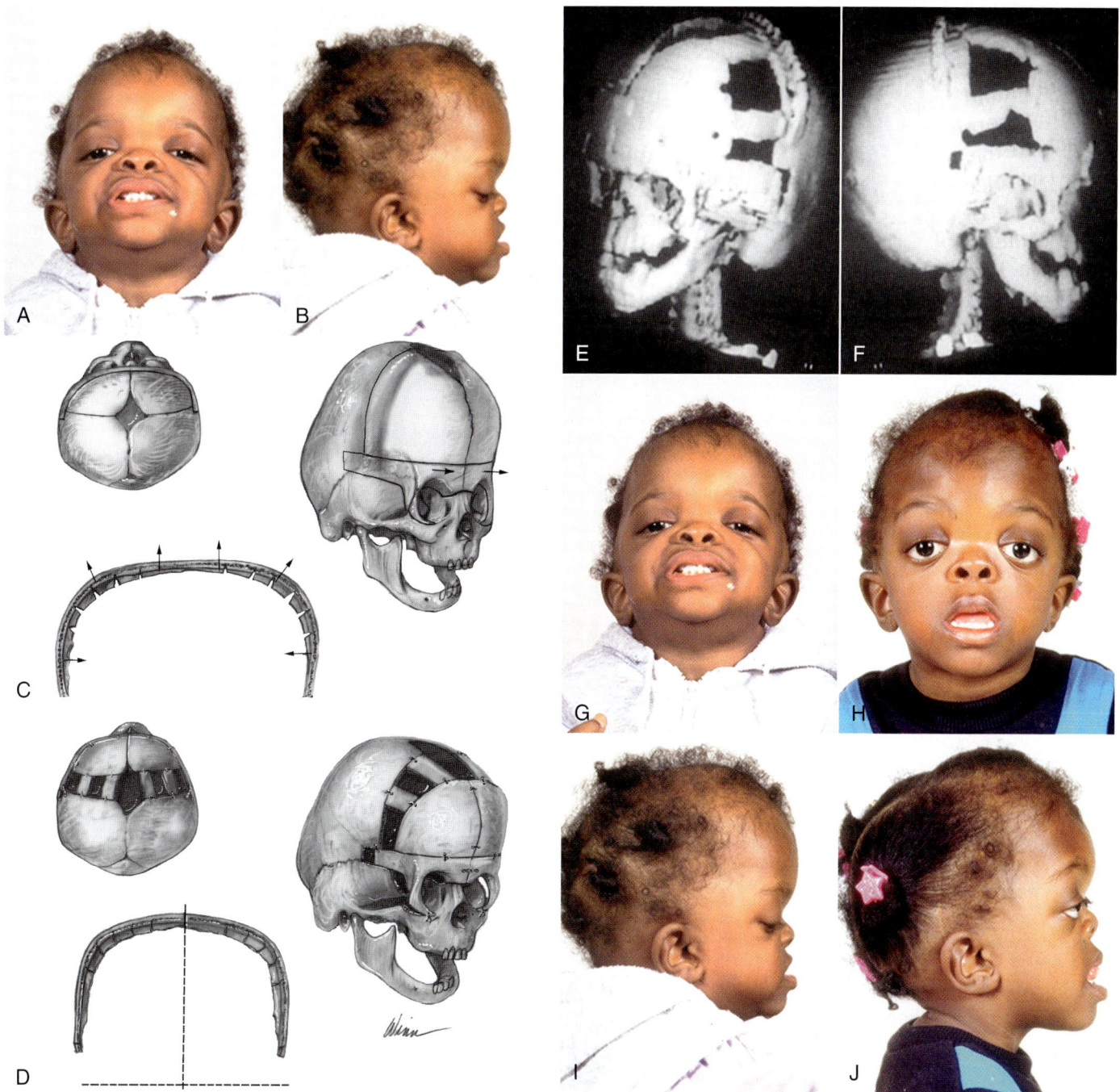

Fig. 91-1 ■ Eighteen-month-old girl with brachycephaly and mid-face deficiency associated with an underlying diagnosis of Crouzon syndrome. Frontal (**A**) and profile (**B**) views before surgery. Craniofacial deformity (**C**) and planned operative procedure (**D**). **E** and **F,** Three-dimensional CT scans of the craniofacial skeleton after fronto-orbital advancement and anterior cranial vault reshaping. Frontal view before surgery (**G**) and 1½ years after undergoing cranio-orbital decompression (**H**). Profile view before surgery (**I**) and 1½ years after undergoing the initial phase of surgery (**J**). (From Posnick JC: Crouzon syndrome: evaluation and staging of reconstruction. In Posnick JC, editor: *Craniofacial and maxillofacial surgery in children and young adults*, vol 1, Philadelphia, 2000, Saunders.)

The "repeat" craniotomy carried out for further decompression and reshaping in a child with Crouzon syndrome is often complicated by brittle cortical bone (which lacks a diploic space and contains sharp spicules piercing the dura), the presence of previously placed fixation devices in the operative field, and convoluted thin dura compressed against (or herniated into) the inner table of the skull. All these problems result in a greater potential for dural tears during calvarectomy than would normally occur during the primary procedure. A greater potential for morbidity should be anticipated when re-elevating the scalp flap, dissecting the dura free of the inner table of the skull and cranial base, and then removing the cranial vault bone.

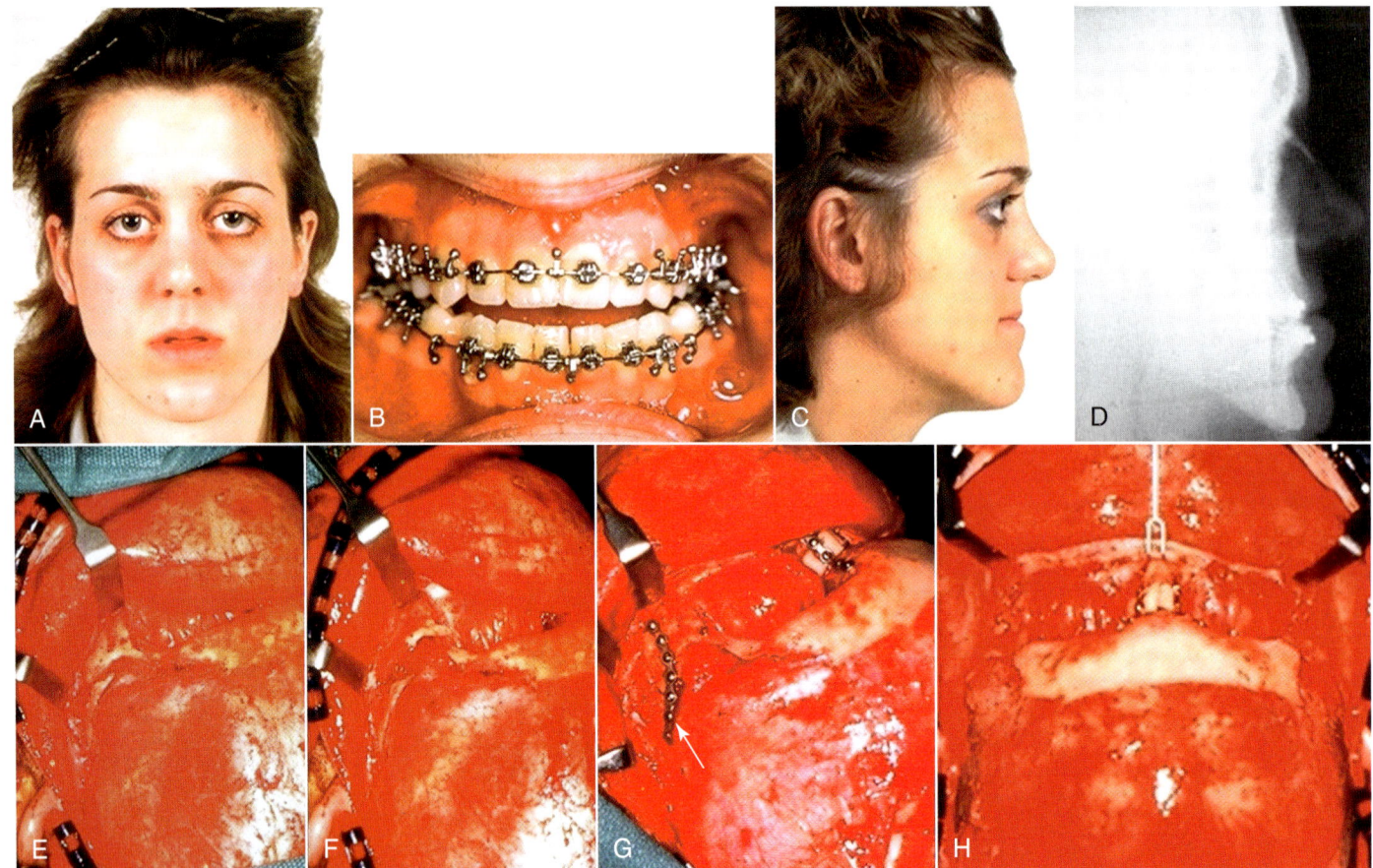

Fig. 91-2 ▪ Fifteen-year-old girl with Crouzon syndrome and mild to moderate mid-face deficiency with retrusion of the infraorbital rims, zygomatic buttresses, and maxilla. Her mid-face deformity was treated with a Le Fort III (extracranial) osteotomy. Frontal (**A**) and occlusal (**B**) views before surgery. Profile view (**C**) and lateral cephalometric radiograph (**D**) before surgery. **E** and **F,** Intraoperative views of the zygomatic complex after osteotomies and disimpaction. Note the potential for an unsightly step-off at the lateral orbital rim. **G** and **H,** Bird's-eye views of the cranio-orbital region after reshaping and stabilization. Note the cranial bone graft placed at the frontonasal region.

Management of the "Total Mid-face" Deformity in Childhood

The type of osteotomies selected to manage a "total mid-face" deficiency/deformity and residual cranial vault dysplasia should depend on the extent and location of the dysmorphology rather than on a fixed universal (tunnel vision) approach to the mid-face malformation. Selection of either a monobloc (with or without additional orbital segmentation), facial bipartition (with or without additional orbital segmental osteotomies), or Le Fort III osteotomy to manage the basic horizontal, transverse, and vertical mid-face deficiencies/deformities in a patient with Crouzon syndrome depends on the patient's initial mid-face and anterior cranial vault morphology. The observed dysmorphology is dependent on the original malformation, the previous procedures carried out, and the effects of ongoing growth.

When evaluating the upper face and mid-face regions in a child born with Crouzon syndrome, if the supraorbital ridge is in good position when viewed from the sagittal plane (the depth of the upper orbits is adequate), the mid-face and forehead have a normal arc of rotation in the transverse plane (not concave), and the root of the nose is of normal width (minimal orbital hypertelorism), there is little need to reconstruct this region (the forehead and upper mid-face) any further. In such patients, the basic residual mid-face deformity is in the lower half of the orbits, zygomatic buttress, and maxilla. If so, the deformity may be managed effectively with an extracranial Le Fort III osteotomy (Fig. 91-2).

If the supraorbital area, anterior cranial base, zygomas, nose, lower orbits, and maxilla all remain deficient in the sagittal plane (horizontal retrusion), a monobloc osteotomy is indicated (Fig. 91-3). In these patients the forehead is generally flat and retruded and will also require reshaping and advancement. If upper mid-face hypertelorism (increased transverse width) and mid-face flattening (horizontal retrusion) with loss of the normal facial curvature (concave arc) are also present, the monobloc unit is split vertically in the midline (facial bipartition), a wedge of interorbital (nasal and ethmoidal) bone is removed, and the orbits and zygomas are repositioned medially while the maxillary posterior arch is widened. Facial bipartition is rarely required in patients with Crouzon syndrome, but monobloc osteotomy is. When a monobloc or facial bipartition osteotomy is carried out as in the "total mid-face" procedure, additional segmentation of the upper and lateral orbits for reconstruction may also be required to normalize the morphology of the orbital esthetic units.

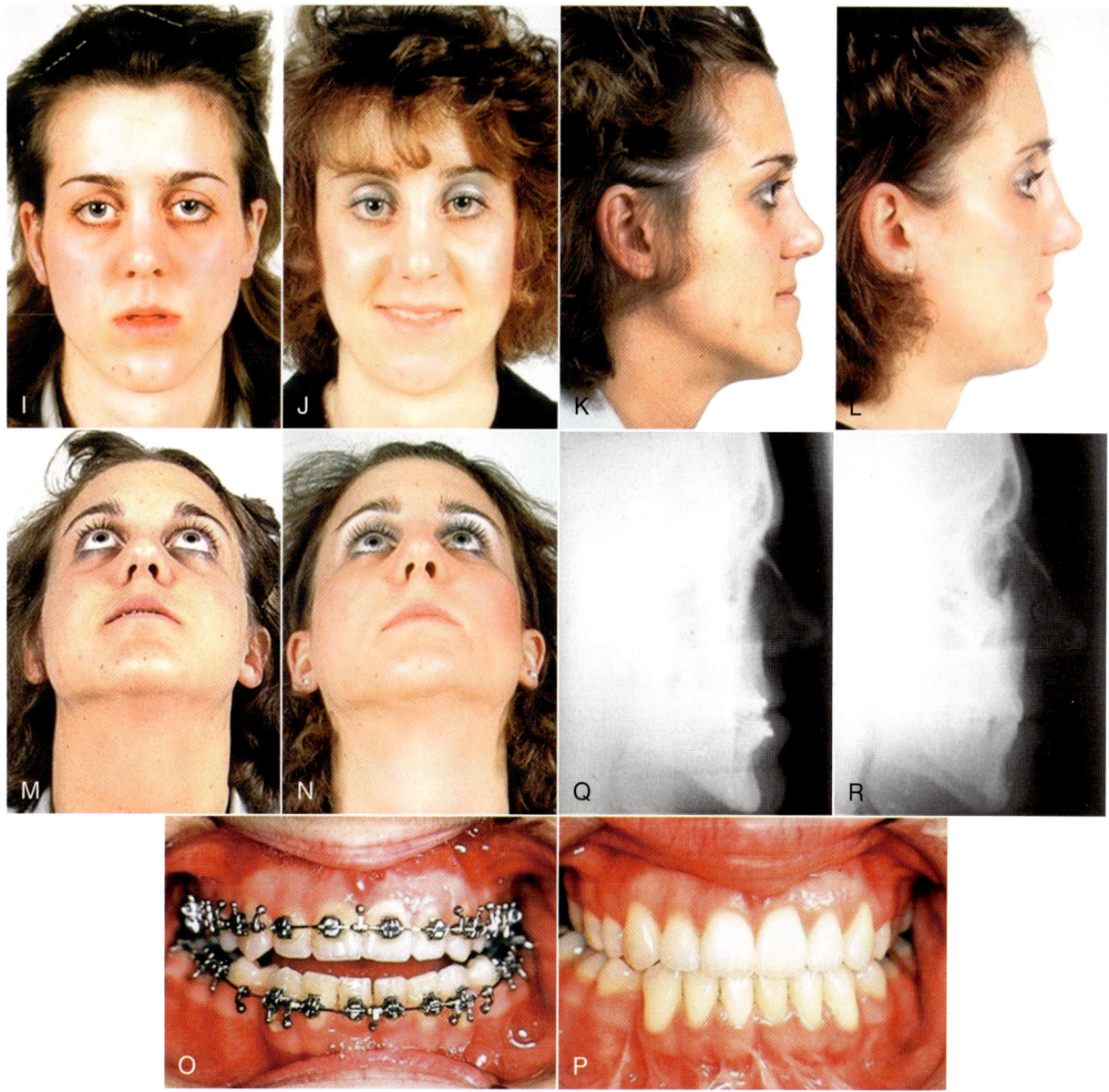

Fig. 91-2, cont'd ■ Frontal views before (**I**) and after Le Fort III (extracranial) osteotomy for midfacial advancement (**J**). Profile views before (**K**) and after surgery (**L**). Worm's-eye view before (**M**) and after surgery (**N**). Occlusal views before (**O**) and after surgery (**P**). Lateral cephalometric radiographs before (**Q**) and after (**R**) surgery. (From Posnick JC: Craniosynostosis: surgical management of the midface deformity. In Bell WH, editor: *Orthognathic and reconstructive surgery*, vol 3, Philadelphia, 1992, Saunders.)

In most cases, an error in judgment will occur if the surgeon attempts to simultaneously adjust the orbits and idealize the occlusion by performing the Le Fort III, monobloc, or facial bipartition osteotomy in isolation without completing a separate Le Fort I osteotomy. The degree of horizontal deficiency observed at the orbits and maxillary dentition is rarely uniform. This further segmentation of the mid-face complex at the Le Fort I level is required to establish normal proportions. If a Le Fort I separation of the "total mid-face" complex is not carried out and the surgeon attempts to achieve a positive overbite and overjet at the incisor teeth, excessive advancement of the orbits and enophthalmos will occur. The Le Fort I osteotomy is generally *not* performed at the time of the "total mid-face" procedure. This will await skeletal maturity and then be combined with orthodontic treatment. Until then, an Angle class III occlusion will remain.

A major esthetic problem specific to the Le Fort III osteotomy when its indications are less than ideal is the creation of irregular step-offs in the lateral orbital rims. This will occur when even a moderate Le Fort III advancement is carried out. These lateral orbital step-offs are unattractive and visible to the casual observer at conversational distance, and later surgical modification is difficult and achieves less than ideal esthetic results. Another problem with the Le Fort III osteotomy is difficulty judging an ideal orbital depth. A frequent result is either residual proptosis or enophthalmos. Simultaneous correction of orbital hypertelorism or correction of a mid-face arc-of-rotation problem is not possible with the Le Fort III

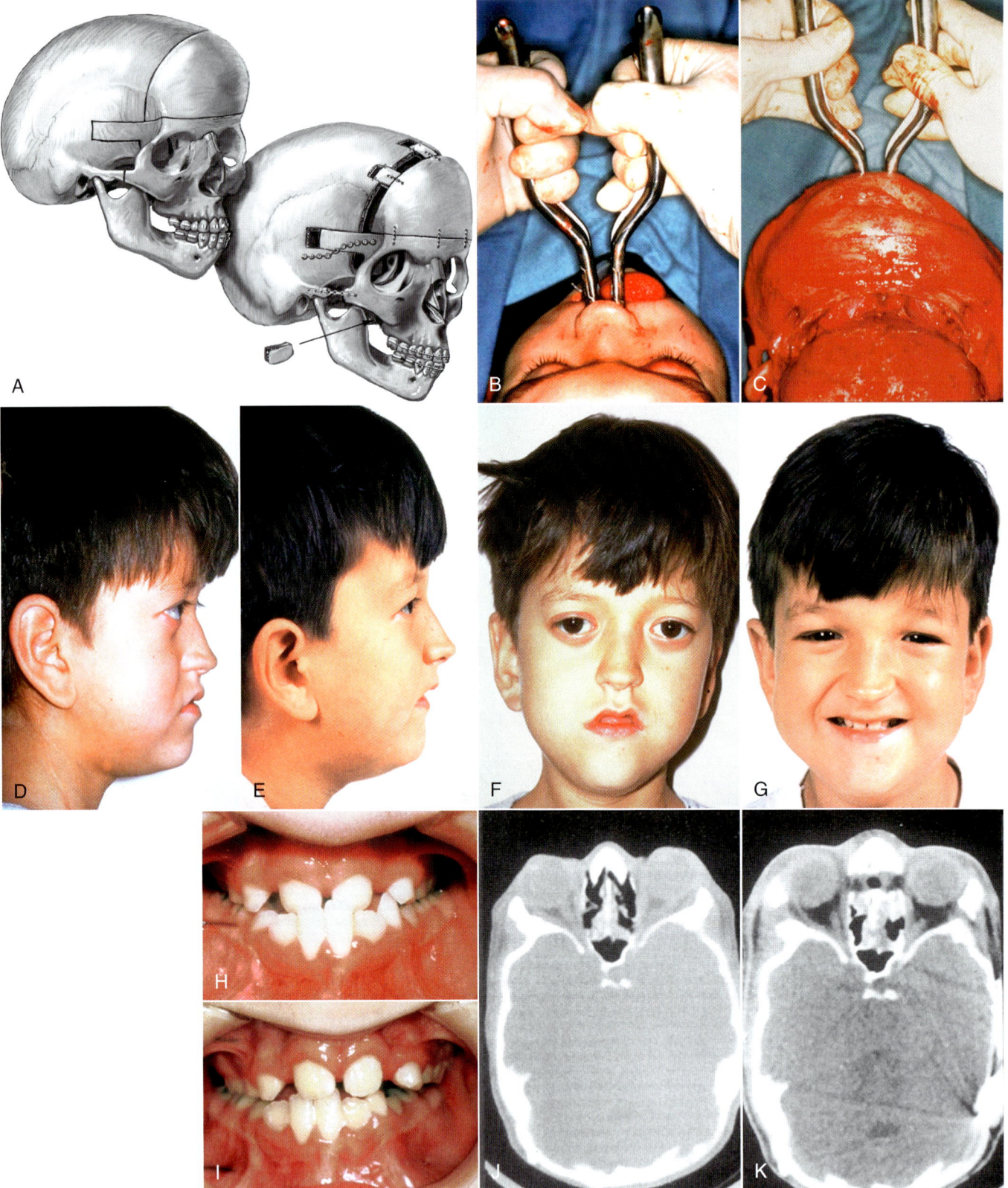

Fig. 91-3 ■ Eight-year-old boy with Crouzon syndrome following an initial phase of cranio-orbital decompression and cranial vault reshaping performed during infancy. He then underwent anterior cranial vault and monobloc osteotomies with advancement to address his total mid-face deficiency. **A,** Craniofacial morphology before and after anterior cranial vault and monobloc osteotomies as described. Osteotomy locations are indicated and stabilization was carried out with miniplates and cranial bone grafts at the osteotomy sites. Intraoperative view of the disimpaction forceps in place, but before disimpaction (**B**), and the same view with the coronal flap turned down (**C**) to indicate the degree of advancement possible at the supraorbital ridge level after mobilization. Profile before (**D**) and after monobloc advancement (**E**). Frontal view before (**F**) and after monobloc advancement (**G**). Occlusal views before (**H**) and after reconstruction (**I**). A comparison of axial CT scans through the mid-orbits before (**J**) and after reconstruction (**K**) shows the resultant increased orbital volume and decreased degree of proptosis. (From Posnick JC: Craniosynostosis: surgical management of the midface deformity. In Bell WH, editor: *Orthognathic and reconstructive surgery*, vol 3, Philadelphia, 1992, Saunders.)

procedure. Excessive lengthening of the nose, accompanied by flattening of the nasofrontal angle, will also occur if the Le Fort III osteotomy is selected when the skeletal morphology favors a monobloc or facial bipartition procedure. It is not possible to later correct the surgically created vertical elongation of the nose.

Final reconstruction of the cranial vault deformities and orbital dystopia in children with Crouzon syndrome can be managed as early as 5 to 7 years of age. By this time the cranial vault and orbits normally attain approximately 85% to 90% of their adult size. When the "upper mid-face" and final cranial vault procedure is carried out after this age, the reconstructive objectives are to approximate adult dimensions in the cranio-orbito-zygomatic region, with the expectation of a stable result (no longer influenced by growth) once healing has occurred. Psychosocial considerations also support the 5- to 7-year age time frame for the upper mid-face and final cranial vault procedure. When the procedure is carried out at this age, the child may enter first grade with a chance for satisfactory self-esteem. Routine orthognathic surgery will be necessary at the time of skeletal maturity to achieve an ideal occlusion, facial profile, and smile.

Orthognathic Procedures for Definitive Occlusal Correction

Although the mandible has normal basic growth potential in children with Crouzon syndrome, the maxilla does not. An Angle class III malocclusion, caused by maxillary retrusion, with an anterior open bite often results. A Le Fort I osteotomy to allow horizontal advancement, transverse widening, and vertical adjustment is generally required in combination with osteoplastic genioplasty (vertical reduction and horizontal advancement) to further correct the lower face deformity. The elective orthognathic surgery is carried out in conjunction with orthodontic treatment planned for completion at the time of early skeletal maturity (approximately 13 to 15 years in girls and 15 to 17 years in boys).

APERT SYNDROME

Apert syndrome has previously been classified on the basis of its clinical findings. Postmortem histologic and radiographic studies suggest that the skeletal deficiencies in a patient with Apert syndrome result from cartilage dysplasia at the cranial base, which leads to premature fusion of the midline sutures from the occiput to the anterior nasal septum. In addition, a component of the syndrome is four-limb symmetry, complex syndactylies of the hands and feet. Fusion and malformation of other joints, including the elbows and shoulders, often occur. The soft tissue drape also varies from that in Crouzon syndrome, with a greater downward lateral slant of the canthi and a distinctive, S-shaped upper eyelid ptosis. The quality of the skin frequently varies from normal, with acne and hyperhidrosis being prominent features. At the molecular level, one of two *FGFR2* mutations involving amino acids (Ser252Trp and Pro253-Arg) has been found to cause Apert syndrome in nearly all patients studied.

STAGING OF RECONSTRUCTION FOR APERT SYNDROME

The treatment approach for primary cranio-orbital decompression and reshaping during infancy is similar to that described for patients with Crouzon syndrome.

Management of the "Total Mid-face" Deformity in Childhood

In almost all patients with Apert syndrome, facial bipartition osteotomies combined with further cranial vault reshaping permit a more complete correction of the abnormal craniofacial skeleton than can be achieved with other mid-face procedures (i.e., monobloc or Le Fort III). When using the facial bipartition approach, a more normal arc of rotation of the mid-face complex is achieved with the midline split (facial bipartition) (Fig. 91-4). This further reduces the stigmata of the preoperative Apert "flat, wide, and retrusive" facial appearance. Facial bipartition also allows the orbits and zygomatic buttresses to shift as units to the midline (correction of hypertelorism) while the maxillary arch is simultaneously widened. Horizontal advancement of the reassembled mid-face complex is then achieved to normalize orbital depth and zygomatic length. The forehead is generally flat, tall, and retruded, with a constricting band just above the supraorbital ridge giving the impression of bitemporal narrowing. Reshaping of the anterior cranial vault is simultaneously carried out. A Le Fort III osteotomy is virtually never adequate for ideal correction of the residual upper face and mid-face deformity seen in patients with Apert syndrome.

PFEIFFER SYNDROME

In 1964, Pfeiffer described a syndrome consisting of craniosynostosis, broad thumbs, broad great toes, and occasionally partial soft tissue syndactyly of the hands. This syndrome is known to have an autosomal dominant inheritance pattern with complete penetrance documented in all recorded two- and three-generation pedigrees. Variable expressivity of the craniofacial and extremity findings is common. Although some authors have found similarities in certain patients with Pfeiffer, Crouzon, and Jackson-Weiss syndromes, the three disorders are nosologically distinct. According to Cohen, the phenotypes of the three conditions do not correlate well with the known molecular findings. Patients with these three syndromes may have similar or even identical mutations in exon B of *FGFR2*, yet they breed true within families, an observation that is as yet unexplained by the molecular findings.

Current thinking suggests that Pfeiffer syndrome is heterogeneous because it is caused by a single recurring mutation (Pro252Arg) of *FGFR1* and by several different mutations affecting *FGFR2*. Cohen has reviewed the literature and further subgrouped Pfeiffer syndrome according to clinical features, associated low-frequency anomalies, and outcome. According to Cohen, Pfeiffer type I corresponds to the classic Pfeiffer syndrome and has a satisfactory prognosis. The type II subgroup is associated with the cloverleaf skull anomaly, whereas type III is not. Both types II and III have a less favorable outcome, with death in infancy frequently seen. The type I variant is frequently manifested as bicoronal craniosynostosis with mid-face involvement. Longitudinal evaluation and staging of reconstruction are dependent on individual variations but are similar to that described for Crouzon syndrome.

CARPENTER SYNDROME

Carpenter syndrome is characterized by craniosynostosis and is often associated with preaxial polysyndactyly of the feet, short fingers with clinodactyly, and variable soft tissue syndactyly; it is sometimes associated with postaxial polydactyly and with other anomalies such as congenital heart defects, short stature, obesity, and mental deficiency. It was first described by Carpenter in 1901 and was later recognized to be an autosomal recessive syndrome. In

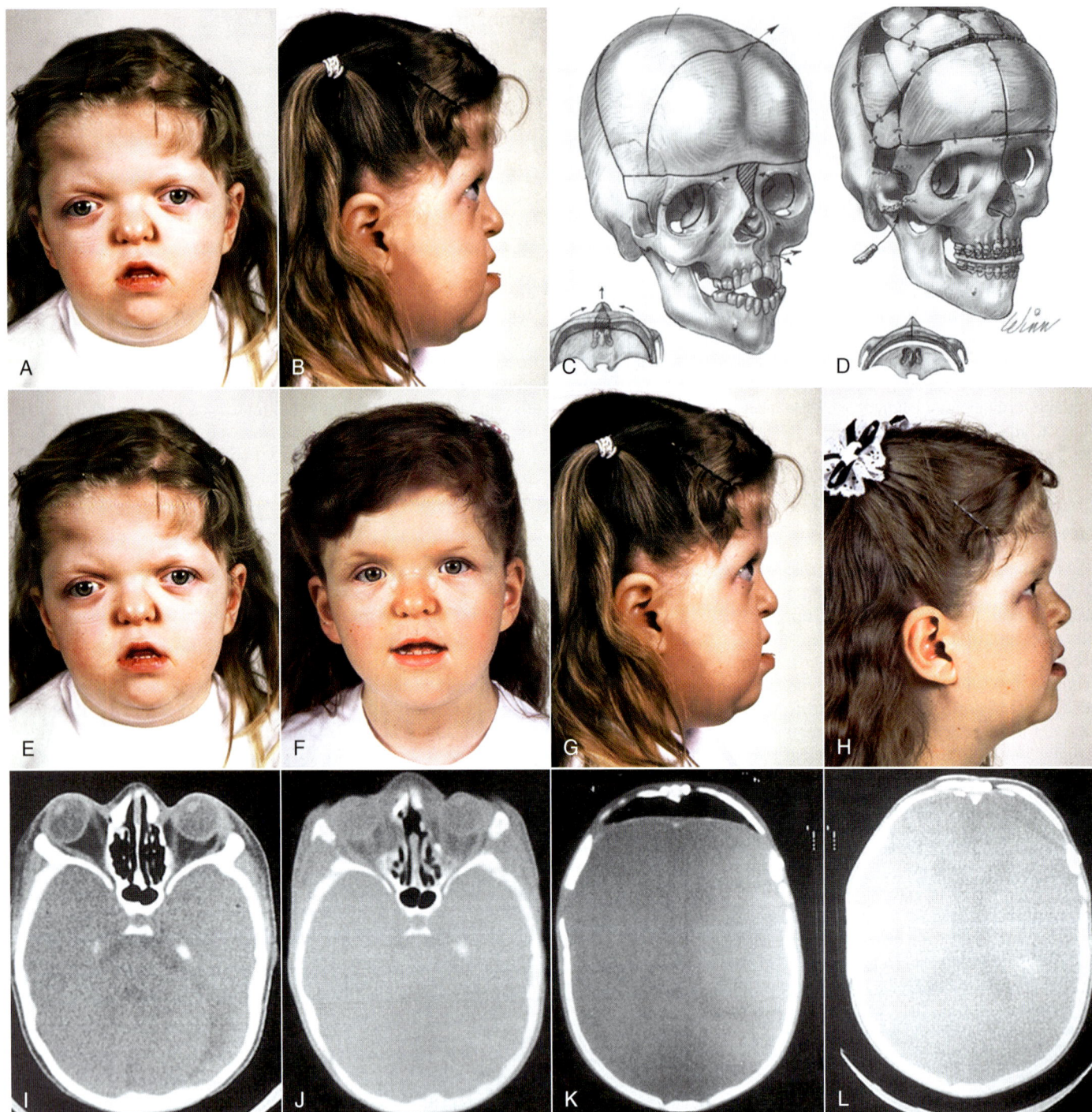

Fig. 91-4 ■ Five-year-old girl with Apert syndrome who underwent decompression and forehead/upper orbital reshaping at 6 months of age. She was then referred with residual deformity requiring cranial vault and facial bipartition osteotomies with reshaping. She will require orthognathic surgery and orthodontic treatment later in the teenage years to complete her reconstruction. Frontal (**A**) and profile (**B**) views before surgery. Illustration of preoperative craniofacial morphology (**C**) and planned and completed osteotomies and reshaping (**D**). Stabilization was achieved with cranial bone grafts and miniplate fixation. Frontal view before (**E**) and 2 years after reconstruction (**F**). Profile view before (**G**) and 2 years after reconstruction (**H**). A comparison of axial-slice CT scans through mid-orbits before (**I**) and after reconstruction (**J**) demonstrates improvement in orbital hypertelorism and orbital depth and diminished eye proptosis. Standard axial CT scans through the cranial vault 1 week after facial bipartition (note the dead space in the retrofrontal region) (**K**) and at 1 year (**L**). Notice that the initial retrofrontal dead space has resolved as a result of brain expansion. (From Posnick JC, editor: *Craniofacial and maxillofacial surgery in children and young adults,* vol 1, Philadelphia, 2000, WB Saunders.)

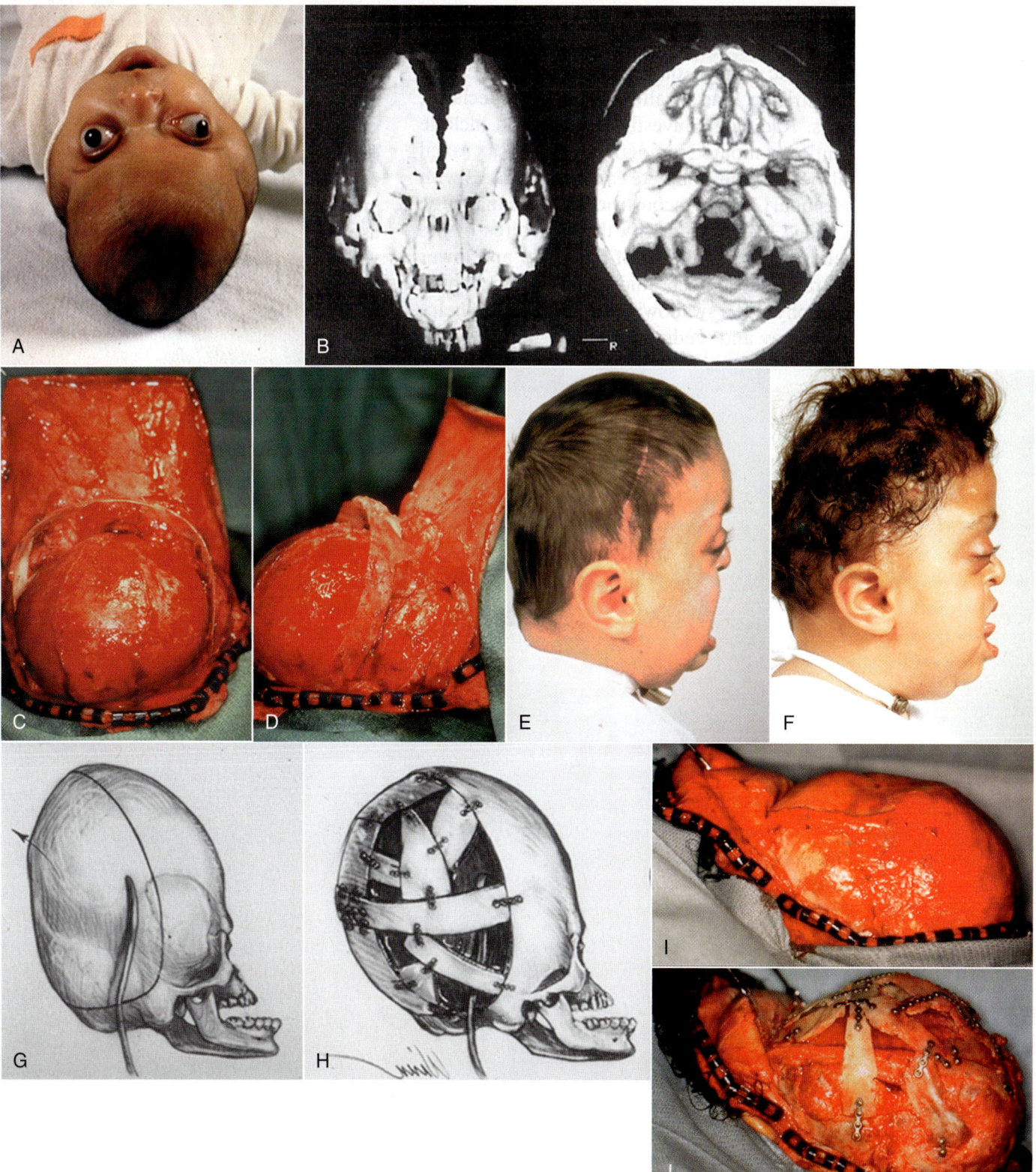

Fig. 91-5 ■ Child with a severe form of cloverleaf skull anomaly. At 10 months of age she underwent first-stage cranial vault and upper orbital decompression with reshaping. She then required a ventriculoperitoneal shunt for the management of hydrocephalus. At 3 ½ years of age, posterior cranial vault decompression with reshaping to increase intracranial volume was performed. At 4 ½ years of age, facial bipartition osteotomies combined with anterior cranial vault reshaping were carried out. After the cranial vault and facial bipartition procedure, nasal airflow improved, and it was possible to remove the tracheostomy tube. The cranial vault reshaping expanded the intracranial volume to provide more space for the brain. The mid-face advancement improved her proptosis and ability to chew and articulate speech. As part of the staged reconstruction, she will require orthognathic surgery combined with orthodontic treatment at the time of early skeletal maturity. Frontal view (**A**) and craniofacial CT scans (**B**) at 10 months of age. Intraoperative lateral (**C**) and bird's-eye (**D**) views at 10 months of age after craniotomy and removal of the upper orbits, followed by the construction of a "bandeau" with 3 cm advancement. Profile view at 2 ½ (**E**) and 3 ½ (**F**) years of age with a flattened posterior cranial vault and severe mid-face deficiency.

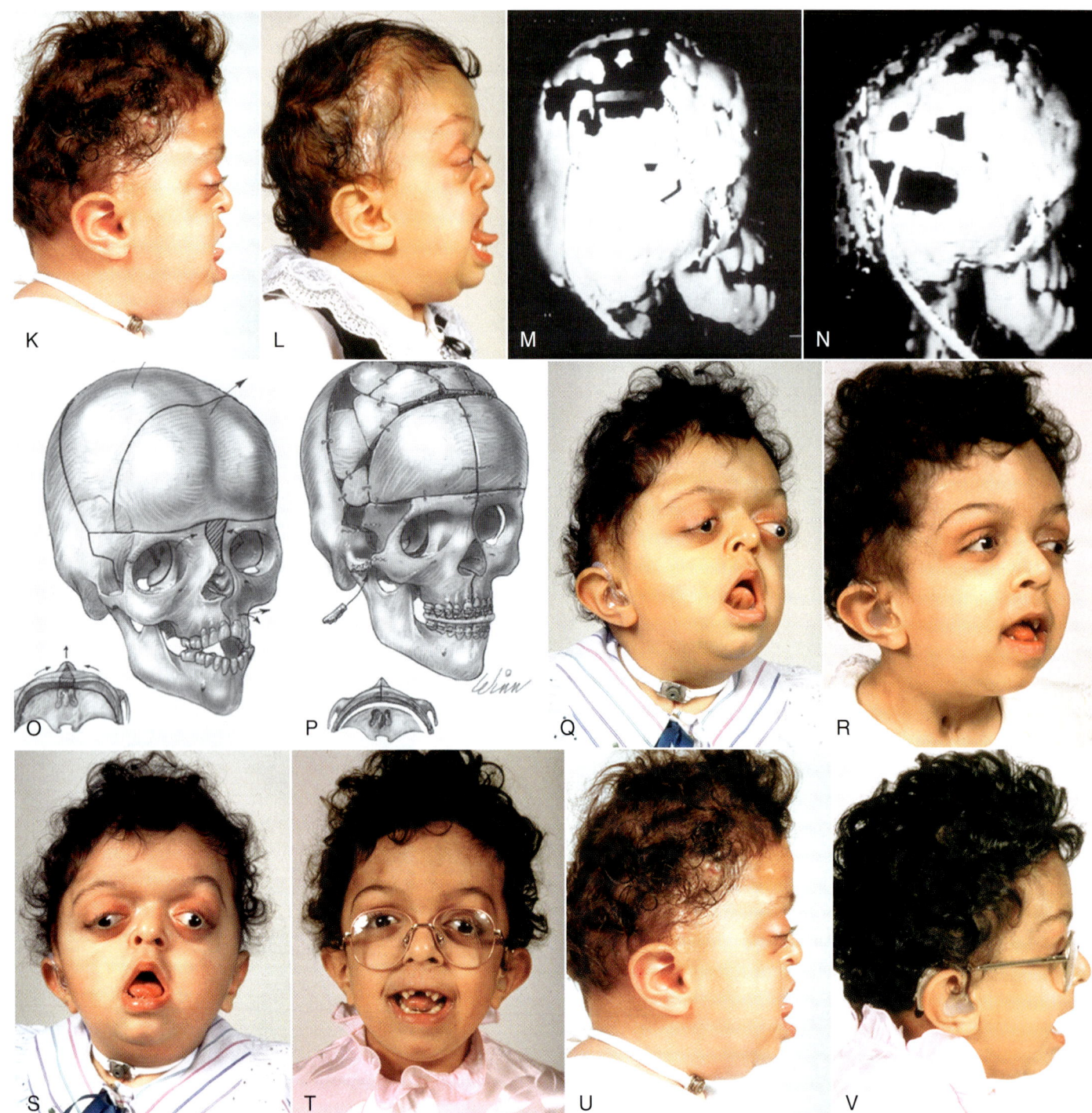

Fig. 91-5, cont'd ■ **G** and **H,** Illustration of the flattened posterior cranial vault. Note the ventriculoperitoneal shunt in place and proposed cranial vault reshaping. Intraoperative side view (patient in the prone position) before (**I**) and after craniotomy and reshaping and fixation of bone segments with miniplates and screws (**J**). The ventriculoperitoneal shunt remains intact and deep to the skull reconstruction. Profile view at 3 ½ years (**K**) and 2 weeks after posterior cranial vault reconstruction (**L**). Comparison of three-dimensional CT scans before (**M**) and just after posterior cranial vault reshaping (**N**). **O** and **P,** Illustrations of the planned facial bipartition and cranial vault reconstruction. Oblique views before (**Q**) and 6 months after facial bipartition osteotomies with reshaping and advancement (**R**). Frontal views before (**S**) and after facial bipartition reconstruction (**T**). Profile view before (**U**) and after facial bipartition reconstruction (**V**).

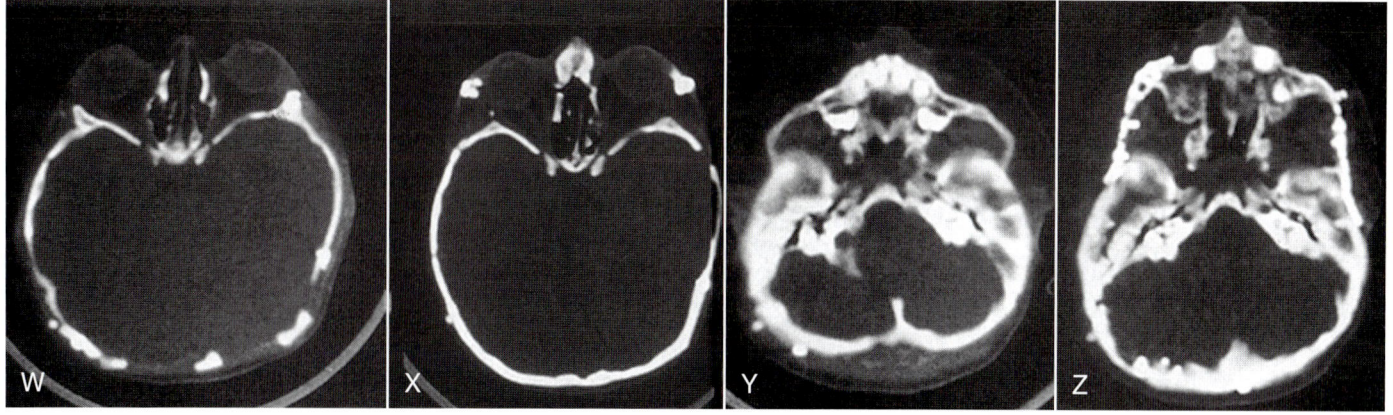

Fig. 91-5, cont'd ▪ Comparison of axial CT slices through the mid-orbits before (**W**) and after reconstruction (**X**). Comparison of axial CT slices through the zygomatic arches before (**Y**) and after reconstruction (**Z**). (From Posnick JC, editor: *Craniofacial and maxillofacial surgery in children and young adults*, vol 1, Philadelphia, 2000, Saunders.)

general, the reconstructive algorithm described for Crouzon syndrome can be followed.

SAETHRE-CHOTZEN SYNDROME

Saethre-Chotzen syndrome has an autosomal dominant inheritance pattern with a high degree of penetrance and expressivity. Its pattern of malformations may include craniosynostosis, low-set frontal hairline, ptosis of the upper eyelids, facial asymmetry, brachydactyly, partial cutaneous syndactyly, and other skeletal anomalies. As part of the reconstruction, cranio-orbital reshaping will almost certainly be required and is similar to that described for Crouzon syndrome. Evaluation and management of the total mid-face deficiency and orthognathic deformities should follow that described for Crouzon syndrome.

CLOVERLEAF SKULL ANOMALY

The kleeblattschädel anomaly (cloverleaf skull) is a trilobular-shaped skull secondary to craniosynostosis (Fig. 91-5). The cloverleaf skull anomaly is known to be both etiologically and pathogenetically heterogeneous. This anomaly is also non-specific; it may occur as an isolated anomaly or together with other anomalies making up various syndromes (i.e., Apert, Crouzon, Carpenter, Pfeiffer, and Saethre-Chotzen). The extent and timing of anterior cranial vault/upper orbital, posterior cranial vault, and mid-face reconstruction are dependent on individual variations in the initial deformity. In general, the protocol described for Crouzon syndrome can be followed.

SUMMARY

The preferred approach for the management of craniofacial dysostosis syndromes is to stage the reconstruction to coincide with facial growth patterns, visceral (brain and eye) function, and psychosocial development. Recognition of the need for a staged reconstruction serves to clarify the objectives of each phase of treatment for the craniofacial surgeon, team, and most importantly, the patient and the patient's family.

By continuing to define our rationale for the timing and extent of surgical intervention and then evaluating both function and esthetic outcomes, we will further improve the quality of life for the many hundreds of children born with syndromic forms of craniosynostosis.

PEARLS AND PITFALLS

- Craniofacial dysostosis syndromes are inherited forms of craniosynostosis in which there is involvement of the cranial vault sutures and sutures of the skull base (premature fusion) and mid-facial skeleton.
- The staged reconstructive approach to craniofacial dysostosis syndromes includes primary cranio-orbital decompression and reshaping (before 1 year of age), surgical management of the total mid-face deficiency (at approximately 5 to 8 years of age), and orthognathic surgery (performed at skeletal maturity).
- In young children in whom signs of increased ICP develop, repeat craniotomy and additional cranial vault expansion may be necessary.
- Management of a total mid-face deficiency usually involves monobloc advancement for patients with Crouzon, Carpenter, Saethre-Chotzen, and Pfeiffer syndromes or a facial bipartition procedure for patients with Apert syndrome.
- Whenever possible, the specific timing of surgery should coincide with facial growth patterns, and early surgery should be avoided unless indicated by specific functional or visceral (brain and eye) conditions.

BIBLIOGRAPHY

Cohen MM Jr: Cloverleaf syndrome update, *Proc Greenwood Gene Center* 6:186-187, 1987.

Cohen MM Jr: Pfeiffer syndrome update, clinical subtypes, and guidelines for differential diagnosis, *Am J Med Genet* 45:300-307, 1993.

Cohen MM Jr: Transforming growth factor βs and fibroblast growth factors and their receptors: role in sutural biology and craniosynostosis, *J Bone Miner Res* 12:322-331, 1997.

Cohen MM Jr, Kreiborg S: The growth pattern in the Apert syndrome, *Clin Genet* 47:617-623, 1993.

Cohen MM Jr, Kreiborg S: Skeletal abnormalities in the Apert syndrome, *Am J Med Genet* 47:624-632, 1993.

Drake AF, Sidman JD: Airway management. In Turvey TA, Vig KWL, Fonseca RJ, editors: *Facial clefts and craniosynostosis: principles and management*, Philadelphia, 1996, WB Saunders, pp 174-182.

Fishman MA, Hogan GR, Dodge PR: The concurrence of hydrocephalus and craniosynostosis, *J Neurosurg* 34:621-629, 1971.

Freide H, Lilja J, Andersson H, et al: Growth of the anterior cranial base after craniotomy in infants with premature synostosis of the coronal suture, *Scand J Plast Reconstr Surg* 17:99-108, 1983.

Gillies H, Harrison SH: Operative correction by osteotomy of recessed malar maxillary compound in case of oxycephaly, *Br J Plast Surg* 3:123-127, 1950.

Hogan GR, Bauman ML: Hydrocephalus in Apert syndrome, *J Pediatr* 79:782-787, 1971.

Jabs EW, Li X, Scott AF, et al: Jackson-Weiss and Crouzon syndromes are allelic with mutations in fibroblast growth factor receptor 2, *Nat Genet* 8:275-279, 1994.

Lajeunie E, Ma HW, Bonaventure J, et al: FGFR2 mutations in Pfeiffer syndrome, *Nat Genet* 9:108, 1995.

Moore MH: Upper airway obstruction in the syndromal craniosynostoses, *Br J Plast Surg* 46:355-362, 1993.

Park WJ, Theda C, Maestri NE, et al: Analysis of phenotypic features and FGFR2 mutations in Apert syndrome, *Am J Hum Genet* 57:321-328, 1995.

Posnick JC: Crouzon syndrome: evaluation and staging of reconstruction. In Posnick JC, editor: *Craniofacial and maxillofacial surgery in children and young adults*, vol 1, Philadelphia, 2000, WB Saunders, pp 271-307.

Posnick JC, al-Qattan MM, Armstrong D: Monobloc and facial bipartition osteotomies reconstruction of craniofacial malformations: a study of extradural dead space, *Plast Reconstr Surg* 97:1118-1128, 1996.

Posnick JC, Farkas LG: The application of anthropometric surface measurements in craniomaxillofacial surgery. In Farkas LG, editor: *Anthropometry of the head and face*, New York, 1994, Raven Press, pp 125-137.

Posnick JC, Ruiz RL: The craniofacial dysostosis syndromes: current surgical thinking and future directions, *Cleft Palate Craniofac J* 37:433, 2000.

Renier D: Intracranial pressure in craniosynostosis: pre- and postoperative recordings. Correlation with functional results. In Persing JA, Jane JA, Edgerton MT, editors: *Scientific foundations and surgical treatment of craniosynostosis*, Baltimore, 1989, Williams & Wilkins, pp 263-269.

Saltz R, Sierra D, Feldman D, et al: Experimental and clinical applications of fibrin glue, *Plast Reconstr Surg* 88:1005-1015, discussion 1016-1017, 1991.

Tessier P: Osteotomies totales de la face: syndrome de Crouzon, syndrome D'Apert: oxycephalies, scaphocephalies, turricephalies, *Ann Chir Plast* 12:273-286, 1967.

Tessier P: Dysostoses cranio-faciales (syndromes de Crouzon et d'Apert): osteotomies totales de la face. In *Transactions of the Fourth International Congress of Plastic and Reconstructive Surgery*, Amsterdam, 1969, p 77.

Tessier P: The definitive plastic surgical treatment of the severe facial deformities of craniofacial dysostosis. Crouzon's and Apert's diseases, *Plast Reconstr Surg* 48:419-442, 1971.

Tessier P: Relationship of craniostenoses to craniofacial dysostoses and to faciostenoses: a study with therapeutic implications, *Plast Reconstr Surg* 48:224-237, 1982.

Turvey TA, Ruiz RL: Craniosynostosis and craniofacial dysostosis. In Fonseca RJ, Baker SB, Wolford LM, editors: *Oral and maxillofacial surgery*, Philadelphia, 2000, WB Saunders, pp 195-220.

Virchow R: Uber den cretinismus, nametlich in Franken, under uber pathologische: Schadelformen. *Verk Phys Med Gessellsch Wurszburg* 2:230-271, 1851.

Chapter 92

Pediatric Head and Neck Tumors: Benign Lesions

Shelly Abramowicz, Bonnie L. Padwa

ODONTOGENIC CYSTS AND TUMORS

ODONTOGENIC CYSTS

A *periapical abscess* forms when inflammatory cells accumulate at the apex of a non-vital tooth. Frequently, the source of the infection is obvious and is associated with a carious lesion or is the result of a previous injury to the tooth and pulpal tissue. When purulent material accumulates at the apex of the tooth, the tooth and the surrounding tissues become tender to palpation and percussion. If the inflammation is contained within the associated bone, an epithelium-lined cyst may form. A periapical cyst consists of a lumen with cellular debris and inflammatory cells. Radiographically, a periapical cyst looks similar to a periapical abscess. There is loss of lamina dura along the associated tooth root and a round, well-circumscribed radiolucency at the tooth apex. Treatment requires removal of the source of the infection (i.e., carious tooth) and débridement of the periapical cyst. If there is an associated infection, incision and drainage of associated spaces with systemic antibiotic treatment may be necessary.

An *eruption cyst* results from expansion of the mucosa overlying the alveolar ridge above an erupting tooth (Fig. 92-1). This lesion is often blue in color and compressible and may bleed on palpation. There is no associated distinct radiolucency, although soft tissue thickening can be visualized radiographically above the erupting tooth. Generally, no treatment is necessary because the tooth will erupt and the cyst will resolve spontaneously. However, if the cyst becomes large, removal of a portion of the overlying gingiva may be necessary to assist with tooth eruption.

A *dentigerous* or *follicular cyst* is the most common type of developmental cyst of the jaws. It develops from proliferation of the enamel organ remnant and grows in size as a result of increased osmotic pressure within the cyst lumen, which causes expansion and bone resorption. The cyst is most commonly associated with impacted third molars and maxillary canines and is frequently attached to the tooth at the cemento-enamel junction. It is usually asymptomatic and often discovered when assessing delayed eruption of a tooth but can sometimes become very large and cause cortical bone expansion and perforation. Radiographically, a dentigerous cyst is a well-defined, unilocular or occasionally multilocular radiolucency associated with the crown of an unerupted tooth. Treatment consists of removal of the associated tooth and enucleation of the cyst. However, if the lesion is associated with an unerupted permanent tooth or it affects a large portion of the jaw, decompression and irrigation allow the cyst to shrink and the teeth to erupt.

The World Health Organization has designated the *odontogenic keratocyst* (OKC) a type of *keratocystic odontogenic tumor* (KCOT). This lesion typically arises from cell rests of the dental lamina of an unerupted tooth. Radiographically, these are well-circumscribed radiolucent lesions that can be multilocular. The histopathology is characterized by (1) a well-defined basal layer with palisading cuboidal or columnar cells, (2) a keratinizing luminal surface that is mostly parakeratin but may be orthokeratin or a mixture of both, (3) an epithelial lining without an inflammatory infiltrate, and (4) a lumen full of keratinaceous debris.

Treatment depends on the size and location of the lesion. When the cyst is small, enucleation with curettage and close radiographic follow-up may be adequate. However, because of the high rate of local recurrence, ranging from 25% to 60%, some advocate peripheral ostectomy, application of Carnoy solution, or liquid nitrogen cryotherapy following curettage. The goal of these adjunctive therapies is to decrease the recurrence rate by eradication of daughter cysts or residual tumor cells in the superficial layers of the bony cavity.

When the lesion is large or there is concern that vital structures (e.g., nerves) may be injured during enucleation, cyst decompression plus irrigation is another option for treatment. After removal of a portion of the cyst wall, an irrigation port is placed into the cyst for twice-daily irrigation with 0.12% chlorhexidine gluconate solution. Depending on the cyst's size, up to 24 months may be needed for the cyst to shrink. A residual cystectomy and peripheral ostectomy are usually required at the end of treatment. August and colleagues found that epithelial dedifferentiation and loss of cytokeratin-10 production occurs with this therapy and may be associated with lower rates of recurrence.

Nevoid basal cell carcinoma syndrome (NBCCS) is an autosomal dominant or spontaneous disorder characterized by multiple cutaneous basal cell carcinomas, odontogenic keratocysts, skeletal anomalies, and facial dysmorphology. Causative mutations for NBCCS occur in the *PTCH1* gene on chromosome 9q22.3-q31, which encodes the principal receptor for the hedgehog signaling pathway. In the setting of this syndrome, the cysts are more aggressive and the recurrence rate after treatment has been reported to be as high as 82%.

Buccal bifurcation cysts develop along the buccal surface of mandibular molars where the roots bifurcate. The proposed cause of this cyst is extension of enamel onto the roots, which results in loss of periodontal attachment along the buccal root surface and extending to the root bifurcation. Radiographically, this cyst is a well-defined radiolucency in the furcation. Enucleation with periodontal scaling and root planing is the recommended treatment without tooth extraction.

ODONTOGENIC TUMORS

The most common odontogenic tumor is an *odontoma*. It arises from the odontogenic epithelium and mesenchyme that produce enamel and dentin. These tumors are usually asymptomatic, slow growing, and often are found incidentally during a routine

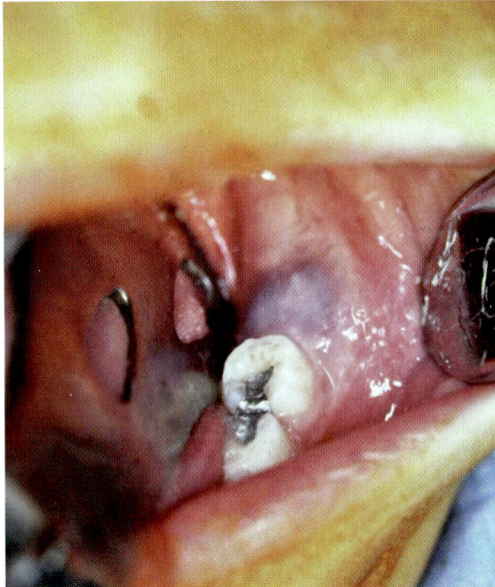

Fig. 92-1 ■ Eruption cyst.

radiographic examination. The radiographic appearance is almost always diagnostic, with the lesions consisting of densely opaque masses of varying size surrounded by a radiolucent line (Fig. 92-2, *A*). These tumors do not typically destroy surrounding bone or resorb adjacent tooth roots. A *complex odontoma* forms an amorphous calcified mass, and a *compound odontoma* is made up of multiple small tooth-like structures. Surgical excision is curative and recurrence is rare (Fig. 92-2, *B*).

An *ameloblastic fibroma* is a mixed tumor of epithelial and mesenchymal origin. The majority (about 80%) of these lesions occur in the posterior mandible, followed by the posterior maxilla; they rarely occur in the anterior region. These tumors are often asymptomatic and they can be associated with an unerupted tooth or may displace developing teeth. Radiographically, they appear as a well-defined unilocular or multilocular radiolucency with a smooth, well-defined margin or sclerotic rim. Histologically, the tumor is composed of mesenchymal tissue resembling primitive dental papilla. Throughout the tumor are long and narrow cords or small discrete islands of odontogenic epithelium that are typically two cells wide and resemble the developing enamel organ. Because this tumor has the potential for recurrence (10% to 20%) and malignant transformation, aggressive curettage or en bloc resection is recommended.

An *ameloblastic fibro-odontoma* resembles an ameloblastic fibroma, but it also contains enamel and dentin. Like an ameloblastic fibroma, it usually occurs in the posterior mandible. Radiographically, it is a well-circumscribed, unilocular mixed radiolucent/radiopaque lesion. It does not typically resorb surrounding bone or adjacent roots. Histologically, this tumor contains varying amounts of dentin-like material, enamel matrix, and even rudimentary tooth buds. This lesion separates from the bone easily, and enucleation plus curettage is curative with rare recurrence.

NON-ODONTOGENIC CYSTS AND TUMORS

NON-ODONTOGENIC CYSTS

A *gingival cyst of the newborn* is a superficial lesion located on the alveolar ridge in infants that arises from remnants of the dental lamina. It is usually smaller than 2 mm and more commonly located

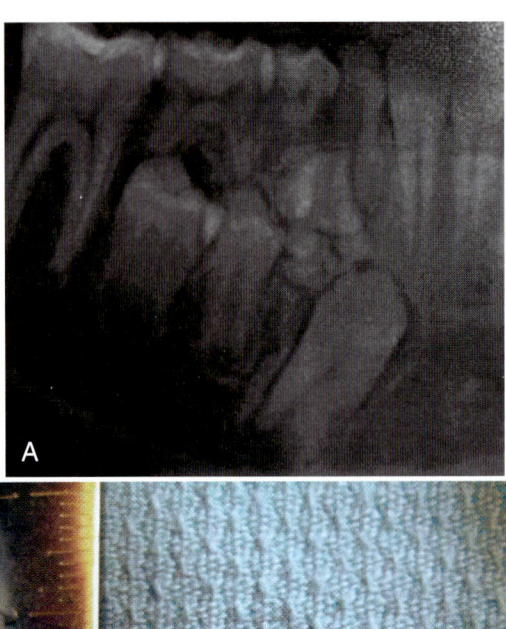

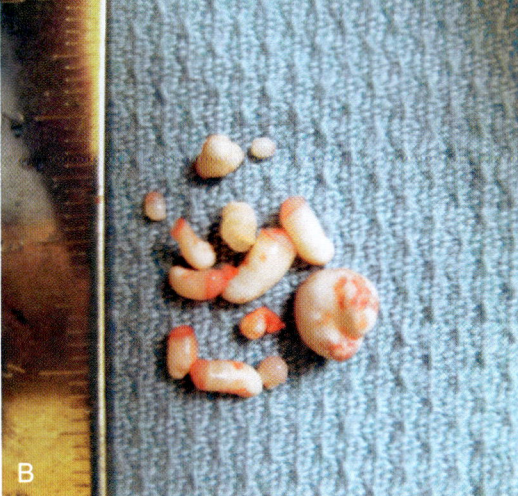

Fig. 92-2 ■ **A,** Radiograph of odontoma. **B,** Odontoma after enucleation.

on the maxillary alveolus. These cysts are filled with keratin and usually disappear once they rupture.

A *nasopalatine duct* or *incisive canal cyst* is the most common non-odontogenic cyst of the oral cavity and occurs in 1% of the population. During embryonic development, the nasopalatine duct connects the oral and nasal cavities. As the palatal processes elevate and fuse in the midline, epithelium that remains in the oral cavity forms this cyst. It appears as a compressible blue swelling on the palatal aspect of the maxillary central incisors (Fig. 92-3, *A*). Radiographically, it is a unilocular, heart-shaped radiolucency that rarely causes root resorption. In an asymptomatic patient, it may be difficult to distinguish between a large incisive foramen and a small nasopalatine duct cyst. If the radiolucency is smaller than 6 mm, it is generally considered a normal foramen. This lesion is treated successfully by reflection of a palatal flap and enucleation, with rare recurrence (Fig. 92-3, *B*). The nasopalatine nerve should be protected to decrease the chance for paresthesia of the anterior palate.

A *traumatic bone cyst* or *simple bone cyst* is an asymptomatic well-circumscribed radiolucency that commonly occurs in the mandible. These lesions are often found on a screening panoramic radiograph before the initiation of orthodontic treatment (Fig. 92-4). Although the etiology and pathogenesis are not known, many patients have a history of trauma to the area. The diagnosis is made at the time of biopsy when an empty cavity is entered and no

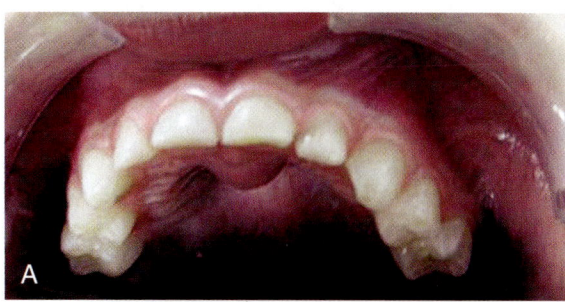

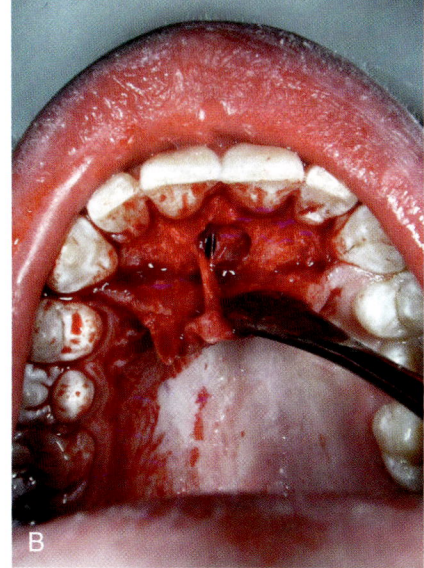

Fig. 92-3 ■ **A,** Nasopalatine duct cyst. **B,** Intraoperative view of a nasopalatine duct cyst.

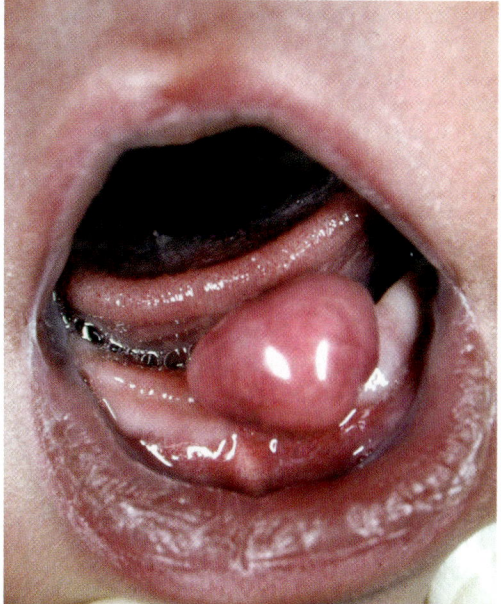

Fig. 92-5 ■ Congenital epulis of the newborn.

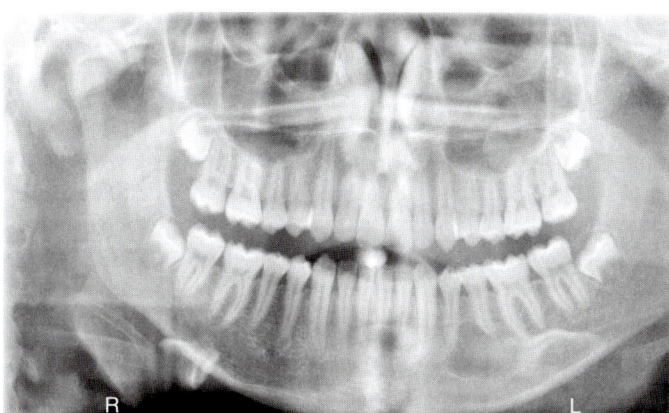

Fig. 92-4 ■ Radiograph of a traumatic bone cyst found as an incidental finding before initiation of orthodontic treatment.

epithelial lining is found. Curettage of the empty cavity provides material for histologic examination and may promote bleeding and callus formation.

An *aneurysmal bone cyst* is similar to a simple bone cyst in that it is not a true cyst with an epithelial lining. The cause of an aneurysmal bone cyst may be a traumatic lesion, vascular malformation, or a neoplasm that disrupts the vasculature of the bone and results in a rapidly enlarging, blood-filled, anomalous vascular condition.

Although it can be found in virtually any bone in the body, when it involves the craniofacial complex, approximately 40% are in the mandible and 25% are in the maxilla. In approximately a third of patients, a contiguous, simultaneously occurring bone lesion such as non-ossifying fibroma, chondroblastoma, giant cell tumor, or fibrous dysplasia is present, in which case it is known as ABC-"plus." Radiographically, the lesion has irregular margins, displaces teeth, and can be unilocular or multilocular. Histologically, there is a fibrous connective tissue stroma with multiple multinucleated giant cells and sinusoidal blood spaces that are lined by fibroblasts and macrophages. Treatment consists of enucleation and curettage. Bleeding can be vigorous until the entire lesion is removed. Recurrence may be related to the biologic behavior of an associated lesion and may require more aggressive treatment dictated by the associated lesion rather than by the cyst.

NON-ODONTOGENIC TUMORS

Congenital epulis of the newborn is a sessile, pink, smooth lesion found on the maxillary alveolar ridge of newborns (Fig. 92-5). It occurs more often in females than in males with a prevalence of 8 : 1. Histologically, the lesion has dense sheets of granular cells in the connective tissue. They are rarely large enough to interfere with feeding, sucking, or breathing but require excision because they do not regress.

A melanotic *neuroectodermal tumor of infancy* is a benign neoplasm of neural crest origin. It has a non-ulcerated, sessile, lobulated appearance with blue or black pigmentation secondary to melanin production by the tumor cells. It has a sudden onset, rapid growth, and a tendency to displace teeth. Radiographically, this tumor may appear as an ill-defined radiolucency with tooth buds floating in space. Histologically, it is characterized by two types of melanin-producing tumor cells in a connective tissue stroma. These cells are reactive for cytokeratin and melanoma-associated antigen (HMB-45). Because of its locally aggressive behavior, this tumor is treated by wide surgical excision with a 5-mm margin.

A *myofibroma* is a solitary, benign proliferation of myofibroblasts that can occur at any age. This lesion is found in soft tissue or bone with a predilection for the head and neck, particularly the mandible. Histologically, it is composed of nodules and fascicles of spindled cells with elongated, tapered, or blunt nuclei and interspersed collagen fibers. Although it can have aggressive clinical features such as rapid growth, a negative desmin stain rules out malignancy. If adjacent bony structures are involved, excision is recommended and enucleation plus curettage is curative for smaller lesions. Recurrence is rare.

Fibrous dysplasia is a benign, progressive condition in which an abnormal increase in the activity of bone protein (G protein) takes place as a result of hormonal changes such as the onset of puberty or pregnancy. Instead of normal bone, immature woven bone within a stroma of abnormal fibrous connective tissue forms and causes expansion and visible deformities. In the majority of patients, the lesions are localized in only one bone (monostotic fibrous dysplasia), whereas others have them in many bones (polyostotic fibrous dysplasia). In about 3% of patients, the condition occurs as a part of the McCune-Albright syndrome, which is caused by a mutation in the *GNAS* gene. Affected patients also have café-au-lait spots, pituitary adenomas, and hormonal abnormalities. Radiographically, fibrous dysplasia has a mixed radiolucent and radiopaque "ground-glass" appearance with expansion of associated bone and displacement of adjacent structures. Histologically, it has an abnormal collagenous matrix surrounding immature bone with irregular distribution and size, also known as "Chinese characters." Treatment depends on each lesion's biologic behavior and includes contour reduction for esthetics, en bloc resection for functional problems, or decompression of adjacent vital structures.

Cherubism is an autosomal dominant disorder with mutations in the gene *SH3BP2*, which has been mapped to chromosome 4p16.3.3, but it can also appear as a part of genetic disorders such as Noonan syndrome, fragile X syndrome, and neurofibromatosis type 1. It is characterized by symmetric enlargement of the mandible, maxilla, or both, which causes rounding of the face with upturned eyes and visible sclera (Fig. 92-6, *A*), premature loss of primary teeth and impaction of permanent teeth. Though usually painless and self-limited, replacement of bone with multilocular cysts composed of fibrotic stromal cells and osteoclast-like cells may cause severe mandibular and maxillary overgrowth with respiratory, vision, speech, and swallowing problem. In adolescence the lesions progress slowly, and in late teens or early twenties the lesions regress and are replaced with normal bone. Radiographic manifestations in the mandible or maxilla consist of bilateral extensive, well-defined multilocular areas of diminished density with few irregular bony septa (Fig. 92-6, *B*). Histologically, the lesions contain numerous multinuclear giant cells in a loose fibrous stroma and eosinophilic cuffing with an increase in osteoid and newly formed bone matrix in the periphery. Because cherubism is expected to regress spontaneously, management consists of longitudinal observation with recontouring for esthetics once the disease becomes quiescent. Surgical intervention is indicated only if functional problems develop.

SOFT TISSUE AND SALIVARY GLAND LESIONS

An *epidermoid* or *sebaceous cyst*, also known as an *epidermal inclusion cyst*, occurs on the face or neck secondary to plugging of hair follicles or traumatic implantation of epithelium into the dermis. A localized build-up of sebum results in a nodular, fluctuant

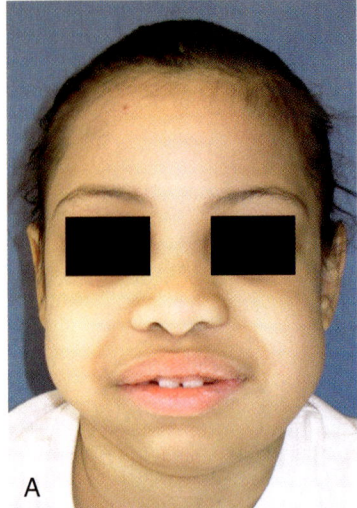

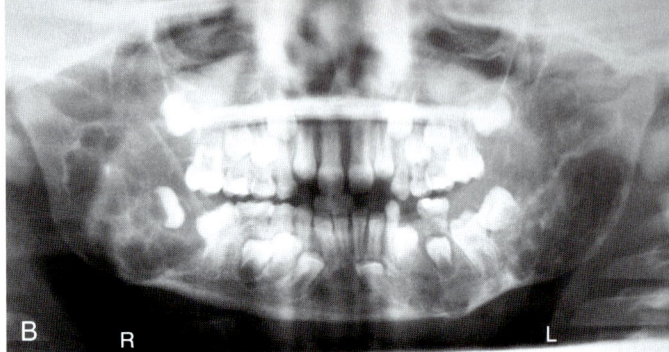

Fig. 92-6 ▪ **A,** Clinical features of a child with cherubism. **B,** Panorex of a child with cherubism.

subcutaneous lesion that may have associated inflammation. It may occur at any age and is most common in acne-prone areas of the head, neck, and back. The lesion is painless, smooth, freely movable, lined by epidermis-like epithelium, and filled with keratin. The cyst can become attached to the overlying dermis and make removal difficult. The incision to remove the cyst should include the drainage point and the hair follicle of origin. This cyst is usually treated by surgical excision, and malignancy is rare. Recurrence is uncommon unless the cyst ruptures during excision, in which case complete excision is less likely and the rate of recurrence is higher.

Dermoid cysts can occur in many areas of the body, including the head and neck. This cyst is developmental in origin and forms as a result of entrapment of skin and undifferentiated ectoderm during fetal development. It may contain sebaceous glands, skin, hair, cartilage, nails, and even teeth. Dermoid cysts can be found in the midline of the floor of the mouth below the mylohyoid muscle and appear as a swelling in the neck. The lesion is typically a painless, doughy, or rubbery mass, and can vary in size from a few millimeters to large lesions that may cause elevation of the tongue and difficulty eating or speaking. Histologically, this cyst is lined by stratified squamous epithelium surrounded by a fibrous connective tissue wall with keratin and sebum in the lumen. Surgical removal is the treatment of choice. Similar to an epidermoid cyst, recurrence is uncommon and malignancy is rare.

A *thyroglossal duct cyst* arises from remnants of the thyroglossal duct, which extends from the foramen cecum at the base of the tongue to the pyramidal lobe of the thyroid gland. The thyroglossal duct tissue usually involutes by the eighth week of intrauterine life, but remnants may lead to cyst formation or ectopic thyroid tissue. These cysts are generally found in the midline over the thyrohyoid membrane (60%), slightly off the midline (15%), within the tongue itself and deep to the foramen cecum (2%), or in the midline below the level of the thyrohyoid membrane (23%). These lesions are doughy, round, and smooth, and they may have a cutaneous fistula that drains pus. Occasionally, the cyst moves with the hyoid bone when the patient swallows. Before excision it is imperative to establish whether the thyroglossal duct cyst contains functioning thyroid tissue so that replacement of thyroid hormone can be coordinated. If discovery of the thyroglossal duct cyst is preceded by an upper respiratory tract infection, a course of antibiotics is recommended with concomitant surgical excision.

Once the cyst is separated from its surrounding tissues, it often remains attached to the body of the hyoid bone. The tract is tied off at its attachment to the hyoid bone, or the body of the hyoid bone is removed along with the cyst itself to eliminate any residual thyroglossal tract epithelium. Recurrence is rare if excision is complete.

A *branchial cleft cyst* originates during embryonic development from invagination or incomplete obliteration of the branchial apparatus. The majority of these cysts (80% to 90%) arise from the second branchial arch and occur along the anterior border of the sternocleidomastoid muscle in close association with the great vessels of the neck. If they arise from the first branchial arch, they may be found in the preauricular area or along the mandible. These cysts are soft, mobile, and non-tender and may be associated with a small skin pit that drains. Unlike a thyroglossal duct cyst, this lesion does not change with head movement or swallowing. The cyst is lined by stratified squamous epithelium with a fibrous wall containing prominent lymphoid tissue with germinal centers. Excision is necessary because spontaneous regression does not occur. Without removal there is a high rate of recurrent infection.

A *melanotic macule* is a pigmented and flat macule of the mucosa (Fig. 92-7). Common locations are the vermilion of the lips, oral mucosa, and gingiva. The presence of multiple macules should raise suspicion for systemic diseases such as Addison disease, Peutz-Jeghers syndrome, or Laugier-Hunziker syndrome. Histologically, the macule is characterized by an accumulation of melanin in the basal keratinocytes and a normal number of melanocytes. In white patients with a lesion on the buccal mucosa, biopsy is necessary to differentiate this lesion from early superficial melanoma.

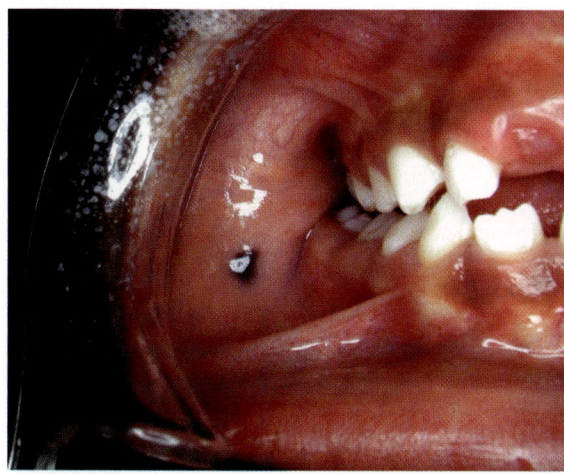

Fig. 92-7 ■ Intraoral photograph of a melanotic macule located on the buccal mucosa.

A *fibroma* is a benign non-tender soft tissue mass that forms in areas of repeated local trauma such as the buccal mucosa adjacent to the occlusal plane. The lesion can usually be excised under local anesthesia, and if there is a traumatic stimulus, it should be eliminated to prevent recurrence.

Verrucous vulgaris and *condyloma acuminatum* are two types of papillomatous lesions caused by strains of human papillomavirus (HPV). Verrucous vulgaris, also known as the common wart, is caused by HPV subtypes 2 and 4. The virus is transmitted through contact with eroded skin or mucosa and it incorporates in the host DNA. This lesion is often found on the labial vermilion or oral mucosa, with similar lesions on the fingers. It is a white lesion with an exophytic, granular or cauliflower-like surface. The other papillomatous lesion is condyloma acuminatum, a sexually transmitted disease caused by HPV subtypes 6 and 11. Though most commonly found on the genitalia, they can be seen in children born to mothers with infected genital tracts. These lesions initially appear as multiple pink or white nodules that can grow and coalesce to form a broad-based, exophytic mass. Although these lesions are asymptomatic, they are unesthetic and may interfere with eating if they become large and involve the oral cavity.

Both lesions have similar histology consisting of thick rete ridges supported by a vascularized connective tissue stroma containing koilocytic cells. The oral lesions should be excised and the bed cauterized to kill any remaining virus. Laser plume containing the virus may cause transmission and hazard to the surgeon. Recurrence is common because the virus remains latent within the cells or is re-inoculated from an infected or untreated person. If condyloma acuminatum is found in a child, sexual activity and possible abuse should be suspected.

A *schwannoma* is a benign proliferation of Schwann cells. It is a smooth and freely movable mass that is commonly found on the tongue or floor of the mouth. It is generally slow growing but can have a sudden increase in size secondary to intralesional hemorrhage. There are two common histologic patterns: spindle cells in palisaded whorls and waves surrounded by an acellular eosinophilic zone (Antoni A pattern) or spindle cells in a haphazard distribution within a fibrillar microcystic matrix (Antoni B pattern). Schwannomas strongly express S-100 protein and are negative for actin and desmin stains. Excision is curative and recurrence is rare.

A *neurofibroma* is an infiltrative lesion arising from a nerve sheath. It is lobulated in appearance with an irregular surface. Histologically, this tumor is made up of spindle-shaped cells with fusiform or wavy nuclei in a myxoid connective tissue matrix scattered with mast cells. A small neurofibroma can be excised with a 1-cm margin. Large neurofibromas, however, are vascular, lack encapsulation, and have multiple prominent projections. Complete excision is not usually possible without morbidity, and debulking is typically the treatment of choice.

Intraoral neurofibromas occur in about 25% of patients with neurofibromatosis, an autosomal dominant trait with variable expressivity. There are nine subtypes with different etiology and clinical manifestation. *Neurofibromatosis type 1* is the most common subtype and is associated with chromosome 17, and *neurofibromatosis type 2* has an association with chromosome 22. Physical findings include axillary or inguinal freckling, Lisch nodules, café-au-lait macules, two or more neurofibromas of any type or one plexiform neurofibroma, optic glioma, distinctive osseous lesion such as sphenoid dysplasia or thinning of long-bone cortex, and a first-degree relative with neurofibromatosis.

A *pyogenic granuloma* is a soft, red or purple mass on the lips, interdental papilla, or buccal mucosa. The cause is thought to be local irritation or trauma in which microorganisms enter the abraded surface and stimulate the proliferation of connective tissue. Histologic evaluation shows granulation tissue with numerous endothelium-lined vascular spaces and fibroblasts. These tumors should be removed because they bleed, become ulcerated, are unesthetic, and can resemble a malignant lesion (e.g., such as leukemia). The lesion can recur if the source of irritation is not removed.

Hemangioma is the most common tumor of infancy. It is usually seen in the head and neck in 4% to 10% of white infants shortly after birth, with an increase in frequency in premature infants. It is three to five times more common in females. Hemangioma is a benign proliferation of blood vessels with raised skin and erythema. Though rare, a large facial hemangioma can be associated with overgrowth of bone. There are three stages in the life cycle of a hemangioma: (1) the proliferating phase (0 to 1 year of age), which occurs as a result of endothelial cell proliferation stimulated by growth factors; (2) the involuting phase (1 to 5 years of age); and (3) the involuted phase (after 5 to 7 years of age), following which they never recur. As the hemangioma involutes, the color fades, nearly normal skin is restored, and the lesion feels softer because of replacement with fat.

Observation is the treatment of choice for hemangiomas unless ulceration (30%), tissue destruction, or pain occurs. If the ulceration is small or superficial, cleansing and daily application of a topical antibiotic are useful. Otherwise, systemic or intralesional corticosteroids or the administration of interferon alfa may be considered. It is important to realize that the clinical outcome of these lesions is extremely unpredictable and that a large and bulky hemangioma can regress completely whereas a flat, superficial hemangioma can irreversibly alter the cutaneous texture, which may result in an atrophic patch. When indicated, a hemangioma can be resected.

A *vascular malformation* is the result of aberrant vessel angiogenesis (capillary, venous, arterial, lymphatic, or a combination) during embryogenesis. Although it may be present at birth, it might not become clinically obvious until late in infancy or childhood. Further proliferation and growth can occur spontaneously or as a result of trauma, infection, or hormonal influences. Vascular malformations are associated with skeletal abnormalities in 35% of cases, such as distortion and hypertrophy with a lymphatic malformation or hypoplasia with a venous malformation. Treatment of vascular malformations is challenging since complete resection of this lesion is not possible. Indications for surgical management include improvement in function, respiration, nutrition, and esthetics. Before surgical intervention, embolization or sclerotherapy is usually necessary to provide temporary occlusion of the nidus. Embolization alone results in only transient improvement because of recruitment of new vessels by the nidus.

A *mucocele* is the most common benign salivary gland lesion in children (Fig. 92-8, *A*). Trauma such as a bite or a fall causes injury to a minor salivary gland, saliva extravagates into the surrounding soft tissue, the fluid becomes walled off, and a pseudocyst forms. If the lesion drains, the fluid is usually thick and viscous, similar to saliva. Although a mucocele sometimes disappears, it generally recurs in the same location. Histologically, it is filled with foamy macrophages and mucoid material surrounded by neutrophils. Definitive treatment of a mucocele is surgical excision and removal of associated minor salivary glands (Fig. 92-8, *B*).

A *ranula* is a bluish, translucent lesion located on the floor of the mouth or below the tongue (Fig. 92-9), and a *plunging ranula* is located below the mylohyoid muscle and may appear as a swelling in the neck. This lesion is sometimes congenital but more often results from trauma to the sublingual gland duct, which causes an

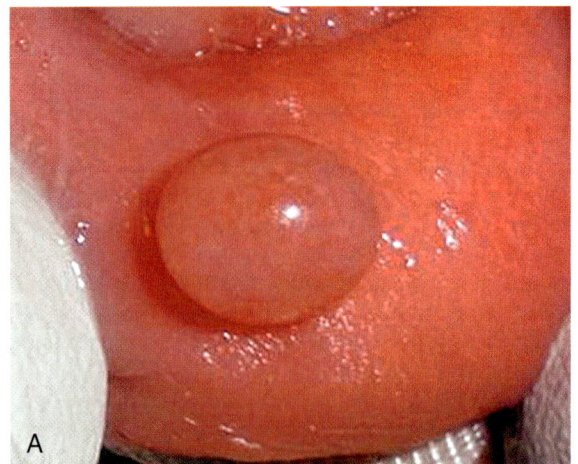
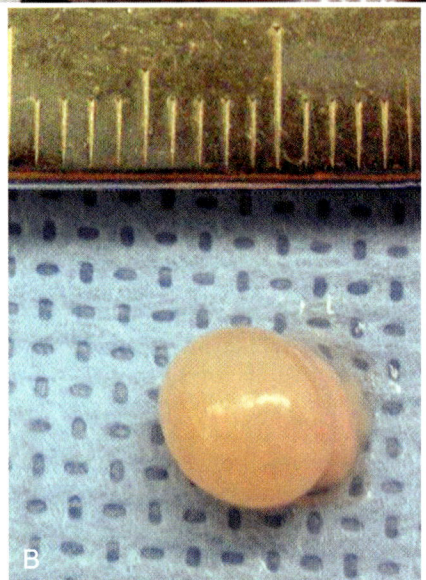

Fig. 92-8 ■ **A,** Mucocele of the lower lip in a 1-year-old child. **B,** Excised mucocele.

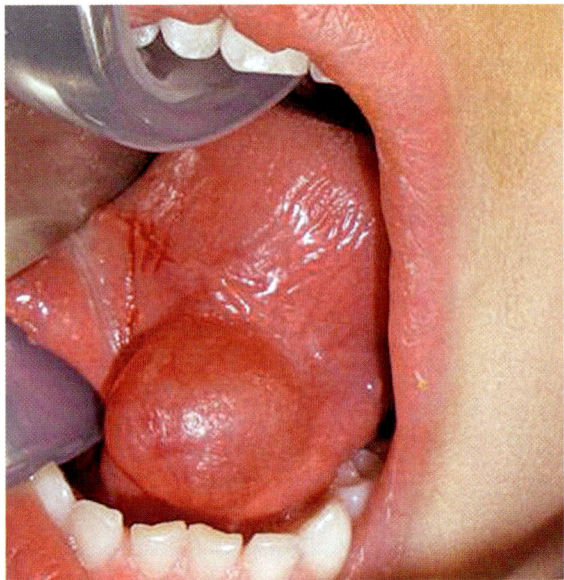

Fig. 92-9 ■ Ranula located below the tongue on the floor of the mouth.

increase in size of the sublingual gland and elevation of the tongue and interferes with swallowing, speech, mastication, or respiration. There are two main techniques in the treatment of a ranula: (1) marsupialization, in which the lining of the lesion is sutured to the mucosal edge to keep the cavity open and form a pathway for continuous drainage, and (2) excision of the ranula and associated sublingual gland via an intraoral approach.

A *pleomorphic adenoma* is a benign, firm, painless, slow-growing salivary gland tumor that is found in the parotid (85%), submandibular (8%), or minor salivary gland (7%). The most common intraoral sites are the palate, upper lip, and buccal mucosa. The multiple histologic combinations of epithelial ducts, tubules, ribbons, or solid sheets and the mesenchymal elements, which are myxoid or hyalinized, are responsible for this lesion's name. Plasmacytoid cells are indicative of this mixed tumor and help eliminate other salivary gland tumors from the differential diagnosis. Treatment presents a therapeutic dilemma. Even though this tumor is benign, recurrences can take place even 30 years after treatment. Although postoperative radiation therapy allows better control of the tumor, the side effects of radiation such as an alteration in facial growth and tooth development must be considered. Therefore, in the parotid gland, excision via superficial or total parotidectomy with preservation of the facial nerve is the treatment of choice.

PEARLS AND PITFALLS

- The behavioral aspects of pediatric care must always be considered when treating a child in an office or hospital setting. These aspects often influence the ultimate treatment of a lesion in a child.
- Benign lesions of the head and neck that occur in children are often different from those in adults. The most common lesions that occur in childhood are odontomas, fibro-osseous lesions, and traumatic bone cysts.
- The frequency of pleomorphic adenoma occurring in a salivary gland decreases with decreasing size of the gland. It is most common in the largest salivary glands.
- Always remember the sequence of eruption and exfoliation of teeth. The etiology of disordered eruption may be unknown in the majority of cases.
- The World Health Organization has designated the odontogenic keratocyst (OKC) a type of benign tumor and has given it the name keratocystic odontogenic tumor (KCOT).
- Hemangioma is a tumor of infancy and is not found in adults. Many other vascular tumors and malformations have been incorrectly termed hemangioma (e.g., cavernous hemangioma). Proper terminology is important because it determines treatment and response to therapy.

BIBLIOGRAPHY

Agaram NP, Collins BM, Barnes L, et al: Molecular analysis to demonstrate that odontogenic keratocysts are neoplastic, *Arch Pathol Lab Med* 128:313-317, 2004.

Amir J, Metzker A, Krikler R, et al: Strawberry hemangioma in preterm infants, *Pediatr Dermatol* 3:331-332, 1986.

August M, Faquin WC, Troulis MJ, et al: Dedifferentiation of odontogenic keratocyst epithelium after cyst decompression, *J Oral Maxillofac Surg* 61:678-683, discussion 683-684, 2003.

Basant Kumar, Sharma SB: Neonatal oral tumors: congenital epulis and epignathus, *J Pediatr Surg* 43:9-11, 2008.

Bodner L, Goldstein J, Sarnat H: Eruption cysts: a clinical report of 24 new cases, *J Clin Pediatr Dent* 28:183-186, 2004.

Boon LM, MacDonald DM, Mulliken JB: Complications of systemic corticosteroid therapy for problematic hemangioma, *Plast Reconstr Surg* 104:1616-1623, 1999.

Boyd JB, Mulliken JB, Kaban LB, et al: Skeletal changes associated with vascular malformations, *Plast Reconstr Surg* 74:789-795, 1984.

Boyne PJ, Hou D, Moretta C, et al: The multifocal nature of odontogenic keratocysts, *J Calif Dent Assoc* 33:961-965, 2005.

Carvalho VM, Perdigão PF, Amaral FR, et al: Novel mutations in the SH3BP2 gene associated with sporadic central giant cell lesions and cherubism, *Oral Dis* 15:106-110, 2009.

Chen WL, Ye JT, Xu LF, et al: A multidisciplinary approach to treating maxillofacial arteriovenous malformations in children, *Oral Surg Oral Med Oral Pathol Oral Radiol Endod* 108:41-47, 2009.

Cobourne MT, Xavier GM, Depew M, et al: Sonic hedgehog signalling inhibits palatogenesis and arrests tooth development in a mouse model of the nevoid basal cell carcinoma syndrome, *Dev Biol* 331:38-49, 2009.

Cohen DM, Bhattacharyya I: Ameloblastic fibroma, ameloblastic fibro-odontoma, and odontoma, *Oral Maxillofac Surg Clin North Am* 16:375-384, 2004.

Davenport M: Lumps and swellings of the head and neck, *BMJ* 312:368-371, 1996.

Dilley DC, Siegel MA, Budnick S: Diagnosing and treating common oral pathologies, *Pediatr Clin North Am* 38:1227-1264, 1991.

Dominguez FV, Keszler A: comparative study of keratocysts, associated and non-associated with nevoid basal cell carcinoma syndrome, *J Oral Pathol* 17:39-42, 1988.

Fletcher CD, Achu P, Van Noorde S, et al: Infantile myofibromatosis: a light microscopic, histochemical and immunohistochemical study suggesting true smooth muscle differentiation, *Histopathology* 11:245-258, 1987.

Foss RD, Ellis GL: Myofibromas and myofibromatosis of the oral region: a clinicopathologic analysis of 79 cases, *Oral Surg Oral Med Oral Pathol Oral Radiol Endod* 89:57-65, 2000.

Gareth D, Evans R: Neurofibromatosis type 2 (NF2): a clinical and molecular review, *Orphanet J Rare Dis* 4:16, 2009.

Gloster HM, Roenigk RK: Risk of acquiring human papillomavirus from the plume produced by the carbon dioxide laser in the treatment of warts, *J Am Acad Dermatol* 32:436-441, 1995.

Gonzalez-Alva P, Tanaka A, Oku Y, et al: Keratocystic odontogenic tumor: a retrospective study of 183 cases, *J Oral Sci* 50:205-212, 2008.

Gosau M, Draenert FG, Müller S, et al: Two modifications in the treatment of keratocystic odontogenic tumors (KCOT) and the use of Carnoy's solution (CS)—a retrospective study lasting between 2 and 10 years, *Clin Oral Investig* 14:27-34, 2010.

Gyulai-Gaál S, Takács D, Szabó G, et al: Mixed odontogenic tumors in children and adolescents, *J Craniofac Surg* 18:1338-1342, 2007.

Hahn H, Wicking C, Zaphiropoulous PG, et al: Mutations of the human homolog of *Drosophila* patched in the nevoid basal cell carcinoma syndrome, *Cell* 85:841-851, 1996.

Kaban LB, Troulis MJ: *Pediatric oral and maxillofacial surgery.* Philadelphia, Saunders, 2004

Kaban LB, Mulliken JB: Vascular anomalies of the maxillofacial region, *J Oral Maxillofac Surg* 44:203-213, 1986.

Kademani D, Costello BJ, Ditty D, et al: An alternative approach to maxillofacial arteriovenous malformations with transosseous direct puncture embolization, *Oral Surg Oral Med Oral Pathol Oral Radiol Endod* 97:701-706, 2004.

Karnes PS: Neurofibromatosis: a common neurocutaneous disorder, *Mayo Clin Proc* 73:1071-1076, 1998.

Madras J, Lapointe H: Keratocystic odontogenic tumour: reclassification of the odontogenic keratocyst from cyst to tumour, *J Can Dent Assoc* 74:165-165h, 2008.

Marler JJ, Mulliken JB: Current management of hemangiomas and vascular malformations, *Clin Plastic Surg* 32:99-116, 2005.

Mehta D, Willging JP: Pediatric salivary gland lesions, *Semin Pediatr Surg* 15:76-84, 2006.

Mulliken JB, Glowacki J: Hemangiomas and vascular malformations in infants and children: a classification based on endothelial characteristics, *Plast Reconstr Surg* 69:412-422, 1982.

Neville B, Damm DD, Allen CM, et al: *Oral and maxillofacial pathology*, ed 3, St Louis, 2009, WB Saunders.

Padwa BL, Denhart BC, Kaban LB: Aneurysmal bone cyst-"plus": a report of three cases, *J Oral Maxillofac Surg* 55:1144-1152, 1997.

Papadaki ME, Troulis MJ, Kaban LB: Advances in diagnosis and management of fibro-osseous lesions, *Oral Maxillofacial Surg Clin Nirth Am* 17:415-434, 2005.

Philipsen HP, Reichart RP, Pratorius F: Mixed odontogenic tumors and odontomas: considerations on interrelationship. Review of the literature and presentation of 134 new cases of odontomas, *Oral Oncol* 33:86-99, 1997.

Pinto A: Pediatric soft tissue lesions, *Dent Clin North Am* 49:241-258, 2005.

Pogrel MA, Jordan RC: Marsupialization as a definitive treatment for the odontogenic keratocyst, *J Oral Maxillofac Surg* 62:651-655, discussion 655-656, 2004. Partial retraction in Pogrel MA: *J Oral Maxillofac Surg* 65:362-363, 2007.

Pompura JR, Sandor GK, Stoneman DW: The buccal bifurcation cyst: a prospective study of treatment outcomes in 44 sites, *Oral Surg Oral Med Oral Pathol Oral Radiol Endod* 83:215-221, 1997.

Regezi JA, Sciubba JJ, Jordan RCK: *Oral pathology: clinical pathologic correlations*, ed 5, St Louis, 2008, WB Saunders.

Rimminucci M, Liu B, Corsi A, et al: The histopathology of fibrous dysplasia of bone in patients with activating mutations of the Gs alpha gene: site-specific patterns and recurrent histological hallmarks, *J Pathol* 187:249-258, 1999.

Rodriguez KH, Vargas S, Robson C, et al: Pleomorphic adenoma of the parotid gland in children, *Int J Pediatr Otorhinolaryngol* 71:1717-1723, 2007.

Scolozzi P, Martinez A, Richter M, et al: A nasopalatine duct cyst in a 7-year-old child, *Pediatr Dent* 30:530-534, 2008.

Selim H, Shaheen S, Barakat K, et al: Melanotic neuroectodermal tumor of infancy: review of literature and case report, *J Pediatr Surg* 43:E25-E29, 2008.

Shohat I, Buchner A, Taicher S: Mandibular buccal bifurcation cyst: enucleation without extraction, *Int J Oral Maxillofac Surg* 32:610-613, 2003.

Silva CE, Silva GC, Vieira TC: Cherubism: clinicoradiographic features, treatment, and long-term follow-up of 8 cases, *J Oral Maxillofac Surg* 62:517-522, 2007.

Tiziani V, Reichenberger E, Buzzo CL, et al: The gene for cherubism maps to chromosome 4p16, *Am J Hum Genet* 65:158-166, 1999.

Trodhal JN: Ameloblastic fibroma: survey of cases from the Armed Forces Institute of Pathology, *Oral Surg Oral Med Oral Pathol* 33:547-558, 1972.

Turkington JRA, Pterson A, Sweeney LE, et al: Neck masses in children, *Br J Radiol* 78:75-85, 2005.

Vazquez E, Enriquez G, Castellote A, et al: US, CT and MR imaging of neck lesions in children, *Radiographics* 15:105-122, 1995.

Vered M, Allon I, Buchner A, et al: Clinicopathologic correlations of myofibroblastic tumors of the oral cavity—myofibroma and myofibromatosis of the oral soft tissues, *J Oral Pathol Med* 36:304-314, 2007.

Welbury RR: Congenital epulis of the newborn, *Br J Oral Surg* 18:238-243, 1980.

Williams VC, Lucas J, Babcock MA, et al: Neurofibromatosis type 1 revisited, *Pediatrics* 123:124-133, 2009.

Yang HG, Yang KC: A new method for facial epidermoid cyst removal with minimal incision, *J Eur Acad Dermatol* 23:887-890, 2009.

Chapter

93

Pediatric Malignant Tumors of the Head and Neck

Sean P. Edwards

Cancer develops in approximately 1 in 350 individuals in the United States by the age of 20 years. Therapeutic advances have enabled 80% of pediatric patients with cancer to survive for 5 years, and most are cured.[1] One in 50 individuals between 20 and 34 years of age are survivors of childhood cancer.[2] Tumors of the head and neck represent only 2% to 5% of all pediatric tumors.[3]

In general, malignant disease in the pediatric population is rare and considerably more so than in the adult population. There are differences in the spectrum of diseases seen in this group and in adults, and when the diseases are similar, there are sometimes differences in their clinical behavior. There are additional management concerns when working with children. Treatment burden is given relatively greater consideration in children since they are growing and developing and treatment may exert untoward influences therein. Furthermore, the greater potential life expectancy in children means that long-term cancer survivors may suffer long-term consequences of treatment that may take decades to become manifested.

There are many rare diseases that may involve the head and neck in the pediatric population. Each of them deserves careful attention by a multidisciplinary tumor board that includes pediatric oncologists, radiation oncologists, dentists, and surgeons. This chapter discusses the general approach to pediatric patients with malignant disease and its management and follow-up.

Several large published reviews have described the incidence of different malignancies in the head and neck in children. Cunningham and associates conducted a 20-year, single-center review of 241 children in whom a malignancy of the head and neck was diagnosed.[3] Lymphomas predominated and accounted for 59% of cases. Soft tissue sarcomas and specifically rhabdomyosarcomas were the next most common at 17.5%. Thyroid carcinomas (10%), neuroblastomas (5%), nasopharyngeal carcinomas (5%), salivary gland malignancies (2.5%), and malignant teratomas (1%) accounted for the remainder of cases. Jaffe and Jaffe reviewed 178 pediatric head and neck malignancies and found that lymphomas accounted for 55%;

rhabdomyosarcomas, 11%; other sarcomas, 10%; thyroid, 5%; and neuroblastomas, 5%.[4] Rapidis and co-authors reviewed 1007 tumors of the head and neck in children. Thirty-one percent of these tumors were malignant, and again, lymphomas (52%) and rhabdomyosarcomas (22%) predominated.[5]

Ord discussed the effect of age on disease prevalence.[6] In the first 3 years of life, retinoblastomas are the most common, with rhabdomyosarcomas and neuroblastomas second and third in incidence, respectively. Between the ages of 3 and 11 years, rhabdomyosarcomas become the most common, followed by lymphomas. From 12 to 20 years of age, lymphomas once again are most common, followed by sarcomas.

Most of these reviews have come from large cancer centers, otolaryngologists, and general pediatric surgeons and may reflect the referral patterns that would be expected in such environments. Oral and maxillofacial surgeons are, in general, more likely to encounter maxillofacial and jaw diseases, especially those requiring surgical management. The incidence of malignant tumors of the jaws in children ranges from 7% to 25%.[7-10] Differences therein may reflect regional referral biases. Sarcoma was the most common diagnosis in each of these reviews. Highlighting both the potential effect of referral bias and the rarity of pediatric oral and maxillofacial malignancies, two large reviews of oral biopsies have been conducted. Shah and colleagues reviewed 5457 biopsy specimens from patients aged 0 to 16 years that were sent to a dental school biopsy service.[11] Only eight of the submissions represented malignant disease. Chen and co-workers reviewed 534 oral biopsy samples and found only 11 (2.1%) to be malignant.[12] Das and Das reviewed 2370 biopsy specimens from patients younger than 20 years and found only 3 to be malignant.[13] Malignant tumors of the head and neck are rare in general, but those involving the jaws and oral cavity would seem to be ever rarer.

GENERAL APPROACH TO PEDIATRIC PATIENTS WITH A MASS IN THE HEAD AND NECK

The differential diagnosis of masses in the head and neck of children includes congenital, infectious, and neoplastic processes. Eighty percent to 90% of head and neck masses in children are benign.

As with adult patients, the clinician should approach these masses with a detailed history and thorough physical examination. In the pediatric population the complaints may be more non-specific, and often much of the history will be derived from a parent. This requires the clinician to interpret the history differently and maintain a high index of suspicion and frequently a lower threshold for ordering further diagnostic studies. Nasopharyngeal tumors, for example, may be accompanied by unilateral nasal obstruction, recurrent epistaxis, otalgia, otorrhea, or cranial nerve deficits.

The history should attempt to elicit the time course of the mass and its effects on the child. Those present at birth, for instance, are more likely to be congenital than neoplastic. Congenital masses need not be manifested in infancy, however, and many cystic lesions may expand later in a child's life, occasionally coincident with an infection. The family history can point to inherited disorders. A child with a mass that is growing who is gaining weight appropriately and is otherwise thriving is less likely to suffer from systemic or disseminated disease.

The physical examination should include the mass and its association with surrounding tissues. Masses that are fixed to surrounding or underlying tissues portend a more grave diagnosis. Cystic lesions may be fluctuant. Movement of a neck mass with swallowing is typical of a thyroglossal duct cyst. Younger children may require examination under anesthesia. When this is the case, multiple general anesthetics can be avoided by combining biopsy and any needed imaging during the same course of anesthesia.

LYMPHOMAS

Lymphomas represent more than 50% of pediatric head and neck malignancies and will most often appear as a neck mass. They are broadly classified as Hodgkin lymphoma (HL) and non-Hodgkin lymphoma (NHL) and are almost equal in frequency.

HL is one of the most common cancers found in children and adolescents; it accounts for 4% and 12% of all invasive cancers in the United States in people between the ages of 0 and 14 and 15 and 30, respectively.[14] HL is rare before the age of 5 years. It is twice as common in boys, and 80% to 90% will involve the neck. A third of children will have constitutional or the so-called B symptoms consisting of fevers, night sweats, and weight loss. The development of HL is associated with Epstein-Barr virus infection and certain immunodeficiency disorders, specifically ataxia-telangiectasia, Wiskott-Aldrich syndrome, and Bloom syndrome.[15]

NHL is also more common in boys than girls (2:1 to 3:1). The incidence of NHL increases steadily throughout life. Roh and associates reviewed 106 lymphomas of the head and neck in children and found that 78% (74/95) of cases of NHL in children occurred in those younger than 10 years. The signs and symptoms are more varied with NHL, and systemic involvement is more common.[15] Burkitt lymphoma accounts for approximately 40% of cases of childhood NHL in the United States. The disease exists in two subtypes. That subtype endemic to Africa frequently involves the maxilla and mandible and is a fast-growing disease. The non-endemic form has a lower tendency to involve the jaws (incidence of 7% to 16%).

Lymphomas in the head and neck can be classified clinically as nodal, extranodal lymphatic, and extralymphatic. The nodal form generally consists of chronically enlarged cervical lymph nodes persisting longer than 6 weeks. Inflammatory adenitis is the primary competing diagnosis. Hodgkin disease in the head and neck will be manifested as enlarged lymph nodes, but enlarged lymph nodes are noted in only 60% of patients with NHL.[15] Extranodal manifestations are essentially limited to NHL and involve the Waldeyer ring of lymphatic tissue. Typical findings include unilateral enlargement of a tonsil, dysphagia, new-onset snoring, rhinolalia, or nasal obstruction.[14] Extralymphatic NHL can involve virtually any portion of the head and neck and requires a higher index of suspicion for prompt diagnosis.

Treatment of both diseases usually consists of multiagent chemotherapy and, in the case of Hodgkin disease, radiotherapy. The surgeon's role is primarily to help establish the diagnosis and procure tissue for histopathologic evaluation, usually through open biopsy. The prognosis for patients with HL and NHL depends on the stage. Hodgkin disease, which is generally detected at stage I or II, has a greater than 90% 5-year survival rate, whereas for NHL, the survival rate is 70% at the same time interval. Systemic dissemination, B symptoms, and central nervous system involvement are negative prognostic indicators.[15]

RHABDOMYOSARCOMA

Rhabdomyosarcoma is the second most common malignant tumor of the head and neck in children and the most common pediatric sarcoma.[16] Approximately 40% of rhabdomyosarcomas appear in the head and neck region. In the head and neck the primary sites include the orbit (25% of head and neck rhabdomyosarcomas) and parameningeal region (40% of head and neck lesions). The remainder occur throughout the head and neck, including the scalp and cheek, parotid bed, and larynx. This last group is the one most likely to be encountered by the oral and maxillofacial surgeon and is generally referred to as non-orbit, non-parameningeal head and neck rhabdomyosarcoma.

Three general pathologic types have been described: embryonal (the most common form), alveolar, and pleomorphic. An undifferentiated subtype has been added by the Intergroup Rhabdomyosarcoma Study (IRS) group. The embryonal group has two further subclassifications, sarcoma botryoides and spindle cell rhabdomyosarcoma, each of which has a better prognosis than the more typical embryonal form.[16]

The work-up includes a complete blood count, electrolyte levels, liver function tests, imaging of the primary site and regional lymph node basins with computed tomography (CT) or magnetic resonance imaging (MRI) (or both), and imaging of the chest for metastatic disease. Bone marrow biopsy is standard. If the tumor involves the parameningeal structures, evaluation for intracranial extension is required. Cerebrospinal fluid should be sampled and MRI performed to detail the extent of disease.

Rhabdomyosarcoma is staged in North America according to the IRS staging classification (Table 93-1). It is based on location, invasiveness, size of the tumor, regional nodal spread, and the presence of metastatic disease. Favorable sites include the orbit and non-parameningeal regions of the head and neck. A parameningeal rhabdomyosarcoma, by virtue of its proximity to the central nervous system and non-specific symptoms, is worse in terms of prognosis. An IRS grouping system is also used to help select adjuvant therapies based on resection margin status and the extent of disease (localized, regional, or distant metastases). Both TNM status and the clinical grouping are used to risk-stratify patients into a grid and help select therapy.

Treatment decisions should be made within the context of a multidisciplinary sarcoma team consisting of surgeons, medical oncologists, radiation therapists, pathologists, and radiologists. Potential for cure and treatment toxicity are of primary concern. Currently, all patients with rhabdomyosarcoma will undergo multiagent chemotherapy.[16] Surgical intervention is aimed at resection with clear margins whenever possible since this offers the best chance for clearance, although this can be difficult for parameningeal disease. Chemotherapy can shrink previously unresectable disease and downgrade a patient's IRS grouping. When surgery is not able to eliminate local disease, radiation therapy is used in an effort to improve local disease control. Radiation therapy, though effective for local control, especially when gross microscopic disease remains, must be balanced against the additional morbidity that would result

from its use versus more aggressive resection. The substantial radiation doses required to improve local control of residual disease are in the range of 50 Gy and carry a risk for acute toxicity, pituitary damage and growth factor deficiency, facial growth restriction, retinal damage, cataracts, lifelong photophobia, dental anomalies, alopecia, and risk for secondary radiation-induced malignancies.

The outcomes of individuals undergoing treatment of rhabdomyosarcoma have continued to improve. They are poorer for children younger than 1 year and older than 9 years. Histology has an important role to play. In IRS-IV, 3-year failure-free survival rates were 83%, 66%, and 55% for embryonal, alveolar, and undifferentiated sarcomas, respectively.[17] Surgical margin status is also important, with IRS grouping 1 and 2 performing better than 3 and 4.[8] Five-year failure-free survival rates for non-orbit, non-parameningeal rhabdomyosarcoma treated by surgery, vincristine, and dactinomycin, with or without cyclophosphamide, were 76% in the IRS-IV trials.[18]

OSTEOSARCOMA

Osteosarcomas of all sites account for approximately 40% to 60% of primary bone tumors. About 10% of osteosarcomas occur in the head and neck, with most being located in the mandible and maxilla.[19,20] The maxilla and mandible are roughly equally affected in most series.[21,22] Osteosarcomas in the head and neck seem to have different biologic behavior than their long-bone counterpart. The peak incidence of maxillary and mandibular lesions is 1 to 2 decades later, they have a lower incidence of metastatic disease, and they are associated with higher survival rates ranging up to 70% to 80%.[21,23,24] Survival seems to be longer in patients younger than 40 years.[22,23]

Osteosarcomas of the jaws typically cause a swelling that may be painful and associated with paresthesias.[25] Evaluation of such a lesion includes an incisional biopsy to confirm the diagnosis and review by a pathologist experienced in sarcoma pathology. Imaging, typically MRI or CT of the head, neck, and chest, is performed to define the extent of disease, search for metastatic lesions, and begin the staging process. MRI may have incremental benefit in evaluating spread of disease to bone marrow. Imaging can demonstrate osteolytic, osteoblastic, or mixed lesions. Periosteal reactions are classically described as "sunburst" in appearance (Fig. 93-1). Typically, cases would be discussed with a multidisciplinary head and neck tumor or sarcoma board and a treatment plan established.

Surgical excision with wide margins is the mainstay of treatment and the single most important factor in determining survival.[21] A

TABLE 93-1	Clinical Grouping Classification of the Intergroup Rhabdomyosarcoma Study
GROUP	**DESCRIPTION**
Group 1	Localized disease, completely resected
Group 2	Grossly resected tumor with microscopic residual disease. Regional disease with involved nodes
Group 3	Gross residual disease
Group 4	Distant metastatic disease present at onset

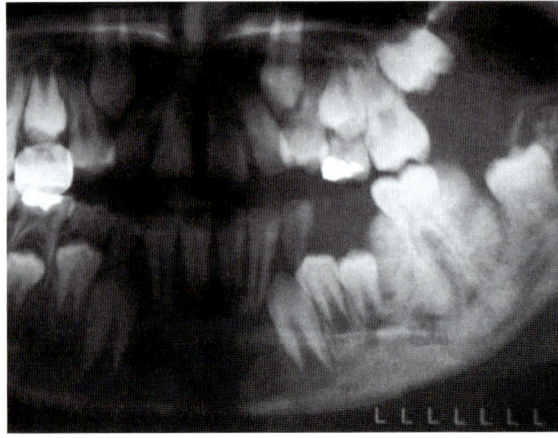

Fig. 93-1 ■ Orthopantomogram demonstrating a sunburst appearance of an osteosarcoma of the left mandible in a child.

retrospective review of 119 jaw and craniofacial osteosarcomas treated at M.D. Anderson Cancer Center demonstrated on multivariate analysis that resection margin status was the only factor found to be predictive of survival. Based on this finding, most surgeons recommend wide, aggressive resection with margins of 2 to 3 cm. Incomplete resection is most often due to technical factors at the skull base and ranges in incidence from 31% to 52%.[26]

Adjuvant therapy for long-bone osteosarcoma has clearly been shown to improve survival rates from 20% in the 1960s to 70% in the 1980s over surgery alone.[27-30] The role of adjuvant chemotherapy in the management of osteosarcomas of the jaws is not as clear, with some studies indicating no benefit from adjuvant therapy.[24,31] This may be due to the fact that although distant metastatic disease is present in as many as 80% of patients with long-bone osteosarcoma, only 18% of jaw osteosarcomas will be accompanied by distant disease.[22] A trend toward benefit has been seen in several large reviews, especially in patients with close or positive margins.[21,23] In their analysis of 119 patients with jaw and craniofacial osteosarcomas, Guadagnolo and colleagues found in a stratified analysis that combined-modality therapy improved the overall survival rate from 31% to 80% over surgery alone when margin status was positive or uncertain.[21]

Osteosarcoma has generally been considered to be radioresistant. Unlike long-bone osteosarcoma, death from jaw osteosarcoma is usually due to local recurrence, thus the interest in the use of radiotherapy to improve local control. Guadagnolo and colleagues specifically addressed the use of radiotherapy in the management of jaw and craniofacial osteosarcomas.[21] They found adjuvant radiotherapy to be of significant benefit in local control, disease-specific survival, and overall survival in patients with positive or uncertain margin status. This benefit was not realized in those with clear surgical margins. Given the potential morbidity of radiotherapy in a growing child, effort should primarily be directed at achieving wide surgical clearance of disease, but when necessary, consideration should be given to the use of radiation therapy when surgical margins are positive or uncertain.

SALIVARY GLAND MALIGNANCIES

Tumors of salivary gland origin represent 5% to 8% of all pediatric head and neck neoplasms.[32] A review of 9993 salivary gland lesions at the Armed Forces Institute of Pathology yielded only 168 pediatric salivary gland tumors, 35 of which were primary epithelial malignancies.[33] A similar review of 1248 salivary gland tumors at M.D. Anderson identified only 16 pediatric cases.[34]

When evaluating a child with a mass in a salivary gland, the clinician must consider a broad differential diagnosis, including infectious and inflammatory conditions, vascular lesions and malformations, congenital lesions, and a myriad of neoplasms. Neoplasms may be epithelial or mesenchymal in origin. Mesenchymal disease includes vascular and lymphatic malformations and more ominous lesions such as rhabdomyosarcoma. Most patients with a salivary gland neoplasm will have a painless, slowly growing mass in the parotid region, where 90% of pediatric salivary tumors occur.[35] Fixation of the overlying skin and facial nerve weakness portend a malignant diagnosis. Involvement of the submandibular and minor salivary glands in most series of pediatric salivary gland tumors seems to be rare and accounts for the remainder of cases. Sublingual gland disease is rarely reported.[35-37] Thirty-five percent to 50% of all pediatric salivary gland masses will be malignant; in adults, the incidence is 15% to 25%.[38,39] Mucoepidermoid carcinoma is the most common malignant salivary gland disease and represents approximately half of the diagnoses.[35] Acinic cell carcinoma is

second in frequency.[35] The outcome of children with malignant salivary gland tumors is good, with overall survival rates of greater than 80%.[36,40]

Evaluation of a suspected salivary gland mass includes CT or MRI to define the tissue characteristics of the mass and the extent of disease. Fine-needle aspiration biopsy can be used to help guide treatment planning preoperatively. Wide excision is the primary mode of therapy with all epithelial salivary gland malignancies. Parotid masses are treated by superficial parotidectomy, and preservation of the facial nerve is accomplished whenever possible. Neck dissection is performed for high-grade disease in children with either existing adenopathy or significant potential for occult disease.[35] Radiation therapy is used only for high-risk disease because of the significant treatment burden and morbidity that result in the pediatric population.

Mucoepidermoid carcinomas in children, as in adults, can have high-, intermediate-, and low-grade histology. In a review by Hicks and Flaitz, 24 of 26 had low- or intermediate-grade histology.[41] Low- and intermediate-grade lesions undergo wide excision, whereas high-grade disease warrants the addition of neck dissection and consideration of adjuvant therapy. As with adults, the prognosis is excellent for those with low- and intermediate-grade lesions and quite poor for those with high-grade lesions.[41]

Sialoblastoma, also known as an embryoma, is a rare malignant lesion of the parotid and submandibular glands.[42] It may develop in infancy or even be diagnosed prenatally. It is considered to be an aggressive disease, although there are relatively few reports of metastatic behavior. Treatment should be directed at complete surgical excision. Some have advocated the use of adjuvant chemotherapy.[43,44]

Minor salivary gland malignant lesions are also predominantly mucoepidermoid carcinoma and fortunately tend to initially be seen with low- to intermediate-grade histology (Fig. 93-2). These lesions have an excellent prognosis, with cure rates of 100% reported in several small series. CT can be useful in assessing palatal lesions for evidence of bone invasion. Caccamese and Ord recommend superficial excision without bone resection in cases of palatal

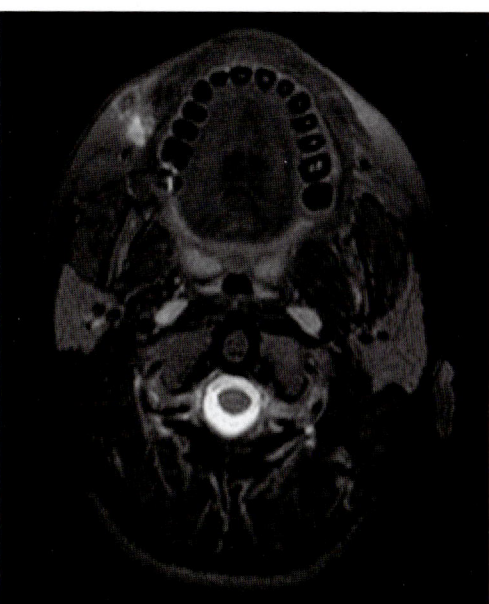

Fig. 93-2 ■ Axial T2-weighted magnetic resonance image demonstrating low-grade mucoepidermoid carcinoma in the cheek of an 8-year-old boy.

mucoepidermoid carcinoma when there is no CT evidence of bone invasion.[45]

LANGERHANS CELL HISTIOCYTOSIS

Langerhans cell histiocytosis (LCH) is a rare proliferative disorder of activated Langerhans cells that exhibits considerable variation in biologic behavior and clinical severity. There is some debate regarding its true nature, but it has the potential for aggressive behavior.[46] Many obsolete terms exist that are synonymous with LCH, including histiocytosis X, eosinophilic granuloma, Letterer-Siwe disease, Hand-Schüller-Christian disease, Hashimoto-Pritzker disease, and many others. The Histiocyte Society has organized the histiocytic disorders into three categories: single-system disease involving a single site, single-system disease that is multifocal, and multisystem disease.[47] The prognosis and treatment are closely linked to the extent of involvement, with solitary lesions being the most indolent. High-risk patients are children younger than 2 years or those with involvement of the liver, spleen, lungs, and hematopoietic system.[46]

LCH is frequently not included in most series of head and neck malignancies in children but is present in most series of malignant jaw tumors. This may represent a referral bias, and though rare, it will probably be seen more often by maxillofacial surgeons.[6] Chuong and Kaban reviewed their series of non-odontogenic jaw tumors and found 5 children with LCH and a mean age of 2.2 years out of a total 47 patients in the series.[8] Approximately 80% of patients will have manifestations in the head and neck,[48] and 10% will have oral manifestations.[49]

The diagnostic workup for a patient with known or suspected disease entails determining the extent of involvement with complete blood counts, liver function tests, and a skeletal survey at a minimum. Serum electrolytes are checked to rule out endocrine disturbances. Skeletal scintigraphy could be used as an alternative to the skeletal survey. Imaging of the maxillofacial lesion is typically done with CT, which will demonstrate lytic lesions with varying degrees of peripheral sclerosis, floating teeth, and widened periodontal ligaments (Fig. 93-3).

Bone is the most common single-organ site of involvement in children. This represents the so-called eosinophilic granuloma. In one review, the jaws were the most common site of involvement at 30%, with the remainder of the lesions occurring in the skull (21%),

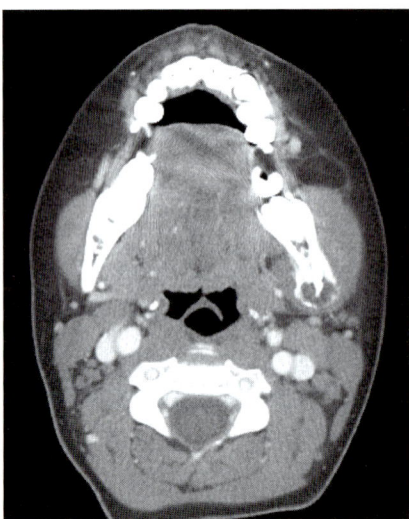

Fig. 93-3 ■ Axial computed tomography scan of 9-year-old boy with Langerhans cell histiocytosis involving the left mandibular ramus.

vertebrae (13%), pelvis (13%), extremities (17%), and ribs (6%).[50] When isolated, these lesions have an excellent prognosis and generally respond well to simple curettage. Disseminated disease is generally treated with chemotherapy, typically vinblastine and prednisone.[46] Several other protocols are under evaluation by the Histiocyte Society (*www.histiocytesociety.org*).

REHABILITATION AND RECONSTRUCTIVE SURGERY

Ablative surgery for a childhood malignancy has the potential to affect mastication, speech, growth, and facial esthetics. Each child and potential defect deserve individual consideration by taking into account the esthetics, function, and psychosocial well-being of the child. Multidisciplinary treatment planning with input from maxillofacial prosthodontists, orthodontists, and speech and language pathologists can be invaluable in optimizing the long-term outcome of their rehabilitation.

The myriad of surgical and prosthetic reconstructive options available for adults are applicable to children with some unique considerations. Non-growing flaps and scar tissue may result in progressive deformities as a child grows. Loss of dentition on one jaw may result in the development of canting in the opposing jaw. Loss of teeth and oral sensation and freely mobile oral tissues may give rise to speech and swallowing difficulties. The younger the patient, the greater the potential for these changes to be significant. Occasionally, these consequences can be avoided or mitigated. For example, a surgeon may choose to obturate a maxillectomy defect in a growing child instead of reconstructing the defect with a flap. Such a prosthesis could be modified on a regular basis to prevent hyper-eruption of the mandibular occlusion and avoid restricting the growth of the remaining maxilla and zygoma. This must be balanced against the burden imposed on a child with an open maxillectomy defect.

Consideration should also be given to the use of dental implants in a growing child. Provision of functional dentition can help with articulation, mastication, and psychosocial well-being and in some instances can be achieved only with dental implants. Younger children are less likely to wear removable prostheses and gain the benefit that would be realized from functional dentition, so consideration should be given to provision of a fixed restoration over a removable prosthesis. The majority of experience that exists in the placement of dental implants in children lies in the hypodontia patient population, but several case reports and small case series have demonstrated successful use of dental implants in children who have been treated for cancer.[51,52] Future growth may result in pseudomigration of a dental implant into a non-restorable position such that it will need to be removed and a definitive reconstruction performed at maturity, but this should not preclude their use in this population.

Free tissue transfer is becoming more frequently advocated for the management of ablative defects of the head and neck. The Microvascular Committee of the American Academy of Otolaryngology–Head and Neck Surgery reported the results of a multi-institution review of the use of microvascular reconstruction.[53] Five centers performed a total of 49 free flaps in patients younger than 21 years (range, 3 to 21). The fibula was the most commonly used flap (21 patients), and the mandible was the site most commonly reconstructed (21 patients). The early results were excellent, with only two flaps (jejunum) lost in the series. No data were presented on the long-term effects on facial growth. Upton and Guo reported on the largest series of pediatric free flaps accumulated over a period of 29 years.[54] Of 433 flaps, 165 were used in head and neck reconstruction. Success and failure rates were comparable to those in adults and were excellent (98% and 2%, respectively). Based on this experience but without specific data, the authors indicated that transferred bone does not grow unless a growth center is transferred as well. Fasciocutaneous flaps did, however, continue to grow with the patient. Overall, donor sites were well tolerated.

LONG-TERM CONSEQUENCES OF RADIATION THERAPY AND CHEMOTHERAPY

Radiation therapy may have significant consequences for children beyond those experienced by adult patients. Radiation therapy can alter craniofacial growth and development and result in dental development anomalies, xerostomia, radiation-induced dental caries, premature tooth loss, wound-healing problems, trismus, and velopharyngeal dysfunction (VPD).[55,56] Doses even as low as 0.72 to 1.22 Gy have been shown to alter tooth and tooth root development.[57] These patients require excellent dental care and can be rehabilitated with dental implants when needed. VPD, most often seen at higher doses (45 to 65 Gy), can be problematic and difficult to manage.[4] VPD may be due to cranial nerve dysfunction or loss of tissue mobility or may be a true tissue deficiency. Its management can be further hampered by the ototoxic effects of radiation therapy and various chemotherapeutic agents. Consideration should be given to both surgical and prosthetic management of these patients. Prosthetic options are typically chosen when treatment effects preclude predictable wound healing and result in poor tissue mobility or significant neuromotor deficits.

Craniofacial growth seems to be sensitive to the effects of radiation therapy, but chemotherapy alone does not seem to have much impact.[58,59] Children treated with cranial irradiation before the age of 5 years and even those treated with whole-body irradiation for myeloablation have experienced attenuation of mandibular growth. It seems that the mandible is four times more sensitive to this effect than the maxilla,[58] probably at least in part because of the cephalocaudal progression of facial growth.

The dental effects attributed to chemotherapy are similar to those from radiation and include enamel hypoplasia, reduced tooth size, and short V-shaped roots (Fig. 93-4). Younger patients (<6 years of age) and those receiving whole-body irradiation are particularly burdened.[60,61] Nasman and associates reported a 19% incidence of shortened tooth roots in children receiving multiagent chemotherapy

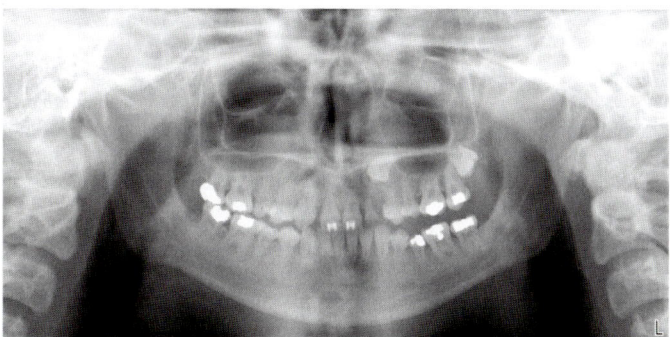

Fig. 93-4 ■ Orthopantomogram demonstrating blunted, V-shaped root apices in an adolescent treated with chemotherapy for neuroblastoma as a child.

versus 94% in those receiving myeloablative whole-body irradiation and cyclophosphamide.[61] The timing of tooth eruption seems to not be affected by chemotherapy.[60]

CHILDHOOD SURVIVORS OF CANCER AND LONG-TERM FOLLOW-UP

Unlike the treatment of many other pediatric conditions, long-term or delayed effects of cancer therapy often accompany survival. Treatment of childhood cancer can have a lasting effect on virtually every organ system in the body, and survivors face many challenges as they transition to adult life. Apart from injury to the various organ systems and their resultant chronic diseases, long-term survivors of childhood cancer may suffer from learning disabilities, posttraumatic stress disorder, and employment and educational difficulties. Their previous diagnosis and the consequences of their treatment can create difficulty in obtaining insurance coverage. The Children's Oncology Group (COG) has made guidelines available online (*www.survivorshipguidelines.org*) to minimize the consequences of these problems through anticipatory guidance and surveillance screening. To assist in this enterprise, many cancer centers have established long-term follow-up clinics. These clinics can help identify adolescents ready to transition to adult care settings, inform the maturing patient and their adult practitioners of the risks associated with cancer treatment, and help deal with the unique psychological issues associated with survivorship. This transition is important and offers the best care model for maturing children. When surveyed, most pediatric oncologists reported being uncomfortable caring for long-term survivors older than 21 years, but at the same time, most adult practitioners are unaware of the consequences and risks associated with cancer therapy.[62] Such specialized clinics can help bridge this gap and optimize the long-term outcomes of children who have survived a malignant disease.

INTEGRATION OF PEDIATRIC PALLIATIVE CARE

Nationally, about a third of childhood deaths are caused by injuries, with the remaining two thirds being attributable to underlying conditions such as prematurity, congenital anomalies, and cancer.[63] With a cancer diagnosis, some children will inevitably fail to respond favorably to treatment efforts and death will ensue. The discussions that surround the end of life are always sensitive and are particularly difficult when the patient is a child. A focus on symptom-directed and supportive care can improve the quality of life experienced by a child with cancer and ease the bereavement for parents and family members.[64] Psychological symptoms, especially anxiety, are a cause of severe suffering for children in the end-of-life care period and should be addressed.

In a study of bereaved parents of children with cancer, parents were more likely to consider care to be of high quality if the physician communicated what to expect in the end-of-life care period.[65] Parents who do not discuss end of life and death with their child before their passing often regret not having done so.[66] Many parents recognize that their child will have an awareness of the impending death, even if they cannot communicate this in clear terms. Furthermore, children with cancer may wish to talk about the meaning of being ill.[67] Recognizing this need and talking directly with children about their disease and its consequences can ease the burden that parents face in initiating these conversations themselves.[64]

Palliative care in pediatrics has undergone a paradigm shift, with the integration of such care being instituted much earlier in the course of treatment. Some experience in adult cancer care would suggest that most families believe that palliative care is instituted too late.[68] Many childhood cancers do not follow a predictable course, and even in those that do, most end with a precipitous decline. Instituting palliative care measures earlier in the course of disease gives patients and families time to prepare adequately. To this end, it has been suggested that palliative care should routinely be integrated into the care of all patients with life-threatening illness.[64] Many children's hospitals have established palliative care teams to help in symptom-directed care and the difficult conversations that must take place. Many of these changes have taken place with the recognition that the institution of symptom management and attention to quality of life and spiritual needs does not preclude therapies with curative intent and can ultimately ease a child's suffering regardless of the outcome.

PEARLS AND PITFALLS

- Pediatric malignant diseases are rare entities. Rare diseases, such as malignancies in children, are best managed in large academic centers where experience with these conditions is concentrated. Each patient should be evaluated and treatment should be planned within the setting of a multidisciplinary tumor board. Many centers will have tumor boards specific for sarcomas, lymphomas, and head and neck tumors.
- Patient age will often dictate the setting of care. For children who need general anesthesia for a biopsy, diagnostic imaging such as CT and MRI can often be accomplished in the same session with a single anesthetic with advance planning.
- Although exceptions do exist, congenital masses are almost never malignant in nature.
- Most pediatric malignant diseases are treated in conjunction with an oncologist, and whenever possible, children should be enrolled in multicenter treatment protocols. Surgeons should endeavor to work with the oncologist to help in accurate staging and classification of the disease for proper enrollment.

- Sarcomas are notoriously difficult to diagnosis and are often misdiagnosed by pathologists without significant experience in their review. It is generally wise to direct pathologic specimens to pathologists with experience in the management of these disease entities.
- Completion of active therapy is not the end of treatment. The burden of therapy must be remembered and incorporated into a long-term care plan. Younger children will bear a disproportionately large burden of treatment-related morbidity. Oral and maxillofacial surgeons have particular expertise in this regard and can help direct care to ensure optimal growth, development, and function of the craniomaxillofacial structures.
- Palliative care teams exist in most large children's hospitals and not only function to support patients and families at the end of life but can also be of benefit to children with significant disabling chronic disease.

REFERENCES

1. Greenlee RT, Murray T, Bolden S, et al: Cancer statistics, *CA Cancer J Clin* 50:7-33, 2000.
2. Hewitt M, Weiner SL, Simone JV, editors: *Childhood cancer survivorship: improving care and quality of life*, Washington, DC, 2003, National Academies Press.
3. Cunningham MJ, Myers EN, Bluestone CD: Malignant tumors of the head and neck in children: a twenty year review, *Int J Pediatr Otorhinolaryngol* 13:279-292, 1987.
4. Jaffe BF, Jaffe N: Head and neck tumors in children, *Pediatrics* 51:731-740, 1973.
5. Rapidis AD, Economidis J, Goumas PD, et al: Tumours of the head and neck in children. A clinico-pathological analysis of 1,007 cases, *J Craniomaxillofac Surg* 16:279-286, 1988.
6. Ord RA: Head and neck malignancies in children. In Kaban LB, Troulis MJ, editors: *Pediatric oral and maxillofacial surgery*, Philadelphia, 2004, WB Saunders, p 247.
7. Bhaskar SN: Oral tumors of infancy and childhood. A survey of 293 cases, *J Pediatr* 63:195-210, 1963.
8. Chuong R, Kaban LB: Diagnosis and treatment of jaw tumors in children, *J Oral Maxillofac Surg* 43:323-332, 1985.
9. Koch H: Statistical evaluation of tumours of the head and neck in infancy and childhood, *J Maxillofac Surg* 2:26-31, 1974.
10. Sato M, Tanaka N, Sato T, et al: Oral and maxillofacial tumours in children: a review, *Br J Oral Maxillofac Surg* 35:92-95, 1997.
11. Shah SK, Le MC, Carpenter WM: Retrospective review of pediatric oral lesions from a dental school biopsy service, *Pediatr Dent* 31:14, 2009.
12. Chen YK, Lin LM, Huang HC, et al: A retrospective study of oral and maxillofacial biopsy lesions in a pediatric population from southern Taiwan, *Pediatr Dent* 20:404-410, 1998.
13. Das S, Das AK: A review of pediatric oral biopsies from a surgical pathology service in a dental school, *Pediatr Dent* 15:208-211, 1993.
14. Gaini RM, Romagnoli M, Sala A, et al: Lymphomas of head and neck in pediatric patients, *Int J Pediatr Otorhinolaryngol* 73(Suppl 1):S65-S70, 2009.
15. Roh JL, Huh J, Moon HN: Lymphomas of the head and neck in the pediatric population, *Int J Pediatr Otorhinolaryngol* 71:1471-1477, 2007.
16. Paulino AC, Okcu MF: Rhabdomyosarcoma, *Curr Probl Cancer* 32:7-34, 2008.
17. Scrable HJ, Witte DP, Lampkin BC, et al: Chromosomal localization of the human rhabdomyosarcoma locus by mitotic recombination mapping, *Nature* 329:645-647, 1987.
18. Pappo AS, Meza JL, Donaldson SS, et al: Treatment of localized nonorbital, nonparameningeal head and neck rhabdomyosarcoma: lessons learned from Intergroup Rhabdomyosarcoma studies III and IV, *J Clin Oncol* 21:638-645, 2003.
19. Wanebo HJ, Koness RJ, MacFarlane JK, et al: Head and neck sarcoma: report of the Head and Neck Sarcoma Registry. Society of Head and Neck Surgeons Committee on Research, *Head Neck* 14:1-7, 1992.
20. Fernandes R, Nikitakis NG, Pazoki A, et al: Osteogenic sarcoma of the jaw: a 10-year experience, *J Oral Maxillofac Surg* 65:1286-1291, 2007.
21. Guadagnolo BA, Zagars GK, Raymond AK, et al: Osteosarcoma of the jaw/craniofacial region: outcomes after multimodality treatment, *Cancer* 115:3262-3270, 2009.
22. Mardinger O, Givol N, Talmi YP, et al: Osteosarcoma of the jaw. The Chaim Sheba Medical Center experience, *Oral Surg Oral Med Oral Pathol Oral Radiol Endod* 91:445-451, 2001.
23. August M, Magennis P, Dewitt D: Osteogenic sarcoma of the jaws: factors influencing prognosis, *Int J Oral Maxillofac Surg* 26:198-204, 1997.
24. Bertoni F, Dallera P, Bacchini P, et al: The Istituto Rizzoli-Beretta experience with osteosarcoma of the jaw, *Cancer* 68:1555-1563, 1991.
25. Chindia ML: Osteosarcoma of the jaw bones, *Oral Oncol* 37:545-547, 2001.
26. Patel SG, Meyers P, Huvos AG, et al: Improved outcomes in patients with osteogenic sarcoma of the head and neck, *Cancer* 95:1495-1503, 2002.

27. Benjamin RS: Regional chemotherapy for osteosarcoma, *Semin Oncol* 16:323-327, 1989.

28. Dorfman HD, Czerniak B: Bone cancers, *Cancer* 75(Suppl):203-210, 1995.

29. Eilber FR, Rosen G: Adjuvant chemotherapy for osteosarcoma, *Semin Oncol* 16:312-322, 1989.

30. Rosen G, Marcove RC, Caparros B, et al: Primary osteogenic sarcoma: the rationale for preoperative chemotherapy and delayed surgery, *Cancer* 43:2163-2177, 1979.

31. Gadwal SR, Gannon FH, Fanburg-Smith JC, et al: Primary osteosarcoma of the head and neck in pediatric patients: a clinicopathologic study of 22 cases with a review of the literature, *Cancer* 91:598-605, 2001.

32. Rush BF, Chambers RG, Ravitch MM: Cancer of the head and neck in children, *Surgery* 53:270-284, 1963.

33. Krolls SO, Trodahl JN, Boyers RC: Salivary gland lesions in children: a survey of 430 cases, *Cancer* 30:459-469, 1972.

34. Callender DL, Frankenthaler RA, Luna MA, et al: Salivary gland neoplasms in children, *Arch Otolaryngol Head Neck Surg* 118:472-476, 1992.

35. Mehta D, Willging JP: Pediatric salivary gland lesions, *Semin Pediatr Surg* 15:76-84, 2006.

36. Guzzo M, Ferrari A, Marcon I, et al: Salivary gland neoplasms in children: the experience of the Istituto Nazionale Tumori of Milan, *Pediatr Blood Cancer* 47:806-810, 2006.

37. Ribeiro Kde C, Kowalski LP, Saba LM, et al: Epithelial salivary glands neoplasms in children and adolescents: a forty-four-year experience, *Med Pediatr Oncol* 39:594-600, 2002.

38. Castro EB, Huvos AG, Strong EW, et al: Tumors of the major salivary glands in children. *Cancer* 29:312-317, 1972.

39. Chong GC, Beahrs OH, Chen ML, et al: Management of parotid gland tumors in infants and children, *Mayo Clin Proc* 50:279-283, 1975.

40. Rogers DA, Rao BN, Bowman L, et al: Primary malignancy of the salivary gland in children, *J Pediatr Surg* 29:44-47, 1994.

41. Hicks J, Flaitz C: Mucoepidermoid carcinoma of salivary glands in children and adolescents: assessment of proliferation markers, *Oral Oncol* 36:454-460, 2000.

42. Cristofaro M, Giudice A, Amentea M, et al: Diagnostic and therapeutic approach to sialoblastoma of submandibular gland: a case report, *J Oral Maxillofac Surg* 66:123-126, 2008.

43. Saribeyoglu ET, Devecioglu O, Karakas Z, et al: How to manage an unresectable or recurrent sialoblastoma, *Pediatr Blood Cancer* 55:374-376, 2010.

44. Williams SB, Ellis GL, Warnock GR: Sialoblastoma: a clinicopathologic and immunohistochemical study of 7 cases, *Ann Diagn Pathol* 10:320-326, 2006.

45. Caccamese JF Jr, Ord RA: Paediatric mucoepidermoid carcinoma of the palate, *Int J Oral Maxillofac Surg* 31:136-139, 2002.

46. Gasent Blesa JM, Alberola Candel V, Solano Vercet C, et al: Langerhans cell histiocytosis, *Clin Transl Oncol* 10:688-696, 2008.

47. Favara BE, Feller AC, Pauli M, et al: Contemporary classification of histiocytic disorders. The WHO Committee on Histiocytic/Reticulum Cell Proliferations. Reclassification Working Group of the Histiocyte Society, *Med Pediatr Oncol* 29:157-166, 1997.

48. Nicollas R, Rome A, Belaich H, et al: Head and neck manifestation and prognosis of Langerhans' cell histiocytosis in children, *Int J Pediatr Otorhinolaryngol* 74:669-673, 2010.

49. Hartman KS: Histiocytosis X: a review of 114 cases with oral involvement, *Oral Surg Oral Med Oral Pathol* 49:38-54, 1980.

50. Baumgartner I, von Hochstetter A, Baumert B, et al: Langerhans'-cell histiocytosis in adults, *Med Pediatr Oncol* 28:9-14, 1997.

51. Genden EM, Buchbinder D, Chaplin JM, et al: Reconstruction of the pediatric maxilla and mandible, *Arch Otolaryngol Head Neck Surg* 126:293-300, 2000.

52. Zwetchkenbaum SR, Oh WS: Prosthodontic management of abnormal tooth development secondary to chemoradiotherapy: a clinical report, *J Prosthet Dent* 98:429-435, 2007.

53. Arnold DJ, Wax MK; Microvascular Committee of the American Academy of Otolaryngology–Head and Neck Surgery: Pediatric microvascular reconstruction: a report from the Microvascular Committee, *Otolaryngol Head Neck Surg* 136:848-851, 2007.

54. Upton J, Guo L: Pediatric free tissue transfer: a 29-year experience with 433 transfers, *Plast Reconstr Surg* 121:1725-1737, 2008.

55. Estilo CL, Huryn JM, Kraus DH, et al: Effects of therapy on dentofacial development in long-term survivors of head and neck rhabdomyosarcoma: the Memorial Sloan-Kettering Cancer Center experience, *J Pediatr Hematol Oncol* 25:215-222, 2003.

56. Jaffe N, Toth BB, Hoar RE, et al: Dental and maxillofacial abnormalities in long-term survivors of childhood cancer: effects of treatment with chemotherapy and radiation to the head and neck, *Pediatrics* 73:816-823, 1984.

57. Rosenberg SW, Kolodney H, Wong GY, et al: Altered dental root development in long-term survivors of pediatric acute lymphoblastic leukemia. A review of 17 cases, *Cancer* 59:1640-1648, 1987.

58. Dahllof G: Craniofacial growth in children treated for malignant diseases, *Acta Odontol Scand* 56:378-382, 1998.

59. Guyuron B, Dagys AP, Munro IR, et al: Effect of irradiation on facial growth: a 7- to 25-year follow-up, *Ann Plast Surg* 11:423-427, 1983.

60. Dahllöf G, Barr M, Bolme P, et al: Disturbances in dental development after total body irradiation in bone marrow transplant recipients, *Oral Surg Oral Med Oral Pathol* 65:41-44, 1988.

61. Nasman M, Forsberg CM, Dahllöf G: Long-term dental development in children after treatment for malignant disease, *Eur J Orthod* 19:151-159, 1997.

62. Henderson TO, Hlubocky FJ, Wroblewski KE, et al: Physician preferences and knowledge gaps regarding the care of childhood cancer survivors: a mailed survey of pediatric oncologists, *J Clin Oncol* 28:878-883, 2010.

63. Arias E, MacDorman MF, Strobino DM, et al: Annual summary of vital statistics—2002, *Pediatrics* 112:1215-1230, 2003.

64. Mack JW, Wolfe J: Early integration of pediatric palliative care: for some children, palliative care starts at diagnosis, *Curr Opin Pediatr* 18:10-14, 2006.

65. Mack JW, Hilden JM, Watterson J, et al: Parent and physician perspectives on quality of care at the end of life in children with cancer, *J Clin Oncol* 23:9155-9161, 2005.

66. Contro NA, Larson J, Scofield S, et al: Hospital staff and family perspectives regarding quality of pediatric palliative care, *Pediatrics* 114:1248-1252, 2004.

67. Hinds PS, Gattuso JS, Fletcher A, et al: Quality of life as conveyed by pediatric patients with cancer, *Qual Life Res* 13:761-772, 2004.

68. Morita T, Akechi T, Ikenaga M, et al: Communication about the ending of anticancer treatment and transition to palliative care, *Ann Oncol* 15:1551-1557, 2004.

Surgical Care of the Hemifacial Microsomia Patient

Stanley Yung-Chuan Liu, Phoebe Good, Janice S. Lee

Hemifacial microsomia (HFM; Online Mendelian Inheritance in Man [OMIM] 164210) is the most common congenital craniofacial anomaly after cleft lip or palate (or both) and occurs in 1 in every 4000 to 5600 children.[1,2] This congenital condition involves the structures of the first and second branchial arches, with variable clinical dysplasia of both skeletal and soft tissues. The five major craniofacial components of HFM include the ear (most consistent finding), mandible (most commonly involved skeletal structure), orbit, cranial nerve VII, and facial soft tissues (including the masticatory muscles) on the affected side. HFM is frequently unilateral; however, bilateral involvement may also occur.[3-5]

ETIOLOGY/PATHOLOGY

The etiology and pathogenesis of HFM are unknown, although it is presumed that there is interference with neural crest cell migration during embryologic development. The condition is believed to be sporadic, but examples of familial transmission have been documented.[6]

CLASSIFICATION

Many classification systems have been used to describe the varying degrees of deformity associated with HFM.[4,7-9] These systems often use the mandible as the cornerstone of the classification since it is frequently affected and treatment of the mandible is typically inevitable. One of the most commonly used classification systems is the modification of the Pruzansky classification described by Kaban and colleagues.[7,10,11] It is based on discrete findings of the presence or absence of critical elements of the mandible, particularly the condyle-ramus-glenoid fossa unit, and it consists of, in order of severity, types I, IIa, IIb, and III (Fig. 94-1). This classification has been instrumental in directing appropriate surgical corrections to achieve mandibular symmetry.

The OMENS classification is also commonly used and is more comprehensive. It includes the five affected facial components of HFM: orbit, mandible, ear, nerve, and soft tissue. Each of the five components is graded 0 to 3 based on the degree of abnormality, with 0 indicating no abnormality and 3 indicating absence or severe deficiency of the structure.[8] This classification system is particularly useful in categorizing the phenotypic variations seen in patients with HFM (Fig. 94-2).

In general, the muscular hypoplasia correlates with the degree of bone deficiency.[8,12] If the coronoid process is missing, the temporalis muscle demonstrates severe hypoplasia and abnormal muscle recruitment; the same relationship holds true between the masseter muscle and the gonial angle.[13] Additionally, the higher the OMENS score, the more likely extra-craniofacial abnormalities are present, including abnormalities of the cardiac, vertebral, central nervous, renal, and pulmonary organ systems.[4] There are developmental correlations between the severity of the mandibular hypoplasia and the other facial anomalies; however, the correlations are weak because of an extremely diverse phenotypic spectrum.[8]

In all patients with HFM, the unilateral impairment in growth causes deviation of the mandibular skeletal midline toward the affected side. Because the mandible is short, retrusive, and narrow on the affected side, downward growth of the maxilla is restricted and a secondary deformity occurs. This results in a vertically short maxilla and an occlusal plane that tilts upward on the affected side.[12]

TREATMENT

Multidisciplinary treatment is required for an ideal outcome.[14] The maxillomandibular complex is often the focus of treatment, with the severity of mandibular deformity dictating the appropriate treatment. The role of the oral and maxillofacial surgeon is critical in establishing the ideal and most stable skeletal foundation that can support the soft tissue augmentation and ear construction. For the purpose of this chapter, we will focus on current therapies related to the skeletal abnormalities associated with HFM and briefly describe therapies to correct the ear and soft tissue abnormalities.

SEQUENCE AND CONTROVERSIES

The main considerations in the surgical management of patients with HFM are timing and the anatomic extent of construction. The ear is typically constructed around the age of 6 years, followed by surgery on the external auditory canal if needed; the maxillomandibular deformities may be addressed while the patient is growing or when skeletal maturation has occurred; and the soft tissue augmentation is performed 6 to 8 months after maxillomandibular correction. The differences in surgical strategy and timing result from inconclusive evidence regarding the progression of mandibular asymmetry in patients with HFM. It is unclear whether there is sustained growth on the affected side that continues at the same rate as on the unaffected side with stable facial asymmetry (constant asymmetry) or whether there is progressive worsening of the facial asymmetry because of the lag in growth of the affected side (progressive asymmetry).

Interestingly, proponents of both the constant versus progressive nature of the mandibular asymmetry have used the same two radiographic studies that monitored longitudinal facial growth in patients with HFM as support for their theory. In radiographic studies by Rune and associates[15] and Polley and co-workers,[16] it was originally concluded that the degree of mandibular asymmetry remains relatively constant throughout craniofacial development, and this was corroborated by clinical observations.[17-19] Based on this theory, correction of the facial deformity is performed after the patient

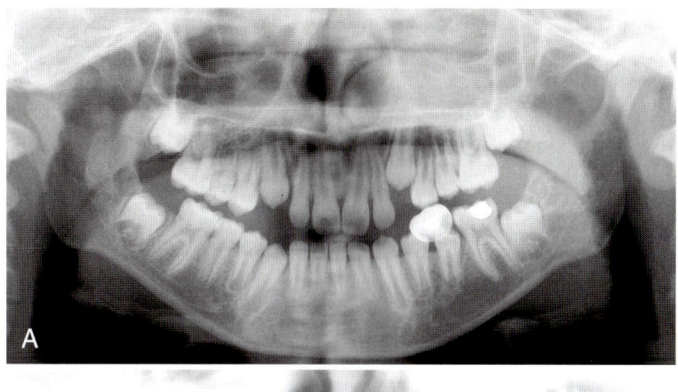

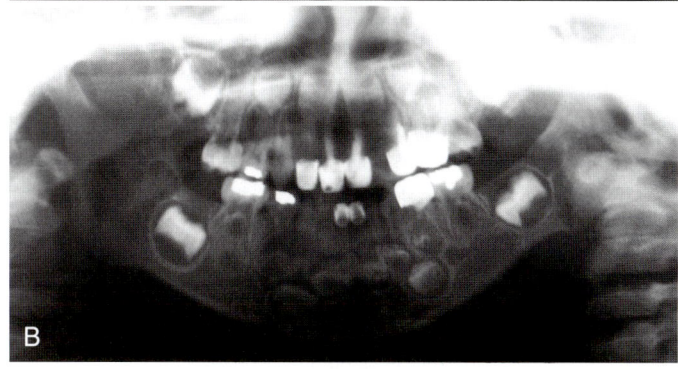

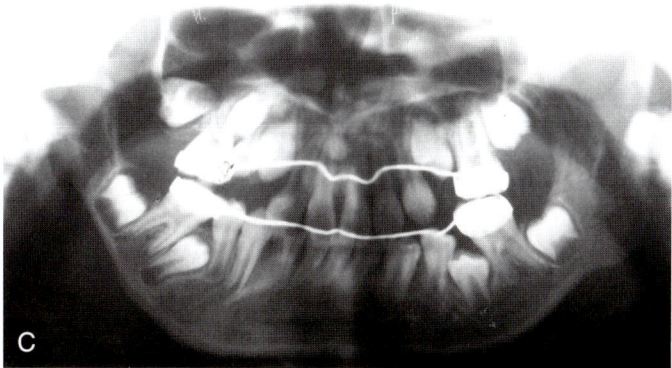

Fig. 94-1 ■ Radiographic demonstrations of type I (**A**), type II (**B**), and type III (**C**) mandibles in patients with hemifacial microsomia.

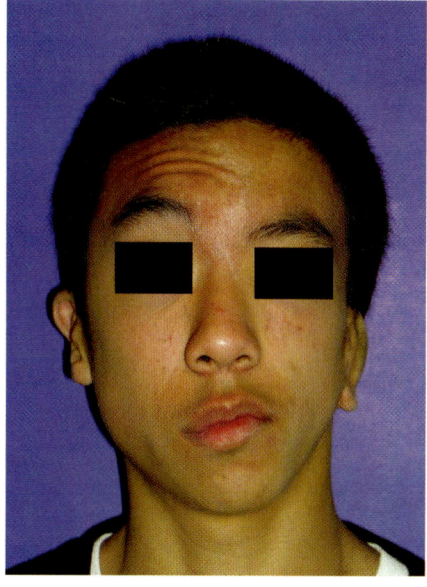

Fig. 94-2 ■ The OMENS classification identifies the five major components of hemifacial microsomia: the orbit, mandible, ear, cranial nerve VII, and soft tissue. This patient demonstrates weakness of cranial nerve VII on the left side.

MANAGEMENT OF THE MAXILLOMANDIBULAR COMPLEX

The hallmark of HFM is facial asymmetry as a result of asymmetric development of the mandible. Treatment of these patients can be grouped into two categories based on the Kaban-Pruzansky classification: types I and IIa are typically treated similarly, and types IIb and III are treated similarly. The timing of treatment is dependent on when the patient and family initiate treatment and whether early or delayed surgical intervention is recommended by the treating craniofacial team or surgeon. Particular goals of treatment are to (1) increase the size of the malformed and underdeveloped mandible and soft tissues, (2) create an articulation between the mandible and the temporal bone, (3) correct the secondary deformities of the maxilla, and (4) establish functional occlusion and optimal facial symmetry.[12,25] When treatment is initiated before completion of craniofacial growth, these goals are accomplished by adhering to the following treatment phases: presurgical orthodontic-orthopedic treatment, mandibular surgery, postsurgical bone induction and secondary correction of the maxillary deformity, final orthodontic treatment, and soft tissue augmentation.[10,25,26]

TREATMENT PLANNING

The combined orthodontic-orthopedic and surgical treatment decisions are based on the patient's clinical findings and craniofacial imaging. Previously, plain films, including a Panorex, posteroanterior cephalogram, and lateral cephalogram, were used to determine the mandibular classification and provide a treatment plan. Currently, computed tomography (CT) with three-dimensional (3D) reconstruction is being used to clearly delineate the asymmetry in patients with HFM because this condition has an impact on the craniofacial skeleton in all three dimensions.[27] These images demonstrate not only the asymmetry of the facial bones but also the extent of cranial base asymmetries and soft tissue deficiencies[28-32] (Fig. 94-3). Composite 3D models of a patient with HFM can be fabricated; however, 3D surgical treatment planning can also be performed with available software, and the 3D models may not be necessary.

has completed growth, as is the case for most orthognathic corrections.

The other possibility is that the affected side lags behind the unaffected side and the patient demonstrates progressive facial asymmetry over time.[10,20-23] Re-interpretation of the data by Rune and colleagues[15] and Polley and co-workers,[16] however, has also been used to support the concept that the mandibular asymmetry is progressive, as reflected by worsening of vertical mandibular skeletal asymmetry and mandibular ramus height ratios.[21] In addition, the degree of progressive asymmetry has been shown to correlate with the severity of mandibular deformity.[10,11,21] Follow-up of a cohort of children after costochondral graft reconstruction also demonstrated that diminished growth of the constructed ramus and condyle (similar to the undergrowth on the untreated affected side) resulted in progressive facial asymmetry with worsening occlusal, piriform, and intergonial canting.[24] Proponents of the second theory favor early treatment of patients with HFM, while they are still growing, to improve facial and mandibular growth, reduce secondary deformities in the maxilla, and enhance the development of a positive body image.

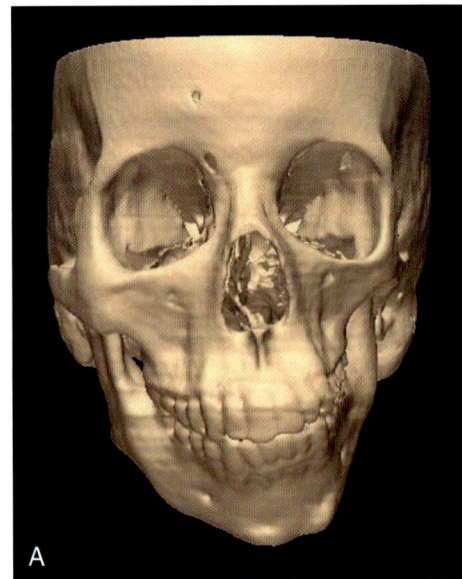

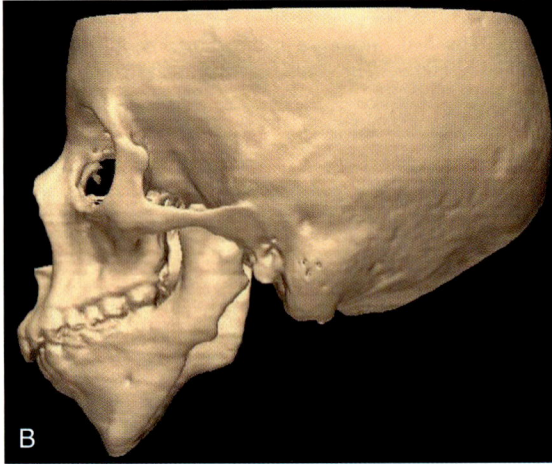

Fig. 94-3 ■ Three-dimensional computed tomography scans of a patient with hemifacial microsomia: frontal (**A**) and profile (**B**) views.

TYPE I AND TYPE IIA

EARLY SURGICAL CORRECTION

For early correction to be effective, a child should be treated during the mixed-dentition stage, and the operation consists of elongation, rotation, and advancement of the hypoplastic mandible to bring the chin point to the midline and create an open bite on the affected side. This can be achieved with mandibular osteotomy, such as bilateral sagittal split osteotomy, or by distraction osteogenesis on the deficient side.[12] Vertical mid-facial growth is complete after eruption of the permanent teeth, and therefore subsequent orthodontically controlled eruption of teeth into the open bite space will not be accompanied by vertical maxillary growth. To maximize the potential for mid-facial growth during the mixed-dentition stage, an orthodontist constructs a functional appliance before surgery to hold the affected side of the mandible in a lowered and forward position. This functional appliance is constructed to train the existing muscles to hold the mandible forward; it can possibly serve as a substitute for the missing condylar cartilage and missing protrusive function of the lateral pterygoid muscle and may stimulate additional length of the mandible. Other benefits derived from this treatment include advancement of the postural position of the mandible, lengthening

of the coronoid process if it is present, increase in size of associated soft tissues, and improvement in cant of the occlusal plane.[14] Particularly in children with type I deformity, a good response to functional appliance therapy may avoid surgical lengthening if the residual occlusal cant is acceptable. For those still needing surgical lengthening, concomitant creation of an open bite during the mixed-dentition stage will maximize vertical growth potential on the affected side and minimize secondary deformity of the maxilla. The open bite is first maintained by a bite block for 3 to 6 months, with subsequent gradual reduction to allow maxillary dental eruption.[12] One of the goals of treatment is to potentially avoid maxillary surgery.

DELAYED SURGICAL CORRECTION

For patients in whom treatment is initiated after growth is complete or if the surgeon's preference is to delay surgical correction until the patient is close to skeletal maturity (13 to 15 years in girls and 15 to 16 years in boys[19]), the surgical treatment plan is similar to conventional orthognathic correction of facial asymmetry. Orthodontic treatment must include appropriate dental decompensation and coordination of the dental arches and possibly extractions. The surgery includes bilateral sagittal split osteotomy for advancement, elongation on the affected side and correction of the cant, and rotation of the midline of the mandible in combination with a Le Fort I osteotomy to lengthen the affected side and ideally level the often steep maxillary occlusal plane. Genioplasty is necessary to correct asymmetry of the chin.

TYPE IIB AND TYPE III

EARLY SURGICAL CORRECTION

Costochondral junction and rib, calvarial, or iliac crest bone grafts can be used to construct the condyle-ramus unit and glenoid fossa before eruption of the permanent dentition. The remainder of the orthodontic management would be the same as for type I and type IIA: use of a bite block and gradual reduction.[12]

Proponents of the theory that there is constant mandibular asymmetry and not progressive asymmetry also support early treatment of patients with type IIb or III deformities if they can derive psychosocial benefit from it.[19] The protocol by Posnick recommends that patients with type IIb undergo mandibular distraction or osteotomy with repositioning of the proximal segment and that patients with type III undergo construction of the absent condyle-ramus unit with a costochondral graft during the mixed-dentition phase.[19] These patients may require additional and definitive orthognathic surgery at skeletal maturity.[19]

For patients in whom construction initially involved autologous bone grafting and who subsequently need repeat reconstruction of the temporomandibular joint (TMJ) complex because of relapse or progressive facial asymmetry, custom-made total TMJ devices have been used with satisfactory results.[33] The advantages of a custom-made alloplastic TMJ over its predecessors include less extensive sacrifice of tissue at the recipient site and ability to simultaneously address the ramus and fossa components[34] (Fig. 94-4).

DELAYED SURGICAL CORRECTION

In our experience with patients who have type IIb or III deformity and in whom treatment is initiated near or at the time of skeletal maturity, a 3D image of the facial CT scan is crucial for designing the treatment plan. The orthodontic preparation is often complex because of the presence of crossbites and significant occlusal canting; however, the basic principles for pre-orthognathic

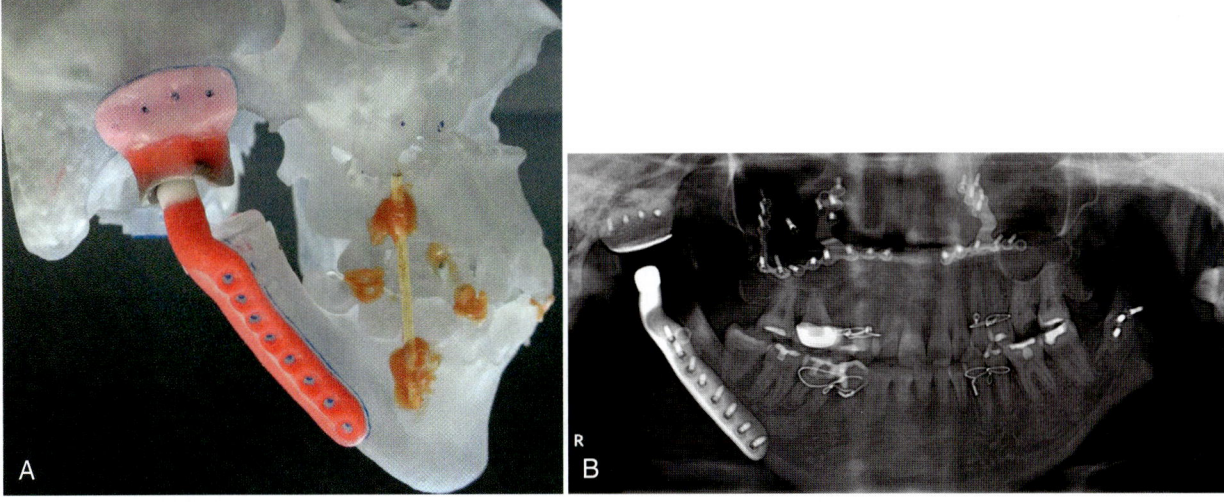

Fig. 94-4 ■ **A,** Custom-made temporomandibular joint prosthesis for a patient with hemifacial microsomia. **B,** Postoperative panoramic radiograph showing the prosthesis in place. Function was excellent after surgery.

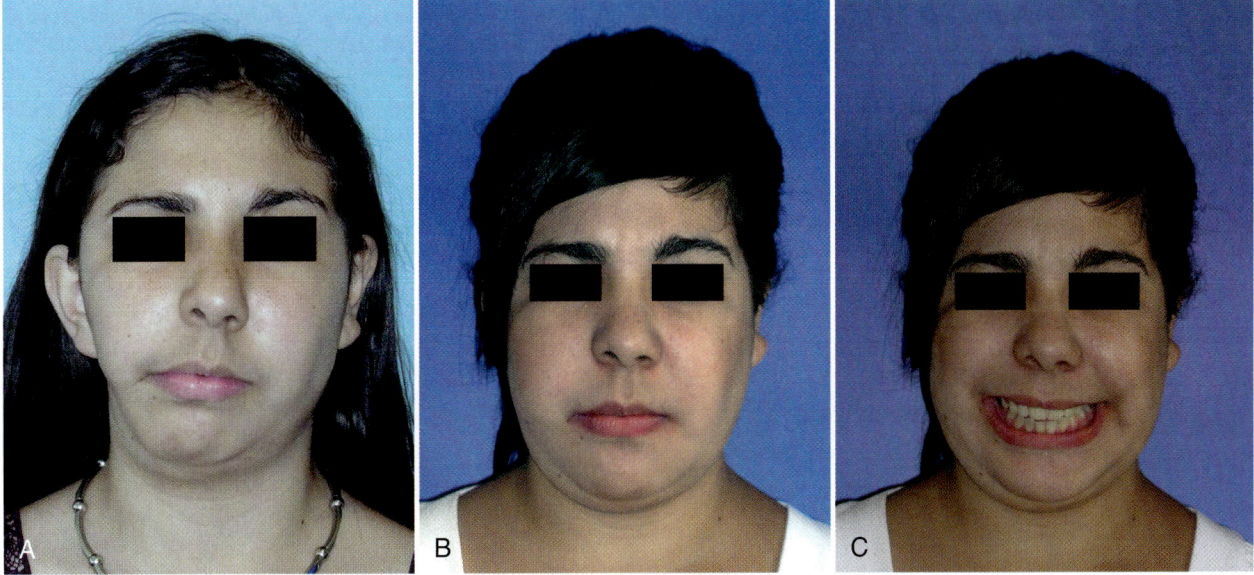

Fig. 94-5 ■ Delayed surgical correction in a patient with type III hemifacial microsomia. This patient required orthognathic procedures and costochondral graft construction of the right condyle-ramus-glenoid fossa unit after reaching skeletal maturity. Soft tissue augmentation of this patient was achieved with injections of fat after skeletal correction. **A,** Before augmentation. **B** and **C,** After augmentation.

preparation, such as dental decompensation and arch coordination, still apply. Once orthodontic treatment has been completed, the goals of surgical treatment are correction of the maxillomandibular cant, leveling of the steep maxillomandibular occlusal plane, and simultaneous construction of the affected condyle-ramus-glenoid fossa unit (Fig. 94-5). In brief, this is achieved by (1) unilateral sagittal split osteotomy (not completely osteotomized) of the unaffected side, (2) Le Fort I osteotomy to correct the maxillary cant and occlusal plane and positioning of the maxilla with an intermediate splint, (3) completion of the sagittal splint osteotomy and placement of the final splint, and (4) construction of the type IIb or III condyle-ramus-glenoid-fossa unit with a costochondral graft or grafts through a sterile and preauricular approach (a submandibular incision may be necessary for rigid fixation of the costochondral graft to the native mandible). The final splint will include a slight

opening of the bite on the affected side to allow costochondral graft remodeling and resorption.

DISTRACTION OSTEOGENESIS

Distraction osteogenesis has been reported to be an effective means of increasing mandibular dimensions in young patients with HFM.[35] However, there remains a lack of statistical evidence to support the use of early distraction osteogenesis as a single-treatment modality for correcting HFM.[36] There is not a great deal of literature regarding long-term follow-up for patients with HFM who have undergone unilateral distraction osteogenesis. Invariably, these studies have limited sample sizes. Furthermore, since measurements of growth are different depending on the study, conclusions are not universal. The most favorable long-term study supporting the use of unilateral distraction osteogenesis was reported by Shetye and colleagues, who followed 12 patients with HFM for 5 years, and 5 of the 12 patients for 10 years.[37] They reported that on average, ramal length increased 13.04 mm in the distracted rami, followed by 3.46 mm of relapse after the first year (27%). In this particular patient population, the average growth rate of ramal height was 0.87 mm per year, as compared to 1.15 mm per year on the normal side (approximate reduction of 25% in growth rate).

However, when mandibular vertical changes were monitored by the height ratio between affected and non-affected rami, Meazzini and colleagues showed 77% relapse to pre-distraction ramal height ratio after 5 years in 8 patients with HFM types I and II.[38] Further significant relapse after use of distraction osteogenesis was reported by Huisinga-Fischer and others using three-dimensional computed tomography imaging to make volumetric measurements of both soft and hard tissue in 8 children with HFM.[39] They found little increase in the volume of the affected side of the masticatory muscles. Also, in approximately 50% of cases there was relapse of bone volume after 1 year of distraction osteogenesis. The relapse had a progressive character when reexamined after 3 years. If distraction osteogenesis is to be considered, it should be considered for type I or IIa. In our experience, a superior and posterior cranial base stop is necessary for an intact proximal segment and successful distal mandibular lengthening. Distraction of a type IIb or III mandible can result in abnormal positioning of the proximal segment with unpredictable projection and rotation of the distal segment. Compliance of the patient and family support are necessary to achieve a successful outcome. Various distraction osteogenesis devices are currently available; the choice should be based on the age and size of the patient and the characteristics of the mandible. In our experience, a curvilinear device has resulted in the best outcome. In any case, movement of the mandible typically occurs in two planes: forward and rotational (to the unaffected side). Unfortunately, the affected side remains quite flat and has little projection laterally.

SOFT TISSUE AUGMENTATION

Soft tissue deficiencies or abnormalities include eyelid-adnexal deficiency, epibulbar dermoid cysts, skin or ear tags, and hypoplasia of the facial soft tissues and muscles on the affected side. At our institution, any soft tissue reconstruction or augmentation involving the eye or orbit is performed by an oculoplastic surgeon, whereas facial soft tissue augmentation is performed by a plastic surgeon. Soft tissue augmentation is normally done 6 to 8 months after the skeletal corrections.

Vascularized free flaps have been used to address preauricular-cheek hypoplasia, which results from diminished thickness of subcutaneous tissue, volume of the muscles of mastication and facial expression, and parotid gland. The anterolateral thigh fasciocutaneous flap, which has a reliable vascular pedicle and relatively thin pliable soft tissue, has been used for patients with HFM with good results.[40] The scapular flap is also commonly used to augment facial soft tissue.[41] More recently, the superficial circumflex iliac artery/superficial inferior epigastric artery–based flap has been used because it offers simultaneous elevation during preparation of the recipient site, wide flap harvesting for a large contour deformity of the face, primary defatting to achieve the necessary thickness, and minimal abdominoplasty scar.[42] In most cases of augmentation using a muscle free flap, debulking and revision are often necessary.

More recently, soft tissue augmentation has been achieved with injections of subcutaneous fat[43,44] (see Fig. 94-5). The technique is associated with fewer complications than seen with a free flap and is a much easier method that can be done in an outpatient setting. Typically, two to three injections have been necessary, and there has been very little evidence of atrophy during our follow-up of up to 5 years in patients who have received fat injections at our institution. The fat injection requires an adequate amount of adipose, typically from the abdomen. This may be difficult to harvest in young, athletic patients, particularly male patients, in whom identifying an adequate amount of fat may not be readily achieved. Once the fat (approximately 60 mL of adipose tissue) is removed through a low-suction syringe aspiration technique, it is centrifuged to consolidate the adipose tissue into a more condensed and injectable mass—approximately 30 mL. The fat is then injected subcutaneously into the affected facial region with a Coleman cannula.[44-46]

EXTERNAL EAR AND ATRESIA REPAIR

The Meurman classification of microtia is used for describing the degree of microtia in patients with HFM.[47] In this classification, grade I microtia includes a malformed auricle and smaller than normal ear. Grade II includes a rudimentary auricle with atresia of the canal. Grade III is a malformed lobule with a missing pinna or completely absent ear (anotia).

Treatment of microtia may follow the four-stage protocol made popular by Brent[48,49] or the two-stage protocol of Nagata.[50] Grafting of a well-sculpted autogenous cartilage framework is done no earlier than 6 years of age. The synchondritic region of the sixth and seventh ribs provides an ample cartilage block to form a framework for the ear (stage I). Later stages include earlobe transposition (stage II), separation of the ear from the head with a skin graft to create the auriculocephalic sulcus (stage III), and tragus construction (stage IV). External ear reconstruction is an integral part of the craniofacial reconstruction because the auricle is often located outside the face mask and projects onto the posterior part of the temporal bone.[51]

Hearing loss in patients with HFM is most often conductive and attributable to stenosis or atresia of the external auditory canal, hypoplasia of the middle ear cavity, or ankylotic ossicles.[52] Hearing devices such as the BAHA soft band may be considered at an early age if there is evidence of conductive hearing loss and auditory stimulation is necessary.[53] A temporal bone CT scan is obtained around the age of 4 to 5 years to determine whether the patient is a candidate for atresia repair. If creation of an external auditory canal is planned, it is typically done after the microtia is repaired and the position of the constructed ear is determined. In general, however, reconstruction of the external auditory canal is not performed if there is adequate hearing in the unaffected ear or a BAHA implant device is preferred.[52,53] The BAHA implant device can be placed at 4 to 5 years of age.

FUTURE DIRECTIONS

The advent of computer-aided surgical simulation (CASS) will probably contribute to the future of complex craniomaxillofacial reconstruction.[27] The ability to simulate surgical correction of such complex conditions as HFM will provide the surgeon with better visualization of the degree of deformity and greater ease in planning and improving the outcome of treatment. Additionally, CT-guided navigational units, such as BrainLAB (Feldkircher, Germany), may allow greater accuracy in the intraoperative execution of these surgical simulations.

Finally, bone and cartilage tissue engineering may permit construction of the abnormal or absent condyle-ramus unit and ear such that grafting and tissue transfers will not be necessary.

PEARLS AND PITFALLS

- In patients with HFM, unilateral growth impairment causes deviation of the mandibular skeletal midline toward the affected side. Since the mandible is short, retrusive, and narrow on the affected side, downward growth of the maxilla is restricted and a secondary deformity occurs and results in a vertically short maxilla and occlusal plane that tilts upward on the affected side. Typically, the maxilla and mandible both require surgical management unless early intervention is initiated with a functional orthodontic appliance during the mixed-dentition stage that will maximize vertical growth potential and minimize secondary deformity of the maxilla.

- Because of the various tissues that are affected and deficient in patients with HFM, both facial skeletal and soft tissue correction is necessary for correction of facial asymmetry. Skeletal correction should be done first, followed by soft tissue augmentation approximately 6 months later.
- Ideal treatment planning for correction of HFM requires 3D analysis using CT imaging; two-dimensional radiographs do not show the extent of the skeletal asymmetry.
- Interdisciplinary management of patients with HFM results in the most ideal outcomes.

REFERENCES

1. Grabb WC: The first and second branchial arch syndrome, *Plast Reconstr Surg* 36:485-508, 1965.
2. Poswillo D: The pathogenesis of the first and second branchial arch syndrome, *Oral Surg Oral Med Oral Pathol* 35:302-328, 1973.
3. Cousley RR, Calvert ML: Current concepts in the understanding and management of hemifacial microsomia, *Br J Plast Surg* 50:536-551, 1997.
4. Horgan JE, Padwa BL, LaBrie RA, et al: OMENS-Plus: analysis of craniofacial and extracraniofacial anomalies in hemifacial microsomia, *Cleft Palate Craniofac J* 32:405-412, 1995.
5. Touliatou V, Fryssira H, Mavrou A, et al: Clinical manifestations in 17 Greek patients with Goldenhar syndrome, *Genet Couns* 17:359-370, 2006.
6. Cousley RR, Wilson DJ: Hemifacial microsomia: developmental consequence of perturbation of the auriculofacial cartilage model? *Am J Med Genet* 42:461-466, 1992.
7. Pruzansky S: Not all dwarfed mandibles are alike, *Birth Defects* 51:120-129, 1969.
8. Vento AR, LaBrie RA, Mulliken JB: The O.M.E.N.S. classification of hemifacial microsomia, *Cleft Palate Craniofac J* 28:68-76, discussion 77, 1991.
9. David DJ, Mahatumarat C, Cooter RD: Hemifacial microsomia: a multisystem classification, *Plast Reconstr Surg* 80:525-535, 1987.
10. Kaban LB, Moses MH, Mulliken JB: Surgical correction of hemifacial microsomia in the growing child, *Plast Reconstr Surg* 82:9-19, 1988.
11. Kaban LB, Mulliken JB, Murray JE: Three-dimensional approach to analysis and treatment of hemifacial microsomia, *Cleft Palate J* 18:90-99, 1981.
12. Kaban LB, Padwa BL, Mulliken JB: Surgical correction of mandibular hypoplasia in hemifacial microsomia: the case for treatment in early childhood, *J Oral Maxillofac Surg* 56:628-638, 1998.
13. Vargervik K, Miller AJ: Neuromuscular patterns in hemifacial microsomia, *Am J Orthod* 86:33-42, 1984.
14. Vargervik K: Mandibular malformations: growth characteristics and management in hemifacial microsomia and Nager syndrome, *Acta Odontol Scand* 56:331-338, 1998.
15. Rune B, Selvik G, Sarnäs KV, et al: Growth in hemifacial microsomia studied with the aid of roentgen stereophotogrammetry and metallic implants, *Cleft Palate J* 18:128-146, 1981.
16. Polley JW, Figueroa AA, Liou EJ, et al: Longitudinal analysis of mandibular asymmetry in hemifacial microsomia, *Plast Reconstr Surg* 99:328-339, 1997.
17. Sarnas KV, Rune B, Aberg M: Maxillary and mandibular displacement in hemifacial microsomia: a longitudinal roentgen stereometric study of 21 patients with the aid of metallic implants, *Cleft Palate Craniofac J* 41:290-303, 2004.
18. Rune B, Sarnäs KV, Selvik G, et al: Roentgen stereometry with the aid of metallic implants in hemifacial microsomia, *Am J Orthod* 84:231-247, 1983.
19. Posnick JC: Surgical correction of mandibular hypoplasia in hemifacial microsomia: a personal perspective, *J Oral Maxillofac Surg* 56:639-650, 1998.
20. Converse JM, Coccaro PJ, Becker M, et al: On hemifacial microsomia. The first and second branchial arch syndrome, *Plast Reconstr Surg* 51:268-279, 1973.
21. Kearns GJ, Padwa BL, Mulliken JB, et al: Progression of facial asymmetry in hemifacial microsomia, *Plast Reconstr Surg* 105:492-498, 2000.
22. Mulliken JB, Kaban LB: Analysis and treatment of hemifacial microsomia in childhood, *Clin Plast Surg* 14:91-100, 1987.
23. Murray JE, Kaban LB, Mulliken JB: Analysis and treatment of hemifacial microsomia, *Plast Reconstr Surg* 74:186-199, 1984.
24. Padwa BL, Mulliken JB, Maghen A, et al: Midfacial growth after costochondral graft construction of the mandibular ramus in hemifacial microsomia, *J Oral Maxillofac Surg* 56:122-127, discussion 127-128, 1998.
25. Vargervik K, Ousterhout DK, Farias M: Factors affecting long-term results in hemifacial microsomia, *Cleft Palate J* 23(Suppl 1):53-68, 1986.
26. Ousterhout DK, Vargervik K: Surgical treatment of the jaw deformities in hemifacial microsomia, *Aust N Z J Surg* 57:77-87, 1987.
27. Gateno J, Xia JJ, Teichgraeber JF, et al: Clinical feasibility of computer-aided surgical simulation (CASS) in the treatment of complex cranio-maxillofacial deformities, *J Oral Maxillofac Surg* 65:728-734, 2007.
28. Ono I, Ohura T, Narumi E, et al: Three-dimensional analysis of craniofacial bones using three-dimensional computer tomography, *J Craniomaxillofac Surg* 20:49-60, 1992.
29. Santos DT, Miyazaki O, Cavalcanti MG: Clinical-embryological and radiological correlations of oculo-auriculo-vertebral spectrum using 3D-CT, *Dentomaxillofac Radiol* 32:8-14, 2003.
30. Troulis MJ, Everett P, Seldin EB, et al: Development of a three-dimensional treatment planning system based on computed tomographic data, *Int J Oral Maxillofac Surg* 31:349-357, 2002.
31. Whyte AM, Hourihan MD, Earley MJ, et al: Radiological assessment of hemifacial microsomia by three-dimensional computed tomography, *Dentomaxillofac Radiol* 19:119-125, 1990.
32. Maki K, Miller AJ, Okano T, et al: Cortical bone mineral density in asymmetrical mandibles: a three-dimensional quantitative computed tomography study, *Eur J Orthod* 23:217-232, 2001.
33. Zanakis NS, Gavakos K, Faippea M, et al: Application of custom-made TMJ prosthesis in hemifacial microsomia, *Int J Oral Maxillofac Surg* 38:988-992, 2009.
34. Saeed NR, Kent JN: A retrospective study of the costochondral graft in TMJ reconstruction, *Int J Oral Maxillofac Surg* 32:606-609, 2003.
35. Molina F, Ortiz Monasterio F: Mandibular elongation and remodeling by distraction: a farewell to major osteotomies, *Plast Reconstr Surg* 96:825-840; discussion 841-842, 1995.
36. Nagy K, Kuijpers-Jagtman AM, Mommaerts MY: No evidence for long-term effectiveness of early osteodistraction in hemifacial microsomia, *Plast Reconstr Surg* 124:2061-2071, 2009.
37. Shetye PR, Grayson BH, Mackool RJ, et al: Long-term stability and growth following unilateral mandibular distraction in growing children with craniofacial microsomia, *Plast Reconstr Surg* 118(4):985-995, 2006.

38. Meazzini MC, Mazzoleni F, Gabriele C, et al: Mandibular distraction osteogenesis in hemifacial microsomia: long-term follow-up, *J Craniomaxillofac Surg* 33(6):370-376, 2005.

39. Huisinga-Fischer CE, Vaandrager JM, Prahl-Andersen B: Longitudinal results of mandibular distraction osteogenesis in hemifacial microsomia, *J Craniofac Surg* 14(6):924-933, 2003.

40. Ji Y, Li T, Shamburger S, et al: Microsurgical anterolateral thigh fasciocutaneous flap for facial contour correction in patients with hemifacial microsomia, *Microsurgery* 22:34-38, 2002.

41. Saadeh PB, Chang CC, Warren SM, et al: Microsurgical correction of facial contour deformities in patients with craniofacial malformations: a 15-year experience, *Plast Reconstr Surg* 121:368e-378e, 2008.

42. Nasir S, Aydin MA, Altuntaş S, et al: Soft tissue augmentation for restoration of facial contour deformities using the free SCIA/SIEA flap, *Microsurgery* 28:333-338, 2008.

43. Kaufman MR, Miller TA, Huang C, et al: Autologous fat transfer for facial recontouring: is there science behind the art? *Plast Reconstr Surg* 119:2287-2296, 2007.

44. Coleman WP 3rd: Fat transplantation, *Dermatol Clin* 17:891-898, viii, 1999.

45. Coleman SR: Structural fat grafting: more than a permanent filler, *Plast Reconstr Surg* 118(3 Suppl):108S-120S, 2006.

46. Coleman KM, Coleman WP 3rd, Benchetrit A: Non-invasive, external ultrasonic lipolysis, *Semin Cutan Med Surg* 28:263-267, 2009.

47. Meurman Y: Congenital microtia and meatal atresia; observations and aspects of treatment, *AMA Arch Otolaryngol* 66:443-463, 1957.

48. Brent B: The correction of microtia with autogenous cartilage grafts: II. Atypical and complex deformities, *Plast Reconstr Surg* 66:13-21, 1980.

49. Brent B: Technical advances in ear reconstruction with autogenous rib cartilage grafts: personal experience with 1200 cases, *Plast Reconstr Surg* 104:319-334, discussion 335-338, 1999.

50. Nagata S: A new method of total reconstruction of the auricle for microtia, *Plast Reconstr Surg* 92:187-201, 1993.

51. Yamada A, Ueda K, Yorozuya-Shibazaki R: External ear reconstruction in hemifacial microsomia, *J Craniofac Surg* 20(Suppl 2):1787-1793, 2009.

52. Brent B: The team approach to treating the microtia atresia patient, *Otolaryngol Clin North Am* 33:1353-1365, viii, 2000.

53. Lustig LR, Arts HA, Brackmann DE, et al: Hearing rehabilitation using the BAHA bone-anchored hearing aid: results in 40 patients, *Otol Neurotol* 22:328-334, 2001.

Chapter 95

Mandibulofacial Dysostosis

Timothy A. Turvey

The spectrum of facial clefting malformations encompasses a group of conditions, including mandibulofacial dysostosis. Within this group are Treacher Collins syndrome, Nager syndrome, Miller syndrome, and others.[1-4] These rare conditions are predominantly autosomal dominant and have varying degrees of expressivity and severity. The conditions are always bilateral, and their expression is typically asymmetric. The cause is unknown, but the pathogenesis has been described in animal models with phenotypes similar to the condition. In animal models, the conditions can be produced by vascular insults to the stapedial artery and by injection of retinoids at specific embryonic intervals.[5-9]

The lateral parts of the face are the targets of these conditions, with the orbits, eyelids, lateral canthus, zygoma, mandibular ramus, skin of the cheek, muscles of mastication, and external and middle ear structures being affected. Displaced hair from the eyelashes and scalp is often observed on the cheek. Because of the hypoplasia of the mandible, the upper airway is commonly narrow at the base of the tongue. Compounding the airway obstruction, choanal atresia can also be observed.[10-13]

The facial phenotype is classic and consists of down-turned lateral palpebral fissures, lateral upper eyelid ptosis, coloboma of the eyelids, lateral and inferior orbital wall hypoplasia, proptosis, overprojection of the nasal dorsum, narrow middle face, short posterior face, elongation of the anterior face, mandibular hypoplasia with retrogenia, and lip incompetence.

The oral findings are variable and include an open bite, cleft palate, and flared mandibular anterior teeth. The occlusion varies depending on the expression of the condition. Apertognathia is also variable. Although mandibular retrognathism and retrogenia are typical, paradoxic class III malocclusion can be observed.

Radiographic findings include a short anterior cranial base, egg-shaped orbits oriented obliquely from medial to lateral, clefts of the zygomatic arch, hypoplastic or aplastic zygomas and mandibular condyles, short ramus height, antegonial notching, retrognathism, and retrogenia. The occlusal and mandibular planes are always steep.

FUNCTIONAL FINDINGS

HEARING

Conductive hearing loss almost always accompanies the condition. The external and middle ear structures are usually involved. For this reason, newborn hearing screening should always be performed, and when abnormal findings are encountered, conductive hearing aids should be applied as soon as possible. Early intervention may improve learning, expressive language, and other communication skills. The middle ear structures can be missing or ankylosed, the ear canal can be atretic or hypoplastic, and the tympanic membrane can be absent. The external ear may also be malformed, ranging from almost complete absence to hypoplasia of the entire external structure.

RESPIRATION

Newborns affected with mandibulofacial dysostosis commonly have respiratory difficulty. This stems from hypoplasia of the nasopharynx and obstruction of the base of the tongue caused by mandibular hypoplasia. The majority respond favorably to prone posturing and avoidance of the supine position. Tracheostomy is an option, but the decision to proceed with it should not be taken lightly. Perinatal tracheostomy may be lifesaving, but postsurgical mortality (up to 15%) can occur with this procedure in neonates and young children. In addition, it places an enormous burden and pressure on families, hospitals, and nursing staff to clean and maintain these devices. When the airway problem is isolated to the base of the tongue and not associated with laryngomalacia, tracheomalacia, or other airway problems, distraction osteogenesis of the mandible is an alternative. This decision, too, should not be taken lightly since it is not a panacea and it will have adverse consequences on the developing dentition, will cause scars, and will require care provider support to activate and keep the appliances clean. Other soft tissue procedures to improve the airway have been described, such as lip-tongue adhesion, but the results are inconsistent. If choanal atresia or hypoplasia accompanies the condition, the nasal airway is additionally compromised. Surgery to relieve the area of obstruction is the only means of treating this condition. The best timing for this surgery is debatable.

FEEDING

Swallowing problems are not typical of this condition; however, most affected neonates have eating problems because of the limited nasal and oropharyngeal space. Neonates are obligate nasal breathers and rely on sucking to assist in the ingestion of milk and fluids. With the airway compromise associated with mandibulofacial dysostosis, feeding is always an issue, and it requires more time and energy than normal. Tube feeding to supplement oral feeding is occasionally helpful. Gastrostomy is an alternative but should be reserved for those with swallowing disorders or failure to thrive. Gastroesophageal reflux is another potential contributor to feeding and airway issues in these patients, and occasionally fundoplication is necessary. Nursing staff and parents must be trained to be patient with feeding.

SPEAKING

Cleft palate occasionally accompanies the mandibulofacial dysostosis conditions. When it does, a cleft palate protocol should be used, except when airway concerns supersede the routine protocols. In general, as the infant gains weight and grows, the mandible advances and the oral pharyngeal space opens, thereby permitting the palate to be repaired at 9 to 18 months of age.

Children with Nager syndrome characteristically have a flaccid, paralyzed, or aplastic soft palate. This condition is one of the most frustrating aspects of cleft care since even obliteration (either surgical or obturation with a prosthesis) has little effect on the hypernasal speech.[14]

When children with mandibulofacial dysostosis have speech problems and the palate is not cleft, it is more likely to be due to hearing issues rather than velopharyngeal dysfunction.

VISION

Many patients with mandibulofacial dysostosis wear corrective lenses. Strabismus, amblyopia, and other visual impairments can accompany these conditions. Other than occasional coloboma of the iris or pupil (or both), there is no typical pattern of visual disturbances with these conditions. Attaching hearing aids to the eyeglass frame avoids wearing a headband to support the aids and encourages the use of both devices simultaneously.

When orbital surgery is performed, diplopia is expected postsurgically, but it usually subsides as the swelling resolves. The diplopia subsides even when bone grafts are placed in the lateral orbital floor to change the shape of the orbit and elevate the level of the globe.

JAW FUNCTION

Ankylosis of the temporomandibular joint has been reported with this condition, but it has never been observed by this author. Most commonly, patients are able to open and close the jaw. Because the muscles of mastication are affected to varying degrees, an inability to excurse laterally or to protrude symmetrically is commonly observed. Reduced biting force is expected because of the abnormal masseter, pterygoid, and temporalis muscles.

Even in the absence of normal temporomandibular joints and with compensatory recruitment of parafunctional muscle activity to open and close the jaw, myofascial pain is infrequent in these conditions.

An inability to incise or masticate efficiently is more associated with malocclusion than with abnormal jaw function.

SURGICAL INTERVENTION

ZYGOMATICOORBITAL RECONSTRUCTION

Surgery can improve the appearance and function of patients with these conditions. The protocol used depends on the expression of the condition. Surgery during infancy should be undertaken to preserve life and vital function. Airway and vision are the two issues that require early intervention. Tracheostomy, distraction osteogenesis, gastrostomy tube placement, fundoplication, choanal atresia repair, and eyelid surgery should be considered to preserve life and vision. If the extent of eyelid absence results in drying and repetitive corneal ulcers, early eyelid reconstruction is indicated. In the absence of globe trauma or drying, eyelid surgery should be reserved for post-skeletal reconstruction. The scarring secondary to eyelid surgery produces scars that can be unsightly (Fig. 95-1).

The initial phase of reconstruction commences at approximately 8 years, depending on the patient and parents' wishes.[10-13,15,16] Orbital

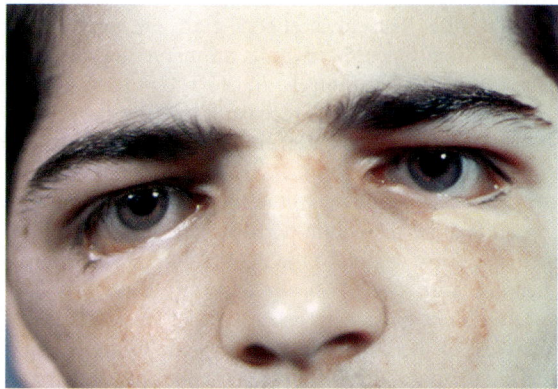

Fig. 95-1 ■ Unsightly eyelid scars from full-thickness skin grafts placed on the inferior lids in the childhood years.

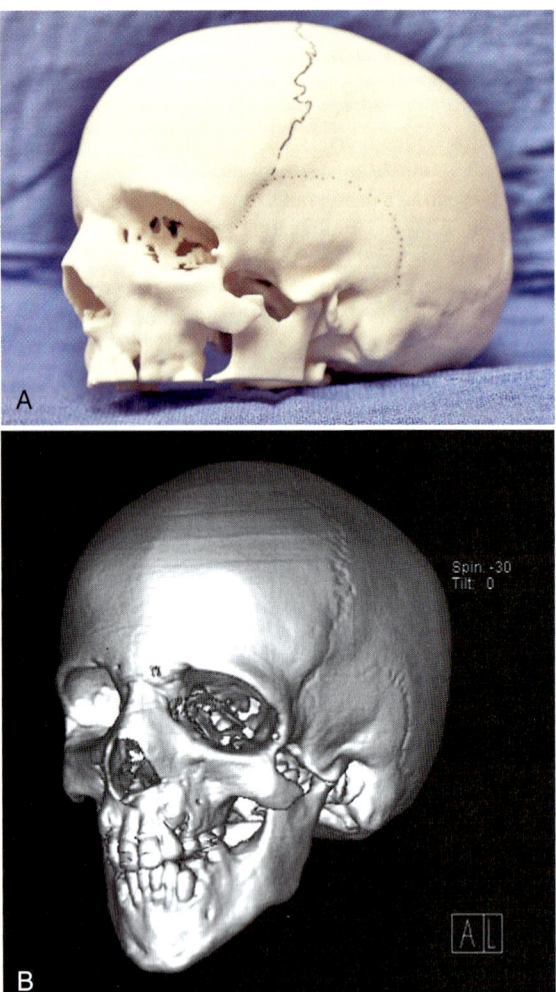

Fig. 95-2 ■ **A,** Stereolithographic model of the skull and face of a patient with Treacher Collins syndrome. **B,** Three-dimensional computed tomography scan of patient with Treacher Collins syndrome.

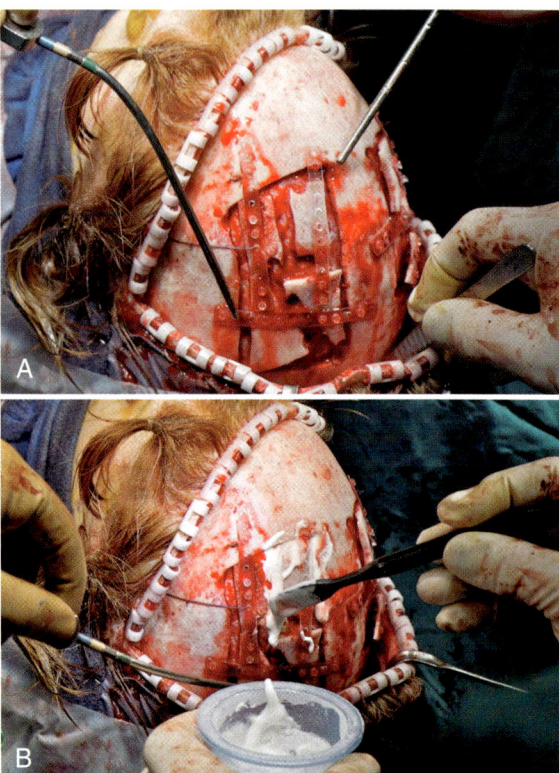

Fig. 95-3 ■ **A,** Reassembling the pieces for coverage of the cranial defect after the graft has been harvested. **B,** Calcium phosphate bone cement placed in the calvarial defects.

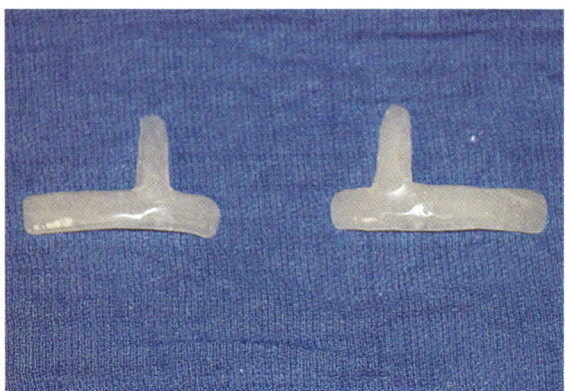

Fig. 95-4 ■ Templates of the desired bone grafts.

and zygomatic reconstruction can be performed with full-thickness temporoparietal bone grafts (large—10 cm). Square blocks can be harvested by conventional neurosurgical methods via burr holes and a craniotome. Selection of the donor site is based on the curvature of the skull and thickness of the bone. Presurgical planning with stereolithographic models, three-dimensional computed tomography (CT), or virtual planning can help determine the best donor site and the precise shape of the defect to be reconstructed (Fig. 95-2).

A coronal incision is used to approach the orbits, zygoma, and lateral orbital walls. The calvarial bone grafts are harvested through this same incision. Once these grafts are harvested, the exact size and shape can be carved from the block. The remaining pieces are then split and the donor site is reconstructed with the remnants. In general, biodegradable mesh is used to reassemble the pieces and to attach the construct to the skull (Fig. 95-3). Through the same incision, the dissection continues to the forehead and orbital region. It is important that the dissection remain subperiosteal over the forehead area and in the region of the zygomas to prevent injury to the facial nerve.

The temporalis muscle is usually intact unless it is elevated during harvest of the cranial bone. The plane of dissection should be under the temporoparietal fascia and either just superficial to or below the superficial layer of the deep temporal fascia. Doing this avoids damage to the facial nerve. This plane of dissection is the same as the subperiosteal plane of the orbit and lateral cheek. The dissection is carried around the infraorbital rim and the lateral maxilla adequately enough to permit insertion of the bone grafts. Subperiosteal dissection of the orbit is limited to the roof, lateral walls, and floor of the orbit. The lateral canthus is always detached. Frequently, the inferior orbital fissure has no anterior or lateral component because of the missing or hypoplastic zygoma. Dissection of tissue over the mid-face must be extensive enough to permit insertion and coverage of the bone graft. Scoring the periosteum with a scalpel helps stretch the soft tissues.

The bone graft is crafted according to the template taken from the stereolithographic model or constructed from virtual planning (Fig. 95-4). The bone graft is inserted and positioned as planned and is then secured with bone screws by anchoring the graft to the lateral orbital wall and to the temporal bone posteriorly. The floor of the orbit on the lateral aspect is usually grafted as well. Once both grafts are secured, the coronal flap is repositioned. The lateral canthus is identified, elevated, and secured to the temporalis fascia with a permanent suture. The flap is then closed in layers while being certain to resuspend the fascial layers to the temporalis fascia or to the calvaria via small burr holes through the outer cortex.

CHIN RECONSTRUCTION

Genioplasty is delayed until the permanent dentition erupts in the anterior mandible, especially the cuspids. This procedure is always performed in patients with mandibulofacial dysostosis conditions. Design of the operation is based on the desired outcome, which usually entails advancement and shortening. Sometimes just projection is required, and sometimes shortening is required. When shortening is desirable, wedge resection should be performed, not amputation of the inferior border. If maximum airway improvement is desired, the osteotomy should be designed to include the genial tubercles. The posterior slope of the anterior surface of the mandible must be considered when planning genioplasty in these conditions. Interpositional bone grafts placed in the posterior wings of the genioplasty will elongate the posterior inferior border and result in further advancement of the chin anteriorly (see Fig. 95-7). Frequently, this is desirable in these conditions.

ORTHOGNATHIC SURGERY

The orthognathic surgical phase of treatment generally commences once the permanent dentition has erupted, but this is also dependent on other factors. Attention to the desires of the patient and the family is of paramount importance in the process. The psychosocial concerns of the patient are the principal drivers of the timing of care, more so than the biologic concerns of the level of skeletal maturity. The patient and family should be made aware of the consequences of engaging in this phase of treatment prematurely and the potential need to reoperate if the patient outgrows the correction.

The orthodontist must decide on the best way to prepare the arches for treatment. Sometimes extractions are required to facilitate arch alignment. In general, if an open bite is present, it should be closed with surgery, not orthodontics. If transverse arch incompatibility is present, it too should be corrected with surgery, not orthodontics.

The orthognathic surgical plan should address the three-dimensional skeletal and occlusal problems identified. Generally, the mandibulofacial dysostosis conditions result in shortness of the posterior face because of hypoplasia of the condyle, ramus, and muscles of mastication. Shortness of the posterior face causes posterior and inferior rotational displacement of the hypoplastic mandible.[17] When this is present, the surgeon should attempt to rotate the posterior face counterclockwise, which will elongate the ramus, project the mandible and chin forward, and thereby shorten the anterior face. To accomplish this, the entire maxilla is mobilized and the posterior maxilla is moved inferiorly to flatten the occlusal plane. This maneuver is difficult and requires the use of bone spreaders to facilitate inferior repositioning (Fig. 95-5). Bone grafting of the defects and bone plate stabilization are necessary. Because of the inferior displacement of the maxilla, the anterior nasal spine and paranasal areas rotate posteriorly, and these areas should be augmented by means of onlay bone grafting. The ramus is elongated with inverted L osteotomies, and the mandible is advanced to its corrected position. This requires extensive stripping of muscle in the subperiosteal plane and traction wires placed at the angles and symphysis to aid in mobilization (Fig. 95-6). The ramus is stabilized

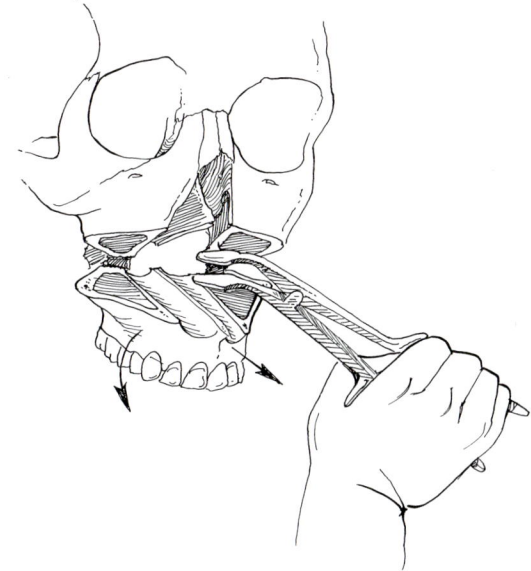

Fig. 95-5 ■ Bone spreaders inserted into the posterior maxilla to facilitate inferior repositioning.

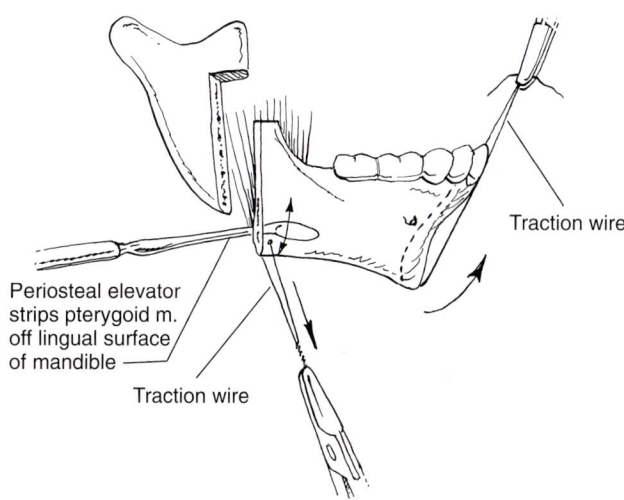

Periosteal elevator strips pterygoid m. off lingual surface of mandible

Traction wire

Traction wire

Fig. 95-6 ■ Wires in the mandibular angles and a circum-mandibular wire in the symphysis permit traction in the directions of movement.

with bone plates and screws, as well as with autogenous bone grafts (Fig. 95-7). The chin is also advanced and shortened via a transoral genioplasty approach. Careful planning is required to maximize the benefits and to achieve the desired result with each of these procedures.

Keys to success in this complex orthognathic surgery include the following:
1. Detailed planning
2. Complete mobilization of the maxilla and mandible to permit adequate elongation of the posterior face
3. Extensive stripping of the muscles of mastication from the ramus and distal segment of the mandible
4. Complete mobilization of the maxilla with down-grafting of the posterior region
5. Complete mobilization of the mandible and overcorrection at the time of surgery
6. Stabilization of the segments with autogenous bone grafts and bone plates and screws

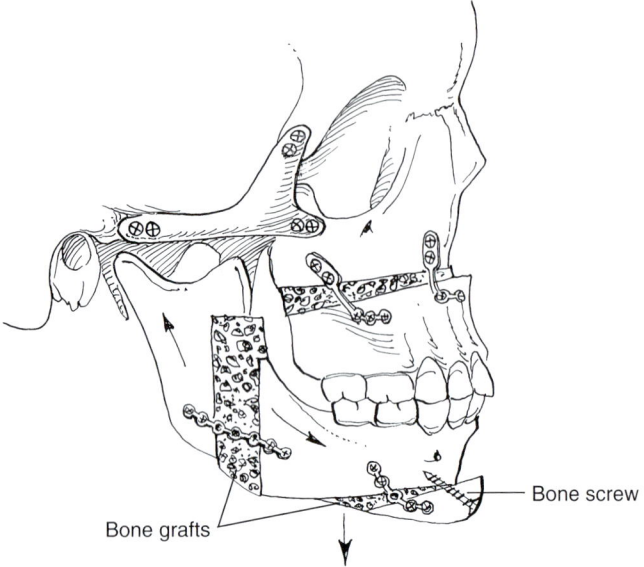

Fig. 95-7 ■ Entire maxillary and mandibular complex with bone grafts in the maxilla and mandible. Stabilization is accomplished with bone plates and screws.

Bone screw

Bone grafts

7. Augmentation of the paranasal areas
8. Control of the postsurgical position of the maxilla and mandible with elastic traction

CASE 1: TREACHER-COLLINS SYNDROME

A 9-year old with Treacher-Collins syndrome had been the victim of ridicule at school and among her peers. She exhibits moderate expression of the condition, including skeletal and soft tissue aberrations consisting of zygomatico-orbital hypoplasia, absence of a complete zygomatic arch, short mandibular ramus, short posterior maxilla, antegonial notching, elongation of the anterior face, retrogenia, overprojection of the nasal dorsum, coloboma of the lower eyelids, down-turned palpebral fissures, anteriorly positioned sideburns, and hearing loss. Oral examination revealed class I mixed dentition with an anterior open bite and absence of a cleft palate. The three-dimensional CT scan and stereolithographic model clearly demonstrate the extent of the skeletal problems (Fig. 95-8, *A* and *B*).

The first stage of reconstruction was offered and accepted by the patient and parents. It consisted of full-thickness cranial bone grafts harvested from the temporoparietal region bilaterally. Templates of the desired bone graft contour were fabricated from the stereolithographic model and taken to surgery to help prepare the correct size

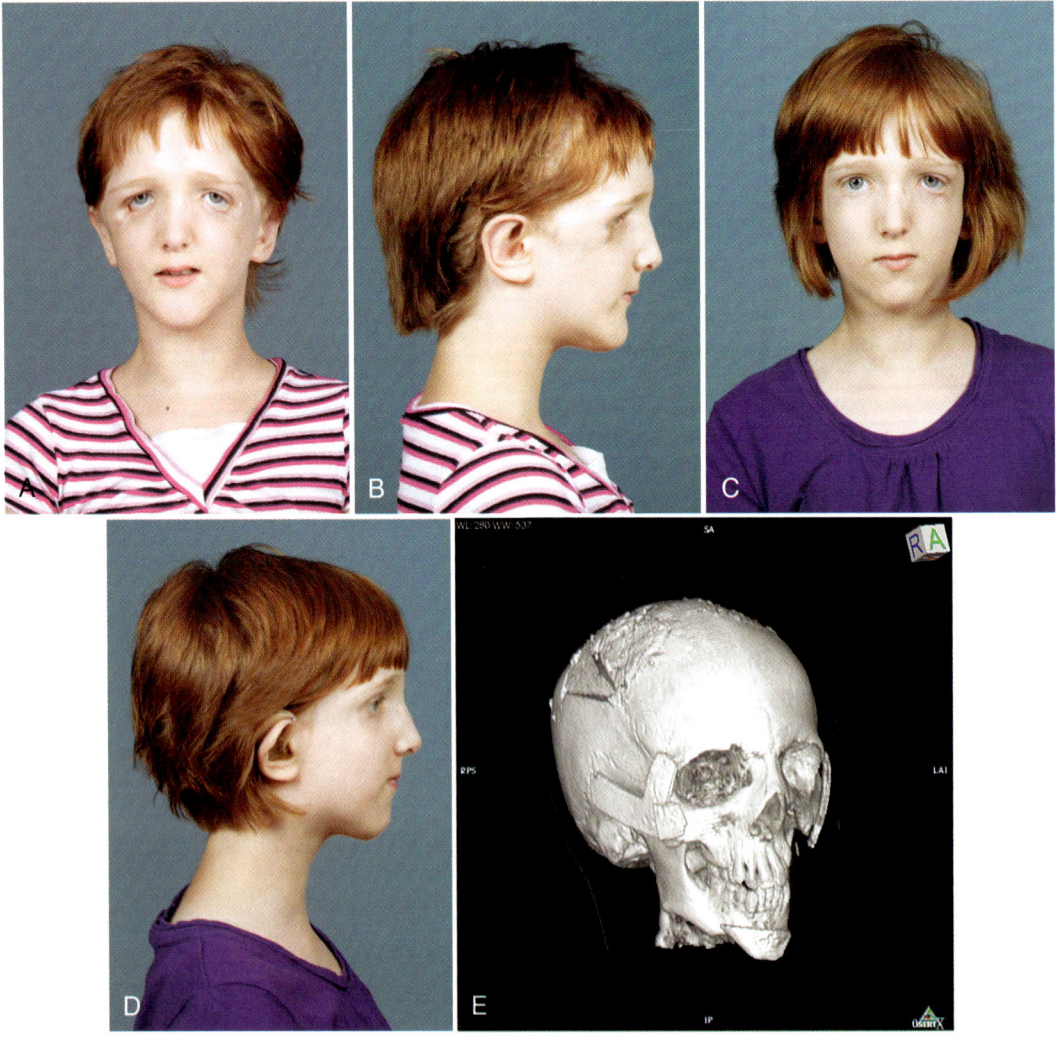

Fig. 95-8 ■ Preoperative frontal (**A**) and profile (**B**) facial views of a 9-year-old girl with Treacher Collins syndrome. Postoperative frontal (**C**) and profile (**D**) views. **E**, Postoperative three-dimensional image.

and shape of the grafts. The bone grafts were fabricated from the 12- × 12-cm harvested blocks. The remaining pieces were then split, and the split pieces were used to reconstruct the skull defect. The pieces were patched together with biodegradable bone plates and screws. The patch network was then fastened to the skull with additional bone plate and screw fixation. The reconstructed site was then further grafted with bone dust taken from the craniectomy holes and with calcium phosphate cement.

Through the same coronal incision, the zygomatico-orbital region was dissected and the extent of the cleft through the zygomatic arch was exposed, as well as the hypoplastic lateral and inferior orbital rims. Through the same incision, the temporal bone was exposed posteriorly at the point where the zygomatic arch articulates with the skull. Dissection must be extensive and carried to the lateral wall of the maxilla to permit insertion of the bone graft. The soft tissues must be stretched intraoperatively. Once the graft is inserted and the position adjusted for symmetry and projection, it is stabilized with biodegradable screws.

The scalp wound is then closed in layers. Lateral canthopexy is performed with the canthus suspended superiorly, and the suture is secured to the fascia above. Several additional suspension sutures are placed to secure the temporoparietal fascia superiorly. The scalp is then closed in two layers.

Simultaneously, augmentation genioplasty was performed to improve the chin/lower lip imbalance. This was performed transorally with a horizontal osteotomy conducted below the mental foramen and stabilized with biodegradable screws. The distal segment was pedicled to the lingual musculature. The decision to offer genioplasty was based on the advanced development and eruption stage of the permanent cuspids. The advantages of performing genioplasty this way in a young patient have been documented, and the potential for complete reformation of the full thickness of the symphysis offers the possibility of additional augmentation later in life.[18]

The patient did well postoperatively and the surgery resulted in improved zygomatico-orbital support and projection of the chin with shortening of the face (Fig. 95-8, *C* to *E*). The periorbital soft tissue deficits become more apparent after surgery and may require repair of the coloboma or cross-eyelid rotational flaps for improvement.

CASE 2: NAGER SYNDROME

A 20-year-old man with Nager syndrome had been monitored since early childhood. He and his family declined an early phase of surgery and elected to delay surgery until this time. Part of that decision was based on the father's untreated identical condition and his attitude that he survived without treatment and his son could

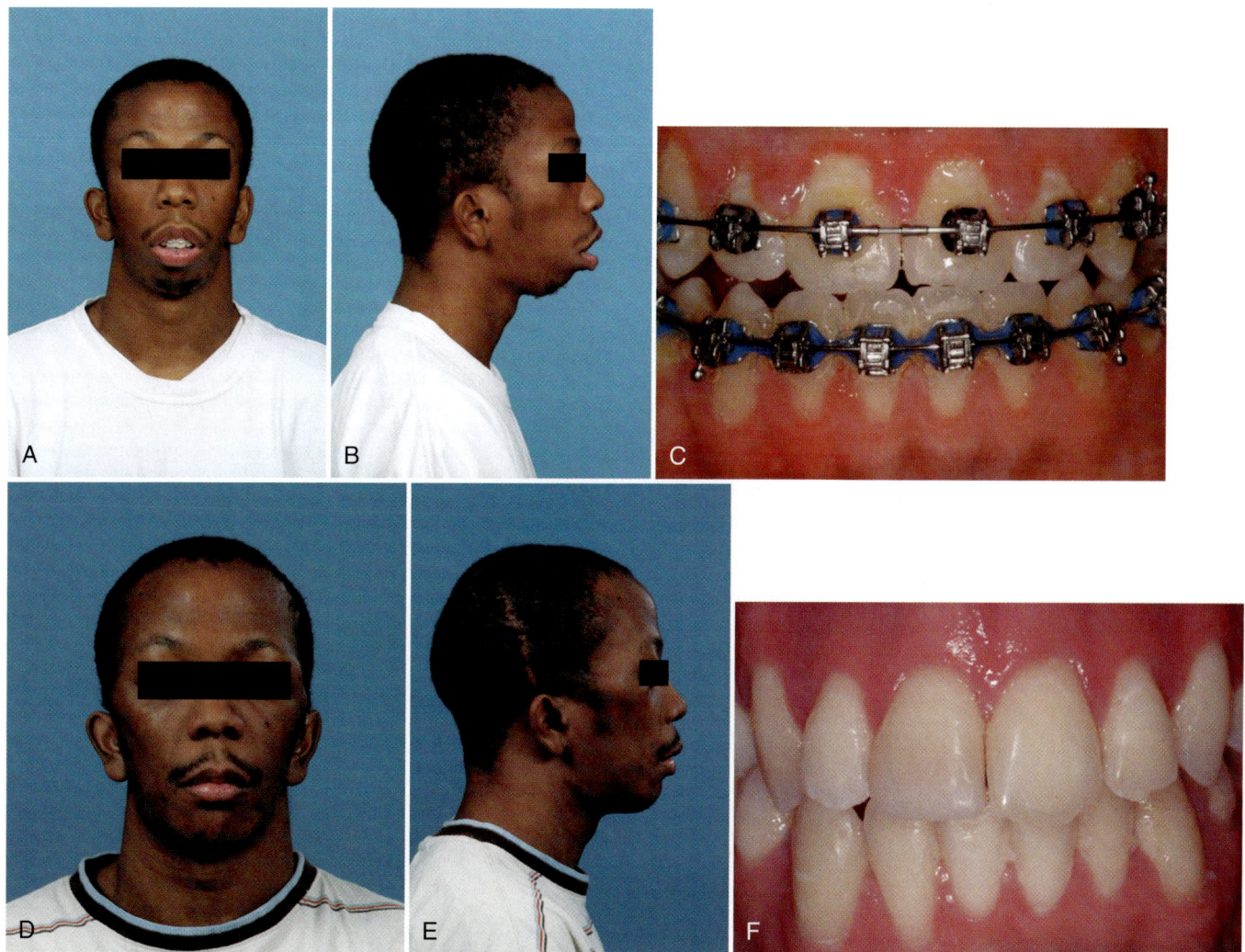

Fig. 95-9 ■ Preoperative frontal (**A**), profile (**B**), and intraoral (**C**) views of a 20-year-old man with Nager syndrome. Postoperative frontal (**D**), profile (**E**), and intraoral (**F**) views.

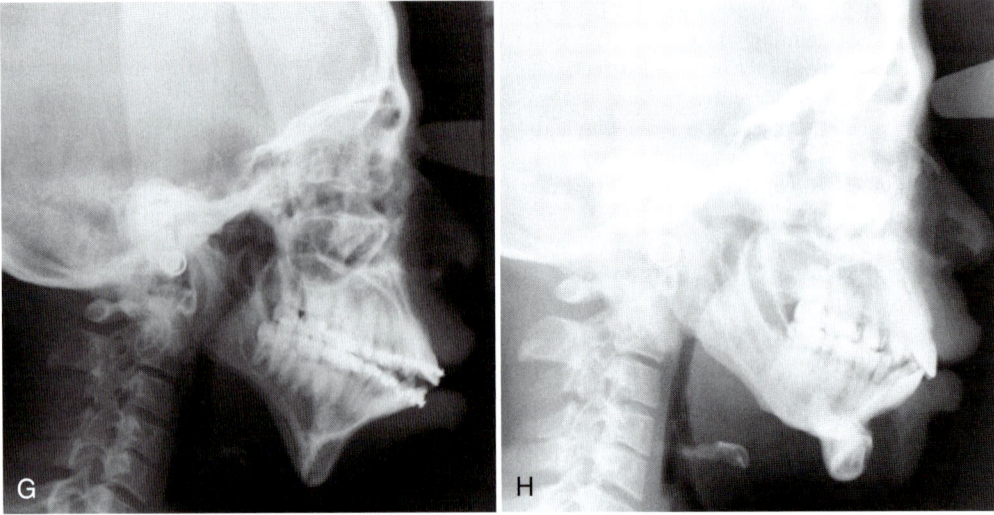

Fig. 95-9, cont'd ■ Preoperative (**G**) and postoperative (**H**) lateral cephalometric radiographs.

persevere as well. At this point the patient elected to proceed with surgery (Fig. 95-9, *A* to *C*).

He underwent orthodontic preparation, which included removal of four premolars. The surgical plan was simultaneous full-thickness cranial bone grafting to the zygomatico-orbital region bilaterally and maxillary and mandibular osteotomies. The cranial bone grafts were harvested and placed at the zygomatico-orbital area through a coronal incision, as previously described.

The objective of the maxillary and mandibular surgery was to rotate the lower face counterclockwise and improve its projection. The maxillary surgery included advancement and inferior positioning of the posterior maxilla with bone grafting. The mandibular surgery consisted of inverted L osteotomies of the ramus to elongate the posterior face and to rotate the symphysis superiorly to shorten the anterior face. This required neck incisions bilaterally, inferior displacement of the posterior border of the mandible greater than 1 cm, and stabilization with bone plates and interpositional autogenous bone grafts. Advancement genioplasty was also performed transorally, and the posterior wings of the pedicle were grafted inferiorly to facilitate further anterior projection of the chin (Fig. 95-9, *D* to *H*).

This surgery is lengthy and difficult but able to be accomplished in a single stage. It must be planned carefully by using articulated study casts, cephalometric tracings, stereolithographic modeling, or computer-guided simulation (alone or in combination).

The airway in many patients with mandibulofacial dysostosis is compromised and requires a plan to avoid tracheostomy. Intubation is a challenge to the anesthesiologist, and fiberoptic nasoendoscopic techniques are frequently necessary to secure an endotracheal tube. This challenge should not be taken casually, and those not familiar with the conditions are often surprised at the abnormal anterior position of the larynx.

PEARLS AND PITFALLS

- Mandibulofacial dysostoses are some of the most challenging facial clefting conditions.
- Skeletal reconstructions should be completed entirely before any soft tissue surgery is initiated in most circumstances.
- Periorbital soft tissue surgery can be performed, but scarring and limited outcomes must be considered before engaging in these procedures.
- Sometimes it is best to accept the soft tissue deficiencies, especially since the skeletal surgery significantly improves the shape of the face and jaws and improves the soft tissue support.

REFERENCES

1. Berry GA: Note on a congenital defect (coloboma) of the lower lid, *R Lond Ophthalmol Hosp Rep* 12:225-257, 1889.
2. Treacher Collins E: Case with symmetric congenital notches in the outer part of each lower lid and defective development of the malar bones, *Trans Ophthalmol Soc U K* 20:190-192, 1900.
3. Nager FR, de Raynier JP: Das Gehororgan bei den angeboranen Kopf-missbildunger, *Pract Otorhinolaryngol* 10(Suppl 2):1-128, 1948.
4. Franceschetti A, Klein D: The mandibulofacial dysostosis: a new hereditary syndrome, *Acta Ophthalmol* 27:143-224, 1949.
5. Poswillo D: The pathogenesis of Treacher Collins syndrome (mandibulofacial dysostosis), *Br J Oral Surg* 13:1-26, 1975.
6. Poswillo D: Otomandibular deformity: pathogenesis as a guide to reconstruction, *J Maxillofac Surg* 2:64-72, 1974.
7. Sulik KK, Johnston MC, Smiley SJ, et al: Mandibulofacial dysostosis (Treacher Collins syndrome): a new proposal for its pathogenesis, *Am J Med Genet* 27:359-372, 1987.
8. Sulik KK, Smiley SJ, Turvey TA, et al: Pathogenesis of cleft palate in Treacher Collins, Nager, and Miller syndromes, *Cleft Palate J* 26:209-216, 1989.
9. Sulik KK, Dehart DB, Rogers JM, et al: Teratogenicity of low dose of all-trans retinoic acid in presomite mouse embryos, *Teratology* 51:398-403, 1995.
10. Rougier J, Tessier P, Hervoust F, et al: *Chirurgie plastique orbito-palpébrale*, Paris, 1977, Masson.
11. Posnick JC, Goldstein JA, Waitzman A: Surgical correction of Treacher Collins malar deficiency: quantitative CT scan analysis of long-term results, *Plast Reconstr Surg* 92:12-22, 1993.
12. Posnick JC: Treacher Collins syndrome: perspectives in evaluation and treatment, *J Oral Maxillofac Surg* 55:1120-1133, 1997.

13. Posnick JC: *Craniofacial and maxillofacial surgery in children and young adults*, Philadelphia, 2000, WB Saunders.

14. Jackson IT, Bauer B, Saleh J, et al: A significant feature of Nager syndrome: palatal agenesis, *Plast Reconstr Surg* 84:219-226, 1989.

15. Freihofer HPM, Borstlap WA: Reconstruction of the zygomatic area. A comparison between osteotomy and onlay techniques, *J Craniomaxillofac Surg* 17:243-248, 1989.

16. Tessier P, Tulasne JF: Management of mandibulofacial synostosis. In Turvey TA, Vig KW, Fonseca RJ, editors: *Facial clefts and craniosynostosis principles and management*, Philadelphia, 1996, WB Saunders.

17. Schendel SA, Tessier P, Tulasne JF: Facial clefting disorders and craniofacial synostosis: skeletal considerations. In Turvey TA, Vig KW, Fonseca RJ, editors: *Facial clefts and craniosynostosis principles and management*, Philadelphia, 1996, WB Saunders.

18. Martinez JT, Turvey TA, Proffit WR: Osseous remodeling following inferior border osteotomy for chin augmentation: an indication for early surgery, *J Oral Maxillofac Surg* 57:1175-1180, 1999.

Pediatric Cranio-maxillofacial Trauma: Mandibular Fractures

Chapter 96

Paul S. Tiwana, Aaron Vickers

Treatment of mandibular fractures in pediatric patients is a challenging, yet rewarding endeavor. Because pediatric patients are experiencing active facial growth and dental development, special considerations must be taken. These complexities require an emphasis on proper planning and conservative treatment. Fundamentally, understanding of complex facial injuries has evolved through experience, both good and bad, with adult patients. Over time, various techniques, such as rigid fixation, were introduced into the pediatric population as well.[1-4] However, one must carefully consider that children are not simply "small adults" and that the application of adult-type treatment can be inappropriate in many circumstances. Furthermore, evolving methods and materials that are impractical for use in adult patients may be better suited for use in the pediatric population.

ETIOPATHOGENESIS/CAUSATIVE FACTORS

For a number of reasons, facial fractures have a lower incidence in children than in adults. For the most part, children reside in a very protective social environment. In the early years of life, parental supervision and a child-friendly environment mitigate the likelihood of serious injury. Although falls during these years are common, their low center of gravity ensures that little harmful force is generated that might cause injury. As children age, they are granted more freedom from the watchful eyes of their parents and begin to engage in activities, such as school and athletics, that increase the risk for injuries.

A number of studies have been conducted over the years to investigate the cause of mandibular fractures in the pediatric population. The Imahara study undertook an extensive review of the National Trauma Data Bank to analyze the incidence and etiology of facial fractures in pediatric patients (Fig. 96-1). The National Trauma Data Bank contains information obtained from more than 600 U.S. trauma centers. This study analyzed 277,008 patients 0 to 18 years of age admitted during the years 2001 to 2005. Of these patients, 12,739 (4.6%) sustained facial fractures. Males were affected about twice as frequently as females. Fractures were progressively more common as patients aged, with a 2.4% incidence in toddlers and infants and increasing to a 6.9% incidence in teens aged 15 to 18 years.

The most common cause of facial fractures in this cohort was motor vehicle accidents (55.1%), followed by assaults (14.5%) and falls (8.6%). Although motor vehicle accidents were the number one cause of facial fractures in all age groups, falls were more common than violence in children aged 0 to 9 years and bicycle accidents were more common than violence in children 5 to 14 years of age. Indeed violence, as a mechanism of injury, was proportionally most common in the 0- to 1-year and 15- to 18-year age groups.[5]

One particular source of injury that any oral and maxillofacial surgeon should always be aware of is child abuse. By its very nature, child abuse is a traumatic act with consequences for the child lingering far beyond healing of the affected soft tissue and bone.[6,7] Unfortunately, most epidemiologic surveys of physical abuse in children show that the abuser is often an immediate family member. Head, neck, and facial injuries account for more than a third of physical abuse–related trauma. Injuries such as burns, lacerations, punctures, and fractures are all seen in abuse cases. Maxillofacial trauma surgeons who care for children should always keep the possibility of child abuse in mind when the history and clinical evaluation of an injury are not consistent. In addition, the discovery of multiple documented injuries at various stages of healing is a very concerning finding. Health care providers are mandated by law to report suspected child abuse in all 50 states.

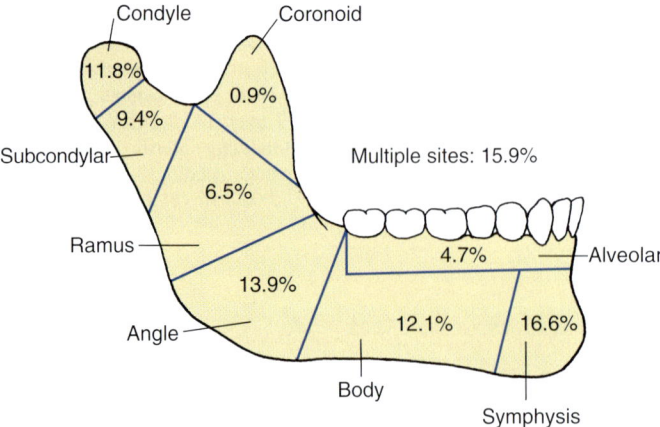

Fig. 96-1 ■ Fracture location in 4169 pediatric patients 0 to 18 years of age with mandibular fractures. (Data from Imahara SD, Hopper RA, Wang J, et al: Patterns and outcomes of pediatric facial fractures in the United States: a survey of the National Trauma Data Bank, *J Am Coll Surg* 207:710-716, 2008.)

DIAGNOSTIC STUDIES

Although there is no substitute for a thorough history and physical examination, modern imaging has provided significant assistance in the detection and treatment-planning stage of mandibular fractures, both in adults and children. Historically, a mandible series consisting of lateral oblique, posteroanterior, and Towne views were obtained to assess mandibular trauma. Later, panoramic radiographs were added by many centers because they were found to have sensitivity and specificity superior to that of the traditional mandible series.[8] Even though the panoramic radiograph is still widely used because of its low cost and widespread availability to maxillofacial surgeons, computed tomography (CT) has replaced plain film radiography as the "gold standard" for the detection of facial trauma.

In a prospective study, confirmed by surgical exploration, Wilson and colleagues found helical CT to have a sensitivity of 100% versus a sensitivity of 86% for panoramic radiography in the detection of mandible fractures.[9] Furthermore, Chacon and associates found the accuracy, sensitivity, and specificity of CT to be superior to that of panoramic radiography for the detection of condylar fractures in a pediatric population.[10]

In addition to improved sensitivity, CT offers other advantages over panoramic radiography as well. Because CT is performed in the supine position, it is ideal when imaging a polytrauma patient who cannot be placed upright for panoramic radiography. Furthermore, this positioning facilitates the use of sedation, which is sometimes necessary in the pediatric population to acquire adequate imaging.[9]

PATHOLOGIC ANATOMY

Critical examination of the stages of gross anatomic craniofacial development leads to several particular issues that have an impact on both the epidemiology and management of pediatric mandibular fractures. First, during infancy and early childhood, rapid brain growth causes a significant increase in head circumference. Head circumference attains greater than 90% of its adult size between 3 and 5 years of age. In addition, the orbits also reach skeletal maturity early in life (5 to 7 years of age). This provides the characteristic appearance of a very prominent forehead and orbits seen in infancy and early childhood. The later-maturing lower facial skeleton remains relatively protected behind these prominent facial features

during this time frame. Consequently, the mid-face and orbits are relatively more prone to injury in early childhood.[8] The bone itself during the early years of development has very high osteogenic potential and is characterized by thick medullary space and thin bony cortices, which results in the bone having a greater likelihood of greenstick fracture. The teeth in the primary dentition have particularly short, bulbous crowns that can make it difficult to achieve stable maxillomandibular fixation (MMF) during fracture reduction and stabilization with traditional techniques.

Development of the craniofacial skeleton during the later childhood years into the mixed-dentition period also yields further insight. During this time the lower two thirds of the face becomes more prominent as a result of forward and downward growth of the face, thus exposing these bones to more injuries. As per the functional matrix theory espoused by Moss and now widely accepted, facial bone growth is guided by the functional requirements of the overlying soft tissue envelope.[11] Accordingly, the mandibular body is lengthened by deposition of bone at the posterior ramus and resorption of bone at the anterior ramus. Downward mandibular growth occurs as the result of endochondral replacement at the mandibular condyles. Skeletal maturity of the maxilla and mandible is attained by approximately 14 to 16 years of age in females and 16 to 18 years of age in males.[12,13]

Early childhood is also characterized by development of the permanent tooth buds, which occupy space in the maxilla and mandible. These unerupted teeth create areas of structural weakness in the bone with a greater probability of sustaining a fracture through them. Furthermore, they must be taken into account when attempting open reduction and internal fixation. In addition, eruption of the permanent teeth in conjunction with loose, exfoliating primary teeth make maxillomandibular wiring and thus fracture reduction and stabilization more difficult. The permanent teeth erupt in a predictable sequence starting with the mandibular central incisors and first molars around 6 years of age. The maxillary incisors and mandibular lateral incisors erupt over the next 2 years or so. Finally, between the ages of 9 and 12, the canines and premolars erupt, followed by the second molars. In most cases the mandibular teeth erupt before their maxillary counterparts, and the teeth erupt from the midline posteriorly with the notable exception of the maxillary first premolar, which often erupts before the maxillary canine.[14] As the permanent dentition becomes fully erupted at about 12 years of age (with the exception of the third molars) and growth continues through the early teenage years, the craniofacial skeleton becomes more adult-like in its form, thereby allowing treatment consistent with that used in adults.[15]

Many times, treatment of pediatric mandibular fractures is dictated by the pattern of injury. In descending order, the most common fracture sites in 4169 patients aged 0 to 18 years with mandibular fractures were the symphysis (16.6%), multiple sites (15.9%), angle (13.9%), body (12.1%), condyle (11.8%), subcondyle (9.4%), ramus (6.5%), alveolus (4.7%), and coronoid (0.9%). When considering these findings, one may group condylar and subcondylar fractures together, which will probably be treated identically, and note that one or the other accounted for more than 20% of the mandibular fractures in that cohort (especially given the propensity for a condylar component in patients with fractures at multiple sites). Similar results have been reported in studies of a smaller scale as well.[16]

TREATMENT/RECONSTRUCTIVE GOALS

The goals of treatment for all patients with mandibular fractures are a return to pre-injury function and appearance. This requires attention to facial symmetry and dental occlusion. Concerns specific to pediatric fractures are the effects of the injury or the treatment on subsequent facial growth and dental development. Finally, whenever possible, patients and surgeons alike prefer to minimize morbidity by shortening the course of treatment.

Pediatric mandibular fractures require thoughtful consideration to avoid further injury to the developing dentition and significant growth disturbance. Most are quite amenable to closed reduction with MMF or the use of splints with skeletal fixation (or both). With the rapid healing and remodeling characteristic of growing pediatric patients, even significant alterations in occlusion and discrepancies in alignment are resolved rapidly. Indications for the use of rigid fixation are not common but do exist. Infants (<1 year of age) with mandibular fractures should be treated by observation. Diet modification is not usually necessary in this age group, and most of these patients will heal in due course with expectant management alone (Fig. 96-2).

SYMPHYSEAL AND PARASYMPHYSEAL MANDIBULAR FRACTURES

For anterior mandibular fractures, closed treatment is usually preferred for a number of reasons. First, these fractures, in isolation, are usually easily reduced, physiologic occlusion is reproduced, and the tremendous bone-healing potential of pediatric patients has an opportunity to take over. Furthermore, open reduction and internal fixation by traditional methods subject the patient to potential damage to unerupted teeth, as well as the possible need for a second surgery to remove the hardware. Finally, in growing patients, postoperative soft tissue scarring may lead to altered or restricted growth in the future.

When MMF alone may not be feasible, two alternative treatments exist. First, construction of a lingual splint from dental models is an elegant but time-consuming technique for reduction and fixation (Fig. 96-3). This technique is completed as follows: (1) alginate dental impressions are taken of both the upper and lower arches, but good-quality impressions may not easily be obtained without significant cooperation from the injured child, and it is therefore sometimes necessary to use an additional anesthetic to take the impressions; (2) stone models are created with the impressions; (3) model surgery is performed on the mandibular model to recreate the pre-injury occlusion; and (4) a lingual acrylic splint is fabricated with holes placed interdentally to hold the splint in place. Once construction of the splint is complete, the patient's mandible is manually reduced and the lingual splint is wired into place. In addition, circum-mandibular wires are sometimes required to further secure the splint. This type of fixation allows anatomic stabilization of the fracture while permitting movement of the mandible, which encourages rehabilitation of condylar fractures, if present. It also avoids the need for an incision and subperiosteal dissection, thus lessening soft tissue scarring.

A second treatment alternative calls for placement of MMF followed by open reduction and internal fixation of the fracture with the use of a miniplate placed at the very *inferior* border of the mandible. The fracture is best approached via a vestibular incision while taking care to provide an adequate soft tissue cuff superiorly and avoiding the mental nerve inferiorly. After good bone reduction, the occlusion is rechecked and a miniplate is secured to the inferior border with monocortical screws. If done properly, this technique poses minimal risk to the unerupted teeth while providing the stability needed for healing. When compared with the use of a lingual splint, two advantages of this option are that this technique does not require the ready availability of a dental laboratory and it is likely to

result in more anatomic reduction than that achieved with a lingual splint. When compared with closed treatment, open treatment facilitates early function and the ability to eat a soft diet as opposed to pureed food or liquids only. The presence of arch wires or bars with elastics facilitates physiologic rehabilitation of patients with a concomitant condylar fracture and also acts as a tension band to augment the mechanical strength of the miniplate. The importance of placing the plate at the very inferior aspect of the mandible must be emphasized. In a young child, the risk of placing screws into the unerupted dentition is great unless this principle is followed (Fig. 96-4).

MANDIBULAR BODY AND ANGLE FRACTURES

Though less common than anterior mandibular fractures, the vast majority of body and angle fracture injuries can likewise be treated with some form of MMF. Sagittal fractures of the mandibular body may also benefit from the placement of a circum-mandibular wire to aid in fracture reduction, as well as fixation (Fig. 96-5). This technique has the decided advantages of semiclosed placement and simple removal. Otherwise, the use of monomaxillary fixation such as with a lingual splint or open reduction of an unstable fracture and placement of a monocortical plate at the inferior border continue to remain options. Adult treatments such as the Champy technique are rarely useful in the pediatric population because of the inherent risks to the unerupted permanent molars. In general, open reduction is reserved solely for badly displaced fractures when closed treatment is unlikely to result in a functionally and cosmetically acceptable result or when these fractures occur in conjunction with condylar fractures. With rare exception, these cases can be done via an intraoral approach with the occasional need for a trocar.

MANDIBULAR CONDYLE FRACTURES

Condylar fractures are a major concern in children for two reasons. First, a relatively significant number of these injuries are never diagnosed, and second, regardless of whether they are diagnosed, condylar fractures can cause significant lower facial asymmetry and masticatory dysfunction, particularly in growing patients. In fact, Proffit and co-authors reported that up to 10% of patients with dentofacial deformities have evidence of previously undiagnosed condylar fractures.[17] The mandible is the last bone in the face to reach skeletal maturity, and consequently, it is vulnerable to injury-related disturbances in growth. This is magnified by the fact that mandibular trauma has a greater incidence in late childhood and adolescence. Classically caused by a fall and commonly heralded by a laceration in the submental region, condylar fractures are characterized by shortening of the ramus on the affected side, which causes deviation of the chin to the affected side. On the unaffected side, open bite and flattening of the body of the mandible are noted. In bilateral fractures of the condyle, posterior displacement of the mandible is seen with an anterior open bite. Occasionally, despite a condylar fracture the child will be able to hold projection, symmetry, and occlusion in the mandible without difficulty. In such cases, observation with diet modification is usually sufficient for treatment. The immediate sequelae of condylar fractures are the same in children and adults. However, the manner in which the fractures propagate can be substantially different. Because the immature mandible has a relatively thick and short condylar neck, children have a propensity for fracture through the condylar head rather than the low neck pattern seen more commonly in adults. In addition,

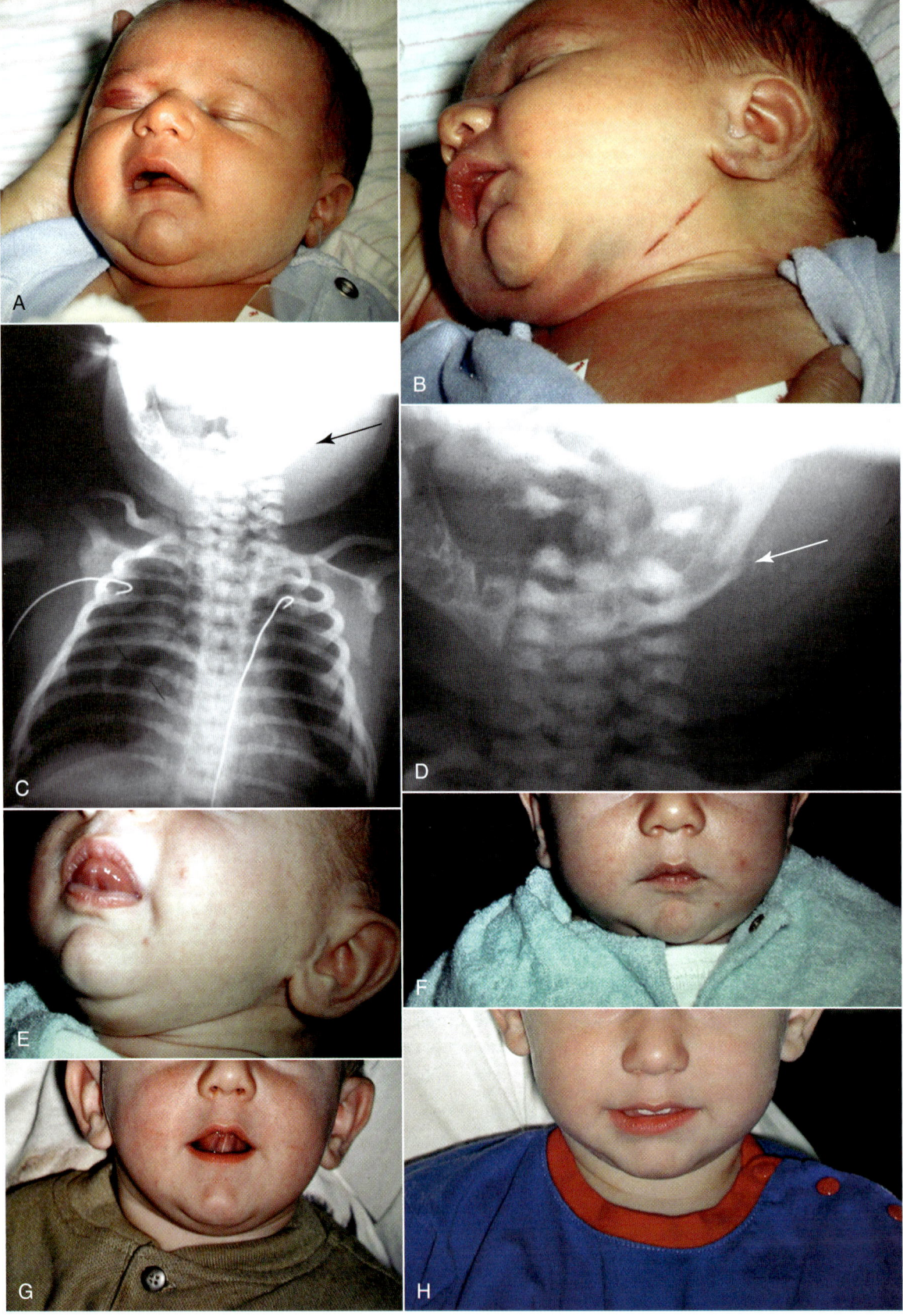

Fig. 96-2 ■ **A,** Facial view of a newborn infant after difficult forceps-assisted delivery. **B,** Facial profile view of the same newborn infant with ecchymosis and facial contusion. **C,** Postnatal chest radiograph showing the mandibular fracture. **D,** Close-up view of a radiograph demonstrating a mandibular fracture secondary to trauma from forceps-assisted delivery. **E,** Lateral facial view at 3 months of life. The mandibular fracture was managed by observation only. **F,** Facial view at 3 months of life. Note the mandibular symmetry. **G,** Facial view of the same child at 18 months of age. The findings on examination were normal. **H,** Facial view of the same child at 3 years of age. Note the continued mandibular symmetry. (From Fonseca R, Marciani R, Turvey T, editors: *Oral and maxillofacial surgery*, vol 2, ed 2, St Louis, 2008, Saunders.)

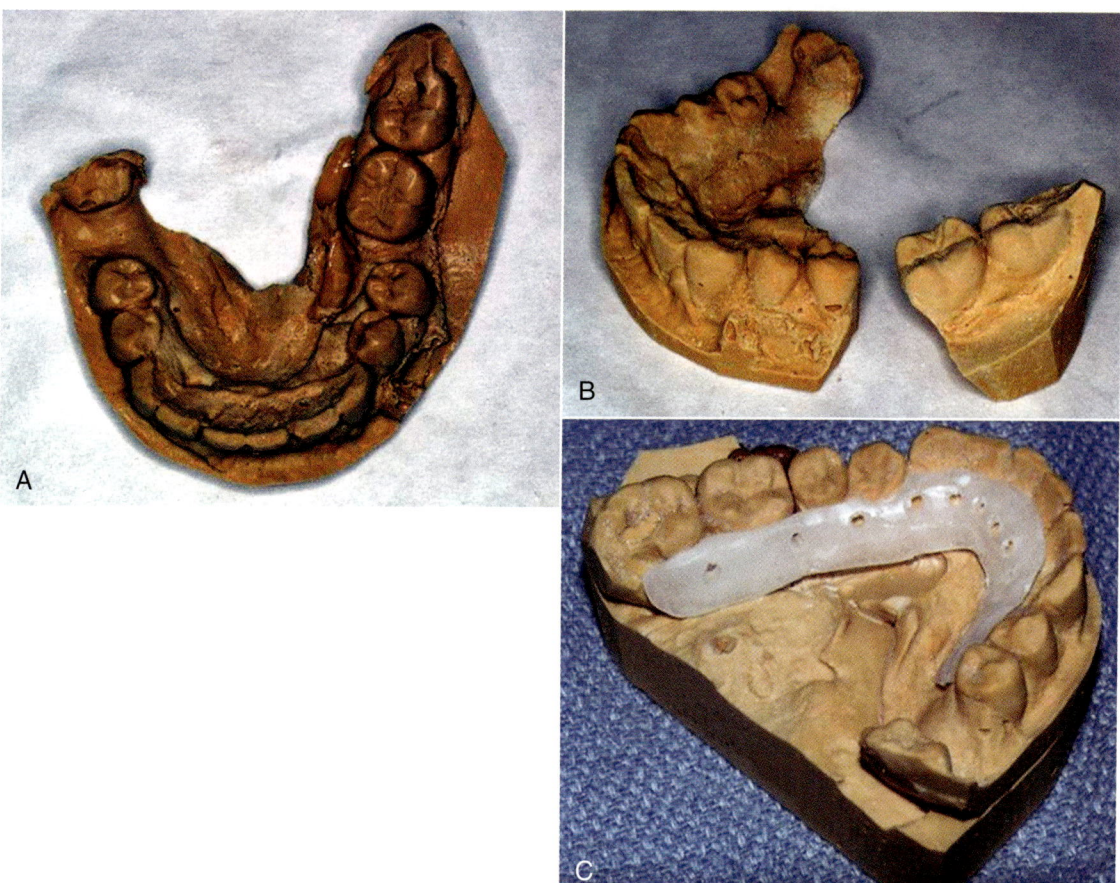

Fig. 96-3 ■ **A,** Stone model of a mandibular arch with a fracture for construction of a lingual splint. **B,** Same model, now sectioned for reduction of occlusion. **C,** Same model now reduced into correct occlusion and mounted on a stone base. A lingual splint was constructed and is in place. Note the holes for placement of wires around the teeth. (From Fonseca R, Marciani R, Turvey T, editors: *Oral and maxillofacial surgery*, vol 2, ed 2, St Louis, 2008, Saunders.)

compression injuries of the fossa and condylar head, as well as medial pole fractures, also occur more commonly in children.

Although the proper treatment of condylar fractures in adults has been the subject of much debate and research, in children open reduction is almost never indicated. Advocacy for closed treatment is biologically based on Walker's primate study and is further documented in the work of Lindahl, Lund, and Gilhuus-Moe.[18-21] In adult patients, closed treatment results in forced adaptation to the altered anatomy, whereas in children, rapid and progressive remodeling of the condylar unit is common. Dramatic evidence of this extensive remodeling can be seen when careful examination of long-term postoperative CT scans is carried out (Fig. 96-6). Although closed reduction of condylar fractures with a *very brief* period of MMF followed by physiotherapy and training elastics is not time or technically demanding, the long-term follow-up required for these injuries is. Despite the fact that ankylosis following condylar fractures is rare in North America (as opposed to the significant incidence in the developing world), children with condylar injuries should be evaluated at regular intervals until the completion of mandibular growth. The assistance of an orthodontist who is familiar with functional appliance therapy for growth modification is invaluable should asymmetry begin to develop in the early postinjury phase. However, if the asymmetry is not or cannot be corrected with growth modification alone, surgical correction with conventional facial osteotomies proceeds once growth is complete.

The amount of time that children with condylar fractures stay in tight elastic MMF before being allowed to function with elastic guidance has been decreasing over time. This is due to the realization that functional movement of the condyle as the bone reacts to the soft tissue forces surrounding it has therapeutic value. Historically, the time frame for tight elastic MMF has been set at approximately 14 days to allow a decrease in swelling and pain before initiating function. However, in our experience, children require only a few days for postinjury pain to subside to the point that function is possible. Given the well-documented capacity for rapid bone healing, the highly osteogenic potential of the facial bones, and the important relationship of the functional soft tissue envelope to the bone in growing patients, this approach remains biologically based.

In instances in which there are accompanying fractures of the mandibular body or symphysis, treatment with a lingual splint for monomaxillary fixation would still allow early mandibular function. Alternatively, closed reduction with wire MMF can be carried out for a brief period, usually 7 to 14 days, followed by elastic guidance to promote function of the joint. The use of monocortical plate fixation at the inferior border, as discussed previously, would also allow immediate mandibular function after combined fractures. Maintenance of mandibular projection, symmetry, and functional occlusion through a closed technique remains the cornerstone in the treatment of condylar fractures in children.

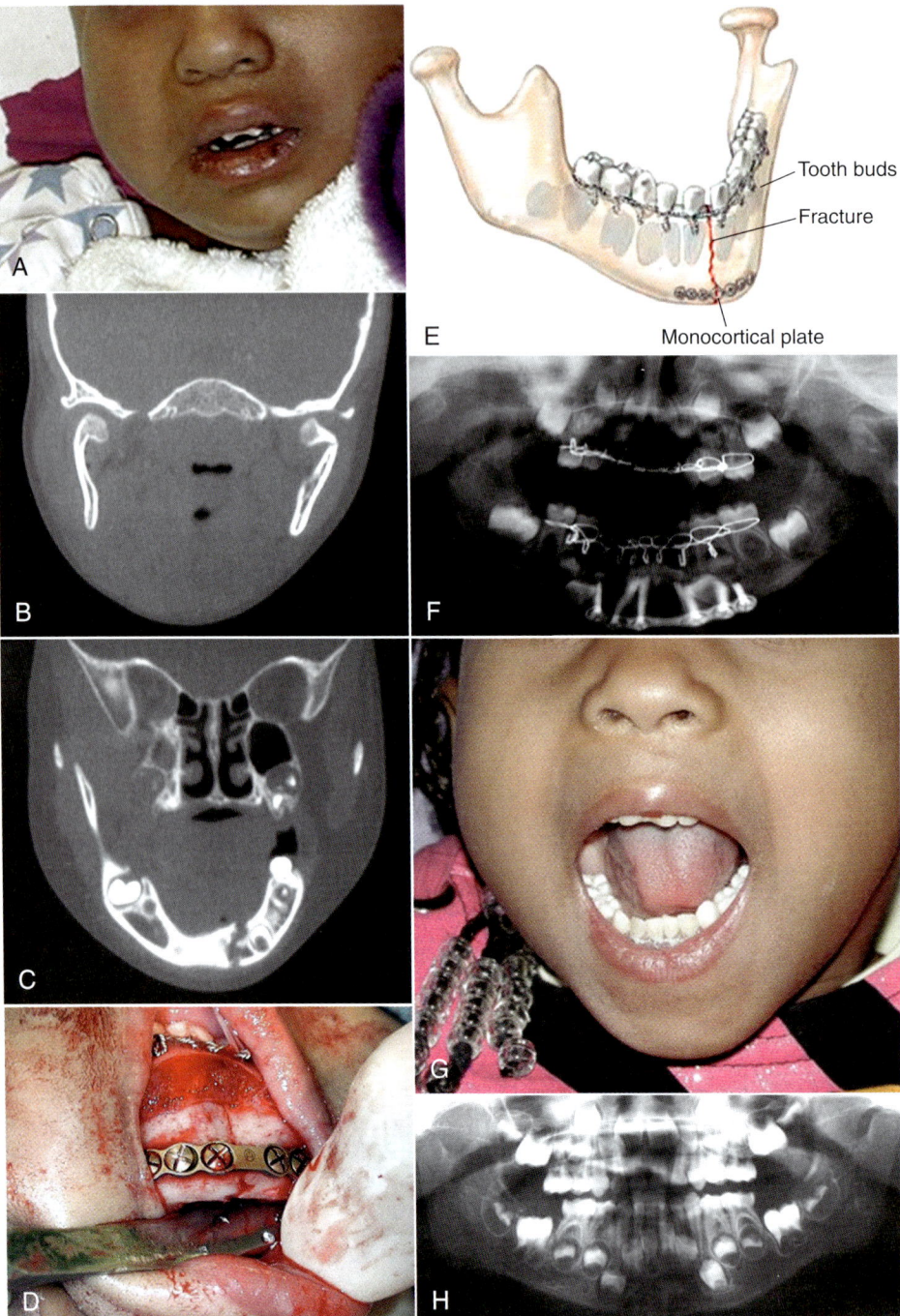

Labels in illustration E: Tooth buds · Fracture · Monocortical plate

Fig. 96-4 ■ **A,** Four-year-old girl with mandibular fractures after a motor vehicle accident. **B,** Coronal computed tomography (CT) scan showing medially displaced bilateral condylar fractures. **C,** Coronal CT scan of the same patient demonstrating a parasymphyseal fracture of the mandible. **D,** Intraoperative view of a monocortical plate placed via an intraoral anterior degloving approach to the mandible. Note the accurate reduction of the lingual cortex. **E,** Illustration of the monocortical plate placement technique for pediatric mandibular fractures. **F,** Postoperative Panorex film demonstrating reduction of the bilateral condylar fractures and the parasymphyseal fracture with a monocortical plate. **G,** Eight-week postoperative facial view showing excellent mouth opening. **H,** Eight-week postoperative Panorex film just after removal of the wire and internal fixation hardware. Note the undisturbed tooth buds in the anterior mandible as a result of placement of the internal fixation and the improvement in mandibular condyle morphology secondary to rapid remodeling promoted by joint function. (From Fonseca R, Marciani R, Turvey T, editors: *Oral and maxillofacial surgery,* vol 2, ed 2, St Louis, 2008, Saunders.)

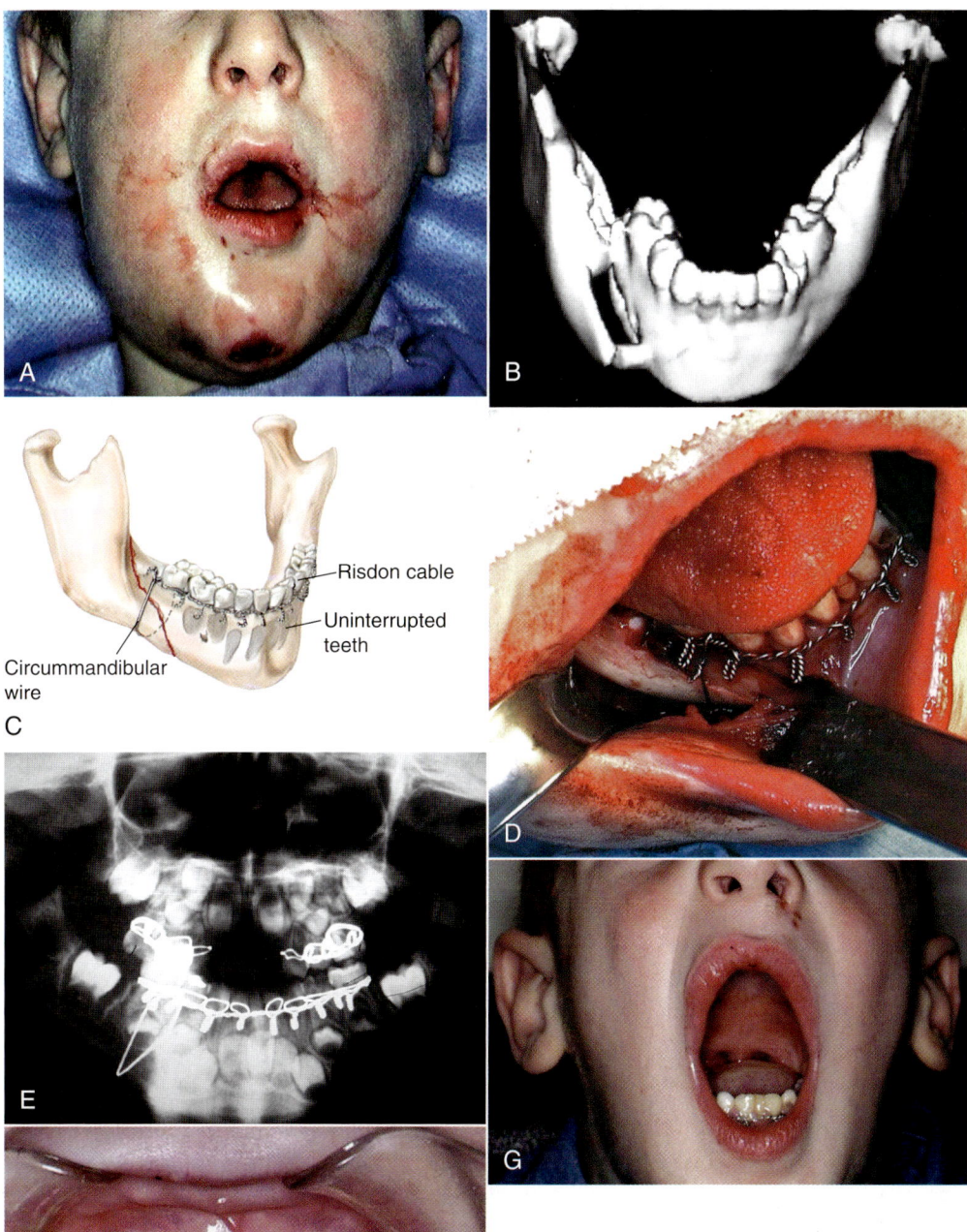

Fig. 96-5 ■ **A,** Facial view of a 5-year-old boy with a mandibular fracture. **B,** Three-dimensional computed tomography scan of the mandible demonstrating a sagittal fracture of the mandibular body with bilateral condylar fractures. **C,** Illustration of the circummandibular wire technique for reduction of sagittal pediatric mandibular fractures. **D,** Intraoperative view showing a circum-mandibular wire in place to stabilize the sagittal fracture of the mandible. **E,** Postoperative Panorex film demonstrating a circum-mandibular wire stabilizing the sagittal fracture of the mandible. **F,** Postoperative occlusion. **G,** Six-week postoperative facial view of the same child with excellent mouth opening. (From Fonseca R, Marciani R, Turvey T, editors: *Oral and maxillofacial surgery,* vol 2, ed 2, St Louis, 2008, Saunders.)

Potential indications for open reduction and internal fixation of pediatric condylar fractures are few. In most cases, conservative treatment of bilateral condylar fractures, as well as fracture-dislocations, still yields acceptable results. One study of fracture-dislocations found that although mild symptoms and radiologic asymmetry were present in more than half of the patients studied, none had clinically apparent facial asymmetry, and symptoms of temporomandibular joint dysfunction were generally mild, especially if one considers the relative impact necessary to cause a fracture-dislocation injury.[22]

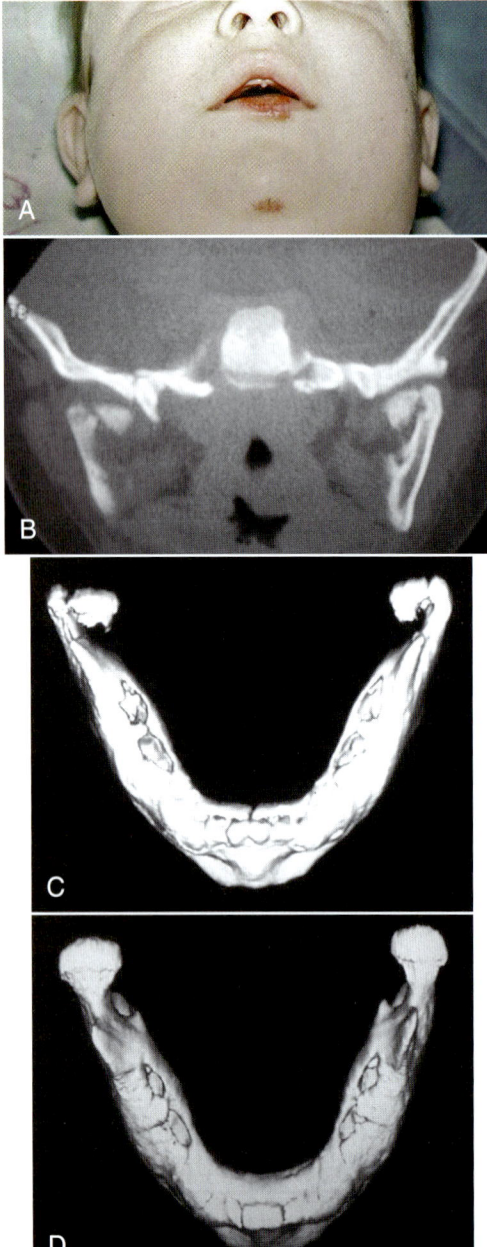

Fig. 96-6 ■ **A,** Facial view of a 3-month-old boy with mandibular fractures after a fall. Note the ecchymosis in the submental region. **B,** Coronal computed tomography (CT) scan of the same patient demonstrating bilateral medially displaced condylar fractures, which were managed by observation only. **C,** Three-dimensional (3D) CT scan of bilateral medially displaced condylar fractures. **D,** 3D CT scan of the same patient 9 weeks after injury demonstrating completely remodeled bilateral condylar fractures of the mandible. (From Fonseca R, Marciani R, Turvey T, editors: *Oral and maxillofacial surgery*, vol 2, ed 2, St Louis, 2008, Saunders.)

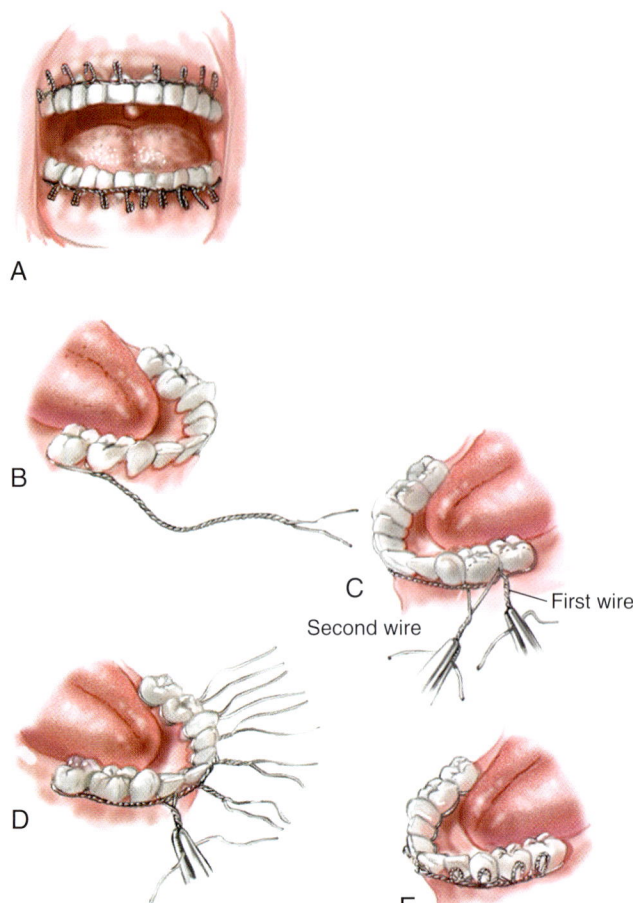

Fig. 96-7 ■ Technique for placement of a Risdon cable for maxillomandibular fixation of pediatric maxillofacial fractures. (From Fonseca R, Marciani R, Turvey T, editors: *Oral and maxillofacial surgery*, vol 2, ed 2, St Louis, 2008, Saunders.)

USE OF THE RISDON CABLE FOR PEDIATRIC MAXILLOFACIAL TRAUMA

The primary and early mixed dentitions have numerous anatomic challenges associated with placement of MMF appliances. The crowns of the teeth are short, squatty, and bulbous and can be loose. In addition, replacement of teeth as a normal process of the succedaneous dentition leads to edentulous areas awaiting full eruption. Various types of arch bars are universally used in the application of MMF during trauma and elective reconstruction of the maxillofacial skeleton. Unfortunately, the design and bulk of these arch bars do not fit the pediatric dentition very well. As a result, the circumdental ligature wires loosen and slide off, and they often do not even survive "struggling" of the child during emergence from anesthesia in the recovery room. To overcome these shortcomings, many advocate the use of skeletal fixation such as circum-mandibular, circumzygomatic, and piriform aperture wires to hold the arch bars in place. This only adds further steps to achieve solid MMF appliances and requires extreme diligence to prevent sawing through the soft bone of the pediatric maxillofacial skeleton when applying the wires.

Use of a modified Risdon cable in the primary and early mixed dentition is efficient in its application, provides excellent stability for elastic fixation, and does not require the additional placement of skeletal fixation. As the name implies, it was first described by Risdon, an otolaryngologist, in 1939.[23] In essence, the traditional arch bar is replaced by a cable of twisted 24-gauge stainless steel wire applied from one side of the dental arch to the other and secured to each tooth with a circumdental 24-gauge stainless steel wire (Fig. 96-7). Alternatively, the cable can be started posteriorly on both sides of the same arch and tied together in the midline for added compression of anterior mandibular fractures. The fundamental advantage is that the cable is thin and can easily be contoured to allow adequate engagement of the circumdental wires. The circumdental wires are then twisted into loops to holding elastics for MMF or guiding functions. Application is rapid in both arches, and very tight MMF can be achieved with elastics alone. During emergence from anesthesia, the elastics "give," thus preventing loss of adequate MMF and requiring a second trip to the operating room to reapply the MMF.

IMPACT OF GROWTH AND DEVELOPMENT ON TREATMENT

The most important concept to understand when treating pediatric mandibular trauma is that children are *not* simply small adults. The treatment algorithms commonly used for the treatment of adult patients are often unacceptable in the pediatric population. Issues such as growth and development, behavior management, and caregiver education are paramount.

Growth and development affect treatment planning in a number of ways. First among them is the effect of unerupted or partially erupted teeth. Extreme care must be taken to avoid damage to developing teeth whenever open reduction is considered. Frequently, the difficulty in achieving an acceptable result forces the provider to suggest closed treatment to prevent damage to the teeth. Furthermore, the titanium plates placed in a growing child are typically removed in 6 to 8 weeks, thus necessitating a second surgery. Traditionally, this has been done to prevent transmigration of the plate through the growing mandible. Even though titanium is thought to be biocompatible, the reality is that a plate that has transmigrated will be difficult to remove later in life should the need arise.

Biodegradable bone plates and screws have been regarded by some as an excellent material for pediatric facial bone surgery.[24,25] In addition, use of these systems has been documented extensively for orthognathic surgery involving the mandible and maxilla by Turvey and associates.[26] However, like distraction osteogenesis of the facial skeleton, biodegradable plates and screws remain a tool in the surgeons' arsenal and should not be considered a panacea.

The evolution of biodegradable plates offers promise; however, biodegradable plating systems have not yet garnered widespread acceptance, particularly for mandibular trauma, because of mechanical limitations, cumbersome size, and difficult handling.[27] To achieve strength comparable to that of titanium plates, biodegradable plates must be significantly larger. Manipulation of the plate typically requires a hot water bath or other heat source. Biodegradable screws are more prone to fracture during placement than their titanium counterparts. Finally, aggressive degradation of the plates and screws has been found on occasion to cause sterile abscesses, which can further complicate healing.

Behavior management and caregiver education are not to be overlooked when treating pediatric patients. Depending on the psychosocial development of the patient, it may not be possible to expect compliance with dietary restrictions and physiotherapy recommendations without an adequate parental support system at home. Indeed, assessing the patient's cognitive abilities and support system during the treatment-planning phase will maximize the likelihood of success.

POSTOPERATIVE TREATMENT

To promote rapid healing and rehabilitation following a mandibular fracture, a number of things can be done. Regardless of whether treatment was performed in closed or open fashion, it is important that the patient be properly educated regarding postoperative wound care and oral hygiene. For pediatric patients, it is critical that the parent or caregiver be involved in this discussion. Patients should be encouraged to continue oral hygiene practice as soon as possible after surgery.[28]

Because the oral cavity is home to a number of potential bacterial pathogens, postoperative wound infection is a significant concern, particularly when using intraoral incisions. As a result, it is common practice to prescribe antibiotics postoperatively to patients undergoing open reduction and internal fixation, as well as those undergoing closed treatment of open fractures. Historically, patients have been prescribed a 5- to 7-day course of antibiotics postoperatively, but recent research has called into question the utility of these extended regimens.[29,30] In reality, in the authors' experience, postoperative infection of pediatric mandibular fractures is extremely rare.

As mentioned previously, one of the cornerstones of successful treatment of pediatric patients with a condylar or subcondylar fracture is early functional rehabilitation. Early function minimizes the likelihood of temporomandibular joint ankylosis and allows the condyle to undergo the rapid remodeling that characterizes healing in pediatric populations. Patients should be encouraged to practice mouth-opening exercises as soon as possible after surgery. A useful exercise is to practice in front of a mirror so that the muscles can be trained to resist deviation on opening. With conscientious attention to rehabilitation, most patients regain unrestricted function.

Not to be overlooked, adequate nutrition and compliance with dietary restrictions are crucial for successful outcomes. For patients who have been treated by open reduction and internal fixation, as well as those undergoing functional treatment of condylar fractures, strict adherence to a soft diet for a period of 4 to 6 weeks will ensure adequate time for the fractures to heal before the mandible is placed under heavy masticatory loads. In addition, it is important to counsel patients and their guardians on the importance of adequate nutrition during the postoperative course. It is a well-established fact that a balanced diet provides the protein and glucose that the body needs to maximize wound healing.[31] Patients should be encouraged to maintain a balanced diet despite functional restrictions such as MMF. Frequently, this will include nutritional supplementation.

PEARLS AND PITFALLS

- Closed treatment is the preferred treatment of anterior mandibular fractures.
- Two alternative treatments to MMF alone are (1) construction of a lingual splint from dental models and (2) placement of MMF followed by open reduction and internal fixation of the fracture with the use of a miniplate placed at the very inferior border of the mandible.
- Open reduction is hardly ever indicated in the treatment of condylar fractures in children.
- Children with condylar injuries should be evaluated at regular intervals until the completion of mandibular growth.
- A modified Risdon cable in the primary and early mixed dentition is efficient in its application, provides excellent stability for elastic fixation, and does not require the additional placement of skeletal fixation.
- The most important concept to understand when treating pediatric mandibular trauma is that children are *not* simply small adults.
- Behavior management and caregiver education are incredibly important when treating pediatric patients.

REFERENCES

1. Posnick JC: The role of plate and screw fixation in the treatment of pediatric facial fractures. In Yaremchuk MJ, Gruss JS, Manson PN, editors: *Rigid fixation of the craniomaxillofacial skeleton*, Stoneham, MA, 1992, Butterworth-Heinemann, pp 396-419.
2. Posnick JC: Craniomaxillofacial fractures in children, *Oral Maxillofac Surg Clin North Am* 1:169-185, 1994.
3. Posnick JC: Management of facial fractures in children and adolescents, *Ann Plast Surg* 33:442-457, 1994.
4. Kaban LB: Diagnosis and treatment of fractures of the facial bones in children, *J Oral Maxillofac Surg* 51:722-779, 1993.
5. Imahara SD, Hopper RA, Wang J, et al: Patterns and outcomes of pediatric facial fractures in the United States: a survey of the National Trauma Data Bank, *J Am Coll Surg* 207:710-716, 2008.
6. Vandeven AM, Newton AW: Update on child abuse, sexual abuse, and prevention, *Curr Opin Pediatr* 18:201-205, 2006.
7. Becker DB, Needleman HL, Kotelchuck M: Child abuse and dentistry: orofacial trauma and its recognition by dentists, *J Am Dent Assoc* 97:24-28, 1978.
8. Chayra GA, Meador LR, Laskin DM: Comparison of panoramic and standard radiographs for the diagnosis of mandibular fractures, *J Oral Maxillofac Surg* 44:677-679, 1986.
9. Wilson IF, Lokeh A, Benjamin CI, et al: Prospective comparison of panoramic tomography (zonography) and helical computed tomography in the diagnosis and operative management of mandibular fractures, *Plast Reconstr Surg* 107:1369-1375, 2001.
10. Chacon GE, Dawson KH, Myall RW, et al: A comparative study of 2 imaging techniques for the diagnosis of condyle fractures in children, *J Oral Maxillofac Surg* 61:668-672, 2003.
11. Moss ML: The functional matrix hypothesis revisited, *Am J Orthod Dentofac Orthop* 112:8-11, 221-226, 338-342, 410-417, 1997.
12. Enlow DH, Hans MG: *Essentials of facial growth*, Philadelphia, 1996, WB Saunders.
13. Proffit WR, Fields HW: *Contemporary orthodontics*, ed 3, St Louis, 2000, CV Mosby.
14. Hosey MT, Duggal M, Welbury R, editors: *Paediatric dentistry*, ed 3, Oxford, 2005, Oxford University Press.
15. Hollinshead WH: *Anatomy for surgeons: the head and neck*, ed 3, Philadelphia, 1982, JB Lippincott.
16. Posnick JC, Wells M, Pron G: Pediatric facial fractures: evolving patterns of treatment, *J Oral Maxillofac Surg* 51:836-844, discussion 844-845, 1993.
17. Proffit WR, Vig KW, Turvey TA: Early fractures of the mandibular condyles: frequently an unsuspected cause of growth disturbances, *Am J Orthod* 78:1-24, 1980.
18. Walker RV: Traumatic mandibular condyle fracture dislocations, effect on growth in the *Macaca rhesus* monkey, *Am J Surg* 100:850-863, 1960.
19. Lindahl L: Condyle fractures of the mandible. IV. Function of the masticatory system, *Int J Oral Surg* 6:195-203, 1977.
20. Lund K: Mandibular growth and remodelling process after condyle fracture, a longitudinal roentgencephalometric study, *Acta Odontol Scand* 32(64):3-117, 1974.
21. Gilhuus-Moe O: Fractures of the mandibular condyle in the growth period, *Acta Odontol Scand* 29:53-63, 1971.
22. Thorén H, Hallikainen D, Iizuka T, et al: Condyle process fractures in children: a follow-up study of fractures with total dislocation of the condyle from the glenoid fossa, *J Oral Maxillofac Surg* 59:768-773, 2001.
23. Risdon F: The surgical treatment of facial injuries, *Can Med Assoc J* 38:(1):33-36, 1938.
24. Eppley BL: Use of resorbable plates and screws in pediatric facial fractures, *J Oral Maxillofac Surg* 63:385-391, 2005.
25. Bell RB, Kindsfater CS: The use of biodegradable plates and screws to stabilize facial fractures, *J Oral Maxillofac Surg* 64:31-39, 2006.
26. Turvey TA, Bell RB, Tejera TJ, et al: The use of self-reinforced biodegradable bone plates and screws in orthognathic surgery, *J Oral Maxillofac Surg* 60:59-65, 2002.
27. Bos RR: Treatment of pediatric facial fractures: the case for metallic fixation, *J Oral Maxillofac Surg* 63:382-384, 2005.
28. Heyden G: Relation between locally high concentration of chlorhexidine and staining as seen in the clinic, *J Periodont Res Suppl* 12:76-80, 1973.
29. Lovato C, Wagner JD: Infection rates following perioperative prophylactic antibiotics versus postoperative extended regimen prophylactic antibiotics in surgical management of mandibular fractures, *J Oral Maxillofac Surg* 67:827-832, 2009.
30. Miles BA, Potter JK, Ellis E 3rd: The efficacy of postoperative antibiotic regimens in the open treatment of mandibular fractures: a prospective randomized trial, *J Oral Maxillofac Surg* 64:576-582, 2006.
31. Guo S, Dipietro LA: Factors affecting wound healing, *J Dent Res* 89:219-229, 2010.

Chapter 97

Pediatric Mid-face Fractures

Clement Qaqish, John F. Caccamese, Jr.

It is universally agreed that maxillofacial trauma is rare in children. Several retrospective reviews have highlighted that the pediatric population accounts for 5% of all facial fractures, with a reported range in the literature of 1.5-15%.[1-8] Mid-facial fractures, in particular, make up an even smaller percentage of fractures, 0.2%-8%, depending on one's anatomic delineation of the middle third of the face.[1-8] It is postulated that the lower incidence of mid-facial injury is related to the anatomic protection of the face afforded by the prominent calvaria of children, as well as the incomplete development of the paranasal sinuses, the flexibility of their osseous suture lines, and their thicker facial adipose tissue.[1,4-6] In addition, it has been suggested that the lower incidence of mid-facial fractures might be the result of under-reporting or outright exclusion of certain injuries, such as dentoalveolar injury and isolated nasal bone fractures as part of the mid-face complex. Nasal and dentoalveolar injuries can often be treated in an outpatient setting and are therefore often presumably excluded from hospital logs. For the purposes of this text, we include in our discussion of fractures of the mid-facial skeleton the following: orbital floor, nasal and naso-orbito-ethmoid complex (NOE), zygomaticomaxillary complex, and Le Fort fractures.

Epidemiologic characterization of facial fractures in children began with the work of Rowe in the 1960s and continued with the work of Kaban and Posnick in the decades that followed.[1-4] Since that time, several authors in varied socioeconomic and geographic situations have broadened our understanding of this process, and some significant trends have emerged from their work and should be mentioned in the foregoing discussion of mid-facial injuries. With respect to pediatric facial trauma in general, children aged 6 to 12 years are most commonly afflicted, with males being more prone to injury than females.[1,2,3-13] Moreover, although there is no consistent etiologic front runner in the retrospective surveys examined, road traffic accidents (RTAs) and falls are among the major causes, depending on the setting of the study. Additionally, the majority of mid-face fractures require operative intervention.[1,2,3-13] Open reduction plus internal fixation appears to be advocated more and more by contemporary surgeons.[1-8] Several authors have expressed the need for accurate reduction and stable internal fixation for complex pediatric facial trauma. This management philosophy is based on the understanding that the secondary reconstruction of residual traumatic deformities can be difficult, as well as a better understanding of the impact of surgery on the growing facial skeleton.

DEVELOPMENTAL ANATOMY AND ITS SURGICAL CONSIDERATIONS

A thorough understanding of craniofacial development will not only aid in appreciating the epidemiologic data presented but also help guide the management of injuries in the pediatric population. During infancy and early childhood there is a significant increase in head circumference to accommodate brain growth. By the end of the sixth year of life, 90% of cranial growth has occurred, the sutures are well articulated, and orbital maturity is almost reached.[14] This provides the characteristic facial appearance in early childhood of a prominent forehead and orbits with a relatively underdeveloped (and protected) lower facial skeleton (Fig. 97-1). Palatal, premaxillary, and midline maxillary suture growth is complete, with obliteration of sutures by the age of 8 to 12.[2-5] The lower two thirds of the face exhibits downward and forward growth, which exposes the bones of the face to injury.[14] Eruption of deciduous teeth occurs in the first 2 years of life, and eruption of the permanent dentition is complete by the age of 12 to 13. Permanent tooth eruption accounts for much of the vertical growth of the lower two thirds of the face.[14] The primary- and mixed-dentition period, or the time between eruption sequences, poses a challenge in terms of pathogenesis and treatment modalities, specifically with respect to fracture patterns and fixation techniques, because of anatomic differences in primary tooth morphology and the presence of tooth buds in the facial skeleton. Permanent tooth buds in the maxilla and mandible create areas of structural weakness in the bone.[5] The presence of tooth buds limits the placement of certain plates and screws for fear of damaging the developing dentition. Furthermore, eruption of the permanent teeth and exfoliation of the primary teeth can also make maxillomandibular fixation (MMF) quite difficult.[9] On the other hand, ongoing growth and eruption of the permanent dentition can often compensate for minor inaccuracies in reduction and fixation. Other general anatomic differences between the adult and pediatric patient populations are that children have a thinner cortex and greater thickness of medullary bone, a higher cranial-to-facial ratio (8 : 1 in infants versus 2 : 1 in adults), more facial adipose tissue (the buccal and labial fat pads), more elastic bone (lending to greenstick fracture), and underdeveloped paranasal sinuses.[1,5,14]

AIRWAY ASSESSMENT AND PERIOPERATIVE MANAGEMENT

Thorough airway assessment of injured pediatric patients is critical, and this cannot be overemphasized in those with facial trauma. The advent of fiberoptic intubation has resulted in a significant decline in the use of tracheostomy for patients with craniofacial trauma, particularly mid-face trauma.[3,4] Additionally, the use of rigid internal fixation has helped expedite postoperative extubation by minimizing the use of MMF. Despite these advances, one must be cognizant of the smaller-caliber airway, shorter trachea, floppy epiglottis, and flaccid oral and pharyngeal soft tissues in younger children, all of which increase the rate of obstruction and airway resistance and thus make intubation more difficult.[1,3,5]

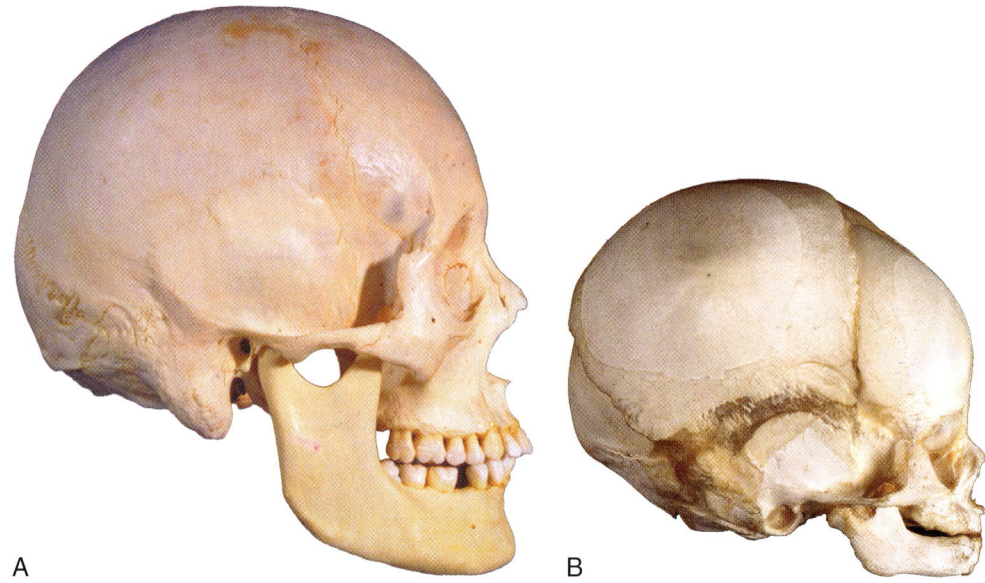

Fig. 97-1 ■ Note the difference in relative proportion of the facial skeleton between pediatric (**A**) and adult (**B**) skulls. (From Liebgott B: *The anatomical basis of disease*, ed 3, St. Louis, 2011, Mosby.)

Resuscitative efforts in children should center on maintaining the airway and avoiding bradycardia.[5] Hypercapnia (and the resultant hypoxemia) depress central nervous system and cardiac function. Because cardiac output is rate-dependent in pediatric patients, bradycardia can result in severe circulatory compromise and should be treated aggressively.[1,5] The lower total body volume in children must also be considered during initial management surveys. Hemorrhage from scalp lacerations and other injuries may lead to clinically significant hypotension and result in precipitous decompensation. It would also behoove the surgeon to have an awareness of associated injuries, particularly after high-velocity blunt trauma, such as those seen with RTAs. Posnick and co-authors reported that 33% of patients who suffered maxillofacial injuries had concurrent injuries to other anatomic sites/organ systems (head, 42%; extremities, 24%; eye, 22%; thorax, 10%; and abdomen, 2%).[4] Kaban reported concurrent injuries in 20% of patients[1,3]; however, the predominant mechanism of injury was not RTA, as in the sample of Posnick and colleagues.

DIAGNOSTIC METHODS

A thorough history and physical examination are critical in both determining a definitive diagnosis and guiding further diagnostic tests, namely, imaging. Determination of the cause, as well as the amount and direction of traumatic force, helps guide the diagnostic evaluation. Particular attention to and documentation of the child's mental status, visual examination, airway status, facial proportions, and occlusion are essential in arriving at a diagnosis. Often by the history and physical examination alone, the type and extent of maxillofacial injury can be characterized. Confirmation of the presence and severity of facial fractures is, however, imperative. Computed tomography (CT), when available, has largely replaced plain film radiography as the modality of choice for the evaluation of trauma patients, both pediatric and adult.[6] With the exception of perhaps panoramic radiographs for evaluation of mandibular fractures, CT is superior to conventional radiography in diagnostic accuracy, anatomic localization of fractures, and detection of occult or greenstick fractures, especially in the context of fractures among tooth buds. Coronal reformatted images are particularly useful in mid-facial

trauma for evaluating changes in facial volume and width, data essential in the evaluation of orbital fractures and NOE fractures. With the advent of multiplanar reformatting and three-dimensional (3D) rendering of CT image data, very precise depiction of anatomic details can be obtained, which will help guide accurate surgical reduction of fractures, as well as fixation. In response to the obvious disadvantage of CT (exposure to radiation), ultrasound (US) has emerged as a safe, inexpensive, and in certain anatomic regions, accurate alternative or adjunctive diagnostic modality.[15] In the depiction of orbitozygomatic complex fractures, US reportedly has a sensitivity and specificity similar to that of CT.[16] It should be noted, however, that edema and soft tissue emphysema both dramatically decrease the sensitivity of US, thus making its broad application less than ideal for a significant proportion of trauma patients.[6] Moreover, US should not be performed on open wounds.[6] That said, US is less widely established, and currently there are not enough data available to support its use as a primary method of diagnosis.

ORBITAL FLOOR FRACTURES

Whether seen in isolation or in association with complex facial trauma patterns, orbital floor fractures are rare in children. The frequency of such fractures does, however, increase with increased pneumatization of the maxillary sinuses.[5] Maxillary sinus development begins between the first and second trimesters, and growth continues until completion of pneumatization after puberty[14] (Fig. 97-2). The usual mechanism of orbital fractures is a direct blow to the eye transmitted through soft tissue down the thin bone of the orbital floor or medial wall. Findings on physical examination may include periorbital edema and ecchymosis, subconjunctival hemorrhage, enophthalmos, diplopia or restriction of ocular movement, and anesthesia or paresthesia along the distribution of the infraorbital nerve. All pertinent physical findings should be documented, and ophthalmologic consultation is suggested in most cases. Aside from actual injury to the globe (which occurs in up to 24% of orbital fractures),[1,3,5] entrapment of extraocular muscle and periorbital tissue is always a concern.[17] Forced duction tests can be difficult on an adult, let alone a pediatric patient, and sedation or even general anesthesia may be required to perform such tests if there is clinical

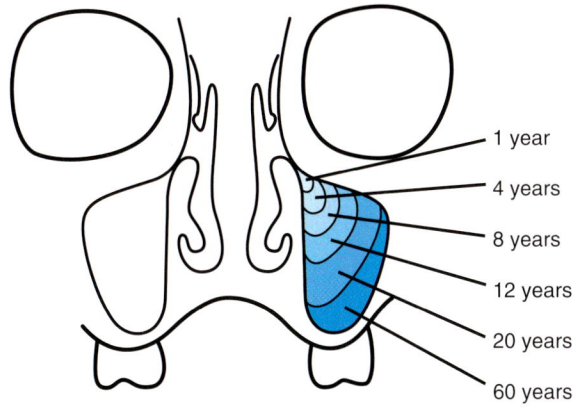

Fig. 97-2 ■ Note the progressive enlargement and pneumatization of the antrum over time. The maxillary sinuses reach maturity after puberty, but pneumatization continues into the alveolar process with age.

1 year
4 years
8 years
12 years
20 years
60 years

suspicion of entrapment. Other signs should alert the clinician to entrapment, including vagally mediated nausea and vomiting or sinus bradycardia, a phenomenon referred to as the oculocardiac or oculovagal reflex.[18]

Fine-cut, 1-mm CT slices with 3D reconstruction provide the most accurate anatomic assessment of the bony orbit.[6] Sagittal and coronal views enable accurate views of the orbital floor and sinus below and highlight changes in volume better than conventional radiography does.[6] Findings on CT may include blow-out or blow-in fractures of the orbit, soft tissue and muscle entrapment, and even retrobulbar hematoma. Retrobulbar hematoma can lead to acute orbital compartment syndrome—a treatable ocular emergency.[1,6] Clinical signs of concern are pain, diplopia, proptosis, loss of pupillary response, and progressive visual deficit. Surgical treatment consists of lateral canthotomy and inferior cantholysis. The diuretics acetazolamide and mannitol might be useful in medical management as well. Intraocular pressure should be monitored before and after treatment.

The most classic (though rare) orbital fracture seen in the pediatric population is the trapdoor fracture (Fig. 97-3). This is a greenstick fracture in which a bone fragment is displaced into the sinus but is attached by a hinge of bone and rebounds toward its premorbid position.[1,6,18,19] The hinge is usually located on the ethmoidal side of the orbital floor. If the fracture segment springs back into its normal anatomic position, any prolapsed orbital contents can become entrapped on the maxillary sinus side of the orbital floor. Of all orbit fractures, these might not exhibit overt signs of trauma, the so-called white-eyed blow-out. In either event, ocular muscle entrapment is an urgent matter that requires surgery as soon as possible to avoid ischemic necrosis of the entrapped muscle.[20] When entrapment has been ruled out, orbital floor repair of large defects can be delayed 7 to 10 days to allow resolution of edema.[6,21] Once ready for definitive treatment, the orbital floor can be approached in a number of ways; the retroseptal transconjunctival approach is advocated by the authors whenever the injury allows. This approach, when combined with lateral canthotomy or transcaruncular extension, provides access to nearly the entire orbital surface area. Exploration enables the surgeon to free entrapped tissue from under the trapdoor or through the continuity defect and either reduce it again or reconstruct it. Endoscopy has been reported as a means of evaluating and even treating orbital floor fractures as well. An endoscope is introduced through the maxillary sinus and the sinus is explored. The orbital floor is then approached and repaired via the anterior

maxillary antrostomy.[22] This enables treatment of the fracture without the esthetic concerns associated with other approaches. It also might afford a better approach to the posterior ledge. In cases of trapdoor fracture, once the orbital floor is reduced, no further treatment is indicated. This technique might be of limited value in some pediatric patients because of the limited size of the maxillary antrum or the position of unerupted teeth with respect to the planned antrostomy site.

NASAL FRACTURES

Apart from dentoalveolar fractures, nasal fractures are the most common pediatric facial fracture.[1-9] Their frequency is probably underestimated because many patients are discharged from emergency rooms and treated as outpatients in ambulatory surgical centers. Poor patient cooperation during physical examination makes a thorough history from the family essential. Questions concerning pre-injury symmetry and appearance may also be helpful, as are pre-injury photographs, if available. Clinical findings suggestive of a nasal fracture include epistaxis, edema, nasal and periorbital ecchymosis, skin or intranasal lacerations, and if the patient permits a speculum examination, the presence of septal ecchymosis, deviation, laceration, or hematoma. Palpable bony irregularities might not be appreciated secondary to edema and compliance with the examination. Moreover, comminution of the resilient nasal bones in a child is uncommon, so crepitus is not a typical finding on examination.[1,3] Intranasal evaluation is critical to rule out a septal hematoma, which would require emergency evacuation because of the risk for septal necrosis and resorption, which could eventually leave the child with a saddle nose deformity.[1,9] CT is a helpful modality to aid in diagnosis and management. If not appreciated clinically, a septal hematoma appears as a subperiosteal, hyperattenuated fluid collection that causes a thickening or bulge in the nasal septum.[6] Lateral blows to the nose result in medial displacement of the ipsilateral nasal bone and cause the contralateral bone to ride over the frontal process of the maxilla.[6] Frontal blows may cause collapse of the nasal bones inward or outward separation of the nasal bones at the midline, the so-called open-book fracture.

Treatment, almost invariably by closed reduction, should be performed within a week to prevent healing of misaligned bones (Fig. 97-4).[1,5] Although some authors believe that sedation with a local anesthetic is sufficient for the treatment of these fractures in older children,[1,3] the current authors advocate general anesthesia for the management of nasal fractures in all age groups to protect the airway from the possibility of posterior nasopharyngeal hemorrhage and improve compliance in this population for more accurate reduction. The nasal bones and septum are typically manipulated with Rowe, Walsham, or Asch forceps or a Boies elevator. Intranasal packing and a splint are used to stabilize the reduction. Closed reduction is obviously not as precise as open reduction, and consequently, revisions are occasionally required. Open reduction, through existing lacerations, enables direct visualization of the reduction and permits fixation (Fig. 97-5). Mustoe and co-authors reported that 3 of 30 treated patients required either revision septoplasty or esthetic rhinoplasty (or both) in the postoperative period for correction of the two most common complications: septal deviation or thickening and widening of the nasal dorsum.[23] None of the patients, however, exhibited signs of maxillary hypoplasia.[1,3-5] This is contrary to the contention of some authors that fracture of the nasomaxillary complex results in mid-facial growth disturbances.[24,25] When external or internal lacerations, or both, are present with comminuted nasal bones, the soft tissue envelope cannot be

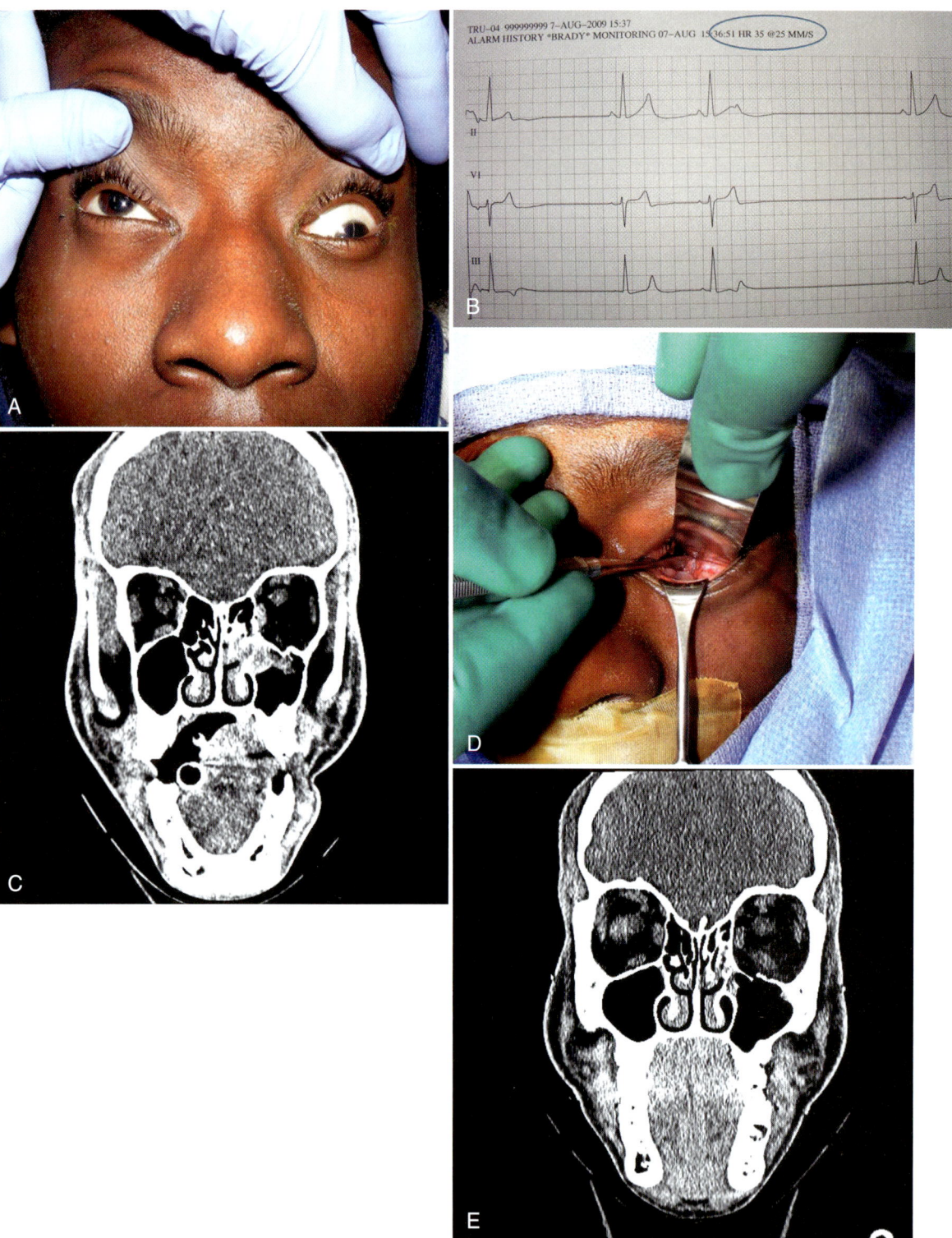

Fig. 97-3 ■ White-eyed orbital floor fracture in a 13-year-old boy after an assault with otherwise unexplained symptomatic bradycardia as a result of the oculocardiac reflex. **A,** Preoperative clinical examination. **B,** Rhythm strip showing bradycardia during the examination. Note the heart rate of 35 beats/min. **C,** Coronal computed tomography (CT) scan showing entrapped infraorbital tissue and absence of the inferior rectus muscle within the orbit. **D,** Intraoperative photograph demonstrating entrapped fibroadipose tissue and muscle. Notice the intact orbital floor and trapdoor fracture, in addition to the ischemic inferior rectus muscle. **E,** Postoperative coronal CT scan demonstrating the reduced inferior rectus muscle.

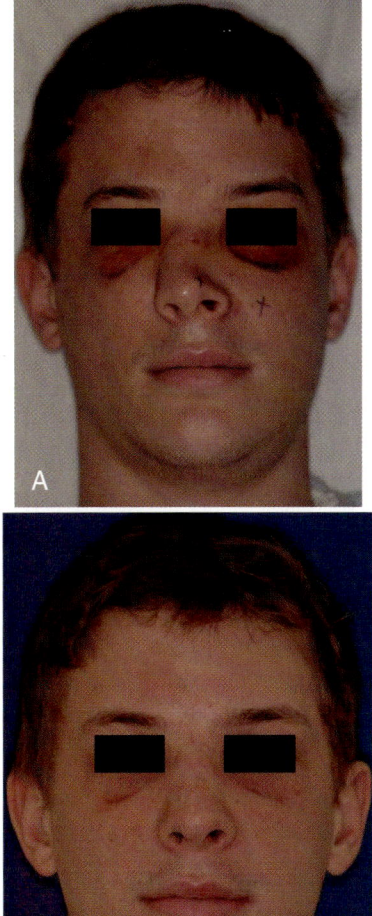

Fig. 97-4 ■ Preoperative (**A**) and postoperative (**B**) photographs of a nasal bone fracture treated by closed reduction.

counted on to support healing or bony union. In these rare cases, open reduction with internal fixation is advocated.

MAXILLARY FRACTURES

Le Fort fractures are quite rare in children and, when they do occur, are typically observed in combination with other complex facial fractures (5-10% of all facial fractures).[1-8] Under-reporting of these fractures may be attributable to the likelihood that the concomitant injuries sustained are often fatal.[1] Most of the few Le Fort fractures reported in published series are suffered in RTAs, usually high-velocity injuries and often with associated intracranial injury.

Physical examination might reveal any of the following: elongation of the middle third of the face, periorbital edema, ecchymosis, and traumatic telecanthus (particularly in comminuted Le Fort II and III fractures) (Fig. 97-6). If patient cooperation permits, intraoral examination may reveal malocclusion and mobility of the maxilla in either the transverse or anteroposterior dimension. Given the complexity of maxillary fractures and their frequent association with other complex injuries (not including maxillofacial injuries), CT with fine-cut 1-mm slices and 3D reconstruction is the imaging modality of choice for evaluation of these fractures.[6]

The developing dentition is often an obstacle to definitive treatment of Le Fort I fractures, which require stabilization of the

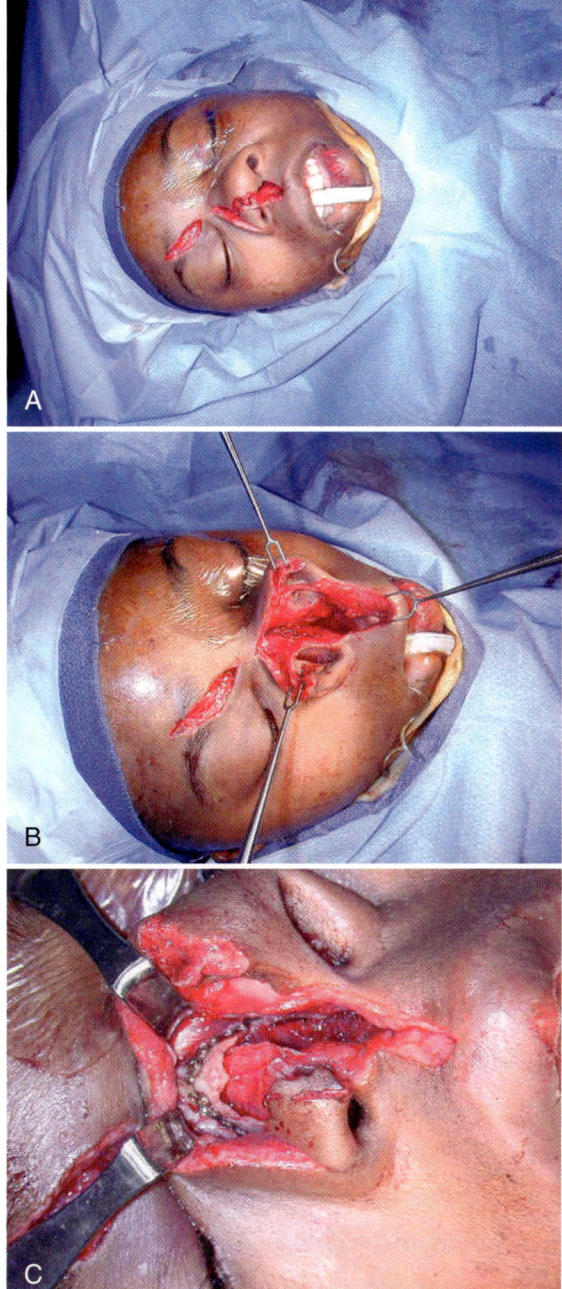

Fig. 97-5 ■ A laceration in the forehead and nasal dorsum provides direct access to the nasal bones for precise reduction and fixation. The soft tissue envelope in this case is insufficient to support closed reduction. **A,** Preoperative view. **B,** Intraoperative defect fully exposed. **C,** Reduction and monocortical fixation with plates and screws.

dentoalveolar complex. This can restrict the use of even monocortical fixation with plates and screws.[1,3-6,9] Additionally, placement of arch bars on patients in the mixed-dentition stage can be difficult. The healing capacity of younger patients makes extended periods of MMF unnecessary. In children younger than 12 years, therefore, these fractures can be treated with MMF. A number of methods have been described to accomplish this, including the use of stout wires or suspension wires from the zygomatic arches or piriform apertures to the mandibular symphysis.[1,9] Le Fort II and III fractures are treated by open reduction and internal fixation with the goal of anatomic reduction and reestablishment of functional

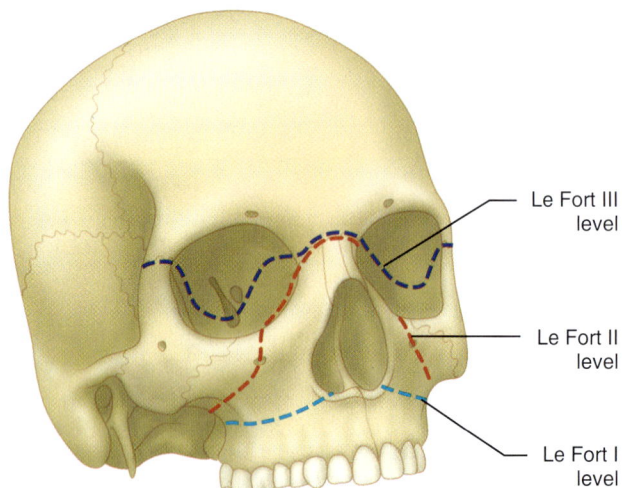

Fig. 97-6 ■ Le Fort fractures displayed as dotted lines. (From Bagheri SC, Jo C: *Clinical review of oral and maxillofacial surgery*, St. Louis, 2008, Mosby.)

occlusion. Access to Le Fort I fractures is achieved largely through a circumvestibular incision in the maxilla, whereas Le Fort II and III fractures are approached via a coronal incision and, if necessary, by approaches to the orbital rims previously mentioned. Reported complications of Le Fort fractures include disruption of the naso-lacrimal system and malocclusion.[1,3,9] Although some authors have reported that trauma to the nasomaxillary complex results in growth restriction and resultant mid-facial hypoplasia,[24,25] these findings are largely inconsistent with patients observed in the majority of published case series.[3-5,7-9]

FRACTURES OF THE ZYGOMATIC COMPLEX

For the purposes of this discussion, zygomatic complex fractures (ZCFs) include those involving the orbitozygomatic and zygomaticomaxillary complex, in addition to the zygomatic arch. ZCFs are common pediatric mid-facial fractures that represent up to 41% of all pediatric mid-facial fractures.[1,2,6] The frontozygomatic and zygomaticotemporal sutures are weak and particularly susceptible to disruption.[6] When a ZCF is suspected, the frontal, maxillary, and temporal processes of the zygoma must all be assessed. Additionally, complex orbitozygomatic fractures commonly involve the floor of the orbit. For this reason, careful ocular examination and mandatory ophthalmologic consultation are recommended. Physical examination might reveal many of the clinical findings seen with orbital floor fractures, including periorbital edema, ecchymosis, subconjunctival hemorrhage, restriction of gaze (with or without muscle entrapment), diplopia, enophthalmos, paresthesia over the distribution of the infraorbital nerve, an antimongoloid slant of the lateral canthus, and palpable step deformities along the suture lines. The cheek can also appear flat, and if the edema is minimal, there may be loss of anteroposterior facial projection. Trismus might also be a clinical finding, particularly in patients with depressed zygomatic arch fractures because of impingement of the arch on the coronoid process.

Clinically significant fractures are treated by open reduction and internal fixation. Moderately to severely displaced fractures are generally treated, whereas minimally or non-displaced fractures can be observed. Treatment should be carried out once the edema resolves and generally no later than 5 to 7 days after injury. Various surgical techniques are used to approach the zygomatic complex for appropriate mobilization, reduction, and fixation. Existing lacerations in the brow can be extended and used to approach fractures. Otherwise, the frontozygomatic suture is best approached via an upper eyelid or supra–tarsal fold incision not unlike that used for upper lid blepharoplasty or a lateral brow incision. Placement of a single monocortical plate for fixation is almost always sufficient at this site.[1,3] Reduction of the zygoma and fracture is easily confirmed at this site as well. Dissection along the medial aspect of the lateral orbital wall reveals the zygomaticosphenoid suture. Evaluation of this site is helpful in confirming appropriate 3D reduction of the zygoma. Approach to the infraorbital rim can be carried out via a subciliary or transconjunctival approach. Either technique provides adequate access to the rim and floor if exploration is warranted, although the transconjunctival approach typically yields better esthetic results. A transoral vestibular incision is used to access the zygomatic buttress of the maxilla. Awareness of the developing permanent maxillary dentition in this region is of value, particularly in children younger than 12 years, when planning plate and screw fixation. High-velocity injuries in which comminution of the zygomatic arch is seen in combination with a ZCF are best approached with a coronal incision in conjunction with the approaches described earlier.[1,3] Reduction of an isolated zygomatic arch fracture can be reasonably achieved with a Gillies approach to the arch. Most often, once the arch is reduced, fixation is unnecessary. However, in the postoperative period, care must be taken to protect the reduced arch from undue pressure, which can result in redisplacement of the fracture segments.

NASO-ORBITO-ETHMOID FRACTURES

Fractures involving the NOE complex are rare in the pediatric population (1-8%).[1-13] These fractures are difficult to treat and are the most potentially disfiguring of all the pediatric facial fractures. When they do occur, they are usually the result of high-velocity injuries such as those seen in RTAs. Given the nature of the insult, an associated head injury is frequently an accompanying finding. Disruption of the internal orbital walls, the ethmoids, the postero-medial canthal region, and the nasal bones is often seen. Physical examination frequently reveals signs of orbital trauma, in addition to telecanthus (Fig. 97-7), depending on the extent of the fracture. Manson's classification of NOE fractures is applicable to this population of patients. Large bone fragments that contain the insertion of the medial canthal ligament characterize type 1 NOE fractures. In type 2 fractures, the segments are smaller and more numerous but the canthal tendon can be found on one of the major fragments. Type 3 fractures are severely comminuted fractures with avulsion of the medial canthus.[26] Avulsion of the canthal tendon cannot usually be detected by imaging alone; definitive integrity of its insertion is generally determined by physical examination and intraoperative inspection. Surgical repair of these fractures is clearly complex and requires proper planning with the aid of accurate diagnostic imaging modalities. CT with 3D reconstruction is invaluable in delineating the degree of comminution of the NOE complex, particularly in and around the lacrimal fossa/medial canthus insertion. CT can also be useful in evaluating the patency of the nasofrontal ducts. Postoperative disruption of the nasofrontal ducts may result in the development of a mucocele in the frontal sinus. Therefore, patency must be verified before definitive reduction and fixation. Nasolacrimal duct and canalicular injury is also common with NOE complex fractures. Acute management might require nasolacrimal intubation with silicone tubes (Crawford tubes or their equivalent).[9] The tubes should be left in place for 3 to 6 months and the nose irrigated with nasal saline.

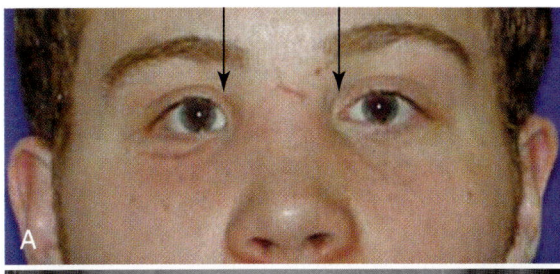

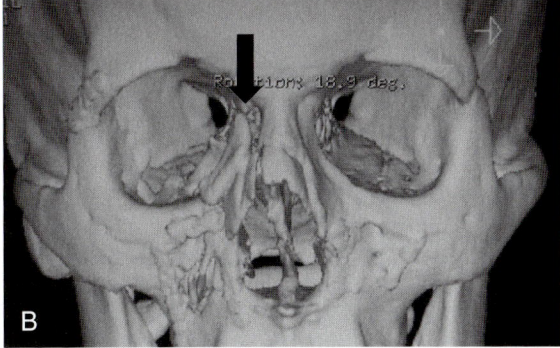

Fig. 97-7 ■ **A,** Postoperative clinical photograph demonstrating traumatic telecanthus in an untreated naso-orbito-ethmoid fracture. **B,** Computed tomography scan demonstrating the untreated fracture.

Chronic or late drainage problems will have to be treated with formal dacryocystorhinostomy.

Treatment is generally advocated within 4 days of injury. Open reduction with internal fixation is the rule. The NOE complex is best approached via the coronal route, with additional access to the orbital rims and floors, if necessary, provided by transconjunctival or subciliary approaches. Precise anatomic reduction is imperative, as is spatial positioning of the insertion of the medial canthal tendon. In cases of medial canthal disruption (type 3 injuries), medial canthopexy will be necessary. This involves resuspension of the insertion of the ligament in a position relatively posterior and superior to its original insertion.[9]

Given the approach to this part of the facial skeleton, some authors have advocated the use of resorbable hardware.[1,3] This mitigates the need for a second coronal flap to remove the plates and screws. Additionally, translocation of titanium implants, particularly in the region of the cranium, makes resorbable plates and screws a more attractive option. The main drawbacks of resorbable fixation in this area are the high plate profile relative to titanium microfixation and the risk for sterile abscess.

RESORBABLE VERSUS METALLIC HARDWARE FIXATION

At present, there is still clinical controversy over the method of fixation for pediatric facial fractures, regardless of anatomic location. Those who advocate the use of bioresorbable hardware argue that biodegradable osteosynthesis negates the need for a second surgery to remove the hardware.[1,27,28] Bioresorbable hardware will not interfere with future imaging interpretation if required.[27-29] Furthermore, growth of the patient and bony inclusion of hardware could be problematic, particularly in view of the drift phenomenon and displacement of intracranial hardware that have been reported.[1,27] The argument that retained hardware might restrict growth has not been clearly substantiated and is therefore less of a reason to opt for resorbable over metallic plate fixation. Those who argue the case for

metallic fixation systems stress that the mechanical properties of resorbable plates are still far inferior to those of titanium.[29] To achieve levels of strength comparable to that of metallic plates and screws, resorbable hardware must be fairly robust and as a consequence is easily palpable and sometimes visible.[29] Moreover, bioresorbable screws also have limited resistance to torsional force,[29] which makes compression of fracture segments difficult. In contrast, metallic screws allow more compression and therefore stability of the fracture segments. The ease of handling of metallic osteosynthesis systems in comparison to biodegradable systems has also been highlighted. Bending of biodegradable plates requires heating, and overheating can weaken the hardware. The subsequent placement of resorbable screws requires both pre-drilling and tapping.[29] Therefore, when compared with traditional metallic systems, fixation with biodegradable systems can be fairly time consuming and technique-sensitive. Unlike titanium plates and screws, the sterilization process with bioresorbable systems is also more elaborate, and most plating systems have a short shelf life.[30]

Clearly, if biodegradable osteosynthesis systems were equivalent, their use would be more widespread, not only in the pediatric population but also in select adult trauma and reconstructive patient cohorts. The reality is that resorbable systems fall short on design, in the context of meeting biomechanical demands, and in ease of use. Long-term follow-up studies to evaluate these plating systems may shed some light on their efficacy in comparison to conventional metallic systems. The development of new techniques and materials may ameliorate some of the shortcomings of current biodegradable systems and make their use more common.

REFERENCES

1. Baumann A, Kaban LB, Troulis MJ: Facial trauma 1: midface fractures. In Kaban LB, Troulis MJ, editors: *Pediatric oral and maxillofacial surgery*, Philadelphia, 2004, WB Saunders, pp 425-440.

2. Rowe NL: Fractures of the jaws of children, *J Oral Surg* 27:497-507, 1969.

3. Kaban LB: Diagnosis and treatment of fractures of the facial bones of children, *J Oral Maxillofac Surg* 51:722-729, 1993.

4. Posnick JC, Wells M, Pron GE: Pediatric facial fractures: evolving patterns of treatment, *J Oral Maxillofac Surg* 51:836-844, 1993.

5. Haug RH, Foss J: Maxillofacial injuries in the pediatric patient, *Oral Surg Oral Med Oral Pathol Oral Radiol* 90:126-134, 2000.

6. Alcalá-Galiano A, Arribas-García IJ, Martin-Pérez MA, et al: Pediatric facial fractures: children are not just small adults, *Radiographics* 28:441-461, quiz, 618, 2008.

7. Eggensperger Wymann NM, Hölzle A, Zachariou Z, et al: Pediatric craniofacial trauma, *J Oral Maxillofac Surg* 66:58-64, 2008.

8. Gassner R, Tuli T, Höchl O, et al: Craniomaxillofacial trauma in children: a review of 3385 cases with 6060 injuries in 10 years, *J Oral Maxillofac Surg* 62:399-407, 2004.

9. Tiwana PS, Kushner GM, Alpert B: Craniomaxillofacial injuries in children. In Marciani RD, Carlson ER, Braun TW, editors: *Oral and maxillofacial surgery*, vol 2, ed 2, Philadelphia, 2008, WB Saunders, pp 352-373.

10. Iida S, Matsuya T: Pediatric maxillofacial fractures: their etiologic characters and fracture patterns, *J Craniomaxillofac Surg* 2:237-241, 2002.

11. Iizuka T, Thóren H, Annino DR Jr, et al: Midfacial fractures in pediatric patients, *Arch Otolaryngol Head Neck Surg* 121:1366-1371, 1995.

12. Bartlett SP, DeLozier JB III: Controversies in the management of pediatric facial fractures, *Clin Plast Surg* 19:245-258, 1992.

13. Chapman VM, Fenton LX, Gao D, et al: Facial fractures in children: unique patterns of injury observed on computed tomography, *J Comput Assist Tomogr* 33:70-72, 2009.

14. Enlow DH: *Facial growth*, ed 3, Philadelphia, 1990, WB Saunders.

15. Freidrich RE, Heiland M, Bartel-Freidrich S: Potential of ultrasound in the diagnosis of midfacial fractures, *Clin Oral Investig* 7:226-229, 2003.

16. McCann PJ, Brockenbank LM, Ayoub AF: Assessment of zygomatico-orbital complex fractures using ultrasonography, *Br J Oral Maxillofac Surg* 38:525-529, 2000.

17. Chandler DB, Rubin PAD: Development in the understanding and management of pediatric orbital fracture, *Int Ophthalmol Clin* 41:87-104, 2001.

18. Sires BS, Stanley RB, Levine LM: Oculocardiac reflex caused by orbital floor trapdoor fracture: and indication for urgent repair, *Arch Ophthalmol* 116:955-956, 1998.

19. Soll DB, Polley BJ: Trapdoor variety of blowout fracture of orbital floor, *Am J Ophthalmol* 60:269-272, 1965.

20. Jordan DR, Allen LH, White J: Intervention within days for some orbital floor fractures: the white-eyed blowout, *Ophthal Plast Recontr Surg* 14:379-390, 1998.

21. Bansagi ZC, Meyer DR: Internal orbital fractures in pediatric age group, characterization and management, *Ophthalmology* 107:829-836, 2000.

22. Chen CT, Chen YR: Endoscopically assisted repair of orbital floor fractures, *Plast Reconstr Surg* 108:2011-2018, 2001.

23. Mustoe TA, Kaban LM, Mulliken JB: Nasal fractures in children, *Br J Plast Surg* 10:135-138, 1987.

24. Precious DS, Delaire JD, Hoffman CD: The effects of nasomaxillary injury on future facial growth, *Oral Surg Oral Med Oral Pathol* 66:525-530, 1988.

25. Ousterhout DK, Vargervik K: Maxillary hypoplasia secondary to midfacial trauma, *Plast Reconstr Surg* 80:491-497, 1987.

26. Leipziger LS, Manson PN: Naso-orbital ethmoid fractures: current concepts and management principles, *Clin Plast Surg* 11:167-193, 1992.

27. Eppley BL: Use of resorbable plates and screws in pediatric facial fractures, *J Oral Maxillofac Surg* 63:385-391, 2005.

28. Eppley BL: Nonmetallic fixation in traumatic midfacial fractures, *J Craniofac Surg* 8:103-109, 1997.

29. Bell RB, Kindsfater CS: The use of biodegradable plates and screws to stabilize facial fractures, *J Oral Maxillofac Surg* 64(1):31-39, 2006.

30. Bos RM: Treatment of pediatric facial fractures: the case for metallic fixation, *J Oral Maxillofac Surg* 63:382-384, 2005.

THE PAST

The diversity of temporomandibular disorders (TMDs) has plagued the profession in the past by engendering a variety of theories and procedures, none of which have completely elucidated the pathophysiology of this most unique joint and associated musculoskeletal apparatus. Historically, most TMDs were treated conservatively, with mixed results, and only in the 1970s and 1980s did the profession embark on routine surgical procedures to address pain, limited opening, joint noises, and even myofascial pain dysfunction. An extensive list of operations were used, including discectomy, condylar shaving, condylotomy, condylectomy, eminectomy, disc plication, arthroscopic lavage, arthrocentesis, flaps, grafts, joint prostheses, and disc replacements (including Proplast Teflon implants [Vitek, Inc., Houston], which resulted in devastating complications). The complications associated with procedures, misdiagnosis, and lack of understanding and the apparent improvement in symptoms with time of many TMDs with more conservative modalities, including minimal intervention, progressively restricted the criteria for surgical intervention during the latter 20 years.

THE PRESENT

Perhaps the most important advancement in this field is that we have "learned what we do not know." Current management of TMDs has progressed to more conservative interventions. Although there is no formal TMD subspecialty, several reputable surgical and non-surgical organizations or groups focus on the science of temporomandibular joint (TMJ) disorders. Surgical interventions continue to have many indications, though with more specific diagnostic criteria. Significant advances have been made in total TMJ reconstruction with custom-made alloplastic/titanium alloys, which are replacing the use of non-vascular (rib) grafting. Microvascular free (fibula) flaps are used routinely for TMJ and mandibular reconstruction after ablative tumor surgery. The pathophysiology of the TMDs has yet to be fully elucidated with regard to etiology, cellular anatomy, inflammatory mediators, and even gender discrepancies. There is a general deficiency of basic science research in our specialty that is also notable in this arena. The intricate and uncertain association of the muscles and occlusion with the TMDs continues to puzzle surgeons and clinicians.

THE FUTURE

Future management of TMDs will embrace the understanding of cellular biology, analysis of synovial fluid, and pathophysiology of the joint and surrounding structures. This will dictate and modify the modern surgical and conservative treatment strategies. The controversies regarding occlusion and the etiopathogenesis of TMJ pain will be elucidated. The technology of total joint reconstruction will improve in both material science and engineering to allow both translation and translocation of prosthetic TMJs. A practical disc replacement material will be identified, thereby reducing the need for local flaps and autogenous disc replacement grafts. In-office diagnosis of TMDs will be enhanced by readily available scanners that allow observation of the TMJ during function without invasive methods (unlike the arthrogram). Minimally invasive techniques will improve and further reduce the need for open joint procedures.

Diagnosis and Management of Temporomandibular Joint Pain and Masticatory Dysfunction

Chapter 98

Franklin M. Dolwick, Shelly Abramowicz, Shahrokh C. Bagheri

Management of patients with masticatory pain and dysfunction is one of the most challenging problems confronting oral and maxillofacial surgeons. The problem exists because of the diverse collection of conditions affecting the masticatory system that have similar symptoms and signs of pain or dysfunction, or both. Several diagnostic classification systems are used but are often non-specific and confusing. Selection of the appropriate treatment protocol is controversial, with treatment decisions being based on one's philosophy of the cause of the condition. Frequently, the approach to diagnosis and treatment of a patient with masticatory pain and dysfunction is more complicated than necessary. Although the pathophysiology of masticatory pain and dysfunction is complex and poorly understood, the approach to most patients should be relatively simple.

The senior author has divided patients with masticatory pain and dysfunction into two general categories, muscular conditions and temporomandibular joint (TMJ) disorders. At the most basic level the surgeon must decide whether the pain or dysfunction, or both, are arising from masticatory muscles or the TMJ. TMJ surgery is not recommended for muscle disorders because it will not decrease the pain and dysfunction and will most likely make them worse. Only patients with pain and dysfunction arising within the TMJ are candidates for TMJ surgery.

BOX 98-1	**Diagnostic Classification of Masticatory Pain and Dysfunction Conditions**

A. Masticatory muscle disorders
   1. Myofascial pain and dysfunction
     a. Nocturnal bruxism
     b. Habitual daytime parafunction
       i. Clenching
       ii. Postural
     c. Trauma—whiplash
   2. Myositis, myospasm, etc.
   3. Neoplasias
B. Temporomandibular joint disorders
   1. Disc derangement disorders (internal derangement)
     a. Anchored disc phenomenon
     b. Disc displacement with reduction
     c. Disc displacement without reduction
     d. Disc perforation
   2. Osteoarthritis (non-inflammatory disorders)
   3. Inflammatory disorders
     a. Capsulitis/synovitis
     b. Polyarthritides
       i. Rheumatoid arthritis
       ii. Juvenile rheumatoid arthritis
       iii. Psoriatic arthritis
       iv. Others
   4. Hypermobility disorders
     a. Subluxation

     b. Dislocation
       i. Acute
       ii. Chronic recurrent
       iii. Chronic
   5. Hypomobility disorders
     a. Extra-articular (pseudo)
     b. Intra-articular (true)
       i. Fibrous
       ii. Osseous
       iii. Combination of fibrous and osseous
   6. Traumatic injuries
     a. Soft tissues
     b. Fractures
       i. Intracapsular
       ii. Extracapsular
   7. Congenital or developmental disorders
     a. Aplasias
     b. Hypoplasias
     c. Hyperplasias
   8. Unusual diseases and disorders
     a. Benign
     b. Malignant
       i. Primary
       ii. Metastatic

The purpose of this chapter is to present a simple practical approach to the diagnosis and management of patients with masticatory pain and dysfunction. Emphasis will be placed on identification of patients who will benefit from surgical intervention and selection of the surgical procedure that will provide the greatest benefit for the patient's specific problem with the least risk for complications.

CLASSIFICATION

Several classifications of conditions associated with masticatory pain and dysfunction have been proposed. Some are based on symptoms and signs, some on disease categories, and others on research criteria. The senior author has used a simple diagnostic classification system that should include most conditions (Box 98-1).

Despite differences in opinion about which operation to perform, there are a group of disorders for which the role of surgery is not disputed, including all of the TMJ disorders except for the disc derangement and arthritic disorders. This chapter focuses on the diagnosis and management of patients with most common masticatory pain and dysfunction disorders who have either masticatory muscle or disc derangement disorders. For the purposes of this chapter, disc derangement disorders and osteoarthritis will be discussed together because they are commonly found together. However, they can certainly occur as distinct disorders.

DIAGNOSIS

At the most basic level, the surgeon must decide whether a patient with masticatory pain and dysfunction has a muscular, joint, or combination of a muscular and joint problem. It is assumed that non-masticatory system causes of the pain have been eliminated. The diagnosis is based on a thorough history, clinical examination, and laboratory and imaging studies.

The history may be the most important part of the evaluation. It should include the chief complaint and a detailed history of the present illness. The clinical examination should be a systematic evaluation of the TMJs for tenderness, joint noise, range of motion with and without pain, and pain on loading. The muscles of mastication and the cervical muscles should be palpated and areas of tenderness noted. Finally, the teeth and occlusion should be assessed. A thorough evaluation of the soft tissues of the oral cavity should also be done. Routine imaging such as a panographic x-ray should be obtained to evaluate the osseous structures of the teeth, their supporting structures, and the TMJs. The need for more advanced imaging or laboratory studies is determined from findings on the preliminary evaluations.

MUSCULAR PAIN AND DYSFUNCTION

The concept of myofascial pain and dysfunction (MPD) was introduced by Laskin in the 1960s. It refers to a group of muscle disorders characterized by diffuse facial pain and limited mouth opening. It can involve problems with the TMJ, muscles of the face, and associated head and neck structures. Frequently, when patients have non-specific signs and symptoms of facial pain of unknown etiology, they are wrongly labeled as having a TMJ problem. In the authors' experience, the majority of patients seen by surgeons with complaints of facial pain and dysfunction have muscular problems.

Recent advances in the understanding of muscular pain and dysfunction have supported the theory that the cause of MPD is often multifactorial. Biologic, behavioral, environmental, social, emotional, and cognitive factors contribute to the development of signs and symptoms. More specifically, there are various predisposing risk factors, such as female gender, anxiety and depression, and a stressful lifestyle. There are multiple perpetuating factors, including acute jaw trauma, sudden changes in occlusion, and excessive jaw activity. Secondary gain such as sympathy or avoidance of an unpleasant activity such as work may also perpetuate the symptoms. The significance of large skeletal discrepancies such as open-bite malocclusion, overjet greater than 6 mm, and missing posterior teeth is unclear, but such discrepancies may predispose patients to MPD.

Although many factors contribute to MPD, the single most commonly identifiable cause is a parafunctional habit such as tooth clenching or grinding, which often occurs secondary to stress and anxiety. In fact, more than 68% of patients treated for MPD report that they clench their teeth. Importantly, bruxism can overload the TMJ and contribute to the development of, perpetuate, and maintain TMJ disc derangements.

Patients with masticatory muscle pain and dysfunction have diffuse, poorly localized pain that is frequently, but not always worse in the morning. Patients generally report sleep disturbances and believe that the pain disrupts their sleep. As noted, more than 68% of patients report that they grind or clench their teeth. They may complain of sore teeth and frequently complain of jaw tiredness and fatigue when eating. They often complain of limited and painful mouth opening. Patients with MPD may also complain of headaches, earaches, and cervical pain. The findings on physical examination are diffuse tenderness to palpation of the masticatory and cervical muscles, especially along the temporalis insertion. The TMJs are either non-tender or minimally tender to palpation, and there is no pain in the TMJ on loading. Mandibular opening may be limited to 30+ mm, and patients will frequently hesitate (guard) during opening, but they can usually be encouraged to open wider. The intraoral examination helps eliminate dental causes as a source of the pain. The number and condition of the teeth, including occlusal wear facets, sore teeth, craze lines, and mobility, are documented. Such findings are an indication that patients are grinding their teeth, although absence of these signs does not eliminate bruxism. Findings on routine radiographic examination are frequently normal, but occasional abnormalities may be observed. The surgeon must remember that patients with severe TMJ signs may occasionally also have MPD as a perpetuating factor.

Because more than 80% of patients with MPD respond favorably to non-surgical interventions, all factors should be addressed with a focus on non-invasive methods that are reversible. The first step should include a thorough explanation of the findings. The patient should be educated and reassured that the pain usually resolves with simple treatment and that a more serious condition does not exist. The patient should be prescribed a home care program that includes jaw rest, a soft diet, limitation of wide mouth opening, and application of warm moist heat. After a period of jaw rest, muscle massage and physical therapy, including stretching and strengthening exercises, should be encouraged. The physical therapy program should be kept simple with exercises consisting of opening and closing the mouth, protrusion, and right and left lateral excursion of the mandible.

Most patients will benefit from an occlusal appliance, especially if they grind their teeth. The appliance should be a simple flat-plane splint that covers all the teeth, and all the teeth should touch the splint evenly in centric occlusion and in a centric relationship. The splint should have a shallow anterior guidance that separates the teeth during excursive movements. The idea is not to reposition the mandible, but to allow the muscles to rest and to decrease TMJ loading. The splint also protects the occlusal surfaces of the teeth from damage during bruxism. It should generally be worn only at night. Frequent adjustments may be necessary, especially when first given to the patient.

Medical therapy should include a non-narcotic analgesic such as a non-steroidal anti-inflammatory medication and, if sleep disturbances exist, a sleep medication such as a low-dose tricyclic antidepressant. Some tricyclic antidepressants have analgesic properties independent of their antidepressant effect and may be useful for patients who have both pain and sleep disturbances. In our experience, cyclobenzaprine has similar benefits. The combination of non-steroidal anti-inflammatory drugs and a low-dose tricyclic antidepressant appears to be most beneficial. Patients who have significant behavioral problems, stress, anxiety, or depression will benefit from psychological evaluation and treatment.

It is important to recognize that the patient's signs and symptoms will resolve slowly over a period of weeks to months and that they will frequently recur. However, most patients with MPD will improve with conservative treatment. It is also important to encourage patients that they will improve and that severe problems rarely occur. If the patient is not improving, re-evaluation should be undertaken to determine whether the diagnosis and treatment are appropriate. TMJ surgery is not recommended for patients with MPD even if the signs and symptoms are severe and persistent. TMJ surgery will not resolve and will usually make it worse.

RELATIONSHIP OF BRUXISM TO INTERNAL DERANGEMENT

Grinding and clenching of the teeth have been shown to adversely load the TMJ. This is especially true of clenching, which causes continued compressive loading of the TMJ tissues. Excessive loading of the joint causes damage to the joint tissues through mechanical, biochemical, and hypoxia-reperfusion mechanisms. In hypoxia-reperfusion injury, the soft tissues become temporarily hypoxic because of excessive loading of the soft tissues, and as reperfusion occurs, free radicals, which are thought to break down hyaluronic acid, are produced. This leads to a failure of the joint lubrication system and results in microscopic changes in articular cartilage, disc stickiness, disc displacement, and eventually degeneration of the articular surfaces of the TMJ.

Though not proven, there is considerable evidence to support this hypothesis. Because MPD may be a significant cause of internal derangement, they are frequently found together. The occurrence of MPD and internal derangement together results in difficulty diagnosing the patient's condition. It is our opinion that failure to recognize this relationship, as well as failure to manage MPD before TMJ surgery for internal derangement, is the primary reason for surgical failure. When MPD is present, it must be managed appropriately if surgical success is to be achieved.

INTERNAL DERANGEMENT

Internal derangement of the TMJ was reintroduced into the literature in the 1970s by Farrar and McCarty. During the 1970s and 1980s it gained wide popularity as the cause of TMJ pain and dysfunction. The primary clinical focus was on TMJ disc displacement and deformity as the cause of TMJ pain and dysfunction, which eventually led to TMJ osteoarthritis. The introduction of TMJ arthroscopy and the recognition that simple lysis and lavage of the upper joint space of the TMJ frequently resulted in decreased pain and improved range of motion led to re-evaluation of the significance of disc position. At the present time, internal derangement is thought to be a dynamic process involving biomechanical, biochemical, and cellular changes, including disc displacement and deformity, synovitis and changes in synovial fluid, degenerative changes in the articular surface, and fibrosis. The shift in thinking from a predominantly mechanical focus to a biologic focus has resulted in a significant change in surgical treatment from mainly open surgery to arthrocentesis and arthroscopy.

Patients with internal derangement have well-localized TMJ pain that is continuous and becomes worse with mandibular functions such as chewing and talking. They report that their TMJ either makes noise (i.e., clicking or crepitus) or previously made noise but no longer does. Patients usually complain that their jaw either does not open smoothly or is limited in its opening. Patients frequently complain of catching or locking sensations. Many patients report that their jaw is locked closed. Clearly, the focus of the patient's complaints is well localized to the TMJ.

Physical examination demonstrates pain and dysfunction that are well localized to the TMJ. The affected TMJ is tender to palpation, and TMJ pain is reported when the joint is loaded. There is interference with smooth joint movement in the form of deviation associated with TMJ clicking or limited opening with pain. Excursive movements are limited toward the unaffected side and usually cause increased pain in the affected joint.

A preliminary diagnosis of internal derangement can generally be made from the clinical examination. Definitive diagnosis and clinical staging of the disc derangement require magnetic resonance imaging (MRI). Based on the clinical findings and MRI, the disc derangement should be classified according to the Wilkes classification system. Classification of the internal derangement is especially important for reporting outcomes of clinical treatment.

MRI of the TMJ is necessary to evaluate the position and shape of the articular disc and to confirm the diagnosis of internal derangement before open TMJ surgery (Fig. 98-1). The absolute indications for MRI are not specific, other than before open TMJ surgery when the diagnosis has not been confirmed by other imaging. MRI does provide valuable information about disc shape that cannot be obtained by other means. MRI also provides information about the presence of joint effusion, marrow edema, and the integrity of the articular surfaces. It is the imaging technique of choice for evaluating the soft tissues of the TMJ. The correlation of TMJ pain with MRI findings is poor, so the diagnosis must always be made from a comparison of the clinical history, physical examination, and findings on MRI. The diagnosis should never be based solely on MRI.

Most patients with pain and dysfunction caused by internal derangement will experience resolution of their symptoms with nonsurgical treatment. In fact, in many patients the symptoms resolve without treatment. Therefore, it is prudent to treat patients with nonsurgical therapies before surgical options are considered.

Non-surgical treatment of TMJ internal derangement is similar to that for MPD. The objectives of treatment are to reduce pain, eliminate inflammation from the joint, eliminate or reduce adverse TMJ loading, and restore TMJ mobility.

The first step in treatment is to educate the patient about internal derangement of the TMJ. The patient should be reassured that the pain and dysfunction usually resolves with simple treatment and that a more serious condition rarely develops. The patient should be provided with a home care program that includes jaw rest, a soft diet, and limitation of jaw opening. Medical therapy should include a non-steroidal anti-inflammatory analgesic. As the pain begins to resolve, simple range-of-motion exercises should be started. These exercises include gentle unforced mandibular opening and excursive movements.

Since bruxism may be an important cause of internal derangement, many patients will require the treatment protocol for MPD; specifically, an occlusal appliance and sleep medications should be provided. The occlusal appliance should be a flat-plane appliance and not a jaw-repositioning device. The objective of treatment with an appliance is to rest the muscles of mastication and reduce adverse loading of the TMJ.

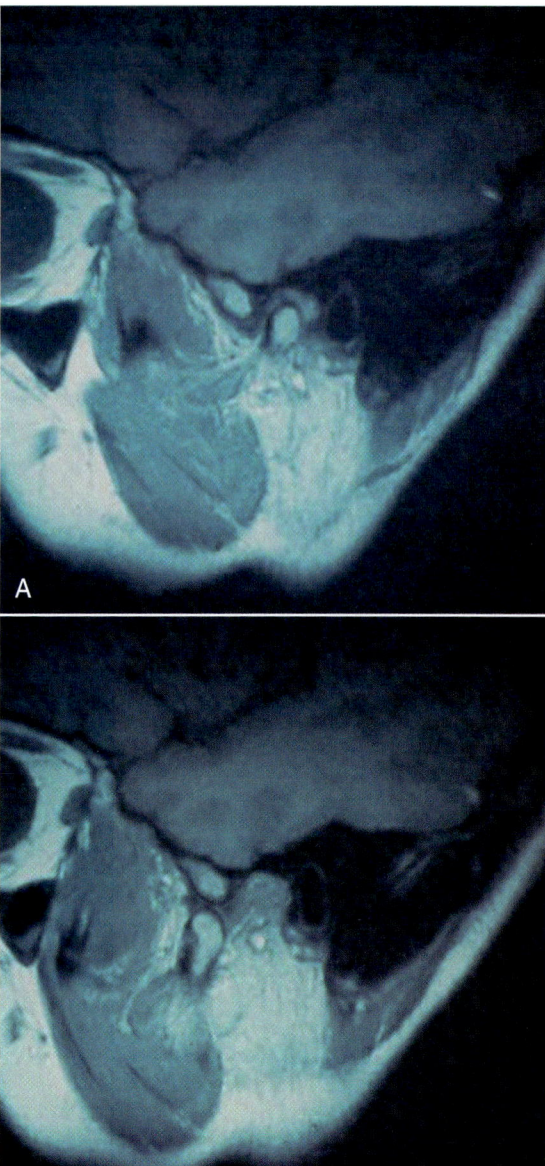

Fig. 98-1 ■ **A,** T1-weighted magnetic resonance image (MRI) in the closed-mouth position showing anterior disc displacement. **B,** T1-weighted MRI in the open-mouth position showing recapture or reduction of the disc.

Most patients will have a decrease in symptoms in about 4 to 6 weeks. Patients who continue to have significant TMJ pain and dysfunction should be re-evaluated for surgical treatment.

SURGICAL TREATMENT

Controversy continues to surround the role of surgery in the management of TMJ pain and dysfunction. Nonetheless, advances have been made with the introduction of new and less invasive techniques such as arthrocentesis and arthroscopy. The role of surgery has evolved since the idea of internal derangement gathered momentum during the 1970s. During this time, renewed interest was focused on the importance of disc displacement and deformity as the cause of TMJ pain and dysfunction. Open joint procedures were developed to reposition and reshape the displaced or deformed disc. Though at first thought to be highly successful, the long-term results proved to be less successful. The success of simpler procedures such as lavage and lysis by arthrocentesis or arthroscopy has raised serious doubts about the pathologic significance of disc position as the cause of TMJ pain and dysfunction. Evidence is accumulating that inflammation of the synovium, changes in synovial fluid, and microscopic changes in the articular surfaces are more significant in causing the pain and dysfunction and may be a cause of the disc displacement.

The successful application of less invasive procedures has established the surgeon's role in the management of TMJ pain and dysfunction. With the increased surgical options available to present-day surgeons, it seems prudent that selection of the surgical procedure with the highest probability of success and the least morbidity should be the objective. Since the likelihood of successful management is determined by the accuracy of the diagnosis, the most important ingredient for success is case selection.

INDICATIONS FOR TEMPOROMANDIBULAR JOINT SURGERY

The indications for TMJ surgery have been consistent for many years, and the criteria are clearly defined:

1. The TMJ is the source of pain or dysfunction that results in significant impairment in daily activities.
2. Non-surgical treatment fails to resolve the problem.
3. A TMJ intracapsular pathologic condition or anatomic derangement is documented that may be a major source of the patient's pain or dysfunction.

Although the indications for surgery may appear clear, they are in fact non-specific. The first criterion, significant pain or dysfunction localized to the TMJ, may be the most important. If the pain or dysfunction is originating within the TMJ, surgical intervention will probably be successful. However, if it is not originally within the joint, not only will surgical intervention be unsuccessful, but the patient's pain or dysfunction may also become worse. Therefore, it is prudent that the surgeon make an accurate diagnosis.

At the most elementary level the surgeon must decide whether the source of the patient's pain and dysfunction is muscle, joint, or a combination of muscle and joint. Unfortunately, the latter seems to be most common. The surgeon must then determine that the muscular pain is manageable with non-surgical treatment before proceeding with surgical intervention. The principal criteria for determining that the pain originates in the TMJ are pain localized to the joint, pain on loading the joint, increased pain during function, pain that is least in the morning and worst in the evening, and evidence of mechanical problems within the joint. It seems clear that the more localized the pain and dysfunction are to the TMJ, the more likely intervention involving the joint will be successful. Conversely, the more diffuse the pain, the less likely that surgical intervention will be successful.

The second criterion, refractory to non-surgical treatment, is also non-specific. There is no clear agreement on a protocol for conservative or non-surgical treatment. However, most surgeons understand what non-surgical treatment involves. It typically includes a combination of patient education, medications, physical therapy, an occlusal appliance, and occasionally behavioral modifications. Because most patients will respond successfully to these treatments or sometimes improve over time without treatment, surgical consideration should be reserved for patients who fail to respond successfully over a reasonable period. Again, it must be emphasized that only patients whose pain and dysfunction are arising from within the TMJ are surgical candidates. Patients whose pain is arising from the muscles of mastication or other non-TMJ sources are not surgical candidates even if their pain and dysfunction are refractory to treatment.

The third criterion, documentation of an intracapsular TMJ pathologic condition or anatomic derangement, generally requires TMJ imaging. The correlation of pain with imaging findings such as disc derangement, dysfunction, and degeneration is poor. Therefore, imaging should be used only to confirm and support the clinical findings. Surgery should not be performed on the basis of imaging alone.

Surgical interventions include arthrocentesis, arthroscopy, condylotomy, and open joint procedures. Randomized clinical trials comparing these procedures do not exist, so the surgeon's experience usually determines the procedure selected. Each procedure has specific benefits, as well as risks. Therefore, the procedure with highest potential for success, the lowest risk, and the most cost-effectiveness should be chosen for the patient's specific condition.

TEMPOROMANDIBULAR JOINT ARTHROCENTESIS

Though included among the surgical procedures, arthrocentesis in reality is a non-surgical procedure. Despite being invasive, the risk for injury to the overlying soft tissues and the joint structures is negligible. Arthrocentesis is the least invasive of the surgical techniques. The concept was based on the observation that simple lysis and lavage of the upper joint space via arthroscopy was highly successful in re-establishing normal range of mouth opening in patients with closed lock of their TMJ.

The technique involves the insertion of two 18-gauge needles into the superior joint space of the TMJ. The procedure is usually performed with intravenous conscious sedation and local anesthesia but can be performed with local anesthesia only. The patient is seated inclined at a 45-degree angle with the head turned to the opposite side to provide an easy approach to the affected joint. After preparation of the preauricular area, the external auditory meatus is blocked with cotton. A line is drawn from the middle of the tragus to the lateral canthus. The posterior needle is inserted along the canthotragal line, 10 mm from the middle of the tragus and 2 mm below the line. Palpation of the glenoid fossa during movement of the condyle confirms the location. After injecting a local anesthetic, the posterior needle is placed by directing it at a 45-degree angle from posterior to anterior and from inferior to superior. The needle is directed toward the middle of the glenoid fossa. Once the lateral aspect of the glenoid fossa is felt, the needle is directed more horizontally and advanced into the middle of the upper joint space. The upper joint space is distended with approximately 2 mL of Ringer solution. Confirmation of placement of the needle into the upper joint space is made by observing the mandible's movement during injection or by backflow into the syringe when pressure is released. The anterior needle is inserted approximately 5 to 10 mm below the canthotragal line. Confirmation of correct placement is made by observing outflow from the posterior needle. Slight adjustment of the needles may need to be made if the outflow is sluggish. The upper joint space is then irrigated with 100 to 300 mL of Ringer solution. The outflow is intermittently occluded during the irrigation to distend the joint space. After completion of the irrigation, medication (steroid or hyaluronic acid) may be placed in the upper joint space. Once the procedure is completed, the mandible is moved through opening, excursive, and protrusive movements. The range of motion and presence of any mechanical interference to movement are noted.

After the procedure the patient is given a mild analgesic and instructed to perform range-of-motion exercises. This is continued for about a week.

Temporary facial nerve weakness or paralysis as a result of the local anesthetic may occur during arthrocentesis. This is transient and disappears in about 30 to 60 minutes. For this reason a short-acting local anesthetic should be used. Other transient complications include preauricular swelling from either extravasation of fluid or hematoma and occlusal changes from distention of the upper joint space. These complications are temporary and generally resolve within 24 hours.

Studies of the outcome of arthrocentesis for painful limited opening have shown consistently improved mouth opening and decreased pain. In groups of patients with disc displacement resistant to conservative treatment, the results of arthrocentesis were not significantly different from those seen with arthroscopic lysis and lavage in decreasing pain and improving mouth opening. Arthrocentesis may also be beneficial in treating any condition involving inflammation in the upper joint space of the TMJ. Since arthrocentesis is a simple outpatient procedure that has no significant complications associated with it and is cost-effective, it is probably the first surgical procedure that should be used in patients with TMJ pain and dysfunction.

The mode of action of arthrocentesis is not known. Its benefit is probably derived from several factors, such as breaking up the stickiness of the disc and fine adhesions by distending the joint and removing inflammatory products from the joint.

TEMPOROMANDIBULAR JOINT ARTHROSCOPY

TMJ arthroscopy developed as a spinoff from the technologic advances made by orthopedic surgeons in arthroscopy of large joints. Miniaturization of the arthroscopic telescope made it possible to apply this technology to the TMJ. TMJ arthroscopy was first introduced into the literature in 1975, but it was not until almost a decade later that the concept of TMJ arthroscopy became popular. Intense interest in TMJ arthroscopy developed in the early 1980s, and it is now widely used.

Arthroscopy is very much an equipment-dependent procedure that relies considerably on complex technology. Despite the minimally invasive nature of arthroscopy, until recently it has been commonly performed under general anesthesia in the operating room. It takes a fair degree of skill and ability to conceptualize a three-dimensional space on a two-dimensional screen image, as well as a high degree of manual dexterity, particularly for operative procedures.

TMJ arthroscopy involves placing an arthroscopic telescope (1.8 to 2.6 mm in diameter) in the upper joint space of the TMJ and then attaching a camera to the arthroscope to project the image onto a television monitor. A second access instrument is placed approximately 10 to 15 mm in front of the arthroscope. This access point provides an outflow portal for irrigation and access for inserting instrumentation into the joint space. The upper joint space is examined systematically starting posteriorly by identifying the posterior attachment tissue. The synovial lining is inspected for the presence of inflammation, such as increased capillary hyperemia. The junction of the posterior band of the disc and posterior attachment tissues can be identified. Movement of the joint allows the identification of clicking or restricted movement of the disc. The articular cartilage of the fossa and eminence can be inspected for degenerative changes such as softness, fibrillation, or tears as the arthroscope is moved through the joint space. The joint space can also be evaluated for the presence of adhesions, loose bodies, or other pathology. The

integrity of the disc and posterior attachment or perforations of the tissue can be identified.

The final step is to move the arthroscope into the anterior part of the upper joint space. Frequently, inflammation and adhesions can be observed in this location. Lysis of adhesions is accomplished by sweeping either the arthroscope or the irrigation cannula through the adhesions and tearing them. After completion of the examination, the joint space is thoroughly irrigated to remove debris, blood clots, and inflammatory products. Before removing the instruments, medications such as steroids may be injected either into the joint space or directly into inflamed tissues.

Sophisticated operative techniques ranging from ablation of adhesions with lasers to plication of the disc with sutures or anchor devices have been developed. These techniques require considerable technical skill, and consequently, only a few surgeons use these advanced techniques.

TMJ arthroscopy is performed as an outpatient procedure, and the patient is discharged after recovery from anesthesia. A pressure dressing is usually placed for 12 to 24 hours postoperatively. Postoperative care includes a non-chewing soft diet for a few days, range-of-motion exercises for several days, an occlusal appliance, and analgesics as necessary for pain control.

Multiple studies have reported 80-90% success rates with arthroscopic lysis and lavage for the management of patients with painful limited mouth opening. The majority of patients have decreased pain and improved mouth opening. Murkami and colleagues have shown in 5- and 10-year follow-up that arthroscopic lysis plus lavage is successful for all stages of internal derangement, and the results are comparable to those reported with open surgery. Data from advanced surgical arthroscopic techniques such as disc repositioning are difficult to interpret, and it is unclear whether the outcomes are better than those achieved with simple lysis and lavage.

The recent development of 1.2-mm arthroscopic telescopes has allowed arthroscopic lysis and lavage to be performed in the office under either conscious intravenous sedation or local anesthesia. The optics of these small arthroscopes are excellent, and superb visualization of the joint structures can be obtained. The techniques are similar to hospital-based arthroscopy. Only lysis and lavage can be performed with the 1.2-mm arthroscope. Use of the 1.2-mm arthroscope provides a technique that has the simplicity of arthrocentesis and many of the advantages of arthroscopy. The preliminary results of office-based arthroscopy are similar to those observed with arthrocentesis and hospital-based arthroscopy for patients with painful limited mouth opening.

MODIFIED CONDYLOTOMY

The modified condylotomy is a variation of the intraoral vertical ramus osteotomy used in orthognathic surgery. The idea of osteotomizing the condylar process for the treatment of TMJ pain was derived from observations that patients who had sustained condylar fractures rarely complained of TMJ problems. In the 1980s, Nickerson developed the modified condylotomy as a means of treating TMJ patients. The aim of the procedure is to surgically reposition the condyle anteriorly and inferiorly beneath the displaced disc, which effectively increases the joint space. Although some authors recommend modified condylotomy for all stages of internal derangement, it seems to be most useful for treating patients with painful TMJ internal derangements and good mouth opening.

The modified condylotomy is performed under general anesthesia, usually as an outpatient procedure, but an overnight stay in the hospital may be required. An incision is made along the anterior border of the mandibular ramus. After exposure of the lateral aspect of the mandibular ramus, a vertical cut is made posterior to the lingual aspect from the coronoid notch to the mandibular angle. Once the condylar segment has been mobilized, the medial ptery-goid muscle is stripped from the inferior aspect of the segment. The mandible is then immobilized with maxillomandibular fixation. Although the surgery is simple, there is a period of fixation for 2 to 3 weeks followed by training elastics so that the occlusion is maintained.

The most significant potential complication of the modified condylotomy of the mandible is excessive condylar sag resulting in malocclusion. Hall reported a complication rate of only 4%, primarily minor occlusal discrepancies.

The reported outcomes have been excellent. Hall reported good pain relief in about 90% of 400 patients treated over a 9-year period. In follow-up studies, a 94% success rate for reduction in patients with disc displacement has been reported. Interestingly, 72% of those patients had normal disc position when evaluated with follow-up MRI studies. The success rate in a group of patients with disc displacement without reduction was slightly less at 88%.

Despite the simplicity of the procedure and its high success rate, it has not become widely used. The reasons for this are unclear but are most likely related to the necessity for maxillomandibular fixation and fear of excessive condylar sag resulting in an unstable occlusion.

OPEN JOINT SURGERY

Open TMJ surgery is the most controversial procedure performed in the TMJ because the outcomes are somewhat unpredictable and open joint surgery has significant potential complications. Open joint surgery is recommended for patients with internal derangement and osteoarthritis who have failed to respond to simpler surgical procedures or have failed previous open surgery. In patients with previous surgery, the surgeon must be hesitant to perform repeated surgery because the success rate is very low; in fact, after two surgeries it may approach zero. The surgeon must be very certain that the source of the pain or dysfunction is arising from within the joint. Severe mechanical interference such as loud, hard clicking with or without intermittent locking is an indication to perform open surgery without performing simpler procedures because experience indicates that simpler procedures are rarely successful in these cases. Open TMJ surgery provides the surgeon with an unlimited scope of procedures ranging from simple lavage and débridement to complete removal of the disc.

Open joint surgery is performed under general anesthesia in the hospital and usually requires a 1- to 2-day stay. The most common surgical approach is via a preauricular endaural incision. Other approaches include the standard preauricular and postauricular incisions. Surgical access to the joint is essentially the same regardless of the site of incision. Exposure of the capsule is performed carefully by using a modified Al-Kayat Bramley approach through the temporal fascia to protect the temporal branches of the facial nerve. After exposure of the capsule, the upper joint space is entered, and it is inspected for the presence of adhesions. The contour and integrity of the fossa and eminence are evaluated, and finally, the disc is visualized. Evaluation of the disc includes assessment of its color, position, mobility, shape, and integrity. After this evaluation of the hard and soft tissues of the joint, a decision is made to either reposition the disc or remove it.

Disc Repositioning

If the disc is intact and can be repositioned without tension, disc repositioning can be performed by removing excess tissue from the superior aspect of the posterior attachment tissues. The lower joint space is not usually entered. The disc is then repositioned and stabilized with sutures. Preoperative MRI of the joint can be useful in evaluating the status of the disc. Disc repositioning is usually performed in patients with Wilkes II or III internal derangements. Bone recontouring of the glenoid fossa or articular eminence (or both) is generally performed, especially in patients with gross mechanical interference. Frequently, the lateral aspect of the articular eminence is very prominent and needs to be reduced. The goal of disc-repositioning surgery is to eliminate mechanical interference to smooth joint function. After completion of the intra-articular procedures, the soft tissues are closed.

Immediately after surgery, the patient may experience swelling in front of the ear and a slight change in occlusion with limited mouth opening. The swelling and change in occlusion resolve in about 2 weeks. Range-of-motion exercises are started immediately and continued until the patient no longer has morning joint stiffness. All patients experience numbness in front of the ear, which resolves in about 6 weeks. Patients normally have moderate discomfort that lasts about 1 to 2 weeks. The most significant complication associated with open surgery is injury to the facial nerve. Even though total facial nerve paralysis is possible, it is rare. An inability to raise the eyebrow is the most commonly observed finding and occurs in about 5% of patients. It generally resolves in about 3 months. A soft diet is recommended for 3 months.

The literature indicates that disc-repositioning surgery is successful in 80-95% of cases; however, experience indicates that this may be an overestimate. Dolwick and Nitzan evaluated 152 patients who underwent TMJ disc-repositioning surgery over a 9-year period between 1980 and 1988 and found a 70-80% rate of improvement in about 90% of the patients up to an 8-year follow-up period. Unfortunately, 5.3% reported that they were worse following surgery. Furthermore, it was also found that the majority of those who did report improvement after surgery continued to experience symptoms of pain, joint noise, and decreased range of motion, though to a far lesser extent than before surgery. Abramowicz reported a 20-year follow-up study on 20 patients from the Dolwick and Nitzan report. All 20 patients were doing well, but most reported some symptoms of pain and decreased range of motion. With MRI, Montgomery evaluated 51 subjects up to 6 years after disc-repositioning surgery and found that disc position was not maintained. Despite this finding, most patients were significantly improved, thus confirming that preservation of a healthy, freely mobile disc is justified.

Discectomy

A diseased or deformed disc that interferes with smooth function of the joint and cannot be repositioned should be removed. Only the portion of the disc that is diseased and deformed needs to be removed. The synovial tissues should be preserved as much as possible. After removal of the disc, just minimal bone recontouring should be performed. Exposure of bone marrow may result in heterotopic bone formation. To minimize the risk for heterotopic bone formation, placement of an interpositional fat graft into the joint space is recommended. The fat graft fills the space created by removal of the disc and prevents the formation of a hematoma. After completion of the intra-articular procedures, the joint space is irrigated and the soft tissues are closed.

The postoperative findings are the same after discectomy as described for disc repositioning. The postoperative recommendations are also the same except that a soft diet is recommended for 6 months.

The complications associated with discectomy are similar to those seen with disc repositioning. Growth of heterotopic bone is more common after discectomy than after other TMJ surgical procedures. This can be a significant complication that results in ankylosis. Occasionally, degeneration of the condyle may occur and result in malocclusion. The frequency of occurrence of heterotopic bone formation and condylar resorption is unclear.

Long-term follow-up data on discectomy procedures have been published. There are four studies with at least 30 years' follow-up in which excellent reduction in pain and improvement of function in most patients have been reported. Bjorland and Larhein found that 10 years after discectomy, 19 of 24 patients reported no pain and had an average mandibular opening of 41.7 mm.

Postoperative imaging studies of patients after discectomy generally show changes in condylar morphology. These changes are thought to be adaptive and not degenerative. Most patients will have crepitant joint noise after discectomy.

PEARLS AND PITFALLS

- Surgery on the TMJ continues to have a small but important role in the management of specific temporomandibular disorders.
- Appropriate case selection is a mandatory requirement for surgical intervention to achieve a successful outcome.
- Past problems with TMJ surgery have been related to indiscriminant aggressive intervention. With the introduction of less invasive surgical techniques, successful outcomes are more predictable and complications are less likely to occur.
- Surgery on the TMJ is best performed by surgeons who maintain the philosophy that surgery should aim to avoid further harm to the joint and err on the side of more conservative procedures. The benefits and limitations of each surgical procedure are readily determined on an individual case basis.
- The goal is to determine the most appropriate technique that will yield the highest probability of success with the lowest morbidity.
- Surgeons should acquaint themselves with the benefits derived from surgery and always keep in mind that a team approach to the management of patients with pain or dysfunction and careful case selection are the most important ingredients for a successful outcome.

BIBLIOGRAPHY

Abramowicz S, Dolwick MF: Twenty-year follow-up study of disc repositioning surgery for temporomandibular joint internal derangement, *J Oral Maxillofac Surg* 68:239-242, 2010.

Al-Belasy FA, Dolwick MF: Arthrocentesis for the treatment of temporomandibular joint closed lock: a review article, *Int J Oral Maxillofac Surg* 36:773-782, 2007.

Alpaslan GH, Alpaslan C: Efficacy of temporomandibular joint arthrocentesis with and without injection of sodium hyaluronate in treatment of internal derangements, *J Oral Maxillofac Surg* 59:613-618, 2001.

Auerbach SM, Laskin DM, Frantsue LM, et al: Depression, pain, exposure to stressful life events, and long-term outcomes in temporomandibular disorder patients, *J Oral Maxillofac Surg* 59:628-633, 2001.

Bjørnland T, Larheim TA: Discectomy of the temporomandibular joint: 3-year follow-up as a predictor of the 10-year outcome, *J Oral Maxillofac Surg* 61(1):55-60, 2003.

Blake DR, Merry P, Unsworth J, et al: Hypoxic-reperfusion injury in the inflamed human joint, *Lancet* 1:289-293, 1989.

Boering G: *Temporomandibular joint arthrosis: an analysis of 400 cases*, Leiden, 1966, Stafleu.

Boyd RL, Gibbs CH, Mahan PE, et al: Temporomandibular joint forces measured at the condyle of *Macaca arctoides*, *Am J Orthod Dentofacial Orthop* 7:472-479, 1990.

Brooks SL, Westesson PL, Erickson L, et al: Prevalence of osseous changes in the temporomandibular joint of asymptomatic persons without internal derangement, *Oral Surg Oral Med Oral Pathol* 3:118-122, 1992.

Carlsson GE: Long-term effects of treatment of craniomandibular disorders, *Cranio* 3:337-342, 1985.

Carlsson GE, Egermark I, Magnusson T: Predictors of bruxism, other oral parafunction, and tooth wear over a 20-year follow-up period, *J Orofac Pain* 17:50-57, 2003.

Carvajal WA, Laskin DM: Long-term evaluation of arthrocentesis for the treatment of internal derangements of the temporomandibular joint, *J Oral Maxillofac Surg* 58:852-855, 2000.

Clark GT: A critical evaluation of orthopedic interocclusal appliance therapy: design, theory and overall effectiveness, *J Am Dent Assoc* 108:359-364, 1984.

Conti PC, dos Santos CN, Koqawa EM, et al: The treatment of painful temporomandibular joint clicking with oral splints: a randomized clinical trial, *J Am Dent Assoc* 137:1108-1114, 2006.

Dahlstrom L: Conservative treatment in craniomandibular disorder, *Swed Dent J* 16:217-230, 1992.

de Bont LG, Boering G, Liam RS, et al: Osteoarthritis and internal derangement of the temporomandibular joint: a light microscopic study, *J Oral Maxillofac Surg* 44:634-643, 1986.

de Leeuw R, Boering G, Stegenga B, et al: Clinical signs of TMJ osteoarthrosis and internal derangement 30 years after nonsurgical treatment, *J Orofac Pain* 8:18-24, 1994.

de Leeuw R, Boering G, Stegenga B, et al: Symptoms of temporomandibular joint osteoarthrosis and internal derangement 30 years after non-surgical treatment, *Cranio* 13:81-88, 1995.

de Leeuw R, Boering G, Stegenga B, et al: Radiographic signs of temporomandibular joint osteoarthrosis and internal derangement 30 years after nonsurgical treatment, *Oral Surg Oral Med Oral Pathol Oral Radiol Endod* 79:382-392, 1995.

de Leeuw R, Boering G, Van der Kuijl B, et al: Hard and soft tissue imaging of the temporomandibular joint 30 years after diagnosis of osteoarthrosis and internal derangement, *J Oral Maxillofac Surg* 54:1270-1280, 1996.

Dimitroulis G: The role of surgery in the management of disorders of the temporomandibular joint: a critical review of the literature; Part 1, *Int J Oral Maxillofac Surg* 34:107-113, 2005.

Dimitroulis G: The role of surgery in the management of disorders of the temporomandibular joint: a critical review of the literature; Part 2, *Int J Oral Maxillofac Surg* 34:231-273, 2005.

Dimitroulis G, Dolwick MF, Martinez A: Temporomandibular joint arthrocentesis and lavage for the treatment of closed lock: a follow-up study, *Br J Oral Maxillofac Surg* 33:23-37, 1995.

Dimitroulis G, McCullough M, Morrison W: Quality of life survey of patients prior to and following temporomandibular joint discectomy, *J Oral Maxillofac Surg* 68:101-106, 2010.

Dolwick MF: Clinical diagnosis of temporomandibular joint internal derangement and myofascial pain and dysfunction, *Oral Maxillofac Surg Clin North Am* 1:1-6, 1989.

Dolwick MF: Intra-articular disc displacement part 1: its questionable role in temporomandibular joint pathology, *J Oral Maxillofac Surg* 53:1069-1072, 1995.

Dolwick MF: The role of temporomandibular joint surgery in the treatment of patients with internal derangement, *Oral Surg Oral Med Oral Pathol Oral Radiol Endod* 83:150-155, 1997.

Dolwick MF: Disc preservation surgery for the treatment of internal derangements of the temporomandibular joints, *J Oral Maxillofac Surg* 59:1047-1050, 2001.

Dolwick MF: Temporomandibular joint surgery for internal derangement, *Dent Clin North Am* 51:195-208, 2007.

Dolwick MF, Aufdemorte TB: Silicone induced foreign-body reaction and lymphadenopathy after temporomandibular joint arthroplasty, *Oral Surg Oral Med Oral Pathol* 59:449-452, 1985.

Dolwick MF, Dimitroulis G: Is there a role for temporomandibular joint surgery? *Br J Oral Maxillofac Surg* 32:307-313, 1994.

Dolwick MF, Dimitroulis G: A re-evaluation of the importance of disc position in temporomandibular disorders, *Aust Dent J* 41:184-187, 1996.

Dolwick MF, Katzberg RW, Helms CA: Internal derangement of the temporomandibular joint: fact or fiction? *J Prosthet Dent* 49:415-418, 1983.

Dolwick MF, Katzberg RW, Helms CA, et al: Arthrotomographic evaluation of the temporomandibular joint, *J Oral Surg* 37:793-799, 1979.

Dolwick MF, Nitzan DW: TMJ disk surgery: 8-year follow-up evaluation, *Fortschr Kiefer Gesichtschir* 35:162-167, 1990.

Dolwick MF, Riggs RR: Diagnosis and treatment of internal derangements of the temporomandibular joint, *Dent Clin North Am* 27:561-572, 1983.

Dolwick MF, Sanders B: *TMJ internal derangement and arthrosis—surgical atlas*, St Louis, 1985, CV Mosby.

Dworkin SF, LeResche L: Research diagnostic criteria for temporomandibular disorders: review, criteria, examinations and specifications, critique, *J Craniomandib Disord* 6:301-355, 1992.

Emshoff R, Brandlmaier I, Bertram S, et al: Relative odds of temporomandibular joint pain as function of magnetic resonance imaging findings of internal derangement, osteoarthrosis, effusion, and bone marrow edema, *Oral Surg Oral Med Oral Pathol Oral Radiol Endod* 95:437-445, 2003.

Emshoff R, Puffer P, Strobl H, et al: Effect of temporomandibular joint arthrocentesis on synovial fluid mediator level of tumor necrosis factor-alpha: implications for treatment outcome, *Int J Oral Maxillofac Surg* 29:176-182, 2000.

Emshoff R, Rudisch A, Bosch R, et al: Effect of arthrocentesis and hydraulic distention on the temporomandibular joint disk position, *Oral Surg Oral Med Oral Pathol Oral Radiol Endod* 89:271-277, 2000.

Emshoff R, Rudisch A, Bosch R, et al: Prognostic indicators of the outcome of arthrocentesis: a short-term follow-up study, *Oral Surg Oral Med Oral Pathol Oral Radiol Endod* 96:12-18, 2003.

Ericksson L, Westesson PL: Long-term evaluation of meniscectomy of the temporomandibular joint, *J Oral Maxillofac Surg* 43:263-269, 1985.

Ericksson L, Westesson PL: Temporomandibular joint discectomy, *Oral Surg Oral Med Oral Pathol* 74:259-272, 1992.

Farrar WB: Diagnosis and treatment of anterior dislocation of articular disc, *N Y J Dent* 41:348-351, 1971.

Farrar WB, McCarty WL: Inferior joint space arthrography and characteristics of condylar paths in internal derangements of TMJ, *J Prosthet Dent* 41:458-463, 1971.

Feinberg SE: Use of composite temporalis muscle flaps for disc replacement, *Oral Maxillofac Surg Clin North Am* 6:335-337, 1994.

Fridrich KL, Wise JM, Zeitler DL: Prospective comparison of arthroscopy and arthrocentesis for temporomandibular joint disorders, *J Oral Maxillofac Surg* 54:816-820, 1996.

Goudot P, Jaquinet AR, Hugonnet S, et al: Improvement of pain and function after arthroscopy and arthrocentesis of the temporomandibular joint: a comparative study, *Craniomaxillofac Surg* 28:39-43, 2000.

Greene CS, Laskin DM: Long-term status of TMJ clicking in patients with myofascial pain and dysfunction, *J Am Dent Assoc* 117:461-465, 1988.

Hall MB: Meniscoplasty of the displaced temporomandibular joint meniscus without violating the inferior joint space, *J Oral Maxillofac Surg* 42:788-792, 1984.

Hall HD: The role of discectomy for treating internal derangements of the temporomandibular joint, *Oral Maxillofac Surg Clin North Am* 6:287-294, 1994.

Hall HD, Indresano AT, Kirk WS, et al: Prospective multicenter comparison of 4 temporomandibular joint operations, *J Oral Maxillofac Surg* 63:1174-1179, 2005.

Hall HD, Link JL: Diskectomy alone and with ear cartilage interposition grafts in joint reconstruction, *Oral Maxillofac Surg Clin North Am* 1:32-40, 1989.

Hall HD, Navarro EZ, Gibbs SJ: One-and three-year prospective outcome study of modified condylotomy for treatment of reducing disc displacement, *J Oral Maxillofac Surg* 58:7-17, 2000.

Hall HD, Navarro EZ, Gibbs SJ: Prospective study of modified condylotomy for treatment on nonreducing disk displacement, *Oral Surg Oral Med Oral Pathol Oral Radiol Endod* 89:147-158, 2000.

Hall HD, Nickerson JW: Is it time to pay more attention to disc position? *J Orofac Pain* 8:90-95, 1994.

Hall HD, Nickerson JW, McKenna SJ: Modified condylotomy for treatment of the painful temporomandibular joint with a reducing disc, *J Oral Maxillofac Surg* 51:133-142, 1993.

Haskin CL, Milam SB, Cameron IL: Pathogenesis of degenerative joint disease in the human temporomandibular joint, *Crit Rev Oral Biol Med* 6:248-277, 1995.

Henny FA, Baldridge OL: Condylectomy for the persistently painful temporomandibular joint, *J Oral Surg* 15:24-27, 1957.

Holmlund AB: Surgery for TMJ internal derangement: evaluation of treatment outcomes and criteria for success, *Int J Oral Maxillofac Surg* 22:75-77, 1993.

Holmlund AB, Gynther GW, Axelsson S: Diskectomy in treatment of internal derangement of the temporomandibular joint. Follow-up at 1, 3 and 5 years, *Oral Surg Oral Med Oral Pathol* 76:266-271, 1993.

Holmlund AB, Gynther GW, Axelsson S: Efficacy of arthroscopic lysis and lavage in patients with chronic locking of temporomandibular joint, *Int J Oral Maxillofac Surg* 23:262-265, 1994.

Huang YL, Pogrel A, Kaban LB: Diagnosis and management of condylar resorption, *J Oral Maxillofac Surg* 55:114-119, 1997.

Indresano AT: Surgical arthroscopy as the preferred treatment for internal derangements of the temporomandibular joint, *J Oral Maxillofac Surg* 59:308-312, 2001.

Ireland VE: The problem of the clicking jaw, *J Prosthet Dent* 3:200-203, 1953.

Israel HA: Current concepts in the surgical management of temporomandibular joint disorders, *J Oral Maxillofac Surg* 52:289-294, 1994.

Israel HA: The use of arthroscopic surgery for the treatment of temporomandibular joint disorders, *J Oral Maxillofac Surg* 57:579-582, 1999.

Katzberg RW, Dolwick MF, Helms CA, et al: Arthrotomography of the temporomandibular joint, *AJR Am J Roetgenol* 134:995-1003, 1980.

Kendell BD, Frost DE: Arthrocentesis, *Atlas Oral Maxillofac Surg Clin North Am* 4:1-14, 1996.

Kiehn CL: Meniscectomy for internal derangement of the temporomandibular joint, *Am J Surg* 83:364-373, 1952.

Kircos LT, Ortendahl DA, Mark AS, et al: Magnetic resonance imaging of the TMJ disc in asymptomatic volunteers, *J Oral Maxillofac Surg* 45:852-854, 1987.

Koslin MG, Martin JC: The use of holmium laser for temporomandibular joint arthroscopic surgery, *J Oral Maxillofac Surg* 51:122-124, 1993.

Kozeniauskas JJ, Ralph WJ: Bilateral arthrographic evaluation of unilateral temporomandibular joint pain and dysfunction, *J Prosthet Dent* 60:98-105, 1988.

Kurita H, Uehara S, Yokochi, et al: A long-term follow-up study of radiographically evident degenerative changes in the temporomandibular joint with different conditions of disk displacement, *Int J Oral Maxillofac Surg* 35:49-54, 2006.

Kurita H, Westesson PL, Yuasa H, et al: Natural course of untreated symptomatic temporomandibular joint disc displacement without reduction, *J Dent Res* 77:361-365, 1998.

Lanz AB: Discitis mandibularis, *Zentralbl Chir* 36:289-291, 1909.

Larheim TA: Role of magnetic resonance imaging in the clinical diagnosis of the temporomandibular joint, *Cells Tissues Organs* 180:6-21, 2005.

Larheim TA, Westesson P, Sano T: Temporomandibular joint disk displacement: comparison in asymptomatic volunteers and patients, *Radiology* 218:428-432, 2001.

Laskin DM: Etiology of the pain and dysfunction syndrome, *J Am Dent Assoc* 79:147-150, 1969.

Lewis EL, Dolwick MF, Abramowicz S, et al: Contemporary imaging of the temporomandibular joint, *Dent Clin North Am* 52:875-890, 2008.

McCain JP: Arthroscopy of the human temporomandibular joint, *J Oral Maxillofac Surg* 46:648-652, 1988.

McCain JP, de la Rua H: Principles and practice of operative arthroscopy of the human temporomandibular joint, *Oral Maxillofac Surg Clin North Am* 1:135-152, 1989.

McCain JP, Podrasky AE, Zabiegalski NA: Arthroscopic disc repositioning and suturing: a preliminary report, *J Oral Maxillofac Surg* 50:568-573, 1992.

McCain JP, Sanders B, Koslin MG, et al: Temporomandibular joint arthroscopy—a 6-year multicenter retrospective study of 4831 joints, *J Oral Maxillofac Surg* 50:926-930, 1992.

McCarty WL, Farrar WB: Surgery for internal derangement of the temporomandibular joint, *J Prosthet Dent* 42:191-196, 1979.

McKenna SJ: Discectomy for the treatment of internal derangements of the temporomandibular joint, *J Oral Maxillofac Surg* 59:1051-1056, 2001.

Mejersjo C, Carlsson GE: Long term results of treatment for temporomandibular pain-dysfunction, *J Prosthet Dent* 49:809-815, 1983.

Mercuri LG: The use of alloplastic prostheses for temporomandibular joint reconstruction, *J Oral Maxillofac Surg* 58:70-75, 2000.

Merrill RG: Historical perspectives and comparisons of temporomandibular joint surgery for internal derangements and arthropathy, *Cranio* 4:74-78, 1986.

Milam SB, Schmitz JP: Molecular biology of temporomandibular joint disorders: proposed mechanisms of disease, *J Oral Maxillofac Surg* 53:1448-1454, 1995.

Montgomery MT, Gordon SM, Van Sickels JE, et al: Changes in signs and symptoms following temporomandibular joint disc repositioning surgery, *J Oral Maxillofac Surg* 50:320-328, 1992.

Moses JJ, Poker I: TMJ arthroscopic surgery: an analysis of 237 patients, *J Oral Maxillofac Surg* 47:790-794, 1989.

Murakami KI, Iizuka T, Matsuki M, et al: Recapturing the persistent anteriorly displaced disk by mandibular manipulation after pumping and applying hydraulic pressure to the upper joint cavity of the temporomandibular joint, *Cranio* 5:17-24, 1987.

Murakami KI, Segami N, Okamoto M, et al: Outcome of arthroscopic surgery for internal derangement of the temporomandibular joint: long-term results covering 10 years, *J Craniomaxillofac Surg* 28:264-271, 2000.

Murakami KI, Tsuboi Y, Bessho K, et al: Outcome of arthroscopic surgery to the temporomandibular joint correlates with stage of internal derangement: five-year follow-up study, *Br J Oral Maxillofac Surg* 36:30-34, 1998.

Nickerson JW: Natural course of osteoarthrosis as it relates to internal derangement of the temporomandibular joint, *Oral Maxillofac Surg Clin North Am* 1:27-46, 1989.

Nitzan DW: The process of lubrication impairment and its involvement in temporomandibular joint disc displacement: a theoretical concept, *J Oral Maxillofac Surg* 59:36-45, 2001.

Nitzan DW, Dolwick MF: An alternative explanation for the genesis of closed-lock symptoms in the internal derangement process, *J Oral Maxillofac Surg* 48:810-815, 1991.

Nitzan DW, Dolwick MF, Heft MW: Arthroscopic lavage and lysis of the temporomandibular joint: a change in perspective, *J Oral Maxillofac Surg* 48:798-801, 1990.

Nitzan DW, Dolwick MF, Martinez GA: Temporomandibular joint arthrocentesis: a simplified treatment for severe limited mouth opening, *J Oral Maxillofac Surg* 49:1163-1167, 1991.

Nitzan DW, Nitzan U, Dan P, et al: The role of hyaluronic acid in protecting surface-active phospholipids from lysis by exogenous phospholipase A(2), *Rheumatology* 40:336-340, 2001.

Nitzan DW, Price A: The use of arthrocentesis for the treatment of osteoarthritic temporomandibular joints, *J Oral Maxillofac Surg* 59:1154-1159, 2001.

Nitzan DW, Samson, Better H: Long-term outcome of arthrocentesis for sudden-onset, persistent, severe closed lock of the temporomandibular joint, *J Oral Maxillofac Surg* 55:151-157, 1997.

Ohnishi M: [Arthroscopy of the temporomandibular joint,] *J Jpn Stomat* 42:207-212, 1975.

Ohnishi M: Arthroscopic laser surgery and suturing for temporomandibular disorders. Techniques and clinical results, *Arthroscopy* 7:212-216, 1991.

Pringle JH: Displacement of the mandibular meniscus and its treatment, *Br J Surg* 6:385-388, 1918.

Quinn PD: Alloplastic reconstruction of the temporomandibular joint, *Selected Readings Oral Maxillofac Surg* 7:1, 2000.

Rasmussen OC: Description of population and progress of symptoms in a longitudinal study of temporomandibular arthropathy, *J Dent Res* 89:196-203, 1981.

Reston JT, Turkelson CM: Meta-analysis of surgical treatments for temporomandibular articular disorders, *J Oral Maxillofac Surg* 61:3-10, 2003.

Sanders B: Arthroscopic surgery of the temporomandibular joint: Treatment of internal derangement with persistent closed lock, *Oral Surg Oral Med Oral Pathol* 62:361-372, 1986.

Sato S, Goto S, Kawamura H, et al: The natural course of nonreducing disc displacement of the TMJ: relationship of clinical findings at initial visit to outcome after 12 months without treatment, *J Orofac Pain* 11:315-320, 1997.

Sato S, Goto S, Nasu F, et al: Natural course of disc displacement with reduction of temporomandibular joint: changes in clinical signs and symptoms, *J Oral Maxillofac Surg* 61:32-34, 2003.

Schiffman EL, Look JO, Hodges JS, et al: Randomized effectiveness study of four therapeutic strategies for TMJ closed lock, *J Dent Res* 86:58-63, 2007.

Schwartz LJ: Pain associated with the TMJ, *J Am Dent Assoc* 51:394-398, 1955.

Silver CML: Long-term results of meniscectomy of the temporomandibular joint, *Cranio* 3:46-57, 1984.

Stengenga B, de Bont LGM, Boering G, et al: Tissue responses to degenerative changes in the temporomandibular joint, *J Oral Maxillofac Surg* 49:1079-1088, 1991.

Takaku S, Toyoda T: Long-term evaluation of discectomy of the temporomandibular joint, *J Oral Maxillofac Surg* 52:722-726, 1994.

Thilander B: Innervation of the temporomandibular disc in man, *Acta Odontol Scand* 22:151-156, 1964.

Toller PA: Osteoarthritis of the mandibular condyle, *Br Dent J* 134:223-231, 1973.

Tolvanen M, Oikarinen VJ, Wolf J: A 30 year follow-up study of temporomandibular joint meniscectomies: a report on five patients, *Br J Oral Maxillofac Surg* 26:311-313, 1988.

Undt G, Murakami I, Rasse M, et al: Open versus arthroscopic surgery for internal derangement of the temporomandibular joint: a retrospective study comparing two centres' results using the Jaw Pain and Function Questionnaire, *J Craniomaxillofac Surg* 34:234-241, 2006.

Westesson PL: Arthrography of the temporomandibular joint, *J Prosthet Dent* 51:535-540, 1984.

Westesson PL, Rohlin M: Internal derangement related to osteoarthrosis in temporomandibular joint autopsy specimens, *Oral Surg Oral Med Oral Pathol* 57:17-22, 1984.

Wilkes C: Internal derangement of the TMJ, *Arch Otolaryngol Head Neck Surg* 115:469-474, 1989.

Temporomandibular Joint: Hypermobility and Ankylosis

Chapter 99

Gary F. Bouloux

The temporomandibular joint (TMJ) is a complicated joint that can be classified as bilateral, diarthrodial, and ginglymoid. It allows both joint rotation and translation. The TMJ is unique in that movement in one joint is associated with movement in the contralateral joint. The TMJ is vulnerable to many pathologic conditions, including ankylosis and hypermobility.

ETIOPATHOGENESIS

HYPERMOBILITY

Hypermobility of the joint can be secondary to trauma, connective tissue disorders, or be idiopathic. The point at which excessive joint mobility becomes problematic is typically when it leads to recurrent joint dislocation. This is characterized by movement of the condyle past the articular eminence and into the infratemporal fossa. The latter may be associated with severe pain and loss of function. Subluxation also involves movement of the condyle past the articular eminence but differs from dislocation in that the condyle can spontaneously relocate to its normal position within the glenoid fossa. TMJ hypermobility may also be associated with an increased prevalence of internal derangement.

ANKYLOSIS

Ankylosis of the TMJ may be defined as fibrous or bony. In either situation, the normal joint anatomy is progressively destroyed and replaced with dense fibrous tissue or bone with a concomitant reduction or loss of joint translation and, ultimately, rotation. Accordingly, the maximal incisal opening (MIO) and lateral excursive movements progressively decrease. The most common causes of ankylosis are trauma, infectious arthritis, autoimmune arthritis, and iatrogenic causes.

PATHOLOGIC ANATOMY

HYPERMOBILITY

A complete understanding of normal joint anatomy is crucial to understanding joint pathology. Hypermobility is often associated with normal joint anatomy. However, the capsule, lateral TMJ ligament, and retrodiscal tissue may be lax and allow excessive condylar movement anterior to the articular eminence. This may result in subluxation or the more problematic dislocation. The one anatomic feature that is most readily identified in patients with subluxation and dislocation is a relatively small articular eminence. Internal derangement may also be associated with hypermobility, but the association between the two is not clearly understood.

ANKYLOSIS

The joint anatomy associated with ankylosis is significantly different from that of a normal joint. Even though the joint capsule and extracapsular ligaments may be present and appear normal, the intraarticular structures are radically altered. This is the case for fibrous ankylosis, in which dense fibrous scar tissue extends from the articulating surface of the vestigial disc to the roof of the glenoid fossa and articular eminence of the temporal bone. Fibrous tissue may also extend from the inferior aspect of the disc to the articulating surface of the condyle. As the fibrosis progresses, the articular disc is typically replaced by fibrous tissue. Extra-articular structures and anatomy are usually unaffected. Bony ankylosis is different and particularly destructive. It often develops from long-standing fibrous ankylosis. Bone extends from the condyle to the glenoid fossa and articular eminence. The disc, retrodiscal tissue, and check ligaments are typically lost as they are replaced by bone. The ankylosis may be extensive and extend anteroposteriorly from the tympanic plate to the infratemporal fossa and mediolaterally from the zygomatic arch to the petrous portion of the temporal bone. The joint capsule is similarly replaced by the expanding bony mass. Extra-articular soft tissues, including nerves, blood vessels, and muscle attachments, may also be displaced.

DIAGNOSTIC STUDIES

HYPERMOBILITY

Hypermobility is easily diagnosed with routine panoramic radiography. The image should demonstrate the condyle anterior to the articular eminence in the infratemporal fossa. Clinical evaluation of the patient should also reveal an anterior open bite of several centimeters and a palpable depression immediately in front of the tragus corresponding to an empty glenoid fossa. However, patients with long-standing TMJ dislocation may not have any appreciable anterior open bite. The same imaging modality can be used to confirm adequate reduction of the dislocation. In the absence of panoramic imaging, computed tomography (CT) can also readily illustrate a condyle that is anterior to the articular eminence. Magnetic resonance imaging (MRI) will provide soft tissue imaging that allows the magnitude of joint translation and disc position to be seen, but it has little to offer in the acute setting.

ANKYLOSIS

Fibrous ankylosis is characterized clinically by limited MIO and, when unilateral, reduced lateral excursion toward the unaffected side. Radiographic features of fibrous ankylosis are conspicuous by their absence. Patients with bony ankylosis have no incisal opening or lateral excursions. Panoramic imaging of bony ankylosis will show heterotopic bone formation and no joint space. However, the ankylosis is best imaged with CT. Axial and coronal images are the most informative, although three-dimensional (3D) reconstructed images provide the most detail. For all but the most simple bony ankyloses, fabrication of a stereolithographic model from the CT scan allows the surgeon to assess the anatomy in detail, plan the surgery, and perform it first on the model. Closely related anatomic structures, including the middle ear, middle cranial fossa, foramen spinosum, jugular fossa, and carotid canal, should be clearly visualized.

RECONSTRUCTIVE GOALS

HYPERMOBILITY

The primary objective is to decrease joint translation and prevent subluxation and dislocation. Normal rotation within the joint should be maintained, but excessive movement of the condyle anterior to the articular eminence must be prevented. When symptomatic internal derangement coexists with hypermobility, disc plication or discectomy can also be performed. Recurrent dislocation can be treated according to one of three basic philosophies. The first is to provide a mechanical barrier to joint translation through bony augmentation of the articular eminence or down-fracture of the root of the zygomatic bone (Dautrey procedure). The second philosophy also reduces joint translation but through plication, imbrication, or scarification of the capsule, ligaments, retrodiscal tissue, and disc. The third philosophy does not limit joint translation but rather eliminates the mechanical barrier to relocating the condyle when it translates past the articular eminence. This is achieved by performing an eminectomy.

ANKYLOSIS

The primary objective is to create a functioning joint that allows some combination of joint rotation or translation. Joint-preserving procedures such as arthroplasty may be possible in patients with fibrous ankylosis if the fibrosis is minimal. If the fibrous ankylosis is more extensive or bony, joint preservation becomes challenging and gap arthroplasty may be needed. This can be combined with the use of interpositional autogenous tissue, alloplastic material, or total joint replacement. Total joint replacement would appear to be the most predictable, but in younger patients it will necessitate subsequent joint replacement over the lifetime of the patient. Total joint replacement is not approved by the Food and Drug Administration for pediatric and adolescent patients who are still growing. In these patients, autogenous tissue may be the preferred treatment because it potentially allows continued growth, although the likelihood of recurrent ankylosis may be increased.

TREATMENT

HYPERMOBILITY

Multiple different approaches to prevent recurrent dislocation have been described. Intra-articular injection of sclerosing agents such as sodium tetradecyl sulfate and sodium morrhuate have been used to create excessive fibrous tissue. Intra-articular injection of blood has also been recommended to promote intra-articular fibrosis. In addition, arthroscopic scarification of the capsule, retrodiscal tissue, and disc with the use of sclerosing agents, cautery, and laser has been reported. These techniques are difficult. The author prefers to manage recurrent TMJ dislocation with one of three surgical procedures, depending on the clinical situation.

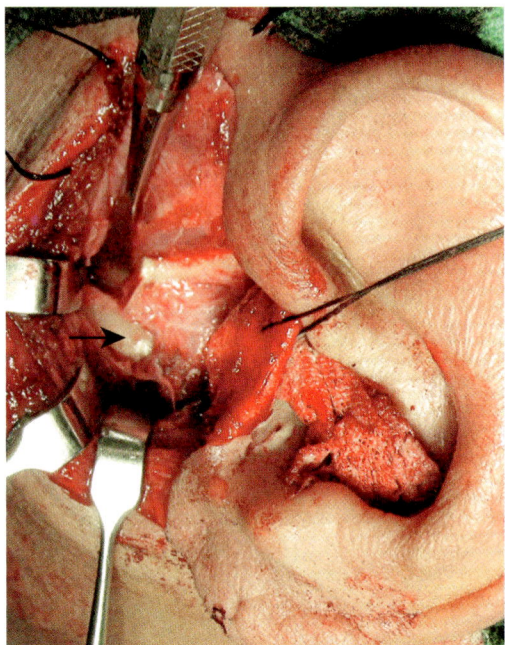

Fig. 99-1 ■ Down-fractured zygomatic arch before medial displacement (*arrow*).

The *Dautrey procedure* (Le Clerc) is a simple extra-articular surgical procedure. It is well suited to patients who have no symptoms of intra-articular pathology. The procedure has been criticized because of bone remodeling and the potential for recurrent dislocation. A standard preauricular incision is used to approach the TMJ capsule. The dissection should be carried forward in a subperiosteal plane to expose the lateral aspect of the articular eminence and root of the zygoma. A periosteal elevator is then used to elevate only the most inferior aspect of the temporalis muscle medial to the root of the zygoma. The same elevator is then passed deep to the root of the zygoma just into the infratemporal fossa to protect the soft tissues. A reciprocating saw is used to osteotomize the root of the zygoma in an oblique manner with the most superior aspect of the cut being posterior to the inferior aspect of the cut. The inferior aspect of the osteotomy should be just anterior to the apex of the articular eminence. The author prefers to displace the root of the zygoma inferiorly and medially with an orthognathic forked nasal septum osteotome. This typically results in a greenstick fracture of the zygomatic arch in a more anterior location (Fig. 99-1). The displaced zygoma usually maintains its new position without any fixation. On rare occasion, the anterior fracture is not greenstick and too much mobility of the displaced zygoma is encountered, which necessitates rigid fixation to the lateral aspect of the eminence with a small bone plate. The condyle must not be able to translate past the apex of the articular eminence at the completion of this procedure.

Arthroplasty provides the opportunity to address intra-articular pathology in addition to hypermobility. It has a role to play in patients with symptomatic internal derangement and recurrent dislocation. The internal derangement should be confirmed with MRI before the surgical procedure. A standard preauricular incision is used to approach the joint capsule. After placement of 0.054 Kirschner wires in the lateral aspect of the articular eminence and neck of the condyle, a Wilkes retractor is activated and the joint distended. Access is then gained to the superior joint space with a curvilinear incision 2 mm below the lip of the fossa. Tenotomy scissors are used to gain access to the inferior joint space by incising

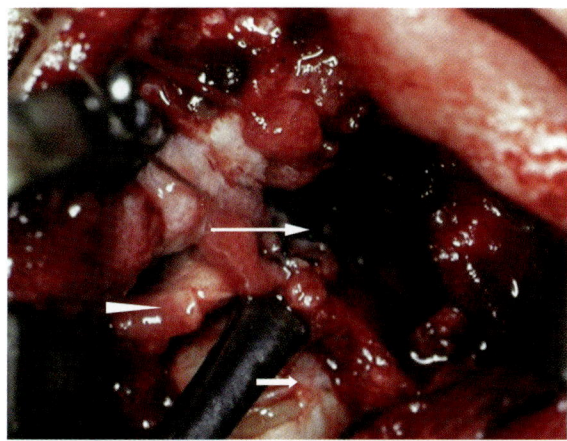

Fig. 99-2 ■ Disc plication (suture line, long *white arrow*; disc, arrow head; condyle, short white arrow).

vertically through the joint capsule and horizontally through the lateral collateral check ligament. This provides excellent access to the superior and inferior joint spaces. The disc can then be mobilized with a periosteal elevator. The areas of adhesion within the superior joint space are often the anterior slope of the eminence or the lateral aspect of the eminence. The most frequent location of adhesions within the inferior joint space is the medial pole. The disc should be able to be passively repositioned when adequate disc mobility has been achieved. The redundant retrodiscal tissue can then be assessed and excised with tenotomy scissors, and plication of the disc to the retrodiscal tissue is begun medially. Several authors advocate the use of a mini–bone anchor to facilitate disc plication, but this is not necessary. Typically, several 5-0 Vicryl sutures (Ethicon, Inc., New Jersey) sutures are placed through the posterior aspect of the disc and the retrodiscal tissue (Fig. 99-2). On the rare occasion when a perforation is present, there may be insufficient tissue to plicate the disc. In this situation the retrodiscal tissue can he horizontally divided as far as the tympanic plate. This transects many of the vertical collagen fibers in the retrodiscal tissue and allows greater forward movement of the tissue. In such circumstances the plication may require a double-layered closure, one for the superior lamina and one for the inferior lamina of the retrodiscal tissue. Alternatively, the retrodiscal tissue can be elevated off the tympanic plate and pedicled inferiorly. Plication can then be completed in single-layered fashion. Lateral plication is performed by attaching the lateral aspect of the disc to the inferior/lateral joint capsule. Three or four horizontal mattress sutures using 4-0 Vicryl are placed in this fashion. The Wilkes retractor is then closed and the lateral aspect of the superior joint space closed with similar suture material. Subsequent to the plication, only a limited degree of joint translation should be possible.

Eminectomy is a procedure that essentially eliminates the articular eminence. It can be combined with arthroplasty, although there is no need to do so. The author reserves eminectomy for rare occasions, but it is useful when other surgical procedures have failed. A standard preauricular approach is used to gain access to the joint capsule. The anterior dissection should extend in a subperiosteal plane anterior to the eminence. After placement of 0.054 Kirschner wires in the lateral aspect of the articular eminence and neck of the condyle, a Wilkes retractor is activated and the joint distended. Entry is again made into the superior joint space with a curvilinear incision 2 mm below the lip of the fossa. A combination of fissure burrs, osteotomes, or a reciprocation rasp can be used to remove the inferior aspect of the articular eminence. On rare occasions, the articular

eminence may be pneumatized and eminectomy then results in exposure of the bony cavities, although this is not a concern. During eminectomy the medial soft tissues envelope should not be breached because of the potential for substantial bleeding. A reciprocating rasp or bone file can then be used to smooth the residual articular eminence. The joint should be irrigated copiously to remove small bone fragments. The superior joint space is then closed as described previously. At the completion of the procedure the condyle should be manipulated. Although translation anterior to the residual eminence will occur, the condyle should easily return to a posterior position within the glenoid fossa without any catching or locking.

ANKYLOSIS

Fibrous ankylosis of the TMJ can generally be treated more conservatively than bony ankylosis, but it does depend on the degree of fibrosis and the residual anatomy of the joint. This is often determined by the degree of movement possible on clinical examination, the number of previous joint procedures, and findings on CT. A standard preauricular approach is used to gain access to the joint capsule. The anterior dissection should extend in a subperiosteal plane anterior to the eminence. After placement of 0.054 Kirschner wires in the lateral aspect of the articular eminence and neck of the condyle, a Wilkes retractor is activated and the joint distended. Entry is again made into the superior joint space with a curvilinear incision 2 mm below the lip of the fossa. The degree of fibrosis is often variable. It may be possible to explore the superior joint space and lyse the adhesions and fibrosis. Access to the inferior joint space is then gained and a similar exploration with lysis performed. If the remaining disc is adequate, it may be possible to leave or plicate it, depending on the disc's position. Frequently, the fibrosis is extensive and the residual disc poorly defined. Discectomy is a reasonable choice should that be the case. A multitude of different autologous tissues, including cartilage, fat, dermis, and temporalis muscle, can be interposed. There is, however, no evidence that disc replacement is superior to discectomy alone. The choice should be made on an individual basis determined more by the degree of fibrosis, the remaining anatomy, and the general appearance of the condyle and glenoid fossa. This author prefers lysis and discectomy alone or the use of a temporalis muscle fascia flap. Postoperative physical therapy is crucial to help prevent recurrence.

Correction of TMJ bony ankylosis is one of the more challenging surgical procedures in oral and maxillofacial surgery. Bony ankylosis requires a gap arthroplasty and reconstruction with autogenous tissue, alloplastic material, or total joint replacement. Autogenous reconstruction has the disadvantage of possible recurrent ankylosis at a rate that may be as high as 20-30%. Recurrent ankylosis requires total joint replacement. Aggressive postoperative physical therapy is the key to reduce this risk for recurrent ankylosis. Gap arthroplasty with autogenous reconstruction should at least be considered in patients with a first episode of ankylosis, particularly pediatric patients, in whom costochondral grafting should be considered. Although gap arthroplasty is common to all procedures, the choice of interpositional material is a little more controversial. Fascia lata, dermis, cartilage, fat, and temporalis fascia/muscle have all been used. The author prefers temporalis fascia/muscle because it is located within the surgical field and is easily harvested and transferred to the surgical site. It can be used with gap arthroplasty alone or combined with costochondral grafts in the pediatric population. Costochondral grafts have the potential to provide additional growth. The supplementary use of low-dose radiation (10 cGy) has been shown to reduce heterotopic bone formation and may be considered in the postoperative period in patients reconstructed with autogenous tissue. A standard preauricular approach is used to gain access to the ankylosis. A subperiosteal plane is developed early and the ankylosis well exposed. Every attempt should be made to develop a subperiosteal plane as far medially as possible. This will also allow the placement of two small channel retractors, one anterior and one posterior to the ankylosis. A 703 fissure burr is then used to remove 2 mm of bone progressing in a lateral to medial direction. The location of the initial osteotomy can be the cleavage plane between the original condyle and glenoid fossa if present. More often than not there is no cleavage plane and the osteotomy should be made more inferior than the original location of the glenoid fossa so that the middle cranial fossa is not breached. The medial extent of the bony ankylosis should not be breached with the burr except in the most anterior and posterior locations, where the channel retractors serve as a mechanical barrier. Final separation of the bone is best achieved with a twist osteotome. These measures provide the best opportunity to avoid damage to the medial soft tissues and the potential for significant bleeding. Although close proximity of the middle meningeal artery , internal jugular vein, and internal carotid artery to the medial lip of the normal glenoid fossa has been reported, the altered anatomy inherent in patients with bony ankylosis makes the potential for bleeding even more of a concern. If reconstruction with a temporalis muscle/fascia flap is planned, only minimal additional bone contouring is required, usually on the medial aspect of the residual condylar stump. If the ankylosis is bilateral, the second joint should be approached in a similar fashion. When using temporalis fascia/muscle flaps, the author does not routinely perform coronoidectomies but rather aggressively mobilizes the mandible. Inability to mobilize the mandible adequately mandates coronoidectomies, however. This does not preclude use of the temporalis fascia/muscle flap, which is vascularized by anterior and posterior deep temporal arteries. Additional scar release, release of the pterygomasseteric sling, or myotomy of the masseter and medial pterygoid muscles is uncommonly performed and requires a retromandibular approach. The temporalis muscle/fascia flap is harvested as a full-thickness flap. It should be kept as long as possible and the width should be sufficient to completely cover the mandibular neo-condyle. The use of several 5-0 Vicryl sutures placed medially and posteriorly through whatever soft tissue remains will provide ample means to secure the flap. It is easier to place these sutures first and leave them untied before swinging the muscle/fascia flap deep to the zygomatic arch and anterior to the articular eminence. Ideally, the periosteal surface of the flap should rest against the residual glenoid fossa. If costochondral reconstruction is planned, removal of more bone is generally mandated to allow the graft to sit against the mandibular ramus with the chondral portion within the glenoid fossa. This is usually combined with a temporalis muscle/fascia flap. In these situations, a second osteotomy is performed approximately 2 cm below the first in a similar fashion, which will result in the delivery of a 2-cm block of bone.

For all cases of recurrent ankylosis and most non-pediatric patients the author prefers total joint replacement. Advantages include early function and a reduced frequency of recurrent ankylosis. Disadvantages include the potential need to replace the joints throughout the life of the patient. Adequate function and longevity with modern joint replacement systems have been established. Stock prostheses (Biomet Microfixation, Jacksonville, Fla) or custom-fit joints (TMJ Concepts, Ventura, Calif) are available. Total joint replacement in patients with ankylosis may be performed as a one- or two-stage surgery. As surgeon experience increases, more cases can be done in one stage. Before surgery a 3D model must be constructed from a standard CT scan. The 3D nature of the ankylosis and the occlusion can readily be assessed. Gap arthroplasty should be performed on the model and then the mandible repositioned to

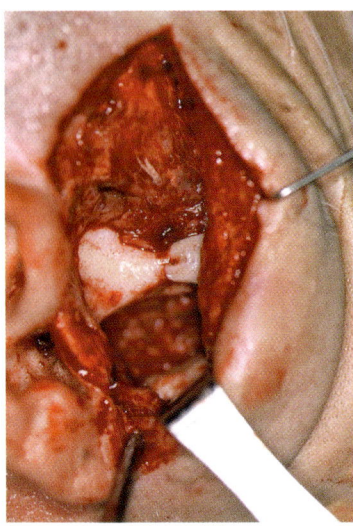

Fig. 99-3 ■ Gap arthroplasty performed on a patient.

create the desired occlusion. An attempt will be made to recreate this on the patient. Ankylosed patients present challenges from an anesthetic perspective, and accordingly, a plan to perform awake fiberoptic intubation or awake tracheostomy should be made. Ivy loops, arch bars, or skeletal wires should then be placed. The intraoral and extraoral procedures must remain separated throughout the surgery. A standard preauricular approach will provide adequate access to the ankylosis. The initial osteotomy should be performed with a 703 burr and twist osteotome with appropriate anterior and posterior medial retractor protection as described previously. A second osteotomy is then performed 2 cm inferior to the first osteotomy in an identical manner, which will result in the delivery of a 2-cm block of bone and creation of a "critical size" gap (Fig. 99-3). Should bleeding be encountered, this is the only opportunity to gain direct access to the source. Coronoidectomies should also be performed from the preauricular approach. Adequate mobility of the mandible should be obtained at this point. If two-stage surgery is planned, the mandible should be placed in the correct occlusion and secured with maxillo-mandibular fixation (MMF). The preauricular surgical field must have sterility maintained during this procedure by placing additional sterile towels over the surgical sites. Before returning to the surgical field, the surgeon should place a towel, OpSite (a transparent adhesive film [Smith & Nephew, London, UK]), or other sterile drape to cover the oral cavity, as well as change gloves. The previous gap arthroplasty sites should be inspected for smooth line angles and hemostasis. A Silastic block can then be carved to fill the gap and placed to maintain space. The wound can then be closed and the patient left in MMF. A postoperative CT scan should be obtained as soon as possible. A 3D model will be made from this scan and a custom TMJ prosthesis made. A second surgical procedure should be planned in 5 or 6 weeks.

Stage II surgery begins with release of the MMF immediately before the procedure. This is important when fiberoptic intubation is planned because it will usually make intubation easier. Prior tracheostomy eliminates this step. A standard preauricular approach will gain access to the previous gap arthroplasty and Silastic block, which is easily removed. The immature peripheral granulation tissue can then be judiciously removed by gentle scraping with a periosteal elevator. Attention can next be directed to the retromandibular incision. The author prefers this approach rather than a transparotid or submandibular approach, both of which tend to be associated with a greater risk for facial nerve injury. This dissection is carried behind

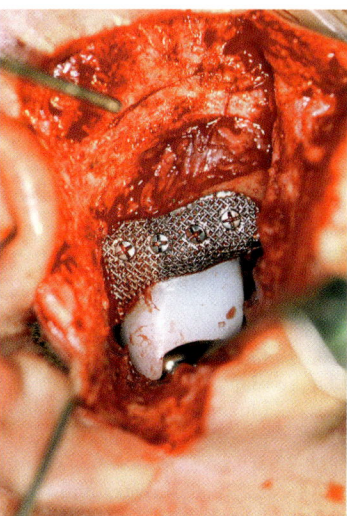

Fig. 99-4 ■ Total joint replacement.

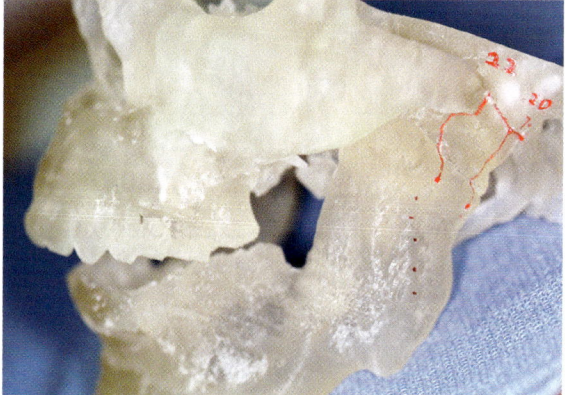

Fig. 99-5 ■ Three-dimensional model of the ankylosis.

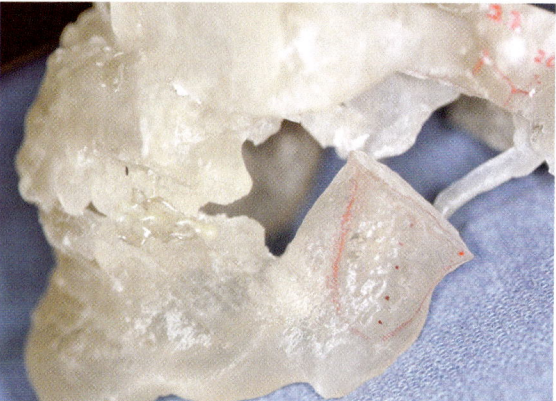

Fig. 99-6 ■ Gap arthroplasty on a three-dimensional model.

the parotid gland anterior to the sternocleidomastoid muscle. Dissection proceeds easily to the level of the posterior belly of the digastric muscle, which defines the medial extent of the dissection. In so doing, the parotid gland and branches of the facial nerve are swept forward and superiorly. Access to the mandibular angle is good, and dissection proceeds laterally in a subperiosteal plane. It is important to expose the entire ramus to facilitate placement of the ramal prosthesis. The fossa and ramus prosthesis may be soaked in a topical antibacterial solution prior to insertion. Attention should next be given to placing the patient back in MMF if it has been released. While maintaining the strictest sterility, attention can then be directed to the preauricular incision. The fossa component can be placed in the correct position and held with either finger pressure or the fossa-holding device through the retromandibular incision. This is then secured with several 2-mm screws. Attention can next be directed to the retromandibular incision. The ramal/condylar component should be positioned appropriately with careful attention to ensure that the condyle is seated in the most posterosuperior position within the fossa (Fig. 99-4). The component is then secured with bicortical 2-mm screws as determined during the planning and manufacture of the joints.

The decision to perform single-stage joint replacement should not be made without careful consideration of the nature of the ankylosis and the remaining anatomy. This requires a preoperative 3D stereolithographic model for planning (Fig. 99-5). Relatively normal anatomy of the mandibular ramus may allow the use of a stock prosthesis after the gap arthroplasty is performed. Stock prostheses require that the anatomy be altered so that the fossa and condyle components fit appropriately. When the anatomy is severely altered, a better choice is a custom-fit joint. This can be made from the preoperative 3D model and inserted during a single-stage surgery. The challenge lies in duplicating the surgery on the model in the patient (Fig. 99-6). The fit of the prosthesis depends on being able to do this with a fair degree of accuracy, which can be more challenging than anticipated.

The potential use of autologous fat should be considered if concern for heterotopic bone formation and recurrent ankylosis is great. The fat is easily harvested from the abdomen and packed around the condyle. The wounds are then closed in standard fashion.

POSTOPERATIVE CARE

HYPERMOBILITY

During the initial postoperative period the patient is encouraged to limit maximal mouth opening. Such limitation often occurs throughout the first few weeks secondary to pain, but the patient should be instructed to limit opening while eating and yawning. There is no advantage to limiting activity after the first 3 weeks, during which time adequate soft tissue healing and scarring will have occurred. Beginning in the fourth week, a structured program of physical activity should be implemented to prevent excessive fibrosis and limited opening. This is critical when arthroplasty or eminectomy has been performed but less important for extra-articular procedures such as the Dautrey procedure. Patients can usually manage their own therapy. Patients should open maximally by using the thumb and middle finger on the incisal edges of the anterior teeth to stretch, and this position should be held for 10 seconds. This should be repeated 10 times. Lateral excursive movements should also be performed. A hand is placed on the lateral aspect of the lower jaw, which is then displaced to the contralateral side to encourage ipsilateral condylar translation. This should also be held for 10 seconds and repeated 10 times. The exercise should be performed bilaterally if surgery was bilateral. All of these exercises should be repeated at least six times a day. These exercises should produce mild discomfort only. The use of moist heat and non-steroidal anti-inflammatory medication before physical therapy can be a tremendous advantage.

ANKYLOSIS

The postoperative period following release of ankylosis is as important as the surgical procedure itself. The physical therapy regimen listed for hypermobility is typically inadequate for ankylosis. Furthermore, it is potentially problematic if patients direct their own physical therapy without close monitoring. It is often advantageous to involve a physical therapist. Several devices have been manufactured to assist patients with physical therapy. All rely on patient compliance, which can be a problem, particularly in the pediatric population. TheraBite (Atos Medical, Inc., West Allis, Wisc.) and Dynasplint (Dynasplint, Severna Park, Maryland) are two mechanical exercises that can greatly improve outcomes by facilitating exercise activity. Despite the simplicity of these devices, regular tongue blades work exceedingly well but are time consuming and difficult to use. Their advantage is that once patients are instructed on how to use the blades, a more accurate picture of their MIO can be obtained by simply recording the number of blades used. In this regard it is easier to set goals and monitor patient progress. Physical therapy should begin in the immediate postoperative period, which means the day of surgery whenever possible. For total joint replacement, this is readily achievable and postoperative pain is often less than might be expected. The use of autogenous tissue for release of ankylosis can be a little more problematic in that pain may be greater and the inherent strength of the reconstruction weaker, at least in the initial postoperative period. This may limit early function, but nevertheless, early and aggressive physical therapy is imperative. Physical therapy should be continued for a minimum of 3 months. There is a group of patients in whom recurrent ankylosis will occur in the mid- and long-term postoperative period and physical therapy may be needed indefinitely. The difficulty is identifying this small patient population, although a previous history of recurrent ankylosis and significant heterotopic bone formation may be risk factors.

PEARLS AND PITFALLS

- Knowledge of normal anatomy is crucial.
- The Dautrey procedure requires that the zygomatic arch be displaced as far medially as possible and the condyle should not be able to subluxate anterior to the eminence when manipulated.
- Adequacy of the eminectomy procedure should be verified by ensuring that the condyle subluxates and easily returns to the glenoid fossa. This must be checked in non–muscle-paralyzed patients.
- When possible, enough bone should be removed from the gap arthroplasty to produce a "critical size" defect, which reduces the likelihood for subsequent recurrent ankylosis.
- Failure to adequately introduce and monitor postoperative physical therapy will probably result in consistently poor outcomes in patients with ankylosis.

BIBLIOGRAPHY

Dautrey J: Reflections sur la chirugie de l'articulation temporomandibulaire, *Acta Stomotol Belg* 72:577-581, 1975.

Dautrey J, Pepersack W: Functional surgery of the temporomandibular joint, *Clin Plast Surg* 9:591-601, 1982.

Guven O: A clinical study on treatment of temporomandibular joint chronic recurrent dislocations by a modified eminoplasty technique, *J Craniofac Surg* 19:1275-1280, 2008.

Kaban LB, Perrott DH, Fisher K: A protocol for management of the temporomandibular joint ankylosis, *J Oral Maxillofac Surg* 48:1145-1151, discussion 1152, 1990.

López AC, MonjeGil F, Fernandez Sanromán J, et al: Glenotemporal osteotomy as a definitive treatment for recurrent dislocation of the jaw, *J Craniomaxillofac Surg* 24:178, 1996.

McKelvey LE: Sclerosing solutions in the treatment of chronic subluxation of the temporomandibular joint, *J Oral Surg* 8:225-236, 1950.

Mercuri LG: The use of alloplastic prostheses for temporomandibular joint reconstruction, *J Oral Maxillofac Surg* 58:70-75, 2000.

Myrhaug H: A new method of operation for habitual dislocation of the mandible. Review of former methods of treatment, *Acta Odontol Scand* 9:247-260, 1951.

Posnick JC, Goldstein JA: Surgical management of temporomandibular joint ankylosis in pediatric population, *Plast Reconstr Surg* 91:791-798, 1993.

Shorey CW, Campbell JH: Dislocation of the temporomandibular joint, *Oral Surg Oral Med Oral Pathol Oral Radiol Endod* 89:662-668, 2000.

Alloplastic Temporomandibular Joint Reconstruction

Chapter **100**

Louis G. Mercuri

Alloplastic temporomandibular joint (TMJ) reconstruction is an entirely biomechanical rather than biologic solution to severe and debilitating anatomic joint disease.[1] Modern reconstructive orthopedic surgery would be unthinkable without the availability of alloplastic total joint prostheses. In the 1960s, posed with the problem that resection arthroplasty was an uncertain procedure with common complications such as recurrent deformity and limited motion, Sir John Charnley developed a successful low-friction total joint replacement (TJR) device.[2] Since that time, with the evolution of surgical techniques, implant materials, and designs, excellent long-term function and improvement in quality of life have been reported, along with device survival rates exceeding 90% after 10 years.[3,4]

Based on evidence from the orthopedic, biomedical engineering, and oral and maxillofacial surgery literature, this chapter discusses the role that total alloplastic reconstruction can play as salvage in the management of patients with severe and debilitating anatomic TMJ disorders to improve mandibular function and overall quality of life.

ETIOPATHOGENESIS/CAUSATIVE FACTORS

The following are the presently accepted indications for TMJ TJR[5]:
1. Inflammatory arthritis involving the TMJ that is not responsive to other modalities of treatment
2. Recurrent fibrosis or ankylosis (or both) not responsive to other modalities of treatment
3. Failed tissue grafts (bone and soft tissue)
4. Failed alloplastic joint reconstruction
5. Loss of vertical mandibular height or occlusal relationships (or both) because of bone resorption, trauma, developmental abnormalities, or pathologic lesions

PATHOLOGIC ANATOMY

Severe pathology associated with mandibular dysfunction and anatomic distortion of the TMJ complex dictates the need for TJR. Because of the multifaceted composition of the TMJ complex and its reliance on coordinated masticatory muscle function, it is an unreasonable expectation that a reconstructed TMJ can be returned to its "normal" premorbid function. Thus, there will always be some functional disability involved in any reconstructed joint, either autogenous or alloplastic.

In a multiply operated patient with an anatomically distorted joint reconstruction, chronic neuropathic pain will be a major component of that patient's disability. Therefore, it is important for both the surgeon and the patient to understand that the primary goal of any type of TMJ reconstruction is restoration of objective mandibular function and form. Any subjective pain relief gained must be considered only of merely secondary benefit.[6]

DIAGNOSTIC STUDIES

A detailed history and head, neck, and oral examination, including evaluation of the occlusion and any oral orthotic devices that the patient has been using, are important. This should be followed by a careful review of any previous imaging (plane films, magnetic resonance imaging, computed tomography) available to determine the need for further imaging to correlate any findings with the chief complaint, history, and clinical examination.

Appropriate laboratory studies may be required, such as in patients suspected of having high inflammatory arthritic disease.[6]

Unmounted and mounted study models are helpful in determining compensatory changes in the occlusion that may necessitate orthodontic management before reconstruction. Severely compromised occlusal or skeletal relationships (or both) must be considered and planned for correction because they will affect mandibular stability after reconstruction and the longevity of alloplastic devices as a result of abnormal wear forces.[7]

Past and recent clinical photographs are helpful in determining the onset of conditions such as unilateral condylar hyperplasia/hypoplasia and apertognathia associated with pathology or previous TMJ surgery.[6]

Present and previous medical and dental records can provide useful information in preparing for future reconstructive surgery and anesthesia, especially in patients with a long history of narcotic use for controlling pain or management in a pain clinic.

If there is any concern regarding the patient's preoperative psychological state, thorough evaluation by a psychologist or psychiatrist familiar with patients with TMJ disorders is essential before any reconstruction is undertaken. Unrealistic expectations of pain control and functional or esthetic results must also be considered and dealt with accordingly.[6]

PRESURGICAL CONSIDERATIONS

Presurgical diagnostic local anesthetic (without vasoconstrictor) blocks of the joint or masticatory muscles (or both) may be performed to try to determine the cause of the pain, as well as to demonstrate the concept of centrally mediated pain to the patient.[6]

Presurgical use of botulinum toxin or muscle relaxants and physical therapy such as ultrasound can be considered, but to date no studies have provided any data that these treatments are helpful in decreasing postoperative masticatory muscle pain in such cases.

TREATMENT/RECONSTRUCTIVE GOALS

Regardless of whether the TMJ is reconstructed with alloplastic, allogeneic, or autogenous material, the following should be the management goals[8]:

1. Improve mandibular function and form
2. Reduce suffering and disability
3. Contain excessive treatment and cost
4. Prevent morbidity

SPECIFIC TREATMENT AND TECHNIQUES

INFLAMMATORY ARTHRITIS INVOLVING THE TEMPOROMANDIBULAR JOINT THAT IS NOT RESPONSIVE TO OTHER MODALITIES OF TREATMENT

Since inflammatory arthritis involves a local synovial-mediated destructive systemic disease process and complete synovectomy cannot be achieved, the orthopedic literature opts for TJR in these cases because the results are very predictable.[9]

In the TMJ, alloplastic reconstruction has been discussed at length.[1,5,8,10-14] All of these authors agree that when the mandibular condyle is extensively damaged, degenerated, or lost, as in arthritic conditions, replacement with either an autogenous graft or alloplastic implant is an acceptable approach to achieve optimal functional and symptomatic improvement.

However, dissatisfaction with some of the facets of autogenous costochondral grafting, particularly in patients with high inflammatory arthritic disease (e.g., rheumatoid arthritis) (Fig. 100-1) and resultant ankylosis, led to the development and use of TMJ TJR devices, and data can be evaluated to support good results with such treatment.[9,12,14]

RECURRENT FIBROSIS OR BONY ANKYLOSIS NOT RESPONSIVE TO OTHER MODALITIES OF TREATMENT

The traditional management of complete bony TMJ ankylosis has been gap arthroplasty with an autogenous tissue graft or alloplastic hemiarthroplasty reconstruction (Fig. 100-2).[5] Although autogenous grafting techniques develop form, mandibular function is typically delayed. Since graft mobility during healing will compromise its incorporation into the host environment or compromise its blood supply, early mandibular mobility often leads to graft-host interface failure[15] and a high incidence of recurrent ankylosis.[16]

For patients with recurrent ankylosis, placing autogenous tissue such as bone into an area where reactive or heterotopic bone is forming intuitively makes no sense. Orthopedic surgeons will typically opt for total alloplastic joint reconstruction in similar situations involving other joints.[17]

Autogenous fat transplantation appears to be a useful adjunct because its use seems to minimize the reoccurrence of joint heterotopic calcification and consequently provides improved and consistent range of mandibular motion.[18]

FAILED TISSUE GRAFTS (BONE AND SOFT TISSUE)

The biology of autogenous tissue grafting requires that the host site have a rich vascular bed for success. Unfortunately, the scar tissue always encountered in a multiply operated patient does not provide an environment conducive to the predictable success of free and occasionally vascularized autogenous tissue grafts. Marx reported that capillaries can penetrate a maximum thickness of 180 to 220 μm of tissue whereas scar tissue surrounding previously operated bone averages 440 μm in thickness.[5] This may account for the clinical observation that free autogenous tissue grafts, such as cartilage, costochondral, and sternoclavicular grafts, often fail in multiply operated patients or those with extreme anatomic architectural discrepancies resulting from pathology (e.g., failed autogenous material).

Therefore, in light of the fundamental biologic issues discussed and reported, TMJ cases involving multiply operated patients, failed previous alloplastic materials, and anatomically distorted and severe intra-articular pathology should be reconstructed with a total alloplastic device to achieve optimal outcomes (Fig. 100-3).

FAILED ALLOPLASTIC JOINT RECONSTRUCTION

Because of osteolysis around failed alloplasts and the resultant anatomic discrepancies in the host bone architecture, it is difficult to adapt and secure autogenous material stably to the distorted anatomic remnants of either the fossa or ramus. Furthermore, the foreign body giant cell reactions associated with failed or failing devices provide a poor environment for the introduction of an autogenous graft.[19]

Orthopedists and biomedical engineers have been studying the effect of failed and failing devices on the long-term outcomes of future implanted alloplastic devices (Fig. 100-4). It is now questioned—and yet to be answered—whether failure of a previously implanted device in some patients results in a cell-mediated immune response that bodes poorly for the outcome of any future implanted alloplastic device.[20,21]

LOSS OF VERTICAL MANDIBULAR HEIGHT OR OCCLUSAL RELATIONSHIP BECAUSE OF BONE RESORPTION, TRAUMA, DEVELOPMENTAL ABNORMALITIES, OR PATHOLOGIC LESIONS

Loss of posterior mandibular vertical dimension because of developmental abnormalities, pathology, and traumatic injury results in a discrepancy in occlusion of the teeth. This is manifested as either an anterior (bilateral loss) or lateral (unilateral loss) open-bite deformity. These situations can be managed by diagnosing the cause of the problem and correcting it at the site of the pathology. In the case of a primary TMJ cause, joint reconstruction rather than osteotomy should be considered.[7] Once again, the reconstructive surgeon must take into consideration the nature of the pathology, the patient's previous local surgical history, and the state of the host bone architecture before deciding on the type of TMJ reconstruction (Fig. 100-5).

POSTOPERATIVE CARE

Returning the joint or joints and muscles of mastication to function as soon as possible postoperatively enhances healing and decreases the development of intra-articular scar tissue that will compromise mandibular range of motion.[22] One of the biggest advantages of alloplastic over autogenous TMJ replacement is the ability to start active physical therapy immediately postoperatively with any of the commercially available jaw-exercising devices (Box 100-1).

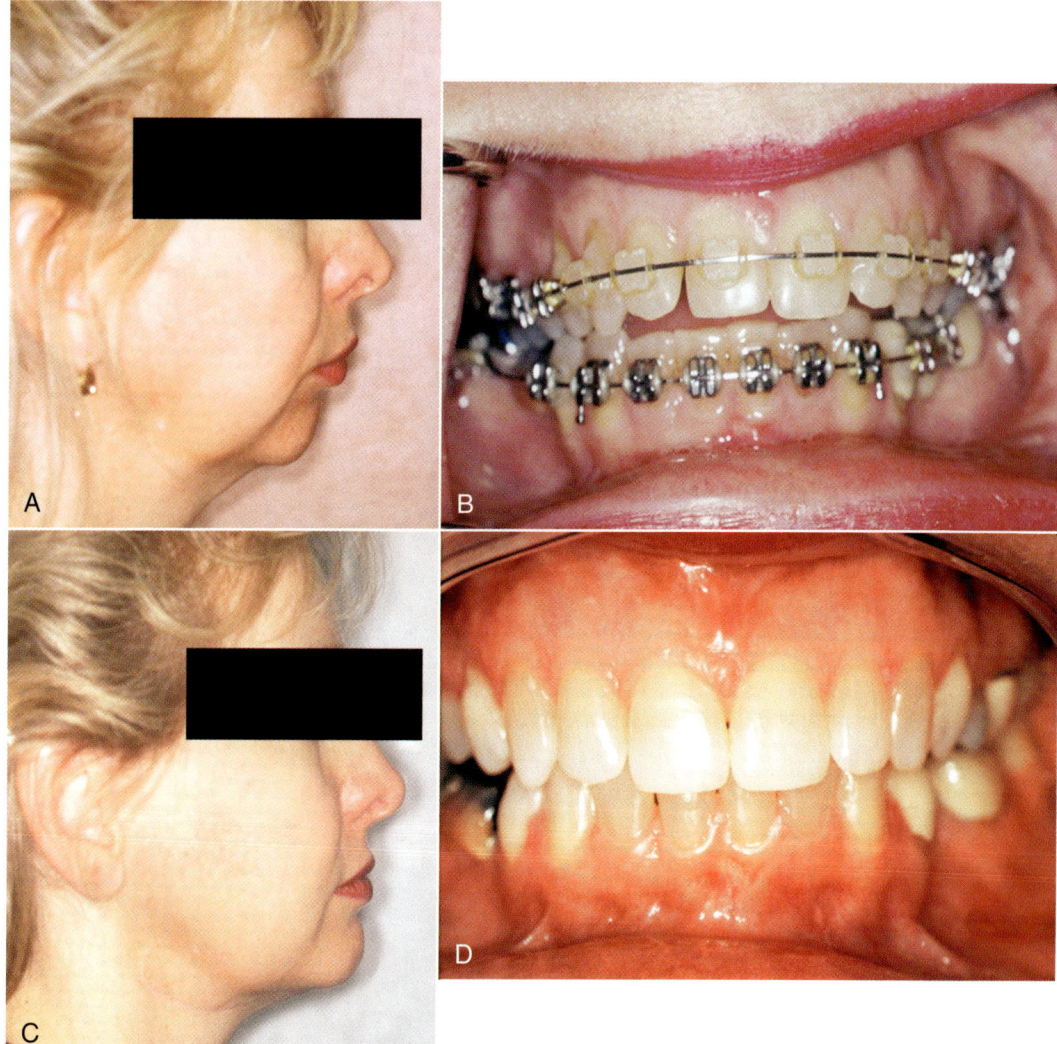

Fig. 100-1 ■ Patient with high inflammatory rheumatoid arthritis. **A** and **B,** Before bilateral total temporomandibular joint replacement (TMJ TJR). **C** and **D,** One year after two-piece Le Fort I maxillary osteotomy and bilateral TMJ TJR.

BOX 100-1	**Instructions for Use of the TheraBite (Atos Medical, West Allis, Wisc.) for Performing Jaw Exercises after Total Temporomandibular Joint Replacement**

1. *Do not* change the settings yourself or have the physical therapist change them.
2. *Do* bring the TheraBite to each follow-up visit. Your doctor will change the settings, depending on your progress.
3. Set aside five times during each day, until told otherwise, during which you can exercise without interruption.
4. Start by applying warm moist heat to the side(s) of your face on which surgery was performed. The heat should be concentrated over the large muscles at the angle(s) of the lower jaw and the side(s) of the head on the same side. This should be done for 20 minutes before exercising. Some patients find it advantageous early in the course of this therapy to take analgesic medication as prescribed at the beginning of this phase of the cycle.
5. Use the TheraBite as you were directed. Do 3 sets of stretch and hold exercises 3 times each for a total of 5 minutes.
6. After completing your exercise sets, apply an ice bag over the same areas that the heat was applied in step 4. Keep the ice in

place for 20 minutes. This step will tend to minimize the swelling that may accompany this exercise regimen, as well as decrease postexercise muscle spasm and pain.

7. While your sutures are in place, be sure that you keep the anti-biotic ointment over the suture line to protect it during steps 4 and 6. At the completion of your exercise regimen, be sure that the incision line is clean and dry. Pat dry with a clean towel and reapply the antibiotic ointment.
8. Immediately following suture removal and for the next 5 days, follow the regimen recommended in step 7. Thereafter, the oint-ment applications can cease, but be sure that the incision line is kept clean.
9. You are to use your TheraBite regimen along with whatever exercises your physical therapist recommends to supplement your convalescence.
10. Call your doctor if you have any questions or if problems arise during or after your Therabite regimen.

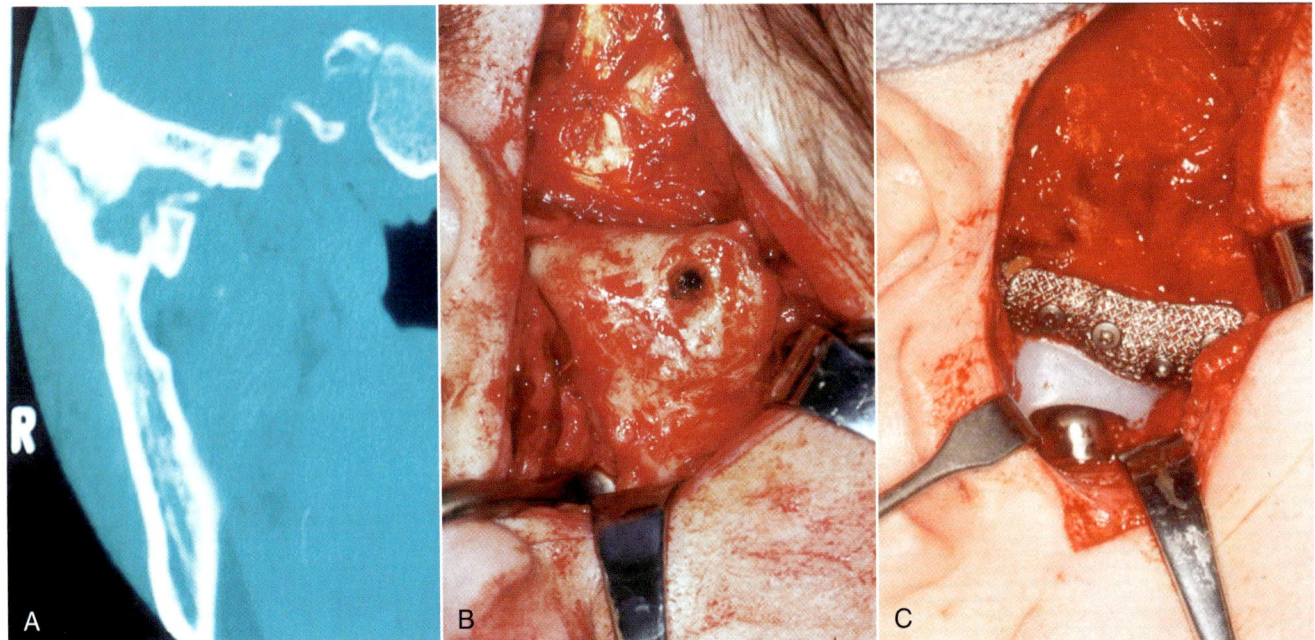

Fig. 100-2 ■ Right temporomandibular joint (TMJ) ankylosis after trauma. **A,** Coronal computed tomography scan before total joint replacement (TJR). **B,** Intraoperative view of the ankylosis. **C,** Patient fitted with a TJR device (TMJ Concepts, Ventura, Calif) on the right TMJ.

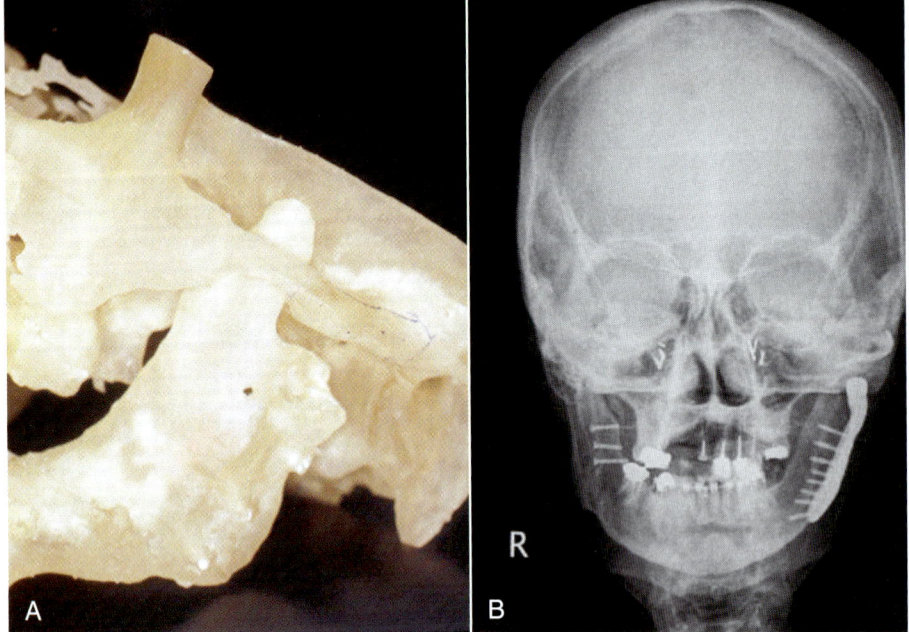

Fig. 100-3 ■ **A,** Stereolaser model of the left temporomandibular joint (TMJ) 3 years after a failed rib graft. Note the coronoid hyperplasia. **B,** Patient fitted with a total joint replacement (TJR) device (TMJ Concepts, Ventura, Calif) on the left TMJ. Note that the ultrahigh-molecular-weight polyethylene component of the fossa is radiolucent.

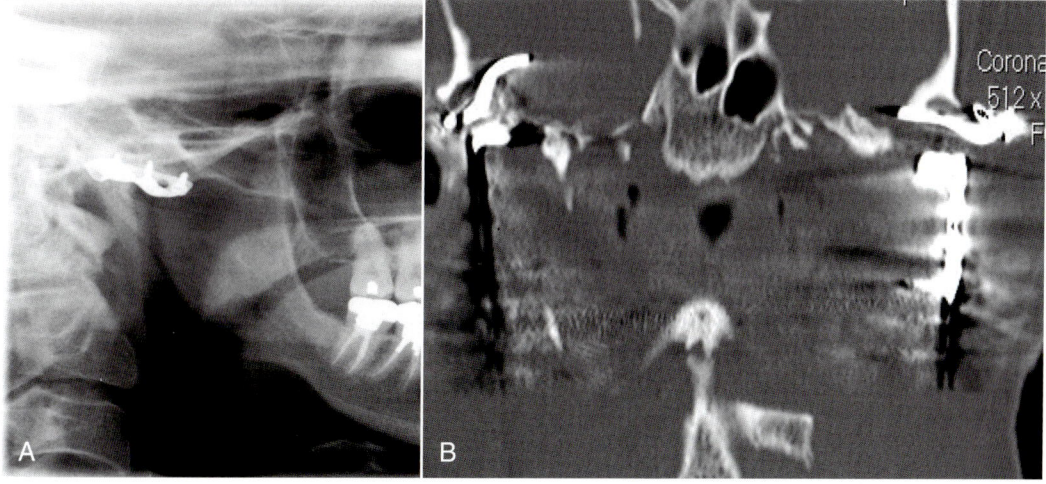

Fig. 100-4 ■ **A,** Failed right temporomandibular joint (TMJ) fossa-eminence device with the condyle-condyloid process of the mandible resorbed 5 years after implantation. **B,** Bilateral metal fossa components of a stock polymethylmethacrylate-on-metal device that migrated into the middle cranial fossa over a 7-year period.

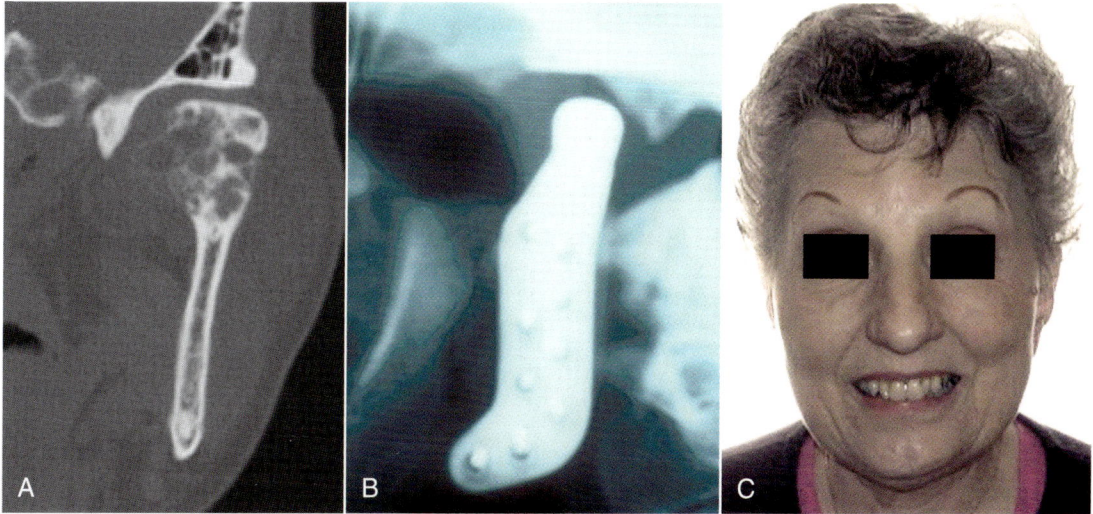

Fig. 100-5 ■ **A,** Coronal computed tomography scan of low-grade fibrosarcoma of the left temporomandibular joint (TMJ). **B,** Orthopantomogram of a patient fitted with a total joint replacement (TJR) device (TMJ Concepts, Ventura, Calif) on the left TMJ after left coronoidectomy. Note that the ultrahigh-molecular-weight polyethylene component of the fossa is radiolucent. **C,** Patient 1 year postoperatively.

Appropriate analgesics, oral antibiotic coverage for 7 to 10 days postoperatively, and muscle relaxants for patients experiencing significant masticatory muscle spasms during jaw exercising are important.

Another advantage of alloplastic TMJ replacement is the ability of patients to escalate the consistency of their diet as their mandibular function increases with the jaw exercises. The only restriction should be chronic gum chewing. The repetitive nature of this action adds additional unnecessary wear potential to the surfaces of these devices over time and provides no apparent functional advantages.

In patients with admitted or clinically identifiable parafunctional habits (i.e., occlusal attrition, scalloped tongue), construction of an oral orthotic to be worn after TMJ reconstruction is essential for maintaining the longevity of these devices. Stress and strain on the components of any alloplastic TMJ device will increase wear and decrease functional life.

PEARLS AND PITFALLS

- Alloplastic TMJ reconstruction is an entirely biomechanical rather than biologic solution to severe and debilitating anatomic joint disease.
- Modern reconstructive orthopedic surgery would be unthinkable without the availability of alloplastic total joint prostheses.
- Alloplastic TMJ reconstruction is a salvage procedure used for the management of patients with severe and debilitating TMJ anatomic disorders to improve mandibular function and their overall quality of life.
- Because of the complex nature of joint function and its related muscle function, it is not a reasonable expectation that a reconstructed joint can be returned to its "normal" premorbid function.
- Both the surgeon and patient must understand that the primary goal of TMJ reconstruction is restoration of objective mandibular function and form; any subjective pain relief gained must be considered only a potential secondary benefit of the reconstruction.
- Severely compromised occlusal relationships must be corrected because they will affect mandibular stability after reconstruction and the longevity of alloplastic devices as a result of abnormal wear forces.

- For patients with recurrent ankylosis, placing autogenous tissue such as bone into an area where reactive or heterotopic bone is forming makes no sense intuitively.
- In light of the fundamental biologic issues discussed and reported, TMJ cases involving multiply operated patients, failed previous alloplastic materials, and anatomically distorted and severe intra-articular pathology should be reconstructed with a total alloplastic device to achieve optimal functional outcomes.
- The biggest advantages of alloplastic over autogenous TMJ replacement are the ability to start active physical therapy immediately postoperatively with any commercially available jaw-exercising device, thus mitigating the healing fibrosis that limits potential mandibular range of motion, and the ability of these devices to provide a predictable and stable reconstruction after restoration of mandibular posterior vertical height lost as a result of joint pathology.
- Stress and strain on the components of any alloplastic TMJ device will increase wear and decrease functional life; therefore, patients with destructive parafunctional habits should use an oral orthotic.

REFERENCES

1. Mercuri LG: The use of alloplastic prostheses for temporomandibular joint reconstruction, *J Oral Maxillofac Surg* 58:70-75, 2000.
2. Charnley J: *Low friction arthroplasty of the hip: theory and practice*, London, 1979, Springer-Verlag.
3. Salvati EA, Wilson PD Jr, Jolley MA, et al: A ten-year follow-up study of our first one hundred consecutive Charnley total hip replacements, *J Bone Joint Surg Am* 63:753-767, 1989.
4. Schulte KR, Callaghan JJ, Kelley SS, et al: The outcomes of Charnley total hip arthroplasty with cement after minimum of twenty-year follow-up. The results of one surgeon, *J Bone Joint Surg Am* 75:961-975, 1993.
5. Mercuri LG: Alloplastic temporomandibular joint reconstruction, *Oral Surg Oral Med Oral Pathol Oral Radiol Endod* 85:631-637, 1998.
6. Mercuri LG: Temporomandibular joint disorders. In Kwon PH, Laskin DM, editors: *Clinician's manual of oral and maxillofacial surgery*, ed 3, Chicago, 2001, Quintessence.
7. de la Coleta KE, Wolford LM, Gonçalves JR, et al: Maxillo-mandibular counter-clockwise rotation and mandibular advancement with TMJ Concepts total joint prostheses. Part I—skeletal and dental stability, *Int J Oral Maxillofac Surg* 38:126-138, 2009.
8. Mercuri LG: The TMJ Concepts patient fitted total temporomandibular joint reconstruction prosthesis. In Donlon WC, editor: *Temporomandibular joint reconstruction, Oral and Maxillofac Surg Clin North Am*, Philadelphia, 2000, Saunders.
9. Mercuri LG: Surgical management of TMJ arthritis. In Laskin DM, Greene CS, Hylander WL, editors: *Temporomandibular joint disorders: an evidence-based approach to diagnosis and treatment*, Chicago, 2006, Quintessence, pp 455-468.
10. McBride KL: Total temporomandibular joint reconstruction. In Worthington P, Evans JR, editors: *Controversies in oral and maxillofacial surgery*, Philadelphia, 1994, WB Saunders.
11. Kent JN, Misiek DJ: Controversies in disc condyle replacement for partial and total temporomandibular joint reconstruction. In Worthington P, Evans JR, editors: *Controversies in oral and maxillofacial surgery*, Philadelphia, 1994, WB Saunders.
12. Donlon WC, editor: *Total temporomandibular joint reconstruction. Oral Maxillofac Surg Clin North Am*, vol 12. Philadelphia, 2000, WB Saunders.
13. Wolford LM, Dingworth DJ, Talwar RM, et al: Comparison of 2 temporomandibular joint prosthesis systems, *J Oral Maxillofac Surg* 61:685-690, discussion 690, 2003.
14. Mercuri LG, Edibam NR, Giobbie-Hurder A: 14-Year follow-up of a patient fitted total temporomandibular joint reconstruction system, *J Oral Maxillofac Surg* 65:1140-1148, 2007.
15. Matsuura H, Miyamoto H, Ishimura J, et al: Effect of partial immobilization on reconstruction of ankylosis of the temporomandibular joint with autogenous costochondral graft, *Br J Oral Maxillofac Surg* 39:196-203, 2001.
16. Saeed NR, Kent JN: A retrospective study of the costochondral graft in TMJ reconstruction, *Int J Oral Maxillofac Surg* 32:606-609, 2003.
17. Petty W, editor: *Total joint replacement*. Philadelphia, 1991, WB Saunders.
18. Mercuri LG, Alcheikh Ali F, Woolson R: Outcomes of total alloplastic replacement with peri-articular autogenous fat grafting for management of re-ankylosis of the temporomandibular joint, *J Oral Maxillofac Surg* 66:1794-1803, 2008.
19. Henry CH, Wolford LM: Treatment outcomes for temporomandibular joint reconstruction after Proplast-Teflon implant failure, *J Oral Maxillofac Surg* 51:352-358, discussion 359-360, 1993.
20. Black J: Systemic effects of biomaterials, *Biomaterials* 5:11-18, 1984.
21. Hallab NJ, Mickecz K, Vermes C: Differential lymphocytic reactivity to serum derived metal-protein complexes produced from cobalt-chrome and titanium based implant alloy degradation, *J Biomed Mater Res* 56: 427-436, 2001.
22. RB Salter: *Continuous passive motion*, Baltimore, 1993, Williams & Wilkins.

Current Treatment of the Effects of Juvenile Idiopathic Arthritis on the Facial Skeleton

Chapter 101

Robert W.T. Myall, R. Bryan Bell

Juvenile idiopathic arthritis (JIA) is a chronic childhood disease that can have a profound effect on growth and development of the facial skeleton. An understanding of the disease and its therapy is necessary before gathering the necessary data to plan therapy and subsequent medical and surgical treatment. This chapter reviews the current knowledge.

ETIOPATHOGENESIS

JIA affects an estimated 300,000 children in the United States and thus constitutes one of the five most common classes of chronic illness in childhood.[1] Diagnosis depends on the medical history, physical examination, and elimination of other diagnoses. Inflammation needs to begin before the patient reaches the age of 16 years, and the symptoms must last from 6 weeks to 3 months with limitation of joint motion accompanied by heat, pain, or tenderness. There are no confirmatory blood tests. JIA is characterized by unpredictable flares during which children may experience an abrupt exacerbation of symptoms.[2] Its effect on growth is multifactorial and includes not only the disease itself but also side effects of medications, altered nutrition, and mechanical problems.[3] Local growth disturbances occur as a result of inflammation and the accompanying increase in vascularity, which may result in either overgrowth or undergrowth of the affected site. In the maxillofacial region, micrognathia, malocclusion, facial asymmetry, and limited mouth opening are known common sequelae. They result mainly from changes in vascularization and destruction of a growth site in the mandibular condyle.[4]

Many names have been ascribed to the pediatric type of chronic arthritis, including juvenile rheumatoid arthritis (JRA), juvenile chronic arthritis (JCA), and JIA. Although JIA is used by most specialists in pediatric rheumatology, other terms, especially JRA, are more common among non-specialist in the United States. There are several subtypes of JIA:

- Oligoarticular pauciarticular: involves fewer than five joints in its first stages and affects about half of all children with arthritis.
- Polyarticular: affects five or more joints and can begin at any age.
- Systemic onset: affects about 10% of children. It begins with repeating fevers with temperatures that can be 103° F or higher and is often accompanied by a pink rash that comes and goes. It may cause inflammation of the internal organs, as well as the joints. Joint swelling may not appear until months or even years after the fevers begin. Anemia and elevated white blood cell counts are also typical findings.
- Psoriatic arthritis: children have both arthritis and psoriasis or a strong family history of psoriasis.
- Enthesitis-related arthritis: a form of JIA that often involves the attachments of ligaments, as well as the spine. It is sometimes called a spondyloarthropathy.

PATHOLOGIC ANATOMY

The most important growth site of the mandible is located in the head of the condyle. Early destruction of its fibrocartilage cap can seriously affect mandibular development. Asymmetry between the two condyles is a common finding in JIA, especially at the onset of the disease.[5]

The relationship between condyle-ramus height, expressed as the condylar ratio, is significantly smaller in children with JIA than in unaffected children with class I or class II malocclusion.[6] The maxilla tends to be smaller in vertical dimensions and is also posteriorly rotated. This can be explained as a reaction to the decreased growth of the mandible or, alternatively, altered loading on the posterior regions of the maxilla.

In patients with unilateral condylar destruction, asymmetry develops with the chin deviating to the affected side and resulting in a shorter vertical dimension on the affected side.[6] A higher degree of mandibular retroposition and smaller mandibular dimensions are found in children with complete destruction of the head of the condyle than in those with partial destruction. Solow and Kreiborg suggested that lack of forward growth of the mandible initiates increased extension of the head in relation to the cervical column to maintain an adequate airway (Fig. 101-1).[7]

They proposed that this increased extension results in soft tissue stretching, which also has a restraining effect on facial development. It is also clear that earlier onset, long duration, and the degree of severity of the disease are directly correlated to extent of the maxillofacial abnormalities. Interestingly, Stabrun and colleagues found reduced mandibular growth in affected children without visible condylar lesions.[8] It is likely that early inflammatory alterations that did not cause any changes on conventional radiography have occurred in the jaw joints of these children. This further underlines the need to consider the use of magnetic resonance imaging (MRI) when jaw growth lags.[9]

Other soft tissue structures that are affected by this disease process are the muscles of mastication. Maximum molar bite force is reduced in children with JIA to about 60% of that recorded in healthy children. This in turn can influence craniofacial morphology during growth.[6]

DIAGNOSTIC STUDIES

The role of imaging has changed over time from not only demonstrating destruction of various portions of the stomatognathic system but also identifying changes with MRI before they are noticeable clinically.[10] It can detect synovial proliferation and joint effusion preceding the development of cartilage destruction and bone erosion. Muller and co-workers found that 63% of their cohort of patients with JIA had involvement of the temporomandibular joint (TMJ) demonstrated when MRI was used with a single dose of gadolinium-based contrast medium.[11] This in turn allows initiation of appropriate therapies at an earlier date with a resultant reduction in condylar destruction.

The most common conventional radiographic signs of arthritis of the TMJ are erosion and flattening of the condyle (Fig. 101-2). This ranges from small erosions on the superior bony surface to almost complete absence of the condylar head. Changes affect the condylar head much more frequently than the glenoid fossa. Reduction of the joint space, anterior displacement of the condyle in the fossa, osteophyte formation, subchondral cysts, and restricted translatory movement have also been described.[12]

Panoramic radiographs and computed tomography (CT) show a higher incidence of lesions in children with polyarticular onset than in those with pauciarticular or systemic-onset types.

MEDICAL TREATMENT

The overall treatment goal is to control symptoms, prevent joint damage, and maintain function. Children with polyarticular JIA whose joint swelling persists and who test positive for rheumatoid factor are more prone to the development of joint damage and may require more aggressive treatment.

The first line of treatment involves a non-steroidal anti-inflammatory drug (NSAID) such as ibuprofen (Motrin or Advil) or

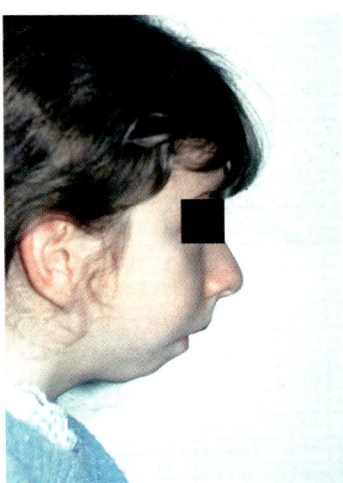

Fig. 101-1 ■ Morphological changes associated with untreated JRA involving the temporomandibular joints. Note severe retrognathism with short posterior facial height and downward and backward rotation of the maxillomandibular complex. Also note increased extension of the head in relation to the cervical column.

naproxen (Naprosyn) administered in a dose appropriate for the child. Younger children may be given liquid preparations or medications that require less frequent use. NSAIDs can cause gastrointestinal distress and should be taken with food.

Disease-modifying antirheumatic drugs (DMARDs) are added as a second-line treatment when the arthritis does not respond to NSAIDs. DMARDs include hydroxychloroquine (Plaquenil), sulfasalazine (Azulfidine), methotrexate (Rheumatrex), and more recently developed medications known as biologics, which include "anti–tumor necrosis factor agents." Nonetheless, because of consistent performance, methotrexate is still considered the "gold standard" against which all other agents are compared.

Control of the disease is of utmost importance when planning surgery because continued destruction of the mandibular condylar growth sites must be arrested before embarking on surgical-orthodontic treatment. This needs to be emphasized to the treating physician, the patient, and the immediate family.

Use of an intra-articular steroid (IAS) injection in joints other than the TMJ with oligoarticular JIA is an accepted therapeutic option. In a recent survey, use of these injections was second only to NSAIDs in the treatment of oligoarticular JIA. These steroids reduce inflammation quickly, and the effect can last for up to a year. Apparently, steroids reduce the amount of inflammation and pannus without adversely affecting hyaline cartilage.[13]

The effect that medical therapy, other than IAS injection, has on the TMJs has been investigated by a number of authors. Ince and associates noted that methotrexate therapy was effective in minimizing TMJ destruction and craniofacial dysmorphology in a group of patients with the polyarticular form of the disease.[3] In 1998, Pedersen reported that the inflammatory activity could be controlled by IAS injections but that there had been no controlled studies of this procedure on the TMJ in growing children.[14] He pointed out that it would be an important modality if inflammation could be detected and treated early, thereby avoiding destruction of the joint, increasing maximal incisal opening (MIO), and allaying other symptoms. He also noted that the TMJ is histologically different from other joints embryologically. It matures, grows, and is loaded differently. Consequently, there was a reluctance to transpose the experience of intra-articular injections in other joints to the TMJs.

Wenneberg and colleagues performed an 8-year study on the effects of IAS injection on the subjective and clinical dysfunction and the radiographic appearance of the TMJ in 16 patients.[15] Subjective symptoms and clinical signs were significantly reduced at follow-up examinations. The erosions of the bony articular margins that could be seen by standard radiographic techniques were found to be remineralized and associated with bony remodeling. These results suggest that IAS injections are beneficial and that

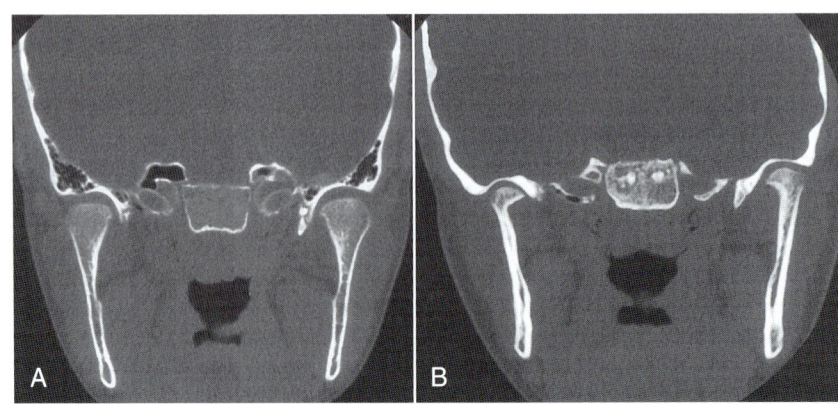

Fig. 101-2 ■ Comparison of normal condylar heads (**A**) with those affected by juvenile rheumatoid arthritis (**B**). (From Ueeck BA, Mahmud NA, Myall RWT: Dealing with the effects of juvenile rheumatoid arthritis in growing children, *Oral Maxillofac Surg Clin North Am* 17:467-473, 2005.)

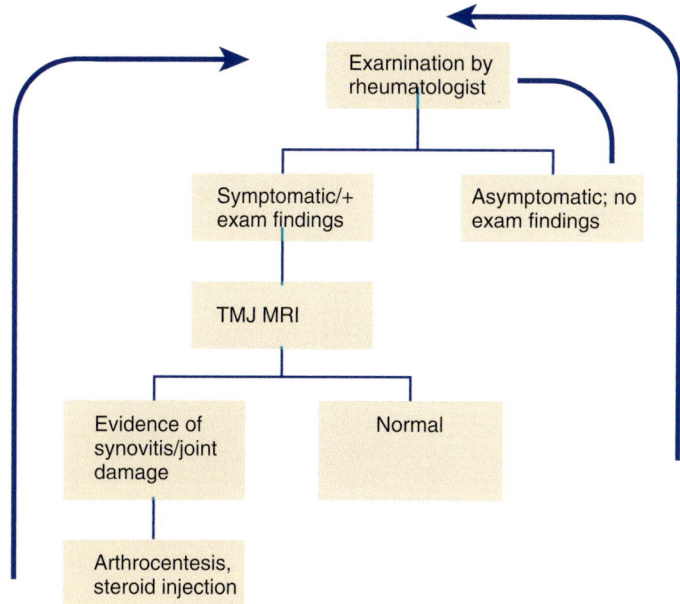

Fig. 101-3 ■ Treatment algorithm detailing the indications for intra-articular steroid injection for the treatment of juvenile idiopathic arthritis with temporomandibular manifestations.

improvement is demonstrated radiographically rather than an adverse effect.[13]

There have been two recent studies on the use of IAS injection. The first by Arabshahi and co-workers showed not only an increase in MIO but also a diminution in patient-reported symptoms.[16] Ringold and co-authors came to the same conclusion but also noted that there was little further improvement with the subsequent use of IAS following the initial injection.[17]

Emboldened by these favorable findings, our group has worked with rheumatologists to develop a protocol for the use of IAS injections to prevent the devastating sequelae of JIA with TMJ manifestations. Four years ago we initiated a protocol that was implemented on rheumatologist examination and clinical findings of TMJ pain, limited incisal opening, joint crepitus, deviation on opening, or other symptoms of TMJ dysfunction (Fig. 101-3). Patients undergo MRI of the TMJs if symptomatic. Evidence of synovitis or joint degeneration prompted arthrocentesis with the injection of 20 mg of triamcinolone hexacetonide. Patients are then examined by repeat MRI 6 months later, and the procedure is repeated until the symptoms and MRI evidence of synovitis are resolved or for a maximum of three to four injections. Preliminary results of this retrospective study suggest that TMJ manifestations are common (about 50% of all patients with JIA) and that IAS injection following arthrocentesis increases MIO and alleviates symptoms. The majority of gain in MIO seems to occur following the first injection, which is a favorable prognostic indicator. Improvement on MRI is typically seen, although complete resolution is not always manifested. Multiple injections seem to be safe in that we have not seen the type of auto-digestion that has been feared in the past. Further long-term studies are needed to assess the long-term benefits and risks associated with this promising new approach.

SURGICAL-ORTHODONTIC TREATMENT

First and most important, it must be established that the general disease process has been halted medically or is in remission. This is accomplished over time through a combination of clinical observation, radiographic imaging, and the use of serial cephalograms. The next important question is when would this individual best be served by surgical-orthodontic intervention. There is no clear-cut answer to this question, and all patients need their own careful assessment. The preponderance of clinicians will wait for cessation of growth. However, in patients with a functional deficit such as sleep apnea or psychosocial issues such as peer teasing, earlier intervention is warranted.[18] There is a small body of opinion favoring early intervention to help use the functional matrix.

Surprisingly little has been written about the orthodontic care of this group of patients. It is complicated by a number of issues, including limited mouth opening, reduced cervical spine motion, and painful large joints, which may prohibit sitting comfortably in the dental chair for protracted periods. Nonetheless, presurgical orthodontics is just as important as it is in patients without disease.

Profitt and colleagues make the point that treatment planning for developmental dentofacial deformities is different from that for acute and chronic disease.[19] They suggest that patients with JIA do not benefit from functional appliance therapy because the forces applied to the joint are more likely to accelerate the degenerative process than to reverse it. Pederson promotes the use of bite splints to gradually unload the joint, guide the mandible into the normal anterior rotational growth pattern, and change the position of the mandible.[14] Wenneberg and Kjellberg point out that others have found value in exercise and training of the soft tissues of the masticatory system.[20]

The next issue to address is anesthesia. Children with JIA have a number of problems that will challenge an anesthetist, and thus preoperative evaluation is mandatory. Restricted neck movement because of fused vertebrae, unstable cervical vertebrae, laxity at the atlantoaxial joint, minimal mouth opening, and micrognathia makes intubation a special challenge. It is suggested that extension and flexion radiographs of the cervical spine have a useful role to play in preoperative assessment (Fig. 101-4).

In patients who are thought to have some instability of the spine at the atlantoaxial joint, the use of intraoperative sand bags or similar means to support the neck and cranium is recommended. At the preoperative visit the anesthetist will also further evaluate the more global problems identified by the surgeon, such as pericarditis, pleuritis, anemia, and the side effects of the medications that the patient might be taking. Finally, comfort of the patient on the table has to be addressed, and pads, rolled towels, sand bags, and other stabilizing material can prevent over-rotation of the neck, overextension of the deformed joints, and neurovascular compression. Not all anesthetists realize that the jaw lengthening will facilitate early extubation postoperatively, and therefore it is well to discuss this early. However, if the anesthetist and surgeon, after conferring, have doubts about the propriety of extubation, the child can be left intubated overnight in the intensive care unit.[21-23] The next day the patient can be extubated over a stylet, thereby facilitating reintubation should it be necessary.

The surgical technique requires thorough understanding of the full spectrum of facial deformity. Every aspect of the problem must be appreciated—the soft tissue, TMJs, dentition, and bone. Furthermore, the variable and chronic nature of JIA can add to the difficulty in predicting and maintaining the inherent stability of this type of surgery. As noted previously, the timing of surgery is a matter of debate, but functional problems such as sleep apnea, as well as psychosocial issues, clearly point to the need to proceed. Otherwise, waiting for the cessation of growth has much to recommend it.

With regard to the mandible, as noted previously, JIA affects the entire mandible in both form and size and the associated soft

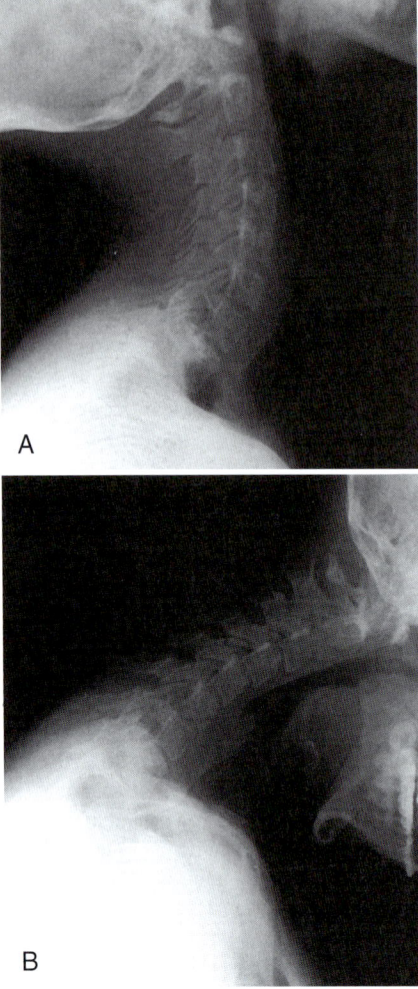

Fig. 101-4 ■ Extension (**A**) and flexion (**B**) radiographic views of the cervical spine. (From Ueeck BA, Mahmud NA, Myall RWT: Dealing with the effects of juvenile rheumatoid arthritis in growing children, *Oral Maxillofac Surg Clin North Am* 17:467-473, 2005.)

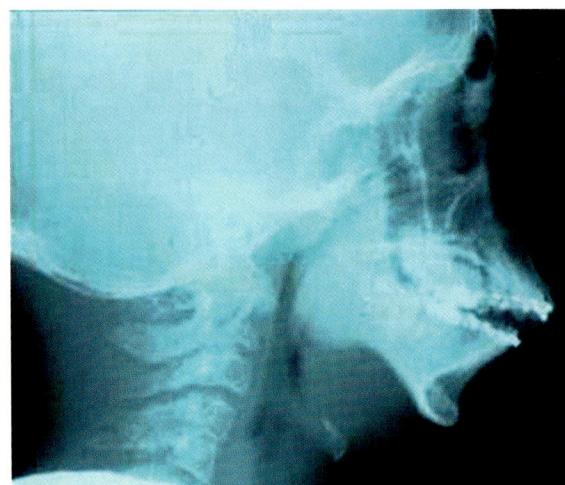

Fig. 101-5 ■ Lateral cephalometric radiograph demonstrating long-term skeletal changes associated with untreated JRA involving the temporomandibular joints. Note short ramus-condyle unit, high mandibular plane angle, and downward and backward rotation of the mandible with skeletal anterior open bite. (From Ueeck BA, Mahmud NA, Myall RWT: Dealing with the effects of juvenile rheumatoid arthritis in growing children, *Oral Maxillofac Surg Clin North Am* 17:467-473, 2005.)

tissues. The cranial base, maxilla, and dentition are also affected secondarily. There is reduced ramal height, a shortened body, retruding chin, steep mandibular plane angle, and frequently antegonial notching (Fig. 101-5).

The deformity progresses with age, and the continued clockwise rotation around the first and second molars results in further steepening of the mandibular plane with subsequent apertognathia and increased lower facial height.

A number of surgical approaches aimed at correcting mandibular micrognathia, either by lengthening the body or by lengthening the ramus, can be used. Standard osteotomies with or without bone grafts, costochondral grafts, and distraction osteogenesis have all been used. Sagittal split osteotomy in this situation was first described by Turpin and West in 1978 when an 11-year-old girl was treated successfully.[24] They have since published the results of her 14-year follow-up.[25] They showed that this technique had acceptable stability over time and most importantly was stable through her teenage years during psychosocial development. Since then, many others have used the sagittal split osteotomy successfully for the treatment of patients with JIA. The goal of the operation includes increasing the vertical height and horizontal length of the mandible.

Counterclockwise rotation of the mandible is often needed to correct the mandibular plane angle and anterior open bite. Rigid internal fixation, either with bicortical screws or with plates, is the fixation of choice.

Inverted L osteotomies with bone grafting can also be performed. This technique is particularly applicable when large movements are required to increase posterior facial height and close a large open bite. It is claimed that the resultant neck scars along with the pain and gait disturbance caused by bone harvest from the hip militate against this approach. The authors believe that a well-placed neck incision that is carefully closed is minimally evident and unsightly. Additionally, placement of a bupivacaine-soaked absorbable sponge in the iliac crest wound, as suggested by Dashow and associates, markedly reduces postoperative pain and decreases the duration of hospital stay and length of time until ambulation.[26]

Genioplasty with an osteotomy technique or augmentation with alloplastic material is required in many of these patients. Older alloplastic materials often led to relapse because they can resorb the underlying mandible. However, newer materials such as polytetrafluoroethylene are used widely in cosmetic surgery.[27] In patients with lack of angle show, augmentation with alloplastic material may be beneficial. These implants can either be custom-made or pre-formed. The decision to place these implants at the time of the initial surgery or as a secondary procedure depends on surgeon and patient preference.

Costochondral grafting attempts to correct the deformity and supply new growth sites, in addition to lengthening the mandible spontaneously. The involved condyles are resected and replaced with costochondral grafts that have a 2- to 3-mm cap of cartilage. However, this approach is not a panacea, as demonstrated in a case series by Svensson and Adell.[28] Not only is there undergrowth and overgrowth of the graft, but asymmetric growth also occurs as a result of the two sides growing at differing rates.

The use of distraction techniques for lengthening both the vertical and horizontal mandibular rami has been reported. Advocates of distraction promote the concept of "histogenesis" and claim that the soft as well as the hard tissues are treated. However, there have been reports of condylar resorption with such treatment.[29,30] The use of distraction for JIA is still evolving, and it should thus be used with caution.

Maxillary surgery can be accomplished at the Le Fort I level in most instances. When excess vertical maxillary growth has occurred, surgery to reduce this effect is performed. Intrusion of the maxilla reduces mid-facial height and is the method most commonly used.

Overall, several conventional techniques have been used successfully for the treatment of JIA. However, there are no randomized clinical trials and few data to guide selection of the technique. The difficulty comes in reconciling the deformity, the disease process, the growth status of the patient, and the planned surgical technique. Keeping in mind the difference between a child with JIA and one who is not afflicted puts the elaborate preoperative assessment, choice of surgical technique, and outcome and stability of surgery in perspective.

PEARLS AND PITFALLS

- JIA is a chronic childhood disease that has a multiplicity of effects on growth and development of the facial skeleton, as well as severe underlying systemic issues.
- Early recognition through careful clinical examination plus the use of CT and MRI leads to timely systemic medical treatment.
- Intra-articular corticosteroid injections can slow or stop condylar destruction and reduce discomfort, thereby allowing patients to continue functioning with the dentofacial deformity.
- In those in whom the effects of JIA on the TMJ have gone unrecognized, the resultant jaw discrepancies are amenable to a variety of surgical-orthodontic approaches.
- Timing is dictated by functional deficits, adverse psychosocial interactions, and control of the underlying disease.
- The care of this group of patients is very much in evolution and relies heavily on case series and extrapolation of standard approaches to dentofacial deformities.

REFERENCES

1. Sandstrom MJ, Schanberg LE: Peer rejection, social behavior, and psychological adjustment in children with juvenile rheumatic disease, *J Pediatr Psychol* 29:29-34, 2004.

2. Weiss JE, Ilowite NT: Juvenile idiopathic arthritis, *Pediatr Clin North Am* 52:413-442, 2005.

3. Ince DO, Ince A, Moore TL: Effect of methotrexate on the temporomandibular joint and facial morphology in juvenile rheumatoid arthritis patients, *Am J Orthod Dentofacial Orthop* 118:75-83, 2000.

4. Ueeck BA: Dealing with the effects of juvenile rheumatoid arthritis in growing children, *Oral Maxillofac Surg Clin North Am* 17:467-473, 2005.

5. Kuseler A, Pedersen TK, Gelineck J, et al: A 2 year followup study of enhanced magnetic resonance imaging and clinical examination of the temporomandibular joint in children with juvenile idiopathic arthritis, *J Rheumatol* 32:162-169, 2005.

6. Kjellberg H: Craniofacial growth in juvenile chronic arthritis, *Acta Odontol Scand* 56:360-365, 1998.

7. Solow B, Kreiborg S: Soft-tissue stretching: a possible control factor in craniofacial morphogenesis, *Scand J Dent Res* 85:505-507, 1977.

8. Stabrun AE, Larheim TA, Hoyeraal HM, et al: Reduced mandibular dimensions and asymmetry in juvenile rheumatoid arthritis. Pathogenetic factors, *Arthritis Rheum* 31:602-611, 1988.

9. Arabshahi B, Cron RQ: Temporomandibular joint arthritis in juvenile idiopathic arthritis: the forgotten joint, *Curr Opin Rheumatol* 18:490-495, 2006.

10. Weiss PF, Arabshahi B, Johnson A, et al: High prevalence of temporomandibular joint arthritis at disease onset in children with juvenile idiopathic arthritis, as detected by magnetic resonance imaging but not by ultrasound, *Arthritis Rheum* 58:1189-1196, 2008.

11. Muller L, Kellenberger CJ, Carnnizzano E, et al: Early diagnosis of temporomandibular joint involvement in juvenile idiopathic arthritis: a pilot study comparing clinical examination and ultrasound to magnetic resonance imaging, *Rheumatology* 48:680-685, 2009.

12. Pedersen TK, Jensen JJ, Melsen B, et al: Resorption of the temporomandibular condylar bone according to subtypes of juvenile chronic arthritis, *J Rheumatol* 28:2109-2115, 2001.

13. Sherry DD, Stein LD, Reed AM, et al: Prevention of leg length discrepancy in young children with pauciarticular juvenile rheumatoid arthritis by treatment with intraarticular steroids, *Arthritis Rheum* 42:2330-2334, 1999.

14. Pedersen TK: Clinical aspects of orthodontic treatment for children with juvenile chronic arthritis, *Acta Odontol Scand* 56:366-368, 1998.

15. Wenneberg B, Kopp S, Grondahl HG: Longterm effect of intra-articular injections of a glucocorticosteroid into the TMJ: a clinical and radiographic 8-year follow-up, *J Craniomandib Disord* 5:11-18, 1991.

16. Arabshahi B, Dewitt EM, Cahill AM, et al: Utility of corticosteroid injection for temporomandibular arthritis in children with juvenile idiopathic arthritis, *Arthritis Rheum* 52:3563-3569, 2005.

17. Ringold S, Torgerson TR, Egbert MA, et al: Intraarticular corticosteroid injections of the temporomandibular joint in juvenile idiopathic arthritis, *J Rheumatol* 35:6:1157-1164, 2008.

18. Leshem D, Tompson B, Britto JA, et al: Orthognathic surgery in juvenile rheumatoid arthritis patients, *Plast Reconstr Surg* 117:1941-1946, 2006.

19. Profitt WR, White RP, Sanver D: *Contemporary treatment of dentofacial deformity*, St Louis, 2003, CV Mosby, pp 200-201.

20. Wenneberg B, Kjellberg H: Effects of masticatory muscle training on craniomandibular disorders and bite force in children with juvenile chronic arthritis, *Clin Exp Rheumatol* 14:462-467, 1996.

21. Kohjitani A, Miyawaki T, Kasuya K, et al: Anesthetic management for advanced rheumatoid arthritis patients with acquired micrognathia undergoing temporomandibular joint replacement, *J Oral Maxillofac Surg* 60:559-566, 2002.

22. Skues MA, Welchew EA: Anaesthesia and rheumatoid arthritis, *Anaesthesia* 48:989-997, 1993.

23. Smith BL: Anaesthesia and Still's disease [letter]. *Anaesthesia* 40:209, 1985.

24. Turpin DL, West RA: Juvenile rheumatoid arthritis: a case report of surgical/orthodontic treatment, *Am J Orthod* 73:312-320, 1978.

25. Turpin DL: Juvenile rheumatoid arthritis: a 14-year posttreatment evaluation, *Angle Orthod* 59:233-238, 1989.

26. Dashow JE, Lewis CW, Hopper RA, et al: Bupivacaine administration and postoperative pain following anterior iliac crest bone graft for alveolar cleft repair, *Cleft Palate Craniofac J* 46:173-178, 2009.

27. Niamtu J III: Advantage of PTFE facial implants in cosmetic facial surgery, *J Oral Maxillofac Surg* 64:543-549, 2006.

28. Svensson B, Adell R: Costochondral grafts to replace mandibular condyles in juvenile chronic arthritis patients: long-term effects on facial growth, *J Craniomaxillofac Surg* 26:275-285, 1998.

29. Van Strijen PJ, Breuning KH, Becking AG, et al: Condylar resorption following distraction osteogenesis: a case report, *J Oral Maxillofac Surg* 59:1104-1107, discussion 1107-1108, 2001.

30. Turvey TA, Simmons K: Orthognathic surgery before completion of growth, *Oral Maxillofac Surg Clin North Am* 6:121-135, 1994.

THE PAST

Facial cosmetic surgery is a relatively new discipline in our field; it has propagated since the 1980s under the auspices of oral and maxillofacial surgery and owes its foundation to our expertise and experience in facial trauma, reconstruction, and orthognathic surgery. In the past the specialty has been challenged with respect to our training and qualifications for performing soft tissue cosmetic surgery. The antiquated arguments suggesting a lack of basic surgical training have been disregarded in view of our ability to perform complex facial reconstructions. The last decade has progressively put to rest the ability of oral and maxillofacial surgeons to safely and effectively perform facial cosmetic procedures given the appropriate additional training. Treatment of bone deformities or injuries bears fundamental differences with regard to soft tissue surgery. However, the facial anatomy is intricately related, and it is the combined knowledge of soft and hard tissue anatomy that has become essential in facial cosmetic surgery.

THE PRESENT

The modern practice of facial cosmetic surgery has not only improved and increased in its repertoire of procedures but has also been redefined by unification of skills within several specialties that encompass traditional soft tissue facial plastic surgery, orthognathic surgery, cosmetic dentistry and implants, dermatology, hair restoration, nutrition, and skin care. This gamut of subspecialties, which is not rooted in any one single specialty, has now been unified under the discipline of facial cosmetic surgery, although the full scope of procedures is seldom practiced by one individual surgeon. Oral and maxillofacial surgeons with the appropriate post-residency training are uniquely positioned to develop a comprehensive approach to facial cosmetics that includes skeletal, dental, and soft tissue esthetics. There are now an increasing number of formal facial cosmetic surgery fellowships in the United States for oral and maxillofacial surgeons that allow training in a wide spectrum of facial surgery, including rhinoplasty and eyelid and face-lift procedures.

THE FUTURE

The full incorporation of facial cosmetic surgery as a subspecialty of oral and maxillofacial surgery will require an output of literature on cosmetic surgery by our profession. The increasing interest in this field by future surgeons will invariably stimulate the academic and private sectors to contribute to the scientific advancement of surgical procedures and hence seat the profession deeper into this discipline. The involvement of the profession in multispecialty cosmetic surgery symposia and organizations on the forefront of cosmetic surgery will be essential. The future will bring improved procedures with less invasive methods, more permanent results, decreased downtime, and reduced risks. An area of significant improvement will be skin care and prevention. There will be an even greater and more effective line of products that slow down or even reverse the effects of cellular aging. Within a short span of time individuals will be able to walk into a laboratory and promptly obtain a map of their genome along with health care information and assessment of their risk for many diseases. This will put on the shoulders of humanity complicated ethical dilemmas; however, for esthetic surgery, it will result in a greater emphasis on prevention and lifestyle.

Chapter

102

Initial Assessment of Facial Cosmetic Surgery Patients

Husain Ali Khan, Shahrokh C. Bagheri

Oral and maxillofacial surgeons are in a unique position to further develop comprehensive skills for performing facial cosmetic surgery. Our expertise in orthognathics and facial bony structures forms the foundation for being able to provide the full scope of facial cosmetic procedures. The authors firmly adhere to the philosophy that evaluation of facial esthetics is deficient without considering both the hard and soft tissue structures of the face. Similarly, adhering exclusively to soft tissue (facial plastic) procedures while ignoring hard tissue (orthognathic) surgical procedures is most often a lack of understanding in modern facial cosmetic surgery.

The full scope of facial cosmetic surgery encompasses three disciplines: orthognathic surgery, dental implantology/prosthetics, and facial plastic surgery with cosmetic dermatology (Fig. 102-1). When possible, adjunctive dermatologic/skin care procedures are used to enhance the surgical results.

The first step in evaluation of a patient is to determine the chief complaint, which may relate to one of three categories:

1. An aging face
2. An acquired deformity of soft or hard tissues
3. A combination of both

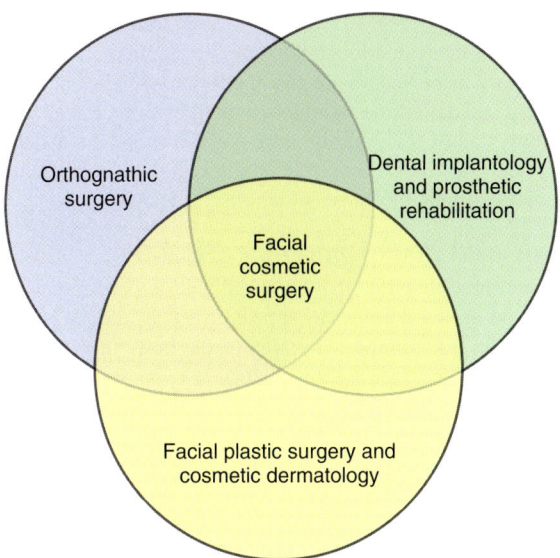

Fig. 102-1 ■ The full scope of facial cosmetic surgery encompasses three disciplines: orthognathic surgery, dental implantology/prosthetics, and facial plastic surgery with cosmetic dermatology.

ETHNIC, CULTURAL, AND GENDER DIFFERENCES

It is often said that beauty is in the eye of the beholder. However, the perception of beauty is continually evolving. As with fashion, our minds adapt to new trends and our eyes progressively break away from traditional patterns. The public often looks to actors, musicians, sports stars, and politicians to set trends in fashion and beauty.

Not unlike the fashion industry, the trends in cosmetic surgery are continually changing, although the general sentiment of youthful appearance is a common denominator. As cosmetic surgeons, it is extremely important to set aside our personal perceptions of beauty and surgical norms and understand the perspective of the patient. Cosmetic parameters for beauty have regional, ethnic, and cultural differences. The surgeon needs to consider the classic norms that pertain to a patient and must never compromise form for function. A successful cosmetic result with compromise of function is a failure.

When consulting with patients of a specific ethnicity, it is important to determine how much of their ethnicity they wish to preserve. In some cases, a patient may want to make only a minimal change in a particular feature (for example, a large dorsal hump or a wide alar base). A surgeon must quickly understand and be comfortable with the patient's expectations and desires for cosmetic surgery.

Today, cosmetic surgeons treat all aspects of the population. In the past, cosmetic surgery was considered to be "in vogue" only by wealthy female patients. Current cosmetic surgery encompasses all socioeconomic classes and genders. In fact, younger patients and male patients are increasingly interested in undergoing cosmetic surgery.

In addition to surgical and dermatologic cosmetic procedures, the surgeon should be an advocate of general preventive health care. The cosmetic consultation allows the opportunity to assess overall wellness, and it is our opinion that performing cosmetic surgery on patients who are not involved in an appropriate wellness program or do not make an active effort to improve their overall health may be counterproductive. Nutrition, exercise, and a healthy lifestyle are the foundations to successful cosmetic surgical interventions. Good nutrition and exercise optimize a person's cardiovascular system and improve cellular turnover. General facial and body appearance often dramatically improves with weight reduction, especially in the younger population. Patients who maintain their body mass index within healthy norms will generally be considered more attractive. In many instances, if overweight patients return to their optimal weight through diet and exercise, their appearance will improve greatly. This will also help the surgeon determine the extent of the cosmetic defect versus excessive weight. It is important for patients to be cautioned that most cosmetic surgical procedures (including body liposuction) are not for weight loss.

INITIAL CONSULTATION

Patient selection is one of the most difficult components of facial cosmetic surgery and is especially important for surgeons with less experience. Being able to understand patients and their needs is one of the most important skills that a surgeon can have. Occasionally, during an initial encounter with a patient, surgeons may be so excited to have a patient showing interest in undergoing a particular procedure that they forget to determine whether the patient is truly a candidate for cosmetic surgery. The surgeon must be thorough in the initial evaluation to determine whether the patient is psychologically and physically stable enough for surgery.

Interpretation of patient desires is the most important factor in determining patient satisfaction. A surgeon can perform a perfect operation, but if the results do not meet the patient's expectations, it will result in an unhappy patient. This is frequently due to inadequate preoperative interpretation of the patient's desire or unreasonable expectations that were not recognized. The ultimate goal is for the patient to be happy and the surgeon to be proud of the work completed.

It is fundamental that during the initial visit a trusting patient-doctor relationship be established to facilitate the patient's comfort and willingness to express goals and concerns regarding cosmetic surgery. Patients should be allowed to freely express their chief complaint without interruption. The presence of an assistant is highly encouraged. Asking open-ended questions such as "How can I help you?" or "What brings you to see us today?" allows patients to express their needs and concerns. Specific questions such as "Are you here to discuss the bump on your nose?" should be avoided. The examination and interview process are best done with access to mirrors to allow improved communication regarding facial anatomic regions.

PAST MEDICAL HISTORY

As with any other surgical procedure, a thorough medical history is imperative. Conditions that have an impact on wound healing (such as diabetes, autoimmune connective tissue disorders, hepatic and renal insufficiency) need to be managed adequately before committing to surgery. The cardiopulmonary status of the patient should be assessed for safe induction of general anesthesia. Uncontrolled hypertension should be managed preoperatively to avoid unstable swings in blood pressure and to aid in homeostasis and prevent hematoma formation.

Psychiatric illnesses should be noted and investigated before any surgical intervention. The following specific conditions and diagnosis should be noted.

Patients with Unrealistic Expectations

Such patients may be grouped into two general categories:
1. Patients who bring pictures of celebrities and request the surgeon to transform their face similar to the image. They may bring

magazine photographs of models with chiseled features or a particular feature that they want the surgeon to mimic.

2. Patients who request drastic changes such that the face would become disproportionate. These patients often seek the opinions of multiple surgeons.

Obsessive-Compulsive Patients

Perfectionists fall into this category. These patients are usually well dressed and are often overly compulsive when arranging the initial examination. They have usually been treated by other surgeons and have complaints about them. They may have a long list of unrealistic questions. These patients magnify any minor imperfection or asymmetry and demand immediate revision surgery. Perfectionist are, by nature, never happy with themselves and will never be happy with the surgical result.

"I Want to Have the Surgery Immediately" Patients

Such patients wish the surgeon to perform the surgery immediately. They feel no need for a proper evaluation and put tight time limits on the surgeon. They generally have little patience with the surgeon's efforts to be thorough during the examination and do not want to hear or care about complications or any possibility of a poor surgical outcome. Usually, these patients have had some previous underlying psychological event.

Indecisive Patients

These patients have often had multiple consultations and are unclear about which procedure they want. They are uncertain whether they really want to undergo a procedure and often prefer the surgeon to take a paternalistic rather than an autonomous approach toward decisions, frequently stating "do whatever you think is best." They are usually seeking cosmetic surgery because of a suggestion of a relative or career advisor. The hallmark of these patients is that they are vague about what would make them happy. Surgery is frequently scheduled, canceled, and rescheduled again.

Rude Patients

Such patients are generally pleasant to the surgeon, but when dealing with office assistants and hospital staff, they can be pushy and demeaning and demand preferential treatment. These unpleasant traits generally surface during the initial evaluation as inappropriate, unpleasant behavior.

Overly Flattering Patients

These patients are generally full of compliments and praise the surgeon's expertise and reputation. With careful probing, the surgeon might determine that the patient has had previous consultations and outcomes that were not satisfactory. They often travel great distances to see the surgeon, with little background knowledge of the doctor or practice. Surgeons should be careful because these patients can quickly turn on them if the surgical outcome has minor imperfections. The compliments may turn to anger.

Patients with a Minimal or Imagined Deformity

At first, most surgeons would agree that a small modification of a minimal deformity might result in a perfect outcome. This may not be the case, though, when dealing with a patient who is overemphasizing a minor deformity. In the mind of this type of patient, a minor deformity can seem as large as a major deformity. These patients are often looking for perfection, and the surgeon must be very careful not to fall into this trap.

Depressed Patients

During the initial evaluation and history, the surgeon must be aware of any history or present diagnosis of depression. The social history of a patient can determine stability in a patient's life. Facial cosmetic surgery may only temporarily improve the mood of a depressed patient, but it rids the patient of the underlying cause. Evaluation by a therapist is prudent in these situations.

Patients with Body Dimorphic Disorders

Body dimorphic disorder (BDD) is defined as preoccupation with an imagined or slight defect in appearance that leads to significant impairment in functioning. Any area of the body may be of center of concern. Some studies show that up to 7% women who seek cosmetic surgery meet the criteria for BDD. There is a 2% prevalence in the general public. Reports have shown that the majority of patients with BDD do not benefit from cosmetic surgery, and in some cases, patients have become violent toward themselves or the surgeon. If a surgeon has any suspicions preoperatively that a patient may suffer from BDD, psychological evaluation may be indicated to rule out BDD.

Patients with Eating Disorders

Patients with anorexia and bulimia generally have a poor self-image and are underweight with altered nutritional status. These patients can be at risk during the perioperative period. Extreme caution has to be taken to screen for this type of patient. When dealing with patients with possible eating disorders, an important question is whether they are happy and satisfied with their current weight. Weight fluctuations in some patients can be very noticeable in the face. Significant weight fluctuations can be due to underlying metabolic or psychological disorders. Red flags should be raised if a patient has lost more than 10 lb in the past year or is constantly changing diets. Some cosmetic surgeons will advise their patients that if they plan to lose more than 10% of their body weight, they should defer surgery until their weight has stabilized. It has been shown that patients who exercise regularly bounce back from surgery much quicker than those who have a sedentary lifestyle. In an aging face, both weight gain and weight loss can give a perception of increased age.

Other Issues

Other important factors include the amount of sun exposure, history of sunburn, and the use of sunscreen. Risk factors for skin cancer should be considered. A history of hypertension and blood dyscrasias must be thoroughly investigated. Postoperative hematoma formation during face-lift procedures, periorbital hematoma and bleeding during blepharoplasty, or postoperative nasal bleeding can be complications of undiagnosed coagulopathies or prolonged uncontrolled elevated blood pressure. Blood dyscrasias can be discovered through the family history or a history of increased bruising or prolonged bleeding after a dental extraction.

In cases in which a patient has undergone a recent traumatic event (loss of job, divorce, loss of a loved one), it may be wise to delay surgery until emotional stability has been achieved. The use of herbal supplementation must be thoroughly investigated since some constituents may affect the coagulation cascade. Patients at high risk for deep venous thrombosis should be recognized, and appropriate preventive protocols should be followed. The use of potent anticoagulants such as warfarin and clopidogrel should be discontinued or the dose reduced in conjunction with the primary care or other involved medical specialist. It is also recommended that aspirin products and non-steroidal anti-inflammatory drugs be discontinued, as well as herbal and health supplementations (e.g.,

TABLE 102-1	Glogau Classification of Photoaging			
GROUP	CLASSIFICATION	TYPICAL AGE	DESCRIPTION	SKIN CHARACTERISTICS
I	Mild	28-35	No wrinkles	Early photoaging: mild pigment changes, no keratosis, minimal wrinkles, minimal or no makeup
II	Moderate	35-50	Wrinkles in motion	Early to moderate photoaging: early brown spots visible, keratosis palpable but not visible, parallel smile lines beginning to appear, wearing some foundation
III	Advanced	50-65	Wrinkles at rest	Advanced photoaging: obvious discolorations, visible capillaries (telangiectases), visible keratosis, wearing heavier foundation always
IV	Severe	60-75	Only wrinkles	Severe photoaging: yellow-gray skin color, previous skin malignancies, wrinkles throughout (no normal skin), cannot wear makeup because it cakes and cracks

vitamin E, *Ginkgo biloba*, St John's wort) 2 weeks before the procedure. Isotretinoin should also be discontinued because it may delay wound healing.

SOCIAL HISTORY

Numerous studies have shown poor wound healing and complications in wound healing to be associated with smoking. Patients should be educated on the importance of smoking cessation. If complete cessation cannot be achieved, a minimum of 2 weeks with no exposure to tobacco products is warranted. A history of alcohol abuse or dependence should be investigated before surgical treatment.

PAST SURGICAL HISTORY

Previous anesthetic and surgical complications are investigated. The number of previous cosmetic surgical procedures, including revisions, should be noted. Patients who have undergone multiple cosmetic procedures, especially for the same anatomic location, should be approached with extreme caution.

PHYSICAL EXAMINATION

Physical examination of the aging face focuses on features different from those in individuals with acquired defects of the face and supporting structures (skeleton, cartilage, muscle, and skin). In this chapter we emphasize the basic concepts since detailed examination of specific facial structures is discussed elsewhere in this text.

Examination of a patient desiring facial cosmetic surgery takes place after a thorough consultation and determination of the patient's chief complaints. We prefer to examine the patient in front of a three-way mirror. A wall mirror with aid of a handheld mirror is also adequate.

Although every surgeon has a different approach, it is recommended that a systematic method that addresses all areas of concern be used. The examination also allows the patient to point out areas of interest that may not have been addressed during the consultation. Once the surgeon understands the patient's needs and complaints, recommendations can be offered that may achieve the patient's goals. Our examination consists of an assessment of the hard tissue (skeletal features) structures (frontal bone, zygoma, maxillomandibular complex). The dentition and occlusion are examined for anterior dental esthetics, dentofacial deformities (e.g., maxillary hypoplasia/hyperplasia), and Angle classification. The soft tissue is examined for signs of laxity, hyperdynamic lines, and fat distribution in the forehead, periorbital areas, mid-face, mandible, and neck.

BOX 102-1	Causes of Facial Aging

- Ultraviolet exposure
- Loss of subcutaneous fat or redistribution of fat
- Changes in the intrinsic muscles of facial expression
- Effects of gravity from loss of elasticity
- Remodeling of the underlying skeleton and cartilage

BOX 102-2	Fitzpatrick's Sun-Reactive Skin Types

- Type I (very white or freckled)—always burn
- Type II (white)—usually burn
- Type III (white to olive) —sometimes burn
- Type IV (brown)—rarely burn
- Type V (dark brown)—very rarely burn
- Type VI (black)—never burn

Finally, the skin is assessed for signs of photoaging, general skin health, and absence of pathology.

Examination of the skin should distinguish photoaging from signs of aging caused by loss and atrophy of subcutaneous fat, redistribution of fat, or atrophy of the muscles of facial expression (Box 102-1). The extent of photoaging can be determined with the Glogau scale (Table 102-1). The Fitzpatrick scale is useful to determine which cosmetic dermatologic procedure is best suited for a particular skin type (Box 102-2). Certain peels and laser treatment work better with certain Fitzpatrick types. Thickness quality and quantity, the amount of mobility, the sebaceous glands, and hypopigmentation/hyperpigmentation are important factors to document when examining the skin. It is also important to make notation of previous surgical scars, and all suspicious precancerous lesions must be thoroughly investigated.

More detailed examination of facial structures is discussed elsewhere in the text. However, the sequence and some important features are emphasized in the following sections.

FACIAL SKELETON

Radiographic views (including panoramic and lateral cephalometric radiographs), along with a full series of photographs, can be obtained to evaluate the facial skeleton. If the surgeon believes that the dentition may play an extensive role in the procedure, obtaining mounted study models will be beneficial in planning treatment. If alloplastic implants are part of the treatment plan, a full dental examination is necessary to rule out any oral or dental pathology. If custom alloplastic implants are part of the treatment plan, a computed tomography scan may be necessary.

When the chief complaint is an acquired facial or dental deformity, the surgeon must first determine whether the underlying pathology involves the skin, cartilage, facial skeleton, or dentition. If a dental deformity is involved, the surgeon should refer the patient to the appropriate dental specialist (e.g., prosthodontist, orthodontist).

HAIR

A basic examination of the hair should be documented. Color, quality, and density should be determined. It is especially important to note hairline position and balding patterns if the treatment plan includes a brow- or face-lift. Sideburn position should also be documented. Asking a few questions about the patient's grooming habits could be helpful in determining future results.

EYES AND NOSE

For periorbital procedures, examination of the eye, orbit, and adnexa is compulsory. The examination should begin with a visual acuity test. For rhinoplasty, many computer software programs are available that can simulate the postoperative results; however, specific outcomes as outlined by the software may be difficult to duplicate precisely. Rhinoplasty truly deals in four dimensions; the fourth dimension is the healing capability of the patient and the changes in soft tissue over time.

LIPS AND TEETH

The size, symmetry, and fullness of the lips should be noted. The position of the lips in repose and while smiling should be precisely documented in reference to the central incisors. Examination of the dentition, including alignment, color and size of the teeth, and previous cosmetic restorations, is noted. The smile line and its relationship to the alar base, gingival tissue, and nasolabial folds are evaluated.

At this point it is a good idea to discuss in detail with patients the likes and dislikes of their dentition and smile. Previous use of fillers and augmentation material for the lips and nasolabial folds can be further investigated at this time.

Mid-face fullness and convexity give the face a youthful appearance. The zygomatic and maxillary facial bones make up the malar eminence and are key facial landmarks. As a person ages, the effects of gravity and atrophy of fat cause the mid-face to descend, which results in deepening of the nasolabial fold. Loss of fat inferior and lateral to the orbital rims accentuates the "hollowed-out" appearance of aging.

Descent of the buccal fat pad as a person ages makes the inferior aspect of the cheeks appear fuller and creates jowling along the jawline. With age the inferior border of the mandible is less sharp, and jowling can be seen when the perimandibular soft tissue and fat descend downward. In edentulous patients this is further pronounced because of the decrease in mandibular width and height. Increased prominence of the submental crease and accumulation of submental fat give the chin a ptotic appearance.

From the lateral view a youthful neck features a cervicomental angle of 90 degrees or less. As a person ages, fat accumulates in the submandibular and submental areas. The increased laxity of skin and descent of the submandibular gland create a blunting of the cervicomental angle. Vertical bands in the anterior aspect of the neck develop as a result of dehiscence of the platysma muscle. This banding can be seen from the submental region to the clavicle.

The location of the hyoid bone should be examined. The ideal location is at the level of C4. An excellent esthetic result is difficult to achieve in patients who have a low hyoid bone or an obtuse cervicomental angle.

RADIOGRAPHS

Panoramic and lateral cephalometric radiographs are quick and economic tools for screening facial cosmetic surgery patients and planning surgical procedures. For example, a lateral cephalogram can aid in visualizing mandibular and chin position and identifying the mandibular plane. Finally, skeletal classification is useful in determining whether a chin implant or mandible-repositioning surgery can be used in conjunction with rhytidectomy or submental liposuction.

PHOTOGRAPHIC DOCUMENTATION

The photographic setup often differs among surgeons. A simple setup consisting of a camera and a clean background is sufficient; however, a sophisticated system with standardized lighting, size, and camera settings is beneficial. The extent of the photographic setup is determined by the specific needs of the surgeon, but most cosmetic surgeons find it extremely valuable to invest in high-quality office photography equipment.

It is the authors' opinion that photographs should be taken by the surgeon or by a trained assistant to ensure standardization of preoperative and postoperative images. Not only is this valuable when dealing with patients, but is also important for academic presentations and for possible publication.

The type of photographs and views required can vary depending on the planned surgical procedure. The authors' standardized set of photographs includes a frontal view, left and right lateral and oblique views, and a worm's eye view (which allows the surgeon to visualize the alae and nostrils). If a hair transplant is part of the treatment plan, views focusing on the hairline and scalp should be obtained. For orthognathic surgery, intraoral views are essential.

SUMMARY

Cosmetic surgery is no longer for just the wealthy sector of the population. In fact, the majority of procedures today are performed on working-class individuals. In the past 10 years there has been an estimated greater than 450% increase in cosmetic surgery. This is in part due to improvements in non-invasive techniques and related products.

The future of cosmetic surgery will continue to be driven by advancements in biocompatible materials, improvement in lasers and resurfacing techniques, improvement in health and wellness techniques, understanding of hormone replacement therapies, genetic manipulation and how it can be applied to hair regeneration, skin reproduction, and weight management. Although many philosophic debates will ensue, it is feasible that in time gene therapy could eliminate obesity and weight-related diseases.

The future for facial cosmetic surgery is exciting for both the patient and the surgeon as the multiple specialties in both medicine and dentistry continue to add to the advancements in the field. There is no one specialty that can meet all the surgical needs for patients, as is evident by the many developing fellowship training programs that cross-train specialists to a common goal.

The true art of cosmetic surgery is matching the correct procedure with the patient. The only way to accomplish this objective is to understand the patient, the patient's personality and expectations, and how one's capabilities can best accomplish the goal.

PEARLS AND PITFALLS

- Surgeons must embrace the fact that cosmetic surgery procedures are elective and that patients who enter their office can continue to live their lives well without the procedure.
- Surgeons must be careful to not talk a patient into any procedure. We should not "push" surgery; patients should request procedures.
- Establishing a comfortable and trustworthy relationship is very important because it will help both the patient and the surgeon through the difficult postoperative period.

- If a surgeon determines that a patient is not mentally or physically able to handle the surgery, procedures must be deferred.
- All surgeon must know their own individual capabilities and plan procedures and operate within these parameters.

BIBLIOGRAPHY

Obagi S, Bridenstine JB: Chemical skin resurfacing, *Oral Maxillofac Surg Clin North Am* 4:541-553, 2000.

Tang H, Brissett AE: Preoperative assessment of the aging patient, *Facial Plast Surg* 22:85-90, 2006.

Tardy EM: *Rhinoplasty: the art and the science*, St Louis, 1996, WB Saunders.

Current Trends in Rhinoplasty

Chapter 103

Shahrokh C. Bagheri, Husain Ali Khan

Like any surgical procedure, the evolution of rhinoplasty is based on improved surgical techniques that survive the test of time and increasing patient expectations. As with most cosmetic procedures, the vast majority of advances in rhinoplasty are derived from teaching surgical experience to younger surgeons through operative training, textbooks, lectures, and symposia. The difficulty of performing randomized or prospective cohort studies and multicenter analysis for cosmetic procedures contributes to the progression of the field via traditional (non–research-based) modes of teaching. Cosmetic surgery is unique among other surgical specialties in that changing trends and racial and regional ethnic preferences drive patients to desire what is considered by them an esthetic result. In no other procedure are such differences as clear as in rhinoplasty. The surgery is individually customized with respect to current ethnic and cultural norms. In modern rhinoplasty, no single procedure or approach can provide such a vast array of patient desires for beauty and functionality. Surgeons must be armed with multiple techniques that are used in concert to give predictable results. Cosmetic rhinoplasty remains one of the most challenging facial cosmetic procedures, and this is unlikely to change despite many advances and changes in this field.

The goal of this chapter is to familiarize readers with the most current basic principles of diagnosis and treatment of rhinoplasty patients. It is not intended as a comprehensive review of the subject but rather to highlight the basic principles, current thinking, and variations in primary rhinoplasty procedures. Revision rhinoplasty is discussed in a separate chapter.

ETIOPATHOGENESIS/CAUSATIVE FACTORS

The desire to undergo rhinoplasty is generally dictated by several factors. Congenitally or acquired (via trauma) nasal deformities such as crooked, deviated, or collapsed nasal structures are common reasons for performing cosmetic rhinoplasty. Such deformities are frequently associated with functional disturbances (most commonly a deviated septum causing impaired airflow) that warrant combined cosmetic and functional septorhinoplasty. Patients' desire for a more attractive or "fashionable" nose is also an important factor. This standard is constantly changing, is largely dictated by media, and crosses all regional and ethnic barriers. Therefore, the need for nasal cosmetic surgery is driven by the combination of preexisting deformities and patients' request for a more esthetic nose.

SURGICAL ANATOMY

The surgical anatomy of the nose can be approached in layers from superficial to deep. The terminology for orientation of nasal anatomy is shown in Figure 103-1. Of distinction is the term *dorsum*, a Latin word that refers to the posterior aspects of a human body part. This is in contrast to the terminology for rhinoplasty, in which dorsum refers to the anterior part of the nasal bridge. The overlying skin of the dorsum and tip can have variable thickness, which can affect the final esthetic outcome. Very thick skin overlying the tip and dorsum can make tip and dorsal refinements less visible. It is important to note that the skin overlying the rhinion is generally thinner than that over the radix or bony dorsum, thus rendering this area susceptible to minor underlying postsurgical irregularities. This overlying skin plus soft tissue envelope (S-STE) has a rich blood supply inferiorly from the angular artery and superiorly from the supratrochlear extension of the angular artery with collateralization from the ophthalmic artery in the medial portion of the orbit. This blood supply is augmented by small branches from the infraorbital artery (itself a branch of the maxillary artery) and inferiorly from branches of the arteries of the nasal septum. There is considerable individual variation in vascular anatomy (especially venous). Venous drainage is via the angular and ophthalmic veins. This rich blood supply renders the nose resilient to vascular compromise despite extensive soft tissue elevation and the use of vasoconstrictors during open rhinoplasty techniques. The lower incidence of postoperative infection following open rhinoplasty using grafts and other alloplastic material in this clean-contaminated area is also evidence of the rich blood supply to this region. Nasal tip dehiscence after open rhinoplasty is rare but is usually due to pressure necrosis from nasal dressings or overzealous subcutaneous debulking of the soft tissue underlying the flap and not due to vasoconstriction. The nose has minor motor nerve innervation to the nostril, dorsum, and glabellar region, which has an impact on facial expression and opening of the nostrils during inspiration.

The sensory supply of the S-STE is bilateral from the infraorbital, supratrochlear, and branches of the ophthalmic nerves. The skin of the nasal tip and the lower nasal structures is innervated by the external nasal branch of the anterior ethmoidal nerve. Complete cutaneous anesthesia can be achieved by regional blocks of these nerves. The transcolumellar open rhinoplasty incision may disrupt the sensory innervations of the nasal tip, although this generally resolves within 1 year postoperatively. Careful subperichondrial dissection over the lower and upper lateral cartilage can minimize this minor functional sequela.

The underlying bony and cartilaginous structure includes the paired nasal bones that articulate with the frontal bone and the nasal processes of the maxilla. The piriform aperture is formed by the maxilla and paired nasal bones. The five major cartilages define the inferior nasal dorsum, tip, nostrils, and columella (Fig. 103-2). The cartilage is covered by a vascular perichondrium and connected via multiple ligaments that support the nasal architecture. Cartilage "memory" and its intrinsic spring mechanism make surgical changes in the lower third of the nose challenging.

DIAGNOSTIC STUDIES

Evaluation of a patient for rhinoplasty involves establishing a trusting relationship with the surgeon and interpretation of the patient's expectations. A large number of patients are unsatisfied because of insufficient preoperative discussion and clarification of their expectations. The surgeon has to be firm in redirecting or denying surgery for expectations that are unreasonable or surgically unobtainable.

Psychological assessment of the patient is also important for the success of cosmetic nasal surgery. The nose is the center of the face and has a significant impact on patient image and self-perception. It is important to realize that the presurgical period is well defined but postsurgical care is "infinite." Therefore, surgeons should use caution with patients who have previous or current psychological conditions that may compromise the results.

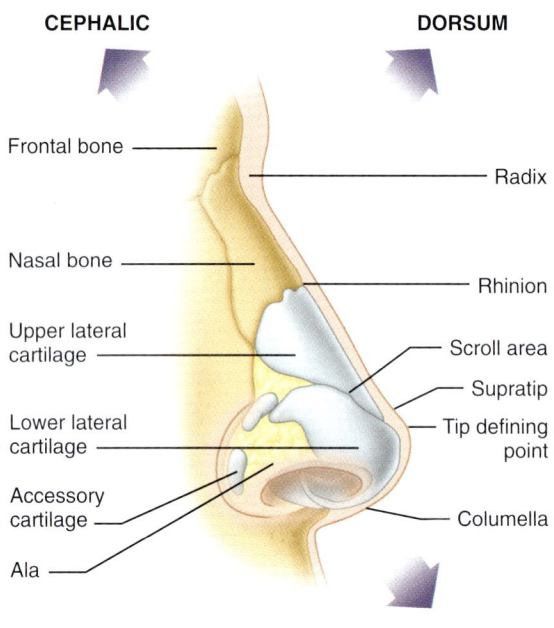

Fig. 103-1 ■ Anatomy of the nasal structures as seen in profile. (From Bagheri SC, Jo C: *Clinical review of oral and maxillofacial surgery,* St Louis, 2008, Mosby.)

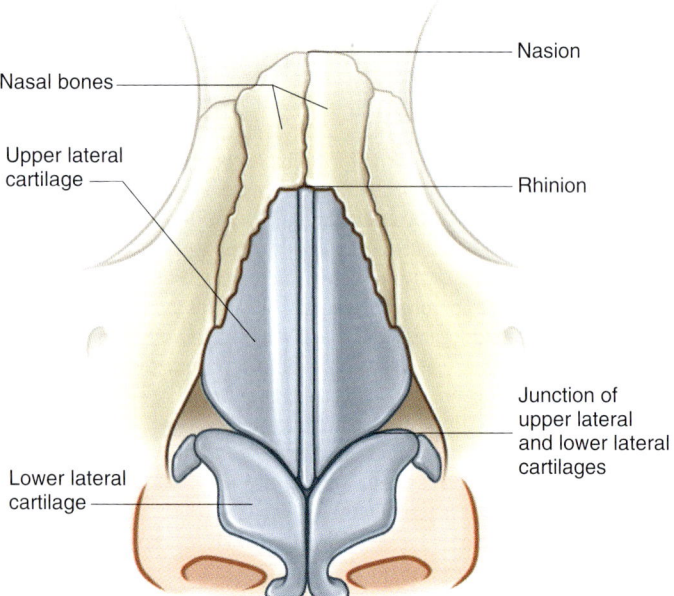

Fig. 103-2 ■ Frontal view of the nose without its skin and soft tissue envelope. (From Aston SJ, Steinbrech DS, Walden JL: *Aesthetic plastic surgery,* Philadelphia, 2009, Saunders.)

Physical examination of the patient includes evaluation of the skin overlying the mid-face. The presence of excessive facial acne, especially over the nasal tip, should be noted since the acne may be exacerbated by elevation of an open rhinoplasty flap. The thickness of the skin also affects the surgical procedure. Thick skin over the nasal tip, especially in a patient with a bulbous nose, can make tip modifications difficult. Debulking of the underlying flap is useful but limited because of compromise of the overlying skin as a result of excessive removal of soft tissue. Conversely, with very thin skin, caution should be exercised with tip modifications. Tip grafting may improve nasal projection; however, with very thin overlying S-STE, the graft may become cosmetically apparent or unappealing, particularly when the skin undergoes age-related changes. The surgeon must see beyond the immediate (1 year) postsurgical results to determine true success.

As with all other surgical procedures, the patient is screened for medical conditions, medications, and allergies that may have an impact on surgery. Appropriate medical judgment should be exercised when considering elective cosmetic rhinoplasty for patients with significant medical co-morbid conditions.

Standard photographic documentation is essential for nasal cosmetic surgery (Fig. 103-3). The nose and face are examined as a single unit to evaluate other facial features such as the cheek bones, chin, lips, and dental esthetics. The nose can be addressed by specific anatomic and functional parameters. The radix, dorsum, tip, nasal base, and septum are used by the authors as specific anatomic

regions that can be surgically modified for cosmetic improvement. This simplistic approach allows the development of a cosmetic treatment plan for each region that is organized into an overall surgical plan (discussed later in this chapter). The anatomy of the septum, turbinates, and overlying mucosa as they relate to nasal function is also noted. When needed, septoplasty and submucous resection of the turbinates are best performed in conjunction with cosmetic rhinoplasty.

TREATMENT/RECONSTRUCTIVE GOALS

Although endless possibilities of surgical techniques and subsequent alterations can be planned, the treatment and reconstructive goals are directly related to patients' desires and surgeons' surgical capabilities. Adherence to strict and careful diagnosis of the nasal deformities and development of a treatment plan will help identify the reconstructive goals. The treatment goals for each anatomic part of the nose are planned. Table 103-1 presents a list of anatomic regions of the nose that are considered in primary rhinoplasty, along with basic characteristics that can be altered by surgery. It should be recognized that surgical alteration of each anatomic area will have an impact on adjacent and all other areas of the nose. For example, reduction of the bony and cartilaginous nasal dorsum can decrease the necessity for nasal tip elevation or radix augmentation and therefore alter the amount of dorsal and tip modifications. The surgical plan is further customized to meet the patient's and surgeon's

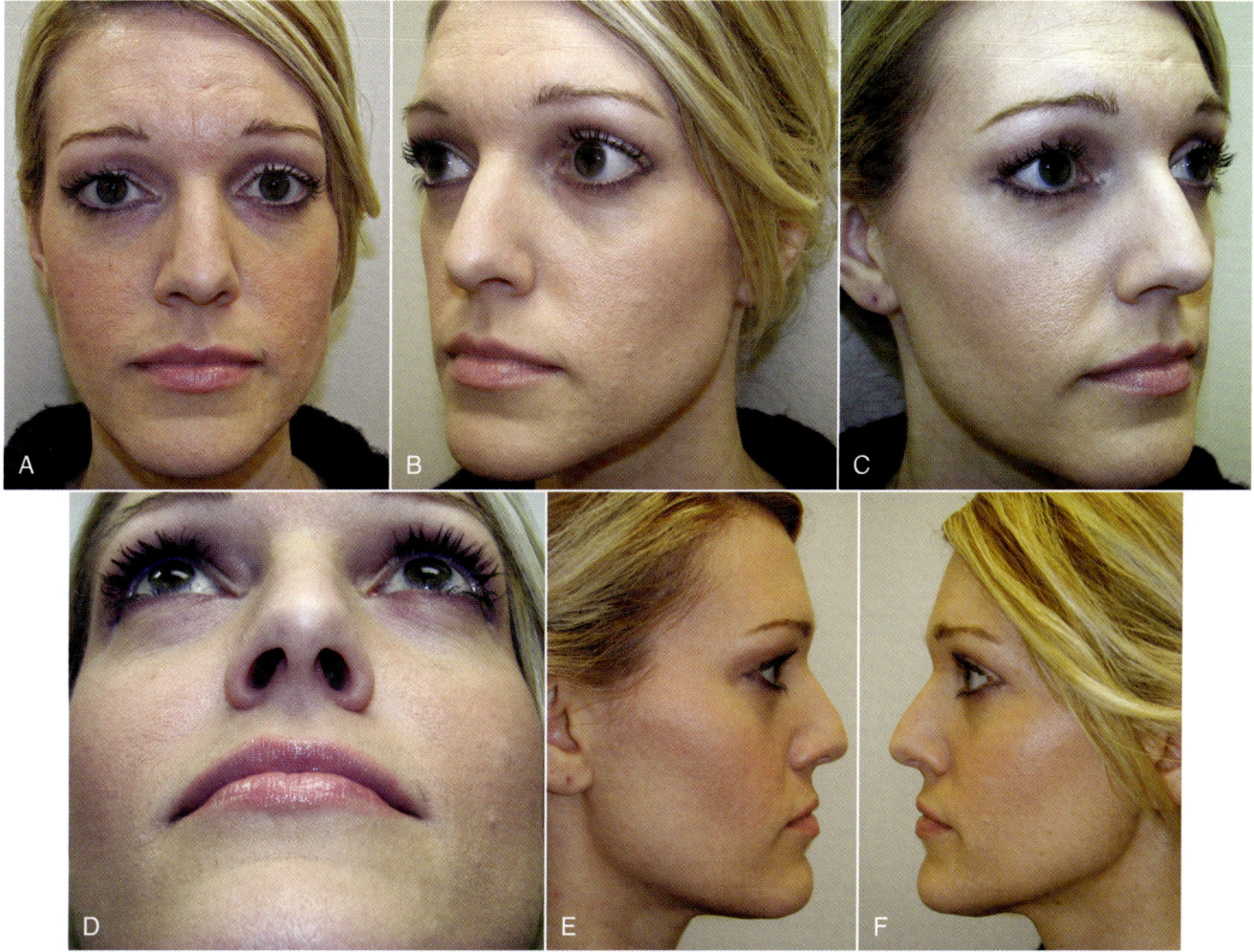

Fig. 103-3 ■ Standard preoperative photographs for rhinoplasty.

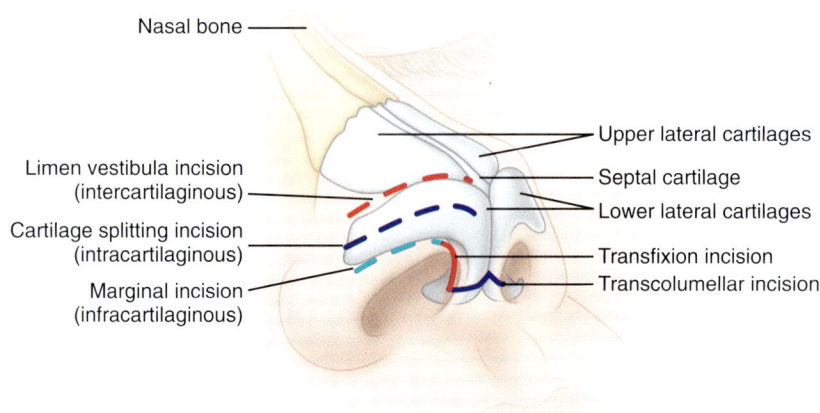

Fig. 103-4 ■ Common sites of incisions for rhinoplasty. (From Bagheri SC, Jo C: *Clinical review of oral and maxillofacial surgery*, St Louis, 2008, Mosby.)

Labels: Nasal bone; Upper lateral cartilages; Septal cartilage; Lower lateral cartilages; Limen vestibula incision (intercartilaginous); Cartilage splitting incision (intracartilaginous); Marginal incision (infracartilaginous); Transfixion incision; Transcolumellar incision

TABLE 103-1	Anatomic Regions of the Nose and Their Main Characteristics for Cosmetic and Functional Rhinoplasty
ANATOMIC REGION	**MAIN CHARACTERISTICS**
Radix	Location, size
Dorsum	Width, size, symmetry
Tip	Volume, projection, shape, definition, rotation, width
Nasal base	Alar base shape, nostril size, columellar anatomy, alar width, symmetry
Septum	Deviation, perforation
Turbinates	Size, obstruction of air flow, inflammation

cosmetic and reconstructive goals. In addition, the assessment of each area is further characterized in detail. For instance, the physician's assessment of a pronounced dorsum should distinguish abnormalities in both the frontal and profile view and can include the bony and cartilaginous components.

The goal of rhinoplasty is to achieve symmetry, nasal balance, and an attractive nose that meets the patient's individual and ethnic norms. Maintaining normal nasal function while achieving the cosmetic alteration cannot be overemphasized.

SPECIFIC TREATMENT AND TECHNIQUES

Regardless of the surgical technique, the success of rhinoplasty is dependent on the final outcome. When possible, surgeons should evaluate their results beyond the first 6 to 12 months, although to a lesser extent the nose will continue to change beyond this period. The stability of the cosmetic result depends on the degree of cartilaginous, ligamentous, bony, and soft tissue disruption and surgically designed structural modifications. Long-term results can be difficult to decipher not only because of the difficulty in sustaining follow-up but also since the nose continues to age along with the other facial structures. Current trends in rhinoplasty advocate key but smaller changes that are more likely to maintain a satisfactory long-term outcome and minimize complications. It should also be emphasized that surgical success is primarily determined by patients' expectations and interpretation of the final outcome. For this reason, preoperative assessment of patients' expectations is of paramount importance.

CLOSED RHINOPLASTY

Rhinoplasty was traditionally developed as a cosmetic procedure to alter the shape of the nose via closed (endonasal) surgical access. This technique has survived the test of time and continues to be a principal approach for many surgeons. In the past 3 decades, though, many surgeons have embraced the open rhinoplasty approach via a transcolumellar incision (Fig. 103-4). Both techniques can provide excellent results. However, major differences in surgical technique, training, visibility, and postoperative outcomes are observed between the methods. Many surgeons strictly adhere to open or closed surgical access for all structural deformities. The authors emphasize a combination of open and closed techniques as the current dictum for modern rhinoplasty surgeons. Although successful outcomes are achieved with both techniques, the authors recommend that students of rhinoplasty acquire the skills to treat and modify the nose with both methods.

In closed rhinoplasty, access to the nasal structures is usually via a combination of partial or complete transfixion incisions along with an intercartilaginous (between the lower and upper lateral cartilage) or intracartilaginous (cartilage splitting) incisions. Simultaneous septoplasty or turbinate reduction can be done through separate incisions. The Killian incision can be used to provide access to the nasal septum when simultaneously using a hemitransfixion incision. The incision is placed at least 5 to 8 mm posterior to the caudal edge of the septal cartilage to avoid compromising the access for hemitransfixion. This allows surgical access to the cartilaginous and bony nasal dorsum for both reduction and augmentation techniques without direct visualization. The nasal tip and columellar structures can also be modified. The cartilage delivery technique is used

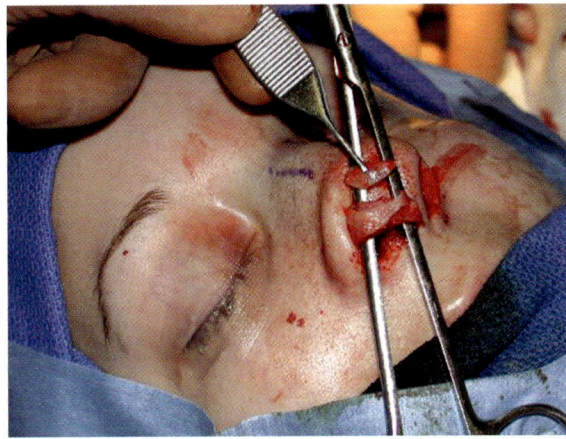

Fig. 103-5 ■ Delivery of the lower lateral cartilage and cephalic strip. Inserting scissors through the intercartilaginous and marginal incisions will expose the lower lateral cartilage. Once it is exposed, a cephalic strip can be taken. (From Fonseca R, Marciani R, Turvey T, editors: *Oral and maxillofacial surgery*, ed 2, St Louis, 2008, Saunders.)

Spreader grafts

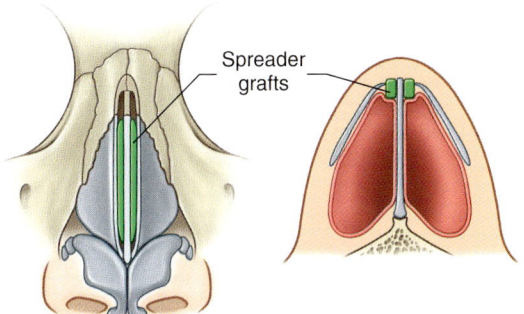

Fig. 103-6 ■ Spreader grafts. (From Guyuron B, Eriksson E, Persing JA: *Plastic surgery: indications and practice*, Philadelphia, 2009, Saunders.)

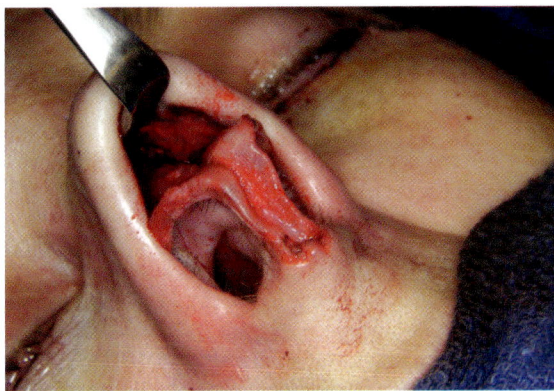

Fig. 103-7 ■ Exposure of nose with an open rhinoplasty incision.

to directly visualize and alter the lower lateral cartilage and tip (Fig. 103-5). The most difficult challenge with the closed rhinoplasty approach is to achieve a predictable and desired alteration of both the bone and cartilage via minimal direct visualization of the altered structures in their anatomic passive relationships. Unlike bone alterations, cartilage has memory, and maintaining cartilage in the desired position is difficult but can be achieved with a variety of cartilage modifications (scoring, transection, repositioning, trimming, suturing, and grafting). Originally, the closed technique was predominantly a reduction technique involving dorsal reduction and nasal osteotomies. Nasal tip modifications were considered difficult and amenable only to minor changes. Although this is still true, equally complex tip modifications can be done via the closed technique, but greater training is required to achieve comfort with the surgical technique and the final esthetic outcomes desired. Grafting of the nasal tip structures can be challenging with the closed approach and requires complex understanding of the tip. Graft movement and stability are among the few problems that the surgeon may encounter.

Advantages of the closed rhinoplasty technique are its speed, less extensive dissection, and absence of a skin incision. It has been suggested that when compared with the closed approach, the open technique (especially without strut grafting) will result in some degree of long-term collapse of the nasal tip because of soft tissue retraction, scarring, and weakening of the foot plates of the lower lateral cartilage. However, as in many areas of cosmetic surgery, this concept has not been validated by long-term prospective cohort studies.

An important addition to functional rhinoplasty was the placement of spreader grafts to preserve or increase the nasal valve angle, which directly correlates with respiratory function of the nose. This can be particularly important, especially with reduction of the width of the dorsum. The graft is usually obtained from the nasal septum (or from the ear cartilage) and is positioned between the nasal septum and the upper lateral cartilage on both sides as needed (Fig. 103-6). Spreader grafts can be placed under direct vision and sutured into place via the open technique. However, placement of grafts via the closed approach is more difficult, and they are potentially less stable. A pocket is created by gentle dissection through the intercartilaginous incision between the nasal septum and the upper lateral cartilage bilaterally. The spreader grafts are positioned in the pocket to achieve the desired effect.

In summary, the endonasal or closed rhinoplasty technique is an effective but highly specialized method, especially with respect to complex nasal tip plastic surgery and augmentation. Mastery of this approach is more difficult. The relative difficulty of the closed technique and the more recent emphasis on the open approach in the literature have made this traditional and important method harder to master for rising rhinoplasty surgeons. It can be safely hypothesized that closed rhinoplasty surgeons can more easily master the open approach than the reverse.

OPEN RHINOPLASTY

A transcolumellar incision with bilateral extension of the margins, also described as the open rhinoplasty technique, has become progressively popular since the 1980s. This access dramatically facilitates the teaching of rhinoplasty and significantly contributes to predictable nasal structural modifications (Fig. 103-7). Achievement of flap viability and the ability to modify and graft cartilage that has been stripped from its supporting perichondrium have contributed to the success of this approach. Previously, students of rhinoplasty would have to learn the complex anatomy and surgical modifications of closed rhinoplasty without visualization of the modified structures. This makes mastery of the technique extremely challenging. The open approach has allowed more rapid understanding of the anatomy by students, which has translated into greater number of surgeons acquiring the skills and interest for this surgery. This flap allows the placement of complex grafts (e.g., shield, columella, tip, supratip, ala, spreader) under direct vision. Although many experienced surgeons may be able to achieve exceptional results and perform grafting via the closed approach, characteristically, this requires a prolonged and sustained learning curve involving years of trial and error that may be achieved only later in one's surgical career. The accelerated learning of nasal modifications via the open approach is a great advantage to novice surgeons and their patients.

The greater visibility associated with open rhinoplasty also facilitates soft tissue modification of the nasal tip. In patients with a bulbous nasal tip secondary to an excessively fibrofatty subcutaneous plane, the flap allows direct access to the underlying tissue for careful removal. In such patients, modifications of the cartilaginous structures can be significantly masked by excessively thick S-STE. Though uncommon, care should be taken to not thin this tissue excessively, which can result in tip dehiscence. Placement of spreader grafts is also greatly facilitated and more accurately performed via the open approach.

Concomitant septoplasty is frequently performed in primary cosmetic rhinoplasty patients. The septal cartilage is approached for functional reasons (deviated septum) or used as a donor site for cartilage reconstruction of the tip, ala, or columellar strut or used in spreader grafts. Traditionally, the septal cartilage is accessed with an endonasal incision (e.g., Killian, transfixion). The septal cartilage can also be approached via the open technique for septoplasty or harvesting of cartilage. As with the endonasal approach, care must be taken to maintain a minimum of 1 cm of dorsal and caudal cartilage for preservation of dorsal support. Collapse of this cartilage can result in a saddle nose deformity. The open approach provides excellent access to the cartilage through subperichondrial dissection of the septal cartilage from above down to the nasal crest of the maxilla. The cartilage can easily be harvested, modified, and repositioned back into its original site.

Open access also allows direct visualization of the nasal bones. Although the majority of reductive nasal modifications can be done through endonasal access, reconstruction and augmentation of the bony and cartilaginous dorsum with autologous (rib, iliac crest) or alloplastic material is greatly facilitated. In summary, rhinoplasty has traditionally been a reductive procedure. The open approach has both facilitated mastering the learning curve for this procedure and enhanced our ability for addition, reduction, and complex reconstruction of the S-STE and bony and cartilaginous structures under direct vision.

Disadvantages of the open rhinoplasty technique include the slightly increased operative time for flap elevation, the presence of a transcolumellar scar, and paresthesia of the nasal tip. The scar is usually well concealed under the nasal tip and is not visible on a frontal view. The inverted V transcolumellar incision allows proper alignment of the flap at closure and also helps camouflage the scar. Surgeons should consider the possibility of keloid formation, especially in African American patients with a previous history of keloids. Paresthesia (hypoesthesia or anesthesia) of the nasal tip is common, particularly after debulking of the underlying S-STE, and can persist for many months postoperatively. Strict adherence to the subperichondrial plane and, when possible, decreased disruption of the flap can minimize this postoperative sequela. However, all patients should be informed about the possibility of prolonged nasal tip paresthesia.

STRATEGIES FOR FOUR ANATOMIC REGIONS OF THE NOSE

Although detailed descriptions of surgical maneuvers for rhinoplasty are beyond the scope of this chapter, here a brief description of the basic strategies for modification of the four anatomic regions of the nose (radix, dorsum, tip, nasal base) follows. These regions are also summarized in Table 103-2.

TABLE 103-2	Outline of Basic Rhinoplasty Maneuvers by Anatomic Location
Radix	
Reduction	Rasp or osteotomy via open or closed techniques.
Augmentation	Augmention can be done with alloplastic (e.g., AlloDerm) or autologous material (bone, cartilage, fascia)
Dorsum	
Reduction	Width reduction with combination of lateral and medial osteotomies. Profile reduction with rasp or osteotome. Excessive dorsal reduction will likely require bilateral nasal osteotomies for closure of open book deformity. Spreader grafts should be considered to maintain the nasal valve angle for preservation of airflow.
Augmentation	Augmentation can be done with alloplastic (e.g., AlloDerm) or autologous material (bone, cartilage, fascia) Bony and cartilaginous augmentation can be done simultaneously.
Tip	
Elevation	Columellar strut, shield and/or tip graft, suturing to nasal septum
Volume Reduction	Cartilage excision or trimming. Use of dome- and tip-defining sutures
Definition	Combination of sutures, grafts, and cartilage excision or trimming
Projection	Graft, suture (dorsum reduction will also affect projection)
Base	
Nostril	Reduction in size is done via nostril sill excision, and the nasal flare and alar base are reduced by alar wedge excision
Ala	Graft to alter alar shape and contour
Columella	Excision or grafting

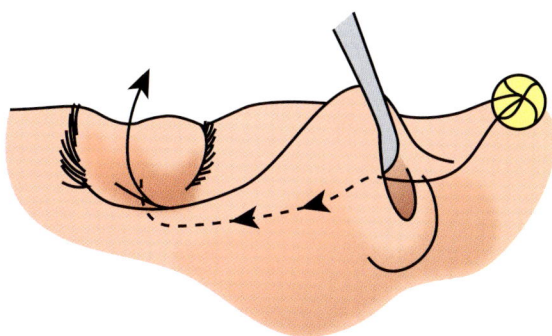

Fig. 103-8 ■ Augmentation of the radix with acellular human dermis or fascia inserted with an attached needle.

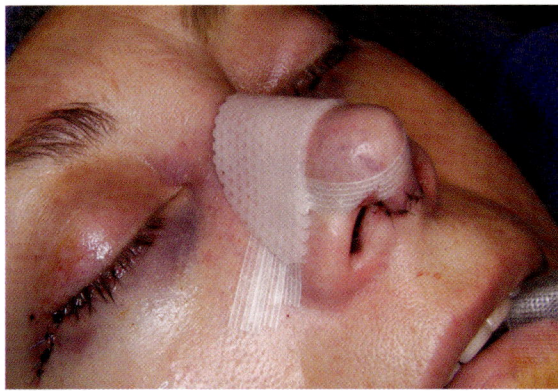

Fig. 103-10 ■ Postoperative placement of a thermoplastic nasal splint after bilateral nasal osteotomies.

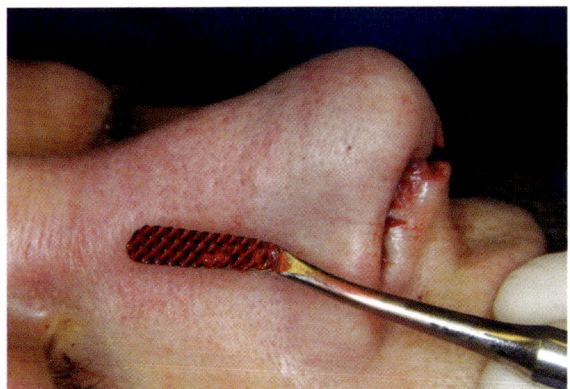

Fig. 103-9 ■ Reduction of the nasal dorsum with a rasp.

RADIX MODIFICATION

The majority of radix modifications involve reduction or augmentation. Reduction has to be done in harmony with dorsum and tip modifications. This is generally achieved by using a rasp or osteotomes via closed or open access. The radix has to be "balanced" to match the dorsum. Reduction of the radix alone will further enhance projection of the nasal dorsum. Augmentation procedures have been performed on this area since the 1930s. Many materials have been used for this purpose, including septal or conchal cartilage, dermis, fascia, and bone. The authors prefer the use of either temporalis fascia or acellular donated human dermis (AlloDerm). Temporalis fascia can easily be harvested via a temporal incision within the hairline. The graft is subsequently inserted at the radix on completion of the rhinoplasty by using an attached needle that is pulled through at the nasion (Fig. 103-8). Overgrafting by 25-30% is recommended to account for subsequent graft resorption and atrophy.

DORSUM MODIFICATION

Traditional rhinoplasty surgeons alter the dorsum to match the esthetics of the nasal tip. Modern rhinoplasty techniques emphasize the concept of a "balanced" nose in which reduction and augmentation strategies are used to achieve harmony between all components and thus attain ideal height of the dorsum. Alterations in the nasal dorsum or the osseocartilaginous vault are complex and involve both cosmetic and functional factors. Reduction of the dorsum is usually done with a rasp or osteotomes (Fig. 103-9). The cartilaginous components (upper lateral and septal cartilage) can be excised with a scalpel or scissors. Depending on the extent of reduction, an open-book deformity may result that can be addressed with lateral nasal osteotomies. Narrowing of the nasal vault will affect the

internal nasal valve angle. Spreader grafts can be used to prevent this complication. The combination of simultaneous medial and lateral osteotomies is less frequently used because of difficulty controlling the mediolateral position of the nasal bone. Lateral nasal osteotomies are also used to decrease the width of the dorsum. These osteotomies are best performed through a small endonasal incision at the inferior and lateral aspect of the piriform rim. However, some surgeons prefer to do this via a small transcutaneous stab incision. A thermoplastic nasal splint is used after nasal osteotomies to stabilize the segments and is kept in place for 1 to 2 weeks (Fig. 103-10).

Augmentation of the dorsum can be achieved with allogeneic or alloplastic material. Septal and ear cartilage can be used for minor augmentation in conjunction with fascia or acellular dermal grafts. Major dorsal reconstruction is best achieved with rib (cartilage and bone) or iliac crest grafts. Alloplastic materials such as silicone or porous polyethylene (Medpor) are less often used because of frequent postoperative complications (graft movement, infection, dehiscence).

TIP MODIFICATION

Nasal tip surgery is the most difficult and challenging aspect of cosmetic rhinoplasty. Adherence to sound surgical techniques and emphasis on minor tip changes allow a more controlled outcome. The nasal tip can be analyzed by six characteristics: volume (based on the size of the lateral crura), width (interdomal distance), shape (broad, bulbous, boxy), projection, rotation, and definition. These characteristics are interrelated and not strictly independently modified (e.g., cephalic lateral crura resection is done primarily to reduce tip volume, but it also increases projection and alters the definition). Understanding of this interrelationship allows the surgeon to better visualize the final outcome. Surgical treatment plans that alter the tip are designed to modify these characteristics. A complete discussion of these techniques is beyond the scope of this chapter, and readers should refer to Suggested Readings for further study. However, basic modifications for each characteristic are summarized in Table 103-3.

NASAL BASE MODIFICATION

When indicated, nasal base modifications should be an integral part of primary cosmetic rhinoplasty. This area is complex and anatomically integrated with the alar base, nostril openings, external nasal valve, columella, and tip. The vast majority of alar base modifications include an alar base wedge excision, a nostril sill/floor excision, or both (Fig. 103-11). The resulting scar is well concealed

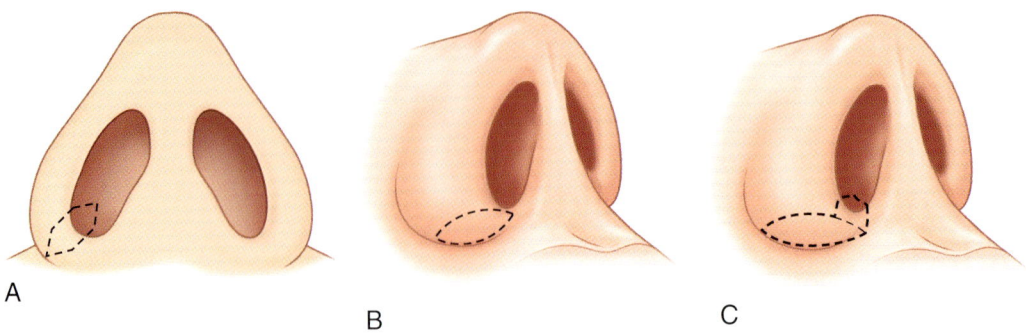

Fig. 103-11 ▪ **A,** Excision of the nostril sill. **B,** Alar wedge excision. **C,** Combined sill/alar excision. (From Daniel RK: *Rhinoplasty: an atlas of surgical techniques*, New York, 2002, Springer.)

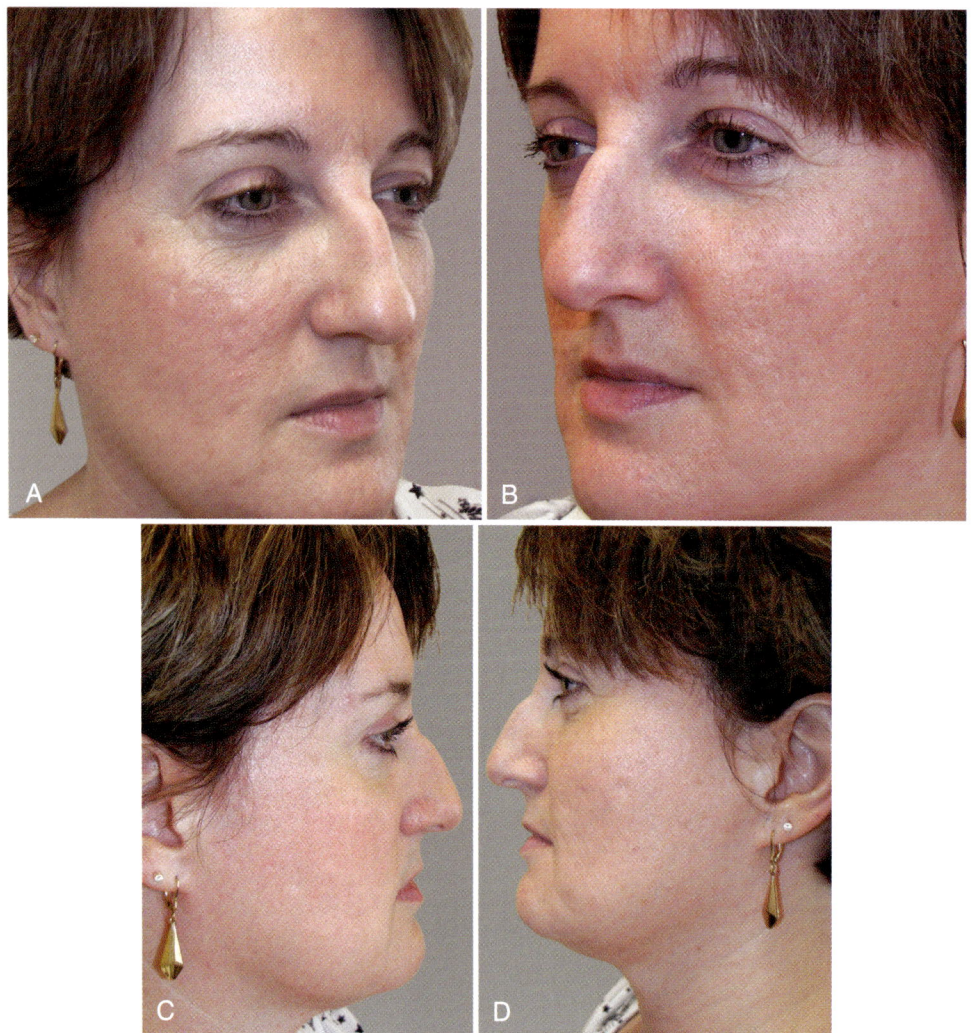

Fig. 103-12 ▪ Preoperative (**A-D**) and postoperative (**E-H**) views after primary cosmetic rhinoplasty.

and infrequently causes complications. The nostril sill excision is extended into the floor of the nose and can be used to reduce the size and visibility of the nostril floor on a frontal view. The alar wedge excision is made in a curvilinear fashion just superior to the alar crease. This excision will reduce the alar flare and is commonly used in rhinoplasty for African Americans. The two incisions can be combined to achieve reduction in alar flare and nostril size. The intraoral alar cinch procedure can also be used to reduce alar width.

GRAFTS

Grafting is an important part of modern rhinoplasty. Multiple autogenous donor sites and several alloplastic grafting materials are available. Most current rhinoplasty surgeons use autogenous cartilage grafts for the majority of primary cosmetic rhinoplasty procedures.

Septal cartilage is the primary choice for most tip, columellar, alar, and dorsal cartilage grafting. In patients in whom septal

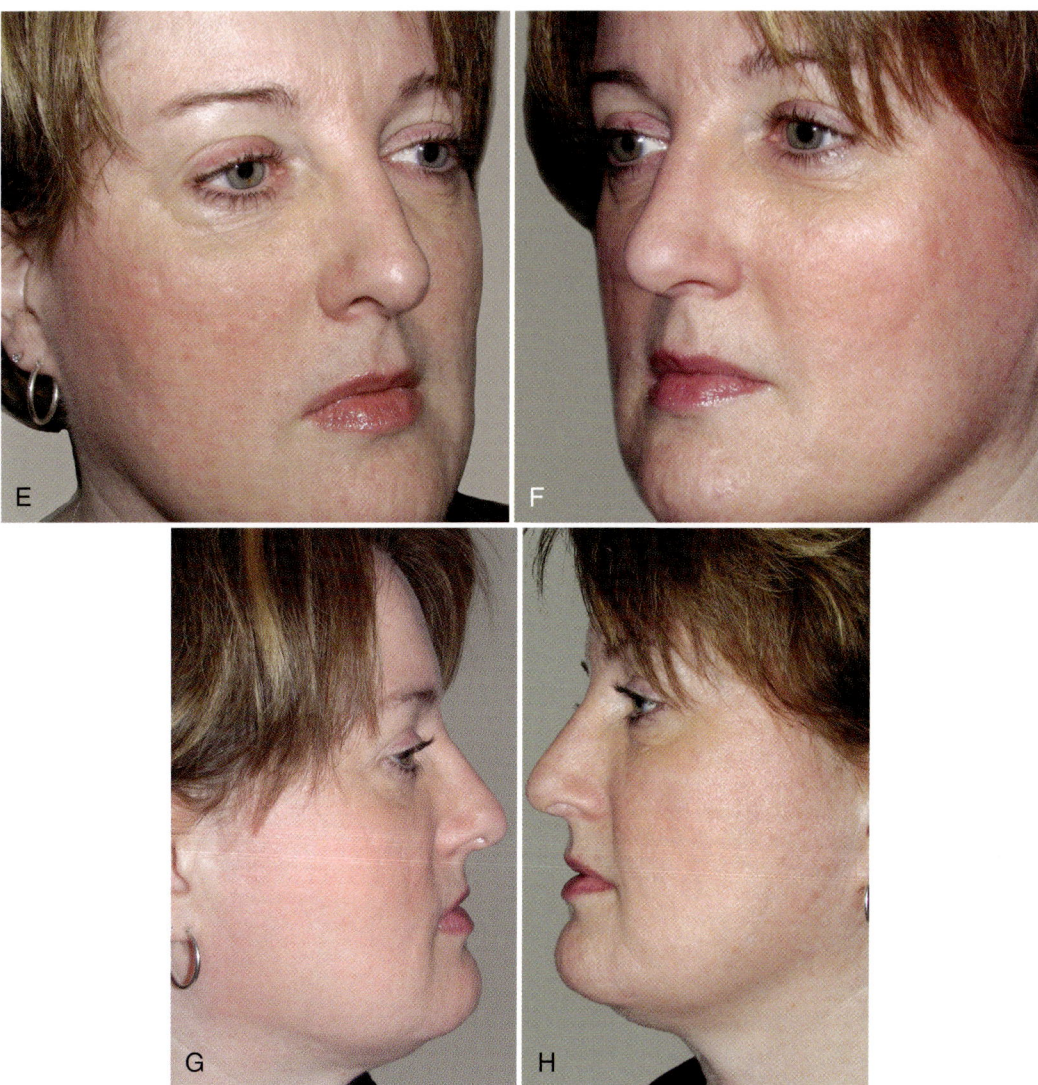

Fig. 103-12, cont'd.

TABLE 103-3	Nasal Tip Characteristics and Possible Surgical Techniques for Modification
ANATOMIC REGION	**PRIMARY MODIFICATION TECHNIQUE**
Volume	Reduction: resection of the cephalic lateral crura Augmentation: shield graft
Width	Reduction: interdomal sutures
Definition	Dome equalization sutures, dome definition sutures, dome creation sutures
Projection	Tip graft, projection suture, columellar strut
Rotation	Rotation suture (to the nasal septum), columellar strut, tip graft
Shape	Graft (tip, ala), cartilage excision/trimming, sutures

cartilage is not available (previous septoplasty or secondary rhinoplasty), the concha can easily be harvested. Temporalis fascia and decellularized human dermis (AlloDerm) are commonly used grafts for the radix or other soft tissue grafting.

Figure 103-12 presents preoperative and postoperative photographs of a patient who underwent cosmetic rhinoplasty and caudal septoplasty. The surgical procedure included dorsal reduction and tip-plasty (cephalic lateral crural resection, interdomal and tip-defining sutures). Lateral osteotomies were not performed on this patient to maintain balance between the tip and dorsal width.

POSTOPERATIVE CARE

Routine postoperative care of rhinoplasty patients should address analgesia, nausea, nutrition, antimicrobial treatment, nasal hygiene, swelling, possible epistaxis, and most important, postoperative visits and support of the patient during the healing process. The authors advocate frequent postoperative visits not only to reinforce wound healing but also for emotional support, especially with respect to the facial edema seen during the immediate postoperative period.

The patient should be instructed to rest in bed with the head elevated and frequent application of a gentle cold compress for the first 24 hours when possible to reduce edema. White gauze is taped or suspended at the nostrils to minimize dripping of blood. Although significant postoperative hemorrhage is uncommon, most patients will have minor epistaxis (especially with nasal osteotomies). Blood clots and mucous secretions can accumulate in intranasal packings and significantly contribute to postoperative discomfort and pain. The intranasal septal packings/splints are sutured to the membranous septum to avoid displacement deeper into the nostril. The authors recommend placing the suture tie at an anterior and visible location for ease of removal.

Patients are encouraged to ambulate early and not remain in bed. This will help minimize edema and reduce postoperative pulmonary complications and deep venous thrombosis. The nostrils can be gently cleansed with normal saline and coated with petroleum jelly. The sutures are removed 7 to 9 days postoperatively. Many patients have significant anxiety related to the postoperative visit (removal of sutures or intranasal splints) and may require encouragement and support. Intravenous sedation can be used in select patients for reduction of anxiety, complete suctioning of the nasal cavity, and removal of old blood clots and sutures. When nasal osteotomies are performed, the nasal cast is removed at 7 to 14 days. The patient is advised to avoid contact with the nasal structures. Postoperative systemic steroids can be used to reduce edema, although this may not be indicated for all patients. Steroids (triamcinolone) can be injected into the nasal tip in the event of prolonged nasal tip edema. The authors recommend at least three injections at 1-week intervals. Similarly, irregularities and depressions can be addressed with injectable fillers after several months have passed. Unfavorable results should be addressed immediately and acknowledged. Unless there are grossly abnormal findings, enough time (8 to 12 months) should elapse before any revision rhinoplasty is considered (see Chapter 104).

PEARLS AND PITFALLS

- The surgeon should fully understand the patient's cosmetic desires and translate them into a surgical procedure to achieve the desired outcome. Failure to comprehend the patient's desires or overestimation of one's ability will result in more frequent unfavorable outcomes.
- With adequate training, oral and maxillofacial surgeons can provide a comprehensive and unique approach to rhinoplasty surgery.
- A successful cosmetic outcome with compromise of nasal function is a failure.
- The goal of primary cosmetic rhinoplasty is to achieve long-term stability (beyond 1 year) of the cosmetic outcome.
- Smaller and more controlled surgical changes provide more predictable outcomes.
- Large and dramatic changes are more difficult to predict.
- Rhinoplasty is a dynamic and individualized procedure for both the patient and the surgeon. A philosophy of open and closed rhinoplasty techniques is emphasized rather than exclusive adherence to one or the other.
- Surgeons should recognize and acknowledge to patients the limitations of the procedure.
- Preoperative visits should address complications in depth.
- Undesired results should be acknowledged with an immediate plan for possible improvement. An informed but disappointed patient is better than an uninformed and angry one.
- There is no one operation suitable for all noses.
- Some patients do not need surgery.

BIBLIOGRAPHY

Bagheri SC, Khan HA, Jahangirian A, et al: An analysis of 101 primary cosmetic rhinoplasties, *J Oral Maxillofac Surg*, August 2011.

Daniel RK: *Rhinoplasty: an atlas of surgical techniques*, New York, 2002, Springer.

Galdino GM, DaSilva And D, Gunter JP: Digital photography for rhinoplasty, *Plast Reconstr Surg* 109:1421-1434, 2002.

Gunter JP: The merits of the open approach in rhinoplasty, *Plast Reconstr Surg* 99:863-867, 1997.

Johnson CM, Toriumi DM: *Open structure rhinoplasty*, Philadelphia, 1990, WB Saunders.

Tardy ME Jr, Dayan S, Hecht D: Preoperative rhinoplasty: evaluation and analysis, *Otolaryngol Clin North Am* 35:1-27, v, 2002.

Toriumi D, Mueller R, Grosch T: Vascular anatomy of the nose and the external rhinoplasty approach, *Arch Otolaryngol Head Neck Surg* 122:24-34, 1996.

Behnam Bohluli, Shahrokh C. Bagheri

Revision rhinoplasty is a general term that deals with the correction of various deformities in a previously operated nose; such deformities range from a subtle irregularity over the nasal tip to a completely distorted nose requiring several reconstructive surgical interventions, including the application of multiple grafts, sutures, and flaps. The present chapter is an overview of the most common deformities, their diagnosis, and current treatment protocols.

ETIOPATHOGENESIS

The need for revision rhinoplasty is multifactorial. The lack of accurate diagnosis and discussion to determine the patient's cosmetic and functional demands is the leading cause of secondary corrective cosmetic nasal surgery. The tendency to make a nose excessively smaller can compromise both the cosmetic and functional outcome. Unrealistic demands by the patient that are unrecognized by the surgeon will probably lead to an unsatisfied patient. Similarly, surgeons should not overestimate their ability and understand the limitations of the applied cosmetic maneuvers. Each surgical procedure has its limitations and standard range of errors. Multiple alterations along with a combination of complex cartilaginous and bony modifications will increase the margin of error in rhinoplasty. Of particular difficulty are patients who have a postoperative result that is deemed satisfactory by the surgeon but yet unsatisfactory by the patients. This is probably due to a lack of initial communication between the surgeon and patient and may pose a significant challenge. All unsatisfactory results must be acknowledged and explored. Rather than ignoring the outcome, discussion and planning should be undertaken for any possible corrective measures.

It is important to distinguish revision rhinoplasty from a staged rhinoplasty in which a second procedure is planned at the primary consultation. For instance, in a patient with a severely crooked nose, precise judgment about the nostrils may be difficult and alar base surgery may be intentionally postponed until a second minor surgery can be performed.

PATHOLOGIC ANATOMY

The anatomy of an operated nose differs completely from its normal counterpart. For this reason, revision surgery requires special attention to anatomy. After the primary operation the skin redrapes over the new framework, followed by a dynamic healing process that extends well beyond the first year and affects the aging nose indefinitely. The result is shrinkage and contracture of skin, which sometimes limits its potential to undergo extensive dissection and major changes in volume. Subcutaneous scars are also inevitably seen in an operated nose. The extent of the scarring depends on the amount of previous surgical manipulations, the presence of dead space, and finally, the biologic behavior of the patient's wound healing.

The osseous and cartilaginous frameworks are subject to many augmentation or reductive procedures in primary rhinoplasty. Therefore, excessive scarring, compromised vascularity, unpredictable healing, over-contoured and excessive reduction of native anatomy, grafts, sutures, and altered mucosa, perichondrium, and periosteum are among the changes seen in a previously operated nose. In particular, a clear path of dissection is not as easily identified in the sub-perichondrial plane at the nasal tip area. Figure 104-1 illustrates open access to a nose previously operated on 5 years previously that demonstrates scarring and altered cartilage anatomy.

Because autografts and alloplastic material are commonly used in primary rhinoplasty, the esthetic surgeon should be ready to confront anatomic changes that are not seen in a normal nose; each of these materials has its own characteristics and frequently provokes unpredictable tissue behavior.

The lower lateral cartilage is often significantly altered by reductive techniques. The continuity of this cartilage may be interrupted in several places. The presence of cartilage and bone grafts will also modify the anatomy. The upper lateral cartilage is usually weakened because of over-resection of the cartilaginous dorsum, which can result in severe esthetic and functional problems. The nasal septum is commonly manipulated in the first surgery to correct septal deviation or to harvest cartilage and is rarely intact in revision cases.

DIAGNOSTIC STUDIES

Proper diagnosis and treatment planning are key to successful revision rhinoplasty and are usually based on three important criteria: psychological evaluation, esthetic analysis, and functional examination. Each of these assessments should be performed before any corrective (or primary) surgery.

PSYCHOLOGICAL EVALUATION

Apart from unsatisfactory esthetic and functional outcomes, patients desiring revision rhinoplasty can be emotionally affected by the unfavorable results of their primary elective surgery. Many revision patients will have a negative memory of their previous surgical experience, which can diminish their confidence and trust in any further esthetic surgery.

Psychological evaluation usually starts with a comprehensive history and a thorough interview. Revision patients seek to fulfill their unmet expectations in their second surgeries. Therefore, all expectations should be listed during the primary interview and any possible unrealistic expectations should be detected. Patients should be gradually prepared for possible outcomes of a well-planned revision surgery that are usually less than ideal. Consideration should

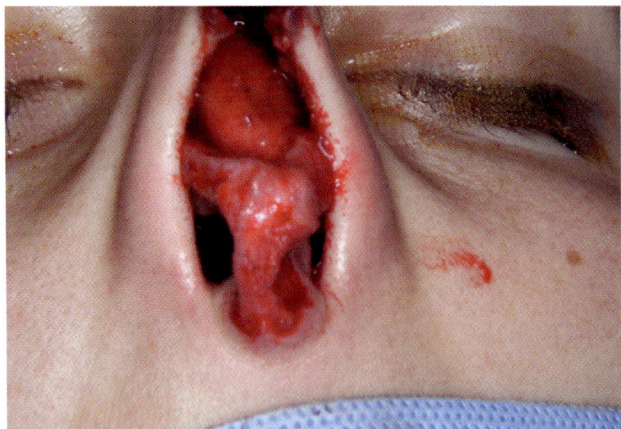

Fig. 104-1 ■ Open access to a nose operated on 5 years previously showing scarring and altered cartilage anatomy.

be given to preoperative psychological consultation. Extensive preoperative consultation will reduce the frequency of postoperative problems related to inadequate communication and misdiagnosis.

ESTHETIC ANALYSIS

Esthetic analysis of patients seeking revision rhinoplasty closely resembles that for primary rhinoplasty (see Chapter 103). Life-size photographs are helpful for rhinometric measurements and analysis of the actual size of the deformities. The use of predictive software will sometimes contribute to the perception of patients and can help esthetic surgeons make correct diagnoses and formulate proper treatment plans, although it can also affect patients' postoperative expectations of the acceptable margin of error related to rhinoplasty surgery.

FUNCTIONAL EXAMINATION

Functional examination begins with visual inspection of the patient while making a deep inspiration. Any possible external valve collapse should be noted. To examine the inner valve, the nasal passages should be visualized with a headlight and nasal speculum. A Cottle test would be informative of the strength of the inner nasal valves and can help detect any valve stenosis.

ANCILLARY DIAGNOSTIC STUDIES

COMPUTED TOMOGRAPHY AND PLAIN RADIOGRAPHS

Most structural abnormalities of the nose can be explored by careful physical examination. Computed tomography (CT) and plain radiographs are sometimes used to assess the condition of the paranasal sinuses or to document septal deformities.

NASAL ENDOSCOPIC EXAMINATION

Nasal endoscopy (rhinoscopic examination) can be used to further assess the nasal mucosa and visualize the nasal septum and associated structures. In the event of any uncertainty, nasal endoscopy will easily reveal even minor septal malformations or can be used to document and assess severe soft tissue complications such as septal perforation.

RHINOMANOMETRY AND ACOUSTIC RHINOMETRY

These techniques are safe, non-invasive diagnostic modalities that are generally used for quantitative measurements of airway patency. Though not routine, they can be used to analyze and compare the effects of surgical corrective procedures with the preoperative parameters.

TREATMENT/RECONSTRUCTIVE GOALS

The main goal of revision rhinoplasty is to restore both esthetic and functional damage caused by the primary surgery or to correct possible deformities that were left untreated in previous surgeries.

To achieve this objective the following minor goals should be taken into consideration: (1) proper diagnosis and treatment planning, (2) determination of the best graft donor site, (3) re-establishment of major and minor tip support, and (4) restoration of form and function of the external and internal nasal valves.

The modern trend in performing revision rhinoplasty is based on augmenting lost tissue, strengthening weakened structures, and precise refining of any possible excess tissue. This can be achieved by an endonasal (closed approach) or open approach (see Chapter 103). The approach depends on the complexity of the corrective surgery and the surgeon's experience; however, minor corrections are usually done via a closed approach, and more complicated cases necessitate an open approach.

AUGMENTATION MATERIAL

Many materials have been introduced for use in primary and revision rhinoplasty and are generally divided into three groups: autogenous grafts, allogeneic grafts, and alloplastic material. Table 104-1 lists the general characteristics and advantages and disadvantages of each augmentation material.

AUTOGENOUS GRAFTS

Autogenous material consists of cartilage, fascia (temporalis fascia, fascia lata), skin, and bone (e.g., calvarial bone and iliac crest). Autogenous cartilage is the most common augmentation material and can be harvested from the nasal septum and auricular and costal cartilage.

Septal Cartilage

Septal cartilage is the donor material of choice for most augmentation procedures. The ease of access within the same surgical field, especially with concomitant septoplasty procedures, is a significant advantage. The cartilage is easily cut and tailored into different shapes and forms, and it can be crushed or morselized to achieve a smooth surface along with elimination of cartilage memory.

The major drawback of septal cartilage is its limited volume, particularly in a previously operated septum. In such cases the risk for septal perforation and inadequate volume of cartilage available make this donor site unacceptable.

Important considerations when harvesting septal cartilage grafts for revision surgery include the following: (1) preservation of a strong "L" framework of septal cartilage (7 to 10 mm in width) is mandatory; (2) severe manipulation of the septum and excessive pressure over the dorsum should be avoided after graft harvesting to prevent dorsal collapse and saddle nose deformity; and (3) if the septal cartilage had been manipulated in previous surgeries, it is best to use an alternative access to the septum. If a transfixion incision was used to gain access to the septum in previous surgeries, a dorsal

TABLE 104-1	Common Augmentation Material in Revision Rhinoplasty and Their Advantages and Disadvantages		
		ADVANTAGES	**DISADVANTAGES**
Autogenous grafts			
Fascia		Resistant to resorption Camouflage the sharp edge of grafts such as crushed cartilage	Donor site morbidity Patient compliance
Cartilage	Septal cartilage	The longitudinal characteristic of this cartilage makes it a favorable choice for spreader grafts	Usually consumed or scarred during primary rhinoplasty, especially the caudal portion
	Auricular cartilage	Excellent alternative choice of autogenous cartilage; the curved nature of auricular contours could be used for alar grafts and composite grafts The remaining subcutaneous portion assists in fixation of the graft	Risk for hematoma Inherent anatomic curvatures Not suitable for crushing and morselizing
	Costochondral cartilage	First choice for massive reconstructions; an abundant amount of cartilage is available	Extensive surgery needed Risk of warping of cartilage and complications at the donor site
Allograft		Available in large quantity Lack of donor site morbidity	Risk of disease transmission Host immune reactions to the graft Resorption Warping
Alloplastic grafts		Available in every size, volume, and hardness Lack of donor site morbidity Easily contorted More favorable in dorsal augmentations	Foreign body reaction or chronic inflammation Infection Extrusion Expensive Unfavorable result in the lower third of the nose and functional structures (e.g., strut, alar grafts, columella) Wound healing complications with subsequent nasal trauma Increased complications in younger patients

open approach in which the upper lateral cartilage is separated from the septum can be used.

Conchal Cartilage

Auricular cartilage is widely used for revision rhinoplasty and can be harvested via anterior (Fig. 104-2) or posterior auricular approaches (Fig. 104-3). The harvested cartilage characteristically possesses a normal anatomic curvature, which can be a favorable or unfavorable characteristic, depending on its planned use. For example, augmentation of the dorsum usually demands a straight cartilage graft, thus making conchal cartilage a difficult choice for this application, whereas for alar and nasal tip reconstruction it can be ideal. The inherent anatomic curvature of auricular cartilage also makes it more resistant to modification by crushing or morselizing.

For surgical access to auricular cartilage the anterior approach is generally preferred, although this is highly variable among surgeons. The posterior approach allows harvest of a greater volume of cartilage, and the donor site scar is more concealed. Attention should be paid to hemostasis and postoperative placement of a pressure dressing to prevent hematoma formation and a subsequent cauliflower deformity.

Rib Cartilage Graft

Rib grafts have recently found great popularity in complex nasal revisions because the rib provides a considerable volume of cartilage with good dimensions. This large bulk of cartilage allows all known

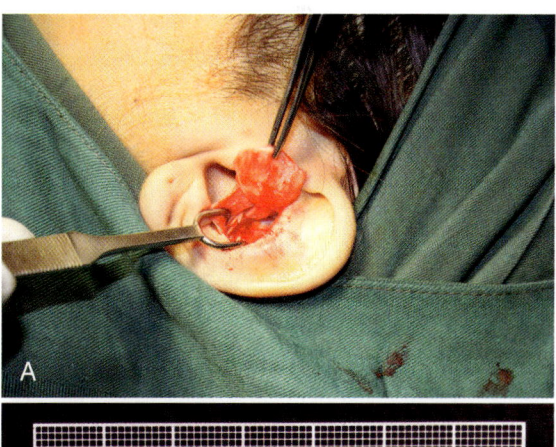
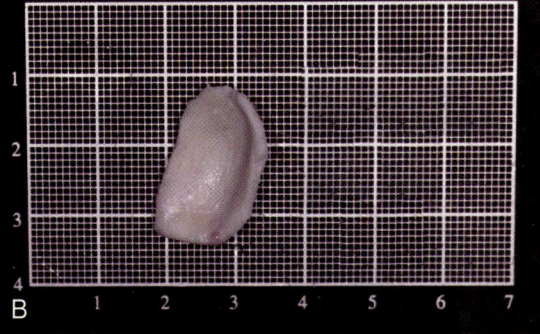

Fig. 104-2 ■ In an anterior approach a 2-cm incision is made 2 to 3 mm deep to the ear bowl (**A**); after wide dissection with scissors, auricular cartilage is harvested (**B**).

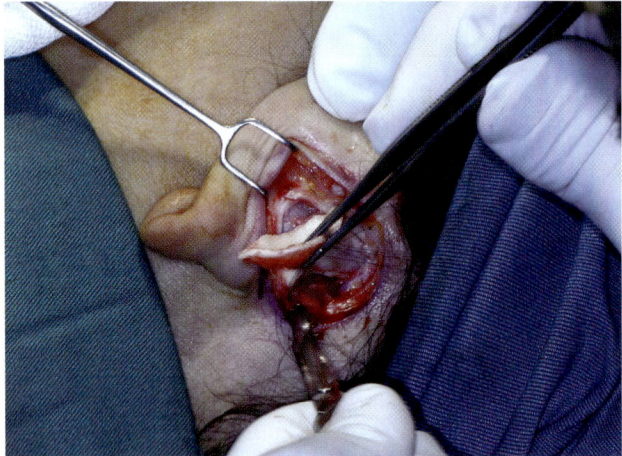

Fig. 104-3 ■ In a posterior approach, dissection and graft harvesting is more difficult, but a larger amount of cartilage can be harvested and the scar is hidden behind the ear.

forms of augmentation reconstruction to be performed without uncertainty regarding the amount of available cartilage. The main drawbacks of rib harvest are difficulty in patient compliance and wound care, postoperative pain, possible visible scars, and risk for pneumothorax.

The fifth, sixth, and seventh ribs are the preferred sites for graft harvesting. In elderly patients, the extent of ossification and the presence of cartilage should be assessed preoperatively with CT or plain radiography of the ribs. The right side is preferred as a donor site to avoid masking possible postoperative chest pain of cardiac origin, especially in the elderly population. Graft warping or distortion is a potential long-term complication of rib grafts. It is generally suggested that a Kirschner wire be inserted in larger rib grafts to reinforce the bulky graft material and help preserve its stability and shape.

HOMOGRAFTS

AlloDerm (donated cellular human dermis) and irradiated costal cartilage are the most commonly used homografts for revision rhinoplasty. The main advantages of homografts are their ease of availability, decreased anesthesia time, and elimination of donor site morbidity. Unpredictable biologic response of the nasal tissues to homografts, cartilage warping, risk for disease transmission, and patient non-compliance are potential limitations of homografts in augmentation rhinoplasty.

ALLOPLASTIC MATERIALS

Alloplastic materials have progressively fallen out of favor and are generally considered a last resource in augmentation rhinoplasty. Silicon, polytetrafluoroethylene, high-density porous polyethylene (Medpor), hyaluronic acid, hydroxyapatite, methylcellulose, polyamides, polyethylene terephthalate, and polypropylene are among the commonly reported alloplastic materials used in rhinoplasty. Infection, graft mobility, migration of the implant, extrusion through nasal skin, chronic inflammatory reactions, and pain over the augmented area have, however, greatly limited their use in rhinoplasty. The esthetic surgeon should be careful when using such material, even if the patient requires massive augmentation and there is a lack of available autogenous sources. It should be emphasized that a previously operated nose has lower vascularity and thinner skin that is more vulnerable to extrusion of alloplastic material.

TIMING OF SURGERY

There is no unanimous consensus regarding the optimal time for revision rhinoplasty, but it is generally believed that such surgery should be delayed for at least 1 year to allow scar maturation and improved visibility of all deformities so that flap reflection can be performed with minimal risk. In the interim, some minor procedures such as alar base resection and unilateral osteotomies that do not require skeletonization may be performed within 6 months postoperatively.

COMMON DEFORMITIES AND TREATMENTS

The following sections describe some commonly seen deformities that may warrant revision rhinoplasty, along with a brief discussion of some standard treatments. A complete analysis of revision rhinoplasty is beyond the scope of this book, and readers should refer to the Suggested Readings for more in-depth information. For ease of discussion, these deformities are classified into three areas based on nasal anatomy: (1) deformities of the upper third involving the bony pyramids, the focus of which is on the bony structures of the nose and problems associated with nasal osteotomies; (2) deformities of the middle third involving the middle vault; and (3) deformities of the lower third of the nose involving the tip, alar base, and columella. It is essential to recognize that in the majority of patients more than one deformity is present and that it is frequently difficult to attribute the deformity to exactly one area only.

DEFORMITIES OF THE BONY PYRAMID

Open Roof Deformity

The presence of an open roof indicates that the lateral osteotomy has failed to sufficiently medialize the nasal bones and a gap exists between the two bony walls. It may also be caused by excessive resection of the bony hump, which makes it impossible to form a new bony pyramid from its short limbs. An open roof deformity may easily be corrected by performing an effective lateral osteotomy and dorsal augmentation in over-resected cases.

Rocker Deformity and Dorsal Irregularities

If the path of the previous nasal osteotomy extends to the thicker, more superior bony pyramid (frontal bone), a bony fulcrum based on this thicker bone will cause protrusion of a bone segment after medial movement of the more inferior nasal bones. The nasal bones will project or "rock" laterally, a condition known as a rocker deformity. If this deformity is minor, a fine bone rasp can easily remove this protrusion. In patients with thin overlying skin, fine irregularities can be covered with a small piece of temporalis fascia (Fig. 104-4) or AlloDerm. In more severe cases or with other concomitant bony irregularities, the osteotomies may need to be repeated to correct the problem.

Several important points need to be emphasized if one intends to correct a rocker deformity with revision nasal osteotomies: (1) The osteotomy should not be extended to the thicker parts of the bony pyramid. It is recommended that the osteotomy be terminated at the level of the medial canthus. (2) It is likely that a previous zero-degree medial osteotomy (Fig. 104-5, *A*) is the second factor (along with the extended lateral osteotomy) that places the patient at risk for the development of a rocker deformity. It is best to limit the use of medial osteotomy to its few indications, and when performed, it should be done at least 15 degrees from the vertical midline (Fig.

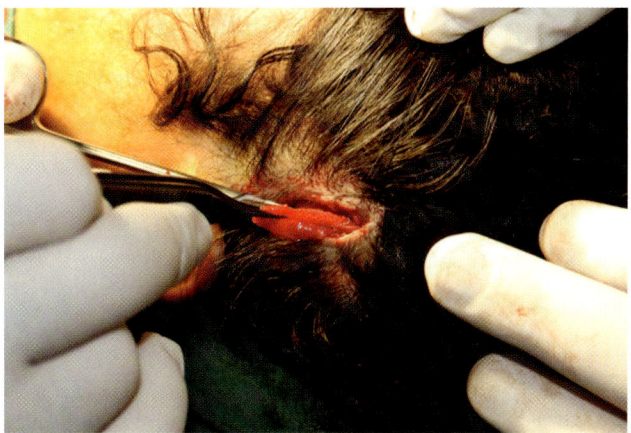

Fig. 104-4 ■ With a small vertical incision over the temporal skin, access to the temporalis fascia is obtained; after dissection an appropriate amount of fascia is harvested.

104-5, *B*). (3) In patients with an existing rocker deformity or if the previous rhinoplasty places them at high risk for the development of this deformity, it is recommended that a deep lateral osteotomy be connected to the medial osteotomies with the use of a 2-mm osteotome through an external stab incision (Fig. 104-5, *C*). This approach allows a more controlled line of osteotomy.

Excessively Wide or Narrow Bony Pyramid

When the bony pyramid is not in ideal balance with the other two thirds, repeating the lateral osteotomy is usually indicated. This osteotomy may be performed via either an external perforated approach or an internal continuous approach. Some surgeons believe that the external approach produces a more controllable greenstick fracture and is therefore preferred for revision rhinoplasty.

In patients with narrow bony pyramids, a precise lateral osteotomy and gentle out-fracture are performed. The key point in extremely narrow bony pyramids is a correct diagnosis. It is important to not confuse the diagnosis with the presence of short nasal bones, which may have the same appearance. In such patients lateral osteotomy is relatively contraindicated and augmentation of the radix will correct this narrow appearance.

Asymmetric Pyramid and Depressed Nasal Bones and Sidewall Steps

Treatment usually involves performing an effective lateral osteotomy. In patients with no concomitant functional problems and with a mild deformity, camouflage grafting of a deficient site or rasping of a protrusion can correct the esthetic problem.

MIDDLE VAULT PROBLEMS

Pollybeak Deformity

A pollybeak deformity is a complication of rhinoplasty in which the typical appearance of the dorsal nasal convexity resembles a parrot's beak. It describes a postoperative condition of disproportionate fullness of the supratip in relation to the tip. This is a paradoxic deformity that occurs with both over-resection and under-resection of the cartilaginous dorsum. In addition, excessive loss of tip projection or columellar collapse will lead to this deformity. Treatment generally depends on correct diagnosis of the underlying causative factor.

In cases of over-resected dorsal humps, the soft tissue fails to adequately redrape over its new cartilaginous framework after the

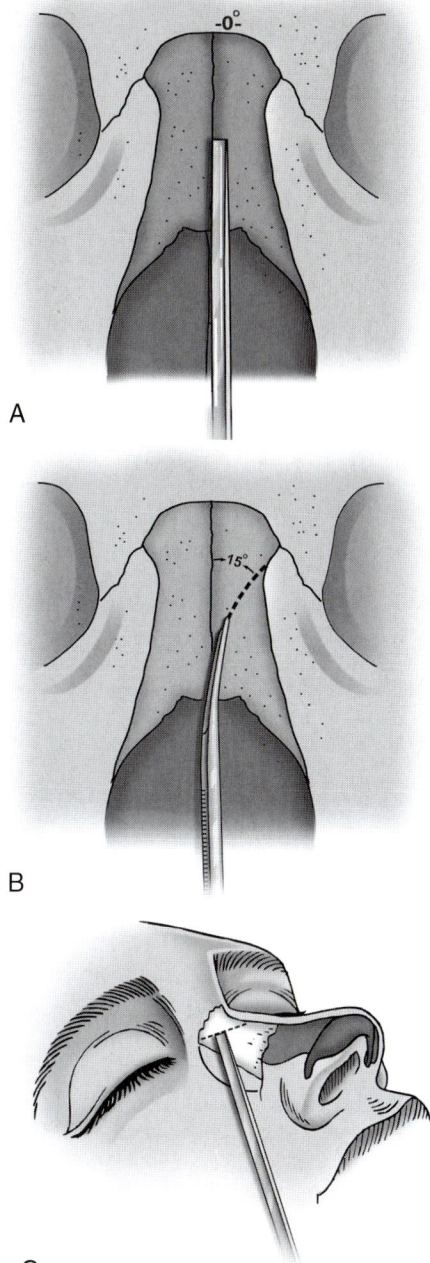

Fig. 104-5 ■ **A,** A zero-degree medial osteotomy may lead to a rocker deformity. **B,** It is suggested that the osteotomy be tilted 15 degrees or curved lateral osteotomes be used instead of straight medial osteotomes. **C,** Sometimes it is appropriate to connect the lateral osteotomy to the medial osteotomy and perform a dotted osteotomy from an extranasal approach.

primary rhinoplasty (Fig. 104-6, *A*). A dead space is formed that is filled with granulation tissue. The result is fullness in the supratip area, and treatment should be focused on restoring the over-resected area (Fig. 104-6, *B*). Treatment consists of dorsal augmentation with septal cartilage, a columellar strut, and alar contouring grafts as needed (Fig. 104-6, *C*). Attempts to trim the supratip granulation tissue without augmentation of the cartilaginous dorsum may result in an exaggerated relapse of this deformity shortly after the operation. Under-resection of the dorsal hump is relatively uncommon (Fig. 104-7). This is corrected by careful trimming or removal of

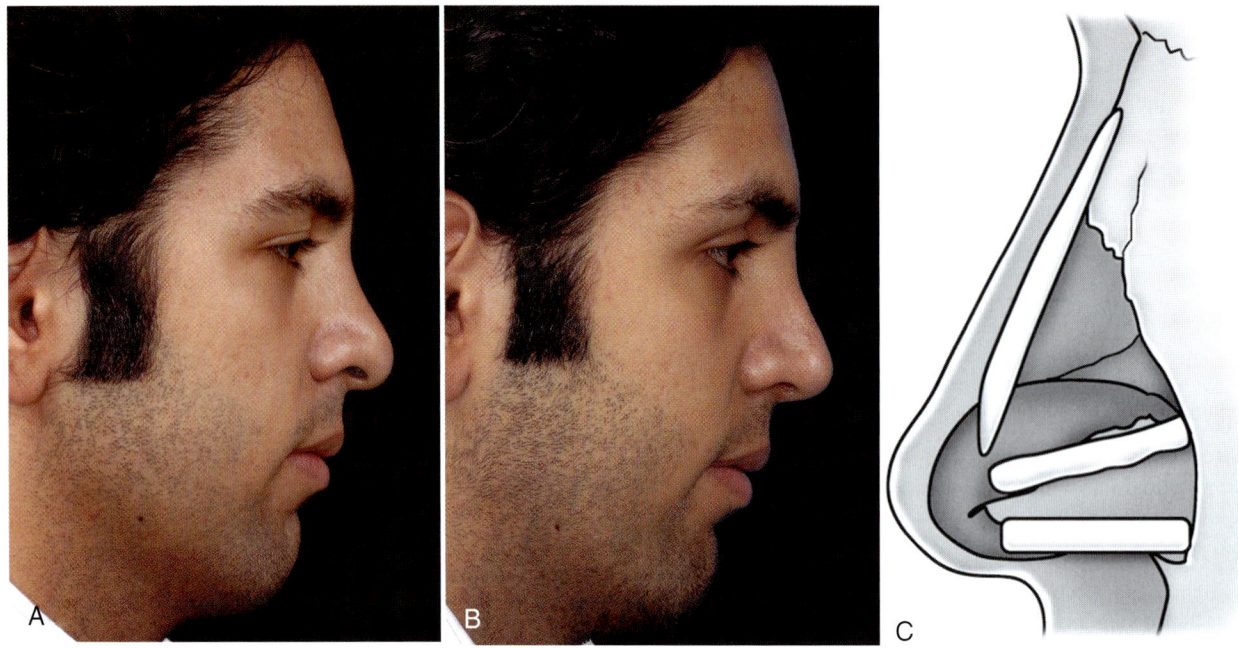

Fig. 104-6 ■ **A,** Pollybeak deformity caused by over-resection and loss of projection. **B** and **C,** Treatment consists of dorsal augmentation with septal cartilage, a columellar strut, and alar contouring grafts.

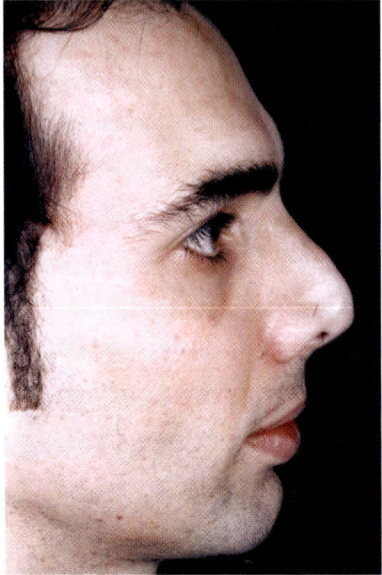

Fig. 104-7 ■ In rare revision patients a pollybeak deformity is a result of under-resection.

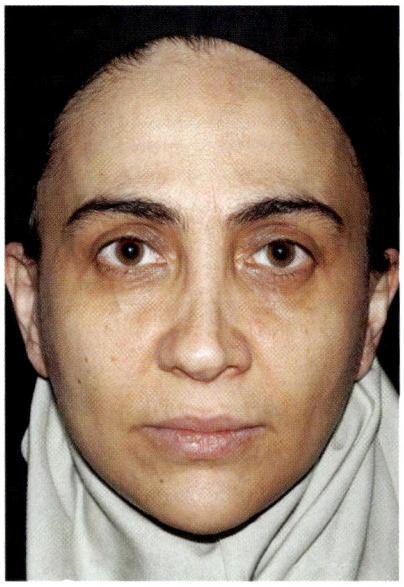

Fig. 104-8 ■ An inverted-V deformity is a result of hump over-resection or inner valve collapse, or both.

the excess bone or cartilage in an incremental manner to avoid over-resection.

Inverted-V Deformity and Weak Middle Vault

An inverted-V deformity refers to a complication of rhinoplasty in which the caudal edge of the nasal bones is apparent, especially on the frontal view. Inadequate support of the upper lateral

cartilage subsequent to dorsal hump reduction can lead to medial and inferior collapse of the upper lateral cartilage and an inverted-V deformity.

The presence of an inverted-V deformity means that caudal edges of the nasal bones are prominent or poorly aligned and make a shadow over the skin in the frontal view (Fig. 104-8). This deformity is most commonly caused by a weakened middle vault as a result of over-resection of the upper lateral cartilage or compromised

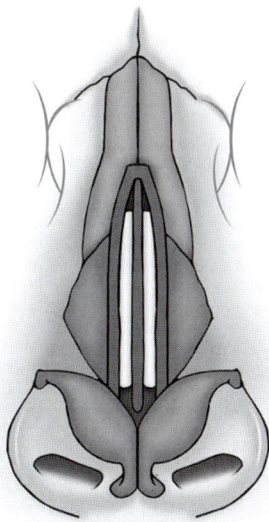

Fig. 104-9 ■ Spreader grafts are placed lateral to the septal cartilage.

integrity of the mucoperichondrium that spans under the junction of the upper lateral cartilage and septum. Correction generally involves reconstruction and strengthening of the middle vault by means of spreader grafts, which is considered the "gold standard" for middle vault reconstruction.

Spreader grafts are usually rectangular pieces of cartilage that are precisely placed in the lateral aspect of the septum (Fig. 104-9) and sutured to it. The cartilage graft can be obtained from septal, auricular, and sometimes rib cartilage. In some patients, several pieces are added on one side of the septum to achieve sufficient strength and width or to assist in correction of a deviated dorsum.

Another complication is improper alignment of the lateral walls of the nasal bones, which will result in a prominent edge on the caudal part of the nasal bones. This problem can be corrected by correct placement of lateral nasal osteotomies.

TIP, ALAR BASE, AND COLUMELLA
Asymmetric Tip

In patients with mild asymmetries, camouflage grafts will usually solve the problem. A small pocket is created in the deficient site, and a small piece of crushed cartilage formed by the fingers is inserted to obtain the ideal symmetric result.

In patients with more severe asymmetries, an open approach is generally preferred. Treatment of such cases usually depends on the correct diagnosis. Figure 104-10 demonstrates the preoperative appearance and postoperative correction of nasal tip asymmetry and irregularity 5 years after the primary cosmetic rhinoplasty. The nasal tip was grafted in selected areas with crushed auricular cartilage. Figure 104-1 shows the anatomy of the nasal tip after reflection of the flap and before any surgical modification.

Asymmetric cephalic trimming, improper tip sutures, and asymmetric dome or lateral crural splitting are among the most common causes of asymmetric nasal tip deformities. Treatment of these complicated conditions entails leveling the asymmetric lower lateral cartilage and covering the sharp edges of the lower lateral cartilage with sutures and cartilage grafts. In patients with a thin skin soft tissue envelope, the sharp edges may be covered with temporalis fascia.

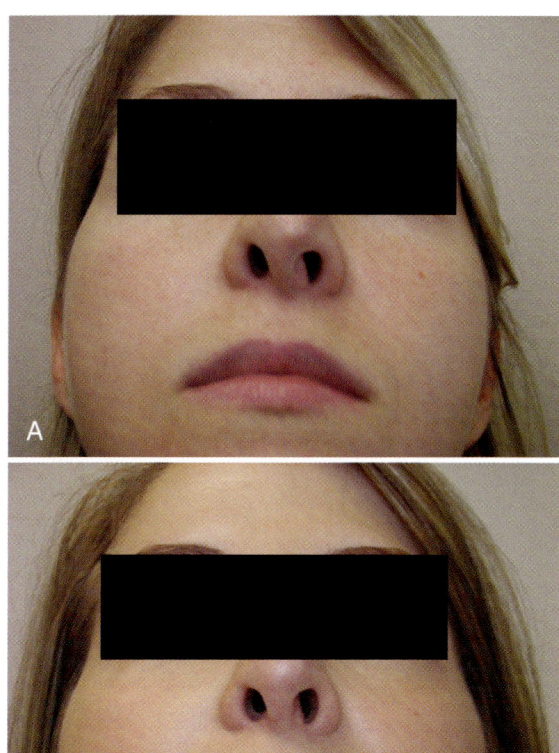

Fig. 104-10 ■ Preoperative (**A**) and postoperative (**B**) photographs showing correction of nasal tip asymmetry and irregularity after primary cosmetic rhinoplasty.

Alar Pinching

Alar pinching is caused by collapse of the lateral nasal tip, which gives the characteristic "pinched" nasal tip appearance. Alar pinching is usually the result of weakened lower lateral cartilage after primary rhinoplasty (Fig. 104-11, *A*). Reduction maneuvers such as extensive cephalic resection, crosshatching of the lateral crura or domes, and dome-splitting maneuvers are the main causes of this deformity, although some conservative procedures, such as tip sutures, may also result in severe pinching when improperly performed. In rare cases a pinch deformity is congenital and becomes exaggerated after primary rhinoplasty or if left untreated.

Mild pinching may easily be corrected via a closed approach. A small rim incision is made, a snug pocket is created in a predetermined pinched area, and a suitable amount of crushed septal cartilage is then inserted to elevate the collapsed tissue. In more severe pinching, lateral crural strut grafts, batten grafts, and alar contouring grafts may be beneficial (Fig. 104-11, *B* to *D*). The name alar batten comes from the word *alar*, which is part of the nasal ala, and *batten*, which implies stiffening as derived from nautical terminology.

To make a batten graft, a suitable piece of septal, auricular, or rib cartilage is cut and placed over the weakened area of the lower lateral cartilage and fixed at two or three points with 5-0 or 6-0 PDS suture; because this graft is placed directly under skin, any sharp edges should be trimmed and beveled carefully. This type of graft should be performed carefully in patient with thin skin.

Lateral crural strut grafts are usually obtained from septal, auricular, or rib cartilage. The piece of cartilage is meticulously cut,

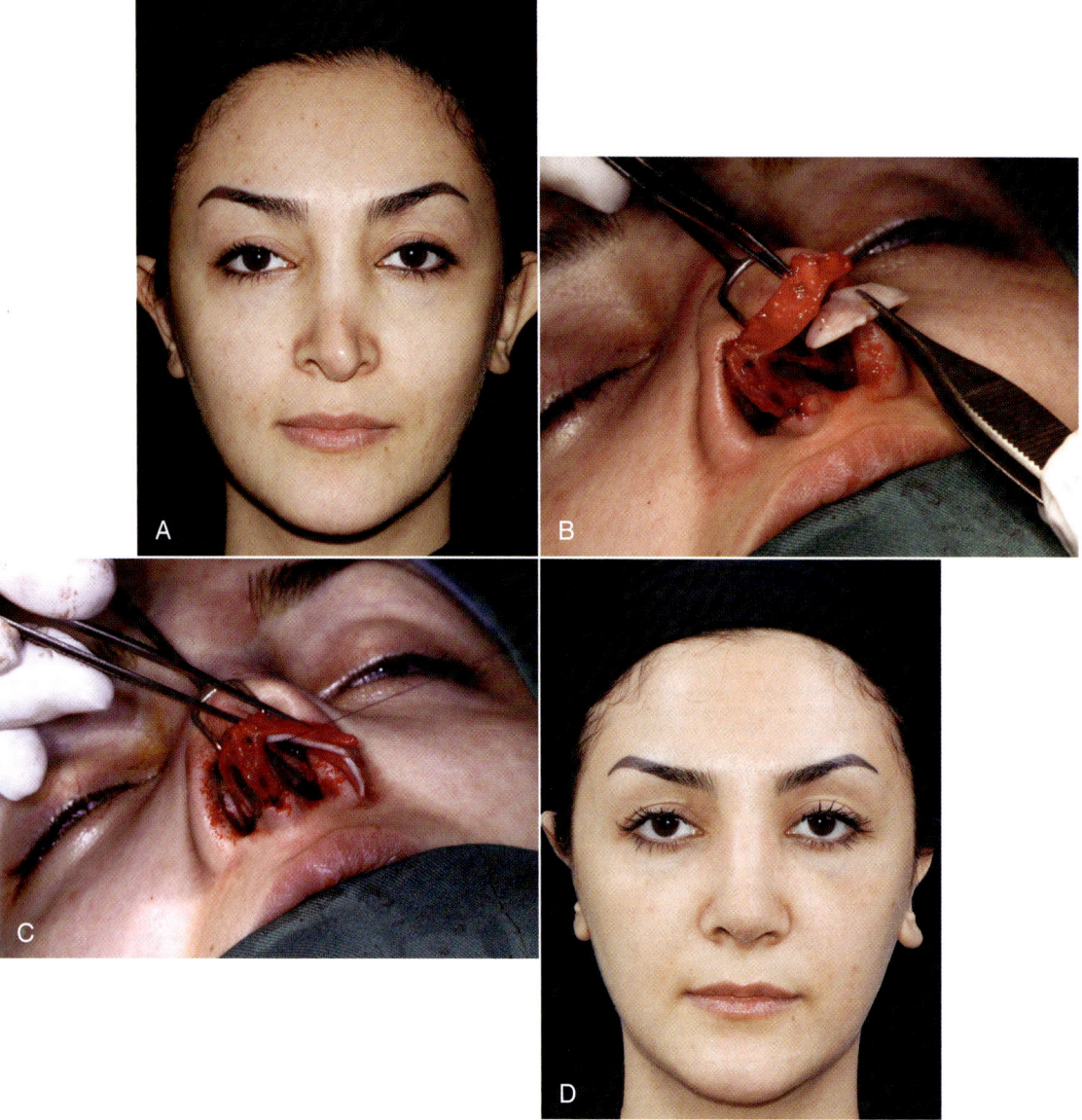

Fig. 104-11 ■ **A,** Severe pinch deformity caused by destruction of the lower lateral cartilage and collapse of the middle nasal vault. **B** and **C,** The remaining segment of lateral crura is dissected from the underlying skin, and a suitable piece of auricular cartilage is fixed under the collapsed lower lateral cartilage. **D,** Postsurgical result.

tailored, and placed under the corresponding lateral crura. This procedure can be performed by making a pocket underneath the lateral crura and the underlying vestibular skin, which forms the interior surface of the nasal external valve, or by raising and stripping the lateral crura from the underlying skin and placement of a strut (see Fig. 104-11, *C* and *D*). The main advantage of the application of a lateral crural strut graft is that it may be helpful in the correction of both pinching and retracted alar deformities, which sometimes occur concomitantly.

Alar spreader grafts are small triangular pieces of cartilage that are placed between the two lateral crura (Fig. 104-12); they help create the normal anatomic distance between the domes and will correct pinching and lower lateral cartilage collapse (Fig. 104-13).

Alar Retraction

Alar rim retraction is a common complication of primary rhinoplasty. It refers to superior retraction of the alar rim that results in excessive nostril and columellar show, most pronounced on the lateral view.

Alar retraction generally occurs after aggressive cephalic resection of the lower lateral cartilage or severe scar formation. If the alar retraction is mild, a small piece of cartilage can be placed caudal to the borders of the involved lateral crura. In more severe cases, alar contouring grafts can make a pleasant contour. Alar contour grafts are quadrangular pieces of cartilage that are cut, tailored, and placed in a pocket that is made in the soft tissue caudal to the lateral crural margins; these types of grafts are positioned in a site that is not filled with cartilage in a normal nose.

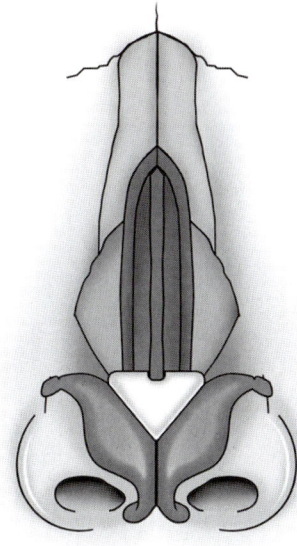

Fig. 104-12 ■ An alar spreader graft is a triangular piece of cartilage that is placed and fixed between the two lateral crura to restore collapsed alar cartilage.

In more severe cases, composite grafts are generally used to compensate for the lost tissue, and these grafts are usually harvested via an external auricular approach. The nasal ala is approached through a small marginal or infracartilaginous incision. The skin and its underlying cartilage are dissected, and the graft is sutured in position.

Hanging Columella

A hanging columella refers to excessive columellar show greater than its esthetically normal range of 2 to 4 mm. Treatment usually consists of resection of small wedges of membranous septum or the caudal portion of the cartilaginous septum. The key point in treating this deformity is correct diagnosis and differentiation between alar retraction and a hanging columella, both of which are characterized by excessive columellar show.

Retracted Columella

Over-resection of the caudal part of the septum or the membranous septum (or both) and excessive scar formation are the main causes of this deformity. Treatment of minor retractions is accomplished by creating a small pocket under the columellar skin and placing small pieces of crushed cartilage to restore the structure. In more severe cases or when a simultaneous columellar strut is needed, the strut is placed caudal to its normal position and the graft extrudes caudally from the medial crura. This extension will increase columellar show.

Under-projected and Over-projected Nasal Tip

Adjustment of tip projection usually follows the same principles that are applied in primary surgery. Loss of tip projection is generally due to the progressive loss of tip support that usually occurs as a result of weakening or destruction of the tip support mechanisms from the primary rhinoplasty. The workhorse for restoring tip projection is the use of a strong columellar strut. This cartilage is typically harvested from septal or rib cartilage. To restore stable tip projection, the columellar strut should span from the anterior nasal spine (or at most 1 to 2 mm from it) to the dome area. This graft should be fixed with several sutures to the medial crural cartilage.

In patients with over-projected tips, which is relatively rare in revision patients, the continuity of the lower lateral cartilage should be eliminated by cutting into the dome or the lateral crural area to reduce the projection. To obtain a stable and predictable projection, it is generally recommended that the excess cartilage be overlapped and resection be avoided when possible. It is preferable to compensate for weakened tip support by using different grafting techniques.

POSTOPERATIVE CARE

The postoperative care of patients undergoing revision procedures closely resembles that for primary surgery (see Chapter 103), although the extent of surgery, the use of several grafts, and possibly the length of surgery may require different considerations regarding the use of antibiotics, corticosteroids, and wound care (e.g., rib graft, ear cartilage grafts).

If there is a possibility of dead space formation or the presence of preexisting granulation tissue, injection of 20 to 40 mg of triamcinolone can be beneficial. It is usually injected over the supratip area every week for at least 4 weeks. A pressure dressing over the supratip area will help the skin redrape over its new cartilaginous framework and assist in resolution of the granulation tissue. If extranasal donor sites such as the ears, rib, or temporalis fascia are used, possible complications should be discussed thoroughly with the patient and the special postoperative issues emphasized.

PEARLS AND PITFALLS

- Revision patients are sometimes psychologically and emotionally disturbed, so before performing any surgical procedure, essential evaluations and consultations should be performed, the limitations of secondary surgery should be discussed, and the patient should be counseled that the result may be acceptable but not ideal.
- Revision rhinoplasty is frequently based on augmentation of improperly lost tissues and strengthening of weakened tissues. Any further resection should be performed with extreme caution.
- Possible donor sites should be examined and discussed with the patient.
- Revision surgery may be the last opportunity for patients to improve their esthetic and functional problems. Any possible future surgeries will be extremely difficult for both the patient and esthetic surgeon. Frequent and complete consultations and adequate time spent on preoperative, intraoperative, and postoperative visits with great attention to detail are essential.
- Postoperative care greatly affects the final outcome of surgery. The use of many pieces of cartilage graft and the presence of contracted and scar tissue in the underlying skin in a patient who has not achieved the desired outcome in the first surgery requires special attention.

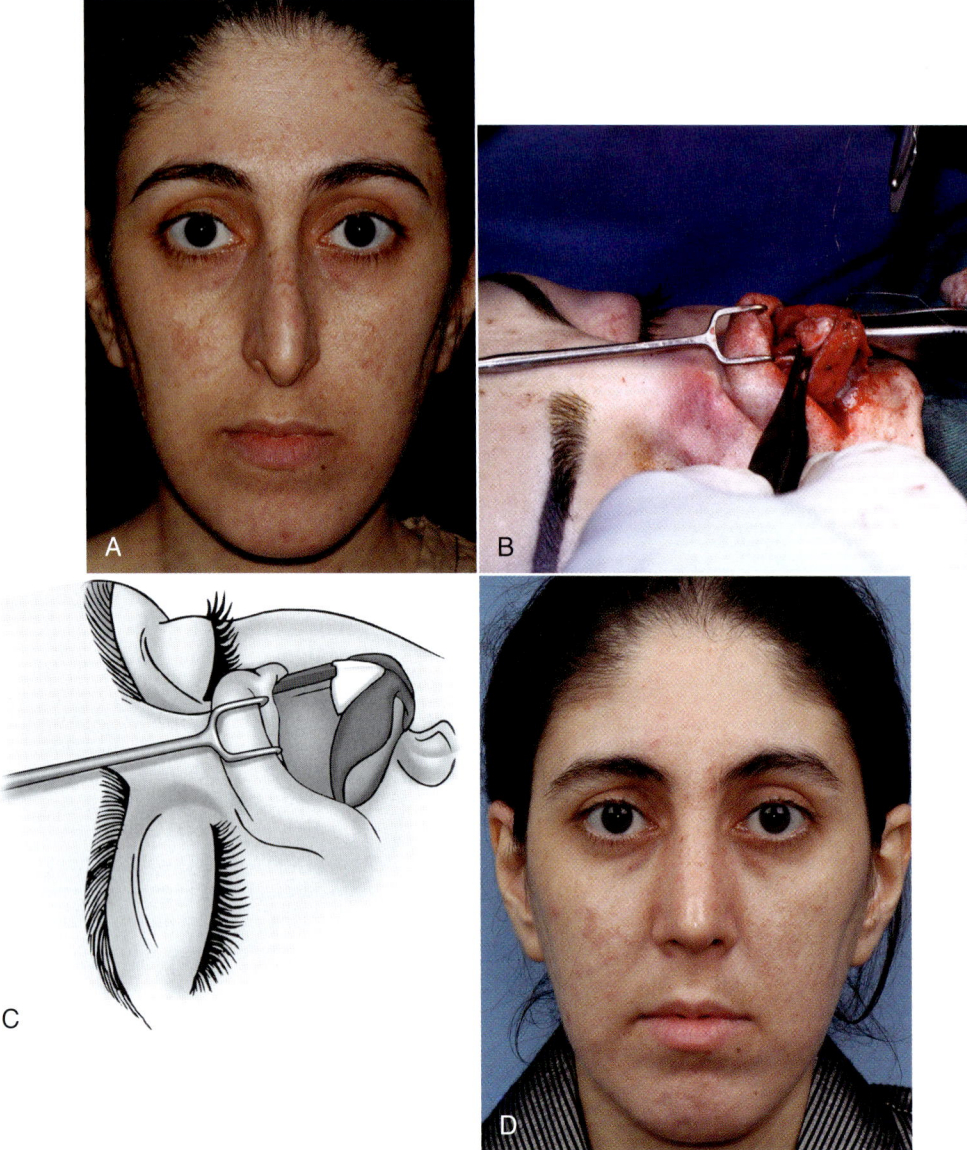

Fig. 104-13 ■ **A,** Patient in whom both the external and internal nasal valves collapsed because of destructive procedures on the lower and upper lateral cartilage. **B** and **C,** Alar spreader graft used to restore the lower lateral cartilage and septal spreaders used for restoration of the middle nasal vault. **D,** Postsurgical result.

BIBLIOGRAPHY

Adamson PA, Litner JA: Psychologic aspects of revision rhinoplasty, *Facial Plast Surg Clin North Am* 14:269-277, v, 2006.

Bagheri SC, Khan HA, Jahangirian A, et al: An analysis of 101 primary cosmetic rhinoplasties, *J Oral Maxillofac Surg*, August 2011.

Baran CN, Tiftikcioglu YO, Baran NK: The use of alloplastic materials in secondary rhinoplasties: 32 years of clinical experience, *Plast Reconstr Surg* 116:1502-1516, 2005.

Boahene KD, Hilger PA: Alar rim grafting in rhinoplasty: indications, technique, and outcomes, *Arch Facial Plast Surg* 11:285-289, 2009.

Bracaglia R, Fortunato R, Gentileschi S: Secondary rhinoplasty, *Aesthetic Plast Surg* 29:230-239, 2005.

Byrd HS, Constantian MB, Guyuron B, et al: Revision rhinoplasty, *Aesthet Surg J* 27:175-187, 2007.

Daniel RK, Calvert JW: Diced cartilage grafts in rhinoplasty surgery, *Plast Reconstr Surg* 113:2156-2171, 2004.

Fedok FG: Revision rhinoplasty, *Facial Plast Surg* 24:269, 2008.

Foda HM: Rhinoplasty for the multiply revised nose, *Am J Otolaryngol* 26:28-34, 2005.

Gunter JP, Cochran CS: Management of intraoperative fractures of the nasal septal "L-strut": percutaneous Kirschner wire fixation, *Plast Reconstr Surg* 117:395-402, 2006.

Kridel RW, Soliemanzadeh P: Tip grafts in revision rhinoplasty, *Facial Plast Surg Clin North Am* 14:331-341, v, 2006.

Romo T 3rd, Kwak ES: Nasal grafts and implants in revision rhinoplasty, *Facial Plast Surg Clin North Am* 14:373-387, vii, 2006.

Romo T 3rd, Sonne J, Choe KS, et al: Revision rhinoplasty, *Facial Plast Surg* 19:299-307, 2003.

Stelter K, Strieth S, Berghaus A: Porous polyethylene implants in revision rhinoplasty: chances and risks, *Rhinology* 45:325-331, 2007.

Toriumi DM, Patel AB, DeRosa J: Correcting the short nose in revision rhinoplasty, *Facial Plast Surg Clin North Am* 14:343-355, vi, 2006.

Weber SM, Baker SR: Alar cartilage grafts, *Clin Plast Surg* 37:253-264, 2010.

Chapter 105

Forehead, Eyebrow, and Upper Eyelid Lifting

Angelo Cuzalina, Tarek Victor Copty

It has been noted that the eyes and brows are the most influential determinants of facial expression. With our continuing pursuit of better understanding of the details of upper facial anatomy, cosmetic surgeons are able to make significant corrections and increase attractiveness of the upper part of the face with relatively minimal invasiveness.

Different regions of the face age at variable rates. The upper third of the face ages in its own unique fashion.[1] Characteristics of the aging brow, temple, eyelids, and face are relatively similar in most people (Fig. 105-1). Gravity, sun exposure, and genetic factors cause the forehead, temple, and glabellar skin to descend. Generally speaking, the aged upper face appears tired, angry, or sad when the changes described take place.[2]

Brow ptosis is a result of inferior migration of the eyebrow below its natural position at the level of the supraorbital bony rim. Clinically, the lateral eyebrow segment almost always becomes ptotic earlier in life than the medial eyebrow segment (Fig. 105-2).[3]

Redundant skin in the upper eyelid (dermatochalasis) is another phenomenon associated with the aging upper face. This "hooding" of the upper eyelids, a result of diminished skin elasticity and tone, can lead to a reduction in visual field acuity and can be cosmetically displeasing to the person affected.[4] Severe upper lid dermatochalasis can lead some patients to constantly exaggerate their elevator muscle action to compensate and maintain as normal a brow position as possible. Raising the forehead is often done subconsciously when the field of vision is being impaired as a result of excessive eyelid laxity over the eye.[2,5] Blepharoplasty or forehead and brow lifting can often relieve the ptosis over the eye and thereby diminish the subconscious forehead wrinkles (Fig. 105-3). These actions cause skin creases horizontally on the forehead. The frontalis muscle causing most of the upper facial rhytides has been the target and the draw to fame of botulinum toxin (Botox) injection.[6]

Elevation and rejuvenation of the forehead, brow, and upper eyelids have been achieved by reducing the forces that cause dynamic wrinkles on the forehead, as well as by repositioning the involved structures to their normal anatomic position. Endoscopic brow lifting was first introduced in 1991 by Keller.[7] The authors' personal experience with this procedure began in 1996. Since then, our patients tend to prefer the endoscopic approach over the other open approaches. In the majority of cases, open techniques may still be preferred in patients with a high hairline or deep forehead rhytides.

Endoscopic forehead and eyebrow lifting has a steep learning curve. Specific instruments, as well as fine surgical skill and dexterity, are needed. Furthermore, this procedure requires intimate knowledge of the anatomy associated with the forehead and periorbital structures. However, once mastered, the procedure offers the patient an elegant surgery with no hair or skin removal and an exceedingly rejuvenated appearance.

ETIOPATHOGENESIS

Facial changes can have an impact on quality of life. Rejuvenating the upper third of the face may be very rewarding to the patient and the cosmetic surgeon. Specific age-related changes in upper facial appearance can be dealt with on an individual basis or by a combination of procedures to result in maximal return of youthfulness.

The endoscopic forehead and brow lift, when properly performed, can address brow ptosis in addition to dynamic muscular problems. Before diagnosing and treating these problems the surgeon must be familiar with the different changes that the aging face experiences, as well as the possible associated causes.

Our basic understanding of the aging process is typically that the forehead, brow, and upper eyelids droop and sink because of gravitational forces and muscle activity or hyperactivity. Pioneering work by several authors has shown that gravity is not the sole determinant of the aging face. These authors have demonstrated that loss of volume, including that of soft tissue and bone, is at least equally important in the pathogenesis of the stigmata of aging (Fig. 105-4).[8] On the one hand, depletion of volume appears to be the major contributor not only to wrinkles but also to descent or sagging of the tissues; on the other hand, recent studies have shown that sun damage is probably just as important in the process of aging as gravity and loss of volume.[9]

We know that photodamage specifically causes considerable collagen deterioration and elastin reorganization, as well as depletion of the water barrier in the stratum corneum. Aged skin shows atrophy of the epidermis with straightening of the rete pegs.[10] There is a moderate decrease in the number of Langerhans cells. Dryness of the skin (xerosis cutis) is a common phenomenon. This was found to be related not to the production of sebum but to lowering of intrinsic epidermal fat and poorer retention of water. Photodamaged dermis has less cellularity and a decrease in elastic fibers, which leads to less skin elasticity.[10,11]

The cumulative effects of gravity on this less elastic skin and decreased volume of subcutaneous tissue evolve into brow ptosis. The development of deep forehead furrows arises from the repeated action of facial mimetic muscles on the overlying skin.[12]

As brow ptosis progresses, dermatochalasis of the upper lids may develop. When a patient is evaluated for blepharoplasty, it is important to consider whether the dermatochalasis is the result of redundant upper eyelid skin, a manifestation of ptotic forehead skin, or both (Fig. 105-5). Failure to recognize the cause of this deformity may result in fixation of the brow in an inappropriate position or incorrectly performing a blepharoplasty, which may result in less than ideal upper eyelid length.

Sun, smoking, nutrition, and dynamic muscle function all contribute to the etiopathogenesis of upper facial aging. However, a genetic predisposition to brow ptosis is one of the most notable

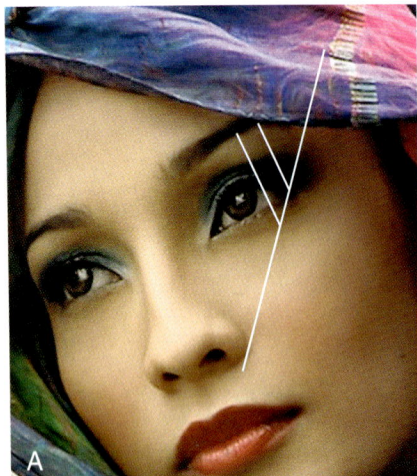

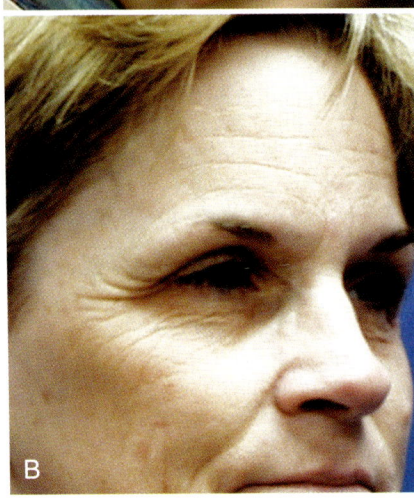

Fig. 105-1 ■ Contrast between a youthful (**A**) and an aged (**B**) upper face. The eyebrow lies above the superior orbital rim, with the lateral third being higher than the medial two thirds. An aged eyebrow shows both medial and lateral descent together with volume loss and hooding over the lateral orbital rim.

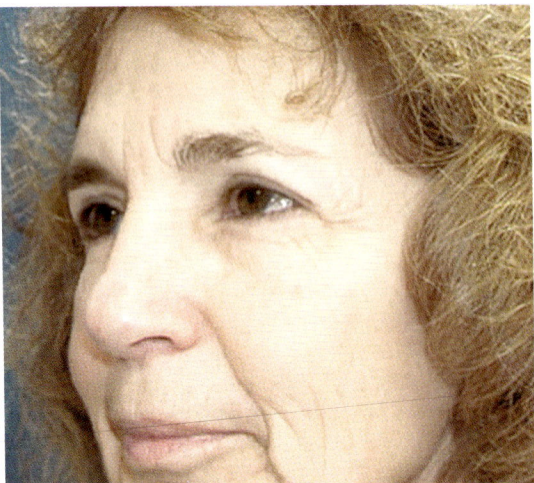

Fig. 105-2 ■ Inferior migration of the eyebrow below its natural position. The lateral brow tends to descend earlier than the medial brow during the aging process. Atrophic changes can also be seen along the entire brow.

causes of premature upper facial third aging that would benefit from cosmetic enhancement.

PATHOLOGIC ANATOMY

To rejuvenate the aging brow, one must have a fundamental understanding of the ideal brow position. In addition, the surgeon must understand the relationships between the skin, subcutaneous adipose tissue, muscle, and the deep fascial layers and their variations throughout the forehead.

Significant differences exist between the eyebrows of men and women (Fig. 105-6). In men, the hairs are embedded in thicker subcutaneous fat, which in turn rests on a prominence created by multiple muscle layers, the brow fat pad, and the underlying bony ridge. The typical male eyebrow should lie at or only slightly above the orbital rim in a more horizontal or uniform arch fashion, whereas the female eyebrow should be arched well above the superior orbital rim, with the highest point of the brow lying on a sagittal line from the lateral canthus.[13,14]

There are classically five layers covering the forehead (Fig. 105-7): skin, a subcutaneous layer of fibrofatty tissue, muscular aponeurosis sheath, loose areolar tissue connecting the galea aponeurosis sheath to the fifth layer, and the deepest layer, the periosteum or pericranium.[15]

Skin is thinner more cephalad and thicker nearer the eyebrow and glabellar areas. The skin lines of the forehead occur in a relatively standard pattern of transverse mid-forehead lines, vertical glabellar lines, and transverse radix lines.[16]

Aged skin is noted to have thinning of the dermis, which makes the skin less elastic and more prone to wrinkling.[17] Subcutaneous tissue is already thin in the upper part of the face, and with normal aging, this layer also becomes comparatively thinner.

Horizontal forehead furrows result from contraction of the underlying frontalis muscle during eyebrow elevation.[18] The frontalis muscle happens to be the only brow elevator. Several other depressor muscles play major roles in facial expression and cause the signs associated with aging skin. These depressor muscles are the corrugator supercilii, procerus, depressor supercilii, and orbicularis oculi muscles (Fig. 105-8).

The procerus muscle is a continuation of the frontalis muscle. It originates on the nasal bones and inserts cephalad into the frontalis muscle fibers and then onto the dermis. Contraction of this pyramidal-shaped muscle creates horizontal rhytides overlying the radix (bunny lines).[12] This muscle is usually transected when performing an endoscopic brow lift.

Similarly, the action of the corrugator supercilii muscle causes inferomedial contraction of the space between the brows and results in vertical and horizontal glabellar wrinkling. The corrugator originates from the inferior edge of the frontal bone, at the junction of the nasal bone and frontal bones, and inserts into the dermis of the medial aspect of the brow. This muscle has two heads, oblique and transverse, both of which need to be addressed when performing a forehead lift procedure.

The depressor supercilii muscle also plays a role in causing the forehead to depress. It originates on the frontal process of the maxilla and inserts into the medial frontalis fibers and dermis just above the medial brow region. Dissection through this muscle during endoscopic brow lifts can be the difference between a successful result and an overly elevated medial brow (Fig. 105-9).[19]

The orbicularis oculi muscle has three parts whose description is based on location: the pretarsal, preseptal, and orbital segments. It arises from the nasal portion of the *frontal bone* and also from the frontal process of the *maxilla* in front of the *lacrimal groove*. When

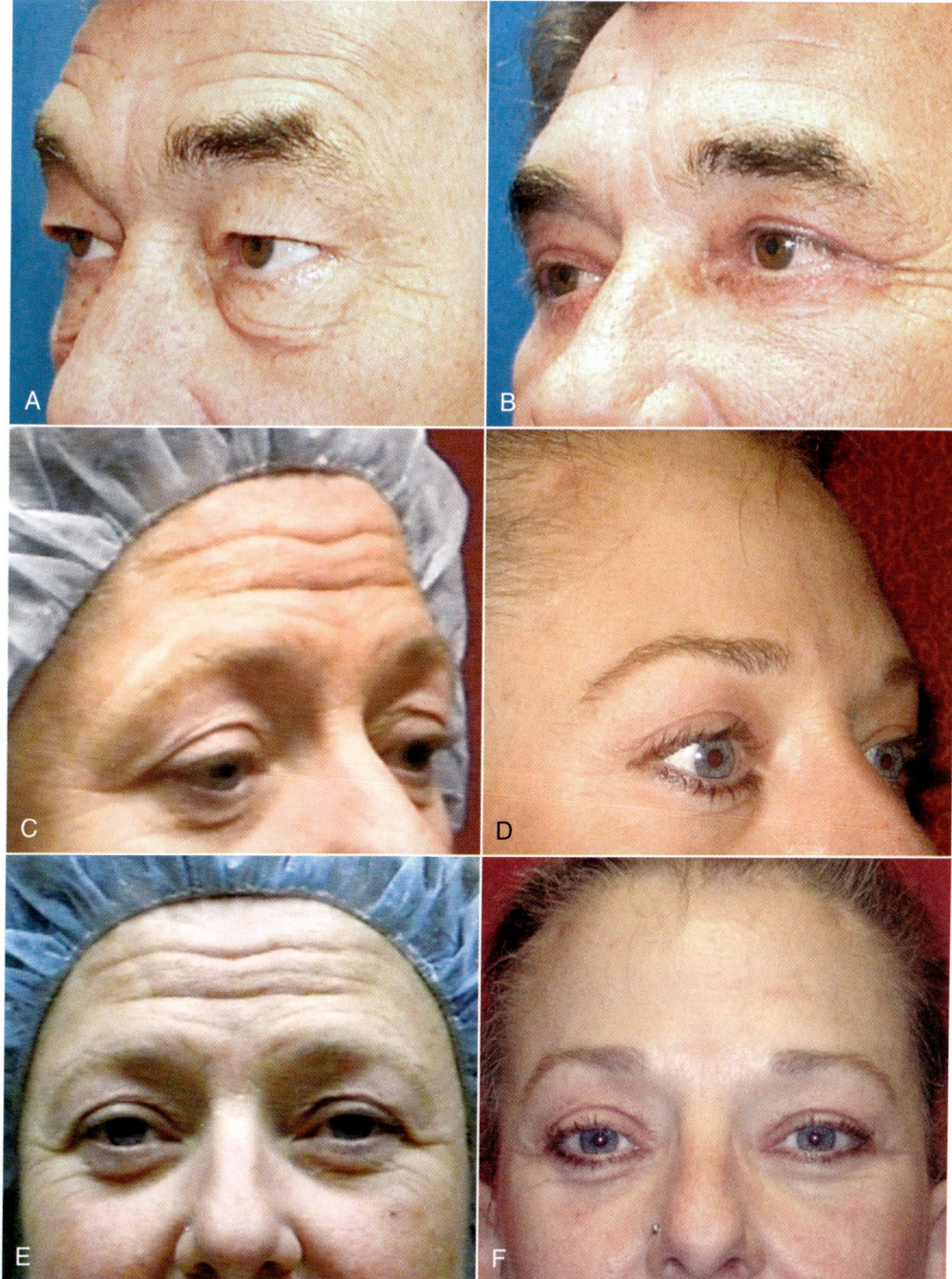

Fig. 105-3 ■ Dermatochalasis or brow ptosis can lead to constant subconscious frontalis activity that gives rise to deep horizontal forehead wrinkles. The two patients shown had different surgical techniques performed (blepharoplasty in **A** and **B**, brow lift in **C** to **F**), yet the resulting removal of laxity over the eye caused the patient to subconsciously quit raising the eyebrows and improved the forehead wrinkles.

the entire muscle is brought into action, the eyebrow, temple, and cheek are drawn toward each other to close the eyelids firmly shut. Transection of the lateral orbital portion of the orbicularis muscle is usually necessary for an adequate upper third face-lift procedure.

The frontalis muscle fibers originate from the deep galeal fascia and insert into the orbital portion of the orbicularis oculi and then into the dermis just below the eyebrow. Laterally in the temporal region, the frontalis muscle fuses into a dense fascial layer known as the zone of adherence. This zone connects the galea of the upper part of the face with the superficial fascial system of the lower part

of the face. Understanding the fascial layers of this confluence is crucial since releasing it is required for the long-term lift desired when performing an endoscopic brow lift.[20,21]

The temporoparietal (spongy) fascia is in continuity with the galea aponeurotica. This layer contains the superficial temporal artery and the frontal branch of the facial nerve (Fig. 105-10). The deep temporal fascia is thicker and has a white glistening appearance. Below the zygomatic arch, this deep temporal fascia splits into two layers called the intermediate temporal and deep temporal fasciae. The temporoparietal fascia is in continuity with

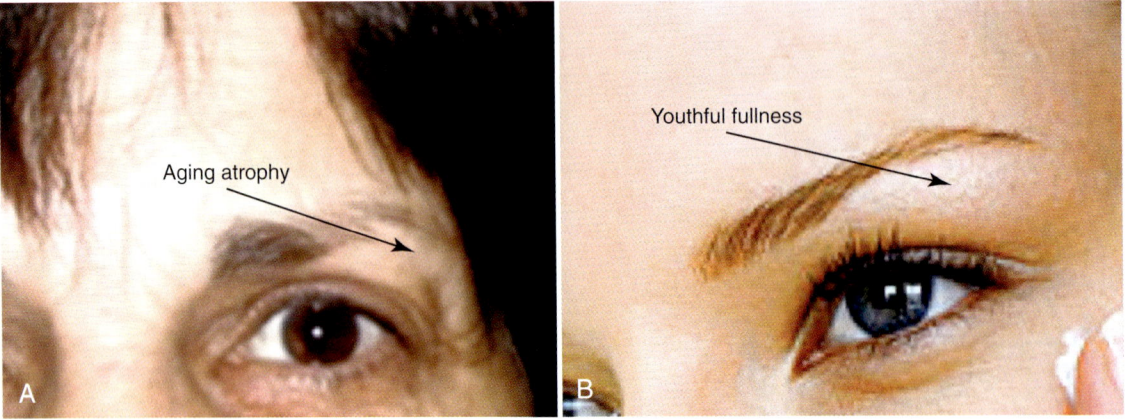

Fig. 105-4 ■ One of the causes of an aging appearance around the eyebrow is loss of volume. Notice the difference in volume associated with the eyebrow when comparing **A** and **B.**

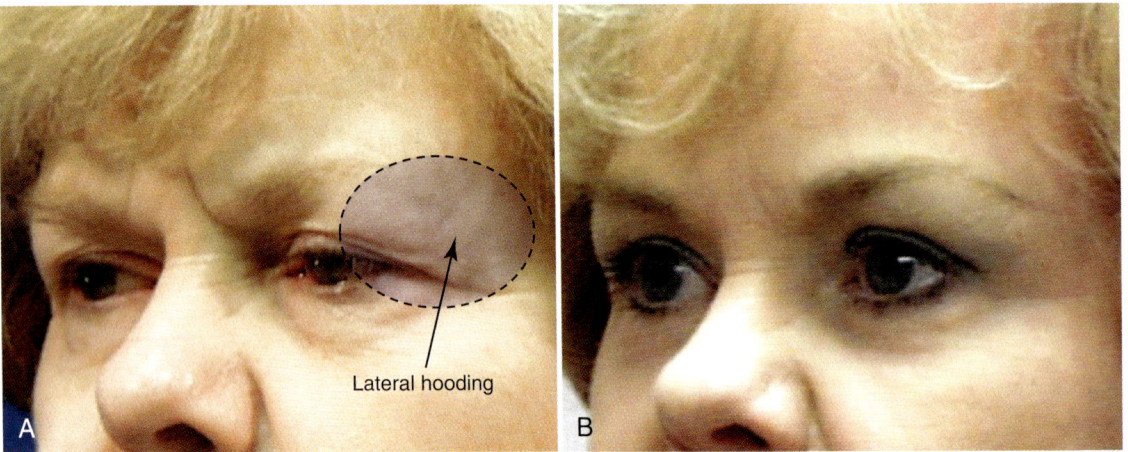

Fig. 105-5 ■ **A,** A brow lift is required for maximum esthetics in patients with lateral hooding and heavy dynamic glabellar rhytides. **B,** A 55-year-old woman 6 months following a brow lift and simultaneous upper and lower blepharoplasty. Blepharoplasty or brow lifting alone would probably have been inadequate treatment to fully improve the extreme laxity and lateral hooding.

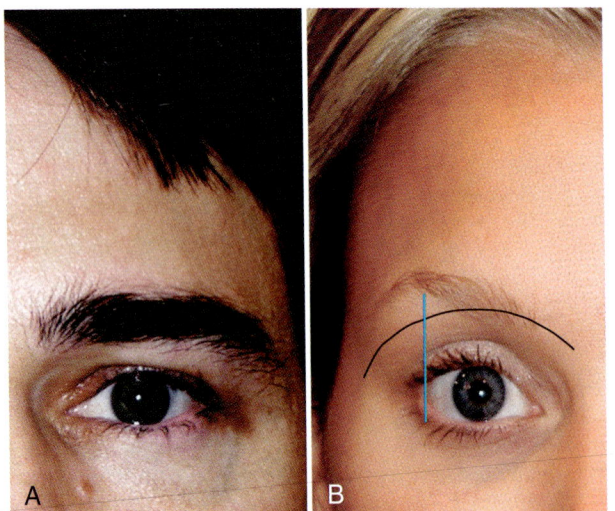

Fig. 105-6 ■ The typical male eyebrow (**A**) should lie at or only slightly above the orbital rim in a more horizontal or uniform arch fashion, whereas the female eyebrow (**B**) should be arched above the superior orbital rim, with the highest point of the brow on a sagittal line from the lateral canthus.

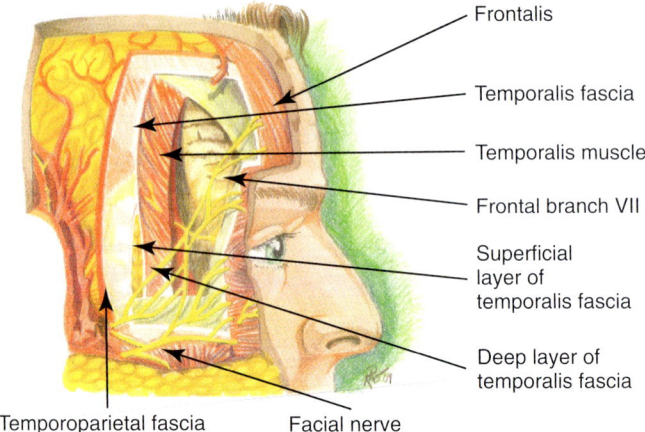

Fig. 105-7 ■ Knowledge of the tissue layers overlying the forehead and temple is critical to avoid nerve injury and perform surgery safely. The frontal nerve lies on the deep side of the temporoparietal fascia.

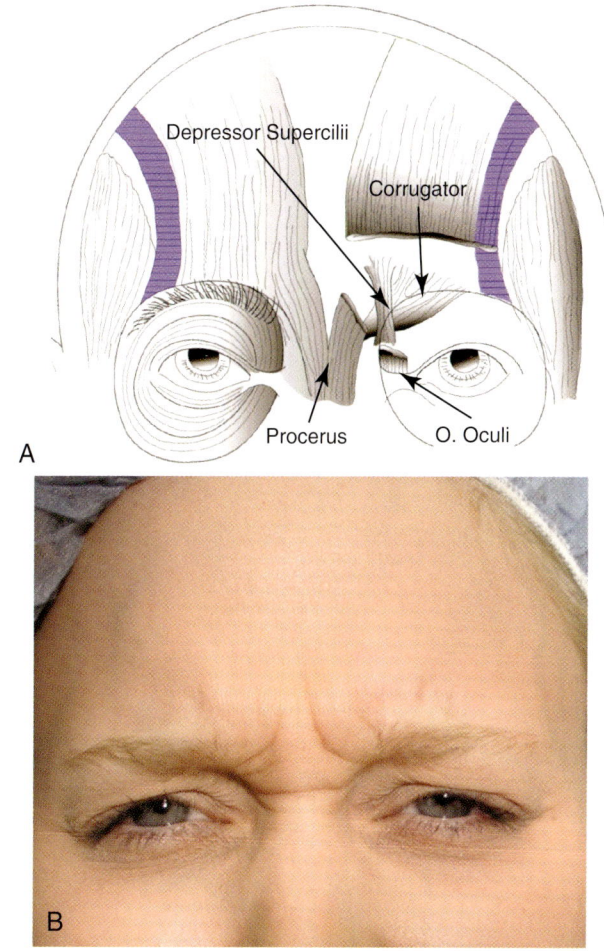

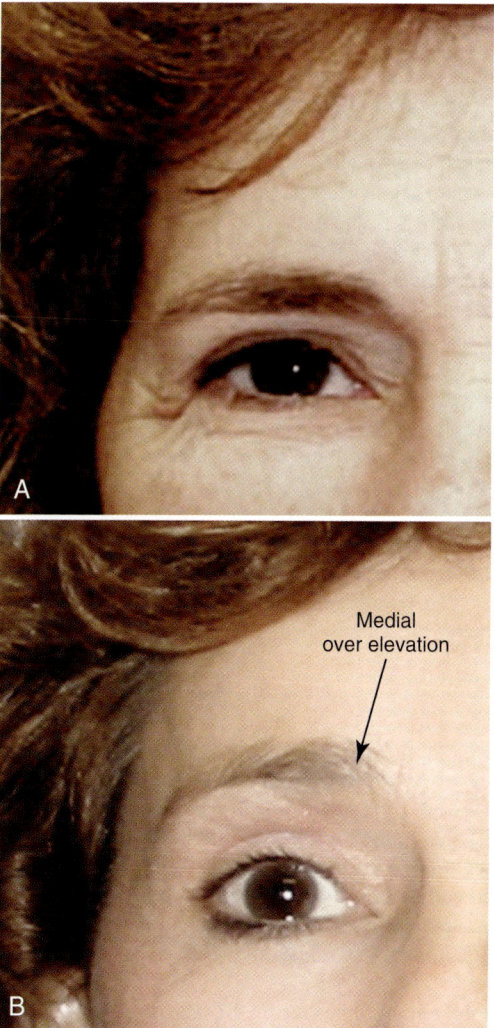

Fig. 105-8 ■ **A,** The major elevator of the eyebrow and forehead is the frontalis muscle. Several depressor muscles are shown through the cut frontalis: the corrugator supercilii, the procerus, the depressor supercilii, and the orbicularis oculi. **B,** The patient demonstrates the classic wrinkles formed from two major depressors. The horizontal (bunny lines) wrinkle is formed by the procerus at the radix. The corrugators form the vertical wrinkles in the glabella.

Fig. 105-9 ■ Overly aggressive dissection through the depressor supercilii can lead to an overly elevated brow appearance. If the medial eyebrow is higher than the lateral brow, the patient will have a "surprised" look, which is not esthetically pleasing.

the superficial musculoaponeurotic system (SMAS) below the zygomatic arch and the galea aponeurotica, which in turn is in continuity with the frontalis muscle.[22]

Detailed understanding of the fascial layers and their relationship to the muscles just described, as well as the relationship of these layers to bones and significant vessels in the region, is essential to perform a safe and successful eyebrow lift procedure.

The frontal bone makes up most of the upper third of the face.[23] The bones involved in brow lift procedures include the frontal, maxillary, zygomatic, temporal, and nasal bones. The suture lines connecting these bones include the coronal, nasofrontal, zygomaticofrontal, and zygomaticotemporal processes. The three bones involved in forming the orbital rim are the frontal, zygomatic, and maxillary bones. The zygomaticofrontal suture line is the landmark for ending most basic brow lift dissections.

Awareness of bone thickness in different locations of the skull is of absolute importance when performing a lifting procedure. If bone tunnels or screws are planned for fixation, the midline should be avoided because of the sagittal sinus, as well as the venous lakes in the mid-frontal area of the cranium. The lateral position of the middle meningeal artery should be noted and avoided near the thin, petrous portion of the parietal bone. The safest placement for tunnels

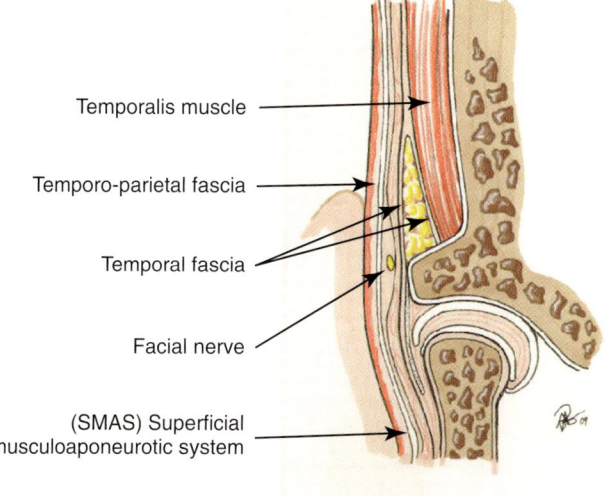

Fig. 105-10 ■ Cross section through the temporomandibular joint and zygomatic arch. The temporal nerve runs immediately below the temporoparietal fascia above the arch, which is the fascia continuous with the superficial musculoaponeurotic system below the arch.

and screws is along a parasagittal line located approximately at the mid-pupil or just anterior to the coronal suture.[24]

Knowledge of the facial nerve is paramount when operating on the face. Endoscopic forehead, temporal, and maxillary dissection provides more opportunity to learn the anatomy of the face from a different perspective. The facial nerve emerges from the substance of the parotid gland in the form of several branches and remains deep to the SMAS.[25] The five branches are the temporal, zygomatic, buccal, mandibular, and cervical nerves.

The temporal (frontal) branch of the facial nerve exits the superior aspect of the parotid gland below the SMAS and eventually crosses the zygomatic arch, usually in multiple branches.[26] Above the arch, the nerve travels in the temporoparietal fascia and enters the lateral part of the frontalis muscle and superior part of the orbicularis oculi. Dissection in this temporal lateral area during a combined forehead lift and face-lift generally requires two planes of dissection. The forehead lift usually involves dissection in the temporal area below the temporoparietal fascia, whereas the face-lift dissection is performed in the subcutaneous plane to avoid injury to the temporal nerve that lies between the two levels of dissection. The temporal and zygomatic branches share the nerve supply to the orbicularis oculi, the corrugator supercilii, and the procerus.[27,28]

It is of importance during dissection to differentiate between the auriculotemporal nerve and the temporal (frontal) nerves. The auriculotemporal nerve (from the trigeminal nerve) supplies sensation to the front of the ear and the skin over the zygomatic arch. This nerve runs 1 cm anterior to the tragus of the ear, whereas the more important temporal branch of the facial nerve runs an average of 2 cm anterior to the tragus when crossing the zygomatic arch. As mentioned earlier, the superficial temporal fascia is continuous with the galea aponeurosis, which contains the superficial temporal artery, the temporal branch of the facial nerve, and the auriculotemporal nerve.[29]

Sensation to the skin covering the face is supplied by the trigeminal nerve. The auriculotemporal nerve supplies the lateral ear and zygoma region with sensation, and the scalp and eyebrow are innervated by the supratrochlear and supraorbital nerves. The supraorbital nerve exits the supraorbital foramen, whereas the supratrochlear nerves exit from around the orbital rim approximately 1 cm medial to the exit of the supraorbital nerve. The supraorbital nerve divides after exiting the cranium into deep and superficial branches. The topographic landmark for the course of the supraorbital nerve at the supraorbital rim reliably lines up with the medial limbus of the iris.[30] The deep (or lateral) division supplies the lateral posterior area of the forehead and scalp, and the superficial (or medial) division enters the frontalis and supplies sensation to the anterior forehead region. The infratrochlear nerves supply sensation to the medial orbital rim and upper part of the nose. These nerves exit just below the supratrochlear nerves (Fig. 105-11).

Since eyelid evaluation and possible intervention play a role in rejuvenating the upper third of the face, the anatomy of the eyelids needs to be addressed. The skin of the eyelid is extremely thin and well vascularized. Typically, the arterial supply runs parallel with the sensory and motor nerves (Fig. 105-12). The upper eyelid skin has very little subcutaneous tissue but is firmly adherent to the underlying orbicularis oculi muscle. The orbicularis muscle is divided into pretarsal, preseptal, and orbital components (Fig. 105-13). Deep to the orbicularis is the orbital septum, a thin fibrous sheet that originates at the orbital rim and is in continuity with the orbital periosteum (Fig. 105-14). The septum fuses with the levator aponeurosis above the superior tarsal border. The tarsal plate and conjunctiva lie deep to the orbital septum (Fig. 105-15).[31,32]

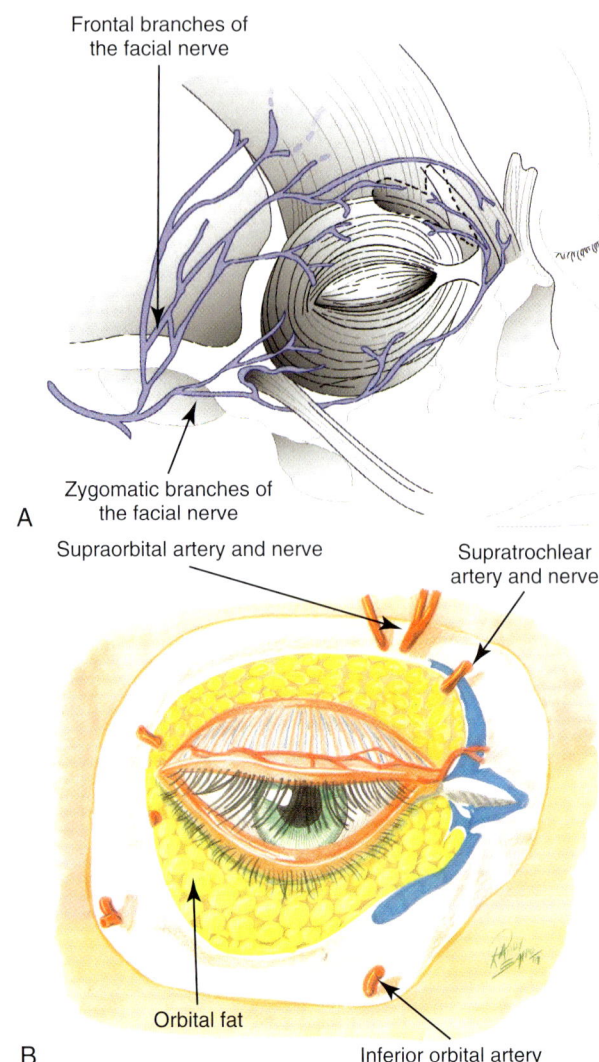

Frontal branches of the facial nerve

Zygomatic branches of the facial nerve

A

Supraorbital artery and nerve

Supratrochlear artery and nerve

Orbital fat

Inferior orbital artery

B

Fig. 105-11 ■ **A,** Location of both the zygomatic and frontal nerves. The corrugator muscle in innervated by both. **B,** Sensory innervation. The supraorbital nerve and supratrochlear nerve can both be seen. The corrugator muscle is not innervated by these sensory nerves despite the fact that they pierce this muscle during their course.

The upper eyelid has two pre-aponeurotic fat pads, the central and medial compartments, that lie between the orbital septum and the levator aponeurosis.[33] The medial fat pads are the most often addressed pads during blepharoplasty. The lacrimal gland occupies the lateral aspect of the orbit and may only rarely need lifting, as in the case of prolapse affecting the visual field. Upper eyelid resection (blepharoplasty) is sometimes combined with a forehead and brow lift for an optimal result (Fig. 105-16).

The levator palpebrae superioris muscle originates at the lesser wing of the sphenoid and inserts into the inferior part of the tarsus and into the orbicularis muscle and skin. This insertion into the skin and muscle of the upper eyelid forms the upper eyelid crease, which falls approximately 1 cm above the upper eyelid margin.[34] The levator and Müller muscle act as the eyelid retractors.

ENDOSCOPIC ANATOMY

Access must be gained by the endoscope for release of the eyebrow from its periosteal attachments. Through incisions to be discussed later in the chapter, blunt dissection is performed in the subperiosteal plane to approximately 2 cm away from the orbital rim and

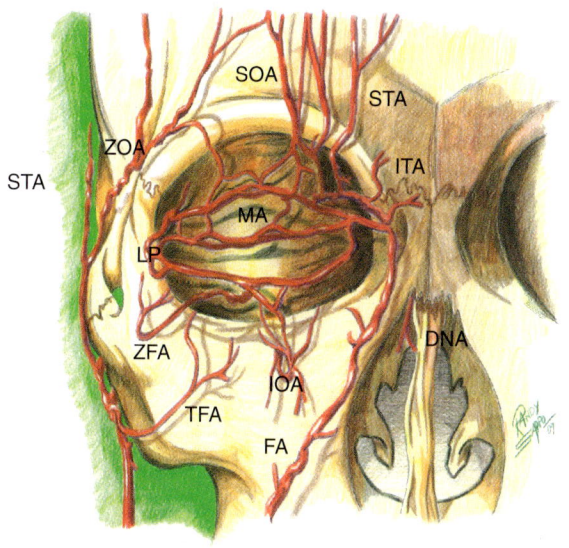

Fig. 105-12 ■ The arterial blood supply to the peri-orbital region is excellent. DNA, dorsal nasal artery; FA, facial artery; ITA, inferior trochlear artery, LP, lateral palpebral artery; MA, meningeal arteries; IOA, inferior orbital artery; SOA, supraorbital artery; STA, superficial temporal artery; STA, supratrochlear artery; TFA, transverse facial artery; ZFA, zygomaticofacial artery; ZOA, zygomatico-orbital artery.

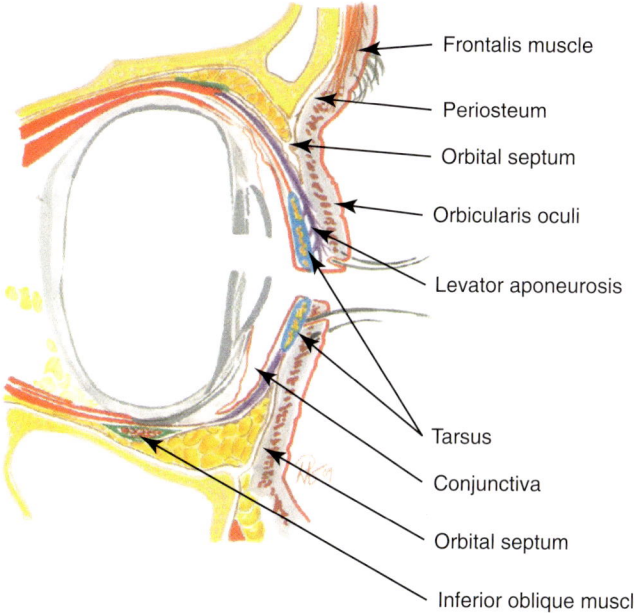

Fig. 105-15 ■ Cross section of the globe. The periosteum is released during an endoscopic brow lift immediately above the point where the orbital septum attaches to bone.

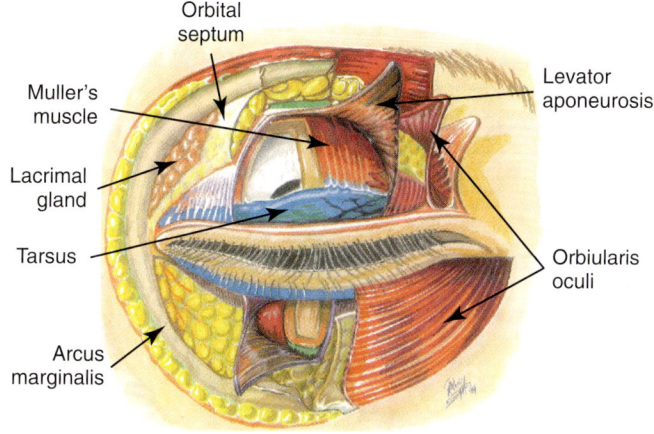

Fig. 105-13 ■ Note the concentrated amount of delicate anatomy in the periorbital region.

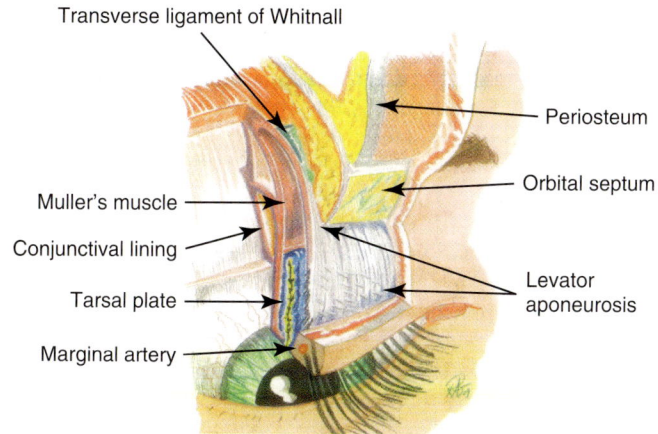

Fig. 105-14 ■ Detailed anatomy of the eyelid and orbit.

zygomatic arch. The last 2 cm needs to be dissected under endo-scopic visual guidance. Laterally, it is the authors' advice to dissect above the superficial temporal fascia through the lateral incisions and connect into the central subperiosteal plane, the "safe zone" (Fig. 105-17). Staying deep to the periosteum prevents injury to the deep divisions and branches of the supraorbital nerve that lie in the subgaleal plane near the zone of fixation. Dissection posteriorly toward the occiput is also performed in the subperiosteal or some-times in the subgaleal plane to create room for scalp elevation and aid in providing space for and maneuverability of the endoscope.[35]

Attention is first directed to the lateral aspect of the elevated forehead flap. The zone of fixation begins at the lateral corner of the superior orbital rim. Again, this is the point where all the fascial layers come together. Dissection laterally in this position to expose the lateral orbicularis oculi and release the zone of fascial conver-gence needs to be precise. The temporal branch of the facial nerve curves medially in this area during its upward path toward the fore-head, and care should be taken to not injure it. Another structure that the cosmetic surgeon will become acquainted with in this lateral corner is the sentinel vein, which is situated approximately 1 cm lateral to the zygomaticofrontal suture line. This vein can be seen going through the temporoparietal fascia at a perpendicular angle. The sentinel vein can be sacrificed, but care must be taken to not cauterize the area where the vein can retract and continue to bleed.[36,37]

The central dissection plane takes the surgeon down to the level of the superior orbital rim, where the entire superior rim should be visualized. The endoscope should provide a good view of the peri-osteum elevated in a relatively bloodless plane. Dissection through the periosteum will reveal the subgaleal fat, except at the supraor-bital nerve level. The nerve, artery, and their branches can be seen penetrating the fascial layers toward the frontalis and subcutaneous tissue and originating from the supraorbital notch in alignment with the medial limbus. While dissecting further superficially toward the muscles of the glabella and medial eyebrow, the surgeon should keep in mind the position of the supraorbital nerve and artery. The supraorbital nerve, as mentioned earlier, runs in line with the medial

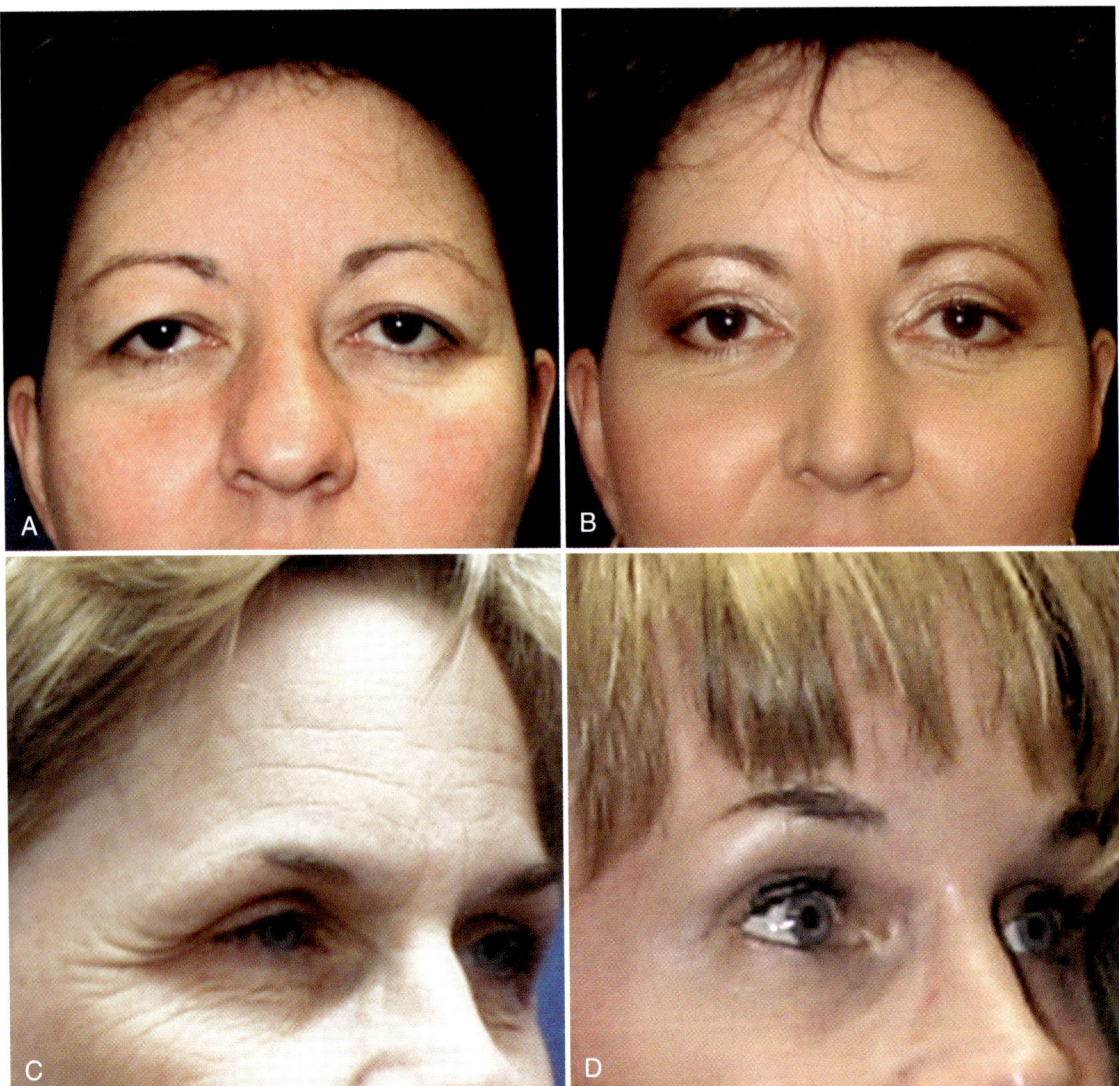

Fig. 105-16 ■ Preoperative (**A**) and postoperative (**B**) photographs of a female patient who has relatively good brow position and obtained a very nice result from upper blepharoplasty alone. Preoperative (**C**) and postoperative (**D**) photographs of female patients who required both brow lifting and blepharoplasty because of severe lateral hooding and laxity of the eyelid skin after lifting the brow.

limbus of the eyebrow.[30] Medial to this nerve bundle, the corrugator supercilii can be seen with its two heads. Once the oblique head of the corrugator is transected, the supratrochlear nerve and depressor supercilii muscle are encountered and should be avoided unless over-elevation is needed by transecting the depressor supercilii muscle (Figs. 105-18 and 105-19). Looking further medially in the glabella will show the procerus muscle, which should also be sacrificed for adequate forehead release while keeping in mind that it is a thin muscle and that an overly aggressive transection technique can penetrate through the skin. Continued dissection toward the skin will then expose the orbicularis oculi, which is typically not disrupted medially unless preoperative evaluation has revealed a need to do so; instead, this muscle will be transected rather laterally to gain lateral eyebrow elevation and a reduction in crow's feet rhytides. In patients with deep horizontal furrows, the periosteum and its overlying fascial layers can be transected along the forehead flap for moderate reduction of these forehead rhytides.

DIAGNOSTIC STUDIES AND PREOPERATIVE EVALUATION

As with all cosmetic surgery, diagnosis and preoperative planning are key. First and foremost, the patient needs to request the cosmetic surgeon to perform eyebrow, eyelid, and forehead restoration. Reasonable expectations and psychological stability need to be the base on which further management is built.

The condition of the skin should be evaluated, especially in patients with significant sun damage and dyschromia. These changes may conceal the results of a good forehead lift. Chemical peels or laser resurfacing may be used in conjunction with a brow lift procedure, as well as with blepharoplasty.

Eyebrow position is assessed while keeping in mind the aforementioned differences between male and female eyebrows. The eyebrow is manually elevated to the expected postoperative position, which may reveal that skin excision may be necessary in some

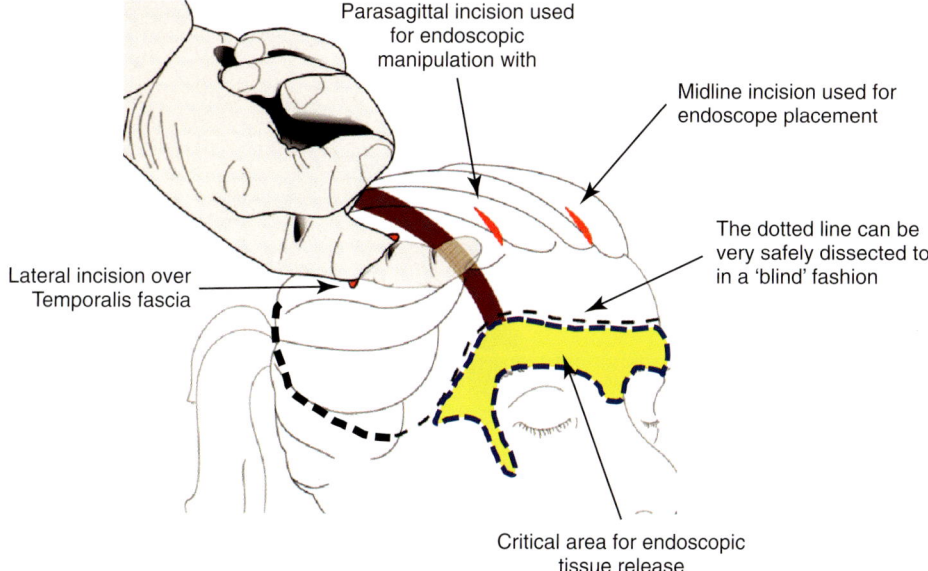

Fig. 105-17 ■ Access gained to the subperiosteal plane via finger dissection after the medial portion of the scalp is elevated with instrument dissection. Blunt and blind dissection can be performed safely down to 1.5 cm above the orbital rims. Further dissection (*yellow shaded area*) should be performed under direct visualization.

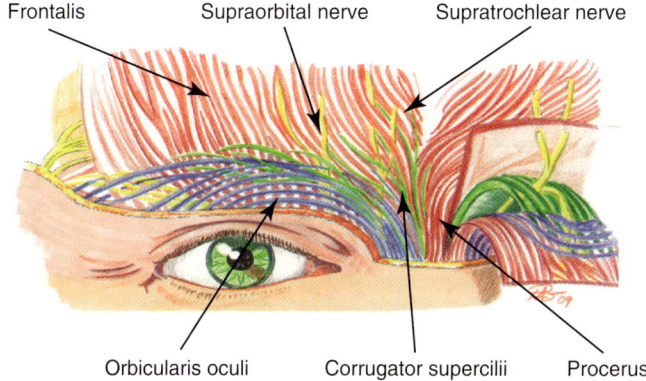

Fig. 105-18 ■ Close relationship between the depressor muscles of the eyebrow and the supraorbital and supratrochlear nerves.

infrequent instances. The forehead distance is then measured. Authors have described the ideal distance from the superior eyebrow to the hairline to be 6 cm. The presence of a long or short forehead may dictate to the surgeon and patient which type of forehead lift will work best. Visual acuity, adequate tear secretion, and eyelid laxity (dermatochalasis) are then assessed. Patients with upper eyelid laxity over their visual field commonly recruit the frontalis muscle to raise their eyebrows in a constant fashion.[38] The eyebrows are ideally evaluated with the frontalis muscle in the most relaxed state. Medial fat pad prominence, orbicularis muscle hypertrophy, and lacrimal gland ptosis are also documented for possible intervention to attain an optimal blepharoplastic result.

Forehead lines, glabellar lines, nasal (bunny) lines, and crow's feet are also noted if present. Some of these age-defining lines are significantly deep and may not be completely eliminated following the lift. Patients' expectations should be realistic, as well as surgeons' understanding of the additive effect of botulinum toxin therapy in the postoperative period. Chronic hyperdynamic action of the brow depressors can lead to muscle hypertrophy, which needs

to be noted for adequate resection or debulking during eyebrow cosmesis.[39]

Finally, bone irregularities are evaluated and calculated into the surgeon's equation for a pleasing cosmetic operative result. Computed tomography or cephalometric radiographs may be needed for detailed evaluation of the bony structure of the patient's forehead, especially if bone reduction and possible involvement of the frontal sinus are to be expected.

All surgical patients must be questioned about their current and past medical history, including previous surgeries, drug allergies, current medications and other over-the-counter drugs, and vitamins that may increase risk for bleeding or deep venous thrombosis. A personal history or family history of bleeding disorders should be noted, as well as labile or uncontrolled hypertension. Certain medications that may increase bleeding time or cause platelet dysfunction should be stopped 2 weeks before surgery and restarted approximately 1 week after surgery.

Preoperative photographs should be taken in different angles to aid in surgical decision making and intraoperative guidance. This is especially helpful since much of the gravitational pull on the eyebrows and eyelids is different in the supine position than when standing or sitting. Such photographs are of absolute importance to the novice cosmetic surgeon. The usual photographs taken include a frontal view, each side view, and a 45-degree picture from each side.

TREATMENT GOALS

Realistic expectations should always be established between cosmetic surgeons and their patients. The different approaches available for surgery should also be discussed.

Four features of the upper third of the face are usually addressed by cosmetic surgeons. One or more of these aspects can be the focus of complaint and thus dictate the treatment goals and surgical approach. The four features are skin quality, rhytides, brow position, and eyelid redundancy/medial fat pat protrusion.

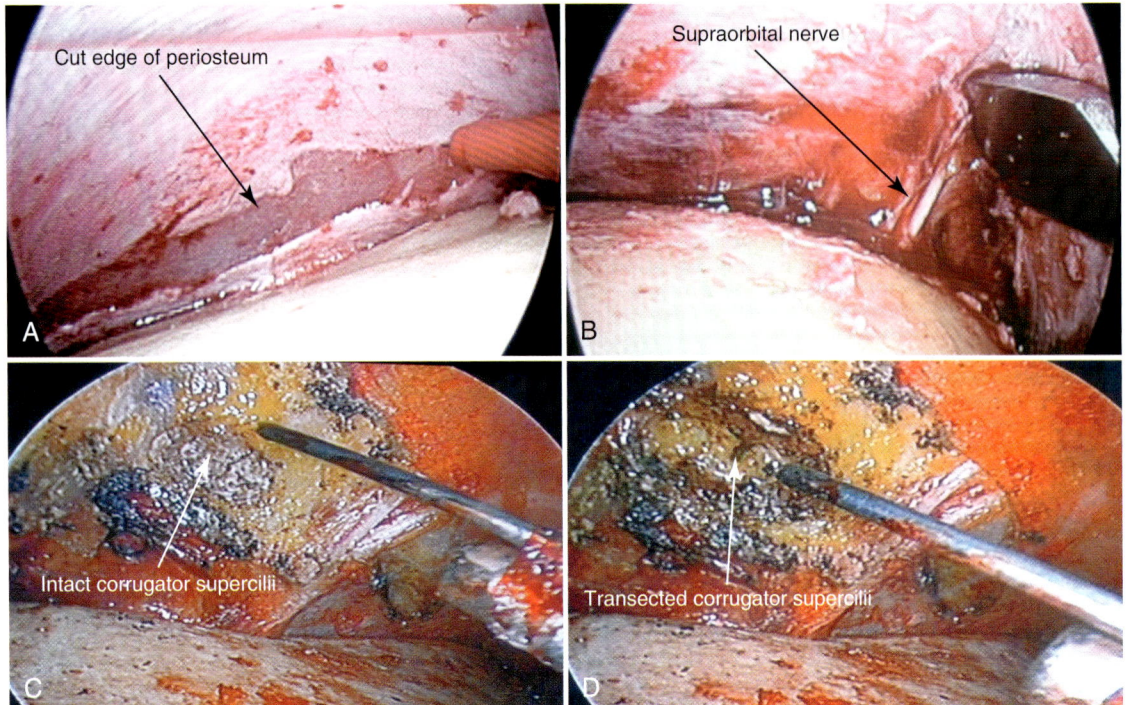

Fig. 105-19 ■ Close relationship between the left corrugator muscle and the supraorbital nerve. The belly of the corrugator lies superficial to the nerve both medially and laterally.

Skin quality, dyschromia, telangiectases, and other skin problems can be improved cosmetically in several ways. Chemical peels, dermabrasion, laser treatments, topical medications, and various injections are all helpful in conjunction with facial cosmetic surgery.[40]

Aging lines and rhytides of the forehead and the periorbital region will be greatly improved with forehead, eyebrow, and eyelid cosmetic surgery. Experienced surgeons will recognize the limitations of surgery when dealing with deep lines and thick skin. Subcutaneous release, laser treatment, botulinum toxin, and filler injections can help deal with these compounding pathologies and can turn the cosmetic result into an exceptional one.

Forehead length, hairline adjustment, and other foci of treatment will require the appropriate procedure for cosmesis of the upper third of the face. The classic coronal lift corrects the eyebrow, forehead, and glabella through a hidden scar in the hairline. Though currently considered to be too large an incision, this technique also moves the hairline posteriorly and may be inappropriate for patients with a long forehead. Patients with a high hairline/long forehead and eyebrow ptosis may best benefit from the trichophytic technique. This procedure allows the surgeon to shorten the forehead but risks the patient having a visible anterior hairline scar.[41]

Eyebrow asymmetry with or without ptosis can be addressed by using a direct eyebrow lift technique, which has the advantage of a lower incidence of postoperative forehead hypoesthesia. The mid-forehead technique can also be used to raise the eyebrows and correct asymmetry. Both the direct and mid-forehead techniques create a probable risk of a visible scar above the eyebrow or in the mid-forehead, respectively.[42]

The endoscopic forehead and eyebrow lift has gained tremendous momentum because of the fact that it is minimally invasive in comparison to the coronal and trichophytic operations. Endoscopically, the cosmetic surgeon can correct eyebrow, forehead, and glabellar signs of aging with less hypoesthesia and chance of alopecia.

Drawbacks include the need for special instrumentation, a significant learning curve, and minor elevation of the patient's hairline.

SPECIFIC TREATMENT AND TECHNIQUES

The lasting effect and minimal morbidity associated with endoscopic upper face-lift have made this procedure sought after by patients and an invaluable tool for every facial cosmetic surgeon.[43] Knowledge of the open techniques is still an absolute necessity for becoming comfortable with the endoscopic technique, as with any minimally invasive procedure. Moreover, the endoscopic approach is not without limitations, and an open procedure may sometimes be needed to correct the patient's specific complaint (Fig. 105-20).

CORONAL FOREHEAD AND BROW LIFT

This technique involves an incision across the hair-bearing scalp approximately 4 to 5 cm behind the hairline and extending from ear to ear. This line can also be connected to a regular face-lift incision at the superior helical attachment of the ear. Dissection is carried down to the subgaleal or subperiosteal level and elevated to the level of the superior orbital rims and laterally into the sub-temporoparietal plane. Correction of any forehead deformity can be addressed with the wide coronal exposure. Deep forehead creases can be reduced with a midline frontalis myotomy, whereas glabellar lines are corrected by transection or resection of the exposed depressor muscles of the eyebrow. Visualization of the supraorbital and supratrochlear nerves is an advantage of this exposure and reduces the risk for injury.

Bone deformities can also be corrected with this approach. This lift can be a great operation for patients with a short forehead (<5 cm), but it can be a significant drawback in those with a normal or long forehead since it elevates the hairline even further. Excision of excess scalp skin is performed after accurate measurement and redraping of the forehead flap. The documented rough estimate is

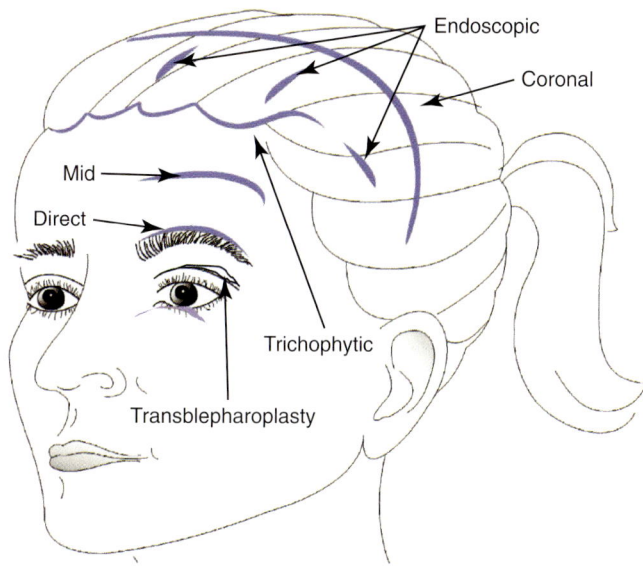

Fig. 105-20 ■ The different incisions and techniques used during forehead and eyebrow lifting.

that 2 cm of scalp must be excised for every 1 cm of brow elevation. As mentioned earlier, this approach can be used for access to the mid-face, but care must be taken to not injure the frontal branches of the facial nerve. This procedure exposes an enormous surgical field and can therefore be a great technique for novice surgeons (Fig. 105-21). It should be kept in mind that other than elevation of the hairline, this procedure poses risk for alopecia, persistent scalp numbness, longer operative time, and excessive blood loss, and results in a long scar.[44]

TRICHOPHYTIC AND PRETRICHIAL FOREHEAD AND BROW LIFT

When it is desirable to shorten the forehead or avoid displacement of the hairline, a trichophytic lift can be the procedure of choice. A trichophytic incision is made just behind the frontal hairline, whereas a pretrichial incision is made in front of the hairline. A modified version of the trichophytic incision involves a beveled incision to cover the scar with hair follicles, as well as creation of a wavy incision to prevent a linear scar.

This technique allows the same excellent exposure that the coronal method provides and has the ability to lower a high forehead or prevent raising it, although limited lateral dissection is usually encountered. Direct visualization of the brow depressor muscles and the associated nerves is gained as with the coronal exposure. Subgaleal or subperiosteal elevation can be used with this method, although a subcutaneous technique is performed more often. Subcutaneous dissection elevates the dermal attachments, releases the deep horizontal creases, and also adds the advantage of reducing posterior scalp sensory loss.

The trichophytic and pretrichial methods are ideal for patients with heavy forehead rhytides, low brow position, or a high forehead. However, patients are discouraged by the visible scar and distorted hairline associated with this technique. As a result, most will opt for the endoscopic approach even if it involves raising the hairline.[45]

ENDOSCOPIC FOREHEAD AND BROW LIFT

The endoscopic technique has become a state-of-the-art approach for dealing with the upper third of the face,[46] mainly because of its benefits, which include no scalp resection, minimal risk for sensory

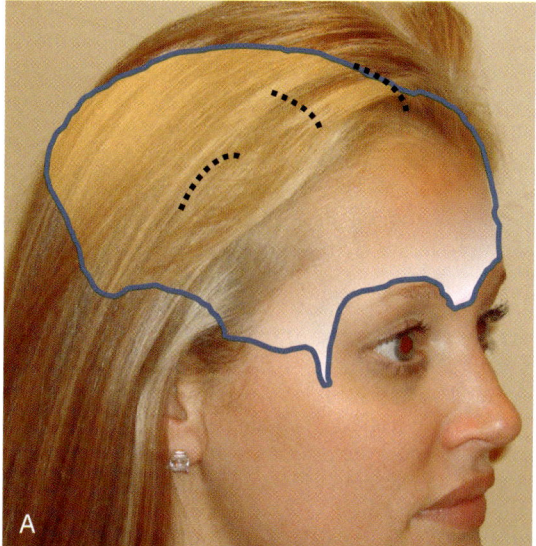
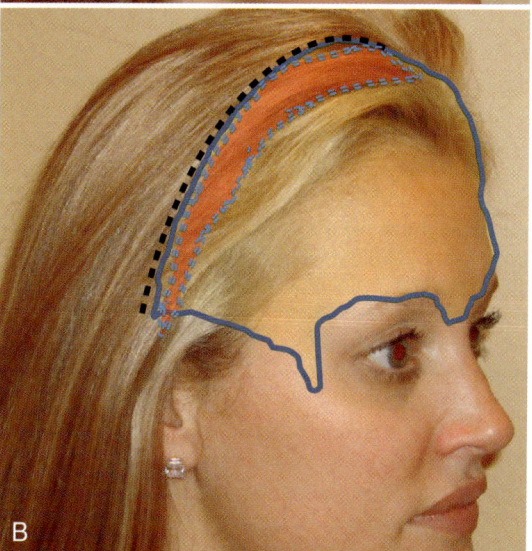
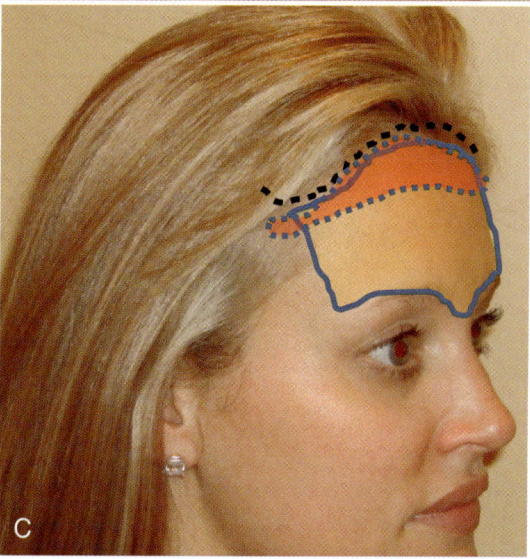

Fig. 105-21 ■ **A,** Endoscopic brow lift. **B,** Coronal brow lift. **C,** Trichophytic brow lift. The dashed lines represent the classic incisions used for each of the common forehead and brow lift procedures shown. The shaded areas with blue outline represent the extent of dissection typically required for each specific technique. The area in red is actual skin excised with each technique.

or motor disruption, less risk for alopecia, small invisible scars, and a shorter and more comfortable recovery period.[47]

The operation begins by making five separate incisions in the hairy scalp. Each incision is approximately 3 cm in length beginning 1 cm posterior to the hairline and extending posteriorly in direction. The first is made in the midline in a sagittal plane, followed by two paramedian incisions made in the parasagittal plane parallel to the midline incision, approximately 3 to 4 cm apart. The vertical alignment of these incisions prevents transection of the sensory nerves to the scalp and allows access to the entire anterior forehead and eyebrows. Care must be taken to not place the parasagittal incisions too laterally over the zone of fixation. These incisions need to be placed over the thick area of the frontal bone in preparation for creation of the bone tunnels or bone screw placement and as far away as possible from the venous lakes of the skull. The last two most lateral incisions are made over the temple in an oblique fashion so that they run parallel to the temporal branch of the facial nerve, as well as the temporal artery and vein. This should reduce the risk for sensory or vascular supply damage to the scalp. The position of the supraorbital nerve is indicated with a marker by following the medial limbus of the iris up to the eyebrow (Figs. 105-22 to 105-24). Dissection is initiated in the central area of the subperiosteal plane while staying medial to the temporal lines. Posterior elevation is performed to approximately 10 cm behind the incisions. Anteriorly, the subperiosteum is elevated to a horizontal line 2 cm above the superior orbital rims and zygomatic arch (Fig. 105-25). Blunt finger dissection can assist in ensuring complete elevation of the forehead and scalp within the limits described. Once this is completed, a connection is created from the lateral incisions to the subperiosteal plane through the upper portion of the zone of fixation. This can be done by blunt finger dissection. Dissection should be avoided below this level where the facial nerve branches lie. The direction of finger placement should be from the lateral incisions toward the central subperiosteal space created and not vice versa, to prevent false tunneling in the spongy temporoparietal fascia. As described earlier, this layer contains the superficial temporal artery and the frontal branch of the facial nerve. The importance of staying directly against the periosteum and temporalis fascia during the initial elevations cannot be emphasized enough (Fig. 105-26).

Direct visualization is necessary to continue the dissection down to the superior orbital rims and the nasofrontal junction. The endoscope is inserted into one of the three median incisions while being careful and delicate in the area of the raised flap. Aggressive retraction can perforate the skin or result in significant postoperative neuropraxia. A smooth and curved periosteal elevator is used to release the periosteum over the superior orbital rims bilaterally, as well as in the nasofrontal area. The dissection should be bimanual while keeping the non-dominant hand over the patient's face to control the tip of the elevator. The endoscope and suction cannula should be held by the assistant. The dissection should be carried laterally over the lateral orbital rim and the zygomatic bone (Figs. 105-27 and 105-28).

The periosteum is then incised with a needle-tipped electrocautery or a laser set at low power. The surgeon must keep in mind the path of the supraorbital vessels toward the frontalis and forehead at the level of the medial limbus on each side.[30] The three ports are used in conjunction for ease of movement of the endoscope, the cautery or laser, and the suction cannula. The temporal incisions can be very helpful as suction ports if the medial ports are too occupied with the endoscope and the cautery device. Cauterization should also be done bimanually because of the relatively small distance that the cautery has to travel to get through the skin, especially in the glabellar area and nasofrontal junction (Figs. 105-29 and 105-30).

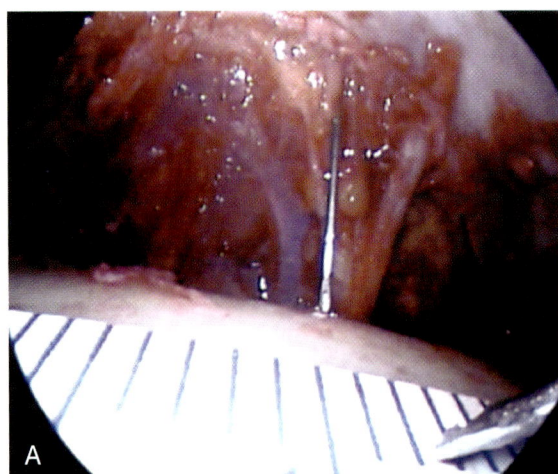

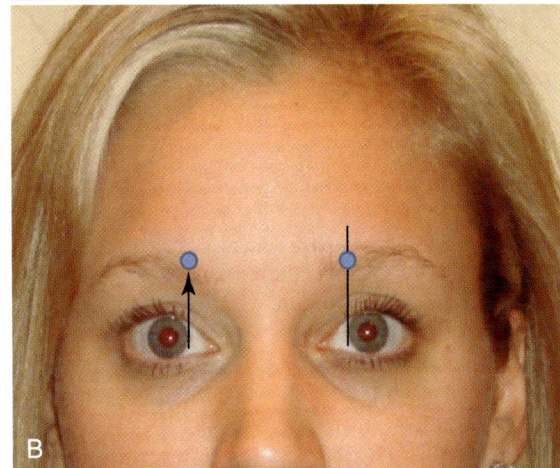

Fig. 105-22 ■ A simple preoperative technique to help locate these important structures is to mark a vertical line through the brow parallel to the medial limbus (iris) while the patient faces forward. The supraorbital vessels and nerves typically lie within 1 mm of this mark at the orbital rim 98% of the time. A study using a needle through the skin mark verifies the stable neurovascular position as seen endoscopically above. The blue dots represent the location of the supraorbital vessels and nerves.

After exposure of the corrugator supercilii and procerus is accomplished, careful transection is done with accurate cauterization. Bleeding muscle edges can be carefully cauterized after external pressure is applied to allow better visualization. Hypertrophy of the depressor muscles can be treated by muscle avulsion. The authors' personal findings are that muscle debulking carries a high risk for nerve damage and postoperative glabellar irregularity. The muscle edges should also be further separated gently with the periosteal elevator by at least 1 cm to aid in release of the arcus marginalis. This can result in a significantly longer elevated brow effect (Fig. 105-31).

Next, dissection along the anterior and inferior aspects of the temporal crest is performed. This line of dissection is carried down to the zygomaticofrontal suture line while keeping in mind the close proximity of the sentinel vein (zygomaticotemporal vein), which runs lateral to the dissection path and may need to be sacrificed for adequate exposure and surgical intervention (Fig. 105-32). The lateral dissection and elevation are key to the extent of elevation and fixation of the eyebrow toward the completion of the endoscopic brow lift (Fig. 105-33).

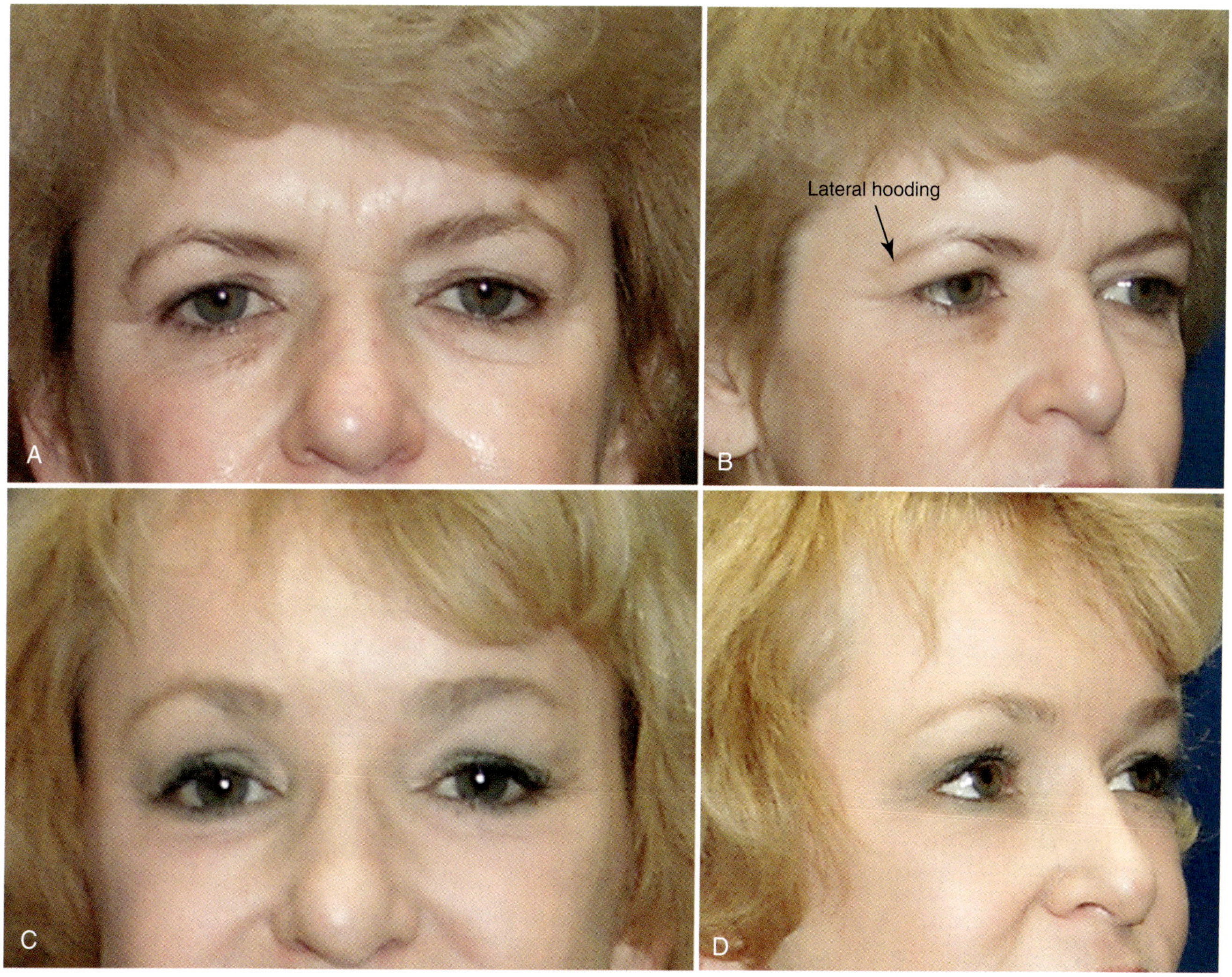

Lateral hooding

Fig. 105-23 ■ **A** and **B,** Preoperative photographs of 54-year-old woman. **C** and **D,** This patient demonstrated the classic improvement seen with a forehead and brow lift 2 months after surgery. The patient did not have upper eyelid surgery performed. Lateral hooding and glabellar rhytides are primary problems best addressed by an endoscopic forehead and brow lift procedure.

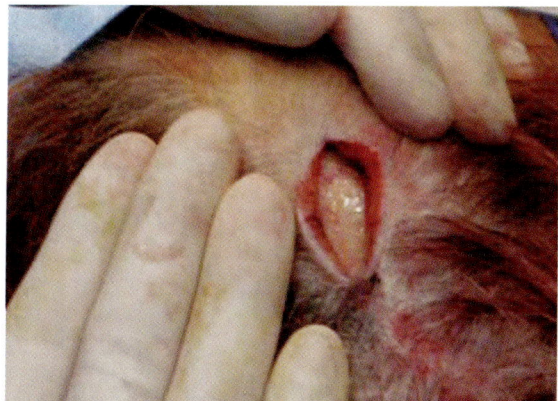

Fig. 105-24 ■ Each of the five incisions for an endoscopic brow lift is typically 3 to 4 cm in length. The three upper incisions are dissected down to bone, and the periosteum is elevated in all directions. One of the parasagittal incisions is shown. No hair is trimmed or removed during endoscopic brow lifting.

This area of dissection is where the endoscopic approach is far and beyond more compatible with other face-lift procedures. If an extended mid-face–lift is intended, the tissue over the zygomatic arch can be elevated between the superficial and deep temporal fascia layers, or abbreviated mid-face–lifts can be assisted by staying in the subperiosteal plane along the lateral orbital rim. Another possibility is a mid-face–lift with intraoral dissection, where the subperiosteal forehead plane can be connected laterally with an intraoral zygoma periosteal plane.

When periosteal dissection and muscle transection are complete, flap elevation and fixation are next. Various approaches have been described for fixating the forehead flap to the underlying bone in its new retracted position (see Fig. 105-31), including suture fixation, bone screws and plates, resorbable screws, bone tunnels, local skin excision, tissue glue, tight head wraps, and temporalis muscle unroofing for added scarring. Even though many of these options are viable and adequate, it must be emphasized that an inadequately released tissue flap will relapse down to its original position even with the "best" fixation technique. The fixation is done through the parasagittal incisions by elevating the lateral third of the brow to

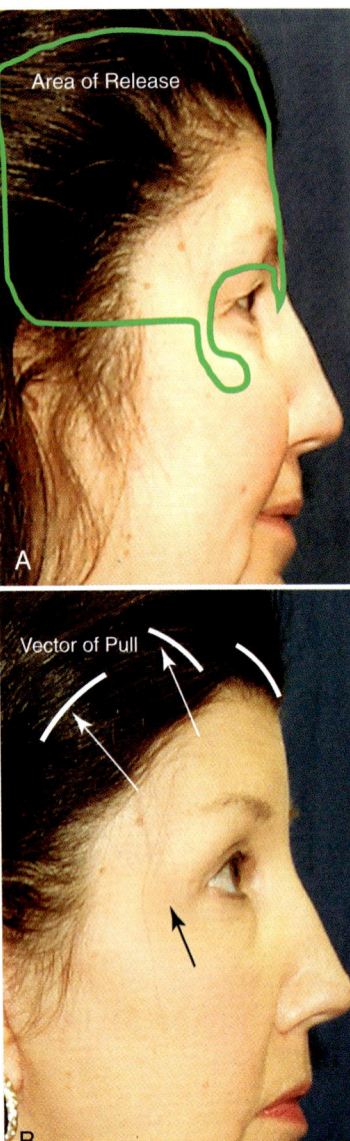

Fig. 105-25 ■ Before (**A**) and after (**B**) photographs of endoscopic fore-head, brow, and mid-face lift show a lateral view of the area of sub-periosteal release and the vector of pull involved in the procedure.

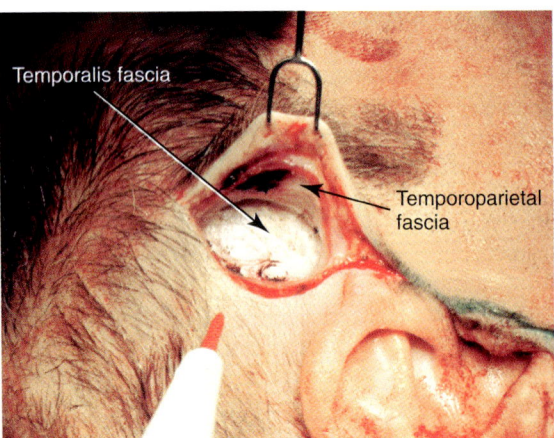

Fig. 105-26 ■ The temporal incisions are made down to the deep temporalis fascia (also known simply as the temporalis fascia), and blunt finger dissection is used to elevate the loose areolar superficial temporoparietal fascia up and off the deeper fascia.

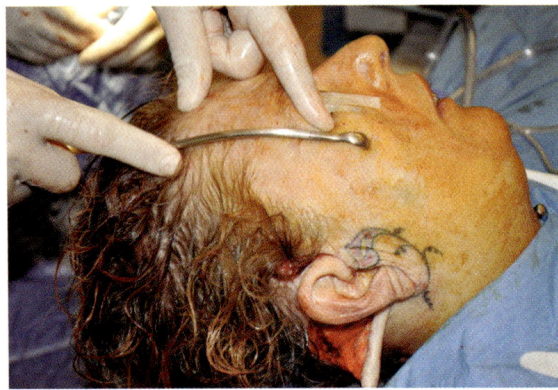

Fig. 105-27 ■ Intraoperative photograph demonstrating how the sub-periosteal dissection is tunneled over the lateral orbital rim into the malar prominence. The elevator is used through a parasagittal incision just behind the hairline. The globe is protected at all times.

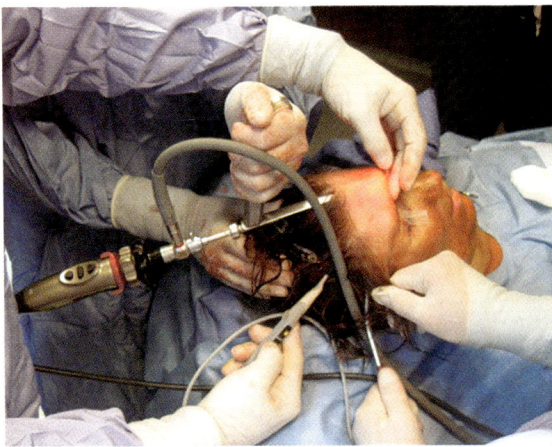

Fig. 105-28 ■ Usual arrangement of surgeon and assistants during an endoscopic brow lift procedure. The surgeon controls the cautery and uses the contralateral hand for counterpressure on the skin to help in control and avoid perforation. The first assistant holds the endoscope and the second assistant (if available) holds the suction device and maintains proper head position.

its maximal elevation and fixating the periosteum to the cranium (Fig. 105-34). The medial brow and glabella will elevate on their own with maximal stretching of the lateral eyebrow. This ensures that the medial brow will remain lower than the lateral side and avoids overcorrection of the medial brow, which would result in an unhappy patient with a long-term surprised expression. Fixation of the lateral tail of the brow by imbrication of the temporoparietal fascia in a posterior and superior direction through the lateral incisions can be done for added effect. This vector can be visualized by a line connecting the outer nasal ala to a point just behind the lateral canthus.

Little relapse is expected in the early postoperative period. Generally, a 1- to 2-mm drop after the first 2 weeks is expected. Different figures have been postulated regarding the amount of time that it takes for the periosteum to adhere to its new position. Recent data show that adequate fusion occurs within 7 to 9 days rather than the older suggestions of 12 weeks. This is proved by the success of transcutaneous bone screws, which are generally removed after 1 week and have excellent long-term retention. The key for a good

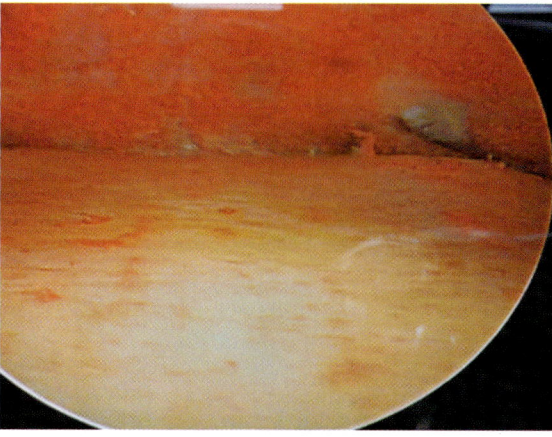

Fig. 105-29 ■ Initial endoscopic view of the periosteum elevated off the frontal bone. Ideally, the periosteum is blunted and elevated over the arcus marginalis without tears before release under direct vision along the orbital rims.

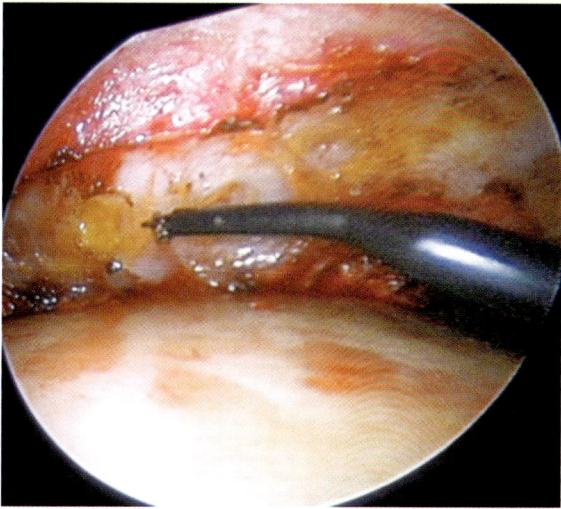

Fig. 105-30 ■ Endoscopic periosteal release via needle-tipped electrocautery demonstrated along the entire arcus marginalis.

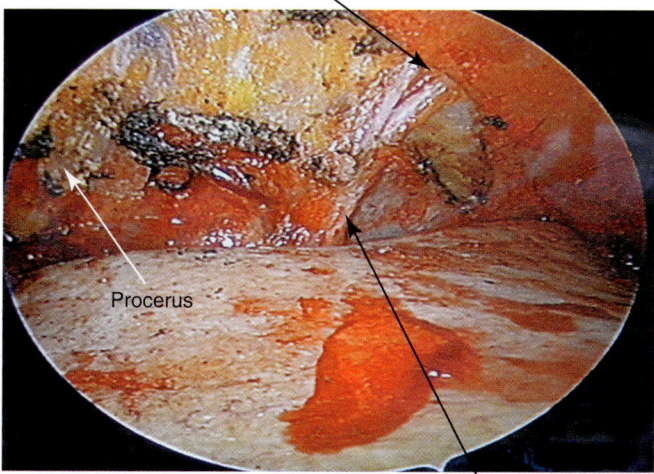

High release at level of SO nerve

Procerus

Right supraorbital nerve root

Fig. 105-31 ■ Periosteal release can be done 1 to 2 cm above the arcus marginalis at the location of the supraorbital nerve as seen in the photograph to avoid accidental transection of the base or trunk of the nerve.

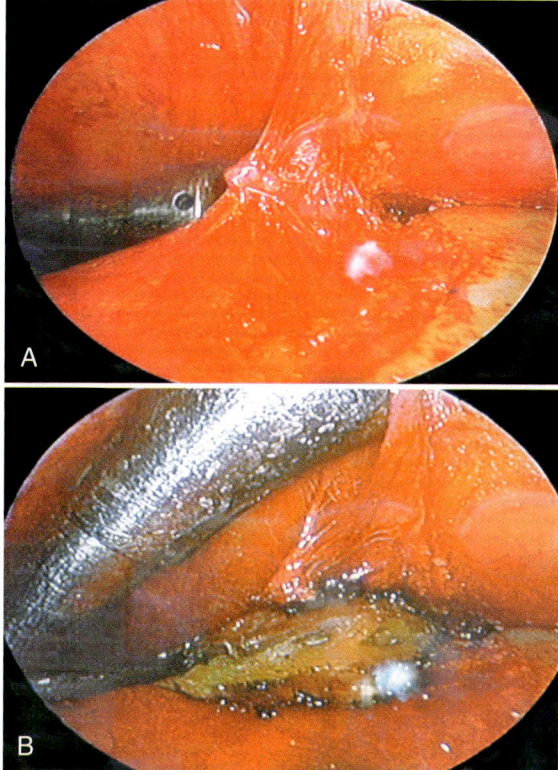

Fig. 105-32 ■ The left lateral orbital ligament (**A**) before release and during initial release (**B**). This ligament is encountered during release over the lateral orbital rim.

long-term result is emphasis on adequate periosteal and ligamentous release along the lateral canthus (Figs. 105-35 to 105-37).

Closure of the incision is done with skin staples, and excellent healing is expected. Forehead flap redundancy disappears by redistribution over the posterior 10 to 20 cm of occipital periosteal elevation. This redistribution accounts for the acceptable minimal raising of the hairline (Fig. 105-38).

DIRECT BROW LIFT

A direct brow lift is considered the simplest of the different approaches to raising the eyebrow. An elliptical skin excision is made just above the superior edge of the eyebrow. The authors' preference is to create a beveled incision to allow some hair follicles to grow over the incision. Dissection is continued in a subcutaneous plane to avoid nerve and vessel injury. Electrocautery is then used to excise the ellipse of tissue.

This type of brow lift is simple and can easily be done with local anesthesia. It can also correct brow asymmetry. Its main disadvantage is the potentially visible scar, although for an elderly patient with heavy wrinkles and thick eyebrows, this could be the procedure of choice.[48]

MID-FOREHEAD AND BROW LIFT

This technique involves mid-forehead and upper forehead elliptical incisions, with the edges and resultant scar lying inside a horizontal forehead crease. Dissection can be carried down to the corrugator and procerus muscles as indicated and allows skin release with excision of excess skin. This is probably the least used of all techniques, but it should be considered when dealing with an elderly patient who has thin eyebrows and deep horizontal rhytides.[49]

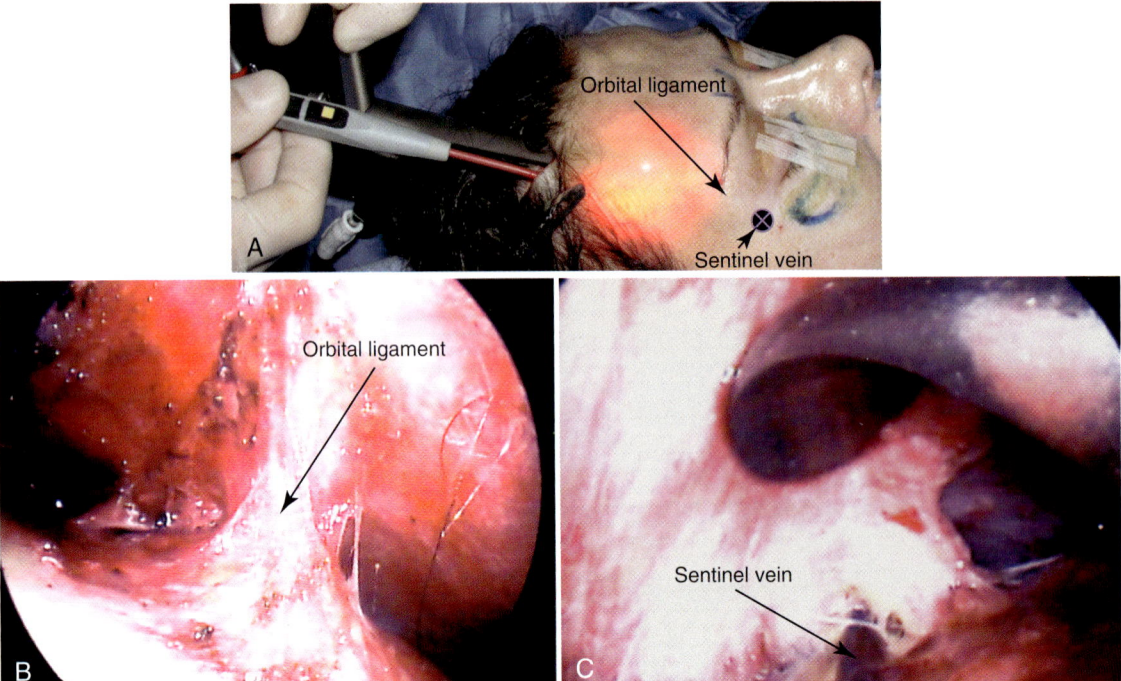

Fig. 105-33 ■ Orbital ligament release is necessary for adequate brow lift stability. Shown here is the endoscopic release of the orbital ligaments to gain access to the lateral orbicularis oculi. The sentinel vein is at the inferior edge of the ligament and can be cauterized, ligated, or avoided.

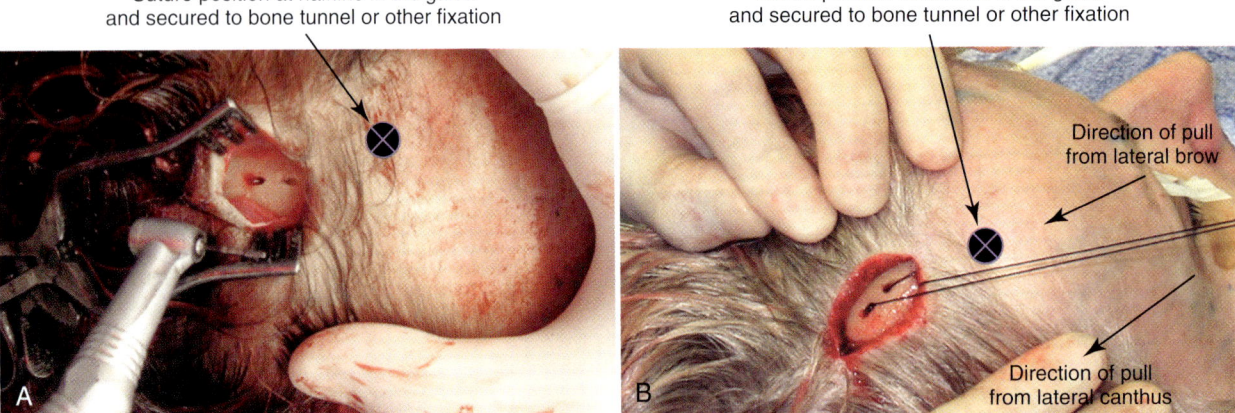

Fig. 105-34 ■ Bone tunnels are one method of fixation. A right parasagittal bone tunnel is shown here near the coronal suture. A secure galeal suture is plicated from the hairline below to the bone tunnel above. The parasagittal skull bone is very thick and allows safe placement of a shallow tunnel.

TRANSPALPEBRAL/TRANSBLEPHAROPLASTY BROW LIFT

Blepharoplasty can be performed in conjunction with any of the brow lift procedures described if indicated. For example, a simple and direct brow lift can be done through a blepharoplasty incision. Dissection can easily expose the corrugator supercilii, the procerus, and the depressor supercilii, each of which can be transected for elevation of the medial eyebrow and reduction of glabellar lines (Fig. 105-39). However, this approach does not address the lateral aspect of the eyebrow in any significant manner.

As mentioned earlier, eyebrow ptosis may be accompanied by dermatochalasis of the upper eyelids, as well as the lower eyelids. Fat pad prominence, orbicularis oculi hypertrophy, and lacrimal gland descent can also make eyelid surgery necessary, with or without forehead and eyebrow lifting. Details regarding eyelid surgery are discussed more extensively elsewhere in this book and should be considered part of one's upper face rejuvenation practice.[50] The supraorbital nerve must be considered with any approach. The location can easily be determined preoperatively.

ADJUNCTIVE PROCEDURES

Autologous Fat Grafting

Facial fat transfer is particularly useful for improving orbital and temporal hollowing, as well as for camouflaging infraorbital rim exposure by malar fat ptosis.[51] Autologous fat grafting has become a very popular adjunct to facial cosmetic surgery, and all

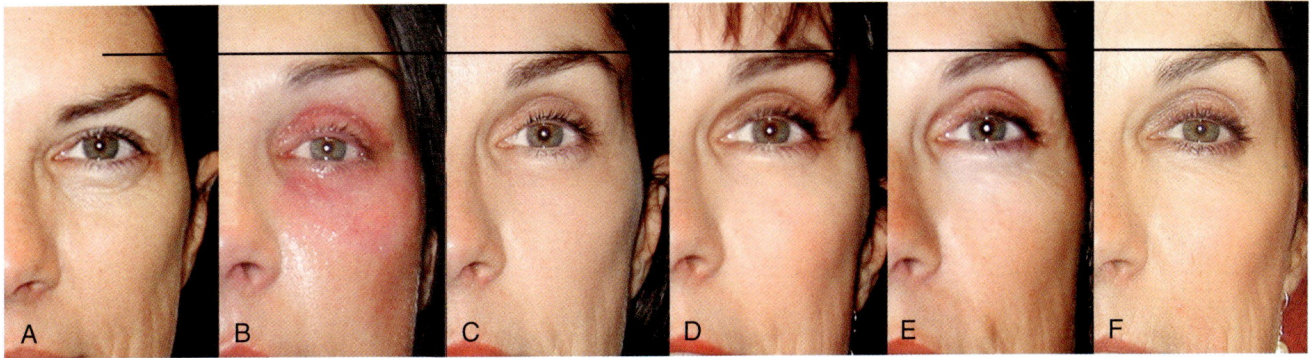

Fig. 105-35 ■ The horizontal line demonstrates the new and stable brow position on a 47-year-old woman following an endoscopic forehead and brow lift procedure. The patient also had upper and lower blepharoplasty performed along with lower laser resurfacing. The key to a good long-term result is adequate tissue dissection and proper fascial release rather than any specific fixation technique. **A,** Preoperative appearance. **B,** Six days after surgery. **C,** Two weeks after surgery. **D,** Two months after surgery. **E,** One year after surgery. **F,** Seven years after surgery.

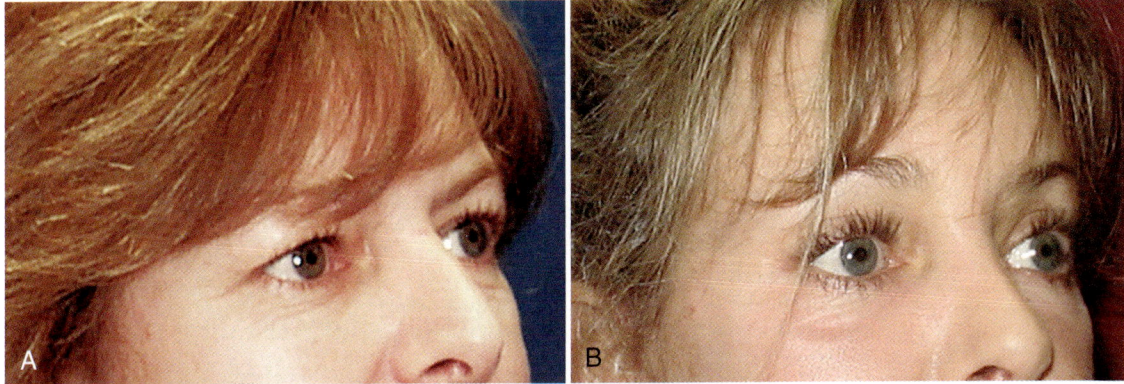

Fig. 105-36 ■ A 51-year-old woman before (**A**) and 4 years following (**B**) endoscopic brow lift and upper blepharoplasty. Her lid laxity required upper blepharoplasty after elevation of the eyebrows. The long-term results are seen and are most related to proper tissue release versus the type of fixation used.

cosmetic surgeons should arm themselves with this powerful tool (Fig. 105-40).

Botulinum Toxin–Assisted Brow Lift

Botulinum toxin has proved to be very effective in reducing visible fine lines and wrinkles of the aging face.[52] With regard to the upper third of the face, reduced frontalis activity, glabellar lines, and lateral orbital crow's feet are all particularly exceptional areas to be "Botoxed." Focusing the injections on the depressor muscles with subsequent unopposed frontalis elevation can lead to brow elevation, hence obtaining a "chemical brow lift."[53]

Botulinum toxin has also been theorized to help in stabilizing the forehead flap elevated during forehead lifting. Injecting the depressor muscles 1 to 2 weeks before surgery is thought to reduce depressor muscle activity postoperatively, which allows the forehead to remain lifted and reduces early postoperative relapse.

Skin Care and Micropigmentation

Several procedures can be used to even out fine wrinkles and dyschromia of the forehead and periorbital skin. Laser resurfacing, dermabrasion, or chemical peels can be used as an adjunct to forehead lift surgery.

The authors' personal experience has led them to treat our patients before any resurfacing procedure with 6 weeks of topical retinoic acid and the addition of hydroquinone for patients with darker skin (Fitzpatrick 3 or higher). Such pretreatment can reduce the risk for post-resurfacing pigment changes and scarring.

Medical micropigmentation is useful to enhance a thin eyebrow, especially in patients with poor hand motor skills. This permanent tattooing can also be used to amplify the lateral contour of the eyebrow in patients with complete thinning of the lateral eyebrow.

POSTOPERATIVE CARE

Once surgical forehead and eyebrow lifting is completed, a compression bandage is applied with a Coban wrap or something similar. It should be wrapped rather tight in the hope of limiting edema and hematoma formation while possibly holding the fixation in place. A drain is not usually needed. Head elevation is beneficial the first week after surgery, as well as the use of cold compresses over the eyes and brows. Exercise should preferably be minimal during the first 2 weeks postoperatively.

The tight head wrap is removed on postoperative day 1, followed by a more comfortable Velcro-type head wrap. Showering with shampoo is allowed after 24 hours, and twice-daily cleaning of the incisions with dilute hydrogen peroxide solution is followed by the application of a thin layer of antibiotic ointment. This is continued

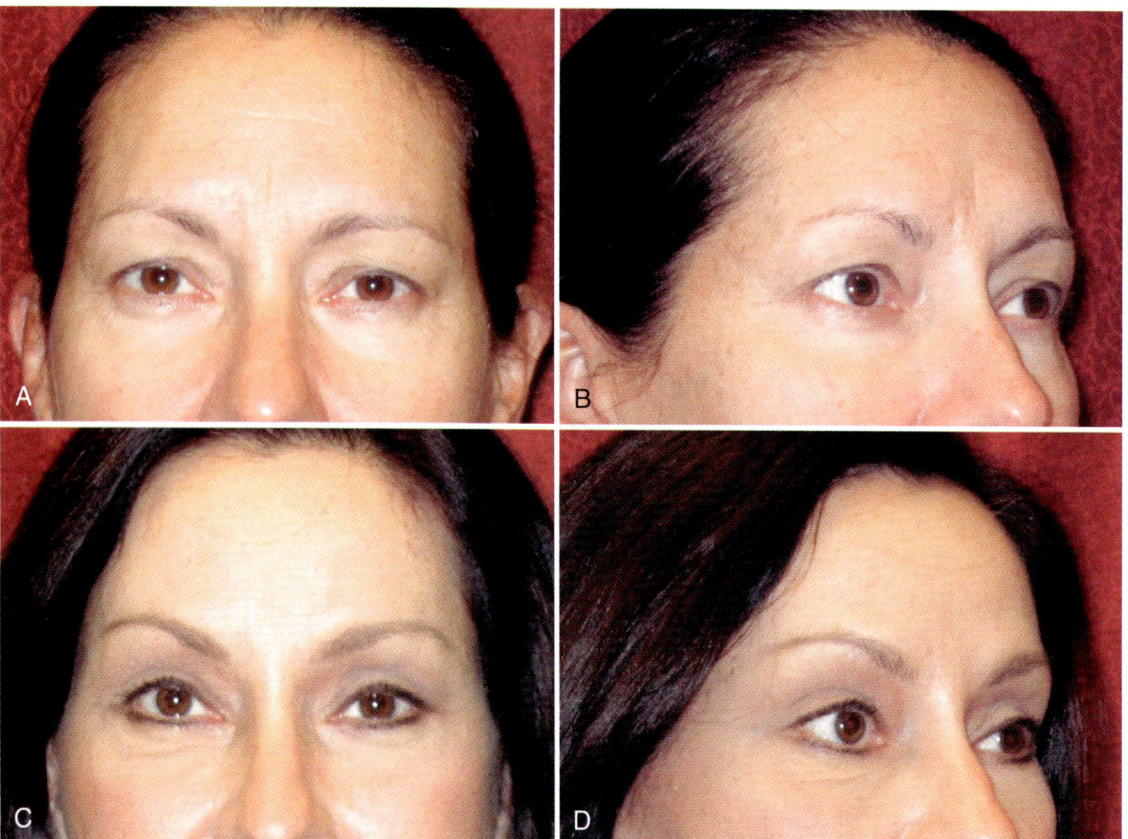

Fig. 105-37 ■ A 60-year-old woman before (**A** and **B**) and 1 year following (**C** and **D**) an endoscopic brow lift procedure. Her lid crease was adequate with lifting of the lateral brow only and was determined preoperatively by raising her outer brow by finger pressure to observe the esthetic effect on the upper lid.

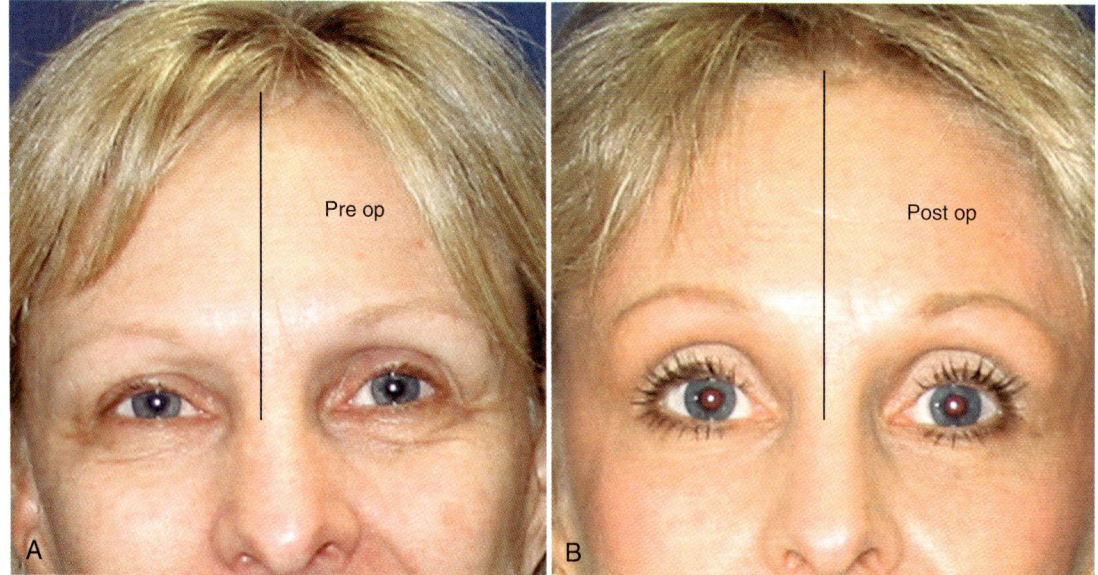

Fig. 105-38 ■ A 53-year-old woman before (**A**) and 1 month following (**B**) an isolated endoscopic brow lift procedure. Hairline elevation can occur following an endoscopic brow lift but is typically minimal, particularly when compared with an open coronal lift, which requires scalp excision and subsequently raises the hairline significantly.

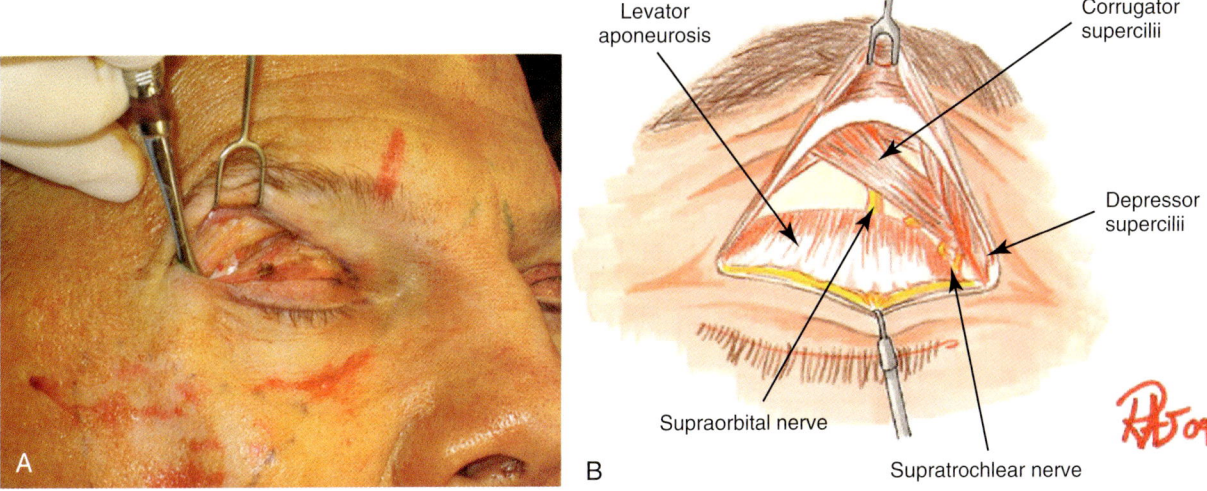

Fig. 105-39 ■ **A,** A 57-year-old man shown during a transblepharoplasty direct brow lift procedure. **B,** Release of the corrugator can be accomplished from the blepharoplasty incision, but care must be taken to avoid injury to the supraorbital nerve, which runs through the muscle.

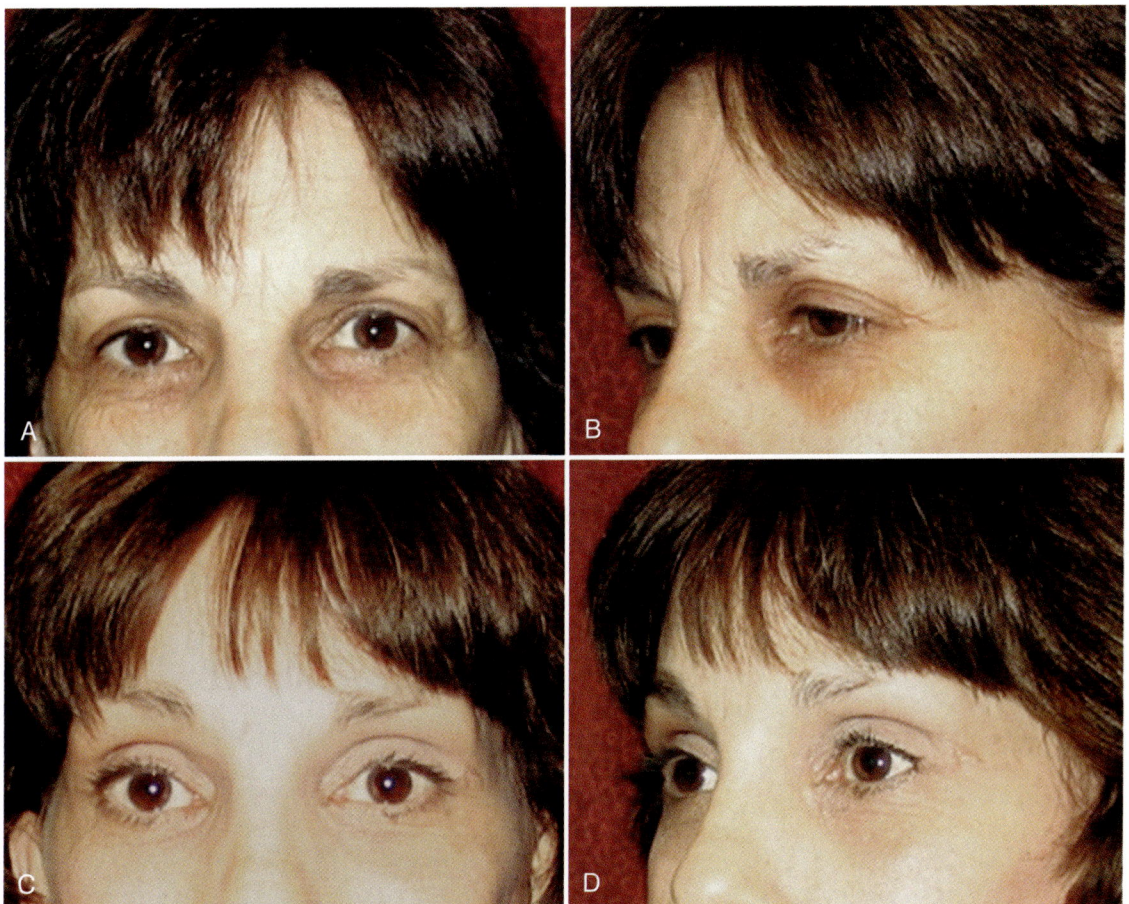

Fig. 105-40 ■ A 58-year-old woman preoperatively (**A** and **B**) and 3 months postoperatively (**C** and **D**) after an endoscopic brow lift procedure along with fat grafting of the eyebrow and lower blepharoplasty. Atrophy of the outer brow is often a major cause of an aged appearance, in addition to brow ptosis.

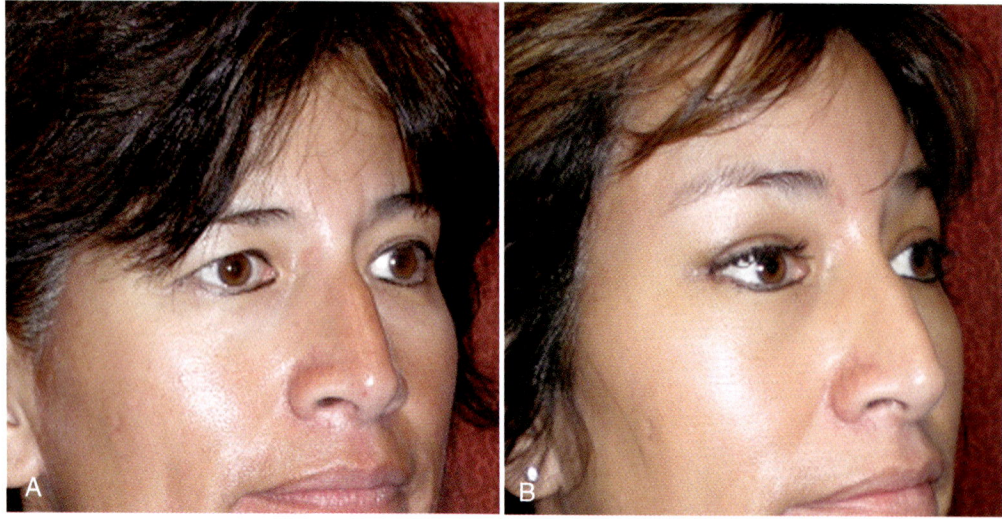

Fig. 105-41 ■ A 55-year-old woman before (**A**) and 1 year following (**B**) an isolated endoscopic brow lift procedure. The patient has a low hairline along with a very low lateral brow position, which makes her an ideal candidate for an endoscopic brow lift.

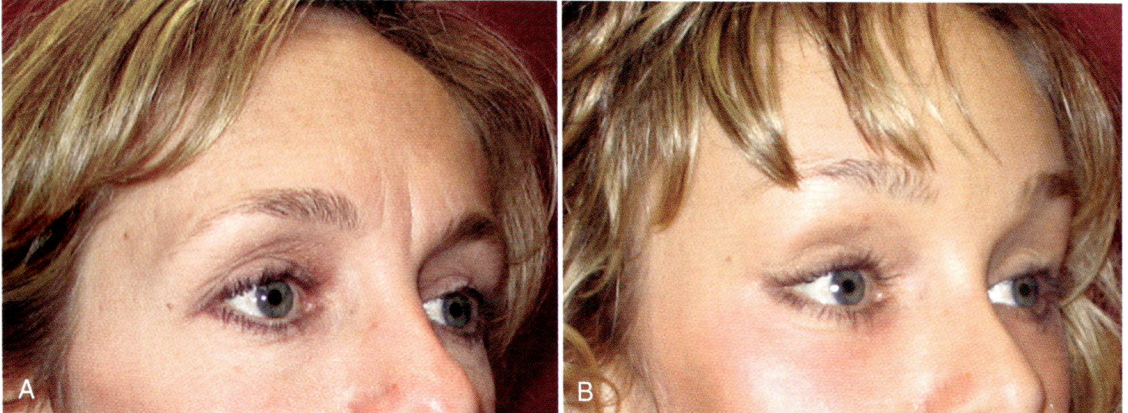

Fig. 105-42 ■ Before (**A**) and after (**B**) effect of an endoscopic brow lift that excessively elevated the lateral canthus. Overly aggressive stripping of the lateral orbital wall in the subperiosteal plane can, on rare occasion, result in a "cat's eye" look by elevating portions of the lateral canthal tendon. Some patients may request exaggerated elevation of the corner of the eye, but most want a much more natural elevation.

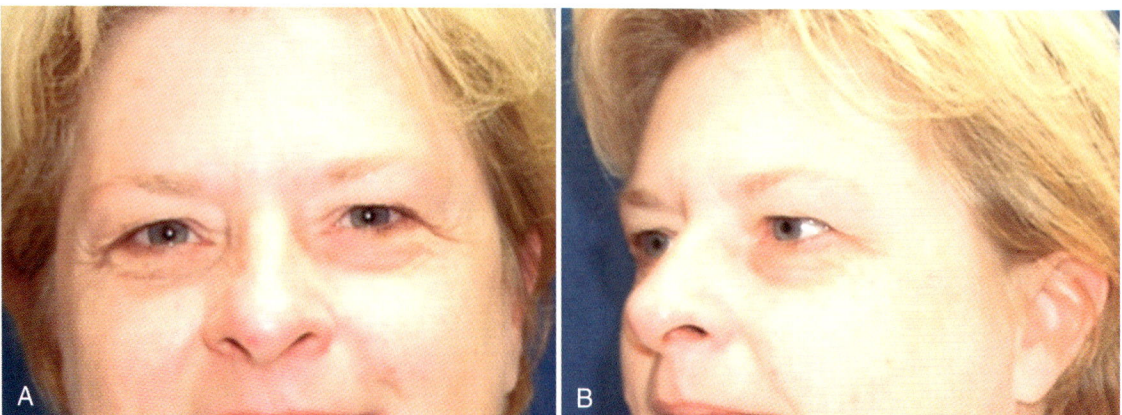

Fig. 105-43 ■ A 52-year-old woman before (**A** and **B**) and 3 months following an endoscopic brow lift procedure and simultaneous upper blepharoplasties (**C** and **D**). When combining procedures, the brow lift is typically performed first so that there is less upper lid laxity that must be cautiously removed subsequently to avoid over-resection and lagophthalmos.

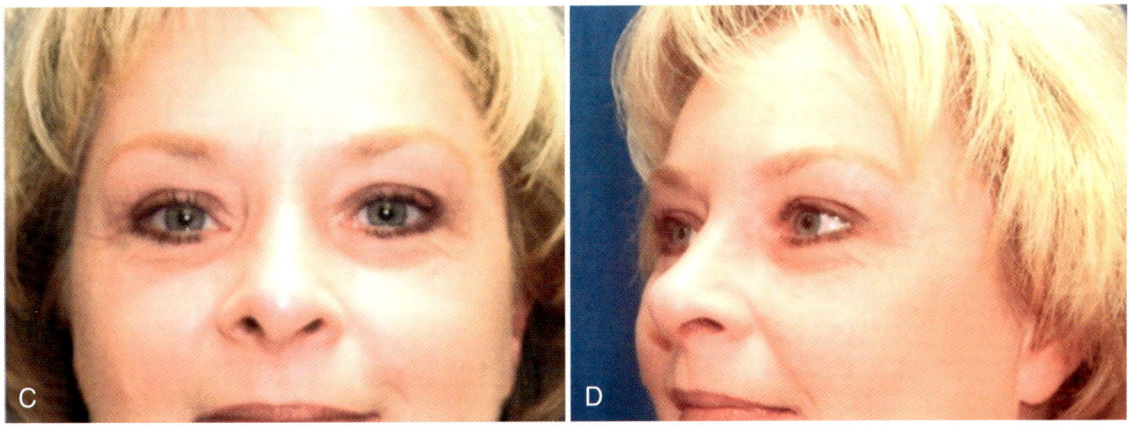

Fig. 105-43, cont'd.

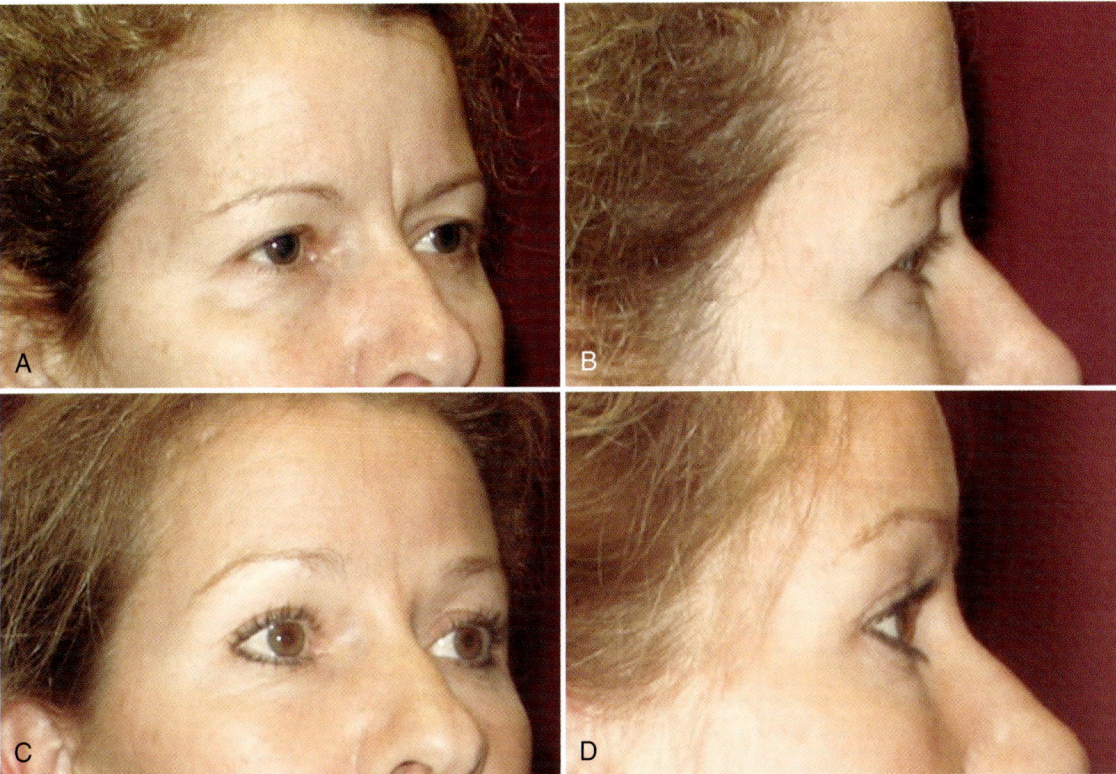

Fig. 105-44 ■ A 49-year-old woman before (**A** and **B**) and 1 year following (**C** and **D**) an isolated endoscopic brow lift procedure. The lateral hooding is treated well with a brow lift, whereas blepharoplasty alone would have produced limited results for this problem.

for 1 week. Hot curling irons and other similar devices must be used with caution since the scalp anesthesia may take several months to resolve.

CONCLUSION

Upper facial rejuvenation has experienced a revolutionary tipping point. The success of minimally invasive brow lifting and chemodenervation (Botox) has made the endoscopic forehead and brow lift the gold standard treatment of brow ptosis. This chapter has discussed how to evaluate the patient's upper facial anatomy and how to treat it, as well as how to recognize brow ptosis with or without associated upper eyelid laxity. Knowledge of the anatomy and location of important nerves has made cosmetic surgery on the upper part of the face safer with excellent long-term results (Fig. 105-41).

Volume repletion also has a role in rejuvenation of the eyebrow and can be a great adjunct to brow lifting. Complications and over-dissection were also discussed, and cosmetic surgeons performing endoscopic brow lifting should be comfortable in dealing with unexpected results (Fig. 105-42).

Rejuvenation of the upper part of the face involves multiple modalities that need to be mastered by the cosmetic surgery. The new era of demands for minimal downtime, as well as minimal invasiveness and expectations of phenomenal results, has brought endoscopic forehead and brow lifting to the forefront of upper facial rejuvenation. This chapter has focused on delivering a safe surgical procedure by extensive knowledge of the anatomy involved and safe application of the endoscopic technique. Finally, the procedure has proved to be safe and consistent and provides good long-term results in the aged ptotic eyebrow (Figs. 105-43 and 105-44).

PEARLS AND PITFALLS

- As with any surgical procedure and skin-undermining procedure, possible complications include but are not limited to wound dehiscence, hematoma, skin edge necrosis, poor wound healing and scar formation, asymmetries, sensory disturbances, facial paralysis, eyelid ptosis, corneal abrasions, dry eye syndrome, hair loss (alopecia), infection, relapse, and irregularities in contour. Most of these rare complications are temporary.
- Hematomas and seromas need to be addressed without delay.
- Wound complications can be dealt with early or late in the healing phase, depending on the severity and location of the problem.
- Asymmetry can be treated early in the postoperative period by external fixation of the skin flaps or, at a later stage, with botulinum toxin or minor surgical revision.
- Facial nerve damage leading to permanent muscle paralysis is the most devastating complication to the surgeon and the patient—extensive anatomic knowledge and proper surgical technique are the most important aspects of preventing such a complication. More often than not, muscle function returns over time, and application of botulinum toxin to the non-paretic side can help achieve symmetry during the recovery period.
- In the authors' experience, forehead sensory changes (esthesia) tend to resolve within 6 to 8 months. During this time the patient may experience a variety of sensory changes ranging from "itching" to "tingling" or "shooting pains." Patient reassurance is important in these situations while attending to the patient's concerns.
- Eye protection is critical during upper face-lift procedures. Corneal abrasions can be painful, as well as dangerous and concerning to the patient. Electrocautery, instruments, and the surgeon's hands are all capable of injuring the globe. Eye lubrication and mechanical coverage/protection need to be addressed before operating on the face, especially the periorbital region.

REFERENCES

1. Pitanguy I: Indications and treatment of frontal and glabellar wrinkles in an analysis of 3,404 consecutive cases of rhytidectomy, *Plast Reconstr Surg* 67:157-166, 1981.
2. Ellis DA, Masai H: The effect of facial animation on the aging upper face, *Arch Otolaryngol Head Neck Surg* 1155:710-713, 1989.
3. Knize D: An anatomically based study of the mechanism of eyebrow ptosis, *Plast Reconstr Surg* 97:1321-1333, 1996.
4. Romo T, Yalamanchili H: Endoscopic forehead lifting, *Dermatol Clin* 23:457-467, 2005.
5. Shorr N, Cohen MS: Cosmetic blepharoplasty, *Ophthalmol Clin North Am* 4:17-33, 1991.
6. Zimbler MS, Nassif PS: Adjunctive applications for botulinum toxin in facial aesthetic surgery, *Facial Plast Surg Clin North Am* 11:477-482, 2003.
7. Keller GS: *Endolaser excision of glabellar frown lines and forehead rhytids*, Paper presented at a meeting of the American Academy of Facial Plastic and Reconstructive Surgery, Los Angeles, February 1, 1992.
8. Lavker RM, Zheng PS, Dong G: Morphology of aged skin, *Clin Geriatr Med* 5:53-67, 1989.
9. Uitto J: The role of elastin and collagen in cutaneous aging: intrinsic aging versus photoexposure, *J Drugs Dermatol* 7(2 Suppl):s12-s16, 2008.
10. Goihman-Yahr: Skin aging and photoaging: an outlook, *Clin Dermatol* 14:153-160, 1996.
11. Uitto J, Bernstein EF: Molecular mechanisms of cutaneous aging: connective tissue alterations in the dermis, *J Investig Dermatol Symp Proc* 3:41-44, 1998.
12. Presti P, Yalamanchili H, Honrado CP: Rejuvenation of the aging upper third of the face, *Facial Plast Surg* 22:91-96, 2006.
13. Huntley JE: *The divine proportion*, New York, 1970, Dover.
14. Rickets RM: Divine proportion of facial aesthetics, *Clin Plast Surg* 9:401-422, 1982.
15. Tolhurst DE, Carstens MH, Greco RJ, et al: The surgical anatomy of the scalp. *Plast Reconst Surg* 87:603-612, discussion 613-614, 1991.
16. Marchac D, Toth B: The axial frontonasal flap revisited, *Plast Reconstr Surg* 76:686-694, 1985.
17. Lavker RM, Zheng PS, Dong G: Morphology of aged skin, *Clin Geriatr Med* 5:53-67, 1989.
18. Guyuron B, Michelow B: Refinements in endoscopic forehead rejuvenation, *Plast Reconstr Surg* 100:154-160, 1997.
19. Knize D: Muscles that act on glabellar skin: a closer look, *Plast Reconstr Surg* 105:350-361, 2000.
20. Knize DM: Reassessment of the coronal incision and subgaleal dissection for the foreheadplasty, *Plast Reconstr Surg* 102:478-489, discussion 490-492, 1998.
21. Grant JCB, editor: *Grant's atlas of anatomy*, ed 6, Baltimore, 1972, Williams & Wilkins.
22. Hoenig JA: Comprehensive management of eyebrow and forehead ptosis, *Otolaryngol Clin North Am* 30:947-984, 2005.
23. Banks P, Brown A: *Fractures of the facial skeleton*, Oxford, 2001, Butterworth-Heinemann.
24. Cuzalina AL: *Peterson's principles of oral and maxillofacial surgery*, vol 2, Philadelphia, 2004, BC Decker.
25. Friedman O: Modern surgery of the aging face, *Facial Plast Surg* 22:120-128, 2006.
26. Gosain AK, Sewall SR, Yousif NJ: The temporal branch of the temporal nerve: how reliably can we predict its path? *Plast Reconstr Surg* 99:1224-1236, 1997.
27. Ellis E, Zide MF: *Surgical approaches to the facial skeleton*, Baltimore, 1995, Williams & Wilkins, pp 59-169.
28. Correia P, Zani R: Surgical anatomy of the facial nerve as related to ancillary operations in rhytidoplasty, *Plast Reconstr Surg* 52:549-552, 1973.
29. Liebman E, Webster R, Berger A, et al: The frontalis nerve in the temporal brow lift, *Arch Otolaryngol Head Neck Surg* 108:232-235, 1982.
30. Cuzalina A, Holmes D: A simple and reliable landmark for identification of the supraorbital nerve in surgery of the forehead: an in vivo anatomical study, *J Oral Maxillofac Surg* 63:25-27, 2005.
31. Seigel R: Surgical anatomy of the upper eyelid fascia, *Ann Plast Surg* 13:263-273, 1984.
32. Putterman AM: *Cosmetic oculoplastic surgery*, ed 3, Philadelphia, 1999, WB Saunders.
33. Ross A, Neal J: Rejuvenation of the aging eyelid, *Facial Plast Surg* 22:97-104, 2006.
34. Fincher EF, Moy RL: Cosmetic blepharoplasty, *Dermatol Clin* 23:431-442, 2005.
35. Isse NG: Endoscopic forehead lift, *Clin Plast Surg* 22:661-673, 1995.
36. Vasconez LO, Core GB, Gamboa-Bobadilla M, et al: Endoscopic techniques in coronal brow lifting, *Plast Reconstr Surg* 94:788-793, 1994.
37. Isse NG: The endoscopic approach to forehead and brow lifting, *Aesthet Surg J* 18:462-464, 1998.
38. Depsey PD, Oneal RM, Ienberg PH: Subperiosteal brow and midface lifts, *Aesthetic Plast Surg* 19:59-68, 1995.
39. Adamson PA, Johnson CM, Anderson JR, et al: The forehead lift: a review, *Arch Otolaryngol Head Neck Surg* 111:325-329, 1985.
40. Buzzel RA: Effects of solar radiation on the skin, *Otolaryngol Clin North Am* 26:1-11, 1993.
41. Maillard JF, Cornette de St. Cyr B, Scheflan M: The subperiosteal bicoronal approach to total facelifting: the DMAS-deep musculoaponeurotic system, *Aesthetic Plast Surg* 15:285-291, 1991.
42. Fett DR, Sutcliffe T, Baylis HI: The coronal eyebrow lift, *Am J Ophthalmol* 96:751-754, 1983.
43. Chajchir A: Endoscopic subperiosteal forehead lift, *Aesthetic Plast Surg* 18:269-274, 1994.

44. Adamson PA, Cormier R, McGraw BL: The coronal forehead lift—modifications and results, *J Otolaryngol* 21:25-29, 1992.

45. Holcomb JD, McCollough EG: Trichophytic incisional approaches to upper facial rejuvenation, *Arch Facial Plast Surg* 3:48-53, 2001.

46. Steinsapir KD, Shorr N, Hoenig JA, et al: The endoscopic forehead lift, *Ophthal Plast Reconstr Surg* 14:107-118, 1998.

47. Jones BM, Grover G: Endoscopic brow lift: a personal review of 538 patients and comparison of fixation techniques, *Plast Reconstr Surg* 113:1242-1250, 2004.

48. Rafarty FM, Goode RL, Abramson NR: The eyebrow lift operation in a man, *Arch Otolaryngol* 104:69-71, 1978.

49. Ellenbogen R: Medial eyebrow lift, *Ann Plast Surg* 5:151-152, 1980.

50. Johnson CM, Waldman SR: Midforehead lift, *Arch Otolaryngol Head Neck Surg* 109:155-159, 1983.

51. Stegman SJ, Chu S, Armstrong RC: Adverse reactions to bovine collagen implant: clinical and histologic features, *J Dermatol Surg Oncol* 14:39-47, 1988.

52. Keen MS, Khosh MM: The role of botulinum toxin A in facial plastic surgery. In Willet JM, editor. *Facial plastic surgery*, Upper Saddle River, NJ, 1997, Prentice Hall, pp 323-329.

53. Frankel AS, Kamer FM: Chemical browlift, *Arch Otolaryngol Head Neck Surg* 124:321-323, 1998.

Micrografting and Hair Transplantation Surgery

Chapter 106

Barry H. Hendler, David C. Stanton

In the last decade or so there has been tremendous increased interest in male pattern baldness (MPB) and hair transplantation surgery. This can be attributed to many factors, primarily improvement in the results of hair transplant surgery through the use of micrografting techniques. In addition, medical therapy for MPB with the use of topical solutions such as minoxidil or the medication finasteride (Propecia) has helped increase public awareness and stimulated the search for other medical approaches to the treatment of MPB. Finally, vastly increased communication between surgeons performing hair transplantation and dramatic changes in medicine affecting cosmetic fields have served to organize and transmit the available knowledge about these procedures.[1]

More than 50 years ago, Norman Orentreich authored a paper on MPB in which his most important observation was that grafts from the hair-bearing rim of the scalp were "donor dominant" and continued to grow hair when implanted into thinning or bald areas.[2] Thus, the concept of multiple scalp grafts for the treatment of baldness has evolved. This movement of hair grafts from genetically preprogrammed, permanently growing sites to balding areas is the foundation of hair transplantation and micrografting as we know it today. This procedure, though used primarily for androgenetic alopecia (MPB), can also be used to cover scars secondary to scalp trauma or previous surgical procedures, radiation and thermal burns, and inactive phases of disease such as scleroderma and other cicatricial processes, as well as for some types of female alopecia. Because MPB is a genetically determined phenomenon, transplantation procedures move permanently growing scalp hair from the sides and back of the head (donor area) to appropriate recipient sites in the frontal, mid-scalp, and vertex regions.[3]

Obviously, hair transplantation requires skill and a strong esthetic sense. Small micrografts and multifollicular grafts must be taken from areas that have excellent prospects for not losing the ability to grow hair during that individual's lifetime. Because hairs grow in specific directions, grafts must be placed in a precise way so that not only does hair growth look full and natural but the pattern of growth also conceals or masks the graft recipient sites and proper angles are achieved for an attractive and complete result. Finally, each individual's characteristics must be evaluated to create the most natural hairline and hair density while fully anticipating facial changes throughout the years.[4]

NORMAL HAIR GROWTH

Hair follicles initially appear in utero. No new follicles are created after birth, and none are lost in adult life. The only factors that change are the density of the follicles (which spread apart as the body surface increases with growth and weight gain) and the type of hair. The first hair to be produced by fetal hair follicles is lanugo hair, which is fine, soft, and unpigmented. This hair is usually shed by the eighth month of gestation.

The first postnatal hair is vellus hair, which is soft, fine, usually pigmented, and seldom more than 2 cm long. Vellus hair remains on the so-called hairless regions of the body such as the forehead and balding scalp. The only completely hairless surfaces are the palms, soles, glans penis, and mucocutaneous junctions.

Hair growth on the human scalp is a kind of mosaic of follicular activity with alternating patterns of growth (anagen) and rest (telogen) separated by a transitional (catagen) phase. Scalp hair grows about 0.3 mm/day, or 6 in/yr. Shedding of 50 to 150 hairs a day is considered normal. When hair is shed, it is replaced by new hair from the same follicle located just below the skin surface. Anagen can be initiated by plucking the telogen hair from a resting follicle or by wounding. Furthermore, certain hormones such as estrogen, progesterone, testosterone, and thyroid hormone influence hair growth.

Hair is composed primarily of keratin protein, the same material found in fingernails and toenails. The most striking feature of the protein of a hair's central cortex is its cysteine content, which is much higher than that of the outer matrix proteins. Hair color depends on the number and type of melanosomes acquired from melanocytes migrating into the hair bulb matrix. In dark hairs, melanosomes are large, ellipsoid, and rich in melanin. In red hairs, they are spherical. White, gray, and blond hairs contain few or minimally pigmented melanosomes.[5]

MALE PATTERN BALDNESS

MPB is the change from terminal hair to vellus hair. The true dimensions and complexity of this process have only recently been appreciated. The progress of MPB is not linear; the condition develops in fits and starts. Terminal hair progresses to vellus hair far past the age at which it was thought that one could delineate the extent of MPB. Surgeons performing hair transplant surgery today realize that it is not the dramatic changes in MPB that occur between the ages of 20 and 35, but what can take place from 40 to 50 years and beyond.

In whites, normal male pattern hair loss is noticeable in about 30% of men by the age of 30 years and in 50% of men by 50 years. Certain racial groups, including the Japanese, Chinese, American Indians, and some tribes of Africans, are relatively immune to the condition, which in whites follows a dominant trait with incomplete penetrance. Expression of this sex-limited gene depends on the level of circulating androgen. This hereditary incidence is noticeable not only in men but also in women who have a strong familial history of baldness.[6]

In men, hair loss can begin as early as the age of 20 years. With normal hair loss, one to several hundred hairs fall each day and are replaced by new hair. In the evolution of MPB, the new hair is fine and thin. Eventually, nothing is left on the scalp but the almost imperceptible fuzz of vellus hair. Simultaneously, hypertrophy of the sebaceous glands and hypersecretion of sebum usually occur and are provoked by androgenetic stimulation of the pilosebaceous follicles, which causes complete loss. MPB usually progresses in a definite pattern. First, the frontal hair regresses, and then loss of the more temporal hair becomes apparent with simultaneous thinning of the vertex. Ultimately, the most severe balding consists of total loss of the frontal and vertex hair. Norwood classified approximately seven different types of MPB.[1] Identification of these types is key to an understanding of proper planning of hair transplantation surgery (Fig. 106-1).

Dihydrotestosterone seems to be the specific hormone responsible for MPB. Genetic predisposition contributes to the topography of MPB because of the number of testosterone receptors on follicular cells and the activity of 5-alpha-reductase enzyme in different areas of the scalp. This enzyme reduces testosterone and inhibits protein synthesis by shortening the anagen phase, thereby producing finer and finer hair until it is eventually lost.[5] Essentially, the hairs are gradually miniaturized in the presence of androgens, with large pigmented terminal hairs being replaced by thin depigmented hairs (vellus-like hairs)

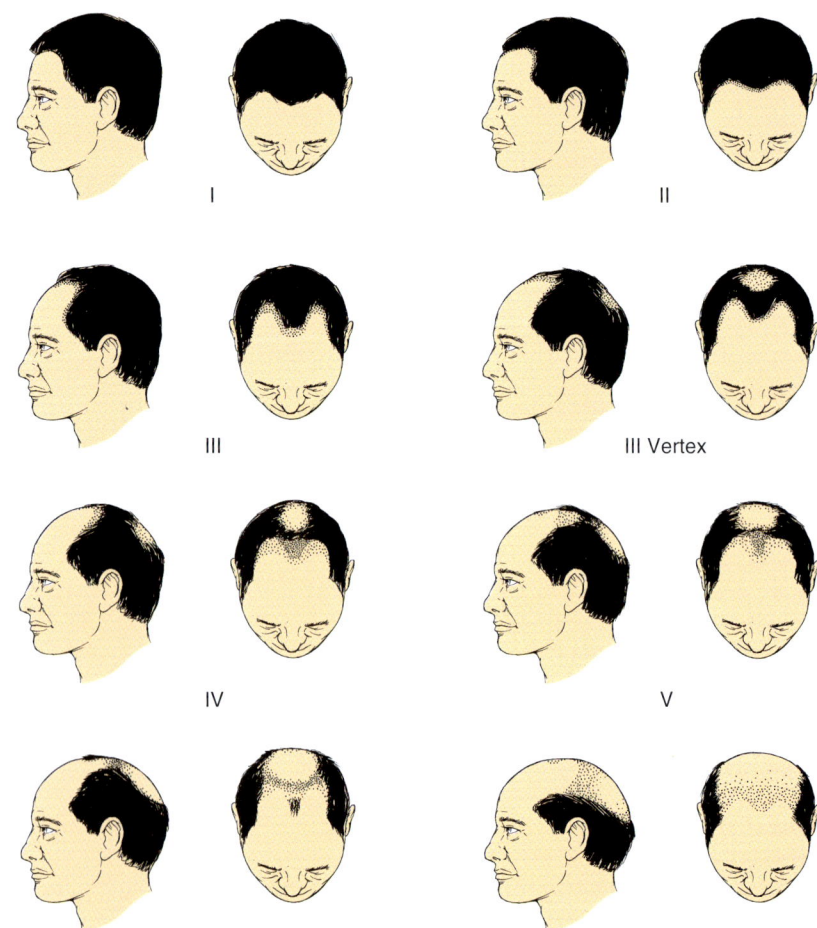

Fig. 106-1 ■ Norwood's classification of male pattern baldness. (Adapted from Norwood OT: Classification and incidence of male pattern baldness. In Norwood OT, Shiell RC, editors: *Hair transplant surgery*, ed 2, Springfield, Ill, 1984, Charles C Thomas, p 6.)

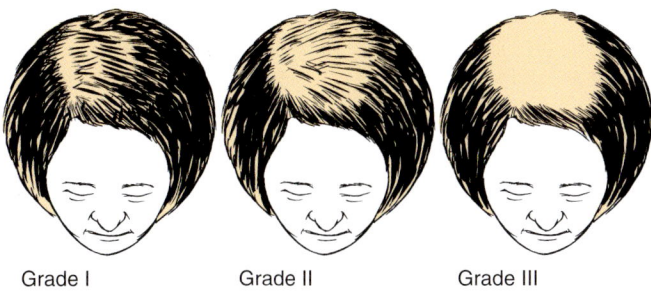

Grade I   Grade II   Grade III

Fig. 106-2 ■ Ludwig's classification of female pattern baldness. (Adapted from Montagna W, Parakkal PF: *The structure and function of the skin*, ed 3, New York, 1974, Academic Press. © 2008 by Johns Hopkins University, Art as Applied to Medicine.)

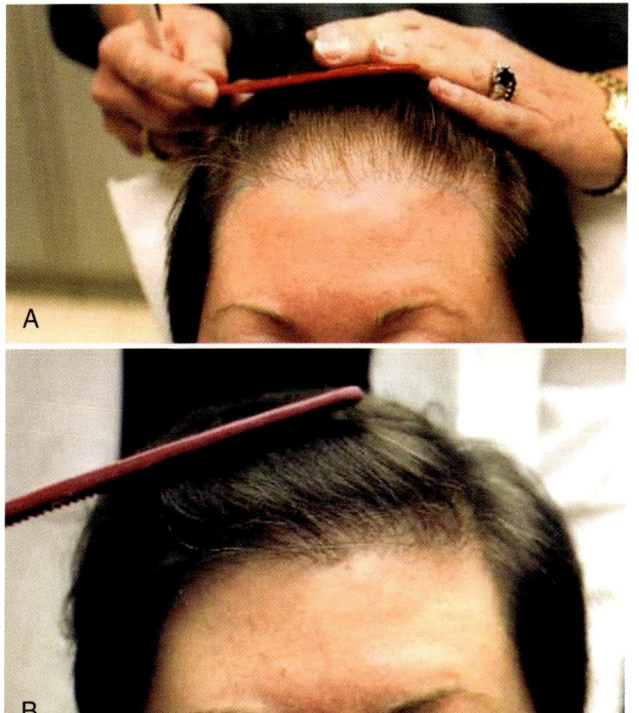

Fig. 106-3 ■ Preoperative (**A**) and postoperative (**B**) female hair restoration. Note the redefinition of the hairline.

FEMALE PATTERN HAIR LOSS

Like MPB, female pattern hair loss is most often due to heredity and aging. Hormonal influences in hereditary hair loss in women may be different from those in men, but researchers are continuing to study it. Unlike men, most women retain some of their natural hairline, which can be thickened to a delicate, yet fuller appearance.

Female pattern hair loss is not as obvious as MPB, but like men, it can be treated effectively. Frequently, women's patterns are more diffuse or spread out over the entire scalp (Fig. 106-2). Whether a female is a candidate for transplantation is determined at the initial consultation. A trained physician can also diagnose whether a woman is experiencing permanent female pattern hair loss and not temporary hair loss related to medical conditions such as pregnancy, disease, or stress.

Significant improvement in hairline definition, hair density, and facial esthetics can be achieved (Figs. 106-3 and 106-4)

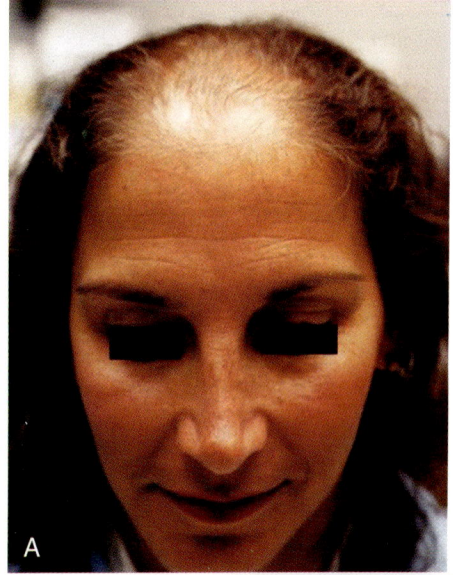

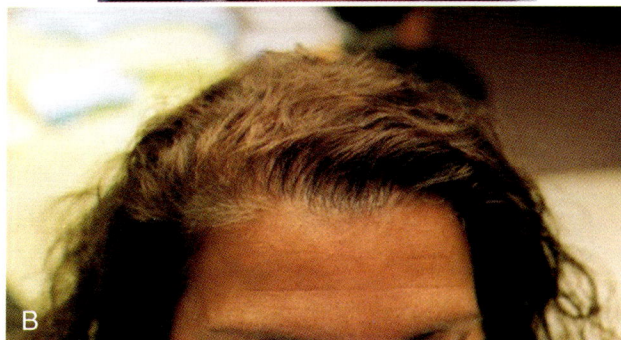

Fig. 106-4 ■ Preoperative (**A**) and postoperative (**B**) female hair restoration. Note the increased hair density.

EYEBROW TRANSPLANTATION

The periorbital region has an important role in the perception of facial esthetics and proportion, and it also imparts volumes to facial expression and nonverbal communication. The causes of eyebrow loss can be mechanical, such as overzealous plucking, electrolysis, or laser hair removal; trauma; or medical conditions such as hormonal imbalance or alopecia universalis.[7]

Hair loss patterns of the eyebrows include decreased density, short overall length of the eyebrow, a size or shape that is too narrow, or a hairless scar. With proper design and surgical technique, it is possible to reconstruct eyebrows with transplanted hairs growing at a natural angle and direction. The surgeon should keep in mind that a female eyebrow generally has a natural peak at the junction of the middle and lateral thirds, approximately at a line tangent to the lateral limbus of the eye. A male eyebrow is generally found to lie over the supraorbital ridge. Patients should participate in the eyebrow design and approve the size, shape, and location preoperatively.

Recipient sites are created with 19- or 20-gauge solid needles and can be placed between existing eyebrow hairs with minimal risk of damage. It is not uncommon for 200 to 350 individual grafts to be placed into one eyebrow. The majority of these grafts will be single-hair grafts, but two-hair grafts can be used in the central portion of the eyebrow, particularly if the donor hair is fine. The authors find that the "stick and place" technique seems to work well for eyebrow reconstruction.

a horseshoe pattern above the ears and neck, and it can be moved to the bald or balding areas. Historically, the usual method of implanting grafts involved three basic types of donor grafts taken from the hair-bearing posterior scalp.

During the initial years of hair restoration surgery, the most common type of graft was a cylindric plug (punch graft) measuring approximately 4 mm and containing 10 to 20 hairs removed from the hair-bearing area and placed in a somewhat smaller cylindric hole in the balding region of the scalp. Depending on the degree of baldness, one to three sessions of transplantation were required per area, with the placement of 50 to 100 grafts at each session. If previous grafts had been done, the later transplants were placed between the previous grafts to create a confluent pattern.

The newest and most recent refinement in hair transplant surgery is follicular unit (FU) transplantation. Studies of horizontal sections of the scalp have revealed that human scalp hairs grow in small compartments or FUs.[8] The FU was first described by Headington in 1984 and was shown to include one to four terminal follicles, one or two vellus follicles, and perifollicular vascular and neural plexuses, all surrounded by concentric layers of collagen fibers.[9] Seager demonstrated that single-hair micrografts, when created by sectioning larger FUs, had less growth than when the FUs were kept intact. This supports the concept of the FU as a physiologic entity rather than just an anatomic one.[10] Consequently, the concept of FU transplantation has developed, with intact FU groupings being dissected under microscopic magnification. Single-FU or multi-FU (two to three FUs) grafts are transplanted.

Micrografts consisting of one to three hairs are implanted along the anterior hairline to eliminate the doll's hair look that cylindric plugs could cause and give the most natural appearance to the hairline.[11] Multi-FUs, which consist of four to six hairs, are placed behind the hairline grafts for added density. These grafts are cut from donor strips taken by ellipse or multiblade knives to allow precise visualization of hair direction and permit careful creation of properly sized grafts (Fig. 106-6).

The tiny full-thickness grafts are then implanted into wounds made with a small (1 to 2 mm) blade (slits) or into puncture receptor sites created by 18-, 19-, or 20-gauge solid needles (Fig. 106-7). In fact, hair replacement surgery is now performed with large quantities (800 to 2500) of micrografts and multi-FUs.

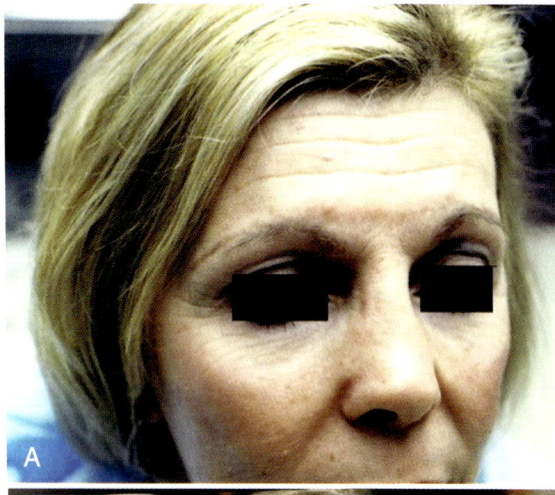
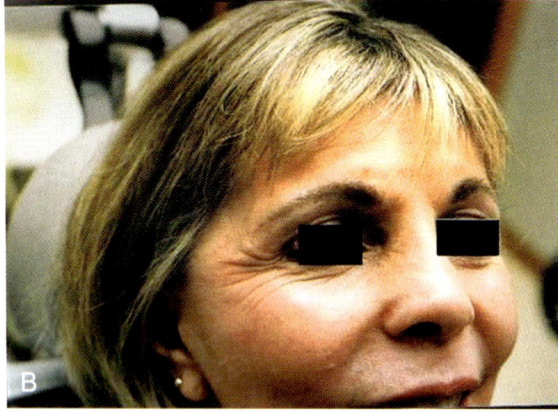

Fig. 106-5 ■ **A,** Preoperative view (lateral portion of the eyebrows drawn in with an eyebrow pencil). **B,** Postoperative eyebrow reconstruction.

The donor area for eyebrow reconstruction is the occipital scalp because this area has tremendous density and often has finer hair. The harvesting technique is as described later, and the donor hairs are dissected under magnification to select hardy single-hair or, occasionally, two-hair grafts.[7] Patients should be informed that the transplanted occipital hair will grow not to a finite length but as though it were still residing on the occipital scalp. Consequently, these transplanted hairs will require trimming.

Ninety percent of the transplanted hairs will grow. Despite proper placement, some of these hairs will grow in a less than optimal direction, such as too vertical or at an obtuse emergence angle from the skin. These hairs can be trained to grow in the proper direction with gels and combing. If these "wild" hairs are unresponsive to training, they can be trimmed short or plucked out.

In the immediate postoperative period, the recipient sites can be gently cleansed with mild soap on postoperative day 1. Application of antibiotic ointment keeps the recipient site moist and can help minimize scabbing (Fig. 106-5).

CYLINDRICAL GRAFTS, MICROGRAFTS, AND MULTIFOLLICULAR GRAFTS

The success of hair transplantation and micrografting results from the fact that hair follicles that are moved from one location on the scalp to another will behave as they did in their original site. For example, even in cases of advanced MPB, hair continues to grow in

HAIRLINE PLACEMENT

Positioning of the anterior frontal hairline is the most critical factor in a successful hair transplantation procedure. Successful placement begins with one's understanding of the concept of facial thirds. The somewhat rounded and tapered frontal hairline is placed with the apex approximately 2 cm above the perceived frontal hairline as defined by dividing the face into thirds. The lateral points of the hairline are made perpendicular to a line drawn to the outer canthus of the eyes. This somewhat posterior placement of the transplanted surgical hairline is a representation of a mature man's hairline through the normal aging process. In anticipating future hair loss, hair transplantation should provide an esthetic result throughout the decades of life.[12] A successfully placed hairline at 30 years of age must also retain the same esthetically pleasing look at age 60 and beyond. Hairlines placed too low will, in most cases, be esthetically unacceptable as the patient reaches the fifth and sixth decades of life. In addition, the retropositioning of the surgically transplanted hairline will limit the number of grafts required for complete fullness and therefore help conserve the amount of donor hair used, especially in individuals with more advanced patterns of balding.

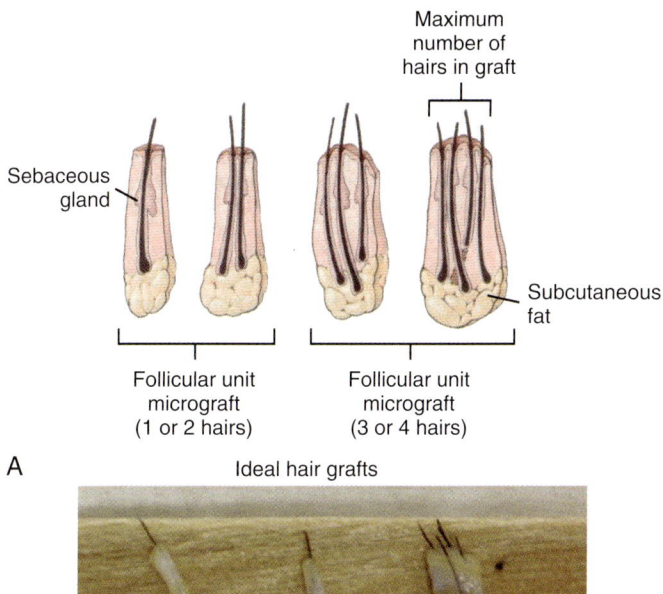

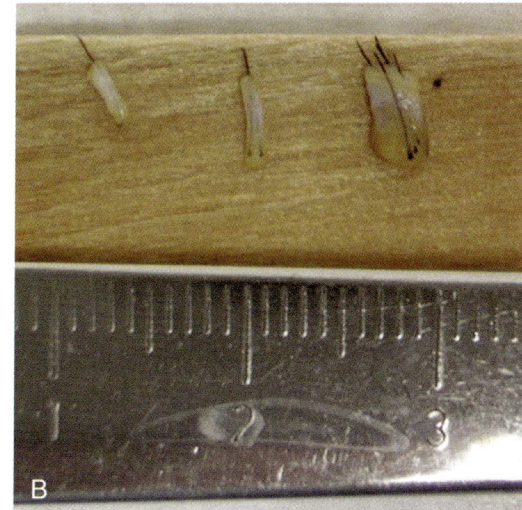

Fig. 106-6 ■ **A,** Micrografts and multifollicular grafts. **B,** Micrografts and multifollicular grafts cut in preparation for implantation. (**A,** From Barrera A: *Hair transplantation: the art of micrografting and minigrafting,* St Louis, 2001, Quality Medical Publishing, p 71.)

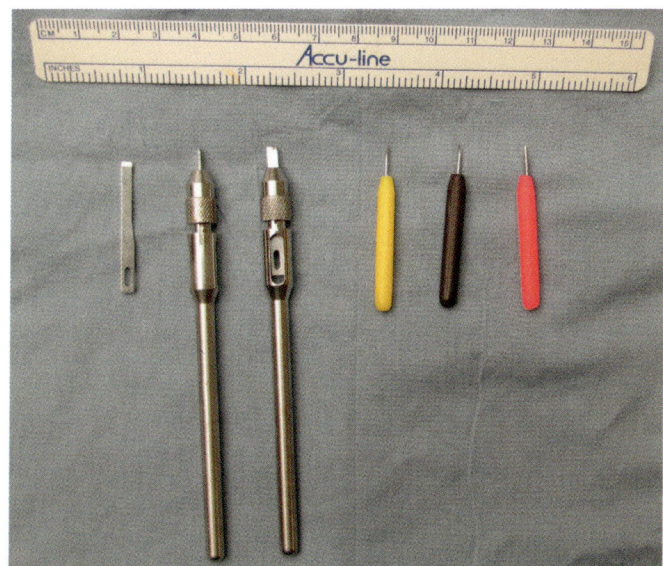

Fig. 106-7 ■ Instruments for recipient site preparation. Slit blade on left. Solid needles on right.

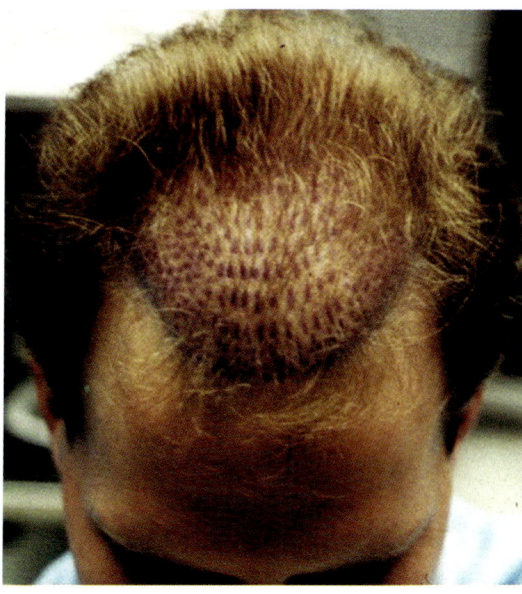

Fig. 106-8 ■ The anticipated hairline—symmetric and rounded. It acts as a guide in this patient for the placement of micrografts and multifollicular grafts in slits.

The anticipated hairline is drawn with an indelible fine-point marking pen. It must be symmetric and properly placed. This is followed by placement of the anticipated recipient sites behind and confluent with the marked hairline in a staggered fashion (Fig. 106-8).

PREOPERATIVE EVALUATION

As with any surgical procedure, it is important to obtain an adequate medical history and perform a careful visual and manual examination of the donor and recipient areas. In patients undergoing procedures for cosmetic purposes or enhancement, the expectations of the patient must be successfully determined and discussed preoperatively. Careful photodocumentation is also advisable.

DONOR SITE SELECTION, PREPARATION, AND ANESTHESIA

After marking the recipient sites, appropriate donor areas are chosen that will match, as closely as possible, the texture and density of the recipient area. In essence, the donor site is hair that would typically exist in a type 6 or 7 pattern.[13] Thus, by visualizing the patient's head from behind, an arbitrary line drawn from the top of the ears would denote an area below which all hair would be genetically programmed to grow indefinitely when transplanted. Similarly, the hair remaining just above and behind the ears would appear to have that same potential.

An area that will provide the needed number of grafts is clipped to a length of approximately 2 mm with either scissors or clippers. One must be able to see the angled direction of the hair growth as it emerges from the scalp to also achieve proper orientation in the recipient area (Fig. 106-9). These hair follicles must also be visualized when using an ellipse or multiblade knife to take a long strip required for micrograft and multifollicular preparation. The area is prepared with an adequate antiseptic solution, either iodophor or alcohol-soaked sponges, to clean and remove any spicules of hair remaining on the surface. With the patient in a sitting position, the

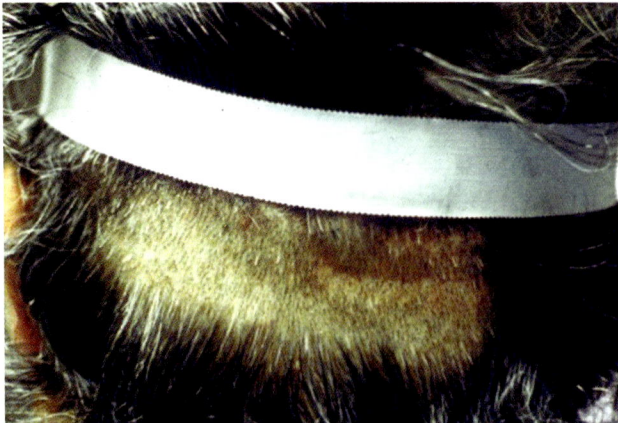

Fig. 106-9 ■ Prepared donor site. Note the minimal scar from a previous procedure.

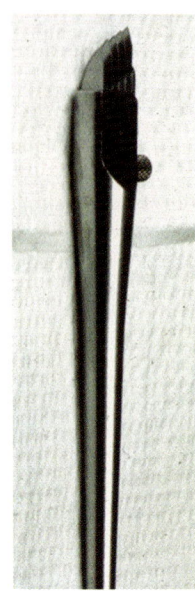

Fig. 106-10 ■ Multiblade knife with spacers to define donor strip width.

donor site is anesthetized with 2% lidocaine with 1:100,000 epinephrine. Use of a vasoconstrictor is usually necessary to aid in hemostasis. A 30-gauge needle is used to achieve a ring block for the recipient sites and subcutaneous infiltration for the donor sites.[3] Nitrous oxide and oxygen or intravenous sedation can also be used during the injection of local anesthetic, which lasts approximately 1 to 2 minutes. Approximately 10 to 15 minutes is required for full vasoconstriction to take place before the procedure is begun.

HARVESTING DONOR STRIPS

Complete preparation of the recipient site involves the use of recipient slit blades and solid needles for micrografts and multi-FUs (i.e., stab wounds or needle punctures at each previously marked position). These wounds are created prior to the dissection for harvesting the grafts so that bleeding will have ceased before one attempts to insert the grafts. The sites are generally created so that the slit or puncture wound is at a right angle to the curvature of the scalp. The only requirement is that the blade or recipient punch pass deep to the skin into subcutaneous tissue. The patient, in a sitting position with the head firmly fixed, has the donor site injected with physiologic saline until maximum turgor is achieved to minimize skin distortion during the procedure.

Because hair transplantation involving micrografts and multifollicular grafting has now evolved into a procedure that generates and moves hundreds or thousands of much smaller grafts, the process adds significant time and complexity to the transplant procedure. To simplify and accelerate the production of grafts, the donor scalp is often harvested as long narrow strips with the aid of a multiblade knife. Grafts of single FUs, two to three FUs, or four to six FUs can easily be visualized and quickly cut from narrow donor strips.

Obtaining donor tissue as long narrow strips with a multiblade knife (Fig. 106-10) has become a mainstay of the transplant procedure for many surgeons, with the ideal strip being defined as one with a full complement of viable intact hairs along the entire length and a minimal number of transected hairs. The two key elements for cutting perfect strips are tumescence and proper angling of the cutting instrument. Maximal tumescence must be obtained by injecting normal saline both subcutaneously and intradermally. The multiblade knife is held by the fingers, and the angle of the knife is constantly changed while maintaining consistent alignment with the hair direction and checking for both parallel alignment of the knife

blade and donor hairs. Depths greater than 6 mm should be avoided in an effort to remain in a dissection plane superficial to the galea, which minimizes the chance of excessive bleeding. After a single pass with the multiblade knife, removal of the strip is accomplished by sharp dissection with super sharp scissors or a scalpel, which is used to cut along a precise plane approximately 1 to 2 mm below the level of the hair follicles. Spacers of 2 to 3 mm define the width of strips, which again are best cut only into the subcutaneous fat layer to avoid the galea aponeurotica (Fig. 106-11). When harvesting of micrografts and multifollicular grafts is complete, the donor site is generally closed in one or two layers to provide a thin scar completely covered by existing hair and actually preserving the amount of donor hair available for subsequent transplant procedures.[14,15]

THE RECIPIENT AREA

The recipient hole is approximately 0.25 mm smaller than the donor graft, and the graft is inserted to test for snugness of fit. A snug fit is essential because revascularization of the graft depends on blood vessels growing from the dermis of the recipient scalp into the dermis of the graft. The recipient site must be acutely angled to match the angle at which the original hair emerged from the scalp. Usually, there is some terminal or lanugo hair to help determine this angle, but essentially all hair is placed in a forward direction (Fig. 106-12).

Such angling of the recipient site improves the direction of hair growth and lengthens the recipient site, thereby better accommodating the graft from the thicker donor skin and preventing elevation of the graft.[11] Micrografts and multifollicular grafts are implanted with a small jeweler's forceps into 1- to 2-mm slits or needle puncture sites.

Inexperienced operators will encounter considerable difficulty at first, and it is important for the recipient sites to have reached the sticky stage of coagulation before implantation is attempted, usually in 5 to 10 minutes. It should be remembered that for micrografts or multifollicular grafts, gentle pressure is applied with a swab or a finger to adjacent grafts while the grafts are inserted. Unquestionably,

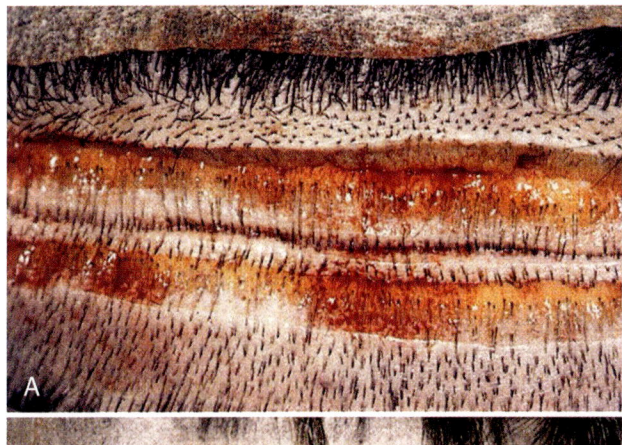

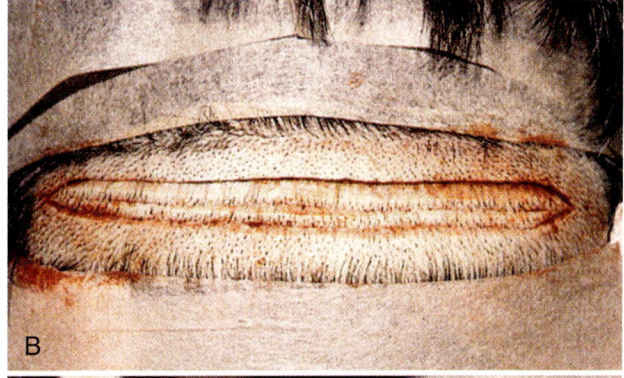

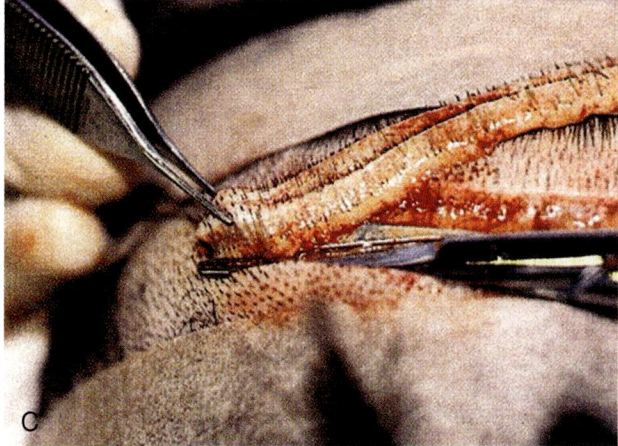

Fig. 106-11 ■ **A** to **C,** Note the direction of the multiblade knife with spacers to define strip width. The harvested strips can be sectioned into grafts of various sizes, usually under at least 2× to 3× magnification or by using a dissecting microscope.

these procedures cannot be performed with consummate expertise and in a timely fashion without using a well-trained transplant team consisting of at least one surgeon who prepares and marks the operative sites and obtains the donor strip and two to three technicians who cut the grafts and place them just as rapidly as they are dissected.

POSTOPERATIVE CARE

The donor and recipient sites may or may not be bandaged. If bandaging is preferred, a nonadhering Telfa (Kendall Company, Boston, Mass) pad coated with antibiotic ointment is placed over the

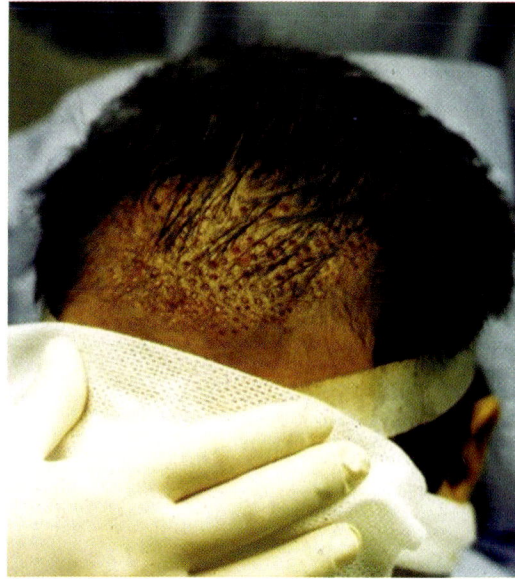

Fig. 106-12 ■ Recipient sites with grafts in place to correct a frontal hair loss pattern.

operative sites. Several layers of flattened gauze sponges (4 × 3 inches) are then used to hold the Telfa in place as the scalp is wrapped with a clean bandage consisting of two to three 4-inch gauze rolls. The dressing is removed the following morning, and the scalp and each graft are cleansed meticulously with a cotton swab and hydrogen peroxide. The hair is washed and styled to cover the operative sites. The patient is mandated to wash the hair twice a day for the first 3 days following each transplant procedure. Suture removal, when necessary, is accomplished 1 to 2 weeks after each procedure. The patient must, of course, be made aware that a lag phase exists before hair growth is initiated. After approximately 3 months, the telogen phase of the implanted grafts ends and anagen begins.

COMPLICATIONS

Bleeding, both during and after the operation, is the most common complication. It usually occurs in patients who have taken aspirin or blood-thinning medications or supplements immediately before surgery. Thus, all patients are asked to abstain from aspirin or aspirin-containing products for at least 10 to 14 days before each transplant procedure. Other blood-thinning medications are adjusted accordingly. Operative bleeding is controlled by pressure, injection of additional epinephrine-containing anesthetic and saline into the bleeding site, or suturing. If adequate control takes place during the procedure, postoperative bleeding is rare.

Edema of the forehead may occur starting on the third or fourth postoperative day. It probably results from excessive anesthetic volume or surgical trauma, and it is particularly disturbing in the frontal area because most patients consider it to be cosmetically annoying. This swelling requires no treatment; however, it is our impression that systemic corticosteroids help eliminate this problem. Our regimen includes 10 mg of dexamethasone intramuscularly at the time of surgery, followed by a 5-day postoperative course of decreasing dexamethasone dosage orally (Decadron 5-13 Pak, Merck, West Point, Pa).

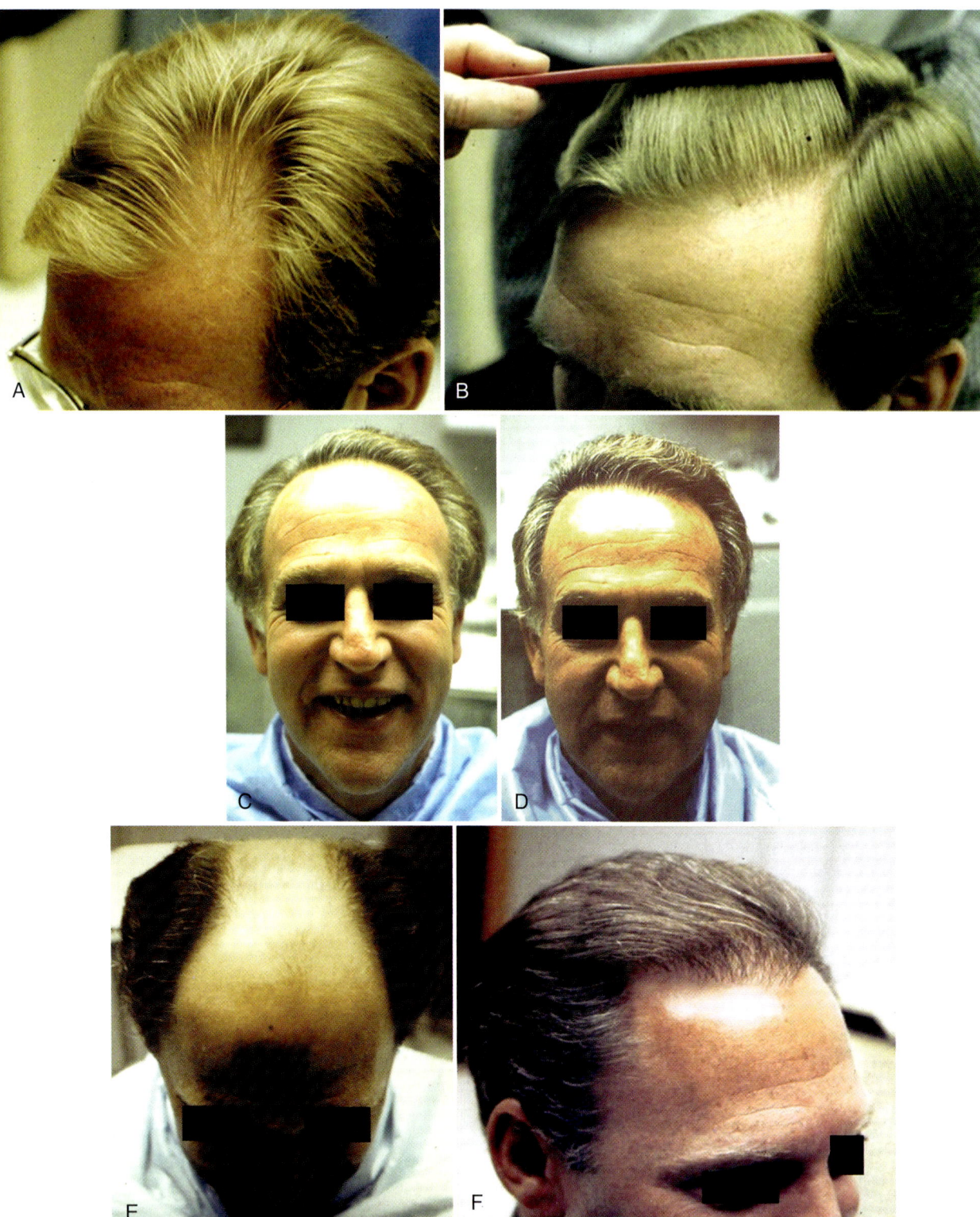

Fig. 106-13 ■ Preoperative and postoperative results in patients with minimal hairline recession (**A** and **B**), a completely restored receding hairline (**C** and **D**), and restoration of a Norwood type 6 extensive hair loss pattern (**E** and **F**).

Infection is a possible complication, although the use of postoperative antibiotics and the requirement that patients wash their hair twice a day for the first 3 days following each surgical procedure virtually eliminates this potential. Patients are given 500 mg of tetracycline for 7 days postoperatively twice a day.

Cobblestoning, or irregular elevation of the grafts, is prevented by proper graft placement and by adequate cleansing postoperatively the morning after each surgical procedure.

Hypertrophic scarring occasionally occurs in patients with a history of poor scar formation. In this case a trial transplant is undertaken with a limited number of different-sized grafts placed in an unobtrusive area while making certain that they fit snugly in the recipient sites. If scarring and poor growth occur, further grafting on that patient should not be done.[3]

With proper patient selection, good hairline design and placement, and meticulous surgical technique, an excellent result can be achieved in most patients (Fig. 106-13).

PEARLS AND PITFALLS

- Adequate tumescence of the donor area is paramount to accurately determine hair shaft angulation.
- Proper angulation of FU grafts maximizes the esthetic result.
- It is better to reconstruct a hairline too high than too low.
- Hairline placement and design are the most important variables for a successful hair restoration procedure.
- Hairline reconstruction should be accomplished with primarily one- or two-FU grafts.
- Adequate moisture helps ensure graft survival; grafts should never be allowed to desiccate.
- The ex vivo time of grafts should be kept to a minimum (2 to 4 hours).
- The novice should start with vertex restoration procedures because this site requires less esthetic and technical subtlety.

REFERENCES

1. Norwood OT: Classification and incidence of male pattern baldness. In Norwood OT, Shiell RC, editors: *Hair transplant surgery*, ed 2, Springfield, Ill, 1984, Charles C Thomas.
2. Orientreich N: Autografts in alopecias and other selected dermatological condition, *Ann N Y Acad Sci* 83:463-479, 1959.
3. Hendler BH: Hair transplantation. In *OMS knowledge update*, vol I, pt. II, Rosemont, Ill, 1995, Esthetic Surgery Section, American Association of Oral and Maxillofacial Surgeons (AAOMS), pp 129-193.
4. Hendler BH: Hair restoration surgery: hair transplantation and micrografting, *Atlas Oral Maxillofac Clin North Am* 6:39-53, 1996.
5. Unger WP, Nordstrom REA, editors: *Hair transplantation*, ed 2. New York, 1988, Marcel Dekker.
6. Stegman SJ, Tromovitch TA: *Cosmetic dermatologic surgery*, Chicago, 1984, Year Book Publishers.
7. Gandleman, M, Epstein, JS: Hair transplantation to the eyebrow, eyelash, and other parts of the body, *Facial Plast Surg Clin North Am* 12:253-261, 2004.
8. Reed M: Hair transplantation. In *Grabb and Smith's plastic surgery*, ed 6, Philadelphia, 2006, Lippincott Williams & Wilkins, pp 562-572.
9. Headington JT: Transverse microscopic anatomy of the human scalp—a basis for a morphometric approach to disorders of the hair follicle, *Arch Dermatol* 120:449-456, 1984.
10. Bernstein RM, Rassman WR: The logic of follicular unit transplantation, *Dermatol Clin* 17:277-295, discussion 296, 1999.
11. Nordstrom REA: "Micrografts" for improvement of the frontal hairline after hair transplantation, *Aesthet Plast Surg* 5:97-101, 1981.
12. Nordstrom REA: The initial interview, *Facial Plast Surg* 2:179-187, 1985.
13. Alt TH: Evaluation of donor harvesting techniques in hair transplantation, *J Dermatol Surg Oncol* 10:799-806, 1984.
14. Morrison ID: An improved method of suturing the donor site in hair transplantation surgery, *Plast Reconstr Surg* 67:378-381, 1981.
15. Pierce HE: Improved method of closure of donor sites in hair transplantation, *J Dermatol Surg Oncol* 6:475-476, 1979.

Chapter 107

Rhytidectomy (Face-Lifting)

Angelo Cuzalina, Tarek Victor Copty, Husain Ali Khan

The face is generally the first to reveal signs of aging. Rejuvenating the aging face has gained tremendous popularity over the last 2 decades. In the past, incisional face-lifting was the main strategy for facial rejuvenation, but during the past decade cosmetic surgeons have revolutionized facial rejuvenation with adjunctive procedures such as alloplastic facial implants, chemodenervation, injectable fillers, and skin resurfacing via laser or chemical exfoliation. Although we now have several weapons to reverse the signs of facial aging, the "modern" face-lift is still the "gold standard" for correcting generalized facial cutis laxa (rhytidosis), jowling, cervicomental redundant skin, and platysmal banding. Facial dyschromia, changes in pigmentation, acne scarring, and deep wrinkles can all be treated with the adjunctive procedures described later in this chapter and in other dedicated chapters in this textbook.

The face-lifts described in the early literature involved skin excision only. Even though the benefit is usually temporary and a rather poor natural appearance results, some surgeons still use this technique for certain patients with unique anatomy or for revision surgery. The current face-lifting techniques are numerous, although most involve manipulation of the superficial musculoaponeurotic system (SMAS). SMAS involvement in face-lifting was first introduced by Mitz and Peyronie in 1976 when their landmark article was published.[1]

Historical details regarding face-lifting are evident from publications in the literature, such as those by Hollander (1912), Lexter (1931), Joseph (1921), Passant (1919), Bourget (1921), and Madam Noel (1926). At that time surgeons and patients were reluctant to make their cosmetic surgical interest public.[2] Hence, technical advances were slow to flourish and propagate (Box 107-1). Even with extensive undermining of skin flaps during face-lifts decades ago, the results were only partially beneficial and did not emphasize pathology of the neck and the platysma. A better understanding of facial anatomy was described by Skoog in 1974, and his manipulation of facial tissue led to the future advancements in face-lifting surgery.[3] Webster and colleagues later added that extensive subcutaneous dissection leads to greater exposure of raw surfaces with an increased risk for complications.[4] Richard Webster was one of the first to recommend a "short flap" with basic SMAS plication and suggested that the skin would advance adequately from its attachment to the elevated deep tissue.

ETIOPATHOGENESIS

Indications for face-lifting cosmetic surgery are numerous and involve the changes that accompany facial aging. First, the patient is identified as seeking facial rejuvenation because of age-related complaints. Upper face-lifting is described in a separate chapter, and our focus here is to target the lower part of the face and neck. Cutis laxa of the jowls and cervical area, deepened nasolabial fissures, and platysmal banding are the main complaints that are targeted by current face-lifting strategies. Genetics, age, and smoking are the key determinants of the cause of signs of facial aging (Fig. 107-1). In general, the average age when patients first seek lower face-lifting and neck lifting can vary widely from 45 to 65 years.

CLINICAL ANATOMY

Surgeons have multiple techniques at their disposal to perform face-lifts, although detailed knowledge of surgical facial anatomy is the key to any cosmetic surgery, regardless of the techniques used (Figs. 107-2 and 107-3). Determining who is best suited for liposuction versus submentoplasty with or without a face-lift is at least half the battle for ultimately producing pleasing esthetic results (Figs. 107-4 to 107-6). Basic neck liposuction for an ideal patient can be dramatic despite being a relatively simple procedure when performed well (Fig. 107-7).

Detailed knowledge of the anatomy in conjunction with the pathology to be corrected is necessary for correct surgical planning and preoperative markings (Fig. 107-8). Marking the skin over the known danger zones can reduce the risk for complications and neurovascular injury (Fig. 107-9). These areas are often obscured when the patient is in the supine position and distorted with local anesthetic.

A surgeon must be mindful of three main danger zones: the mid-zygomatic temporal region, the malar eminence region, and the area at the inferior border of the mandible near the angle. The mid-zygomatic arch area contains the temporal or frontal branch of the facial nerve (Fig. 107-10). The nerve crosses over the arch approximately 2 cm from the external auditory meatus.[5] It can be easily injured in the area over the bony prominence where there is less soft tissue.

The second zone is at the zygomatic/malar eminence, which contains both a plexus of vessels connecting the transverse facial artery and the facial artery proper and the zygomatic branch of the facial nerve, which crosses cephalad near the lateral canthus of the eye (Fig. 107-11). This area is known as the "MacGregor patch" and is named for the strong zygomatico-dermal fibrous attachments present here.

The third zone lies at the inferior border of the mandible a short distance anterior to the angle. The marginal mandibular branch of the facial nerve courses just below the inferior border of the mandible approximately 20-50% of the time, but it can be situated as much as 1.5 cm below the inferior border.[6] Initial dissection over the platysma avoids injury to the marginal mandibular nerve, and

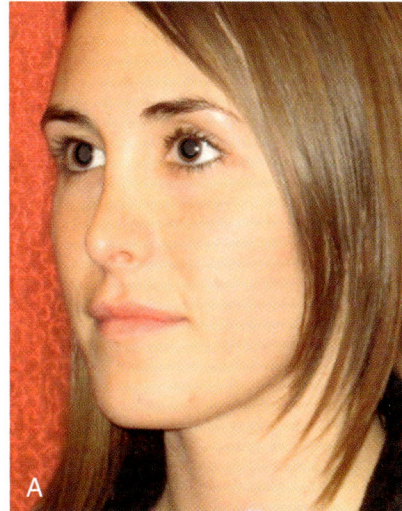

Malar fat pad descent

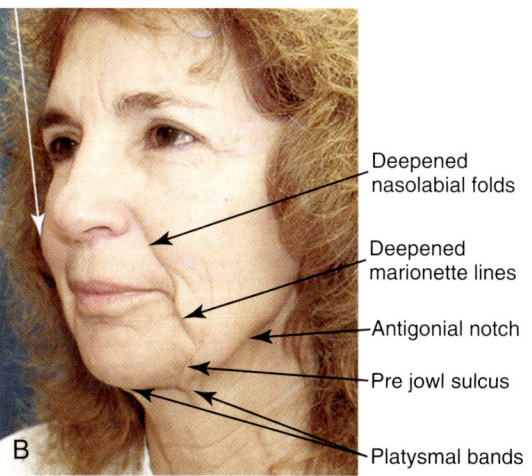

Deepened
nasolabial folds

Deepened
marionette lines

Antigonial notch

Pre jowl sulcus

Platysmal bands

Fig. 107-1 ■ The facial features of a youthful, 25-year-old woman (**A**) are contrasted with those of a somewhat aged, 55-year-old woman (**B**). Their lower facial and mid-face regions are vastly different because of the aging process. The malar fat pad and jowls descend secondary to gravity and loss of tissue integrity. The prejowl sulcus deepens, and bone resorption taking place along the mandibular border accentuates the cutis laxa that occurs with age. The aged eyebrow shows both: medial and lateral descent with loss of volume and hooding over the lateral orbital rim.

BOX 107-1	Face-lift History (Abbreviated List)

- Subcutaneous rhytidectomy (Lexar, 1916)
- Subcutaneous and platysma (Skoog, 1974)
- Subcutaneous with description of the superficial musculoaponeurotic system (Mitz and Peyronie, 1976)
- Musculofascial plane described (Jost and Levet, 1984)
- Subperiosteal technique (Tessier, 1990; Psilakis, 1988; Ramirez, 1991)
- Deep-plane technique (Hamra, 1984)
- Composite technique (Hamra, 1990)
- Mini-lifts, e.g., S-lift (Saylan and others, 2003)
- "Lifestyle or Quick Lift": just patented "mini"-lifts
- "MACS lift," minimal-access cranial suspension (Tonnard and Verpaele, 2004)

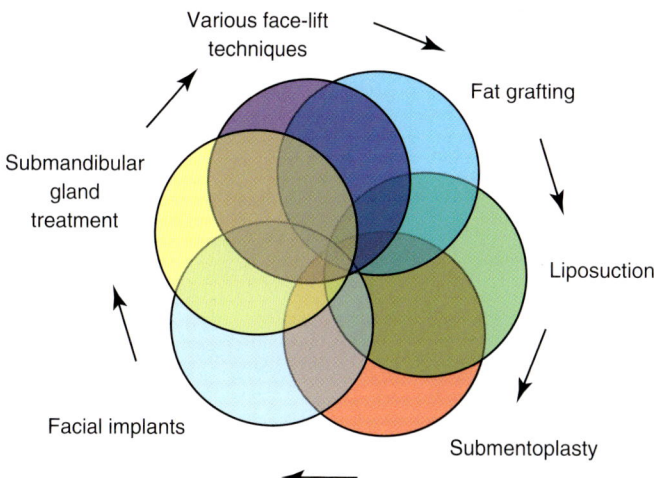

Fig. 107-2 ■ Multiple techniques can be used to perform face-lifts. Detailed knowledge of surgical facial anatomy is the key to any cosmetic surgery regardless of the techniques used. Selection of the most ideal technique or techniques is based on a correct working diagnosis along with realistic expectations and desires of the patient.

later dissection below the platysma must be done with greater care to maintain integrity of the nerve.

Several other landmarks and surface anatomy must be identified and noted. The great auricular nerve and accessory nerves are found in the posterior triangle of the neck approximately 6 cm below the earlobe along the posterior border of the sternocleidomastoid; this area is also known as the "Erb point" by some. However, the Erb point was not originally used for this description. The point, also known as the punctum nervosum, was originally used to describe the spot where the four cutaneous branches of the cervical plexus exited. Regardless of names, the great auricular nerve is typically 6 to 7 cm below the ear canal just posterior to the sternocleidomastoid muscle, and care must be taken to avoid inadvertent injury to this large sensory nerve during a face-lift.[7] Flap elevation in the cervical region should therefore be kept above the sternocleidomastoid fascia to avoid these nerves (Fig. 107-12).

The facial artery is a major provider of the blood supply to the face. This artery originates from the external carotid artery in the neck and then crosses the mandible at the antegonial notch adjacent to the anterior edge of the masseter muscle. Other contributors to the blood supply of the face include the supraorbital and supratrochlear arteries from the internal carotid system and the external carotid artery, which terminates as the superficial temporal artery and the internal maxillary artery.[8]

The facial nerve has three main components: visceral motor, sensory, and special sensory. The visceral motor component stimulates the lacrimal gland, salivary gland, mucosal membranes, and palate. The general sensory component supplies the skin over the conchal bowl and a small component of skin in the posterior auricular area and provides sensation to the wall of the external auditory canal, as well as the tympanic membrane. The special sensory component innervates the anterior two thirds of the tongue and both the hard and soft palate. The brachial motor component supplies motor innervation to the muscles responsible for facial expression. The frontalis and occipitalis are supplied by both sides of the motor cortex, and the remaining muscles of facial expression are supplied by only one side.

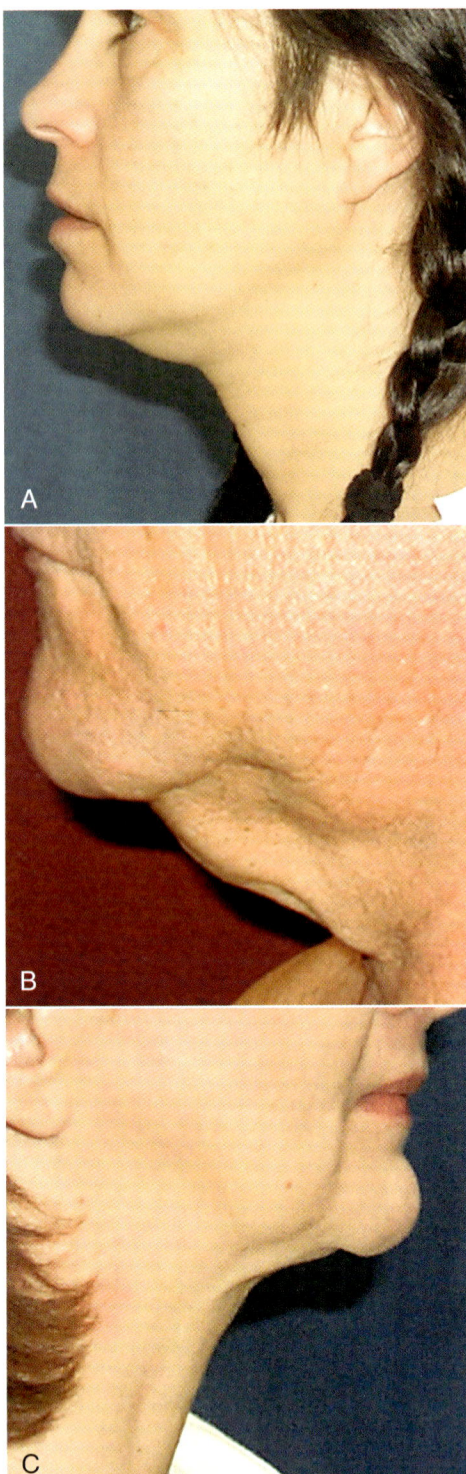

Fig. 107-3 ■ Patient assessment should look at skin tone/laxity, platysmal banding, amount of fat and location, jowling, jaw bone structure, submandibular gland ptosis, and hyoid position. **A,** A good candidate for liposuction. **B,** A good candidate for submentoplasty and face-lift. **C,** A bad candidate.

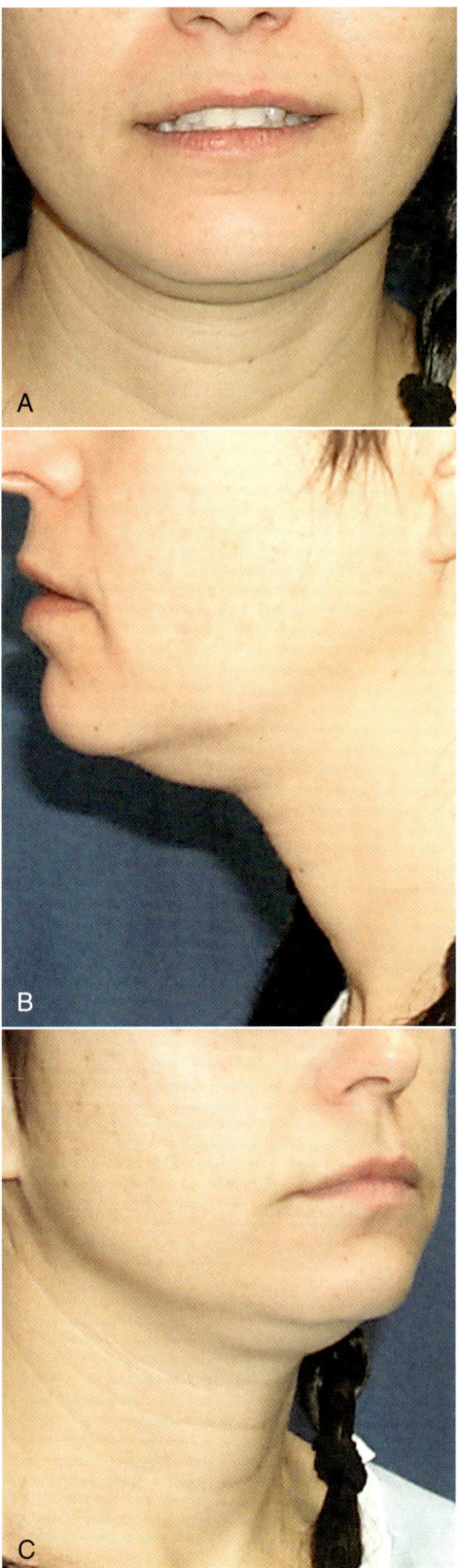

Fig. 107-4 ■ Preoperative photographs showing ideal neck anatomy for basic submental liposuction only.

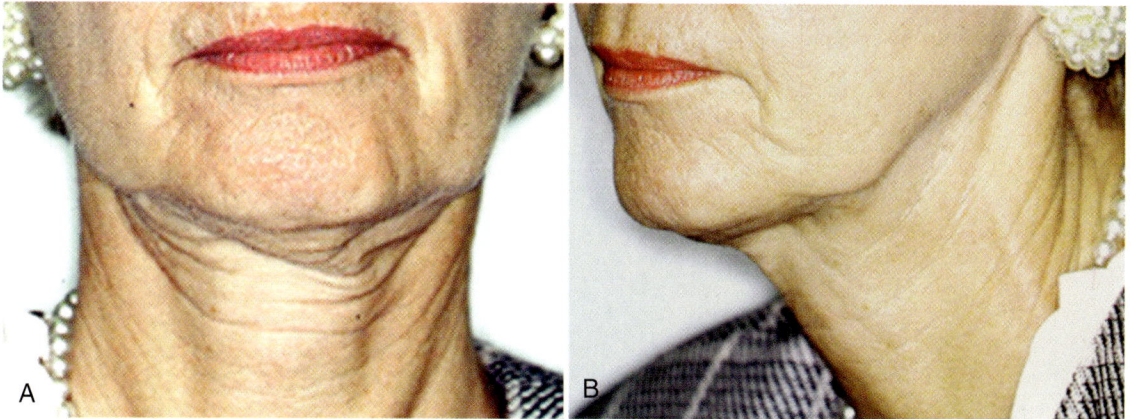

Fig. 107-5 ■ **A,** Ideal neck anatomy for a basic face-lift includes loose skin, thin/average frame, minor banding, normal hyoid, no gland ptosis, good bone structure, and normal digastrics. Preoperative photographs show ideal neck anatomy for a basic face-lift. Frequently, submentoplasty may not be required with this type of patient. **B,** Postoperative view.

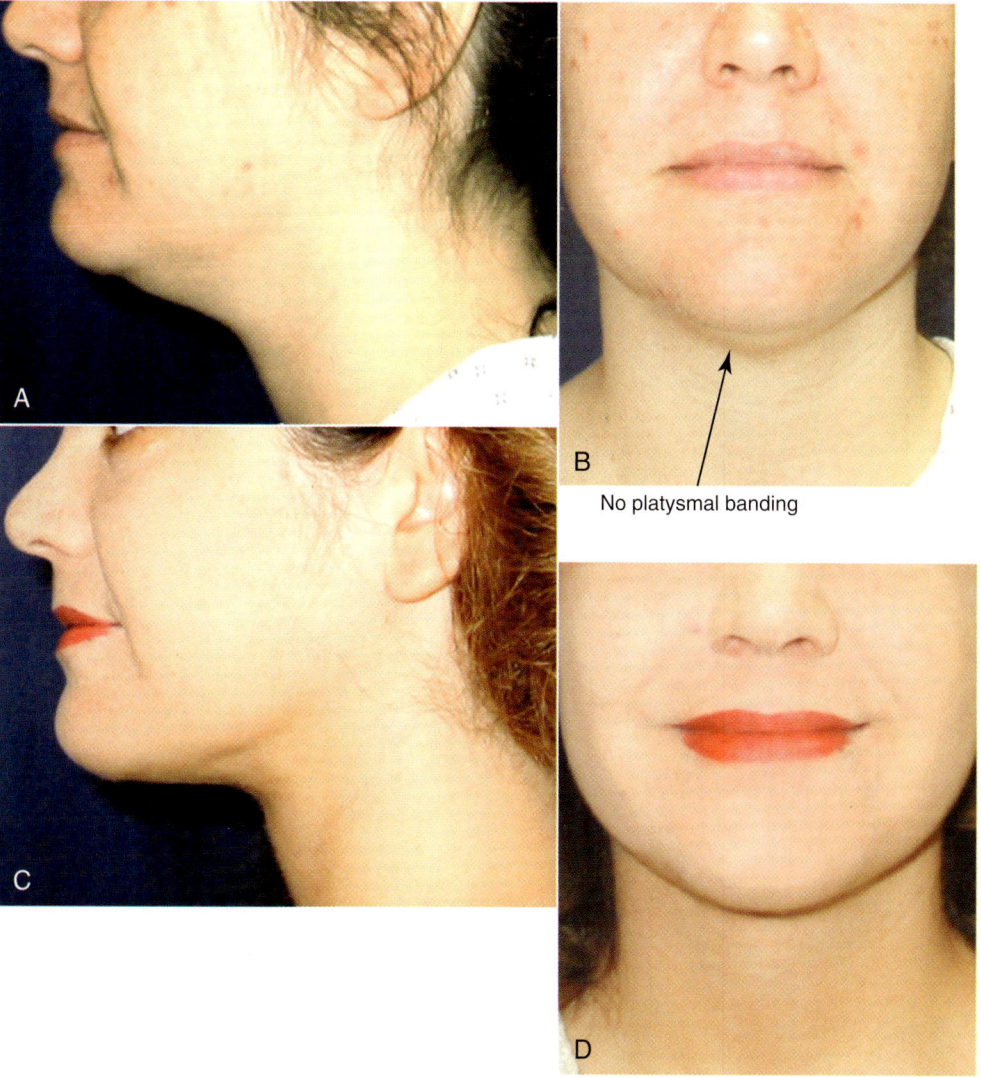

No platysmal banding

Fig. 107-6 ■ Ideal neck criteria include good skin elasticity, adequate excess *superficial* fat, minimal muscle laxity and no banding, good bone structure, and a patient who understands the limitations of the procedure. Side (**A**) and facial (**B**) preoperative views of the "ideal" neck. Side (**C**) and facial (**D**) views 6 months following basic neck liposuction only.

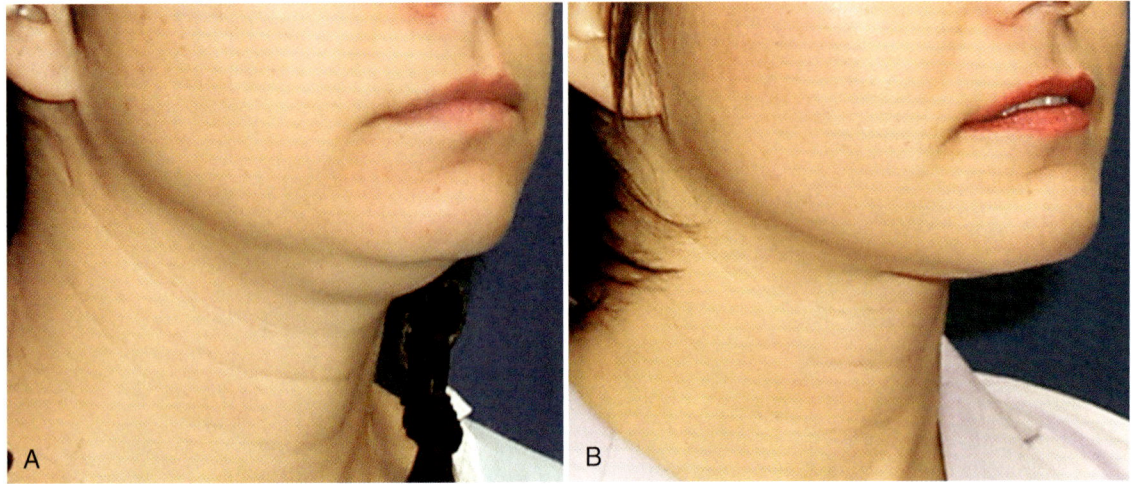

Fig. 107-7 ■ "Ideal" neck in a 41-year-old woman. **A,** Preoperatively. **B,** Four months following basic neck liposuction and a small chin implant.

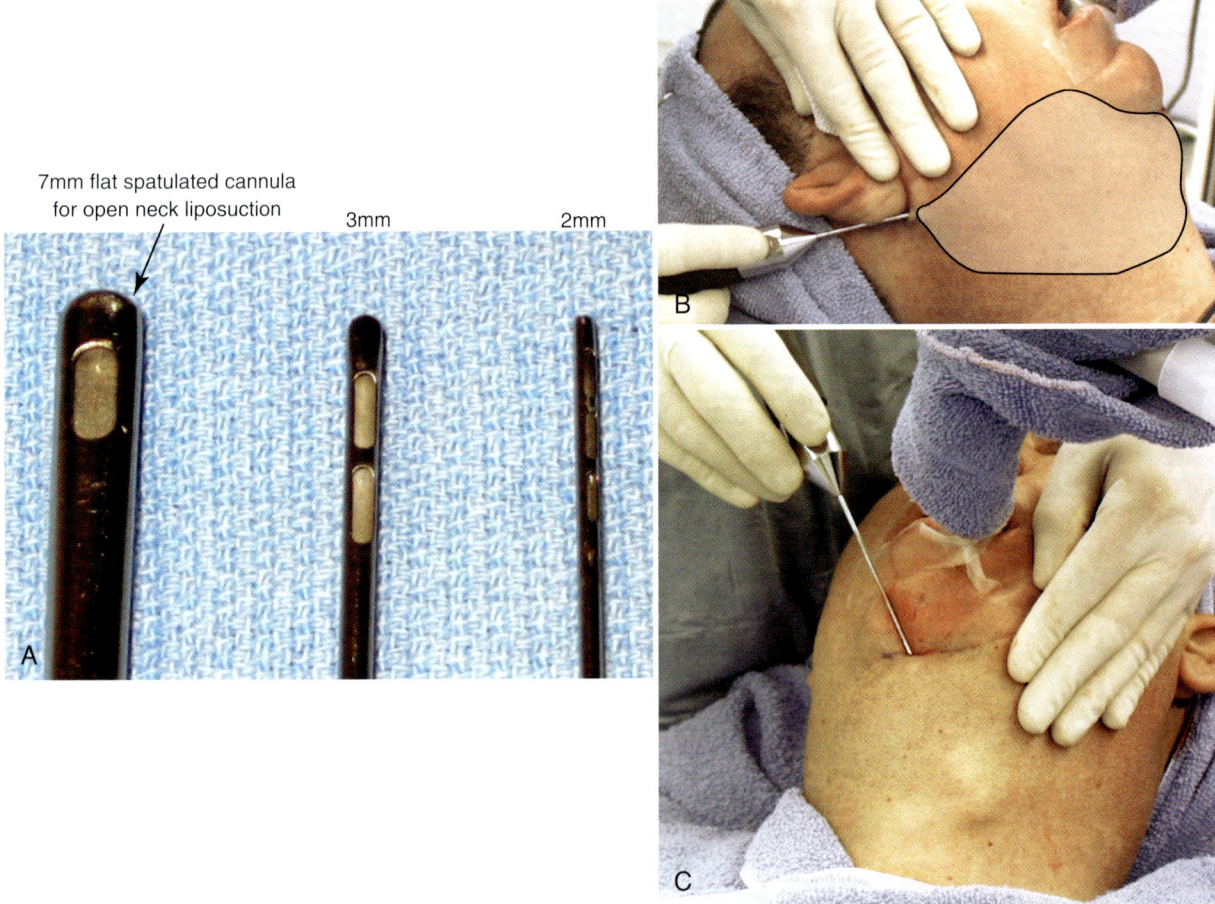

7mm flat spatulated cannula for open neck liposuction

3mm

2mm

Fig. 107-8 ■ **A,** Small (2 to 3 mm) microcannulas are ideal for a basic liposuction technique in the neck. Larger, flat cannulas may be used safely with an "open" technique, such as submentoplasty. **B,** Cervical liposuction from the retroauricular area. **C,** Submental liposuction from the submental crease.

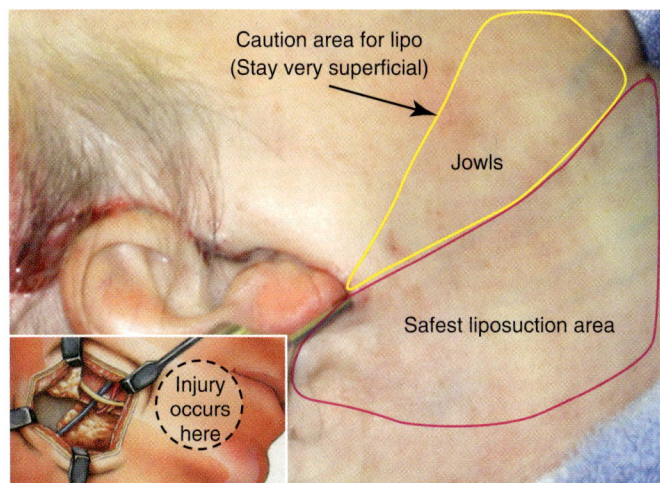

Fig. 107-9 ■ Liposuction of the cervical and jowl regions. Caution must be used in the jowl region to avoid injury to the marginal mandibular nerve. Tumescent local anesthesia provides anesthesia, as well as vasoconstriction and hydrodissection, when injected properly. The tumescent solution consists of 500 mL of normal saline, 1.5 mg of epinephrine, and 30 mL of 2% lidocaine (600 mg). A 0.12% lidocaine solution with 1:333,333 epinephrine is injected with a 22-gauge spinal needle.

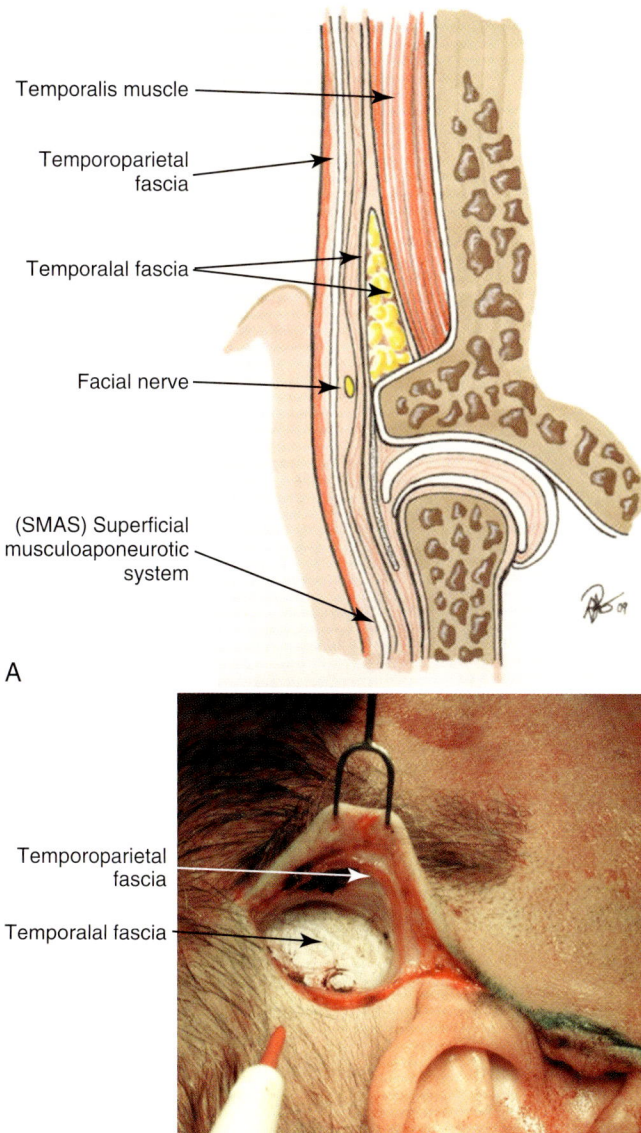

Fig. 107-10 ■ **A,** Cross section through the temporomandibular joint and zygomatic arch. The temporal nerve runs immediately below the temporoparietal fascia above the arch, which is the fascia continuous with the superficial musculoaponeurotic system below the arch. **B,** Clinical photograph demonstrating one technique used in the temporal region in which dissection is carried out below the frontal nerve above the arch.

The facial nerve exits from the stylomastoid foramen. Small branches of the facial trunk first innervate the stylohyoid and posterior belly of the digastric muscle. A branch also travels with the posterior auricular nerve to innervate the occipitalis muscle. The main trunk of the facial nerve enters the parotid and divides the gland into deep and upper lobes. The main trunk splits into two divisions, the temporofacial and cervicofacial. The temporofacial divides into temporal, zygomatic, and buccal branches. The cervicofacial divides into lower buccal, marginal mandibular, and cervical branches.[9]

In Stuzin and colleagues' classic article in 1989, the temporal branch of the facial nerve was found to consistently be located in the temporoparietal fascia.[10] Dissection is therefore carried out directly on top of the superficial layer of the deep temporal fascia. The recommended path of dissection to the arch is within the subaponeurotic plane to 2 cm above the arch, and then dissection deepens to penetrate the superficial layer of the deep temporal fascia.

Once the zygomatic and buccal branches of the facial nerve exit the parotid gland, they course deep to the masseteric fascia and travel on the external surface of the buccal fat pad and its fascia. The terminal branches of the zygomatic and buccal branches perforate the anterior masseteric fascia and enter the buccal fat pad compartment. The terminal end of the zygomatic branch travels to the deep surface of the orbicularis oculi, zygomaticus, levator quadratus, and orbicularis oris muscles. The buccal branch terminates deep to the surface of the orbicularis oris and triangularis muscles. Because of the location of the zygomatic and buccal branches of the facial nerve, dissection anterior to the parotid in a sub-SMAS plane can damage the buccal and zygomatic branches.

After the marginal mandibular branch leaves the anterior inferior border of the parotid gland it courses deep to the platysma. Variations of the nerve and its position relative to the inferior border of the mandible have been reported. The marginal mandibular branch of the facial nerve posterior to the facial artery has been reported by Dingman and Grabb to be below the inferior border of the mandible 19% of the time. However, Baker and Conley found that the marginal mandibular branch was always 1 to 2 cm below the inferior border of the mandible.[6] In patients with excessive skin laxity, the marginal mandibular nerve lies even more inferiorly.

Several other anatomic landmarks should be identified on the patient's skin before planning treatment, such as the shape and consistency of the temporal tuft of hair, the postauricular hairline, the external anatomy of the ear, the nasolabial fold, the amount of submental fat, and the position of the hyoid bone. Most women have a "double tuft" of hair in the temporal and preauricular area (Figs. 107-13 to 107-15). The level of the temporal hair tuft should be preserved. Surgeons must take care to keep the temporal tuft flap trimmed and be mindful of the fact that any hair excised may result

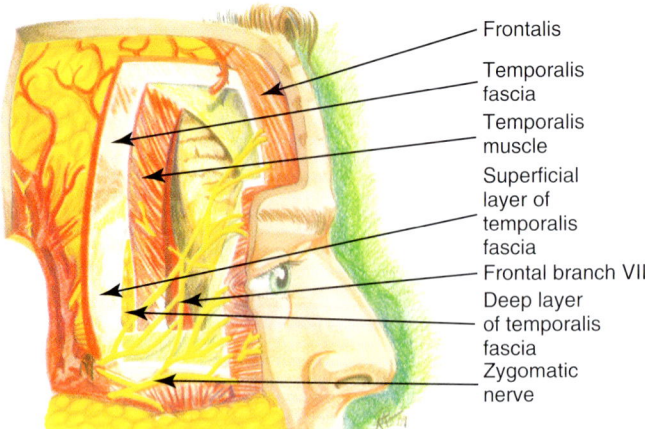

Frontalis
Temporalis fascia
Temporalis muscle
Superficial layer of temporalis fascia
Frontal branch VII
Deep layer of temporalis fascia
Zygomatic nerve

Fig. 107-11 ■ The tissue layers overlying the forehead and temple are critical to understand for avoiding nerve injury and providing safe surgery. The frontal nerve lies on the deep side of the temporoparietal fascia and superficial to the temporalis fascia.

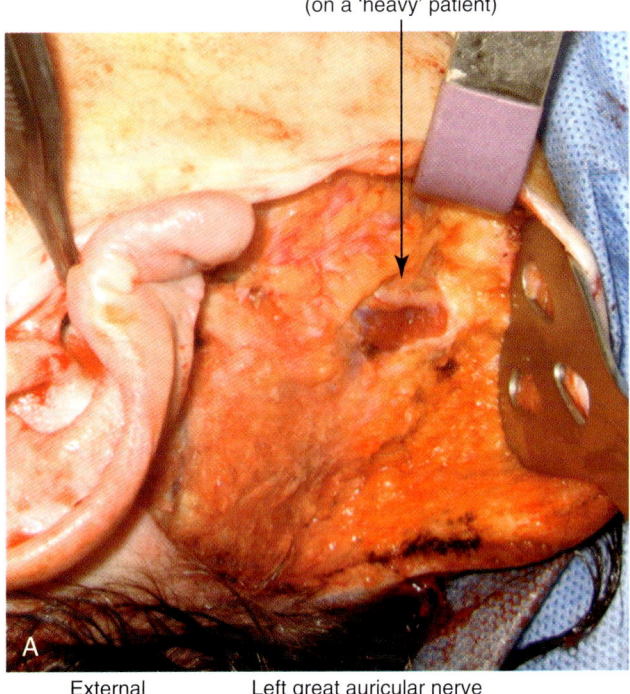

Right great auricular nerve (on a 'heavy' patient)

A

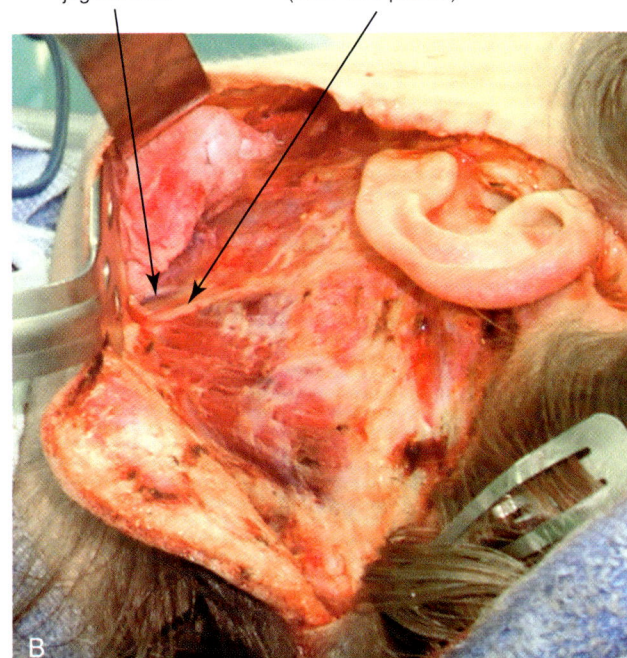

External jugular vein

Left great auricular nerve (on a 'thin' patient)

B

Fig. 107-12 ■ The great auricular nerve is the most commonly injured nerve during a face-lift because of its relatively superficial location.

in an abnormally high tuft. Postauricularly, the point at which the hairline crosses the helix of the ear is generally considered to be the superior extent of the postauricular incision before curving into the hair-bearing scalp. A *thicker* flap can be maintained posteriorly when elevating a face-lift flap from within the occipital hair (Fig. 107-16). Postauricular skin is less at risk for ischemia with this technique versus those with incisions along the hairline. Finally, other face-lift techniques can be used to provide greater lift in the mid-face (minimal-access cranial suspension [MACS] lift), but the basic face-lift is used primarily to elevate the jowls and neck in the majority of patients (Figs. 107-17 to 107-19).

The level and location of the hyoid bone, the amount and size of jowling, the degree of submental adiposity, and the presence of platysmal bands must all be assessed to determine the extent of submental liposuction, as well as the amount of platysmal resection and plication. It should also be realized that retrognathia and a high or anterior hyoid position can prevent achievement of a "perfect" face-lift result (Figs. 107-20 to 107-22).

The anterior extent of dissection is usually marked and identified preoperatively to limit the anterior extent of flap elevation. This is done to protect the vascularity of the skin flap, as well as to avoid injury to the facial nerve or one of its main branches. Some surgeons prefer to dissect 4 to 6 cm anteriorly and inferiorly from the preauricular incision. This is an approximation, however, and may not always be accurate. Most surgeons dissect subcutaneously until there is enough release for maximal lift and esthetics (Figs. 107-23 and 107-24). In most patients the anterior extent of dissection near the commissure of the mouth can be marked to avoid dissection past the modiolus or closer than 2 cm to the commissure. This also avoids injury to the marginal mandibular nerve, which is subplatysmal until approximately 2 cm lateral to the corner of the mouth, at which point it becomes superficial and penetrates the undersurface of the facial mimetic muscles. Limiting anterior dissection to a point short of the commissure can prevent the unwanted "windswept" look that is sometimes seen following skin-only face-lifts or in patients undergoing multiple surgeries.

The anterior extent in the malar region typically extends just shy of the MacGregor patch region, which is found around the most prominent portion of the zygoma. However, certain composite face-lift techniques extend to the lateral canthal region. The temporal region over the zygomatic arch is one of the danger zones, and anterior dissection in this area is often carried out only halfway between the anterior aspect of the ear and the lateral canthus of the eye. Dissection in this area must remain in the subcutaneous plane because of the thinness of the tissue over the zygomatic arch and the potential risk for injury to the temporal branch of the facial nerve. Above the zygomatic arch region, the anterior extent of dissection is dependent on whether significant lifting of the mid-facial region is required and whether a simultaneous forehead and brow

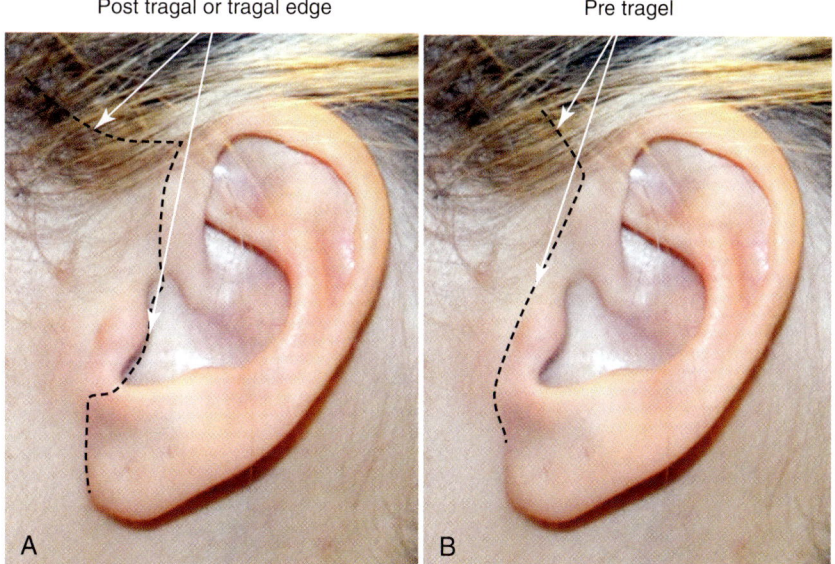

Post tragal or tragal edge   Pre tragel

Fig. 107-13 ▪ Female versus male face-lift incisions. **A,** Female incision. **B,** Male incision.

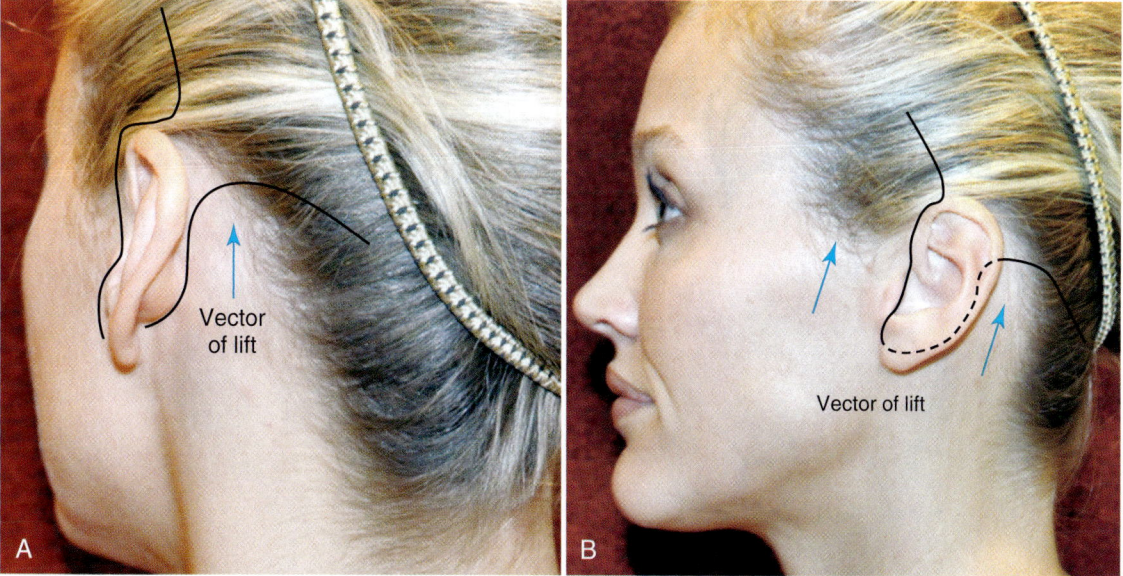

Vector of lift

Vector of lift

Fig. 107-14 ▪ Total intra-hairline incisions. Advantages include well-hidden scars and less risk for ischemia because of thicker flaps at the incisions. Disadvantages include elevation of the temporal hair tuft and more challenging alignment of the posterior hairline.

lift will be performed. If both face-lift and brow lift procedures are being performed, biplanar dissection must be done. Neck dissection in the subcutaneous plane can be variable, but with a short flap, subcutaneous dissection is often carried out only to the posterior border of the jowling area. The occipital region may require dissection superiorly 1 to 2 cm to help align the hair after advancement. More extensive undermining anteriorly and inferiorly is used to clearly view the posterior border of the platysma (Figs. 107-25 and 107-26).

Knowledge of surface anatomy and skin landmarks is absolutely essential to formulate a thorough surgical treatment plan. Attention to detail even before the initial incision can help avoid future complications.

DIAGNOSTIC STUDIES

Patients being evaluated for rhytidectomy who are likely to have the best results are those with a small amount of excess adipose tissue and a significant amount of skin laxity in the submental, cervical, and jowl areas. Younger, healthy, non-smoking patients with a fair complexion and good underlying bone structure typically have the best results and fewest complications. Unfortunately, most patients do not fit into this category and have co-morbid conditions that need to be addressed carefully during the preoperative assessment.

In the past, most patients seeking face-lifts were in their 60s or 70s. Today, cosmetic surgery is more accessible and socially more accepted. The current average age of the typical face-lift patient is

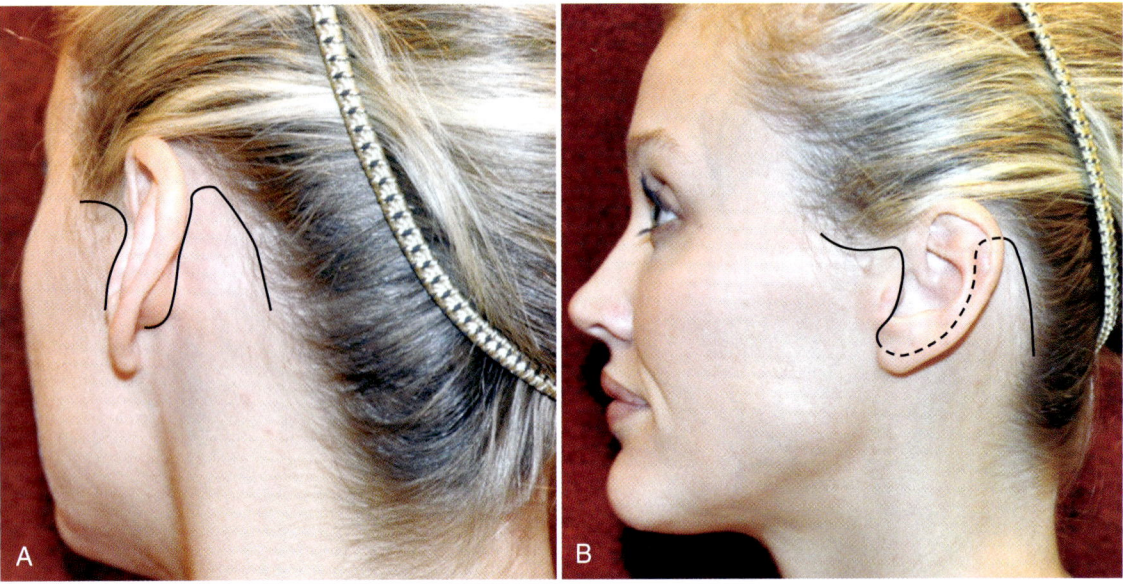

Fig. 107-15 ■ Alternate choices for face-lift incisions. Advantages include an uncomplicated technique and no changes in the hairline. Disadvantages include the potential for visible scars and ischemia in the thin occipital area.

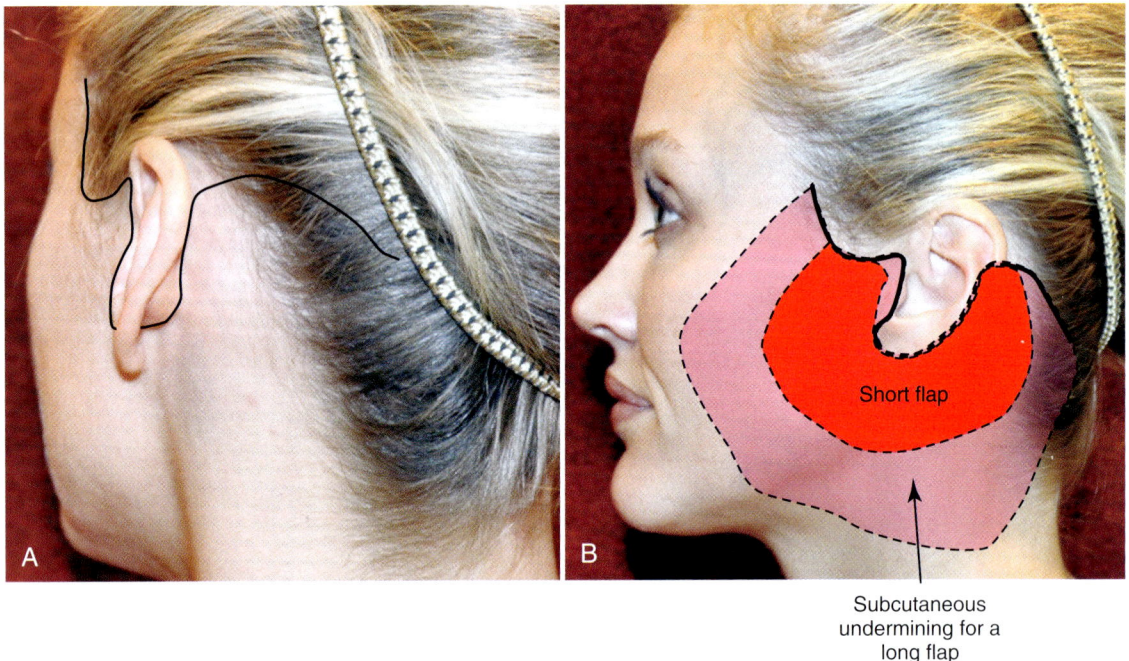

Short flap

Subcutaneous
undermining for a
long flap

Fig. 107-16 ■ Extended flap with mixed periauricular incisions. Advantages include great access for major lifting in the jowls and neck, less risk for ischemia because of thicker flaps by the ears, and no elevation of the temporal tuft. Disadvantages include a slightly longer operative time and more challenging alignment of the posterior hairline.

closer to 50 years.[11] Facial skin laxity and wrinkles usually become noticeable around the third decade of life. There are no present age restrictions for face-lifting, but it should be considered when establishing a treatment plan for patients older than 40 years.

Rhytidectomy is elective, and thus each patient must be analyzed and evaluated with regard to the risks versus benefits associated with

the procedure. Many common medical conditions may be relative contraindications if they are poorly controlled, including diabetes, hypertension, chronic obstructive pulmonary disease, collagen vascular disease, and bleeding dyscrasias.

Some surgeons regard smoking as an absolute contraindication, yet most strongly advise patients to stop smoking at least 3 weeks

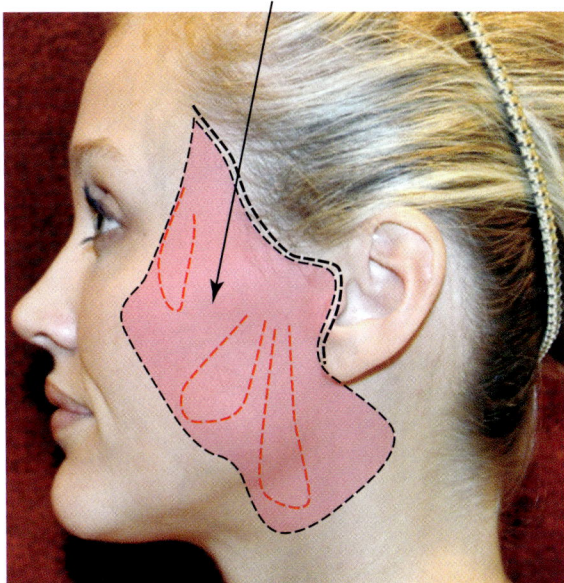

Area of subcutaneous
undermining

Fig. 107-17 ▪ Minimal-access cranial suspension (MACS) lift. Advantages include great access to the mid-face and jowls, no postauricular incisions, and no elevation of the temporal tuft. Disadvantages include a slightly longer operating time and potentially visible scars.

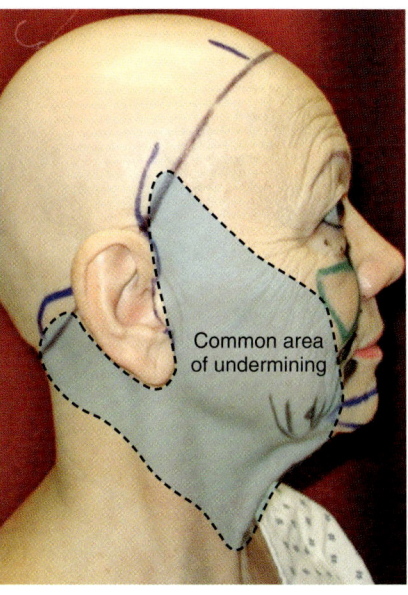

Common area
of undermining

Fig. 107-18 ▪ Typical areas of improvement or lack of improvement with a "classic" lower face-lift and neck lift. The average area of dissection shown limits how much improvement can be achieved in the perioral area beyond the jowls and neck. The improvement attained with a basic lower face-lift and neck lift is good for the jowls/jaw lines, good for the submental area and neck, fair for malar ptosis, poor for the nasolabial area, poor for marionette lines, and none for the lip lines.

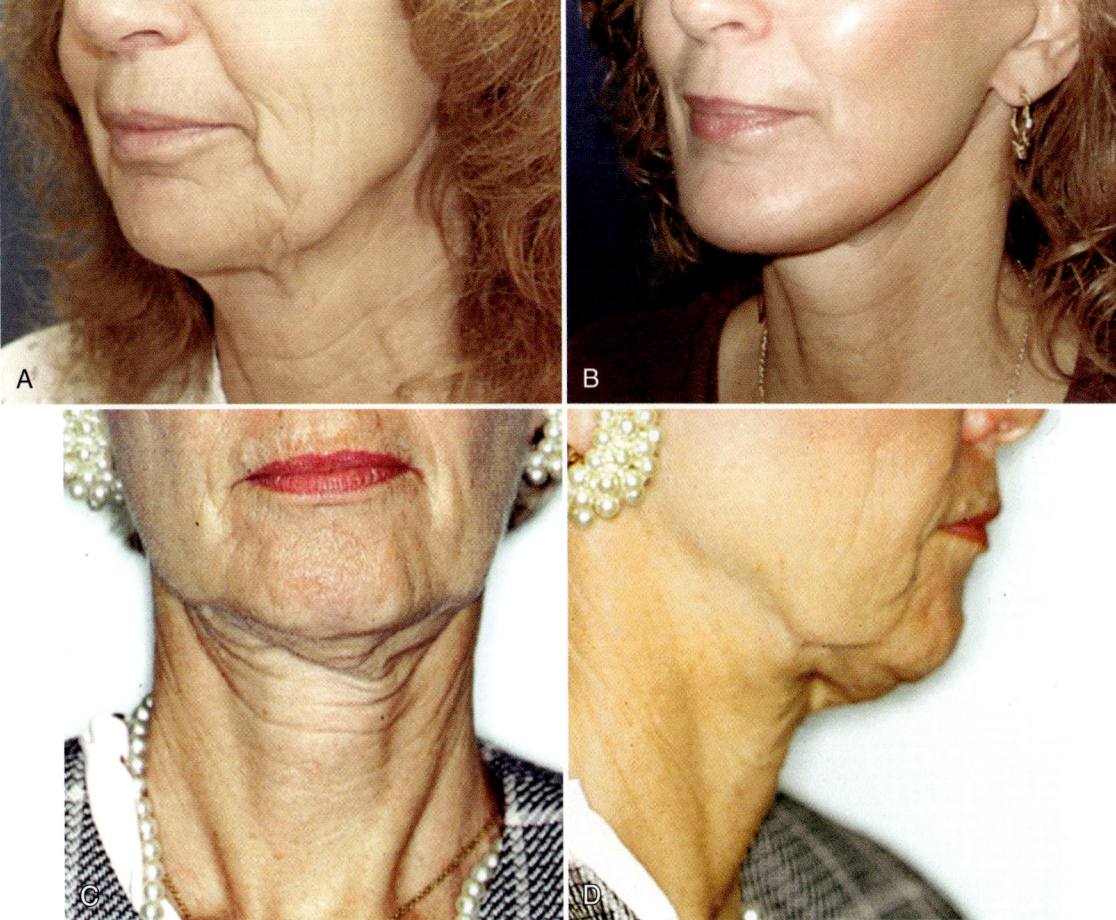

Fig. 107-19 ▪ "Ideal" necks shown in preoperative views and 1 year following a basic lower face-lift and chin implant. **A** and **B,** Fifty-seven-year-old woman preoperatively (**A**) and postoperatively (**B**). **C-F,** Fifty-five-year-old woman preoperatively (**C** and **D**) and postoperatively (**E** and **F**).

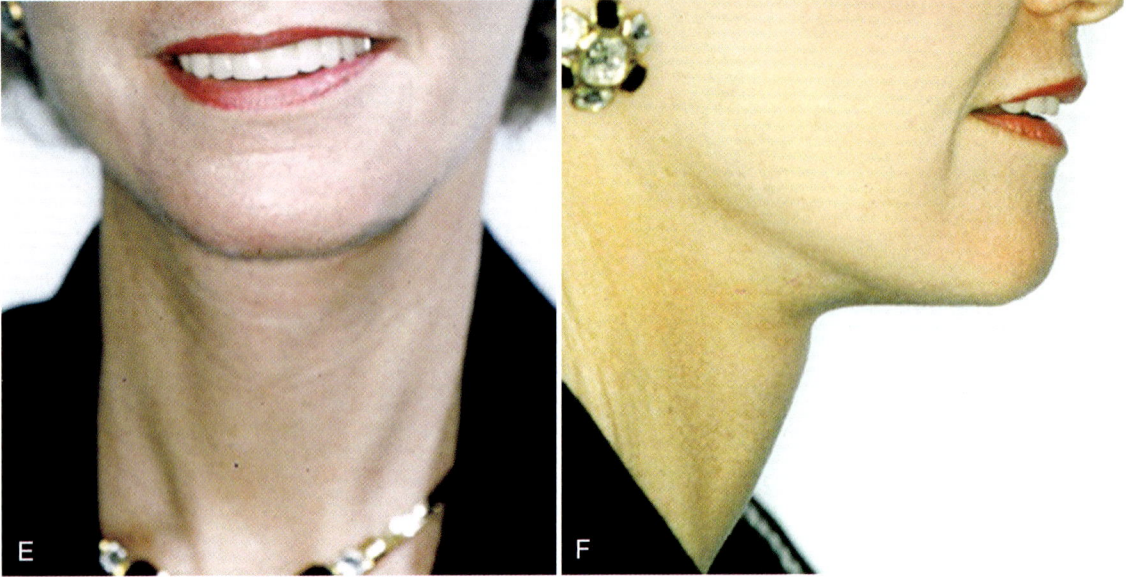

Fig. 107-19, cont'd.

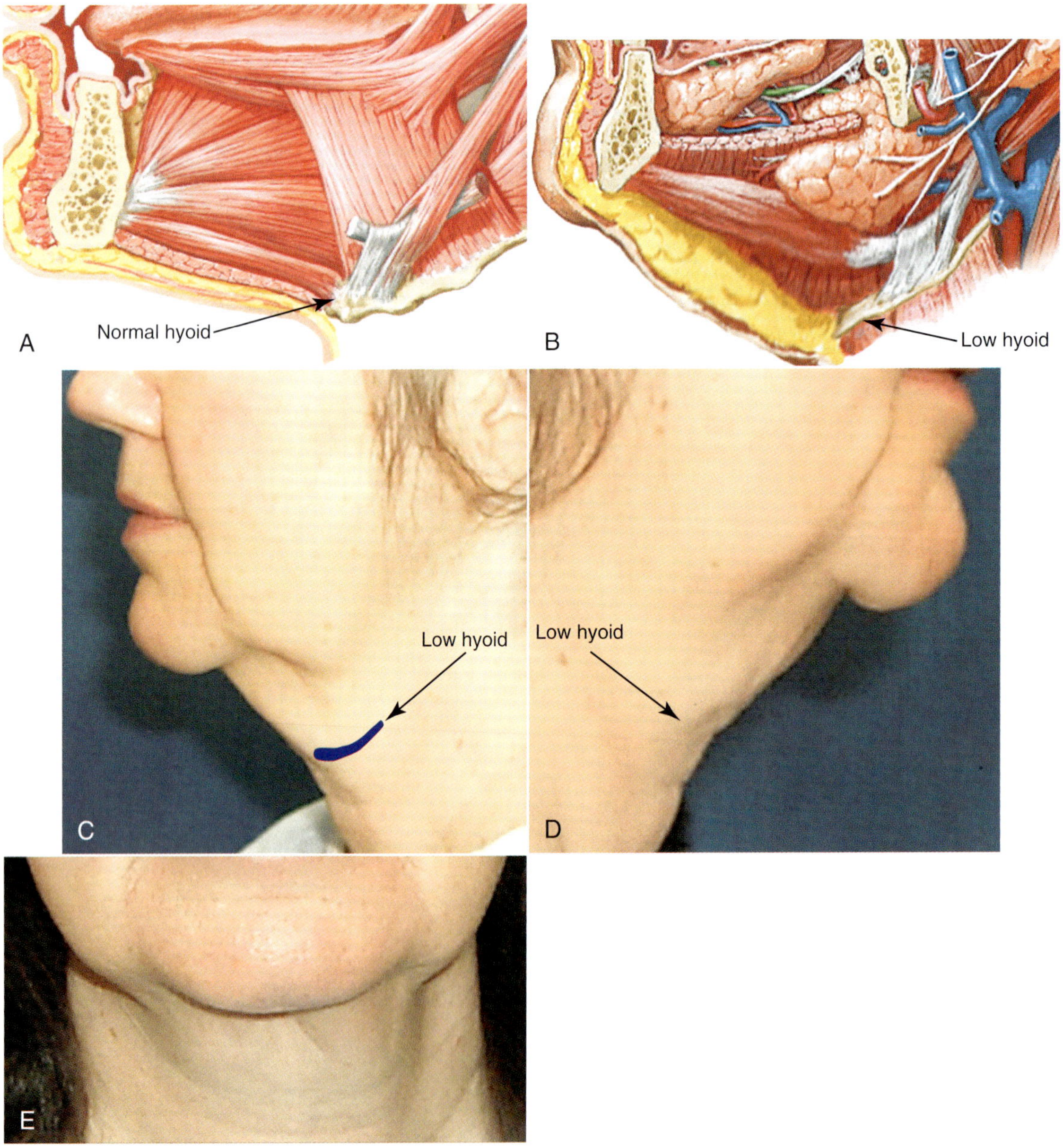

A Normal hyoid

B Low hyoid

C Low hyoid

D Low hyoid

E

Fig. 107-20 ▪ Hypertrophic digastric muscles and a low hyoid position are the two most difficult anatomic variants to improve during face-lifting. These variants often go unnoticed until after a face-lift. It is critical to inform patients of the limitations of treatment.

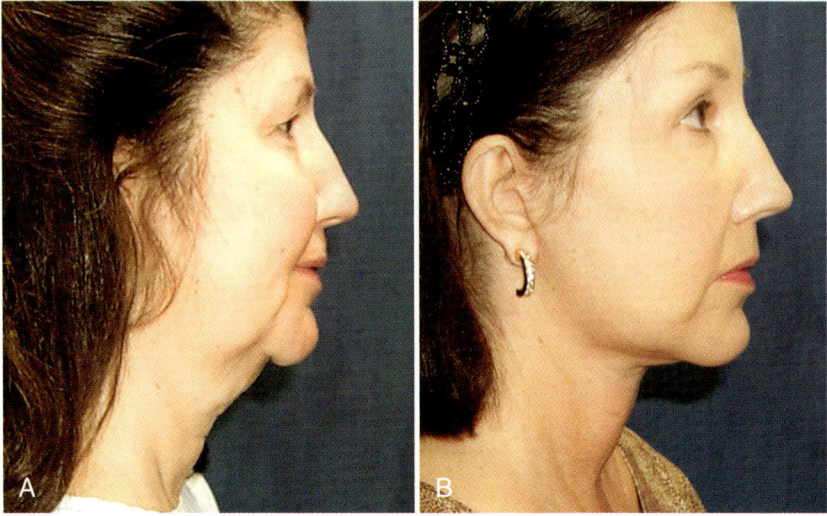

Fig. 107-21 ■ Low hyoid position and digastric hypertrophy. **A,** Fifty-two-year-old before a face-lift and submentoplasty with excision of deep fat, minor reduction of the digastric muscle, platysmal back cuts with undermining, and anterior plication. **B,** Six months postoperatively.

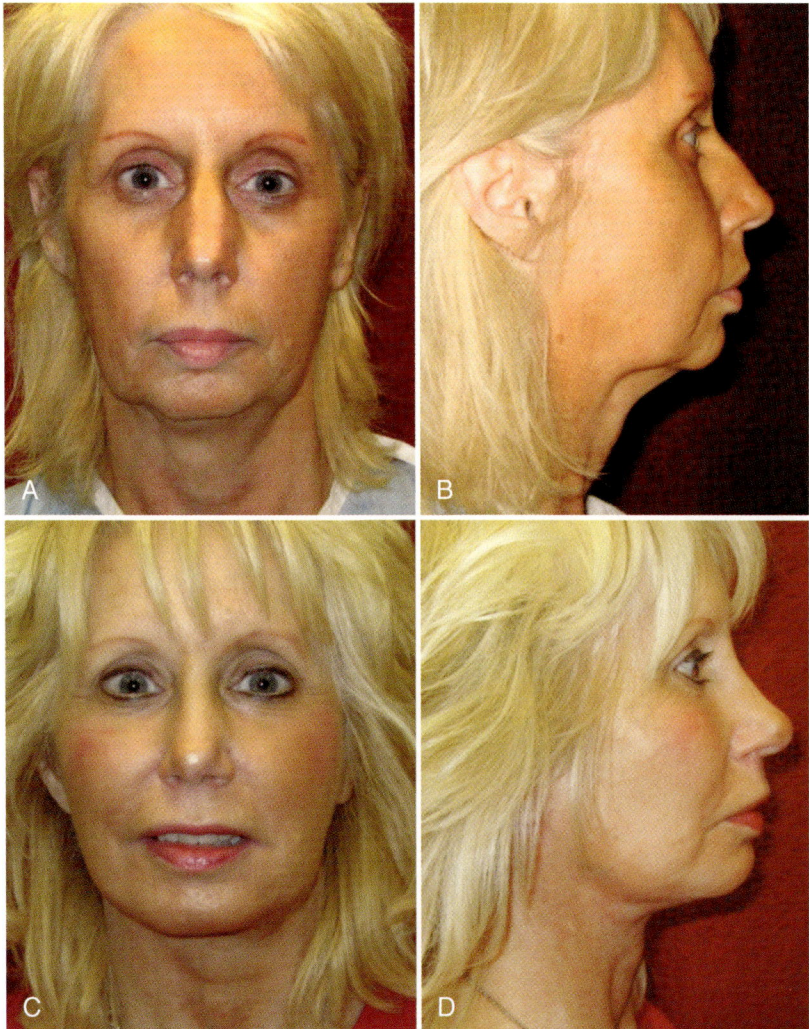

Fig. 107-22 ■ Frontal (**A**) and side (**B**) views before surgery. Frontal (**C**) and side (**D**) views 6 months after a face-lift, submentoplasty, fat grafting, rhinoplasty, and a chin implant in a patient with poor hyoid position because of severe mandibular hypoplasia. Orthognathic surgery was an option but not desired by the patient; therefore, total correction of problems in the lower facial third is limited.

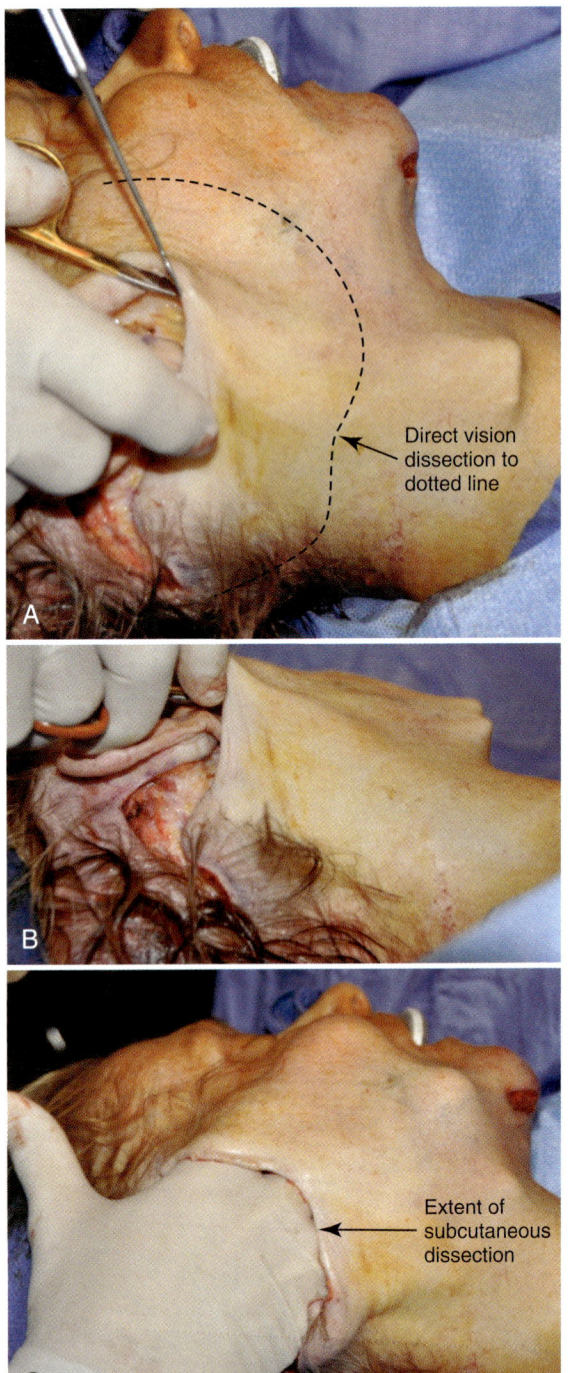

Fig. 107-23 ■ The extent of dissection is variable among surgeons. Dissection (*dashed line* in **A**) can easily be performed under direct vision for the first 5 cm from the ear. When undermining in the occipital region, dissection is kept as deep as possible but over the sternocleidomastoid muscle and its investing fascia. Blind dissection is more likely to injure the great auricular nerve or external jugular vein.

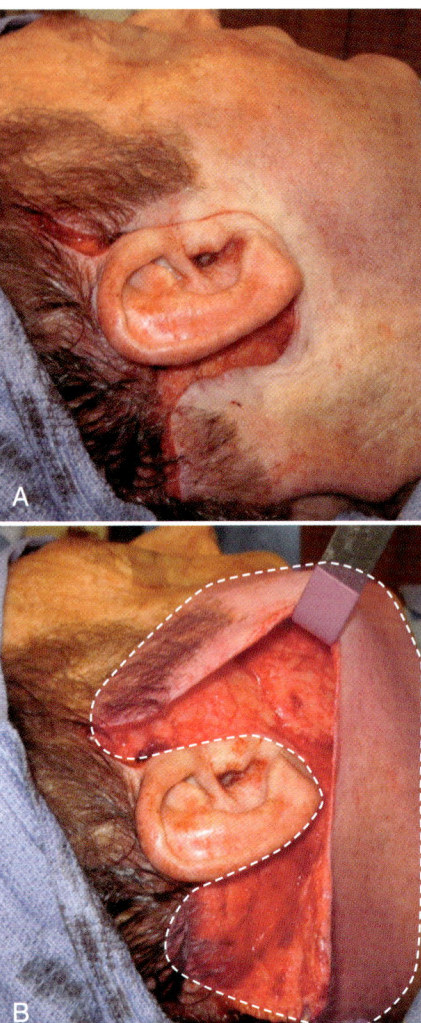

Fig. 107-24 ■ The typical male face-lift incision shown can be hidden in the hair at each end but is usually placed in front of the tragus (pretragal) to avoid pulling hair-bearing skin onto the ear. Deep tissue elevation can be performed once the entire subcutaneous flap is elevated. **A,** Standard male face-lift incisions. **B,** The extent of undermining is variable.

before surgery and for an additional 3 weeks afterward. The reported skin slough rate is as high as 13 times greater in smokers than in non-smoking patients after face-lifts.[12] If surgery is to be performed on a smoking patient, a modest short-flap "mini–face-lift" can be done to reduce the risk for skin necrosis, or a subperiosteal lift can also be performed.

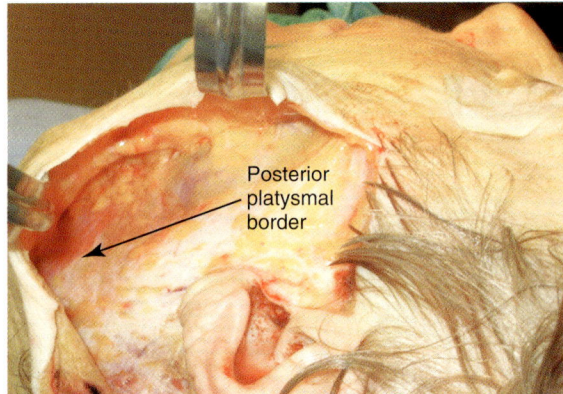

Fig. 107-25 ■ A lengthy subcutaneous face-lift flap is elevated to view the posterior platysmal border. The edge of the posterior platysma is a common location for suture elevation with or without deep plane elevation.

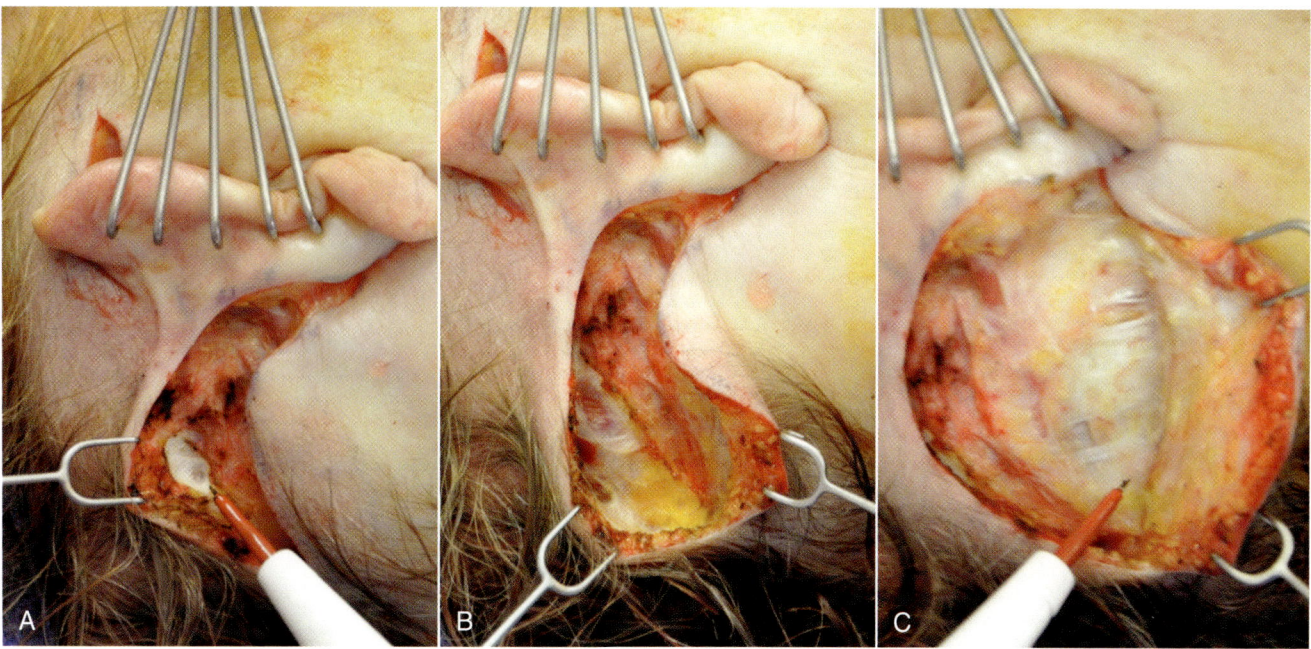

Fig. 107-26 ■ A, Minor superior undermining in the occipital region helps in redraping the tissue during closure to match up the posterior hairline. **B** and **C,** Dissection is kept as deep as possible over the sternocleidomastoid muscle and its investing fascia.

Indications for face-lift surgery in the majority of patients relate to aging of the lower part of the face and neck (Fig. 107-27). Cutis laxa of the jowls and cervical area is usually the most common complaint. It should also be noted that face-lifts may not improve the nasolabial folds. This particular problem does not require the ability to perform every face-lifting technique proficiently. In fact, most leading cosmetic surgeons use one particular technique for the majority of their face-lifts.[13] Repetition usually breeds confidence and expertise. The key is understanding the indications for and limitations of a technique and explaining them to the patient.

PATIENT PREPARATION

As with any surgical procedure, informed consent and adequate documentation must be obtained before proceeding. Ideally, the written consent form is reviewed by the patient well in advance of the day of surgery.

Based on the patient's medical history, certain laboratory tests may be required. A 12-lead electrocardiogram, urinalysis, and hematocrit are indicated for all patients older than 40 years. The decision to order other advanced testing such as electrolytes, prothrombin time, partial thromboplastin time, or chest radiography depends on the findings obtained from a detailed history and physical examination.

Patients should be warned to avoid aspirin and non-steroidal anti-inflammatory drugs. Vitamin E should also be stopped 2 weeks before surgery to minimize platelet dysfunction and unwanted bleeding.

Most patients do not realize that instructions to take nothing by mouth should not prevent them from taking their regular morning blood pressure medications with a sip of water. Patients with no history of hypertension but with borderline blood pressure preoperatively may benefit from clonidine preoperatively. A small dose of clonidine before surgery has been shown to stabilize intraoperative and postoperative blood pressure, thereby decreasing the risk for hemorrhage.[14]

Other preoperative measures include thorough washing of the hair and face with germicidal soap by the patient on the morning of surgery. Certain patients may benefit from preoperative sedation with a mild benzodiazepine the night before and the morning of surgery.

The patient should have the incision site marked and the hair taped, shaved, or braided before being transported to the operating room. Following sedation or general anesthesia, paper tape is wrapped around the patient's hair and head immediately posterior to the incision sites in the temporal and mastoid regions. The hair anterior to the temporal incision site may be twisted together and held with a rubber band or paper tape. With incisions planned entirely in front of the hairline, no hair need be shaved. Using paper tape to wrap the patient's hair can be extremely helpful in avoiding the nuisance of loose hair while attempting to suture. K-Y jelly or Polysporin ointment is helpful during surgery if the hair begins to creep into the wounds.

A light alcohol or povidone-iodine (Betadine) preparation is recommended just before infiltration of local anesthetic. During skin preparation, the patient can receive 1 g of cefazolin and 8 mg of dexamethasone (Decadron) intravenously. Because it takes 15 minutes to achieve the maximal benefit of local vasoconstriction, it may be done before the surgeon scrubs and drapes.

ANESTHESIA

Face-lifting may be performed with various anesthetic techniques. Because of the length of surgery, intravenous sedation with longer-acting medications such as diazepam (Valium) rather than midazolam (Versed) is advocated. However, the use of midazolam combined with fentanyl and a continuous propofol infusion drip works well.

Regardless of the type of sedation or general anesthetic used, the key to successful and smooth surgery is effective local anesthesia.

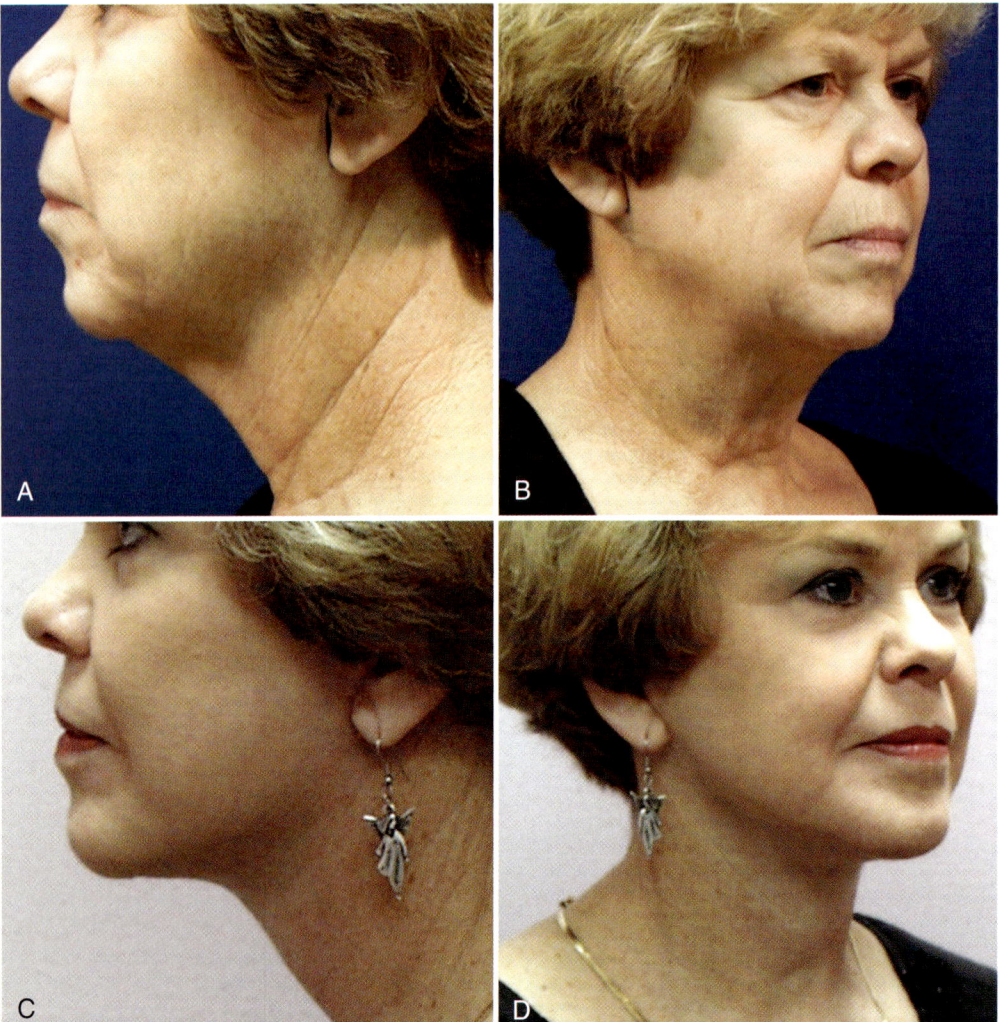

Fig. 107-27 ■ **A** and **B,** This patient exhibits the classic anatomy for which a lower face-lift and neck lift would be cosmetically beneficial. Major sagging in the jowls and neck usually requires a face-lift for correction. **C** and **D,** Eighteen months after surgery. The patient had additional age-related issues that were simultaneously corrected with other procedures: endoscopic forehead and brow lift, face-lift/neck lift, submentoplasty and minor liposuction, upper and lower blepharoplasties, full-face laser skin resurfacing, chin implant, and injection of botulinum toxin.

Adequate local infiltration into the subdermal plexus and subcutaneous tissue provides the necessary vasoconstriction for proper surgical technique. Regional nerve blocks are also helpful when using intravenous sedation to improve pain control.

The local anesthetic used may vary. Tumescent or standard bottle solutions can be used. One tumescent solution that works particularly well is a combination consisting of 50 mL of 2% lidocaine and 0.5 mL of 1 : 1000 epinephrine mixed in 250 mL of normal saline. This yields a solution consisting of 0.4% lidocaine and 1 : 500,000 epinephrine. Typically, the entire 250 mL is infiltrated throughout the patient's face and neck as needed. The injection is easily performed with a 20- or 22-gauge spinal needle connected to an auto-refilling syringe or an automatic pump. A standard syringe and needle can work well, but it takes much more time to inject the entire amount.

A non-tumescent technique that typically uses less than 50 mL of an anesthetic solution injected via standard needles on 10-mL syringes is a combination of 1% lidocaine with 1 : 100,000 epinephrine mixed evenly with 0.5% bupivacaine (Marcaine) with 1 : 200,000 epinephrine. The resulting epinephrine concentration is 1 : 150,000,

and the concentration of lidocaine is decreased to 0.5% in an attempt to avoid toxicity because of the significant volume of anesthetic needed to infiltrate the entire face and neck. Bupivacaine has its own toxic properties but allows adequate working time when the patient is not under general anesthesia. Bupivacaine is injected at a concentration of 0.25%, which must be kept in mind because of its relationship to the total dosing volume.

Fortunately, even with the larger volumes of anesthetic solution required, complications related to local anesthesia are rare. It cannot be overstated how critical the local anesthetic is for proper face-lift technique. Inadequate infiltration increases surgical time and complications and can also devastate a surgical treatment plan.

SPECIFIC TREATMENT AND TECHNIQUES

SUBMENTOPLASTY

Even though we believe that submentoplasty is almost always a necessity if simultaneously performing a face-lift, it is not necessarily performed by many face-lift surgeons (Fig. 107-28). There are

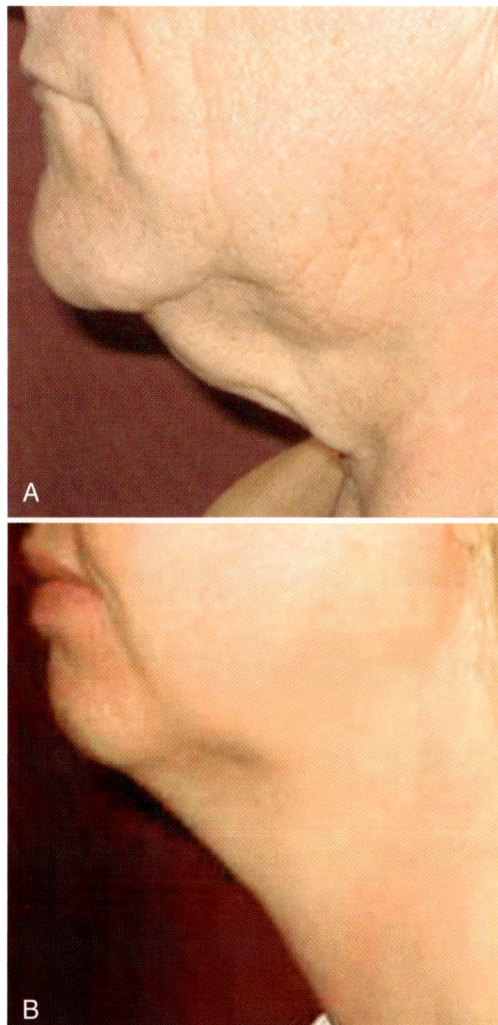

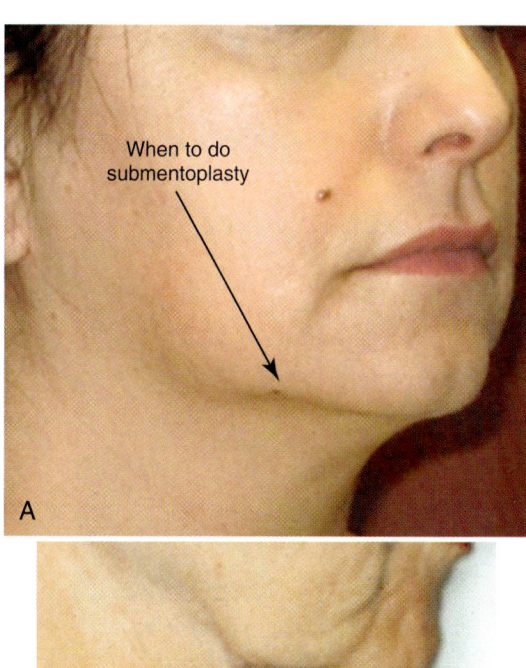

When to do
submentoplasty

A

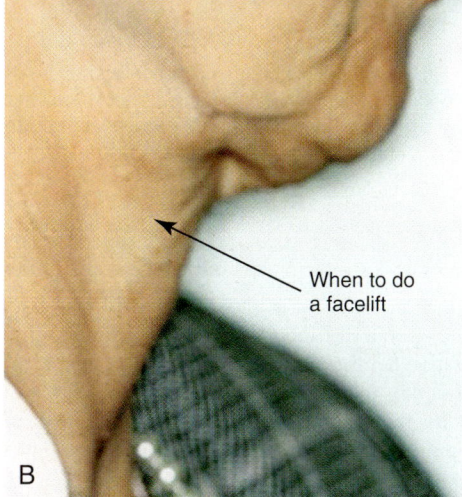

When to do
a facelift

B

Fig. 107-28 ■ There are two main reasons why submentoplasty is used in cosmetic surgery: (1) to *enhance face-lift* results in patients with major submental problems (shown in part **A**) and (2) as an *isolated* procedure in patients with adequate skin tone who need more than liposuction but require no lifting of the jowls (shown in part **B**).

Fig. 107-29 ■ Two patients demonstrate the two main reasons why submentoplasty may be selected as a cosmetic procedure. **A,** Submentoplasty candidate—platysmal banding, mild skin laxity at most, large volume of subplatysmal fat, as part of a standard face-lift, and hypertrophic submandibular glands. **B,** Facelift candidate—jowling and significant skin laxity.

two prevalent reasons for not performing submentoplasty simultaneously with a face-lift. First, some believe that it is not worth the time because the posterior SMAS pull improves the anterior neck tissues alone. Of course, this may be true for some necks initially, but it inevitably leads to relapse of tissue laxity in the anterior aspect of the neck 4 to 6 months following the face-lift. The indications for performing submentoplasty are based on the amount of deep platysmal fat present, the amount of platysmal laxity, the quality of the skin, and the desires of the patient (Figs. 107-29 to 107-33).

Second, midline platysmal plication may compromise some of the elevation that a surgeon could otherwise obtain in the jowl region because the anterior pull is partially competing with the SMAS elevation from the face-lift. This may be partially true when using a short-flap technique but is not an issue with a combined long-flap face-lift and submentoplasty technique. The goal of any cosmetic rejuvenation procedure is a more youthful appearance that is both natural and long-lasting. Combining anterior platysmaplasty with a face-lift is usually necessary to achieve the latter.

When doing a platysmaplasty, we do not perform liposuction first because we believe that it is essential to maintain an even thickness

of superficial fat attached to the dermis (Figs. 107-34 to 107-36). Thus, when the skin is redraped, there is less chance of an uneven appearance and skin rippling. Face-lift scissors are used to undermine the skin while leaving an even layer of subdermal fat (Figs. 107-37 and 107-38). The dissection is carried inferiorly as far as the lower border of the thyroid cartilage and laterally to the posterior border of the mandible. Wide skin undermining is necessary to allow proper skin redraping after treatment of the deep tissues has been addressed. Inadequate skin undermining will inevitably lead to bunching after midline plication of the platysma. If skin elasticity is deemed to be inadequate during the preoperative visit, a face-lift combined with a submentoplasty is usually required (Fig. 107-39).

A flat spatulated cannula can then be used to perform liposuction on the fat overlying the platysma under direct vision. A lighted Aufricht retractor improves visualization through the small submental incision. Any excess submental fat is then resected. A Kelly clamp or large hemostat is placed in the midline to hold the platysma and fat while a needle-tipped cautery or scissors is used to resect it. It is at this point that the anterior jugular veins may be encountered.

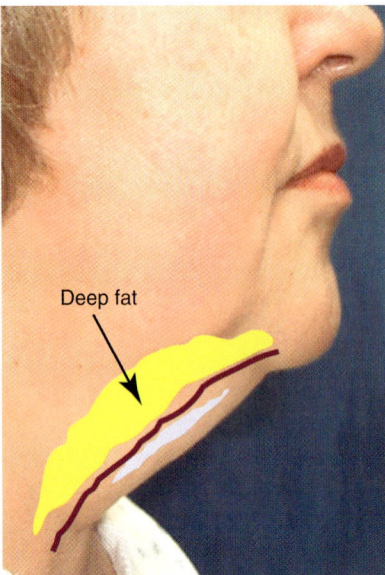

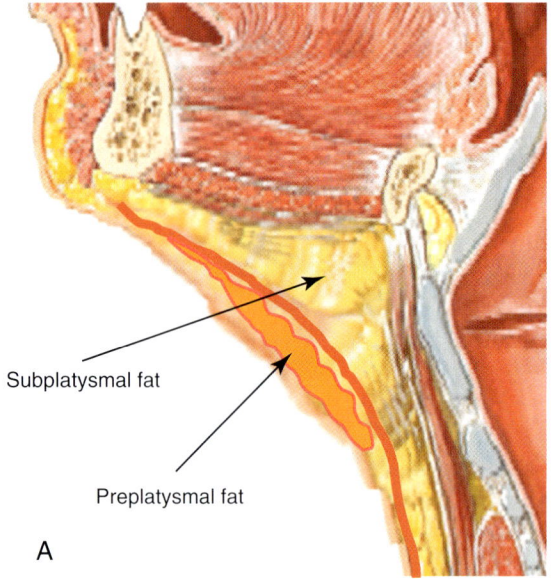

Fig. 107-30 ■ Difficult neck anatomy. Submentoplasty is often required during a face-lift in patients with challenging necks such as those with the following problems: heavy (thick) necks, poor muscle tone, low hyoid, ptotic or large glands, weak chin, digastric hypertrophy, and poor jaw structure.

Proper hemostasis must be achieved or it will be very difficult to complete the operation properly and there will be a greater chance of postoperative hematoma.

After resecting the midline fat, the anterior borders of the platysma and the hyoid bone are identified. The platysma is then backcut beginning at the level of the hyoid bone (Figs. 107-40 to 107-44). The backcut is carried an average of 5 to 7 cm and stays parallel to the inferior border of the mandible and well below the inferior extent of the submandibular gland. When making this incision through the platysma, care should be taken to not injure the facial vessels or nerve. The platysma is undermined superior to the backcut area. If submandibular gland ptosis or gland enlargement is recognized, we often manage this problem by resecting the superficial portion of the gland with the needle-tipped cautery. This procedure is difficult to perform and is not recommended for novice surgeons (Figs. 107-45 to 107-49). Bleeding can be encountered, which is often difficult to control because of such a small incision and poor access.

After mobilizing the platysma bilaterally, a corset platysmaplasty is then performed. We use running 2-0 Vicryl suture to accomplish this. The inferior platysmal edges are plicated at the midline to the fascia over the hyoid bone. If a chin implant is to be used to camouflage a poor cervicomental angle related to a low hyoid position, it is placed at this time. Dissection is carried to the periosteum of the mandible in the midline. A subperiosteal pocket is then created at the lower border of the mandible, and a solid silicone implant is placed into the pocket. It is secured to the periosteum of the inferior border of the mandible with a single 4-0 Vicryl suture. After ensuring strict hemostasis, the skin is closed with 4-0 Monocryl deep and 5-0 plain gut suture on the skin.

CHIN ENHANCEMENT

Left untreated, microgenia can make a good face-lift appear unfinished. When a patient has a weak chin, horizontal neck length is less than ideal and neck appearance is somewhat more obtuse in shape

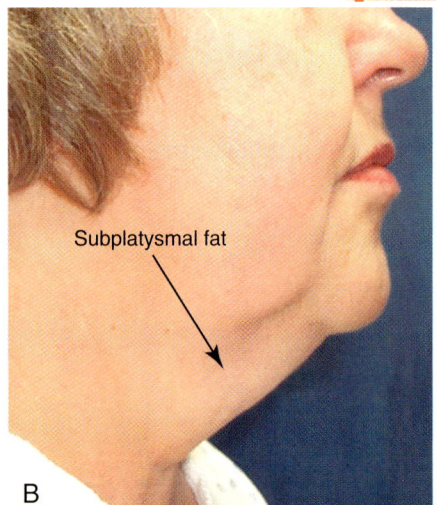

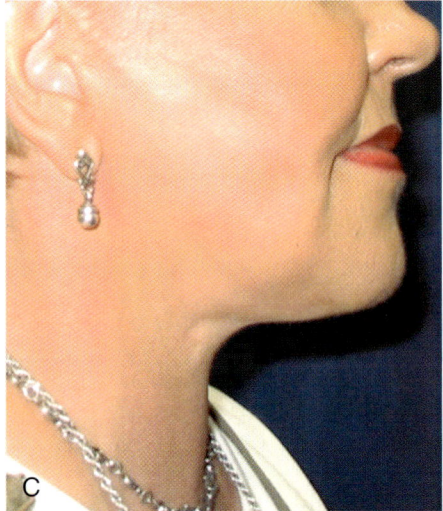

Fig. 107-31 ■ "Heavy" necks often require face-lifting with associated aggressive subplatysmal fat excision: removal of fat above and below the platysmal muscle and open jowl and neck liposuction. Adequate fat should be left on the skin to allow aggressive deep fat removal via submentoplasty. The patient should be warned of the limitations of the procedure. A diet/weight loss is recommended before and after surgery. **A,** Preplatysmal and subplatysmal fat. **B,** Subplatysmal fat on a patient before surgery. **C,** Appearance 1½ years after a face-lift with aggressive submentoplasty.

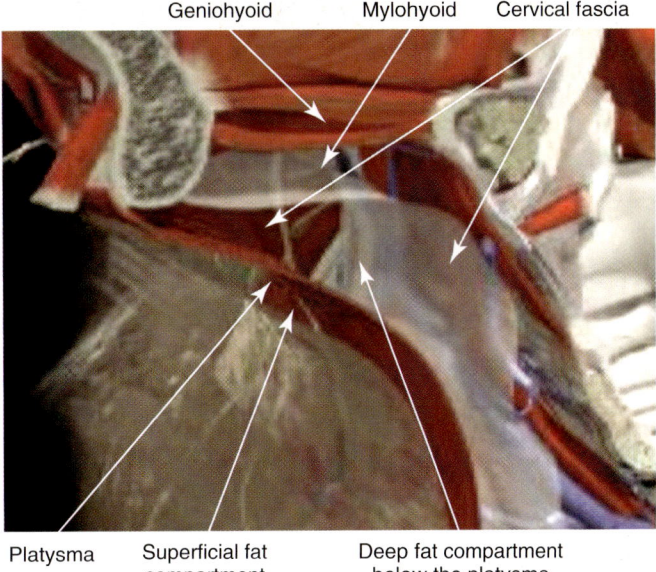

Genioglossus   Mylohyoid   Cervical fascia

Platysma   Superficial fat   Deep fat compartment
            compartment   below the platysma

Fig. 107-32 ▪ Slightly heavy or "obtuse" chin-neck angle in which the majority of neck fat is stored in the "subplatysmal" compartment. Heavy patients or those with a genetic predisposition for a poor chin-neck angle also have a high percentage of deep fat that must be directly excised. Liposuction alone significantly treats only the fat *above* the platysma.

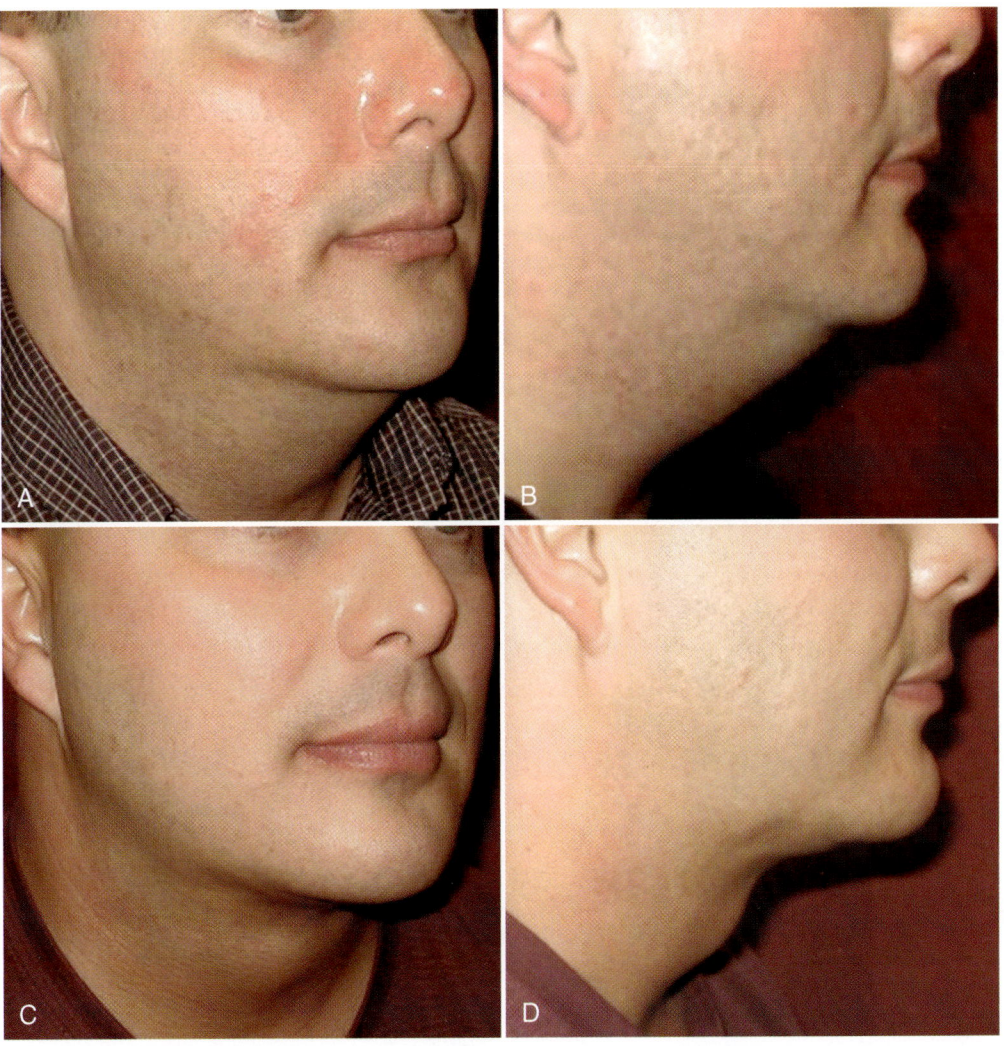

Fig. 107-33 ▪ Multiple techniques are used by surgeons when performing face-lifts. Detailed knowledge of surgical facial anatomy is key to any cosmetic surgery regardless of the techniques used. This 37-year-old man was treated successfully with submentoplasty alone because of preoperative assessment of deep subplatysmal fat but excellent skin tone. **A** and **B,** Before surgery. **C** and **D,** Four months postoperatively following isolated submentoplasty.

versus the nearly 90-degree shape seen during youth. Adding a silicone chin implant through a submental incision during a submentoplasty or face-lift can dramatically improve the overall results and is a relatively simple procedure (Figs. 107-50 to 107-54). In addition to improving neck length, new "anatomically" shaped chin implants improve the deepened prejowl sulcus that commonly develops with age (Figs. 107-55 and 107-56). The jaw line as well as neck length are improved with appropriately placed chin implants and can improve many face-lift results.

RHYTIDECTOMY INCISIONS

The temporal incision may extend directly superior from the preauricular sulcus incision, or it may be stepped around the anterior edge of the temporal tuft of hair. The latter is particularly useful if the temporal tuft is high, as in patients who have previously undergone face-lifts. The superior extent curves slightly anteriorly but stays well hidden in the thickest temporal hair. It also extends superiorly into the hair as far as necessary (usually 3 to 4 cm) to allow some degree of lifting of the mid-face region (Fig. 107-57). The hair incision should parallel the hair follicles, or the superior edge should be beveled so that hair growth will hide the resulting scar.

The continuous incision of the typical face-lift can be divided into three main portions: temporal, periauricular, and mastoid. For men, the incision is made in the preauricular sulcus anterior to the tragus to prevent hair growth over the tragus postoperatively. This same incision can be used in women, but most surgeons position the preauricular incision at the posterior edge of the tragus to further camouflage the scar.

Retroauricular or mastoid incisions may be placed in the hair-bearing scalp or immediately in front of the hairline. Either technique begins at the superior extent of the retroauricular sulcus incision at the level of the external auditory canal or at the point where the postauricular hair crosses the perimeter of the ear helix. The angle of skin incision should be approximately 90 degrees to avoid skin necrosis. Incisions in front of the mastoid hairline are simple and avoid postoperative changes in the hairline or hair loss but may leave a noticeable, widened scar if undue skin tension is present on closure. Fortunately, even short hairstyles will grow to cover this incision. When incisions are carried directly into the hair, the result is a well-hidden scar but also probably hair loss and difficulties in vectors of pull to reapproximate the hairline.

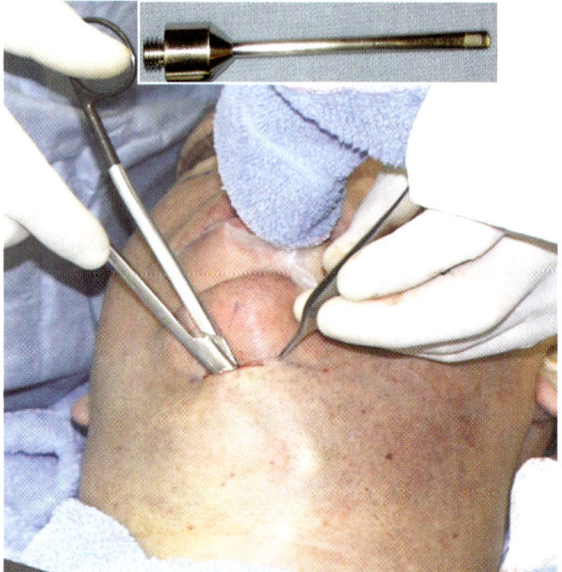

Fig. 107-34 ■ Platysmal manipulation of any kind requires wide access and meticulous wide submental flap elevation. A large 7-mm open spatula cannula (*inset photograph*) is used for liposuction only *after* skin elevation and is directed toward the platysma to clearly expose the platysmal muscle.

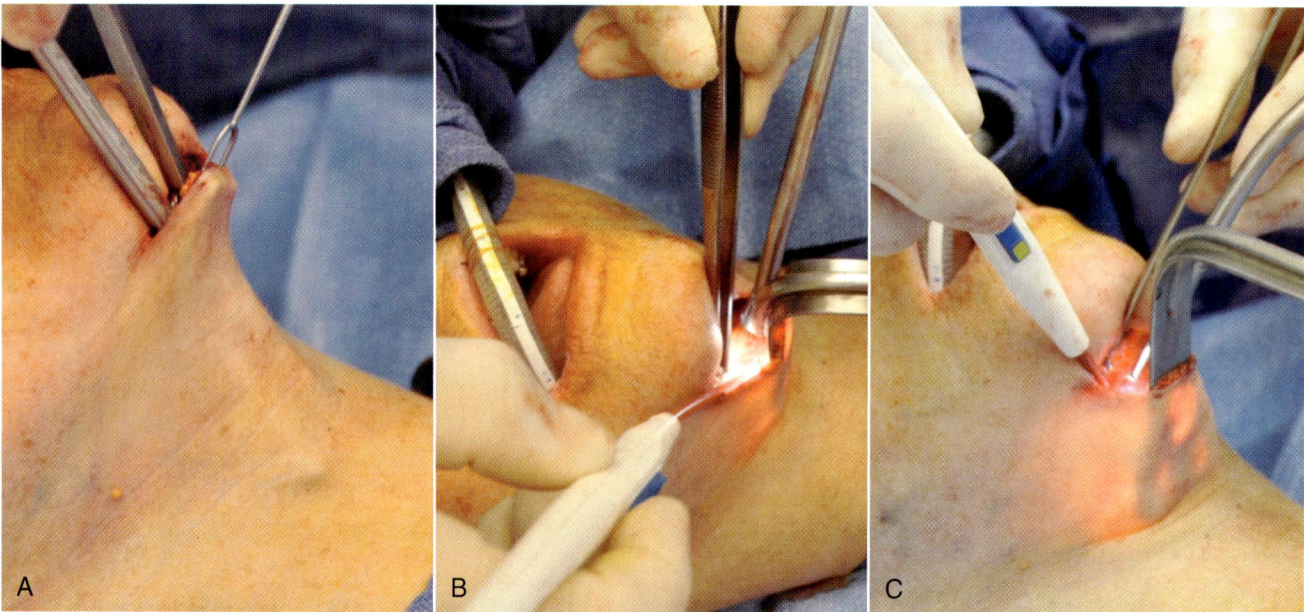

Fig. 107-35 ■ A submental skin flap is made through an incision in the submental crease (**A**) and elevated sharply with face-lift scissors. **B** and **C,** Lighted equipment and retraction required when working through a small opening. A fiberoptic "sweetheart"-type retractor and Yankauer suction are needed for performing submentoplasty.

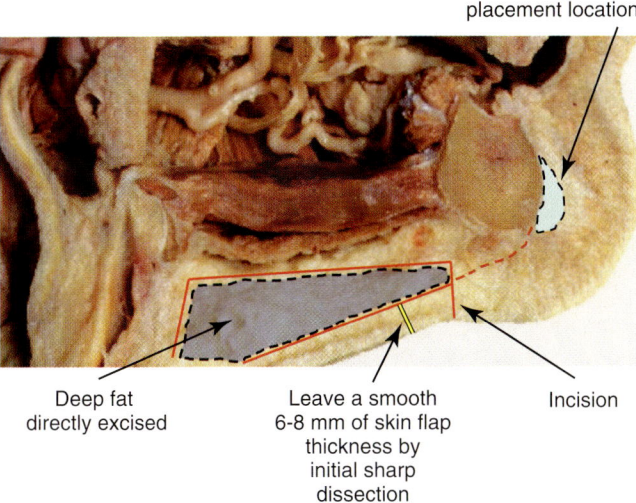

Chin implant
placement location

Deep fat
directly excised

Leave a smooth
6-8 mm of skin flap
thickness by
initial sharp
dissection

Incision

Fig. 107-36 ■ It is critical to maintain an even, healthy layer of fat on the skin surface when planning direct excision of deep fat. Platysmal plication, resection, or chin implant placement can be performed simultaneously. The red lines indicate the place where a smooth plane of dissection must be made to avoid irregularities or skin fibrosis. Damage or exposure to the dermis or deep muscle should be avoided if at all possible.

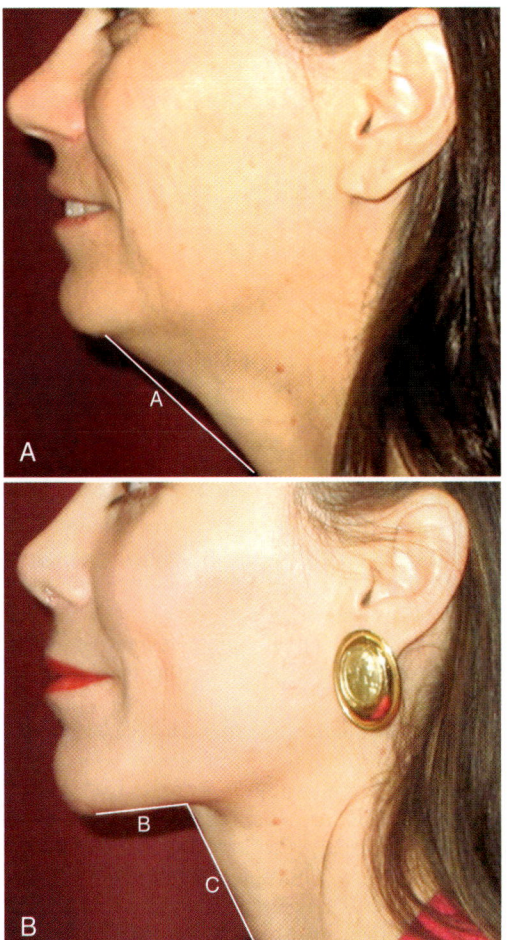

Fig. 107-37 ■ A < (B + C) = No skin excision if the patient has good skin elasticity. The patient is shown preoperatively (**A**) and 6 months following isolated submentoplasty (no face-lift) with partial platysmal resection and deep fat excision (**B**). A submentoplasty alone can be performed in patients *who have good skin tone* and minimal jowling because the excess skin is required for normal redraping over the increased deep surface area, as shown above.

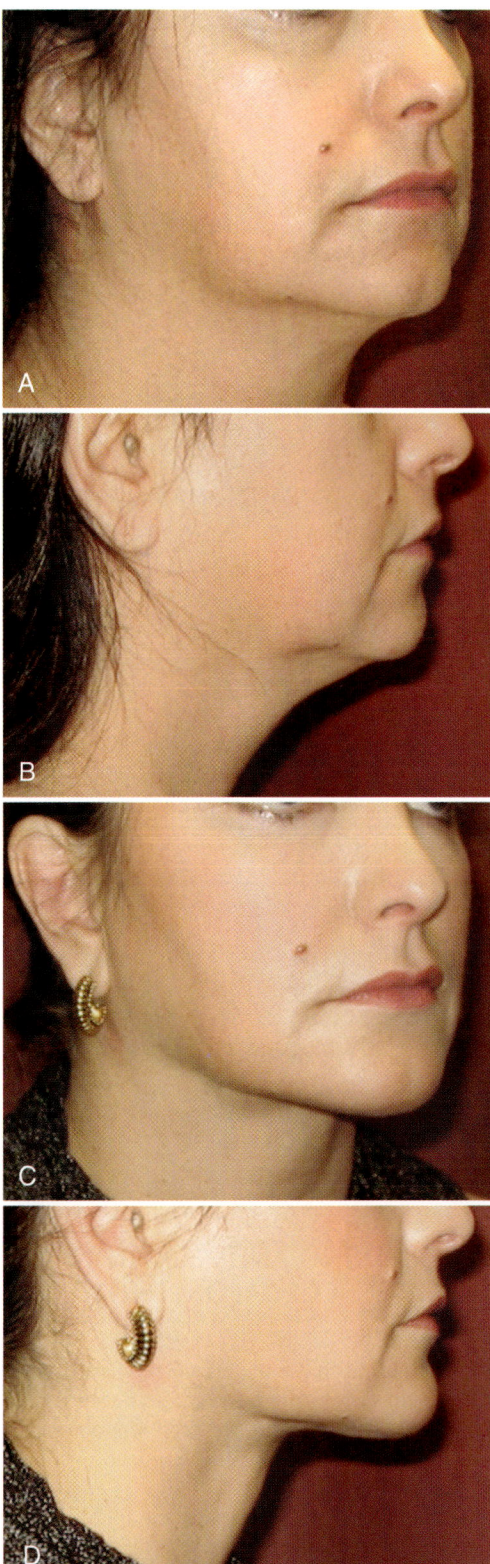

Fig. 107-38 ■ Isolated submentoplasty involving a platysmal backcut, undermining, and anterior plication technique. Minor irregularities can be seen in the submandibular triangle where skin retraction developed as a result of minor internal fibrosis and skeletonization. **A** and **B,** Before surgery. **C** and **D,** Two years after surgery.

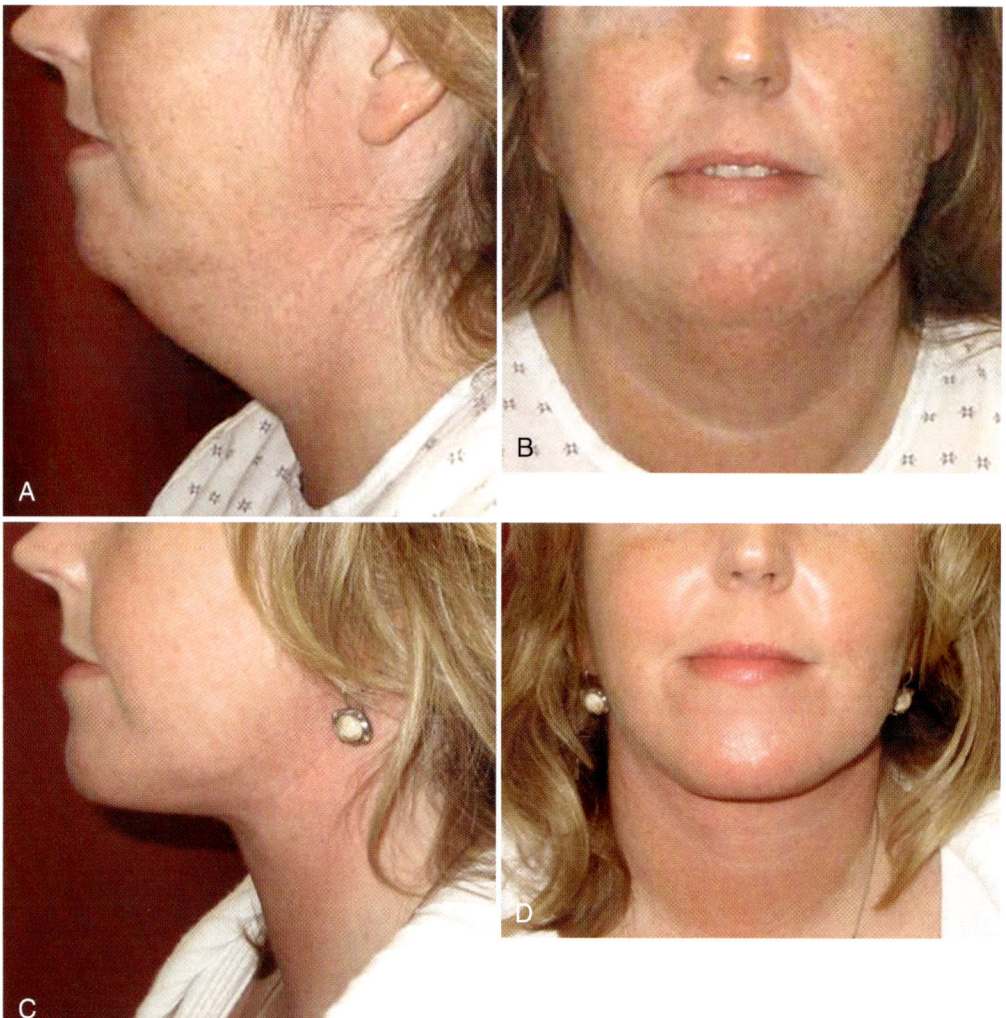

Fig. 107-39 ■ A submentoplasty involving a platysmal backcut, undermining, and anterior plication technique is shown, in addition to a face-lift and a small chin implant. A face-lift was performed in addition to submentoplasty because of the significant skin laxity remaining after major fat excision. **A** and **B,** Before surgery, note the very obtuse chin-neck angle. **C** and **D,** After surgery.

FLAP UNDERMINING AND PLICATION OF THE SUPERFICIAL MUSCULOAPONEUROTIC SYSTEM

The operative technique described is the common SMAS plication, or short-flap face-lift. Too many varieties of face-lifts exist today to describe each in detail. Third-generation or subperiosteal face-lifts constitute only a minority of the face-lifts being performed.[15] The technique chosen should be determined by the patient's diagnosis.

Even though variations of the incision for different face-lift techniques have just minor differences, the SMAS can be dealt with in quite different ways to achieve the required result. The SMAS can be elevated off the parotid fascia in the so-called deep-plane technique. Simple plication can be done as described in detail later versus the "double–purse-string" technique used by many facial cosmetic surgeons. Following subcutaneous flap elevation, several types of SMAS or deep tissue lifting techniques exist, including SMASectomy and imbrications (Figs. 107-58 and 107-59). Several other techniques can be found in the literature. In the following paragraphs we discuss our personal choice of technique and describe it in detail.

Undermining carried out from the incisions should be in the subcutaneous plane with approximately 4 to 5 mm of subcutaneous fat left attached to the skin flap to maintain adequate vascularity of the flap. Novice surgeons have a tendency to begin too thin. The short flap is usually close to 5 cm in length from the incisions but may vary if the patient's anatomy requires more or less release for optimal esthetics and safety. This means that the flap will stop short of the oral commissure by 2 cm. Eversion of the flap beyond the masseter does nothing but increase edema and dead space. Dissection is also limited near the lateral edge of the eye by stopping close to the edge of the orbicularis oculi.

The zygomatic eminence is another limiting landmark of dissection. The level of temporal dissection may be changed to the sub-temporoparietal fascial plane just on top of the glistening white temporalis fascia. Use of a deep plane above the zygomatic arch is necessary to avoid damage to the frontal nerve. Undermining in the mastoid region and hair-bearing area should be done below the hair follicles to minimize alopecia. Dissection inferior to the lobe of the ear must be done cautiously to stay superficial to the sternocleidomastoid fascia and platysmal muscles. During posterior undermining, one should remain immediately above the fascia of

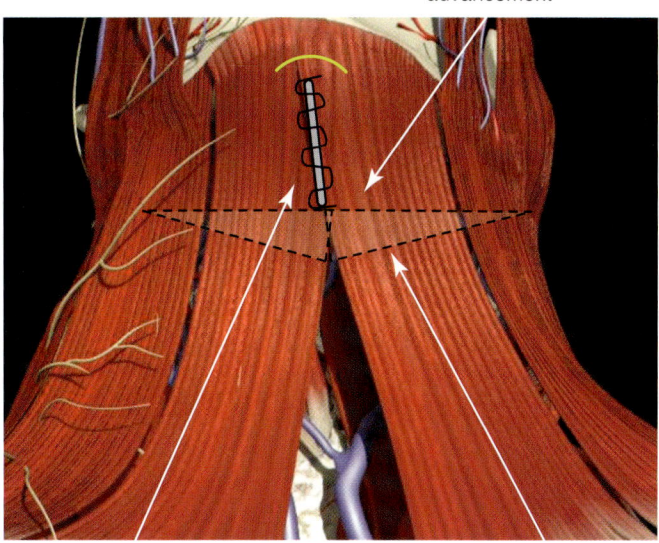

Platysmal flap advancement

Inferior and medial corner of each residual platysmal edge plicated together at the hyoid

Back cutting of platysma (optional)

Fig. 107-40 ■ Submentoplasty involving a platysmal backcut, undermining, and anterior plication technique. An anterior "corset" platysmaplasty is optional, as well as not using a backcut.

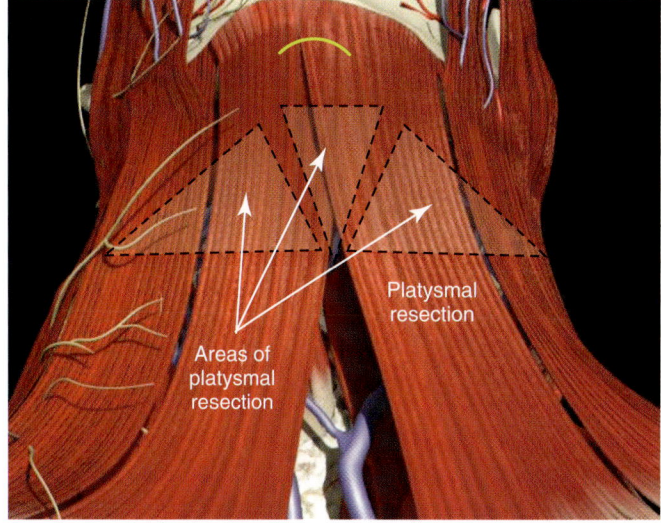

Areas of platysmal resection

Platysmal resection

Alternate treatment of platysma

Fig. 107-41 ■ Submentoplasty performed with a platysmal partial resection technique. Care must be taken to leave a smooth and uniform layer of fat attached to the skin surface if resecting the platysma.

the sternocleidomastoid to avoid injury to the great auricular nerve. Following subcutaneous flap elevation, a second layer (biplane flap) can be elevated over the parotid and below the cervical platysma (Figs. 107-60 and 107-61). The deep-plane flap typically extends horizontally at the arch and can be used to help elevate the malar fat pad. Elevation of a deep flap is more risky than simple plication but has much less chance of bunching or causing irregularities under the skin. A composite face-lift elevates a deep

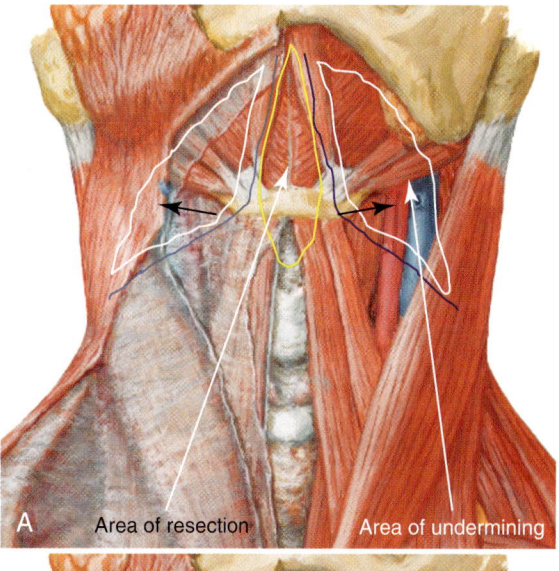

A Area of resection Area of undermining

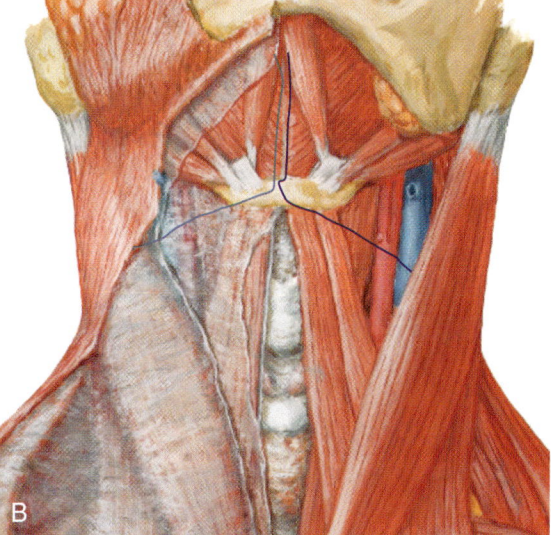

B

Anterior plication with 2-0 vicryl

Fig. 107-42 ■ Submentoplasty involving a platysmal backcut, undermining, and anterior plication technique. The plication is performed in the midline from the hyoid to the mandible.

flap off the parotid without performing extended subcutaneous elevation (Fig. 107-62). A composite lift provides the best blood supply to the skin since the deep tissue remains attached. This technique, however, is more challenging than the more traditional techniques.

The actual dissection can be facilitated by subdermal infiltration of anesthetic, as well as microcannular liposuction, which is done routinely from submental and infralobular punctures. This creates tunnels that make later sharp dissection easier. The final undermining is usually performed with "face-lift" scissors in pushing and cutting movements. Dissection is facilitated by countertraction on the flap with the use of skin hooks at the edge of the flap and distal tightening by the assistant. Bleeding should be controlled carefully during the process with cauterization. In addition, open suction-assisted lipectomy at this time over the parotid area defines the more fibrous portion of the SMAS needed for plication.

Plication, as described by Webster and colleagues, is the act of suturing fascial tissue folded over itself.[16] This differs from

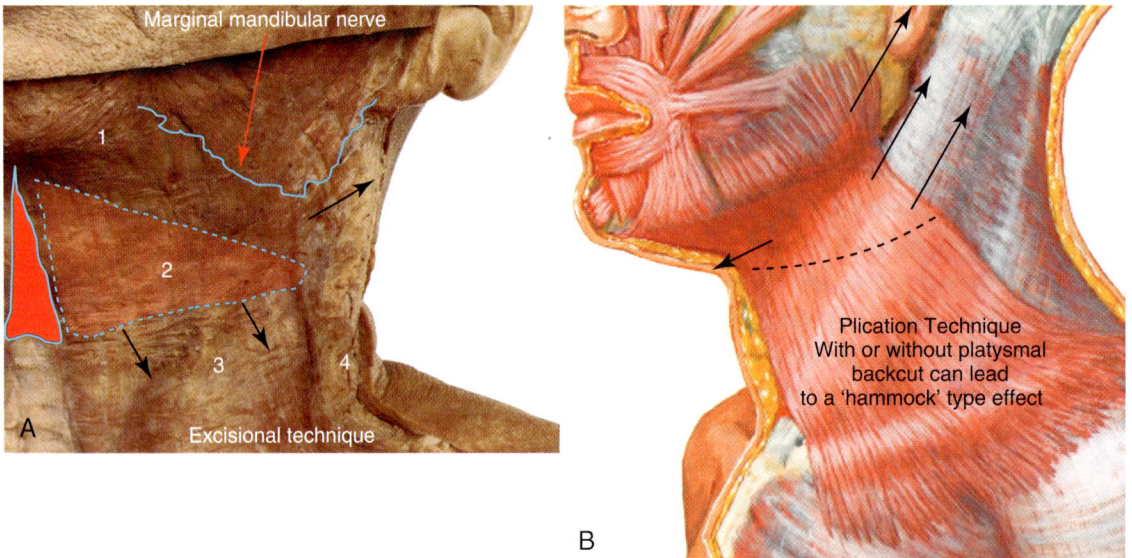

Fig. 107-43 ■ Dueling face-lift and anterior platysmal plication may compete, but some surgeons believe that it may also create a positive "hammock" effect on the neck.

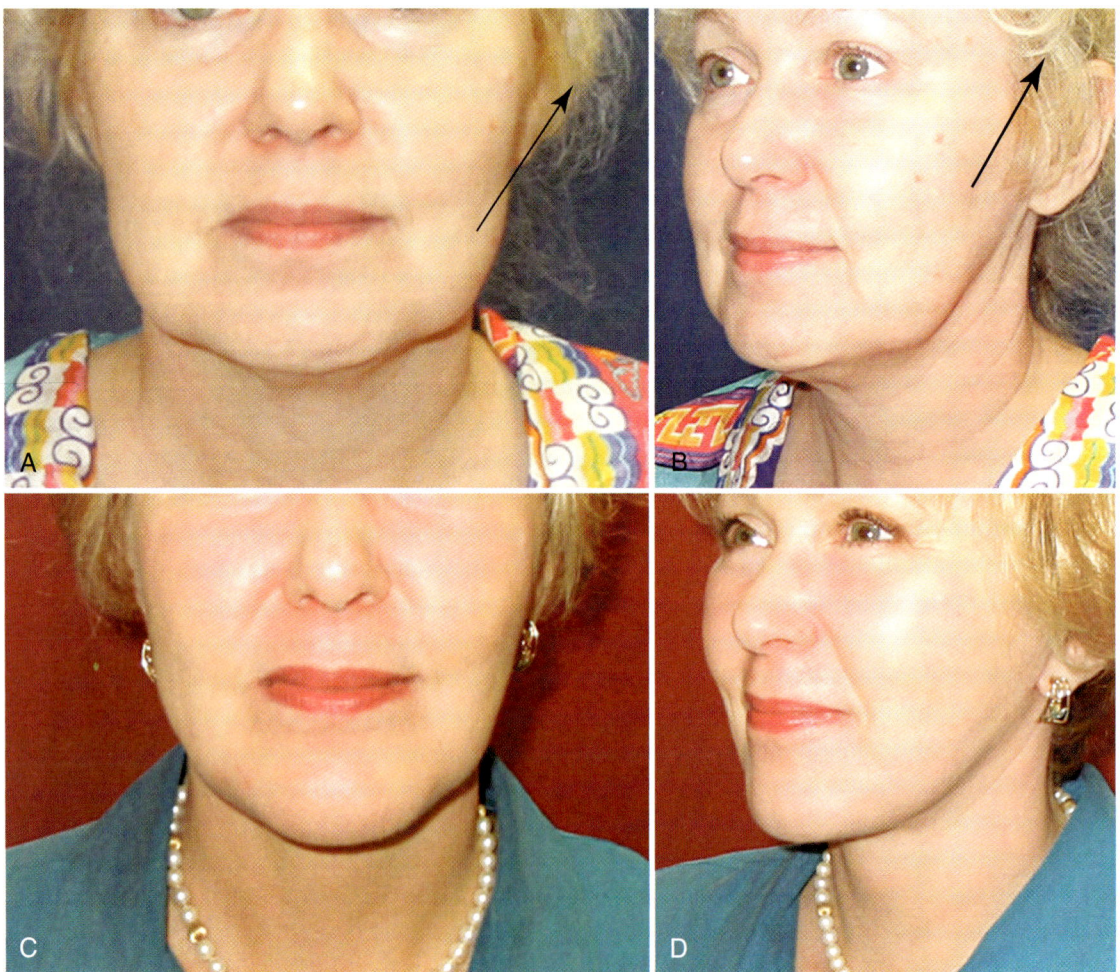

Fig. 107-44 ■ Platysmal backcut without plication. The 54-year-old patient shown underwent a face-lift to treat her "jowling" and a platysmal backcut only (no anterior plication) in the hope of achieving maximal posterior and superior lift of her jowls. **A** and **B,** Before surgery. **C** and **D,** Six months after surgery. The patient underwent a face-lift, submentoplasty/liposuction, chin implant, upper blepharoplasties, lower blepharoplasties, buccal fat pad excision, and periorbital laser resurfacing.

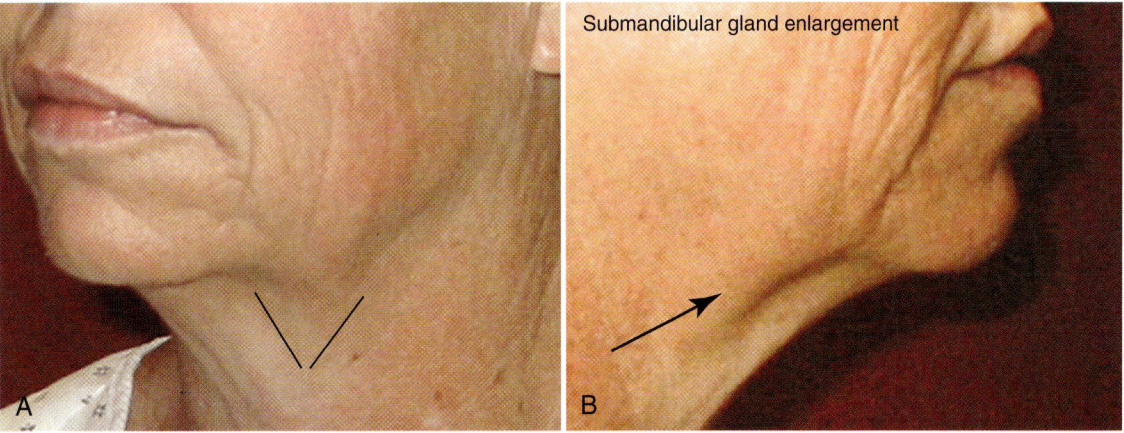

Fig. 107-45 ■ Neck sagging and fullness in a "V" shape 2 to 3 cm below the mandibular border (**A**) are often due to an enlarged gland (**B**) rather than jowling as a result of skin laxity alone.

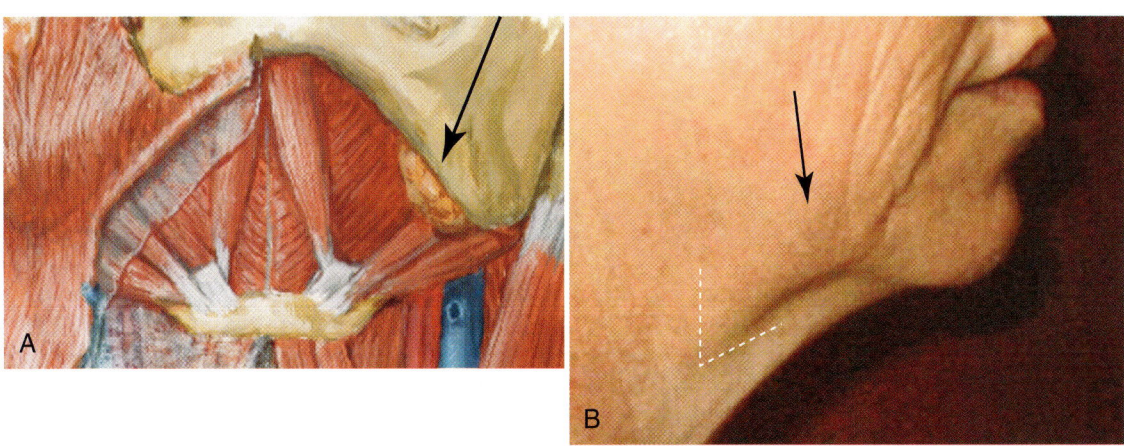

Fig. 107-46 ■ Ptotic/enlarged submandibular salivary glands are often noticed after a face-lift (*triangle shape* below the jowl). Options available for correcting submandibular gland/neck fullness include partial surgical *resection* (difficult) and surgical *slings* (relapse often). Patients should be informed of this limitation.

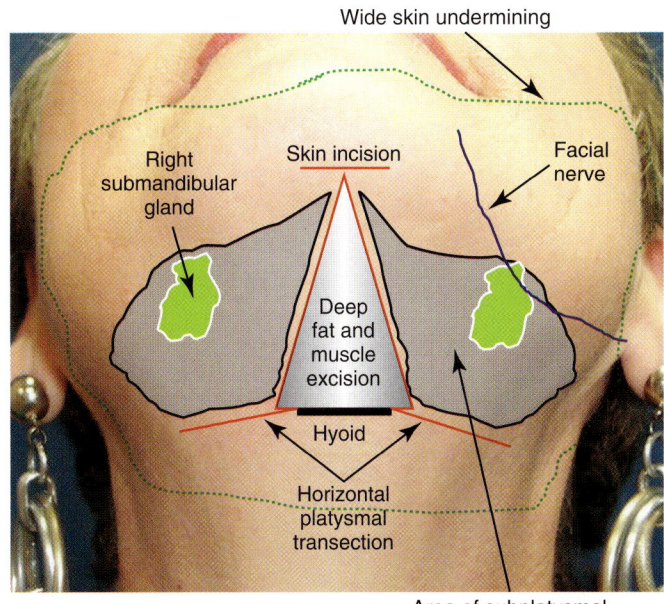

Fig. 107-47 ■ Partial surgical resection of the submandibular glands can be performed cautiously via an incision in the submental crease.

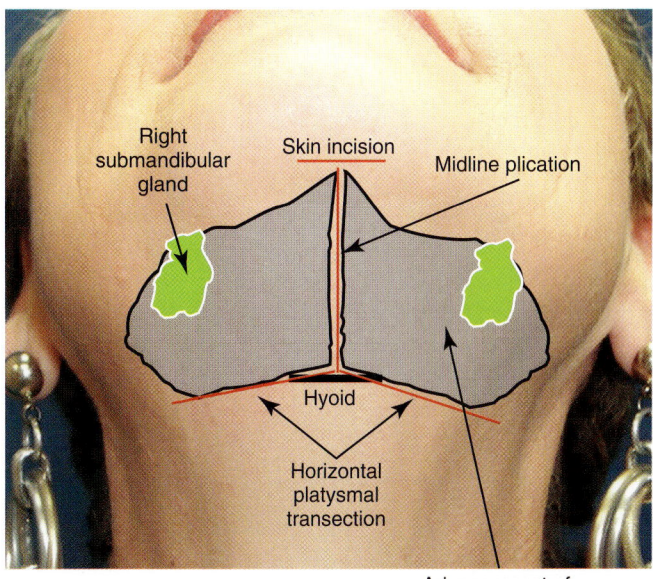

Fig. 107-48 ■ Cervical fascia is closed directly over the gland (to lessen the risk for sialocele) before the advancement of flaps and midline plication.

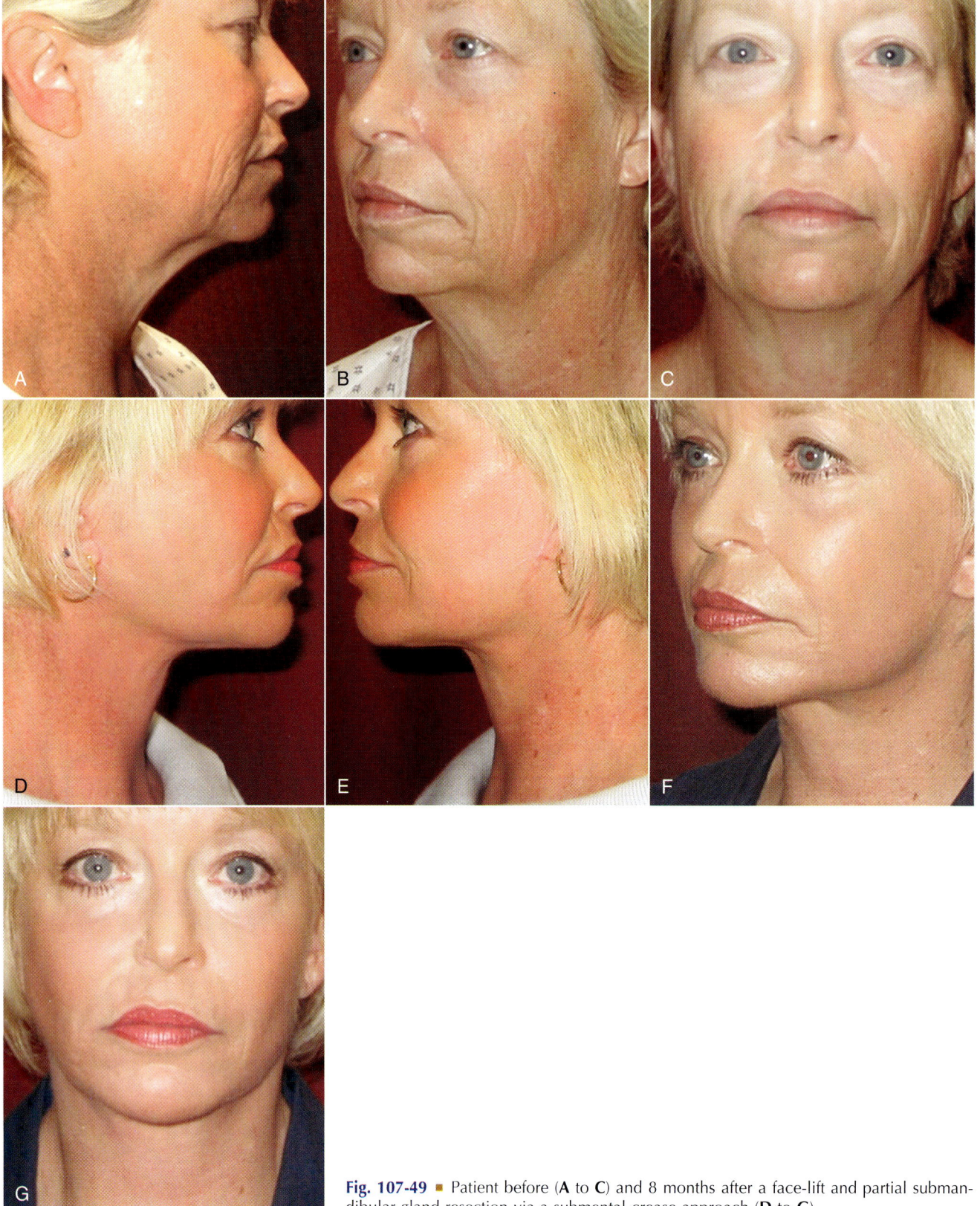

Fig. 107-49 ■ Patient before (**A** to **C**) and 8 months after a face-lift and partial submandibular gland resection via a submental crease approach (**D** to **G**).

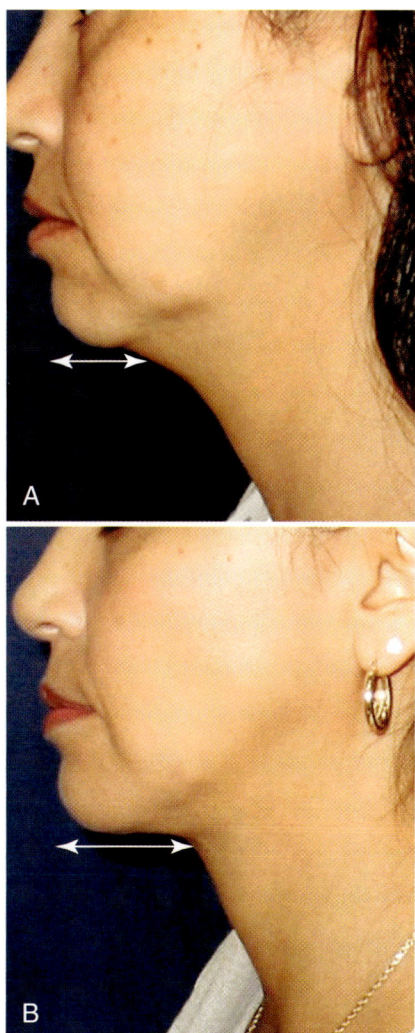

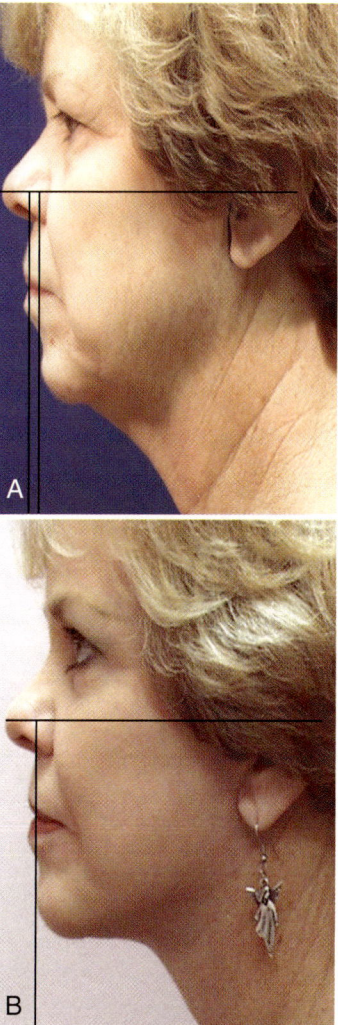

Fig. 107-50 ■ The benefits of a chin implant or submentoplasty (or both) are tremendous for some preoperative anatomic variants. Because horizontal neck length increases with placement of a chin implant, chin augmentation when microgenia is present improves the appearance of the neck. This patient was treated with a chin implant and isolated submentoplasty.

Fig. 107-51 ■ Chin position is assessed by dropping a line perpendicular to the Frankfort line through the vermilion border of the lower lip. The difference in distance between another perpendicular line drawn through the current chin position gives a good estimate of the size of the chin implant and millimeters of projection required.

imbrication, which is suturing a flap over deeper-lying tissue. Hence, SMAS plication involves simply folding the tissue on itself with sutures, whereas SMAS imbrication requires resection followed by pulling the anterior edge over the posterior tissue against which it will be sutured. Webster and colleagues reported no significant difference in results when using either method of SMAS fixation. More recently, the anatomy and viscoelastic properties of the SMAS have been studied more closely in the hope of finding a technique that will provide the best and longest-lasting effects.[17]

Once the skin flap is complete, SMAS plication is performed to elevate predominantly the sagging tissue of the jowls, cheek, and neck. It should also be noted that excessive subdermal dissection defeats the cosmetic skin support of the SMAS. The direction of pull is generally in a posterior to superior direction, but vectors are slightly different in front of and behind the ear to obtain the most natural and esthetic appearance. Deep wrinkles and sun damage require a more posterior pull, whereas aging is corrected more superiorly. One should recognize that a young face is not a tight face. The first key skin closure suture is placed at the base of the ear after determining how much skin should be excised by making a vertical

cut in the skin flap to this level based on redraping appearance (Fig. 107-63). Key initial plication sutures include one from the mandibular angle to the base of the tragus and another from the edge of the platysma to the mastoid fascia.[18] Sutures are placed with the knot buried to decrease foreign body reactions on the skin. Additional plication sutures are placed around the ear as needed. Plication sutures are also used to pull the temporoparietal fascia of the temporal skin flap posterosuperiorly and are attached to the strong temporalis fascia below. Limited subcutaneous dissection combined with SMAS plication reduces the dead space of the flap.

SKIN EXCISION AND WOUND CLOSURE

Following plication, the skin is redraped over the ear. Any minor skin dimpling or folds should be corrected before proceeding. Additional skin release is occasionally necessary. The skin is then incrementally excised to achieve primary closure with minimal tension. It is best to begin limited skin excision at the earlobe, with care being taken to avoid any downward tension on the earlobe. Next, separate vectors are used for the remaining preauricular and

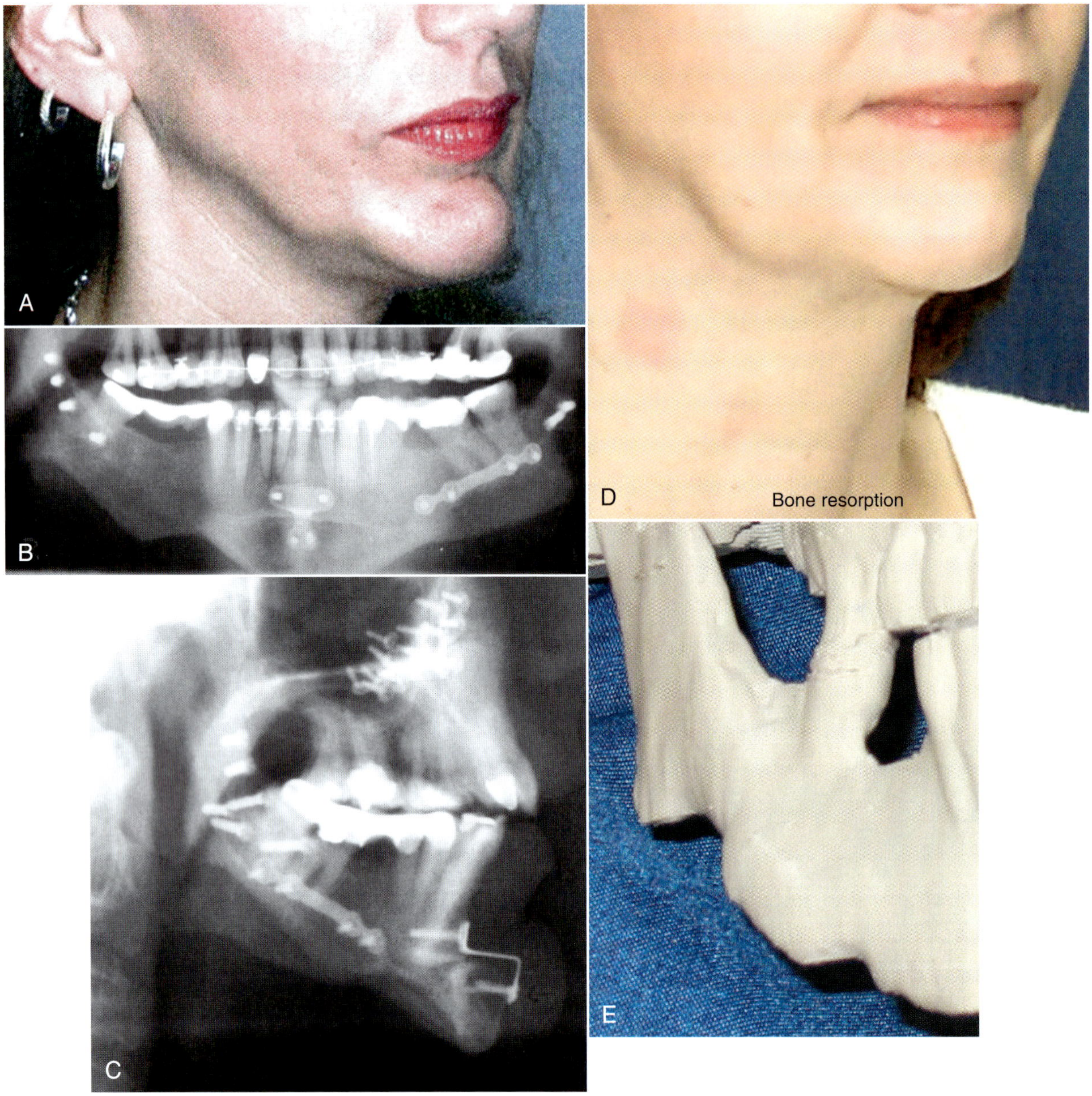

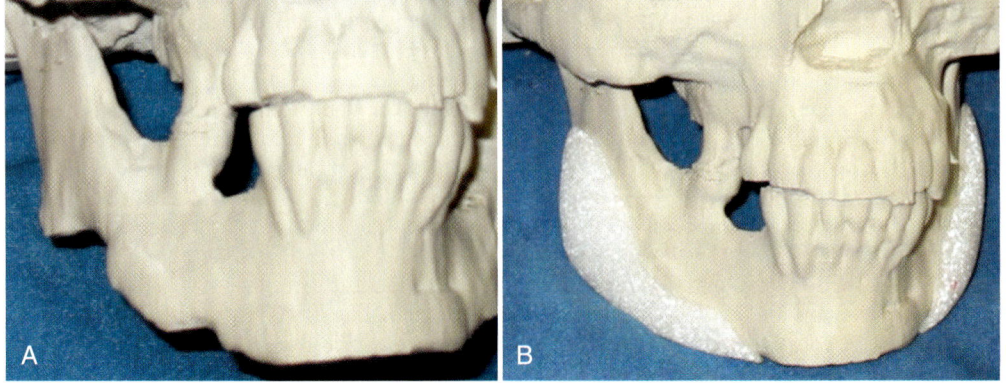

Fig. 107-52 ■ Caution should be exercised if planning a face-lift after orthognathic surgery since major bone resorption can occur years later and be more notable after a face-lift. Bone resorption on two patients: 8 years following jaw surgery (**A** and **B**) and bone resorption 12 years following jaw surgery (**C** to **E**).

Fig. 107-53 ■ Following three-dimensional computed tomography (**A**), custom mandibular angle implants with prejowl implant extensions (**B**) and submentoplasty (no face-lift) were used to improve the neck anatomy dilemma in this patient.

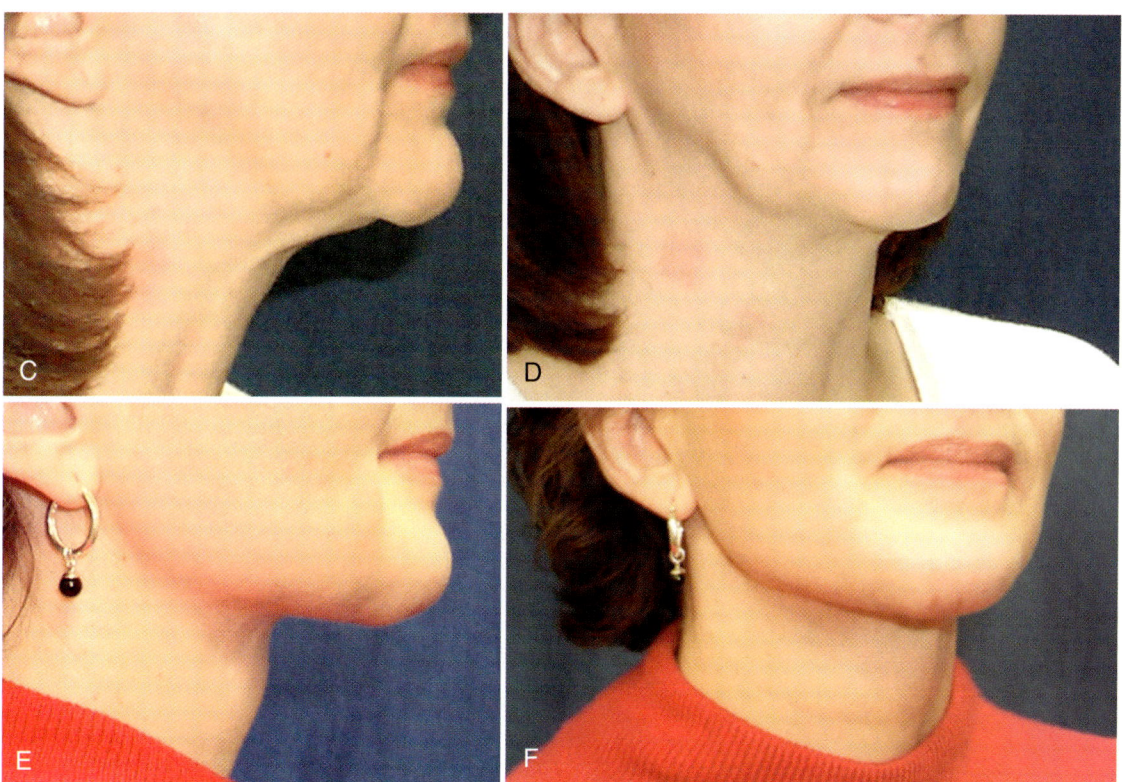

Fig. 107-53, cont'd ▪ **C** and **D,** Preoperative views. **E** and **F,** Postoperative views.

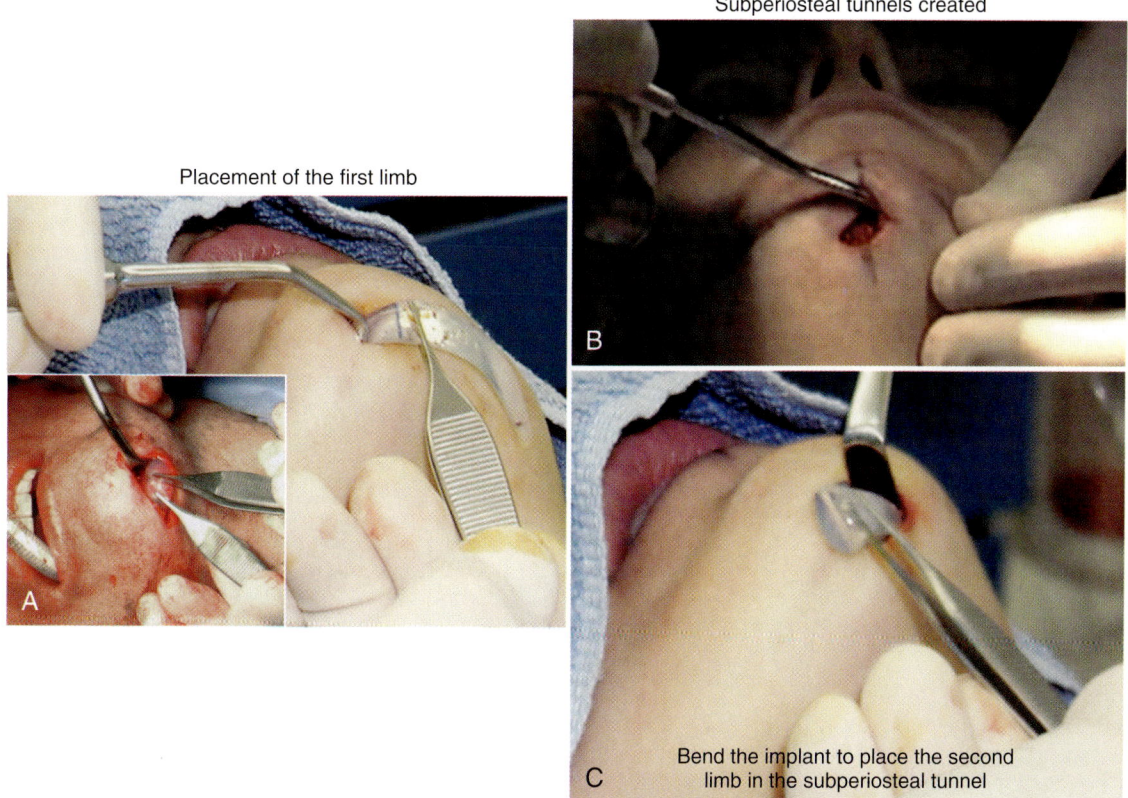

Subperiosteal tunnels created

Placement of the first limb

Bend the implant to place the second limb in the subperiosteal tunnel

Fig. 107-54 ▪ An extraoral chin implant placement technique. Advantages of the extraoral (incision in the submental crease) technique over intraoral approaches include lower risk for infection, less trauma, and improved stability of position. **A,** Placement of the first limb. **B,** Subperiosteal tunnels created. **C,** Bending the implant to place the second limb in the subperiosteal tunnel.

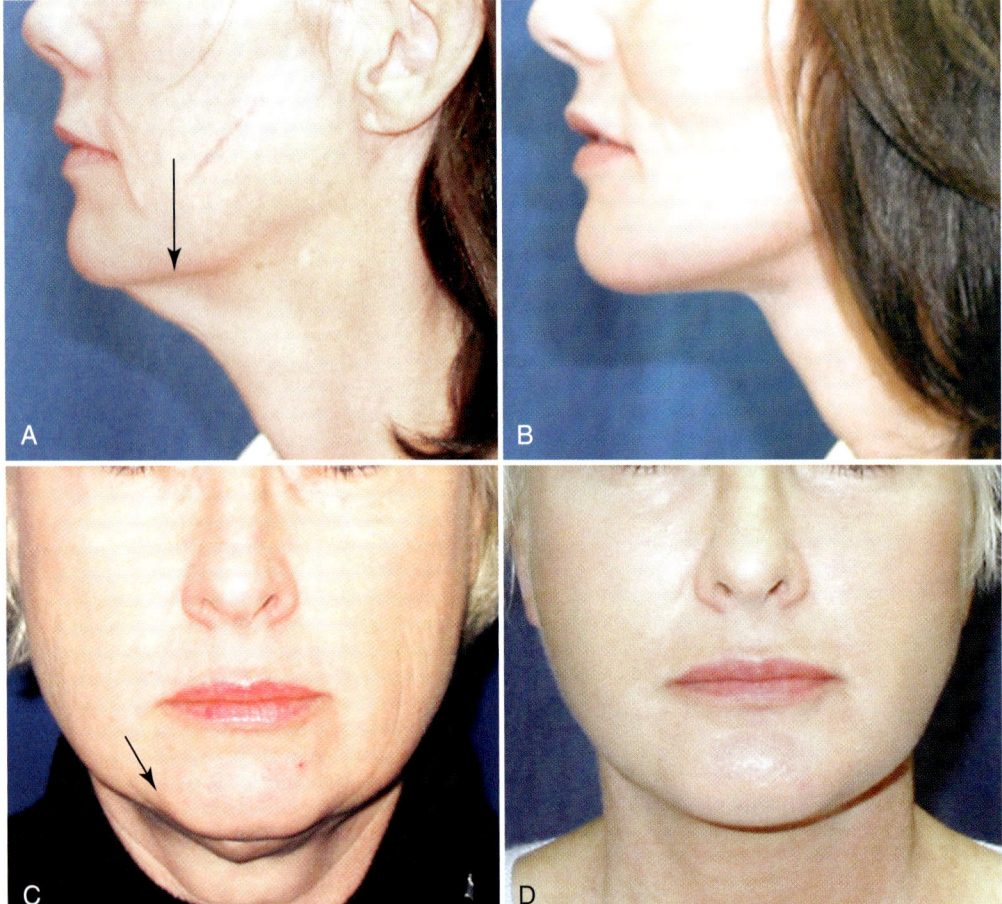

Fig. 107-55 ■ Chin implants were placed at the same time as a face-lift was performed. The prejowl region was considerably improved as a result of the implant filling in these areas, which further improved the shape of the jaw line. **A** and **B,** Face-lift, submentoplasty, and prejowl implant. **C** and **D,** Face-lift, submentoplasty, and chin implant.

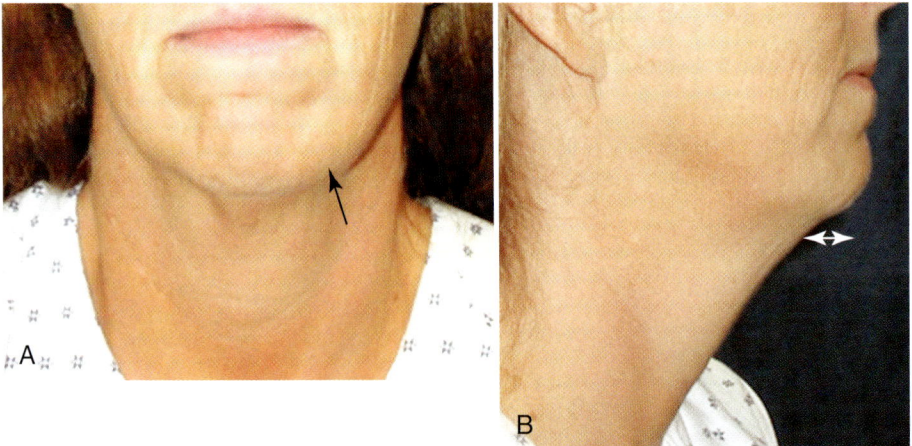

Fig. 107-56 ■ Chin implants were placed at the same time as a face-lift, submentoplasty, and perioral fat grafting. The prejowl region was significantly improved along with neck length. **A** and **B,** Preoperative views.

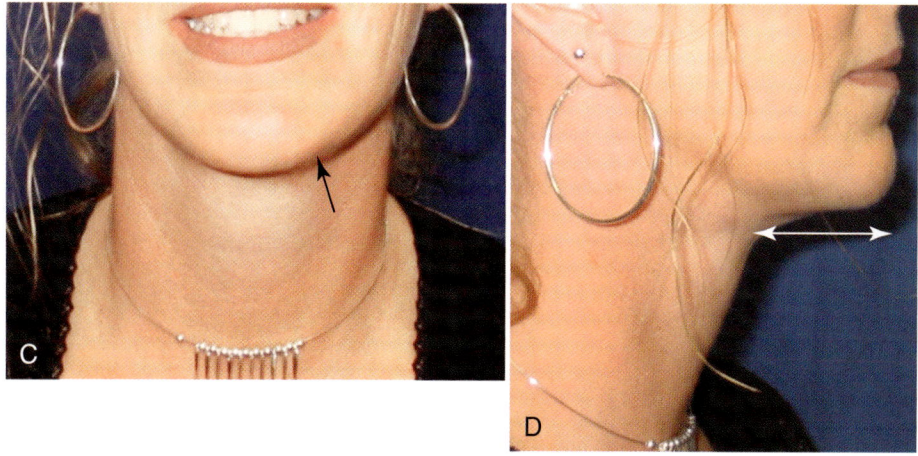

Fig. 107-56, cont'd ■ **C** and **D,** One year postoperatively.

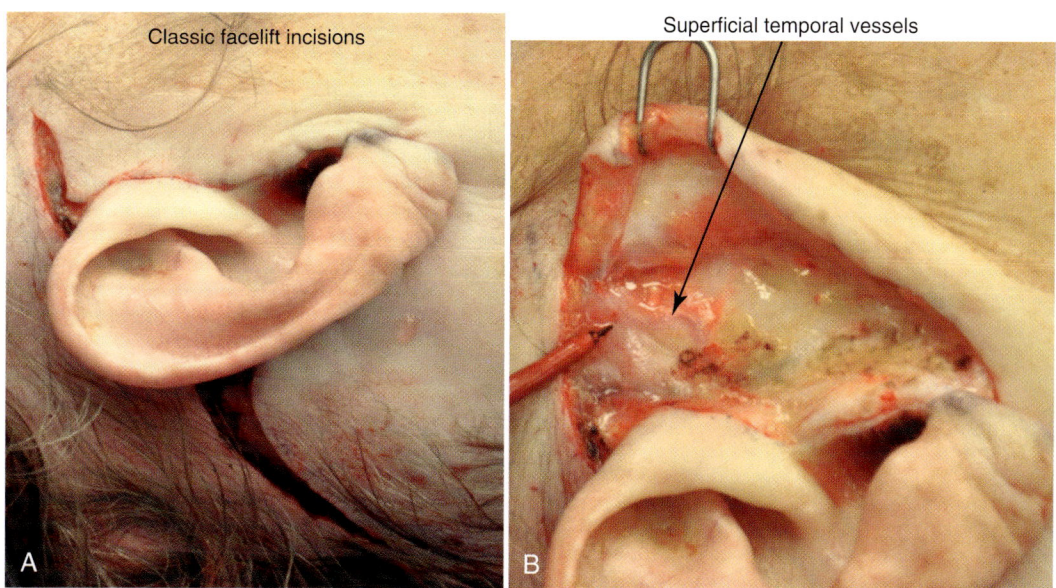

Fig. 107-57 ■ Classic pretrichial temporal (**A**) and intratrichial posterior face-lift (**B**) incisions are shown. Subcutaneous dissection in front of the ear can avoid vessels (*arrow* in part **B**) if kept in an ideal plane.

postauricular skin, and initial staples or sutures are placed for alignment. Heavy, permanent sutures such as 1-Nurolon can be used with a thick occipital flap to perform major neck lifting and decrease tension on the nearby thinner postauricular skin. If the hairline was crossed with the initial incisions, it must be realigned at this point (Fig. 107-64). Isolated staples at a few key points during skin excision help avoid over-trimming and dog-ear formation. Subcutaneous sutures then are placed with enough room left in the postauricular sulcus to insert a closed suction drain behind each ear and down into the neck if desired. Many surgeons, including us, do not use drains but leave a portion of the postauricular incision minimally open to allow drainage of minor fluid accumulations. Staples are placed in the hair-bearing incisions. The preauricular incisions are closed with 6-0 nylon or plain gut suture following careful skin excision beginning at the earlobe and working toward the temple (Figs. 107-65 to 107-67). Before final closure of the preauricular incisions, other procedures such as fat grafting through the flap can easily be

performed (Fig. 107-68). Malar implants placed via an intraoral route to fill the mid-face should be performed following final face-lift closure since it is not an entirely sterile procedure (Fig. 107-69). Consistency in sequencing of a face-lift and associated procedures will help make the procedure go more smoothly and efficiently (Box 107-2). Polysporin ointment is applied to the incisions after suture placement. Finally, if dressings are to be placed, they are applied with only mild pressure to avoid compromising the vascularity of the skin flaps.

A dressing consisting of 3M Reston foam 1563L (3M Medical-Surgical, St. Paul, Minn) and a Nexcare Coban (3M Medical-Surgical) head wrap is then placed over the submental region. It is worn for 24 hours. When the patient returns the following day postoperatively, the wrap is removed and the patient wears a compression garment such as a face-lift bra. This is to be worn as much as possible, day and night, during the first week. After 1 week, the patient is to wear the garment at night only for 2 more weeks.

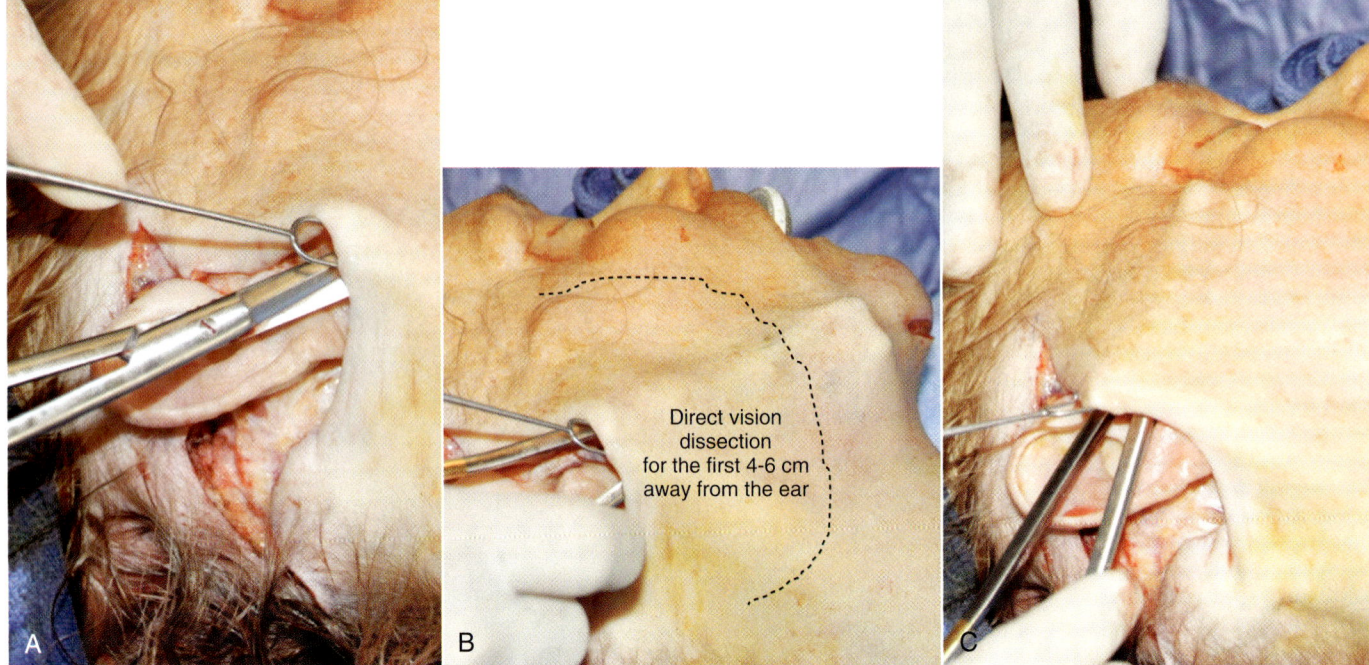

Fig. 107-58 ■ Following dissection under direct vision, an extended subcutaneous face-lift flap can be elevated beginning along the border of the mandible and proceeding out toward the jowl regions (**A** and **B**). Subcutaneous dissection with scissors in the malar region (**C**) must be performed cautiously.

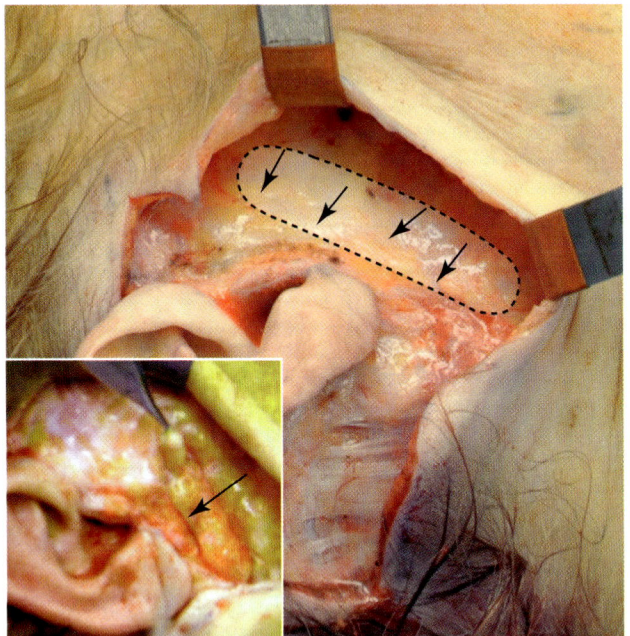

Fig. 107-59 ■ Multiple techniques can be used to elevate the musculofascial tissues deep to the elevated subcutaneous face-lift flap. A simple superficial musculoaponeurotic system strip excision technique is shown in which tissue in front of the ear is excised and then the edges are plicated together with a face-lift.

BOX 107-2	Sequencing of Face-Lift and Associated Procedures

Surgical Technique (Order of Treatment)
- Initial preparation, tumescent injection, second preparation, and draping
- Submental flap elevation (if indicated)
- Open microsuction or microliposuction (if indicated)
- Completion of submentoplasty (platysma treatment)
- Chin implant placement (if indicated)
- Face-lift, superficial musculoaponeurotic system techniques, and closure

Postoperative Care
- Neck foam and loose wrap for 24 hours (optional)
- Elastic head wrap (Velcro and easily removable)
  - 20 h/day for 1 week
  - At night for weeks 2 and 3
- Staples in hair removed in 7 days
- Normal hair shampoo daily

POSTOPERATIVE CARE

Patients may go home after adequate recovery from anesthesia. However, they should be instructed that a full-time sitter is required should they go home or stay in an overnight guest suite. They are given a postoperative care instruction sheet and told to call immediately if asymmetric swelling or severe pain develops. Some surgeons leave dressings off the first night so that hematomas can be discovered early. Patients are to sleep at a 45-degree angle to limit postoperative edema. Ice may be used as tolerated the first night. Prescriptions usually include narcotic analgesics, a 3- to 5-day course of antibiotics, and a few promethazine (Phenergan) suppositories in the event that nausea develops. The patient is told to continue all preoperative blood pressure medications.

Patients should return for removal of the dressing on the next day. The incisions are cleaned with dilute peroxide and water. Any drains that were placed are removed at this time. The home care

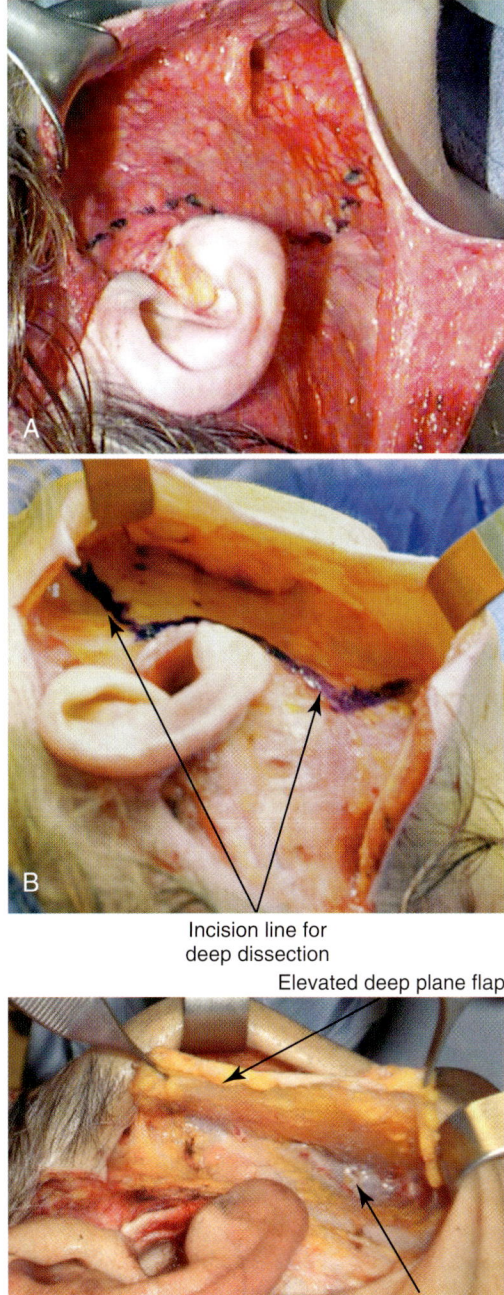

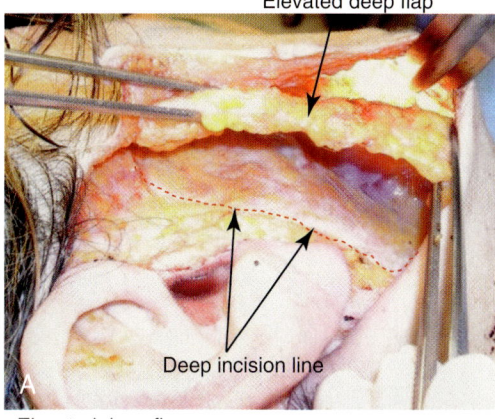

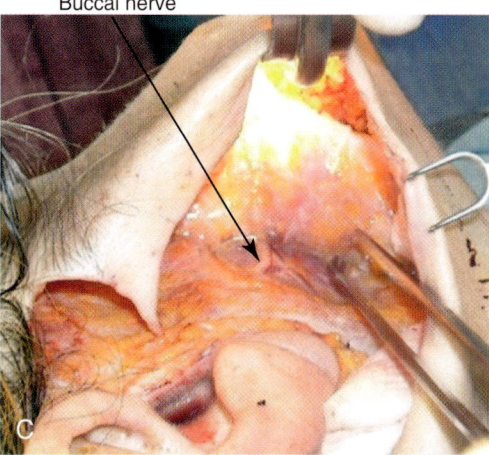

Fig. 107-61 ■ Advantages of a biplane face-lift include good skin redraping from a long subcutaneous flap and significant deep tissue elevation with proper technique.

Fig. 107-60 ■ A deep biplanar flap elevated off the parotid fascia can be used to provide smooth elevation of the face. The double-plane lift is associated with a greater risk for nerve injury than are short-flap and plication-only techniques.

develop. Patients are warned to avoid driving because of the risk associated with sudden turning of the neck, which should be avoided. Smoking is prohibited for at least 2 weeks after surgery.

INTRAOPERATIVE COMPLICATIONS

UNEXPECTED BLEEDING

Unexpected intraoperative bleeding, though rarely a major problem, can be a significant nuisance to the surgeon and may lead to more serious postoperative problems when it compromises the surgical

instructions are reiterated, and an elastic chin-neck wrap is placed. Patients can and should shower later that same day. They should wear the elastic neck strap as much as possible the first week. Sutures in the preauricular region are removed 5 days after surgery. Final staple removal occurs at 8 to 10 days. The next follow-up appointment is usually scheduled 1 month later if no complications

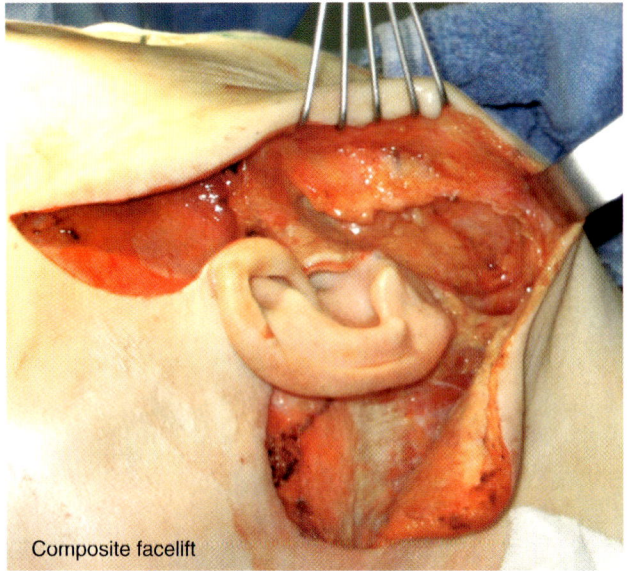

Fig. 107-62 ▪ The composite face-lift was popularized by Dr. Sam T. Hamra in 1990. Multiple tissue planes are elevated *as one unit*, such as the orbicularis oculi; minor subcutaneous undermining may be needed to theoretically improve blood supply to the skin. A composite face-lift is demonstrated in a patient with alopecia totalis. The subcutaneous flap is only 1 cm away from the ear when the flap is carried down to a deep layer over the parotid to elevate the remaining flap as one unit of skin, fat, and musculofascial tissue.

technique. Excessive hemorrhage from the flaps can often be prevented by avoiding aspirin products and vitamin E for 10 to 14 days before surgery. Hypertension can also add to the blood loss during a procedure, and hematoma formation can result from even brief episodes of hypertension. Patients should therefore be advised to continue their antihypertensive medications before surgery. Some surgeons prescribe clonidine the night and morning before surgery to minimize hypertensive episodes, even in patients without a history of hypertension. Good technique for both local anesthesia and sedation is vital. Allowing 15 minutes after the injection of a local anesthetic with epinephrine before making the initial incision is critical for maintaining hemostasis.

Once the incisions have been made and the flaps elevated, any small areas of bleeding are easily controlled with careful use of bipolar cautery. However, indiscriminant deep cauterization must be limited to avoid thermal injury to branches of the facial nerve. Larger vessels that are not easily cauterized should be carefully clamped and tied. Two regions of the face that are a particular nuisance with respect to vascular disruption are the vascular plexus over the zygomatic prominence, also known as the MacGregor patch, and the area of the external jugular vein that crosses over the sternocleidomastoid muscle. These regions will not be violated as long as the skin flap remains superficial to the cervical fascia.

ANESTHETIC COMPLICATIONS

Complications resulting from poor anesthetic technique can be frustrating and increase the likelihood of other surgical problems. Anesthetic techniques vary, but if an intravenous sedation technique

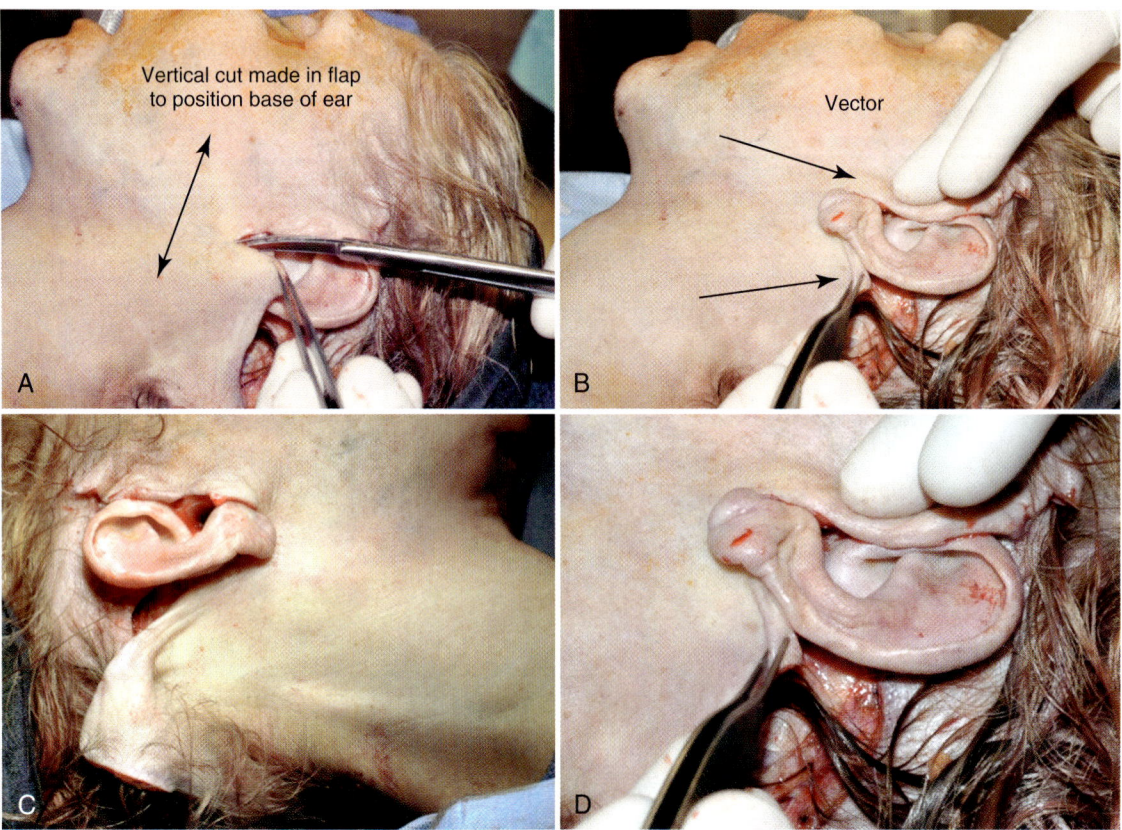

Fig. 107-63 ▪ Setting the base of the ear is critical after the deep work is complete. The vector of lift is determined by what looks best and most natural on the table. The location of the base of the ear with respect to the flap is critical to allow normal redraping and for posterior hair alignment. Cutting too far one way or the other can cause major closure problems.

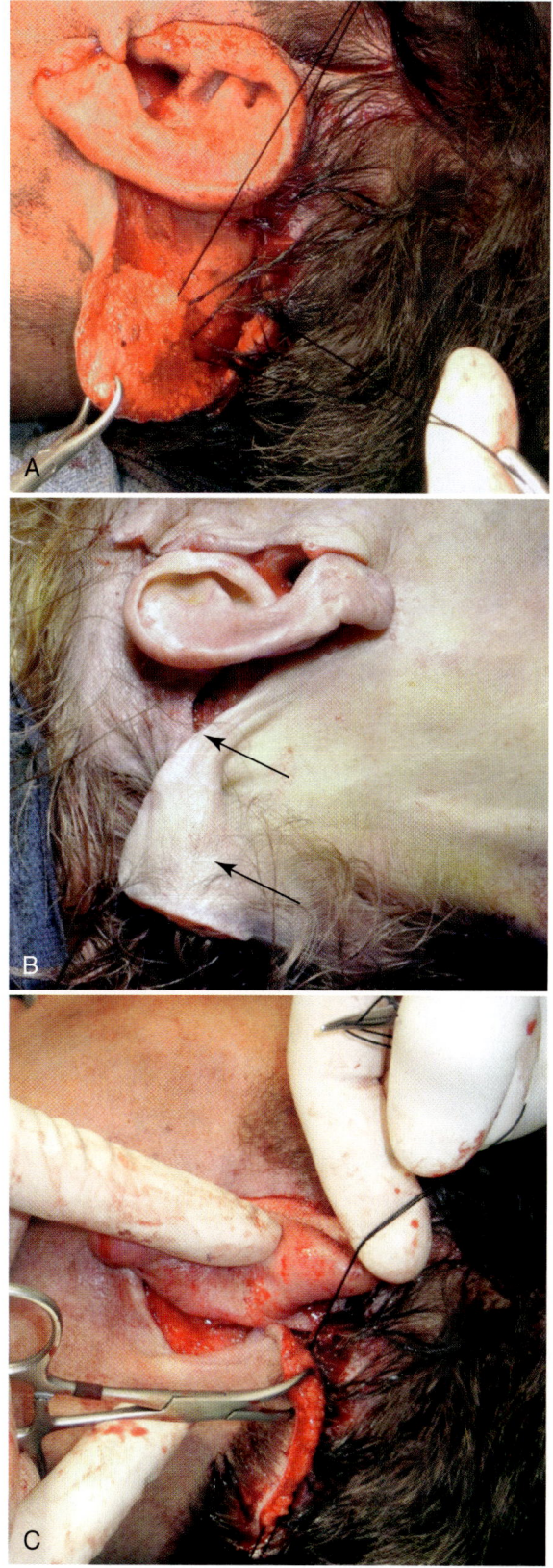

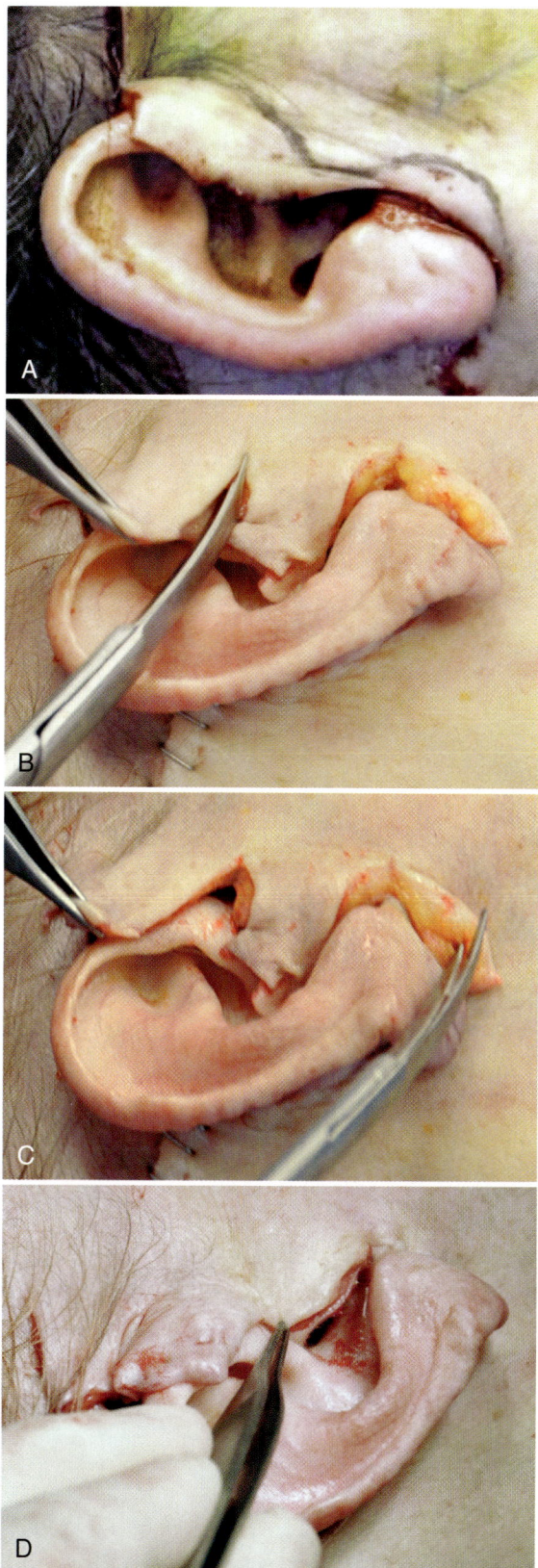

Fig. 107-64 ■ Elevation of occipital tissue with two deep 1-Nurolon sutures supports the ear and prevents migration of the incision, as well as preventing ischemic problems in adjacent thinner tissues.

Fig. 107-65 ■ Trimming of skin around the tragus is critical. It is ideal to work from the bottom up. Horizontal pre-cuts on each side of the tragus are an easy way to trim excess skin and avoid skin tension.

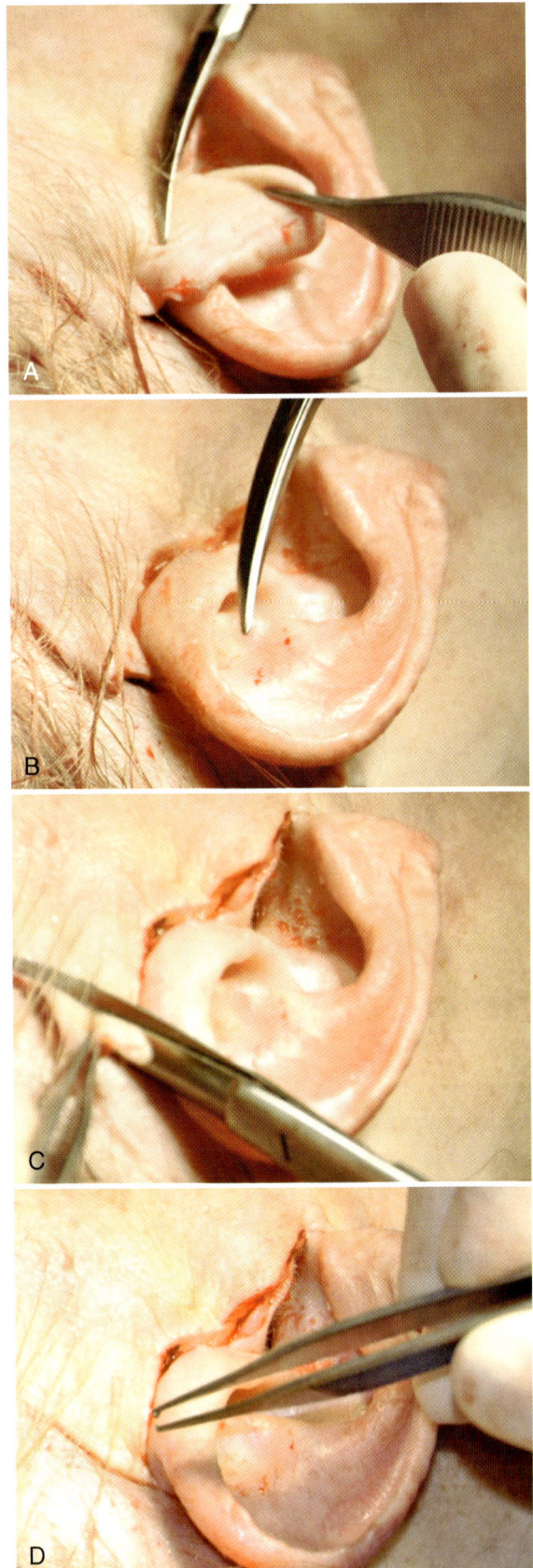

Fig. 107-66 ■ Trimming the remaining skin above the tragus is best performed near the end by using the curve of the scissors to excise skin around the helix. The pretrichial skin is trimmed last since any irregularities at that point can be adjusted easier in the hair than the earlobe.

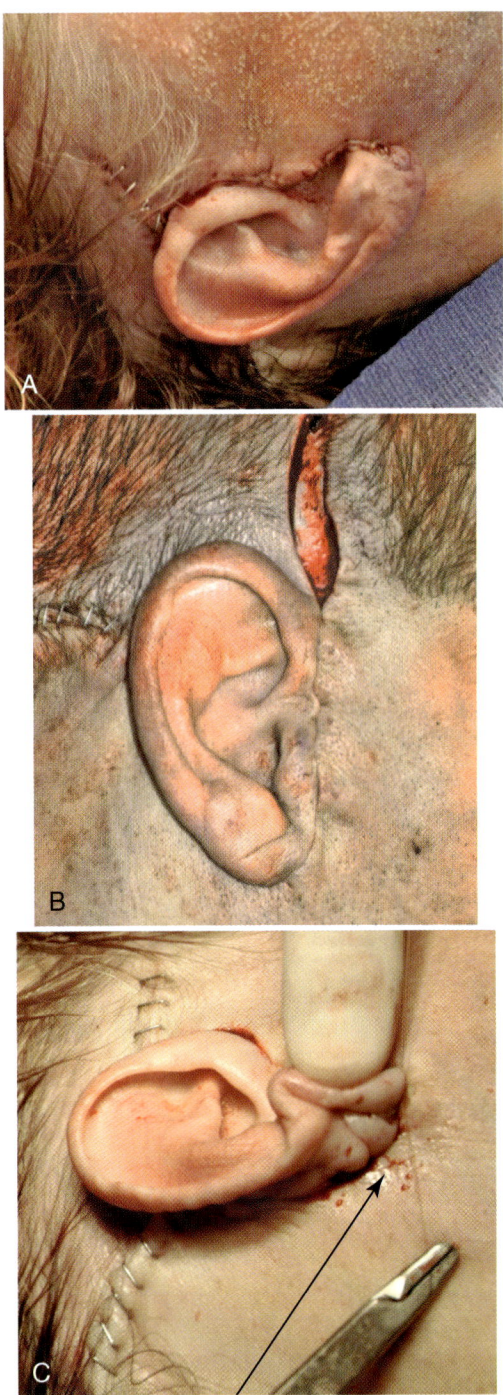

Base of ear most likely to dehisce
so extra sutures are used at ear base

Fig. 107-67 ■ Face-lift closure in males is typically easier than in women when a pretragal incision is used. Nonetheless, incisions around the earlobe in men or women require meticulous closure since this is the most common area for the wound to pull apart. The base of the ear is most likely to dehisce, so extra sutures are used at the ear base (see *arrow* in part **C**).

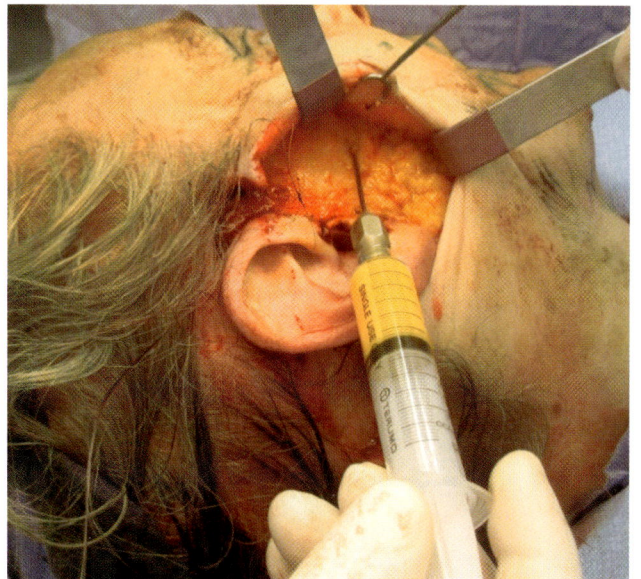

Fig. 107-68 ■ Fat grafting in the mid-face, which can be done through the face-lift flap before final closure.

is planned rather than general anesthesia, longer-acting intravenous medications will help "smooth" the anesthesia. During a procedure that may take longer than 2 hours, substituting diazepam for midazolam is one such example. In addition, maintaining normal to low-normal blood pressure throughout the procedure is critical; therefore, techniques such as a propofol drip infusion can greatly improve the patient's sedation. Maintaining well-administered sedation or general anesthesia decreases the chance for postoperative bleeding and hematoma formation by avoiding sporadic and rapid elevations in blood pressure.

With regard to local anesthesia, many techniques can be used. Local anesthetic toxicity occurs more frequently with face-lift surgery than with other types of facial surgery because of the greater amounts of anesthetic required. Use of tumescent anesthesia with a dilute solution of lidocaine and epinephrine is one method of reducing this risk. Vasoconstriction can be excellent, but large volumes of fluid need to be infused into the subcutaneous tissue. The tumescent technique seems to distort the tissue initially, but tissue distortion is minimal 15 minutes after the infusion. The results have been good with this technique, with minimal adverse effects.

Non-tumescent local anesthesia for face-lifting results in a higher lidocaine blood level (see the section on anesthesia), and the surgeon must be aware of the maximal limits to avoid toxicity. Non-tumescent

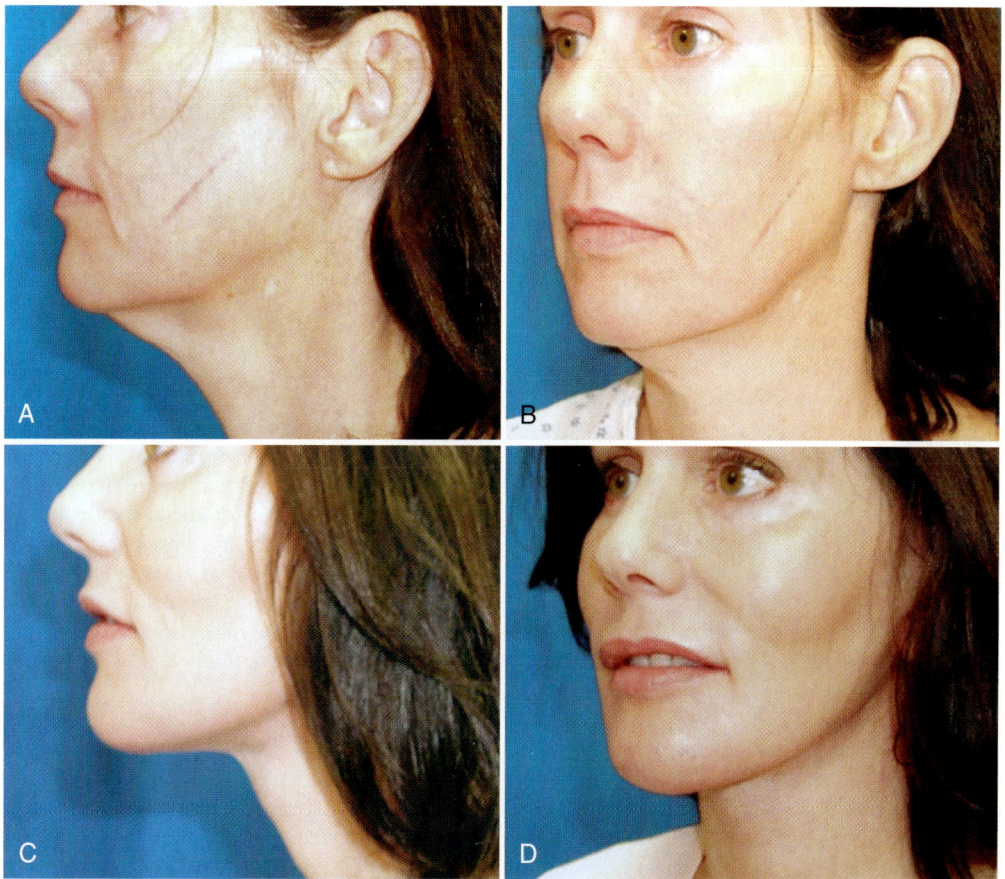

Fig. 107-69 ■ Placement of cheek implants during a face-lift should be performed after final closure of the face-lift since intraoral cheek implant placement is a non-sterile procedure: before (**A** and **B**) and after (**C** and **D**) face-lift and cheek implants.

anesthetic injection can be performed in stages by waiting to inject the opposite side of the face. Although toxicity is rare even with non-tumescent anesthesia, staged anesthetic injections can help avoid the problem.

PTOTIC SUBMANDIBULAR GLAND

With age, the submandibular gland becomes ptotic despite coverage by the superficial cervical fascia that contains the gland. Unfortunately, because older patients also have skin laxity and jowling, a ptotic submandibular gland may not be recognized preoperatively. Intraoperatively, this condition may be recognized when the SMAS layer is being pulled tightly. Overaggressive tension in this region sometimes pulls the submandibular gland laterally and creates a bulge at the antegonial notch area. Some surgeons recommend placement of a submandibular sling to elevate the gland superiorly and medially. This technique is not always successful, and the best course of action is often redirection and manipulation of the SMAS.

CYANOTIC FLAP

Skin flaps that become bruised or cyanotic during surgery are certainly worrisome; although this is not a complication itself, it is a warning sign that venous congestion or vascular compromise has occurred. Mild discoloration during surgery is common, but significant cyanosis appearing along the mandibular margin or high in the postauricular area may eventually develop into true skin necrosis, particularly in smokers and thin-skinned elderly patients. It is also seen more frequently when performing long-flap face-lifts. Recognition of these warning signs should cause the surgeon to avoid longer flaps and undue skin tension at closure.

IRREGULARITY

Irregularities during face-lift surgery may be the result of excessive tension on the SMAS or skin. They can also be caused by malpositioned sutures pulling on the sternocleidomastoid or the wrong vector of pull. Frequently, they are simply secondary to inadequate flap release or irregular fat deposits. The problem is best corrected at the time of surgery by removing sutures as needed and redirecting the flaps. The posterior margin of the platysma muscle may become bulky at the anterior edge of the sternocleidomastoid. Open suction lipectomy performed in the preauricular region down to the white glistening fascia reduces adiposity and helps in identifying the SMAS. It also aids in keeping the tissue smooth during plication or imbrication.

EARLY POSTOPERATIVE COMPLICATIONS

HEMATOMA

Hematoma is the most common early postoperative complication and occurs in approximately 5% of face lift patients. Fortunately, only 1% of hematomas are considered major, or rapidly expanding hematomas that require immediate surgical treatment (Fig. 107-70).[19] Most hematomas are minor collections of blood that can easily be handled in the outpatient setting. Frequently, they require only evacuation by "milking" the skin flap to express blood from behind the ear through a small open incision site. Should a major hematoma occur, immediate surgical treatment is required to avoid overlying skin necrosis. Opening the entire incision with proper lighting and sterility, meticulous irrigation, and hemostasis should be achieved following surgical evacuation of the hematoma.

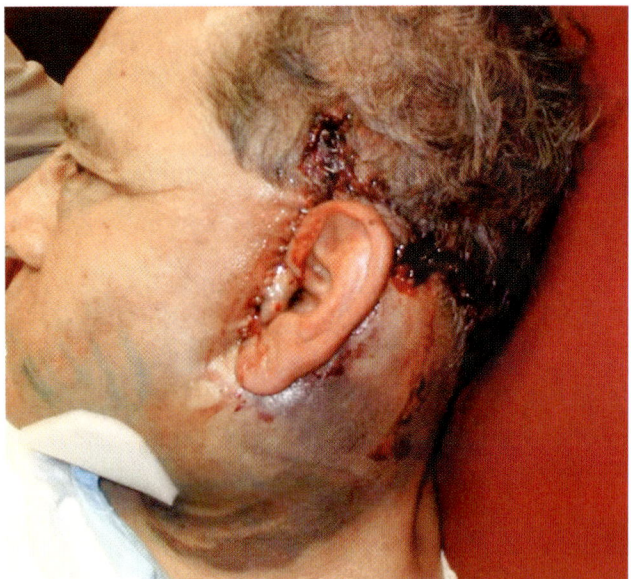

Fig. 107-70 ■ An acute hematoma a few hours after a face-lift requires immediate surgical treatment. In addition, control of blood pressure is essential since postoperative pain and hypertension are leading causes of post–face-lift hematomas.

INFECTION

Infection following face-lift surgery is extremely rare, but the risk for a skin infection warrants safeguards. As with all surgery, sterile surgical technique should be used. In addition, preoperative administration of a first-generation cephalosporin, such as 1 g cefazolin intravenously, has been shown to further decrease the incidence of postoperative infections. Similar to most postoperative infections, face-lift infections tend to occur 2 to 5 days postoperatively and begin along the incision sites. Treatment involves local wound care, drainage, antibiotics, and culture swabs for identification of the organism. Immunocompromised patients might need more aggressive intravenous antibiotic therapy. True, rapidly progressing fasciitis is rare but has been reported and can be disfiguring if left undetected.

WOUND DEHISCENCE

Breakdown of wound margins is not uncommon. The usual cause of dehiscence along incision sites is inadequate deep sutures, excessive skin tension, or removal of superficial sutures or staples too early. Most surgeons recommend removal of peri-auricular sutures (if non-reabsorbable) 5 days postoperatively. Staples in the hairline, temporally and postauricularly, should remain in place for 8 to 10 days. Avoidance of excessive skin excision and redraping at low tension are also crucial in decreasing the incidence of wound dehiscence and help achieve the best possible wound healing.

SKIN FLAP NECROSIS

Skin flap necrosis is rare but does occur at a higher frequency in patients who smoke or those in whom large hematomas develop postoperatively. Vascular compromise of the flaps leads to early cyanosis from venous congestion or pallor from compromised arterial supply. If skin cyanosis or pallor is noted at the time of surgery, serious thought should be given to re-evaluating flap thickness and halting further undermining.

As with most complications, the best treatment is prevention. Maintaining adequate flap thickness is critical, particularly in patients who smoke. Leaving 4 to 5 mm of subcutaneous fat is considered adequate for most patients. A short flap is warranted in heavy smokers for the same reason. In many cases, surgeons refuse to treat heavy smokers. If surgery is to be performed on patients who smoke, a period of abstinence for 2 weeks before and after surgery is advocated. Nicotine's effect on vasoconstriction is profound in the immediate postoperative period. Patients should be thoroughly counseled before proceeding with surgery. It has been documented that skin flap necrosis occurs 80% of the time in patients who smoke more than one pack per day. Skin sloughing of any amount is 12 times more common in smokers than in non-smokers.[11]

Skin necrosis is usually managed conservatively by local wound care. Oral antibiotics along with topical Polysporin ointment and daily cleansing are recommended. Most small areas of skin necrosis (<1 cm) tend to heal well within 2 months. Even larger areas may heal with only minor residual scarring. The most common areas are the preauricular and postauricular regions secondary to a thin flap or excessive skin tension. Meticulous surgical technique, as well as preoperative counseling of smokers, will help reduce this difficult problem.

MOTOR NERVE DYSFUNCTION

Injury to the facial nerve causing paralysis is rare. It has been reported to occur in 0.53-2.6% of patients, with the most commonly affected branches being the marginal mandibular and the temporal nerves. Eighty-five percent of motor nerve injuries resolve spontaneously. The causes of neurapraxia are excessive tension on the SMAS during plication, overzealous electrocautery, and indiscriminant dissection. The most superficial locations of the temporal branch and the marginal mandibular branch are over the zygomatic arch and mandibular angle, respectively. It should be noted that certain variations in surgical technique may be more likely to damage other branches of the facial nerves.[10] For instance, composite and other deep-plane techniques are associated with a greater incidence of buccal nerve and zygomatic nerve injury than are superficial techniques, particularly when the zygomaticus major or orbicularis oculi muscles are manipulated.

Regrettably, treatment of motor nerve injuries is limited. Usually, the location of the injury is unknown, and therefore reanastomosis is not advocated. The majority of injuries occur distal to a vertical line drawn from the lateral canthus of the eye. Fortunately, most nerve function returns with time. Immediate postoperative paralysis is most often due to the anesthetic and resolves within hours. Nerve repair and muscle nerve transfer have been attempted with only mediocre success. In-depth knowledge of facial anatomy and nerve location is the best way to avoid the problem of nerve injury in face-lift surgery.

SENSORY NERVE INJURY

The great auricular nerve is the most common sensory nerve injured during rhytidectomy.[20] The anesthesia at the inferior portion of the ear and surrounding skin usually resolves in 2 to 4 months. The most likely cause is temporary neurapraxia related to distortion of the nerve within tightly plicated tissue over the sternocleidomastoid muscle. However, if transection of the nerve occurs, permanent sensory loss and neuroma formation are possible. Transection is best treated by immediate microanastomosis.

The preauricular and postauricular skin is the most common site for a sensory deficit. It is caused by injury to the terminal branches of the great auricular and auriculotemporal nerves. Fortunately, sensory loss in these regions is rarely permanent and sensation returns with time.

LATE POSTOPERATIVE COMPLICATIONS

ABNORMAL WOUND HEALING OR HYPERTROPHIC SCARS

Widening of skin incisions is a result of excessive skin tension, inadequate deep sutures, or too early removal of sutures. Some patients may simply be more prone to hypertrophic scarring or keloid formation. The most common location for scar widening is the postauricular region. Careful placement of deep sutures helps eliminate this possibility. Other hypertrophic scarring may be secondary to complications such as skin flap necrosis or hematoma. Persistent scarring 2 to 3 months postoperatively may require steroid injections or revision surgery. Minor revision surgery on hypertrophic scars should be delayed for 1 year. However, poorly healing wounds caused by stitch abscesses, wound breakdown and infection, or poor alignment may be treated earlier if the tissue can be closed without tension.

EARLOBE DISTORTION

Earlobe deformities may be seen when excessive tension is placed inferior to the lobe. With time, the downward contraction pulls the earlobe and creates what is known as a "bat wing deformity," "devil's ear," or "elfin ear deformity."[21] The deformity is a blending of the helix into the neck with no distinctive lobe. This can be avoided by backcutting of the skin incision under the lobe and reduced skin tension. Reconstruction of an elfin ear requires a V-Y plasty or nearly complete revision face-lift with SMAS plication to reduce tension and significant skin undermining (Fig. 107-71).

ALOPECIA OR CHANGES IN THE HAIRLINE

Alopecia or hair loss after face-lift surgery is rare but has been reported in the temporal tuft region in 2.8% of patients.[4] Unusual tension is the most common cause of this complication. Most surgeons advocate incisions parallel to the hair shaft and reduced skin tension on the wound. Recent articles have advised oblique incisions across the follicle in the hope of obtaining hair growth on both sides of the incision to improve scar camouflage. Although oblique cuts may allow hair growth to hide scars better, proper wound reapproximation is more difficult and a wider scar may result if there is undue tension.

Unfavorable changes in the hairline are usually related to poor planning of the incision in the preauricular and postauricular regions.[22] Incisions that follow immediately in front of the hairline avoid this problem, but a scar may be visible if widening occurs. Retroauricular incisions that extend into the hairline conceal the scar better, but the hairline must be realigned properly before wound closure. This occasionally creates problems with the vector of pull in the lower part of the neck and compromises the proper direction of lift to align the hair. Temporal tuft hair loss is a problem that has been well documented following face-lift surgery, particularly when the incision extends straight up from the tragus with no consideration for skin excision.

Two traditional options exist: stepping the incision around the temporal tuft of hair or using a separate transverse incision to lay back a new temporal tuft during a straight vertical extension from the tragus. A third option is to not excise the skin but allow bunching of the redundant temporal skin, which dissipates over a period of several months. If hair loss should occur in this region, micrografting of hair can be performed. Other unfavorable hair changes in men involve facial hair growth on the tragus. Standard post-tragal incisions are used for men to keep the tragus free of hair.

Elfin ear deformity caused by improper
tension at base of ear during prior closure

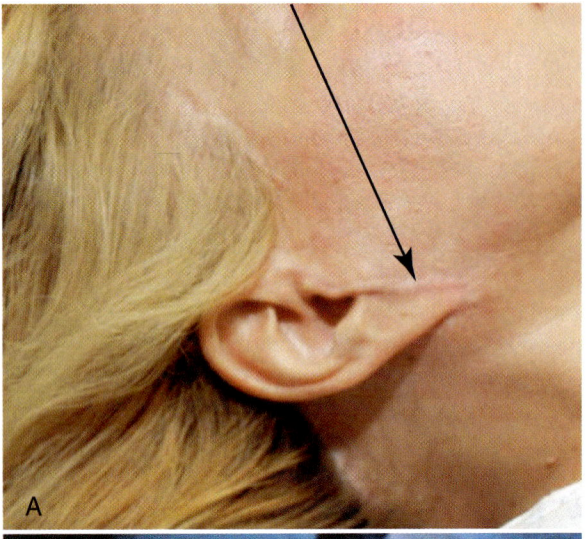

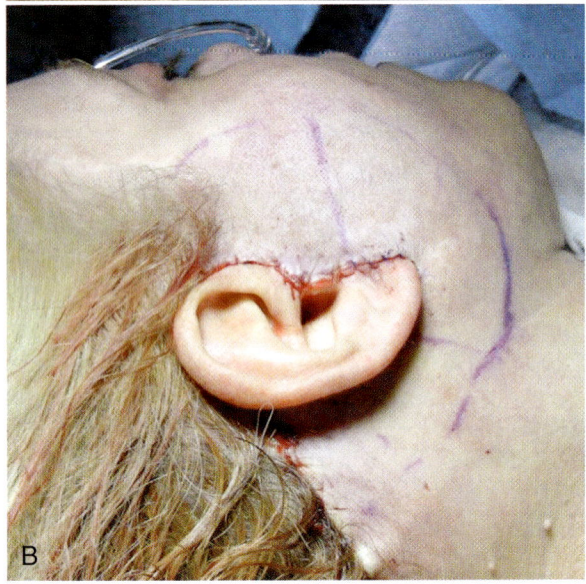

Fig. 107-71 ■ Revision of a pixie or elfin earlobe (*arrow* in part **A**) often requires a "mini-lift" for complete correction (**B**).

PLATYSMAL BANDING

Persistent platysmal banding is a problem in patients with preoperative neck skin laxity and platysmal banding. A corset platysmaplasty has been recommended for patients with severe platysmal banding anteriorly at the time of face-lift surgery. Unfortunately, even with ideal platysmal treatment, postoperative neck irregularities may occur.

Anterior plication during a face-lift may decrease the benefit gained with respect to the cervical facial angle. Instead, anterior border resection of the platysma through a submental incision at the time of face-lift surgery is easily performed and in most cases yields better results. Severe general laxity of the platysma in a heavy neck may best be treated by platysmal resection to help avoid postoperative bands (Fig. 107-72).

Should banding develop postoperatively, gentle massage by the patient can be helpful. Although the benefit of massage is unknown, it allows progressive healing and gives the patient an active role in treatment. Thick bands cannot be improved by this method and may require steroid injections or eventual revision by resection.

Botulinum toxin (Botox) injections have recently been advocated for platysmal banding. The medication is safe when properly used to paralyze isolated superficial muscles, but the effects last only 3 to 4 months before reinjection is required.

HYPERVASCULARITY AND CHANGES IN PIGMENTATION

Changes in pigmentation may occasionally occur after unusual inflammation, infection, or skin sloughing, especially in patients with darker skin tone, because of stimulation of melanocytes as occurs following laser skin resurfacing. The opposite of this is melanocyte death, which results in hypopigmentation, but this is a less common result. Initial treatment is reassurance of the patient unless the changes are severe. Avoidance of the sun is critical, and use of bleaching creams such as hydroquinones may be necessary if the hyperpigmented changes persist.

Hypervascular regions of the skin flap may become apparent postoperatively, particularly after minor infections or inflammatory reactions. Again, reassurance is advocated initially. If the hypervascular or telangiectatic regions persist, treatment can be performed with a small-gauge needle and electrocautery. If available, selective laser treatment specific for the hemoglobin molecule may be beneficial. CO_2 lasers are rarely beneficial in patients with postoperative hypervascularity.

CHRONIC PAIN OR TRAUMATIC TIC

Fortunately, this is an extremely rare complication. Initial treatment with non-steroidal anti-inflammatory drugs, muscle relaxants, and drugs used to treat conditions such as tic douloureux or postoperative neurogenic pain syndrome may be indicated. Regional nerve blocks may help in the diagnosis. Regional injection of local anesthetic and a mild steroid solution is needed to aid in pain control. In addition, increasing dosages of amitriptyline (Elavil) or gabapentin (Neurontin) may be helpful. Most chronic pain resolves with time. However, a true tic may require neurectomy if medication fails.

PAROTID FISTULA

Iatrogenic dissection into the parotid gland substance may lead to a parotid fistula. Careful attention to anatomy and the proper surgical plane will avoid this problem, but should it occur, oversewing of the defect with the overlying musculofascial aponeurosis will help prevent a fistula from forming. If a parotid fistula does occur or is suspected to have occurred, a moderate pressure dressing over the region may allow spontaneous remission. Most fistulas resolve spontaneously after a few weeks of persistent moderate swelling. Rarely is surgical exploration needed with layered overclosure.

THE DISSATISFIED PATIENT

Patient dissatisfaction following face-lift surgery is usually a result of unrealistic expectations. Thorough preoperative evaluation and honest discussion regarding the risks, benefits, and prognosis should take place. Patients with unreasonable expectations and unattainable goals should be avoided or managed carefully.

Once a dissatisfied patient has voiced a complaint, the surgeon must be attentive, listen closely, and not be defensive. Frank discussion about realistic means of correcting the problem should take place. Maintaining good rapport with patients is critical to help them

Text continued on p. 985

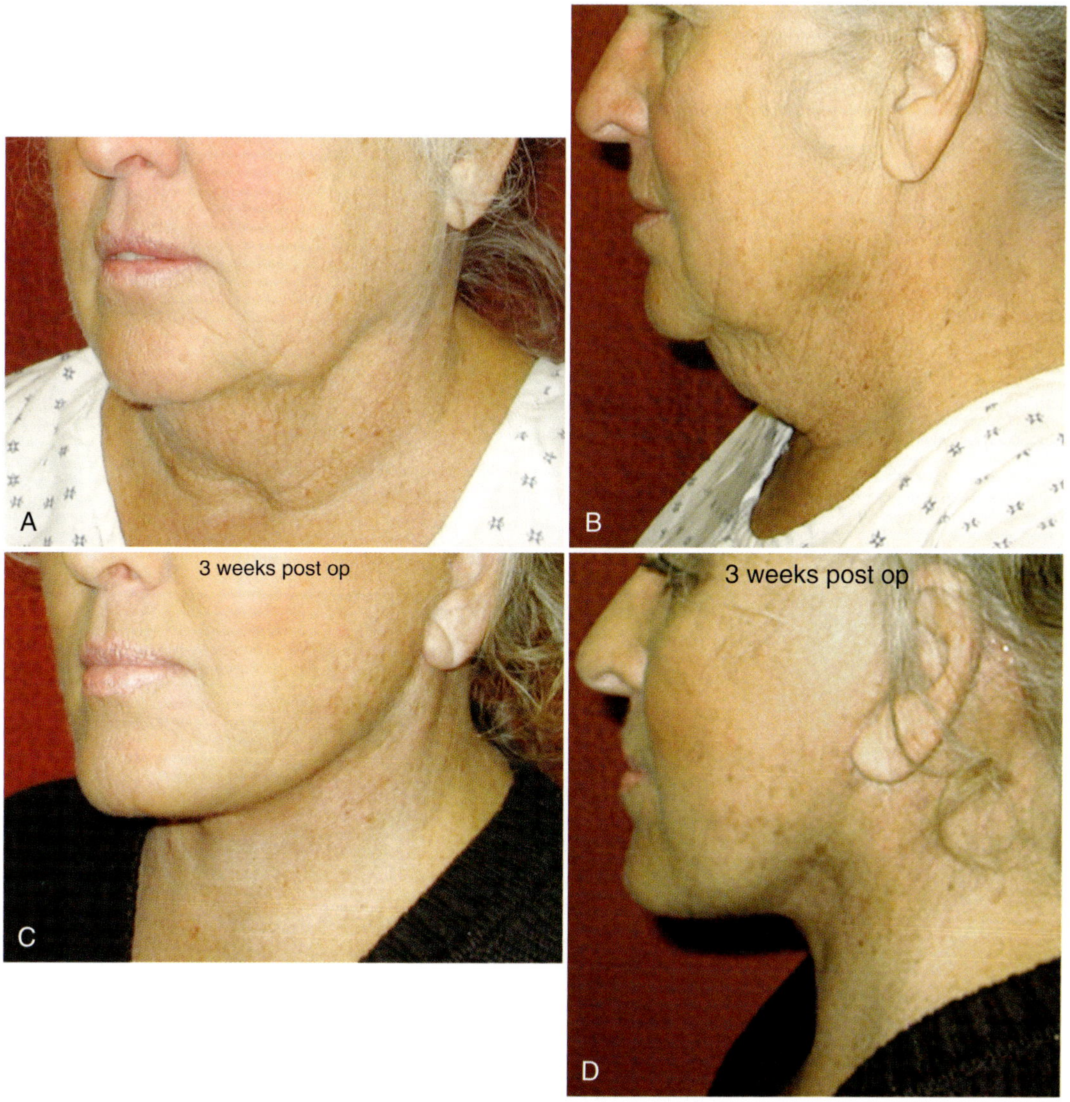

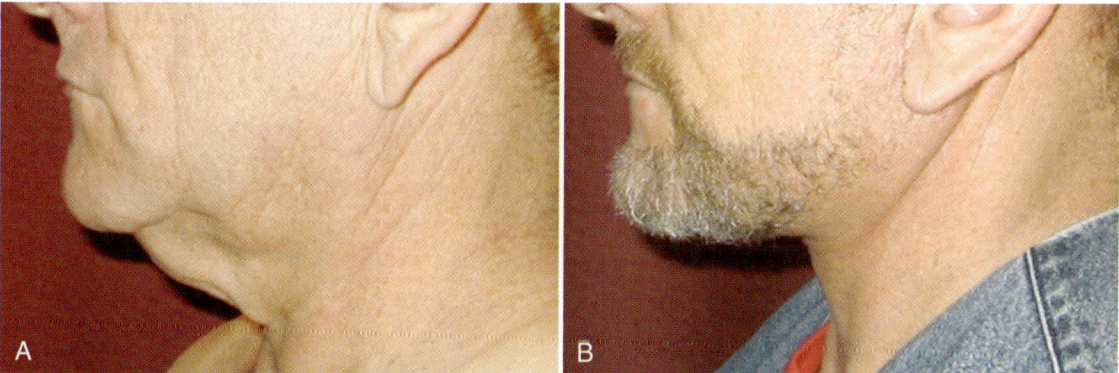

3 weeks post op

3 weeks post op

Fig. 107-72 ■ Seventy-year-old woman preoperatively (**A** and **B**) and 3 weeks postoperatively (**C** and **D**) following a lower face-lift and neck lift with associated submentoplasty. Significant deep (subplatysmal) fat was excised along with excision of redundant platysmal muscle. Both techniques are required when extreme skin laxity exists together with a large, heavy neck.

Fig. 107-73 ■ Extreme cutis laxa (**A**) requires a full lower face-lift and neck lift, often combined with aggressive submentoplasty. **B,** The results in this type of patient can be dramatic and have the potential to give the patient a very nice improvement.

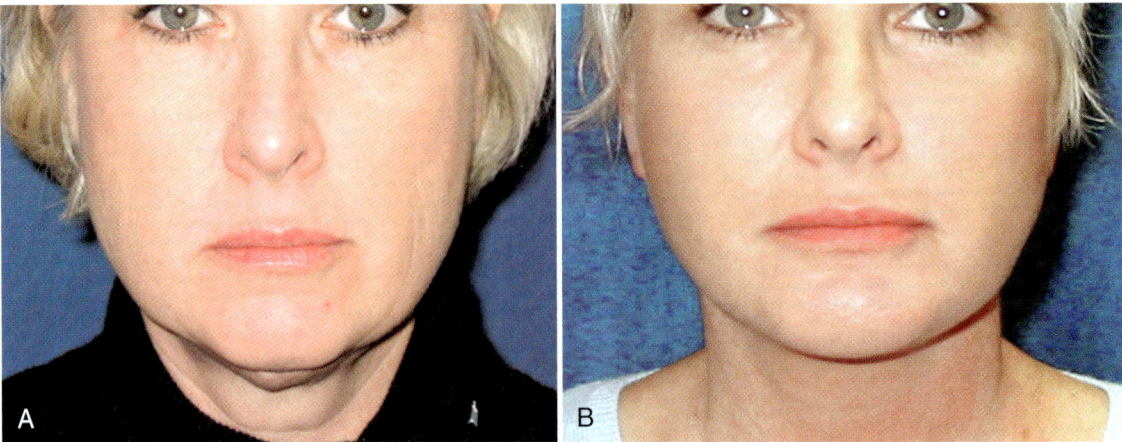

Fig. 107-74 ■ Lower face-lift and neck lift surgery offers significant rejuvenation, particularly in the jowls and submental areas: before (**A**) and after (**B**) a face-lift and chin implant.

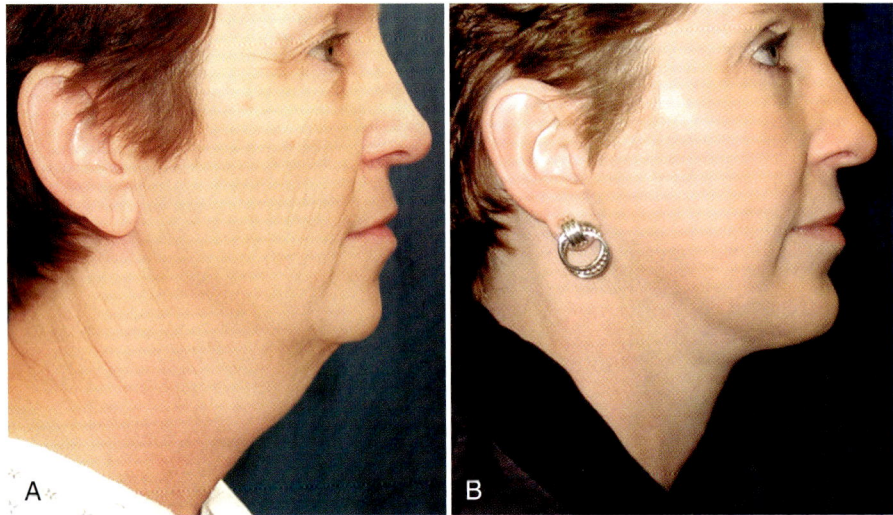

Fig. 107-75 ■ Patient before (**A**) and 1 year following a face-lift, submentoplasty, chin implant, and laser skin resurfacing (**B**). The face-lift, submentoplasty, and chin implant were used to give the dramatic change in neck profile appearance.

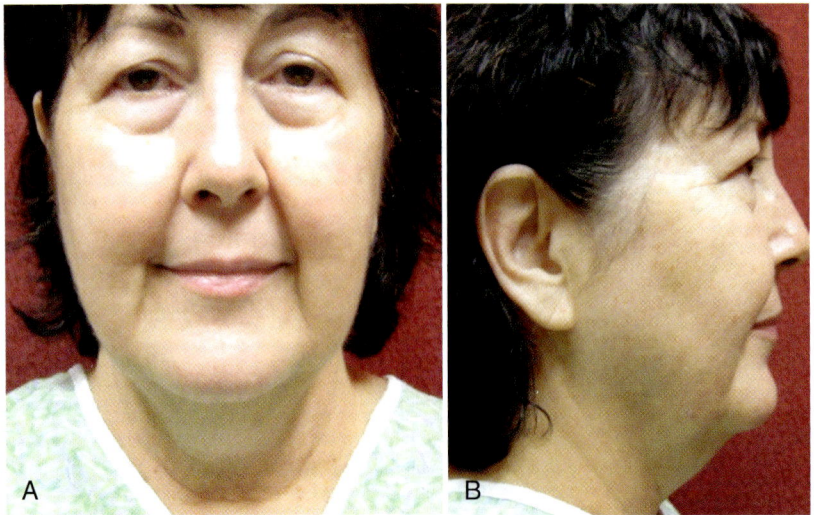

Fig. 107-76 ■ Patient before (**A** and **B**) and 2 months following a face-lift, submentoplasty, and blepharoplasties (**C** and **D**).

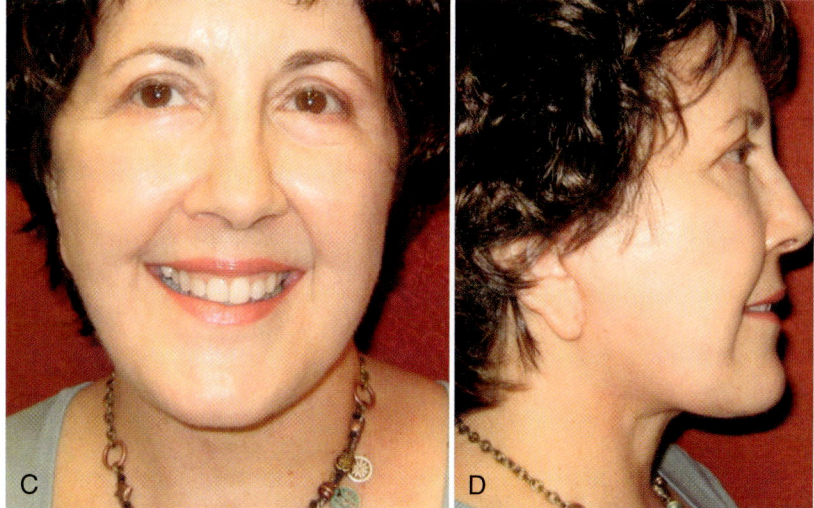

Fig. 107-76, cont'd.

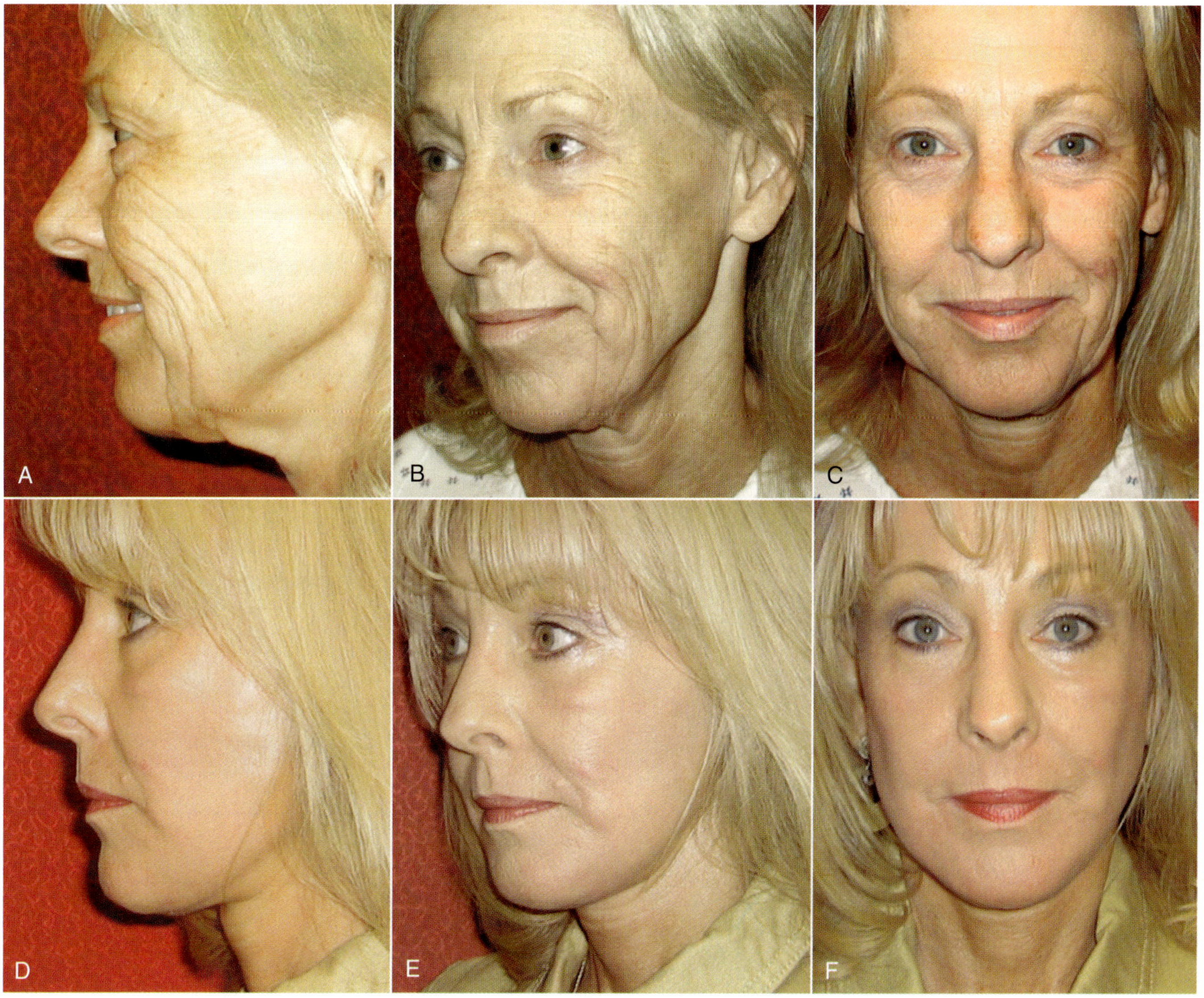

Fig. 107-77 ■ Patient before (**A** to **C**) and 6 months following a face-lift, fat grafting, and laser skin resurfacing (**D** to **F**).

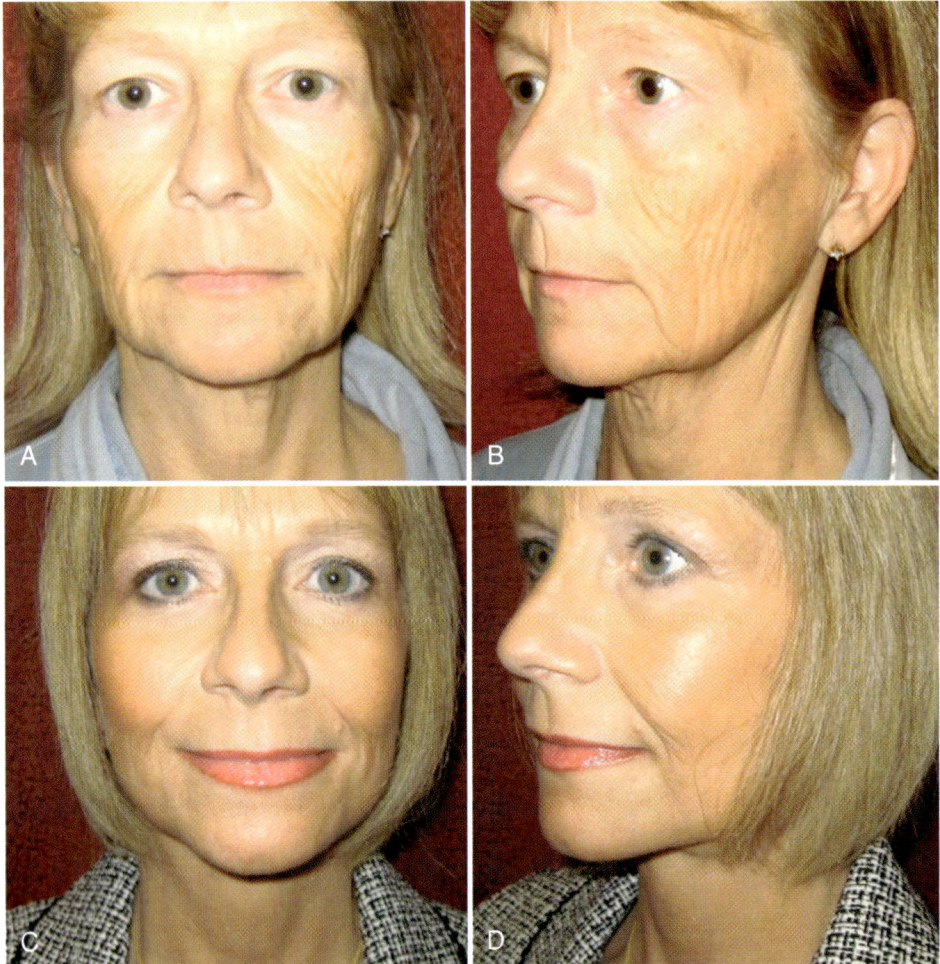

Fig. 107-78 ■ Patient before (**A** and **B**) and 6 months following a face-lift, fat grafting, cheek implants, and laser skin resurfacing (**C** and **D**).

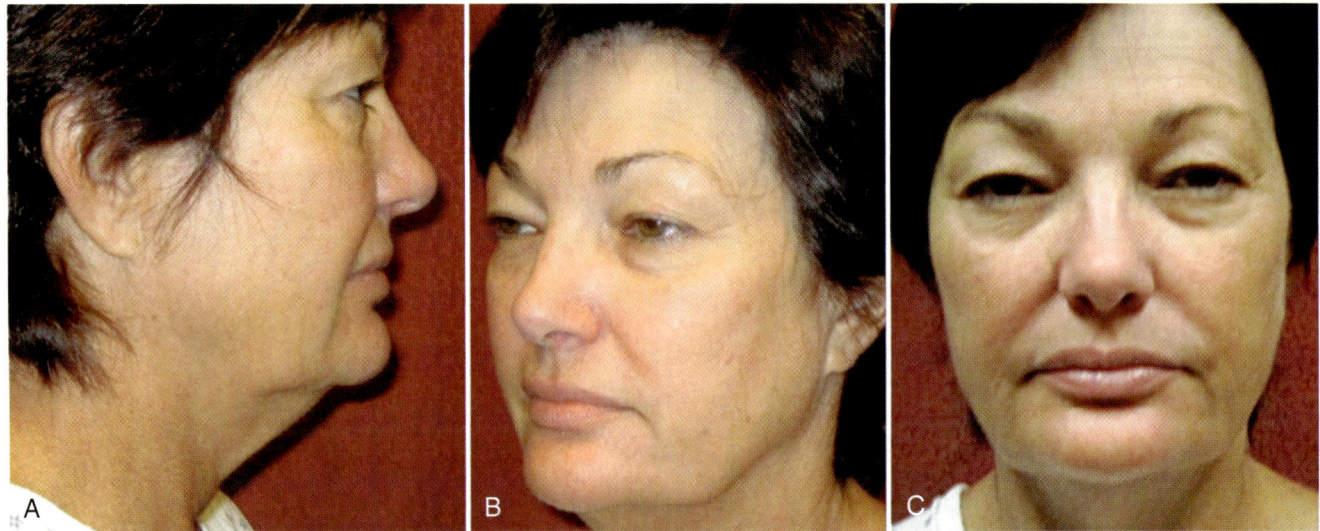

Fig. 107-79 ■ Patient before (**A** to **C**) and 6 months following a face-lift and blepharoplasties (**D** to **F**). Her neck improvement is significant but is not noticed as much as the major eyelid change.

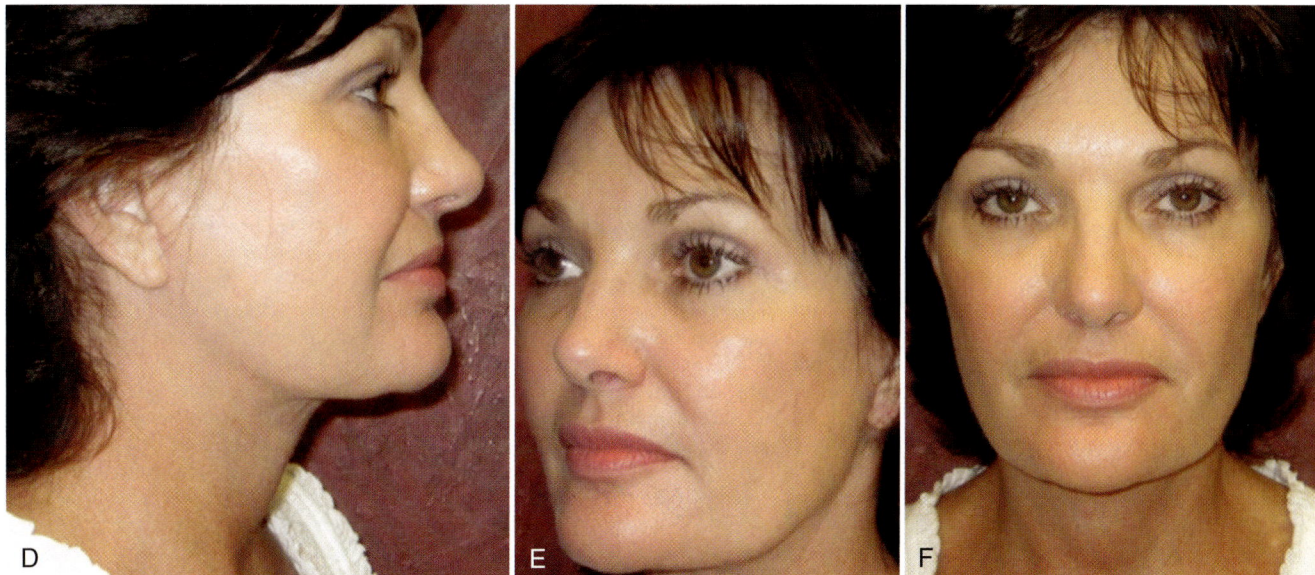

Fig. 107-79, cont'd.

through a difficult time. If revision surgery is contemplated, allowing adequate time for healing will improve the result, as well as avoid a surgical situation that appears panicky or rushed. Maintaining a positive attitude and empathizing with the patient are always helpful. Many dissatisfied patients seek other surgeons after the primary surgeon brushes off the complaint without paying attention or showing concern to the stressed patient.

CONCLUSION

Fortunately, patient satisfaction following face-lift surgery is high (more than 90% are pleased with the results). Selecting ideal patients with anatomy that would most benefit from jowl and neck lifting improves any surgeon's rate of successful outcomes (Figs. 107-73 to 107-75). Patients who would probably improve by minimal amounts or appear unrealistic are best avoided. Finally, face-lifting alone may not provide the improvement that a particular patient hopes to achieve. Assessing patients' goals for total facial rejuvenation and educating them on what can be achieved are

necessary to have a totally satisfied patient in many cases (Figs. 107-76 to 107-79). Knowing your limitations and working openly with patients can help prevent dissatisfaction (Box 107-3). Developing an ideal treatment plan based on the patient's chief complaint and a thorough examination and history of the present illness is just as important as performing the actual procedures.

BOX 107-3	Keys for Success in Lower Face-Lift Surgery

- Know your own limitations and learn to recognize which patients are difficult and *which are easy*!
- Be gentle and meticulous with soft tissues.
- Use your oral and maxillofacial surgical expertise to fully evaluate soft tissue and bone (*use implants* when helpful).
- Inform the patient of limitations and perform *only techniques* that will make a *significant difference* with the lowest risk possible.

PEARLS AND PITFALLS

- Thorough preoperative planning and preparation decrease the chance for complications. Should a problem occur, prompt attention and treatment are required to prevent further complications. Complications may be recognized intraoperatively, in the early postoperative period, or even months postoperatively.
- Cosmetic surgery patients are happy with their results when their preoperative expectations are met. Therefore, informed consent at the consultation visit must divulge to the patient what can reasonably be expected, as well as what potential problems may arise. Patient dissatisfaction is more often a result of lack of disclosure during the preoperative visit than a suboptimal cosmetic result. A patient whose unrealistic goals were not addressed will be dissatisfied despite what would be considered an acceptable surgical result.

- Complications can occur with any operation and should be dealt with candidly. Denying that a problem exists, no matter how trivial to the surgeon, can cause major dissatisfaction in the patient. Conversely, a problem that is dealt with in a straightforward manner benefits both the surgeon and patient. The patient should understand that additional surgery is sometimes necessary, strictly because of the nature of the surgery and the variability of patient healing.
- The potential face-lift complications are many. However, of the complications covered in this chapter, less than 4% are considered major problems that require reoperation.[18] The objective of the surgeon is to discern when a patient has a problem that requires immediate attention.

REFERENCES

1. Mitz V, Peyronie M: The superficial musculo-aponeurotic system (SMAS) in the parotid and cheek area, *Plast Reconstr Surg* 58:80-88, 1976.

2. Larrabee W, Ridenour B: Rhytidectomy: technique and complications, *Am J Otolaryngol* 13:1-15, 1992.

3. Skoog T: *Plastic surgery: new methods and refinements*, vol. 6, Philadelphia, 1974, WB Saunders, pp 300-330.

4. Webster RC, Davidson TM, White MF, et al: Conservative face-lift surgery, *Arch Otolaryngol* 102:657-662, 1976.

5. Ellis E, Zide MF: *Surgical approaches to the facial skeleton*, Baltimore, 1995, Williams & Wilkins.

6. Baker PC, Conley J: Avoiding facial nerve injuries in rhytidectomy. Anatomical variations and pitfalls, *Plast Reconstr Surg* 64:78-795, 1979.

7. Bernstein G: Surface landmarks for the identification of key anatomic structures of the face and neck, *J Dermatol Surg Oncol* 12:722-726, 1986.

8. Bentsianov B, Blitzer A: Facial anatomy, *Clin Dermatol* 22:3-13, 2004.

9. Burnham MA, Niamtu J. Facial nerves relevant to cosmetic surgery, *Oral Maxillofac Surg Clin North Am* 12:613-621, 2000.

10. Stuzin JM, Wagstrom L, Kawamoto HK, et al: Anatomy of the frontal branch of the facial nerve: the significance of the temporal fat pad, *Plast Reconstr Surg* 83:265-271, 1989.

11. Waite PO, Cuzalina LA: Rhytidectomy (face-lift), In Fonseca R, editor: *Oral and maxillofacial surgery*, Philadelphia, 2000, WB Saunders, pp 365-381.

12. Knobloch K, Gohritz A, Reuss E, et al: Nicotine in plastic surgery: a review, *Chirurg* 79:956-962, 2008.

13. McCullough EG, Beeson WH, Webster RC: Face-lift. In Beeson WH, McCollough EG, editors: *Aesthetic surgery of the aging face*, St Louis, 1986, CV Mosby, pp 71-128.

14. Man D: Premedication with oral clonidine for facial rhytidectomy, *Plast Reconstr Surg* 94:214-215, 1994.

15. Ramirez OM: The subperiosteal rhytidectomy: the third-generation face-lift, *Ann Plast Surg* 28:218-234, 1992.

16. Webster R, Smith R, Smith K. Face-lift, part IV: use of superficial musculoaponeurotic system suspending sutures, *Head Neck Surg* 6:780-791, 1984.

17. Har-Shai Y, Bodner SR, Egozy-Golan D, et al: Viscoelastic properties of the superficial musculoaponeurotic system SMAS: a microscopic and mechanical study, *Aesthetic Plast Surg* 21:219-224, 1997.

18. Beeson WH. Face-lift, *Facial Plast Surg Clin North Am* 131-277, 1993.

19. Pitanguy I, Ceravolo MP: Hematoma post-rhytidectomy: how we treat it, *Plast Reconstr Surg* 4:526-528, 1981.

20. Baker TJ, Gordon HL, Mesienko P: Rhytidectomy, *Plast Reconstr Surg* 59:24-30, 1977.

21. Goldwyn RM: Late bleeding after rhytidectomy from injury to the superficial temporal vessels, *Plast Reconstr Surg* 88:443-445, 1991.

22. Alexander RW: Cosmetic alterations of the aging neck: rhytidectomy, *Oral Maxillofac Surg Clin North Am* 2:247-257, 1990.

Chapter **108**

Blepharoplasty

Joseph D. Walrath, Brent R. Hayek, Ted Wojno

Upper and lower blepharoplasty is performed to treat prominent orbital fat, redundant skin and muscle, and other esthetic problems in the periocular region. Frequently, upper blepharoplasty is performed to remove excess skin that partially occludes the visual axis. Lower blepharoplasty is rarely indicated to treat a functional abnormality of the lower lids; rather, it is overwhelmingly cosmetic. Both procedures can have a dramatic impact on appearance and facial expression. Blepharoplasty can significantly alter the interaction, real or perceived, of patients within their social contexts; it can also disrupt specific ethnic features that are important in self-identity. When not performed carefully, blepharoplasty can lead to decreased vision, discomfort, deformity, and reoperation. Therefore, both careful patient selection and precise surgical technique are essential in the performance of upper and lower blepharoplasty.

ETIOPATHOGENESIS/CAUSATIVE FACTORS

Many potential factors can lead to the real or perceived prominence of orbital fat and excessive periocular skin and muscle. Studies have shown that orbital fat volume may increase with age. This process of orbital fat expansion can also be observed in an exaggerated fashion in a subset of patients with thyroid ophthalmopathy. Involutional changes in the orbital septum may further enhance the prominence of the orbital fat compartments. Skin can lose fixation to the underlying tissues and be stretched by the expanding or prolapsing orbital fat compartments. The lateral and medial canthal tendons can become lax as a result of senile changes or excessive

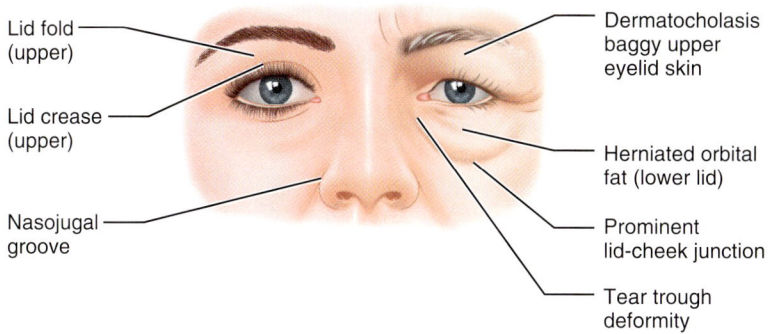

Lid fold (upper)

Lid crease (upper)

Nasojugal groove

Dermatocholasis baggy upper eyelid skin

Herniated orbital fat (lower lid)

Prominent lid-cheek junction

Tear trough deformity

Fig. 108-1 ■ Surface anatomy of the periocular region of a typical non-Asian patient in the youthful (*left*) and aging (*right*) state.

manipulation. Descent of the brows may occur and lead to the perception of excess skin between the brow and upper eyelashes. In addition, recurrent inflammatory or traumatic insults to the upper and lower eyelids can result in thinning of the tissues, redundancy of skin and muscle, loss of skin fixation, and laxity of the tendinous supporting structures of the upper and lower eyelids.

PATHOLOGIC ANATOMY

THE UPPER EYELID AND SURROUNDING TISSUE

Many excellent publications have detailed the anatomy of the periocular soft tissues. The upper eyelid crease and fold are essential elements of upper eyelid surface anatomy (Fig. 108-1); inattention to these aspects of anatomy can foil the surgical goal of a youthful appearance or, worse, alter important ethnic features. The upper eyelid crease is formed by the anterior attachments of the levator aponeurosis that pass through the orbicularis and insert onto the dermis; it is modulated by the mass of pre-aponeurotic orbital fat. This fat is confined by the orbital septum, which inserts variably onto the levator aponeurosis or superior tarsus. In non-Asians, the crease usually adopts a semilunar shape; in Asians, the crease is generally much flatter in curvature.

The eyelid fold is defined by the eyelid crease. It functions to provide tissue for recruitment when the eyelid closes, thereby preventing corneal exposure. Similar to the eyelid crease, it has significant ethnic variation. The eyelid fold is also modulated by the relative position of the brow; as the brow descends, the fold can become more prominent as the skin beneath the brow becomes redundant. Redundant upper eyelid skin is referred to as dermatochalasis. More subtly, there are patients with *apparent* excess skin who simply have lost deep fixation of the lid crease and consequently have a poorly defined lid-fold complex; not uncommonly, these patients have previously undergone eyelid surgery (Fig. 108-2).

The lid fold may or may not join smoothly into an epicanthal fold, a redundant bridge of skin that joins the upper and lower eyelids medially. There are several variants of epicanthal folds; in general, alteration of the structure of these folds should be avoided unless that is the specific surgical goal.

Contributing to the bulky appearance of the upper eyelid are the orbicularis oculi muscle, the pre-aponeurotic orbital fat, the lacrimal gland, and the retro–orbicularis oculi fat (ROOF). The pre-aponeurotic fat is composed of two distinct pockets, a larger central fat pocket and a smaller medial fat pocket. The medial pocket is deeper and whitish in appearance and contains the medial palpebral artery. Deeper structures that are easily avoided during upper blepharoplasty are the supraorbital bundle and the trochlea (Fig. 108-3). The lacrimal gland, however, is often encountered and is easily dealt

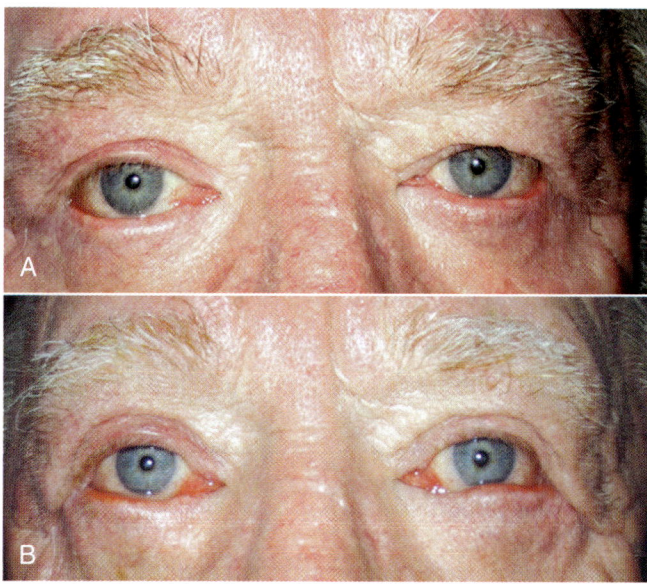

Fig. 108-2 ■ Poor crease fixation. **A,** Preoperatively, the patient demonstrates loss of crease fixation in the left upper lid that gives the appearance of excess skin. **B,** Surgical restoration of the skin crease without any actual skin removal.

with. The ROOF is preseptal and is partially responsible for the appearance of "heaviness" of the sub-brow tissue in some patients (Fig. 108-4). In Asians, the ROOF often extends inferiorly toward the pretarsal space.

THE LOWER EYELID AND SURROUNDING TISSUE

The surface anatomy of the lower eyelid has several important cosmetic elements (see Fig. 108-1). The lid-cheek junction delineates the inferior orbital rim and is accentuated by the orbital septum, arcus marginalis, and orbitomalar ligament. A prominent nasojugal groove, known as a tear trough deformity, can be of cosmetic importance and is often the target for periocular injectable fillers or fat repositioning. Younger patients may also have lower eyelid folds. Nasally, an epicanthal fold may extend from the lower lid toward the upper lid.

There are three anterior orbital fat pockets in the lower lid. The medial and central fat pockets are separated by the inferior oblique muscle, which is frequently encountered during lower blepharoplasty and should be left untouched. The arcuate expansion of the inferior oblique separates the central and lateral pockets and can be violated without consequence. The lacrimal sac is deep and medial to the nasal fat pocket and is easily avoided. The medial palpebral

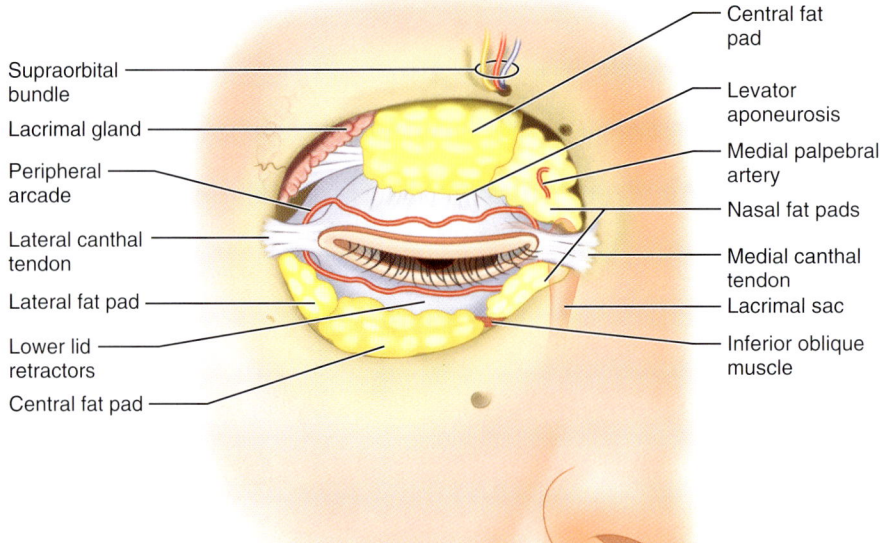

Fig. 108-3 ▪ Anatomy of the anterior orbit. The surgeon will often encounter the lacrimal gland and the inferior oblique muscle during upper and lower blepharoplasty. The former can be repositioned, and the latter should be left untouched.

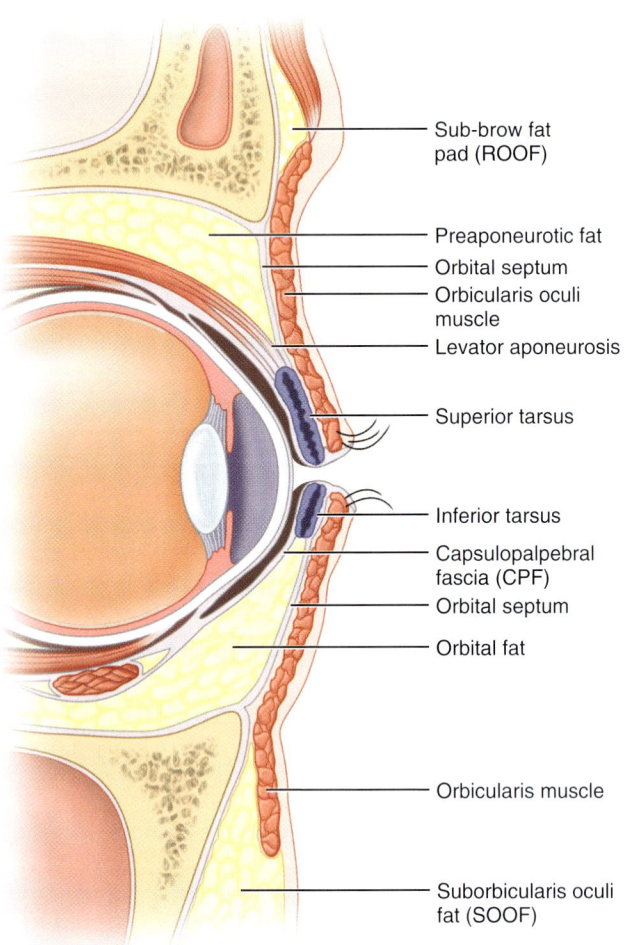

Fig. 108-4 ▪ Cross-sectional anatomy of the anterior orbit.

artery is often encountered in the medial fat pocket and frequently requires attention (see Fig. 108-3).

DIAGNOSTIC STUDIES

When upper blepharoplasty is performed for functional, vision-limiting purposes, visual field documentation is required for reimbursement by most insurers. A technician manually maps a patient's visual field for each eye in the native state with the use of a Goldmann perimeter (Fig. 108-5). The technician then tapes the redundant lid skin up and repeats the test to demonstrate the functional improvement achieved when tissue is withdrawn from the visual axis. This test can also be performed with an automated perimeter.

Generally speaking, in patients with abnormalities of eyelid position or function, it is inappropriate to perform blepharoplasty unless the clinician is prepared to diagnose and treat these problems as well. Additionally, there are many patients who seek referral for "puffiness" of the upper eyelids who have subclinical thyroid eye disease. The most common abnormality on physical examination in these patients is mild upper or lower eyelid retraction, which may or may not result in a thyroid eye disease "stare." The upper eyelids normally rest 1 to 2 mm below the superior border of the cornea. Any white "scleral show" above the limbus when the eyelids are at rest is abnormal and should prompt an ophthalmologic evaluation. If there is an abnormal amount of sub-brow tissue or if the sub-brow fullness varies diurnally, serologic evaluation of the patient's thyroid status and possibly a medical or ophthalmic evaluation are warranted. Operating on a patient with active thyroid eye disease can lead to significant inflammation, which can occasionally be vision threatening.

Finally, if the patient has a history of a bleeding disorder, this needs to be fully evaluated before surgery. The most feared complication of blepharoplasty is loss of vision, and in the rare instance of this complication, the proximal cause is usually orbital hemorrhage. We insist that patients stop taking aspirin and non-steroidal anti-inflammatory drugs for 2 weeks, clopidogrel for 7 days, and warfarin for 5 days before surgery. Patients are also told to abstain from other substances that adversely affect bleeding time, such as vitamin

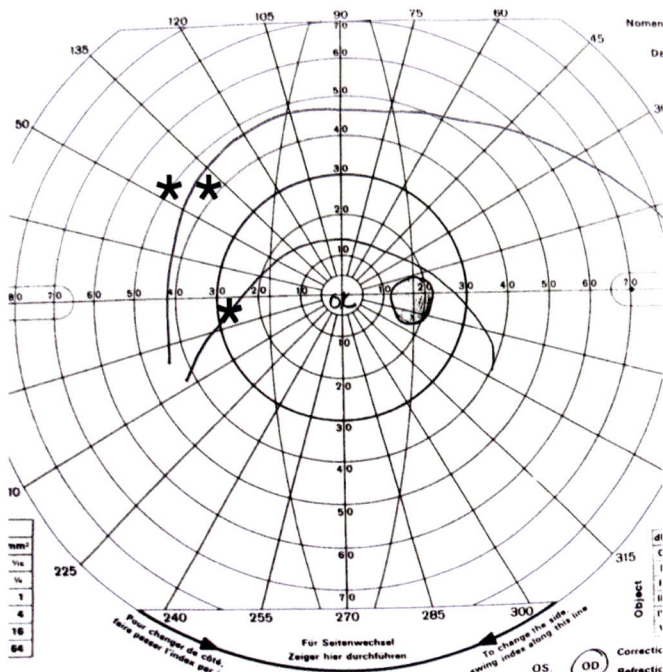

Fig. 108-5 ■ Visual field demonstrating the functional significance of dermatochalasis. This field has been mapped from the right eye of a patient by a technician trained in use of the Goldmann perimeter. The lower arc (*) delineates the extent of the visual field with the upper eyelid in its native state. When the excess lid skin is taped up, the visual field is significantly increased (**). The blind spot is seen to the right of the fixation point.

E, omega-3 fatty acids, and certain types of ethnic medicinal substances, such as Reishi mushrooms (known as *ling zhi* in China).

TREATMENT/RECONSTRUCTIVE GOALS

There is some debate about the features of the ocular adnexa that make a face appear youthful. Although our surgical approach in the upper eyelids is often to remove tissue from the lids, orbit, and sub-brow space, many think that this fullness of the upper eyelid and sub-brow space evokes a youthful appearance. However, most would agree that in older patients, when the skin becomes atrophic and loses some of its deep attachments, the orbital fat pockets prolapse, and the brow descends, the resultant fullness in the sub-brow space is not evocative of youthfulness.

In the lower lids, prominent inferior orbital fat pockets and "baggy" lids can make a patient appear old or tired. Conversely, a prominent lid-cheek junction, a "hollow" look, can also make a patient appear skeletonized and elderly. Notwithstanding the clinician's bias, it is most important to recognize that patients themselves usually have specific cosmetic and functional complaints and that a well-executed surgery that does not address these complaints is destined to be a failure.

SPECIFIC TREATMENT AND TECHNIQUES

UPPER BLEPHAROPLASTY

The Preoperative Evaluation

Before performing upper blepharoplasty, a careful evaluation needs to be conducted to determine the underlying functional and/or cosmetic issues important to the patient. Specifically, if true

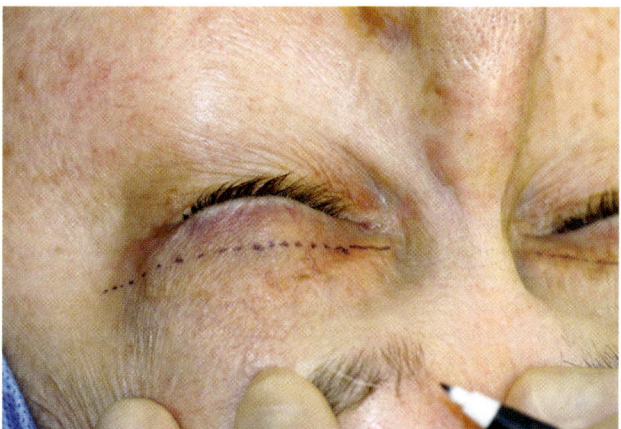

Fig. 108-6 ■ The crease is marked and the incision is extended nasally no further than the visible extent of the medial canthal tendon and temporally to a variable degree, depending on the amount of excess skin.

blepharoptosis is noted, it needs to be addressed surgically at the time of blepharoplasty. Similarly, if significant brow ptosis is found, it might also need to be addressed at the time of blepharoplasty. Several other components of the upper eyelid esthetic examination need to be addressed, including the degree of excess skin (if any), the degree of excess anterior orbital fat (if any), the quality of the skin fixation, the height and quality of the skin crease, the presence or absence of epicanthal folds, and the position of the lacrimal gland. It is often helpful to simulate the surgical end point for the patient by using a blunt instrument or cotton-tipped applicator to gather up the sub-brow skin in front of a handheld mirror. The right and left sides should be compared for symmetry.

Patient Preparation and Marking

In the preoperative holding area, the office findings are reviewed and confirmed. For procedures performed in a surgical center, we prefer to mark the patient with a sterile marking pen after the full face preparation has been completed while the patient is supine. It can be helpful to make a mental note of the difference in the appearance of the lids when the patient is supine and when seated upright. Occasionally, a medial canthal web or prominent fat pocket will be visible only in the upright position. It is important to limit irritating stimuli while measuring and marking the skin excision by keeping surgical lamps turned away and placing drops of an ophthalmic topical anesthetic in both eyes before face preparation.

Patients are asked to open and close their eyes, which will highlight the position of the skin crease. If the crease is strong, the incision will occasionally be marked along that skin crease. As a general rule, in non-Asian adults the authors mark the incision 10 mm from the lid margin centrally, 9 mm from the lid margin temporally, and 6 mm from the lid margin nasally. In general, this corresponds to the top of the tarsal plate and will become the new lid crease. A smooth curve connects the three points (Fig. 108-6). This curve continues medially for a few millimeters, parallel to and above the medial canthal tendon. It extends temporally to a variable distance beyond the lateral orbital rim, depending on the degree of excess tissue that will be removed. In patients with well-defined creases preoperatively, it is reasonable to utilize these creases. However, right and left should still be measured to ensure symmetry. In the Asian upper eyelid, the crease mark is usually placed at the top of the tarsal plate; however, the tarsal plate is much shorter in Asians, so the values are significantly less. In some cases, Asian patients prefer a crease that is even lower. Typically, the crease has a flatter curvature as well. The position and shape of the skin crease need to be negotiated before surgery on Asian patients.

The amount of skin to be removed varies greatly from patient to patient and, uncommonly, between the right and left sides of the same patient. In general, the residual skin between the thick skin of the brow (which typically is present several millimeters below the brow hairs) and incision line should be at least 1 cm, but it may be 1.5 cm or more, depending on the patient. It should also be noted that many patients modify their brow positions artificially by hair removal or brow painting, and these modifications may disguise inherent brow asymmetry or descent. Utilizing the transition point between the thick skin of the brow and the thin skin of the eyelid, instead of the brow hairs, is more reliable when determining the extent of the skin excision. It is important to negotiate with the patient and to occasionally review photographs from the patient's youth to help establish the specific surgical end point.

The width of the planned skin excision is marked over the central eyelid with the use of Green forceps, which gently gather up the loose skin between the previously marked lid crease incision and the brow. There should be no tension on the lid margin when the excess skin is gathered to prevent overly aggressive skin excision and possible lagophthalmos. Green forceps are again used over the temporal eyelid. A smooth line is traced from markings and tapered medially and laterally to connect with the lid crease marking (Fig. 108-7). Depending on the degree of excess skin, the excision can be carried into a crow's foot quite far laterally, perhaps a centimeter or more beyond the lateral orbital rim. It is sometimes useful to mark the temporal extent of the dermatochalasis while the patient is sitting up in the holding area, to aid in this determination. Nasally, the skin excision should not extend more than a millimeter or two nasal to the puncta, to avoid web formation or unsightly scarring in this critical area. Care again needs to be taken when designing the skin excision in Asian patients because it is usually significantly less than in non-Asian patients. In these patients the amount of skin excision should be carefully negotiated preoperatively. It is safer to excise less tissue and revise in the office later in these patients.

If repair of brow ptosis is to be performed, it is done before blepharoplasty. The area of eyelid skin designated for removal is less than it would be for the same patient undergoing blepharoplasty alone. The upper lid skin excision can be marked beforehand while manually fixating the brow in the desired position before the start of the procedure. It is helpful to mark the upper lid before surgically fixating the brow because significant lid edema may develop intraoperatively during the brow portion of the surgery and make it more difficult to determine the appropriate skin excision.

In some patients the skin excision should be marked more conservatively than our standard approach. In patients with significant prolapsed orbital fat that is going to be excised, removal of the fat sculpts a relative concavity, which will require maintenance of a larger surface area for the residual skin. Finally, it has been our experience that the skin excision in many patients with a history of Graves orbitopathy should be more conservative than in other patients because of their "thicker" skin and subcutaneous tissue. It is self-evident that a conservative skin excision can be increased quite easily, whereas the situation is much more difficult after an overly aggressive skin excision.

In general, the skin excision for the contralateral upper eyelid is marked in similar fashion, with the exception that the overall size of the skin incision can usually be transposed from the first eyelid. The surgeon can compare the distance between the inferior border of the brow and the upper edge of the proposed skin excision to verify the symmetry of the markings. Additionally, observing the markings while having the patient look up and down will further confirm the symmetry of the proposed skin excision.

The Dissection

After marking the skin, a total of about 1 to 1.5 mL of local anesthetic is injected subcutaneously into each upper lid during a brief period of monitored sedation. The authors use a 50/50 mixture of 2% lidocaine (with 1:100,000 epinephrine) and 0.75% bupivacaine, with hyaluronidase added in a ratio of 1 mL per 9 mL of anesthetic. Hyaluronidase, combined with gentle massage, distributes the anesthetic evenly and lessens the tissue distortion and turgor caused by the injection.

A No. 15 blade is used for the skin incision. Skin and orbicularis muscle are then sharply excised with Westcott scissors. Care is taken when excising along the inferior skin edge to avoid disruption of the underlying levator aponeurosis. Following skin-muscle excision, the orbital septum with underlying pre-aponeurotic fat should be visible (Fig. 108-8). The septum is opened widely with Westcott scissors. If the orbital septum and fat are not easily visible because of residual overlying orbicularis, the surgeon applies digital pressure with the ring finger to retropulse the globe and prolapse the fat anteriorly beneath the orbicularis; the resultant bulge is the pre-aponeurotic fat, which lies superior to the levator and is the target for sharp dissection. After the septum is opened, the capsule surrounding the pre-aponeurotic fat (the "second septum") is sharply incised.

An assistant provides downward traction on the upper lid to moderately stretch the levator aponeurosis. The surgeon grasps and

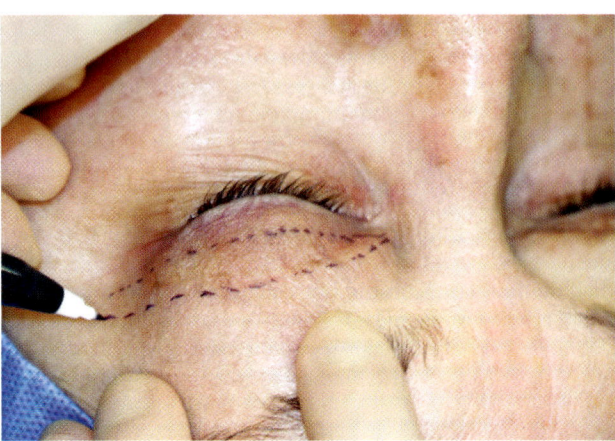

Fig. 108-7 ■ The desired skin excision is marked.

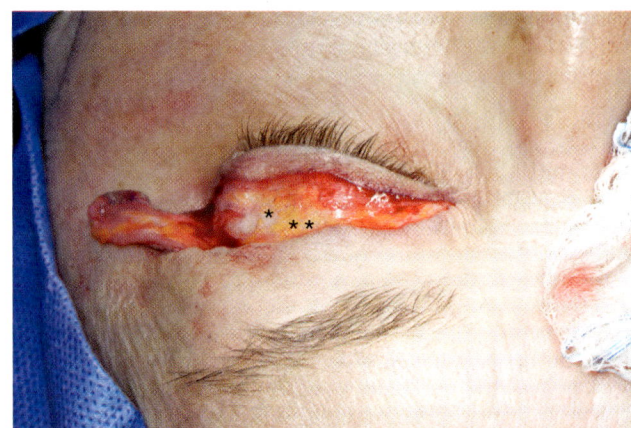

Fig. 108-8 ■ Dissection to the orbital septum. The skin and orbicularis are reflected, along with a portion of the orbital septum. The levator aponeurosis (*) is whitish and visible deep to the orbital fat (**).

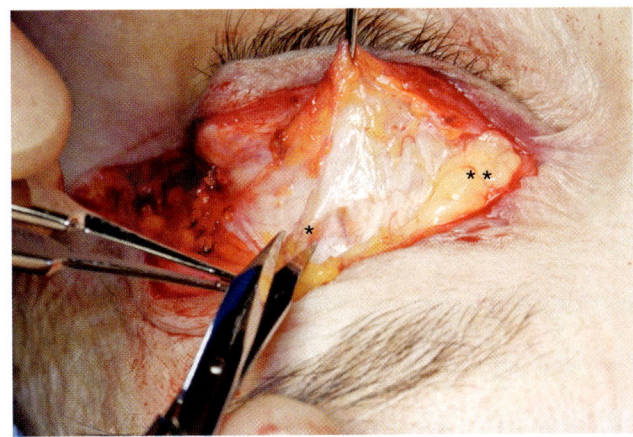

Fig. 108-9 ■ Fat is dissected free from the underlying levator aponeurosis. Numerous fine attachments (*) are present in the natural plane between fat and the levator. The nasal fat pocket is exposed (**).

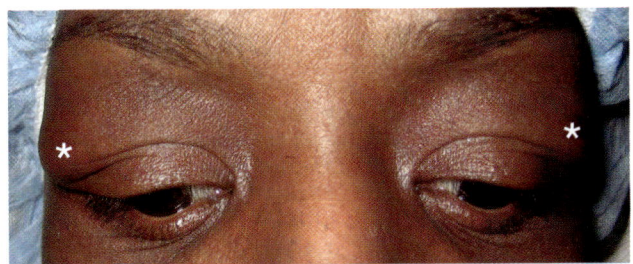

Fig. 108-10 ■ A patient with prominent lacrimal glands (*). The excess tissue in the pre-aponeurotic space creates multiple lid creases temporally. A tissue deficit in this space can also cause multiple lid creases. During blepharoplasty, lacrimal gland biopsy was performed.

lifts the pre-aponeurotic fat directly while snipping the wispy bands between the central fat pocket and the levator aponeurosis (Fig. 108-9). If need be, the central fat pocket is sharply dissected from the grayish lobular tissue of the lacrimal gland laterally; this often requires additional local anesthetic injected directly into the gland and nearly always necessitates additional cautery as well. The central fat is then clamped with a mosquito hemostat, cut, cauterized with bipolar cautery, and released. Next, the medial fat pocket is identified; this usually requires additional dissection and possibly slight extension of the skin incision medially. There is a potential for brisk bleeding from the medial palpebral artery, which can be controlled with bipolar cautery. The medial pocket is recognizable because it is characteristically much whiter than the central fat pocket. It is also often sensitive to manipulation, thus requiring supplemental local anesthetic injected directly into the fat. The nasal fat is decapsulated with Westcott scissors, clamped with a mosquito hemostat, trimmed, and cauterized.

Small amounts of residual fat will often retract with point applications of cautery, which will shrink the fat capsule. This same approach can shrink a mildly prominent or anteriorly displaced lacrimal gland. Occasionally, the gland is located too far anteriorly and needs to be surgically repositioned (Fig. 108-10). The upper skin edge of the blepharoplasty incision is elevated with a rake or Desmarres retractor, and sharp dissection is carried down to the superolateral orbital rim; because there are no vital structures to avoid during this dissection, it can be performed rapidly. A single 6-0 braided non-absorbable suture can be passed through the substance of the gland and secured directly to the periosteum of the inner aspect of the superolateral rim, thereby repositioning the gland. If the glands are enlarged, biopsy is warranted. This is the same dissection that one performs when executing a browpexy, except that the lateral third of the brow is fixated to the periosteum superior to the orbital rim.

Skin Closure

It is critical to recreate a lid crease during closure; failure to do so can lead to the late appearance of excess "baggy" skin, which in fact is not redundant but rather poorly fixated (see Fig. 108-2). The authors prefer 6-0 braided non-absorbable suture for crease augmentation. The basic principle is to replicate the native slips of levator aponeurosis that pass anteriorly into the pretarsal orbicularis in the unoperated state. The lower skin edge (pretarsal) is gently smoothed out and placed where it will rest when the skin closure is complete. The skin is then secured in this position, directly to the levator, at two paracentral sites. For each site the authors use forceps to lift the levator aponeurosis beneath the presumptive site of skin fixation, pass a 6-0 non-absorbable suture through the aponeurosis, and then secure it to the skin edge in a subcuticular pass. The knot is buried.

The most difficult part of the skin closure involves the nasal aspect, where excess skin results in focal "puffiness" and skin shortage results in medial canthal webbing. Surgical alteration of this region, as well as right-left asymmetry, can have a dramatic cosmetic effect. The natural quality of the patient's skin fixation medially, combined with surgical dissection and tissue edema, can lead to poor fixation over the nasal fat pocket. Frequently, removal of the underlying nasal fat pocket leaves a relative concavity underlying the medial skin that contributes to the focal appearance of skin excess. To line this concavity and deeply fixate the skin, the authors often use one or two interrupted 6-0 fast-absorbing plain gut stitches to close the nasal aspect of the skin incision. The closure incorporates a bite of the medial levator aponeurosis or the medial fat capsule, and the skin is pulled down into the recess to eliminate some of the "puffiness." The remaining skin incision can be closed with running 6-0 non-absorbable suture such as polypropylene, which is removed in 5 to 7 days. It is helpful to use a bolster on the medial aspect of the closure, usually a sterile segment of rubber band, because the area can become quite swollen and make suture removal difficult and painful for the patient.

In Asian patients, significantly more attention is paid to the crease. Four or five buried non-absorbable sutures are inserted to form the crease in the manner described previously. In addition, several interrupted 6-0 silk sutures that incorporate bites of the levator aponeurosis are placed for the skin closure. The inflammatory silk sutures lead to good adhesion between the levator and the skin edge. The remaining skin is closed with running 6-0 polypropylene. The sutures are removed in 5 to 7 days.

LOWER BLEPHAROPLASTY

The Preoperative Evaluation

Redressing skin excess is often part of the surgical plan when performing lower blepharoplasty, particularly in older patients. Adequate stability of lid position in the event of potential skin excision should be ensured, usually with horizontal tightening of the lower lids. The need for some degree of additional skin excision and redraping is the reason why the authors infrequently perform blepharoplasty via a transconjunctival approach alone. However, in many younger patients with youthful skin and good lid tone, transconjunctival blepharoplasty is appropriate.

In most patients, fat excision will also be part of the surgical plan. However, in patients with mild to moderate fat prolapse and a prominent lid-cheek junction, the authors sometimes choose to reset

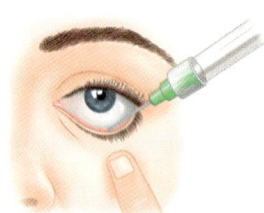

A Needle injects from underside of eyelid, ballooning up the subconjunctival space.

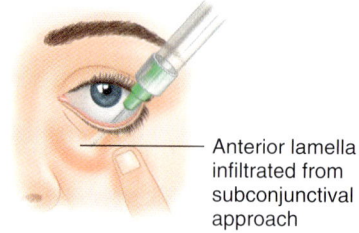

Anterior lamella infiltrated from subconjunctival approach

B Then needle is advanced, and injection is carried out in the suborbicularis space.

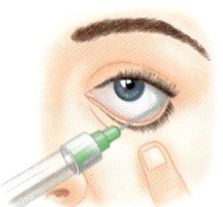

C Needle injects outside corner of eyelid, transconjunctivally.

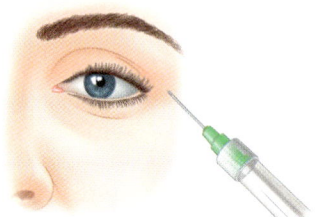

D Needle injects straight down onto lateral orbital rim.

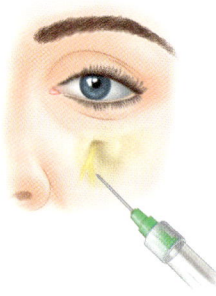

E Needle performs infraorbital block for septal reset variation.

Fig. 108-11 ■ Injecting the lower lids to prepare for blepharoplasty. Transconjunctival injection is performed through the lower eyelid to balloon the subconjunctival space. The needle is then advanced and further injection is carried out in the suborbicularis space. The lateral canthus is also injected transconjunctivally.

the orbital septum anteriorly, with little or no fat removal. This creates a smoother transition from lid to cheek. Fat can also be positioned in the preperiosteal plane to lessen the tear trough deformity.

The Dissection

During a brief period of monitored sedation, transconjunctival injection of local anesthetic is performed, initially subconjunctivally and then deeper into the subcutaneous space. The lateral canthus is also injected transconjunctivally. A supplemental percutaneous injection is performed onto the lateral orbital rim. A total of roughly 3 mL can be used for each side. In general, the lower eyelids require more extensive infiltration with local anesthetic than do the uppers. If septal reset is being considered, an infraorbital block is performed (Fig. 108-11).

When performing simultaneous upper and lower blepharoplasty, it is important to keep the incisions separated laterally by approximately 1 cm to avoid lateral webbing. In such cases the surgeon angles the lower skin incision inferiorly (Fig. 108-12). The surgeon

starts by making a 1- to 2-cm-long incision lateral to the orbital rim and adjacent to but not including the lateral canthus. The incision is made through skin and muscle. Hemostasis is achieved with bipolar cautery. Stevens scissors are used for blunt dissection in the suborbicularis (preseptal) plane along the entire length of the lower lid; this is a natural plane and the dissection can be performed rapidly (Fig. 108-13). The Stevens scissors are then used to incise the skin-muscle flap in a subciliary line. This incision is beveled so that a cuff of orbicularis is left on the remaining lid margin. It is best to make this incision approximately 1 to 2 mm below the lashes. If closer to the lash line than this, closure may result in sutures being too close to the surface of the eye.

An assistant retracts the skin-muscle flap inferiorly while hemostasis is achieved. At this point the orbital septum and underlying fat should easily be visible (Fig. 108-14). In a manner analogous to upper blepharoplasty, the surgeon cuts into the inferior orbital fat directly while avoiding the underlying lower lid retractors (the analogue to the levator aponeurosis of the upper lid). The three inferior fat pockets are exposed; the nasal fat pocket is the deepest. It is not

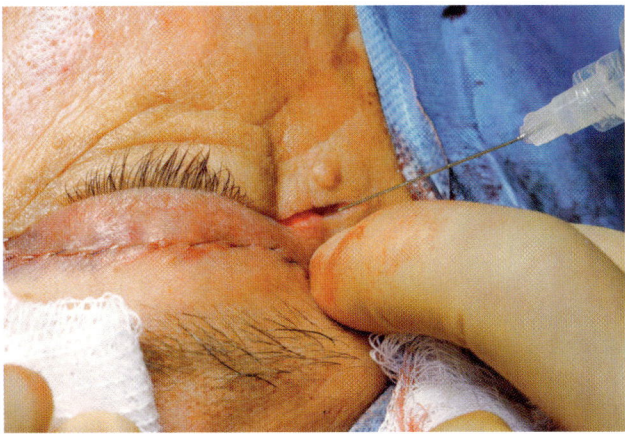

Fig. 108-12 ■ Lower lid incision demonstrated. The incision is angled inferiorly away from the upper lid incision.

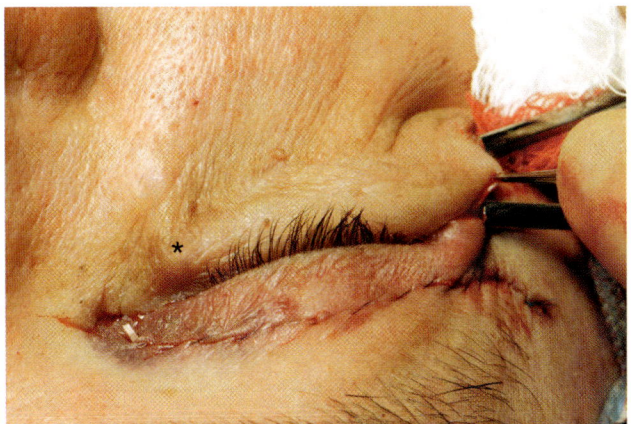

Fig. 108-13 ■ Undermining the skin muscle flap. The tips of Stevens scissors can be seen beneath the flap medially (*).

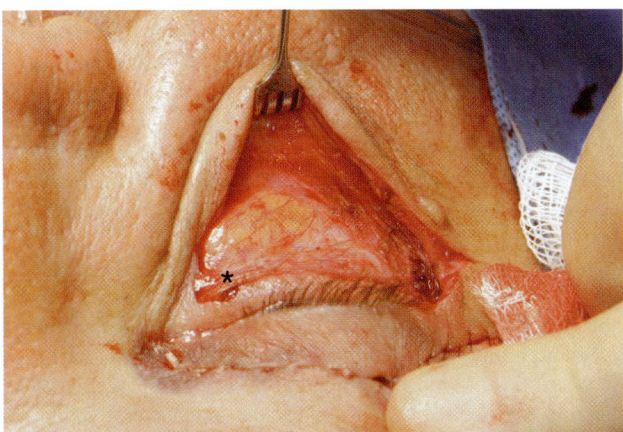

Fig. 108-14 ■ Skin-muscle flap reflected. The underlying orbital septum and fat are easily visualized. A cuff of orbicularis remains on the lid (*).

unusual to see the inferior oblique as it courses between the nasal and central fat pockets. Damage to this muscle can lead to torsional diplopia, which can be disabling. Similar to the upper nasal fat pocket, the lower nasal fat pocket contains a medial palpebral artery that can bleed briskly. In addition, this fat pocket also often needs a supplemental injection of local anesthetic. Fat is clamped, cut, and cauterized.

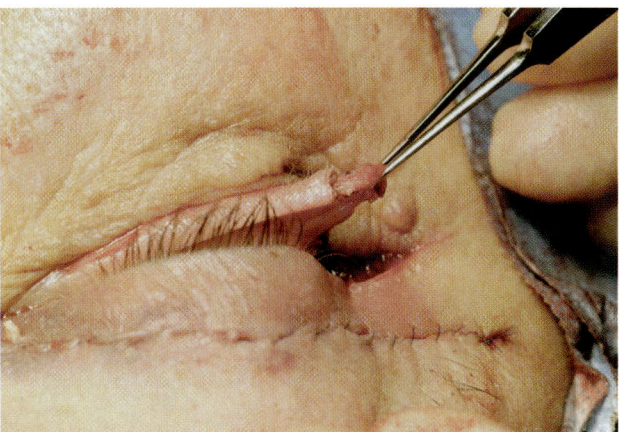

Fig. 108-15 ■ Lateral tarsal strip completed.

In anticipation of vertical shortening of the lid skin-muscle flap after redraping, it is important to anchor the lower lid firmly to prevent any resultant lower lid retraction. This is accomplished by horizontally shortening the lower lid and refixating it to the lateral orbital rim, a process referred to as canthoplasty. Blunt Westcott scissors are used to perform a full-thickness canthotomy. This will connect to the previously made skin-muscle incision just outside the lateral canthus. The periosteum of the lateral orbital rim is exposed with the Westcott scissors. Lower crus cantholysis is performed while the surgeon distracts the lower lid inferiorly and feels for complete release of the lid with each snip. In general, the cantholysis can be carried out just beneath the inferior border of the lateral tarsus. The lateral end of the lid is then grasped with forceps and pulled toward the lateral orbital rim so that an estimate of the requisite amount of horizontal shortening can be made.

The surgeon then prepares the lower eyelid for reattachment to the lateral orbital rim. Sharp Westcott scissors are used to excise the mucous membrane that forms the margin of the lower lid, as well as the skin and muscle anterior to the tarsus in the region to be reattached to the rim (Fig. 108-15). Light bipolar cautery is usually necessary. The lid is then anchored to the inner aspect of the lateral orbital rim periosteum with 4-0 absorbable or non-absorbable suture material (Fig. 108-16). It is helpful to distract the globe and orbital contents medially with a cotton-tipped applicator to allow some room for this suture pass. A second suture is placed to further support the lid to the periosteum of the outer aspect of the rim. The excess length of tarsal strip is removed, if any.

The position along the lateral rim at which the lower lid is repositioned is critical. In a patient with eyes of average prominence, the lid should be snug against the globe such that grasping it with forceps centrally can distract it only 1-2 mm from the globe. However, it is difficult to attain this degree of tension in patients with prominent eyes because doing so will cause the lids to "bowstring" beneath the eye. In these patients the end point is one of less tension, with the lid being anchored slightly superiorly onto the lateral orbital rim. Occasionally, the lower lid retractors will need to be incised to allow greater elevation of the lower lid. In the most prominent eyes, a spacer graft such as autogenous ear cartilage or one of the numerous commercially available xenografts is interposed within the lower lid retractors to provide further vertical support.

Lateral Canthopexy Variation

Some surgeons advocate canthopexy, as opposed to canthoplasty, for horizontally supporting the lid. This procedure simply involves passing a 4-0 suture through the tarsus of the lateral lid and

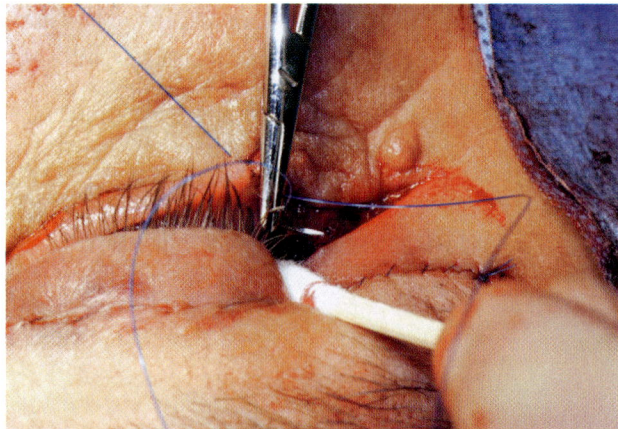

Fig. 108-16 ▪ Lateral tarsal strip reattached. The strip is secured to the inner aspect of the lateral orbital rim periosteum.

anchoring it to the periosteum of the inner aspect of the lateral orbital rim, without any true lid shortening. It may be possible to achieve appropriate tension in the lower lid in many cases with this technique.

Septal Reset Variation

In patients with prominent lid-cheek junctions, the authors occasionally perform a septal reset in which the septum is opened only inferiorly and secured across the anterior face of the inferior orbital rim. The inferior orbital rim is exposed beneath the skin-muscle flap, which is developed in the usual manner. Needle-tipped monopolar cautery is used to lyse the orbitomalar ligament along the length of the orbital rim while the surgeon feels for release. The inferior-most aspect of the orbital septum is then incised along its length. It may or may not be advisable to remove some fat at this point, depending on the patient. After the lid is horizontally tightened, the surgeon then oversews the septum directly to periosteum anterior to the inferior rim with running 5-0 polyglactin, all the while observing the lower lid margin to ensure that excess downward tension does not develop. Monopolar cautery can be used to gently create small foci of scarring in the septum to tighten it and possibly prevent or delay subsequent herniation of additional orbital fat.

Skin Closure

The superolateral aspect of the skin-muscle flap is anchored to the lateral orbital rim periosteum with a buried suture to provide further support. Usually, limited excision of the height of the skin-muscle flap is required, typically just a few millimeters. A lateral dog-ear of skin and muscle is also invariably removed. The skin is then closed loosely with a running 6-0 polypropylene suture. Unlike the upper lid, the running passes directly beneath the lower lid can be spaced out such that only four or five passes are required to traverse the lid. It is helpful to use a bolster medially, instead of a knot, to aid in suture removal. The suture is removed in 5 to 7 days.

The lateral palpebral commissure may or may not need to be reformed during closure, for which there are several techniques. One simple method that is often satisfactory is to pass a 5-0 or 6-0 plain gut suture full-thickness through each lid, starting on the external upper lid and externalizing on the lower lid. Another method is to pass fast-absorbing suture starting from within the lateral incision, exiting on the lid margin, and then passing back through the lid margin of the other lid, with the knot eventually being tied and buried within the surgical incision site laterally (Fig. 108-17).

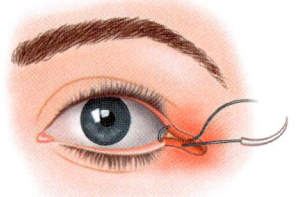

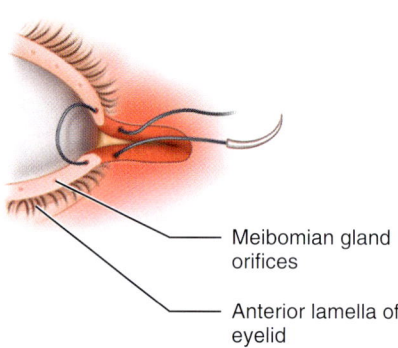

Meibomian gland orifices

Anterior lamella of eyelid

Fig. 108-17 ▪ Lateral canthal reapproximation. A rapidly absorbable suture such as plain gut is used.

Performing lateral commissure reformation with a long-lasting suture is likely to cause irritation and is not recommended.

POSTOPERATIVE CARE

The authors instruct patients to apply a washcloth soaked in ice water frequently for the first 2 days postoperatively. Activity is to be limited for the 2 weeks following surgery; there should be minimal straining, no heavy lifting, and no exercise that significantly increases the heart rate. These precautions are aimed at minimizing the risk for postoperative bleeding. The authors instruct patients to resume normal bathing immediately, to apply a mild ophthalmic antibiotic ointment, usually erythromycin, to the sutures two times per day, and to return for suture removal in 5 to 7 days. After the sutures are removed, the authors instruct patients to continue to use the ointment for another day or two. Prolonged direct sun exposure is discouraged to prevent hyperpigmentation of the incisional scar.

Lower blepharoplasty invariably results in some degree of conjunctival chemosis, for which there is no treatment of well-established efficacy. It resolves after the disrupted lymphatics are given enough time to reestablish themselves, which can take weeks to months. Restoration of lymphatic flow may be accelerated by massaging the lateral wound against the bony lateral orbital rim, making small semicircles with the index finger, and pressing the thickened scar tissue directly onto the bony rim. It is important that this be demonstrated properly to patients so that they do not rub the lower eyelid vigorously and cause lateral dehiscence of the eyelid or increased lower lid laxity. This process can be started 1 week after suture removal.

ACKNOWLEDGMENT

The authors would like to thank Debora Jordan for her expertise in obtaining clinical photographs for this chapter.

PEARLS AND PITFALLS

- Keep the drapes loose on the face. Tight drapes along the forehead will artificially elevate the brow. Tight drapes along the cheeks will confound any attempts to redrape the skin and muscle or establish proper lid position.
- Care should be taken when revising lids in patients with facial nerve dysfunction. There is not generally unilateral skin excess. The apparent skin excess is due to brow depression, as well as an inability to completely lower the eyelid. Lid skin excision is not therapeutic in these patients and may "lock in" their lagophthalmic state.
- Injection of both lower lids will occasionally lead to some degree of asymmetric paralysis of the inferior rectus muscles, which may cause hypertropia. This should be taken into account when judging lower lid positions. Observing only the position where the lid meets the inferior cornea will lead to asymmetric results in these instances. Patients should be reassured that the double vision will resolve when the anesthesia wears off.
- Upper lid height can vary during blepharoplasty because of epinephrine in the local anesthetic, which stimulates the sympathetically activated Müller muscle. Do not be alarmed if one of the lids ends up 2 mm higher than its starting point, but make sure that the skin excision is not aggressive.

BIBLOGRAPHY

Chen WP: *Asian blepharoplasty and the eyelid crease*, ed 2, Oxford, 2006, Butterworth-Heinemann.

Hamra ST: Arcus marginalis release and orbital fat preservation in midface rejuvenation, *Plast Reconstr Surg* 96:354-362, 1999.

McCord CD, Codner MA: *Eyelid and periorbital surgery*, St Louis, 2008, Quality Medical Publishing.

Morax S, Touitou V: Complications of blepharoplasty, *Orbit* 25:303-318, 2006.

Ablative Facial Resurfacing Chapter 109

Matthew R. Hlavacek

Facial resurfacing has been used as a modality of therapy as far back as 1500 BC when it was practiced by the ancient Egyptians. It has evolved through chemical and abrasive techniques to include different laser technologies. Technical advancements have heralded improved results with less morbidity, which has led to a great surge in the popularity of facial resurfacing. As a surgical treatment, ablative facial resurfacing will be the focus of this chapter. It primarily includes dermabrasion, chemical peeling, and laser resurfacing. The primary focus of treatments will be on the most common dermatopathologic entities that can be improved by resurfacing. Finally, a brief review of potential complications and their prevention will be presented.

ETIOPATHOGENESIS/CAUSATIVE FACTORS

The primary causative factors for which patients seek facial resurfacing include intrinsic age-related and extrinsic environmentally associated changes which cause dyspigmentation, dyskeratosis, and cutis laxa. Additionally, facial resurfacing is commonly sought for the treatment of facial scars, including acne scarring. Resurfacing has also been used for many dermatopathologic entities, such as keloids, rhinophyma, xanthelasma, seborrheic keratosis, and actinic keratosis.

As patients age, *intrinsic changes* result in the epidermis becoming more fragile with weaker cell adhesion and a thinner stratum corneum. Deeper dermal changes include flattening of the papillary dermis, decreased number of appendages and sensory organs, and decreased vascularity. Age-related degradation and disorganization in elastin and collagen and decreased ground substance lead to less resilient skin that is more lax and prone to rhytidosis. These changes are compounded in women after menopause with the depletion of estrogenic support (1) This all contributes to decreased water content, which results in increased surface roughness and xerosis. Senile decrease in melanocytes and dysfunction of these cells give rise to areas of uneven color. Additionally, as women cycle through hormonal exposure, including pregnancy, birth control, and hormone replacement therapy, melanocytes can be stimulated to produce more melanin when exposed to the sun, This results in areas of hyperpigmentation.

TABLE 109-1	Fitzpatrick Classification				
SKIN TYPE	**HAIR**	**EYE**	**SKIN**	**RESPONSE TO ULTRAVIOLET LIGHT EXPOSURE**
I	Red	Green	Fair	Always burns
II	Blond	Blue	Fair	Burns with some tans
III	Brown	Brown	Medium	Tans with some burns
IV	Dark brown	Brown	Medium dark	Tans easily, rarely burns
V	Black	Black	Dark	Tans easily, vary rarely burns
VI	Black	Black	Black	Does not burn

In regards to *extrinsic factors,* as sun exposure occurs, the ultraviolet (UV) radiation associated damage accumulates. Interestingly, up to 50% of a person's exposure to UV radiation occurs before the age of 18.[2] Repeated sun exposure causes cellular abnormality and decreased healing ability. The pathognomonic changes include accentuation of elastotic changes in the upper dermis.[3] Basically, sun exposure accelerates intrinsic aging.

Finally, with regard to scarring, up to 95% of patients with acne will have some extent of scarring. This is due to inflammation and necrosis of the pilosebaceous unit, which can cause "ice pick" type scars. Alternatively, wider-spread inflammation in the subcuticular layer can result in more diffuse fat necrosis and larger crater-like defects.[4]

PATHOLOGIC ANATOMY

Among its other functions, the skin serves as a barrier to insult from the harsh external environment. The skin is divided microscopically into different layers based on its cellular content. The epidermis is the "superficial" layer of the skin and includes a layer of continuously regenerating squamous epithelial cells. Additionally, this layer contains melanocytes, which are responsible for pigmentation; Langerhans cells, which are responsible for macrophage activity; and Merkel cells, which have sensory function. Thus, this layer is largely responsible for the color and texture of the skin. It has no collagen fibers and little inherent strength.

Underneath the epidermis is the dermis with its more superficial papillary layer and deeper reticular layer. The papillary layer is loosely arranged with a vascular arcade. The reticular layer forms the bulk of the dermis with its interlacing collagen and elastic fibers. The main cell of the dermis is the fibroblast, which produces the ground substance and the collagen and elastin. The dermis serves to support and provide nourishment to the epidermis.[5]

Finally, underneath the dermis is loose subcutaneous tissue that contains adipose tissue and larger vessels. Most of the adnexal structures, including hair follicles and sweat glands, originate from this layer (Fig. 109-1).

DIAGNOSTIC STUDIES

A good subjective history, including the goals of the patient, and the physical examination are perhaps the most important diagnostic resources. Besides determining how realistic the patient's goals are, other important subjective history includes the patient's sun exposure history, skin care regimen, co-morbid conditions, medication history, and skin cancer history.

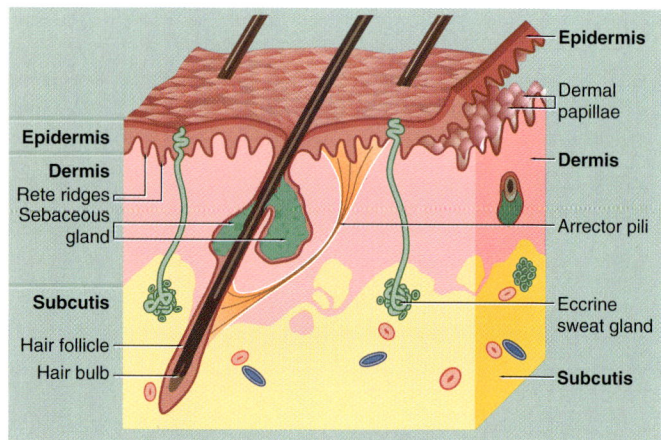

Fig. 109-1 ■ Architecture of skin. Observe how the adenexal structures, which are responsible for re-epithelialization, are located in the subcutaneous layer.

Evaluation of the skin includes complexion, texture, thickness, oiliness, and degree of photoaging, specfically the severity of rhytidosis and laxity. The Fitzpatrick and Glogau classifications are very useful for guidance toward these ends. Matching the patient's skin type and complexion with the appropriate treatment will maximize the resurfacing effect while minimizing postoperative complications. The Fitzpatrick classification system ranks the skin's tendency to tan or burn in association with the patient's skin, hair, and eye color. This is illustrated in Table 109-1. Patients in classes I to III with more sun-reactive skin types tend to have better results than darker skinned patients. These patients have lighter hair, eye, and/or skin color and usually burn easier when exposed to the sun. They have a lower incidence of post-treatment hyperpigmentation but a higher incidence of post-treatment hypopigmentation. They will also be prone to premature skin aging without proper UV protection. Patients with a type IV or greater complexion are at higher risk for unfavorable post laser pigmentary changes and may be more suitable candidates for non-ablative techniques. Patients with darker skin types who desire resurfacing first require a test spot behind the ear or in an inconspicuous area to evaluate the results. Even normal healing here does not guarantee the final overall skin response. The transitional patients may require multiple less aggressive treatments to obtain the same endpoint goal as the Asian patient in Fig. 109-2. Luckily, the darker patients rarely seek resurfacing treatment because their skin is more resistant to photoaging. Although the Fitzpatrick classification is useful, probably the simplest criterion for judging the patient's skin type is its response to sun exposure.[6]

TABLE 109-2	Glogau Classification				
SKIN TYPE	PHOTOAGING	CHANGES IN PIGMENTATION	PATHOLOGY	WRINKLES	AGE
I	Early	Mild	None	Minimal	20-35
II	Moderate	Senile lentigines	Non-visible dyskeratosis	Dynamic	35-45
III	Advanced	Marked dyschromia	Visible dyskeratosis, telangiectasia	Static	50s
III	Senile	Yellow-gray	Actinic keratosis ± malignancy	Severe	60s

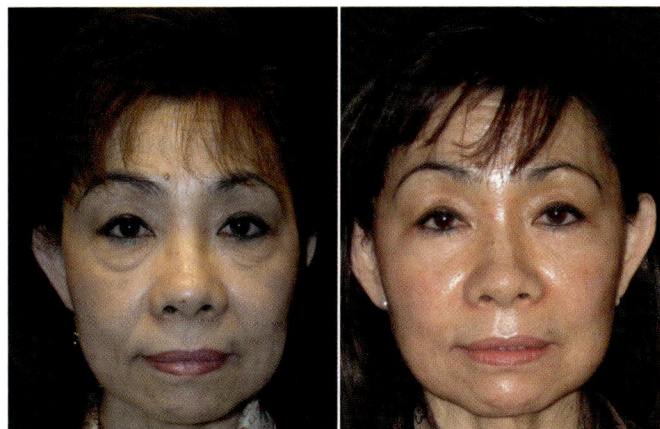

Fig. 109-2 ■ Darker Fitzpatrick skin type. This patient required multiple conservative laser treatments instead of a single, more aggressive treatment to avoid complications.

The degree of degenerative changes in the dermis and epidermis and the severity of photoaging are ranked to classify and guide treatment decisions in the Glogau classification scheme. This is shown in Table 109-2. Patients classified as types III and IV are the best candidates for ablation with their marked dyspigmentation and dyskeratosis. These patients have the greatest margin for improvement but should be warned that moderate to severe skin laxity requires a lifting procedure for correction.

An alternative part of the diagnostic phase of treatment of these patients is recognizing which patients are *not* good candidates for these procedures. Such patients include those with collagen vascular diseases and those who are immunosuppressed. In addition, patients with compromised integrity of the adnexal structures, including those with a history of isotretinoin (Accutane) use within the last 6 months, those with a history of facial irradiation, and patients with burn scars, are not good candidates. Some relative contraindications include patients with multiple co-morbid conditions or poorly controlled health issues and those taking anticoagulation medications.

Resurfacing can cause activation of preexisting dermatopathologic entities such as eczema, rosacea, or atopic dermatitis. Caution is warranted in patients prone to hypertrophic or keloid scarring. Patients who have previously undergone facial surgery, including lower eyelid blepharoplasty, may also be poor candidates for resurfacing. These patients may be at increased risk for ectropion. As mentioned previously, darkly complected patients should be warned regarding their increased risk for postoperative hyperpigmentation or hypopigmentation. Of course, patients with a tendency toward body dysmorphia or secondary gain or those with unrealistic expectations should not be acceptable candidates for any cosmetic surgery. Finally, skin pathology suspicious for malignant changes should undergo biopsy and be treated before resurfacing.

TREATMENT/RECONSTRUCTIVE GOALS

Goals of treatment include rejuvenated skin with less dyskeratosis, rhytidosis, and dyschromia. In addition, with regard to scarring, goals include lightening and reduction of the scarring. It is common to achieve only 50% improvement with ablative resurfacing when treating moderate to severe acne scarring. Another goal should be avoidance of complications through proper patient evaluation and selection of treatment.

SPECIFIC TREATMENT AND TECHNIQUES

PRETREATMENT CONDITIONING

Although there is some controversy regarding the necessity for pre-treating skin, most practitioners would agree that pre-treatment with tretinoin and a bleaching agent speeds re-epithelialization and decreases the incidence of postoperative hyperpigmentation. Tretinoin, which is retinoic acid, acts by decreasing cellular adhesiveness and increasing cell turnover to restore normal epidermal thickness. The thinning of the stratum corneum allows better penetration of the resurfacing agent. Tretinoin also encourages collagen synthesis.[7,8] Patients with thicker oilier skin tolerate and benefit from retinoic acid to a greater degree. Patients with thin atrophic skin may experience more dehydration and irritation. When patients cannot tolerate tretinoin, daily application of glycolic acid or weekly alpha-hydroxyl acid peels for 4 to 6 weeks can be substituted.

Hydroquinone and kojic acid are bleaching agents that stabilize melanocytes and reduce dyspigmentation before laser treatment. They also decrease the risk for postoperative inflammatory hyperpigmentation. The mechanism of action includes inhibition of tyrosinase, which decreases melanin formation and increases melanin degradation. This is especially useful in patients with darker skin types.[9]

Retinoic acid and hydroquinone have a synergistic effect on each other in that retinoic acid increases penetration of the hydroquinone and also works to suppress melanocyte metabolism. To be most effective, the bleaching agent should be applied twice daily and retinoic acid applied at bedtime. A mild steroid can be prescribed initially with the tretinoin to attenuate the irritation that the skin undergoes during the 2- to 4-week acclimation period. Additionally, patients can apply tretinoin every other day instead of every day until the dermatitis period resolves. Patients should use a sun block in the morning, including a moisturizer, preferably with UVA and UVB protection. The minimal amount of time necessary for patients to maximize the conditioning is typically 4 to 6 weeks because the epidermal cell cycle extends roughly this long.

PREOPERATIVE MEDICATIONS

In the more immediate pretreatment period, patients require additional preparation. Ablative facial resurfacing typically necessitates some form of anesthesia, and thus patients require the appropriate pre-anesthesia instructions for sedation or general anesthesia as per recommendations of the American Society of Anesthesiology. Patients are asked to wash with an antimicrobial cleanser such as Hibiclens the night before and also the morning of the treatment. In a further attempt to reduce microbial load, the patient is given a preoperative dose of appropriate antibiotics, which is continued for 5-7 days postoperatively. Many studies have suggested benefit of antibiotic prophylaxis.[10-12] This should especially be a consideration when an occlusive dressing is used.

Prophylactic administration of a nucleoside analogue antiviral has been demonstrated to prevent outbreaks and decrease the duration and severity of postoperative herpes simplex virus. infection.[13] Up to 70% of patients without a previous history have a positive titer.[14] The incidence of outbreaks in patients without a previous history has been shown to be as high as 10% in untreated patients undergoing resurfacing and 50% in those with a positive history.[15] The antiviral should be started the day before and continued postoperatively until the skin is reepithelialized, usually in 10 to 14 days, depending on the depth of resurfacing. The antiviral inhibits viral replication only in intact epidermal cells, and thus the drug must be at a therapeutic level before the skin begins to reepithelialize.[15] Some recommend prophylactic antifungal coverage, but studies have not found the incidence of post-resurfacing fungal infections to be high enough to warrant this additional therapeutic measure.

DERMABRASION

Dermabrasion is thought by many to be the most effective mode of treatment of facial scars, including acne and the post-traumatic variety. It is also very popular for the treatment of perioral rhytides and rhinophyma (Fig. 109-3). It can be used for treating appropriate dermatopathologic conditions located from a superficial level to a mid-reticular level. Originally described by the Egyptians and performed with sandpaper, modern techniques have evolved through a wire brush to what is probably most commonly used today, a diamond fraise.

Dermabrasion is performed with a hand piece that rotates up to the 35,000-rpm range and has a variety of shapes, sizes, and coarseness of fraise tips. The procedure is usually done with the patient under sedation or general anesthesia, including tumescent or cryogenic preparation. The latter technique increases the rigidity of the tissue and control of the resurfacing. Increasing the rigidity of the surface allows more even abrasion and decreases "grabbing" of the skin by the fraise or brush.[16] Hanke and associates recommend avoiding lowering the skin temperature below −30° C because this increases the risk for tissue necrosis.[17]

A diamond fraise is a better selection for neophytes since it offers a larger margin of safety and is not as aggressive as the brush. The different shapes are very useful for the different contours of the face. Brushes are capable of more efficient removal of skin but have a greater tendency to "run" on the skin. They require a greater level of expertise.

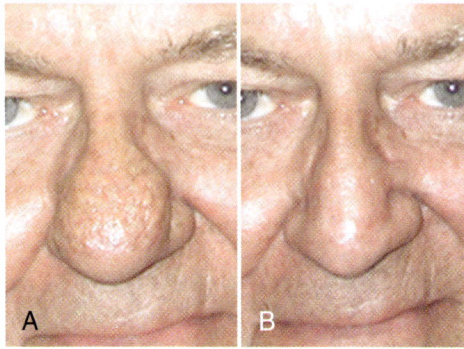

Fig. 109-3 ■ Rhinophyma pre- and post-laser resurfacing.

As with other methods of resurfacing, it is best to perform this therapy stepwise in a subunit basis over the entire face. It is best to begin in dependent areas to avoid pooling of blood in adjacent facial subunits. The depth of punctate facial scars and deep rhytides should be marked to assist in determining the depth of abrasion needed. One should always dermabrade toward orifices rather than away. Furthermore, care should be taken to avoid crossing the hairline so that iatrogenic alopecia does not develop. The orbital rim and inferior border of the mandible are technically sensitive areas because these can be areas of increased scarring. Besides thinner skin, there is a paucity of pilosebaceous units on the neck.

The long axis of the fraise or bush should be held parallel to the surface of the skin to avoid gouging. The dermabrasion is performed to the desired depth, which is usually the papillary dermis. Punctate bleeding from the capillary loops is encountered at this level. The appearance of small parallel strands of collagen signifies passage into the reticular dermis. The tops of the sebaceous lobules can be visualized when approaching the mid-reticular dermis, which is at least a stopping point if not a danger zone. This is because increased scarring occurs below this depth.[18] After treatment, the skin should be débrided with cotton gauze. Application of a solution of dilute epinephrine is useful to diminish oozing. Needless to say, appropriate precautionary measures should be taken as microdroplets of blood and tissue are aerosolized throughout the procedure, thereby increasing the risk for exposure to blood-borne pathogens.

CHEMICAL PEELS

When compared with other modalities, chemical peels have a long-standing safety and efficacy record, are low in cost and easily performed. They are also associated with a relatively quick recovery time. They treat intrinsic and extrinsic aging but are less effective in treating vascular lesions and deep acne scarring. As described by Obagi, chemical peeling agents can be split by mechanism of action into keratolytic agents and protein-denaturing agents.[16] Keratolytics are primarily used for superficial peeling procedures, whereas denaturants are for superficial or deep peels. Besides the potential efficiency of the peeling agent, many other factors help control the depth of the peel. These include concentration, amount applied, skin thickness and oiliness, duration of treatment, and preconditioning. Because this chapter focuses on ablative resurfacing, keratolytics such as glycolic and salicylic acid will not be discussed. The more common denaturants, include trichloroacetic acid (TCA), with or without Jessner solution and phenol peels.

Peels have classically been described as superficial, medium, or deep according to the depth of dermis that they treat, as shown in Table 109-3. Superficial peels are limited to the epidermis. Medium-depth peels are limited to the upper reticular dermis and deep peels extend to the mid-reticular dermis (Fig. 109-4)[19] Before peeling it is important to remove the excess oil debris and excess stratum corneum to increase the efficiency of the chemicals. Most use acetone on a 4 × 4-inch pad to lightly scrub and débride the skin. Some start with a Septisol keratolytic scrub. After the skin is débrided, defatted, and degreased, the peel will have a more even penetration to the desired depth.

Medium-depth peels treat down into the papillary dermis in a single setting. These peels are used for the treatment of acne, post-inflammatory erythema, melasma, and actinic damage, including epidermal dysplasia. They are also used to treat fine rhytides, mild acne scarring, and deeper hyperpigmentation. Note the improvement in the fine perioral and nasolabial ford rhytids as well as in the skin texture in the patient in (Fig. 109-5). The prototypic agent for this level of treatment is 35% TCA, which causes protein denaturation and coagulation. It is helpful because it has less effect on melanocyte

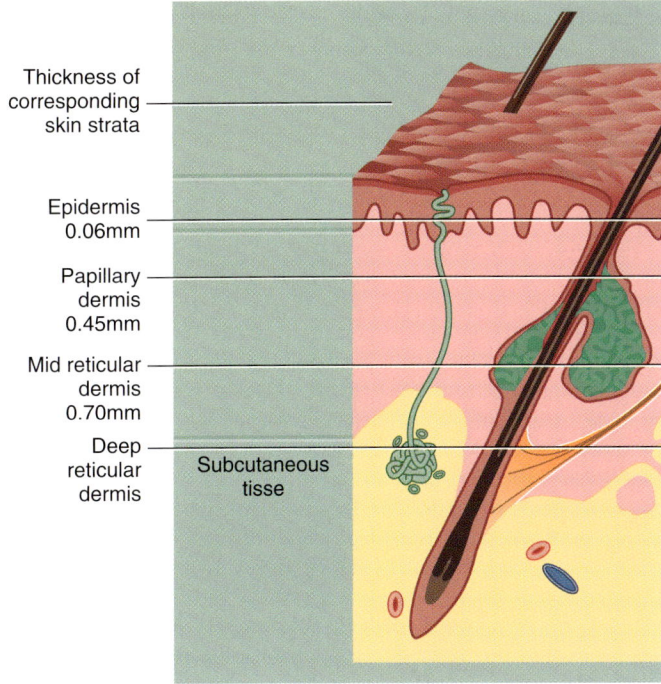

Thickness of corresponding skin strata

Epidermis 0.06mm

Papillary dermis 0.45mm

Mid reticular dermis 0.70mm

Deep reticular dermis

Subcutaneous tisse

Fig. 109-4 ▪ Thickness of skin strata. Avoid resurfacing to the deep reticular dermis or deeper to prevent complications.

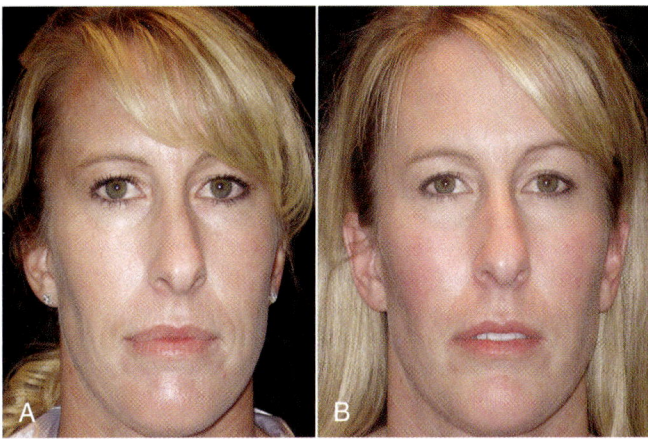

Fig. 109-5 ▪ Chemical peel pre- and post-treatment.

TABLE 109-3	**Types of Peels**	
SUPERFICIAL	**MEDIUM**	**DEEP**
15% TCA		

Jessner solution
  14% Resorcinol
	35% TCA
	Jessner solution +
	  35% TCA
		55% TCA
		Baker-Gordon
		  solution

14% Salicylic acid		3 mL 88% phenol
14% Lactic acid 100 mL Ethanol		2 mL tap water 3 Drops croton oil
Unna paste Resorcinol Zinc oxide		8 Drops Septisol
Salicylic acid		
Alpha-hydroxyl acids		

TCA, Trichloroacetic acid.

metabolism and therefore less chance of unfavorably bleaching skin. It can be used for Fitzpatrick type III and possibly type IV patients with the appropriate preconditioning regimen. When the area is pretreated with either Jessner solution, glycolic acid, or solid carbon dioxide, TCA achieves quicker and deeper penetration. Jessner solution is a keratolytic solution that consists of a combination of 14% each of salicylic acid, resorcinol, and lactic acid mixed in ethanol.

The peeling agents should be applied with cotton gauze or cotton-tipped applicators and the patient's head elevated to avoid pooling of the agent in concavities of the face. The face is treated from the forehead down as described for dermabrasion, except that the

periorbital area is last because this area is the most difficult to treat. The eyelids are treated with only dampened applicators while staying 2 to 3 mm from the palpebral fissure in an attempt to avoid exposure of the eye to the agent. Tears should not be allowed to roll on the face because they can move to the neck and carry solution and thereby potentially cause a postpeel defect. Application while stretching areas of deeper wrinkles and scars will ensure proper exposure. Feathering the application over the mandibular border will help prevent a line of demarcation.

Penetration into the papillary dermis causes a deep white frost, penetration deep to this and into the reticular dermis causes an opaque dense white frost, and penetration deeper yet into the dermis and subcutaneous tissues will cause a gray appearance. This is undesirable because the risk for prolonged erythema and scarring increases.

Jessner solution will cause a faint pink frosting on the face. After it has dried, the 35% TCA solution is applied evenly. The agent will penetrate at around 2 minutes, at which point cool compresses can be applied if needed. The peel creates a burning sensation that can be tolerated without anesthesia by some, but topical or local anesthesia and more frequently, sedation are usually required.

Deep peels are used for treatment of the aforementioned dermatopathology but also for deeper wrinkles, acne scarring, and skin laxity to a mild degree. This peeling is prototypically completed with the Baker-Gordon phenol peel. It can produce profound changes in severely actinically damaged and intrinsically aged skin on a consistent basis. It causes a second-degree chemical burn, which results in a new stratified collagen layer. It is also associated with longer postoperative morbidity, including an increased risk for postoperative complications. This specifically, includes hypopigmentation, scarring, or textural changes.[20] The best candidates are those with severe damage and age-related changes and also lighter Fitzpatrick skin types.

The Baker-Gordon peel permits deeper penetration than pure phenol. This is because Septisol is a surfactant that reduces skin tension and allows more even penetration, and croton oil is an epidermolytic that enhances absorption. The phenol is absorbed, detoxified in the liver, and excreted renally. It takes only small levels to cause cardiac arrhythmias, which are most commonly manifested as premature ventricular contractions but could potentially include lethal arrhythmias. Thus, a metabolic profile and renal evaluation in addition to an electrocardiogram are recommended preoperatively. Good hydration of the patient before, during, and after the peel promotes the excretion of phenol and helps prevent toxicity. To further prevent cardiotoxic serum levels while also increasing control of the peel, the face needs to be treated in subunits with 15-minute intervals between each cosmetic unit. The phenol absorbed from the skin has a higher correlation to the surface area exposed than the concentration used.[21] As with other peels, the eyes are treated last. If peeling solution gets in the eyes, mineral oil rather than water should be used for flushing because water can increase penetration. The solution should be blended lightly over the mandibular border. Some practitioners select to occlude these peels to increase the efficiency of the peel. Occlusion increases the risk for attaining cardiotoxic levels versus unoccluded peels as a result of the tape preventing evaporation of the phenol solution.

The peel causes enough discomfort that regional local anesthetic blocks in addition to at least intravenous sedation or general anesthesia are required. After the application, the skin turns a frosty white color. The burning can be intense for the first 30 seconds, the phenol anesthetizes the skin, and then the pain returns again in 30 minutes and lasts for the rest of the day.

LASER RESURFACING

Laser resurfacing has waxed and waned in popularity since its development. This has been due to the significant clinical results but also the marked postoperative morbidity. The continuous-mode laser became popular starting in the 1970s but produced excessive scarring because of adjacent thermal damage. This led to the development of a superpulsed laser with shortened thermal exposure and consequently to ultrapulsed lasers, which deliver very high energy over a shortened period. This spares the surrounding skin. Fractional laser resurfacing was created to deliver the results of an ablative resurfacing effort with a non-ablative postoperative course. This includes faster re-epithelialization, less erythema and discomfort, and ultimately, less downtime. This technology ablates only part of the skin while leaving "micro" islands of non-ablated tissue in between. Thus, the same surface area receives the effect of ablation with more healing potential for quicker re-epithelialization. As with all resurfacing wounds, these wounds originate from non-damaged adjacent adnexal structures. Advantages of the laser primarily include greater control and predictability of the intended treatment, but also lack of aerosolization of blood associated with dermabrasion and lack of the toxic profile of phenol.

Laser is an acronym for light amplification by the stimulated emission of radiation. Lasers act by emitting a specific wavelength of energy, or light, in the form of photons, which are preferentially absorbed by a specific chromophore in the skin. This is otherwise known as selective photothermolysis. The laser light is monochromatic and coherent. The energy is measured in joules, and the amount delivered per unit area is the fluence (J/cm^2). The pulse width, or duration, is the time over which the set energy is delivered. If the pulse duration exceeds the capacity of energy that the particle can absorb, more energy is transferred to the surrounding tissue and thereby increases the thermal damage to this tissue. Thus, to affect the particular chromophore while minimizing damage to surrounding tissue, it is important to not exceed or overheat the particle. This illustrates the idea of the thermal relaxation time,[22] which has specifically been defined as the time needed for a heated object to cool to half its elevated temperature. If the pulse duration does not exceed the thermal relaxation time, necrosis will be minimized to the intended treatment zone. From superficial to deep, the laser creates characteristic zones of injury, including the zone of ablated tissue, charred tissue, heat-denatured collagen, and finally, collagen shrinkage.[16] Post-resurfacing healing time, erythema, pigment loss, and scarring are related to the depth of coagulation necrosis.

The lasers discussed in this chapter to demonstrate the principles of ablative laser resurfacing include the carbon dioxide and erbium:yttrium aluminum garnet (Erb:YAG) lasers. These lasers produce a wavelength of energy that has specificity for the water molecule. The thermal relaxation time of water is 1 ms. Its threshold for ablation is 5 J/cm^2. At this energy fluence, delivery of a 1-ms energy pulse will ablate 30 μm of tissue and leave up to 120 μm of residual thermal damage.[23]

The CO_2 laser emits a wavelength of 10,600 nm and is available as a continuous and pulsed laser, in addition to a fractionated option. At standard settings, the pulsed laser uses 90% of the light to ablate the first 20 to 30 μm of tissue. Using a high-energy pulse lasting less than 1 ms provides precisely controlled tissue vaporization, minimal thermal damage, hemostasis, and heat shrinkage of collagen in the dermis. This results in skin tightening. Overlapping passes of the computer pattern generator (CPG) and multiple passes over the same area result in pulse stacking. Although this increases the ablative effect and depth, it also increases the potential for prolonged postoperative recovery and complications. Ablative CO_2 resurfacing will always contribute to a "refreshed" look when combined with other procedures such as a blepharoplasty Figs. 109-6 and 109-7. However, it is the treatment of choice for severe age-related changes (Fig. 109-8).

Erb:YAG lasers were created in an attempt to allay the prolonged healing of the CO_2 laser but give comparable results. The wavelength of this laser is 2940 nm, and these lasers have 16 times the affinity for water, which results in more absorption, less coagulation necrosis, and less penetration per pass. This laser ablates at a fraction of the CO_2 laser with roughly a quarter of the residual thermal damage.[24] Pulse stacking with this laser does not increase the

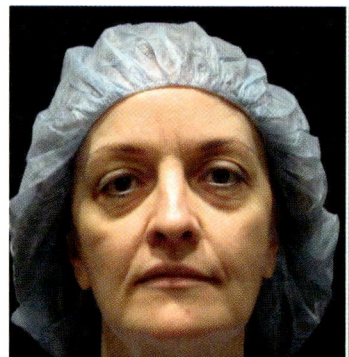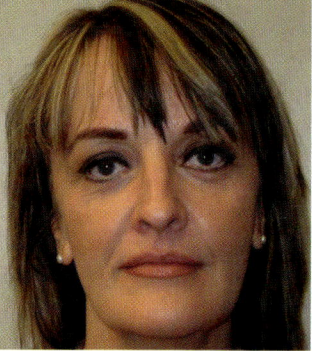

Fig. 109-6 ■ Ablative laser resurfacing pre- and post-treatment. Note improvement in skin tone and texture.

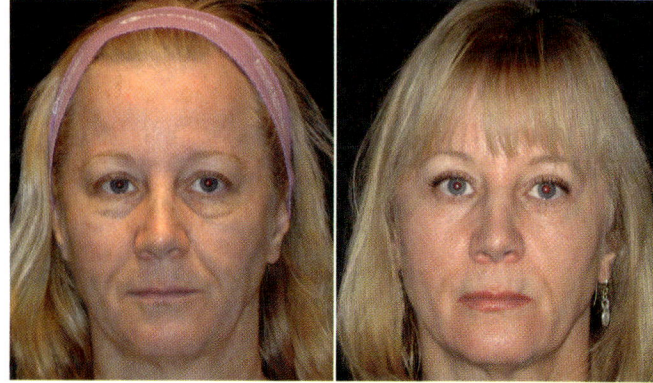

Fig. 109-7 ■ Ablative laser resurfacing pre- and post-treatment. Note treatment of the fine lower eyelid sun damage as well as minor tightening of the skin and lightening of the nasolabial furrows.

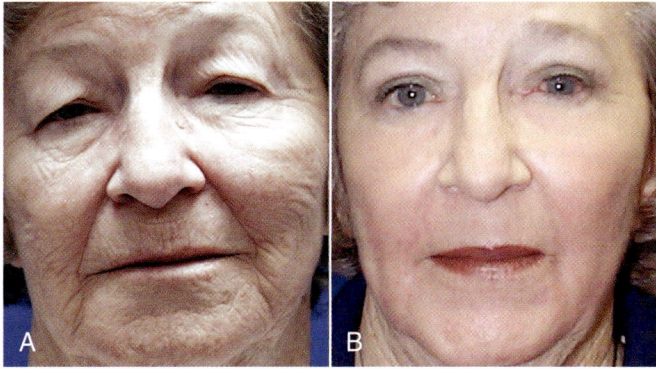

Fig. 109-8 ■ Ablative laser resurfacing pre- and post-treatment. Note dramatic improvement when combined with other surgical procedures such as blepharoplasty.

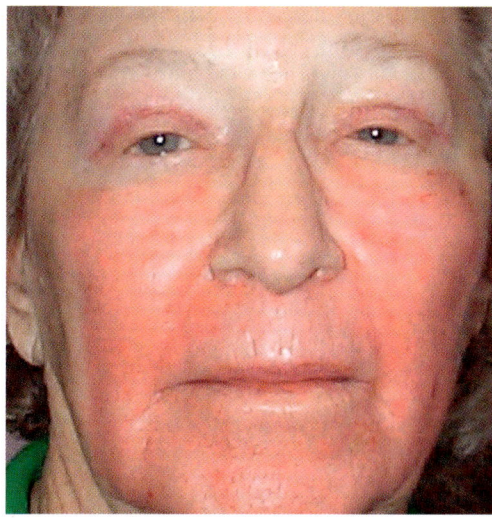

Fig. 109-9 ■ Postoperative ablative resurfacing appearance. The patient will appear with red and "raw" skin for the first 7 to 10 days after the treated skin is sloughed.

thickness of thermal damage, and there is not enough energy to induce the immediate contraction seen with the CO_2 technology.[25] Multiple passes may be needed to achieve the desired response.

The Erb:YAG laser is available in variable pulsed modes, short and long. The short mode of treatment provides good results for more superficial pathology with less healing time, but also less collagen shrinkage. The long-pulse mode approaches the results achieved with CO_2 laser resurfacing but with intermediate healing time. The Erb:YAG laser results in more bleeding because, as mentioned previously, it does not share the coagulative effects of CO_2 laser resurfacing.

Laser treatment requires special precautionary measures to be performed in the safest manner possible. Laser resurfacing requires protection of the patient's eyes with laser-resistant intraocular shields. Additionally, fire precautions need to be in place, including management of the oxygen that the patient is receiving. Signs should be placed on entryways to the room, and the staff needs to observe the measures needed to prevent unplanned laser injury. Water should obviously be immediately available in the event of a fire.

Because many different systems are available at present, it is difficult to provide parameters of use, but generally speaking, the periorbital area and the inferior mandible undergo laser treatment at two thirds the power used for the rest of the face. The pattern should be overlapped as little as possible, especially with the CO_2 laser, to achieve homogeneous resurfacing. The face is treated in subunits as described previously, and it is always preferable to treat the entire face. The periorbital area is treated last, as is feathering of the mandible, because these areas are more technically sensitive. Feathering from the lower part of the mandible into the neck can be done by defocusing the laser and also lasering at a 45-degree angle to the skin surface. Alternatively, this can be accomplished by decreasing the fluence on the laser.

Problematic areas such as the perioral region or other areas with deeper rhytides and ice pick scars can undergo multiple passes. If multiple passes are to be used with the CO_2 laser, some advocate removing the char in between passes with wet gauze. The char may interfere with the efficacy of the laser and also act as a heat sink potentially causing more residual damage, erythema, and scarring. It is important to dry the skin after débridement since water is the chromophore for the laser and it may block the interaction of the laser with the skin. Removal of the char is debatable, with a recent study by Niamtu revealing decreased postoperative erythema and less postoperative discomfort, in addition to a lack of hypertrophic scarring, when multiple passes are used without débridement of char.[26] It is also important to keep the skin dry with the Erb:YAG laser, but removal of the char is not required.

The end point of laser treatment is effacement of the rhytides and smoothing of the photoaged skin. Alternatively, reaching the yellowish hue of the mid-reticular dermis is a stopping point to prevent scarring and hypopigmentation. Laser treatment past this point is difficult with the Erb:YAG laser because bleeding may preclude further treatment.

POSTOPERATIVE CARE

After an ablative resurfacing injury, the skin goes through stages of healing, including an inflammatory stage, re-epithelialization, fibroplasia, and collagen remodeling.[23] With dermabrasion and lasering, the wound will be exudative with weeping and crusting for the first 5 to 7 days. This is reflected in Fig. 109-9. Chemical peels will cause the skin to take on a dusky look over the first 12 to 24 hours. Over the following 3 days the skin will acquire a leathery look and begin to "shed." Around 5 to 7 days after treatment the new pinkish underlying epithelium is revealed. The skin is typically re-epithelialized by around post-treatment day 10 regardless of modality.

Edema and pain occur in the first 24 to 48 hours and peak around the third postoperative day. The swelling can be controlled with head elevation, ice packs, and corticosteroids if severe. The face may be numb, so the patient should be cautioned to use the ice packs appropriately. The burning and pain in the first week are controlled with narcotics, non-steroidal anti-inflammatory drugs, ice, and misting spray. Some prefer occlusive dressings to speed up re-epithelialization and improve patient comfort for the first couple of days.[27] These dressings can be cumbersome to remove and may become a source of infection. Prolonged occlusion can lead to acne.

After ablation, patients should continue their medications as prescribed, including antiviral and antibiotic agents. They should wash their face gently or soak it three to four times a day. This action assists in débriding serous crust and sloughing skin, and also prevents infection. Vinegar solution is also recommended for soaking or a mist spray on the face because the acetic acid promotes epithelialization and inhibits bacterial growth. Cleaning is followed by the application of an emollient such as Aquaphor. This coats the skin and forms a bio-occlusive dressing that gives the patient comfort and encourages epithelialization. Antibiotic ointments are avoided because they can cause mild allergic dermatitis.[28] Itching is typical as the skin reepithelializes and is usually treated adequately with antihistamines, steroid ointment, or both. Ice packs can also help alleviate the pruritus. To avoid scarring, patients should be specifically instructed to not "pick" off sloughing skin and also to not let scabbing form in the case of dermabrasion and laser treatment.

After resurfacing there will be a variable period of post-treatment erythema. Depending on the mode of treatment and the depth, this erythema can last from around 2 weeks to 4 months but can take up to 6 months to resolve for deeper ablation. Mineral-based make-up can be worn after the skin is re-epithelialized to camouflage the erythema. Skin conditioning, including retinoids and bleaching agents, can be restarted at 2 to 4 weeks post treatment, depending on what is tolerated. Additionally, a sun block and moisturizer should also be restarted. If hyperpigmentation is suspected, the tretinoin and hydroquinone should be restarted as soon as possible. Sun avoidance is paramount to prevent postinflammatory hyperpigmentation.

COMPLICATIONS

Complications are typically caused by poor intraoperative technique, failure of the patient to adhere to the postoperative recovery regimen, and insufficiently evaluated variability in each patient, such as the Fitzpatrick type, degree of sun exposure, amount of preconditioning, and any medical co-morbid conditions. The best way to avoid complications with ablative facial resurfacing is proper patient assessment and application of the appropriate technique. Additionally, it is very important to ensure that the patient has realistic expectations because no resurfacing technique will return the skin to its perfect state. Failed patient expectations are a common complication, especially for less experienced practitioners.

Complications can be categorized into infectious, cicatricial, pigmentary, and inflammatory.[29] After the skin has been denuded of its outer protective layer, it becomes susceptible to bacterial, fungal, and viral infections. The incidence of bacterial infections in these patients is 4-8% with the use of prophylactic antibiotics.[30] The most common infectious organism cultured is *Staphylococcus aureus*, but other frequently cultured organisms include *Streptococcus* and *Pseudomonas*. Viral infections occur in 2-7% of patients who have received prophylaxis, with the most common virus being herpes simplex. *Candida* is the most common fungal pathogen. To make things complex, these organisms can all be present in infectious concentrations simultaneously. Bacterial infections are usually associated with weeping, crusting, and pruritus. Viral infections are characterized by marked pain and a distinct pattern of erythematous erosions. Fungal infections will also be pruritic with white patches. Infections that occur up to a month after the resurfacing should be suspected of being caused by atypical mycobacteria.

The first step in resolution is to identify the pathogen by culture or KOH preparation (or both), followed by thorough cleansing and appropriate broad-spectrum antimicrobial treatment. After the results of bacterial cultures and sensitivity testing are obtained, a more specific antibiotic can be selected. In the case of a viral infection, the maximum dose of the previously prescribed prophylactic agent should be used or a switch made to a different antiviral. Fungal infections are treated with systemic antifungals. Infections can lead to scarring and uneven results, and thus early detection, proper treatment, and close follow-up are key to preventing permanent sequelae. Dissemination or systemic spread would be an indication for hospital admission and intravenous therapy.

Cicatricial complications usually result from poor patient evaluation preoperatively, such as resurfacing a patient prone to scarring or overly aggressive resurfacing. Examples include extending the ablation too deep or, in the case of laser resurfacing, using excessively high energy densities and stacking pulses. Additionally, patients who experience postoperative wound infection or contact dermatitis or those with a propensity toward hypertrophic scars or keloid formation are at increased risk. This can become evident as early as the first week and is usually preempted by inappropriately tender erythema. Initial treatment includes topical steroids, silicone sheeting, and massage. Treatment of more extreme or persistent scars includes triamcinolone (Kenalog) or 5-fluorouracil injections and consideration of pulsed dye lasering.[31] If the scarring is resistant, excision and primary closure are an option.

Postinflammatory hyperpigmentation is the most common adverse effect of laser resurfacing and has been reported in up to 36% of patients.[32] It is more common in patients with Fitzpatrick type III and greater skin categories and is more common in patients who experience higher levels of sun exposure after treatment. It usually appears in 3 to 4 weeks after the procedure but can occur as soon as 10 to 14 days afterward. Its incidence is decreased by pretreatment conditioning with retinoic acid and a bleaching agent. With appropriate treatment, the hyperpigmentation will generally resolve within months. For those who do not respond, non-ablative laser treatments can be performed to better blend the skin.

Hypopigmentation is a relatively rare problem. It usually develops 6 to 12 months after resurfacing and is more common with dermabrasion and chemical peels than with laser resurfacing. Hypopigmentation can occur postoperatively in up to 16% of patients.[31] Again, its occurrence is related to the depth of penetration of the ablation. It is made more noticeable by resurfacing only subunits and especially when contrasted against more advanced photodamage, a condition otherwise known as pseudo-hypopigmentation. It is best to allow multiple months for resolution. Attempts at treatment can include re-resurfacing to stimulate migration of functional melanocytes into the area or UV light therapy to stimulate melanogenesis.[33] Without improvement, the condition is unlikely to resolve and the patient is unfortunately left to camouflage the hypopigmentation with make-up.

The duration of post-treatment erythema is directly associated with the depth of resurfacing. Erythema occurs more often with laser resurfacing than with chemical peeling or dermabrasion. It can last multiple months following treatment and is treated conservatively with topical steroids and reassurance. It is important to consider other causes, including wound infection, dermatitis, flare-up of rosacea, and incipient scar formation. Additionally, pulsed dye lasering may be an option, especially for scar formation.

Other inflammatory postoperative problems include milia, acne, and contact dermatitis. Milia form as a result of reepithelialization of follicles and subsequent microcyst formation. It usually occurs around 3 weeks after the procedure and is more common with laser resurfacing and dermabrasion. Milia can be removed with the tip of a large-bore needle and manual expression or, alternatively, with frequent facial cleansing and treatment with retinoic acid. Patients with a previous history of acne formation are at an increased risk for a flare-up 1 to 2 weeks postoperatively. Resolution generally occurs after the use of occlusive ointment and dressings is discontinued. Contact dermatitis is relatively common and manifested as diffuse, intense facial erythema and pruritus. It is usually due to exposure of the deepithelialized tissue to an irritant such as the ingredients in fragrances, topical ointments, soaps, moisturizers, or cosmetics. The most common offending agents are topical antibiotics. Treatment includes discontinuation of the offending agent, use of antihistamines, and potentially, topical and/or oral steroids, depending on the intensity.

PEARLS AND PITFALLS

- Resurfacing will not return the skin to a pre-aged state.
- Patients must have realistic goals for the treatment to be successful.
- Ablative resurfacing treats rhytides, dyskeratosis, and dyschromias, but only lifting procedures will treat moderate to severe skin laxity.
- A good subjective history, including reactivity to sun, and physical examination are the most diagnostic resources.
- Patients with lighter Fitzpatrick skin types have a lower incidence of post-treatment hyperpigmentation and a higher incidence of post-treatment hypopigmentation.
- Treatment of acne scarring is difficult, and it is common to achieve only 50% improvement with ablative resurfacing.
- Preconditioning with tretinoin and a bleaching agent speed re-epithelialization and decrease the incidence of postoperative hyperpigmentation.

- Ablative resurfacing should be avoided in darker Fitzpatrick skin types to prevent complications.
- The full face rather than subunits should be treated when possible to avoid lines of demarcation.
- Overly aggressive ablation causes prolonged erythema and increases the risk for hypopigmentation and scarring.
- Exposure to sun after ablation causes postinflammatory hyperpigmentation.
- Patients should be specifically instructed to not "pick" the sloughing skin off in the case of peeling or to not let scabbing form in the case of dermabrasion and lasering to avoid scarring.
- The best way to avoid complications with ablative facial resurfacing is proper patient assessment and application of the appropriate technique.

REFERENCES

1. Vaillant L, Callens A: Hormone replacement therapy and skin aging, *Therapy* 51:67-70, 1996.
2. Baker J: Dermabrasion. In Nahai F, editor: *Art of aesthetic surgery principles and techniques*, St Louis, 2005, Quality Medical Publishing, pp 367-382.
3. Uitto J, Fazio MJ, Olsen DR: Molecular mechanisms of cutaneous aging, *J Am Acad Dermatol* 21:614-622, 1989.
4. Robertson KM: Acne vulgaris, *Facial Plastic Surg Clin North Am* 12:347-355, 2004.
5. Burkitt HG: Skin. In Burkitt HG, Young B, Heath JW, editors: *Wheaters's functional histology*, ed 3, Edinborough, 1993, Churchill Livingstone, pp 152-169.
6. Stuzin JM, Baker TJ, Nahai F. Chemical Peel. In Nahai F, editor: *The art of aesthetic surgery—principles and techniques*, St Louis, 2005, Quality Medical Publishing, pp 384-448.
7. Hevia O, Nemeth AJ, Taylor JR: Tretinoin accelerates healing after trichloroacetic acid chemical peel, *Arch Dermatol* 127:678-682, 1991.
8. Weinstein GD, Nigra TP, Pochi PE, et al: Topical tretinoin treatment for photodamaged skin—a multicenter study, *Arch Dermatol* 127:659-665, 1991.
9. Rubin MG: Reversal of photodamage with chemical nonpeel techniques. In Rubin MG, editor: *Manual of chemical peels*, editors Winters R, James M, & Caputo G. Philadelphia, 1995, JB Lippincott, pp 27-43.
10. Nanni CA, Alster TS: Complication of carbon dioxide laser resurfacing, *Dermatol Surg* 24:315-320, 1998.
11. Bernstein LJ, Kauvar AB, Grossman MC, et al: The short and long term side effects of carbon dioxide laser resurfacing, *Dermatol Surg* 23:519-525, 1997.

12. Gaspar Z, Vincuillo C, Elliot T: Antibiotic prophylaxis for full face laser resurfacing, *Arch Dermatol* 137:313-315, 2001.
13. Dutzler P: Antiviral therapy of herpes simplex and varicella zoster virus infections, *Intervirology* 40:343-356, 1997.
14. Beeson WH, Rachel J: Valacyclovir prophylaxis for herpes simplex virus infection recurrence following laser skin resurfacing, *Dermatol Surg* 28:331-336, 2002.
15. Apfelberg DB: Perioperative considerations in laser resurfacing, *Int J Aesthetic Restor Surg* 5:21-28, 1997.
16. Obagi S, Chaudhary-Patel M, Overview of skin resurfacing modalities. In Gutff R, Katowitz JA, editors: *Essentials in ophthalmology—oculoplastics and orbit*, Berlin, 2007, Springer, pp 261-269.
17. Hanke CW, Roenigk HH, Pinski JB. Complications of dermabrasion resulting from excessively cold skin refrigeration, *J Dermatol Surg Oncol* 11:896-900, 1985.
18. Alt TH: Dermabrasion. In Krause CJ, editor: *Aesthetic facial surgery*, Philadelphia, 1991, JB Lippincott, pp 623-640.
19. Rubin MG: What are skin peels? In Rubin MG, editor: *Manual of chemical peels*, editors Winters R, James M, & Caputo G. Philadelphia, 1995, JB Lippincott, p 22.
20. Coleman WP, Futel JM: The glycolic acid and trichloroacetic acid peel, *J Dermatol Surg Oncol* 20:76-80, 1985.
21. Brody HJ: *Deep peeling, chemical peeling and resurfacing*, St Louis, 1997, CV Mosby, pp 137-160.
22. Anderson RR, Parish RR: Selective photothermolysis: precise microsurgery by selective absorption of pulsed radiation, *Science* 220:524-527, 1983.
23. Yang CC, Chai CY: Animal study of skin resurfacing utilizing the ultrapulse carbon

dioxide laser, *Ann Plast Surg* 35:154-158, 1995.
24. Vogler K, Reindl M: Erbium laser parameters for new medical applications, *Biophotonics Int* Nov/Dec:40-47, 1996.
25. Freeberg IM, Eisen AZ, Wolff K et al: Skin resurfacing—laser. In Herd R, Dover JS, Arndt KA, editors: *Dermatology in general medicine*, New York, 1999, McGraw-Hill, pp 2950-2958.
26. Niamtu J: To debride or not to debride? That is the question: rethinking char removal in ablative CO_2 laser skin resurfacing, *Dermatol Surg* 34:1200-1211, 2008.
27. Collawn SS: Re-epithelialization of the skin following CO_2 laser resurfacing, *J Cosmet Laser Ther* 3:123-127, 2001.
28. Fitzpatrick RE, Goldman MP, Sripachya-Anunt S: Resurfacing of photodamage on the neck with an Ultrapulse carbon dioxide laser, *Lasers Surg Med* 28:145-149, 2001.
29. Sabini P: Classifying, diagnosing and treating the complications of resurfacing the facial skin, *Facial Plast Surg Clin North Am* 12:357-361, 2004.
30. Manuskiatti W, Fitzpatrick RE, Goldman MP: Prophylactic antibiotics in patients undergoing laser resurfacing of the skin, *J Am Acad Dermatol* 40:77-84, 1999.
31. Airan LE, Hruza G: Current lasers in skin resurfacing, *Facial Plast Surg Clin North Am* 13:127-139, 2005.
32. Alster TS, West TB: Resurfacing of atrophic facial acne scars with high energy, pulsed carbon diode laser, *Dermatol Surg* 22:151-154, 1996.
33. Fulton JE, Rahimi AD, Mansoor S, et al: The treatment of hypopigmentation after skin resurfacing, *Dermatol Surg* 30:95-101, 2004.

Jill M. Weber, Jonathan S. Bailey

Management of non-melanoma skin cancer (NMSC) can be challenging for the oral and maxillofacial surgeon. The incidence of skin cancer is increasing with the aging population, and treatment decisions must be individualized for every patient. Surgical excision remains the 'gold standard' treatment of basal cell carcinoma (BCC) and squamous cell carcinoma (SCC). Once the cutaneous malignancy is completely excised, multiple reconstructive options exist. Reconstructive goals include preservation of facial function and cosmesis. Facial reconstruction can be achieved with a variety of surgical options that camouflage defects and preserve important anatomic structures. Postoperatively, careful wound management and close follow-up can minimize long-term complications and recurrence.

ETIOPATHOGENESIS/CAUSATIVE FACTORS

With more than 1 million cases diagnosed each year, NMSC has become the most common malignancy in the United States. Recent studies have indicated that patients with NMSC are younger and have multiple lesions throughout their lifetime. Approximately 80% of all skin cancer diagnoses are BCC, with a BCC/SCC ratio of 4:1 (Fig. 110-1). The cause of NMSC is multifactorial. Frequent exposure to ultraviolet radiation, which is capable of inducing DNA mutations in the p53 tumor suppressor gene, is the primary causative factor. Other well-documented risk factors include fair skin, light eyes and hair, older age, male sex, and immunosuppression. Patients with a diagnosis of NMSC are also at high risk for the development of a second lesion. Meta-analysis of subsequent NMSC diagnoses has demonstrated a 44% chance of subsequent BCCs developing and an 18% chance for subsequent SCCs. Finally, actinic keratoses and Bowen disease (SCC in situ) are common precursors of SCC in patients with increased sun exposure. These patches of irregular, scaly plaques serve as an indication for long-term skin surveillance.

PATHOLOGIC ANATOMY

Surgical excision in the head and neck region requires careful preoperative planning and a thorough understanding of reconstructive options. Facial anatomy, sensation, and function should be preserved while ensuring complete removal of the malignant lesion. The skin is composed of both a superficial and deep vascular plexus between the dermis and subcutaneous fat (Fig. 110-2).

The blood supply to the face is derived from branches of the external and internal carotid arteries with rich collateral networks. Although the face is highly vascularized and adaptable, limitations do exist. The surrounding skin color, texture, hair growth, and

anatomic structures must be carefully considered. Reconstruction of a wound should not compromise function, esthetics, or blood supply.

Facial cutaneous defects can be categorized into well-known esthetic units: forehead, periorbita, nose, cheek, lip, chin, ear, and scalp (Fig. 110-3). These units have both advantages and limitations in surgical reconstruction that must be considered preoperatively.

The skin also adapts to repetitive contracture of facial muscles by forming relaxed skin tension lines (RSTLs). These lines or creases correspond to the insertion of facial musculature into the overlying dermis (Fig. 110-4). Careful placement of incisions within subunit margins and RSTLs can skillfully mask an oncologic reconstruction.

DIAGNOSTIC STUDIES

Laboratory tests and radiographic imaging studies are often not indicated for simple NMSC of the head and neck region. A diagnosis of NMSC must be obtained from a biopsy of the lesion. Ideally, the specimen chosen is from the most representative area of the lesion. Surgical diagnostic options include shave, punch, incisional, and excisional biopsy. If the lesion is suspected to violate deep structures such as muscle or periosteum, computed tomography with intravenous contrast enhancement is warranted (Fig. 110-5). The incidence of metastasis in patients with NMSC is less than 1% for BCC but can be as high as 20% for cutaneous SCC of the head and neck region. Larger, invasive lesions require aggressive surgical excision and possibly lymph node dissection.

Shave biopsies are useful for exophytic lesions in the epidermis or superficial dermis (Fig. 110-6). A punch biopsy includes dermis and subcutaneous fat for extended histologic examination. Three-millimeter to 4-mm punch biopsies are usually adequate to obtain an appropriate histologic sampling of a suspicious skin lesion. Incisional and excisional biopsies are often used for larger lesions or inflammatory/ulcerative lesions in which comparison to normal skin is desirable. These excisions are usually elliptic in nature. Once a diagnosis of NMSC has been made, surgical treatment options can be considered.

TREATMENT GOALS

The goals of treatment are to completely remove the malignant lesion and preserve normal function and appearance of the face. Although surgical excision of NMSC is the gold standard, ablative options also include cryotherapy, curettage and electrodesiccation, laser ablation, photodynamic therapy, radiation therapy, topical 5-fluorouracil, and Mohs micrographic surgery. Surgical excision of a BCC or SCC involves removal of the lesion along with adequate margins of normal tissue to ensure complete removal of malignant pathology. Reported recommendations for adequate surgical margins

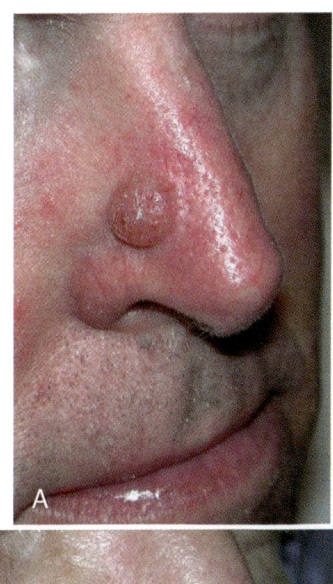

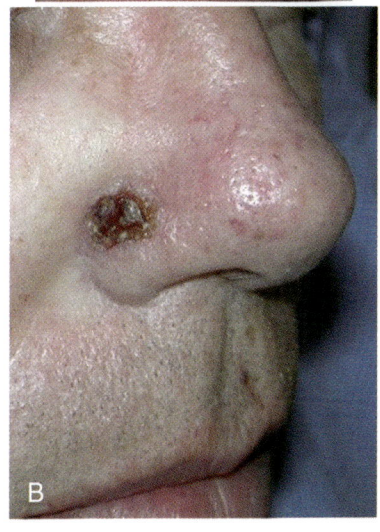

Fig. 110-1 ■ **A,** Typical pearlescent basal cell carcinoma nodule with central telangiectasias and superficial skin crusting. **B,** Typical squamous cell carcinoma lesion with erythematous, rolled margins and overlying ulceration.

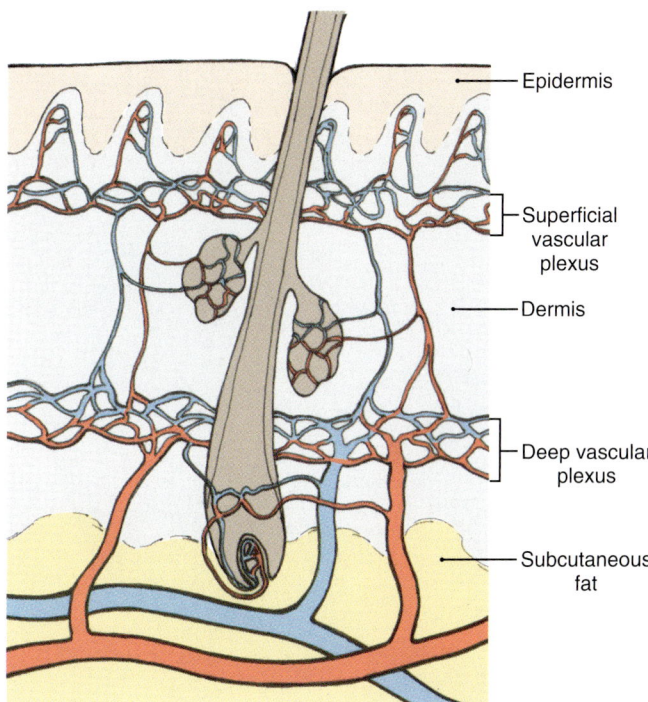

Fig. 110-2 ■ Cutaneous dermal vascular supply. (From Baker SR: *Local flaps in facial reconstruction*, ed 2, Philadelphia, 2007, Mosby.)

vary from 2 to 10 mm. For lesions smaller than 2 cm, studies have demonstrated that more than 96% are completely excised with 4-mm margins. Smaller lesions can be excised with slightly smaller margins, whereas lesions larger than 2 cm require margins up to 1 cm.

Histologic variants of BCC can influence the recommended excision margins as well. Although nodular, pigmented, and superficially spreading BCCs are managed conservatively, morpheaform BCC requires wider surgical margins. A histologic diagnosis of morpheaform BCC requires at least 7-mm margins with frozen sections or Mohs micrographic surgery. Recommended margins for excision are included in Table 110-1. Surgical excisions must always be correlated with final pathology to confirm negative margins.

SPECIFIC RECONSTRUCTIVE TREATMENT AND TECHNIQUES

Repair of facial cutaneous defects should start with a reconstructive algorithm for the least invasive method to maintain cosmesis and function. Generally, the "ladder" of reconstruction includes healing by secondary intention, primary closure (immediate or delayed),

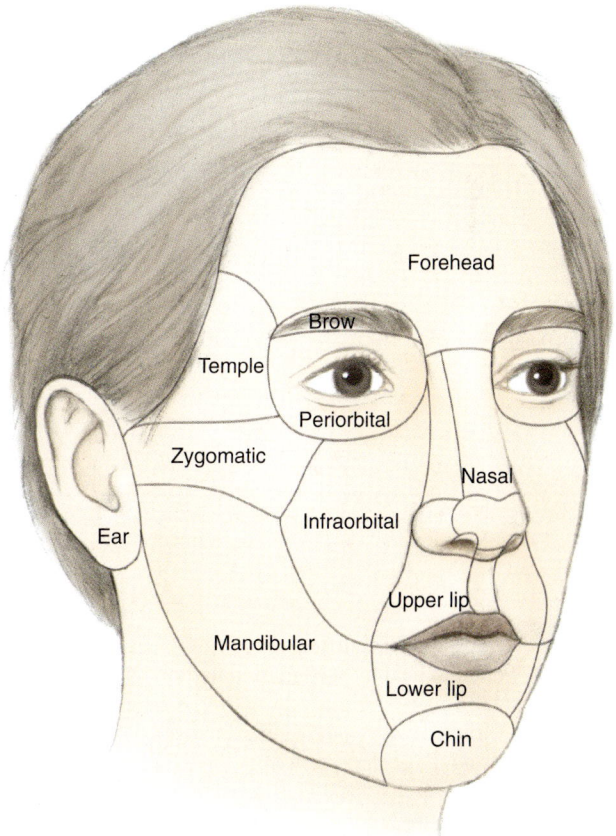

Fig. 110-3 ■ Facial esthetic subunits. (From Baker SR: *Local flaps in facial reconstruction*, ed 2, Philadelphia, 2007, Mosby.)

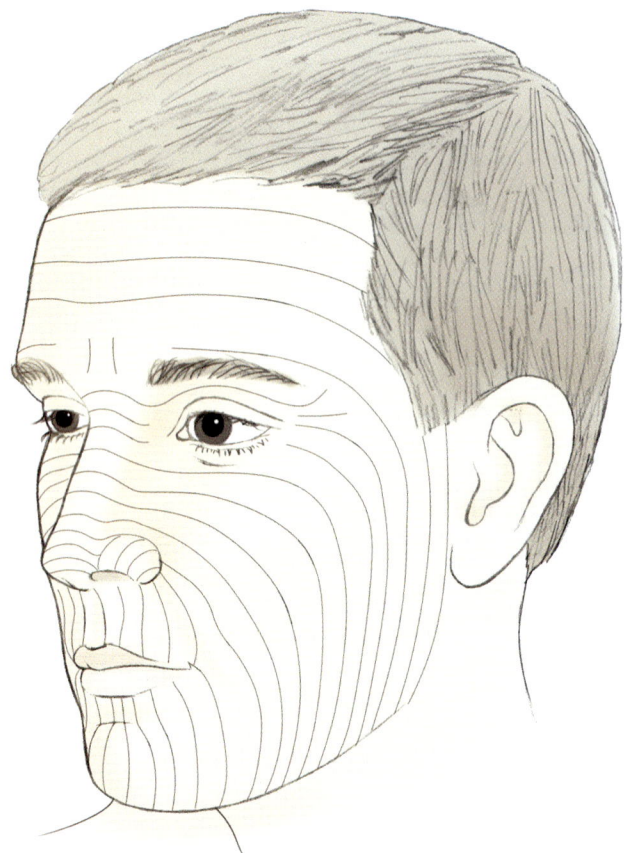

Fig. 110-4 ■ Facial relaxed skin tension lines. These lines deepen with age and incisions should be parallel to them to decrease visible scars. (From Baker SR: *Local flaps in facial reconstruction*, ed 2, Philadelphia, 2007, Mosby.)

TABLE 110-1	Authors' Recommended Margins for Excision of Cutaneous Non-melanoma Skin Cancer
LESION SIZE	**MARGINS**
<1 cm	2-3 mm
1-2 cm	3-5 mm
>2 cm	10 mm or Mohs surgery
Morpheaform basal cell carcinoma	7-10 mm or Mohs surgery

Data from Bailey JS, Goldwasser MS: Surgical management of facial skin cancer, *Oral Maxillofac Surg Clin North Am* 17:205-233, 2005.

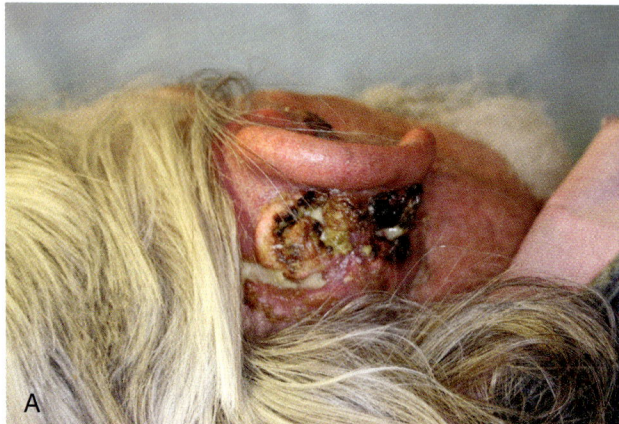

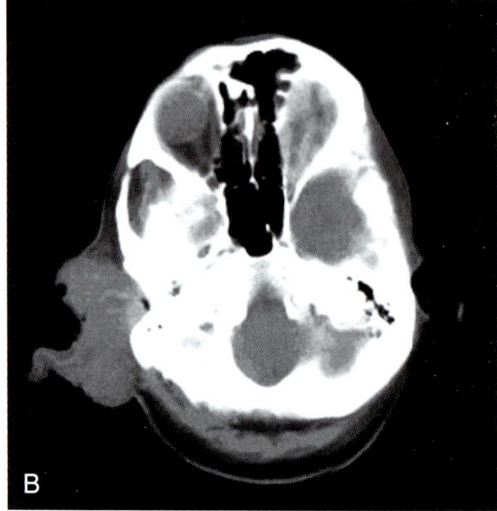

Fig. 110-5 ■ **A,** Large, ulcerative squamous cell carcinoma of the right helix and postauricular region. **B,** Computed tomography scan with contrast enhancement demonstrating a skin lesion with invasion of the temporal bone.

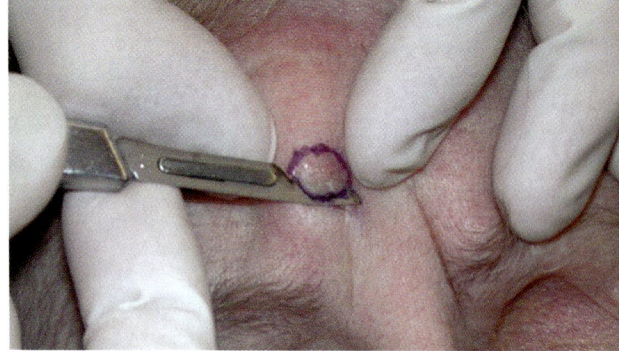

Fig. 110-6 ■ Shave biopsy of forehead basal cell carcinoma.

skin grafts, local flaps, distant flaps, and microvascular free flaps. Allowing a wound to heal by secondary intention may be useful for defects too small to graft or close primarily. Small elliptic defects may be reconstructed with simple, linear closure. A well-planned excision will camouflage the scar within the RSTLs of the face.

When planned properly, local flaps provide excellent color match and adequate blood supply for reconstruction. Flaps can be classified according to their blood supply (random or axial), configuration (bilobe, rhomboid), location (local, distant), movement (rotation, transposition), and tissue type (skin, skin/muscle) (Fig. 110-7). Most facial flaps are randomly patterned to include a blood supply from the highly vascular superficial and deep plexus of the face. Once stabilized, a random flap receives blood supply through its base. Neovascularization of the flap begins 3 to 7 days after transfer to the surrounding tissue bed. Axial flaps are based on blood supply by a direct vessel that is incorporated into the flap. However, most axial flaps have some random blood supply at their distal end.

Facial reconstruction is often achieved with rotation, advancement, or transposition flaps. Rotation flaps move tissue around a

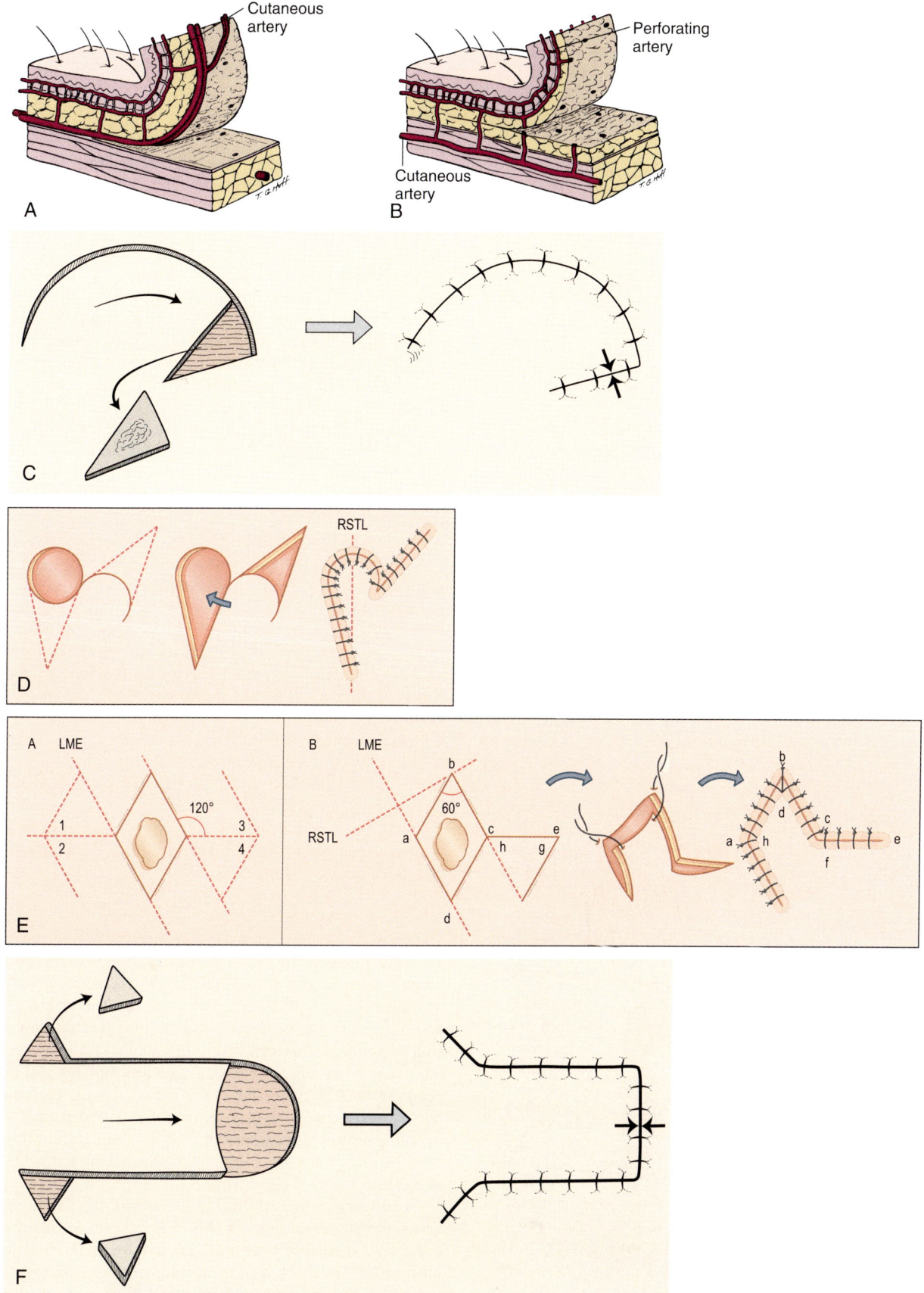

Fig. 110-7 ■ **A,** Axial flap. **B,** Random flap. **C,** Rotational flap. **D,** Transposition flap. **E,** Advancement flap. **F,** Rhomboid flap. (**A** and **B,** From Browner BD, Jupiter JB, Levine AM, et al: *Skeletal trauma,* ed 4, Philadelphia, 2009, Saunders; **C** and **F,** From Baker SR: *Local flaps in facial reconstruction,* ed 2, Philadelphia, 2007, Mosby; **D** and **E,** From Albert DM, Miller JW, Azar DT, et al: *Albert & Jakobiec's principles and practice of ophthalmology,* ed 3, Philadelphia, 2008, Saunders.)

central pivot point from the donor site to the surgical defect. Examples of rotation flaps include rhomboid and bilobe flaps. The classic rhomboid flap has sides of equal length and opposing 60- and 120-degree angles (see Fig. 110-7, *F*). The flap can be rotated in four directions to determine the most cosmetic options for closure. Advancement flaps have a linear configuration and are directly moved into an adjacent defect. Examples of advancement flaps include single (melolabial, dorsal nasal, cervicofacial), bipedicle, or V-Y. Transposition flaps are created to move the donor site to the defect about a pedicle. The tissue beneath the flap remains undisturbed while the flap is allowed to heal. Several days later, the flap is inset and the pedicle is removed.

With knowledge of facial subunits and restorative options, one can carefully plan a cosmetic and functional reconstruction. No single flap or graft is ideal for every defect. Common reconstructive options for facial subunits are provided in the following sections.

FOREHEAD

The forehead unit extends from the hairline superiorly to the eyebrows and nasion inferiorly. Laterally, two convex subunits extend from the lateral orbital rim to the hairline at the level of the zygomatic arch. Within this esthetic unit, the frontalis and corrugator muscles form the horizontal and vertical RSTLs of the forehead. The temporal branch of the facial nerve crosses the zygomatic arch and inserts deep to the frontalis muscle no more than 2 cm above the lateral aspect of the eyebrow. The adjacent hairline and eyebrows provide potential areas for scar camouflage. Care must be taken to prevent brow asymmetry and cause a permanent surprised or menacing look.

Smaller excisions (<1 cm) within the forehead and glabella should be oriented parallel to RSTLs and be closed primarily (Fig. 110-8). Larger defects in this region can be reconstructed with advancement or rotation flaps. Unilateral or bilateral advancement flaps, such as H-plasty, can be designed along RSTLs. These flaps

are undermined in the mid to deep subcutaneous planes and advanced superficial to the underlying muscle. Large defects may also be reconstructed with split-thickness or full-thickness skin grafts, but color mismatch and deformities in contour often result.

PERIORBITA

The periorbital units include the upper and lower eyelids and the medial and lateral canthus subunits. The margins of the upper lid include the brow superiorly and the gray line of the upper lid inferiorly. The lower lid is bounded by the gray line of the lower lid superiorly and the infraorbital rim inferiorly. The lids can be divided into anterior and posterior lamellae. The anterior lamella consists of thin periorbital skin, minimal subcutaneous fat, and the orbicularis oculi muscle. The muscle originates medially from the medial orbital rim and canthal tendon and passes laterally in concentric loops over the lid. It is innervated on its deep surface by the facial nerve. The posterior lamella includes the tarsal plate, orbital septum, lid retractors, and conjunctiva. The orbital septum, continuous with the periosteum of the orbit, inserts into the levator aponeurosis of the upper lid and the tarsal plate of the lower lid.

The canthus subunits include the orbital rims and canthal ligaments. The medial canthal ligament separates into anterior and posterior limbs inserting onto the anterior and posterior lacrimal crests. The medial canthus subunit also includes the superior and inferior lacrimal puncta and canalicular system. The lateral canthal ligament also separates into anterior and posterior limbs that insert onto the lateral orbital periosteum and Whitnall tubercle.

Small partial-thickness lid defects can be reconstructed with primary closure. The wound must be free of tension to avoid lid traction and resultant ectropion. Larger defects can be reconstructed with full-thickness skin grafts or local rotation, advancement, or transposition flaps. Lateral advancement flaps can be useful and hidden within lid creases to advance the skin medially. This avoids vertical tension and ectropion as well. Adequate donor sites for full-thickness grafting include preauricular or postauricular, upper lid, and supraclavicular and medial upper extremity skin. Full-thickness defects less than 25% of the lid can be reconstructed with primary closure. Defects less than 50% often require cantholysis for closure, whereas larger defects necessitate specialized pedicled or transposition flaps.

NOSE

The boundaries of the nasal unit include the nasion superiorly, the ala and columella inferiorly, and the intersection of the medial cheek subunit with the lateral dorsum laterally. The nasal subunits include the lateral nasal wall, dorsum, ala, and tip. The skin overlying the nose varies in thickness and ease of mobility. The dorsum and lateral wall subunits are covered with thin, mobile skin. The nasal tip and inferior nasal subunits are thicker with less mobility and more sebaceous glands. Deep to the subcutaneous tissues, the paired nasal bones provide bony support for the nose. The dorsum is supported by the upper lateral cartilage and nasal septum. Inferiorly, the nasal tip consists of the lower lateral cartilage and the fibroadipose tissue of the ala.

Small surgical defects within the lateral nasal wall and dorsum can be closed primarily within RSTLs. The excision along the lateral nasal wall should be oriented vertically for camouflage within the junction of the cheek and nose. Moderate defects may be reconstructed with local cheek advancement flaps or a dorsal nasal flap. The dorsal nasal flap is a rotation-advancement flap that maintains excellent color match and skin consistency within the subunits of the nose. The flap can be randomly oriented or designed with an axial pedicle from the angular artery.

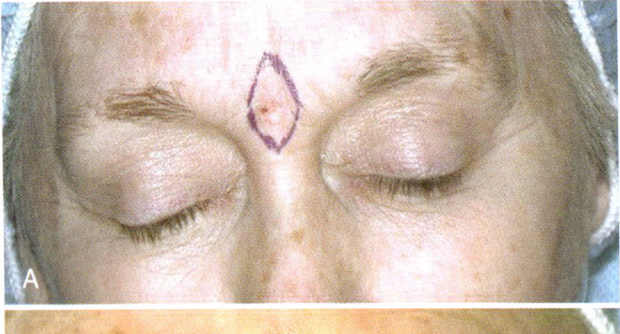
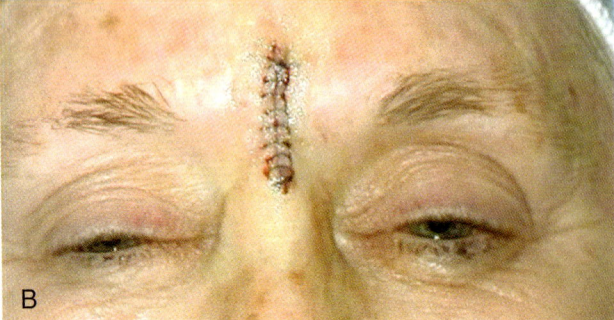

Fig. 110-8 ■ **A,** Planned elliptic excision of a midline forehead basal cell carcinoma. **B,** Primary closure of a small surgical defect parallel to relaxed skin tension lines.

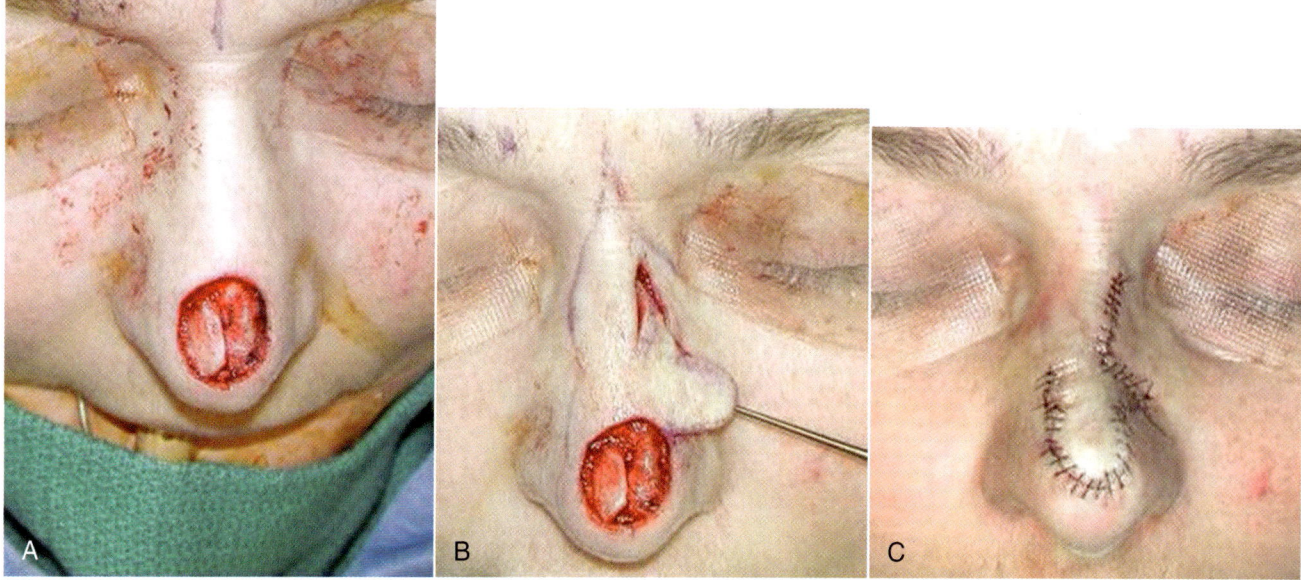

Fig. 110-9 ■ **A,** Nasal tip defect after excision of squamous cell carcinoma. **B,** Elevation and rotation of a bilobe flap. **C,** Insertion of the flap.

Defects of the lower third of the nose are difficult to close primarily. Nasal tip defects may be closed with a full-thickness skin graft. However, cosmetic outcomes may be compromised because of poor skin color and consistency match. Common donor sites include preauricular or postauricular and supraclavicular skin. The nasal tip can often be reconstructed with a bilobe flap (Fig. 110-9). The random rotation flap can be based medially or laterally for defects less than 1.5 cm. The flaps are rotated into the surgical defect at 45 to 60 degrees from the axis of rotation for a total arc of 90 to 120 degrees. Small wedge excisions can be completed to decrease flap redundancy at the turning point of the flap. Each flap is 10-20% smaller than the surgical defect that it restores. The superior flap is usually harvested from the lateral nasal wall with a resultant well-hidden vertical scar. Care should be taken to avoid alar retraction with a defect less than 1 cm from the alar margin.

The alar subunit can be more difficult to reconstruct. Superficial defects limited to the ala can be managed with local advancement flaps, such as the melolabial flap. The random flaps may be designed with either superior or inferior pedicles. Full-thickness lesions require cartilage grafting to prevent contracture or nasal valve collapse. Composite grafts may be used for small defects. Skin, subcutaneous tissue, and cartilage may be harvested from the helical rim or conchal bowl to provide alar support. Donor size is limited to approximately 2 cm to ensure revascularization of the graft.

Larger nasal defects involving the dorsum, lateral nasal wall, and tip can be reconstructed with a paramedian forehead flap. This axial pattern flap is based on the supratrochlear artery and provides excellent color match. The supratrochlear artery exits the orbit and travels superiorly in a subcutaneous plane 1.7 to 2.2 cm from the midline of the forehead. Intraoperatively, Doppler ultrasound is used to identify the vessel and mark the course of the pedicle. The defect size can be transferred to the forehead for size match. The proximal flap is elevated to include the frontalis muscle, superficial to the periosteum. The distal flap may be elevated in a subdermal plane because the vessels run more superficially. Once elevated, the transpositional flap is rotated and inset. The forehead defect is closed primarily by skin undermining and advancement. Three weeks after primary repair, the flap is separated, thinned, and inset for optimal cosmetic results.

CHEEK

The cheek esthetic units extend from the zygomatic arches and infraorbital rims superiorly to the inferior border of the mandible inferiorly. Medially, they are bounded by the nasolabial and melolabial folds, as well as by the lateral dorsum of the nose. The cheek unit extends laterally to the preauricular crease. Within this esthetic unit, RSTLs are more vertical posteriorly and diagonal in the anterior perioral region. The skin in the anterior subunit is thicker and more mobile, whereas the preauricular region is much thinner. This skin covers the superficial musculoaponeurotic system, which is continuous with the temporoparietal fascia superiorly and the platysma inferiorly. The deeper parotidomasseteric fascia encloses the facial nerve as it divides the parotid gland into superficial and deep lobes.

Cheek reconstruction can be categorized by subunits: suborbital and perioral medial cheek, mid-cheek, and temporal/preauricular. Small medial cheek defects can be closed primarily and camouflaged along RSTLs or the melolabial fold. Larger defects often require advancement or rotation flaps, such as a cervicofacial advancement flap (Fig. 110-10). The flaps can be extended into the neck or postauricular regions to use the skin mobility within this region. Mid-cheek defects can be closed primarily along RSTLs as well. The final orientation should be more vertical than within the perioral region. Larger defects may require skin grafting or cervicofacial advancement. Care must be taken to avoid vertical tension with resultant lower eyelid ectropion.

The temporal/preauricular skin has less laxity than the rest of the cheek. However, small defects may be advanced primarily to follow the vertical RSTLs and parallel the hairline. Larger defects may require local advancement flaps. Care must be taken to not advance hair-bearing regions onto the subunits of the face.

LIP

The lip unit can be divided into three subunits: upper lip, lower lip, and mental unit. The boundaries of the upper lip include the ala and columella superiorly, the wet/dry line inferiorly, and the nasolabial grooves laterally. The lower lip boundaries include the wet/dry line superiorly, the mentolabial groove inferiorly, and the melolabial groove laterally. The chin is bounded by the mentolabial groove and

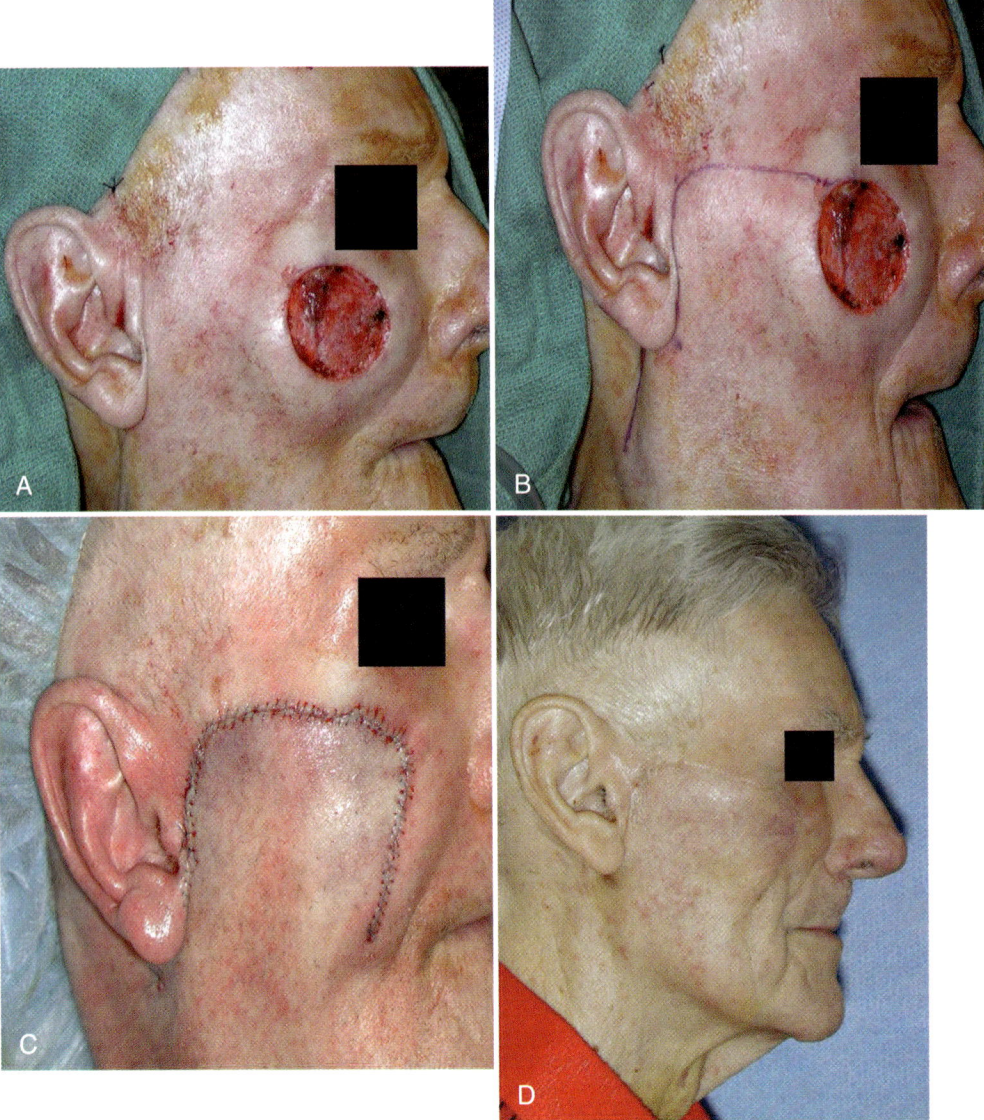

Fig. 110-10 ■ **A,** Large mid-cheek defect after excision of squamous cell carcinoma. **B,** Posteriorly based cervicofacial advancement flap designed between the temporal and mid-cheek subunits. **C,** Advancement and inset along the right preauricular skin crease. **D,** Postoperative lateral view.

extends inferiorly to the jawline. Deep to the subcutaneous tissues, the orbicularis oris forms the sphincter of the mouth. The upper lip functions in speech and animation, whereas the lower lip is more important as a competent sphincter. The upper lip also contains the philtrum, a subunit that should be preserved or reconstructed for optimal cosmesis. Surrounding muscle groups insert into the orbicularis to elevate or depress the upper or lower lip. The blood supply to the lip unit includes branches of the external carotid artery: superior labial artery, inferior labial artery, and mental artery.

The main goals of lip reconstruction include maintaining oral competence, adequate mouth opening, and normal anatomy for speech. Small partial-thickness defects that do not violate the orbicularis may be reconstructed with primary closure. Care must be taken to closely reapproximate the white roll and vermilion border; even small discrepancies will be noticeable to the patient. Small partial-thickness or full-thickness defects of the lips (<30%) can be reconstructed with primary closure. A simple wedge excision with layered closure of mucosa, orbicularis, and skin is well tolerated. Larger partial-thickness defects of the upper lip can also be reconstructed with an inferiorly based melolabial flap (Fig. 110-11).

Large full-thickness defects of the upper or lower lip (>30-40%) require two-stage lip flaps or large advancement flap reconstruction. Abbe and Estlander flaps are lip-switch flaps that borrow pedicled tissue from the opposing lip. The flaps are designed with a height equal to the defect and a width approximately half that of the defect. The flaps are elevated with care to include and preserve the labial artery within the subcutaneous tissue. Two to three weeks after the primary surgery, the flap is divided. Karapandzic flaps can also be used for large lower lip defects. The perioral incisions create bilateral skin and muscle flaps for rotation and advancement. Although neurovascular and sphincter function is well maintained, the patient must be prepared for postoperative microstomia.

EAR

The external ear consists of thin skin and subcutaneous tissue over flexible fibrocartilage. The auricular subunit can be divided into the helix, antihelix, conchal bowl, and triangular fossa. The lobule subunit is dense in connective tissue and fat without underlying cartilage. Reconstruction of small, partial-thickness defects can be managed with primary closure over intact perichondrium. Larger

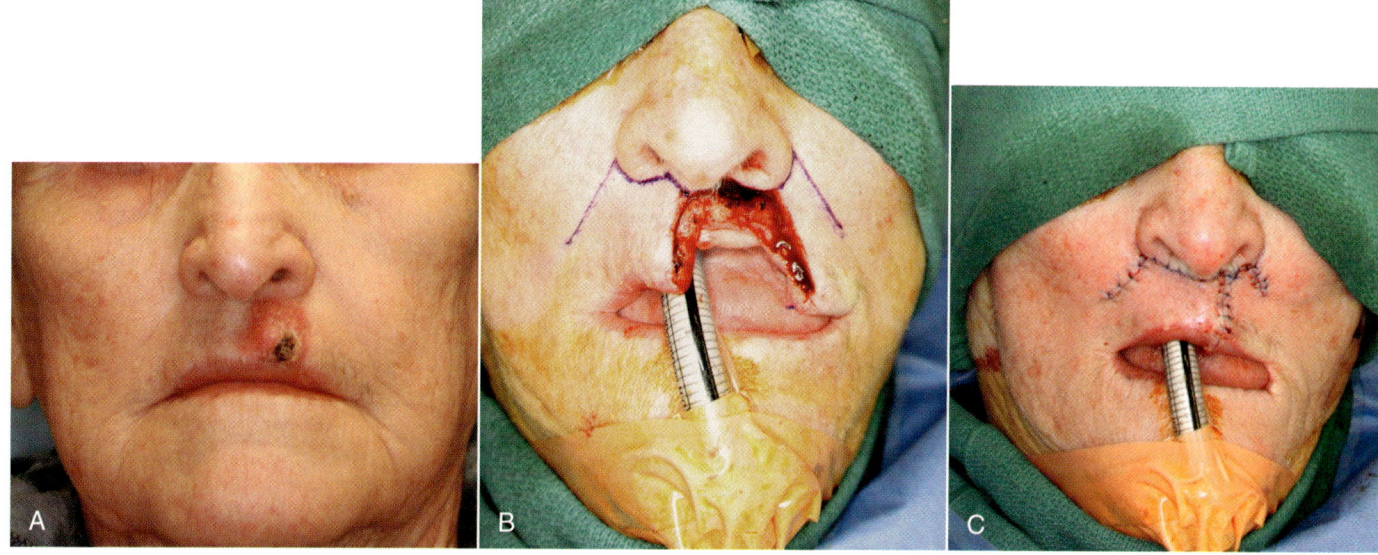

Fig. 110-11 ■ **A,** Large invasive squamous cell carcinoma of the upper lip. **B,** Full-thickness excision with an inferiorly based melolabial advancement flap design. **C,** Flap insertion.

partial-thickness defects can be reconstructed with full-thickness skin grafts over cartilage and perichondrium. If the perichondrium is resected, cartilage can be excised with placement of a full-thickness graft along the underlying posterior dermis. Partial-thickness defects along the helix may also be managed with wedge excision or helical advancement and primary closure. Lesions within the lobule subunit can often be closed primarily with minimal cosmetic deformity.

SCALP

The scalp can be divided into layers from superficial to deep: skin, subcutaneous tissue, musculoaponeurotic layer, loose areolar tissue, and pericranium. Its rich blood supply is derived from the supra-orbital, supratrochlear, superficial temporal, postauricular, and occipital arteries. The skin and subcutaneous tissues of the scalp are closely adherent and surgically indivisible. The musculoaponeurotic layer is formed by a continuous fusion of the frontalis, occipitalis, and auricular muscles. The galea is the dense fibrous sheet connecting these muscles in the midline. Deep to the aponeurosis, the loose areolar tissue can easily be mobilized from the pericranium for surgical dissection and reconstruction.

Small scalp defects (<2 to 3 cm) can be repaired by primary closure. Undermining within the loose areolar plane allows greater mobility and advancement beneath the rigid galeal layer. Other reconstructive options include skin grafting or healing by secondary intention. Cosmetic outcomes are often unacceptable with these techniques because of the lack of hair and poor color match within the reconstructed defect. Larger scalp defects can be reconstructed with advancement, rotation, or transposition flaps. Skin may be advanced with multiple, bilateral flaps to close up to 20% of the scalp. With larger defects, tissue expansion or free flap reconstruction should be considered.

ANTISEPSIS AND ANTIBIOTIC THERAPY

The incidence of postoperative wound infections in patients undergoing elective skin procedures performed in a surgical environment is less than 1%. Surgical antisepsis is achieved by cleansing the skin, isolating a surgical field, using sterile equipment, and preparing the surgeon and staff. Wounds on intact skin can be cleansed with povidone-iodine solution, chlorhexidine, or isopropyl alcohol. Standard antibiotic hand washes are adequate to reduce the bacterial load for clean dermatologic procedures. The facial wounds can then be draped with care to ensure comfort of the patient. Exposure of a patient's hair, mouth, or nose does not statistically increase infection rates. Patients undergoing simple skin excision are not routinely given preoperative or postoperative antibiotic therapy. However, antibiotics may benefit the patient if nasal or oral mucosa is involved or the surgery entails extensive duration and dissection. Adequate coverage for the common skin bacterium *Staphylococcus aureus* can be achieved with first-generation cephalosporins administered 30 to 60 minutes before the procedure.

POSTOPERATIVE CARE

Postoperative care includes meticulous cleansing of the wound until the sutures are removed. Placement of dressings on facial wounds is often unnecessary. Pressure or bolster dressings may be applied to free grafts or to nose or ear reconstructions to prevent graft movement or hematoma formation. Wounds should be cleansed with a 1:1 mixture of hydrogen peroxide and water every 8 hours until the sutures are removed. A thin layer of topical antibiotic ointment is recommended after cleansing for 2 to 3 days. Facial sutures are typically removed 4 to 7 days postoperatively; scalp sutures and staples can be removed in 7 to 14 days, depending on wound size and tension. If desired, wounds can be supported with adhesive strips after suture removal for increased tensile strength. Patients are discouraged from exposing the wound to direct shower spray or water submersion before suture removal. If delayed reconstruction is planned, the wound is routinely treated with wet-to-dry dressings that are changed two to three times daily until reconstruction takes place. After removal of the sutures, patients are instructed on gentle cleansing of the wound, minimization of sun exposure, and routine use of sunscreen.

PEARLS AND PITFALLS

- Reconstruction of a defect across facial subunits or RSTLs often results in poor cosmesis. Scar revision may be necessary for realignment.
- A biopsy should avoid necrotic or ulcerative tissue samples to obtain an accurate histologic diagnosis.
- Mohs micrographic surgery is a conservative ablation technique that minimizes tissue loss in challenging reconstructive areas such as the eyelids, bridge of the nose, or ala.
- Delayed reconstruction is an excellent option for practitioners without access to frozen section pathology. The patient can often

maintain dressing changes with minimal instruction. The treatment interval also ensures complete excision and allows more time for planning surgery.
- The elasticity of skin should not be underestimated, especially in the elderly. Planning for reconstruction should include careful observation of the mobility of surrounding skin. The skin can be widely undermined to achieve greater rotation or advancement.
- Wound care instructions for the patient should be regimented and clear. This will often avoid confusion, patient hesitation, and dirty postoperative wounds.

BIBLIOGRAPHY

Bailey J, Goldwasser M: Surgical management of facial skin cancer, *Oral Maxillofac Surg Clin North Am* 17:205-233, 2005.

Baker SR: *Local flaps in facial reconstruction,* ed 2, St Louis, 2007, CV Mosby.

Bruce AJ, Brodland DG: Overview of skin cancer detection and prevention for the primary care physician, *Mayo Clin Proc* 75:491-500, 2000.

Ellis E, Zide M: *Surgical approaches to the facial skeleton,* ed 2, Baltimore, Lippincott Williams & Wilkins, 1995.

Fahrner L III: Mohs micrographic surgery for mucocutaneous malignancies, *Oral Maxillofac Surg Clin North Am* 17:161-171, 2005.

Ghauri RR, Gunter AA, Weber RA: Frozen section analysis in the management of skin cancers, *Ann Plast Surg* 43:156-160, 1999.

Herford A, Zide M: Reconstruction of superficial skin cancer defects of the nose, *J Oral Maxillofac Surg* 59:760-767, 2001.

Kanjilal S, Strom SS, Clayman GL, et al: p53 mutations in nonmelanoma skin cancer of the head and neck: molecular evidence for field cancerization, *Cancer Res* 55:3604-3609, 1995.

Manstein ME, Manstein CH, Smith R: How accurate is frozen section for skin cancers? *Ann Plast Surg* 50:607-609, 2003.

Martinez JC, Otley CC: The management of non-melanoma skin cancer: a review for the primary care physician, *Mayo Clin Proc* 76:1253-1265, 2001.

Poulson M, Burmeister B, Kennedy D: Preservation of form and function in the

management of head and neck skin cancer, *World J Surg* 27:868-874, 2003.

Reddy L, Zide M: Reconstruction of skin cancer defects of the auricle, *J Oral Maxillofac Surg* 62:1457-1471, 2004.

Thomas DJ, King AR, Peat BG: Excision margins for nonmelanotic skin cancer, *Plast Reconstr Surg* 112:57-63, 2003.

Wolf DJ, Zitelli JA: Surgical margins for basal cell carcinoma, *Arch Dermatol* 123:340-344, 1987.

Zide M, Adnot J: Delayed treatment of patients with multiple facial skin cancer defects: the effect of setting, *J Oral Maxillofac Surg* 66:1545-1550, 2008.

Chapter **111**

Evaluation and Management of Maxillofacial Vascular Lesions

Edward T. Lahey III, Leonard B. Kaban

In order to develop a rational plan for management of oral and maxillofacial vascular anomalies, clinicians must have a basic understanding of the biology of these lesions and the nomenclature and classification system used to characterize them. Often referred to as birthmarks, vascular lesions are often as misunderstood by the medical community as they are by the lay community. While a standard classification system has been adopted, the medical literature is replete with archaic terminology that persists and continues to be passed on to new generations of clinicians. Outdated terms such as "stork bite," "angioma simplex," or the indiscriminately applied "hemangioma" were derived from classification systems

that were either descriptive, pathological, or embryological in nature. A biologically based classification system of vascular lesions proposed by Mulliken and Glowacki in 1982 was accepted as the standard classification system by the International Society for the Study of Vascular Anomalies in 1996. This binary system designates vascular lesions as either tumors or malformations based on endothelial cell kinetics and clinical behavior. Vascular malformations are relevant to the daily practice of most oral and maxillofacial surgeons and will be the focus of this chapter. Vascular tumors will be discussed only in the context of differentiating them from malformations.

ETIOPATHOGENESIS

The innermost cell layer of hematic and lymphatic vessels, the endothelium, has a relatively slow turnover time. A vascular lesion that demonstrates endothelial hyperplasia (enlargement due to increased cell number), with mitotic figures and short doubling times, is categorized as a *vascular tumor*. The most commonly encountered vascular tumor (and, for that matter, most common tumor of infancy) is the infantile hemangioma. This tumor generally appears at or shortly after birth (most commonly in the craniofacial area) and rapidly grows for the first year of life, then slowly involutes over the next 5 to 7 years until an end-stage, involuted lesion remains. It occurs more commonly in premature and female neonates, does not occur intraosseously, and while it rarely (<1%) can lead to deformational changes in adjacent bone, it has no direct physiological influence on osseous growth. In turn, a vascular lesion that exhibits a normal rate of endothelial turnover but structural and morphological anomalies due to errors in embryogenesis is termed a *vascular malformation*. Vascular malformations are always present (though not always seen) at birth, do not proliferate but instead demonstrate slow, relentless expansion, and do not involute. The reader may question this statement, having experienced abrupt changes in the presentation of a long-standing vascular malformation. Trauma, sepsis, hormonal modulation, and changes in blood or lymph flow and/or pressure may indeed temporarily speed up a malformation's expansion, but this is due to hypertrophy (enlargement due to an increase in size of existing structures) and not hyperplasia. Vascular malformations have equal sex distribution, can occur intraosseously, and in up to a third of the cases produce secondary skeletal changes. This last point is of particular importance to the oral and maxillofacial surgeon.

Vascular malformations can usually be differentiated from hemangiomas by clinical exam and history with an accuracy of 90% (Fig. 111-1). In the rare situation where the diagnosis is equivocal, additional studies can be obtained. Histological studies of a biopsy specimen should be obtained, especially if a rare or possibly malignant vascular tumor is suspected. Lawley et al. demonstrated that the Wilms tumor 1 (WT1) gene as detected in mRNA of endothelium is expressed in the endothelium of hemangiomas but not in vascular malformations. Leon-Villapalos et al. also confirmed that the erythrocyte-type glucose transporter protein GLUT-1 is usually expressed in hemangiomas but not vascular malformations. Serum and urine markers are less helpful in differentiating between the two anomalies.

The etiology of vascular malformation development is incompletely understood but molecular studies suggest abnormalities in signaling processes that regulate cellular proliferation and apoptosis, differentiation, maturation, and adhesion are possible causes. While several families demonstrating autosomal dominant inheritance of vascular malformations have been identified and are being studied, the overwhelming majority of vascular malformations occur sporadically and lack any Mendelian pattern of inheritance. Vascular malformations are known components of several syndromes involving the maxillofacial region. The most germane are mentioned in the following sections of this chapter. It is interesting to note that a recent study found that individuals with Down syndrome have an 80% risk reduction of vascular anomalies.

SUBCLASSIFICATION OF VASCULAR MALFORMATIONS

Vascular malformations are described and classified by the vessels involved and their flow characteristics. Anatomically, malformations may be composed of capillaries, lymphatic vessels, veins, arteries, or a combination of the above and are named accordingly (e.g., capillary malformation, lymphatic malformation, venous-lymphatic malformation, arterio-venous malformation, etc.). Dynamically, malformations may demonstrate slow or fast fluid flow. Slow-flow malformations include capillary, lymphatic, and venous malformations alone or in any combination. Fast-flow malformations are any that contain an arterial component (e.g., arterial or arteriovenous malformations).

Understanding the nature and behavior of vascular malformations based on the Mulliken and Glowacki classification has allowed surgeons to develop rational treatment strategies that have improved safety and care of patients with these difficult lesions. Evaluation and treatment of each type of malformation is detailed later. It should be noted that combination vascular malformations are treated based on the characteristics of the predominant, deeper malformation.

SLOW-FLOW MALFORMATIONS: CAPILLARY, LYMPHATIC, VENOUS

Slow-flow malformations are listed in ascending order of frequency and flow characteristics:

CAPILLARY MALFORMATIONS

Capillary malformations (CMs) consist of postcapillary venules that have a decreased density of precapillary neurons, leading to the theory that diminished neural modulation of vascular tone may play a role in their development. They have frequently been referred to as "port-wine stains" and have a birth prevalence of 0.3% with equal sex distribution. They often occur in dermatomal distributions. On the face (a common location for CMs), 45% of lesions are restricted to one of the three trigeminal dermatomes. The remaining 55% of facial CMs may occur in overlapping ipsilateral dermatomes or they may cross the facial midline in a bilateral distribution. CMs are usually evident at birth and are often confused with the common vascular birthmark termed the *nevus flammeus neonatorum*. Nevus flammeus occurs in 50% of white newborns and is named according to its location ("angel kiss" when on the upper face and "stork bite" when on the nuchal area). These vascular birthmarks have an unknown etiology, are harmless, and typically disappear within a year. If they persist beyond a year, then reevaluation of the presumed diagnosis is required.

CMs occur sporadically with rare familial cohorts demonstrating an inheritance pattern and are associated with several syndromes. Sturge-Weber is the most common syndrome associated with CMs. The ophthalmic (V1) dermatome of the trigeminal nerve is always involved with possible additional involvement of the maxillary (V2) and mandibular (V3) distributions and ipsilateral ocular and leptomeningeal vascular anomalies. If extensive, intracranial vascular anomalies can cause refractory seizures, contralateral hemiplegia, and delayed motor and cognitive development.

Clinical Features

CMs present at birth as macular, pink/red cutaneous stains that blanch with pressure. Unlike CMs of the trunks and limbs, facial CMs typically develop a deeper hue and are prone to nodular fibrovascular overgrowth in adulthood. It has been noted that patients with facial CMs do not develop acne in the area of the malformation. There is often enlargement of the soft tissue and underlying skeleton, most notably in the maxillofacial region. In the oral and maxillofacial surgery literature, these malformations are often erroneously reported as "hemangiomas." When an underlying skeletal deformity caused by a CM is treated by orthognathic surgery, the case is then

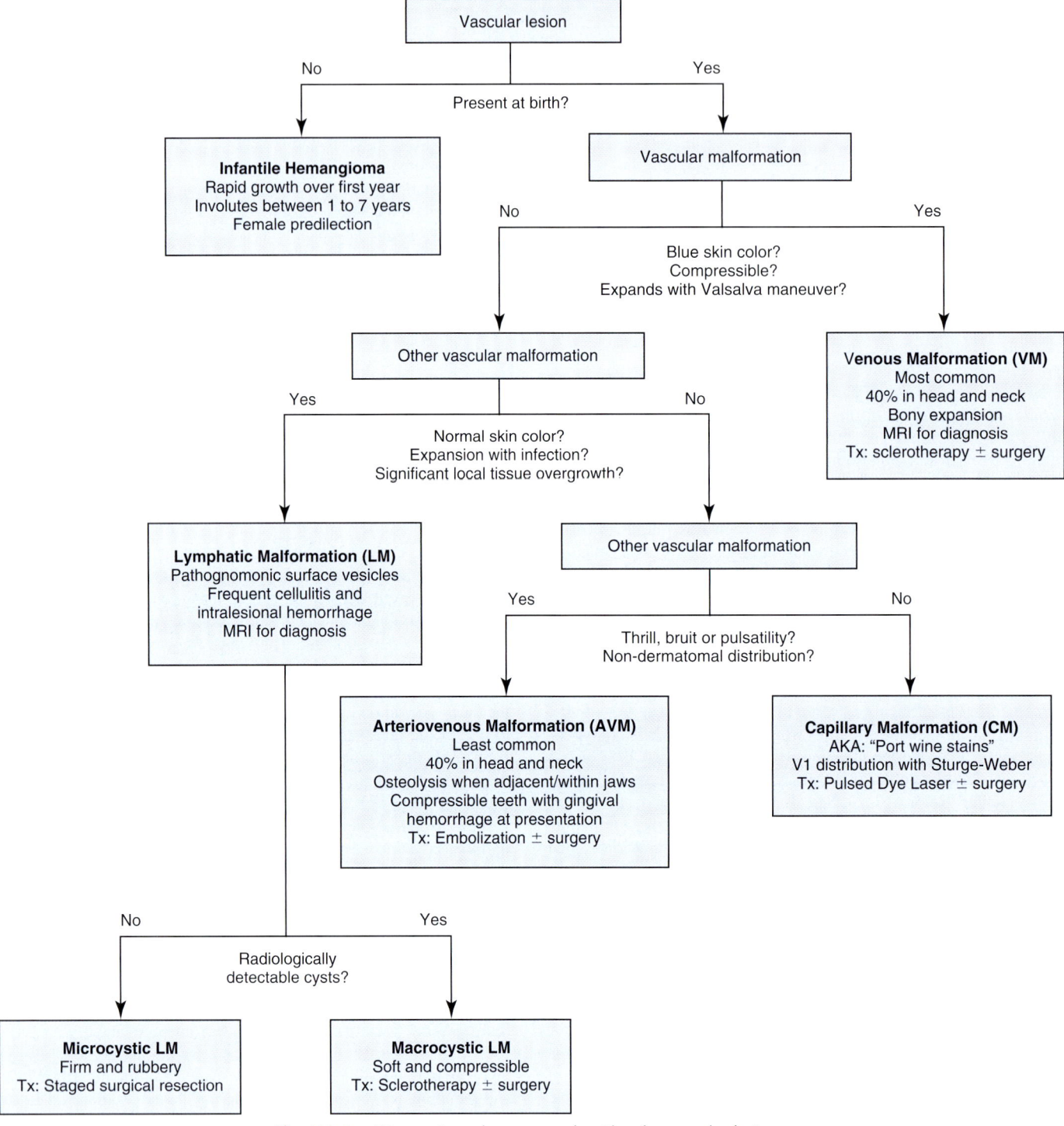

Fig. 111-1 ■ Diagnostic and treatment algorithm for vascular lesions.

reported incorrectly as orthognathic surgery in the setting of a "hemangioma" of the jaw(s).

Diagnostic Studies

No specific laboratory tests are required for CMs. Radiological studies such as MRI or Doppler ultrasound are performed to rule out other associated vascular anomalies that may be deep to the superficial capillary malformation.

Treatment

CMs are treated for esthetic purposes or to prevent overgrowth of adjacent tissue such as the maxillofacial skeleton. Prior to the advent of lasers, camouflage with flesh color tattooing or coagulation by electrocauterization was commonly used to manage CMs. Pulsed dye lasers, which have organic molecules pumped by an argon laser, are now considered the treatment of choice. They work best on lateral facial CMs in persons with fair skin who tan poorly

(Fitzpatrick types I and II). Using wavelengths of 577 nm to 585 nm with a spot size of 5 to 10 mm and energy of 6 to 8 joules/cm^2 at short pulse durations (0.45 to 3 milliseconds) allows selective thermolysis by targeting hemoglobin (the chromophore) to a depth no more than 1.2 mm. This produces little damage to surrounding tissue. The skin is generally cooled with cool air, ice, or 10 to 50 millisecond spurts of cryogen immediately prior to laser exposure. This reduces epidermal melanin absorption. Ten percent overlap of treatment areas ensures the best result.

There is controversy with regard to treatment timing, with some advocating treatment in infancy and others believing age makes no difference. If not anesthetized, patients can expect to feel a "snap" and warm sensation at the treatment area followed by an itch that can last up to 30 minutes. Multiple treatments are necessary, especially in older patients with more mature CMs. Successful lightening occurs in up to 80% of lesions.

The small fibrovascular nodules that can occur are excised, and contour resections of adjacent soft tissue hypertrophy as well as osseous overgrowths can also be completed. Skeletal overgrowth resulting in malocclusion is treated with presurgical orthodontics and orthognathic surgery. The latter is not contraindicated in the setting of pure CMs and is usually performed using hypotensive anesthesia. Mucosal incisions for orthognathic surgery in the presence of CMs can be expected to bleed more profusely than usual but can be easily managed. Dental extractions may also be performed with use of local hemostatic measures.

Posttreatment Care

After laser treatment, the area undergoes stages of color change: initially, a blue-gray discoloration, followed by darkening to almost black over the next 24 hours. This lasts between 10 to 14 days, after which the treated area will appear red. Fading or lightening of the CM becomes evident during the next 2 to 4 weeks (about a month after treatment). Patients will have postoperative discomfort akin to sunburn for which analgesics are prescribed. Ice should be applied to the treated areas for the first 24 hours to reduce swelling. Both hyperpigmentation and hypopigmentation can occur after treatment, though hyperpigmentation generally fades in 8 to 12 weeks. Aloe or Aquaphor (Beiersdorf AG, Hamburg, Germany), can be applied daily until the skin lightens. Hypopigmentation is usually temporary. All patients should be reminded to wear sunscreen throughout the year, and in up to 50% of patients the lesion darkens again in 3 to 4 years.

LYMPHATIC MALFORMATIONS

Lymphatic malformations (LMs) consist of lymphatic spaces filled with eosinophilic, protein-rich fluid and are further subdivided into microcystic, macrocystic, or combined lesions. An LM is considered macrocystic when radiologically detectable cysts are present. This was previously referred to as a "cystic hygroma." The microcystic LM has no radiologically detectable cysts and was known as a "lymphangioma." LMs have been associated with several syndromes, including Noonan and trisomy 13. The incidence of LMs is not known, but they account for 2.8 of every 100,000 hospital admissions. LMs are usually noted between birth and 2 years of age but macrocystic LMs can be diagnosed prenatally by the late first and early second trimesters. If a bilateral cervical LM is diagnosed prenatally, an ex utero intrapartum treatment (EXIT) procedure to secure the newborn's airway may be necessary. The infant is partially delivered via cesarean section and while the placenta and umbilical cord are still intact, the airway is examined and either endotracheal intubation or tracheostomy is completed as needed. Once the airway is secured, the delivery is completed and the umbilical cord clamped. This is an important concept to understand as LMs occur most commonly in the cervicofacial region, with the macrocystic subtype dominating.

LMs are particularly morbid, with patients often developing cellulitis and spontaneous intralesional hemorrhage (in up to 17% of LMs). These problems are often chronic in nature and may require prolonged treatment.

Clinical Features

Patients with LMs most commonly present with a complaint of swelling. The overlying skin is either normal or bluish in color. Dermal involvement can lead to puckering of the overlying skin while involvement of the subcutis or submucosa presents as pathognomonic vesicles resembling minute blisters. If intralesional hemorrhage occurs, the vesicles will appear dark red. In addition, LMs often swell during a viral or bacterial infection anywhere in the body. Macrocystic LMs are soft on palpation, while microcystic LMs are rubbery and firm and, unlike venous malformations (VMs, discussed later), LMs cannot be manually decompressed.

Local tissue overgrowth is characteristically present. LMs of the forehead and orbit cause proptosis, ptosis, restrictive eye movement, and localized overgrowth. Facial LMs lead to macrochilia, macrotia, and macromala, while in the lower face and oral cavity LMs can result in mandibular overgrowth and macroglossia. The tongue and mandibular overgrowth individually or in combination lead to a class III skeletal malocclusion often with an anterior open bite. Cervical LMs most frequently occur in the anterior cervical triangle, sometimes leading to speech and swallowing impairment and/or oropharyngeal airway obstruction.

Diagnostic Studies

MRI is the most useful diagnostic imaging technique. LMs are hyperintense on T2-weighted sequences and hypointense on T1-weighted sequences. Macrocystic LMs often have "fluid-fluid" levels due to layering of protein or old blood, while microcystic LMs typically appear as diffuse "sheets" of bright signal on T2-weighted images.

Plain radiographs and computed tomographic (CT) scans are of limited diagnostic assistance but they are used for planning treatment of skeletal changes caused by LMs. Ultrasound is helpful to differentiate between macrocystic and microcystic LMs. Macrocystic lesions demonstrate anechoic cysts, often containing internal debris and internal septations with no flow, while microcystic LMs are ill-defined echogenic masses showing diffuse involvement of surrounding tissue.

Blood cultures taken in the setting of systemic illness from an infected LM rarely provide insight on the offending organism(s).

Treatment

Treatment is directed at the sequelae of LMs, such as bleeding, infection, contour defects, and malocclusion, and improving function and esthetics. Spontaneous intralesional hemorrhage leading to enlargement and discoloration is treated with pain medication, rest, and serial observation. If a large collection of intralesional blood is noted, preventive antibiotics may be indicated. Long-term prophylactic antibiotics are not generally used. Judicious dental care is a critical preventive maneuver in management of cervicofacial LMs. Patients should be placed on antibiotics active against oral pathogens at the first sign of maxillofacial LM infection. If frank cellulitis develops, patients will require hospital admission for intravenous antibiotic therapy that is often continued for 6 to 8 weeks.

Treatment of macrocystic LMs differs from treatment of microcystic LMs, highlighting the need for accurate subtype identification. Macrocystic LMs are treated most often with sclerotherapy.

Introduction of a sclerosing agent into the lymphatic macrocyst leads to inflammation, fibrosis, and eventual scarring, obliteration, and shrinkage of the LM. The most common sclerosants used in the United States are ethanol, doxycycline, bleomycin, and sodium tetradecyl sulfate. OK-432 (Picibanil), a derivative from a killed strain of group A *Streptococcus pyogenes* in a penicillin suspension that works by an unclear mechanism, is used in many countries outside the United States.

Sclerotherapy is directed at the individual cysts. Each cyst is cannulated with an angiocatheter (or pigtail catheter for large cysts) under ultrasound guidance. The cystic fluid is aspirated and measured, and the cyst is then injected with the sclerosant (e.g., doxycycline at a concentration of 10 mg/mL). For very large cysts, the pigtail catheter is secured and the cyst is injected and drained sequentially for several days.

Sclerotherapy is ineffective for treatment of microcystic LMs, which are best addressed by excision. Staged excision is necessary with total excision rarely being possible. Each resection should concentrate on a defined anatomic region that is dissected as thoroughly as possible with constant nerve monitoring when appropriate. Blood loss should be limited to less than the patient's total blood volume. Upper eyelid LMs are removed through upper tarsal fold incisions, with hemifacial LMs being resected through preauricular incisions or via a transoral route. Labial LMs are resected through a transverse mucosal incision without violation of the vermilion border. Macroglossia is addressed with reduction glossoplasty and excisions from the floor of the mouth and submandibular tissues. Cervical LMs require exploration of the neck with complete dissection of all neurovascular structures.

Skeletal malocclusions are treated with presurgical orthodontic therapy followed by orthognathic surgery. Orthognathic correction is carried out after the completion of skeletal growth, often with adjunctive contour reduction of the bone and partial glossectomy. Tongue reduction is necessary to allow corrective positioning of the mandible with a setback procedure.

Dental extractions may safely be completed though as noted above, judicious use of pre- and postoperative antibiotics is required. Incision and drainage of odontogenic abscesses is also not contraindicated, but the surgeon must be aware of the need for prolonged antibiotic therapy and intensive wound care. Floor of the mouth and cervical LMs that necessitate tracheostomy placement at birth are generally not treated until the newborn is at least a year old.

Post-treatment Care

Although sclerotherapy of LMs results in post-treatment edema, this is usually not severe enough to compromise the airway. There is a significant risk of infection; therefore, patients are treated with prophylactic antibiotics during treatment, that is continued for 7 to 10 days after treatment. Cyst involution is assessed approximately 6 weeks after treatment with additional sessions being scheduled at 6- to 8-week intervals.

Meticulous postoperative wound care is essential because wound complications such as prolonged drainage, swelling, seroma formation, and infection are common. Prolonged suction drainage is necessary with cystic areas often needing to be tapped repeatedly after operation to remove serous fluid and to allow the cutaneous flaps to adhere. Postoperative recurrence secondary to lymphatic regeneration and re-expansion occurs with a frequency up to 40%.

VENOUS MALFORMATIONS

Venous malformations (VMs) are the most common slow-flow malformations, accounting for 50% of referrals to vascular anomalies centers. They are believed to have an incidence of 1/10,000 live births, and 40% are located in the head and neck. VMs are sporadic in 95% of cases. The other 5% make up a subtype known as glomuvenous malformations (GVMs). GVMs are caused by a known genetic defect that follows an autosomal dominant inheritance pattern. Multifocal VMs of the extremities, including the soles and palms, and the gastrointestinal tract are the hallmark of the blue rubber bleb nevus syndrome. This syndrome can include the oral mucosa and is important to identify as the gastrointestinal VMs often lead to chronic anemia.

Clinical Features

VMs present as bluish, soft, compressible masses with no bruit, thrill, or radiant heat. In the head and neck they are usually unilateral and are often more extensively involved than they initially appear. Measures to increase venous pressure (such as Valsalva maneuver or dependent positioning) can temporarily enlarge VMs and help confirm the diagnosis. While usually painless, phleboliths and thrombosis can occur leading to stiffness and pain. VMs of the head and neck are often more painful on awakening in the morning, presumably because of stasis and swelling. GVMs are usually superficial, appearing as painful blue-purple papules and nodules with a "pebbly" surface.

VMs involve bone primarily or secondarily and produce distortion of both shape and size leading to facial asymmetry and malocclusion. They are found more commonly in the mandible than the maxilla and likely represent what was, and still often is, incorrectly referred to as "intraosseous hemangiomas" in the oral and maxillofacial surgery literature. While speech and swallowing are rarely impeded by VM of the tongue, cheek, and palate, oropharyngeal and hypopharyngeal involvement can compress and distort the airway and lead to development of obstructive sleep apnea.

Diagnostic Studies

After history and physical examination, MRI is the most useful radiographic technique. Pre- and postcontrast T1- and T2-weighted images with fat suppression are crucial. VMs are hyperintense on T2-weighted sequences and differ from LMs by enhancement of contents on T1-weighted images. Phleboliths and thrombi are seen as signal voids on all MRI sequences. MR angiography, venography, and lymphangiography contribute little to the diagnosis of low-flow anomalies.

Plain films are of limited diagnostic assistance for VMs. Phleboliths may be seen and in cases of intraosseous involvement, the skeleton will have a soap-bubble or honeycomb appearance. Ultrasonography may be helpful as an initial screening of vascular malformations of unclear diagnosis. VMs reveal low-flow, heterogenous lesions with mixed echogenicity with hypoechoic lacunae and occasional calcifications.

Coagulation studies are required preoperatively in patients with extensive VMs or a history of easy bruising or bleeding during procedures. PT and PTT are often normal, while D-dimer and fibrin split products are elevated and fibrinogen and platelet levels are decreased secondary to localized intravascular coagulopathy, which is found in up to 42% of patients.

Treatment

Treatment of VMs is indicated for alleviation of pain, prevention or treatment of skeletal deformities, and correction of functional and esthetic problems. Pain secondary to phleboliths is treated with aspirin, which can be continued prophylactically on a daily basis.

The primary treatment modality of VMs is sclerotherapy with surgery being reserved as an adjunctive procedure in certain cases. Several different agents are available, with the most commonly used agent being absolute ethanol, which instantly precipitates endothelial proteins, inducing rapid thrombosis. While ethanol is the most potent sclerosing agent, it also has the highest risk of side effects and the most serious complications. These risks include soft-tissue necrosis, local cranial nerve damage, and systemic effects such as central nervous system depression, acute pulmonary hypertension, thromboembolism, cardiac arrhythmias, and cardiovascular collapse and death. The risks may be dose-related and the total dose should never exceed 1 mL/kg (with a maximum of 60 mL) per session. Alternative detergent agents for sclerosis such as sodium tetradecyl sulfate (STS), polidocanol, sodium morrhuate, and ethanolamine have milder and less frequent side effects. These agents are particularly useful in superficial lesions or lesions with nerve involvement. Foaming of the detergents by agitating air with 10 mL of 3% STS with 2 mL of Ethiodol is thought to increase efficacy by increasing surface area contact between endothelium and the sclerosant microbubbles. Outside the United States, bleomycin, an antibiotic with cytotoxic properties, has been advocated in the treatment of VMs because of its effectiveness with little postprocedural edema. Concerns about its association with pulmonary fibrosis when used for chemotherapeutic purposes (at a dose far greater than that used for sclerotherapy) have limited its use within the United States.

If a coagulopathy is detected before treatment, it should first be corrected with subcutaneous low-molecular-weight heparin starting 10 days prior to the procedure and continued for 10 to 14 days afterward. Fibrinogen and D-dimer levels should be followed.

Small cutaneous and mucosal VMs can be injected with a mild sclerosant such as 1% STS. Large VMs require formal percutaneous sclerotherapy completed under general anesthesia by an experienced interventional radiologist. In brief review, during percutaneous sclerotherapy the lesion is cannulated using an angiocatheter under fluoroscopic guidance, confirmed by blood or lymph return. Contrast is injected to allow evaluation of the position of the needle, communication between the different components of the VM, and the local vascular anatomy (most importantly the lesion's venous drainage). The volume of sclerosant is estimated from the amount of contrast required to visualize the lesion. If rapid venous drainage is noted in the VM, the lesion's outflow must be slowed with direct compression during sclerosing to prevent systemic spread of the agent. Typically, the risk of systemic spread of the sclerosant is reduced after 2 to 3 minutes but attempts can be made to aspirate back the sclerosing agent and then compression is relieved under fluoroscopic visualization. In some VMs, venous drainage cannot be compressed so the drainage system must first be disrupted. This is accomplished by injection of platinum coils or a liquid polymer such as N-butyl-cyanoacrylate or ethylene vinyl alcohol copolymer (Onyx, ev3 Endovascular, Inc., Plymouth, Minn) to occlude the draining vessel. Occlusion of arteries feeding VMs is not an alternative treatment as this could lead to a large area of necrosis, and reported outcomes have been less successful than with sclerosant therapy. The success with sclerotherapy is high (as much as 76% success in one series), though repeated treatment (at least 6 to 8 weeks after the first treatment) may be necessary.

In cases of recalcitrant VMs that fail to reach satisfactory reduction, surgical resection of the remaining malformation is generally completed several weeks after sclerotherapy. Surgical intervention is also indicated for VMs near critical nerves, VMs involving thrombus, as well as small, focal, cutaneous or mucosal VMs.

Extraction of teeth and the management of odontogenic infections and skeletal malocclusions in the setting of a VM differ depending on whether the VM is intraosseous or extraosseous. If the VM is extraosseous, teeth can safely be extracted and orthodontic treatment and orthognathic procedures can be completed without

excessive bleeding. An odontogenic infection is treated with antibiotics and drainage of obvious abscesses. If the VM is intraosseous and a dental extraction is required, the patient should first undergo sclerotherapy (or embolization of a feeding artery if emergent treatment is required) followed by extraction of the tooth in the operating room under hypotensive general anesthesia with judicious use of local hemostatic measures such as a collagen sponge (Avitene Ultrafoam, C.R. Bard, Inc., Murray Hill, NJ) wrapped in a collagen sheet packed into the extraction site, which is then oversewn. Orthognathic procedures are often contraindicated in the setting of an intraosseous VM due to the risk of major intraoperative hemorrhage.

Post-treatment Care

Despite a 0.1 mg/kg pretreatment dose of dexamethasone, post-sclerotherapy edema can be significant. Edema begins soon after injection, peaks within 24 hours, and lasts for up to 2 weeks. Elevation of the head of the bed and judicious use of ice packs can help during the first 24 hours. This is most important with VMs of the airway. In cases involving the upper airway, the patient may need to remain intubated in the post-treatment period until edema resolves. Completion of a tracheostomy is the most prudent course if repeated treatments are necessary.

Sclerosants cause immediate local hemolysis and subsequent hemoglobinuria, which is managed by doubling maintenance intravenous fluid (IVF) for at least 4 hours posttreatment. A Foley catheter is used to monitor urinary output in all cases except for superficial lesions in which only a few milliliters of sclerosant are used. If gross hemoglobinuria occurs, the urine is alkalinized by replacing standard IVF with 75 mEq of sodium bicarbonate per liter of 5% dextrose. Locally, antibiotic ointment is applied to puncture sites and a loose dressing is placed. If a treated VM is large or deep, patients are kept in the hospital overnight; otherwise most can be discharged home after 4 to 8 hours of monitoring in the day surgical recovery room. Postoperative pain, which is more severe when ethanol sclerosant is used, is treated with narcotic pain medication.

FAST-FLOW MALFORMATIONS: ARTERIOVENOUS, ARTERIAL

ARTERIOVENOUS MALFORMATIONS

Arteriovenous malformations (AVMs) are rare in comparison to the low flow vascular malformations. They occur most commonly in the head and neck area as intracranial (the most common presentation) or extracranial lesions. Pure arterial malformations are exceedingly rare and are managed in a fashion similar to the management of AVMs. On the face, AVMs occur most commonly (in descending order of frequency) in the cheek, ear, nose, mandible, and maxilla, with a slightly higher female-to-male ratio (1.5:1). Most AVMs are sporadic, but they can be associated with known syndromes such as hereditary hemorrhagic telangiectasia (Rendu-Osler-Weber syndrome), which often involves the mucosa of the oral cavity. Histologically, arteries and veins directly communicate without intervening arterioles, venules, or capillary beds in AVMs. The AVM epicenter is referred to as the "nidus," and it is supplied by multiple feeding arteries. This rerouting of blood under arterial pressure and flow into a venous system is the mechanism of the lesion's pathophysiology. Spontaneous hemorrhage due to venous rupture as well as intranodal aneurysms can occur. Additionally, the shunting of blood may cause either a localized "steal" phenomenon leading to chronically ischemic tissue that is painful, frequently infected, and ulcerated or, if large enough, AVMs can lead to high output cardiac failure.

Clinical Features

AVMs are often misdiagnosed as CMs or vascular birthmarks at birth due to their innocuous presentation. The fast flow nature of the lesion usually first presents within the first 2 decades of life as local warmth and pulsations with both a thrill and bruit being noted. Later changes include ulceration, pain, and hemorrhage. AVM evolution through these presentations is unpredictable, so a clinical, four-stage system was introduced by Robert Schobinger in 1990 at the International Society for the Study of Vascular Anomalies (ISSVA) meeting. The classification is stage I (quiescence): warm, pink stain; stage II (expansion): same as stage I, plus enlargement, pulsations, thrill, bruit, and tense/tortuous veins; stage III (destruction): same as stage II, plus dystrophic skin changes, ulceration, tissue necrosis, bleeding, and persistent pain; stage IV (decompensation): same as stage III, plus cardiac failure. Changes due both to primary bony involvement (true intraosseous AVMs) as well as secondary bony involvement (soft tissue AVMs adjacent to bone) present as bone destruction (osteolysis). Primary bony involvement of AVMs of the head and neck occurs only in the tooth-bearing areas. Patients with intraosseous AVMs of the jaws present with mobile, depressible teeth with hemorrhage from the gingival sulci, stained mucosa, and gingival hypertrophy.

Diagnostic Studies

Plain radiographs demonstrate radiolucencies reflecting osteolysis of bone as well as displaced teeth. CT scans with contrast allow further evaluation of the bony changes and also display a highly enhancing lesion. Ultrasound shows a heterogeneous lesion with numerous hypoechoic lacunae, with Doppler US demonstrating a high-flow lesion with arterial pulsatile flow.

T1- and T2-weighted MRI images are characterized by low signal intensity due to the "flow void" phenomenon of rapid blood flow and turbulence. Angiography is an invaluable tool but it is not used diagnostically. Instead, angiography is an integral part of the armamentarium of AVM management.

Treatment

AVMs are one of the most difficult malformations to treat, and cure is not often possible. Treatment is indicated for palliation of pain, bleeding, or cardiac failure as well as in preparation for surgery in the area of AVMS, such as tooth extraction. Treatment is also indicated when AVMs demonstrate evolution to higher stages.

The mainstays of management are embolization, sclerotherapy, surgical resection and reconstruction or some combination of these modalities. Prior to the availability of interventional radiologic therapy, treatment consisted of angiography to identify feeding vessels which were then ligated. This was then followed by resection of the AVM. This treatment invariably led to a worsened presentation as the lesion rarely was completely excised and collateral flow was recruited from nearby arteries, resulting in an even more complicated AVM. Intravascular therapy via percutaneous or endovascular intervention has advanced the treatment of AVMs. The feeding vessel should never be embolized (except in cases of life-threatening hemorrhage) as this will always lead to recruitment and deny access for future therapy. The best chance for a complete cure is via preoperative "super-selective" embolization targeted at the nidus and venous outflow of the AVM followed by surgical resection 1 to 3 days (no later than 7 to 10 days) after the embolization.

Preoperative embolization can be completed with temporary occlusive agents such as Gelfoam, PVAs (polyvinyl alcohol particles), or biospheres (all of which are phagocytosed within weeks of placement) or permanent liquid agents such as absolute ethanol, nBCA (N-butyl 2-cyanoacrylate), or the afore mentioned Onyx. The handling properties of Onyx have made it a commonly used product with a drawback being its black color, leading to discoloration of the treatment site. In the maxillofacial skeleton, use of most permanent agents has been associated with foreign-body reactions and bone infections, especially at extraction sites. Because of this noted increase in inflammation and bone infection, it is the preference of the authors to combine embolization with direct platinum coil injection into the intraosseous AVM. Early studies suggest that Onyx may lead to fewer occurrences of foreign-body reaction and bone infection.

A deep space odontogenic abscess in the setting of an AVM should also be treated with assistance of interventional radiology, which can provide not only vascular management but also image-guided drainage of the abscess if necessary.

Surgical intervention is always completed with use of hypotensive anesthesia, along with multiple, large bore IV access and properly cross-matched blood products. If tissue resection is indicated after embolization, knowing the extent of the wide resection can be difficult. Intraoperative frozen sections from the resection margins can be helpful, with observation of the pattern of bleeding of the wound edges perhaps being the most helpful guide. The wounds are closed primarily, and unaffected overlying skin can be spared. Primary bony involvement requires bony resection (with possible immediate reconstruction), while secondary bony involvement does not necessitate bony excision. Angiography allows distinction between primary and secondary bony involvement. If complete resection is not achievable, then super-selective arterial embolization of a targeted area of the AVM to allow control of bleeding or local surgical intervention is the treatment of choice.

Dental extractions can be completed following embolization with placement of local hemostatic agents and primary closure of the extraction site. Once the tooth is extracted, primary mucosal coverage is attempted with the intention of achieving complete separation of the intraosseous AVM from the oral cavity.

Stage I and II lesions are often treated conservatively with yearly clinical and radiological reevaluation and no intervention until they become symptomatic. This being said, embolization followed by surgery is most successful with stage I and localized stage II lesions and is primarily palliative in stage III and IV lesions. It is the authors' experience that teeth in the presence of an intraosseous AVM invariably lead to progression of the lesion to higher stages. Edentulating the affected jaw using the previously detailed technique halts and/or reverses the progression and in three cases has maintained the AVM in stage I for 3 to 20 years.

PEARLS AND PITFALLS

- The first step in management of a vascular lesion is to determine if it is a tumor or a malformation.
- Not all vascular malformations are the same; they each carry their own management issues.
- Sclerotherapy and embolization is directed at lesions and their outflow vessels but not the feeding vessels.
- Treatment of vascular malformations rarely can be managed by a single clinician in isolation and are usually best treated collaboratively at centers with appropriate resources.

BIBLIOGRAPHY

Berenguer B, Burrows PE, Zurakowski D, Mulliken JB: Sclerotherapy of craniofacial venous malformations: complications and results, *Plast Reconstr Surg* 104:1-11, 1999.

Boyd JB, Mulliken JB, Kaban LB, et al: Skeletal changes associated with vascular malformations, *Plast Reconstr Surg* 74:789-795, 1984.

Choi DJ, Alomari AI, Chaudry G, Orbach DB: Neurointerventional management of low-flow vascular malformations of the head and neck, *Neuroimag Clin N Am* 19:199-218, 2009.

Dubois J, Garel L, Grignon A, et al: Imaging of hemangiomas and vascular malformations in children, *Acad Radiol* 5:390-400, 1998.

Ethunandan M, Mellor TK: Haemangiomas and vascular malformations of the maxillofacial region: a review, *Br J Oral Maxillofac Surg* 44:263-272, 2006.

Fishman SJ, Smithers J, Folkman J, et al: Blue rubber bleb nevus syndrome: surgical eradication of gastrointestinal bleeding, *Ann Surg* 241:523-528, 2005.

Garzon MC, Huang JT, Enjolras O, Frieden IJ: Vascular malformations part I, *J Am Acad Dermatol* 56:353-370, 2007.

Greene AK, Kim S, Rogers GF, et al: Risk of vascular anomalies with Down syndrome, *Pediatrics* 121:e135-e140, 2008.

Kaban LB, Blaeser B, Perrott DH: Head and neck vascular anomalies, *Oral Maxillofac Surg* 5:4-18, 1997.

Kaban LB, Mulliken JB: Maxillofacial vascular anomalies. In Kaban LB, Troulis MJ: *Pediatric oral and maxillofacial surgery*, Philadelphia, 2004, Saunders, pp 259-285.

Kaban LB, Mulliken JB: Vascular anomalies of the maxillofacial region, *J Oral Maxillofac Surg* 44:203-213, 1986.

Lawley LP, Cerimele F, Weiss SW, et al: Expression of Wilms tumor 1 gene distinguishes vascular malformations from proliferative endothelial lesions, *Arch Dermatol* 141:1297-1300, 2005.

Marler JJ, Fishman SJ, Kilroy SM, et al: Increased expression of urinary matrix metalloproteinases parallels the extent and activity of vascular anomalies, *Pediatrics* 116:38-45, 2005.

Marler JJ, Mulliken JB: Current management of hemangiomas and vascular malformations, *Clin Plastic Surg* 32:99-116, 2005.

Mulliken JB: Hemangiomas and vascular malformations. In McCarthy JG, Galiano RD, Boutros SG, editors: *Current therapy in plastic surgery*, Philadelphia, 2005, Saunders, pp 53-59.

Mulliken JB, Fishman SJ, Burrows PE: Vascular anomalies, *Curr Probl Surg* 37:517-584, 2000.

Mulliken JB, Glowacki J: Hemangiomas and vascular malformations in infants and children: a classification based on endothelial characteristics, *Plast Reconstr Surg* 69(3):412-422, 1982.

Niimi Y, Song JK, Berenstein A: Current endovascular management of maxillofacial vascular malformations, *Neuroimag Clin N Am* 17:223-237, 2007.

Sexton J: Laser management of vascular and pigmented lesions. In Catone GA, Alling CC: *Laser applications in oral and maxillofacial surgery*, Philadelphia, 1997, W.B. Saunders, pp 167-179.

Tan OT: Pulsed dye laser treatment of adult port-wine stains. In *Management and treatment of benign cutaneous vascular lesions*, Malvern, Pa, 1992, Lea & Febiger, pp 83-106.

Vikkula M, Boon LM, Mulliken JB, Olsen BR: Molecular basis of vascular anomalies, *Trends Cardiovasc Med* 8:281-292, 1998.

Wu IC, Orbach DB: Neurointerventional management of high-flow vascular malformations of the head and neck, *Neuroimag Clin N Am* 19:219-240, 2009.

THE PAST

Obstructive sleep apnea syndrome (OSAS) is a relatively new syndrome first reported in the medical literature in 1965, although William Osler recognized the clinical stigmata in the early 1900s and named the trait "Pickwickian syndrome" after a character in a Charles Dickens novel. In the early days, tracheostomy was the recommended treatment. It was not until 1981 that continuous positive airway pressure (CPAP) was introduced. Since the 1980s, a variety of surgical and nonsurgical treatments have emerged in attempts to cure this condition without a tracheostomy. The use of oral appliances to open the airway and advance the mandible developed along with procedures to increase airway space including septoplasty, tonsillectomy, turbinectomy, uvulopalatopharyngoplasty (UPPP), somnoplasty, tongue reduction, maxillomandibular advancement, genial tubercle advancement, and hyoid suspension. The diversity of procedures and the multispecialty involvement in this syndrome is evidence of the lack of understanding toward a specific diagnosis for an anatomic area of obstruction.

THE PRESENT

OSAS is recognized as a significant health hazard with several surgical and nonsurgical specialties devoted to its remedy. Advanced training in sleep disorders and board certification in sleep medicine has become well established, although there has been little interest by oral and maxillofacial surgeons to obtain this certification. There continue to be challenges in the definitive diagnosis of the exact anatomic cause of OSAS. When indicated, maxillomandibular advancement significantly improves OSAS, although this procedure has not been widely recommended by the other treating specialties despite convincing clinical evidence. This is in part due to the perceived complexity of this procedure, the potential need for orthodontic involvement, and the relative absence of our specialty in many medical and surgical societies, especially outside the academic centers. The current management of OSAS is best performed though a multidisciplinary team composed of several specialists, including oral and maxillofacial surgeons, to avoid unnecessary surgeries or delayed treatment of clinically obvious nasopharyngeal or maxillofacial deformities. Although there are some comprehensive sleep apnea teams, the multidisciplinary team concept has not been widely adapted in practice, mostly because of limited time commitments by multiple physicians and cost. Therefore, patients are often shuffled between specialists. Despite these difficulties, treatment has become more standardized with greater collaboration between clinicians.

THE FUTURE

This field is in its infancy. The treatment and diagnosis of OSAS will become more standardized and elucidated. Advances in imaging, including live three-dimensional imaging of the airway during sleep, will shed further information. With more specific diagnosis of the cause of obstruction, surgical interventions will become more effective and predictable. Sleep centers will become more prevalent, and a greater portion of the population will be diagnosed and treated. Specialists will become more involved in the relevant societies to achieve more recognition in the sleep medicine community and to establish themselves as authorities in the surgical treatment of OSAS. With time, the need for fellowship training for OMFS in sleep medicine and surgery will become obvious.

Chapter

112

Obstructive Sleep Apnea: Evaluation and Treatment Planning

Reginald H.B. Goodday

Oral and maxillofacial surgeons play an important role in the primary surgical treatment of patients with obstructive sleep apnea syndrome (OSAS). These surgical specialists have considerable experience and expertise in the diagnosis and treatment of dentofacial deformities. Application of the same surgical principles and procedures in patients who have anatomic abnormalities that contribute to narrowing or obstruction of the pharyngeal airway during sleep will produce predictable and successful outcomes.

INCIDENCE

Patients with obstructive sleep apnea experience repeated complete and partial blockages of the upper airway during sleep. Such blockages are referred to as apneas and hypopneas. An obstructive apnea is defined as the absence of breathing for 10 seconds or more, despite an effort to breathe. The clinical definition of hypopnea is a 30% reduction in thoraco-abdominal movement or airflow as compared with baseline lasting at least 10 seconds, with 4% or more oxygen desaturation.[1]

The severity of obstructive sleep apnea (OSA) is measured using the apnea-hypopnea index (AHI), which assesses the total number of apneas and hypopneas per hour of sleep. Obstructive sleep apnea syndrome is defined as an AHI $\geq$ 5 along with excessive daytime sleepiness reported by the patient. Guidelines produced by the Institute for Clinical Systems Improvement (ICSI) state that a diagnosis of mild OSA requires an AHI score of 5 to 15; AHI scores of 16 to 30 indicate moderate OSA; and those greater than 30 indicate severe OSA.[2]

OSAS is a common disorder with an incidence of 4% and 2% among middle-aged (30 to 60 years) men and women, respectively. Estimates for elderly men range from 28% to 67% and from 20% to 54% for elderly women.[3] The prevalence of sleep-disordered breathing, which is defined as an AHI of at least 5, is 24% of adult men and 9% of adult women.[4]

There is a disparity between the estimated prevalence of obstructive sleep apnea and daytime sleepiness, and the number of patients whose conditions are recognized and treated. Young and colleagues reported that at least 80% of the cases of moderate and severe OSA in adults aged 30 to 60 years in the general population go undiagnosed.[5] Kapur et al. have reported that the true prevalence of OSA and associated daytime sleepiness may be three times higher than the number of patients diagnosed with this sleep disorder.[6] The significant health and social consequences of OSAS and the recent finding that it is a relatively common condition that frequently remains undiagnosed make it an important public health issue.

RISK/CAUSATIVE FACTORS

The fundamental problem associated with obstructive sleep apnea is the inability to maintain upper airway (UAW) patency when sleeping, which can result in reduction (hypopnea) or cessation (apnea) of breathing. The obstruction can occur at multiple levels in the airway, and it is critical to diagnose the site of occlusion. Patency of the UAW is maintained mostly by the activation of pharyngeal muscles in the underlying soft tissue structures,[7] which depends on the facial skeleton and muscle tone.

Factors associated with the patient's craniofacial anatomy can alter the mechanical properties of the upper airway and increase its propensity to collapse during sleep. Static cephalometric analysis using radiography, computerized tomography, and magnetic resonance imaging (MRI) has revealed a number of skeletal and soft tissue structural differences during wakefulness between individuals with and without obstructive sleep apnea. Features such as repositioning of the maxilla and mandible, enlarged tongue or soft palate, and decreased posterior airway space can narrow upper airway dimensions and promote the occurrence of apnea and hypopneas during sleep.[8] Even in the absence of clinically obvious craniofacial abnormalities, subtle differences in maxillary and mandibular size or position can increase the vulnerability for obstructive sleep apnea. A meta-analysis of studies investigating the craniofacial risk factors show that mandibular body length is the craniofacial measure with the strongest association with increased risk for OSA.[9] In the Wisconsin Cohort of Sleep Disordered Breathing Study, two thirds or more of the variability of the apnea-hypopnea index was explained by facial structure and obesity.[10] In nonobese subjects, the major contributor was facial structure.

The size and the position of the tongue are important considerations in OSA. In the supine position, the tongue projects posteriorly and is counteracted by the tone of the genioglossal muscle. MRI volumetric studies have identified tongue size as a major predictor of OSA. With advancing age, sleep-related difficulties, including excessive daytime sleepiness secondary to obstructive sleep apnea, become increasingly common.[11-14] Data from the community-based Sleep Heart Health Study have shown that OSA prevalence increases steadily with age and reaches a plateau after the age of 60 years.[15] Mechanisms proposed for the age-related increase in prevalence include increased deposition of fat in the parapharyngeal area, lengthening of the soft palate, and changes in body structure surrounding the pharynx.[5,16]

Epidemiologic studies from around the world have consistently identified body weight as the strongest risk factor for obstructive

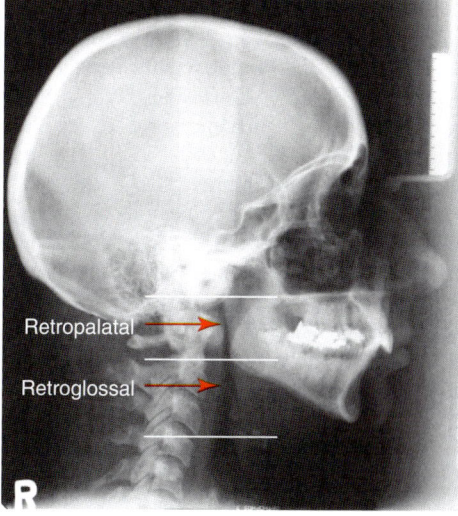

Fig. 112-1 ■ OSAS patients have multiple sites of airway obstruction during episodes of apnea and hypopnea. The two major sites of obstruction are in the retropalatal and retroglossal regions.

sleep apnea.[4,13,14,17-25] In the Wisconsin Sleep Cohort Study, a one standard deviation difference in body mass index (BMI) was associated with a fourfold increase in disease prevalence.[4] It has long been recognized that men have greater vulnerability than women toward developing obstructive sleep apnea. Clinic-based studies have shown that, in patients referred for clinical evaluation, the ratio of men to women is in the range from 5 to 8 to 1.[26] The male predisposition for the sleep disorder has been attributed to sex differences in anatomic and functional properties of the upper airway and in the ventilatory response to arousals from sleep.[27,28] Hormonal influences are also likely to have an important role in the pathogenesis of obstructive sleep apnea, as disease prevalence is higher in post- versus premenopausal women.[14]

Studies to localize the site of functional obstruction in the upper airway have shown that there is rarely a single anatomic site of occlusion; more commonly there are multiple sites of UAW obstruction during episodes of hypopnea and apnea.[29] The two major sites of obstruction are in the retropalatal and retroglossal regions[30] (Fig. 112-1). Positional factors that may exacerbate upper airway resistance during sleep include mouth opening (which increases collapsibility or decreases efficacy of dilator muscles)[31] and a supine posture (which facilitates the gravitational forces that posteriorly displace the tongue and soft palate).[32,33]

Upper airway competence involves complex interactions between anatomy and physiology. For most, OSA is an abnormality of a structurally small and abnormally collapsible upper airway interacting with normal physiologic mechanisms.[34]

HARMFUL EFFECTS OF OSAS

The physiologic changes that accompany each obstructive event in patients with OSAS include hypoxemia, hypercapnia, fluctuations in intrathoracic pressure caused by increased respiratory effort, arousal from sleep, and increased sympathetic tone. On a repetitive basis, these physiologic events are believed to result in long-term comorbidities such as hypertension, cardiac-related death while sleeping, coronary artery disease, stroke, depression, diabetes mellitus, and glaucoma.[35-39] Results demonstrating that effective treatment of OSAS can abort and even reverse the atherogenic process suggest that it should be diagnosed and treated as early as possible to prevent cardiovascular sequelae.[36,40-46] Deficits affecting attention, concentration, vigilance, manual dexterity, visual motor skills, memory, verbal fluency, and executive function have been reportedly associated with OSAS.[47] Excessive daytime sleepiness can undoubtedly influence one's driving performance. Prospectively gathered motor vehicle accident rates in OSAS patients have been found to be 1.3 to 7 times higher than those in the general population.[48-50] There is evidence indicating an increased risk of occupational accidents for those with OSAS.[51] Patients suffering from excessive daytime sleepiness (EDS) will often complain of a lack of daytime energy, decreased feeling of well-being, and decreased libido and sexual performance.

OSAS is a life-threatening disease that predisposes the patient to physical harm, significant social discord, and poor quality of life.

EVALUATION OF OBSTRUCTIVE SLEEP APNEA

The diagnosis of obstructive sleep apnea is based on findings acquired by a clinical history, physical examination, imaging studies, and polysomnography.

Clinical symptoms of OSA include very loud snoring, choking at night, witnessed apneas, frequent arousals, excessive daytime sleepiness, poor concentration, poor memory, mood changes, irritability, headaches upon awakening, absence of dreams, and symptoms of depression. Although many of these symptoms are very sensitive, they are not always specific to obstructive sleep apnea. The best predictor of obstructive sleep apnea is the triad of symptoms that includes loud snoring, apnea witnessed by a bed partner, and excessive daytime sleepiness.[52] In the primary care setting, the Epworth Sleepiness Scale (ESS) is the most frequently used questionnaire-based measure of excess daytime somnolence; it is a subjective, eight-item, self-reported questionnaire that is simple to use and takes less than 2 minutes to complete (Fig. 112-2). Not only can the ESS confirm pathologic sleepiness, but it can also be used to validate posttreatment improvement in patients with OSA. An ESS score of 10 or greater is considered abnormal.

Clinical examination has been shown to be useful in the prediction of OSA and its severity.[53-57] During the clinical examination, the patient's height, weight, BMI, and blood pressure are recorded. The patient's facial profile is noted, with special attention paid to the chin-neck angle and nasolabial angle. Examination of the oral cavity includes documentation of the presence/size of tonsils, soft palate tissue redundancy, uvula length and thickness, and size and presence of indentations of the tongue. Although many authors recommend nasopharyngoscopy in conjunction with the Müller maneuver to identify the site of obstruction, several recent articles suggest that, because multiple factors are involved in the dynamics of OSA that are not fully understood, the likelihood of surgical success does not correlate with the clinical finding on Müller's maneuver.[58-60] A recent clinical review of airway evaluation in obstructive sleep apnea patients by Stuck found that the reliability of the Müller maneuver remains highly questionable, as the evaluation used by this technique seems subjective and hard to reproduce. He concluded that the Müller maneuver does not facilitate patient selection for the varying surgical interventions used in OSA patients.[61]

Lateral x-ray cephalometry is one of the standard diagnostic tools used for patients with sleep-disordered breathing (SDB), especially with regard to the evaluation of the skeletal craniofacial morphology. It is regarded as a mandatory assessment tool and its value is not questioned.[61] Although beneficial effects of CT scanning on treatment selection and thereby treatment outcome have been

Epworth Sleepiness Scale

Name: _____

Date: _____

Your age: (Yr) _____   Your sex: ☐ Male ☐ Female

How likely are you to doze off or fall asleep in the situations described below, in contrast to feeling just tired?

This refers to your usual way of life in recent times.

Even if you haven't done some of these things recently try too work out how they would have affected you.

Use the following scale to choose the most appropriate number for each situation:

0 = Would never doze
1 = Slight chance of dozing
2 = Moderate chance of dozing
3 = High chance of dozing

Situation	Chance of dozing
Sitting and reading..	☐
Watching TV..	☐
Sitting, inactive in a public place (e.g., a theatre or a meeting)..........	☐
As a passenger in a car for an hour without a break........	☐
Lying down to rest in the afternoon when circumstances permit.......	☐
Sitting and talking to someone...	☐
Sitting quietly after a lunch without alcohol............................	☐
In a car, while stopped for a few minutes in the traffic.................	☐
Total...	☐

Score:
0-10 Normal range
10-12 Borderline
12-24 Abnormal

Fig. 112-2 ■ The Epworth Sleepiness Scale is a self-reported questionnaire that can be used to confirm pathologic sleepiness and validate posttreatment improvement in patients with OSA. A score above 10 is considered to be abnormal.

repeatedly postulated, the literature does not demonstrate its clinical use to date.[61] Only a small number of authors have attempted to establish distinct protocols for the use of MRI of the upper airway in SDB. Hardly any consensual standards exist for this indication. MRI has not become a standard procedure, neither in the diagnostic workup for patients with SDB nor in management of the disease in terms of surgical or nonsurgical treatment.

Overnight polysomnography conducted in a sleep laboratory identifies sleep apnea caused by obstructive or central events and remains the gold standard for the diagnosis of sleep apnea. Central sleep apnea (CSA) is characterized by a lack of drive to breathe during sleep, resulting in insufficient or absent ventilation and compromised gas exchange. In contrast to OSA, in which ongoing respiratory efforts are observed, CSA is defined by a lack of respiratory effort during cessation of airflow. CSA, like OSA, is associated with important complications including frequent nighttime wakenings, excessive daytime sleepiness, and an increased risk of adverse cardiovascular outcomes. CSA is relatively uncommon and may affect less than 5% of patients referred to a sleep clinic.[62] Usually, CSA is considered to be the primary diagnosis when greater than 50% of apneas are scored as central in origin (i.e., greater than 10-second cessation of breathing in the absence of respiratory effort).[63] Typically, these patients are thinner and snore less than patients with OSA, although male predominance is likely a common trait. The underlying mechanisms for this disorder are not fully understood. Given the range of pathophysiologic factors contributing to the varied forms of CSA, treatment approaches also vary considerably and do not include surgery. Noninvasive ventilation such as continuous positive airway pressure (CPAP) has been shown to be effective in some patients with CSA. The mechanism for improvement in these patients is not clear but may relate to the prevention of inhibitory reflex mechanisms that arise during airway closure and potentially to CPAP-induced increases in lung volume and oxygen stores.[64]

Overnight polysomnography involves the use of electro-encephalogram (EEG), electro-oculogram (EOG), electromyogram (EMG), electrocardiogram (ECG), microphone measurement of snoring, pulse oxymetry, respiratory inductance plethysmography, airflow measurement, and recording of body position by infrared imaging. The stage of sleep is determined by a combination of EEG, EOG, and EMG. Episodes of apnea and hypopnea are determined from a reduction in airflow in combination with oxygen desaturation.

TREATMENT OPTIONS

To assist the patient in making an informed decision regarding treatment choices, the oral and maxillofacial surgeon must be familiar with the risks and benefits of common treatment options. OSAS can be managed nonsurgically or surgically. The recommended treatment should target potential contributing factors identified by history, physical examination, and UAW imaging. The severity of the patient's condition should also be considered when treatment options are reviewed.

In 2009, a literature search in PubMed under the heading "obstructive sleep apnea and treatment" yielded approximately 7,200 articles. The same search in 2005 resulted in approximately 3,400 articles. This demonstrates that the interest in this condition is increasing in an exponential fashion, but it also suggests that there is not a clear-cut approach to the management of these patients. A breakdown of these articles reveals approximately 13 nonsurgical options. Surgical options total approximately 19 procedures and deal with surgery in eight regions of the head and neck, which include the pharynx, hyoid, tonsil, tongue, palate, turbinates, nasal septum, and nasal valve. To recommend the best treatment option, the surgeon needs to understand the underlying pathology and recommend treatment based on the correction of an anatomic abnormality.

Nonsurgical management options included behavioral interventions, CPAP devices, and oral appliances. Because obesity is a risk factor for OSAS, a reduction in body weight can reduce the number of obstructive apneas. In the Wisconsin Sleep Cohort Study, a 10% weight gain predicted a 32% increase in AHI, whereas a 10% weight loss predicted a 26% decrease in AHI.[7] It should be noted, however, that the recurrence of OSAS has been reported after surgically induced weight loss, even though the weight was not regained.[65] Although patients may be advised to lose weight, they will have difficulty doing so, particularly in the more severe cases, because excess daytime somnolence and fatigue may discourage the patient from exercising. It is also important to note that approximately 30% of people with OSAS are not obese, and these patients most often have an underlying craniofacial deformity.[66] Mild OSA may be improved with avoidance of alcohol and sedatives and by sleeping in a more upright or lateral position.[67-69] Patients with OSA who sleep on their backs (the supine position) often have prolonged respiratory events, greater oxygen desaturation, longer arousals from sleep, and louder snoring than those who sleep laterally.[33] When sleep posture is altered to a more lateral position through the use of pillows or body belts, changes occur in the patient's lung volume, neurovascular activity, and airway size, so as to support the airway with reduced collapsibility. However, long-term randomized trials are lacking for this intervention, and a number of small studies have reported that AHI scores are only partially reduced by lateral sleep posture.[70] Nasal dilators do not appear to alleviate the symptoms or decrease the severity of OSA.[71,72]

The most successful nonsurgical treatment of OSAS is continuous positive airway pressure (CPAP) applied by a nasal or full face mask. CPAP therapy maintains upper airway patency during sleep by acting as a pneumatic splint and opening the airways, thus abolishing apnea, hypopnea, and snoring, and improving sleep quality. The pressure required to achieve this is titrated at a sleep laboratory during the polysomnography. CPAP is a sound, evidence-based treatment option that has been shown to decrease daytime sleepiness and improve mood and quality of life.[73-76] Unfortunately, because of physical discomfort associated with wearing the unit, drying of the nasal and oral mucous membranes, dislodgement during sleep, noise, and the inconvenience of transporting the unit, the long-term compliance with CPAP use on a nightly basis can be as low as 25%.[77] It is prudent to advise all patients to undergo a trial of CPAP therapy before considering irreversible treatment options such as surgery.

The American Academy of Sleep Medicine (AASM) currently recommends oral appliances for the treatment of mild to moderate OSA in patients who prefer them to CPAP therapy or who do not respond to the CPAP therapy.[78] Treatment of OSA with dental devices is generally viewed as being less efficacious than treatment with CPAP.[79-82] Overall, oral appliances are felt to be successful in cases of mild OSAS but relatively less effective in more severe cases.[83-89] One of the factors limiting wider application of oral appliance treatment is the inability to identify those patients who will have a successful outcome before investing the time and resources necessary to implement this treatment. The significant potential negative long-term effects of oral appliances are temporomandibular joint pain and detrimental changes to the patient's occlusion.[90] An important concern is that a dental appliance may eliminate or decrease snoring in certain patients but their sleep apnea persists, and the patient is not aware of the potential need to seek further treatment.

Surgical treatment options include tracheostomy, uvulopalato-pharyngoplasty (UPPP), isolated hard or soft tissue surgery, and maxillo-mandibular advancement (MMA). Tracheostomy was the first successful surgical treatment for OSAS and has a virtually 100% success rate because it bypasses the level of obstruction in the UAW completely.[91] Medical and obvious social problems associated with tracheostomy stimulated the search for alternate treatment.

A common surgical treatment is the UPPP, originally described in 1981 by Fujita and, at that time, recommended as the sole treatment for OSAS.[92] It continues to be popular despite reviews that report improvement in less than 50% of patients and complete control of OSAS in less than 25% of patients.[93] The reason for the very low success rate of this procedure is that it addresses only one site of a multisite problem. Soft tissue changes are unpredictable—in fact, the changes can be detrimental because they cause narrowing of the pharyngeal airway. Clinical examination of the UPPP patient reveals that the soft palate appears shorter and has a firm scar band on the inferior surface. More important, however, is that lateral cephalometric radiographs reveal that although the soft palate is much shorter, it is also much thicker, and this can result in a narrower retropalatal pharyngeal airway as seen on cephalometric radiographs (Fig. 112-3). This could explain why the AHI *increases* in approximately 30% of patients after UPPP.[94]

The presence of tonsil or adenoid hypertrophy physically reduces the dimensions of the pharyngeal airway, and, when present, surgery to remove this excess tissue should be considered as first-stage

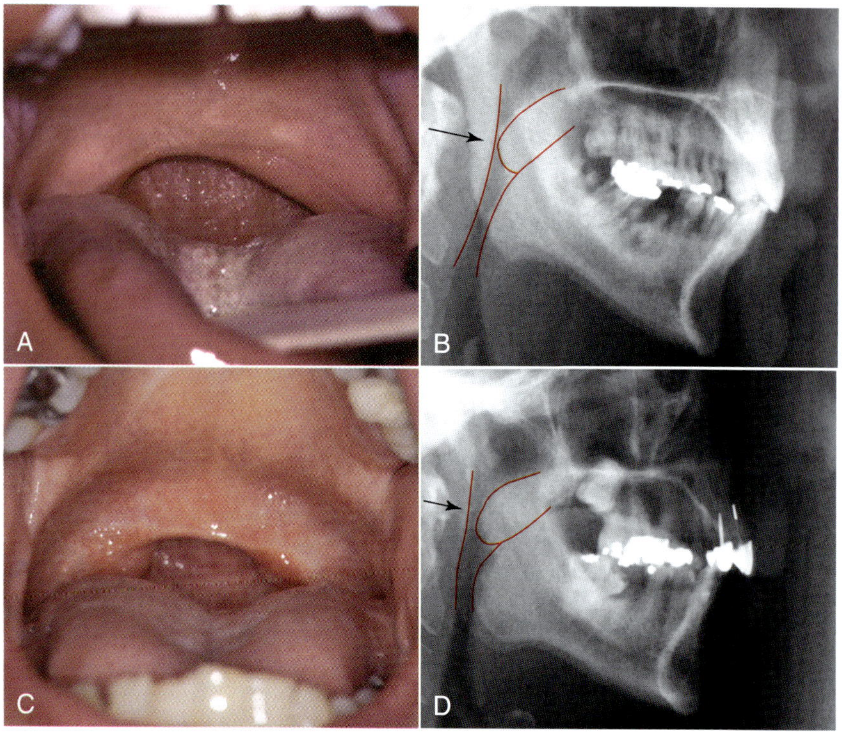

Fig. 112-3 ■ Clinical views (**A** and **C**) of the soft palate with corresponding radiographs (**B** and **D**) in two patients who have undergone uvulopalatopharyngoplasty that failed to treat their OSAS. The soft palate is now shorter and thicker than normal and the retropalatal pharyngeal airway has not improved.

treatment. If septal deviation or exostosis and turbinate enlargement are present, these abnormalities can be addressed at the same time as the performance of a maxillary advancement procedure. Treatments isolated to these areas in the nasal cavity have not proven to significantly benefit the patient, and ultimately the patient requires additional surgical procedures including orthognathic surgery.

Maxillo-mandibular advancement surgery (MMA) has been considered in the treatment of sleep apnea since the late 1970s and is considered the most successful surgical alternative to tracheostomy for the treatment of OSA.[95,96] Of significance, is the realization that MMA is the one procedure that can address anatomic abnormalities in all of the anatomic regions of the head and neck identified as the surgical objective in each of the 19 surgical procedures commonly discussed in the literature. The major biologic basis of this treatment relates to how MMA improves the dimensions and stability of the pharyngeal airway. When a mandibular advancement is performed, the anterior belly of the digastric, the mylohyoid, the genioglossus, and the geniohyoid muscles help pull the tongue forward and upward away from the pharynx. Performing a maxillary advancement pulls the soft tissue of the palate forward and upward and also pulls the palatoglossal muscles, which increases tongue support. Both movements have a positive influence on the pharyngeal airway (Fig. 112-4). Fiberoptic nasopharyngoscopy after MMA reveals a decrease in airway collapsibility secondary to improvement in lateral pharyngeal wall stability.[97] Analysis of the morphologic changes of the pharyngeal airway in obstructive sleep apnea patients by helical computed tomography scanning following maxillo-mandibular advancement surgery revealed a significant enlargement of lateral and anteroposterior (AP) airway dimensions for all patients, at all levels.[98]

TREATMENT PLANNING

A criticism of most surgical treatment protocols for MMA surgery in patients with OSAS is the rather "abstract" selection process for surgical candidates.[99] This criticism highlights the need for the use

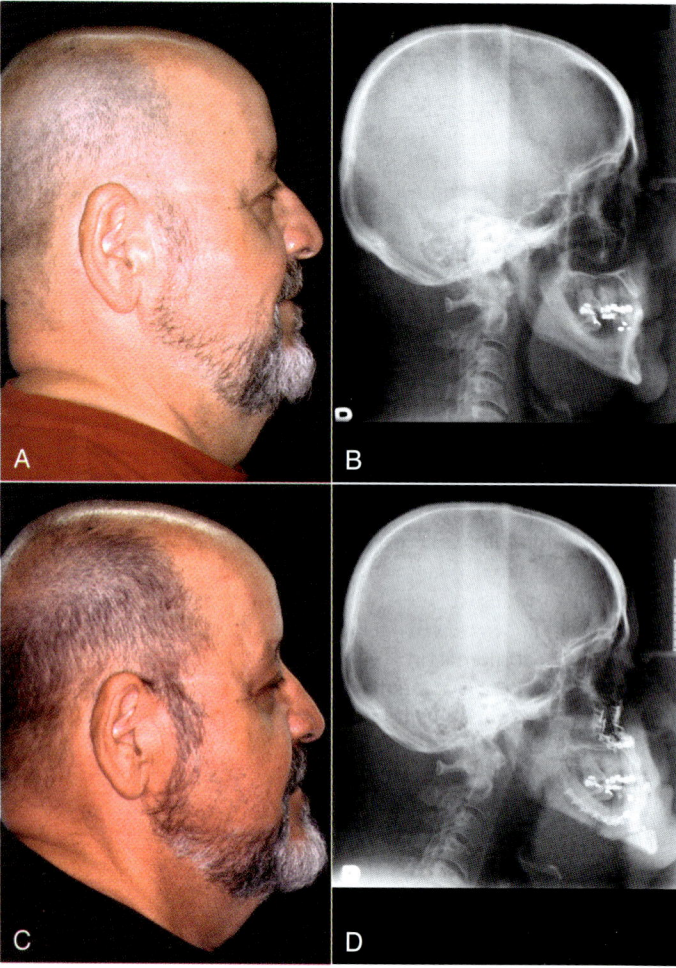

Fig. 112-4 ■ Preoperative (**A**) and postoperative (**C**) clinical profile views with corresponding cephalometric radiographs (**B** and **D**) of an OSAS patient demonstrating significant improvement in the pharyngeal airway after maxillo-mandibular advancement surgery.

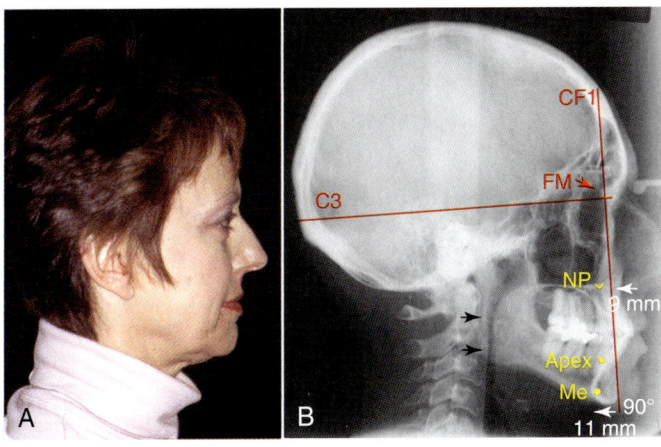

Fig. 112-5 ■ Sleep apnea patient who clinically does not have an obvious skeletal abnormality. Cephalometric analysis, however, demonstrates that the maxilla and mandible can be advanced approximately 10 mm and the patient will remain within the range of normal facial balance. **A,** Clinical profile view. **B,** Lateral cephalometric radiograph with Delaire's lines of anterior facial balance and demonstrating a narrow pharyngeal airway.

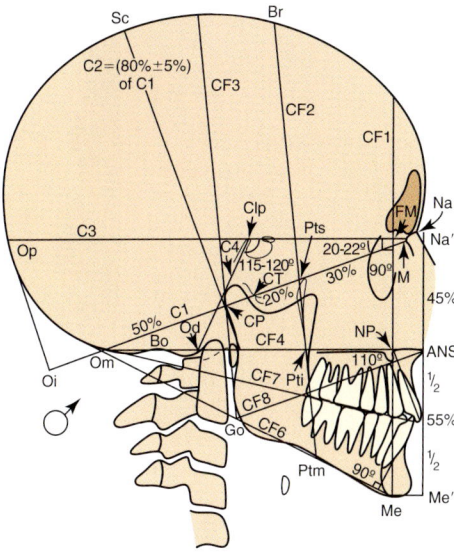

Fig. 112-6 ■ Delaire's architectural and structural craniofacial cephalometric analysis, which constructs a visual treatment objective and is useful to predict movements of the maxilla and the mandible that can be achieved to enlarge the pharyngeal airway while staying within the range of normal facial balance.

of a cephalometric radiograph and the appropriate cephalometric analysis that will identify bony and soft tissue abnormalities related to the soft palate, pharyngeal airway, and maxillo-mandibular complex influencing the multiple sites of obstruction. If the radiographic and clinical examinations of the soft tissues of the pharynx reveal a narrow airway in conjunction with retrognathia of the maxilla and mandible, then the patient should be a candidate for MMA surgery. Because an underlying skeletal abnormality is sometimes hard to detect clinically, it is reasonable for an oral and maxillofacial surgeon to assess these patients (Fig. 112-5).

The surgeon's goal is to optimize the advancement of the deficient structures while maintaining normal facial balance for each individual patient. To do this, the surgeon should use a cephalometric analysis that clearly demonstrates all the maxillofacial abnormalities, as well as provide a visual treatment objective. An example of such an analysis is the Architectural and Structural Craniofacial Analysis of Delaire (Fig. 112-6).[100] Delaire has constructed an analysis that is based on mutual balance of the cranial and facial bony structures and allows the face to be studied in relation to the cranium and cranial spinal articulation. Statistical averages are avoided, and individual proportions influenced by the unique features of each skeleton are relied on. This analysis is very useful to the oral and maxillofacial surgeon, as it (1) allows the clinician to determine the shape the abnormal structure should have had, (2) allows examination of the constitution of skeletal abnormalities graphically, and (3) constructs a visual treatment objective. The surgeon can predict the movement of the maxilla and mandible that can be achieved to enlarge the pharyngeal airway while staying within the range of normal facial balance for each individual. The objective of treating the abnormal airway is not made at a cost of poor esthetics. In fact, movement of abnormal structures into a more normal position tends to result in a favorable change in facial appearance (Fig. 112-7).[101]

Because of the life-threatening effects of OSA, the severity of the patient's airway problem may determine the magnitude of the advancement of the maxilla or mandible. In these cases, the patients should be advised before surgery if the surgeon believes the required movements fall outside the range of normal facial balance.

The lines of the Delaire Analysis that analyze the AP balance of the face include lines C3 and CF1 (Fig. 112-8). Line C3 is drawn from the M point through the apex of the clinoid process and extends posteriorly until it intersects the external surface of the occipital bone. The M point is situated at the junction of the frontonasal and maxillonasal sutures and is always situated just in front of the bony opacity formed by the summit of the ascending nasal maxillary process. Line C3 normally passes just over and parallel to the cribriform plate, then close to the upper lip to the upper chiasmal groove, and then by the anterior clinoid process. Line CF1 is the anterior line of craniofacial balance. It is traced passing through the frontomaxillary (FM) point, which anatomically corresponds to the middle of the upper border of the ascending nasal process of the maxilla and its sutural articulation of the frontal bone. This point lies on C3 and resides at the center of the bony opacity created by the superior extremity of the ascending nasal process of the maxilla. It can be located directly below the ridge of reinforcement, which forms part of the base of the frontal sinus. Line CF1 is extended upward to its intersection with the external frontal cortical bone and downward, passing below the bony Menton. Angle C3 to CF1 takes different values depending on the age and sex of the patient. After pubescent growth is complete, the normal values are 85° to 90° in females and 90° to 95° in males. Normally, line CF1 passes through the frontal sinus, the FM point, the anterior border of the nasopalatine canal (NP point), the distal slope of the occlusal edge of the crown of the upper canine, the apex of the lower central incisor, and Menton (ME point), which is the osseous point of contact between the posterior border of the symphysis and the inferior border of the mandible (Fig. 112-9). The presence of an anatomic abnormality is suggested when line CF1 does not pass through these points.

When the NP point does not coincide with CF1, then a new CF1 can be constructed by drawing this line at an angle 90° (female) or 95° (male) to C3, through the FM point and extended beyond the ME point. The surgeon can then measure the distance between the NP point and line CF1, knowing that if the maxilla is advanced so that the NP point lies on CF1, the maxilla will be within the limit

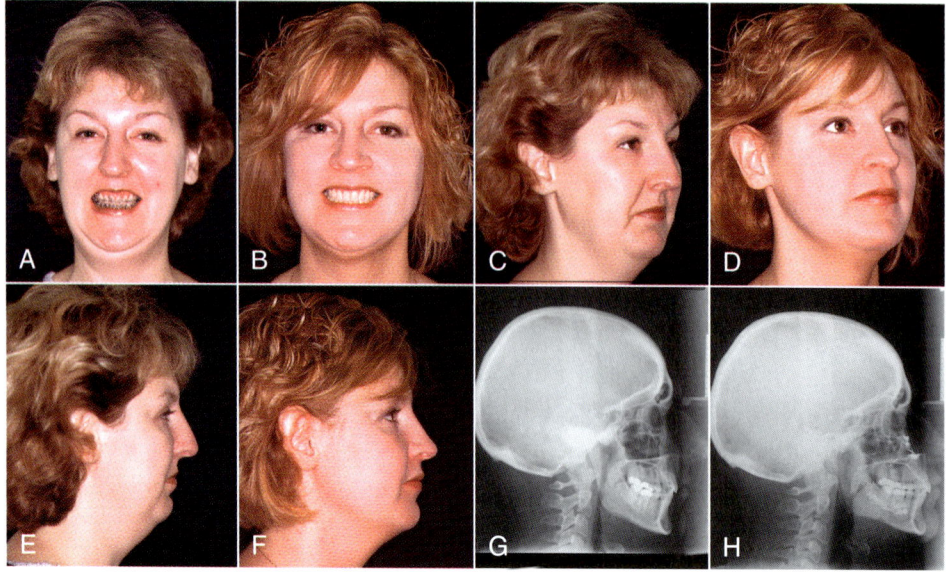

Fig. 112-7 ■ The surgical advancement of the maxilla and mandible (MMA) to a position of normal facial balance will result in a favorable change in facial appearance. **A,** Frontal view before MMA. **B,** Frontal view after MMA. **C,** Oblique view before MMA. **D,** Oblique view after MMA. **E,** Profile view before MMA. **F,** Profile view after MMA. **G,** Lateral cephalometric radiograph before MMA. **H,** Lateral cephalometric radiograph after MMA, showing improvement in the pharyngeal airway.

Fig. 112-8 ■ Lines of the Delaire analysis that analyze the anteroposterior balance of the face. **A,** Lines C3 and CF1. **B,** M point is situated at the junction of the frontonasal and maxillonasal sutures and is always situated just in front of the bony opacity formed by the summit of the ascending nasomaxillary process. **C,** FM point anatomically corresponds to the middle of the upper border of the ascending nasal process of the maxilla and its sutural articulation of the frontal bone. This point lies on C3 and resides at the center of the bony opacity created by the superior extremity of the ascending nasal process of the maxilla. **D,** Line CF1 is extended through FM point upward to its intersection with the frontal cortical bone and downward, passing below the bony Menton. After pubescent growth is complete, the normal values are 85° to 90° in females and 90° to 95° in males.

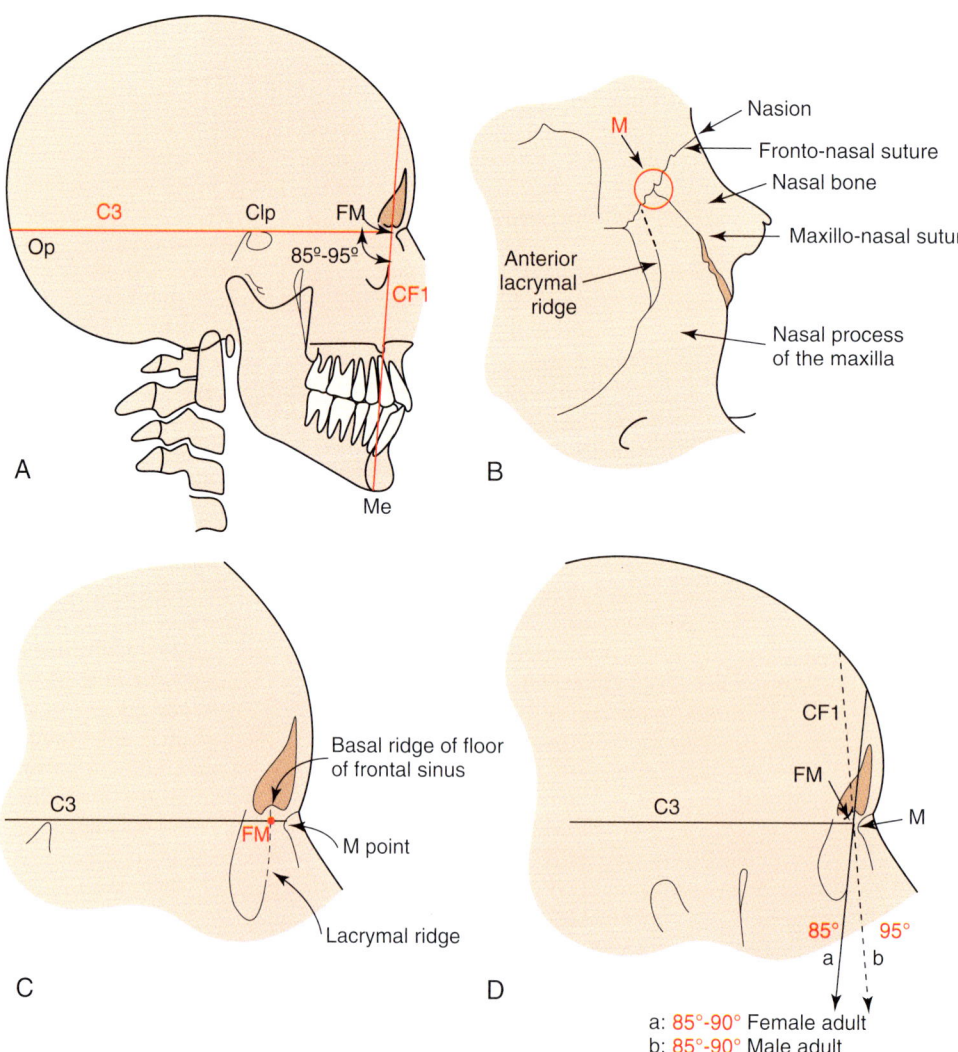

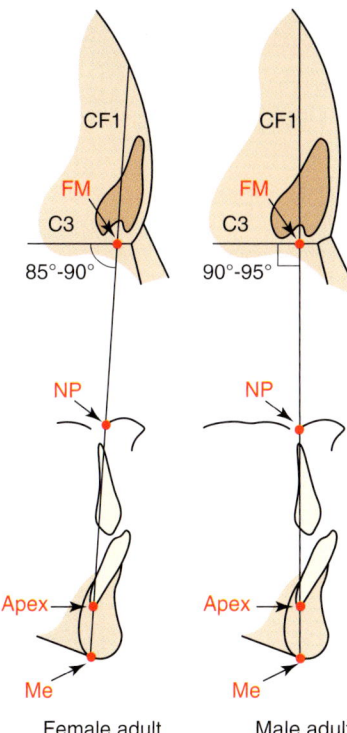

Fig. 112-9 ■ In patients with normal facial balance, line CF1 passes through the frontal sinus, FM, NP point, distal slope of the occlusal edge of the crown of the upper canine, the apex of the lower central incisor, and Menton (Me point).

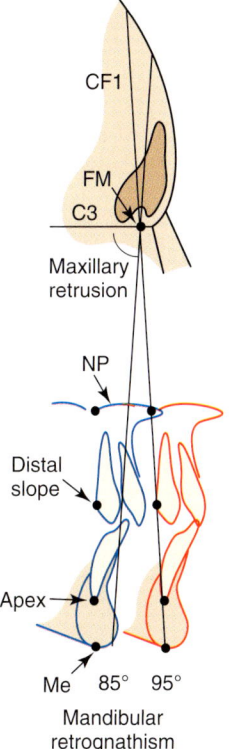

Fig. 112-10 ■ In patients with dentofacial deformities, CF1 can be constructed by drawing this line at an angle (up to) 95 degrees to C3 through the FM point. The surgeon can then measure the distance between the NP point and line CF1, knowing that if the maxilla is advanced so that the NP point lies on the line CF1, the maxilla will be within the limits of normal facial balance. The surgeon should also measure the distance between the ME point and CF1, knowing that this is the amount of surgical advancement that can be performed while keeping the mandible within the limits of normal facial balance.

of normal facial balance. The surgeon should also measure the distance between the ME point and CF1, knowing that this is the amount of surgical advancement that can be performed while keeping the mandible within the limits of normal facial balance (Fig. 112-10). If the Menton lies behind CF1 and the line passes through the apex of the lower incisor tooth, then a genioplasty is required to advance the chin and associated muscles to both improve the pharyngeal airway and achieve facial balance (Fig. 112-11). Thus, the following can be viewed objectively and eventually measured: the degree of maxillary retrognathia, the degree of mandibular retrognathia, microgenia, and the degree of AP displacement between the maxilla and the mandible in relation to both the "ideal" and to each other.

After determining the required movements based on the cephalometric analysis, the maxillary and mandibular advancement can be achieved using a LeFort 1 maxillary osteotomy and a bilateral saggital split osteotomy of the mandible, respectively. Unless there is a class II or III malocclusion being corrected at the same time as the surgery, synchronous advancement of the maxilla and mandible can be performed to maintain presurgical occlusion. A concomitant advancement genioplasty is performed in cases of anterior mandibular deficiency as determined by the preoperative cephalometric tracing (Fig. 112-12). Based on a visual treatment objective, the prediction tracing is completed and the definitive movements are decided before surgery. To guarantee that the movements are achieved during the operation, it is necessary to perform model surgery that accurately produces the planned surgical cuts. The unique features of each case determine whether the maxilla or mandible is first advanced and fixated, to then be used as the guide for positioning of the other jaw. With the use of rigid fixation, it is possible to advance the mandible the predetermined amount, fixate

using titanium plates or bicortical screws, and then advance the maxilla using the operative mandible as the guide. If there is a flat occlusal plane, the mandible can be advanced in a predictable manner. If the patient has an accentuated curve of Spee, it is more accurate to advance the maxilla first.

Occasionally a cephalometric radiograph will reveal constriction of the retropalatal airway, yet the maxilla cannot be significantly advanced and remains within the range of normal facial balance. In these patients, an examination of the facial soft tissue may reveal an acute nasolabial angle, which would limit the magnitude of maxillary advancement. An option is to perform a segmental LeFort I with the removal of a transverse segment of bone that either contains the first bicuspid teeth or consists of approximately 7 mm of bone if the patient is edentulous. This will allow an advancement of the posterior maxilla and its attached soft tissue, in addition to the advancement of the anterior segment that keeps the face within normal facial balance. This segmental surgery involves the removal of bone from the maxillary sinus and floor of the nose (Fig. 112-13).

PATIENT OUTCOMES

Cases to illustrate the use of MMA to treat OSA patients are found in Fig. 112-14. The Delaire cephalometric analysis was used in each case to determine the advancements required for the maxilla and mandible. Confirmation of achieving the planned surgical

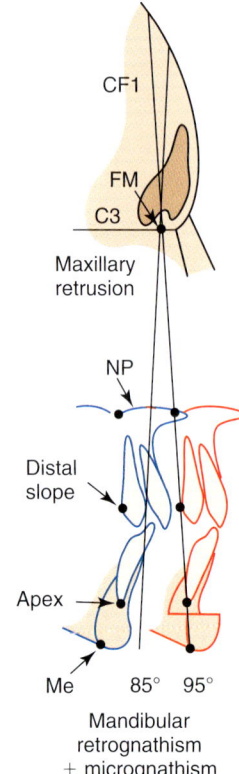

Fig. 112-11 ■ Me point (Menton). If Menton lies behind CF1 when the line passes through the apex of the lower central incisor tooth, then a genioplasty is required to advance the chin and associated muscles to improve the pharyngeal airway and achieve facial balance.

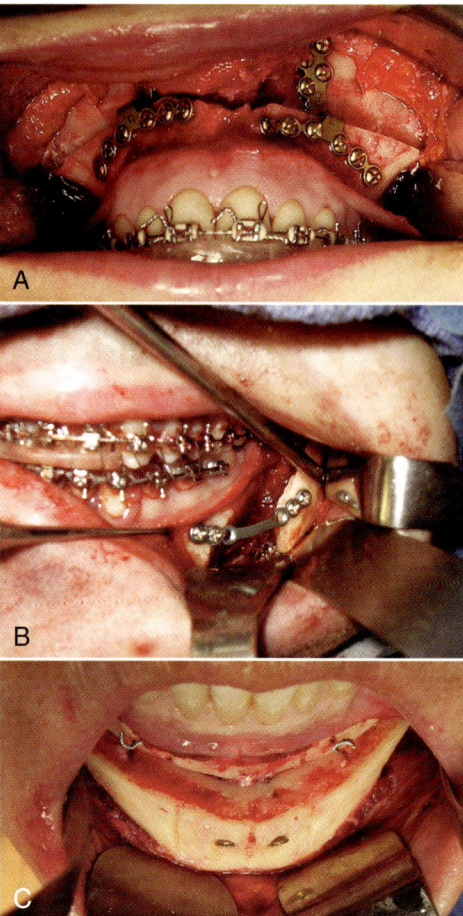

Fig. 112-12 ■ **A,** LeFort I maxillary osteotomy with a 9-mm advancement. **B,** Bilateral sagittal split osteotomy with a 17-mm advancement. **C,** Genioplasty with a 12-mm advancement.

movements is observed by placing the presurgical cephalometric tracing over the post-surgical radiograph, noting the position of the anatomic landmarks to CF1. Ideally, the points (FM, NP, apex, ME) will fall on this line of anterior facial balance.

The following outcome studies of OSAS patients treated using the Delaire analysis to plan surgical movements have demonstrated positive results.

In a prospective study to compare the effectiveness of MMA to continuous positive airway pressure in patients who could not tolerate CPAP, the results revealed that the mean AHI decreased significantly with CPAP and remained low after MMA surgery. Subjective ratings of sleepiness did not significantly improve until *after* surgery. Self-reported measures of depressive symptoms showed improvement, with significantly greater decrease in symptoms after surgery, compared with CPAP. These results confirm previous reports of the effectiveness of CPAP in the treatment of OSAS. However, outcomes after MMA appear as positive or better, particularly in self-reported mood and sleepiness symptoms.[102]

Another study demonstrated a significant reduction between the preoperative and postoperative Epworth Sleepiness scores, which represented an improvement in daytime sleepiness from levels seen in severe OSAS to levels similar to those in normal controls. Statistically significant reductions were observed in the number of patients reporting problems with memory, concentration, and stress. Of patients who snored preoperatively, 90% either stopped snoring (45%) or reported a reduction in snoring severity (45%). The surgery was considered a worthwhile experience by 83.3% of the patients.[103] These results were confirmed in a second study in which the elimination of excess daytime sleepiness, snoring, and witnessed apneas

were found to be statistically significant. Ninety percent of the patients reported that they would undergo MMA again, and all patients would recommend the treatment to others with OSAS. This is a testimony to the success of MMA as a surgical option to treat OSAS. Such a high level of patient satisfaction should be encouraging to those patients who are considering this treatment option.[104] In the same group of patients, objective measurements to determine treatment outcomes revealed a significant decrease in the mean AHI from 46.5% to 9.3% following MMA surgery.[104] A similar study looked at the effectiveness of maxillo-mandibular advancement surgery for treating patients with severe OSAS. Subjective and objective treatment outcomes following MMA surgery were evaluated in twelve patients who had a preoperative respiratory disturbance index (RDI) greater than 100. In this group, the mean RDI was 119.2. The postoperative polysomnography, performed an average of 8.5 months following the surgery, revealed a mean RDI of 17.3. The postoperative RDI was less than 5 for five of the twelve patients, and four patients had an RDI between 5 and 15. In this study, subjective data in the form of a postsurgery Epworth Sleepiness Scale were available for eight patients and revealed a mean value of 5 compared to 12.7 before surgery. All eight patients considered the surgery to be a worthwhile experience.[105]

A positive outcome following MMA surgery is the elimination of the need for CPAP postsurgery. A review of 59 patients who had used CPAP before MMA surgery, revealed that all patients expressed

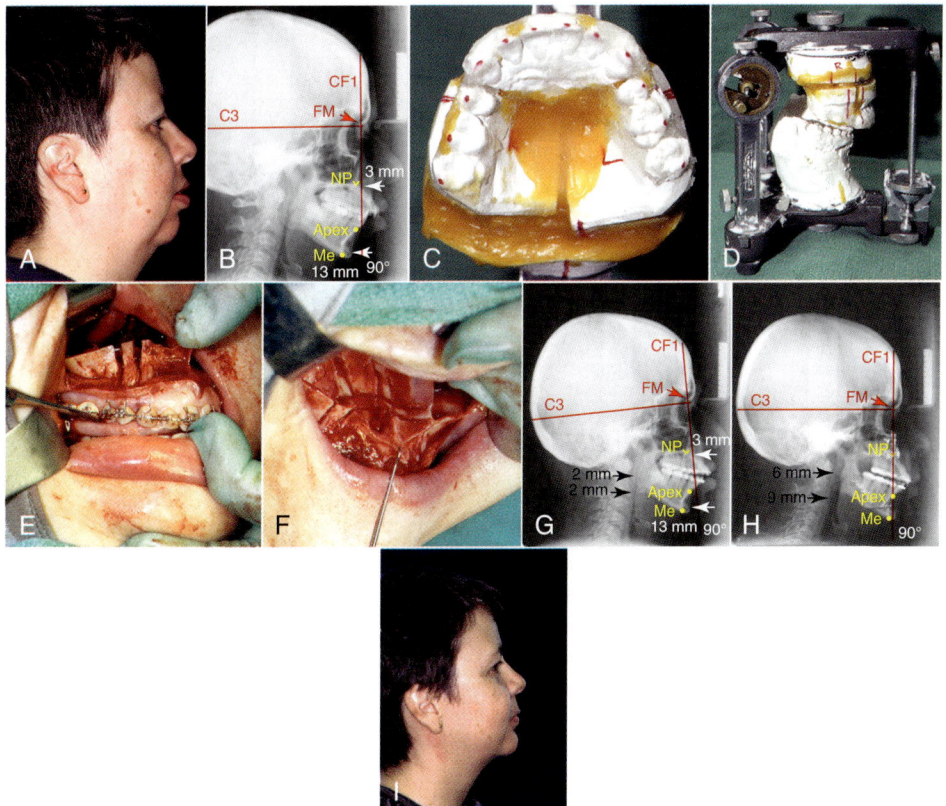

Fig. 112-13 ■ Presurgical profile view of patient with severe obstructive sleep apnea syndrome. The cephalometric radiograph reveals constriction of both the retropalatal and retroglossal airways. Clinical examination reveals an acute nasolabial angle, and cephalometric analysis confirms that the maxilla can be advanced only 3 mm. The Menton, however, can be moved anteriorly 13 mm. Model surgery confirms that the removal of a transverse segment of bone containing the first bicuspid teeth will allow a 7-mm advancement of the posterior maxilla in addition to the 3-mm advancement of the anterior segment, for an overall 10-mm advancement of the posterior border of the hard palate. **A,** Pretreatment profile view. **B,** Pretreatment cephalometric analysis. **C,** Model surgery with the first bicuspids removed and the posterior segment advanced. **D,** Articulated models used for an intermediate splint showing much greater advancement of the posterior segment compared with anterior movement. **E,** Intraoperative view of vertical osteotomy cuts to allow removal of the bony segment from the first bicuspid region. **F,** Intraoperative view of transverse cuts to allow removal of bone from the floor of the nose. **G,** Presurgical cephalometric radiograph confirming the surgical movement necessary to achieve facial balance and revealing the constricted oropharyngeal airway. **H,** Postsurgical cephalometric radiograph demonstrating that the surgical objectives have been achieved, with the patient having normal facial balance and the pharyngeal airway having improved significantly. **I,** Postsurgical profile view.

dissatisfaction with using CPAP. In fact, the reason for seeking alternative treatment in almost all cases of OSA patients was to eliminate the need for CPAP. The most common question asked by a patient when discussing the risks and benefits of MMA is "If I have this done, will I still need to use CPAP?" In this study, 55 patients (93%) did not require CPAP after surgery, and only 4 patients required its continuous use.[106] This finding identifies a major benefit that the patient can consider when choosing a treatment option.

Anesthetists in many surgical centers are concerned about potential airway obstruction after MMA surgery in sleep apnea patients. Both the anesthetist and surgeon should know if immediate postoperative changes in the pharyngeal airway after this procedure subjects the OSA patient to increased risks of airway obstruction during the perioperative period. A study assessing the radiographic changes in the pharynx of OSA patients during the period of maximum edema after orthognathic surgery revealed an increase in the mean distance from the posterior pharyngeal wall to the soft palate and base of the tongue of over 5 mm and 6 mm, respectively. This study concluded that postoperative edema did not affect the AP dimension of the cephalometric radiograph and supports favorable changes in the pharyngeal airway during the immediate postoperative period after orthognathic surgery.[107] These findings are supported by another study, which assessed the immediate postoperative airway using pulse oximetry data. In 19 MMA patients, presurgery pulse oximetry data were compared with data gathered over the 48 hours immediately after surgery. Desaturation was defined as at least a 5% decrease for 10 seconds. These OSA patients had an average of 15.2

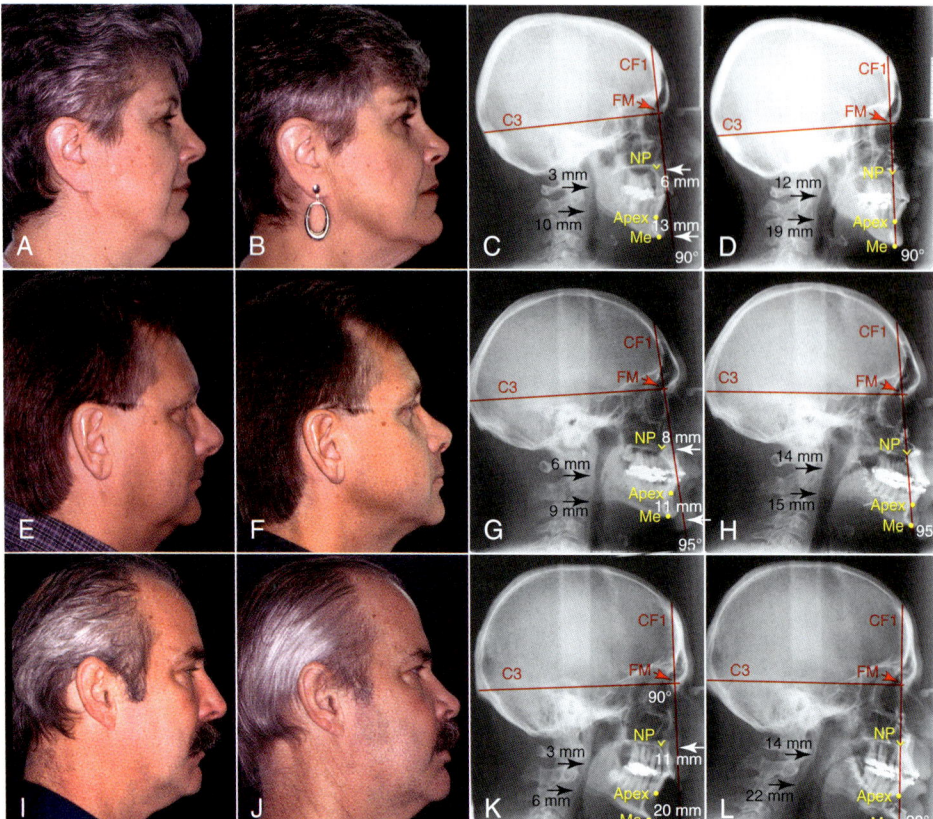

Fig. 112-14 ■ Patients with obstructive sleep apnea syndrome treated with maxillo-mandibular advancement using the Delaire cephalometric analysis to determine the magnitude of movement of the maxilla and mandible. **A-D,** Female patient balanced at 90° CF1/C3. **E-H,** Male patient balanced at 95° CF1/C3. **I-J,** Male patient balanced at 90° CF1/C3. **A, E,** and **I** show profile views presurgery. **B, F,** and **J** show profile views postsurgery. **C, G,** and **K** show presurgery cephalometric radiographs. **D, H,** and **L** show postsurgery cephalometric radiographs. Note the significant improvement in the retropalatal and retropharyngeal airways and normal facial balance demonstrated by the alignment of points (FM, NP, apex, Me) on the line of anterior facial balance, CF1, following surgery.

desaturations per hour presurgery, which dropped to an average of 1.3 per hour immediately postsurgery.[108]

Review of lateral cephalometric radiographs of OSAS patients who had previous UPPP typically reveals a short, thick soft palate. In patients in whom UPPP failed to eliminate symptoms of OSAS, this anatomic alteration may potentially contribute to velopharyngeal insufficiency in OSA patients after MMA. A review of 14 MMA patients who had previously undergone an unsuccessful UPPP revealed a statistically significant reduction in excess daytime sleepiness, snoring, and witnessed apneas after MMA surgery. Two patients experienced occasional nasal regurgitation after MMA, which resolved within 1 year. Only one subject reported slightly hyper nasal speech after MMA. Although UPPP is often promoted as a simple procedure with minimal pain and morbidity, it is interesting that 66% of these patients felt that UPPP was more painful and recovery more difficult than with the MMA procedure. One hundred percent of the subjects reported that they would undergo MMA again, and only one of the 14 patients would undergo UPPP again

(and that was because the patient felt UPPP decreased the frequency of his sore throat).[109] This finding, plus the low success rate of UPPP, calls into question the use of UPPP as a first-stage surgical treatment.

SUMMARY

Obstructive sleep apnea syndrome is a relatively common condition that predisposes the patient to physical harm, significant social discord, and poor quality of life.

Treatment by advancing the maxilla and mandible is a surgical option that should be considered for OSAS patients who have demonstrable retrognathia and narrowing of the pharyngeal airway. This option follows a principle based on scientific rationale rather than trial and error, and, in most cases, will negate the need for multiple surgeries.

MMA is a stable, predictable procedure that results in significant improvement and a high level of patient satisfaction.

PEARLS AND PITFALLS

- Surgical treatment of OSAS should be based on a specific diagnosis of an anatomic area of obstruction. Accurate diagnosis of abnormal anatomy that can be treated with one surgery should avoid multiple unnecessary procedures.
- Studies to localize the site of functional obstruction in the upper airway have shown that there is rarely a single anatomic site of occlusion, but more commonly multiple sites of upper airway obstruction during episodes of hypopnea in apnea. The two major sites of obstruction are in the retropalatal and retroglossal regions.
- Maxillomandibular advancement surgery is the one procedure that can address anatomic abnormalities in all the anatomic regions of the head and neck identified in each of the 19 most common surgical procedures discussed in the literature. MMA surgery can have a direct or indirect effect on the nasal valve, nasal septum, nasal turbinates, palate, tongue, tonsillar pillar region, hyoid bone, and pharynx.
- Studies investigating craniofacial risk factors show that mandibular body length is a craniofacial measure with the strongest association with increased risk for OSA. Two thirds or more of the variability of the apnea hypopnea index was explained by facial structure and obesity. Thirty percent of obstructive sleep apnea patients are nonobese, and in these patients the major contributing risk factor is facial structure.
- A common surgical treatment of OSAS is the uvulopalatopharyngoplasty (UPPP); however, review of the literature reports improvement in fewer than 50% of patients and complete control of OSAS in fewer than 25% of patients. The reason for the low success rate of this procedure is that it addresses only one site of a multisite problem. Soft tissues changes are unpredictable; in fact, the changes can be detrimental because they cause narrowing of the pharyngeal airway. Clinical examination of UPPP patients reveals that the soft palate appears shorter and has a firm scar band on the inferior surface. More important, however, is that lateral cephalometric radiographs reveal that although the soft palate is much shorter, it is also much thicker, which can result in a narrower retropalatal pharyngeal airway as seen on cephalometric radiographs. This could explain why the AHI increases in approximately 30% after UPPP.
- The best predictor of obstructive sleep apnea is the triad of symptoms, which include loud snoring, apnea witnessed by a bed partner, and excessive daytime sleepiness. In the primary care setting, the Epworth Sleepiness Scale (ESS) is the most frequently used questionnaire-based measure of excess daytime somnolence, consisting of a subjective, eight-item, self-reported questionnaire that is simple to use and takes less than 2 minutes to complete. Not only can the ESS confirm pathologic sleepiness, but it can also be used to validate post-treatment improvement in patients with OSA. An ESS score of ≥10 is considered abnormal.
- A criticism of most surgical treatment protocols for MMA surgery in patients with OSAS is the rather "abstract" selection process for surgical candidates. This criticism highlights the need for the use of a cephalometric radiograph and the appropriate cephalometric analysis that will identify bony and soft tissue abnormalities related to the soft palate, pharyngeal airway, and maxillomandibular complex influencing the multiple sites of obstruction. If the radiographic and clinical examination of the soft tissue of the pharyngeal reveal a narrow airway in conjunction with the retrognathia of the maxilla and mandible, then the patient should be a candidate for MMA surgery.
- Oral and maxillofacial surgeons have considerable experience and expertise in the diagnosis and treatment of dentofacial deformities. Application of the same surgical principles and procedures in patients with anatomic abnormalities that contribute to narrowing or obstruction of the pharyngeal airway during sleep will produce predictable and successful outcomes.

REFERENCES

1. Kushida CA, Littner MR, Morgenthaler T, et al: Practice parameters for the indications for polysomnography and related procedures: an update for 2005, *Sleep* 28:499, 2005.
2. Institute for Clinical Systems Improvement web site: *Healthcare guideline: Diagnosis and treatment of obstructive sleep apnea in adults*, ed 6, 2008.
3. Goodday RH: Nasal respiration, nasal airway resistance, and obstructive sleep apnea syndrome, *Oral Maxillofac Surg Clin North Am* 9:167-177, 1997.
4. Young T, Palta M, Dempsey J, et al: The occurrence of sleep-disordered breathing among middle-aged adults, *N Engl J Med* 328:1230-1235, 1993.
5. Young T, Evans L, Finn L, Palta M: Estimation of the clinically diagnosed proportion of sleep apnea syndrome in middle-aged men and women, *Sleep* 20:705-707, 1997.
6. Kapur V, Strohl KP, Redline S, et al: Underdiagnosis of sleep apnea syndrome in US communities, *Sleep Breath* 6:49-54, 2002.
7. Peppard PE, Young T, Palta M, et al: Longitudinal study of moderate weight change and sleep-disordered breathing, *JAMA* 284:3015-3021, 2000.

8. Cistulli PA: Craniofacial abnormalities in obstructive sleep apnoea: implications for treatment, *Respirology* 1:167-174, 1996.
9. Miles PG, Vig PS, Weyant RJ, et al: Craniofacial structure and obstructive sleep apnea syndrome: a qualitative analysis and meta-analysis of the literature, *Am J Orthod Dentofacial Orthop* 109:163-172, 1996.
10. Dempsey JA, Skatrud JB, Jacques AJ, et al: Anatomical determinates of sleep disordered breathing across the spectrum of clinical and non-clinical subjects, *Chest* 122:840-851, 2002.
11. Ford DE, Kamerow DB: Epidemiologic study of sleep disturbances and psychiatric disorders: an opportunity for prevention? *JAMA* 262:1479-1484, 1989.
12. Gislason T, Reynisdottir H, Kristbjarnson H, Benediktsdottir B: Sleep habits and sleep disturbances among the elderly: an epidemiological survey, *J Intern Med* 234:31-39, 1993.
13. Bixler EO, Vgontzas AN, Ten Have T, et al: Effects of age on sleep apnea in men: I. Prevalence and severity, *Am J Respir Crit Care Med* 157:144-148, 1998.
14. Bixler EO, Vgontzas AN, Lin HM, et al: Prevalence of sleep-disordered breathing in women: effects of gender, *Am J Respir Crit Care Med* 163:608-613, 2001.
15. Young T, Shahar E, Nieto FJ, et al: Predictors of sleep-disordered breathing in community-dwelling adults: the Sleep Heart Health Study, *Arch Intern Med* 162:893-900, 2002.
16. Flegel KM, Carroll MD, Ogden CL, Johnson CL: Prevalence and trends in obesity among US adults, 1999-2000, *JAMA* 288:1723-1727, 2002.
17. Eikermann M, Jordan AS, Chamberlin NL, et al: The influence of aging on pharyngeal collapsibility during sleep, *Chest* 131:1702-1709, 2007.
18. Bearpark H, Elliott L, Grunstein R, et al: Snoring and sleep apnea: a population study in Australian men, *Am J Respir Crit Care Med* 151:1459-1465, 1995.
19. Duran J, Esnaola S, Rubio R, Iztueta A: Obstructive sleep apnea-hypopnea and related clinical features in a population-based sample of subjects aged 30 to 70 yr, *Am J Respir Crit Care Med* 163:685-689, 2001.
20. Ip MS, Lam B, Lauder IJ, et al: A community study of sleep-disordered breathing in middle-aged Chinese men in Hong Kong, *Chest* 119:62-69, 2001.

21. Ip MS, Lam B, Tang LC, et al: A community study of sleep-disordered breathing in middle-aged Chinese women in Hong Kong: prevalence and gender differences, *Chest* 125:127-134, 2004.

22. Kim J, In K, Kim J, et al: Prevalence of sleep-disordered breathing in middle-aged Korean men and women, *Am J Respir Crit Care Med* 170:1108-1113, 2004.

23. Udwadia ZF, Doshi AV, Lonkar SG, Singh CI: Prevalence of sleep-disordered breathing and sleep apnea in middle-aged urban Indian men, *Am J Respir Crit Car Med* 169:168-173, 2004.

24. Newman AB, Foster G, Givelber R, et al: Progression and regression of sleep-disordered breathing with changes in weight: the Sleep Heart Health Study, *Arch Intern Med* 165:2408-2413, 2005.

25. Tishler PV, Larkin EK, Schluchter MD, Redline S: Incidence of sleep disordered breathing in an urban adult population: the relative importance of risk factors in the development of sleep-disordered breathing, *AJMA* 289:2230-2237, 2003.

26. Strohl KP, Redline S: Recognition of obstructive sleep apnea, *Am J Respir Crit Care Med* 154:279-289, 1996.

27. Jordan AS, McEvoy RD: Gender differences in sleep apnea: epidemiology, clinical presentation and pathogenic mechanisms, *Sleep Med Rev* 7:377-389, 2003.

28. Jordan AS, McEvoy RD, Edwards JK, et al: The influence of gender and upper airway resistance on the ventilatory response to arousal in obstructive sleep apnoea in humans, *J Physiol* 558:993-1004, 2004.

29. Rama AN, Tekwani SH, Kushida CA: Sites of obstruction in obstructive sleep apnea, *Chest* 122:1139, 2002.

30. Schellenberg JB, Maislin G, Schwab RJ: Physical findings and the risk for obstructive sleep apnea: the importance of oropharyngeal structures, *Am J Respir Crit Care Med* 162:740, 2000.

31. Meurice JC, Marc I, Carrier G, et al: Effects of mouth opening on upper airway collapsibility in normal sleeping subjects, *Am J Respir Crit Care Med* 153:255; 1996.

32. Malhotra A, Trinder J, Fogel R, et al: Postural effects on pharyngeal protective mechanisms, *Sleep* 27:1105, 2004.

33. Oksenberg A, Khamaysi I, Silverberg DS, et al: Association of body position with severity of apneic events in patients with severe nonpositional obstructive sleep apnea, *Chest* 118:1018-1024, 2000.

34. Woodson BT, Franco R: Physiology of sleep disordered breathing, *Otolaryngol Clin North Am* 40:691-711, 2007.

35. Sharabi Y, Dagan Y, Gorssman E: Sleep apnea as a risk factor for hypertension, *Curr Opin Nephrol Hypertens* 13:359, 2004.

36. Gami AS, Howard DE, Olson EJ, et al: Day-night pattern of sudden death in obstructive sleep apnea, *N Engl J Med* 352:1206-1214, 2005.

37. Punjabi NM, Shahar E, Redline S, et al: Sleep-disordered breathing, glucose intolerance, and insulin resistance: the sleep heart health study, *Am J Epidemiol* 160:521, 2004.

38. Hirshkowitz M: The clinical consequences of obstructive sleep apnea and associated excessive sleepiness, *J Fam Pract* 57(suppl. 8):S9-S16, 2008.

39. Mojon DS, Hess CW, Goldblum D, et al: Normal-tension glaucoma is associated with sleep apnea syndrome, *Ophthalmologica* 216:180-184, 2002.

40. Drager LF, Bortolotto LA, Pedrose RP, et al: Left atrial diameter is independently associated with arterial stiffness in patients with obstructive sleep apnea: potential implications for atrial fibrillation, *Int J Cardiol* 144:257-259, 2009.

41. Durán-Cantolla J, Aizpuru F, Martinez-Null C, Barbé F: Obstructive sleep apnea/hypopnea and systemic hypertension, *Sleep Med Rev* 13:323-331, 2009.

42. Friedman O, Logan AG: The price of obstructive sleep apnea-hypopnea: hypertension and other ill effects, *Am J Hypertens* 22(5):474-483, 2009.

43. Garvey JF, Taylor CT, McNichols WT: Cardiovascular disease in obstructive sleep apnoea syndrome; the role of intermittent hypoxia and inflammation, *Eur Respir J* 33(5):1195-1205, 2009.

44. Kario K: Obstructive sleep apnea syndrome and hypertension: ambulatory blood pressure, *Hypertens Res* 32:428-432, 2009.

45. Martinez-Garcia MA, Soler-Cataluna JJ, Ejarque-Martinez L, et al: Continuous positive airway pressure treatment reduces mortality in patients with ischemic stroke and obstructive sleep apnea: a 5-year follow-up study, *Am J Respir Crit Care Med* 180:36-49, 2009.

46. Yaggi H, Cancato J, Kernan W, et al: Obstructive sleep apnea as a risk factor for stroke and death, *N Engl J Med* 353:2034-2041, 2005.

47. Engleman H, Joffe D: Neuropsychological function in obstructive sleep apnea, *Sleep Med Rev* 3:59, 1999.

48. Barbe F, Pericas J, Munoz A, et al: Automobile accidents in patients with sleep apnea syndrome: an epidemiologic and mechanistic study, *Am J Respir Crit Care Med* 158:18, 1998.

49. Findley LJ, Unverzagt ME, Suratt PM: Automobile accidents involving patients with obstructive sleep apnea, *Am Rev Respir Dis* 138:337, 1998.

50. George CR, Smiley A: Sleep apnea and automobile crashes, *Sleep* 22:790, 1999.

51. Lindberg E, Carter N, Gislason T, Janson C: Role of snoring and daytime sleepiness in occupational accidents, *Am J Respir Crit Care Med* 164:2031-2035, 2001.

52. Woodson BT, Han JK: Relationship of snoring and sleepiness as presenting symptoms in a sleep clinic population, *Ann Otol Rhinol Laryngol* 114(10):762-767, 2005.

53. Friedman M, Tanyeri H, La Rosa M, et al: Clinical predictors of obstructive sleep apnea, *Laryngoscope* 109:1901-1907, 1999.

54. Kushida CA, Efron B, Guilleminault C: A predictive morphometric model for OSAS, *Ann Intern Med* 127:581-587, 1997.

55. Tsai WH, Remmers JE, Brant R, et al: A decision rule for the diagnostic testing in OSA, *Am J Respir Crit Care Med* 167:1427-1432, 2003.

56. el-Ganzouri AR, McCarthy RJ, Tuman KJ, et al: Preoperative airway assessment: predictive value of a multivariate risk index, *Anesth Analg* 82:1197-1204, 1996.

57. Pang KRIP, Terris DJ, Podolsky R: Severity of obstructive sleep apnea: correlation with clinical examination and patient perception, *Otolaryngol Head Neck Surg* 135:555-560, 2006.

58. Katsontonis GP, Maas CS, Walsh JK: The predictive efficacy of the Muller maneuver in uvulopalatopharyngoplasty, *Laryngoscope* 99:677-680, 1989.

59. Doghramji K, Jabourian ZH, Pilla M, et al: Predictors of outcome for uvulopalatopharyngoplasty, *Laryngoscope* 105:311-314, 1995.

60. Petri N, Suadicani P, Wildschiodtz G, et al: Predictive value of Muller maneuver, cephalometry and clinical features for the outcome of uvulopalatopharyngoplasty: evaluation of predictive factors using discriminant analysis in 30 sleep apnea patients, *Acta Otolaryngol* 114:565-571, 1994.

61. Stuck BA, Maurer JT: Airway evaluation in obstructive sleep apnea, *Sleep Med* 12:411-436, 2008.

62. Malhotra A, Berry RB, White DP: Central sleep apnea. In Carney PR, Berry RB, Geyer D, editors: *Clinical sleep disorders*, Philadelphia, 2004, Lippincott Williams & White.

63. Eckert DJ, Jordan AS, Merchia P, Malhotra A: Central sleep apnea: pathophysiology and treatment, *Chest* 131:595, 2007.

64. Krachman SL, Crocetti J, Berger TJ, et al: Effects of nasal continuous positive airway pressure on oxygen body stores in patients with Cheyne-Stokes respiration and congestive heart failure, *Chest* 123:59, 2003.

65. Pillar G, Peled R, Lavie P: Recurrence of sleep apnea without concomitant weight increase 7.5 years after weight reduction surgery, *Chest* 106:1702, 1994.

66. Strelzow VV, Blanks RH, Basile A, Strerzlow AE: Cephalometric airway analysis in obstructive sleep apnea syndrome, *Laryngoscope* 98:1149, 1988.

67. Barvaux VA, Aubert G, Rodenstein DO: Weight loss as a treatment for obstructive sleep apnoea, *Sleep Med Rev* 4:435-452, 2000.

68. Heath M: Management of obstructive sleep apnoea, *Br J Nurs* 2:802-804, 1993.

69. Lugaresi E, Cirignotta F, Montagna P: Pathogenic aspects of snoring and obstructive apnea syndrome, *Schweiz Med Wochenschr* 118:1018-1024, 1988.

70. Chan ASL, Lee RWW, Cistulli PA: Non-positive airway pressure modalities: mandibular advancement devices/positional

therapy, *Proc Am Thorac Soc* 5:179-184, 2008.

71. Höijer U, Ejnell H, Hedner J, et al: The effects of nasal dilation on snoring and obstructive sleep apnea, *Arch Otolaryngol Head Neck Surg* 118:281-284, 1992.

72. Kohler M, Bloch KE, Stradling JR: The role of the nose in the pathogenesis of obstructive sleep apnoea and snoring, *Eur Respir J* 30:1208-1215, 2007.

73. Sullivan CE, Issa FG, Berthon-Jones M, Eves L: Reversal of obstructive sleep apnoea by continuous positive airway pressure applied through the nares, *Lancet* 1:862-865, 1981.

74. Weaver TE, Chasens ER: Continuous positive airway pressure treatment for sleep apnea in older adults, *Sleep Med Rev* 11:99-111, 2007.

75. Engleman HM, Kingshott RN, Wraith PK, et al: Randomized placebo-controlled cross-over trial of continuous positive airway pressure for mild sleep apnea/hypopnea syndrome, *Am J Respir Crit Care Med* 159:461, 1999.

76. Jenkinson C, Davies RJ, Mullins R, Stradling JR: Comparison of therapeutic and subtherapeutic nasal continuous positive airway pressure for obstructive sleep apnoea: a randomized prospective parallel trial, *Lancet* 353:2100, 1999.

77. Kribbs NB, Redline S, Smith PL: Objective monitoring of nasal CPAP usage in OSAS patients, *Sleep Res* 20:270, 1991.

78. Kushida CA, Morgenthaler TI, Littner MR, et al: Practice parameters for the treatment of snoring and obstructive sleep apnea with oral appliances: an update for 2005, *Sleep* 29:240-243, 2006.

79. Ferguson KA, Cartwright R, Rogers R, Schmidt-Nowara W: Oral appliances for snoring and obstructive sleep apnea: a review, *Sleep* 29:244-262, 2006.

80. Barnes M, McEvoy RD, Banks S, et al: Efficacy of positive airway pressure and oral appliance in mild to moderate obstructive sleep apnea, *Am J Respir Crit Care Med* 170:656-664, 2004.

81. Engleman HM, McDonald JP, Graham D, et al: Randomized crossover trial of two treatments for sleep apnea/hypopnea syndrome: continuous positive airway pressure and mandibular repositioning splint, *Am J Respir Crit Care Med* 166:855-859, 2002.

82. Tan YK, L'Estrange PR, Luo YM, et al: Mandibular advancement splints and continuous positive airway pressure in patients with obstructive sleep apnoea: a randomized crossover trial, *Eur J Orthod* 24:239-249, 2002.

83. Schmidt-Nowara WW, Lowe A, Wegand L, et al: Oral appliances for the treatment of snoring and obstructive sleep apnea: a review, *Sleep* 18:501, 1995.

84. Ferguson KA, Ono T, Lowe AA, et al: A randomized crossover study of an oral appliance vs nasal-continuous positive airway pressure in the treatment of mild-moderate obstructive sleep apnea, *Chest* 109:1269, 1996.

85. Mehta A, Qian J, Petocz P, et al: A randomized, controlled study of a mandibular advancement splint for obstructive sleep apnea, *Am J Respir Crit Care Med* 163:1457, 2001.

86. Gotsopoulos H, Chen C, Qian J, Cistulli PA: Oral appliance therapy improves symptoms in obstructive sleep apnea: a randomized, controlled trial, *Am J Respir Crit Care Med* 166:743, 2002.

87. Johnston CD, Gleadhill IC, Cinnamond MJ, et al: Mandibular advancement appliances and obstructive sleep apnoea: a randomized clinical trial, *Eur J Orthod* 24:251, 2002.

88. Randerath WJ, Heise M, Hinz R, Ruehle KH: An individually adjustable oral appliance vs continuous positive airway pressure in mild-to-moderate obstructive sleep apnea syndrome, *Chest* 122:569, 2002.

89. Millman RP, Rosenburg CL, Kramer NR: Oral appliances in the treatment of snoring and sleep apnea, *Otolaryngol Clin North Am* 31:1039, 1999.

90. Almeida FR, Lowe AA, Otsuka R, et al: Long-term sequelae of oral appliance therapy in obstructive sleep apnea patients: Part 2. Study-model analysis, *Am J Orthod Dentofacial Orthop* 129:205, 2006.

91. Fee WE, Ward PH: Permanent tracheostomy: a new surgical technique, *Ann Otol Rhinol Laryngol* 86:635, 1977.

92. Fujita S, Conway W, Zorick F, Roth T: Surgical correction of anatomic abnormalities in obstructive sleep apnea syndrome: uvulopalatopharyngoplasty, *Otolaryngol Head Neck Surg* 89:923-934, 1981.

93. Sher AE, Schechtman KB, Piccirillo JF: An American Sleep Disorders Association review: the efficacy of surgical modifications of the upper airway in adults with obstructive sleep apnea syndrome, *Sleep* 19:156, 1996.

94. Hessel NS, DeVries N: Increase of the apnoea-hypopnoea index after uvulopalatopharyngoplasty: analysis of failure, *Clin Otolaryngol* 29:682, 2004.

95. Prinsell J: Maxillomandibular advancement surgery in a site-specific treatment approach for obstructive sleep apnea in 50 consecutive patients, *Chest* 116:1519, 1999.

96. Pirsig W, Verse T: Long-term results in the treatment of obstructive sleep apnea, *Eur Arch Otorhinolaryngol* 257:570, 2000

97. Li KK, Guilleminault C, Riley RW, Powell NB: Obstructive sleep apnea and maxillomandibular advancement: an assessment of airway changes using radiographic and nasopharyngoscopic examinations, *J Oral Maxillofac Surg* 60:526, 2002.

98. Fairburn SC, Waite PD, Vilos G, et al: Three-dimensional changes in upper airways of patients with obstructive sleep apnea following maxillomandibular advancement, *J Oral Maxillofac Surg* 65:6-12, 2007.

99. Hoekma A, deLange J, Stegenga B, de Bond LGM: Oral appliances and maxillomandibular advancement surgery: an alternative treatment protocol for the obstructive sleep apnea-hypopnea syndrome, *J Oral Maxillofac Surg* 64:886-891, 2006.

100. Delaire J, Schendel SA, Tulasne JF: An architectural and structural craniofacial analysis: a new lateral cephalometric analysis, *Oral Surg Oral Med Oral Pathol* 52:226, 1981.

101. Goodday R, Gregoire C: Facial appearance following surgical treatment for obstructive sleep apnea syndrome, *Gen Dent*, May 2008, Special Issue.

102. Rajda M, Eskes G, Morrison D, et al: *Effects of obstructive sleep apnea and subsequent treatment on mood and cognition*. World Association of Sleep Medicine, First Congress, Berlin, Germany, October 13-15, 2005.

103. Robertson C: Subjective evaluation of orthognathic surgical outcomes in OSAS patients, *J Oral Maxillofac Surg* 58 (suppl 1):57, 2000.

104. Robertson CG, Goodday RH, Rajda M, et al: Subjective and objective treatment outcomes of maxillomandibular advancement for the treatment of obstructive sleep apnea syndrome, *J Oral Maxillofac Surg* 61 (suppl 1):76, 2003,

105. Goodday R, Conrod S: Treatment outcomes following maxillomandibular advancement surgery for treatment of severe obstructive sleep apnea with respiratory disturbance indices (RDIs) greater than 100, *J Oral Maxillofac Surg* 67 (suppl 2):42, 2009.

106. Gregoire C, Goodday R, Robertson C: The effect of maxillomandibular advancement surgery on controlled positive airway pressure (CPAP) use in patients with obstructive sleep apnea, *J Oral Maxillofac Surg* 63 (suppl 1):48, 2005.

107. Robertson C, Goodday RH, Precious DS, Morrison AD: Post-surgical pharyngeal airway changes following orthognathic surgery in OSAS patients, *J Oral Maxillofac Surg* 57 (suppl 1):80, 1999.

108. Powell J, Yim D, Morrison A, Goodday R: Oxygen saturations in patients undergoing maxillomandibular advancement surgery for obstructive sleep apnea: a preoperative to postoperative comparison, *J Oral Maxillofac Surg* 62 (suppl 1):57, 2004.

109. Robertson CG, Goodday RH, Precious DS, Morrison AD: Risks and benefits of maxillomandibular advancement in OSAS patients with previous UPPP, *J Oral Maxillofac Surg* 60 (suppl 1):64, 2002.

113

Obstructive Sleep Apnea—Surgical Treatment: Part I, UPPP, Genioglossus Advancement, Hyoid Suspension

Robert A. Strauss, Adam P. McCormick

Obstructive sleep apnea (OSA) and obstructive sleep apnea syndrome (OSAS), apneas with clinical symptoms, are potentially fatal diseases that have a myriad of causes.[1] The two main types of sleep apnea are obstructive and central (i.e., apnea caused by centrally induced respiratory depression and not due to obstruction), although a combination of the two is common. Surgeons are generally called upon to manage the OSA subset, because there is no good surgical option for central sleep apnea.

Understanding that the source and level of obstruction causing OSA can occur anywhere in the airway from the tip of the nose to the vocal cords, surgical management of OSAS is predicated on finding the source of anatomic constriction and either surgically dilating it or at least preventing it from collapsing or constricting during sleep. Once the diagnosis has been made using clinical history, physical examination, diagnostic nasopharyngoscopy, and objective polysomnography, a treatment plan is constructed to treat one or more of these areas of the airway.

Surgical management of OSAS has historically been divided into a group of clinical phases. This is based on the theory that one should start with the lowest morbidity procedures (phase I) and work up to more major surgery (phase II) as necessary, based on the response of the simpler procedures. Although this does make some sense, it is evident now that these "simpler" procedures are also not likely to cure patients with high levels of apnea. Therefore many surgeons now proceed immediately to more major and clinically effective phase II surgery when the severity of the clinical situation warrants it (i.e., maxillomandibular advancement in patients with high level of disease). Phase II procedures generally affect multiple areas over a larger cross section of the airway at one time and represent the best opportunity to effectively treat the disease process occurring throughout the airway. In patients with a lower apnea-hypopnea index (AHI), however, the use of phase I treatments (those that target an isolated area) are commonly still used, often in a stepwise fashion, until the OSAS is controlled or phase II treatment is indicated. Of course, this is based on the assumption that the targeted area is, in fact, the anatomic area of obstruction within the airway. With the advent of three-dimensional imaging (and hopefully with increasing use of more accurate dynamic imaging while the patient is sedated), it may be possible in the near future to better predict what treatment will have the greatest effect with the least morbidity.

Phase I treatment options are quite varied, and the choice of which one or ones to use is based on the anatomic source suspected by the clinician. The choice of surgical procedures is often also affected by the training, comfort, and experience of the surgeon. An ear, nose, and throat (ENT) surgeon might consider an early septoplasty, whereas an oral and maxillofacial surgeon (OMFS) might choose a genial osteotomy in the same patient based on their comfort in treating these anatomic areas, the medical history, and anesthetic risk of the patient.

The purpose of this chapter is to discuss the various options available for phase I treatment. With phase I treatment, as with any therapy, the most conservative approach yielding the highest increase in oxygenation and reduction of the AHI should always be considered.

WEIGHT LOSS

Although not universal, the vast majority of patients with OSA are obese, and there is a direct correlation between this disease and body mass index (BMI).[2] The BMI is defined as the weight in kilograms divided by the height in meters squared (kg/m^2). A BMI of more than 25 kg/m^2 is defined as overweight, whereas a BMI of more than 30 kg/m^2 is considered obese. Not only does obesity lead to adverse systemic conditions, such as cardiovascular disease, diabetes, and certain cancers, mechanically the increased weight in the cervical region increases the likelihood of obstruction. With weight gain, there is a subsequent increase in neck circumference, which constricts the hypopharynx and oropharynx. Increased fatty deposits in the peripharyngeal area also leads to constriction of the airway. It is generally recognized that any male patient with a neck size greater than 18.5, or a female with a neck size greater than 17.5, has OSA until proven otherwise.[3-6]

Weight loss, even in moderate amounts, can greatly affect the degree of apnea.[7,8] A recent study by Tuomilehto et al[9] showed a low calorie diet with lifestyle modifications resulted in significant reductions in patients with moderate OSA. Therefore it is prudent for any overweight patient diagnosed with OSA to initiate a weight loss program as part of the first line of defense against this disease. This may require medical supervision, and proper referral should be made by the surgeon to a clinician with experience in this area. In extreme cases, bariatric surgery may be indicated before any airway surgery.

CONTINUOUS POSITIVE AIRWAY PRESSURE

Continuous positive airway pressure (CPAP) is almost always initiated as part of first-line treatment of OSA and has been the mainstay of therapy for decades.[10] CPAP acts as a pneumatic splint for the airway by pushing air under pressure into the pharynx and preventing collapse of the soft tissues of the airway during sleep. This is accomplished through an air pump and a tight-fitting nasal mask that the patient wears nightly for the duration of their life (Fig. 113-1). In general, only pressurized room air is used, and oxygen is not necessary or indicated.

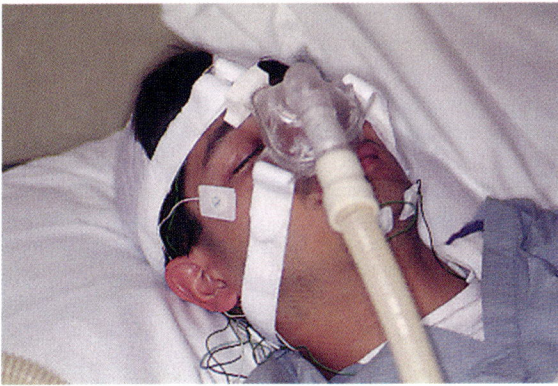

Fig. 113-1 ■ A patient using a CPAP mask. This is connected to an air pump and may be continuous at one pressure level, or the pressure can be stepped during inspiration and expiration (BiPAP) to make use more comfortable.

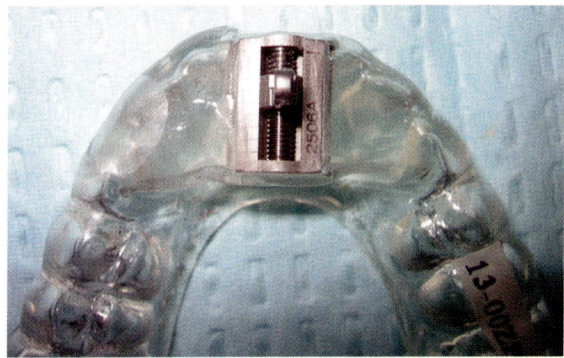

Fig. 113-2 ■ A mandibular repositioning appliance. Most current oral appliances have some mechanism to adjust the degree of advancement. This one uses a jackscrew.

CPAP has been shown to reduce blood pressure, decrease AHI, decrease the results of the Epworth Sleepiness Scale (ESS), improve sleep efficiency, and decrease oxygen desaturation.[11]

When first receiving CPAP, the patient is evaluated by polysomnography while undergoing CPAP titration, increasing the air pressure until respiratory events are maximally diminished. The CPAP trial study can be done on the same night as a shortened-duration standard polysomnography ("split-night study") or as a separate titration, allowing for longer titration times and the chance for more accurate diagnosis and titration.

Despite the success of CPAP in preventing the symptoms associated with OSA, tolerance of the delivery system is difficult for many people. Patient compliance has been reported to be only 65% to 80%, with 8% to 15% terminating treatment after the first night.[12-14] Many patients either cannot tolerate the mask or lose it inadvertently during the night. In this situation, other types of delivery systems are available (e.g., nasal prongs and pillows) that may work better for any individual patient, and proper referral to an experienced sleep disorders physician is highly recommended.

The advantages of CPAP are that it provides immediate treatment of the apnea (as opposed to surgery which may take several weeks to relieve apnea), can be totally curative, is titrated to an objective effect, has low morbidity, and is portable. Its disadvantages, other than the common lack of tolerance, are some potential dermatologic effects of the mask, airway drying, and possible barotrauma. For those that can tolerate its use, however, CPAP is still the most common and effective form of phase I treatment for OSA. It is generally when there is failure to tolerate the CPAP, or when patients electively choose to seek surgical options to eliminate the need for CPAP, that surgical treatments are explored.

POSITIONING DEVICES

Sleep apnea is often accentuated in the supine position because of gravitational effects on the airway. A simple and conservative approach to reduction of symptoms is sleep positioning. Various devices can be used to force the patient into sleep positions other than supine. A recent study by Skinner et al[15] compared CPAP to the classic "tennis ball technique," where patients wear a halter top with a tennis ball sewn into the back, preventing them from rolling onto their backs during sleep. This study revealed 13 of 18 patients with mild OSA using the tennis ball technique had a reduction in their AHI to less than 10, which was deemed a success compared to 16 of 18 patients using CPAP. Although not as effective as CPAP, this conservative approach shows some promising results in mild to moderate OSA of positional origin. Other similar devices include special pillows and foam wedges. The avoidance of the supine posture during sleep seems a logical management strategy for position-dependent mild OSA, and several studies have shown the effectiveness of this conservative treatment.[16-18] The disadvantage to the tennis ball technique is that few patients are willing to use such devices over the long term, and it works only in mild cases where the supine position accounts for the majority of respiratory events.

ORAL APPLIANCES

Oral appliances are also considered an acceptable first-line therapy in the treatment of mild to moderate levels of OSA for patients unable to tolerate CPAP or who prefer oral appliance therapy, as indicated in the 2009 Guidelines Publication of the American Academy of Sleep Medicine.[19] Recent data show oral appliances to be effective replacements for patients unable to tolerate CPAP (or who prefer this to CPAP) with mild to moderate sleep apnea.[20-23]

The basic concept is the same for each of these mandibular repositioning appliances—to prevent retropositioning of the mandible and the hypopharyngeal tongue base when a patient's musculature relaxes during sleep. In some cases this is accomplished by actually advancing the mandible from its centric occlusion position, whereas others merely maintain the centric occlusion position during sleep (i.e., just preventing retropositioning but not advancing). In addition, they increase the muscular tonus, which may also prevent airway collapse.

There are currently over 70 appliances used to treat OSA and it is beyond the scope of this chapter to detail each one. They differ in terms of material, range of mandibular movement, amount of dental coverage, rigidity, amount of mandibular advancement, and bite opening. The prime difference is whether the device is fixed, or adjustable and titratable, usually using a jackscrew appliance or class II elastics of varying sizes placed between the arches to control the degree of advancement (Fig. 113-2). Most oral appliances now allow the practitioner to vary the degree of advancement to maximize effect on the apnea while minimizing potential temporomandibular joint (TMJ) and occlusal damage (Fig. 113-3). Some appliances have been designed to attach to the CPAP mask the patient wears at night to facilitate simultaneous use.

The process of providing a patient with this device involves obtaining an alginate impression of the dental arches, along with an occlusal record, and construction of the splint by a commercial

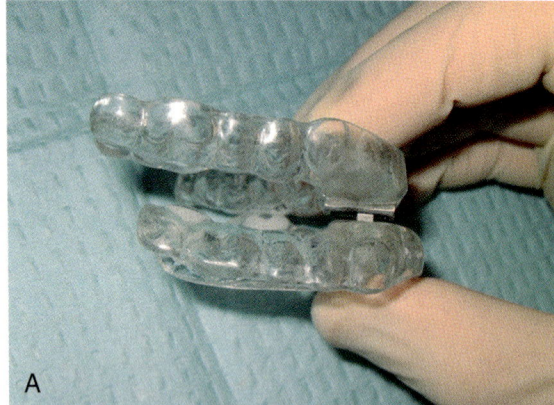

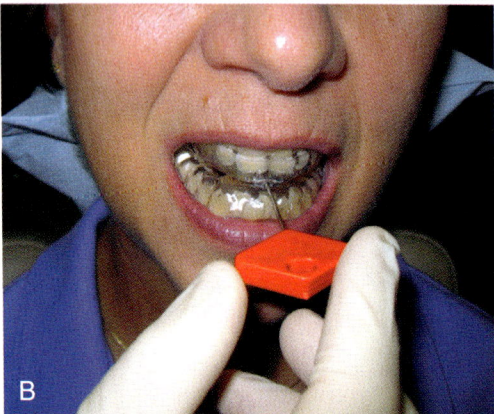

Fig. 113-3 ▪ A, The mandibular hook fits into the maxillary jackscrew to lock the two devices together. There should be posterior contacts to limit TMJ issues. **B,** A key is used to rotate and advance the jackscrew, thus adjusting the amount of repositioning.

laboratory. Once returned, the device must be inserted and adjusted according to the manufacturer's recommendation. At that time, it is imperative to insure a proper fit to prevent damage to the teeth, and appropriate bilateral contacts and excursions without interference to prevent myofascial pain symptoms. As the device is worn, intermittent adjustments are required, and the device will likely need to be replaced every year or two.

Once placed, the degree of advancement obtained by the elastics or the jackscrew should be initiated at the centric occlusion level and advanced every few days until the patient's symptoms disappear or the patient begins to experience significant TMJ discomfort. Maintaining the patient in centric occlusion may be adequate for many patients, because it still prevents the patient's tongue base from receding during sleep. In some cases, however, it will be necessary to advance beyond the centric occlusion position by 2 to 5 mm to obtain adequate results.

Mandibular advancement devices are currently the most commonly used appliances. However, other devices have been used with varying degrees of success. Tongue-retaining devices that physically hold the tongue in a forward position, as well as palatal lift appliances, have also been used. These appliances only address obstruction at the level of the tongue and soft palate, respectively, and currently have little place in the management of OSA.

Because these appliances can lead to severe TMJ and occlusal disturbances, it is important that oral appliances only be fitted by qualified dental personnel with training and experience in sleep medicine and sleep-related disorders, TMJ disorders, dental occlusion, and associated structures.[24] Even in the best of circumstances, some TMJ tightness may occur in the morning from the chronic

advancement, and this may require morning muscle exercises or the use of bite tab stabilizers to assist in replacement of the condyle-disk complex into the fossa. Many courses are now available to general dentists to provide the necessary training. It is imperative, however, that a general dentist work in tandem with a qualified sleep physician and OMFS to provide proper and complete care to the patient.

The success of an oral appliance should allow the patient to feel more alert with fewer arousals, less snoring, and improved breathing. In mild to moderate OSA, the AHI should be reduced by 50% or dropped to a level of ten or fewer events per hour to signal effective use of the device. It is important that placement of the appliance is followed by a repeat PSG to determine effectiveness. This can be done effectively with either a laboratory PSG or with a portable monitoring device. The appliance should also fit comfortably and minimize any dental or skeletal changes through their continued use. Patients often complain of muscle stiffness, TMJ pain, and dry mouth from use of the oral appliances, and unless addressed, these will lead the patient to stop using the device.

These appliances have been shown to be an effective alternative to CPAP, which may be advantageous when noncompliance with CPAP is an issue.[25] In many patients, the use of oral appliances is easier and less intrusive than CPAP, and when applicable, may be substituted.

PALATAL PILLARS

Patients suffering from snoring with mild to minimal OSA may benefit from the placement of palatal pillars. Pillars are woven polyester tubes approximately 1 inch long that, when placed in the soft palate, can cause scarring and stiffen the tissue to prevent drooping of the palate and subsequent obstruction at this level. Patient selection is of utmost importance in increasing the likelihood this procedure will decrease snoring or manage mild apnea. Obstructions found to be localized in the palate via clinical exam, nasopharyngoscopy and cephalometric analysis, are amenable to this procedure. Patients with a BMI less than 25, small uvulas and flaccid, bulky soft palates are also ideal candidates for this procedure. Importantly, patients should be advised this surgery usually does not completely eliminate snoring, but may change the intensity significantly, allowing the bed partner to remain asleep throughout the night. The devices are also approved by the U.S. Food and Drug Administration for mild sleep apnea management, but most surgeons limit their use to pure snoring or only very mild OSAS at most.

Palatal pillars are easily placed in the office with local anesthesia, and placement takes about 10 minutes. During the procedure, a specially designed, preloaded, injection gun is used to place three implants into the muscular soft palate centered around the midline and 1 cm on each side of the midline (Fig. 113-4, *A* and *B*). It is imperative that the implants be placed within the muscle so that they do not extrude over time (Fig. 113-4, *C*). Once placed, fibrosis ensues, thereby stiffening and adding support to the soft palate. This technique has been shown to be moderately effective in reducing snoring and daytime somnolence.[26]

Following the procedure, patients are placed on a diet of soft, cold foods for 24 hours, after which they are able to return to a general diet. Patients may complain of temporary fullness at the back of the throat and some mild soreness for 1 to 2 days but should be assured that this will be very short-lived. Most patients are relatively asymptomatic and return to work the next morning. Close follow-up is essential to monitor rejection of the implant or extrusion through the mucosa within the first few weeks postoperatively. The stiffening process may take up to 90 days for maximum effect to be noticed.

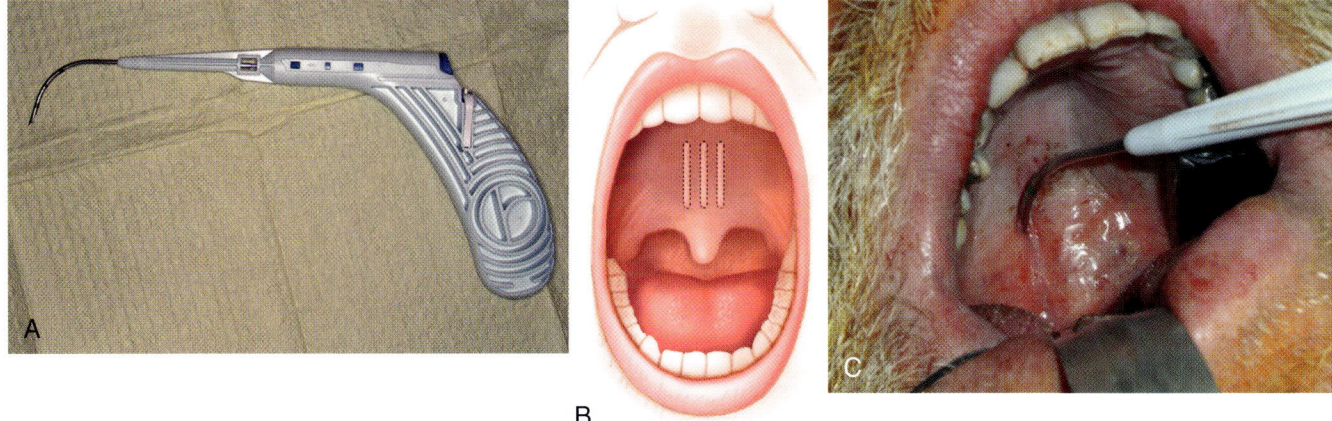

Fig. 113-4 ▪ **A,** A palatal pillar placement device. **B,** Three pillars are placed within the muscle near the midline of the palate. **C,** Palatal pillars being placed in the palate. (**B** from Walker RP: Palatal implants for snoring and sleep apnea. Oper Tech Otolaryngol Head Neck Surg 17(4):238-241, 2006.)

RADIOFREQUENCY ABLATION

Radiofrequency devices use radiofrequency energy to cauterize and create a series of known and controlled submucosal volumetric lesions, which lead to thermal contraction and ablation within tissue. This method has been used for more than a century, and more specifically for the treatment of OSA, for the past decade with varying degrees of success in the tongue, nasal turbinates, and in the soft palate. Initially, surgical electrocautery and lasers were used within the tissue; however, because of the charring and lack of control over tissue effects, there was significant scarring and excessive contraction. Studies have shown that a lower temperature, with longer duration and repeated procedures, has a higher success rate with minimal tissue necrosis.[27]

In this procedure, temperatures from 120° F to 200° F are delivered to the tissues via a handpiece electrode. The sheathed electrode allows for the tip to work deep within the tissue, preventing superficial loss of tissue. The surrounding tissues undergo vacuolar degeneration with subsequent internal scarring. This scarring causes the tissue to stiffen, and its size and flaccidity are diminished.

A small to moderate amount of local anesthesia (approximately 2 mL) with a vasoconstrictor is delivered to the soft palate by injection after the area has been topically anesthetized with benzocaine, butamben/tetracaine/benzocaine (Cetacaine), or lidocaine. The electrode is placed into the soft palate with the tip of the electrode positioned just superior to the uvula and inserted to a depth such that the sheathed part of the electrode protects the superficial mucosa. The exposed electrode is inserted solidly into the submucosal tissues, where the tip reaches a temperature of 120° F within approximately 10 seconds. A single lesion in the palate is created and the electrode is then removed from the tissue. In the tongue, a midline lesion is created and two additional sites are placed lateral to the initial midline lesion to complete the ablation.

Postprocedure, patients may feel a sense of fullness at the back of their throats and complain of a sore throat. Nonopioid analgesics are generally sufficient for any postoperative pain. The healing process may take 3 to 4 months with the need for additional procedures before the patient notices stiffening and volume reduction. Patients often tend to notice a diminished intensity of snoring after the first procedure, however. A second procedure is typically necessary if snoring continues 6 months after the initial ablation.[28]

Although many of these radiofrequency devices were sold, the procedure is not used as often as when it was introduced because of its lack of predictability.

UVULOPALATOPHARYNGOPLASTY

Uvulopalatopharyngoplasty (UPPP) has been historically, along with nasal septoplasty, the most commonly used procedure to treat OSA. This was primarily because it was the only viable surgical procedure available until relatively recently, when the surgical options for OSA treatment expanded. In fact, this procedure was never truly a very effective surgery unless the primary site of obstruction was the soft palate. Since we now know that the majority of obstructions occur at multiple levels within the airway, targeted procedures such as UPPP are now generally considered only a single component of a more complex phase I treatment plan and are rarely done alone.

As with any targeted procedure, thorough examination, imaging, and nasopharygoscopy should be performed to determine if the likely source of obstruction is in the soft palate. The nasopharyngoscopy aids the surgeon not only in determining the level or levels of obstruction, but also in ruling out any neoplastic or pathologic processes, which though unlikely, may be present and causing the obstruction.[29] Only when the level or levels of obstruction are ascertained can the surgeon determine if UPPP will be a viable treatment option (either as the sole procedure or in combination with other procedures) for the patient with OSA.

UPPP has traditionally been performed in the hospital operating room under general anesthesia and has been reported to have varying degrees of complications ranging from velopharyngeal insufficiency, dysphagia (difficulty swallowing), voice changes, and death from general anesthesia.[30]

First developed by Ikematsu, who followed habitual snorers for several years, the procedure entailed performing an adenoidectomy, tonsillectomy, and uvulectomy and excising the redundant lateral pharyngeal wall mucosa. The original technique has been modified to varying degrees, but the goal of shortening the palate and thereby widening the airway has remained consistent.

If the tonsils are to be removed a tonsillectomy may be performed by any standard technique. The uvula is then grasped with an Allis forceps and everted to expose the posterior aspect. A curvilinear incision is made at the base of the uvula extending to each tonsillar

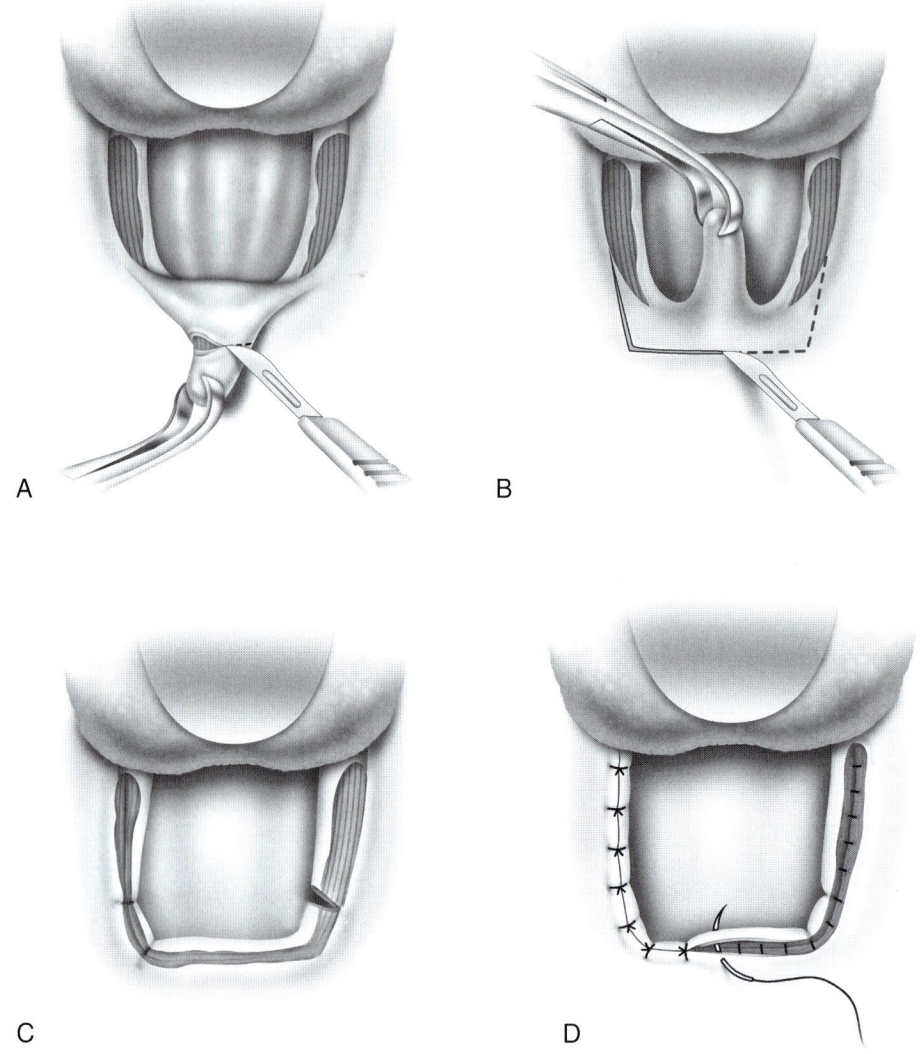

A

B

C

D

Fig. 113-5 ■ Uvulopalatopharyngoplasty (UPPP). **A,** After tonsillectomy, if needed, the uvula is picked up and incised posteriorly. **B** and **C,** The anterior soft palate is then excised and the resulting two flaps are closed (**D**) primarily to shorten the palate and stretch the pharyngeal walls. (From Friedman M. Sleep Apnea and Snoring: Surgical and Non-Surgical Therapy, Philadelphia, 2009, Saunders.)

pillar bilaterally. A trapezoid-shaped incision is outlined in the mucosa of the anterior soft palate that extends above the uvula (Fig. 113-5). The uvula is then excised, which then allows the posterior soft palate to be closed to the anterior soft palate superiorly. The posterior and anterior tonsillar pillars bilaterally are closed primarily (Fig. 113-6).[31]

LASER-ASSISTED UVULOPALATOPLASTY

In the early 1990's, Kamami[32] described a simpler and less morbid variation of the standard scalpel UPPP. The laser-assisted uvulopalatoplasty (LAUP) was initially described as a treatment for simple snoring only, but using the laser for its many surgical advantages. This procedure is generally done in the office with local or IV sedation anesthesia. The laser is fitted with a specially designed backstop handpiece to prevent inadvertent damage to the pharyngeal wall. The procedure begins with full-thickness incisions on either side of the uvula extending into the palate just short of the insertion of the levator palatinus muscle (approximately 1 cm in length) (Fig. 113-7,

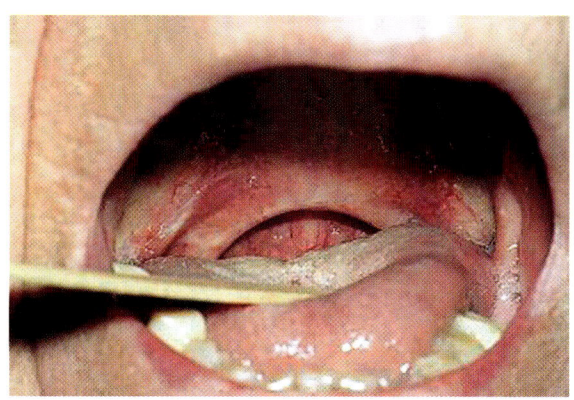

Fig. 113-6 ■ Postoperative result after UPPP. Note the taught palatal band.

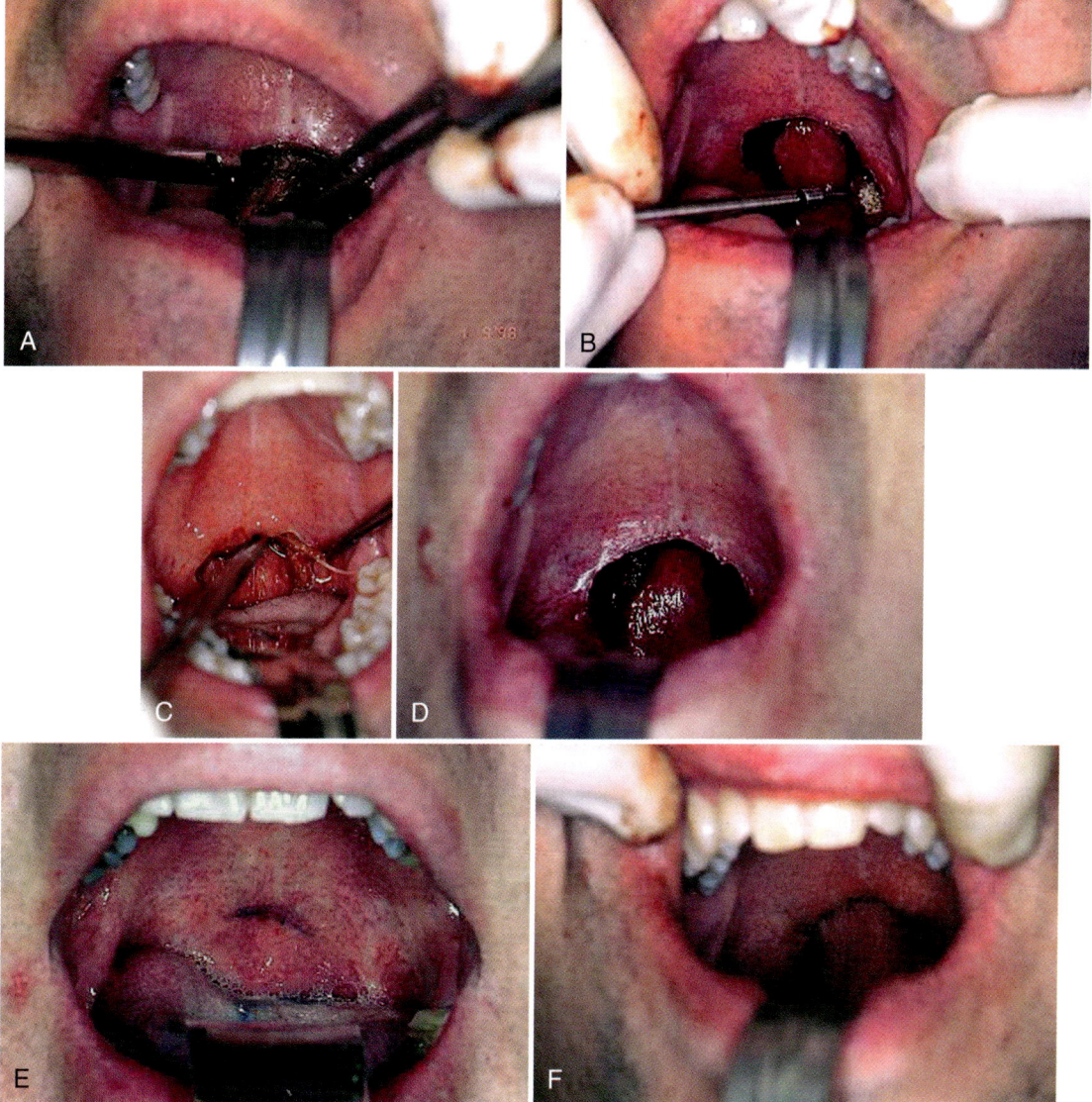

Fig. 113-7 ■ Laser-assisted uvulopalatoplasty (LAUP). **A,** A backstop handpiece is used to create the vertical cut in the palate without damaging the pharyngeal wall. The cut should extend just short of the levator palatinus muscle. **B,** The levator insertion should be marked with a surgical pen or with methylene blue on a 25 gauge needle. **C,** The handpiece is turned sideways and the cuts connected in the midline to remove the uvula and a portion of the soft palate. **D,** After the removal of the uvula and a portion of the soft palate. **E and F,** Preoperative and postoperative views of a LAUP procedure.

A). The muscle should not be violated to prevent postoperative velopharyngeal insufficiency. This is prevented by marking the levator insertion dimpling during flexion of the palate with phonation or gagging. This can be accomplished using either a surgical marking pen or a 25-gauge needle dipped in half-strength methylene blue (Fig. 113-7, *B*). These vertical "trenches" are then connected horizontally to remove the uvula and a portion of the soft palate (Fig. 113-7, *C* to *F*). The laser of choice is generally the carbon dioxide (CO_2), which is used in continuous wave (CW) mode at high power densities (usually 14 to 18 W with a less than 1.0-mm spot size) to create rapid and deep incisions. Although some charring does occur, which can increase postoperative discomfort, the end result of this lateral thermal effect is bloodless surgery.

The procedure proved to be quick and simple with low morbidity and is still an effective treatment for snoring.[32] It is accompanied, however, with a week or more of a significantly sore throat and dysphagia. When studied for the treatment of sleep apnea, the LAUP proved less beneficial as a stand-alone procedure, much like the standard UPPP.[33,34] The degree of postoperative scar contracture and the minimal tissue excision results in only minimal expansion of the airway. Although still a useful if somewhat painful treatment for snoring, the LAUP is generally not considered a particularly good treatment for OSA.

UVULOPALATOPHARYNGOPLASTY—LASER ASSISTED

A modification to the scalpel UPPP and the simple LAUP was described in 1994. A CO_2 laser is used to perform a more invasive procedure than a LAUP via a minor modification of the standard

UPPP, which is called uvulopalatopharyngoplasty–laser assisted (UPPP-LA).[35] Like the UPPP, the UPPP-LA is similarly used to correct obstructions at the palatal and oropharyngeal level by removing the uvula, modifying redundant pharyngeal and palatal tissues, and performing a primary closure of the posterior and anterior pillars. This enlarges the retropalatal airway and tightens the redundant pharyngeal tissues. The procedure begins much like a LAUP with lateral trenches and a horizontal excision, but the vertical trenches are placed further laterally to approximate the tonsillar pillars (Fig. 113-8, *A*). After the incisions are made, the area of the front surface of the anterior pillar is ablated to deepithelialize the surface (Fig. 113-8, *B* and *C*), and the posterior pillar is then sutured to this portion of the anterior pillar, thereby tightening the pharyngeal tissues. The soft palate that remains after the horizontal excision is also undermined to allow closure of the posterior side of the palate to the anterior side. Approximately six to eight resorbable sutures are used[35] (Fig. 113-8, *D*). If the patient has small tonsils they can be ablated with the laser before or during the procedure, but if they are larger than a standard scalpel, UPPP is performed with simultaneous tonsillectomy. The results of UPPP-LA are similar to scalpel UPPP but with lower morbidity (Fig. 113-8, *E* to *G*).[36]

If the surgeon finds the obstruction is occurring at the level of the palate, then a UPPP-LA may be performed on an inpatient or outpatient basis (based on the severity of the OSA and the medical history of the patient) with local anesthetic, sedation, or general anesthesia. If the degree of sleep apnea is significant, an inpatient procedure and a monitored overnight bed is often appropriate. This is especially true when this procedure is performed in concert with other airway and OSA procedures. In a retrospective study by Strocker et al,[37] 36 of 40 patients were discharged to home without morbidity. Three patients were hospitalized for nonmedical reasons and one was an inpatient for unrelated medical reasons.

Some studies have shown UPPP and UPPP-LA to be only 40% effective in eliminating symptoms (snoring) associated with OSA.[34,38] Others have reported up to 70% success if patients are selected correctly based on the anatomy and level of obstruction.[39] Li et al[40] found up to 78% success if patients are correctly selected based on their anatomy and level of obstruction. Classifying the area of obstruction on imaging or nasopharyngoscopy is imperative for optimal outcomes associated with UPPP, UPPP-LA, or any other palatal procedure.

FUJITA CLASSIFICATION SYSTEM

The classification system of Fujita is commonly used to illustrate the extent of obstruction at the nasopharynx, oropharynx, and/or hypopharynx on diagnostic nasopharyngoscopy. This is accomplished using a Mueller maneuver, visualizing closure at the level of the soft palate and hypopharynx during inspiration with a closed nose and mouth.[41] This approximates closure during obstructive events during sleep (Fig. 113-9). Obstructions that are predominately at the level of the nasopharynx and oropharynx are classified as a Fujita I obstruction. Fujita II obstructions, those that occur further down the airway and are a combination of obstructions at the oropharynx and hypopharynx, are further subdivided into IIa and IIb; the IIa is mainly at the level of the oropharnyx and IIb at the level of the hypopharynx. A Fujita III classification describes obstruction at the level of the hypopharynx. Patients that are being considered for a palatal procedure alone should be Fujita I or IIa, whereas Fujita IIb and III patients should be considered for surgery that targets this area, multiple phase I procedures, or phase II therapy.[42]

COMPLICATIONS

All of the palatal procedures have the same disadvantages and complications. Because of the muscular incisions, pain is universal and lasts from 8 to 10 days after surgery. Velopharyngeal insufficiency with nasal speech and nasal reflux is less common, occurring in 1% to 13% of patients, and is generally temporary.[43] However, when this occurs long-term it is a problematic and disappointing complication. Bleeding occurs more commonly with UPPP than with UPPP-LA, and can be quite profuse on occasion. The use of the laser makes bleeding much less common. Finally, globus, a sensation of something in the back of the throat, is relatively common and may last up to 1 year after surgery. Thus all patients should be warned of this preoperatively.[44]

ANTERIOR MANDIBULAR OSTEOTOMY

Because the tongue is held forward by its connection to the genial tubercle, it stands to reason that advancing this portion of the mandible should help to alleviate the obstruction of the airway by the tongue base at the level of the hypopharynx. There are several different surgical options for this purpose.

INFERIOR GENIAL OSTEOTOMY WITH HYOID MYOTOMY

A procedure originally described by Riley and Powell,[45] the inferior genial osteotomy with hyoid myotomy, consists of a high horizontal genioplasty, including the tubercle on the inner cortex of the mandible, done with a hyoid myotomy and suspension. The main concept of this procedure is forward advancement of the anteroinferior aspect of the mandible with its associated musculature while maintaining the general continuity of the mandible. This allows for repositioning the segment attached to the genioglossus more anteriorly, advancing the tongue base forward, and improving the hypopharyngeal airway. Hendler et al[46] showed patients with moderate OSA (AHI 21 to 40) did well with AMO, with 86% of patients achieving success. In patients with moderately severe OSA (AHI 41 to 60), the success rate decreased to 64%. In patients with severe OSA (AHI 61 or more), the procedure was successful only 15% of the time. It is also clear that the success was highest in those patients with a normal or near-normal BMI when compared with those patients with mild or morbid obesity. The success achieved in patients with a normal BMI was 60%. This decreased to 43% in those patients with obesity. The criteria for success were determined as follows: an RDI of less than 20 as well as a minimum 50% reduction in RDI from preoperative levels.[45]

Complications of this procedure, however, include paresthesia of the mental nerves and fracture of the mandible within the diminished midline alveolus.

Concurrent with this procedure, the infrahyoid musculature is often transected, allowing the hyoid bone to be elevated anteriorly and superiorly during the AMO. Many surgeons avoid the genial advancement with hyoid myotomy (GAHM) procedure because of the higher incidence of postoperative problems with deglutition and speech. With the advent of newer hyoid suspension techniques, the classic hyoid myotomy and suspension has become less common.

Riley et al[45] showed a 67% success rate in patients who underwent inferior mandibular osteotomy with hyoid myotomy. The 33% who were nonresponders were found to be more obese and have more mandibular deficiencies than the responders. Of course, this depends on where the primary obstruction is located.

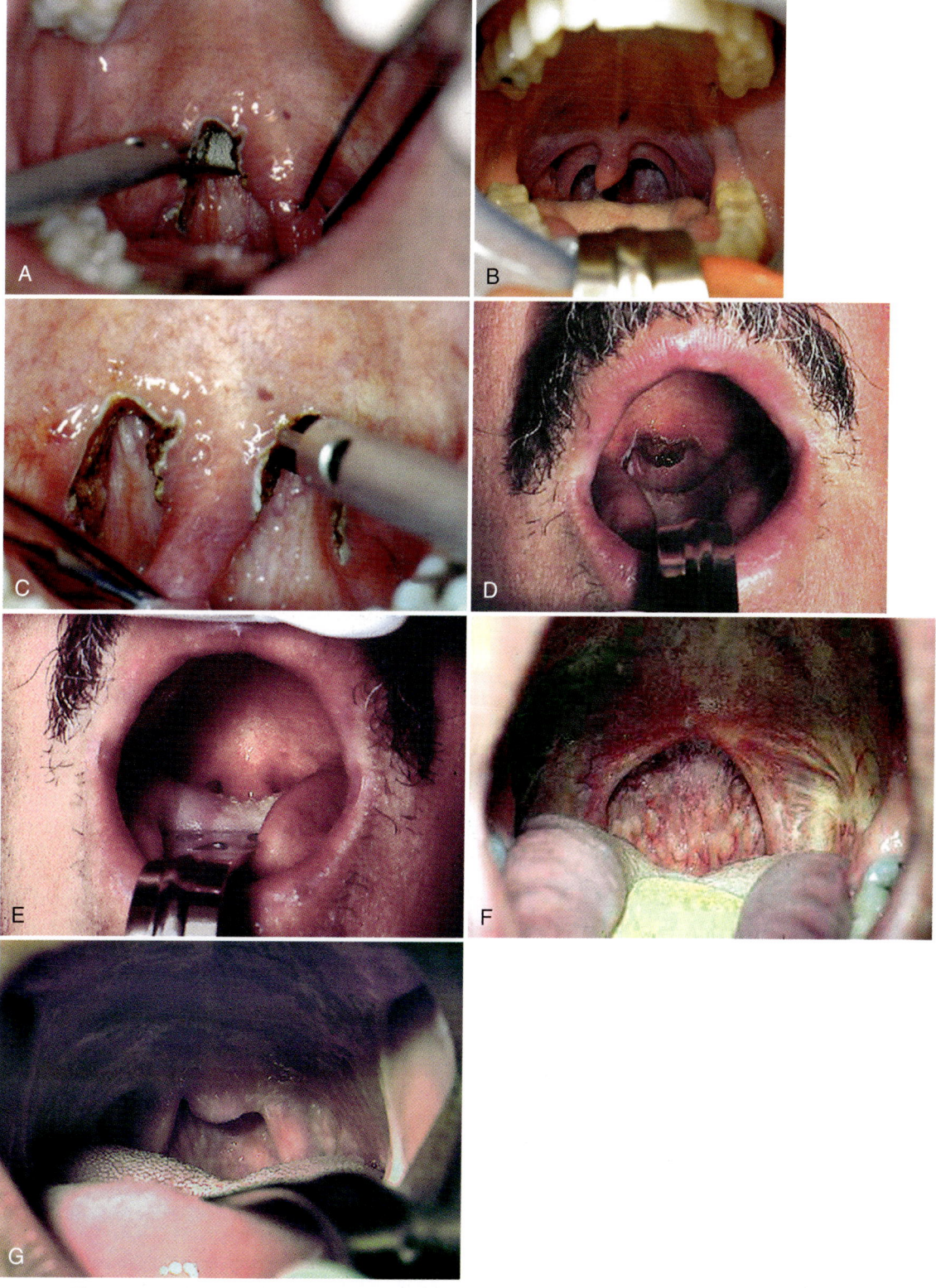

Fig. 113-8 ■ Uvulopalatopharyngoplasty–laser assisted (UPPP-LA). **A,** The procedure begins with a wide excision of the soft palate to the tonsillar pillars. The tissue is removed just short of the levator insertion. **B,** The anterior and posterior tonsillar pillars are minimally excised or ablated. **C,** The tonsillar pillars after ablation and removal of the soft palatal segment. **D,** The posterior pillar and posterior portion of the soft palate are advanced and sutured to the anterior pillars and soft palatal flap using a resorbable suture. **E,** Preoperative view of UPPP-LA. **F,** Immediate postoperative view. **G,** Long-term result.

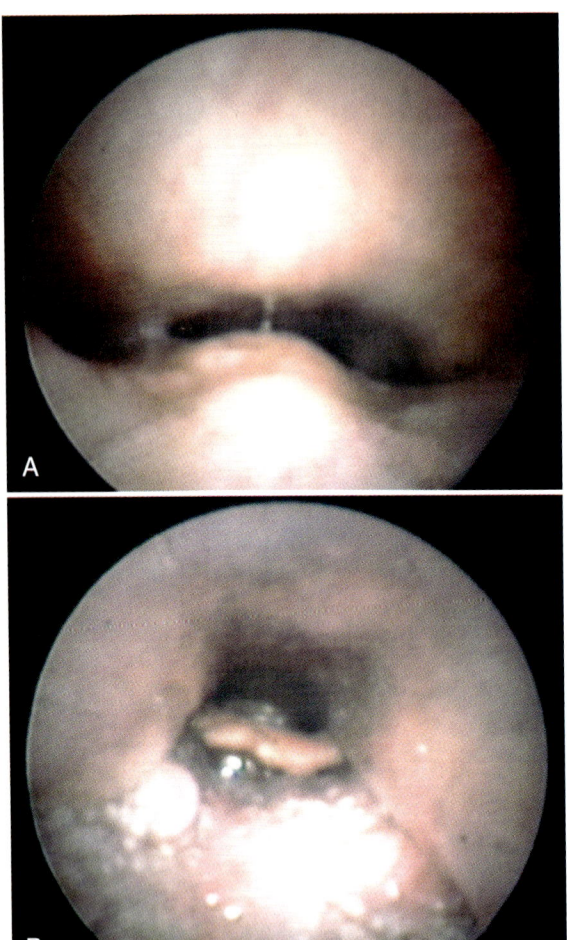

Fig. 113-9 ■ **A,** Mueller maneuver at level of soft palate. **B,** Mueller maneuver at level of the base of the tongue. The degree of closure is noted and applied to the Fujita classification system.

GENIAL TUBERCLE ADVANCEMENT

Another technique used for genioglossus muscle stabilization is the genial tubercle advancement (GTA). This technique entails a bicortical, rectangular osteotomy that includes the genial tubercles. A 2-mm bicortical bone screw is placed at the midpoint of the genial prominence on the facial surface of the mandible giving the surgeon a guide for a symmetric osteotomy. The rectangular osteotomy is outlined between the canines, 5 mm below the roots of the teeth and 7 mm above the inferior border to prevent root damage and mandible fracture, respectively (Fig. 113-10, *A*). The osteotomy is carried through the thickness of the mandible until the segment is totally free other than the attachment of the genioglossus on the lingual side. The screw also allows the surgeon to grasp and pull the block anteriorly. The lingual cortical plate will now be anterior to the buccal cortical plate (Fig. 113-10, *B*). For cosmetic reasons, the buccal cortical plate and medullary bone are osteotomized, leaving only the lingual cortical plate attached to the genioglossus muscle (Fig. 113-10, *C*). Alternatively, the buccal rectangular window can be removed first, then the medullary bone removed with a large round bur to expose the lingual cortex. The screw is then placed in the lingual cortex and the remainder of the procedure continues in the same fashion (Fig. 113-10, *D* to *F*). This has the advantage of better visualization, easier access, and less likelihood of making the lingual window smaller than the buccal window, thereby increasing

the likelihood of missing the muscle and making stabilization more difficult. In either case, the segment is then stabilized with a small bone plate and secured with screws (Fig. 113-10, *G*). This technique can advance the genioglossus attachment the full thickness of the anterior mandible, approximately 10 mm. One potential complication of this is that the genioglossus is placed under significant tension and can avulse off the tubercle.[47]

TREPHINE OSTEOTOMY

Another variation to this procedure is the trephine osteotomy genial bone advancement trephine (GBAT system) (Stryker Leibinger Inc., Kalamazoo, Mich). With this technique, the operator places a circular guide on the buccal bone overlying the genial tubercle location, and a bicortical hole is drilled to depth and measured. The guide plate is then secured with bicortical screws (Fig. 113-11, *A*). A trephine is then used to make the osteotomy over the guide plate through the mandible (Fig. 113-11, *B*). Upon completion of the osteotomy, the guide plate and attached bony core are pulled anteriorly. The medullary bone is grasped with special bone-holding forceps, and the guide plate is removed from the block (Fig. 113-11, *C*). For cosmetic reasons, the buccal cortical plate and medullary bone are removed with an oscillating saw. A specially designed prefitted plate is then secured with two additional bicortical screws to hold the segment in the new advanced position (Fig. 113-11, *D*). The GBAT system performed with UPPP has been shown to significantly reduce RDI and AI while improving oxygen desaturation and enlarging the posterior airway space.[48] The advantage of this procedure over the standard window osteotomy is that it allows a more standardized osteotomy and has a simplified and predictable fixation technique.

REPOSE GENIOGLOSSUS ADVANCEMENT SYSTEM

Another novel procedure is the Repose genioglossus advancement system (Medtronic, Inc., Minneapolis, Minn). The objective of this procedure is to create a suspension or "hammock" suture in the tongue so that when the patient is supine and sleeping, the tongue cannot move posteriorly, thus preventing collapse of the airway space. Studies have shown the effects of genioglossus advancement on its own have been very effective in select patients with mild to moderate OSAS who have isolated tongue base issues,[49] and also with UPPP when other areas are involved.[50,51]

Repose genioglossus advancement is accomplished via an intraoral or extraoral approach. The extraoral approach entails making a 2-cm submental incision approximately 2 cm from the inferior border of the mandible. The lingual, inferior mandible, just below the genial tubercle, is exposed by blunt dissection. The intraoral approach is accomplished by making a lingual gingival sulcular incision with a full-thickness mucoperiosteal flap to expose the genial tubercle. A specially designed right-angle screw drill is then placed in the incision and a single, titanium bone screw is placed in the inferior lingual mandible at the level of or slightly below the genial tubercle (Fig. 113-12).

The screw has a double-ended polypropylene suture built into the head, and the thread is tailed out of the wound. A temporary loop suture is then attached to a proprietary "suture passer," which resembles a preloaded mandibular awl. This is used to enter the incision and is then directed to one side of the base of the tongue, 1 cm off midline at the level of the circumvallate papillae. The temporary suture is then freed from the suture passer at the base of the tongue. One of the tails attached to the screw is loaded into the suture passer and is placed into the incision with the tip directed to the contralateral base of the tongue, 1 cm off midline, at or below the level of the circumvallate papillae. This end is then freed from the suture

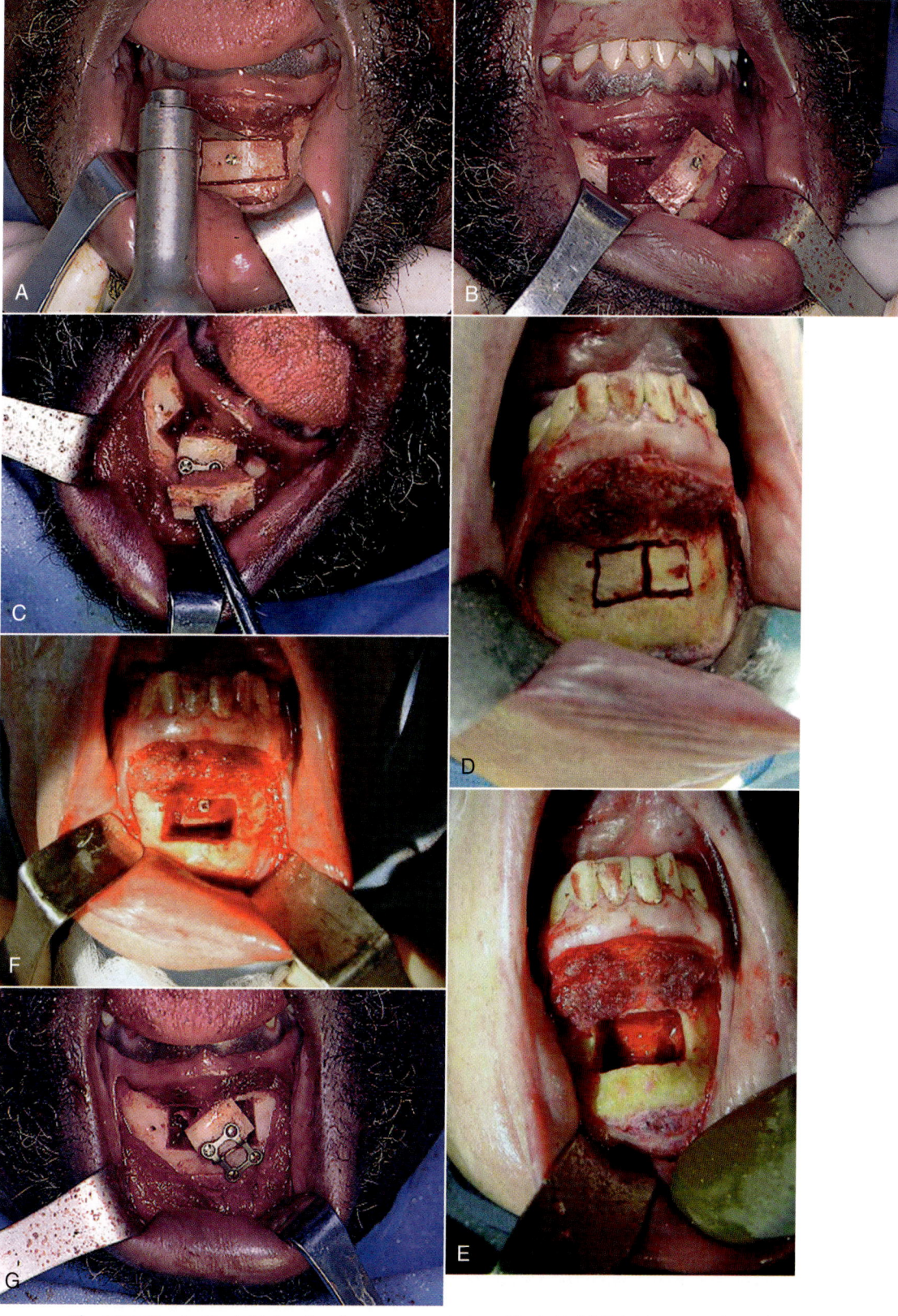

Fig. 113-10 ■ **A,** Genial tubercle advancement window. The initial full-thickness cut is made with an oscillating saw to avoid the roots and approximately 7 mm from the inferior border. **B,** The segment can be advanced and fixed with either a screw or a bone plate. Note the muscle attached to the back of the segment. Overrotation of the segment should be avoided to prevent dislocation of the muscle. **C,** For cosmetic reasons (unless the patient is retrogenic), the anterior cortex and medullary bone can be removed and the plate affixed to the lingual plate. **D,** Instead of doing a full-thickness osteotomy, the buccal plate and medullary bone can be removed initially to expose the lingual plate. This makes it easier to obtain a uniform size of the osteotomy from buccal to lingual. **E,** The lingual plate is then osteotomized and advanced. **F,** The lingual segment is then pulled anteriorly using a screw placed in the segment. **G,** The segment is then fixed with a bone plate.

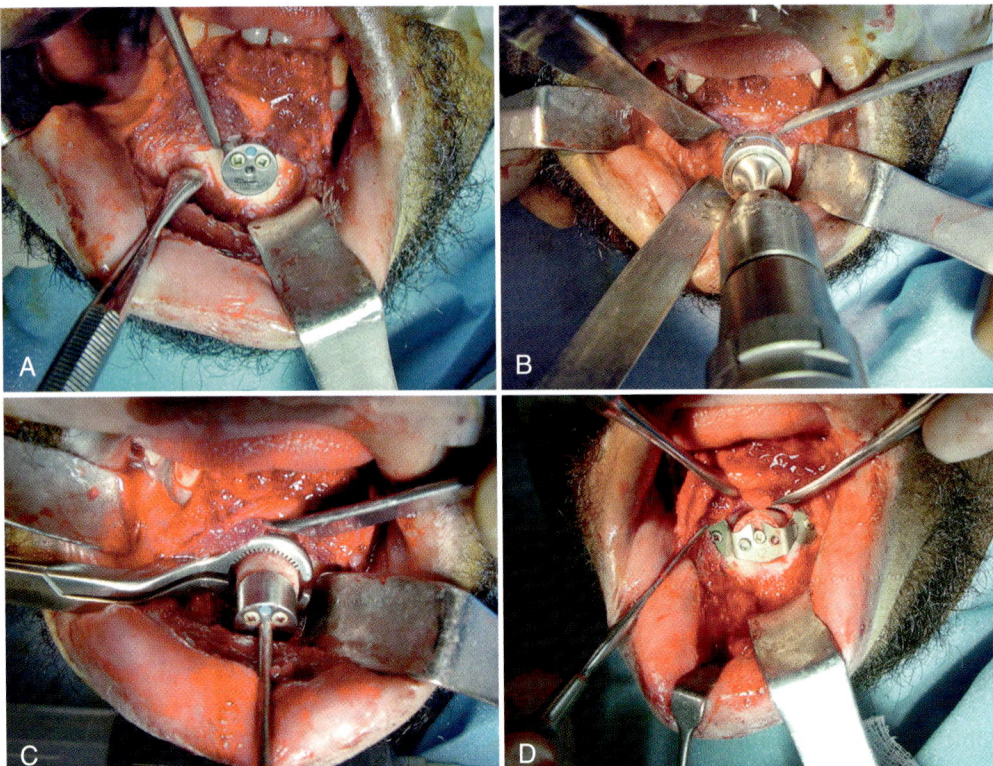

Fig. 113-11 ■ A, The GBAT system. A metal disc is first attached to the genial area overlying the muscle. **B,** A trephine is then used over the disc and used to cut through the entire thickness of the mandible. **C,** Once osteotomized with the trephine, the segment is advanced and held by a specially designed forceps. Once grasped, the anterior portion of the segment can be osteotomized and removed for cosmetic reasons. **D,** The segment is then held in place using a specially designed bone plate. The degree of advancement can be controlled using different sizes of prebent plates.

passer and attached to a large, free curved needle. The needle is directed toward the temporary loop suture, where the first exit hole was created at the base of tongue, taking a 2-mm bite of the base of tongue tissue. The suture is removed from the needle, placed in the temporary loop suture, and pulled back through the tongue toward the incision. This maneuver internalizes and triangulates the suture into the tongue. The surgeon's hand is then used intraorally to palpate the base of tongue while the other hand pulls on the sutures, thus tightening and causing the base of tongue to have a slight midline dimple (see Fig. 113-12, *C*). Once adequate suspension is obtained, the sutures are tied and the wound is closed in a layered fashion. Over time the suture will obtain additional stability through fibrosis around the foreign body suture.

The procedure is generally performed in the operating room and takes about 60 minutes. Potential complications include lingual nerve and hypoglossal nerve damage, fracture of the inferior border of the mandible, breakage of the suture prematurely, and infection.

COMPLICATIONS

The problem with all of the genioglossus advancement procedures is the likelihood that relapse of the muscle position will occur over time. Standard muscle advancement procedures (i.e., genial windows) definitely show some relapse that result from the inevitable muscular tension.[47,52] Some procedures, such as the Repose system rely on scarring over time to hold the muscle forward. Although initial studies seem to indicate that long-term results are possible with genioglossus muscle advancement,[52] more definitive

and longer term studies will be required to more accurately determine the effectiveness of these procedures.

HYOID SUSPENSION

Hyoid myotomy with suspension is a procedure that is used to advance the hyoglossus muscle connection to the hyoid bone, thereby increasing the posterior airway space in the hypopharynx. Several variations of this procedure have been described, varying primarily on whether the hyoid is suspended to the inferior border of the mandible or to the superior aspect of the larynx. As with many OSA-related surgeries, the approach taken seems to correlate with the anatomic comfort zone of the surgeon (i.e., OMFSs generally suspend to the mandible, whereas ENT surgeons use the larynx).[53-55]

Although the concept seems good, it is clear in the literature that hyoid myotomy and suspension, as with most phase I treatment, is not very successful when done alone. In a recent study, only 17% of patients who underwent a hyoid suspension alone to correct their OSA were found to have a decrease in their AHI to a clinically significant level.[56]

Hence, hyoid myotomy is typically combined with genioglossus advancement and sometimes with UPPP or UPPP-LA for multilevel obstructions. Studies have shown hyoid suspension combined with the aforementioned techniques has a 40% to 80% success rate in patients with mild to moderate sleep apnea, but surgical success declined to 42% when patients had severe OSAS.[44,57]

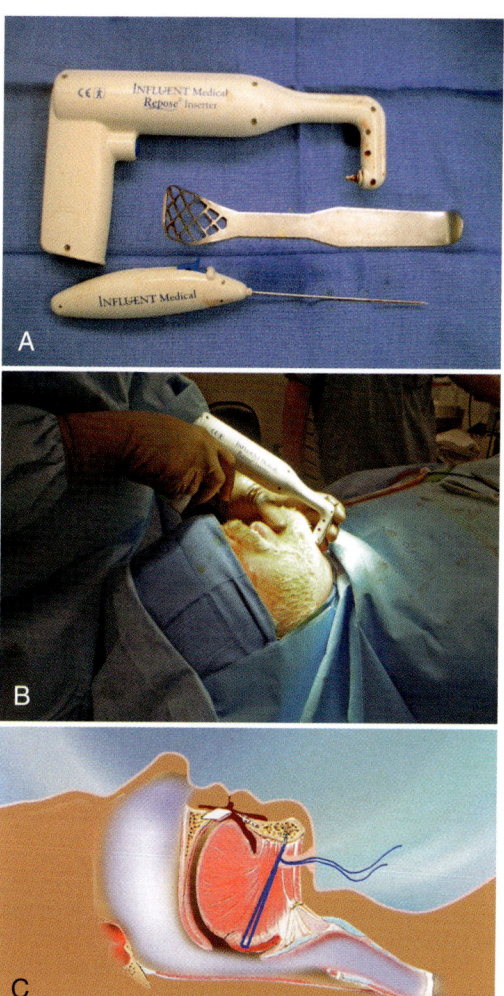

Fig. 113-12 ■ **A,** The Repose System. **B,** A right-angle screwdriver is used to place the screw and its attached suture into the lingual side of the mandible from an extraoral approach. This can also be done intraorally. **C,** The suture is placed through one side of the base of the tongue and then retracted back to the screw from the other side using a custom trocar. The suture is then tied to the soft tissue overlying the screw to advance and tighten the base of the tongue. (**C** courtesy Medtronic, Inc, Minneapolis, Minn.)

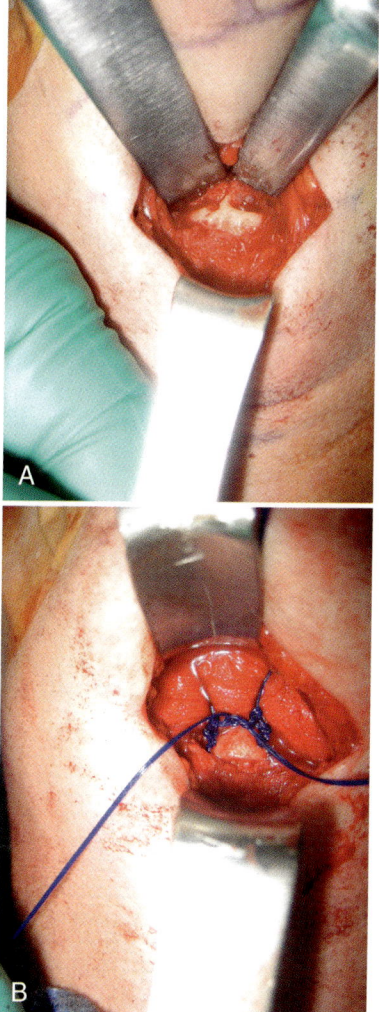

Fig. 113-13 ■ **A,** The hyoid bone is exposed for hyoid suspension using the Repose System. **B,** The sutures coming from the screws placed at the inferior border bilaterally using the right-angle driver are then tied around the hyoid and to each other.

The procedure entails making a horizontal midline incision in the neck, and dissection is carried down to expose the superior aspect of the hyoid bone (Fig. 113-13, *A*). An Alice clamp is used to grasp the hyoid bone to assess appropriate mobility of the hyoid. Additional dissection and sometimes myotomy of the infrahyoid musculature may be needed to increase mobility of the hyoid. At this point the larynx can be exposed inferiorly, or the inferior border of the mandible can be dissected out superiorly to view the intended suspension site. A nonresorbable suture or other sling material (e.g., fascia lata) is then wrapped around the lateral side of the hyoid and sutured to the larynx or affixed to the mandible with a screw (Fig. 113-13, *B*).

REPOSE HYOID SUSPENSION

A relatively new variation of this procedure is the repose system for hyoid suspension (Medtronic, Inc.). This procedure is usually combined with a repose genioglossus advancement as described earlier in this chapter. The procedure involves the same dissection as for traditional hyoid suspension. Attention is then directed to exposing the lingual aspect of the mandible and using the right angle Repose bone screw inserter to place two screws at the inferior-lingual border of the mandible just under the canines. These screws come preloaded with sutures fused to the back end. The inserter is removed from the site with the sutures tailing from the back end of the screw (Fig. 113-14, *A*). An Alice clamp is then used to grasp the hyoid bone with an upward lift toward the chin to hyperextend the inferior musculature, thereby facilitating suture passage around the hyoid. Using a French eye needle, the nonresorbable Repose suture is then passed from the inferior musculature under the hyoid to exit on the superior aspect, approximately 1 cm off midline. This same pass is done a second time slightly medial to the first. The suture is then tied to the contralateral screw tails, which have been passed in the opposite direction (superior to inferior) while the hyoid is being held in the new advanced position. It is important that this be done with

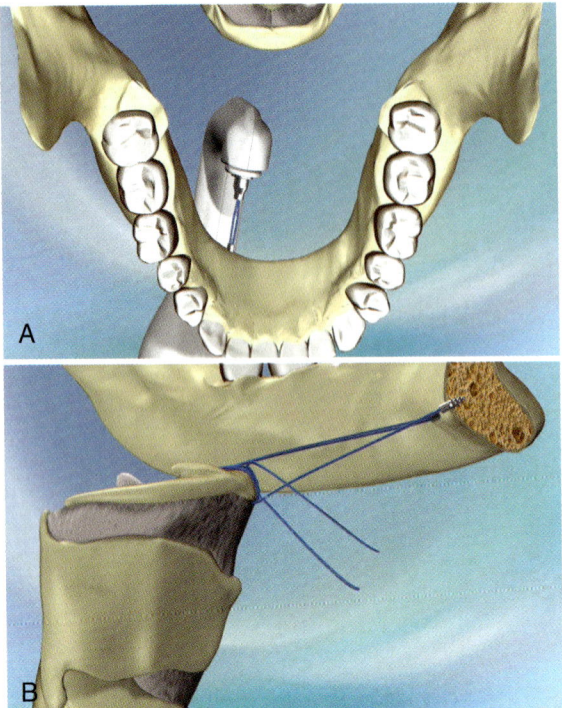

Fig. 113-14 ■ **A** and **B,** During placement, the hyoid is advanced anteriorly and superiorly. (Courtesy Medtronic, Inc., Minneapolis, Minn.)

a surgeon's knot with the help of an assistant holding the knot until it is double thrown (to prevent loosening). This maneuver elevates the hyoid and subsequently pulls the infrahyoid musculature very tightly (Fig. 113-14, *B*). The free ends are cut and the wound is then irrigated and closed in a layered fashion.

The advantage of the Repose system lies in its relative ease of use. The placement of the screws is made easier by the use of the right-angle inserter, and it is not necessary to tie the suture to a free screw placed in the mandible, which has a high likelihood of breaking with time. However, the end result is identical to the traditional method of suspension.[58]

SEPTOPLASTY

Because of the increased airspeed and diminished airflow resulting from tissue collapse, a deviated septum can be another point of obstruction in OSA.[59] Septoplasty may be performed to correct this obstruction and has been shown to improve the AHI for mild OSA.[60] Because it is a relatively easy procedure and commonly performed by otolaryngologists, it was for many years frequently chosen to manage OSA. Although it can be done alone in some cases, it is usually combined with another procedure, usually UPPP. As we now better understand the anatomic and multifactorial nature of OSA, this procedure is somewhat less frequently performed and is primarily reserved for cases where obvious and significant deviation contributes to OSA.

Septoplasty identifies the specific area of septal deviation and targets that area for resection. Hydrodissection is carried out with local anesthesia, lifting the perichondrium and mucosa from the

cartilage. The location of the deformity dictates the type and placement of the incision in the mucosa. A Joseph or Freer elevator is used to reflect the perichondrium and mucosa from the cartilage. Once the septum is skeletonized, the cartilage can be resected, or the deformity can be removed with a bur, forceps, curette, or file. It is imperative that a 1-cm rim of cartilage be left on the septum at all times to prevent nasal collapse. In addition, care should be taken in insuring that the mucosa on both sides remains intact to prevent a septal perforation and a subsequent whistle deformity.

In addition to septoplasty, turbinate reduction and radiofrequency ablation of the turbinates has also shown to be successful in decreasing apneas and hypopneas. Because these procedures are easily performed and carry low morbidity, they should be performed with septoplasty whenever indicated.

A retrospective study by Lorente[60] included 34 patients with nasal respiratory insufficiency and chronic snoring. The mean AHI was reduced from 46 to 32 and their minimal mean oxygen saturation was increased from 76 to 83 with septoplasty and turbinate reduction. Conversely, a randomized trial of nasal surgery by Koutsourelakis et al[61] failed to demonstrate significant improvement in 49 patients with fixed nasal obstructions.

It would seem evident that, like most other phase I targeted treatments, isolation of likely sources of obstruction would increase the likelihood of success.

CONCLUSION

Phase I treatment for OSA is the first step in the progressive treatment plan for management of this disease. Many such treatments are available and all are useful to some degree. However, because they are all targeted to one anatomic area, and because we now know that most OSA patients have multilevel obstructions, it would seem evident that no single procedure is likely to be curative except in mild cases or in situations where one anatomic area is responsible. A critical look at the literature bears this out. The only exception to this is CPAP, which does treat the entire airway and can be curative. CPAP is, therefore, justifiably used as the initial treatment for most if not all OSA patients.

When combined together, however, it does seem that many mild to moderate cases of OSA can be managed or cured with phase I treatments. The object is to attempt to delineate the principle source or sources of obstruction and then choose the procedure or procedures that will correct those anatomic areas.

Unfortunately, it also appears that phase I treatments are not likely going to be long-term cures for severe OSA. It is for this reason that phase II treatment such as MMA may ensue, or be used primarily if the clinician feels that phase I treatments are likely to fail and wishes to avoid the time delay and potential complications that pursuing phase I would require.

PEARLS AND PITFALLS

- Phase I therapy is generally directed at a specific area identified on clinical exam.
- Phase I therapy is likely only effective in mild to moderate OSAS.
- Severe OSAS generally is not amenable to phase I therapy.
- Multiple phase I therapies may be combined to address certain areas of obstruction.

REFERENCES

1. Punjabi NM, Caffo BS, Goodwin JL, Gottlieb DJ, Newman AB, et al: Sleep-disordered breathing and mortality: A prospective cohort study, *PLoS Med* 6(8):e1000132, 2009.

2. Madani M, Farideh M: The pandemic of obesity and its relationship to sleep apnea, *Atlas Oral Maxillofac Surg Clin North Am* 81-88, 2007.

3. Davies RJO, Stradling JR: The relationship between neck circumference, radiographic pharyngeal anatomy, and the obstructive sleep apnea syndrome, *Eur Respir J* 3:509-514, 1990.

4. Stradling JR, Crosby JH: Predictors and prevalence of obstructive sleep apnea and snoring in 1001 middle aged men, *Thorax* 46:85-90, 1991.

5. Katz I, Stradling J, Slutsky AS, Zamel N, Hoffstein V: Do patients with obstructive sleep apnea have thick necks? *Am Rev Respir Dis* 141:1228-1231, 1990.

6. Hoffstein V, Mateika S: Differences in abdominal and neck circumferences in patients with and without obstructive sleep apnea, *Eur Respir J* 5:377-381, 1992.

7. Kajaste S: Effects of cognitive–behavioral weight loss program on overweight obstructive sleep apnea, *J Sleep Res* 3:245-249, 1994.

8. Kansanen M: The effects of a very low-calorie diet–induced weight loss on the severity of obstructive sleep apnea and autonomic nervous function in obese patients with obstructive sleep apnea syndrome, *Clin Physiol* 4:377-385, 1998.

9. Tuomilehto HP: Lifestyle intervention with weight reduction: first-line treatment in mild obstructive sleep apnea, *Am J Respir Crit Care Med* 179(4):320-327, 2009.

10. Sanders MH, Redline S: Obstructive sleep apnea/hypopnea syndrome, *Curr Treat Options Neurol* 1(4):279-290, 1999.

11. Giles TL: Continuous positive airways pressure for obstructive sleep apnea in adults. *Cochrane Database Syst Rev Oct* 18(4): CD005308, 2006.

12. Waldhorn RE, TW Herrick, MC Nguyen, AE O'Donnell, J Sordero, Potolicchio SJ: Long term compliance with nasal continuous positive airway pressure therapy of obstructive sleep apnea, *Chest* 97:33-38, 1990.

13. Weaver TE, Maislin G, Dinges DF, Younger J, Cantor C, McCloskey S: Self-efficacy in sleep apnea: instrument development and patient perceptions of obstructive sleep apnea risk, treatment benefit, and volition to use continuous positive airway pressure, *Sleep* 26(6):727-732, 2003.

14. Wells RD, Freedland KE, Carney RM, Duntley SP, Stepanski EJ: Adherence, reports of benefits, and depression among patients treated with continuous positive airway pressure, *Psychosomatic Medicine* 69(5):449-454, 2007.

15. Skinner MA: Efficacy of the "tennis ball technique" versus nCPAP in the management of position-dependent obstructive sleep apnea syndrome, *Respirology* 13:708-715, 2008.

16. Cartwright RD: Effect of sleep position on sleep apnea severity, *Sleep* 7:110-114, 1984.

17. Oksenberg A, Silverberg DS, Arons E, Radwan H: Positional vs nonpositional obstructive sleep apnea patients: anthropomorphic, nocturnal polysomnographic, and multiple sleep latency test data, *Chest* 112: 629-639, 1997.

18. Richard W, Kox D, den Herder C, Laman M, van Tinteren H: The role of sleep position in obstructive sleep apnea syndrome, *Eur Arch Otorhinolaryngol* 263:946-950, 2006.

19. Epstein LJ, Kristo D, Strollo PJ Jr, Friedman N, Malhotra A, Patil SP, Ramar K, Rogers R, Schwab RJ, Weaver EM, Weinstein MD: Clinical guideline for the evaluation, management and long-term care of obstructive sleep apnea in adults. Adult Obstructive Sleep Apnea Task Force of the American Academy of Sleep Medicine, *J Clin Sleep Med* 5(3):263-276, 2009.

20. Barnes M: Efficacy of positive airway pressure and oral appliance in mild to moderate obstructive sleep apnea, *Am J Respir Crit Care Med* 170(6):656-664, 2004.

21. Bloch KE: Alternatives to CPAP in the treatment of the obstructive sleep apnea syndrome, *Swiss Med Wkly* 136(17-18):261-267, 2006.

22. Lim J: Oral appliances for obstructive sleep apnea, *Cochrane Database Syst Rev* 25(1): CD004435, 2006.

23. Thickett EM: A prospective evaluation assessing the effectiveness of the "Dynamax" mandibular appliance in the management of obstructive sleep apnea, *Surgeon* 7(1):14-17, 2009.

24. Kushida C, Morgenthaler T, Littner M: Practice parameters for the treatment of snoring and obstructive sleep apnea with oral appliances: an update for 2005, *Sleep* 29(2): 240-243, 2006.

25. Winfried RJ, Heise M, Hinz R, Ruchle K: An individually adjustable oral appliance vs. continuous positive airway pressure in mild-to-moderate obstructive sleep apnea syndrome, *Sleep* 29(2):240-243, 2006.

26. Ho WK, Wei WI, Chung KF: Managing disturbing snoring with palatal implant, *Arch Otolaryngol Head Neck Surg* 130:753-758, 2004.

27. Bäck LJ: Radiofrequency surgery of the soft palate in the treatment of mild obstructive sleep apnea is not effective as a single-stage procedure: A randomized single-blinded placebo-controlled trial, *Laryngoscope* 119 (8):1621-1627, 2009.

28. Ceylan K: First-choice treatment in mild to moderate obstructive sleep apnea single-stage, multilevel, temperature-controlled radiofrequency tissue volume reduction or nasal continuous positive airway pressure, *Arch Otolaryngol Head Neck Surg* 135(9): 915-919, 2009.

29. Strauss R: Flexible Endoscopic nasopharyngoscopy, *Atlas Oral Maxillofac Surg Clin North Am* 15:111-128, 2007.

30. Kezirian EJ: Incidence of serious complications after uvulopalatopharyngoplasty, *Laryngoscope* 114(3):450-453, 2004.

31. Tiner BD, Waite P: *Surgical and Nonsurgical Management of Obstructive Sleep Apnea.* Peterson's Principles of Oral and Maxillofacial Surgery, ed 2, Ch. 63, pp.1305-1306.

32. Kamami YV: Outpatient treatment of snoring with CO_2 laser: laser-assisted UPPP, *J Otolaryngol* 23(6):391-394, 1994.

33. Ryan CF, Love LL: Unpredictable results of laser assisted uvulopalatoplasty in the treatment of obstructive sleep apnea, *Thorax* 55(5):399-404, 2000.

34. Lyngkaran T, Kanaglaingam J, Rajeswaran R, Georgalas C, Kotecha B: Long-term outcomes of laser-assisted uvulopalatoplasty in 168 patients with snoring, *J Laryngol Otol* 120(11):932-938, 2006.

35. Madani M: Laser assisted uvulopalatopharyngoplasty (LA-UPPP) for the treatment of snoring and mild to moderate obstructive sleep apnea, *Atlas Oral Maxillofac Surg Clin North Am* 15(2):129-137, 2007.

36. Finkestein Y, Shapiro-Feinberg M, Stein G: Uvulopalatopharyngoplasty vs. laser-assisted uvulopalatoplasty: anatomical considerations, *Arch Otolaryngol Head Neck Surg* 123:265-276, 1997.

37. Strocker AM, Cohen AN, Wang MB: The safety of outpatient UPPP for obstructive sleep apnea: a retrospective review of 40 cases, *Ear Nose Throat J* 87(8):466-468, 2008.

38. Walenczak I, Sie kiewicz A, Rogowski M, Swietek M: The evaluation of the effectiveness of uvulopalatopharyngoplasy in the treatment of selected patients with mild to moderate obstructive sleep apnea—one year of postoperative follow up, *Pol Merkur Lekarski* 22(132):529-531, 2007.

39. Madani M: Complications of laser-assisted uvulopalatopharyngoplasty (LA-UPPP) and radiofrequency treatments of snoring and chronic nasal congestion: a 10-year review of 5,600 patients, *J Oral Maxillofac Surg* 62(11):1351-1362, 2004.

40. Li HY, Wang PC, Lee LA, Chen NH, Fang TJ: Prediction of uvulopalatopharyngoplasty outcome: anatomy-based staging system versus severity-based staging system, *Sleep* 29(12):1537-1541, 2006.

41. Fujita S: Obstructive sleep apnea syndrome: pathophysiology, upper airway evaluation and surgical treatment, *Ear Nose Throat J* 72(1):67-72, 75-6, 1993.

42. Sher AE, Thorpy MJ, Shprintzen RJ, Spielman AJ, Burack B, McGregor PA: Predictive value of Muller maneuver in selection of patients for uvulopalatopharyngoplasty, *Laryngoscope* 95(12):1483-1487, 1985.

43. Franklin KA: Effects and side-effects of surgery for snoring and obstructive sleep apnea—a systematic review, *Sleep* 32(1):27-36, 2009.

44. Riley RW, Powell NB, Guilleminault C: Obstructive sleep apnea syndrome: a review of 306 consecutively treated surgical patients,

Otolaryngol Head Neck Surg 108:117-125, 1993.

45. Riley RW, Powell NB, Guilleminault C: Inferior mandibular osteotomy and hyoid myotomy suspension for obstructive sleep apnea: a review of 55 patients, *J Oral Maxillofac Surg* 47(2):159-164, 1989.

46. Hendler BH, Costello BJ, Silverstein KE: An analysis of uvulopalatopharyngoplasty, genioglossus advancement and maxillomandibular advancement for the treatment of obstructive sleep apnea, *J Oral Maxillofac Surg* 59:892-897, 2001.

47. McAndrew BP, Strauss RA: Delayed muscle detachment after genial tubercle advancement in a patient with obstructive sleep apnea, *J Oral Maxillofac Surg* 58(9):1040-1043, 2000.

48. Miller FR, Watson D, Boseley M: The role of the Genial Bone Advancement Trephine system in conjunction with uvulopalatopharyngoplasty in the multilevel management of obstructive sleep apnea, *Otolaryngol Head Neck Surg* 130(1):73-79, 2004.

49. Hamans F: Adjustable tongue advancement for obstructive sleep apnea: A pilot study, *Ann Otol Rhinol Laryngol* 117(11):815-823, 2008.

50. Pang KP, Terris DJ: Operative Techniques in Otolaryngology, *Elsevier* 17:252-256, 2006.

51. Thomas AJ: Preliminary findings from a prospective, randomized trial of two tongue-base surgeries for sleep-disordered breathing, *Otolaryngol Head Neck Surg* 129:529-546 (Nov), 2003.

52. Neruntarat C: Genioglossus advancement and hyoid myotomy: short-term and long-term results, *J Laryngol Otol* 117(6):482-486, 2003.

53. Dattilo DJ: Modification of the anterior mandibular osteotomy for genioglossus advancement with hyoid suspension for obstructive sleep apnea, *J Oral Maxillofac Surg* 65(9):1876-1879, 2007.

54. Neruntarat C: Hyoid myotomy with suspension under local anesthesia for obstructive sleep apnea syndrome, *Eur Arch Otorhinolaryngol* 260(5):286-290, 2003.

55. Hörmann K: Modified hyoid suspension for therapy of sleep related breathing disorders. operative technique and complications, *Laryngorhinootologie* 80(9):517-521, 2001.

56. Bowden MT, Kezirian EJ, Utley D, Goode RL: Outcomes of hyoid suspension for the treatment of obstructive sleep apnea, *Arch Otolaryngol Head Neck Surg* 131(5):440-445, 2005.

57. Baisch A, Maurer JT, Hörmann K: The effect of hyoid suspension in a multilevel surgery concept for obstructive sleep apnea, *Otolaryngol Head Neck Surg* 134(5):856-861, 2006.

58. Miller FR: Role of the tongue base suspension suture with The Repose System bone screw in the multilevel surgical management of obstructive sleep apnea, *Otolaryngol Head Neck Surg* 126(4):392-398, 2002.

59. Nowak C, Bourgin P, Portier F, Genty E, Escourrou P, Bobin S: Nasal obstruction and compliance to nasal positive airway pressure, *Ann Otolaryngol Chir Cervicofac* 120(3):161-166, 2003.

60. Lorente J: Effects of functional septoplasty in obstructive sleep apnea syndrome, *Med Clin (Barc)* 125(8):290-292, 2005.

61. Koutsourelakis I, Georgeopoulos G, Perraki E, Vagiakis E: Randomized trial of nasal surgery for fixed nasal obstruction in obstructive sleep apnea, *Eur Respir J* 31(1):110-117, 2008.

Chapter **114**

Obstructive Sleep Apnea—Surgical Treatment: Part II, Maxillomandibular Advancement for Adults

Jeffrey R. Prinsell

Surgery for obstructive sleep apnea (OSA) is indicated when applicable conservative therapies are unsuccessful or intolerable and for patients with an underlying specific surgically correctable abnormality that is causing the OSA.[1] It can provide definitive treatment and, thus, eliminate issues of patient compliance with other therapies, but only if performed competently, both in terms of technical skill and on the correctly identified area(s) of upper airway (UA) obstruction.

Maxillomandibular advancement (MMA) with adjunctive extrapharyngeal procedures is the most effective acceptable (excludes tracheostomy) surgical treatment of OSA, with a therapeutic efficacy equal to nasal continuous positive airway pressure (nCPAP). Like nCPAP that pneumatically splints open the UA, MMA "pulls forward" the anterior pharyngeal tissues (e.g., soft palate and tongue) attached to the maxilla, mandible, and hyoid to structurally enlarge the entire velo-orohypopharyngeal airway; and enhance the neuromuscular tone of the pharyngeal dilator musculature (e.g., tensor veli palatini and genioglossus), via an extrapharyngeal operation with minimal risks of postoperative edema-induced UA embarrassment or pharyngeal dysfunction.[2]

ETIOPATHOGENESIS

OSA is part of a continuum of sleep-related breathing disorders (SBD) that also includes snoring and upper airway resistance syndrome, which results from repetitive collapse or obstruction of the UA during sleep that is caused by a complex array of physiologic and anatomic abnormalities. Snoring is the "warning bell" of partial or impending airway collapse, whereas OSA occurs with a complete airway obstruction lasting longer than 10 seconds. Resultant reduced oxyhemoglobin levels to the brain, heart, and other vital organs can lead to a myriad of signs and symptoms, including daytime hypersomnolence, memory loss, morning headaches, irritability, depression, decreased libido, and impaired concentration. Left untreated,

OSA can cause hypertension, stroke, cardiovascular dysrhythmias, myocardial infarction, and sudden death while asleep.

OSA is a very common but potentially life-threatening medical disorder. An estimated prevalence of SBD is 24% and 9% of adult males and females, respectively,[3] and an estimated 50 to 70 million Americans suffer from chronic sleep disorders. Daytime sleepiness alone costs $150 billion annually in lost productivity and mishaps, and another $48 billion in medical costs related to motor vehicle accidents that involve drowsy drivers; 20% of all serious car crashes are associated with daytime hypersomnolence, independent of alcohol.[4] Factors that can precipitate or exacerbate OSA include advancing age, weight gain, sedative-hypnotic medications and alcoholic beverages within 2 hours of sleep, and supine sleep.

PATHOLOGIC ANATOMY

Disproportionate UA anatomy in OSA may include specific structures or multiple sites or areas that can be diffusely complex, which varies between different patients. OSA surgical procedures can be classified anatomically as intrapharyngeal or extrapharyngeal. Intrapharyngeal procedures are performed on soft tissues that compose or lie within the velo-orohypopharyngeal airway wall or lumen, whereas extrapharyngeal surgery involves skeletal structures that lie outside the UA. Common intrapharyngeal sites include an elongated or retropositioned soft palate in the velopharynx, and hypertrophied tonsils and macroglossia or a retropositioned tongue base in the orohypopharynx. Hypoplastic or retropositioned extrapharyngeal lower facial skeletal structures, including the maxilla, mandible, and hyoid, may also be causative of OSA because they support or stabilize these velo-orohypopharyngeal soft tissues. In contrast to extrapharyngeal surgery, intrapharyngeal procedures can produce life-threatening UA edema in the immediate postoperative period[5] and are often subtherapeutic because they address isolated sites or limited areas of an often diffusely complex, narrowed velo-orohypopharyngeal airway.[6]

DIAGNOSTIC STUDIES

POLYSOMNOGRAPHY

OSA, as well as other SBD, is diagnosed by overnight polysomnography (PSG), which is a sleep study usually performed in a sleep laboratory. Multiple physiologic parameters are recorded to establish the diagnosis and quantitate severity. An apnea-hypopnea index (AHI) greater than 10 (events per hour of sleep), an apnea index (AI) greater than 5, and a lowest arterial oxyhemoglobin saturation (LSAT) less than 90% are pathologic. PSG is also performed to assess the therapeutic efficacy of OSA treatments, which include nCPAP, oral appliances, weight loss, positional therapy, and surgery.

CEPHALOMETRIC ANALYSIS

Clinical examination alone is inadequate to evaluate the UA. In comparison with other reputable diagnostic modalities (e.g., nasopharyngolaryngoscopy, intraluminal pressure transducers, somnofluoroscopy, computed tomography scans, and magnetic resonance imaging), lateral cephalometry (though limited to a static, lateral, two-dimensional view of the head and neck in awake erect patients), is comfortably noninvasive, safe with minimal radiation exposure, easy to perform in an outpatient setting, and inexpensive. It produces results that are objective, standardized, and reproducible, and therefore has been utilized extensively in the OSA literature.

If cephalometry (Fig. 114-1) is to be employed for diagnostic imaging of the UA in OSA patients, two modifications are

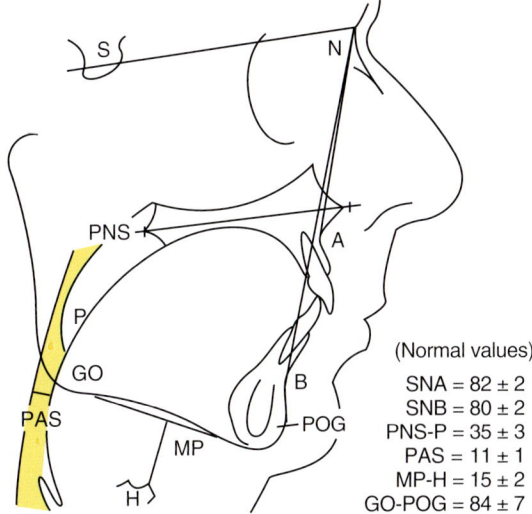

(Normal values)

SNA = 82 ± 2
SNB = 80 ± 2
PNS-P = 35 ± 3
PAS = 11 ± 1
MP-H = 15 ± 2
GO-POG = 84 ± 7

Fig. 114-1 ■ Lateral cephalometric analysis. (Adapted from Prinsell JR: Maxillomandibular advancement surgery in a site-specific treatment approach for obstructive sleep apnea in 50 consecutive patients, *Chest* 1999;116(6):1519-1529, Figure 1.)

recommended. First, because pharyngeal volume fluctuates with phases of respiration, cephalometry should be standardized by obtaining films at both end-tidal volume (ETV) and during a modified Mueller maneuver (forced inspiration against a closed mouth and nose, to simulate UA collapse associated with negative inspiratory forces generated during OSA events). Second, because the most critical site of orohypopharyngeal closure may vary, the cephalometric posterior airway space (PAS) should be measured at the narrowest level of hypopharyngeal collapse, rather than a level determined by skeletal landmarks.[2]

ORAL APPLIANCES AS PREDICTORS OF MANDIBULAR ADVANCEMENT

It is difficult to predict therapeutic efficacy of any surgical treatment for OSA. However, unlike the maxilla, the mandible can be reversibly protruded and the UA imaged (e.g., with lateral cephalometry) to view and measure velo-orohypopharyngeal enlargement. Custom-fabricated oral appliances worn during sleep can be tested with overnight PSG to document therapeutic efficacy of mandibular advancement for OSA.[7] If mandibular advancement appliances are subtherapeutic (e.g., because there are multiple sites of UA narrowing or severe orohypopharyngeal narrowing not fully relieved by sole mandibular advancement due to limitations of temporomandibular joint condylar translation), or therapeutic but intolerable with required nightly use, then MMA might be a reasonable alternative. Although oral appliances are generally therapeutic for mild to moderate OSA,[8,9] MMA may be necessary for more severe OSA and for those who cannot tolerate wearing devices while asleep.

TREATMENT GOALS

All OSA surgery should (strive to) accomplish the following general goals[10]: be safe, with minimal morbidity; cause minimal pain, disfigurement, and dysfunction; be therapeutic; be cost-effective; and be comprehensive, ideally addressing all sites of UA obstruction in one operation (Box 114-1).

Patients may be evaluated for OSA surgery when four prerequisites are satisfied.[10] First, they exhibit OSA diagnosed by PSG

From Prinsell JR: Maxillomandibular advancement (MMA) in a site-specific treatment approach for obstructive sleep apnea: A surgical algorithm. *Sleep Breath* 2000;4(4):147-154, Table 1.

From Prinsell JR. Maxillomandibular advancement (MMA) in a site-specific treatment approach for obstructive sleep apnea: A surgical algorithm. *Sleep Breath* 2000;4(4):147-154, Table 2.

(inclusion criteria of an AHI greater than 15 or an AI greater than 5 and an LSAT less than 90%) that is clinically significant (inclusion criterion of excessive daytime sleepiness). Second, all applicable conservative therapies (e.g., nCPAP, weight loss, positional therapy, reduction of late evening sedative-hypnotic medications or alcoholic beverages, oral appliances or other devices) have been unsuccessful or intolerable. Third, they are medically and psychologically stable, and, fourth, are willing to proceed with surgery (Box 114-2).

The selection of surgical procedures should not be market driven or specialty- or stage-specific; rather, selection should be "site-specific,"[2] based on each patient's specific sites of UA obstruction. For specific sites or segmental areas that are distinctly identifiable, treat with appropriate procedures that address these specific sites or areas. If a staged approach is recommended and desired, treat the most severe or critical site or area first. For those patients with diffusely complex or multiple sites or areas that are not easily identified, extrapharyngeal skeletal advancement procedures (e.g., MMA) may be performed initially (see Box 114-2).[2]

(NOTE: Parameters used by different authors to measure OSA surgical "success" vary in the literature. The primary inclusion criterion for the case series in Tables 114-1 to 114-3 and Figure 114-6 is reported preoperative and postoperative AHI or occasionally the respiratory disturbance index (RDI), which are used synonymously though slight differences currently exist. The reader is referred to the source documents, because these definitions have varied over time. Unless otherwise stated, "success" is generally defined as a postoperative AHI less than 20 and/or greater than 50% reduction in AHI. To standardize results of the AHI data, the primary outcome measure for comparison of surgical procedures is the **mean percentage (%) reduction in AHI** [from preoperative to postoperative].)

SURGICAL TREATMENT AND MMA TECHNIQUES

TELEGNATHIC SURGERY

Although the surgical techniques are similar, the treatment goals and criteria for success differ for MMA as telegnathic (derived from the Greek words *tele*, which means "over a distance," and *gnathis*, which relates to the jaws) surgery versus orthognathic (derived from the Greek words *ortho*, which means "to straighten," and *gnathis*) surgery. Whereas orthognathic surgery includes maxillary and mandibular osteotomies to treat malocclusion to improve mastication, speech, and esthetics, telegnathic surgery includes skeletal (i.e., maxillary, mandibular, and hyoid) advancement to anatomically enlarge and physiologically stabilize the pharyngeal airway to treat OSA. Ideally, MMA may harmoniously satisfy the goals and be successful as both orthognathic and telegnathic surgery. However, this may not always be feasible. Accordingly it should not be viewed as failure, but rather, accepted as known limitations of this type of surgery.[11]

For example, telegnathic MMA may be therapeutic for OSA, but yet maintain an existing, albeit "untreated," malocclusion in a patient who elects not to pursue concomitant orthodontic therapy. On the other hand, orthognathic mandibular setback surgery to successfully treat a Class III malocclusion might create hypopharyngeal narrowing and frank OSA.[12] Another case scenario is sole mandibular advancement to correct a Class II malocclusion, but yet is subtherapeutic for existing OSA in that maxillary advancement was also required to enlarge and stabilize the entire velo-orohypopharyngeal airway.

In addition to malocclusion, other dental problems such as severe periodontal disease or compromised fixed bridgework may be relative contraindications for elective orthognathic surgery, but yet not (contraindications) for telegnathic surgery to treat the potentially life-threatening medical disorder of OSA. In cases of hypopharyngeal narrowing in the absence of skeletal hypoplasia (i.e., a normal profile), MMA might create an unesthetic facial appearance in terms of bimaxillary protrusion with alar base flaring and nasal tip rotation.

Unlike the relatively healthy and younger orthognathic patient, the typical OSA patient (who finally presents for telegnathic MMA after years of failed prior therapies) has a health status that is often compromised by morbid obesity, hypertension, and other medical problems, as well as depression and cognitive dysfunction. Hence, the perioperative management is often more intensive, and the associated risks higher, for telegnathic (versus orthognathic) surgery.

SURGICAL PRINCIPLES AND MANAGEMENT

Telegnathic MMA (Figs. 114-2 and 114-3) is a technically tedious and difficult operation that is best performed under hypotensive anesthesia (to control blood loss) in a hospital operating room with both a surgeon and assistant surgeon. Bilateral sagittal split ramus osteotomies (BSSRO) with rigid internal and/or maxillomandibular fixation (MMF) are performed for mandibular advancement. A Le Fort I osteotomy (LF) with bone graft and rigid internal fixation (RIF) is performed for maxillary advancement to anterosuperiorly reposition and stabilize the attached soft palate for velopharyngeal enlargement (thereby perhaps eliminating invasive soft palatal surgery), and to maintain a functional occlusal relationship with the synchronously advanced mandibular dentition (thereby preserving the functions of mastication and speech articulation).

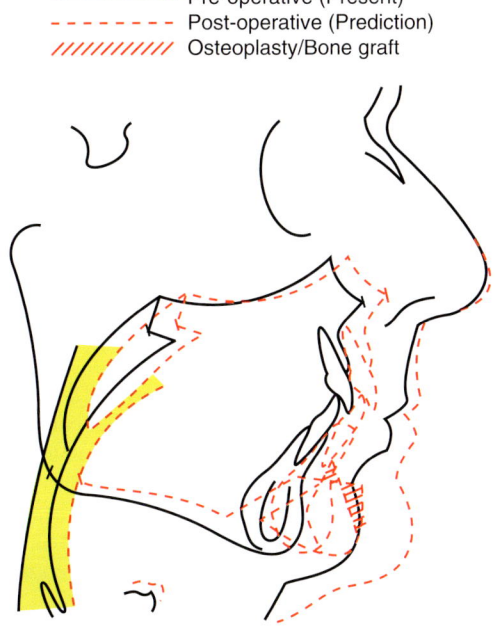

Legend:
——— Pre-operative (Present)
- - - - - - - Post-operative (Prediction)
/////////// Osteoplasty/Bone graft

Fig. 114-2 ■ Lateral cephalometric prediction of MMA. (Adapted from Prinsell JR: Maxillomandibular advancement surgery in a site-specific treatment approach for obstructive sleep apnea in 50 consecutive patients, *Chest* 1999;116(6):1519-1529, Figure 2.)

The soft palate is a tissue organ whose known primary function is to prevent reflux of air and liquids into the nasopharynx during speech and swallowing, respectively. Also, its role in snoring may be a self-protection warning sign, or "bell" (to the bed partner), of partial or impending UA obstruction, which may progress to OSA. A dysmorphic or abnormal-looking soft palate may be an anatomic variant of normal that ensures compensatory functioning and, therefore, may not always be a cause of OSA. Retropalatal narrowing and collapse, often induced by swallowing (e.g., during nasopharyngolaryngoscopy), should be understood as normal velopharyngeal closure, rather than perhaps misinterpreted as a site of obstruction dictating surgery.[2] Surgical ablation or distortion may produce dysfunction, such as velopharyngeal insufficiency (VPI); velopharyngeal stenosis; voice changes; dysphagia; and, in cases of "social" snoring amelioration, may produce "silent" apnea—either of immediate or delayed (with advancing age and/or weight gain) onset. In addition, pain, hemorrhage, and UA obstruction in the immediate postoperative period may occur because of velopharyngeal edema which, particularly if compounded with coexisting untreated hypopharyngeal narrowing, can result in death.[5,13-16]

MMA preserves the functional integrity of the pharyngeal tissues. Edema from the intraoral labial vestibular MMA incisions is anatomically shielded from the UA by the underlying bony structures and, thus, is confined to the facial soft tissues. Although this extraosseous edema may produce a frightfully swollen face, it does not typically extend to the UA. The entire velo-orohypopharyngeal airway is more patent at the moment of skeletal advancement, (i.e., like the immediate UA opening produced by a CPR "jaw-thrust" maneuver). Hence, early endotracheal tube (ETT) extubation is encouraged (serving to minimize ETT-induced glottic edema) and usually accomplished in the operating room at the conclusion of the operation. Centrally acting opiate and opioid narcotics (which can cause respiratory depression and therefore are to be used judiciously) may not be necessary because, first of all, rigidly fixated MMA bony segments (unlike operated pharyngeal soft tissues) do not move and accordingly are not painful during swallowing, coughing, and vocalization; and second, trigeminal (sensory) nerve branches encased

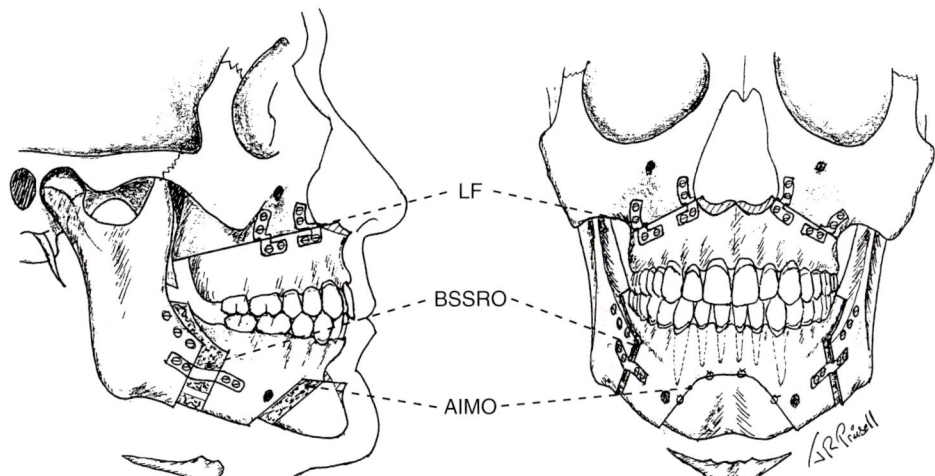

Fig. 114-3 ■ Maxillomandibular advancement (MMA). Abbreviations: *LF,* Le Fort I osteotomy with bone graft and rigid internal fixation for advancement of the maxilla with anterosuperior repositioning of the soft palate; *BSSRO,* bilateral sagittal split ramus osteotomies with rigid internal fixation for mandibular advancement; *AIMO,* anterior inferior mandibular osteotomy with bone graft and osteotomy for additional advancement of the genial tubercles with attached muscles, tongue base, and indirect hyoid suspension. (From Prinsell JR: Maxillomandibular advancement surgery in a site-specific treatment approach for obstructive sleep apnea in 50 consecutive patients, *Chest* 1999;116(6):1519-1529, Figure 3.)

within bony canals are usually surgically traumatized, resulting in numbness rather than severe pain.[2]

COUNTERCLOCKWISE ROTATIONAL ADVANCEMENT

The amount of mandibular advancement is usually the main determinant of the therapeutic efficacy of MMA for OSA, because the most critical site of UA obstruction is usually hypopharyngeal. (The hypopharynx is the common "bottleneck" from the nasal and oral inspiratory pathways.) However, the limiting factor for the amount of MMA advancement is the degree of maxillary protrusion, which thins the upper lip and results in excessive maxillary incisor show, alar base flaring (even with compensatory nasal base cinch sutures and V-Y advancement closure of the vestibular tissues), and upward nasal tip rotation. Hence, the LF is usually performed before the BSSROs. Osteoplasty of the anterior nasal spine minimizes excessive nasal tip rotation. The piriform rims are enlarged, the caudal edge of the nasal septum relieved, and the inferior turbinates out-fractured to minimize iatrogenic nasal obstruction. The amount of anterior maxillary impaction is determined by the degree of maxillary incisor show with lips in repose. Resultant telescoping of the inferior over the superior edges of the osteotomized anterior maxillary walls provides a trough for placement of corticocancellous bone, which prevents soft tissue ingress and promotes a uniform and stable bony union.[2]

Counterclockwise rotation of the maxillomandibular complex allows for maximum mandibular advancement to enlarge the hypopharynx[2,17] for therapeutic efficacy while minimizing the unesthetic affects of excessive maxillary advancement.[2] Other esthetic enhancements of counterclockwise rotational advancement include elimination of excessive maxillary incisal show at rest or gummy smile and lip incompetence in dolichocephalic facies, increased horizontal and vertical dimension of the lower face with accentuation of the lower jawline and hyoid elevation that raises the chin–neck angle in mandibular retrognathism cases (Fig. 114-4), and tightening or rejuvenation of neck skin laxity in relatively older patients (Fig. 114-5).

PREVENTION OF SKELETAL AND AIRWAY RELAPSE

Counterclockwise rotation with anterior maxillary impaction allows for greater mandibular advancement. For example, the resultant mandibular advancement following 6 mm maxillary advancement and 3 mm anterior impaction might be 15 mm. Posteroinferiorly directed forces from the intact tongue-related (e.g., genioglossus) and suprahyoid (e.g., geniohyoid and anterior digastric) musculature on the distal mandibular osteotomy segments may cause skeletal instability and relapse. In contrast to conventional orthognathic surgery, it is critical that anteroinferior mandibular myotomies not be performed in telegnathic MMA, because intact tongue-related and suprahyoid musculature is necessary for orohypopharyngeal enlargement to treat OSA. However, release of the deep tendons of the temporalis and masseteric sling at the inferior border and vertical scoring of the inelastic periosteum lateral to the BSSROs facilitates this counterclockwise rotational advancement.[2]

To minimize skeletal and attached anterior pharyngeal tissue relapse, RIF must be reinforced, for example, with bicortical screws and unicortical bone plates at the superior and inferior borders, respectively, of BSSROs (see Fig. 114-3). Corticocancellous block bone grafts wedged between all osteotomy advancement "gaps" will minimize soft tissue ingress and, thus, promote more uniform and esthetic bony unions. Temporary MMF with anteriorly directed elastic ligatures around orthodontic appliances or arch bars facilitates advancement and stability of the distal mandibular segment for

RIF placement. Dental implants may facilitate MMF in cases of periodontally unstable dentitions and partial or complete edentulism. Once healed to a bony union, the advanced maxillomandibular complex is stable,[2,18] with an expanded velo-orohypopharyngeal airway in all three dimensions.[19]

ANTERIOR INFERIOR MANDIBULAR OSTEOTOMY

An extrapharyngeal anterior inferior mandibular osteotomy (AIMO) produces additional advancement of the tongue-related and suprahyoid musculature (an indirect hyoid suspension) for additional enlargement and stabilization of the orohypopharyngeal airway. It is critical that the height, width, and thickness of the distal segment be large enough to include all muscle insertions that may extend beyond the genial tubercles superiorly, laterally, and inferiorly.[2] In contrast to AIMO, a sliding genioplasty made with a single horizontal cut may be too low, and a rectangular pull-through "window" segment that does not include the inferior border may be too small, respectively, to capture all of the muscle insertions, and a 90-degree torsion of this distal segment (for structural stabilization) may precipitate tendon rupture or necrosis and detachment of this soft tissue pedicle.[70]

A wide inferiorly based trapezoid-shaped AIMO should extend to within 5 mm of the teeth apices, at least 10 mm anterior to the mental foramina, and include the inferior mandibular border. The distal segment is advanced the full bicortical thickness and stabilized by overlapping the superior edge of the lingual cortex anterior to the buccal cortex of the proximal (tooth-bearing) segment before placement of RIF. Aggressive osteoplasty of the distal segment's buccal cortex will allow a tension-free vestibular closure, as well as reshape an otherwise unesthetic prognathic chin. Corticocancellous bone grafting will minimize soft tissue ingress, promote a more uniform bony union, and lessen an otherwise unesthetic deep mentolabial fold[2] (see Figs. 114-2, 114-3, 114-4, and 114-5).

DISTRACTION OSTEOGENESIS

Although used extensively for transverse maxillary expansion in children and adults, and reported in the pediatric literature for single-jaw (e.g., mandibular and midfacial) and, less commonly, staged two-jaw lengthening, the potential application of distraction osteogenesis (DO) for simultaneous maxillary and mandibular advancement for OSA is challenging and promising.[21-23]

Telegnathic surgery utilizing DO offers three advantages over conventional osteotomies. First, DO may be performed before skeletal maturation to treat OSA in younger patients (e.g., children and infants). Second, DO allows greater advancement of hard and accompanying soft tissues to treat more severe cases of skeletal hypoplasia, including craniofacial syndromes and/or soft tissue inelasticity. The surgical technique involves less tissue dissection, and bone grafting is not needed. The gradual soft tissue accommodation associated with incremental skeletal advancement may improve skeletal stability in terms of minimizing skeletal relapse due to muscle tension or soft tissue inelasticity. Third, the amount of jaw advancement may be titrated to optimal therapeutic positioning, as confirmed by serial PSG, analogous to the titration of nCPAP and oral appliance therapy.[11,23]

On the other hand, telegnathic surgery utilizing DO has three disadvantages, in comparison with conventional osteotomies. First, patients may be intolerant of the extraosseous fixation devices and noncompliant with the required multiple office visits for serial adjustments of these devices. Second, inherent difficulties with parallel alignment of distraction devices and subsequent coordination of vectors of skeletal advancement, particularly in bimaxillary cases, may result in higher incidences of malocclusion and facial

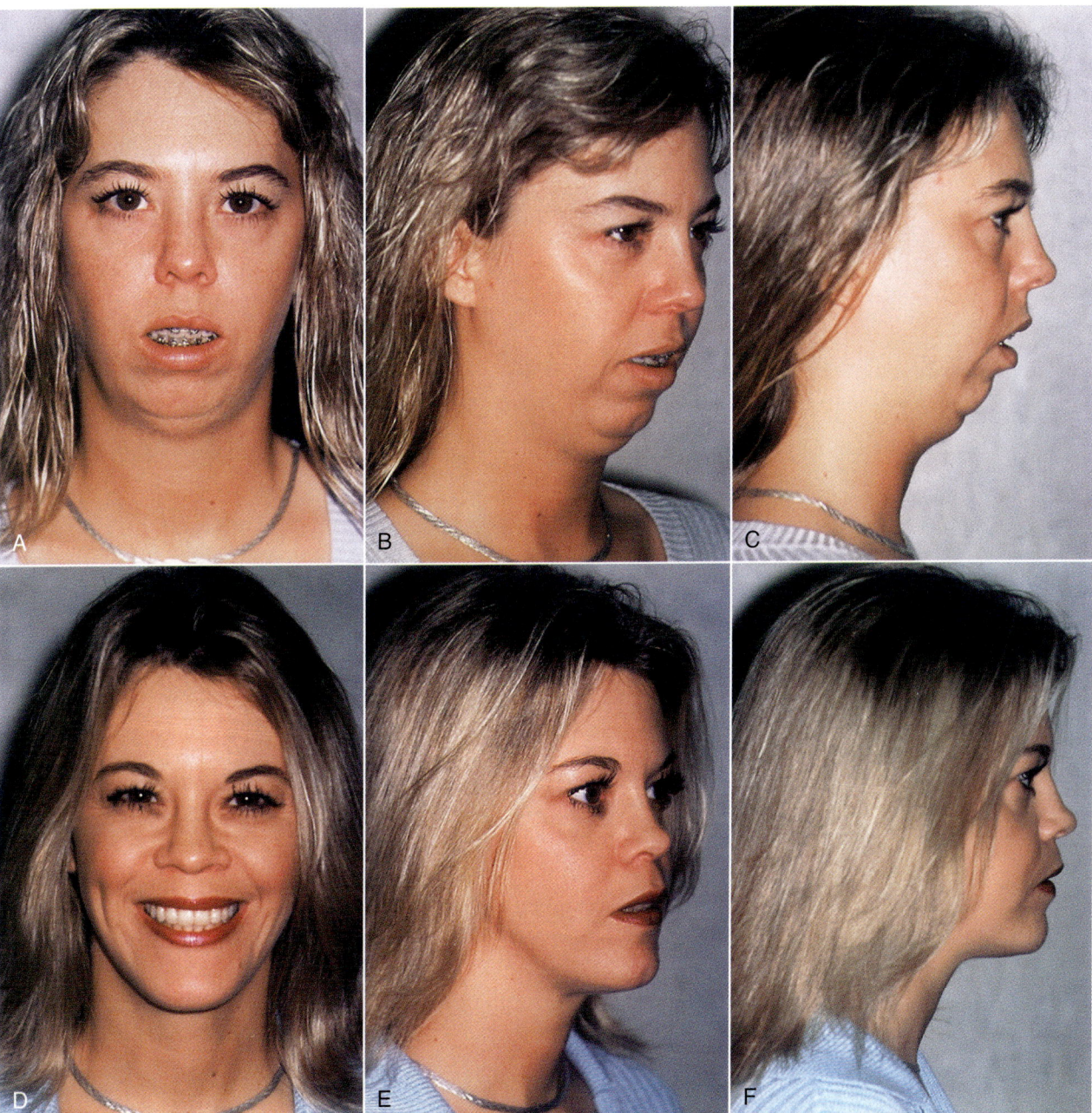

Fig. 114-4 ■ MMA case with counterclockwise rotation, AIMO with indirect hyoid suspension, and submental suction lipectomy. Preoperative (**A** to **C**) and postoperative (**D** to **F**) photographs.

asymmetry. Third, financial costs of the hardware, additional surgery (e.g., for hardware removal), and labor intensive postoperative care are higher than conventional osteotomies. These limitations should lessen with technical improvements (e.g., miniaturized and bioresorble distraction devices) and refined clinical expertise.[11] The indications for telegnathic DO will become more clearly defined with additional scientific studies.

SURGICAL STAGING WITH UNILEVEL AND MULTILEVEL OPERATIONS

Although MMA is known to be highly therapeutic for OSA, its indications and staging protocols remain unsettled. This is partly because of existing diagnostic dilemmas such as: identifying and ranking (in terms of severity) the often diffusely complex or multiple sites of obstruction; and knowing when and how to prioritize and combine the numerous available surgical procedures in one or more stages, which may be influenced (and perhaps biased) by the surgeon's education, training, and experience.[2] One approach is to perform certain procedures stepwise according to a methodical sequential (staging) protocol, such as uvulopalatopharyngoplasty (UPPP) and other procedures first; then, if unsuccessful, an MMA. However, this may result in unnecessary additional intrapharyngeal surgery with potentially life-threatening UA edema that may be painful, dysfunctional, expensive, subtherapeutic, and ultimately a deterrent for patients to seek definitive surgical treatment. (Note: "Phase" and "stage" are synonymous and thus are used interchangeably.)

In general, multilevel (surgical procedures performed concomitantly to address multiple levels of UA narrowing)[20,24-48] and unilevel

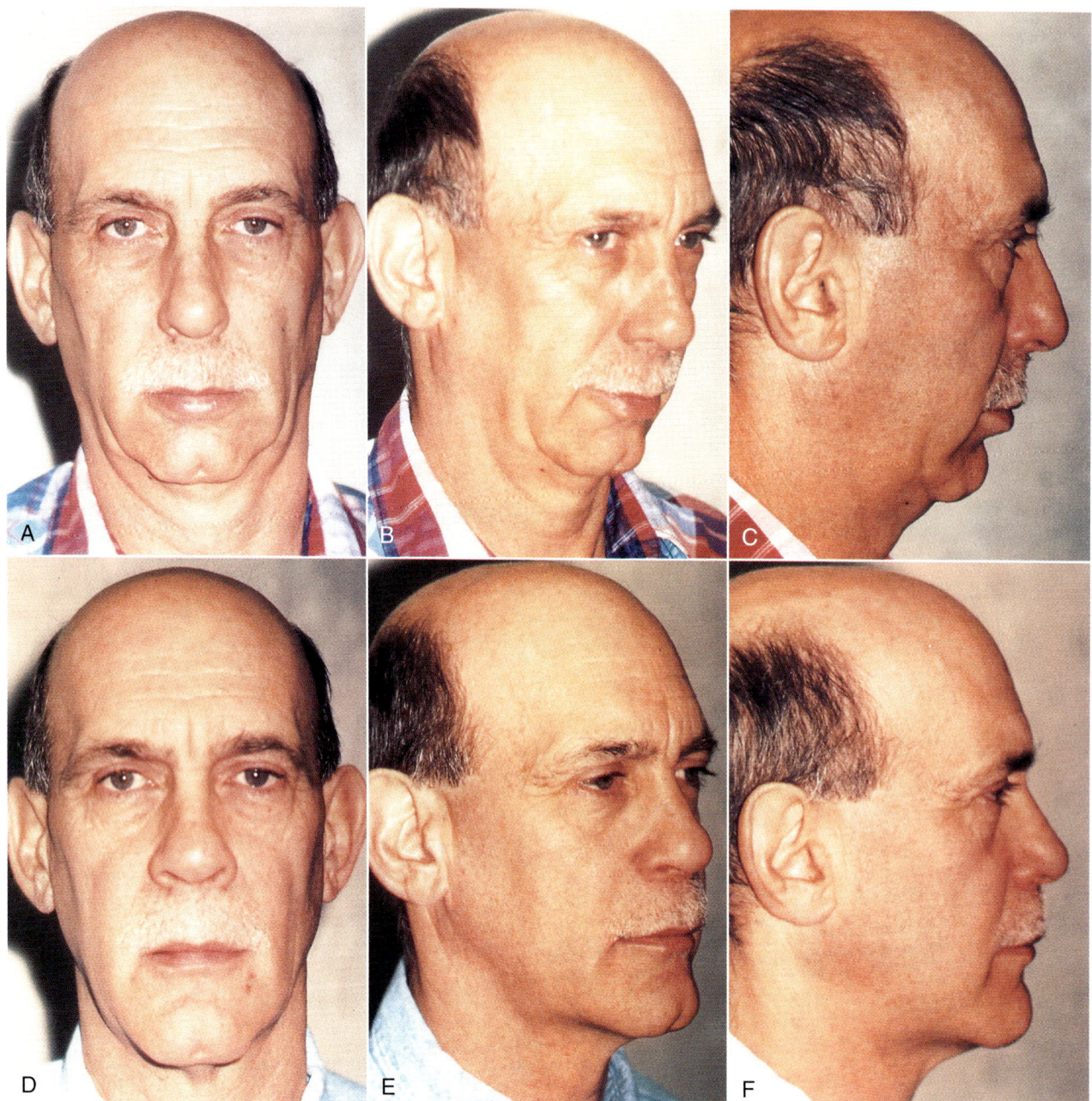

Fig. 114-5 ■ MMA case with counterclockwise rotation and AIMO with indirect hyoid suspension. Preoperative (**A** to **C**) and postoperative (**D** to **F**) photographs.

(surgery to address single levels of UA narrowing) operations are less therapeutic than MMA. Riley et al[24] reported a success rate of 60% (145 of 239 cases) and only 42% (44 of 104 cases with severe OSA) for phase I surgery, which consisted of UPPP and/or genioglossus advancement with hyoid myotomy (GAHM) suspension in the largest multilevel series. Sher et al[5] reported 41% success (137 of 337 cases from 37 series) of UPPP, which is the most commonly performed OSA surgery. Elshaug et al[49] reported success rates of 52% (92 of 178 cases from 7 subsequent series) for UPPP, 49% (35 of 72 cases from 3 series) for laser-assisted uvuloplasty (LAUP), and 61% (22 of 36 cases from 2 series) for radiofrequency (RF) tissue reduction. Kezirian et al[50] reported that many hypopharyngeal procedures are also relatively subtherapeutic, including 62% success (56 of 91 cases from 4 series) of GA, 55% success (180 of 328 cases from 5 series) of GAHM, 35% success (95 of 269 cases from 11

series) of RF tongue base (RFTB), 35% success (27 of 77 cases from 6 series) of tongue base suspension (TBS) via a bone screw–anchored sling stitch; 50% success (37 of 74 cases from 5 series) of midline glossectomy (MLG); and 50% success (51 of 101 cases from 4 series) of hyothyroidopexy (HSThy).

In general, most patients do not pursue additional (i.e., staged) OSA surgery, despite the knowledge that MMA is highly therapeutic. Riley et al[24] reported that only 26% (24 of 94) of their stage I (UPPP and/or GAHM) failures, Bettega et al[20] reported that only 38% (13 of 34) of their stage I (UPPP, tonsillectomy [Tons], HSThy, and GA or inferior sagittal osteotomy [ISO]) failures, and Lee et al[41] reported that only 27% (3 of 11) of their stage I (UPPP and ISO or AIMO) failures, proceeded to stage II (MMA). None of the 9 and 18 multilevel surgical failures from Dattilo et al[29] (UPPP, LAUP, or uvulopalatal flap; hyoid suspension [HS], GA, and

Tons) and Hendler et al[42] (UPPP and anterior mandibular osteotomy [AMO]) participated in their respective MMA series.

PRIMARY AND SECONDARY MMA

Fifteen MMA case series (inclusion criterion of more than 5 cases) performed in adult OSA patients (pediatric and DO cases were excluded) are listed in Table 114-1. Eleven "primary" MMA series were performed initially as a definitive (single-staged) operation[2,29,42,51-58]; and four "secondary" (e.g., phase II) MMA series followed unilevel or multilevel (e.g., phase I) surgery as part of two-phase protocols.[20,24,59,60] MMA was highly therapeutic with summary mean percent reductions in AHI of 86.5% (88.4% for case series with no concomitant intrapharyngeal, and 92.1% with extrapharyngeal procedures) for primary, and 86.6% for secondary MMA. Significantly, no additional stages of surgery were reported following any MMA series.

Riley et al[24] reported the largest MMA series in which 89 of 91 OSA cases were treated successfully, for a success rate of 98%. However, it is perhaps misleading that MMA was labeled phase II in that 67 of 91 did not participate in phase I of their two-phase protocol. In contrast, Dattilo et al[29] reported 93% success (14 of 15 cases),and Hochban et al[51] reported 97% success (37 of 38 cases) of MMA as a primary single-stage surgery without concomitant adjunctive procedures or prior phase I procedures. In Hochban's series of healthy nonobese patients with specific cranioskeletal deformities and pharyngeal narrowing, a stepwise algorithm of staged procedures was "not justified."

All MMA series reported significant UA enlargement (measured by PAS) and maxillary and mandibular advancement (measured by SNA, SNB, and Go-Pog). The hyoid elevated (measured by MP-H) in most cases. Table 114-2 provides definitions of these standard cephalometric abbreviations. In an earlier report of their MMA series, Hochban et al[61] showed that PAS enlarged at all four levels of measurement: the uvula tip, maxillary plane, occlusal plane, and mandibular plane; and Dekeister et al[52] reported retropalatal and retrolingual enlargement following MMA. Prinsell[2] showed that OSA due to UA narrowing can sometimes occur in the absence of skeletal hypoplasia, and Li et al[59] reported 92% success (23 of 25 cases) of MMA performed in the absence of maxillomandibular hypoplasia (e.g., normal SNA and SNB). Goh et al[54] reported 91% success (10 of 11 cases) of MMA modified by anterior maxillomandibular segmental subapical dentoalveolar setback osteotomies following premolar extractions with ostectomies to minimize potential unesthetic bimaxillary protrusive facial profiles in Asian males.

All MMA series reported significant improvements in mean PSG parameters of AHI, LSAT, (see Table 114-1), number of desaturations less than 90%, percent sleep efficiency, percent stage 3 + 4 sleep, and percent REM sleep (Table 114-3). Improvements in daytime hypersomnolence and cognitive performance were measured by vigilance tests[53] and Epworth Sleepiness Scales[29,52,55] and other quality of life parameters.[2,58,59,61-63] Mean systolic and diastolic blood pressures improved from 138.9 to 123.9 mm Hg and 89.9 to 80.2 mm Hg, respectively[2] (Table 114-3), and several patients no longer required antihypertension medications following MMA.[54,62]

EXTRAPHARYNGEAL VERSUS INTRAPHARYNGEAL ADJUNCTIVE PROCEDURES WITH MMA

Therapeutic efficacy of MMA is generally lower in MMA cases that employ concomitant adjunctive intrapharyngeal procedures (see Table 114-1, Fig. 114-6). Smatt et al[57] reported 83% success (15 of 18 cases) of uvuloplasty and MLG with MMA and advancement genioplasty (Genio). Waite et al[56] reported 74% success (17 of 23 cases) of

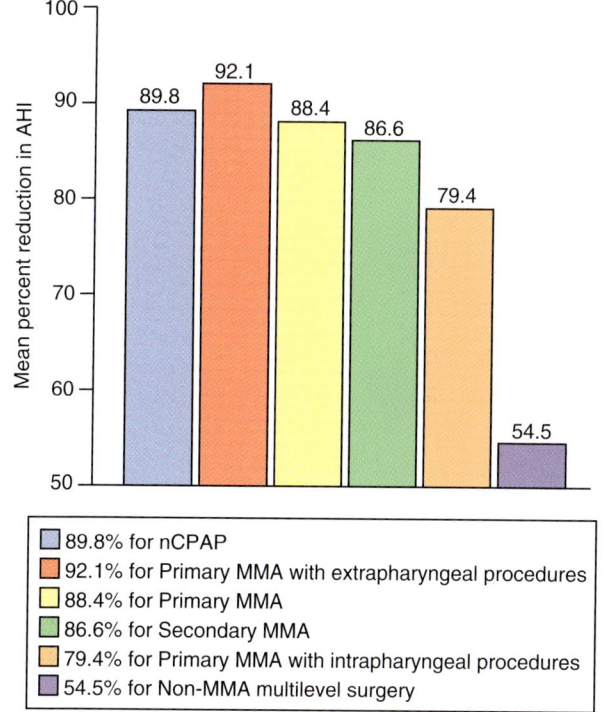

Fig. 114-6 ■ Mean percent reduction in AHI for different surgeries compared with nCPAP.

UPPP and MLG with MMA, septoplasty/turbinate reduction (S/TR) and Genio. Lye et al[58] reported 87% success (13 of 15 cases) of UPPP with MMA, S/TR, and Genio. Hendler et al[42] reported a 57% success (4 of 7 cases) of UPPP with MMA, AMO and tracheostomy. Li et al[60] reported 83% success (19 of 23 MMA cases) of morbidly obese patients with OSA (baseline mean BMI of 45 and AHI of 83) who failed phase I (UPPP, GA and/or HS and tracheostomy). Bettega et al[20] reported 75% success (15 of 20 MMA cases) that included 13 phase I failures of UPPP, Tons, S/TR, and GA via a 90-degree rotated rectangular genial tubercle advancement osteotomy.

Intrapharyngeal procedures should, in general, probably not be performed concomitantly with MMA for several reasons. First, intrapharyngeal postoperative edema may cause UA embarrassment that may be difficult to manage, particularly in the setting of temporary MMF and coexisting extrapharyngeal edema from MMA. These cases may require temporary tracheostomy, prolonged endotracheal intubation, or autotitrating CPAP with risk of barotrauma-induced intrapharyngeal hemorrhage. Second, intrapharyngeal pain, particularly when compounded with that of MMA, may require excessive use of centrally acting opiates and opioids that may precipitate narcotic-induced respiratory depression. Third, intrapharyngeal pain may impede swallowing of liquids and pureed nutrition, which is already difficult for patients following MMA. Fourth, intrapharyngeal procedures may compromise the therapeutic efficacy of MMA. LF maxillary advancement may create excessive tension on concurrent operated soft palatal tissue that may exacerbate velopharyngeal cicatricial scarring and stenosis, as well as VPI and other dysfunction. Permanent suturing of the hyoid inferiorly to the thyroid (e.g., HS via hyothyroidopexy) may impede anterosuperior hyoid repositioning that otherwise occurs with the mandibular component of MMA.

Extrapharyngeal procedures, whose postoperative edema and scarring does not typically affect the velo-orohypopharygneal airway, can be performed concomitantly with MMA as a safe

Text continued on p. 1060

TABLE 114-1 Primary and Secondary MMA, With and Without Adjunctive Procedures

REF #	PRIMARY AUTHOR YR	# CASES % SUCCESS (AHI <20)	ADJUNCTIVE PROCEDURES (IN ADDITION TO LF & BSSRO)	BMI (KG/M²)	AGE (YR)	% MALE	AHI PRE-OP	AHI POST-OP	AHI CPAP	% REDUCTIONS IN AHI SURG	% REDUCTIONS IN AHI CPAP	LSAT PRE-OP	LSAT POST-OP	LSAT CPAP	# DAYS HOSPITAL
Primary MMA															
51	Hochban, 1997	37/38 = 97.4% (AHI <10)			42.8	36 = 94.7	45.2	2.5		94.5					
52	Dekiester, 2006	25		28.0 (3.4)	48.0		45.0 (19.0)	7.0 (7.0)		84.4					
53	Conradt, 1998	24		26.7 (2.9)	42.7 (10.7)	24 = 100	59.3 (24.1)	5.6 (9.6)	5.3 (6.0)	90.6	91.1				
29	Dattilo, 2004	14/15 = 93.3%			44.2	12 = 80	76.2	12.6		83.5					
54	Goh, 2003	10/11 = 90.9%	AMMSSSO after premolar extractions	29.4 (4.6)	42.8	11 = 100	70.7 (15.9)	11.4 (7.4)		83.9		58.6 (12.3)	83.9 (8.8)		4.2
55	Kessler, 2007	6		28.0	46.9	4 = 67	37.0	4.0		89.2		78.0	89.0		
		119								88.4					
Primary MMA with Extrapharyngeal Procedures															
2	Prinsell, 1999	50/50 = 100% (AHI <15)	AIMO-50, S/TR = 28/26, Lipo-26, Sinus-13, Tori-1	30.7 (4.5)	42.7 (9.3)	44 = 88	59.2 (28.4)	4.7 (5.9)	5.4 (6.8)	92.1	90.9	72.7 (13.6)	88.6 (3.9)	88.6 (6.3)	1.7 (0.5)
		50								92.1					
Primary MMA with Intrapharyngeal Procedures															
56	Waite, 1989	17/23 = 73.9%	UPPP-17, MLG-8, S/TR-23, Genio-15		45.0	21 = 91.3	63.0	15.0		76.2					7.8
57	Smatt, 2005	15/18 = 83.3% (AHI <15)	Uvuloplasty, MLG, Genio	29.2 (4.1)	46.6 (6.1)	15 = 83.3	54.0 (20.7)	9.7 (6.7)		82.0					
58	Lye, 2008	13/15 = 86.7%	UPPP-12, S/TR-12, Genio-12	32.1	47.9	13 = 86.7	69.1	13.9		79.9		76.5	85.0		
42	Hendler, 2001	4/7 = 57.1	UPPP-7, AMO-5, Trach-4	36.3	47.0 (6.2)	6 = 85.7	90.1 (31.6)	16.5 (62.0)		81.7		64.9 (16.3)	88.2 (5.1)		

REF #	PRIMARY AUTHOR YR	# CASES % SUCCESS (AHI <20)	ADJUNCTIVE PROCEDURES (IN ADDITION TO LF & BSSRO)	BMI (KG/M²)	AGE (YR)	% MALE	AHI PRE-OP	AHI POST-OP	AHI CPAP	% REDUCTIONS IN AHI SURG	% REDUCTIONS IN AHI CPAP	LSAT PRE-OP	LSAT POST-OP	LSAT CPAP	# DAYS HOSPITAL
		63								79.4					
	Total all Primary MMA	232								86.5					
Secondary MMA															
24	Riley, 1993	89/91 = 97.8%	(67/91 did not participate in Phase I) (Prior UPPP and/or HS)	31.1 (6.3)	43.5	81 = 89	68.3 (23.3)	8.4 (5.9)	7.6 (5.9)	87.7	88.9	63.2 (17.5)	86.6 (3.4)	87.0 (3.9)	2.4 (0.7)
59	Li, K 2000	23/25 = 92.0%	(Prior UPPP, GA, and/or HS)	32.4	43.7	21 = 84.0	60.6	8.6		85.8		75.2	88.0		
60	Li, K 2000	19/23 = 82.6%	(5/23 did not participate in Phase I) (Prior UPPP-23, GA and/or HS-16, Trach-11)	45.0 (5.4)	42.6 (7.9)	15 = 65.2	83.0 (30.1)	10.6 (10.8)		87.2		63.9 (17.7)	86.0 (7.9)		
20	Bettega, 2000	15/20 = 75.0% (AHI <15)	(7 did not participate in Phase I) (Prior UPPP, GAHM, HSThy, ISO, S/TR, Tons)	26.9 (4.3)	44.4	18 = 90.0	59.3 (29.0)	11.1 (8.9)		81.3		82.0 (11.0)	90.0 (7.0)		7.0
		159								86.6					
	Total all Primary & Secondary MMA	391								86.5					

AIMO, anterior inferior mandibular osteotomy; *AMMSSO*, anterior maxillary and mandibular segmental subapical setback osteotomies; *AMO*, anterior maxillary and mandibular segmental subapical setback osteotomy; *EUPF*, extended uvulopalatal flap; *GA*, genioglossus advancement; *GAHM*, genioglossus advancement hyoid myotomy; *Genio*, advancement genioplasty; *HS*, hyoid suspension; *HSMd*, HS to mandible; *HSThy*, HS to thyroid or hyothyroidopexy; *ISO*, inferior sagittal osteotomy; *Lipo*, cervicofacial or submental suction lipectomy; *MLG*, midline glossectomy; *RFTB*, radiofrequency reduction of tongue base; *S/TR*, septoplasty/turbinate reduction; *Sinus*, maxillary sinus curettage; *TBS*, tongue base suspension via bone screw-anchored sling stitch; *Tons*, tonsillectomy; *Trach*, tracheostomy; *Tori*, mandibular lingual tori removal; *UPPP*, uvulopalatopharyngoplasty; *LAUP*, laser-assisted uvuloplasty; *UFlap*, uvuloflap; *UPFlap*, uvulopalatal flap.

All values are mean #s with standard deviations in parenthesis, e.g., (SD)
N is the # of cases.
% success is the # of cases/total # of cases that met the primary criteria of success, which is an AHI <20 (unless otherwise listed, e.g., AHI <15) and/or >50% reduction in AHI.
BMI is body mass index, kg/m².
AHI is apnea hypopnea index, which is also substituted for RDI (respiratory disturbance index) data.
LSAT is lowest arterial oxyhemoglobin saturation.
Pre-op is preoperative, and Post-op (or PO) is postoperative.
nCPAP is nasal continuous positive airway pressure.

TABLE 114-2　MMA: Lat Cephalometric Analysis

REF #	PRIMARY AUTHOR	N		PAS PRE-OP	PAS POST-OP	PAS CHANGE (MM)	SNA PRE-OP	SNA POST-OP	SNB PRE-OP	SNB POST-OP	GO-POG PRE-OP	GO-POG POST-OP	GO-POG CHANGE (MM)	MP-H PRE-OP	MP-H POST-OP
52	Dekeister	25	EVP	5.0 (2.0)	10.0 (2.0)	5.0	80.0 (5.0)	86.0 (5.0)	78.0 (5.0)	81.0 (5.0)				21.0 (5.0)	21.0 (5.0)
			ELP	8.0 (3.0)	14.0 (3.0)	6.0									
51	Hochban	38											10.6		
61	Hochban	21	Uvula	7.0 (2.2)	11.8 (3.6)	4.8	79.6 (3.4)	85.2 (4.5)	75.2 (4.0)	80.7 (3.8)					
			Mx	25.7 (4.1)	32.1 (4.4)	6.4									
			Occl	7.4 (2.6)	11.3 (3.9)	3.9									
			Md	8.3 (2.0)	15.2 (3.9)	6.9									
2	Prinsell	50	ETV	5.1 (2.4)	11.6 (3.4)	6.5	79.0 (4.2)	86.4 (4.1)	74.7 (4.1)	81.6 (4.1)	72.1 (4.7)	86.5 (5.7)	14.4	24.3 (5.8)	22.4 (6.0)
			MM	0.8 (1.5)	5.7 (3.9)	4.9								37.1 (10.6)	33.7 (9.0)
56	Waite	23				7.0							12.5		
57	Smatt	18											10.7 (2.8)		
24	Riley	91		4.3 (1.8)	9.4 (2.2)	5.1	74.0 (8.2)	76.7 (6.2)							
59	Li	25		5.1 (2.4)	9.7 (3.1)	4.6	85.6 (3.5)	93.1 (4.2)	81.1 (1.7)	87.5 (3.4)				24.3 (7.7)	17.5 (7.7)
60	Li	23		7.0 (4.6)	11.2 (3.8)	4.2	82.1 (5.0)	90.3 (6.8)	78.0 (5.1)	84.8 (5.4)				27.6 (10.2)	21.9 (8.2)
42	Hendler	7											10.2 (2.3)		

PAS, Posterior airway space, mm; *EVP*, retropalatal PAS; *ELP*, retrolingual PAS; *Uvula*, PAS at uvula tip; *Mx*, PAS at maxillary plane; *Occl*, PAS at occlusal plane; *Md*, PAS at mandibular plane; *ETV*, PAS at End Tidal Volume; *MM*, PAS during a modified Muller Maneuver; *SNA*, Sella – Nasion – A point of maxilla, degrees; *SNB*, Sella – Nasion – B point of mandible, degrees; *Go-Pog*, gonion – pogonion, mm; *MP-H*, mandibular plane – hyoid, mm.

TABLE 114-3   MMA: Blood Pressure and Sleep Staging Parameters

REF #	PRIMARY AUTHOR, YR	N	BLOOD PRESSURE (MM HG)		% SLEEP EFFICIENCY			% STAGE 3 & 4 SLEEP			% REM SLEEP			EPWORTH SLEEPINESS SCALE	
			PRE-OP	POST-OP	PRE-OP	POST-OP	CPAP	PRE-OP	POST-OP	CPAP	PRE-OP	POST-OP	CPAP	PRE-OP	POST-OP
61	Hochban, 1994	21						8.4 (5.9)	15.1 (5.3)						
52	Dekeister, 2006	25						8.0 (6.0)	15.0 (12.0)					11.0 (5.0)	6.0 (4.0)
53	Conradt, 1998	24			80.2 (9.9)	84.2 (9.3)	85.2 (6.5)	8.0 (6.1)	14.4 (7.3)	18.2 (12.8)	19.6 (7.4)	21.3 (5.6)	12.2 (6.3)		
29	Dattilo, 2004	15												17.9	4.7
55	Kessler, 2007	6												11.0	4.0
2	Prinsell, 1999	50	138.9/89.9 (15.6)/(12.3)	123.9/80.2 (13.8)/(11.1)	83.2 (11.9)	86.7 (9.9)	83.1 (16.7)	6.2 (13.6)	9.0 (13.6)	10.1 (14.1)	9.9 (7.7)	16.5 (7.4)	23.1 (19.5)		
24	Riley, 1993	91						2.9 (4.4)	8.2 (7.7)	12.0 (13.6)	8.9 (4.0)	19.1 (6.0)	20.8 (8.8)		
20	Bettega, 2000	20						4.0 (4.0)	8.0 (5.0)		21 (10)	27 (7)			

N, Number of cases; *CPAP*, continuous positive airway pressure; *REM*, rapid eye movement.

single-stage operation. Prinsell[2] reported 100% success (50 of 50 consecutive cases, some morbidly obese and some without skeletal hypoplasia) of MMA performed with the following extrapharyngeal procedures in a site-specific approach (the selection of adjunctive procedures depended on the sites of disproportionate UA that varied between different patients): AIMO for additional advancement of tongue-related and suprahyoid musculature (an indirect HS without invasive hyoid surgery); S/TR and removal of antral polyps performed via direct access while the maxilla was downfractured; removal of prominent anterior mandibular lingual tori to increase tongue space in the floor of the mouth; and cervicofacial or submental suction-assisted lipectomy to debulk "weight" on the underlying anterior pharyngeal tissues against the orohypopharyngeal airway, particularly during supine sleep.[2]

MMA VERSUS CPAP AND OTHER MULTILEVEL SURGERY

Nasal CPAP is generally accepted as a first-line treatment of OSA because of its high therapeutic efficacy and convenience of pneumatically splinting open the velo-orohypopharyngeal airway without having to identify the specific sites of disproportionate anatomy in individual patients. However, many patients are noncompliant with required nightly use at home due to intolerance issues,[64-67] which essentially negates therapeutic efficacy recorded in the sleep lab. Compliance rates defined by ratio formulas whose denominators are only several hours of use per day[64,66,67] are inherently flawed in that any time interval of nCPAP nonuse, particularly during the remaining latter hours of "deeper" sleep when OSA often worsens, leaves the UA unsplinted and the patient at risk for deleterious events. A more accurate method of calculating compliance might employ continuous (24 hours per day) monitoring at home with nCPAP "chips" and electroencephalography to measure time of use while asleep divided by total sleep time. (Analogy: Like seat belts, nCPAP saves lives only when utilized.) Nevertheless, nCPAP is widely considered the gold standard to which all other therapies, including surgery, are compared.

MMA, which permanently enlarges the velo-orohypopharyngeal airway, has a therapeutic efficacy equal to and without the compliance problems of nCPAP. In several case series in which the same respective cohorts of patients were treated with nCPAP before MMA, the mean percent reduction in AHI was 89.8% for nCPAP, versus 89.5% following MMA,[2,24,53] versus 92.1% following primary MMA with extrapharyngeal procedures.[2] The increase (improvement) in mean percent sleep efficiency (a PSG measure of how well one sleeps) was 1.9% with nCPAP versus 4.5% following MMA.[2,53] MMA and nCPAP also showed similar marked improvements in daytime vigilance tests as objective measures of daytime hypersomnolence and cognitive performance.[53]

Figure 114-6 compares the summary **mean percent reduction in AHI** (primary standardized outcome measure of therapeutic efficacy) totals in all case series listed by surgical category versus nCPAP: 89.8% for nCPAP;[2,23,54] 92.1% for primary MMA with extrapharyngeal procedures;[2] 88.4% for primary MMA;[29,51-55] 86.6% for secondary MMA;[20,24,59,60] 79.4% for primary MMA with intrapharyngeal procedures[42,56-58] (see Table 114-1); and 54.5% for non-MMA multilevel surgery (1,077 cases from 29 series).[20,24-48]

INDICATIONS FOR MMA

MMA should satisfy the general goals and guidelines for OSA surgery, including the four surgical prerequisites (see Boxes 114-1 and 114-2). Box 114-3 lists the indications and contraindications for MMA. The primary anatomic criterion for MMA is hypopharyngeal

---

| BOX 114-3 | **Maxillomandibular Advancement (MMA): Indications & Contraindications** |

Indications
1. Surgical prerequisites (see Box 114-2) are satisfied
2. Hypopharyngeal narrowing (i.e., Fujita type III) (e.g., cephalometric posterior airway space [PAS] <9 mm at end-tidal volume [ETV])
3. Velo-orohypopharyngeal (VOH) narrowing (i.e., Fujita type II)
4. May combine with adjunctive extrapharyngeal procedures (whose postoperative edema does not affect the VOH airway)
5. Even in absence of dentocraniofacial skeletal deformities (e.g., retrognathia)
6. Diffusely complex or multiple sites of disproportionate upper airway anatomy that include (VO)H narrowing (e.g., ETV PAS <9 mm) as a:
   a. Primary single-stage definitive operation, or
   b. Stage 1 operation to enlarge and stabilize entire VOH to minimize risk of potential edema-induced airway embarrassment associated with subsequent intrapharyngeal surgery, if necessary, for clinically significant residual OSA

Contraindications
1. Surgical prerequisites (see Box 114-2) not satisfied
2. Absence of hypopharyngeal narrowing (e.g., ETV PAS >9 mm), such as sole velopharyngeal narrowing (e.g., Fujita type I)

From Prinsell JR. Maxillomandibular advancement (MMA) in a site-specific treatment approach for obstructive sleep apnea: A surgical algorithm. *Sleep Breath* 2000;4(4):147-154, Table 4.

(retrolingual) narrowing (Fujita type III airway obstruction), which can be measured by the cephalometric ETV PAS less than 9 mm. (Specific measurements for other imaging modalities as inclusion criteria for MMA have not been published.) In the setting of hypopharyngeal narrowing, coexistent velopharyngeal narrowing (Fujita type II obstruction), as well as nonpharyngeal sites, may also be treated with MMA. Patients with sites of obstruction in the absence of hypopharyngeal narrowing, such as sole velopharyngeal (retropalatal) narrowing (Fujita type I obstruction) should not receive MMA, but may be considered for other procedures, such as UPPP.[10]

Although most OSA cases with velo-orohypopharyngeal narrowing occur in the setting (and perhaps as a result) of maxillomandibular hypoplasia, exceptions have been reported.[2,59] Hence, skeletal measurements (e.g., lateral cephalometric SNA, SNB, and Go-Pog) are not the primary diagnostic anatomic determinants for MMA, but rather are certainly useful for quantifying the amount of skeletal advancement that produces the velo-oropharyngeal enlargement (e.g., PAS).

MMA may be performed initially for selected cases of diffusely complex or multiple sites of velo-orohypopharyngeal obstruction, including coexisting soft palatal dysmorphism and mild to moderate tonsillar hypertrophy. This is done to enlarge and stabilize the entire velo-orohypopharyngeal UA to either definitively treat the OSA and obviate the need for invasive segmental intrapharyngeal procedures (which may be painful, dysfunctional, and subtherapeutic), or decrease the risk of postoperative edema-induced airway embarrassment after subsequent intrapharyngeal surgery, which may be necessary in cases of clinically significant residual OSA that may occur with advancing age and/or weight gain.[2]

COMPLICATIONS OF MMA

The most common complication of MMA is neurosensory deficit (consensus of many surgeons via verbal communication, and Riley et al[24] with published numerical data: 12.5% cases with permanent

IAN anesthesia). Waite et al[56] reported a 44% incidence of minor malocclusion treated with occlusal equilibration. Less commonly reported complications by Riley et al[24] include superficial wound infection (5%), removal of hardware (2.5%) and TMJ disorder (2.5%). There have been no reported cases of pharyngeal dysfunction, postoperative hemorrhage, or deaths due to edema-induced airway embarrassment. Mean hospital stays following MMA include 7.8 days by Waite et al,[56] 7 days by Bettega et al,[20] 4.2 days by Goh et al,[54] 2.4 days by Riley et al,[24] and 1.7 days by Prinsell.[2]

Riley et al[63] reported relatively stable long-term therapeutic efficacy of MMA for OSA. The two most significant variables affecting outcome were BMI and the amount of skeletal advancement. Progressive recurrence of OSA resulted from significant weight gain (5%) and mandibular skeletal relapse (2.5%; in one early case in which BSSRO utilized wire osteosynthesis and MMF, instead of RIF).

ROLE OF MMA

MMA satisfies the general goals of OSA surgery (see Box 114-1) and is the most successful (excluding tracheostomy) acceptable surgical treatment for OSA, with a therapeutic efficacy comparable to nCPAP. In general, MMA therapeutic efficacy may be enhanced with concomitant extrapharyngeal procedures such as AIMO, but without intrapharyngeal procedures such as UPPP. As a comprehensive, safe, nondysfunctional, extrapharyngeal operation that structurally enlarges and physiologically stabilizes the entire velo-orohypopharyngeal UA, MMA may eliminate the need for (and thus circumvent the staging dilemmas associated with) multiple, segmental, less successful, and invasive intrapharyngeal procedures. In accordance with the general guidelines for OSA surgery (see Box 114-2) in which a site-specific approach is advocated, MMA should not be limited to cases of severe OSA or dentocraniofacial skeletal deformities, or as a last resort when other surgeries have failed; but rather, it is also indicated as the initial surgical treatment of choice for (velo-oro) hypopharyngeal narrowing, even in the setting of relatively mild OSA and in the absence of retrognathism.[2]

MMA as a potentially definitive primary single-stage surgical treatment of OSA, particularly when performed in a relatively young adult population, may result in a significant improvement in quality of life[2,53,58,59,61-63] and a reduction in OSA-related health risks (e.g., hypertension, cardiovascular dysrhythmias, stroke, myocardial infarction, hypersomnolence-induced injuries such as those caused by motor vehicle accidents, and neuropsychiatric disorders such as depression and cognitive dysfunction) that, when projected over an average normal lifetime, should result in considerable financial savings for the health care system.[68]

Nevertheless, MMA should not be used indiscriminately, because it is technically difficult to perform and laden with potential morbidity. Although skeletal osteotomies, when healed to a bony union, are stable with no significant relapse, and the relatively long-term results of MMA are promising,[63] the effect of soft-tissue laxity that occurs with natural aging (with or without weight gain) in terms of possible progressive velo-orohypopharyngeal narrowing and worsening of residual OSA, is unknown. Additional studies are warranted, with larger numbers of cases and longer follow-up periods.

POSTOPERATIVE CARE

Following surgery, MMA patients must be carefully monitored in an intensive care unit (ICU). Portable monitoring with continuous transcutaneous pulse oximetry and sleep staging parameters is essential to document whether sleep does in fact occur in these patients, who often lie awake in fear of facial swelling, possible

apnea, and the intimidating ICU environment (e.g., noisy monitors and bright lights, which should be minimized especially in the early morning hours to promote sleep) in order to assess the postoperative OSA status to be expected later in the patient's home. Minor desaturations are permissible without CPAP while the patient is being weaned off supplemental oxygen onto room air, provided the lower limit established for each individual is significantly higher than their preoperative diagnostic PSG LSAT. Full overnight diagnostic PSG is necessary when fully recovered from surgery, typically at 2 months,[2] to document therapeutic efficacy.

The frightful facial edema from this extrapharyngeal surgery (that does not typically compromise the pharyngeal airway) is lessened with IV corticosteroids. In the setting of temporary MMF and anticipated nasal congestion and lip edema, oral breathing can be enhanced (and air hunger minimized) by placement of semirigid bilateral airway tubes (e.g., 3-inch-long modified pieces of the extubated ETT) inserted at the lip commissures. Hemostats or wire cutters and an Allis clamp must be kept at bedside for possible emergency release of MMF and tongue base advancement for airway access, respectively.

To minimize risk of narcotic-induced respiratory depression, centrally acting opiates and opioids must be used judiciously and perhaps replaced with nonnarcotic analgesics, as well as a long-acting local anesthetic such as bupivacaine injected into the operated tissues at the conclusion of the surgery for pain management. Sequential leg compression devices placed at the start of surgery (to minimize risk of deep venous thrombosis) are not removed until the patient ambulates. The bladder catheter that was inserted at the start of the surgery is removed later that evening to encourage voiding by the morning of the first postoperative day. Nutritional counseling for clear liquids the first week, followed by a strict nonchewing diet for 2 months, is recommended. Most otherwise healthy patients may be discharged from the hospital on the first postoperative day and return to their normal activities, with physical restrictions, in 2 weeks.

PEARLS AND PITFALLS

- The selection of OSA surgical procedures should be determined by the correctly identified site(s) or level(s) of disproportionate UA anatomy, which varies between patients.
- The primary anatomic criterion for MMA is hypopharyngeal narrowing (e.g., ETV PAS less than 9 mm), which usually but not always occurs in the setting of skeletal hypoplasia.
- Counterclockwise rotational advancement of the maxillomandibular complex allows for maximum orohypopharyngeal enlargement (to enhance therapeutic efficacy) and an esthetically acceptable facial appearance. The maxilla is the limiting factor in the amount of MMA advancement.
- Anteroinferior mandibular myotomies are to be avoided because intact tongue-related and suprahyoid musculature are necessary for UA enlargement to treat the OSA. Hence, reinforced RIF (e.g., bicortical screws and bone plates at the superior and inferior portions of BSSROs), AIMO distal segment buccal cortex osteoplasty and other modifications) are necessary to prevent skeletal and corresponding UA and OSA relapse.
- MMA has high therapeutic efficacy as either a primary or secondary operation and may be safely combined with adjunctive extrapharyngeal procedures (whose surgical edema does not compromise the UA and scarring does not disrupt pharyngeal function) as a safe, single-staged, definitive operation for OSA.

REFERENCES

1. Practice parameters for the treatment of obstructive sleep apnea in adults: the efficacy of surgical modifications of the upper airway. Report of the American Sleep Disorders Association, *Sleep* 19(2):152-155, 1996.

2. Prinsell JR: Maxillomandibular advancement surgery in a site-specific treatment approach for obstructive sleep apnea in 50 consecutive patients, *Chest* 116(6):1519-1529, 1999.

3. Young T, Palta M, Dempsey J, Skatrud J, Weber S, Badr S: The occurrence of sleep-disordered breathing among middle-aged adults, *N Engl J Med* 29(328):1230-1235, 1993.

4. Institute of Medicine Report: Sleep disorders and sleep deprivation: an unmet public health problem, (http://nap.edu) April 2006.

5. Sher AE, Schechtman KB, Piccirillo JF: The efficacy of surgical modifications of the upper airway in adults with obstructive sleep apnea syndrome, *Sleep* 19(2):156-177, 1996.

6. Prinsell JR: Maxillomandibular advancement surgery for obstructive sleep apnea surgery, *JADA* 133:1489-1497, 2002.

7. Hoekema A, Lange J, Stegenga B, de Bont LG: Oral appliances and maxillomandibular advancement surgery: an alternate treatment protocol for the obstructive sleep apnea-hypopnea syndrome, *J Oral Maxillofac Surg* 64:886-891, 2006.

8. Kushida CA, Morgenthaler TI, Littner MR, et al: Practice parameters for the treatment of snoring and obstructive sleep apnea with oral appliances: an update for 2005, *Sleep* 29:240-243, 2006.

9. Ferguson KA, Cartwright R, Rogers R, Schmidt-Nowara W: Oral appliances for snoring and obstructive sleep apnea: A review, *Sleep* 29:244-262, 2006.

10. Prinsell JR: Maxillomandibular advancement (MMA) in a site-specific treatment approach for obstructive sleep apnea: a surgical algorithm, *Sleep Breath* 4(4):147-154, 2000.

11. Prinsell JR: Telegnathic surgery for obstructive sleep apnea syndrome, *AAOMS Oral & Maxillofacial Surgery Update* 4:88-97, 2006.

12. Chen F, Terada K, Hua Y, Saito I: Effects of bimaxillary surgery and mandibular setback surgery on patients with Class III skeletal deformities, *Am J Orthod Dentofacial Orthop* 131:372-377, 2007.

13. Fairbanks DN: Uvulopalatopharyngoplasty complications and avoidance strategies, *Otolaryngol Head Neck Surg* 102:239-245, 1990.

14. Zohar Y, Finkelstein Y, Talmi YP, Bar-Ilan Y: Uvulopalatopharyngoplasty: evaluation of postoperative complications, sequelae, and results, *Laryngoscope* 101:775-779, 1991.

15. Haavisto L, Suonpaa J: Complications of uvulopalatopharyngoplasty, *Clin Ototlaryngol* 19:243-247, 1994.

16. Kezirian EJ, Weaver EM, Yueh B, Deyo RA, Khuri SF, Daley J, Henders W: Incidence of serious complications after uvulopalatopharyngoplasty, *Laryngoscope* 114:450-453, 2004.

17. Mehra P, Downie M, Pita MC, Wolford LM: Pharyngeal airway space changes after counterclockwise rotation of the maxillomandibular complex, *Am J Orthod Dentofacial Orthop* 120(2):154-159, 2001.

18. Goncalves JR, Cassano DS, Wolford LM, Santos-Pinto A, Marquez IM: Postsurgical stability of counterclockwise maxillomandibular advancement surgery: affect of articular disc repositioning, *J Oral Maxillofac Surg* 66:724-738, 2008.

19. Fairburn SC, Waite PD, Vilos G, Harding SM, Bernreuter W, Cure J, Cherala S: Three-dimensional changes in upper airways of patients with obstructive sleep apnea following maxillomandibular advancement, *J Oral Maxillofac Surg* 65:6-12, 2007.

20. Bettega, G, Pepin JL, Veal D, Deschaux C, Raphael B, Levy P: Obstructive sleep apnea syndrome. Fifty-one consecutive patients treated by maxillofacial surgery, *Am J Respir Crit Care Med* 162:641-649, 2000.

21. Cohen SR, Simms C, Burstein FD: Mandibular distraction osteogenesis in the treatment of upper airway obstruction in children with craniofacial deformities, *Plast Reconstr Surg* 101:312-318, 1998.

22. Li KK, Powell NB, Riley RW, Guilleminault C: Distraction osteogenesis in adult obstructive sleep apnea surgery: a preliminary report, *J Oral Maxillofac Surg* 60:6-10, 2002.

23. Thompson SH, Quinn M, Helman JI, Baur DA: Maxillomandibular distraction osteogenesis advancement for the treatment of obstructive apnea, *J Oral Maxillofac Surg* 65:1427-1429, 2007.

24. Riley RW, Powell NB, Guilleminalt C: Obstructive sleep apnea syndrome: a review of 306 consecutively treated surgical patients, *Otolaryngol Head Neck Surg* 108(2):117-125, 1993.

25. Hsu PP, Brett RH: Multiple level pharyngeal surgery for obstructive sleep apnoea, *Singapore Med J* 42(4):160-164, 2001.

26. Neruntarat C: Genioglossus advancement and hyoid myotomy: short-term and long-term results, *J Laryngol Otol* 117(6):482-486, 2003.

27. Ramirez SG, Loube DI: Inferior sagittal osteotomy with hyoid bone suspension for obese patients with sleep apnea, *Arch Otolaryngol Head Neck Surg* 122:953-957, 1996.

28. Bowden MT, Kezirian EJ, Utley D, Goode RL: Outcomes of hyoid suspension for the treatment of obstructive sleep apnea, *Arch Otolaryngol Head Neck Surg* 131(5):440-445, 2005.

29. Dattilo DJ, Drooger SA: Outcome assessment of patients undergoing maxillofacial procedures for the treatment of sleep apnea: comparison of subjective and objective results, *J Oral Maxillofac Surg* 62:164-168, 2004.

30. Vilaseca I, Morello A, Montserrat JM, Santamaria J, Iranzo A: Usefulness of uvulopalatopharyngoplasty with genioglossus and hyoid advancement in the treatment of obstructive sleep apnea, *Arch Otolaryngol Head Neck Surg* 128:435-440, 2002.

31. Chabolle F, Wagner I, Blumen MB, Sequert C, Fleury B, DeDieuleveult T: Tongue base reduction with hyoepiglottoplasty: A treatment for severe obstructive sleep apnea, *Laryngoscope* 109(8):1273-1280, 1999.

32. Jacobowitz O: Palatal and tongue base surgery for surgical treatment of obstructive sleep apnea: a prospective study, *Otolaryngol Head Neck Surg* 135(2):258-264, 2006.

33. Richard W, Kox D, Herder C, Tinteren H, Vries N: One stage multilevel surgery (uvulopalatopharyngoplasty, hyoid suspension, radiofrequency ablation of tongue base with/without genioglossus advancement) in obstructive sleep apnea syndrome, *Eur Arch Otorhinolaryngol* 264:439-444, 2007.

34. Baisch A, Maurer JT, Hormann K: The effect of hyoid suspension in a multilevel surgery concept for obstructive sleep apnea, *Otolaryngol Head Neck Surg* 134(5):856-861, 2006.

35. Verse T, Baisch A, Maurer JT, Stuck BA, Hormann K: Multilevel surgery for obstructive sleep apnea: short-term results, *Otolaryngol Head Neck Surg* 134(4):571-577, 2006.

36. Nelson LM: Combined temperature-controlled radiofrequency tongue reduction and UPPP in apnea surgery, *Ear Nose Throat J* 80(9):640-644, 2001.

37. Friedman M, Ibrahim H, Lee G, Joseph NJ: Combined uvulopalatopharyngoplasty and radiofrequency tongue base reduction for treatment of obstructive sleep apnea/hypopnea syndrome, *Otolaryngol Head Neck Surg* 129(6):611-621, 2003.

38. Vicente E, Marin JM, Carrizo S, Naya MJ: Tongue-base suspension in conjunction with uvulopalatopharyngoplasty for treatment of severe obstructive sleep apnea: long-term follow-up results, *Laryngoscope* 116(7):1223-1227, 2006.

39. Sorrenti G, Piccin O, Latini G, Scaramuzzino G, Mondini S, Ceroni R: Tongue base suspension technique in obstructive sleep apnea: personal experience, *Arch Otorhinolaryngol Ital* 23:274-280, 2003.

40. Miller FR, Watson D, Malis D: Role of the tongue base suspension suture with the Repose system bone screw in the multilevel surgical management of obstructive sleep apnea, *Otolaryngol Head Neck Surg* 126:392-398, 2002.

41. Lee NR, Givens CD, Wilson J, Robins RB: Staged surgical treatment of obstructive sleep apnea syndrome: a review of 35 patients, *J Oral Maxillofac Surg* 57:382-385, 1999.

42. Hendler BH, Costello BJ, Silverstein K, Yen D, Goldberg A: A protocol for uvulopalatopharyngoplasty, mortised genioplasty, and maxillomandibular advancement in patients with obstructive sleep apnea: an analysis of 40 cases, *J Oral Maxillofac Surg* 59:892-897, 2001.

43. Johnson NT, Chinn J: Uvulopalatopharyngoplasty and inferior sagittal mandibular osteotomy with genioglossus advancement for treatment of obstructive sleep apnea, *Chest* 101(1):278-283, 1994.

44. Miller FR, Watson D, Boseley M: The role of the genial bone advancement trephine system in conjunction with uvulopalatopharyngoplasty in the multilevel management of obstructive sleep apnea, *Otolaryngol Head Neck Surg* 130:73-79, 2004.

45. Li HY, Wang PC, Hsu CY, Lee SW, Chen NH, Liu SA: Combined nasal-palatopharyngeal surgery for obstructive sleep apnea: simultaneous or staged? *Acta Otolaryngol* 125(3):298-303, 2005.

46. Li HY, Wang PC, Hsu CY, Chen NH, Lee LA, Fang TJ: Same-stage palatopharyngeal and hypopharyngeal surgery for severe obstructive sleep apnea, *Acta Otolaryngol* 124(7):820-826, 2004.

47. Elasfour A, Miyazaki S, Itasaka Y, Yamakawa K, Ishikawa K, Togawa K: Evaluation of uvulopalatopharyngoplasty in treatment of obstructive sleep apnea syndrome, *Acta Otolaryngol Suppl* 537:52-56, 1998.

48. Mickelson SA, Rosenthal L: Midline glossectomy and epiglottidectomy for obstructive sleep apnea syndrome, *Laryngoscope* 107(5):614-619, 1997.

49. Elshaug AG, Moss JR, Southcott AM, Hiller JE: Redefining success in airway surgery for obstructive sleep apnea: a meta analysis and synthesis of the evidence, *Sleep* 30:461-467, 2007.

50. Kezirian EJ, Goldberg AN: Hypopharyngeal surgery in obstructive sleep apnea, *Arch Otolaryngol Head Neck Surg* 32:206-213, 2006.

51. Hochban W, Conradt R, Bradenburg U, Heitmann J, Peter JH: Surgical maxillofacial treatment of obstructive sleep apnea, *Plast Reconstr Surg* 99:619-626, 1997.

52. Dekeister C, Lacassagne L, Tiberge M, Montemayor T, Migureres M, Paoli JR: Mandibular advancement surgery in patients with severe obstructive sleep apnea uncontrolled by continuous positive airway pressure. A retrospective review of 25 patients between 1998 and 2004, *Rev Mal Respir* 23:430-437, 2006.

53. Conradt R, Hochban W, Heitmann J, et al: Sleep fragmentation and daytime vigilance in patients with OSA treated by surgical maxillomandibular advancement compared to CPAP therapy, *J Sleep Res* 7(3):217-223, 1998.

54. Goh YH, Lim KA: Modified maxillomandibular advancement for the treatment of obstructive sleep apnea: A preliminary report, *Laryngoscope* 113:1577-1582, 2003.

55. Kessler P, Ruberg F, Obbarius H, Iro H, Neukam FW: Surgical management of obstructive sleep apnea, *Mund Kiefer Gesichts Chir* 11(2):81-88, 2007.

56. Waite PD, Wooten V, Lachner J, Guyette RF: Maxillomandibular advancement surgery in 23 patients with obstructive sleep apnea syndrome, *J Oral Maxillofac Surg* 47:1256-1261, 1989.

57. Smatt Y, Ferri J: Retrospective study of 18 patients treated by maxillomandibular advancement with adjunctive procedures for obstructive sleep apnea syndrome, *J Craniofac Surg* 16(5):770-777, 2005.

58. Lye KW, Waite PD, Meara D, Wang D: Quality of life evaluation of maxillomandibular advancement surgery for treatment of obstructive sleep apnea, *J Oral Maxillofac Surg* 66:968-972, 2008.

59. Li KK, Riley RW, Powell NB, Guilleminault C: Maxillomandibular advancement for persistent obstructive apnea after phase I surgery in patients without maxillomandibular deficiency, *Laryngoscope* 110:1684-1688, 2000.

60. Li KK, Powell NB, Riley RW, Zonato A, Gervacio L, Guilleminault C: Morbidly obese patients with severe obstructive sleep apnea: is airway reconstructive surgery a viable treatment option? *Laryngoscope* 110:982-987, 2000.

61. Hochban W, Brandenburg U, Peter JH: Surgical treatment of obstructive sleep apnea by maxillomandibular advancement, *Sleep* 17(7):624-629, 1994.

62. Riley RW, Powell NB, Guilleminault C: Maxillary, mandibular, and hyoid advancement for treatment of obstructive sleep apnea: a review of 40 patients, *J Oral Maxillofac Surg* 48:20-26, 1990.

63. Riley RW, Powell NB, Li KK, Troell RJ, Guilleminault C: Surgery and obstructive sleep apnea: long-term clinical outcomes, *Otolaryngol Head Neck Surg* 122:415-421, 2000.

64. Kribbs NB, Pack AI, Kline LR, et al: Objective measurement of patterns of nasal CPAP use by patients with obstructive sleep apnea, *Am Rev Respir Dis* 147:887-895, 1993.

65. Reeves-Hoche MK, Meck R, Zwillich CW: Nasal CPAP: an objective evaluation of patient compliance, *Am J Respir Crit Care Med* 149:149-154, 1994.

66. Sin DD, Mayers I, Man GC, Pauluk L: Long-term compliance rates to continuous positive airway pressure in obstructive sleep apnea, *Chest* 121:430-435, 2002.

67. Gay P, Weaver T, Loube D, Iber C: Evaluation of positive airway pressure treatment for sleep related breathing disorders in adults, *Sleep* 29(3):381-401, 2006.

68. Kapur V, Blough DK, Sandblom RE, et al: The medical cost of undiagnosed sleep apnea, *Sleep* 22(6):749-755, 1999.

Obstructive Sleep Apnea—Surgical Treatment: Part III, Mandibular Advancement for Children

Brinda Thimmappa, Stephen A. Schendel

Respiratory compromise in patients with congenital craniofacial anomalies is usually secondary to retrognathia and the resultant glossoptosis of the tongue base. Severe airway obstruction, termed obstructive sleep apnea (OSA) or sleep disorder breathing (SDB), is associated with significant morbidity and mortality in infants and children. They exhibit frequent episodes of oxygen desaturation, hypoxemia, acidosis, inspiratory stridor, sternal retraction, and poor feeding. Infants and children with long-term airway obstruction exhibit failure to thrive, daytime somnolence, hemodynamic changes (including cor pulmonale and pulmonary hypertension), developmental disabilities, insufficient weight gain, malnutrition, increased pulmonary morbidity, and death.

Numerous modalities have been used to treat obstructive sleep apnea, including prone positioning, nasopharyngeal airways, tongue-lip adhesion, mandibular distraction, and tracheostomy. Mandibular distraction has proven to be an effective method for airway management in children. Its application relieves the source of obstruction and eliminates the risks of delayed speech, feeding difficulties, mucus plugging, and tracheomalacia associated with tracheostomy. In a relatively short time, the family is able to care for an affected child at home without the aid of monitors, nasal tubes, or frequent repositioning.

ETIOPATHOGENESIS

Patients with congenital retrognathia and glossoptosis, with or without cleft palate, are diagnosed with Pierre Robin sequence (Fig. 115-1). This group represents the majority of children who may benefit from mandibular distraction. Additional findings of ocular abnormalities and one of several defined mutations in collagen production lead to the diagnosis of Stickler syndrome. Children with mandibulofacial dysostosis disorders such as Treacher Collins syndrome, Nager syndrome, and bilateral hemifacial microsomia often suffer from obstructive apnea and may also benefit from mandibular distraction.

PATHOLOGIC ANATOMY

Common to the syndromes just discussed is the presence of hypoplasia of the mandible. Mandibular retrognathia, with or without the presence of micrognathia, positions the base of the tongue posteriorly, resulting in glossoptosis. On physical examination, significant mandibular-maxillary discrepancy is noted, as measured from the apex of the mandibular alveolar ridge and the apex of the maxillary alveolar ridge in the midline, and is especially pronounced when the patient is supine, with the force of gravity acting on it, or while feeding. The tongue base abuts the posterior pharyngeal wall. The result is an infant with labored, noisy breathing, rapid development of fatigue, and costal retractions. Surgical techniques such as

glossopexy or tongue-lip adhesion, that position the tongue forward, are often criticized in that only the soft tissue is addressed and not the underlying skeletal problem.

DIAGNOSTIC STUDIES

Evaluation of mandibular retrognathia includes a polysomnogram, pH probe study or modified barium swallow, laryngoscopy, and maxillofacial CT scan.

The polysomnogram, performed in the supine position, records central apneas, obstructive apneas, and hypopneas. Central apneas are characterized by an absence or decrease in respiratory effort. In contrast, obstructive episodes are associated with an increased respiratory effort while airflow decreases. Hypopnea refers to a decrease in airflow by 30% to 50% from baseline. It is important to exclude central apnea as a cause of respiratory distress, as this neurologic condition will not benefit from skeletal advancement. Normal values of the calculated apnea-hypopnea index (AHI) in children are different from those of adults. Studies of normal children have suggested that an AHI greater than 1 is abnormal, with AHI 1 to 4 classified as mild OSA; AHI 5 to 10, moderate OSA; and AHI greater than 10, severe OSA. Cohen and colleagues demonstrated an improvement of mean AHI from 25.24 to 1.72 following mandibular distraction.

The polysomnogram also provides data on sleep architecture. Obstructive events may worsen during rapid eye movement (REM) sleep as muscle tone decreases. The result is frequent awakenings and less time spent in REM sleep. In growing children, the result may be decreased secretion of growth hormone and other chemical signals released during REM sleep, which can contribute to developmental delays.

Feeding difficulties often accompany respiratory distress in this population, even in the absence of associated cleft palate. A pH probe study may be performed at the time of polysomnogram and allows diagnosis of gastroesophageal reflux that may limit oral feeds. Gastroenterologists or feeding therapists may recommended a modified barium swallow when there is concern the child is at risk for aspiration with oral feeds.

Laryngobronchoscopy, which in many infants and children can be performed without anesthesia or intubation, confirms the absence of underlying laryngomalacia, tracheomalacia, or vocal cord paralysis before surgical intervention. The presence of glossoptosis as a source of obstruction may also be confirmed (Fig. 115-2).

Maxillofacial CT scan provides anatomic data on the amount and quality of bone available and degree of obstruction. Ideally, 2 cm of bone measured at the angle of the mandible will provide adequate bone stock for device placement. Maxillary-mandibular discrepancy, as well as the area of the airway, may be calculated with greater accuracy. The development of the temporomandibular

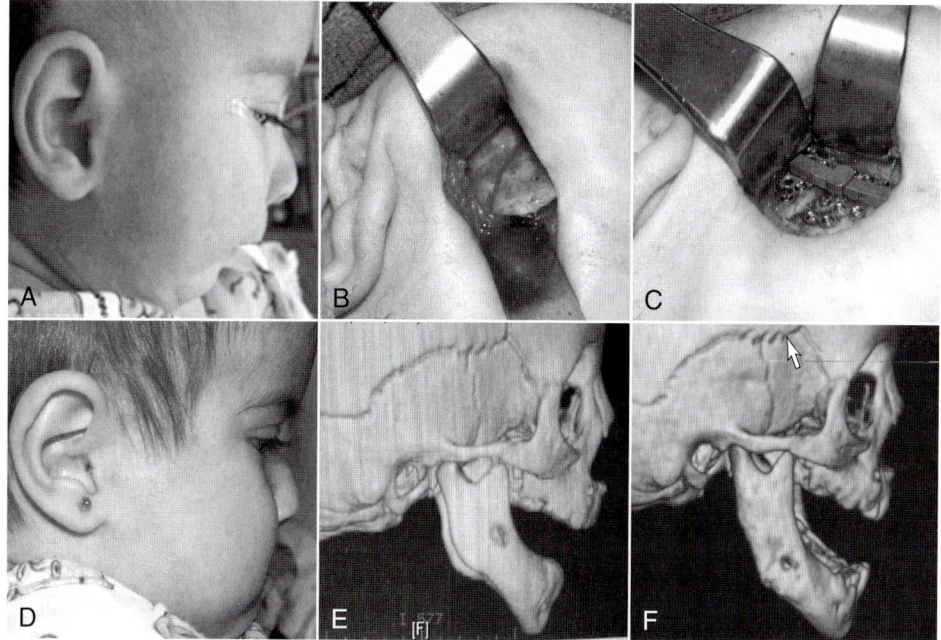

Fig. 115-1 ■ **A,** Six-month-old infant with isolated Pierre Robin sequence. **B,** Lateral corticotomy performed just posterior to mandibular angle. **C,** Distractor placement. **D,** Postoperative lateral photograph. **E,** Preoperative CT scan. **F,** Postoperative CT scan with curvilinear regenerate of ramus and body of mandible.

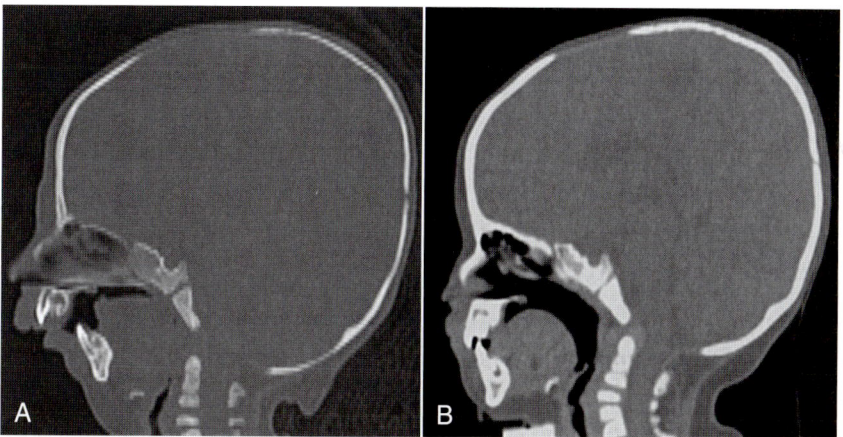

Fig. 115-2 ■ Preoperative sagittal (**A**) views demonstrating glossoptosis and airway obstruction. Following completion of distraction and consolidation period (**B**).

joint and location of tooth follicles are also obtained from CT data.

RECONSTRUCTIVE GOALS

The goal of treatment is to relieve airway obstruction by advancing the mandible, carrying with it the tongue base and thereby relieving airway obstruction. The type of device, location of osteotomies, and distraction vectors are chosen to limit complications such as damage to nerves or developing teeth and creation of an open bite. Secondary goals reported in the literature include avoidance or early removal of tracheostomy, improvement in feeding, and accelerated growth, even in the absence of feeding interventions.

SPECIFIC TREATMENT AND TECHNIQUES

Many distraction devices exist today. Infant mandibular distraction was first done with an external device. Advantages of an external device include ability to adjust the vector during the course of distraction, reduced subperiosteal dissection that may interrupt blood supply to the regenerate, and removal of device without a return to the operating room. Alternatively, internal devices are less cumbersome to patient and caregivers, are less prone to external trauma or pin site irritation, and minimize torque, with less chance of device loosening. Resorbable internal devices also offer the benefit of a single-stage distraction. Horizontal ramus osteotomy, vertical ramus osteotomy, angle osteotomy, and mandibular body osteotomy have all been reported effective in relieving airway obstruction.

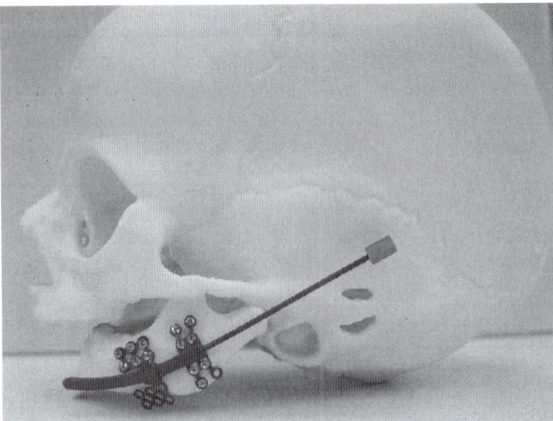

Fig. 115-3 ■ Infant curvilinear mandibular distractor (OsteoMed, Addison, Tex).

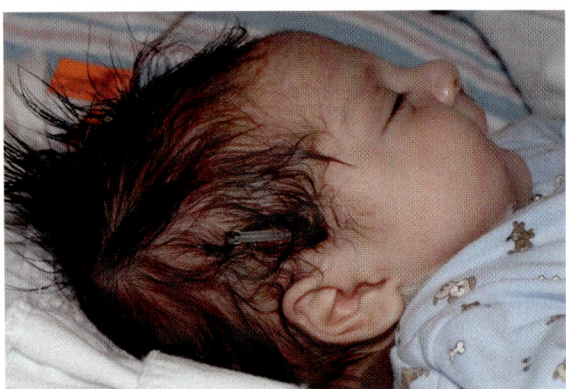

Fig. 115-4 ■ Activator rods in place.

It is the preferred technique of the senior author to use an internal curvilinear device (Fig. 115-3). Its design produces a curvilinear vector that models the logarithmic pattern of normal human mandibular growth. It avoids an anterior open bite, which may be created after distraction in a single vector. Coupled with an oblique osteotomy at the angle of the mandible, impingement of the coronoid process on the zygomatic arch with distraction is avoided. An ideal radius of curvature of 52 mm has been determined from clinical and radiographic studies of the infant mandible.

After induction of general anesthesia, the patient is intubated orally. Intravenous antibiotics are given, and the endotracheal tube is secured to the maxillary alveolus with a 2-0 silk suture.

Incisions are marked 1.5 to 2.0 cm in length and slightly inferior and parallel to the inferior mandibular border. After identifying the platysma muscle, division of the muscle and further dissection is performed with the aid of a nerve stimulator until the mandible is reached. Subperiosteal exposure of the mandibular ramus, angle, and body is necessary for device placement. If present on preoperative CT scan, identification of the sigmoid notch before osteotomy prevents inadvertent damage to the temporomandibular joint or entrance of the inferior alveolar nerve. The distractor device is then introduced into the wound and the osteotomy site is marked. The device is then removed and a lateral corticotomy is performed with a reciprocating saw. An osteotome is used to complete the osteotomy, while taking care to preserve the inferior alveolar nerve. Blunt dissection is then carried up toward the temporal scalp and a stab incision is made for the introduction of the activation arm (Fig. 115-4). Bony stabilization is then performed with 8-mm length screws. A minimum of three screws in each footplate is recommended. Complete osteotomy of the mandible is confirmed intraoperatively by turning the activation rod and observing movement of the segments. The incision is closed in layers, with approximation of the of the platysma muscle as a distinct layer.

An alternative method for surgical planning is with the aid of a skull fabricated from 3-D CT data. Model surgery, including osteotomies, contouring of footplates to the bone surface, and removal of excess screw holes, can be carried out and the device then sterilized for intraoperative use.

POSTOPERATIVE CARE

Patients are transferred to the intensive care unit postoperatively and in general remain intubated. The ideal rate and rhythm of distraction in infants and children has not been established. Prospective studies that provide guidelines for distraction in the craniofacial skeleton are also lacking. It is accepted that bone growth is much more robust in children and even more so in infants, so that a reduced latency period is necessary to prevent premature consolidation. In addition, a greater rate of distraction is well tolerated, relative to the studies of distraction osteogenesis in the appendicular skeleton. At our institution, distraction is started the next day at a rate of 2 mm per day (1 mm twice daily). Distraction is continued until overcorrection is achieved with a slight class III relation. The average length of distraction has been 19 mm in our series, with an associated three times increase in cross-sectional area of the retroglossal oropharyngeal airway. Activation rods are removed at bedside and the pin exit wounds are allowed to heal by secondary intention. Intravenous antibiotics are continued for 5 days postoperatively with topical antibiotics at the pin sites.

Within 5 postoperative days, most children are ready for extubation. This correlates with 10 mm of mandibular movement. Oral feeding is introduced under the direction of the occupational therapist. Patients are typically planned for discharge from the hospital once a stable airway is maintained and a feeding regimen determined. Patients are scheduled for device removal after a minimum consolidation period of 2 to 3 months, although this may be delayed in infants with associated cleft palates until the time of palatoplasty. Device removal is considered necessary in skeletally immature individuals so that growth is not restricted by the device. However, no human or animal study to date has addressed this theoretical concern.

PEARLS AND PITFALLS

- Patient selection is critical to success. A complete workup is necessary to first identify the patients who will benefit from this procedure and then optimize surgical planning. The chances of eventually requiring tracheostomy in patients with components of central apnea, neurologic dysfunction, or subglottic areas of obstruction must be discussed with families before intervention.

- Possible complications include malunion, hardware failure, and infection. The enhanced blood supply of the craniofacial skeleton and regenerative ability of the infant make malunion a rare occurrence. The soft quality of neonatal and infant bone and the limited amount of bone available for fixation can lead to hardware failure, which is increased in external devices. This may be diagnosed during the course of distraction as asymmetric advancement of the mandible or little or no resistance encountered during turning of the activation rods. Hardware failure itself increases the chances of infection and may require prolonged antibiotic therapy for treatment of osteomyelitis. CT scan is useful in diagnosis of each of these.

- Facial nerve palsy, manifest as an asymmetric cry or ptosis of eyelids, may be encountered in the immediate postoperative period. The submandibular dissection places the marginal mandibular branch at greatest risk of transaction. Care must be coordinated with the anesthesia team to ensure that paralytic agents are not administered to the patient, which may interfere with use of a nerve stimulator during dissection. For the same reason, local anesthesia must be infiltrated in a subcutaneous plane superficial to the platysma muscle. The most common cause of postoperative palsy however is neuropraxia secondary to retraction necessary for device placement. The family should be reassured that this generally resolves within 6 weeks without treatment.

- Patients with severe mandibular-maxillary discrepancy may require repeated distraction for management of airway or oral rehabilitation. The anatomic classification of the mandibular hypoplasia, condyles, and temporomandibular joint affect the outcome with regard to feeding, speech, and respiration. Postoperative polysomnograms assess the success of the surgery and identify those children still at risk of obstructive apnea and its sequelae.

- Although limited published data indicate that distraction offers improved feeding in a greater number of patients than surgical interventions such as tongue-lip adhesion, nearly all patients require the assistance of feeding therapists for several weeks postoperatively.

BIBLIOGRAPHY

Cohen SR, Simms C, Burstein FD: Mandibular distraction osteogenesis in the treatment of upper airway obstruction in children with craniofacial deformities, *Plast Reconstr Surg* 101:312, 1998.

Denny AD, Talisman R, Hanson PR et al: Mandibular distraction osteogenesis in very young patients to correct airway obstruction, *Plast Reconstr Surg* 108:302, 2001.

Isadi K, Yellon R, Mandell DL et al: Correction of upper airway obstruction in the newborn with internal mandibular distraction osteogenesis, *J Craniofac Surg* 14:493, 2003.

Looby JF, Schendel SA, Lorenz HP et al: Airway analysis: with bilateral distraction of the infant mandible, *J Craniofac Surg* 20:131-146, 2009.

Miller JJ, Kahn DK, Lorenz HP, Schendel SA: Infant mandibular distraction with an internal curvilinear device, *J Craniofac Surg* 18:1403, 2007.

Monasterio F, Molina F, Berlanga F et al: Swallowing disorders in Pierre Robin sequence: its correction by distraction, *J Craniofac Surg* 15:934, 2004.

THE PAST

Infections of the head and neck, especially those of odontogenic origin, are among the oldest conditions treated by our surgical specialty. Despite all interventions many patients have suffered dire consequences. Elimination of infection by removal of the source is an ancient surgical concept; however, the development of local and general anesthesia have facilitated painless surgery. The two basic principles of infection management—establishing drainage and removing the source—received a boost from the discovery of the "wonder drug" penicillin by Alexander Fleming in 1928 (although it was not used until the 1940s). In spite of the monumental discovery of antibiotics, the principal treatment of odontogenic infections remains surgical, and except for historic advances in preventative measures (such as water fluoridation), this is unlikely to change in the foreseeable future. Further identification of the oral microbial flora in parallel with the constant but often lagging discovery of new and improved antibiotics has resulted in an ongoing battle between antimicrobial resistance and microbiologists. The identification of nonbacterial (e.g., viral, fungal) infections affecting the head and neck, especially in the immunocompromised patient, has and continues to challenge our profession.

THE PRESENT

Modern management of oral and maxillofacial infections has mastered the anatomy of the potential spaces of the head and neck along with techniques for effective and safe surgical access. Recognition of a compromised patient and prompt establishment of a secure airway using advanced intubation techniques, such as fiber-optics or tracheostomy, have become essential in severe infections. Developments in anesthesiology intubation techniques, critical care medicine, infectious diseases, and antimicrobial therapy have significantly reduced the complications and fatalities. Improved imaging technology has enhanced our detection and execution of surgical therapy. Despite all advances, infections of the maxillofacial area from odontogenic sources or as a complication of other surgical interventions remain prevalent and comprise a notable part of most surgical practices. Attention to infection control protocols and use of prophylactic antibiotics and other preventive measures have reduced the incidence of infections.

THE FUTURE

Infectious pathogens will remain a worthy "adversary" in the surgical care of the future. The excessive use of antibiotics and the emergence of highly resistant organisms are likely to pose an even greater problem. With the global population explosion, the public health measures will become more challenging. Technology will bring new tools to combat infections that will include improved diagnostic modalities, effective vaccines, less invasive and more rapid culture and sensitivity studies to guide antibiotic therapy, and more selective antimicrobial delivery technology. Laboratory science will develop specific and sensitive tests to diagnose and follow progression of therapy. Surgery will remain an essential tool for treatment of many infections. New imaging technologies, minimally invasive surgical techniques, molecular methods for diagnosis and selection of antibiotics, and new antibacterial and antiviral drugs may improve the available treatments in the future.

Chapter

116

Antimicrobial Treatment of Head and Neck Infections

Thomas R. Flynn

The microbiology of head and neck infections is constantly changing. This continual dynamic evolution of the microflora of oral and head and neck infections is due to rapid genetic change in the microorganisms that cause them. Oral bacteria can reproduce as frequently as every 20 minutes. This rapid genetic turnover affords pathogens the ability to respond quickly to environmental pressures, such as antiseptics and antibiotics. In addition, our understanding of the molecular biology of oral pathogens is progressing at an ever-increasing rate. As a result, the nomenclature of oral pathogens is constantly changing as well. All of these factors necessitate constant study of the microbiology and antimicrobial treatment of head and neck infections.

The rapid ability of bacteria to respond to antibiotic selection pressure enables them to adapt to the therapeutic milieu that we as health care providers establish. For example, increasing penicillin-resistance rates were noted among the oral flora in the decade of the 1990s. This prompted a change from penicillin to clindamycin as the empirical antibiotic of choice for orofacial infections. On the other hand, since 2000 the virtually indiscriminate use of clindamycin may have resulted in increasing numbers of clindamycin-resistant oral streptococci. These same organisms have remained generally penicillin-sensitive. Thus many clinicians believe that in the nonallergic patient, penicillin and amoxicillin have returned to the status of first empirical antibiotics of choice in the treatment of odontogenic infections.

As our experience with new and even older antibiotics continues to mount, we become aware of new complications and the mechanisms of previously recognized complications of antibiotic therapy.

For example, antibiotic-associated colitis has now been associated with the exotoxin elaborated by *Clostridium difficile.* Once the cause of antibiotic-associated colitis was identified, we were able to establish diagnostic and treatment methods for this antibiotic complication. Among the fluoroquinolones, the propensity of moxifloxacin, for example, to prolong the cardiac Q-T interval has limited its usefulness and necessitated an increased awareness of the potential for drug interactions associated with antibiotic therapy. The fluoroquinolones, as a class of drugs, interfere with proper development of growing cartilage. Therefore they are not used in patients younger than 18 years.

Thus all of these considerations require oral and maxillofacial surgeons to remain constantly abreast of new developments in the microbiology and antibiotic therapy of head and neck infections.

ETIOPATHOGENESIS AND CAUSATIVE FACTORS

Most infections of the head and neck are initiated by streptococci and perpetuated by anaerobes. This pattern probably applies to non-odontogenic as well as odontogenic abscess-forming head and neck infections. The streptococci are able to elaborate hyaluronidases that lyse the ground substance of connective tissue, allowing the bacteria to spread through soft tissue planes. Then, these bacteria are able to synthesize nutrients upon which the anaerobic members of the infecting flora depend. Further, the streptococci are able to consume local oxygen supplies, and by their acidic by-products, reduce the pH of the infected site. In this manner, the invading streptococci are able to create a favorable environment for the later growth of obligate anaerobic bacteria. Thus, in the first 3 days of symptoms, a predominantly aerobic or facultative flora is cultivated from head and neck infections. Thereafter, a mixed flora of aerobic or facultative organisms plus anaerobes can be isolated. Once an infection matures and the local oxygen supplies have been consumed, such as within an abscess cavity, a purely anaerobic flora is often identified.

Many of the anaerobic bacteria, however, are able to synthesize penicillinases. This capability allows the anaerobic members of the infecting flora to "return the favor" to the invading species by neutralizing many β-lactam antibiotics, such as penicillin, providing protection for otherwise penicillin-sensitive organisms. This phenomenon has been demonstrated in a recent case series of severe odontogenic infections requiring hospitalization, in which penicillin therapy failed in 21% of patients receiving it and in 60% of the cases in which one or more penicillin-resistant organisms was isolated.[1,2]

The usual pathogens of head and neck infections are listed in Table 116-1. The similarities among the pathogens associated with the various types of head and neck infection lend further credence to the concept that the primary pathogenic agents of head and neck infections are streptococci plus anaerobes. One may add to that list certain respiratory pathogens, such as *Haemophilus influenzae,* and

TABLE 116-1	Major Pathogens of Head and Neck Infections	
TYPE OF INFECTION		**MICROORGANISMS**
Odontogenic cellulitis/abscess		*Streptococcus milleri* group Peptostreptococci *Prevotella* and *Porphyromonas* Fusobacteria
Rhinosinusitis	Acute	*Streptococcus pneumoniae* *Haemophilus influenzae* Head and neck anaerobes (*Peptostreptococcus, Prevotella,* *Porphyromonas, Fusobacterium*) GABHS (group A beta-hemolytic streptococci) *Staphylococcus aureus* *Moraxella catarrhalis* Viruses
	Chronic	Head and neck anaerobes
	Fungal	*Aspergillus* *Rhizopus* spp. (*Mucor*)
	Nosocomial (esp. if intubated)	Enterobacteriaceae (esp. *Pseudomonas, Acinetobacter, Escheria coli*) *Staphylococcus aureus* Yeasts (*Candida* spp.)
Osteomyelitis of the jaws	Acute	Odontogenic flora *Staphylococcus aureus* and skin flora in trauma *Salmonella* in sickle cell disease
	Chronic	*Actinomyces* spp.
Necrotizing fasciitis		Streptococcal (Groups A, C, G) Polymicrobial (aerobes + anaerobes) Clostridial Community-associated MRSA
Fungal	Mucosal or disseminated Soft tissue	*Candida* spp. *Histoplasma* spp. *Blastomyces* sp.
	Sinus	*Aspergillus* *Rhizopus* (*Mucor*)

TABLE 116-2	Clinical Features of Tuberculous versus Nontuberculous Head and Neck Infections	
CLINICAL FEATURE	TUBERCULOUS	NONTUBERCULOUS
Cervical lymphadenitis	Posterior, supraclavicular, multiple, bilateral	Enlarging mass around the mandible
Constitutional symptoms (fever, weight loss, fatigue)	Present	Absent
History of tuberculosis or TB contact	Present	Absent
Sinus formation	High	Low
Age	Adult	Child
Tuberculin skin test (PPD)	Positive	Intermediate or negative
Chest x-ray	Signs of active or previous tuberculosis	Normal

Adapted from Bayazıt YA, Bayazıt N, Namiduru M: Mycobacterial cervical lymphadenitis. ORL J Otorhinolaryngol Relat Spec 66:275-280, 2004.

Staphylococcus aureus for skin-related or nosocomial infection, such as poststernotomy osteomyelitis of the sternum. Necrotizing fasciitis occurs in four types, according to the microbial etiology. In the head and neck, the polymicrobial and the streptococcal types occur most frequently.

Some head and neck infections are caused by pathogens other than bacteria. Of course, there are viral infections such as herpes simplex stomatitis and herpangina. Fungal infections, such as mucormycosis and noma, may also occur in the immunosuppressed or malnourished patient. Mycobacterial infections are divided into tuberculous and nontuberculous types. Table 116-2 lists the comparative diagnostic features of tuberculous and nontuberculous infections of the head and neck. This information may assist the clinician in choosing diagnostic maneuvers for identifying mycobacterial infections.

A new association between syphilis and HIV among men who have sex with men (MSM) may present as orofacial infection. There has been a dramatic increase in syphilis among MSM in the United States in recent years. This spread of syphilis has been facilitated by the misconception that unprotected oral sex is safe, since HIV is not carried in saliva at infective levels. On the other hand, the syphilitic chancre and the mucus patches of secondary syphilis are highly infective with *Treponema pallidum*. The ulcerated lesions of primary and secondary syphilis serve as very effective portals of entry for HIV. In this manner, syphilis may serve as a potentiating cofactor in the spread of HIV infection. An oral chancre is illustrated in Figure 116-1.

PATHOLOGIC ANATOMY

The usual pathogens of head and neck infections are the oral streptococci and anaerobes. Both of these groups are excellent abscess-formers, and when these organisms are introduced deeply into the tissues, such as in a dental periapical infection, the infection tends to pass through the stages of infection. These are inoculation, the spread of bacteria into soft tissue spaces; edema, the initial inflammatory response to bacteria and their by-products; cellulitis, a highly inflamed spreading induration; abscess, characterized by central fluctuance and suppuration; and finally resolution, when spontaneous or surgical drainage is achieved. Further, the infection tends to spread through recognized anatomic compartments, such as bone, fascial spaces, the paranasal sinuses, or vascular structures, especially the valveless head and neck veins. The anatomic presentation of various head and neck infections is presented later, in the chapter on the surgical therapy of head and neck infections.

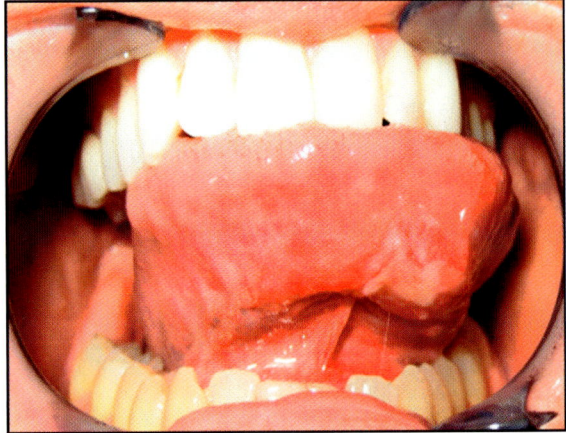

Fig. 116-1 ■ A primary chancre of syphilis on the ventral surface of the tongue. (From Flynn TR, Hunter GJ, Johnson MM. Case records of the Massachusetts General Hospital. Case 6-2010. A 37-year-old man with a lesion on the tongue. N Engl J Med. Feb 25;362:740-748, 2010.)

Other types of head and neck infections, however, also follow characteristic anatomic patterns. For example, viruses and treponemes tend to cause spreading surface mucosal infections, such as herpes and syphilis. The superficial form of necrotizing fasciitis follows the platysma muscle from the inferior border of the mandible down the neck and onto the chest wall. This phenomenon is illustrated in Figure 116-2, which depicts the end result of necrotizing fasciitis, osteomyelitis; and split-thickness skin grafting in a patient with uncontrolled HIV infection, multiple periapical abscesses, and osteomyelitis of the mandible.

Fungal infections tend to follow microvascular patterns. Their propensity to invade and occlude capillaries and other small vascular channels causes the necrosis seen in mucormycosis and other related infections. On the other hand, bacterial infections may occasionally follow the larger vascular pathways. Odontogenic cavernous sinus thrombosis, as illustrated in Figure 116-3, follows recognized venous pathways from the face into the cranium. Small emissary veins that perforate the inner table of the cranium may allow bacteria from chronic sinusitis to pass into the brain, causing brain abscess, as illustrated in Figure 116-4. Sometimes these small emissary veins also allow infection to pass through paper-thin layers of bone from the sinuses into the orbit, as illustrated in Figure 116-5, in which a maxillary and ethmoid sinusitis passed through the lamina papyracea into the orbit, causing orbital subperiosteal abscess.

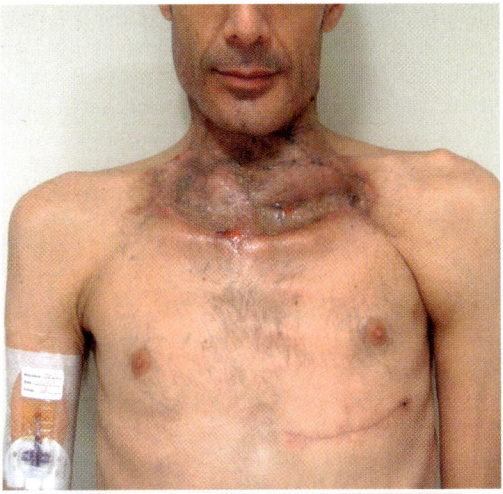

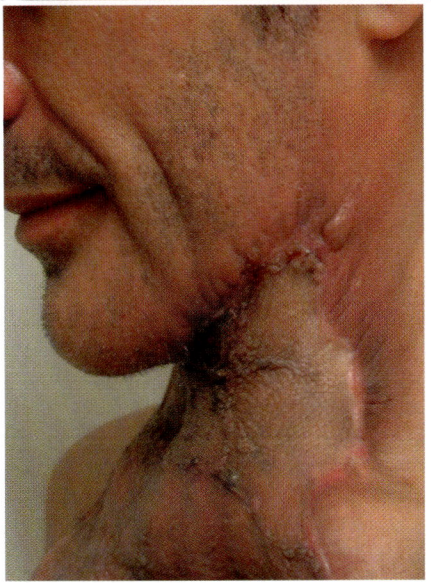

Fig. 116-2 ■ Clinical result of odontogenic abscess, mandibular osteo-myelitis, necrotizing fasciitis, and skin grafting in a 37-year-old male with previously uncontrolled HIV infection.

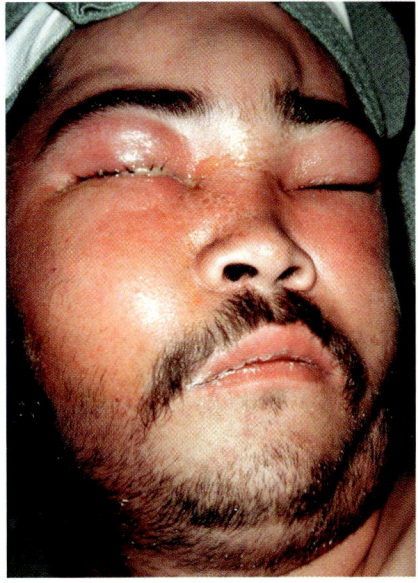

Fig. 116-3 ■ Cavernous sinus thrombosis due to an upper right first molar. (From Flynn TR, Topazian RG: Infections of the oral cavity. In Waite D, editor: Textbook of practical oral and maxillofacial surgery. Philadelphia, 1987, Lea & Febiger.)

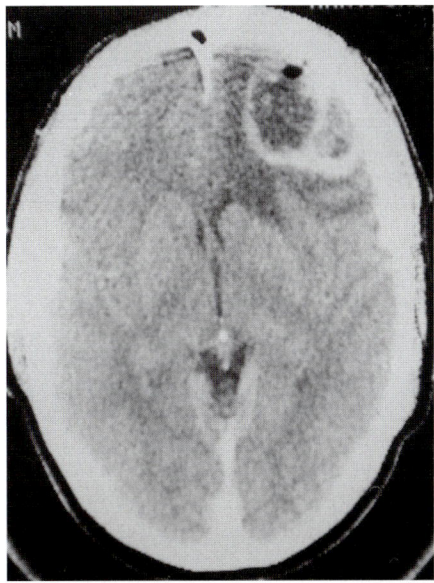

Fig. 116-4 ■ CT of frontal lobe brain abscess caused by nearby frontal sinusitis.

Necrotizing fasciitis may also have a deep anatomic pattern. Cases historically described as descending necrotizing mediastinitis may represent the same process as necrotizing fasciitis, only on a deeper anatomic plane. Rapidly developing cases of mediastinitis, characterized by necrotic tissue found deep in the neck at surgical exploration, may simply be cases of necrotizing fasciitis that have followed the deep fascial planes of the neck into the danger space and from there into the mediastinum.[3]

DIAGNOSTIC STUDIES

The Gram stain is a simple and rapidly available diagnostic test that can quickly identify broad categories of bacteria. This test indicates the ability of the sampled bacteria to bind Gram's iodide stain. The cell morphology and the growth pattern of the bacteria, such as cocci or rods, and distribution in pairs, chains, or clumps can also be observed.

The most widely used and currently dependable method for diagnosing bacterial infections is culture and sensitivity. Since 94% of odontogenic infections contain anaerobic bacteria, it is important for the clinician to identify both aerobic and anaerobic bacteria by using culture swabs for each type. Certain types of swab culture systems, however, are capable of preserving both aerobic and anaerobic bacteria, at least for reasonably brief periods of time. The surgeon should check the expiration date of culture swabs before using them because of their short shelf life.

A major limitation of conventional culture methods is that approximately 60% of the oral flora, for example, are not yet culturable by available methods. Therefore a large proportion of the species found in a given specimen may not be identified. On the other hand, it is reassuring to note that conventional culture methods do seem to yield clinically useful information. Another limitation of conventional culture methods is the time required for identification of fastidious organisms such as the slow-growing oral pathogens.

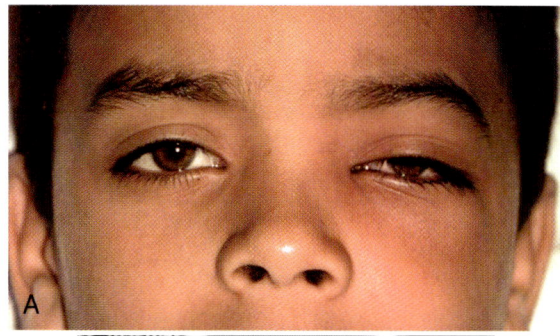

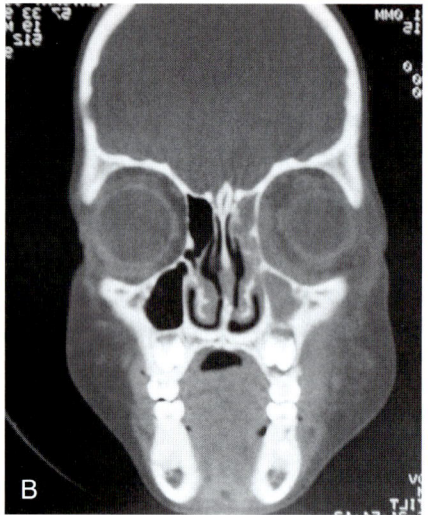

Fig. 116-5 ■ Subperiosteal orbital abscess. **A,** Clinical view. **B,** CT demonstrating left maxillary and ethmoid sinusitis, soft tissue thickening along the left medial orbital wall, and lateral displacement of the globe. (From Simos C, Flynn TR, Piecuch JF, Topazian RG: Infections of the oral cavity. In Feigin RD, Cherry JD, Demmler-Harrison GL, et al, editors: Textbook of pediatric infectious diseases, ed 6. Philadelphia, 2009, Lippincott.)

TABLE 116-3	Indications for Culture and Sensitivity Testing in Head and Neck Infections
INDICATION	**EXAMPLE**
Potentially serious or life-threatening infection	Infection in the masticator, perimandibular, or deep neck spaces
Need for inpatient care	Poorly controlled systemic disease, e.g. diabetes
Immunologic compromise	Cancer chemotherapy
Failed prior treatment	Therapeutic failure of prior course of antibiotic
Recurrent infection	Recurrent osteomyelitis
Hospital-acquired infection	Sinusitis after prolonged intubation

Often, species identification cannot be made until 7 days or more after sampling. By this time, the patient's clinical course has usually either improved or deteriorated dramatically. Antibiotic sensitivity testing may require up to another 7 days in the case of slow-growing organisms. More timely availability of culture and sensitivity results would be most useful to clinicians. Practical clinical indications for culture and sensitivity testing are listed in Table 116-3.

In the future, molecular methods that use the polymerase chain reaction (PCR) to identify infecting pathogens by their genetic content will be used increasingly to speed the availability of culture and sensitivity data. In research studies, molecular methods are able to identify oral pathogens within 1 to 2 days after sampling, and methods that directly identify antibiotic resistance genes are now being developed. Molecular tests are currently available clinically to aid in diagnosis of tuberculosis, HIV, and various head and neck infections.

TREATMENT GOALS

The ideal antibiotic would have a spectrum of coverage specific to the pathogens causing a given clinical manifestation, no toxicity to the host, no liability to bacterial resistance, and low cost. Clearly the currently available antibiotics fail to meet these goals.

For example, the spectrum of imipenem is too broad to be widely useful in head and neck infections, since the gram-negative enteric rods are susceptible to it, in addition to the usual head and neck pathogens. On the other hand, clindamycin has an excellent spectrum, covering the oral streptococci and anaerobes; however, *Eikenella corrodens* is inherently resistant to clindamycin. *E. corrodens* is an occasional pathogen in severe odontogenic infections. Except for potentially fatal allergic reactions, the penicillins are not toxic drugs; whereas the new fourth generation fluoroquinolones, such as moxifloxacin, while providing an excellent spectrum of coverage for head and neck infections, have the liability of many drug interactions involving the cytochrome P450 liver microsomal enzyme system, which can result in fatal cardiac dysrhythmias.

A treatment algorithm for the overall use of antibiotics in oral and maxillofacial surgery is shown in Figure 116-6. The current costs of commonly used antibiotics that are appropriate for head and neck infections are listed in Table 116-4 (oral preparations) and Table 116-5 (intravenous preparations).

Less frequent dosing of intravenous antibiotics offsets the cost of the drug itself. Although the cost per dose of penicillin is much less than that of moxifloxacin, the daily expense for moxifloxacin, given only once per day, is less than half the expense of penicillin, as shown in Table 116-5. Table 116-4 compares the costs of commonly used antibiotics to that of amoxicillin. Table 116-5 compares them to penicillin G and clindamycin.

Antibiotic resistance is a growing problem, even in head and neck infections. Over the decade of the 1990s, several studies demonstrated an increasing incidence of subjects carrying one or more penicillin-resistant strains from 33% in the early 1990s to 54% in 1999. The *Streptococcus milleri* group (*Streptococcus intermedius, S. constellatus,* and *S. anginosus*), which is responsible for abscess-forming odontogenic infections, has developed an increasing rate of resistance to clindamycin, of up to 17% of strains. Clinicians have recently seen significantly more frequent therapeutic failures of clindamycin in the treatment of severe odontogenic infections. Similarly, the widespread use of the cephalosporins has been associated with increasing hospital-acquired infections due to enterococci, which have high resistance to this family of antibiotics.

The enterococci are inhabitants of the oropharynx. They have an unusual ability to pass antibiotic resistance genes to bacteria of other species. Occupying their strategic position at the oropharyngeal entryway to the aerodigestive tract, the enterococci have the potential to dramatically worsen the problem of antibiotic resistance. Vancomycin-resistant enterococci and other highly resistant organisms possessing the ability to pass their antibiotic resistance genes to oropharyngeal pathogens pose a significant threat to the security

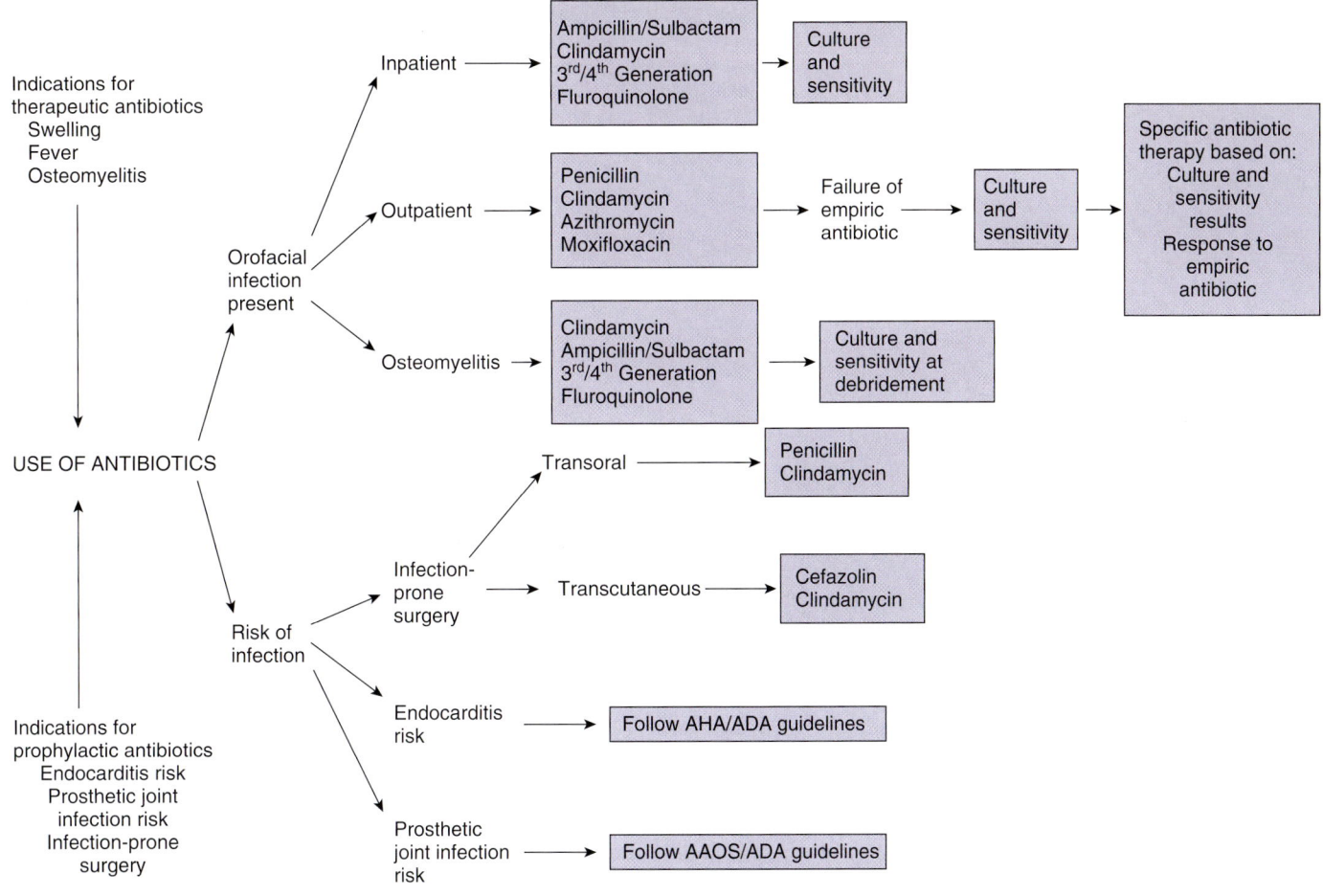

Fig. 116-6 ■ Algorithm for the use of antibiotics in oral and maxillofacial surgery. (Modified from Flynn TR: Use of antibiotics. In Laskin DM, Abubaker AO, editors: Decision making in oral and maxillofacial surgery. Chicago, 2007, Quintessence.)

with which oral and maxillofacial surgeons have customarily prescribed the usual antibiotics of choice for head and neck infections.

The overuse of antibiotics following lax indications, such as the take-home prescription for an antibiotic following the extraction of erupted teeth, is a significant contributor to the problem of antibiotic resistance. Clinicians should be aware that by giving a prescription to a patient they select for antibiotic-resistant organisms, not only in the patient, but also in the patient's family. After a 1-week course of penicillin for strep throat, Brook and colleagues[4] found an increased carriage of penicillin-resistant organisms in the siblings and parents of the pediatric patients. This antibiotic resistance level did not decrease to baseline at 3 months postadministration. Brook and co-workers[5] also found a monthly variation in the carriage of penicillin-resistant organisms among school children in the Washington, D.C., public school system. Following a trough in September, the carriage of penicillin-resistant organisms increased until March, when resistance levels started to decline. This occurred during 2 consecutive years. Apparently, as the winter weather develops, more and more children are given courses of antibiotics for upper respiratory infections. These children then pass antibiotic-resistant strains of bacteria to each other within their school community. By administering a course of antibiotics to patients, we are selecting for the survival of antibiotic-resistant organisms, not only in our patients, but also in their families and in entire communities.

Table 116-6 lists indications and contraindications for antibiotic therapy in oral and maxillofacial surgery practice.

The problem of antibiotic resistance is compounded by the use of massive amounts of antibiotics in animal agriculture. The tonnage of antibiotics found in animal feed dwarfs the amount used for therapeutic purposes in animals and humans. These supplements are used to combat infections caused by the unsanitary conditions and unnatural diets regularly used in industrial methods of raising of food animals for human consumption. The passage of highly resistant bacteria from food animals to humans has recently been documented.

Because of the mounting problem of antibiotic resistance, the American Dental Association (ADA) Council on Scientific Affairs has published a policy on antibiotic use by dentists, which is summarized in Table 116-7. Although the policy does not define simple and complex infections, the surgeon can use the criteria listed in Box 116-1 to differentiate complex from simple infections. The essence of the ADA policy is that broad-spectrum antibiotics as defined in Table 116-7 should be used for complex infections, and narrow-spectrum antibiotics should be used for simple infections. Deviation from the ADA policy may pose a problem unless the clinician is able to document a valid rationale for noncompliance.[6]

The use of prophylactic antibiotics for the prevention of bacterial endocarditis and late prosthetic joint infections (LPJI) is well accepted. On the other hand, significant systematic analyses of the available literature indicate that the evidence supporting even these

TABLE 116-4   **Costs of Oral Antibiotics**

ANTIBIOTIC	USU. DOSE	USU. INTRVL	WHLSALE COST '09*	WHLSALE COST '10*	1 WK RET'L COST '09†	1 WK RET'L COST 10†	AMOXICILLIN COST RATIO
Penicillins							
Amoxicillin	500 mg	8 hr	$0.37	$0.37	$10.99	$11.99	1.00
Penicillin V	500 mg	6 hr	$0.38	$0.74	$12.29	$12.29	1.03
Augmentin	875 mg	12 hr	$5.05	$5.05	$51.99	$51.99	4.34
Augmentin XR	2 g	12 hr	$8.62	$7.38	$137.99	$108.99	9.09
Dicloxacillin	500 mg	6 hr	$1.20	$1.20	$24.99	$25.59	2.13
Cephalosporins (Generation)							
Cephalexin caps (1st)	500 mg	6 hr	$1.38	$1.23	$15.99	$15.19	1.27
Cefadroxil (1st)	500 mg	12 hr	$3.60	$3.60	$49.49	$49.49	4.13
Cefuroxime (2nd)	500 mg	8 hr	$8.02	$8.02	$84.99	$84.99	7.09
Cefaclor ER (generic)	500 mg	12 hr	$3.79	$4.15	$55.59	$64.59	5.39
Cefdinir (3rd)	600 mg	24 hr	$10.23	$10.22	$76.99	$65.59	5.47
Erythromycins							
Erythromycin base	500 mg	6 hr	$0.30	$0.30	$17.29	$17.99	1.50
Clarithromycin (Biaxin XL)	500 mg	24 hr	$4.52	$5.01	$38.39	$34.69	2.89
Azithromycin (Zithromax)	250 mg	12 hr	$7.78	$7.78	$120.99	$120.99	10.09
Telithromycin (Ketek)	800 mg	24 hr	$12.00	$11.52	$106.99	$102.99	8.59
Antianaerobic							
Clindamycin (generic)	150 mg	6 hr	$1.19	$1.19	$31.79	$31.79	2.65
Clindamycin (2 T generic)	300 mg	6 hr	$2.38	$2.38	$59.99	$59.99	5.00
Clindamycin (generic)	300 mg	6 hr	$3.76	$3.76	$87.59	$87.59	7.31
Metronidazole	500 mg	6 hr	$0.73	$0.73	$34.49	$34.49	2.88
Other							
Trimethoprim/sulfameth	160/800 mg	12 hr	$0.91	$0.66	$110.99	$11.99	1.00
Vancomycin	125 mg	6 hr	$21.16	$29.10	$627.99	$849.99	70.89
Ciprofloxacin	500 mg	12 hr	$5.38	$5.31	$13.49	$13.49	1.13
Moxifloxacin (Avelox)	400 mg	24 hr	$17.04	$16.35	$138.99	$138.99	11.59
Doxycycline	100 mg	12 hr	$1.14	$1.14	$10.99	$11.99	1.00
Linezolid (Zyvox)	600 mg	12 hr	$91.24	$91.97	$1,312.99	$1,322.99	110.34

Usual doses and intervals are for moderate infections, and are not to be considered prescriptive.
Amoxicillin cost ratio = Retail cost of antibiotic for 1 wk/retail cost of amoxicillin for 1 wk.
*Source: Wholesale price per pill paid by a large pharmacy chain in the Boston region. Courtesy of Aaron von Dolson, CPHT.
†Retail Cost/1 wk = Retail price charged for a 1 week prescription at a large pharmacy chain in the Boston region. Courtesy of Aaron von Dolson, CPHT.

| TABLE 116-5 | Costs of Intravenous Antibiotics |

ANTIBIOTIC	USUAL DOSE	USUAL INTRVL	PHARMACY COST '08	PHARMACY COST '09*	TOTAL COST 24 HOURS	TOTAL COST FOR 7 DAYS	PENICILLIN G COST RATIO	CLINDA COST RATIO
Penicillins								
Penicillin G	2 m.u.	4 hr	$16.80	$13.19	$103.13	$721.89	1.00	3.39
Ampicillin	1 g	6 hr	$7.38	$7.38	$45.52	$318.64	0.44	1.50
Unasyn	3 g	6 hr	$15.00	$14.40	$73.60	$515.20	0.71	2.42
Oxacillin	2 g	6 hr	$20.11	$20.11	$96.44	$675.08	0.94	3.17
Ticarcillin	3 g	4 hr	$12.38	$12.37	$98.25	$687.72	0.95	3.23
Timentin	3 g	4 hr	$16.00	$16.31	$116.86	$853.02	1.18	4.01
Cephalosporins (Generation)								
Cefazolin (1st)	1 g	8 hr	$2.60	$2.61	$19.83	$138.81	0.19	0.65
Cefotetan (2nd)	1 g	12 hr	$13.50	$13.50	$35.00	$245.00	0.34	1.15
Cefuroxime (2nd)	1.5 g	8 hr	$13.46	$7.08	$33.24	$232.68	0.32	1.09
Ceftazidime (3rd)	2 g	8 hr	$21.00	$28.45	$97.35	$681.45	0.94	3.20
Ceftriaxone (3rd)	1 g	24 hr	$6.60	$6.29	$10.29	$72.03	0.10	0.34
Cefepime (4th)	2 g	12 hr	$36.59	$40.35	$88.70	$620.90	0.86	2.92
Monobactam								
Aztreonam	1 g	8 hr	$30.00	$40.77	$134.31	$940.17	1.30	4.42
Carbapenem								
Imipenem-cilastatin	0.5 g	6 hr	$39.00	$41.25	$181.00	$1,267.00	1.76	5.96
Meropenem	1 g	8 hr	$68.00	$75.91	$239.73	$1,678.11	2.32	7.89
Penicillin-Allergy								
Erythromycin	1 g	6 hr	$16.72	$21.07	$100.28	$701.96	0.97	3.30
Azithromycin	0.5 g	24 hr	$33.00	$19.80	$23.80	$166.60	0.23	0.78
Vancomycin	0.5 g	6 hr	$3.88	$4.42	$33.68	$235.76	0.33	1.11
Vancomycin	1.0 g	12 hr	$7.75	$7.62	$23.24	$162.68	0.23	0.76
Antianaerobic								
Clindamycin	0.9 g	8 hr	$6.24	$6.13	$30.39	$212.73	0.29	1.00
Metronidazole	0.5 g	6 hr	$32.75	$2.56	$26.24	$183.68	0.25	0.86
Other								
Doxycycline	0.1 g	12 hr	$14.75	$14.75	$37.50	$262.50	0.36	1.23
Levofloxacin[†]	750 mg	24 hr	$58.00	$58.16	$62.16	$435.12	0.60	2.05
Moxifloxacin[†]	400 mg	24 hr	$42.00	$42.00	$46.00	$322.00	0.45	1.51
Linezolid	600 mg	12 hr	$82.00	$114.38	$236.76	$1,657.32	2.30	7.79

Total Cost of Therapy includes $1.00 for infusion materials and $3.00 labor cost, per dose
Penicillin Cost Ratio = 24 Hr. Cost of Antibiotic/24 Hr. cost of Penicillin G.
Usual doses and intervals are for moderate infections, and are not to be considered prescriptive.
*Source: 2010 Red Book, Physicians' Desk Reference, Thomson Reuters, Montvale, NJ, 2010 Prices are average wholesale price, generic when available.
[†]Fluoroquinolones IV are for NPO patients only, due to excellent oral absorption.

TABLE 116-6	Indications and Contraindications for Use of Antibiotics

THERAPEUTIC INDICATIONS	PROPHYLACTIC INDICATIONS
Swelling beyond the alveolar process	Endocarditis prophylaxis (follow published guidelines)
Lymphadenopathy	Late prosthetic joint infection prophylaxis (follow published guidelines)
Fever >101° F	Cancer chemotherapy
	Third molar surgery
Osteomyelitis	Poorly controlled diabetes (HbA1c >8)
QUESTIONABLE THERAPEUTIC INDICATIONS	**QUESTIONABLE PROPHYLACTIC INDICATIONS**
Severe pain	Dental implant placement, with or without bone grafting
Patient demand	Periodontal surgery
Patient wishes to postpone definitive treatment	Apicoectomy
Doctor wishes to postpone definitive treatment	Sinus exposure during dental extraction

False Therapeutic Indications

Multiple dental extractions, with or without periapical pathosis, periodontitis

As a substitute for definitive treatment

BOX 116-1	Simple and Complex Infections

Simple Infections
Swelling limited to the alveolar process and/or vestibular space
First attempt at treatment
Nonimmunocompromised patient

Complex Infections
Swelling extending beyond the vestibular space
Failed prior treatment
Immunocompromised patient
Inpatient care necessary

Data from Flynn TR: Principles of management and prevention of odontogenic infections. In Ellis E, Hupp JR, Tucker MR, editors: Contemporary oral and maxillofacial surgery, ed 5. St. Louis, 2008, Mosby, pp 291-315.

indications is weak. Lockhart and colleagues[7] have found convincing evidence to support antibiotic prophylaxis for dental procedures only in the additional case of concurrent or recent cancer chemotherapy. Ren and Malmstrom[8] performed a meta-analysis of antibiotic prophylaxis of wound infection following third molar surgery. Their review found evidence to support the use of a preoperative antibiotic dose for the removal of impacted mandibular third molars

TABLE 116-7	Narrow and Broad Spectrum Antibiotics for Oral Infections

NARROW SPECTRUM ANTIBIOTICS	COMMENT
Penicillin V	For outpatient infections; better aerobic coverage than amoxicillin
Metronidazole	Obligate anaerobes only; effective as a sole antibiotic, however
Clindamycin	For penicillin-allergic patients
Broad Spectrum Antibiotics	
Amoxicillin	Better anaerobic coverage than penicillin V
Amoxicillin/clavulanate	For sinusitis
Cephalexin	Fair-poor anaerobic coverage
Cephradine	Longer duration than cephalexin
Azithromycin	Effective in odontogenic infections
Doxycycline	Many oral flora are now resistant

Data selected from ADA Council on Scientific Affairs: Combating antibiotic resistance, J Am Dent Assoc 135:484-487, 2004.

and weaker evidence of additional benefit obtained by continuing the antibiotic course for up to 4 days postoperatively. Halpern and Dodson[9] found similar supportive evidence in a prospective randomized clinical trial.

SPECIFIC TREATMENT AND TECHNIQUES

The empirical antibiotics of choice for various head and neck infections are listed in Table 116-8. In making this initial antibiotic selection, the clinician must consider multiple factors, including medical history, potential drug interactions, previous antibiotic therapy, and the location and severity of the clinical presentation.

In odontogenic infections, a 3-day course of amoxicillin, combined with the appropriate surgical treatment, was associated with the same excellent outcomes as a 7-day course. Similar results have been found with other antibiotics. Longer courses have not shown additional benefit.[10] These data are consistent with other findings that patient compliance with antibiotic therapy generally lasts for 3 to 4 days and that short courses of antibiotics select for resistant bacteria less than longer courses. In osteomyelitis, the duration of antibiotic therapy is often determined by the normalization of tests that indicate inflammation or bone metabolism. C-reactive protein (CRP) level, erythrocyte sedimentation rate (ESR), and urinary lysylpyridinoline level have been used for this purpose. In actinomycotic osteomyelitis, however, antibiotics may need to be continued for 6 months or more.

The major potential causes for treatment failure in head and neck infections are listed in Table 116-9. The causes of treatment failure related to antibiotic therapy include noncompliance with the prescribed regimen, lack of vascularity or antibiotic distribution to the infected site, decreased antibiotic absorption, incorrect bacterial diagnosis, bacterial resistance to the chosen antibiotic, incorrect choice of empirical antibiotic therapy, and incorrect antibiotic dosage regimen.

TABLE 116-8	Empiric Antibiotics of Choice for Head And Neck Infections

TYPE OF INFECTION		EMPIRICAL ANTIBIOTIC OF CHOICE
Odontogenic Infections		
Outpatient		Amoxicillin
		Clindamycin
		Azithromycin
	Penicillin allergy	Clindamycin
		Azithromycin
		Moxifloxacin (over 18 years of age)
Inpatient		Ampicillin + sulbactam
		Clindamycin
		Ampicillin + metronidazole
	Penicillin allergy	Clindamycin
		Ceftriaxone (avoid in anaphylactic type of PCN allergy)
		Moxifloxacin (over 18 years of age)
		Vancomycin + metronidazole ± moxifloxacin
Rhinosinusitis		
Acute (after failed 7-day trial of antihistamine-decongestant, with persistent facial pain, nasal purulent drainage; if severe may treat sooner)		Amoxicillin
		Amoxicillin/clavulanate
		Cefdinir, cefpodoxime, or cefprozil
		Moxifloxacin (over 18 years of age)
	Penicillin allergy	Clarithromycin or azithromycin
		Telithromycin
		Moxifloxacin (over 18 years of age)
Chronic		Antibiotics not effective: ENT consultation
Intubated		Doripenem, imipenem, or meropenem
		Ticarcillin or piperacillin
		Ceftazidime + vancomycin
		Cefepime + vancomycin
Fungal		Posaconazole
		Amphotericin B
Osteomyelitis of the jaw		Clindamycin
		Ampicillin + sulbactam
		Ampicillin + metronidazole
	Penicillin allergy	Clindamycin
		Moxifloxacin (over 18 years of age)
Histoplasmosis and blastomycosis		Itraconazole
		Fluconazole
		Amphotericin B (systemic or disseminated)
Candidiasis		
Oral, non-AIDS		Nystatin or clotrimazole
		Fluconazole or itraconazole
Oral, AIDS		Fluconazole or itraconazole
		Posaconazole or amphotericin B

Modified from Gilbert DN, Moellering RC Jr, Eliopoulos GM, et al: The Sanford guide to antimicrobial therapy 2010, ed 40. Sperryville, VA, 2010, Antimicrobial Therapy, Inc.

Compliance with antibiotic therapy is a complex problem involving multiple factors that the clinician must take into account when choosing an antibiotic. For example, the cost of a given antibiotic may be prohibitive for certain patients. Therefore a general knowledge of the costs of various antibiotics, as listed in Table 116-4, plus a frank discussion with the patient about those costs can be most helpful in improving compliance. Other factors related to patient compliance include the number of doses per day, unpleasant side effects, and the duration of therapy. In general, decreased

dosage frequency and shorter antibiotic courses improve compliance. Patients will often stop taking an antibiotic soon after they begin to feel better. Selection of antibiotics of equal therapeutic value but with better taste, for example, in the liquid form can also improve compliance. The liquid form of most cephalosporins tastes better than that of the penicillins, and clotrimazole lozenges have better taste than nystatin lozenges.

The success of antibiotic therapy depends upon the ability of a given antibiotic to penetrate the infected site. The vascularity of

TABLE 116-9	Causes of Treatment Failure
CAUSE	EXAMPLE
Inadequate surgery	Undrained loculation of pus
Depressed host defenses	Poorly controlled diabetes
Foreign body	Bone plate, dental implant
Tumor	Squamous cell carcinoma
Obstruction of anatomic drainage	Sialolithiasis, sinusitis
Antibiotic problems	
• Selection	Incorrect choice of empiric antibiotic
• Compliance	Patient cannot afford prescription
• Absorption	Dairy products interfere with fluoroquinolones
• Dosage	Incorrect dosage prescribed
• Allergy	Penicillin allergy
• Toxicity	Antibiotic-associated colitis
Superinfection	Candidiasis following antibiotic prescription
Reinfection	Relapse of actinomycosis

TABLE 116-10	Criteria for Changing Antibiotics
CRITERION	EXAMPLE
Allergy	Hives or rash with penicillin
Toxic reaction	Nausea or vomiting with erythromycin
Postoperative CT demonstrating adequate surgery	All loculations have drains in place
Repeated surgery unsuccessful	Worsening swelling, fever, WBC, C-reactive protein
At least 48 hours of IV antibiotic	Allowing for clinical effect to become evident
At least 72 hours of oral antibiotic	Serum level following oral administration is significantly less than intravenous
Culture and sensitivity report indicating antibiotic resistance	*Eikenella corrodens* cultured from a patient taking clindamycin
Diagnosis of necrotizing fasciitis is made	Broad-spectrum antibiotic therapy indicated until culture reports are received

abscess cavities is much reduced relative to normal tissues. For example, the penetration of clindamycin into abscess cavities is the best of all currently available antibiotics, at 33% of its concentration in the serum. Other antibiotics do not penetrate abscesses as well. Therefore incision and drainage must accompany antibiotic therapy for abscess-causing infections.

Certain antibiotics, such as the fluoroquinolones and linezolid, are equally well absorbed by the oral and intravenous routes. Accordingly, these antibiotics are administered parenterally only when the oral route is unavailable. This property can be used to the patient's advantage, thus preventing the complications of prolonged intravenous antibiotic administration. For example, moxifloxacin can be used orally for osteomyelitis of the jaw. This prevents the complications of prolonged intravenous therapy, such as embolism, thrombophlebitis, catheter dislodgement, and infection. The cost of care is reduced also. In a recent case, the author was able to eliminate the additional risks of narcotic overdose and septic endocarditis by using moxifloxacin to treat osteomyelitis in a patient with concomitant intravenous drug abuse.

The criteria for changing antibiotics are listed in Table 116-10. They include, of course, an allergic or toxic reaction to the drug. The clinician should also allow 2 days of intravenous therapy and 3 days of oral therapy for the clinical effect of a given antibiotic to be evident. If the clinical signs of fever, increased white blood cell count, wound drainage, swelling, induration, and pain continue to worsen after incision and drainage plus antibiotic therapy, the surgeon should evaluate whether the deterioration is due to antibiotic failure or inadequate surgical therapy.

The use of postoperative CT scans has been shown to be effective in eliminating mortality in cases of mediastinitis. In a case series by Freeman and co-workers,[11] the historical mortality of approximately 20% in mediastinitis was reduced to 0% in 10 cases. The therapeutic

approach included the use of postoperative CT scans every 48 to 72 hours, or for clinical deterioration. This diagnostic approach enabled the authors to reestablish dependent drainage, repeatedly debride necrotic tissues, and identify collections of purulent material in previously unsuspected locations.

If, however, postoperative CT indicates adequate surgical drainage, and 48 to 72 hours of antibiotic therapy have proven unsuccessful, the clinician is justified in changing the antibiotic regimen before culture and sensitivity results are available. If these results indicate that an organism resistant to the current antibiotic regimen has been isolated, then the selection of an effective antibiotic is indicated.

Necrotizing fasciitis justifies an empirical change to broad-spectrum antibiotics, because of the polymicrobial nature of this infection and the rapid destruction of large amounts of tissue. Four types of necrotizing fasciitis have been identified: streptococcal (group A, C, or G); clostridial (gas gangrene); polymicrobial (aerobes and anaerobes); and community-acquired MRSA. Odontogenic head and neck necrotizing fasciitis is usually polymicrobial, with streptococci and anaerobes, but especially because staphylococci are frequently isolated in necrotizing fasciitis, broad coverage should be maintained until culture results are received. Currently, a carbapenem (imipenem, meropenem, ertapenem, or doripenem) plus vancomycin are used. In suspected odontogenic or clostridial cases, penicillin plus clindamycin may be used, alternatively or in addition to the carbapenem plus vancomycin.[12]

Finally, the clinician should bear in mind that the bacterial diagnosis, based on culture and sensitivity testing, may change over time. This may be due to an actual change in the infecting flora, or it may be due to the loss of the causative pathogens that were in the previous specimen. Repeat cultures are useful in cases that are failing to respond to appropriate surgical and antimicrobial therapies.

PEARLS AND PITFALLS

- Recently, an increased rate of clindamycin resistance has been identified among the viridans streptococci. In a recent unpublished case series at our hospital, fairly severe and recalcitrant infections have occurred despite the use of clindamycin. Some of these cases were postoperative infections in which clindamycin was used as a prophylactic antibiotic. In fact, some of the postoperative infection cases included patients not allergic to penicillin in whom clindamycin was used prophylactically. Fortunately, in these cases a penicillin was effective. Therefore, at our hospital, the penicillins are used as prophylactic antibiotics in nonallergic patients. Clindamycin is reserved for patients who are allergic to penicillin. Similarly, in severe odontogenic infections requiring hospitalization, ampicillin/sulbactam (Unasyn) has seen increasing use as the empirical antibiotic of choice.

- *Eikenella corrodens* is a pathogen that occasionally causes head and neck infections. This organism is inherently resistant to clindamycin, metronidazole, and the macrolides. It is susceptible to high doses of the penicillins, but its penicillin resistance rate is increasing. The fluoroquinolones, trimethoprim/sulfamethoxazole, second- or third-generation cephalosporins, doxycycline, and imipenem are effective.

- Many infectious disease specialists recommend levofloxacin in odontogenic infections, but moxifloxacin may be preferable among the fluoroquinolones because of its added activity against oral anaerobes.

- Even though the oral and maxillofacial surgeon must continually devote considerable study to the latest developments in the microbiology and antibiotic therapy of head and neck infections, the surgeon must be aware that the primary treatment of abscess-forming head and neck infections is surgical incision and drainage to remove the cause of the infection. Our improved understanding of the role of biofilms in head and neck infections, including odontogenic infections, osteomyelitis, and necrotizing fasciitis underscores the necessity for surgical debridement, removal of the cause of infection, and sometimes repeated debridement and drainage.

- In 1940, Ashbel Williams published a series of 37 cases of Ludwig angina with a mortality rate of 54%. The surgical protocol was incision and drainage only for the identification of a fluctuant abscess and emergency tracheotomy if the airway became threatened. Only 3 years later, in 1943, Dr. Williams and Dr. Walter Guralnick published a series of 20 cases of Ludwig angina in which they had reduced the mortality of this dreaded infection to 10%. This dramatic improvement in mortality occurred before penicillin, the first true antibiotic, became available. This lifesaving advance occurred because of a changed surgical protocol in which the airway was secured by endotracheal intubation or urgent or elective tracheotomy, and all anatomic spaces affected by abscess or cellulitis were aggressively treated early in the course of infection with wide surgical drainage.

- Therefore we as surgeons must maintain that the primary treatment of abscess-forming infections of the head and neck is to establish a secure airway and then aggressively drain all affected anatomic fascial spaces. This is followed by removal of the anatomic cause of infection, such as an infected tooth.[13,14]

REFERENCES

1. Flynn TR, Shanti RM, Levy M, et al: Severe odontogenic infections, part one: prospective report. *J Oral Maxillofac Surg* 64:1093-1103, 2006.

2. Flynn TR, Shanti RM, Hayes C. Severe odontogenic infections, part two: prospective outcomes study. *J Oral Maxillofac Surg* 64:1104-1113, 2006.

3. Flynn TR. Anatomy of oral and maxillofacial infections. In Topazian RG, Goldberg MH, Hupp JR, editors: *Oral and maxillofacial infections*, ed 4. Philadelphia, 2002, Saunders, pp 188-213.

4. Brook I: Emergence and persistence of beta-lactamase-producing bacteria in the oropharynx following penicillin treatment. *Arch Otolaryngol Head Neck Surg* 114:667-670, 1988.

5. Brook I, Gober AE: Monthly changes in the rate of recovery of penicillin-resistant organisms from children. *Pediatr Infect Dis J* 16:255-257, 1997.

6. American Dental Association Council on Scientific Affairs. Combating antibiotic resistance. *J Am Dent Assoc.* 135:484-487, 2004.

7. Lockhart PB, Loven B, Brennan MT, Fox PC: The evidence base for the efficacy of antibiotic prophylaxis in dental practice. *J Am Dent Assoc* 138:458-474, 2007.

8. Ren Y-F, Malmstrom HS: Effectiveness of antibiotic prophylaxis in third molar surgery: A meta-analysis of randomized controlled clinical trials. *J Oral Maxillofac Surg* 65: 1909-1921, 2007.

9. Halpern LR, Dodson TB: Does prophylactic administration of systemic antibiotics prevent postoperative inflammatory complications after third molar surgery? *J Oral Maxillofac Surg* 65:177-185, 2007.

10. Chardin H, Yasukawa K, Nouacer N, et al: Reduced susceptibility to amoxicillin of oral streptococci following amoxicillin exposure. *J Med Microbiol* 58:1092-1097, 2009.

11. Freeman RK, Vallieres E, Verrier ED, et al: Descending necrotizing mediastinitis: an analysis of the effects of serial surgical debridement on patient mortality. *J Thorac Cardiovasc Surg* 119:260-267, 2000.

12. Gilbert DN, Moellering RC, Eliopoulos GM, et al: *The Sanford guide to antimicrobial therapy 2009*, ed 39. Sperryville, VA, 2009, Antimicrobial Therapy.

13. Williams AC: Ludwig's angina. *Surg Gynecol Obstet* 70:140-149, 1940.

14. Williams AC, Guralnick WC: The diagnosis and treatment of Ludwig's angina: a report of twenty cases. *N Engl J Med* 228:443-450, 1943.

Principles and Surgical Management of Head and Neck Infections

Thomas R. Flynn

Thanks to water fluoridation, improved medical and dental care, and the availability of antibiotics the incidence of severe head and neck infections is decreasing. Nonetheless, serious and life threatening infections still occur at unpredictable times. Therefore, the oral and maxillofacial surgeon must remain continually up to date by periodic study of the evolving diagnostic studies, surgical principles, and treatment techniques for infections. Conscientious application of the principles discussed below may not guarantee a favorable outcome of every serious case of head and neck infection that we may encounter; but by using them, surgeons may rest assured that their treatment has met the standard of care.

ETIOPATHOGENESIS—CAUSATIVE FACTORS

In a recent study of severe odontogenic infections, caries and resulting periapical infection was the most frequent predisposing dental disease, most frequently arising in the mandibular posterior teeth. In contrast to other studies, pterygomandibular space infection was diagnosed more frequently than the submandibular space (59% versus 54% of cases). The lateral pharyngeal space was involved in a surprising 43% of cases, by extension from the pterygomandibular space.

Odontogenic and sinus infections tend to cause deeply seated abscesses because they introduce abscess-forming bacteria into deep structures that do not have natural drainage pathways. In the case of sinusitis, for example, the natural drainage pathways can become obstructed due to mucosal edema, thus setting up the cascade of infection, soft tissue edema, tissue necrosis within a closed compartment, resorption of bone, and finally the spread of infection into surrounding soft tissue compartments.

The spread of dental infection from the jaws is determined by the relationship of the tooth apex to the nearby muscle attachments. For example, as shown in Figure 117-1, *A*, periapical infection may pass through the bony cortical plate superior to the attachment of the buccinator muscle to form a buccal space abscess. If the perforation is on the inferior side of the buccinator muscle (Figure 117-1, *B*), then the infection will spread into the vestibular space.

PATHOLOGIC ANATOMY

The deep fascial spaces of the head and neck can be divided into five related groups of spaces as outlined in Table 117-1. The anatomic boundaries and relationships of the individual spaces are described in Tables 117-2 and 117-3.

The subcutaneous space contains all tissues between the skin and the superficial layer of the deep cervical fascia. In the face, this includes the buccal and infraorbital spaces as well. The buccal space lies between the buccinator muscle and the skin. The infraorbital space lies between two heads of the quadratus labii superioris muscle, the levator labii superioris, and the levator anguli oris. It communicates laterally with the buccal space. Infection can pass around the medial or lateral side of the levator labii superioris at the infraorbital rim to enter the periorbital space, another portion of the subcutaneous space. Infection in the infraorbital space may therefore pass freely into the periorbital, buccal, and even the superficial temporal spaces by following the leaflet of the buccal fat pad that rises superiorly into the superficial temporal space. Such an infection is illustrated in Figure 117-2.

The perimandibular spaces were originally described as the submaxillary space by Grodinsky and Holyoke. Infectious involvement of all the perimandibular spaces (submandibular, submental, and sublingual) has been termed Ludwig's angina. Infection in one of the perimandibular spaces may rapidly spread into the others by passing around the muscles that divide these spaces. In Figure 117-3, the left submandibular space infection in this patient has spread around the anterior belly of the digastric muscle to involve the submental space.

The masticator space was originally described as a unitary compartment. Clinically, however, infections usually involve only one of its four components (submasseteric, pterygomandibular, superficial temporal, deep temporal.) Nonetheless, the masticator space, taken as a whole, was the most frequently involved deep fascial space in a recent study, at 78% of cases.

A clinical photograph of an infection involving each of these components, along with a corresponding CT image of infection in that component is seen in Figures 117-4 to 117-6.

The deep neck spaces (lateral pharyngeal, retropharyngeal, and pretracheal) were described as Space 3 by Grodinsky and Holyoke. These potential anatomic spaces lie superficial to the visceral division of the middle layer of the deep cervical fascia. The visceral division of this fascia surrounds the trachea, esophagus, and thyroid gland inferior to the hyoid bone, as shown in Figure 117-7. Superior to the hyoid bone, the visceral division is known as buccopharyngeal fascia. This fascial layer lies on the superficial (skin) side of the pharyngeal constrictor muscles. The fascial layers defining the lateral pharyngeal space are illustrated in Figure 117-8.

The lateral pharyngeal space lies between the buccopharyngeal fascia and the medial pterygoid muscle. In this region, the aponeurosis of Zuckerkandl and Testut separates the lateral pharyngeal space into anterior and posterior compartments. The anterior compartment contains only areolar connective tissue, and can be safely drained intraorally. The posterior compartment contains the carotid sheath, and its lateral border is the parotid gland. The inferior extent of the lateral pharyngeal space is at the hyoid bone, where swelling may be externally visible.

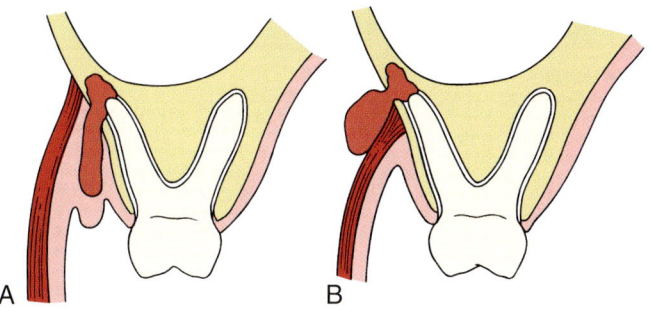

Fig. 117-1 ■ **A,** A periapical infection that has eroded through the lateral cortical plate of the maxilla superior to the attachment of the buccinator muscle, causing a buccal space infection. **B,** A similar infection that has eroded through the lateral cortical plate inferior to the attachment of the buccinator, causing a vestibular space infection. (From Hupp JR, Ellis E, Tucker MR: Contemporary oral and maxillofacial surgery, ed 5. St. Louis, 2008, Mosby.)

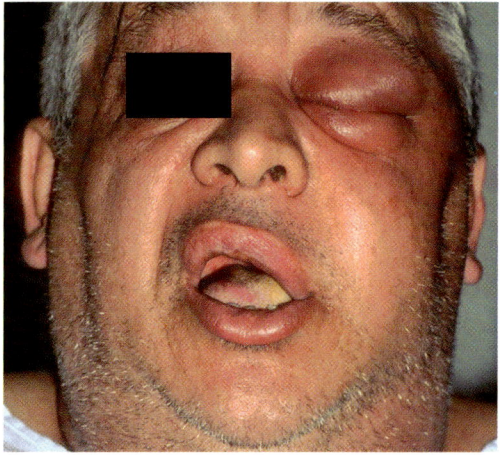

Fig. 117-2 ■ A buccal space infection that has followed the extensions of the buccal fat pad into the infraorbital, periorbital, and superficial temporal spaces. (From Flynn TR: Surgical management of orofacial infections. Atlas Oral Maxillofac Surg Clin North Am 8:77, 2000.)

TABLE 117-1	Related Groups of the Deep Fascial Spaces of the Head and Neck
GROUP OF SPACES	**COMPONENT SPACES**
Subcutaneous	Subcutaneous Infraorbital Buccal
Perioral	Vestibular Space of the body of the mandible Palatal
Perimandibular	Submandibular Sublingual Submental
Masticator	Submasseteric Pterygomandibular Superficial temporal Deep temporal (including infratemporal)
Deep neck spaces	Lateral pharyngeal (parapharyngeal) Retropharyngeal Pretracheal
Mediastinal	Danger space Superior mediastinum Anterior mediastinum Middle mediastinum Posterior mediastinum

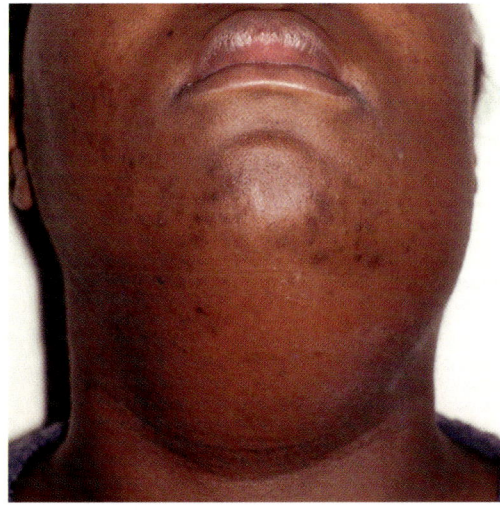

Fig. 117-3 ■ A left submandibular space infection that has passed around the anterior belly of the digastric muscle to involve the submental space. (From Flynn TR: Surgical management of orofacial infections. Atlas Oral Maxillofac Surg Clin North Am 8:77, 2000.)

The retropharyngeal space lies between the buccopharyngeal (above the hyoid bone) or retropharyngeal fascia (below the hyoid bone) and the alar fascia, as shown in Figure 117-9. The retropharyngeal fascia fuses with the alar fascia at a variable level between the 6th cervical and 4th thoracic vertebrae, forming the bottom of the retropharyngeal space. When an infectious process contacts this anatomic barrier, it may rupture through the alar fascia and enter the danger space.

The pretracheal space is not frequently involved in head and neck infections. It is the potential space between the trachea and the thyroid gland and the more superficial cervical strap muscles. It communicates laterally with the retropharyngeal space between the inferior thyroid artery and the thyroid cartilage. Importantly, however, the inferior portion of the pretracheal space communicates

with the superior mediastinum, and below that the anterior mediastinum.

Head and neck infections can also spread via vascular channels, especially the valveless veins of the head and neck. Septic thrombophlebitis may thus ascend into the dural venous sinuses counter to the normal flow pattern. Cavernous sinus thrombosis may rarely arise from infection in facial and neck veins. The anterior route involves the angular vein, passing through the infraorbital space, or the ophthalmic veins in orbital infections. Odontogenic or maxillary sinus infections may enter the angular vein in the face, and ethmoid sinus infections may pass through the lamina papyracea on the medial wall of the orbit to enter one of the ophthalmic veins. From there, infectious thrombophlebitis can follow the ophthalmic vein through the superior orbital fissure into the cavernous sinus.

The posterior route to the cavernous sinus involves the posterior facial vein, possibly due to buccal or infratemporal space infection. The posterior facial vein drains into the pterygoid plexus, from which emissary veins pass through the foramina of Vesalius, ovale,

TABLE 117-2	Borders of the Deep Spaces of the Head and Neck					
	BORDERS					
SPACE	**ANTERIOR**	**POSTERIOR**	**SUPERIOR**	**INFERIOR**	**SUPERFICIAL OR MEDIAL***	**DEEP OR LATERAL[†]**
Buccal	Corner of mouth	Masseter m Pterygomandibular Sp.	Maxilla Infraorbital Space	Mandible	Subcutaneous tissue and skin	Buccinator m
Infraorbital	Nasal cartilages	Buccal space	Quadratus labii superioris m	Oral mucosa	Quadratus labii superioris m	Levator anguli oris m Maxilla
Submandibular	Ant belly digastric m	Post. belly digastric m. Stylohyoid m Stylopharyngeus m.	Inf. and medial surfaces of mandible	Digastric tendon	Platysma m, Investing fascia	Mylohyoid Hyoglossus sup constrictor muscles
Submental	Inf border of mandible	Hyoid bone	Mylohyoid m	Investing fascia	Investing fascia	Ant bellies digastric mm.[†]
Sublingual	Lingual surface of mandible	Submandibular space	Oral mucosa	Mylohyoid m	Muscles of tongue*	Lingual surface of mandible[†]
Pterygomandibular	Buccal space	Parotid gland	Lateral pterygoid m	Inf border of mandible	Med pterygoid muscle*	Ascending ramus of mandible[†]
Submasseteric	Buccal space	Parotid gland	Zygomatic arch	Inf. border of mandible	Ascending ramus of mandible*	Masseter m[†]
Lateral pharyngeal	Sup and mid pharyngeal constrictor mm	Carotid sheath and scalene fascia	Skull base	Hyoid bone	Pharyngeal constrictors and retropharyngeal space	Medial pterygoid m[†]
Retropharyngeal	Sup and mid pharyngeal constrictor mm	Alar fascia	Skull base	Fusion of alar and prevertebral fasciae at C6-T4		Carotid sheath and lateral pharyngeal space[†]
Pretracheal	Sternothyroid-thyrohyoid fascia	Retropharyngeal space	Thyroid cartilage	Superior mediastinum	Sternothyroid-thyrohyoid fascia	Visceral fascia over trachea and thyroid gland

Ant, Anterior; *Inf,* inferior; *Lat,* lateral; *m,* muscle; *Med,* medial; *mm,* muscles; *Post,* posterior; *Sp,* space; *Sup,* superior.
*Lateral border.
[†]Medial border.
From Flynn TR, Topazian RG: Infections of the oral cavity. In Waite D, editor: Textbook of practical oral and maxillofacial surgery. Philadelphia, 1987, Lea & Febiger.

and lacerum to join the inferior petrosal sinus and then the cavernous sinus.

Recently, Lemierre syndrome has been described as a cause of cavernous sinus thrombosis via the internal jugular vein, which drains the inferior petrosal sinus. Lemierre syndrome is a septic thrombophlebitis of the internal jugular vein, usually resulting from peritonsillar infection. Odontogenic infection may also cause Lemierre syndrome by involvement of the lateral pharyngeal space. The usual presentation of Lemierre syndrome is due to septic emboli that follow the usual flow pattern to the heart, where they are distributed to the lungs, liver, bone, and joints, causing metastatic abscesses. *Fusobacterium necrophorum* is the most frequently identified pathogen. More recently, however, other bacteria, especially of the genus *Fusobacterium,* have been associated with this condition. Anticoagulation and appropriate surgical therapy are used.

Although dental infections have been implicated in central nervous system (CNS) infections, such as cavernous sinus thrombosis and brain abscess, the majority of CNS infections arise from the paranasal sinuses. The most frequent cause of cavernous sinus thrombosis is sphenoid sinusitis, via emissary veins that perforate the thin layer of bone separating these two structures. In similar fashion, most brain abscesses are caused by infection of the paranasal air cavities lying directly opposite the site of brain abscess.

DIAGNOSTIC STUDIES

Contrast-enhanced CT (CECT) is the preferred method for identification of and delineation of the anatomic spread of severe deep fascial space infections. Although CT may not be necessary when infection involves only the more superficial spaces, infection involving the deeper structures can be significantly more difficult to delineate using clinical methods alone. CECT demonstrates the hypervascular capsule that may surround a well-established abscess

TABLE 117-3	Relations of Deep Spaces in Infections			
SPACE	**LIKELY CAUSES**	**CONTENTS**	**NEIGHBORING SPACES**	**APPROACH FOR I & D**
Buccal	Upper bicuspids Upper molars Lower bicuspids	Parotid duct Ant. facial a. and v. Transverse facial artery & vein Buccal fat pad	Infraorbital Pterygomandibular Infratemporal	Intraoral (small) Extraoral (large)
Infraorbital	Upper cuspid	Angular a. and v. Infraorbital n.	Buccal	Intraoral
Submandibular	Lower molars	Submandibular gland Facial a. and v. Lymph nodes	Sublingual Submental Lateral pharyngeal Buccal	Extraoral
Submental	Lower anteriors Fracture of symphysis	Ant. jugular v. Lymph nodes	Submandibular (on either side)	Extraoral
Sublingual	Lower bicuspids Lower molars Direct trauma	Sublingual glands Wharton's ducts Lingual n. Sublingual a. and v.	Submandibular Lateral pharyngeal Visceral (trachea and esophagus)	Intraoral Intraoral-extraoral
Pterygomandibular	Lower 3rd molars Fracture of angle of mandible	Mandibular div. of trigeminal n. Inf. alveolar a. and v.	Buccal Lateral pharyngeal Submasseteric Deep temporal Parotid Peritonsillar	Intraoral Intraoral-extraoral
Submasseteric	Lower 3rd molars Fracture of angle of mandible	Masseteric a. and v.	Buccal Pterygomandibular Superficial temporal Parotid	Intraoral Intraoral-extraoral
Infratemporal & deep temporal	Upper molars	Pterygoid plexus Int. max. a. and v. Mand. div. of trigeminal n. Skull base foramina	Buccal Superf. temporal Inf. petrosal sinus	Intraoral Extraoral Intraoral-extraoral
Superficial temporal	Upper molars Lower molars	Temporal fat pad Temporal branch of facial n.	Buccal Deep temporal	Intraoral Extraoral Intraoral-extraoral
Lateral pharyngeal	Lower third molars Tonsils Infection in neighboring spaces	Carotid a. Internal jugular v. Vagus n. Cervical sympathetic chain	Pterygomandibular Submandibular Sublingual Peritonsillar Retropharyngeal	Intraoral Intraoral-extraoral

Ant, Anterior; *Inf*, inferior; *Int*, internal; *Superf*, superficial; *a*, artery; *v.*, vein; *n.* nerve; *div.*, division; *max.*, maxillary; *mand*, mandibular.
From Flynn TR, Topazian RG: Infections of the oral cavity. In Waite D, editor: Textbook of practical oral and maxillofacial surgery. Philadelphia, 1987, Lea & Febiger.

cavity, seen as ring enhancement. The combination of CECT and experienced clinical examination was able to identify clinically significant loculations of pus in the head and neck in 85% of cases.

Magnetic resonance imaging (MRI) has also been used for the diagnosis of deep fascial space infections. However, since head and neck infections commonly involve bone and dental structures, the superiority of CT in imaging hard tissues has made it the more versatile and clinically useful examination.

Radionuclide scans using technetium, gallium, and indium-tagged white blood cells have been used to identify deep infections, especially osteomyelitis. Technetium tends to accumulate in bone that has an increased metabolic rate. Gallium selectively collects in inflammatory cells, thus identifying inflamed areas. Similarly indium-tagged white blood cells tend to accumulate in areas of

abscess and infection. However, the diagnostic utility of bone scanning in the identification of osteomyelitis has been limited by the lack of specificity. For example, technetium may accumulate in hypermetabolic areas of bone that are not infected, such as healing fractures and sites of tooth extraction. Similarly, gallium and indium-tagged white blood cells accumulate in areas of inflammation, but not necessarily infection. Bone scans generally remain positive for at least 1 year following surgical or traumatic insult, often confounding the diagnosis.

Ultrasound, especially color-enhanced Doppler ultrasound, has been used to identify abscesses clinically. Ultrasound, however, is most useful in superficial infections, which are also readily identified by clinical examination. Thus CECT remains the most useful diagnostic tool in deeply seated infections of the head and neck.

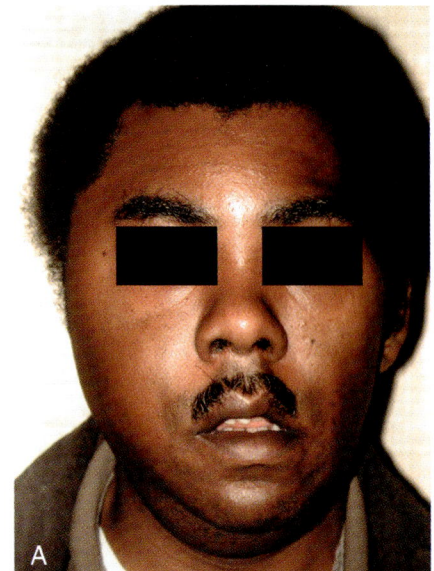

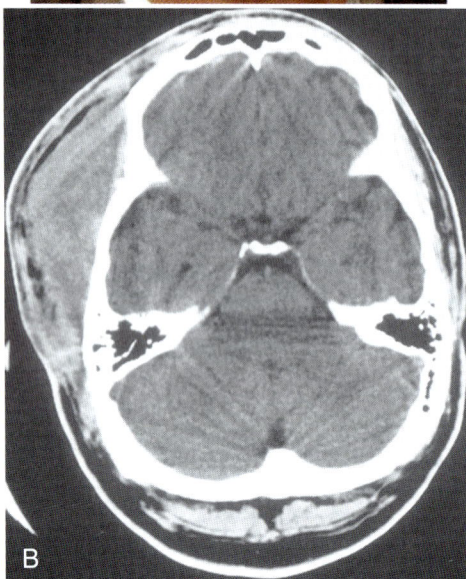

Fig. 117-4 ▪ **A,** Infection involving all of the components of the right masticator space, of 60 days' duration. **B,** CT of the right temporal space abscess in this patient, from which 60 mL of pus was aspirated. (**A** from Flynn TR: The swollen face. Emerg Med Clin North Am 15:481, 2000. **B** from Flynn TR: Anatomy of oral and maxillofacial infections. In Topazian RG, Goldberg MH, Hupp JR, editors: Oral and maxillofacial infections, ed 4. Philadelphia, 2002, Saunders.)

TREATMENT AND RECONSTRUCTIVE GOALS

The eight steps to guide treatment of severe odontogenic infections are listed in Box 117-1.

The first three steps, to determine the severity of the infection, to evaluate host defenses, and to decide upon the treatment setting, can be accomplished within the first 5 minutes of the initial patient encounter.

The severity of infection is determined by its location and rate of progression. Infection in the various deep fascial spaces can be classified as low, moderate, and high severity, as outlined in Box 117-2. Low severity infections, such as those involving the

BOX 117-1	Eight Steps in the Management of Severe Head and Neck Infections
1	Determine severity
2	Evaluate host defenses
3	Decide: Inpatient vs. outpatient
4	Treat surgically
5	Support medically
6	Choose antibiotic appropriately
7	Administer antibiotic appropriately
8	Reevaluate frequently

BOX 117-2	Severity of Deep Fascial Space Infections
Severity	**Anatomic Space**
Low	Vestibular
	Palatal
	Space of the body of the mandible
	Infraorbital
	Buccal
	Subcutaneous
Moderate	Submandibular
	Submental
	Sublingual
	Pterygomandibular
	Submasseteric
	Superficial temporal
	Deep temporal (or infratemporal)
High	Lateral pharyngeal
	Retropharyngeal
	Pretracheal
Extreme	Danger space
	Mediastinum
	Intracranial infection

vestibular and subcutaneous spaces, have low potential of threatening the airway or vital structures. Usually these infections can be treated on an outpatient basis, barring significant comorbidities. Moderate severity infections have the potential to hinder access to the airway, making endotracheal intubation difficult. For example, masticator space infections cause trismus, due to inflammation in the muscles of mastication. Perimandibular infections can elevate the tongue and cause swelling of the epiglottis, hindering intubation. High severity infections have the potential to directly compress or deviate the airway, or to damage vital structures such as the brain and the heart. For example, the child in Figure 117-10 has a lateral pharyngeal space infection on the left, which is deviating the trachea toward the right. In order to straighten his airway, this young patient has repositioned his head toward the right shoulder. The CT scan in Figure 117-11 demonstrates how a lateral and retropharyngeal space infection has deviated and effaced the airway.

A rapidly progressing infection, such as the one illustrated in Figure 117-12, can create a surgical emergency. The right infraorbital and periorbital swelling has extended during 4 hours to involve the opposite eye, the forehead, and the right deep temporal space. In addition, dilation of the retinal veins on the left side has elicited

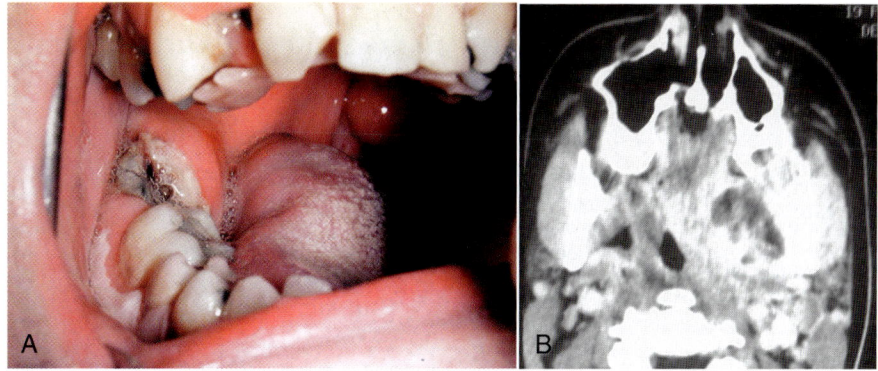

Fig. 117-5 ■ **A,** Pterygomandibular space infection due to an infected fracture of the mandible involving a partially erupted and carious right lower third molar. Note the deviation of the uvula to the opposite side and the swelling of the right anterior tonsillar pillar. **B,** CT of a pterygoman-dibular space abscess, with a collection of fluid lying between the ascending ramus of the mandible and the medially displaced medial pterygoid muscle. (**A** from Flynn TR, Topazian RG: Infections of the oral cavity. In Waite D, editor: Textbook of practical oral and maxillofacial surgery. Philadelphia, 1987, Lea & Febiger. **B** from Flynn TR: The swollen face. Severe odontogenic infections. Emerg Med Clin North Am 15:481, 2000.)

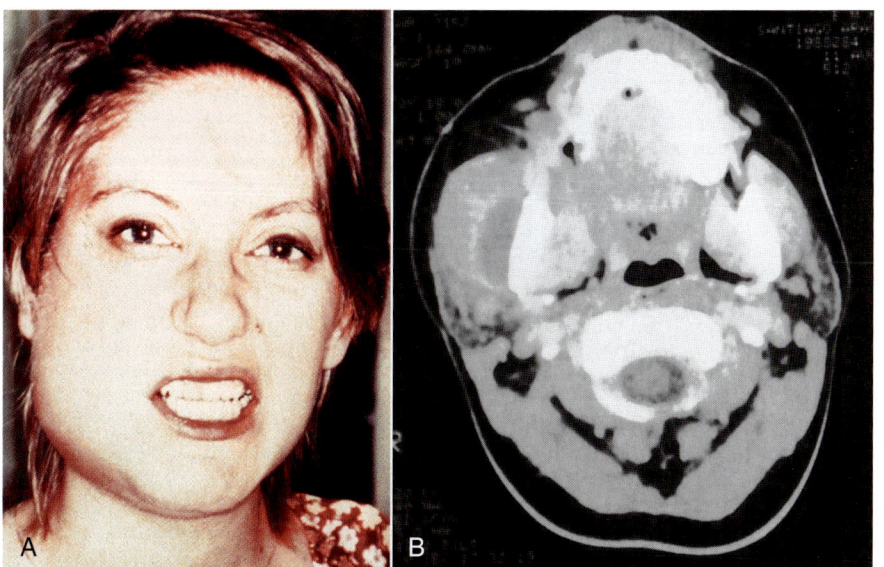

Fig. 117-6 ■ **A,** A submasseteric space infection, causing swelling over the right mandibular ascending ramus and severe trismus. **B,** CT of a submasseteric space abscess, with a collection of pus lying between the ascending ramus of the mandible and the overlying edematous masseter muscle. (**A** from Goldberg MH: Odontogenic infections. In Topazian RG, Goldberg MH, Hupp JR, editors: Oral and maxillofacial infections, ed 4. Philadelphia, 2002, Saunders. **B** from Flynn TR: Anatomy of oral and maxillofacial infections. In Topazian RG, Goldberg MH, Hupp JR, editors: Oral and maxillofacial infections, ed 4. Philadelphia, 2002, Saunders.)

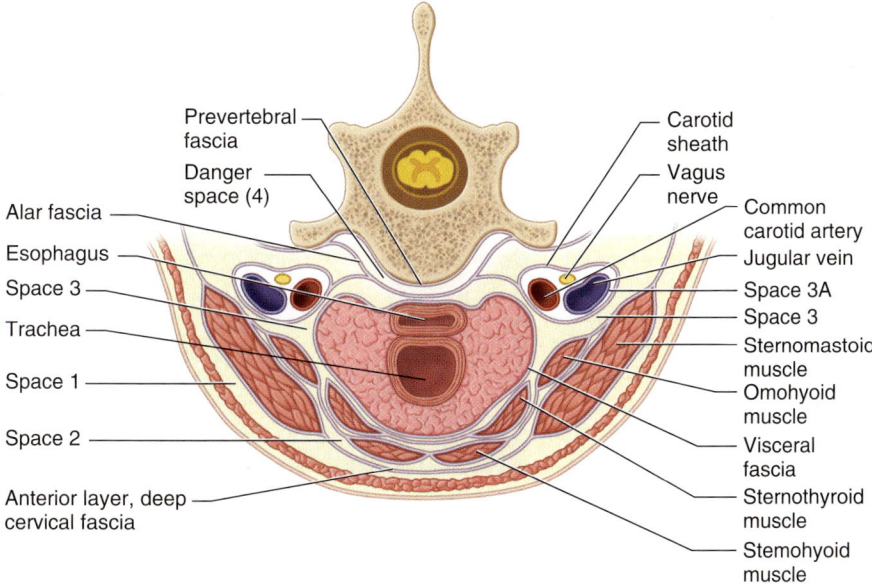

Fig. 117-7 ■ Axial section of the neck at the level of the 6th cervical vertebra illustrating the pretracheal and retropharyngeal spaces, lying just superficial to the visceral division of the middle layer of the deep cervical fascia, which encircles the trachea, esophagus, and thyroid gland. The numbered spaces of Grodinsky and Holyoke are also shown.

Fig. 117-8 ■ Oblique section through the ascending ramus of the mandible illustrating the anterior and posterior compartments of the lateral pharyngeal space, separated by the aponeurosis of Zuckerkandl and Testut. (From Flynn TR: Anatomy and surgery of deep fascial space infections. In Kelly JJ, editor: *Oral and maxillofacial surgery knowledge update 1994.* Rosemont, IL, 1994, American Association of Oral and Maxillofacial Surgeons.)

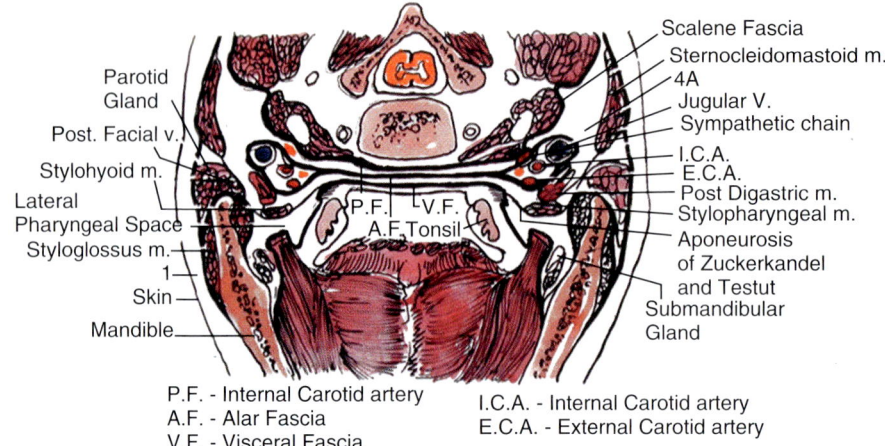

P.F. - Internal Carotid artery
A.F. - Alar Fascia
V.F. - Visceral Fascia

I.C.A. - Internal Carotid artery
E.C.A. - External Carotid artery

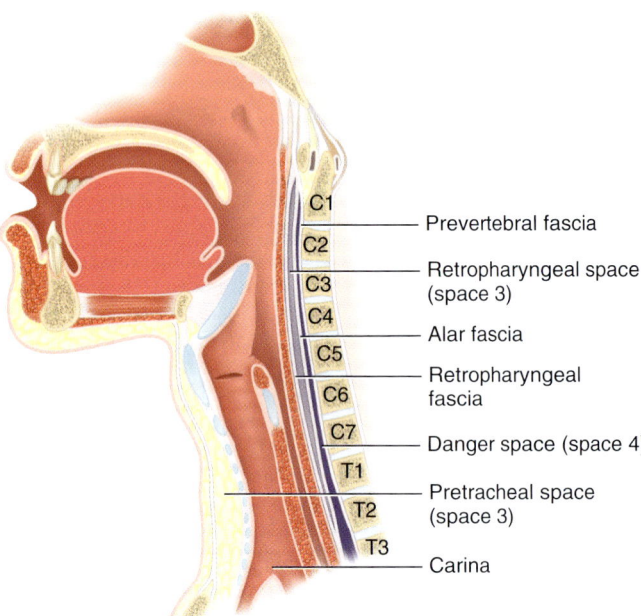

Fig. 117-9 ■ Sagittal section of the neck illustrating the light blue retropharyngeal space lying between the visceral division of the middle layer of the deep cervical fascia (called the retropharyngeal fascia in this location) and the alar fascia. These two layers fuse at a level between the 6th cervical and 4th thoracic vertebrae to form the bottom of the retropharyngeal space.

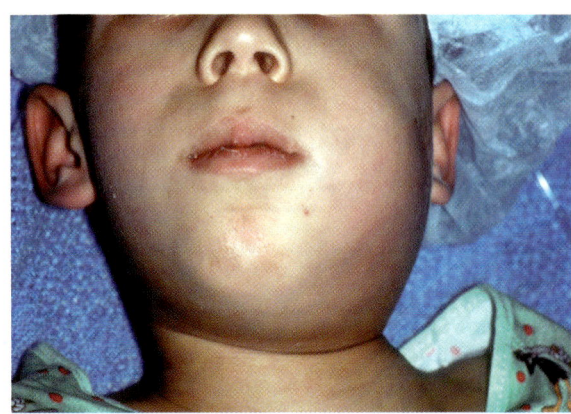

Fig. 117-10 ■ A child with left buccal, submandibular, and lateral pharyngeal space infection. Note that the head is deviated to the opposite side to position the upper airway over the laterally deviated trachea. (From Simos C, Flynn TR, Piecuch JF, Topazian RG: Infections of the oral cavity. In Feigin RD, Cherry JD, Demmler-Harrison GL, et al, editors: Textbook of pediatric infectious diseases, ed 6. Philadelphia, 2009, Saunders.)

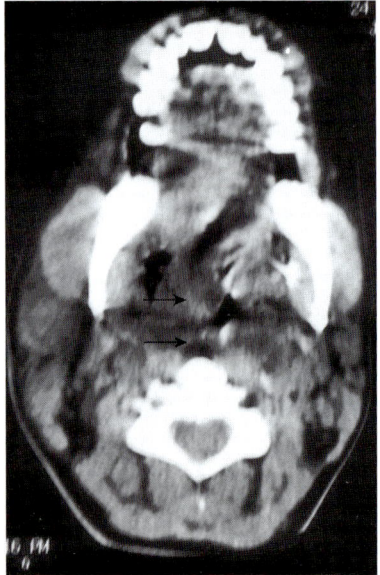

Fig. 117-11 ■ CT of the neck demonstrating lateral and anterior displacement of the airway by the mass effect of a lateral and retropharyngeal space infection (*arrows*). (From Flynn TR: The swollen face. Emerg Med Clin North Am 15:481, 2000.)

the first clinical sign of cavernous sinus thrombosis. Obstruction of the venous outflow of the retinal veins on the unaffected side occurs early in cavernous sinus thrombosis, because the right and left cavernous sinuses have multiple venous interconnections across the midline. On the other hand, the patient shown in Figure 117-4 has a history of 60 days of right facial swelling. Although the swelling is large, his infection has clearly not followed a fulminant course.

Evaluation of host defenses is accomplished primarily by carefully taking a history. Box 117-3 lists the most common immunocompromising diseases. Of special concern is diabetes. Recently the common use of the hemoglobin A1C test has afforded an easily quantifiable method for assessing diabetes control. A hemoglobin A1C level of 7 or lower indicates good control of diabetes; levels of 9 or greater indicate poor control.

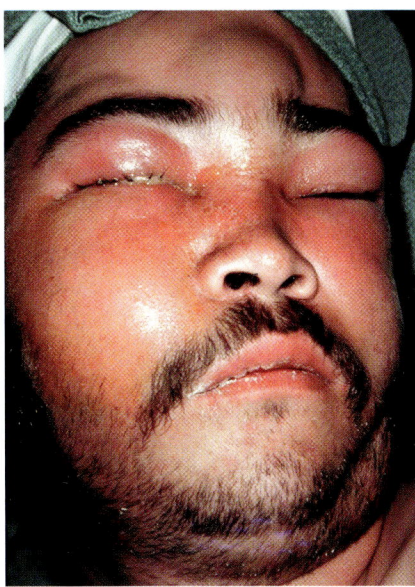

Fig. 117-12 ■ A patient with a 3-day-old right buccal, infraorbital, and periorbital swelling due to an upper right first molar. The swelling has extended to the opposite periorbital space, the forehead, and the deep temporal space via the buccal and infratemporal spaces. The cavernous sinus is also involved. (From Flynn TR, Topazian RG: Infections of the oral cavity. In Waite D, editor: Textbook of practical oral and maxillofacial surgery. Philadelphia, 1987, Lea & Febiger.)

BOX 117-3   Immunocompromising Diseases

- Diabetes
- Steroid therapy
- Organ transplants
- End-stage renal disease
- Malignancy
- Chemotherapy
- Malnutrition
- Alcoholism
- End-stage AIDS

BOX 117-4   Indications for Hospitalization

- T >101° F
- Dehydration
- Impending airway compromise or threat to vital structures
- Infection of deep neck spaces or masticator space
- Need for general anesthesia
- Need for inpatient control of systemic disease

The surgeon is wise also to evaluate the patient's systemic reserve. For example, subclinical levels of heart disease in the elderly patient may diminish cardiac reserve, reducing the physiologic tolerance to fever and the stresses of general anesthesia and surgery. Therefore the level of control of cardiac, respiratory, and metabolic diseases should be considered in the decision for or against hospital admission.

The fourth step is to determine the setting of care: inpatient or outpatient. The indications for hospitalization of the patient with head and neck infection are listed in Box 117-4. In uncertain cases, it is wise to err on the side of inpatient care for the infected patient, since continuous airway monitoring, advanced imaging techniques, and consultation with other specialists are available.

The fifth step in the treatment of severe odontogenic infections is to perform the appropriate surgery. The surgical goals in head and neck infections are to secure the airway, to establish dependent drainage and to remove the cause of infection, such as a carious tooth. Incision and drainage decreases the bacterial load the immune system must confront by physically removing pus. In addition, the dead space of the abscess cavity is collapsed, enhancing vascular flow to the region, at least partially by reducing the pressure exerted by the expanding abscess cavity against surrounding tissue. Removal of the cause of infection also reduces the load of necrotic tissue and eliminates the substrate for continued bacterial growth and invasion of surrounding tissues, especially in biofilm-mediated infections, such as odontogenic infections, osteomyelitis, and osteonecrosis.

Step six is to support the patient medically. This includes reestablishing adequate nutrition as soon as possible. Other supportive measures include rehydration and control of systemic diseases, such as diabetes, hypertension, and cardiac and pulmonary disease. Often, medical consultation is indicated in this regard.

The two steps that deal with antibiotic therapy are discussed fully in the previous chapter. The reader is referred to Table 116-8 in that chapter, which lists the empiric antibiotics of choice for given head and neck infections.

The final step in the treatment of severe head and neck infections is frequent reevaluation. For outpatients, the appropriate follow-up period is from 1 to 4 days, depending upon the severity of the infection. Most are seen on the second day following surgical treatment, as long as the patient does not notice any symptomatic deterioration. At 2 days, the improvement is usually marked and obvious, and the surgical drain can be removed. Barring unforeseen complications, a final follow-up visit can occur 5 to 7 days following drain removal.

For hospitalized patients, daily follow up is the general rule. The progress of the infection is monitored by temperature, white blood cell count, dysphagia, and dyspnea. On palpation, the infected site should be softening and decreasing in size by 2 to 3 days following surgery.

Failure of improvement in any of these parameters may justify a postoperative CT scan to verify proper drain placement or to detect a spreading infection or undrained abscess. Failure to improve clinically despite adequate surgical drainage as documented by postoperative CT is an indication to change the current antibiotic. Ylijoki and colleagues found that a rising C-reactive protein (CRP) level on the second day following incision and drainage indicated the need for reoperation in a case series of severe odontogenic infections. Diabetes mellitus and elevated CRP level also predict severity and complications in mediastinitis. Flynn and co-workers found that the only predictors of the length of hospital stay were variables that measured the severity of the infection, such as the number of infected spaces and operating time; and complications, such as therapeutic failure of the empiric antibiotic, and reoperation. In contrast to other studies, the white blood cell count at admission, immune system compromise, and infection of the deep neck spaces did not predict the length of hospital stay.

The decision to extubate after surgery can at times be difficult. In severe head and neck infections, the source of respiratory failure is generally upper airway obstruction, as opposed to inadequate pulmonary function. The available ventilatory parameters of respiratory rate, vital capacity, negative inspiratory force, minute ventilation, and blood gases do not evaluate airway obstruction.

The air leak test is the most dependable method for predicting successful extubation. It is performed by preoxygenating the patient, suctioning fluids from the oropharynx and endotracheal tube (ETT),

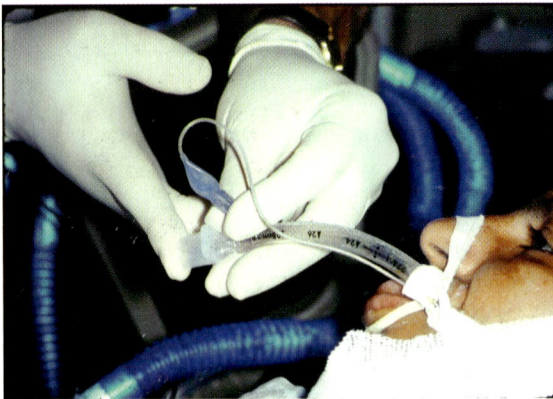

Fig. 117-13 ■ Air leak test. After preoxygenation and suction of fluids from the mouth, pharynx, and endotracheal tube, the cuff is deflated. Then a finger obstructs the endotracheal tube to determine whether the patient can breathe around the tube.

BOX 117-5	Criteria for Hospital Discharge

- Extubation
- T <100° F for 24 hours
- Oral intake >10 mL/kg/shift for 2 shifts
- All drains out
- Swelling decreasing
- Minimal or no drainage
- Adequate control of systemic disease
- Ambulation

deflating the ETT cuff, and then obstructing the ETT with a finger (Figure 117-13). If the patient is able to breathe around the obstructed ETT without becoming restless or hypoxic, then a successful air leak test can be recorded. For the actual extubation procedure, it is wise to preoxygenate the patient, suction the airway and the ETT, and then extubate over a stylet or tube changer. The surgeon may consider extubation in the operating room.

The decision on hospital discharge can be made when the criteria in Box 117-5 are met. Thus the patient should have been afebrile for the previous 24 hours, the oral intake and excretory functions should be normal, the swelling should be decreasing in size and softening, and the wound discharge should be minimal or have ceased. Further, any concomitant systemic disease should be under adequate control.

SPECIFIC TREATMENT TECHNIQUES

The general principles of surgical drainage of severe head and neck infections include primarily the establishment of a secure airway, early and aggressive incision and drainage of all spaces affected by cellulitis or abscess, exploration, debridement, and removal of the cause of infection.

In the 1940s Williams and Guralnick reduced the mortality of Ludwig's angina from 54% to 10% by establishing a policy of immediate airway security by intubation or tracheotomy and aggressive, thorough exploration of all infected anatomic spaces. All of this was accomplished before penicillin became available to civilians. Although CECT and clinical examination can detect a collection of more than 2 mL of pus, the presence or absence of pus at incision and drainage does not predict length of hospital stay or complications. Incision and drainage of an area with cellulitis does

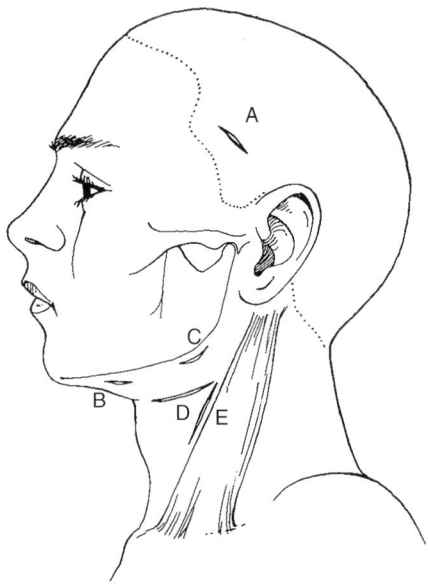

Fig. 117-14 ■ **A** through **E:** Extraoral incision placement for drainage of head and neck infections. (From Flynn TR: Surgical management of orofacial infections. Atlas Oral Maxillofac Surg Clin North Am 8:77, 2000.)

not appear to spread the infection, as previously feared. Instead, early incision and drainage aborts the predictable spread of severe infection from one anatomic space to another.

The usual sites for extraoral incision and drainage of head and neck infections are illustrated in Figure 117-14. Intraoral incisions are generally made in the oral vestibule at the point of maximum swelling. An incision over the pterygomandibular raphé allows intraoral drainage of the pterygomandibular or submasseteric spaces or the anterior compartment of the lateral pharyngeal space.

The extraoral incision at *A* in Figure 117-14 can be used to drain the superficial or deep temporal space. Dependent drainage can be directed intraorally by making a second incision in the maxillary posterior vestibule. Blunt dissection can then be carried from the extraoral to the intraoral incision on either side of the temporalis muscle. The incision at *C* can be used to drain the submasseteric space, and incisions at *B* and *C* allow through-and-through drainage of the submandibular space. The submental space can be drained in a through-and-through manner by using bilateral incisions at *B*.

The incision at *D* in Figure 117-14 can allow the simultaneous exploration and drainage of the submandibular and lateral pharyngeal spaces. It is similar to a Risdon incision except that it is placed more inferiorly, just superior to the level of the hyoid bone. Drainage of the lateral pharyngeal space is illustrated in Figure 117-15. The incision is carried through skin, subcutaneous tissue, superficial fascia, and the platysma muscle, while looking for and protecting the marginal mandibular branch of the facial nerve. The anterior layer of the deep cervical fascia overlying the submandibular gland can then be incised to allow blunt dissection of the submandibular space. The lateral pharyngeal space is explored by blunt dissection posterior to the angle of the mandible and anterior to the sternocleidomastoid muscle. Blunt finger dissection into the lateral pharyngeal space at this point allows identification of the pulsatile carotid sheath posteriorly, the transverse processes of the cervical vertebrae posteromedially, the styloid process medially, and the medial surface of the ascending ramus of the mandible, covered by the medial pterygoid muscle anterolaterally. If drainage of the retropharyngeal space is desired, the dissection can be continued until

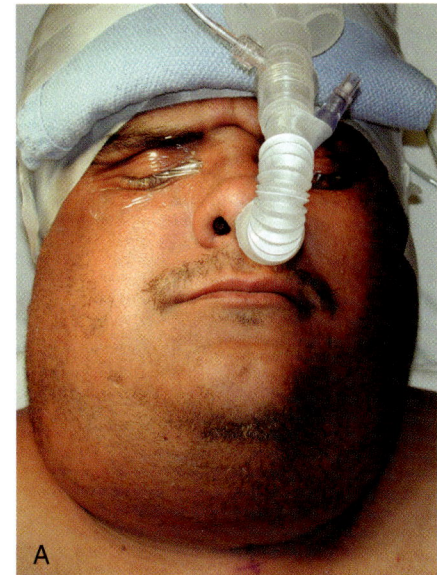

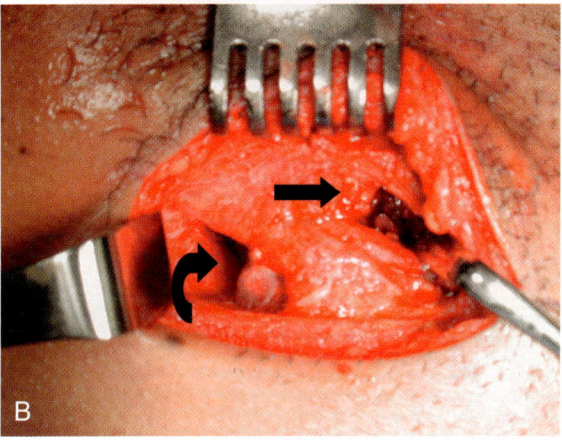

Fig. 117-15 ■ **A,** A patient with right submandibular and lateral pharyngeal space abscess. **B,** Drainage of the submandibular space by incision through the anterior layer of the deep cervical fascia just superior to the submandibular gland (*straight arrow*), and drainage of the lateral pharyngeal space by incision of that fascia and blunt dissection between the anterior border of the sternocleidomastoid muscle and the angle of the mandible (*curved arrow*). (**A** from Flynn TR: Complex odontogenic infections. In Ellis E, Hupp JR, Tucker MR, editors: Contemporary oral and maxillofacial surgery, ed 5. St. Louis, 2008, Mosby.)

the vertebral bodies and the contralateral transverse processes of the cervical vertebrae can be palpated. Anteriorly, the surgeon should be able to palpate the endotracheal tube as well.

If the retropharyngeal space must be explored to its inferior extent, then the incisions at *D* and *E* in Figure 117-14 can be combined. This allows a more extensive exposure of the sternocleidomastoid muscle and the carotid sheath. These structures can then be retracted posteriorly and laterally to allow blunt exploration of the entire retropharyngeal space. The pretracheal space and the anterior and superior mediastinum can be explored from an apron incision, which consists of bilateral incisions at *E* in Figure 117-14 that are connected horizontally across the midline, just superior to the suprasternal notch.

Until recently, the mortality of mediastinitis has been reported at about 20% of cases. Factors that predict mortality and unfavorable outcomes include age, delay of diagnosis, and concomitant systemic disease. However, Freeman and colleagues reported no mortality in a series of 10 cases by using the following treatment regimen. Immediate incision and drainage was performed using a thoracotomy incision and open direct exploration, debridement, irrigation, and drainage of the mediastinum. Cervical incisions were used to explore and debride infection in the neck when necessary. Postoperative CT scans were obtained every 48 to 72 hours, or more frequently if the clinical condition deteriorated. The postoperative CTs were used to guide additional surgeries to aggressively drain any new loculations of pus. In fact, extension of the infection into the abdomen through the diaphragm was found in 30% of cases. The subjects underwent a mean of six operations and six CT scans. The length of hospital stay ranged from 14 to 113 days, with a mean of 46 days. Thus in cases of mediastinitis, early, aggressive, and additional surgeries combined with frequent postoperative CTs reduced the mortality of mediastinitis from 20% to 0% in a small case series.

The diagnosis of osteomyelitis of the jaws remains as challenging as its surgical treatment. Ultimately, the diagnosis is determined by the surgeon's clinical judgment. Multiple sources of information, including bone cultures harvested at surgery, histopathologic confirmation of necrotic bone, radiographic imaging, clinical examination, past medical history, and the surgical finding of avascular bone at debridement must be evaluated. For example, a spicule of necrotic bone exfoliating after tooth extraction may appear on culture and histopathologic examination to be infected necrotic bone. However, if the simple removal of the necrotic spicule results in rapid healing, prolonged antibiotic therapy and extensive surgical debridement are not indicated.

The treatment of acute suppurative osteomyelitis of the jaws involves incision and drainage of any soft tissue involvement, plus debridement of necrotic bone and foreign material found within the infected area (e.g., teeth, bone plates, bullet fragments, or dental implants.)

At the time of debridement and sequestrectomy, the surgeon should remove bone that is not clearly vascularized. The surgeon will recognize viable bone by small bleeding points within freshly irrigated cortical bone. Medullary bone should be more vascular and bleed more readily, and it should have grossly recognizable calcified trabeculae within the soft tissue of the medullary space. The medullary soft tissue should have good strength and vascularity; it should not be friable or have suppuration or a slimy coating suggestive of a bacterial biofilm. Once the debridement has encountered viable bone at all of its margins, wide corticotomy by removal of the lateral cortical plate or perforation of the cortex with burr holes may enhance blood flow to the remaining medullary bone, promoting healing.

The surgeon should consider placing a rigid fixation device, such as a reconstructive bone plate, to prevent or to treat pathologic fracture. If pathologic fracture or segmental resection is likely, the surgeon may adapt and partially fixate the bone plate to the mandible before the bony debridement. The bone plate and fixation screws can be resterilized during debridement, before they are replaced at the final stages of the operation. This process is illustrated in Figure 117-16.

If possible, the oral mucosa should be closed in watertight fashion after surgical debridement. Any new wound drainage can be directed extraorally with a drain brought out through the skin via a separate, inferiorly placed stab incision. This will allow wound irrigation and gravity-dependent drainage. An irrigating drain may be placed in through-and-through fashion in the surgical wound. However, the use of active suction drains should be avoided, since the active drain may pull contaminated oral fluids through the oral incision into the surgical wound.

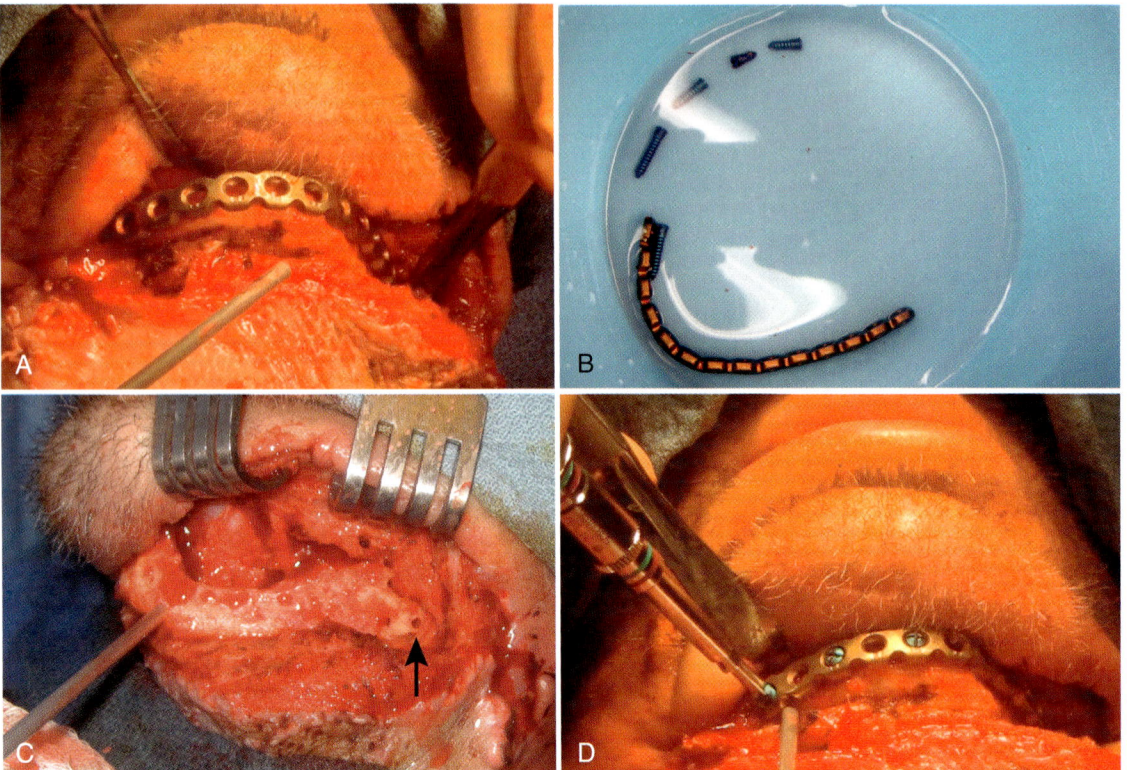

Fig. 117-16 ■ **A,** Adaptation and partial fixation of a rigid reconstruction plate to the mandible before debridement of osteomyelitis. **B,** The contoured bone plate and fixation screws are sent for resterilization. **C,** Completed debridement of the mandible, showing empty screw holes (*arrow*). **D,** After resterilization, the plate and screws are replaced, and fixation is completed with additional screws.

Although a comprehensive discussion of the treatment of sinusitis is beyond the scope of this chapter, the oral and maxillofacial surgeon should be aware that approximately 20% of sinusitis is odontogenic. Tooth extraction in the setting of acute maxillary sinusitis can be problematic, since an immediate closure of oroantral communication may fail. Therefore the surgeon may wish to treat acute maxillary sinusitis medically before extracting the tooth that is causing the infection.

The treatment of chronic, recurrent sinusitis with open surgical approaches has been supplanted by functional endoscopic sinus surgery. This minimally invasive approach to sinusitis is aimed at restoring the anatomic drainage pathways for the involved sinuses without the removal of healthy portions of the lining respiratory mucosa. Retention of this functional mucosa is important in achieving long-term functional restoration of sinus health. Another important treatment principle in sinusitis is evaluation of all of the paranasal sinuses. Treatment of one of the sinuses in an isolated fashion carries a high risk of failure when multiple sinuses are involved.

Although odontogenic causes of brain abscesses and cavernous sinus thrombosis are extremely rare, the oral and maxillofacial surgeon may be called upon to evaluate oral infection as a potential cause of CNS infection. CNS infections usually require prolonged antibiotic therapy to prevent recurrence or chronicity. In cavernous sinus thrombosis, anticoagulation therapy may also be necessary.

POSTOPERATIVE CARE

Surgical drains should be removed when the drainage ceases. In odontogenic infection, drains can usually be removed 2 to 4 days after surgery. Beyond that period, the antigenic nature of latex drains can generate some wound drainage by themselves. There has been no evidence-based research to support or refute the use of postoperative irrigation via surgical drains. When accomplished using aseptic technique, however, irrigation appears to be an opportunity to reduce the bioburden of bacteria and necrotic tissue within the surgical wound. Partial removal of drains, allowing the soft tissue pathway of the drain to gradually collapse behind the drain, similarly has no evidence-based support. This practice may be of benefit, however, with long drains or recalcitrant infections.

It would be ideal to have a laboratory test that would confirm the resolution of osteomyelitis of the jaws. Historically, the erythrocyte sedimentation rate has been used, but the lack of specificity of this test causes many false-positive results. More recently however, the CRP test has been relied upon by infectious disease experts to assess recovery from osteomyelitis. However, this author has personally experienced a case of osteomyelitis following partial odontectomy that was caused by *Actinomyces odontolyticus*. Even though actinomycotic osteomyelitis is usually caused by *Actinomyces israelii* or *Actinomyces naeslundii*, when the parenteral antibiotic therapy was abruptly discontinued after normalization of CRP level, pain and paresthesia returned. Successful treatment occurred only when this case was treated as a true actinomycotic osteomyelitis of the jaw with 6 weeks of parenteral ampicillin/sulbactam, followed by 6 months of oral amoxicillin/clavulanate.

Recently, Springer and co-workers used urinary lysylpyridinoline (LP) levels to assess severity and monitor recovery from osteomyelitis of the jaws. Urinary LP levels rise with bone destruction and gradually fall with bone repair. Recurrence or worsening of the osteomyelitis is also associated with a rise of LP. This test holds promise for use in diagnosis and therapeutic monitoring. Its clinical use, however, is not yet widespread.

CASES IN POINT

POINT 1

A patient presented to an oral and maxillofacial surgeon with a submandibular, submental, and sublingual swelling, plus swelling of the anterior tonsillar pillar and deviation of the uvula to the opposite side. The causative tooth appeared to be a partially erupted mandibular third molar. At the initial visit, the patient stated, "I would rather die than go to the hospital."

Over the ensuing 5 days, the oral and maxillofacial surgeon performed incision and drainage, extraction of the mandibular third molar, and repeated incision and drainage in the office under deep sedation, using oral antibiotic therapy. The day following the second incision and drainage was a Saturday. That afternoon, the patient told his wife that he was not feeling so well. He lay down on the couch. About an hour later his wife could not arouse him. He was declared dead upon arrival at the hospital, due to airway obstruction by an infected swelling.

One lesson in this case is that there may be times when the surgeon may not be able, in conscience, to comply with a patient demand. Often a sincere, concerned discussion with the patient may convince him or her to accept the surgeon's recommendation. If this fails, an informed refusal of consent may protect the surgeon from civil liability.

POINT 2

In a recently reported case series of 37 severe odontogenic infections, all requiring hospitalization according to the criteria in Box 117-4, none of the patients died. There were no instances of mediastinitis. There were only two cases in which reoperation was required. Even though the antibiotic regimen used (penicillin G in 33 cases) would now be considered out of date, the complication rate in this study was very low. The surgical protocol was aggressive incision and drainage of all anatomic deep spaces affected by cellulitis or abscess as soon as medically possible. This study appears to confirm the findings of Williams and Guralnick from 1943: immediate establishment of a secure airway and aggressive surgery reduces mortality in head and neck infections.

PEARLS AND PITFALLS

- It is very important for an oral and maxillofacial surgeon to be up-to-date on the current diagnostic studies, surgical principles, and treatment techniques for infections.
- The primary treatment of abscess-forming head and neck infections is surgery.
- Antibiotics are supportive but not curative care.
- The primary principles of the treatment of such infections are airway protection, early and aggressive incision and drainage, and removal of the cause of infection.
- An informed refusal of consent may protect the surgeon from civil liability.

BIBLIOGRAPHY

Bennett JD, Flynn TR: Anesthetic considerations in orofacial infections. In Topazian RG, Goldberg MH, Hupp JR, editors: *Oral and maxillofacial infections*, ed 4, Philadelphia, 2002, Saunders.

Flynn TR: Anatomy of oral and maxillofacial infections. In Topazian RG, Goldberg MH, Hupp JR, editors: *Oral and maxillofacial infections*, ed 4, Philadelphia, 2002, Saunders, pp 188-213.

Flynn TR, Shanti RM, Hayes C: Severe odontogenic infections, part two: prospective outcomes study, *J Oral Maxillofac Surg* 64:1104, 2006.

Flynn TR, Shanti RM, Levy M, Adamo AK, et al: Severe odontogenic infections, part one: prospective report, *J Oral Maxillofac Surg* 64: 1093, 2006.

Freeman RK, Vallieres E, Verrier ED, et al: Descending necrotizing mediastinitis: an analysis of the effects of serial surgical debridement on patient mortality, *J Thorac Cardiovasc Surg* 119:260, 2000.

Grodinsky M, Holyoke E: The fascia and fascial spaces of the head and neck regions, *Am J Anat* 63:367-407, 1938.

Springer IN, Wiltfang J, Dunsche A, Lier GC, et al: A new method of monitoring osteomyelitis, *Int J Oral Maxillofac Surg* 36:527, 2007.

Williams AC: Ludwig's angina, *Surg Gynecol Obstet* 70:140, 1940.

Williams AC, Guralnick WC: The diagnosis and treatment of Ludwig's angina: a report of twenty cases, *N Engl J Med* 228:443, 1943.

Ylijoki S, Suuronen R, Jousimies-Somer H, Meurman JH, Lindqvist C. Differences between patients with or without the need for intensive care due to severe odontogenic infections, *J Oral Maxillofac Surg* 59(8):867-872, 2001.

118

Ludwig's Angina

Sam E. Farish

Ludwig's angina is a term for a rapidly progressive cellulitis of the floor of the mouth and neck with induration and bilateral submandibular, sublingual, and submental space involvement with an infectious process; dysphagia and respiratory obstruction may ensue. Typically no abscess or lymphadenopathy is seen in the classic description, but progression to abscess formation within the involved space and contiguous spaces is most often the case. Angina derives from the Latin term *angere*, meaning "to strangle."[1] Grodinsky stated in a 1939 paper that Ludwig's angina was a unique deep neck abscess characterized by (1) occurrence bilaterally in more than one space, (2) production of gangrenous serosanguineous infiltration with or without pus, (3) involvement of connective tissue and muscle but not glandular structures, (4) spread by continuity, not via lymphatics.[2] The eponymous condition named after Wilhelm Frederick von Ludwig may have been the cause of the author's own death, because he died at the age of 75 years, days after developing an inflammation of the neck.[3] It should be noted that the early descriptions of the condition were based on clinical and necropsy findings of patients whose fate "despite the most skillful therapy is almost always fatal."[4] Mortality and morbidity associated with the condition are greatly reduced in the modern era of antibiotics, improved imaging, and airway management.

ETIOPATHOGENESIS

The most common cause of Ludwig's angina is odontogenic. More specifically the lower second and third molars are implicated because their roots extend below the mylohyoid muscle, and periapical abscesses of these teeth result in lingual cortical penetration with an ensuing submandibular infection. The submandibular space is subdivided into the sublingual space above the mylohyoid and the submaxillary space below it. These two divisions freely communicate with each other over the posterior border of the digastric muscle. The submandibular space communicates with the submental space anteriorly past the anterior belly of the digastric muscle. Ludwig's angina, when critically reviewed using modern diagnostic and imaging techniques, anaerobic cultures, and contemporary patient management protocols, is not distinct from other space infections. It is, in fact, an extensive spread of infection throughout the mouth floor and neck caused by the same organisms responsible for less morbid head and neck infections.[5] Although Ludwig's angina is odontogenic in up to 90% of cases,[6,7] oral lacerations,[8] mandible fracture,[9] infections of oral malignancy,[10] and bilateral sialolithiasis-related submandibular gland infection[11] have also been implicated. The bacterial isolates of Ludwig's angina are varied, but are mostly aerobes and anaerobes, including α-hemolytic streptococci, staphylococci, and bacteroides.[12] In addition, other anaerobes such as peptostreptococci, peptococci,[13-15] *Fusobacterium nucleatum*, *Viellonella* species, and spirochetes[6] have also been isolated in cultures from patients with Ludwig's angina. Gram-negative organisms such as *Neisseria catarrhalis*, *Escherichia coli*, *Pseudomonas aeruginosa*, and *Haemophilus influenzae* have also been reported.[13] A recent article reported a fatal case of Ludwig's angina associated with *Gemella morbillorum*, a facultative anaerobic organism.[16] In summary most deep neck infections are caused by oral flora and most are polymicrobial, of which 75% are obligate anaerobes.[12] Results of blood cultures from patients with Ludwig's angina are generally negative.[15]

PATHOLOGIC ANATOMY

To adequately treat Ludwig's angina, the anatomy of the fascial spaces of the neck where the infection is contained and where it may spread must be thoroughly understood. Fascia is a band of connective tissue that surrounds structures (e.g., muscles) and by its nature of layering gives rise to potential spaces that allow for the spread of infection.[17,18] The superficial fascia is located immediately deep to the skin. It contains fat and is continuous from the base of the neck into the face; that is, it traverses the length of the face and neck. Infections in this space are superficial and easily observed early on. The deep cervical fascia lies deep to the superficial fascia under the platysma muscle.

The deep cervical fascia assists muscle movement because it limits the muscle volume contained within, it provides attachments for some muscles, and it also encloses nerves and blood vessels. It is subdivided in the neck into four layers (Box 118-1). An understanding of these divisions is at the heart of the knowledge necessary for effective infection management. The superficial layer of the deep cervical fascia lies immediately deep to the superficial fascia and platysma muscle. It encircles the neck completely, and as it approaches the sternocleidomastoid and trapezius muscles, it splits to lie on their superficial and deep surfaces. It is attached anteriorly to the chin, hyoid bone, and sternum. Posteriorly it attaches to the spinous processes of the cervical vertebrae. Superiorly it attaches to the occipital protuberance, superior nuchal line, mastoid process, inferior border of the zygomatic arch, and the inferior border of the mandible from the angle to the midline (Fig. 118-1). Inferiorly it attaches to the sternum where it splits into anterior and posterior parts, and it also attaches to the clavicle and the acromium of the scapula.

The middle layer of the deep cervical fascia consists of a **muscular portion**, which surrounds the strap muscles; a **visceral portion or buccopharyngeal portion**, which lies deep to the superficial layer of the deep cervical fascia posterior to the pharynx; and a **pretracheal layer**, which covers the thyroid gland, esophagus, and trachea. The muscular portion attaches superiorly at the hyoid bone and thyroid cartilage, and inferiorly at the medial sternum. The visceral portion of the middle layer of the deep cervical covers the

1. Superficial layer of the deep cervical fascia (investing layer)
2. Middle layer of the deep cervical fascia
3. Deep layer of the deep cervical fascia
4. Carotid sheath (made up of all three layers of the deep cervical fascia)

muscular layer of the pharynx and is continued forward onto the buccinator muscle. It lies posterior to the pharynx and is attached to the base of the skull above, and then runs inferiorly into the mediastinum where it fuses with the alar fascia (see later). The pretracheal layer attaches superiorly to the larynx and inferiorly into the fibrous pericardium in the superior mediastinum and encircles the thyroid gland (see Fig. 118-1).

The deep layer of the deep cervical fascia consists of a prevertebral layer and the alar fascia. The prevertebral layer of the deep cervical fascia completely encircles the cervical portions of the prevertebral muscles and the postvertebral muscles. It is attached above at the skull base and inferiorly at the coccyx. The alar fascia is a portion of the prevertebral fascia found between the middle layer of the deep cervical fascia and the prevertebral layers of the deep cervical fascia. It is attached above at the base of the skull, and inferiorly it fuses with the visceral portion of the middle layer of the deep cervical fascia at the level of T2. The alar fascia separates the retropharyngeal space from the "danger space." The danger space is a subdivision of the retropharyngeal space, extending from the base of the skull to the level of the diaphragm; it provides a route for the spread of infection from the pharynx to the mediastinum.

The carotid sheath, which contains the carotid artery, the internal jugular vein, and the vagus nerve, is enclosed within a sheath composed of contributions from the superficial, middle, and deep layers of the deep cervical fascia. It is attached above to the base of the skull and merges below with tissues surrounding the aortic arch.

The submandibular space is composed of two potential spaces that span the region from the mucosa of oral cavity to the superficial layer of the deep cervical fascia. It encloses the area between the mandible and the hyoid bone (Fig. 118-2). The mylohyoid muscle originates on the mylohyoid line on the lingual surface of the mandible and inserts on the symphysis menti, the mylohyoid raphe, and the body of the hyoid bone posteriorly. This muscle horizontally divides the submandibular space into the sublingual space above (supramylohyoid compartment) and the submandibular or submaxillary space below (inframylohyoid compartment) (Fig. 118-3). Most refer to the combined space as the submandibular space, whose two components communicate freely along the posterior aspect of the mylohyoid muscle. The supramylohyoid compartment of the submandibular space contains loose areolar tissue, sublingual glands, submandibular glands, Wharton duct, the lingual artery and vein, geniohyoid muscles, and the lingual and hypoglossal nerves. The inframylohyoid compartment contains the anterior bellies of the digastric muscles, submandibular glands, lymph nodes, and the facial artery and vein. The portion of the inframylohyoid compartment confined between the anterior bellies of the digastric muscles is referred to as the submental space (see Fig. 118-2). Infections involving the submental and sublingual spaces can result in elevation and protrusion of the tongue, which compromises the airway. The submandibular space communicates freely with the lateral pharyngeal space and by extension the retropharyngeal space. From the retropharyngeal space, which lies between the buccopharyngeal

layer of the middle layer of the deep cervical fascia covering the pharynx and esophagus and the anterior alar fascia (see Fig. 118-1), infections can spread into the danger space by perforation. The danger space, which lies posterior to the alar fascia and where the alar fascia and the middle layer of the cervical fascia fuse and anterior to the prevertebral fascia, extends from the base of the skull to the diaphragm. This is the pathway for mediastinal and lung involvement with neck infections. The carotid sheath is another pathway for infection from the submandibular space to spread to the mediastinum (see Fig. 118-1).

DIAGNOSTIC STUDIES

Clinical examination including pertinent vital signs is supplemented by panoramic radiographs and CT scans. There is really no rationale for anything other than CT with contrast, because anything of interest to those treating such infections is seen better with contrast. The CT scan should be ordered as fine cuts from the aortic bulb to the top of the head.[19] Renal disease and allergy to contrast are the limited contraindications to CT contrast. Figure 118-4 is a CT scan with contrast of a patient with Ludwig's angina. A white blood cell count is valuable as a baseline and to follow the progress of treatment in the postoperative period. Cultures and aspirates should be obtained as soon as possible. If aspiration can be performed before initiation of empirical antibiotic therapy it is preferable. C-reactive protein levels can be used to monitor response to treatment. The microbiology of Ludwig's angina is commonly polymicrobial and anaerobic organisms predominate. Anaerobic organisms are increasingly resistant to penicillin because of the production of β-lactamases.[20,21] *Eikenella corrodens*, an anaerobe frequently isolated in young people and IV drug abusers, is universally resistant to clindamycin and metronidazole, but is sensitive to penicillin and aminoglycosides.[22,23] Methicillin-resistant *Staphylococcus aureus* (MRSA) has been seen with increasing prevalence in community-acquired deep neck infections in IV drug abusers, immunocompromised patients, and the young.[24,25] *Klebsiella pneumoniae* is a consistent cause of deep neck infections in patients with poorly controlled diabetes.[26,27]

TREATMENT GOALS

Treatment of Ludwig's angina is based on four principles[12]:
1. Sufficient airway management
2. Early and aggressive antibiotic therapy
3. Incision and drainage for any who fail medical management or form localized abscesses
4. Adequate nutrition and hydration support

Sufficient airway management is initiated by maintaining the patient in a sitting position and giving supplemental oxygen by mask or nasal prongs. Inability to protrude the tongue is a hallmark of floor of mouth swelling as is seen in Ludwig's angina (Fig. 118-5). Suction apparatus at bedside for patient and attendant use is essential. Patients with Ludwig's angina who have not been intubated or had a surgical airway should never be left unattended. Har-El and colleagues[15] reported that up to 67% of patients with Ludwig's angina required anticipatory or emergent intubation. Airway observation can be considered if oxygen saturations are being maintained adequately and aggressive antimicrobial therapy has been initiated. It seems that observation can be a very good strategy in children with Ludwig's angina, because only 10% of children in a retrospective study required airway control, whereas 52% of patients older than 15 years had a tracheostomy.[28] Stridor, difficulty managing secretions, and cyanosis are late signs of impending airway

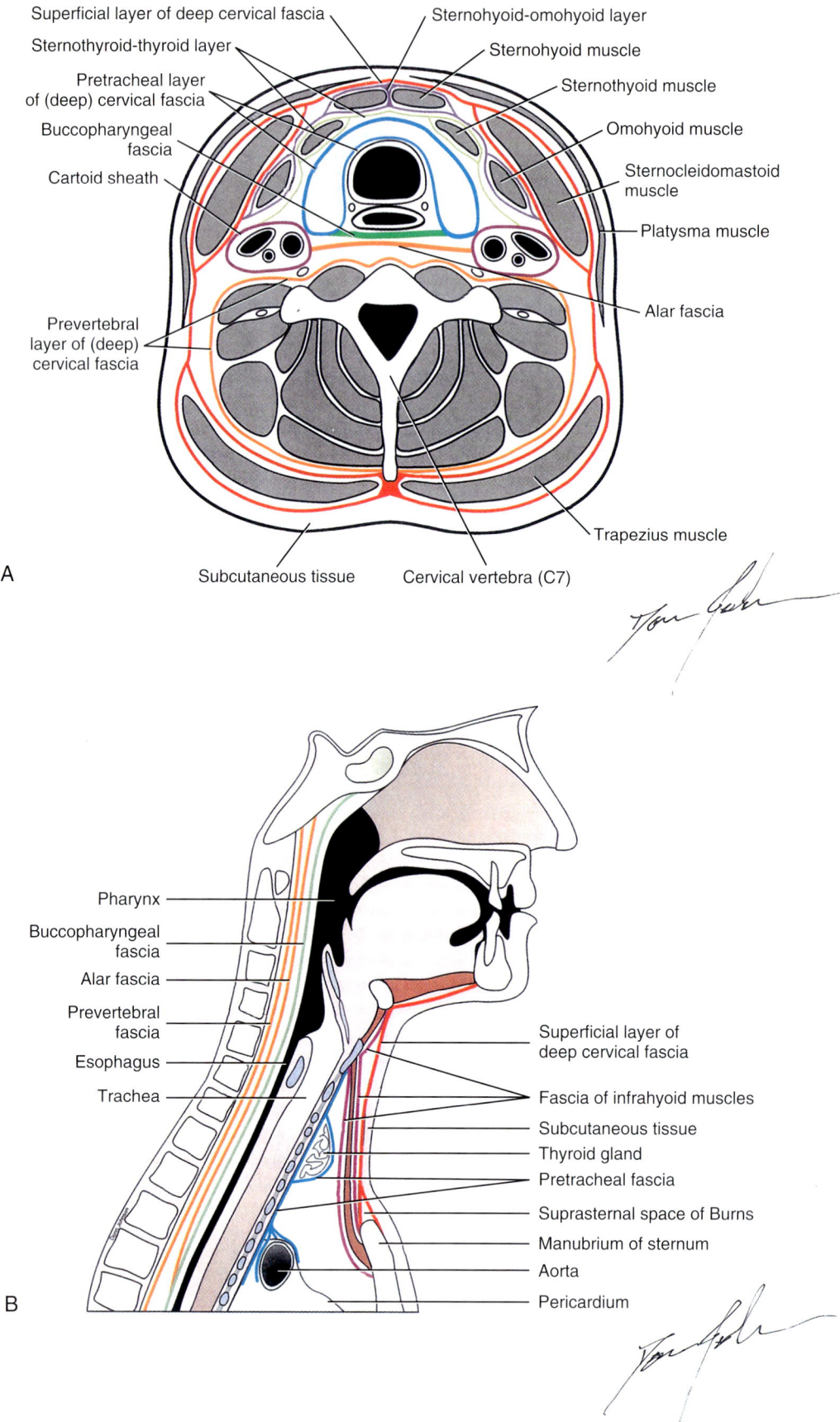

Fig. 118-1 ■ **A** and **B**, Fascia of the neck. (Copyright Donn Johnson at Atlanta VA Medical Center Art Department.)

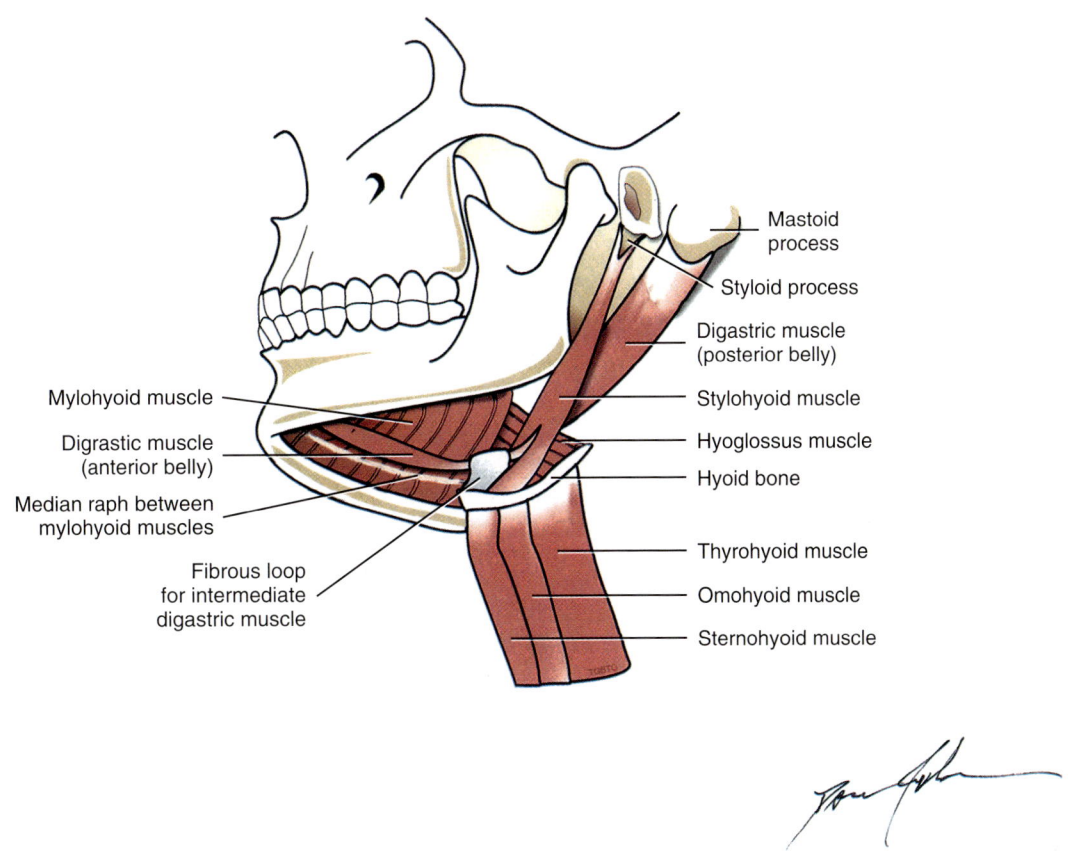

Fig. 118-2 ■ Submandibular space from below the mylohyoid muscle. (Copyright Donn Johnson at Atlanta VA Medical Center Art Department.)

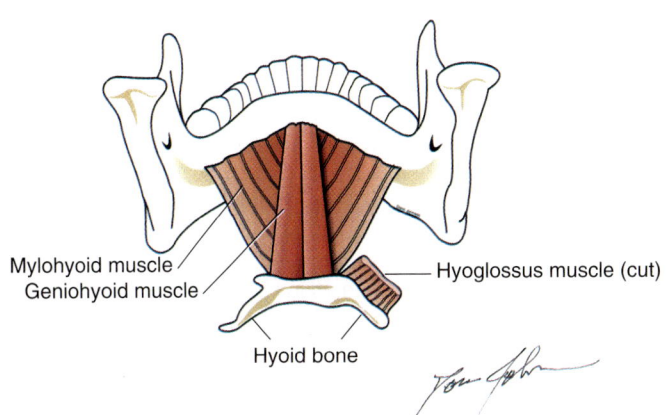

Fig. 118-3 ■ Submandibular space from above the mylohyoid muscle. (Copyright Donn Johnson at Atlanta VA Medical Center Art Department.)

obstruction and must be managed aggressively. Airway management in the presurgical setting should be tailored to the condition of the patient and the experience of the treating practitioner.[29,30]

Antibiotic therapy is empirical until culture and sensitivity results are obtained. The empirical therapy planned should be effective against the aerobic and anaerobic bacteria species commonly involved, and after culture and sensitivity results are obtained, therapy can be tailored accordingly. Adequate empirical coverage consists of either penicillin with a β-lactamase inhibitor (amoxicillin or ticarcillin with clavulanic acid) or a β-lactamase–resistant antibiotic (cefoxitin, cefuroxime, imipenumm, or meropenem) in combination with a drug that is effective against most anaerobes (clindamycin or metronidazole).[20,27,30,31] Treatment including vancomycin should be considered for IV drug abusers and immunocompromised patients who are likely candidates for MRSA infections.[20,32] Addition of gentamicin to the empirical therapy should be strongly considered for diabetic patients.[20,27] Parenteral antibiotics should be used until the patient is afebrile for at least 48 hours; after this time, oral therapy can be continued for 2 weeks, using amoxicillin with clavulanic acid, clindamycin, ciprofloxacin, trimethoprim-sulfamethoxazole, or metronidazole.[20,21,32]

Surgical incision and drainage are the mainstay for severe and complicated deep neck infections that do not respond to medical management within 48 hours. Surgery is indicated in cases of airway compromise, septicemia, deteriorating condition, descending infection, diabetes mellitus, and palpable or radiographic evidence of abscess formation.

Adequate nutrition and hydration is important in any patient with a head and neck infection. Malnutrition is well documented in the literature, with rates up to 50% in certain surgical populations. A prospective study of 500 patients admitted to an acute care teaching hospital in England determined that 40% of patients were undernourished on presentation, and patients lost an average of 5.4% of their body weight during their hospital stay.[33] When decreased or nonexistent oral intake secondary to pain and difficulty eating or swallowing in a patient with Ludwig's angina is added to the substandard baseline many patients are known to maintain, serious nutrition and hydration issues can be manifest. It is widely known that malnutrition affects outcomes in surgical patients, with increased

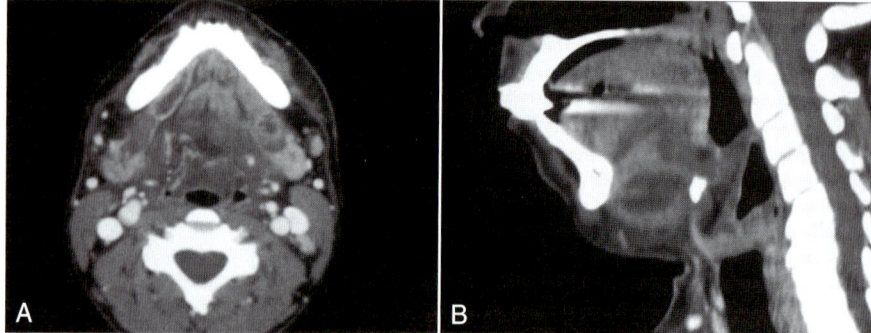

Fig. 118-4 ■ CTs with contrast of a patient with Ludwig's angina. (Courtesy Dr. Edwin Granite, Wilmington, Dele.)

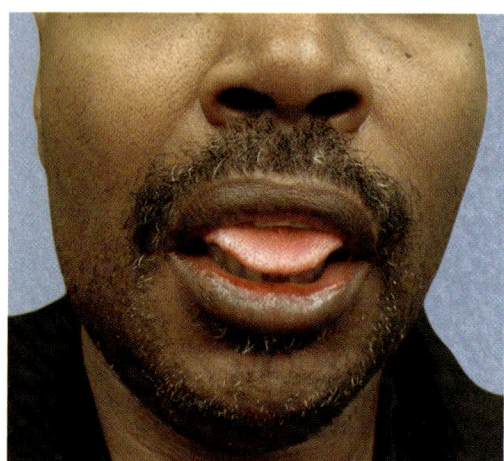

Fig. 118-5 ■ Inability to protrude the tongue is a sign of an infectious process involving the floor of the mouth. (Courtesy Dr. Edwin Granite, Wilmington, Dele.)

mortality and morbidity seen in the malnourished. Nutritional support is frequently initiated for malnourished patients undergoing surgery, but the indications are not sufficiently clear as to when to intervene.[34] The reduction of food intake results in loss of fat, muscle, skin, and, late in the process, bone and viscera. There is weight loss and associated increase in extracellular fluid volume. As nutritional requirements fall when body mass is lost, what is ingested is more efficiently used and work at the cellular level is decreased. The decreased tissue mass and decreased work capacity at the cellular level reduce homeostatic responses to stressors such as infection and surgery. Surgical and infection stresses increase protein and energy requirements due to a hypermetabolic, catabolic state.[34] Nutrients are redistributed from reserves such as fat and muscle to more active tissues such as the liver, bone, and visceral organs, and protein caloric malnutrition occurs within a few days. Consequences of malnutrition include increased susceptibility to infection, immune system dysfunction, and poor wound healing.[35]

SPECIFIC TREATMENT AND TECHNIQUES

Because airway management is the most important factor in patients with Ludwig's angina, most treatment strategies center on this element. Treatments ranging from conservative airway management, consisting of close observation and intravenous antibiotics, to airway intervention with endotracheal intubation or tracheostomy have been considered. In a recent paper, Greenberg and colleagues[36]

suggested that there is a subset of patients with Ludwig's angina who can be treated safely with conservative management. They reported that 72% of patients treated over a 9-year period responded adequately to conservative airway management, and only one of these patients deteriorated and required emergency intubation. Of those treated nonconservatively, seven of eight patients were able to be intubated using fiber-optic nasendoscopy and one required a tracheostomy under local anesthesia.[36]

If the plan is for an incision and drainage, the airway management for general anesthesia becomes a major consideration. Frequently patients with Ludwig's angina are not trismatic, and this can lead an inexperienced anesthesiology practitioner to conclude that the intubation will not be difficult and that the patient can be paralyzed before attempted intubation. Because the swelling in the floor of the mouth prevents the anterior and inferior displacement of the tongue with the laryngoscope blade, the glottis cannot be visualized. Incision and drainage procedures planned for the operating room with general anesthesia should be preceded by consultation with the anesthesiologist about suspected airway problems at intubation. Awake fiber-optic techniques are suggested for achieving an airway in such patients. A tracheostomy set should always be in the room, in case there is a need for local tracheostomy or an emergent cricothyrotomy.

Surgical drainage in Ludwig's angina should include bilateral submandibular incisions as well as a midline submental incision. Entry into the supramylohyoid spaces bilaterally can be obtained by blunt dissection through the mylohyoid muscle from below. Penrose drains should be placed in both supramylohyoid and inframylohyoid spaces bilaterally as well as through and through drains from the submandibular space to the submental space from both sides. A patient with Ludwig's who has had an incision and drainage (I & D) is shown in Figure 118-6. Debridement of necrotic tissue and copious irrigation complete the I & D procedure. Drains should be marked so their location can be determined and sutured with loops so they can be advanced without having to reanesthetize the patient while drains are resutured to the skin. Absorbent dressings are then applied, and use of tape can be avoided if a bandnet dressing retainer is constructed. The oral cavity is then entered, indicated teeth are removed, and any other intraoral procedures are completed.

POSTOPERATIVE CARE

Intubation with ventilatory assistance is indicated until a patent airway is ensured in the postoperative period. The respiratory support team must be convinced that the patient has no pulmonary problems, but rather only needs his airway protected until the swelling allows extubation. To plan extubation, sedation is decreased and a weaning period is instigated. Most consider the ability to breath adequately around an uncuffed tube with the lumen blocked

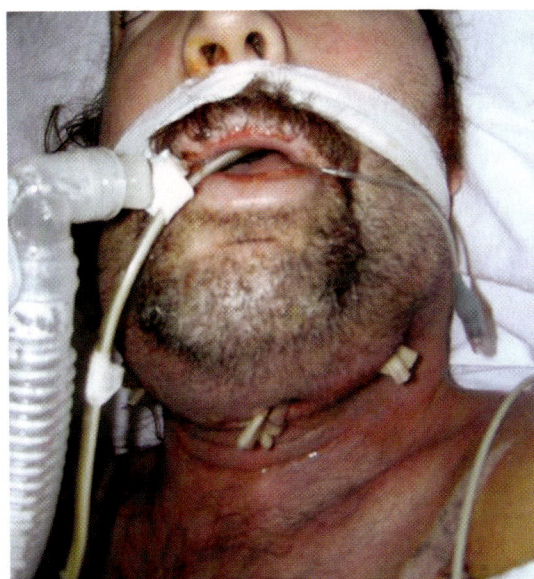

Fig. 118-6 ■ Typical patient with Ludwig's angina after I & D, intubated with drains in place.

is indicative of an adequate airway. Extubation in the early morning over a stylet with the availability of a tracheostomy set is highly recommended.

Empirical antibiotic therapy is continued until results of cultures and sensitivity tests are reported, at which time appropriate adjustments can be made in therapeutic regimens. The patient's body temperature should be carefully monitored for signs of steady decrease as expected with infection control, or spikes or increases suggestive of therapeutic failures. White blood cell counts should also show a downward trend if treatment has been effective, whereas spikes can indicate progression or inadequate drainage. Clinical examination for such changes as dysphonia, dysphagia, increased swelling, or increased pain assist in discovery of insufficient response to treatment or extension of the infection to additional spaces. Abrupt deterioration of a patient's condition can herald extension into the parapharyngeal or visceral space. Repeat CT scans with contrast will reveal extension of the infectious process to additional anatomic areas or verify clinical impression of improving status.

Parenteral antibiotics should be used until the patient is afebrile for at least 48 hours, after which oral therapy can be continued for 2 weeks, using amoxicillin with clavulanic acid, clindamycin, ciprofloxacin, trimethoprim-sulfamethoxazole, or metronidazole.[20,32] Drains can be removed when nonproductive or when the need to irrigate the involved spaces appears to be diminished.

PEARLS AND PITFALLS

- Ludwig's angina is a submandibular space abscess with an extensive spread of infection throughout the floor of the mouth and the neck; it is caused by the same organisms responsible for less morbid head and neck infections.
- Because the floor of the mouth is affected in Ludwig's angina, endotracheal intubation is much more difficult because the tongue cannot be moved forward and down by the laryngoscope blade to allow visualization of the glottis.
- Airway management is the number one priority in cases of Ludwig's angina.
- A certain subset of patients with Ludwig's angina can be managed conservatively without airway intervention.
- CT with contrast from the aortic bulb to the top of the head is indicated in all head and neck infections.
- Planned empirical therapy for Ludwig's angina should be effective against the aerobic and anaerobic bacteria species commonly involved; after results of culture and sensitivity tests are obtained, therapy can be adjusted accordingly.
- Adequate empiric antibiotic coverage consists of either penicillin with a β-lactamase inhibitor (amoxicillin or ticarcillin with clavulanic acid) or a β-lactamase-resistant antibiotic (cefoxitin, cefuroxime, imipenumm, or meropenem) in combination with a drug which is effective against most anerobes (clindamycin or metronidazole).
- Consideration should be given to the use of Vancomycin in IV drug abusers and immunocompromised patients who are likely candidates for MRSA infections.
- Gentamicin addition to the empiric therapy should be a strong consideration in diabetic patients.
- Parenteral antibiotics should be used until the patient is afebrile for at least 48 hours, following which oral therapy can be continued for 2 weeks using amoxicillin with clavulanic acid, clindamycin, ciprofloxacin, trimethoprim-sulfamethoxazole, or metranidazole.

REFERENCES

1. Britt JC, Josephson GD, Gross CW: Ludwig's angina in the pediatric population: a report of a case and review of the literature, *Int J Pediatr Otorhinolaryngol* 52:79-87, 2000.
2. Grodinsky M: Ludwig's angina: an anatomical and clinical study with review of the literature, *Surgery* 5:678-696, 1939.
3. Wasson J, Hopkins C, Bowdler D: Did Ludwig's angina kill Ludwig? *J Laryngol Otol* 120:363-365, 2006.
4. Burke J: Angina Ludovici: a translation, together with a biography of Wilhelm F.V. Ludwig, *Bull Hist Med* 7:1115-1126, 1939.
5. Marciani RD: Clinical considerations in head and neck infections. In Peterson LJ, Indresano AT, Marciani RD, Roser SM, editors: *Principles of oral and maxillofacial surgery,* Philadelphia, 1992, Lippincott, p 175.
6. Moreland LW, Corey J, McKinzie R: Ludwig's angina: report of a case and review of the literature, *Arch Intern Med* 148:461-466, 1988.
7. Sethi DS, Stanley RE: Deep neck abscesses—changing trends, *J Laryngol Otol* 108:138-143, 1994.
8. Gross SJ, Nieburg PI: Ludwig's angina in childhood, *Am J Dis Child* 131:291-292, 1977.
9. Rosen EA, Shulman RH, Shaw AS: Ludwig's angina: a complication of a bilateral mandibular fracture: report of a case, *J Oral Surg* 30:196-200, 1972.
10. Fischmann GE, Graham BS: Ludwig's angina resulting from the infection of an oral malignancy, *J Oral Maxillofac Surg* 43:795-796, 1985.
11. Honrado CP, Lam SM, Karen M: Bilateral submandibular gland infection presenting as Ludwig's angina: first report of a case, *Ear Nose Throat J* 80:217-223, 2001.
12. Chou Y Lee Y, Chao H: An upper airway obstruction emergency: Ludwig's angina, *Pediatr Emerg Care* 23:892-896, 2007.
13. Busch RF, Shah D: Ludwig's angina: improved treatment, *Otolaryngol Head Neck Surg* 117:S172-S175, 1997.
14. Hartmann RW Jr: Ludwig's angina in children, *Am Fam Physician* 60:109-112, 1999.
15. Har-EL G, Aroesty JH, Shaha A, et al: Changing trends in deep neck abscess. A retrospective study of 110 patients, *Oral Surg Oral Med Oral Pathol Oral Radiol Endod* 77:446-450, 1994.

16. Sofianou D, Peftoulidou, Manolis EN, et al: A fatal case of Ludwig's angina and mediastinitis caused by an unusual microorganism, *Gemella morbillorum, Scand J Infect Dis* 37:367-369, 2005.

17. Norton NS: *Netter's head and neck anatomy for dentistry,* Philadelphia, 2007, Saunders Elsevier, p 460.

18. Grodinsky M, Holyoke EA: The fascia and fascial spaces of the head, neck and adjacent regions, *Am J Anat* 63;367-407, 1938.

19. Personal communication, Pat Hudgins, Professor of Radiology, Emory University School of Medicine, February 29, 2009.

20. Vieira F, Allen SM, Stocks RS, Thompson JW: Deep neck infection, *Otolaryngol Clin North Am* 41:459-483, 2008.

21. Brook I: Anaerobic bacteria in upper respiratory tract and other head and neck infections, *Ann Otol Rhinol Laryngol* 111:430-440, 2002.

22. Lee K, Tami T, Echavez M, et al: Deep neck infections in patients at risk for acquired immunodeficiency syndrome, *Laryngoscope* 100:915-919, 1990.

23. Coticchia J, Getnick G, Yun R, et al: Age-, site-, and time-specific differences in pediatric deep neck abscesses, *Arch Otolaryngol Head Neck Surg* 130:201-207, 2004.

24. Miller L, Perdreau-Remington F, Rieg G, et al: Necrotizing fasciitis caused by community-associated methicillin-resistant *Staphylococcus aureus* in Los Angeles, *N Engl J Med* 352:1445-1453, 2005.

25. Huang T, Liu T, Chen P, et al: Deep neck infection: analysis of 210 cases, *Head Neck* 26:854-860, 2004.

26. Lee J, Kin H, Lim S: Predisposing factors of complicated deep neck infection: an analysis of 158 cases, *Yonsei Med J* 48:55-62, 2007.

27. Wang L, Kuo W, Tsai S, et al: Characterizations of life-threatening deep cervical space infections: a review of one hundred ninety-six cases, *Am J Otolaryngol* 24:111-117, 2003.

28. Kurien M, Matthew J, Job A, et al: Ludwig's angina, *Clin Otolaryngol* 22:263-265, 1997.

29. Marple BF: Ludwig's angina: a review of current airway management, *Arch Otolaryngol Head Neck Surg* 125:596-599, 1999.

30. Neff SPW, Mery AF, Anderson B: Airway management in Ludwig's angina, *Anaesth Intensive Care* 27:659-661, 1999.

31. Stalfors J, Adielsson A, Ebenfelt A, et al: Deep neck space infections remain a surgical challenge; a study of 72 patients, *Acta Otolaryngol* 124:1191-1196, 2004.

32. Weed HG, Forest LA: Deep neck infection. In Cummings CW, Flint PW, Harker LA, et al, editors: *Otolaryngology: head and neck surgery,* vol 3, ed 4. Philadelphia, 2005, Elsevier Mosby, pp 2515-2524.

33. McWhirter JP, Pennington CR: Incidence and recognition of malnutrition in hospital, *Br Med J* 308:945, 1994.

34. Kiyama T, Witte MB, Thornton FJ, Barbul A: The route of nutrition support affects the early phase of wound healing, *JPEN J Parenter Enteral Nutr* 22:276, 1998.

35. Kinney JM, Weissman C: Forms of malnutrition in stressed and unstressed patients, *Clin Chest Med* 7:19, 1986.

36. Greenberg SLL, Huang J, Chang RSK, Ananda SN: Surgical management of Ludwig's angina, *Aust N Z J Surg* 77:540-543, 2007.

INDEX

Note: Page numbers followed by f refer to figures; page numbers followed by t refer to tables; page numbers followed by b refer to boxes.